STUDENT'S SOLUTIONS MANUAL

DAVID ATWOOD
Rochester Community and Technical College

A GRAPHICAL APPROACH TO PRECALCULUS WITH LIMITS

A UNIT CIRCLE APPROACH

SIXTH EDITION

John Hornsby
University of New Orleans

Margaret L. Lial
American River College

Gary Rockswold
Minnesota State University, Mankato

PEARSON

Boston Columbus Indianapolis New York San Francisco Upper Saddle River
Amsterdam Cape Town Dubai London Madrid Milan Munich Paris Montreal Toronto
Delhi Mexico City São Paulo Sydney Hong Kong Seoul Singapore Taipei Tokyo

The author and publisher of this book have used their best efforts in preparing this book. These efforts include the development, research, and testing of the theories and programs to determine their effectiveness. The author and publisher make no warranty of any kind, expressed or implied, with regard to these programs or the documentation contained in this book. The author and publisher shall not be liable in any event for incidental or consequential damages in connection with, or arising out of, the furnishing, performance, or use of these programs.

Reproduced by Pearson from electronic files supplied by the author.

Copyright © 2015, 2011, 2007 Pearson Education, Inc.
Publishing as Pearson, 75 Arlington Street, Boston, MA 02116.

All rights reserved. No part of this publication may be reproduced, stored in a retrieval system, or transmitted, in any form or by any means, electronic, mechanical, photocopying, recording, or otherwise, without the prior written permission of the publisher. Printed in the United States of America.

ISBN-13: 978-0-321-91558-0
ISBN-10: 0-321-91558-5

2 3 4 5 6 OPM 17 16 15

www.pearsonhighered.com

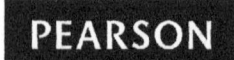

Contents

Chapter 1	Linear Functions, Equations, and Inequalities	1
Chapter 2	Analysis of Graphs and Functions	41
Chapter 3	Polynomial Functions	91
Chapter 4	Rational, Power, and Root Functions	159
Chapter 5	Inverse, Exponential, and Logarithmic Functions	211
Chapter 6	Systems and Matrices	261
Chapter 7	Analytic Geometry and Nonlinear Systems	335
Chapter 8	The Unit Circle and the Functions of Trigonometry	377
Chapter 9	Trigonometric Identities and Equations	447
Chapter 10	Applications of Trigonometry; Vectors	501
Chapter 11	Further Topics in Algebra	553
Chapter 12	Limits, Derivatives, and Definite Integrals	591
Chapter R	Reference: Basic Algebraic Concepts	615
Appendice	B,C,D	629

Chapter 1: Linear Functions, Equations, and Inequalities

1.1: Real Numbers and the Rectangular Coordinate System

1. (a) The only natural number is 10.

   (b) The whole numbers are 0 and 10.

   (c) The integers are $-6, -\frac{12}{4}$ (or -3), 0, 10.

   (d) The rational numbers are $-6, -\frac{12}{4}$ (or -3), $-\frac{5}{8}, 0, .31, .\overline{3}$, and 10.

   (e) The irrational numbers are $-\sqrt{3}, 2\pi$ and $\sqrt{17}$.

   (f) All of the numbers listed are real numbers.

   (f) All of the numbers listed are real numbers.

3. (a) There are no natural numbers listed.

   (b) There are no whole numbers listed.

   (c) The integers are $-\sqrt{100}$ (or -10) and -1.

   (d) The rational numbers are $-\sqrt{100}$ (or -10), $-\frac{13}{6}, -1, 5.23, 9.\overline{14}, 3.14,$ and $\frac{22}{7}$.

   (e) There are no irrational numbers listed.

   (f) All of the numbers listed are real numbers..

5. The number 16,351,000,000,000 is a natural number, integer, rational number, and real number.

7. The number -25 is an integer, rational, and real number.

9. The number $\frac{7}{3}$ is a rational and real number.

11. The number $5\sqrt{2}$ is a real number.

13. Natural numbers would be appropriate because population is only measured in positive whole numbers.

15. Rational numbers would be appropriate because shoes come in fraction sizes.

17. Integers would be appropriate because temperature is given in positive and negative whole numbers.

19. [number line with points at $-4, -3, -2, -1, 0, 1$]

21. [number line with points at $-.5, .75, 0, \frac{5}{3}, 3.5$]

23. A rational number can be written as a fraction, $\frac{p}{q}, q \neq 0,$ where p and q are integers. An irrational number cannot be written in this way.

25. The point $\left(2, \frac{5}{7}\right)$ is in Quadrant I. See Figure 25-33.

2 Chapter 1 Linear Functions, Equations, and Inequalities

27. The point $(-3,-2)$ is in Quadrant III. See Figure 25-33.

29. The point $(0,5)$ is located on the y-axis, therefore is not in a quadrant. See Figure 25-33.

31. The point $(-2,4)$ is in Quadrant II. See Figure 25-33.

33. The point $(-2,0)$ is located on the x-axis, therefore is not in a quadrant. See Figure 25-33.

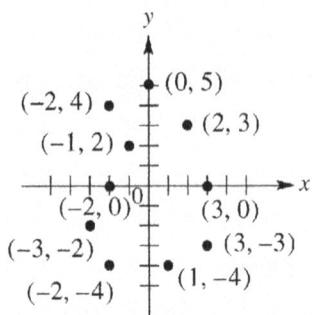

Figure 25-33

35. If $xy>0$, then either $x>0$ and $y>0 \Rightarrow$ Quadrant I, or $x<0$ and $y<0 \Rightarrow$ Quadrant III.

37. If $\dfrac{x}{y}<0$, then either $x>0$ and $y<0 \Rightarrow$ Quadrant IV, or $x<0$ and $y>0 \Rightarrow$ Quadrant II.

39. Any point of the form $(0,b)$ is located on the y-axis.

41. $[-5,5]$ by $[-25,25]$

43. $[-60,60]$ by $[-100,100]$

45. $[-500,300]$ by $[-300,500]$

47. See Figure 47.

49. See Figure 49.

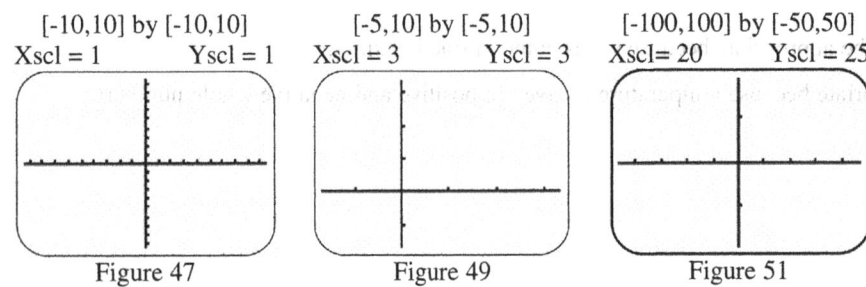

Figure 47 Figure 49 Figure 51

51. See Figure 51.

53. There are no tick marks, which is a result of setting Xscl and Yscl to 0.

55. $\sqrt{58} \approx 7.615773106 \approx 7.616$

57. $\sqrt[3]{33} \approx 3.20753433 \approx 3.208$

59. $\sqrt[4]{86} \approx 3.045261646 \approx 3.045$

61. $19^{1/2} \approx 4.35889844 \approx 4.359$

63. $46^{1.5} \approx 311.9871792 \approx 311.987$

65. $(5.6-3.1)/(8.9+1.3) \approx .25$

67. $\sqrt{(\pi\wedge 3 + 1)} \approx 5.66$

69. $3(5.9)^2 - 2(5.9) + 6 = 98.63$

71. $\sqrt{(4-6)^2 + (7+1)^2} \approx 8.25$

73. $\sqrt{(\pi-1)}/\sqrt{(1+\pi)} \approx .72$

75. $2/(1-\sqrt[3]{5}) \approx -2.82$

77. $a^2 + b^2 = c^2 \Rightarrow 8^2 + 15^2 = c^2 \Rightarrow 64 + 225 = c^2 \Rightarrow 289 = c^2 \Rightarrow c = 17$

79. $a^2 + b^2 = c^2 \Rightarrow 13^2 + b^2 = 85^2 \Rightarrow 169 + b^2 = 7225 \Rightarrow b^2 = 7056 \Rightarrow b = 84$

81. $a^2 + b^2 = c^2 \Rightarrow 5^2 + 8^2 = c^2 \Rightarrow 25 + 64 = c^2 \Rightarrow 89 = c^2 \Rightarrow c = \sqrt{89}$

83. $a^2 + b^2 = c^2 \Rightarrow a^2 + (\sqrt{13})^2 = (\sqrt{29})^2 \Rightarrow a^2 + 13 = 29 \Rightarrow a^2 = 16 \Rightarrow a = 4$

85. (a) $d = \sqrt{(2-(-4))^2 + (5-3)^2} = \sqrt{(6)^2 + (2)^2} = \sqrt{36+4} = \sqrt{40} = 2\sqrt{10}$

    (b) $M = \left(\dfrac{-4+2}{2}, \dfrac{3+5}{2}\right) = \left(\dfrac{-2}{2}, \dfrac{8}{2}\right) = (-1, 4)$

87. (a) $d = \sqrt{(6-(-7))^2 + (-2-4)^2} = \sqrt{(13)^2 + (-6)^2} = \sqrt{169+36} = \sqrt{205}$

    (b) $M = \left(\dfrac{-7+6}{2}, \dfrac{4+(-2)}{2}\right) = \left(\dfrac{-1}{2}, \dfrac{2}{2}\right) = \left(-\dfrac{1}{2}, 1\right)$

89. (a) $d = \sqrt{(2-5)^2 + (11-7)^2} = \sqrt{(-3)^2 + (4)^2} = \sqrt{9+16} = \sqrt{25} = 5$

    (b) $M = \left(\dfrac{5+2}{2}, \dfrac{7+11}{2}\right) = \left(\dfrac{7}{2}, \dfrac{18}{2}\right) = \left(\dfrac{7}{2}, 9\right)$

91. (a) $d = \sqrt{(-3-(-8))^2 + ((-5)-(-2))^2} = \sqrt{(5)^2 + (-3)^2} = \sqrt{25+9} = \sqrt{34}$

    (b) $M = \left(\dfrac{-8+(-3)}{2}, \dfrac{-2+(-5)}{2}\right) = \left(\dfrac{-11}{2}, \dfrac{-7}{2}\right) = \left(-\dfrac{11}{2}, -\dfrac{7}{2}\right)$

93. (a) $d = \sqrt{(6.2-9.2)^2 + (7.4-3.4)^2} = \sqrt{(-3)^2 + (4)^2} = \sqrt{9+16} = \sqrt{25} = 5$

    (b) $M = \left(\dfrac{9.2+6.2}{2}, \dfrac{3.4+7.4}{2}\right) = \left(\dfrac{15.4}{2}, \dfrac{10.8}{2}\right) = (7.7, 5.4)$

95. (a) $d = \sqrt{(6x-13x)^2 + (x-(-23x))^2} = \sqrt{(-7x)^2 + (24x)^2} = \sqrt{49x^2 + 576x^2} = \sqrt{625x^2} = 25x$

    (b) $M = \left(\dfrac{13x+6x}{2}, \dfrac{-23x+x}{2}\right) = \left(\dfrac{19x}{2}, \dfrac{-22x}{2}\right) = \left(\dfrac{19}{2}x, -11x\right)$

4   Chapter 1 Linear Functions, Equations, and Inequalities

97. Using the midpoint formula we get: $\left(\dfrac{7+x_2}{2}, \dfrac{-4+y_2}{2}\right) = (8,5) \Rightarrow \left(\dfrac{7+x_2}{2}\right) = 8 \Rightarrow 7+x_2 = 16 \Rightarrow x_2 = 9$ and

$\dfrac{-4+y_2}{2} = 5 \Rightarrow -4+y_2 = 10 \Rightarrow y_2 = 14$. Therefore the coordinates are: $Q(19,14)$.

99. Using the midpoint formula we get: $\left(\dfrac{5.64+x_2}{2}, \dfrac{8.21+y_2}{2}\right) = (-4.04, 1.60) \Rightarrow \dfrac{5.64+x_2}{2} = -4.04 \Rightarrow$

$5.64 + x_2 = -8.08 \Rightarrow x_2 = -13.72$ and $\dfrac{8.21+y_2}{2} = 1.60 \Rightarrow 8.21 + y_2 = 3.20 \Rightarrow y_2 = -5.01$. Therefore the

coordinates are: $Q(-13.72, -5.01)$.

101. $M = \left(\dfrac{2007+2011}{2}, \dfrac{17+36}{2}\right) = \left(\dfrac{4018}{2}, \dfrac{53}{2}\right) = (2009, 26.5)$; the revenue was about \$26.5 billion.

103. In 2005, $M = \left(\dfrac{2003+2007}{2}, \dfrac{18,810+21,203}{2}\right) = \left(\dfrac{4010}{2}, \dfrac{40,013}{2}\right) = (2005, 20,006.5)$; poverty level

was approximately \$20,007. In 2009, $M = \left(\dfrac{2007+2011}{2}, \dfrac{21,203+22,350}{2}\right) = \left(\dfrac{4018}{2}, \dfrac{43,553}{2}\right) =$

$(2009, 21,776.5)$; poverty level was approximately \$21,777.

105. (a) See Figure 105.
(b) $d = \sqrt{(50-0)^2 + (0-40)^2} = \sqrt{(50)^2 + (-40)^2} = \sqrt{2500+1600} = \sqrt{4100} \approx 64.0$ miles.

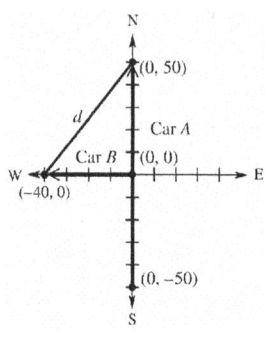

Figure 105

107. Using the area of a square produces: $(a+b)^2 = a^2 + 2ab + b^2$. Now, using the sum of the small

square and the four right triangles produces $c^2 + 4\left(\dfrac{1}{2}ab\right) = c^2 + 2ab$. Therefore $a^2 + 2ab + b^2 = c^2 + 2ab$,

and subtracting $2ab$ from both sides produces $a^2 + b^2 = c^2$.

1.2: Introduction to Relations and Functions

1. The interval is $(-1, 4)$.

3. The interval is $(-\infty, 0)$.

5. The interval is $[1,2)$.

7. $(-4,3) \Rightarrow \{x \mid -4 < x < 3\}$

9. $(-\infty, -1] \Rightarrow \{x \mid x \leq -1\}$

11. $\{x \mid -2 \leq x < 6\}$

13. $\{x \mid x \leq -4\}$

15. A parenthesis is used if the symbol is $<$, $>$, $-\infty$, or ∞ or. A square bracket is used if the symbol is $\leq$ or $\geq$.

17. See Figure 17

19. See Figure 19

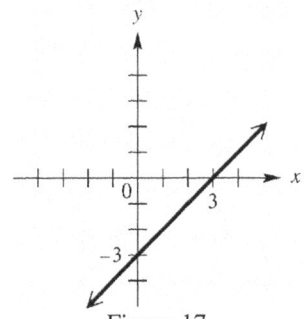

Figure 17

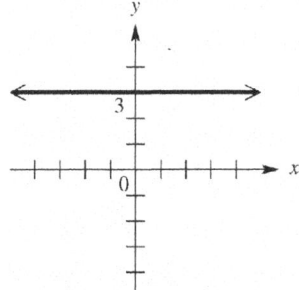

Figure 19

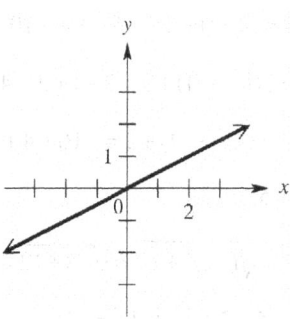

Figure 21

21. See Figure 21

23. See Figure 23

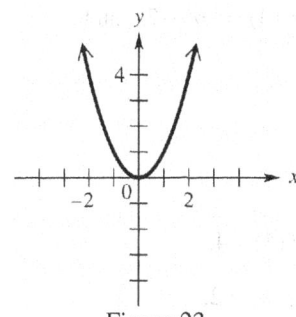

Figure 23

25. The relation is a function. Domain: $\{5,3,4,7\}$ Range: $\{1,2,9,6\}$.

27. The relation is a function. Domain: $\{1,2,3\}$, Range: $\{6\}$.

29. The relation is not a function. Domain: $\{4,3,-2\}$, Range: $\{1,-5,3,7\}$.

31. The relation is a function. Domain: $\{11,12,13,14\}$, Range: $\{-6,-7\}$.

33. The relation is a function. Domain: $\{0,1,2,3,4\}$, Range: $\{\sqrt{2}, \sqrt{3}, \sqrt{5}, \sqrt{6}, \sqrt{7}\}$.

35. The relation is a function. Domain: $(-\infty, \infty)$, Range: $(-\infty, \infty)$.

37. The relation is not a function. Domain: $[-4,4]$, Range: $[-3,3]$.

39. The relation is a function. Domain: $[2,\infty)$, Range: $[0,\infty)$.

41. The relation is not a function. Domain: $[-9,\infty)$, Range: $(-\infty,\infty)$.

43. The relation is a function. Domain: $\{-5,-2,-1,-.5,0,1.75,3.5\}$, Range: $\{-1,2,3,3.5,4,5.75,7.5\}$.

45. The relation is a function. Domain: $\{2,3,5,11,17\}$ Range: $\{1,7,20\}$.

47. From the diagram, $f(-2) = 2$.

49. From the diagram, $f(11) = 7$.

51. $f(1)$ is undefined since 1 is not in the domain of the function.

53. $f(-2) = 3(-2) - 4 = -6 - 4 = -10$

55. $f(1) = 2(1)^2 - (1) + 3 = 2 - 1 + 3 = 4$

57. $f(4) = -(4)^2 + (4) + 2 = -16 + 4 + 2 = -10$

59. $f(9) = 5$

61. $f(-2) = \sqrt{(-2)^3 + 12} = \sqrt{-8+12} = \sqrt{4} = 2$

63. $f(8) = |5 - 2(8)| = |-11| = 11$

65. Given that $f(x) = 5x$, then $f(a) = 5a$, $f(b+1) = 5(b+1) = 5b+5$, and $f(3x) = 5(3x) = 15x$

67. Given that $f(x) = 2x - 5$, then $f(a) = 2a - 5$, $f(b+1) = 2(b+1) - 5 = 2b + 2 - 5 = 2b - 3$, and
$f(3x) = 2(3x) - 5 = 6x - 5$

69. Given that $f(x) = 1 - x^2$, then $f(a) = 1 - a^2$, $f(b+1) = 1 - (b+1)^2 = 1 - (b^2 + 2b + 1) = -b^2 - 2b$, and
$f(3x) = 1 - (3x)^2 = 1 - 9x^2$

71. Since $f(-2) = 3$, the point $(-2, 3)$ lies on the graph of f.

73. Since the point $(7, 8)$ lies on the graph of f, $f(7) = 8$.

75. From the graph: (a) $f(-2) = 0$, (b) $f(0) = 4$, (c) $f(1) = 2$, and (d) $f(4) = 4$.

77. From the graph: (a) $f(-2)$ is undefined, (b) $f(0) = -2$, (c) $f(1) = 0$, and (d) $f(4) = 2$.

79. (a) – (f) Answers will vary. Refer to the definitions in the text.

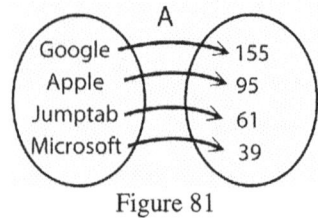

Figure 81

81. (a) $A = \{(\text{Google}, 155), (\text{Apple}, 95), (\text{Jumptab}, 61), (\text{Microsoft}, 39)\}$, The U.S. mobile advertising revenue in 2011 for Google was $155,000,000 dollars.

(b) See Figure 81.

(c) $D = \{\text{Google, Apple, Jumptab, Microsoft}\}$, $R = \{155, 95, 61, 39\}$

Reviewing Basic Concepts (Sections 1.1 and 1.2)

1. See Figure 1.

2. The distance is $d = \sqrt{(6-(-4))^2 + (-2-5)^2} = \sqrt{100+49} = \sqrt{149}$.

   The midpoint is $M = \left(\dfrac{-4+6}{2}, \dfrac{5-2}{2}\right) = \left(1, \dfrac{3}{2}\right)$.

3. $\dfrac{\sqrt{5}+\pi}{(\sqrt[3]{3}+1)} \approx 1.168$

4. $d = \sqrt{(12-(-4))^2 + (-3-27)^2} = \sqrt{256+900} = \sqrt{1156} = 34$

5. Using Pythagorean Theorem, $11^2 + b^2 = 61^2 \Rightarrow b^2 = 61^2 - 11^2 \Rightarrow b^2 = 3600 \Rightarrow b = 60$ inches.

6. The set $\{x \mid -2 < x \leq 5\}$ is the interval $(-2, 5]$. The set $\{x \mid x \geq 4\}$ is the interval $[4, \infty)$.

7. The relation is not a function because it does not pass the vertical line test. Domain: $[-2, 2]$, Range: $[-3, 3]$.

8. See Figure 8.

9. Given $f(x) = 3 - 4x$ then $f(-5) = 3 - 4(-5) = 23$ and $f(a+4) = 3 - 4(a+4) = 3 - 4a - 16 = -4a - 13$

10. From the graph, $f(2) = 3$ and $f(-1) = -3$.

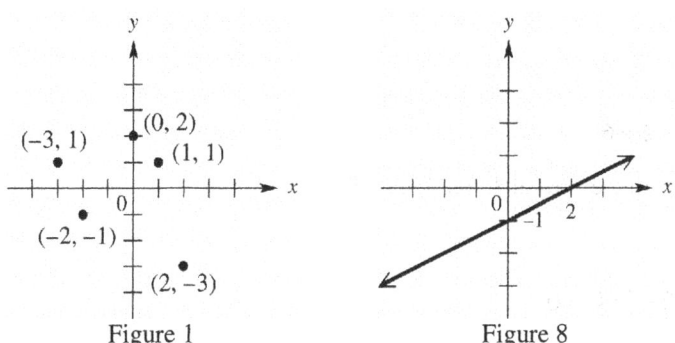

Figure 1   Figure 8

1.3: Linear Functions

1. The graph is shown in Figure 1.

   (a) x-intercept: 4 (b) y-intercept: -4 (c) Domain: $(-\infty, \infty)$ (d) Range: $(-\infty, \infty)$

   (e) The equation is in slope-intercept form, therefore $m = 1$.

3. The graph is shown in Figure 3.

   (a) x-intercept: 2 (b) y-intercept: -6 (c) Domain: $(-\infty, \infty)$ (d) Range: $(-\infty, \infty)$

8   Chapter 1 Linear Functions, Equations, and Inequalities

(e) The equation is in slope-intercept form, therefore $m = 3$.

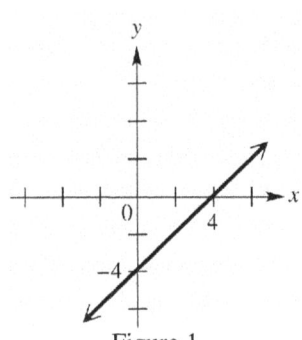
Figure 1

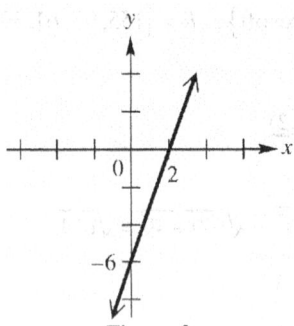
Figure 3

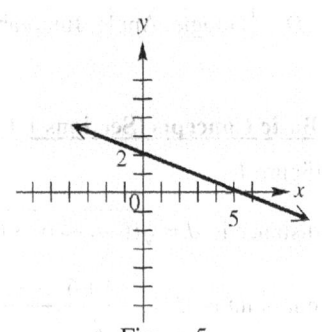
Figure 5

5. The graph is shown in Figure 5.

   (a) x-intercept: 5   (b) y-intercept: 2   (c) Domain: $(-\infty, \infty)$ (d) Range: $(-\infty, \infty)$

   (e) The equation is in slope-intercept form, therefore $m = -\dfrac{2}{5}$.

7. The graph is shown in Figure 7.

   (a) x-intercept: 0   (b) y-intercept: 0   (c) Domain: $(-\infty, \infty)$ (d) Range: $(-\infty, \infty)$

   (e) The equation is in slope-intercept form, therefore $m = 3$.

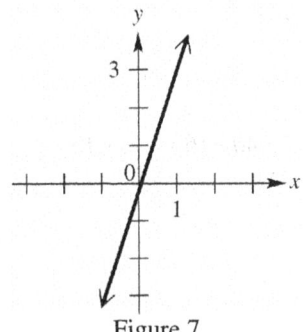
Figure 7

9. (a) $f(-2) = (-2) + 2 = 0$ and $f(4) = (4) + 2 = 6$

   (b) The x-intercept is -2 and corresponds to the zero of f. See Figure 9.

   (c) $x + 2 = 0 \Rightarrow x = -2$

11. (a) $f(-2) = 2 - \dfrac{1}{2}(-2) = 3$ and $f(4) = 2 - \dfrac{1}{2}(4) = 0$

    (b) The x-intercept is 4 and corresponds to the zero of f. See Figure 11.

    (c) $2 - \dfrac{1}{2}x = 0 \Rightarrow \dfrac{1}{2}x = 2 \Rightarrow x = 4$

Section 1.3   9

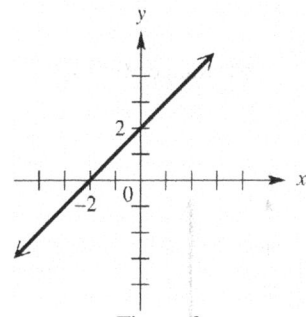
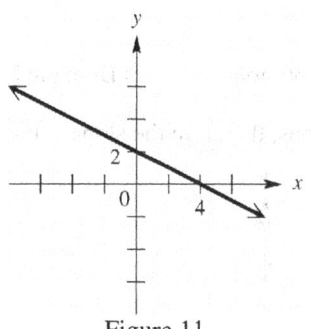
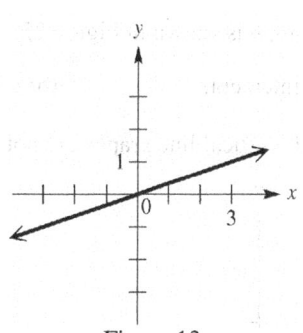

Figure 9   Figure 11   Figure 13

13. (a) $f(-2) = \frac{1}{3}(-2) = -\frac{2}{3}$ and $f(4) = \frac{1}{3}(4) = \frac{4}{3}$

   (b) The x-intercept is 0 and corresponds to the zero of f. See Figure 13.

   (c) $\frac{1}{3}x = 0 \Rightarrow x = 0$

15. (a) $f(-2) = .4(-2) + .15 = -.65$ and $f(4) = .4(4) + .15 = 1.75$

   (b) The x-intercept is $-.375$ and corresponds to the zero of f. See Figure 15.

   (c) $.4x + .15 = 0 \Rightarrow .4x = -.15 \Rightarrow x = -.375$

17. (a) $f(-2) = \frac{2-(-2)}{4} = 1$ and $f(4) = \frac{2-(4)}{4} = -\frac{1}{2}$

   (b) The x-intercept is 2 and corresponds to the zero of f. See Figure 17.

   (c) $\frac{2-x}{4} = 0 \Rightarrow 2 - x = 0 \Rightarrow x = 2$

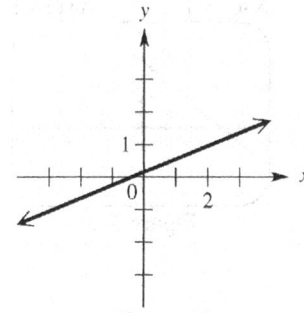
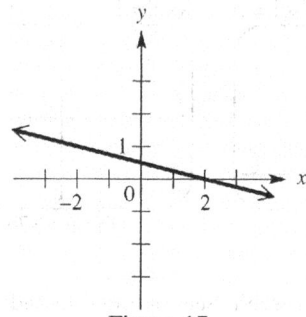
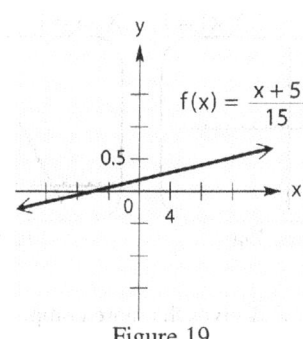

Figure 15   Figure 17   Figure 19

19. (a) $f(-2) = \frac{-2+5}{15} = \frac{3}{15} = \frac{1}{5}$ and $f(4) = \frac{4+5}{15} = \frac{9}{15} = \frac{3}{5}$

   (b) The x-intercept is –5 and corresponds to the zero of f. See Figure 19

   (c) $\frac{x+5}{15} = 0 \Rightarrow x + 5 = 0 \Rightarrow x = -5$

21. The graph of $y = ax$ always passes through (0, 0).

23. The graph is shown in Figure 23.

   (a) x-intercept: none   (b) y-intercept: –3   (c) Domain: $(-\infty, \infty)$ (d) Range: $\{-3\}$

   (e) The slope of all horizontal line graphs or constant functions is $m = 0$.

Copyright © 2015 Pearson Education, Inc

10   Chapter 1 Linear Functions, Equations, and Inequalities

25. The graph is shown in Figure 25.

   (a) *x*-intercept: −1.5   (b) *y*-intercept: none   (c) Domain: $\{-1.5\}$ (d) Range: $(-\infty, \infty)$

   (e) All vertical line graphs are not functions, therefore the slope is undefined.

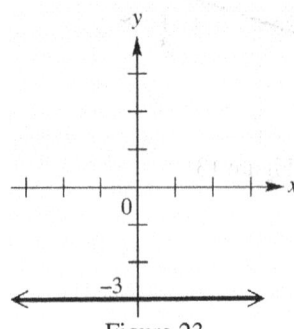
Figure 23

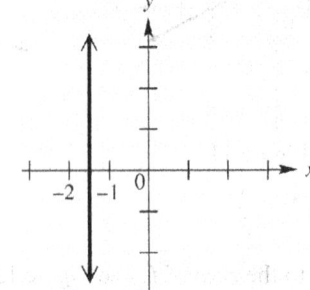
Figure 25

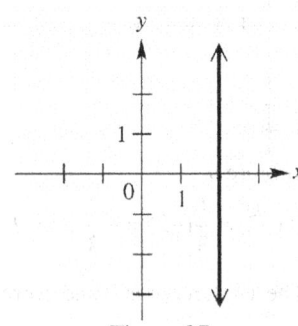
Figure 27

27. The graph is shown in Figure 27.

   (a) *x*-intercept: 2   (b) *y*-intercept: none   (c) Domain: $\{2\}$

   (d) Range: $(-\infty, \infty)$ (e) All vertical line graphs are not functions, therefore the slope is undefined.

29. All functions in the form *f*(*x*) = *a* are constant functions.

31. This is a horizontal line graph, therefore *y* = 3.

33. This is a vertical line graph on the *y*-axis, therefore *x* = 0.

35. Window B gives the more comprehensive graph. See Figures 35a and 35b.

[-10,10] by [-10,10]   [-10,10] by [-5,25]   [-3,3] by [-5,5]   [-5,5] by [-10,14]
Xscl = 1   Yscl = 1   Xscl = 1   Yscl = 5   Xscl= 1   Yscl = 1   Xscl = 1   Yscl= 2

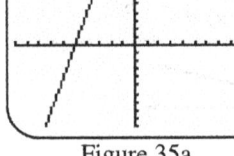
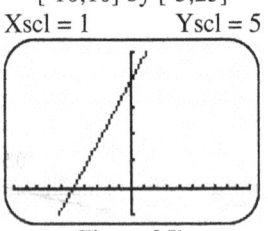
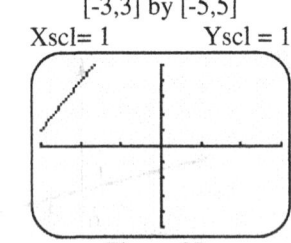
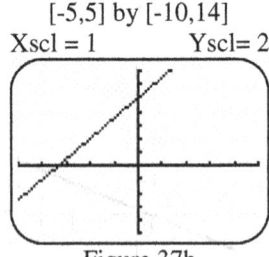

Figure 35a   Figure 35b   Figure 37a   Figure 37b

37. Window B gives the more comprehensive graph. See Figures 37a and 37b.

39. $m = \dfrac{6-1}{3-(-2)} = \dfrac{5}{5} = 1$

41. $m = \dfrac{4-(-3)}{8-(-1)} = \dfrac{7}{9}$

43. $m = \dfrac{5-3}{-11-(-11)} = \dfrac{2}{0} \Rightarrow$ undefined slope

45. $m = \dfrac{9-9}{\frac{1}{2}-\frac{2}{3}} = \dfrac{0}{-\frac{1}{6}} \Rightarrow 0$

47. $m = \dfrac{-\dfrac{2}{3} - \dfrac{1}{6}}{\dfrac{1}{2} - \left(-\dfrac{3}{4}\right)} = \dfrac{-\dfrac{5}{6}}{\dfrac{5}{4}} \Rightarrow -\dfrac{2}{3}$

49. The average rate of change is evaluated as $m = \dfrac{y_2 - y_1}{x_2 - x_1} = \dfrac{20-4}{0-4} = -\dfrac{16}{4} = -4$. The value of the machine is decreasing $4000 each year during these years.

51. The average rate of change is evaluated as $m = \dfrac{y_2 - y_1}{x_2 - x_1} = \dfrac{3-3}{4-0} = \dfrac{0}{4} = 0$. The percent of pay raise is not changing but will remain constant at 3% per year.

53. Since $m = 3$ and $b = 6$, graph A most closely resembles the equation.

55. Since $m = -3$ and $b = -6$, graph C most closely resembles the equation.

57. Since $m = 3$ and $b = 0$, graph H most closely resembles the equation.

59. Since $m = 0$ and $b = 3$, graph B most closely resembles the equation.

61. (a) The graph passes through $(0,1)$ and $(1,-1) \Rightarrow m = \dfrac{-1-1}{1-0} = \dfrac{-2}{1} = -2$. The y-intercept is $(0,1)$ and the x-intercept is $\left(\dfrac{1}{2}, 0\right)$.

   (b) Using the slope and y-intercept, the formula is $f(x) = -2x + 1$.

   (c) The x-intercept is the zero of $f \Rightarrow \dfrac{1}{2}$.

63. (a) The graph passes through $(0, 2)$ and $(3,1) \Rightarrow m = \dfrac{1-2}{3-0} = \dfrac{-1}{3} = -\dfrac{1}{3}$. The y-intercept is $(0,2)$ and the x-intercept is $(6,0)$.

   (b) Using the slope and y-intercept, the formula is $f(x) = -\dfrac{1}{3}x + 2$.

   (c) The x-intercept is the zero of $f \Rightarrow 6$.

65. (a) The graph passes through $(0, 300)$ and $(2, -100) \Rightarrow m = \dfrac{-100 - 300}{2 - 0} = \dfrac{-400}{2} = -200$.

   The y-intercept is $(0, 300)$ and the x-intercept is $\left(\dfrac{3}{2}, 0\right)$.

   (b) Using the slope and y-intercept, the formula is $f(x) = -200x + 300$.

   (c) The x-intercept is the zero of $f \Rightarrow \dfrac{3}{2}$.

67. Using $(0, 2)$ and $(1, 6)$, $m = \dfrac{6-2}{1-0} = \dfrac{4}{1} = 4$. From the table, the y-intercept is $(0,2)$. Using these two answers and slope-intercept form, the equation is $f(x) = 4x + 2$.

12 Chapter 1 Linear Functions, Equations, and Inequalities

69. Using (0, –3.1) and (.2, –3.38), $m = \dfrac{-3.38 - (-3.1)}{.2 - 0} = \dfrac{-.28}{.2} = -1.4$. From the table, the y-intercept is $(0, -3.1)$. Using these two answers and slope-intercept form, the equation is $f(x) = -1.4x - 3.1$.

71. The graph of a constant function with positive k is a horizontal graph above the x-axis. Graph A

73. The graph of an equation of the form x = k with k > 0 is a vertical line right of the y-axis. Graph D

75. Using (–1, 3) with a rise of 3 and a run of 2, the graph also passes through (1, 6). See Figure 75.

77. Using (3, –4) with a rise of –1 and a run of 3, the graph also passes through (6, –5). See Figure 77.

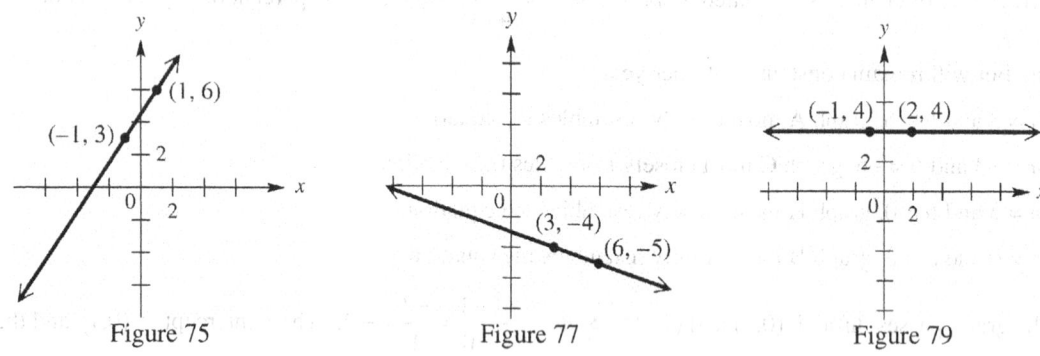

Figure 75   Figure 77   Figure 79

79. Using (–1, 4) with slope of 0, the graph is a horizontal line which also passes through (2, 4). See Figure 79.

81. Using (0, –4) with a rise of 3 and a run of 4, the graph also passes through (4, –1). See Figure 81.

83. Using (–3, 0) with undefined slope, the graph is a vertical line which also passes through (–3, 2). See Figure 83.

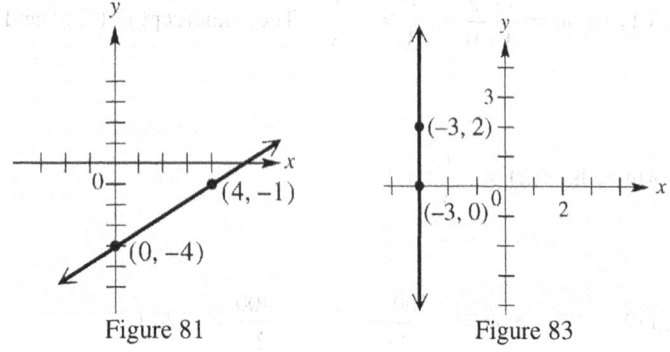

Figure 81   Figure 83

85. (a) Using the points (0, 2000) and (4, 4000), $m = \dfrac{4000 - 2000}{4 - 0} = \dfrac{2000}{4} = 500$. The y-intercept is $(0, 2000)$. The formula is $f(x) = 500x + 2000$.

    (b) Water is entering the pool at a rate of 500 gallons per hour. The pool contains 2000 gallons initially.

    (c) From the graph $f(7) = 5500$ gallons. By evaluating, $f(7) = 500(7) + 2000 = 5500$ gallons.

87. (a) The rain fell at a rate of $\frac{1}{4}$ inches per hour, so $m = \frac{1}{4}$. The initial amount of rain at noon was 3 inches, so $b = 3$. The equation $f(x) = \frac{1}{4}x + 3$.

(b) By 2:30 P.M. ($x = 2.5$), the total rainfall was $f(2.5) = \frac{1}{4}(2.5) + 3 = 3.625$ in.

89. (a) $f(15) = \frac{15}{5} = 3$, The delay of a bolt of lightning 3 miles away is 15 seconds.

(b) See Figure 89.

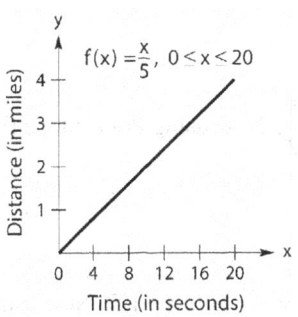

Figure 89

91. $f(x) = 0.075x$, $f(86) = 0.075(86) = 6.45$, The tax on $86 is $6.45.

93. The increase of $192 per credit can be shown as the slope and the fixed fees of $275 can be shown as the y-intercept. The function is $f(x) = 192x + 275$. $f(11) = 192(11) + 275 = \$2387$

95. (a) Since the average rate of change has been 0.9 degrees per decade we will write the slope as 0.09 degrees per year. The function is $W(x) = 0.09x$.

(b) $W(15) = 0.09(15) = 1.35$, In 15 years the Antarctic has warmed 1.35 degrees farenheit, on average.

1.4: Equations of Lines and Linear Models

1. Using Point-Slope Form yields $y - 3 = -2(x - 1) \Rightarrow y - 3 = -2x + 2 \Rightarrow y = -2x + 5$.

3. Using Point-Slope Form yields $y - 4 = 1.5(x - (-5)) \Rightarrow y - 4 = 1.5x + 7.5 \Rightarrow y = 1.5x + 11.5$.

5. Using Point-Slope Form yields $y - 1 = -.5(x - (-8)) \Rightarrow y - 1 = -.5x - 4 \Rightarrow y = -.5x - 3$.

7. Using Point-Slope Form yields $y - (-4) = 2\left(x - \frac{1}{2}\right) \Rightarrow y + 4 = 2x - 1 \Rightarrow y = 2x - 5$.

9. Using Point-Slope Form yields $y - \frac{2}{3} = \frac{1}{2}\left(x - \frac{1}{4}\right) \Rightarrow y - \frac{2}{3} = \frac{1}{2}x - \frac{1}{8} \Rightarrow y = \frac{1}{2}x + \frac{13}{24}$.

14   Chapter 1 Linear Functions, Equations, and Inequalities

11. Use the points to (−4, −6) and (6, 2) find the slope: $m = \dfrac{2-(-6)}{6-(-4)} \Rightarrow m = \dfrac{4}{5}$. Now using Point-Slope Form yields $y - 2 = \dfrac{4}{5}(x - 6) \Rightarrow y - 2 = \dfrac{4}{5}x - \dfrac{24}{5} \Rightarrow y = \dfrac{4}{5}x - \dfrac{14}{5}$.

13. Use the points (−12, 8) and (8, −12) to find the slope: $m = \dfrac{-12-8}{8-(-12)} \Rightarrow m = \dfrac{-20}{20} \Rightarrow m = -1$. Now using Point-Slope Form yields $y - 8 = -1(x + 12) \Rightarrow y - 8 = -x - 12 \Rightarrow y = -x - 4$.

15. Use the points (4, 8) and (0, 4) to find the slope: $m = \dfrac{4-8}{0-4} \Rightarrow m = \dfrac{-4}{-4} \Rightarrow m = 1$. Now using Slope-Intercept Form yields $b = 4 \Rightarrow y = x + 4$.

17. Use the points (3, −8) and (5, −3) to find the slope: $m = \dfrac{-3-(-8)}{5-3} \Rightarrow m = \dfrac{5}{2}$. Now using Point-Slope Form yields $y - (-8) = \dfrac{5}{2}(x - 3) \Rightarrow y + 8 = \dfrac{5}{2}x - \dfrac{15}{2} \Rightarrow y = \dfrac{5}{2}x - \dfrac{31}{2}$.

19. Use the points (2, 3.5) and (6, −2.5) to find the slope: $m = \dfrac{-2.5-3.5}{6-2} \Rightarrow m = \dfrac{-6}{4} \Rightarrow m = -1.5$. Now using Point-Slope Form yields $y - 3.5 = -1.5(x - 2) \Rightarrow y - 3.5 = -1.5x + 3 \Rightarrow y = -1.5x + 6.5$.

21. Use the points (0, 5) and (10, 0) to find the slope: $m = \dfrac{0-5}{10-0} \Rightarrow m = \dfrac{-5}{10} \Rightarrow m = -\dfrac{1}{2}$. Now using Point-Slope Form yields $y - 5 = -\dfrac{1}{2}(x - 0) \Rightarrow y - 5 = -\dfrac{1}{2}x \Rightarrow y - \dfrac{1}{2}x + 5$.

23. Use the points (−5, −28) and (−4, −20) to find the slope: $m = \dfrac{-20-(-28)}{-4-(-5)} \Rightarrow m = \dfrac{8}{1} \Rightarrow m = 8$. Now using Point-Slope Form yields $y - (-20) = 8(x - (-4)) \Rightarrow y + 20 = 8x + 32 \Rightarrow y = 8x + 12$.

25. Use the points (2, −5) and (4, −11) to find the slope: $m = \dfrac{-11-(-5)}{4-2} \Rightarrow m = \dfrac{-6}{2} \Rightarrow m = -3$. Now using Point-Slope Form yields $y - (-5) = -3(x - 2) \Rightarrow y + 5 = -3x + 6 \Rightarrow y = -3x + 1$.

27. To find the x-intercept set $y = 0$, then $x - 0 = 4 \Rightarrow x = 4$. Therefore (4, 0) is the x-intercept. To find the y-intercept set $x = 0$, then $0 - y = 4 \Rightarrow y = -4$. Therefore (0, −4) is the y-intercept. See Figure 27.

29. To find the x-intercept set $y = 0$, then $3x - 0 = 6 \Rightarrow 3x = 6 \Rightarrow x = 2$. Therefore (2, 0) is the x-intercept. To find the y-intercept set $x = 0$, then $3(0) - y = 6 \Rightarrow y = -6$. Therefore (0, −6) is the y-intercept. See Figure 29.

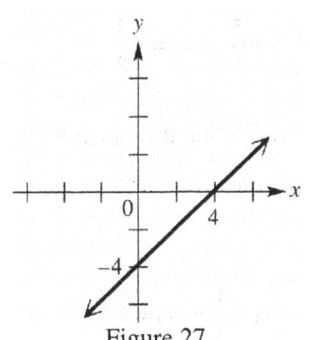

Figure 27

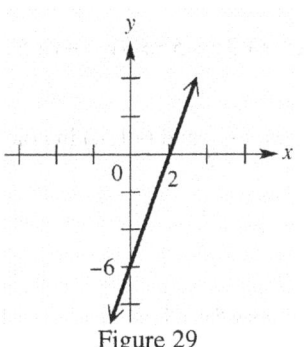

Figure 29

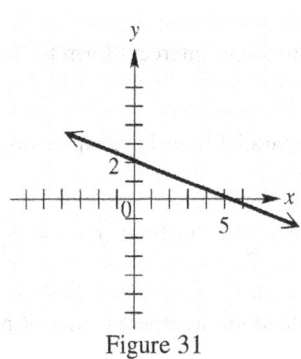

Figure 31

31. To find the *x*-intercept: set $y = 0$, then $2x + 5(0) = 10 \Rightarrow 2x = 10 \Rightarrow x = 5$. Therefore $(5, 0)$ is the *x*-intercept. To find the *y*-intercept: set $x = 0$, then $2(0) + 5y = 10 \Rightarrow 5y = 10 \Rightarrow y = 2$. Therefore $(0, 2)$ is the *y*-intercept. See Figure 31.

33. To find a second point set $x = 1$, then $y = 3(1) \Rightarrow y = 3$. A second point is $(1, 3)$. See Figure 33.

35. To find a second point set $x = 4$, then $y = -.75(4) \Rightarrow y = -3$. A second point is $(4, -3)$. See Figure 35.

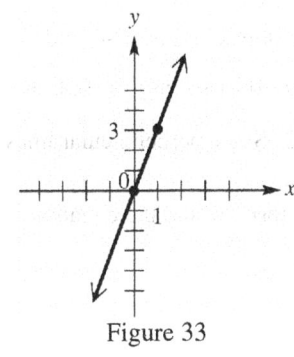

Figure 33

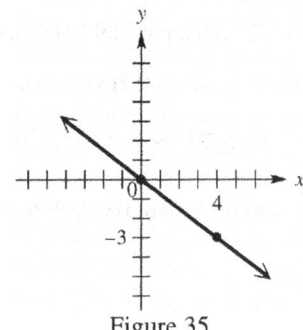

Figure 35

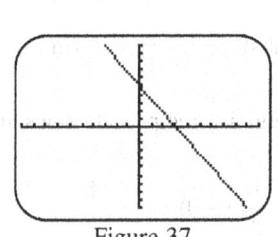

Figure 37

37. $5x + 3y = 15 \Rightarrow 3y = -5x + 15 \Rightarrow y = -\dfrac{5}{3}x + 5$. See Figure 37.

39. $-2x + 7y = 4 \Rightarrow 7y = 2x + 4 \Rightarrow y = \dfrac{2}{7}x + \dfrac{4}{7}$. See Figure 39.

41. $1.2x + 1.6y = 5.0 \Rightarrow 12x + 16y = 50 \Rightarrow 16y = -12x + 50 \Rightarrow y = -\dfrac{12}{16}x + \dfrac{50}{16} \Rightarrow y = -\dfrac{3}{4}x + \dfrac{25}{8}$. See Figure 41.

[-5,5] by [-5,5]
Xscl = 1   Yscl = 1

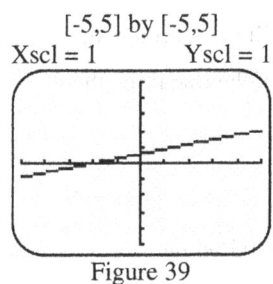

Figure 39

[-6,6] by [-4,4]
Xscl = 1   Yscl = 1

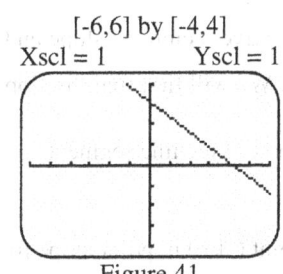

Figure 41

16 Chapter 1 Linear Functions, Equations, and Inequalities

43. Put into slope-intercept form to find slope: $x + 3y = 5 \Rightarrow 3y = -x + 5 \Rightarrow y = -\frac{1}{3}x + \frac{5}{3} \Rightarrow m = -\frac{1}{3}$.

    Since parallel lines have equal slopes, use $m = -\frac{1}{3}$ and $(-1, 4)$ in point-slope form to find the equation:

    $y - 4 = -\frac{1}{3}(x - (-1)) \Rightarrow y - 4 = -\frac{1}{3}x - \frac{1}{3} \Rightarrow y = -\frac{1}{3}x + \frac{11}{3}$.

45. Put into slope-intercept form to find slope: $3x + 5y = 1 \Rightarrow 5y = -3x + 1 \Rightarrow y = -\frac{3}{5}x + \frac{1}{5} \Rightarrow m = -\frac{3}{5}$. Since

    perpendicular lines have negative reciprocal slopes, use $m = \frac{5}{3}$ and $(1, 6)$ in point-slope form to find the

    equation: $y - 6 = \frac{5}{3}(x - 1) \Rightarrow y - 6 = \frac{5}{3}x - \frac{5}{3} \Rightarrow y = \frac{5}{3}x + \frac{13}{3}$.

47. The equation $y = -2$ has a slope $m = 0$. A line perpendicular to this would have an undefined slope which would have an equation in the form $x = a$. An equation in the form $x = a$ through $(-5, 7)$ is $x = -5$.

49. The equation $y = -.2x + 6$ has a slope $m = -0.2$. Since parallel lines have equal slopes, use $m = -.2$ and $(-5, 8)$ in point-slope form to find the equation $y - 8 = -0.2(x - (-5)) \Rightarrow y - 8 = -0.2x - 1 \Rightarrow y = -0.2x + 7$.

51. Put into slope-intercept form to find slope: $2x + y = 6 \Rightarrow y = -2x + 6 \Rightarrow m = -2$. Since perpendicular lines

    have negative reciprocal slopes, use $m = \frac{1}{2}$ and the origin $(0, 0)$ in point-slope form to find the equation

    $y - 0 = \frac{1}{2}(x - 0) \Rightarrow y = \frac{1}{2}x$.

53. The equation $x = 3$ has an undefined slope. A line perpendicular to this would have a slope $m = 0$, which would have an equation in the form $y = b$. An equation in the form $y = b$ through $(1, 2)$ is $y = 2$.

55. We will first find the slope of the line through the given points: $m = \dfrac{\frac{2}{3} - \frac{1}{2}}{-3 - (-5)} = \dfrac{\frac{1}{6}}{2} \Rightarrow m = \frac{1}{12}$. Since

    perpendicular lines have negative reciprocal slopes, use $m = -12$ and the point $(-2, 4)$ in point-slope form to find the equation $y - 4 = -12(x - (-2)) \Rightarrow y = -12x - 20$.

57. The slope of the perpendicular bisector will have a negative reciprocal slope and will pass through the midpoint of the line segment joined by the two points. We will first find the slope of the line through the

    given points: $m = \frac{10 - 2}{2 - (-4)} = \frac{8}{6} \Rightarrow m = \frac{4}{3}$. The midpoint of the line segment

    is $\left(\frac{-4 + 2}{2}, \frac{2 + 10}{2}\right) = (-1, 6)$. Use $m = -\frac{3}{4}$ and the point $(-1, 6)$ in point-slope form to find the

    equation $y - 6 = -\frac{3}{4}(x - (-1)) \Rightarrow y = -\frac{3}{4}x + \frac{21}{4}$.

59. (a) The Pythagorean Theorem and its converse.

Section 1.4   17

(b) Using the distance formula from $(0, 0)$ to $(x_1, m_1 x_1)$ yields: $d(0,P) = \sqrt{(x_1)^2 + (m_1 x_1)^2}$.

(c) Using the distance formula from $(0, 0)$ to $(x_2, m_2 x_2)$ yields: $d(0,Q) = \sqrt{(x_2)^2 + (m_2 x_2)^2}$.

(d) Using the distance formula from $(x_1, m_1 x_1)$ to $(x_2, m_2 x_2)$ yields:

$d(P,Q) = \sqrt{(x_2 - x_1)^2 + (m_2 x_2 - m_1 x_1)^2}$.

(e) Using Pythagorean Theorem yields: $[d(0,P)]^2 + [d(0,Q)]^2 = [d(P,Q)]^2 \Rightarrow$

$(x_1)^2 + (m_1 x_1)^2 + (x_2)^2 + (m_2 x_2)^2 = (x_1 - x_2)^2 + (m_1 x_1 - m_2 x_2)^2 \Rightarrow (x_1)^2 + (m_1 x_1)^2 + (x_2)^2 + (m_2 x_2)^2 =$

$(x_1)^2 - 2x_1 x_2 + (x_2)^2 + (m_1 x_1)^2 - 2 m_1 m_2 x_1 x_2 + (m_2 x_2)^2 \Rightarrow 0 = -2 m_1 m_2 x_1 x_2 - 2x_1 x_2$.

(f) $0 = -2 x_1 x_2 - 2 m_1 m_2 x_1 x_2 \Rightarrow 0 = -2 x_1 x_2 (1 + m_1 m_2)$

(g) By the zero-product property, for $-2 x_1 x_2 (1 + m_1 m_2) = 0$ either $-2 x_1 x_2 = 0$ or $1 + m_1 m_2 = 0$.

Since $x_1 \neq 0$ and $x_2 \neq 0$, $-2 x_1 x_2 \neq 0$, and it follows that $1 + m_1 m_2 = 0 \Rightarrow m_1 m_2 = -1$.

(h) The product of the slopes of two perpendicular lines, neither of which is parallel to an axis, is -1.

61. (a) Use the given points to find slope, then $m = \dfrac{161 - 128}{4 - 1} = \dfrac{33}{3} \Rightarrow m = 11$. Now use point-slope form to

find the equation: $y - 128 = 11(x - 1) \Rightarrow y - 128 = 11x - 11 \Rightarrow y = 11x + 117$.

(b) From the slope the biker is traveling 11 mph.

(c) At $x = 0$, $y = 11(0) + 117 \Rightarrow y = 117$, therefore 117 miles from the highway.

(d) Since at 1 hour and 15 minutes $x = 1.25$, then $y = 11(1.25) + 117 \Rightarrow y = 130.75$, so 130.75 miles away.

63. (a) Use the points $(2007, 18)$, $(2010, 24)$ to find slope, then $m = \dfrac{24 - 18}{2010 - 2007} = \dfrac{6}{3} \Rightarrow m = 2$. Now use

point-slope form to find the equation: $y - 18 = 2(x - 2007) \Rightarrow y - 18 = 2x - 4014 \Rightarrow y = 2x - 3996$.

(b) $y = 2(2013) - 3996 = 30$. There was approximately \$30 billion in betting revenue in 2013.

65. (a) Since the plotted points form a line, it is a linear relation. See Figure 65.

(b) Using the first two points find the slope: $m = \dfrac{0 - (-40)}{32 - (-40)} = \dfrac{40}{72} = \dfrac{5}{9}$, now use slope-intercept form to

find the function: $C(x) - 0 = \dfrac{5}{9}(x - 32) \Rightarrow C(x) = \dfrac{5}{9}(x - 32)$. The slope of $\dfrac{5}{9}$ means that the Celsius

temperature changes $5°$ for every $9°$ change in Fahrenheit temperature.

(c) $C(83) = \dfrac{5}{9}(83 - 32) = 28\dfrac{1}{3}°C$

67. (a) The slope is $\dfrac{37 - 6}{2011 - 2005} = \dfrac{31}{6}$ ∴ Using point-slope form produces the equation:

$y - 6 = \dfrac{31}{6}(x - 2005)$.

(b) Every year from 2005 to 2011, Google advertising revenue increased by about \$5.2 billion on average.

(c) 2007 Revenue: $y - 6 = \frac{31}{6}(2007 - 2005) \Rightarrow y = \frac{31}{6}(2) + 6 \Rightarrow y \approx 16.3$ billion

2009 Revenue: $y - 6 = \frac{31}{6}(2009 - 2005) \Rightarrow y = \frac{31}{6}(4) + 6 \Rightarrow y \approx 26.67$ billion

The 2007 value compares favorably and the 2009 value is too high.

69. (a) Enter the years in L_1 and enter tuition and fees in L_2. The regression equation is:
$y \approx 586.89x - 1,147,738$.

(b) See Figure 69.

(c) At $x = 2005$, $y \approx 586.89(2005) - 1,147,738 \Rightarrow \$28,976$ this is close to the actual value of $\$29,307$.

[-50,250] by [-50,110]
Xscl = 50   Yscl = 50

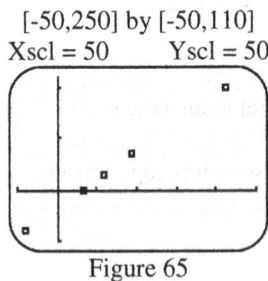

Figure 65

[1975,2015] by [13000,32000]
Xscl = 10   Yscl = 10

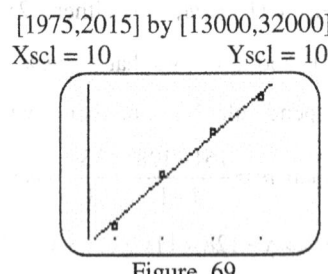

Figure 69

71. (a) Enter the distance in L_1 and enter velocity in L_2. The regression equation is: $y \approx 0.06791x - 16.32$.

(b) At $y = 37,000$, $y \approx 0.06791(37,000) - 16.32 \approx 2500$ or approximately 2500 light-years.

73. Enter the Gestation Period in L_1 and enter Life Span in L_2. The regression equation is: $y \approx .101x + 11.6$ and the correlation coefficient is: $r \approx .909$. There is a strong positive correlation, because .909 is close to 1.

Reviewing Basic Concepts (Sections 1.3 and 1.4)

1. Since $m = 1.4$ and $b = -3.1$, slope-intercept form gives the function: $f(x) = 1.4x - 3.1$.
$f(1.3) = 1.4(1.3) - 3.1 \Rightarrow f(1.3) = -1.28$

2. See Figure 2. x-intercept: $\frac{1}{2}$, y-intercept: 1, slope: −2, domain: $(-\infty, \infty)$, range: $(-\infty, \infty)$

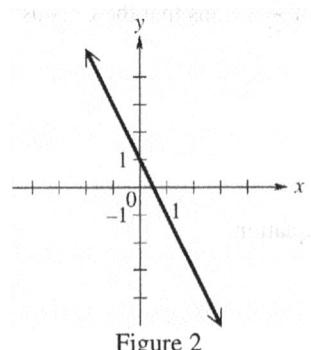

Figure 2

3. $m = \dfrac{6-4}{5-(-2)} = \dfrac{2}{7}$

4. Vertical line graphs are in the form $x = a$; through point $(-2, 10)$ would be $x = -2$.

   Horizontal line graphs are in the form $y = b$; through point $(-2, 10)$ would be $y = 10$.

5. See Figures 5a and 5b.

[-10,10] by [-10,10]
Xscl = 1   Yscl = 1

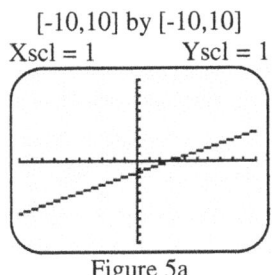

Figure 5a

[-10,10] by [-10,10]
Xscl = 1   Yscl = 1

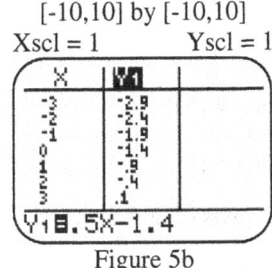

Figure 5b

[1940,2020] by [2,4]
Xscl= 10   Yscl = .5

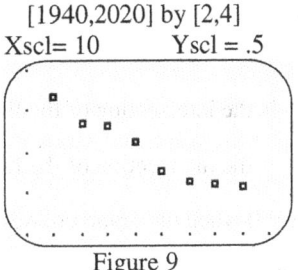

Figure 9

6. The line of the graph rises 2 units for each 1 unit to the right, therefore the slope is: $m = \dfrac{2}{1} = 2$.

   The y-intercept is: $b = -3$. The slope-intercept form of the equation is: $y = 2x - 3$.

7. The slope is: $m = \dfrac{4-2}{(-2)-5} = \dfrac{2}{-7} = -\dfrac{2}{7}$; now using point-slope form the equation is:

   $y - 4 = -\dfrac{2}{7}(x+2) \Rightarrow y - 4 = -\dfrac{2}{7}x - \dfrac{4}{7} \Rightarrow y = -\dfrac{2}{7}x + \dfrac{24}{7}$.

8. Find the given equation in slope-intercept form: $3x - 2y = 5 \Rightarrow -2y = -3x + 5 \Rightarrow y = \dfrac{3}{2}x - \dfrac{5}{2}$.

   The slope of this equation is $m = \dfrac{3}{2}$, therefore the slope of a perpendicular line will be the negative

   reciprocal: $m = -\dfrac{2}{3}$. Using point-slope form yields the equation:

   $y - 3 = -\dfrac{2}{3}(x+1) \Rightarrow y - 3 = -\dfrac{2}{3}x - \dfrac{2}{3} \Rightarrow y = -\dfrac{2}{3}x + \dfrac{7}{3}$.

9. (a) See Figure 9.

   (b) As x increases, y decreases, therefore a negative correlation coefficient.

   (c) Enter the years in L_1 and enter people per household in L_2. The regression equation is:
   $y \approx -0.0165x + 35.6$ and the correlation coefficient is: $r = -0.9648$

   (d) The regression equation is: $y \approx -0.0165(1975) + 35.6 \Rightarrow y \approx 3.01$, which is close to the actual value 2.94.

1.5: Linear Equations and Inequalities

1. $-3x - 12 = 0 \Rightarrow -3x = 12 \Rightarrow x = -4$

3. $5x = 0 \Rightarrow x = 0$

5. $2(3x-5)+8(4x+7)=0 \Rightarrow 6x-10+32x+56=0 \Rightarrow 38x=-46 \Rightarrow x=-\dfrac{46}{38} \Rightarrow x=-\dfrac{23}{19}$

7. $3x+6(x-4)=0 \Rightarrow 3x+6x-24=0 \Rightarrow 9x=24 \Rightarrow x=\dfrac{24}{9} \Rightarrow x=\dfrac{8}{3}$

9. $1.5x+2(x-3)+5.5(x+9)=0 \Rightarrow 1.5x+2x-6+5.5x+49.5=0 \Rightarrow 9x=-43.5 \Rightarrow$
   $x=\dfrac{-43.5}{9} \Rightarrow x=-\dfrac{29}{6}$

11. The solution to $y_1=y_2$ is the intersection of the lines or $x=\{10\}$.

13. The solution to $y_1=y_2$ is the intersection of the lines or $x=\{1\}$.

15. When $y_1=y_2$, $y=0$. $y=0$ when the graph crosses the x-axis or at the zero $x=\{3\}$.

17. When $x=10$ is substituted into each function the result is 20.

19. There is no real solution if y_1-y_2 yields a contradiction, $y=b$, where $b \neq 0$. This equation is called a contradiction and the solution set is: $\emptyset$.

21. $2x-5=x+7 \Rightarrow x-5=7 \Rightarrow x=12$ **Check:** $2(12)-5=12+7 \Rightarrow 19=19$ The graphs of the left and right sides of the equation intersect when $x=12$. The solution set is $\{12\}$.

23. $0.01x+3.1=2.03x-2.96 \Rightarrow 3.1=2.02x-2.96 \Rightarrow 6.06=2.02x \Rightarrow x=3$
    Check: $0.01(3)+3.1=2.03(3)-2.96 \Rightarrow .03+3.1=6.09-2.96 \Rightarrow 3.13=3.13$
    The graphs of the left and right sides of the equation intersect when $x=3$. The solution set is $\{3\}$.

25. $-(x+5)-(2+5x)+8x=3x-5 \Rightarrow -x-5-2-5x+8x=3x-5 \Rightarrow 2x-7=3x-5 \Rightarrow -2=x$
    Check: $-(-2+5)-(2+5(-2))+8(-2)=3(-2)-5 \Rightarrow -2-5-2+10-16=-6-5 \Rightarrow -11=-11$. The graphs of the left and right sides of the equation intersect when $x=-2$. The solution set is $\{-2\}$.

27. $\dfrac{2x+1}{3}+\dfrac{x-1}{4}=\dfrac{13}{2} \Rightarrow 12\left(\dfrac{2x+1}{3}+\dfrac{x-1}{4}\right)=12\left(\dfrac{13}{2}\right) \Rightarrow 8x+4+3x-3=78 \Rightarrow 11x+1$
    $=78 \Rightarrow 11x=77 \Rightarrow x=7$ **Check:** $\dfrac{2(7)+1}{3}+\dfrac{7-1}{4}=\dfrac{13}{2} \Rightarrow 5+\dfrac{6}{4}=\dfrac{13}{2} \Rightarrow \dfrac{13}{2}=\dfrac{13}{2}$
    The graphs of the left and right sides of the equation intersect when $x=7$. The solution set is $\{7\}$.

29. $\dfrac{1}{2}(x-3)=\dfrac{5}{12}+\dfrac{2}{3}(2x-5) \Rightarrow 12\left[\dfrac{1}{2}(x-3)=\dfrac{5}{12}+\dfrac{2}{3}(2x-5)\right] \Rightarrow 6x-18=5+16x-40 \Rightarrow$
    $-10x=-17 \Rightarrow x=\dfrac{17}{10}$ **Check:** $\dfrac{1}{2}\left(\dfrac{17}{10}-3\right)=\dfrac{5}{12}+\dfrac{2}{3}\left(2\left(\dfrac{17}{10}\right)-5\right) \Rightarrow \dfrac{1}{2}\left(-\dfrac{13}{10}\right)=\dfrac{5}{12}+\dfrac{2}{3}\left(-\dfrac{16}{10}\right)$
    $\Rightarrow -\dfrac{13}{20}=\dfrac{5}{12}+\left(-\dfrac{32}{30}\right) \Rightarrow -\dfrac{78}{120}=\dfrac{50}{120}+\left(-\dfrac{128}{120}\right) \Rightarrow -\dfrac{78}{120}=-\dfrac{78}{120}$. The graphs of the left and right sides of the equation intersect when $x=\dfrac{17}{10}$. The solution set is $\left\{\dfrac{17}{10}\right\}$.

31. $0.1x - 0.05 = -0.07x \Rightarrow 0.17x = 0.05 \Rightarrow 17x = 5 \Rightarrow x = \dfrac{5}{17}$

    Check: $1\left(\dfrac{5}{17}\right) - 0.05 = -0.07\left(\dfrac{5}{17}\right) \Rightarrow 10\left(\dfrac{5}{17}\right) - 5 = -7\left(\dfrac{5}{17}\right) \Rightarrow \dfrac{50}{17} - 5 = -\dfrac{35}{17} = -\dfrac{35}{17}$

    The graphs of the left and right sides of the equation intersect when $x = \dfrac{5}{17}$. The solution set is $\left\{\dfrac{5}{17}\right\}$.

33. $0.40x + 0.60(100 - x) = 0.45(100) \Rightarrow 0.40x + 60 - 0.60x = 45 \Rightarrow -0.20x = -15 \Rightarrow 20x = -1500 \Rightarrow x = 75$

    Check: $0.40(75) + 0.60(100 - 75) = 0.45(100) \Rightarrow 30 + 15 = 45 \Rightarrow 45 = 45$. The graphs of the left and right sides of the equation intersect when $x = 75$. The solution set is $\{75\}$.

35. $2[x - (4 + 2x) + 3] = 2x + 2 \Rightarrow 2[x - 4 - 2x + 3] = 2x + 2 \Rightarrow 2[-x - 1] = 2x + 2 \Rightarrow$

    $-2x - 2 = 2x + 2 \Rightarrow -4x = 4 \Rightarrow x = -1$

    Check: $2[-1 - (4 + 2(-1)) + 3] = 2(-1) + 2 \Rightarrow 2[-1 - 2 + 3] = 0 \Rightarrow 2[0] = 0 \Rightarrow 0 = 0$

    The graphs of the left and right sides of the equation intersect when $x = -1$. The solution set is $\{-1\}$.

37. $\dfrac{5}{6}x - 2x + \dfrac{1}{3} = \dfrac{1}{3} \Rightarrow 6\left(\dfrac{5}{6}x - 2x + \dfrac{1}{3} = \dfrac{1}{3}\right) \Rightarrow 5x - 12x + 2 = 2 \Rightarrow -7x = 0 \Rightarrow x = 0$

    Check: $\dfrac{5}{6}(0) - 2(0) + \dfrac{1}{3} = \dfrac{1}{3} \Rightarrow \dfrac{1}{3} = \dfrac{1}{3}$

    The graphs of the left and right sides of the equation intersect when $x = 0$. The solution set is $\{0\}$.

39. $5x - (8 - x) = 2[-4 - (3 + 5x - 13)] \Rightarrow 6x - 8 = 2[-5x + 6] \Rightarrow 6x - 8 = -10x + 12 \Rightarrow$

    $16x = 20 \Rightarrow x = \dfrac{20}{16} = \dfrac{5}{4}$

    Check: $5\left(\dfrac{5}{4}\right) - \left(8 - \dfrac{5}{4}\right) = 2\left[-4 - \left(3 + 5\left(\dfrac{5}{4}\right) - 13\right)\right] \Rightarrow \dfrac{25}{4} - \dfrac{27}{4} = 2\left[-4 - \left(\dfrac{25}{4}\right) - 10\right] \Rightarrow$

    $-\dfrac{2}{4} = 2\left[6 - \dfrac{25}{4}\right] \Rightarrow -\dfrac{1}{2} = 2\left[-\dfrac{1}{4}\right] \Rightarrow -\dfrac{1}{2} = -\dfrac{1}{2}$. The graphs of the left and right sides of the equation

    intersect when $x = \dfrac{5}{4}$. The solution set is $\left\{\dfrac{5}{4}\right\}$.

41. When $x = 4$, both Y_1 and Y_2 have a value of 8. Therefore the solution set is $\{4\}$.

43. Graph $Y_1 = 4(0.23 + \sqrt{5})$ and $Y_2 = \sqrt{2}x + 1$ as shown in Figure 43. The graphs intersect when $x \approx 16.07$.

    Therefore the solution set is $\{16.07\}$.

45. Graph $Y_1 = 2\pi x + \sqrt[3]{4}$ and $Y_2 = 0.5\pi x - \sqrt{28}$ as shown in Figure 45. The graphs intersect when $x \approx -1.46$.

    Therefore the solution set is $\{-1.46\}$.

[-10,30] by [-10,30]   [-15,5] by [-15,5]   [-10,10] by [-10,10]

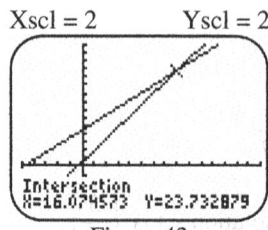
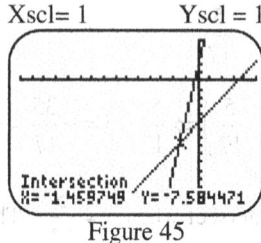
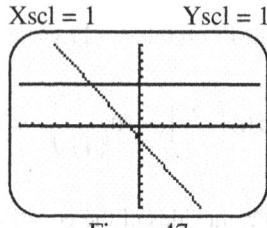

Figure 43   Figure 45   Figure 47

47. Graph $Y_1 = 0.23(\sqrt{3}+4x)-0.82(\pi x+2.3)$ and $Y_2 = 5$ as shown in Figure 47. The graphs intersect when $x \approx -3.92$. Therefore the solution set is $\{-3.92\}$.

49. $5x+5 = 5(x+3)-3 \Rightarrow 5x+5 = 5x+15-3 \Rightarrow 5x+5 = 5x+12 \Rightarrow 5 = 12 \Rightarrow$ Contradiction. The solution set is $\varnothing$ The table of $Y_1 = 5x+5$ and $Y_2 = 5(x+3)-3$ never produces the same answers, therefore supports the Contradiction.

51. $6(2x+1) = 4x+8\left(x+\dfrac{3}{4}\right) \Rightarrow 12x+6 = 4x+8x+6 \Rightarrow 12x+6 = 12x+6 \Rightarrow 6=6 \Rightarrow$ Identity. The solution set is $(-\infty, \infty)$ The table of $Y_1 = 6(2x+1)$ and $Y_2 = 4x+8\left(x+\dfrac{3}{4}\right)$ produces all the same answers, therefore supports the Identity.

53. $7x-3[5x-(5+x)] = 1-4x \Rightarrow 7x-3[4x-5] = 1-4x \Rightarrow 7x-12x+15 = 1-4x \Rightarrow$
$-5x+15 = 1-4x \Rightarrow -x = -14 \Rightarrow x = 14 \Rightarrow$ Conditional.
The solution set is 14. The table of $Y_1 = 7x-3[5x-(5+x)]$ and $Y_2 = 1-4x$ shows that the answers are the same when $x = 14$.

55. $0.2(5x-4)-0.1(6-3x) = 0.4 \Rightarrow x-0.8-0.6+0.3x = 0.4 \Rightarrow 1.3x-1.4 = 0.4 \Rightarrow 1.3x = 1.8 \Rightarrow$
$x = \dfrac{18}{13} \Rightarrow$ Conditional. The solution set is $\dfrac{18}{13}$ The table of $Y_1 = 0.2(5x-4)-0.1(6-3x)$ and $Y_2 = 0.4$ shows that the answers are the same when $x = \dfrac{18}{13}$.

57. $-4[6-(-2+3x)] = 21+12x \Rightarrow -4[8-3x] = 21+2x \Rightarrow -32+12x = 21+2x \Rightarrow -32 = 21 \Rightarrow$
Contradiction. The solution set is $\varnothing$. The table of $Y_1 = -4[6-(-2+3x)]$ and $Y_2 = 21+12x$ never produces the same answers, therefore supports the Contradiction.

59. $\dfrac{1}{2}x-2(x-1) = 2-\dfrac{3}{2}x \Rightarrow \dfrac{1}{2}x-2x+2 = 2-\dfrac{3}{2}x \Rightarrow -\dfrac{3}{2}+2 = -\dfrac{3}{2}+2 \Rightarrow 2=2 \Rightarrow$ Identity.
The solution set is $(-\infty, \infty)$. The table of $Y_1 = \dfrac{1}{2}x-2(x-1)$ and $Y_2 = 2-\dfrac{3}{2}x$ produces all the same answers, therefore supports the Identity.

61. $\dfrac{x-1}{2} = \dfrac{3x-2}{6} \Rightarrow 6\left[\dfrac{x-1}{2} = \dfrac{3x-2}{6}\right] \Rightarrow 3(x-2) = 3x-2 \Rightarrow 3x-6 = 3x-3 \Rightarrow -6 = -3 \Rightarrow$

   Contradiction. The solution set is ∅. The table of $Y_1 = \dfrac{x-1}{2}$ and $Y_2 = \dfrac{3x-2}{6}$ never produces the same answers, therefore supports the Contradiction.

63. For the given functions, $f(x) = g(x)$ when the graphs intersect or when $x = 3$. The solution is {3}.

65. For the given functions, $f(x) < g(x)$ when the graph of $f(x)$ is below the graph of $g(x)$ or when $x > 3$. The solution is $(3, \infty)$.

67. For the given inequality, $y_1 - y_2 \geq 0 \Rightarrow f(x) - g(x) \geq 0 \Rightarrow f(x) \geq g(x)$ when the graph of $f(x)$ is above or intersects the graph of $g(x)$ or when $x \leq 3$. The solution is $(-\infty, 3]$.

69. For the given functions, $f(x) \leq f(x)$ when the graph of is $f(x)$ below or intersects the graph $g(x)$ of or when $x \geq 3$. The solution is $[3, \infty)$.

71. For the given functions, $f(x) \leq 2$ when the graph of $f(x)$ is below or equal to 2 or when $x \geq 3$. The solution is $[3, \infty)$.

73. (a) The function $f(x) > 0$ when the graph is above the x-axis for the interval $(20, \infty)$.

   (b) The function $f(x) < 0$ when the graph is below the x-axis for the interval $(-\infty, 20)$.

   (c) The function $f(x) \geq 0$ when the graph intersects or is above the x-axis for the interval $[20, \infty)$.

   (d) The function $f(x) \leq 0$ when the graph intersects or is below the x-axis for the interval $(-\infty, 20]$.

75. (a) If the solution set of $f(x) \geq g(x)$ is $[4, \infty)$, then $f(x) = g(x)$ at the intersection of the graphs, $x = 4$ or {4}.

   (b) If the solution set of $f(x) \geq g(x)$ is $[4, \infty)$, then $f(x) > g(x)$ is the same, but does not include the intersection of the graphs for the interval $(4, \infty)$.

   (c) If the solution set of $f(x) \geq g(x)$ is $[4, \infty)$, then $f(x) < g(x)$ is left of the intersection of the graphs for the interval: $(-\infty, 4)$.

77. (a) $3x - 6 = 0 \Rightarrow 3x = 6 \Rightarrow x = 2$, Interval Notation : {2}

   (b) $3x - 6 > 0 \Rightarrow 3x > 6 \Rightarrow x > 2$, Interval Notation : $(2, \infty)$

   (c) $3x - 6 < 0 \Rightarrow 3x < 6 \Rightarrow x < 2$, Interval Notation : $(-\infty, 2)$

79. (a) $1 - 2x = 0 \Rightarrow -2x = -1 \Rightarrow x = \dfrac{1}{2}$, Interval Notation : $\left\{\dfrac{1}{2}\right\}$

   (b) $1 - 2x \leq 0 \Rightarrow -2x \leq -1 \Rightarrow x \geq \dfrac{1}{2}$, Interval Notation : $\left[\dfrac{1}{2}, \infty\right)$

(c) $1-2x \geq 0 \Rightarrow -2x \geq -1 \Rightarrow x \leq \dfrac{1}{2}$, Interval Notation : $\left(-\infty, \dfrac{1}{2}\right]$

81. (a) $x+12 = 4x \Rightarrow -3x = -12 \Rightarrow x = 4$, Interval Notation : $\{4\}$

   (b) $x+12 > 4x \Rightarrow -3x > -12 \Rightarrow x < 4$, Interval Notation : $(-\infty, 4)$

   (c) $x+12 < 4x \Rightarrow -3x < -12 \Rightarrow x > 4$, Interval Notation : $(4, \infty)$

83. (a) $9-(x+1) < 0 \Rightarrow -x+8 < 0 \Rightarrow -x < -8 \Rightarrow x > 8 \Rightarrow$ the interval is $(8, \infty)$. The graph of $y_1 = 9-(x+1)$ is below the x-axis for the interval $(8, \infty)$.

   (b) If $9-(x+1) < 0$ for $(8, \infty)$, then $9-(x+1) \geq 0$ for the interval $(-\infty, 8]$. The graph of $y_1 = 9-(x+1)$ intersects or is above the x-axis for the interval $(-\infty, 8]$.

85. (a) $2x-3 > x+2 \Rightarrow x-3 > 2 \Rightarrow x > 5 \Rightarrow$ the interval is $(5, \infty)$. The graph of $y_1 = 2x-3$ is above the graph of $y_2 = x+2$ for the interval $(5, \infty)$.

   (b) If $2x-3 > x+2$ for $(5, \infty)$, then $2x-3 \leq x+2$ for the interval $(-\infty, 5]$. The graph $y_1 = 2x-3$ intersects or is below the graph $y_2 = x+2$ for the interval $(-\infty, 5]$.

87. (a) $10x+5-7x \geq 8(x+2)+4 \Rightarrow 3x+5 \geq 8x+20 \Rightarrow -5x \geq 15 \Rightarrow x \leq -3 \Rightarrow$ the interval is $(-\infty, -3]$. The graph of $y_1 = 10x+5-7x$ intersects or is above the graph of $y_2 = 8(x+2)+4$ for the interval $(-\infty, -3]$.

   (b) If $10x+5-7x \geq 8(x+2)+4$ for $(-\infty, -3)$, then $10x+5-7x < 8(x+2)+4$ for the interval $(-3, \infty)$. The graph of $y_1 = 10x+5-7x$ is below the graph of $y_2 = 8(x+2)+4$ for the interval $(-3, \infty)$.

89. (a) $x+2(-x+4)-3(x+5) < -4 \Rightarrow x-2x+8-3x-15 < -4 \Rightarrow -4x < 3 \Rightarrow x > -\dfrac{3}{4} \Rightarrow$ the interval is $\left(-\dfrac{3}{4}, \infty\right)$. The graph of $y_1 = x+2(-x+4)-3(x+5)$ is below the graph of $y_2 = -4$ for the interval $\left(-\dfrac{3}{4}, \infty\right)$.

   (b) If $x+2(-x+4)-3(x+5) < -4$ for $\left(-\dfrac{3}{4}, \infty\right)$, then $x+2(-x+4)-3(x+5) \geq -4$ for the interval $\left(-\infty, -\dfrac{3}{4}\right]$. The graph of $y_1 = x+2(-x+4)-3(x+5)$ intersects or is above the graph $y_2 = -4$ for the interval $\left(-\infty, -\dfrac{3}{4}\right]$.

91. $\frac{1}{3}x - \frac{1}{5}x \le 2 \Rightarrow \left[\frac{1}{3}x - \frac{1}{5}x \le 2\right] \Rightarrow 5x - 3x \le 30 \Rightarrow 2x \le 30 \Rightarrow x \le 15 \Rightarrow (-\infty, 15]$. The graph of

$y_1 = \frac{1}{3}x - \frac{1}{5}x$ intersects or is below the graph of $y_2 = 2$ for the interval $(-\infty, 15]$.

93. $\frac{x-2}{2} - \frac{x+6}{3} > -4 \Rightarrow 6\left[\frac{x-2}{2} - \frac{x+6}{3} > -4\right] \Rightarrow 3x - 6 - (2x+12) > -24 \Rightarrow$

$x - 18 > -24 \Rightarrow x > -6 \Rightarrow (-6, \infty)$. The graph of $y_1 = \frac{x-2}{2} - \frac{x+6}{3}$ is above the graph of

$y_2 = 5$ for the interval: $(-6, \infty)$.

95. $0.6x - 2(0.5x + .2) \le 0.4 - 0.3x \Rightarrow .6x - 1x - 0.4 \le 0.4 - 0.3x \Rightarrow 10[0.6x - 1x - 0.4 \le 0.4 - 0.3x] \Rightarrow$

$6x - 10x - 4 \le 4 - 3x \Rightarrow -4x - 4 \le 4 - 3x \Rightarrow -x \le 8 \Rightarrow x \ge -8 \Rightarrow [-8, \infty)$. The graph of

$y_1 = 0.6x - 2(0.5x + .2)$ intersects or is below the graph of $y_2 = 0.4 - 0.3x$ for the interval $[-8, \infty)$.

97. $-\frac{1}{2}x + 0.7x - 5 > 0 \Rightarrow 10\left[-\frac{1}{2}x + 0.7x - 5 > 0\right] \Rightarrow -5x + 7x - 50 > 0 \Rightarrow 2x > 50 \Rightarrow$

$x > 25 \Rightarrow (25, \infty)$. The graph of $y_1 = -\frac{1}{2}x + .7x - 5$ is above the graph of $y_2 = 0$ for the interval $(25, \infty)$.

99. $-4(3x+2) \ge -2(6x+1) \Rightarrow -12x - 8 \ge -12x - 2 \Rightarrow -8 \ge -2$; since this is false the solution is $\emptyset$.

The graph of $y_1 = -4(3x+2)$ never intersects or is above the graph of $y_2 = -2(6x+1)$, therefore the solution is $\emptyset$.

101. (a) As time increases, distance increases, therefore the car is moving away from Omaha.
 (b) The distance function $f(x)$ intersects the 100 mile line at 1 hour and the 200 mile line at 3 hours.
 (c) Using the answers from (b) the interval is [1, 3].
 (d) Because x hours is $0 \le x \le 6$, the interval is (1, 6].

103. $4 \le 2x + 2 \le 10 \Rightarrow 2 \le 2x \le 8 \Rightarrow 1 \le x \le 4 \Rightarrow [1, 4]$ The graph of $y_2 = 2x + 2$ is between the graphs of $y_1 = 4$ and $y_3 = 10$ for the interval [1, 4].

105. $-10 > 3x + 2 > -16 \Rightarrow -12 > 3x > -18 \Rightarrow -4 > x > -6 \Rightarrow -6 < x < -4 \Rightarrow (-6, -4)$

The graph of $y_2 = 3x + 2$ is between the graphs of $y_1 = -10$ and $y_3 = -16$ for the interval $(-6, -4)$.

107. $-3 \le \frac{x-4}{-5} < 4 \Rightarrow 15 \ge x - 4 > -20 \Rightarrow 19 \ge x > -16 \Rightarrow -16 < x \le 19 \Rightarrow (-16, 19]$ The graph of

$y_2 = \frac{x-4}{-5}$ is between the graphs of $y_1 = -3$ and $y_3 = 4$ for the interval $(-16, 19]$.

109. $-\dfrac{1}{2} < x - 4 < \dfrac{1}{2} \Rightarrow \dfrac{7}{2} < x < \dfrac{9}{2} \Rightarrow \left(\dfrac{7}{2}, \dfrac{9}{2}\right)$. The graph of $y_2 = x - 4$ is between $y_1 = -\dfrac{1}{2}$ and $y_3 = \dfrac{1}{2}$ for the interval $\left(\dfrac{7}{2}, \dfrac{9}{2}\right)$.

111. $-4 \leq \dfrac{1}{2}x - 5 \leq 4 \Rightarrow 1 \leq \dfrac{1}{2}x \leq 9 \Rightarrow 2 \leq x \leq 18 \Rightarrow [2, 18]$. The graph of $y_2 = \dfrac{1}{2}x - 5$ is on or between $y_1 = -4$ and $y_3 = 4$ for the interval $(2, 18)$.

113. $\sqrt{2} \leq \dfrac{2x+1}{3} \leq \sqrt{5} \Rightarrow 3\sqrt{2} \leq 2x + 1 \leq 3\sqrt{5} \Rightarrow 3\sqrt{2} - 1 \leq 2x \leq 3\sqrt{5} - 1 \Rightarrow$

$\dfrac{3\sqrt{2} - 1}{2} \leq x \leq \dfrac{3\sqrt{5} - 1}{2} \Rightarrow \left[\dfrac{3\sqrt{2} - 1}{2}, \dfrac{3\sqrt{5} - 1}{2}\right]$; The graph of $y_2 = \dfrac{2x + 1}{3}$ is on or between the graphs of

$y_1 = \sqrt{2}$ and $y = \sqrt{5}$. for the interval $\left[\dfrac{3\sqrt{2} - 1}{2}, \dfrac{3\sqrt{5} - 1}{2}\right]$.

115. (a) The graph of $T(x) = 65 - 19x$ intersects the graph of $D(x) = 50 - 5.8x$ at $\approx (1.136, 43.41)$. Since the x-coordinate is altitude, the clouds will not form below 1.14 miles or for the interval: $[0, 1.14)$.

(b) Clouds will not form when air temperature is above dew point temperature or $T(x) > D(x)$.

Then $65 - 19x > 50 - 5.8x \Rightarrow -13.2x > -15 \Rightarrow x < \dfrac{15}{13.2}$ for the interval $\left[0, \dfrac{15}{13.2}\right)$.

117. Since $C = 2\pi r$ and radius is in the range $1.99 \leq r \leq 2.01$, circumference is in the range $2\pi(1.99) \leq 2\pi r \leq 2\pi(2.01) \Rightarrow 3.98\pi \leq C \leq 4.02\pi$.

119. The graph of $y_1 = 3.7x - 11.1$ crosses the x-axis at $x = 3$. There is one solution to this equation. Because a linear equation can only cross the x-axis in one location, there is only one solution to any linear equation.

120. $3.7x - 11.1 < 0 \Rightarrow 3.7x < 11.1 \Rightarrow x < 3 \Rightarrow (-\infty, 3)$ $3.7x - 11.1 > 0 \Rightarrow 3.7x > 11.1 \Rightarrow x > 3 \Rightarrow (3, \infty)$

The value of $x = 3$ given by the equation represents the boundary between the sets of real numbers given by the inequality solutions $(-\infty, 3)$ and $(3, \infty)$.

121. The graph of $y_1 = -4x + 6$ crosses the x-axis at $x = 1.5$.

$-4x + 6 < 0 \Rightarrow -4x < -6 \Rightarrow x > \dfrac{-6}{-4} \Rightarrow x > 1.5 \Rightarrow (1.5, \infty)$

$-4x + 6 > 0 \Rightarrow -4x > -6 \Rightarrow x < \dfrac{-6}{-4} \Rightarrow x > 1.5 \Rightarrow (-\infty, 1.5)$

122. (a) If $a \neq 0$, then $ax + b = 0 \Rightarrow ax = -b \Rightarrow x = -\dfrac{b}{a}$

(b) If $a > 0$, a positive slope, then $ax + b < 0 \Rightarrow ax < -b \Rightarrow x < \dfrac{-b}{a} \Rightarrow \left(-\infty, \dfrac{-b}{a}\right)$

If $a>0$, a positive slope, then $ax+b<0 \Rightarrow ax>-b \Rightarrow x>\frac{-b}{a} \Rightarrow \left(\frac{-b}{a},\infty\right)$

(c) If $a<0$, a negative slope, then $ax+b<0 \Rightarrow ax<-b \Rightarrow x>\frac{-b}{a} \Rightarrow \left(\frac{-b}{a},\infty\right)$

If $a<0$, a positive slope, then $ax+b>0 \Rightarrow ax>-b \Rightarrow x<\frac{-b}{a} \Rightarrow \left(-\infty,\frac{-b}{a}\right)$

1.6: Applications of Linear Functions

1. $.75(40) = 30L$

3. When combining a 26% acid solution to a 32% acid solution the result will be a solution with between 26% and 32% acid. (A) 36% is not in between these percent values and not a possible concentration.

5. If x is the second number, then $6x-3$ is the first number. The equation with the sum of these two numbers equal to 32 is: (D) $(6x-3)+x=32$.

7. If $P = 2L+2W$ then $P = 2L+2(19) \Rightarrow 98 = 2L+38 \Rightarrow 60 = 2L \Rightarrow L = 30$ cm.

9. Let x = width and $2x-2.5$ = length. If $P = 2W+2L$, then
$40.6 = 2x+2(2x-2.5) \Rightarrow 40.6 = 6x-5 \Rightarrow 45.6 = 6x \Rightarrow x = 7.6$. The width is 7.6 cm.

11. Let x = the original square side length and $2x-3$ = the new square side length. If $P = 4s$, then
$4(x+3) = 2x+40 \Rightarrow 4x+12 = 2x+40 \Rightarrow 2x = 28 \Rightarrow x = 14$. The original side length is 14 cm.

13. With an aspect ratio of 4:3, let x = width and $\frac{4}{3}x$ = length. If $P = 2W+2L$, then
$98 = 2x+2\left(\frac{4}{3}x\right) \Rightarrow 98 = 2x+\frac{8}{3}x \Rightarrow 98 = \frac{14}{3}x \Rightarrow 294 = 14x \Rightarrow x = 21$. The width is 21 inches and the length is $\frac{4}{3}(21) = 28$ inches. Use the Pythagorean theorem to find the diagonal
$c^2 = (21)^2 + (28)^2 \Rightarrow c^2 = 441+784 \Rightarrow c^2 = 1225 \Rightarrow c = 35$. The television is advertised as a 35 inch screen.

15. Let x = the short side length and $2x$ = the longer two side lengths. If $P = s+s+s$, then
$30 = x+2x+2x \Rightarrow 30 = 5x \Rightarrow x = 6$. The shortest side is 6 cm long.

17. Let x = the number of hours traveled at 70 mph, and (6-x) = the number of hours traveled at 55 mph. Since D = RT and the total distance traveled by the car was 372 miles, then $55(6-x) + 70x = 372 \Rightarrow 330 - 55x + 70x = 372 \Rightarrow 15x = 42 \Rightarrow x = 2.8$. The car traveled for 2.8 hours at 70 mph and (6-2.8)=3.2 hours at 55 mph.

19. Let x = gallons of 5% acid solution. Then
$5(.10)+x(.05) = (x+5)(.07) \Rightarrow .50+.05x = .07x+.35 \Rightarrow .15 = .02x \Rightarrow 15 = 2x \Rightarrow x = 7.5$.

Mix in 7.5 gallons of 5% acid solution.

21. Let $x =$ gallons of pure alcohol. Then

    $20(.15) + x(1.00) = (x + 20)(.25) \Rightarrow 3 + x = .25x + 5 \Rightarrow .75x = 2 \Rightarrow x = 2.67$ or $2\frac{2}{3}$.

    Mix in $2\frac{2}{3}$ gallons of pure alcohol.

23. Let $x =$ milliliters of water. Then $8(.06) + x(0) = (x + 8)(.04) \Rightarrow .48 = .04x + .32 \Rightarrow$

    $0.16 = 0.04 \Rightarrow 4x = 16 \Rightarrow x = 4$. Mix in 4 milliliters of water.

25. Let $x =$ liters of fluid to be drained and pure antifreeze added. The $16(0.80) - x(0.80) + x(1.00) = 16(0.90) \Rightarrow$

    $12.8 - 0.80x + x = 14.4 \Rightarrow 0.20x = 1.6 \Rightarrow 20x = 160 \Rightarrow x = 8$. Drain and add in 8 liters of antifreeze.

27. Let $x =$ gallons of 94-octane gasoline. Then

    $400(0.99) + x(0.94) = (x + 400)(0.97) \Rightarrow 396 + 0.94x = 0.97x + 388$

    $8 = 0.03x \Rightarrow 3x = 800 \Rightarrow x = 266.67$ or $266\frac{2}{3}$. Mix in $266\frac{2}{3}$ gallons of 94-octane gasoline.

29. (a) $F(2008) = -\frac{5}{44}(2008) + 276.18 \approx 48$, IN 2008 the winning men's 100-meter freestyle time was about

    48 seconds.

    (b) $53 = -\frac{5}{44}x + 276.18 \Rightarrow x \approx 1963.98$. The years would have been from 1948 to about 1964.

31. (a) Use the points (2011, 192) and (2014, 249) to find the slope, $m = \frac{249 - 192}{2014 - 2011} = \frac{57}{3} = 19$ and the

    point (2014, 249) to find the equation of the line. $S(x) - 249 = 19(x - 2014) \Rightarrow S(x) = 19x - 38017$

    (b) Sales increased, on average by $19 billion per year.

    (c) $325 = 19x - 38017 \Rightarrow x = 2018$ The sales will reach $325 billion in 2018.

33. (a) If the fixed cost = $200 and the variable cost = $.02 the cost function is: $C(x) = 0.02x + 200$.

    (b) If she gets paid $.04 per envelope stuffed and $x =$ number of envelopes, the revenue function

    is $R(x) = 0.04x$.

    (c) $R(x) = C(x)$ when $0.02x + 200 = 0.04x \Rightarrow 200 = 0.02x \Rightarrow x = 10,000$.

    (d) Graph $C(x)$ and $R(x)$, see Figure 33. Rebecca takes a loss when stuffing less than 10,000

    envelopes and makes a profit when stuffing over 10,000 envelopes.

35. (a) If the fixed cost = $2300 and the variable cost = $3.00 the cost function is: $C(x) = 3.00x + 2300$.

    (b) If he gets paid $5.50 per delivery and $x =$ number of deliveries, the revenue function is: $R(x) = 5.50x$.

    (c) $R(x) = C(x)$ when $3.00x + 2300 = 5.50x \Rightarrow 2300 = 2.50x \Rightarrow x = 920$.

    (d) Graph $C(x)$ and $R(x)$. See Figure 35. Tom takes a loss when making fewer than 920 deliveries and

    makes a profit when making over 920 deliveries.

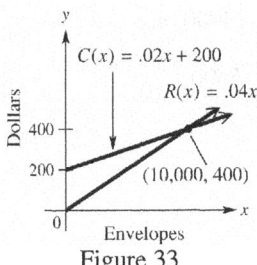
Figure 33

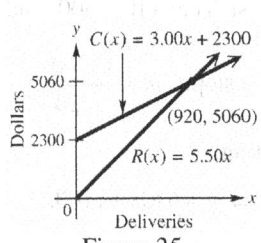
Figure 35

37. If $y = kx$, $x = 3$, and $y = 7.5$, then $7.5 = k(3) \Rightarrow k = 2.5$. Now, with

$k = 2.5$ and $x = 8$, $y = 2.5(8) \Rightarrow y = 20$ when $x = 8$.

39. If $y = kx$, $x = 25$, and $y = 1.5$, then $1.50 = k(25) \Rightarrow k = 0.06$. Now, with $k = 0.06$

and $y = 5.10$, $5.10 = 0.06x \Rightarrow x = \$85$ when $y = \$5.10$

41. Let y = pressure and x = depth for the direct proportion: $y = kx$. Then $13 = k(30) \Rightarrow k = \dfrac{13}{30}$.

Now use $k = \dfrac{13}{30}$ and a depth of 70 feet to find the pressure: $y = \dfrac{13}{30}(70) \Rightarrow y = \dfrac{91}{3} \Rightarrow y = 30\dfrac{1}{3}$ lb/in^2.

43. Let t = tuition and c = credits taken for the direct proportion $t = kc$. Then

$720.50 = k(11) \Rightarrow k = 65.5$. Now use the constant of variation $k = 65.5$ and 16 credits to find the

tuition: $y = 65.5(16) \Rightarrow y = \$1048$.

45. First use proportion to find the radius of the water at a depth of 44 feet $\dfrac{5}{11} = \dfrac{x}{6} \Rightarrow 11x = 30 \Rightarrow x \approx 2.727$.

Now use the cone volume formula to find the water's volume:

$V = \dfrac{1}{3}\pi r^2 h \Rightarrow V = \dfrac{1}{3}\pi(2.727)^2(6) \approx 46.7$ ft^3.

47. Since the triangles are similar, use a proportion to solve: $\dfrac{1.75}{2} = \dfrac{45}{x} \Rightarrow 1.75x = 90 \Rightarrow x \approx 51.43$ or

$x = 51\dfrac{3}{7}$ feet tall.

49. Let w = weight, d = distance, and use the direct proportion $w = kd$ to find k:

$3 = k(2.5) \Rightarrow k = 1.2$. Now use $k = 1.2$ and a weight of 17 pounds to find the stretch

length: $17 = 1.2(d) \Rightarrow d = 14.17$ or $14\dfrac{1}{6}$ in.

51. With direct proportion $y_1 = kx_1$ and $y_2 = kx_2$, then $k = \dfrac{y_1}{x_1} = \dfrac{y_2}{x_2}$. Now let $y_1 = 250$ tagged

trout, $y_2 = 7$ tagged trout, $x_2 = 350$ sample trout, and x_1 = total trout. Therefore

$\dfrac{250}{x_1} = \dfrac{7}{350} \Rightarrow 7x_1 = 87{,}500 \Rightarrow x_1 = 12{,}500$ is the estimate for total population of trout.

53. (a) Let x = number of heaters produced and y = cost. Then (10, 7500) and (20, 13900) are two points on the graph of the linear function. Find the slope: $m = \dfrac{13900 - 7500}{20 - 10} = \dfrac{6400}{10} = 640$.

Now use point-slope form to find the linear function:

$y - 7500 = 640(x - 10) \Rightarrow y - 7500 = 640x - 640 \Rightarrow y = 640x + 1100$.

(b) $y = 640(25) + 1100 \Rightarrow y = 16,000 + 1100 \Rightarrow y = \$17,100$.

(c) Graph $y = 640x + 1100$ and locate the point (25, 17,100) on the graph.

55. (a) Let x = number of years after 2002 and y = value, then (0, 120,000) and (10, 146,000) are two points on the graph of the linear function. Find the slope: $m = \dfrac{146,000 - 120,000}{10 - 0} = \dfrac{26,000}{10} = 2,600$.

The y-intercept is: 120,000. Therefore the linear function is: $y = 2,600x + 120,000$.

(b) $y = 2,600(7) + 120,000 \Rightarrow y = 18200 + 120,000 \Rightarrow y = \$138,200$ value of the house.

(c) The value of the house increased, on average, \$2,600 per year.

57. (a) Surface area = $4\pi r^2 \Rightarrow 4\pi(3960)^2 \approx 197,000,000 \text{ mi}^2$.

(b) $(197,000,000)(0.71) \approx 140,000,000 \text{ mi}^2$

(c) $\dfrac{680,000}{140,000,000} \approx 0.00486$ miles. Converted to feet is $(0.00486)(5280) \approx 25.7$ feet.

(d) Since this height is greater than the heights of both Boston and San Diego these cities would be flooded.

(e) We know from above that oceans cover approximately 140,000,000 square miles of the earth. The Antarctic ice cap contains 6,300,000 cubic miles of water.

$\dfrac{6,300,000}{140,000,000} = 0.045$ miles. Converted to feet is $(0.045)(5280) \approx 238$ feet.

59. (a) $y = \dfrac{5}{3}(27) + 455 \Rightarrow y = 45 + 455 \Rightarrow y = 500 \text{ cm}^3$.

(b) $605 = \dfrac{5}{3}x + 455 \Rightarrow 150 = \dfrac{5}{3}x \Rightarrow x = 90° \text{ C}$.

(c) $0 = \dfrac{5}{3}x + 455 \Rightarrow -455 = \dfrac{5}{3}x \Rightarrow x = -273° \text{C}$.

61. $I = PRT \Rightarrow \dfrac{I}{RT} = P$ or $P = \dfrac{I}{RT}$

63. $P = 2L + 2W \Rightarrow P - 2L = 2W \Rightarrow W = \dfrac{P - 2L}{2}$ or $W = \dfrac{P}{2} - L$

65. $A = \dfrac{1}{2}h(b_1 + b_2) \Rightarrow 2A = h(b_1 + b_2) \Rightarrow h = \dfrac{2A}{b_1 + b_2}$

Section 1.6   31

67. $S = 2LW + 2WH + 2HL \Rightarrow S - 2LW = H(2W + 2L) \Rightarrow \dfrac{S - 2LW}{2W + 2L}$

69. $V = \dfrac{1}{3}\pi r^2 h \Rightarrow 3V = \pi r^2 h \Rightarrow h = \dfrac{3V}{\pi r^2}$

71. $S = \dfrac{n}{2}(a_1 + a_n) \Rightarrow 2S = n(a_1 + a_n) \Rightarrow n = \dfrac{2S}{a_1 + a_n}$

73. $s = \dfrac{1}{2}gt^2 \Rightarrow 2s = gt^2 \Rightarrow g = \dfrac{2s}{t^2}$

75. Let P = the amount put into the short-term note, then $240,000 - P$ = the amount put into the long-term note. With $13,000 one year interest income, solve:
$P(.06)(1) + (240,000 - P)(0.05)(1) = 13,000 \Rightarrow 0.06P + 120,000 - 0.05P = 13,000 \Rightarrow$
$0.01P = 1,000 \Rightarrow P \Rightarrow 100,000$. The short-term note was $100,000 and the long-term was $140,000.

77. Let P = the amount deposited at 2.5% interest rate, then $2P$ = the amount deposited at 3% interest rate. With a one year interest income of $850, solve:
$0.025P(1) + 0.03(2P)(1) = 850 \Rightarrow 0.025P + 0.06P = 850 \Rightarrow 0.085P = 850 \Rightarrow P = 10,000$.
Therefore, $10,000 was deposited at 2.5% and $20,000 was deposited at 3%.

79. After taxes, Marietta was able to invest 70% of the original winnings. This is $0.70(200,000) = \$140,000$.
Now let P = amount invested at 1.5%, then $140,000 - P$ = the amount invested at 4%. With a one year interest income of $4350, solve: $0.015P + 0.04(140,000 - P) = 4350 \Rightarrow 0.015P + 5600 - 0.04P = 4350 \Rightarrow$
$-0.025P = -1250 \Rightarrow P = 50,000$. Therefore, $50,000 was invested at 1.5% and $90,000 was invested at 4%.

Reviewing Basic Concepts (Sections 1.5 and 1.6)

1. $3(x-5) + 2 = 1 - (4 + 2x) \Rightarrow 3x - 15 + 2 = 1 - 4 - 2x \Rightarrow 3x - 13 = -2x - 3 \Rightarrow 5x = 10 \Rightarrow x = 2$. The graphs of the left and right sides of the equation intersect at $x = 2$; this supports the solution set: {2}.

2. Graph $y_1 = \pi(1-x)$ and $y_2 = .6(3x-1)$. See Figure 2. The graphs intersect at $x = .757$.

3. $0 = \dfrac{1}{3}(4x-2) + 1 \Rightarrow 0 = \dfrac{4}{3}x - \dfrac{2}{3} + 1 \Rightarrow -\dfrac{1}{3} = \dfrac{4}{3}x \Rightarrow -\dfrac{1}{4}$. Graph $y_1 = \dfrac{1}{3}(4x-2) + 1$. See Figure 3.

   The graph intersects the x-axis at $x = -\dfrac{1}{4}$.

[-10,10] by [-10,10]   [-10,10] by [-10,10]
Xscl = 1   Yscl = 1   Xscl = 1   Yscl = 1

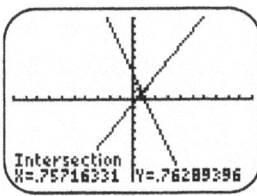
Figure 2

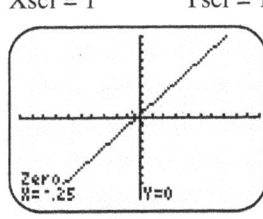
Figure 3

32   Chapter 1 Linear Functions, Equations, and Inequalities

4. (a) $4x-5=-2(3-2x)+3 \Rightarrow 4x-5=-6+4x+3 \Rightarrow -5=-3$. Since this is false, the equation is a contradiction and the solution set is: $\emptyset$.

   (b) $5x-9=5(-2+x)+1 \Rightarrow 4x-5=-6+4x+3 \Rightarrow -5=-3$. Since this is true the equation is an identity and the solution set is: $(-\infty,\infty)$.

   (c) $5x-4=3(6-x) \Rightarrow 5x-4=18-3x \Rightarrow 8x=22 \Rightarrow x=\dfrac{11}{4}$. The equation is a conditional equation and the solution set is: $\left\{\dfrac{11}{4}\right\}$.

5. $2x+3(x+2)<1-2x \Rightarrow 2x+3x+6<1-2x \Rightarrow 7x<-5 \Rightarrow x<-\dfrac{5}{7}$. The solution set is: $\left(-\infty,\dfrac{5}{7}\right)$.

   Graph $y_1=2x+3(x+2)$ and $y_2=1-2x$; the graph of y_1 is below the graph of y_2 when $x<-\dfrac{5}{7}$, which supports the original solution.

6. $-5\leq 1-2x<6 \Rightarrow -6 \Rightarrow -2x<5 \Rightarrow 3\geq x>-\dfrac{5}{2} \Rightarrow -\dfrac{5}{2}<x\leq 3 \Rightarrow \left(-\dfrac{5}{2},3\right]$

7. (a) The graphs intersect at $x=2 \Rightarrow \{2\}$

   (b) The graph of $f(x)$ intersects or is below the graph of $g(x)$ for $x\geq 2$, on $[2,\infty)$.

8. Since the triangles formed by the shadows are similar, use proportion to solve.

   $\dfrac{x}{27}=\dfrac{6}{4} \Rightarrow 4x=162 \Rightarrow x=40.5$ ft.

9. (a) Since the income from each disc is $5.50, a function R for revenue from selling x discs is: $R(x)=5.50x$.

   (b) Since the cost of producing each disc is $1.50 and there is a one-time equipment cost of $800, a function C for cost of recording x discs is: $C(x)=1.50x+800$.

   (c) Solve $R(x)=C(x)$: $5.5x=1.5x+800 \Rightarrow 4x=800 \Rightarrow x=200$ discs.

10. $V=\pi r^2 h \Rightarrow h=\dfrac{V}{\pi r^2}$

Chapter 1 Review Exercises

1. Use the distance formula: $d=\sqrt{(-1-5)^2+(16-(-8))^2} \Rightarrow d \Rightarrow \sqrt{(-6)^2+24^2} \Rightarrow d=\sqrt{36+576} \Rightarrow d=\sqrt{612}=6\sqrt{17}$.

2. Use the midpoint formula: Midpoint $=\left(\dfrac{-1+5}{2},\dfrac{16-8}{2}\right)=(2,4)$.

3. Use the slope formula: $m = \dfrac{16-(-8)}{-1-5} \Rightarrow m = \dfrac{24}{-6} = -4$.

4. Use point-slope form and slope from ex. 3: $y-16 = -4(x-(-1)) \Rightarrow y-16 = -4x-4 \Rightarrow y = -4x+12$.

5. Change to slope-intercept form: $3x+4y = 144 \Rightarrow 4y = -3x+144 \Rightarrow y = -\dfrac{3}{4}x+36 \Rightarrow m = -\dfrac{3}{4}$.

6. For the x-intercept, $y = 0$. Therefore, $3x + 4(0) = 144 \Rightarrow 3x = 144 \Rightarrow x = 48$.

7. For the y-intercept, $x = 0$. Therefore, $3(0) + 4y = 144 \Rightarrow 4y = 144 \Rightarrow y = 36$.

8. One possible window is: $[-10, 50]$ by $[-40, 40]$.

9. Since $f(3) = 6$ and $f(-2) = 1$, $(3,6)$ and $(-2,1)$ are points on the graph of the line. Using these points, find the slope: $m = \dfrac{6-1}{3-(-2)} = \dfrac{5}{5} = 1$. Use point-slope form to find the function:

    $f(x) - 6 = 1(x-3) \Rightarrow f(x) - 6 = x - 3 \Rightarrow f(x) = x + 3$. Now solve for $f(8)$: $f(8) = 8 + 3 = 11$.

10. The slope of the given equation is -4. A line perpendicular to this will have a slope of $\dfrac{1}{4}$. Using this and

    point-slope form produces: $y - 4 = \dfrac{1}{4}(x-(-2)) \Rightarrow y - 4 = \dfrac{1}{4}x + \dfrac{1}{2} \Rightarrow y = \dfrac{1}{4}x + \dfrac{9}{2}$.

11. (a) $m = \dfrac{-4-5}{2-(-1)} \Rightarrow m = \dfrac{-9}{3} = -3$

    (b) Use point-slope form: $y - 5 = -3(x-(-1)) \Rightarrow y - 5 = -3x - 3 \Rightarrow y = -3x + 2$

    (c) Midpoint $= \left(\dfrac{-1+2}{2}, \dfrac{5+(-4)}{2}\right) = \left(\dfrac{1}{2}, \dfrac{1}{2}\right)$ or $(0.5, 0.5)$

    (d) $d = \sqrt{(2-(-1))^2 + (-4-5)^2} \Rightarrow d\sqrt{3^2+(-9)^2} \Rightarrow d = \sqrt{9+81} = \sqrt{90} = 3\sqrt{10}$

12. (a) $m = \dfrac{1.5-(-3.5)}{-1-(-3)} \Rightarrow m = \dfrac{5}{2} = 2.5$

    (b) Use point-slope form: $y - 1.5 = 2.5(x-(-1)) \Rightarrow y - 1.5 = 2.5x + 2.5 \Rightarrow y = 2.5x + 4$

    (c) Midpoint $= \left(\dfrac{-1+(-3)}{2}, \dfrac{1.5+(-3.5)}{2}\right) = \left(-\dfrac{4}{2}, -\dfrac{2}{2}\right) = (-2, -1)$

    (d) $d = \sqrt{(-1-(-3))^2 + (1.5-(-3.5))^2} \Rightarrow d = \sqrt{2^2+(5)^2} \Rightarrow d = \sqrt{4+25} = \sqrt{29}$

13. C most closely represents: $m < 0, b < 0$.

14. F most closely represents: $m > 0, b < 0$.

15. A most closely represents: $m < 0, b > 0$.

16. B most closely represents: $m > 0, b > 0$.

17. E most closely represents: $m = 0$.

18. D most closely represents: $b = 0$.

34 Chapter 1 Linear Functions, Equations, and Inequalities

19. The rate of change is evaluated as $m = \dfrac{62.9 - 66.7}{2009 - 2001} = -\dfrac{3.8}{8} = -0.475$. The graph confirms that the line through the ordered pairs falls from left to right and therefore has a negative slope. Thus, the number of basic cable subscribers decreased by an average of 0.475 million (or 475,000) each year from 2001 to 2009. See Figure 19.

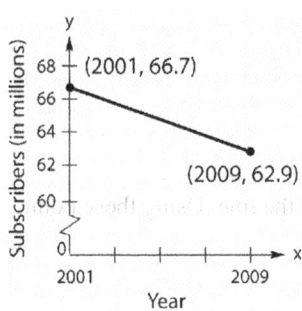

Figure 19

20. False, the slopes are different. Although the difference is small, the lines are not parallel and will intersect.

21. $f(x) = g(x)$ when the graphs intersect or when $x = -3$. I $\{-3\}$ is the best match.

22. $f(x) > g(x)$ when the graph of $f(x)$ is above the graph of $g(x)$ or when $x > -3$. K $(-3, \infty)$ is the best match.

23. $f(x) < g(x)$ when the graph of $f(x)$ is below the graph of $g(x)$ or when $x < -3$. B $(-\infty, 3)$ is the best match.

24. $g(x) \geq f(x)$ when the graph of $g(x)$ intersects or is above the graph of $f(x)$ or when $x \leq -3$. A $(-\infty, -3]$ is the best match.

25. $y_2 - y_1 = 0 \Rightarrow y_2 = y_1 \Rightarrow g(x) = f(x)$ when the graphs intersect or when $x = -3.1$. I $\{-3\}$ is the best match.

26. $f(x) < 0$ when the graph of $f(x)$ is below the x-axis or when $x < -5$. M $(-\infty, -5)$ is the best match.

27. $g(x) > 0$ when the graph of $g(x)$ is above the x-axis or when $x < -2$. O $(-\infty, -2)$ is the best match.

28. $y_2 - y_1 < 0 \Rightarrow y_2 < y_1 \Rightarrow g(x) < f(x)$ when the graph of $g(x)$ is below the graph of $f(x)$ or when $x > -3$. K $(-3, \infty)$ is the best match.

29. $5[3 + 2(x - 6)] = 3x + 1 \Rightarrow 5[2x - 9] = 3x + 1 \Rightarrow 10x - 45 = 3x + 1 \Rightarrow 7x = 46 \Rightarrow x = \dfrac{46}{7}$.

 The graphs of $y_1 = 5[3 + 2(x - 6)]$ and $y_2 = 3x + 1$ intersect at: $\left\{\dfrac{46}{7}\right\}$, which supports the result.

30. $\dfrac{x}{4} - \dfrac{x+4}{3} = -2 \Rightarrow 12\left[\dfrac{x}{4} - \dfrac{x+4}{3} = -2\right] \Rightarrow 3x - 4(x+4) = -24 \Rightarrow -x - 16 = -24 \Rightarrow -x = -8 \Rightarrow x = 8$.

 The graphs of $y_1 = \dfrac{x}{4} - \dfrac{x+4}{3}$ and $y_2 = -2$ intersect at: $\{8\}$, which supports the result.

31. $-3x-(4x+2)=3 \Rightarrow -7x-2=3 \Rightarrow -7x=5 \Rightarrow x=-\dfrac{5}{7}$. The graphs

 of $y_1=-3x-(4x+2)$ and $y_2=3$ intersect at: $\left\{-\dfrac{5}{7}\right\}$, which supports the result.

32. $-2x+9+4x=2(x-5)-3 \Rightarrow 2x+9=2x-10 \Rightarrow 9=-10$. This is false, therefore this is a

 contradiction and the solution is: $\varnothing$. The graphs of $y_1=-2x+9+4x$ and $y_2=2(x-5)-3$ are

 parallel and do not intersect, therefore no solution, $\varnothing$, which supports the result.

33. $0.5x+0.7(4-3x)=0.4x \Rightarrow 0.5x+2.8-2.1x=0.4x \Rightarrow 5x+28-21x=4x \Rightarrow -20x=-28 \Rightarrow$

 $x=\dfrac{7}{5}$. The graphs of $y_1=.5x+.7(4-3x)$ and $y_2=.4x$ intersect at: $\left\{\dfrac{7}{5}\right\}$, which supports the result.

34. $\dfrac{x}{4}-\dfrac{5x-3}{6}=2-\dfrac{7x+18}{12} \Rightarrow 12\left[\dfrac{x}{4}-\dfrac{5x-3}{6}=2-\dfrac{7x+18}{12}\right] \Rightarrow 3x-2(5x-3)=$

 $24-(7x+18) \Rightarrow -7x+6=-7x+6 \Rightarrow 6=6$. This is true, therefore an identity and the solution is:

 $(-\infty,\infty)$. The graphs of $y_1=\dfrac{x}{4}-\dfrac{5x-3}{6}$ and $y_2=2-\dfrac{7x+18}{12}$ are the same line; the solution is

 $(-\infty,\infty)$, which supports the result.

35. $x-8<1-2x \Rightarrow 3x<9 \Rightarrow x<3$. The graph of $y_1=x-8$ is below the graph of $y_2=1-2x$ for

 the interval: $(-\infty,3)$, which supports the result.

36. $\dfrac{4x-1}{3} \geq \dfrac{x}{5}-1 \Rightarrow 15\left[\dfrac{4x-1}{3} \geq \dfrac{x}{5}-1\right] \Rightarrow 5(4x-1) \geq 3x-15 \Rightarrow 20x-5 \geq 3x-15 \Rightarrow$

 $17x \geq -10 \Rightarrow x \geq -\dfrac{10}{17}$. The graph of $y_1=\dfrac{4x-1}{3}$ intersects or is above the graph of $y_2=\dfrac{x}{5}-1$

 for the interval: $\left[-\dfrac{10}{17},\infty\right)$, which supports the result.

37. $-6 \leq \dfrac{4-3x}{7}<2 \Rightarrow -42 \leq 4-3x<14 \Rightarrow -46 \leq -3x<10 \Rightarrow \dfrac{46}{3} \geq x > -\dfrac{10}{3} \Rightarrow -\dfrac{10}{3}<x \leq \dfrac{46}{3}$ or

 for the interval: $\left(-\dfrac{10}{3},\dfrac{46}{3}\right]$.

38. (a) Graph $y_1=5\pi+(\sqrt{3})x-6.24(x-8.1)+(\sqrt[3]{9})x$. See Figure 38. Find the x-intercept: $x \approx \{-3.81\}$.

 (b) $f(x)<0$ when the graph of $f(x)$ is below the x-axis. This happens for the interval: $(-\infty,-3.81)$.

 (c) $f(x) \geq 0$ when the graph of $f(x)$ intersects or is above the x-axis. This happens for the interval:

 $[-3.81,\infty)$.

[-10,10] by [-10,10]
Xscl = 1   Yscl = 1

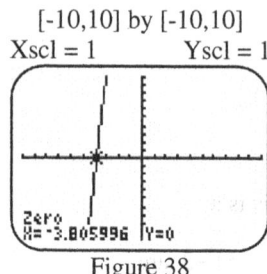

Figure 38

39. It costs $30 to produce each CD and there is a one-time advertisement cost, therefore: $C(x) = 30x + 150$.

40. Each tape is sold for $37.50, therefore: $R(x) = 37.50x$.

41. $C(x) = R(x)$ when $30x + 150 = 37.50x \Rightarrow 150 = 7.50x \Rightarrow x = 20$.

42. When the graph of $R(x)$ is below $C(x)$ the company is losing money, when $R(x)$ intersects $C(x)$ the company breaks even, and when $R(x)$ is above $C(x)$ the company makes money. This happens as follows: losing money when $x < 20$, breaking even when $x = 20$, and making money when $x > 20$.

43. $A = \dfrac{24f}{B(p+1)} \Rightarrow AB(p+1) = 24f \Rightarrow f = \dfrac{AB(p+1)}{24}$.

44. $A = \dfrac{24f}{B(p+1)} \Rightarrow AB(p+1) = 24f \Rightarrow B = \dfrac{24f}{A(p+1)}$.

45. (a) $f(x) = -3.52(5) + 58.6 \Rightarrow f(x) = -17.6 + 58.6 = 41°$ F.

    (b) $-15 = -3.52x + 58.6 \Rightarrow -73.6 = -3.52x \Rightarrow x \approx 20.9$ or about 21,000 feet.

    (c) Graph $y_1 = -3.52x + 58.6$. Find the coordinates of the point where $x = 5$ to support the answer in (a). Find the coordinates of the point where $y = -15$ to support the answer in (b).

46. (a) Linear regression gives the model: $f(x) \approx 0.12331x - 244.75$. Answers may vary.

    (b) $f(1990) \approx 0.12331x - 244.75 = \$0.63$ million The cost of a 30 second Super Bowl ad in 1990 was approximately $0.63 million. This value is within about 0.17 million of the actual cost.

    (c) $4 \approx 0.12331x - 244.75 \Rightarrow x \approx 2017$ Thus, the cost for a 30 second Super Bowl ad could reach $4 million 2017.

47. Let x = bat speed and y = ball travel distance; then (50, 320) and (80, 440) are two points on the graph of the function. Use the points to find slope: $m = \dfrac{440 - 320}{80 - 50} \Rightarrow m = \dfrac{120}{30} = 4$. Now use point-slope form to find the equation for the model: $y - 320 = 4(x - 50) \Rightarrow y - 320 = 4x - 200 \Rightarrow y = 4x + 120$. Because the slope is 4, the ball will travel 4 feet further for each additional 1 mph in bat speed.

48. Since surface area is: $A = 2(lw) + 2(lh) + 2(wh)$ we can solve

    $496 = 2(18)(8) + 2(18)h + 2(8)h \Rightarrow 496 = 288 + 36h + 16h \Rightarrow 208 = 52h \Rightarrow h = 4$. The height of the box is 4 feet.

49. Since there are 5280 feet in a mile, there are $5280 \times 26.2 = 138,336$ feet in a marathon. Since there are 3.281 feet in a meter, there are $100 \times 3.281 = 328.1$ feet in a 100 meter dash. Now use a proportion to solve:

    $\dfrac{9.58}{328.1} = \dfrac{x}{138,336} \Rightarrow 328.1x = 1325258.88 \Rightarrow x \approx 4039.19$ seconds to run a marathon. Divide by 60 to get minutes run: $4039.19 \div 60 = 67.32$ minutes run or 1 hour 7 minutes and 19 seconds.

50. $C = \dfrac{5}{9}(864 - 32) \Rightarrow C = \dfrac{5}{9}(832) \Rightarrow C = \dfrac{4160}{9} \Rightarrow 462\dfrac{2}{9}\,°\text{C}.$

51. Find the constant of variation: $4k = 3000 \Rightarrow k = 750$. Use this to find the pressure: $10(750) = 7500$ kg/m^2.

52. (a) Use any two points to find slope: $m = \dfrac{1.8 - 3}{1 - 0} \Rightarrow m = \dfrac{-1.2}{1} = -1.2$ Now use point-slope form to find the equation: $y - 3 = -1.2(x - 0) \Rightarrow y = -1.2x + 3$.

    (b) $y = -1.2(-1.5) + 3 \Rightarrow y = 1.8 + 3 \Rightarrow y = 4.8$ when $x = -1.5$.

    $y = -1.2(3.5) + 3 \Rightarrow y = -4.2 + 3 \Rightarrow y = -1.2$ when $x = 3.5$.

53. (a) Enter the years in L_1 and enter test scores in L_2. The regression equation is: $f(x) = 1.2x - 1886.4$

    (b) $y = 1.2(2012) - 1886.4 \Rightarrow y = 2414.4 - 1886.4 \Rightarrow y = 528$.

    (c) Over time data can change its pattern or character. Answers may vary.

54. Let x = the amount of 5% solution to be added, then solve:

    $120(.20) + x(.05) = (120 + x)(.10) \Rightarrow 24 + .05x = 12 + .10x \Rightarrow 12 = .05x \Rightarrow x = 240$ mL of 5% solution needs to be added.

55. The company will at least break even when $R(x) \geq C(x)$, therefore solve:

    $8x \geq 3x + 1500 \Rightarrow 5x \geq 1500 \Rightarrow x \geq 300$ or for the interval: $[300, \infty)$. 300 or more DVD's need to be sold to at least break even.

56. Let m = mental age and c = chronological age, then $IQ = \dfrac{100m}{c}$.

    (a) $130 = \dfrac{100m}{7} \Rightarrow 910 = 100m \Rightarrow m = 9.1$ years.

    (b) $IQ = \dfrac{100(20)}{16} \Rightarrow IQ = \dfrac{2000}{16} \Rightarrow IQ = 125$ years.

57. (a) Enter the heights in L_1 and enter weights in L_2. The regression equation is: $y \approx 4.512x - 154.4$

    (b) $y = 4.51(75) - 154.4 \Rightarrow y = 338.25 - 154.4 \Rightarrow y \approx 184$.

58. (a) Enter the heights in L_1 and enter weights in L_2. The regression equation is: $y \approx 4.465x - 133.3$

    (b) $y = 4.465(80) - 133.3 \Rightarrow y = 357.2 - 133.3 \Rightarrow y \approx 224$.

38   Chapter 1 Linear Functions, Equations, and Inequalities

Chapter 1 Test

1. (a) The number $\frac{4}{2} = 2$ is a natural number, integer, rational number, and real number.

    (b) The number π is a real number.

    (c) The number $\sqrt{2}$ is a real number.

    (d) The number $0.25 = \frac{1}{4}$ is a rational number and real number.

2. Use technology to approximate the following.

    (a) $\sqrt{5} \approx 2.236$

    (b) $\sqrt[3]{7} \approx 1.913$

    (c) $3^{1/4} \approx 1.316$

    (d) $\frac{1-1.1^2}{2+\pi^2} \approx -0.018$

3. $d = \sqrt{(-2-4)^2 + (4-(-3))^2} = \sqrt{6^2 + 7^2} = \sqrt{36+49} = \sqrt{85}$, $M = \left(\frac{-2+4}{2}, \frac{4+(-3)}{2}\right) = \left(\frac{2}{2}, \frac{1}{2}\right) = \left(1, \frac{1}{2}\right)$

4. (a) $f(-2) = 4 - 7(-2) = 4 + 14 = 18$

    (b) $f(b) = 4 - 7b$

    (c) $f(a+h) = 4 - 7(a+h) = 4 - 7a - 7h$

5. The set of ordered pairs $\{(3,4),(2,-5),(1,0),(4,-5)\}$ represents a function since each x-coordinate corresponds to only one y-coordinate.

6. (a) $m = \frac{4-1}{1-(-5)} = \frac{3}{6} = \frac{1}{2}$

    (b) $m = \frac{9-3}{4-4} = \frac{6}{0} \Rightarrow$ undefined

    (c) $m = \frac{5-5}{1.7-1.2} = \frac{0}{0.5} = 0$

7. (a) Domain: $(-\infty, \infty)$, Range: $[2, \infty)$, x-intercept: none, y-intercept: $(0, 3)$

    (b) Domain: $(-\infty, \infty)$, Range: $(-\infty, 0]$, x-intercept: $(3,0)$, y-intercept: $(0,-3)$

    (c) Domain: $[-4, \infty)$, Range: $[0, \infty)$, x-intercept: $(-4, 0)$, y-intercept: $(0, 2)$

8. (a) $f(x) = g(x)$ when the graph of $f(x)$ intersects the graph of $g(x)$ therefore $\{-4\}$.

    (b) $f(x) < g(x)$ when the graph of $f(x)$ is below the graph of $g(x)$, for the interval: $(-\infty, -4)$.

    (c) $f(x) \geq g(x)$ when the graph of $f(x)$ intersects or is above the graph of $g(x)$, for the interval: $[-4, \infty)$.

    (d) $f(y_2 - y_1) = 0 \Rightarrow y_2 = y_1 \Rightarrow g(x) = f(x)$ when the graph of $g(x)$ intersects the graph of $f(x)$, therefore $\{-4\}$.

Section 1.T   39

9. (a) $y_1 = 0$ when the graph of $f(x)$ intersects the x-axis, therefore $\{5.5\}$.

   (b) $y_1 < 0$ when the graph of $f(x)$ is below the x-axis, for the interval $(-\infty, 5.5]$.

   (c) $y_1 > 0$ when the graph of $f(x)$ is above the x-axis, for the interval $(5.5, \infty)$.

   (d) $y_1 \leq 0$ when the graph of $f(x)$ intersects or is below the x-axis, for the interval $(-\infty, 5.5]$.

10. (a) $3(x-4) - 2(x-5) = -2(x+1) - 3 \Rightarrow 3x - 12 - 2x + 10 = -2x - 2 - 3 \Rightarrow x - 2 = -2x - 5$

    $\Rightarrow 3x = -3 \Rightarrow x = -1$. Check: $3(-1-4) - 2(-1-5) = -2(-1+1) - 3 \Rightarrow$

    $3(-5) - 2(-6) = -2(0) - 3 \Rightarrow -15 + 12 = 0 - 3 \Rightarrow -3 = -3$

   (b) Graph $y_1 = 3(x-4) - 2(x-5)$ and $y_2 = -2(x+1) - 3$. See Figure 10. $f(x) > g(x)$ for the

    interval: $(-1, \infty)$ because the graph of $y_1 = f(x)$ is above the graph of $y_2 = g(x)$ for domain values

    greater than -1.

   (c) See Figure 10. $f(x) < g(x)$ for the interval $(-\infty, -1)$ because the graph of $y_1 = f(x)$ is below the graph

    of $y_2 = g(x)$ for domain values less than -1.

11. (a) $-\frac{1}{2}(8x+4) + 3(x-2) = 0 \Rightarrow -4x - 2 + 3x - 6 = 0 \Rightarrow -x - 8 = 0 \Rightarrow x = -8$ or $\{-8\}$.

   (b) $-\frac{1}{2}(8x+4) + 3(x-2) \leq 0 \Rightarrow -4x - 2 + 3x - 6 \leq 0 \Rightarrow -x - 8 \leq 0 \Rightarrow x \geq -8$ or for the

    interval: $[-8, \infty)$.

   (c) Graph $y_1 - \frac{1}{2}(8x+4) + 3(x-2)$. See Figure 11. The x-intercept is -8 supporting the result in part (a).

    The graph of the linear function lies below or on the x-axis for domain values greater than or equal to

    -8, supporting the results in part (b).

[-10,10] by [-10,10]
Xscl = 1   Yscl = 1

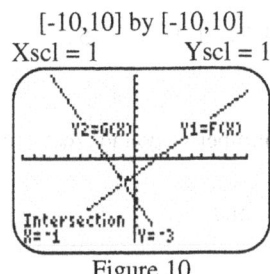
Figure 10

[-15,5] by [-10,10]
Xscl = 1   Yscl = 1

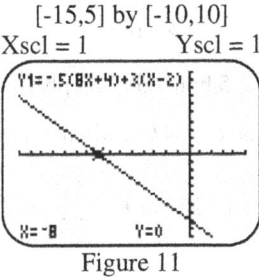
Figure 11

12. (a) Since x represents the number of years since 2007, we will use the points $(0, 13837)$ and

    $(5, 15082)$ find the slope: $a = \dfrac{15,082 - 13,837}{5 - 0} = \dfrac{1245}{5} = 249$. The y-intercept is the point $(0, 13837)$

    thus the value of b is 13837. The linear function is $f(x) = 249x + 13,837$.

   (b) The number of stations increased, on average, by 249 per year.

Copyright © 2015 Pearson Education, Inc

40 Chapter 1 Linear Functions, Equations, and Inequalities

(c) Since x represents the number of years since 2007 we will let $x = 7$.
$f(7) = 249(7) + 13,837 = 15,580$. The number of radio stations in 2014 is about 15,580.

13. (a) Since the given line has a slope of -2 and parallel lines have equal slopes, our new line has a slope of -2. Now use point-slope form: $y - 5 = -2(x - (-3)) \Rightarrow y - 5 = -2x - 6 \Rightarrow y = -2x - 1$.

    (b) The equation: $-2x + y = 0 \Rightarrow y = 2x$ has a slope of 2. Since perpendicular lines have slopes whose product equals -1, our new line has a slope of $-\frac{1}{2}$. Now use point-slope form:
    $y - 5 = -\frac{1}{2}(x - (-3)) \Rightarrow y - 5 = -\frac{1}{2}x - \frac{3}{2} \Rightarrow y = -\frac{1}{2}x + \frac{7}{2}$.

14. For the x-intercept $y = 0$, therefore: $3x - 4(0) = 6 \Rightarrow 3x = 6 \Rightarrow x = 2$. The x-intercept is $(2, 0)$. For the y-intercept $x = 0$, therefore: $3(0) - 4y = 6 \Rightarrow -4y = 6 \Rightarrow y = -\frac{6}{4} = -\frac{3}{2}$. The y-intercept is: $\left(0, -\frac{3}{2}\right)$. Using the intercepts: $\left(0, -\frac{3}{2}\right)$ and $(2, 0)$, the slope is $m = \dfrac{0 - \left(-\frac{3}{2}\right)}{2 - 0} = \dfrac{\frac{3}{2}}{2} \Rightarrow m = \dfrac{3}{4}$.

15. The equation of the horizontal line passing through $(-3, 7)$ is $y = 7$. The equation of the vertical line passing through $(-3, 7)$ is $x = -3$.

16. (a) Enter the wind speed in L_1 and enter degrees in L_2. The regression equation is: $Y \approx -.246x + 35.7$ and the correlation coefficient is: $r \approx -.96$.

    (b) $y \approx -.246(40) + 35.7 \Rightarrow y \approx -9.84 + 35.7 \Rightarrow y \approx 25.9\ °F$.

17. Let x be the number of hours the car traveled at 60 mph and then $4 - x$ will be the number of hours the car traveled at 74 mph. Using the formula $D = RT$, we know the distance traveled at 60 mph is $60x$, and the distance traveled at 74 mph is $74(4 - x)$. Since the total distance traveled is 275 miles we have the equation $60x + 74(4 - x) = 275 \Rightarrow 60x + 296 - 74x = 275 \Rightarrow -14x = -21 \Rightarrow x = 1.5$ and $4 - x = 2.5$. Therefore, the car traveled for 1.5 hours at 60 mph and 2.5 hours at 74 mph.

18. Since the load is directly proportional to the width we have $y = kx$, where y is the number of pounds that can be supported and x is the width in inches. Then, $510 = k(2.25) \Rightarrow k = \dfrac{510}{2.25} = 226\dfrac{2}{3}$ and $y = \left(226\dfrac{2}{3}\right)(3.1) = 702\dfrac{2}{3}$ pounds.

Chapter 2: Analysis of Graphs and Functions

2.1: Graphs of Basic Functions and Relations; Symmetry

1. $(-\infty, \infty)$.

3. $(0,0)$

5. increases

7. x-axis

9. odd

11. The domain can be all real numbers; therefore, the function is continuous for the interval $(-\infty, \infty)$.

13. The domain can only be values where $x \geq 0$; therefore, the function is continuous for the interval $[0, \infty)$.

15. The domain can be all real numbers except -3; therefore, the function is continuous for the interval $(-\infty, -3) \cup (-3, \infty)$.

17. (a) The function is increasing for the interval $(3, \infty)$

    (b) The function is decreasing for the interval $(-\infty, 3)$

    (c) The function is never constant; therefore, none.

    (d) The domain can be all real numbers; therefore, the interval $(-\infty, \infty)$.

    (e) The range can only be values where $y \geq 0$; therefore, the interval $[0, \infty)$.

19. (a) The function is increasing for the interval $(-\infty, 1)$

    (b) The function is decreasing for the interval $(4, \infty)$

    (c) The function is constant for the interval $(1, 4)$

    (d) The domain can be all real numbers; therefore, the interval $(-\infty, \infty)$.

    (e) The range can only be values where $y \leq 3$; therefore, the interval $(-\infty, 3]$.

21. (a) The function is never increasing; therefore, none

    (b) The function is decreasing for the intervals $(-\infty, -2)$ and $(3, \infty)$

    (c) The function is constant for the interval $(-2, 3)$.

    (d) The domain can be all real numbers; therefore, the interval $(-\infty, \infty)$.

    (e) The range can only be values where $y \leq 1.5$ or $y \geq 2$; therefore, the interval $(-\infty, 1.5] \cup [2, \infty)$.

23. Graph $f(x) = x^5$. See Figure 23. As x increases for the interval $(-\infty, \infty)$, y increases; therefore, the function is increasing.

25. Graph $f(x) = x^4$. See Figure 25. As x increases for the interval $(-\infty, 0)$ y decreases; therefore, the function is decreasing on $(-\infty, 0)$

42   Chapter 2: Analysis of Graphs of Functions

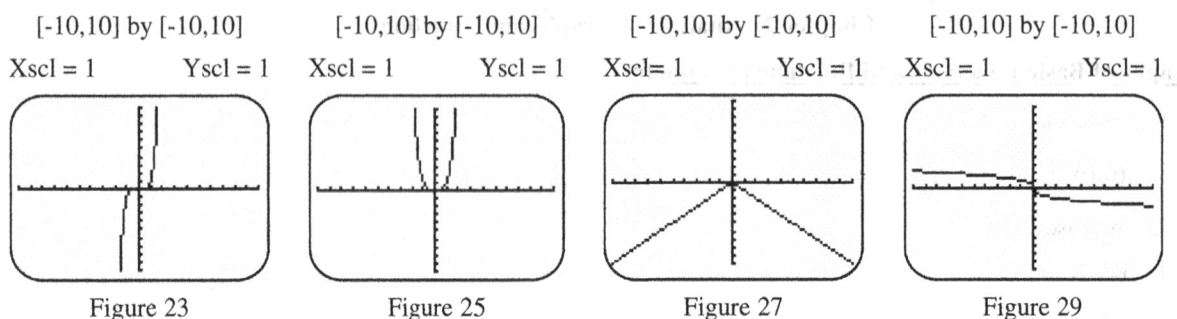

Figure 23   Figure 25   Figure 27   Figure 29

27. Graph $f(x) = -|x|$. See Figure 27. As x increases for the interval $(-\infty, 0)$, y increases; therefore, the function is increasing on $(-\infty, 0)$.

29. Graph $f(x) = -\sqrt[3]{x}$. See Figure 29. As x increases for the interval $(-\infty, \infty)$, y decreases; therefore, the function is decreasing.

31. Graph $f(x) = 1 - x^3$. See Figure 31. As x increases for the interval $(-\infty, \infty)$, y decreases; therefore, the function is decreasing.

33. Graph $f(x) = 2 - x^2$. See Figure 33. As x increases for the interval $(-\infty, 0)$ y increases; therefore, the function is increasing on $(-\infty, 0)$.

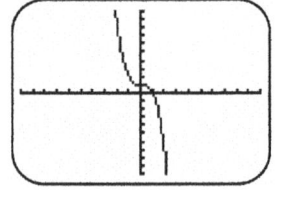

Figure 31   Figure 33

35. (a) No (b) Yes (c) No
37. (a) Yes (b) No   (c) No
39. (a) Yes (b) Yes (c) Yes
41. (a) No (b) No   (c) Yes
43. (a) Since $f(-x) = f(x)$, this is an even function and is symmetric with respect to the y-axis. See Figure 43a.
    (b) Since $f(-x) = -f(x)$, this is an odd function and is symmetric with respect to the origin. See Figure 43b.

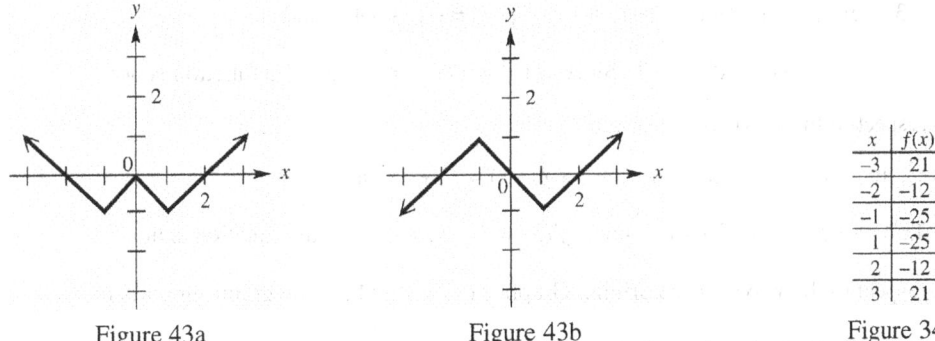

Figure 43a Figure 43b Figure 34

45. If f is an even function then $f(-x) = f(x)$ or opposite domains have the same range. See Figure 45

47. This is an even function since opposite domains have the same range.

49. This is an odd function since opposite domains have the opposite range.

51. This is neither even nor odd since the opposite domains are neither the opposite or same range.

53. If $f(x) = x^4 - 7x^2 + 6$, then $f(-x) = (-x)^4 - 7(-x)^2 + 6 \Rightarrow f(-x) = x^4 - 7x^2 + 6$. Since $f(-x) = f(x)$, the function is even.

55. If $f(x) = 3x^3 - x$, then $f(-x) = 3(-x)^3 - (-x) \Rightarrow f(-x) = -3x^3 + x$ and $-f(x) = -(3x^3 - x) \Rightarrow -f(x) = -3x^3 + x$. Since $f(-x) = -f(x)$, the function is odd.

57. If $f(x) = x^6 - 4x^4 + 5$ then $f(-x) = (-x)^6 - 4(-x)^4 + 5 \Rightarrow f(-x) = x^6 - 4x^4 + 5$. Since $f(-x) = f(x)$, the function is even.

59. If $f(x) = 3x^5 - x^3 + 7x$, then $f(-x) = 3(-x)^5 - (-x)^3 + 7(-x) \Rightarrow f(-x) = -3x^5 + x^3 - 7x$ and $-f(x) = -(3x^5 - x^3 + 7x) \Rightarrow -f(x) = -3x^5 + x^3 - 7x$. Since $f(-x) = -f(x)$, the function is odd.

61. If $f(x) = |5x|$, then $f(-x) = |5(-x)| \Rightarrow f(-x) = |5x|$. Since $f(-x) = f(x)$, the function is even.

63. If $(-3, 11)$ and $(2, 9)$ then $f(-x) = \frac{1}{2(-x)} \Rightarrow f(-x) = -\frac{1}{2x}$ and $-f(x) = -\left(\frac{1}{2x}\right) \Rightarrow -f(x) = -\frac{1}{2x}$. Since $f(-x) = -f(x)$, the function is odd.

65. If $f(x) = -x^3 + 2x$, then $f(-x) = -(-x)^3 + 2(-x) \Rightarrow f(-x) = x^3 - 2x$ and $-f(x) = -(-x^3 + 2x) \Rightarrow -f(x) = x^3 - 2x$. Since $f(-x) = -f(x)$, the function is symmetric with respect to the origin. Graph $f(x) = -x^3 + 2x$; the graph supports symmetry with respect to the origin.

67. If $f(x) = 0.5x^4 - 2x^2 + 1$, then $f(-x) = 0.5(-x)^4 - 2(-x)^2 + 1 \Rightarrow f(-x) = 0.5x^4 - 2x^2 + 1$. Since $f(-x) = f(x)$, the function is symmetric with respect to the y-axis. Graph $f(x) = 0.5x^4 - 2x^2 + 1$; the graph supports symmetry with respect to the y-axis.

44   Chapter 2: Analysis of Graphs of Functions

69. If $f(x) = x^3 - x + 3$, then $f(-x) = (-x)^3 - (-x) + 3 \Rightarrow f(-x) = -x^3 + x + 3$ and $-f(x) = -(x^3 - x + 3) \Rightarrow -f(x) = -x^3 + x - 3$. Since $f(x) \neq f(-x) \neq -f(x)$, the function is not symmetric with respect to the y-axis or the origin.

71. If $f(x) = x^6 - 4x^3$, then $f(-x) = (-x)^6 - 4(-x)^3 \Rightarrow f(-x) = x^6 + 4x^3$ and $-f(x) = -(x^6 - 4x^3) \Rightarrow -f(x) = -x^6 + 4x^3$. Since $f(x) \neq f(-x) \neq -f(x)$, the function is not symmetric with respect to the y-axis or the origin. Graph $f(x) = x^6 - 4x^3$; the graph supports no symmetry with respect to the y-axis or the origin.

73. If $f(x) = -6$, then $f(-x) = -6$, Since $f(-x) = f(x)$, the function is symmetric with respect to the y-axis. Graph $f(x) = -6$; the graph supports symmetry with respect to the y-axis.

75. If $f(x) = \dfrac{1}{4x^3}$, then $f(-x) = \dfrac{1}{4(-x)^3} \Rightarrow f(-x) = -\dfrac{1}{4x^3}$ and $-f(x) = -\left(\dfrac{1}{4x^3}\right) \Rightarrow -f(x) = -\dfrac{1}{4x^3}$. Since $f(-x) = -f(x)$, the function is symmetric with respect to the origin. Graph $f(x) = \dfrac{1}{4x^3}$; the graph supports symmetry with respect to the origin.

2.2: Vertical and Horizontal Shifts of Graphs

1. The equation $y = x^2$ shifted 3 units upward is $y = x^2 + 3$.

3. The equation $y = \sqrt{x}$ shifted 4 units downward is $y = \sqrt{x} - 4$.

5. The equation $y = |x|$ shifted 4 units to the right is $y = |x - 4|$.

7. The equation $y = x^3$ shifted 7 units to the left is $y = (x + 7)^3$.

9. The equation $y = x^2$ shifted 2 units downward and 3 units right is $y = (x - 3)^2 - 2$.

11. The equation $y = \sqrt{x}$ shifted 3 units upward and 6 units to the left is $y = \sqrt{x + 6} + 3$.

13. The equation $y = x^2$ shifted 500 units upward and 2000 units right is $y = (x - 2000)^2 + 500$.

15. Shift the graph of f 4 units upward to obtain the graph of g.

17. The equation $y = x^2 - 3$ is $y = x^2$ shifted 3 units downward; therefore, graph B.

19. The equation $y = (x + 3)^2$ is $y = x^2$ shifted 3 units to the left; therefore, graph A.

21. The equation $y = |x + 4| - 3$ is $y = |x|$ shifted 4 units to the left and 3 units downward; therefore, graph B.

23. The equation $y = (x - 3)^3$ is $y = x^3$ shifted 3 units to the right; therefore, graph C.

25. The equation $y = (x + 2)^3 - 4$ is $[-a, -b]$. shifted 2 units to the left and 4 units downward; therefore, graph B.

27. Using $Y_2 = Y_1 + k$ and $x = 0$, we get $-5 = -3 + k \Rightarrow k = -2$.

Section 2.2   45

29. From the graphs, $(6,2)$ is a point on Y_1 and $(6,-1)$ a point on Y_2. Using $Y_2 = Y_1 + k$ and $x = 6$, we get $-1 = 2 + k \Rightarrow k = -3$.

31. For the equation $y = x^2$, the Domain is $(-\infty, \infty)$ and the Range is $[0, \infty)$. Shifting this 3 units downward gives us: (a) Domain: $(-\infty, \infty)$ (b) Range: $[-3, \infty)$.

33. For the equation $y = |x|$, the Domain is $(-\infty, \infty)$ and the Range is $[0, \infty)$. Shifting this 4 units to the left and 3 units downward gives us: (a) Domain: $(-\infty, \infty)$ (b) Range: $[-3, \infty)$.

35. For the equation $y = x^3$, the Domain is $(-\infty, \infty)$ and the Range is $(-\infty, \infty)$. Shifting this 3 units to the right gives us: (a) Domain: $(-\infty, \infty)$ (b) Range: $(-\infty, \infty)$

37. For the equation $y = x^2$, the Domain is $(-\infty, \infty)$ and the Range is $[0, \infty)$. Shifting this 1 unit to the right and 5 units downward gives us: (a) Domain: $(-\infty, \infty)$ (b) Range: $[-5, \infty)$.

39. For the equation $y = \sqrt{x}$, the Domain is $[0, \infty)$. and the Range is $[0, \infty)$. Shifting this 4 units to the right gives us: (a) Domain: $[4, \infty)$. (b) Range: $[0, \infty)$.

41. For the equation $y = x^3$, the Domain is $(-\infty, \infty)$ and the Range is $(-\infty, \infty)$. Shifting this 1 unit to the right and 4 units upward gives us: (a) Domain: $(-\infty, \infty)$ (b) Range: $(-\infty, \infty)$

43. The graph of $y = f(x)$ is the graph of the equation $y = x^2$ shifted 1 unit to the right. See Figure 43.

45. The graph of $y = x^3 + 1$ is the graph of the equation $y = x^3$ shifted 1 unit upward. See Figure 45.

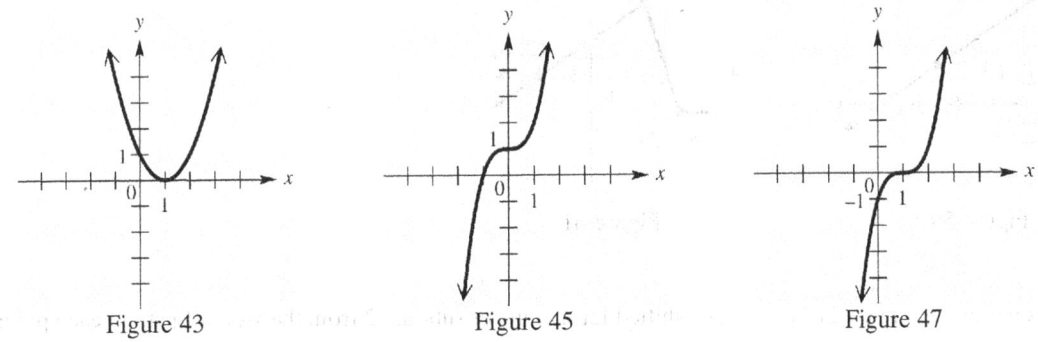

Figure 43   Figure 45   Figure 47

47. The graph of $y = (x-1)^3$ is the graph of the equation $y = x^3$ shifted 1 unit to the right. See Figure 47.

49. The graph of $y = \sqrt{x-2} - 1$ is the graph of the equation $y = \sqrt{x}$ shifted 2 units to the right and 1 unit downward. See Figure 49.

51. The graph of $f(x)$ is the graph of the equation $y = x^2$ shifted 2 units to the left and 3 units upward. See Figure 51.

46　Chapter 2: Analysis of Graphs of Functions

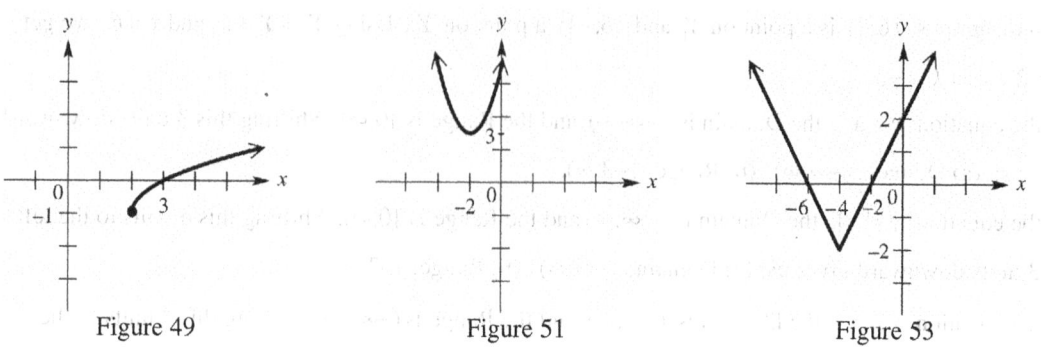

Figure 49　　　Figure 51　　　Figure 53

53. The graph of $y = |x+4| - 2$ is the graph of the equation $y = |x|$ shifted 4 units to the left and 2 units downward. See Figure 53.

55. Since h and k are positive, the equation is $y = x^2$ shifted to the right and down; therefore, B.

57. Since h and k are positive, the equation is $y = x^2$ shifted to the left and up; therefore, A.

59. The equation $y = f(x) + 2$ is $y = f(x)$ shifted up 2 units or add 2 to the y-coordinate of each point as follows: $(-3, 2) \Rightarrow (-3, 0); (-1, 4) \Rightarrow (-1, 6); (5, 0) \Rightarrow (5, 2)$. See Figure 59.

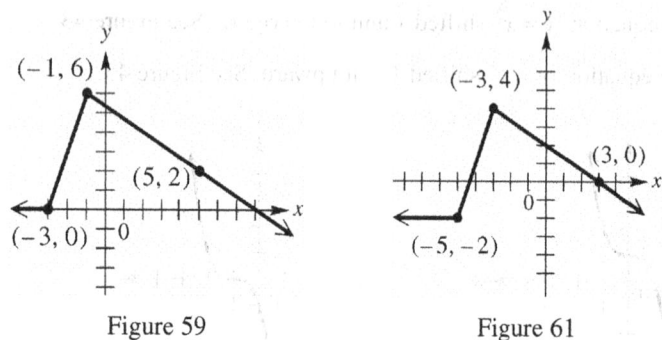

Figure 59　　　Figure 61

61. The equation $y = f(x+2)$ is $y = f(x)$ shifted left 2 units or subtract 2 from the x-coordinate of each point as follows: $(-3, -2) \Rightarrow (-5, -2); (-1, 4) \Rightarrow (-3, 4); (5, 0) \Rightarrow (3, 0)$. See Figure 61.

63. The graph is the basic function $y = x^2$ translated 4 units to the left and 3 units up; therefore, the new equation is $y = (x+4)^2 + 3$. The equation is now increasing for the interval: (a) $(-4, \infty)$ and decreasing for the interval: (b) $(-\infty, -4)$.

65. The graph is the basic function $y = x^3$ translated 5 units down; therefore, the new equation is $y = x^3 - 5$. The equation is now increasing for the interval: (a) $(-\infty, \infty)$ and does not decrease; therefore: (b) none.

67. The graph is the basic function $y = \sqrt{x}$ translated 2 units to the right and 1 unit up; therefore, the new equation is $y = \sqrt{x-2} + 1$. The equation is now increasing for the interval: (a) $(2, \infty)$ and does not decrease; therefore: (b) none.

69. (a) $f(x) = 0$: $\{3, 4\}$

(b) $f(x) > 0$: for the intervals $(-\infty, 3) \cup (4, \infty)$.

(c) $f(x) < 0$: for the interval $(3, 4)$.

71. (a) $f(x) = 0$: $\{-4, 5\}$

    (b) $f(x) \geq 0$: for the intervals $(-\infty, -4] \cup [5, \infty)$

    (c) $f(x) \leq 0$: for the interval $[-4, 5]$.

72. (a) $f(x) = 0$: never; therefore: $\emptyset$.

    (b) $f(x) \geq 0$: for the interval $[1, \infty)$.

    (c) $f(x) \leq 0$: never; therefore: $\emptyset$.

73. The translation is 3 units to the left and 1 unit up; therefore, the new equation is $y = |x + 3| + 1$. The form $y = |x - h| + k$ will equal $y = |x + 3| + 1$ when: $h = -3$ and $k = 1$.

74. The equation $y = x^2$ has a Domain: $(-\infty, \infty)$ and a Range: $[0, \infty)$. After the translation the Domain is still: $(-\infty, \infty)$ but now the Range is $(38, \infty)$, a positive or upward shift of 38 units. Therefore, the horizontal shift can be any number of units, but the vertical shift is up 38. This makes h any real number and $k = 38$.

75. (a) $B(4) = 66.25(4) + 160 = 425$; In 2010, 425,000 bankruptcies were filed.

    (b) We will use the point (2006, 160) and the slope of 66.25 in the point slope form for the equation of a line. $y - y_1 = m(x - x_1) \Rightarrow y - 160 = 66.25(x - 2006) \Rightarrow y = 66.25(x - 2006) + 160$

    (c) $y = 66.25(2010 - 2006) + 160 = 66.25(4) + 160 = 425$, In 2010, 425,000 bankruptcies were filed.

    (d) $293 = 66.25(x - 2006) + 160 \Rightarrow 133 = 66.25(x - 2006) \Rightarrow \frac{133}{66.25} = x - 2006 \Rightarrow x = 2006 + \frac{133}{66.25}$.

    There will be 293 thousand bankruptcies in 2008.

77. $U(2011) = 13(2011 - 2006)^2 + 115 = 13(25) + 115 = 440$; The average U.S. household spent $440 on Apple products in 2011.

79. (a) Enter the year in L_1 and enter tuition and fees in L_2. The year 2000 corresponds to $x = 0$ and so on. The regression equation is $y \approx 402.5x + 3460$.

    (b) Since $x = 0$ corresponds to 2000, the equation when the exact year is entered is
    $y = 402.5(x - 2000) + 3460$

    (c) $y \approx 402.5(2009 - 2000) + 3460 \Rightarrow y \approx \$7100$

81. See Figure 81.

48   Chapter 2: Analysis of Graphs of Functions

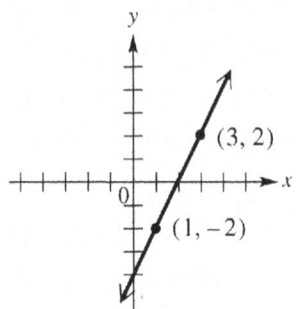

Figure 81

82. $m = \dfrac{2-(-2)}{3-1} \Rightarrow m = \dfrac{4}{2} = 2$

83. Using slope-intercept form yields: $y_1 - 2 = 2(x-3) \Rightarrow y_1 - 2 = 2x - 6 \Rightarrow y_1 = 2x - 4$

84. $(1, -2+6)$ and $(3, 2+6) \Rightarrow (1, 4)$ and $(3, 8)$

85. $m = \dfrac{8-4}{3-1} \Rightarrow m = \dfrac{4}{2} = 2$

86. Using slope-intercept form yields: $y_2 - 4 = 2(x-1) \Rightarrow y_2 - 4 = 2x - 2 \Rightarrow y_2 = 2x + 2$.

87. Graph $y_1 = 2x - 4$ and $y_2 = 2x + 2$ See Figure 87. The graph y_2 can be obtained by shifting the graph of y_1 upward 6 units. The constant 6, comes from the 6 we added to each y-value in Exercise 84.

[-10,10] by [-10,10]
Xscl = 1   Yscl = 1

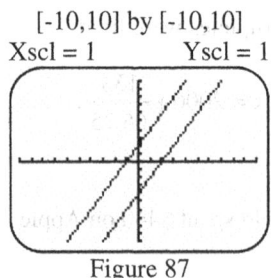

Figure 87

88. c; c; the same as; c; upward (or positive vertical)

2.3: Stretching, Shrinking, and Reflecting Graphs

1. The function $y = x^2$ vertically stretched by a factor of 2 is $y = 2x^2$.

3. The function $y = \sqrt{x}$ reflected across the y-axis is $y = \sqrt{-x}$.

5. The function $y = |x|$ vertically stretched by a factor of 3 and reflected across the x-axis is $y = -3|x|$.

7. The function $y = x^3$ vertically shrunk by a factor of 0.25 and reflected across the y-axis is $y = 0.25(-x^3)$ or $y = -0.25x^3$.

9. Graph $y_1 = x$, $y_2 = x + 3$ (y_1 shifted up 3 units), and $y_3 = x - 3$ (y_1 shifted down 3 units). See Figure 9.

11. Graph $y_1 = |x|$, $y_2 = |x - 3|$ (y_1 shifted right 3 units), and $y_3 = |x + 3|$ (y_1 shifted left 3 units). See Figure 11

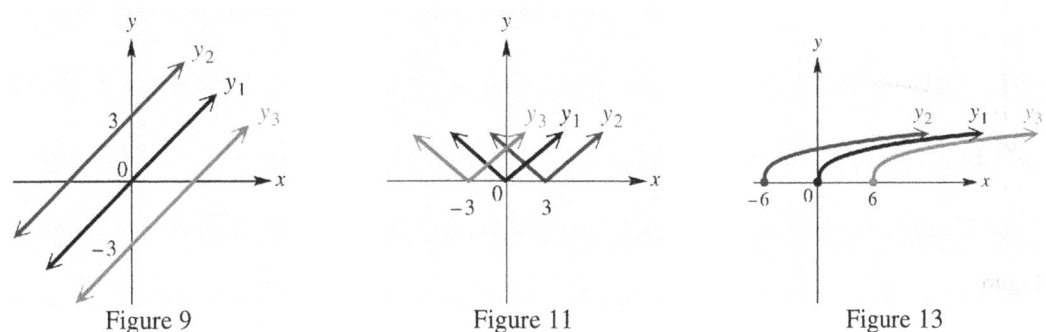

Figure 9   Figure 11   Figure 13

13. Graph $y_1 = \sqrt{x}$, $y_2 = \sqrt{x+6}$ (y_1 shifted left 6 units), and $y_3 = \sqrt{x-6}$ (y_1 shifted right 6 units). See Figure 13.

15. Graph $y_1 = \sqrt[3]{x}$, $y_2 = -\sqrt[3]{x}$ (y_1 reflected across the x-axis), and $y_3 = -2\sqrt[3]{x}$ (y_1 reflected across the x-axis and stretched vertically by a factor of 2). See Figure 15.

17. Graph $y_1 = |x|$, $y_2 = -2|x-1|+1$ (y_1 reflected across the x-axis, stretched vertically by a factor of 2, shifted right 1 unit, and shifted up 1 unit), and $y_3 = -\frac{1}{2}|x|-4$ (y_1 reflected across the x-axis, shrunk by factor of $\frac{1}{2}$, and shifted down 4 units). See Figure 17.

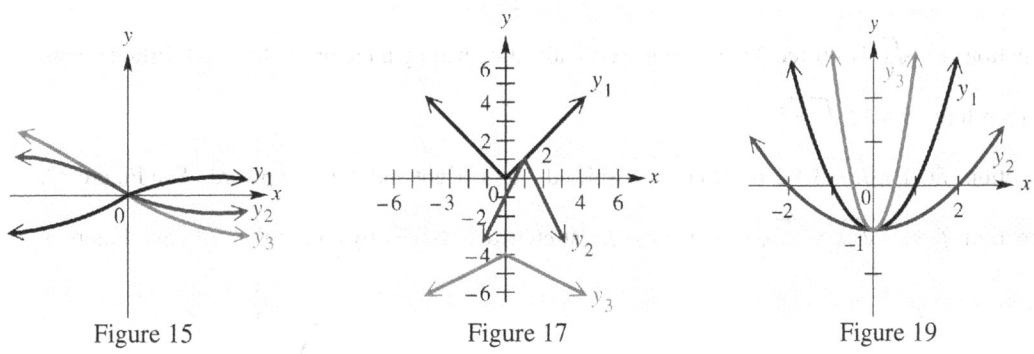

Figure 15   Figure 17   Figure 19

19. Graph $y_1 = x^2 - 1$ (which is $y = x^2$ shifted down 1 unit), $y_2 = \left(\frac{1}{2}x\right)^2 - 1$ (y_1 shrunk vertically by A factor of $\frac{1}{2}$), and $y_3 = (2x)^2 - 1$ (y_1 stretched vertically by a factor of 2^2 or 4). See Figure 19.

21. Graph $y_1 = \sqrt[3]{x}$, $y_2 = \sqrt[3]{-x}$ (y_1 reflected across the y-axis), and $y_3 = \sqrt[3]{-(x-1)}$ (y_1 reflected across the y-axis and shifted right 1 unit). See Figure 21.

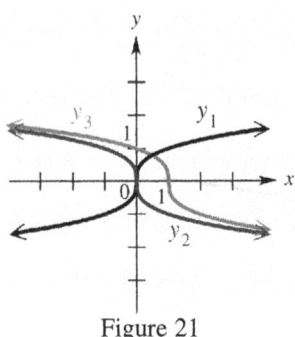

Figure 21

23. The graph $y = f(x) = x^2$ has been reflected across the x-axis, shifted 5 units to the right, and shifted 2 units downward; therefore, the equation of $g(x)$ is $g(x) = -(x-5)^2 - 2$.

25. The graph $y = f(x) = \sqrt{x}$ has been reflected across the y-axis and shifted 1 unit upward; therefore, the equation of $g(x)$ is $g(x) = \sqrt{-x} + 1$.

27. 4; x

29. 2; left; $\frac{1}{4}$; x; 3; downward (or negative)

31. 3; right; 6

33. The function $y = x^2$ is vertically shrunk by a factor of $\frac{1}{2}$ and shifted 7 units down; therefore, $y = \frac{1}{2}x^2 - 7$.

35. The function $y = \sqrt{x}$ is shifted 3 units right, vertically stretched by a factor of 4.5, and shifted 6 units down; therefore, $y = 4.5\sqrt{x-3} - 6$.

37. The function $f(x) = \sqrt{x-3} + 2$ is $f(x) = \sqrt{x}$ shifted 3 units right and 2 units upward. See Figure 37.

39. The function $f(x) = \sqrt{2x} = \sqrt{2}\sqrt{x}$ is $f(x) = \sqrt{x}$ stretched vertically by a factor of $\sqrt{2}$. See Figure 39.

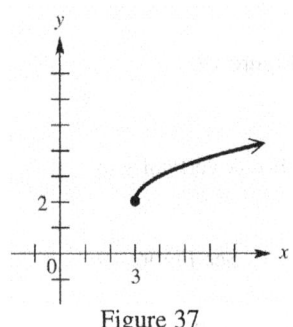
Figure 37

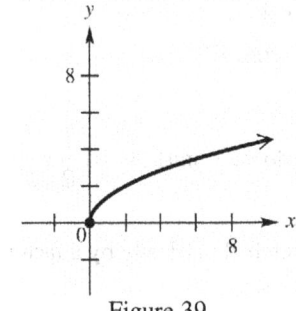
Figure 39

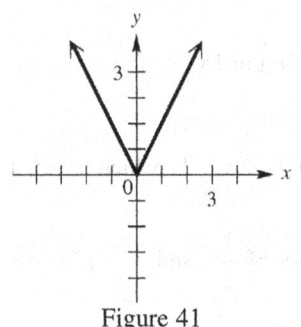
Figure 41

41. The function $f(x) = |2x| = 2|x|$ is $f(x) = |x|$ stretched vertically by a factor of 2. See Figure 41.

43. The function $f(x) = 1 - \sqrt{x}$ is $f(x) = \sqrt{x}$ reflected across the x-axis and shifted 1 unit upward. See Figure 43.

45. The function $f(x) = -\sqrt{1-x} = -\sqrt{-(x-1)}$ is $f(x) = \sqrt{x}$ reflected across both the x-axis, the y-axis and shifted 1 unit right. See Figure 45.

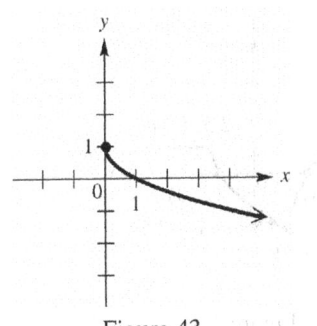
Figure 43

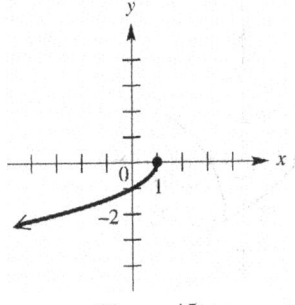
Figure 45

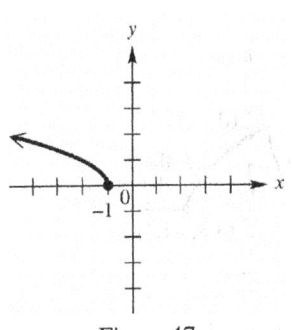
Figure 47

47. The function $f(x) = \sqrt{-(x+1)}$ is $f(x) = \sqrt{x}$ reflected across the y-axis and shifted 1 unit left. See Figure 47.

49. The function $f(x) = (x-1)^3$ is $f(x) = x^3$ shifted 1 unit right. See Figure 49.

51. The function $f(x) = -x^3$ is $f(x) = x^3$ reflected across the x-axis. See Figure 51.

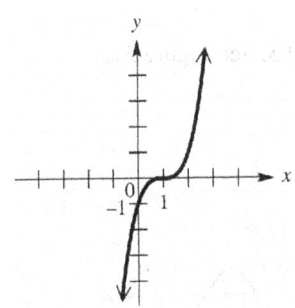
Figure 49

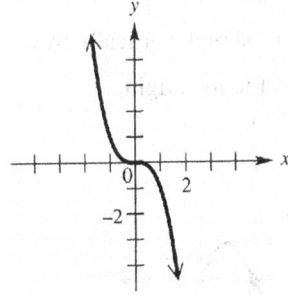
Figure 51

53. (a) The equation $y = -f(x)$ is $y = f(x)$ reflected across the x-axis. See Figure 53a.

(b) The equation $y = f(-x)$ is $y = f(x)$ reflected across the y-axis. See Figure 53b.

(c) The equation $y = 2f(x)$ is $y = f(x)$ stretched vertically by a factor of 2. See Figure 53c.

(d) From the graph $f(0) = 1$.

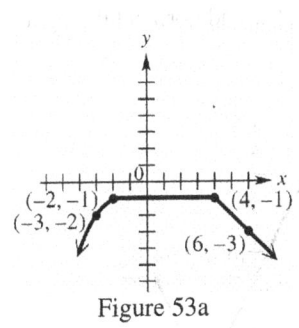
Figure 53a

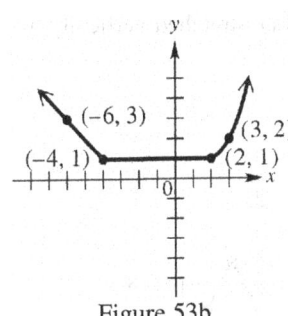
Figure 53b

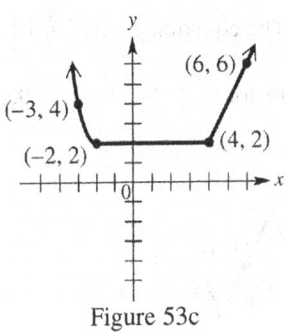
Figure 53c

55. (a) The equation $f(x)$ is $y = f(x)$ reflected across the x-axis. See Figure 55a.

(b) The equation $y = f(-x)$ is $y = f(x)$ reflected across the y-axis. See Figure 55b.

(c) The equation $y = f(x+1)$ is $y = f(x)$ shifted 1 unit to the left. See Figure 55c.

(d) From the graph, there are two x-intercepts, $(-1, 0)$ and $(4, 0)$.

52 Chapter 2: Analysis of Graphs of Functions

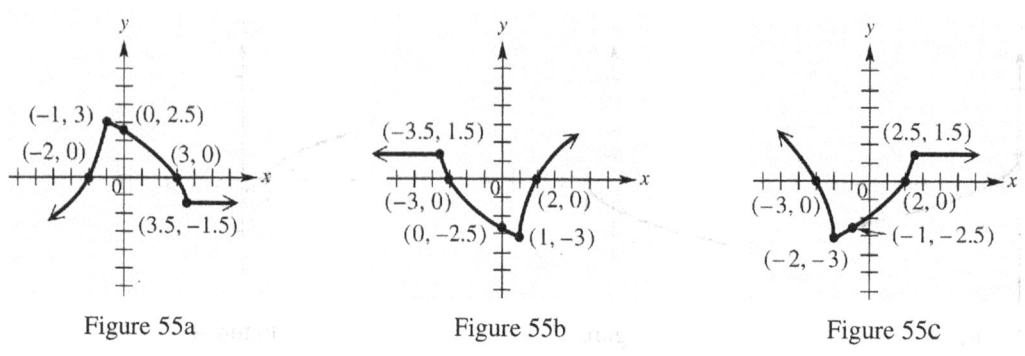

Figure 55a   Figure 55b   Figure 55c

57. (a) The equation $y = -f(x)$ is $y = f(x)$ reflected across the x-axis. See Figure 57a.

(b) The equation $y = f\left(\dfrac{1}{3}x\right)$ is $y = f(x)$ stretched horizontally by a factor of 3. See Figure 57b.

(c) The equation $y = 0.5f(x)$ is $y = f(x)$ shrunk vertically by a factor of 0.5. See Figure 57c.

(d) From the graph, symmetry with respect to the origin.

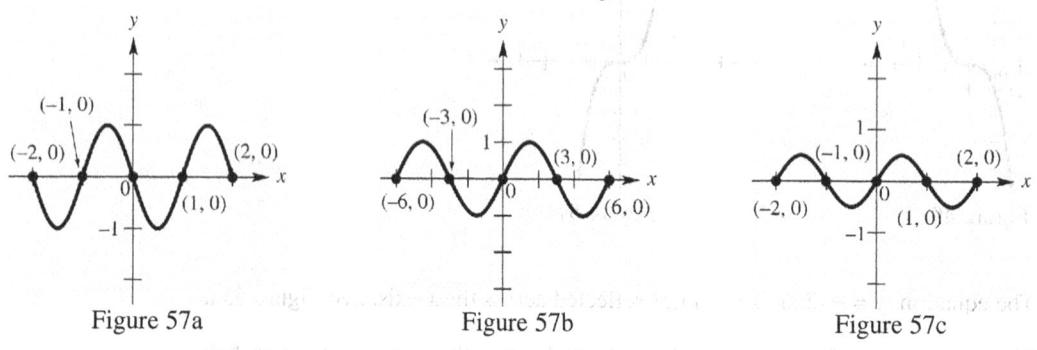

Figure 57a   Figure 57b   Figure 57c

59. (a) The equation $y = f(x)+1$ is $y = f(x)$ shifted 1 unit upward. See Figure 59a.

(b) The equation $-30°$ is $y = f(x)$ reflected across the x-axis and shifted 1 unit down. See Figure 59b.

(c) The equation $y = 2f\left(\dfrac{1}{2}x\right)$ is $y = f(x)$ stretched vertically by a factor of 2 and horizontally by a factor of 2. See Figure 59c.

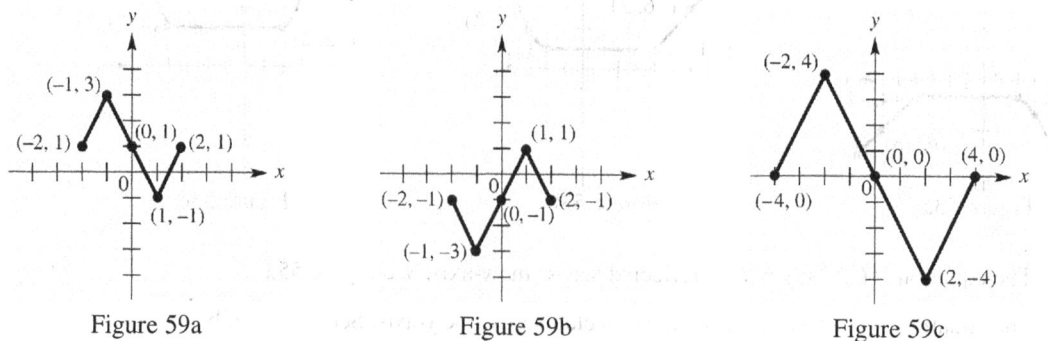

Figure 59a   Figure 59b   Figure 59c

61. (a) The equation $y = f(2x)+1$ is x shrunk horizontally by a factor of $\{2\}$ and shifted 1 unit upward. See Figure 61a.

(b) The equation $y = 2f\left(\dfrac{1}{2}x\right)+1$ is $y = f(x)$ stretched vertically by a factor of 2, stretched horizontally by a factor of 2, and shifted 1 unit upward. See Figure 61b.

(c) The equation $y = \dfrac{1}{2}f(x-2)$ is $y = f(x)$ shrunk vertically by a factor of $\dfrac{1}{2}$ and shifted 2 units to the right. See Figure 61c.

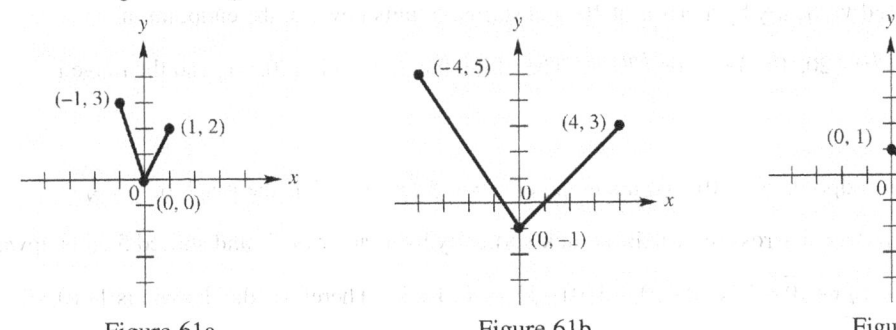

Figure 61a　　　　　　　Figure 61b　　　　　　　Figure 61c

63. (a) If $(r, 0)$ is the x-intercept of $y = f(x)$ and $y = -f(x)$ is $y = f(x)$ reflected across the x-axis, then $(r, 0)$ is also the x-intercept of $y = -f(x)$.

(b) If $(r, 0)$ is the x-intercept of $y = f(x)$ and $y = f(-x)$ is $f(x)$ reflected across the y-axis, then $(-r, 0)$ is the x-intercept of $y = -f(x)$

(c) If $(r, 0)$ is the x-intercept of $y = f(x)$ and $y = -f(-x)$ is $y = f(x)$ reflected across both the x-axis and y-axis, then $(-r, 0)$, is the x-intercept of $y = -f(-x)$.

65. Since $y = f(x-2)$ is $y = f(x)$ shifted 2 units to the right, the domain of $f(x-2)$ is $[-1+2, 2+2]$ or $[1,4]$, and the range is the same: $[0,3]$.

67. Since $-f(x)$ is $f(x)$ reflected across the x-axis, the domain of $-f(x)$ is the same: $[-1,2]$, and the range is $[-3,0]$. .

69. Since $f(2x)$ is $f(x)$ shrunk horizontally by a factor of $\dfrac{1}{2}$, the domain of $f(2x)$ is $\left[\dfrac{1}{2}(-1), \dfrac{1}{2}(2)\right]$ or $\left[-\dfrac{1}{2}, 1\right]$, and the range is the same: $[0,3]$.

71. Since $3f\left(\dfrac{1}{4}x\right)$ is $f(x)$ stretched horizontally by a factor of 4, the domain of $3f\left(\dfrac{1}{4}x\right)$ is $[4(-1), 4(2)]$ or $[-4,8]$, and stretched vertically by a factor of 3, the range is $[3(0), 3(3)]$ or $[0,9]$.

73. Since $f(-x)$ is $f(x)$ reflected across the y-axis, the domain of $f(-x)$ is $[-(-1), -(2)] = [1,-2]$ or $[-2,1]$; and the range is the same: $[0,3]$.

75. Since $f(-3x)$ is $f(x)$ reflected across the y-axis and shrunk horizontally by a factor of $\frac{1}{3}$, the domain of $f(-3x)$ is $\left[-\frac{1}{3}(-1), -\frac{1}{3}(2)\right] = \left[\frac{1}{3}, -\frac{2}{3}\right]$ or $\left[-\frac{2}{3}, \frac{1}{3}\right]$, and the range is the same: $[0,3]$.

77. Since $y = \sqrt{x}$ has an endpoint of (0, 0), and the graph of $y = 10\sqrt{x-20} + 5$ is the graph of $y = \sqrt{x}$ shifted 20 units right, stretched vertically by a factor of 10, and shifted 5 units upward, the endpoint of $y = 10\sqrt{x-20} + 5$ is $(0+20, 10(0)+5)$ or $(20,5)$. Therefore, the domain is $[20, \infty)$, and the range is $[5, \infty)$.

79. Since $y = \sqrt{x}$ has an endpoint of (0, 0), and the graph of $y = -.5\sqrt{x+10} + 5$ is the graph of $y = \sqrt{x}$ shifted 10 units left, reflected across the x-axis, shrunk vertically by a factor of .5, and shifted 5 units upward, the endpoint of $y = -.5\sqrt{x+10} + 5$ is $(0-10, -.5(0)+5)$ or $(-10, 5)$. Therefore, the domain is $[-10, \infty)$, and the range, because of the reflection across the x-axis, is $(-\infty, 5]$.

81. The graph of $y = -f(x)$ is $y = f(x)$ reflected across the x-axis; therefore, $y = -f(x)$ is decreasing for the interval (a,b).

83. The graph of $y = -f(-x)$ is $y = f(x)$ reflected across both the x-axis and y-axis; therefore, $y = -f(-x)$ is increasing for the interval $(-b, -a)$

85. (a) the function is increasing for the interval: $(-1, 2)$.

    (b) the function is decreasing for the interval: $(-\infty, -1)$.

    (c) the function is constant for the interval: $(2, \infty)$.

87. (a) the function is increasing for the interval: $(1, \infty)$.

    (b) the function is decreasing for the interval: $(-2, 1)$.

    (c) the function is constant for the interval: $(-\infty, -2)$.

89. From the graph, the point on y_2 is approximately $(8, 10)$.

91. Use two points on the graph to find the slope. Two points are $(-2, -1)$ and $(-1, 1)$; therefore, the slope is $m = \frac{1-(-1)}{-1-(-2)} = \frac{2}{1} \Rightarrow m = 2$. The stretch factor is 2 and the graph has been shifted 2 units to the left and 1 unit down; therefore, the equation is $y = 2|x+2| - 1$.

93. Use two points on the graph to find the slope. Two points are $(0, 2)$ and $(1, -1)$; therefore, the slope is $m = \frac{-1-2}{1-0} = \frac{-3}{1} \Rightarrow m = -3$. The stretch factor is 3, the graph has been reflected across the x-axis, and shifted 2 units upward; therefore, the equation is $y = -3|x| + 2$.

95. Use two points on the graph to find the slope. Two points are (0,-4) and (3,0); therefore, the slope is $m = \dfrac{-4-0}{0-3} = \dfrac{4}{3} \Rightarrow m = \dfrac{4}{3}$. The stretch factor is $\dfrac{4}{3}$ and the graph has been shifted 4 units down.; therefore, the equation is $y = \dfrac{4}{3}|x| - 4$.

97. Since $y = f(x)$ is symmetric with respect to the y-axis, for every (x, y) on the graph, $(-x, y)$ is also on the graph. Reflection across the y-axis reflect onto itself and will not change the graph. It will be the same.

Reviewing Basic Concepts (Sections 2.1—2.3)

1. (a) The function $f(x) = |x|$ shifted up one unit yields the function $f(x) = |x| + 1$. Therefore, this function has a domain of $(-\infty, \infty)$ and a range of of $[1, \infty)$. The function is increasing from $(0, \infty)$ and decreasing from $(-\infty, 0)$.

    (b) The function $f(x) = x^2$ shifted to the right 2 units yields the function $f(x) = (x-2)^2$. Therefore, this function has a domain of $(-\infty, \infty)$ and a range of of $[0, \infty)$. The function is increasing from $(2, \infty)$ and decreasing from $(-\infty, 2)$.

    (c) The function $f(x) = \sqrt{x}$ reflected over the x-axis yields the function $f(x) = -\sqrt{x}$. Therefore, this function has a domain of $[0, \infty)$ and a range of of $(-\infty, 0]$. The function is never increasing and decreasing from $(0, \infty)$.

2. (a) If $y = f(x)$ is symmetric with respect to the origin, then another function value is $f(-3) = -6$.

    (b) If $y = f(x)$ is symmetric with respect to the y-axis, then another function value is $f(-3) = 6$.

    (c) If $f(-x) = -f(x)$, $y = f(x)$ is symmetric with respect to both the x-axis and y-axis, then another function value is $f(-3) = -6$.

    (d) If $y = f(-x)$, $y = f(x)$ is symmetric with respect to the y-axis, then another function value is $f(-3) = 6$.

3. (a) The equation $y = (x-7)^2$ is $y = x^2$ shifted 7 units to the right: B.

    (b) The equation $y = x^2 - 7$ is $y = x^2$ shifted 7 units downward: D.

    (c) The equation $y = 7x^2$ is $y = x^2$ stretches vertically by a factor of 7: E.

    (d) The equation $y = (x+7)^2$ is $y = x^2$ shifted 7 units to the left: A.

    (e) The equation $y = \left(\dfrac{1}{3}x\right)^2$ is $y = x^2$ stretches horizontally by a factor of 3: C.

4. (a) The equation $y = x^2 + 2$ is $y = x^2$ shifted 2 units upward: B.

    (b) The equation $y = x^2 - 2$ is $y = x^2$ shifted 2 units downward: A.

    (c) The equation $y = (x+2)^2$ is $y = x^2$ shifted 2 units to the left: G.

    (d) The equation $y = (x-2)^2$ is $y = x^2$ shifted 2 units to the right: C.

56 Chapter 2: Analysis of Graphs of Functions

(e) The equation $y = 2x^2$ is $y = x^2$ stretched vertically by a factor of 2: F.

(f) The equation $y = -x^2$ is $y = x^2$ reflected across the x-axis D.

(g) The equation $y = (x-2)^2 + 1$ is $y = x^2$ shifted 2 units to the right and 1 unit upward: H.

(h) The equation $y = (x+2)^2 + 1$ is $y = x^2$ shifted 2 units to the left and 1 unit upward: E.

5. (a) The equation $y = |x| + 4$ is $y = |x|$ shifted 4 units upward. See Figure 5a.

(b) The equation $y = |x+4|$ is $y = |x|$ shifted 4 units to the left. See Figure 5b.

(c) The equation $y = |x-4|$ is $y = |x|$ shifted 4 units to the right. See Figure 5c.

(d) The equation $y = |x+2| - 4$ is $y = |x|$ shifted 2 units to the left and 4 units down. See Figure 5d.

(e) The equation $y = -|x-2| + 4$ is $y = |x|$ reflected across the x-axis, shifted 2 units to the right, and 4 units upward. See Figure 5e.

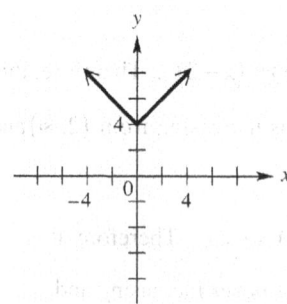

Figure 5a

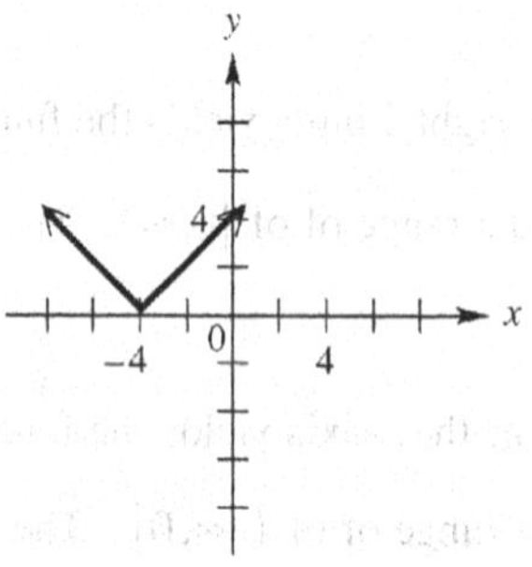

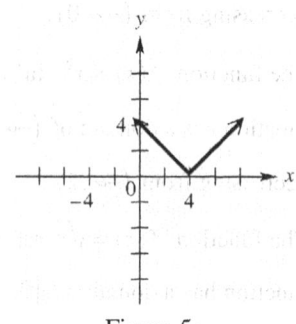

Figure 5b

Figure 5c

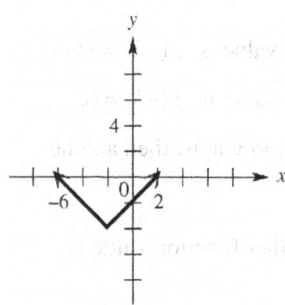

Figure 5d

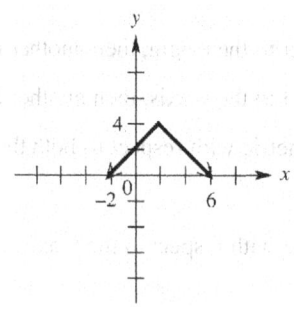

Figure 5e

6. (a) The graph is the function $f(x) = |x|$ reflected across the x-axis, shifted 1 unit left and 3 units upward. Therefore, the equation is $y = -|x+1| + 3$.

(b) The graph is the function $g(x) = \sqrt{x}$ reflected across the x-axis, shifted 4 units left and 2 units upward. Therefore, the equation is $y = -\sqrt{x+4} + 2$.

(c) The graph is the function $g(x) = \sqrt{x}$ stretches vertically by a factor of 2, shifted 4 units left and 4 units downward. Therefore, the equation is $y = 2\sqrt{x+4} - 4$.

(d) The graph is the function $f(x) = |x|$ shrunk vertically by a factor of $\frac{1}{2}$, shifted 2 units right and 1 unit downward. Therefore, the equation is $y = \frac{1}{2}|x-2| - 1$.

7. (a) The graph of $g(x)$ is the graph $f(x)$ shifted 2 units upward. Therefore, $c = 2$.

   (b) The graph of $g(x)$ is the graph $f(x)$ shifted 4 units to the left. Therefore, $c = 4$.

8. The graph of $y = F(x+h)$ is a horizontal translation of the graph of $y = F(x)$. The graph of $y = F(x) + h$ is not the same as the graph of $y = F(x+h)$, because the graph of $y = F(x) + h$ is a vertical translation of the graph of $y = F(x)$.

9. (a) If f is even, then $f(x) = f(-x)$. See Figure 9a.

   (b) If f is odd, then $f(-x) = -f(-x)$. See Figure 9b.

x	$f(x)$
-3	4
-2	-6
-1	5
1	5
2	-6
3	4

Figure 9a

x	$f(x)$
-3	4
-2	-6
-1	5
1	-5
2	6
3	-4

Figure 9b

10. (a) $R(x) = 5(7) + 2 = 37$, In 2011, Google's ad revenues were $37 billion.

    (b) Using the point (2004, 2) and the slope of 5 with the point slope formula we will have
    $y - 2 = 5(x - 2004) \Rightarrow y = 5(x - 2004) + 2$.

    (c) $y = 5(2011 - 2004) + 2 = 5(7) + 2 = 37$, In 2011, Google's ad revenues were $37 billion.

    (d) $27 = 5(x - 2004) + 2 \Rightarrow 25 = 5(x - 2004) \Rightarrow 5 = x - 2004 \Rightarrow x = 2009$

2.4: Absolute Value Functions

1. We reflect the graph of $y = f(x)$ across the x-axis for all points for which $y < 0$. Where $y \geq 0$, the graph remains unchanged. See Figure 1.

3. We reflect the graph of $y = f(x)$ across the x-axis for all points for which $y < 0$. Where $y \geq 0$, the graph remains unchanged. See Figure 3.

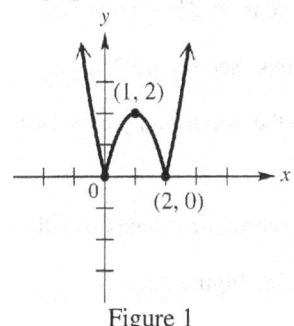

Figure 1

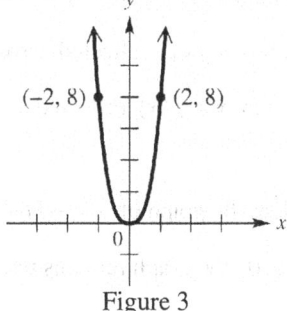

Figure 3

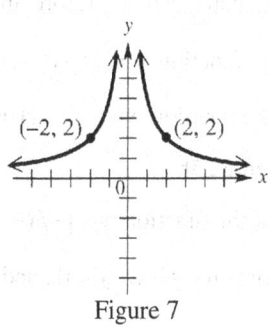

Figure 7

5. Since for all y, $y \geq 0$, the graph remains unchanged. That is, $y = |f(x)|$ has the same graph as $y = f(x)$.

7. We reflect the graph of $y = f(x)$ across the x-axis for all points for which $y < 0$. Where $y \geq 0$, the graph remains unchanged. See Figure 7.

9. We reflect the graph of $y = f(x)$ across the x-axis for all points for which $y < 0$. Where $y \geq 0$, the graph remains unchanged. See Figure 9.

58   Chapter 2: Analysis of Graphs of Functions

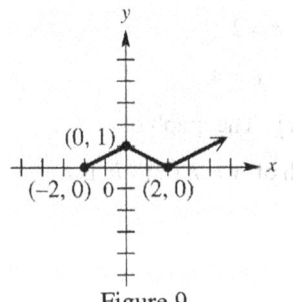

Figure 9

11. If $f(a) = -5$, then $|f(a)| = |-5| = 5$.

13. If $f(x) = -x^2$, then $y = |f(x)| \Rightarrow y = |-x^2| \Rightarrow y = x^2$. Therefore, the range of $y = |f(x)|$ is $[0, \infty)$.

15. If the range of $y = f(x)$ is $(-\infty, -2]$, the range of $y = |f(x)|$ is $[2, \infty)$ since all negative values of y are reflected across the x-axis.

17. From the graph of $y = (x+1)^2 - 2$ the domain of $f(x)$ is $(-\infty, \infty)$, and the range is $[-2, \infty)$.

    From the graph of $y = |(x+1)^2 - 2|$ the domain of $|f(x)|$ is $(-\infty, \infty)$, and the range is $[0, \infty)$.

19. From the graph of $y = -1 - (x-2)^2$ the domain of $f(x)$ is $(-\infty, \infty)$, and the range is $(-\infty, -1]$. From the graph of $y = |-1 - (x-2)^2|$ the domain of $|f(x)|$ is $(-\infty, \infty)$, and the range is $[1, \infty)$.

21. From the graph, the domain of $f(x)$ is $[-2, 3]$, and the range is $[-2, 3]$. For the function $y = |f(x)|$, we reflect the graph of $y = f(x)$ across the x-axis for all points for which $y < 0$, and, where $y \geq 0$, the graph remains unchanged. Therefore, the domain of $y = |f(x)|$ is $[-2, 3]$, and the range is $[0, 3]$.

23. From the graph, the domain of $f(x)$ is $[-2, 3]$, and the range is $[-3, 1]$. For the function $y = |f(x)|$, we reflect the graph of $y = f(x)$ across the x-axis for all points for which $y < 0$, and, where $y \geq 0$, the graph remains unchanged. Therefore, the domain of $y = |f(x)|$ is $[-2, 3]$, and the range is $[0, 3]$.

25. (a) The function $y = f(-x)$ is the function $y = f(x)$ reflected across the y-axis. See Figure 25a.

    (b) The function $y = -f(-x)$ is the function $y = f(x)$ reflected across both the x-axis and y-axis. See Figure 25b.

    (c) For the function $y = |-f(-x)|$ we reflect the graph of $y = -f(-x)$ (ex. b) across the x-axis for all points for which $y < 0$, and where $y \geq 0$, the graph remains unchanged. See Figure 25c.

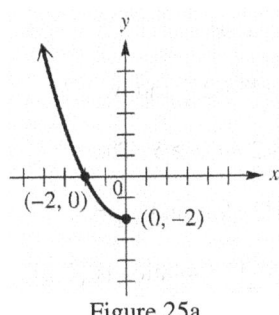

Figure 25a

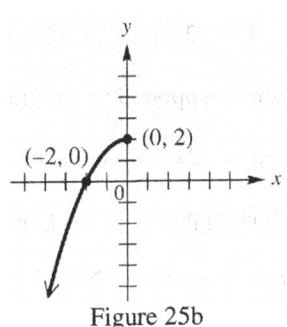

Figure 25b

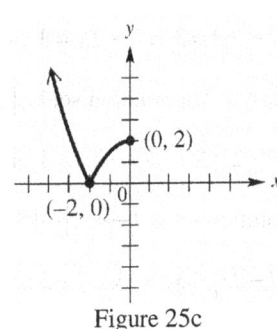

Figure 25c

27. The graph of $y = |f(x)|$ can not be below the x-axis; therefore, Figure A shows the graph of $y = f(x)$, while Figure B shows the graph of $y = |f(x)|$.

29. (a) From the graph, $y_1 = y_2$ at the coordinates $(-1, 5)$ and $(6, 5)$; therefore, the solution set is $\{-1, 6\}$.

    (b) From the graph, $y_1 < y_2$ for the interval $(-1, 6)$.

    (c) From the graph, $y_1 > y_2$ for the intervals $(-\infty, -1) \cup (6, \infty)$.

31. (a) From the graph, $y_1 = y_2$ at the coordinate $(4, 1)$; therefore, the solution set is $\{4\}$.

    (b) From the graph, $y_1 < y_2$ never occurs; therefore, the solution set is $\varnothing$.

    (c) From the graph, $y_1 > y_2$ for all values for x except 4; therefore, the solution set is the intervals $(-\infty, 4) \cup (4, \infty)$.

33. The V-shaped graph is that of $f(x) = |.5x + 6|$, since this is typical of the graphs of absolute value functions of the form $f(x) = |ax + b|$

34. The straight line graph is that of $g(x) = 3x - 14$ which is a linear function.

35. The graphs intersect at $(8, 10)$, so the solution set is $\{8\}$.

36. From the graph, $f(x) > g(x)$ for the interval $(-\infty, 8)$.

37. From the graph, $f(x) < g(x)$ for the interval $(8, \infty)$.

38. If $|.5x + 6| - (3x - 14) = 0$ then $|.5x + 6| = 3x - 14$. Therefore, the solution is the intersection of the graphs, or $\{8\}$.

39. (a) $|x + 4| = 9 \Rightarrow x + 4 = 9$ or $x + 4 = -9 \Rightarrow x = 5$ or $x = -13$. The solution set is $\{-13, 5\}$, which is supported by the graphs of $y_1 = |x + 4|$ and $y_2 = 9$.

    (b) $|x + 4| > 9 \Rightarrow x + 4 > 9$ or $x + 4 < -9 \Rightarrow x > 5$ or $x < -13$. The solution is $(-\infty, -13) \cup (5, \infty)$, which is supported by the graphs of $y_1 = |x + 4|$ and $y_2 = 9$.

    (c) $|x + 4| < 9 \Rightarrow -9 < x + 4 < 9 \Rightarrow -13 < x < 5$. The solution is $(-13, 5)$, which is supported by the graphs of $|x + 4|$ and $y_2 = 9$.

41. (a) $|7-2x|=3 \Rightarrow 7-2x=3$ or $7-2x=-3 \Rightarrow -2x=-4$ or $-2x=-10 \Rightarrow x=2$ or $x=5$. The solution set is $\{2,5\}$, which is supported by the graphs of $y_1=|7-2x|$ and $y_2=3$.

(b) $|7-2x|\geq 3 \Rightarrow 7-2x\geq 3$ or $7-2x\leq -3 \Rightarrow -2x\geq -4$ or $-2x\leq -10 \Rightarrow x\leq 2$ or $x\geq 5$. The solution set is $(-\infty,2]\cup[5,\infty)$, which is supported by the graphs of $y_1=|7-2x|$ and $y_2=3$.

(c) $|7-2x|\leq 3 \Rightarrow -3\leq 7-2x\leq 3 \Rightarrow -10\leq -2x\leq -4 \Rightarrow 5\geq x\geq 2$ or $2\leq x\leq 5$. The solution is $[2,5]$, which is supported by the graphs of $y_1=|7-2x|$ and $y_2=3$.

43. (a) $|2x+1|+3=5 \Rightarrow 2x+1=2$ or $2x+1=-2 \Rightarrow 2x=1$ or $2x=-3 \Rightarrow x=\dfrac{1}{2}$ or $x=-\dfrac{3}{2}$. The solution set is $\left\{-\dfrac{3}{2},\dfrac{1}{2}\right\}$, which is supported by the graphs of $y_1=|2x+1|+3$ and $y_2=5$.

(b) $|2x+1|+3\leq 5 \Rightarrow -2\leq 2x+1\leq 2 \Rightarrow -3\leq 2x\leq 1 \Rightarrow -\dfrac{3}{2}\leq x\leq \dfrac{1}{2}$. The solution is $\left[-\dfrac{3}{2},\dfrac{1}{2}\right]$, which is supported by the graphs of $y_1=|2x+1|+3$ and $y_2=5$.

(c) $|2x+1|+3\geq 5 \Rightarrow 2x+1\geq 2$ or $2x+1\leq -2 \Rightarrow 2x\geq 1$ or $2x\leq -3 \Rightarrow x\geq \dfrac{1}{2}$ or $x\leq -\dfrac{3}{2}$. The solution is $\left(-\infty,-\dfrac{3}{2}\right]\cup\left[\dfrac{1}{2},\infty\right)$, which is supported by the graphs of $y_1=|2x+1|+3$ and $y_2=5$.

45. (a) $|5-7x|=0 \Rightarrow 5-7x=0 \Rightarrow 7x=5 \Rightarrow x=\dfrac{5}{7}$. The solution set is $\left\{\dfrac{5}{7}\right\}$, which is supported by the graphs of $y_1=|5-7x|$ and $y_2=0$.

(b) $|5-7x|\geq 0 \Rightarrow 5-7x\geq 0$ or $5-7x\leq 0 \Rightarrow 7x\geq 5$ or $7x\leq 5 \Rightarrow x\geq \dfrac{5}{7}$ or $x\leq \dfrac{5}{7}$. The solution is $(-\infty,\infty)$, which is supported by the graphs of $y_1=|5-7x|$ and $y_2=0$.

(c) $|5-7x|\leq 0 \Rightarrow 0\leq 5-7x\leq 0 \Rightarrow 5\geq 7x\geq 5 \Rightarrow \dfrac{5}{7}\geq x\geq \dfrac{5}{7}$. The solution set is $\left\{\dfrac{5}{7}\right\}$, which is supported by the graphs of $y_1=|5-7x|$ and $y_2=0$.

47. (a) Absolute value is always positive; therefore, the solution set is $\emptyset$, which is supported by the graphs of $y_1=\left|\sqrt{2x}-3.6\right|$ and $y_2=-1$.

(b) Absolute value is always positive, and so cannot be less than or equal to -1; therefore, the solution set is $\emptyset$, which is supported by the graphs of $y_1=\left|\sqrt{2x}-3.6\right|$ and $y_2=-1$.

(c) Absolute value is always positive, and so is always greater than -1; therefore, the solution is $(-\infty,\infty)$, which is supported by the graphs of $y_1=\left|\sqrt{2x}-3.6\right|$ and $y_2=-1$.

49. $3|4-3x|-4=8 \Rightarrow 3|4-3x|=12 \Rightarrow |4-3x|=4 \Rightarrow 4-3x=4$ or $4-3x=-4 \Rightarrow -3x=0$ or

$-3x=-8 \Rightarrow x=0$ or $x=\frac{8}{3}$. Therefore, the solution set is $\left\{0,\frac{8}{3}\right\}$.

51. $\frac{1}{2}\left|-2x+\frac{1}{2}\right|=\frac{3}{4} \Rightarrow \left|-2x+\frac{1}{2}\right|=\frac{3}{2} \Rightarrow -2x+\frac{1}{2}=\frac{3}{2}$ or $-2x+\frac{1}{2}=-\frac{3}{2} \Rightarrow -2x=1$ or

$-2x=-2 \Rightarrow x=-\frac{1}{2}$ or $x=1$. Therefore, the solution set is $\left\{-\frac{1}{2},1\right\}$.

53. $4.2|.5-x|+1=3.1 \Rightarrow 4.2|.5-x|=2.1 \Rightarrow |.5-x|=.5 \Rightarrow .5-x=.5$ or $.5-x=-.5 \Rightarrow -x=0$ or

$-x=-1 \Rightarrow x=0$ or $x=1$. Therefore, the solution set is $\{0,1\}$.

55. $|15-x|<7 \Rightarrow -7<15-x<7 \Rightarrow 22>x>8$ or $8<x<22$. Therefore, the solution is $(8,22)$.

57. $|2x-3|>1 \Rightarrow 2x-3>1$ or $2x-3<-1 \Rightarrow 2x>4$ or $\left(\frac{f}{g}\right)(-3) = \frac{-3(-3)-4}{(-3)^2} = \frac{5}{9}$. or $x<1$. Therefore,

the solution is $(-\infty,1) \cup (2,\infty)$.

59. $|-3x+8| \geq 3 \Rightarrow -3x+8 \geq 3$ or $-3x+8 \leq -3 \Rightarrow -3x \geq -5$ or $-3x \leq -11 \Rightarrow x \leq \frac{5}{3}$ or $x \geq \frac{11}{3}$.

Therefore, the solution is $\left(-\infty,\frac{5}{3}\right] \cup \left[\frac{11}{3},\infty\right)$.

61. $\left|6-\frac{1}{3}x\right|>0 \Rightarrow 6-\frac{1}{3}x>0$ or $6-\frac{1}{3}x<0 \Rightarrow -\frac{1}{3}x>-6$ or $-\frac{1}{3}x<-6 \Rightarrow x<18$ or $x>18$. Therefore,

the solution is every real number except 18: $(-\infty,18) \cup (18,\infty)$.

63. Absolute value is always positive, and so cannot be less than or equal to -6; therefore, the solution set is $\emptyset$.

65. Absolute value is always positive, and so is always greater than -5; therefore, the solution is $(-\infty,\infty)$.

67. (a) $3x+1=2x-7 \Rightarrow x+1=-7 \Rightarrow x=-8$ $3x+1=-(2x-7) \Rightarrow 3x+1=-2x+7 \Rightarrow 5x=6 \Rightarrow x=\frac{6}{5}$.

Therefore, the solution set is $\left\{-8,\frac{6}{5}\right\}$.

(b) Graph $y_1 = |3x+1|$ and $y_2 = |2x-7|$. See Figure 67. From the graph, $|f(x)|>|g(x)|$ when $y_1 > y_2$

which is for the interval $(-\infty,-8) \cup \left(\frac{6}{5},\infty\right)$.

(c) Graph $y_1 = |3x+1|$ and $y_2 = |2x-7|$ See Figure 67. From the graph, $|f(x)|<|g(x)|$ when $y_1 < y_2$

which is for the interval $\left(-8,\frac{6}{5}\right)$.

[-20,20] by [-10,50]
Xscl = 2   Yscl = 5

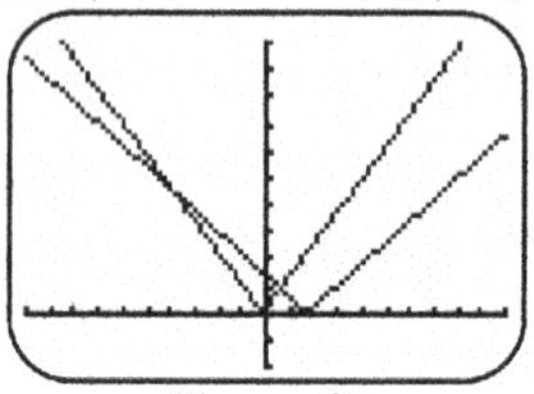

[-10,10] by [-4,16]
Xscl = 1   Yscl = 1

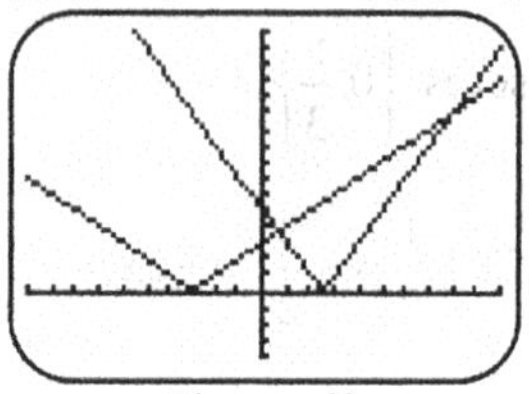

Figure 67   Figure 69

69. (a) $-2x+5 = x+3 \Rightarrow -3x = -2 \Rightarrow x = \dfrac{2}{3}$ or $-2x+5 = -(x+3) \Rightarrow -2x+5 = -x-3 \Rightarrow$

$-x = -8 \Rightarrow x = 8$. Therefore, the solution set is $\left\{\dfrac{2}{3}, 8\right\}$.

(b) Graph $y_1 = |-2x+5|$ and $y_2 = |x+3|$. See Figure 69. From the graph, $|f(x)| > |g(x)|$ when $y_1 > y_2$, which it is for the interval $\left(-\infty, \dfrac{2}{3}\right) \cup (8, \infty)$.

(c) Graph $y_1 = |-2x+5|$ and $y_2 = |x+3|$. See Figure 69. From the graph, $|f(x)| < |g(x)|$ when $y_1 < y_2$, which it is for the interval $\left(\dfrac{2}{3}, 8\right)$.

[-6,6] by [-2,10]
Xscl = 1   Yscl = 1

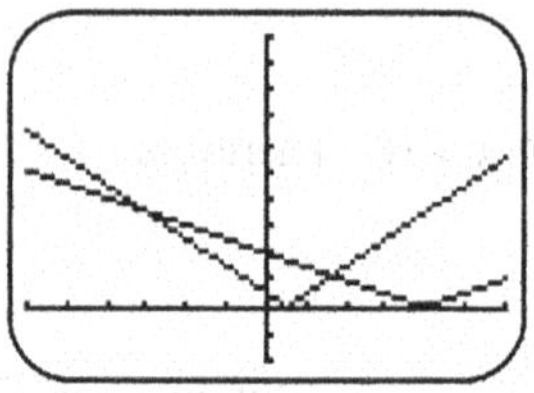

[-10,10] by [-4,16]
Xscl = 1   Yscl = 2

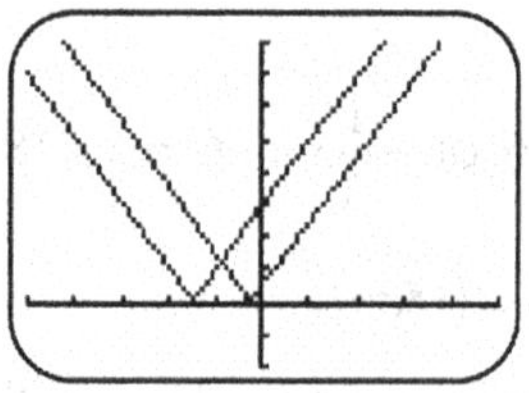

Figure 71   Figure 73

71. (a) $x - \dfrac{1}{2} = \dfrac{1}{2}x - 2 \Rightarrow \dfrac{1}{2}x = -\dfrac{3}{2} \Rightarrow x = -3$ or $x - \dfrac{1}{2} = -\left(\dfrac{1}{2}x - 2\right) \Rightarrow x - \dfrac{1}{2} = -\dfrac{1}{2}x + 2 \Rightarrow$

$\dfrac{3}{2}x = \dfrac{5}{2} \Rightarrow x = \dfrac{5}{3}$. Therefore, the solution set is $\left\{-3, \dfrac{5}{3}\right\}$.

(b) Graph $y_1 = \left|x - \dfrac{1}{2}\right|$ and $y_2 = \left|\dfrac{1}{2}x - 2\right|$. From the graph, $|f(x)| > |g(x)|$ when $y_1 > y_2$, which it is for the interval $(-\infty, -3) \cup \left(\dfrac{5}{3}, \infty\right)$.

(c) Graph $y_1 = \left|x - \dfrac{1}{2}\right|$ and $y_2 = \left|\dfrac{1}{2}x - 2\right|$. See Figure 71. From the graph $|f(x)| < |g(x)|$ when $y_1 < y_2$, which it is for the interval $\left(-3, \dfrac{5}{3}\right)$.

Section 2.4   63

73. (a) $4x+1=4x+6 \Rightarrow 1=6 \Rightarrow \emptyset$ or $4x+1=-(4x+6) \Rightarrow 4x=1=-4x-6 \Rightarrow 8x=-7 \Rightarrow -\frac{7}{8}$.

Therefore, the solution set is $\left\{-\frac{7}{8}\right\}$.

(b). Graph $y_1=|4x+1|$ or $y_2=|4x+6|$. See Figure 73. From the graph $|f(x)|>|g(x)|$ when $y_1>y_2$, which it is for the interval $\left(-\infty, \frac{7}{8}\right)$.

(c) Graph $y_1=|4x+1|$ or $y_2=|4x+6|$. See Figure 73. From the graph, $|f(x)|<|g(x)|$ when $y_1>y_2$, which is for the interval $\left(-\frac{7}{8}, \infty\right)$.

75. (a) $0.25x+1=0.75x-3 \Rightarrow -0.50x=-4 \Rightarrow x=8$ or $0.25x+1=-(0.75x-3) \Rightarrow 0.25x+1=-0.75x+3 \Rightarrow$
$x=2$. Therefore, the solution set is $\{2,8\}$.

(b) Graph $y_1=|.25x+1|$ and $y_2=|.75x-3|$. See Figure 75. From the graph, $|f(x)|>|g(x)|$ when $y_1<y_2$, which it is for the interval $(2,8)$.

(c) Graph $y_1=|.25x+1|$ and $y_2=|.75x-3|$. See Figure 75. From the graph, $|f(x)|<|g(x)|$
when $y_1<y_2$, which it is for the interval $(-\infty, 2) \cup (8, \infty)$.

[-20,20] by [-4,16]
Xscl = 2   Yscl = 1

[-10,10] by [-10,10]
Xscl= 1   Yscl = 1

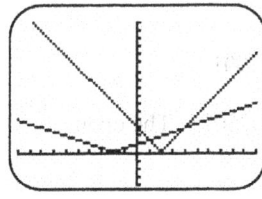

Figure 75   Figure 77

77. (a) $3x+10=-(-3x-10) \Rightarrow 3x+10=3x+10 \Rightarrow$ there are an infinite number of solutions.

Therefore, the solution set is $(-\infty, \infty)$.

(b) Graph $y_1=|3x+10|$ and $y_2=|-3x-10|$. See Figure 77. From the graph, $|f(x)|>|g(x)|$
when $y_1>y_2$, for which there is no solution.

(c) Graph $y_1=|3x+10|$ and $y_2=|-3x-10|$. See Figure 77. From the graph, $|f(x)|<|g(x)|$
when $y_1<y_2$, for which there is no solution.

79. Graph $y_1=|x+1|+|x-6|$ and $y_2=11$. See Figure 79. From the graph, the lines intersect at $(-3,11)$
and $(2,9)$. Therefore, the solution set is $\{-3,8\}$.

81. Graph $y_1=|x|+|x-4|$ and $y_2=8$. See Figure 81. From the graph, the lines intersect at $(-2,8)$ and $(6,8)$.
Therefore, the solution set is $\{-2,6\}$.

Copyright © 2015 Pearson Education, Inc

64   Chapter 2: Analysis of Graphs of Functions

[-10,10] by [-4,16]
Xscl = 1   Yscl = 1

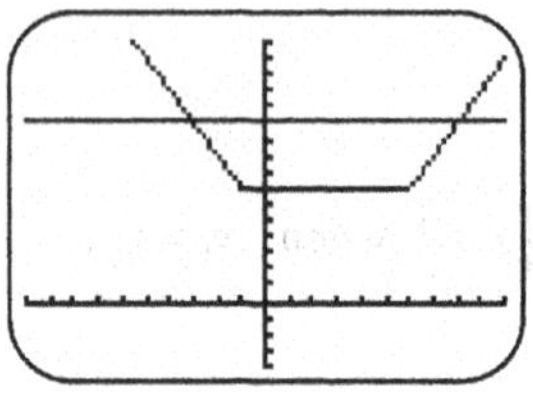

Figure 79

[-10,10] by [-4,16]
Xscl= 1   Yscl = 1

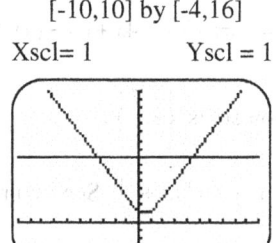

Figure 81

83. (a) $|T-50| \le 22 \Rightarrow -22 \le T-50 \le 22 \Rightarrow 28 \le T \le 72$.

   (b) The average monthly temperatures in Boston vary between a low of $28°$ F and a high of $72°$ F. The monthly averages are always within $22°$ of $50°$ F.

85. (a) $|T-61.5| \le 12.5 \Rightarrow -12.5 \le T-61.5 \le 12.5 \Rightarrow 49 \le T \le 74$..

   (b) The average monthly temperatures in Buenos Aires vary between a low of $49°$ F (possibly in July) and a high of $74°$ F (possibly in January). The monthly averages are always within $12.5°$ of $61.5°$ F.

87. $|x-8.0| \le 1.5 \Rightarrow -1.5 \le x-8.0 \le 1.5 \Rightarrow 6.5 \le x \le 9.5$; therefore, the range is the interval $[6.5, 9.5]$.

89. (a) $P_d = |116-125| \Rightarrow P_d = |-9| = 9$.

   (b) $17 = |P-130| \Rightarrow P-130 = 17 \text{ or } P-130 = -17 \Rightarrow P = 147 \text{ or } P = 113$.

91. If the difference between y and 1 is less than .1, then $|y-1| < .1 \Rightarrow |2x+1-1| < .1 \Rightarrow$ $|2x| < .1 \Rightarrow -.1 < 2x < .1 \Rightarrow -.05 < x < .05$. The open interval of x is $(-.05, .05)$.

93. If the difference between y and 3 is less than .001, then $|y-3| < .001 \Rightarrow |4x-8-3| < .001 \Rightarrow$ $|4x-11| < .001 \Rightarrow -.001 < 4x-11 < .001 \Rightarrow 10.999 < 4x < 11.001 \Rightarrow 2.74975 < x < 2.75025$. The open interval of x is $(2.74975, 2.75025)$.

95. If $|2x+7| = 6x-1$ then $|2x+7|-(6x-1) = 0$. Graph $y_1 = |2x+7|-(6x-1)$, See Figure 95. The x-intercept is 2; therefore, the solution set is $\{2\}$.

97. If $|x-4| > .5x-6$ then $|x-4|-(.5x-6) > 0$. Graph $y_1 = |x-4|-(.5x-6)$, See Figure 97. The equation is > 0, or the graph is above the x-axis, for the interval: $(-\infty, \infty)$.

[-10,10] by [-10,10]
Xscl = 1   Yscl = 1

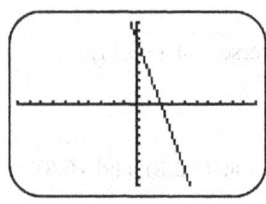

Figure 95

[-10,10] by [-10,10]
Xscl = 1   Yscl = 1

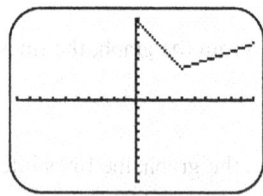

Figure 97

[-10,10] by [-1,6]
Xscl= 1   Yscl = 1

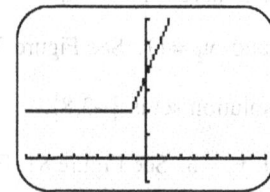

Figure 99

99. If $|3x+4| < -3x-14$ then $|3x+4| - (-3x-14) < 0$. Graph $y_1 = |3x+4| - (-3x-14)$, See Figure 99. The equation is < 0, or the graph is below the x-axis, never or for the solution set: $\varnothing$.

2.5: Piecewise-Defined Functions

1. (a) From the graph, the speed limit is 40 mph.
   (b) From the graph, the speed limit is 30 mph for 6 miles.
   (c) From the graph, $f(5) = 40$ mph; $f(13) = 30$ mph; and $f(19) = 55$ mph.
   (d) From the graph, the graph is discontinuous at $x = 4, 6, 8, 12,$ and 16. The speed limit changes at each discontinuity.

3. (a) From the graph, the Initial amount was: 50,000 gal.; and the final amount was: 30,000 gal.
   (b) From the graph, during the first and fourth days.
   (c) From the graph, $f(2) = 45,000$ gal; $f(4) = 40,000$ gal.
   (d) From the graph, between days 1 and 3 the water dropped: $\dfrac{50,000 - 40,000}{2} = \dfrac{10,000}{2} = 5,000$ gal./day.

5. (a) $f(-5) = 2(-5) = -10$ (b) $f(-1) = 2(-1) = -2$
   (c) $f(0) = 0 - 1 = -1$ (d) $f(3) = 3 - 1 = 2$

7. (a) $f(-5) = 2 + (-5) = -3$ (b) $f(-1) = -(-1) = 1$
   (c) $f(0) = -(0) = 0$ (d) $f(3) = 3(3) = 9$

9. Yes, continuous. See Figure 9.

11. Not continuous. See Figure 11

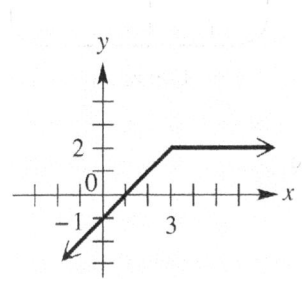
Figure 9

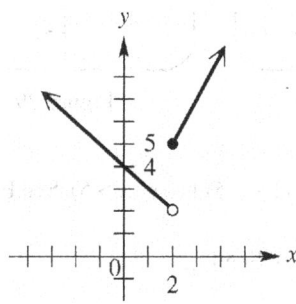
Figure 11

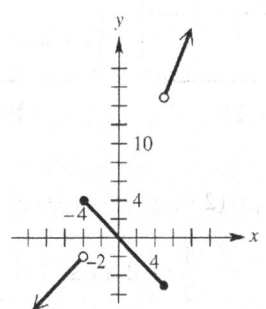
Figure 13

13. Not continuous. See Figure 13.
15. Not continuous. See Figure 15.
17. Yes, continuous. See Figure 17.

66 Chapter 2: Analysis of Graphs of Functions

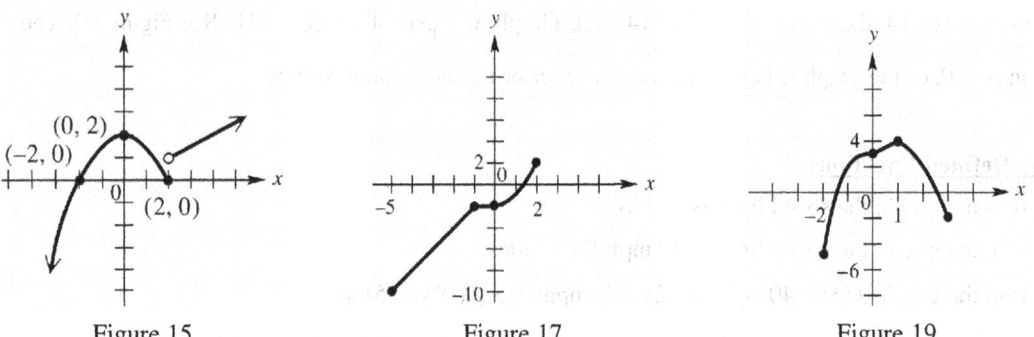

Figure 15   Figure 17   Figure 19

19. Yes, continuous. See Figure 19.

21. Look for a $y = x^2$ graph if $x \geq 0$; and a linear graph if $x < 0$. Therefore: B.

23. Look for a horizontal graph above the x-axis if $x \geq 0$; and a horizontal graph below the x-axis if $x < 0$. Therefore: D.

25. Graph $y_1 = (x-1)(x \leq 3) + (2)(x > 3)$, See Figure 25.

27. Graph $y_1 = (4-x)(x < 2) + (1+2x)(x \geq 2)$, See Figure 27.

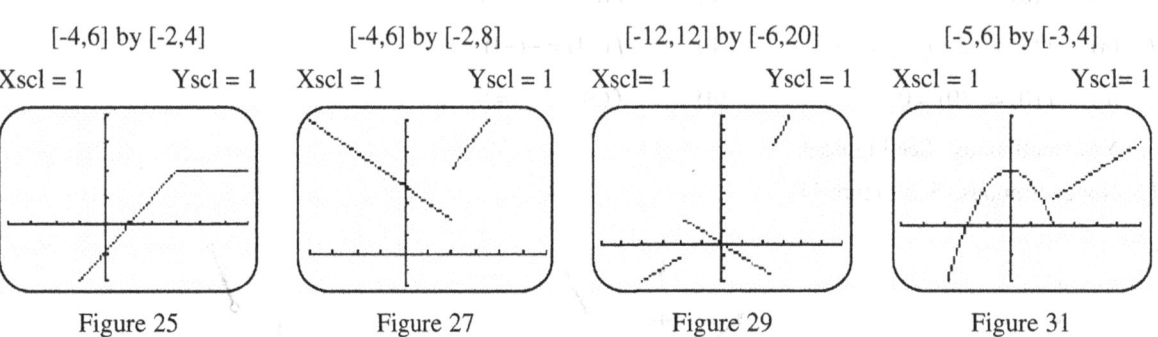

Figure 25   Figure 27   Figure 29   Figure 31

29. Graph $y_1 = (2+x)(x < -4) + (-x)(-4 \leq x \text{ and } x \leq 5) + (3x)(x > 5)$, See Figure 29.

31. Graph $y_1 = \left(-\dfrac{1}{2}x + 2\right)(x \leq 2) + \left(\dfrac{1}{2}x\right)(x > 2)$, See Figure 31.

33. From the graph, the function is $f(x) = \begin{cases} 2 & \text{if } x \leq 0 \\ -1 & \text{if } x > 1 \end{cases}$; domain: $(-\infty, 0] \cup (1, \infty)$; range: $\{-1, 2\}$.

35. From the graph, the function is $f(x) = \begin{cases} x & \text{if } x \leq 0 \\ 2 & \text{if } x > 0 \end{cases}$; domain: $(-\infty, \infty)$; range: $(-\infty, 0] \cup \{2\}$.

37. From the graph, the function is $f(x) = \begin{cases} \sqrt[3]{x} & \text{if } x < 1 \\ x+1 & \text{if } x \geq 1 \end{cases}$; domain: $(-\infty, \infty)$; range: $(-\infty, 1) \cup [2, \infty)$.

39. There is an overlap of intervals since the number 4 satisfies both conditions. To be a function, every x-value is used only once.

41. The graph of $y = [\![x]\!]$ is shifted 1.5 units downward.

43. The graph of $y = [\![x]\!]$ is reflected across the x-axis.

45. Graph $y = [\![x]\!] - 1.5$, See Figure 45.

47. Graph $y = -[\![x]\!]$, See Figure 47.

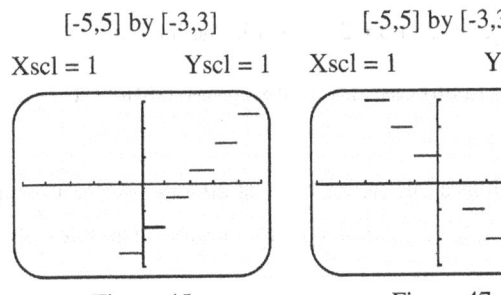

Figure 45   Figure 47

49. When $0 \le x \le 3$ the slope is 5, which means the inlet pipe is open and the outlet pipe is closed; when $3 < x \le 5$ the slope is 2, which means both pipes are open; when $5 < x \le 8$ the slope is 0, which means both pipes are closed; when $8 < x \le 10$ the slope is -3, which means the inlet pipe is closed and the outlet pipe is open.

51. (a) $f(1.5) = 1.12, f(3) = 1.32$, It costs $1.12 to mail 1.5 oz and $1.32 to mail 3 oz.

    (b) Domain: $(0, 5]$; Range: $\{0.92, 1.12, 1.32, 1.52, 1.72\}$. See figure 51.

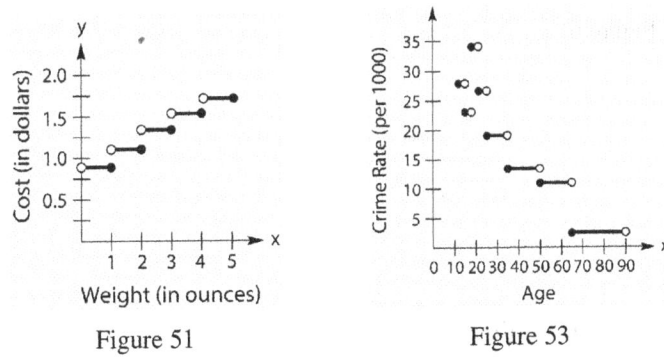

Figure 51   Figure 53

53. (a) From the table, graph the piecewise function. See Figure 53.

    (b) The likelihood of being a victim peaks from age 16 up to age 20, then decreases.

55. (a) From the graph, the highest speed is 55 mph and the lowest speed is 30 mph.

    (b) There are approximately 12 miles of highway with a speed of 55 mph.

    (c) Fromt the graph, $f(4) = 40; f(12) = 30; f(18) = 55$.

57. (a) A 3.5 minute call would round up to 4 minutes. A 4 minute call would cost: $.50 + 3(.25) = \$1.25$.

    (b) We use a piecewise defined function where the cost increases after each whole number as follows:

68   Chapter 2: Analysis of Graphs of Functions

$$f(x) = \begin{cases} .50 & \text{if } 0 < x \le 1 \\ .75 & \text{if } 1 < x \le 2 \\ 1.00 & \text{if } 2 < x \le 3 \\ 1.25 & \text{if } 3 < x \le 4 \\ 1.50 & \text{if } 4 < x \le 5 \end{cases}$$ Another possibility is $f(x) = \begin{cases} .50 & \text{if } 0 < x \le 1 \\ .50 - .25[\![1-x]\!] & \text{if } 1 < x \le 5 \end{cases}$.

59. For x in the interval $(0,2]$, $y = 25$. For x in the interval $(2,3]$, $y = 25 + 3 = 28$. For x in the interval $(3,4]$, $y = 28 + 3 = 31$ and so on. The graph is a step function. In this case, the first step has a different width. See Figure 59.

61. Sketch a piecewise function that fills a tank at a rate of 5 gallons a minute for the first 20 minutes (the time it takes to fill the 100 gallon tank) and then drains the tank at a rate of 2 gallons per minute for 50 minutes (the time it takes to drain the 100 gallon tank). See Figure 61.

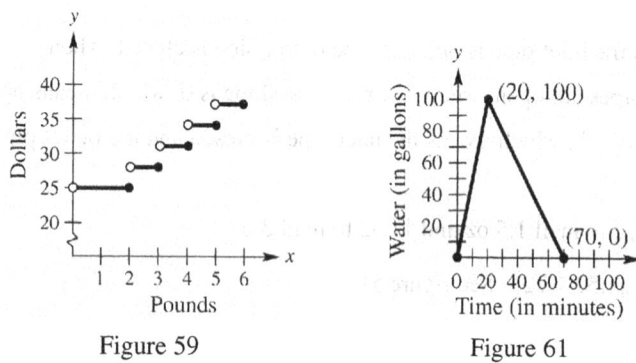

Figure 59   Figure 61

2.6: Operations and Composition

1. $x^2 + (2x - 5) = x^2 + 2x - 5 \Rightarrow E$.

3. $x^2(2x - 5) = 2x^3 - 5x^2 \Rightarrow F$.

5. $(2x - 5)^2 = 4x^2 - 20x + 25 \Rightarrow A$.

7. $(f \circ g)(3) = f(g(3)) = f(2(3) - 1) = f(5) = 5^2 + 3(5) = 40$

9. $(f \circ g)(x) = f(g(x)) = f(2x - 1) = (2x - 1)^2 + 3(2x - 1) = 4x^2 - 4x + 1 + 6x - 3 = 4x^2 + 2x - 2$

11. $(f + g)(3) = f(3) + g(3) = ((3)^2 + 3(3)) + (2(3) - 1) = 23$

13. $(f \cdot g)(4) = f(4) \cdot g(4) = ((4)^2 + 3(4)) \cdot (2(4) - 1) = 196$

15. $\left(\dfrac{f}{g}\right)(-1) = \dfrac{f(-1)}{g(-1)} = \dfrac{(-1)^2 + 3(-1)}{2(-1) - 1} = \dfrac{2}{3}$

17. $(f - g)(2) = f(2) - g(2) = ((2)^2 + 3(2)) - (2(2) - 1) = 7$

19. $(g - f)(-2) = g(-2) - f(-2) = (2(-2) - 1) - ((-2)^2 + 3(-2)) = -3$

21. $\left(\dfrac{g}{f}\right)(0) = \dfrac{g(0)}{f(0)} = \dfrac{2(0) - 1}{(0)^2 + 3(0)} = \dfrac{-1}{0} \Rightarrow$ undefined

23. (a) $(f+g)(x) = (4x-1)+(6x+3) = 10x+2$, $(f-g)(x) = (4x-1)-(6x+3) = -2x-4$

    $(fg)(x) = (4x-1)(6x+3) = 24x^2+12x-6x-3 = 24x^2+6x-3$

    (b) All values can replace x in all three equations; therefore, the domain is $(-\infty, \infty)$ in all cases.

    (c) $\left(\dfrac{f}{g}\right)(x) = \dfrac{4x-1}{6x+3}$; all values can replace x, except $-\dfrac{1}{2}$; therefore, the domain is $\left(-\infty, -\dfrac{1}{2}\right) \cup \left(-\dfrac{1}{2}, \infty\right)$.

    (d) $(f \circ g)(x) = f[g(x)] = 4(6x+3)-1 = 24x+12-1 = 24x+11$; all values can be input for x; therefore, the domain is $(-\infty, \infty)$

    (e) $(g \circ f)(x) = g[f(x)] = 6(4x-1)+3 = 24x-6+3 = 24x-3$; all values can replace x; therefore, the domain is $(-\infty, \infty)$.

25. (a) $(f+g)(x) = |x+3|+2x$, $(f-g)(x) = |x+3|-2x$, $(fg)(x) = |x+3|(2x)$

    (b) All values can replace x in all three equations; therefore, the domain is $(-\infty, \infty)$ in all cases.

    (c) $\left(\dfrac{f}{g}\right)(x) = \dfrac{|x+3|}{2x}$; all values can replace x, except 0; therefore, the domain is $(-\infty, 0) \cup (0, \infty)$

    (d) $(f \circ g)(x) = f[g(x)] = |(2x)+3| = |2x+3|$; all values can replace x; therefore, the domain is $(-\infty, \infty)$.

    (e) $(g \circ f)(x) = g[f(x)] = 2(|x+3|) = 2|x+3|$; all values can replace x; therefore, the domain is $(-\infty, \infty)$

27. (a) $(f+g)(x) = \sqrt[3]{x+4}+(x^3+5) = \sqrt[3]{x+4}+x^3+5$, $(f-g)(x) = \sqrt[3]{x+4}-(x^3+5) = \sqrt[3]{x+4}-x^3-5$

    $(fg)(x) = \left(\sqrt[3]{x+4}\right)(x^3+5)$

    (b) All values can replace x in all three equations; therefore, the domain is $(-\infty, \infty)$ in all cases.

    (c) $\left(\dfrac{f}{g}\right)(x) = \dfrac{\sqrt[3]{x+4}}{(x^3+5)}$ all values can replace x, except $\sqrt[3]{-5}$, so the domain is $(-\infty, \sqrt[3]{-5}) \cup (\sqrt[3]{-5}, \infty)$.

    (d) $(f \circ g)(x) = f[g(x)] = \sqrt[3]{(x^3+5)+4} = \sqrt[3]{x^3+9}$; all values can replace x, so the domain is $(-\infty, \infty)$.

    (e) $(g \circ f)(x) = g[f(x)] = \left(\sqrt[3]{x+4}\right)^3+5 = x+4+5 = x+9$; all values can replace x, so the domain is $(-\infty, \infty)$.

29. (a) $(f+g)(x) = \sqrt{x^2+3}+(x+1) = \sqrt{x^2+3}+x+1$, $(f-g)(x) = \sqrt{x^2+3}-(x+1) = \sqrt{x^2+3}-x-1$

    $(fg)(x) = \left(\sqrt{x^2+3}\right)(x+1)$

    (b) All values can replace x in all three equations; therefore, the domain is $(-\infty, \infty)$ in all cases.

    (c) $\left(\dfrac{f}{g}\right)(x) = \dfrac{\sqrt{x^2+3}}{(x+1)}$; all values can replace x, except -1; therefore, the domain is $(-\infty, -1) \cup (-1, \infty)$.

    (d) $(f \circ g)(x) = f[g(x)] = \sqrt{(x+1)^2+3} = \sqrt{x^2+2x+1+3} = \sqrt{x^2+2x+4}$; all values can replace x; therefore, the domain is $(-\infty, \infty)$.

70   Chapter 2: Analysis of Graphs of Functions

  (e) $(g \circ f)(x) = g[f(x)] = \left(\sqrt{x^2+3}\right) + 1 = \sqrt{x^2+3} + 1$; all values can replace x; therefore, the domain is, $(-\infty, \infty)$.

31. (a) From the graph, $4 + (-2) = 2$.

  (b) From the graph, $1 - (-3) = 4$.

  (c) From the graph, $(0)(-4) = 0$.

  (d) From the graph, $\dfrac{1}{-3} = -\dfrac{1}{3}$.

33. (a) From the graph, $0 + 3 = 3$.

  (b) From the graph, $-1 - 4 = -5$.

  (c) From the graph, $(2)(1) = 2$.

  (d) From the graph, $\dfrac{3}{0} \Rightarrow$ undefined.

35. (a) From the table, $7 + (-2) = 5$.

  (b) From the table, $10 - 5 = 5$.

  (c) From the table, $(0)(6) = 0$.

  (d) From the table, $\dfrac{5}{0} =$ undefined.

37. See Table 37.

x	$(f+g)(x)$	$(f-g)(x)$	$(fg)(x)$	$\left(\dfrac{f}{g}\right)(x)$
-2	6	-6	0	0
0	5	5	0	undefined
2	5	9	-14	-3.5
4	15	5	50	2

  Figure 37

39. $M(2004) \approx 260$ and $F(2004) \approx 400 \Rightarrow T(2004) = M(2004) + F(2004) = 260 + 400 = 660$

41. The slopes of the line segments for the period 2000-2004 are much steeper than the slopes of the corresponding line segments for the period 2004-2008. Thus, the number of associate's degrees increased more rapidly during the period 2000-2004.

43. $(T - S)(2000) = T(2000) - S(2000) = 19 - 13 = 6$. This represents the billions of dollars spent for general science in 2000.

45. In space and other technologies spending was almost static in the years 1995-2000.

47. (a) $(f \circ g)(4) = f[g(4)]$, so from the graph find $g(4) = 0$. Now find $f(0) = -4$; therefore, $(f \circ g)(4) = -4$.

  (b) $(g \circ f)(3) = g[f(3)]$, so from the graph find $f(3) = 2$. Now find $g(2) = 2$; therefore, $(g \circ f)(3) = 2$.

  (c) $(f \circ f)(2) = f[f(2)]$, so from the graph find $f(2) = 0$. Now find $f(0) = -4$; therefore, $(f \circ f)(2) = -4$.

49. (a) $(f \circ g)(1) = f[g(1)]$, so from the graph find $g(1) = 2$. Now find $f(2) = -3$; therefore, $(f \circ g)(1) = -3$.

(b) $(g \circ f)(-2) = g[f(-2)]$, so from the graph find $f(-2) = -3$. Now find $g(-3) = -2$; therefore, $(g \circ f)(-2) = -2$.

(c) $(g \circ g)(-2) = g[g(-2)]$, so from the graph find $g(-2) = -1$. Now find $g(-1) = 0$; therefore, $(g \circ g)(-1) = 0$.

51. (a) $(g \circ f)(1) = g[f(1)]$, so from the table find $f(1) = 4$. Now find $g(4) = 5$; therefore, $(g \circ f)(1) = 5$.

(b) $(f \circ g)(4) = f[g(4)]$, so from the table find $g(4) = 5$. $f(5)$ is undefined; therefore, $(f \circ g)(4)$ is undefined.

(c) $(f \circ f)(3) = f[f(3)]$, so from the table find $f(3) = 1$. Now find $f(1) = 4$; therefore, $(f \circ f)(3) = 4$.

53. From the table, $g(3) = 4$ and $f(4) = 2$.

55. Since $Y_3 = Y_1 \circ Y_2$ and $X = -1$, we solve $Y_1[Y_2(-1)]$. First solve $Y_2 = (-1)^2 = 1$, now solve $Y_1 = 2(1) - 5 = -3$; therefore, $Y_3 = -3$.

57. Since $Y_3 = Y_1 \circ Y_2$ and $X = 7$, we solve $Y_1[Y_2(7)]$. First solve $Y_2 = (7)^2 = 49$, now solve $Y_1 = 2(49) - 5 = 93$; therefore, $Y_3 = 93$.

59. (a) $(f \circ g)(x) = f[g(x)] = (x^2 + 3x - 1)^3$; all values can be input for x; therefore, the domain is $(-\infty, \infty)$.

(b) $(g \circ f)(x) = g[f(x)] = (x^3)^2 + 3(x^3) - 1 = x^6 + 3x^3 - 1$; all values can be input for x; therefore, the domain is $(-\infty, \infty)$.

(c) $(f \circ f)(x) = f[f(x)] = (x^3)^3 = x^9$; all values can be input for x; therefore, the domain is $(-\infty, \infty)$.

61. (a) $(f \circ g)(x) = f[g(x)] = (\sqrt{1-x})^2 = 1 - x$; all values can be input for x; therefore, the domain is $(-\infty, \infty)$.

(b) $(g \circ f)(x) = g[f(x)] = (\sqrt{1-(x^2)}) = \sqrt{1-x^2}$; only values where $x^2 \leq 1$ can be input for x; therefore, the domain is $[-1, 1]$.

(c) $(f \circ f)(x) = f[f(x)] = (x^2)^2 = x^4$; all values can be input for x; therefore, the domain is $(-\infty, \infty)$.

63. (a) $(f \circ g)(x) = f[g(x)] = \dfrac{1}{(5x)+1} = \dfrac{1}{5x+1}$; all values can be input for x, except $-\dfrac{1}{5}$; therefore, the domain is $\left(-\infty, -\dfrac{1}{5}\right) \cup \left(-\dfrac{1}{5}, \infty\right)$.

(b) $(g \circ f)(x) = g[f(x)] = 5\left(\dfrac{1}{x+1}\right) = \dfrac{5}{x+1}$; all values can be input for x, except -1; therefore, the domain is $(-\infty, -1) \cup (-1, \infty)$.

(c) $(f \circ f)(x) = f[f(x)] = \dfrac{1}{\left(\dfrac{1}{x+1}\right)+1} = \dfrac{1}{\dfrac{1}{x+1}+\dfrac{x+1}{x+1}} = \dfrac{1}{\dfrac{x+2}{x+1}} = \dfrac{x+1}{x+2}$; all values can be input for x, except

those that make $\dfrac{x+1}{x+2} = 0$ or undefined. That would be -1 and -2; therefore, the domain is

$(-\infty, -2) \cup (-2, -1) \cup (-1, \infty)$.

65. (a) $(f \circ g)(x) = f[g(x)] = 2(4x^3 - 5x^2) + 1 = 8x^3 - 10x^2 + 1$; all values can be input for x; therefore, the domain is $(-\infty, \infty)$.

(b) $(g \circ f)(x) = g[f(x)] = 4(2x+1)^3 - 5(2x+1)^2 = 4(8x^3 + 12x^2 + 6x + 1) - 5(4x^2 + 4x + 1) =$
$32x^3 + 48x^2 + 24x + 4 - (20x^2 + 20x + 5) = 32x^3 + 28x^2 + 4x - 1$; all values can be input for x; therefore, the domain is $(-\infty, \infty)$.

(c) $(f \circ f)(x) = f[f(x)] = 2(2x+1) + 1 = 4x + 3$; all values can be input for x; therefore, the domain is $(-\infty, \infty)$.

67. (a) $(f \circ g)(x) = f(g(x)) = f(5) = 5$, all values can be input for x, thefore the domain is $(-\infty, \infty)$.

(b) $(g \circ f)(x) = g(f(x)) = g(5) = 5$, all values can be input for x, therefore the domain is $(-\infty, \infty)$.

(c) $(f \circ f)(x) = f(f(x)) = f(5) = 5$, all values can be input for x, therefore the domain is $(-\infty, \infty)$.

69. $(f \circ g)(x) = f[g(x)] = 4\left(\dfrac{1}{4}(x-2)\right) + 2 = x - 2 + 2 = x$, $(g \circ f)(x) = g[f(x)] = \dfrac{1}{4}((4x+2) - 2) = \dfrac{1}{4}(4x) = x$

71. $(f \circ g)(x) = f[g(x)] = \sqrt[3]{5\left(\dfrac{1}{5}x^3 - \dfrac{4}{5}\right) + 4} = \sqrt[3]{(x^3 - 4) + 4} = \sqrt[3]{x^3} = x$

$(g \circ f)(x) = g[f(x)] = \dfrac{1}{5}\left(\sqrt[3]{5x+4}\right)^3 - \dfrac{4}{5} = \dfrac{1}{5}(5x+4) - \dfrac{4}{5} = x + \dfrac{4}{5} - \dfrac{4}{5} = x$

73. Graph $y_1 = \sqrt[3]{x-6}$, $y_2 = x^3 + 6$, and $y_3 = x$ in the same viewing window. See Figures 73. The graph of y_2 can be obtained by *reflecting* the graph of y_1 across the line $y_3 = x$.

[-10,10] by [-10,10]
Xscl = 1   Yscl = 1

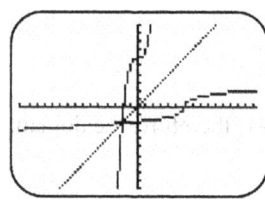

Figure 73

75. $f(x) = x^2 - 4 \Rightarrow f(x+h) = (x+h)^2 - 4 = x^2 + 2xh + h^2 - 4$;
$f(x) + f(h) = (x^2 - 4) + (h^2 - 4) = x^2 + h^2 - 8$

77. $f(x) = 3x - x^2 \Rightarrow f(x+h) = 3(x+h) - (x+h)^2 = 3x + 3h - (x^2 + 2xh + h^2) = -x^2 - 2xh + 3x - h^2 + 3h$;

$f(x) + f(h) = (3x - x^2) + (3h - h^2) = -x^2 + 3x - h^2 + 3h$

79. Using $\dfrac{f(x+h) - f(x)}{h}$ gives: $\dfrac{4(x+h) + 3 - (4x+3)}{h} = \dfrac{4x + 4h + 3 - 4x - 3}{h} = \dfrac{4h}{h} = 4$.

81. Using $\dfrac{f(x+h) - f(x)}{h}$ gives: $\dfrac{-6(x+h)^2 - (x+h) + 4 - (-6x^2 - x + 4)}{h}$

$= \dfrac{-6(x^2 + 2xh + h^2) - x - h + 4 + 6x^2 + x - 4}{h} = \dfrac{-6x^2 - 12xh - 6h^2 - x - h + 4 + 6x^2 + x - 4}{h}$

$= \dfrac{-12xh - 6h^2 - h}{h} = -12x - 6h - 1$.

83. Using $\dfrac{f(x+h) - f(x)}{h}$ gives: $\dfrac{(x+h)^3 - x^3}{h} = \dfrac{x^3 + 3x^2h + 3xh^2 + h^3 - x^3}{h} = \dfrac{3x^2h + 3xh^2 + h^3}{h} = 3x^2 + 3xh + h^2$.

85. Using $\dfrac{f(x+h) - f(x)}{h}$ gives: $\dfrac{1 - (x+h)^2 - (1 - x^2)}{h} = \dfrac{1 - (x^2 + 2xh + h^2) - 1 + x^2}{h} =$

$\dfrac{1 - x^2 - 2xh - h^2 - 1 + x^2}{h} = \dfrac{-2xh - h^2}{h} = -2x - h$

87. Using $\dfrac{f(x+h) - f(x)}{h}$ gives: $\dfrac{3(x+h)^2 - (3x^2)}{h} = \dfrac{3(x^2 + 2xh + h^2) - 3x^2}{h} =$

$\dfrac{3x^2 + 6xh + 3h^2 - 3x^2}{h} = \dfrac{6xh + 3h^2}{h} = 6x + 3h$

89. Using $\dfrac{f(x+h) - f(x)}{h}$ gives: $\dfrac{\dfrac{1}{2(x+h)} - \dfrac{1}{2x}}{h} = \dfrac{\dfrac{2x - (2x + 2h)}{2x(2x+2h)}}{h} = \dfrac{\dfrac{-2h}{2x(2x+2h)}}{h} = \dfrac{-1}{2x(x+h)}$

91. One possible solution is $f(x) = x^2$ and $g(x) = 6x - 2$. Then $(f \circ g)(x) = f[g(x)] = (6x - 2)^2$.

93. One possible solution is $f(x) = \sqrt{x}$ and $g(x) = x^2 - 1$. Then $(f \circ g)(x) = f[g(x)] = \sqrt{x^2 - 1}$.

95. One possible solution is $f(x) = \sqrt{x} + 12$ and $g(x) = 6x$. Then $(f \circ g)(x) = f[g(x)] = \sqrt{6x} + 12$.

97. (a) With a cost of $10 to produce each item and a fixed cost of $500, the cost function is $C(x) = 10x + 500$.

(b) With a selling price of $35 for each item, the revenue function is $R(x) = 35x$.

(c) The profit function is $P(x) = R(x) - C(x) \Rightarrow P(x) = 35x - (10x + 500) \Rightarrow P(x) = 25x - 500$.

(d) A profit is shown when $P(x) > 0 \Rightarrow 25x - 500 > 0 \Rightarrow 25x > 500 \Rightarrow x > 20$. Therefore, 21 items must be produced and sold to realize a profit.

(e) Graph $y_1 = 25x - 500$. The smallest whole number for which $P(x) > 0$ is 21. Use a window of $[0, 30]$ by $[-1000, 500]$, for example.

99. (a) With a cost of $100 to produce each item and a fixed cost of $2700, the cost function is $C(x) = 100x + 2700$.

(b) With a selling price of $280 for each item, the revenue function is $R(x) = 280x$.

(c) The profit function is $P(x) = R(x) - C(x) \Rightarrow P(x) = 280x - (100x + 2700) \Rightarrow P(x) = 180x - 2700$.

74 Chapter 2: Analysis of Graphs of Functions

(d) A profit is shown when $P(x) > 0 \Rightarrow 180x - 2700 > 0 \Rightarrow 180x > 2700 \Rightarrow x > 15$. Therefore, 16 items must be produced and sold to realize a profit.

(e) Graph $y_1 = 180x - 2700$, the smallest whole number for which $P(x) > 0$ is 16. Use a window of $[0, 30]$ by $[-3000, 500]$, for example.

101. (a) If $V(r) = \frac{4}{3}\pi r^3$, then a 3 inch increase would be $V(r) = \frac{4}{3}\pi(r+3)^3$, and the volume gained would be
$V(r) = \frac{4}{3}\pi(r+3)^3 - \frac{4}{3}\pi r^3$.

(b) Graph $y_1 = \frac{4}{3}\pi(x+3)^3 - \frac{4}{3}\pi x^3$ in the window $[0,10]$ by $[0,1500]$. See Figure 101. Although this appears to be a portion of a parabola, it is actually a cubic function.

(c) From the graph in exercise 91b, an input value of $x = 4$ results in a gain of $y \approx 1168.67$.

(d) $V(4) = \frac{4}{3}\pi(4+3)^3 - \frac{4}{3}\pi(4)^3 = \frac{4}{3}\pi(343) - \frac{4}{3}\pi(64) = \frac{1372}{3}\pi - \frac{256}{3}\pi = \frac{1116}{3}\pi = 372\pi \approx 1168.67$.

103. (a) If x = width, then $2x$ = length. Since the perimeter formula is $P = 2W + 2L$ our perimeter function is $P(x) = 2(x) + 2(2x) = 2x + 4x \Rightarrow P(x) = 6x$. This is a linear function.

(b) Graph $P(x) = 6x$ in the window $[0,10]$ by $[1,100]$. See Figure 103b. From the graph when $x = 4, y = 24$. The 4 represents the width of a rectangle and 24 represents the perimeter.

(c) If $x = 4$ is the width of a rectangle then $2x = 8$ is the length. See Figure 103c. Using the standard perimeter formula yields $P = 2(4) + 2(8) = 24$. This compares favorably with the graph result in part b.

(d) (Answers may vary.) If the perimeter y of a rectangle satisfying the given conditions is 36, then the width x is 6. See Figure 103d.

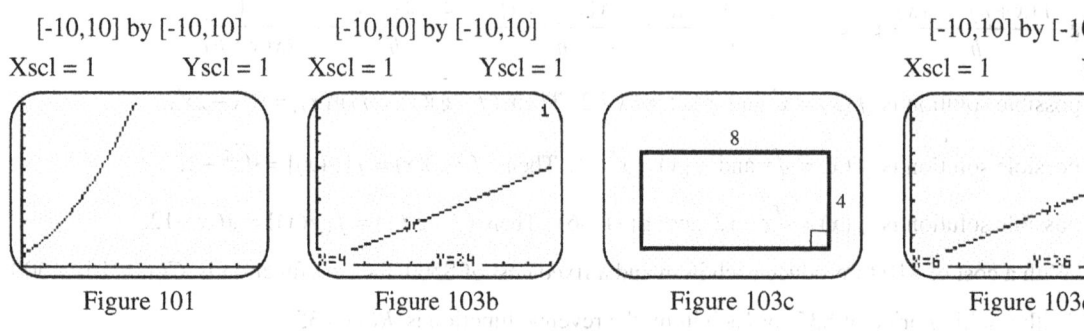

Figure 101   Figure 103b   Figure 103c   Figure 103d

105. (a) $A(2x) = \frac{\sqrt{3}}{4}(2x)^2 = \frac{\sqrt{3}}{4}(4x^2) \Rightarrow A(2x) = \sqrt{3}x^2$

(b) $A(x) = \frac{\sqrt{3}}{4}(16)^2 = \frac{\sqrt{3}}{4}(256) \Rightarrow A(x) = 64\sqrt{3}$ square units.

(c) On the graph of $y = \frac{\sqrt{3}}{4}x^2$, locate the point where $x = 16$ to find $y \approx 110.85$, an approximation for $64\sqrt{3}$.

107. (a) $A(2100) = 42$, ; The average age of a person in 2100 is projected to be 42 years. $T(2100) = 430$, In 2100, the living world's population will have a combined life experience of 430 billion years.

(b) $\dfrac{T(2100)}{A(2100)} = \dfrac{430}{42} \approx 10.2$, The world population will be about 10.2 billion in 2100.

(c) $P(x)$ gives the world's population during year x.

109. (a) $(f+g)(2010) = 13.0 + 74.3 = 87.3$

(b) The function $(f+g)(x)$ computes the total SO_2 and Carbon Monoxide during year x.

(c) Add functions f and g.

x	1970	1980	1990	2000	2010
$(f+g)(x)$	235.2	211.3	177.3	130.8	87.3

111. (a) The function h is the subtraction of function f from g. Therefore, $h(x) = g(x) - f(x)$.

(b) $h(1996) = g(1996) - f(1996) = 841 - 694 = 147$, $h(2006) = g(2006) = f(2006) = 1165 - 1012 = 153$

(c) Using the points (1996, 147) and (2006, 153) from part b, the slope is $m = \dfrac{153-147}{2006-1996} = \dfrac{6}{10} = .6$. Now using point slope form: $y - 147 = .6(x - 1996) \Rightarrow y = .6(x - 1996) + 147$.

Reviewing Basic Concepts (Sections 2.4—2.6)

1. (a) $\left|\dfrac{1}{2}x+2\right| = 4 \Rightarrow \dfrac{1}{2}x+2 = 4 \Rightarrow \dfrac{1}{2}x = 2 \Rightarrow x = 4$ or $\dfrac{1}{2}x+2 = -4 \Rightarrow \dfrac{1}{2}x = -6 \Rightarrow x = -12$.

Therefore, the solution set is $\{-12, 4\}$.

(b) $\left|\dfrac{1}{2}x+2\right| > 4 \Rightarrow \dfrac{1}{2}x+2 > 4 \Rightarrow \dfrac{1}{2}x > 2 \Rightarrow x > 4$ or $\dfrac{1}{2}x+2 < -4 \Rightarrow \dfrac{1}{2}x < -6 \Rightarrow x < -12$. Therefore, the solution interval is $(-\infty, -12) \cup (4, \infty)$.

(c) $\left|\dfrac{1}{2}x+2\right| \leq 4 \Rightarrow -4 \leq \dfrac{1}{2}x+2 \leq 4 \Rightarrow -6 \leq \dfrac{1}{2}x \leq 2 \Rightarrow -12 \leq x \leq 4$.

Therefore, the solution interval is $[-12, 4]$.

2. For the graph of $y = |f(x)|$, we reflect the graph of $y = f(x)$ across the x-axis for all points for which $y < 0$. Where $y \geq 0$, the graph remains unchanged. See Figure 2.

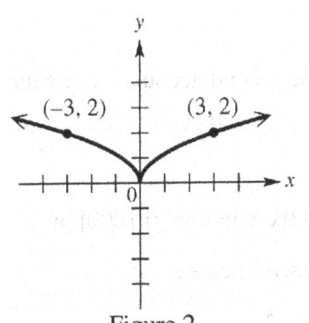

Figure 2

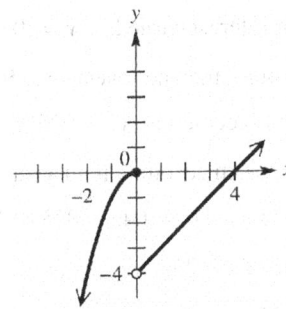

Figure 5a

3. $|2x+4| = |1-3x| \Rightarrow 2x+4 = 1-3x \Rightarrow 5x = -3 \Rightarrow x = -\dfrac{3}{5}$ or $2x+4 = -(1-3x) \Rightarrow 2x+4 = 3x-1 \Rightarrow 5 = x$

76   Chapter 2: Analysis of Graphs of Functions

The solution set is $\left\{-\dfrac{3}{5}, 5\right\}$.

4. (a) $f(-3) = 2(-3) + 3 = -3$ (b) $f(0) = (0)^2 + 4 = 4$ (c) $f(2) = (2)^2 + 4 = 8$

5. (a) See Figure 5a.

   (b) Graph $y_1 = (-x^2)*(x \le 0) + (x-4)*(x > 0)$ in the window [-10,10] by [-10,10]. See Figure 5b.

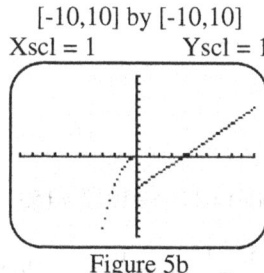

[-10,10] by [-10,10]
Xscl = 1   Yscl = 1

Figure 5b

6. (a) $(f+g)(x) = (-3x-4) + (x^2) = x^2 - 3x - 4$. Therefore, $(f+g)(1) = (1)^2 - 3(1) - 4 = -6$.

   (b) $(f-g)(x) = (-3x-4) - (x^2) = -x^2 - 3x - 4$. Therefore, $(f-g)(3) = -(3)^2 - 3(3) - 4 = -22$.

   (c) $(fg)(x) = (-3x-4)(x^2) = -3x^3 - 4x^2$. Therefore, $(fg)(1) = -3(-2)^3 - 4(-2)^2 = 24 - 16 = 8$.

   (d) $\left(\dfrac{f}{g}\right)(x) = \dfrac{-3x-4}{x^2}$. Therefore, $\left(\dfrac{f}{g}\right)(-3) = \dfrac{-3(-3)-4}{(-3)^2} = \dfrac{5}{9}$.

   (e) $(f \circ g)(x) = f[g(x)] = -3(x)^2 - 4 \Rightarrow (f \circ g)(x) = -3x^2 - 4$

   (f) $(g \circ f)(x) = g[f(x)] = (-3x-4)^2 \Rightarrow (g \circ f)(x) = 9x^2 + 24x + 16$

7. One of many possible solutions for $(f \circ g)(x) = h(x)$ is $f(x) = x^4$ and $g(x) = x + 2$. Then $(f \circ g)(x) = f[g(x)] = (x+2)^4$.

8. $\dfrac{-2(x+h)^2 + 3(x+h) - 5 - (-2x^2 + 3x - 5)}{h} = \dfrac{-2(x^2 + 2xh + h^2) + 3x + 3h - 5 + 2x^2 - 3x + 5}{h} =$

   $\dfrac{-2x^2 - 4xh - 2h^2 + 3x + 3h - 5 + 2x^2 - 3x + 5}{h} = \dfrac{-4xh - 2h^2 + 3h}{h} = -4x - 2h + 3$.

9. (a) At 4% simple interest the equation for interest earned is $y_1 = .04x$.

   (b) If he invested x dollars in the first account, then he invested $x+500$ in the second account. The equation for the amount of interest earned on this account is $y_2 = .025(x+500) \Rightarrow y_2 = .025x + 12.5$.

   (c) It represents the total interest earned in both accounts for 1 year.

   (d) Graph $y_1 + y_2 = .04x + (.025x + 12.5) \Rightarrow y_1 + y_2 = .04x + .025x + 12.5$ in the window [0,1000] by [0,100]. See Figure 9. An input value of $x = 250$, results in $28.75 earned interest.

   (e) At $x = 250$, $y_1 + y_2 = .04(250) + .025(250) + 12.5 = 10 + 6.25 + 12.5 = 28.75.

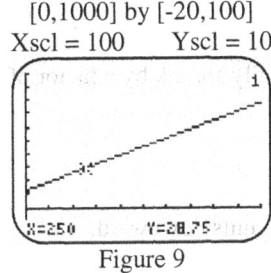

[0,1000] by [-20,100]
Xscl = 100   Yscl = 10

Figure 9

10. If the radius is r, then the height is $2r$ and the equation is
$$S = \pi r\sqrt{r^2 + (2r)^2} = \pi r\sqrt{r^2 + 4r^2} = \pi r\sqrt{5r^2} \Rightarrow S = \pi r^2\sqrt{5}.$$

Chapter 2 Review Exercises

The graphs for exercises 1–10 can be found in the "Function Capsule" boxes located in section 2.1 in the text.

1. True Both $f(x) = x^2$ and $f(x) = |x|$ have the interval: $[0, \infty)$ as the range.

2. True Both $f(x) = x^2$ and $f(x) = |x|$ increase on the interval: $[0, \infty)$.

3. False The function $f(x) = \sqrt{x}$ has the domain: $[0, \infty)$ and $f(x) = \sqrt[3]{x}$ the domain: $(-\infty, \infty)$.

4. False The function $f(x) = \sqrt[3]{x}$ increases on its entire domain.

5. True The function $f(x) = x$ has a domain and range of: $(-\infty, \infty)$

6. False The function $f(x) = \sqrt{x}$ is not defined on $(-\infty, 0)$, so certainly cannot be continuous.

7. True All of the functions show increases on the interval: $[0, \infty)$

8. True Both $f(x) = x$ and $f(x) = x^3$ have graphs that are symmetric with respect to the origin.

9. True Both $f(x) = x^2$ and $f(x) = |x|$ have graphs that are symmetric with respect to the y-axis.

10. True No graphs are symmetric with respect to the x-axis.

11. Only values where $x \geq 0$ can be input for x, therefore the domain of $f(x) = \sqrt{x}$ is: $[0, \infty)$

12. Only positive solution are possible in absolute value functions, therefore the range of $f(x) = \sqrt{x}$ is: $[0, \infty)$

13. All solution are possible in cube root functions, therefore the range of $f(x) = \sqrt[3]{x}$ is: $(-\infty, \infty)$.

14. All values can be input for x, therefore the domain of $f(x) = x^2$ is: $(-\infty, \infty)$.

15. The function $f(x) = \sqrt[3]{x}$ increases for all inputs for x, therefore the interval is: $(-\infty, \infty)$.

16. The function $f(x) = |x|$ increases for all inputs where $x \geq 0$, therefore the interval is: $[0, \infty)$

17. The equation is the equation $y = \sqrt{x}$. Only values where $x \geq 0$ can be input for x, therefore the domain of $y = \sqrt{x}$ is: $[0, \infty)$

18. The equation $y^2 = x$ is the equation $y = \sqrt{x}$ Square root functions have both positive and negative solutions and all solution are possible, therefore the range of $y = \sqrt{x}$ is: $(-\infty, \infty)$.

19. The graph of $f(x) = (x+3) - 1$ is the graph $y = x$ shifted 3 units to the left and 1 unit downward.

78   Chapter 2: Analysis of Graphs of Functions

See Figure 19.

20. The graph of $f(x) = -\frac{1}{2}x + 1$ is the graph reflected $y = x$ across the x-axis, vertically shrunk by a factor of $\frac{1}{2}$, and shifted 1 unit upward. See Figure 20.

21. The graph of $f(x) = (x+1)^2 - 2$ is the graph $y = x^2$ shifted 1 unit to the left and 2 units downward. See Figure 21.

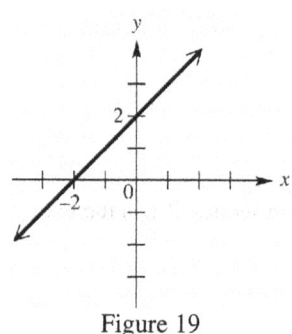
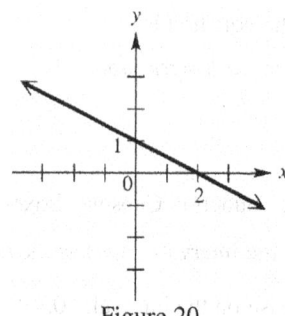
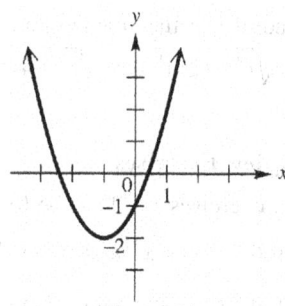

Figure 19   Figure 20   Figure 21

22. The graph of $f(x) = -2x^2 + 3$ is the graph $y = x^2$ reflected across the x-axis, vertically stretched by a factor of 2, and shifted 3 units upward. See Figure 22.

23. The graph of $f(x) = -x^3 + 2$ is the graph $y = x^3$ reflected across the x-axis and shifted 2 units upward. See Figure 23.

24. The graph of $f(x) = (x-3)^3$ is the graph $y = x^3$ shifted 3 units to the right. See Figure 24.

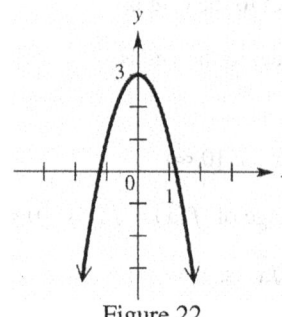
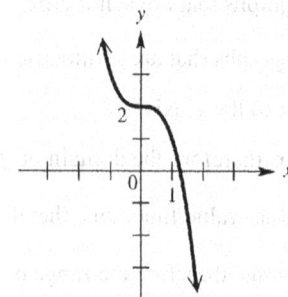
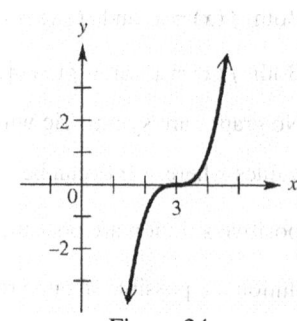

Figure 22   Figure 23   Figure 24

25. The graph of $f(x) = \sqrt{\frac{1}{2}x}$ is the graph $y = \sqrt{x}$ horizontally stretched by a factor of 2. See Figure 25.

26. The graph of $f(x) = \sqrt{x-2} + 1$ is the graph $y = \sqrt{x}$ shifted 2 units to the right and 1 unit upward. See Figure 26.

27. The graph of $f(x) = 2\sqrt[3]{x}$ is the graph $y = \sqrt[3]{x}$ vertically stretched by a factor of 2. See Figure 27.

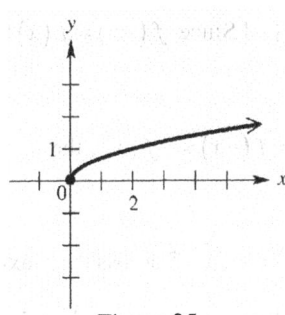
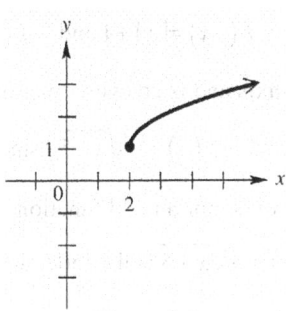
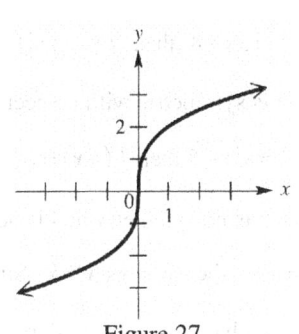

Figure 25   Figure 26   Figure 27

28. The graph of $f(x) = \sqrt[3]{x} - 2$ is the graph $y = \sqrt[3]{x}$ shifted 2 units downward. See Figure 28.

29. The graph of $f(x) = |x-2|+1$ is the graph $y = |x|$ shifted 2 units right and 1 unit upward. See Figure 29.

30. The graph of $f(x) = |-2x+3|$ is the graph $y = |x|$ horizontally shrunk by a factor of $\frac{1}{2}$, shifted $\left(\frac{1}{2}\right)(3)$ or $\frac{3}{2}$ units to the left, and reflected across the y-axis. See Figure 30.

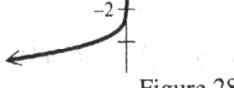
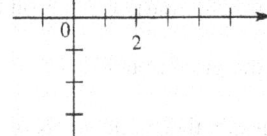
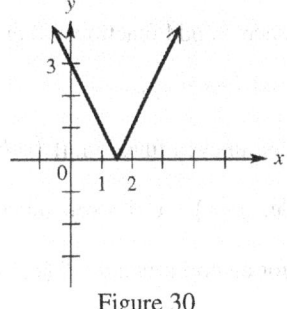

Figure 28   Figure 29   Figure 30

31. (a) From the graph, the function is continuous for the intervals: $(-\infty, -2), [-2, 1]$ and $(1, \infty)$

    (b) From the graph, the function is increasing for the interval: $[-2, 1]$

    (c) From the graph, the function is decreasing for the interval: $(-\infty, -2)$

    (d) From the graph, the function is constant for the interval: $(1, \infty)$

    (e) From the graph, all values can be input for x, therefore the domain is: $(-\infty, \infty)$

    (f) From the graph, the possible values of y or the range is: $\{-2\} \cup [-1, 1] \cup (2, \infty)$

32. $x = y^2 - 4 \Rightarrow y^2 = x+4 \Rightarrow y = \sqrt{x+4}$ and $y = -\sqrt{x+4}$.

33. From the graph, the relation is symmetric with respect to the x-axis, y-axis, and origin. The relation is not a function since some inputs x have two outputs y.

34. If $F(x) = x^3 - 6$, then $F(-x) = (-x)^3 - 6 \Rightarrow F(-x) = -x^3 - 6$ and $-F(x) = -(x^3 - 6) \Rightarrow -F(x) = -x^3 + 6$.

    Since $F(x) \neq F(-x) \neq -F(x)$ the function has no symmetry and is neither an ever nor an odd function.

35. If $f(x) = |x| + 4$, then $f(-x) = |(-x)| + 4 \Rightarrow f(-x) = |x| + 4$ and $-f(x) = -|x| - 4$ Since $f(-x) = f(x)$ the function is symmetric with respect to the y-axis and is an even function.

36. If $f(x) = \sqrt{x-5}$ then $f(-x) = \sqrt{(-x)-5}$ and $-f(x) = -\sqrt{x-5}$. Since $f(x) \neq f(-x) \neq -f(x)$, the function has no symmetry and is neither an even nor an odd function.

37. If $y^2 = x - 5$ then $y = \pm\sqrt{x-5}$. Since $f(x) = -\sqrt{x-5}$ is the reflection of $f(x) = -\sqrt{x-5}$ across the x-axis, the relation has symmetry with respect to the x-axis. Also, one x inputs can produce two y outputs the relation is not a function.

38. If $f(x) = 3x^4 + 2x^2 + 1$ then $f(-x) = 3(-x)^4 + 2(-x)^2 + 1 \Rightarrow f(-x) = 3x^4 + 2x^2 + 1$ and $-f(x) = -3x^4 - 2x^2 - 1$. Since $f(-x) = f(x)$ the function is symmetric with respect to the y-axis and is an even function.

39. True, a graph that is symmetrical with respect to the x-axis means that for every (x, y) there is also $(x, -y)$.

40. True, since an even function and one that is symmetric with respect to the y-axis both contain the points (x, y) and $(-x, y)$.

41. True, since an odd function and one that is symmetric with respect to the origin both contain the points (x, y) and $(-x, -y)$.

42. False, for an even function, if (a, b) is on the graph, then $(-a, b)$ is on the graph and not $(a, -b)$. For example, $f(x) = x^2$ is even, and (2, 4) is on the graph, but (2, −4) is not.

43. False, for an odd function, if (a, b) is on the graph, then $(-a, -b)$ is on the graph and not $(-a, b)$ For example, $f(x) = x^3$ is odd, and $(2, 8)$ is on the graph, but $(-2, 8)$ is not.

44. True, if $(x, 0)$ is on the graph of $f(x) = 0$ then $(-x, 0)$ is on the graph.

45. The graph of $y = -3(x+4)^2 - 8$ is the graph of $y = x^2$ shifted 4 units to the left, vertically stretched by a factor of 3, reflected across the x-axis, and shifted 8 units downward.

46. The equation $y = \sqrt{x}$ reflected across the y-axis is: $f(x) = \sqrt{-x}$ then reflected across the x-axis is: $y = -\sqrt{-x}$ now vertically shrunk by a factor of $\frac{2}{3}$ is: $y = -\frac{2}{3}\sqrt{-x}$, and finally shifted 4 units upward is: $y = -\frac{2}{3}\sqrt{-x} + 4$.

47. Shift the function f upward 3 units. See Figure 47.
48. Shift the function f to the right 2 units. See Figure 48.
49. Shift the function f to the left 3 units and downward 2 units. See Figure 49.

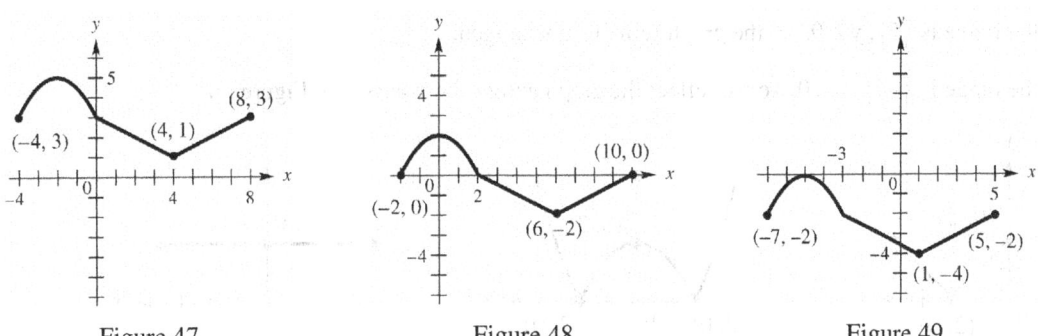

Figure 47   Figure 48   Figure 49

50. For values where $f(x) > 0$ the graph remains the same. For values where $f(x) < 0$ reflect the graph across the x-axis. See Figure 50.

51. Horizontally shrink the function f by a factor of $\frac{1}{4}$. See Figure 51.

52. Horizontally stretch the function f by a factor of 2. See Figure 52.

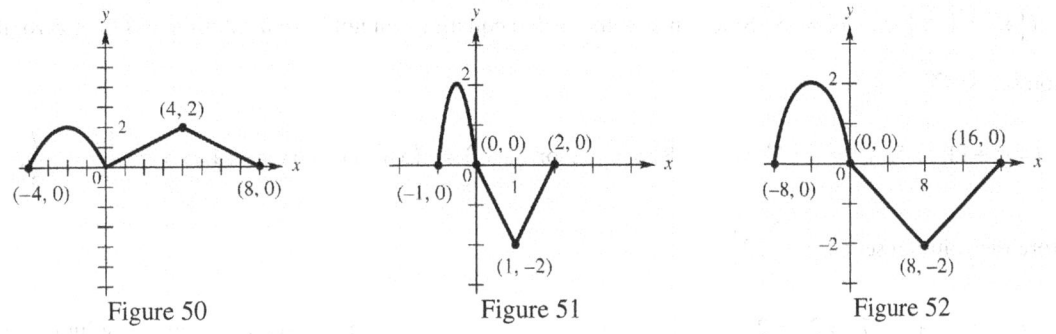

Figure 50   Figure 51   Figure 52

53. The function is shifted upward 4 units, therefore the domain remains the same: $[-3, 4]$ and the range is increased by 4 and is: $[2, 9]$.

54. The function is shifted left 10 units, therefore the domain is decreased by 10 and is $[-13, -6]$; and the function is stretched vertically by a factor of 5, therefore the range is multiplied by 5 and is: $[-10, 25]$.

55. The function is horizontally shrunk by a factor of $\frac{1}{2}$, therefore the domain is divided by 2 and is: $\left[-\frac{3}{2}, 2\right]$; and the function is reflected across the x-axis, therefore the range is opposites of the original and is: $[-5, 2]$.

56. The function is shifted right 1 unit, therefore the domain is increased by 1 and is: $[-2, 5]$; and the function is also shifted upward 3 units, therefore the range is increased by 3 and is: $[1, 8]$.

57. We reflect the graph of $y = f(x)$ across the x-axis for all points for which $y < 0$. Where $y \geq 0$, the graph remains unchanged. See Figure 57.

58. We reflect the graph of $y = f(x)$ across the x-axis for all points for which < 0. Where $y \geq 0$, the graph remains unchanged. See Figure 58.

82 Chapter 2: Analysis of Graphs of Functions

59. Since the range is $\{2\}, y \geq 0$, so the graph remains unchanged.

60. Since the range is $\{-2\}, y < 0$, so we reflect the graph across the x-axis. See Figure 60.

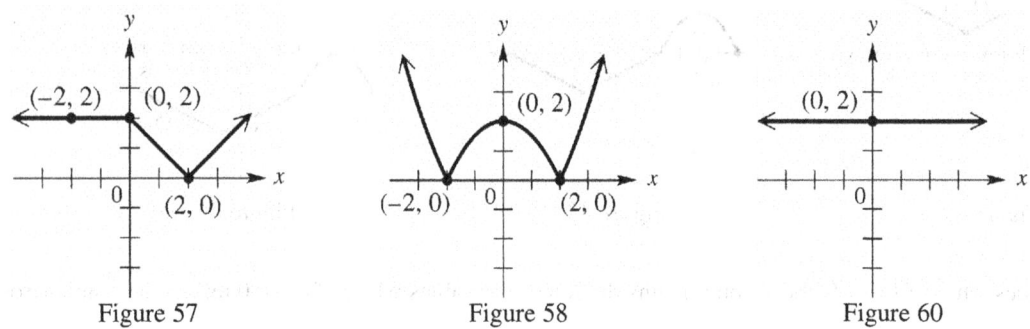

Figure 57   Figure 58   Figure 60

61. $|4x+3|=12 \Rightarrow 4x+3=12 \Rightarrow 4x=9 \Rightarrow x=\dfrac{9}{4}$ or $4x+3=-12 \Rightarrow 4x=-15 \Rightarrow x=-\dfrac{15}{4}$, therefore the solution set is: $\left\{-\dfrac{15}{4},\dfrac{9}{4}\right\}$.

62. $|-2x-6|+4=1 \Rightarrow |-2x-6|=-3$. Since an absolute value equation can not have a solution less than zero, the solution set is: $\varnothing$

63. $|5x+3|=|x+11| \Rightarrow 5x+3=x+11 \Rightarrow 4x=8 \Rightarrow x=2$ or $5x+3=-(x+11) \Rightarrow 6x=-14 \Rightarrow x=-\dfrac{14}{6}=-\dfrac{7}{3}$, therefore the solution set is: $\left\{-\dfrac{7}{3},2\right\}$.

64. $|2x+5|=7 \Rightarrow 2x+5=7 \Rightarrow 2x=2 \Rightarrow x=1$ or $2x+5=-7 \Rightarrow 2x=-12 \Rightarrow x=-6$, therefore the solution set is: $\{-6,1\}$.

65. $|2x+5|\leq 7 \Rightarrow -7\leq 2x+5\leq 7 \Rightarrow -12\leq 2x\leq 2 \Rightarrow -6\leq x\leq 1$, therefore the interval is: $\{-6,1\}$.

66. $|2x+5|\geq 7 \Rightarrow 2x+5\geq 7 \Rightarrow 2x\geq 2 \Rightarrow x\geq 1$ or $2x+5\leq -7 \Rightarrow 2x\leq -12 \Rightarrow x\leq -6$, therefore the solution is the interval: $(-\infty,-6]\cup[1,\infty)$.

67. $|5x-12|0 \Rightarrow 5x-12>0 \Rightarrow 5x>12 \Rightarrow x>\dfrac{12}{5}$ or $5x-12<0 \Rightarrow 5x=12 \Rightarrow x<\dfrac{12}{5}$, therefore the solution is the interval: $\left(-\infty,\dfrac{12}{5}\right)\cup\left(\dfrac{12}{5},\infty\right)$ or $\left\{x\,|\,x\neq\dfrac{12}{5}\right\}$.

68. Since an absolute value equation can not have a solution less than zero, the solution set is: $\varnothing$

69. $2|3x-1|+1=21 \Rightarrow 2|3x-1|=20 \Rightarrow |3x-1|=10 \Rightarrow 3x-1=10 \Rightarrow 3x=11 \Rightarrow x=\dfrac{11}{3}$ or $3x-1=-10 \Rightarrow 3x=-9 \Rightarrow x=-3$, therefore the solution set is: $\left\{-3,\dfrac{11}{3}\right\}$.

Copyright © 2015 Pearson Education, Inc

70. $|2x+1| = |-3x+1| \Rightarrow 2x+1 = -3x+1 \Rightarrow 5x = 0 \Rightarrow x = 0$ or $2x+1 = -(-3x+1) \Rightarrow -x = -2 \Rightarrow x = 2$, therefore the solution set is: $\{0, 2\}$.

71. The x-coordinates of the points of intersection of the graphs are -6 and 1. Thus, $\{-6, 1\}$ is the solution set of $y_1 = y_2$ The graph of y_1 lies on or below the graph of y_2 between -6 and 1, so the solution set of $y_1 \leq y_2$ is $[-6, 1]$ The graph of y_1 lies above the graph of y_2 everywhere else, so the solution set of $y_1 \geq y_2$ is $(-\infty, -6] \cup [1, \infty)$.

72. Graph $y_1 = |x+1| + |x-3|$ and $\{-3, -1\}$ See Figure 72. The intersections are $x = -3$ and $x = 5$, therefore the solution set is: $\{-3, 5\}$. **Check:** $|(-3)+1| + |(-3)-3| = 8 \Rightarrow |-2| + |-6| = 8 \Rightarrow 2 + 6 = 8 \Rightarrow 8 = 8$ and $|(5)+1| + |(5)-3| = 8 \Rightarrow |6| + |2| = 8 \Rightarrow 6 + 2 = 8 \Rightarrow 8 = 8$

[-10,10] by [-4,16]

Xscl = 1   Yscl = 1

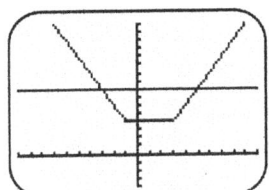

Figure 72

73. Initially, the car is at home. After traveling 30 mph for 1 hr, the car is 30 mi away from home. During the second hour the car travels 20 mph until it is 50 mi away. During the third hour the car travels toward home at 30 mph until it is 20 mi away. During the fourth hour the car travels away from home at 40 mph until it is 60 mi away from home. During the last hour, the car travels 60 mi at 60 mph until it arrives home.

74. See Figure 74

75. See Figure 75

76. See Figure 76

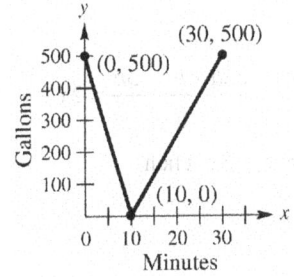

Figure 74

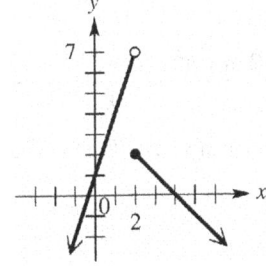

Figure 75

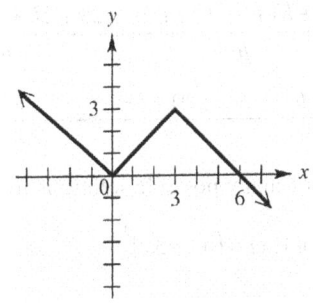

Figure 76

84   Chapter 2: Analysis of Graphs of Functions

77. Graph $y_1 = (3x+1)*(x<2)+(-x+4)*(x\geq 2)$ in the window $[-10,10]$ by

    $|4x+8|>4 \Rightarrow 4x+8>4 \Rightarrow 4x>-4 \Rightarrow -1$ See Figure 77.

78. See Figure 78.

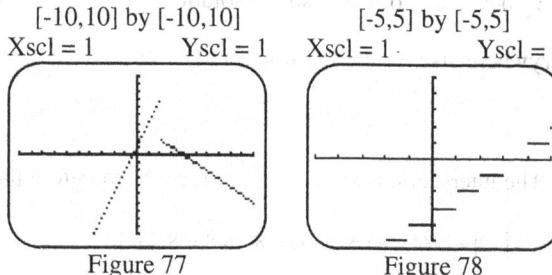

  Figure 77   Figure 78

79. From the graphs $(f+g)(1) = 2+3 = 5$

80. From the graphs $(f-g)(0) = 1-4 = -3$

81. From the graphs $(fg)(-1) = (0)(3) = 0$

82. From the graphs $\left(\dfrac{f}{g}\right)(2) = \dfrac{3}{2}$

83. From the graphs $(f \circ g)(2) = f[g(2)] = f(2) = 3$

84. From the graphs $(g \circ f)(2) = g[f(2)] = g(3) = 2$

85. From the graphs $(g \circ f)(-4) = g[f(-4)] = g(2) = 2$

86. From the graphs $(f \circ g)(-2) = f[g(-2)] = f(2) = 3$

87. From the table $(f+g)(1) = 7+1 = 8$

88. From the table $(f-g)(3) = 9-1 = 0$

89. From the table $(fg)(-1) = (3)(-2) = -6$

90. From the table $\left(\dfrac{f}{g}\right)(0) = \dfrac{5}{0}$, which is undefined.

91. From the tables $(g \circ f)(-2) = g[f(-2)] = g(1) = 2$

92. From the graphs $(f \circ g)(3) = f[g(3)] = f(-2) = 1$

93. $\dfrac{2(x+h)+9-(2x+9)}{h} = \dfrac{2x+2h+9-2x-9}{h} = \dfrac{2h}{h} = 2$

94. $\dfrac{(x+h)^2-5(x+h)+3-(x^2-5x+3)}{h} = \dfrac{x^2+2xh+h^2-5x-5h+3-x^2+5x-3}{h} = \dfrac{2xh+h^2-5h}{h} = 2x+h-5$

95. One of many possible solutions for $(f \circ g)(x) = h(x)$ is: $f(x) = x^2$ and $g(x) = x^3 - 3x$ Then

    $(f \circ g)(x) = \left(x^3 - 3x\right)^2$.

96. One of many possible solutions for $(f \circ g)(x) = h(x)$ is $f(x) = \dfrac{1}{x}$ and $g(x) = x - 5$ Then

    $$(f \circ g)(x) = f[g(x)] = \dfrac{1}{x-5}$$

97. If $V(r) = \dfrac{4}{3}\pi r^3$, then a 4 inch increase would be: $V(r) = \dfrac{4}{3}\pi(r+4)^3$, and the volume gained would be:

    $$V(r) = \dfrac{4}{3}\pi(r+4)^3 - \dfrac{4}{3}\pi r^3.$$

98. (a) Since $h = d, r = \dfrac{d}{2}$ and the formula for the volume of a can is: $V = \pi r^2 h$, the function is:

    $$V(d) = \pi\left(\dfrac{d}{2}\right)^2 d \Rightarrow V(d) = \dfrac{\pi d^3}{4}$$

    (b) Since $h = d, r = \dfrac{d}{2}, c = 2\pi r$ and the formula for the surface area of a can is: $A = 2\pi r h + 2\pi r^2$, the

    function is: $S(d) = 2\pi\left(\dfrac{d}{2}\right)d + 2\pi\left(\dfrac{d}{2}\right)^2 \Rightarrow S(d) = \pi d^2 + \dfrac{\pi d^2}{2} \Rightarrow S(d) = \dfrac{3\pi d^2}{2}$

99. The function for changing yards to inches is: $f(x) = 36x$ and the function for changing miles to yards is:

    $g(x) = 1760x$ The composition of this which would change miles into inches is:

    $f[g(x)] = 36[1760(x)] \Rightarrow (f \circ g)(x) = 63,360x$.

100. If $x =$ width, then length $= 2x$ A formula for Perimeter can now be written as: $P = x + 2x + x + 2x$ and the function is: $P(x) = 6x$ This is a linear function.

Chapter 2 Test

1. (a) D, only values where $x \geq 0$ can be input into a square root function.
   (b) D, only values where $y \geq 0$ can be the solution to a square root function.
   (c) C, all values can be input for x in a squaring function.
   (d) B, only values where $y \geq 3$ can be the solution to $f(x) = x^2 + 3$
   (e) C, all values can be input for x in a cube root function.
   (f) C, all values can be a solution in a cube root function.
   (g) C, all values can be input for x in an absolute value function.
   (h) D, only values where $y \geq 0$ can be the solution to an absolute value function.
   (i) D, if $x = y^2$ then $y = \sqrt{x}$ and only values where $x \geq 0$ can be input into a square root function.
   (j) C, all values can be a solution in this function.

2. (a) This is $f(x)$ shifted 2 units upward. See Figure 2a.
   (b) This is $f(x)$ shifted 2 units to the left. See Figure 2b.
   (c) This is $f(x)$ reflected across the x-axis. See Figure 2c.
   (d) This is $f(x)$ reflected across the y-axis. See Figure 2d.
   (e) This is $f(x)$ vertically stretched by a factor of 2. See Figure 2e.

86 Chapter 2: Analysis of Graphs of Functions

(f) We reflect the graph of $y = f(x)$ across the x-axis for all points for which $2.75 Where $y \geq 0$ the graph remains unchanged. See Figure 2f.

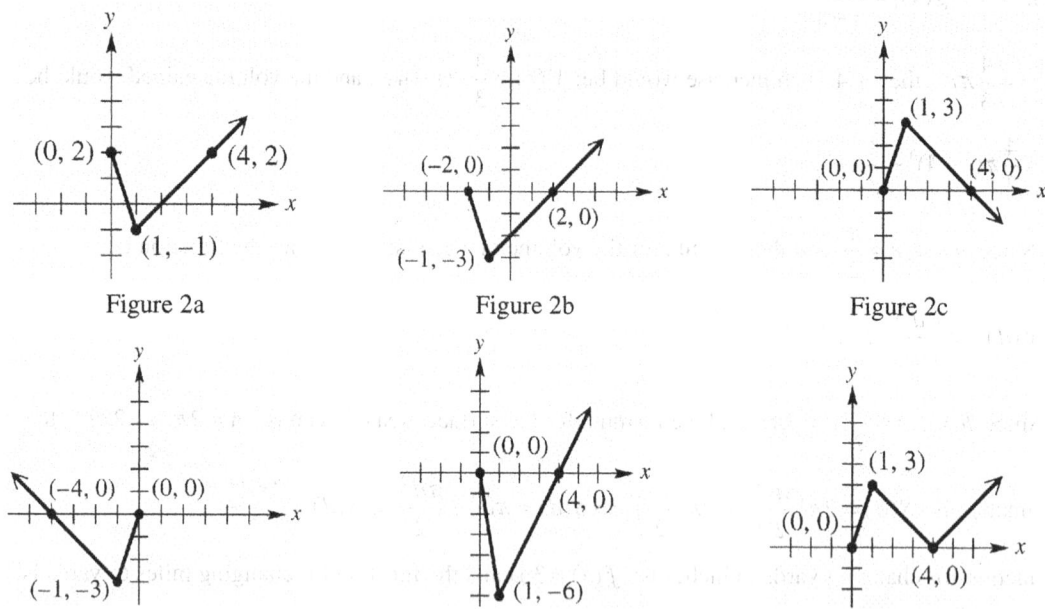

Figure 2a   Figure 2b   Figure 2c

Figure 2d   Figure 2e   Figure 2f

3. (a) Since $y = f(2x)$ is $y = f(x)$ horizontally shrunk by a factor of $\frac{1}{2}$, the point $(-2, 4)$ on $y = f(x)$ becomes the point $(-1, 4)$ on the graph of $y = f(2x)$.

    (b) Since $y = f\left(\frac{1}{2}x\right)$ is $y = f(x)$ horizontally stretched by a factor of 2, the point $(-2, 4)$ on $y = f(x)$ becomes the point $(-4, 4)$ on the graph of $y = f\left(\frac{1}{2}x\right)$.

4. (a) The graph of $f(x) = -x(x-2)^2 + 4$ is the basic graph $f(x) = x^2$ reflected across the x-axis, shifted 2 units to the right, and shifted 4 units upward. See Figure 4a.

    (b) The graph of $f(x) = -2\sqrt{-x}$ is the basic graph $f(x) = \sqrt{x}$ reflected across the y-axis and vertically stretched by a factor of 2. See Figure 4b.

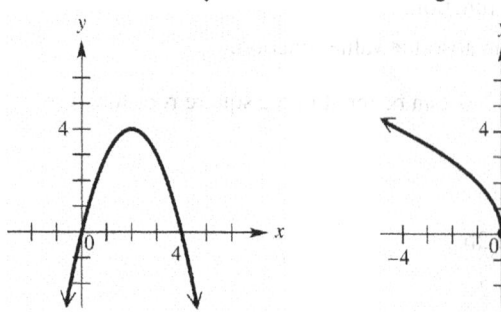

Figure 4a 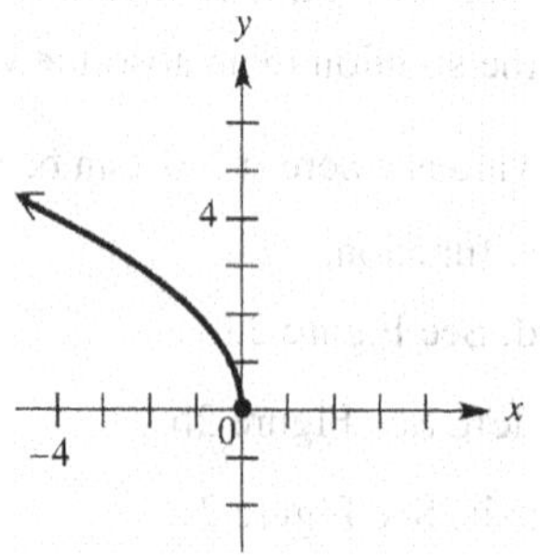   Figure 4b

Copyright © 2015 Pearson Education, Inc

5. (a) If the graph is symmetric with respect to the y-axis, then $(x, y) \Rightarrow (-x, y)$ therefore $(3, 6) \Rightarrow (-3, 6)$.

    (b) If the graph is symmetric with respect to the x-axis, then $(x, y) \Rightarrow (-x, -y)$ therefore $(3, 6) \Rightarrow (-3, -6)$.

    (c) See Figure 5. We give an actual screen here. The drawing should resemble it.

[-4,4] by [0,]
Xscl = 1   Yscl = 1

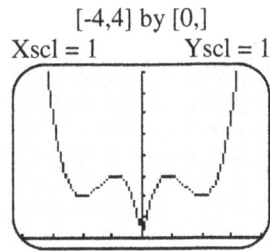

Figure 5

6. (a) Shift the graph of $y = \sqrt[3]{x}$ to the left 2 units, vertically stretch by a factor of 4, and shift 5 units downward.

    (b) Graph $y = |x|$ reflected across the x-axis, vertically shrunk by a factor of $\frac{1}{2}$ shifted 3 units to the right, and shifted up 2 units. See Figure 6. From the graph the domain is: $(-\infty, \infty)$; and the range is: $(-\infty, 2]$.

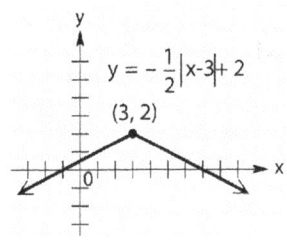

Figure 6

7. (a) From the graph, the function is increasing for the interval: $(-\infty, -3)$

    (b) From the graph, the function is decreasing for the interval: $(4, \infty)$

    (c) From the graph, the function is constant for the interval: $(-3, 4)$

    (d) From the graph, the function is continuous for the intervals: $(-\infty, -3), (-3, 4), (4, \infty)$.

    (e) From the graph, the domain is: $(-\infty, \infty)$

    (f) From the graph, the range is: $(-\infty, 2)$

8. (a) $|4x+8| = 4 \Rightarrow 4x+8 = 4 \Rightarrow 4x = -4 \Rightarrow x = -1$ or $4x+8 = -4 \Rightarrow 4x = -12 \Rightarrow x = -3$, therefore the solution set is: $\{-3, -1\}$

    (b) $|4x+8| < 4 \Rightarrow -4 < 4x+8 < 4 \Rightarrow -12 < 4x < -4 \Rightarrow -3 < x < -1$, therefore the solution is: $(-3, -1)$.

    (c) $|4x+8| > 4 \Rightarrow 4x+8 > 4 \Rightarrow 4x > -4 \Rightarrow x > -1$ or $4x+8 < -4 \Rightarrow 4x < -12 \Rightarrow x < -3$ therefore the solution is: $(-\infty, -3) \cup (-1, \infty)$.

9. (a) $(f-g)(x) = 2x^2 - 3x + 2 - (-2x+1) \Rightarrow (f-g)(x) = 2x^2 - x + 1$

88   Chapter 2: Analysis of Graphs of Functions

(b) $\left(\dfrac{f}{g}\right)(x) = \dfrac{2x^2 - 3x + 2}{-2x + 1}$

(c) The domain can be all values for x, except any that make $g(x) = 0$. Therefore

$-2x + 1 \neq 0 \Rightarrow -2x \neq -1 \Rightarrow x \neq \dfrac{1}{2}$ or the interval: $\left(-\infty, \dfrac{1}{2}\right) \cup \left(\dfrac{1}{2}, \infty\right)$

(d) $(f \circ g)(x) = f[g(x)] = 2(-2x + 1)^2 - 3(-2x + 1) + 2 = 2(4x^2 - 4x + 1) + 6x - 3 + 2 =$

$8x^2 - 8x + 2 + 6x - 3 + 2 = 8x^2 - 2x + 1$

(e) $(g \circ f)(x) = g[f(x)] = -2(2x^2 - 3x + 2) + 1 = -4x^2 + 6x - 4 + 1 = -4x^2 + 6x - 3$

(f) $\dfrac{2(x+h)^2 - 3(x+h) + 2 - (2x^2 - 3x + 2)}{h} = \dfrac{2(x^2 + 2xh + h^2) - 3x - 3h + 2 - 2x^2 + 3x - 2}{h} =$

$\dfrac{2x^2 + 4xh + 2h^2 - 3x - 3h + 2 - 2x^2 + 3x - 2}{h} = \dfrac{4xh + 2h^2 - 3h}{h} = 4x + 2h - 3$

10. (a) See Figure 10a.

(b) Graph $y_1 = (-x^2 + 3) * (x \leq 1) + \left(\sqrt[3]{x} + 2\right) + \left(\sqrt[3]{x} + 2\right) * (x > 1)$ in the window $[-4.7, 4.7]$ by $[-5.1, 5.1]$

See Figure 10b.

(c) The graph is not connected at $x = 1$ and thus f is not continuous when $x = 1$.

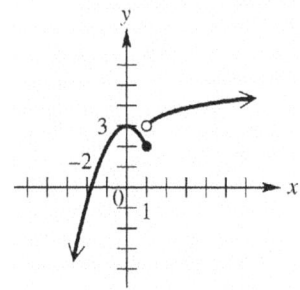

Figure 10a

[-4.7,4.7] by [-5.1,5.1]
Xscl = 1   Yscl = 1

[0,10] by [0,6]
Xscl = 1   Yscl = 1

[0,1,000] by [-4,000,4000]
Xscl = 50   Yscl = 500

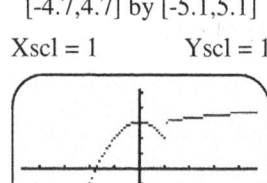 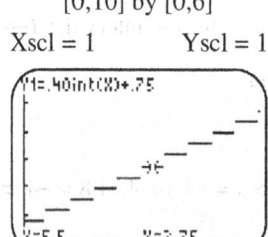 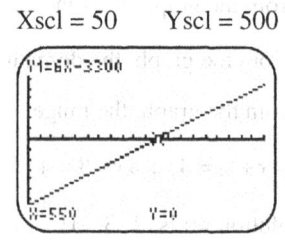

Figure 10b   Figure 11   Figure 12

11. (a) See Figure 11.

(b) Set $x = 5.5$ then $\$2.75$ is the cost of a 5.5 minute call. See the display at the bottom of the screen.

12. (a) With an initial set-up cost of $\$3300$ and a production cost of $\$4.50$ the function is: $C(x) = 3300 + 4.50x$

(b) With a selling price of $\$10.50$ the revenue function is: $R(x) = 10.50x$

(c) $P(x) = R(x) - C(x) \Rightarrow P(x) = 10.50x - (3300 + 4.50x) \Rightarrow P(x) = 6x - 3300$

(d) To make a profit $P(x) > 0$, therefore $6x - 3300 > 0 \Rightarrow 6x > 3300 \Rightarrow x > 550$
Tyler needs to sell 551 before he earns a profit.

(e) Graph $y_1 = 6x - 3300$, See Figure 12. The first integer x-value for which $P(x) > 0$ is 551

Chapter 3: Polynomial Functions

3.1: Complex Numbers

1. The complex number $-9i$ can be written $0-9i$.

   (a) The real part is 0. (b) The imaginary part is -9. (c) The number is pure imaginary.

3. The complex number π can be written $\pi + 0i$.

   (a) The real part is π. (b) The imaginary part is 0. (c) The number is real.

5. The complex number $3+7i$ is written in standard form.

   (a) The real part is 3. (b) The imaginary part is 7. (c) The number is nonreal complex.

7. The complex number $i\sqrt{7}$ can be written $0+\sqrt{7}i$.

   (a) The real part is 0. (b) The imaginary part is $\sqrt{7}$. (c) The number is pure imaginary.

9. The complex number $\sqrt{-7}$ can be written $0+\sqrt{7}i$.

   (a) The real part is 0. (b) The imaginary part is $\sqrt{7}$. (c) The number is pure imaginary.

11. $3i+5i = (3+5)i = 8i$

13. $(-7i)(1+i) = -7i - 7i^2 = -7i - 7(-1) = 7 - 7i$

15. True

17. True

19. False. *Every* real number is a complex number.

21. $\sqrt{-100} = i\sqrt{100} = 10i$

23. $-\sqrt{-400} = -i\sqrt{400} = -20i$

25. $-\sqrt{-39} = -i\sqrt{39}$

27. $5+\sqrt{-4} = 5+i\sqrt{4} = 5+2i$

29. $9-\sqrt{-50} = 9-i\sqrt{50} = 9-i\sqrt{25 \cdot 2} = 9-5i\sqrt{2}$

31. $i\sqrt{-9} = i^2\sqrt{9} = -3$

33. $\sqrt{-13} \cdot \sqrt{-13} = i\sqrt{13} \cdot i\sqrt{13} = 13i^2 = -13$

35. $\sqrt{-3} \cdot \sqrt{-8} = i\sqrt{3} \cdot i\sqrt{8} = \sqrt{24}i^2 = -2\sqrt{6}$

37. $\dfrac{\sqrt{-30}}{\sqrt{-10}} = \dfrac{i\sqrt{30}}{i\sqrt{10}} = \dfrac{i\sqrt{10 \cdot 3}}{i\sqrt{10}} = \dfrac{i\sqrt{10} \cdot \sqrt{3}}{i\sqrt{10}} = \sqrt{3}$

39. $\dfrac{\sqrt{-24}}{\sqrt{8}} = \dfrac{i\sqrt{24}}{\sqrt{8}} = \dfrac{i\sqrt{8 \cdot 3}}{\sqrt{8}} = \dfrac{i\sqrt{8} \cdot \sqrt{3}}{\sqrt{8}} = i\sqrt{3}$

41. $\dfrac{\sqrt{-10}}{\sqrt{-40}} = \dfrac{i\sqrt{10}}{i\sqrt{40}} = \dfrac{i\sqrt{10}}{i\sqrt{10 \cdot 4}} = \dfrac{i\sqrt{10}}{i\sqrt{10} \cdot \sqrt{4}} = \dfrac{1}{\sqrt{4}} = \dfrac{1}{2}$

43. $\dfrac{\sqrt{-6} \cdot \sqrt{-2}}{\sqrt{3}} = \dfrac{i\sqrt{6} \cdot i\sqrt{2}}{\sqrt{3}} = \dfrac{i^2\sqrt{3} \cdot \sqrt{2} \cdot \sqrt{2}}{\sqrt{3}} = \dfrac{i^2\sqrt{2} \cdot \sqrt{2}}{1} = -\sqrt{4} = -2$

45. $(3+2i)+(4-3i) = (3+4)+(2-3)i = 7-i$

47. $(-2+3i)-(-4+3i) = (-2-(-4))+(3-3)i = 2+0i = 2$

49. $(3-8i)+(2i+4) = (3+4)+(-8+2)i = 7-6i$

51. $(2-5i)-(3+4i)-(-2+i) = 2-5i-3-4i+2-i = (2-3+2)+(-5i-4i-i) = 1-10i$

53. $(-6+5i)+(4-4i)+(2-i) = (-6+4+2)+(5+(-4)+(-1))i = 0+0i = 0$

55. $(2+i)(3-2i) = 6-4i+3i-2i^2 = 6-i-2(-1) = 8-i$

57. $(2+4i)(-1+3i) = -2+6i-4i+12i^2 = -2+2i+12(-1) = -14+2i$

59. $(-3+2i)^2 = (-3+2i)(-3+2i) = 9-6i-6i+4i^2 = 9-12i+4(-1) = 5-12i$

61. $(3+i)(-3-i) = -9-3i-3i-i^2 = -9-6i-(-1) = -8-6i$

63. $(2+3i)(2-3i) = 4-9i^2 = 4-9(-1) = 13$

65. $\left(\sqrt{6}+i\right)\left(\sqrt{6}-i\right) = 6-i^2 = 6-(-1) = 7$

67. $i(3-4i)(3+4i) = i(9-16i^2) = i(9-16(-1)) = 25i$

69. $3i(2-i)^2 = 3i(4-4i+i^2) = 3i(4-4i+(-1)) = 3i(3-4i) = 9i-12i^2 = 9i-12(-1) = 12+9i$

71. $(2+i)(2-i)(4+3i) = (4-i^2)(4+3i) = (4-(-1))(4+3i) = 5(4+3i) = 20+15i$

73. $i^5 = i^4 \cdot i^1 = 1^1 \cdot i = i$

75. $i^{15} = (i^4)^3 \cdot i^3 = 1^3 \cdot (-i) = -i$

77. $i^{64} = (i^4)^{16} = 1^{16} = 1$

79. $i^{-6} = (i^6)^{-1} = [(i^4)^1 \cdot i^2]^{-1} = [1^1 \cdot (-1)]^{-1} = (-1)^{-1} = -1$

81. $\dfrac{1}{i^9} = i^{-9} = (i^9)^{-1} = [(i^4)^2 \cdot i]^{-1} = [1^2 \cdot i]^{-1} = (i)^{-1} = \dfrac{1}{i} = \dfrac{1}{i} \cdot \dfrac{i}{i} = \dfrac{i}{i^2} = \dfrac{i}{-1} = -i$

83. $\dfrac{1}{i^{-51}} = i^{51} = (i^4)^{12} \cdot i^3 = 1^{12} \cdot (-i) = -i$

85. $\dfrac{-1}{-i^{12}} = \dfrac{1}{i^{12}} = \dfrac{1}{(i^4)^3} = \dfrac{1}{1^3} = \dfrac{1}{1} = 1$

87. $\left(\dfrac{\sqrt{2}}{2}+\dfrac{\sqrt{2}}{2}i\right)^2 = \left(\dfrac{\sqrt{2}}{2}\right)^2 + 2\left(\dfrac{\sqrt{2}}{2}\right)\left(\dfrac{\sqrt{2}}{2}i\right) + \left(\dfrac{\sqrt{2}}{2}i\right)^2 = \dfrac{2}{4}+\dfrac{2}{2}i+\dfrac{2}{4}i^2 = \dfrac{1}{2}+i-\dfrac{1}{2} = i$

89. The conjugate of $5-3i$ is $5+3i$.

91. The conjugate of $-18i = 0-18i$ is $0+18i = 18i$.

93. The conjugate of $-\sqrt{8} = -\sqrt{8}+0i$ is $-\sqrt{8}-0i = -\sqrt{8}$.

95. $\dfrac{3}{-i} = \dfrac{3}{-i} \cdot \dfrac{i}{i} = \dfrac{3i}{-i^2} = \dfrac{3i}{-(-1)} = \dfrac{3i}{1} = 3i$

97. $\dfrac{-10}{i} = \dfrac{-10}{i} \cdot \dfrac{-i}{-i} = \dfrac{10i}{-(-1)} = \dfrac{10i}{1} = 10i$

99. $\dfrac{1-3i}{1+i} = \dfrac{1-3i}{1+i} \cdot \dfrac{1-i}{1-i} = \dfrac{1-i-3i+3i^2}{1^2-i^2} = \dfrac{-2-4i}{1-(-1)} = \dfrac{-2-4i}{2} = -1-2i$

101. $\dfrac{-3+4i}{2-i} = \dfrac{-3+4i}{2-i} \cdot \dfrac{2+i}{2+i} = \dfrac{-6-3i+8i+4i^2}{2^2-i^2} = \dfrac{-10+5i}{4-(-1)} = \dfrac{-10+5i}{5} = -2+i$

103. $\dfrac{4-3i}{4+3i} = \dfrac{4-3i}{4+3i} \cdot \dfrac{4-3i}{4-3i} = \dfrac{16-12i-12i+9i^2}{4^2-(3i)^2} = \dfrac{7-24i}{16-(-9)} = \dfrac{7-24i}{25} = \dfrac{7}{25} - \dfrac{24}{25}i$

105. The method involves multiplying by 1, the multiplicative identity.

3.2: Quadratic Functions and Graphs

1. Since $a > 0$, the parabola opens upward. The vertex is $(4,-3)$. The graph is shown in B.

3. Since $a > 0$, the parabola opens upward. The vertex is $(-4,-3)$. The graph is shown in D.

5. (a) $P(x) = x^2 - 2x - 15 \Rightarrow P(x) + 15 = x^2 - 2x \Rightarrow P(x) + 15 + 1 = x^2 - 2x + 1 \Rightarrow$

    $P(x) + 16 = (x-1)^2 \Rightarrow P(x) = (x-1)^2 - 16$

    (b) The vertex is $(1,-16)$.

    (c) See Figure 5a and 5b.

7. (a) $P(x) = -x^2 - 3x + 10 \Rightarrow -P(x) = x^2 + 3x - 10 \Rightarrow -P(x) + 10 = x^2 + 3x \Rightarrow$

    $-P(x) + 10 + \dfrac{9}{4} = x^2 + 3x + \dfrac{9}{4} \Rightarrow -P(x) + \dfrac{49}{4} = \left(x + \dfrac{3}{2}\right)^2 \Rightarrow -P(x) = \left(x + \dfrac{3}{2}\right)^2 - \dfrac{49}{4} \Rightarrow$

    $P(x) = -\left(x + \dfrac{3}{2}\right)^2 + \dfrac{49}{4}$

    (b) The vertex is $\left(-\dfrac{3}{2}, \dfrac{49}{4}\right)$ or $(-1.5, 12.25)$.

    (c) See Figure 7a and 7b.

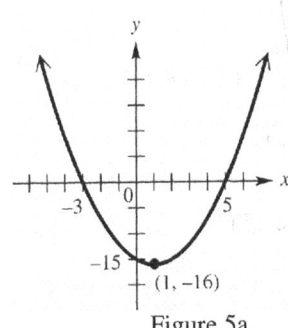

Figure 5a

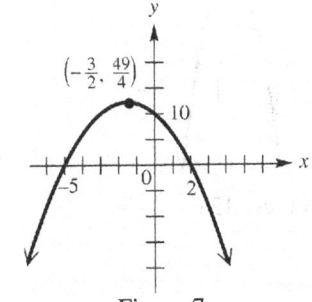

Figure 7a

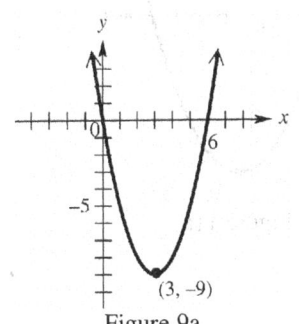

Figure 9a

94　CHAPTER 3　Polynomial Functions

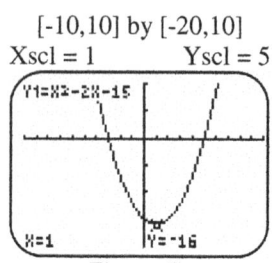

Figure 5b

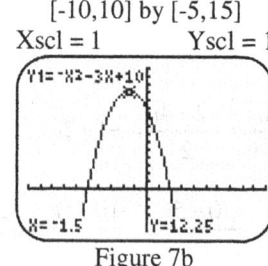

Figure 7b

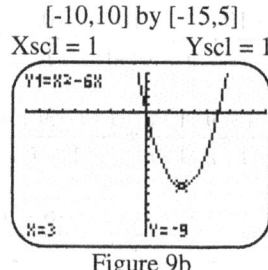

Figure 9b

9. (a) $P(x) = x^2 - 6x \Rightarrow P(x) + 9 = x^2 - 6x + 9 \Rightarrow P(x) + 9 = (x-3)^2 \Rightarrow P(x) = (x-3)^2 - 9$

(b) The vertex is $(3, -9)$.

(c) See Figure 9a and 9b.

11. (a). $P(x) = 2x^2 - 2x - 24 \Rightarrow \dfrac{P(x)}{2} = x^2 - x - 12 \Rightarrow \dfrac{P(x)}{2} + 12 = x^2 - x \Rightarrow$

$\dfrac{P(x)}{2} + 12 + \dfrac{1}{4} = x^2 - x + \dfrac{1}{4} \Rightarrow \dfrac{P(x)}{2} + \dfrac{49}{4} = \left(x - \dfrac{1}{2}\right)^2 \Rightarrow \dfrac{P(x)}{2} = \left(x - \dfrac{1}{2}\right)^2 - \dfrac{49}{4} \Rightarrow P(x) = 2\left(x - \dfrac{1}{2}\right)^2 - \dfrac{49}{2}$

(b) The vertex is $\left(\dfrac{1}{2}, -\dfrac{49}{2}\right)$ or $(0.5, -24.5)$.

(c) See Figure 11a and 11b.

13. (a) $P(x) = -2x^2 + 6x \Rightarrow \dfrac{P(x)}{-2} = x^2 - 3x \Rightarrow \dfrac{P(x)}{-2} + \dfrac{9}{4} = x^2 - 3x + \dfrac{9}{4} \Rightarrow$

$\dfrac{P(x)}{-2} + \dfrac{9}{4} = \left(x - \dfrac{3}{2}\right)^2 \Rightarrow \dfrac{P(x)}{-2} = \left(x - \dfrac{3}{2}\right)^2 - \dfrac{9}{4} \Rightarrow P(x) = -2\left(x - \dfrac{3}{2}\right)^2 + \dfrac{9}{2}$

(b) The vertex is $\left(\dfrac{3}{2}, \dfrac{9}{2}\right)$ or $(1.5, 4.5)$.

(c) See Figure 13a and 13b.

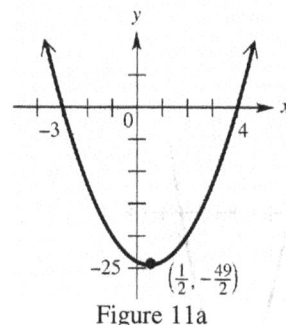

Figure 11a

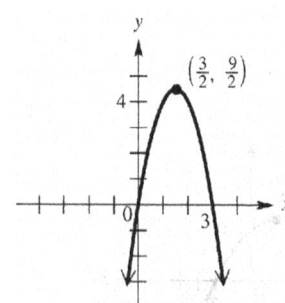

Figure 13a

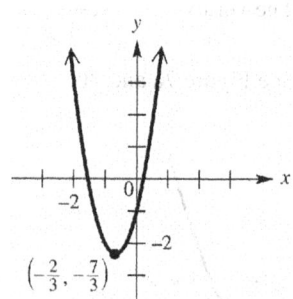

Figure 15a

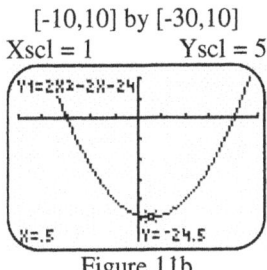
[-10,10] by [-30,10]
Xscl = 1   Yscl = 5
Figure 11b

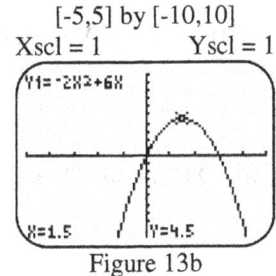
[-5,5] by [-10,10]
Xscl = 1   Yscl = 1
Figure 13b

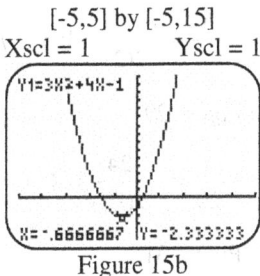
[-5,5] by [-5,15]
Xscl = 1   Yscl = 1
Figure 15b

15. (a) $P(x) = 3x^2 + 4x - 1 \Rightarrow \dfrac{P(x)}{3} = x^2 + \dfrac{4}{3}x - \dfrac{1}{3} \Rightarrow \dfrac{P(x)}{3} + \dfrac{1}{3} = x^2 + \dfrac{4}{3}x \Rightarrow$

$\dfrac{P(x)}{3} + \dfrac{1}{3} + \dfrac{4}{9} = x^2 + \dfrac{4}{3}x + \dfrac{4}{9} \Rightarrow \dfrac{P(x)}{3} + \dfrac{7}{9} = \left(x + \dfrac{2}{3}\right)^2 \Rightarrow \dfrac{P(x)}{3} = \left(x + \dfrac{2}{3}\right)^2 - \dfrac{7}{9} \Rightarrow P(x) = 3\left(x + \dfrac{2}{3}\right)^2 - \dfrac{7}{3}$

(b). The vertex is $\left(-\dfrac{2}{3}, -\dfrac{7}{3}\right)$ or $(-0.67, -2.33)$.

(c) See Figure 15a and 15 b.

17. (a) Since $a > 0$, the parabola opens upward. The vertex is $(4, -2)$. The graph is given in D.

(b) Since $a > 0$, the parabola opens upward. The vertex is $(2, -4)$. The graph is given in B.

(c) Since $a < 0$, the parabola opens downward. The vertex is $(4, -2)$. The graph is given in C.

(d) Since $a < 0$, the parabola opens downward. The vertex is $(2, -4)$. The graph is given in A.

19. (a) $(2, 0)$ (b) $D: (-\infty, \infty), R: [0, \infty)$ (c) $x = 2$ (d) $[2, \infty)$ (e) $(-\infty, 2]$ (f) Min.: $P(2) = 0$

21. (a) $(-3, -4)$ (b) $D: (-\infty, \infty), R: [-4, \infty)$ (c) $x = -3$ (d) $[-3, \infty)$ (e) $(-\infty, -3]$ (f) Min.: $f(-3) = -4$

23. (a) $(-3, 2)$ (b) $D: (-\infty, \infty), R: (-\infty, 2]$ (c) $x = -3$ (d) $(-\infty, -3]$ (e) $[-3, \infty)$ (f) Max.: $P(-3) = 2$

25. (a) $x = -\dfrac{b}{2a} = -\dfrac{-10}{2(1)} = 5;\ y = P(5) = (5)^2 - 10(5) + 21 = -4 \Rightarrow$ Vertex: $(5, -4)$

(b) See Figure 25.

27. (a) $x = -\dfrac{b}{2a} = -\dfrac{4}{2(-1)} = 2;\ y = -(2)^2 + 4(2) - 2 = 2 \Rightarrow$ Vertex: $(2, 2)$

(b) See Figure 27.

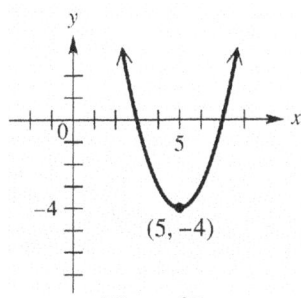
Figure 25

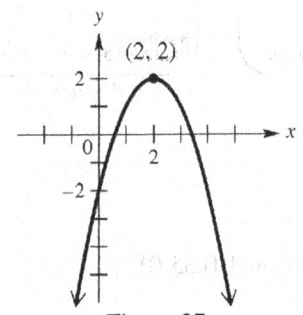
Figure 27

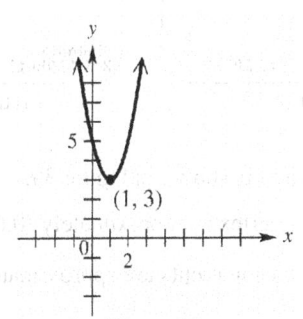
Figure 29

29. (a) $x = -\dfrac{b}{2a} = -\dfrac{(-4)}{2(2)} = 1;\ y = f(1) = 2(1)^2 - 4(1) + 5 = 3 \Rightarrow$ Vertex: $(1, 3)$

(b) See Figure 29.

31. (a) $x = -\dfrac{b}{2a} = -\dfrac{24}{2(-3)} = 4;\ y = f(4) = -3(4)^2 + 24(4) - 46 = 2 \Rightarrow$ Vertex: $(4, 2)$

(b) See Figure 31.

33. (a) $x = -\dfrac{b}{2a} = -\dfrac{-2}{2(2)} = \dfrac{1}{2};\ y = f\left(\dfrac{1}{2}\right) = 2\left(\dfrac{1}{2}\right)^2 - 2\left(\dfrac{1}{2}\right) + 1 = \dfrac{1}{2} \Rightarrow$ Vertex: $\left(\dfrac{1}{2}, \dfrac{1}{2}\right)$.

(b) See Figure 33.

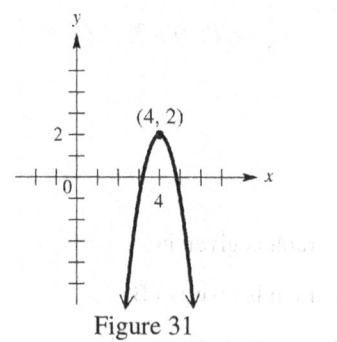
Figure 31

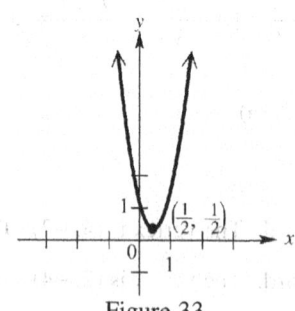
Figure 33

35. The graph is shown in Figure 35.

(a) The vertex is approximately $(2.71, 5.20)$

(b) The x-intercepts are approximately $(-1.33, 0)$ and $(6.74, 0)$.

37. The graph is shown in Figure 37.

(a) The vertex is approximately $(1.12, 0.56)$.

(b) There are no x-intercepts.

[-10,10] by [-10,10]
Xscl = 1   Yscl = 1

[-5,5] by [-5,5]
Xscl = 1   Yscl = 1

[-5,5] by [-5,5]
Xscl = 1   Yscl = 1

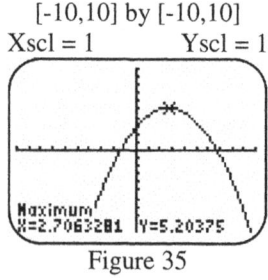
Figure 35

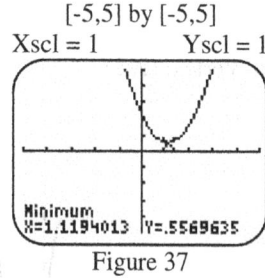
Figure 37

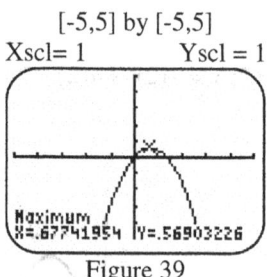
Figure 39

39. The graph is shown in Figure 39.

(a) The vertex is approximately $(0.68, 0.57)$.

(b) The x-intercepts are approximately $(0, 0)$ and $(1.35, 0)$.

41. The minimum value of 3 is found at the vertex.

43. The graph would not intersect the line $y = 1$. There are no solutions to $f(x) = 1$.

45. (a) From the symmetry of the y-values in the table, the vertex is $(4,-12)$.

    (b) Since all other y-values are larger than -12, the vertex is a minimum point.

    (c) The minimum value of the function is -12 and is located at the vertex.

    (d) Since the function is quadratic with a minimum value of -12, the range is $[-12,\infty)$.

47. (a) From the symmetry of the y-values in the table, the vertex is $(1.5, 2)$.

    (b) Since all other y-values are smaller than 2, the vertex is a maximum point.

    (c) The maximum value of the function is 2 and is located at the vertex.

    (d) Since the function is quadratic with a maximum value of 2, the range is $(-\infty, 2]$.

49. Since the data are in the shape of a parabola that opens downward, a quadratic model with $a < 0$ is appropriate.

51. Since the data are in the shape of a parabola that opens upward, a quadratic model with $a > 0$ is appropriate.

53. Since the data are in the shape of a line that rises from left to right, a linear model with $m > 0$ is appropriate.

55. Let $h = -1$, $k = -4$, $x = 5$ and $P(x) = 104$ in $P(x) = a(x-h)^2 + k$ and determine the value of a.

    $104 = a(5+1)^2 - 4 \Rightarrow 104 = a(6)^2 - 4 \Rightarrow 108 = 36a \Rightarrow a = 3$

    $P(x) = 3(x+1)^2 - 4 \Rightarrow P(x) = 3(x^2 + 2x + 1) - 4 \Rightarrow P(x) = 3x^2 + 6x - 1$

57. Let $h = 8$, $k = 3$, $x = 10$ and $P(x) = 5$ in $P(x) = a(x-h)^2 + k$ and determine the value of a.

    $5 = a(10-8)^2 + 3 \Rightarrow 5 = a(2)^2 + 3 \Rightarrow 2 = 4a \Rightarrow a = 0.5$. $P(x) = 0.5(x-8)^2 + 3 \Rightarrow$

    $P(x) = 0.5(x^2 - 16x + 64) + 3 \Rightarrow P(x) = 0.5x^2 - 8x + 35$ or $P(x) = \frac{1}{2}x^2 - 8x + 35$

59. Let $h = -4$, $k = -2$, $x = 2$ and $P(x) = -26$ in $P(x) = a(x-h)^2 + k$ and determine the value of a.

    $-26 = a(2+4)^2 - 2 \Rightarrow -26 = a(6)^2 - 2 \Rightarrow -24 = 36a \Rightarrow a = -\frac{2}{3}$

    $P(x) = -\frac{2}{3}(x+4)^2 - 2 \Rightarrow P(x) = -\frac{2}{3}(x^2 + 8x + 16) - 2 \Rightarrow P(x) = -\frac{2}{3}x^2 - \frac{16}{3}x - \frac{38}{3}$

61. (a) Since the parabola opens upward and the vertex is $(4,90)$, the function decreases from 0 to 4 and increases from 4 to 8. Therefore, the heart rate decreases during the first 4 minutes and increases during the next 4 minutes.

    (b) Since parabola opens upward the minimum occurs at the vertex $(4, 90)$. Therefore, the minimum heart rate is 90 bpm after 4 minutes.

63. (a) The data are not linear since the data increase and then decrease.

    (b) Using coordinate $(2, 120)$, $f(x) = a(x-2)^2 + 120$. To find, use $(0, 84) \Rightarrow$

    $84 = a(0-2)^2 + 120 \Rightarrow -36 = a(4) \Rightarrow a = -9$; $f(x) = -9(x-2)^2 + 120$.

    (c) $D = \{x \mid 0 \leq x \leq 4\}$

65. (a) The value of t cannot be negative because t represents elapsed time after the rock is launched.

    (b) The original height of the rock is $s_0 = 0$ which represents ground level.

98 CHAPTER 3 Polynomial Functions

(c) Since $v_0 = 90$ and $s_0 = 0$, $s(t) = -16t^2 + v_0 t + s_0 \Rightarrow s(t) = -16t^2 + 90t$.

(d) $s(1.5) = -16(1.5)^2 + 90(1.5) = 99$ feet

(e) $x = -\dfrac{b}{2a} = -\dfrac{90}{2(-16)} = 2.8125$; $y \approx s(2.8125) = -16(2.8125)^2 + 90(2.8125) = 126.5625$. The vertex is (2.8125, 126.5625). The rock reaches a maximum height of 126.5625 feet after 2.8125 seconds. A graph of $y = -16x^2 + 90x$ (not shown) also gives a vertex of (2.8125, 126.5625).

(f) A graph of $y = -16x^2 + 90x$ (not shown) has x-intercepts at (0, 0) and (5.625, 0). The rock will hit the ground after 5.625 seconds.

67. (a) The graphs of $-16x^2 + 150x$ and $y_2 = 355$ are shown in Figure 67a. The graphs do not intersect, which indicates that the ball does not reach a height of 355 feet.

(b) The graphs of $y_1 = -16x^2 + 250x + 30$ and $y_2 = 355$ are shown in Figure 67b. The graphs intersect when $x \approx 1.43$ and $x \approx 14.19$ which indicates that the ball is 355 feet high at about 1.4 and 14.2 seconds.

[0,20] by [3,400]
Xscl = 1   Yscl = 10

[0,20] by [0,1200]
Xscl = 5   Yscl = 100

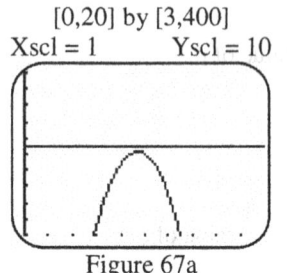
Figure 67a

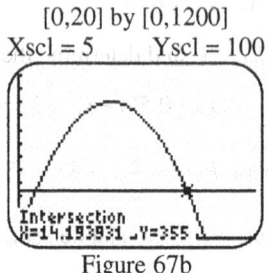
Figure 67b

69. See Figure 69.
71. See Figure 71.

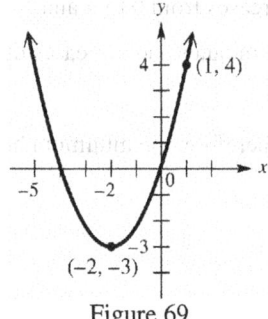
Figure 69

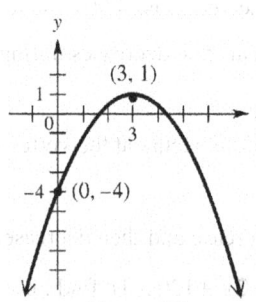
Figure 70

3.3: Quadratic Equations and Inequalities

1. $x^2 = 4 \Rightarrow \sqrt{x^2} = \sqrt{4} \Rightarrow x = \pm 2$; therefore, G.

3. $x^2 + 2 = 0 \Rightarrow x^2 = -2 \Rightarrow \sqrt{x^2} = \sqrt{-2} \Rightarrow x = \pm i\sqrt{2}$; therefore, C.

5. $x^2 = -8 \Rightarrow \sqrt{x^2} = \sqrt{-8} \Rightarrow x = \pm 2i\sqrt{2}$; therefore, H.

7. $x - 2 = 0 \Rightarrow x = 2$; therefore, D.

9. Equation D, which is in the form $ab = 0$, is set up for the zero product property. Either $3x + 1 = 0 \Rightarrow x = -\frac{1}{3}$ or $x - 7 = 0 \Rightarrow x = 7$. The solution set is $\left\{-\frac{1}{3}, 7\right\}$.

11. Equation C, which has an x^2 coefficient of 1, does not require step 1 of the method of completing the square.
$x^2 + x = 12 \Rightarrow x^2 + x + \frac{1}{4} = 12 + \frac{1}{4} \Rightarrow \left(x + \frac{1}{2}\right)^2 = \frac{49}{4} \Rightarrow x + \frac{1}{2} = \pm\frac{7}{2} \Rightarrow x = -\frac{1}{2} \pm \frac{7}{2}$. The solution set is $\{-4, 3\}$.

13. $x^2 = 16 \Rightarrow x = \pm\sqrt{16} \Rightarrow x = \{\pm 4\}$; For graphical support, show that the graphs of $y_1 = x^2$ and $y_2 = 16$ intersect when $x = \pm 4$.

15. $2x^2 = 90 \Rightarrow x^2 = 45 \Rightarrow x = \pm\sqrt{45} \Rightarrow x = \pm 3\sqrt{5}$; For graphical support, show that the graphs of $y_1 = 2x^2$ and $y_2 = 90$ intersect when $x = \pm 3\sqrt{5} \approx \pm 6.7$.

17. $x^2 = -16 \Rightarrow x = \pm i\sqrt{16} \Rightarrow x = \pm 4i$; For graphical support, show that the graphs of $y_1 = x^2$ and $y_2 = -16$ do not intersect; therefore, no real solutions.

19. $x^2 = -18 \Rightarrow x = \pm i\sqrt{18} \Rightarrow x = \pm 3i\sqrt{2}$; For graphical support, show that the graphs of $y_1 = x^2$ and $y_2 = -18$ do not intersect; therefore, no real solutions.

21. $(3x - 1)^2 = 12 \Rightarrow 3x - 1 = \pm\sqrt{12} \Rightarrow 3x - 1 = \pm 2\sqrt{3} \Rightarrow 3x = \pm 2\sqrt{3} + 1 \Rightarrow x = \frac{1 \pm 2\sqrt{3}}{3}$. For graphical support, show that the graphs of $y_1 = (3x - 1)^2$ and $y_2 = 12$ intersect when $x = \frac{1 \pm 2\sqrt{3}}{3}$; $x \approx -0.8$ or 1.5.

23. $(5x - 3)^2 = -3 \Rightarrow 5x - 3 = \pm\sqrt{-3} \Rightarrow 5x - 3 = \pm i\sqrt{3} \Rightarrow 5x = \pm i\sqrt{3} + 3 \Rightarrow x = \frac{3}{5} \pm \frac{\sqrt{3}}{5}i$. For graphical support, show that the graphs of $y_1 = (5x - 3)^2$ and $y_2 = -3$ do not intersect; therefore, there are no real solutions.

25. $x^2 = 2x + 24 \Rightarrow x^2 - 2x - 24 = 0 \Rightarrow (x - 6)(x + 4) = 0 \Rightarrow x - 6 = 0$ or $x + 4 = 0 \Rightarrow x = -4$ or 6. For graphical support, show that the graph of $y_1 = x^2 - 2x - 24 = 0$ has x-intercepts $x = -4$ and 6.

27. $3x^2 - 2x = 0 \Rightarrow x(3x - 2) = 0 \Rightarrow x = 0$ or $3x - 2 = 0 \Rightarrow x = 0$ or $\frac{2}{3}$. For graphical support, show that the graph of $y_1 = 3x^2 - 2x$ has x-intercepts $x = 0$ and $\frac{2}{3}$.

29. $x(14x + 1) = 3 \Rightarrow 14x^2 + x - 3 = 0 \Rightarrow (2x + 1)(7x - 3) = 0 \Rightarrow 2x + 1 = 0$ or $7x - 3 = 0 \Rightarrow x = -\frac{1}{2}$ or $\frac{3}{7}$. For graphical support, show that the graph of $y_1 = 14x^2 + x - 3$ has x-intercepts $x = -\frac{1}{2}$ and $\frac{3}{7}$.

31. $-4+9x-2x^2 = 0 \Rightarrow (-4+x)(1-2x) = 0 \Rightarrow -4+x = 0$ or $1-2x = 0 \Rightarrow x = \frac{1}{2}$ or 4. For graphical support, show that the graph of $y_1 = -4+9x-2x^2$ has x-intercepts $x = \frac{1}{2}$ and 4.

33. $\frac{1}{3}x^2 - \frac{1}{6}x = 24 \Rightarrow \frac{1}{3}x^2 + \frac{1}{3}x - 24 = 0 \Rightarrow x^2 - x - 72 = 0 \Rightarrow (x-9)(x+8) = 0 \Rightarrow x-9 = 0$ or $x+8 = 0 \Rightarrow x = -8$ or 9. For graphical support, show that the graph of $y_1 = \frac{1}{3}x^2 - \frac{1}{3}x - 24$ has x-intercepts $x = -8$ and 9.

35. $(x+2)(x-1) = 7x+5 \Rightarrow x^2 + x - 2 = 7x+5 \Rightarrow x^2 - 6x - 7 = 0 \Rightarrow (x-7)(x+1) = 0 \Rightarrow x-7 = 0$ or $x+1 = 0 \Rightarrow x = -1$ or 7. For graphical support, show that the graph of $y_1 = x^2 - 6x - 7$ has x-intercepts $x = -1$ and 7.

37. Use the quadratic formula to solve $x^2 - 2x - 4 = 0$; therefore, $a = 1$, $b = -2$ and $c = -4$

$x = \frac{-(-2) \pm \sqrt{(-2)^2 - 4(1)(-4)}}{2(1)} = \frac{2 \pm \sqrt{4+16}}{2} = \frac{2 \pm \sqrt{20}}{2} = \frac{2 \pm 2\sqrt{5}}{2} = \frac{2(1 \pm \sqrt{5})}{2} \Rightarrow x = 1 \pm \sqrt{5}$. For graphical support, show that the graph of $y_1 = x^2 - 2x - 4$ has x-intercepts $x = 1 \pm \sqrt{5}$; $x \approx -1.24$ and 3.24.

39. Use the quadratic formula to solve $y_1 = 2x^2 + 2x = -1 \Rightarrow 2x^2 + 2x + 1 = 0$; therefore, $a = 2$, $b = 2$ and $c = 1$

$x = \frac{-2 \pm \sqrt{(2)^2 - 4(2)(1)}}{2(2)} = \frac{-8 \pm \sqrt{4-8}}{4} = \frac{-2 \pm \sqrt{-4}}{4} = \frac{-2 \pm 2i}{4} = \frac{2(-1 \pm i)}{4} \Rightarrow x = -\frac{1}{2} \pm \frac{1}{2}i$. For graphical support, show that the graph of $y_1 = 2x^2 + 2x + 1$ has no x-intercepts; therefore, there are no real solutions.

41. Use the quadratic formula to solve $x(x-1) = 1 \Rightarrow x^2 - x - 1 = 0$; therefore, $a = 1$, $b = -1$ and $c = -1$

$x = \frac{-(-1) \pm \sqrt{(-1)^2 - 4(1)(-1)}}{2(1)} = \frac{1 \pm \sqrt{1+4}}{2} \Rightarrow x = \frac{1 \pm \sqrt{5}}{2}$. For graphical support, show that the graph of $y_1 = x^2 - x - 1$ has x-intercepts $x = \frac{1 \pm \sqrt{5}}{2}$; $x \approx -0.62$ and 1.62.

43. Use the quadratic formula to solve $x^2 - 5x = x - 7 \Rightarrow x^2 - 6x + 7 = 0$; therefore, $a = 1$, $b = -6$, and $c = 7$.

$x = \frac{-(-6) \pm \sqrt{(-6)^2 - 4(1)(7)}}{2(1)} = \frac{6 \pm \sqrt{36-28}}{2} = \frac{6 \pm \sqrt{8}}{2} = \frac{6 \pm 2\sqrt{2}}{2} = \frac{2(3 \pm \sqrt{2})}{2} \Rightarrow x = 3 \pm \sqrt{2}$. For graphical support, show that the graph of $y_1 = x^2 - 6x + 7$ has x-intercepts $x = 3 \pm \sqrt{2}$; $x \approx 1.59$ and 4.41.

45. Use the quadratic formula to solve $4x^2 - 12x = -11 \Rightarrow 4x^2 - 12x + 11 = 0$; therefore, $a = 4$, $b = -12$ and $c = 11$. $x = \frac{-(-12) \pm \sqrt{(-12)^2 - 4(4)(11)}}{2(4)} = \frac{12 \pm \sqrt{144-176}}{8} = \frac{12 \pm \sqrt{-32}}{8} = \frac{12 \pm 4i\sqrt{2}}{8} = \frac{4(3 \pm i\sqrt{2})}{8} \Rightarrow$

$x = \dfrac{3}{2} \pm \dfrac{\sqrt{2}}{2}i$. For graphical support, show that the graph of $y_1 = 4x^2 - 12x + 11$ has no x-intercepts; therefore, there are no real solutions.

47. Use the quadratic formula to solve $\dfrac{1}{3}x^2 + \dfrac{1}{4}x - 3 = 0 \Rightarrow 12\left(\dfrac{1}{3}x^2 + \dfrac{1}{4}x - 3 = 0\right) \Rightarrow 4x^2 + 3x - 36 = 0$; therefore, $a = 4, b = 3$ and $c = -36$. $x = \dfrac{-3 \pm \sqrt{(3)^2 - 4(4)(-36)}}{2(4)} = \dfrac{-3 \pm \sqrt{9 + 576}}{8} = \dfrac{-3 \pm \sqrt{585}}{8} \Rightarrow x = \dfrac{-3 \pm 3\sqrt{65}}{8}$. For graphical support, show that the graph of $y_1 = 4x^2 + 3x - 36$ has x-intercepts $x = \dfrac{-3 \pm 3\sqrt{65}}{8}$; $x \approx -3.4$ and 2.6.

49. Use the quadratic formula to solve $(3 - x)^2 = 25 \Rightarrow 9 - 6x + x^2 = 25 \Rightarrow x^2 - 6x - 16 = 0$; therefore, $a = 1, b = -6$ and $c = -16$. $x = \dfrac{-(-6) \pm \sqrt{(-6)^2 - 4(1)(-16)}}{2(1)} = \dfrac{6 \pm \sqrt{36 + 64}}{2} = \dfrac{6 \pm \sqrt{100}}{2} \Rightarrow \dfrac{6 \pm 10}{2} \Rightarrow$ $x = -2$ or 8. For graphical support, show that the graph of $y_1 = x^2 - 6x - 16$ has x-intercepts $x = -2$ and 8.

51. Use the quadratic formula to solve $2x^2 - 4x = 1 \Rightarrow 2x^2 - 4x - 1 = 0$; therefore $a = 2, b = -4$ and $c = -1$. $x = \dfrac{-(-4) \pm \sqrt{(-4)^2 - 4(2)(-1)}}{2(2)} = \dfrac{4 \pm \sqrt{16 + 8}}{4} = \dfrac{4 \pm \sqrt{24}}{4} \Rightarrow \dfrac{4 \pm 2\sqrt{6}}{4} = \dfrac{2(2 \pm \sqrt{6})}{4} \Rightarrow x = \dfrac{2 \pm \sqrt{6}}{2}$. For graphical support, show that the graph of $y_1 = 2x^2 - 4x - 1$ has x-intercepts $x = \dfrac{2 \pm \sqrt{6}}{2}$; $x \approx -0.2$ and 2.2.

53. Use the quadratic formula to solve $x^2 = -1 - x \Rightarrow x^2 + x + 1 = 0$; therefore, $a = 1, b = 1$ and $c = 1$. $x = \dfrac{-1 \pm \sqrt{(1)^2 - 4(1)(1)}}{2(1)} = \dfrac{-1 \pm \sqrt{1 - 4}}{2} = \dfrac{-1 \pm \sqrt{-3}}{2} \Rightarrow x = -\dfrac{1}{2} \pm \dfrac{\sqrt{3}}{2}i$. For graphical support, show that the graph of $y_1 = x^2 + x + 1$ has no x-intercepts; therefore, there are no real solutions.

55. Use the quadratic formula to solve $4x^2 - 20x + 25 = 0$; therefore, $a = 4, b = -20$ and $c = 25$. $x = \dfrac{-(-20) \pm \sqrt{(-20)^2 - 4(4)(25)}}{2(4)} = \dfrac{20 \pm \sqrt{400 - 400}}{8} = \dfrac{20 \pm 0}{8} \Rightarrow x = \dfrac{20}{8} = \dfrac{5}{2}$. For graphical support, show that the graph of $y_1 = 4x^2 - 20x + 25$ has x-intercept $x = \dfrac{5}{2} = 2.5$.

57. Use the quadratic formula to solve $-3x^2 + 4x + 4 = 0$; therefore, $a = -3, b = 4$ and $c = 4$. $x = \dfrac{-4 \pm \sqrt{(4)^2 - 4(-3)(4)}}{2(-3)} = \dfrac{-4 \pm \sqrt{16 + 48}}{-6} = \dfrac{-4 \pm \sqrt{64}}{-6} = \dfrac{-4 \pm 8}{-6} = \dfrac{-2(2 \pm 4)}{-6} = \dfrac{2 \pm 4}{3} \Rightarrow x = -\dfrac{2}{3}$ or 2. For graphical support, show that the graph of $y_1 = -3x^2 + 4x + 4$ has x-intercepts $x = -\dfrac{2}{3}$ or 2; $x \approx -0.7$ and 2.

59. Use the quadratic formula to solve $(x+5)(x-6)=(2x-1)(x-4) \Rightarrow x^2-x-30=2x^2-9x+4 \Rightarrow$

$x^2-8x+34=0$; therefore, $a=1$, $b=-8$, and $c=34$. $x=\dfrac{-(-8)\pm\sqrt{(-8)^2-4(1)(34)}}{2(1)}=\dfrac{8\pm\sqrt{64-136}}{2}=$

$\dfrac{8\pm\sqrt{-72}}{2}=\dfrac{8\pm 6i\sqrt{2}}{2}=\dfrac{2(4\pm 3i\sqrt{2})}{2} \Rightarrow x=4\pm 3i\sqrt{2}$. For graphical support, show that the graph of

$y_1=2x^2-9x+4$ has no x-intercepts; therefore, there are no real solutions.

61. $x^2-2x=2 \Rightarrow x^2-2x+1=2+1 \Rightarrow (x-1)^2=3 \Rightarrow x-1=\pm\sqrt{3} \Rightarrow x=1\pm\sqrt{3}$

63. $2x^2+6x-3=0 \Rightarrow x^2+3x-\dfrac{3}{2}=0 \Rightarrow x^2+3x=\dfrac{3}{2} \Rightarrow x^2+3x+\dfrac{9}{4}=\dfrac{3}{2}+\dfrac{9}{4} \Rightarrow \left(x+\dfrac{3}{2}\right)^2=\dfrac{15}{4} \Rightarrow$

$\left(x+\dfrac{3}{2}\right)=\pm\sqrt{\dfrac{15}{4}} \Rightarrow x=-\dfrac{3}{2}\pm\dfrac{\sqrt{15}}{2} \Rightarrow x=\dfrac{-3\pm\sqrt{15}}{2}$

65. $x(x-1)=3 \Rightarrow x^2-x=3 \Rightarrow x^2-x+\dfrac{1}{4}=3+\dfrac{1}{4} \Rightarrow \left(x-\dfrac{1}{2}\right)^2=\dfrac{13}{4} \Rightarrow x-\dfrac{1}{2}=\pm\sqrt{\dfrac{13}{4}} \Rightarrow x=\dfrac{1\pm\sqrt{13}}{2}$

67. $2x^2-x+3=0 \Rightarrow x^2-\dfrac{1}{2}x+\dfrac{3}{2}=0 \Rightarrow x^2-\dfrac{1}{2}x=-\dfrac{3}{2} \Rightarrow x^2-\dfrac{1}{2}x+\dfrac{1}{16}=-\dfrac{3}{2}+\dfrac{1}{16} \Rightarrow \left(x-\dfrac{1}{4}\right)^2=\dfrac{-23}{16} \Rightarrow$

$\left(x-\dfrac{1}{4}\right)=\pm\sqrt{\dfrac{-23}{16}} \Rightarrow x=\dfrac{1}{4}\pm i\dfrac{\sqrt{23}}{4}$

69. For the equation $x^2+8x+16=0$; $a=1$, $b=8$, and $c=16$; therefore, the discriminant is

$(8)^2-4(1)(16)=64-64=0$. Because the discriminant is 0, there is 1 real solution. Since a, b, and c are

nonzero integers and the discriminant is a square of an integer the solution is rational.

71. For the equation $4x^2=6x+3 \Rightarrow 4x^2-6x-3=0$; $a=4$, $b=-6$, and $c=-3$; therefore, the discriminant is

$(-6)^2-4(4)(-3)=36+48=84$. Because the discriminant is positive, there are 2 real solutions. Since a, b,

and c are nonzero integers and the discriminant is not the square of an integer, the solutions are irrational.

73. For the equation $9x^2+11x+4=0$; $a=9$, $b=11$, and $c=4$; therefore, the discriminant is

$(11)^2-4(9)(4)=121-144=-23$. Because the discriminant is negative, there are no real solutions.

75. If $x=4$ or 5, then $(x-4)(x-5)=0 \Rightarrow x^2-9x+20=0$; and $a=1$, $b=-9$, and $c=20$.

77. If $x=1-\sqrt{2}$ or $1+\sqrt{2}$, then $\left(x-(1-\sqrt{2})\right)\left(x-(1+\sqrt{2})\right)=0 \Rightarrow (x-1+\sqrt{2})(x-1-\sqrt{2})=0 \Rightarrow$

$x^2-x-x\sqrt{2}-x+1+\sqrt{2}+x\sqrt{2}-\sqrt{2}-2=0 \Rightarrow x^2-2x-1=0$; and $a=1$, $b=-2$, and $c=-1$.

79. If $x=2i$ or $-2i$, then $(x-2i)(x+2i)=0 \Rightarrow x^2-4i^2=0 \Rightarrow x^2+4=0$; and $a=1$, $b=0$, $c=4$.

81. If $x=2-\sqrt{5}$ or $2+\sqrt{5}$, then $\left(x-(2-\sqrt{5})\right)\left(x-(2+\sqrt{5})\right)=0 \Rightarrow (x-2+\sqrt{5})(x-2-\sqrt{5})=0 \Rightarrow$

$x^2-2x-x\sqrt{5}-2x+4+2\sqrt{5}+x\sqrt{5}-2\sqrt{5}-5=0 \Rightarrow x^2-4x-1=0$; and $a=1$, $b=-4$, $c=-1$.

83. The graph of the function $f(x) = ax^2 + bx + c$ is a parabola, $a < 0$ will make the parabola open downward, and $b^2 - 4ac = 0$ gives us 1 real solution or 1 x-intercept. See Figure 83.

85. The graph of the function $f(x) = ax^2 + bx + c$ is a parabola, $a < 0$ will make the parabola open downward, and $b^2 - 4ac < 0$ gives us no real solutions or no x-intercepts. See Figure 85.

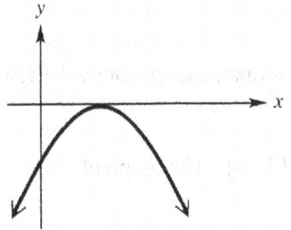

Figure 83

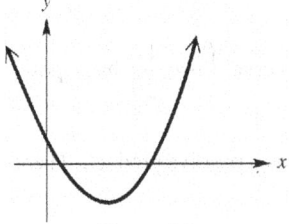

Figure 85   Figure 87

87. The graph of the function $f(x) = ax^2 + bx + c$ is a parabola, $a > 0$ will make the parabola open upward, and $b^2 - 4ac > 0$ gives us 2 real solutions or 2 x-intercepts. See Figure 87.

89. From the graph, $f(x) = 0$ when 2 or 4.

91. From the graph, $f(x) > 0$ for the interval $(-\infty, 2) \cup (4, \infty)$.

93. From the graph, $g(x) < 0$ for the interval $(-\infty, 3) \cup (3, \infty)$.

95. From the graph, $h(x) > 0$ always, but no x-intercepts; therefore, the solution is $(-\infty, \infty)$.

97. From the graph, $h(x) = 0$ has no real solutions, because $h(x)$ has no x-intercepts. The graph is completely above the x-axis; therefore, there are two nonreal complex solutions.

99. The x-coordinate of the vertex of the graph of $y = f(x)$ is the midpoint of the x-intercepts or $\frac{2+4}{2} = 3$.

101. From the graph, $y = g(x)$ will have a y-intercept and it will be negative.

103. (a) First, set $x^2 + 4x + 3 = 0$, then $(x+1)(x+3) = 0$ and the endpoints will be $x = \{-3, -1\}$. The numbers -3 and -1 divide the number line into 3 intervals. The interval $(-\infty, -3)$ has a positive product, the interval $(-3, -1)$ has a negative product, and the interval $(-1, \infty)$ has a positive product. Therefore, $x^2 + 4x + 3 \geq 0$ for the interval $(-\infty, -3] \cup [-1, \infty)$. The graph of $y_1 = x^2 + 4x + 3$ intersects or is above the x-axis for the interval $(-\infty, -3] \cup [-1, \infty)$.

(b) First, set $x^2 + 4x + 3 = 0$, then $(x+1)(x+3) = 0$ and the endpoints will be $x = \{-3, -1\}$. The numbers -3 and -1 divide the number line into 3 intervals. The interval $(-\infty, -3)$ has a positive product, the interval $(-3, -1)$ has a negative product, and the interval $(-1, \infty)$ has a positive product. Therefore,

104 CHAPTER 3 Polynomial Functions

$x^2+4x+3<0$ for the interval $(-3,-1)$. The graph of $y_1 = x^2+4x+3$ is below the x-axis for the interval $(-3,-1)$.

105. (a) First, $2x^2-9x>-4 \Rightarrow 2x^2-9x+4>0$, now set $2x^2-9x+4=0$ then $(2x-1)(x-4)=0$ and the endpoints will be $x=\frac{1}{2}$ and $x=4$. The numbers $\frac{1}{2}$ and 4 divide the number line into 3 intervals. The interval $\left(-\infty,\frac{1}{2}\right)$ has a positive product, the interval $\left(\frac{1}{2},4\right)$ has a negative product, and the interval $(4,\infty)$ has a positive product. Therefore, $2x^2-9x>-4$ for the interval $\left(-\infty,\frac{1}{2}\right)\cup(4,\infty)$. The graph of $y_1 = 2x^2-9x+4$ is above the x-axis for the interval $\left(-\infty,\frac{1}{2}\right)\cup(4,\infty)$.

(b) First, $2x^2-9x\leq-4 \Rightarrow 2x^2-9x+4\leq 0$, now set $2x^2-9x+4=0$ then $(2x-1)(x-4)=0$ and the endpoints will be $x=\frac{1}{2}$ and $x=4$. The numbers $\frac{1}{2}$ and 4 divide the number line into 3 intervals. The interval $\left(-\infty,\frac{1}{2}\right)$ has a positive product, the interval $\left(\frac{1}{2},4\right)$ has a negative product, and the interval $(4,\infty)$ has a positive product. Therefore, $2x^2-9x\leq-4$ for the interval $\left(\frac{1}{2},4\right)$. The graph of $y_1 = 2x^2-9x+4$ intersects or is below the x-axis for the interval $\left[\frac{1}{2},4\right]$.

107. (a) First, set $-x^2-x=0$, then $-x(x+1)=0$ and the endpoints will be $x=-1$ and $x=0$. The numbers -1 and 0 divide the number line into 3 intervals. The interval $(-\infty,-1)$ has a negative product, the interval $(-1,0)$ has a positive product, and the interval $(0,\infty)$ has a negative product. Therefore, $-x^2-x\leq 0$ for the interval $(-\infty,-1]\cup[0,\infty)$. The graph of $y_1 = -x^2-x$ intersects or is below the x-axis for the interval $(-\infty,-1]\cup[0,\infty)$.

(b) First, set $-x^2-x=0$, then $-x(x+1)=0$ and the endpoints will be $x=-1$ and $x=0$. The numbers -1 and 0 divide the number line into 3 intervals. The interval $(-\infty,-1)$ has a negative product, the interval $(-1,0)$ has a positive product, and the interval $(0,\infty)$ has a negative product. Therefore, $-x^2-x>0$ for the interval $(-1,0)$. The graph of $y_1 = -x^2-x$ is above the x-axis for the interval $(-1,0)$.

109. (a) First, set $x^2-x+1=0$, then by the quadratic formula $x=\frac{-(-1)\pm\sqrt{(-1)^2-4(1)(1)}}{2(1)}=\frac{1\pm\sqrt{-3}}{2} \Rightarrow x=\frac{1}{2}\pm\frac{\sqrt{3}}{2}i$. The inequality has no real solutions, the graph is a parabola opening upward

which does not intersect, but is completely above the x-axis. Therefore, $x^2 - x + 1 < 0$ never happens and the solution is $\emptyset$.

(b) First, set $x^2 - x + 1 = 0$, then by the quadratic formula $x = \dfrac{-(-1) \pm \sqrt{(-1)^2 - 4(1)(1)}}{2(1)} = \dfrac{1 \pm \sqrt{-3}}{2} \Rightarrow x = \dfrac{1}{2} \pm \dfrac{\sqrt{3}}{2}i$. The graph of this equation is a parabola opening upward, has no real solutions, and does not intersect, but is completely above the x-axis. Therefore, $x^2 - x + 1 \geq 0$ for all values of x and the solution is the interval $(-\infty, \infty)$.

111. (a) First, $2x + 1 \geq x^2 \Rightarrow x^2 - 2x - 1 \leq 0$, now set $x^2 - 2x - 1 = 0$, then by the quadratic formula

$x = \dfrac{-(-2) \pm \sqrt{(-2)^2 - 4(1)(-1)}}{2(1)} = \dfrac{2 \pm \sqrt{8}}{2} = \dfrac{2(1 \pm \sqrt{2})}{2} \Rightarrow x = 1 \pm \sqrt{2}$, and the endpoints will be

$x = 1 - \sqrt{2}$ and $x = 1 + \sqrt{2}$. The numbers $1 - \sqrt{2}$ and $1 + \sqrt{2}$ divide the number line into 3 intervals. The interval $(-\infty, 1 - \sqrt{2})$ has a positive product, the interval $(1 - \sqrt{2}, 1 + \sqrt{2})$ has a negative product, and the interval $(1 + \sqrt{2}, \infty)$ has a positive product. Therefore, $x^2 - 2x - 1 \leq 0$ for the interval $[1 - \sqrt{2}, 1 + \sqrt{2}]$.

The graph of $y_1 = x^2 - 2x - 1$ intersects or is below the x-axis for the interval $[1 - \sqrt{2}, 1 + \sqrt{2}]$.

(b) First, $2x + 1 < x^2 \Rightarrow x^2 - 2x - 1 > 0$, now set $x^2 - 2x - 1 = 0$, then by the quadratic formula

$x = \dfrac{-(-2) \pm \sqrt{(-2)^2 - 4(1)(-1)}}{2(1)} = \dfrac{2 \pm \sqrt{8}}{2} = \dfrac{2(1 \pm \sqrt{2})}{2} \Rightarrow x = 1 \pm \sqrt{2}$, and the endpoints will be

$x = 1 - \sqrt{2}$ and $x = 1 + \sqrt{2}$. The numbers $1 - \sqrt{2}$ and $1 + \sqrt{2}$ divide the number line into 3 intervals. The interval $(-\infty, 1 - \sqrt{2})$ has a positive product, the interval $(1 - \sqrt{2}, 1 + \sqrt{2})$ has a negative product, and the interval $(1 + \sqrt{2}, \infty)$ has a positive product. Therefore, $x^2 - 2x - 1 > 0$ for the interval

$(-\infty, 1 - \sqrt{2}) \cup (1 + \sqrt{2}, \infty)$. The graph of $y_1 = x^2 - 2x - 1$ is above the x-axis for the interval

$(-\infty, 1 - \sqrt{2}) \cup (1 + \sqrt{2}, \infty)$.

113. (a) First, $x - 3x^2 > -1 \Rightarrow 3x^2 - x - 1 < 0$, now set $3x^2 - x - 1 = 0$, then by the quadratic formula

$x = \dfrac{1 \pm \sqrt{(-1)^2 - 4(3)(-1)}}{2(3)} \Rightarrow x = \dfrac{1 \pm \sqrt{13}}{6}$, and the endpoints will be $x = \dfrac{1 - \sqrt{13}}{6}$ and

$x = \dfrac{1 + \sqrt{13}}{6}$. The numbers $\dfrac{1 - \sqrt{13}}{6}$ and $\dfrac{1 + \sqrt{13}}{6}$ divide the number line into 3 intervals. The

interval $\left(-\infty, \dfrac{1 - \sqrt{13}}{6}\right)$ has a positive product, the interval $\left(\dfrac{1 - \sqrt{13}}{6}, \dfrac{1 + \sqrt{13}}{6}\right)$ has a negative

106   CHAPTER 3   Polynomial Functions

product, and the interval $\left(\dfrac{1+\sqrt{13}}{6},\infty\right)$ has positive product. Therefore, $3x^2-x-1<0$ for the interval $\left(\dfrac{1-\sqrt{13}}{6},\dfrac{1+\sqrt{13}}{6}\right)$. The graph of $y_1=3x^2-x-1$ is below the x-axis for the interval $\left(\dfrac{1-\sqrt{13}}{6},\dfrac{1+\sqrt{13}}{6}\right)$.

(b) First, $x-3x^2\le -1 \Rightarrow 3x^2-x-1\ge 0$, now set $3x^2-x-1=0$, then by the quadratic formula

$x=\dfrac{1\pm\sqrt{(-1)^2-4(3)(-1)}}{2(3)} \Rightarrow x=\dfrac{1\pm\sqrt{13}}{6}$, and the endpoints will be $x=\dfrac{1-\sqrt{13}}{6}$ and

$x=\dfrac{1+\sqrt{13}}{6}$. The numbers $\dfrac{1-\sqrt{13}}{6}$ and $\dfrac{1+\sqrt{13}}{6}$ divide the number line into 3 intervals. The

interval $\left(-\infty,\dfrac{1-\sqrt{13}}{6}\right)$ has a positive product, the interval $\left(\dfrac{1-\sqrt{13}}{6},\dfrac{1+\sqrt{13}}{6}\right)$ has a negative

product, and the interval $\left(\dfrac{1+\sqrt{13}}{6},\infty\right)$ has positive product. Therefore, $3x^2-x-1\ge 0$ for the

intervals $\left(-\infty,\dfrac{1-\sqrt{13}}{6}\right)$ or $\left(\dfrac{1+\sqrt{13}}{6},\infty\right)$. The graph of $y_1=3x^2-x-1$ is above the x-axis for the

interval $\left(-\infty,\dfrac{1-\sqrt{13}}{6}\right)\cup\left(\dfrac{1+\sqrt{13}}{6},\infty\right)$.

115. $s=\dfrac{1}{2}gt^2 \Rightarrow \dfrac{2s}{g}=t^2 \Rightarrow t=\pm\sqrt{\dfrac{2s}{g}} \Rightarrow t=\pm\dfrac{\sqrt{2sg}}{g}$

117. $a^2+b^2=c^2 \Rightarrow a^2=c^2-b^2 \Rightarrow a=\pm\sqrt{c^2-b^2}$

119. $S=4\pi r^2 \Rightarrow \dfrac{S}{4\pi}=r^2 \Rightarrow r=\pm\sqrt{\dfrac{S}{4\pi}} \Rightarrow r=\pm\dfrac{\sqrt{S\pi}}{2\pi}$

121. $V=e^3 \Rightarrow e=\sqrt[3]{V}$

123. $F=\dfrac{kMv^4}{r} \Rightarrow \dfrac{Fr}{kM}=v^4 \Rightarrow v=\pm\sqrt[4]{\dfrac{Fr}{kM}} \Rightarrow v=\pm\dfrac{\sqrt[4]{FrkMkMkM}}{kM} \Rightarrow v=\pm\dfrac{\sqrt[4]{Frk^3M^3}}{kM}$

125. $P=\dfrac{E^2R}{(r+R)^2} \Rightarrow P(r+R)^2=E^2R \Rightarrow P(r^2+2rR+R^2)-E^2R=0 \Rightarrow Pr^2+2\,Pr\,R+PR^2-E^2R=0$

$\Rightarrow PR^2+(2\,Pr-E^2)R+Pr^2=0$. Now use the quadratic formula:

$$R = \frac{-(2Pr - E^2) \pm \sqrt{4P^2r^2 - 4E^2 Pr + E^4 - 4(P)(Pr^2)}}{2(P)} = \frac{E^2 - 2Pr \pm \sqrt{E^4 - 4E^2 Pr}}{2P} \Rightarrow$$

$$R = \frac{E^2 - 2Pr \pm E\sqrt{E^2 - 4Pr}}{2P}$$

127. Use the quadratic formula: $x = \frac{-y \pm \sqrt{y^2 - 4(1)(y^2)}}{2(1)} = \frac{-y \pm \sqrt{-3y^2}}{2} \Rightarrow x = -\frac{y}{2} \pm \frac{\sqrt{3}}{2} yi.$ For $y^2 + xy + x^2 = 0$

 use the quadratic formula: $y = \frac{-x \pm \sqrt{x^2 - 4(1)(x^2)}}{2(1)} = \frac{-x \pm \sqrt{-3x^2}}{2} \Rightarrow y = -\frac{x}{2} \pm \frac{\sqrt{3}}{2} xi.$

129. $3y^2 + 4xy - 9x^2 = -1 \Rightarrow -9x^2 + 4yx + (3y^2 + 1) = 0$. Now use the quadratic formula:

$$x = \frac{-4y \pm \sqrt{(4y)^2 - 4(-9)(3y^2 + 1)}}{2(-9)} = \frac{-4y \pm \sqrt{16y^2 + 108y^2 + 36}}{-18} =$$

$$\frac{-4y \pm \sqrt{124y^2 + 36}}{-18} = \frac{-4y \pm \sqrt{4(31y^2 + 9)}}{-18} = \frac{-4y \pm 2\sqrt{31y^2 + 9}}{-18} \Rightarrow x = \frac{2y \pm \sqrt{31y^2 + 9}}{9}$$

$3y^2 + 4xy - 9x^2 = -1 \Rightarrow 3y^2 + 4xy + (-9x^2 + 1) = 0$. Now use the quadratic formula:

$$x = \frac{-4x \pm \sqrt{(4x)^2 - 4(3)(-9x^2 + 1)}}{2(3)} = \frac{-4x \pm \sqrt{16x^2 + 108x^2 - 12}}{6} =$$

$$\frac{-4x \pm \sqrt{124x^2 - 12}}{6} = \frac{-4x \pm \sqrt{4(31x^2 - 3)}}{6} = \frac{-4x \pm 2\sqrt{31x^2 - 3}}{6} \Rightarrow y = \frac{-2x \pm \sqrt{31x^2 - 3}}{3}$$

131. (a) $f(0) = \frac{4}{5}(0-10)^2 + 80 = 160$ and $f(2) = \frac{4}{5}(2-10)^2 + 80 = 131.2$. Initially when the person stops exercising the heart rate is 160 beats per minute, and after 2 minutes the heart rate has dropped to about 131 beats per minute.

 (b) Graph $Y_1 = 100$, $Y_2 = 0.8(x-10)^2 + 80$ and $Y_3 = 120$ (Not shown). The person's heart rate is between 100 and 120 when the graph of Y_2 is between Y_1 and Y_3. This occurs between approximately 2.9 minutes and 5 minutes after the person stops exercising.

Reviewing Basic Concepts (Sections 3.1—3.3)

1. $(5+6i) - (2-4i) - 3i = 5 + 6i - 2 + 4i - 3i = 3 + 7i$

2. $i(5+i)(5-i) = i(25 - i^2) = i(25 - (-1)) = 26i$

3. $\frac{-10-10i}{2+3i} \cdot \frac{2-3i}{2-3i} = \frac{-20 + 30i - 20i + 30i^2}{4 - 9i^2} = \frac{-20 + 10i - 30}{4+9} = -\frac{50}{13} + \frac{10}{13}i$

4. See Figure 4.

[-10,10] by [-10,10]
Xscl = 1   Yscl = 1

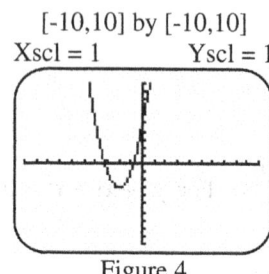

Figure 4

5. Use the vertex formula: $\dfrac{-b}{2a} = \dfrac{-8}{2(2)} = -2,$ now input $x = -2$ into the equation: $2(-2)^2 + 8(-2) + 5 = -3.$ The vertex is $(-2,-3)$ and it is a minimum because $a = 2,$ which is positive; therefore, the parabola opens up.

6. Since the vertex is $(-2,-3)$ and the graph is a parabola opening up, the axis of symmetry is $x = -2.$

7. From the graph, the domain is $(-\infty, \infty)$ and the range is $[-3, \infty).$

8. $9x^2 = 25 \Rightarrow x^2 = \dfrac{25}{9} \Rightarrow x = \pm\dfrac{5}{3}$

9. $3x^2 - 5x = 2 \Rightarrow 3x^2 - 5x - 2 = 0 \Rightarrow (3x+1)(x-2) = 0 \Rightarrow 3x+1 = 0$ or $x - 2 = 0 \Rightarrow x = -\dfrac{1}{3}$ and $x = 2.$

10. For $-x^2 + x + 3 = 0$ use the quadratic formula: $x = \dfrac{-1 \pm \sqrt{1^2 - 4(-1)(3)}}{2(-1)} = \dfrac{-1 \pm \sqrt{13}}{-2} \Rightarrow x = \dfrac{1 \pm \sqrt{13}}{2}.$

11. First, set $3x^2 - 5x - 2 = 0,$ then $g(x)$ and the endpoints will be $x = -\dfrac{1}{3}$ and $x = 2.$ The numbers $-\dfrac{1}{3}$ and 2 divide the number line into 3 intervals. The interval $\left(-\infty, -\dfrac{1}{3}\right)$ has a positive product, the interval $\left(-\dfrac{1}{3}, 2\right)$ has a negative product, and the interval $(2, \infty)$ has a positive product. Therefore, $3x^2 - 5x - 2 \leq 0$ for the interval $\left[-\dfrac{1}{3}, 2\right].$ The graph of $y_1 = 3x^2 - 5x - 2$ intersects or is below the x-axis for the interval $\left[-\dfrac{1}{3}, 2\right].$

12. First, set $x^2 - x - 3 = 0$ then by the quadratic formula $x = \dfrac{-(-1) \pm \sqrt{(-1)^2 - 4(1)(-3)}}{2(1)} \Rightarrow x = \dfrac{1 \pm \sqrt{13}}{2}$ and the endpoints will be $x = \dfrac{1 - \sqrt{13}}{2}$ and $x = \dfrac{1 + \sqrt{13}}{2}.$ The numbers $\dfrac{1 - \sqrt{13}}{2}$ and $\dfrac{1 + \sqrt{13}}{2}$ divide the number line into 3 intervals. The interval $\left(-\infty, \dfrac{1 - \sqrt{13}}{2}\right)$ has a positive product, the interval $\left(\dfrac{1 - \sqrt{13}}{2}, \dfrac{1 + \sqrt{13}}{2}\right)$ has a negative product, and the interval $\left(\dfrac{1 + \sqrt{13}}{2}, \infty\right)$ has a positive product. Therefore, $x^2 - x - 3 > 0$ for the

interval $\left(-\infty, \frac{1-\sqrt{13}}{2}\right) \cup \left(\frac{1+\sqrt{13}}{2}, \infty\right)$. The graph of $y_1 = x^2 - x - 3$ is above the x-axis for the interval $\left(-\infty, \frac{1-\sqrt{13}}{2}\right) \cup \left(\frac{1+\sqrt{13}}{2}, \infty\right)$.

13. First, $x(3x-1) \leq -4 \Rightarrow 3x^2 - x + 4 \leq 0$, now set $3x^2 - x + 4 = 0$, then by the quadratic formula $x = \frac{-(-1) \pm \sqrt{(-1)^2 - 4(3)(4)}}{2(3)} = \frac{1 \pm \sqrt{-47}}{6} \Rightarrow x = \frac{1}{6} \pm \frac{\sqrt{47}}{6}i$. The inequality has no real solutions, the graph is a parabola opening upward which does not intersect, but is completely above the x-axis. Therefore, $3x^2 - x + 4 \leq 0$ never happens and the solution is $\emptyset$.

Section 3.4 Applications of Quadratic Functions and Models

1. The y-coordinate of the vertex is maximum y-value. Using the vertex formula yields:
$x = -\frac{b}{2a} = -\frac{32}{2(-16)} = 1$. If $x = 1$, then $y = -16(1)^2 + 32(1) + 100 = 116 \Rightarrow$ the maximum y-value is 116.

3. The y-coordinate of the vertex is minimum y-value. Using the vertex formula yields:
$x = -\frac{b}{2a} = -\frac{-24}{2(3)} = 4$. If $x = 4$, then $y = 3(4)^2 - 24(4) + 50 = 2 \Rightarrow$ the minimum y-value is 2.

5. $-4x^2 + 5x = 1 \Rightarrow 4x^2 - 5x + 1 = 0 \Rightarrow (4x-1)(x-1) = 0 \Rightarrow (4x-1) = 0 \Rightarrow x = \frac{1}{4}$ and $(x-1) = 0 \Rightarrow x = 1$.

7. $\frac{1}{2}x^2 + 3 = 6x \Rightarrow \frac{1}{2}x^2 - 6x + 3 = 0$. Using the quadratic equation we have the following:
$\frac{6 \pm \sqrt{(-6)^2 - 4\left(\frac{1}{2}\right)(3)}}{2\left(\frac{1}{2}\right)} = 6 \pm \sqrt{30}$

9. A, The area of a rectangle is $L \cdot W = A \Rightarrow x(2x+2) = 40,000$.

11. (a) $30 - x$ would be the other number.

    (b) Since both numbers are positive and their sum is 30, the restrictions are $0 < x < 30$.

    (c) Multiplying $x(30-x)$ would give the function $P(x) = 30x - x^2 \Rightarrow P(x) = -x^2 + 30x$.

    (d) Using the Vertex formula yields $x = \frac{-b}{2a} = \frac{-30}{2(-1)} \Rightarrow x = 15$. If $x = 15$, then $y = 30 - (15) \Rightarrow y = 15$.

    Also, if $x = 15$ the maximum product is $P(15) = -(15)^2 + 30(15) = -225 + 450 = 225$. The graph of $y = -x^2 + 30x$ has a vertex point of $(15, 15)$, which supports the result.

13. Perimeter of fence $= 2l + 2w = 1000 \Rightarrow l = 500 - w$. If $A = l \cdot w$ then $A = (500-w)w = 500w - w^2$. This is a parabola opening downward and by the vertex formula, the maximum area occurs when $w = -\frac{b}{2a} = -\frac{500}{2(-1)} = 250$.

The dimensions that maximize area are 250 ft. by 250 ft.

15. (a) $640-2x$ would be the other side.

(b) Since all three numbers are positive, their sum is 640, and two of them are x, the restrictions are $0 < 2x < 640 \Rightarrow 0 < x < 320$.

(c) Multiplying $x(640-2x)$ would give the function $A(x) = 640x - 2x^2 \Rightarrow A(x) = -2x^2 + 640x$.

(d) See Figure 15. From the graph, between 57.04 ft and 85.17 ft or between 234.17 ft and 262.96 ft, will give an area between 30,000 and 40,000 feet.

(e) Using the Vertex formula yields $x = \dfrac{-b}{2a} = \dfrac{-640}{2(-2)} \Rightarrow x = 160$. If $x = 160$, then $y = 640 - 2(160) \Rightarrow y = 320$. Also, if $x = 160$, the maximum product is $A(160) = -2(160)^2 + 640(160) = -51,200 + 102,400 \Rightarrow A(x) = 51,200$. The graph of $y = -2x^2 + 640x$ has a vertex point of $(160, 320)$, which supports the result.

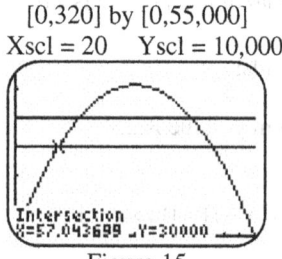

[0,320] by [0,55,000]
Xscl = 20   Yscl = 10,000

Figure 15

17. (a) $s(1) = -16(1)^2 + 44(1) + 4 = 32$; the baseball is 32 feet high after 1 second.

(b) For $s(t) = -16t^2 + 44t + 4$, the vertex formula gives $t = -\dfrac{b}{2a} = -\dfrac{44}{2(-16)} = 1.375$ and $f(1.375) = -16(1.375)^2 + 44(1.375) + 4 = 34.25$; the maximum height is 34.25 feet.

19. The height when it hits the ground will be $0 \Rightarrow 75 - 16t^2 = 0 \Rightarrow 16t^2 = 75 \Rightarrow t^2 = \dfrac{75}{16} \Rightarrow$
$t = \sqrt{\dfrac{75}{16}} \Rightarrow t = \dfrac{\sqrt{75}}{4} \Rightarrow t \approx 2.2$ seconds.

21. (a) If the width is x units long, then the length is twice the width or $2x$ units long.

(b) The width will be $x - 2(2) = x - 4$ units long, and the length will be $2x - 2(2) = 2x - 4$ units long. Since both measurements are positive and 4 inches are removed from each measurement, the restrictions are $x > 4$.

(c) Since volume for the box is $V = L \cdot W \cdot H, V = (2x-4)(x-4)(2)$ and the function is $V(x) = 4x^2 - 24x + 32$.

(d) $320 = 4x^2 - 24x + 32 \Rightarrow 4x^2 - 24x - 288 = 0 \Rightarrow 4(x^2 - 6x - 72) = 0 \Rightarrow 4(x-12)(x+6) = 0$

$\Rightarrow x = -6$ or 12. Since length cannot be negative, $x = 12$. If $x = 12$, the dimensions are 8 in by 20 in. From the graph of $y = 4x^2 - 24x + 32$, when $x = 12$, $y = 320$. This support our analytical result.

(e) From the graph (not shown) of $y = 4x^2 - 24x + 32$, when $400 < y < 500, 13.0 < x < 14.2$ in.

23. The surface area of the can is $V = \pi r^2 + \pi r^2 + 2\pi r(h) \Rightarrow 54.19 = 2\pi r^2 + 2(4.25)\pi r \Rightarrow$

$6.28x^2 + 26.69x - 54.19 = 0$ now use the quadratic formula: $\dfrac{-26.69 \pm \sqrt{(26.69)^2 - 4(6.28)(-54.19)}}{2(6.28)} =$

$\dfrac{-26.69 \pm \sqrt{2073.6}}{12.56} = \dfrac{-26.69 \pm 45.537}{12.56} \Rightarrow r = -5.751$ or 1.5. Since length cannot be negative, $r = 1.5$ in.

25. If $A = s^2$, then $800 = s^2 \Rightarrow s = \sqrt{800} = 20\sqrt{2}$. Since the lawn is square, the diagonal of the lawn would equal $d^2 = (20\sqrt{2})^2 + (20\sqrt{2})^2 \Rightarrow d^2 = 1600 \Rightarrow d = 40$. The radius of the circular pattern is half the diagonal; therefore, the radius is $r = 20$ ft.

27. If we use Pythagorean Theorem, we get $h^2 + 12^2 = (2h+3)^2 \Rightarrow$

$h^2 + 144 = 4h^2 + 12h + 9 \Rightarrow 3h^2 + 12h - 135 = 0 \Rightarrow (3h + 27)(h - 5) = 0 \Rightarrow x = -9.5$. Since length cannot be negative, the height of the dock is 5 ft.

29. If we use Pythagorean Theorem, we get $(8+2)^2 + (9+4)^2 = x^2 \Rightarrow 100 + 169 = x^2 \Rightarrow$

$x^2 = 269 \Rightarrow x = \sqrt{269} \Rightarrow x \approx 16.4$. Since a 16 ft ladder will be too short, the ladder must be at least 17 ft.

31. Let $x =$ length of the picture and let $(x - 4) =$ the width of the picture. Then $A = l \cdot w \Rightarrow A = x(x - 4) \Rightarrow$

$320 = x^2 - 4x \Rightarrow x^2 - 4x - 320 = 0. \Rightarrow (x - 20)(x + 16) = 0 \Rightarrow x = 20$. Thus, the length and width of the picture is 20 and 16 inches respectively. The dimensions of the frame will include an additional 4 inches to both the length and width to yield the final dimensions of 20 inches by 24 inches.

33. (a) Since x equals the loss of 1 apartment for each $20 increase, the number of apartments rented is $80 - x$.

(b) Since each increase is $20 and x equals the number of increases, the rent per apartment is $400 + 20x$.

(c) Since revenue is the number of apartments rented times rent per apartment, we multiply a and b.

$(80 - x)(400 + 20x) = 32,000 + 1200x - 20x^2 \Rightarrow R(x) = -20x^2 + 1200x + 32,000$.

(d) $37,500 = -20x^2 + 1200x + 32,000 \Rightarrow -20x^2 + 1200x - 5,500 = 0 \Rightarrow$

$-20(x^2 - 60x + 275) = 0 \Rightarrow -20(x - 55)(x - 5) = 0 \Rightarrow x = 5$ or 55.

(e) Use the vertex formula: $x = \dfrac{-b}{2a} = \dfrac{-1200}{-40} = 30$. If $x = 30$, then the rent per apartment is

$r(30) = 400 + 20(30) = 400 + 600 = \$1000$.

35. (a) If $f(x) = 10$ and $x = 15$, then $10 = \dfrac{-16(15)^2}{0.434v^2} + 1.15(15) + 8 \Rightarrow 10 = \dfrac{-3600}{0.434v^2} + 25.25 \Rightarrow$

$-15.25 = \dfrac{-3600}{0.434v^2} \Rightarrow -6.6185v^2 = -3600 \Rightarrow v^2 = \dfrac{3600}{6.6185} \Rightarrow v \approx 23.32 \text{ft/sec}.$

(b) If $v = 23.32$, then $y = \dfrac{-16x^2}{0.434(23.32)^2} + 1.15x + 8 \Rightarrow y = -.06779x^2 + 1.15x + 8$. Graph this equation, the graph does pass through points $(0,8)$ and $(15,10)$.

(c) Use the vertex formula: $x = \dfrac{-b}{2a} = \dfrac{-1.15}{2(-0.06779)} \approx 8.48$. If $x \approx 8.48$, then the maximum height is

$f(8.48) = -0.06779(8.48)^2 + 1.15(8.48) + 8 \Rightarrow f(8.48) = 12.88 \text{ ft}.$

37. (a) If $x = 2$, then $h(2) = -0.5(2)^2 + 1.25(2) + 3 = -2 + 2.5 + 3 \Rightarrow h(2) = 3.5 \text{ ft}$.

(b) If $h(x) = 3.25$ then $3.25 = -0.5x^2 + 1.25x + 3 \Rightarrow -0.5x^2 + 1.25x - 0.25 = 0 \Rightarrow$

$4(-0.5x^2 + 1.25x + 0.25 = 0) \Rightarrow -2x^2 + 5x - 1 = 0 \Rightarrow 2x^2 - 5x + 1 = 0$ Now use the quadratic

formula: $x = \dfrac{5 \pm \sqrt{(-5)^2 - 4(2)(1)}}{2(2)} = \dfrac{5 \pm \sqrt{17}}{4} \Rightarrow x = 0.219$ or 2.281. Therefore, the frog is 3.25 feet above the ground at approximately 0.2 ft and 2.3 ft.

(c) Using the vertex formula yields $x = \dfrac{-b}{2a} = \dfrac{-1.25}{2(-0.5)} \Rightarrow x = 1.25$ ft as the horizontal distance.

(d) From part (c) the maximum height was reached when the horizontal distance was $x = 1.25$; therefore,

$h(1.25) = -0.5(1.25)^2 + 1.25(1.25) + 3 = -0.78125 + 1.5625 + 3 \Rightarrow h(1.25) \approx 3.78$ ft high.

39. If $f(x) = 800$, then $800 = \dfrac{1}{10}x^2 - 3x + 22 \Rightarrow .1x^2 - 3x - 778 - 0$. Now use the quadratic formula:

$x = \dfrac{3 \pm \sqrt{9 - 4(0.1)(-778)}}{2(0.1)} = \dfrac{3 \pm \sqrt{320.2}}{0.2} \Rightarrow x \approx 104.5$ ft/sec. Converted is $x = \dfrac{104.5(60)(60)}{5280} = 71.25$ mph.

41. (a) See Figure 41a.

(b) Using the defined function and the vertex (7, 12) yields $f(x) = a(x-7) + 12$. Now use (1, 108) to find the function; $108 = a(1-7)^2 + 12 \Rightarrow 96 = 36a \Rightarrow a = \dfrac{8}{3}$; therefore, the function is $f(x) = \dfrac{8}{3}(x-7)^2 + 12$.

(c) See Figure 41c. From the graph, we see that there is a good fit.

(d) Using the regression feature yields $g(x) \approx 2.72x^2 - 38.93x + 149.46$.

(e) For February, $x = 2$. Therefore, $f(2) = \dfrac{8}{3}(2-7)^2 + 12 \approx 79$, and

$g(2) = 2.72(2)^2 - 38.93(2) + 149.46 \approx 82$.

For June, $x = 6$. Therefore, $f(6) = \dfrac{8}{3}(6-7)^2 + 12 \approx 15$, and $g(6) = 2.72(6)^2 - 38.93(6) + 149.46 \approx 14$.

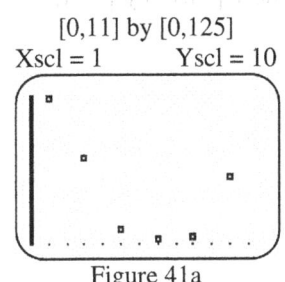

Figure 41a

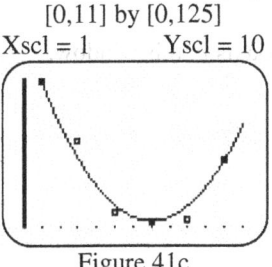

Figure 41c

43. (a) See Figure 43a.

(b) $f(45) = 0.056057(45)^2 + 1.06657(45) = 113.515425 + 47.99565 \Rightarrow x \approx 161.5$ feet. When the speed is 45 mph, the stopping distance is 161.5 feet.

(c) See Figure 43c. The model is quite good, although the stopping distances are a little low for the higher speeds.

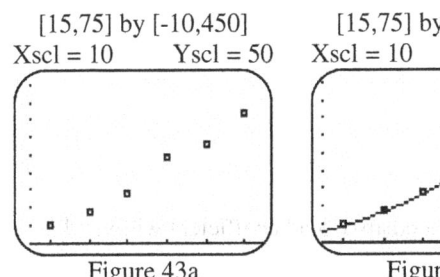

Figure 43a   Figure 43c

3.5: Higher-Degree Polynomial Functions and Graphs

1. With three extrema, the minimum degree of f is 4.

3. The points (a,b) and (c,d) are local maxima, and (e,t) is a local minimum.

5. The highest point of the graph, (a, b) is an absolute maximum.

7. The function f, has local maximum values of b and d; a local minimum value of t; and an absolute maximum value of b.

9. $P(x)$ is a positive odd-degree polynomial graph; therefore, ⌐

11. $P(x)$ is a negative odd-degree polynomial graph; therefore, ⌐

13. $P(x)$ is a positive even-degree polynomial graph; therefore, ⌣

15. $P(x)$ is a negative even-degree polynomial graph; therefore, ⌢

17. $P(x)$ is a positive even-degree polynomial graph; therefore, ⌣

19. $P(x)$ is a negative odd-degree polynomial graph; therefore, ⌐

21. The graph of $f(x) = x^n$ for $n \in$ {positive odd integers} will take the shape of the graph of $f(x) = x^3$, but gets steeper as n and x increase.

114 CHAPTER 3 Polynomial Functions

23. See Figure 23. As the odd exponent *n* gets larger, the graph *flattens out* in the window $[-1,1]$ by $[-1,1]$.

The graph of $y = x^7$ will be between $y = x^5$ and the *x*-axis in this window.

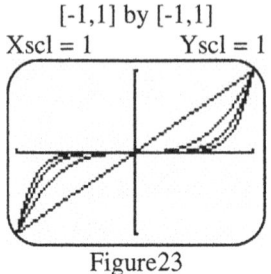

[-1,1] by [-1,1]
Xscl = 1   Yscl = 1

Figure 23

25. Graphing in various windows produces a local maximum of (2, 3.67), and a local minimum of (3, 3.5).

27. Graphing in various windows produces a local maximum of (−3.33, −1.85), and a local minimum of (−4, −2).

29. Graphing in various windows produces two *x*-intercepts, $(2.10, 0)$ and $(2.15, 0)$.

31. Graphing in various windows produces no *x*-intercept.

33. $P(x)$ is a positive odd-degree polynomial graph; therefore, D

35. $P(x)$ is a negative even-degree polynomial graph; therefore, B

37. A. The third-degree function can have at most 2 local extrema and a positive lead coefficient will yield a right side end behavior opening up.

39. From the graph, the function graphed in C has 1 real zero.

41. B and D. A third-degree function can have at most 2 local extrema.

43. From the graph, the function graphed in A has 1 *negative* real zero.

45. From the graph, the function graphed in B has a range of approximately $[-100, \infty)$.

47. False. A polynomial function of degree 3 will have at most 3 *x*-intercepts.

49. True. With a positive *y*-intercept and negative even-degree end behavior, it must have 2 *x*-intercepts.

51. True. With a negative even-degree end behavior, which is shifted up 5 units, it will have 2 *x*-intercepts.

53. False. With odd-degree end behavior, it will have at least 1 and at most 5 *x*-intercepts. Thus it may have only 1.

55. Shift the graph of $y = x^4$ three units to the left, stretch vertically by a factor of 2, and shift downward 7 units. See Figures 55a and 55b.

56. Shift the graph of $y = x^4$ one unit to the left, stretch vertically by a factor of 3, reflect across the *x*-axis, and shift upward 12 units. See Figures 56a and 56b.

Copyright © 2015 Pearson Education, Inc

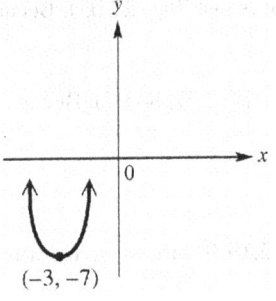

Figure 55a

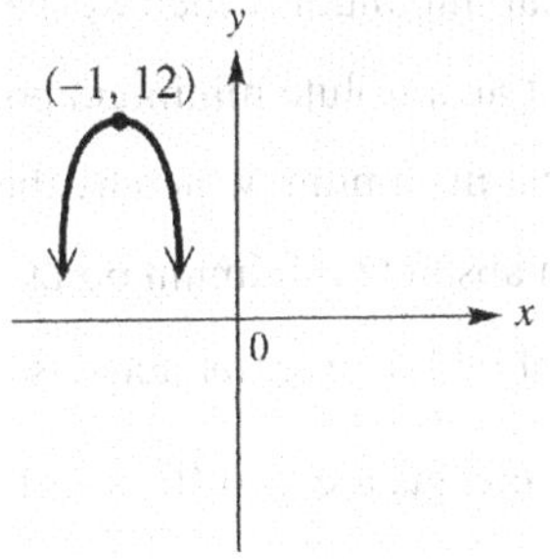

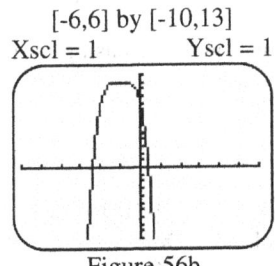

Figure 56a

[-10,10] by [-10,10]
Xscl = 1   Yscl = 1

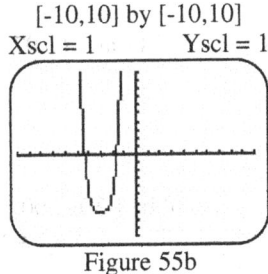

Figure 55b

[-6,6] by [-10,13]
Xscl = 1   Yscl = 1

Figure 56b

57. Shift the graph of $y = x^3$ one unit to the right, stretch vertically by a factor of 3, reflect across the x-axis, and shift upward 12 units. See Figures 57a and 57b.

58. Shift the graph of $y = x^5$ one unit to the right, stretch vertically by a factor of .5, and shift upward 13 units. See Figures 58a and 58b.

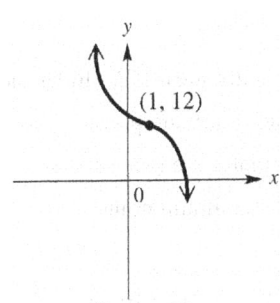

Figure 57a

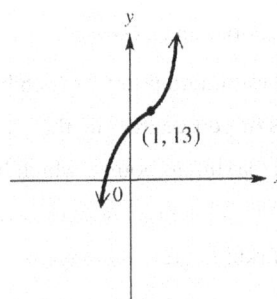

Figure 58a

[-6,6] by [-100,100]
Xscl = 1   Yscl = 10

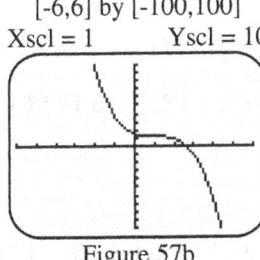

Figure 57b

[-6,6] by [-100,100]
Xscl = 1   Yscl = 10

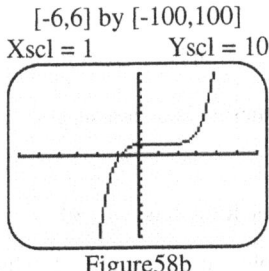

Figure 58b

59. See Figure 59 for the graph of this function.

(a) Because it is a polynomial function, its domain is $(-\infty, \infty)$.

(b) From the graph of P, there is one local minimum, which by the calculator is (−4.74, −27.03). Because the function is of odd-degree, it is not an absolute minimum point.

(c) From the graph of P, there is one local maximum, which by the calculator is (0.07, 84.07). Because the function is of odd-degree, it is not an absolute minimum point.

(d) Because the polynomial function is of odd-degree, its range is $(-\infty, \infty)$.

(e) Using the calculator we find the *x*-intercepts are $(-6, 0)$, $(-3.19, 0)$ and $(2.19, 0)$; the *y*-intercept is $(0, 84)$.

(f) From the graph and our results, the function is increasing for the interval $(-4.74, 0.07)$.

(g) From the graph and our results, the function is decreasing for the intervals $(-\infty, -4.74)$ and $(0.07, \infty)$. $(-\infty, -1.52)$ and $(2.85, \infty)$.

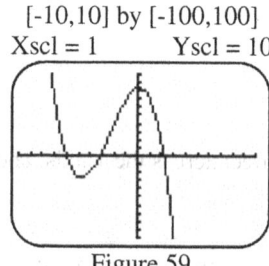
[-10,10] by [-100,100]
Xscl = 1   Yscl = 10
Figure 59

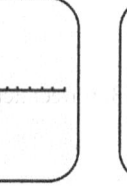

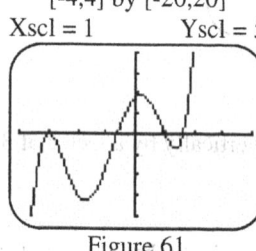
[-4,4] by [-20,20]
Xscl = 1   Yscl = 5
Figure 61

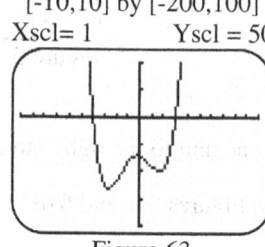
[-10,10] by [-200,100]
Xscl = 1   Yscl = 50
Figure 63

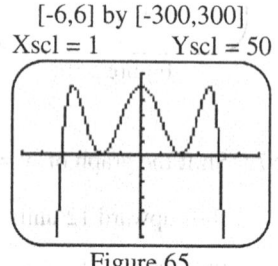
[-6,6] by [-300,300]
Xscl = 1   Yscl = 50
Figure 65

61. See Figure 61 for the graph of this function.

    (a) Because it is a polynomial function, its domain is $(-\infty, \infty)$.

    (b) From the graph of P, there are 2 local minimum points, which by the calculator are (−1.73, −16.39) and (1.35, −3.49). Because the function is of odd-degree, neither is an absolute minimum point.

    (c) From the graph of P, there are 2 local maximum points, which by the calculator are (−3, 0) and (0.17, 9.52). Because the function is of odd-degree, neither is an absolute maximum point.

    (d) Because the polynomial function is of odd-degree, its range is $(-\infty, \infty)$.

    (e) Using the calculator, we find the *x*-intercepts are $(-3, 0)$, $(-0.62, 0)$, $(1, 0)$, and $(1.62, 0)$; the *y*-intercept is $(0, 9)$.

    (f) From the graph and our results, the function is increasing on $(-\infty, -3), (-1.73, 0.17)$ and $(1.35, \infty)$.

    (g) From the graph and our results, the function is decreasing for the intervals $(-3, -1.73)$ and $(0.17, 1.35)$.

63. See Figure 63 for the graph of this function.

    (a) Because it is a polynomial function, its domain is $(-\infty, \infty)$.

    (b) From the graph of P, there is one absolute minimum point, which by the calculator is (−2.63, −132.69), and one local minimum point, which by the calculator is (1.68, −99.90).

    (c) From the graph of P, there is one local maximum point, which by the calculator is (−0.17, −71.48). Because the function is of positive even-degree, there is not an absolute maximum point.

(d) Because the positive even-degree function has an absolute minimum, given in (b), its range is $(-132.69, \infty)$.

(e) Using the calculator, we find the x-intercepts are $(-4, 0)$, and $(3, 0)$; the y-intercept is $(0, -72)$.

(f) From the graph and our results, the function is increasing for the intervals, $(-2.63, -0.17)$ and $(1.68, \infty)$.

(g) From the graph and our results, the function is decreasing for the intervals, $(-\infty, -2.63)$ and $(-0.17, 1.68)$.

65. See Figure 65 for the graph of this function.

(a) Because it is a polynomial function, its domain is $(-\infty, \infty)$.

(b) From the graph of P, there is two local minimum points, which by the calculator are $(-2, 0)$ and $(2, 0)$. Because the function is of negative even-degree, there is not an absolute minimum point.

(c) From the graph of P, there are 3 absolute maximum points, which by the calculator are $(-3.46, 256)$, $(0, 256)$, and $(3.46, 256)$.

(d) Because the negative even-degree function has an absolute maximum, its range is $(-\infty, 256]$.

(e) Using the calculator we find the x-intercepts are $(-4, 0)$, $(-2, 0)$, $(2, 0)$, and $(4, 0)$; the y-intercept is $(0, 256)$.

(f) From the graph and our results, the function is increasing on $(-\infty, -3.46)$, $(-2, 0)$ and $(2, 3.46)$.

(g) From the graph and our results, the function is decreasing on $(-3.46, -2)$, $(0, 2)$, and $(3.46, \infty)$.

67. There are many possible valid windows, through experimentation one window is [−10, 10] by [−40, 10].

69. There are many possible valid windows, through experimentation one window is [−10, 20] by [−1500, 500].

71. There are many possible valid windows, through experimentation one window is [−10, 10] by [−20, 500].

73. (a) Let x = 3 correspond to March. $f(3) = 0.0145(3)^4 - 0.426(3)^3 + 3.53(3)^2 - 6.23(3) + 72 \approx 74.8$. The average high temperature in March is $74.8°$.

Let x = 7 correspond to July. $f(7) = 0.0145(7)^4 - 0.426(7)^3 + 3.53(7)^2 - 6.23(7) + 72 \approx 90.1$ The average high temperature in July is $90.1°$.

(b) From the graph of $f(x)$ we can see that the average temperature is 80 in April and October.

Reviewing Basic Concepts (Sections 3.4 and 3.5)

1. (a) The total length of the fence must equal $2L + 2x = 300 \Rightarrow 2L = 300 - 2x \Rightarrow L = 150 - x$.

(b) Since width equals x and length equals $150 - x$, the function is $A(x) = x(150 - x)$.

(c) Since length and width must both be positive, the restrictions are $0 < x < 150$.

(d) $5000 = x(150 - x) \Rightarrow x^2 - 150x + 5000 = 0 \Rightarrow (x - 50)(x - 100) = 0 \Rightarrow x = 50$ or 100. Using either value will yield a garden, which is 50 m by 100 m.

2. (a) See Figure 2a.

(b) Using the defined function and the point (51, .1) yields $f(x) = a(x-51)+0.1$. Now use (101, 4.7) to find the function: $4.7 = a(101-51)^2 + 0.1 \Rightarrow 4.6 = 2500a \Rightarrow a = 0.0018$; therefore, the function is $f(x) = 0.0018(x-51)^2 + 0.1$.

(c) Using the regression feature yields $g(x) \approx 0.0026x^2 - 0.3139x + 9.426$.

(d) Graph the data and two equations from (b) and (c), See Figure 2d. The regression function fits better because it passes through more data points. Neither function would fit the data for $x < 51$.

3. $P(x)$ is a positive odd-degree polynomial graph; therefore, ⌒.

4. A polynomial of degree 3 can have at most 2 extrema, and at most 3 x-intercepts.

5. $P(x)$ is a positive even-degree polynomial graph; therefore, ⌣.

6. See Figure 6.

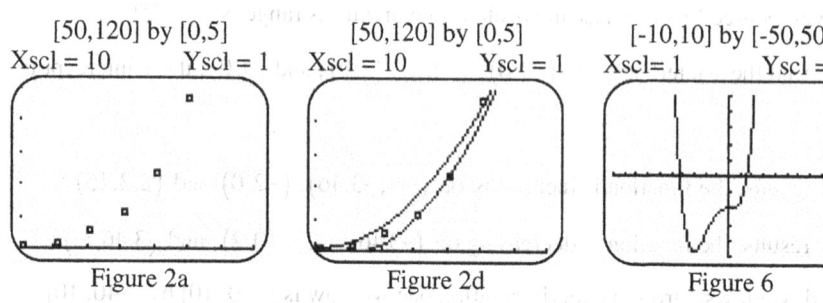

Figure 2a Figure 2d Figure 6

7. From the graph of P, there is one extrema, an absolute minimum point, which by the calculator is $(-3, -47)$.

8. Using the calculator, we find the x-intercepts are $(-4.26, 0)$ and $(1.53, 0)$; the y-intercept is $(0, -20)$.

3.6: Topics in the Theory of Polynomial Functions (I)

1. $\dfrac{10x^6}{5x^3} = 2x^3$

3. $\dfrac{8x^9}{3x^7} = \dfrac{8}{3}x^2$

5. $\dfrac{2x^6 + 3x^3}{2x} = \dfrac{2x^6}{2x} + \dfrac{3x^3}{2x} = x^5 + \dfrac{3}{2}x^2$

7. $\dfrac{8x^3 - 5x}{2x} = \dfrac{8x^3}{2x} - \dfrac{5x}{2x} = 4x^2 - \dfrac{5}{2}$

9. $P(1) = 3(1)^2 - 2(1) - 6 \Rightarrow P(1) = -5$ and $P(2) = 3(2)^2 - 2(2) - 6 \Rightarrow P(2) = 2$. These answers differ in sign; therefore, there is a real zero between them. Graphed on a calculator, the real zero is approximately 1.79.

11. $P(2) = 2(2)^3 - 8(2)^2 + (2) + 16 \Rightarrow P(2) = 2$ and $P(2.5) = 2(2.5)^3 - 8(2.5)^2 + (2.5) + 16 \Rightarrow P(2.5) = -0.25$.

These answers differ in sign; therefore, there is a real zero between them. By graphing on the calculator, the real zero is approximately 2.39.

13. $P(1.5) = 2(1.5)^4 - 4(1.5)^2 + 3(1.5) - 6 \Rightarrow P(1.5) = -0.375$ and $P(2) = 2(2)^4 - 4(2)^2 + 3(2) - 6 \Rightarrow P(2) = 16$.

These answers differ in sign; therefore, there is a real zero between them. By graphing on the calculator, the real zero is approximately 1.52.

15. $P(2.7) = -(2.7)^4 + 2(2.7)^3 + (2.7) + 12 \Rightarrow P(2.7) = 0.9219$ and $P(2.8) = -(2.8)^4 + 2 \cdot (2.8)^3 + (2.8) + 12 \Rightarrow$

$P(2.8) = -2.7616$. These answers differ in sign; therefore, there is a real zero between them. By graphing on the calculator, the real zero is approximately 2.73.

17. $P(-1.6) = (-1.6)^5 - 2(-1.6)^3 + 1 \Rightarrow P(-1.6) = -1.29376$ and $P(-1.5) = (-1.5)^5 - 2(-1.5)^3 + 1 \Rightarrow$

$P(-1.5) = 0.15625$. These answers differ in sign; therefore, there is a real zero between them. By graphing on the calculator, the real zero is approximately -1.51.

19. There is at least one zero between 2 and 2.5.

21. $x+5 \overline{\smash{\big)}\, x^3 + 2x^2 - 17x - 10} \Rightarrow \dfrac{x^3 + 2x^2 - 17x - 10}{x+5} = x^2 - 3x - 2$

$$\begin{array}{r} x^2 - 3x - 2 \\ x+5 \overline{\smash{\big)}\, x^3 + 2x^2 - 17x - 10} \\ \underline{x^3 + 5x^2} \\ -3x^2 - 17x - 10 \\ \underline{-3x^2 - 15x} \\ -2x - 10 \\ \underline{-2x - 10} \\ 0 \end{array}$$

23. $x-5 \overline{\smash{\big)}\, 3x^3 - 11x^2 - 20x + 3} \Rightarrow \dfrac{3x^3 - 11x^2 - 20x + 3}{x-5} = 3x^2 + 4x + \dfrac{3}{x-5}$

$$\begin{array}{r} 3x^2 + 4x \\ x-5 \overline{\smash{\big)}\, 3x^3 - 11x^2 - 20x + 3} \\ \underline{3x^3 - 15x^2} \\ 4x^2 - 20x + 3 \\ \underline{4x^2 - 20x} \\ 3 \end{array}$$

25.
$$\require{enclose}
\begin{array}{r}
x^3-x^2-6x \\
x-2 \enclose{longdiv}{x^4-3x^3-4x^2+12x} \\
\underline{x^4-2x^3} \\
-x^3-4x^2+12x \\
\underline{-x^3+2x^2} \\
-6x^2+12x \\
\underline{-6x^2+12x} \\
0
\end{array}$$

$\Rightarrow \dfrac{x^4-3x^3-4x^2+12x}{x-2} = x^3-x^2-6x$

27.
$$\begin{array}{r}
x^2+3x+3 \\
x-1 \enclose{longdiv}{x^3+2x^2+0x-3} \\
\underline{x^3-x^2} \\
3x^2+0x-3 \\
\underline{3x^2-3x} \\
3x-3 \\
\underline{3x-3} \\
0
\end{array}$$

$\Rightarrow \dfrac{x^3+2x^2-3}{x-1} = x^2+3x+3$

29.
$$\begin{array}{r}
-2x^2+2x-3 \\
x+1 \enclose{longdiv}{-2x^3+0x^2-x-2} \\
\underline{-2x^3-2x^2} \\
2x^2-x-2 \\
\underline{2x^2+2x} \\
-3x-2 \\
\underline{-3x-3} \\
1
\end{array}$$

$\Rightarrow \dfrac{-2x^3-x-2}{x+1} = -2x^2+2x-3+\dfrac{1}{x+1}$

31.
$$\begin{array}{r}
x^4+x^3+x^2+x+1 \\
x-1 \enclose{longdiv}{x^5+0x^4+0x^3+0x^2+0x-1} \\
\underline{x^5-x^4} \\
x^4+0x^3+0x^2+0x-1 \\
\underline{x^4-x^3} \\
x^3+0x^2+0x-1 \\
\underline{x^3-x^2} \\
x^2+0x-1 \\
\underline{x^2-x} \\
x-1 \\
\underline{x-1} \\
0
\end{array}$$

$\Rightarrow \dfrac{x^5-1}{x-1} = x^4+x^3+x^2+x+1$

33.
$$3\overline{)\begin{array}{ccc} 1 & -4 & 3 \\ & 3 & -3 \\ \hline 1 & -1 & 0 \end{array}}$$
Therefore, $P(3) = 0$.

35.
$$-2\overline{)\begin{array}{cccc} 5 & 2 & -1 & 5 \\ & -10 & 16 & -30 \\ \hline 5 & -8 & 15 & -25 \end{array}}$$
Therefore, $P(-2) = -25$.

37.
$$2\overline{)\begin{array}{ccc} 1 & -5 & 1 \\ & 2 & -6 \\ \hline 1 & -3 & -5 \end{array}}$$
Therefore, $P(2) = -5$.

39.
$$0.5\overline{)\begin{array}{cccc} 1 & 0 & -1 & 4 \\ & 0.5 & 0.25 & -.375 \\ \hline 1 & 0.5 & -0.75 & 3.625 \end{array}}$$
Therefore, $P(0.5) = 3.625$.

41.
$$\sqrt{2}\,\overline{)\begin{array}{cccc} 1 & 0 & -1 & 0 & -3 \\ & \sqrt{2} & 2 & \sqrt{2} & 2 \\ \hline 1 & \sqrt{2} & 1 & \sqrt{2} & -1 \end{array}}$$
Therefore, $P(\sqrt{2}) = -1$.

43.
$$\sqrt[3]{4}\,\overline{)\begin{array}{cccc} -1 & 0 & 1 & 4 \\ & -\sqrt[3]{4} & -\sqrt[3]{16} & \sqrt[3]{4}-4 \\ \hline -1 & -\sqrt[3]{4} & 1-\sqrt[3]{16} & \sqrt[3]{4} \end{array}}$$
Therefore, $P(\sqrt[3]{4}) = \sqrt[3]{4}$.

45.
$$2\overline{)\begin{array}{ccc} 1 & 2 & -8 \\ & 2 & 8 \\ \hline 1 & 4 & 0 \end{array}}$$
Yes; since $P(2) = 0$, 2 is a zero.

47.
$$4\overline{)\begin{array}{ccc} 2 & -6 & -9 & 6 \\ & 8 & 8 & -4 \\ \hline 2 & 2 & -1 & 2 \end{array}}$$
No; since $P(4) \neq 0$, 4 is not a zero.

49.
$$-0.5\overline{)\begin{array}{ccc} 4 & 12 & 7 & 1 \\ & -2 & -5 & -1 \\ \hline 4 & 10 & 2 & 0 \end{array}}$$
Yes; since $P(-0.5) = 0$, -0.5 is a zero.

51.
$$-5\overline{)\begin{array}{ccc} 8 & 50 & 47 & 15 \\ & -40 & -50 & 15 \\ \hline 8 & 10 & -3 & 30 \end{array}}$$
No; since $P(-5) \neq 0$, -5 is not a zero.

53.
$$\sqrt{6}\,\overline{)\begin{array}{ccccccc} -2 & 0 & 5 & 0 & -3 & 0 & 270 \\ & -2\sqrt{6} & -12 & -7\sqrt{6} & -42 & -45\sqrt{6} & -270 \\ \hline -2 & -2\sqrt{6} & -7 & -7\sqrt{6} & -45 & -45\sqrt{6} & 0 \end{array}}$$
Yes; since $P(\sqrt{6}) = 0$, $\sqrt{6}$ is a zero.

122   CHAPTER 3   Polynomial Functions

55. Since the x-intercepts are -3, 1, and 4, the linear factors are $(x-(-3)), (x-1), (x-4)$ or $(x+3), (x-1), (x-4)$.

56. Since the x-intercepts are -3, 1, and 4, the solutions to $P(x) = 0$ are -3, 1, and 4.

57. Since the x-intercepts are -3, 1 and 4; the zeros are -3, 1, and 4

58. Use synthetic division and divide by 2:

    $$\begin{array}{r|rrrr} 2 & 1 & -2 & -11 & 12 \\ & & 2 & 0 & -22 \\ \hline & 1 & 0 & -11 & -10 \end{array}$$

    The remainder is -10; therefore, $P(2) = -10$.

59. Using the x-intercepts and graph, $P(x) > 0$ for the $(-3, 1) \cup (4, \infty)$.

60. Using the x-intercepts and graph, $P(x) < 0$ for the $(-\infty, -3) \cup (1, 4)$.

61. First, use synthetic division to factor out the given zero.

    $$\begin{array}{r|rrrr} 3 & 1 & -2 & -5 & 6 \\ & & 3 & 3 & -6 \\ \hline & 1 & 1 & -2 & 0 \end{array}$$

    Now completely factor the resulting quadratic expression: $x^2 + x - 2 \Rightarrow (x-1)(x+2)$.

    The other zeros are -2 and 1.

63. First, use synthetic division to factor out the given zero.

    $$\begin{array}{r|rrrr} 1 & 1 & 0 & -2 & 1 \\ & & 1 & 1 & -1 \\ \hline & 1 & 1 & -1 & 0 \end{array}$$

    Now solve the quadratic equation, $x^2 + x - 1 = 0$, using the quadratic formula:

    $x = \dfrac{-1 \pm \sqrt{1^2 - 4(1)(-1)}}{2(1)} = \dfrac{-1 \pm \sqrt{5}}{2}$ The other zeros are $\dfrac{-1-\sqrt{5}}{2}$ and $\dfrac{-1+\sqrt{5}}{2}$.

65. First, use synthetic division to factor out the given zero.

    $$\begin{array}{r|rrrr} -2 & 3 & 5 & -3 & -2 \\ & & -6 & 2 & 2 \\ \hline & 3 & -1 & -1 & 0 \end{array}$$

    Now solve the quadratic equation, $3x^2 - x - 1 = 0$, using the quadratic formula:

    $x = \dfrac{1 \pm \sqrt{(-1)^2 - 4(3)(-1)}}{2(3)} = \dfrac{1 \pm \sqrt{13}}{6}$ The other zeros are $\dfrac{1-\sqrt{13}}{6}$ and $\dfrac{1+\sqrt{13}}{6}$.

67. First, use synthetic division to factor out the first given zero. Then use synthetic division to factor out the second given zero from the resulting expression: $x^3 - 6x^2 - 5x + 30$.

$$\begin{array}{r|rrrrr} -6) & 1 & 0 & -41 & 0 & 180 \\ & & -6 & 36 & 30 & -180 \\ \hline & 1 & -6 & -5 & 30 & 0 \end{array} \Rightarrow \begin{array}{r|rrrr} 6) & 1 & -6 & -5 & 30 \\ & & 6 & 0 & -30 \\ \hline & 1 & 0 & -5 & 0 \end{array}$$

Finally, solve the resulting equation $x^2 - 5 = 0 \Rightarrow x^2 = 5 \Rightarrow x = \pm\sqrt{5}$.

Therefore, the other zeros are $-\sqrt{5}$ and $\sqrt{5}$.

69. First, use synthetic division to factor out the given zero.

$$\begin{array}{r|rrrr} 8) & -1 & 8 & 3 & -24 \\ & & -8 & 0 & 24 \\ \hline & -1 & 0 & 3 & 0 \end{array}$$

Now solve the resulting equation: $-x^2 + 3 = 0 \Rightarrow -x^2 = -3 \Rightarrow x^2 = 3 \Rightarrow x = \pm\sqrt{3}$

Therefore, the other zeros are $-\sqrt{3}$ and $\sqrt{3}$.

71. First, use synthetic division to factor out the given zero.

$$\begin{array}{r|rrrr} 2) & 2 & -3 & -17 & 30 \\ & & 4 & 2 & -30 \\ \hline & 2 & 1 & -15 & 0 \end{array}$$

Now completely factor the resulting quadratic expression: $2x^2 + x - 15 \Rightarrow (2x-5)(x+3)$.

The linear factors are $P(x) = (x-2)(2x-5)(x+3)$.

73. First, use synthetic division to factor out the given zero.

$$\begin{array}{r|rrrr} -4) & 6 & 25 & 3 & -4 \\ & & -24 & -4 & 4 \\ \hline & 6 & 1 & -1 & 0 \end{array}$$

Now completely factor the resulting quadratic expression: $6x^2 + x - 1 \Rightarrow (3x-1)(2x+1)$. Therefore, the linear factors are $P(x) = (x+4)(3x-1)(2x+1)$.

75. First, use synthetic division to factor out the given zero.

$$\begin{array}{r|rrrr} -3) & -6 & -13 & 14 & -3 \\ & & 18 & -15 & 3 \\ \hline & -6 & 5 & -1 & 0 \end{array}$$

Now completely factor the resulting quadratic expression: $-6x^2 + 5x - 1 \Rightarrow (-3x+1)(2x-1)$.

The linear factors are $P(x) = (x+3)(-3x+1)(2x-1)$.

77. First, use synthetic division to factor out the given zero.

124 CHAPTER 3 Polynomial Functions

$$\begin{array}{r|rrrr} -5) & 1 & 5 & -3 & -15 \\ & & -5 & 0 & 15 \\ \hline & 1 & 0 & -3 & 0 \end{array}$$

Now completely factor the resulting quadratic expression: $x^2 - 3 = (x+\sqrt{3})(x-\sqrt{3})$.

The linear factors are $P(x) = (x+5)(x+\sqrt{3})(x-\sqrt{3})$.

79. First, use synthetic division to factor out the given zero.

$$\begin{array}{r|rrrr} -1) & 1 & -2 & -7 & -4 \\ & & -1 & 3 & 4 \\ \hline & 1 & -3 & -4 & 0 \end{array}$$

Now completely factor the resulting quadratic expression: $x^2 - 3x - 4 \Rightarrow (x-4)(x+1)$.

The linear factors are $P(x) = (x+1)(x-4)(x+1)$ or $(x+1)^2(x-4)$.

81.
$$\begin{array}{r} x^3 + 2 \\ 3x-7 \overline{\smash{\big)}\, 3x^4 - 7x^3 + 6x - 16} \\ \underline{3x^4 - 7x^3} \\ 6x - 16 \\ \underline{6x - 14} \\ -2 \end{array}$$
$\Rightarrow \dfrac{3x^4 - 7x^3 + 6x - 16}{3x-7} = x^3 + 2 + \dfrac{-2}{3x-7}$

83.
$$\begin{array}{r} 5x^2 - 12 \\ x^2+2 \overline{\smash{\big)}\, 5x^4 - 2x^2 + 6} \\ \underline{5x^4 + 10x^2} \\ -12x^2 + 6 \\ \underline{-12x^2 - 24} \\ 30 \end{array}$$
$\Rightarrow \dfrac{5x^4 - 2x^2 + 6}{x^2+2} = 5x^2 - 12 + \dfrac{30}{x^2+2}$

85.
$$\begin{array}{r} 4x + 5 \\ 2x^2-3 \overline{\smash{\big)}\, 8x^3 + 10x^2 - 12x - 15} \\ \underline{8x^3 - 12x} \\ 10x^2 - 15 \\ \underline{10x^2 - 15} \\ 0 \end{array}$$
$\Rightarrow \dfrac{8x^3 + 10x^2 - 12x - 15}{2x^2+3} = 4x + 5$

87.
$$\begin{array}{r} x^2-2x+4 \\ 2x^2+3x+2 \overline{) 2x^4-x^3+4x^2+8x+7} \\ \underline{2x^4+3x^3+2x^2} \\ -4x^3+2x^2+8x \\ \underline{-4x^3-6x^2-4x} \\ 8x^2+12x+7 \\ \underline{8x^2+12x+8} \\ -1 \end{array}$$
$\Rightarrow \dfrac{2x^4-x^3+4x^2+8x+7}{2x^2+3x+2} = x^2-2x+4+\dfrac{-1}{2x^2+3x+2}$

89.
$$\begin{array}{r} \frac{1}{2}x \\ 2x+1 \overline{) x^2+\frac{1}{2}x-1} \\ \underline{x^2+\frac{1}{2}x} \\ -1 \end{array}$$
$\Rightarrow \dfrac{x^2+\frac{1}{2}x-1}{2x+1} = \dfrac{1}{2}x+\dfrac{-1}{2x+1}$

91.
$$\begin{array}{r} \frac{1}{2}x-\frac{1}{2} \\ 2x^2-1 \overline{) x^3-x^2+0x+1} \\ \underline{x^3 \quad\;-\frac{1}{2}x} \\ -x^2+\frac{1}{2}x+1 \\ \underline{-x^2 \quad\;+\frac{1}{2}} \\ \frac{1}{2}x+\frac{1}{2} \end{array}$$
$\Rightarrow \dfrac{x^3-x^2+1}{2x^2-1} = \dfrac{1}{2}x-\dfrac{1}{2}+\dfrac{\frac{1}{2}x+\frac{1}{2}}{2x^2-1}$

3.7: Topics in the Theory of Polynomial Functions (II)

1. With the given zeros 4 and $2+i$, the conjugate of $2+i$ or $2-i$ is also a zero. Therefore,

   $P(x) = (x-4)(x-(2+i))(x-(2-i)) = (x-4)(x-2-i)(x-2+i) = (x-4)(x^2-4x+5)$

   $= x^3-4x^2+5x-4x^2+16x-20 \Rightarrow P(x) = x^3-8x^2+21x-20.$

3. With the given zeros 5 and i, the conjugate of i or $-i$ is also a zero. Therefore,

   $P(x) = (x-5)(x-i)(x-(-i)) = (x-5)(x^2-i^2) = (x-5)(x^2+1) \Rightarrow P(x) = x^3-5x^2+x-5.$

5. With the given zeros 0 and $3+i$, the conjugate of $3+i$ or $3-i$ is also a zero. Therefore,

   $P(x) = (x-0)(x-(3+i))(x-(3-i)) = (x)(x-3-i)(x-3+i) = (x)(x^2-6x+10)$

   $\Rightarrow P(x) = x^3-6x^2+10x.$

7. With the given zeros $-3, -1,$ and 4, the function $P(x)$ is $P(x) = a(x-(-3))(x-(-1))(x-4) =$

   $a(x+3)(x+1)(x-4) = a(x+3)(x^2-3x-4) \Rightarrow P(x) = a(x^3-13x-12)$

Since $P(2) = 5$ we can solve for a:

$$5 = a((2)^3 - 13(2) - 12) \Rightarrow 5 = a(8 - 26 - 12) \Rightarrow -30a = 5 \Rightarrow a = -\frac{5}{30} = -\frac{1}{6}$$

Therefore, $P(x) = -\frac{1}{6}(x^3 - 13x - 12) \Rightarrow P(x) = -\frac{1}{6}x^3 + \frac{16}{3}x + 2$.

9. With the given zeros $-2, 1$ and 0, the function $P(x)$ is

$$P(x) = a(x-(-2))(x-1)(x-0) = a(x+2)(x-1)(x) \Rightarrow P(x) = ax(x^2 + x - 2)$$

Since $P(-1) = -1$, we can solve for a: $-1 = a(-1)((-1)^3 + (-1) - 2) \Rightarrow -1 = -a(1 - 1 - 2)$

$\Rightarrow -a(-2) = -1 \Rightarrow 2a = -1 \Rightarrow a = -\frac{1}{2}$. Therefore, $P(x) = -\frac{1}{2}x(x^2 + x - 2) \Rightarrow P(x) = -\frac{1}{2}x^3 - \frac{1}{2}x^2 + x$.

11. With the given zeros $4, 1+i$, and the conjugate of $1+i$ or $1-i$ also a zero, the function $P(x)$ is

$$P(x) = a(x-4)(x-(1+i))(x-(1-i)) = a(x-4)(x-1-i)(x-1+i) =$$

$a(x-4)(x^2 - 2x + 2) = a(x^3 - 2x^2 + 2x - 4x^2 + 8x - 8) \Rightarrow P(x) = a(x^3 - 6x^2 + 10x - 8)$. Since $P(2) = 4$,

we can solve for a: $4 = a((2)^3 - 6(2)^2 + 10(2) - 8) \Rightarrow 4 = a(8 - 24 + 20 - 8) \Rightarrow -4a = 4 \Rightarrow a = -\frac{1}{1} = -1$.

Therefore, $P(x) = -1(x^3 - 6x^2 + 10x - 8) \Rightarrow P(x) = -x^3 + 6x^2 - 10x + 8$.

13. First, use synthetic division to factor out the given zero.

```
3 | 1   -1   -4   -6
  |      3    6    6
  |_____
    1    2    2    0
```

Now solve the resulting quadratic equation, $x^2 + 2x + 2 = 0$, using the

quadratic formula: $x = \frac{-2 \pm \sqrt{(2)^2 - 4(1)(2)}}{2(1)} = \frac{-2 \pm \sqrt{-4}}{2} = \frac{-2 \pm 2i}{2} = -1 \pm i$.

Therefore, the other zeros are $-1-i$ and $-1+i$.

15. First, use synthetic division to factor out the first given zero. Then use synthetic division to factor out the second given zero from the resulting expression $x^3 - x^2 - 7x + 3$

```
-3 | 1   2  -10  -18   9           3 | 1  -1  -7   3
   |     -3   33   21  -9  =>        |     3   6  -3
   |_____         |_____
     1  -1   -7    3   0              1   2  -1   0
```

Finally, solve the resulting quadratic equation, $x^2 + 2x - 1 = 0$, using the quadratic formula:

$$x = \frac{-2 \pm \sqrt{(2)^2 - 4(1)(-1)}}{2(1)} = \frac{-2 \pm \sqrt{8}}{2} = \frac{-2 \pm 2\sqrt{2}}{2} = -1 \pm \sqrt{2}.$$

Therefore, the other zeros are $-1+\sqrt{2}$ and $-1-\sqrt{2}$.

SECTION 3.7   127

17. With the given zero $3i$, the conjugate $-3i$ is also a zero. Use synthetic division to factor out these zeros.

$$3i\overline{)\begin{array}{cccc} 1 & -1 & 10 & -9 & 9 \\ & 3i & -9-3i & 9+3i & -9 \end{array}} \Rightarrow \quad -3i\overline{)\begin{array}{cccc} 1 & -1+3i & 1-3i & 3i \\ & -3i & 3i & -3i \end{array}}$$
$$\phantom{3i\overline{)}}\begin{array}{cccc} 1 & -1+3i & 1-3i & 3i & 0 \end{array} \qquad \phantom{-3i\overline{)}}\begin{array}{cccc} 1 & -1 & 1 & 0 \end{array}$$

Finally, solve the resulting quadratic equation, $x^2 - x + 1 = 0$, using the quadratic formula:

$$x = \frac{1 \pm \sqrt{(-1)^2 - 4(1)(1)}}{2(1)} = \frac{1 \pm \sqrt{-3}}{2} = \frac{1}{2} \pm \frac{\sqrt{3}}{2}i.$$

Therefore, the other zeros are $-3i$, $\frac{1}{2} + \frac{\sqrt{3}}{2}i$, and $\frac{1}{2} - \frac{\sqrt{3}}{2}i$.

19. With the given zeros 5 and -4, $P(x) = a(x-5)(x-(-4)) = a(x-5)(x+4) \Rightarrow P(x) = a(x^2 - x - 20)$.

There are many possible solutions. For example, when $a = 1$, $P(x) = x^2 - x - 20$.

21. With the given zeros $-3, 2, i$, the conjugate of i or $-i$ is also zero. The function $P(x)$ is

$$P(x) = a(x-(-3))(x-2)(x-i)(x-(-i)) = a(x+3)(x-2)(x-i)(x+i) =$$

$$\Rightarrow P(x) = a(x^2 + x - 6)(x^2 + 1) = a(x^4 + x^3 - 5x^2 + x - 6).$$ There are many possible solutions. For

example, when $a = 1$, $P(x) = x^4 + x^3 - 5x^2 + x - 6$.

23. With the given zeros $1 + \sqrt{3}$, $1 - \sqrt{3}$, and 1,

$$P(x) = a\left(x - \left(1 + \sqrt{3}\right)\right)\left(x - \left(1 - \sqrt{3}\right)\right)(x-1) = a\left(x - 1 - \sqrt{3}\right)\left(x - 1 + \sqrt{3}\right)(x-1) =$$

$$a\left(x^2 - x + \sqrt{3}x - x + 1 - \sqrt{3} - \sqrt{3}x + \sqrt{3} - 3\right)(x-1) = a(x^2 - 2x - 2)(x-1) =$$

$$a(x^3 - x^2 - 2x^2 + 2x - 2x + 2) \Rightarrow P(x) = a(x^3 - 3x^2 + 2).$$ There are many possible solutions. For example,

when $a = 1$, $P(x) = x^3 - 3x^2 + 2$.

25. With the given zeros $-1, 2$, and $3 + 2i$, the conjugate of $3 + 2i$ or $3 - 2i$ is also a zero.

$$P(x) = a(x-(3+2i))(x-(3-2i))(x-(-1))(x-2) = a(x-3-2i)(x-3+2i)(x+1)(x-2) =$$

$$a(x^2 - 3x + 2ix - 3x + 9 - 6i - 2ix + 6i - 4i^2)(x^2 - x - 2) = a(x^2 - 6x + 13)(x^2 - x - 2) =$$

$$a(x^4 - x^3 - 2x^2 - 6x^3 + 6x^2 + 12x + 13x^2 - 13x - 26) \Rightarrow P(x) = a(x^4 - 7x^3 + 17x^2 - x - 26).$$ There are

many possible solutions. For example, when $a = 1$, $P(x) = x^4 - 7x^3 + 17x^2 - x - 26$.

27. With the given zeros -1, and $6 - 3i$, the conjugate of $6 - 3i$ or $6 + 3i$ also a zero. The function is

$$P(x) = a(x-(6-3i))(x-(6+3i))(x-(-1)) = a(x-6+3i)(x-6-3i)(x+1) =$$

$$a(x^2 - 6x - 3ix - 6x + 36 + 18i + 3ix - 18i - 9i^2)(x+1) = a(x^2 - 12x + 45)(x+1) =$$

$a(x^3 -12x^2 +45x+x^2 -12x+45) \Rightarrow P(x) = a(x^3 -11x^2 +33x+45)$. There are many possible solutions. For example, when $a=1$, $P(x) = x^3 -11x^2 +33x+45$.

29. With the given zeros -3 (multiplicity 2) and $2+i$, the conjugate of $2+i$ or $2-i$ also a zero.

$P(x) = a(x-(2+i))(x-(2-i))(x-(-3))^2 = a(x-2-i)(x-2+i)(x+3)^2 =$

$a(x^2 -2x+ix-2x+4-2i-ix+2i-i^2)(x^2 +6x+9) = a(x^2 -4x+5)(x^2 +6x+9) =$

$a(x^4 +6x^3 +9x^2 -4x^3 -24x^2 -36x+5x^2 +30x+45) \Rightarrow P(x) = a(x^4 +2x^3 -10x^2 -6x+45)$. There are many possible solutions. For example, when $a=1$, $P(x) = x^4 +2x^3 -10x^2 -6x+45$.

31 - 39. See Figures 31-39

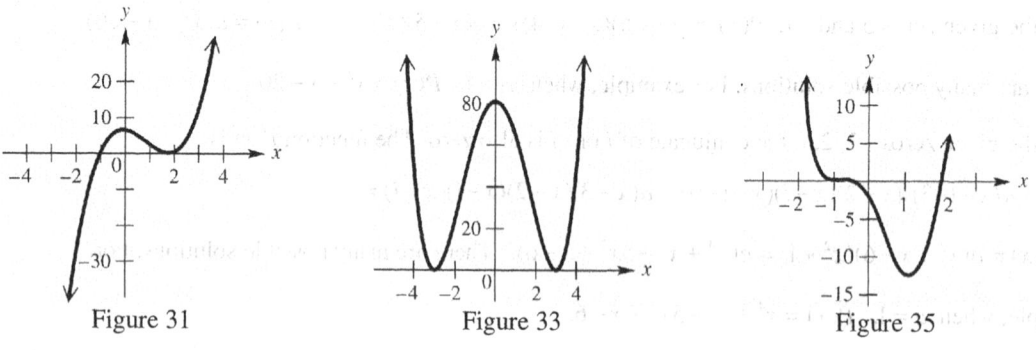

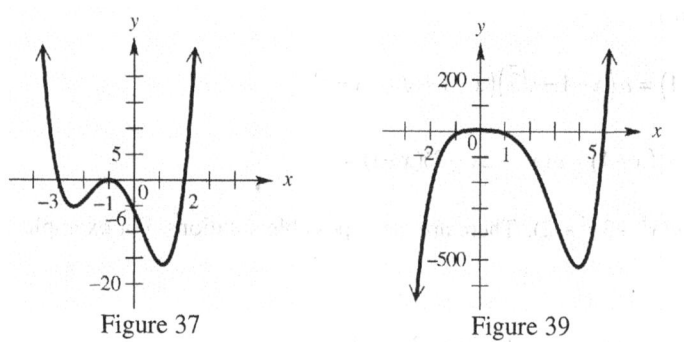

41. Since the graph crosses the x-axis at $(-1,0), (0,0)$, and $(2,0)$ and by the factor theorem the three factors are $(x-(-1))$, $(x-0)$, and $(x-2)$. The general form of the function is $f(x) = a(x)(x+1)(x-2)$. We will find the value of a using the point $(1, 2)$. $2 = a(1)(1+1)(1-2) \Rightarrow 2 = -2a \Rightarrow a = -1$. The function is $f(x) = -(x)(x+1)(x-2)$.

43. Since the graph crosses the x-axis at $(-2,0), (-1,0)$, and $(1,0)$ and by the factor theorem the three factors are $(x-(-2))$, $(x-(-1))$, and $(x-1)$. The general form of the function is $f(x) = a(x+2)(x+1)(x-1)$. We will find the value of a using the point $(0, -1)$. $-1 = a(0+2)(0+1)(0-1) \Rightarrow -1 = -2a \Rightarrow a = \frac{1}{2}$. The function is $f(x) = \frac{1}{2}(x+2)(x+1)(x-1)$.

45. Since the graph crosses the x-axis at $(-4,0), (-1,0), (1,0)$, and $(2,0)$ and by the factor theorem the four factors are $(x-(-4)), (x-(-1)), (x-1), (x-2)$. The general form of the function is $f(x) = a(x+4)(x+1)(x-1)(x-2)$. We will find the value of a using the point $(0, 2)$.

    $2 = a(0+4)(0+1)(0-1)(0-2) \Rightarrow 2 = 8a \Rightarrow a = \dfrac{1}{4}$. The function is

    $f(x) = \dfrac{1}{4}(x+4)(x+1)(x-1)(x-2)$.

47. First, use synthetic division to factor out the first –2. Then use synthetic division to factor out the second –2 from the resulting expression: $x^3 + 0x^2 - 7x - 6$.

    $$\begin{array}{r|rrrr} -2 & 1 & 2 & -7 & -20 & -12 \\ & & -2 & 0 & 14 & 12 \\ \hline & 1 & 0 & -7 & -6 & 0 \end{array} \Rightarrow \begin{array}{r|rrrr} -2 & 1 & 0 & -7 & -6 \\ & & -2 & 4 & 6 \\ \hline & 1 & -2 & -3 & 0 \end{array}$$

    Finally, completely factor the resulting quadratic expression: $x^2 - 2x - 3 = (x-3)(x+1)$. Therefore, the zeros are –2, 3, and –1, and the factored form is $P(x) = (x+2)^2(x-3)(x+1)$.

49. Since non real complex zeros occur in pairs, there will be 0, 2, or 4 non real complex zeros, leading to 5, 3, or 1 real zeros.

51. (a) Not Possible. With a zero of $1+i$, its conjugate $1-i$ must also be a zero, and this would give 4 zeros to a degree 3 function, which is not possible.

    (b) Possible. Since non real complex zeros occur in pairs, there can be 4 non real complex zeros.

    (c) Not Possible. We cannot have a multiplicity of 6 for a degree 5 function.

    (d) Possible. With $1+2i$ having a multiplicity of 2, its conjugate $1-2i$ must also have a multiplicity of 2. This means the function has a minimum of 4 zeros which is possible.

53. (a) Using the Rational Zeros Theorem yields $\dfrac{p}{q} = \pm\dfrac{1,2,5,10}{1} = \pm 1 \pm 2 \pm 5 \pm 10$.

    (b) A graph (not shown) would indicate that there are no zeros less than -2 or greater than 5.

    (c) First, use synthetic division to factor using values discovered in steps (a) and (b)

    $$\begin{array}{r|rrrr} -2 & 1 & -2 & -13 & -10 \\ & & -2 & 8 & 10 \\ \hline & 1 & -4 & -5 & 0 \end{array}$$

    Now completely factor the resulting quadratic expression: $x^2 - 4x - 5 \Rightarrow (x-5)(x+1)$. Therefore, the rational zeros are $-2, -1$ and 5.

    (d) The factored form of $P(x)$ is $P(x) = (x+2)(x+1)(x-5)$.

130 CHAPTER 3 Polynomial Functions

55. (a) Using the Rational Zeros Theorem yields $\dfrac{p}{q} = \pm\dfrac{1,2,3,5,6,10,15,30}{1}$

   (b) A graph (not shown) would indicate that there are no zeros less than -5 or greater than 2.

   (c) First, use synthetic division to factor using values discovered in steps (a) and (b).

   $$\begin{array}{r|rrrr} -5) & 1 & 6 & -1 & -30 \\ & & -5 & -5 & 30 \\ \hline & 1 & 1 & -6 & 0 \end{array}$$

   Now completely factor the resulting quadratic expression: $x^2 + x - 6 \Rightarrow (x+3)(x-2)$. Therefore, the rational zeros are $-5, -3$ and 2.

   (d) The factored form of $P(x)$ is $P(x) = (x+5)(x+3)(x-2)$.

57. (a) Using the Rational Zeros Theorem yields

   $\dfrac{p}{q} = \pm\dfrac{1,2,3,4,6,12}{1,2,3,6} = \pm 1, \pm 2, \pm 3, \pm 4, \pm 6, \pm 12, \pm\dfrac{1}{2}, \pm\dfrac{3}{2}, \pm\dfrac{1}{3}, \pm\dfrac{2}{3}, \pm\dfrac{4}{3}, \pm\dfrac{1}{6}$.

   (b) A graph (not shown) would indicate that there are no zeros less than -4 or greater than $\dfrac{3}{2}$.

   (c) First, use synthetic division to factor using values discovered in steps (a) and (b).

   $$\begin{array}{r|rrrr} -4) & 6 & 17 & -31 & -12 \\ & & -24 & 28 & 12 \\ \hline & 6 & -7 & -3 & 0 \end{array}$$

   Now completely factor the resulting quadratic expression: $6x^2 - 7x - 3 \Rightarrow (3x+1)(2x-3)$. Therefore, the rational zeros are $-4, -\dfrac{1}{3}$, and $\dfrac{3}{2}$.

   (d) The factored form of $P(x)$ is $P(x) = (x+4)(3x+1)(2x-3)$.

59. Using the Rational Zeros Theorem yields

   $\dfrac{p}{q} = \pm\dfrac{1,2,3,6}{1,2,3,4,6,12} = \pm 1, \pm 2, \pm 3, \pm 6, \pm\dfrac{1}{2}, \pm\dfrac{3}{2}, \pm\dfrac{1}{3}, \pm\dfrac{2}{3}, \pm\dfrac{1}{6}, \pm\dfrac{1}{12}, \pm\dfrac{1}{4}, \pm\dfrac{3}{4}$. Use synthetic division to factor using values from above.

   $$\begin{array}{r|rrrr} -\dfrac{3}{2}) & 12 & 20 & -1 & -6 \\ & & -18 & -3 & 6 \\ \hline & 12 & 2 & -4 & 0 \end{array}$$

   Now completely factor the resulting quadratic expression: $12x^2 + 2x - 4 \Rightarrow 2(2x-1)(3x+2)$. The factored form of $P(x)$ is $P(x) = (3x+2)(2x+3)(2x-1)$.

SECTION 3.7   131

61. Using the Rational Zeros Theorem yields $\dfrac{p}{q} = \pm \dfrac{1,2,3,4,6,12}{1,2,3,4,6,8,12,24} =$

$\pm 1, \pm 2, \pm 3, \pm 4, \pm 6, \pm 12, \pm \dfrac{1}{2}, \pm \dfrac{3}{2}, \pm \dfrac{1}{3}, \pm \dfrac{2}{3}, \pm \dfrac{4}{3}, \pm \dfrac{1}{4}, \pm \dfrac{3}{4}, \pm \dfrac{1}{6}, \pm \dfrac{1}{8}, \pm \dfrac{3}{8}, \pm \dfrac{1}{12}, \pm \dfrac{1}{24}$.

Factor out a 2, $P(x) = 24x^3 + 40x^2 - 2x - 12 \Rightarrow P(x) = 2(12x^3 + 20x^2 - x - 6)$. Now use synthetic division to factor using values from above.

$$\begin{array}{r|rrrr} -\tfrac{3}{2} & 12 & 20 & -1 & -6 \\ & & -18 & -3 & 6 \\ \hline & 12 & 2 & -4 & 0 \end{array}$$

Now completely factor the resulting quadratic expression: $12x^2 + 2x - 4 \Rightarrow 2(3x+2)(2x-1)$. The factored form of $P(x)$ is $P(x) = 2(2x+3)(3x+2)(2x-1)$.

63. To eliminate the fractions, multiply the function by 2; therefore, $P(x) = 2\left(x^3 + \dfrac{1}{2}x^2 - \dfrac{11}{2}x - 5\right) =$

$2x^3 + x^2 - 11x - 10$. Now, use the Rational Zeros Theorem to identify possible zeros:

$\dfrac{p}{q} = \pm 10, \pm 5, \pm 1, \pm \dfrac{1}{2}, \pm \dfrac{5}{2}$. Next, from the calculator graph of the equation, we choose to check -1 by synthetic division.

$$\begin{array}{r|rrr} -1 & 2 & 1 & -11 & -10 \\ & & -2 & 1 & 10 \\ \hline & 2 & -1 & -10 & 0 \end{array}$$

Now, completely factor the resulting quadratic expression: $2x^2 - x - 10 \Rightarrow (2x-5)(x+2)$. Therefore, the rational zeros are $-2, -1,$ and $\dfrac{5}{2}$.

65. To eliminate the fractions, multiply the function by 12; therefore,

$P(x) = 12\left(\dfrac{1}{6}x^4 - \dfrac{11}{12}x^3 + \dfrac{7}{6}x^2 - \dfrac{11}{12}x + 1\right) = 2x^4 - 11x^3 + 14x^2 - 11x + 12$. Now, use the Rational Zeros

Theorem to identify possible zeros: $\dfrac{p}{q} = \pm 1, \pm 2, \pm 3, \pm 4, \pm 6, \pm 12, \pm \dfrac{1}{2}, \pm \dfrac{3}{2}$. Next, from the calculator,

graph of the equation, we choose to check $\dfrac{3}{2}$ and 4 by synthetic division. (The second from the result of the first)

$\dfrac{3}{2} \big) \begin{array}{cccc} 2 & -11 & 14 & -11 & 12 \\ & 3 & -12 & 3 & -12 \\ \hline 2 & -8 & 2 & -8 & 0 \end{array}$ $\Rightarrow$ $4 \big) \begin{array}{cccc} 2 & -8 & 2 & -8 \\ & 8 & 0 & 8 \\ \hline 2 & 0 & 2 & 0 \end{array}$

Now, completely factor the resulting quadratic expression: $2x^2 + 2 \Rightarrow 2(x^2 + 1) \Rightarrow x^2 = -1 \Rightarrow x = \pm i$.

Since $\pm i$ are not real numbers, the rational zeros are $\dfrac{3}{2}$ and 4.

67. $P(x) = 6x^4 - 5x^3 - 11x^2 + 10x - 2$. Now use the Rational Zeros Theorem to identify possible zeros: $\dfrac{p}{q} = \pm 1, \pm 2, \pm \dfrac{1}{2}, \pm \dfrac{1}{3}, \pm \dfrac{2}{3}, \pm \dfrac{1}{6}$. Next, from the calculator, graph of the equation, we choose to check $\dfrac{1}{2}$ and $\dfrac{1}{3}$ by synthetic division. (The second from the result of the first)

$\dfrac{1}{2} \big) \begin{array}{cccc} 6 & -5 & -11 & 10 & -2 \\ & 3 & -1 & -6 & 2 \\ \hline 6 & -2 & -12 & 4 & 0 \end{array}$ $\Rightarrow$ $\dfrac{1}{3} \big) \begin{array}{cccc} 6 & -2 & -12 & 4 \\ & 2 & 0 & -4 \\ \hline 6 & 0 & -12 & 0 \end{array}$

Now completely factor the resulting quadratic expression: $6x^2 - 12 \Rightarrow 6(x^2 - 2) \Rightarrow x^2 = 2 \Rightarrow x = \pm\sqrt{2}$

The factored form of $P(x)$ is $P(x) = (2x-1)(3x-1)(x-\sqrt{2})(x+\sqrt{2})$.

69. $P(x) = 21x^4 + 13x^3 - 103x^2 - 65x - 10$. Now use the Rational Zeros Theorem to identify possible zeros:

$\dfrac{p}{q} = \pm 1, \pm 2, \pm 5, \pm 10, \pm \dfrac{5}{21}, \pm \dfrac{5}{7}, \pm \dfrac{5}{3}, \pm \dfrac{2}{21}, \pm \dfrac{2}{7}, \pm \dfrac{2}{3}, \pm \dfrac{10}{21}, \pm \dfrac{10}{7}, \pm \dfrac{10}{3}, \pm \dfrac{1}{21}, \pm \dfrac{1}{7}, \pm \dfrac{1}{3}$. Next, from the calculator, graph of the equation, we choose to check $-\dfrac{2}{7}$ and $-\dfrac{1}{3}$ by synthetic division. (The second from the result of the first)

$-\dfrac{2}{7} \big) \begin{array}{cccc} 21 & 13 & -103 & -65 & -10 \\ & -6 & -2 & 30 & 10 \\ \hline 21 & 7 & -105 & -35 & 0 \end{array}$ $\Rightarrow$ $-\dfrac{1}{3} \big) \begin{array}{cccc} 21 & 7 & -105 & -35 \\ & -7 & 0 & 35 \\ \hline 21 & 0 & -105 & 0 \end{array}$

Now completely factor the resulting quadratic expression: $21x^2 - 105 \Rightarrow 21(x^2 - 5) \Rightarrow x^2 = 5 \Rightarrow x = \pm\sqrt{5}$

The factored form of $P(x)$ is $P(x) = (7x+2)(3x+1)(x-\sqrt{5})(x+\sqrt{5})$.

71. With the given zero i, the conjugate $-i$ is also a zero. Now use synthetic division to factor out these zeros.

$$\begin{array}{r|rrrrr} i) & 1 & -1 & 5 & -5 & 4 & -4 \\ & & i & -1-i & 1+4i & -4+4i & 4 \\ \hline & 1 & -1+i & 4-i & -4+4i & -4i & 0 \end{array} \Rightarrow \begin{array}{r|rrrrr} -i) & 1 & -1+i & 4-i & -4+4i & -4i \\ & & -i & i & -4i & 4i \\ \hline & 1 & -1 & 4 & -4 & 0 \end{array}$$

From the graph of the resulting polynomial we can see that 1 is a zero.

$$\begin{array}{r|rrrr} 1) & 1 & -1 & 4 & -4 \\ & & 1 & 0 & 4 \\ \hline & 1 & 0 & 4 & 0 \end{array}$$

The resulting polynomial $x^2 + 4 \Rightarrow x = \pm 2i$. The factors of P(x) are $(x-1)(x-i)(x+i)(x-2i)(x+2i)$.

73. With the given zero $-2i$, the conjugate $2i$ is also a zero. Now use synthetic division to factor out these zeros.

$$\begin{array}{r|rrrrr} -2i) & 1 & 1 & 2 & 4 & -8 \\ & & -2i & -4-2i & -4+4i & 8 \\ \hline & 1 & 1-2i & -2-2i & 4i & 0 \end{array} \Rightarrow \begin{array}{r|rrrr} 2i) & 1 & 1-2i & -2-2i & 4i \\ & & 2i & 2i & -4i \\ \hline & 1 & 1 & -2 & 0 \end{array}$$

Factoring the resulting polynomial we have $x^2 + x - 2 = (x+2)(x-1)$. The factors of P(x) are $(x+2)(x-1)(x-2i)(x+2i)$.

75. With the given zero $1+i$, the conjugate $1-i$ is also a zero. Now use synthetic division to factor out these zeros.

$$\begin{array}{r|rrrrr} 1+i) & 1 & -2 & 3 & -2 & 2 \\ & & 1+i & -2 & 1+i & -2 \\ \hline & 1 & -1+i & 1 & -1+i & 0 \end{array} \Rightarrow \begin{array}{r|rrrr} 1-i) & 1 & -1+i & 1 & -1+i \\ & & 1-i & 0 & 1-i \\ \hline & 1 & 0 & 1 & 0 \end{array}$$

Factoring the resulting polynomial we have $x^2 + 1 \Rightarrow x = \pm i$. The factors of P(x) are $(x-(1+i))(x-(1-i))(x-i)(x+i)$.

77. Because the function $P(x)$ has coefficient signs: $+ - + +$, which is 2 sign changes, the function has 2 or 0 possible positive real zeros. Because $P(-x) = 2(-x)^3 - 4(-x)^2 + 2(-x) + 7 = -2x^3 - 4x^2 - 2x + 7$ has coefficient signs: $- - - +$, which is 1 sign change, the function has 1 negative real zero. From graphing the function, $P(x)$ actually has 0 positive and 1 negative real zeros.

79. Because the function $P(x)$ has coefficient signs: $+ + + -$, which is 1 sign change, the function has 1 positive real zero. Because $P(-x) = 5(-x)^4 + 3(-x)^2 + 2(-x) - 9 = 5x^4 + 3x^2 - 2x - 9$ has coefficient signs: $+ + - -$, which is 1 sign change, the function has 1 negative real zero.

81. Because the function $P(x)$ has coefficient signs: $+ + - + +$, which is 2 sign changes, the function has 2 or 0 possible positive real zeros. Because $P(-x) = (-x)^5 + 3(-x)^4 - (-x)^3 + 2(-x) + 3 =$

$-x^5+3x^4+x^3-2x+3$ has coefficient signs: $-++-+$, which is 3 sign changes, the function has 3 or 1 possible negative real zeros. From graphing the function, $P(x)$ actually has 0 positive and 1 negative real zero.

83. Using the Boundedness Theorem, we divide synthetically by $x-2$.

$$\begin{array}{r|rrrrr} 2) & 1 & -1 & 3 & -8 & 8 \\ & & 2 & 2 & 10 & 4 \\ \hline & 1 & 1 & 5 & 2 & 12 \end{array}$$

The result is all nonnegative; therefore, no real zero greater than 2.

85. Using the Boundedness Theorem, we divide synthetically by $x-(-2)$.

$$\begin{array}{r|rrrrr} -2) & 1 & 1 & -1 & 0 & 3 \\ & & -2 & 2 & -2 & 4 \\ \hline & 1 & -1 & 1 & -2 & 7 \end{array}$$

The result alternates in sign; therefore, no real zero less than -2.

87. Using the Boundedness Theorem, we divide synthetically by $x-1$.

$$\begin{array}{r|rrrr} 1) & 3 & 2 & -4 & 1 & -1 \\ & & 3 & 5 & 1 & 2 \\ \hline & 3 & 5 & 1 & 2 & 1 \end{array}$$

The result is all nonnegative; therefore, no real zero greater than 1.

89. Using the Boundedness Theorem, we divide synthetically by $x-2$.

$$\begin{array}{r|rrrrrr} 2) & 1 & 0 & -3 & 0 & 1 & 2 \\ & & 2 & 4 & 2 & 4 & 10 \\ \hline & 1 & 2 & 1 & 2 & 5 & 12 \end{array}$$

The result is all nonnegative; therefore, no real zero greater than 2.

91. From the graph, the function has zeros $-6, 2$ and 5, the function $P(x)$ is

$P(x) = a(x-(6))(x-2)(x-5) = a(x+6)(x-2)(x-5) = a(x+6)(x^2-7x+10) \Rightarrow$

$P(x) = a(x^3 - x^2 - 32x + 60)$. Since $P(0) = 30$, we can solve for a:

$30 = a((0)^3 - (0)^2 - 42(0) + 60) \Rightarrow 30 = a(0-0-0+60) \Rightarrow 60a = 30 \Rightarrow a = \dfrac{30}{60} = \dfrac{1}{2}$.

Therefore, $P(x) = \dfrac{1}{2}(x^3 - x^2 - 32x + 60) \Rightarrow P(x) = \dfrac{1}{2}x^3 - \dfrac{1}{2}x^2 - 16x + 30$.

93. (a) Because the function $P(x)$ has coefficient signs: $--++$, which is 1 sign change, the function has 1 positive real zero. Because $P(-x) = -2(-x)^4 - (-x)^3 + (-x) + 2 = -2x^4 + x^2 - x + 2$ has coefficient signs: $-+-+$, which is 3 sign changes, the function has 3 or 1 negative real zero.

(b) By the Rational Zero Theorem, the possible rational zeros are $\dfrac{p}{q} = \pm\dfrac{1,2}{1,2} = \pm 1, \pm 2, \pm\dfrac{1}{2}$.

(c) From part (b) and a calculator graph of the equation, we choose 1 and −1 to check by synthetic division. (The second from the result of the first)

$$1\overline{)\begin{array}{ccccc}-2 & -1 & 0 & 1 & 2\end{array}} \qquad -1\overline{)\begin{array}{cccc}-2 & -3 & -3 & -2\end{array}}$$
$$\underline{\begin{array}{ccccc} & -2 & -3 & -3 & -2\end{array}} \Rightarrow \underline{\begin{array}{cccc} & 2 & 1 & 2\end{array}}$$
$$\begin{array}{ccccc}-2 & -3 & -3 & -2 & 0\end{array} \qquad \begin{array}{cccc}-2 & -1 & -2 & 0\end{array}$$

The resulting polynomial $-2x^2 - x - 2$ has no real zeros, so the rational zeros are 1 and −1.

(d) No other real zeros, the remaining zeros are imaginary.

(e) Using the quadratic equation yields

$$x = \frac{-(-1) \pm \sqrt{(-1)^2 - 4(-2)(-2)}}{2(-2)} = \frac{1 \pm \sqrt{-15}}{-4} \Rightarrow x = -\frac{1}{4} + i\frac{\sqrt{15}}{4} \text{ and } -\frac{1}{4} - i\frac{\sqrt{15}}{4}.$$

(f) The rational zeros are the x-intercepts; therefore, $(1, 0)$ and $(-1, 0)$.

(g) Find $P(0)$: $P(0) = -2(0)^4 - (0)^3 + (0) + 2 \Rightarrow P(0) = 2$. The y-intercept is $(0, 2)$.

(h) $$4\overline{)\begin{array}{ccccc}-2 & -1 & 0 & 1 & 2\end{array}}$$
$$\underline{\begin{array}{ccccc} & -8 & -36 & -144 & -572\end{array}} \qquad \text{Therefore, } f(4) = -570; (4, -570).$$
$$\begin{array}{ccccc}-2 & -9 & -36 & -143 & -570\end{array}$$

(i) $P(x)$ is an negative even-degree polynomial graph; therefore, ⌢

(j) See Figure 93.

94. (a) Because the function $P(x)$ has coefficient signs: + + + + +, which is 0 sign changes, the function has 0 positive real zeros. Because $P(-x) = 4(-x)^5 + 8(-x)^4 + 9(-x)^3 + 27(-x)^2 + 27(-x) =$
$-4x^5 + 8x^4 - 9x^3 + 27x^2 - 27x$ has coefficient signs: − + − + −, which is 4 sign changes, the function has 4, 2, or 0 negative real zeros.

(b) By using the Rational Zero Theorem, after factoring out an x, the possible rational zeros are
$$\frac{p}{q} = \pm\frac{1,3,9,27}{1,2,4} = 0, \pm 1, \pm 3, \pm 9, \pm 27, \pm\frac{1}{2}, \pm\frac{3}{2}, \pm\frac{9}{2}, \pm\frac{27}{2}, \pm\frac{1}{4}, \pm\frac{3}{4}, \pm\frac{9}{4}, \pm\frac{27}{4}.$$

(c) Factoring out the x gives 0 as one of the zeros, now from part (b) and a calculator graph of the equation, we choose $-\frac{3}{2}$ (multiplicity 2, because it appears tangent) to check by synthetic division. (The second from the result of the first)

$$-\frac{3}{2}\overline{)\begin{array}{cccc}4 & 8 & 9 & 27 & 27\end{array}} \qquad -\frac{3}{2}\overline{)\begin{array}{cccc}4 & 2 & 6 & 18\end{array}}$$
$$\underline{\begin{array}{cccc} & -6 & -3 & -9 & -27\end{array}} \Rightarrow \underline{\begin{array}{cccc} & -6 & 6 & -18\end{array}}$$
$$\begin{array}{cccc}4 & 2 & 6 & 18 & 0\end{array} \qquad \begin{array}{cccc}4 & -4 & 12 & 0\end{array}$$

The resulting polynomial $4x^2 - 4x + 12$ has no real zeros, so the rational zeros are 0 and $-\frac{3}{2}$ (multiplicity 2).

(d) No other real zeros, the remaining zeros are imaginary.

136   CHAPTER 3   Polynomial Functions

(e) Using the quadratic formula after factoring $4(x^2 - x + 3)$ yields

$$x = \frac{-(-1) \pm \sqrt{(-1)^2 - 4(1)(3)}}{2(1)} = \frac{1 \pm \sqrt{-11}}{2} \Rightarrow x = \frac{1}{2} + i\frac{\sqrt{11}}{2} \text{ and } \frac{1}{2} - i\frac{\sqrt{11}}{2}.$$

(f) The rational zeros are the x-intercepts; therefore, $(0, 0)$ and $\left(-\frac{3}{2}, 0\right)$.

(g) Find $P(0)$: $P(0) = 4(0)^5 + 8(0)^4 + 9(0)^3 + 27(0)^2 + 27(0) \Rightarrow P(0) = 0$. The y-intercept is $(0, 0)$.

(h)
```
4)4   8    9    27    27    0
      16   96   420   1788  7260
      4    24   105   447   1815  7260
```
Therefore, $f(4) = 7260$; $(4, 7260)$.

(i) $P(x)$ is an positive odd-degree polynomial graph; therefore, ⌒

(j) See Figure 94.

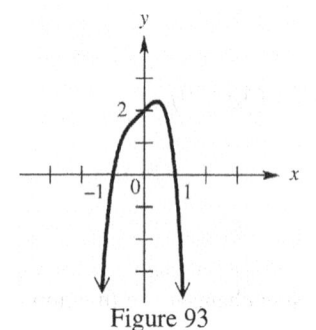
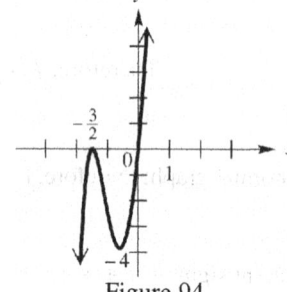

Figure 93   Figure 94

95. (a) Because the function $P(x)$ has coefficient signs: + − −, which is 1 sign change, the function has 1 positive real zero. Because $P(-x) = 3(-x)^4 - 14(-x)^2 - 5 = 3x^4 - 14x^2 - 5$ has coefficient signs: + − −, which is 1 sign change, the function has 1 negative real zero.

(b) By the Rational Zeros Theorem, the possible rational zeros are $\frac{p}{q} = \pm\frac{1,5}{1,3} = \pm 1, \pm 5, \pm\frac{1}{3}, \pm\frac{5}{3}$.

(c) Set equal to 0 and factor the function: $0 = 3x^4 - 14x^2 - 5 \Rightarrow 0 = (3x^2 + 1)(x^2 - 5)$. The factor $3x^2 + 1$ will yield imaginary zeros and $x^2 - 5$ yields irrational zeros; therefore, there are no rational zeros.

(d) From part (c), the factor $\left\{\pm\frac{5}{2}, \pm 1\right\} = \{-2.5, -1, 1, 2.5\}$; therefore, $-\sqrt{5}$ and $\sqrt{5}$ are real zeros.

(e) Using the quadratic formula on the factor $3x^2 + 1 = 0$ found in part (c), yields

$$x = \frac{-(0) \pm \sqrt{(0)^2 - 4(3)(1)}}{2(3)} = \frac{0 \pm \sqrt{-12}}{6} = \frac{\pm 2i\sqrt{3}}{6} \Rightarrow x = -i\frac{\sqrt{3}}{3} \text{ and } i\frac{\sqrt{3}}{3}.$$

(f) The rational zeros are the x-intercepts; therefore, 1 and $\left(-\sqrt{5}, 0\right)$ and $\left(\sqrt{5}, 0\right)$.

(g) Find $P(0)$: $P(0) = 3(0)^4 - 14(0)^2 - 5 \Rightarrow P(0) = -5$. The y-intercept is $(0, -5)$.

(h)
$$\begin{array}{r|rrrrr} 4) & 3 & 0 & -14 & 0 & -5 \\ & & 12 & 48 & 136 & 144 \\ \hline & 3 & 12 & 34 & 136 & 536 \end{array}$$
Therefore, $f(4) = 539$; $(4, 539)$.

(i) $P(x)$ is a positive even-degree polynomial graph; therefore, $\smile$

(j) See Figure 95.

96. (a) Because the function $P(x)$ has coefficient signs: $--++--$, which is 2 sign changes, the function has 2 or 0 positive real zeros. Because $P(-x) = -(-x)^5 - (-x)^4 + 10(-x)^3 + 10(-x)^2 - 9(-x) - 9 = x^5 - x^4 - 10x^3 + 10x^2 + 9x - 9$ has coefficient signs: $+--++-$, which is 3 sign changes, the function has 3 or 1 negative real zeros.

(b) By using the Rational Zeros Theorem, the possible rational zeros are $\dfrac{p}{q} = \pm \dfrac{1, 3, 9}{1} = \pm 1, \pm 3, \pm 9$.

(c) From part (b) and a calculator graph of the equation, we choose $-3, 1$ and 3 to check by synthetic division.

$$\begin{array}{r|rrrrrr} -3) & -1 & -1 & 10 & 10 & -9 & -9 \\ & & 3 & -6 & -12 & 6 & 9 \\ \hline & -1 & 2 & 4 & -2 & -3 & 0 \end{array} \Rightarrow \begin{array}{r|rrrrr} 1) & -1 & 2 & 4 & -2 & -3 \\ & & -1 & 1 & 5 & 3 \\ \hline & -1 & 1 & 5 & 3 & 0 \end{array} \Rightarrow$$

$$\begin{array}{r|rrrr} 3) & -1 & 1 & 5 & 3 \\ & & 0 & -3 & -6 & -3 \\ \hline & -1 & -2 & -1 & 0 \end{array}$$

Factor the resulting expression to obtain the last 2 zeros. $-x^2 - 2x - 1 = -(x+1)(x+1) = 0 \Rightarrow x = -1$ (multiplicity 2). Therefore, the rational zeros are $-3, -1$ (multiplicity 2), and 3.

(d) No other real zeros, all are rational and given in part (c).

(e) No complex zeros, all are rational.

(f) The rational zeros are the x-intercepts; therefore, $(-3, 0), (-1, 0)$ (multiplicity 2), and $(3, 0)$.

(g) Find $P(0)$: $P(0) = -(0)^5 - (0)^4 + 10(0)^3 + 10(0)^2 - 9(0) - 9 \Rightarrow P(0) = -9$. The y-intercept is $(0, -9)$.

(h)
$$\begin{array}{r|rrrrrr} 4) & -1 & -1 & 10 & 10 & -9 & -9 \\ & & -4 & 20 & -40 & -120 & -516 \\ \hline & -1 & -5 & -10 & -30 & -129 & -525 \end{array}$$
Therefore, $f(4) = -525$; $(4, -525)$.

(i) $P(x)$ is a negative odd-degree polynomial graph; therefore, $\curvearrowright$

(j) See Figure 96.

97. (a) Because the function $P(x)$ has coefficient signs, $-+-+-$, which is 4 sign changes, the function has 4, 2 or 0 positive real zeros. Because $P(-x) = -3x^4 - 22x^3 - 55x^2 - 52x - 12$ has coefficient signs, $-----$, which is 0 sign changes, the function has 0 negative real zeros.

(b) By the Rational Zeros Theorem, the possible rational zeros are

$\dfrac{p}{q} = \pm \dfrac{1, 2, 3, 4, 6, 12}{1, 3} = \pm 1, \pm 2, \pm 3, \pm 4, \pm 6, \pm 12, \pm \dfrac{1}{3}, \pm \dfrac{2}{3}, \pm \dfrac{4}{3}$

138   CHAPTER 3   Polynomial Functions

(c) From part (b) and a calculator graph of the equation we choose $\frac{1}{3}$ and 3 to check by synthetic division.

$$\frac{1}{3}\overline{\smash{\big)}\begin{array}{rrrrr} -3 & 22 & -55 & 52 & -12 \\ & -1 & 7 & -16 & 12 \\ \hline -3 & 21 & -48 & 36 & 0 \end{array}} \Rightarrow 3\overline{\smash{\big)}\begin{array}{rrrr} -3 & 21 & -48 & 36 \\ & -90 & 36 & -36 \\ \hline -3 & 12 & -12 & 0 \end{array}}$$

Factor the resulting expression to obtain the last 2 zeros. $-3x^2 + 12x - 12 = -3(x-2)(x-2) = 0 \Rightarrow x = 2$ (with a multiplicity of 2). Therefore, the rational zeros are $\left(\frac{1}{3}, 0\right)$, $(2, 0)$ (multiplicity 2), and $(3, 0)$.

(d) No other real zeros, all are rational.

(e) No complex zeros, all are rational.

(f) The rational zeros are the *x*-intercepts; therefore, the answers are $\frac{1}{3}$, 2 (multiplicity 2), and 3.

(g) Find $P(0)$: $P(0) = -3(0)^4 + 22(0)^3 - 55(0)^2 + 52(0) - 12 \Rightarrow P(0) = -12$. The *y*-intercept is -12.

(h) $$4\overline{\smash{\big)}\begin{array}{rrrrr} -3 & 22 & -55 & 52 & -12 \\ & -12 & 40 & -60 & -32 \\ \hline -3 & 10 & -15 & -8 & -44 \end{array}}$$ Therefore, $f(4) = -44$; $(4, -44)$.

(i) $P(x)$ is a negative even-degree polynomial graph; therefore, it is ⌢

(j) See Figure 97.

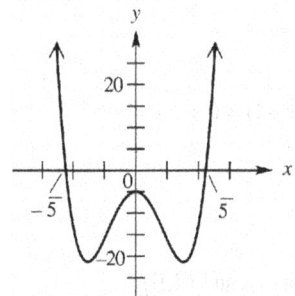
Figure 95

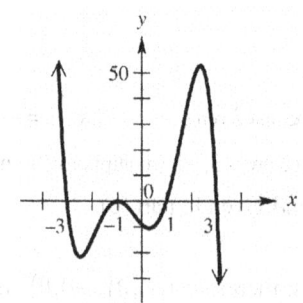
Figure 96

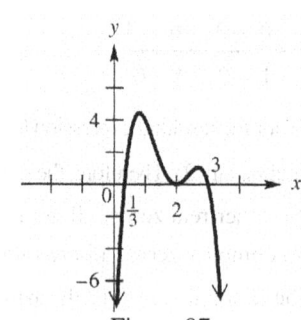
Figure 97

98. The function has 2 irrational zeros of $\pm\sqrt{5}$, which can be approximated to ± 2.236.

3.8: Polynomial Equations and Inequalities; Further Applications and Models

1. $x^3 - 25x = 0 \Rightarrow x(x^2 - 25) = 0 \Rightarrow x(x+5)(x-5) = 0 \Rightarrow x = 0, (x+5) = 0, (x-5) = 0 \Rightarrow x = 0, x = -5, x = 5$.

3. $x^4 - x^2 = 2x^2 + 4 \Rightarrow x^4 - 3x^2 - 4 = 0 \Rightarrow (x^2 - 4)(x^2 + 1) = 0 \Rightarrow (x^2 - 4) = 0, (x^2 + 1) = 0 \Rightarrow$
   $x = \pm 2$. The solution to $x^2 + 1$ is not a real number.

5. $x^3 - 3x^2 - 18x = 0 \Rightarrow x(x^2 - 3x - 18) = 0 \Rightarrow x(x-6)(x+3) = 0 \Rightarrow x = 0, (x-6) = 0, (x+3) = 0 \Rightarrow$
   $x = 0, x = 6, x = -3$

7. $2x^3 = 4x^2 - 2x \Rightarrow 2x^3 - 4x^2 + 2x = 0 \Rightarrow 2x(x^2 - 2x + 1) = 0 \Rightarrow 2x(x-1)^2 = 0 \Rightarrow 2x = 0, (x-1)^2 = 0 \Rightarrow x = 0, x = 1$.

9. $12x^3 = 17x^2 + 5x \Rightarrow 12x^3 - 17x^2 - 5x = 0 \Rightarrow x(12x^2 - 17x - 5) = 0 \Rightarrow x(4x+1)(3x-5) = 0 \Rightarrow$

   $x = 0, x = -\dfrac{1}{4}, x = \dfrac{5}{3}$.

11. $2x^3 + 4 = x(x+8) \Rightarrow 2x^3 + 4 = x^2 + 8x \Rightarrow 2x^3 - x^2 - 8x + 4 = 0 \Rightarrow x^2(2x-1) - 4(2x-1) = 0 \Rightarrow (x^2 - 4)(2x-1) = 0$

    $\Rightarrow (x^2 - 4) = 0, (2x-1) = 0 \Rightarrow x = \pm 2, x = \dfrac{1}{2}$.

13. First, factor the equation: $7x^3 + x = 0 \Rightarrow x(7x^2 + 1) = 0 \Rightarrow x = 0$ and $7x^2 + x = 0$. Now solve:

    $7x^2 + 1 = 0 \Rightarrow 7x^2 = -1 \Rightarrow x^2 = -\dfrac{1}{7} \Rightarrow x = \pm\dfrac{\sqrt{-1}}{\sqrt{7}} \Rightarrow x = \pm\dfrac{i}{\sqrt{7}} \Rightarrow x = \pm\dfrac{i}{\sqrt{7}} \cdot \dfrac{\sqrt{7}}{\sqrt{7}} \Rightarrow x = \pm\dfrac{i\sqrt{7}}{7}$. The solution

    set is $\left\{0, \pm\dfrac{i\sqrt{7}}{7}\right\}$.

15. First, factor the equation.

    $3x^3 + 2x^2 - 3x - 2 = 0 \Rightarrow x^2(3x+2) - 1(3x+2) = 0 \Rightarrow (x^2 - 1)(3x+2) = 0 \Rightarrow (x+1)(x-1)(3x+2) = 0$.

    Now solve. $x+1 = 0 \Rightarrow x = -1$; $x-1 = 0 \Rightarrow x = 1$; $3x+2 = 0 \Rightarrow x = -\dfrac{2}{3}$. The solution set is $\left\{-1, -\dfrac{2}{3}, 1\right\}$.

17. First, factor the equation: $x^4 - 11x^2 + 10 = 0 \Rightarrow (x^2 - 1)(x^2 - 10) = 0 \Rightarrow (x+1)(x-1)(x^2 - 10) = 0$. Now

    solve: $x+1 = 0 \Rightarrow x = -1$; $x-1 = 0 \Rightarrow x = 1$; $x^2 - 10 = 0 \Rightarrow x^2 = 10 \Rightarrow x = \pm\sqrt{10}$. The solution set is

    $\left\{\pm 1, \pm\sqrt{10}\right\}$.

19. First, factor the equation: $4x^4 - 25x^2 + 36 = 0 \Rightarrow (4x^2 - 9)(x^2 - 4) = 0$. Now solve:

    $4x^2 - 9 = 0 \Rightarrow 4x^2 = 9 \Rightarrow x^2 = \dfrac{9}{4} \Rightarrow x = \pm\sqrt{\dfrac{9}{4}} \Rightarrow x = \pm\dfrac{3}{2}$; $x^2 - 4 = 0 \Rightarrow x^2 = 4 \Rightarrow x = \pm\sqrt{4} \Rightarrow x = \pm 2$. The

    solution set is $\left\{\pm\dfrac{3}{2}, \pm 2\right\} = \{-2, -1.5, 1.5, 2\}$. When graphed on the calculator, these values are supported as

    the x-intercepts of $y = 4x^4 - 29x^2 + 25$.

21. First, factor the equation: $x^4 - 15x^2 - 16 = 0 \Rightarrow (x^2 - 16)(x^2 + 1) = 0$. Now solve:

    $x^2 - 16 = 0 \Rightarrow x^2 = 16 \Rightarrow x = \pm\sqrt{16} \Rightarrow x = \pm 4$; $x^2 + 1 = 0 \Rightarrow x^2 = -1 \Rightarrow x = \pm\sqrt{-1} \Rightarrow x = \pm i$. The solution set

    is $\{-4, 4, -i, i\}$. When graphed on the calculator, the real values -4 and 4 are supported as the only x-

    intercepts of $y = x^4 - 15x^2 - 16$.

23. First, factor the equation: $x^3 - x^2 - 64x + 64 = 0 \Rightarrow x^2(x-1) - 64(x-1) = 0 \Rightarrow$

    $(x^2 - 64)(x-1) = 0 \Rightarrow (x+8)(x-8)(x-1) = 0$. Now solve: $x+8 = 0 \Rightarrow x = -8$; $x-8 = 0 \Rightarrow x = 8$;

    $x-1 = 0 \Rightarrow x = 1$. The solution set is $\{-8, 1, 8\}$. When graphed on the calculator, these values are supported

    as the x-intercepts of $y = x^3 - x^2 - 64x + 64$.

25. First, factor the equation: $-2x^3 - x^2 + 3x = 0 \Rightarrow -x(2x^2 + x - 3) = 0 \Rightarrow -x(2x+3)(x-1) = 0$. Now solve:

    $-x = 0 \Rightarrow x = 0$; $2x + 3 = 0 \Rightarrow x = -\dfrac{3}{2}$; $x - 1 = 0 \Rightarrow x = 1$. The solution set is $\{-1.5, 0, 1\}$. When graphed on the calculator, these values are supported as the x-intercepts of $-2x^3 - x^2 + 3x = 0$.

27. First, factor the equation: $x^3 + x^2 - 7x - 7 = 0 \Rightarrow x^2(x+1) - 7(x+1) = 0 \Rightarrow (x^2 - 7)(x+1) = 0$. Now solve:

    $x + 1 = 0 \Rightarrow x = -1$; $x^2 - 7 = 0 \Rightarrow x^2 = 7 \Rightarrow x = \pm\sqrt{7}$. The solution set is $\{-1, \pm\sqrt{7}\}$, When graphed on the calculator, these values are supported as the x-intercepts of $y = x^3 + x^2 - 7x - 7$.

29. First, factor the equation by $-x$: $-3x^3 - x^2 + 6x = 0 \Rightarrow -x(3x^2 + x - 6) = 0$. Now one solution is $-x = 0 \Rightarrow x = 0$, and we use the quadratic formula on the remaining factor to find the other solutions:

    $x = \dfrac{-1 \pm \sqrt{1^2 - 4(3)(-6)}}{2(3)} \Rightarrow x = \dfrac{-1 \pm \sqrt{73}}{6}$. The solution set is $\left\{0, \dfrac{-1-\sqrt{73}}{6}, \dfrac{-1+\sqrt{73}}{6}\right\}$. When graphed on the calculator, these values are supported as the x-intercepts of $y = -3x^3 - x^2 + 6x$.

31. First, factor the equation by $3x$: $3x^3 + 3x^2 + 3x = 0 \Rightarrow 3x(x^2 + x + 1) = 0$. Now one solution is $3x = 0 \Rightarrow x = 0$ and we use the quadratic formula on the remaining factor to find the other solutions:

    $x = \dfrac{-1 \pm \sqrt{1^2 - 4(1)(1)}}{2(1)} \Rightarrow x = \dfrac{-1 \pm \sqrt{-3}}{2} \Rightarrow x = \dfrac{-1 \pm i\sqrt{3}}{2}$. The solution set is $\left\{0, -\dfrac{1}{2} - \dfrac{\sqrt{3}}{2}i, -\dfrac{1}{2} + \dfrac{\sqrt{3}}{2}i\right\}$.

    When graphed on the calculator, the real value 0 is the only x-intercept of $y = 3x^3 + 3x^2 + 3x$.

33. First, factor the equation: $x^4 + 17x^2 + 16 = 0 \Rightarrow (x^2 + 16)(x^2 + 1) = 0$. Now solve: $x^2 + 16 = 0 \Rightarrow$

    $x^2 = -16 \Rightarrow x = \pm\sqrt{-16} \Rightarrow x = \pm 4i$; $x^2 + 1 = 0 \Rightarrow x^2 = -1 \Rightarrow x = \pm\sqrt{-1} \Rightarrow x = \pm i$. The solution set is $\{-4i, -i, i, 4i\}$. There are no real solutions, a conclusion which is supported when graphed on the calculator, with no x-intercepts for $y = x^4 + 17x^2 + 16$.

35. First, factor the equation: $x^6 + 19x^3 - 216 = 0 \Rightarrow (x^3 - 8)(x^3 + 27) = 0 \Rightarrow$

    $(x - 2)(x^2 + 2x + 4)(x + 3)(x^2 - 3x + 9) = 0$. Now solve: $x - 2 = 0 \Rightarrow x = 2$; $x + 3 = 0 \Rightarrow x = -3$. We use the quadratic formula on the remaining factors to find the other solutions:

    $x = \dfrac{-2 \pm \sqrt{2^2 - 4(1)(4)}}{2(1)} = \dfrac{-2 \pm \sqrt{-12}}{2} = \dfrac{-2 \pm 2i\sqrt{3}}{2} \Rightarrow -1 \pm i\sqrt{3}$;

    $x = \dfrac{-(-3) \pm \sqrt{(-3)^2 - 4(1)(9)}}{2(1)} = \dfrac{3 \pm \sqrt{-27}}{2} \Rightarrow x = \dfrac{3 \pm 3i\sqrt{3}}{2} = \dfrac{3}{2} \pm \dfrac{3\sqrt{3}}{2}i$. The solution set is

    $\left\{-3, 2, -1 - i\sqrt{3}, -1 + i\sqrt{3}, \dfrac{3}{2} - \dfrac{3\sqrt{3}}{2}i, \dfrac{3}{2} + \dfrac{3\sqrt{3}}{2}i\right\}$. When graphed on the calculator, the real values -3 and 2 are supported as the only x-intercepts of $y = x^6 + 19x^3 - 216$.

SECTION 3.8   141

37. See Figure 37. From the graph the following is found:
   (a) $P(x) = 0: \{-2, 1, 4\}$.
   (b). $P(x) < 0: (-\infty, -2) \cup (1, 4)$.
   (c). $P(x) > 0: (-2, 1) \cup (4, \infty)$.

39. See Figure 39. From the graph the following is found:
   (a). $P(x) = 0: \{-2.5, 1, 3 \text{ (multiplicity 2)}\}$.
   (b). $P(x) < 0: (-2.5, 1)$.
   (c). $P(x) > 0: (-\infty, -2.5) \cup (1, 3) \cup (3, \infty)$.

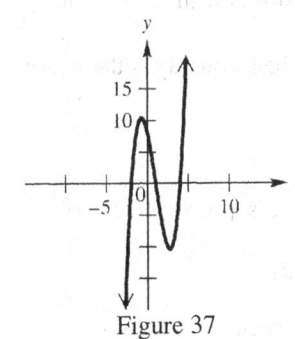
Figure 37

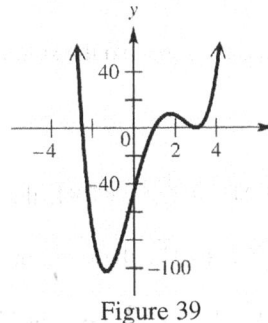
Figure 39

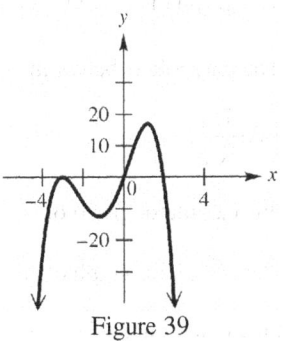
Figure 39

41. See Figure 41. From the graph the following is found:
   (a) $P(x) = 0: \{-3 \text{ (multiplicity 2)}, 0, 2\}$.
   (b) $P(x) \geq 0: [-3] \cup [0, 2]$.
   (c) $P(x) \leq 0: (-\infty, 0] \cup [2, \infty)$.

43. (a) $3(x^2 + 4) + 2x(3x - 12) = 0 \Rightarrow 3x^2 + 12 + 6x^2 - 24x = 0 \Rightarrow 9x^2 - 24x + 12 = 0 \Rightarrow$

   $3(3x^2 - 8x + 4) = 0 \Rightarrow (3x - 2)(x - 2) = 0 \Rightarrow 3x - 2 = 0 \text{ or } x - 2 = 0 \Rightarrow x = \frac{2}{3}, 2$

   (b) The graph of $y = 3(x^2 + 4) + 2x(3x - 12)$ or equivalently $y = 9x^2 - 24x + 12$ is a parabola that opens upward with zeros $\frac{2}{3}$ and 2. The parabola is below the x-axis between its zeros, so the solution set to the inequality is the interval $\left(\frac{2}{3}, 2\right)$. Note that it is not necessary to actually graph the parabola to solve the inequality.

45. (a) $3(x+1)^2 (2x-1)^4 + 8(x+1)^3 (2x-1)^3 = 0 \Rightarrow \left[(x+1)^2 (2x-1)^3\right] [3(2x-1) + 8(x+1)] = 0 \Rightarrow$

   $\left[(x+1)^2 (2x-1)^3\right] [(6x-3) + (8x+8)] = 0 \Rightarrow (x+1)^2 (2x-1)^3 (14x+5) = 0 \Rightarrow$

   $(x+1)^2 = 0, (2x-1)^3 = 0, (14x+5) = 0 \Rightarrow x = -1, -\frac{5}{14}, \frac{1}{2}$

Copyright © 2015 Pearson Education, Inc

(b) The graph of $y = (x+1)^2 (2x-1)^3 (14x+5)$ is a degree six polynomial that is above the x-axis from $\left(-\infty, -\frac{5}{14}\right)$ and $\left(\frac{1}{2}, \infty\right)$. The solution set to the inequality is the interval $\left(-\infty, -\frac{5}{14}\right] \cup \left[\frac{1}{2}, \infty\right)$. Note that it is helpful to actually graph the cubic to solve the inequality.

47. (a) $3kx^2 - 7x = 0 \Rightarrow x(3kx - 7) = 0 \Rightarrow x = 0$ or $3kx - 7 = 0 \Rightarrow 3kx = 7 \Rightarrow x = \frac{7}{kx}$,

    The solution set is $\left\{0, \frac{7}{3k}\right\}$.

    (b) The graph of $y = 3kx^2 - 7x$ is a parabola that opens upward (since k is positive) with zeros 0 and $\frac{7}{3k}$. The parabola is below the x-axis between the zeros, so the solution set to the inequality is the interval $\left(0, \frac{7}{3k}\right)$.

49. From the calculator graph of $y_1 = 0.86x^3 - 5.24x^2 + 3.55x + 7.84$, the solution set is $\{-0.88, 2.12, 4.86\}$.

51. From the calculator graph of $y_1 = -\sqrt{7}x^3 + \sqrt{5}x^2 + \sqrt{17}$, the solution set is $\{1.52\}$.

53. Given the equation $2.45x^4 - 3.22x^3 = -0.47x^2 + 6.54x + 3$, rearrange to get the calculator graph of $y_1 = 2.54x^4 - 3.22x^3 + 0.47x^2 - 6.54x - 3$. The solution set is $\{-0.40, 2.02\}$.

55. $x^2 = -1 \Rightarrow x = \pm\sqrt{-1} \Rightarrow x = \pm i \Rightarrow \{-i, i\}$.

57. First, factor the equation $x^3 = -1 \Rightarrow x^3 + 1 = 0 \Rightarrow (x+1)(x^2 - x + 1) = 0$. Now one solution is $x + 1 = 0 \Rightarrow x = -1$, and we use the quadratic formula on the remaining factor to find the other solutions.

    $x = \frac{-(-1) \pm \sqrt{(-1)^2 - 4(1)(1)}}{2(1)} \Rightarrow x = \frac{1 \pm i\sqrt{3}}{2}$. The solution set is $\left\{-1, \frac{1}{2} - \frac{\sqrt{3}}{2}i, \frac{1}{2} + \frac{\sqrt{3}}{2}i\right\}$.

59. First, factor the equation $x^3 = 27 \Rightarrow x^3 - 27 = 0 \Rightarrow (x-3)(x^2 + 3x + 9) = 0$. Now one solution is $x - 3 = 0 \Rightarrow x = 3$. We use the quadratic formula on the remaining factor to find the other solutions.

    $x = \frac{-3 \pm \sqrt{3^2 - 4(1)(9)}}{2(1)} \Rightarrow x = \frac{-3 \pm \sqrt{-27}}{2} = \frac{-3 \pm 3i\sqrt{3}}{2}$. The solution set is $\left\{3, -\frac{3}{2} - \frac{3\sqrt{3}}{2}i, -\frac{3}{2} + \frac{3\sqrt{3}}{2}i\right\}$.

61. First, factor the equation $x^4 = 16 \Rightarrow x^4 - 16 = 0 \Rightarrow (x^2 - 4)(x^2 + 4) = 0 \Rightarrow (x-2)(x+2)(x^2 + 4) = 0$. Now two solutions are $x - 2 = 0 \Rightarrow x = 2$, and $x + 2 = 0 \Rightarrow x = -2$. We solve the remaining factor for the last two solutions. $x^2 + 4 = 0 \Rightarrow x^2 = -4 \Rightarrow x = \pm\sqrt{-4} \Rightarrow x = \pm 2i$. The solution set is $\{-2, 2, -2i, 2i\}$.

63. First, factor the equation $x^3 = -64 \Rightarrow x^3 + 64 = 0 \Rightarrow (x+4)(x^2 - 4x + 16) = 0$. Now one solution is $x + 4 = 0 \Rightarrow x = -4$. We use the quadratic formula on the remaining factor to find the other solutions.

    $x = \frac{-(-4) \pm \sqrt{(-4)^2 - 4(1)(16)}}{2(1)} = \frac{4 \pm \sqrt{-48}}{2} \Rightarrow x = \frac{4 \pm 4i\sqrt{3}}{2} = 2 \pm 2i\sqrt{3}$. The solution set is $\{-4, 2 - 2i\sqrt{3}, 2 + 2i\sqrt{3}\}$.

65. $x^2 = -18 \Rightarrow x = \sqrt{-18} \Rightarrow x = \pm 3i\sqrt{2} \Rightarrow \{-3i\sqrt{2}, 3i\sqrt{2}\}$.

67. (a) First, find f(x) for $d = 0.8$. $f(x) = \frac{\pi}{3}x^3 - 5\pi x^2 + \frac{500\pi(0.8)}{3} \Rightarrow f(x) = \frac{\pi}{3}x^3 - 5\pi x^2 + \frac{400\pi}{3}$. Now graph this equation on a graphing calculator. We find the smallest positive zero is at $x \approx 7.1286$ cm. or $x \approx 7.13$ cm. The ball floats partly above the surface.

   (b) First, find $f(x)$ for $d = 2.7$. $f(x) = \frac{\pi}{3}x^3 - 5\pi x^2 + \frac{500\pi(2.7)}{3} \Rightarrow f(x) = \frac{\pi}{3}x^3 - 5\pi x^2 + \frac{1350\pi}{3}$. Now graph this equation on a graphing calculator. We find the graph has no zero; the sphere sinks below the surface because it is more dense than water.

   (c) First, find $f(x)$ for $d = 1$. $f(x) = \frac{\pi}{3}x^3 - 5\pi x^2 + \frac{500\pi(1)}{3} \Rightarrow f(x) = \frac{\pi}{3}x^3 - 5\pi x^2 + \frac{500\pi}{3}$. Now graph this equation on a graphing calculator. We find the smallest positive zero is at $x = 10$ cm; the balloon floats even with the surface.

69. (a) Since the box has sides $x > 0$ and since the box must have some width, we have $12 - 2x > 0 \Rightarrow -2x > -12 \Rightarrow x < 6$. Therefore, the restrictions are $0 < x < 6$.

   (b) Since $V = lwh$, length $= 18 - 2x$, and width $= 12 - 2x$, the function is
   $V(x) = (18 - 2x)(12 - 2x)(x) \Rightarrow V(x) = x(4x^2 - 60x + 216) \Rightarrow V(x) = 4x^3 - 60x^2 + 216x$.

   (c) By graphing the function from (b) on a graphing calculator, we can find that the maximum volume is at $x \approx 2.35$ in., which produces a volume of $V(2.35) \approx 4(2.35)^3 - 60(2.35)^2 + 216(2.35) \approx 228.16$ in^3.

   (d) By graphing the function from (b) on a graphing calculator, we can find the volume to be greater than 80 in^3 for the interval $0.42 < x < 5$.

71. By graphing the equation on a graphing calculator, we find the smallest positive zero which is less than 10 is $x \approx 2.61$ in.

73. (a) A length 1 inch less than the hypotenuse (x) is $x - 1$.

   (b) Using the Pythagorean Theorem yields $l^2 + (x-1)^2 = x^2 \Rightarrow l^2 = x^2 - (x-1)^2 \Rightarrow$
   $l^2 = x^2 - (x^2 - 2x + 1) \Rightarrow l^2 = 2x - 1 \Rightarrow l = \sqrt{2x - 1}$.

   (c) Since $A = \frac{1}{2}bh = 84$, the equation is $\frac{1}{2}(\sqrt{2x-1})(x-1) = 84 \Rightarrow$
   $(\sqrt{2x-1})(x-1) = 168 \Rightarrow [(\sqrt{2x-1})(x-1)]^2 = 168^2 \Rightarrow (2x-1)(x-1)^2 = 28,224 \Rightarrow$
   $(2x-1)(x^2 - 2x + 1) = 28,224 \Rightarrow 2x^3 - 5x^2 + 4x - 28,225 = 0$.

   (d) By graphing the equation from (c) on a graphing calculator, we get an x-intercept of 25. Therefore, the hypotenuse is $x = 25$ in., one leg is $x - 1 = 24$ in., and the other leg is $\sqrt{2x-1} = \sqrt{49} = 7$ in.

75. (a) Since $l = 11 - 2x$, $w = 8.5 - 2x$, $h = x$, and $V = lwh$, we get an equation of
   $V = (11 - 2x)(8.5 - 2x)(x) \Rightarrow V = (93.5 - 17x - 22x + 4x^2)(x) \Rightarrow V = 4x^3 - 39x^2 + 93.5x$. Because all sides of the box must be positive, the restrictions on this equation will be $8.5 - 2x > 0 \Rightarrow -2x > -8.5 \Rightarrow$

$x < 4.25 \Rightarrow 0 < x < 4.25$. Now using the table feature on the graphing calculator yields a maximum value, within the restrictions, of $x \approx 1.59$. The volume is $4(1.59)^3 - 39(1.59)^2 + 93.5(1.59) \approx 66.15$ in^3.

(b) Using the table feature on the graphing calculator for the equation $V = 4x^3 - 39x^2 + 93x$ yields a volume greater than 40 in^3 when x is in the following range: 0.54 in $< x <$ 2.92 in.

77. (a) See Figure 77a.

(b) From the regression feature, the best-fitting quadratic function is $C(x) \approx 0.0035x^2 - 49x + 22$. See Figure 77b.

(c) From the regression feature, the best-fitting cubic function is
$C(x) \approx 0.000068x^3 + 0.00987x^2 - 0.653x + 23$. See Figure 77c.

(d) Using the graphs of each, the cubic function is a slightly better fit.

(e) Using the cubic function and graph, $C(x) > 10$ when $0 \le x < 31.92$.

[-5,70] by [-5,25] [-5,70] by [-5,25] [-5,70] by [-5,25]
Xscl = 5 Yscl = 5   Xscl = 5 Yscl = 5   Xscl = 5 Yscl = 5

Figure 77a   Figure 77b   Figure 77c

Reviewing Basic Concepts (Sections 3.6—3.8)

1. $P(3) = 2(3)^4 - 7(3)^3 + 29(3) - 30 \Rightarrow P(3) = 162 - 189 + 87 - 30 \Rightarrow P(3) = 30$.

2. Since $P(2) = 2(2)^4 - 7(2)^3 + 29(2) - 30 \Rightarrow P(2) = 32 - 56 + 58 - 30 \Rightarrow P(2) = 4$, $P(2)$ is not a zero.

3. Since $2 + i$ is a zero, its conjugate $2 - i$ is also a zero. First, use synthetic division to factor out these two zeros from the equation and the resulting equation.

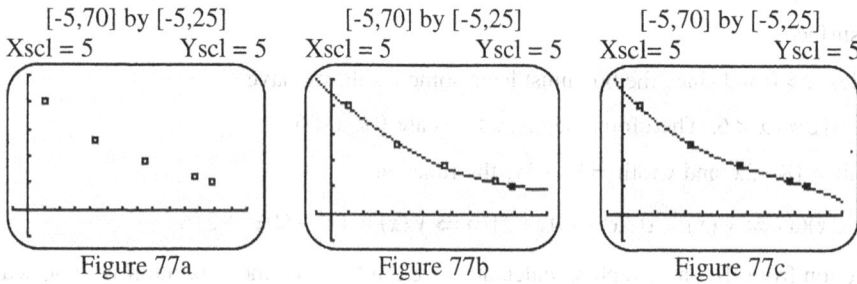

Now completely factor the resulting expression, $2x^2 + x - 6 = (2x - 3)(x + 2)$. The linear factors are $P(x) = (2x - 3)(x + 2)(x - 2 - i)(x - 2 + i)$.

4. Since the zeros are $\frac{3}{2}$, and i, and the conjugate of i is $-i$, the function is $P(x) = a\left(x - \frac{3}{2}\right)(x - i)(x + i) \Rightarrow$

$P(x) = a\left(x - \frac{3}{2}\right)(x^2 + 1) \Rightarrow P(x) = a\left(x^3 - \frac{3}{2}x^2 + x - \frac{3}{2}\right)$. If $P(x) = 15$, then $15 = a\left(3^3 - \frac{3}{2}(3)^2 + 3 - \frac{3}{2}\right) \Rightarrow$

$15 = a\left(27 - \frac{27}{2} + 3 - \frac{3}{2}\right) \Rightarrow 15 = a(30 - 15) \Rightarrow 15 = 15a \Rightarrow a = 1$. Therefore, the function is

$P(x) = x^3 - \frac{3}{2}x^2 + x - \frac{3}{2}$.

5. Since the zeros are $-4, -4, 1+2i$, and its conjugate $1-2i$, the function is
$P(x) = a(x+4)^2(x-1-2i)(x-1+2i) \Rightarrow P(x) = a(x^2+8x+16)(x^2-2x+5) \Rightarrow$
$P(x) = a(x^4+6x^3+5x^2+8x+80)$. If $a = 1$, then $P(x) = x^4+6x^3+5x^2+8x+80$. (Answers may vary).

6. For the function the possible zeros are $x = \pm \dfrac{1, 2, 5, 10}{1, 2} \Rightarrow x = \pm 1, \pm 2, \pm 5, \pm 10, \pm \dfrac{1}{2}, \pm \dfrac{5}{2}$. From a calculator graph, we can choose $x = -2$ to check by synthetic division.

$$\begin{array}{r|rrr} -2 & 2 & 1 & -11 & -10 \\ & & -4 & 6 & 10 \\ \hline & 2 & -3 & -5 & 0 \end{array}$$

Now solve the resulting quadratic equation: $2x^2 - 3x - 5 = 0 \Rightarrow (2x-5)(x+1) = 0 \Rightarrow 2x-5 = 0$ and $x+1 = 0 \Rightarrow$
$x = \dfrac{5}{2}, -1,$ and -2.

7. Use the quadratic formula on the equation $x^2 = \dfrac{12 \pm \sqrt{(-12)^2 - 4(3)(1)}}{2(3)} = \dfrac{12 \pm \sqrt{132}}{6} = \dfrac{12 \pm 2\sqrt{33}}{6} = \dfrac{6 \pm \sqrt{33}}{3}$.

Therefore, $x = \pm \sqrt{\dfrac{6 \pm \sqrt{33}}{3}}$.

8. (a) From the regression feature, the best-fitting quadratic function is
$P(x) \approx 0.0004815x^3 + 0.0303x^2 - 0.1989x + 3.1$.

   (b) $P(34) \approx 0.0004815(34)^3 + 0.0303(34)^2 - 0.1989(34) + 3.1 \approx 50.3$ This value is within 300 of the actual value of 50 thousand.

   (c) Using calculator graphs of $y_1 = 0.0004815x^3 + 0.0303x^2 - 0.1989x + 3.1$ and $y_2 = 100$, the intersection is $x \approx 45$ or approximately the year 2005.

Chapter 3 Review Exercises

1. $(17-i) + (1-3i) = 18-4i$.

2. $(17-i) - (1-3i) = 17-i-1+3i = 16+2i$.

3. $(17-i)(1-3i) = 17-51i-i+3i^2 = 17-52i-3 = 14-52i$.

4. $(17-i)^2 = (17-i)(17-i) = 289-17i+i^2 = 289-34i-1 = 288-34i$.

5. $\dfrac{1}{1-3i} \cdot \dfrac{1+3i}{1+3i} = \dfrac{1+3i}{1-9i^2} = \dfrac{1+3i}{1-9i^2} = \dfrac{1+3i}{10} = \dfrac{1}{10} + \dfrac{3}{10}i$.

6. $\dfrac{17-i}{1-3i} \cdot \dfrac{1+3i}{1+3i} = \dfrac{17+51i-i-3i^2}{1-9i^2} = \dfrac{20+50i}{10} = 2+5i$.

7. Since all real numbers can be input for x, the domain is $(-\infty, \infty)$.

8. By using the vertex formula, we first find the x-coordinate of the vertex. $x = \dfrac{-b}{2a} = \dfrac{-(-6)}{2(2)} = \dfrac{6}{4} = \dfrac{3}{2}$. Now solve for y. $P\left(\dfrac{3}{2}\right) = 2\left(\dfrac{3}{2}\right)^2 - 6\left(\dfrac{3}{2}\right) - 8 \Rightarrow P\left(\dfrac{3}{2}\right) = \dfrac{9}{2} - \dfrac{18}{2} - \dfrac{16}{2} = -\dfrac{25}{2}$. The vertex is $\left(\dfrac{3}{2}, -\dfrac{25}{2}\right)$.

9. Since the function is a positive even-degree equation, the end behavior is ⌣

10. At the x-intercept, $P(x) = 0$. Therefore, $2x^2 - 6x - 8 = 0 \Rightarrow x^2 - 3x - 4 = 0 \Rightarrow$ $(x-4)(x+1) = 0 \Rightarrow x = -1, 4$. The x-intercepts are $(-1, 0)$ and $(4, 0)$.

11. At the y-intercept, $x = 0$. Therefore, $P(0) = 2(0)^2 - 6(0) - 8 \Rightarrow P(0) = -8$. The y-intercept is $(-8, 0)$.

12. From a calculator graph of $P(x) = 2x^2 - 6x - 8$, the range is $\left[-\dfrac{25}{2}, \infty\right)$.

13. From a calculator graph of $P(x) = 2x^2 - 6x - 8$, the graph is increasing for the interval $\left[\dfrac{3}{2}, \infty\right)$, and decreasing for the interval $\left(-\infty, \dfrac{3}{2}\right]$.

14. (a) $2x^2 - 6x - 8 = 0 \Rightarrow x^2 - 3x - 4 = 0 \Rightarrow (x-4)(x+1) = 0 \Rightarrow x = -1$ or 4.

    (b) First, set $2x^2 - 6x - 8 = 0$, then $x^2 - 3x - 4 = 0 \Rightarrow (x-4)(x+1) = 0$, and the solution set will be $\{-1, 4\}$. The numbers -1 and 4 divide the number line into 3 intervals. The interval $(-\infty, -1)$ has a positive product, the interval $(-1, 4)$ has a negative product, and the interval $(4, \infty)$ has a positive product. Therefore, $2x^2 - 6x - 8 > 0$ for the interval $(-\infty, 1) \cup (4, \infty)$.

    (c) First, set $2x^2 - 6x - 6 - 8 = 0$, then $x^2 - 3x - 4 = 0 \Rightarrow (x-4)(x+1) = 0$ and the solution set will be $\{-1, 4\}$. The numbers -1 and 4 divide the number line into 3 intervals. The interval $(-\infty, -1)$ has a positive product, the interval $(-1, 4)$ has a negative product, and the interval $(4, \infty)$ has a positive product. Therefore, $2x^2 - 6x - 8 \leq 0$ for the interval $[-1, 4]$.

15. The graph intersects the x-axis at -1 and 4, supporting the answer in (a). It lies above the x-axis when $x < -1$ or $x > 4$, supporting the answer in (b). It lies below the x-axis when x is between -1 and 4 inclusive, supporting the answer in (c).

16. From problem 8, we know the vertex of $P(x) = 2x^2 - 6x - 8$ is $\left(\dfrac{3}{2}, -\dfrac{25}{2}\right)$. The vertical line of symmetry through this point has the equation $x = \dfrac{3}{2}$.

17. The discriminate is $b^2 - 4ac = (5.47)^2 - 4(-2.64)(3.54) = 29.9209 + 37.3824 = 67.3033$. Since the discriminant is greater than 0, there are two x-intercepts.

18. From the calculator graph of $P(x) = -2.64x^2 + 5.47x + 3.54$, the x-intercepts are $x = 0.52$ and 2.59.

19. From the calculator graph of $P(x) = -2.64x^2 + 5.47x + 3.54$, the vertex is $(1.04, 6.37)$.

20. Using the vertex formula yields $x = \dfrac{-b}{2a} = \dfrac{-5.47}{2(-2.64)} \approx 1.04$. Now solve for

    $P(1.04) = -2.64(1.04)^2 + 5.47(1.04) + 3.54 \approx 6.37$. The vertex is $(1.04, 6.37)$.

21. (a) From the graph, the maximum value of $f(x)$ is 4.

    (b) From the graph, the maximum value of 4 is reached when $x = 1$.

    (c) From the graph, there would be two intersections with $y = 2$; therefore, there are two real solutions.

    (d) From the graph, there would be no intersections with $y = 6$; therefore, there are no real solutions.

22. At zero seconds, the height is $s(0) = -16(0)^2 + 800(0) + 600 = 600$. The projectile was fired from 600 feet.

23. From the calculator graph of the equation, the vertex is $(25, 10600)$. The maximum height is reached after 25 sec.

24. From the calculator graph of the equation, the vertex is $(25, 10600)$. The maximum height is 10,600 feet.

25. From the calculator graph of the equation, and $y = 5000$, the graph of the equation is above $y = 5000$ for the interval $(6.3, 43.7)$. Therefore, the projectile is above 5,000 feet between 6.3 seconds and 43.7 seconds.

26. From the calculator graph of the equation, the x-intercept (when the projectile hits the ground) is $x = 50.739$. The projectile will be in the air for approximately 50.7 seconds.

27. (a) Let $x = $ the width and $3x = $ the length of the cardboard. Then the base of the box will be $w = (x-8)$, and $l = (3x-8)$, and its height is $h = 4$. Since $v = lwh$, we get a function

    $V(x) = (x-8)(3x-8)(4) \Rightarrow V(x) = (3x^2 - 32x + 64)(4) \Rightarrow V(x) = 12x^2 - 128x + 256$.

    (b) If the volume is 2496, then $2496 = 12x^2 - 128x + 256 \Rightarrow 0 = 12x^2 - 128x - 2240 \Rightarrow$

    $0 = 3x^2 - 32x - 560$. Using the quadratic formula to solve this yields

    $x = \dfrac{-(-32) \pm \sqrt{(-32)^2 - 4(3)(-560)}}{2(3)} = \dfrac{32 \pm 88}{6} \Rightarrow x = 20, -\dfrac{28}{3}$. Since we can not have a negative distance we throw out $x = -\dfrac{28}{3}$. Therefore, the original dimensions are 20 in. by 60 in.

    (c) Graphing $y_1 = V(x)$ and $y_2 = 2496$ on a graphing calculator shows that the graphs intersect at $x = 20$.

28. (a) See Figure 28.

    (b) Using the form $P(x) = a(x-h)^2 + k$ and a vertex of $(0, 353)$ yields $P(x) = a(x-0)^2 + 353$. Now solve for a using a second point of $(285, 2000)$. $2000 = a(285-0)^2 + 353 \Rightarrow$

    $1647 = 81225a \Rightarrow a \approx 0.0203$. Therefore, the function is $P(x) = 0.0203x^2 + 353$.

    (c) Using the regression feature of the graphing calculator for the data yields

[-28.5, 313.5] by [73, 2280]

Xscl = 50   Yscl = 100

148   CHAPTER 3   Polynomial Functions

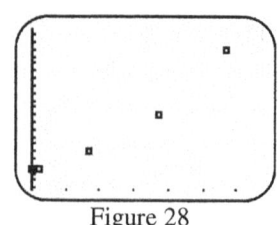

Figure 28

29. First, find $P(-2) = -3(-2)^3 - (-2)^2 + 2(-2) - 4 = 24 - 4 - 4 - 4 \Rightarrow P(-2) = 12$ and

$P(-1) = -3(-1)^3 - (-1)^2 + 2(-1) - 4 = 3 - 1 - 2 - 4 \Rightarrow P(-1) = -4$. Since $P(-2) = 12$ and $P(-1) = -4$ differ in sign, the intermediate value theorem assures us that there is a real zero between -2 and -1.

30. (a) $\quad 3\overline{)1 \quad 1 \quad -11 \quad -10}$ Therefore, $Q(x) = x^2 + 4x + 1;\ R = -7$.
    $\quad\quad\quad\quad\quad 3 \quad 12 \quad 3$
    $\quad\quad\quad\overline{\quad 1 \quad 4 \quad 1 \quad -7}$

    (b) $\quad -2\overline{)3 \quad 8 \quad 5 \quad 10}$ Therefore, $Q(x) = 3x^2 + 2x + 1;\ R = 8$.
    $\quad\quad\quad\quad\quad -6 \ -4 \ -2$
    $\quad\quad\quad\overline{\quad 3 \quad 2 \quad 1 \quad 8}$

31. $3x+1\overline{\smash{\big)}6x^3 - 4x^2 + 4x + 3}$ with quotient $2x^2 - 2x + 2$ $\Rightarrow \dfrac{6x^3 - 4x^2 + 4x + 3}{3x+1} = 2x^2 - 2x + 2 + \dfrac{1}{3x+1}$

$\quad\quad\quad\underline{6x^3 + 2x^2}$
$\quad\quad\quad\quad\ -6x^2 + 4x$
$\quad\quad\quad\quad\ \underline{-6x^2 - 2x}$
$\quad\quad\quad\quad\quad\quad 6x + 3$
$\quad\quad\quad\quad\quad\quad \underline{6x + 2}$
$\quad\quad\quad\quad\quad\quad\quad\quad 1$

32. $x^2 - 3x + 1\overline{\smash{\big)}2x^3 - 5x^2 + 0x + 1}$ with quotient $2x+1$ $\Rightarrow \dfrac{2x^3 - 5x^2 + 1}{x^2 - 3x + 1} = 2x + 1 + \dfrac{x}{x^2 - 3x + 1}$

$\quad\quad\quad\underline{2x^3 - 6x^2 + 2x}$
$\quad\quad\quad\quad\quad x^2 - 2x + 1$
$\quad\quad\quad\quad\quad \underline{x^2 + 3x + 1}$
$\quad\quad\quad\quad\quad\quad\quad\quad x$

33. $2\overline{)-1 \quad 5 \quad -7 \quad 1}$ Therefore, $P(2) = -1$.
    $\quad\quad\quad -2 \quad 6 \quad -2$
    $\overline{\ -1 \quad 3 \ -1 \ -1}$

34. $2\overline{)2 \quad -3 \quad 7 \quad -12}$ Therefore, $P(2) = 6$.
    $\quad\quad\quad 4 \quad 2 \quad 18$
    $\overline{\ 2 \quad 1 \quad 9 \quad 6}$

Copyright © 2015 Pearson Education, Inc

35.
```
2)5   0  -12   2  -8
     10   20  16  36
   ─────────────────────
    5  10    8  18  28
```
Therefore, $P(2) = 28$.

36.
```
2)1  0  0   4  -2  -4
      2  4   8  24  44
   ────────────────────
    1  2  4  12  22  40
```
Therefore, $P(2) = 40$.

37. The conjugate of $7+2i$ must also be a zero; therefore, $7-2i$ is also a zero.

38. With the given zeros of $-1, 4,$ and 7, the function $P(x)$ is

    $P(x) = a(x-(-1))(x-4)(x-7) = a(x+1)(x-4)(x-7) = a(x+1)(x^2-11x+28) \Rightarrow$

    $P(x) = a(x^3-10x^2+17x+28)$. One of many possible functions, if $a=1$, is $P(x) = x^3-10x^2+17x+28$.

39. With the given zeros of $8, 2,$ and 3, the function $P(x)$ is

    $P(x) = a(x-8)(x-2)(x-3) = a(x-8)(x-2)(x-3) = a(x-8)(x^2-5x+6) \Rightarrow$

    $P(x) = a(x^3-13x^2+46x-48)$. One of many possible functions, if $a=1$, is $P(x) = x^3-13x^2+46x-48$.

40. With the given zeros of $\sqrt{3}, -\sqrt{3}, 2,$ and 3, the function $P(x)$ is

    $P(x) = a(x-\sqrt{3})(x-(-\sqrt{3}))(x-2)(x-3) = a(x-\sqrt{3})(x+\sqrt{3})(x-2)(x-3) =$

    $a(x^2-3)(x^2-5x+6) \Rightarrow a(x^4-5x^3+3x^2+15x-18)$. One of many possible functions, if $a=1$, is

    $P(x) = x^4-5x^3+3x^2+15x-18$.

41. With the given zeros of $-2+\sqrt{5}, -2-\sqrt{5}, -2$ and 1, the function $P(x)$ is

    $P(x) = a(x-(-2+\sqrt{5}))(x-(-2-\sqrt{5}))(x-(-2))(x-1) =$
    $a(x+2-\sqrt{5})(x+2+\sqrt{5})(x+2)(x-1) = a(x^2+4x-1)(x^2+x-2) = a(x^4+5x^3+x^2-9x+2)$. One of many

    possible functions, if $a=1$, is $P(x) = x^4+5x^3+x^2-9x+2$.

42. Use synthetic division to check if -1 is a zero.

    ```
    -1)2  1  -4   3   1
         -2   1   3  -6
       ─────────────────
        2 -1  -3   6  -5
    ```
    Since $P(-1) = -5$ and not 0, -1 is not a zero.

43. Use synthetic division to check if $x+1$ or $x=-1$ is a zero.

    ```
    -1)1  2  3  2
         -1 -1 -2
       ──────────
        1  1  2  0
    ```
    Since $P(-1) = 0$, -1 or $x+1$ is a factor.

44. With the given zeros $3, 1, -1-3i$, the conjugate of $-1-3i$ is also a zero, so the function $P(x)$ is

    $P(x) = a(x-3)(x-1)(x-(-1-3i))(x-(-1+3i)) =$

    $a(x-3)(x-1)(x+1+3i)(x+1-3i) = a(x^2-4x+3)(x^2+2x+10) = a(x^4-2x^3+5x^2-34x+30)$.

Since $P(2) = -36$, we can solve for a.

$-36 = a((2)^4 - 2(2)^3 + 5(2)^2 - 34(2) + 30) \Rightarrow -36 = a(16 - 16 + 20 - 68 + 30) \Rightarrow -18a = -36 \Rightarrow a = 2$.

Therefore, $P(x) = 2(x^4 - 2x^3 + 5x^2 - 34x + 30) \Rightarrow P(x) = 2x^4 - 4x^3 + 10x^2 - 68x + 60$.

45. With the given zero $1-i$, the conjugate $1+i$ is also a zero. Use synthetic division to factor out these zeros.

$$\begin{array}{r|rrrrr} 1-i) & 1 & -3 & -8 & 22 & -24 \\ & & 1+i & -3+i & -10+12i & 24 \\ \hline & 1 & -2-i & -11+i & 12+12i & 0 \end{array} \Rightarrow \begin{array}{r|rrrr} 1+i) & 1 & -2-i & -11+i & 12+12i \\ & & 1+i & -1-i & -12-12i \\ \hline & 1 & -1 & -12 & 0 \end{array}$$

Finally, solve the resulting quadratic equation, $x^2 - x - 12 = 0 \Rightarrow x^2 - x - 12 = 0 \Rightarrow$

$(x-4)(x+3) = 0 \Rightarrow x = -3, 4$. The zeros are $x = \{-3, 4, 1-i, 1+i\}$.

46. With the given zeros 1 and $2i$, the conjugate of $2i$, or $-2i$, is also a zero. Use synthetic division to factor out these zeros.

$$\begin{array}{r|rrrrr} 1) & 2 & -1 & 7 & -4 & -4 \\ & & 2 & 1 & 8 & 4 \\ \hline & 2 & 1 & 8 & 4 & 0 \end{array} \Rightarrow \begin{array}{r|rrrr} 2i) & 2 & 1 & 8 & 4 \\ & & 4i & -8+2i & -4 \\ \hline & 2 & 1+4i & 2i & 0 \end{array} \Rightarrow \begin{array}{r|rrr} -2i) & 2 & 1+4i & 2i \\ & & -4i & -2i \\ \hline & 2 & 1 & 0 \end{array}$$

Finally, solve the resulting linear equation: $2x + 1 = 0 \Rightarrow 2x = -1 \Rightarrow x = -\dfrac{1}{2}$. The zeros are

$x = -\dfrac{1}{2}, 1, 2i, -2i$.

47. Using the Rational Zeros Theorem, the possible zeros are

$x = \pm\dfrac{1, 2, 4, 8}{1, 3} = \pm 1, \pm 2, \pm 4, \pm 8, \pm\dfrac{1}{3}, \pm\dfrac{2}{3}, \pm\dfrac{4}{3}, \pm\dfrac{8}{3}$. From graphing the equation, we choose to check

possible zeros -2, 4, and $\dfrac{1}{3}$ by synthetic division.

$$\begin{array}{r|rrrrr} 2) & 3 & -4 & -26 & -21 & -14 & 8 \\ & & -6 & 20 & 12 & 18 & 8 \\ \hline & 3 & -10 & -6 & -9 & 4 & 0 \end{array} \Rightarrow \begin{array}{r|rrrrr} 4) & 3 & -1 & -6 & -9 & 4 \\ & & 12 & 8 & 8 & -4 \\ \hline & 3 & 2 & 2 & -1 & 0 \end{array} \Rightarrow \begin{array}{r|rrrr} \frac{1}{3}) & 3 & 2 & 2 & -1 \\ & & 1 & 1 & 1 \\ \hline & 3 & 3 & 3 & 0 \end{array}$$

Finally, solve the resulting quadratic equation, $x^2 + x + 1 = 0$, using the quadratic formula:

$x = \dfrac{-1 \pm \sqrt{1^2 - 4(1)(1)}}{2(1)} = \dfrac{-1 \pm \sqrt{-3}}{2}$. This results in non-real solutions; therefore, the rational solutions

are $x = -2, \dfrac{1}{3}$, and 4.

48. Because the function $P(x)$ has coefficient signs, $++---$, which is 1 sign change, the function has 1

positive real zero. Because $P(-x) = 3(-x)^4 + (-x)^3 - (-x)^2 - 2(-x) - 1 = 3x^4 - x^3 - x^2 + 2x - 1$ has

coefficient signs, $+--+-$, which is 3 sign changes, the function has 3 or 1 possible negative real zeros.

49. Using the Boundedness Theorem, we divide synthetically by $x-2$.

$$\begin{array}{r|rrrr} 2) & 2 & 3 & -5 & 8 & -10 \\ & & 4 & 14 & 18 & 52 \\ \hline & 2 & 7 & 9 & 26 & 42 \end{array}$$

The result is entirely non-negative; therefore, there can be no real zero greater than 2. Again using the Boundedness Theorem, we divide synthetically by $x-(-4)$.

$$\begin{array}{r|rrrr} -4) & 2 & 3 & -5 & 8 & -10 \\ & & -8 & 20 & -60 & 208 \\ \hline & 2 & -5 & 15 & -52 & 198 \end{array}$$ The result alternates in sign; therefore, there is no real zero less than -4.

50. Graphing the equation on a calculator shows x-intercepts of $-1.62, 0.62,$ and 3. Therefore, there are 3 real solutions and the integer root is 3.

51. Using synthetic division we can factor out the root 3.

$$\begin{array}{r|rrrr} 3) & 1 & -2 & -4 & 3 \\ & & 3 & 3 & -3 \\ \hline & 1 & 1 & -1 & 0 \end{array}$$ Using the result of the synthetic division the factors are $(x-3)(x^2+x-1)$.

52. The remaining zeros can be found by solving, $x^2+x-1=0$, using the quadratic formula.

$$x=\frac{-1\pm\sqrt{1^2-4(1)(-1)}}{2(1)}=\frac{-1\pm\sqrt{5}}{2}.$$ The solution set is $\left\{\frac{-1-\sqrt{5}}{2},\frac{-1+\sqrt{5}}{2}\right\}$.

53. The x-intercepts from the graph are approximately equal to the solutions found in #50. $\frac{-1-\sqrt{5}}{2}\approx -1.62$, and $\frac{-1+\sqrt{5}}{2}\approx 0.62$.

54. (a) From the graph and the answers of #50, $P(x)>0$ for the interval $\left(\frac{-1-\sqrt{5}}{2},\frac{-1+\sqrt{5}}{2}\right)\cup(3,\infty)$.

(b) From the graph and the answers of #50, $P(x)\leq 0$ for the interval $\left(-\infty,\frac{-1-\sqrt{5}}{2}\right]\cup\left[\frac{-1+\sqrt{5}}{2},3\right]$.

55. First, factor out an x. $x^3-2x^2+5x=0 \Rightarrow x(x^2-2x+5) \Rightarrow x=0$ is a zero. Now solve the quadratic equation using the quadratic formula: $x=\frac{-2\pm\sqrt{2^2-4(1)(5)}}{2(1)}=\frac{-2\pm\sqrt{-16}}{2}=\frac{-2\pm 4i}{2}=-1\pm 2i$. Since two of the zeros are not real, the only x-intercept is $(0,0)$.

56. The zeros are $-2, 1,$ and 3. The 3 has multiplicity 2, because it appears tangent to the x-axis. The factored form is now: $P(x)=(x+2)(x-1)(x-3)^2$.

57. Since its end behavior has both ends going in the same direction, either up or down, the degree is even.

58. Since its end behavior has one end going up and the other going down, the degree is odd.

59. Since its end behavior has the right end approaching positive infinity, the lead coefficient is positive.

60. Since $g(x)$ has no x-intercepts, it has no real solutions.

61. From the graph, $f(x) < 0$ is true for the interval $(-\infty, a) \cup (b, c)$.

62. From the graph, $f(x) > g(x)$ is true for the interval (d, h).

63. If $f(x) - g(x) = 0$ then $f(x) = g(x)$. This happens at the intersection of the graphs, which is at $\{d, h\}$.

64. If $r + pi$ is a solution, then its conjugate $r - pi$ is also a solution.

65. Since $f(x)$ has three real zeros, and a polynomial of degree 3 can have at most three zeros, there can be no other zeros, real or non-real complex.

66. False. A 7th degree function can have at most 7 x-intercepts.

67. True. A 7th degree function can have at most 6 local extrema.

68. True. $f(0) = 3(0)^7 - 8(0)^6 + 9(0)^5 + 12(0)^4 - 18(0)^3 + 26(0)^2 - (0) + 500 \Rightarrow f(0) = 500$.

69. True. The end behavior of an odd-degree polynomial with a positive lead coefficient is down to the left. Because the function has a positive y-intercept, the graph of the equation must cross the negative x-axis at least one time. Therefore, it must have at least one negative x-intercept.

70. True. An even-degree polynomial with a positive lead coefficient will have the end behavior of both ends going upward; therefore, a graph with a negative y-intercept must cross the x-axis at least 2 times and will have at least 2 real zeros.

71. False. The conjugate must also be a zero, but the conjugate of $-\frac{1}{2} + i\frac{\sqrt{3}}{2}$ is $-\frac{1}{2} - i\frac{\sqrt{3}}{2}$, and not $\frac{1}{2} + i\frac{\sqrt{3}}{2}$.

72. From the graph, there are two local maxima.

73. From the graph, there is one local minimum that lies on the x-axis. It has coordinates $(2, 0)$.

74. Use synthetic division to factor out $x - 5$.

    $$\begin{array}{r|rrrrrr} 5 & -2 & 15 & -21 & -32 & 60 & 0 \\ & & -10 & 25 & 20 & -60 & 0 \\ \hline & -2 & 5 & 4 & -12 & 0 & 0 \end{array}$$

    From this result, the quotient is the equation $Q(x) = -2x^4 + 5x^3 + 4x^2 - 12x$.

75. Because all real numbers can be input for x, the range is $(-0.97, -54.15)$.

76. Using the calculator functions, this local minimum point has coordinates $(-0.97, -54.15)$.

77. We first factor by grouping and then solve. $3x^3 + 2x^2 - 21x - 14 = 0 \Rightarrow x^2(3x + 2) - 7(3x + 2) = 0 \Rightarrow$
    $(3x + 2)(x^2 - 7) = 0 \Rightarrow 3x + 2 = 0 \Rightarrow 3x = -2 \Rightarrow x = -\frac{2}{3}$ or $x^2 - 7 = 0 \Rightarrow x^2 = 7 \Rightarrow x = \pm\sqrt{7}$. Therefore, the solution set is $\left\{-\sqrt{7}, -\frac{2}{3}, \sqrt{7}\right\}$. Graphing this equation shows x-values of ± 2.65 and -0.67, which are equal to the solution set, and therefore support our analytic solution.

78. An even-degree polynomial with a negative lead coefficient has an end behavior of ⌒. The function has zeros $x = -1$ (multiplicity 2,) 2, and 3; therefore, there are x-intercepts at those values of x.

The graph will be tangent to the x-axis at $x = -1$ (multiplicity 2) and the y-intercept is $y = -6$.
See Figure 78.

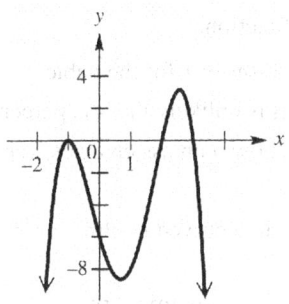

Figure 78

(a) $P(x) = 0$ at the x-intercepts; therefore, $x = \{1, 2, 3\}$.

(b) From the graph, $P(x) > 0$ for the interval $(2, 3)$.

(c) From the graph, $P(x) < 0$ for the interval $(-\infty, -1) \cup (-1, 2) \cup (3, \infty)$.

79. If $x =$ cube side length and $V = s^3$, the volume of the cube after the top is cut off is
$V = (x)(x)(x-2) = 32 \Rightarrow x^3 - 2x^2 - 32 = 0$. After graphing for possible roots, we use synthetic division to check 4 as a root.

$$4)\overline{1 \quad -2 \quad 0 \quad -32}$$
$$\quad\quad 4 \quad 8 \quad 32$$
$$\overline{1 \quad 2 \quad 8 \quad 0}$$

Now solve the resulting equation, $x^2 - 2x + 8 = 0$. $x = \dfrac{-2 \pm \sqrt{2^2 - 4(1)(8)}}{2(1)} = \dfrac{-2 \pm \sqrt{-28}}{2}$. Both of these roots are non-real; therefore, the only real root is 4, and the dimensions of the original cube are 4 in. by 4 in. by 4 in.

80. (a) Since, from a calculator graph of the equation, the zero is at approximately 9.26. Therefore, the restrictions on t are $0 \le t \le 9.26$.

(b) See Figure 80.

(c) From the graph, the object reaches its highest point at approximately $t = 4.08$ seconds.

(d) From the graph, the object reaches its highest point at approximately $s(t) = 131.63$ meters.

(e) The object reaches the ground when $s(t) = 0$; therefore, the equation is $-4.9t^2 + 40t + 50 = 0$. We solve this using the quadratic formula.

$t = \dfrac{-40 \pm \sqrt{40^2 - 4(-4.9)(50)}}{2(-4.9)} = \dfrac{-40 \pm \sqrt{2580}}{-9.8}$; $t \approx -1.10$ or 9.26. Since we cannot have negative time, the object reaches the ground in approximately 9.26 sec.

81. For the year 2010 $x = 45$; therefore, $y = -0.00002(45)^3 + 0.0022(45)^2 - 0.096(45) + 3.05 \approx 1.36$ million.

82. (a) See Figure 82a.

(b) Using the capabilities of the graphing calculator, the quadratic function is
$f(x) \approx -0.011x^2 + 0.869x + 11.9$.

154   CHAPTER 3   Polynomial Functions

(c) Using the capabilities of the calculator, the cubic function is
$f(x) \approx -0.00087x^3 + 0.0456x^2 - 0.219x + 17.8$.

(d) See Figure 82b, for the quadratic function, and Figure 82c, for the cubic function.

(e) Both functions approximate the data well. Although the value of R^2 is closer to 1 for the cubic function, the quadratic function is probably better for prediction because it is unlikely that the percent of out-of-pocket spending would decrease after 2025 (as the cubic function shows) unless changes were made in Medicare law.

(f) A linear model would not really be appropriate because the data points lie in a curved nonlinear path.

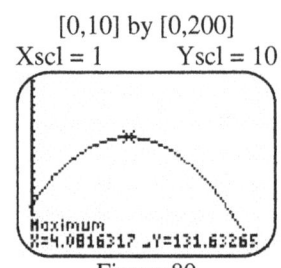
[0,10] by [0,200]
Xscl = 1   Yscl = 10
Figure 80

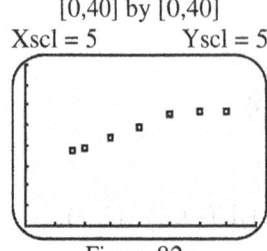
[0,40] by [0,40]
Xscl = 5   Yscl = 5
Figure 82a

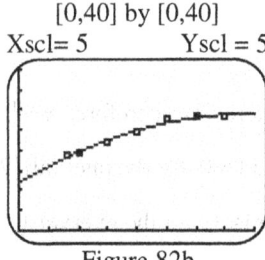
[0,40] by [0,40]
Xscl = 5   Yscl = 5
Figure 82b

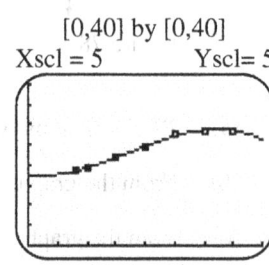
[0,40] by [0,40]
Xscl = 5   Yscl = 5
Figure 82c

83. Answers will vary. Example, given 7; x^7

84. Answers will vary.

85. Answers will vary.

86. Answers will vary. Domain: $(-\infty, \infty)$; Range: $(-\infty, \infty)$.

Chapter 3 Test

1. (a) $(8 - 7i) - (-12 + 2i) = 20 - 9i$.

   (b) $\dfrac{11 + 10i}{2 + 3i} \cdot \dfrac{2 - 3i}{2 - 3i} = \dfrac{22 - 33i + 20i - 30i^2}{4 - 9i^2} = \dfrac{22 - 13i + 30}{4 + 9} = \dfrac{52 - 13i}{13} = 4 - i$.

   (c) $i^{65} = (i^4)^{16}(i) = 1^{16}(i) = i$.

   (d) $2i(3-i)^2 = 2i(9 - 6i + i^2) = 2i(9 - 6i - 1) = 2i(8 - 6i) = 16i - 12i^2 = 12 + 16i$.

   (e) $\sqrt{-36} = \sqrt{36}\sqrt{-1} = 6i$

   (f) $\sqrt{-5} \cdot \sqrt{-20} = \sqrt{5} \cdot \sqrt{-1} \cdot \sqrt{4} \cdot \sqrt{5} \cdot \sqrt{-1} = \sqrt{5} \cdot i \cdot 2 \cdot \sqrt{5} \cdot i = 5 \cdot 2 \cdot (-1) = -10$

2. (a) Use the vertex formula to find the x-coordinate. $x = -\dfrac{b}{2a} = -\dfrac{-4}{2(-2)} = -1$. Now solve for $f(-1)$ to find the y-coordinate of the vertex. $f(-1) = -2(-1)^2 - 4(-1) + 6 = -2 + 4 + 6 = 8$. The vertex is $(-1, 8)$.

   (b) See Figure 2b. Finding the maximum on the graph gives the vertex: $(-1, 8)$.

   (c) First, we find the zeros by factoring.
   $-2x^2 - 4x + 6 = 0 \Rightarrow -2(x^2 + 2x - 3) = 0 \Rightarrow -2(x+3)(x-1) = 0 \Rightarrow x = -3$ or 1. Now support this on the graphing calculator using a graph and a table, See Figure 2c.

(d) For the y-intercept we let $x = 0$; therefore, $f(0) = -2(0) - 4(0) + 6 \Rightarrow f(0) = 6$.

(e) All values can be input for x. The domain is $(-\infty, \infty)$; since $(-1, 8)$ is a maximum, the range is $(-\infty, 8]$.

(f) From the graph, the function is increasing for the interval $(-\infty, -1]$, and decreasing for the interval $[-1, \infty)$.

3. $6x^2 - 15x + 6 = 0 \Rightarrow 3(2x^2 - 5x + 2) = 0 \Rightarrow (2x-1)(x-2) = 0 \Rightarrow x = \frac{1}{2}, 2$

4. $x^2 - 4x = 2 \Rightarrow x^2 - 4x + 4 = 2 + 4 \Rightarrow (x-2)^2 = 6 \Rightarrow x - 2 = \pm\sqrt{6} \Rightarrow x = 2 \pm \sqrt{6}$

5. (a) We solve the equation using the quadratic formula. $x = \frac{-3 \pm \sqrt{3^2 - 4(3)(-2)}}{2(3)} = \frac{-3 \pm \sqrt{9+24}}{6} \Rightarrow$
$x = \left\{\frac{-3-\sqrt{33}}{6}, \frac{-3+\sqrt{33}}{6}\right\}$.

(b) See Figure 5. From this graph, (i) $f(x) < 0$ for the interval $\left(\frac{-3-\sqrt{33}}{6}, \frac{-3+\sqrt{33}}{6}\right)$, and (ii) $f(x) \geq 0$
for the interval $\left(-\infty, \frac{-3-\sqrt{33}}{6}\right] \cup \left[\frac{-3+\sqrt{33}}{6}, \infty\right)$.

[-9.4,9.4] by [-4.1,8.1]   [-9.4,9.4] by [-4.1,8.1]   [-4.7,4.7] by [-3.1,3.1]
Xscl = 1   Yscl = 1   Xscl = 1   Yscl = 1   Xscl= 1   Yscl = 1

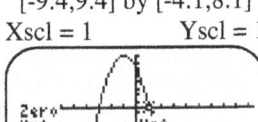
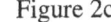
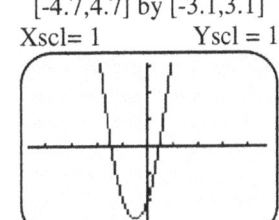

Figure 2b   Figure 2c   Figure 5

6. Since $V = lwh$, $720 = (11+x)(3x)(x) \Rightarrow 720 = 3x^3 + 33x^2 \Rightarrow 0 = 3x^3 + 33x^2 - 720 \Rightarrow 0 = x^3 + 11x^2 - 240$.

After graphing on a calculator, we use synthetic division to check 4 as a factor.

```
4) 1   11    0   -240
        4   60    240
   ─────────────────────
   1   15   60     0
```

Now solve the resulting equation, $x^2 + 15x + 60 = 0$, using the quadratic formula:

$x = \frac{-15 \pm \sqrt{15^2 - 4(1)(60)}}{2(1)} = \frac{-15 \pm \sqrt{-15}}{2}$. These solutions will both be nonreal; therefore, the only real solution is 4, and the dimensions are $11 + 4$, $3(4)$, and 4 or 15 in. by 12 in. by 4 in.

7. (a) Using the capabilities of the graphing calculator, the quadratic function is
$f(x) = 0.00019838x^2 - 0.79153x + 791.46$

156   CHAPTER 3   Polynomial Functions

(b). $f(1975) \approx 1.99$, This value is very close to the actual value of 2.01.

8. (a) Use synthetic division to factor out the given zeros.

$$\begin{array}{r|rrrrrr} 3 & 1 & -5 & 3 & 1 & 40 & -24 & -72 \\ & & 3 & -6 & -9 & -24 & 48 & 72 \\ \hline & 1 & -2 & -3 & -8 & 16 & 24 & 0 \end{array} \quad \begin{array}{r|rrrrrr} 3 & 1 & -2 & -3 & -8 & 16 & 24 \\ & & 3 & 3 & 0 & -24 & -24 \\ \hline & 1 & 1 & 0 & -8 & -8 & 0 \end{array} \Rightarrow$$

$$\begin{array}{r|rrrr} -1 & 1 & 1 & 0 & -8 & -8 \\ & & -1 & 0 & 0 & 8 \\ \hline & 1 & 0 & 0 & -8 & 0 \end{array} \Rightarrow \quad \begin{array}{r|rrrr} 2 & 1 & 0 & 0 & -8 \\ & & 2 & 4 & 8 \\ \hline & 1 & 2 & 4 & 0 \end{array}$$

Now solve the resulting equation, $x^2 + 2x + 4 = 0$, using the quadratic formula.

$x = \dfrac{-2 \pm \sqrt{2^2 - 4(1)(4)}}{2(1)} = \dfrac{-2 \pm \sqrt{-12}}{2} = \dfrac{-2 \pm 2i\sqrt{3}}{2} = -1 \pm i\sqrt{3}$. The other zeros of $f(x)$ are

$x = -1 - i\sqrt{3}, -1 + i\sqrt{3}$.

(b) An even-degree polynomial with a positive lead coefficient has end-behavior ⌣. See Figure 8.

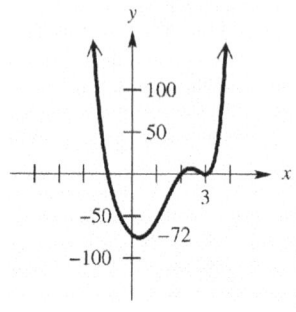

Figure 8

9. (a) We can find the zeros by factoring. $4x^4 - 21x^2 - 25 = 0 \Rightarrow (4x^2 - 25)(x^2 + 1) = 0 \Rightarrow$

$4x^2 - 25 = 0 \Rightarrow 4x^2 = 25 \Rightarrow x^2 = \dfrac{25}{4} \Rightarrow x = \pm\sqrt{\dfrac{25}{4}} = \pm\dfrac{5}{2}$ or

$x^2 + 1 = 0 \Rightarrow x^2 = -1 \Rightarrow x = \pm\sqrt{-1} \Rightarrow x = \pm i$. The zeros are $x = -\dfrac{5}{2}, \dfrac{5}{2}, -i, i$.

(b) Use a graph and table to support the results. See Figure 9.

(c) It is symmetric with respect to the y-axis.

(d) From the graph and the results, (i) $f(x) \geq 0$ for the interval $\left(-\infty, -\dfrac{5}{2}\right] \cup \left[\dfrac{5}{2}, \infty\right)$, and (ii) $f(x) < 0$

for the interval $\left(-\dfrac{5}{2}, \dfrac{5}{2}\right)$.

[-4,4] by [-60,60]

Xscl = 1   Yscl = 10

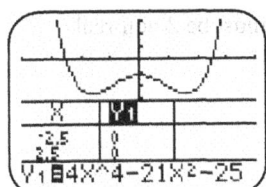

Figure 9

10. (a) Using the Rational Zeros Theorem, the possible zeros are $x = \pm \dfrac{1, 2, 11, 22}{1, 3} =$

    $\pm 1, \pm 2, \pm 11, \pm 22, \pm \dfrac{1}{3}, \pm \dfrac{2}{3}, \pm \dfrac{11}{3}$, and $\pm \dfrac{22}{3}$.

    (b) From a calculator graph of the equation, we choose to check -2 and $\dfrac{1}{3}$ by synthetic division.

    $$\begin{array}{r|rrrrr} -2 & 3 & 5 & -35 & -55 & 22 \\ & & -6 & 2 & 66 & -22 \\ \hline & 3 & -1 & -33 & 11 & 0 \end{array} \Rightarrow \begin{array}{r|rrrr} \frac{1}{3} & 3 & -1 & -33 & 11 \\ & & 1 & 0 & -11 \\ \hline & 3 & 0 & -33 & 0 \end{array}$$

    Now solve the resulting equation. $3x^2 - 33 = 0 \Rightarrow x^2 - 11 = 0 \Rightarrow x^2 = 11 \Rightarrow x = \pm\sqrt{11}$. Since these are not rational, the rational zeros are $-2, \dfrac{1}{3}$.

    (c) Since $f(3) = 3(3)^4 + 5(3)^3 + 35(3)^2 - 55(3) + 22 = -80$ and

    $f(4) = 3(4)^4 + 5(4)^3 + 35(4)^2 - 55(4) + 22 = 330$ differ in sign, the intermediate value theorem assures us that there is a real zero between 3 and 4.

    (d) Because the function has coefficient signs $++--+$, which is 2 sign changes, the function has 2 or 0 positive real zeros. Because $f(-x) = 3(-x)^4 + 5(-x)^3 - 35(-x)^2 - 55(-x) + 22 =$

    $3x^4 - 5x^3 - 35x^2 + 55x + 22$ has coefficient signs, $+--++$, which is 2 sign changes, the function has 2 or 0 possible negative real zeros.

    (e) Using the Boundedness Theorem we divide synthetically by $x-(-5)$.

    $$\begin{array}{r|rrrrr} -5 & 3 & 5 & -35 & -55 & 22 \\ & & -15 & 50 & -75 & 650 \\ \hline & 3 & -10 & 15 & -130 & 672 \end{array}$$

    The result alternates signs; therefore, there is no real zero less than -5. Also using the Boundedness Theorem, we divide synthetically by $x-4$.

    $$\begin{array}{r|rrrrr} 4 & 3 & 5 & -35 & -55 & 22 \\ & & 12 & 68 & 132 & 308 \\ \hline & 3 & 17 & 33 & 77 & 330 \end{array}$$

    The result is all non-negative; therefore, there is no real zero greater than 4.

11. (a) Using the capabilities of the calculator and graphing the equation yields real solutions of $\{0.189, 1, 3.633\}$.

(b) A 5th degree equation has 5 solutions. Since there are 3 real solutions, there must be 2 non-real complex solutions.

12. (a) $\dfrac{8x^3 - 4x^2}{2x} = \dfrac{8x^3}{2x} - \dfrac{4x^2}{2x} = 4x^2 - 2x$

(b)
$$x-1 \overline{\smash{\big)}\, 3x^3 - 5x^2 + 0x + 6} \qquad \text{quotient: } 3x^2 - 2x - 2$$
$$\underline{3x^3 - 3x^2}$$
$$-2x^2 + 0x$$
$$\underline{-2x^2 + 2x}$$
$$-2x + 6$$
$$\underline{-2x + 2}$$
$$4$$

$\Rightarrow \dfrac{3x^3 - 5x^2 + 6}{x-1} = 3x^2 - 2x - 2 + \dfrac{4}{x-1}$

(c)
$$2x-1 \overline{\smash{\big)}\, 2x^4 - x^3 + 4x^2 - 4x + 3} \qquad \text{quotient: } x^3 + 2x - 1$$
$$\underline{2x^4 - x^3}$$
$$4x^2 - 4x$$
$$\underline{-4x^2 - 2x}$$
$$-2x + 3$$
$$\underline{-2x + 1}$$
$$2$$

$\Rightarrow \dfrac{2x^4 - x^3 + 4x^2 - 4x + 3}{2x-1} = x^3 + 2x - 1 + \dfrac{2}{2x-1}$

(d)
$$x^2+2 \overline{\smash{\big)}\, x^4 + 0x^2 - 2x + 6} \qquad \text{quotient: } x^2 - 2$$
$$\underline{x^4 + 2x^2}$$
$$-2x^2 - 2x$$
$$\underline{-2x^2 \quad\;\; -4}$$
$$-2x + 4 + 6$$

$\Rightarrow \dfrac{x^4 - 2x + 6}{x^2+2} = x^2 - 2 + \dfrac{-2x + 10}{x^2+2}$

13. The cubic polynomial has zeros of 4 and $2i$ will also have $-2i$ (conjugate pairs theorem). Therefore, we will have $f(x) = a(x-4)(x-(2i))(x-(-2i)) = a(x-4)(x-2i)(x+2i)$. Now use the given point to find the value of a, $-15 = a(1-4)(1-2i)(1+2i) \Rightarrow -15 = a(-3)(5) \Rightarrow a = 1$. The polynomial is $f(x) = (x-4)(x-2i)(x+2i) = (x-4)(x^2+4) = x^3 - 4x^2 + 4x - 16$

14. $x^3 + 3x = 0 \Rightarrow x(x^2+3) = 0 \Rightarrow x = 0 \text{ or } (x^2+3) = 0 \Rightarrow x^2 = -3 \Rightarrow x = \pm i\sqrt{3}$ The solution set is $\{0, \pm i\sqrt{3}\}$.

Chapter 4: Rational, Power, and Root Functions

4.1: Rational Functions and Graphs I

1. The only value for x that cannot be used as input is 0. The domain is $(-\infty, 0) \cup (0, \infty)$.

   It is not possible for this function to output the value 0. The range is $(-\infty, 0) \cup (0, \infty)$.

3. The function decreases everywhere it is defined, $(-\infty, 0) \cup (0, \infty)$. It never increases and is never constant.

5. Because the function is undefined when $x = 3$, the vertical asymptote has the equation $x = 3$. As $|x|$ increases without bound, the graph of the function will move closer and closer to the graph of $y = 2$.

7. Because $f(-x) = f(x)$, the function is even. The graph has symmetry with respect to the y-axis.

9. Graphs A, B, and C have domain $(-\infty, 3) \cup (3, \infty)$ because each has a vertical asymptote at $x = 3$.

11. Graph A has range $(-\infty, 3) \cup (3, \infty)$ because it exists above and below the horizontal asymptote at $y = 0$.

13. The only graph that would intersect the line $y = 3$ exactly one time is graph A.

15. Graphs A, C, and D have the x-axis as a horizontal asymptote.

17. Let $g(x) = y = \dfrac{1}{x}$, then $f(x) = 2g(x)$. To obtain the graph of f, stretch the graph of $y = \dfrac{1}{x}$ vertically by a factor of 2. See Figures 17a and 17b. The domain is $(-\infty, 0) \cup (0, \infty)$. The range is $(-\infty, 0) \cup (0, \infty)$.

19. Let $g(x) = y = \dfrac{1}{x}$, then $f(x) = g(x+2)$. To obtain the graph of f, shift the graph of $y = \dfrac{1}{x}$ to the left 2 units. See Figures 19a and 19b. The domain is $(-\infty, -2) \cup (-2, \infty)$. The range is $(-\infty, 0) \cup (0, \infty)$.

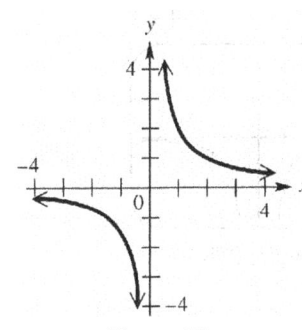
Figure 17a

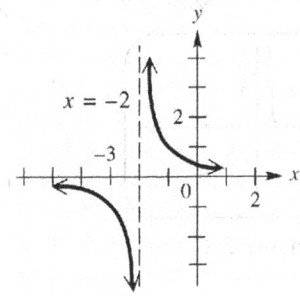
Figure 19a

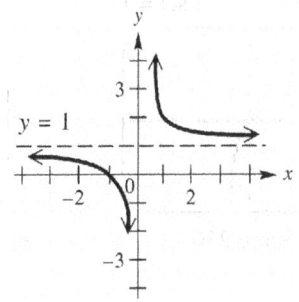
Figure 21a

[-4.7,4.7] by [-3.1,31.]
Xscl = 1   Yscl = 1

[-6.7,2.7] by [-3.1,3.1]
Xscl = 1   Yscl = 1

[-4.7,4.7] by [-2.1,4.1]
Xscl = 1   Yscl = 1

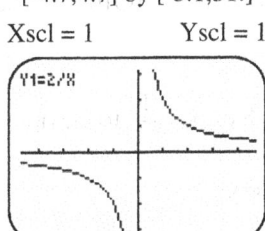
Figure 17b

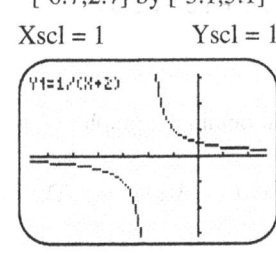
Figure 19b

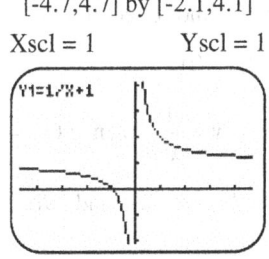
Figure 21b

21. Let $g(x) = y = \dfrac{1}{x}$, then $f(x) = g(x) + 1$. To obtain the graph of f, shift the graph of $y = \dfrac{1}{x}$ upward 1 unit. See Figures 21a and 21b. The domain is $(-\infty, 0) \cup (0, \infty)$. The range is $(-\infty, 1) \cup (1, \infty)$.

23. Let $g(x) = y = \dfrac{1}{x}$, then $f(x) = g(x-1) + 1$. To obtain the graph of f, shift the graph of $y = \dfrac{1}{x}$ to the right 1 unit and upward 1 unit. See Figures 23a and 23b. The domain is $(-\infty, 1) \cup (1, \infty)$. The range is $(-\infty, 1) \cup (1, \infty)$.

25. Let $g(x) = y = \dfrac{1}{x^2}$, then $f(x) = g(x) - 2$. To obtain the graph of f, shift the graph of $y = \dfrac{1}{x^2}$ downward 2 units. See Figures 25a and 25b. The domain is $(-\infty, 0) \cup (0, \infty)$. The range is $(-2, \infty)$.

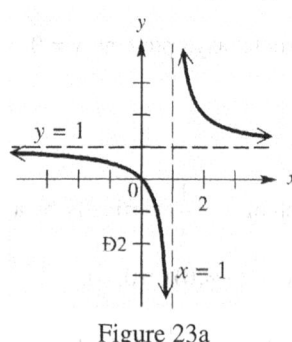
Figure 23a

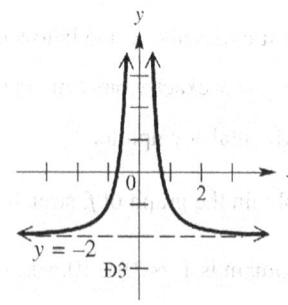
Figure 25a

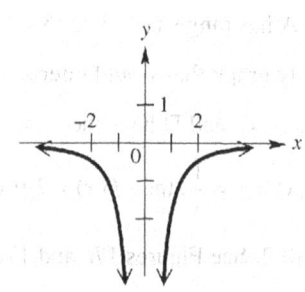
Figure 27a

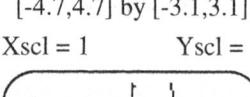
[-4.7,4.7] by [-3.1,3.1]
Xscl = 1   Yscl = 1

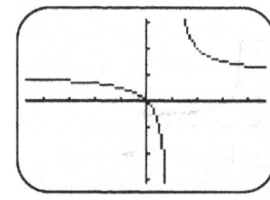
Figure 23b

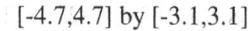
[-4.7,4.7] by [-3.1,3.1]
Xscl = 1   Yscl = 1

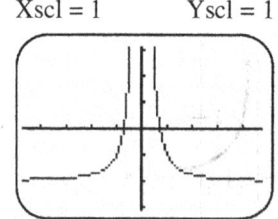
Figure 25b

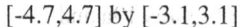
[-4.7,4.7] by [-3.1,3.1]
Xscl = 1   Yscl = 1

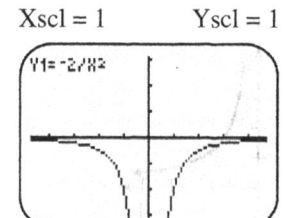
Figure 27b

27. Let $g(x) = y = \dfrac{1}{x^2}$, then $f(x) = -2g(x)$. To obtain the graph of f, stretch the graph of $y = \dfrac{1}{x^2}$ vertically by a factor of 2 and reflect it across the x-axis. See Figures 27a and 27b. The domain is $(-\infty, 0) \cup (0, \infty)$. The range is $(-\infty, 0)$

29. Let $g(x) = y = \dfrac{1}{x^2}$, then $f(x) = g(x-3)$. To obtain the graph of f, shift the graph of $y = \dfrac{1}{x^2}$ to the right 3 units. See Figures 29a and 29b. The domain is $(-\infty, 3) \cup (3, \infty)$. The range is $(0, \infty)$.

31. Let $g(x) = y = \dfrac{1}{x^2}$, then $f(x) = -g(x+2) - 3$. To obtain the graph of f, shift the graph of $y = \dfrac{1}{x^2}$ to the left 2 units, reflect it across the x-axis and shift it downward 3 units. See Figures 31a and 31b. The domain is $(-\infty, -2) \cup (-2, \infty)$. The range is $(-\infty, -3)$.

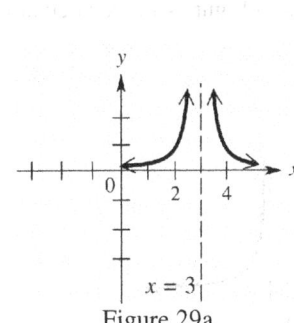
Figure 29a

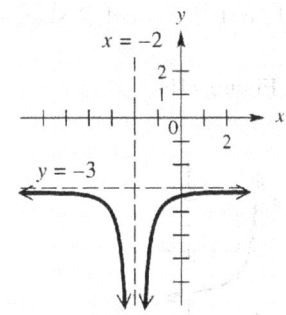
Figure 31a

[-1.7,7.7] by [-1.1,5.1]
Xscl = 1   Yscl = 1

[-6.7,2.7] by [-5.1,1.1]
Xscl = 1   Yscl = 1

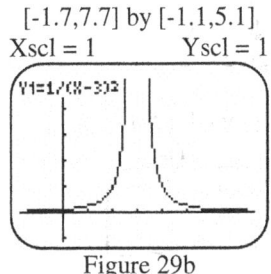
Figure 29b

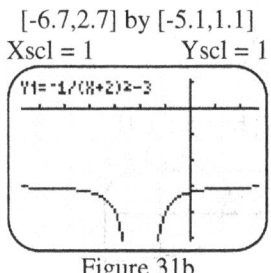
Figure 31b

33. The graph of f is obtained by shifting the graph of $y = \dfrac{1}{x^2}$ to the right 2 units. This is shown in graph C.

35. The graph of f is obtained by shifting the graph of $y = \dfrac{1}{x}$ to the right 2 units and reflecting it across the x-axis. This is shown in graph B.

37. The vertical asymptote shifts 2 units left to $x = -1$. The horizontal asymptote shifts 1 unit down to $y = 1$. The domain shifts 2 units left to $(-\infty, -1) \cup (-1, \infty)$. The range shifts 1 unit down to $(-\infty, 1) \cup (1, \infty)$.

39. Perform long division: $x - 2 \overline{) x - 1}$ $\Rightarrow$ $\dfrac{x-1}{x-2} = 1 + \dfrac{1}{x-2}$. The graph of $y = 1 + \dfrac{1}{x-2}$ is obtained by
    $\underline{x - 2}$
    1

shifting the graph of $y = \dfrac{1}{x}$ to the right 2 units and 1 unit upward. A sketch is shown in Figure 39a. A calculator graph of $y_1 = (x-1)/(x-2)$ is shown in Figure 39b.

41. Perform long division: $x+3 \overline{\smash{)}\begin{array}{r}-2\\-2x-5\\\underline{-2x-6}\\1\end{array}}$ $\Rightarrow \dfrac{-2x-5}{x+3} = -2 + \dfrac{1}{x+3}$. The graph of $y = -2 + \dfrac{1}{x+3}$ is obtained by shifting the graph of $y = \dfrac{1}{x}$ to the left 3 units and 2 units downward. A sketch is shown in Figure 41a. A calculator graph of $y_1 = (-2x-5)/(x+3)$ is shown in Figure 41b.

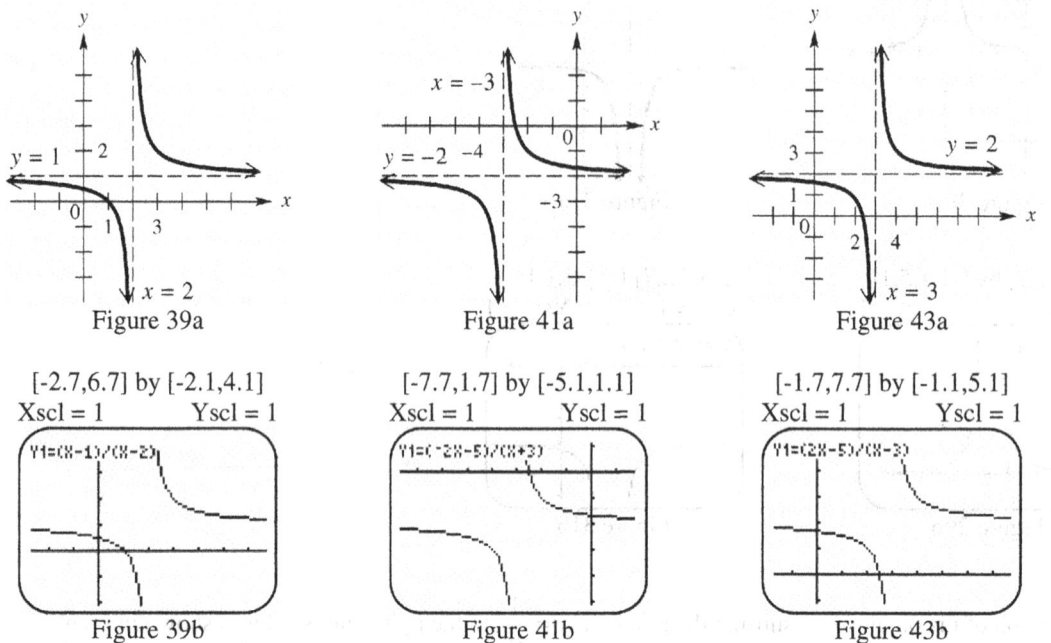

Figure 39a   Figure 41a   Figure 43a

[-2.7,6.7] by [-2.1,4.1]   [-7.7,1.7] by [-5.1,1.1]   [-1.7,7.7] by [-1.1,5.1]
Xscl = 1   Yscl = 1   Xscl = 1   Yscl = 1   Xscl = 1   Yscl = 1

Figure 39b   Figure 41b   Figure 43b

43. Perform long division: $x-3 \overline{\smash{)}\begin{array}{r}2\\2x-5\\\underline{2x-6}\\1\end{array}}$ $\Rightarrow \dfrac{2x-5}{x-3} = 2 + \dfrac{1}{x-3}$. The graph of $y = 2 + \dfrac{1}{x-3}$ is obtained by shifting the graph of $y = \dfrac{1}{x}$ to the right 3 units and 2 units upward. A sketch is shown in Figure 43a. A calculator graph of $y_1 = (2x-5)/(x-3)$ is shown in Figure 43b.

4.2: Rational Functions and Graphs II

1. Because -1 is a zero of the denominator but not of the numerator, the line $x = -1$ is a vertical asymptote: D.

3. The degree of the numerator is less than the degree of the denominator, so the x-axis is a horizontal asymptote: G.

5. Because $f(x) = \dfrac{x^2 - 16}{x+4} = \dfrac{(x-4)(x+4)}{x+4} = x - 4$ for all $x \neq -4$, there is a hole at $x = -4$: E.

7. Because $f(x) = \dfrac{x^2 + 3x + 4}{x - 5} = x + 8 + \dfrac{44}{x - 5}$, the line $y = x + 8$ is an oblique asymptote: F.

9. Since 5 is a zero of the denominator but not of the numerator, the line $x = 5$ is a vertical asymptote and the domain is $(-\infty, 5) \cup (5, \infty)$. Since $f(x) \to 0$ as $|x| \to \infty$, the line $y = 0$ is a horizontal asymptote. Since the degree of the numerator is less than the degree of the denominator, there is no oblique asymptote.

11. Since $-\dfrac{1}{2}$ is a zero of the denominator but not of the numerator, the line $x = -\dfrac{1}{2}$ is a vertical asymptote and the domain is $\left(-\infty, -\dfrac{1}{2}\right) \cup \left(-\dfrac{1}{2}, \infty\right)$. Since the degrees of the numerator and denominator are equal, the horizontal asymptote is $y = \dfrac{-3}{2} = -\dfrac{3}{2}$. Since the degree of the numerator is equal to the degree of the denominator, there is no oblique asymptote.

13. Since -3 is a zero of the denominator but not of the numerator, the line $x = -3$ is a vertical asymptote and the domain is $(-\infty, -3) \cup (-3, \infty)$. Since the degree of the numerator is greater than the degree of the denominator, there is no horizontal asymptote. Since $\dfrac{x^2 - 1}{x + 3} = x - 3 + \dfrac{8}{x + 3}$, the oblique asymptote is $y = x - 3$.

15. Since -2 and $\dfrac{5}{2}$ are zeros of the denominator but not of the numerator, the lines $x = -2$ and $x = \dfrac{5}{2}$ are vertical asymptotes and the domain is $(-\infty, -2) \cup \left(-2, \dfrac{5}{2}\right) \cup \left(\dfrac{5}{2}, \infty\right)$. Since the degrees of the numerator and denominator are equal, the horizontal asymptote is $y = \dfrac{1}{2}$. Since the degree of the numerator is equal to the degree of the denominator, there is no oblique asymptote.

17. Function A, because the denominator can never be equal to 0.

19. From the graph, the vertical asymptote is $x = 2$, the horizontal asymptote is $y = 4$, and there is no oblique asymptote. The function is defined for all $x \neq 2$, therefore the domain is $(-\infty, 2) \cup (2, \infty)$.

21. From the graph, the vertical asymptotes are $x = -2$ and $x = 2$, the horizontal asymptote is $y = -4$, and there is no oblique asymptote. The function is defined for all $x \neq \pm 2$, therefore the domain is $(-\infty, -2) \cup (-2, 2) \cup (2, \infty)$.

23. From the graph, the vertical asymptote is $x = 1$, the horizontal asymptote is $y = 0$ and there is no oblique asymptote. The function is defined for all $x \neq 1$, therefore the domain is $(-\infty, 1) \cup (1, \infty)$.

25. From the graph, the vertical asymptote is $x = -1$, there is no horizontal asymptote, and the oblique asymptote passes through the points $(0, -1)$ and $(1, 0)$. Thus, the equation of the oblique asymptote is $y = x - 1$. The function is defined for all $x \neq -1$, therefore the domain is $(-\infty, -1) \cup (-1, \infty)$.

164 CHAPTER 4 Rational, Power, and Root Functions

27. From the graph, there is no vertical asymptote, the horizontal asymptote is $y = 0$, and there is no oblique asymptote. The function is defined for all *x*, therefore the domain is $(-\infty, \infty)$.

29. See Figure 29.

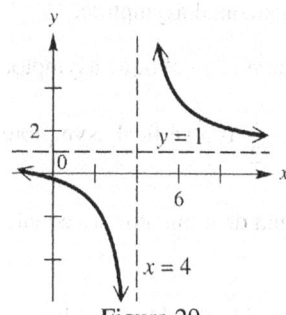
Figure 29

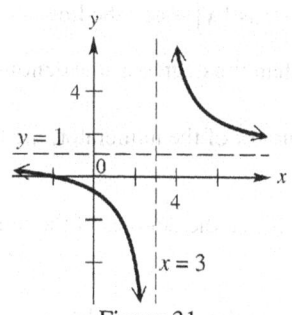
Figure 31

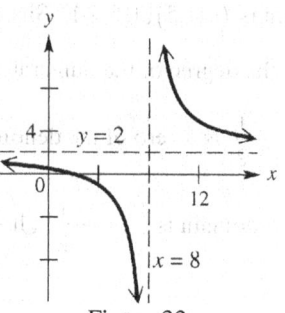
Figure 33

31. See Figure 31.
33. See Figure 33.
35. See Figure 35.
37. See Figure 37.

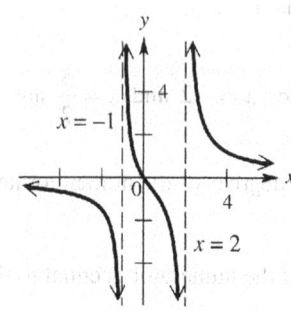
Figure 35

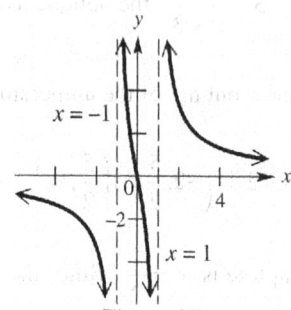
Figure 37

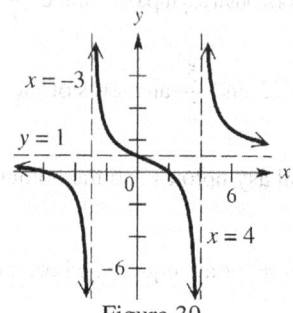
Figure 39

39. See Figure 39.
41. See Figure 41.
43. See Figure 43.

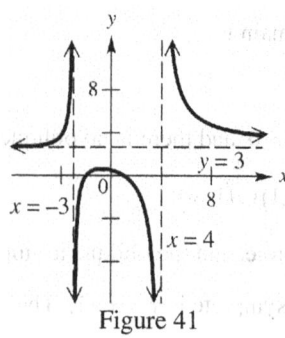
Figure 41

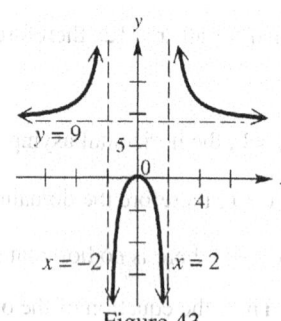
Figure 43

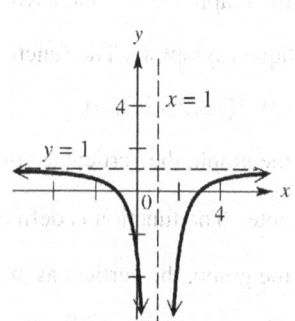
Figure 45

45. See Figure 45.

Copyright © 2015 Pearson Education, Inc

47. See Figure 47.
49. See Figure 49.

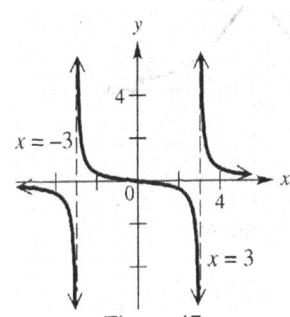
Figure 47

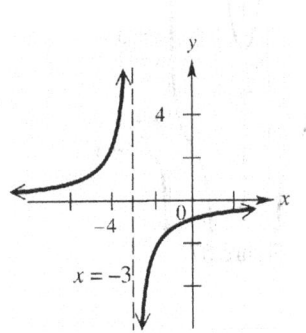
Figure 49

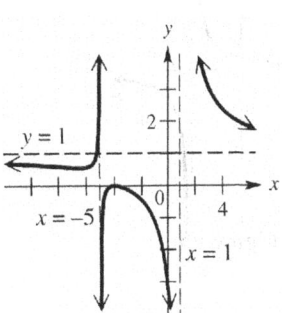
Figure 51

51. See Figure 51.
53. See Figure 53.
55. See Figure 55.

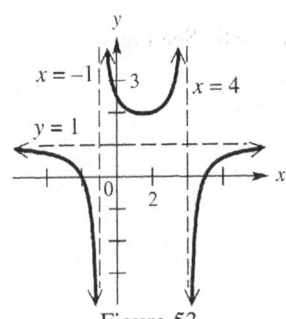
Figure 53

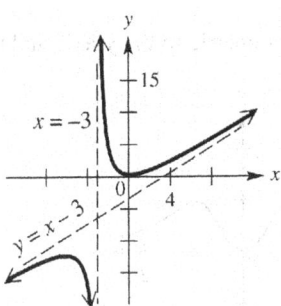
Figure 55

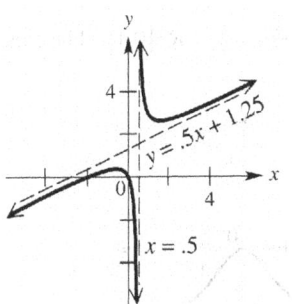
Figure 57

57. See Figure 57.
59. See Figure 59.
61. See Figure 61

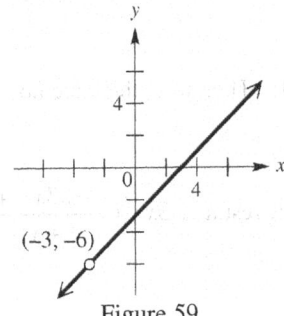
Figure 59

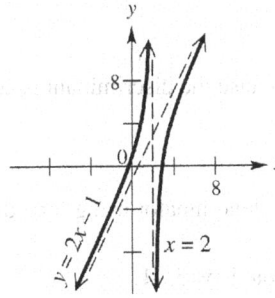
Figure 61

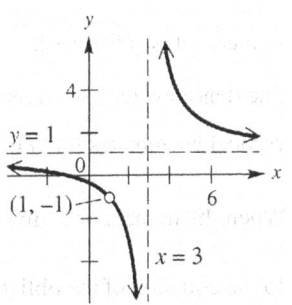
Figure 63

63. See Figure 63.
65. See Figure 65.
67. See Figure 67.

166   CHAPTER 4   Rational, Power, and Root Functions

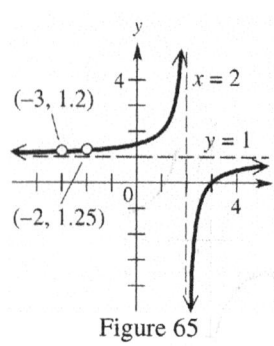
Figure 65

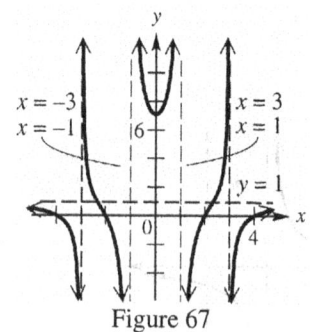
Figure 67

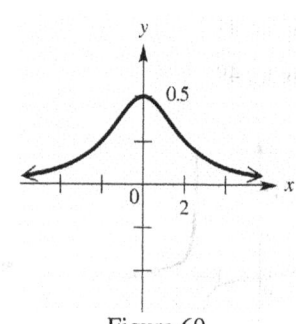
Figure 69

69. The domain is $(-\infty,\infty)$ because the denominator as no real zeros, the range is the interval $\left(0,\dfrac{1}{2}\right]$, and the graph is symmetric with respect to the y-axis. There are no vertical asymptotes and the x-axis is the horizontal asymptote. See Figure 69.

71. $D:(-\infty,\infty)$, $R:(-1,0]$ The function is symmetric to the y-axis and the HA is y = -1. See Figure 71.

73. $D:(-\infty,\infty)$, $R:[0,1]$ The function is symmetric to the y-axis and the HA is y = 0. See Figure 73.

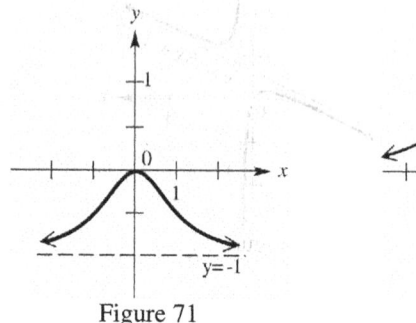
Figure 71

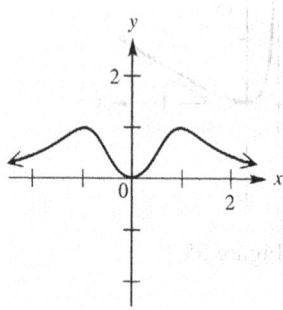
Figure 73

75. (a) The x-intercepts are the solutions of $3x^3+2x^2-12x-8=0 \Rightarrow (3x+2)(x^2-4)=0 \Rightarrow x=-\dfrac{2}{3},\pm 2$. The y-intercept is $f(0)=-2$.

    (b) The denominator has no real zeros because the discriminant is equal to -15. Therefore, there are no vertical asymptotes for $f(x)$.

    (c) When the numerator is divided by the denominator using long division the result is $3x-1+\dfrac{-23x-4}{x^2+x+4}$, so the equation of the oblique asymptote is y=3x-1.

    (d) The graph in Figure 75 correctly suggests that both the domain and range are both $(-\infty,\infty)$.

77. (a) The x-intercepts are the solutions of $x^3+4x^2-x-4=0 \Rightarrow (x-4)(x^2-1)=0 \Rightarrow x=4,\pm 1$. The y-intercept is $f(0)=1$.

    (b) The denominator has no real zeros because the discriminant is equal to -28. Therefore, there are no vertical asymptotes for $f(x)$.

Section 4.2   167

(c) When the numerator is divided by the denominator using long division the result is
$-\dfrac{1}{2}x - \dfrac{3}{2} + \dfrac{-2x-10}{-2x^2-2x-4}$, so the equation of the oblique asymptote is $-\dfrac{1}{2}x - \dfrac{3}{2}$.

(d) The graph in Figure 77 correctly suggests that both the domain and range are both $(-\infty, \infty)$.

[-4.7,4.7] by [-3.1,3.1]   [-4.7,4.7] by [-3.1,3.1]
Xscl = 1   Yscl = 1   Xscl = 1   Yscl = 1

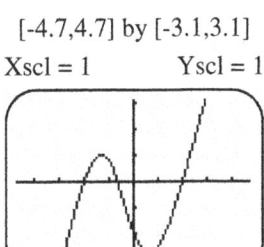
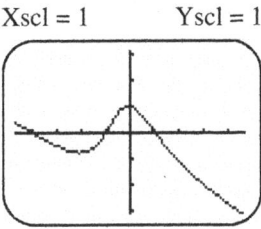

Figure 75   Figure 77

79. The expression is equal to 0 when $x = 4$, thus $p = 4$. The expression is undefined when $x = 2$, thus $q = 2$.

81. The expression is equal to 0 when $x = -2$, thus $p = -2$. The expression is undefined when $x = -1$, thus $q = -1$.

83. A vertical asymptote of $x = 2$ indicates that the denominator should contain the factor $(x-2)$. A hole at $x = -2$ indicates that both the numerator and denominator should contain the factor $(x+2)$. An x-intercept of 3 indicates that the numerator should contain the factor $(x-3)$. One possible equation for the function is
$f(x) = \dfrac{(x-3)(x+2)}{(x-2)(x+2)} = \dfrac{x^2-x-6}{x^2-4}$. Other functions are possible.

85. Vertical asymptotes of $x = 0$ and $x = 4$ indicate that the denominator should contain the factors x and $(x-4)$. An x-intercept of 2 indicates that the numerator should contain the factor $(x-2)$. Since there is a horizontal asymptote at $y = 0$, the degree of the numerator should be less than the degree of the denominator. One possible equation for the function is $f(x) = \dfrac{x-2}{x(x-4)} = \dfrac{x-2}{x^2-4x}$. Other functions are possible.

87. (a) Reflect the graph across the x-axis. See Figure 87a.
    (b) Reflect the graph across the y-axis. See Figure 87b.

88. (a) Reflect the graph across the x-axis. See Figure 88a.
    (b) Reflect the graph across the y-axis. See Figure 88b.

89. (a) Reflect the graph across the x-axis. See Figure 89a.
    (b) Reflect the graph across the y-axis. See Figure 89b.

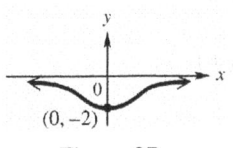

Figure 87a   Figure 88a   Figure 89a

Copyright © 2015 Pearson Education, Inc

168 CHAPTER 4 Rational, Power, and Root Functions

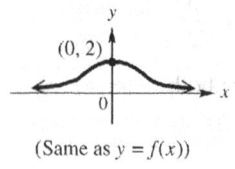

(Same as $y = f(x)$)

Figure 87b

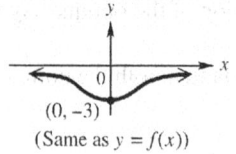

(Same as $y = f(x)$)

Figure 88b

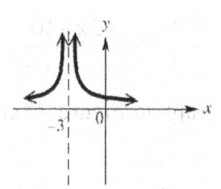

Figure 89b

90. (a) Reflect the graph across the x-axis. See Figure 90a.

(b) Reflect the graph across the y-axis. See Figure 90b.

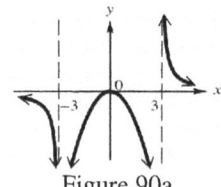

Figure 90a

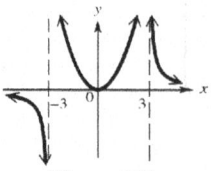

Figure 90b

91. Perform long division:
$$-x+4 \overline{\smash{\big)}\,2x^2+0x+3} \atop \underline{2x^2-8x}\atop 8x+3 \atop \underline{8x-32}\atop 35}^{-2x-8} \Rightarrow \frac{2x^2+3}{4-x} = -2x-8 + \frac{35}{4-x}$$

The oblique asymptote is $y = -2x-8$.

The graphs of $y_1 = (2x^2+3)/(4-x)$ and $y_2 = -2x-8$ are shown in Figure 91.

93. Perform long division:

$$x+2 \overline{\smash{\big)}\,-x^2+x+0} \atop \underline{-x^2-2x} \atop 3x+0 \atop \underline{3x+6} \atop -6}^{-x+3} \Rightarrow \frac{x-x^2}{x+2} = -x+3 + \frac{-6}{x+2}$$

The oblique asymptote is $y = -x+3$.

The graphs of $y_1 = (x-x^2)/(x+2)$ and $y_2 = -x+3$ are shown in Figure 93.

[-18.8,18.8] by [-50,25]
Xscl = 1   Yscl = 1

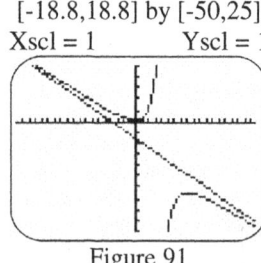

Figure 91

[-3,8] by [-10,10]
Xscl = 1   Yscl = 1

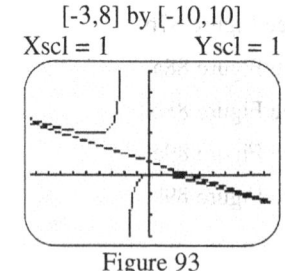

Figure 93

[-50,50] by [0,1000]
Xscl = 10   Yscl = 100

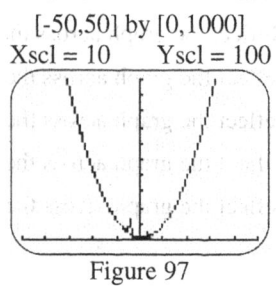

Figure 97

95. (a) Disregard the remainder to get the equation of the oblique asymptote, $y = x+1$.

Copyright © 2015 Pearson Education, Inc

(b) Set the original function equal to the expression for the oblique asymptote and solve:

$$\frac{x^5+x^4+x^2+1}{x^4+1}=x+1 \Rightarrow x^5+x^4+x^2+1=(x^4+1)(x+1) \Rightarrow$$

$$x^5+x^4+x^2+1=x^5+x^4+x+1 \Rightarrow x^2+1=x+1 \Rightarrow x^2-x=0 \Rightarrow x(x-1)=0 \Rightarrow x=0,1.$$

The graph crosses the oblique asymptote at $x=0$ and $x=1$

(c) For large values of x, $x+1 < \frac{x^5+x^4+x^2+1}{x^4+1}$. Thus, the function approaches its asymptote from above.

97.

$$x^2+x-12 \overline{\smash{\big)}\, x^4+0x^3-5x^2+0x+4}$$ with quotient x^2-x+8

$$\frac{x^4-5x^2+4}{x^2+x-12}=x^2-x+8+\frac{-20x+100}{x^2+x-12}$$

Long division steps:
$x^4+x^3-12x^2$
$-x^3+7x^2+0x$
$-x^3-x^2+12x$
$8x^2-12x+4$
$8x^2+8x-96$
$-20x+100$

The graphs of $y_1=(x^4-5x^2+4)/(x^2+x-12)$ and $y_2=x^2-x+8$ are shown in figure 97. In this window, the two graphs seem to overlap (coincide), suggesting that as $|x| \to \infty$, the graph of f approaches the graph of g, giving an asymptotic effect.

4.3: Rational Equations, Inequalities, Models and Applications

1. (a) The graph never intersects the x-axis. The solution set of $f(x)=0$ is $\emptyset$.

   (b) The graph is below the x-axis on the interval $(-\infty,-2)$. Thus $f(x)<0$ on $(-\infty,-2)$.

   (c) The graph is above the x-axis on the interval $(-2,\infty)$. Thus $f(x)>0$ on $(-2,\infty)$.

3. (a) The graph intersects the x-axis at $x=-1$. The solution set of $f(x)=0$ is $\{-1\}$.

   (b) The graph is below the x-axis on the interval $(-1,0)$. Thus $f(x)<0$ on $(-1,0)$.

   (c) The graph is above the x-axis on the interval $(-\infty,-1)\cup(0,\infty)$. Thus $f(x)>0$ on $(-\infty,-1)\cup(0,\infty)$.

5. (a) The graph intersects the x-axis at $x=0$. The solution set of $f(x)=0$ is $\{0\}$.

   (b) The graph is below the x-axis on the interval $(-2,0)\cup(2,\infty)$. Thus $f(x)<0$ on $(-2,0)\cup(2,\infty)$.

   (c) The graph is above the x-axis on the interval $(-\infty,-2)\cup(0,2)$. Thus $f(x)>0$ on $(-\infty,-2)\cup(0,2)$.

7. (a) The graph intersects the x-axis at $x=0$. The solution set of $f(x)=0$ is $\{0\}$.

   (b) The graph is below the x-axis on the interval $(-1,0)\cup(0,1)$. Thus $f(x)<0$ on $(-1,0)\cup(0,1)$.

   (c) The graph is above the x-axis on the interval $(-\infty,-1)\cup(1,\infty)$. Thus $f(x)>0$ on $(-\infty,-1)\cup(1,\infty)$.

9. (a) The graph intersects the x-axis at $x=0$. The solution set of $f(x)=0$ is $\{0\}$.

(b) The graph is below the x-axis on the interval $(1,2) \cup (2,3)$. Thus $f(x) < 0$ on $(1,2) \cup (2,3)$.

(c) The graph is above the x-axis on the interval $(-\infty,-2) \cup (-2,0) \cup (0,1) \cup (3,\infty)$. Thus $f(x) > 0$ on the interval $(-\infty,-2) \cup (-2,0) \cup (0,1) \cup (3,\infty)$.

11. (a) The graph intersects the x-axis at $x = 2.5$. The solution set of $f(x) = 0$ is $\{2.5\}$.

(b) The graph is below the x-axis on the interval $(2.5, 3)$. Thus $f(x) < 0$ on $(2.5, 3)$.

(c) The graph is above the x-axis on the interval $(-\infty, 2.5) \cup (3, \infty)$. Thus $f(x) > 0$ on $(-\infty, 2.5) \cup (3, \infty)$.

13. Multiply through by the LCD, $(x-1)(x+1)$. $\dfrac{2x}{x^2-1} \cdot (x-1)(x+1) = \dfrac{2}{x+1} \cdot (x-1)(x+1) - \dfrac{1}{x-1} \cdot (x-1)(x+1) \Rightarrow$

$2x = 2(x-1) - (x+1) \Rightarrow 2x = 2x - 2 - x - 1 \Rightarrow 2x = x - 3 \Rightarrow x = -3$. The solution set is $\{-3\}$.

15. Multiply through by the LCD, $x(x-3)(x+3)$.

$\dfrac{4}{x^2-3x} \cdot x(x-3)(x+3) - \dfrac{1}{x^2-9} \cdot x(x-3)(x+3) = 0 \cdot x(x-3)(x+3) \Rightarrow 4(x+3) - x = 0 \Rightarrow$

$4x + 12 - x = 0 \Rightarrow 3x = -12 \Rightarrow x = -4$. The solution set is $\{-4\}$.

17. Multiply through by the LCD, x^2.

$1 \cdot x^2 - \dfrac{13}{x} \cdot x^2 + \dfrac{36}{x^2} \cdot x^2 = 0 \cdot x^2 \Rightarrow x^2 - 13x + 36 = 0 \Rightarrow (x-4)(x-9) = 0 \Rightarrow x = 4 \text{ or } 9$.

The solution set is $\{4, 9\}$.

19. Multiply through by the LCD, x^2.

$1 \cdot x^2 + \dfrac{3}{x} \cdot x^2 = \dfrac{5}{x^2} \cdot x^2 \Rightarrow x^2 + 3x = 5 \Rightarrow x^2 + 3x - 5 = 0 \Rightarrow$

$x = \dfrac{-3 \pm \sqrt{3^2 - 4(1)(-5)}}{2(1)} = \dfrac{-3 \pm \sqrt{29}}{2}$. The solution set is $\left\{\dfrac{-3 \pm \sqrt{29}}{2}\right\}$.

21. Multiply through by the LCD, $x(2-x)$.

$\dfrac{x}{2-x} \cdot x(2-x) + \dfrac{2}{x} \cdot x(2-x) - 5 \cdot x(2-x) = 0 \cdot x(2-x) \Rightarrow x^2 + 2(2-x) - 5x(2-x) = 0 \Rightarrow$

$6x^2 - 12x + 4 = 0 \Rightarrow 3x^2 - 6x + 2 = 0$.

$x = \dfrac{-(-6) \pm \sqrt{(-6)^2 - 4(3)(2)}}{2(3)} = \dfrac{6 \pm \sqrt{12}}{6} = \dfrac{2(3 \pm \sqrt{3})}{2(3)} = \dfrac{3 \pm \sqrt{3}}{3}$. The solution set is $\left\{\dfrac{3 \pm \sqrt{3}}{3}\right\}$.

23. Rewrite the equation as $\dfrac{1}{x^4} - \dfrac{3}{x^2} - 4 = 0$ and multiply through by the LCD, x^4.

$\dfrac{1}{x^4} \cdot x^4 - \dfrac{3}{x^2} \cdot x^4 - 4 \cdot x^4 = 0 \cdot x^4 \Rightarrow 1 - 3x^2 - 4x^4 = 0 \Rightarrow 4x^4 + 3x^2 - 1 = 0 \Rightarrow$

$(4x^2 - 1)(x^2 + 1) = 0 \Rightarrow (2x+1)(2x-1)(x^2+1) = 0 \Rightarrow 2x + 1 = 0 \text{ or } 2x - 1 = 0 \text{ or } x^2 + 1 = 0 \Rightarrow$

$2x = -1$ or $2x = 1$ or $x^2 = -1 \Rightarrow x = -\dfrac{1}{2}$ or $x = \dfrac{1}{2}$ or $x = \pm i$. The solution set is $\left\{\pm\dfrac{1}{2}, \pm i\right\}$.

25. Multiply through by the LCD, $(x+2)(x+7)$.

$\dfrac{1}{x+2} \cdot (x+2)(x+7) + \dfrac{3}{x+7} \cdot (x+2)(x+7) = \dfrac{5}{x^2+9x+14} \cdot (x+2)(x+7) \Rightarrow$

$1(x+7) + 3(x+2) = 5 \Rightarrow x + 7 + 3x + 6 = 5 \Rightarrow 4x = -8 \Rightarrow x = -2$.

This solution is extraneous. The solution set is $\varnothing$.

27. Multiply through by the LCD, $(x-3)(x+3)$.

$\dfrac{x}{x-3} \cdot (x-3)(x+3) + \dfrac{4}{x+3} \cdot (x-3)(x+3) = \dfrac{18}{x^2-9} \cdot (x-3)(x+3) \Rightarrow$

$x(x+3) + 4(x-3) = 18 \Rightarrow x^2 + 3x + 4x - 12 = 18 \Rightarrow x^2 + 7x - 30 = 0 \Rightarrow (x+10)(x-3) = 0 \Rightarrow x = -10$ or $x = 3$.

The solution $x = 3$ is extraneous. The solution set is $\{-10\}$.

29. Rewrite the equation as $\dfrac{9}{x} + \dfrac{4}{6x-3} = \dfrac{2}{6x-3}$ and multiply through by the LCD, $x(6x-3)$.

$\dfrac{9}{x} \cdot x(6x-3) + \dfrac{4}{6x-3} \cdot x(6x-3) = \dfrac{2}{6x-3} \cdot x(6x-3) \Rightarrow 9(6x-3) + 4x = 2x \Rightarrow$

$54x - 27 + 4x = 2x \Rightarrow 56x = 27 \Rightarrow x = \dfrac{27}{56}$. The solution set is $\left\{\dfrac{27}{56}\right\}$.

31. (a) $\dfrac{x-3}{x+5} = 0 \Rightarrow x - 3 = 0(x+5) \Rightarrow x - 3 = 0 \Rightarrow x = 3$. The solution set is $\{3\}$.

(b) Graph $y_1 = (x-3)/(x+5)$ as shown in Figure 31. With vertical asymptote $x = -5$, the graph is below or intersects the x-axis on the interval $(-5, 3]$. The solution set is $(-5, 3]$.

(c) Graph $y_1 = (x-3)/(x+5)$ as shown in Figure 31. With vertical asymptote $x = -5$, the graph is above or intersects the x-axis on the interval $(-\infty, -5) \cup [3, \infty)$. The solution set is $(-\infty, -5) \cup [3, \infty)$.

33. (a) $\dfrac{x-1}{x+2} = 1 \Rightarrow x - 1 = 1(x+2) \Rightarrow x - 1 = x + 2 \Rightarrow -1 = 2$ (false). The solution set is $\varnothing$.

(b) Graph $y_1 = (x-1)/(x+2) - 1$ as shown in Figure 33. With vertical asymptote $x = -2$, the graph is above the x-axis on the interval $(-\infty, -2)$. The solution set is $(-\infty, -2)$.

(c) Graph $y_1 = (x-1)/(x+2) - 1$ as shown in Figure 33. With vertical asymptote $x = -2$, the graph is below the x-axis on the interval $(-2, \infty)$. The solution set is $(-2, \infty)$.

[-10,10] by [-5,8]   [-10,10] by [-5,10]   [-5,5] by [-5,5]   [-3,3] by [-20,20]
Xscl = 1   Yscl = 1   Xscl = 1   Yscl = 1   Xscl = 1   Yscl = 1   Xscl = 1   Yscl = 5

172   CHAPTER 4   Rational, Power, and Root Functions

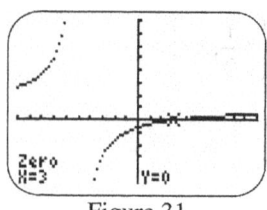

Figure 31   Figure 33   Figure 35   Figure 37

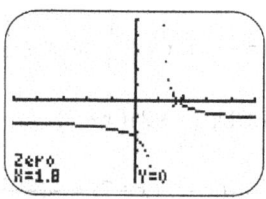

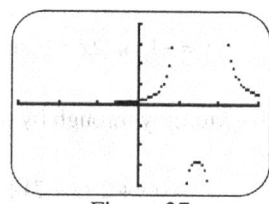

35. (a) $\dfrac{1}{x-1} = \dfrac{5}{4} \Rightarrow 5(x-1) = 4(1) \Rightarrow 5x - 5 = 4 \Rightarrow 5x = 9 \Rightarrow x = \dfrac{9}{5}$. The solution set is $\left\{\dfrac{9}{5}\right\}$.

   (b) Graph $y_1 = 1/(x-1) - 5/4$ as shown in Figure 35. With vertical asymptote $x = 1$, the graph is below the x-axis on the interval $(-\infty, 1) \cup \left(\dfrac{9}{5}, \infty\right)$. The solution set is $(-\infty, 1) \cup \left(\dfrac{9}{5}, \infty\right)$.

   (c) Graph $y_1 = 1/(x-1) - 5/4$ as shown in Figure 35. With vertical asymptote $x = 1$, the graph is above the x-axis on the interval $\left(1, \dfrac{9}{5}\right)$. The solution set is $\left(1, \dfrac{9}{5}\right)$.

37. (a) $\dfrac{4}{x-2} = \dfrac{3}{x-1} \Rightarrow 4(x-1) = 3(x-2) \Rightarrow 4x - 4 = 3x - 6 \Rightarrow x = -2$. The solution set is $\{-2\}$.

   (b) Graph $y_1 = 4/(x-2) - 3/(x-1)$ as shown in Figure 37. With vertical asymptotes $x = 1$ and $x = 2$, the graph is below or intersects the x-axis on $(-\infty, -2] \cup (1, 2)$. The solution set is $(-\infty, -2] \cup (1, 2)$.

   (c) Graph $y_1 = 4/(x-2) - 3/(x-1)$ as shown in Figure 37. With vertical asymptotes $x = 1$ and $x = 2$, the graph is above or intersects the x-axis on $[-2, 1) \cup (2, \infty)$. The solution set is $[-2, 1) \cup (2, \infty)$.

39. (a) $\dfrac{1}{(x-2)^2} = 0 \Rightarrow 1 = 0(x-2)^2 \Rightarrow 1 = 0$ (false). The solution set is $\varnothing$.

   (b) Graph $y_1 = 1/(x-2)^2$ as shown in Figure 39. The graph is never below the x-axis. The solution set is $\varnothing$.

   (c) Graph $y_1 = 1/(x-2)^2$ as shown in Figure 39. With vertical asymptote $x = 2$, the graph is above the x-axis on the interval $(-\infty, 2) \cup (2, -\infty)$. The solution set is $(-\infty, 2) \cup (2, \infty)$.

41. (a) $\dfrac{5}{x+1} = \dfrac{12}{x+1} \Rightarrow 5(x+1) = 12(x+1) \Rightarrow 5x + 5 = 12x + 12 \Rightarrow -7x = 7 \Rightarrow x = -1$. This solution is extraneous. The solution set is $\varnothing$.

   (b) Graph $y_1 = 5/(x+1) - 12/(x+1)$ as shown in Figure 41. With vertical asymptote $x = -1$, the graph is above the x-axis on the interval $(-\infty, -1)$. The solution set is $(-\infty, -1)$.

   (c) Graph $y_1 = 5/(x+1) - 12/(x+1)$ as shown in Figure 41. With vertical asymptote $x = -1$, the graph is below the x-axis on the interval $(-1, \infty)$. The solution set is $(-1, \infty)$.

[-5,10] by [-5,10]
Xscl = 1   Yscl = 1

[-10,10] by [-10,10]
Xscl = 1   Yscl = 1

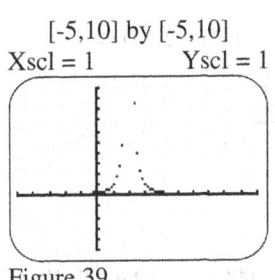
Figure 39

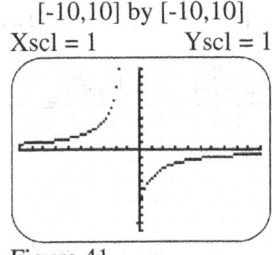
Figure 41

43. (a) The equation $\dfrac{(x-2)(2)-(2x+1)(1)}{(x-2)^2}=0$ is true only when $(x-2)(2)-(2x+1)(1)=0$. Solving we have

$(x-2)(2)-(2x+1)(1)=0 \Rightarrow 2x-4-2x-1=0 \Rightarrow -5 \neq 0$, The solution is $\varnothing$.

(b) The quotient changes sign only when x-values make the numerator or denominator 0. From part (a) we know that there are no x-values that make the numerator equal to 0. Solve $(x-2)^2 = 0$ to find the value(s) that make the denominator 0. $(x-2)^2 = 0 \Rightarrow x-2=0 \Rightarrow x=2$

Interval	Test Value	Positive or Negative Result
$(-\infty, 2)$	0	Negative
$(2, \infty)$	3	Negative

The solution is $(-\infty, 2) \cup (2, \infty)$.

45. (a) The equation $\dfrac{(x^2+1)(2x)-(x^2-1)(2x)}{(x^2+1)^2}=0$ is true only when $(x^2+1)(2x)-(x^2-1)(2x)=0$.

Solving we have $(x^2+1)(2x)-(x^2-1)(2x)=0 \Rightarrow (2x)(x^2+1-x^2+1)=0 \Rightarrow (2x)(2)=0 \Rightarrow x=0$

The solution is 0.

(b) The quotient changes sign only when x-values make the numerator or denominator 0. From part (a) we know that $x=0$. Solve $(x^2+1)^2 = 0$ to find the value(s) that make the denominator 0.

$(x^2+1)^2 = 0 \Rightarrow x^2+1=0 \Rightarrow x^2 = -1 \Rightarrow x = \pm i$ Thus, there are no real numbers that make the denominator equal to zero.

Interval	Test Value	Positive or Negative Result
$(-\infty, 0]$	-2	Negative
$[0, \infty)$	2	Positive

The solution is $[0, \infty)$.

47. (a) The equation $\dfrac{(2x+1)(2x)-(x^2+1)(2)}{(2x+1)^2}=0$ is true only when $(2x+1)(2x)-(x^2+1)(2)=0$.

Solving we have $(2x+1)(2x) - (x^2+1)(2) = 0 \Rightarrow 4x^2 + 2x - 2x^2 - 2 = 0 \Rightarrow 2x^2 + 2x - 2 = 0 \Rightarrow$

$$x = \frac{-(2) \pm \sqrt{(2)^2 - 4(2)(-2)}}{2(2)} = \frac{-2 \pm \sqrt{4+16}}{4} = \frac{-2 \pm \sqrt{20}}{4} = \frac{-2 \pm 2\sqrt{5}}{4} = \frac{-1 \pm \sqrt{5}}{2}$$

The solution is $\frac{-1 \pm \sqrt{5}}{2}$.

(b) The quotient changes sign only when x-values make the numerator or denominator 0. From part (a) we know that $x = \frac{-1 \pm \sqrt{5}}{2}$. Solve $(2x+1)^2 = 0$ to find the value(s) that make the denominator 0.

$(2x+1)^2 = 0 \Rightarrow 2x+1 = 0 \Rightarrow 2x = -1 \Rightarrow x = -\frac{1}{2}$.

Interval	Test Value	Positive or Negative Result
$\left(-\infty, \frac{-1-\sqrt{5}}{2}\right)$	-2	Positive
$\left(\frac{-1-\sqrt{5}}{2}, -\frac{1}{2}\right)$	-1	Negative
$\left(-\frac{1}{2}, \frac{-1+\sqrt{5}}{2}\right)$	0	Negative
$\left(\frac{-1+\sqrt{5}}{2}, \infty\right)$	2	Positive

The solution is $\left(\frac{-1-\sqrt{5}}{2}, -\frac{1}{2}\right) \cup \left(-\frac{1}{2}, \frac{-1+\sqrt{5}}{2}\right)$.

49. The numerator is negative and the denominator is always positive; therefore, the quotient is always negative. Because the inequality requires that the rational expression be less than 0, the solution set is $(-\infty, \infty)$.

51. The numerator is negative and the denominator is always positive; therefore, the quotient is always negative. Because the inequality requires that the rational expression be greater than 0, the solution set is $\varnothing$.

53. The numerator is always positive and the denominator is negative; therefore, the quotient is always negative. Because the inequality requires that the rational expression be greater than or equal to 0, the solution set is $\varnothing$.

55. The numerator is always positive and the denominator is always positive; therefore, the quotient is always positive. Because the inequality requires that the rational expression be greater than 0, the solution set is $(-\infty, \infty)$.

57. The numerator is always positive or zero and the denominator is always positive; therefore, the quotient is always positive or zero. Because the inequality requires that the rational expression be less than or equal to 0, the solution set is $\{1\}$. Note that when $x = 1$, the rational expression equals 0 and the inequality is satisfied.

59. The graph of $y_1 = (3-2x)/(1+x)$ has a vertical asymptote at $x = -1$ and an x-intercept at $x = \frac{3}{2}$. The graph of y_1 is below the x-axis on the interval $(-\infty, -1) \cup \left(\frac{3}{2}, \infty\right)$.

61. The graph of $y_1 = \frac{(x+1)(x-2)}{x+3}$ has a vertical asymptote at $x = -3$ and x-intercepts at $x = -1$ and $x = 2$. The graph of $P(3) = 0$ is below the x-axis on the interval $(-\infty, -3) \cup (-1, 2)$.

63. The graph of $y_1 = (x+1)^2/(x-2)$ has a vertical asymptote at $x = 2$ and an x-intercept at $x = -1$. The graph of y_1 intersects or is below the x-axis on the interval $(-\infty, 2)$. Note that 2 can not be included.

65. The graph of $y_1 = \frac{2x-5}{(x+1)(x-1)}$ has vertical asymptotes at $x = -1$ and $x = 1$ and an x-intercept at $x = \frac{5}{2}$.

    The graph of y_1 is on or above the x-axis on the interval $(-1, 1) \cup \left[\frac{5}{2}, \infty\right)$.

67. First, rewrite the inequality: $\frac{1}{x-3} \leq \frac{5}{x-3} \Rightarrow \frac{1}{x-3} - \frac{5}{x-3} \leq 0 \Rightarrow \frac{-4}{x-3} \leq 0$

    The graph of $y_1 = -4/(x-3)$ has a vertical asymptote at $x = 3$ and no x-intercept.

    The graph of y_1 intersects or is below the x-axis on the interval $(3, \infty)$. Note that 3 can not be included.

69. First, rewrite the inequality: $2 - \frac{5}{x} + \frac{2}{x^2} \geq 0 \Rightarrow \frac{2x^2 - 5x + 2}{x^2} \geq 0 \Rightarrow \frac{(2x-1)(x-2)}{x^2} \geq 0$

    The graph of $y_1 = (2x-1)(x-2)/x^2$ has a vertical asymptote at $x = 0$ and x-intercepts of $x = \frac{1}{2}$ and $x = 2$.

    The graph of y_1 intersects or is above the x-axis on the interval $(-\infty, 0) \cup \left(0, \frac{1}{2}\right] \cup [2, \infty)$.

71. (a) The graph of $y_1 = (\sqrt{2}x+5)/(x^3 - \sqrt{3})$ is shown in Figure 71. The x-intercept is approximately -3.54. The solution set of the equation is $\{-3.54\}$.

    (b) There is a vertical asymptote when $x^3 - \sqrt{3} = 0 \Rightarrow x^3 = \sqrt{3} \Rightarrow x = \sqrt[3]{\sqrt{3}} \approx 1.20$. Thus, the graph is above the x-axis on the interval $(-\infty, -3.54) \cup (1.20, \infty)$. See Figure 71.

    (c) The graph is below the x-axis on the interval $(-3.54, 1.20)$. See Figure 71.

73. (a) The graph is shown in Figure 73. The equation of the horizontal asymptote is $y = \frac{10}{1} \Rightarrow y = 10$.

    (b) The initial insect population occurs when $x = 0$. Here $f(0) = \frac{10(0)+1}{(0)+1} = 1$ million insects.

    (c) After several months, the insect population levels off at 10 million insects.

    (d) The horizontal asymptote $y = 10$ represents the limiting population after a long time.

176   CHAPTER 4   Rational, Power, and Root Functions

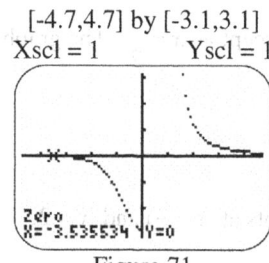

Figure 71

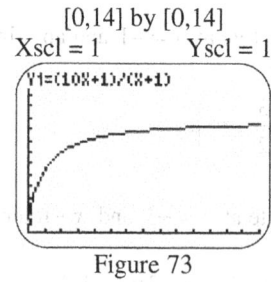

Figure 73

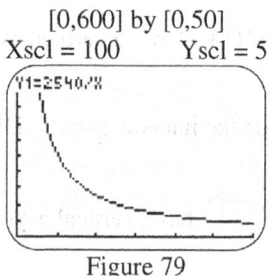

Figure 79

75. (a) $0.25 = \dfrac{x-5}{x^2-10x} \Rightarrow 0.25(x^2-10x) = x-5 \Rightarrow 0.25x^2 - 2.5x = x-5 \Rightarrow 0.25x^2 - 3.5x + 5 = 0 \Rightarrow$

$x = \dfrac{-(-3.5) \pm \sqrt{(-3.5)^2 - 4(0.25)(5)}}{2(0.25)} = \dfrac{3.5 \pm \sqrt{7.25}}{0.5} \approx 1.6 \text{ or } 12.4;$ Since $x > 10$, $x \approx 12.4$ cars/min.

(b) Since 2 attendants can serve only 10 cars/min, 3 attendants are needed.

77. A surface area of 280 square inches indicates that $2\,lw + 2\,lh + 2\,hw = 280$ or $lw + lh + hw = 140$. Solving this equation for h gives $h = \dfrac{140 - lw}{l+w}$. Since the length is twice the width, $l = 2w$. Then, by substitution,

$h = \dfrac{140 - (2w)w}{2w + w} \Rightarrow h = \dfrac{140 - 2w^2}{3w}$. Since the volume is 196 cubic inches, $lwh = 196$. Substituting for l and h

yields $(2w)w\left(\dfrac{140 - 2w^2}{3w}\right) = 196 \Rightarrow \dfrac{280w - 4w^3}{3} = 196 \Rightarrow 280w - 4w^3 = 588 \Rightarrow$

$4w^3 - 280w + 588 = 0 \Rightarrow w^3 - 70w + 147 = 0$. Graphing this equation as $y_1 = x\wedge 3 - 70x + 147$ in [0,10] by $[-150, 450]$ shows the possible values for the width as the x-intercepts (figure not shown). The possible values for the width are 7 inches and approximately 2.266 inches.

If $w \approx 2.266$, then $l \approx 2(2.266) \approx 4.532$ and $h = \dfrac{140 - 2(2.266)^2}{3(2.266)} \approx 19.084$. In this case, the dimensions are

approximately 2.266 by 4.532 by 19.084 inches. If $w = 7$, then $l = 14$ and $h = \dfrac{140 - 2(7)^2}{3(7)} = 2$ inches. In

this case the dimensions are 7 by 14 by 2 inches.

79. (a) $f(400) = \dfrac{2540}{400} = 6.35$ in. A curve designed for 60 miles per hour with a radius of 400 feet should have the outer rail elevated 6.35 inches.

(b) See Figure 79. As the radius x of the curve increases, the elevation of the outer rail decreases.

(c) The horizontal asymptote is $y = 0$. As the radius of the curve increases without bound ($x \to \infty$), the tracks become straight and no elevation or banking ($y \to 0$) is necessary.

(d) $12.7 = \dfrac{2540}{x} \Rightarrow 12.7x = 2540 \Rightarrow x = \dfrac{2540}{12.7} = 200$ ft.

Copyright © 2015 Pearson Education, Inc

81. (a) $D(0.05) = \dfrac{2500}{30(0.3+0.05)} \approx 238$. The braking distance for a car going 50 mph on a 5% uphill grade is about 238 ft.

(b) As the uphill grade x increases, the braking distance decreases. This agrees with driving experience.

(c) $220 = \dfrac{2500}{30(0.3+x)} \Rightarrow 6600(0.3+x) = 2500 \Rightarrow 0.3 + x = \dfrac{2500}{6000} \Rightarrow x = \dfrac{2500}{6600} - 0.3 \Rightarrow x \approx 0.079$. The grade associated with a braking distance of 220 feet is about 7.9% uphill.

83. Here $r = \dfrac{km^2}{s}$. By substitution, $12 = \dfrac{k(6)^2}{4} \Rightarrow 48 = 36k \Rightarrow k = \dfrac{48}{36} \Rightarrow k = \dfrac{4}{3}$. That gives $r = \dfrac{\frac{4}{3}m^2}{s}$. When $m = 4$ and $s = 10$, $r = \dfrac{\frac{4}{3}(4)^2}{10} = \dfrac{\frac{64}{3}}{10} = \dfrac{64}{30} = \dfrac{32}{15}$.

85. Here $a = \dfrac{kmn^2}{y^3}$. By substitution, $9 = \dfrac{k(4)(9)^2}{(3)^3} \Rightarrow 243 = 324k \Rightarrow k = \dfrac{243}{324} \Rightarrow k = \dfrac{3}{4}$. That gives $a = \dfrac{\frac{3}{4}mn^2}{y^3}$. When $m = 6$, $n = 2$ and $y = 5$, $a = \dfrac{\frac{3}{4}(6)(2)^2}{(5)^3} = \dfrac{18}{125}$.

87. For $k > 0$, if y varies directly as x, when x increases, y increases, and when x decreases, y decreases.

89. If y is inversely proportional to x, $y = \dfrac{k}{x}$. If x doubles, $y = \dfrac{k}{2x} \Rightarrow y = \dfrac{1}{2} \cdot \dfrac{k}{x}$. That is, y becomes half as much.

91. If y is directly proportional to the third power of x, $y = kx^3$. If x triples, $y = k(3x)^3 \Rightarrow y = 27 \cdot kx^3$. That is, y becomes 27 times as much.

93. Here $BMI = \dfrac{kw}{h^2}$. By substitution, $24 = \dfrac{k(177)}{(72)^2} \Rightarrow 177k \Rightarrow k = \dfrac{124{,}416}{177} \Rightarrow k \approx 703$. That gives $BMI \approx \dfrac{703w}{h^2}$. When $w = 130$ and $h = 66$, $BMI \approx \dfrac{703(130)}{(66)^2} \approx 21$.

95. Here $R = \dfrac{k}{d^2}$. By substitution, $0.5 = \dfrac{k}{(2)^2} \Rightarrow 2 = k$. That gives $R = \dfrac{2}{d^2}$. When $d = 3$, $R = \dfrac{2}{(3)^2} \approx \dfrac{2}{9}$ ohm.

97. Here $W = \dfrac{k}{d^2}$. By substitution, $160 = \dfrac{k}{(4000)^2} \Rightarrow 2{,}560{,}000{,}000 = k$. That gives $W = \dfrac{2{,}560{,}000{,}000}{d^2}$. Note that 8000 miles above Earth's surface, $d = 12{,}000$. When $d = 12{,}000$, $W = \dfrac{2{,}560{,}000{,}000}{(12{,}000)^2} = 17.8$ lb.

99. Here $V = kr^2h$. By substitution, $300 = k(3)^2(10.62) \Rightarrow \dfrac{300}{95.58} = k \Rightarrow k \approx 3.1387$. That gives $V = 3.1387r^2h$. When $r = 4$ and $h = 15.92$, $V \approx 3.1387(4)^2(15.92) \approx 799.5$. (Note that the actual value of k is π.)

178   CHAPTER 4   Rational, Power, and Root Functions

101. Tooney can clean the entire mess in 15 minutes and can complete $\frac{t}{15}$ of the mess in t minutes. Mudcat can clean the entire mess in 12 minutes and can complete $\frac{t}{12}$ of the mess in t minutes. Together they can complete $\frac{t}{15}+\frac{t}{12}$ of the mess in t minutes. The job is complete when the fraction of the mess reaches 1.

$\frac{t}{15}+\frac{t}{12}=1 \Rightarrow 12t+15t=180 \Rightarrow 27t=180 \Rightarrow t=6$ minutes and 40 seconds.

103. Mrs. Schmulen can grade tests in 5 hours and can complete $\frac{t}{5}$ of the tests in t hours. Mr. Elwyn and Mrs. Schmulen can grade the tests together in 3 hours and can complete $\frac{t}{3}$ of the tests in t hours.

The job is complete when the fraction of the completed tests reaches 1.

$\frac{t}{3}-\frac{t}{5}=1 \Rightarrow 5t-3t=15 \Rightarrow 2t=15 \Rightarrow t=7$ hours and 30 minutes.

105. The inlet pipe can fill the vat in 5 hours and can fill $\frac{t}{5}$ of the vat in t hours. The outlet pipe can empty the vat in 10 hours and can empty $\frac{t}{10}$ of the vat in t hours. The job is complete when the fraction of the full tank reaches 1. $\frac{t}{5}-\frac{t}{10}=1 \Rightarrow 10t-5t=50 \Rightarrow 5t=50 \Rightarrow t=10$ hours.

107. Let x = the amount of time required to empty the pool then (x-20) will be the amount of time required to fill the pool. Then the rate of emptying the pool is given by $\frac{1}{x}$ and the rate of filling of the pool is $\frac{1}{x-20}$.

When both pipes are open it takes 4 hours (or 240 minutes) to fill the pool. The rate of filling the pool when both pipes are open is given by $\frac{1}{240}$.

$\frac{1}{x-20}-\frac{1}{x}=\frac{1}{240} \Rightarrow 240x-240(x-20)=x(x-20) \Rightarrow x^2-20x-4800=0 \Rightarrow (x-80)(x+60)=0 \Rightarrow x=80$.

Therefore, it will take 80 minutes to empty with the outlet pipe and 60 minutes to fill with the inlet pipe.

Reviewing Basic Concepts (Sections 4.1—4.3)

1. A sketch of the graph is shown in Figure 1a. A graph of $y_1 = 1/(x+2)-3$ is shown in Figure 1b.

2. For the function to be defined, the denominator cannot equal 0. $x^2-1 \neq 0 \Rightarrow x^2 \neq 1 \Rightarrow x \neq \pm 1$. The domain is $(-\infty,-1) \cup (-1,1) \cup (1,\infty)$.

3. A vertical asymptote occurs when the denominator equals 0. $x-6=0 \Rightarrow x=6$.

4. Since the degrees of the numerator and the denominator are the same, the ratio of the leading coefficients of the numerator and denominator is used to find the equation of the horizontal asymptote. $y=\frac{1}{1} \Rightarrow y=1$.

5. Perform long division:

$$\begin{array}{r} x-2 \\ x+3 \overline{)x^2 + x + 5} \\ \underline{x^2+3x} \\ -2x+5 \\ \underline{-2x-6} \\ 11 \end{array}$$

$\Rightarrow \dfrac{x^2+x+5}{x+3} = x-2+\dfrac{11}{x+3}$

The oblique asymptote is $y = x-2$.

6. A sketch of the graph is shown in Figure 6a. A graph of $y_1 = (3x+6)/(x-4)$ $y_1 = 1/(x+2)-3$ is shown in Figure 6b.

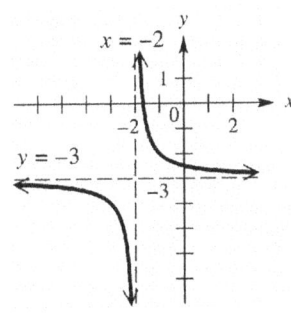

Figure 1a

[-6.7, 2.7] by [-8.2, 1]
Xscl = 1   Yscl = 1

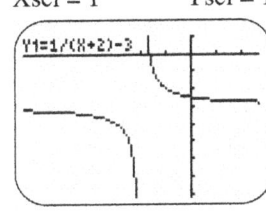

Figure 1b

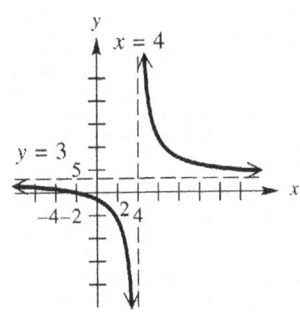

Figure 6a

[-6.2, 12.4] by [-18.6, 18.6]
Xscl = 1   Yscl=1

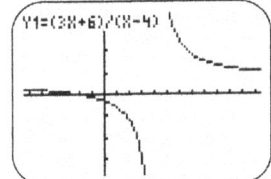

Figure 6b

7. (a) The graph intersects the x-axis at $x = -4$. The solution set is $\{-4\}$.

   (b) The graph is above the x-axis on the interval $(-\infty, -4) \cup (2, \infty)$. The solution set is $(-\infty, -4) \cup (2, \infty)$.

   (c) The graph is below the x-axis on the interval $(-4, 2)$. The solution set is $(-4, 2)$.

8. First, rewrite the inequality. $\dfrac{x+4}{3x+1} > 1 \Rightarrow \dfrac{x+4}{3x+1} - 1 > 0 \Rightarrow \dfrac{x+4-3x-1}{3x+1} > 0 \Rightarrow \dfrac{-2x+3}{3x+1} > 0$. The graph of $y_1 = (-2x+3)/(3x+1)$ has a vertical asymptote at $x = -\dfrac{1}{3}$ and an x-intercept at $x = \dfrac{3}{2}$. The graph of y_1 is above the x-axis on the interval $\left(-\dfrac{1}{3}, \dfrac{3}{2}\right)$.

9. The base of the parallelogram varies inversely as its height. The constant of variation is 24.

180   CHAPTER 4   Rational, Power, and Root Functions

10. Here $S = \dfrac{kWT^2}{L}$ By substitution, $600 = \dfrac{k(4)(4)^2}{50} = \dfrac{64k}{50} \Rightarrow k = 468.75$. When $W = 2$, $T = 2$, $L = 50$

$S = \dfrac{468.75(2)(2)^2}{(50)^2} = 75$ pounds.

4.4: Functions Defined by Powers and Roots

1. Since $13^2 = 169, \sqrt{169} = 13$.

3. Since $(-2)^5 = -32, \sqrt[5]{-32} = -2$.

5. $81^{3/2} = (\sqrt{81})^3 = 9^3 = 729$.

7. $125^{-2/3} = \dfrac{1}{125^{2/3}} = \dfrac{1}{\left(\sqrt[3]{125}\right)^2} = \dfrac{1}{5^2} = \dfrac{1}{25}$.

9. $(-1000)^{2/3} = (\sqrt[3]{-1000})^2 = (-10)^2 = 100$.

11. $8^{2/3} = (8^{1/3})^2 = 2^2 = 4$.

13. $16^{3/4} = (16^{1/4})^{-3} = (2)^{-3} = \dfrac{1}{2^3} = \dfrac{1}{8}$.

15. $-81^{0.5} = -81^{1/2} = -\sqrt{81} = -9$.

17. $64^{1/6} = \sqrt[6]{64} = 2$.

19. $(-9^{3/4})^2 = (9^{3/4})^2 = 9^{3/2} = (\sqrt{9})^3 = 3^3 = 27$.

21. $\sqrt[3]{2x} = (2x)^{1/3}$.

23. $\sqrt[3]{z^5} = z^{5/3}$.

25. $(\sqrt[4]{y})^{-3} = (y^{1/4})^{-3} = y^{-3/4} = \dfrac{1}{y^{3/4}}$.

27. $\sqrt{x} \cdot \sqrt[3]{x} = x^{1/2} \cdot x^{1/3} = x^{1/2 + 1/3} = x^{5/6}$.

29. $\sqrt{y \cdot \sqrt{y}} = (y \cdot y^{1/2})^{1/2} = (y^{3/2})^{1/2} = y^{3/4}$.

31. $\sqrt[3]{(-4)} \approx -1.587401052$.

33. $\sqrt[3]{(-125)} = -5$.

35. $\sqrt[3]{(-17)} \approx -2.571281591$.

37. $\sqrt[6]{(\pi^2)} \approx 1.464591888$.

39. $13^{-1/3} \approx 0.4252903703$.

41. $32^{0.2} = 2$.

43. $(5/6)^{-1.3} \approx 1.267463962$.

45. $\pi^{-3} \approx 0.0322515344$.

47. $f(x) = x^{1.62} \Rightarrow f(1.2) = 1.2^{1.62} \approx 1.34$.

49. $f(x) = x^{3/2} - x^{1/2} \Rightarrow f(50) = 50^{3/2} - 50^{1/2} \approx 346.48$.

51. See Figure 51.

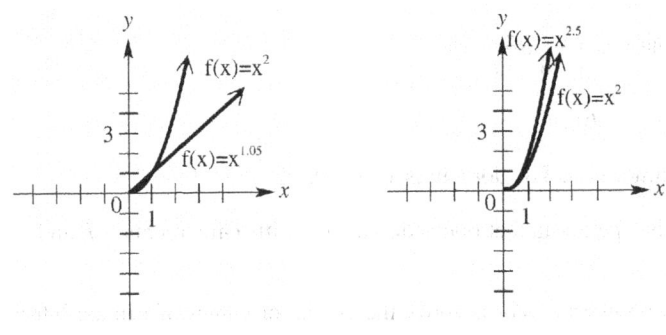

Figure 51   Figure 53

53. See Figure 53.

55. (a) $16^{-3/4} = \dfrac{1}{16^{3/4}} = \dfrac{1}{(\sqrt[4]{16})^3} = \dfrac{1}{(2)^3} = \dfrac{1}{8} = 0.125$.

    (b) $16^{-3/4} = (\sqrt[4]{16})^{-3} = 0.125$ and $16^{-3/4} = \sqrt[4]{16^{-3}} = 0.125$. Other expressions are possible.

    (c) A calculator will show that $0.125 = \dfrac{1}{8}$.

57. See Figure 57.
58. See Figure 58.
59. See Figure 59.
60. See Figure 60.

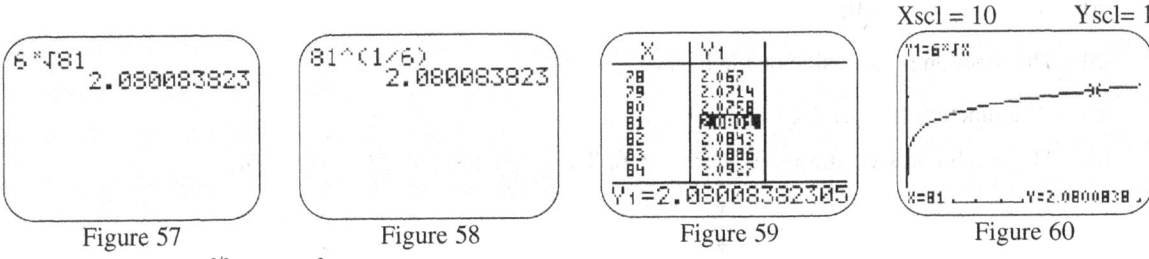

Figure 57   Figure 58   Figure 59   Figure 60

61. $S(4) = 1.27(4)^{2/3} \approx 3.2 \ ft^2$.

63. $f(15) = 15^{1.5} \approx 58.1 \ yr$.

65. (a) From the hint, $a(1)^b = 1960 \Rightarrow a = 1960$.

    (b) Since $f(3) = 525, 1960(3)^b = 525 \Rightarrow 3^b = \dfrac{525}{1960} \Rightarrow 3^b \approx 0.278$. By trial and error, $b \approx -1.2$.

182   CHAPTER 4   Rational, Power, and Root Functions

(c) $f(4) = 1960(4)^{-1.2} \approx 371$. If the zinc ion concentration reaches 371 mg per L, a rainbow trout will survive, on average, 4 min.

67. $f(2) = 0.445(2)^{1.25} \approx 1.06$ g.

69. Using the Power Regression feature on a graphing calculator yields $a \approx 874.54$ and $b \approx -0.49789$.

71. $S(0.5) = 0.2(0.5)^{\frac{2}{3}} \approx 0.126$. The surface area of the wings of a 0.5 kg bird is approximately 0.126 sq. meters.

73. $5 + 4x \geq 0 \Rightarrow 4x \geq -5 \Rightarrow x \geq -\frac{5}{4}$. The domain is $\left[-\frac{5}{4}, \infty\right)$.

75. $6 - x \geq 0 \Rightarrow 6 \geq x \Rightarrow x \leq 6$. The domain is $(-\infty, 6)$.

77. The cube root function is defined for all values of x. The domain is $(-\infty, \infty)$.

79. The graph of $y = 49 - x^2 = (7 + x)(7 - x)$ is a parabola that opens downward with x-intercepts -7 and $8 = \frac{k(1^4)}{9^2} \Rightarrow 648 = k \Rightarrow k = 648$. This graph intersects or is above the x-axis for values of x in the interval $[-7, 7]$. That is, $49 - x^2 \geq 0$ on the interval $[-7, 7]$. The domain is $[-7, 7]$.

81. The graph of $y = x^3 - x = x(x+1)(x-1)$ is a cubic graph with x-intercepts $-1, 0$ and 1. This graph intersects or is above the x-axis for values of x in the interval $[-1, 0] \cup [1, \infty)$. That is, $x^3 - x \geq 0$ on the interval $[-1, 0] \cup [1, \infty)$. The domain is $[-1, 0] \cup [1, \infty)$.

83. The graph is shown in Figure 83.
    (a) The range is $[0, \infty)$.
    (b) The function is increasing on the interval $\left(-\frac{5}{4}, \infty\right)$.
    (c) The function is never decreasing.
    (d) The graph intersects the x-axis when $x = -1.25$. The solution set of $f(x) = 0$ is $\{-1.25\}$.

85. The graph is shown in Figure 85.
    (a) The range is $(-\infty, 0]$.
    (b) The function is increasing on the interval $(-\infty, 6)$.
    (c) The function is never decreasing.
    (d) The graph intersects the x-axis when $x = 6$. The solution set of $f(x) = 0$ is $\{6\}$.

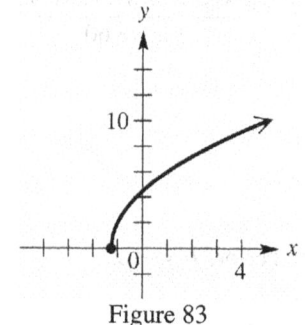
Figure 83

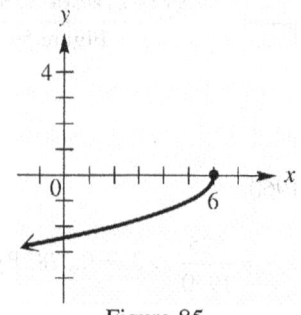
Figure 85

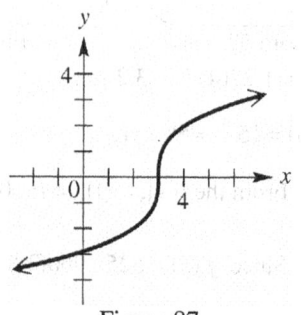
Figure 87

87. The graph is shown in Figure 87.
    (a) The range is $(-\infty, \infty)$.
    (b) The function is increasing on the interval $(-\infty, \infty)$.
    (c) The function is never decreasing.
    (d) The graph intersects the x-axis when $x = 3$. The solution set of $f(x) = 0$ is $\{3\}$.

89. The graph is shown in Figure 89.
    (a) The range is $[0, 7]$.
    (b) The function is increasing on the interval $(-7, 0)$.
    (c) The function is decreasing on the interval $(0, 7)$.
    (d) The graph intersects the x-axis when $x = -7$ or $x = 7$. The solution set of $f(x) = 0$ is $\{-7, 7\}$.

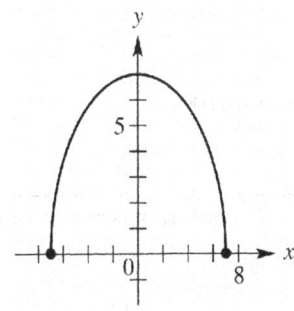
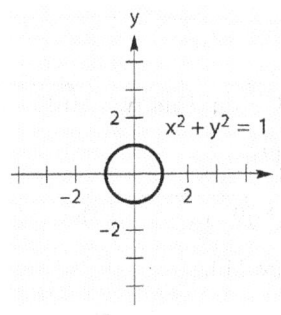
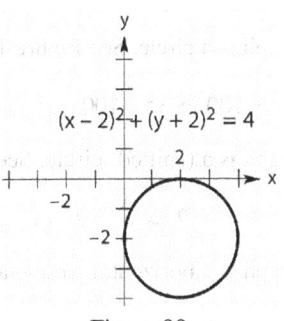

Figure 89 Figure 97 Figure 99

91. Since $y = \sqrt{9x+27} = \sqrt{9(x+3)} = 3\sqrt{x+3}$, the graph can be obtained by shifting the graph of $y = \sqrt{x}$ to the left 3 units and vertically stretching by a factor of 3.

93. Since $y = \sqrt{4x+16} + 4 = \sqrt{4(x+4)} + 4 = 2\sqrt{x+4} + 4$, the graph can be obtained by shifting the graph of $y = \sqrt{x}$ to the left 4 units, vertically stretching by a factor of 2, and shifting upward 4 units.

95. Since $y = \sqrt{18-9x} + 1 = \sqrt{9(2-x)} + 1 = 3\sqrt{2-x} + 1$ the graph can be obtained by reflecting the graph of $y = \sqrt{x}$ across the y-axis, shifting 2 units to the right, vertically stretching by a factor of 3, and shifting upward 1 unit.

97. See Figure 97.

99. See Figure 99.

101. See Figure 101.

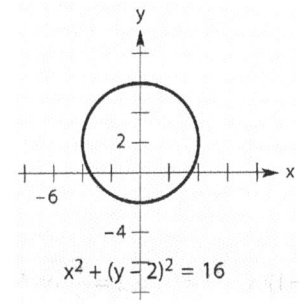
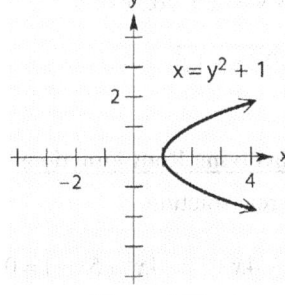
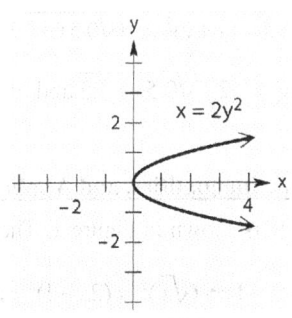

Figure 101 Figure 103 Figure 105

103. See Figure 103.

105. See Figure 105.

107. See Figure 107.

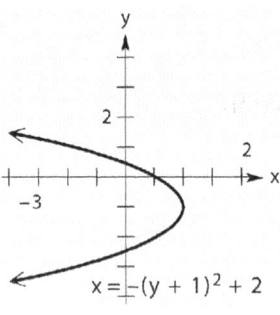

Figure 107

109. The graph is a circle. See Figure 109.

$x^2 + y^2 = 100 \Rightarrow y^2 = 100 - x^2 \Rightarrow y = \pm\sqrt{100 - x^2}$; Thus $y_1 = \sqrt{100 - x^2}$ and $y_2 = -\sqrt{100 - x^2}$.

111. The graph is a (shifted) circle. See Figure 111.

$(x-2)^2 + y^2 = 9 \Rightarrow y^2 = 9 - (x-2)^2 \Rightarrow y = \pm\sqrt{9 - (x-2)^2}$; Thus $y_1 = \sqrt{9 - (x-2)^2}$ and $y_1 = -\sqrt{9 - (x-2)^2}$.

113. The graph is a horizontal parabola. See Figure 113.

$x = y^2 + 6y + 9 \Rightarrow x = (y+3)^2 \Rightarrow \pm\sqrt{x} = y+3 \Rightarrow y = -3 \pm \sqrt{x}$; Thus $y_1 = -3 + \sqrt{x}$ and $y_2 = -3 - \sqrt{x}$.

[-15,15] by [-10,10]   [-9.4,9.4] by [-6.2,6.2]   [-10,10] by [-10,10]   [-10,10] by [-10,10]
Xscl = 1   Yscl = 1   Xscl = 1   Yscl = 1   Xscl = 1   Yscl = 1   Xscl = 1   Yscl = 1

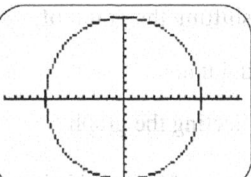 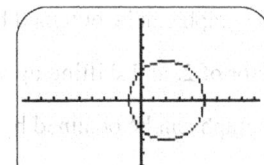 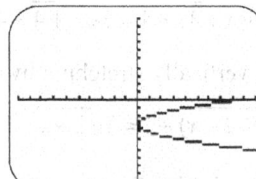 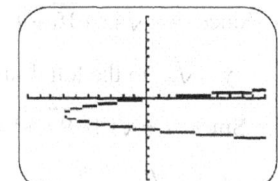

Figure 109   Figure 111   Figure 113   Figure 115

115. The graph is a horizontal parabola. See Figure 115.

$x = 2y^2 + 8y + 1 \Rightarrow 0.5x = y^2 + 4y + 0.5 \Rightarrow 0.5x = (y^2 + 4y + 4) + 0.5 - 4 \Rightarrow 0.5x = (y+2)^2 - 3.5 \Rightarrow$

$0.5x + 3.5 = (y+2)^2 \Rightarrow \pm\sqrt{0.5x + 3.5} = y + 2 \Rightarrow y = -2 \pm \sqrt{0.5x + 3.5}$

Thus $y_1 = -2 + \sqrt{0.5x + 3.5}$ and $y_2 = -2 - \sqrt{0.5x + 3.5}$.

4.5: Equations, Inequalities, and Applications Involving Root Functions

1. A sketch is shown in Figure 1. There is one real solution.

$\sqrt{x} = 2x - 1 \Rightarrow (\sqrt{x})^2 = (2x-1)^2 \Rightarrow x = 4x^2 - 4x + 1 \Rightarrow 4x^2 - 5x + 1 = 0 \Rightarrow (4x-1)(x-1) = 0 \Rightarrow x = \frac{1}{4}$ or 1.

The solution set is {1}. The value $\frac{1}{4}$ is extraneous.

Section 4.5   185

3. A sketch is shown in Figure 3. There is one real solution.

   $\sqrt{x} = -x+3 \Rightarrow (\sqrt{x})^2 = (-x+3)^2 \Rightarrow x = x^2 - 6x + 9 \Rightarrow x^2 - 7x + 9 = 0 \Rightarrow$

   $x = \dfrac{-(-7) \pm \sqrt{(-7)^2 - 4(1)(9)}}{2(1)} = \dfrac{7 \pm \sqrt{13}}{2}.$

   The solution set is $\{11\}$. The value $\left\{\dfrac{7-\sqrt{13}}{2}\right\}$ is extraneous.

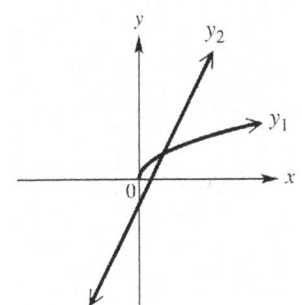
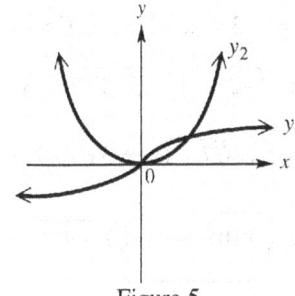

   Figure 1   Figure 3   Figure 5

5. A sketch is shown in Figure 5. There are two real solutions. There are no extraneous values.

   $\sqrt[3]{x} = x^2 \Rightarrow (\sqrt[3]{x})^3 = (x^2)^3 \Rightarrow x = x^6 \Rightarrow x^6 - x = 0 \Rightarrow x(x^5 - 1) = 0 \Rightarrow x = 0$ or 1.

   The solution set is $\{0, 1\}$.

7. Substitute $x = \dfrac{3}{2}$: $15\left(\dfrac{3}{2}\right)^{-2} - 19\left(\dfrac{3}{2}\right)^{-1} + 6 = 0 \Rightarrow 15\left(\dfrac{2}{3}\right)^2 - 19\left(\dfrac{2}{3}\right) + 6 = 0 \Rightarrow 15\left(\dfrac{4}{9}\right) - 19\left(\dfrac{2}{3}\right) + 6 = 0 \Rightarrow$

   $\left(\dfrac{20}{3}\right) - \left(\dfrac{38}{3}\right) + \left(\dfrac{18}{3}\right) = 0 \Rightarrow \dfrac{0}{3} = 0$ The value of $x = \dfrac{3}{2}$ is a correct solution.

   Substitute $x = \dfrac{5}{3}$: $15\left(\dfrac{5}{3}\right)^{-2} - 19\left(\dfrac{5}{3}\right)^{-1} + 6 = 0 \Rightarrow 15\left(\dfrac{3}{5}\right)^2 - 19\left(\dfrac{3}{5}\right) + 6 = 0 \Rightarrow 15\left(\dfrac{9}{25}\right) - 19\left(\dfrac{3}{5}\right) + 6 = 0 \Rightarrow$

   $\left(\dfrac{27}{5}\right) - \left(\dfrac{57}{5}\right) + \dfrac{30}{5} = 0 \Rightarrow \dfrac{0}{5} = 0$ The value of $x = \dfrac{5}{3}$ is a correct solution.

9. $\sqrt{3x-8} = x - 4 \Rightarrow 3x - 8 = (x-4)^2 \Rightarrow 3x - 8 = x^2 - 8x + 16 \Rightarrow x^2 - 11x + 24 = 0 \Rightarrow$

   $(x-8)(x-3) = 0 \Rightarrow x = 8$ or 3

   Check: $\sqrt{3(8)-8} = 8 - 4 \Rightarrow \sqrt{16} = 4 \Rightarrow 4 = 4.$

   Check: $\sqrt{3(3)-8} = 3 - 4 \Rightarrow \sqrt{1} = -1 \Rightarrow 1 \ne -1.$ The solution set is $\{8\}$.

11. $\sqrt{x+5} + 1 = x \Rightarrow \sqrt{x+5} = x - 1 \Rightarrow x + 5 = (x-1)^2 \Rightarrow$

    $x + 5 = x^2 - 2x + 1 \Rightarrow x^2 - 3x - 4 = 0 \Rightarrow (x-4)(x+1) = 0 \Rightarrow x = -1$ or $x = 4$.

    Check: $\sqrt{-1+5} + 1 = -1 \Rightarrow \sqrt{4} + 1 = -1 \Rightarrow x = -1 \Rightarrow 3 \ne -1$ (not a solution).

    Check: $\sqrt{4+5} + 1 = 4 \Rightarrow \sqrt{9} + 1 = 4 \Rightarrow 4 = 4.$ The solution set is $\{4\}$.

13. $\sqrt{2x+3} - \sqrt{x+1} = 1 \Rightarrow \sqrt{2x+3} = \sqrt{x+1} + 1 \Rightarrow 2x+3 = \left(\sqrt{x+1}+1\right)^2 \Rightarrow$

    $2x+3 = x+12\sqrt{x+1}+1 \Rightarrow 2x+3 = x+2+2\sqrt{x+1} \Rightarrow x+1 = 2\sqrt{x+1} \Rightarrow$

    $(x+1)^2 = 4(x+1) \Rightarrow x^2+2x+1 = 4x+4 \Rightarrow x^2-2x-3 = 0 \Rightarrow (x-3)(x+1) = 0 \Rightarrow x = -1 \text{ or } x = 3$

    Check: $\sqrt{2(-1)+3} - \sqrt{(-1)+1} = 1 \Rightarrow \sqrt{1} - \sqrt{0} = 1 \Rightarrow 1 = 1$.

    Check: $\sqrt{2(3)+3} - \sqrt{3+1} = 1 \Rightarrow \sqrt{9} - \sqrt{4} = 1 \Rightarrow 3-2 = 1 \Rightarrow 1 = 1$; The solution set is $\{-1, 3\}$.

15. $\sqrt[3]{x+1} = -3 \Rightarrow x+1 = (-3)^3 \Rightarrow x+1 = -27 \Rightarrow x = -28$.

    Check: $\sqrt[3]{-28+1} = \sqrt[3]{-27} = -3$. The solution set is $\{-28\}$.

17. $\sqrt[3]{3x^2+7} = \sqrt[3]{7-4x} \Rightarrow 3x^2+7 = 7-4x \Rightarrow 3x^2+4x = 0 \Rightarrow x(3x+4) = 0 \Rightarrow x = 0 \text{ or } x = -\dfrac{4}{3}$

    Check: $\sqrt[3]{3(0)^2+7} = \sqrt[3]{7-4(0)} \Rightarrow \sqrt[3]{7} = \sqrt[3]{7}$

    Check: $\sqrt[3]{3\left(-\dfrac{4}{3}\right)^2+7} = \sqrt[3]{7-4\left(-\dfrac{4}{3}\right)} \Rightarrow \sqrt[3]{\dfrac{37}{3}} = \sqrt[3]{\dfrac{37}{3}}$ The solution set is $\left\{0, -\dfrac{4}{3}\right\}$.

19. $\sqrt[4]{x-2}+4 = 6 \Rightarrow \sqrt[4]{x-2} = 2 \Rightarrow x-2 = (2)^4 \Rightarrow x-2 = 16 \Rightarrow x = 18$.

    Check: $\sqrt[4]{18-2}+4 = 6 \Rightarrow \sqrt[4]{16}+4 = 6 \Rightarrow 6 = 6$. The solution set is $\{18\}$.

21. $x^{2/5} = 4 \Rightarrow (x^{2/5})^{5/2} = 4^{5/2} \Rightarrow x = (\sqrt{4})^5 \Rightarrow x = (\pm 2)^5 \Rightarrow x = \pm 32$.

    Check: $(\pm 32)^{2/5} = (\sqrt[5]{\pm 32})^2 = (\pm 2)^2 = 4$. The solution set is $\{-32, 32\}$.

23. $2x^{1/3} - 5 = 1 \Rightarrow 2x^{1/3} = 6 \Rightarrow x^{1/3} = 3 \Rightarrow (x^{1/3})^3 = 3^3 \Rightarrow x = 27$.

    Check: $2(27)^{1/3} - 5 = 2\sqrt[3]{27} - 5 = 2(3) - 5 = 6 - 5 = 1$. The solution set is $\{27\}$.

25. $x^{-2} + 3x^{-1} + 2 = 0 \Rightarrow (x^{-1})^2 + 3(x^{-1}) + 2 = 0$, let $u = x^{-1}$, then $u^2 + 3u + 2 = 0 \Rightarrow (u+2)(u+1) = 0 \Rightarrow u = -2$

    or $u = -1$. Because $u = x^{-1}$, it follows that $x = u^{-1}$. Thus $x = (-2)^{-1} \Rightarrow x = \dfrac{1}{(-2)} \Rightarrow x = -\dfrac{1}{2}$ or

    $x = (-1)^{-1} \Rightarrow x = \dfrac{1}{(-1)} = -1$. Therefore, $x = -1$ or $-\dfrac{1}{2}$.

    Check: $(-1)^{-2} + 3(-1)^{-1} + 2 = 1 - 3 + 2 = 0$; $\left(-\dfrac{1}{2}\right)^{-2} + 3\left(-\dfrac{1}{2}\right)^{-1} + 2 = 4 - 6 + 2 = 0$.

    The solution set is $\left\{-1, -\dfrac{1}{2}\right\}$.

27. $5x^{-2} + 13x^{-1} = 28 \Rightarrow 5(x^{-1})^2 + 13(x^{-1}) - 28 = 0$, let $u = x^{-1}$, then

$5u^2 +13u-28=0 \Rightarrow (5u-7)(u+4)=0 \Rightarrow u = \dfrac{7}{5}$ or $u=-4$. Because $u=x^{-1}$, it follows that $x=u^{-1}$. Thus

$x = \left(\dfrac{7}{5}\right)^{-1} \Rightarrow x = \dfrac{5}{7}$ or $x = (-4)^{-1} \Rightarrow x = -\dfrac{1}{4}$. Therefore, $x = -\dfrac{1}{4}$ or $\dfrac{5}{7}$.

Check: $5\left(-\dfrac{1}{4}\right)^{-2} + 13\left(-\dfrac{1}{4}\right)^{-1} = 80 - 52 = 28$; $5\left(\dfrac{5}{7}\right)^{-2} + 13\left(\dfrac{5}{7}\right)^{-1} = \dfrac{49}{5} + \dfrac{91}{5} = \dfrac{140}{5} = 28$.

The solution set is $\left\{-\dfrac{1}{4}, \dfrac{5}{7}\right\}$.

29. $x^{2/3} - x^{1/3} - 6 = 0 \Rightarrow (x^{1/3})^2 - x^{1/3} - 6 = 0$; let $u = x^{1/3}$, then $u^2 - u - 6 = 0 \Rightarrow (u-3)(u+2) = 0 \Rightarrow u = -2$ or $u = 3$. Because $u = x^{1/3}$, it follows that $x = u^3$. Thus $x = (-2)^3 \Rightarrow x = -8$ or $x = 3^3 \Rightarrow x = 27$. Therefore, $x = -8$ or 27.

Check: $(-8)^{2/3} - (-8)^{1/3} - 6 = 4 + 2 - 6 = 0$; $(27)^{2/3} - (27)^{1/3} - 6 = 9 - 3 - 6 = 0$. The solution set is $\{-8, 27\}$.

31. $x^{3/4} - x^{1/2} - x^{1/4} + 1 = 0 \Rightarrow (x^{1/4})^3 - (x^{1/4})^2 - (x^{1/4}) + 1 = 0$; let $u = x^{1/4}$, then

$u^3 - u^2 - u + 1 = 0 \Rightarrow (u^3 - u^2) - (u-1) = 0 \Rightarrow u^2(u-1) - 1(u-1) = 0 \Rightarrow$

$(u^2 - 1)(u-1) = 0 \Rightarrow (u+1)(u-1)(u-1) = 0 \Rightarrow u = -1$ or $u = 1$. Because $u = x^{1/4}$ it follows that $x = u^4$. Thus $x = (-1)^4 \Rightarrow x = 1$ or $x = (1)^4 \Rightarrow x = 1$. Therefore, $x = 1$.

Check: $(1)^{3/4} - (1)^{1/2} - (1)^{1/4} + 1 = 1 - 1 - 1 + 1 = 0$; The solution set is $\{1\}$.

33. (a) $\sqrt{3x+7} = 2 \Rightarrow (\sqrt{3x+7})^2 = 2^2 \Rightarrow 3x+7 = 4 \Rightarrow 3x = -3 \Rightarrow x = \dfrac{-3}{3} \Rightarrow x = -1$. The solution set is $\{-1\}$.

A graph of $y_1 = \sqrt{3x+7}$ and $y_2 = 2$ is shown in Figure 33.

(b) From the graph, $y_1 > y_2$ on the interval $(-1, \infty)$.

(c) Since the graph of y_1 begins when $3x+7 = 0 \Rightarrow x = -\dfrac{7}{3}$, $y_1 < y_2$ on the interval $\left[-\dfrac{7}{3}, -1\right)$.

35. (a) $\sqrt{4x+13} = 2x-1 \Rightarrow (\sqrt{4x+13})^2 = (2x-1)^2 \Rightarrow 4x+13 = 4x^2 - 4x + 1 \Rightarrow$

$4x^2 - 8x - 12 = 0 \Rightarrow x^2 - 2x - 3 = 0 \Rightarrow (x+1)(x-3) = 0 \Rightarrow x = -1$ or 3 (-1 is extraneous). The solution set is $\{3\}$. A graph of $y_1 = \sqrt{4x+13}$ and $y_2 = 2x-1$ is shown in Figure 35.

(b) Since the graph of y_1 begins when $4x+13 = 0 \Rightarrow x = -\dfrac{13}{4}$, $y_1 > y_2$ on the interval $\left[-\dfrac{13}{4}, 3\right)$.

(c) From the graph, $y_1 < y_2$ on the interval $(3, \infty)$.

[-4.7,4.7] by [-2.1,4.1]
Xscl = 1   Yscl = 1
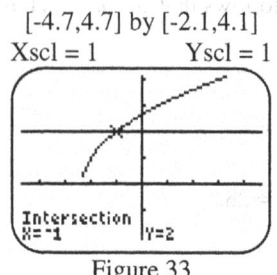
Figure 33

[-4.7,4.7] by [-4.2,8.2]
Xscl = 1   Yscl = 1
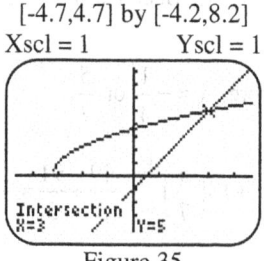
Figure 35

[-2.7,6.7] by [-3.2,9.2]
Xscl= 1   Yscl = 1
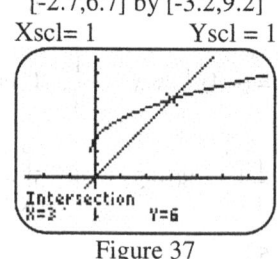
Figure 37

[-3.4,15.4] by [-2.2,10.2]
Xscl = 1   Yscl= 1
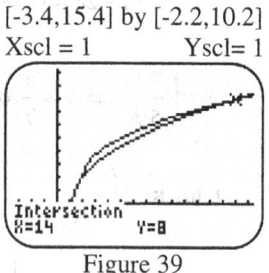
Figure 39

37. (a) $\sqrt{5x+1}+2=2x \Rightarrow \sqrt{5x+1}=2x-2 \Rightarrow (\sqrt{5x+1})^2=(2x-2)^2 \Rightarrow$

$5x+1=4x^2-8x+4 \Rightarrow 4x^2-13x+3=0 \Rightarrow (4x-1)(x-3)=0 \Rightarrow x=\frac{1}{4}$ or 3 ($\frac{1}{4}$ is extraneous).

The solution set is {3}. A graph of $y_1=\sqrt{5x+1}+2$ and $y_2=2x$ is shown in Figure 37.

(b) Since the graph of y_1 begins when $5x+1=0 \Rightarrow x=-\frac{1}{5}$, $y_1 > y_2$ on the interval $\left[-\frac{1}{5},3\right)$.

(c) From the graph, $y_1 < y_2$ on the interval $(3,\infty)$.

39. (a) $\sqrt{3x-6}+2=\sqrt{5x-6} \Rightarrow (\sqrt{3x-6}+2)^2=(\sqrt{5x-6})^2 \Rightarrow$

$3x-6+4\sqrt{3x-6}+4=5x-6 \Rightarrow 4\sqrt{3x-6}=2x-4 \Rightarrow (4\sqrt{3x-6})^2=(2x-4)^2 \Rightarrow$

$16(3x-6)=4x^2-16x+16 \Rightarrow 48x-96=4x^2-16x+16 \Rightarrow 4x^2-64x+112=0 \Rightarrow$

$x^2-16x+28=0 \Rightarrow (x-2)(x-14)=0 \Rightarrow x=2$ or 14. The solution set is {2,14}. A graph of

$y_1=\sqrt{3x-6}+2$ and $y_2=\sqrt{5x-6}$ is shown in Figure 39.

(b) From the graph, $y_1 > y_2$ on the interval (2,14).

(c) From the graph, $y_1 < y_2$ on the interval $(14,\infty)$.

41. (a) $\sqrt[3]{x^2-2x}=\sqrt[3]{x} \Rightarrow (\sqrt[3]{x^2-2x})^3=(\sqrt[3]{x})^3 \Rightarrow x^2-2x=x \Rightarrow x^2-3x=0 \Rightarrow x(x-3)=0 \Rightarrow x=0$ or $x=3$.

The solution set is {0,3}. A graph of $y_1=\sqrt[3]{x^2-2x}$ and $y_2=\sqrt[3]{x}$ is shown in Figure 41.

(b) From the graph, $y_1 > y_2$ on the interval $(-\infty,0) \cup (3,\infty)$.

(c) From the graph, $y_1 < y_2$ on the interval (0,3).

43. (a) $\sqrt[4]{3x+1}=1 \Rightarrow (\sqrt[4]{3x+1})^4=1^4 \Rightarrow 3x+1=1 \Rightarrow 3x=0 \Rightarrow x=0$. The solution set is {0}. A graph of

$y_1=\sqrt[4]{3x+1}$ and $y_2=1$ is shown in Figure 43.

(b) From the graph, $y_1 > y_2$ on the interval $(0,\infty)$.

(c) Since the graph of y_1 begins when $3x+1=0 \Rightarrow x=-\frac{1}{3}$, $y_1 < y_2$ on the interval $\left[-\frac{1}{3},0\right)$.

[-4.7,4.7] by [-3.1,3.1]
Xscl = 1   Yscl = 1

[-4.7,4.7] by [-3.1,3.1]
Xscl = 1   Yscl = 1

[-4.7,4.7] by [-3.1,3.1]
Xscl= 1   Yscl = 1

[-5,45] by [-1,3]
Xscl = 5   Yscl= 1

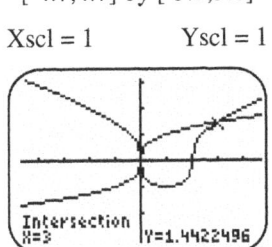
Figure 41

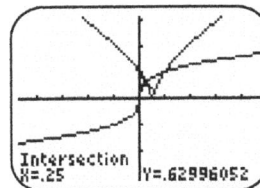
Figure 42

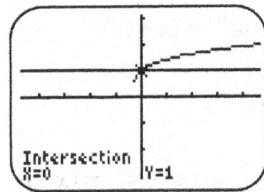
Figure 43

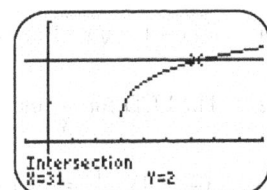
Figure 44

45. (a) $(2x-5)^{1/2} - 2 = (x-2)^{1/2} \Rightarrow [(2x-5)^{1/2} - 2]^2 = [(x-2)^{1/2}]^2 \Rightarrow$

$2x - 5 - 4(2x-5)^{1/2} + 4 = x - 2 \Rightarrow x + 1 = 4(2x-5)^{1/2} \Rightarrow (x+1)^2 = [4(2x-5)^{1/2}]^2 \Rightarrow$

$x^2 + 2x + 1 = 16(2x-5) \Rightarrow x^2 + 2x + 1 = 32x - 80 \Rightarrow x^2 - 30x + 81 = 0 \Rightarrow (x-3)(x-27) = 0 \Rightarrow x = 3$ or 27 (3 is extraneous). The solution set is $\{27\}$. A graph of $y_1 = (2x-5)^{1/2} - 2$ and $y_2 = (x-2)^{1/2}$ is shown in Figure 45.

(b) From the graph, $y_1 \geq y_2$ on the interval $[27, \infty)$.

(c) Since the graph of y_1 begins when $2x - 5 = 0 \Rightarrow x = \dfrac{5}{2}$, $y_1 \leq y_2$ on the interval $\left[\dfrac{5}{2}, 27\right]$.

47. (a) $(x+6x)^{1/4} = 2 \Rightarrow [(x^2+6x)^{1/4}]^4 = 2^4 \Rightarrow x^2 + 6x = 16 \Rightarrow x^2 + 6x - 16 = 0 \Rightarrow (x+8)(x-2) = 0 \Rightarrow x = -8$ or 2. The solution set is $\{-8, 2\}$. A graph of $y_1 = (x^2+6x)^{1/4}$ and $y_2 = 2$ is shown in Figure 47.

(b) From the graph, $y_1 > y_2$ on the interval $(-\infty, -8) \cup (2, \infty)$.

(c) Since $x^2 + 6x = 0 \Rightarrow x(x+6) = 0 \Rightarrow x = 0$ or -6, the graph of y_1 has endpoints when $x = -6$ and 0. From the graph, $y_1 < y_2$ on the interval $(-8, -6] \cup [0, 2)$.

[-5,45] by [-2,8]
Xscl = 5   Yscl = 2

[-11,5] by [-1,4]
Xscl = 1   Yscl = 1

[-2,2] by [-2,2]
Xscl= 1   Yscl = 1

[5,10] by [-100,100]
Xscl= 1   Yscl = 10

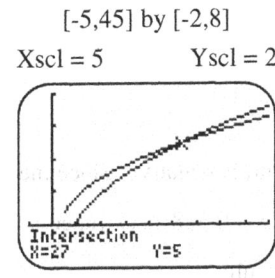
Figure 45

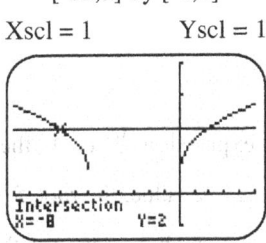
Figure 47

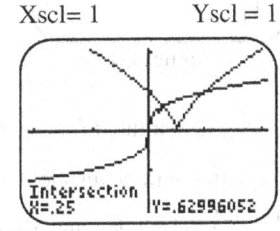
Figure 49

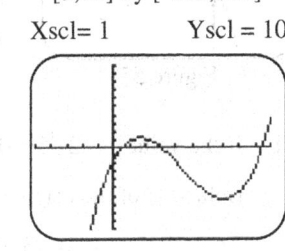
Figure 55

49. (a) $(2x-1)^{2/3} = x^{1/3} \Rightarrow [(2x-1)^{2/3}]^3 = (x^{1/3})^3 \Rightarrow (2x-1)^2 = x$

$\Rightarrow 4x^2 - 4x + 1 = x \Rightarrow 4x^2 - 5x + 1 = 0 \Rightarrow (4x-1)(x-1) = 0 \Rightarrow x = \dfrac{1}{4}$ or 1. The solution set is $\left\{\dfrac{1}{4}, 1\right\}$.

A graph of $y_1 = (2x-1)^{2/3}$ and $y_2 = x^{1/3}$ is shown in Figure 49.

(b) From the graph, $y_1 > y_2$ on the interval $\left(-\infty, \dfrac{1}{4}\right) \cup (1, \infty)$.

190   CHAPTER 4   Rational, Power, and Root Functions

(c) From the graph, $\sqrt{18-2} = \sqrt{16} = 4 \neq 14-18$; on the interval $\left(\frac{1}{4}, 1\right)$.

51. $\sqrt[3]{4x-4} = \sqrt{x+1} \Rightarrow (4x-4)^{1/3} = (x+1)^{1/2}$.

52. The LCD for $\frac{1}{3}$ and $\frac{1}{2}$ is 6.

53. $\left[(4x-4)^{1/3}\right]^6 = \left[(x+1)^{1/2}\right]^6 \Rightarrow (4x-4)^2 = (x+1)^3$.

54. $(4x-4)^2 = (x+1)^3 \Rightarrow 16x^2 - 32x + 16 = x^3 + 3x^2 + 3x + 1 \Rightarrow x^3 - 13x^2 + 35x - 15 = 0$.

55. The graph crosses the x-axis 3 times so the equation has 3 real roots. See Figure 55.

56. $3\overline{)\begin{array}{cccc} 1 & -13 & 35 & -15 \\ & 3 & -30 & 15 \\ \hline 1 & -10 & 5 & 0 \end{array}}$ The value in the remainder position is 0; therefore, $P(3) = 0$.

57. From the synthetic division shown above, $P(x) = (x-3)(x^2 - 10x + 5)$.

58. If $x^2 - 10x + 5 = 0$, then $x = \dfrac{-(-10) \pm \sqrt{(-10)^2 - 4(1)(5)}}{2(1)} = \dfrac{10 \pm \sqrt{80}}{2} = 5 \pm 2\sqrt{5} \Rightarrow \{5 \pm 2\sqrt{5}\}$.

59. The three solutions are $3, 5+2\sqrt{5}$, and $5-2\sqrt{5}$.

60. The graph of $y_3 = y_1 - y_2$, where $y_1 = \sqrt[3]{4x-4}$, and $y_2 = \sqrt{x+1}$ is shown in Figure 60. There are 2 real solutions.

[-5,10] by [-100,100]
Xscl = 1   Yscl = 10

[-2,20] by [-0.5,0.5]
Xscl = 1   Yscl = 0.1

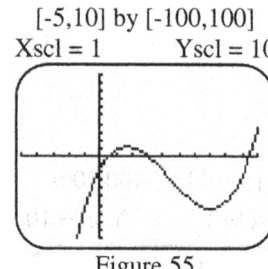

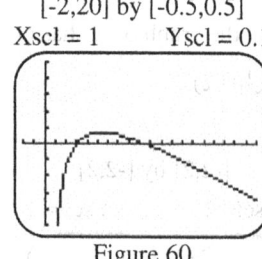

Figure 55   Figure 60

61 If the value $5 - 2\sqrt{5} \approx 0.528$ is substituted for x in the expression $\sqrt[3]{4x-4}$, the result is negative. Since the right side of the original equation will never yield a negative value, the root $5 - 2\sqrt{5} \approx 0.528$ is extraneous. The solution set is $\{3, 5+2\sqrt{5}\}$. The calculator figure shown above supports this result.

62. The solution set of the original equation is a subset of the solution set found in the previous exercise. The extraneous solution was obtained when each side of the original equation was raised to the sixth power.

63. (a) $\dfrac{\frac{2}{3}(x-2)x^{-1/3} - x^{2/3}}{(x-2)^2} = \dfrac{3}{1} \left| \dfrac{\frac{2}{3}(x-2)x^{-1/3} - x^{2/3}}{(x-2)^2} \right| \cdot \dfrac{\frac{1}{3}}{\frac{3}{1}} = \dfrac{2(x-2)x^{-1/3} - 3x^{2/3}}{3(x-2)^2} = \dfrac{x^{-1/3}[2(x-2) - 3x]}{3(x-2)^2} =$

$\dfrac{2x-4-3x}{3x^{1/3}(x-2)^2} = \dfrac{-x-4}{3x^{1/3}(x-2)^2}$

(b) Starting with the simplified expression from part (a) we will solve $\dfrac{-x-4}{3x^{1/3}(x-2)^2}=0$. The expression $\dfrac{-x-4}{3x^{1/3}(x-2)^2}$ will equal 0 only when the numerator is equal to 0. $-x-4=0 \Rightarrow x=-4$

65. (a) $\dfrac{\frac{1}{3}(x^2+1)x^{-2/3}-2x^{4/3}}{(x^2+1)^2} = \dfrac{3}{\frac{3}{1}}\left[\dfrac{\frac{1}{3}(x^2+1)x^{-2/3}-2x^{4/3}}{(x^2+1)^2}\right] = \dfrac{(x^2+1)x^{-2/3}-6x^{4/3}}{3(x^2+1)^2} =$

$\dfrac{(x^2+1)x^{-2/3}-6x^{4/3}}{3(x^2+1)^2} = \dfrac{x^{-2/3}\left[(x^2+1)-6x^2\right]}{3(x^2+1)^2} = \dfrac{\left[(x^2+1)-6x^2\right]}{3x^{2/3}(x^2+1)^2} = \dfrac{1-5x^2}{3x^{2/3}(x^2+1)^2}$

(b) Starting with the simplified expression from part (a) we will solve $\dfrac{1-5x^2}{3x^{2/3}(x^2+1)^2}=0$. The expression $\dfrac{1-5x^2}{3x^{2/3}(x^2+1)^2}$ will equal 0 only when the numerator is equal to 0. Solve as follows:

$1-5x^2=0 \Rightarrow 5x^2=1 \Rightarrow x^2=\dfrac{1}{5} \Rightarrow x=\pm\sqrt{\dfrac{1}{5}}$

67. (a) $\dfrac{x^{1/4}-x^{-3/4}}{x} = \dfrac{x^{-3/4}[x-1]}{x} = \dfrac{x-1}{x^{3/4}(x)} = \dfrac{x-1}{x^{7/4}}$

(b) Starting with the simplified expression from part (a) we will solve $\dfrac{x-1}{x^{7/4}}=0$. The expression $\dfrac{x-1}{x^{7/4}}$ will equal 0 only when the numerator is equal to 0. $x-1=0 \Rightarrow x=1$

69. (a) $\dfrac{(x^2+1)^{1/2}-\frac{1}{2}x(x^2+1)^{-1/2}(2x)}{x^2+1} = \dfrac{2}{\frac{2}{1}}\left[\dfrac{(x^2+1)^{1/2}-\frac{1}{2}x(x^2+1)^{-1/2}(2x)}{x^2+1}\right]=$

$\dfrac{2(x^2+1)^{1/2}-x(x^2+1)^{-1/2}(2x)}{2(x^2+1)} = \dfrac{(x^2+1)^{-1/2}\left[2(x^2+1)-x(2x)\right]}{2(x^2+1)} = \dfrac{\left[2(x^2+1)-x(2x)\right]}{2(x^2+1)^{1/2}(x^2+1)} =$

$\dfrac{\left[(2x^2+2)-(2x^2)\right]}{2(x^2+1)^{1/2}(x^2+1)} = \dfrac{2}{2(x^2+1)^{1/2}(x^2+1)} = \dfrac{1}{(x^2+1)^{3/2}}$

(b) Starting with the simplified expression from part (a) we will solve $\dfrac{1}{(x^2+1)^{3/2}}=0$. The expression

$\dfrac{1}{(x^2+1)^{3/2}}$ will equal 0 only when the numerator is equal to 0. Since the numerator is a constant there is no solution to this equation.

71. $\sqrt{\sqrt{x}} = x \Rightarrow x^{1/4} = x \Rightarrow \left[x^{1/4}\right]^4 = x^4 \Rightarrow x = x^4 \Rightarrow x - x^4 = 0 \Rightarrow x(1-x^3) = 0 \Rightarrow x = 0$ or 1.

The solution set is $\{0,1\}$.

73. $\sqrt{\sqrt{28x+8}} = \sqrt{3x+2} \Rightarrow (28x+8)^{1/4} = (3x+2)^{1/2} \Rightarrow \left[(28x+8)^{1/4}\right]^4 = \left[(3x+2)^{1/2}\right]^4 \Rightarrow$

$28x+8 = (3x+2)^2 \Rightarrow 28x+8 = 9x^2+12x+4 \Rightarrow 9x^2-16x-4 = 0 \Rightarrow (9x+2)(x-2) = 0 \Rightarrow x = -\dfrac{2}{9}$ or 2. The

solution set is $\left\{-\dfrac{2}{9}, 2\right\}$.

75. $\sqrt[3]{\sqrt{32x}} = \sqrt[3]{x+6} \Rightarrow (32x)^{1/6} = (x+6)^{1/3} \Rightarrow \left[(32x)^{1/6}\right]^6 = \left[(x+6)^{1/3}\right]^6 \Rightarrow 32x = (x+6)^2 \Rightarrow$

$32x = x^2+12x+36 \Rightarrow x^2-20x+36 = 0 \Rightarrow (x-2)(x-18) = 0 \Rightarrow x = 2$ or 18. The solution set is $\{2,18\}$.

77. $v = \dfrac{350}{\sqrt{6000}} \approx 4.5$ km per sec

79. $p = 2\pi\sqrt{\dfrac{5}{32}} \approx 2.5$ sec

81. $s = 30\sqrt{\dfrac{900}{97}} \approx 91$ mph

83. (a) Since the distance from C to D is 20 feet, the distance from P to C is $20-x$.

(b) The value must be between 0 and 20. That is, $0 < x < 20$.

(c) $(AP)^2 = (DP)^2 + (AD)^2 \Rightarrow (AP)^2 = x^2 + 12^2 \Rightarrow AP = \sqrt{x^2+12^2}$;

$(BP)^2 = (CP)^2 + (BC)^2 \Rightarrow (BP)^2 = (20-x)^2 + 16^2 \Rightarrow BP = \sqrt{(20-x)^2+16^2}$

(d) $f(x) = \sqrt{x^2+12^2} + \sqrt{(20-x)^2+16^2}$, $0 < x < 20$.

(e) The graph of $y_1 = \sqrt{x^2+12^2} + \sqrt{(20-x)^2+16^2}$ is shown in Figure 73. Here $f(4) \approx 35.28$. When the stake is 4 feet from the 12-foot pole, approximately 35.28 feet of wire will be required.

(f) Using the calculator, $f(x)$ is a minimum (about 34.41 feet) when $x \approx 8.57$ feet.

(g) This problem examined how the total amount of wire used can be expressed in terms of the distance from the stake at P to the base of the 12-foot pole. We find that the amount of wire used can be minimized when the stake is approximately 8.57 feet from the 12-foot pole.

[0,20] by [0,50]
Xscl = 1   Yscl = 10

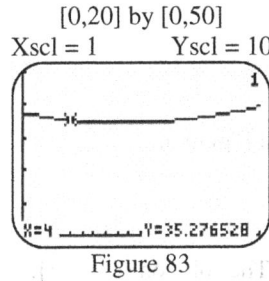

Figure 83

85. Using the Pythagorean theorem, the diagonal distance traveled on the river is $d = \sqrt{x^2 + 3^2}$. Noting that the rate of travel on land is 5 mph, the rate of travel on water is 2 mph, and that $t = \dfrac{d}{r}$, the time needed to travel on land is $\dfrac{8-x}{5}$ and the time needed to travel on the river is $\dfrac{\sqrt{x^2+9}}{2}$. The total travel time is given by the function $y_1 = \dfrac{8-x}{5} + \dfrac{\sqrt{x^2+9}}{2}$. By graphing this function (not shown), we find that the minimum value for time occurs when $x \approx 1.31$. The hunter should travel $8 - 1.31 = 6.69$ miles along the river.

87. We will refer to the original position of the *Inspiration* as the origin. At time x hours past noon, the *Celebration* is $60 - 30x$ miles south of the origin and the *Inspiration* is $20x$ miles west of the origin. Using the Pythagorean theorem, the distance between the ships is given by the function $y_1 = \sqrt{(60-30x)^2 + (20x)^2}$. By graphing this function (not shown), we find that the distance between the ships is a minimum when $x \approx 1.38$ hours. At the time 1.38 hours past noon (about 1:23 P.M.) the ships are about 33.28 miles apart.

Reviewing Basic Concepts (Sections 4.4 and 4.5)

1. As the exponent increases in value, the curve rises more rapidly for $x \geq 1$. See Figure 1.
2. $S(0.75) = 0.3(0.75)^{3/4} \approx 0.24 \, m^2$
3. See Figure 3a and Figure 3b.

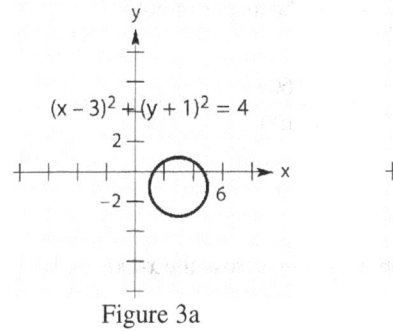

Figure 3a

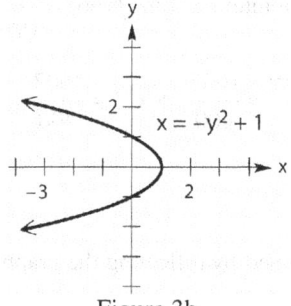

Figure 3b

4. Solving the equation for y yields $x^2 + y^2 = 16 \Rightarrow y^2 = 16 - x^2 \Rightarrow y = \pm\sqrt{16-x^2}$. The expressions are $y_1 = \sqrt{16-x^2}$ and $y_2 = -\sqrt{16-x^2}$ which are graphed in a square window in Figure 4.

194 CHAPTER 4 Rational, Power, and Root Functions

5. Solving the equation for y yields $x = y^2 + 4y + 4 + 2 \Rightarrow x - 2 = (y+2)^2 \Rightarrow$

    $\pm\sqrt{x-2} = y + 2 \Rightarrow -2 \pm \sqrt{x-2} = y \Rightarrow y = -2 \pm \sqrt{x-2}$. The expressions are

    $y_1 = -2 + \sqrt{x-2}$ and $y_2 = -2 - \sqrt{x-2}$ which are graphed in a square window in Figure 5.

6. $\sqrt{3x+4} = 8 - x \Rightarrow \left(\sqrt{3x+4}\right)^2 = (8-x)^2 \Rightarrow 3x + 4 = 64 - 16x + x^2 \Rightarrow$

    $x^2 - 19x + 60 = 0 \Rightarrow (x-4)(x-15) = 0 \Rightarrow x = 4, 15$. The solution 15 is extraneous. The solution set is $\{4\}$.

7. The graph of $y_1 = \sqrt{3x+4}$ is above the graph of $y_2 = 8 - x$ on the interval $(4, \infty)$. See Figure 7-8.

[0,10] by [0,10]
Xscl = 1   Yscl = 1

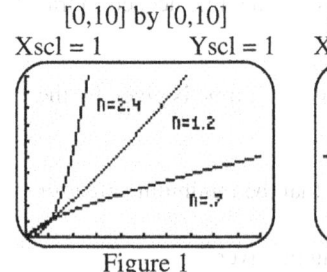

Figure 1

[-9.4,9.4] by [-6.2,6.2]
Xscl = 1   Yscl = 1

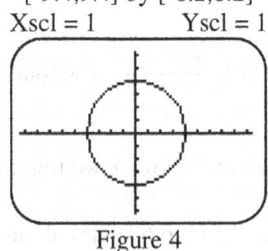

Figure 4

[-9.4,9.4] by [-6.2,6.2]
Xscl = 1   Yscl = 1

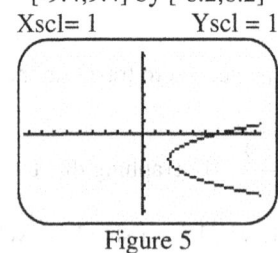

Figure 5

[-3,12] by [-3,12]
Xscl = 1   Yscl = 1

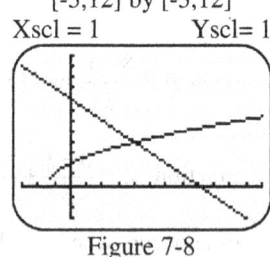

Figure 7-8

8. Noting that the graph of $y_1 = \sqrt{3x+4}$ does not start until $3x + 4 = 0 \Rightarrow 3x = -4 \Rightarrow x = -\dfrac{4}{3}$, the graph of

    $y_1 = \sqrt{3x+4}$ is below the graph of $y_2 = 8 - x$ on the interval $\left[-\dfrac{4}{3}, 4\right]$. See Figure 7-8.

9. $\sqrt{3x+4} + \sqrt{5x+6} = 2 \Rightarrow \sqrt{3x+4} = 2 - \sqrt{5x+6} \Rightarrow \left(\sqrt{3x+4}\right)^2 = \left(2 - \sqrt{5x+6}\right)^2 \Rightarrow$

    $3x + 4 = 4 - 4\sqrt{5x+6} + 5x + 6 \Rightarrow 4\sqrt{5x+6} = 2x + 6 \Rightarrow \left(4\sqrt{5x+6}\right)^2 = (2x+6)^2 \Rightarrow$

    $16(5x+6) = 4x^2 + 24x + 36 \Rightarrow 80x + 96 = 4x^2 + 24x + 36 \Rightarrow 4x^2 - 56x - 60 = 0 \Rightarrow$

    $x^2 - 14x - 15 = 0 \Rightarrow (x+1)(x-15) = 0 \Rightarrow x = -1, 15$. The solution 15 is an extraneous solution.

    The solution set is $\{-1\}$.

10. (a) cat: $f(24) = \dfrac{1607}{\sqrt[4]{24^3}} \approx 148$ beats per minute; person: $f(66) = \dfrac{1607}{\sqrt[4]{66^3}} \approx 69$ beats per minute

    (b) $400 = \dfrac{1607}{\sqrt[4]{66^3}} \Rightarrow 400\sqrt[4]{x^3} = 1607 \Rightarrow \sqrt[4]{x^3} = \dfrac{1607}{400} \Rightarrow x^{3/4} = \dfrac{1607}{400} \Rightarrow x = \left(\dfrac{1607}{400}\right)^{4/3} \approx 6.4$ inches.

Chapter 4 Review Exercises

1. (a) The graph of $y = -\dfrac{1}{x} + 6$ can be obtained by reflecting the graph of $y = \dfrac{1}{x}$ across the x-axis and shifting upward 6 units.

   (b) A sketch of the graph is shown in Figure 1b.

   (c) A calculator graph is shown in Figure 1c.

2. (a) The graph of $y = \dfrac{4}{x} - 3$ can be obtained by stretching the graph of $y = \dfrac{1}{x}$ by a factor of 4 and shifting downward 3 units.

(b) A sketch of the graph is shown in Figure 2b.
(c) A calculator graph is shown in Figure 2c.

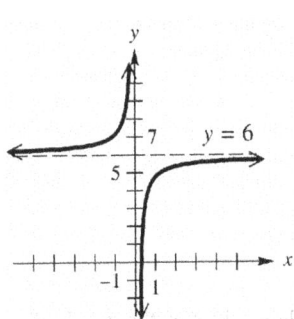

Figure 1b

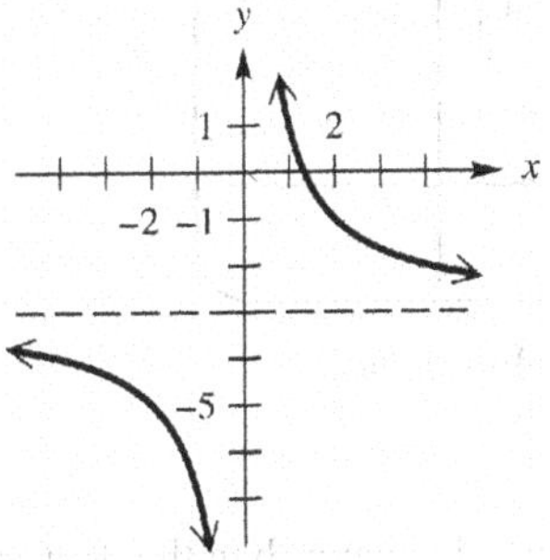

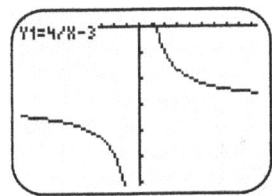

Figure 2b

[-4.7,4.7] by [-3.1,12.4]

Xscl = 1   Yscl = 1

[-9.4,9.4] by [-6.1,0.1]

Xscl = 1   Yscl = 1

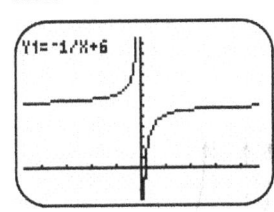

Figure 1c

Figure 2c

3. (a) The graph of $y = -\dfrac{1}{(x-2)^2}$ can be obtained by reflecting the graph of $y = \dfrac{1}{x^2}$ across the x-axis and shifting to the right 2 units.

(b) A sketch of the graph is shown in Figure 3b.

(c) A calculator graph is shown in Figure 3c.

4. (a) The graph of $y = \dfrac{2}{x^2} + 1$ can be obtained by stretching the graph of $y = \dfrac{1}{x^2}$ by a factor of 2 and shifting upward 1 unit.

(b) A sketch of the graph is shown in Figure 4b.

(c) A calculator graph is shown in Figure 4c.

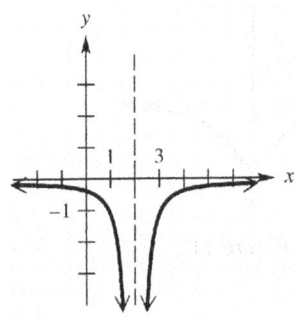

Figure 3b

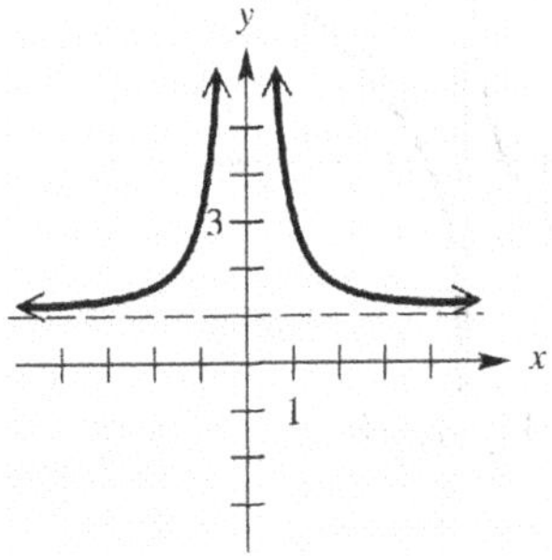

Figure 4b

Copyright © 2015 Pearson Education, Inc

196   CHAPTER 4 Rational, Power, and Root Functions

[-2.7,6.7] by [-3.1,3.1]
Xscl = 1   Yscl = 1

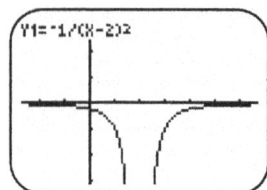

Figure 3c

[-9.4,9.4] by [-6.1,0.1]
Xscl = 1   Yscl = 1

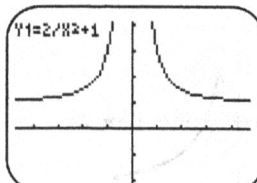

Figure 4c

5. When the degree of the numerator is exactly 1 greater than the degree of the denominator, the graph of a rational function defined by an expression written in lowest terms will have an oblique asymptote.

6. See Figure 6.
7. See Figure 7.
8. See Figure 8.

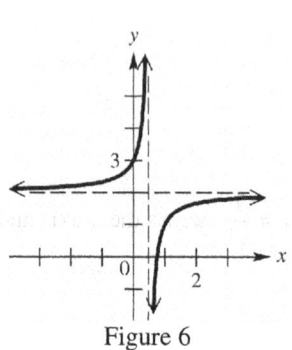

Figure 6

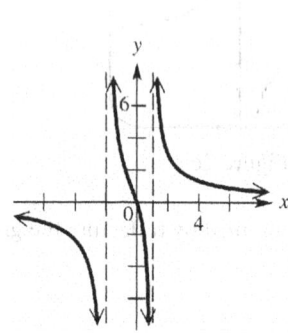

Figure 7

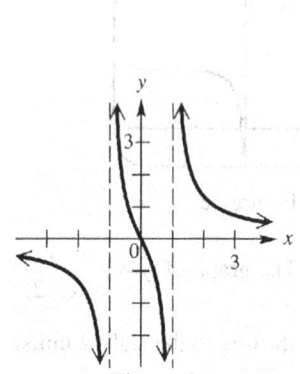

Figure 8

9. See Figure 9.
10. See Figure 10.
11. See Figure 11.

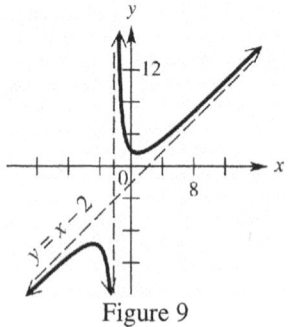

Figure 9

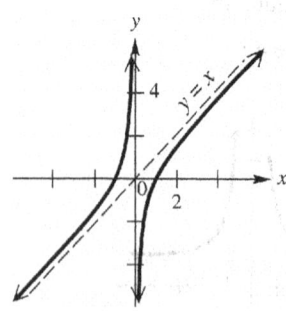

Figure 10

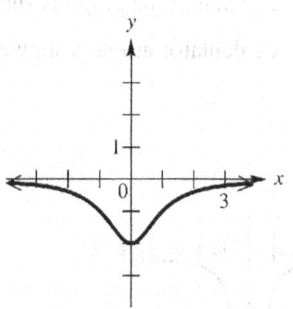

Figure 11

12. See Figure 12.
13. See Figure 13.

Copyright © 2015 Pearson Education, Inc

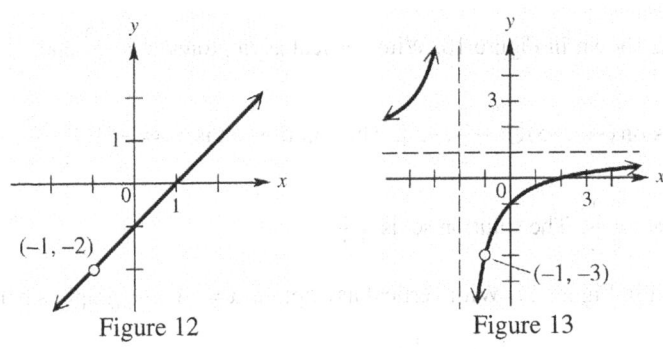

Figure 12   Figure 13

14. A vertical asymptote of $x = 0$ indicates that the denominator should contain the factor x. Since there are no x-intercepts, the numerator can never equal zero. Since there is a horizontal asymptote at $y = 0$, the degree of the numerator is less than the degree of the denominator. The end behavior of the graph suggests that the degree of the denominator is even. Since the graph passes through the point $\left(2, \dfrac{1}{4}\right)$, one possible equation for the function is $f(x) = \dfrac{1}{x^2}$. Other functions are possible.

15. A vertical asymptote of $x = 1$ indicates that the denominator should contain the factor $(x-1)$. A horizontal asymptote of $y = -3$ indicates that the degrees of the numerator and denominator should be equal and the leading coefficient of the numerator should be -3 times that of the denominator. An x-intercept of 2, indicates that the numerator should contain the factor $(x-2)$. One possible equation for the function is $f(x) = \dfrac{-3(x-2)}{x-1} = \dfrac{-3x+6}{x-1}$. Other functions are possible.

16. An x-intercept of -2 indicates that the numerator should contain the factor $(x+2)$. A "hole" when $x = 2$ indicates that both the numerator and denominator should contain the factor $(x-2)$. One possible equation for the function is $f(x) = \dfrac{(x+2)(x-2)}{x-2} = \dfrac{x^2-4}{x-2}$. Other functions are possible.

17. Since there are no x-intercepts the numerator can never equal zero. Since there is a horizontal asymptote at $y = 0$, the degree of the numerator is less than the degree of the denominator. The end behavior of the graph suggest that the degree of the denominator is even. Since the graph goes through (0,-1) a possible graph is $y = -\dfrac{1}{x^2+1}$.

18. (a) $\dfrac{5}{2x+5} = \dfrac{3}{x+2} \Rightarrow 5(x+2) = 3(2x+5) \Rightarrow 5x+10 = 6x+15 \Rightarrow x = -5$; the solution set is $\{-5\}$.

    (b) Graph $y_1 = 5/(2x+5) - 3/(x+2)$ as shown in Figure 18. With vertical asymptotes $x = -\dfrac{5}{2}$ and $x = -2$, the graph is below the x-axis on $\left(-5, -\dfrac{5}{2}\right) \cup (-2, \infty)$. The solution set is $\left(-5, -\dfrac{5}{2}\right) \cup (-2, \infty)$.

198   CHAPTER 4   Rational, Power, and Root Functions

(c) Graph $y_1 = 5/(2x+5) - 3/(x+2)$ as shown in Figure 18. With vertical asymptotes $x = -\frac{5}{2}$ and

$x = -2$, the graph is above the x-axis on $(-\infty, -5) \cup \left(-\frac{5}{2}, -2\right)$. The solution set is $(-\infty, -5) \cup \left(-\frac{5}{2}, -2\right)$.

19. (a) $\dfrac{3x-2}{x+1} = 0 \Rightarrow 3x - 2 = 0 \Rightarrow 3x = 2 \Rightarrow x = \dfrac{2}{3}$. The solution set is $\left\{\dfrac{2}{3}\right\}$.

(b) Graph $y_1 = (3x-2)/(x+1)$ as shown in Figure 17. With vertical asymptote $x = -1$, the graph is below

the x-axis on the interval $\left(-1, \dfrac{2}{3}\right)$. The solution set is $\left(-1, \dfrac{2}{3}\right)$.

(c) Graph $y_1 = (3x-2)/(x+1)$ as shown in Figure 17. With vertical asymptote $x = -1$, the graph is above

the x-axis on the interval $(-\infty, -1) \cup \left(\dfrac{2}{3}, \infty\right)$. The solution set is $(-\infty, -1) \cup \left(\dfrac{2}{3}, \infty\right)$.

20. (a) Multiply through by the LCD, x^2.

$1 \cdot x^2 - \dfrac{5}{x} \cdot x^2 + \dfrac{6}{x^2} \cdot x^2 = 0 \cdot x^2 \Rightarrow x^2 - 5x + 6 = 0 \Rightarrow (x-2)(x-3) = 0 \Rightarrow x = 2, 3$

This solution set is $\{2, 3\}$.

(b) Graph $y_1 = 1 - 5/x + 6/x^2$ as shown in Figure 20. With vertical asymptote $x = 0$, the graph is below or

intersects the x-axis on $[2, 3]$. The solution set is $[2, 3]$.

(c) Graph $y_1 = 1 - 5/x + 6/x^2$ as shown in Figure 20. With vertical asymptote $x = 0$, the graph is above or

intersects the x-axis on $(-\infty, 0) \cup (0, 2] \cup [3, \infty)$. The solution set is $(-\infty, 0) \cup (0, 2] \cup [3, \infty)$.

21. (a) Multiply through by the LCD, $(x-2)(x+1)$.

$\dfrac{3}{x-2} \cdot (x-2)(x+1) + \dfrac{1}{x+1} \cdot (x-2)(x+1) = \dfrac{1}{x^2 - x - 2} \cdot (x-2)(x+1) \Rightarrow$

$3(x+1) + 1(x-2) = 1 \Rightarrow 3x + 3 + x - 2 = 1 \Rightarrow 4x = 0 \Rightarrow x = 0$; This solution set is $\{0\}$.

(b) Graph $y_1 = \dfrac{3}{x-2} + \dfrac{1}{x+1} - \dfrac{1}{x^2 - x - 2}$ as shown in Figure 19. With vertical asymptotes $x = -1$ and

$x = 2$, the graph is below or intersects the x-axis on $(-\infty, -1) \cup [0, 2)$. The solution set is

$(-\infty, -1) \cup [0, 2)$.

(c) Graph $y_1 = \dfrac{3}{x-2} + \dfrac{1}{x+1} - \dfrac{1}{x^2 - x - 2}$ as shown in Figure 19. With vertical asymptotes

$x = -1$ and $x = 2$, the graph is above or intersects the x-axis on $(-1, 0] \cup (2, \infty)$. The solution set is

$(-1, 0] \cup (2, \infty)$.

[-6.9,2.5] by [-10,30]
Xscl = 1   Yscl = 5

[-9.4,9.4] by [-3.1,6.2]
Xscl = 1   Yscl = 1

[-9.4,9.4] by [-6.2,6.2]
Xscl = 1   Yscl = 1

[-9.4,9.4] by [-6.2,6.2]
Xscl = 1   Yscl= 1

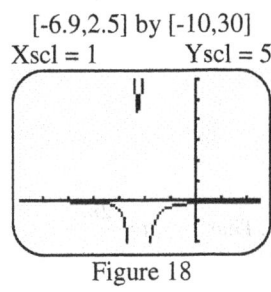
Figure 18

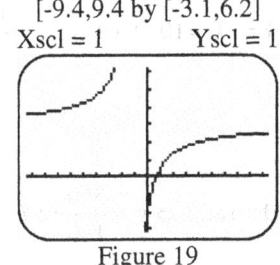
Figure 19

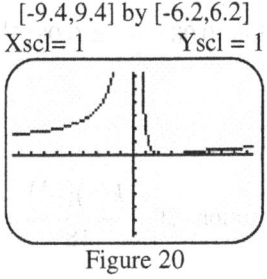
Figure 20

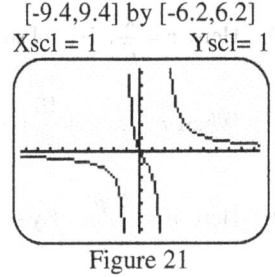
Figure 21

22. The graph intersects the x-axis when $x = -2$. The solution set is $\{-2\}$.

23. The graph is below the x-axis on the interval $(-2,-1)$. The solution set is $(-2,-1)$.

24. The graph is above the x-axis on the interval $(-\infty,-2)\cup(-1,\infty)$. The solution set is $(-\infty,-2)\cup(-1,\infty)$.

25. $|f(x)|>0$ for all $x \neq -2$ and $x \neq -1$. The solution set is $(-\infty,-2)\cup(-2,-1)\cup(-1,\infty)$.

26. (a) See Figure 26.

    (b) 127.3 thousand dollars or $127,300

[0,100] by [0,150]
Xscl = 10   Yscl = 10

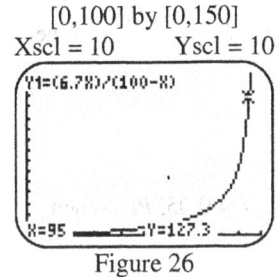
Figure 26

27. (a) Since $0 \leq x < 40,$ the denominator is positive. Multiplying by the LCD will not change the inequality.

$\dfrac{x^2}{1600-40x} \leq 8 \Rightarrow x^2 \leq 8(1600-40x) \Rightarrow x^2 \leq 12{,}800-320x \Rightarrow x^2+302x-12{,}800 \leq 0$ The left side of

this inequality is a quadratic polynomial whose positive zero can be obtained using the quadratic formula. The zero is approximately 35.96. The graph of this parabola is below the x-axis for values of x in the interval [0, 36]. Note that rounding to a whole number is appropriate since x represents a number of cars. The solution set is [0, 36].

    (b) The average line length is less than or equal to 8 cars when the average arrival rate is 36 cars per hour or less.

28. (a) When the coefficient of friction becomes smaller, the braking distance increases.

    (b) Since $0 < x \leq 1,$ the denominator is positive. Multiplying by the LCD will not change the inequality.

$\dfrac{120}{x} \geq 400 \Rightarrow 120 \geq 400x \Rightarrow \dfrac{120}{400} \geq x \Rightarrow x \leq 0.3;$ The solution set is $(0,0.3]$.

29. Here $y = \dfrac{k}{x}$. By substitution, $5 = \dfrac{k}{6} \Rightarrow k = 30.$ That is, $y = \dfrac{30}{x}.$ When $x = 15,$ $y = \dfrac{30}{15} = 2.$

30. Here $z = \dfrac{k}{t^3}$. By substitution, $0.08 = \dfrac{k}{5^3} \Rightarrow 0.08(5^3) = k \Rightarrow k = 10$. That is, $z = \dfrac{10}{t^3}$.

    When $t = 2$, $z = \dfrac{10}{2^3} = 1.25$.

31. Here $m = \dfrac{knp^2}{q}$. By substitution, $20 = \dfrac{k(5)(6^2)}{18} \Rightarrow 360 = 180k \Rightarrow k = \dfrac{360}{180} \Rightarrow k = 2$. That is, $m = \dfrac{2np^2}{q}$.

    When $n = 7$, $p = 11$, and $q = 2$, $m = \dfrac{2(7)(11^2)}{2} = 847$.

32. The height of this cone varies *inversely* as the *square* of the *radius* of its base. The constant of variation is $\dfrac{300}{\pi}$.

33. Here $I = \dfrac{k}{d^2}$. By substitution, $70 = \dfrac{k}{5^2} \Rightarrow 70(5^2) = k \Rightarrow k = 1750$. That is, $I = \dfrac{1750}{d^2}$.

    When $d = 12$, $I = \dfrac{1750}{12^2} \approx 12.15$ candela.

34. Here $R = \dfrac{k}{d^2}$. By substitution, $0.4 = \dfrac{k}{0.01^2} \Rightarrow 0.4(0.01^2) = k \Rightarrow k = 0.00004$. That is, $R = \dfrac{0.00004}{d^2}$. When $d = 0.03$, $I = \dfrac{0.00004}{0.03^2} = \dfrac{0.00004}{0.0009} = \dfrac{4}{90} = \dfrac{2}{45}$ ohm.

35. Here $I = kPt$. By substitution, $110 = k(1000)(2) \Rightarrow \dfrac{110}{2000} = k \Rightarrow k = 0.055$. That is, $I = 0.055Pt$. When $P = 5000$ and $t = 5$, $I = 0.055(5000)(5) = \$1375$.

36. Here $F = \dfrac{kws^2}{r}$. By substitution, $3000 = \dfrac{k(2000)(30^2)}{500} \Rightarrow 1{,}500{,}000 = 1{,}800{,}000k \Rightarrow k = \dfrac{1.5}{1.8} \Rightarrow k = \dfrac{5}{6}$.

    That is, $F = \dfrac{\frac{5}{6}ws^2}{r}$. When $w = 2000$, $s = 60$, and $r = 800$, $F = \dfrac{\frac{5}{6}(2000)(60^2)}{(800)} = 7500$ lb.

37. Here $L = \dfrac{kd^4}{h^2}$. By substitution, $8 = \dfrac{k(1^4)}{9^2} \Rightarrow k = 648$. That is, $L = \dfrac{648d^4}{h^2}$. When $h = 12$, and $d = \dfrac{2}{3}$,

    $L = \dfrac{648\left(\frac{2}{3}\right)^4}{12^2} = \dfrac{128}{144} = \dfrac{8}{9}$ metric tons.

38. Here $L = \dfrac{kwh^2}{l}$. By substitution, $400 = \dfrac{k(12)(15)^2}{8} \Rightarrow 3200 = 2700k \Rightarrow k = \dfrac{3200}{2700} = \dfrac{32}{27}$. That is,

    $L = \dfrac{\frac{32}{27}wh^2}{l}$. When $l = 16, w = 24$ and $h = 8$, $L = \dfrac{\frac{32}{27}(24)(8^2)}{16} = \dfrac{\frac{49{,}152}{27}}{16} = \dfrac{49{,}152}{432} = \dfrac{1024}{9} = 113\dfrac{1}{9}$ kg.

39. Here $w = \dfrac{k}{d^2}$. By substitution, $90 = \dfrac{k}{6400^2} \Rightarrow 90(6400^2) = k \Rightarrow k = 3{,}686{,}400{,}000$.

That is, $w = \dfrac{3{,}686{,}400{,}000}{d^2}$. When $d = 7200$, $w = \dfrac{3{,}686{,}400{,}000}{7200^2} = \dfrac{3{,}686{,}400{,}000}{51{,}840{,}000} = \dfrac{640}{9} = 71\dfrac{1}{9}$ kg.

40. Louise can clean the site in 5 hours and can complete $\dfrac{t}{5}$ of the grooming in t hours. Keith can clean the site in 7 hours and can complete $\dfrac{t}{7}$ of the grooming in t hours. Together they can complete $\dfrac{t}{7} + \dfrac{t}{7}$ of the cleaning in t hours. The job is complete when the fraction of the cleaning reaches 1. $\dfrac{t}{5} + \dfrac{t}{7} = 1 \Rightarrow 7t + 5t = 35 \Rightarrow 12t = 35 \Rightarrow t = 2\dfrac{11}{12}$ or 2 hours and 55 minutes.

41. Terry and Carrie can clean the house in 7 hours and can clean $\dfrac{t}{7}$ of the hours in t hours. Daniel can make a mess of the house in 2 hours and can make a mess of $\dfrac{t}{2}$ of the house in t hours. The job is complete when the fraction of the messy house reaches 1. $\dfrac{t}{2} - \dfrac{t}{7} = 1 \Rightarrow 7t - 2t = 14 \Rightarrow 5t = 14 \Rightarrow t = 2\dfrac{4}{5}$ or 2 hours and 48 minutes.

42. Jack and Kevin can clean the dishes in 15 minutes and can clean $\dfrac{t}{15}$ of the dishes in t minutes. Jack can clean the dishes in 35 minutes and can clean $\dfrac{t}{35}$ of the dishes in t minutes. The job is complete when the fraction of the clean dishes reaches 1. $\dfrac{t}{15} - \dfrac{t}{35} = 1 \Rightarrow 35t - 15t = 525 \Rightarrow 20t = 525 \Rightarrow t = 26\dfrac{1}{4}$ or 26 minutes and 15 seconds.

43. This function yields the cube root graph shifted a units to the left. See Figure 43.

44. This function yields the square root graph stretched and reflected across the x-axis. See Figure 44.

45. This function yields the cube root graph shifted up b units. See Figure 45.

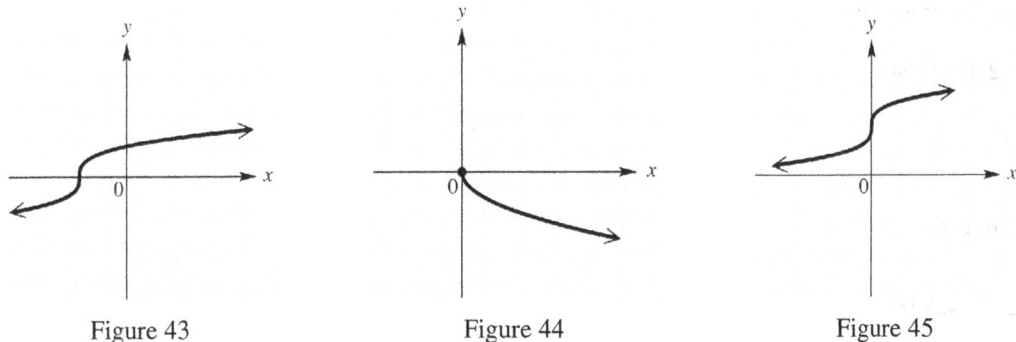

Figure 43   Figure 44   Figure 45

46. This function yields the cube root graph shifted a units to the right. See Figure 46.

202 CHAPTER 4 Rational, Power, and Root Functions

47. This function yields the cube root graph stretched, reflected across the x-axis, and shifted down b units. See Figure 47.

48. This function yields the square root graph shifted a units to the left and b units up. See Figure 48.

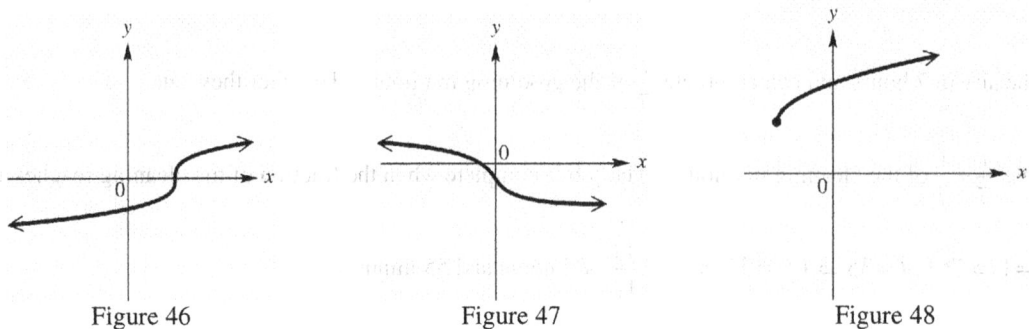

Figure 46   Figure 47   Figure 48

49. Since $12^2 = 144$, $\sqrt{144} = 12$.

50. Since $(-4)^3 = -64$, $\sqrt[3]{-64} = -4$.

51. Since $\left(\dfrac{1}{3}\right)^3 = \dfrac{1}{27}$, $\sqrt[3]{\dfrac{1}{27}} = \dfrac{1}{3}$.

52. Since $3^4 = 81$, $\sqrt[4]{81} = 3$.

53. Since $\left(-\dfrac{2}{3}\right)^5 = -\dfrac{32}{243}$, $\sqrt[5]{\dfrac{32}{243}} = -\dfrac{2}{3}$.

54. Since $(-2)^5 = -32$, $(-32)^{1/5} = -2$. Therefore, $-(-32)^{1/5} = -(-2) = 2$.

55. $36^{-3/2} = \dfrac{1}{36^{3/2}} = \dfrac{1}{\left(\sqrt{36}\right)^3} = \dfrac{1}{6^3} = \dfrac{1}{216}$

56. $-1000^{2/3} = -\left(\sqrt[3]{1000}\right)^2 = -(10)^2 = -100$

57. $(-27)^{-4/3} = \dfrac{1}{(-27)^{4/3}} = \dfrac{1}{\left(\sqrt[3]{-27}\right)^4} = \dfrac{1}{(-3)^4} = \dfrac{1}{81}$

58. $16^{3/4} = \left(\sqrt[4]{16}\right)^3 = 2^3 = 8$

59. $\sqrt[4]{84.6} \approx 2.429260411$

60. $\sqrt[4]{\dfrac{1}{16}} = 0.5$

61. $\left(\dfrac{1}{8}\right)^{4/3} = 0.0625$

62. $12^{1/3} \approx 2.289428485$

63. $2x - 4 \geq 0 \Rightarrow 2x \geq 4 \Rightarrow x \geq \dfrac{4}{2} \Rightarrow x \geq 2$; The domain is $[2, \infty)$.

64. The graph of f is a square root graph reflected across the x-axis. The range is $(-\infty, 0]$.

65. (a) None. The function is never increasing.

    (b) The function is decreasing over its entire domain, $(2, \infty)$.

66. Solving the equation for y yields $x^2 + y^2 = 25 \Rightarrow y^2 = 25 - x^2 \Rightarrow y = \pm\sqrt{25 - x^2}$. The expressions are $y_1 = \sqrt{25 - x^2}$ and $y_2 = -\sqrt{25 - x^2}$ which are graphed in a square window in Figure 66.

67. (a) $\sqrt{5 + 2x} = x + 1 \Rightarrow \left(\sqrt{5 + 2x}\right)^2 = (x+1)^2 \Rightarrow 5 + 2x = x^2 + 2x + 1 \Rightarrow$

    $x^2 - 4 = 0 \Rightarrow (x+2)(x-2) = 0 \Rightarrow x = -2$ or 2 (-2 is extraneous)

    The solution set is $\{2\}$. A graph of $y_1 = \sqrt{5 + 2x}$ and $y_2 = x + 1$ is shown in Figure 67.

    (b) Since the graph of y_1 begins when $5 + 2x = 0 \Rightarrow x = -2.5$, $y_1 > y_2$ on the interval $[-2.5, 2)$.

    (c) From the graph, $y_1 < y_2$ on the interval $(2, \infty)$.

68. (a) $\sqrt{2x + 1} - \sqrt{x} = 1 \Rightarrow \sqrt{2x + 1} = \sqrt{x} + 1 \Rightarrow \left(\sqrt{2x+1}\right)^2 = \left(\sqrt{x} + 1\right)^2 \Rightarrow$

    $2x + 1 = x + 2\sqrt{x} + 1 \Rightarrow x = 2\sqrt{x} \Rightarrow x^2 = \left(2\sqrt{x}\right)^2 \Rightarrow x^2 = 4x \Rightarrow x^2 - 4x = 0 \Rightarrow x(x - 4) = 0 \Rightarrow x = 0$ or 4

    The solution set is $\{0, 4\}$. A graph of $y_1 = \sqrt{2x + 1} - \sqrt{x}$ and $y_2 = 1$ is shown in Figure 68.

    (b) From the graph, $y_1 > y_2$ on the interval $(4, \infty)$.

    (c) From the graph, $y_1 < y_2$ on the interval $(0, 4)$.

69. (a) $\sqrt[3]{6x + 2} = \sqrt[3]{4x} \Rightarrow \left(\sqrt[3]{6x + 2}\right)^3 = \left(\sqrt[3]{4x}\right)^3 \Rightarrow 6x + 2 = 4x \Rightarrow 2x = -2 \Rightarrow x = -1$

    The solution set is $\{-1\}$. A graph of $y_1 = \sqrt[3]{6x + 2}$ and $y_2 = \sqrt[3]{4x}$ is shown in Figure 69.

    (b) From the graph, $y_1 \geq y_2$ on the interval $[-1, \infty)$.

    (c) From the graph, $y_1 \leq y_2$ on the interval $(-\infty, -1]$.

[-9.4,9.4] by [-6.1,6.1]   [-9.4,9.4] by [-6.1,6.1]   [-2.7,6.7] by [-2,2]   [-4.7,4.7] by [-3.1,3.1]
Xscl = 1   Yscl = 1   Xscl = 1   Yscl = 1   Xscl= 1   Yscl = 1   Xscl = 1   Yscl= 1

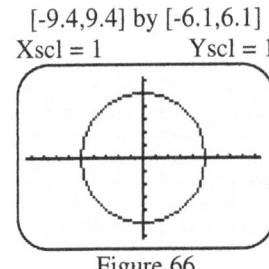
Figure 66

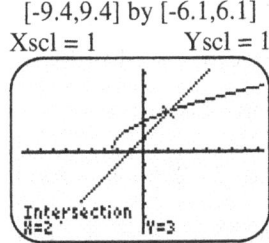
Figure 67

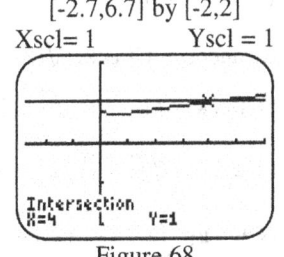
Figure 68

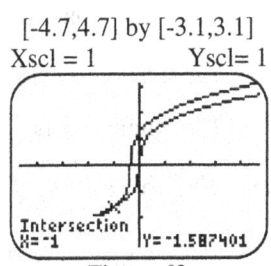
Figure 69

70. (a) $(x - 2)^{2/3} - x^{1/3} = 0 \Rightarrow (x - 2)^{2/3} = x^{1/3} \Rightarrow \left[(x - 2)^{2/3}\right]^3 = \left[x^{1/3}\right]^3 \Rightarrow$

    $(x - 2)^2 = x \Rightarrow x^2 - 4x + 4 = x \Rightarrow x^2 - 5x + 4 = 0 \Rightarrow (x - 1)(x - 4) = 0 \Rightarrow x = 1, 4$

    The solution set is $\{1, 4\}$. A graph of $y_1 = (x - 2)^{2/3}$ and $y_2 = 0$ is shown in Figure 70.

204   CHAPTER 4   Rational, Power, and Root Functions

(b) From the graph, $y_1 \geq y_2$ on the interval $(-\infty, 1] \cup [4, \infty)$.

(c) From the graph, $y_1 \leq y_2$ on the interval $[1, 4]$.

[-2.7, 6.7] by [-6.2, 6.2]
Xscl = 1   Yscl = 1

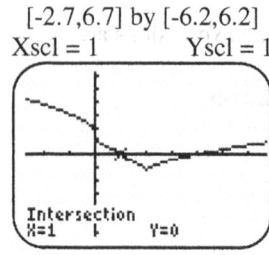

Figure 70

71. $x^5 = 1024 \Rightarrow (x^5)^{1/5} = 1024^{1/5} \Rightarrow x = 4$ The solution set is $\{4\}$. **Check:** $4^5 = 1024$

72. $x^{1/3} = 4 \Rightarrow (x^{1/3})^3 = 4^3 \Rightarrow x = 64$ The solution set is $\{64\}$. **Check:** $64^{1/3} = 4$

73. $\sqrt{x-2} = x-4 \Rightarrow (\sqrt{x-2})^2 = (x-4)^2 \Rightarrow x-2 = x^2 - 8x + 16 \Rightarrow x^2 - 9x + 18 = 0 \Rightarrow$
$(x-3)(x-6) = 0 \Rightarrow x = 3$ or 6

The solution $x = 3$ is extraneous. **Check:** $\sqrt{3-2} = \sqrt{1} = 1 \neq 3 - 4$

The solution set is $\{6\}$. **Check:** $\sqrt{6-2} = \sqrt{4} = 2 = 6 - 4$

74. $x^{3/2} = 27 \Rightarrow (x^{3/2})^{2/3} = 24^{2/3} \Rightarrow x = 9$ The solution set is $\{9\}$. **Check:** $9^{3/2} = 27$

75. $2x^{1/4} + 3 = 6 \Rightarrow 2x^{1/4} = 3 \Rightarrow x^{1/4} = \frac{3}{2} \Rightarrow (x^{1/4})^4 \Rightarrow x = \frac{81}{16}$ The solution set is $\left\{\frac{81}{16}\right\}$.

Check: $2\left(\frac{81}{16}\right)^{1/4} + 3 = 2\left(\frac{3}{2}\right) + 3 = 3 + 3 = 6$

76. $\sqrt{x-2} = 14 - x \Rightarrow (\sqrt{x-2})^2 = (14-x)^2 \Rightarrow x - 2 = 196 - 28x + x^2 \Rightarrow$
$x^2 - 29x + 198 = 0 \Rightarrow (x-11)(x-18) = 0 \Rightarrow x = 11$ or 18

The solution $x = 18$ is extraneous. **Check:** $\sqrt{18-2} = \sqrt{16} = 4 \neq 14 - 18$

The solution set is $\{11\}$. **Check:** $\sqrt{11-2} = \sqrt{9} = 3 = 14 - 11$

77. $\sqrt[3]{2x-3} + 1 = 4 \Rightarrow \sqrt[3]{2x-3} = 3 \Rightarrow (\sqrt[3]{2x-3})^3 = 3^3 \Rightarrow 2x - 3 = 27 \Rightarrow 2x = 30 \Rightarrow x = 15$

The solution set is $\{15\}$. **Check:** $\sqrt[3]{2(15)-3} + 1 = \sqrt[3]{30-3} + 1 = \sqrt[3]{27} + 1 = 3 + 1 = 4$

78. $x^{1/3} + 3x^{1/3} = -2 \Rightarrow 4x^{1/3} = -2 \Rightarrow x^{1/3} = -\frac{1}{2} \Rightarrow (x^{1/3})^3 = \left(-\frac{1}{2}\right)^3 \Rightarrow x = -\frac{1}{8}$

The solution set is $\left\{-\frac{1}{8}\right\}$. **Check:** $\left(-\frac{1}{8}\right)^{1/3} + 3\left(-\frac{1}{8}\right)^{1/3} = -\frac{1}{2} + 3\left(-\frac{1}{2}\right) = -\frac{1}{2} - \frac{3}{2} = -\frac{4}{2} = -2$

79. $2x^{-2} - 5x^{-1} = 3 \Rightarrow 2(x^{-1})^2 - 5(x^{-1}) = 3$

Let $u = x^{-1}$, then $2u^2 - 5u - 3 = 0 \Rightarrow (2u+1)(u-3) = 0 \Rightarrow u = -\dfrac{1}{2}$ or 3.

If $u = x^{-1}$, then $x = u^{-1}$, thus $x = -2$ or $\dfrac{1}{3}$

The solution set is $\left\{-2, \dfrac{1}{3}\right\}$. **Check:** $2(-2)^{-2} - 5(-2)^{-1} = 3 \Rightarrow 2\left(\dfrac{1}{4}\right) - 5\left(-\dfrac{1}{2}\right) = 3 \Rightarrow \dfrac{1}{2} + \dfrac{5}{2} = 3$;

$2\left(\dfrac{1}{3}\right)^{-2} - 5\left(\dfrac{1}{3}\right)^{-1} = 3 \Rightarrow 2(9) - 5(3) = 3 \Rightarrow 18 - 15 = 3$

80. $x^{-3} + 2x^{-2} + x^{-1} = 0 \Rightarrow (x^{-1})^3 + 2(x^{-1})^2 + (x^{-1}) = 0$

Let $u = x^{-1}$, then $u^3 + 2u^2 + u = 0 \Rightarrow u(u^2 + 2u + 1) = 0 \Rightarrow u(u+1)(u+1) = 0 \Rightarrow u = -1$ or 0.

If $u = x^{-1}$, then $x = u^{-1}$, thus $x = (-1)^{-1}$ or $(0)^{-1} \Rightarrow x = \dfrac{1}{-1}$ or $\dfrac{1}{0}$ Since $\dfrac{1}{0}$ is undefined, $x = -1$.

The solution set is $\{-1\}$. **Check:** $(-1)^{-3} + 2(-1)^{-2} + (-1)^{-1} = 0 \Rightarrow -1 + 2 + (-1) = 0 \Rightarrow 0 = 0$

81. $x^{2/3} - 4x^{1/3} - 5 = 0 \Rightarrow (x^{1/3})^2 - 4(x^{1/3}) - 5 = 0$

Let $u = x^{1/3}$, then $u^2 - 4u - 5 = 0 \Rightarrow (u-5)(u+1) = 0 \Rightarrow u = -1$ or 5.

If $u = x^{1/3}$, then $x = u^3$, thus $x = -1$ or 125.

The solution set is $\{-1, 125\}$. **Check:** $(-1)^{2/3} - 4(-1)^{1/3} - 5 = 0 \Rightarrow 1 - (-4) - 5 = 0 \Rightarrow 0 = 0$;

$(125)^{2/3} - 4(125)^{1/3} - 5 = 0 \Rightarrow 25 - 4(5) - 5 = 0 \Rightarrow 0 = 0$

82. $x^{3/4} - 16x^{1/4} = 0 \Rightarrow (x^{1/4})^3 - 16(x^{1/4}) = 0$

Let $u = x^{1/4}$, then $u^3 - 16u = 0 \Rightarrow u(u^2 - 16) = 0 \Rightarrow u(u+4)(u-4) = 0 \Rightarrow u = -4, 0, 4$.

If $u = x^{1/4}$, then $x = u^4$; thus $x = 0$ or 256.

The solution set in $\{0, 256\}$. **Check:** $(0)^{3/4} - 16(0)^{1/4} = 0 \Rightarrow 0 - 0 = 0$;

$(256)^{3/4} - 16(256)^{1/4} = 0 \Rightarrow 64 - 16(4) = 0 \Rightarrow 0 = 0$

83. $\sqrt{x+1} + 1 = \sqrt{2x} \Rightarrow (\sqrt{x+1} + 1)^2 = 2x \Rightarrow x + 1 + 2\sqrt{x+1} + 1 = 2x \Rightarrow 2\sqrt{x+1} = x - 2 \Rightarrow$

$4(x+1) = x^2 - 4x + 4 \Rightarrow 4x + 4 = x^2 - 4x + 4 \Rightarrow x^2 - 8x = 0 \Rightarrow x(x-8) = 0 \Rightarrow x = 0$ or 8

The solution $x = 0$ is extraneous. **Check:** $\sqrt{0+1} + 1 = \sqrt{2(0)} \Rightarrow 1 + 1 = 0 \Rightarrow 2 \neq 0$

The solution set is $\{8\}$. **Check:** $\sqrt{8+1} + 1 = \sqrt{2(8)} \Rightarrow \sqrt{9} + 1 = \sqrt{16} \Rightarrow 4 = 4$

84. $\sqrt{x-2} = 5 - \sqrt{x+3} \Rightarrow (\sqrt{x-2})^2 = (5 - \sqrt{x+3})^2 \Rightarrow x - 2 = 25 - 10\sqrt{x+3} + x + 3 \Rightarrow$

$-30 = -10\sqrt{x+3} \Rightarrow (-30)^2 = \left(-10\sqrt{x+3}\right)^2 \Rightarrow 900 = 100(x+3) \Rightarrow 9 = x + 3 \Rightarrow x = 6$

The solution set is $\{6\}$. **Check:** $\sqrt{6-2} = 5 - \sqrt{6+3} \Rightarrow \sqrt{4} = 5 - \sqrt{9} \Rightarrow 2 = 5 - 3 \Rightarrow 2 = 2$

85. (a) If the length L of the pendulum increases, so does the period of oscillation T.

(b) There are a number of ways to find n and k. One way is to realize that $k = \dfrac{L}{T^n}$ for some integer n. The ratio should be the constant k for each data point when the correct n is found. Another way is to use regression.

(c) By trial and error, $k \approx 0.81$; $n = 2$.

(d) $5 = 0.81(T^2) \Rightarrow \dfrac{5}{0.81} = T^2 \Rightarrow \sqrt{\dfrac{5}{0.81}} = T \Rightarrow T \approx 2.48$ sec

(e) Since $T = \sqrt{\dfrac{L}{k}}$, when length doubles T increases by a factor of $\sqrt{2} \approx 1.414$.

86. Since the volume is $\pi r^2 h = 27\pi$, solving for h yields $h = \dfrac{27}{r^2}$. Substituting this value in the formula for surface area yields $S = 2\pi r\left(\dfrac{27}{r^2}\right) + \pi r^2 \Rightarrow S = \dfrac{54\pi}{r} + \pi r^2$. By graphing $y_1 = \dfrac{54\pi}{r} + \pi r^2$ (not shown), the minimum value for surface area occurs when $r = 3$ inches.

Chapter 4 Test

1. (a) See Figure 1a.

    (b) The graph is obtained by reflecting the graph of $y = \dfrac{1}{x}$ across the x-axis or the y-axis.

    (c) See Figure 1c.

2. (a) See Figure 2a.

    (b) The graph is obtained by reflecting the graph of $y = \dfrac{1}{x^2}$ across the x-axis and shifting it downward 3 units.

    (c) See Figure 2c

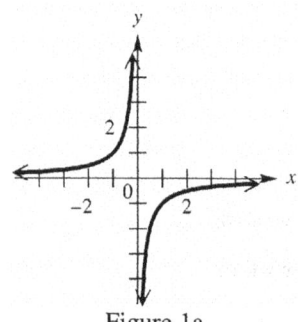
Figure 1a

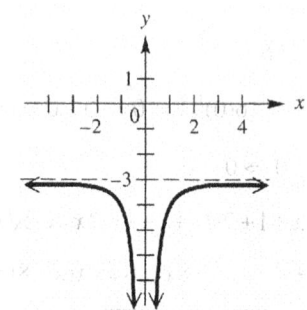
Figure 2a

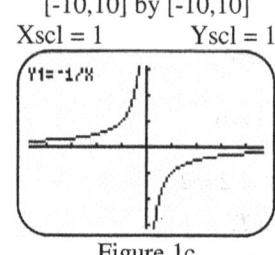
Figure 1c

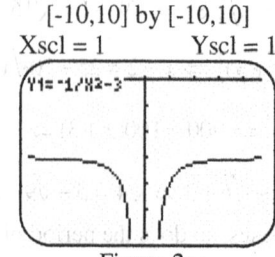
Figure 2c

3. (a) The domain is the set of values that do not make the denominator equal to zero.
   $x^2 - 3x - 4 = 0 \Rightarrow (x-4)(x+1) = 0 \Rightarrow x = 4, -1$ The domain is $(-\infty, -1) \cup (-1, 4) \cup (4, \infty)$.

   (b) Vertical asymptotes occur for values of x that make the denominator equal to zero, $x = -1$ and $x = 4$.

   (c) Since the degrees of the numerator and denominator are equal, the horizontal asymptote can be found using the ratio of the leading coefficients, $y = \frac{1}{1} = 1$.

   (d) The y-value of the y-intercept occurs at $f(0) = \frac{0^2 + 0 - 6}{0^2 - 3(0) - 4} = 1.5$. The intercept is $(0, 1.5)$.

   (e) The x-intercepts occur for values of x that make the numerator equal to zero, -3 and 2. The intercepts are $(-3, 0)$ and $(2, 0)$

   (f) $\frac{x^2 + x - 6}{x^2 - 3x - 4} = 1 \Rightarrow x^2 + x - 6 = x^2 - 3x - 4 \Rightarrow x - 6 = -3x - 4 \Rightarrow 4x = 2 \Rightarrow x = 0.5$
   The coordinates of the intersection point are (0.5, 1).

   (g) See Figure 3.

4. (a) Since $\frac{2x^2 + x - 3}{x - 2} = 2x + 5 + \frac{7}{x - 2}$, the oblique asymptote is $y = 2x + 5$.

   (b) See Figure 4.

5. (a) Since $\frac{x^2 - 16}{x + 4} = \frac{(x+4)(x-4)}{x+4} = x - 4$ for $x \neq -4$, The "hole" occurs when $x = -4$.

   (b) See Figure 5.

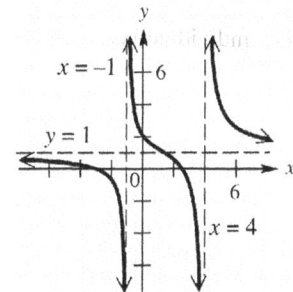

Figure 3

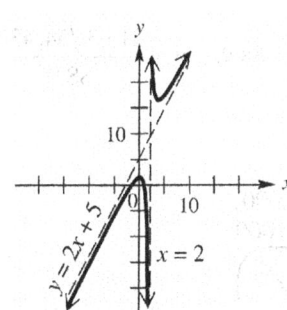

Figure 4

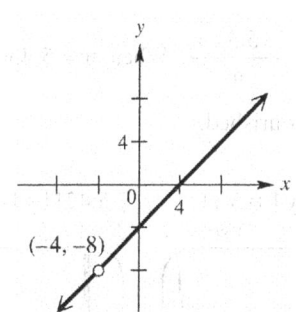

Figure 5

6. (a) Multiply each side of the equation by the LCD, $(x - 2)(x + 2)$.

   $(x-2)(x+2) \cdot \frac{3}{x-2} + (x-2)(x+2) \cdot \frac{21}{x^2 - 4} = \frac{14}{x+2} \cdot (x-2)(x+2) \Rightarrow$

   $3(x+2) + 21 = 14(x-2) \Rightarrow 3x + 6 + 21 = 14x - 28 \Rightarrow 11x = 55 \Rightarrow x = 5$. The solution set is $\{5\}$.

   (b) Graph $y_1 = 3/(x-2) + 21/(x^2 - 4) - 14/(x+2)$ as shown in Figure 6. With vertical asymptotes $x = -2$ and $x = 2$, and x-intercept 5, the graph is above or intersects the x-axis on the interval $(-\infty, -2) \cup (2, 5]$. The solution set is $(-\infty, -2) \cup (2, 5]$.

[-9.4,9.4] by [-20,10]
Xscl = 1   Yscl = 2

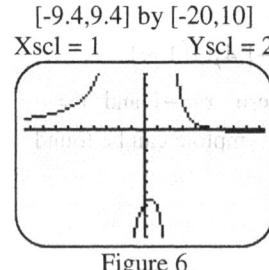

Figure 6

7. (a) $W(30) = \dfrac{1}{40-30} = \dfrac{1}{10}$; $W(39) = \dfrac{1}{40-39} = \dfrac{1}{1} = 1$; $W(39.9) = \dfrac{1}{40-39.9} = \dfrac{1}{0.1} = 10$.

When the rate is 30 vehicles per minute, the average wait time is $\dfrac{1}{10}$ minute (6 seconds). The other results are interpreted similarly.

(b) The vertical asymptote occurs when the denominator equals zero, at $x = 40$. As x approaches 40, W gets larger and larger without bound. See Figure 7.

(c) $5 = \dfrac{1}{40-x} \Rightarrow 5(40-x) = 1 \Rightarrow 200 - 5x = 1 \Rightarrow 5x = 199 \Rightarrow x = \dfrac{199}{5} = 39.8$

8. Here $p = \dfrac{k\sqrt[3]{w}}{h}$. By substitution, $100 = \dfrac{k\sqrt[3]{48,820}}{78.7} \Rightarrow 7870 = \sqrt[3]{48,820}\,k \Rightarrow k = \dfrac{7870}{\sqrt[3]{48,820}} \Rightarrow k \approx 215.3$. That is, $p = \dfrac{215.3\sqrt[3]{w}}{h}$. When $w = 5,430$ and $h = 88.9$, $p = \dfrac{215.3\sqrt[3]{54,430}}{88.9} \approx 92$. The individual is undernourished.

[0,40] by [-0.5,1]   [-5,42] by [-1000,10,000]
Xscl = 5   Yscl = 1   Xscl = 5   Yscl = 1000

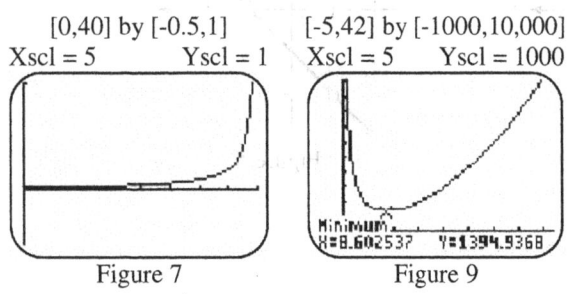

Figure 7   Figure 9

9. Graph $y_1 = (8000 + 2\pi x^3)/x$ as shown in Figure 9. When the radius is approximately 8.6 cm, the amount of aluminum needed will be a minimum of approximately 1394.9 cm^2.

10. (a) $\sqrt[3]{-27} = \sqrt[3]{-1^3 \cdot 3^3} = -3$

(b) $25^{-\frac{3}{2}} = \left(25^{\frac{1}{2}}\right)^{-3} = 5^{-3} = \dfrac{1}{5^3} = \dfrac{1}{125}$

11. $\left(\sqrt[3]{x}\right)^{-4} = x^{-\frac{4}{3}} = \dfrac{1}{x^{4/3}}$

12. See Figure 12a and Figure 12b.

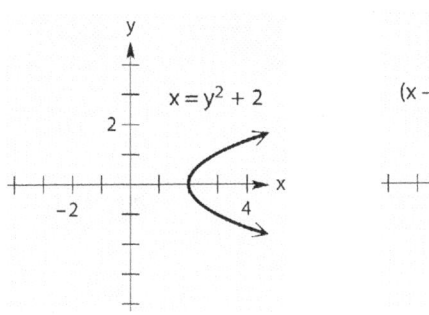
Figure 12a

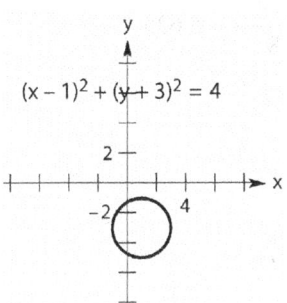
Figure 12b

13. The graph of $y_1 = -\sqrt{5-x}$ is shown in Figure 13.

    (a) $5 - x \geq 0 \Rightarrow 5 \geq x \Rightarrow x \leq 5$; The domain is $(-\infty, 5]$.

    (b) From the graph, the range is $(-\infty, 0]$.

    (c) This function *increases* over its entire domain.

    (d) The graph intersects the x-axis when $x = 5$. The solution set is $\{5\}$.

    (e) The graph below the x-axis for all values in the domain except 5. The solution set is $(-\infty, 5)$.

14. (a) $\sqrt{4-x} = x+2 \Rightarrow \left(\sqrt{4-x}\right)^2 = (x+2)^2 \Rightarrow 4-x = x^2 + 4x + 4 \Rightarrow x^2 + 5x = 0 \Rightarrow x(x+5) = 0 \Rightarrow x = 0, -5$.

    The solution $x = -5$ is extraneous. The solution set is $\{0\}$. The graph of $y_1 = \sqrt{4-x}$ and $y_2 = x+2$ shown in Figure 14 supports this result.

    (b) The graph of y_1 is above the graph of y_2 on the interval $(-\infty, 0)$. The solution set is $(-\infty, 0)$.

    (c) The graph of y_1 is below or intersects the graph of y_2 on the interval $[0, 4]$. The solution set is $[0, 4]$.

[-10,10] by [-10,10]
Xscl = 1   Yscl = 1

[-10,10] by [-10,10]
Xscl = 1   Yscl = 1

[0,600] by [70,0000,100,000]
Xscl = 100   Yscl = 10,000

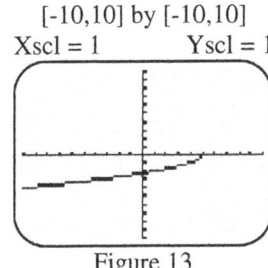
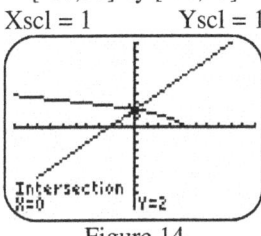
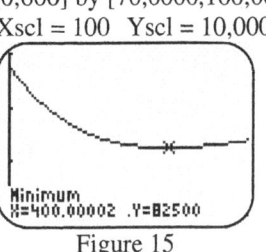

Figure 13   Figure 14   Figure 15

15. Let S be a point on land between Q and R such that the distance from Q to S is x yards. Then the distance from S to R is given by $600 - x$. By the Pythagorean theorem, the distance from P to S is $\sqrt{x^2 + 300^2}$. The total cost of the cable is given by $C = 125\sqrt{x^2 + 300^2} + 100(600 - x)$. The graph of this function is shown in Figure 15. The minimum cost is achieved when the cable is laid underwater from P to S, which is located 400 yards away from Q in the direction of R.

Copyright © 2015 Pearson Education, Inc

16. $z = \dfrac{kx^2}{y} \Rightarrow 10 = \dfrac{k(4^2)}{2} \Rightarrow k = \dfrac{5}{4}, \ z = \dfrac{\frac{5}{4}(6)^2}{8} = 5.625$

Chapter 5: Inverse, Exponential, and Logarithmic Functions

5.1: Inverse Functions

1. Different x-values always produce different y-values; therefore, yes, it is one-to-one.

3. Choosing 2 and -2 as values for x yields $f(2) = 2^2 = 4$ and $f(-2) = (-2)^2 = 4$. Since different values of x produce the same value for $f(x)$, the function is not one-to-one.

5. Choosing 6 and -6 as values for x yields $f(6) = \sqrt{36-6^2} = 0$ and $f(-6) = \sqrt{36-(6)^2} = 0$. Since different values of x produce the same value for $f(x)$, the function is not one-to-one.

7. Every horizontal line will intersect the graph at exactly one point; therefore, yes, it is one-to-one.

9. There are horizontal lines that will intersect the graph at more than one point; therefore, it is not one-to-one.

11. Every horizontal line will intersect the graph at exactly one point; therefore, yes, it is one-to-one.

13. A certain horizontal line intersects the whole horizontal graph (more than one point); therefore, it is not one-to-one.

15. Every horizontal line will intersect the graph at exactly one point; therefore, yes, it is one-to-one.

17. Choosing 4 and 0 as values for x yields $f(4) = (4-2)^2 = 4$ and $f(0) = (0-2)^2 = 4$. Since different values of x produce the same value for $f(x)$, the function is not one-to-one.

19. Different x-values always produce different y-values; therefore, yes, it is one-to-one.

21. Different x-values always produce different y-values; therefore, yes, it is one-to-one.

23. Different x-values always produce different y-values; therefore, yes, it is one-to-one.

25. Since different x-values greater than zero all produce the same $f(x) = 3$, it is not one-to-one.

27. For a function to have an inverse, it must be one-to-one.

29. If f and g are inverses, then $(f \circ g)(x) = x$, and $(g \circ f)(x) = x$.

31. If the point (a,b) lies on the graph of f, and f has an inverse, then the point (b,a) lies on the graph f^{-1}.

33. If the function f has an inverse, then the graph of f^{-1} may be obtained by reflecting the graph of f across the line with equation $y = x$.

35. If $f(-4) = 16$ and $f(4) = 16$, then f does not have an inverse because it is not one-to-one.

37. $(f \circ g)(x) = 3\left(\dfrac{x+7}{3}\right) - 7 = x + 7 - 7 = x$ and $(g \circ f)(x) = \dfrac{(3x-7)+7}{3} = \dfrac{3x}{3} = x$. Since $(f \circ g)(x) = x$ and $(g \circ f)(x) = x$, the function f and g are inverses.

39. $(f \circ g)(x) = \left(\sqrt[3]{x-4}\right)^3 + 4 = x - 4 + 4 = x$ and $(g \circ f)(x) = \sqrt[3]{(x^3+4)-4} = \sqrt[3]{x^3} = x$. Since $(f \circ g)(x) = x$ and $(g \circ f)(x) = x$, the function f and g are inverses.

41. $(f \circ g)(x) = -(-\sqrt[5]{x})^5 = -(-x) = x$ and $(g \circ f)(x) = -\sqrt[5]{(-x^5)} = -(-x) = x$. Since $(f \circ g)(x) = x$ and $(g \circ f)(x) = x$, the function f and g are inverses.

43. Every x-value in f corresponds to only one y-value, and every y-value corresponds to only one x-value, so f is a one-to-one function. The inverse function is found by interchanging the x- and y-values in each ordered pair; therefore, $f^{-1} = \{(4,10),(5,20),(6,30),(7,40)\}$.

45. Every x-value in f corresponds to only one y-value. However, the y-value 5 corresponds to two x-values, 1 and 3. Because some y-values corresponds to more than one x-value, f is not one-to-one.

47. Every x-value in f corresponds to only one y-value, and every y-value corresponds to only one x-value, so f is a one-to-one function. The inverse function is found by interchanging the x- and y-values in each ordered pair. Therefore, $f^{-1} = \{(0^2,0),(1^2,1),(2^2,2),(3^2,3),(4^2,4)\}$.

49. Untying your shoelaces

51. Leaving a room

53. Unwrapping a package

55. For the function $y = 3x - 4$, the inverse is $x = 3y - 4 \Rightarrow x + 4 = 3y \Rightarrow y = \frac{x+4}{3} \Rightarrow f^{-1}(x) = \frac{x+4}{3}$. For the graphs, see Figure 55. Since all real numbers can be input for x in f and f^{-1}, and since all real numbers can be solutions for $f(x)$ and $f^{-1}(x)$, the domain and range of both f and f^{-1} are $(-\infty, \infty)$.

57. For the function $y = x^3 + 1$, the inverse is $x = y^3 + 1 \Rightarrow x - 1 = y^3 \Rightarrow y = \sqrt[3]{x-1} \Rightarrow f^{-1}(x) = \sqrt[3]{x-1}$. For the graphs, see Figure 57. Since all real numbers can be input for x in f and f^{-1}, and all real numbers can be solutions for $f(x)$ and $f^{-1}(x)$, the domain and range of both f and f^{-1} are $(-\infty, \infty)$.

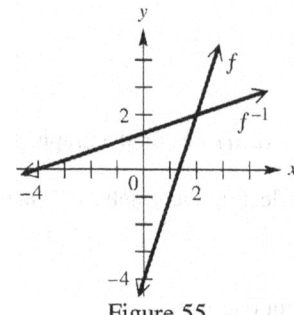
Figure 55

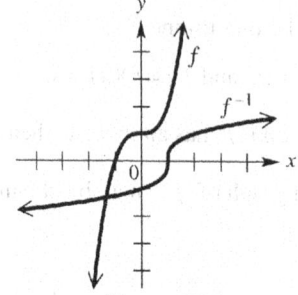
Figure 57

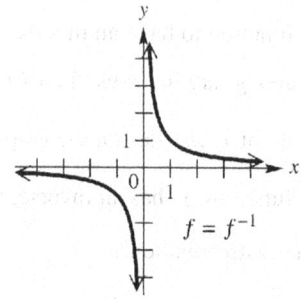
Figure 61

59. Since when $y = 4$, $x = -2$ or 2, the function is not one-to-one.

61. For the function $y = \frac{1}{x}$, the inverse is $x = \frac{1}{y} \Rightarrow y = \frac{1}{x} \Rightarrow f^{-1}(x) = \frac{1}{x}$ For the graphs, see Figure 61. Since all real numbers except 0 can be input for x in f and f^{-1}, and all real numbers except 0 can be solutions for $f(x)$, the domain and range of both f and f^{-1} are $(-\infty, 0) \cup (0, \infty)$.

63. For the function $y = \dfrac{2}{x+3}$, the inverses is $x = \dfrac{2}{y+3} \Rightarrow (y+3)x = 2 \Rightarrow y+3 = \dfrac{2}{x} \Rightarrow y = \dfrac{2}{x} - 3 \Rightarrow$ $y = \dfrac{2-3x}{x} \Rightarrow f^{-1}(x) = \dfrac{2-3x}{x}$. For the graphs, see Figure 63. All real numbers except -3 can be input for x in f and all real numbers except 0 can be input for x in f^{-1}. Therefore, the domain of f is equal to the range of $f^{-1} = (-\infty, -3) \cup (-3, \infty)$, and the domain of f^{-1} is equal to the range of $f = (-\infty, 0) \cup (0, \infty)$.

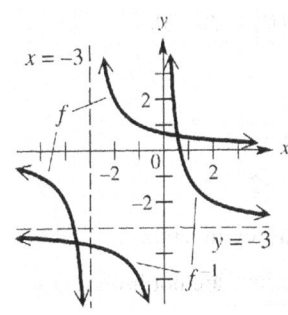
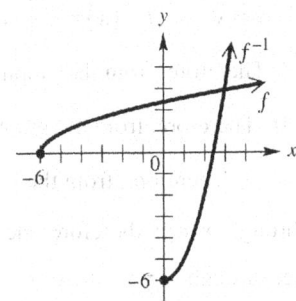

Figure 63   Figure 65

65. For the function $f(x) = \sqrt{6+x}$, $x \geq -6$, the inverse is $x = \sqrt{6+y}$, $x \geq 0$ (A square root can not equal a negative number.) $\Rightarrow x^2 = 6 + y \Rightarrow y = x^2 - 6 \Rightarrow f^{-1}(x) = x^2 - 6$, $x \geq 0$. For the graph, see Figure 65. All real numbers $x \geq -6$ can be input for x in x and all real numbers $x \geq 0$ can be input for x in f^{-1}. Also, all real numbers $x \geq 0$ can be a solution for f and all real numbers $x \geq -6$ can be a solution for f^{-1}. Therefore, the domain of f is equal to the range of $f^{-1} = [-6, \infty)$, and the domain of f^{-1} is equal to the range of $f = [0, \infty)$.

67. $y = \dfrac{4x}{x+1} \Rightarrow y(x+1) = 4x \Rightarrow xy + y = 4x \Rightarrow xy - 4x = -y \Rightarrow x(y-4) = -y \Rightarrow x = \dfrac{-y}{y-4} \Rightarrow$
$f^{-1}(x) = \dfrac{-x}{x-4} \Rightarrow f^{-1}(x) = \dfrac{x}{4-x}$

69. $y = \dfrac{1-2x}{3x} \Rightarrow 3xy = 1 - 2x \Rightarrow 3xy + 2x = 1 \Rightarrow x(3y+2) = 1 \Rightarrow x = \dfrac{1}{3y+2} \Rightarrow f^{-1}(x) = \dfrac{1}{3x+2}$

71. $y = \sqrt{x^2 - 4}, x \geq 2 \Rightarrow y^2 = x^2 - 4 \Rightarrow x^2 = y^2 + 4 \Rightarrow x = \sqrt{y^2 + 4} \Rightarrow f^{-1}(x) = \sqrt{x^2 + 4}$

73. $y = 5x^3 - 7 \Rightarrow 5x^3 = y + 7 \Rightarrow x^3 = \dfrac{y+7}{5} \Rightarrow x = \sqrt[3]{\dfrac{y+7}{5}} \Rightarrow f^{-1}(x) = \sqrt[3]{\dfrac{x+7}{5}}$

75. $y = \dfrac{x}{4+3x} \Rightarrow y(4+3x) = x \Rightarrow 4y + 3xy = x \Rightarrow 3xy - x = -4y \Rightarrow x(3y-1) = -4y \Rightarrow$
$x = \dfrac{-4y}{3y-1} \Rightarrow f^{-1}(x) = \dfrac{-4x}{3x-1}$

77. $y = \dfrac{3-x}{2x+1} \Rightarrow y(2x+1) = 3-x \Rightarrow 2xy + y = 3-x \Rightarrow 2xy + x = 3-y \Rightarrow x(2y+1) = 3-y \Rightarrow x = \dfrac{3-y}{2y+1} \Rightarrow$

$f^{-1}(x) = \dfrac{3-x}{2x+1}$

79. $f(2) = (2)^3 = 8.$

81. $f(-2) = (-2)^3 = -8.$

83. If $f(x) = x^3$, then the inverse is $x = y^3 \Rightarrow y = \sqrt[3]{x} \Rightarrow f^{-1}(x) = \sqrt[3]{x}$, and $f^{-1}(0) = \sqrt[3]{0} = 0.$

85. For inverses, when $f^{-1}(4)$, then $f(x) = 4$ Therefore, from the graph, $x = 4.$

87. For inverses, when $f^{-1}(0)$, then $f(x) = 0$. Therefore, from the graph $x = 2.$

89. For inverses, when $f^{-1}(-3)$, then $f(x) = -3$. Therefore, from the graph $x = -2.$

91. The graphs are reflections of each other through $x = y$; therefore, the functions are inverses.

93. The graphs are not reflections of each other through $x = y$; therefore, the functions are not inverses.

95. Yes, for $f(x) = 2x + 4$ the inverse is $x = 2y + 4 \Rightarrow x - 4 = 2y \Rightarrow \dfrac{x-4}{2} = y \Rightarrow f^{-1}(x) = \dfrac{1}{2}x - 2,$ which is equal to $g(x).$

97. Since $(x_1, y_1) = (y_2, x_2)$, the x's and y's are switched, and the screen suggest that they are linear functions.

99. Reflect the graph across the line $y = x$. See Figure 99.

101. Reflect the graph across the line $y = x$. See Figure 101.

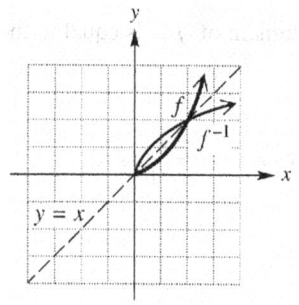
Figure 99

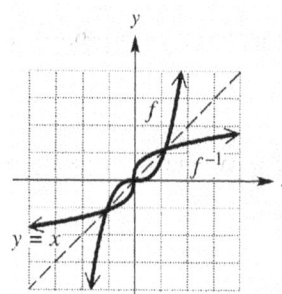
Figure 101

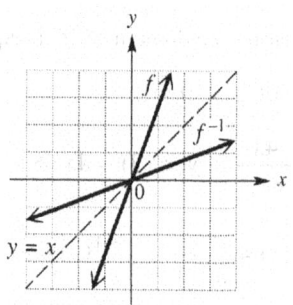
Figure 103

103. Reflect the graph across the line $y = x$. See Figure 103.

105. It represents the cost in dollars of building 1000 cars.

107. With $m = a = \dfrac{a}{1}$, the inverse function will switch the x and y terms and the graph of the inverse is a reflection across the line $y = x$ which will have the slope $m = \dfrac{1}{a}.$

109. From the graph of the function in the given window, the function fails the horizontal line test and is not one-to-one. See Figure 109.

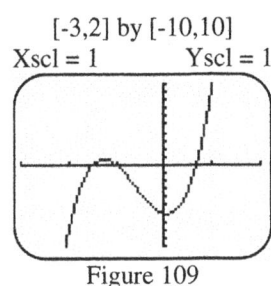

Figure 109

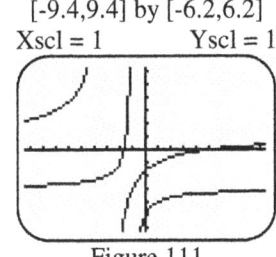

Figure 111

111. From the graph of the function in the given window, the function passes the horizontal line test and is one-to-one. The inverse is $x = \dfrac{y-5}{y+3} \Rightarrow xy + 3x = y - 5 \Rightarrow xy - y = -3x - 5 \Rightarrow y(x-1) = -3x - 5 \Rightarrow y = \dfrac{-3x-5}{x-1} \Rightarrow$

$f^{-1}(x) = \dfrac{-3x-5}{x-1}$. For both graphs, see Figure 111.

113. If $f(x) = 4x - 1$, then the inverse is $x = 4y - 1 \Rightarrow x + 1 = 4y \Rightarrow y = \dfrac{x+1}{4} \Rightarrow f^{-1}(x) = \dfrac{x+1}{4}$. Inputting the numbers given yields numbers that correspond to the letters: TREASURE HUNT IS ON.

115. Using the function $f(x) = x^3 + 1$ on the letters NO PROBLEM or the corresponding numbers 14, 15, 16, 18, 15, 2, 12, 5, and 13, yields the numbers 2745, 3376, 4097, 5833, 3376, 9, 1729, 126, and 2198. The inverse is $x = y^3 + 1 \Rightarrow x - 1 = y^3 \Rightarrow \sqrt[3]{x-1} = y \Rightarrow f^{-1}(x) = \sqrt[3]{x-1}$.

117. From the graph on a calculator, one possible answer that passes the horizontal line test is the domain $[0, \infty)$.

119. From the graph on a calculator, one possible answer that passes the horizontal line test is the domain $[6, \infty)$.

121. From the graph on a calculator, one possible answer that passes the horizontal line test is the domain $[0, \infty)$.

123. If $f(x) = -x^2 + 4$, $x \geq 0$, then the inverse is $x = -y^2 + 4$, $y \geq 0 \Rightarrow x - 4 = -y^2 \Rightarrow$
$4 - x = y^2 \Rightarrow y = \sqrt{4-x} \Rightarrow f^{-1}(x) = \sqrt{4-x}$.

125. If $f(x) = |x - 6|$, $x \geq 6$, then the inverse is $x = |y - 6|$, $y \geq 6 \Rightarrow x = y - 6 \Rightarrow x + 6 = y \Rightarrow$
$f^{-1}(x) = x + 6$, $x \geq 0$.

5.2: Exponential Functions

1. See Figure 1
3. See Figure 3

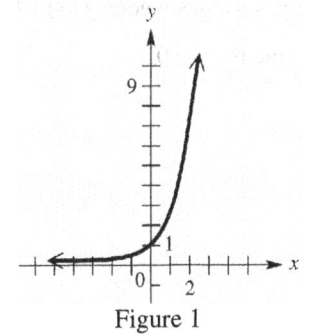

Figure 1

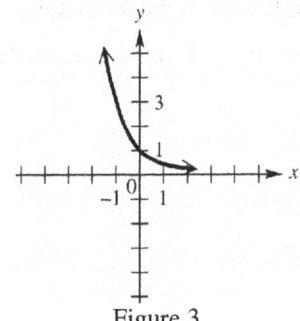

Figure 3

5. $4^x = 2 \Rightarrow (2^2)^x = 2^1 \Rightarrow 2^{2x} = 2^1 \Rightarrow 2x = 1 \Rightarrow x = \dfrac{1}{2}.$

7. $\left(\dfrac{1}{2}\right)^x = 4 \Rightarrow (2^{-1})^x = 2^2 \Rightarrow 2^{-x} = 2^2 \Rightarrow -x = 2 \Rightarrow x = -2.$

9. From the calculator, $2^{\sqrt{10}} \approx 8.952419619.$

11. From the calculator, $\left(\dfrac{1}{2}\right)^{\sqrt{2}} \approx 0.3752142272.$

13. From the calculator, $4.1^{-\sqrt{3}} \approx 0.0868214883.$

15. From the calculator, $\sqrt{7}^{\sqrt{7}} \approx 13.1207791$

17. From the calculator, the point $\left(\sqrt{10}, 8.9524196\right)$ lies on the graph of $y = 2^x.$

19. From the calculator, the point $(\sqrt{2}, 0.37521423)$ lies on the graph of $y = \left(\dfrac{1}{2}\right)^x.$

21. See Figure 21. All values can be input for x; therefore, the domain is $(-\infty, \infty)$. Only values where $f(x) > 0$ are possible solutions; therefore, the range is $(-\infty, 0)$. From the graph, the asymptote is $y = 0.$

23. See Figure 23. All values can be input for x; therefore, the domain is $(-\infty, \infty)$. Only values where $f(x) > 0$ are possible solutions; therefore, the range is $(0, \infty)$. From the graph, the asymptote is $y = 0.$

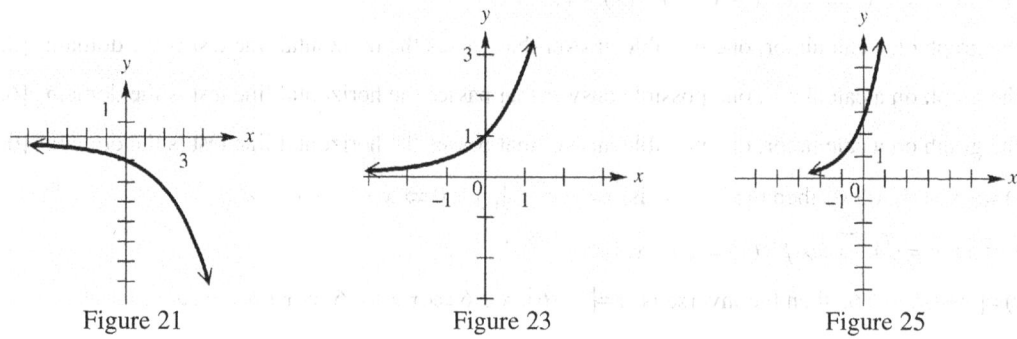

Figure 21   Figure 23   Figure 25

25. See Figure 25. All values can be input for x; therefore, the domain is $(-\infty, \infty)$. Only values where $f(x) > 0$ are possible solutions; therefore, the range is $(0, \infty)$. From the graph, the asymptote is $y = 0.$

27. See Figure 27. All values can be input for x; therefore, the domain is $(-\infty, \infty)$. Only values where $f(x) > 0$ are possible solutions; therefore, the range is $(0, \infty)$. From the graph, the asymptote is $y = 0.$

29. See Figure 29. All values can be input for x; therefore, the domain is $(-\infty, \infty)$. Only values where $f(x) > 0$ are possible solutions; therefore, the range is $(0, \infty)$. From the graph, the asymptote is $y = 0.$

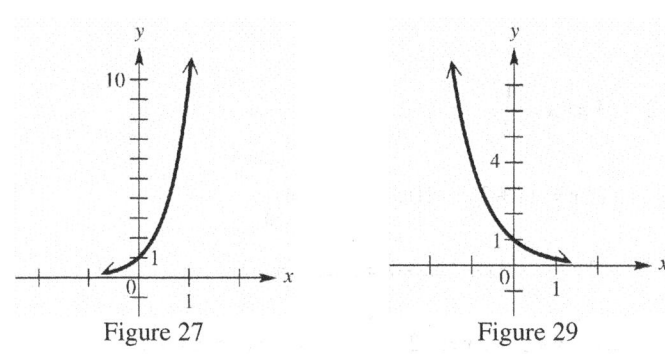

Figure 27   Figure 29

31. (a) Since the graph goes up to the right, $a > 1$.
    (b) From the graph, the domain is $(-\infty, \infty)$, the range is $(0, \infty)$, and the asymptote is $y = 0$.
    (c) Reflect f(x) across the *x*-axis. See Figure 31c.
    (d) From the graph, the domain is $(-\infty, \infty)$, the range is $(-\infty, 0)$, and the asymptote is $y = 0$.
    (e) Reflect f(x) across the *y*-axis. See Figure 31e.
    (f) From the graph, the domain is $(-\infty, \infty)$, the range is $(0, \infty)$, and the asymptote is $y = 0$.

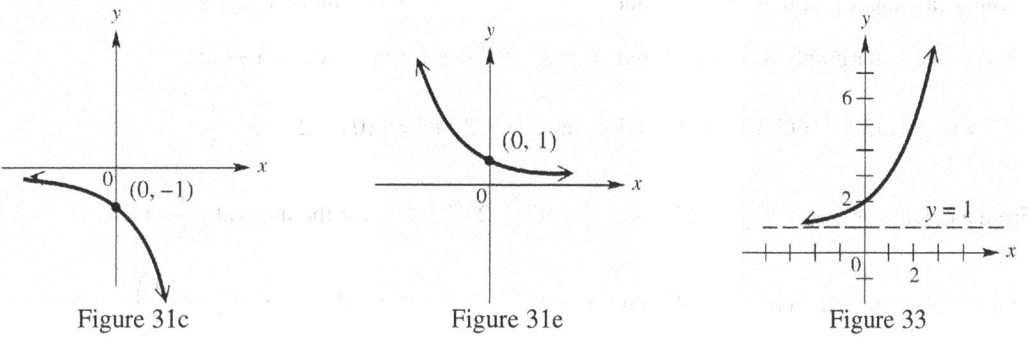

Figure 31c   Figure 31e   Figure 33

33. Shift the original graph (not shown) 1 unit upward. See Figure 33.
35. Shift the original graph (not shown) 1 unit left. See Figure 35.

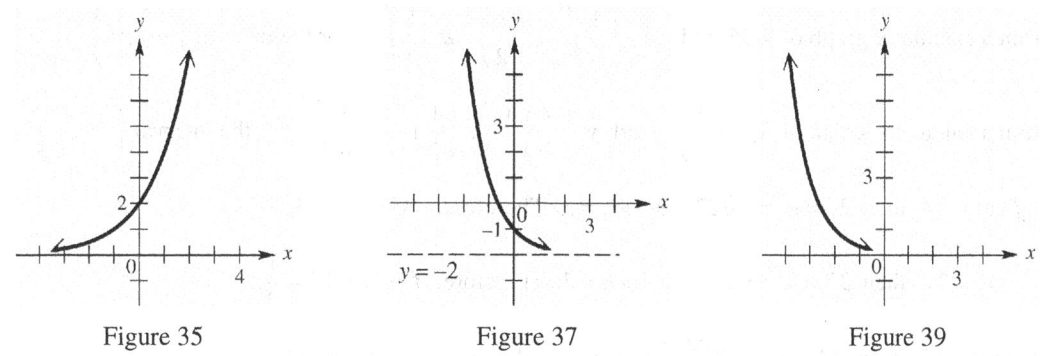

Figure 35   Figure 37   Figure 39

37. Shift the original graph (not shown) 2 units downward. See Figure 37.
38. Shift the original graph (not shown) 4 units upward. See Figure 38.
39. Shift the original graph (not shown) 2 units left. See Figure 39.
41. $2^{3-x} = 8 \Rightarrow 2^{3-x} = 2^3 \Rightarrow 3 - x = 3 \Rightarrow -x = 0 \Rightarrow x = 0$.

43. $12^{x-3} = 1 \Rightarrow 12^{x-3} = 12^0 \Rightarrow x-3 = 0 \Rightarrow x = 3$.

45. $e^{4x-1} = (e^2)^x \Rightarrow e^{4x-1} = e^{2x} \Rightarrow 4x-1 = 2x \Rightarrow 2x = 1 \Rightarrow x = \frac{1}{2}$.

47. $27^{4x} = 9^{x+1} \Rightarrow (3^3)^{4x} \Rightarrow (3^2)^{x+1} \Rightarrow 3^{12x} = 3^{2x+2} \Rightarrow 12x = 2x+2 \Rightarrow 10x = 2 \Rightarrow x = \frac{1}{5}$.

49. $4^{x-2} = 2^{3x+3} \Rightarrow (2^2)^{x-2} = 2^{3x+3} \Rightarrow 2^{2x-4} = 2^{3x+3} \Rightarrow 2x-4 = 3x+3 \Rightarrow -7 = x \Rightarrow x = -7$.

51. $(\sqrt{2})^{x+4} = 4^x \Rightarrow (2^{1/2})^{x+4} = (2^2)^x \Rightarrow 2^{\frac{1}{2}x+2} = 2^{2x} \Rightarrow \frac{1}{2}x+2 = 2x \Rightarrow 2 = \frac{3}{2}x \Rightarrow 4 = 3x \Rightarrow x = \frac{4}{3}$.

53. $(\sqrt{2})^{-2x} = \left(\frac{1}{2}\right)^{2x+3} \Rightarrow (2^{1/2})^{-2x} = (2^{-1})^{2x+3} \Rightarrow 2^{-x} = 2^{-2x-3} \Rightarrow -x = -2x-3 \Rightarrow x = -3$

55. $(6)^{1-x} = \left(\frac{1}{36}\right)^{2x} \Rightarrow (6)^{1-x} = (6^{-2})^{2x} \Rightarrow (6)^{1-x} = (6)^{-4x} \Rightarrow 1-x = -4x \Rightarrow 3x = -1 \Rightarrow x = -\frac{1}{3}$

57. (a) $2^{x+1} = 8 \Rightarrow 2^{x+1} = 2^3 \Rightarrow x+1 = 3 \Rightarrow x = 2$.

(b) From a calculator graph of $y_1 = 2^{x+1}$ and $y_2 = 8$, $2^{x+1} < 8$ for the interval $(2, \infty)$.

(c) From a calculator graph of $y_1 = 2^{x+1}$ and $y_2 = 8$, $2^{x+1} < 8$ for the interval $(-\infty, 2)$.

59. (a) $27^{4x} = 9^{x+1} \Rightarrow (3^3)^{4x} = (3^2)^{x+1} \Rightarrow 3^{12x} = 3^{2x+2} \Rightarrow 12x = 2x+2 \Rightarrow 10x = 2 \Rightarrow x = \frac{1}{5}$.

(b) From a calculator graph of $y_1 = 27^{4x}$ and $y_2 = 9^{x+1}$, $27^{4x} > 9^{x+1}$ for the interval $\left(\frac{1}{5}, \infty\right)$.

(c) From a calculator graph of $y_1 = 27^{4x}$ and $y_2 = 9^{x+1}$, $27^{4x} < 9$ for the interval $\left(-\infty, \frac{1}{5}\right)$.

61. (a) $\left(\frac{1}{2}\right)^{-x} = \left(\frac{1}{4}\right)^{x+1} \Rightarrow (2^{-1})^{-x} = (2^{-2})^{x+1} \Rightarrow 2^x = 2^{-2x-2} \Rightarrow x = -2x-2 \Rightarrow 3x = -2 \Rightarrow x = -\frac{2}{3}$.

(b) From a calculator graph of $= \emptyset$ and $y_2 = \left(\frac{1}{4}\right)^{x+1}$, $\left(\frac{1}{2}\right)^{-x} \geq \left(\frac{1}{4}\right)^{x+1}$ for the interval $\left[-\frac{2}{3}, \infty\right)$.

(c) From a calculator graph of $y_1 = \left(\frac{1}{2}\right)^{-x}$ and $y_2 = \left(\frac{1}{4}\right)^{x+1}$, $\left(\frac{1}{2}\right)^{-x} \leq \left(\frac{1}{4}\right)^{x+1}$ for the interval $\left(-\infty, -\frac{2}{3}\right]$.

63. (a) If $f(x) = 27$, then $27 = a^3 \Rightarrow \sqrt[3]{27} = a \Rightarrow a = 3$. Therefore, $f(1) = 3^1 = 3$.

(b) If $f(x) = 27$, then $27 = a^3 \Rightarrow \sqrt[3]{27} = a \Rightarrow a = 3$. Therefore, $f(-1) = 3^{-1} = \frac{1}{3}$.

(c) If $f(x) = 27$, then $27 = a^3 \Rightarrow \sqrt[3]{27} = a \Rightarrow a = 3$. Therefore, $f(2) = 3^2 = 9$.

(d) If $f(x) = 27$, then $27 = a^3 \Rightarrow \sqrt[3]{27} = a \Rightarrow a = 3$. Therefore, $f(0) = 3^0 = 1$.

65. If point $(-3, 64)$ in on the graph of $f(x) = a^x$, then $64 = \frac{1}{a^3} \Rightarrow \frac{1}{64} = a^3 \Rightarrow \sqrt[3]{\frac{1}{64}} \Rightarrow a = \frac{1}{4}$. The equation is $f(x) = \left(\frac{1}{4}\right)^x$.

67. $f(t) = \left(\dfrac{1}{3}\right)^{1-2t} = \left(\dfrac{1}{3}\right)^{1} \cdot \left(\dfrac{1}{3}\right)^{-2t} = \left(\dfrac{1}{3}\right)\left(\left(\dfrac{1}{3}\right)^{-2}\right)^{t} = \left(\dfrac{1}{3}\right)(3^2)^t \Rightarrow f(t) = \left(\dfrac{1}{3}\right)9^t$.

69. (a) Use the formula $A = p\left(1+\dfrac{r}{n}\right)^{nt}$ to find the amount in the account.

$A = 20000\left(1+\dfrac{0.03}{1}\right)^{(1)(4)} = 20000(1.03)^4 \Rightarrow A = \$22,510.18$.

(b) Use the formula $A = p\left(1+\dfrac{r}{n}\right)^{nt}$ to find the amount in the account.

$A = 20000\left(1+\dfrac{0.03}{2}\right)^{(2)(4)} = 20000(1.015)^8 \Rightarrow A = \$22,529.85$.

71. (a) Use the formula to find the $A = p\left(1+\dfrac{r}{n}\right)^{nt}$ amount in the account.

$A = 27500\left(1+\dfrac{0.0395}{365}\right)^{(365)(5)} = 27500(1.000108219)^{1825} \Rightarrow A = \$33,504.34$.

(b) Use the formula $A = Pe^{rt}$ to find the amount in the account.

$A = 27500\left(e^{(0.0395)(5)}\right) = 27500e^{0.1975} \Rightarrow A = \$33,504.71$.

73. Plan A: $A = 40000\left(1+\dfrac{0.025}{4}\right)^{(4)(3)} = 40000(1.00625)^{12} \Rightarrow A = \$43,105.30$.

Plan B: $A = 40000e^{(0.024)(3)} = 40000e^{(0.072)} \Rightarrow A = \$42,986.21$ Plan A is better by $119.09.

75. Set $y_1 = 1000\left(1+\dfrac{0.05}{1}\right)^{x} \Rightarrow y_1 = 1000(1.05)^x$, and $y_2 = 1000\left(1+\dfrac{0.05}{12}\right)^{12x}$.

Graphing each on the same calculator screen shows the line y_2 slightly above line y_1. Also, using the table function for y_1, y_2 and $y_2 - y_1$ yields the following differences: (1 year) – $1.16, (2 years) – $2.44, (5 years) – $7.08, (10 years) – $18.12, (20 years) –$59.34, (30 years) – $145.80, and (40 years) – $318.43.

77. (a) See Figure 77a.
(b) Exponential would be better because the average rate of change between data points is not constant.
(c) See Figure 77c.
(d) $p(1500) = 1013e^{-0.0001341(1500)} = 828.4210207 \Rightarrow p(1500) \approx 828$ mb.

$p(11,000) = 1013e^{-0.0001341(11,000)} = 231.7296764 \Rightarrow p(11,000) \approx 232$ mb. $p(1500)$ is slightly lower than the actual, and $p(11,000)$ is slightly higher than the actual.

220   CHAPTER 5   Inverse, Exponential, and Logarithmic Functions

[-1000,11000] by [0,1200]   [-1000,11000] by [0,1200]   [0,60] by [0,1.2]
Xscl = 1000   Yscl = 100   Xscl = 1000   Yscl = 100   Xscl= 10   Yscl = 0.2

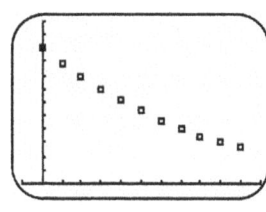 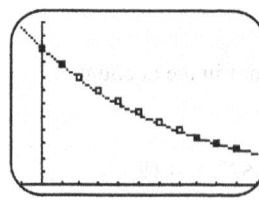 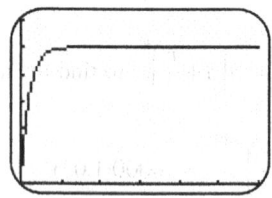

Figure 77a   Figure 77c   Figure 79

79. (a) $f(2) = 1 - e^{-5(2)} = 1 - 0.367879441 = 0.632120559 \Rightarrow f(2) \approx 0.63$. There is a 63% chance that at least one car will enter the intersection during a 2-minute period.

(b) See Figure 79. As time progresses, the probability increases and begins to approach 1. That is, it is almost certain that at least one car will enter the intersection during a 60-minute period.

81. With $a > 0$, all inputs for x yield different solutions. The function is one-to-one and an inverse function exists.

82. See Figure 82.

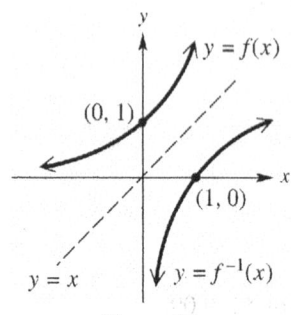

Figure 82

83. To find the inverse, switch the x and y, $x = a^y$.

84. If $a = 10$ then $x = a^y$ will be $x = 10^y$.

85. If $a = e$ then $x = a^y$ will be $x = e^y$.

86. If (p, q) is on f then switching the x and y means (q, p) will be on f^{-1}.

5.3: Logarithms and Their Properties

1. (a) By the definitions of logarithms, $2^4 = 16$ is equivalent to $\log_2 16 = 4$; it matches with C.

(b) By the definitions of logarithms, $3^0 = 1$ is equivalent to $\log_3 1 = 0$; it matches with A.

(c) By the definitions of logarithms, $10^{-1} = \frac{1}{10} = 0.1$ is equivalent to $\log_{10} 0.1 = -1$; it matches with E.

(d) By the definitions of logarithms, $2^{1/2} = \sqrt{2}$ is equivalent to $\log_2 \sqrt{2} = \frac{1}{2}$; it matches with B.

(e) By the definitions of logarithms, $e^{-2} = \frac{1}{e^2}$ is equivalent to $\log_e \frac{1}{e^2} = -2$; it matches with F.

(f) By the definitions of logarithms, $\left(\dfrac{1}{2}\right)^{-3} = 8$ is equivalent to $\log_{1/2} 8 = -3$; it matches with D.

3. By the definitions of logarithms, $3^4 = 81$ is equivalent to $\log_3 81 = 4$.

5. By the definitions of logarithms, $\left(\dfrac{1}{2}\right)^{-4} = 16$ is equivalent to $\log_{1/2} 16 = -4$.

7. By the definitions of logarithms, $10^{-4} = 0.0001$ is equivalent to $\log 0.0001 = -4$.

9. By the definitions of logarithms and natural logarithms, $e^0 = 1$ is equivalent to $\ln 1 = 0$.

11. By the definitions of logarithms, $\log_6 36 = 2$ is equivalent to $6^2 = 36$.

13. By the definitions of logarithms, $\log_{\sqrt{3}} 81 = 8$ is equivalent to $\left(\sqrt{3}\right)^8 = 81$.

15. By the definitions of logarithms, $\log_{10} 0.001 = -3$ is equivalent to $10^{-3} = 0.001$.

17. By the definitions of logarithms, $\log \sqrt{10} = 0.5$ is equivalent to $10^{0.5} = \sqrt{10}$.

19. By the definitions of logarithms, $\log_5 125 = x \Rightarrow 5^x = 125$. Since we know $5^3 = 125$, it follows that $x = 3$.

21. By the definitions of logarithms, $\log_x 3^{12} = 24 \Rightarrow x^{24} = 3^{12} \Rightarrow \left(x^2\right)^{12} = 3^{12}$. Since $x^2 = 3$, it follows that $x = \sqrt{3}$.

23. By the definitions of logarithms, $\log_6 x = -3 \Rightarrow x = 6^{-3} \Rightarrow x = \dfrac{1}{6^3} \Rightarrow x = \dfrac{1}{216}$.

25. By the definitions of logarithms, $\log_x 16 = \dfrac{4}{3} \Rightarrow x^{4/3} = 16 \Rightarrow \left(x^{4/3}\right)^{3/4} = 16^{3/4} \Rightarrow x = \sqrt[4]{16^3} \Rightarrow x = 8$.

27. By the definitions of logarithms, $\log_2(x+1) = 3 \Rightarrow x + 1 = 2^3 \Rightarrow x + 1 = 8 \Rightarrow x = 7$

29. By the definitions of logarithms, $\log_9 \dfrac{\sqrt[4]{27}}{3} = x \Rightarrow 9^x = \dfrac{\sqrt[4]{27}}{3} \Rightarrow (3^2)^x = \dfrac{3^{3/4}}{3} \Rightarrow 3^{2x} = 3^{-1/4}$. Since $3^{2x} = 3^{-1/4}$, $2x = -\dfrac{1}{4} \Rightarrow x = -\dfrac{1}{8}$.

31. (a) Using the properties of logarithms, $3^{\log_3 7} = 7$.

    (b) Using the properties of logarithms, $4^{\log_4 9} = 9$.

    (c) Using the properties of logarithms, $12^{\log_{12} 4} = 4$.

    (d) Using the properties of logarithms, $a^{\log_a k} \, (k > 0, a > 0, a \neq 1) = k$.

33. (a) Using the properties of logarithms, $\log_3 1 = 0$.

    (b) Using the properties of logarithms, $\log_4 1 = 0$.

    (c) Using the properties of logarithms, $\log_{12} 1 = 0$.

    (d) Using the properties of logarithms, $\log_a 1 \, (a > 0, a \neq 1) = 0$.

35. By properties of logarithms, $\log 10^{1.5} = \log_{10} 10^{1.5} = 1.5$.

37. By properties of logarithms, $\log 10^{\sqrt{5}} = \log_{10} 10^{\sqrt{5}} = \sqrt{5}$.

39. By properties of logarithms, $\ln e^{2/3} = \frac{2}{3}$.

41. By properties of logarithms, $\ln e^{\pi} = \pi$.

43. By properties of logarithms, $\sqrt{7} \ln e^{\sqrt{7}} = \sqrt{7}\left(\sqrt{7}\right) = 7$.

45. From the calculator, $\log 43 \approx 1.633468456$.

47. From the calculator, $\log 0.783 \approx -1.062382379$.

49. From the calculator, $\log 28^3 = 3\log 28 = 3(1.447158031) \approx 4.341474094$.

51. From the calculator, $\ln 43 \approx 3.761200116$.

53. From the calculator, $\ln 0.783 \approx -0.244622583$.

55. From the calculator, $\ln 28^3 = 3\ln 28 = 3(3.33220451) \approx 9.996613531$.

57. Since $\text{pH} = -\log[H_3O^+]$ and grapefruit has $H_3O^+ = 6.3 \times 10^{-4}$, $\text{pH} = -\log(6.3 \times 10^{-4}) \approx 3.20066 \approx 3.2$.

59. Since $\text{pH} = -\log[H_3O^+]$ and crackers have $H_3O^+ = 3.9 \times 10^{-9}$, $\text{pH} = -\log(3.9 \times 10^{-9}) \approx 8.408935 \approx 8.4$.

61. Since $\text{pH} = -\log[H_3O^+]$ and soda pop has a $\text{pH} = 2.7$,

    $2.7 = -\log[H_3O^+] \Rightarrow -2.7 = \log[H_3O^+] \Rightarrow H_3O^+ = 10^{-2.7} \Rightarrow H_3O^+ \approx 0.001995 \approx 2 \times 10^{-3}$.

63. Since $\text{pH} = -\log[H_3O^+]$ and beer has a $\text{pH} = 4.8$,

    $4.8 = -\log[H_3O^+] \Rightarrow -4.8 = \log[H_3O^+] \Rightarrow H_3O^+ = 10^{-4.8} \Rightarrow H_3O^+ \approx 0.00001585 \approx 1.6 \times 10^{-5}$.

65. $\log_3 \frac{2}{5} = \log_3 2 - \log_3 5$.

67. $\log_2 \frac{6x}{y} = \log_2 6 + \log_2 x - \log_2 y$.

69. $\log_5 \frac{5\sqrt{7}}{3m} = \log_5 5 + \log_5 7^{1/2} - (\log_5 3 + \log_5 m) = 1 + \frac{1}{2}\log_5 7 - \log_5 3 - \log_5 m$.

71. $\log_4 (2x + 5y)$ cannot be rewritten.

73. $\log_k \frac{pq^2}{m} = \log_k p + \log_k q^2 - \log_k m = \log_k p + 2\log_k q - \log_k m$.

75. $\log_m \sqrt{\frac{r^3}{5z^5}} = \log_m \left(\frac{r^3}{5z^5}\right)^{1/2} = \frac{1}{2}[\log_m r^3 - (\log_m 5 + \log_m z^5)] = \frac{1}{2}(3\log_m r - \log_m 5 - 5\log_m z)$ or

    $\frac{3}{2}\log_m r - \frac{1}{2}\log_m 5 - \frac{5}{2}\log_m z$

77. $\log_a x + \log_a y - \log_a m = \log_a \frac{xy}{m}$

79. $2\log_m a - 3\log_m b^2 = \log_m a^2 - \log_m (b^2)^3 = \log_m \dfrac{a^2}{b^6}$

81. $2\log_a (z-1) + \log_a (3z+2),\ z > 0 \Rightarrow \log_a (z-1)^2 + \log_a (3z+2) = \log_a \left((z-1)^2 (3z+2)\right)$

83. $-\dfrac{2}{3}\log_5 5m^2 + \dfrac{1}{2}\log_5 25m^2 \Rightarrow \log_5 \left(5m^2\right)^{-2/3} + \log_5 \left(25m^2\right)^{1/2} \Rightarrow \log_5 \left(5^{-2/3} m^{-4/3}\right) + \log_5 5m \Rightarrow$

$\log_5 \left(5^{-2/3} m^{-4/3}\right)(5m) \Rightarrow \log_5 \left(5^{1/3} m^{-1/3}\right)$ or $\log_5 \sqrt[3]{\dfrac{5}{m}}$

85. $3\log x - 4\log y = \log x^3 - \log y^4 = \log \dfrac{x^3}{y^4}$

87. $\ln(a+b) + \ln a - \dfrac{1}{2}\ln 4 = \ln(a+b) + \ln a - \ln\sqrt{4} = \ln \dfrac{(a+b)a}{2}$

89. $\log_5 10 = \dfrac{\log 10}{\log 5} \approx 1.430676558$

91. $\log_{15} 5 = \dfrac{\log 5}{\log 15} \approx 0.5943161289$

93. $\log_{100} 83 = \dfrac{\log 83}{\log 100} \approx 0.9595390462$

95. $\log_{2.9} 7.5 = \dfrac{\log 7.5}{\log 2.9} \approx 1.892441722$

97. To get the graph of $y = -3^x + 7$, reflect the graph of $y = 3^x$ across the x-axis and shift 7 units upward.

98. See Figure 98.

    [-5,5] by [-10,10]

    Xscl = 1   Yscl = 1

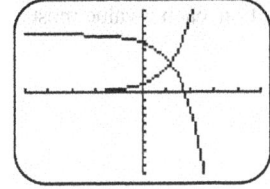

Figure 98

99. From the calculator's capabilities, the x-intercept of $y_2 = -3^x + 7$ is $x \approx 1.7712437492$.

100. If $0 = -3^x + 7$ then $3^x = 7$. Now using base 3 logarithm yields $\log_3 3^x = \log_3 7 \Rightarrow x = \log_3 7$.

101. $\log_3 7 = \dfrac{\log 7}{\log 3} = 1.77124374916$

102. The approximations are close enough to support the conclusion that the x-intercept is equal to $\log_3 7$.

224 CHAPTER 5 Inverse, Exponential, and Logarithmic Functions

103. $\ln\left|x+\sqrt{x^2+3}\right|+\ln\left|x-\sqrt{x^2+3}\right|=\ln 3 \Rightarrow \ln\left(\left|x+\sqrt{x^2+3}\right|\left|x-\sqrt{x^2+3}\right|\right)=\ln 3 \Rightarrow$

$\ln\left|x^2+x\sqrt{x^2+3}-x\sqrt{x^2+3}-\left(\sqrt{x^2+3}\right)^2\right|=\ln 3 \Rightarrow \ln\left|\left(x^2-x^2-3\right)\right|=\ln 3 \Rightarrow$

$\ln|-3|=\ln 3 \Rightarrow \ln 3 = \ln 3$

105. $\frac{1}{3}\ln\left(\frac{x^2+1}{5}\right)-\frac{1}{3}\ln\left(\frac{x^2+4}{5}\right)=\ln\sqrt[3]{\frac{x^2+1}{x^2+4}} \Rightarrow \ln\left(\sqrt[3]{\frac{x^2+1}{5}}\right)-\ln\left(\sqrt[3]{\frac{x^2+4}{5}}\right)=\ln\sqrt[3]{\frac{x^2+1}{x^2+4}} \Rightarrow$

$\ln\left(\frac{\sqrt[3]{\frac{x^2+1}{5}}}{\sqrt[3]{\frac{x^2+4}{5}}}\right)=\ln\sqrt[3]{\frac{x^2+1}{x^2+4}} \Rightarrow \ln\sqrt[3]{\frac{x^2+1}{x^2+4}} = \ln\sqrt[3]{\frac{x^2+1}{x^2+4}}$

107. With a total of 100 individuals and 50 individuals of each species, $P_1=\frac{50}{100}=\frac{1}{2}$ and $P_2=\frac{50}{100}=\frac{1}{2}$. Now

using the index of diversity, $H=-\left(\frac{1}{2}\log_2\left(\frac{1}{2}\right)+\frac{1}{2}\log_2\left(\frac{1}{2}\right)\right)=-\log_2\left(\frac{1}{2}\right)=-(-1) \Rightarrow H=1.$

109. (a) $S(100)=0.36\ln\left(1+\frac{100}{0.36}\right) \approx 2.0269 \approx 2$

(b) $S(200)=0.36\ln\left(1+\frac{200}{0.36}\right) \approx 2.2758 \approx 2$

(c) $S(150)=0.36\ln\left(1+\frac{150}{0.36}\right) \approx 2.1725 \approx 2$

(d) $S(10)=0.36\ln\left(1+\frac{10}{0.36}\right) \approx 1.2095 \approx 1$

Reviewing Basic Concepts (Sections 5.1—5.3)

1. No, because the x-values -2 and 2 both correspond to the y-value 4. In a one-to-one function, each y-value must correspond to exactly one x-value (and each x-value to exactly one y-value).

2. (a) Interchange the x- and y-values:

x	12	21	32	45
y	7	8	9	10

(b) For $f(x)=\frac{x+5}{4}$ the inverse is $x=\frac{y+5}{4} \Rightarrow 4x=y+5 \Rightarrow y=4x-5 \Rightarrow f^{-1}(x)=4x-5.$

3. Graph $f(x)=2x+3$ and reflect it across the line $y=x$. See Figure 3.

4. See Figure 4.

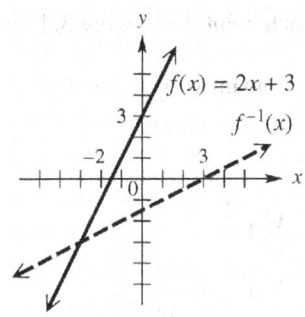
Figure 3

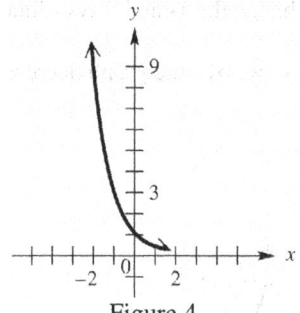
Figure 4

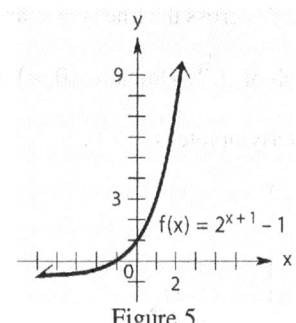
Figure 5

5. See Figure 5.

   (a) It is shifted 1 unit left and 1 unit downward.

   (b) Domain: $(-\infty, \infty)$ Range: $(-1, \infty)$

   (c) $y = -1$

   (d) The graph of the line passes the horizontal line test and is a one to one function.

6. $4^{2x} = 8 \Rightarrow (2^2)^{2x} = 2^3 \Rightarrow 2^{4x} = 2^3 \Rightarrow 4x = 3 \Rightarrow x = \dfrac{3}{4}$.

7. Using $A = P\left(1 + \dfrac{r}{n}\right)^{nt}$, we get $A = 600\left(1 + \dfrac{0.04}{4}\right)^{4(3)} = 600(1.01)^{12} = 676.10$.

   The interest earned is $676.10 - 600 = 76.10$.

8. (a) $\log\left(\dfrac{1}{\sqrt{10}}\right) = \log_{10} 10^{-1/2} = -\dfrac{1}{2}$

   (b) $2\ln e^{1.5} = \ln e^{2(1.5)} = \log_e e^3 = 3$

   (c) $\log_2 4 = 2$ because we know that $2^2 = 4$.

9. From the properties of logarithms, $\log \dfrac{3x^2}{5y} = \log 3 + \log x^2 - (\log 5 + \log y) = \log 3 + 2\log x - \log 5 - \log y$.

10. From the properties of logarithms, $\ln 4 + \ln x - 3\ln 2 = \ln 4 + \ln x - \ln 2^3 = \ln \dfrac{4x}{8} = \ln \dfrac{x}{2}$.

5.4: Logarithmic Functions

1. Reflect f across the line $y = x$ and interchange the x- and y-coordinates for each point. See Figure 1. From the graph of f^{-1}, Domain: $(0, \infty)$; Range: $(-\infty, \infty)$; the graph increases on its domain $(0, \infty)$; and the vertical asymptote is $x = 0$.

3. Reflect f across the line $y = x$ and interchange the x- and y-coordinates for each point. See Figure 3. From the graph of f^{-1}, Domain: $(0,\infty)$; Range: $(-\infty,\infty)$; the graph decreases on its domain $(0,\infty)$; and the vertical asymptote is $x = 0$.

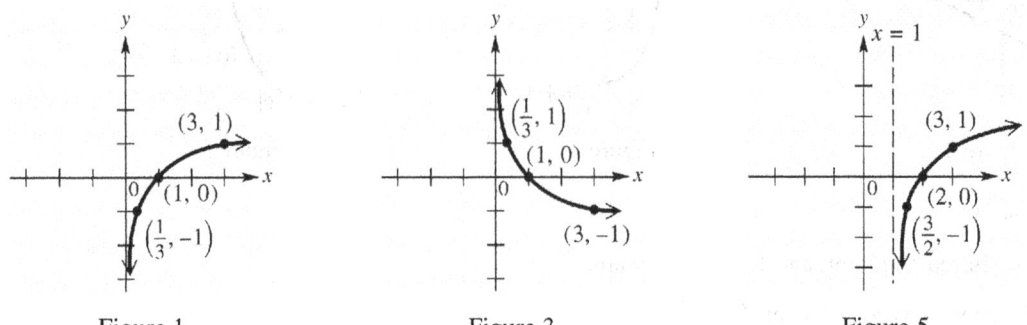

Figure 1   Figure 3   Figure 5

5. Reflect f across the line $y = x$ and interchange the x- and y-coordinates for each point. See Figure 5. From the graph of f^{-1}, Domain: $(1,\infty)$; Range: $(-\infty,\infty)$; the graph increases on its domain $(1,\infty)$; and the vertical asymptote is $x = 1$.

7. Logarithmic

9. Since the argument of a logarithm must be positive, $2x > 0 \Rightarrow x > 0$. The domain is $(0,\infty)$.

11. Since the argument of a logarithm must be positive, $(-x) > 0 \Rightarrow x < 0$. The domain is $(-\infty, 0)$.

13. Since the argument of a natural logarithm must be positive, $(x^2 + 7) > 0$, this is true for all values of x, therefore the domain is $(-\infty,\infty)$.

15. Since the argument of a natural logarithm must be positive, $(-x^2 + 4) > 0$. Now set $(-x^2 + 4) = 0 \Rightarrow$ $x^2 - 4 = 0 \Rightarrow x^2 = 4 \Rightarrow x = -2, 2$. The endpoints -2 and 2 divide the number line into 3 intervals. The interval $(-\infty, -2)$ has a negative solution; the interval $(-2, 2)$ has a positive solution; and the interval $(2, \infty)$ has a negative solution. Therefore, $(-x^2 + 4) > 0$ for the interval $(-2, 2)$ and the domain is $y = x$

17. Since the argument of a natural logarithm must be positive, $(x^2 - 4x - 21) > 0$. Now set $x^2 - 4x - 21 = 0 \Rightarrow (x - 7)(x + 3) = 0 \Rightarrow x = -3, 7$. The endpoints -3 and 7 divide the number line into 3 intervals. The interval $(-\infty, -3)$ has a positive product; the interval $(-3, 7)$ has a negative product; and the interval $(7, \infty)$ has a positive product. Therefore, $x^2 - 4x - 21 > 0$ for the interval $(-\infty, -3) \cup (7, \infty)$ and the domain is $(-\infty, -3) \cup (7, \infty)$.

19. Since the argument of a natural logarithm must be positive, $(x^3 - x) > 0$. Now set $x^3 - x = 0 \Rightarrow x(x^2 - 1) = 0 \Rightarrow x(x+1)(x-1) = 0 \Rightarrow x = -1, 0, 1$. The endpoints $-1, 0,$ and 1 divide the

number line into 4 intervals. The interval $(-\infty,-1)$ has a negative product; the interval $(-1,0)$ has a positive product; the interval $(0,1)$ has a negative product; and the interval $(1,\infty)$ has a positive product. Therefore, $x^3-x>0$ for the interval $(-1,0)\cup(1,\infty)$ and the domain is $(-1,0)\cup(1,\infty)$.

21. Since the argument of a natural logarithm must be positive, $\frac{x+3}{x-4}>0$. Now set both $x+3=0$ and $x-4=0 \Rightarrow x=-3, 4$. The endpoints -3 and 4 divide the number line into 3 intervals. The interval $(-\infty,-3)$ has a positive product; the interval $(-3,4)$ has a negative product; and the interval $(4,\infty)$ has a positive product. Therefore, $\frac{x+3}{x-4}>0$ for the interval $(-\infty,-3)\cup(4,\infty)$ and the domain is $(-\infty,-3)\cup(4,\infty)$.

23. Since the argument of a natural logarithm must be positive, $|3x-7|>0$. Since this is true for all real x-values except when $3x-7=0$, we solve for $3x-7=0 \Rightarrow 3x=7 \Rightarrow x=\frac{7}{3}$. Therefore, $|3x-7|>0$ for the interval $\left(-\infty,\frac{7}{3}\right)\cup\left(\frac{7}{3},\infty\right)$, and the domain is $\left(-\infty,\frac{7}{3}\right)\cup\left(\frac{7}{3},\infty\right)$.

25. Shift the graph of $f(x)=\log_2 x$ upward 3 units to sketch the graph of $f(x)=(\log_2 x)+3$. See Figure 25.

27. Shift the graph of $f(x)=\log_2 x$ left 3 units and reflect all negative y-values across the x-axis to sketch the graph of $f(x)=|\log_2(x+3)|$. See Figure 27.

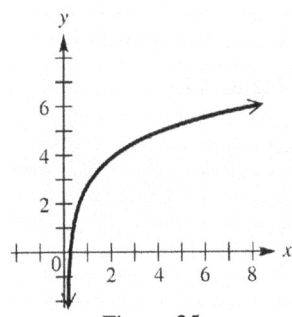
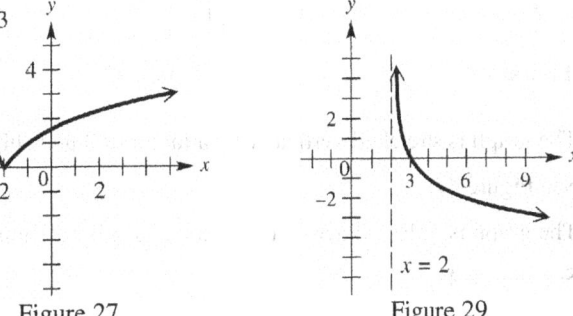

Figure 25   Figure 27   Figure 29

29. Shift the graph of $f(x)=\log_{1/2} x$ right 2 units to sketch the graph of $f(x)=\log_{1/2}(x-2)$. See Figure 29.

31. The graph of $y=e^x+3$ is the graph of $y=e^x$ shifted 3 units upward. The correct graph is B.

33. The graph of $y=e^{x+3}$ is similar to the graph of $y=e^x$ with a y-intercept of $(0,e^3)$. The correct graph is D.

35. The graph of $y=\ln x+3$ is the graph of $y=\ln x$ passing through $(1,-3)$. The correct graph is A.

37. The graph of $y=\ln(x-3)$ is the graph of $y=\ln x$ shifted 3 units right. The correct graph is C.

39. Graph a logarithmic function with base greater than 1 that has an asymptote at $x=0$ and passes through $(1,0)$ and $(5,1)$. See Figure 39.

228   CHAPTER 5   Inverse, Exponential, and Logarithmic Functions

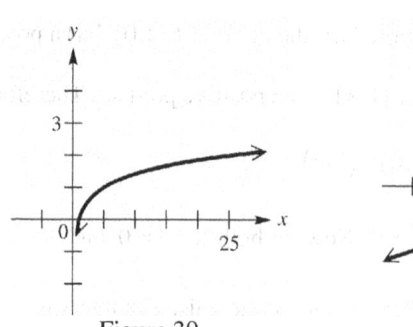
Figure 39

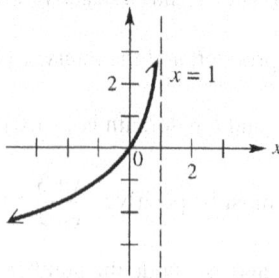
Figure 41

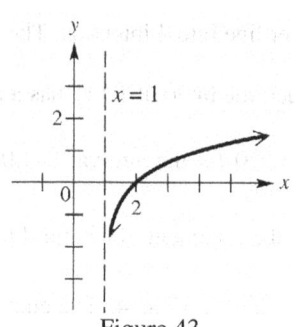
Figure 43

41. Graph a logarithmic function with base between 0 and 1 that is shifted 1 unit left then reflected across the y-axis, has an asymptote at $x=1$, and passes through $(0,0)$ and $(-1,-1)$. See Figure 41.

43. Graph a logarithmic function with base greater than 1 that is shifted 1 unit right, has an asymptote at $x=1$, and passes through $(2,0)$ and $(4,1)$. See Figure 43.

45. (a) The graph is shifted 4 units to the left.
    (b) See Figure 45.

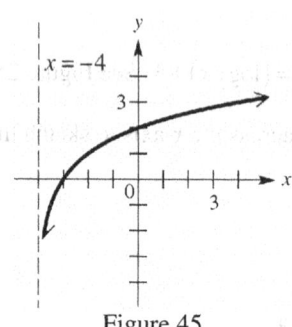
Figure 45

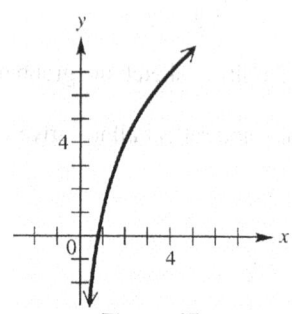
Figure 47

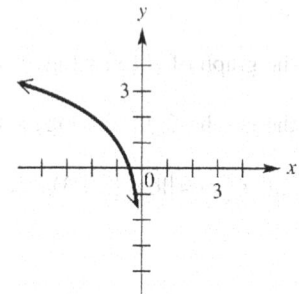
Figure 49

47. (a) The graph is stretched vertically by a factor of 3 and shifted 1 unit upward.
    (b) See Figure 47.

49. (a) The graph is reflected across the y-axis and shifted 1 unit upward.
    (b) See Figure 49.

51. The graphs are not the same because the domain of $y = \log x^2$ is $(-\infty, 0) \cup (0, \infty)$ while the domain of $y = 2\log x$ is $(0, \infty)$. The power rule does not apply if the argument is nonpositive.

53. (a) If $\log_9 27 = x$ then $9^x = 27 \Rightarrow (3^2)^x = 27 \Rightarrow 3^{2x} = 3^3 \Rightarrow 2x = 3 \Rightarrow x = \frac{3}{2}$.

    (b) By the change of base rule, $\log_9 27 = \frac{\log 27}{\log 9}$, then by calculator, $\frac{\log 27}{\log 9} \approx \frac{1.43136}{0.95424} = 1.5 = \frac{3}{2}$.

    (c) The point $\left(27, \frac{3}{2}\right)$ is on the graph of $y = \log_9 27$, which supports the answer in part a.

55. (a) If $\log_{16} \frac{1}{8} = x$ then $16^x = \frac{1}{8} \Rightarrow (2^4)^x = \frac{1}{2^3} \Rightarrow 2^{4x} = 2^{-3} \Rightarrow 4x = -3 \Rightarrow x = -\frac{3}{4}$.

(b) By the change of base rule, $\log_{16}\dfrac{1}{8}=\dfrac{\log\dfrac{1}{8}}{\log 16}$, then by calculator, $\dfrac{\log\dfrac{1}{8}}{\log 16}\approx\dfrac{-0.90309}{1.20412}=-0.75=-\dfrac{3}{4}$.

(c) The point $\left(\dfrac{1}{8},-\dfrac{3}{4}\right)$ is on the graph of $y=\log_{16}\dfrac{1}{8}$, which supports the answer in part a.

57. For the function $f(x)=4^{x}-3$, the inverse is found by interchanging the *x*- and *y*-values.

$x=4^{y}-3\Rightarrow x+3=4^{y}\Rightarrow \log_{4}(x+3)=\log_{4}4^{y}\Rightarrow \log_{4}(x+3)=y$

Therefore, $f^{-1}(x)=\log_{4}(x+3)$. Graph f and f^{-1} in the same window. See Figure 57.

59. For the function $f(x)=-10^{x}+4$, the inverse is found by interchanging the *x*- and *y*-values.

$x=-10^{y}+4\Rightarrow x-4=-10^{y}\Rightarrow -x+4=10^{y}\Rightarrow \log(-x+4)=\log 10^{y}\Rightarrow \log(-x+4)=y$

Therefore, $f^{-1}(x)=\log(4-x)$. Graph f and f^{-1} in the same window. See Figure 59.

[-4.7,4.7] by [-3.1,3.1]   [-6,6.] by [-4.,4.]
Xscl = 1   Yscl = 1   Xscl = 1   Yscl = 1

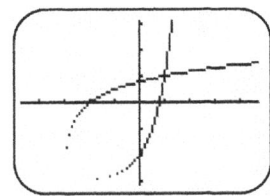
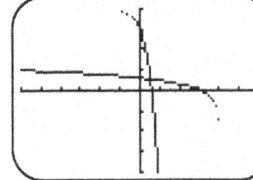

Figure 57   Figure 59

61. (a) First, find *a*. Using the given information, $2=\log_{a}3\Rightarrow a^{2}=3\Rightarrow a=\sqrt{3}$.

Then, $f\left(\dfrac{1}{9}\right)=\log_{\sqrt{3}}\left(\dfrac{1}{9}\right)=x\Rightarrow \left(\sqrt{3}\right)^{x}=\dfrac{1}{9}\Rightarrow 3^{1/2x}=3^{-2}\Rightarrow \dfrac{1}{2}x=-2\Rightarrow x=-4$.

(b) Since $a=\sqrt{3}$ from part a, $f(27)=\log_{\sqrt{3}}27=x\Rightarrow \left(\sqrt{3}\right)^{x}=27\Rightarrow 3^{\frac{1}{2}x}=3^{3}\Rightarrow \dfrac{1}{2}x=3\Rightarrow x=6$.

(c) Since $a=\sqrt{3}$ from part a, find f^{-1} for the function $f(x)=\log_{\sqrt{3}}x$. The inverse is found by interchanging the *x*- and *y*-values: $x=\log_{\sqrt{3}}y\Rightarrow \left(\sqrt{3}\right)^{x}=y\Rightarrow f^{-1}(x)=\left(\sqrt{3}\right)^{x}$.

Now $f^{-1}(-2)=\left(\sqrt{3}\right)^{-2}=\dfrac{1}{3}$.

(d) Since $a=\sqrt{3}$ from part a, find f^{-1} for the function $f(x)=\log_{\sqrt{3}}x$. The inverse is found by interchanging the *x*- and *y*-values: $x=\log_{\sqrt{3}}y\Rightarrow \left(\sqrt{3}\right)^{x}=y\Rightarrow f^{-1}(x)=\left(\sqrt{3}\right)^{x}$.

Now, $f^{-1}(0)=\left(\sqrt{3}\right)^{0}=1$.

63. Graphing $y_{1}=2^{-x}$ and $y_{2}=\log_{10}x$ in the same window yields the intersection point $(1.87,0.27)$. Therefore, the solution is $x\approx 1.87$.

65. (a) The left side is a reflection of the right side with respect to the axis of the tower.

The graph of $f(-x)$ is the reflection of $f(x)$ with respect to the y-axis.

(b) Since the horizontal line on the top has one-half on each side of the y-axis, the x-coordinate on the right side will be $x = \frac{1}{2}(15.7488) \Rightarrow x = 7.8744$. Using $f(7.8744) = -301\ln\left(\frac{7.8744}{207}\right) \approx 984$ feet.

(c) Graphing $y_1 = -301\ln\left(\frac{x}{207}\right)$ and $y_2 = 500$ in the same window yields the approximate intersection point $(39.31, 500)$. Therefore, the height is approximately 39 feet.

67. (a) Using $x = 9$, yields $f(9) = 27 + 1.105\log(9+1) = 27 + 1.105\log 10 = 28.105$ in.

(b) It tells us that at 99 miles from the eye of a typical hurricane, the barometric pressure is 29.21 inches.

5.5: Exponential and Logarithmic Equations and Inequalities

1. $3e^{2x} + 1 = 5 \Rightarrow 3e^{2x} = 4 \Rightarrow e^{2x} = \frac{4}{3} \Rightarrow 2x = \ln\frac{4}{3} \Rightarrow x = \frac{1}{2}\ln\frac{4}{3}$

3. $2(10^x) = 14 \Rightarrow 10^x = 7 \Rightarrow x = \log 7$

5. $\frac{1}{2}\log_2 x = \frac{3}{4} \Rightarrow \log_2 x = \frac{3}{2} \Rightarrow x = 2^{3/2}$

7. $4\ln 3x = 8 \Rightarrow \ln 3x = 2 \Rightarrow 3x = e^2 \Rightarrow x = \frac{1}{3}e^2$

9. (a) $3^x = 7 \Rightarrow \log 3^x = \log 7 \Rightarrow x\log 3 = \log 7 \Rightarrow x = \frac{\log 7}{\log 3}$ (Other forms of the answer are possible.)

(b) From the calculator, the solution is $x \approx 1.771$.

11. (a) $\left(\frac{1}{2}\right)^x = 5 \Rightarrow \log\left(\frac{1}{2}\right)^x = \log 5 \Rightarrow x\log\left(\frac{1}{2}\right) = \log 5 \Rightarrow x = \frac{\log 5}{\log(1/2)}$

(Other forms of the answer are possible.)

(b) From the calculator, the solution is $x \approx -2.322$.

13. (a) $0.8^x = 4 \Rightarrow \log 0.8^x = \log 4 \Rightarrow x\log 0.8 = \log 4 \Rightarrow x = \frac{\log 4}{\log 0.8}$ (Other forms of the answer are possible.)

(b) From the calculator, the solution is $x \approx -6.213$.

15. (a) $4^{x-1} = 3^{2x} \Rightarrow \log 4^{x-1} = \log 3^{2x} \Rightarrow (x-1)\log 4 = (2x)\log 3 \Rightarrow x\log 4 - \log 4 = 2x\log 3 \Rightarrow$

$x\log 4 - 2x\log 3 = \log 4 \Rightarrow x(\log 4 - 2\log 3) = \log 4 \Rightarrow x = \frac{\log 4}{\log 4 - 2\log 3}$

(Other forms of the answer are possible.)

(b) From the calculator, the solution is $x \approx -1.710$.

17. (a) $6^{x+1} = 4^{2x-1} \Rightarrow \log 6^{x+1} = \log 4^{2x-1} \Rightarrow (x+1)\log 6 = (2x-1)\log 4 \Rightarrow x\log 6 + \log 6 = 2x\log 4 - \log 4 \Rightarrow$

$x\log 6 - 2x\log 4 = -\log 6 - \log 4 \Rightarrow x(\log 6 - 2\log 4) = -\log 6 - \log 4 \Rightarrow x = \frac{-\log 6 - \log 4}{\log 6 - 2\log 4}$

(Other forms of the answer are possible.)

(b) From the calculator, the solution is $x \approx 3.240$.

19. (a) No real number value for x can produce a negative solution. Therefore, the solution set is $\emptyset$.

21. (a) $e^{x-3} = 2^{3x} \Rightarrow \ln e^{x-3} = \ln 2^{3x} \Rightarrow (x-3)\ln e = 3x \ln 2 \Rightarrow x - 3 = 3x \ln 2 \Rightarrow$

$x - 3x \ln 2 = 3 \Rightarrow x(1 - 3\ln 2) = 3 \Rightarrow x = \dfrac{3}{1 - 3\ln 2}$ (Other forms of the answer are possible.)

(b) From the calculator, the solution is $x \approx -2.779$.

23. (a) No real number value for x can produce a negative solution. Therefore, the solution set is $\emptyset$.

25. (a) $0.05(1.15)^x = 5 \Rightarrow \log 0.05 + \log(1.15)^x = \log 5 \Rightarrow x \log 1.15 = \log 5 - \log 0.05 \Rightarrow$

$x \log 1.15 = \log \dfrac{5}{0.05} \Rightarrow x \log 1.15 = \log 100 \Rightarrow x \log 1.15 = 2 \Rightarrow x = \dfrac{2}{\log 1.15}$

(Other forms of the answer are possible.)

(b) From the calculator, the solution is $x \approx 32.950$.

27. (a) $3(2)^{x-2} + 1 = 100 \Rightarrow 3(2)^{x-2} = 99 \Rightarrow \log 3 + \log 2^{x-2} = \log 99 \Rightarrow (x-2)\log 2 = \log 99 - \log 3 \Rightarrow$

$x \log 2 - 2\log 2 = \log 99 - \log 3 \Rightarrow x \log 2 = \log 99 - \log 3 + 2\log 2 \Rightarrow$

$x \log 2 = \log\left(\dfrac{99}{3}\right) + 2\log 2 \Rightarrow x = \dfrac{\log 33}{\log 2} + \dfrac{2\log 2}{\log 2} \Rightarrow x = 2 + \dfrac{\log 33}{\log 2}$

(Other forms of the answer are possible.)

(b) From the calculator, the solution is $x \approx 7.044$.

29. (a) $2(1.05)^x + 3 = 10 \Rightarrow 2(1.05)^x = 7 \Rightarrow \log 2 + \log 1.05^x = \log 7 \Rightarrow x \log 1.05 = \log 7 - \log 2 \Rightarrow$

$x \log 1.05 = \log\left(\dfrac{7}{2}\right) \Rightarrow x = \dfrac{\log 3.5}{\log 1.05}$. (Other forms of the answer are possible.)

(b) From the calculator, the solution is $x \approx 25.677$.

31. (a) $5(1.015)^{x-1980} = 8 \Rightarrow 1.015^{x-1980} = \dfrac{8}{5} \Rightarrow (x - 1980)\log 1.015 = \log 1.6 \Rightarrow$

$x - 1980 = \dfrac{\log 1.6}{\log 1.015} \Rightarrow x = 1980 + \dfrac{\log 1.6}{\log 1.015}$ (Other forms of the answer are possible.)

(b) From the calculator, the solution is $x \approx 2011.568$.

33. $5\ln x = 10 \Rightarrow \ln x = \dfrac{10}{5} \Rightarrow \ln x = 2 \Rightarrow e^{\ln x} = e^2 \Rightarrow x = e^2$

35. $\ln(4x) = 1.5 \Rightarrow e^{\ln 4x} = e^{1.5} \Rightarrow 4x = e^{1.5} \Rightarrow x = \dfrac{e^{1.5}}{4}$

37. $\log(2 - x) = 0.5 \Rightarrow 10^{\log(2-x)} = 10^{0.5} \Rightarrow 2 - x = \sqrt{10} \Rightarrow -x = \sqrt{10} - 2 \Rightarrow x = 2 - \sqrt{10}$

39. $\log_6(2x + 4) = 2 \Rightarrow 6^{\log_6(2x+4)} = 6^2 \Rightarrow 2x + 4 = 36 \Rightarrow 2x = 32 \Rightarrow x = 16$

41. $\log_4(x^3 + 37) = 3 \Rightarrow 4^{\log_4(x^3 - 37)} = 4^3 \Rightarrow x^3 + 37 = 64 \Rightarrow x^3 = 27 \Rightarrow \sqrt[3]{x^3} = \sqrt[3]{27} \Rightarrow x = 3$

43. $\ln x + \ln x^2 = 3 \Rightarrow \ln x(x^2) = 3 \Rightarrow \ln x^3 = 3 \Rightarrow e^{\ln x^3} = e^3 \Rightarrow x^3 = e^3 \Rightarrow \sqrt[3]{x^3} = \sqrt[3]{e^3} \Rightarrow x = e$

45. $2\ln(x-1)+30=34 \Rightarrow 2\ln(x-1)=4 \Rightarrow \ln(x-1)=2 \Rightarrow x-1=e^2 \Rightarrow x=e^2+1$

47. $5\log(x^2-1)+7=12 \Rightarrow 5\log(x^2-1)=5 \Rightarrow \log(x^2-1)=1 \Rightarrow x^2-1=10 \Rightarrow x^2=11 \Rightarrow x=\pm\sqrt{11}$

49. $3\log_2(3x^2+2)+1=2 \Rightarrow 3\log_2(3x^2+2)=1 \Rightarrow \log_2(3x^2+2)=\dfrac{1}{3} \Rightarrow 3x^2+2=2^{1/3} \Rightarrow x^2=\dfrac{2^{1/3}-2}{3} \Rightarrow x$ is $\emptyset$

51. $\log x + \log(x-21)=2 \Rightarrow \log x(x-21)=2 \Rightarrow \log(x^2-21x)=2 \Rightarrow 10^{\log(x^2-21x)}=10^2 \Rightarrow$

    $x^2-21x=100 \Rightarrow x^2-21x-100=0 \Rightarrow (x-25)(x+4)=0 \Rightarrow x=-4,\ 25$

    Since the argument of a logarithm can not be negative, the solution is $x=25$

53. $\ln(4x-2)-\ln 4 = -\ln(x-2) \Rightarrow \ln(4x-2)+\ln(x-2)=\ln 4 \Rightarrow \ln(4x-2)(x-2)=\ln 4 \Rightarrow$

    $\ln(4x^2-10x+4)=\ln 4 \Rightarrow e^{\ln(4x^2-10x+4)}=e^{\ln 4} \Rightarrow 4x^2-10x+4=4 \Rightarrow 4x^2-10x=0 \Rightarrow$

    $(2x)(2x-5)=0 \Rightarrow x=0,\ \dfrac{5}{2}$

    Since the argument of a logarithm cannot be zero, the solution is $x=2.5$.

55. $\log_5(x+2)+\log_5(x-2)=1 \Rightarrow \log_5(x+2)(x-2)=1 \Rightarrow \log_5(x^2-4)=1 \Rightarrow 5^{\log_5(x^2-4)}=5^1 \Rightarrow$

    $x^2-4=5 \Rightarrow x^2=9 \Rightarrow x=-3,\ 3$

    Since the argument of a logarithm cannot be negative, the solution is $x=3$.

57. $\log_7(4x)-\log_7(x+3)=\log_7 x \Rightarrow \log_7 4x = \log_7 x + \log_7(x+3) \Rightarrow \log_7 4x = \log_7 x(x+3) \Rightarrow$

    $\log_7 4x = \log_7(x^2+3x) \Rightarrow 7^{\log_7 4x} = 7^{\log_7(x^2+3x)} \Rightarrow 4x=x^2+3x \Rightarrow x^2-x=0 \Rightarrow x(x-1)=0 \Rightarrow x=0,\ 1$

    Since the argument of a logarithm can not be zero, the solution is $x=1$.

59. $\ln e^x - 2\ln e = \ln e^4 \Rightarrow x-2(1)=4 \Rightarrow x=6$

61. $\log x = \sqrt{\log x} \Rightarrow (\log x)^2 = (\sqrt{\log x})^2 \Rightarrow (\log x)^2 = \log x \Rightarrow (\log x)^2 - \log x = 0 \Rightarrow \log x(\log x - 1)=0$,

    then $\log x = 0 \Rightarrow x=1$ or $\log x - 1 = 0 \Rightarrow \log x = 1 \Rightarrow x=10$. The solution are $x=1,\ 10$.

63. (a) Graph on a calculator $y_1 = e^{-2\ln x}$ and $y_2 = \dfrac{1}{16}$. The graphs intersect at $x=4$.

    (b) From the graph, $e^{-2\ln x} < \dfrac{1}{16}$ for the interval $(4,\infty)$.

    (c) From the graph, $e^{-2\ln x} > \dfrac{1}{16}$ for the interval $(0,4)$.

65. The statement is incorrect. We must reject any solution that is not in the domain of any logarithmic function in the equation.

67. If $1.5^{\log x}=e^5$ then $1.5^{\log x}-e^5=0$. From a calculator graph of $y_1=1.5^{\log x}-e^5$, the x-intercept or solution is $x\approx 19.106$.

69. $r=p-k\ln t \Rightarrow r-p=-k\ln t \Rightarrow \dfrac{r-p}{-k}=\ln t \Rightarrow \ln t = \dfrac{p-r}{k} \Rightarrow e^{\ln t}=e^{(p-r)/k} \Rightarrow t=e^{(p-r)/k}$

71. $T = T_0 + (T_1 - T_0)10^{-kt} \Rightarrow T - T_0 = (T_1 - T_0)10^{-kt} \Rightarrow \dfrac{T - T_0}{T_1 - T_0} = 10^{-kt} \Rightarrow$

$\log\left(\dfrac{T - T_1}{T_1 - T_0}\right) = \log 10^{-kt} \Rightarrow \log\left(\dfrac{T - T_1}{T_1 - T_0}\right) = -kt \Rightarrow t = -\dfrac{1}{k}\log\left(\dfrac{T - T_1}{T_1 - T_0}\right)$

73. $A = T_0 + Ce^{-kt} \Rightarrow A - T_0 = Ce^{-kt} \Rightarrow \dfrac{A - T_0}{C} = e^{-kt} \Rightarrow \ln\left(\dfrac{A - T_0}{C}\right) = \ln e^{-kt} \Rightarrow$

$-kt = \ln\left(\dfrac{A - T_0}{C}\right) \Rightarrow k = \dfrac{\ln\left(\dfrac{A - T_0}{C}\right)}{-t}$

75. $y = A + B(1 - e^{-Cx}) \Rightarrow y = A + B - Be^{-Cx} \Rightarrow y - A - B = -Be^{-Cx} \Rightarrow \dfrac{-y + A + B}{B} = e^{-Cx} \Rightarrow$

$\ln\left(\dfrac{A + B - y}{B}\right) = \ln e^{-Cx} \Rightarrow \ln\left(\dfrac{A + B - y}{B}\right) = -Cx \Rightarrow x = -\dfrac{\ln\left(\dfrac{A + B - y}{B}\right)}{C}$

77. $\log A = \log B - C\log x \Rightarrow \log A = \log B - \log x^C \Rightarrow \log A = \log \dfrac{B}{x^C} \Rightarrow 10^{\log A} = 10^{\log(B/x^C)} \Rightarrow A = \dfrac{B}{x^C}$

79. $A = P\left(1 + \dfrac{r}{n}\right)^{nt} \Rightarrow \dfrac{A}{P} = \left(1 + \dfrac{r}{n}\right)^{nt} \log\left(\dfrac{A}{P}\right) = \log\left(1 + \dfrac{r}{n}\right)^{nt} \Rightarrow \log\left(\dfrac{A}{P}\right) = nt\log\left(1 + \dfrac{r}{n}\right) \Rightarrow t = \dfrac{\log\left(\dfrac{A}{P}\right)}{n\log\left(1 + \dfrac{r}{n}\right)}$

81. $e^{2x} - 6e^x + 8 = 0 \Rightarrow (e^x - 4)(e^x - 2) = 0 \Rightarrow (e^x - 4) = 0 \text{ or } (e^x - 2) = 0 \Rightarrow x = \{\ln 4, \ln 2\}$.

83. $2e^{2x} + e^x = 6 \Rightarrow 2e^{2x} + e^x - 6 = 0 \Rightarrow (2e^x - 3)(e^x + 2) = 0 \Rightarrow (2e^x - 3) = 0 \text{ or } (e^x + 2) = 0 \Rightarrow x = \{\ln \dfrac{3}{2}\}$.

85. $\dfrac{1}{2}e^{2x} + e^x = 1 \Rightarrow \dfrac{1}{2}e^{2x} + e^x - 1 = 0.$ Let $a = e^x \Rightarrow \dfrac{1}{2}a^2 + a - 1 = 0$ and use the quadratic formula to solve:

$a = \dfrac{-1 \pm \sqrt{1^2 - (4)(\frac{1}{2})(-1)}}{(2)(\frac{1}{2})} = \dfrac{-1 \pm \sqrt{1 + 2}}{1} = -1 \pm \sqrt{3} \Rightarrow a = \sqrt{3} - 1 \Rightarrow \sqrt{3} - 1 = e^x \Rightarrow x = \ln\left(\sqrt{3} - 1\right)$

87. $3^{2x} + 35 = 12(3^x) \Rightarrow 3^{2x} - 12(3^x) + 35 = 0 \Rightarrow (3^x - 7)(3^x - 5) = 0 \Rightarrow (3^x - 7) \text{ or } (3^x - 5) = 0 \Rightarrow$

$x = \{\log_3 7, \log_3 5\}$

89. $(\log_2 x)^2 + \log_2 x = 2 \Rightarrow (\log_2 x)^2 + \log_2 x - 2 = 0.$ Let $a = \log_2 x \Rightarrow a^2 + a - 2 = 0 \Rightarrow$

$(a + 2)(a - 1) = 0 \Rightarrow a = 1, -2.$ $1 = \log_2 x \Rightarrow x = 2 \text{ or } -2 = \log_2 x \Rightarrow x = \dfrac{1}{4} \Rightarrow x = \{2, \dfrac{1}{4}\}$.

91. $(\ln x)^2 + 16 = 10\ln x \Rightarrow (\ln x)^2 - 10\ln x + 16 = 0.$ Let $a = \ln x \Rightarrow a^2 - 10a + 16 = 0 \Rightarrow$

$(a - 8)(a - 2) = 0 \Rightarrow a = 8, 2.$ $8 = \ln x \Rightarrow x = e^8 \text{ or } 2 = \ln x \Rightarrow x = e^2 \Rightarrow x = \{e^8, e^2\}$

93. $-2e^x + 5 = 0 \Rightarrow -2e^x = -5 \Rightarrow e^x = \dfrac{5}{2} \Rightarrow x = \ln\dfrac{5}{2}$. From the graph $f(x) < 0$ when x is in the interval $\left(\ln\dfrac{5}{2}, \infty\right)$ and $f(x) \geq 0$ when x is in the interval $\left(-\infty, \ln\dfrac{5}{2}\right]$.

95. $2(3^x) - 18 = 0 \Rightarrow 2(3^x) = 18 \Rightarrow 3^x = 9 \Rightarrow x = 2$. From the graph $f(x) < 0$ when x is in the interval $(-\infty, 2)$ and $f(x) \geq 0$ when x is in the interval $[2, \infty)$.

97. $3^{2x} - 9^{x+1} = 0 \Rightarrow 3^{2x} = 9^{x+1} \Rightarrow 3^{2x} = 3^{2x+2} \Rightarrow 2x = 2x + 2 \Rightarrow$ No solution. From the graph $f(x) < 0$ when x is in the interval $(-\infty, \infty)$ and $f(x) \geq 0$ for no values of x.

99. $8 - 4\log_5(x) = 0 \Rightarrow 8 = 4\log_5(x) \Rightarrow 2 = \log_5(x) \Rightarrow x = 25$. From the graph $f(x) < 0$ when x is in the interval $(25, \infty)$ and $f(x) \geq 0$ for values of x in the interval $(0, 25]$.

101. $\ln(x+2) = 0 \Rightarrow x + 2 = 1 \Rightarrow x = -1$. From the graph $f(x) < 0$ when x is in the interval $(-2, -1)$ and $f(x) \geq 0$ for values of x in the interval $[-1, \infty)$.

103. $7 - 5\log x = 0 \Rightarrow 5\log x = 7 \Rightarrow \log x = \dfrac{7}{5} \Rightarrow x = 10^{7/5}$. From the graph $f(x) < 0$ when x is in the interval $\left(10^{7/5}, \infty\right)$ and $f(x) \geq 0$ for values of x in the interval $\left(0, 10^{7/5}\right]$.

105. For $x^2 = 2^x$, graph on a calculator $y_1 = x^2 - 2^x$. From the calculator, the x-intercepts or solutions are -0.767, 2, and 4.

107. For $\log x = x^2 - 8x + 14$, graph on a calculator $y_1 = \log x - x^2 + 8x - 14$, From the calculator the x-intercepts or solutions are 2.454 and 5.659.

109. For $e^x = \dfrac{1}{x+2}$, graph on a calculator $y_1 = e^x - \dfrac{1}{x+2}$. From the calculator, the x-intercept or solution is -0.443.

111. $\log_2 \sqrt{2x^2} - 1 = 0.5 \Rightarrow \log_2 \sqrt{2x^2} = 1.5 \Rightarrow 2^{\log_2 \sqrt{2x^2}} = 2^{3/2} \Rightarrow \sqrt{2x^2} = \sqrt{2^3} \Rightarrow$
$2x^2 = 2^3 \Rightarrow 2x^2 = 8 \Rightarrow x^2 = 4 \Rightarrow x = -2, 2.$

113. $\ln(\ln e^{-x}) = \ln 3 \Rightarrow \ln(-x) = \ln 3 \Rightarrow -x = 3 \Rightarrow x = -3$

115. If $y = 2$, then $2 = \dfrac{2 - \log(100 - x)}{0.42} \Rightarrow 2(0.42) = 2 - \log(100 - x) \Rightarrow$
$0.84 = 2 - \log(100 - x) \Rightarrow -1.16 = -\log(100 - x) \Rightarrow 1.16 = \log(100 - x) \Rightarrow$
$10^{1.16} = 10^{\log(100-x)} \Rightarrow 14.454398 \approx 100 - x \Rightarrow -85.5 \approx -x \Rightarrow x \approx 85.5\%$

117. If $f(x) = 33$, then $33 = 31.5 + 1.1\log(x+1) \Rightarrow 1.5 = 1.1\log(x+1) \Rightarrow \dfrac{1.5}{1.1} = \log(x+1) \Rightarrow$
$10^{1.5/1.1} = 10^{\log(x+1)} \Rightarrow 23.1013 \approx x + 1 \Rightarrow x \approx 22.1013 \Rightarrow x \approx 22$.

Reviewing Basic Concepts (Sections 5.4 and 5.5)

1. If $f(x) = 3^x$ and $f(x) \approx 10.98(1.14)^x$ then f and g are inverse functions, and their graphs are symmetric with respect to the line with equation $y = x$. The domain of f is the range of g and vice versa.

2. See Figure 2.

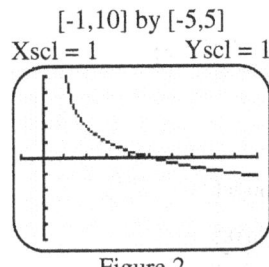

[-1,10] by [-5,5]
Xscl = 1   Yscl = 1

Figure 2

3. From the graph, the asymptote is $x = 5$ the x-intercept is $(5, 0)$; and there is no y-intercept.

4. The graph of $f(x)$ is the same as the graph of $g(x)$, reflected across the x-axis, shifted 1 unit to the right, and shifted two units upward.

5. For $f(x) = 2 - \log_2(x-1)$, the inverse is determined by interchanging x and y:

$$x = 2 - \log_2(y-1) \Rightarrow x - 2 = -\log_2(y-1) \Rightarrow 2 - x = \log_2(y-1) \Rightarrow 2^{(2-x)} = 2^{\log(y-1)} \Rightarrow$$

$$2^{(2-x)} = y - 1 \Rightarrow y = 1 + 2^{(2-x)} \Rightarrow f^{-1}(x) = 1 + 2^{2-x}$$

6. $3^{2x-1} = 4^x \Rightarrow \log 3^{2x-1} = \log 4^x \Rightarrow (2x-1)\log 3 = x \log 4 \Rightarrow 2x \log 3 - \log 3 = x \log 4 \Rightarrow$

$$2x \log 3 - x \log 4 = \log 3 \Rightarrow x(2\log 3 - \log 4) = \log 3 \Rightarrow x = \frac{\log 3}{2\log 3 - \log 4} = \frac{\log 3}{\log \frac{9}{4}}$$

7. $\ln 5x - \ln(x+2) = \ln 3 \Rightarrow \ln\left(\frac{5x}{x+2}\right) = \ln 3 \Rightarrow \frac{5x}{x+2} = 3 \Rightarrow 3(x+2) = 5x \Rightarrow 3x + 6 = 5x \Rightarrow 6 = 2x \Rightarrow x = 3$

8. $10^{5\log x} = 32 \Rightarrow \log 10^{5\log x} = \log 32 \Rightarrow 5\log x = \log 32 \Rightarrow \log x^5 = \log 32 \Rightarrow x^5 = 32 \Rightarrow x = 2$

9. $H = 1000(1 - e^{-kn}) \Rightarrow \frac{H}{1000} = 1 - e^{-kN} \Rightarrow 1 - \frac{H}{1000} = e^{-kN} \Rightarrow \ln\left(1 - \frac{H}{100}\right) = \ln e^{-kN} \Rightarrow$

$$\ln\left(1 - \frac{H}{1000}\right) = -kN \Rightarrow N = -\frac{1}{k}\ln\left(1 - \frac{H}{1000}\right)$$

10. If $f(x) = 2300$, then $2300 = 280\ln(x+1) + 1925 \Rightarrow 375 = 280\ln(x+1) \Rightarrow$

$$e^{375/280} = e^{\ln(x+1)} \Rightarrow e^{375/280} = x + 1 \Rightarrow x = e^{375/280} - 1 \Rightarrow x \approx 2.8 \text{ acres}$$

5.6: Further Applications & Modeling with Exponential & Logarithmic Functions

1. Using the given function, $\frac{1}{3}A_0 = A_0 e^{-0.0001216t} \Rightarrow \frac{1}{3} = e^{-0.0001216t} \Rightarrow \ln\frac{1}{3} = \ln e^{-0.0001216t} \Rightarrow$

   $\ln\frac{1}{3} = -0.0001216t \Rightarrow t = \dfrac{\ln\left(\frac{1}{3}\right)}{-0.0001216} \Rightarrow t \approx 9034.6 \approx 9{,}000$ years ago.

3. Using the given function, $0.15 A_0 = A_0 e^{-0.0001216t} \Rightarrow 0.15 = e^{-0.0001216t} \Rightarrow \ln 0.15 = \ln e^{-0.0001216t} \Rightarrow$

   $\ln 0.15 = -0.0001216t \Rightarrow t = \dfrac{\ln(0.15)}{-0.0001216} \Rightarrow t \approx 15601.3 \approx 16{,}000$ years old.

5. (a) With a half-life of 21.7 years and using the exponential decay function, our model is

   $\frac{1}{2} A_0 = A_0 e^{-21.7k} \Rightarrow 0.5 = e^{-21.7k} \Rightarrow \ln 0.5 = \ln e^{-21.7k} \Rightarrow \ln 0.5 = -21.7k \Rightarrow k = \dfrac{\ln 0.5}{-21.7}$

   $k \approx 0.032$. The exponential decay model is $A(t) = A_0 e^{-0.032t}$.

   (b) $400 = 500 e^{-0.032t} \Rightarrow \dfrac{400}{500} = e^{-0.032t} \Rightarrow \ln 0.8 = \ln e^{-0.032t} \Rightarrow \ln 0.8 = -0.032t \Rightarrow \dfrac{\ln 0.8}{-0.032} = t \Rightarrow t \approx 6.97$ yr.

   (c) $A(10) = 500 e^{-0.032(10)} \Rightarrow A(10) = 500 e^{-0.32} \Rightarrow A(10) \approx 363$ grams.

7. (a) Since the amount remaining is less than half of the original 2 milligrams, the half-life is less than 200 days.

   (b) Using the exponential decay function, $A_0 = 2$, and the ordered pair $(100, 1.22)$ from the table, yields the formula: $1.22 = 2e^{-100k} \Rightarrow 0.61 = e^{-100k} \Rightarrow \ln 0.61 = \ln e^{-100k} \Rightarrow$

   $\ln 0.61 = -100k \Rightarrow k = \dfrac{\ln 0.61}{100} \Rightarrow k \approx .005$. The formula that models the data is $A = 2e^{-0.005t}$.

   (c) Graph $y_1 = 2e^{-0.005t}$ and $y_2 = 1$ on the calculator. The intersection of the graphs is the approximate half-life: 140 days.

9. (a) $R(x) = \log \dfrac{I}{I_0} \Rightarrow 7.4 = \log \dfrac{I}{I_0} \Rightarrow \dfrac{I}{I_0} = 10^{7.4} \Rightarrow I = 10^{7.4} I_0 \approx 25{,}118{,}864 I_0$

   (b) $R(x) = \log \dfrac{I}{I_0} \Rightarrow 6.3 = \log \dfrac{I}{I_0} \Rightarrow \dfrac{I}{I_0} = 10^{6.3} \Rightarrow I = 10^{6.3} I_0 \approx 1{,}995{,}262 I_0$

   (c) $\dfrac{10^{7.4}}{10^{6.3}} = 10^{1.1} \approx 12.6$ times more intense.

11. Use the equation to find the intensity of a star magnitude 1:

    $1 = 6 - \dfrac{5}{2}\log \dfrac{I}{I_0} \Rightarrow -5 = -\dfrac{5}{2}\log \dfrac{I}{I_0} \Rightarrow \log \dfrac{I}{I_0} \Rightarrow 10^2 = 10^{\log I/I_0} \Rightarrow 100 = \dfrac{I}{I_0} \Rightarrow I = 100 I_0$. Now use the equation to find the intensity of a star magnitude 3:

$3 = 6 - \frac{5}{2}\log\frac{I}{I_0} \Rightarrow -3 = -\frac{5}{2}\log\frac{I}{I_0} \Rightarrow \frac{6}{5} = \log\frac{I}{I_0} \Rightarrow 10^{6/5} = 10^{\log I/I_0} \Rightarrow 10^{6/5} = \frac{I}{I_0} \Rightarrow I \approx 15.85 I_0$. Comparing

intensities of the magnitude 1 star to the magnitude 3 star yields $\frac{100 I_0}{15.85 I_0} \approx 6.31$. The magnitude 1 star is

approximately 6.3 times more intense then the magnitude 3 star.

13. (a) First solve for k, using $f(x) = 60, T_0 = 20, t = 1 C = 100 - 20 = 80; 60 = 20 + 80e^{-k(1)} \Rightarrow$

$40 = 80e^{-k} \Rightarrow 0.5 = e^{-k} \Rightarrow \ln 0.5 = \ln e^{-k} \Rightarrow \ln 0.5 = -k \Rightarrow k = -\ln 0.5 \Rightarrow k \approx 0.693$. The equation

is $f(t) = 20 + 80x^{-0.693t}$.

(b) $f(0.5) = 20 + 80e^{-0.693(0.5)} \Rightarrow f(0.5) \approx 76.6°C$.

(c) Solve for t, with $f(t) = 50, 50 = 20 + 80e^{-0.693t} \Rightarrow 30 = 80e^{-0.69et} \Rightarrow \frac{30}{80} = e^{-0.693t} \Rightarrow$

$\ln 0.375 = \ln e^{-0.693t} \Rightarrow \ln 0.375 = -0.693t \Rightarrow t = \frac{\ln 0.375}{-0.693} \Rightarrow t \approx 1.415$ or about 1 hour 25 minutes.

15. (a) Set $L_1 \to$ Year and $L_2 \to$ CFC 12(ppb) and use the exponential regression capabilities of the calculator

to find the equation: $y \approx 0.72(1.041)^x$. Therefore the values are $C \approx 0.72$ and $a \approx 1.041$.

(b) Use the equation from part a, to find $f(13): f(13) = 0.72(1.041)^{13} \Rightarrow f(13) \approx 1.21$.

17. (a) $A(3) = 1000(1.025)^3 = \$1076.89$

(b) $A(10) = 1000(1.025)^{10} = \$1280.08$

(c) $1900 = 1000(1.025)^x \Rightarrow 1.9 = 1.025^x \Rightarrow \ln(1.9) = x \ln 1.025 \Rightarrow x = \frac{\ln 1.9}{\ln 1.025} \approx 26$ years

19. (a) $B(1) = 3.5e^{0.02(1)} \approx 3.57$ million/mL

(b) $B(6.5) = 3.5e^{0.02(6.5)} \approx 3.99$ million/mL

(c) $3.5e^{0.02x} = 6 \Rightarrow e^{0.02x} = \frac{12}{7} \Rightarrow 0.02x = \ln\frac{12}{7} \Rightarrow x = \frac{\ln 12/7}{0.02} \approx 27$ hours

21. $3000 = 2500e^{0.0375t} \Rightarrow e^{0.0375t} = 1.2 \Rightarrow 0.0375t = \ln 1.2 \Rightarrow t = \frac{\ln 1.2}{0.0375} \approx 4.9$ years

23. $5000 = 2500e^{0.05t} \Rightarrow e^{0.05t} = 2 \Rightarrow 0.05t = \ln 2 \Rightarrow t = \frac{\ln 2}{0.05} \approx 13.9$ years

25. (a) The domain for this scenario would be $A \geq 1000$. The amount in the account must always be greater than or equal to the principal.

(b) $T(1200) = 50 \ln \frac{1200}{1000} \approx 9.1$ years

(c) $50 \ln \frac{A}{1000} = 23.5 \Rightarrow \ln \frac{A}{1000} = \frac{23.5}{50} \Rightarrow e^{23.5/50} = \frac{A}{1000} \Rightarrow A = 1000 e^{23.5/50} \approx \$1600$

27. (a) Use the Compound Interest Formula

238   CHAPTER 5   Inverse, Exponential, and Logarithmic Functions

$$A = P\left(1+\frac{r}{n}\right)^{nt}, \quad 5000 = 1000\left(1+\frac{0.035}{4}\right)^{4t} \Rightarrow 5 = 1.00875^{4t} \Rightarrow \log 5 = \log 1.00875^{4t} \Rightarrow$$

$$t = \frac{\log 5}{4\log 1.00785} \Rightarrow \approx 46.2 \text{ years.}$$

(b) Use the Continuous Compound Interest Formula

$$A = Pe^{rt}, \quad 5000 = 1000e^{0.035t} \Rightarrow 5 = e^{0.035t} \Rightarrow \ln 5 = \ln e^{0.035t} \Rightarrow \ln 5 = 0.035t \Rightarrow$$

$$t = \frac{\ln 5}{0.035} \Rightarrow t \approx 46.0 \text{ years.}$$

29. Use the Compound Interest Formula

$$A = P\left(1+\frac{r}{n}\right)^{nt}, \quad 30000 = 27000\left(1+\frac{0.023}{4}\right)^{4t} \Rightarrow \frac{30000}{27000} = 1.00575^{4t} \Rightarrow \frac{10}{9} = 1.00575^{4t} \Rightarrow$$

$$\log\frac{10}{9} = \log 1.00575^{4t} \Rightarrow \log\frac{10}{9} = 4t \cdot \log 1.00575 \Rightarrow t = \frac{\log\frac{10}{9}}{4\log 1.00575} \Rightarrow t \approx 4.6 \text{ years.}$$

31. Use the Compound Interest Formula

$$A = P\left(1+\frac{r}{n}\right)^{nt}, \quad A = 60000\left(1+\frac{0.02}{4}\right)^{4(5)} \Rightarrow A = 60000(1.005)^{20} \Rightarrow A = \$66293.73$$

Now use the Continuous Compound Interest Formula $A = Pe^{rt}$, $A = 60000e^{0.018(5)} \Rightarrow A \approx \$65650.48$
The better investment is the 2% rate compounded quarterly; it will earn $643.27 more.

33. $R = \left(1+\frac{0.03}{4}\right)^{4} - 1 \Rightarrow R \approx 1.075^4 - 1 \Rightarrow R \approx 0.030339$ or $R \approx 3.03\%$.

35. $P = 10,000\left(1+\frac{0.03}{2}\right)^{-2(5)} \Rightarrow P = 10,000(1.015)^{-10} \Rightarrow P = \$8616.67.$

37. $25000 = 30416\left(1+\frac{r}{1}\right)^{-1(5)} \Rightarrow \frac{25000}{30416} = (1+r)^{-5} \Rightarrow \left(\frac{25000}{30416}\right)^{-1/5} = 1+r \Rightarrow r \approx 0.03993$ or about 4%.

39. (a) Using $R = \dfrac{P}{\dfrac{1-(1+i)^{-n}}{i}}$, and $n = 12(4) = 48$, $i = \dfrac{0.075}{12} = 0.00625$ yields

$$R = \frac{8500}{\frac{1-(1+0.00625)^{-48}}{0.00625}} \Rightarrow R \approx \$205.52.$$

(b) The total interest paid will be $I = nR - P \Rightarrow I = 48(205.52) - 8500 \Rightarrow I \approx \$1364.96.$

41. (a) Using $R = \dfrac{P}{\dfrac{1-(1+i)^{-n}}{i}}$, and $n = 12(30) = 360$, $i = \dfrac{0.0725}{12}$ yields

$$R = \frac{125000}{\frac{1-(1+0.0725/12)^{-360}}{0.0725/12}} \Rightarrow R \approx \$852.72.$$

(b) The total interest paid will be $I = nR - P \Rightarrow I = 360(852.72) - 125000 \Rightarrow I \approx \$181,979.20.$

Section 5.6   239

43. (a) First enter $y_1 = 1500\left(1 + \dfrac{0.0575}{365}\right)^{365t}$ into the calculator, now using the table feature, the investment will triple when $y_1 = 4500$. From the table, $t \approx 19.1078 \Rightarrow t \approx 19$ years $+ 0.1078(365)$ days $\Rightarrow t \approx 19$ years, 39 days. Analytically, for $y = 4500$, the solution is

$$4500 = 1500\left(1 + \dfrac{0.0575}{365}\right)^{365t} \Rightarrow 3 = (1.000157534)^{365t} \Rightarrow \ln 3 = 365t \ln 1.000157534$$

$$\Rightarrow t = \dfrac{\ln 3}{365 \ln 1.000157534} \Rightarrow t \approx 19.1078 \text{ or 19 years and 39 days.}$$

(b) First enter $y_1 = 2000\left(1 + \dfrac{0.08}{365}\right)^{365t}$ into the calculator, now using the table feature, the investment will triple when $y_1 = 2000$. From the table, $t \approx 11.455 \Rightarrow t \approx 11$ years $+ 0.455(365)$ days $\Rightarrow t \approx 11$ years 166 days.

45. (a) $A(5) = 2,400,000 e^{0.023(5)} \Rightarrow A(5) \approx 2,692,496 \Rightarrow A(5) \approx 2,700,000.$

(b) $A(10) = 2,400,000 e^{0.023(5)} \Rightarrow A(10) \approx 3,020,640 \Rightarrow A(10) \approx 3,000,000.$

(c) $A(60) = 2,400,000 e^{0.023(5)} \Rightarrow A(60) \approx 9,539,764 \Rightarrow A(60) \approx 9,500,000.$

47. (a) $42(2)^x = 400 \Rightarrow 2^x = \dfrac{200}{21} \Rightarrow x \ln 2 = \ln \dfrac{200}{21} \Rightarrow x = \dfrac{\ln 200/21}{\ln 2} \approx 3.25$, The result is in the third year.

(b) See Figure 47.

(c) $42(2)^x = 1000 \Rightarrow 2^x = \dfrac{500}{21} \Rightarrow x \ln 2 = \ln \dfrac{500}{21} \Rightarrow x = \dfrac{\ln 500/21}{\ln 2} \approx 4.57$, The result is in the fourth year.

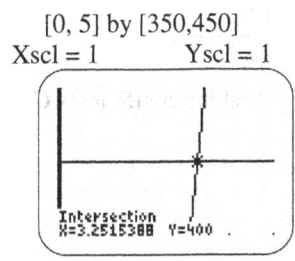

Figure 47

49. (a) Use the coordinate (2012, 17) to find the coefficient C: $17 = Ca^{(2012-2012)} \Rightarrow 17 = Ca^0 \Rightarrow 17 = C$,

Use (2060, 31) and $C = 17$ to find a: $31 = 17a^{(2060-2012)} \Rightarrow 31 = 17a^{48} \Rightarrow a^{48} = \dfrac{31}{17} \Rightarrow a = \sqrt[48]{\dfrac{31}{17}} \approx 1.0126$

The value of a is greater than or equal to one since the percentage is increasing.

(b) $P(2030) = 17(1.0126)^{2030-2012} = 17(1.0126)^{18} \approx 21.3\%$

(c) $17(1.0126)^{x-2012} = 25 \Rightarrow 1.0126^{x-2012} = \dfrac{25}{17} \Rightarrow (x-2012)\ln 1.0126 = \ln \dfrac{25}{17} \Rightarrow$

$x - 2012 = \dfrac{\ln \dfrac{25}{17}}{\ln 1.0126} \Rightarrow x = \dfrac{\ln \dfrac{25}{17}}{\ln 1.0126} + 2012 \approx 2042.8$

51. $N(t) = 100,000e^{rt} \Rightarrow 200,000 = 100,000e^{r(2)} \Rightarrow 2 = e^{r(2)} \Rightarrow \ln 2 = 2r \Rightarrow r = \dfrac{\ln 2}{2} \Rightarrow r \approx 0.3466$.

$350,000 = 100,000e^{0.3466t} \Rightarrow 3.5 = e^{0.3466t} \Rightarrow \ln 3.5 = 0.3466t \Rightarrow t = \dfrac{\ln 3.5}{0.3466} \Rightarrow t \approx 3.6$ hours.

53. Since x represents the number of years after 1980, we will use the coordinate (0, 30) to find the coefficient C: $30 = Ca^0 \Rightarrow 30 = C$, The cost for each year after 1980 was 75% of the year prior and we have the coordinate (1, 22.5): $22.5 = 30a^{(1)} \Rightarrow 22.5 = 30a \Rightarrow a = \dfrac{22.5}{30} \Rightarrow a = 0.75$

The function is $f(x) = 30(0.75)^x$. Let $f(x) = 1$ to find the year when the price was $1.

$30(0.75)^x = 1 \Rightarrow 0.75^x = \dfrac{1}{30} \Rightarrow x \ln 0.75 = \ln \dfrac{1}{30} \Rightarrow x = \dfrac{\ln \dfrac{1}{30}}{\ln 0.75} \approx 11.8$, Since x represents the number of years after 1980, the result is about 1992.

55. (a)

X	0	15	30	45	60	75	90	125
G(x)	7	21	57	111	136	158	164	178

(b) Since there are 261 people in the village the equation is $g(x) = 261 - f(x)$.

(c) Graph the data on the same calculator graph as $y_1 = \dfrac{171}{1+18.6e^{-0.0747x}}$ and $y_2 = 18.3(1.024)^x$.

From the graph, y_1 is the better fit.

(d) Using $g(x) = 261 - f(x)$ and $g(x) = \dfrac{171}{1+18.6e^{-0.0747x}}$ yields $f(x) = 261 - \dfrac{171}{1+18.6e^{-0.0747x}}$.

57. (a) Use the capabilities of the exponential regression calculator and L_1 and L_2, to find the coefficients C and a: $C \approx 5.772$, $a \approx 1.277 \Rightarrow f(x) = 5.772(1.277)^{x-2008}$

(b) See Figure 57.

[2005,2015] by [2,20]

Xscl = 1   Yscl = 1

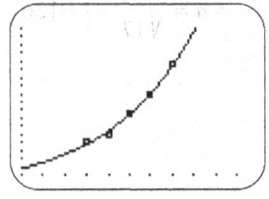

Figure 57

59. (a) $f(25) = \dfrac{9}{1+271e^{-0.122(25)}} \Rightarrow f(25) \approx 0.065$; and $f(65) = \dfrac{9}{1+271e^{-0.122(25)}} \Rightarrow f(65) \approx 0.82$. Among people age 25, 6.5% have some CHD, while among people age 65, 82% have some CHD.

(b) $0.50 = \dfrac{0.9}{1+271e^{-0.122x}} \Rightarrow 0.5(1+271e^{-0.122x}) = 0.9 \Rightarrow 1+271e^{-0.122x} = \dfrac{0.9}{0.5} \Rightarrow$

$271e^{-0.122x} = \dfrac{0.9}{0.5} - 1 \Rightarrow e^{-0.122x} = \dfrac{\frac{0.9}{0.5}-1}{271} \Rightarrow \ln e^{-0.122x} = \ln\left(\dfrac{\frac{0.9}{0.5}-1}{271}\right) \Rightarrow$

$-0.122x = \ln\left(\dfrac{\frac{0.9}{0.5}-1}{271}\right) \Rightarrow x = \dfrac{\ln\left(\dfrac{\frac{0.9}{0.5}-1}{271}\right)}{-0.122} \Rightarrow x \approx 47.75$. The likelihood is 50% at about age 48.

Summary Exercises on Functions: Domains and Defining Equations and Composition

1. Choice A can be written as a function of x. $3x+2y=6 \Rightarrow y = f(x) = -\frac{3}{2}x+3$

3. Choice C can be written as a function of x. $x^3+y^3=5 \Rightarrow y = f(x) = \sqrt[3]{5-x^3}$

5. Choice A can be written as a function of x. $x = \frac{2-y}{y+3} \Rightarrow y = f(x) = \frac{2-3x}{x+1}$

7. Choice D can be written as a function of x. $2x = \frac{1}{y^3} \Rightarrow y = f(x) = \sqrt[3]{\frac{1}{2x}}$

9. Choice C can be written as a function of x. $\frac{x}{4} - \frac{y}{9} = 0 \Rightarrow y = f(x) = \frac{9x}{4}$

11. Domain: $(-\infty, \infty)$

13. Domain: $(-\infty, \infty)$

15. Domain: $(-\infty, \infty)$ The domain is the set of all real numbers that make the denominator not equal to zero.

17. Domain: $(-\infty, -3) \cup (-3, 3) \cup (3, \infty)$ The domain is the set of all real numbers that make the denominator not equal to zero.

19. Domain: $(-4, 4)$ The domain is the set of all real numbers that make $16 - x^2 > 0$.

21. Domain: $(-\infty, -1] \cup [8, \infty)$ The domain is the set of all real numbers that make $x^2 - 7x - 8 \geq 0$.

242 CHAPTER 5 Inverse, Exponential, and Logarithmic Functions

Interval	Test Point	Value of x^2-7x-8	Sign of x^2-7x-8
$(-\infty, -1)$	-2	10	Positive
$(-1, 8)$	0	-8	Negative
$(8, \infty)$	10	22	Positive

23. Domain: $(-\infty, \infty)$ The domain is the set of all real numbers that make the denominator not equal to zero.

25. Domain: $[1, \infty)$ The domain is the set of all real numbers that make $x^3 - 1 \geq 0$.

27. Domain: $(-\infty, \infty)$ The domain is the set of all real numbers that make $x^2 + x + 4$ a real number.

29. Domain: $(-\infty, 1)$ The domain is the set of all real numbers that make the denominator not equal to zero or $\dfrac{-1}{x^3-1} \geq 0$.

Interval	Test Point	Value of $\frac{-1}{x^3-1}$	Sign of $\frac{-1}{x^3-1}$
$(-\infty, 1)$	0	1	Positive
$(1, \infty)$	2	$-\frac{1}{7}$	Negative

31. Domain: $(-\infty, \infty)$ The domain is the set of all real numbers that make $x^2 + 1 > 0$.

33. Domain: $(-\infty, -2) \cup (-2, 3) \cup (3, \infty)$ Since $\left(\dfrac{x+2}{x-3}\right)^2 \geq 0$ for all real numbers, the domain of $f(x)$ is the set of all real numbers such that $\dfrac{x+2}{x-3} \neq 0$.

35. Domain: $(-\infty, 0) \cup (0, \infty)$ The domain is the set of all real numbers such that $\dfrac{1}{x}$ is defined.

37. Domain: $(-\infty, \infty)$

39. Domain: $[-2, 2]$ The domain is the set of all real numbers such that $16 - x^4 \geq 0$.

Interval	Test Point	Value of $16-x^4$	Sign of $16-x^4$
$(-\infty, -2)$	-3	-65	Negative
$(-2, 2)$	0	16	Positive
$(2, \infty)$	3	-65	Negative

41. Domain: $(-\infty, -7] \cup (-4, 3) \cup [9, \infty)$ The domain is the set of real numbers such that $\frac{x^2-2x-63}{x^2+x-12} \geq 0$.

$\frac{x^2-2x-63}{x^2+x-12}$ is not defined for $x^2+x-12=0 \Rightarrow (x+4)(x-3)=0 \Rightarrow x \neq -4$ or $x \neq 3$. Solve $\frac{x^2-2x-63}{x^2+x-12}=0$

to find the test intervals: $\frac{x^2-2x-63}{x^2+x-12}=0 \Rightarrow x^2-2x-63=0 \Rightarrow (x-9)(x+7)=0 \Rightarrow x=9$ or $x=-7$.

Interval	Test Point	Value of $\frac{x^2-2x-63}{x^2+x-12}$	Sign
$(-\infty, -7)$	-10	$\frac{19}{26}$	Positive
$(-7, -4)$	-5	$-\frac{7}{2}$	Negative
$(-4, 3)$	0	$\frac{21}{4}$	Positive
$(3, 9)$	5	$-\frac{8}{3}$	Negative
$(9, \infty)$	10	$\frac{17}{98}$	Positive

43. Domain: $(-\infty, 5]$ The domain is the set of real numbers such that $5-x \geq 0 \Rightarrow 5 \geq x$

45. Domain: $(-\infty, 4) \cup (4, \infty)$ The domain is the set of real numbers such that

$\left|\frac{1}{4-x}\right| > 0 \Rightarrow \frac{1}{4-x} > 0 \Rightarrow 4-x > 0 \Rightarrow 4 > x$ or $-\frac{1}{4-x} < 0 \Rightarrow -4+x < 0 \Rightarrow x < 4$

47. Domain: $(-\infty, -5] \cup [5, \infty)$ The domain is the set of real numbers such that $\sqrt{x^2-25}$ is a real number.
$x^2-25 \geq 0 \Rightarrow x^2 \geq 25 \Rightarrow x \geq 5$ or $x \leq -5$

49. Domain: $(-2, 6)$ The domain is the set of real numbers such that $\frac{-3}{(x+2)(x-6)} > 0$ and $(x+2)(x-6) \neq 0 \Rightarrow$
$x \neq -2$ or $x \neq 6$.

Interval	Test Point	Value of $\frac{-3}{(x+2)(x-6)}$	Sign of $\frac{-3}{(x+2)(x-6)}$
$(-\infty, -2)$	-3	$-\frac{1}{3}$	Negative
$(-2, 6)$	0	$\frac{1}{4}$	Positive
$(6, \infty)$	7	$-\frac{1}{3}$	Negative

51. (a) $(f \circ g)(x) = f(g(x)) = f(5x+7) = -6(5x+7)+9 = -30x-42+9 = -30x-33$

    The domain and range of both f and g are $(-\infty, \infty)$, so the domain of $f \circ g$ is $(-\infty, \infty)$.

    (b) $(g \circ f)(x) = g(f(x)) = g(-6x+9) = 5(-6x+9)+7 = -30x+45+7 = -30x+52$

    The domain of $g \circ f$ is $(-\infty, \infty)$.

53. (a) $(f \circ g)(x) = f(g(x)) = f(x+3) = \sqrt{x+3}$ The domain and range of g are $(-\infty, \infty)$, however, the domain and range of f are $[0, \infty)$. So, $x+3 \geq 0 \Rightarrow x \geq -3$. Therefore, the domain of $f \circ g$ is $[-3, \infty)$.

    (b) $(g \circ f)(x) = g(f(x)) = g(\sqrt{x}) = \sqrt{x}+3$ The domain and range of g are $(-\infty, \infty)$, however, the domain and range of f are $[0, \infty)$. Therefore, the domain of $g \circ f$ is $[0, \infty)$.

55. (a) $(f \circ g)(x) = f(g(x)) = f(x^2+3x-1) = (x^2+3x-1)^3$

    The domain and range of f and g are $(-\infty, \infty)$, so the domain of $f \circ g$ is $(-\infty, \infty)$.

    (b) $(g \circ f)(x) = g(f(x)) = g(x^3) = (x^3)^2 + 3(x^3) - 1 = x^6 + 3x^3 - 1$

    The domain and range of f and g are $(-\infty, \infty)$, so the domain of $g \circ f$ is $(-\infty, \infty)$.

57. (a) $(f \circ g)(x) = f(g(x)) = f(3x) = \sqrt{3x-1}$ The domain and range of g are $(-\infty, \infty)$, however, the domain and range of f are $[1, \infty)$. So, $3x-1 \geq 0 \Rightarrow x \geq \frac{1}{3}$. Therefore, the domain of $f \circ g$ is $\left[\frac{1}{3}, \infty\right)$.

    (b) $(g \circ f)(x) = g(f(x)) = g(\sqrt{x-1}) = 3\sqrt{x-1}$ The domain and range of g are $(-\infty, \infty)$, however, the range of f is $[0, \infty)$. So $x-1 \geq 0 \Rightarrow x \geq 1$. Therefore, the domain of $g \circ f$ is $[1, \infty)$.

59. (a) $(f \circ g)(x) = f(g(x)) = f(x+1) = \frac{2}{x+1}$ The domain and range of g are $(-\infty, \infty)$, however, the domain of f is $(-\infty, 0) \cup (0, \infty)$. So, $x+1 \neq 0 \Rightarrow x \neq -1$. Therefore, the domain of $f \circ g$ is $(-\infty, -1) \cup (-1, \infty)$.

(b) $(g \circ f)(x) = g(f(x)) = g\left(\frac{2}{x}\right) = \frac{2}{x} + 1$ The domain and range of f is $(-\infty, 0) \cup (0, \infty)$, however, the domain and range of g are $(-\infty, \infty)$. So $x \neq 0$. Therefore, the domain of $g \circ f$ is $(-\infty, 0) \cup (0, \infty)$.

61. (a) $(f \circ g)(x) = f(g(x)) = f\left(-\frac{1}{x}\right) = \sqrt{-\frac{1}{x} + 2}$ The domain and range of g are $(-\infty, 0) \cup (0, \infty)$, however, the domain of f is $[-2, \infty)$. So, $-\frac{1}{x} + 2 \geq 0 \Rightarrow x < 0$ or $x \geq \frac{1}{2}$ (using test intervals). Therefore, the domain of $f \circ g$ is $(-\infty, 0) \cup \left[\frac{1}{2}, \infty\right)$.

(b) $(g \circ f)(x) = g(f(x)) = g\left(\sqrt{x+2}\right) = -\frac{1}{\sqrt{x+2}}$ The domain of f is $[-2, \infty)$ and its range is $(-\infty, \infty)$. The domain and range of g are $(-\infty, 0) \cup (0, \infty)$. So $x + 2 > 0 \Rightarrow x > -2$. Therefore, the domain of $g \circ f$ is $(-2, \infty)$.

63. (a) $(f \circ g)(x) = f(g(x)) = f\left(\frac{1}{x+5}\right) = \sqrt{\frac{1}{x+5}}$ The domain of g is $(-\infty, -5) \cup (-5, \infty)$, and the range of g is $(-\infty, 0) \cup (0, \infty)$. The domain of f is $[0, \infty)$. Therefore, the domain of $f \circ g$ is $(-5, \infty)$.

(b) $(g \circ f)(x) = g(f(x)) = g\left(\sqrt{x}\right) = \frac{1}{\sqrt{x}+5}$ The domain and range of f is $[0, \infty)$. The domain of g is $(-\infty, -5) \cup (-5, \infty)$. Therefore, the domain of $g \circ f$ is $[0, \infty)$.

65. (a) $(f \circ g)(x) = f(g(x)) = f\left(\frac{1}{x}\right) = \frac{1}{1/x - 2} = \frac{x}{1-2x}$ The domain and range of g are $(-\infty, 0) \cup (0, \infty)$. The domain of f is $(-\infty, -2) \cup (-2, \infty)$, and the range of f is $(-\infty, 0) \cup (0, \infty)$. So, $\frac{x}{1-2x} < 0 \Rightarrow x < 0$ or $0 < x < \frac{1}{2}$ or $x > \frac{1}{2}$ (using test intervals). Thus, $x \neq 0$ and $x \neq \frac{1}{2}$. Therefore, the domain of $f \circ g$ is $(-\infty, 0) \cup \left(0, \frac{1}{2}\right) \cup \left(\frac{1}{2}, \infty\right)$.

(b) $(g \circ f)(x) = g(f(x)) = g\left(\frac{1}{x-2}\right) = \frac{1}{1/(x-2)} = x - 2$ The domain and range of g are $(-\infty, 0) \cup (0, \infty)$. The domain of f is $(-\infty, -2) \cup (-2, \infty)$, and the range of f is $(-\infty, 0) \cup (0, \infty)$. Therefore, the domain of $g \circ f$ is $(-\infty, -2) \cup (-2, \infty)$.

67. (a) $(f \circ g)(x) = f(g(x)) = f\left(\sqrt{x}\right) = \log\left(\sqrt{x}\right)$ The domain of g is $(-\infty, \infty)$ and range of g is $[0, \infty)$. The domain of f is $(0, \infty)$, and the range of f is $(-\infty, \infty)$. So the domain of $f \circ g$ is $(0, \infty)$.

(b) $(g \circ f)(x) = g(f(x)) = g(\log x) = \sqrt{\log x}$ The domain of g is $(-\infty, \infty)$ and range of g is $[0, \infty)$. The domain of f is $(0, \infty)$, and the range of f is $(-\infty, \infty)$. So the domain of $g \circ f$ is $[1, \infty)$.

69. (a) $(f \circ g)(x) = f(g(x)) = f(\sqrt{x}) = e^{\sqrt{x}}$ The domain of g is $(-\infty, \infty)$ and range of g is $[0, \infty)$. The domain of f is $(-\infty, \infty)$, and the range of f is $(0, \infty)$. So the domain of $f \circ g$ is $[0, \infty)$.

(b) $(g \circ f)(x) = g(f(x)) = g(e^x) = \sqrt{e^x}$ The domain of g is $(-\infty, \infty)$ and range of g is $[0, \infty)$. The domain of f is $(-\infty, \infty)$, and the range of f is $(0, \infty)$. So the domain of $g \circ f$ is $(-\infty, \infty)$.

71. (a) $(f \circ g)(x) = f(g(x)) = f(\ln \sqrt{x}) = -(\ln \sqrt{x})^2$ The domain g is $(0, \infty)$. The domain of f is $(-\infty, \infty)$ So the domain of $f \circ g$ is $(0, \infty)$.

(b) $(g \circ f)(x) = g(f(x)) = g(-x^2) = \ln \sqrt{-x^2}$ The function is undefined for negative values. So the domain of $g \circ f$ is $\emptyset$.

73. (a) $(f \circ g)(x) = f(g(x)) = f\left(\dfrac{x}{x-2}\right) = 5\left(\dfrac{x}{x-2}\right) - 2 = \dfrac{3x+4}{x-2}$ The domain g is $(-\infty, 2) \cup (2, \infty)$. The domain of f is $(-\infty, \infty)$ So the domain of $f \circ g$ is $(-\infty, 2) \cup (2, \infty)$.

(b) $(g \circ f)(x) = g(f(x)) = g(5x-2) = \dfrac{5x-2}{5x-2-2} = \dfrac{5x-2}{5x-4}$ The domain g is $(-\infty, 2) \cup (2, \infty)$. The domain of f is $(-\infty, \infty)$ So the domain of $g \circ f$ is $\left(-\infty, \dfrac{4}{5}\right) \cup \left(\dfrac{4}{5}, \infty\right)$.

Chapter 5 Review Exercises

1. The function is not one-to-one, the graph fails the horizontal line test.

2. The function is not one-to-one, the graph fails the horizontal line test.

3. The function is not one-to-one, the graph fails the horizontal line test.

4. The function is one-to-one, different x-values always produce different y-values.

5. The function is not one-to-one, the graph fails the horizontal line test.

6. The function is not one-to-one, the graph fails the horizontal line test.

7. All real numbers can be input for x, therefore the domain is $(-\infty, \infty)$.

8. All real numbers can be solutions to $f(x)$, therefore the range is $(-\infty, \infty)$.

9. Since f is one-to-one, it has an inverse.

10. For $f(x)=\sqrt[3]{2x-7}$ the inverse is

$$x=\sqrt[3]{2y-7} \Rightarrow x^3=2y-7 \Rightarrow x^3+7=2y \Rightarrow y=\frac{x^3+7}{2} \Rightarrow f^{-1}(x)=\frac{x^3+7}{2}.$$

11. See Figure 11. The graphs are reflections across the line $y=x$.

[10,70] by [0,60]

Xscl = 10   Yscl = 10

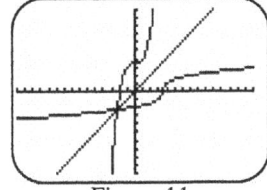

Figure 11

12. $(f \circ f^{-1})(x)=\sqrt[3]{2\left(\frac{x^3+7}{2}\right)-7}=\sqrt[3]{x^3}=x$ and $(f^{-1} \circ f)(x)=\frac{\left(\sqrt[3]{2x-7}\right)^3+7}{2}=\frac{2x-7+7}{2}=\frac{2x}{2}=x$.

13. $y=a^{x+2}$ is the graph of $y=a^x$ shifted 2 units left with a y-intercept of a^2. Therefore, it matches C.

14. $y=a^x+2$ is the graph of $y=a^x$ shifted 2 units upward with a y-intercept of 3. Therefore, it matches A.

15. $y=-a^x+2$ is the graph of $y=a^x$ reflected across the x-axis, then shifted 2 units upward, with a y-intercept of 1. Therefore, it matches D.

16. $y=a^{-x}+2$ is the graph of $y=a^x$ reflected across the y-axis, then shifted 2 units upward, with a y-intercept of 3. Therefore, it matches B.

17. Because the graph goes up to the left, the value of a is $0<x<1$.

18. All real numbers can be input for x, therefore the domain is $(-\infty,\infty)$.

19. From the graph, only values where $f(x)>0$, are possible solutions. Therefore, the range is $(0,\infty)$.

20. Since every real number a raised to the zero power equals 1, $f(0)=a^0=1$.

21. Reflect $f(x)$ across the line $y=x$. See Figure 21.

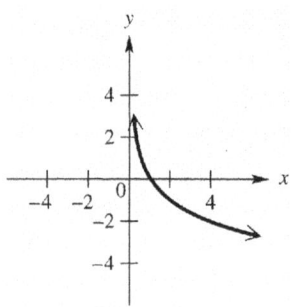

Figure 21

22. For $f(x) = a^x$, the inverse is, $x = a^y \Rightarrow y = \log_a x \Rightarrow f^{-1}(x) = \log_a x$.

23. See Figure 23. From the graph, the domain is $(-\infty, \infty)$; and the range is $(0, \infty)$.

24. See Figure 24. From the graph, the domain is $(-\infty, \infty)$; and the range is $(2, \infty)$.

25. See Figure 25. From the graph, the domain is $(-\infty, \infty)$; and the range is $(-\infty, 0)$.

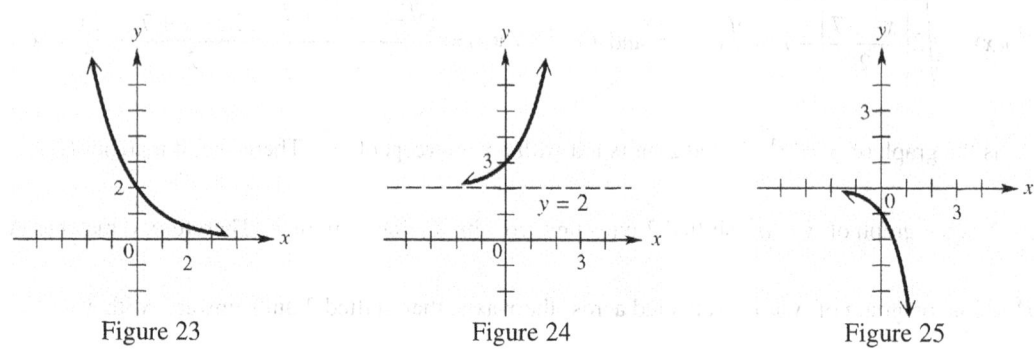

Figure 23   Figure 24   Figure 25

26. The graph of $f(x) = a^x$ with $0 < x < 1$ would have a range that decreases as the domain increases. Since the negative is on the exponent for $f(x) = a^{-x}$, the graph is reflected across the y-axis and is therefore now increasing as the domain increases. It is increasing on its domain.

27. (a) $\left(\dfrac{1}{8}\right)^{-2x} = 2^{x+3} \Rightarrow (2^{-3})^{-2x} = 2^{x+3} \Rightarrow 2^{6x} = 2^{x+3} \Rightarrow 6x = x+3 \Rightarrow 5x = 3 \Rightarrow x = \dfrac{3}{5}$

  (b) If $\left(\dfrac{1}{8}\right)^{-2x} \geq 2^{x+3}$, then $\left(\dfrac{1}{8}\right)^{-2x} - 2^{x+3} \geq 0$. Now graph $y_1 = \left(\dfrac{1}{8}\right)^{-2x} - 2^{x+3}$ on a calculator, use the answer from part (a), and from the graph the solution to $\left(\dfrac{1}{8}\right)^{-2x} - 2^{x+3} \geq 0$ is the interval $\left[\dfrac{3}{5}, \infty\right)$.

28. (a) $3^{-x} = \left(\dfrac{1}{27}\right)^{1-2x} \Rightarrow 3^{-x} = (3^{-3})^{1-2x} \Rightarrow 3^{-x} = 3^{-3+6x} \Rightarrow -x = -3+6x \Rightarrow 3 = 7x \Rightarrow x = \dfrac{3}{7}$

(b) If $3^{-x} < \left(\frac{1}{27}\right)^{1-2x}$, then $3^{-x} - \left(\frac{1}{27}\right)^{-2x} < 0$. Now graph $y_1 = 3^{-x} - \left(\frac{1}{27}\right)^{1-2x}$ on a calculator, use the answer from part (a), and from the graph the solution to $3^{-x} - \left(\frac{1}{27}\right)^{1-2x} < 0$ is the interval $\left(\frac{3}{7}, \infty\right)$.

29. (a) $0.5^{-x} = 0.25^{x+1} \Rightarrow 0.5^{-x} = (0.5^2)^{x+1} \Rightarrow 0.5^{-x} = 0.5^{2x+2} \Rightarrow -x = 2x+2 \Rightarrow -2 = 3x \Rightarrow x = -\frac{2}{3}$

(b) If $0.5^{-x} > 0.25^{x+1}$, then $0.5^{-x} - 0.25^{x+1} > 0$. Now graph $y_1 = 0.5^{-x} - 0.25^{x+1}$ on a calculator, use the answer from part (a), and from the graph the solution to $0.5^{-x} - 0.25^{x+1} > 0$ is the interval $\left(-\frac{2}{3}, \infty\right)$.

30. (a) $0.4x = 2.5^{1-x} \Rightarrow \log 0.4^x = \log 2.5^{1-x} \Rightarrow x \log 0.4 = (1-x)\log 2.5 \Rightarrow x \log 0.4 = \log 2.5 - x \log 2.5 \Rightarrow$

$x \log 0.4 + x \log 2.5 = \log 2.5 \Rightarrow x(\log 0.4 + \log 2.5) = \log 2.5 \Rightarrow x = \frac{\log 2.5}{\log 0.4 + \log 2.5}$, using a

calculator, this is equal to $\frac{\log 2.5}{0}$, which is undefined. The solution is $\varnothing$.

(b) If $0.4^x < 2.5^{1-x}$ then $0.4x - 2.5^{1-x} < 0$. Now graph $y_1 = 0.4x - 2.5^{1-x}$ on a calculator, from the graph the solution to $0.4x - 2.5^{1-x} < 0$ is the interval $(-\infty, \infty)$.

31. We can find the intersection points of $y = x^2$ and $y = 2^x$ by using the intersection of graphs method and graph the equation $y_1 = x^2 - 2^x$ to finding the x-intercepts. Using the calculator the intercepts are $2, 4$, and -0.766664696. The missing point in common is $(-0.766664696, 0.58777475603)$.

32. Using the intersection of graphs method, graph $y = 3^x - \pi$ and find the x-intercept. From the calculator, the x-intercepts is $x = \{1.041978046\}$.

33. From the calculator, $\log 58.3 \approx 1.7656685547633 \approx 1.7657$.

34. From the calculator, $\log 0.00233 \approx -2.63264407897 \approx -2.6326$.

35. From the calculator, $\ln 58.3 \approx 4.06560209336 \approx 4.0656$.

36. From the calculator, $\log_2 0.00233 = \frac{\log 0.00233}{\log 2} = -8.7455$.

37. By the definitions of logarithms, $\log_{13} 1 = x \Rightarrow 13^x = 1$ since we know $13^0 = 1$ it follows that $x = 0$.

38. By the properties of logarithms, $\ln e^{\sqrt{6}} = \log_e e^{\sqrt{6}} = \sqrt{6}$.

39. By the properties of logarithms, $\log_5 5^{12} = 12$.

40. By the properties of logarithms, $7^{\log_7 13} = 13$.

41. By the properties of logarithms, $3^{\log_3 5} = 5$.

42. By the change of base rule, $\log_4 9 = \dfrac{\log 9}{\log 4} \approx 1.58496250072 \approx 1.5850$.

43. The x-intercept is 1, and the graph is increasing. The correct graph is E.

44. Since $f(x) = \log_2(2x) = \log_2 2 + \log_2 x = 1 + \log_2 x$, the graph will be similar to that of $f(x) = \log_2 x$, but will have a vertical shift up 1. The x-intercept will be $\dfrac{1}{2}$, since $\log_2 2\left(\dfrac{1}{2}\right) = \log_2 1 = 0$.

    The correct graph is D.

45. Since $f(x) = \log_2\left(\dfrac{1}{x}\right) = \log_2 x^{-1} = -\log_2 x$, the graph will be similar to that of $f(x) = \log_2 x$, but will be reflected across the x-axis. The x-intercept is 1. The correct graph is B.

46. Since $f(x) = \log_2\left(\dfrac{x}{2}\right) = \log_2\left(\dfrac{1}{2}x\right) = \log_2\left(\dfrac{1}{2}\right) + \log_2 x = -1 + \log_2 x$, the graph will be similar to that of $f(x) = \log_2 x$, but will have a vertical shift down 1 unit. The x-intercept will be 2, since $\log_2\left(\dfrac{2}{2}\right) = \log_2 1 = 0$. The correct graph is C.

47. With $f(x) = \log_2(x-1)$, the graph will be similar to that of $f(x) = \log_2 x$, but will be shifted 1 unit to the right; the x-intercept will be 2. The correct graph is F.

48. With $f(x) = \log_2(-x)$, the graph will be similar to that of $f(x) = \log_2 x$, but will be reflected across the y-axis. The x-intercept is -1, since $\log_2(-(-1)) = \log_2 1 = 0$. The correct graph is A.

49. See Figure 49. From the graph, the domain is $(0, \infty)$ and the range is $(-\infty, \infty)$.

50. See Figure 50. From the graph, the domain is $(2, \infty)$ and the range is $(-\infty, \infty)$.

51. See Figure 51. From the graph, the domain is $(-\infty, 0)$ and the range is $(-\infty, \infty)$.

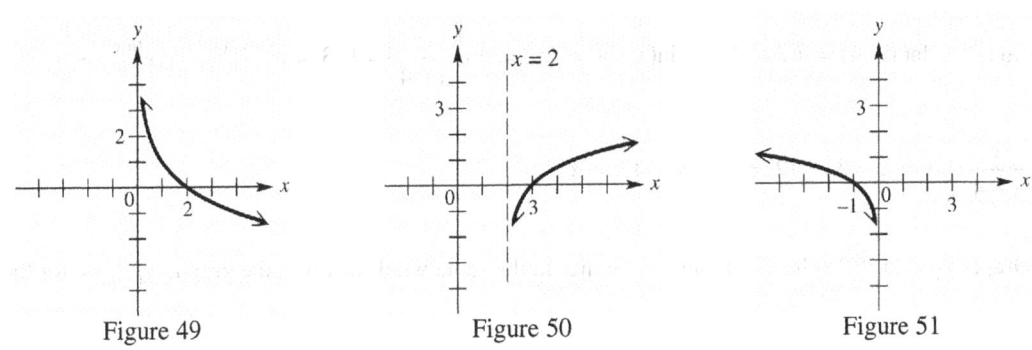

Figure 49   Figure 50   Figure 51

52. The functions in Exercises 49, 50, and 51 are the inverses, respectively, of those in Exercises 23, 24, and 25.

53. If the function has a point $(81,4)$, then $f(81)=4$. Therefore, $\log_a 81 = 4 \Rightarrow a^4 = 81 \Rightarrow a^4 = 3^4 \Rightarrow a = 3$. The base is 3.

54. If the function has a point $\left(-4, \dfrac{1}{16}\right)$, then $f(-4) = \dfrac{1}{16}$. Therefore, $a^{-4} = \dfrac{1}{16} \Rightarrow a^{-4} = 2^{-4} \Rightarrow a = 2$. The base is 2.

55. $\log_3 \dfrac{mn}{5r} = \log_3 mn - \log_3 5r = \log_3 m + \log_3 n - (\log_3 5 + \log_3 r) = \log_3 m + \log_3 n - \log_3 5 - \log_3 r$

56. $\log_2 \dfrac{\sqrt{7}}{15} = \log_2 \sqrt{7} - \log_2 15 = \log_2 7^{1/2} - \log_2 15 = \dfrac{1}{2}\log_2 7 - \log_2 15.$

57. $\log_5(x^2 y^4 \sqrt[5]{m^3 p}) = \log_5 x^2 + \log_5 y^4 + \log_5(m^3 p)^{1/5} = 2\log_5 x + 4\log_5 y + \dfrac{1}{5}\log_5(m^3 p) =$

$2\log_5 x + 4\log_5 y + \dfrac{1}{5}(\log_5 m^3 + \log_5 p) = 2\log_5 x + 4\log_5 y + \dfrac{3}{5}\log_5 m + \dfrac{1}{5}\log_5 p$

58. The properties of logarithms do not apply to polynomials.

59. (a) $\log(x+3) + \log x = 1 \Rightarrow \log(x+3)(x) = 1 \Rightarrow 10^{\log(x+3)(x)} = 10^1 \Rightarrow (x+3)(x) = 10 \Rightarrow$
$x^2 + 3x - 10 = 0 \Rightarrow (x+5)(x-2) = 0 \Rightarrow x = -5, 2.$

Since the argument of a logarithm cannot be negative, the solution is $x = 2$.

(b) Graph $y_1 = \log(x+3) + \log x$ and $y_2 = 1$ in the same window. From the graph, $y_1 > y_2$ for the interval $(2, \infty)$.

60. (a) $\ln e^{\ln e} - \ln(x-4) = \ln 3 \Rightarrow \ln x - \ln(x-4) = \ln 3 \Rightarrow \ln\left(\dfrac{x}{x-4}\right) = \ln 3 \Rightarrow e^{\ln(x/x-4)} = e^{\ln x} \Rightarrow$

$\dfrac{x}{x-4} = 3 \Rightarrow x = 3x - 12 \Rightarrow -2x = -12 \Rightarrow x = 6$

(b) Graph $y_1 = \ln e^{\ln x} - \ln(x-4)$ and $y_2 = \ln 3$ in the same window. From the graph, $y_1 \leq y_2$ for the interval $[6, \infty)$.

61. (a) $\ln e^{\ln 2} - \ln(x-1) = \ln 5 \Rightarrow \ln 2 - \ln(x-1) = \ln 5 \Rightarrow \ln\left(\dfrac{2}{x-1}\right) = \ln 5 \Rightarrow e^{\ln(2/x-1)} = e^{\ln 5} \Rightarrow$

$\dfrac{2}{x-1} = 5 \Rightarrow 2 = 5x - 5 \Rightarrow 5x = 7 \Rightarrow x = \dfrac{7}{5}$ or 1.4

(b) Graph $y_1 = \ln e^{\ln 2} - \ln(x-1)$ and $y_2 = \ln 5$ in the same window. From the graph, $y_1 \geq y_2$ for the interval $(1, 1.4]$.

62. (a) $8^x = 32 \Rightarrow (2^3)^x = 2^5 \Rightarrow 2^{3x} = 2^5 \Rightarrow 3x = 5 \Rightarrow x = \dfrac{5}{3}$

63. (a) $\dfrac{8}{27} = x^{-3} \Rightarrow \left(\dfrac{2}{3}\right)^3 = x^{-3} \Rightarrow \left(\dfrac{2}{3}\right)^3 = \left(\dfrac{1}{x}\right)^3 \Rightarrow \dfrac{2}{3} = \dfrac{1}{x} \Rightarrow 2x = 3 \Rightarrow x = \dfrac{3}{2}$

64. (a) $10^{2x-3} = 17 \Rightarrow \log 10^{2x-3} = \log 17 \Rightarrow (2x-3)\log 10 = \log 17$

$\Rightarrow 2x - 3 = \log 17 \Rightarrow 2x = 3 + \log 17 \Rightarrow x = \dfrac{3 + \log 17}{2}$

(b) From the calculator the solutions is $x \approx 2.115$.

65. (a) $e^{x+1} = 10 \Rightarrow \ln e^{x+1} = \ln 10 \Rightarrow (x+1)\ln e = \ln 10 \Rightarrow x + 1 = \ln 10 \Rightarrow x = -1 + \ln 10$

(Other forms of the answer are possible.)

(b) From the calculator, the solutions is $x \approx 1.303$.

66. (a) $\log_{64} x = \dfrac{1}{3} \Rightarrow 64^{\log_{64} x} = 64^{1/3} \Rightarrow x = 64^{1/3} \Rightarrow x = 4$

67. (a) $\ln(6x) - \ln(x+1) = \ln 4 \Rightarrow \ln\dfrac{6x}{x+1} = \ln 4 \Rightarrow e^{\ln 6x/x+1} = e^{\ln 4} \Rightarrow \dfrac{6x}{x+1} = 4 \Rightarrow 4x + 4 = 6x \Rightarrow$

$4 = 2x \Rightarrow x = 2$

68. (a) $\log_{12}(2x)+\log_{12}(x-1)=1 \Rightarrow \log_{12}(2x)(x-1)=1 \Rightarrow \log_{12} 2x^2-2x=1 \Rightarrow$

$12^{\log_{12} 2x^2-2x}=12^1 \Rightarrow 2x^2-2x=12 \Rightarrow 2x^2-2x-12=0 \Rightarrow 2(x^2-x-6)=0 \Rightarrow$

$2(x-3)(x+2)=0 \Rightarrow x=-2, 3$. Since the argument of a logarithm cannot be negative, the solution is $x=3$.

69. (a) $\log_{16}\sqrt{x+1}=\frac{1}{4} \Rightarrow 16^{\log_{16}\sqrt{x+1}}=16^{1/4} \Rightarrow \sqrt{x+1}=16^{1/4} \Rightarrow x+1=(16^{1/4})^2 \Rightarrow$

$x+1=16^{1/2} \Rightarrow x+1=4 \Rightarrow x=3$

70. (a) $\ln x + 3\ln 2 = \ln\frac{2}{x} \Rightarrow \ln x + \ln 2^3 = \ln\frac{2}{x} \Rightarrow \ln[(x)(2^3)] = \ln\frac{2}{3} \Rightarrow$

$\ln 8x = \ln\frac{2}{x} \Rightarrow e^{\ln 8x} = e^{\ln 2/x} \Rightarrow 8x = \frac{2}{x} \Rightarrow 8x^2 = 2 \Rightarrow x^2 = \frac{2}{8} \Rightarrow x^2 = \frac{1}{4} \Rightarrow x = -\frac{1}{2}, \frac{1}{2}$

Since the argument of a natural logarithm can not be negative, the solution is $x=\frac{1}{2}$.

71. (a) $\ln[\ln(e^{-x})] = \ln 3 \Rightarrow \ln(-x) = \ln 3 \Rightarrow e^{\ln(-x)} = e^{\ln 3} \Rightarrow -x=3 \Rightarrow x=-3$

72. (a) $\ln e^x - \ln e^3 = \ln e^5 \Rightarrow x-3=5 \Rightarrow x=8$

73. No real number value for x can produce a negative solution; therefore, $x=\varnothing$.

74. $N=a+b\ln\left(\frac{c}{d}\right) \Rightarrow N-a=b\ln\left(\frac{c}{d}\right) \Rightarrow \frac{N-a}{b}=\ln\left(\frac{c}{d}\right) \Rightarrow$

$e^{(N-a)/b}=e^{\ln(c/d)} \Rightarrow e^{(N-a)/b}=\frac{c}{d} \Rightarrow c=de^{(N-a)/b}$

75. $y=y_0 e^{-kt} \Rightarrow \frac{y}{y_0}=e^{-kt} \Rightarrow \ln\left(\frac{y}{y_0}\right)=\ln e^{-kt} \Rightarrow \ln\left(\frac{y}{y_0}\right)=-kt \Rightarrow t=\frac{\ln(y/y_0)}{-k}$

76. Graph $y_1 = \log_{10} x$ and $y_2 = x-2$ in the same window. By the capabilities of the calculator, the x-coordinates of the intersections are $x \approx 0.010$ and $x \approx 2.376$.

77. Graph $y_1 = 2^{-x}$ and $y_2 = \log_{10} x$ in the same window. By the capabilities of the calculator, the x-coordinate of the intersection is $x \approx 1.874$.

78. Graph $y_1 = x^2 - 3$ and $y_2 = \log x$ in the same window. By the capabilities of the calculator, the x-coordinates of the intersections are $x \approx 0.001$ and $x \approx 1.805$.

79. Use the Compound Interest Formula: $A = P\left(\dfrac{1+r}{n}\right)^{nt}$ with $A = \$4613$, $P = \$3500$, $t = 10$, and $n = 1$.

$$4613 = 3500\left(1+\dfrac{r}{1}\right)^{1(10)} \Rightarrow \dfrac{4613}{3500} = (1+r)^{10} \Rightarrow \left(\dfrac{4613}{3500}\right)^{0.1} = 1+r \Rightarrow r = \left(\dfrac{4613}{3500}\right)^{0.1} - 1 \Rightarrow$$

$r \approx 0.027996$. The annual interest rate, rounded to the nearest tenth, is 2.8%.

80. Use the Compound Interest Formula: $A = P\left(1+\dfrac{r}{n}\right)^{nt}$ with $A = \$58344$, $P = \$48000$, $r = 0.05$, and $n = 2$.

$$58,344 = 48,000\left(1+\dfrac{0.05}{2}\right)^{2t} \Rightarrow 58,344 = 48,000(1.025)^{2t} \Rightarrow \left(\dfrac{58,344}{48,000}\right) = 1.025^{2t} \Rightarrow 1.2155 = 1.025^{2t}$$

$$\Rightarrow \ln 1.2155 = \ln 1.025^{2t} \Rightarrow \ln 1.2155 = 2t \ln 1.025 \Rightarrow t = \dfrac{\ln 1.2155}{2 \ln 1.025} \Rightarrow t \approx 3.951698 \text{ or about 4 years.}$$

81. For the first 8 years, use the Compound Interest Formula:

$A = P\left(1+\dfrac{r}{n}\right)^{nt}$ with $P = \$12000$, $t = 8$, $r = 0.05$, and $n = 1$.

$$A = 12,000\left(1+\dfrac{0.05}{1}\right)^{8(1)} \Rightarrow A = 12,000(1.05)^8 \Rightarrow A \approx \$17,729.47$$

Now for the second 6 years, use the Compound Interest Formula:

$A = P\left(1+\dfrac{r}{n}\right)^{nt}$ with $P = \$17,729.47$, $t = 6$, $r = 0.06$, and $n = 1$.

$$A = 17,729.47\left(1+\dfrac{0.06}{1}\right)^{1(6)} \Rightarrow A = 17,729.47(1.06)^6 \Rightarrow A \approx \$25,149.59$$

At the end of the 14 year period, $\$25,149.59$ would be in the account.

82. (a) Use the Compound Interest Formula: $A = P\left(1+\dfrac{r}{n}\right)^{nt}$ with $P = \$2000$, $r = .03$, $t = 5$, and $n = 4$.

$$A = 2000\left(1+\dfrac{0.03}{4}\right)^{4(5)} \Rightarrow A = 2000(1.0075)^{20} \Rightarrow A \approx \$2,322.37$$

(b) Use the Continuous Compound Interest Formula: $A = Pe^{rt}$, with $P = \$2000$, $r = 0.03$, and $t = 5$.

$A = 2000e^{(0.03)(.5)} \Rightarrow A \approx \$2323.67$.

(c) Use the Continuous Compound Interest Formula:

$A = Pe^{rt}$ with $A = \$6000$, $P = \$2000$, and $r = 0.03$.

$6000 = 2000e^{0.03t} \Rightarrow 3 = e^{0.03t} \Rightarrow \ln 3 = \ln e^{0.03t} \Rightarrow \ln 3 = 0.03t \Rightarrow t = \dfrac{\ln 3}{0.03} \Rightarrow t \approx 36.6204$

It would take about 36.6 years to triple.

83. (a) See Figure 83. Since L is increasing, heavier planes require longer runways.

(b) We can find the answer by solving $L(10)$ and $L(100)$. $L(10) = 3\log 10 = 3(1) = 3$ or 3000 feet; $L(100) = 3 \log 100 = 3(2) = 6$ or 6000 feet. No, it does not increase by a factor of 10, but rather it increases by a factor of 2 to 6000 feet.

84. $2200 = 280\ln(x+1) + 1925 \Rightarrow 275 = 280(x+1) \Rightarrow \dfrac{275}{280} = \ln(x+1) \Rightarrow e^{275/280} = e^{\ln(x+1)} \Rightarrow$

$e^{275/280} = x+1 \Rightarrow x = e^{275/280} - 1 \Rightarrow x \approx 1.67$ acres.

85. (a) $P(0.5) = 0.04e^{-4(0.5)} \Rightarrow P(0.5) \approx 0.0054$ grams/liter

(b) $P(1) = 0.4e^{-4(1)} \Rightarrow P(1) \approx 0.00073$ grams/liter

(c) $P(2) = 0.04e^{-4(2)} \Rightarrow P(2) \approx 0.000013$ grams/liter

(d) $0.002 = 0.04e^{-4x} \Rightarrow 0.05 = e^{-4x} \Rightarrow \ln 0.05 = \ln e^{-4x} \Rightarrow \ln 0.05 = -4x \Rightarrow$

$x = \dfrac{\ln 0.05}{-4} \Rightarrow x \approx 0.75$ miles.

86. (a) $p(2) = 250 - 120(2.8)^{-0.5(2)} \Rightarrow p(2) \approx 207$

(b) $p(10) = 250 - 120(28)^{-0.5(10)} \Rightarrow p(10) \approx 249$

(c) See Figure 86. When $x = 2$, the graph supports the answer of 207 from part (a).

[0,50] by [0,6]   [0,10] by [0,300]
Xscl = 10   Yscl = 1   Xscl = 1   Yscl = 50

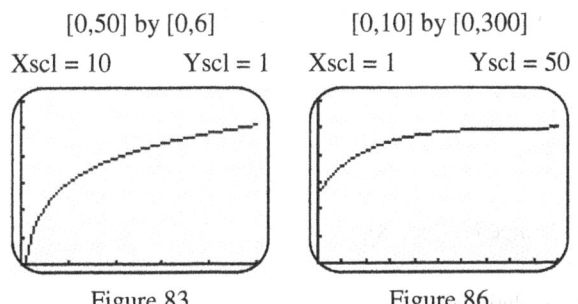

Figure 83   Figure 86

87. Find t when $v(t) = 147$.

$$147 = 176\left(1 - e^{-0.18t}\right) \Rightarrow \frac{147}{176} = 1 - e^{-0.18t} \Rightarrow e^{-0.18t} = 1 - \frac{147}{176} \Rightarrow e^{-0.18t} = \frac{29}{176} \Rightarrow$$

$$\ln e^{-0.18t} = \ln\left(\frac{29}{176}\right) \Rightarrow -0.18t = \ln\left(\frac{29}{176}\right) \Rightarrow t = \frac{\ln\left(\frac{29}{176}\right)}{-0.18} = t \approx 10.017712$$

It will take the skydiver about 10 seconds to attain the speed of 147 feet/second (100 mph)

Chapter 5 Test

1. (a) This function has a decreasing graph with a y-axis asymptote. This matches with B.

   (b) This function has an increasing graph with a y-intercept of 1. This matches with A.

   (c) This function has an increasing graph with a y-axis asymptote. This matches with C.

   (d) This function has a decreasing graph with a y-intercept of 1. This matches with D.

2. (a) Since the graph of $f(x) = 3 - 4x$ passes the horizontal line test the function is one-to-one.

   By definition, a function has an inverse if and only if it is one to one, therefore this function has an inverse.

   (b) Since the graph of $f(x) = x^2 - 3x$ does not pass the horizontal line test the function is not one-to-one. By definition, a function has an inverse if and only if it is one to one, therefore this function does not have an inverse.

   (c) Since the graph of $f(x) = 5(2)^x$ passes the horizontal line test the function is one-to-one. By definition, a function has an inverse if and only if it is one to one, therefore this function has an inverse.

3. (a) $f(x) = 5x - 7 \Rightarrow y = 5x - 7 \Rightarrow y + 7 = 5x \Rightarrow \frac{y+7}{5} = x \Rightarrow f^{-1}(x) = \frac{x+7}{5}$

   (b) $f(x) = 2\log x \Rightarrow y = 2\log x \Rightarrow \frac{y}{2} = \log x \Rightarrow 10^{y/2} = x \Rightarrow f^{-1}(x) = 10^{x/2}$

   (c) $f(x) = \frac{x+1}{x-2} \Rightarrow y = \frac{x+1}{x-2} \Rightarrow y(x-2) = x+1 \Rightarrow xy - 2y = x+1 \Rightarrow xy - x = 2y + 1 \Rightarrow$
   $x(y-1) = 2y+1 \Rightarrow x = \frac{2y+1}{y-1} \Rightarrow f^{-1}(x) = \frac{2x+1}{x-1}$

4. (a) See Figure 4.

   (b) From the graph, the domain is $(-\infty, \infty)$, and the range is $(-\infty, 8)$.

   (c) From the graph, it has a horizontal asymptote with equation $y = 8$.

(d) Set $y = 0$ to find the x-intercept. $0 = -2^{x-1} + 8 \Rightarrow 2^{x-1} = 8 \Rightarrow 2^{x-1} = 2^3 \Rightarrow x - 1 = 3 \Rightarrow x = 4$.

The x-intercept is (4, 0). Set $x = 0$ to find the y-intercept. $y = -2^{0-1} + 8 \Rightarrow y = -\frac{1}{2} + 8 \Rightarrow y = 7.5$.

The y-intercept is (0, 7.5).

(e) To find the inverse, interchange the x and y variables and solve for y. $x = -2^{y-1} + 8 \Rightarrow$

$x - 8 = -2^{y-1} \Rightarrow 8 - x = 2^{y-1} \Rightarrow \log(8 - x) = \log 2^{y-1} \Rightarrow \log(8 - x) = (y - 1) \log 2 \Rightarrow$

$\log(8 - x) = y \log 2 - 1 \log 2 \Rightarrow \log(8 - x) + \log 2 = y \log 2 \Rightarrow y = \dfrac{\log(8-x) + \log 2}{\log 2}$ or

$y = \dfrac{\log(8-x)}{\log 2} + 1$.

[-10,10] by [-10,10]

Xscl = 1   Yscl = 1

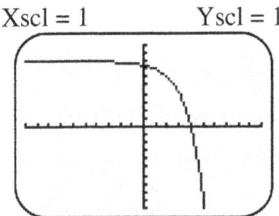

Figure 4

5. $(\frac{1}{8})^{2x+3} = 16^{x+1} \Rightarrow (2^{-3})^{2x-3} = (2^4)^{x+1} \Rightarrow 2^{-6x+9} = 2^{4x+4} \Rightarrow -6x + 9 = 4x + 4 \Rightarrow 5 = 10x \Rightarrow x = \dfrac{1}{2}$

or $x = 0.5$.

6. (a) Use the Compound Interest Formula $A = P\left(1 + \dfrac{r}{n}\right)^{nt}$, with $P = \$10000$, $r = 0.035$, $t = 4$, and $n = 4$.

$A = 10000\left(1 + \dfrac{0.035}{4}\right)^{4(4)} \Rightarrow A \approx \$11,495.74$.

(b) Use the Continuous Compound Interest Formula $A = Pe^{rt}$, with $P = \$10000$, $r = 0.035$, and $t = 4$.

$A = 10,000e^{0.035(4)} \Rightarrow A \approx \$11,502.74$.

7. The expression, $\log_5 27$, is the exponent to which 5 must be raised in order to obtain 27. To find an

approximation with a calculator, use the change-of-base rule: $\log_5 27 = \dfrac{\log 27}{\log 5}$.

8. (a) From the calculator, $\log 45.6 \approx 1.659$.

(b) From the calculator, $\ln 470 \approx 6.153$.

258 CHAPTER 5 Inverse, Exponential, and Logarithmic Functions

(c) From the calculator, $\log_3 769 = \dfrac{\log 769}{\log 3} \approx 6.049$.

9. $\log \dfrac{m^3 n}{\sqrt{y}} = \log m^3 + \log n - \log \sqrt{y} = \log m^3 + \log n - \log y^{1/2} \Rightarrow 3\log m + \log n - \dfrac{1}{2}\log y$.

10. $2\log x + \dfrac{1}{2}\log y - 4\log z = \log x^2 + \log y^{1/2} - \log z^4 = \log \dfrac{x^2 \sqrt{y}}{z^4}$

11. By the inverse property of logarithms $\ln e^y = y \Rightarrow \ln e^{2x} = 2x$

    By the inverse property of logarithms $10^{\log y} = y \Rightarrow 10^{\log x^2} = x^2$

12. The domain of the function $f(x) = \ln(x)$ is $x > 0$. Therefore, the domain of the function

    $f(x) = \ln(2x+1)$ will be $2x+1 > 0 \Rightarrow 2x > -1 \Rightarrow x > -\dfrac{1}{2}$. The domain in interval notation

    is $\left(-\dfrac{1}{2}, \infty\right)$.

13. $A = Pe^{rt} \Rightarrow \dfrac{A}{P} = e^{rt} \Rightarrow \ln \dfrac{A}{P} = \ln e^{rt} \Rightarrow \ln A - \ln P = rt \Rightarrow t = \dfrac{\ln A - \ln P}{r}$.

14. (a) $\log_2 x + \log_2 (x+2) = 3;\ x > 0 \Rightarrow \log_2 [x(x+2)] = 3 \Rightarrow 2^{\log_2 [x(x+2)]} = 2^3 \Rightarrow x(x+2) = 2^3 \Rightarrow$

    $x^2 + 2x - 8 = 0 \Rightarrow (x+4)(x-2) = 0 \Rightarrow x = -4, 2$. Since the argument of a logarithm can not be

    negative, the solution cannot be the extraneous solution -4, so the solution is $x = 2$.

    (b) Using the change-of-base rule on $y_1 = \log_2 x + \log_2 (x+2) - 3$ yields $y_1 = \dfrac{\log x}{\log 2} + \dfrac{\log(x+2)}{\log 2} - 3$.

    Graph the equation. See Figure 14. The x-intercept is $x = 2$.

    (c) From the graph, $\log_2 x + \log_2 (x+2) > 3$ for the interval $(2, \infty)$.

[-10,10] by [-10,10]
Xscl = 1   Yscl = 1

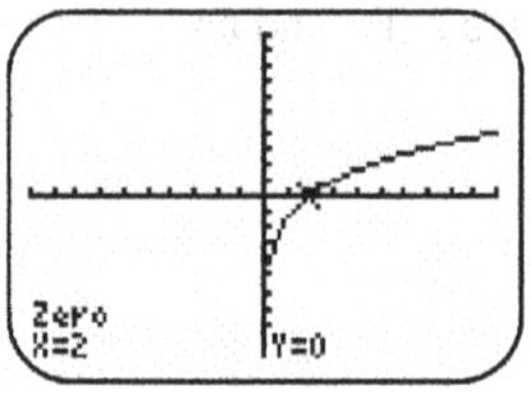

Figure 14

Section 5.T   259

15. (a) $2e^{5x+2} = 8 \Rightarrow e^{5x+2} = 4 \Rightarrow \ln e^{5x+2} = \ln 4 \Rightarrow 5x+2 = \ln 4 \Rightarrow 5x = \ln 4 - 2 \Rightarrow x = \dfrac{\ln 4 - 2}{5}$.

   (Other forms of the answer are possible.)

   (b) From the calculator, the solution is $x = -0.123$.

16. (a) $6^{2-x} = 2^{3x+1} \Rightarrow \log 6^{2-x} = \log 2^{3x+1} \Rightarrow (2-x)\log 6 = (3x+1)\log 2 \Rightarrow$
   $2\log 6 - x\log 6 = 3x\log 2 + \log 2 \Rightarrow 2\log 6 - \log 2 = 3x\log 2 + x\log 6 \Rightarrow$
   $\log \dfrac{6^2}{2} = x(\log(2^3)(6)) \Rightarrow \log 18 = x(\log 48) \Rightarrow x = \dfrac{\log 18}{\log 48}$.

   (b) From the calculator, the solution is $x = 0.747$.

17. (a) $\log(\ln x) = 1 \Rightarrow 10^{\log(\ln x)} = 10^1 \Rightarrow \ln x = 10 \Rightarrow e^{\ln x} = e^{10} \Rightarrow x = e^{10}$.

   (b) From the calculator, the solution is $x = 22{,}026.466$.

18. (a) The 2 in the equation is the original population; tripling this would yield $y = 3 \cdot 2$ The match is B.

   (b) In this function, $y = 3$; therefore, the match is D.

   (c) In this function, $t = 3$; therefore, the match is C.

   (d) Since 4 month equals $\dfrac{1}{3}$ year, in this function $t = \dfrac{1}{3}$; therefore, the match is A.

19. (a) See Figure 19a.   (b) See Figure 19b.
    (c) See Figure 19c.   (d) See Figure 19d.

   Function (c) is the best at describing $A(t)$ because it starts at 350 and gradually decreases as time increases.

[0,10] by [0,500]   [0,10] by [0,500]   [0,10] by [0,500]   [0,10] by [0,500]
Xscl = 1   Yscl = 100   Xscl = 1   Yscl = 100   Xscl = 1   Yscl = 100   Xscl = 1   Yscl = 100

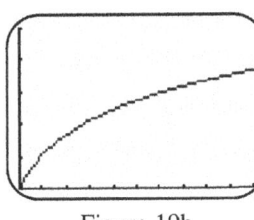
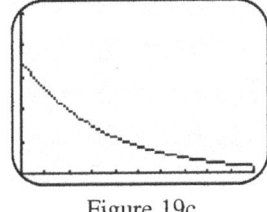
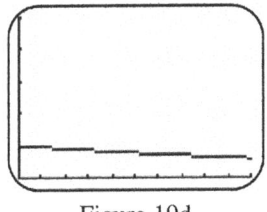

Figure 19a   Figure 19b   Figure 19c   Figure 19d

20. (a) Using the exponential decay model $A(t) = A_0 e^{-kt}$, we can solve for k with $A_0 = 2$ and $t = 1600$.

   $\dfrac{1}{2}(2) = 2e^{-k(1600)} \Rightarrow 1 = 2e^{-k(1600)} \Rightarrow \dfrac{1}{2} = e^{-k(1600)} \Rightarrow \ln \dfrac{1}{2} = \ln e^{-k(1600)} \Rightarrow \ln \dfrac{1}{2} = -k(1600) \Rightarrow$

   $k = \dfrac{\ln(5)}{-1600} \Rightarrow k \approx 0.000433$. The model is $A(t) = 2e^{-0.000433t}$.

Copyright © 2015 Pearson Education, Inc

(b)　$A(9600) = 2e^{-0.000433(9600)} \Rightarrow A(9600) \approx 0.03$ grams.

(c)　$0.5 = 2e^{-0.000433t} \Rightarrow 0.25 = e^{-0.000433t} \Rightarrow \ln 0.25 = \ln e^{-0.000433t} \Rightarrow$

$\ln 0.25 = -0.000433t \Rightarrow t = \dfrac{\ln 0.25}{-0.000433} \Rightarrow t \approx 3200$ years.

Chapter 6: Systems and Matrices

6.1: Systems of Equations

1. From the graph, the population is greater in Jacksonville than in New Orleans from 2006 to 2009.

3. Approximately (2005, 1.26)

5. year, population (in millions)

7. From the graph, the solution is $(2,2)$. Using substitution, first solve [equation 1] for x, $x - y = 0 \Rightarrow x = y$ [equation 3]. Substitute y for x in [equation 2]: $y + y = 4 \Rightarrow 2y = 4 \Rightarrow y = 2$. Now substitute 2 for y in [equation 3]: $x = y \Rightarrow x = 2$. The solution is $(2,2)$.

9. From the graph, the solution is $\left(\dfrac{1}{2}, -2\right)$. Using substitution, first solve [equation 2] for x:

   $2x - 3y = 7 \Rightarrow 2x = 3y + 7 \Rightarrow x = \dfrac{3}{2}y + \dfrac{7}{2}$ [equation 3]. Substitute $\dfrac{3}{2}y + \dfrac{7}{2}$ for x in [equation 1]:

   $6\left(\dfrac{3}{2}y + \dfrac{7}{2}\right) + 4y = -5 \Rightarrow 9y + 21 + 4y = -5 \Rightarrow 13y = -26 \Rightarrow y = -2$. Now substitute -2 in for y in

   [equation 3]: $x = \dfrac{3}{2}(-2) + \dfrac{7}{2} \Rightarrow x = -3 + \dfrac{7}{2} \Rightarrow x = \dfrac{1}{2}$. The solution is $\left(\dfrac{1}{2}, -2\right)$.

11. Since $y = x$ in [equation 2], we can use substitution. Substitute x for y in [equation 1]:

    $6x - (x) = 5 \Rightarrow 5x = 5 \Rightarrow x = 1$. Now substitute 1 for x in [equation 2]: $y = x \Rightarrow y = 1$. The solution is $(1,1)$.

13. Using substitution, first solve [equation 1] for x, $x + 2y = -1 \Rightarrow x = -2y - 1$ [equation 3]. Substitute $-2y - 1$ for x in [equation 2]: $2(-2y - 1) + y = 4 \Rightarrow -3y - 2 = 4 \Rightarrow -3y = 6 \Rightarrow y = -2$. Now substitute -2 for y in [equation 3]: $x = -2(-2) - 1 \Rightarrow x = 3$. The solution is $(3, -2)$.

15. Since $y = 2x + 3$ in [equation 1], we can use substitution. Substitute $2x + 3$ for y in [equation 2]:

    $3x + 4(2x + 3) = 78 \Rightarrow 11x + 12 = 78 \Rightarrow 11x = 66 \Rightarrow x = 6$. Now substitute 6 for x in [equation 1]: $y = 2(6) + 3 \Rightarrow y = 15$. The solution is $(6, 15)$.

17. Using substitution, first solve [equation 1] for x: $3x - 2y = 12 \Rightarrow 3x = 2y + 12 \Rightarrow x = \dfrac{2}{3}y + 4$ [equation 3].

    Substitute $\dfrac{2}{3}y + 4$ for x in [equation 2]: $5\left(\dfrac{2}{3}y + 4\right) = 4 - 2y \Rightarrow \dfrac{10}{3}y + 2y = 4 - 20 \Rightarrow \dfrac{16}{3}y = -16$

    $\Rightarrow y = -3$. Now substitute -3 for y in [equation 3]: $x = \dfrac{2}{3}(-3) + 4 \Rightarrow x = 2$. The solution is $(2, -3)$.

19. Using substitution, first solve [equation 2] for y: $2x + y = 5 \Rightarrow y = -2x + 5$ [equation 3]. Substitute $-2x + 5$ for y in [equation 1]: $4x - 5(-2x + 5) = -11 \Rightarrow 4x + 10x - 25 = -11 \Rightarrow 14x = 14 \Rightarrow x = 1$. Now substitute 1 for y in [equation 3]: $y = -2(1) + 5 \Rightarrow y = 3$. The solution is $(1, 3)$.

21. Using substitution, first solve [equation 2] for y: $9y = 31 + 2x \Rightarrow y = \dfrac{31 + 2x}{9}$ [equation 3]. Substitute

$\dfrac{31+2x}{9}$ for y in [equation 1]: $4x + 5\left(\dfrac{31+2x}{9}\right) = 7 \Rightarrow 9\left[4x + 5\left(\dfrac{31+2x}{9}\right) = 7\right] \Rightarrow$

$36x + 5(31 + 2x) = 63 \Rightarrow 36x + 155 + 10x = 63 \Rightarrow 46x = -92 \Rightarrow x = -2$.

Now substitute -2 for x in [equation 3]: $y = \dfrac{31 + 2(-2)}{9} \Rightarrow y = 3$. The solution is $(-2, 3)$.

23. Using substitution, first solve [equation 1] for x: $3x - 7y = 15 \Rightarrow 3x = 7y + 15 \Rightarrow x = \dfrac{7y+15}{3}$ [equation 3].

Substitute $\dfrac{7y+15}{3}$ for x in [equation 2]: $3\left(\dfrac{7y+15}{3}\right) + 7y = 15 \Rightarrow 7y + 15 + 7y = 15 \Rightarrow 14y = 0 \Rightarrow y = 0$.

Now substitute 0 for y in [equation 3]: $x = \dfrac{7(0)+15}{3} \Rightarrow x = 5$. The solution is $(5, 0)$.

25. Using substitution, first solve [equation 1] for x: $2x - 7y = 8 \Rightarrow 2x = 7y + 8 \Rightarrow x = \dfrac{7y+8}{2}$ [equation 3].

Substitute $\dfrac{7y+8}{2}$ for x in [equation 2]: $-3\left(\dfrac{7y+8}{2}\right) + \dfrac{21}{2}y = 5 \Rightarrow 2\left[-3\left(\dfrac{7y+8}{2}\right) + \dfrac{21}{2}y = 5\right] \Rightarrow$

$-3(7y+8) + 21y = 10 \Rightarrow -21y - 24 + 21y = 10 \Rightarrow -24 = 10$.

Since this is a false statement, the solution set is $\varnothing$.

27. Using substitution, first solve [equation 1] for x: $x - 2y = 4 \Rightarrow x = 4 + 2y$ [equation 3]. Substitute

$x = 4 + 2y$ for x in [equation 2]: $-2(4+2y) + 4y = -8 \Rightarrow -8 - 4y + 4y = -8 \Rightarrow -8 = -8$. Since this is

a true statement, the system is dependent and the solutions are $(4+2y, y)$ or $\left(x, \dfrac{x-4}{2}\right)$.

29. Multiply the first equation by 3 and add to eliminate the y-variable:

$9x - 3y = -12$
$x + 3y = 12$
$\overline{10x = 0} \Rightarrow x = 0$. Substitute 0 for x in the second equation: $(0) + 3y = 12 \Rightarrow y = 4$. The

solution is $(0, 4)$.

31. Multiply the second equation by 2, and subtract to eliminate the x-variable:

$4x + 3y = -1$
$4x + 10y = 6$
$\overline{ -7y = -7} \Rightarrow y = 1$. Substitute 1 for y in the first equation: $4x + 3(1) = -1 \Rightarrow 4x = -4 \Rightarrow x = -1$.

The solution is $(-1, 1)$.

33. Multiply the second equation by 4, and subtract to eliminate the x-variable:

$$12x - 5y = 9$$
$$12x - 32y = -72$$
$$\overline{\;27y = \;\;81}$$ ⇒ $y = 3$. Substitute 3 for y in the first equation: $12x - 5(3) = 9 \Rightarrow 12x = 24 \Rightarrow x = 2$.

The solution is $(2, 3)$.

35. Multiply the first equation by 2 and add to eliminate both variables.

$$8x - 2y = 18$$
$$-8x + 2y = -18$$
$$\overline{\;0 = \;\;0}$$ ⇒ infinite number of solutions. Therefore, the solutions have the following

relationship: $4x - y = 9 \Rightarrow -y = -4x + 9 \Rightarrow y = 4x - 9$. The solution set is $\{(x, 4x - 9)\}$ or $\left\{\left(\dfrac{y+9}{4}, y\right)\right\}$.

37. Multiply the first equation by 2 and add to eliminate both variables:

$$18x - 10y = 2$$
$$-18y + 10y = 1$$
$$\overline{\;0 = 3}$$ ⇒ ∅

39. Multiply the first equation by 2 and subtract to eliminate both variables:\

$$6x + 2y = 12$$
$$6y + 2y = 1$$
$$\overline{\;0 = 13}$$ ⇒ ∅

41. First, multiplying both equations by 6 yields $3x + 2y = 48$ and $4x + 9y = 102$. Now multiply the first equation by 4, the second equation by 3, and subtract to eliminate the x-variable:

$$12x + 8y = 192$$
$$12x + 27y = 306$$
$$\overline{\;-19y = -114}$$ ⇒ $y = 6$. Substitute 6 for y in the first equation (multiplied by 6):

$3x + 2(6) = 48 \Rightarrow 3x = 36 \Rightarrow x = 12$. The solution is $(12, 6)$.

43. Multiplying the first equation by 12 and the second by 6 yields $8x + 3y = 46$ and $x + 2y = 9$. Now multiply the second equation by 8, and subtract to eliminate the x-variable:

$$8x + 3y = 46$$
$$8x + 16y = 72$$
$$\overline{\;-13y = -26}$$ ⇒ $y = 2$. Substitute 2 for y in the second equation (multiplied by 6):

$x + 2(2) = 9 \Rightarrow x = 5$. The solution is $(5, 2)$.

45. Graph each function in the same window. The intersection or solution is $(0.138, -4.762)$.

47. Graph each function in the same window. The intersection or solution is $(-8.708, -15.668)$.

49. An inconsistent system will conclude with no variables and a false statement, such as $0 = 1$. A system with dependent equations will conclude with no variables and a true statement, such as $0 = 0$.

From these equations, when we subtract, we will get the result $0 = 0$ when $k = -6$, and the result $0 = (-6 - k)$ when $k \neq -6$. Therefore, the system will have no solution when $k \neq -6$, and system will have infinitely many solutions when $k = -6$.

51. See Figure 51.

53. See Figure 53

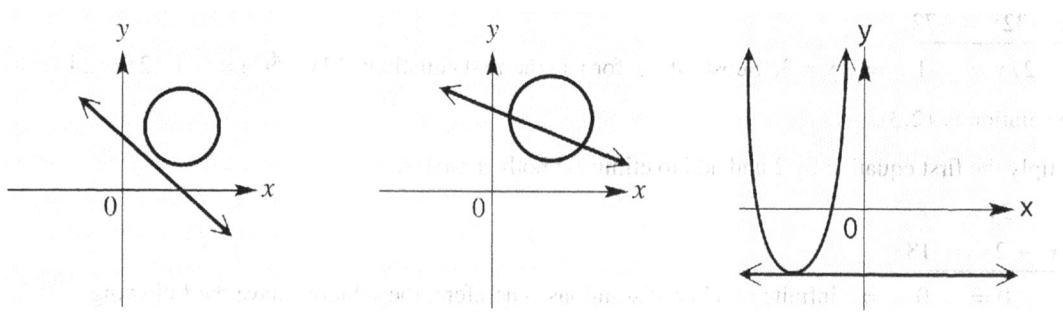

Figure 51   Figure 53   Figure 55

55. See Figure 55.

57. See Figure 57.

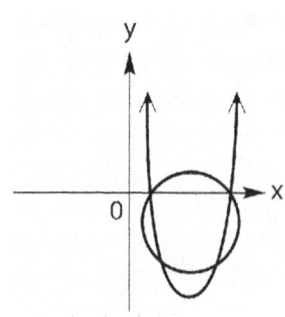 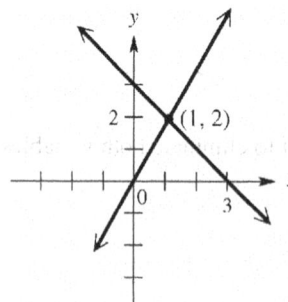 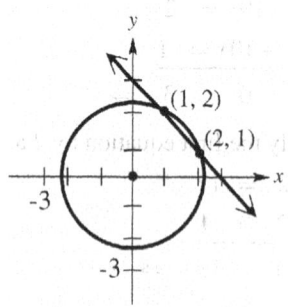

Figure 57   Figure 59   Figure 61

59. Check: $1+2=3 \Rightarrow 3=3$, $2(1)-2=0 \Rightarrow 0=0$. See Figure 59.

61. Check: $1^2+2^2=5 \Rightarrow 5=5$, $2=3-1 \Rightarrow 2=2$, $2^2+1^2=5 \Rightarrow 5=5$, $1=3-2 \Rightarrow 1=1$.

63. Check: $1=(-1)^2 \Rightarrow 1=1$, $(-1)^2+1^2=2$, $1=1^2 \Rightarrow 1=1$, $1^2+1^2=2 \Rightarrow 2=2$.

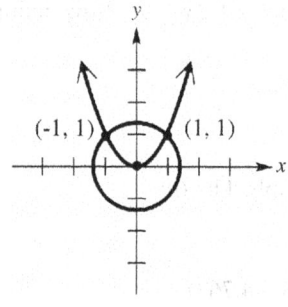 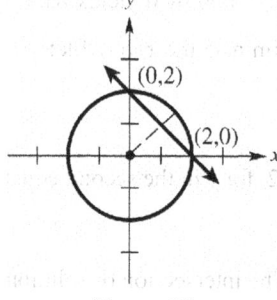

Figure 63   Figure 65

65. Check: $0^2+2^2=4 \Rightarrow 0+4=4 \Rightarrow 4=4$, $0+2=2 \Rightarrow 2=2$.

    $2^2+0^2=4 \Rightarrow 4+0=4 \Rightarrow 4=4$, $2+0=2 \Rightarrow 2=2$.

67. Since [equation 1] is solved for y, we substitute $-x^2+2$ for y in [equation 2]:

    $x-(-x^2+2)=0 \Rightarrow x^2+x-2 \Rightarrow (x+2)(x-1)=0 \Rightarrow x=-2$ or 1. Substituting these values into [equation 1] yields $y = -(-2)^2 + 2 \Rightarrow y = -4 + 2 \Rightarrow y = -2$ and $y = -(1)^2 + 2 \Rightarrow y = -1 + 2 \Rightarrow y = 1$.

The solution set is $\{(-2,-2),(1,1)\}$.

69. First solve [equation 2] for x: $x - y = 1 \Rightarrow x = y + 1$ [equation 3]. Now substitute $y + 1$ for x in

    [equation 1]: $(y+1)^2 + y^2 = 5 \Rightarrow (y^2 + 2y + 1) + y^2 = 5 \Rightarrow y^2 + 2y + 1 + y^2 - 5 = 0 \Rightarrow$

    $2y^2 + 2y - 4 = 0 \Rightarrow 2(y-1)(y+2) = 0 \Rightarrow y = 1$ or -2. Substituting these values into [equation 3]

    yields $x = (1) + 1 \Rightarrow x = 2$ and $x = (-2) + 1 \Rightarrow x = -1$. The solution set is $\{(-1,-2),(2,1)\}$.

71. First solve [equation 2] for x^2: $-x^2 + y = -4 \Rightarrow x^2 = y + 4$ [equation 3]. Now substitute $y + 4$ for x^2 in

    [equation 1]: $(y+4) + y^2 = 10 \Rightarrow y^2 + y + 4 - 10 = 0 \Rightarrow y^2 + y - 6 = 0 \Rightarrow (y-2)(y+3) = 0 \Rightarrow y = 2$

    or -3. Substituting these values into [equation 3] yields $x^2 = 2 + 4 \Rightarrow x = \pm\sqrt{6}$ and $x^2 = -3 + 4 \Rightarrow x = \pm 1$.

    The solution set is $\{(-1,-3),(1,-3),(-\sqrt{6},2),(\sqrt{6},2)\}$.

73. Graph each function in the same window. The intersections or solutions are $(-0.79, 0.62)$ and $(0.88, 0.77)$.

75. Graph each function in the same window. The intersection or solution is $(0.06, 2.88)$.

77. (a) Let x represent the amount spent in 2012, and let y represent the amount spent in 2011.
    The required system of equations is $x + y = 1858$ and $x - y = 226$.

    (b) Adding the two equations results in $2x = 2084 \Rightarrow x = 1042$. From the first equation,
    $1042 + y = 1858 \Rightarrow y = 816$. The solution set is $\{(1042, 816)\}$.

    (c) The amount spent in 2012 was $1042 million and the amount spent in 2011 was $816 million.

79. Let x be the selling price in 2010 and y be the selling price in 2012. Then, $0.7x = y$ and $x - y = 195$. By

    substitution we have $x - 0.7x = 195 \Rightarrow 0.3x = 195 \Rightarrow x = 650$. Substitute $x = 650$ into $x - y = 195 \Rightarrow$

    $650 - y = 195 \Rightarrow y = 455$. In 2010 the average price was $650 and in 2012 the average price was $455.

81. Let x = the width of the base; therefore, the length $2x$, and let y = the height of the box. Since the volume is

    588 in^2, $2x^2 y = 588$ and so $y = \dfrac{588}{2x^2} = \dfrac{294}{x^2}$. Since the surface area is 448 in^2,

    $2(2x)(x) + 2(x)(y) + 2(2x)(y) = 448 \Rightarrow 4x^2 + 6xy = 448$. Substituting for y in this equation yields

    $4x^2 + 6x \cdot \dfrac{294}{x^2} = 448$. Simplifying we get $4x^3 - 448x + 1764 = 0$. By graphing the left side of the equation,

    the x-intercepts are approximately 5.17 and 7. See Figure 81. When $x \approx 5.17$, the dimensions are 5.17 by

    $2(5.17) \approx 10.34$ by $\dfrac{294}{(5.17)^2} \approx 11.00$ inches. When $x = 7$, the dimensions are 7 by $2(7) = 14$

    by $\dfrac{294}{(7)^2} = 6$ inches.

266   CHAPTER 6   Systems and Matrices

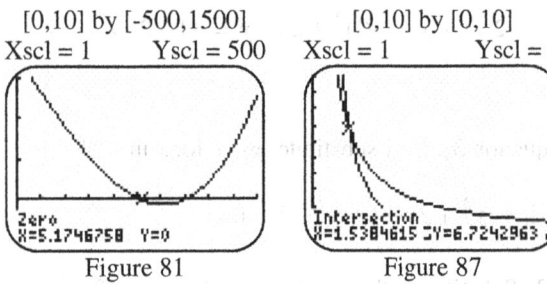

Figure 81   Figure 87

83. First let $H = 180$ in each equation and solve for y:

$$180 = 0.491x + 0.468y + 11.2 \Rightarrow 0.468y = 180 - 11.2 - 0.491x \Rightarrow y_1 = \frac{168.8 - 0.491x}{0.468}$$

$$180 = -0.981x + 1.872y + 26.4 \Rightarrow 1.872y = 180 - 26.4 - 0.981x \Rightarrow y_2 = \frac{153.6 + 0.981x}{1.872}.$$ Now graph each

equation in the same window and the intersection is approximately $(177.1, 174.9)$. This means that if an athlete's maximum heart rate is 180 beats per minute (bpm), then it will be about 177 bpm after 5 seconds and 175 bpm after 10 seconds.

85. (a) Let x = the amount spent by Apple and y = the amount spent by Samsung. Then

$x + y = 293$ and $x - y = 93$

(b) $x + y = 293$
$\underline{x - y = 93}$
$2x = 386 \Rightarrow x = 193.$

Then, $x - y = 93 \Rightarrow 193 - y = 93 \Rightarrow y = 100$ The solution is $(193, 100)$.

(c) From January to June 2012, Apple spent $193 million and Samsung spent $100 million.

87. If $V = \pi r^2 h$ and $V = 50$ then $50 = \pi r^2 h$; and $S.A = 2\pi rh$ and $S.A. = 65$ then $65 = 2\pi rh$. Now solve each for h: $50 = \pi r^2 h \Rightarrow h_1 = \frac{50}{\pi r^2}$; and $65 = 2\pi rh \Rightarrow h_2 = \frac{65}{2\pi r}$. Graph each equation in the same window. See Figure 87. The intersection is approximately: $(1.538, 6.724)$; therefore, $r \approx 1.538$ and $h \approx 6.724$.

89. Add the equations to eliminate the w_2-variable: $w_1 + \sqrt{2}w_2 = 300$
$\underline{\sqrt{3}w_1 - \sqrt{2}w_2 = 0}$
$(1 + \sqrt{3})w_1 = 300 \quad \Rightarrow w_1 = \frac{300}{(1+\sqrt{3})} \approx 109.8.$

Now substitute 109.8 for w_1 in the first equation:

$$\left(\frac{300}{(1+\sqrt{3})}\right) + \sqrt{2}w_2 = 300 \Rightarrow \sqrt{2}w_2 = 300 - \frac{300}{(1+\sqrt{3})} \Rightarrow \sqrt{2}w_2 = \frac{300(1+\sqrt{3}) - 300}{1+\sqrt{3}} \Rightarrow$$

Section 6.1   267

$\sqrt{2}\,w_2 = \dfrac{300\sqrt{3}}{1+\sqrt{3}} \Rightarrow w_2 = \dfrac{300\sqrt{3}}{1+\sqrt{3}} \times \dfrac{1}{\sqrt{2}} = \dfrac{300\sqrt{3}}{\sqrt{2}+\sqrt{6}} \Rightarrow w_2 \approx 134.5$. The solution is (109.8, 134.5).

91. The total number of vehicles entering intersection A is $500+150 = 650$ vehicles per hour. The expression $x+y$ represents the number of vehicles leaving intersection A each hour. Therefore, we have $x+y = 650$. The total number of vehicles leaving intersection B is $50+400 = 450$ vehicles per hour. There are 100 vehicles entering intersection B from the south and y vehicles entering intersection B from the west. Thus $y+100 = 450 \Rightarrow y = 350$. Using substitution, substitute 350 in for y into the equation $x+y = 650$: $x+350 = 650 \Rightarrow x = 300$. At intersection A, a stoplight should allow for 300 vehicles per hour to travel south and 350 vehicles per hour to continue traveling east.

93. (a) $p = \dfrac{1}{10}q \Rightarrow p = \dfrac{1}{10}(15) \Rightarrow p = 1.5$, The price will be $1.50 for a supply of 15 units.

    $p = 15 - \dfrac{2}{3}q \Rightarrow p = 15 - \dfrac{2}{3}(15) \Rightarrow p = 5$, The price will be $5 for a demand of 15 units.

    (b) Since the two equations $p = \dfrac{1}{10}q$ and $p = 15 - \dfrac{2}{3}q$ are already solved for p we will set the two equations equal to each other and solve for q.

    $\dfrac{1}{10}q = 15 - \dfrac{2}{3}q \Rightarrow 3q = 450 - 20q \Rightarrow 23q = 450 \Rightarrow q \approx 19.57 \approx 20$ units.

    Substitute $q = 20$ into $p = \dfrac{1}{10}(19.57) \Rightarrow p = 1.96$. The equilibrium price is $1.96 with a demand of about 20 units.

95. Find where $C = R, 20x+10,000 = 30x-11,000 \Rightarrow 21,000 = 10x \Rightarrow x = 2,100$. Now substitute 2,100 in for x into the first equation: $C = 20(2,100)+10,000 = 42,000+10,000 \Rightarrow C = 52,000$. When $x = 2,100;\ R = C = \$52,000$.

97. If $t = \dfrac{1}{x}$ and $u = \dfrac{1}{y}$, then $5\left(\dfrac{1}{x}\right)+15\left(\dfrac{1}{y}\right) = 16 \Rightarrow 5t+15u = 16$ and $5\left(\dfrac{1}{x}\right)+4\left(\dfrac{1}{y}\right) = 5 \Rightarrow 5t+4u = 5$. The equations are $5t+4u = 16$ and $5t+4u = 5$.

98. Subtract the two equations to eliminate the x-variable:

    $5t+15u = 16$
    $5t+\ 4u = \ \ 5$
    $\overline{\ \ \ \ 11u = 11}\ \ \Rightarrow u = 1$.

    Now substitute 1 for u in the first equation: $5t+15(1) = 16 \Rightarrow 5t = 1 \Rightarrow t = \dfrac{1}{5}$. Therefore, $u = 1$ and $t = \dfrac{1}{5}$.

99. If $t = \dfrac{1}{x}$ and $t = \dfrac{1}{5}$, then $\dfrac{1}{x} = \dfrac{1}{5}$ and $x = 5$. If $u = \dfrac{1}{y}$ and $u = 1$, then $\dfrac{1}{y} = 1 \Rightarrow y = 1$.

268 CHAPTER 6 Systems and Matrices

100. $\dfrac{5}{x}+\dfrac{15}{y}=16 \Rightarrow xy\left(\dfrac{5}{x}+\dfrac{15}{y}=16\right) \Rightarrow 5y+15x=16xy \Rightarrow 5y-16xy=-15x \Rightarrow$

$y(5-16x)=-15x \Rightarrow y=\dfrac{-15x}{5-16x}.$

101. $\dfrac{5}{x}+\dfrac{4}{y}=5 \Rightarrow xy\left(\dfrac{5}{x}+\dfrac{4}{y}=5\right) \Rightarrow 5y+4x=5xy \Rightarrow 5y-5xy=-4x \Rightarrow y(5-5x)=-4x \Rightarrow y=\dfrac{-4x}{5-5x}.$

102. See Figure 102. The graphs intersect at (5, 1), which supports the indicated exercise.

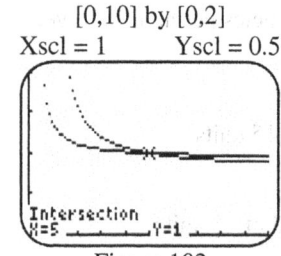

Figure 102

103. If we let $t=\dfrac{1}{x}$ and $u=\dfrac{1}{y}$, then our new equations are $2t+u=\dfrac{3}{2}$ and $3t-u=1$. Add these to eliminate the u-variable:

$2t+u=\dfrac{3}{2}$

$\underline{3t-u=1}$

$5t \quad =\dfrac{5}{2} \Rightarrow t=\dfrac{1}{2}$. If $t=\dfrac{1}{x}$ and $t=\dfrac{1}{2}$, then $\dfrac{1}{x}=\dfrac{1}{2} \Rightarrow x=2$. Now substitute $t=\dfrac{1}{2}$ into $2t+u=\dfrac{3}{2}$,

which yields $2\left(\dfrac{1}{2}\right)+u=\dfrac{3}{2} \Rightarrow u=\dfrac{1}{2}$. If $u=\dfrac{1}{y}$ and $u=\dfrac{1}{2}$, then $\dfrac{1}{y}=\dfrac{1}{2} \Rightarrow y=2$. The solution is (2,2)

105. If we let $t=\dfrac{1}{x}$ and $u=\dfrac{1}{y}$, then our new equations are $2t+3u=18$ and $4t-5u=-8$. Multiply the first equation by 2 and subtract to eliminate the t-variable.

$4t+6u=36$

$\underline{4t-5u=-8}$

$11u=44 \Rightarrow u=4.$

If $u=\dfrac{1}{y}$ and $u=4$, then $\dfrac{1}{y}=4 \Rightarrow 4y=1 \Rightarrow y=\dfrac{1}{4}$. Now substitute $u=4$ into $2t+3u=18$, which yields

$2t+3(4)=18 \Rightarrow 2t=6 \Rightarrow t=3$. If $t=\dfrac{1}{x}$ and $t=3$, then $\dfrac{1}{x}=3 \Rightarrow 3x=1 \Rightarrow x=\dfrac{1}{3}.$

The solution is $\left(\dfrac{1}{3},\dfrac{1}{4}\right)$.

6.2: Solution of Linear Systems in Three Variables

1. For $2x+y-z=-1$ and $(-3,6,1)$: $2(-3)+(6)-1=-1 \Rightarrow -6+6-1=-1 \Rightarrow -1=-1$.

   For $x-y+3z=-6$ and $(-3,6,1)$: $(-3)-6+3(1)=-6 \Rightarrow -3-6+3=-6 \Rightarrow -6=-6$.

   For $-4x+y+z=19$ and $(-3,6,1)$: $-4(-3)+6+1=19 \Rightarrow 12+6+1=19 \Rightarrow 19=19$.

3. For $5x-y+2z=-0.4$ and $(-0.2,0.4,0.5)$: $5(-0.2)-(0.4)+2(0.5)=-0.4 \Rightarrow$

   $-1-0.4+1=0.4 \Rightarrow -0.4=-0.4$.

   For $x+4z=1.8$ and $(-0.2,0.4,0.5)$: $(-0.2)+4(0.5)=1.8 \Rightarrow -0.2+4(0.5)=1.8 \Rightarrow$

   $-0.2+2.0=1.8 \Rightarrow 1.8=1.8$.

   For $-3y+z=-0.7$ and $(-0.2,0.4,0.5)$: $-3(0.4)+(0.5)=-0.7 \Rightarrow -1.2+0.5=-0.7 \Rightarrow -0.7=-0.7$.

5. For $x-y+z=-2$ and $(-2,-1,3)$: $(-2)-(-1)+(3)=2 \Rightarrow -2+1+3=2 \Rightarrow 2=2$.

   For $3x-2y+z=-1$ and $(-2,-1,3)$: $3(-2)-2(-1)+(3)=-1 \Rightarrow -6+2+3=-1 \Rightarrow -1=-1$.

   For $x+y=-3$ and $(-2,-1,3)$: $(-2)+(-1)=-3 \Rightarrow -2+(-1)=-3 \Rightarrow -3=-3$.

7. First add [equation 1] and [equation 2] to eliminate z and produce [equation 4]. Second add [equation 2] and [equation 3] to eliminate y and z and produce [equation 5].

   $$\begin{array}{rl} x+y+z=2 & [1] \\ 2x+y-z=5 & [2] \\ \hline 3x+2y=7 & [4] \end{array} \qquad \begin{array}{rl} 2x+y-z=5 & [2] \\ x-y+z=-2 & [3] \\ \hline 3x=3 & [5] \end{array}$$

   Solve [equation 5] for x: $3x=3 \Rightarrow x=1$. Substitute $x=1$ into [equation 4] to solve for y:

   $3(1)+2y=7 \Rightarrow 2y=4 \Rightarrow y=2$. Finally, substitute $x=1$ and $y=2$ into [equation 1] to solve for z:

   $(1)+(2)+z=2 \Rightarrow z=-1$. The solution is $(1,2,-1)$.

9. First, add [equation 1] and [equation 2] to eliminate y and produce [equation 4]. Second, multiply [equation 3] by 3 and add [equation 1] to eliminate y and produce [equation 5].

   $$\begin{array}{rl} x+3y+4z=14 & [1] \\ 2x-3y+2z=10 & [2] \\ \hline 3x+6z=24 & [4] \end{array} \qquad \begin{array}{rl} 9x-3y+3z=27 & 3[3] \\ x+3y+4z=14 & [1] \\ \hline 10x+7z=41 & [5] \end{array}$$

   Next multiply [equation 4] by 10 and add to [equation 5] multiplied by -3 to eliminate x and produce [equation 6]

   $$\begin{array}{rl} 30x+60z=240 & 10[4] \\ -30x-21z=-123 & -3[5] \\ \hline 39z=117 & [6] \end{array}$$

   Solve [equation 6] for z: $39z=117 \Rightarrow z=3$. Substitute $z=3$ into [equation 4] to solve for x:

   $3x+6(3)=24 \Rightarrow 3x+6 \Rightarrow x=2$. Finally, substitute $x=2$ and $z=3$ into [equation 1] to solve for y:

   $(2)+3y+4(3)=14 \Rightarrow 3y=0 \Rightarrow y=0$. The solution is $(2,0,3)$.

11. First, multiply [equation 1] by 2 and add [equation 3] to eliminate all the variables.

270 CHAPTER 6 Systems and Matrices

$$\begin{array}{rcl} 2x + 4y + 6z &=& 16 \quad 2[1] \\ -2x - 4y - 6z &=& 5 \quad\;\; [3] \\ \hline 0 &=& 21 \end{array}$$

Since this is false, the solution set is ∅.

13. First, add [equation 1] and [equation 2] to eliminate z and produce [equation 4]. Second, multiply [equation 1] by 3 and add [equation 3] to eliminate z and produce [equation 5].

$$\begin{array}{rcl} x + 4y - z &=& 6 \quad [1] \\ 2x - y + z &=& 3 \quad [2] \\ \hline 3x + 3y &=& 9 \quad [4] \end{array} \qquad \begin{array}{rcl} 3x + 12y - 3z &=& 18 \quad 3[1] \\ 3x + 2y + 3z &=& 16 \quad\;\; [2] \\ \hline 6x + 14y &=& 34 \quad\;\; [5] \end{array}$$

Next multiply [equation 4] by -2 and add to [equation 5] to eliminate x and produce [equation 6].

$$\begin{array}{rcl} -6x - 6y &=& -18 \quad -2[4] \\ 6x + 14y &=& 34 \quad\;\; [5] \\ \hline 8y &=& 16 \quad\;\; [6] \end{array}$$

Solve [equation 6] for y: y: $8y = 16 \Rightarrow y = 2$. Substitute $y = 2$ into [equation 4] to solve for x: $3x + 3(2) = 9 \Rightarrow 3x = 3 \Rightarrow x = 1$. Finally, substitute $x = 1$ and $y = 2$ into [equation 1] to solve for z: $(1) + 4(2) - z = 6 \Rightarrow -z = -3 \Rightarrow z = 3$. The solution is $(1, 2, 3)$.

15. First, multiply [equation 1] by -3 and add [equation 2] to eliminate y and produce [equation 4]. Second, multiply [equation 1] by 2 and add [equation 3] to eliminate y and produce [equation 5]

$$\begin{array}{rcl} -15x - 3y + 9z &=& 18 \quad -3[1] \\ 2x + 3y + z &=& 5 \quad\;\; [2] \\ \hline -13x + 10z &=& 23 \quad\;\; [4] \end{array} \qquad \begin{array}{rcl} 10x + 2y - 6z &=& -12 \quad 2[1] \\ -3x - 2y + 4z &=& 3 \quad\;\; [3] \\ \hline 7x - 2z &=& -9 \quad\;\; [5] \end{array}$$

Next multiply [equation 5] by 5 and add [equation 4] to eliminate z and produce [equation 6]

$$\begin{array}{rcl} 35x - 10z &=& -45 \quad 5[5] \\ -13x + 10z &=& 23 \quad\;\; [4] \\ \hline 22x &=& -22 \quad\;\; [6] \end{array}$$

Solve [equation 6] for x: $22x = -22 \Rightarrow x = -1$. Substitute $x = -1$ into [equation 4] to solve for z: $-13(-1) + 10z = 23 \Rightarrow 10z = 10 \Rightarrow z = 1$. Finally, substitute $x = -1$ and $z = 1$ into [equation 1] to solve for y: $5(-1) + y - 3(1) = -6 \Rightarrow y = 2$. The solution is $(-1, 2, 1)$.

17. First, add [equation 1] and [equation 3] to eliminate x and produce [equation 4]. Second, multiply [equation 3] by 3 and add [equation 2] to eliminate x and produce [equation 5].

$$\begin{array}{rcl} x - 3y - 2z &=& -3 \quad [1] \\ -x - y + 4z &=& 3 \quad [3] \\ \hline -4y + 2z &=& 0 \quad [4] \end{array} \qquad \begin{array}{rcl} -3x - 3y + 12z &=& 9 \quad 3[3] \\ 3x + 2y - z &=& 12 \quad\;\; [2] \\ \hline -y + 11z &=& 21 \quad\;\; [5] \end{array}$$

Next multiply [equation 5] by -4 and add [equation 4] to eliminate y and produce [equation 6].

$$\begin{array}{rcl} 4y - 44z &=& -84 \quad -4[5] \\ -4y + 2z &=& 0 \quad\;\; [4] \\ \hline -42z &=& -84 \quad\;\; [6] \end{array}$$

Solve [equation 6] for z: $-42z = -84 \Rightarrow z = 2$. Substitute $z = 2$ into [equation 4] to solve for y: $-4y+2(2)=0 \Rightarrow -4y=-4 \Rightarrow y=1$. Finally, substitute $y=1$ and $z=2$ into [equation 1] to solve for x: $x-3(1)-2(2)=-3 \Rightarrow x=4$. The solution is $(4,1,2)$.

19. First eliminate x by multiplying [equation 1] by -2 and adding [equation 2].

$$\begin{array}{rl} -2x+4y-6z=-12 & -2\,[1] \\ \underline{2x-y+2z=5} & [2] \\ 3y-4z=-7 & \end{array}$$

Now solve this for y. $3y-4z=-7 \Rightarrow 3y=4z-7 \Rightarrow y=\dfrac{4z-7}{3}$. Now substitute this into [equation 2].

$2x-\dfrac{4z-7}{3}+2z=5 \Rightarrow 3\left(2x-\dfrac{4z-7}{3}+2z=5\right) \Rightarrow 6x-4z+7+6z=15 \Rightarrow$

$6x+2z=8 \Rightarrow x=\dfrac{8-2z}{6} \Rightarrow x=\dfrac{4-z}{3}$. We have infinitely many solutions $\left(\dfrac{4-z}{3},\dfrac{4z-7}{3},z\right)$.

21. First eliminate x by adding [equation 1] to [equation 2] multiplied by -3:

$$\begin{array}{rl} 3x+4y-z=13 & [1] \\ \underline{-3x-3y-6z=-45} & -3\,[2] \\ y-7z=-32 & \end{array}$$

Now solve this for y: $y-7z=-32 \Rightarrow y=7z-32$. Now substitute this into [equation 2].

$x+(7z-32)+2z=15 \Rightarrow x+9z=47 \Rightarrow x=47-9z$.

We have infinitely many solutions $(47-9z, 7z-32, z)$.

23. First, multiply [equation 1] by 3 and add [equation 2] to eliminate y and produce [equation 4], then simplify. Second, multiply [equation 3] by 3 and add [equation 2] to eliminate y and produce [equation 5] then simplify.

$$\begin{array}{rl} 24x-9y+18z=-6 & 3[1] \\ \underline{4x+9y+4z=18} & [2] \\ 28x+22z=12 & [4] \\ =14x+11z=6 & [4a] \end{array} \qquad \begin{array}{rl} 36x-9y+24z=-6 & 3[2] \\ \underline{4x+9y+4z=18} & [2] \\ 40x+28z=12 & [5] \\ =10x+7z=3 & [5a] \end{array}$$

Next multiply [equation 4a] by 5 and add [equation 5a] multiplied by -7 to eliminate x and produce [equation 6].

$$\begin{array}{rl} 70x+55z=30 & 5[4a] \\ \underline{-70x-49z=-21} & -7[5a] \\ 6z=9 & [6] \end{array}$$

Solve [equation 6] for z: $6z=9 \Rightarrow z=\dfrac{3}{2}$. Substitute $z=\dfrac{3}{2}$ into [equation 5a] to solve for x:

$10x+7\left(\dfrac{3}{2}\right)=3 \Rightarrow 2\left[10x+7\left(\dfrac{3}{2}\right)=3\right] \Rightarrow 20x+21=6 \Rightarrow 20x=-15 \Rightarrow x=-\dfrac{3}{4}$. Finally, substitute $x = -\frac{3}{4}$ and $z = \frac{3}{2}$ into [equation 2] to solve for y: $4\left(-\frac{3}{4}\right) + 9y + 4\left(\frac{3}{2}\right) = 18 \Rightarrow$

$-3 + 9y + 6 = 18 \Rightarrow 9y = 15 \Rightarrow y = \frac{15}{9} = \frac{5}{3}$. The solution is $\left(-\frac{3}{4}, \frac{5}{3}, \frac{3}{2}\right)$.

25. First, add [equation 1] and [equation 2] multiplied by -1 to eliminate x and produce [equation 4]. Second, add [equation 3] and [equation 4] to eliminate y and produce [equation 5].

$$\begin{array}{rl} x - z = & 2 \quad [1] \\ -x - y = & 3 \quad -1[2] \\ \hline -y - z = & 5 \quad [4] \end{array} \qquad \begin{array}{rl} y - z = & 1 \quad [3] \\ -y - z = & 5 \quad [4] \\ \hline -2z = & 6 \quad [5] \end{array}$$

Solve [equation 5] for z: $-2z = 6 \Rightarrow z = -3$. Substitute $z = -3$ into [equation 1] to solve for x: $x - (-3) = 2 \Rightarrow x = -1$. Finally, substitute $z = -3$ into [equation 3] to solve for y: $y - (-3) = 1 \Rightarrow y = -2$. The solution is $(-1, -2, -3)$.

27. First, multiply [equation 1] by 3 and add [equation 2] multiplied by -2 to eliminate y and produce [equation 4]. Second, add [equation 4] and [equation 3] multiplied by -9 to eliminate x.

$$\begin{array}{rl} 9x + 6y - 3z = & -3 \quad 3[1] \\ -6y - 2z = & -24 \quad -2[2] \\ \hline 9x \quad - 5z = & -27 \quad [4] \end{array} \qquad \begin{array}{rl} 9x - 5z = & -27 \quad [4] \\ -9x + 27z = & 27 \quad [3] \\ \hline 22z = & 0 \Rightarrow z = 0. \end{array}$$

Substitute $z = 0$ to solve [equation 2] for y: $3y + 0 = 12 \Rightarrow y = 4$. Finally, substitute $z = 0$ into [equation 3] to solve for x: $x - 3(0) = -3 \Rightarrow x = -3$. The solution is $(-3, 4, 0)$.

29. First eliminate y by adding [equation 1] to [equation 2].

$$\begin{array}{rl} x - y + z = & -6 \\ 4x + y + z = & 7 \\ \hline 5x \quad + 2z = & 1 \end{array}$$

Now solve this for x. $5x + 2z = 1 \Rightarrow 5x = 1 - 2x \Rightarrow x = \frac{1 - 2x}{5}$. Now substitute this into [equation 1].

$\frac{1 - 2z}{5} - y + z = -6 \Rightarrow 5\left(\frac{1 - 2z}{5} - y + z = -6\right) \Rightarrow 1 - 2z - 5y + 5z = -30 \Rightarrow -5y + 3z = -31 \Rightarrow$

$-5y = -3z - 31 \Rightarrow y = \frac{3z + 31}{5}$. We have infinitely many solutions $\left(\frac{1 - 2z}{5}, \frac{3z + 31}{5}, z\right)$.

31. First, multiply [equation 1] by -3 and add [equation 2] to eliminate x and produce [equation 4]. Second, add [equation 4] and [equation 3] to eliminate y.

$$\begin{array}{rl} -6x - 9y - 12z = & -9 \quad -3[1] \\ 6x + 3y + 8z = & 6 \quad -2[2] \\ \hline -6y - 4z = & -3 \quad [4] \end{array} \qquad \begin{array}{rl} -6y - 4z = & -3 \quad [4] \\ 6y - 4z = & 1 \quad [3] \\ \hline -8z = & -2 \Rightarrow z = \frac{1}{4}. \end{array}$$

Substitute $z = \dfrac{1}{4}$ to solve [equation 3] for y: $6y - 4\left(\dfrac{1}{4}\right) = 1 \Rightarrow 6y = 2 \Rightarrow y = \dfrac{1}{3}$. Finally, substitute $y = \dfrac{1}{3}$

and $z = \dfrac{1}{4}$ into [equation 1] to solve for x: $2x + 3\left(\dfrac{1}{3}\right) + 4\left(\dfrac{1}{4}\right) = 3 \Rightarrow 2x = 1 \Rightarrow x = \dfrac{1}{2}$.

The solution is $\left(\dfrac{1}{2}, \dfrac{1}{3}, \dfrac{1}{4}\right)$.

33. If we let $t = \dfrac{1}{x}$, $u = \dfrac{1}{y}$, and $v = \dfrac{1}{z}$, then our new equations are $t + u - v = \dfrac{1}{4}$ [1], $2t - u + 3v = \dfrac{9}{4}$ [2], and

    $-t - 2u + 4v = 1$ [3]. First, add [equation 1] and [equation 3] to eliminate t and produce [equation 4].

    Second, add [equation 2] and [equation 3] multiplied by 2 to eliminate t and produce [equation 5].

    $x^2 - 3x = 4 \Rightarrow x^2 - 3x - 4 = 0 \Rightarrow x = (x-4)(x+1) = 0 \Rightarrow x = 4, -1$.

    $\begin{array}{ll} t + u - v = \dfrac{1}{4} & [1] \\ -t - 2u + 4v = 1 & [2] \\ \hline -u + 3v = \dfrac{5}{4} & [4] \end{array}$
    $\quad\quad$
    $\begin{array}{ll} 2t - u + 3v = \dfrac{4}{9} & [2] \\ -2t - 4u + 8v = 2 & 2[3] \\ \hline -5u + 11v = \dfrac{17}{4} & [5] \end{array}$

    Next multiply [equation 4] by -5 and add [equation 5] to eliminate u and produce [equation 6].

    $\begin{array}{ll} 5u - 15v = -\dfrac{25}{4} & -5[4] \\ -5u + 11v = \dfrac{17}{4} & [5] \\ \hline -4v = -\dfrac{8}{4} & [6] \end{array}$

    Solve [equation 6] for v. $-4v = -2 \Rightarrow v = \dfrac{1}{2}$. If $v = \dfrac{1}{2}$ and $v = \dfrac{1}{z}$, then $\dfrac{1}{2} = \dfrac{1}{z} \Rightarrow z = -2$.

    Substitute $v = \dfrac{1}{2}$ into [equation 4] to solve for u. $-u + 3\left(\dfrac{1}{2}\right) = \dfrac{5}{4} \Rightarrow -u = -\dfrac{1}{4}$. If $u = \dfrac{1}{4}$ and $u = \dfrac{1}{y}$ then

    $\dfrac{1}{4} = \dfrac{1}{y} \Rightarrow y = 4$. Finally, substitute $v = \dfrac{1}{2}$ and $u = \dfrac{1}{4}$ into [equation 3] to solve for t.

    $-t - 2\left(\dfrac{1}{4}\right) + 4\left(\dfrac{1}{2}\right) = 1 \Rightarrow -2t - 1 + 4 = 2 \Rightarrow -2t = -1 \Rightarrow t = \dfrac{1}{2}$.

    If $t = \dfrac{1}{2}$ and $t = \dfrac{1}{x}$ then $\dfrac{1}{2} = \dfrac{1}{x} \Rightarrow x = 2$. The solution is $(2, 4, 2)$.

35. If we let $t = \dfrac{1}{x}$, $u = \dfrac{1}{y}$, and $v = \dfrac{1}{z}$ then our new equations are $2t - 2u + v = -1$ [1], $4t + u - 2v = -9$ [2],

    and $t + u - 3v = -9$ [3]. First, add [equation 1] and [equation 2] multiplied by 2 to eliminate u and produce

    [equation 4]. Second, add [equation 1] and [equation 3] multiplied by 2 to eliminate u and produce [equation 5].

274   CHAPTER 6   Systems and Matrices

$$\begin{array}{rl} 2t-2u+v=-1 & [1] \\ 8t+2u-4v=-18 & 2[2] \\ \hline 10t-3v=-19 & [4] \end{array}$$

$$\begin{array}{rl} 2t-2u+v=-1 & [1] \\ 8t+2u-6v=-18 & 2[3] \\ \hline 4t-5v=-19 & [5] \end{array}$$

Next multiply [equation 4] by 2 and add [equation 5] multiplied by -5 to eliminate t and produce [equation 6].

$$\begin{array}{rl} 20t-6v=-38 & 2[2] \\ -20t+25v=95 & -5[5] \\ \hline 19v=57 & [6] \Rightarrow v=3 \end{array}$$

If $v=3$ and $v=\dfrac{1}{z}$ then $3=\dfrac{1}{z}\Rightarrow 3z=1\Rightarrow z=\dfrac{1}{3}$. Substitute $v=3$ into [equation 5] to solve for t.

$4t+5(3)=-19\Rightarrow 4t=-4\Rightarrow t=-1$. If $t=-1$ and $t=\dfrac{1}{x}$ then $-1=\dfrac{1}{x}\Rightarrow -x=1\Rightarrow x=-1$. Finally, substitute $v=3$ and $t=-1$ into [equation 1] to solve for u. $2(-1)-2u+(3)=-1\Rightarrow -2u=-2\Rightarrow u=1$.

If $u=1$ and $=\dfrac{1}{y}$ then $1=\dfrac{1}{y}\Rightarrow y=1$. The solution is $\left(-1,1,\dfrac{1}{3}\right)$.

37. Add [equation 1] and [equation 2] to eliminate z and produce [equation 4].

$$\begin{array}{rl} x-4y+2z=-2 & [1] \\ x+2y-2z=-3 & [2] \\ \hline 2x-2y=-5 & [4] \end{array}$$

Add [equation 4] to [equation 3] multiplied by -2.

$$\begin{array}{rl} 2x-2y=-5 & [4] \\ -2x+2y=-8 & -2[3] \\ \hline 0=-13 & \end{array}$$

Since this is a false statement, the solution is ∅.

39. Subtract [equation 3] from [equation 1] to eliminate x and produce equation [4].

$$\begin{array}{rl} x+y+z=0 & [1] \\ x+3y+3z=5 & [3] \\ \hline -2y-2z=-5 & [4] \end{array}$$

Subtract [equation 3] from [equation 2] to eliminate x and produce equation [5].

$$\begin{array}{rl} x-y-z=3 & [2] \\ x+3y+3z=5 & [3] \\ \hline -4y-4z=-2 & [5] \end{array}$$

Multiply [equation 4] by 2 and subtract [equation 5].

$$\begin{array}{rl} -4y-4z=-10 & 2[4] \\ -4y-4z=-2 & [5] \\ \hline 0=-8 & \end{array}$$

Since this is a false statement, the solution is ∅.

41. Add the first two equations.

$$2x - y + 2z = 6$$
$$\underline{-x + y + z = 0}$$
$$x + 3z = 6$$

Add this equation to the third equation.

$$x + 3z = 6$$
$$\underline{-x - 3z = -6}$$
$$0 = 0$$

Therefore, we have infinitely many solutions. $x + 3z = 6 \Rightarrow x = -3z + 6$.

Multiply the second equation by 2 and add to the first equation: \

$$2x - y + 2z = 6$$
$$\underline{-2x + 2y + 2z = 0}$$
$$y + 4z = 6 \Rightarrow y = -4z + 6.$$

We have infinitely many solutions $(-3z + 6, -4z + 6, z)$.

43. First, add [equation 2] and [equation 3] multiplied by -1 to eliminate y and produce [equation 4]. Second, add [equation 1] and [equation 3] multiplied by -20 to eliminate y.

$$4x + 2y + 3z = 280 \quad [2]$$
$$\underline{-3x - 2y - z = -180 \quad -1[3]}$$
$$x + 2z = 100 \quad [4]$$

$$25x + 40y + 20z = 2200 \quad [1]$$
$$\underline{-60x - 40y - 20z = -3600 \quad -20[3]}$$
$$-35x = -1400 \Rightarrow x = 40$$

Substitute $x = 40$ to solve [equation 4] for z. $40 + 2z = 100 \Rightarrow 2z = 60 \Rightarrow z = 30$. Finally, substitute $x = 40$ and $z = 30$ into [equation 3] to solve for y. $3(40) + 2y + 30 = 180 \Rightarrow 2y = 30 \Rightarrow y = 15$.

The solution is $(40, 15, 30)$.

45. Let x = number of gallons of \$9 grade, y = number of gallons of \$3 grade, and z = number of gallons of \$4.50 grade. From the information the equations are $x + y + z = 300$ [1], $9x + 3y + 4.5z = 6(300)$ [2], and $z = 2y$ [3]. Substitute [equation 3] into both [equation 1] and [equation 2] to produce equations [4] and [5]. [3] into [1] produces $x + y + 2y = 300 \Rightarrow x + 3y = 300$ [4]. [3] into [2] produces $9x + 3y + 4.5(2y) = 1800 \Rightarrow 9x + 12y = 1800$ [5]. Now add [equation 5] to [equation 4] multiplied by -9.

$$9x + 12y = 1800 \quad [5]$$
$$\underline{-9x - 27y = -2700 \quad -9[4]}$$
$$-15y = -900 \quad \Rightarrow y = 60$$

Substitute $y = 60$, into [3]. $z = 2(60) \Rightarrow z = 120$. Finally, substitute $y = 60$, and $z = 120$ into [1]. $x + 60 + 120 = 300 \Rightarrow x = 120$. She should use 120 gallons of \$9 water, 60 gallons of \$3 water, and 120 gallons of \$4.50 water.

276 CHAPTER 6 Systems and Matrices

47. Let x = price of the senior ticket, y = price of adult ticket, and z = price of student ticket. From the information given the equations are $2x+y+2z = 51$ [1], $y+5z = 55$ [2], and $2x+2y+7z = 75$ [3]. First solve [equation 2] for y and substitute into [equation 1] and create [equation 4].
$2x+55-5z+2z = 51 \Rightarrow 2x-3z = -4$ Now substitute [equation 2] into [equation 3] and create [equation 5] $2x+2(55-5z)+7z = 75 \Rightarrow 2x+110-10z+7z = 75 \Rightarrow 2x-3z = -35$.

Subtracting [equation 4] from [equation 5] we will eliminate both the x and z variables.
$$\begin{aligned} 2x-3z &= -35 \\ 2x-3z &= -4 \\ \hline 0 &= -31 \end{aligned}$$

This shows that there is no solution to this system of equations. The ticket pricing was inconsistent.

49. Let x = measure of the largest angle, y = measure of the medium angle, and z = measure of the smallest angle. From the information the equations are $a+b+c = 180$ [1], $a = 2b-55$ [2], and $c = b-25$ [3]. Substitute both [2] and [3] into [1]. $(2b-55)+b+(b-25) = 180 \Rightarrow 4b-80 = 180 \Rightarrow 4b = 260 \Rightarrow b = 65$. Substitute $b = 65$ into [3]. $c = 65-25 \Rightarrow c = 40$, and substitute $b = 65$ into [2]. $a = 2(65)-55 \Rightarrow a = 130-55 \Rightarrow a = 75$. The angles are $75°$, $65°$, and $40°$.

51. Let x = the amount invested at 4%, y = the amount invested at 4.5%, and z = the amount invested at 2.5%. From the information the equations are $x+y+z = 10000$ [1], $0.04x+0.025y+0.045z = 415$ [2], and $y = 2x$ [3]. Substitute [equation 3] into [equation 1] and [equation 3] into [equation 2] multiplied by 1000, to produce equations [4] and [5]. [3] into [1] $\Rightarrow x+2x+z = 10000 \Rightarrow 3x+z = 10000$ [4]. [3] into $1000[2] \Rightarrow 40x+45(2x)+25z = 415000 \Rightarrow 130x+25z = 415000 \Rightarrow 26x+5z = 83000$ [5]. Now multiply [equation 4] by -5 and add to [equation 5].

$$\begin{aligned} -15x-5y &= -50000 & -5[4] \\ 26x+5y &= 83000 & [5] \\ \hline 11x &= 33000 & \Rightarrow x = 3000 \end{aligned}$$

Substitute $x = 3000$, into [3]. $y = 2(3000) \Rightarrow y = 6000$. Finally, substitute $x = 3000$ and $y = 6000$ into [1]. $3000+6000+z = 10000 \Rightarrow z = 1000$. He invested $3000 at 4%, $6000 at 4.5%, and $1000 at 2.5%.

53. Let x = the number of EZ models, y = the number of Compact models, and z = the number of Commercial models. From the information, the two equations are derived:
(weight) $10x+20y+60z = 440$ [1] and (volume) $10x+8y+28z = 248$ [2]. First, subtract [2] from [1].
$$\begin{aligned} 10x+20y+60z &= 440 & [1] \\ 10x+8y+28z &= 248 & [2] \\ \hline 12y+32z &= 192 & \Rightarrow 12y = -32z+192 \Rightarrow y = -\frac{8}{3}z+16. \end{aligned}$$

Now substitute into [1]: $10x+20\left(-\frac{8}{3}z+16\right)+60z = 440 \Rightarrow 3\left[10x+20\left(-\frac{8}{3}z+16\right)+60z = 440\right] \Rightarrow$

$30x - 160z + 960 + 180z = 1320 \Rightarrow 30x = -20z + 360 \Rightarrow x = -\frac{2}{3}z + 12$. From the equations for x and y, z must be a multiple of 3 for x and y to be whole numbers. There are three possibilities:

If $z = 0$, then $y = -\frac{8}{3}(0) + 16 = 16$ and $x = -\frac{2}{3}(0) + 12 = 12$. Therefore, 12 EZ, 16 Comp., and 0 Comm.

If $z = 3$, then $y = -\frac{8}{3}(3) + 16 = 8$ and $x = -\frac{2}{3}(3) + 12 = 10$. Therefore, 10 EZ, 8 Comp, and 3 Comm.

If $z = 6$, then $y = -\frac{8}{3}(6) + 16 = 0$ and $x = -\frac{2}{3}(6) + 12 = 8$. Therefore, 8 EZ, 0 Comp., and 6 Comm.

If $z \geq 9$, then y is less than zero; therefore, no solution is possible.

55. (a) $a + 20b + 2c = 190$
$a + 5b + 3c = 320$
$a + 40b + c = 50$

(b) Using technology, the solution is (30, –2, 100). So the equation is $P = 30 - 2A + 100S$.

(c) When A = 10 and S = 2500, P = 30 – 2(10) + 100(2.5) = $260,000.

57. Using the form $y = ax^2 + bx + c$ and the given points yields the following equations.

For $(-3, 0)$: $0 = a(-3)^2 + b(-3) + c \Rightarrow 9a - 3b + c = 0$. [equation 1]

For $(0, -3)$: $-3 = a(0)^2 + b(0) + c \Rightarrow c = -3$. [equation 2]

For $(1, 0)$: $0 = a(1)^2 + b(1) + c \Rightarrow a + b + c = 0$. [equation 3]

First, substitute $c = -3$ into [equation 1] and [equation 3] and then add the two equations to eliminate b.

$9a - 3b - 3 = 0$ [1] $9a - 3b = 3$ [1]
$a + b - 3 = 0$ [3] $\Rightarrow$ $3a + 3b = 9$ 3[3]
                                $12a = 12 \Rightarrow a = 1$

Substitute $a = 1$ into [3]. $1 + b - 3 = 0 \Rightarrow b = 2$ The equation is $y = x^2 + 2x - 3$.

59. Using the form $y = ax^2 + bx + c$ and the given points yields the following equations.

For $(1.5, 6.25)$: $6.25 = a(1.5)^2 + b(1.5) + c \Rightarrow 2.25a + 1.5b + c = 6.25$. [equation 1]

For $(0, -2)$: $-2 = a(0)^2 + b(0) + c \Rightarrow c = -2$. [equation 2]

For $(-1.5, 3.25)$: $3.25 = a(-1.5)^2 + b(-1.5) + c \Rightarrow 2.25a - 1.5b + c = 3.25$. [equation 3]

Substitute $c = -2$ into [1]. $2.25a + 1.5b - 2 = 6.25 \Rightarrow 2.25a + 1.5b = 8.25$. [equation 4]

Substitute $c = -2$ into [3]. $2.25a - 1.5b - 2 = 3.25 \Rightarrow 2.25a - 1.5b = 5.25$. [equation 5]

Now add [equation 4] and [equation 5]

$2.25a + 1.5b = 8.25$ [4]
$2.25a - 1.5b = 5.25$ [5]
$4.5a = 13.5 \Rightarrow a = 3$

Finally, substitute $a = 3$ and $c = -2$ into [1]. $6.25 = 2.25(3) + 1.5b + (-2) \Rightarrow b = 1$.

The equation is $y = 3x^2 + x - 2$.

61. Using the form $y = ax^2 + bx + c$, and the given points yields the following equations.

278   CHAPTER 6   Systems and Matrices

For $(-1, 4)$: $4 = a(-1)^2 + b(-1) + c \Rightarrow a - b + c = 4$. [equation 1]

For $(1, 2)$: $2 = a(1)^2 + b(1) + c \Rightarrow a + b + c = 2$. [equation 2]

For $(3, 8)$: $8 = a(3)^2 + b(3) + c \Rightarrow 9a + 3b + c = 8$. [equation 3]

First, add [equation 1] and [equation 2] multiplied to eliminate both b.

Second, add [equation 2] and [equation 3] multiplied by –3 to eliminate b and produce [equation 5].

```
 a - b + c = 4    [1]        -3a - 3b - 3c = -6   -3[2]
 a + b + c = 2    [2]         9a + 3b +  c =  8    [3]
─────────────                 ──────────────────
 2a    + 2c = 6   [4]         6a       - 2c = 2    [5]
```

```
 2a + 2c = 6     [4]
 6a - 2c = 2     [5]
─────────────
 8a      = 8     ⇒ a = 1
```

Finally, substitute a = 1 into [5]. $6(1) - 2c = 2 \Rightarrow c = 2$.

Finally, substitute a = 1 and c = 2 into [1]. $(1) - b + (2) = 4 \Rightarrow -b = 1 \Rightarrow b = -1$.

The equation is $y = x^2 - x + 2$.

63. Using the form $y = ax^2 + bx + c$, and the given points yields the following equations.

For $(0, 1)$: $1 = a(0)^2 + b(0) + c \Rightarrow c = 1$. [equation 1]

For $(1, 0)$: $0 = a(1)^2 + b(1)^2 + c \Rightarrow a + b + c = 0$. [equation 2]

For $(2, -5)$: $-5 = a(2)^2 + b(2) + c \Rightarrow 4a + 2b + c = -5$. [equation 3]

Substitute c = 1 into [1]. $a + b + 1 = 0 \Rightarrow a + b = -1$. [equation 4]

Substitute c = 1 into [3]. $4a + 2b + 1 = -5 \Rightarrow 4a + 2b = -6$. [equation 5]

Now add [equation 4] and [equation 5] multiplied by -2.

```
 -2a - 2b =  2    -2[4]
  4a - 2b = -6      [5]
─────────────
  2a      = -4    ⇒ a = -2
```

Finally, substitute a = -2 and c = 1 into [1]. $(-2) + b + (1) = 0 \Rightarrow b = 1$.

The equation is $y = -2x^2 + x + 1$.

65. Using the form $x^2 + y^2 + ax + by + c = 0$ and the given points yields the following equations.

For $(1, 4)$: $(1)^2 + (4)^2 + a(1) + b(4) + c = 0 \Rightarrow 1 + 16 + a + 4b + c = 0 \Rightarrow a + 4b + c = -17$.
[equation 1]

For $(5, 2)$: $(5)^2 + (2)^2 + a(5) + b(2) + c = 0 \Rightarrow 25 + 4 + 5a + 2b + c = 0 \Rightarrow 5a + 2b + c = -29$.
[equation 2]

For $(-3, -4)$: $(-3)^2 + (-4)^2 + a(-3) + b(-4) + c = 0 \Rightarrow 9 + 16 - 3a - 4b + c = 0 \Rightarrow -3a - 4b + c = -25$.
[equation 3]

Now, add [equation 1] multiplied by -1 to [equation 2] to eliminate c and produce [equation 4].
Then, add [equation 3] multiplied by -1 to [equation 2] to eliminate c and produce [equation 5].

$$\begin{array}{ll} 5a+2b+c=-29 & [2] \\ \underline{-a-4b-c=17} \quad -1\,[1] \\ 4a-2b=-12 & [4] \end{array} \qquad \begin{array}{ll} 5a+2b+c=-29 & [2] \\ \underline{3a+4b-c=25} \quad -1\,[3] \\ 8a+6b=-4 & [5] \end{array}$$

Next multiply [equation 4] by 3 and add [equation 5] to eliminate b.

$$\begin{array}{ll} 12a-6b=-36 & 3\,[4] \\ \underline{8a+6b=-4} & [5] \\ 20a=-40 & \Rightarrow a=-2 \end{array}$$

Substitute $a=-2$ into [4]. $4(-2)-2b=-12 \Rightarrow -8-2b=-12 \Rightarrow -2b=-4 \Rightarrow b=2$. Finally, substitute $a=-2$ and $b=2$ into [1]. $(-2)+4(2)+c=-17 \Rightarrow c=-23$. The equation is $x^2+y^2-2x+2y-23=0$.

67. Using the form $x^2+y^2+ax+by+c=0$ and the given points yields the following equations.

    For $(-1,3)$: $(-1)^2+(3)^2+a(-1)+b(3)+c=0 \Rightarrow 1+9-a+3b+c=0 \Rightarrow -a+3b+c=-10$.
    [equation 1]

    For $(6,2)$: $(6)^2+(2)^2+a(6)+b(2)+c=0 \Rightarrow 36+4+6a+2b+c=0 \Rightarrow 6a+2b+c=-40$.
    [equation 2]

    For $(-2,-4)$: $(-2)^2+(-4)^2+a(-2)+b(-4)+c=0 \Rightarrow 4+16-2a-4b+c=0 \Rightarrow -2a-4b+c=-20$.
    [equation 3]

    Now, subtract [equation 1] from [equation 2] to eliminate c and produce [equation 4].
    Then, subtract [equation 3] from [equation 2] to eliminate c and produce [equation 5].

    $$\begin{array}{ll} 6a+2b+c=-40 & [2] \\ \underline{a-3b-c=10} \quad -1\,[1] \\ 7a-b=-30 & [4] \end{array} \qquad \begin{array}{ll} 6a+2b+c=-40 & [2] \\ \underline{2a+4b-c=20} \quad -1\,[3] \\ 8a+6b=-20 & [5] \end{array}$$

    Next multiply [equation 4] by 6 and add [equation 5] to eliminate b.

    $$\begin{array}{ll} 42a-6b=-180 & 6\,[4] \\ \underline{8a+6b=-20} & [5] \\ 50a=-200 & \Rightarrow a=-4 \end{array}$$

    Substitute $a=-4$ into [4]. $7(-4)-b=-30 \Rightarrow -b=-2 \Rightarrow b=2$. Finally, substitute $a=-4$ and $b=2$ into [1]. $-(-4)+3(2)+c=-10 \Rightarrow c=-20$. The equation is $x^2+y^2-4x+2y-20=0$.

69. Using the form $x^2+y^2+ax+by+c=0$ and the given points yields the following equations.

    For $(2,1)$: $(2)^2+(1)^2+a(2)+b(1)+c=0 \Rightarrow 4+1+2a+b+c=0 \Rightarrow 2a+b+c=-5$. [equation 1]

    For $(-1,0)$: $(-1)^2+(0)^2+a(-1)+b(0)+c=0 \Rightarrow 1+0-a+0b+c=0 \Rightarrow -a+c=-1$. [equation 2]

    For $(3,3)$: $(3)^2+(3)^2+a(3)+b(3)+c=0 \Rightarrow 9+9+3a+3b+c=0 \Rightarrow 3a+3b+c=-18$. [equation 3]

    Now, multiply [equation 1] by -3 and add [equation 3] to eliminate b and produce [equation 4].

Next multiply [equation 2] by 2 and add [equation 4] to eliminate c.

$$\begin{array}{rl} -6a-3b-3c=15 & -3\ [1] \\ \underline{3a+3b+c=-18} & [3] \\ -3a-2c=-3 & [4] \end{array}$$

$$\begin{array}{rl} -2a+2c=-2 & 2\ [2] \\ \underline{-3a-2c=-3} & [4] \\ -5a=-5 & \Rightarrow a=1. \end{array}$$

Substitute $a=1$ into [2]. $-(1)+c=-1 \Rightarrow c=0$. Finally, substitute $a=1$ and $c=0$ into [1].

$2(1)+b+0=-5 \Rightarrow b=-7$. The equation is $x^2+y^2+x-7y=0$.

71. Using the form $s(t)=at^2+bt+c$ and the given points yields the following equations.

   For $(0,5)$: $5=a(0)^2+b(0)+c \Rightarrow c=5$.

   For $(1,23)$: $23=a(1)^2+b(1)+c \Rightarrow a+b+c=23$. [equation 1]

   For $(2,37)$: $37=a(2)^2+b(2)+c \Rightarrow 4a+2b+c=37$. [equation 2]

   First, multiply [equation 1] by -2 and add [equation 2] to eliminate b and produce [equation 3].

$$\begin{array}{rl} -2a-2b-2c=-46 & -2\ [1] \\ \underline{4a+2b+c=37} & [2] \\ 2a-c=-9 & [3] \end{array}$$

   Substitute $c=5$ into [3]. $2a-(5)=-9 \Rightarrow 2a=-4 \Rightarrow a=-2$.

   Finally, substitute $a=-2$ and $c=5$ into [1]. $(-2)+b+(5)=23 \Rightarrow b=20$.

   The equation is $s(t)=-2t^2+20t+5$, and $s(8)=-2(8)^2+20(8)+5=-128+160+5=37$.

6.3: Solution of Linear Systems by Row Transformations

1. For $\begin{bmatrix} 2 & 4 \\ 4 & 7 \end{bmatrix}$, $\frac{1}{2}R_1 \to \begin{bmatrix} 1 & 2 \\ 4 & 7 \end{bmatrix}$.

3. For $\begin{bmatrix} 1 & 5 & 6 \\ -2 & 3 & -1 \\ 4 & 7 & 0 \end{bmatrix}$, $2R_1+R_2 \to \begin{bmatrix} 1 & 5 & 6 \\ 0 & 13 & 11 \\ 4 & 7 & 0 \end{bmatrix}$.

5. For $\begin{bmatrix} -3 & 1 & -4 \\ 2 & 1 & 3 \\ 10 & 5 & 2 \end{bmatrix}$, $-5R_2+R_3 \to \begin{bmatrix} -3 & 1 & -4 \\ 2 & 1 & 3 \\ 0 & 0 & -13 \end{bmatrix}$.

7. The augmented matrix is $\begin{bmatrix} 2 & 3 & | & 11 \\ 1 & 2 & | & 8 \end{bmatrix}$.

9. The augmented matrix is $\begin{bmatrix} 1 & 5 & | & 6 \\ 1 & 0 & | & 3 \end{bmatrix}$.

11. The augmented matrix is $\begin{bmatrix} 2 & 1 & 1 & | & 3 \\ 3 & -4 & 2 & | & -7 \\ 1 & 1 & 1 & | & 2 \end{bmatrix}$.

13. The augmented matrix is $\begin{bmatrix} 1 & 1 & 0 & | & 2 \\ 0 & 2 & 1 & | & -4 \\ 0 & 0 & 1 & | & 2 \end{bmatrix}$.

15. The system of equations is $2x + y = 1$
    $3x - 2y = -9$.

17. The system of equations is $x = 2$
    $y = 3$
    $z = -2$.

19. The system of equations is $3x + 2y + z = 1$
    $2y + 4z = 22$
    $-x - 2y + 3z = 15$

21. The system can be written as $x + 2y = 3$ and $y = -1$. Substituting $y = -1$ into the first equation gives $x + 2(-1) = 3 \Rightarrow x = 5$. The solution is $(5, -1)$.

23. The system can be written as $x - 5y = 6$ and $0 = 0$. The solution is $(5y + 6, y)$.

25. The system can be written as $x + y - z = 4$, $y - z = 2$, and $z = 1$. Substituting $z = 1$ into the second equation gives $y - (1) = 2 \Rightarrow y = 3$ Substituting $y = 3$ and $z = 1$ into the first equation gives $x + (3) - (1) = 4 \Rightarrow x = 2$. The solution is $(2, 3, 1)$.

27. The system can be written as $x + 2y - z = 5$, $y - 2z = 1$, and $0 = 0$. Since $0 = 0$, there are an infinite number of solutions. The second equation gives $y = 1 + 2z$. Substituting this into the first equation gives $x + 2(1 + 2z) - z = 5 \Rightarrow x = 3 - 3z$. The solution can be written as $\{(3 - 3z, 1 + 2z, z) \mid z \text{ is a real number}\}$.

29. The system can be written as $x + 2y + z = -3$, $y - 3z = \frac{1}{2}$, and $0 = 4$. Since $0 = 4$ is false, there are no solutions.

31. Using the Row Echelon Method, the given system of equations yields the matrix $\begin{bmatrix} 1 & 1 & | & 5 \\ 1 & -1 & | & -1 \end{bmatrix}$, which by

    $-R_1 + R_2 \to \begin{bmatrix} 1 & 1 & | & 5 \\ 0 & -2 & | & -6 \end{bmatrix} \Rightarrow \left(-\frac{1}{2}R_2\right) \to \begin{bmatrix} 1 & 1 & | & 5 \\ 0 & 1 & | & 3 \end{bmatrix}$. From this matrix, we have the resulting equation $y = 3$.

    Now substitute $y = 3$ into the resulting R_1 equation. $x + (3) = 5 \Rightarrow x = 2$. The solution is $(2, 3)$.

33. Using the Row Echelon Method, the given system of equations yields the matrix $\begin{bmatrix} 1 & 1 & | & -3 \\ 2 & -5 & | & -6 \end{bmatrix}$, which by

    $-2R_1 + R_2 \to \begin{bmatrix} 1 & 1 & | & -3 \\ 0 & -7 & | & 0 \end{bmatrix} \Rightarrow \left(-\frac{1}{7}R_2\right) \to \begin{bmatrix} 1 & 1 & | & -3 \\ 0 & 1 & | & 0 \end{bmatrix}$. From this matrix, we have the resulting equation

    $y = 0$. Now substitute $y = 0$ into the resulting R_1 equation. $x + (0) = -3 \Rightarrow x = -3$.
    The solution is $(-3, 0)$.

35. Using the Row Echelon Method, the given system of equations yields the matrix $\begin{bmatrix} 2 & -3 & | & 10 \\ 2 & 2 & | & 5 \end{bmatrix}$, which by

$-R_1 + R_2 \to \begin{bmatrix} 2 & -3 & | & 10 \\ 0 & 5 & | & -5 \end{bmatrix} \Rightarrow \left(\frac{1}{2}R_1\right)$ and $\left(\frac{1}{5}R_2\right) \to \begin{bmatrix} 1 & -\frac{3}{2} & | & 5 \\ 0 & 1 & | & -1 \end{bmatrix}$. From this matrix, we have the resulting

equation $y = -1$. Now substitute $y = -1$ into the resulting R_1 equation.

$x - \frac{3}{2}(-1) = 5 \Rightarrow 2x + 3 = 10 \Rightarrow 2x = 7 \Rightarrow x = \frac{7}{2}$. The solution is $\left(\frac{7}{2}, -1\right)$.

37. Using the Row Echelon Method, the given system of equations yields the matrix $\begin{bmatrix} 2 & -3 & | & 2 \\ 4 & -6 & | & 1 \end{bmatrix}$, which by

$-2R_1 + R_2 \to \begin{bmatrix} 2 & -3 & | & 2 \\ 0 & 0 & | & -3 \end{bmatrix}$. Since this matrix yields the equation $0 = -3$, which is false; therefore,

the solution is $\varnothing$.

39. Using the Row Echelon Method, the given system of equations yields the matrix $\begin{bmatrix} 6 & -3 & | & 1 \\ -12 & 6 & | & -2 \end{bmatrix}$, which by

$2R_1 + R_2 \to \begin{bmatrix} 6 & -3 & | & 1 \\ 0 & 0 & | & 0 \end{bmatrix}$. The matrix yields the equation $0 = 0$. Since this is true, there are ∞ solutions.

From the resulting R_1, the solutions have the relationship: $-3y = 1 - 6x \Rightarrow y = \frac{6x-1}{3}$; $\left[\text{or } x = \frac{3y+1}{6}\right]$.

The solution is $\left(x, \frac{6x-1}{3}\right)$ or $\left(\frac{3y+1}{6}, y\right)$.

41. Using the Row Echelon Method, the given system of equations yields the matrix $\begin{bmatrix} 1 & 1 & 0 & | & -1 \\ 0 & 1 & 1 & | & 4 \\ 1 & 0 & 1 & | & 1 \end{bmatrix}$, which by

$-R_1 + R_3 \to \begin{bmatrix} 1 & 1 & 0 & | & -1 \\ 0 & 1 & 1 & | & 4 \\ 0 & -1 & 1 & | & 2 \end{bmatrix} \Rightarrow R_2 + R_3 \to \begin{bmatrix} 1 & 1 & 0 & | & -1 \\ 0 & 1 & 1 & | & 4 \\ 0 & 0 & 2 & | & 6 \end{bmatrix} \Rightarrow \left(\frac{1}{2}R_3\right) \to \begin{bmatrix} 1 & 1 & 0 & | & -1 \\ 0 & 1 & 1 & | & 4 \\ 0 & 0 & 1 & | & 3 \end{bmatrix}$. From this matrix,

we have the resulting equation $z = 3$. Now use back-substitution. Substituting $z = 3$ into the resulting R_2 yields

$y + 3 = 4 \Rightarrow y = 1$. Finally, substituting $y = 1$ and $z = 3$ into the resulting R_1 yields $x + 1 = -1 \Rightarrow x = -2$.

The solution is $(-2, 1, 3)$.

43. Using the Row Echelon Method, the given system of equations yields the matrix $\begin{bmatrix} 1 & 1 & -1 & | & 6 \\ 2 & -1 & 1 & | & -9 \\ 1 & -2 & 3 & | & 1 \end{bmatrix}$, which

by $(-2R_1 + R_2)$ and $(-R_1 + R_3) \to \begin{bmatrix} 1 & 1 & -1 & | & 6 \\ 0 & -3 & 3 & | & -21 \\ 0 & -3 & 4 & | & -5 \end{bmatrix} \Rightarrow -R_2 + R_3 \to \begin{bmatrix} 1 & 1 & -1 & | & 6 \\ 0 & -3 & 3 & | & -21 \\ 0 & 0 & 1 & | & 16 \end{bmatrix} \Rightarrow$

$\left(-\frac{1}{3}R_2\right) \to \begin{bmatrix} 1 & 1 & -1 & | & 6 \\ 0 & 1 & -1 & | & 7 \\ 0 & 0 & 1 & | & 16 \end{bmatrix}$. From this matrix, we have the resulting equation $z = 16$. Now use back

substitution, substituting $z = 16$ into the resulting R_2. This yields $y - 16 = 7 \Rightarrow y = 23$. Finally, substituting $y = 23$ and $z = 16$ into the resulting R_1 yields $x + 23 - 16 = 6 \Rightarrow x = -1$. The solution is $(-1, 23, 16)$.

45. Using the Row Echelon Method, the given system of equations yields the matrix $\begin{bmatrix} -1 & 1 & 0 & | & -1 \\ 0 & 1 & -1 & | & 6 \\ 1 & 0 & 1 & | & -1 \end{bmatrix}$, which

by $R_1 + R_3 \to \begin{bmatrix} -1 & 1 & 0 & | & -1 \\ 0 & 1 & -1 & | & 6 \\ 0 & 1 & 1 & | & -2 \end{bmatrix} \Rightarrow -R_2 + R_3 \to \begin{bmatrix} -1 & 1 & 0 & | & -1 \\ 0 & 1 & -1 & | & 6 \\ 0 & 0 & 2 & | & -8 \end{bmatrix} \Rightarrow$

$(-R_1)$ and $\left(\frac{1}{2}R_2\right) \to \begin{bmatrix} 1 & -1 & 0 & | & 1 \\ 0 & 1 & -1 & | & 6 \\ 0 & 0 & 1 & | & -4 \end{bmatrix}$. From this matrix, we have the resulting equation $z = -4$. Now use

back-substitution. Substituting $z = -4$ into the resulting R_2 yields $y + 4 = 6 \Rightarrow y = 2$. Finally, substituting $y = 2$ and $z = -4$ into the resulting R_1 yields $-x + 2 = -1 \Rightarrow x = 3$. The solution is $(3, 2, -4)$.

47. Using the Row Echelon Method, the given system of equations yields the matrix $\begin{bmatrix} 2 & -1 & 3 & | & 0 \\ 1 & 2 & -1 & | & 5 \\ 0 & 2 & 1 & | & 1 \end{bmatrix}$, which by

$R_1 \leftrightarrow R_2 \to \begin{bmatrix} 1 & 2 & -1 & | & 5 \\ 2 & -1 & 3 & | & 0 \\ 0 & 2 & 1 & | & 1 \end{bmatrix} \Rightarrow -2R_1 + R_2 \to \begin{bmatrix} 1 & 2 & -1 & | & 5 \\ 0 & -5 & 5 & | & -10 \\ 0 & 2 & 1 & | & -1 \end{bmatrix} \Rightarrow 2R_2 + 5R_3 \to \begin{bmatrix} 1 & 2 & -1 & | & 5 \\ 0 & -5 & 5 & | & -10 \\ 0 & 0 & 15 & | & -15 \end{bmatrix} \Rightarrow$

$\left(-\frac{1}{5}R_2\right) + \left(\frac{1}{15}R_3\right) \to \begin{bmatrix} 1 & 2 & -1 & | & 5 \\ 0 & 1 & -1 & | & 2 \\ 0 & 0 & 1 & | & -1 \end{bmatrix}$. From this matrix, we have the resulting equation $z = -1$. Now use

back-substitution. Substituting $(x+1)(x-3) \Rightarrow 5x - 3 = A(x-3) + B(x+1)$. into the resulting R_2 yields $y + 1 = 2 \Rightarrow y = 1$. Finally, substituting $y = 1$ and $x = 3 \Rightarrow 12 = B(4) \Rightarrow B = 3$. into the resulting R_1 yields $x + 2 + 1 = 5 \Rightarrow x = 2$. The solution is $(2, 1, -1)$.

49. Using the Row Echelon Method, the given system of equations yields the matrix $\begin{bmatrix} 1 & 1 & -2 & | & -6 \\ 1 & -1 & 1 & | & 4 \\ 2 & 0 & -1 & | & -1 \end{bmatrix}$, which

by $(R_1 - R_2) \to R_2$ $\begin{bmatrix} 1 & 1 & -2 & | & -6 \\ 0 & 2 & -3 & | & -10 \\ 2 & 0 & -1 & | & -1 \end{bmatrix} \Rightarrow (-2R_1 + R_3) \to R_3$ $\begin{bmatrix} 1 & 1 & -2 & | & -6 \\ 0 & 2 & -3 & | & -10 \\ 0 & -2 & 3 & | & 11 \end{bmatrix} \Rightarrow$

$(R_2 + R_3) \to R_3$ $\begin{bmatrix} 1 & 1 & -2 & | & -6 \\ 0 & 2 & -3 & | & -10 \\ 0 & 0 & 0 & | & 1 \end{bmatrix}$ From this matrix, we have the resulting equation $0 = 1$.

There is not solution to this system of equations.

51. Using the capabilities of the calculator, the Reduced Row Echelon Method of

$\begin{bmatrix} 0.07 & 0.23 & | & 9 \\ -1.25 & 0.33 & | & 2.4 \end{bmatrix}$ The solution is approximately $(7.785, 36.761)$.

53. Using the capabilities of the calculator, the Reduced Row Echelon Method of

$\begin{bmatrix} 2.1 & 0.5 & 1.7 & | & 4.9 \\ -2 & 1.5 & -1.7 & | & 3.1 \\ 5.8 & -4.6 & 0.8 & | & 9.3 \end{bmatrix} = \begin{bmatrix} 1 & 0 & 0 & | & 5.21127 \\ 0 & 1 & 0 & | & 3.73944 \\ 0 & 0 & 1 & | & -4.65493 \end{bmatrix}$. The solution is approximately $(5.211, 3.739, -4.655)$.

55. Using the capabilities of the calculator, the Reduced Row Echelon Method of

$\begin{bmatrix} 53 & 95 & 12 & | & 108 \\ 81 & -57 & -24 & | & -92 \\ -9 & 11 & -78 & | & 21 \end{bmatrix} = \begin{bmatrix} 1 & 0 & 0 & | & -0.24997 \\ 0 & 1 & 0 & | & 1.2838 \\ 0 & 0 & 1 & | & -0.05934 \end{bmatrix}$. The solution is approximately $(-0.250, 1.284, -0.059)$.

57. In both cases, we simply write the coefficients and do not write the variables. This is possible because we agree on the order in which the variables appear (descending degree).

59. The given system of equations yields the matrix, $\begin{bmatrix} 1 & -3 & 2 & | & 10 \\ 2 & -1 & -1 & | & 8 \end{bmatrix}$, which by

$-2R_1 + R_2 \to \begin{bmatrix} 1 & -3 & 2 & | & 10 \\ 0 & 5 & -5 & | & -12 \end{bmatrix} \Rightarrow \frac{1}{5}R_2 \begin{bmatrix} 1 & -3 & 2 & | & 10 \\ 0 & 1 & -1 & | & -\frac{12}{5} \end{bmatrix}$. Since we cannot eliminate more than one

coefficient there are an infinite number of solutions and they will be in the following relationship. From the

result of R_2, $y - z = -\frac{12}{5} \Rightarrow 5y - 5z = -12 \Rightarrow 5y = 5z - 12 \Rightarrow y = \frac{5z - 12}{5}$. Now substitute this into the

result of R_1: $x - 3\left(\frac{5z-12}{5}\right) + 2z = 10 \Rightarrow 5x - 5z + 36 + 10z = 50 \Rightarrow 5x - 5z = 14 \Rightarrow$

$5x = 5z + 14 \Rightarrow x = \frac{5z + 14}{5}$. The solution is $\left(\frac{5z+14}{5}, \frac{5z-12}{5}, z\right)$.

Section 6.3   285

61. The given system of equations yields the matrix $\begin{bmatrix} 1 & 2 & -1 & | & 0 \\ 3 & -1 & 1 & | & 6 \\ -2 & -4 & 2 & | & 0 \end{bmatrix}$, which by

$(-3R_1 + R_2)$ and $(2R_1 + R_3) \to \begin{bmatrix} 1 & 2 & -1 & | & 0 \\ 0 & -7 & 4 & | & 6 \\ 0 & 0 & 0 & | & 0 \end{bmatrix}$ since $-\dfrac{32}{11}z = -\dfrac{96}{11} \Rightarrow z = 3$. is $0 = 0$, there are

infinitely many solutions and the solutions are in the following relationship: From the result of R_2,

$-7y + 4z = 6 \Rightarrow -7y = 6 - 4z \Rightarrow y = \dfrac{4z - 6}{7}$. Now substitute this into the result of R_1:

$x + 2\left(\dfrac{4z-6}{7}\right) - z = 0 \Rightarrow 7x + 8z - 12 - 7z = 0 \Rightarrow 7x + z = 12 \Rightarrow 7x = 12 - z \Rightarrow x = \dfrac{12-z}{7}$.

The solution is $\left(\dfrac{12-z}{7}, \dfrac{4z-6}{7}, z\right)$.

63. The given system of equations yields the matrix $\begin{bmatrix} 1 & -2 & 1 & | & 5 \\ -2 & 4 & -2 & | & 2 \\ 2 & 1 & -1 & | & 2 \end{bmatrix}$. By $(2R_1 + R_2)$ and

$(-2R_1 + R_3) \to \begin{bmatrix} 1 & -2 & 1 & | & 5 \\ 0 & 0 & 0 & | & 12 \\ 0 & 5 & -3 & | & -8 \end{bmatrix}$. Since R_2 is $0 = 12$, there is no solution or $\varnothing$.

65. The given system of equations yields the matrix $\begin{bmatrix} 1 & 3 & -2 & -1 & | & 9 \\ 4 & 1 & 1 & 2 & | & 2 \\ -3 & -1 & 1 & -1 & | & -5 \\ 1 & -1 & -3 & -2 & | & 2 \end{bmatrix}$, which by $\begin{matrix} -4R_1 + R_2 \\ 3R_1 + R_3 \\ -R1 + R_4 \end{matrix} \to$

$\begin{bmatrix} 1 & 3 & -2 & -1 & | & 9 \\ 0 & -11 & 9 & 6 & | & -34 \\ 0 & 8 & -5 & -4 & | & 22 \\ 0 & -4 & -1 & -1 & | & -7 \end{bmatrix} \Rightarrow \begin{matrix} R_3 + 2R_4 \\ 8R_2 + 11R_3 \end{matrix} \to \begin{bmatrix} 1 & 3 & -2 & -1 & | & 9 \\ 0 & -11 & 9 & 6 & | & -34 \\ 0 & 0 & 17 & 4 & | & -30 \\ 0 & 0 & -7 & -6 & | & 8 \end{bmatrix} \Rightarrow$

$7R_3 + 17R_4 \to \begin{bmatrix} 1 & 3 & -2 & -1 & | & 9 \\ 0 & -11 & 9 & 6 & | & -34 \\ 0 & 0 & 17 & 4 & | & -30 \\ 0 & 0 & 0 & -74 & | & -74 \end{bmatrix} \Rightarrow \begin{matrix} -\frac{1}{11}R_2 \\ -\frac{1}{17}R_3 \\ -\frac{1}{74}R_4 \end{matrix} \to \begin{bmatrix} 1 & 3 & -2 & -1 & | & 9 \\ 0 & 1 & \frac{-9}{11} & \frac{-6}{11} & | & \frac{34}{11} \\ 0 & 0 & 1 & \frac{4}{17} & | & -\frac{30}{17} \\ 0 & 0 & 0 & 1 & | & 1 \end{bmatrix}$. From this matrix, we

have the resulting equation $w = 1$. Now use back-substitution. Substituting $w = 1$ into the resulting R_3 yields

$z + \dfrac{4}{17}(1) = -\dfrac{30}{17} \Rightarrow z = -\dfrac{34}{17} \Rightarrow z = -2$. Substituting $w = 1$ and $z = -2$ into the resulting R_2 yields

$y - \frac{9}{11}(-2) - \frac{6}{11}(1) = \frac{34}{11} \Rightarrow y + \frac{18-6}{11} = \frac{34}{11} \Rightarrow y = \frac{34-12}{11} = \frac{22}{11} \Rightarrow y = 2$. Finally, substitute

$y = 2, z = -2,$ and $w = 1$ into $R_1: x + 3(2) - 2(-2) - 1 = 9 \Rightarrow x + 9 = 9 \Rightarrow x = 0$.

The solution is $(0, 2, -2, 1)$.

67. (a) Using the given equation model, the given system of equations and the capabilities of the calculator, the

Reduced Row Echelon Method of: $\begin{bmatrix} 1800 & 5000 & 1 & | & 1300 \\ 3200 & 12000 & 1 & | & 5300 \\ 4500 & 13000 & 1 & | & 6500 \end{bmatrix} = \begin{bmatrix} 1 & 0 & 0 & | & 0.5714286 \\ 0 & 1 & 0 & | & 0.4571429 \\ 0 & 0 & 1 & | & -2014.2857 \end{bmatrix}$.

Therefore, the equation is $F = 0.5714N + 0.4571R - 2014$.

(b) Let $N = 3500$ and $R = 12{,}500$. Then $F = 0.5714(3500) + 0.4571(12{,}500) - 2014 \Rightarrow F \approx 5699.65$.

This model predicts monthly food costs of approximately $5700.

69. Let x represent the number of model A, and y the number of model B. Using the information yields

$\begin{cases} 2x + 3y = 34 \\ 25x + 30y = 365 \end{cases} \rightarrow \begin{bmatrix} 2 & 3 & | & 34 \\ 25 & 30 & | & 365 \end{bmatrix}$, which by $\begin{matrix} \frac{1}{2}R_1 \\ \frac{1}{5}R_2 \end{matrix} \rightarrow \begin{bmatrix} 1 & \frac{3}{2} & | & 17 \\ 5 & 6 & | & 73 \end{bmatrix} \Rightarrow -5R_1 + R_2 \rightarrow$

$\begin{bmatrix} 1 & \frac{3}{2} & | & 17 \\ 0 & -\frac{3}{2} & | & -12 \end{bmatrix} \Rightarrow -\frac{2}{3}R_2 \rightarrow \begin{bmatrix} 1 & \frac{3}{2} & | & 17 \\ 0 & 1 & | & 8 \end{bmatrix}$. From this matrix, we have the resulting equation $y = 8$. Now

substituting $y = 8$ into R_1 yields $x + \frac{3}{2}(8) = 7 \Rightarrow x + 12 = 17 \Rightarrow x = 5$. The maximum number is Model A:

5 bicycles, and Model B: 8 bicycles.

71. Let $x =$ the amount of money at 2%, $y =$ the amount of money at 3%, and $z =$ the amount of money at

2.5%. Using the information yields $\begin{cases} x + y + z = 12{,}500 \\ y = 1000 + \frac{1}{2}x \Rightarrow -\frac{1}{2}x + y = 1000 \\ 0.02x + 0.03y + 0.025z = 305 \end{cases}$. This system yields

$\begin{bmatrix} 1 & 1 & 1 & | & 12{,}500 \\ -0.5 & 1 & 0 & | & 1{,}000 \\ 0.02 & 0.03 & 0.025 & | & 305 \end{bmatrix}$, which by $\frac{1}{2}R_1 + R_2$ and $-2R_1 + 100R_3$, $\begin{bmatrix} 1 & 1 & 1 & | & 12{,}500 \\ 0 & 1.5 & 0.5 & | & 7{,}250 \\ 0 & 1 & 0.5 & | & 5{,}500 \end{bmatrix}$ and

$-\frac{2}{3}R_2 + R_3 \rightarrow \begin{bmatrix} 1 & 1 & 1 & | & 12{,}500 \\ 0 & 1.5 & 0.5 & | & 7{,}250 \\ 0 & 0 & \frac{1}{6} & | & \frac{4000}{6} \end{bmatrix} \Rightarrow 6R_3 \rightarrow \begin{bmatrix} 1 & 1 & 1 & | & 12{,}500 \\ 0 & 1.5 & 0.5 & | & 7{,}250 \\ 0 & 0 & 1 & | & 4000 \end{bmatrix}$

From this matrix, we have the resulting equation $z = 4{,}000$ and $1.5y + 0.5z = 7{,}250$. Substitute $z = 4000$

into $1.5y + 0.5z = 7{,}250 \Rightarrow 1.5y + 0.5(4000) = 7250 \Rightarrow y = 3500$. Finally, substitute $z = 4000$ and $y = 3500$

into $R_1: x + y + z = 12{,}500 \Rightarrow x + 3500 + 4000 = 12{,}500 \Rightarrow x = 5000$. The loans

were: $5,000 at 2%, $3500 at 3%, and $4000 at 2.5%.

73. (a) The three equations can be written as: $25 = 0^2 + 0 + c, 260 = 2^2a + 2b + c$, and

$695 = 4^2a + 4b + c \Rightarrow 16a + 4b + c = 695, 4a + 2b + c = 260,$ and $c = 25$.

Therefore, the matrix is: $\begin{bmatrix} 16 & 4 & 1 & | & 695 \\ 4 & 2 & 1 & | & 260 \\ 0 & 0 & 1 & | & 25 \end{bmatrix}$

(b) Using technology, $a = 25, b = 67.5, c = 25$. $f(x) = 25x^2 + 67.5x + 25$.

(c) See Figure 73

(d) For example, in 2014 the predicted sales is $f(6) = 25(6)^2 + 67.5(6) + 25 = 1330$ Answers may vary.

75. (a) Using $f(x) = ax^2 + bx + c$ and the data from the table yields:

From the point $(1990, 11)$: $11 = a(1990)^2 + b(1990) + c \Rightarrow 1990^2 a + 1990b + c = 11$.

From the point $(2010, 10)$: $10 = a(2010)^2 + b(2010) + c \Rightarrow 2010^2 a + 2010b + c = 10$.

From the point $(2030, 6)$: $6 = a(2030)^2 + b(2030) + c \Rightarrow 2030^2 a + 2030b + c = 6$.

(b) Now using the capabilities of the calculator, the Reduced Row Echelon Method of:

$\begin{bmatrix} 1990^2 & 1990 & 1 & | & 11 \\ 2010^2 & 2010 & 1 & | & 10 \\ 2030^2 & 2030 & 1 & | & 6 \end{bmatrix} = \begin{bmatrix} 1 & 0 & 0 & | & -0.00375 \\ 0 & 1 & 0 & | & 14.95 \\ 0 & 0 & 1 & | & -14,889.125 \end{bmatrix}$.

Therefore, the equation is $f(x) = -0.00375x^2 + 14.95x - 14889.125$.

(c) See Figure 75.

(d) Answers will vary, for example in 2015 the predicted ratio is $f(2015) \approx 9.3$.

[0,5] by [20,725]
Xscl = 1   Yscl = 5

[1983,2035] by [5,12]
Xscl = 5   Yscl = 1

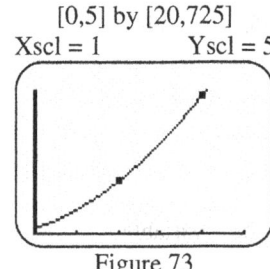
Figure 73

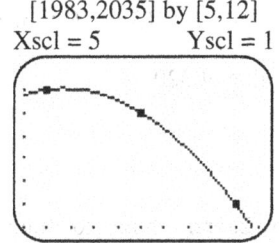
Figure 75

77. (a) At intersection A, incoming traffic is equal to $x + 5$. The outgoing traffic is given by $y + 7$. Therefore, $x + 5 = y + 7$. The incoming traffic at intersection B is $z + 6$ and the outgoing traffic is $x + 3$, so $z + 6 = x + 3$. Finally, at intersection C, the incoming flow is $y + 3$ and the outgoing flow is $z + 4$, so $y + 3 = z + 4$.

(b) The three equations are $\begin{cases} x+5 = y+7 \Rightarrow x-y = 2 \\ z+6 = x+3 \Rightarrow x-z = 3 \\ y+3 = z+4 \Rightarrow y-z = 1 \end{cases}$ which can be represented by $\begin{bmatrix} 1 & -1 & 0 & | & 2 \\ 1 & 0 & -1 & | & 3 \\ 0 & 1 & -1 & | & 1 \end{bmatrix}$.

Then by $-R_1 + R_2 \rightarrow \begin{bmatrix} 1 & -1 & 0 & | & 2 \\ 0 & 1 & -1 & | & 1 \\ 0 & 1 & -1 & | & 1 \end{bmatrix} \Rightarrow -R_2 + R_3 \rightarrow \begin{bmatrix} 1 & -1 & 0 & | & 2 \\ 0 & 1 & -1 & | & 1 \\ 0 & 0 & 0 & | & 0 \end{bmatrix}$. Since in the result of

R_3 $0 = 0$, there are infinite solutions. They are $y - z = 1 \Rightarrow y = z + 1$ and $x - z = 3 \Rightarrow x = z + 3$. The solution is $(z+3, z+1, z)$, where $z \geq 0$.

(c) There are infinitely many solutions since some cars could be driving around the block continually.

79. (a) Using the given model and information from the table the equations are

$x = \dfrac{Dx}{D} = \dfrac{-114}{-114} = 1$, $y = \dfrac{Dy}{D} = \dfrac{228}{-114} = -2$,

(b) The equations can be represented by $\begin{bmatrix} 1 & 871 & 11.5 & 3 & | & 239 \\ 1 & 847 & 12.2 & 2 & | & 234 \\ 1 & 685 & 10.6 & 5 & | & 192 \\ 1 & 969 & 14.2 & 1 & | & 343 \end{bmatrix}$. Using the capabilities of the calculator,

the Reduced Row Echelon Method produces the solutions $a \approx -715.457$, $b \approx 0.34756$, $c \approx 48.6585$, and $d \approx 30.71951$.

(c) The equation is $F = -715.457 + 0.34756A + 48.6585P + 30.71951W$.

(d) Input the given data into the equation.

$F = -715.457 + 0.34756(960) + 48.6585(12.6) + 30.71951(3) \Rightarrow F \approx 323.45623$. This is

approximately 323, which is close to the actual value of 320.

Reviewing Basic Concepts (Section 6.1-6.3)

1. Multiply the first equation by 5, the second equation by 2, and subtract to eliminate the x-variable.

    $10x - 15y = 90$
    $10x + 4y = 14$
    $\overline{}$
    $-19y = 76 \Rightarrow y = -4$ Substitute (-4) for y in the second equation:

    $10x + 4(-4) = 14 \Rightarrow 10x = 30 \Rightarrow x = 3$. The solution is $\{(3, -4)\}$.

2. The equations are: $2x + y = -4 \Rightarrow y_1 = -2x - 4$ and $-x + 2y = 2 \Rightarrow 2y = x + 2 \Rightarrow y = \dfrac{x+2}{2} \Rightarrow$

    $y_2 = \dfrac{1}{2}x + 1$. Graph y_1 and y_2 in the same window, the intersection is $\{(-2, 0)\}$. See Figure 2.

3. Using substitution, first solve [equation 2] for x, $x + 2y = 2 \Rightarrow x = -2y + 2$ [equation 3]. Substitute $(-2y+2)$ in for x, in [equation 1]: $5(-2y+2) + 10y = 10 \Rightarrow -10y + 10 + 10y = 10 \Rightarrow 10 = 10$. Since this is true, there is an infinite number of solutions given as $(-2y+2, y)$ or $\left(x, \dfrac{2-x}{2}\right)$.

4. Subtract [equation 2] from [equation 1] to eliminate both variables.
$x - y = 6$
$x + y = 4$
$0 = 2 \Rightarrow$ Since this is false the solution is $\varnothing$.

5. First solve [equation 1] for y and substitute into [equation 2]: $6x + 2y = 10 \Rightarrow 2y = 10 - 6x \Rightarrow y = 5 - 3x$. Now substitute: $2x^2 - 3(-3x + 5) = 11 \Rightarrow 2x^2 + 9x - 15 = 11 \Rightarrow 2x^2 + 9x - 26 = 0 \Rightarrow$ $(2x + 13)(x - 2) = 0 \Rightarrow x = -6.5$ and $x = 2$. If $x = -6.5$, then by substitution: $y = -3(-6.5) + 5 \Rightarrow y = 19.5 + 5 \Rightarrow y = 24.5$. If $x = 2$, then by substitution $y = -3(2) + 5 \Rightarrow y = -1$.
The solution is: $\{(2, -1), (-6.5, 24.5)\}$. See Figure 5 for graphical support.

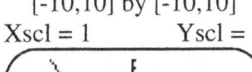

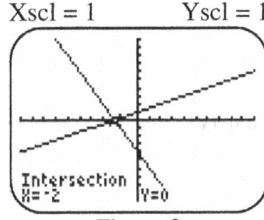

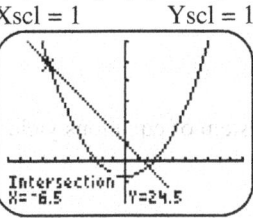

Figure 2   Figure 5

6. The equations can be represented by: $\begin{bmatrix} 1 & 1 & 1 & | & 1 \\ -1 & 1 & 1 & | & 5 \\ 0 & 1 & 2 & | & 5 \end{bmatrix} . R_1 + R_2 \rightarrow \begin{bmatrix} 1 & 1 & 1 & | & 1 \\ 0 & 2 & 2 & | & 6 \\ 0 & 1 & 2 & | & 5 \end{bmatrix} \Rightarrow$

$R_2 - 2R_1 \rightarrow \begin{bmatrix} 1 & 1 & 1 & | & 1 \\ 0 & 2 & 2 & | & 6 \\ 0 & 0 & -2 & | & -4 \end{bmatrix}$.

Now solve the resulting equation $R_3 : -2z = -4 \Rightarrow z = 2$. Substitute $z = 2$ into the resulting equation R_2: $2y + 2(2) = 6 \Rightarrow 2y = 2 \Rightarrow y = 1$. Finally, substitute $y = 1$ and $z = 2$ into R_1: $x + (1) + (2) = 1 \Rightarrow x = -2$. The solution is $\{(-2, 1, 2)\}$.

7. Using the Reduced Row Echelon method, the given system of equations yields the matrix, $\begin{bmatrix} 2 & 4 & 4 & | & 4 \\ 1 & 3 & 1 & | & 4 \\ -1 & 3 & 2 & | & -1 \end{bmatrix}$.

Using the capabilities of the calculator, the Reduced Row Echelon Method produces the solutions $x = 2$, $y = 1$, and $z = -1$.

290   CHAPTER 6   Systems and Matrices

8. Solve the augmented matrix $\begin{bmatrix} 2 & 1 & 2 & | & 10 \\ 1 & 0 & 2 & | & 5 \\ 1 & -2 & 2 & | & 1 \end{bmatrix}$, which by $\begin{matrix} R_1 - 2R_2 \\ R_1 - 2R_3 \end{matrix} \rightarrow \begin{bmatrix} 2 & 1 & 2 & | & 10 \\ 0 & 1 & -2 & | & 0 \\ 0 & 5 & -2 & | & 8 \end{bmatrix} \Rightarrow$

$-5R_2 + R_3 \rightarrow \begin{bmatrix} 2 & 1 & 2 & | & 10 \\ 0 & 1 & -2 & | & 0 \\ 0 & 0 & 8 & | & 8 \end{bmatrix}$. Now solve the resulting equation $R_3: 8z = 8 \Rightarrow z = 1$. Substitute $z = 1$

into the resulting equation $R_2: y - 2(1) = 0 \Rightarrow y = 2$. Finally, substitute $y = 2$ and $z = 1$ into R_1:

$2x + (2) + 2(1) = 10 \Rightarrow 2x = 6 \Rightarrow x = 3$. The solution is $(3, 2, 1)$.

9. Let x represent the number of LCD monitors and y represent the number of CRT monitors.

Then from the information the equations are $\begin{matrix} x + y = 133 & [1] \\ x - y = 43 & [2] \end{matrix}$ Add [equation 1] and [equation 2]:

$2x = 176 \Rightarrow x = 88$. Substitute $x = 88$ into [1]: $88 + y = 143 \Rightarrow y = 45$. There were approximately 88 million LCD monitors sold and 45 million CRT monitors sold in 2006.

10. Let x = amount at 2%, y = amount at 3%, and x = amount at 4%. Then from the information:

$x + y + z = 5000$

$0.02x + 0.03y + 0.04z = 165$

$z = x + y \Rightarrow x + y - z = 0$

Using the Reduced Row Echelon method, the given system of equations yields the matrix

$\begin{bmatrix} 1 & 1 & 1 & | & 5000 \\ 0.02 & 0.03 & 0.04 & | & 165 \\ 1 & 1 & -1 & | & 0 \end{bmatrix}$.

Using the capabilities of the calculator, the Reduced Row Echelon Method produces the solutions $x = 1000$, $y = 1500$, and $z = 2500$.

There was $1000 invested at 2%, $1500 invested at 3%, and $2500 invested at 4%.

6.4: Matrix Properties and Operations

1. Because the number of rows equals the number of columns, this is a 2×2 square matrix.

3. This is a 3×4 matrix.

5. Because there is only one column, this is a 2×1 column matrix.

7. Because the number of rows equals the number of columns, there is only one row and column, this is a 1×1 square matrix (one row and one column).

9. For $\begin{bmatrix} w & x \\ y & z \end{bmatrix} = \begin{bmatrix} 3 & 2 \\ -1 & 4 \end{bmatrix}$, $w = 3$, $x = 2$, $y = -1$, and $z = 4$.

11. For $\begin{bmatrix} 0 & 5 & x \\ -1 & 3 & y+2 \\ 4 & 1 & z \end{bmatrix} = \begin{bmatrix} 0 & w+3 & 6 \\ -1 & 3 & 0 \\ 4 & 1 & 8 \end{bmatrix}$, $w + 3 = 5 \Rightarrow w = 2$, $x = 6$, $y + 2 = 0 \Rightarrow y = -2$, and $z = 8$.

13. For $\begin{bmatrix} z & 4r & 8s \\ 6p & 2 & 5 \end{bmatrix} + \begin{bmatrix} -9 & 8r & 3 \\ 2 & 7 & 4 \end{bmatrix} = \begin{bmatrix} 2 & 36 & 27 \\ 20 & 7 & 12a \end{bmatrix}$,

    $z - 9 = 2 \Rightarrow z = 11$; $4r + 8r = 36 \Rightarrow r = 3$; $8s + 3 = 27 \Rightarrow 8s = 24 \Rightarrow s = 3$

    $6p + 2 = 20 \Rightarrow 6p = 18 \Rightarrow p = 3$; $5 + 4 = 12a \Rightarrow 9 = 12a \Rightarrow a = \dfrac{3}{4}$

15. The two matrices must have the same dimensions. To find the sum, add the corresponding entries. The sum will be a matrix with the same dimension.

17. $\begin{bmatrix} 6 & -9 & 2 \\ 4 & 1 & 3 \end{bmatrix} + \begin{bmatrix} -8 & 2 & 5 \\ 6 & -3 & 4 \end{bmatrix} = \begin{bmatrix} 6-8 & -9+2 & 2+5 \\ 4+6 & 1-3 & 3+4 \end{bmatrix} = \begin{bmatrix} -2 & -7 & 7 \\ 10 & -2 & 7 \end{bmatrix}$

19. $\begin{bmatrix} -6 & 8 \\ 0 & 0 \end{bmatrix} - \begin{bmatrix} 0 & 0 \\ -4 & -2 \end{bmatrix} = \begin{bmatrix} -6-0 & 8-0 \\ 0-(-4) & 0-(-2) \end{bmatrix} = \begin{bmatrix} -6 & 8 \\ 4 & 2 \end{bmatrix}$

21. $\begin{bmatrix} 6 & -2 \\ 5 & 4 \end{bmatrix} + \begin{bmatrix} -1 & 7 \\ 7 & -4 \end{bmatrix} = \begin{bmatrix} 6-1 & -2+7 \\ 5+7 & 4-4 \end{bmatrix} = \begin{bmatrix} 5 & 5 \\ 12 & 0 \end{bmatrix}$

23. $\begin{bmatrix} -8 & 4 & 0 \\ 2 & 5 & 0 \end{bmatrix} + \begin{bmatrix} 6 & 3 \\ 8 & 9 \end{bmatrix}$ Matrices must be the same size to add or subtract. We cannot add $(2 \times 3) + (2 \times 2)$.

25. $\begin{bmatrix} 9 & 4 & 1 & -2 \\ 5 & -6 & 3 & 4 \\ 2 & -5 & 1 & 2 \end{bmatrix} - \begin{bmatrix} -2 & 5 & 1 & 3 \\ 0 & 1 & 0 & 2 \\ -8 & 3 & 2 & 1 \end{bmatrix} + \begin{bmatrix} 2 & 4 & 0 & 3 \\ 4 & -5 & 1 & 6 \\ 2 & -3 & 0 & 8 \end{bmatrix} =$

    $\begin{bmatrix} 9+2+2 & 4-5+4 & 1-1+0 & -2-3+3 \\ 5-0+4 & -6-1-5 & 3-0+1 & 4-2+6 \\ 2+8+2 & -5-3-3 & 1-2+0 & 2-1+8 \end{bmatrix} = \begin{bmatrix} 13 & 3 & 0 & -2 \\ 9 & -12 & 4 & 8 \\ 12 & -11 & -1 & 9 \end{bmatrix}$

27. $2\begin{bmatrix} 2 & -1 \\ 5 & 1 \\ 0 & 3 \end{bmatrix} + \begin{bmatrix} 5 & 0 \\ 7 & -3 \\ 1 & 1 \end{bmatrix} - \begin{bmatrix} 9 & -4 \\ 4 & 4 \\ 1 & 6 \end{bmatrix} = \begin{bmatrix} 4+5-9 & -2+0+4 \\ 1+7-4 & 2-3-4 \\ 0+1-1 & 6+1-6 \end{bmatrix} = \begin{bmatrix} 0 & 2 \\ 13 & -5 \\ 0 & 1 \end{bmatrix}$

29. $2\begin{bmatrix} 2 & -1 & -1 \\ -1 & 2 & -1 \\ -1 & -1 & 2 \end{bmatrix} + 3\begin{bmatrix} 1 & 2 & 3 \\ 2 & 1 & 3 \\ 2 & 3 & 1 \end{bmatrix} = \begin{bmatrix} 4+3 & -2+6 & -2+9 \\ -2+6 & 4+3 & -2+9 \\ -2+6 & -2+9 & 4+3 \end{bmatrix} = \begin{bmatrix} 7 & 4 & 7 \\ 4 & 7 & 7 \\ 4 & 7 & 7 \end{bmatrix}$.

31. $3\begin{bmatrix} 6 & -1 & 4 \\ 2 & 8 & -3 \\ -4 & 5 & 6 \end{bmatrix} + 5\begin{bmatrix} -2 & -8 & -6 \\ 4 & 1 & 3 \\ 2 & -1 & 5 \end{bmatrix} = \begin{bmatrix} 18 & -3 & 12 \\ 6 & 24 & -9 \\ -12 & 15 & 18 \end{bmatrix} + \begin{bmatrix} -10 & -40 & -30 \\ 20 & 5 & 15 \\ 10 & -5 & 25 \end{bmatrix} =$

    $\begin{bmatrix} 18-10 & -3-40 & 12-30 \\ 6+20 & 24+5 & -9+15 \\ -12+10 & 15-5 & 18+25 \end{bmatrix} = \begin{bmatrix} 8 & -43 & -18 \\ 26 & 29 & 6 \\ -2 & 10 & 43 \end{bmatrix}$

33. $2[A] = 2\begin{bmatrix} -2 & 4 \\ 0 & 3 \end{bmatrix} = \begin{bmatrix} -4 & 8 \\ 0 & 6 \end{bmatrix}$

35. $2[A] - [B] = 2\begin{bmatrix} -2 & 4 \\ 0 & 3 \end{bmatrix} - \begin{bmatrix} -6 & 2 \\ 4 & 0 \end{bmatrix} = \begin{bmatrix} -4+6 & 8-2 \\ 0-4 & 6-0 \end{bmatrix} = \begin{bmatrix} 2 & 6 \\ -4 & 6 \end{bmatrix}$

37. $5[A]+0.5[B]=5\begin{bmatrix}-2 & 4\\ 0 & 3\end{bmatrix}+0.5\begin{bmatrix}-6 & 2\\ 4 & 0\end{bmatrix}=\begin{bmatrix}-10-3 & 20+1\\ 0+2 & 15+0\end{bmatrix}=\begin{bmatrix}-13 & 21\\ 2 & 15\end{bmatrix}$

39. $[A]=([A]+[B])-[B]=\begin{bmatrix}6 & 12 & 0\\ -10 & -4 & 11\end{bmatrix}-\begin{bmatrix}4 & 6 & -5\\ -6 & 3 & 2\end{bmatrix}=\begin{bmatrix}6-4 & 12-6 & 0+5\\ -10+6 & -4-3 & 11-2\end{bmatrix}=\begin{bmatrix}2 & 6 & 5\\ -4 & -7 & 9\end{bmatrix}$

41. A is 4×2 and B is 2×4. For AB, the number of columns of A is the same as the number of rows of B; therefore, AB has dimensions: $4(\text{rows of }A)\times 4(\text{columns of }B)$ or AB is 4×4. For BA, the number of columns of B is the same as the number of rows of A; therefore, BA has dimensions: $2(\text{rows of }B)\times 2(\text{columns of }A)$ or BA is 2×2.

43. A is 3×5 and B is 5×2. For AB, the number of columns of A is the same as the number of rows of B; therefore, AB has dimensions: $3(\text{rows of }A)\times 2(\text{columns of }B)$ or AB is 3×2. For BA, the number of columns of B is not the same as the number of rows of A; therefore, BA is not defined.

45. A is 4×3 and B is 2×5. For AB, the number of columns of A is not the same as the number of rows of B; therefore, AB is not defined. For BA, the number of columns of B is not the same as the number of rows of A; therefore, BA is also not defined.

47. ... the number of columns of M equal the number of rows of N.

49. A and B are both 2×2 so AB and BA are also both 2×2.

$AB=\begin{bmatrix}1 & -1\\ 2 & 0\end{bmatrix}\begin{bmatrix}-2 & 3\\ 1 & 2\end{bmatrix}=\begin{bmatrix}-3 & 1\\ -4 & 6\end{bmatrix}; BA=\begin{bmatrix}-2 & 3\\ 1 & 2\end{bmatrix}\begin{bmatrix}1 & -1\\ 2 & 0\end{bmatrix}=\begin{bmatrix}4 & 2\\ 5 & -1\end{bmatrix}$

51. Since both A and B are 2×3, the number of rows in B is not equal to the number of columns in A, so AB is undefined. Also, the number of rows in A is not equal to the number of columns in B so BA is undefined.

53. $AB=\begin{bmatrix}3 & -1\\ 1 & 0\\ -2 & -4\end{bmatrix}\begin{bmatrix}-2 & 5 & -3\\ 9 & -7 & 0\end{bmatrix}=$

$\begin{bmatrix}3(-2)+(-1)(9) & 3(5)+(-1)(-7) & 3(-3)+(-1)(0)\\ 1(-2)+0(9) & 1(5)+0(-7) & 1(-3)+0(0)\\ -2(-2)+(-4)(9) & -2(5)+(-4)(-7) & -2(-3)+(-4)(0)\end{bmatrix}\Rightarrow AB=\begin{bmatrix}-15 & 22 & -9\\ -2 & 5 & -3\\ -32 & 18 & 6\end{bmatrix}$

$BA=\begin{bmatrix}-2 & 5 & -3\\ 9 & -7 & 0\end{bmatrix}\begin{bmatrix}3 & -1\\ 1 & 0\\ -2 & -4\end{bmatrix}=\begin{bmatrix}-2(3)+5(1)+(-3)(-2) & -2(-1)+5(0)+(-3)(-4)\\ 9(3)+(-7)(1)+0(-2) & 9(-1)+(-7)(0)+0(-4)\end{bmatrix}\Rightarrow BA=\begin{bmatrix}5 & 14\\ 20 & -9\end{bmatrix}$

55. AB is undefined, we cannot multiply a 3×3 by a 2×3.

$BA=\begin{bmatrix}-1 & 3 & -1\\ 7 & -7 & 1\end{bmatrix}\begin{bmatrix}1 & -1 & 0\\ 2 & -1 & 5\\ 6 & 1 & -4\end{bmatrix}=$

$\begin{bmatrix}-1(1)+3(2)+(-1)(6) & -1(-1)+3(-1)+(-1)(1) & -1(0)+3(5)+(-1)(-4)\\ 7(1)+(-7)(2)+1(6) & 7(-1)+-7(-1)+1(1) & 7(0)+(-7)(-5)+1(-4)\end{bmatrix}\Rightarrow BA=\begin{bmatrix}-1 & -3 & 19\\ -1 & 1 & -39\end{bmatrix}$

57. $\begin{bmatrix} 3 & -4 & 1 \\ 5 & 0 & 2 \end{bmatrix} \begin{bmatrix} -1 \\ 4 \\ 2 \end{bmatrix} = \begin{bmatrix} 3(1)-4(4)+1(2) \\ 5(-1)+0(4)+2(2) \end{bmatrix} = \begin{bmatrix} -3-16+2 \\ -5+0+4 \end{bmatrix} = \begin{bmatrix} -17 \\ -1 \end{bmatrix}$

59. $\begin{bmatrix} 5 & 2 \\ -1 & 4 \end{bmatrix} \begin{bmatrix} 3 & -2 \\ 1 & 0 \end{bmatrix} = \begin{bmatrix} 5(3)+2(1) & 5(-2)+2(0) \\ -1(3)+4(1) & -1(-2)+4(0) \end{bmatrix} = \begin{bmatrix} 15+2 & -10+0 \\ -3+4 & 2+0 \end{bmatrix} = \begin{bmatrix} 17 & -10 \\ 1 & 2 \end{bmatrix}$

61. $\begin{bmatrix} 2 & 2 & -1 \\ 3 & 0 & 1 \end{bmatrix} \begin{bmatrix} 0 & 2 \\ -1 & 4 \\ 0 & 2 \end{bmatrix} = \begin{bmatrix} 2(0)+2(-1)+(-1)(0) & 2(2)+2(4)+(-1)(2) \\ 3(0)+0(-1)+1(0) & 3(2)+0(4)+1(2) \end{bmatrix} = \begin{bmatrix} 0-2+0 & 4+8-2 \\ 0+0+0 & 6+0+2 \end{bmatrix} = \begin{bmatrix} -2 & 10 \\ 0 & 8 \end{bmatrix}$

63. $\begin{bmatrix} -2 & -3 & -4 \\ 2 & -1 & 0 \\ 4 & -2 & 3 \end{bmatrix} \begin{bmatrix} 0 & 1 & 4 \\ 1 & 2 & -1 \\ 3 & 2 & -2 \end{bmatrix} =$

$\begin{bmatrix} -2(0)+(-3)(1)+(-4)(3) & -2(1)+(-3)(2)+(-4)(2) & -2(4)+(-3)(-1)+(-4)(-2) \\ 2(0)+(-1)(1)+0(3) & 2(1)+(-1)(2)+0(2) & 2(4)+(-1)(-1)+0(-2) \\ 4(0)+(-2)(1)+3(3) & 4(1)+(-2)(2)+3(2) & 4(4)+(-2)(-1)+3(-2) \end{bmatrix} =$

$\begin{bmatrix} 0-3-12 & -2-6-8 & -8+3-8 \\ 0-1+0 & 2-2+0 & 8+1+0 \\ 0-2+9 & 4-4+6 & 16+2-6 \end{bmatrix} = \begin{bmatrix} -15 & -16 & 3 \\ -1 & 0 & 9 \\ 7 & 6 & 12 \end{bmatrix}$

65. $\begin{bmatrix} -2 & 4 & 1 \end{bmatrix} \begin{bmatrix} 3 & -2 & 4 \\ 2 & 1 & 0 \\ 0 & -1 & 4 \end{bmatrix} = \begin{bmatrix} -2(3)+4(2)+1(0) & -2(-2)+4(1)+1(-1) & -2(4)+4(0)+1(4) \end{bmatrix} =$
$\begin{bmatrix} -6+8+0 & 4+4-1 & -8+0+4 \end{bmatrix} = \begin{bmatrix} 2 & 7 & -4 \end{bmatrix}$

67. $\begin{bmatrix} p & q \\ r & s \end{bmatrix} \begin{bmatrix} a & c \\ b & d \end{bmatrix} = \begin{bmatrix} pa+qb & pc+qd \\ ra+sb & rc+sd \end{bmatrix}$

69. $BA = \begin{bmatrix} 5 & 1 \\ 0 & -2 \\ 3 & 7 \end{bmatrix} \begin{bmatrix} 4 & -2 \\ 3 & 1 \end{bmatrix} = \begin{bmatrix} 5(4)+1(3) & 5(-2)+1(1) \\ 0(4)+(-2)(3) & 0(-2)+(-2)(1) \\ 3(4)+7(3) & 3(-2)+7(1) \end{bmatrix} = \begin{bmatrix} 23 & -9 \\ -6 & -2 \\ 33 & 1 \end{bmatrix}$

71. $BC = \begin{bmatrix} 5 & 1 \\ 0 & -2 \\ 3 & 7 \end{bmatrix} \begin{bmatrix} -5 & 4 & 1 \\ 0 & 3 & 6 \end{bmatrix} = \begin{bmatrix} 5(-5)+1(0) & 5(4)+1(3) & 5(1)+1(6) \\ 0(-5)-2(0) & 0(4)-2(3) & 0(1)-2(6) \\ 3(-5)+7(0) & 3(4)+7(3) & 3(1)+7(6) \end{bmatrix} = \begin{bmatrix} -25 & 23 & 11 \\ 0 & -6 & -12 \\ -15 & 33 & 45 \end{bmatrix}$

73. We cannot multiply A and B because we cannot multiply a (2×2) by a (3×2).

75. $A^2 = \begin{bmatrix} 4 & -2 \\ 3 & 1 \end{bmatrix} \begin{bmatrix} 4 & -2 \\ 3 & 1 \end{bmatrix} = \begin{bmatrix} 4(4)-2(3) & 4(-2)-2(1) \\ 3(4)+1(3) & 3(-2)+1(1) \end{bmatrix} = \begin{bmatrix} 10 & -10 \\ 15 & -5 \end{bmatrix}$

77. $AB \neq BA; BC \neq CB; AC \neq CA$. Matrix multiplication is not commutative.

79. (a) From the information the matrix is $\begin{bmatrix} 50 & 100 & 30 \\ 10 & 90 & 50 \\ 60 & 120 & 40 \end{bmatrix}$.

294 CHAPTER 6 Systems and Matrices

(b) The income matrix is $\begin{bmatrix} 12 \\ 10 \\ 15 \end{bmatrix}$.

(c) $\begin{bmatrix} 50 & 100 & 30 \\ 10 & 90 & 50 \\ 60 & 120 & 40 \end{bmatrix} \begin{bmatrix} 12 \\ 10 \\ 15 \end{bmatrix} = \begin{bmatrix} 50(12) + 100(10) + 30(15) \\ 10(12) + 90(10) + 50(15) \\ 60(12) + 120(10) + 40(15) \end{bmatrix} = \begin{bmatrix} 2050 \\ 1770 \\ 2520 \end{bmatrix}$

(d) $2050 + 1770 + 2520 = \$6340$

81. (a) From R_2 the equation is $d_{n+1} = -0.05 m_n + 1.05 d_n$ (hundredths). The deer population will grow at 5 %/year.

(b) Let $m_n = 2000$ and $d_n = 5000$ and multiply the given matrices:

$\begin{bmatrix} m_{n+1} \\ d_{n+1} \end{bmatrix} = \begin{bmatrix} 0.51 & 0.4 \\ -0.05 & 1.05 \end{bmatrix} \begin{bmatrix} 2000 \\ 5000 \end{bmatrix} = \begin{bmatrix} 1020 + 2000 \\ -100 + 5250 \end{bmatrix} = \begin{bmatrix} 3020 \\ 5150 \end{bmatrix}$

After 1 year there will be 3020 mountain lions and 515,000 deer.

Now multiply this 1 year matrix by the given matrix to find year 2.

$\begin{bmatrix} m_{n+2} \\ d_{n+2} \end{bmatrix} = \begin{bmatrix} 0.51 & 0.4 \\ -0.05 & 1.05 \end{bmatrix} \begin{bmatrix} 3020 \\ 5150 \end{bmatrix} = \begin{bmatrix} 1540.2 + 2060 \\ -151 + 5407.5 \end{bmatrix} = \begin{bmatrix} 3600.2 \\ 5256.5 \end{bmatrix}$

After 2 years there will be 3600 mountain lions and approximately 525,700 deer.

(c) Let $m_n = 4000$ and $d_n = 5000$ and multiply the given matrices:

$\begin{bmatrix} m_{n+1} \\ d_{n+1} \end{bmatrix} = \begin{bmatrix} 0.51 & 0.4 \\ -0.05 & 1.05 \end{bmatrix} \begin{bmatrix} 4000 \\ 5000 \end{bmatrix} = \begin{bmatrix} 2040 + 2000 \\ -200 + 5250 \end{bmatrix} = \begin{bmatrix} 4040 \\ 5050 \end{bmatrix}$

After 1 year there will be 4040 mountain lions and 505,000 deer. Now multiply this 1 year matrix by the given matrix to find year 2. $\begin{bmatrix} m_{n+2} \\ d_{n+2} \end{bmatrix} = \begin{bmatrix} 0.51 & 0.4 \\ -0.05 & 1.05 \end{bmatrix} \begin{bmatrix} 4040 \\ 5050 \end{bmatrix} = \begin{bmatrix} 2060.4 + 2020 \\ -202 + 5302.5 \end{bmatrix} = \begin{bmatrix} 4080.4 \\ 5100.5 \end{bmatrix}$

After 2 years there will be 4080 mountain lions and approximately 510,050 deer. Mountain Lions: after 1 year $= \dfrac{4040}{4000} = 1.01$; after 2 years $= \dfrac{4080}{4040} = 1.01$

Deer: after 1 year $= \dfrac{505,000}{500,000} = 1.01$; after 2 years $= \dfrac{510,050}{500,000} = 1.01$

83. $A + B = B + A$: $A + B = \begin{bmatrix} a_{11} + b_{11} & a_{12} + b_{12} \\ a_{21} + b_{21} & a_{22} + b_{22} \end{bmatrix} = B + A$.

85. $(AB)C = A(BC)$:

$(AB)C = \begin{bmatrix} a_{11}b_{11} + a_{12}b_{21} & a_{11}b_{12} + a_{12}b_{22} \\ a_{21}b_{11} + a_{22}b_{21} & a_{21}b_{12} + a_{22}b_{22} \end{bmatrix} \begin{bmatrix} c_{11} & c_{12} \\ c_{21} & c_{22} \end{bmatrix} =$

$\begin{bmatrix} (a_{11}b_{11}c_{11} + a_{12}b_{21}c_{11}) + (a_{11}b_{12}c_{21} + a_{12}b_{22}c_{21}) & (a_{11}b_{11}c_{12} + a_{12}b_{21}c_{12}) + (a_{11}b_{12}c_{22} + a_{12}b_{22}c_{22}) \\ (a_{21}b_{11}c_{11} + a_{22}b_{21}c_{11}) + (a_{21}b_{12}c_{21} + a_{22}b_{22}c_{21}) & (a_{21}b_{11}c_{12} + a_{22}b_{21}c_{12}) + (a_{21}b_{12}c_{22} + a_{22}b_{22}c_{22}) \end{bmatrix}$

$$A(BC) = \begin{bmatrix} a_{11} & a_{12} \\ a_{21} & a_{22} \end{bmatrix} \begin{bmatrix} b_{11}c_{11}+b_{12}c_{21} & b_{11}c_{12}+b_{12}c_{22} \\ b_{21}c_{11}+b_{22}c_{21} & b_{21}c_{12}+b_{22}c_{22} \end{bmatrix} =$$

$$\begin{bmatrix} (a_{11}b_{11}c_{11}+a_{11}b_{12}c_{21})+(a_{12}b_{21}c_{11}+a_{12}b_{22}c_{21}) & (a_{11}b_{11}c_{12}+a_{11}b_{12}c_{22})+(a_{12}b_{21}c_{12}+a_{12}b_{22}c_{22}) \\ (a_{21}b_{11}c_{11}+a_{21}b_{21}c_{21})+(a_{22}b_{21}c_{11}+a_{22}b_{22}c_{21}) & (a_{21}b_{11}c_{12}+a_{21}b_{12}c_{22})+(a_{22}b_{21}c_{12}+a_{22}b_{22}c_{22}) \end{bmatrix}$$

Therefore, $(AB)C = A(BC)$.

87. $c(A+B) = cA + cB$:

$$c(A+B) = \begin{bmatrix} c(a_{11}+b_{11}) & c(a_{12}+b_{12}) \\ c(a_{21}+b_{21}) & c(a_{22}+b_{22}) \end{bmatrix} = \begin{bmatrix} ca_{11}+cb_{11} & ca_{12}+cb_{12} \\ ca_{21}+cb_{21} & ca_{22}+cb_{22} \end{bmatrix} = cA + cB$$

89. $(cA)d = (cd)A$:

$$(cA)d = \begin{bmatrix} ca_{11} & ca_{12} \\ ca_{21} & ca_{22} \end{bmatrix} \cdot d = \begin{bmatrix} cda_{11} & cda_{12} \\ cda_{21} & cda_{22} \end{bmatrix} = (cd)A.$$

6.5: Determinants and Cramer's Rule

1. $\det \begin{bmatrix} -5 & 9 \\ 4 & -1 \end{bmatrix} = 5 - 36 = -31$

3. $\det \begin{bmatrix} -1 & -2 \\ 5 & 3 \end{bmatrix} = -3 - (-10) = 7$

5. $\det \begin{bmatrix} 9 & 3 \\ -3 & -1 \end{bmatrix} = -9 - (-9) = 0$

7. $\det \begin{bmatrix} 3 & 4 \\ 5 & -2 \end{bmatrix} = -6 - 20 = -26$

9. Use $A_{ij} = (-1)^{i+j} \cdot M_{ij}$, to find the cofactor of each element a.

   For a_{21}, find $A_{21} = (-1)^{2+1} \cdot \left(\det \begin{bmatrix} 0 & 1 \\ 2 & 1 \end{bmatrix} \right) = -1(0-2) = 2$

   For a_{22}, find $A_{22} = (-1)^{2+2} \cdot \left(\det \begin{bmatrix} -2 & 1 \\ 4 & 1 \end{bmatrix} \right) = 1(-2-4) = -6$

   For a_{23}, find $A_{23} = (-1)^{2+3} \cdot \left(\det \begin{bmatrix} -2 & 0 \\ 4 & 2 \end{bmatrix} \right) = -1(-4-0) = 4$

11. Use $A_{ij} = (-1)^{i+j} \cdot M_{ij}$, to find the cofactor of each element a.

    For a_{21}, find $A_{21} = (-1)^{2+1} \cdot \left(\det \begin{bmatrix} 2 & -1 \\ 4 & 1 \end{bmatrix} \right) = -1(2+4) = -6$

    For a_{22}, find $A_{22} = (-1)^{2+2} \cdot \left(\det \begin{bmatrix} 1 & -1 \\ 1 & 1 \end{bmatrix} \right) = 1(1-1) = 0$

For a_{23}, find $A_{23} = (-1)^{2+3} \cdot \left(\begin{bmatrix} 1 & 2 \\ -1 & -4 \end{bmatrix} \right) = -1(4+2) = -6$

13. Evaluate, expand by the second row. Therefore, $\det = (-)(a_{21})(M_{21}) + (a_{22})(M_{22}) - (a_{23})(M_{23})$:

$-2\left(\det \begin{bmatrix} -7 & 8 \\ 3 & 0 \end{bmatrix}\right) + 1\left(\det \begin{bmatrix} 4 & 8 \\ -6 & 0 \end{bmatrix}\right) - 3\left(\det \begin{bmatrix} 4 & -7 \\ -6 & 3 \end{bmatrix}\right) = -2(-24) + 1(48) - 3(-30) = 48 + 48 + 90 = 186.$

15. Evaluate, expand by the first column. Therefore, $\det = (a_{11})(M_{11}) - (a_{21})(M_{21}) + (a_{31})(M_{31})$:

$1\left(\det \begin{bmatrix} 2 & -1 \\ 1 & 4 \end{bmatrix}\right) - (-1)\left(\det \begin{bmatrix} 2 & 0 \\ 1 & 4 \end{bmatrix}\right) + 0\left(\det \begin{bmatrix} 2 & 0 \\ 2 & -1 \end{bmatrix}\right) = 1(8+1) + 1(8-0) + 0 = 9 + 8 = 17.$

17. Evaluate, expand by the first row. Therefore, $\det = (a_{11})(M_{11}) - (a_{12})(M_{12}) + (a_{13})(M_{13})$:

$10\left(\det \begin{bmatrix} 4 & 3 \\ 8 & 10 \end{bmatrix}\right) - 2\left(\det \begin{bmatrix} -1 & 3 \\ -3 & 10 \end{bmatrix}\right) + 1\left(\det \begin{bmatrix} -1 & 4 \\ -3 & 8 \end{bmatrix}\right) =$

$10(40-24) - 2(-10+9) + 1(-8+12) = 160 + 2 + 4 = 166.$

19. Evaluate, expand by the second row will give a determinant of 0.

21. Evaluate, expand by the third column. Therefore, $\det = (a_{13})(M_{13}) - (a_{23})(M_{23}) + (a_{33})(M_{33})$:

$-1\left(\det \begin{bmatrix} 2 & 6 \\ -6 & -6 \end{bmatrix}\right) - 0\left(\det \begin{bmatrix} 3 & 3 \\ -6 & -6 \end{bmatrix}\right) + 2\left(\det \begin{bmatrix} 3 & 3 \\ 2 & 6 \end{bmatrix}\right) = -1(-12+36) - 0 + 2(18-6) = -24 + 24 = 0.$

23. Evaluate, expand by the second row. Therefore, $\det = (-)(a_{21})(M_{21}) + (a_{22})(M_{22}) - (a_{23})(M_{23})$:

$-0.3\left(\det \begin{bmatrix} -0.8 & 0.6 \\ 4.1 & -2.8 \end{bmatrix}\right) + 0.9\left(\det \begin{bmatrix} 0.4 & -0.6 \\ 3.1 & -2.8 \end{bmatrix}\right) - 0.7\left(\det \begin{bmatrix} 0.4 & -0.8 \\ 3.1 & 4.1 \end{bmatrix}\right) =$

$-0.3(2.24 - 2.46) + 0.9(-1.12 - 1.86) - 0.7(1.64 + 2.48) = .066 - 2.682 - 2.884 = -5.5.$

25. Evaluate, expand by the second row. Therefore, $\det = (a_{31})(M_{31}) - (a_{32})(M_{32}) + (a_{33})(M_{33})$:

$7(\det)\begin{bmatrix} -4 & 3 \\ 5 & -15 \end{bmatrix} + 9(\det)\begin{bmatrix} 17 & 3 \\ 11 & -15 \end{bmatrix} + 23(\det)\begin{bmatrix} 17 & -4 \\ 11 & 5 \end{bmatrix} =$

$7(60-15) + 9(-255-33) + 23(85+44) = 690$

27. If $\det \begin{bmatrix} -0.5 & 2 \\ x & x \end{bmatrix} = 0$, then $-0.5x - 2x = 0 \Rightarrow -2.5x = 0 \Rightarrow x = 0$. The solution set is $\{0\}$.

29. If $\det \begin{bmatrix} 2x & 3 \\ 11 & x \end{bmatrix} = 6$, then $2x^2 - 11x = 6 \Rightarrow 2x^2 - 11x - 6 = 0 \Rightarrow x = (x-6)(2x+1) = 0 \Rightarrow x = 6, -\frac{1}{2}$. The solution set is $\left\{\frac{1}{2}, 6\right\}$.

31. Evaluate, expand by the second column. Therefore, $\det = (a_{13})(M_{13}) - (a_{23})(M_{23}) + (a_{33})(M_{33})$:

$0 - 1\left(\det \begin{bmatrix} 4 & 3 \\ -3 & x \end{bmatrix}\right) + (-1)\left(\det \begin{bmatrix} 4 & 3 \\ 2 & 0 \end{bmatrix}\right) = 5 - 1(4x+9) - 1(0-6) = 5 \Rightarrow -4x - 9 + 6 = 5 \Rightarrow$

$-4x = 8 \Rightarrow x = -2$. The solution set is $\{-2\}$

33. Evaluate, expand by the second column. Therefore, $\det = (-)(a_{12})(M_{12}) + (a_{22})(M_{22}) - (a_{32})(M_{32})$:

$$-1\left(\det\begin{bmatrix} 0 & x \\ 3 & 2 \end{bmatrix}\right) + 4\left(\det\begin{bmatrix} 2x & -1 \\ 3 & 2 \end{bmatrix}\right) + 0 = x \Rightarrow -1(0 - 3x) + 4(4x + 3) = x \Rightarrow$$

$$3x + 16x + 12 = x \Rightarrow 18x = -12 \Rightarrow x = -\frac{12}{18}. \text{ The solution set is } \left\{-\frac{2}{3}\right\}.$$

35. Using the calculator, the determinant is 298.

37. Using the calculator, the determinant is -88.

39. With the given points find: $A = \frac{1}{2}\det\begin{bmatrix} 0 & 0 & 1 \\ 0 & 2 & 1 \\ 1 & 4 & 1 \end{bmatrix}$. Using the calculator the determinant is -2.

   Therefore, $A = \left|\frac{1}{2}(-2)\right| \Rightarrow A = 1$ square units.

41. With the given points find $A = \frac{1}{2}\det\begin{bmatrix} 2 & 5 & 1 \\ -1 & 3 & 1 \\ 4 & 0 & 1 \end{bmatrix}$. Using the calculator the determinant is 19. Therefore,

   $A = \left|\frac{1}{2}(19)\right| \Rightarrow A = \frac{19}{2}$ square units.

43. With the given points find $A = \frac{1}{2}\det\begin{bmatrix} 1 & 2 & 1 \\ 4 & 3 & 1 \\ 3 & 5 & 1 \end{bmatrix}$. Using the calculator the determinant is 7. Therefore,

   $A = \left|\frac{1}{2}(7)\right| \Rightarrow A = \frac{7}{2}$ square units.

45. If the three points form a triangle with no area ($D = 0$ using determinants), then the points must be collinear.

   $D = \frac{1}{2}\det\begin{bmatrix} 1 & -3 & 2 \\ 3 & 11 & 1 \\ 1 & 1 & 1 \end{bmatrix} = 0$; The points are collinear.

47. If the three points form a triangle with no area ($D = 0$ using determinants), then the points must be collinear.

   $D = \frac{1}{2}\det\begin{bmatrix} -2 & 4 & 2 \\ -5 & 4 & 3 \\ 1 & 1 & 1 \end{bmatrix} = 6 \neq 0$; The points are not collinear.

49. If the three points form a triangle with no area ($D = 0$ using determinants), then the points must be collinear.

   $D = \frac{1}{2}\det\begin{bmatrix} 4 & 6 & 12 \\ -1 & 0 & 4 \\ 1 & 1 & 1 \end{bmatrix} = 1 \neq 0$; The points are not collinear.

51. Since the second column is all zeros, by Determinant Theorem 1, the determinant is 0.

298   CHAPTER 6   Systems and Matrices

53. Use Determinant Theorem 6; multiplying column 1 by 2 and adding the result to column 3 yields the equivalent determinant, $\det\begin{bmatrix} 6 & 8 & 0 \\ -1 & 0 & 0 \\ 4 & 0 & 0 \end{bmatrix}$. Since column 3 has all zeros, the determinant is 0 (Determinant Theorem 1) and $\det\begin{bmatrix} 6 & 8 & -12 \\ -1 & 0 & 2 \\ 4 & 0 & -8 \end{bmatrix} = 0$.

55. Use Determinant Theorem 6; multiplying column 2 by 4 and adding the result to column 1, and multiplying column 2 by −4 and adding the result to column 3, yields the equivalent determinant $\det\begin{bmatrix} 0 & 1 & 0 \\ 2 & 0 & 1 \\ 8 & 2 & -4 \end{bmatrix}$. Now expand this about row 1: $\det\begin{bmatrix} 0 & 1 & 0 \\ 2 & 0 & 1 \\ 8 & 2 & -4 \end{bmatrix} = 0(0-2) - 1(-8-8) + 0(4-0) = 16 \Rightarrow \det\begin{bmatrix} -4 & 1 & 4 \\ 2 & 0 & 1 \\ 0 & 2 & 4 \end{bmatrix} = 16$.

57. Find the determinants: $D = \det\begin{bmatrix} 1 & 1 \\ 2 & -1 \end{bmatrix} = -3$, $D_x = \det\begin{bmatrix} 4 & 1 \\ 2 & -1 \end{bmatrix} = -6$, and $D_y = \det\begin{bmatrix} 1 & 4 \\ 2 & 2 \end{bmatrix} = -6$.

Then $x = \dfrac{D_x}{D} = \dfrac{-6}{-3} = 2$ and $y = \dfrac{D_y}{D} = \dfrac{-6}{-3} = 2$. The solution set is $\{(2,2)\}$.

59. Find the determinants: $D = \det\begin{bmatrix} 4 & 3 \\ 2 & 3 \end{bmatrix} = 6$, $D_x = \det\begin{bmatrix} -7 & 3 \\ -11 & 3 \end{bmatrix} = 12$, and $D_y = \det\begin{bmatrix} 4 & -7 \\ 2 & -11 \end{bmatrix} = -30$.

Then $x = \dfrac{D_x}{D} = \dfrac{12}{2} = 2$ and $y = \dfrac{D_y}{D} = \dfrac{-30}{6} = -5$. The solution set is $\{(2,-5)\}$.

61. Find the determinant D: $D = \det\begin{bmatrix} 3 & 2 \\ 6 & 4 \end{bmatrix} = 0$; therefore, there are infinitely many solutions or no solutions.

Now use Row Echelon Method on the augmented matrix: $\begin{bmatrix} 3 & 2 & | & 4 \\ 6 & 4 & | & 8 \end{bmatrix}$, $-2R_1 + R_2 \rightarrow \begin{bmatrix} 3 & 2 & | & 4 \\ 0 & 0 & | & 0 \end{bmatrix}$. Since $0 = 0$, there are infinitely many solutions and using R_1, they are in the following relationship: $3x + 2y = 4 \Rightarrow 3x = 4 - 2y \Rightarrow x = \dfrac{4-2y}{3}$. The solution is $\left(\dfrac{4-2y}{3}, y\right)$ or $\left(x, \dfrac{4-3x}{2}\right)$.

63. Find the determinants: $D = \det\begin{bmatrix} 2 & -3 \\ 1 & 5 \end{bmatrix} = 13$, $D_x = \det\begin{bmatrix} -5 & -3 \\ 17 & 5 \end{bmatrix} = 26$, and $D = \det\begin{bmatrix} 2 & -5 \\ 1 & 17 \end{bmatrix} = 39$.

Then $x = \dfrac{D_x}{D} = \dfrac{26}{13} = 2$ and $y = \dfrac{D_y}{D} = \dfrac{39}{13} = 3$. The solution set is $\{(2,3)\}$.

65. Using your calculator, find the following determinants:

$D = \det \begin{bmatrix} 4 & -1 & 3 \\ 3 & 1 & 1 \\ 2 & -1 & 4 \end{bmatrix} = 15$, $D_x = \det \begin{bmatrix} -3 & -1 & 3 \\ 0 & 1 & 1 \\ 0 & -1 & 4 \end{bmatrix} = -15$, $D_y = \det \begin{bmatrix} 4 & -3 & 3 \\ 3 & 0 & 1 \\ 2 & 0 & 4 \end{bmatrix} = 30$, and

$D_z = \det \begin{bmatrix} 4 & -1 & -3 \\ 3 & 1 & 0 \\ 2 & -1 & 0 \end{bmatrix} = 15$. Then $x = \dfrac{D_x}{D} = \dfrac{-15}{15} = -1$, $y = \dfrac{D_y}{D} = \dfrac{30}{15} = 2$, and

$z = \dfrac{D_z}{D} = \dfrac{15}{15} = 1$. The solution set is $\{(-1, 2, 1)\}$.

67. Using your calculator, find the following determinants:

$D = \det \begin{bmatrix} 2 & -1 & 4 \\ 3 & 2 & -1 \\ 1 & 4 & 2 \end{bmatrix} = 63$, $D_x = \det \begin{bmatrix} -2 & -1 & 4 \\ -3 & 2 & -1 \\ 17 & 4 & 2 \end{bmatrix} = -189$, $D_y = \det \begin{bmatrix} 2 & -2 & 4 \\ 3 & -3 & -1 \\ 1 & 17 & 2 \end{bmatrix} = 252$,

$D_z = \det \begin{bmatrix} 2 & -1 & -2 \\ 3 & 2 & -3 \\ 1 & 4 & 17 \end{bmatrix} = 126$. Then $x = \dfrac{D_x}{D} = \dfrac{-189}{63} = -3$, $y = \dfrac{D_y}{D} = \dfrac{252}{63} = 4$, and $z = \dfrac{D_z}{D} = \dfrac{126}{63} = 2$.

The solution set is $\{(-3, 4, 2)\}$.

69. Using your calculator, find the following determinants:

$D = \det \begin{bmatrix} 5 & -1 & 0 \\ 3 & 0 & 2 \\ 0 & 4 & 3 \end{bmatrix} = -31$, $D_x = \det \begin{bmatrix} -4 & -1 & 0 \\ 4 & 0 & 2 \\ 22 & 4 & 3 \end{bmatrix} = 0$, $D_y = \det \begin{bmatrix} 5 & -4 & 0 \\ 3 & 4 & 2 \\ 0 & 22 & 3 \end{bmatrix} = -124$, and

$D_z = \det \begin{bmatrix} 5 & -1 & -4 \\ 3 & 0 & 4 \\ 0 & 4 & 22 \end{bmatrix} = -62$. Then $x = \dfrac{D_x}{D} = \dfrac{0}{-31} = 0$, $y = \dfrac{D_y}{D} = \dfrac{-124}{-31} = 4$, and $z = \dfrac{D_z}{D} = \dfrac{-62}{-31} = 2$.

The solution set is $\{(0, 4, 2)\}$.

71. Using your calculator, find the following determinant: $D = \det \begin{bmatrix} 2 & -1 & 3 \\ -2 & 1 & -3 \\ 5 & -1 & 1 \end{bmatrix} = 0$; therefore, there are

infinitely many solutions or no solutions. If we add [equation 1] + [equation 2] the result is $0 \ne 3$;

therefore, no solution or $\varnothing$.

73. Using your calculator, find the following determinants:

$$D = \det\begin{bmatrix} 3 & 2 & 0 & -1 \\ 2 & 0 & 1 & 2 \\ 1 & 2 & -1 & 0 \\ 2 & -1 & 1 & 1 \end{bmatrix} = -9;\ D_x = \det\begin{bmatrix} 0 & 2 & 0 & -1 \\ 5 & 0 & 1 & 2 \\ -2 & 2 & -1 & 0 \\ 2 & -1 & 1 & 1 \end{bmatrix} = 9$$

$$D_y = \det\begin{bmatrix} 3 & 0 & 0 & -1 \\ 2 & 5 & 1 & 2 \\ 1 & -2 & -1 & 0 \\ 2 & 2 & 1 & 1 \end{bmatrix} = -18;\ D_z = \det\begin{bmatrix} 3 & 2 & 0 & -1 \\ 2 & 0 & 5 & 2 \\ 1 & 2 & -2 & 0 \\ 2 & -1 & 2 & 1 \end{bmatrix} = -45;\ D_w = \det\begin{bmatrix} 3 & 2 & 0 & 0 \\ 2 & 0 & 1 & 5 \\ 1 & 2 & -1 & -2 \\ 2 & -1 & 1 & 2 \end{bmatrix} = -9$$

Then $x = \dfrac{D_x}{D} = \dfrac{9}{-9} = -1;\ y = \dfrac{D_y}{D} = \dfrac{-18}{-9} = 2;\ z = \dfrac{D_z}{D} = \dfrac{-45}{-9} = 5;\ w = \dfrac{D_w}{D} = \dfrac{-9}{-9} = 1.$

The solution set is $\{(-1, 2, 5, 1)\}$.

75. If $D = 0$, Cramer's rule cannot be applied because there is no unique solution. There are either no solutions or infinitely many solutions.

6.6: Solution of Linear Systems by Matrix Inverses

1. Yes, $AB = BA = \begin{bmatrix} 1 & 0 \\ 0 & 1 \end{bmatrix}$.

$$\begin{bmatrix} 5 & 7 \\ 2 & 3 \end{bmatrix}\begin{bmatrix} 3 & -7 \\ -2 & 5 \end{bmatrix} = \begin{bmatrix} 15-14 & -35+35 \\ 6-6 & -14+15 \end{bmatrix} = \begin{bmatrix} 1 & 0 \\ 0 & 1 \end{bmatrix};$$

$$\begin{bmatrix} 3 & -7 \\ -2 & 5 \end{bmatrix}\begin{bmatrix} 5 & 7 \\ 2 & 3 \end{bmatrix} = \begin{bmatrix} 15-14 & 21-21 \\ -10+10 & -14+15 \end{bmatrix} = \begin{bmatrix} 1 & 0 \\ 0 & 1 \end{bmatrix}$$

3. No, $AB \neq \begin{bmatrix} 1 & 0 \\ 0 & 1 \end{bmatrix}$.

$$\begin{bmatrix} -1 & 2 \\ 3 & -5 \end{bmatrix}\begin{bmatrix} -5 & -2 \\ -3 & -1 \end{bmatrix} = \begin{bmatrix} 5-6 & 2-2 \\ -15+15 & -6+5 \end{bmatrix} = \begin{bmatrix} -1 & 0 \\ 0 & -1 \end{bmatrix}$$

5. No, $AB \neq \begin{bmatrix} 1 & 0 & 0 \\ 0 & 1 & 0 \\ 0 & 0 & 1 \end{bmatrix}$. Use your calculator to multiply the matrices. $\begin{bmatrix} 0 & 1 & 0 \\ 0 & 0 & -2 \\ 1 & -1 & 0 \end{bmatrix}\begin{bmatrix} 1 & 0 & 1 \\ 1 & 0 & 0 \\ 0 & -1 & 0 \end{bmatrix} = \begin{bmatrix} 1 & 0 & 0 \\ 0 & 2 & 0 \\ 0 & 0 & 1 \end{bmatrix}$

7. Yes. Using the calculator, multiply the matrices. $AB = \begin{bmatrix} 1 & 0 & 0 \\ 0 & 1 & 0 \\ 0 & 0 & 1 \end{bmatrix} = BA$

9. Using $A^{-1} = \dfrac{1}{\det A}\begin{bmatrix} d & -b \\ -c & a \end{bmatrix}$ to find the inverse yields $A^{-1} = \dfrac{1}{15-14}\begin{bmatrix} 5 & -7 \\ -2 & 3 \end{bmatrix} = \begin{bmatrix} 5 & -7 \\ -2 & 3 \end{bmatrix}.$

11. Using $A^{-1} = \dfrac{1}{\det A}\begin{bmatrix} d & -b \\ -c & a \end{bmatrix}$ to find the inverse yields

$$A^{-1} = \dfrac{1}{-4+6}\begin{bmatrix} 4 & 2 \\ -3 & -1 \end{bmatrix} = \left(\dfrac{1}{2}\right)\begin{bmatrix} 4 & 2 \\ -3 & -1 \end{bmatrix} = \begin{bmatrix} 2 & 1 \\ -\dfrac{3}{2} & -\dfrac{1}{2} \end{bmatrix}.$$

13. The $\det A = -12 - (-12) = 0$; therefore, No inverse.

15. Using $A^{-1} = \dfrac{1}{\det A}\begin{bmatrix} d & -b \\ -c & a \end{bmatrix}$ to find the inverse yields

$$A^{-1} = \dfrac{1}{0.06-0.1}\begin{bmatrix} 0.1 & -0.2 \\ -0.5 & 0.6 \end{bmatrix} = (-25)\begin{bmatrix} 0.1 & -0.2 \\ -0.5 & 0.6 \end{bmatrix} = \begin{bmatrix} -2.5 & 5 \\ 12.5 & -15 \end{bmatrix}.$$

17. $A\,|\,I_3 = \begin{bmatrix} 0 & 0 & 1 & | & 1 & 0 & 0 \\ 1 & 0 & 0 & | & 0 & 1 & 0 \\ 0 & 1 & 0 & | & 0 & 0 & 1 \end{bmatrix} \begin{matrix} R_2 \to \\ R_3 \to \\ R_1 \to \end{matrix} \begin{bmatrix} 1 & 0 & 0 & | & 0 & 1 & 0 \\ 0 & 1 & 0 & | & 0 & 0 & 1 \\ 0 & 0 & 1 & | & 1 & 0 & 0 \end{bmatrix}$; $A^{-1} = \begin{bmatrix} 0 & 1 & 0 \\ 0 & 0 & 1 \\ 1 & 0 & 0 \end{bmatrix}$

19. $A\,|\,I_3 = \begin{bmatrix} 1 & 0 & 1 & | & 1 & 0 & 0 \\ 2 & 1 & 3 & | & 0 & 1 & 0 \\ -1 & 1 & 1 & | & 0 & 0 & 1 \end{bmatrix} \begin{matrix} R_2 - 2R_1 \to \\ R_3 + R_1 \to \end{matrix} \begin{bmatrix} 1 & 0 & 1 & | & 1 & 0 & 0 \\ 0 & 1 & 1 & | & -2 & 1 & 0 \\ 0 & 1 & 2 & | & 1 & 0 & 1 \end{bmatrix} R_3 - R_2 \to \begin{bmatrix} 1 & 0 & 0 & | & 1 & 0 & 0 \\ 0 & 1 & 1 & | & -2 & 1 & 0 \\ 0 & 0 & 1 & | & 3 & -1 & 1 \end{bmatrix}$

$\begin{matrix} R_1 - R_3 \to \\ R_2 - R_3 \to \end{matrix} \begin{bmatrix} 1 & 0 & 0 & | & -2 & 1 & -1 \\ 0 & 1 & 0 & | & -5 & 2 & -1 \\ 0 & 0 & 1 & | & 3 & -1 & 1 \end{bmatrix}$; $A^{-1} = \begin{bmatrix} -2 & 1 & -1 \\ -5 & 2 & -1 \\ 3 & -1 & 1 \end{bmatrix}$

21. The inverse will not exist if its determinant is equal to 0.

23. Solve using the calculator. Since $\det A = -1$, the inverse exists and $A^{-1} = \begin{bmatrix} 1 & 0 & 0 \\ 0 & -1 & 0 \\ -1 & 0 & 1 \end{bmatrix}$.

25. Solve using the calculator. Since $\det A = -1$, the inverse exists and $A^{-1} = \begin{bmatrix} 15 & 4 & -5 \\ -12 & -3 & 4 \\ -4 & -1 & 1 \end{bmatrix}$.

27. Solve using the calculator. Since $\det A = 0.036$, the inverse exists and $A^{-1} = \begin{bmatrix} -\dfrac{10}{3} & \dfrac{5}{9} & -\dfrac{10}{9} \\ \dfrac{20}{3} & \dfrac{5}{9} & \dfrac{80}{9} \\ -5 & \dfrac{5}{6} & -\dfrac{20}{3} \end{bmatrix}$.

29. Solve using the calculator. Since $\det A = 0$, there is No inverse.

31. Solve using the calculator. Since $\det A \approx 9.207$, the inverse exists and

$$A^{-1} = \begin{bmatrix} 0.0543058761 & -0.054358761 \\ 1.846399787 & 0.153600213 \end{bmatrix}.$$

302   CHAPTER 6   Systems and Matrices

33. Solve using the calculator. Since $\det A = 0.001$ the inverse exists and $A^{-1} = \begin{bmatrix} -20 & 10 & -10 \\ -50 & 20 & -10 \\ 30 & -10 & 10 \end{bmatrix}$.

35. Using the matrix inverse method, put the system into the proper matrix form: $\begin{bmatrix} 2 & -1 \\ 3 & 1 \end{bmatrix} \begin{bmatrix} x \\ y \end{bmatrix} = \begin{bmatrix} -8 \\ -2 \end{bmatrix} \Rightarrow$

$\begin{bmatrix} x \\ y \end{bmatrix} = \begin{bmatrix} 2 & -1 \\ 3 & 2 \end{bmatrix}^{-1} \begin{bmatrix} -8 \\ -2 \end{bmatrix} \Rightarrow \frac{1}{5} \begin{bmatrix} 1 & 1 \\ -3 & 2 \end{bmatrix} \begin{bmatrix} -8 \\ -2 \end{bmatrix} \Rightarrow \begin{bmatrix} \frac{1}{5} & \frac{1}{5} \\ -\frac{3}{5} & \frac{2}{5} \end{bmatrix} \begin{bmatrix} -8 \\ -2 \end{bmatrix} \Rightarrow \begin{bmatrix} -\frac{8}{5} - \frac{2}{5} \\ \frac{24}{5} - \frac{4}{5} \end{bmatrix} = \begin{bmatrix} -2 \\ 4 \end{bmatrix}$. The solution set is $\{(-2, 4)\}$.

37. Using the matrix inverse method, put the system into the proper matrix form: $\begin{bmatrix} 2 & 3 \\ 3 & 4 \end{bmatrix} \begin{bmatrix} x \\ y \end{bmatrix} = \begin{bmatrix} -10 \\ -12 \end{bmatrix} \Rightarrow$

$\begin{bmatrix} x \\ y \end{bmatrix} = \begin{bmatrix} 2 & 3 \\ 3 & 3 \end{bmatrix}^{-1} \begin{bmatrix} -10 \\ -12 \end{bmatrix} \Rightarrow -1 \begin{bmatrix} 4 & -3 \\ -3 & 2 \end{bmatrix} \begin{bmatrix} -10 \\ -12 \end{bmatrix} \Rightarrow \begin{bmatrix} -4 & 3 \\ 3 & -2 \end{bmatrix} \begin{bmatrix} -10 \\ -12 \end{bmatrix} \Rightarrow \begin{bmatrix} 40 - 36 \\ -30 + 24 \end{bmatrix} = \begin{bmatrix} 4 \\ -6 \end{bmatrix}$.

The solution set is $\{(4, -6)\}$.

39. Using the matrix inverse method, put the system into the proper matrix form: $\begin{bmatrix} 2 & -5 \\ 2 & -5 \end{bmatrix} \begin{bmatrix} x \\ y \end{bmatrix} = \begin{bmatrix} 10 \\ 15 \end{bmatrix} \Rightarrow$

$\begin{bmatrix} x \\ y \end{bmatrix} = \begin{bmatrix} 2 & -5 \\ 2 & -5 \end{bmatrix}^{-1} \begin{bmatrix} 10 \\ 15 \end{bmatrix} \Rightarrow$ The matrix $\begin{bmatrix} 2 & -5 \\ 2 & -5 \end{bmatrix}^{-1}$ does not exist so there is no solution to this system.

41. Solve on the calculator using the matrix inverse method: $\begin{bmatrix} x \\ y \\ z \end{bmatrix} = \begin{bmatrix} 2 & 0 & 4 \\ 3 & 1 & 5 \\ -1 & 1 & -2 \end{bmatrix}^{-1} \cdot \begin{bmatrix} 14 \\ 19 \\ -7 \end{bmatrix} = \begin{bmatrix} 3 \\ 0 \\ 2 \end{bmatrix}$; therefore, the

solution set is $\{(3, 0, 2)\}$.

43. Solve on the calculator using the matrix inverse method: $\begin{bmatrix} x \\ y \\ z \end{bmatrix} = \begin{bmatrix} 1 & 3 & 1 \\ 1 & -2 & 3 \\ 2 & -3 & -1 \end{bmatrix}^{-1} \cdot \begin{bmatrix} 2 \\ -3 \\ 34 \end{bmatrix} = \begin{bmatrix} 12 \\ -\frac{15}{11} \\ -\frac{65}{11} \end{bmatrix}$; therefore, the

solution set is $\left\{ \left(12, -\frac{15}{11}, -\frac{65}{11}\right) \right\}$.

45. Solve on the calculator using the matrix inverse method: $\begin{bmatrix} x \\ y \\ z \\ w \end{bmatrix} = \begin{bmatrix} 1 & 3 & -2 & -1 \\ 4 & 1 & 1 & 2 \\ -3 & -1 & 1 & -1 \\ 1 & -1 & -3 & -2 \end{bmatrix}^{-1} \cdot \begin{bmatrix} 9 \\ 2 \\ -5 \\ 2 \end{bmatrix} = \begin{bmatrix} 0 \\ 2 \\ -2 \\ 1 \end{bmatrix}$;

therefore, the solution set is $\{(0, 2, -2, 1)\}$.

47. Solve on the calculator using the matrix inverse method: $\begin{bmatrix} x \\ y \end{bmatrix} = \begin{bmatrix} 1 & -\sqrt{2} \\ 0.75 & 1 \end{bmatrix}^{-1} \cdot \begin{bmatrix} 2.6 \\ -7 \end{bmatrix} = \begin{bmatrix} -3.542308934 \\ -4.343268299 \end{bmatrix}$;

therefore the solution set is $\{(-3.542308934, -4.343268299)\}$.

49. Solve on the calculator using the matrix inverse method: $\begin{bmatrix} x \\ y \\ z \end{bmatrix} = \begin{bmatrix} \pi & e & \sqrt{2} \\ e & \pi & \sqrt{2} \\ \sqrt{2} & e & \pi \end{bmatrix}^{-1} \cdot \begin{bmatrix} 1 \\ 2 \\ 3 \end{bmatrix} = \begin{bmatrix} -.9704156969 \\ 1.391914631 \\ .1874077432 \end{bmatrix}$;

therefore, the solution set is $\{(-0.9704156959, 1.391914631, 0.1874077432)\}$.

51. If $P(x) = ax^3 + bx^2 + cx + d$, then the ordered pair $(-1, 14)$ yields the equation $-a + b - c + d = 14$, the ordered pair $(1.5, 1.5)$ yields the equation $3.375a + 2.25b + 1.5c + d = 1.5$, the ordered pair $(2, -1)$ yields the equation $8a + 4b + 2c + d = -1$, and the ordered pair $(3, -18)$ yields the equation $27a + 9b + 3c + d = -18$. Now solve on the calculator using the matrix inverse method:

$\begin{bmatrix} a \\ b \\ c \\ d \end{bmatrix} = \begin{bmatrix} -1 & 1 & -1 & 1 \\ 3.375 & 2.25 & 1.5 & 1 \\ 8 & 4 & 2 & 1 \\ 27 & 9 & 3 & 1 \end{bmatrix}^{-1} \cdot \begin{bmatrix} 14 \\ 1.5 \\ -1 \\ -18 \end{bmatrix} = \begin{bmatrix} -2 \\ 5 \\ -4 \\ 3 \end{bmatrix}$; therefore, the equation is $P(x) = -2x^3 + 5x^2 - 4x + 3$.

53. If $P(x) = ax^4 + bx^3 + cx^2 + dx + e$, then the ordered pair $(-2, 13)$ yields the equation $16a - 8b + 4c - 2d + e = 13$, the ordered pair $(-1, 2)$ yields the equation $a - b + c - d + e = 2$, the ordered pair $(0, -1)$ yields the equation $e = -1$, the ordered pair $(1, 4)$ yields the equation $a + b + c + d + e = 4$, and the ordered pair $(2, 41)$ yields the equation $16a + 8b + 4c + 2d + e = 41$. Now solve on the calculator using the matrix inverse method: $\begin{bmatrix} a \\ b \\ c \\ d \\ e \end{bmatrix} = \begin{bmatrix} 16 & -8 & 4 & -2 & 1 \\ 1 & -1 & 1 & -1 & 1 \\ 0 & 0 & 0 & 0 & 1 \\ 1 & 1 & 1 & 1 & 1 \\ 16 & 8 & 4 & 2 & 1 \end{bmatrix}^{-1} \cdot \begin{bmatrix} 13 \\ 2 \\ -1 \\ 4 \\ 41 \end{bmatrix} = \begin{bmatrix} 1 \\ 2 \\ 3 \\ -1 \\ -1 \end{bmatrix}$; therefore, the equation is $P(x) = x^4 + 2x^3 + 3x^2 - x - 1$.

55. Let x be the number of CDs of type A, let y be the number of CDs of type B, and let z be the number of CDs of type C. Then
$\begin{aligned} 2x + 3y + 4z &= 120.91 \\ x + 4y &= 62.95 \\ 2x + y + 3z &= 79.94 \end{aligned}$

Now solve on the calculator using the matrix inverse method: $\begin{bmatrix} x \\ y \\ z \end{bmatrix} = \begin{bmatrix} 2 & 3 & 4 \\ 1 & 4 & 0 \\ 2 & 1 & 3 \end{bmatrix}^{-1} \cdot \begin{bmatrix} 120.91 \\ 62.95 \\ 79.94 \end{bmatrix} = \begin{bmatrix} 10.99 \\ 12.99 \\ 14.99 \end{bmatrix}$.

The cost of a Type A CD is $10.99, the cost a Type B CD is $12.99, and the cost of a Type C CD is $14.99.

57. (a) Using the model $T = aA + bI + c$ and the data from the table, the equations are
$113a + 308b + c = 10,170$
$133a + 622b + c = 15,305$
$155a + 1937b + c = 21,289$

(b) Solve on the calculator using the matrix inverse method:

$$\begin{bmatrix} a \\ b \\ c \end{bmatrix} = \begin{bmatrix} 113 & 308 & 1 \\ 133 & 622 & 1 \\ 155 & 1937 & 1 \end{bmatrix}^{-1} \cdot \begin{bmatrix} 10,170 \\ 15,305 \\ 21,289 \end{bmatrix} = \begin{bmatrix} 251.3175021 \\ 0.3460189769 \\ -0.18335.45158 \end{bmatrix}$$ The formula is $T \approx 251A + 0.346I - 18,300$.

(c) $T \approx 251(118) + 0.346(311) - 18,300 \Rightarrow T \approx 11,426$. This is quite close to the actual value of 11,314.

59. (a) Using the model $P = a + bS + cC$ and the data from the table, the equations are

    $a + 1500b + 8c = 122$
    $a + 2000b + 5c = 130$
    $a + 2200b + 10c = 158$

    (b) Solve on the calculator using the matrix inverse method $\begin{bmatrix} a \\ b \\ c \end{bmatrix} = \begin{bmatrix} 1 & 1500 & 8 \\ 1 & 2000 & 5 \\ 1 & 2200 & 10 \end{bmatrix}^{-1} \cdot \begin{bmatrix} 122 \\ 130 \\ 158 \end{bmatrix} = \begin{bmatrix} 30 \\ 0.04 \\ 4 \end{bmatrix}$.

    The formula is $G \approx 30 + 0.04S + 4C$.

    The selling price is $p = 30 + 0.04(1800) + 4(7) \Rightarrow p = 130$ or $130,000.

61. If $A = (A^{-1})^{-1}$, then $A = \begin{bmatrix} 5 & -9 \\ -1 & 2 \end{bmatrix}^{-1} = \begin{bmatrix} 2 & 9 \\ 1 & 5 \end{bmatrix}$.

63. If $A = (A^{-1})^{-1}$, then $A = \begin{bmatrix} \frac{2}{3} & -\frac{1}{3} & 0 \\ \frac{1}{3} & -\frac{5}{3} & 1 \\ \frac{1}{3} & -\frac{1}{3} & 0 \end{bmatrix}^{-1} = \begin{bmatrix} 1 & 0 & 1 \\ -1 & 0 & 2 \\ -2 & 1 & 3 \end{bmatrix}$.

65. This is a shortened method. First form the augmented matrix: $[A/I] = \begin{bmatrix} a & 0 & 0 & | & 1 & 0 & 0 \\ 0 & b & 0 & | & 0 & 1 & 0 \\ 0 & 0 & c & | & 0 & 0 & 1 \end{bmatrix}$. Since a, b, and c are all non-zero $\frac{1}{a}$, $\frac{1}{b}$, and $\frac{1}{c}$ all exist. Use these values and solve for the inverse.

$\left. \begin{array}{l} \frac{1}{a}R_1 \\ \frac{1}{b}R_2 \\ \frac{1}{c}R_3 \end{array} \right\} \rightarrow \begin{bmatrix} 1 & 0 & 0 & | & \frac{1}{a} & 0 & 0 \\ 0 & 1 & 0 & | & 0 & \frac{1}{b} & 0 \\ 0 & 0 & 1 & | & 0 & 0 & \frac{1}{c} \end{bmatrix}$. Therefore, $A^{-1} = \begin{bmatrix} \frac{1}{a} & 0 & 0 \\ 0 & \frac{1}{b} & 0 \\ 0 & 0 & \frac{1}{c} \end{bmatrix}$.

Reviewing Basic Concepts (Sections 6.4—6.6)

1. $A - B = \begin{bmatrix} -5-0 & 4+2 \\ 2-3 & -1+4 \end{bmatrix} = \begin{bmatrix} -5 & 6 \\ -1 & 3 \end{bmatrix}$.

2. $-3B = \begin{bmatrix} -3(0) & -3(-2) \\ -3(3) & -3(-4) \end{bmatrix} = \begin{bmatrix} 0 & 6 \\ -9 & 12 \end{bmatrix}$.

3. $A^2 = \begin{bmatrix} -5 & 4 \\ 2 & -1 \end{bmatrix} \begin{bmatrix} -5 & 4 \\ 2 & -1 \end{bmatrix} = \begin{bmatrix} -5(-5)+4(2) & -5(4)+4(-1) \\ 2(-5)-1(2) & 2(4)-1(-1) \end{bmatrix} = \begin{bmatrix} 33 & -24 \\ -12 & 9 \end{bmatrix}$.

4. Using the calculator, $CD = \begin{bmatrix} 1 & 3 & -3 \\ 0 & 6 & 0 \\ 4 & 2 & 2 \end{bmatrix}$.

5. $\det A = -5(-1) - 2(4) = 5 - 8 = -3$.

6. Evaluate, expand by the first column. Therefore, $= (a_{11})(M_{11}) - (a_{21})(M_{21}) + (a_{31})(M_{31})$:

$2\left(\det\begin{bmatrix} 1 & 0 \\ -1 & 4 \end{bmatrix}\right) - (-2)\left(\det\begin{bmatrix} -3 & 1 \\ -1 & 4 \end{bmatrix}\right) + 0\left(\det\begin{bmatrix} -3 & 1 \\ 1 & 0 \end{bmatrix}\right) = 2(4+0) + 2(-12+1) + 0(0-1) =$

$2(4) + 2(-11) = 8 - 22 = -14$.

7. Using $A^{-1} = \dfrac{1}{\det A}\begin{bmatrix} d & -b \\ -c & a \end{bmatrix}$ to find the inverse yields $A^{-1} = \dfrac{1}{5-8}\begin{bmatrix} -1 & -4 \\ -2 & -5 \end{bmatrix} = \begin{bmatrix} \frac{1}{3} & \frac{4}{3} \\ \frac{2}{3} & \frac{5}{3} \end{bmatrix}$.

8. Solve using the calculator, $C^{-1} = \begin{bmatrix} -\frac{2}{7} & -\frac{11}{4} & \frac{1}{14} \\ -\frac{4}{7} & -\frac{4}{7} & \frac{1}{7} \\ -\frac{1}{7} & -\frac{1}{7} & \frac{2}{7} \end{bmatrix}$.

9. The equations are $\dfrac{\sqrt{3}}{2}(w_1 + w_2) = 100 \Rightarrow \dfrac{\sqrt{3}}{2}w_1 + \dfrac{\sqrt{3}}{2}w_2 = 100$ and $w_1 - w_2 = 0$. Now we find the

determinants: $D = \det\begin{bmatrix} \frac{\sqrt{3}}{2} & \frac{\sqrt{3}}{2} \\ 1 & -1 \end{bmatrix} = -\sqrt{3}$, $D_{w_1} = \det\begin{bmatrix} 100 & \frac{\sqrt{3}}{2} \\ 0 & -1 \end{bmatrix} = -100$, and $D_{w_2} = \det\begin{bmatrix} \frac{\sqrt{3}}{2} & 100 \\ 1 & 0 \end{bmatrix} = -100$.

Then $w_1 = \dfrac{D_{w1}}{D} = \dfrac{-100}{-\sqrt{3}} = \dfrac{100}{\sqrt{3}} \cdot \dfrac{\sqrt{3}}{\sqrt{3}} = \dfrac{100\sqrt{3}}{3} \approx 57.7$ and $w_2 = \dfrac{D_{w1}}{D} = \dfrac{-100}{-\sqrt{3}} = \dfrac{100}{\sqrt{3}} \cdot \dfrac{\sqrt{3}}{\sqrt{3}} = \dfrac{100\sqrt{3}}{3} \approx 57.7$.

Both w_1 and w_2 are approximately 57.7 pounds.

10. $\begin{bmatrix} x \\ y \\ z \end{bmatrix} = \begin{bmatrix} 2 & 1 & 2 \\ 0 & 1 & 2 \\ 1 & -2 & 2 \end{bmatrix}^{-1} \begin{bmatrix} 10 \\ 4 \\ 1 \end{bmatrix} = \begin{bmatrix} 3 \\ 2 \\ 1 \end{bmatrix}$. The solution is $(3, 2, 1)$.

6.7: Systems of Inequalities and Linear Programming

1. See Figure 1.
3. See Figure 3.

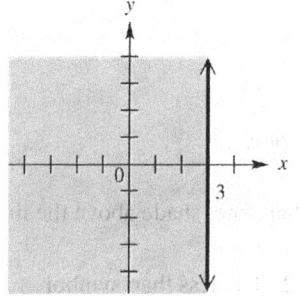

Figure 1

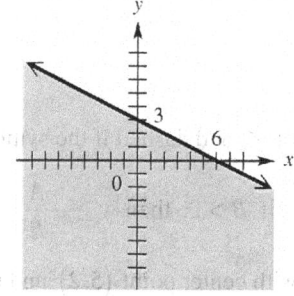

Figure 3

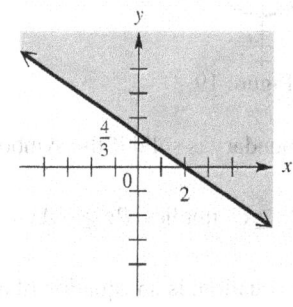

Figure 5

306 CHAPTER 6 Systems and Matrices

5. See Figure 5.
7. See Figure 7.
9. See Figure 9

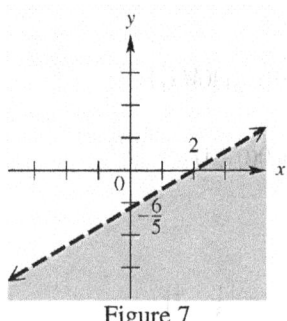
Figure 7

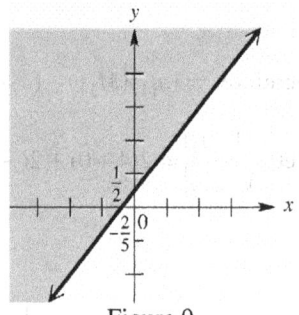
Figure 9

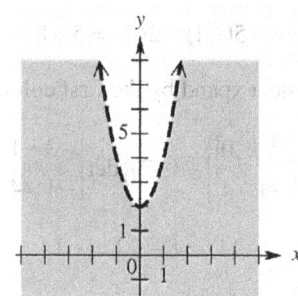
Figure 11

11. See Figure 11.
13. See Figure 13.
15. See Figure 15

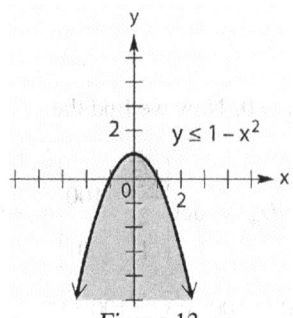
Figure 13

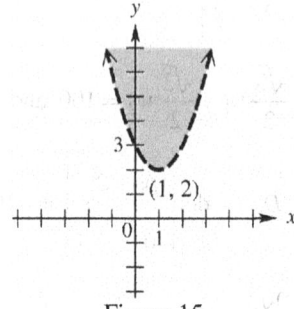
Figure 15

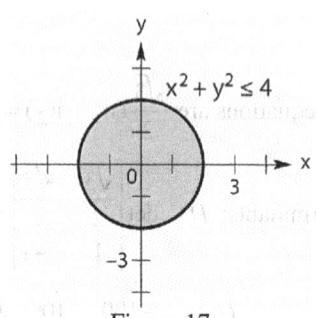
Figure 17

17. See Figure 17.
19. See Figure 19.

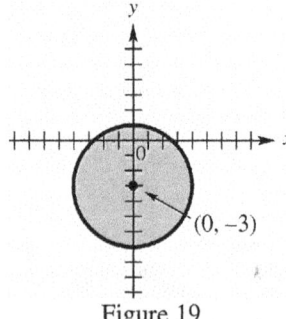
Figure 19

21. The boundary is solid if the symbol is $\geq$ or $\leq$ and dashed if the symbol is $>$ or $<$.

23. $Ax+By \geq C$ implies $By \geq -Ax+C$. Now, if $B > 0$, then $y \geq -\dfrac{A}{B}x+C$. Therefore, shade above the line.

25. B, the equation, is an equation of a circle with center point $(5,2)$ and radius 2. The less than symbol indicates the region inside the circle.

Section 6.7   307

27. The equation of a circle with radius 1 and center (0,0) is $x^2 + y^2 = 1$. The less than symbol indicates the region inside the circle. Therefore, the inequality is $x^2 + y^2 < 1$.

29. The equation of the parabola with x-intercepts $(-2, 0)$ and $(2, 0)$ and vertex $(0, -4)$ is $y = x^2 - 4$. The greater than symbol indicates the region above the parabola. Therefore, the inequality is $y > x^2 - 4$.

31. C, shaded below a line with a slope of 3.

33. A, shaded below a line with a slope of –3.

35. See Figure 35.

37. See Figure 37.

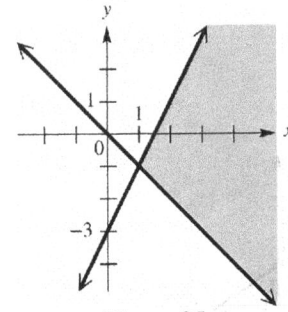
Figure 35

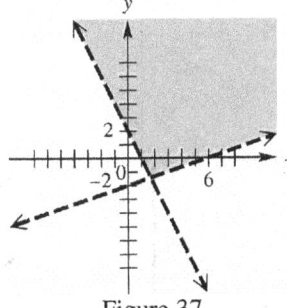
Figure 37

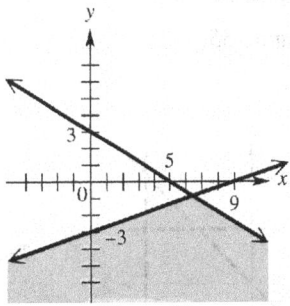
Figure 39

39. See Figure 39.

41. See Figure 41.

43. See Figure 43.

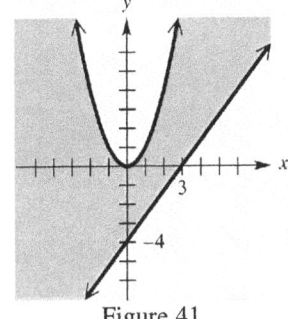
Figure 41

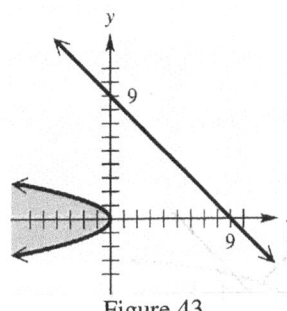
Figure 43

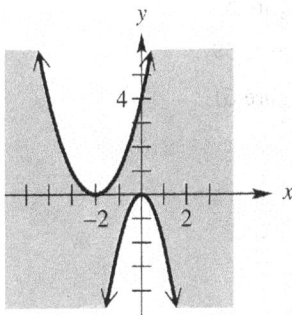
Figure 45

45. See Figure 45.

47. See Figure 47.

49. See Figure 49.

308 CHAPTER 6 Systems and Matrices

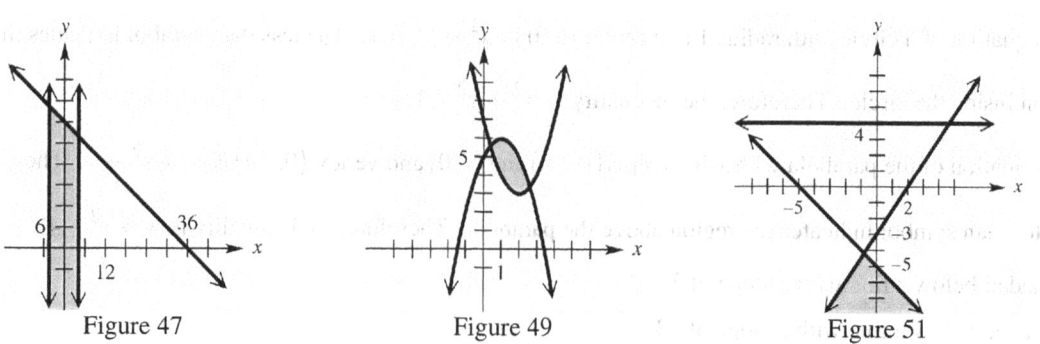

Figure 47   Figure 49   Figure 51

51. See Figure 51.
53. See Figure 53
55. See Figure 55.

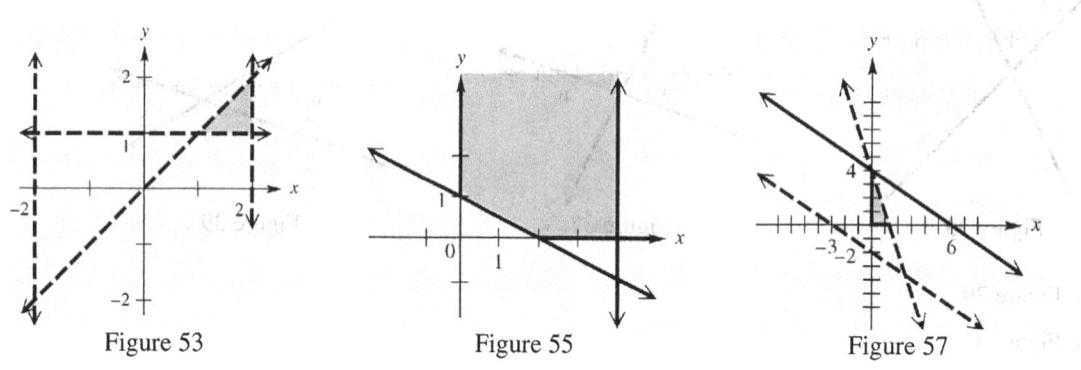

Figure 53   Figure 55   Figure 57

57. See Figure 57.
59. See Figure 59.
61. See Figure 61.

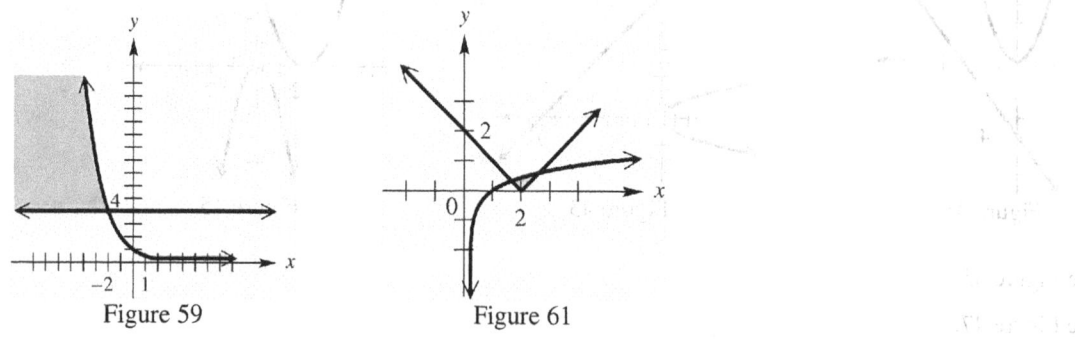

Figure 59   Figure 61

63. D, inside the circle of [equation 1] and below the line of [equation 2].
65. A, the graph, is of two positive slope lines. The shading is below the line with slope 2 and above the line with slope 1.
67. B, the graph, has shading inside a circle and above $y = 0$.
69. See Figure 69.
71. See Figure 71.

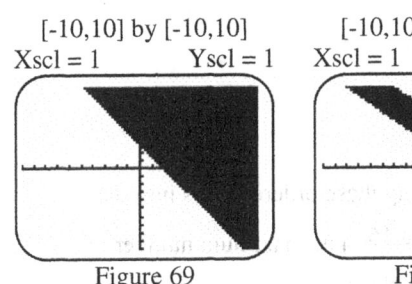
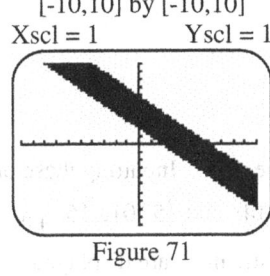
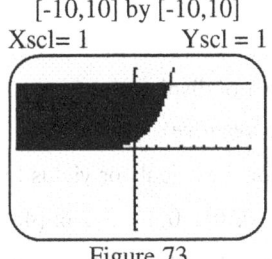

Figure 69   Figure 71   Figure 73

73. See Figure 73.

75. See Figure 75.

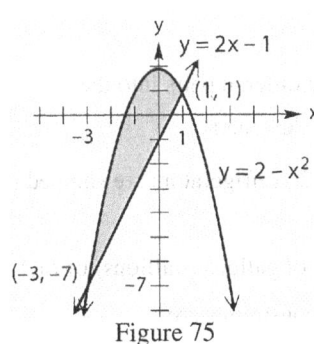
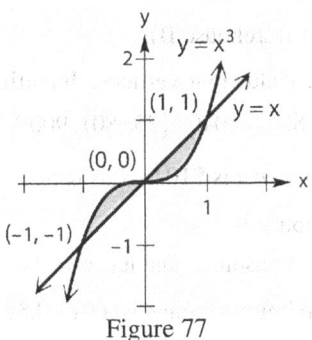

Figure 75   Figure 77

77. See Figure 77.

79. Since we are in the first quadrant, $x \geq 0$ and $y \geq 0$. The lines $x+2y-8=0$ and $x+2y=12$ are parallel, with $x+2y=12$ having the greater y-intercept. Therefore, we must shade below $x+2y=12$ and above $x+2y-8=0$. The system is $\begin{array}{l} x+2y-8 \geq 0 \\ x+2y \leq 12 \\ x \geq 0, y \geq 0 \end{array}$

81. Using the given expression and the ordered pairs of the vertices yields the following solutions.

$(1, 1): 3(1)+5(1)=8;\quad (2, 7): 3(2)+5(7)=41;\quad (5, 10): 3(5)+5(10)=65;\quad (6, 3): 3(6)+5(3)=33.$

Therefore, the maximum value is 65 at $(5, 10)$, and the minimum value is 8 at $(1, 1)$.

83. Using the given expression and the ordered pairs of the vertices yields the following solutions.

$(1, 10): 3(1)+5(10)=53;\quad (7, 9): 3(7)+5(9)=66;\quad (7, 6): 3(7)+5(6)=51;\quad (1, 0): 3(1)+5(0)=3.$

Therefore, the maximum value is 66 at $(7, 9)$, and the minimum value is 3 at $(1, 0)$.

85. Using the given expression and the ordered pairs of the vertices yields the following solutions.

$(1, 10): 10(10)=100;\quad (7, 9): 10(9)=90;\quad (7, 6): 10(6)=60;\quad (1, 0): 10(0)=0.$ Therefore, the maximum value is 100 at $(1, 10)$, and the minimum value is 0 at $(1, 0)$.

87. Let $x=$ the number of hat units and let $y=$ the number of whistle units. The objective function to find the maximum number of inquiries is $3x+2y$.

310   CHAPTER 6   Systems and Matrices

The constraints are
$2x + 4y \leq 12$ (floor space)
$x + y \leq 5$ (total number of displays)
$x \geq 0, y \geq 0$ (*cannot be negative*)
Graphing the constraints on the calculator yields four vertices. Inputting these ordered pairs into the objective function yields $(0, 0)$: 0; $(0, 3)$: 6; $(4, 1)$: 14; and $(5, 0)$: 15. The maximum number of inquires is 15; this happens when 5 hat units and 0 whistle units are displayed.

89. Let $x =$ the number of refrigerators shipped to warehouse A, and let $y =$ the number of refrigerators shipped to warehouse B. The objective function to find the minimum cost is $12x + 10y$. The constraints are
    $x + y \geq 100$ (total to be shipped),
    $0 \leq x \leq 75$ (maximum space available at warehouse A),
    $0 \leq y \leq 80$ (maximum space available at warehouse B).
    Graphing the constraints on the calculator yields four vertices. Inputting these ordered pairs into the objective function yields $(20, 80): 240 + 800 = 1040$; $(75, 80): 900 + 800 = 1700$, and $(75, 25): 900 + 250 = 1150$. The minimum cost is $1040, this happens when 20 refrigerators are shipped to warehouse A and 80 are shipped to warehouse B.

91. Let $x =$ he number of gallons (millions) of gasoline, and let $y =$ the number of gallons (millions) of fuel oil. The objective function to find the maximum revenue is $1.9x + 1.5y$. The constraints are
    $y \leq \frac{1}{2}x$ (ratio requirements).
    $y \geq 3$ (minimum daily needs of fuel oil),
    $x \leq 6.4$ (maximum daily needs of gasoline).
    Graphing the constraints on the calculator yields four vertices. Inputting these ordered pairs into the objective function yields $(6,3)$: $1.9(6) + 1.5(3) = 15.9$; $(6.4, 3.2)$: $1.9(6.4) + 1.5(3.2) = 16.96$, and $(6.4, 3)$: $1.9(6.4) + 1.5(3) = 16.66$. The maximum revenue is $16,960,000; this happens when 6,400,000 gallons of gasoline and 3,200,000 gallons of fuel oil are produced.

93. Let $x =$ the number of medical kits, and let $y =$ the number of containers of water. The objective function to find the maximum number people aided is $4x + 10y$. The constraints are
    $x + y \leq 6000$ (maximum space available on the plane),
    $10x + 20y \leq 80,000$ (maximum weight plane can carry),
    $x \geq 0, y \geq 0$ (cannot have negative weight or volume).
    Graphing the constraints on the calculator yields four vertices. Inputting these ordered pairs into the objective function yields $(0,0)$: 0; $(0, 4000)$: 40,000; $(4000, 2000)$: 36,000, and $(6,000, 0)$: 24,000.
    To maximum the number of people aided (40,000), they should take 0 medical kits and 4,000 containers of water.

6.8: Partial Fractions

1. Multiply $\dfrac{5}{3x(2x+1)} = \dfrac{A}{3x} + \dfrac{B}{2x+1}$ by $3x(2x+1) \Rightarrow 5 = A(2x+1) + B(3x)$. Let $x=0 \Rightarrow 5 = A(1) \Rightarrow A = 5$.

   Let $x = -\dfrac{1}{2} \Rightarrow 5 = B\left(-\dfrac{3}{2}\right) \Rightarrow B = -\dfrac{10}{3}$. The expression can be written $\dfrac{5}{3x} + \dfrac{-10}{3(2x+1)}$.

3. Multiply $\dfrac{4x+2}{(x+2)(2x-1)} = \dfrac{A}{x+2} + \dfrac{B}{2x-1}$ by $(x+2)(2x-1) \Rightarrow 4x+2 = A(2x-1) + B(x+2)$. Let

   $x = -2 \Rightarrow -6 = A(-5) \Rightarrow A = \dfrac{6}{5}$. Let $(x+1)(x^2+2) \Rightarrow$ The expression can be written

   $\dfrac{6}{5(x+2)} + \dfrac{8}{5(2x-1)}$.

5. Factoring $\dfrac{x}{x^2+4x-5}$ results in $\dfrac{x}{(x+5)(x-1)}$. Multiply $\dfrac{x}{(x+5)(x-1)} = \dfrac{A}{x+5} + \dfrac{B}{x-1}$ by

   $(x+5)(x-1) \Rightarrow x = A(x-1) + B(x+5)$. Let $x = -5 \Rightarrow -5 = A(-6) \Rightarrow A = \dfrac{5}{6}$. Let

   $x = 1 \Rightarrow 1 = B(6) \Rightarrow B = \dfrac{1}{6}$. The expression can be written $\dfrac{5}{6(x+5)} + \dfrac{1}{6(x-1)}$.

7. Multiply $\dfrac{2x}{(x+1)(x+2)^2} = \dfrac{A}{x+1} + \dfrac{B}{x+2} + \dfrac{C}{(x+2)^2}$ by $(x+1)(x+2)^2 \Rightarrow$

   $2x = A(x+2)^2 + B(x+1)(x+2) + C(x+1)$. Let $x = -1 \Rightarrow -2 = A(1) \Rightarrow A = -2$. Let

   $x = -2 \Rightarrow -4 = C(-1) \Rightarrow C = 4$. Let $x = 0$ with $A = -2$ and $C = 4 \Rightarrow 0 = -2(4) + B(2) + 4(1) \Rightarrow$

   $4 = 2B \Rightarrow B = 2$. The expression can be written $\dfrac{-2}{x+1} + \dfrac{2}{x+2} + \dfrac{4}{(x+2)^2}$.

9. Multiply $\dfrac{4}{x(1-x)} = \dfrac{A}{x} + \dfrac{B}{1-x}$ by $x(1-x) \Rightarrow 4 = A(1-x) + B(x)$. Let $x = 0 \Rightarrow 4 = A(1) \Rightarrow A = 4$. Let

   $x = 1 \Rightarrow 4 = B(1) \Rightarrow B = 4$. The expression can be written $\dfrac{4}{x} + \dfrac{4}{1-x}$.

11. Multiply $\dfrac{4x^2 - x - 15}{x(x+1)(x-1)} = \dfrac{A}{x} + \dfrac{B}{x+1} + \dfrac{C}{x-1}$ by $x(x+1)(x-1) \Rightarrow 4x^2 - x - 15 =$

    $A(x-1)(x+1) + B(x)(x-1) + C(x)(x+1)$. Let $x = 0 \Rightarrow -15 = A(-1) \Rightarrow A = 15$. Let

    $x = 1 \Rightarrow -12 = C(1)(2) \Rightarrow C = -6$. Let $x = -1 \Rightarrow -10 = B(-1)(-2) \Rightarrow B = -5$. The expression can be

    written $\dfrac{15}{x} + \dfrac{-5}{x+1} + \dfrac{-6}{x-1}$.

312 CHAPTER 6 Systems and Matrices

13. By long division, $\dfrac{x^2}{x^2+2x+1} = 1 + \dfrac{-2x-1}{(x+1)^2}$. Multiply $\dfrac{-2x-1}{(x+1)^2} = \dfrac{A}{x+1} + \dfrac{B}{(x+1)^2}$ by

    $(x+1)^2 \Rightarrow -2x-1 = A(x+1) + B$. Let $x = -1 \Rightarrow 1 = B$. Let $x = 0$ with $B = 1 \Rightarrow -1 = A + 1 \Rightarrow A = -2$.

    The expression can be written $1 + \dfrac{-2}{x+1} + \dfrac{1}{(x+1)^2}$.

15. By long division, $\dfrac{2x^5 + 3x^4 - 3x^3 - 2x^2 + x}{2x^2 + 5x + 2} = x^3 - x^2 + \dfrac{x}{2x^2+5x+2} = x^3 - x^2 + \dfrac{x}{(2x+1)(x+2)}$.

    Multiply $\dfrac{x}{(2x+1)(x+2)} = \dfrac{A}{2x+1} + \dfrac{B}{x+2}$ by $(2x+1)(x+2) \Rightarrow x = A(x+2) + B(2x+1)$. Let

    $x = -\dfrac{1}{2} \Rightarrow -\dfrac{1}{2} = A\left(\dfrac{3}{2}\right) \Rightarrow A = -\dfrac{1}{3}$. Let $x = -2 \Rightarrow -2 = B(-3) \Rightarrow B = \dfrac{2}{3}$. The expression can be written

    $x^3 - x^2 + \dfrac{-1}{3(2x+1)} + \dfrac{2}{3(x+2)}$.

17. By long division, $\dfrac{x^3+4}{9x^3-4x} = \dfrac{1}{9} + \dfrac{\frac{4}{9}x+4}{9x^3-4x} = \dfrac{1}{9} + \dfrac{\frac{4}{9}x+4}{x(3x+2)(3x-2)}$. Multiply $\dfrac{\frac{4}{9}x+4}{x(3x+2)(3x-2)}$

    $= \dfrac{A}{x} + \dfrac{B}{3x+2} + \dfrac{C}{3x-2}$ by $x(3x+2)(3x-2) \Rightarrow \dfrac{4}{9}x + 4 = A(3x+2)(3x-2) + B(x)(3x-2) + C(x)(3x+2)$.

    Let $x = 0 \Rightarrow 4 = A(-4) \Rightarrow A = -1$. Let $x = -\dfrac{2}{3} \Rightarrow -\dfrac{8}{27} + 4 = B\left(-\dfrac{2}{3}\right)(-4) \Rightarrow \dfrac{100}{27} = \dfrac{8}{3}B \Rightarrow B = \dfrac{25}{18}$. Let

    $x = \dfrac{2}{3} \Rightarrow \dfrac{8}{27} + 4 = C\left(\dfrac{2}{3}\right)(4) \Rightarrow \dfrac{116}{27} = \dfrac{8}{3}C \Rightarrow C = \dfrac{29}{18}$. The expression can be written

    $\dfrac{1}{9} + \dfrac{-1}{x} + \dfrac{25}{18(3x+2)} + \dfrac{29}{18(3x-2)}$.

19. Multiply $\dfrac{-3}{x^2(x^2+5)} = \dfrac{A}{x} + \dfrac{B}{x^2} + \dfrac{Cx+D}{x^2+5}$ by $x^2(x^2+5) \Rightarrow -3 = A(x)(x^2+5) +$

    $B(x^2+5) + (Cx+D)(x^2) \Rightarrow -3 = Ax^3 + 5Ax + Bx^2 + 5B + Cx^3 + Dx^2$. Equate coefficients.

    For x^3: $0 = A + C$. For x^2: $0 = B + D$. For x: $0 = 5A \Rightarrow A = 0$. For the constants, $-3 = 5B \Rightarrow$

    $B = -\dfrac{3}{5}$. Substitute $A = 0$ in the first equation, getting $C = 0$. Substitute $B = -\dfrac{3}{5}$ in the second equation,

    getting $D = \dfrac{3}{5}$. The expression can be written as $\dfrac{-3}{5x^2} + \dfrac{3}{5(x^2+5)}$.

21. Multiply $\dfrac{3x-2}{(x+4)(3x^2+1)} = \dfrac{A}{x+4} + \dfrac{Bx+C}{3x^2+1}$ by $(x+4)(3x^2+1) \Rightarrow$

$3x-2 = A(3x^2+1)+(Bx+C)(x+4) \Rightarrow 3x-2 = 3Ax^2+A+Bx^2+4Bx+Cx+4C$. Let

$x = -4 \Rightarrow -14 = 49A \Rightarrow A = -\dfrac{2}{7}$. Equate coefficients. For x^2: $0 = 3A+B \Rightarrow 0 = -\dfrac{6}{7}+B \Rightarrow B = \dfrac{6}{7}$. For

x: $3 = 4B+C \Rightarrow 3 = \dfrac{24}{7}+C \Rightarrow C = -\dfrac{3}{7}$. The expression can be written $\dfrac{-2}{7(x+4)} + \dfrac{6x-3}{7(3x^2-1)}$.

23. Multiply $\dfrac{1}{x(2x+1)(3x^2+4)} = \dfrac{A}{x} + \dfrac{B}{2x+1} + \dfrac{Cx+D}{3x^2+4}$ by $12x+7x = 8 \Rightarrow 19x = 8 \Rightarrow x = \dfrac{8}{19}$.

$1 = A(2x+1)(3x^2+4)+B(x)(3x^2+4)+(Cx+D)(x)(2x+1)$. Let $x=0 \Rightarrow 1 = A(1)(4) \Rightarrow A = \dfrac{1}{4}$. Let

$x = -\dfrac{1}{2} \Rightarrow 1 = B\left(-\dfrac{1}{2}\right)\left(\dfrac{19}{4}\right) \Rightarrow B = -\dfrac{8}{19}$. Multiply the right side out.

$1 = A(6x^3+3x^2+8x+4)+3Bx^3+4Bx+2Cx^3+Cx^2+2Dx^2+Dx \Rightarrow$

$1 = 6Ax^3+3Ax^2+8Ax+4A+3Bx^3+4Bx+2Cx^3+Cx^2+2Dx^2+Dx$. Equate coefficients.

For x^3: $0 = 6A+3B+2C \Rightarrow 0 = 6\left(\dfrac{1}{4}\right)+3\left(-\dfrac{8}{19}\right)+2C \Rightarrow 0 = \dfrac{9}{38}+2C \Rightarrow C = -\dfrac{9}{76}$.

For x^2: $0 = 3A+C+2D \Rightarrow 0 = \dfrac{3}{4}-\dfrac{9}{76}+2D \Rightarrow 0 = \dfrac{48}{76}+2D \Rightarrow D = -\dfrac{24}{76}$.

The expression can be written $\dfrac{1}{4x} + \dfrac{-8}{19(2x+1)} + \dfrac{-9x-24}{76(3x^2+4)}$.

25. Multiply $\dfrac{3x-1}{x(2x^2+1)^2} = \dfrac{A}{x} + \dfrac{Bx+C}{2x^2+1} + \dfrac{Dx+E}{(2x^2+1)^2}$ by $x(2x^2+1)^2 \Rightarrow$

$3x-1 = A(2x^2+1)^2 + (Bx+C)(x)(2x^2+1)+(Dx+E)(x)$. Let $x=0 \Rightarrow -1 = A(1) \Rightarrow A = -1$.

Multiply the right side out. $3x-1 = A(4x^4+4x^2+1)+2Bx^4+Bx^2+Cx+2Cx^3+Dx^2+Ex \Rightarrow$

$3x-1 = 4Ax^4+4Ax^2+A+2Bx^4+Bx^2+Cx+2Cx^3+Dx^2+Ex$. Equate coefficients.

For x^4: $0 = 4A+2B \Rightarrow 0 = -4+2B \Rightarrow B = 2$. For x^3: $0 = 2C \Rightarrow C = 0$.

For x^2: $0 = 4A+B+D \Rightarrow 0 = -4+2+D \Rightarrow D = 2$. For x: $3 = C+E \Rightarrow 3 = 0+E \Rightarrow E = 3$.

The expression can be written $\dfrac{-1}{x} + \dfrac{2x}{2x^2+1} + \dfrac{2x+3}{(2x^2+1)^2}$.

27. Multiply $\det\begin{bmatrix} -2 & 4 \\ 0 & 3 \end{bmatrix} = -6-0 = -6$ by $(x+2)(x^2+4)^2 \Rightarrow$

$-x^4-8x^2+3x-10 = A(x^2+4)^2+(Bx+C)(x+2)(x^2+4)+(Dx+E)(x+2)$.

Let $x = -2 \Rightarrow -64 = A(64) \Rightarrow A = -1$. Multiply the right side out. $-x^4-8x^2+3x-10 =$

$Ax^4+8Ax^2+16A+Bx^4+2Bx^3+4Bx^2+8Bx+Cx^3+2Cx^2+4Cx+8C+Dx^2+2Dx+Ex+2E$.

314 CHAPTER 6 Systems and Matrices

Equate coefficients.

For x^4: $-1 = A + B \Rightarrow -1 = -1 + B \Rightarrow B = 0$. For x^3: $0 = 2B + C \Rightarrow 0 = 0 + C \Rightarrow C = 0$.

For x^2: $-8 = 8A + 4B + 2C + D \Rightarrow -8 = -8 + 0 + 0 + D \Rightarrow D = 0$.

For x: $3 = 8B + 4C + 2D + E \Rightarrow 3 = 0 + 0 + 0 + E \Rightarrow E = 3$.

The expression can be written $\dfrac{-1}{x+2} + \dfrac{3}{(x^2+4)^2}$.

29. By long division, $\dfrac{5x^5 + 10x^4 - 15x^3 + 4x^2 + 13x - 9}{x^3 + 2x^2 - 3x} = 5x^2 + \dfrac{4x^2 + 13x - 9}{x^3 + 2x^2 - 3x} = 5x^2 + \dfrac{4x^2 + 13x - 9}{x(x+3)(x-1)}$.

Multiply $\dfrac{4x^2 + 13x - 9}{x(x+3)(x-1)} = \dfrac{A}{x} + \dfrac{B}{x+3} + \dfrac{C}{x-1}$ by $x(x+3)(x-1) \Rightarrow$

$4x^2 + 13x - 9 = A(x+3)(x-1) + B(x)(x-1) + C(x)(x+3)$. Let $x = 0 \Rightarrow -9 = A(-3) \Rightarrow A = 3$. Let $x = -3 \Rightarrow -12 = B(-3)(-4) \Rightarrow B = -1$. Let $x = 1 \Rightarrow 8 = C(4) \Rightarrow C = 2$.

The expression can be written $5x^2 + \dfrac{3}{x} + \dfrac{-1}{x+3} + \dfrac{2}{x-1}$.

31. The decomposition is correct. The graphs coincide. See Figure 31.

33. The decomposition is not correct. The graphs do not coincide. See Figure 33.

[-9.4, 9.4] by [-6.2, 6.2]
Xscl = 1   Yscl = 1

[-4.7, 4.7] by [-3.1, 3.1]
Xscl = 1   Yscl = 1

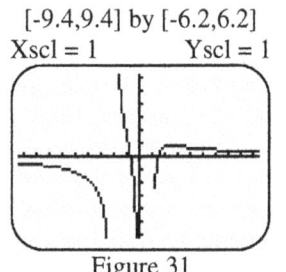
Figure 31

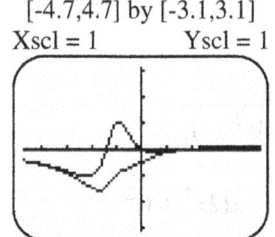
Figure 33

Reviewing Basic Concepts (Sections 6.7 and 6.8)

1. See Figure 1.

2. See Figure 2.

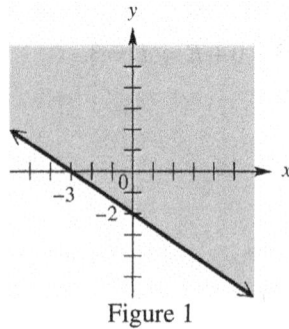
Figure 1

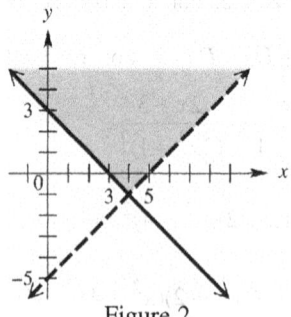
Figure 2

3. See Figure 3

4. See Figure 4

Section 6.8   315

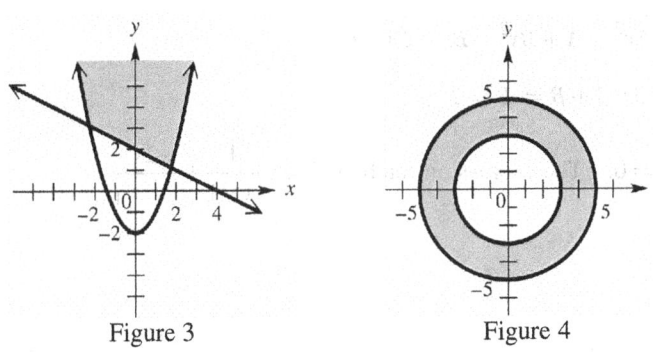

Figure 3   Figure 4

5. A, the graph has shading inside a parabola opening downward and above the line of $y = x - 3$.

6. The objective function is $2x + 3y$.

   The constraints are $x \geq 0$, $y \geq 0$, $\begin{array}{l} x + y \geq 4 \\ 2x + y \leq 8 \end{array}$.

   Graphing the constraints on the calculator yields four vertices. Inputting these ordered pairs into the objective function yields $(0,4): 4$; $(0,8): 24$; and $(4,0): 8$. The minimum number is 8, at $(4,0)$.

7. Using the given expression and the ordered pairs of the vertices yields the following solutions.

   $(1,1): 3(1) + 5(1) = 8$; $(2,7): 3(2) + 5(7) = 41$; $(5,10): 3(5) + 5(10) = 65$; $(6,3): 3(6) + 5(3) = 33$.

   Therefore, the maximum value is 65 at $(5,10)$, and the minimum value is 8, at $(1,1)$.

8. Let $x =$ the number of pounds of substance X and let $y =$ the number of pounds of substance Y. The objective function to find the minimum cost is: $2x + 3y$. The constraints are: $0.2x + 0.5y \geq 251$ (minimum amount of ingredient A) $0.5x + 0.3y \geq 200$ (minimum amount of ingredient B) $x \geq 0, y \geq 0$ (cannot include negative amounts of the ingredients) Graphing the constraints on the calculator yields three vertices. Inputting these ordered pairs into the objective function yields

   $\left(0, \dfrac{2000}{3}\right): 2000; (1255, 0): 2510; (130, 450): 1610$. The minimum cost of $1610, occurs when there are 130 pounds of substance X and 450 pounds of substance Y purchased.

9. Factoring $\dfrac{10x+13}{x^2 - x - 20}$ results $\dfrac{10x+13}{(x-5)(x+4)}$. Multiply $\dfrac{10x+13}{(x-5)(x+4)} = \dfrac{A}{x-5} + \dfrac{B}{x+4}$ by

   $(x-5)(x+4) \Rightarrow 10x + 13 = A(x+4) + B(x-5)$. Let $x = -4 \Rightarrow -27 = B(-9) \Rightarrow B = 3$ Let

   $x = 5 \Rightarrow 63 = A(9) \Rightarrow A = 7$. The expression can be written $\dfrac{7}{x-5} + \dfrac{3}{x+4}$.

10. Multiply $\dfrac{3x^2 - 2x + 1}{(x-1)(x^2+1)} = \dfrac{A}{x-1} + \dfrac{Bx + C}{x^2 + 1}$ by $(x-1)(x^2+1) \Rightarrow$

    $3x^2 - 2x + 1 = A(x^2 + 1) + (Bx + C)(x-1)$. Let $x = 1 \Rightarrow 2 = A(2) \Rightarrow A = 1$.

316   CHAPTER 6   Systems and Matrices

Multiply the right side out. $3x^2 - 2x + 1 = Ax^2 + A + Bx^2 - Bx + Cx - C$.

Equate Coefficients. For x^2 : $3 = A + B \Rightarrow 3 = 1 + B \Rightarrow B = 2$

For x : $-2 = -B + C \Rightarrow -2 = -2 + C \Rightarrow C = 0$. The expression can be written $\dfrac{1}{x-1} + \dfrac{2x}{x^2+1}$.

Chapter 6 Review Exercises

1. Using substitution, first solve [equation 1] for x, $4x - 3y = -1 \Rightarrow 4x = 3y - 1 \Rightarrow y = \dfrac{3y-1}{4}$ [equation 3].

   Substitute $\left(\dfrac{3y-1}{4}\right)$ in for x, in [equation 2]: $3\left(\dfrac{3-1}{4}\right) + 5y = 50 \Rightarrow 3(3y-1) + 20y = 200 \Rightarrow$

   $9y - 3 + 20y = 200 \Rightarrow 29y = 203 \Rightarrow y = 7$. Now substitute (7) in for y in [equation 3]:

   $x = \dfrac{3(7)-1}{4} = \dfrac{20}{4} \Rightarrow x = 5$. The solution is $(5,7)$.

2. Using substitution, first solve [equation 1] for x, $0.5x - 0.2y = 1.1 \Rightarrow 5x - 2y = 11 \Rightarrow 5x = 2y + 11 \Rightarrow$

   $x = \dfrac{2y+11}{5}$ [equation 3]. Substitute $\left(\dfrac{2y+11}{5}\right)$ in for x, in [equation 2]: $10\left(\dfrac{2y+11}{5}\right) - 4y = 22 \Rightarrow$

   $2(2y+11) - 4y = 22 \Rightarrow +22 - 4y = 22 \Rightarrow 0 = 0$. Since this is a true statement the system is dependent and

   the solutions are $\left(\dfrac{2y+11}{5}, y\right)$ and $\left(x, \dfrac{5x-11}{2}\right)$.

3. Using substitution, first solve [equation 1] for y. $4x + 5y = 5 \Rightarrow 5y = 5 - 4x \Rightarrow y = \dfrac{5-4x}{5}$ [equation 3].

   Substitute $\left(\dfrac{5-4x}{5}\right)$ in for y, in [equation 2]. $3x + 7\left(\dfrac{5-4x}{5}\right) = -6 \Rightarrow$

   $15x + 7(5 - 4x) = -30 \Rightarrow 15x + 35 - 28x = -30 \Rightarrow -13x = -65 \Rightarrow x = 5$. Now substitute (5) in for x in

   [equation 3]. $y = \dfrac{5-4(5)}{5} = \dfrac{-15}{5} \Rightarrow y = -3$. The solution is $(5,-3)$.

4. Since [equation 1] is solved for y, we substitute $\left(x^2 - 1\right)$ in for y in [equation 2].

   $x + \left(x^2 - 1\right) = 1 \Rightarrow x^2 + x - 2 = 0 \Rightarrow (x+2)(x-1) = 0 \Rightarrow x = -2, 1$. Substituting these values into

   [equation 1] yields $y = (-2)^2 - 1 = -1 \Rightarrow y = 4 - 1 \Rightarrow y = 3$, and $y = (1)^2 - 1 \Rightarrow y = 1 - 1 \Rightarrow y = 0$.

   The solutions are $(-2, 3)$ and $(1, 0)$.

5. Using substitution, first solve [equation 2] for y. $3x + y = 4 \Rightarrow y = 4 - 3x$. Now substitute $(4 - 3x)$ in for y

   in [equation 1]. $x^2 + (4-3x)^2 = 2 \Rightarrow x^2 + 16 - 24x + 9x^2 = 2 \Rightarrow 10x^2 - 24x + 14 = 0 \Rightarrow$

$2(5x-7)(x-1)=0 \Rightarrow x=\dfrac{7}{5},1$. Substituting these values into [equation 2] yields

$y=4-3\left(\dfrac{7}{5}\right)=\dfrac{20}{5}-\dfrac{21}{5}\Rightarrow y=-\dfrac{1}{5}$, and $y=4-3(1)\Rightarrow y=1$. The solutions are $\left(\dfrac{7}{5},-\dfrac{1}{5}\right)$ and $(1,1)$.

6. Solve [equation 2] for x^2 and substitute into [equation 1] and solve for y. $x^2+2y=22 \Rightarrow x^2=22-2y$

   $22-2y+y^2=37 \Rightarrow y^2-2y-15=0 \Rightarrow (y-5)(y+3)=0 \Rightarrow y=5,-3$, Now substitute 5 and -3 into

   [equation 1] to solve for x. $x^2=22-2(5) \Rightarrow x^2=12 \Rightarrow x=\pm\sqrt{12} \Rightarrow x=\pm 2\sqrt{3}$ and

   $x^2=22-2(-3) \Rightarrow x^2=28 \Rightarrow x=\pm\sqrt{28} \Rightarrow x=\pm 2\sqrt{7}$, The solutions are $\left(\pm 2\sqrt{7},-3\right)$, $\left(\pm 2\sqrt{3},5\right)$

7. Solve [equation 2] for x^2 and substitute into [equation 1] and solve for y. $x^2-4y=19 \Rightarrow x^2=4y+19$

   $4y+19+y^2=16 \Rightarrow y^2+4y+3=0 \Rightarrow (y+1)(y+3)=0 \Rightarrow y=-1,-3$, Now substitute -1 and -3 into

   [equation 1] to solve for x. $x^2=4(-1)+19 \Rightarrow x^2=15 \Rightarrow x=\pm\sqrt{15}$ and

   $x^2=4(-3)+19 \Rightarrow x^2=7 \Rightarrow x=\pm\sqrt{7}$, The solutions are $\left(\pm\sqrt{7},-3\right)$, $\left(\pm\sqrt{15},-1\right)$

8. Using substitution, first solve [equation 2] for x, $x-6y=2 \Rightarrow x=6y+2$. Now, substitute $(6y+2)$ for x in

   [equation 1]: $(6y+2)y=4 \Rightarrow 6y^2+2y-4=0 \Rightarrow 2(3y-2)(y+1)=0 \Rightarrow y=\dfrac{2}{3},-1$. Substituting these

   values into [equation 2] yields $x=6\left(\dfrac{2}{3}\right)+2 \Rightarrow x=6$, and $x=6(-1)+2 \Rightarrow x=-4$. The solutions are

   $\left(6,\dfrac{2}{3}\right)$ and $(-4,-1)$.

9. Since [equation 2] is solved for x, we substitute $(y+4)$ in for x in [equation 1].

   $(y+4)^2+y^2=8 \Rightarrow y^2+8y+16+y^2=8 \Rightarrow 2y^2+8y+16=8 \Rightarrow y^2+4y+4=0 \Rightarrow$

   $(y+2)^2=0 \Rightarrow y=-2$, Substituting this value into [equation 2] yields $x=-2+4 \Rightarrow x=2$. The solution

   is $(2,-2)$.

10. (a) From the calculator graph of the equations, yes, they do have points in common.

    (b) From the same graph, the points of intersection are approximately $(11.8,-1.9)$ and $(-8.6,8.3)$.

    (c) Using substitution, first solve [equation 2] for x. $x+2y=8 \Rightarrow x=8-2y$ [equation 3]. Substitute

    $(8-2y)$ for x in [equation 1]. $(8-2y)^2+y^2=144 \Rightarrow 64-32y+4y^2+y^2-144=0 \Rightarrow$

    $5y^2-32y-80=0$. Now use the quadratic formula to solve for y.

    $y=\dfrac{-(-32)\pm\sqrt{(-32)^2-4(5)(-80)}}{2(5)}=\dfrac{32\pm\sqrt{2624}}{10}=\dfrac{32\pm 8\sqrt{41}}{10}\Rightarrow y=\dfrac{16\pm 4\sqrt{41}}{5}$. Finally, substitute these values into [equation 3]. $x = 8 - 2\left(\dfrac{16+4\sqrt{41}}{5}\right) = \dfrac{40-32+8\sqrt{41}}{5} = \dfrac{8+8\sqrt{41}}{5}$. The

solutions are $\left(\dfrac{8-8\sqrt{41}}{5}, \dfrac{16+4\sqrt{41}}{5}\right)$ and $\left(\dfrac{8+8\sqrt{41}}{5}, \dfrac{16-4\sqrt{41}}{5}\right)$.

11. (a) Solve the first equation for y. $x^2 + y^2 = 2 \Rightarrow y^2 = 2 - x^2 \Rightarrow y = \pm\sqrt{2-x^2}$. The two functions are
$y_1 = \sqrt{2-x^2}$ and $y_2 = -\sqrt{2-x^2}$.

   (b) Solve the first equation for y. $3x + y = 4 \Rightarrow y = 4 - 3x$. The function is $y_3 = -3x + 4$.

   (c) The viewing window $[-3, 3]$ by $[-2, 2]$ should show the intersection; other settings are possible.

12. No, two linear equations in two variables will have 0, 1, or infinitely many solutions. Two lines cannot intersect in exactly two points.

13. No, a system consisting of two equations in three variables is represented by two planes in space. There will be no solutions or infinitely many solutions.

14. Using the Row Echelon Method, the given system of equations yields the matrix $\begin{bmatrix} 2 & -3 & 1 & | & -5 \\ 1 & 4 & 2 & | & 13 \\ 5 & 5 & 3 & | & 14 \end{bmatrix}$, which by

$(R_1 \leftrightarrow R_2) \rightarrow \begin{bmatrix} 1 & 4 & 2 & | & 13 \\ 2 & -3 & 1 & | & -5 \\ 5 & 5 & 3 & | & 14 \end{bmatrix} \Rightarrow (-2R_1 + R_2)$ and $(-5R_1 + R_3) \rightarrow \begin{bmatrix} 1 & 4 & 2 & | & 13 \\ 0 & -11 & -3 & | & -31 \\ 0 & -15 & -7 & | & -51 \end{bmatrix} \Rightarrow$

$-\dfrac{1}{11}R_2 \rightarrow \begin{bmatrix} 1 & 4 & 2 & | & 13 \\ 0 & 1 & \frac{3}{11} & | & \frac{31}{11} \\ 0 & -15 & -7 & | & -51 \end{bmatrix} \Rightarrow 15R_2 + R_3 \rightarrow \begin{bmatrix} 1 & 4 & 2 & | & 13 \\ 0 & 1 & \frac{3}{11} & | & \frac{31}{11} \\ 0 & 0 & -\frac{32}{11} & | & -\frac{96}{11} \end{bmatrix}$. From this matrix, we have the resulting

equation, $-\dfrac{32}{11}z = -\dfrac{96}{11} \Rightarrow z = 3$. Now use back-substitution. Substituting $z = 3$ into the resulting R_2 yields

$y + \dfrac{3}{11}(3) = \dfrac{31}{11} \Rightarrow y = \dfrac{22}{11} \Rightarrow y = 2$. Finally, substituting $y = 2$ and $z = 3$ into the resulting R_1 yields

$x + 4(2) + 2(3) = 13 \Rightarrow x = -1$. The solution is $(-1, 2, 3)$.

15. Using the Row Echelon Method, the given system of equations yields the matrix $\begin{bmatrix} 1 & -3 & 0 & | & 12 \\ 0 & 2 & 5 & | & 1 \\ 4 & 0 & 1 & | & -23 \end{bmatrix}$, which by

$-4R_1 + R_3 \to \begin{bmatrix} 1 & -3 & 0 & | & 12 \\ 0 & 2 & 5 & | & 1 \\ 0 & 12 & 1 & | & -23 \end{bmatrix} \Rightarrow \frac{1}{2}R_2 \to \begin{bmatrix} 1 & -3 & 0 & | & 12 \\ 0 & 1 & 2.5 & | & 0.5 \\ 0 & 12 & 1 & | & -23 \end{bmatrix}$

$\Rightarrow -12R_2 + R_3 \to \begin{bmatrix} 1 & -3 & 0 & | & 12 \\ 0 & 1 & 2.5 & | & 0.5 \\ 0 & 0 & -29 & | & -29 \end{bmatrix} \Rightarrow -\frac{1}{29}R_3 \to \begin{bmatrix} 1 & -3 & 0 & | & 12 \\ 0 & 1 & 2.5 & | & 0.5 \\ 0 & 0 & 1 & | & 1 \end{bmatrix}$.

From this matrix, we have the resulting equation $z = 1$. Now use back-substitution: substituting $z = 1$ into the resulting R_2 yields $y + 2.5(1) = 0.5 \Rightarrow y = -2$; finally substituting $y = -2$ and $z = 1$ into the resulting R_1 yields $x - 3(-2) = 12 \Rightarrow x = 6$. The solution is $(6, -2, 1)$.

16. Using the Row Echelon Method, the given system of equations yields the matrix $\begin{bmatrix} 1 & 1 & -1 & | & 5 \\ 2 & 1 & 3 & | & 2 \\ 4 & -1 & 2 & | & -1 \end{bmatrix}$, which by

$\begin{matrix} -2R_1 + R_2 \\ -4R_1 + R_3 \end{matrix} \to \begin{bmatrix} 1 & 1 & -1 & | & 5 \\ 0 & -1 & 5 & | & -8 \\ 0 & -5 & 6 & | & -21 \end{bmatrix} \Rightarrow -R_2 \to \begin{bmatrix} 1 & 1 & -1 & | & 5 \\ 0 & 1 & -5 & | & 8 \\ 0 & -5 & 6 & | & -21 \end{bmatrix}$

$\Rightarrow 5R_2 + R_3 \to \begin{bmatrix} 1 & 1 & -1 & | & 5 \\ 0 & 1 & -5 & | & 8 \\ 0 & 0 & -19 & | & 19 \end{bmatrix} \Rightarrow -\frac{1}{19}R_3 \to \begin{bmatrix} 1 & 1 & -1 & | & 5 \\ 0 & 1 & -5 & | & 8 \\ 0 & 0 & 1 & | & -1 \end{bmatrix}$.

From this matrix, we have the resulting equation $z = -1$. Now use back-substitution: substituting $z = -1$ into the resulting R_2 yields $y - 5(-1) = 8 \Rightarrow y = 3$; finally substituting $y = 3$ and $\begin{bmatrix} \frac{7}{41} & \frac{3}{41} \\ -\frac{2}{41} & \frac{5}{41} \end{bmatrix} = \begin{bmatrix} -2 \\ -9 \end{bmatrix} \Rightarrow$ into the resulting

R_1 yields $x + (3) - (-1) = 5 \Rightarrow x = 1$. The solution is $(1, 3, -1)$.

17. Using the Row Echelon Method, the given system of equations yields the matrix $\begin{bmatrix} 5 & -3 & 2 & | & -5 \\ 2 & 1 & -1 & | & 4 \\ -4 & -2 & 2 & | & -1 \end{bmatrix}$, which

by $\frac{1}{5}R_1 \to \begin{bmatrix} 1 & -0.6 & 0.4 & | & -1 \\ 2 & 1 & -1 & | & 4 \\ -4 & -2 & 2 & | & -1 \end{bmatrix} \Rightarrow (-2R_1 + R_2)$ and

$(4R_1 + R_3) \to \begin{bmatrix} 1 & -0.6 & 0.4 & | & -1 \\ 0 & 2.2 & -1.8 & | & 6 \\ 0 & -4.4 & 3.6 & | & -5 \end{bmatrix} \Rightarrow \frac{5}{11}R_2 \to \begin{bmatrix} 1 & -0.6 & 0.4 & | & -1 \\ 0 & 1 & -\frac{9}{11} & | & \frac{30}{11} \\ 0 & -4.4 & 3.6 & | & -5 \end{bmatrix} \Rightarrow$

320   CHAPTER 6   Systems and Matrices

$4.4R_2+R_3 \to \begin{bmatrix} 1 & -0.6 & 0.4 & | & -1 \\ 0 & 1 & -\frac{9}{11} & | & \frac{30}{11} \\ 0 & 0 & 0 & | & 7 \end{bmatrix}$. Since R_3 yields $0=7$, which is never true the system is inconsistent

and the solution is ∅.

18. Using the Reduced Row Echelon Method, the given system of equations yields the matrix $\begin{bmatrix} 2 & 3 & | & 10 \\ -3 & 1 & | & 18 \end{bmatrix}$,

which by $\frac{1}{2}R_1 \to \begin{bmatrix} 1 & \frac{3}{2} & | & 5 \\ -3 & 1 & | & 18 \end{bmatrix}$, $3R_1+R_2 \to \begin{bmatrix} 1 & \frac{3}{2} & | & 5 \\ 0 & \frac{11}{2} & | & 33 \end{bmatrix} \Rightarrow \frac{2}{11}R_2 \to \begin{bmatrix} 1 & \frac{3}{2} & | & 5 \\ 0 & 1 & | & 6 \end{bmatrix} \Rightarrow -\frac{3}{2}R_2+R_1 \to \begin{bmatrix} 1 & 0 & | & -4 \\ 0 & 1 & | & 6 \end{bmatrix}$.

From this Reduced Row matrix, we have the solution $(-4,6)$.

19. Using the Reduced Row Echelon Method, the given system of equations yields the matrix $\begin{bmatrix} 3 & 1 & | & -7 \\ 1 & -1 & | & -5 \end{bmatrix}$,

which by $R_2+R_1 \to \begin{bmatrix} 4 & 0 & | & -12 \\ 1 & -1 & | & -5 \end{bmatrix} \Rightarrow \frac{1}{4}R_1 \to \begin{bmatrix} 1 & 0 & | & -3 \\ 1 & -1 & | & -5 \end{bmatrix} \Rightarrow R_1-R_2 \to \begin{bmatrix} 1 & 0 & | & -3 \\ 0 & 1 & | & 2 \end{bmatrix}$. From this Reduced Row

matrix, we have the solution $(-3,2)$.

20. Using the Reduced Row Echelon Method, the given system of equations yields the matrix $\begin{bmatrix} 1 & 0 & -1 & | & -3 \\ 0 & 1 & 1 & | & 6 \\ 2 & 0 & -3 & | & -9 \end{bmatrix}$, which

by $-2R_1+R_3 \to \begin{bmatrix} 1 & 0 & -1 & | & -3 \\ 0 & 1 & 1 & | & 6 \\ 0 & 0 & -1 & | & -3 \end{bmatrix} \Rightarrow -R_3 \to \begin{bmatrix} 1 & 0 & -1 & | & -3 \\ 0 & 1 & 1 & | & 6 \\ 0 & 0 & 1 & | & 3 \end{bmatrix} \Rightarrow \begin{matrix} R_3+R_1 \\ -R_3+R_2 \end{matrix} \begin{bmatrix} 1 & 0 & 0 & | & 0 \\ 0 & 1 & 0 & | & 3 \\ 0 & 0 & 1 & | & 3 \end{bmatrix}$. From this Reduced

Row matrix, we have the solution $(0,3,3)$.

21. Using the Reduced Row Echelon Method, the given system of equations yields the matrix

$\begin{bmatrix} 1 & 2 & 1 & | & 0 \\ 3 & 2 & -1 & | & 4 \\ -1 & 2 & 3 & | & -4 \end{bmatrix}$, which by $\begin{matrix} -3R_1+R_2 \\ R_1+R_3 \end{matrix} \to \begin{bmatrix} 1 & 2 & 1 & | & 0 \\ 0 & -4 & -4 & | & 4 \\ 0 & 4 & 4 & | & -4 \end{bmatrix} \Rightarrow$

$-\frac{1}{4}R_2 \to \begin{bmatrix} 1 & 2 & 1 & | & 0 \\ 0 & 1 & 1 & | & -1 \\ 0 & 4 & -4 & | & -4 \end{bmatrix} \Rightarrow -4R_2+R_3 \to \begin{bmatrix} 1 & 2 & 1 & | & 0 \\ 0 & 1 & 1 & | & -1 \\ 0 & 0 & 0 & | & 0 \end{bmatrix} \Rightarrow$

From this Reduced Row matrix, we have $y+z=-1 \Rightarrow y=-1-z$. Solve for x from Row 1.

$x+2(-1-z)+z=0 \Rightarrow x-2-z=0 \Rightarrow x=z+2$. The system is dependent and the solution is

given by $\{(z+2,-z-1,z)\}$.

22. $\begin{bmatrix} -5 & 4 & 9 \\ 2 & -1 & -2 \end{bmatrix} + \begin{bmatrix} 1 & -2 & 7 \\ 4 & -5 & -5 \end{bmatrix} = \begin{bmatrix} -5+1 & 4-2 & 9+7 \\ 2+4 & -1-5 & -2-5 \end{bmatrix} = \begin{bmatrix} -4 & 2 & 16 \\ 6 & -6 & -7 \end{bmatrix}$.

Copyright © 2015 Pearson Education, Inc

23. $\begin{bmatrix} 3 \\ 2 \\ 5 \end{bmatrix} - \begin{bmatrix} 8 \\ -4 \\ 6 \end{bmatrix} + \begin{bmatrix} 1 \\ 0 \\ 2 \end{bmatrix} = \begin{bmatrix} 3-8+1 \\ 2+4+0 \\ 5-6+2 \end{bmatrix} = \begin{bmatrix} -4 \\ 6 \\ 1 \end{bmatrix}$.

24. $\begin{bmatrix} 2 & 5 & 8 \\ 1 & 9 & 2 \end{bmatrix} - \begin{bmatrix} 3 & 4 \\ 7 & 1 \end{bmatrix}$. We cannot subtract matrices of unlike size $(2 \times 3) - (2 \times 3)$, the solution is $\varnothing$.

25. $3 \begin{bmatrix} 2 & 4 \\ -1 & 4 \end{bmatrix} - 2 \begin{bmatrix} 5 & 8 \\ 2 & -2 \end{bmatrix} = \begin{bmatrix} 6 & 12 \\ -3 & 12 \end{bmatrix} - \begin{bmatrix} 10 & 16 \\ 4 & -4 \end{bmatrix} = \begin{bmatrix} 6-10 & 12-16 \\ -3-4 & 12+4 \end{bmatrix} = \begin{bmatrix} -4 & -4 \\ -7 & 16 \end{bmatrix}$.

26. $-1 \begin{bmatrix} 3 & -5 & 2 \\ 1 & 7 & -4 \end{bmatrix} + 5 \begin{bmatrix} 0 & 2 \\ -1 & 3 \end{bmatrix}$. We cannot add matrices of unlike size $(2 \times 3) + (2 \times 2)$, the solution is $\varnothing$.

27. $10 \begin{bmatrix} 2x & y \\ 5y & 6x \end{bmatrix} + 2 \begin{bmatrix} -3x & 6y \\ 2y & 5x \end{bmatrix} = \begin{bmatrix} 20x & 10y \\ 50y & 60x \end{bmatrix} + \begin{bmatrix} -6x & 12y \\ 4y & 10x \end{bmatrix} = \begin{bmatrix} 20x-6x & 10y+12y \\ 50y+4y & 60x+10x \end{bmatrix} = \begin{bmatrix} 14x & 22y \\ 54y & 70x \end{bmatrix}$

28. The sum of two $m \times n$ matrices A and B is founded by adding corresponding elements.

29. $\begin{bmatrix} -8 & 6 \\ 5 & 2 \end{bmatrix} \begin{bmatrix} 3 & -1 \\ 7 & 2 \end{bmatrix} = \begin{bmatrix} -8(3)+6(7) & -8(-1)+6(2) \\ 5(3)+2(7) & 5(-1)+2(2) \end{bmatrix} = \begin{bmatrix} -24+42 & 8+12 \\ 15+14 & -5+4 \end{bmatrix} = \begin{bmatrix} 18 & 20 \\ 29 & -1 \end{bmatrix}$.

30. $\begin{bmatrix} 3 & 2 & -1 \\ 4 & 0 & 6 \end{bmatrix} \begin{bmatrix} -2 & 0 \\ 0 & 2 \\ 3 & 1 \end{bmatrix} = \begin{bmatrix} 3(-2)+2(0)-1(3) & 3(0)+2(2)-1(1) \\ 4(-2)+0(0)+6(3) & 4(0)+0(2)+6(1) \end{bmatrix} = \begin{bmatrix} -9 & 3 \\ 10 & 6 \end{bmatrix}$.

31. $\begin{bmatrix} 1 & -2 & 4 & 2 \\ 0 & 1 & -1 & 8 \end{bmatrix} \begin{bmatrix} -1 \\ 2 \\ 0 \\ 1 \end{bmatrix} = \begin{bmatrix} 1(-1)-2(2)+4(0)+2(1) \\ 0(-1)+1(2)-1(0)+8(1) \end{bmatrix} = \begin{bmatrix} -3 \\ 10 \end{bmatrix}$.

32. $\begin{bmatrix} 1 & 2 & 5 \\ -3 & 4 & 7 \\ 0 & 2 & -1 \end{bmatrix} \begin{bmatrix} 4 & 2 & 3 \\ 10 & -5 & 6 \end{bmatrix} = $ We cannot multiply matrices of size $(3 \times 3) \times (2 \times 3)$, the solution is $\varnothing$.

33. $\begin{bmatrix} 4 & 2 & 3 \\ 10 & -5 & 6 \end{bmatrix} \begin{bmatrix} 1 & 2 & 5 \\ -3 & 4 & 7 \\ 0 & 2 & -1 \end{bmatrix} = \begin{bmatrix} 4-6+0 & 8+8+6 & 20+14-3 \\ 10+15+0 & 20-20+12 & 50-35-6 \end{bmatrix} = \begin{bmatrix} -2 & 22 & 31 \\ 25 & 12 & 9 \end{bmatrix}$.

34. $\begin{bmatrix} 3 & -1 & 0 \end{bmatrix} \begin{bmatrix} 1 & 3 & 2 \\ 2 & -4 & 0 \\ 5 & 7 & 3 \end{bmatrix} = \begin{bmatrix} 3-2+0 & 9+4+0 & 6+0+0 \end{bmatrix} = \begin{bmatrix} 1 & 13 & 6 \end{bmatrix}$.

35. Yes; $AB = \begin{bmatrix} 3 & 2 \\ 13 & 9 \end{bmatrix} \begin{bmatrix} 9 & -2 \\ -13 & 3 \end{bmatrix} = \begin{bmatrix} 27-26 & -6+6 \\ 117-117 & -26+27 \end{bmatrix} = \begin{bmatrix} 1 & 0 \\ 0 & 1 \end{bmatrix}$.

$BA = \begin{bmatrix} 9 & -2 \\ -13 & 3 \end{bmatrix} \begin{bmatrix} 3 & 2 \\ 13 & 9 \end{bmatrix} = \begin{bmatrix} 27-26 & 18-18 \\ -39+39 & -26+27 \end{bmatrix} = \begin{bmatrix} 1 & 0 \\ 0 & 1 \end{bmatrix}$.

36. Yes; $AB = \begin{bmatrix} 1 & 0 \\ 2 & -3 \end{bmatrix} \begin{bmatrix} 1 & 0 \\ \frac{2}{3} & -\frac{1}{3} \end{bmatrix} = \begin{bmatrix} 1+0 & 0+0 \\ 2-2 & 0+1 \end{bmatrix} = \begin{bmatrix} 1 & 0 \\ 0 & 1 \end{bmatrix}$ $BA = \begin{bmatrix} 1 & 0 \\ \frac{2}{3} & -\frac{1}{3} \end{bmatrix} \begin{bmatrix} 1 & 0 \\ 2 & -3 \end{bmatrix} = \begin{bmatrix} 1+0 & 0+0 \\ \frac{2}{3}-\frac{2}{3} & 0+1 \end{bmatrix} = \begin{bmatrix} 1 & 0 \\ 0 & 1 \end{bmatrix}$.

37. No; $AB = \begin{bmatrix} 2 & 0 & 6 \\ 0 & 1 & 0 \\ 1 & 0 & 1 \end{bmatrix} \begin{bmatrix} -1 & 0 & \frac{3}{2} \\ 0 & 1 & 0 \\ \frac{1}{4} & 0 & -1 \end{bmatrix} = \begin{bmatrix} -2+0+\frac{3}{2} & 0+0+0 & 3+0-6 \\ 0+0+0 & 0+1+0 & 0+0+0 \\ -1+0+\frac{1}{4} & 0+0+0 & \frac{3}{2}+0-1 \end{bmatrix} = \begin{bmatrix} -\frac{1}{2} & 0 & -3 \\ 0 & 1 & 0 \\ -\frac{3}{4} & 0 & \frac{1}{2} \end{bmatrix}$.

38. Yes; $AB = \begin{bmatrix} 1 & 0 & 2 \\ 0 & 2 & 4 \\ 0 & 0 & 1 \end{bmatrix} \begin{bmatrix} 1 & 0 & -2 \\ 0 & \frac{1}{2} & -2 \\ 0 & 0 & 1 \end{bmatrix} = \begin{bmatrix} 1+0+0 & 0+0+0 & -2+0+2 \\ 0+0+0 & 0+1+0 & 0-4+4 \\ 0+0+0 & 0+0+0 & 0+0+1 \end{bmatrix} = \begin{bmatrix} 1 & 0 & 0 \\ 0 & 1 & 0 \\ 0 & 0 & 1 \end{bmatrix}$.

$BA = \begin{bmatrix} 1 & 0 & -2 \\ 0 & \frac{1}{2} & -2 \\ 0 & 0 & 1 \end{bmatrix} \begin{bmatrix} 1 & 0 & 2 \\ 0 & 2 & 4 \\ 0 & 0 & 1 \end{bmatrix} = \begin{bmatrix} 1+0+0 & 0+0+0 & 2+0-2 \\ 0+0+0 & 0+1+0 & 0+2-2 \\ 0+0+0 & 0+0+0 & 0+0+1 \end{bmatrix} = \begin{bmatrix} 1 & 0 & 0 \\ 0 & 1 & 0 \\ 0 & 0 & 1 \end{bmatrix}$.

39. $\det A = 30 - 30 = 0$. Since the determinant is equal to 0, A^{-1} does not exist.

40. Using $A^{-1} = \frac{1}{\det A} \begin{bmatrix} d & -b \\ -c & a \end{bmatrix}$ to find the inverse yields $A^{-1} = \begin{bmatrix} -4 & 2 \\ 0 & 3 \end{bmatrix}^{-1} = -\frac{1}{12} \begin{bmatrix} 3 & -2 \\ 0 & -4 \end{bmatrix} = \begin{bmatrix} -\frac{1}{4} & \frac{1}{6} \\ 0 & \frac{1}{3} \end{bmatrix}$.

41. Using $A^{-1} = \frac{1}{\det A} \begin{bmatrix} d & -b \\ -c & a \end{bmatrix}$ to find the inverse yields $A^{-1} = \begin{bmatrix} 2 & 0 \\ -1 & 5 \end{bmatrix}^{-1} = \frac{1}{10} \begin{bmatrix} 5 & 0 \\ 1 & 2 \end{bmatrix} = \begin{bmatrix} \frac{1}{2} & 0 \\ \frac{1}{10} & \frac{1}{5} \end{bmatrix}$.

42. Solve using the calculator, $A^{-1} = \begin{bmatrix} \frac{1}{4} & \frac{1}{2} & \frac{1}{2} \\ \frac{1}{4} & -\frac{1}{2} & \frac{1}{2} \\ \frac{1}{8} & -\frac{1}{4} & -\frac{1}{4} \end{bmatrix} = \begin{bmatrix} 0.25 & 0.5 & 0.5 \\ 0.25 & -0.5 & 0.5 \\ 0.125 & -0.25 & -0.25 \end{bmatrix}$.

43. Solve using the calculator $A^{-1} = \begin{bmatrix} \frac{2}{3} & 0 & -\frac{1}{3} \\ \frac{1}{3} & 0 & -\frac{2}{3} \\ -\frac{2}{3} & 1 & \frac{1}{3} \end{bmatrix}$.

44. Solve using the calculator, the determinant of $A = 0$; therefore, there is no inverse.

45. Using the matrix inverse method, put the system into the proper matrix form:

$\begin{bmatrix} 1 & 1 \\ 2 & 3 \end{bmatrix} \begin{bmatrix} x \\ y \end{bmatrix} = \begin{bmatrix} 4 \\ 10 \end{bmatrix} \Rightarrow \begin{bmatrix} x \\ y \end{bmatrix} = \begin{bmatrix} 1 & 1 \\ 2 & 3 \end{bmatrix}^{-1} \begin{bmatrix} 4 \\ 10 \end{bmatrix} \Rightarrow \begin{bmatrix} 3 & -1 \\ -2 & 1 \end{bmatrix} \begin{bmatrix} 4 \\ 10 \end{bmatrix} \Rightarrow \begin{bmatrix} 12-10 \\ -8+10 \end{bmatrix} = \begin{bmatrix} 2 \\ 2 \end{bmatrix}$. The solution is $(2,2)$.

46. Using the matrix inverse method, put the system into the proper matrix form:

$\begin{bmatrix} 5 & -3 \\ 2 & 7 \end{bmatrix} \begin{bmatrix} x \\ y \end{bmatrix} = \begin{bmatrix} -2 \\ -9 \end{bmatrix} \Rightarrow \begin{bmatrix} x \\ y \end{bmatrix} = \begin{bmatrix} 5 & -3 \\ 2 & 7 \end{bmatrix}^{-1} \begin{bmatrix} -2 \\ -9 \end{bmatrix} \Rightarrow \begin{bmatrix} \frac{7}{41} & \frac{3}{41} \\ -\frac{2}{41} & \frac{5}{41} \end{bmatrix} \begin{bmatrix} -2 \\ -9 \end{bmatrix} \Rightarrow \begin{bmatrix} -\frac{14}{41} - \frac{27}{41} \\ \frac{4}{41} - \frac{45}{41} \end{bmatrix} = \begin{bmatrix} -1 \\ -1 \end{bmatrix}$.

The solution is $(-1, -1)$.

47. Using the matrix inverse method, put the system into the proper matrix form:

$\begin{bmatrix} 2 & 1 \\ 3 & -2 \end{bmatrix} \begin{bmatrix} x \\ y \end{bmatrix} = \begin{bmatrix} 5 \\ 4 \end{bmatrix} \Rightarrow \begin{bmatrix} x \\ y \end{bmatrix} = \begin{bmatrix} 2 & 1 \\ 3 & -2 \end{bmatrix}^{-1} \begin{bmatrix} 5 \\ 4 \end{bmatrix} \Rightarrow \begin{bmatrix} \frac{2}{7} & \frac{1}{7} \\ \frac{3}{7} & -\frac{2}{7} \end{bmatrix} \begin{bmatrix} 5 \\ 4 \end{bmatrix} \Rightarrow \begin{bmatrix} \frac{10}{7} + \frac{4}{7} \\ \frac{15}{7} - \frac{8}{7} \end{bmatrix} = \begin{bmatrix} 2 \\ 1 \end{bmatrix}$. The solution is $(2,1)$.

48. Using the matrix inverse method, put the system into the proper matrix form:

$\begin{bmatrix} 1 & -2 \\ 3 & 1 \end{bmatrix} \begin{bmatrix} x \\ y \end{bmatrix} = \begin{bmatrix} 7 \\ 7 \end{bmatrix} \Rightarrow \begin{bmatrix} x \\ y \end{bmatrix} = \begin{bmatrix} 1 & -2 \\ 3 & 1 \end{bmatrix}^{-1} \begin{bmatrix} 7 \\ 7 \end{bmatrix} \Rightarrow \begin{bmatrix} \frac{1}{7} & \frac{2}{7} \\ -\frac{3}{7} & \frac{1}{7} \end{bmatrix} \begin{bmatrix} 7 \\ 7 \end{bmatrix} \Rightarrow \begin{bmatrix} \frac{7}{7} + \frac{14}{7} \\ -\frac{21}{7} + \frac{7}{7} \end{bmatrix} = \begin{bmatrix} 3 \\ -2 \end{bmatrix}$. The solution is $(3, -2)$.

49. Solve on the calculator using the matrix inverse method:

$\begin{bmatrix} x \\ y \\ z \end{bmatrix} = \begin{bmatrix} 1 & 2 & 0 \\ 0 & 3 & -1 \\ 1 & 2 & -1 \end{bmatrix}^{-1} \cdot \begin{bmatrix} -1 \\ -5 \\ -3 \end{bmatrix} = \begin{bmatrix} 1 \\ -1 \\ 2 \end{bmatrix}$; therefore, the solution is $(1, -1, 2)$.

50. The determinant of the coefficient matrix is $\det \begin{bmatrix} 3 & -2 & 4 \\ 4 & 1 & -5 \\ -6 & 4 & -8 \end{bmatrix} = 0$; therefore, infinitely many solutions or no solutions. Now use Row Echelon Method on the augmented matrix:

$\begin{bmatrix} 3 & -2 & 4 & | & 1 \\ 4 & 1 & -5 & | & 2 \\ -6 & 4 & -8 & | & -2 \end{bmatrix} \Rightarrow 2R_1 + R_3 \rightarrow \begin{bmatrix} 3 & -2 & 4 & | & 1 \\ 4 & 1 & -5 & | & 2 \\ 0 & 0 & 0 & | & 0 \end{bmatrix}$. Since $0 = 0$, the equation has an infinite number of

solutions. Continue to use Row Echelon Method to find these solutions: $R_1 + 2R_2 \rightarrow \begin{bmatrix} 3 & -2 & 4 & | & 1 \\ 11 & 0 & -6 & | & 5 \\ 0 & 0 & 0 & | & 0 \end{bmatrix}$.

Now solve for R_2 for x: $11x - 6z = 5 \Rightarrow 11x = 6z + 5 \Rightarrow x = \dfrac{6z+5}{11}$. Now substitute $x = \dfrac{6z+5}{11}$ into R_1 and solve for y:

$3\left(\dfrac{6z+5}{11}\right) - 2y + 4z = 1 \Rightarrow 18z + 15 - 22y + 44z = 11 \Rightarrow -22y = -62z - 4 \Rightarrow y = \dfrac{62z+4}{22} = \dfrac{31z+2}{11}$.

The solution is $\left(\dfrac{6z+5}{11}, \dfrac{31z+2}{11}, z\right)$. Other forms are possible.

51. Solve on the calculator using the matrix inverse method:

$\begin{bmatrix} x \\ y \\ z \end{bmatrix} = \begin{bmatrix} 1 & 1 & 1 \\ 2 & -1 & 0 \\ 0 & 3 & 1 \end{bmatrix}^{-1} \cdot \begin{bmatrix} 1 \\ -2 \\ 2 \end{bmatrix} = \begin{bmatrix} -1 \\ 0 \\ 2 \end{bmatrix}$; therefore, the solution is $(-1, 0, 2)$.

52. Solve on the calculator using the matrix inverse method:

$\begin{bmatrix} x \\ y \\ z \end{bmatrix} = \begin{bmatrix} 1 & 0 & 0 \\ 0 & 1 & 1 \\ 2 & 0 & -3 \end{bmatrix}^{-1} \cdot \begin{bmatrix} -3 \\ 6 \\ -9 \end{bmatrix} = \begin{bmatrix} -3 \\ 5 \\ 1 \end{bmatrix}$; therefore, the solution is $(-3, 5, 1)$.

53. Solve on the calculator using the matrix inverse method:

$\begin{bmatrix} x \\ y \\ z \end{bmatrix} = \begin{bmatrix} 2 & -4 & 4 \\ 1 & -3 & 2 \\ 1 & -1 & 2 \end{bmatrix}^{-1} \cdot \begin{bmatrix} 0 \\ -3 \\ 1 \end{bmatrix} \Rightarrow \emptyset$. Since the inverse of the 3×3 matrix does not exist this system is inconsistent.

54. One solution to the solution set $\{(4-y, y)\}$ is $\{(4-1, 1)\} \Rightarrow \{(3, 1)\}$. Answers may vary.

55. $\det \begin{bmatrix} -1 & 8 \\ 2 & 9 \end{bmatrix} = -9 - 16 = -25.$

56. $\det \begin{bmatrix} -2 & 4 \\ 0 & 3 \end{bmatrix} = -6 - 0 = -6.$

57. Evaluate, expand by the second column. Therefore, $\det = (-)(a_{12})(M_{12}) + (a_{22})(M_{22}) - (a_{32})(M_{32})$:

$-4 \left(\det \begin{bmatrix} 3 & 2 \\ -1 & 3 \end{bmatrix} \right) + 0 - 0 = -4(9+2) = -4(11) = -44.$

58. Evaluate, expand by the second column. Therefore, $\det = (-)(a_{12})(M_{12}) + (a_{22})(M_{22}) - (a_{32})(M_{32})$:

$-2 \left(\det \begin{bmatrix} 4 & 3 \\ 5 & 2 \end{bmatrix} \right) + 0 - (-1) \left(\det \begin{bmatrix} -1 & 3 \\ 4 & 3 \end{bmatrix} \right) = -2(8-15) + 1(-3-12) = -2(-7) + 1(-15) = 14 - 15 = -1.$

59. If $\det \begin{bmatrix} -3 & 2 \\ 1 & x \end{bmatrix} = 5$, then $-3x - 2 = 5 \Rightarrow -3x = 7 \Rightarrow x = \dfrac{7}{-3}$. The solution set is $\left\{ -\dfrac{7}{3} \right\}$.

60. If $\det \begin{bmatrix} 3x & 7 \\ -x & 4 \end{bmatrix} = 8$, then $12x + 7x = 8 \Rightarrow 19x = 8 \Rightarrow x = \dfrac{8}{19}$. The solution set is $\left\{ \dfrac{8}{19} \right\}$.

61. Evaluate, expand by the third column. Therefore, $\det = (a_{13})(M_{13}) - (a_{23})(M_{23}) + (a_{33})(M_{33})$:

$0 - (-1) \left(\det \begin{bmatrix} 2 & 5 \\ 0 & 2 \end{bmatrix} \right) + 0 = 4 \Rightarrow 4 = 4.$ Since this is always true, all real numbers can be input for x.

62. Evaluate, expand by the first row. Therefore, $\det = (a_{11})(M_{11}) - (a_{12})(M_{12}) + (a_{13})(M_{13})$:

$6x \left(\det \begin{bmatrix} 5 & 3 \\ 2 & -1 \end{bmatrix} \right) - 2 \left(\det \begin{bmatrix} 1 & 3 \\ x & -1 \end{bmatrix} \right) + 0 = 2x \Rightarrow 6x(-5-6) - 2(-1-3x) = 2x \Rightarrow$

$-66x + 2 + 6x = 2x \Rightarrow -60x + 2 = 2x \Rightarrow -62x = -2 \Rightarrow x = \dfrac{-2}{-62}.$ The solution set is $\left\{ \dfrac{1}{31} \right\}$.

63. (a) $D = \det \begin{bmatrix} 3 & -1 \\ 2 & 1 \end{bmatrix} = 5.$

(b) $D_x = \det \begin{bmatrix} 28 & -1 \\ 2 & 1 \end{bmatrix} = 30.$

(c) $D_y = \det \begin{bmatrix} 3 & 28 \\ 2 & 2 \end{bmatrix} = -50.$

(d) $x = \dfrac{D_x}{D} = \dfrac{30}{5} = 6;\ y = \dfrac{D_y}{D} = \dfrac{-50}{5} = -10.$ The solution is $(6, -10)$.

64. (a) $A =$ the coefficient matrix: $A = \begin{bmatrix} 3 & -1 \\ 2 & 1 \end{bmatrix}.$

(b) $B =$ the answer matrix: $B = \begin{bmatrix} 28 \\ 2 \end{bmatrix}.$

(c) To solve for x and y, multiply A^{-1} by B: $\begin{bmatrix} x \\ y \end{bmatrix} = A^{-1}B = \begin{bmatrix} 6 \\ -10 \end{bmatrix}$; therefore, the solution is $(6,-10)$.

65. If $D = 0$, there would be division by 0, which is undefined. The system will have no solutions or infinitely many solutions.

66. Find the determinants $D = \det\begin{bmatrix} 3 & 1 \\ 5 & 4 \end{bmatrix} = 7$, $D_x = \det\begin{bmatrix} -1 & 1 \\ 10 & 4 \end{bmatrix} = -14$, and $D_y = \det\begin{bmatrix} 3 & -1 \\ 5 & 10 \end{bmatrix} = 35$. Then

$x = \dfrac{D_x}{D} = \dfrac{-14}{7} = -2$ and $y = \dfrac{D_y}{D} = \dfrac{35}{7} = 5$. The solution is $(-2, 5)$.

67. Find the determinants $D = \det\begin{bmatrix} 3 & 7 \\ 5 & -1 \end{bmatrix} = -38$, $D_x = \det\begin{bmatrix} 2 & 7 \\ -22 & -1 \end{bmatrix} = 152$, and $D_y = \det\begin{bmatrix} 3 & 2 \\ 5 & -22 \end{bmatrix} = -76$.

Then $x = \dfrac{D_x}{D} = \dfrac{152}{-38} = -4$ and $y = \dfrac{D_y}{D} = \dfrac{-76}{-38} = 2$. The solution is $(-4, 2)$.

68. Find the determinants $D = \det\begin{bmatrix} 2 & -5 \\ 3 & 4 \end{bmatrix} = 23$, $D_x = \det\begin{bmatrix} 8 & -5 \\ 10 & 4 \end{bmatrix} = 82$, and $D_y = \det\begin{bmatrix} 2 & 8 \\ 3 & 10 \end{bmatrix} = -4$. Then

$x = \dfrac{D_x}{D} = \dfrac{82}{23}$ and $y = \dfrac{D_y}{D} = \dfrac{-4}{23}$. The solution is $\left(\dfrac{82}{23}, -\dfrac{4}{23}\right)$.

69. Using your calculator, find the following determinants:

$D = \det\begin{bmatrix} 3 & 2 & 1 \\ 4 & -1 & 3 \\ 1 & 3 & -1 \end{bmatrix} = 3$, $D_x = \det\begin{bmatrix} 2 & 2 & 1 \\ -16 & -1 & 3 \\ 12 & 3 & -1 \end{bmatrix} = -12$, $D_y = \det\begin{bmatrix} 3 & 2 & 1 \\ 4 & -16 & 3 \\ 1 & 12 & -1 \end{bmatrix} = 18$, and

$D_z = \det\begin{bmatrix} 3 & 2 & 2 \\ 4 & -1 & -16 \\ 1 & 3 & 12 \end{bmatrix} = 6$ Then $x = \dfrac{D_x}{D} = \dfrac{-12}{3} = -4$, $y = \dfrac{D_y}{D} = \dfrac{18}{3} = 6$, and $z = \dfrac{D_z}{D} = \dfrac{6}{3} = 2$.

The solution is $(-4, 6, 2)$.

70. The determinant of the coefficient matrix is $\det\begin{bmatrix} 5 & -2 & -1 \\ -5 & 2 & 1 \\ 1 & -4 & -2 \end{bmatrix} = 0$; therefore, infinitely many or no

solutions. Now use Row Echelon Method on the augmented matrix: $\begin{matrix} R_3 \to R_1 \\ R_2 \to R_3 \end{matrix} \to \begin{bmatrix} 1 & -4 & -2 & | & 0 \\ 5 & -2 & -1 & | & 8 \\ -5 & 2 & 1 & | & -8 \end{bmatrix} \Rightarrow$

Since $R_2 + R_3$ produces $0 = 0$, there are infinitely many solutions and they are dependent solutions.

Continue to use Row Echelon Method to find these solutions: $R_1 + 2R_3 \to \begin{bmatrix} 1 & -4 & -2 & | & 0 \\ 5 & -2 & -1 & | & 8 \\ -9 & 0 & 0 & | & -16 \end{bmatrix}$.

Solve for x using R_3: $-9x = -16 \Rightarrow x = \dfrac{16}{9}$. Now substitute $x = \dfrac{16}{9}$ into R_1 and solve for y:

$\dfrac{16}{9} - 4y - 2z = 0 \Rightarrow 16 - 36y - 18z = 0 \Rightarrow -36y = 18z - 16 \Rightarrow y = \dfrac{18z - 16}{-36} = \dfrac{8 - 9z}{18}$.

The solution is $\left(\dfrac{16}{9}, \dfrac{8 - 9z}{18}, z \right)$.

71. Using your calculator, find the following determinants:

$D = \det \begin{bmatrix} -1 & 3 & -4 \\ 2 & 4 & 1 \\ 3 & 0 & -1 \end{bmatrix} = 67; \quad D_x = \det \begin{bmatrix} 2 & 3 & -4 \\ 3 & 4 & 1 \\ 9 & 0 & -1 \end{bmatrix} = 172; \quad D_y = \det \begin{bmatrix} -1 & 2 & -4 \\ 2 & 3 & 1 \\ 3 & 9 & -1 \end{bmatrix} = -14;$

$D_z = \det \begin{bmatrix} -1 & 3 & 2 \\ 2 & 4 & 3 \\ 3 & 0 & 9 \end{bmatrix} = -87$. Then $x = \dfrac{D_x}{D} = \dfrac{172}{67}$, $y = \dfrac{D_y}{D} = \dfrac{-14}{67}$, and $z = \dfrac{D_z}{D} = \dfrac{-87}{67}$.

The solution is $\left(\dfrac{172}{67}, -\dfrac{14}{67}, -\dfrac{87}{67} \right)$.

72. Let x = the amount of rice in cups and y = the amount of soybeans in cups. Then from the information the system of equations is $15x + 22.5y = 9.5$ [equation 1] and $810x + 270y = 324$ [equation 2]. Multiply [equation 1] by -12 and add [equation 2] to eliminate y:

$-180x - 270y = -114$
$\underline{810x + 270y = 324}$
$630x = 210 \Rightarrow x = \dfrac{210}{630} = \dfrac{1}{3}$. Now substitute $x = \dfrac{1}{3}$ into [equation 1] and solve for y:

$15\left(\dfrac{1}{3}\right) + 22.5y = 9.5 \Rightarrow 5 + 22.5y = 9.5 \Rightarrow 2.5y = 4.5 \Rightarrow y = 0.20 \text{ or } \dfrac{1}{5}$.

The meal should include $\dfrac{1}{3}$ cup of rice and $\dfrac{1}{5}$ cup of soybeans.

73. Let x = the number of CD's and y = the number of plastic holders. From the information the system of equations is obtained: $x + y = 100$ [equation 1] and $0.40x + 0.30y = 38.00$ [equation 2]. Multiply [equation 1] by -30 and add [equation 2] multiplied by 100 to eliminate y:

$-30x - 30y = -3000$
$\underline{40x + 30y = 3800}$
$10x = 800 \Rightarrow x = 80$. Now substitute $x = 80$ into [equation 1] and solve for y:

$80 + y = 100 \Rightarrow y = 20$. They should send 80 CD's and 20 holders.

74. Let x = the number pounds of $4.60 tea, y = the number of pounds of $5.75 tea, and z = the number of pounds of $6.50 tea. From the information, the system of equations is obtained: $x + y + z = 20$ [equation 1],

$4.6x + 5.75y + 6.5z = 20(5.25) = 105$ and $x = y + z \Rightarrow x - y - z = 0$. Now create the coefficient matrix and solve on the calculator using the matrix inverse method:

$A = \begin{bmatrix} 1 & 1 & 1 \\ 4.6 & 5.75 & 6.5 \\ 1 & -1 & -1 \end{bmatrix}$. Therefore, $\begin{bmatrix} x \\ y \\ z \end{bmatrix} = \begin{bmatrix} 1 & 1 & 1 \\ 4.6 & 5.75 & 6.5 \\ 1 & -1 & -1 \end{bmatrix}^{-1} \cdot \begin{bmatrix} 20 \\ 105 \\ 0 \end{bmatrix} = \begin{bmatrix} 10 \\ 8 \\ 2 \end{bmatrix}$.

They should use 10 pounds of $4.60 tea, 8 pounds of $5.75 tea, and 2 pounds of $6.50 tea.

75. Let $x =$ the amount of 5% solution (ml), $y =$ the amount of 15% solution (ml), and $z =$ the amount of 10% solution (ml). Then from the information, the system of equations is $x + y + z = 20$ [equation 1],

$0.05x + 0.15y + 0.10z = 0.08(20) = 1.6$, and $x = y + z + 2 \Rightarrow x - y - z = 2$. Now create the coefficient matrix and solve on the calculator using the matrix inverse method:

$A = \begin{bmatrix} 1 & 1 & 1 \\ 5 & 15 & 10 \\ 1 & -1 & -1 \end{bmatrix}$; therefore, $\begin{bmatrix} x \\ y \\ z \end{bmatrix} = \begin{bmatrix} 1 & 1 & 1 \\ 5 & 15 & 10 \\ 1 & -1 & -1 \end{bmatrix}^{-1} \cdot \begin{bmatrix} 20 \\ 160 \\ 2 \end{bmatrix} = \begin{bmatrix} 11 \\ 3 \\ 6 \end{bmatrix}$.

They should use 11 ml of 5% solution, 3 ml of 15% solution, and 6 ml of 10% solution.

76. (a) Using $P = a + bA + cW$ and the data from the table yields,

$a + 39b + 142c = 113$
$a + 53b + 181c = 138$
$a + 65b + 191c = 152$

Now using the capabilities of the calculator and the Reduced Row Echelon Method:

$\begin{bmatrix} 1 & 39 & 142 & | & 113 \\ 1 & 53 & 181 & | & 138 \\ 1 & 65 & 191 & | & 152 \end{bmatrix} = \begin{bmatrix} 1 & 0 & 0 & | & 32.780488 \\ 0 & 1 & 0 & | & 0.9024390 \\ 0 & 0 & 1 & | & 0.3170732 \end{bmatrix}$.

Therefore, the equation is $P \approx 32.78 + 0.9024A + 0.3171W$.

(b) Using $A = 55$ and $W = 175$ yields $P \approx 32.78 + 0.9024(55) + 0.3171(175) \Rightarrow P \approx 138$.

77. Using the equation for a polynomial of degree 3 and given points yields:

$(-2, 1):\quad -8a + 4b - 2c + d = 1$

$(-1, 6):\quad -a + b - c + d = 6$

$(2, 9):\quad 8a + 4b + 2c + d = 9$

$(3, 26):\quad 27a + 9b + 3c + d = 26$

The equations can be represented by $\begin{bmatrix} -8 & 4 & -2 & 1 & | & 1 \\ -1 & 1 & -1 & 1 & | & 6 \\ 8 & 4 & 2 & 1 & | & 9 \\ 27 & 9 & 3 & 1 & | & 26 \end{bmatrix}$.

Using the capabilities of the calculator, the Reduced Row Echelon Method produces the solutions: $a = 1$, $b = 0$, $c = -2$, $d = 5$. The equation is $P(x) = x^3 - 2x + 5$.

78. Using $f(x) = ax^2 + bx + c$ and the data from the graph yields:

From the point $(-6, 4)$: $36a - 6b + c = 4$.

From the point $(-4, -2)$: $16a - 4b + c = -2$.

From the point $(2, 4)$: $4a + 2b + c = 4$.

Now using your calculator, find the following determinants:

$D = \det \begin{bmatrix} 36 & -6 & 1 \\ 16 & -4 & 1 \\ 4 & 2 & 1 \end{bmatrix} = -96; D_a = \det \begin{bmatrix} 4 & -6 & 1 \\ -2 & -4 & 1 \\ 4 & 2 & 1 \end{bmatrix} = -48; D_b = \det \begin{bmatrix} 36 & 4 & 1 \\ 16 & -2 & 1 \\ 4 & 4 & 1 \end{bmatrix} = -192;$

$D_c = \det \begin{bmatrix} 36 & -6 & 4 \\ 16 & -4 & -2 \\ 4 & 2 & 4 \end{bmatrix} = 192$ Then $a = \dfrac{D_a}{D} = \dfrac{-48}{-96} = \dfrac{1}{2}, b = \dfrac{D_b}{D} = \dfrac{-192}{-96} = 2$, and

$c = \dfrac{D_c}{D} = \dfrac{192}{-96} = -2$. The equation is $P(x) = \dfrac{1}{2}x^2 + 2x - 2$.

79. See Figure 79.
80. See Figure 80.

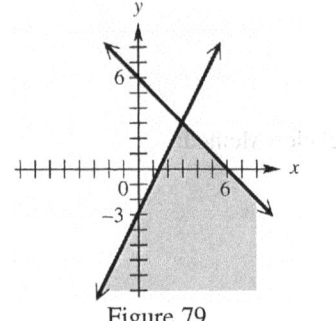
Figure 79

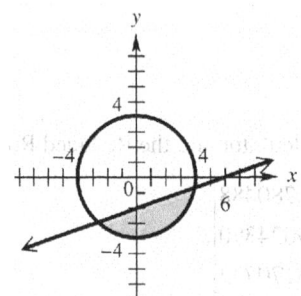
Figure 80

81. Graphing $x \geq 0$, $y \geq 0$, $3x + 2y \leq 12$ and $5x + y \geq 5$ in the same window yields four vertices. Using the given expression and the ordered pairs of the vertices yields the following solutions:

$(0, 5)$: $2(0) + 4(5) = 20$

$(0, 6)$: $2(0) + 4(6) = 24$

$(1, 0)$: $2(1) + 4(0) = 2$

$(4, 0)$: $2(4) + 4(0) = 8$

Therefore, the maximum value is 24 at $(0, 6)$.

82. Graphing $x \geq 0$, $y \geq 0$, $x + y \leq 50$, $2x + y \geq 20$ and $x + 2y \geq 30$ in the same window yields five vertices. Using the given expression and the ordered pairs of the vertices yields the following solutions:

$(0,50): 4(0)+2(50)=100$

$(0,20): 4(0)+2(20)=40$

$\left(\dfrac{10}{3},\dfrac{40}{3}\right): 4\left(\dfrac{10}{3}\right)+2\left(\dfrac{40}{3}\right)=40$

$(30,0): 4(30)+2(0)=120$

$(50,0): 4(50)+2(0)=200$

Therefore, the minimum value is 40 at (0,20) and $\left(\dfrac{10}{3},\dfrac{40}{3}\right)$

Note: values on the line $2x+y=20$ also give minimums of 40 between the two points.

83. Let x = the number radios produced daily and let y = the number of Blu-ray players produced daily. The objective function to find the maximum profit is $15x+35y$.

   The constraints are

   $5 \leq x \leq 25$ (radio production restrictions)

   $0 \leq y \leq 30$ (Blu-ray player maximum production)

   $x \leq y$ (radio production less than or equal to Blu-ray player production)

   Graphing the constraints on the calculator yields four vertices. Inputting these ordered pairs into the objective function yields (5,30): 1125, (5,5): 250, (25,30): 1425, and (25,25): 1250.

   The maximum profit is $1425, this happens when 25 radios and 30 Blu-ray players are manufactured.

84. Factoring $\dfrac{5x-2}{x^2-4}$ results in $\dfrac{5x-2}{(x-2)(x+2)}$. Multiply $\dfrac{5x-2}{(x-2)(x+2)} = \dfrac{A}{x-2} + \dfrac{B}{x+2}$ by

    $(x-2)(x+2) \Rightarrow 5x-2 = A(x+2) + B(x-2)$. Let $x = -2 \Rightarrow -12 = B(-4) \Rightarrow B = 3$.

    Let $x = 2 \Rightarrow 8 = A(4) \Rightarrow A = 2$. The expression can be written $\dfrac{2}{x-2} + \dfrac{3}{x+2}$.

85. Factoring $\dfrac{x+2}{x^3+2x^2+x}$ results in $\dfrac{x+2}{x(x+1)^2}$. Multiply $\dfrac{x+2}{x^3-x^2+4x} = \dfrac{A}{x} + \dfrac{B}{x+1} + \dfrac{C}{(x+1)^2}$ by

    $x(x+1)^2 \Rightarrow x+2 = A(x+1)^2 + Bx(x+1) + Cx$. Let $x = 0 \Rightarrow 2 = A(1) \Rightarrow A = 2$. Let

    $x = -1 \Rightarrow 1 = C(-1) \Rightarrow C = -1$. Let $x = 1$, $A = 2$, $C = -1 \Rightarrow$

    $3 = 2(4) + B(1)(2) - 1 \Rightarrow 3 = 8 = 2B - 1 \Rightarrow B = -2$

    The expression can be written $\dfrac{2}{x} + \dfrac{-2}{x+1} + \dfrac{-1}{(x+1)^2}$ or $\dfrac{2}{x} - \dfrac{2}{x+1} - \dfrac{1}{(x+1)^2}$.

86. Factoring $\dfrac{x+2}{x^3-x^2+4x}$ results in $\dfrac{x+2}{x(x^2-x+4)}$. Multiply $\dfrac{x+2}{x(x^2-x+4)} = \dfrac{A}{x} + \dfrac{Bx+C}{x^2-x+4}$ by

    $x(x^2-x+4) \Rightarrow x+2 = A(x^2-x+4) + (Bx+C)(x) \Rightarrow x+2 = (A+B)x^2 + (C-A)x + 4A$.

By equating coefficients $A+B=0$, $C-A=1$, and $4A=2 \Rightarrow A=\frac{1}{2}$. Since $A+B=0$ and

$A=\frac{1}{2}$, $B=-\frac{1}{2}$. Since $C-A=1$ and $A=\frac{1}{2}$, $C=\frac{3}{2}$.

The expression can be written $\frac{\frac{1}{2}}{x}+\frac{-\frac{1}{2}x+\frac{3}{2}}{x^2-x+4}=\frac{1}{2x}+\frac{-x+3}{2(x^2-x+4)}$.

87. Factoring $\frac{6x^2-x-3}{x^3-x}=\frac{6x^2-x-3}{x(x^2-1)}=\frac{6x^2-x-3}{x(x-1)(x+1)}$. Multiply $\frac{6x^2-x-3}{x(x-1)(x+1)}=\frac{A}{x}+\frac{B}{x-1}+\frac{C}{x+1}$ by

$x(x-1)(x+1) \Rightarrow 6x^2-x-3 = A(x-1)(x+1)+(B)(x)(x+1)+(C)x(x-1)$.

Let $x=0 \Rightarrow -3=-A \Rightarrow A=3$. Let $x=1 \Rightarrow 2=2B \Rightarrow B=1$. Let $x=-1 \Rightarrow 4=2C \Rightarrow C=2$.

The expression can be written $\frac{3}{x}+\frac{1}{x-1}+\frac{2}{x+1}$.

Chapter 6 Test

1. (a) The first is the equation of a circle; the second is the equation of a line.

   (b) A circle and a line could intersect in 0, 1, or 2 points.

   (c) First solve the second equation for y: $2x-y=0 \Rightarrow y=2x$. Now substitute $y=2x$ into

   Equation 1: $x^2+(2x)^2=5 \Rightarrow x^2+4x^2=5 \Rightarrow 5x^2=5 \Rightarrow x^2=1 \Rightarrow x=\pm 1$

   Now substitute these values into $y=2x$: $y=2(1) \Rightarrow y=2$, and $y=2(-1) \Rightarrow y=-2$

   The solutions are $(-1,-2)$ and $(1,2)$.

   (d) Graph on a calculator shows two points of intersection. See Figure 1.

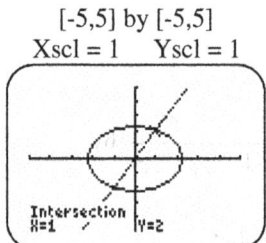
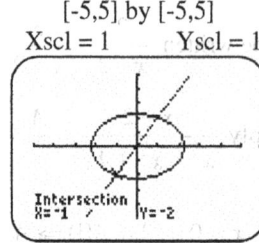

Figure 1

2. (a) First solve [equation 1] for x and substitute the result into [equation 2]. $x-2y=1 \Rightarrow x=1+2y$

   $2(1+2y)+y=7 \Rightarrow 2+4y+y=7 \Rightarrow 5y=5 \Rightarrow y=1$. Now substitute this value into [equation 1]

   $x=1+2(1) \Rightarrow x=3$, The solution set is $\{(3,1)\}$.

   (b) First solve [equation 1] for y and substitute the result into [equation 2]. $3x-y=1 \Rightarrow y=3x-1$

$-6x+2(3x-1)=-2 \Rightarrow -6x+6x+-2=-2 \Rightarrow -2=-2$. This implies that we have an infinite number of solutions. We will show the solution set as $\{(x,3x-1)\}$ or $\left\{\left(\dfrac{y+1}{3},y\right)\right\}$.

3. (a) Multiply [equation 2] by -3 and add it to [equation 1] to eliminate the x variable.

   $3x-4y=7$ [1]

   $-3x-9y=\dfrac{-27}{2}$ $-3[2]$

   _____

   $-13y=-\dfrac{13}{2} \Rightarrow y=\dfrac{1}{2}$

   Now substitute this y-value into [equation 1] to solve for x. $x+3\left(\dfrac{1}{2}\right)=\dfrac{9}{2} \Rightarrow x=\dfrac{6}{2}=3$.

   The solution set is $\left\{\left(3,\dfrac{1}{2}\right)\right\}$.

   (b) Multiply [equation 1] by 2 and add it to [equation 2] to eliminate the x variable.

   $2x-2y=10$ $2[1]$

   $-2x+2y=1$ [2]

   _____

   $0=11 \Rightarrow$ No solution

   We have found that there is no solution to this system of equations. The solution set is $\varnothing$.

4. First solve [equation 1] for x^2 and substitute the result into [equation 2]. $x^2-y=5 \Rightarrow x^2=y+5$

   $y+5+y^2=11 \Rightarrow y^2+y-6=0 \Rightarrow (y+3)(y-2)=0 \Rightarrow y=-3,2$, Now substitute these values into [equation 1] to find the values of x: $x^2=(-3)+5 \Rightarrow x^2=2 \Rightarrow x=\pm\sqrt{2}$, and

   $x^2=(2)+5 \Rightarrow x^2=7 \Rightarrow x=\pm\sqrt{7}$, The solution set is $\{(-\sqrt{2},-3),(\sqrt{2},-3),(-\sqrt{7},2),(\sqrt{7},2)\}$.

5. (a) Using the Row Echelon Method, the given system of equations yields the matrix,

   $\begin{bmatrix} 2 & 1 & 1 & | & 3 \\ 1 & 2 & -1 & | & 3 \\ 3 & -1 & 1 & | & 5 \end{bmatrix}$, which by $(R1 \leftrightarrow R2) \rightarrow \begin{bmatrix} 1 & 2 & -1 & | & 3 \\ 2 & 1 & 1 & | & 3 \\ 3 & -1 & 1 & | & 5 \end{bmatrix} \Rightarrow (-2R_1+R_2)$ and

   $\Rightarrow (-3R_1+R_3) \rightarrow \begin{bmatrix} 1 & 2 & -1 & | & 3 \\ 0 & -3 & 3 & | & -3 \\ 0 & -7 & 4 & | & -4 \end{bmatrix} \Rightarrow (7R_2-3R_3) \rightarrow \begin{bmatrix} 1 & 2 & -1 & | & 3 \\ 0 & -3 & 3 & | & -3 \\ 0 & 0 & 9 & | & -9 \end{bmatrix}$. From this matrix, we have

   the resulting equation, $9z=-9 \Rightarrow z=-1$. Now use back-substitution: $z=-1$ substituting into the resulting $x=2: -12=C(4) \Rightarrow C=-3$. yields, $-3y+3(-1)=-3 \Rightarrow -3y=0 \Rightarrow y=0$;

   finally substituting $y=0$ and $z=-1$ into the resulting R_1 yields, $x+2(0)-(-1)=3 \Rightarrow x=2$.

   The solution is $\{(2,0,-1)\}$.

(b) First subtract [equation 1] from [equation 3] to eliminate the x variable and create [equation 4]. Then add -2 multiplied by [equation 1] to [equation 2] to eliminate the x variable and create [equation 5].

$$\begin{array}{rl} x+2y+2z=5 & \quad [3] \\ -x-y+z=-1 & \quad -1[1] \\ \hline y+3z=4 & \quad [4] \end{array} \qquad \begin{array}{rl} 2x+3y+z=6 & \quad [2] \\ -2x-2y+2z=-2 & \quad -2[1] \\ \hline y+3z=4 & \quad [5] \end{array}$$

Note that equations [4] and [5] are the same and this implies that we have an infinite number of solutions. Solve [equation 4] for y and substitute into [equation 1] to solve for x:

$y+3z=4 \Rightarrow y=4-3z$ then $x+(4-3z)-z=1 \Rightarrow x=4z-3$. The solution set is $\{(4z-3, 4-3z, z)\}$.

6. (a) $3\begin{bmatrix} 2 & 3 \\ 1 & -4 \\ 5 & 9 \end{bmatrix} - \begin{bmatrix} -2 & 6 \\ 3 & -1 \\ 0 & 8 \end{bmatrix} = \begin{bmatrix} 6 & 9 \\ 3 & -12 \\ 15 & 27 \end{bmatrix} - \begin{bmatrix} -2 & 6 \\ 3 & -1 \\ 0 & 8 \end{bmatrix} = \begin{bmatrix} 6+2 & 9-6 \\ 3-3 & -12+1 \\ 15-0 & 27-8 \end{bmatrix} = \begin{bmatrix} 8 & 3 \\ 0 & -11 \\ 15 & 19 \end{bmatrix}$.

(b) Cannot add $(1\times 2)+(1\times 2)+(2\times 2)$; therefore, the solution set is $\varnothing$.

(c) $\begin{bmatrix} 2 & 1 & -3 \\ 4 & 0 & 5 \end{bmatrix} \begin{bmatrix} 1 & 3 \\ 2 & 4 \\ 3 & -2 \end{bmatrix} = \begin{bmatrix} 2+2-9 & 6+4+6 \\ 4+0+15 & 12+0-10 \end{bmatrix} = \begin{bmatrix} -5 & 16 \\ 19 & 2 \end{bmatrix}$.

7. (a) AB can be found; it will be $n \times n$

(b) BA can be found; it will be $n \times n$

(c) $AB = BA$ is not necessarily true, since matrix multiplication is not commutative.

(d) Since the number of rows of the first matrix is not equal to the number of columns of the second matrix, AC cannot be found.

Since the number of rows of the first matrix is equal to the number of columns of the second matrix, CA can be found; it will be $m \times n$.

8. (a) $\det \begin{bmatrix} 4 & 9 \\ -5 & -11 \end{bmatrix} = -44+45 = 1$

(b) Evaluate, expand by the second column. Therefore, $\det = (-)(a_{12})(M_{12}) + (a_{22})(M_{22}) - (a_{32})(M_{32})$:

$0\left(\det\begin{bmatrix} -1 & 9 \\ 12 & -3 \end{bmatrix}\right) + 7\left(\det\begin{bmatrix} 2 & 8 \\ 12 & -3 \end{bmatrix}\right) - 5\left(\det\begin{bmatrix} 2 & 8 \\ -1 & 9 \end{bmatrix}\right) = 0 + 7(-6-96) - 5(18+8) \Rightarrow$

$7(-102) - 5(26) = -844$

9. Find the determinants: $D = \det\begin{bmatrix} 2 & -3 \\ 4 & 5 \end{bmatrix} = 22$, $D_x = \det\begin{bmatrix} -33 & -3 \\ 11 & 5 \end{bmatrix} = -132$, and $D_y = \det\begin{bmatrix} 2 & -33 \\ 4 & 11 \end{bmatrix} = 154$.

Then $x = \dfrac{D_x}{D} = \dfrac{-132}{22} = -6$ and $y = \dfrac{D_y}{D} = \dfrac{154}{22} = 7$. The solution set is $\{(-6, 7)\}$.

10. (a) For the system: $A = \begin{bmatrix} 1 & 1 & -1 \\ 2 & -3 & -1 \\ 1 & 2 & 2 \end{bmatrix}$, $X = \begin{bmatrix} x \\ y \\ z \end{bmatrix}$, and $B = \begin{bmatrix} -4 \\ 5 \\ 3 \end{bmatrix}$.

(b) Solve using the calculator, $A^{-1} = \begin{bmatrix} \frac{1}{4} & \frac{1}{4} & \frac{1}{4} \\ \frac{5}{16} & -\frac{3}{16} & \frac{1}{16} \\ -\frac{7}{16} & \frac{1}{16} & \frac{5}{16} \end{bmatrix}$.

(c) $\begin{bmatrix} x \\ y \\ z \end{bmatrix} = \begin{bmatrix} 1 & 1 & -1 \\ 2 & -3 & -1 \\ 1 & 2 & 2 \end{bmatrix}^{-1} \begin{bmatrix} -4 \\ 5 \\ 3 \end{bmatrix} = \begin{bmatrix} 1 \\ -2 \\ 3 \end{bmatrix}$. The solution is $\{(1, -2, 3)\}$.

(d) For the new system: $A = \begin{bmatrix} 0.5 & 1 & 1 \\ 2 & -3 & -1 \\ 1 & 2 & 2 \end{bmatrix}$ and by the calculator, $\det A = 0$. Since the determinant equals zero, there is no inverse and the matrix inverse method cannot be used.

11. (a) Using $f(x) = ax^2 + bx + c$ and the data from the table yields

$(0, 1.3): 0^2 a + 0b + c = 1.3$

$(100, 2.5): 100^2 a + 100b + c = 2.5$

$(200, 8.9): 200^2 a + 200b + c = 8.9$

Now using the capabilities of the calculator and the Reduced Row Echelon Method:

$\begin{bmatrix} 0 & 0 & 1 & | & 1.3 \\ 100^2 & 100 & 1 & | & 2.5 \\ 200^2 & 200 & 1 & | & 8.9 \end{bmatrix} = \begin{bmatrix} 1 & 0 & 0 & | & 0.000264 \\ 0 & 1 & 0 & | & -0.014 \\ 0 & 0 & 1 & | & 1.3 \end{bmatrix}$.

Therefore, the equation is $f(x) = 0.00026x^2 - 0.014x + 1.3$.

(b) Using the functions of the calculator we see that that the population will reach 8 billion in about 2040. See Figure 11.

[-5,250] by [0,15]
Xscl = 5   Yscl = 1

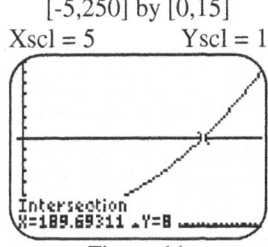

Figure 11

12. B, the graph is shaded above the line; therefore, $y > 2 - x$ and outside the parabola; therefore, $y < x^2 - 5$.

13. Let x = the number type X cabinets and let y = the number of type Y cabinets.

The objective function to find the maximum storage space is $8x + 12y$. The constraints are,

334 CHAPTER 6 Systems and Matrices

$100x + 200y \leq 1400$ (cost of cabinets), $6x + 8y \leq 72$ (floor space), and $x \geq 0$ and $y \geq 0$ (cannot have a negative number of cabinets). Graphing the constraints on the calculator yields four vertices. Inputting these ordered pairs into the objective function yields,

$(0,0)$: $8(0) + 12(0) = 0$

$(12,0)$: $8(12) + 12(0) = 96$

$(8,3)$: $8(8) + 12(3) = 100$

$(0,7)$: $8(0) + 12(7) = 84$

The maximum storage is 100 cubic feet, when there are 8 cabinets of type X and 3 cabinets of type Y.

14. Factoring $\dfrac{7x-1}{x^2-x-6}$ results in $\dfrac{7x-1}{(x-3)(x+2)}$. Multiply $\dfrac{7x-1}{(x-3)(x+2)} = \dfrac{A}{x-3} + \dfrac{B}{x+2}$ by $(x-3)(x+2) \Rightarrow 7x-1 = A(x+2) + B(x-3)$.

Let $x = -2 \Rightarrow -15 = B(-5) \Rightarrow B = 3$. Let $x = 3 \Rightarrow 20 = A(5) \Rightarrow A = 4$.

The expression can be written $\dfrac{4}{x-3} + \dfrac{3}{x+2}$.

15. The expression $\dfrac{x^2-11x+6}{(x+2)(x-2)^2}$ is factored. Multiply $\dfrac{x^2-11x+6}{(x+2)(x-2)^2} = \dfrac{A}{x+2} + \dfrac{B}{x-2} + \dfrac{C}{(x-2)^2}$ by $(x+2)(x-2)^2 \Rightarrow x^2 - 11x + 6 = A(x-2)^2 + B(x-2)(x+2) + C(x+2)$.

Let $x = -2 \Rightarrow 32 = A(16) \Rightarrow A = 2$. Let $x = 2$: $-12 = C(4) \Rightarrow C = -3$.

Let $x = 0$, $A = 2$, $C = -3$: $6 = 4(2) - 4B + 2(-3) \Rightarrow$

$6 = 8 - 4B - 6 \Rightarrow 6 = 2 - 4B \Rightarrow 4 = -4B \Rightarrow B = -1$.

The expression can be written $\dfrac{2}{x+2} + \dfrac{-1}{x-2} + \dfrac{-3}{(x-2)^2}$.

Chapter 7: Analytic Geometry and Nonlinear Systems

7.1: Circles and Parabolas

1. E. Since $x = 2y^2$ is equivalent to $y^2 = 4\left(\frac{1}{8}\right)x$, this is a parabola that opens to the right $(c > 0)$.

3. H. Since $x^2 = -3y$ is equivalent to $x^2 = 4\left(-\frac{3}{4}\right)y$, this is a parabola that opens downward $(c < 0)$.

5. F. This is the equation of a circle centered at the origin with radius $\sqrt{5}$.

7. D. This is the equation of a circle centered at the point $(-3, 4)$ with radius $\sqrt{25} = 5$.

9. Here $h = 1$, $k = 4$ and $r^2 = 3^2 = 9$. The equation is $(x-1)^2 + (y-4)^2 = 9$.

11. A circle that is centered at the origin with $r^2 = 1^2 = 1$ has equation $x^2 + y^2 = 1$.

13. Here $h = \frac{2}{3}$, $k = -\frac{4}{5}$ and $r^2 = \left(\frac{3}{7}\right)^2 = \frac{9}{49}$. The equation is $\left(x - \frac{2}{3}\right)^2 + \left(y + \frac{4}{5}\right)^2 = \frac{9}{49}$.

15. The radius is the distance between $(-1, 2)$ and $(2, 6)$: $r = \sqrt{(2-(-1))^2 + (6-2)^2} = \sqrt{9+16} = 5$. Here $h = -1$, $k = 2$ and $r^2 = 5^2 = 25$. The equation is $(x+1)^2 + (y-2)^2 = 25$.

17. If the center is $(-3, -2)$, the circle must touch the x-axis at the point $(-3, 0)$. The radius is 2. Here $h = -3$, $k = -2$ and $r^2 = 2^2 = 4$. The equation is $(x+3)^2 + (y+2)^2 = 4$.

19. The equation is that of a circle with center (3, 3) and radius 0. That is, the graph is the point (3, 3).

21. Midpoint: $\left(\frac{5+(-1)}{2}, \frac{-9+3}{2}\right) = (2, -3) \Rightarrow$ The center of the circle is (2,-3).

    Distance: $d = \sqrt{(2-5)^2 + (-3-(-9))^2} = \sqrt{9+36} = \sqrt{45} \Rightarrow$ The radius of the circle is $\sqrt{45}$ units. The equation of the circle is $(x-2)^2 + (y+3)^2 = 45$.

23. Midpoint: $\left(\frac{-5+(1)}{2}, \frac{-7+1}{2}\right) = (-2, -3) \Rightarrow$ The center of the circle is (-2,-3).

    Distance: $d = \sqrt{(-2-1)^2 + (-3-(1))^2} = \sqrt{9+16} = \sqrt{25} = 5 \Rightarrow$ The radius of the circle is 5 units. The equation of the circle is $(x+2)^2 + (y+3)^2 = 25$.

25. Midpoint: $\left(\frac{-5+(5)}{2}, \frac{0+0}{2}\right) = (0, 0) \Rightarrow$ The center of the circle is (0,0).

    Distance: $d = \sqrt{(0-(-5))^2 + (0-0)^2} = \sqrt{25} = 5 \Rightarrow$ The radius of the circle is 5 units.

    The equation of the circle is $(x)^2 + (y)^2 = 25$.

27. In a circle, the radius is the distance from the center to any point on the circle.

336 CHAPTER 7 Analytic Geometry and Nonlinear Systems

29. This is the equation of a circle centered at the origin with radius $\sqrt{4} = 2$. See Figure 29. From the figure, the domain is $[-2, 2]$, and the range is $[-2, 2]$.

31. This is the equation of a circle centered at the origin with radius $\sqrt{0} = 0$. The graph is only the point (0, 0). See Figure 31. From the figure, the domain is $\{0\}$, and the range is $\{0\}$.

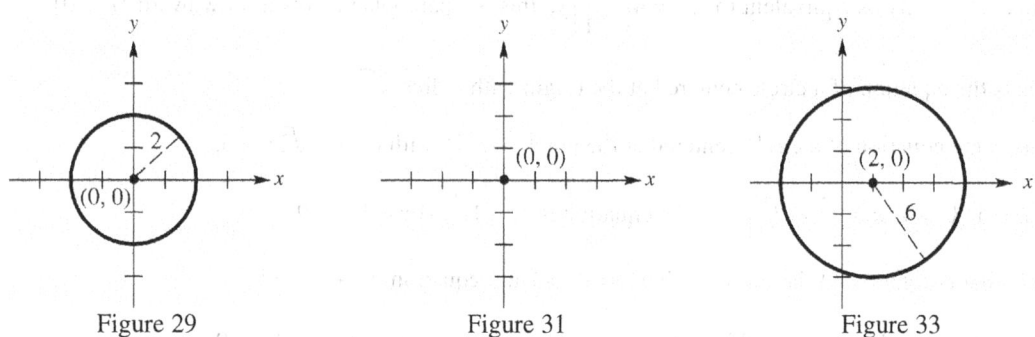

Figure 29   Figure 31   Figure 33

33. This is the equation of a circle centered at $(2, 0)$ with radius $\sqrt{36} = 6$. See Figure 33. From the figure, the domain is $[-4, 8]$, and the range is $[-6, 6]$.

35. This is the equation of a circle centered at $(5, -4)$ with radius $\sqrt{49} = 7$. See Figure 35. From the figure, the domain is $[-2, 12]$, and the range is $[-11, 3]$.

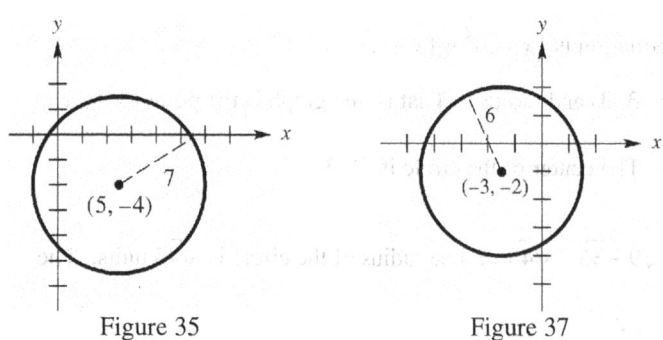

Figure 35   Figure 37

37. This is the equation of a circle centered at $(-3, -2)$ with radius $\sqrt{36} = 6$. See Figure 37. From the figure, the domain is $[-9, 3]$, and the range is $[-8, 4]$.

39. $x^2 + (y-2)^2 + 10 = 9 \Rightarrow x^2 + (y-2)^2 = -1$. This is the equation of a circle centered at $(0, 2)$ with radius $\sqrt{-1}$. No such graph exists. The domain is $\varnothing$ and the range is $\varnothing$.

41. $x^2 + y^2 = 81 \Rightarrow y^2 = 81 - x^2 \Rightarrow y = \pm\sqrt{81 - x^2}$ Graph $y_1 = \sqrt{81 - x^2}$ and $y_2 = \sqrt{81 - x^2}$ as shown in Figure 41. From the figure, the domain is $[-9, 9]$, and the range is $[-9, 9]$.

Copyright © 2015 Pearson Education, Inc

43. $(x-3)^2 + (y-2)^2 = 25 \Rightarrow (y-2)^2 = 25 - (x-3)^2 \Rightarrow y - 2 = \pm\sqrt{25-(x-3)^2} \Rightarrow y = 2 \pm \sqrt{25-(x-3)^2}$.

Graph $y_1 = 2 - \sqrt{25-(x-3)^2}$ and $y_2 = 2 + \sqrt{25-(x-3)^2}$ as shown in Figure 43. From the figure, the domain is $[-2, 8]$, and the range is $[-3, 7]$.

[-14.1, 14.1] by [-9.3, 9.3]
Xscl = 1   Yscl = 1

[-9.4, 9.4] by [-4.2, 8.2]
Xscl = 1   Yscl = 1

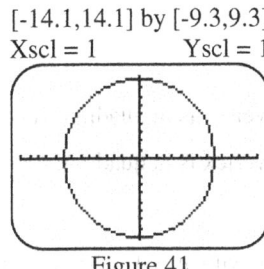
Figure 41

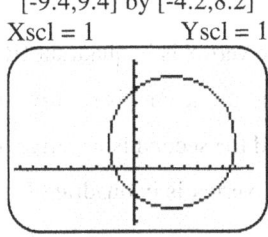
Figure 43

45. $x^2 + 6x + y^2 + 8y + 9 = 0 \Rightarrow (x^2 + 6x + 9) + (y^2 + 8y + 16) = -9 + 9 + 16 \Rightarrow (x+3)^2 + (y+4)^2 = 16$. The graph is a circle with center $(-3, -4)$, and radius $r = 4$.

47. $x^2 - 4x + y^2 + 12y = -4 \Rightarrow (x^2 - 4x + 4) + (y^2 + 12y + 36) = -4 + 4 + 36 \Rightarrow (x-2)^2 + (y+6)^2 = 36$.

The graph is a circle with center $(2, -6)$, and radius $r = 6$.

49. $4x^2 + 4x + 4y^2 - 16y - 19 = 0 \Rightarrow 4\left(x^2 + x + \dfrac{1}{4}\right) + 4(y^2 - 4y + 4) = 19 + 1 + 16 \Rightarrow$

$4\left(x + \dfrac{1}{2}\right)^2 + 4(y-2)^2 = 36 \Rightarrow \left(x + \dfrac{1}{2}\right)^2 + (y-2)^2 = 9$. The graph is a circle with center $\left(-\dfrac{1}{2}, 2\right)$, and radius $r = 3$.

51. $x^2 + 2x + y^2 - 6y + 14 = 0 \Rightarrow (x^2 + 2x + 1) + (y^2 - 6y + 9) = -14 + 1 + 9 \Rightarrow (x+1)^2 + (y-3)^2 = -4$. The graph does not exist since the value for the radius is not a real number.

53. $x^2 - 2x + y^2 + 4y = 0 \Rightarrow (x^2 - 2x + 1) + (y^2 + 4y + 4) = 1 + 4 \Rightarrow (x-1)^2 + (y+2)^2 = 5$. The graph is a circle with center $(1, -2)$ and radius $r = \sqrt{5}$.

55. $b^2 = \dfrac{1}{2}$. $(x+2)^2 + y^2 = \dfrac{4}{9}$. The graph is a circle with center $(-2, 0)$, and radius $r = \dfrac{2}{3}$.

57. D. Since $(x-4)^2 = y + 2$ is equivalent to $(x-4)^2 = 4\left(\dfrac{1}{4}\right)(y+2)$, the parabola has vertex $(4, -2)$, and it opens upward $(c > 0)$.

59. C. Since $y + 2 = -(x-4)^2$ is equivalent to $(x-4)^2 = 4\left(-\dfrac{1}{4}\right)(y+2)$, the parabola has vertex $(4, -2)$, and it opens downward $(c < 0)$.

61. F. Since $(y-4)^2 = x+2$ is equivalent to $(y-4)^2 = 4\left(\dfrac{1}{4}\right)(x+2)$, the parabola has vertex $(-2,4)$, and it opens to the right $(c>0)$.

63. E. Since $x+2 = -(y-4)^2$ is equivalent to $(y-4)^2 = 4\left(-\dfrac{1}{4}\right)(x+2)$, the parabola has vertex $(-2,4)$, and it opens to the left $(c<0)$.

65. (a) If both coordinates of the vertex are negative, the vertex is in quadrant III.
    (b) If the first coordinate of the vertex is negative and the second is positive, the vertex is in quadrant II.
    (c) If the first coordinate of the vertex is positive and the second is negative, the vertex is in quadrant IV.
    (d) If both coordinates of the vertex are positive, the vertex is in quadrant I.

67. Since $x^2 = 16y$ is equivalent to $x^2 = 4(4)y$, the equation is in the form $x^2 = 4cy$ with $c=4$. The focus is $(0,4)$, and the equation of the directrix is $y=-4$. The axis is $x=0$, or the y-axis.

69. Since $x^2 = -\dfrac{1}{2}y$ is equivalent to $x^2 = 4\left(-\dfrac{1}{8}\right)y$, the equation is in the form $x^2 = 4cy$ with $c=-\dfrac{1}{8}$. The focus is $\left(0,-\dfrac{1}{8}\right)$, and the equation of the directrix is $y=\dfrac{1}{8}$. The axis is $x=0$, or the y-axis.

71. Since $y^2 = \dfrac{1}{16}x$ is equivalent to $y^2 = 4\left(\dfrac{1}{64}\right)x$, the equation is in the form $y^2 = 4cx$ with $c=\dfrac{1}{64}$. The focus is $\left(\dfrac{1}{64},0\right)$, and the equation of the directrix is $x=-\dfrac{1}{64}$. The axis is $y=0$, or the x-axis.

73. Since $y^2 = -16x$ is equivalent to $y^2 = 4(-4)x$, the equation is in the form $y^2 = 4cx$ with $c=-4$. The focus is $(-4,0)$, and the equation of the directrix is $x=4$. The axis is $y=0$, or the x-axis.

75. If the vertex is $(0,0)$ and the focus is $(0,-2)$, then the parabola opens downward and $c=-2$. The equation is $x^2 = 4cy \Rightarrow x^2 = -8y$.

77. If the vertex is $(0,0)$ and the focus is $\left(-\dfrac{1}{2},0\right)$, then the parabola opens to the left and $c=-\dfrac{1}{2}$. The equation is $y^2 = 4cx \Rightarrow y^2 = -2x$.

79. If the vertex is $(0,0)$ and the parabola opens to the right, the equation is in the form $y^2 = 4cx$. Find the value or c by using the fact that the parabola passes through $(2,-2\sqrt{2})$. Thus, $(-2\sqrt{2})^2 = 4c(2) \Rightarrow c=1$. The equation is $y^2 = 4cx \Rightarrow y^2 = 4x$.

81. If the vertex is (0, 0) and the parabola opens downward, the equation is in the form $x^2 = 4cy$. Find the value of c by using the fact that the parabola passes through $\left(\sqrt{10}, -5\right)$. Thus, $\left(\sqrt{10}\right)^2 = 4c(-5) \Rightarrow c = -\frac{1}{2}$. The equation is $x^2 = 4cy \Rightarrow x^2 = -2y$.

83. If the vertex is (0, 0) and the parabola has y-axis symmetry, the equation is in the form $x^2 = 4cy$. Find the value of c by using the fact that the parabola passes through $(2, -4)$. Thus, $(2)^2 = 4c(-4) \Rightarrow c = -\frac{1}{4}$. The equation is $x^2 = 4cy \Rightarrow x^2 = -y$.

85. If the focus is (0,2) and the vertex is (0,1), the parabola opens upward and $c = 1$. Substituting in $(x-h)^2 = 4c(y-k)$, we get $(x-0)^2 = 4(1)(y-1)$ or $x^2 = 4(y-1)$.

87. If the focus is (0,0) and the directrix has equation $x = -2$, the vertex is (-1,0) and $c = 1$. The parabola opens to the right. Substituting in $(y-k)^2 = 4c(x-h)$, we get $(y-0)^2 = 4(1)(x-(-1))$ or $y^2 = 4(x+1)$.

89. If the focus is (-1,3) and the directrix has equation $y = 7$, the vertex is (-1,5) and $c = -2$. The parabola opens downward. Substituting in $(y-k)^2 = 4c(x-h)$, we get $(x+1)^2 = 4(-2)(y-5)$ or $(x+1)^2 = -8(y-5)$.

91. Since the parabola has a horizontal axis, the equation is in the form $(y-k)^2 = 4c(x-h)$. Find the value of c by using the fact that the parabola passes through (-4,0) and the vertex is (-2,3). Substituting $x = -4$, $y = 0$, $h = -2$, and $k = 3$ yields $(0-3)^2 = 4c(-4-(-2)) \Rightarrow c = -\frac{9}{8}$. The equation is $(y-3)^2 = -\frac{9}{2}(x+2)$.

93. The equation $y = (x+3)^2 - 4$ can be written as $(x+3)^2 = 4\left(\frac{1}{4}\right)(y+4)$. The vertex is $(-3,-4)$. The vertical axis has equation $x = -3$, and the parabola opens upward. See Figure 93. From the figure, the domain is $(-\infty, \infty)$, and the range is $[-4, \infty)$.

95. The equation $y = -2(x+3)^2 + 2$ can be written as $(x+3)^2 = 4\left(-\frac{1}{8}\right)(y-2)$. The vertex is (-3,2). The vertical axis has equation $x = -3$, and the parabola opens downward. See Figure 95. From the figure, the domain is $(-\infty, \infty)$, and the range is $(-\infty, 2]$.

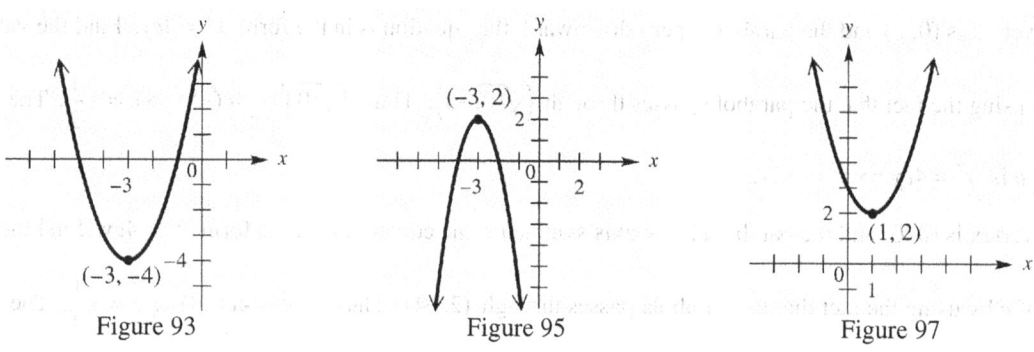

Figure 93   Figure 95   Figure 97

97. Rewrite the equation: $y = x^2 - 2x + 3 \Rightarrow y - 3 + 1 = x^2 - 2x + 1 \Rightarrow y - 2 = (x-1)^2$. The equation $y - 2 = (x-1)^2$ can be written as $(x-1)^2 = 4\left(\dfrac{1}{4}\right)(y-2)$. The vertex is (1,2). The vertical axis has equation $x = 1$, and the parabola opens upward. See Figure 97. From the figure, the domain is $(-\infty, \infty)$, and the range is $[2, \infty)$.

99. Rewrite the equation: $y = 2x^2 - 4x + 5 \Rightarrow y - 5 + 2 = 2(x^2 - 2x + 1) \Rightarrow y - 3 = 2(x-1)^2$. The equation $y - 3 = 2(x-1)^2$ can be written as $(x-1)^2 = 4\left(\dfrac{1}{8}\right)(y-3)$. The vertex is (1,3). The vertical axis has equation $x = 1$, and the parabola opens upward. See Figure 99. From the figure, the domain is $(-\infty, \infty)$, and the range is $[3, \infty)$.

101. The equation $x = y^2 + 2$ can be written as $(y-0)^2 = 4\left(\dfrac{1}{4}\right)(x-2)$. The vertex is (2,0). The horizontal axis has equation $y = 0$, and the parabola opens to the right. See Figure 101. From the figure, the domain is $[2, \infty)$ and the range is $(-\infty, \infty)$.

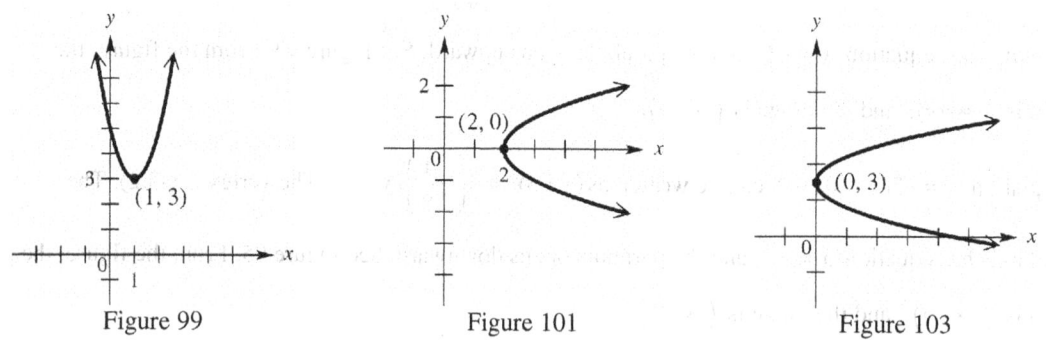

Figure 99   Figure 101   Figure 103

103. The equation $x = (y-3)^2$ can be written as $(y-3)^2 = 4\left(\dfrac{1}{4}\right)(x-0)$. The vertex is (0,3). The horizontal axis has equation $y = 3$, and the parabola opens to the right. See Figure 103. From the figure, the domain is $[0, \infty)$, and the range is $(-\infty, \infty)$.

105. The equation $x = (y-4)^2 + 2$ can be written as $(y-4)^2 = 4\left(\frac{1}{4}\right)(x-2)$. The vertex is (2,4). The horizontal axis has equation $y = 4$, and the parabola opens to the right. See Figure 105. From the figure, the domain is $[2, \infty)$, and the range is $(-\infty, \infty)$.

107. Rewrite the equation: $x = \frac{2}{3}y^2 - 4y + 8 \Rightarrow \frac{3}{2}x = y^2 - 6y + 12 \Rightarrow \frac{3}{2}x - 12 + 9 = y^2 - 6y + 9 \Rightarrow$

$\frac{3}{2}x - 3 = (y-3)^2 \Rightarrow \frac{3}{2}(x-2) = (y-3)^2$. The equation $\frac{3}{2}(x-2) = (y-3)^2$ can be written

$(y-3)^2 = 4\left(\frac{3}{8}\right)(x-2)$. The vertex is (2,3). The horizontal axis has equation $y = 3$ and the parabola opens to the right. See Figure 107. From the figure, the domain is $[2, \infty)$ and the range is $(-\infty, \infty)$.

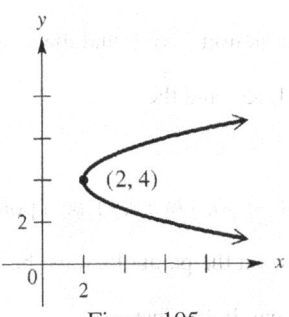
Figure 105

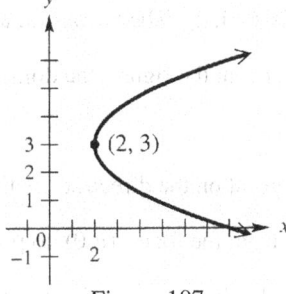
Figure 107

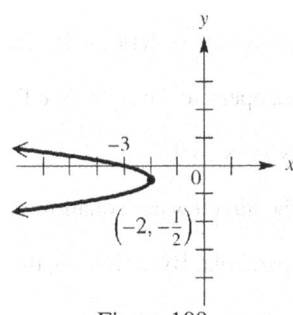
Figure 109

109. Rewrite the equation: $x = -4y^2 - 4y - 3 \Rightarrow x + 3 - 1 = -4\left(y^2 + y + \frac{1}{4}\right) \Rightarrow x + 2 = -4\left(y + \frac{1}{2}\right)^2$. The

equation $x + 2 = -4\left(y + \frac{1}{2}\right)^2$ can be written $\left(y + \frac{1}{2}\right)^2 = 4\left(-\frac{1}{16}\right)(x+2)$. The vertex is $\left(-2, -\frac{1}{2}\right)$. The

horizontal axis has equation $y = -\frac{1}{2}$ and the parabola opens to the left. See Figure 109. From the figure, the

domain is $(-\infty, -2]$ and the range is $(-\infty, \infty)$.

111. Rewrite the equation: $x = 2y^2 - 4y + 6 \Rightarrow x - 6 + 2 = 2(y^2 - 2y + 1) \Rightarrow x - 4 = 2(y-1)^2$. The equation

$x - 4 = 2(y-1)^2$ can be written $(y-1)^2 = 4\left(\frac{1}{8}\right)(x-4)$. The vertex is (4,1). The horizontal axis has

equation $y = 1$ and the parabola opens to the right. See Figure 111. From the figure, the domain is $[4, \infty)$

and the range is $(-\infty, \infty)$.

113. Rewrite the equation: $2x = y^2 - 2y + 9 \Rightarrow 2x - 9 + 1 = y^2 - 2y + 1 \Rightarrow 2(x-4) = (y-1)^2$. The equation

$2(x-4) = (y-1)^2$ can be written $(y-1)^2 = 4\left(\frac{1}{2}\right)(x-4)$. The vertex is (4, 1). The horizontal axis has

342   CHAPTER 7   Analytic Geometry and Nonlinear Systems

equation $y = 1$ and the parabola opens to the right. See Figure 113. From the figure, the domain is $[4, \infty)$ and the range is $(-\infty, \infty)$.

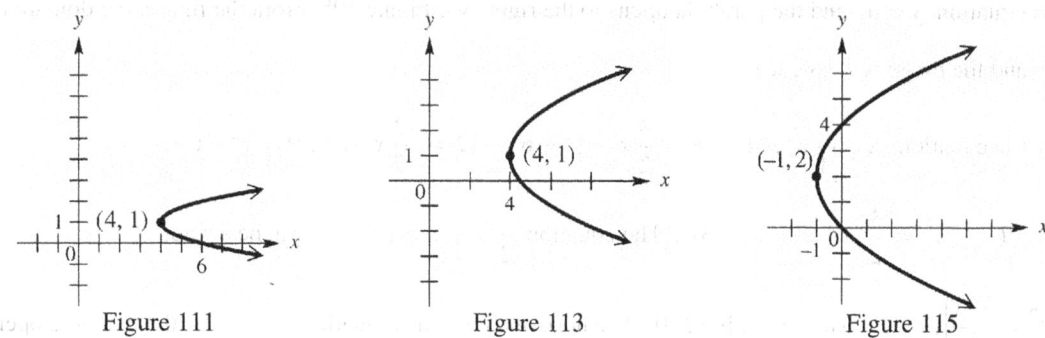

Figure 111   Figure 113   Figure 115

115. Rewrite the equation: $y^2 - 4y + 4 = 4x + 4 \Rightarrow (y-2)^2 = 4(x+1)$. The equation $(y-2)^2 = 4(x+1)$ can be written $(y-2)^2 = 4(1)(x+1)$. The vertex is $(-1, 2)$. The horizontal axis has equation $y = 2$ and the parabola opens to the right. See Figure 115. From the figure, the domain is $[-1, \infty)$ and the range is $(-\infty, \infty)$.

117. Since the directrix has equation $x = -c$, a point on the directrix has the form $(-c, y)$. Let (x, y) be a point on the parabola. By definition, the distance from the focus $(c, 0)$ to point (x, y) on the parabola, must be equal to the distance from point $(-c, y)$ on the directrix to point (x, y) on the parabola. That is

$\sqrt{(x-c)^2 + (y-0)^2} = \sqrt{(x+c)^2 + (y-y)^2} \Rightarrow$

$(x-c)^2 + y^2 = (x+c)^2 \Rightarrow x^2 - 2xc + c^2 + y^2 = x^2 + 2xc + c^2 \Rightarrow -2xc + y^2 = 2xc \Rightarrow y^2 = 4xc$.

119. (a) For Mars, $y = \dfrac{19}{11}x - \dfrac{12.6}{3872}x^2$. For the moon, $y = \dfrac{19}{11}x - \dfrac{5.2}{3872}x^2$. Graph

$y_1 = (19/11)x - (12.6/3872)x^2$ and $y_2 = (19/11)x - (5.2/3872)x^2$ as shown in Figure 119.

(b) From the graph, the ball thrown on Mars reaches a maximum height of $y \approx 229$ and the ball thrown on the moon reaches a maximum height of $y \approx 555$.

[0,1500] by [0,1000]
Xscl = 500   Yscl = 500

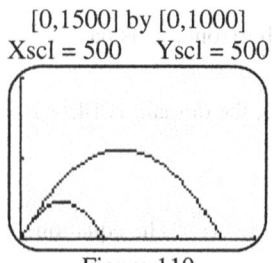

Figure 119

121. $y = -\dfrac{5 \times 10^{-9}}{2(10^7)}(0.4)^2 = -4 \times 10^{-17}$; the alpha particle is deflected 4×10^{-17} meter downward.

Copyright © 2015 Pearson Education, Inc

123. Let the vertex of the parabola be (0, 12). The equation of the parabola is of the form $(x-h)^2 = 4c(y-k)$.

By substitution, the equation is $(x-0)^2 = 4c(y-12) \Rightarrow x^2 = 4c(y-12)$. Since the parabola passes through the point (6, 0), the value of c can be found by substitution:

$6^2 = 4c(0-12) \Rightarrow 36 = 4c(-12) \Rightarrow -3 = 4c \Rightarrow c = -\frac{3}{4}$. The equation is $x^2 = -3(y-12)$. Noting that the y-coordinate 9 feet up is 9, half the width can be found by substitution: $x^2 = -3(9-12) \Rightarrow x^2 = 9 \Rightarrow x = 3$; The width is 6 feet.

7.2: Ellipses and Hyperbolas

1. G. This is an ellipse with $a^2 = 16$, $b^2 = 4$, and $c = \sqrt{16-4} = \sqrt{12} = 2\sqrt{3}$. The Foci are $(0, \pm 2\sqrt{3})$.

3. F. This is a hyperbola centered at (0, 0) with a horizontal transverse axis.

5. E. Since $h = -2$ and $k = 4$, this is an ellipse centered at $(-2, 4)$.

7. D. Since $h = -2$ and $k = 4$, this is a hyperbola centered at $(-2, 4)$.

9. A circle can be interpreted as an ellipse whose foci have the same coordinates. The "coinciding foci" give the center of the circle.

11. $\frac{x^2}{9} + \frac{y^2}{4} = 1 \Rightarrow a = 3$ and $b = 2$. $a^2 - b^2 = 3^2 - 2^2 = 5 = c^2 \Rightarrow c = \sqrt{5}$. The foci are $(\pm\sqrt{5}, 0)$. The endpoints of the major axis (vertices) are $(\pm 3, 0)$ so the domain is $[-3, 3]$. The endpoints of the minor axis are $(0, \pm 2)$, so the range is $[-2, 2]$. The ellipse is graphed in Figure 11.

13. $9x^2 + 6y^2 = 54 \Rightarrow \frac{x^2}{6} + \frac{y^2}{9} = 1 \Rightarrow a = 3$ and $b = \sqrt{6}$. $a^2 - b^2 = 9 - 6 = 3 = c^2 \Rightarrow c = \sqrt{3}$. The foci are $(0, \pm\sqrt{3})$. The endpoints of the major axis (vertices) are $(0, \pm 3)$ so the range is $[-3, 3]$. The endpoints of the minor axis are $(\pm\sqrt{6}, 0)$ so the domain is $[-\sqrt{6}, \sqrt{6}]$. The ellipse is graphed in Figure 13.

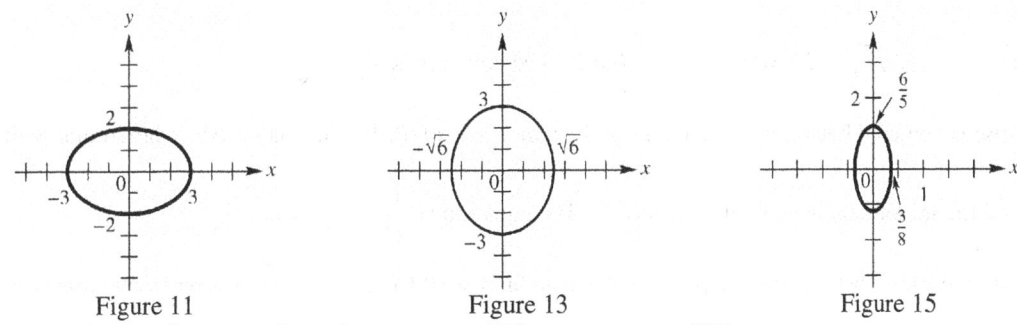

Figure 11   Figure 13   Figure 15

15. $\frac{25y^2}{36} + \frac{64x^2}{9} = 1 \Rightarrow \frac{y^2}{\frac{36}{25}} + \frac{x^2}{\frac{9}{64}} = 1 \Rightarrow a = \sqrt{\frac{36}{25}} = \frac{6}{5}$ and $b = \sqrt{\frac{9}{64}} = \frac{3}{8}$

344 CHAPTER 7 Analytic Geometry and Nonlinear Systems

The endpoints of the major axis (vertices) are $\left(0, \pm \frac{6}{5}\right)$ so the range is $\left[-\frac{6}{5}, \frac{6}{5}\right]$. The endpoints of the minor axis are $\left(\pm \frac{3}{8}, 0\right)$ so the domain is $\left[-\frac{3}{8}, \frac{3}{8}\right]$. See Figure 15.

17. The ellipse is centered at $(1,-3)$. The major axis is vertical and has length $2a = 10$. The length of the minor axis is $2b = 6$. The graph is shown in Figure 17. The domain is $[-2,4]$ and the range is $[-8, 2]$.

19. The ellipse is centered at $(2, 1)$. The major axis is horizontal and has length $2a = 8$. The length of the minor axis is $2b = 6$. The graph is shown in Figure 19. The domain is $[-2,6]$ and the range is $[-2,4]$.

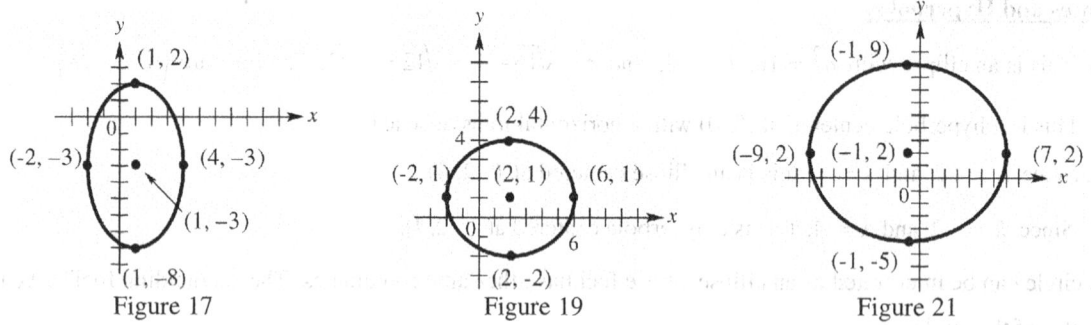

Figure 17   Figure 19   Figure 21

21. The ellipse is centered at $(-1,2)$. The major axis is horizontal and has length $2a = 16$. The length of the minor axis is $2b = 14$. The graph is shown in Figure 21. The domain is $[-9,7]$ and the range is $[-5,9]$.

23. The ellipse is centered between the foci at $(0,0)$. The major axis is horizontal with $a = 4$. Since the foci are $(\pm 2, 0)$, we know that $c = 2$. Since $c^2 = a^2 - b^2$, the value of b can be found by substitution:

$b^2 = a^2 - c^2 = 4^2 - 2^2 = 16 - 4 = 12 \Rightarrow b = \sqrt{12}$. The equation is $\frac{x^2}{16} + \frac{y^2}{12} = 1$.

25. The ellipse is centered between the foci at $(0,0)$. The major axis is vertical with $a = 2\sqrt{2}$. Since the foci are $(0, \pm 2)$, we know that $c = 2$. Since $c^2 = a^2 - b^2$, the value of b can be found by substitution:

$b^2 = a^2 - c^2 = \left(2\sqrt{2}\right)^2 - 2^2 = 8 - 4 = 4 \Rightarrow b = 2$. The equation is $\frac{x^2}{4} + \frac{y^2}{8} = 1$.

27. The ellipse is centered between the endpoint of the major axis of $(0,0)$. The major axis is horizontal with $a = 4$ and the minor axis is vertical with $b = 2$. The equation is $\frac{x^2}{16} + \frac{y^2}{4} = 1$.

29. The ellipse is centered between the endpoints of the major axis at $(0,0)$. The major axis is horizontal with $a = 6$. Since $c^2 = a^2 - b^2$, the value of b can be found by substitution:

$b^2 = a^2 - c^2 = 6^2 - 4^2 = 36 - 16 = 20 \Rightarrow b = \sqrt{20}$. The equation is $\frac{x^2}{36} + \frac{y^2}{20} = 1$.

31. Since the center is $(3,-2)$, we know that $h=3$ and $k=-2$. Since $c^2=a^2-b^2$, the value of b can be found by substitution: $b^2=a^2-c^2=5^2-3^2=25-9=16 \Rightarrow b=4$. The major axis is vertical so the equation is $\dfrac{(x-3)^2}{16}+\dfrac{(y+2)^2}{25}=1$.

33. The ellipse is centered between the foci at $(0,0)$. The major axis is vertical with $a=3$. Since the foci are $(0,\pm 2)$, we know that $c=2$. Since $c^2=a^2-b^2$, the value of b can be found by substitution: $b^2=a^2-c^2=3^2-2^2=9-4=5 \Rightarrow b=\sqrt{5}$. The equation is $\dfrac{y^2}{9}+\dfrac{x^2}{5}=1$.

35. Since the center is $(5,2)$, we know that $h=5$ and $k=2$. Since the minor axis is horizontal and has length 8, $b=4$. Since $c^2=a^2-b^2$ and $c=3$, the value of a can be found by substitution: $3^2+4^2=a^2 \Rightarrow a^2=25 \Rightarrow a=5$. The equation is $\dfrac{(x-5)^2}{25}+\dfrac{(y-2)^2}{16}=1$.

37. The ellipse is centered between the vertices at $(4,5)$ and $a=\dfrac{9-1}{2}=4$. The major axis is vertical. Since the minor axis has length 6, $b=3$. The equation is $\dfrac{(x-4)^2}{9}+\dfrac{(y-5)^2}{16}=1$.

39. $9x^2+18x+4y^2-8y-23=0 \Rightarrow 9(x^2+2x)+4(y^2-2y)=23 \Rightarrow 9(x^2+2x+1)+4(y^2-2y+1)=23+9+4 \Rightarrow 9(x+1)^2+4(y-1)^2=36 \Rightarrow \dfrac{(x+1)^2}{4}+\dfrac{(y-1)^2}{9}=1$

    The center is $(-1,1)$. The vertices are $(-1,1-3),(-1,1+3)$ or $(-1,-2),(-1,4)$.

41. $4x^2+8x+y^2+2y+1=0 \Rightarrow 4(x^2+2x)+(y^2+2y)=-1 \Rightarrow 4(x^2+2x+1)+(y^2+2y+1)=-1+4+1 \Rightarrow 4(x+1)^2+(y+1)^2=4 \Rightarrow \dfrac{(x+1)^2}{1}+\dfrac{(y+1)^2}{4}=1$

    The center is $(-1,-1)$. The vertices are $(-1,-1-2),(-1,-1+2)$ or $(-1,-3),(-1,1)$.

43. $4x^2+16x+5y^2-10y+1=0 \Rightarrow 4(x^2+4x)+5(y^2-2y)=-1 \Rightarrow 4(x^2+4x+4)+5(y^2-2y+1)=-1+16+5 \Rightarrow 4(x+2)^2+5(y-1)^2=20 \Rightarrow \dfrac{(x+2)^2}{5}+\dfrac{(y-1)^2}{4}=1$

    The center is $(-2,1)$. The vertices are $(-2-\sqrt{5},1),(-2+\sqrt{5},1)$.

45. $16x^2-16x+4y^2+12y=51 \Rightarrow 16(x^2-x)+4(y^2+3y)=51 \Rightarrow 16\left(x^2-x+\dfrac{1}{4}\right)+4\left(y^2+3y+\dfrac{9}{4}\right)=51+4+9 \Rightarrow 16\left(x-\dfrac{1}{2}\right)^2+4\left(y+\dfrac{3}{2}\right)^2=64 \Rightarrow \dfrac{\left(x-\dfrac{1}{2}\right)^2}{4}+\dfrac{\left(y+\dfrac{3}{2}\right)^2}{16}=1$

The center is $\left(\frac{1}{2}, -\frac{3}{2}\right)$. The vertices are $\left(\frac{1}{2}, -\frac{3}{2}-4\right), \left(\frac{1}{2}, -\frac{3}{2}+4\right)$ or $\left(\frac{1}{2}, -\frac{11}{2}\right), \left(\frac{1}{2}, \frac{5}{2}\right)$.

47. The transverse axis is horizontal with $a = 4$ and $b = 3$. The asymptotes are $y = \pm\frac{3}{4}x$. See Figure 47. The domain is $(-\infty, -4] \cup [4, \infty)$ and the range is $(-\infty, \infty)$.

49. $49y^2 - 36x^2 = 1764 \Rightarrow \frac{y^2}{36} - \frac{x^2}{49} = 1$ The transverse axis is vertical with $a = 6$ and $b = 7$. The asymptotes are $y = \pm\frac{6}{7}x$. See Figure 49. The domain is $(-\infty, \infty)$ and the range is $(-\infty, -6] \cup [6, \infty)$.

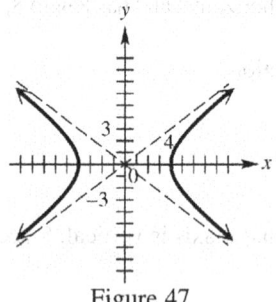
Figure 47

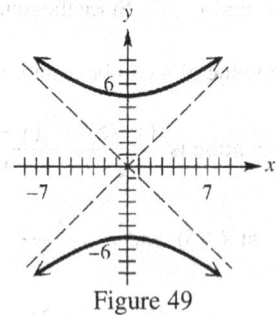
Figure 49

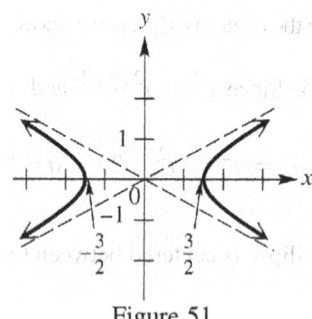
Figure 51

51. $\frac{4x^2}{9} - \frac{25y^2}{16} = 1 \Rightarrow \frac{x^2}{\frac{9}{4}} - \frac{y^2}{\frac{16}{25}} = 1$. The transverse axis is horizontal with $a = \frac{3}{2}$ and $b = \frac{4}{5}$. The asymptotes are $y = \pm\frac{18}{15}x$. See Figure 51. The domain is $\left(-\infty, -\frac{3}{2}\right] \cup \left[\frac{3}{2}, \infty\right)$ and the range is $(-\infty, \infty)$.

53. $9x^2 - 4y^2 = 1 \Rightarrow \frac{x^2}{\frac{1}{9}} - \frac{y^2}{\frac{1}{4}} = 1$. The transverse axis is horizontal with $a = \frac{1}{3}$ and $b = \frac{1}{2}$. The asymptotes are $y = \pm\frac{3}{2}x$. See Figure 53. The domain is $\left(-\infty, -\frac{1}{3}\right] \cup \left[\frac{1}{3}, \infty\right)$ and the range is $(-\infty, \infty)$.

55. The center is $(1, -3)$ and the transverse axis is horizontal with $a = 3$ and $b = 5$. See Figure 55. The domain is $(-\infty, -2] \cup [4, \infty)$ and the range is $(-\infty, \infty)$.

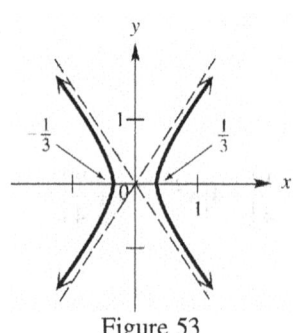
Figure 53

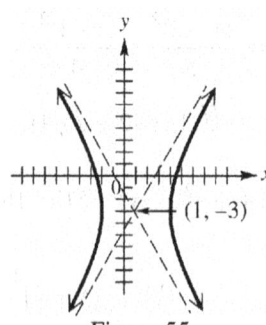
Figure 55

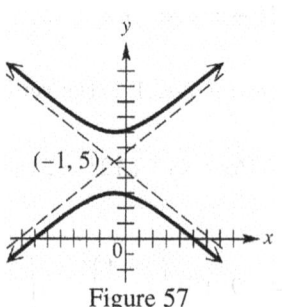
Figure 57

Section 7.2   347

57. The center is $(-1,5)$ and the transverse axis is vertical with $a=2$ and $b=3$. See Figure 57. The domain is $(-\infty,\infty)$ and the range is $(-\infty,3]\cup[7,\infty)$.

59. $16(x+5)^2-(y-3)^2=1 \Rightarrow \dfrac{(x+5)^2}{\frac{1}{16}}-\dfrac{(y-3)^2}{1}=1$ The center is $(-5, 3)$ and the transverse axis is horizontal with $a=\dfrac{1}{4}$ and $b=1$. See Figure 59. The domain is $\left(-\infty,-5-\dfrac{1}{4}\right]\cup\left[-5+\dfrac{1}{4},\infty\right)$ or $\left(-\infty,-\dfrac{21}{4}\right]\cup\left[-\dfrac{19}{4},\infty\right)$ and the range is $(-\infty,\infty)$.

61. $9(x-2)^2-4(y+1)^2=36 \Rightarrow \dfrac{(x-2)^2}{4}-\dfrac{(y+1)^2}{9}=1$. The center is $(2, -1)$ and the transverse axis is vertical with $a=2$ and $b=3$. See Figure 61. The domain is $(-\infty,0]\cup[4,\infty)$ and the range is $(-\infty,\infty)$.

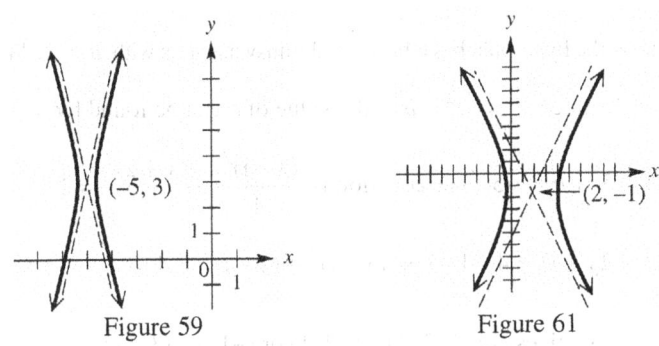

Figure 59   Figure 61

63. The hyperbola has a horizontal transverse axis with $c=4$. The x-intercepts coincide with the vertices, so $a=3$. The center is located between the foci at $(0, 0)$. Since $c^2=a^2+b^2$, the value of b can be found by substitution: $b^2=c^2-a^2=4^2-3^2=16-9=7 \Rightarrow b=\sqrt{7}$. The equation is $\dfrac{x^2}{9}-\dfrac{y^2}{7}=1$.

65. The asymptotes intersect at the origin so the center is $(0, 0)$. The hyperbola has a vertical transverse axis and the y-intercepts coincide with the vertices so $a=3$. From the asymptotes, $\dfrac{a}{b}=\dfrac{3}{5}$ with $a=3 \Rightarrow b=5$. The equation is $\dfrac{y^2}{9}-\dfrac{x^2}{25}=1$.

67. The center is located between the vertices at $(0, 0)$. The hyperbola has a vertical transverse axis with $a=6$. From the asymptotes, $\dfrac{a}{b}=\dfrac{1}{2}$ with $a=6 \Rightarrow b=12$. The equation is $\dfrac{y^2}{36}-\dfrac{x^2}{144}=1$.

69. The center is located between the vertices at $(0, 0)$. The hyperbola has a horizontal transverse axis with $a=3$. The equation is of the form $\dfrac{x^2}{a^2}-\dfrac{y^2}{b^2}=1$. By substitution using the point $(6, 1)$,

$\dfrac{6^2}{3^2} - \dfrac{1^2}{b^2} = 1 \Rightarrow \dfrac{36}{9} - 1 = \dfrac{1}{b^2} \Rightarrow 3 = \dfrac{1}{b^2} \Rightarrow b^2 = \dfrac{1}{3}$. The equation is $\dfrac{x^2}{3^2} - \dfrac{y^2}{\frac{1}{3}} = 1$ or $\dfrac{x^2}{9} - 3y^2 = 1$.

71. The center is located between the foci at (0, 0). The hyperbola has a vertical transverse axis with $c = \sqrt{13}$. From the asymptotes, $\dfrac{a}{b} = 5$. Also, from $c^2 = a^2 + b^2 \Rightarrow a^2 + b^2 = 13$. Solving these equations simultaneously results in $a^2 = \dfrac{25}{2}$ and $b^2 = \dfrac{1}{2}$. The equation is $\dfrac{y^2}{\frac{25}{2}} - \dfrac{x^2}{\frac{1}{2}} = 1$ or $\dfrac{2y^2}{25} - 2x^2 = 1$.

73. The center is located between the vertices at (4, 3). The hyperbola has a vertical transverse axis with $a = 2$. From the asymptotes, $\dfrac{a}{b} = 7$ with $a = 2 \Rightarrow b = \dfrac{2}{7}$. The equation is $\dfrac{(y-3)^2}{4} - \dfrac{(x-4)^2}{\frac{4}{49}} = 1$ or

$\dfrac{(y-3)^2}{4} - \dfrac{49(x-4)^2}{4} = 1$.

75. With center $(1, -2)$ and vertex $(3, -2)$, we know the hyperbola has a horizontal transverse axis with $a = 2$. With center $(1, -2)$ and focus $(4, -2)$, we know $c = 3$. Since $c^2 = a^2 + b^2$, the value of b can be found by substitution: $b^2 = c^2 - a^2 = 3^2 - 2^2 = 9 - 4 = 5 \Rightarrow b = \sqrt{5}$. The equation is $\dfrac{(x-1)^2}{4} - \dfrac{(y+2)^2}{5} = 1$.

77. $x^2 - 2x - y^2 + 2y = 4 \Rightarrow (x^2 - 2x + 1) - (y^2 - 2y + 1) = 4 + 1 - 1 \Rightarrow (x-1)^2 - (y-1)^2 = 4 \Rightarrow$

$\dfrac{(x-1)^2}{4} - \dfrac{(y-1)^2}{4} = 1$. The center is (1, 1). The vertices are (1–2, 1), (1+2, 1) or (–1, 1), (3, 1).\

79. $3y^2 + 24y - 2x^2 + 12x + 24 = 0 \Rightarrow 3(y^2 + 8y) - 2(x^2 - 6x) = -24 \Rightarrow$

$3(y^2 + 8y + 16) - 2(x^2 - 6x + 9) = -24 + 48 - 18 \Rightarrow 3(y+4)^2 - 2(x-3)^2 = 6 \Rightarrow \dfrac{(y+4)^2}{2} - \dfrac{(x-3)^2}{3} = 1$.

The center is (3, 4). The vertices are $(3, -4 - \sqrt{2})$, $(3, -4 + \sqrt{2})$.

81. $x^2 - 6x - 2y^2 + 7 = 0 \Rightarrow (x^2 - 6x + 9) - 2y^2 = -7 + 9 \Rightarrow (x-3)^2 - 2(y-0)^2 = 2 \Rightarrow$

$\dfrac{(x-3)^2}{2} - \dfrac{(y-0)^2}{1} = 1$. The center is $(3, 0)$. The vertices are $(3 - \sqrt{2}, 0), (3 + \sqrt{2}, 0)$.

83. $4y^2 + 32y - 5x^2 - 10x + 39 = 0 \Rightarrow 4(y^2 + 8y) - 5(x^2 + 2x) = -39 \Rightarrow$

$4(y^2 + 8y + 16) - 5(x^2 + 2x + 1) = -39 + 64 - 5 \Rightarrow 4(y+4)^2 - 5(x+1)^2 = 20 \Rightarrow \dfrac{(y+4)^2}{5} - \dfrac{(x+1)^2}{4} = 1$.

The center is $(-1, -4)$. The vertices are $(-1, -4 - \sqrt{5}), (-1, -4 + \sqrt{5})$.

85. If the focus is (0,2) and the vertex is (0,1), the parabola opens upward and $c = 1$. Substituting in $(x-h)^2 = 4c(y-k)$, we get $(x-0)^2 = 4(1)(y-1)$ or $x^2 = 4(y-1)$.

86. If the focus is (-1,2) and the vertex is (3,2), the parabola opens to the left and $c = -4$. Substituting in $(y-k)^2 = 4c(x-h)$, we get $(y-2)^2 = -16(x-3)$.

87. If the focus is (0,0) and the directrix has equation $x = -2$, the vertex is (-1,0) and $c = 1$. The parabola opens to the right. Substituting in $(y-k)^2 = 4c(x-h)$, we get $(y-0)^2 = 4(1)(x-(-1))$ or $y^2 = 4(x+1)$.

88. If the focus is (2,1) and the directrix has equation $x = -1$, the vertex is $\left(\frac{1}{2}, 1\right)$ and $c = \frac{3}{2}$. The parabola opens to the right. Substituting in $(y-k)^2 = 4c(x-h)$, we get $(y-1)^2 = 4\left(\frac{3}{2}\right)\left(x - \frac{1}{2}\right)$ or $(y-1)^2 = 6\left(x - \frac{1}{2}\right)$.

89. If the focus is (-1,3) and the directrix has equation $y = 7$, the vertex is (-1,5) and $c = -2$. The parabola opens downward. Substituting in $(y-k)^2 = 4c(x-h)$, we get $(x+1)^2 = 4(-2)(y-5)$ or $(x+1)^2 = -8(y-5)$.

90. If the focus is (1,2) and the directrix has equation $y = 4$, the vertex is (1,3) and $c = -1$. The parabola opens downward. Substituting in $(x-h)^2 = 4c(y-k)$, we get $(x-1)^2 = 4(-1)(y-3)$ or $(x-1)^2 = -4(y-3)$.

91. The patient and the emitter are 12 units apart. These positions represent the foci of the ellipse so $c = 6$. With the minor axis measuring 16 units, $b = 8$. Since $c^2 = a^2 - b^2$, the value of a can be found by substitution: $a^2 = b^2 + c^2 = 6^2 + 8^2 = 36 + 64 = 100 \Rightarrow a = 10$. The equation is $\frac{x^2}{100} + \frac{y^2}{64} = 1$.

93. A major axis measuring 620 feet indicates that $a = 310$. A minor axis measuring 513 feet indicates that $b = 256.5$. Then $5c^2 = a^2 - b^2 = 310^2 - 256.5^2 \Rightarrow c = \sqrt{310^2 - 256.5^2} \approx 174.1$. The distance between the foci is $2c \approx 2(174.1) \approx 348.2$ feet.

95. Using a vertical major axis, $a = 15$. The minor axis has length 20, so $b = 10$. The equation is $\frac{y^2}{225} + \frac{x^2}{100} = 1$. Assuming the truck drives exactly in the middle of the road, we want to find y when $x = 6$. $\frac{y^2}{225} + \frac{6^2}{100} = 1 \Rightarrow \frac{y^2}{225} = 1 - \frac{36}{100} \Rightarrow y^2 = 225\left(1 - \frac{36}{100}\right) \Rightarrow y = \sqrt{225\left(1 - \frac{36}{100}\right)} = 12$. The truck must be just under 12 feet high to pass through.

97. (a) Since $c = \sqrt{a^2 - b^2} = \sqrt{4465^2 - 4462^2} \approx 163.6$, one focus is located at the point (163.6, 0). The graph representing Earth is a circle with radius 3960 with center (163.6, 0). The equation for Earth is $(x - 163.6)^2 + y^2 = 3690^2$. To graph this equation, solve for y and graph two parts. $(x - 163.6)^2 + y^2 = 3690^2 \Rightarrow y^2 = 3690^2 - (x - 163.6)^2 \Rightarrow y = \pm\sqrt{3690^2 - (x - 163.6)^2}$ To graph the

350 CHAPTER 7 Analytic Geometry and Nonlinear Systems

ellipse, solve for y and graph two parts.

$$\frac{x^2}{4465^2}+\frac{y^2}{4462^2}=1 \Rightarrow \frac{y^2}{4462^2}=1-\frac{x^2}{4465^2} \Rightarrow y^2 = 4462^2\left(1-\frac{x^2}{4465^2}\right) \Rightarrow y = \pm\sqrt{4462^2\left(1-\frac{x^2}{4465^2}\right)}$$

The graphs are shown in Figure 97.

(b) The minimum distance is $4465-(3960+163.6) \approx 341$ miles. The maximum distance is $4465-(3960+163.6) \approx 669$ miles.

[-6750,6750] by [-4500,4500]
Xscl = 1000 Yscl = 1000

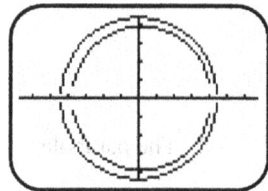

Figure 97

99. (a) Find a and b in the equation $\dfrac{x^2}{a^2}-\dfrac{y^2}{b^2}=1$. Because the equations of the asymptotes of a hyperbola with horizontal transverse axes are $y=\pm\dfrac{b}{a}x$, and the given asymptotes are $y=\pm x$, it follows that $\dfrac{a}{b}=1$ or $a=b$. Since the line $y=x$ intersects the x-axis at a 45° angle, the triangle shown in the third quadrant is a 45°- 45°- 90° right triangle and both legs must have length d. Then, by the Pythagorean theorem, $c^2 = d^2 + d^2 = 2d^2$. That gives $c=d\sqrt{2}$. Also, for a hyperbola $c^2 = a^2 + b^2$, and since $a=b$, $c^2 = a^2 + a^2 = 2a^2$. That gives $c=a\sqrt{2}$. From these two equations, $a\sqrt{2}=d\sqrt{2}$ and so $a=d$. That is, $a=b=d=5\times10^{-14}$. Thus the equation of the trajectory of A, where $x>0$, is given by $\dfrac{x^2}{\left(5\times10^{-14}\right)^2}-\dfrac{y^2}{\left(5\times10^{-14}\right)^2}=1$. Solving for x yields $x^2-y^2=\left(5\times10^{-14}\right)^2 \Rightarrow$ $x^2 = y^2 + 2.5\times10^{-27} \Rightarrow x=\sqrt{y^2+2.5\times10^{-27}}$. This equation represents the right half of the hyperbola, as shown in the textbook.

(b) Since $a=5\times10^{-14}$, the distance from the origin to the vertex is 5×10^{-14}. The distance from N to the origin can be found using the Pythagorean theorem. Let h represent this distance, then $h^2 = d^2 + d^2$. That is, $h^2 = \left(5\times10^{-14}\right)^2 + \left(5\times10^{-14}\right)^2 \Rightarrow h^2 = 5\times10^{-27} \Rightarrow h \approx 7\times10^{-14}$. The minimum distance between the centers of the alpha particle and the gold nucleus is $5\times10^{-14}+7\times10^{-14} \approx 1.2\times10^{-13}$.

101. Let (x,y) be any point on the ellipse and start with the distance formula.

$\sqrt{(x+3)^2+y^2}+\sqrt{(x-3)^2+y^2}=10$ Given Equation.

$\sqrt{(x+3)^2+y^2}=10-\sqrt{(x-3)^2+y^2}$ Subtract $\sqrt{(x-3)^2+y^2}$.

$(x+3)^2 + y^2 = 100 - 20\sqrt{(x-3)^2 + y^2} + (x-3)^2 + y^2$	Square each side.
$(x+3)^2 - (x-3)^2 - 100 = -20\sqrt{(x-3)^2 + y^2}$	Subtract $(x-3)^2$ and 100.
$x^2 + 6x + 9 - x^2 + 6x - 9 - 100 = -20\sqrt{(x-3)^2 + y^2}$	Expand the binomials.
$12x - 100 = -20\sqrt{(x-3)^2 + y^2}$	Simplify.
$25 - 3x = 5\sqrt{(x-3)^2 + y^2}$	Divide each side by -4.
$625 - 150x + 9x^2 = 25(x^2 - 6x + 9 + y^2)$	Square each side.
$625 - 150x + 9x^2 = 25x^2 - 150x + 225 + 25y^2$	Multiply the right side.
$-16x^2 - 25y^2 = -400$	Simplify.
$\dfrac{-16x^2}{-400} + \dfrac{-25y^2}{-400} = \dfrac{-400}{-400}$	Divide each side by $x = \ln(t-1) \Rightarrow t = e^x + 1$.
$\dfrac{x^2}{25} + \dfrac{y^2}{16} = 1$	Simplify.

Reviewing Basic Concepts (Sections 7.1 and 7.2)

1. (a) The circle is defined in B.
   (b) The parabola is defined in D.
   (c) The ellipse is defined in A.
   (d) The hyperbola is defined in C.

2. $12x^2 - 4y^2 = 48 \Rightarrow \dfrac{x^2}{4} - \dfrac{y^2}{12} = 1$. The transverse axis is horizontal with $a = 2$ and $b = \sqrt{12}$. The asymptotes are $y = \pm \dfrac{\sqrt{12}}{2} x$. See Figure 2.

3. Rewrite the equation. $y = 2x^2 + 3x - 1 \Rightarrow y + 1 + \dfrac{9}{8} = 2\left(x^2 + \dfrac{3}{2}x + \dfrac{9}{16}\right) \Rightarrow y + \dfrac{17}{8} = 2\left(x + \dfrac{3}{4}\right)^2$. The equation $y + \dfrac{17}{8} = 2\left(x + \dfrac{3}{4}\right)^2$ can be written $y + \dfrac{17}{8} = 4\left(\dfrac{1}{2}\right)\left(x + \dfrac{3}{4}\right)^2$. The vertex is $\left(-\dfrac{3}{4}, \dfrac{17}{8}\right)$. See Figure 3.

352   CHAPTER 7   Analytic Geometry and Nonlinear Systems

4. $x^2 + y^2 - 2x + 2y - 2 = 0 \Rightarrow (x^2 - 2x + 1) + (y^2 + 2y + 1) = 2 + 1 + 1 \Rightarrow (x-1)^2 + (y+1)^2 = 4$. The graph is a circle with center $(1,-1)$ and radius $\left(-4 + \dfrac{1}{16}, 1\right) \Rightarrow \left(-\dfrac{63}{16}, -1\right)$ See Figure 4.

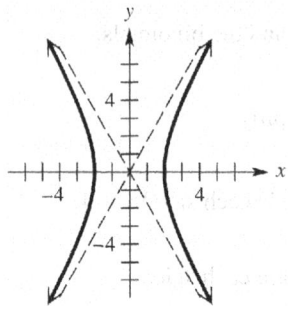

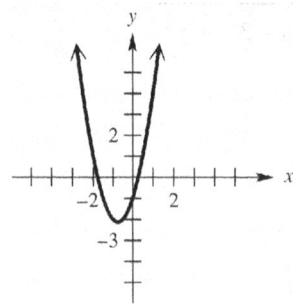

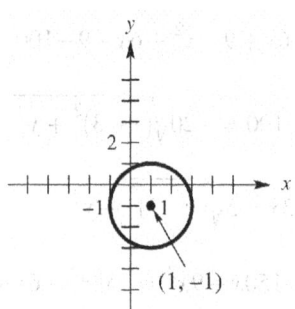

Figure 2   Figure 3   Figure 4

5. $4x^2 + 9y^2 = 36 \Rightarrow \dfrac{x^2}{9} + \dfrac{y^2}{4} = 1 \Rightarrow a = 3$ and $b = 2$. The ellipse is graphed in Figure 5.

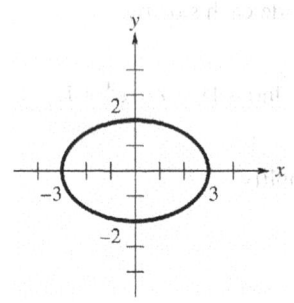

Figure 5

6. If $c < a$, it is an ellipse. If $c > a$, it is a hyperbola.

7. A circle with center $(2,-1)$ and radius 3 has equation $(x-2)^2 + (y+1)^2 = 9$.

8. The ellipse is centered between the foci at $(0,0)$. The major axis is horizontal with $a = 6$. Since the foci are $(\pm 4, 0)$, we know that $c = 4$. Since $c^2 = a^2 - b^2$, the value of b can be found by substitution: $b^2 = a^2 - c^2 = 6^2 - 4^2 = 36 - 16 = 20 \Rightarrow b = \sqrt{20}$. The equation is $\dfrac{x^2}{36} + \dfrac{y^2}{20} = 1$.

9. The hyperbola has a vertical transverse axis with $c = 4$. The vertices are $(0, \pm 2)$ so $a = 2$. The center is located between the foci at $(0,0)$. Since $c^2 = a^2 + b^2$, the value of b can be found by substitution: $b^2 = c^2 - a^2 = 4^2 - 2^2 = 16 - 4 = 12 \Rightarrow b = \sqrt{12}$. The equation is $\dfrac{y^2}{4} - \dfrac{x^2}{12} = 1$.

10. If the vertex is $(0,0)$ and the focus is $\left(0, \frac{1}{2}\right)$, then the parabola opens upward and $c = \frac{1}{2}$. The equation is

    $x^2 = 4cy \Rightarrow x^2 = 2y$.

7.3: The Conic Sections and Nonlinear Systems

1. $x^2 + y^2 = 144 \Rightarrow (x-0)^2 + (y-0)^2 = 12^2$ The graph of this equation is a circle with center $(0,0)$ and radius 12. Also, note in our original equation, the x^2- and y^2-terms have the same positive coefficient.

3. $y = 2x^2 + 3x - 4 \Rightarrow y = 2\left(x^2 + \frac{3}{2}x\right) - 4 \Rightarrow y = 2\left(x^2 + \frac{3}{2}x + \frac{9}{16} - \frac{9}{16}\right) - 4 \Rightarrow y = 2\left(x + \frac{3}{4}\right)^2 + 2\left(-\frac{9}{16}\right) - 4$

   $\Rightarrow y = 2\left(x + \frac{3}{4}\right)^2 - \frac{9}{8} - 4 \Rightarrow y = 2\left(x + \frac{3}{4}\right)^2 - \frac{41}{8} \Rightarrow y - \left(-\frac{41}{8}\right) = 2\left[x - \left(-\frac{3}{4}\right)\right]^2$ The graph of this equation is a parabola opening upwards with a vertex of $\left(-\frac{3}{4}, -\frac{41}{8}\right)$. Also, note our original equation has an x^2- term, but no y^2-term.

5. $x - 1 = -3(y - 4)^2$ The graph of this equation is a parabola opening to the left with a vertex of $(1, 4)$. Also, note when expanded, our original equation has a y^2-term, but no x^2-term.

7. $\frac{x^2}{49} + \frac{y^2}{100} = 1 \Rightarrow \frac{x^2}{7^2} + \frac{y^2}{10^2} = 1$ The graph of this equation is an ellipse centered at the origin and x-intercepts of 7 and –7, and y-intercepts of 10 and –10. Also, note in our original equation, the x^2- and y^2-terms both have different positive coefficients.

9. $\frac{x^2}{4} - \frac{y^2}{16} = 1 \Rightarrow \frac{x^2}{2^2} - \frac{y^2}{4^2} = 1$ The graph of this equation is a hyperbola centered at the origin with x-intercepts of 2 and –2, and asymptotes of $y = \pm \frac{4}{2}x = \pm 2x$. Also, note in our original equation, the x^2- and y^2-terms have coefficient that are opposite in sign.

11. $\frac{x^2}{25} - \frac{y^2}{25} = 1 \Rightarrow \frac{x^2}{5^2} - \frac{y^2}{5^2} = 1$ The graph of this equation is a hyperbola centered at the origin with x-intercepts of 5 and –5, and asymptotes of $y = \pm \frac{5}{5}x = \pm x$. Also, note in our original equation, the x^2- and y^2-terms have coefficients that are opposite in sign.

13. $\dfrac{x^2}{4} = 1 - \dfrac{y^2}{9} \Rightarrow \dfrac{x^2}{4} + \dfrac{y^2}{9} = 1 \Rightarrow \dfrac{(x-0)^2}{2^2} + \dfrac{(y-0)^2}{3^2} = 1$ The equation is of the form $\dfrac{(x-h)^2}{b^2} + \dfrac{(y-k)^2}{a^2} = 1$

with $a = 3$, $b = 2$, $h = 0$, and $k = 0$, so the graph of the given equation is an ellipse.

15. $\dfrac{(x+3)^2}{16} + \dfrac{(y-2)^2}{16} = 1 \Rightarrow (x+3)^2 + (y-2)^2 = 16 \Rightarrow [x-(-3)]^2 + (y-2)^2 = 4^2$ The equation is of the

form $(x-h)^2 + (y-k)^2 = r^2$ with $r = 4$, $h = -3$, and $k = 2$, so the graph of the given equation is a circle.

17. $x^2 - 6x + y = 0 \Rightarrow y = -x^2 + 6x \Rightarrow y = -(x^2 - 6x + 9 - 9) \Rightarrow y = -(x-3)^2 + 9 \Rightarrow y - 9 = -(x-3)^2$

The equation is of the form $y - k = a(x-h)^2$ with $a = -1$, $h = 3$, and $k = 9$, so the graph of the given equation is a parabola.

19. $4(x-3)^2 + 3(y+4)^2 = 0 \Rightarrow \dfrac{4(x-3)^2}{12} + \dfrac{3(y+4)^2}{12} = 0 \Rightarrow \dfrac{(x-3)^2}{3} + \dfrac{[y-(-4)]^2}{4} = 0$

The graph is the point $(3, -4)$.

21. $x - 4y^2 - 8y = 0 \Rightarrow x = 4y^2 + 8y \Rightarrow x = 4(y^2 + 2y + 1 - 1) \Rightarrow x = 4(y+1)^2 - 4 \Rightarrow x - (-4) = 4[y - (-1)]^2$

The equation is of the form $x - h = a(y-k)^2$ with $a = 4$, $h = -4$, and $k = -1$, so the graph of the given equation is a parabola.

23. $6x^2 - 12x + 6y^2 - 18y + 25 = 0 \Rightarrow 6(x^2 - 2x + 1 - 1) + 6\left(y^2 - 3y + \tfrac{9}{4} - \tfrac{9}{4}\right) = -25 \Rightarrow$

$6(x^2 - 2x + 1) - 6 + 6\left(y^2 - 3y + \tfrac{9}{4}\right) - \tfrac{27}{2} = -25 \Rightarrow 6(x-1)^2 + 6\left(y - \tfrac{3}{2}\right)^2 = -25 + 6 + \tfrac{27}{2}$

$6(x-1)^2 + 6\left(y - \tfrac{3}{2}\right)^2 = -\tfrac{50}{2} + \tfrac{12}{2} + \tfrac{27}{2} \Rightarrow 6(x-1)^2 + 6\left(y - \tfrac{3}{2}\right)^2 = -\tfrac{11}{2} \Rightarrow (x-1)^2 + \left(y - \tfrac{3}{2}\right)^2 = -\tfrac{11}{12}$

A sum of squares can never be negative. This equation has no graph.

25. $x^2 = 4y - 8 \Rightarrow x^2 = 4(y-2) \Rightarrow y - 2 = \tfrac{1}{4}(x-0)^2$ The equation is of the form $y - k = a(x-h)^2$ with

$a = \tfrac{1}{4}$, $h = 0$, and $k = 2$, so the graph of the given equation is a parabola with vertex $(0, 2)$ and vertical axis

$x = 0$ (the y-axis). Use the vertex and axis and plot a few additional points.

27. $x^2 = 25 + y^2 \Rightarrow x^2 - y^2 = 25 \Rightarrow \dfrac{x^2}{25} - \dfrac{y^2}{25} = 1 \Rightarrow \dfrac{(x-0)^2}{5^2} - \dfrac{(y-0)^2}{5^2} = 1$ The equation is of the form

$\dfrac{(x-h)^2}{a^2} - \dfrac{(y-k)^2}{b^2} = 1$ with $a = 5$, $b = 5$, $h = 0$, and $k = 0$, so the graph of the given equation is a hyperbola

with center $(0, 0)$, vertices $(-5, 0)$ and $(5, 0)$, and asymptotes $y = \pm x$.

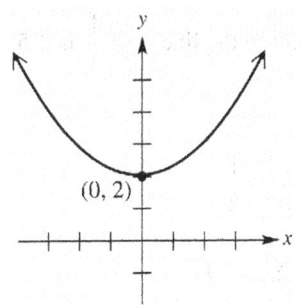

Figure 25

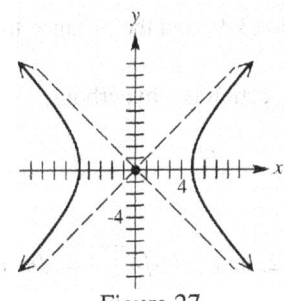

Figure 27

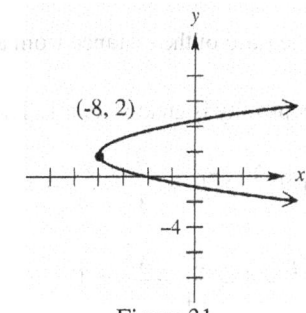

Figure 31

29. $\dfrac{x^2}{4}+\dfrac{y^2}{4}=-1 \Rightarrow x^2+y^2=-4$ A sum of squares can never be negative. This equation has no graph.

31. $y^2-4y=x+4 \Rightarrow y^2-4y+4-4=x+4 \Rightarrow (y-2)^2-4=x+4 \Rightarrow x+8=(y-2)^2 \Rightarrow$

    $x-(-8)=(y-2)^2$ The equation is of the form $x-h=a(y-k)^2$ with $a=1$, $h=-8$, and $k=2$, so the graph of the given equation is a parabola with vertex (−8, 2) and horizontal axis $y=2$.

33. $3x^2+6x+3y^2-12y=12 \Rightarrow x^2+2x+y^2-4y=4 \Rightarrow (x^2+2x+1-1)+(y^2-4y+4-4)=4$

    $(x+1)^2-1+(y-2)^2-4=4 \Rightarrow (x-1)^2+(y-2)^2=4+1+4 \Rightarrow (x+1)^2+(y-2)^2=9$

    $\Rightarrow [x-(-1)]^2+(y-2)^2=3^2$ The equation is of the form $(x-h)^2+(y-k)^2=r^2$ with $r=3$, $h=-1$, and $k=2$, so the graph of the given equation is a circle with center (−1, 2) and radius 3.

35. $4x^2-8x+9y^2-36y=-4 \Rightarrow 4(x^2-2x+1-1)+9(y^2-4y+4-4)=-4 \Rightarrow$

    $4(x-1)^2-4+9(y-2)^2-36=-4 \Rightarrow 4(x-1)^2+9(y-2)^2=36 \Rightarrow$

    $\dfrac{4(x-1)^2}{36}+\dfrac{9(y-2)^2}{36}=1 \Rightarrow \dfrac{(x-1)^2}{9}+\dfrac{(y-2)^2}{4}=1 \Rightarrow \dfrac{(x-1)^2}{3^2}+\dfrac{(y-2)^2}{2^2}=1$

    The equation is of the form $\dfrac{(x-h)^2}{a^2}+\dfrac{(y-k)^2}{b^2}=1$ with $a=3$, $b=2$, $h=1$, and $k=2$, so the graph of the given equation is an ellipse with center (1, 2) and vertices (−2, 2), (4, 2), (1, 0) and (1, 4).

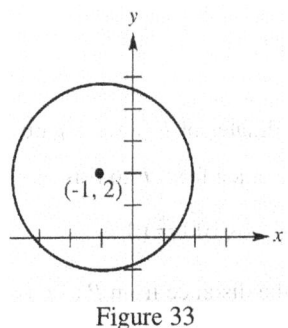

Figure 33

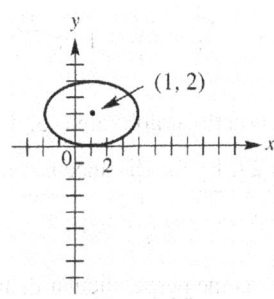

Figure 35

37. Since the sum of the distances from two points (foci) is a constant, the conic section is an ellipse.

356 CHAPTER 7 Analytic Geometry and Nonlinear Systems

39. Since the ratio of the distance from a point to (3, 0) and the distance from a point to the line $x = \frac{4}{3}$ is 1.5, the eccentricity is greater than 1. The conic section is a hyperbola.

41. $12x^2 + 9y^2 = 36 \Rightarrow \frac{x^2}{3} + \frac{y^2}{4} = 1 \Rightarrow a = 2, b = \sqrt{3}$, and $c = \sqrt{4-3} = 1$; $d = \frac{c}{a} = \frac{1}{2}$.

43. $x^2 - y^2 = 4 \Rightarrow \frac{x^2}{4} - \frac{y^2}{4} = 1 \Rightarrow a = 2, b = 2$, and $c = \sqrt{4+4} = \sqrt{8}$; $e = \frac{c}{a} = \frac{\sqrt{8}}{2} = \sqrt{2}$.

45. $4x^2 + 7y^2 = 28 \Rightarrow \frac{x^2}{7} + \frac{y^2}{4} = 1 \Rightarrow a = \sqrt{7}, b = 2$, and $c = \sqrt{7-4} = \sqrt{3}$; $e = \frac{c}{a} = \frac{\sqrt{3}}{\sqrt{7}} = \frac{\sqrt{21}}{7}$.

47. $x^2 - 9y^2 = 18 \Rightarrow \frac{x^2}{18} - \frac{y^2}{2} = 1 \Rightarrow a = \sqrt{18}, b = \sqrt{2}$, and $c = \sqrt{18+2} = \sqrt{20}$; $e = \frac{c}{a} = \frac{\sqrt{20}}{\sqrt{18}} = \frac{\sqrt{10}}{3}$.

49. Since $e = 1$, the conic is a parabola. With center $(0,0)$ and focus $(0,8)$, the equation is
$x^2 = 4cy \Rightarrow x^2 = 32y$.

51. Since $0 < e < 1$, the conic is an ellipse with $c = 3$. Now $\frac{c}{a} = e \Rightarrow \frac{3}{a} = \frac{1}{2} \Rightarrow a = 6$. For an ellipse,
$b^2 = a^2 - c^2 = 36 - 9 = 27$. The equation is $\frac{x^2}{36} + \frac{y^2}{27} = 1$.

53. Since $e > 1$, the conic is a hyperbola with $a = 6$. Now $\frac{c}{a} = e \Rightarrow \frac{c}{6} = 2 \Rightarrow c = 12$. For a hyperbola,
$b^2 = c^2 - a^2 = 144 - 36 = 108$. The equation is $\frac{x^2}{36} - \frac{y^2}{108} = 1$.

55. Since $e = 1$, the conic is a parabola. With center $(0,0)$ and focus $(0,-1)$, the equation is
$x^2 = 4cy \Rightarrow x^2 = -4y$.

57. Since $0 < e < 1$, the conic is an ellipse with $a = 3$. Now $\frac{c}{a} = e \Rightarrow \frac{c}{3} = \frac{4}{5} \Rightarrow c = \frac{12}{5}$. For an ellipse,
$b^2 = a^2 - c^2 = 9 - \frac{144}{25} = \frac{81}{25}$. The equation is $\frac{x^2}{\frac{81}{25}} + \frac{y^2}{9} = 1$ or $\frac{25x^2}{81} + \frac{y^2}{9} = 1$.

59. From the graph, the coordinates of P (a point on the graph) are $(-3, 8)$, the coordinates of F (a focus) are $(3, 0)$, the equation of L (the directrix) is $x = 27$. By the distance formula, the distance from P to F is
$\sqrt{(x_2 - x_1)^2 + (y_2 - y_1)^2} = \sqrt{[3-(-3)]^2 + (0-8)^2} = \sqrt{6^2 + (-8)^2} = \sqrt{36 + 64} = \sqrt{100} = 10$

The distance from a point to a line is defined as the perpendicular distance, so the distance from P to L is $|27 - (-3)| = 30$. Thus, $e = \frac{\text{Distance of } P \text{ from } F}{\text{Distance of } P \text{ from } L} = \frac{10}{30} = \frac{1}{3}$.

61. From the graph, we see that $F = \left(\sqrt{2}, 0\right)$ and L is the vertical line $x = -\sqrt{2}$. Choose $(0,0)$, the vertex of the parabola, as P. Distance of P from $F = \sqrt{2}$, and distance of P from $L = \sqrt{2}$. Thus, we have
$e = \frac{\text{Distance of } P \text{ from } F}{\text{Distance of } P \text{ from } L} = \frac{\sqrt{2}}{\sqrt{2}} = 1.$

63. From the graph, we see that $P = (9, -7.5)$, $F = (9, 0)$ and L is the vertical line $x = 4$. Distance of P from $F = 7.5$, and distance of P from $L = 5$. Thus, $e = \frac{\text{Distance of } P \text{ from } F}{\text{Distance of } P \text{ from } L} = \frac{7.5}{5} = 1.5.$

65. Add the equations to eliminate the y^2:

$x^2 + y^2 = 10$
$\underline{2x^2 - y^2 = 17}$
$3x^2 \quad\quad = 27 \Rightarrow x^2 = 9 \Rightarrow x = \pm 3.$

Substituting these values into [equation 1] yields $(-3)^2 + y^2 = 10 \Rightarrow y^2 = 1 \Rightarrow y = \pm 1$ and $(3)^2 + y^2 = 10 \Rightarrow y^2 = 1 \Rightarrow y = \pm 1$. The solution set is $\{(-3,1),(-3,-1),(3,1),(3,-1)\}$.

67. Multiply [equation 1] by 3 and subtract to eliminate the x^2:

$3x^2 + 6y^2 = 27$
$\underline{3x^2 - 4y^2 = 27}$
$\quad\quad 10y^2 = 0 \Rightarrow 10y^2 = 0 \Rightarrow y = 0.$

Substituting 0 into [equation 1] for y, yields $x^2 + 2(0)^2 = 9 \Rightarrow x^2 = 9 \Rightarrow x = \pm 3$. The solution set is $\{(3,0),(-3,0)\}$.

69. Multiply [equation 1] by 3 and [equation 2] by 2 and subtract to eliminate both x^2 and y^2:

$6x^2 + 6y^2 = 60$
$\underline{6x^2 + 6y^2 = 60}$
$\quad\quad 0 \quad\quad = 0 \Rightarrow$ infinite number of solutions. The solutions have the following relationship:
$2x^2 + 2y^2 = 20 \Rightarrow 2y^2 = 20 - 2x^2 \Rightarrow y^2 = 10 - x^2 \Rightarrow y = \pm\sqrt{10-x^2}$. The solution set is
$\left\{\left(x, -\sqrt{10-x^2}\right), \left(x, \sqrt{10-x^2}\right)\right\}$.

71. First solve [equation 2] for x: $x - y = -2 \Rightarrow x = y - 2$ [equation 3]. Now substitute $y - 2$ for x in
[equation 1]: $3(y-2)^2 + 2y^2 = 5 \Rightarrow 3(y^2 - 4y + 4) + 2y^2 = 5 \Rightarrow 3y^2 - 12y + 12 + 2y^2 - 5 = 0 \Rightarrow$
$5y^2 - 12y + 7 = 0 \Rightarrow (5y - 7)(y - 1) = 0 \Rightarrow y = 1$ or $\frac{7}{5}$. Substituting these values into [equation 3]
yields $x = (1) - 2 \Rightarrow x = -1$ and $x = \left(\frac{7}{5}\right) - 2 \Rightarrow x = -\frac{3}{5}$. The solution set is $\left\{\left(-\frac{3}{5}, \frac{7}{5}\right), (-1,1)\right\}$.

73. Add the equations to eliminate the y^2:

$x^2 + y^2 = 8$
$\underline{x^2 - y^2 = 0}$
$2x^2 = 8 \Rightarrow x^2 = 4 \Rightarrow x = \pm 2$.

Substituting these values into [equation 2] yields $(-2)^2 - y^2 = 0 \Rightarrow y^2 = 4 \Rightarrow y = \pm 2$ and $(2)^2 - y^2 = 0 \Rightarrow y^2 = 4 \Rightarrow y = \pm 2$ The solution set is $\{(-2,-2),(-2,2),(2,-2),(2,2)\}$.

75. Subtract the equations to eliminate both x^2 and y^2

$x^2 + xy + y^2 = 3$
$\underline{x^2 - xy + y^2 = 1}$
$ 2xy = 2 \Rightarrow y = \dfrac{1}{x}$

Substituting this result into [equation 2] yields $x^2 - x\left(\dfrac{1}{x}\right) + \left(\dfrac{1}{x}\right)^2 = 1 \Rightarrow x^2 - 1 + \dfrac{1}{x^2} = 1 \Rightarrow$

$x^4 - x^2 + 1 = x^2 \Rightarrow x^4 - 2x^2 + 1 = 0 \Rightarrow (x^2 - 1)(x^2 - 1) = 0 \Rightarrow x = \pm 1$. Substitute these values into

$y = \dfrac{1}{x}$ yields $y = \dfrac{1}{-1} = -1$ and $y = \dfrac{1}{1} = 1$ The solution set is $\{(1,1),(-1,-1)\}$.

77. Add the equations to eliminate both xy and y^2

$x^2 - xy + y^2 = 5$
$\underline{2x^2 + xy - y^2 = 10}$
$3x^2 = 15 \Rightarrow x^2 = 5 \Rightarrow x = \pm\sqrt{5}$

Substituting these results into [equation 1] yields $\left(-\sqrt{5}\right)^2 - \left(-\sqrt{5}\right)y + y^2 = 5 \Rightarrow 5 + \sqrt{5}y + y^2 = 5 \Rightarrow$

$y^2 + \sqrt{5}y = 0 \Rightarrow y(y + \sqrt{5}) = 0 \Rightarrow y = 0, -\sqrt{5}$ and $\left(\sqrt{5}\right)^2 - \left(\sqrt{5}\right)y + y^2 = 5 \Rightarrow 5 - \sqrt{5}y + y^2 = 5 \Rightarrow$

$y^2 - \sqrt{5}y = 0 \Rightarrow y(y - \sqrt{5}) = 0 \Rightarrow y = 0, \sqrt{5}$.

The solution set is $\{(\sqrt{5},0),(-\sqrt{5},0),(\sqrt{5},\sqrt{5}),(-\sqrt{5},-\sqrt{5})\}$.

79. First solve [equation 3] for y and substitute into [equation 2]:
$\begin{array}{l} 2x^2 + y^2 + 3z^2 = 3 \\ 2x + y - z = 1 \\ x + y = 0 \end{array}$

$x + y = 0 \Rightarrow y = -x$: $2x - x - z = 1 \Rightarrow x - z = 1 \Rightarrow z = x - 1$, Substituting $y = -x$ and $z = x - 1$ into

[equation 1] yields: $2x^2 + (-x)^2 + 3(x-1)^2 = 3 \Rightarrow 2x^2 + x^2 + 3x^2 - 6x + 3 = 3 \Rightarrow 6x^2 - 6x = 0 \Rightarrow$

$6x(x-1) = 0 \Rightarrow x = 0, 1$. Substitute these values to find y and z. $y = -(0) = 0$, $z = 0 - 1 = -1$ and

$y = -(1) = -1$, $z = 1 - 1 = 0$, The solution set is $\{(0,0,-1),(1,-1,0)\}$.

81. See Figure 81.

83. See Figure 83.

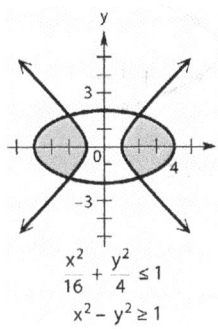
$\frac{x^2}{16} + \frac{y^2}{4} \leq 1$
$x^2 - y^2 \geq 1$
Figure 81

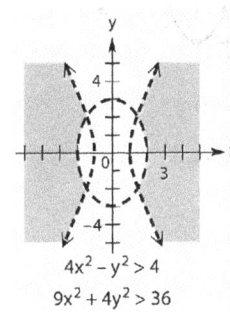
$4x^2 - y^2 > 4$
$9x^2 + 4y^2 > 36$
Figure 83

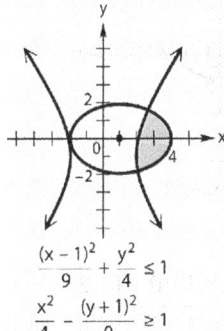
$\frac{(x-1)^2}{9} + \frac{y^2}{4} \leq 1$
$\frac{x^2}{4} - \frac{(y+1)^2}{9} \geq 1$
Figure 85

85. See Figure 85.

87. For an ellipse, $c = \sqrt{a^2 - b^2} = \sqrt{5013 - 4970} = \sqrt{43}$. The eccentricity is $e = \frac{c}{a} = \frac{\sqrt{43}}{\sqrt{5013}} \approx .093$.

89. (a) Earth orbits every $365 \cdot 24 \cdot 60 \cdot 60 = 31{,}536{,}000$ seconds. Thus $\frac{y^2}{16} - \frac{x^2}{9} = 1$ The maximum velocity of Earth is $v_{max} = \frac{2\pi(1.496 \times 10^8)}{31{,}536{,}000} \sqrt{\frac{1+.0167}{1-.0167}} \approx 30.3$ km per sec. The maximum velocity of Earth is $v_{min} = \frac{2\pi(1.496 \times 10^8)}{31{,}536{,}000} \sqrt{\frac{1+.0167}{1-.0167}} \approx 29.3$ km per sec.

(b) The minimum and maximum velocities are equal. Therefore, the planet's velocity is constant.

(c) A planet is at its maximum and minimum distances from a focus when it is located at the vertices of the ellipse. Thus the minimum and maximum velocities of a planet will occur at the vertices of the elliptical orbit, which are $a+c$ for the minimum and $a-c$ for the maximum.

91. Here $a+c = 94.6$ and $a-c = 91.4$. Solving these equations simultaneously results in $a = 93$ and $c = 1.6$. The eccentricity is $e = \frac{c}{a} = \frac{1.6}{93} \approx 0.0172$.

7.4: Parametric Equations

1.
t	-2	-1	0	1	2
x	-3	-1	1	3	5
y	-4	-3	-2	-1	0

3.
t	-2	-1	0	1	2
x	-1	0	1	2	3
y	3	0	-1	0	3

360 CHAPTER 7 Analytic Geometry and Nonlinear Systems

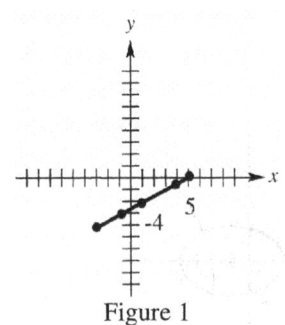
Figure 1

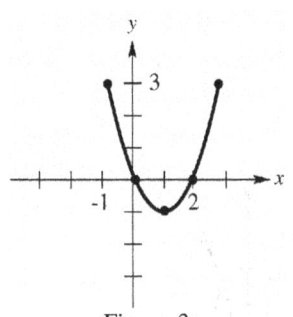
Figure 3

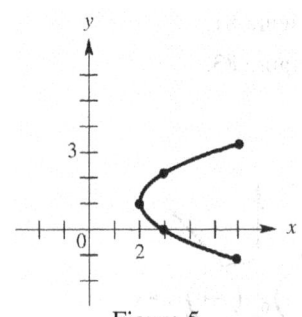
Figure 5

5.

t	-2	-1	0	1	2
x	6	3	2	3	6
y	3	2	1	0	1

7. See Figure 7. From the first equation, $x = 2t \Rightarrow t = \dfrac{1}{2}x$. By substitution in the second equation, $y = \dfrac{1}{2}x + 1$.

   When t is in $[-2, 3]$, the range of $x = 2t$ is x in $[-4, 6]$.

9. See Figure 9. From the first equation, $x = \sqrt{t} \Rightarrow t = x^2$. By substitution in the second equation,

   $y = 3x^2 - 4$. When t is in $[0, 4]$, the range of $x = \sqrt{t}$ is x in $[0, 2]$.

[-8,8] by [-8,8]
Xscl = 1   Yscl = 1

[-6,6] by [-6,10]
Xscl = 1   Yscl = 1

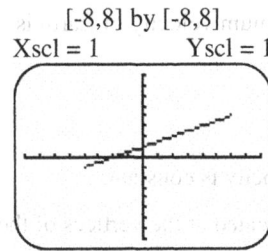
Figure 7

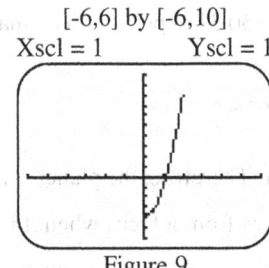
Figure 9

11. See Figure 11. From the first equation, $x = t^3 + 1 \Rightarrow t^3 = x - 1$. By substitution in the second equation,

    $y = x - 2$. When t is in $[-3, 3]$, the range of $x = t^3 + 1$ is x in $[-26, 28]$.

13. See Figure 13. From the second equation, $y = \sqrt{3t - 1} \Rightarrow t = \dfrac{y^2 + 1}{3}$. By substitution in the second equation,

    $x = 2^{(y^2+1)/3}$. When t is in $\left[\dfrac{1}{3}, 4\right]$, the range of $y = \sqrt{3t = -1}$ is y in $[0, \sqrt{11}]$.

| [-30,30] by [-30,30] | [-2,30] by [-2,10] | [-6,6] by [-4,4] | [-6,6] by [-4,4] |
| Xscl = 2   Yscl = 2 | Xscl = 1   Yscl = 1 | Xscl = 1   Yscl = 1 | Xscl = 1   Yscl = 1 |

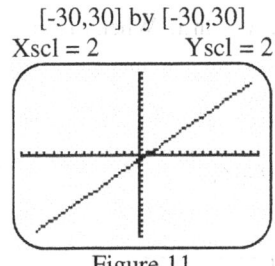 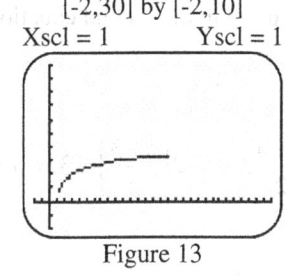 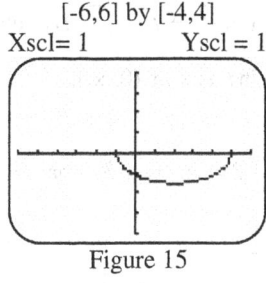 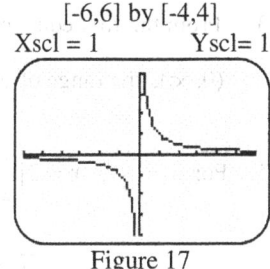

Figure 11 Figure 13 Figure 15 Figure 17

15. See Figure 15. From the first equation, $x = t + 2 \Rightarrow t = x - 2$. By substitution in the second equation, $y = -\frac{1}{2}\sqrt{9 - (x-2)^2}$. When t is in $[-3,3]$, the range of $x = t + 2$ is x in $[-1,5]$.

17. See Figure 17. From the first equation, $x = t \Rightarrow t = x$. By substitution in the second equation, $y = \frac{1}{x}$. When t is in $(-\infty, 0) \cup (0, \infty)$, the range of $x = t$ is x in $(-\infty, 0) \cup (0, \infty)$.

19. From the first equation, $x = 3t \Rightarrow t = \frac{1}{3}x$. By substitution in the second equation, $y = \frac{1}{3}x - 1$. When t is in $(-\infty, \infty)$, the range of $x = 3t$ is x in $(-\infty, \infty)$.

21. From the second equation, $y = t + 1 \Rightarrow t = y - 1$. By substitution in the first equation, $x = 3(y - 1)^2$. When t is in $(-\infty, \infty)$, the range of $y = t + 1$ is y in $(-\infty, \infty)$.

23. From the second equation, $y = 4t^3 \Rightarrow t = \sqrt[3]{\frac{y}{4}}$. By substitution in the first equation, $x = 3\left(\frac{y}{4}\right)^{2/3}$. When t is in $(-\infty, \infty)$, the range of $y = 4t^3$ is y in $(-\infty, \infty)$.

25. From the first equation, $x = t \Rightarrow t = x$. By substitution in the second equation, $y = \sqrt{x^2 + 2}$. When t is in $(-\infty, \infty)$, the range of $x = t$ is x in $(-\infty, \infty)$.

27. From the first equation, $x = e^t \Rightarrow t = \ln x$. By substitution in the second equation, $y = \frac{1}{x}$. When t is in $(-\infty, \infty)$, the range of $x = e^t$ is x in $(0, \infty)$.

29. From the first equation, $x = \frac{1}{\sqrt{t+2}} \Rightarrow t = \frac{1}{x^2} - 2$. By substitution in the second equation, $y = 1 - 2x^2$. When t is in $(-2, \infty)$, the range of $x = \frac{1}{\sqrt{t+2}}$ is x in $(0, \infty)$.

31. From the first equation, $x = t + 2 \Rightarrow t = x - 2$. By substitution in the second equation, $y = \frac{1}{x}$. When t has the restriction $t \neq 2$, the range of $x = t + 2$ has the restriction $x \neq 0$.

362   CHAPTER 7   Analytic Geometry and Nonlinear Systems

33. From the first equation, $x = t^2 \Rightarrow t = \sqrt{x}$. By substitution in the second equation, $y = \ln x$. When t is in $(0, \infty)$, the range of $x = \ln t$ is x in $(0, \infty)$.

35. For $x = \frac{1}{2}t$, $y = 2\left(\frac{1}{2}t\right) + 3 \Rightarrow y = t + 3$. For $x = \frac{t+3}{2}$, $y = 2\left(\frac{t+3}{2}\right) + 3 \Rightarrow y = t + 6$.

37. For $x = \frac{1}{3}t$, $y\sqrt{3\left(\frac{1}{3}t\right) + 2} \Rightarrow y = \sqrt{t+2}$ for t in $[-2, \infty)$. For $x = \frac{t-2}{3}$, $y = \sqrt{3\left(\frac{t-2}{3}\right) + 2} \Rightarrow y = \sqrt{t}$ for t in $[0, \infty)$.

39. For $x = t^3 + 1$, $t^3 + 1 = y^3 + 1 \Rightarrow y = t$. For $x = t$, $t = y^3 + 1 \Rightarrow y = \sqrt[3]{t-1}$.

41. For $x = \sqrt{t+1}$, $\sqrt{t+1} = \sqrt{y+1} \Rightarrow y = t$ for t in $[-1, \infty)$. For $x = \sqrt{t}$, $\sqrt{t} = \sqrt{y+1} \Rightarrow y+1 = t \Rightarrow y = t-1$ for t in $[0, \infty)$.

43. (a) Find t when $y = 0$. $400 \cdot \frac{\sqrt{2}}{2} t - 16t^2 = 0 \Rightarrow 16t^2 - 200\sqrt{2} t = 0 \Rightarrow t(16t - 200\sqrt{2}) = 0 \Rightarrow$

$16t - 200\sqrt{2} = 0 \Rightarrow 16t = 200\sqrt{2} \Rightarrow t = \frac{200\sqrt{2}}{16} \approx 17.7$ seconds.

(b) Find x when $t \approx 17.7$. $x = 400 \cdot \frac{\sqrt{2}}{2}(17.7) \approx 5000$ feet.

(c) Find y when $x \approx 8.85$ (half the total time). $y = 400 \cdot \frac{\sqrt{2}}{2}(8.85) - 16(8.85)^2 \approx 1250$ feet.

45. See Figure 45. From the first equation, $x = 60t \Rightarrow t = \frac{x}{60}$. By substitution in the second equation,

$y = 80\left(\frac{x}{60}\right) - 16\left(\frac{x}{60}\right)^2 \Rightarrow y = \frac{4}{3}x - \frac{x^2}{225}$.

[0,300] by [0,200]
Xscl = 50   Yscl = 50

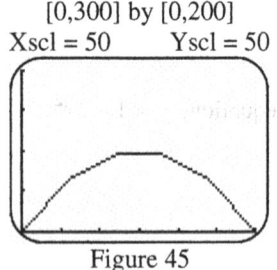

Figure 45

47. From the first equation, $x = v_0 \frac{\sqrt{2}}{2} t \Rightarrow t = \frac{2x}{v_0 \sqrt{2}}$. By substitution in the second equation,

$$y = v_0 \frac{\sqrt{2}}{2} \left(\frac{2x}{v_0 \sqrt{2}} \right) - 16 \left(\frac{2x}{v_0 \sqrt{2}} \right)^2 \Rightarrow y = x - \frac{32}{(v_0)^2} x^2.$$

49. A line through (x_1, y_1) with slope m is given by $y - y_1 = m(x - x_1)$. For $x = t$, $y - y_1 = m(t - x_1)$.

    For $t = x - x_1$, $y - y_1 = mt \Rightarrow y = mt + y_1$. Many answers are possible.

Reviewing Basic Concepts (Sections 7.3 and 7.4)

1. $3x^2 + y^2 - 6x + 6y = 0 \Rightarrow 3(x^2 - 2x + 1) + (y^2 + 6y + 9) = 0 + 3 + 9 \Rightarrow$

   $3(x-1)^2 + (y+3)^2 = 12 \Rightarrow \frac{(x-1)^2}{4} + \frac{(y+3)^2}{12} = 1$; ellipse centered at $(1, -3)$.

2. $y^2 - 2x^2 + 8y - 8x - 4 = 0 \Rightarrow (y^2 + 8y + 16) - 2(x^2 + 4x + 4) = 4 + 16 - 8 \Rightarrow$

   $(y+4)^2 - 2(x+2)^2 = 12 \Rightarrow \frac{(y+4)^2}{12} - \frac{(x+2)^2}{6} = 1$; hyperbola centered at $(-4, -2)$.

3. $3y^2 + 12y + 5x = 3 \Rightarrow 3(y^2 + 4y + 4) = -5x + 3 + 12 \Rightarrow 3(y+2)^2 = -5(x-3) \Rightarrow (y+2)^2 = \frac{5}{3}(x-3)$;

   parabola with center $(3, -2)$ that opens to the left.

4. $x^2 + 25y^2 = 25 \Rightarrow \frac{x^2}{25} + \frac{y^2}{1} = 1 \Rightarrow a = 5$, $b = 1$, and $c = \sqrt{25-1} = \sqrt{24}$. $e = \frac{c}{a} = \frac{\sqrt{24}}{5} = \frac{2\sqrt{6}}{5}$.

5. $8y^2 - 4x^2 = 8 \Rightarrow \frac{y^2}{1} - \frac{x^2}{2} = 1 \Rightarrow a = 1$, $b = \sqrt{2}$, and $c = \sqrt{1+2} = \sqrt{3}$. $e = \frac{c}{a} = \frac{\sqrt{3}}{1} = \sqrt{3}$.

6. $3x^2 + 4y^2 = 108 \Rightarrow \frac{x^2}{36} + \frac{y^2}{27} = 1 \Rightarrow a = 6$, $b = \sqrt{27}$, and $c = \sqrt{36-27} = \sqrt{9}$. $e = \frac{c}{a} = \frac{3}{6} = \frac{1}{2}$.

7. Since $e = 1$, the conic is a parabola. With center $(0, 0)$ and focus $(-2, 0)$, the equation is

   $y^2 = 4cx \Rightarrow y^2 = -8x$.

8. The ellipse is centered between the foci at $(0,0)$. The major axis is horizontal with $a = 5$. Since the foci are $(\pm 3, 0)$, we know that $c = 3$. Since $c^2 = a^2 - b^2$, the value of b can be found by substitution.

   $b^2 = a^2 - c^2 = 5^2 - 3^2 = 25 - 9 = 16 \Rightarrow b = 4$. The equation is $\dfrac{x^2}{25} + \dfrac{y^2}{16} = 1$.

9. The hyperbola has a vertical transverse axis with $c = 5$. The vertices are $(0, \pm 4)$, so $a = 4$. The center is located between the foci at $(0,0)$. Since $c^2 = a^2 + b^2$, the value of b can be found by substitution.

   $b^2 = c^2 - a^2 = 5^2 - 4^2 = 25 - 16 = 9 \Rightarrow b = 3$. The equation is $\dfrac{y^2}{16} - \dfrac{x^2}{9} = 1$.

10. The center is located between the vertices at $(0, 0)$. The hyperbola has a horizontal transverse axis with $a = 3$. From the asymptotes, $\dfrac{b}{a} = \dfrac{2}{3}$ with. $a = 3 \Rightarrow b = 2$. The equation is $\dfrac{x^2}{9} - \dfrac{y^2}{4} = 1$.

11. Add 2 multiplied by [equation 1] to equation 2 to eliminate x^2:

    $4x^2 + 2y^2 = 18$
    $-4x^2 + 3y^2 = 27$
    $\overline{5y^2 = 45} \Rightarrow y^2 = 9 \Rightarrow y = \pm 3$

    Substitute these values into [equation 1] to solve for x: $2x^2 + (3)^2 = 9 \Rightarrow 2x^2 = 0 \Rightarrow x = 0$,

    $2x^2 + (-3)^2 = 9 \Rightarrow 2x^2 = 0 \Rightarrow x = 0$, The solution set is $\{(0, -3), (0, 3)\}$.

12. See Figure 12.

13. Using a vertical minor axis, $b = 9$. The major axis has length 30, so $a = 15$. The equation is

    $\dfrac{x^2}{225} + \dfrac{y^2}{81} = 1$. When $x = 6$, $\dfrac{6^2}{225} + \dfrac{y^2}{81} = 1 \Rightarrow \dfrac{y^2}{81} = 1 - \dfrac{36}{225} \Rightarrow y^2 = 81\left(1 - \dfrac{36}{225}\right) \Rightarrow$

    $y = \sqrt{81\left(1 - \dfrac{36}{225}\right)} \approx 8.25$ feet.

14. (a) See Figure 14.

(b) From the first equation, $x = 2t \Rightarrow t = \dfrac{x}{2}$. By substitution in the second equation, $y = \sqrt{\dfrac{x^2}{4} + 1}$.

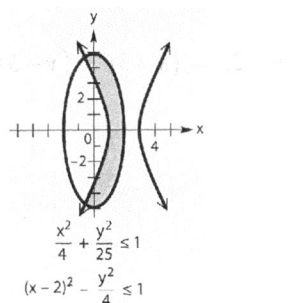

Figure 12

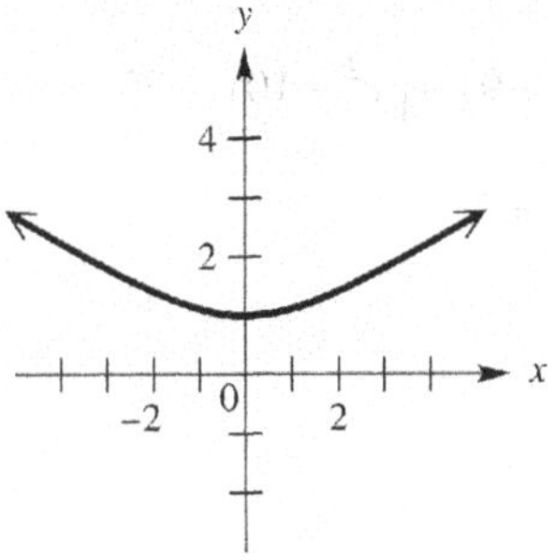

Figure 14

Chapter 7 Review Exercises

1. Here $h = -2$, $k = 3$, and $r^2 = 5^2 = 25$. The equation is $(x+2)^2 + (y-3)^2 = 25$. See Figure 1. From the figure, the domain is $[-7, 3]$, and the range is $[-2, 8]$.

2. Here $h = \sqrt{5}$, $k = -\sqrt{7}$, and $r^2 = \left(\sqrt{3}\right)^2 = 3$. The equation is $\left(x - \sqrt{5}\right)^2 + \left(y + \sqrt{7}\right)^2 = 3$. See Figure 2. From the figure, the domain is $\left[\sqrt{5} - \sqrt{3}, \sqrt{5} + \sqrt{3}\right]$, and the range is $\left[-\sqrt{7} - \sqrt{3}, -\sqrt{7} + \sqrt{3}\right]$.

3. The radius is the distance between $(-8, 1)$ and $(0, 16)$. $r = \sqrt{(0 - (-8))^2 + (16 - 1)^2} = \sqrt{64 + 225} = 17$. Here $h = -8$, $k = 1$, and $r^2 = 17^2 = 289$. The equation is $(x+8)^2 + (y-1)^2 = 289$. See Figure 3. From the figure, the domain is $[-25, 9]$, and the range is $[-16, 18]$.

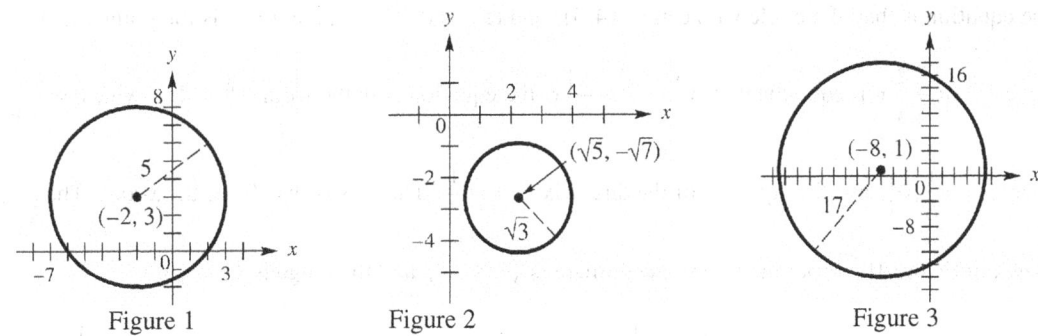

Figure 1   Figure 2   Figure 3

4. If the center is $(3, -6)$, the circle must touch the x-axis at the point $(3, 0)$. The radius is 6. Here $h = 3$, $k = -6$, and $r^2 = 6^2 = 36$. The equation is $(x-3)^2 + (y+6)^2 = 36$. See Figure 4. From the figure, the domain is $[-3, 9]$, and the range is $[-12, 0]$.

5. $x^2 - 4x + y^2 + 6y + 12 = 0 \Rightarrow (x^2 - 4x + 4) + (y^2 + 6y + 9) = -12 + 4 + 9 \Rightarrow (x-2)^2 + (y+3)^2 = 1.$

   The circle has center $(2, -3)$, and radius $r = 1$.

6. $x^2 - 6x + y^2 - 10y + 30 = 0 \Rightarrow (x^2 - 6x + 9) + (y^2 - 10y + 25) = -30 + 9 + 25 \Rightarrow (x-3)^2 + (y-5)^2 = 4.$

   The circle has center $(3, 5)$, and radius $r = 2$.

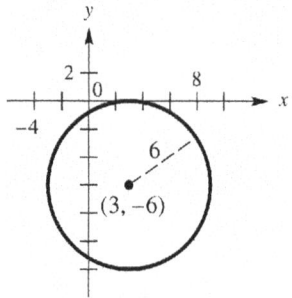

Figure 4

7. $2x^2 + 14x + 2y^2 + 6y = -2 \Rightarrow x^2 + 7x + y^2 + 3y = -1 \Rightarrow$

   $\left(x^2 + 7x + \frac{49}{4}\right) + \left(y^2 + 3y + \frac{9}{4}\right) = -1 + \frac{49}{4} + \frac{9}{4} \Rightarrow \left(x + \frac{7}{2}\right)^2 + \left(y + \frac{3}{2}\right)^2 = \frac{54}{4}.$

   The circle has center $\left(-\frac{7}{2}, -\frac{3}{2}\right)$, and radius $r = \frac{\sqrt{54}}{2} = \frac{3\sqrt{6}}{2}$.

8. $3x^2 + 3y^2 + 33x - 15y = 0 \Rightarrow x^2 + 11x + y^2 - 5 = 0 \Rightarrow$

   $\left(x^2 + 11x + \frac{121}{4}\right) + \left(y^2 - 5y + \frac{25}{4}\right) = 0 + \frac{121}{4} + \frac{25}{4} \Rightarrow \left(x + \frac{11}{2}\right)^2 + \left(y - \frac{5}{2}\right)^2 = \frac{146}{4}.$

   The circle has center $\left(-\frac{11}{2}, \frac{5}{2}\right)$, and radius $r = \frac{\sqrt{146}}{2}$.

9. The equation is that of a circle with center $(4, 5)$, and radius 0. That is, the graph is the point $(4, 5)$.

10. Since $y^2 = -\frac{2}{3}x$ is equivalent to $y^2 = 4\left(-\frac{1}{6}\right)x$, the equation is in the form $y^2 = 4cx$ with $c = -\frac{1}{6}$. The focus is $\left(-\frac{1}{6}, 0\right)$, and the equation of the directrix is $x = \frac{1}{6}$. The axis is $y = 0$, or the x-axis. The graph is shown in Figure 10. From the figure, the domain is $(-\infty, 0]$, and the range is $(-\infty, \infty)$.

11. Since $y^2 = 2x$ is equivalent to $y^2 = 4\left(\frac{1}{2}\right)x$, the equation is in the form $y^2 = 4cx$ with $c = \frac{1}{2}$. The focus is $\left(\frac{1}{2}, 0\right)$, and the equation of the directrix is $x = -\frac{1}{2}$. The axis is $y = 0$, or the x-axis. The graph is shown in Figure 11. From the figure, the domain is $[0, \infty)$, and the range is $(-\infty, \infty)$.

12. Since $3x^2 - y = 0$ is equivalent to $x^2 = 4\left(\dfrac{1}{12}\right)y$, the equation is in the form $x^2 = 4cy$ with $c = \dfrac{1}{12}$. The focus is $\left(0, \dfrac{1}{12}\right)$, and the equation of the directrix is $y = -\dfrac{1}{12}$. The axis is $x = 0$, or the y-axis. The graph is shown in Figure 12. From the figure, the domain is $(-\infty, \infty)$, and the range is $[0, \infty)$.

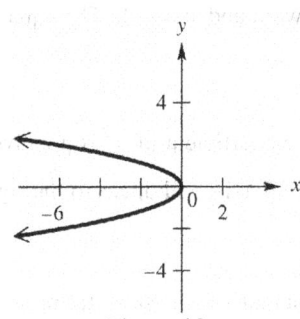
Figure 10

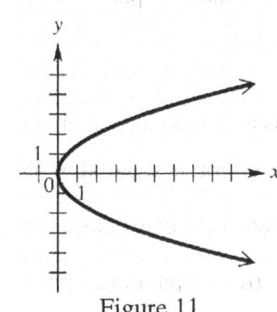
Figure 11

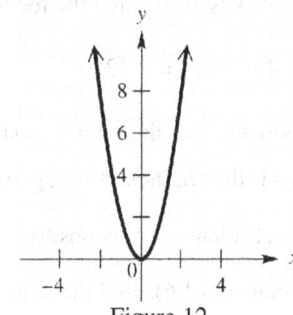
Figure 12

13. Since $x^2 + 2y = 0$ is equivalent to $x^2 = 4\left(-\dfrac{1}{2}\right)y$, the equation is in the form $x^2 = 4cy$ with $c = -\dfrac{1}{2}$. The focus is $\left(0, -\dfrac{1}{2}\right)$, and the equation of the directrix is $y = \dfrac{1}{2}$. The axis is $x = 0$, or the y-axis. The graph is shown in Figure 13. From the figure, the domain is $(-\infty, \infty)$, and the range is $(-\infty, 0]$.

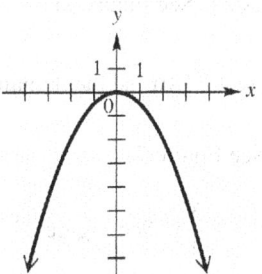
Figure 13

14. If the vertex is $(0,0)$, and the focus is $(4,0)$, then the parabola opens to the right and $c = 4$. The equation is

$$y^2 = 4cx \Rightarrow y^2 = 16x.$$

15. If the vertex is $(0,0)$, and the parabola opens to the right, the equation is in the form $y^2 = 4cx$. Find the value of c by using the fact that the parabola passes through $(2,5)$. Thus, $(5)^2 = 4c(2) \Rightarrow c = \dfrac{25}{8}$. The equation is $y^2 = 4cx \Rightarrow y^2 = \dfrac{25}{2}x$.

16. If the vertex is $(0,0)$, and the parabola opens downward, the equation is in the form $x^2 = 4cy$. Find the value of c by using the fact that the parabola passes through $(3,-4)$. Thus, $(3)^2 = 4c(-4) \Rightarrow c = -\frac{9}{16}$. The equation is $x^2 = 4cy \Rightarrow x^2 = -\frac{9}{4}y$.

17. If the vertex is $(0,0)$, and the focus is $(0,-3)$, then the parabola opens downward and $c = -3$. The equation is $x^2 = 4cy \Rightarrow x^2 = -12y$.

18. If the equation has the x-term squared, it has a vertical axis, and opens up if the coefficient of x^2 is positive or down if the coefficient is negative. If the y-term is squared, it has a horizontal axis, and opens to the right if the coefficient of y^2 is positive or to the left if the coefficient is negative.

19. If the focus is $(2,6)$, and the vertex is t$(-5,6)$, the parabola opens to the right and $c = 7$. Substituting in $(y-k)^2 = 4c(x-h)$, we get $(y-6)^2 = -28(x+5)$.

20. If the focus is $(4,5)$, and the vertex is $(4,3)$, the parabola opens upward and $c = 2$. Substituting in $(x-h)^2 = 4c(y-k)$, we get $(x-4)^2 = 8(y-3)$.

21. $\frac{x^2}{5} + \frac{y^2}{9} = 1 \Rightarrow a = 3$ and $b = \sqrt{5}$. The endpoints of the major axis (vertices) are $(0,\pm 3)$, so the range is $[-3,3]$, The endpoints of the minor axis are $(\pm\sqrt{5},0)$, so the domain is $[-\sqrt{5},\sqrt{5}]$. See Figure 21.

22. $\frac{x^2}{16} + \frac{y^2}{4} = 1 \Rightarrow a = 4$ and $b = 2$. The endpoints of the major axis (vertices) are $(\pm 4,0)$, so the domain is $[-4,4]$. The endpoints of the minor axis are $(0,\pm 2)$, so the range is $[-2,2]$. See Figure 22.

23. The transverse axis is horizontal with $a = 8$ and $b = 6$. The asymptotes are $y = \pm\frac{3}{4}x$. See Figure 23. The domain is $(-\infty,-8]\cup[8,\infty)$, and the range is $(-\infty,\infty)$. The vertices are $(-8,0)$ and $(8,0)$.

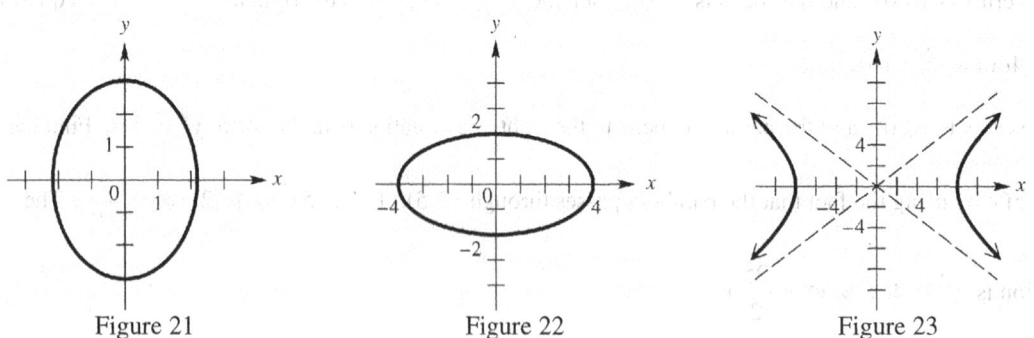

Figure 21   Figure 22   Figure 23

24. The transverse axis is vertical with $a = 5$ and $b = 3$. The asymptotes are $y = \pm\frac{5}{3}x$. See Figure 24. The domain is $(-\infty,\infty)$, and the range is $(-\infty,-5]\cup[5,\infty)$. The vertices are $(0,-5)$ and $(0,5)$.

25. The ellipse is centered at $(3,-1)$. The major axis is horizontal and has length $2a = 4$, so the vertices are $(1,-1)$ and $(5,-1)$. The length of the minor axis is $2b = 2$. The graph is shown in Figure 25. The domain is $[1,5]$, and the range is $[-2,0]$.

26. The ellipse is centered at $(2,-3)$. The major axis is horizontal and has length $2a = 6$, so the vertices are $(-1,-3)$ and $(5,-3)$. The length of the minor axis is $2b = 4$. The graph is shown in Figure 26. The domain is $[-1,5]$ and the range is $[-5,-1]$.

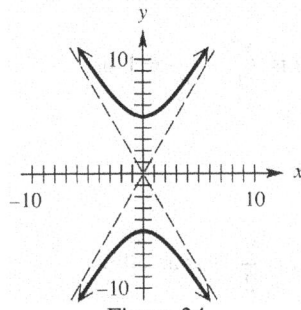
Figure 24

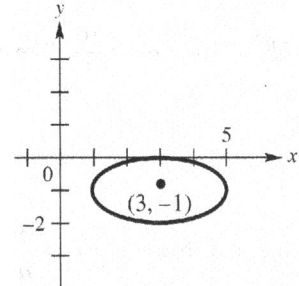
Figure 25

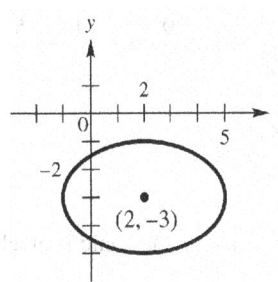
Figure 26

27. The center is $(-3,-2)$ and the transverse axis is vertical with $a = 2$ and $b = 3$. See Figure 27. The domain is $(-\infty,\infty)$ and the range is $(-\infty,-4] \cup [0,\infty)$. The vertices are $(-3,-4)$ and $(-3,0)$.

28. The center is $(-1,2)$ and the transverse axis is horizontal with $a = 4$ and $b = 2$. See Figure 28. The domain is $(-\infty,-5] \cup [3,\infty)$ and the range is $(-\infty,\infty)$. The vertices are $(-5,2)$ and $(3,2)$.

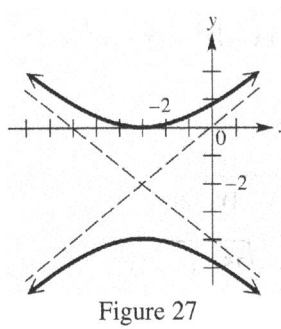
Figure 27

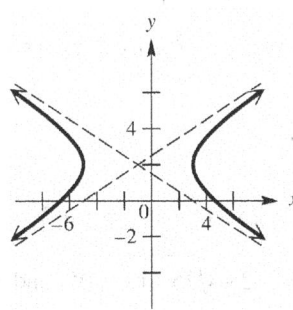
Figure 28

29. The major axis is vertical with $a = 4$. Since one focus is $(0,2)$, we know that $c = 2$. Since $c^2 = a^2 - b^2$, the value of b can be found by substitution: $b^2 = a^2 - c^2 = 4^2 - 2^2 = 16 - 4 = 12 \Rightarrow b = \sqrt{12}$. The equation is $\dfrac{x^2}{12} + \dfrac{y^2}{16} = 1$.

30. The major axis is horizontal with $a = 6$. Since one focus is $(-2,0)$, we know that $c = 2$. Since $c^2 = a^2 - b^2$, the value of b can be found by substitution: $b^2 = a^2 - c^2 = 6^2 - 2^2 = 36 - 4 = 32 \Rightarrow b = \sqrt{32}$. The equation is $\dfrac{x^2}{36} + \dfrac{y^2}{32} = 1$.

370 CHAPTER 7 Analytic Geometry and Nonlinear Systems

31. The hyperbola has a vertical transverse axis with $c = 5$. The y-intercepts coincide with the vertices so $a = 4$.

    Since $c^2 = a^2 + b^2$, the value of b can be found by substitution:

    $b^2 = c^2 - a^2 = 5^2 - 4^2 = 25 - 16 = 9 \Rightarrow b = 3$. The equation is $\dfrac{y^2}{16} - \dfrac{x^2}{9} = 1$.

32. The hyperbola has a vertical transverse axis. The y-intercept coincides with a vertex so $a = 2$. The equation

    is of the form $\dfrac{y^2}{a^2} - \dfrac{x^2}{b^2} = 1$. By substitution using the point (2, 3):

    $\dfrac{3^2}{2^2} - \dfrac{2^2}{b^2} = 1 \Rightarrow \dfrac{9}{4} - 1 = \dfrac{4}{b^2} \Rightarrow \dfrac{5}{4} = \dfrac{4}{b^2} \Rightarrow 5b^2 = 16 \Rightarrow b^2 = \dfrac{16}{5}$. The equation is $\dfrac{y^2}{4} - \dfrac{x^2}{\frac{16}{5}} = 1$ or

    $\dfrac{y^2}{4} - \dfrac{5x^2}{16} = 1$.

33. Since $0 < e < 1$, the conic is an ellipse with $c = 3$. Now $\dfrac{c}{a} = e \Rightarrow \dfrac{3}{a} = \dfrac{2}{3} \Rightarrow a = \dfrac{9}{2}$. For an ellipse,

    $b^2 = a^2 - c^2 = \dfrac{81}{4} - 9 = \dfrac{45}{4}$. The equation is $\dfrac{x^2}{\frac{45}{4}} + \dfrac{y^2}{\frac{81}{4}} = 1$ or $\dfrac{4x^2}{45} + \dfrac{4y^2}{81} = 1$.

34. Since $e > 1$, the conic is a hyperbola with $c = 5$. Now $\dfrac{c}{a} = e \Rightarrow \dfrac{5}{a} = \dfrac{5}{2} \Rightarrow a = 2$. For a hyperbola,

    $b^2 = c^2 - a^2 = 25 - 4 = 21$. The equation is $\dfrac{x^2}{4} - \dfrac{y^2}{21} = 1$.

35. (a) $x^2 + y^2 + 2x + 6y - 15 = 0 \Rightarrow x^2 + 2x + 1 + y^2 + 6y + 9 = 15 + 9 + 1 \Rightarrow (x+1)^2 + (y+3)^2 = 25$;

    The center is $(-1, -3)$.

    (b) The radius is $r = \sqrt{25} = 5$.

    (c) $(x+1)^2 + (y+3)^2 = 25 \Rightarrow (y+3)^2 = 25 - (x+1)^2 \Rightarrow y + 3 = \pm\sqrt{25 - (x+1)^2} \Rightarrow$

    $y = -3 \pm \sqrt{25 - (x+1)^2}$; Graph $y = -3 - \sqrt{25 - (x+1)^2}$ and $y = -3 + \sqrt{25 - (x+1)^2}$.

36. D. $4x^2 + y^2 = 36 \Rightarrow \dfrac{x^2}{9} + \dfrac{y^2}{36} = 1$; This is an ellipse with major axis on the y-axis.

37. E. $x = 2y^2 + 3 \Rightarrow 4\left(\dfrac{1}{8}\right)(x - 3) = (y - 0)^2$; This is a parabola that opens to the right.

38. A. $(x-1)^2 + (y+2)^2 = 36$; This is a circle with center $(1, -2)$ and radius 6.

39. C. $\dfrac{x^2}{36} + \dfrac{y^2}{9} = 1$; This is an ellipse with major axis on the x-axis.

40. B. $(y-1)^2 - (x-2)^2 = 36 \Rightarrow \dfrac{(y-1)^2}{36} - \dfrac{(x-2)^2}{36} = 1$; This is a hyperbola with center $(2, 1)$.

41. F. $y^2 = 36 + 4x^2 \Rightarrow y^2 - 4x^2 = 36 \Rightarrow \dfrac{y^2}{36} - \dfrac{x^2}{9} = 1$; This is a hyperbola with transverse axis on the y-axis.

42. $4x^2+8x+25y^2-250y=-529 \Rightarrow 4(x^2+2x)+25(y^2-10y)=-529 \Rightarrow$

$4(x^2+2x+1)+25(y^2-10y+25)=-529+4+625 \Rightarrow 4(x+1)^2+25(y-5)^2=100 \Rightarrow$

$\dfrac{(x+1)^2}{25}+\dfrac{(y-5)^2}{4}=1$; The center is $(-1,5)$. The vertices are $(-1-5,5),(-1+5,5)$ or $(-6,5),(4,5)$.

43. $5x^2+20x+2y^2-8y=-18 \Rightarrow 5(x^2+4x)+2(y^2-4y)=-18 \Rightarrow$

$5(x^2+4x+4)+2(y^2-4y+4)=-18+20+8 \Rightarrow 5(x+2)^2+2(y-2)^2=10 \Rightarrow$

$\dfrac{(x+2)^2}{2}+\dfrac{(y-2)^2}{5}=1$; The center is $(-2,2)$. The vertices are $\left(-2,2-\sqrt{5}\right),\left(-2,2+\sqrt{5}\right)$.

44. $x^2+4x-4y^2+24y=36 \Rightarrow (x^2+4x+4)-4(y^2-6y+9)=36+4-36 \Rightarrow$

$(x+2)^2-4(y-3)^2=4 \Rightarrow \dfrac{(x+2)^2}{4}-\dfrac{(y-3)^2}{1}=1$. The center is $(-2,3)$. The vertices are

$(-2-2,3),(-2+2,0)$ or $(-4,3),(0,3)$.

45. $4y^2+8y-3x^2+6x=11 \Rightarrow 4(y^2+2y+1)-3(x^2-2x+1)=11+4-3 \Rightarrow$

$4(y+1)^2-3(x-1)^2=12 \Rightarrow \dfrac{(y+1)^2}{3}-\dfrac{(x-1)^2}{4}=1$. The center is $(1,-1)$.

The vertices are $\left(1,-1-\sqrt{3}\right),\left(1,-1+\sqrt{3}\right)$.

46. $9x^2+25y^2=225 \Rightarrow \dfrac{x^2}{25}+\dfrac{y^2}{9}=1 \Rightarrow a=5, b=3$, and $c=\sqrt{25-9}=4; e=\dfrac{c}{a}=\dfrac{4}{5}$

47. $4x^2+9y^2=36 \Rightarrow \dfrac{x^2}{9}+\dfrac{y^2}{4}=1 \Rightarrow a=3, b=2$, and $c=\sqrt{9-4}=\sqrt{5}; e=\dfrac{c}{a}=\dfrac{\sqrt{5}}{3}$

48. $9x^2-y^2=9 \Rightarrow \dfrac{x^2}{1}-\dfrac{y^2}{9}=1 \Rightarrow a=1, b=3$, and $c=\sqrt{1+9}=\sqrt{10}; e=\dfrac{c}{a}=\dfrac{\sqrt{10}}{1}=\sqrt{10}$

49. The parabola opens to the right so the equation has the form $(y-k)^2=4c(x-h)$. With vertex $(-3,2)$ and

y-intercept $(0,5)$, $(5-2)^2=4c(0+3) \Rightarrow 9=12c \Rightarrow c=\dfrac{3}{4}$. The equation is $(y-2)^2=3(x+3)$. This can

also be written $x=\dfrac{1}{3}(y-2)^2-3$.

50. The center is located between the foci at $(0, 0)$. The hyperbola has a vertical transverse axis with $c=12$.

From the asymptotes, $\dfrac{a}{b}=1$. Also $c^2=a^2+b^2 \Rightarrow a^2+b^2=144$. Solving these equations simultaneously

results in $a^2=72$ and $b^2=72$. The equation is $\dfrac{y^2}{72}-\dfrac{x^2}{72}=1$.

372   CHAPTER 7   Analytic Geometry and Nonlinear Systems

51. The foci are (0, 0) and (4, 0), so the center is (2, 0) and $c = 2$. The sum of the distances is 8 so $2a = 8 \Rightarrow a = 4$. For an ellipse, $b^2 = a^2 - c^2 = 16 - 4 = 12$. The equation is $\dfrac{(x-2)^2}{16} + \dfrac{y^2}{12} = 1$.

52. The foci are (0, 0) and (0, 4), so the center is (0, 2) and $c = 2$. The difference of the distances is 2 so $2a = 2 \Rightarrow a = 1$. For a hyperbola, $b^2 = c^2 - a^2 = 4 - 1 = 3$. The equation is $\dfrac{(y-2)^2}{1} - \dfrac{x^2}{3} = 1$.

53. Add the two equations to eliminate the y^2: $\begin{array}{r} 2x^2 - y^2 = 8 \\ 4x^2 + y^2 = 16 \\ \hline 6x^2 = 24 \end{array} \Rightarrow x^2 = 4 \Rightarrow x = \pm 2$

Substitute these values into [equation 2] to find the value of y: $4(2)^2 + y^2 = 16 \Rightarrow y^2 = 0 \Rightarrow y = 0$, $4(-2)^2 + y^2 = 16 \Rightarrow y^2 = 0 \Rightarrow y = 0$, The solution set is $\{(2,0),(-2,0)\}$.

54. See Figure 54.

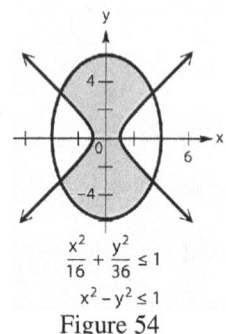

$\dfrac{x^2}{16} + \dfrac{y^2}{36} \le 1$
$x^2 - y^2 \le 1$
Figure 54

55. See Figure 55.
56. See Figure 56.

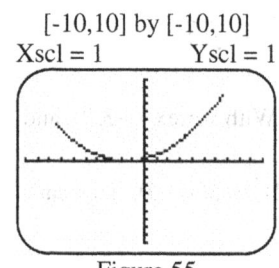 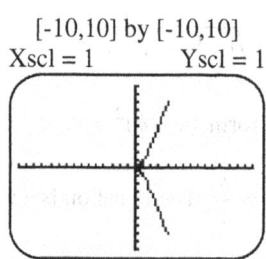

Figure 55   Figure 56

57. From the 1st equation, $x = \sqrt{t-1} \Rightarrow t = x^2 + 1$. By substitution in the 2nd equation $y = \sqrt{x^2 + 1}$. This is equivalent to $y^2 - x^2 = 1$. When t is in $[1, \infty)$, the range of $x = \sqrt{t-1}$ is x in $[0, \infty)$.

58. From the 1st equation, $x = 3t + 2 \Rightarrow t = \dfrac{x-2}{3}$. By substitution in the 2nd equation $y = \dfrac{x-2}{3} - 1$. This is equivalent to $x - 3y = 5$. When t is in $[-5, 5]$, the range of $x = 3t + 2$ is x in $[-13, 17]$.

59. Since the major axis has length 134.5 million miles, $2a = 134.5 \Rightarrow a = 67.25$. From the given eccentricity, $\dfrac{c}{a} = 0.006775 \Rightarrow \dfrac{c}{67.25} = 0.006775 \Rightarrow c = 67.25(0.006775) = 0.4456$ million miles. The smallest distance is $67.25 - 0.4456 \approx 66.8$ million miles and the largest distance is $67.25 + 0.4456 \approx 67.7$ million miles.

60. Since the smallest distance between the comet and the sun is 89 million miles, $a - c = 89$. The given eccentricity provides the equation $\dfrac{c}{a} = 0.964$. Solving these two equations simultaneously gives $a \approx 2472.222$ and $c \approx 2383.222$. Then $b^2 = a^2 - c^2 \Rightarrow b^2 = 2472.222 - 2383.222 \Rightarrow b^2 \approx 432{,}135$. The equation is $\dfrac{x^2}{a^2} + \dfrac{y^2}{b^2} = 1 \Rightarrow \dfrac{x^2}{6{,}111{,}882} + \dfrac{y^2}{432{,}135} = 1$.

61. The value of $\dfrac{k}{\sqrt{D}}$ is $\dfrac{2.82 \times 10^7}{\sqrt{42.5 \times 10^6}} \approx 4326$. Since $2090 < 4326$, $V < \dfrac{k}{\sqrt{D}}$. The trajectory is elliptic.

62. The velocity must be more than 4326 m per sec. The minimum increase is $4326 - 2090 \approx 2236$ m per sec.

63. The required increase in velocity is less when D is larger.

64. $Ax^2 + Cy^2 + Dx + Ey + F = 0 \Rightarrow A\left(x^2 + \dfrac{D}{A}x\right) + C\left(y^2 + \dfrac{E}{C}y\right) = -F \Rightarrow$

$A\left(x^2 + \dfrac{D}{A}x + \dfrac{D^2}{4A^2}\right) + C\left(y^2 + \dfrac{E}{C}y + \dfrac{E^2}{4C^2}\right) = -F + \dfrac{D^2}{4A} + \dfrac{E^2}{4C} \Rightarrow A\left(x + \dfrac{D}{2A}\right)^2 + C\left(y + \dfrac{E}{2C}\right)^2$

$= \dfrac{CD^2 + AE^2 - 4ACF}{4AC} \Rightarrow \dfrac{\left(x + \frac{D}{2A}\right)^2}{\frac{CD^2 + AE^2 - 4ACF}{4A^2C}} + \dfrac{\left(y + \frac{E}{2C}\right)^2}{\frac{CD^2 + AE^2 - 4ACF}{4AC^2}} = 1$. The center is $\left(-\dfrac{D}{2A}, -\dfrac{E}{2C}\right)$.

Chapter 7 Test

1. (a) B. This is a hyperbola with center $(-3, -2)$.

   (b) A. This is a circle with center $(3, 2)$ and radius 4.

   (c) D. This is a circle with center $(-3, 2)$ and radius 4.

   (d) E. This is a parabola that opens downward.

   (e) F. This is a parabola that opens to the right.

   (f) C. This is an ellipse with center $(-3, -2)$.

2. $y^2 = \dfrac{1}{8}x \Rightarrow (y - 0)^2 = 4\left(\dfrac{1}{32}\right)(x - 0)$; this is a parabola with vertex $(0, 0)$ that opens to the right. Since $c = \dfrac{1}{32}$, the focus is located at $\left(\dfrac{1}{32}, 0\right)$ and the equation of the directrix is $x = -\dfrac{1}{32}$.

3. See Figure 3. This is the graph of a function with domain $[-6, 6]$ and range $[-1, 0]$.

374 CHAPTER 7 Analytic Geometry and Nonlinear Systems

[-9,9] by [-3,3]
Xscl = 1   Yscl = 1

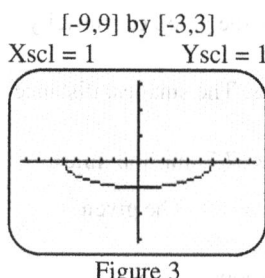

Figure 3

4. $\dfrac{x^2}{25}-\dfrac{y^2}{49}=1 \Rightarrow \dfrac{y^2}{49}=\dfrac{x^2}{25}-1 \Rightarrow y^2=49\left(\dfrac{x^2}{25}-1\right) \Rightarrow y=\pm\sqrt{49\left(\dfrac{x^2}{25}-1\right)} \Rightarrow y=\pm 7\sqrt{\dfrac{x^2}{25}-1}$ The equations are $y_1=7\sqrt{\dfrac{x^2}{25}-1}$ and $y_2=-7\sqrt{\dfrac{x^2}{25}-1}$.

5. This is a hyperbola with vertical transverse axis. Here $a=2$ and $b=3$. The asymptotes are $y=\pm\dfrac{2}{3}x$. See Figure 5. Since $c=\sqrt{a^2+b^2}=\sqrt{2^2+3^2}=\sqrt{13}$, the foci are $(0,-\sqrt{13})$ and $(0,\sqrt{13})$. The center is $(0,0)$. The vertices are $(0,-2)$ and $(0,2)$.

6. $x^2+4y^2+2x-16y+17=0 \Rightarrow x^2+2x+1+4(y^2-4y+4)=-17+1+16 \Rightarrow (x+1)^2+4(y-2)^2=0$; The only point that satisfies this equation is $(-1,2)$. See Figure 6.

7. $y^2-8y-2x+22=0 \Rightarrow y^2-8y+16=2x-22+16 \Rightarrow (y-4)^2=2(x-3) \Rightarrow (y-4)^2=4\left(\dfrac{1}{2}\right)(x-3)$;

   This is a parabola with vertex $(3, 4)$ and focus $(3.5, 4)$. See Figure 7.

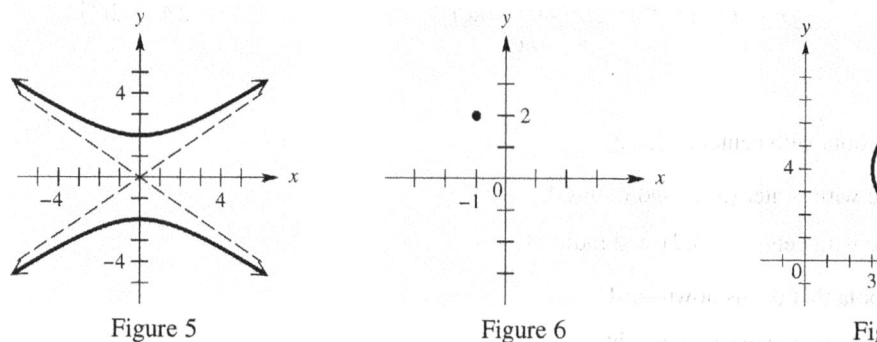

Figure 5   Figure 6   Figure 7

8. $x^2+(y-4)^2=9 \Rightarrow (x-0)^2+(y-4)^2=9$; This is a circle with center $(0, 4)$ and radius 3. See Figure 8.

9. This is an ellipse with horizontal major axis. Here $a=7$ and $b=4$ so $c=\sqrt{7^2-4^2}=\sqrt{33}$. The center is $(3,-1)$. The vertices are $(3-7,-1)$ and $(3+7,-1)$ or $(-4,-1)$ and $(10,-1)$. The foci are $\left(3+\sqrt{33},-1\right)$ and $\left(3-\sqrt{33},-1\right)$. See Figure 9.

Copyright © 2015 Pearson Education, Inc

10. From the 2nd equation $y = t-1 \Rightarrow t = y+1$. Substituting in the 1st equation yields $x = 4(y+1)^2 - 4$. This equation can be written $(y+1)^2 = 4\left(\dfrac{1}{16}\right)(x+4)$. This is a parabola that opens to the right. The vertex is $(-4, -1)$ and the focus is $\left(-4 + \dfrac{1}{16}, -1\right) \Rightarrow \left(-\dfrac{63}{16}, -1\right)$. See Figure 10.

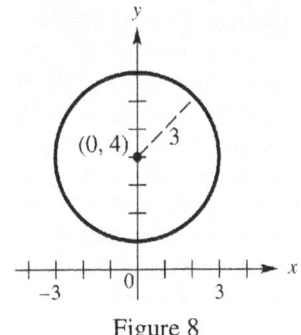

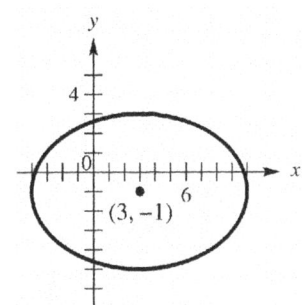

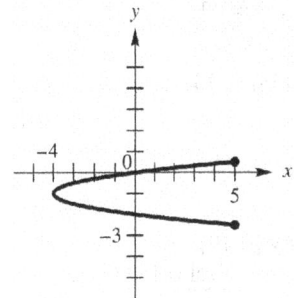

Figure 8   Figure 9   Figure 10

11. (a) Since $e = 1$, the conic is a parabola. With center $(0, 0)$ and focus $(0, -2)$, we know that $c = -2$. The equation is $x^2 = 4cy \Rightarrow x^2 = -8y \Rightarrow y = -\dfrac{1}{8}x^2$.

    (b) Since $0 < e < 1$, the conic is an ellipse with $a = 3$. Now $\dfrac{c}{a} = e \Rightarrow \dfrac{c}{3} = \dfrac{5}{6} \Rightarrow c = \dfrac{15}{6}$. For an ellipse, $b^2 = a^2 - c^2 = 9 - \dfrac{225}{36} = \dfrac{11}{4}$. The equation is $\dfrac{x^2}{\frac{11}{4}} + \dfrac{y^2}{9} = 1$ or $\dfrac{4x^2}{11} + \dfrac{y^2}{9} = 1$.

12. Using a vertical minor axis, $b = 12$. The major axis has length 40 so $a = 20$. The equation is $\dfrac{x^2}{400} + \dfrac{y^2}{144} = 1$. When $x = 10$, $\dfrac{10^2}{400} + \dfrac{y^2}{144} = 1 \Rightarrow \dfrac{y^2}{144} = 1 - \dfrac{1}{4} \Rightarrow y^2 = 144\left(\dfrac{3}{4}\right) \Rightarrow y = 12\sqrt{\dfrac{3}{4}} \approx 10.39\, ft.$

13. Add 4 multiplied by [equation 1] and 3 multiplied by [equation 2] to eliminate x^2:

    $12x^2 + 8y^2 = 20$
    $-12x^2 + 9y^2 = -3$
    $\overline{}$
    $17y^2 = 17 \Rightarrow y^2 = 1 \Rightarrow y = \pm 1$

    Substitute these values into [equation 1] to find the values of x: $3(1)^2 + 2y^2 = 5 \Rightarrow 2y^2 = 2 \Rightarrow y = \pm 1$, $3(-1)^2 + 2y^2 = 5 \Rightarrow 2y^2 = 2 \Rightarrow y = \pm 1$, The solution set is $\{(1,1),(1,-1),(-1,1),(-1,-1)\}$.

14. See Figure 14.

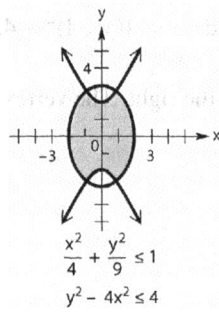

$$\frac{x^2}{4} + \frac{y^2}{9} \leq 1$$
$$y^2 - 4x^2 \leq 4$$

Figure 14

15. See Figure 15.

[-5,5] by [0,10]
Xscl = 1   Yscl = 1

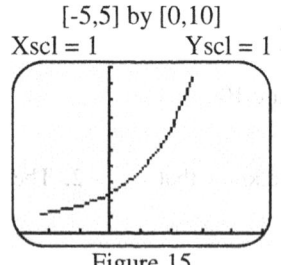

Figure 15

16. $x = \dfrac{1}{t+3} \Rightarrow t = \dfrac{1}{x} - 3$. Substituting this in $y = t + 3 \Rightarrow y = \dfrac{1}{x}, x \neq 0$.

Chapter 8: The Unit Circle and the Functions of Trigonometry

8.1: Angles, Arcs and Their Measures

1. An angle of $360°$ has an equivalent radian measure of 2π.

3. The least positive angle coterminal with $-180°$ has degree measure $180°$.

5. The formula relating $r, \theta,$ and s is $s = r\theta$.

7. (a) $c + 30° = 90° \Rightarrow c = 60°$

   (b) $s + 30° = 180° \Rightarrow s = 150°$

9. (a) $c + 45° = 90° \Rightarrow c = 45°$

   (b) $s + 45° = 180° \Rightarrow s = 135°$

11. (a) Since $90° = \dfrac{\pi}{2}$ radians, $c + \dfrac{\pi}{4} = \dfrac{\pi}{2} \Rightarrow c = \dfrac{2\pi}{4} - \dfrac{\pi}{4} \Rightarrow c = \dfrac{\pi}{4}$.

    (b) Since $180° = \pi$ radians, $s + \dfrac{\pi}{4} = \pi \Rightarrow s = \dfrac{4\pi}{4} - \dfrac{\pi}{4} \Rightarrow s = \dfrac{3\pi}{4}$.

13. (a) Since a complete revolution is $360°$, then $\dfrac{180°}{360°} = \dfrac{1}{2}$ of a revolution.

    (b) Since a complete revolution is $360°$, then $\dfrac{40°}{360°} = \dfrac{1}{9}$ of a revolution.

    (c) Since a complete revolution is $360°$, then $\dfrac{1°}{360°} = \dfrac{1}{180}$ of a revolution.

15. (a) $c + x° = 90° \Rightarrow c = (90 - x)°$

    (b) $s + x° = 180° \Rightarrow s = (180 - x)°$

17. Since $360° \div 12° = 30°$, every 5 minute section is $30°$. Therefore 5 o'clock equals $5 \cdot 30° = 150°$.

19. Since $360° \div 60° = 6°$, every 1 minute section is $6°$. Therefore 3:15 equals 1 minute $+ \left(\dfrac{1}{4} \cdot 6 \text{ minutes}\right)$ or $1.25 \cdot 6° = 7°30'$

21. $7x + 11x = 180 \Rightarrow 18x = 180 \Rightarrow x = 10$, therefore the angles are: $7(10) = 70°$ and $11(10) = 110°$.

23. $(5k + 5) + (3k + 5) = 90 \Rightarrow 8k + 10 = 90 \Rightarrow 8k = 80 \Rightarrow k = 10$, therefore the angles are: $5(10) + 5 = 55°$ and $3(10) + 5 = 35°$.

25. $(6x - 4) + (8x - 12) = 180 \Rightarrow 14x - 16 = 180 \Rightarrow 14x = 196 \Rightarrow x = 14$, therefore the angles are: $6(14) - 4 = 80°$ and $8(14) - 12 = 100°$.

27. $62°18' + 21°41' = 83°59'$

29. $71°18' - 47°29' = 70°78' - 47°29' = 23°49'$

31. $90° - 72°58'11'' = 89°59'60'' - 72°58'11'' = 17°1'49''$

33. $20°54' = \left(20\dfrac{54}{60}\right)° = 20.9°$

378   Chapter 8: The Unit Circle and the Functions of Trigonometry

35. $91°35'54" = 91°35'\dfrac{54}{60} = 91°35.9' = \left(91\dfrac{35.9}{60}\right)° = 91.598°$

37. $31.4296° = 31° + .4296(60') = 31°25.776' = 31°25'.776(60") = 31°25'47"$

39. $89.9004° = 89° + .9004(60') = 89°54.024' = 89°54'.024(60") = 89°54'1"$

41. See Figure 41. The coterminal angles are: $75° + 360° = 435°$ and $75° - 360° = -285°$, are in quadrant I.

43. See Figure 43. The coterminal angles are: $174° + 360° = 534°$ and $174° - 360° = -186°$, are in quadrant II.

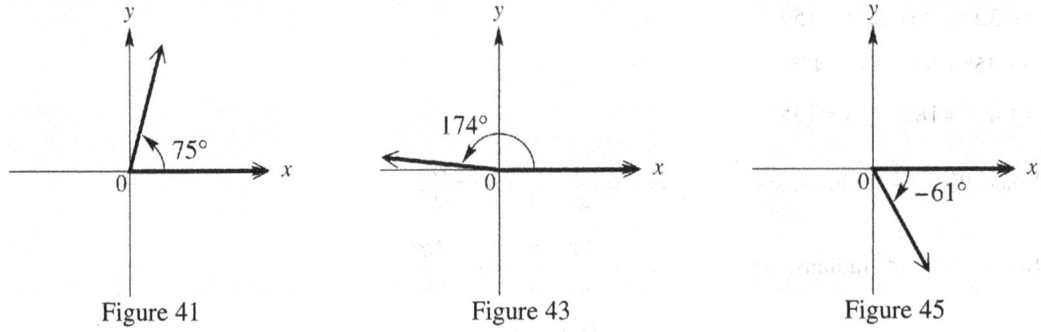

Figure 41   Figure 43   Figure 45

45. See Figure 45. The coterminal angles are: $-61° + 360° = 299°$ and $-61° - 360° = -421°$ are in quadrant IV.

47. The smallest positive degree measure of the coterminal angle is: $-40° + 360° = 320°$.

49. The smallest positive degree measure of the coterminal angle is: $450° - 360° = 90°$.

51. The smallest positive radian measure of the coterminal angle is: $-\dfrac{\pi}{4} + 2\pi = -\dfrac{\pi}{4} + \dfrac{8\pi}{4} = \dfrac{7\pi}{4}$.

53. The smallest positive radian measure of the coterminal angle is: $-\dfrac{3\pi}{2} + 2\pi = -\dfrac{3\pi}{2} + \dfrac{4\pi}{2} = \dfrac{\pi}{2}$.

55. All degree measure coterminal angles will be multiples of $360°$, therefore: $30° + n \cdot 360°$.

57. All degree measure coterminal angles will be multiples of $360°$, therefore: $-90° + n \cdot 360°$.

59. All radian measure coterminal angles will be multiples of 2π, therefore: $\dfrac{\pi}{4} + n \cdot 2\pi \Rightarrow \dfrac{\pi}{4} + 2n\pi$.

61. All radian measure coterminal angles will be multiples of 2π, therefore: $-\dfrac{3\pi}{4} + n \cdot 2\pi \Rightarrow -\dfrac{3\pi}{4} + 2n\pi$.

63. $60° \cdot \dfrac{\pi}{180} = \dfrac{\pi}{3}$ radians.

65. $150° \cdot \dfrac{\pi}{180} = \dfrac{5\pi}{6}$ radians.

67. $-45° \cdot \dfrac{\pi}{180} = -\dfrac{\pi}{4}$ radians.

69. $\dfrac{\pi}{3} \cdot \dfrac{180}{\pi} = 60°$

71. $\dfrac{7\pi}{4} \cdot \dfrac{180}{\pi} = 315°$

73. $\dfrac{11\pi}{6} \cdot \dfrac{180}{\pi} = 330°$

75. $39° \dfrac{\pi}{180} = \dfrac{39}{180} \cdot \pi = .68$

77. $139°10' = \left(139\dfrac{10}{60}\right)° = 139.167° \Rightarrow 139.167° \cdot \dfrac{\pi}{180} = \dfrac{139.167}{180} \cdot \pi = 2.43$

79. $64.29° \cdot \dfrac{\pi}{180} = \dfrac{64.29}{180} \cdot \pi = 1.12$

81. $2 \cdot \dfrac{180}{\pi} = \dfrac{360}{\pi} = 114.592° = 114° + .592(60') = 114°35'$

83. $1.74 \cdot \dfrac{180}{\pi} = \dfrac{313.2}{\pi} = 99.695° = 99° + .695(60') = 99°42'$

85. $-1.3 \cdot \dfrac{180}{\pi} = \dfrac{-234}{\pi} = -74.485° = -74° + .485(60') = -74°29'$

87. Going around the circle counterclockwise and starting at $0° = 0$ radians; $30° = \dfrac{\pi}{6}$ radians; $45° = \dfrac{\pi}{4}$ radians; $60° = \dfrac{\pi}{3}$ radians; $90° = \dfrac{\pi}{2}$ radians; $120° = \dfrac{2\pi}{3}$ radians; $135° = \dfrac{3\pi}{4}$ radians; $150° = \dfrac{5\pi}{6}$ radians; $180° = \pi$ radians; $210° = \dfrac{7\pi}{6}$ radians; $225° = \dfrac{5\pi}{4}$ radians; $240° = \dfrac{4\pi}{3}$ radians; $270° = \dfrac{3\pi}{2}$ radians; $300° = \dfrac{5\pi}{3}$ radians; $315° = \dfrac{7\pi}{3}$ radians; and $330° = \dfrac{11\pi}{6}$ radians.

89. Since arc length is found by the formula $s = r\theta$, the arc length is: $s = 4 \cdot \dfrac{\pi}{2} \Rightarrow s = 2\pi$.

91. Since arc length is found by the formula $s = r\theta$, the radius is: $6\pi = r \cdot \dfrac{3\pi}{4} \Rightarrow r = 6\pi \cdot \dfrac{4}{3\pi} \Rightarrow r = 8$.

93. Since arc length is found by the formula $s = r\theta$, the central angle is: $3 = 3\theta \Rightarrow \theta = \dfrac{3}{3} \Rightarrow \theta = 1$.

95. Since arc length is found by the formula $s = r\theta$, the arc length is: $s = 12.3\left(\dfrac{2\pi}{3}\right) \Rightarrow s = 8.2\pi \Rightarrow s \approx 25.76$ cm.

97. Since $60° = 60 \cdot \dfrac{\pi}{180} = \dfrac{\pi}{3}$ radians and arc length is found by the formula $s = r\theta$, the arc length is:

$s = 4.82\left(\dfrac{\pi}{3}\right) \Rightarrow s \approx 1.607\pi \Rightarrow s \approx 5.05$ m.

99. Since $44° - 33° = 11°$, $11° \cdot \dfrac{\pi}{180} \approx .06111\pi$ radians, and arc length is found by the formula $s = r\theta$, the arc length is: $s = 6400(.06111\pi) \Rightarrow s \approx 391.1\pi \Rightarrow s \approx 1200$ km.

101. Since $41+12=53°$, $53°\cdot\dfrac{\pi}{180}\approx 0.29444\pi$ radians, and arc length is found by the formula $s=r\theta$, the arc length is: $s=6400(.29444\pi)\Rightarrow s\approx 1884.42\pi \Rightarrow s\approx 5900$ km.

103. Using $w=\dfrac{\theta}{t}$ yields: $w=\dfrac{\frac{3\pi}{4}}{8}=\dfrac{3\pi}{4}\cdot\dfrac{1}{8}\Rightarrow w=\dfrac{3\pi}{32}$ radians per second.

105. Using $w=\dfrac{\theta}{t}$ yields: $\dfrac{5\pi}{27}=\dfrac{\frac{2x}{9}}{t}\Rightarrow 5\pi t=\dfrac{27}{1}\cdot\dfrac{2\pi}{9}\Rightarrow 5\pi t=6\pi\Rightarrow t=\dfrac{6\pi}{5\pi}\Rightarrow t=\dfrac{6}{5}$ minutes.

107. Using $s=rwt$ yields: $s=6\left(\dfrac{\pi}{3}\right)(9)\Rightarrow s=18\pi$ cm.

109. Using $s=rwt$ yields: $6\pi=2\left(\dfrac{\pi}{4}\right)t\Rightarrow 6\pi=\dfrac{\pi}{2}t\Rightarrow 6\pi\cdot\dfrac{2}{\pi}=t\Rightarrow t=12$ sec.

111. (a) The weight will rise the same distance as the arc length of the rotation. Therefore since arc length is found by the formula $s=r\theta$, the arc length is: $s=9.27\left(71+\dfrac{50}{60}\right)\cdot\dfrac{\pi}{180}\Rightarrow 9.27(71.83)\dfrac{\pi}{180}\Rightarrow s\approx 11.6$

   (b) The weight will rise the same distance as the arc length of the rotation. Therefore since arc length is found by the formula $s=r\theta$, the angle is: $6=9.27(\theta)\Rightarrow \theta=.647$ Changing this to degree measure yields: $.647\cdot\dfrac{180}{\pi}=\dfrac{116.505}{\pi}\approx 37.085°\approx 37°+.085(60')\approx 37°5'$.

113. First find the arc length that the smaller wheel rotates, arc length is found by the formula $s=r\theta$ the arc length is: $s=5.23\left(60\cdot\dfrac{\pi}{180}\right)\Rightarrow s\approx 1.743\Rightarrow s\approx 5.477$ cm Now the larger wheel travels the same arc length, therefore the angle of rotation is: $5.477\approx 8.16\theta\Rightarrow \theta\approx .671$ Changing this to degree measure yields: $0.671\cdot\dfrac{180}{\pi}=\dfrac{120.78}{\pi}\approx 38.5°$

115. First find the arc length that the pedal wheel rotates, arc length is found by the formula $s=r\theta$ the arc length is: $s=4.72\left(180\cdot\dfrac{\pi}{180}\right)\Rightarrow s\approx 4.72\pi\Rightarrow s\approx 14.828$ in. Now the smallest wheel travels the same arc length, therefore the angle of rotation is: $14.828=1.38\theta\Rightarrow \theta\approx 10.745$. Finally, using this radian rotation calculate the distance traveled with a wheel radius of 13.6 inches: $s\approx 13.6(10.745)\Rightarrow s\approx 146$ in.

117. Using the area of a sector formula $A=\dfrac{1}{2}r^2\theta$ yields: $A=\dfrac{1}{2}(29.2)^2\left(\dfrac{5\pi}{6}\right)\Rightarrow A\approx 1120\,\text{m}^2$.

119. Using the area of a sector formula $A=\dfrac{1}{2}r^2\theta$ yields: $A=\dfrac{1}{2}(12.7)^2\left(81°\cdot\dfrac{\pi}{180}\right)\Rightarrow A\approx 114\,\text{cm}^2$.

121. First find using $s = r\theta$ yields: $2\pi = 6\theta \Rightarrow \theta = \dfrac{\pi}{3}$. Now using the area of a sector formula $A = \dfrac{1}{2}r^2\theta$ yields:

    $A = \dfrac{1}{2}(6)^2\left(\dfrac{\pi}{3}\right) \Rightarrow A \approx \dfrac{36\pi}{6} = 6\pi$.

123. Since the area scanned in 1 second would yield: $\theta = \dfrac{1}{48} \cdot 2\pi = \dfrac{\pi}{24}$ radians, we can solve for area

    using $A = \dfrac{1}{2}r^2\theta$. Therefore, $A = \dfrac{1}{2}(240)^2\left(\dfrac{\pi}{24}\right) \Rightarrow A \approx 3800\,\text{mi}^2$.

125. To find the portion cleaned we will find the 10 inch radius sector and subtract the inside 3 inch radius sector.

    The 10 in radius is: $A = \dfrac{1}{2}10^2\left(95° \cdot \dfrac{\pi}{180}\right) \Rightarrow A \approx 82.9\,\text{in}^2$. The 3 in radius is:

    $A = \dfrac{1}{2}3^2\left(95° \cdot \dfrac{\pi}{180}\right) \Rightarrow A \approx 7.5\,\text{in}^2$. Subtracting these yields: $82.9 - 7.5 \approx 75.4\,\text{in}^2$.

127. (a) Each sector is: $360° \div 26 = 13.85°$.

    (b) Using the area of a sector formula $A = \dfrac{1}{2}r^2\theta$ and $r = \dfrac{50}{2} \Rightarrow r = 25$ yields:

    $A = \dfrac{1}{2}25^2\left(13.85° \cdot \dfrac{\pi}{180}\right) \Rightarrow A \approx 76\,\text{m}^2$.

129. If the diameter is 26, then the radius is 13, therefore 15 radians per second of rotation would have a linear speed of: $v = rw \Rightarrow v = 13.15 = 195$ inches per second which is equal to $195 \div 12 = 16\dfrac{1}{4}$ feet per second. This is equal to: $(16.25 \div 5280) \cdot 60 \cdot 60 \approx 11.1$ mph.

131. First we need to find inches: $15\,\text{mph} = 15.5280.12 = 950,400$ inches. Next we need to find θ using the arc length formula and a radius of : $r = \dfrac{2.25}{2} = 1.125 : 950,400 = 1.125\theta \Rightarrow \theta = 844,800$. Now use the angular

    speed formula: $w = \dfrac{844,800}{(60)(60)} \Rightarrow w = 234.67$ radians per second.

133. (a) The radian angle formed by 1 day is: $\theta = \dfrac{1}{365}(2\pi) \Rightarrow \theta = \dfrac{2\pi}{365}$ radians per day.

    (b) With $\theta = \dfrac{2\pi}{365}$ per day and $t = 24$ hours per day, the angular speed is: $V = \dfrac{\theta}{t} \Rightarrow v = \dfrac{\frac{2\pi}{365}}{24} \Rightarrow v = \dfrac{\pi}{4380}$

    radians per hour.

    (c) With $r = 93,000,000$ and $\theta = \dfrac{\pi}{4380}$ radians per hour, the linear speed is:

    $v = rw \Rightarrow v = 93,000,000\left(\dfrac{\pi}{4380}\right) \Rightarrow v = 66,700$ mph.

382   Chapter 8: The Unit Circle and the Functions of Trigonometry

135. With a radius of $r = \dfrac{10}{2} = 5$, a θ of 5000 revolutions per minute, and a time of 60 seconds in a minute, the

angular speed is: $w = \dfrac{\theta}{t} \Rightarrow w = \dfrac{5000(2\pi)}{60} \Rightarrow w = \dfrac{500\pi}{3}$ radians per second and the linear speed is is:

$v = rw \Rightarrow v = 5\left(\dfrac{500\pi}{3}\right) \Rightarrow v = \dfrac{2500\pi}{3}$ inches per second.

137. First find the radian measure of $7°12'$: $\theta = \dfrac{7(60)+12}{360(60)} \cdot 2\pi \Rightarrow \theta \approx .1257$ radians. Next use $\theta = .12566$ and the

arc length formula to find the radius: $496 = r(.12566) \Rightarrow r = 3947$ miles. Now we can find the

circumference: $C = 2r\pi \Rightarrow C = 2(3947)\pi \Rightarrow C \approx 24{,}800$ miles.

Section 8.2: The Unit Circle and its Functions

1. $\dfrac{\frac{\pi}{3}}{2\pi} = \dfrac{\pi}{3} \cdot \dfrac{1}{2\pi} = \dfrac{1}{6}$

3. $\dfrac{\frac{\pi}{4}}{2\pi} = \dfrac{\pi}{4} \cdot \dfrac{1}{2\pi} = \dfrac{1}{8}$

5. $\dfrac{\frac{\pi}{6}}{2\pi} = \dfrac{\pi}{6} \cdot \dfrac{1}{2\pi} = \dfrac{1}{12}$

7. $\dfrac{3\pi}{2\pi} = \dfrac{3}{2}$

9. $\dfrac{\frac{3\pi}{2}}{2\pi} = \dfrac{3\pi}{2} \cdot \dfrac{1}{2\pi} = \dfrac{3}{4}$

11. $\dfrac{\frac{5\pi}{4}}{2\pi} = \dfrac{5}{8}$

13. Since $\sin s = y$ and $\cos s = x$; $\tan s = \dfrac{y}{x}$, $\sin s = \dfrac{3}{5}$, $\cos s = \dfrac{4}{5}$, $\tan s = \dfrac{3}{4}$

15. Since $\sin s = y$ and $\cos s = x$; $\tan s = \dfrac{y}{x}$, $\sin s = -\dfrac{5}{13}$, $\cos s = \dfrac{12}{13}$, $\tan s = -\dfrac{5}{12}$

17. Since $\sin s = y$ and $\cos s = x$; $\tan s = \dfrac{y}{x}$, $\sin s = \dfrac{21}{29}$, $\cos s = -\dfrac{20}{29}$, $\tan s = -\dfrac{21}{20}$

19. From the figure, the point is $(-1, 0)$. Since $\sin s = y$ and $\cos s = x$, $\sin s = 0$ and $\cos s = -1$. Finally, since $y = 0$. cosecant and cotangent are undefined.

21. From the figure, the point is $(1, 0)$. Since $\sin s = y$ and $\cos s = x$, $\sin s = 0$ and $\cos s = 1$. Finally, since $y = 0$ cosecant and cotangent are undefined.

23. From the figure, the point is $(0,-1)$. Since $\sin s = y$ and $\cos s = x$, $\sin s = -1$ and $\cos s = 0$. Finally, since $x = 0$, secant and tangent are undefined.

25. From the figure, the point is $(0,1)$ Since $\sin s = y$ and $\cos s = x$, $\sin s = 1$ and $\cos s = 0$. Finally, since $x = 0$, secant and tangent are undefined.

27. From the figure, a point on the unit circle is $(-1,0)$. Since $x = -1$ and $y = 0$, the six functions are:

    $\cos s = x \Rightarrow \cos s = -1$ $\qquad$ $\sin s = y \Rightarrow \sin s = 0$ $\qquad$ $\tan s = \dfrac{y}{x} \Rightarrow \tan s = \dfrac{0}{-1} = 0$

    $\cot s = \dfrac{x}{y} = \dfrac{-1}{0} \Rightarrow$ undefined $\qquad$ $\sec s = \dfrac{1}{x} \Rightarrow \sec s = \dfrac{1}{-1} = -1$ $\qquad$ $\csc s = \dfrac{1}{y} = \dfrac{1}{0} \Rightarrow$ undefined

29. From the figure, a point on the unit circle is $(1,0)$. Since $x = 1$ and $y = 0$, the six functions are:

    $\cos s = x \Rightarrow \cos s = 1$ $\qquad$ $\sin s = y \Rightarrow \sin s = 0$ $\qquad$ $\dfrac{\pi}{\left(\frac{1}{4}\right)} = 8\pi$

    $\cot s = \dfrac{x}{y} = \dfrac{1}{0} \Rightarrow$ undefined $\qquad$ $\sec s = \dfrac{1}{x} \Rightarrow \sec s = \dfrac{1}{1} = 1$ $\qquad$ $\csc s = \dfrac{1}{y} = \dfrac{1}{0} \Rightarrow$ undefined

31. From the figure, a point on the unit circle is $(0,1)$. Since $x = 0$ and $y = -1$, the six functions are:

    $\cos s - x \Rightarrow \cos s = 0$ $\qquad$ $\sin s = y \Rightarrow \sin s = -1$ $\qquad$ $\tan s = \dfrac{y}{x} = \dfrac{-1}{0} \Rightarrow$ undefined

    $\cot s = \dfrac{x}{y} \Rightarrow \cot s = \dfrac{0}{-1} = 0$ $\qquad$ $\sec s = \dfrac{1}{x} = \dfrac{1}{0} \Rightarrow$ undefined $\qquad$ $\csc s = \dfrac{1}{y} \Rightarrow \csc s = \dfrac{1}{-1} = -1$

33. From the figure, a point on the unit circle is $(0,1)$. Since $x = 0$ and $y = 1$, the six functions are:

    $\cos s = x \Rightarrow \cos s = 0$ $\qquad$ $\sin s = y \Rightarrow \sin s = 1$ $\qquad$ $\tan s = \dfrac{y}{x} = \dfrac{1}{0} \Rightarrow$ undefined

    $\cot s = \dfrac{0}{1} = 0$ $\qquad$ $\sec s = \dfrac{1}{x} = \dfrac{1}{0} \Rightarrow$ undefined $\qquad$ $\csc s = \dfrac{1}{y} \Rightarrow \csc s = \dfrac{1}{1} = 1$

35. Because $\cos s = x$ and $\sin s = y$, it follows that $x = \dfrac{12}{13}$ and $y = \dfrac{5}{13}$. Thus x is positive and y is positive, so (x, y) is located in quadrant I.

37. Because $\cos s = x$ and $\sin s = y$, it follows that $x = -\dfrac{4}{5}$ and $y = -\dfrac{3}{5}$. Thus x is negative and y is negative, so (x, y) is located in quadrant III.

39. Because $\cos s = x$ and $\sin s = y$, it follows that $x = -\dfrac{84}{85}$ and $y = \dfrac{13}{85}$. Thus x is negative and y is positive, so (x, y) is located in quadrant II.

384 Chapter 8: The Unit Circle and the Functions of Trigonometry

41. (a) Because $\frac{\pi}{2} \approx 1.57$, it follows that $0 \leq s \leq \frac{\pi}{2}$. Thus, s corresponds to a point (x, y) in quadrant I.

   (b) In quadrant I, $x > 0$ and $y > 0$. Because $\cos s = x$ and $\sin s = y$ it follows that $\cos s$ is positive and $\sin s$ is positive.

43. (a) Because $\frac{\pi}{2} \leq \frac{3\pi}{4} \leq \pi$ and the negative indicates that we are moving in a negative direction from zero. Thus, s corresponds to a point (x, y) in quadrant III.

   (b) In quadrant III, $x < 0$ and $y < 0$. Because $\cos s = x$ and $\sin s = y$ it follows that $\cos s$ is negative and $\sin s$ is negative.

45. (a) Because $\frac{\pi}{2} \leq 2.3 \leq \pi$, s corresponds to a point (x, y) in quadrant II.

   (b) In quadrant I, $x < 0$ and $y > 0$. Because $\cos s = x$ and $\sin s = y$ it follows that $\cos s$ is positive and $\sin s$ is negative.

47. (a) Because $-\frac{5\pi}{2} \leq -7 \leq 2\pi$ and the negative indicates that we are moving in a negative direction from zero. Thus, we will move more than a full rotation in the negative direction and s corresponds to a point (x, y) in quadrant IV.

   (b) In quadrant IV, $x > 0$ and $y < 0$. Because $\cos s = x$ and $\sin s = y$ it follows that $\cos s$ is positive and $\sin s$ is negative.

49. Because $0 < 0.75 < \frac{\pi}{2}$, s is found in quadrant I. Now from the calculator (radian mode):

   $\cos s \approx .7316888689$ $\sin s \approx .68163876$ $\tan s \approx .9315964599$

   $\cot s = \frac{1}{\tan s} \approx 1.073426149$ $\sec s = \frac{1}{\cos s} \approx 1.366701125$ $\csc s = \frac{1}{\sin s} \approx 1.4670527724$

51. Because $-\pi < -4.25 < -\frac{3\pi}{2}$, s is found in quadrant II. Now from the calculator (radian mode):

   $\cos s \approx .4460874899$ $\sin s \approx .8949893582$ $\tan s \approx -2.0066309028$

   $\cot s = \frac{1}{\tan s} \approx .4984277029$ $\sec s = \frac{1}{\cos s} \approx 2.241712719$ $\csc s = \frac{1}{\sin s} \approx 1.117331721$

53. Because $-\frac{\pi}{2} < -2.25 < -\pi$, s is found in quadrant III. Now from the calculator (radian mode):

   $\cos s \approx -.6281736227$ $\sin s \approx -.77807361969$ $\tan s \approx 1.238627616$

   $\cot s = \frac{1}{\tan s} \approx .8073451511$ $\sec s = \frac{1}{\cos s} \approx -1.591916572$ $\csc s = \frac{1}{\sin s} \approx -1.285226125$

55. Because $\frac{3\pi}{2} < 5.5 < 2\pi$, s is found in quadrant IV. Now from the calculator (radian mode):

    $\cos s \approx .7086697743$ $\qquad\qquad$ $\sin s \approx -.7055403256$ $\qquad\qquad$ $\tan s \approx -.9955840522$

    $\cot s = \dfrac{1}{\tan s} \approx -1.004435535$ $\qquad$ $\sec s = \dfrac{1}{\cos s} \approx 1.411094471$ $\qquad$ $\csc s = \dfrac{1}{\sin s} \approx -1.417353429$

57. For exercises 57 - 62 answers will vary depending on the name used. Suppose the first name is Shannon. Then $s = 7$ and $\cos 7 \approx .7539022543$.

58. For exercises 57 - 62 answers will vary depending on the name used. Suppose the last name is Mulkey. Then $n = 6$, and $\cos(7 + 2(6)\pi) \approx .7539022543$.

59. They are the same. The real numbers s and $s + 2n\pi$ correspond to the same point on the unit circle, because its circumference is 2π.

60. For exercises 57 - 62 answers will vary depending on the name used. Suppose the last name is Castellucio. Then $s = 11$ and $s = 11 \approx -.9999902066$.

61. For exercises 57 - 62 answers will vary depending on the name used. Suppose the first name is Frankie. Then $n = 7$, and $\sin(11 + 2(7)\pi) \approx -.9999902066$.

62. They are the same. The real numbers s and $s + 2n\pi$ correspond to the same point on the unit circle, because its circumference is 2π.

63. The point $\left(-\dfrac{\sqrt{3}}{2}, -\dfrac{1}{2}\right)$ corresponds to $\dfrac{7\pi}{6}$ on the unit circle. Since the function is sine, we use the y-value of the point to obtain $\sin\dfrac{7\pi}{6} = -\dfrac{1}{2}$.

65. The point $\left(\dfrac{\sqrt{2}}{2}, \dfrac{\sqrt{2}}{2}\right)$ corresponds to $\dfrac{3\pi}{3}$ on the unit circle. Since the function is tangent and by definition

    $\tan s = \dfrac{y}{x}$, $\tan\dfrac{3\pi}{4} = \dfrac{\frac{\sqrt{2}}{2}}{-\frac{\sqrt{2}}{2}} = \dfrac{\sqrt{2}}{2} \cdot \left(-\dfrac{2}{\sqrt{2}}\right) = -1$.

67. The point $\left(-\dfrac{1}{2}, \dfrac{\sqrt{3}}{2}\right)$ corresponds to $\dfrac{2\pi}{6}$ on the unit circle. The function is secant and by definition

    $\sec s = \dfrac{1}{\cos s}$, therefore, $\sec\dfrac{2\pi}{3} = \dfrac{1}{\cos\dfrac{2x}{3}}$. Since the function is cosine, we use the x-value of the point to

    obtain $\sec\dfrac{2\pi}{3} = \dfrac{1}{-\frac{1}{2}} = -2$.

69. The point $\left(-\dfrac{\sqrt{3}}{2}, \dfrac{1}{2}\right)$ corresponds to $\dfrac{5\pi}{6}$ on the unit circle. The function is cotangent and by definition

    $\cot s = \dfrac{1}{\tan s}$, therefore, $\cot \dfrac{5\pi}{6} = \dfrac{1}{\tan \dfrac{5\pi}{6}}$. Since the function is tangent and by definition

    $\tan s = \dfrac{y}{x}$, $\cot \dfrac{5\pi}{6} = \dfrac{1}{\tan \dfrac{5\pi}{6}} = 1 \div \left(\dfrac{\frac{1}{2}}{-\frac{\sqrt{3}}{2}}\right) = 1 \div \left(\dfrac{1}{2} \cdot \left(-\dfrac{2}{\sqrt{3}}\right)\right) = 1 \div \left(-\dfrac{1}{\sqrt{3}}\right) = -\sqrt{3}.$

71. The point on the unit circle for $s = -\dfrac{5\pi}{6}$ is the same as that for $\dfrac{7\pi}{6}$. The point $\left(-\dfrac{\sqrt{3}}{2}, -\dfrac{1}{2}\right)$ corresponds to

    $\dfrac{7\pi}{3}$ on the unit circle. Since the function is sine, we use the y-value of the point to obtain

    $\sin\left(-\dfrac{5\pi}{6}\right) = \sin\dfrac{7\pi}{6} = -\dfrac{1}{2}.$

73. The point on the unit circle for $s = \dfrac{23\pi}{6}$ is the same as that for $\dfrac{11\pi}{6}$. The point $\left(\dfrac{\sqrt{3}}{2}, \dfrac{1}{2}\right)$ corresponds to

    $\dfrac{11\pi}{6}$ on the unit circle. The function is secant and by definition $\sec s = \dfrac{1}{\cos s}$, therefore, $\sec\dfrac{11\pi}{6} = \dfrac{1}{\cos\dfrac{11\pi}{6}}$.

    Since the function is cosine, we use the x-value of the point to obtain $\sec\dfrac{23\pi}{6} = \sec\dfrac{11\pi}{6} = \dfrac{1}{\frac{\sqrt{3}}{2}} = \dfrac{2}{\sqrt{3}} = \dfrac{2\sqrt{3}}{3}.$

75. The point on the unit circle for $s = -\dfrac{13\pi}{6}$ is the same as that for $-\dfrac{\pi}{6}$. The point $\left(\dfrac{\sqrt{3}}{2}, -\dfrac{1}{2}\right)$ corresponds to

    $\dfrac{11\pi}{6}$ on the unit circle. Since the function is cosine, we use the x-value of the point to obtain

    $\cos\left(-\dfrac{13\pi}{6}\right) = \cos\dfrac{11\pi}{6} = \dfrac{\sqrt{3}}{2}.$

77. The point on the unit circle for $s = -\dfrac{13\pi}{4}$ is the same as that for $-\dfrac{5\pi}{4}$, which is the same as that for $\dfrac{3\pi}{4}$.

    The point $\left(-\dfrac{\sqrt{2}}{2}, -\dfrac{\sqrt{2}}{2}\right)$ corresponds to $\dfrac{3\pi}{4}$ on the unit circle. Since the function is tangent and by

    definition $\tan s = \dfrac{y}{x}$, $\tan\left(-\dfrac{13\pi}{4}\right) = \dfrac{\frac{\sqrt{2}}{2}}{-\frac{\sqrt{2}}{2}} = \dfrac{\sqrt{2}}{2} \cdot \left(-\dfrac{\sqrt{2}}{2}\right) = -1.$

79. Since $\cos s = x$ and $\sin s = y$, the identity $\cos^2 s + \sin^2 s = 1$ would yield:

$\left(\dfrac{3}{5}\right)^2 + y^2 = 1 \Rightarrow y^2 = 1 - \dfrac{9}{25} \Rightarrow y^2 = \dfrac{16}{25} \Rightarrow y = \pm\dfrac{4}{5}$, but $y > 0$, therefore $y = \dfrac{4}{5}$. Now using $x = \dfrac{3}{5}$ and

$y = \dfrac{4}{5}$, the six trigonometric functions are:

$\cos s = x = \dfrac{3}{5}$ $\qquad\qquad\qquad\qquad \cot s = \dfrac{1}{\tan s} = \dfrac{1}{\dfrac{4}{3}} = \dfrac{3}{4} \qquad\qquad\qquad \sin s = y = \dfrac{4}{5}$

$\sec s = \dfrac{1}{\cos x} = \dfrac{1}{\dfrac{3}{5}} = \dfrac{5}{3} \qquad\qquad \tan s = \dfrac{y}{x} = \dfrac{4}{5} \cdot \dfrac{5}{3} = \dfrac{4}{3} \qquad\qquad \csc s = \dfrac{1}{\sin s} = \dfrac{1}{\dfrac{4}{5}} = \dfrac{5}{3}$

81. Since $\cos s = x$ and $\sin s = y$, the identity $\cos^2 s + \sin^2 s = 1$ would yield:

$x^2 + \left(\dfrac{24}{25}\right)^2 = 1 \Rightarrow x^2 = 1 - \dfrac{576}{625} \Rightarrow x^2 = \dfrac{49}{625} \Rightarrow y = \pm\dfrac{7}{25}$, but $x < 0$, therefore $x = -\dfrac{7}{25}$. Now using

$x = -\dfrac{7}{25}$ and $y = \dfrac{24}{25}$, the six trigonometric functions are:

$\cos s = x = -\dfrac{7}{25} \qquad\qquad\qquad \sin s = y = \dfrac{24}{25} \qquad\qquad\qquad \tan s = \dfrac{y}{x} = \dfrac{24}{25} \cdot \left(-\dfrac{25}{7}\right) = -\dfrac{24}{7}$

$\cot s = \dfrac{1}{\tan s} = \dfrac{1}{-\dfrac{24}{7}} = -\dfrac{7}{24} \quad \sec s = \dfrac{1}{\cos s} = \dfrac{1}{-\dfrac{7}{25}} = -\dfrac{25}{7} \quad \csc s = \dfrac{1}{\sin s} = \dfrac{1}{\dfrac{24}{25}} = \dfrac{25}{24}$

83. Since $\cos s = x$ and $\sin s = y$, the identity $\cos^2 s + \sin^2 s = 1$ would

yield: $\left(-\dfrac{1}{3}\right)^2 + y^2 = 1 \Rightarrow y^2 = 1 - \dfrac{1}{9} \Rightarrow y^2 = \dfrac{8}{9} \Rightarrow y = \pm\dfrac{2\sqrt{2}}{3}$, but $y < 0$, therefore $y = -\dfrac{2\sqrt{2}}{3}$. Now using

$x = -\dfrac{1}{3}$ and $y = -\dfrac{2\sqrt{2}}{3}$, the six trigonometric functions are:

$\cos s = x = -\dfrac{1}{3} \qquad\qquad\qquad \sin s = y = -\dfrac{2\sqrt{2}}{3} \qquad\qquad \tan s = \dfrac{y}{x} = \left(-\dfrac{2\sqrt{2}}{3}\right)\cdot\left(-\dfrac{3}{1}\right) = 2\sqrt{2}$

$\cot s = \dfrac{1}{\tan s} = \dfrac{1}{2\sqrt{2}} = -\dfrac{\sqrt{2}}{4} \quad \sec s = \dfrac{1}{\cos s} = \dfrac{1}{-\dfrac{1}{3}} = -3 \quad \csc s = \dfrac{1}{\sin s} = \dfrac{1}{-\dfrac{2\sqrt{2}}{3}} = -\dfrac{3}{2\sqrt{2}} = -\dfrac{3\sqrt{2}}{4}$

85. If $\sin s = \dfrac{1}{2}$ and $\cos s = \dfrac{\sqrt{3}}{2}$, then we can find the trigonometric functions as follows:

$\tan s = \dfrac{\sin s}{\cos s} = \dfrac{1}{2} \cdot \dfrac{2}{\sqrt{3}} = \dfrac{1}{\sqrt{3}} = \dfrac{\sqrt{3}}{3} \qquad\qquad \cot s = \dfrac{1}{\tan s} = \dfrac{1}{\dfrac{\sqrt{3}}{3}} = \dfrac{3}{\sqrt{3}} = \dfrac{3\sqrt{3}}{3} = \sqrt{3}$

$$\sec s = \frac{1}{\cos s} = \frac{1}{\frac{\sqrt{3}}{2}} = \frac{2}{\sqrt{3}} = \frac{2\sqrt{3}}{3} \qquad \csc s = \frac{1}{\sin s} = \frac{1}{\frac{1}{2}} = 2$$

87. If $\sin s = \frac{4}{5}$ and $\cos s = -\frac{3}{5}$, then we can find the trigonometric functions as follows:

$$\tan s = \frac{\sin s}{\cos s} = \frac{4}{5} \cdot \left(-\frac{5}{3}\right) = -\frac{4}{3} \qquad \cot s = \frac{1}{\tan s} = \frac{1}{-\frac{4}{3}} = -\frac{3}{4}$$

$$\sec s = \frac{1}{\cos s} = \frac{1}{-\frac{3}{5}} = -\frac{5}{3} \qquad \csc s = \frac{1}{\sin s} = \frac{1}{\frac{4}{5}} = \frac{5}{4}$$

89. If $\sin s = -\frac{\sqrt{3}}{2}$ and $\cos s = \frac{1}{2}$, then we can find the trigonometric functions as follows:

$$\tan s = \frac{\sin s}{\cos s} = \left(-\frac{\sqrt{3}}{2}\right) \cdot \frac{2}{1} = -\sqrt{3} \qquad \cot s = \frac{1}{\tan s} = \frac{1}{-\sqrt{3}} = -\frac{\sqrt{3}}{3}$$

$$\sec s = \frac{1}{\cos s} = \frac{1}{\frac{1}{2}} = 2 \qquad \csc s = \frac{1}{\sin s} = \frac{1}{-\frac{\sqrt{3}}{2}} = -\frac{2}{\sqrt{3}} = -\frac{2\sqrt{3}}{3}$$

91. Since $\sin s = y$ and $\sin s > 0$, s is in either quadrant I or II.

Since $\cos s = x$ and $\cos s < 0$, s is in either quadrant II or III. The point s is found in quadrant II.

93. Since $\sin \frac{11\pi}{6} = -\sin \frac{\pi}{6} = \frac{1}{2}$ and $\sec s < 0$, s is in either quadrant II or III.

Since $\csc s = \frac{1}{y}$ and $\csc s < 0$, s is in either quadrant III or IV. The point s is found in quadrant III.

95. Since $\cos s = x$ and $\cos s > 0$, s is in either quadrant I or IV.

Since $\sin s = y$ and $\sin s < 0$, s is in either quadrant III or IV. The point s is found in quadrant IV.

97. $1 + \tan^2 s = 1 + \frac{\sin^2 s}{\cos^2 s} = \frac{\cos^2 s + \sin^2 s}{\cos^2 s} = \frac{1}{\cos^2 s} = \sec^2 s$

99. If s is a real number corresponding to point (a,b), then $\sin s = y \Rightarrow \sin s = b$ and $\cos s = x \Rightarrow \cos s = a$.

$\cos s = x \Rightarrow \cos(s - 2\pi) = x \Rightarrow \cos(s - 2\pi) = a$.

101. If s is a real number corresponding to point (a,b), then and $s - 6\pi$ would be a coterminal angle to an angle with measure s. Therefore $\sin s = y \Rightarrow \sin(s - 6\pi) = y \Rightarrow \sin(s - 6\pi) = b$ and

$\cos s = x \Rightarrow \cos(s - 6\pi) = x \Rightarrow \cos(s - 6\pi) = a$.

103. If s is a real number corresponding to point (a,b), then $-s$ would be an angle that intersects the unit circle at the point $(a,-b)$. Therefore, $\sin -s = y \Rightarrow \sin -s = -b$ and $\cos -s = x \Rightarrow \cos -s = a$.

105. If s is a real number corresponding to point (a,b), then $s - \frac{\pi}{2}$ would be an angle with an additional negative one-quarter turn with a terminal side intersecting the unit circle at the point $(b,-a)$. Therefore,

$$\sin\left(s - \frac{\pi}{2}\right) = y \Rightarrow \sin\left(s - \frac{\pi}{2}\right) = -a \text{ and } \cos\left(s - \frac{\pi}{2}\right) = x \Rightarrow \cos\left(s - \frac{\pi}{2}\right) = b.$$

Reviewing Basic Concepts (Sections 8.1 and 8.2)

1. (a) complement: $c + 35° = 90° \Rightarrow c = 55°$ supplement: $s + 35° = 180° \Rightarrow s = 145°$

    (b) complement, since $90° = \frac{\pi}{2}$ radians, $c + \frac{\pi}{4} = \frac{\pi}{2} \Rightarrow c = \frac{2\pi}{4} - \frac{\pi}{4} \Rightarrow c = \frac{\pi}{4}$.

    supplement, since $180° = \pi$ radians, $s + \frac{\pi}{4} = \pi \Rightarrow s = \frac{4\pi}{4} - \frac{\pi}{4} \Rightarrow s = \frac{3\pi}{4}$.

2. $32.25° = 32° + .25°(60)' = 32°15'0"$.

3. $59°35'30" = \left(59 + \frac{35}{60} + \frac{30}{(60)(60)}\right)° = 59.59\overline{16}°$.

4. (a) The smallest positive degree measure of the coterminal angle is: $560° - 360° = 200°$.

    (b) The smallest positive radian measure of the coterminal angle is: $-\frac{2\pi}{3} + 2\pi = -\frac{2\pi}{3} + \frac{6\pi}{3} = \frac{4\pi}{3}$.

5. (a) $240° \cdot \frac{\pi}{180} = \frac{4\pi}{3}$ (b) $\frac{3\pi}{4} \cdot \frac{180}{\pi} = 135°$

6. (a) Since $120° = 120° \cdot \frac{\pi}{180} = \frac{2\pi}{3}$ and arc length is found by the formula $s = r\theta$, the arc length is:

    $s = 3\left(\frac{2\pi}{3}\right) \Rightarrow s = 2\pi$ cm.

    (b) Using the area of a sector formula $A = \frac{1}{2}r^2\theta$ yields: $A = \frac{1}{2}(3)^2\left(\frac{2\pi}{3}\right) \Rightarrow A = 3\pi$ cm².

7. (a) An angle of $s = -2\pi$ radians intersects the unit circle at the point $(1,0)$.

    (b) From the properties of $45°-45°$ right triangles, an angle of $s = \frac{5\pi}{4}$ radians intersects the unit circle at the point $\left(-\frac{\sqrt{2}}{2}, -\frac{\sqrt{2}}{2}\right)$.

    (c) An angle of $s = \frac{5\pi}{2}$ radians intersects the unit circle at the point $(0,1)$

390 Chapter 8: The Unit Circle and the Functions of Trigonometry

8. An angle of $\csc 270° = -1$ radians intersects the unit circle at the point $(0, -1)$. Therefore, since:

$\left\{x \mid x \neq \dfrac{\pi}{2} + n\pi, \text{where } n \text{ is an integer}\right\}$; $\theta = -\dfrac{7\pi}{6} = 2\pi - \dfrac{7\pi}{6} = \dfrac{12\pi}{6} - \dfrac{7\pi}{6} = \dfrac{5\pi}{6}$

$\tan s = \dfrac{y}{x}, \tan \dfrac{5\pi}{2} = \dfrac{-1}{0} = $ undefined $\csc s = \dfrac{1}{y}, \csc \dfrac{5\pi}{2} = \dfrac{1}{-1} = -1$

$\sec s = \dfrac{1}{x}, \sec \dfrac{5\pi}{2} = \dfrac{1}{0} = $ undefined $\cot s = \dfrac{x}{y}, \cot \dfrac{5\pi}{2} = \dfrac{0}{-1} = 0$

9. (a) From the properties of $30°-60°$ right triangles, an angle of $s = \dfrac{7\pi}{6}$ radians intersects the unit circle at

the point $\left(-\dfrac{\sqrt{3}}{2}, -\dfrac{1}{2}\right)$. Therefore, since: $\sin s = y, \sin \dfrac{7\pi}{6} = -\dfrac{1}{2}$

$\csc s = \dfrac{1}{y}, \csc \dfrac{7\pi}{6} = \dfrac{1}{-\dfrac{1}{2}} = -2$ $\cos s = x, \cos \dfrac{7\pi}{6} = -\dfrac{\sqrt{3}}{2}$ $\sec s = \dfrac{1}{x}, \sec \dfrac{7\pi}{6} = \dfrac{1}{-\dfrac{\sqrt{3}}{2}} = -\dfrac{2}{\sqrt{3}} = -\dfrac{2\sqrt{3}}{3}$

$\tan s = \dfrac{y}{x}, \tan \dfrac{7\pi}{6} = \dfrac{-\dfrac{1}{2}}{-\dfrac{\sqrt{3}}{2}} = -\dfrac{1}{2}\cdot\left(-\dfrac{2}{\sqrt{3}}\right) = \dfrac{\sqrt{3}}{3}$ $\cot s = \dfrac{x}{y}, \cot \dfrac{7\pi}{6} = \dfrac{-\dfrac{\sqrt{3}}{2}}{-\dfrac{1}{2}} = -\dfrac{\sqrt{3}}{2}\cdot\left(-\dfrac{2}{1}\right) = \sqrt{3}$ \

(b) From the properties of $30°-60°$ right triangles, an angle of $s = -\dfrac{2\pi}{3}$ radians intersects the unit circle

at the point $\left(-\dfrac{1}{2}, -\dfrac{\sqrt{3}}{2}\right)$. Therefore, since: $\sec \theta \leq -1$ $45°$

$\cos s = x, \cos -\dfrac{2\pi}{3} = -\dfrac{1}{2}$ $\sec s = \dfrac{1}{x}, \sec -\dfrac{2\pi}{3} = \dfrac{1}{-\dfrac{1}{2}} = -2$

$\tan s = \dfrac{y}{x}, \tan -\dfrac{2\pi}{3} = \dfrac{-\dfrac{\sqrt{3}}{2}}{-\dfrac{1}{2}} = -\dfrac{\sqrt{3}}{2}\cdot\dfrac{2}{1} = \sqrt{3}$ $\cot s = \dfrac{x}{y}, \cot -\dfrac{2\pi}{3} = \dfrac{-\dfrac{1}{2}}{-\dfrac{\sqrt{3}}{2}} = -\dfrac{1}{2}\cdot\dfrac{2}{\sqrt{3}} = \dfrac{1}{\sqrt{3}} = \dfrac{\sqrt{3}}{3}$

10. Using the calculator (radian mode),

$(360° - 300°) = 60°$ $\tan 2.25 \approx -1.238627616; \csc 2.25 \approx 1.285226125; \sec 2.25 \approx -1.591916572;$ and

$\cot 2.25 \approx -.8073451511$.

8.3: Graphs of the Sine and Cosine Functions

1. Since $\sin 0 = 0$, $\sin \dfrac{\pi}{2} = 1$, the amplitude is 1, and the period is $\dfrac{2\pi}{(1)} = 2\pi$, the graph is G.

3. Since $-\sin 0 = 0$, $-\sin \dfrac{\pi}{2} = -1$, the amplitude is 1, and the period is $\dfrac{2\pi}{(1)} = 2\pi$, the graph is E.

Copyright © 2015 Pearson Education, Inc

Section 8.3   391

5. Since $\sin 2(0) = 0$, $\sin 2\left(\dfrac{\pi}{4}\right) = \sin \dfrac{\pi}{2} = 1$, the amplitude is 1, and the period is $\dfrac{2\pi}{(2)} = \pi$, the graph is B.

7. Since $2\sin 0 = 2(0) = 0$, $2\sin \dfrac{\pi}{2} = 2(1) = 2$, the amplitude is 2, and the period is $\dfrac{2\pi}{(1)} = 2\pi$, the graph is F.

9. The graph of $y = \sin\left(x - \dfrac{\pi}{4}\right)$ is the graph of $y = \sin x$ translated $\dfrac{\pi}{4}$ units to the right, therefore the graph is D.

11. The graph of $y = \cos\left(x - \dfrac{\pi}{4}\right)$ is the graph of $y = \cos x$ translated $\dfrac{\pi}{4}$ units to the right, therefore the graph is H.

13. The graph of $y = 1 + \sin x$ is the graph of $y = \sin x$ translated 1 unit upward, therefore the graph is B.

15. The graph of $y = 1 + \cos x$ is the graph of $y = \cos x$ translated 1 unit upward, therefore the graph is F.

17. The equation $y = 3\sin(2x - 4)$ has an amplitude 3; a period of $\dfrac{2\pi}{(2)} = \pi$; and a phase shift $\dfrac{4}{2} = 2$, therefore B.

19. The equation $y = 4\sin(3x - 2)$ has an amplitude 4; a period of $\dfrac{2\pi}{(3)}$; and a phase shift $\dfrac{2}{3}$ therefore C.

21. See Figure 21. From the equation, the amplitude is 2.

23. See Figure 23. From the equation, the amplitude is $\dfrac{2}{3}$.

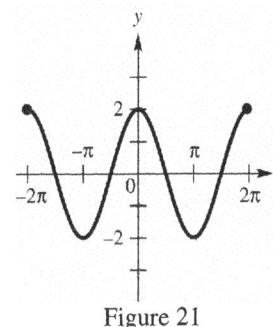

Figure 21

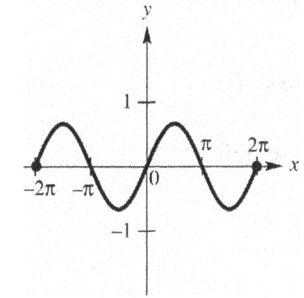

Figure 23

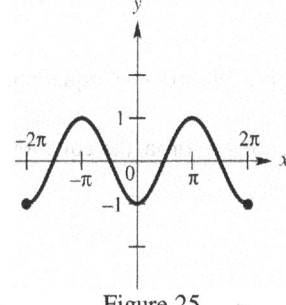

Figure 25

25. See Figure 25. From the equation, the amplitude is 1.

27. See Figure 27. From the equation, the amplitude is 2.

29. See Figure 29. From the equation, the period is and the amplitude is 1.

392   Chapter 8: The Unit Circle and the Functions of Trigonometry

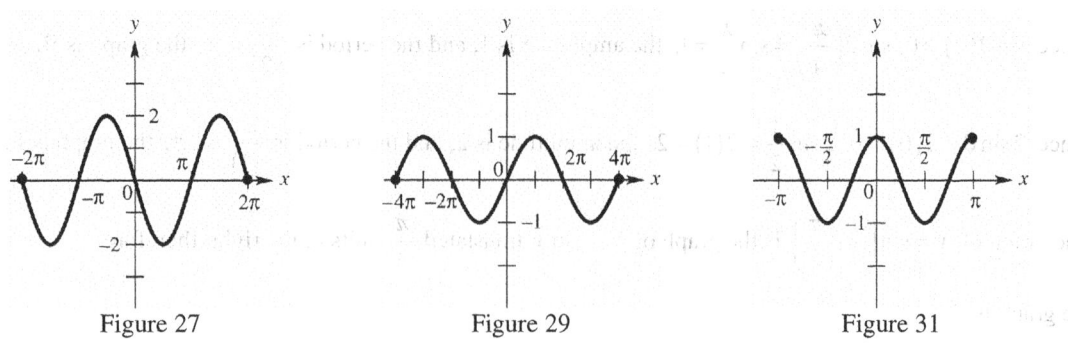

Figure 27   Figure 29   Figure 31

31. See Figure 31. From the equation, the period is π and the amplitude is 1.

33. See Figure 33. From the equation, the period is 8π and the amplitude is 2.

35. See Figure 35. From the equation, the period is $\dfrac{2\pi}{3}$ and the amplitude is 2.

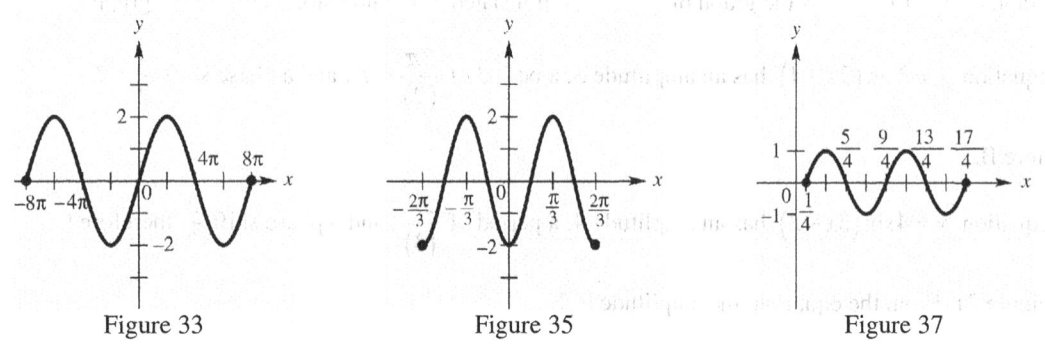

Figure 33   Figure 35   Figure 37

37. See Figure 37. From the equation, the phase shift is $\dfrac{\pi}{4}$.

39. See Figure 39. From the equation, the phase shift is $\dfrac{\pi}{3}$.

41. See Figure 41. From the equation, the phase shift is $-\pi$.

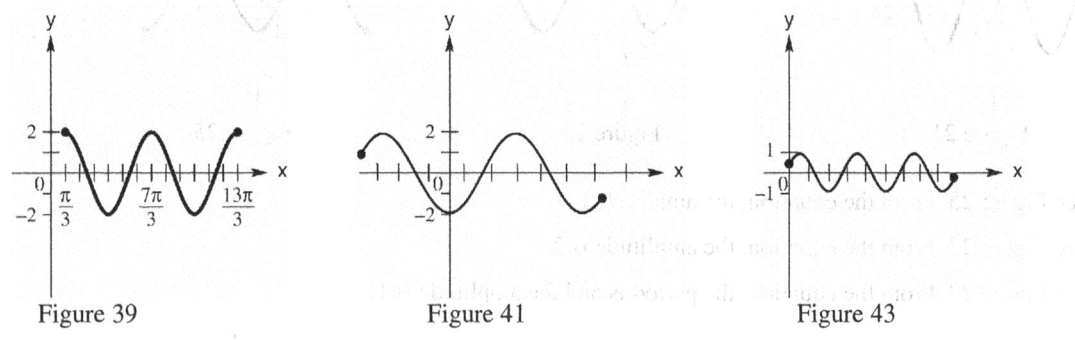

Figure 39   Figure 41   Figure 43

43. See Figure 43. Note that $y = \sin\left(2x + \dfrac{\pi}{4}\right)$ can be written as $y = \sin\left(2\left(x + \dfrac{\pi}{8}\right)\right)$ and the phase shift is $-\dfrac{\pi}{8}$.

45. (a) From the equation, the amplitude is: $|-4| = 4$.

Copyright © 2015 Pearson Education, Inc

(b) From the equation, the period is: $\theta = \dfrac{2\pi}{2} = \pi$

(c) Since $y = -4\sin(2x - \pi) \Rightarrow y = -4\sin\left[2\left(x - \dfrac{\pi}{2}\right)\right]$, the phase shift is: $\dfrac{\pi}{2}$.

(d) No vertical translation.

(e) The range is: $[-4, 4]$. See Figure 45.

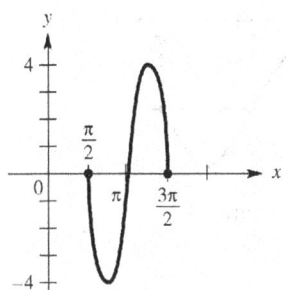

Figure 45

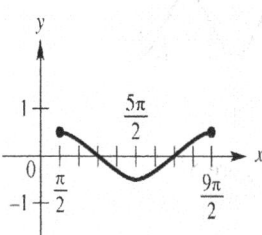

Figure 47

47. (a) From the equation, the amplitude is: $\dfrac{1}{2}$.

(b) From the equation, the period is: $\dfrac{2\pi}{\dfrac{1}{2}} = 4\pi$.

(c) Since $y = \dfrac{1}{2}\cos\left(\dfrac{1}{2}x - \dfrac{\pi}{4}\right) \Rightarrow y = \dfrac{1}{2}\cos\left[\dfrac{1}{2}\left(x - \dfrac{\pi}{2}\right)\right]$, the phase shift is: $\dfrac{\pi}{2}$.

(d) No vertical translation.

(e) The range is: $\left[-\dfrac{1}{2}, \dfrac{1}{2}\right]$. See Figure 47.

49. (a) From the equation, the amplitude is: $\left|-\dfrac{2}{3}\right| = \dfrac{2}{3}$.

(b) From the equation, the period is: $\dfrac{2\pi}{\left(\dfrac{3}{4}\right)} = \dfrac{8\pi}{3}$.

(c) From the equation, there is no phase shift.

(d) From the equation, the vertical translation is: upward 1 unit.

(e) The range is: $\left[-\dfrac{2}{3}, \dfrac{2}{3}\right]$ translated upward 1 unit, therefore, $\left[\dfrac{1}{3}, \dfrac{5}{3}\right]$. See Figure 49.

51. (a) From the equation, the amplitude is: $|-2| = 2$.

(b) From the equation, the period is: $\dfrac{2\pi}{\left(\frac{1}{2}\right)} = 4\pi$.

(c) From the equation, there is no phase shift.

(d) From the equation, the vertical translation is: upward 1 unit.

(e) The range is: $[-2, 2]$ translated upward 1 unit, therefore, $[-1, 3]$. See Figure 51.

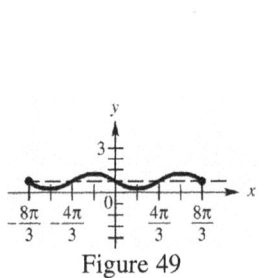
Figure 49

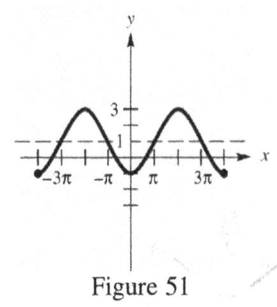
Figure 51

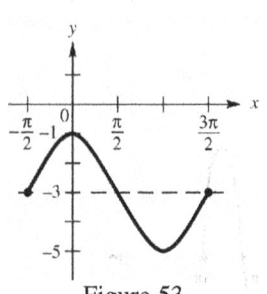
Figure 53

53. (a) From the equation, the amplitude is: 2.

(b) From the equation, the period is: $\dfrac{2\pi}{(1)} = 2\pi$.

(c) From the equation, the phase shift is: $-\dfrac{\pi}{2}$.

(d) From the equation, the vertical translation is: downward 3 unit.

(e) The range is: $[-2, 2]$ translated downward 3 units, therefore, $[-5, -1]$. See Figure 53.

55. (a) From the equation, the amplitude is: 1.

(b) From the equation, the period is: $\dfrac{2\pi}{(2)} = \pi$.

(c) From the equation, the phase shift is: $-\dfrac{\pi}{4}$.

(d) From the equation, the vertical translation is: upward $\dfrac{1}{2}$ unit.

(e) The range is: $[-1, 1]$ translated upward $\dfrac{1}{2}$ unit, therefore, $\left[-\dfrac{1}{2}, \dfrac{3}{2}\right]$. See Figure 55.

57. (a) From the equation, the amplitude is: 2.

(b) From the equation, the period is: $\cos T = 2\pi$

(c) From the equation, the phase shift is: π.

(d) From the equation, there is no vertical translation.

(e) The range is: $[-2, 2]$. See Figure 57.

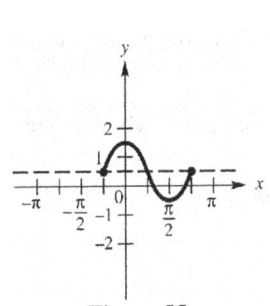

Figure 55

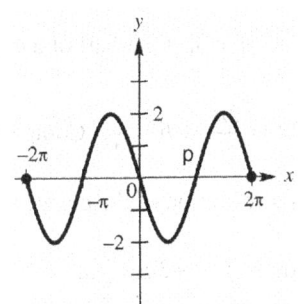

Figure 57

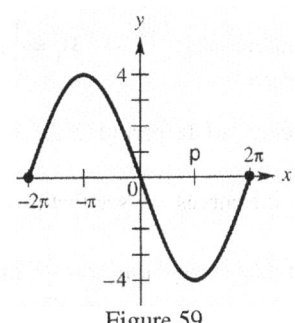

Figure 59

59. (a) From the equation, the amplitude is: 4.

(b) From the equation, the period is: $\dfrac{2\pi}{\left(\frac{1}{2}\right)} = 4\pi$.

(c) Since $y = 4\cos\left(\dfrac{1}{2}x + \dfrac{\pi}{2}\right) \Rightarrow y = 4\cos\left[\dfrac{1}{2}(x+\pi)\right]$, the phase shift is: $-\pi$.

(d) From the equation, there is no vertical translation.

(e) The range is: $[-4, 4]$. See Figure 59.

61. (a) From the equation, the amplitude is: $|-1| = 1$.

(b) From the equation, the period is: $\dfrac{2\pi}{(3)}$.

(c) Since $y = 2 - \sin\left(3x - \dfrac{\pi}{5}\right) \Rightarrow y = 2 - \sin\left[3\left(x - \dfrac{\pi}{15}\right)\right]$, the phase shift is: $\dfrac{\pi}{15}$.

(d) From the equation, the vertical translation is: upward 2 units.

(e) The range is: $[-1,1]$. translated upward 2 units, therefore, $[1,3]$. See Figure 61.

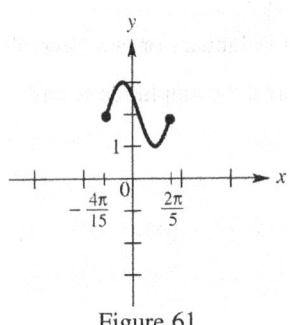

Figure 61

63. The amplitude is $\dfrac{1}{2}[2-(-2)] = \dfrac{1}{2}(4) = 2$, so $a = 2$. One complete cycle of the graph is achieved in π units, so the period $\pi = \dfrac{2\pi}{b} \Rightarrow b = 2$. Comparing the given graph with the general and cosine curves, we see that this graph is a cosine curve. Substituting $a = 2$ and $b = 2$, the function is $y = 2\cos 2x$.

65. The amplitude is $\frac{1}{2}[3-(-3)] = \frac{1}{2}(6) = 3$, so $a = 3$. One-half of a complete cycle of the graph is achieved in 2π units, so the period $2 \cdot 2\pi = 4\pi \Rightarrow 4\pi = \frac{2\pi}{b} \Rightarrow b = \frac{1}{2}$. Comparing the given graph with the general and cosine curves, we see that this graph is a reflection of the cosine curve. Thus $a = -3$. Substituting $a = -3$ and $b = \frac{1}{2}$, the function is $y = -3\cos\frac{1}{2}x$.

67. The amplitude is $\frac{1}{2}[3-(-3)] = \frac{1}{2}(6) = 3$, so $a = 3$. One complete cycle of the graph is achieved in $\frac{\pi}{2}$ units, so the period $\frac{\pi}{2} = \frac{2\pi}{b} \Rightarrow b = 4$. Comparing the given graph with the general and cosine curves, we see that this graph is a sine curve. Substituting $a = 3$ and $b = 4$, the function is $y = 3\sin 4x$.

69. This is the sine curve shifted down one unit, so the equation is $y = -1 + \sin x$.

71. The maximum is at $\left(\frac{\pi}{3}, 1\right)$, so the cosine curve has been shifted $\frac{\pi}{3}$ units to the right. Thus, the equation is $y = \cos\left(x - \frac{\pi}{3}\right)$.

73. (a) From the graph, the maximum is 40°F and the minimum is −40°F.

(b) From the graph, the amplitude is 40 and the period is 12. Since there is no vertical translation, the amplitude will help us find the maximum and minimum average temperature values of 40° and −40° and the period represents the 12 months of the calendar year. The monthly average temperatures vary by 80°F over a 12-month period.

(c) The x-intercepts represents the two months when the average temperature is 0°F.

75. (a) From the graph, the maximum is 87°F in July, and the minimum is 62°F in January or late December.

(b) Since a minimum temperature 50° would increase the range of temperatures, the amplitude would increase. See Figure 75.

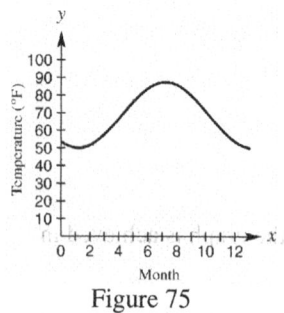

Figure 75

77. The graph repeats each day, so the period is 24 hours.

Section 8.3   397

79. (a) From the equation, the amplitude is 34; the period is $\frac{\pi}{6} = \frac{2\pi}{b} \Rightarrow b = 12$, and the phase shift is 4.3.

  (b) May corresponds to $x = 5$, $f(5) = 34\sin\left[\frac{\pi}{6}(5-4.3)\right] \approx 12.2°\,F$

  December corresponds to $x = 12$, $f(12) = 34\sin\left[\frac{\pi}{6}(12-4.3)\right] \approx -26.4°\,F$

  (c) Since half of the months have average temperatures above zero and half have average temperatures below zero, we would conjecture that the average yearly temperature is $0°\,F$.

81. (a) We predict the average yearly temperature by finding the mean of the average monthly temperatures:

  $\frac{51+55+63+67+77+86+90+84+71+59+52}{12} = \frac{845}{12} = 70.4°F$.

  This is very close to the actual value of $70.4°F$.

  (b) See Figure 81b.

  (c) Since amplitude $a \approx \frac{90-51}{2} \Rightarrow c = 70.5$; the period is 12 months or $b = \frac{2\pi}{(12)} = \frac{\pi}{6}$; the vertical translation is $c = \frac{51+90}{2} \Rightarrow c = 70.5$; and the phase shift can be found by using the minimum temperature value. Since the coldest month is January, when $x = 1$, $b = (1-d)$ must equal $(-\pi + 2\pi n)$, where n is an integer, since the cosine function is a minimum at these values. Letting $n = 0$, we can solve for d: $\frac{\pi}{6}(1-d) = -x \Rightarrow 1-d = -6 \Rightarrow d = 7$. The table shows that temperatures are actually a little warmer after July than before, so we choose for a better approximation. Now using a, b, c, and d yields: $f(x) = 19.5\cos\left[\frac{\pi}{6}(x-7.2)\right] + 70.5$.

  (d) See Figure 81d. The function gives an excellent model for the given data.

  (e) Set the calculator to the nearest hundredth and the regression equation is, see Figure 81e.

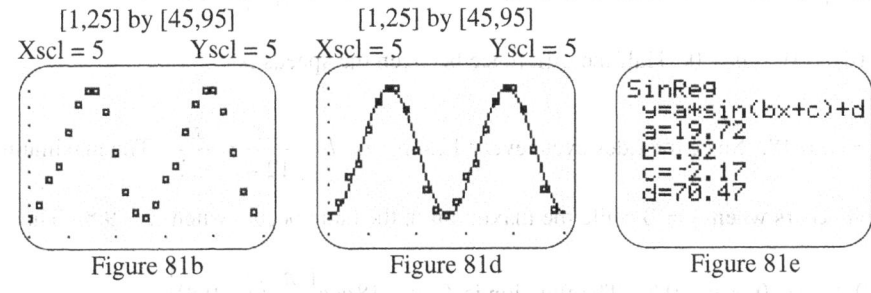

Figure 81b   Figure 81d   Figure 81e

83. (a) See Figure 83a.

398 Chapter 8: The Unit Circle and the Functions of Trigonometry

(b) The maximum monthly average temperature is 68° and the minimum is 40°. The midpoint of these values is $\frac{1}{2}(68+40) = 50 \Rightarrow d = 50$. Half the difference between the temperatures is $\frac{1}{2}(68-40) = 14 \Rightarrow a = 14$. Since the temperatures cycle every 12 months, $b = \frac{2\pi}{12} = \frac{\pi}{6}$. The maximum of the $y = \sin x$ graph occurs when $x = \frac{\pi}{2}$ while the maximum in the table occurs when $x = 7$. Thus $\frac{\pi}{6}(7-c) = \frac{\pi}{2} \Rightarrow 7-c = 3 \Rightarrow c = 4$. The function is $f(x) = 14\sin\left[\frac{\pi}{6}(x-4)\right] + 50$.

(c) See Figure 83c.

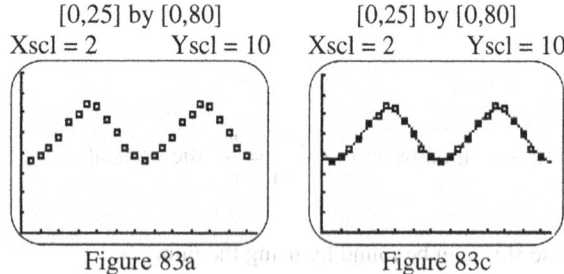

Figure 83a   Figure 83c

85. (a) The maximum monthly average temperature is 92° and the minimum is 58°. The midpoint of these values is $\frac{1}{2}(92+58) = 75 \Rightarrow d = 50$. Half the difference between the temperatures is $\frac{1}{2}(92-58) = 17 \Rightarrow a = 17$. Since the temperatures cycle every 12 months, $b = \frac{2\pi}{12} = \frac{\pi}{6}$. The maximum of the $y = \cos x$ graph occurs when $x = 0$ while the maximum in the table occurs when $x = 7$. Thus $\frac{\pi}{6}(7-c) = 0 \Rightarrow 7-c = 0 \Rightarrow c = 7$. The function is $f(x) = 17\cos\left[\frac{\pi}{6}(x-7)\right] + 75$.

(b) Yes, different values of c are possible of the form $c = 7 + 12n$ where n is an integer.

87. (a) The maximum current speed is $18bk$ and the minimum is $-18bk$. The midpoint of these values is $\frac{1}{2}(18+(-18)) = 0 \Rightarrow d = 0$. Half the difference between the speeds is $\frac{1}{2}(18-(-18)) = 18 \Rightarrow a = 18$. Since the tides cycle every 12.4 hours, $b = \frac{2\pi}{12.4} = \frac{\pi}{6.2}$. The maximum of the $y = \cos x$ graph occurs when $x = 0$ while the maximum in the table occurs when $x = 9.8$. Thus $\frac{\pi}{6.2}(9.8-c) = 0 \Rightarrow 9.8-c = 0 \Rightarrow c = 9.8$. The function is $f(x) = 18\cos\left[\frac{\pi}{6.2}(x-9.8)\right]$.

(b) The canal contains the most water at 3.7 and 16.1 hours after midnight (high tides). At these points water is rushing out of the canal at 18bk. The canal contains the least water at 9.8 and 22.2 hours after midnight (low tides). At these points water is rushing into the canal at 18bk. See Figure 87.

89. (a) See Figure 89.

(b) If $x = 1970$ corresponds to 1970 then the equation is:

$$c(x) = .4(x-1970)^2 + .6(x-1970) + 330 + 7.5 \sin\left[2\pi(x-1970)\right].$$

[0,24] by [-20,20]
Xscl = 4   Yscl = 5

[5,25] by [320,380]
Xscl = 5   Yscl = 10

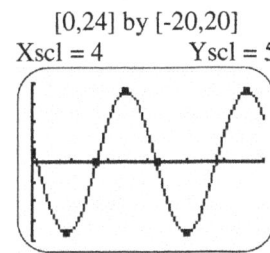

Figure 87

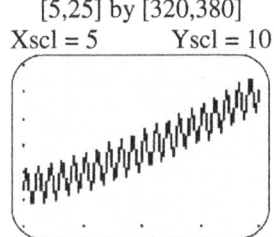

Figure 89

91. $-1 \le y \le 1 \Rightarrow$ Amplitude : 1 , Period: 8 squares $= 8(30°) = 240° = \dfrac{4\pi}{3}$

93. (a) No. The graphs are different. We can say that in general $\sin bx \ne b \sin x$ for $x \ne 1$.

(b) No. The graphs are different. We can say that in general $\cos bx \ne b \cos x$ for $x \ne 1$.

8.4 Graphs of the Other Circular Functions

1. The basic cosecant graph reflected across the x-axis, therefore graph B.

3. The basic tangent graph reflected across the x-axis, therefore graph E.

5. The basic tangent graph translated $\dfrac{\pi}{4}$ units to the right, therefore graph D.

7. True, $x = \dfrac{\pi}{2}$ is the smallest positive asymptote of the tangent function.

9. False, secant values are undefined when $x = \dfrac{\pi}{2} + \pi k$ while cosecant values are undefined when $x = \pi k$.

11. $\sec(-x) = \dfrac{1}{\cos(-x)} = \dfrac{1}{\cos x} = \sec x$

13. $\tan(-x) = \dfrac{\sin(-x)}{\cos(-x)} = \dfrac{-\sin x}{\cos x} = -\tan x$

15. (a) From the equation, the period is: $\dfrac{2\pi}{\left(\dfrac{1}{2}\right)} = 4\pi.$

(b) From the equation, there is no phase shift.

(c) From the equation, the range is $(-\infty, -2] \cup [2, \infty)$.

400   Chapter 8: The Unit Circle and the Functions of Trigonometry

17. (a) From the equation, the period is: $\dfrac{2\pi}{(1)} = 2\pi$.

   (b) From the equation, the phase shift is: $-\dfrac{\pi}{2}$ units to the right.

   (c) From the equation, the range is $(-\infty, -2] \cup [2, \infty)$.

19. (a) From the equation, the period is: $\dfrac{\pi}{\left(\dfrac{1}{3}\right)} = 3\pi$ (The phase shift for the basic cotangent function is π.)

   (b) From the equation, the phase shift is: $\left(\dfrac{\pi}{2}\text{ units to the right}\right)$

   (c) The range of all cotangent functions is $(-\infty, \infty)$.

21. (a) From the equation, the period is: $\dfrac{2\pi}{(2)} = \pi$.

   (b) From the equation, the phase shift is: $-\dfrac{\pi}{2}$. $\left(\dfrac{\pi}{2}\text{ units to the left}\right)$

   (c) From the equation, the range is $\left(-\infty, -\dfrac{1}{2}\right] \cup \left[\dfrac{1}{2}, \infty\right)$.

23. (a) From the equation, the period is: $\dfrac{\pi}{(1)} = \pi$. (The phase shift for the basic tangent function is π.)

   (b) From the equation, the phase shift is: $-\dfrac{\pi}{4}$.

   (c) The range of all tangent functions is $(-\infty, \infty)$.

25. Graph a secant function with a period of 2π a range of $(-\infty, -1] \cup [1, \infty)$ and no phase shift. See Figure 25.

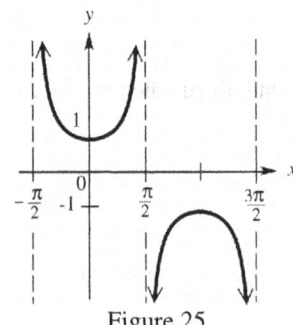
Figure 25

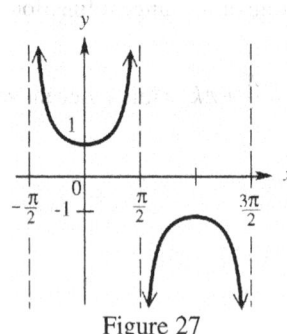
Figure 27

27. Graph a secant function with a period of 2π a range of $(-\infty, -1] \cup [1, \infty)$ and a phase shift of 2π to the right. See Figure 27.

29. Graph a secant function with a period of $\dfrac{\pi}{\left(\dfrac{1}{4}\right)} = 8\pi$ a range of $(-\infty, -3] \cup [3, \infty)$ and no phase shift.

   See Figure 29.

Section 8.4   401

31. Graph a cosecant function with a period of $\frac{2\pi}{(1)} = 2\pi$, a range $\left(-\infty, -\frac{1}{2}\right] \cup \left[\frac{1}{2}, \infty\right)$, of reflected across the x-axis, and a phase shift $\frac{\pi}{2}$ units to the left. See Figure 31.

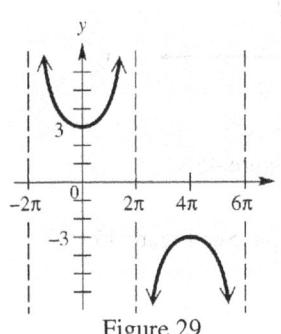
Figure 29

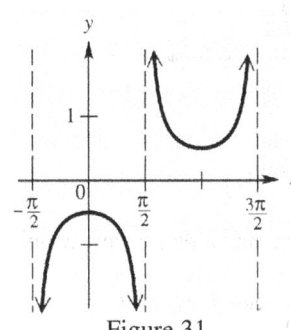
Figure 31

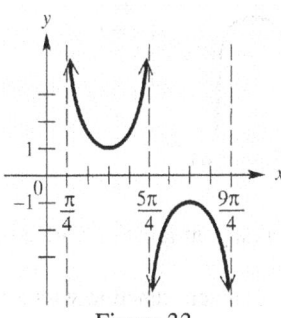
Figure 33

33. Graph a cosecant function with a period of $\frac{2\pi}{(1)} = 2\pi$, and a phase shift $\frac{\pi}{4}$ units to the right. See Figure 33.

35. Graph a secant function with a period of $\frac{2\pi}{(1)} = 2\pi$, and a phase shift $\frac{\pi}{4}$ units to the left. See Figure 35.

37. Since $y = \sec\left(\frac{1}{2}x + \frac{\pi}{3}\right) \Rightarrow y = \sec\frac{1}{2}\left(x + \frac{2\pi}{3}\right)$, graph a secant function with a period $\frac{2\pi}{\left(\frac{1}{2}\right)} = 4\pi$, and a phase shift $\frac{2\pi}{3}$ units to the left. See Figure 37.

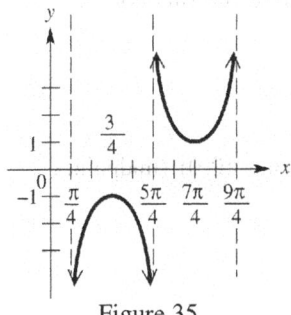
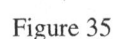
Figure 35

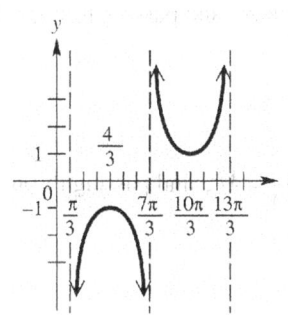
Figure 37

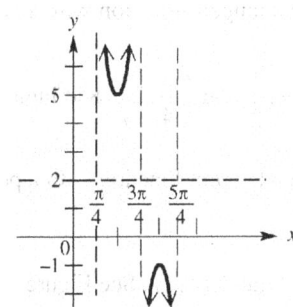
Figure 39

39. Since $y = 2 + 3\sec(2x - \pi) \Rightarrow y = 2 + 3\sec 2\left(x - \frac{\pi}{2}\right)$, graph a secant function with a period $\frac{2\pi}{(2)} = \pi$ a vertical shift 2 units upward therefore a range of $(-\infty, -1] \cup [5, \infty)$, and a phase shift $\frac{\pi}{2}$ units to the right.

41. Graph a cosecant function with a period $\frac{2\pi}{(1)} = 2\pi$, reflected across the x-axis, a vertical shift 1 unit upward therefore a range of $\left(-\infty, -\frac{1}{2}\right] \cup \left[\frac{3}{2}, \infty\right)$, and a phase shift $\frac{3\pi}{4}$ units to the right. See Figure 41.

43. Graph a tangent function with a period of π, and no phase shift. See Figure 43.

402 Chapter 8: The Unit Circle and the Functions of Trigonometry

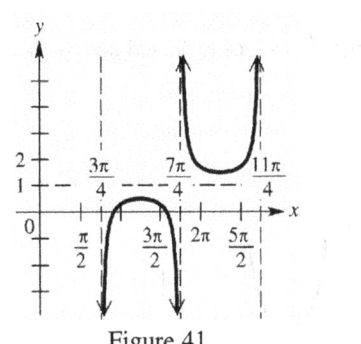

Figure 41

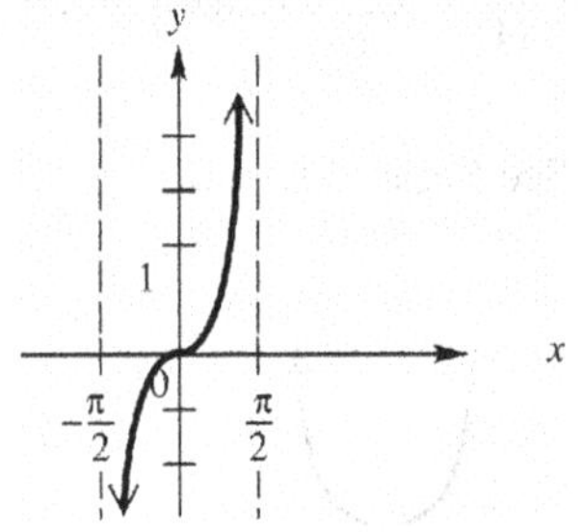

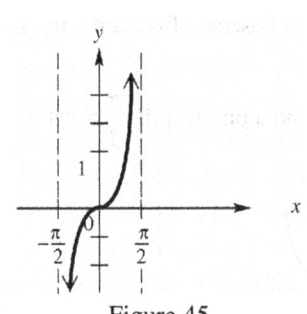

Figure 43

Figure 45

45. Graph a tangent function with a period of π, and a phase shift π units to the right. See Figure 45.

47. Graph a tangent function with a period $\dfrac{\pi}{(4)}$. See Figure 47.

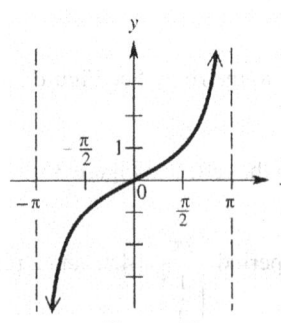

Figure 47

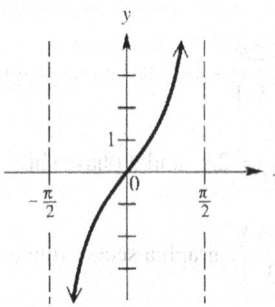

Figure 49

49. Graph a tangent function with a period $\dfrac{\pi}{(1)} = \pi$; and passing through the points $(0,0)$ (midpoint), $\left(-\dfrac{\pi}{4},-2\right)$ and $\left(\dfrac{\pi}{4},2\right)$. See Figure 49.

51. Graph a tangent function with a period $\dfrac{\pi}{\left(\dfrac{1}{4}\right)} = 4\pi$; and passing through the points $(0,0)$ (midpoint), $(-\pi,-2)$, and $(\pi,2)$. See Figure 51.

53. Graph a cotangent function with a period $\dfrac{\pi}{(3)}$; and passing through the points $\left(\dfrac{\pi}{6},0\right)$ (midpoint), $\left(\dfrac{\pi}{12},1\right)$, and $\left(\dfrac{\pi}{4},-1\right)$. See Figure 53.

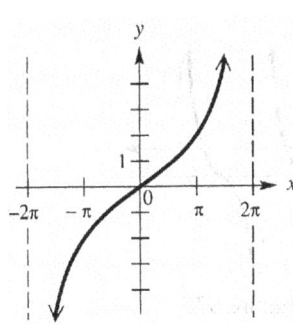

Figure 51

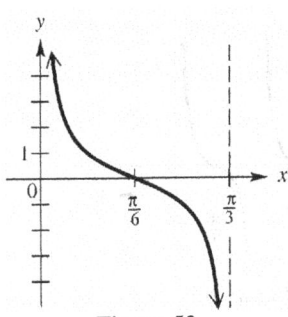

Figure 53

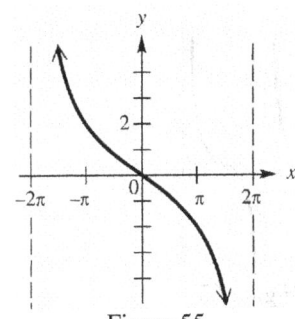

Figure 55

55. Graph a tangent function with a period $\dfrac{\pi}{\left(\frac{1}{4}\right)} = 4\pi$, is reflected across the x-axis, and passes through the points $(0,0)$ (midpoint), $(-\pi, 2)$, and $(\pi, -2)$. See Figure 55.

57. Graph a cotangent function with a period $\dfrac{\pi}{(4)}$; and passing through the points $\left(\dfrac{\pi}{8}, 0\right)$ (midpoint), $\left(\dfrac{\pi}{16}, \dfrac{1}{2}\right)$, and $\left(\dfrac{3\pi}{16}, -\dfrac{1}{2}\right)$. See Figure 57.

59. Since $y = \tan(2x - \pi) \Rightarrow y = \tan 2\left(x - \dfrac{\pi}{2}\right)$, graph a tangent function, over a two period interval, with a period $\dfrac{\pi}{(2)}$ and a phase shift of $\dfrac{\pi}{2}$ units to the right. See Figure 59.

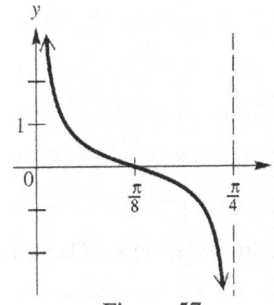

Figure 57

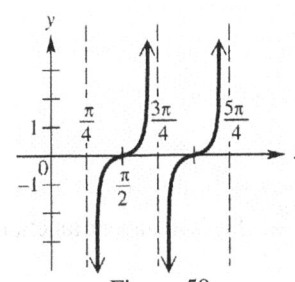

Figure 59

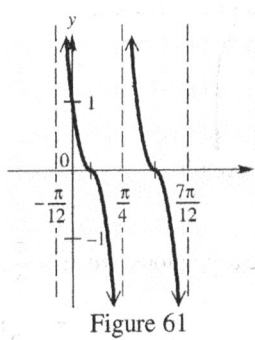

Figure 61

61. Since $y = \cot\left(3\pi + \dfrac{x}{4}\right) \Rightarrow y = \cot 3\left(x + \dfrac{\pi}{12}\right)$, graph a cotangent function, over a two period interval, with a period $\dfrac{\pi}{(3)}$ and a phase shift of $\dfrac{\pi}{12}$ units to the left. See Figure 61.

63. Graph a tangent function with a period $\dfrac{\pi}{(1)} = \pi$ and vertical shift 1 unit upward. See Figure 63.

65. Graph a cotangent function with a period $\dfrac{\pi}{(1)} = \pi$, is reflected across the x-axis, and vertical shift 1 unit upward. See Figure 65.

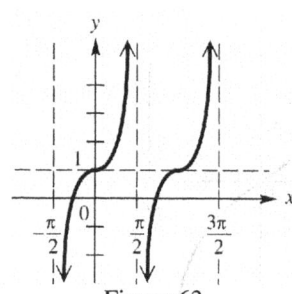
Figure 63

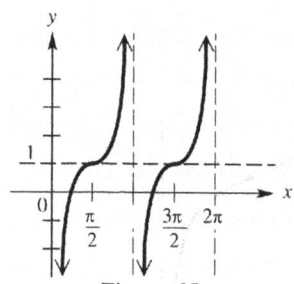
Figure 65

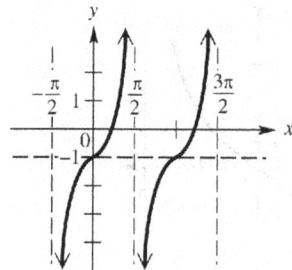
Figure 67

67. Graph a tangent function with a period $\dfrac{\pi}{(1)} = \pi$, and vertical shift 1 unit downward, and passes through the points $(0,-1)$ (midpoint), $\left(-\dfrac{\pi}{4},-3\right)$ and $\left(\dfrac{\pi}{4},1\right)$ See Figure 67.

69. Since $y = -1 + \dfrac{1}{2}\cot(2x - 3\pi) \Rightarrow y = -1 + \dfrac{1}{2}\cot 2\left(x - \dfrac{3\pi}{2}\right)$, graph a cotangent function, over a two period interval, with a period $\dfrac{\pi}{(2)}$, a phase shift of $\dfrac{3\pi}{2}$ units to the right, has a vertical shift 1 unit downward, and passes through the points $\left(\dfrac{3\pi}{4},-1\right)$ (midpoint), $\left(\dfrac{5\pi}{8},-\dfrac{1}{2}\right)$ and $\left(\dfrac{7\pi}{8},-\dfrac{3}{2}\right)$. See Figure 69.

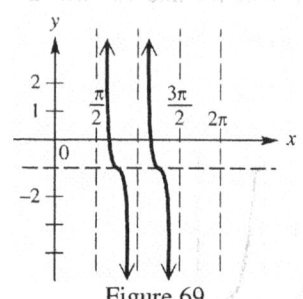
Figure 69

71. Since the asymptotes are at $-\dfrac{\pi}{2}, \dfrac{\pi}{2}$, and $\dfrac{3\pi}{2}$, this is a tangent function of the form $y = a\tan x$. The graph passes through the point $\left(\dfrac{\pi}{4},-2\right)$. Substituting these values into the equation above gives

$y = a\tan x \Rightarrow -2 = a\tan \dfrac{\pi}{4} \Rightarrow -2 = a\cdot 1 \Rightarrow -2 = a$ Thus, the equation of the graph is $y = -2\tan x$.

73. Since the asymptotes are at $0, \dfrac{\pi}{3}$, and $\dfrac{2\pi}{3}$, this is a tangent function of the form $y = a\tan bx$. The period of the function is $\dfrac{\pi}{b} = \dfrac{\pi}{3} \Rightarrow b = 3$. The graph passes through the point $\left(\dfrac{\pi}{12},1\right)$. Substituting these values into the equation above gives $y = a\cot bx \Rightarrow 1 = a\cot\left(3\cdot\dfrac{\pi}{12}\right) \Rightarrow 1 = a\cot\dfrac{\pi}{4} \Rightarrow 1 = a$.

Thus, the equation of the graph is $y = \cot 3x$.

75. Since the asymptotes are at multiples of π, this is a cotangent function of the form $y = a \cot x$. The graph passes through the point $\left(\dfrac{\pi}{4}, -3\right)$. Substituting these values into the equation above gives

$y = a \cot x \Rightarrow -3 = a \cot \dfrac{\pi}{4} \Rightarrow -3 = a \cdot 1 \Rightarrow -3 = a$ Thus, the equation of the graph is $y = -3 \cot x$.

77. Since the graph crosses the y-axis at $(0,1)$, this is a secant graph with $a = 1$. The period is $\left| -\dfrac{\pi}{4} - \dfrac{\pi}{4} \right| = \dfrac{\pi}{2}$.

Thus, $b = \dfrac{2\pi}{\dfrac{\pi}{2}} \Rightarrow b = 4$. The equation of the graph is $y = \sec 4x$.

79. This is the graph of $y = \csc x$ translated two units down. Thus, the equation of the graph is $y = -2 + \csc x$.

Reviewing Basic Concepts (Sections 8.3 and 8.4)

1. From the equation, the amplitude is $|-1| = 1$ and the period is $\dfrac{2\pi}{(1)} = 2\pi$ See Figure 1.

2. From the equation, the amplitude is 3, the period is $\dfrac{2\pi}{(\pi)} = 2$, and the phase shift is $-\dfrac{\pi}{\pi} = -1$ See Figure 2

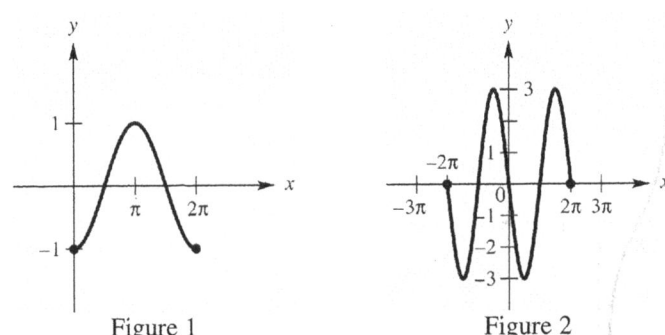

Figure 1   Figure 2

3. (a) Since the amplitude is 6.5 and the vertical shift is 12.4, the maximum number of daylight hours is $6.5 + 12.4 = 18.9$ hours and the minimum is $-6.5 + 12.4 = 5.9$ hours.

   (b) The amplitude represents half the difference in the daylight hours between the longest and shortest days. The period represents 12 months or one year.

4. From the equation, the period is: $\dfrac{2\pi}{(1)} = 2\pi$; the phase shift is: $x + y$ or $\dfrac{\pi}{4}$ units to the right; the domain is:

   $\left\{ x \middle| x \neq \dfrac{\pi}{4} + n\pi, \text{ where } n \text{ is an integer} \right\}$; and the range is: $(-\infty, -1] \cup [1, \infty)$. See Figure 4.

5. From the equation, the period is: $\dfrac{2\pi}{(1)} = 2\pi$; the phase shift is: $-\dfrac{\pi}{4}$ or $\dfrac{\pi}{4}$ units to the left; the domain is:

406 Chapter 8: The Unit Circle and the Functions of Trigonometry

$\left\{ x \mid x \neq \dfrac{\pi}{4} + n\pi, \text{ where } n \text{ is an integer} \right\}$; and the range is: $(-\infty, -1] \cup [1, \infty)$. See Figure 5.

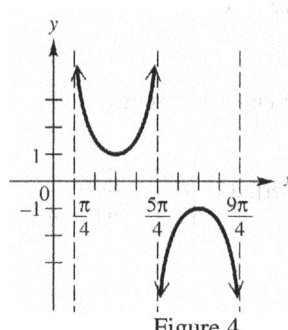
Figure 4

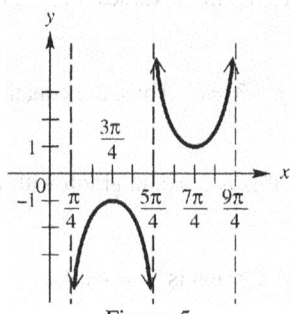
Figure 5

6. From the equation, the period is: $\dfrac{\pi}{(1)} = \pi$; the domain is: $\left\{ x \mid x \neq \dfrac{\pi}{2} + n\pi, \text{ where } n \text{ is an integer} \right\}$; and the range is: $(-\infty, \infty)$. See Figure 6.

7. From the equation, the period is: $\dfrac{\pi}{(1)} = \pi$; the domain is: $\left\{ x \mid x \neq n\pi, \text{ where } n \text{ is an integer} \right\}$; and the range is: $(-\infty, \infty)$. See Figure 7.

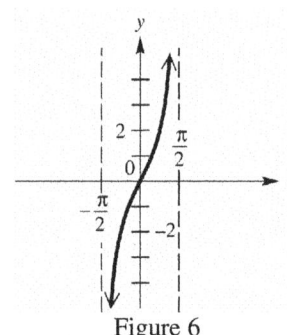
Figure 6

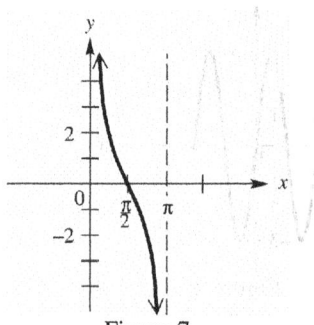
Figure 7

8.5: Functions of Angles and Fundamental Identities

1. $x = 5, y = 12 \Rightarrow r = \sqrt{x^2 + y^2} = \sqrt{5^2 + (12)^2} = \sqrt{169} = 13$,

   $\sin \theta = \dfrac{y}{r} = \dfrac{12}{13}; \cos \theta = \dfrac{x}{r} = \dfrac{5}{13}; \tan \theta = \dfrac{y}{x} = \dfrac{12}{5}; \csc \theta = \dfrac{r}{y} = \dfrac{13}{12}; \sec \theta = \dfrac{r}{x} = \dfrac{13}{5}; \cot \theta = \dfrac{y}{x} = \dfrac{5}{12}$.

3. They are the same for each trigonometric function. They are coterminal angles.

5. $x = 5, y = -12 \Rightarrow r = \sqrt{x^2 + y^2} = \sqrt{5^2 + (-12)^2} = \sqrt{169} = 13$, See Figure 5.

   $\sin \theta = \dfrac{y}{r} = \dfrac{-12}{13} = -\dfrac{12}{13}; \cos \theta = \dfrac{x}{r} = \dfrac{5}{13}; \tan \theta = \dfrac{y}{x} = \dfrac{-12}{5} = -\dfrac{12}{5}$

   $\csc \theta = \dfrac{r}{y} = \dfrac{13}{-12} = -\dfrac{13}{12}; \sec \theta = \dfrac{r}{x} = \dfrac{13}{5}; \cot \theta = \dfrac{5}{-12} = -\dfrac{5}{12}$.

7. $x = -3, y = 4 \Rightarrow r = \sqrt{x^2 + y^2} = \sqrt{(-3)^2 + (4)^2} = \sqrt{25} = 5$ See Figure 7.

$\sin\theta = \dfrac{y}{r} = \dfrac{4}{5}; \cos\theta = \dfrac{x}{r} = \dfrac{-3}{5} = -\dfrac{3}{5}; \tan\theta = \dfrac{y}{x} = \dfrac{4}{-3} = -\dfrac{4}{3}$

$\csc\theta = \dfrac{r}{y} = \dfrac{5}{4}; \sec\theta = \dfrac{r}{x} = \dfrac{5}{-3} = -\dfrac{5}{3}; \cot\theta = \dfrac{-3}{4} = -\dfrac{3}{4}.$

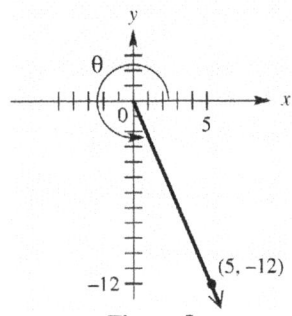
Figure 5

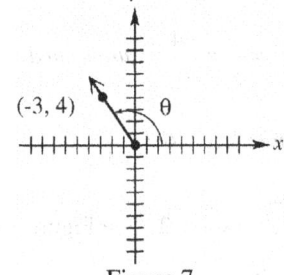
Figure 7

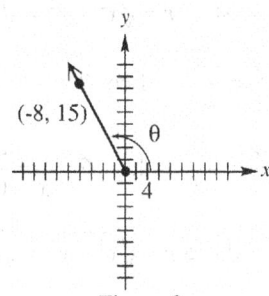
Figure 9

9. $x = -8, y = 15 \Rightarrow r = \sqrt{x^2 + y^2} = \sqrt{(-8)^2 + (15)^2} = \sqrt{289} = 17$ See Figure 9.

$\sin\theta = \dfrac{y}{r} = \dfrac{15}{17}; \cos\theta = \dfrac{x}{r} = \dfrac{-8}{17} = -\dfrac{8}{17}; \tan\theta = \dfrac{y}{x} = \dfrac{15}{-8} = -\dfrac{15}{8}$

$\csc\theta = \dfrac{r}{y} = \dfrac{17}{15}; \sec\theta = \dfrac{r}{x} = \dfrac{17}{-8} = -\dfrac{17}{8}; \cot\theta = \dfrac{-8}{15} = -\dfrac{8}{15}.$

11. $x = 7, y = -24 \Rightarrow r = \sqrt{x^2 + y^2} = \sqrt{(7)^2 + (-24)^2} = \sqrt{625} = 25$ See Figure 11.

$\sin\theta = \dfrac{y}{r} = \dfrac{-24}{25} = -\dfrac{24}{25}; \cos\theta = \dfrac{x}{r} = \dfrac{7}{25}; \tan\theta = \dfrac{y}{x} = \dfrac{-24}{7} = -\dfrac{24}{7}$

$\csc\theta = \dfrac{r}{y} = \dfrac{25}{-24} = -\dfrac{25}{24}; \sec\theta = \dfrac{r}{x} = \dfrac{25}{7}; \cot\theta = \dfrac{-7}{24} = -\dfrac{7}{24}.$

13. $x = 0, y = 2 \Rightarrow r = \sqrt{x^2 + y^2} = \sqrt{(0)^2 + (2)^2} = \sqrt{4} = 2$ See Figure 13.

$\sin\theta = \dfrac{y}{r} = \dfrac{2}{2} = 1; \cos\theta = \dfrac{x}{r} = \dfrac{0}{2} = 0; \tan\theta = \dfrac{y}{x} = \dfrac{2}{0} \Rightarrow undefined.$

$\csc\theta = \dfrac{r}{y} = \dfrac{2}{2} = 1; \sec\theta = \dfrac{r}{x} = \dfrac{2}{0} \Rightarrow undefined;; \cot\theta = \dfrac{0}{2} = 0.$

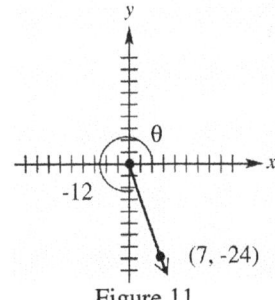
Figure 11

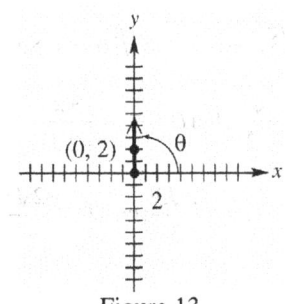
Figure 13

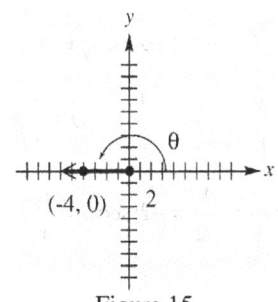
Figure 15

15. $x = -4, y = 0 \Rightarrow r = \sqrt{x^2 + y^2} = \sqrt{(-4)^2 + (0)^2} = \sqrt{16} = 4$ See Figure 15.

$\sin\theta = \dfrac{y}{r} = \dfrac{0}{4} = 0; \cos\theta = \dfrac{x}{r} = \dfrac{-4}{4} = -1; \tan\theta = \dfrac{y}{x} = \dfrac{0}{-4} = 0$

$\csc\theta = \dfrac{r}{y} = \dfrac{4}{0} \Rightarrow undefined; \sec\theta = \dfrac{r}{x} = \dfrac{4}{-4} = -1; \cot\theta = \dfrac{-4}{0} \Rightarrow undefined.$

17. $x = 0, y = -4 \Rightarrow r = \sqrt{x^2 + y^2} = \sqrt{(0)^2 + (-4)^2} = \sqrt{16} = 4$ See Figure 17.

$\sin\theta = \dfrac{y}{r} = \dfrac{-4}{4} = -1; \cos\theta = \dfrac{x}{r} = \dfrac{0}{4} = 0; \tan\theta = \dfrac{y}{x} = \dfrac{-4}{0} \Rightarrow undefined.$

$\csc\theta = \dfrac{r}{y} = \dfrac{4}{-4} = -1; \sec\theta = \dfrac{r}{x} = \dfrac{4}{0} \Rightarrow undefined; ; \cot\theta = \dfrac{0}{-4} = 0.$

19. $x = 1, y = \sqrt{3} \Rightarrow r = \sqrt{x^2 + y^2} = \sqrt{(1)^2 + (\sqrt{3})^2} = \sqrt{4} = 2$ See Figure 19.

$\sin\theta = \dfrac{y}{r} = \dfrac{\sqrt{3}}{2}; \cos\theta = \dfrac{x}{r} = \dfrac{1}{2}; \tan\theta = \dfrac{y}{x} = \dfrac{\sqrt{3}}{1} = \sqrt{3}$

$\csc\theta = \dfrac{r}{y} = \dfrac{2}{\sqrt{3}} = \dfrac{2}{\sqrt{3}} \cdot \dfrac{\sqrt{3}}{\sqrt{3}} = \dfrac{2\sqrt{3}}{3}; \sec\theta = \dfrac{r}{x} = \dfrac{2}{1} = 2; \cot\theta = \dfrac{1}{\sqrt{3}} = \dfrac{1}{\sqrt{3}} \cdot \dfrac{\sqrt{3}}{\sqrt{3}} = \dfrac{\sqrt{3}}{3}.$

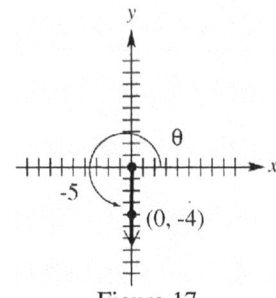
Figure 17

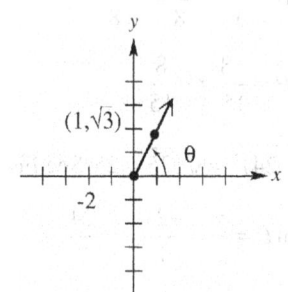
Figure 19

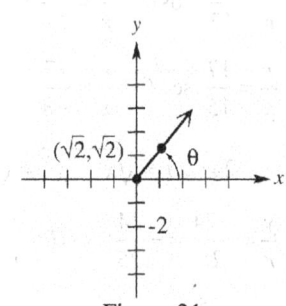
Figure 21

21. $x = -\sqrt{2}, y = -\sqrt{2} \Rightarrow r = \sqrt{x^2 + y^2} = \sqrt{(-\sqrt{2})^2 + (-\sqrt{2})^2} = \sqrt{4} = 2$ See Figure 21.

$\sin\theta = \dfrac{y}{r} = \dfrac{\sqrt{2}}{2}; \cos\theta = \dfrac{x}{r} = \dfrac{\sqrt{2}}{2} =; \tan\theta = \dfrac{y}{x} = \dfrac{\sqrt{2}}{\sqrt{2}} = 1$

$\csc\theta = \dfrac{r}{y} = \dfrac{2}{\sqrt{2}} = \dfrac{2}{\sqrt{2}} \cdot \dfrac{\sqrt{2}}{\sqrt{2}} = \sqrt{2}; \sec\theta = \dfrac{r}{x} = \dfrac{2}{\sqrt{2}} = \dfrac{2}{\sqrt{2}} \cdot \dfrac{\sqrt{2}}{\sqrt{2}} = \sqrt{2}; \cot\theta = \dfrac{\sqrt{2}}{\sqrt{2}} = 1.$

23. $x = -2\sqrt{3}, y = -2 \Rightarrow r = \sqrt{x^2 + y^2} = \sqrt{(-2\sqrt{3})^2 + (-2)^2} = \sqrt{16} = 4$ See Figure 23.

$\sin\theta = \dfrac{y}{r} = \dfrac{-2}{4} = -\dfrac{1}{2}; \cos\theta = \dfrac{x}{r} = \dfrac{-2\sqrt{3}}{4} = -\dfrac{\sqrt{3}}{2}; \tan\theta = \dfrac{y}{x} = \dfrac{-2}{-2\sqrt{3}} = \dfrac{1}{\sqrt{3}} = \dfrac{\sqrt{3}}{3}$

$\csc\theta = \dfrac{r}{y} = \dfrac{4}{-2} = -2; \sec\theta = \dfrac{r}{x} = \dfrac{4}{-2\sqrt{3}} = -\dfrac{2}{\sqrt{3}} = -\dfrac{2\sqrt{3}}{3}; \cot\theta = \dfrac{-2\sqrt{3}}{-2} = \sqrt{3}.$

Section 8.5   409

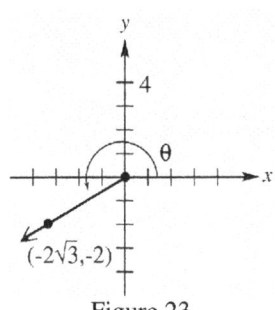

Figure 23

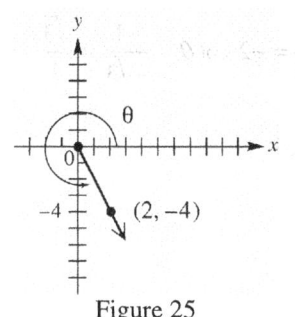

Figure 25

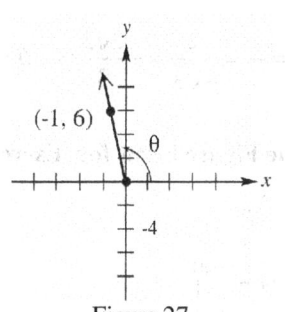

Figure 27

25. Let $x = 2, y = -4 \Rightarrow r = \sqrt{x^2 + y^2} = \sqrt{(2)^2 + (-4)^2} = \sqrt{20} = 2\sqrt{5}$ See Figure 25.

$\sin\theta = \dfrac{y}{r} = \dfrac{-4}{2\sqrt{5}} = -\dfrac{2}{\sqrt{5}} = -\dfrac{2\sqrt{5}}{5}; \cos\theta = \dfrac{x}{r} = \dfrac{2}{2\sqrt{5}} = \dfrac{1}{\sqrt{5}} = \dfrac{\sqrt{5}}{5}; \tan\theta = \dfrac{y}{x} = \dfrac{-4}{2} = -2$

$\csc\theta = \dfrac{r}{y} = \dfrac{2\sqrt{5}}{-4} = -\dfrac{\sqrt{5}}{2}; \sec\theta = \dfrac{r}{x} = \dfrac{2\sqrt{5}}{2} = \sqrt{5}; \cot\theta = \dfrac{2}{-4} = -\dfrac{1}{2}.$

27. Let $x = -1, y = 6 \Rightarrow r = \sqrt{x^2 + y^2} = \sqrt{(-1)^2 + (6)^2} = \sqrt{37}$ See Figure 27.

$\sin\theta = \dfrac{y}{r} = \dfrac{6}{\sqrt{37}} = \dfrac{6\sqrt{37}}{37}; \cos\theta = \dfrac{x}{r} = \dfrac{-1}{\sqrt{37}} = -\dfrac{\sqrt{37}}{37}; \tan\theta = \dfrac{y}{x} = \dfrac{6}{-1} = -6$

$\csc\theta = \dfrac{r}{y} = \dfrac{\sqrt{37}}{6}; \sec\theta = \dfrac{r}{x} = \dfrac{\sqrt{37}}{-1} = -\sqrt{37}; \cot\theta = \dfrac{-1}{6} = -\dfrac{1}{6}.$

29. Let $x = -7, y = -4 \Rightarrow r = \sqrt{x^2 + y^2} = \sqrt{(-7)^2 + (-4)^2} = \sqrt{65}$ See Figure 29.

$\sin\theta = \dfrac{y}{r} = \dfrac{-4}{\sqrt{65}} = -\dfrac{4\sqrt{65}}{65}; \cos\theta = \dfrac{x}{r} = \dfrac{-7}{\sqrt{65}} = -\dfrac{7\sqrt{65}}{65}; \tan\theta = \dfrac{y}{x} = \dfrac{-4}{-7} = \dfrac{4}{7}$

$\csc\theta = \dfrac{r}{y} = \dfrac{\sqrt{65}}{-4} = -\dfrac{\sqrt{65}}{4}; \sec\theta = \dfrac{r}{x} = \dfrac{\sqrt{65}}{-7} = -\dfrac{\sqrt{65}}{7}; \cot\theta = \dfrac{-7}{-4} = \dfrac{7}{4}.$

31. Let $x = 2, y = -2 \Rightarrow r = \sqrt{x^2 + y^2} = \sqrt{(2)^2 + (-2)^2} = \sqrt{8} = 2\sqrt{2}.$ See Figure 31.

$\sin\theta = \dfrac{y}{r} = \dfrac{-2}{2\sqrt{2}} = -\dfrac{1}{\sqrt{2}} = -\dfrac{\sqrt{2}}{2}; \cos\theta = \dfrac{x}{r} = \dfrac{2}{2\sqrt{2}} = \dfrac{1}{\sqrt{2}} = \dfrac{\sqrt{2}}{2}; \tan\theta = \dfrac{y}{x} = \dfrac{-2}{2} = -1$

$\csc\theta = \dfrac{r}{y} = \dfrac{2\sqrt{2}}{-2} = -\sqrt{2}; \sec\theta = \dfrac{r}{x} = \dfrac{2\sqrt{2}}{2} = \sqrt{2}; \cot\theta = \dfrac{2}{-2} = -1.$

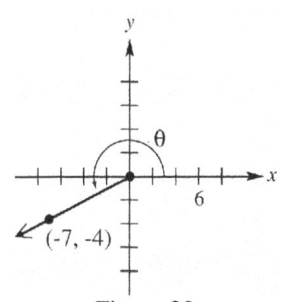

Figure 29

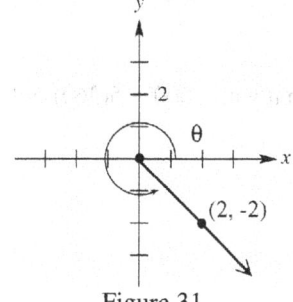

Figure 31

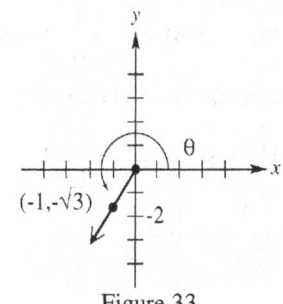

Figure 33

33. Let $x = -1, y = -\sqrt{3} \Rightarrow r = \sqrt{x^2 + y^2} = \sqrt{(-1)^2 + (-\sqrt{3})^2} = \sqrt{4} = 2.$ See Figure 33.

$\sin\theta = \dfrac{y}{r} = \dfrac{-\sqrt{3}}{2} = -\dfrac{\sqrt{3}}{2}; \cos\theta = \dfrac{x}{r} = \dfrac{-1}{2} = -\dfrac{1}{2}; \tan\theta = \dfrac{y}{x} = \dfrac{-\sqrt{3}}{-1} = \sqrt{3}$

$$\csc\theta = \frac{r}{y} = \frac{2}{-\sqrt{3}} = -\frac{2\sqrt{3}}{3}; \sec\theta = \frac{r}{x} = \frac{2}{-1} = -2; \cot\theta = \frac{-1}{-\sqrt{3}} = \frac{\sqrt{3}}{3}.$$

Use the Figure below for Exercises 35-51.

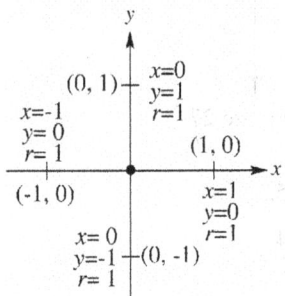

Figure 35-51

35. $\cos 90° = \dfrac{x}{r} = \dfrac{0}{1} = 0$

37. $\tan 180° = \dfrac{y}{x} = \dfrac{0}{-1} = 0$

39. $\sec 180° = \dfrac{r}{x} = \dfrac{1}{-1} = -1$

41. The quadrantal angle $\theta = -270°$ is coterminal with $-270° + 360° = 90°$. $\sin(-270)° = \sin 90° = \dfrac{y}{r} = \dfrac{1}{1} = 1$

43. The quadrantal angle $\theta = 540°$ is coterminal with $540° - 360° = 180°$.
$\cot 540° = \cot 180° = \dfrac{x}{y} = \dfrac{-1}{0} \Rightarrow$ undefined.

45. The quadrantal angle $\theta = -450°$ is coterminal with $720° - 450° = 270°$.
$\csc(-450)° = \csc 270° = \dfrac{r}{y} = \dfrac{-1}{1} = -1$

47. The quadrantal angle $\theta = 1800°$ is coterminal with $1800° - 5(360)° = 0°$.
$\sin(1800)° = \sin 0° = \dfrac{y}{r} = \dfrac{0}{1} = 0$

49. The quadrantal angle $\theta = 1800°$ is coterminal with $1800° - 5(360)° = 0°$.
$\csc(1800)° = \csc 0° = \dfrac{r}{y} = \dfrac{1}{0} \Rightarrow$ undefined.

51. The quadrantal angle $\theta = 1800°$ is coterminal with $1800° - 5(360)° = 0°$.
$\sec(1800)° = \sec 0° = \dfrac{r}{x} = \dfrac{1}{1} = 1$

53. $\sec\theta = \dfrac{1}{\cos\theta} = \dfrac{1}{\tfrac{2}{3}} = \dfrac{3}{2}$

55. $\csc\theta = \dfrac{1}{\sin\theta} = \dfrac{1}{-\tfrac{3}{7}} = -\dfrac{7}{3}$

57. $\cot\theta = \dfrac{1}{\tan\theta} = \dfrac{1}{5}$

59. $\cos\theta = \dfrac{1}{\sec\theta} = \dfrac{1}{-\dfrac{5}{2}} = -\dfrac{2}{5}$

61. $\sin\theta = \dfrac{1}{\csc\theta} = \dfrac{1}{\sqrt{2}} = \dfrac{\sqrt{2}}{2}$

63. $\tan\theta = \dfrac{1}{\cot\theta} = \dfrac{1}{-2.5} = -0.4$

65. This angle is a quadrantal angle whose terminal side lies either on the positive part of the y-axis or the negative part of the y-axis. Any point on these terminal sides would have the form $(0,k)$, where k is a real number, $k \neq 0$. $\cos\left[(2n+1)\cdot 90°\right] = \dfrac{x}{r} = \dfrac{0}{\sqrt{0^2 + k^2}} = \dfrac{0}{\sqrt{k^2}} = 0$.

67. This angle is a quadrantal angle whose terminal side lies either on the positive part of the x-axis or the negative part of the x-axis. Any point on these terminal sides would have the form $(k,0)$, where k is a real number, $k \neq 0$. $\cos\left[(2n+1)\cdot 180°\right] = \dfrac{x}{r} = \dfrac{-k}{\sqrt{0^2 + k^2}} = -1$

69. Since $\sin\theta > 0, \csc > 0$. The functions are greater than 0 (positive) in quadrants I and II.

71. Since $\sin\theta > 0$ in quadrants I and II and $\cos\theta > 0$ in quadrants I and IV. Both conditions are met only in quadrant I.

73. Since $\tan\theta < 0$ in quadrants II and IV and $\cos\theta < 0$ in quadrants II and III. Both conditions are met only in quadrant II.

75. Since $\sec\theta > 0$ in quadrants I and IV and $\csc\theta > 0$ in quadrants I and II. Both conditions are met only in quadrant I.

77. Since $\sec\theta < 0$ in quadrants II and III and $\csc\theta < 0$ in quadrants III and IV. Both conditions are met only in quadrant III.

79. Since $\sin\theta < 0 \Rightarrow \csc\theta < 0$ in quadrants III and IV. Both functions are less than 0 in quadrants III and IV.

81. The answers to 71 and 75 are the same because functions in exercise 71 are the reciprocals of the function in exercise 75.

83. Impossible because the range of $\sin\theta$ is $[-1,1]$.

85. Possible because the range of $\cos\theta$ is $[-1,1]$.

87. Possible because the range of $\tan\theta$ is $(-\infty,\infty)$

89. Impossible because the range of $\sec\theta$ is $(-\infty,-1]\cup[-1,\infty)$.

91. Possible because the range of $\csc\theta$ is $(-\infty,-1]\cup[-1,\infty)$.

93. Possible because the range of $\cot\theta$ is $(-\infty,\infty)$.

95. Possible because the range of $\sin\theta$ is $[-1,1]$ and the range of $\csc\theta$ is $(-\infty,-1]\cup[-1,\infty)$.

97. Impossible because the range of $\cos\theta$ is $[-1,1]$.

99. $\tan\theta = \dfrac{15}{-8}$ with θ in quadrant II, $\tan\theta = \dfrac{y}{x} \Rightarrow x = -8, y = 15$.

$x^2 + y^2 = r^2 \Rightarrow (-8)^2 + (15)^2 = r^2 \Rightarrow r^2 = 289 \Rightarrow r = 17$.

$\sin\theta = \dfrac{y}{r} = \dfrac{15}{17}, \cos\theta = \dfrac{x}{r} = \dfrac{-8}{17} = -\dfrac{8}{17}, \tan\theta = \dfrac{y}{x} = \dfrac{15}{-8} = -\dfrac{15}{8}$

$\csc\theta = \dfrac{r}{y} = \dfrac{17}{15}, \sec\theta = \dfrac{r}{x} = \dfrac{17}{-8} = -\dfrac{17}{8}, \cot\theta = \dfrac{x}{y} = \dfrac{-8}{15} = -\dfrac{8}{15}$

101. $\sin\theta = \dfrac{\sqrt{5}}{7}$ with θ in quadrant I, $\sin\theta = \dfrac{y}{r} \Rightarrow y = \sqrt{5}, r = 7$.

$x^2 + y^2 = r^2 \Rightarrow x^2 + \left(\sqrt{5}\right)^2 = (7)^2 \Rightarrow x^2 = 44 \Rightarrow x = \pm 2\sqrt{11}$. θ is in quadrant I, let $x = 2\sqrt{11}$.

$\sin\theta = \dfrac{y}{r} = \dfrac{\sqrt{5}}{7}, \cos\theta = \dfrac{x}{r} = \dfrac{2\sqrt{11}}{7}, \tan\theta = \dfrac{y}{x} = \dfrac{\sqrt{5}}{2\sqrt{11}} = \dfrac{\sqrt{55}}{22}$

$\csc\theta = \dfrac{r}{y} = \dfrac{7}{\sqrt{5}} = \dfrac{7\sqrt{5}}{5}, \sec\theta = \dfrac{r}{x} = \dfrac{7}{2\sqrt{11}} = \dfrac{7\sqrt{11}}{22}, \cot\theta = \dfrac{x}{y} = \dfrac{2\sqrt{11}}{\sqrt{5}} = \dfrac{2\sqrt{55}}{5}$

103. $\cot\theta = \dfrac{\sqrt{3}}{8}$ with θ in quadrant I, $\cot\theta = \dfrac{x}{y} \Rightarrow x = \sqrt{3}, y = 8$.

$x^2 + y^2 = r^2 \Rightarrow \left(\sqrt{3}\right)^2 + (8)^2 = r^2 \Rightarrow r^2 = 67 \Rightarrow r = \sqrt{67}$.

$\sin\theta = \dfrac{y}{r} = \dfrac{8}{\sqrt{67}} = \dfrac{8\sqrt{67}}{67}, \cos\theta = \dfrac{x}{r} = \dfrac{\sqrt{3}}{\sqrt{67}} = \dfrac{\sqrt{201}}{67}, \tan\theta = \dfrac{y}{x} = \dfrac{8}{\sqrt{3}} = \dfrac{8\sqrt{3}}{3}$

$\csc\theta = \dfrac{r}{y} = \dfrac{\sqrt{67}}{8}, \sec\theta = \dfrac{r}{x} = \dfrac{\sqrt{67}}{\sqrt{3}} = \dfrac{\sqrt{201}}{3}, \cot\theta = \dfrac{x}{y} = \dfrac{\sqrt{3}}{8}$

105. $\sin\theta = \dfrac{\sqrt{2}}{6}$ with $\cos\theta < 0$, θ in quadrant II, $\sin\theta = \dfrac{y}{r} \Rightarrow y = \sqrt{2}, r = 6$.

$x^2 + y^2 = r^2 \Rightarrow x^2 + \left(\sqrt{2}\right)^2 = (6)^2 \Rightarrow x^2 = 34 \Rightarrow x = \pm\sqrt{34}$. θ is in quadrant II, let $x = -\sqrt{34}$.

$\sin\theta = \dfrac{y}{r} = \dfrac{\sqrt{2}}{6}, \cos\theta = \dfrac{x}{r} = -\dfrac{\sqrt{34}}{6}, \tan\theta = \dfrac{y}{x} = -\dfrac{\sqrt{2}}{\sqrt{34}} = -\dfrac{\sqrt{68}}{34} = -\dfrac{\sqrt{17}}{17}$

$\csc\theta = \dfrac{r}{y} = \dfrac{6}{\sqrt{2}} = 3\sqrt{2}, \sec\theta = \dfrac{r}{x} = -\dfrac{6}{\sqrt{34}} = -\dfrac{6\sqrt{34}}{34} = -\dfrac{3\sqrt{34}}{17}, \cot\theta = \dfrac{x}{y} = -\dfrac{\sqrt{34}}{\sqrt{2}} = -\dfrac{\sqrt{68}}{2} = -\sqrt{17}$

107. $\sec\theta = -4$ with $\sin\theta > 0$, θ in quadrant II, $\sec\theta = \dfrac{r}{x} \Rightarrow x = -1, r = 4$.

$x^2 + y^2 = r^2 \Rightarrow (-1)^2 + y^2 = (4)^2 \Rightarrow y^2 = 15 \Rightarrow y = \pm\sqrt{15}$. θ is in quadrant II, let $y = \sqrt{15}$.

$\sin\theta = \dfrac{y}{r} = \dfrac{\sqrt{15}}{4}, \cos\theta = \dfrac{x}{r} = -\dfrac{1}{4}, \tan\theta = \dfrac{y}{x} = -\dfrac{\sqrt{15}}{1} = -\sqrt{15}$

$$\csc\theta = \frac{r}{y} = \frac{4}{\sqrt{15}} = \frac{4\sqrt{15}}{15}, \sec\theta = \frac{r}{x} = -4 = -\frac{6\sqrt{34}}{34} = -\frac{3\sqrt{34}}{17}, \cot\theta = \frac{x}{y} = -\frac{1}{\sqrt{15}} = -\frac{\sqrt{15}}{15}$$

109. Use the Pythagorean Identity $\sin^2\theta + \cos^2\theta = 1$ to write $\cos\theta, \sin^2\theta + \cos^2\theta = 1 \Rightarrow \cos^2 = 1 - \sin^2\theta \Rightarrow$ $\cos\theta = \pm\sqrt{1-\sin^2\theta}$. Since θ is acute, it is in quadrant I and $\cos\theta = \sqrt{1-\sin^2\theta}$.

111. First use the Pythagorean Identity $1 + \cot^2\theta = \csc^2\theta$ to write $\csc\theta, 1 + \cot^2\theta = \csc^2\theta \Rightarrow$ $\csc\theta = \pm\sqrt{1+\cot^2\theta}$ since θ is in quadrant III, $\csc\theta = -\sqrt{1+\cot^2\theta}$. Substituting this into the Reciprocal Identity $\sin\theta = \frac{1}{\csc\theta}$ yields: $\sin\theta = -\frac{1}{\sqrt{1+\cot^2\theta}}$ or $-\frac{\sqrt{1+\cot^2\theta}}{1+\cot^2\theta}$.

113. Use the Pythagorean Identity $\sin^2\theta + \cos^2\theta = 1$ to write $\cos\theta, \sin^2\theta + \cos^2\theta = 1 \cos^2 = 1 - \sin^2\theta \Rightarrow$ $\cos\theta = \pm\sqrt{1-\sin^2\theta}$. Since θ is in quadrant I or IV, $\cos\theta = \sqrt{1-\sin^2\theta}$. Now substituting this into the Quotient Identity $\tan\theta = \frac{\sin\theta}{\cos\theta}$ yields $\tan\theta = \frac{\sin\theta}{\sqrt{1-\sin^2\theta}}$ or $\frac{\sin\theta\sqrt{1-\sin^2\theta}}{1-\sin^2\theta}$.

115. Dividing $x^2 + y^2 = r^2$ by y^2 yields: $\frac{x^2}{y^2} + \frac{y^2}{y^2} = \frac{r^2}{y^2}$ which is equal to: $\cot^2\theta + 1 = \csc^2\theta \Rightarrow 1 + \cot^2\theta = \csc^2\theta$.

117. False $\sin\theta + \cos\theta \neq 1$ for all values of θ. For example, if $\theta = 30°$, then $\sin 30° + \cos 30° = \frac{1}{2} + \frac{\sqrt{3}}{2} = \frac{1+\sqrt{3}}{2} \neq 1$.

118. False; if $\cot\theta = \frac{\cos\theta}{\sin\theta}$ and $\cot\theta = \frac{1}{2}$, this does not imply that $\sin\theta = 2$ since $\sin\theta \leq 1$ for all θ.

119. (a) The slope of the line is .03, so when x increases by 100 feet, y increases by 3 feet. Thus the highway has a grade of 3%.

   (b) Using the point from part (a), $(100, 3)$ we first solve for r and then find $\sin\theta$:
   $r = \sqrt{100^2 + 3^2} \Rightarrow r = \sqrt{10,009}$, then $\sin\theta = \frac{y}{r} = \frac{-6}{10,009}$. Now use the formula $R = W(\sin\theta)$, to find grade resistance $R = 25,000\left(\frac{3}{\sqrt{10,009}}\right) \approx 750$ pounds.

121. (a) $d = 4\tan(2\pi)(0) \Rightarrow d = 0$ m.

   (b) $d = 4\tan(2\pi)(.2) \Rightarrow d \approx 12.3$ m.

   (c) $d = 4\tan(2\pi)(.2) \Rightarrow d \approx 12.3$m.

   (d) $d = 4\tan(2\pi)(.2) \Rightarrow d \approx 12.3$m.

   (e) The value $t = .25$ yields: $d = 4\tan(2\pi)(.25) \Rightarrow d = 4\tan\frac{\pi}{2}$. Since $\tan\frac{\pi}{2}$ is undefined, .25 is a meaningless value for t.

8.6: Evaluating Trigonometric Functions

1. $\sin A = \dfrac{\text{opp}}{\text{hyp}} = \dfrac{21}{29}$ $\cos A = \dfrac{\text{adj}}{\text{hyp}} = \dfrac{20}{29}$ $\tan A = \dfrac{\text{opp}}{\text{adj}} = \dfrac{21}{20}$

   $\csc A = \dfrac{\text{hyp}}{\text{opp}} = \dfrac{29}{21}$ $\sec A = \dfrac{\text{hyp}}{\text{adj}} = \dfrac{29}{20}$ $\cot A = \dfrac{\text{adj}}{\text{opp}} = \dfrac{20}{21}$

3. $\sin A = \dfrac{\text{opp}}{\text{hyp}} = \dfrac{n}{p}$ $\cos A = \dfrac{\text{adj}}{\text{hyp}} = \dfrac{m}{p}$ $\tan A = \dfrac{\text{opp}}{\text{adj}} = \dfrac{n}{m}$

   $\csc A = \dfrac{\text{hyp}}{\text{opp}} = \dfrac{p}{n}$ $\sec A = \dfrac{\text{hyp}}{\text{adj}} = \dfrac{p}{m}$ $\cot A = \dfrac{\text{adj}}{\text{opp}} = \dfrac{m}{n}$

5. Using the 30°-60° right triangle rules, for a 30° angle the hypotenuse $= 2$, the opposite side $= 1$, and the adjacent side $= \sqrt{3}$, therefore $\tan 30° = \dfrac{1}{\sqrt{3}} = \dfrac{\sqrt{3}}{3}$ and $\cot 30° = \dfrac{\sqrt{3}}{1} = \sqrt{3}$.

7. Using the 30°-60° right triangle rules, for a 60° angle the hypotenuse $= 2$, the opposite side $= \sqrt{3}$, and the adjacent side $= 1$, therefore $\sin 60° = \dfrac{\sqrt{3}}{2}$; $\cot 60° = \dfrac{1}{\sqrt{3}} = \dfrac{\sqrt{3}}{3}$; and $\csc 60° = \dfrac{2}{\sqrt{3}} = \dfrac{2\sqrt{3}}{3}$.

9. First find the reference angle: $(180° - 135°) = 45°$. Using 45°-45° right triangle rules, for a 45° angle the hypotenuse $= \sqrt{2}$, the opposite side $= 1$, and the adjacent side $= 1$. Since $\theta = 135°$ is in quadrant II, x is negative and cosine, secant, tangent, and cotangent are negative, therefore $\tan 135° = -\tan 45° = -\dfrac{1}{1} = -1$; and $\cot 135° = -\cot 45° = -\dfrac{1}{1} = -1$.

11. First find the reference angle: $(210° - 180°) = 30°$. Using 30°-60° right triangle rules, for a 30° angle the hypotenuse $= 2$, the opposite side $= 1$, and the adjacent side $= \sqrt{3}$. Since $\theta = 210°$ is in quadrant III, x is negative and sine, cosine, secant, and cotangent are negative, therefore $\cos 210° = -\cos 30° = -\dfrac{\sqrt{3}}{2}$; and $\sec 210° = -\sec 30° = -\dfrac{2}{\sqrt{3}} = -\dfrac{2\sqrt{3}}{3}$.

13. (a) Using the 30°-60° right triangle rules, for a 30° angle the hypotenuse $= 2$, the opposite side $= 1$, and the adjacent side $= \sqrt{3}$, therefore $\tan 30° = \dfrac{1}{\sqrt{3}} = \dfrac{\sqrt{3}}{3}$.

    (b) Using the calculator, $\tan 30° = \dfrac{\sqrt{3}}{3} \approx .5773502692$

15. (a) Using the 30°-60° right triangle rules, for a 30° angle the hypotenuse $= 2$, the opposite side $= 1$ and the adjacent side $= \sqrt{3}$, therefore $\sin 30° = \dfrac{1}{2}$.

    (b) $\sin 30° = \dfrac{1}{2}$ is a rational number.

17. (a) Using the 30°-60° right triangle rules, for a 30° angle the hypotenuse = 2, the opposite side = 1, and the adjacent side = $\sqrt{3}$, therefore $\sec 30° = \dfrac{2}{\sqrt{3}} = \dfrac{2\sqrt{3}}{3}$.

    (b) Using the calculator, $\sec 30° = (\cos 30°)^{-1} = \dfrac{2\sqrt{3}}{3} \approx 1.154700538$

19. (a) Using the 45°-45° right triangle rules, for a 45° angle the hypotenuse = $\sqrt{2}$, the opposite side = 1, and the adjacent side = 1, therefore $\csc 45° = \dfrac{\sqrt{2}}{1} = \sqrt{2}$.

    (b) Using the calculator, $\csc 45° = (\sin 45°)^{-1} = \sqrt{2} \approx 1.414213562$

21. (a) Using the 45°-45° right triangle rules, for a 45° angle the hypotenuse = $\sqrt{2}$, the opposite side = 1, and the adjacent side = 1, therefore $\cos 45° = \dfrac{1}{\sqrt{2}} = \dfrac{\sqrt{2}}{2}$.

    (b) Using the calculator, $\cos 45° = \dfrac{\sqrt{2}}{2} \approx .7071067812$

23. (a) Because $\theta = \dfrac{\pi}{3} = 60°$ we use the 30°-60° right triangle rules, for a 60° angle the hypotenuse = 2, the opposite side = $\sqrt{3}$, and the adjacent side = 1, therefore $\sin \dfrac{\pi}{3} = \sin 60° = \dfrac{\sqrt{3}}{2}$.

    (b) $\sin \dfrac{\pi}{3} = \sin 60° = \dfrac{\sqrt{3}}{2} = .8660254038$

25. (a) Because $\theta = \dfrac{\pi}{3} = 60°$ we use the 30°-60° right triangle rules, for a 60° angle the hypotenuse = 2, the opposite side = $\sqrt{3}$, and the adjacent side = 1, therefore $\tan \dfrac{\pi}{3} = \tan 60° = \dfrac{\sqrt{3}}{1} = \sqrt{3}$.

    (b) $\tan \dfrac{\pi}{3} = \tan 60° = \dfrac{\sqrt{3}}{1} = \sqrt{3} = 1.732050808$

27. (a) Because $\theta = \dfrac{\pi}{6} = 30°$ we use the 30°-60° right triangle rules, for a 30° angle the hypotenuse = 2, the opposite side = 1, and the adjacent side = $\sqrt{3}$, therefore $\csc \dfrac{\pi}{6} = \csc 30° = \dfrac{2}{1} = 2$.

    (b) $\csc \dfrac{\pi}{6} = \csc 30° = 2$ is a rational number.

29. (a) Because $\theta = \dfrac{\pi}{3} = 60°$ we use the 30°-60° right triangle rules, for a 60° angle the hypotenuse = 2, the opposite side = $\sqrt{3}$, and the adjacent side = 1, therefore $\csc \dfrac{\pi}{3} = \csc 60° = \dfrac{2}{\sqrt{3}} = \dfrac{2\sqrt{3}}{3}$.

    (b) $\csc \dfrac{\pi}{3} = \csc 60° = \left(\sin \dfrac{\pi}{3}\right)^{-1} = (\sin 60°)^{-1} = \dfrac{2\sqrt{3}}{3} = 1.154700538$

31. The exact value of $\sin 45°$ is $\dfrac{\sqrt{2}}{2}$. The decimal value given is an approximation.

33. $\cot 73° = \tan(90° - 73°) = \tan 17°$.

35. $\sin 38° = \cos(90° - 38°) = \cos 52°$.

37. $\tan 25°43' = \cot(90° - 25°43') = \cot(89°60' - 25°43') = \cot 64°17'$

39. $\cos\dfrac{\pi}{5} = \sin\left(\dfrac{\pi}{2} - \dfrac{\pi}{5}\right) = \sin\left(\dfrac{5\pi}{10} - \dfrac{2\pi}{10}\right) = \sin\dfrac{3\pi}{10}$

41. $\tan 0.5 = \cot\left(\dfrac{\pi}{2} - 0.5\right)$

43. $\cos 1 = \sin\left(\dfrac{\pi}{2} - 1\right)$

45. If $\theta = 98°$ then $\theta' = 180° - 98° = 82°$

47. If $\theta = 230°$ then $\theta' = 230° - 180° = 50°$

49. If $\theta = -135°$ then $\theta' = 180° + (-135°) = 45°$

51. If $\theta = 750°$ then $\theta' = 750° - 720° = 30°$

53. If $\theta = \dfrac{4\pi}{3}$ then $\theta' = \dfrac{4\pi}{3} - \pi = \dfrac{4\pi}{3} - \dfrac{3\pi}{3} = \dfrac{\pi}{3}$.

55. If $\theta = -\dfrac{4\pi}{3} = 2\pi - \dfrac{4\pi}{3} = \dfrac{6\pi}{3} - \dfrac{4\pi}{3} = \dfrac{2\pi}{3}$ then $\theta' = \pi - \dfrac{2\pi}{3} = \dfrac{3\pi}{3} - \dfrac{2\pi}{3} = \dfrac{\pi}{3}$

57. It is easy to find one-half of 2, which is 1. This is, then, the measure of the side opposite the $30°$ angle, and the ratios are easily found. Yes, any positive number could have been used.

59. First find the reference angle: $(360° - 300°) = 60°$. Using $30°$-$60°$ right triangle rules, for a $60°$ angle the hypotenuse $= 2$, the opposite side $= \sqrt{3}$, and the adjacent side $= 1$. Since $\theta = 300°$ is in quadrant IV, y is negative and sine, tangent, cotangent, and cosecant are negative, therefore:

$\sin 300° = -\sin 60° = -\dfrac{\sqrt{3}}{2}$ $\qquad$ $\csc 300° = -\csc 60° = -\dfrac{2}{\sqrt{3}} = -\dfrac{2\sqrt{3}}{3}$

$\cos 300° = \cos 60° = \dfrac{1}{2}$ $\qquad$ $\sec 300° = \sec 60° = \dfrac{2}{1} = 2$

$\tan 300° = -\tan 60° = -\dfrac{\sqrt{3}}{1} = -\sqrt{3}$ $\qquad$ $\cot 300° = -\cot 60° = -\dfrac{1}{\sqrt{3}} = -\dfrac{\sqrt{3}}{3}$

61. First find the reference angle: $(405° - 360°) = 45°$. Using the $45°$-$45°$ right triangle rules, for a $45°$ angle the hypotenuse $= \sqrt{2}$, the opposite side $= 1$, and the adjacent $= 1$. Since $\theta = 405°$ is in quadrant I, all functions are positive, therefore:

$\sin 405° = \sin 45° = \dfrac{1}{\sqrt{2}} = \dfrac{\sqrt{2}}{2}$ $\qquad$ $\csc 405° = \csc 45° = \dfrac{\sqrt{2}}{1} = \sqrt{2}$

$\cos 405° = \cos 45° = \dfrac{1}{\sqrt{2}} = \dfrac{\sqrt{2}}{2}$ $\qquad$ $\sec 405° = \sec 45° = \dfrac{\sqrt{2}}{1} = \sqrt{2}$

$\tan 405° = \tan 45° = \dfrac{1}{1} = 1$ 　　　　　　　　　　$\cot 405° = \cot 45° = \dfrac{1}{1} = 1$

63. First find the reference angle: $\left(2\pi - \dfrac{11\pi}{6}\right) = \dfrac{\pi}{6}$. Since $\dfrac{\pi}{6}$ radians is equal to 30° we use the 30°-60° right triangle rules, for a 30° angle the hypotenuse $= 2$, the opposite side $= 1$, and the adjacent side $= \sqrt{3}$. Since $\theta = \dfrac{11\pi}{6}$ is in quadrant IV, y is negative and sine, tangent, cotangent, and cosecant are negative, therefore:

$\sin\dfrac{11\pi}{6} = -\sin\dfrac{\pi}{6} = -\dfrac{1}{2}$ 　　　　　　　$\csc\dfrac{11\pi}{6} = -\csc\dfrac{\pi}{6} = -\dfrac{2}{1} = -2$

$\cos\dfrac{11\pi}{6} = \cos\dfrac{\pi}{6} = \dfrac{\sqrt{3}}{2}$ 　　　　　　　$\sec\dfrac{11\pi}{6} = \sec\dfrac{\pi}{6} = \dfrac{2}{\sqrt{3}} = \dfrac{2\sqrt{3}}{3}$

$\tan\dfrac{11\pi}{6} = -\tan\dfrac{\pi}{6} = -\dfrac{1}{\sqrt{3}} = -\dfrac{\sqrt{3}}{3}$ 　　$\cot\dfrac{11\pi}{6} = -\cot\dfrac{\pi}{6} = -\dfrac{\sqrt{3}}{1} = -\sqrt{3}$

65. First find the reference angle: $\left(2\pi - \dfrac{7\pi}{4}\right) = \dfrac{\pi}{4}$ Since $\dfrac{\pi}{4}$ radians is equal to 45° we use the 45°-45° right triangle rules, for a 45° angle the hypotenuse $= \sqrt{2}$, the opposite side $= 1$, and the adjacent $= 1$. Since $\theta = -\dfrac{7\pi}{4}$ is in quadrant I, all functions are positive, therefore:

$\sin-\dfrac{7\pi}{4} = \sin\dfrac{\pi}{4} = \dfrac{1}{\sqrt{2}} = \dfrac{\sqrt{2}}{2}$ 　　　　　$\csc-\dfrac{7\pi}{4} = \csc\dfrac{\pi}{4} = \dfrac{\sqrt{2}}{1} = \sqrt{2}$

$\cos-\dfrac{7\pi}{4} = \cos\dfrac{\pi}{4} = \dfrac{1}{\sqrt{2}} = \dfrac{\sqrt{2}}{2}$ 　　　　　$\sec-\dfrac{7\pi}{4} = \sec\dfrac{\pi}{4} = \dfrac{\sqrt{2}}{1} = \sqrt{2}$

$\tan-\dfrac{7\pi}{4} = \tan\dfrac{\pi}{4} = \dfrac{1}{1} = 1$ 　　　　　　　$\cot-\dfrac{7\pi}{4} = \cot\dfrac{\pi}{4} = \dfrac{1}{1} = 1$

67. First find the reference angle: $\left(4\pi - \dfrac{19\pi}{6}\right) = \dfrac{5\pi}{6}$, then $\theta = \pi - \dfrac{5\pi}{6} = \dfrac{\pi}{6}$. Since $\dfrac{\pi}{6}$ radians is equal to 30° we use the 30°-60° right triangle rules, for a 30° angle the hypotenuse $= 2$, the opposite side $= 1$, and the adjacent side $= \sqrt{3}$. Since $\theta = -\dfrac{19\pi}{6}$ is in quadrant II, x is negative and cosine, secant, tangent, and cotangent are negative, therefore:

$\sin-\dfrac{19\pi}{6} = \sin\dfrac{\pi}{6} = \dfrac{1}{2}$ 　　　　　　　$\csc-\dfrac{19\pi}{6} = \csc\dfrac{\pi}{6} = \dfrac{2}{1} = 2$

$\cos-\dfrac{19\pi}{6} = -\cos\dfrac{\pi}{6} = -\dfrac{\sqrt{3}}{2}$ 　　　　　$\sec-\dfrac{19\pi}{6} = -\sec\dfrac{\pi}{6} = -\dfrac{2\sqrt{3}}{3}$

$\tan-\dfrac{19\pi}{6} = -\tan\dfrac{\pi}{6} = -\dfrac{1}{\sqrt{3}} = -\dfrac{\sqrt{3}}{3}$ 　$\cot-\dfrac{19\pi}{6} = -\cot\dfrac{\pi}{6} = -\dfrac{\sqrt{3}}{1}$

69. Calculate in degree mode: $\tan 29° \approx .5543090515$

71. Calculate in degree mode: $\cot 41°24' = \cot 41\frac{24}{60}° = \cot 41.4° = (\tan 41.4°)^{-1} \approx 1.134277349$

73. Calculate in degree mode: $\sec 183°48' = \sec 145\frac{48}{60}° = \sec 183.8° = (\cos 183.8°)^{-1} \approx -1.002203376$

75. Calculate in degree mode: $\tan(-80°6') = \tan\left(-80\frac{6}{60}°\right) \approx \tan(-80.1°) \approx -5.729741647$

77. Calculate in radian mode: $\sin 2.5 \approx .5984721441$

79. Calculate in radian mode: $\tan 5 \approx -3.3805155006$

81. (a) Find the reference angle: $\theta' = \left(\frac{7\pi}{6} - \pi\right) = \frac{\pi}{6}$. Since $\theta = \frac{7\pi}{6}$ is in quadrant III, sine is negative and the reference angle function is: $-\sin\frac{\pi}{6}$

    (b) Since $\frac{\pi}{6}$ radians is equal to $30°$ we use the $30°$-$60°$ right triangle rules, for a $30°$ angle the hypotenuse $= 2$, the opposite side $= 1$, and the adjacent side $= \sqrt{3}$, therefore $-\sin\frac{\pi}{6} = -\frac{1}{2}$.

    (c) Calculate in radian mode: $\sin\frac{7\pi}{6} = -0.5$, which is equal to $-\sin\frac{\pi}{6} = -\frac{1}{2}$.

83. (a) Find the reference angle: $\cos\frac{\pi}{3} = \frac{1}{2}$. Since $\theta = \frac{3\pi}{4}$ is in quadrant II, tangent is negative and the reference angle function is: $-\tan\frac{\pi}{4}$.

    (b) Since $\frac{\pi}{4}$ radians is equal to $45°$ we use the $45°$-$45°$ right triangle rules, for a $45°$ angle the hypotenuse $= \sqrt{2}$, the opposite side $= 1$, and the adjacent $= 1$. therefore $-\tan\frac{\pi}{4} = -\frac{1}{1} = -1$.

    (c) Calculate in radian mode: $\tan\frac{3\pi}{4} = -1$, which is equal to $-\tan\frac{\pi}{4} = -\frac{1}{1} = -1$.

85. (a) Find the reference angle: $\theta' = \left(\frac{7\pi}{6} - \pi\right) = \frac{\pi}{6}$. Since $\sin A = \frac{opp}{hyp} = \frac{60}{61}$ is in quadrant III, cosine is negative and the reference angle function is: $-\cos\frac{\pi}{6}$.

    (b) Since $\frac{\pi}{6}$ radians is equal to $30°$. we use the $30°$-$60°$ right triangle rules, for a $30°$ angle the hypotenuse $= 2$, the opposite side $= 1$, and the adjacent side $= \sqrt{3}$, therefore $-\cos\frac{\pi}{6} = -\frac{\sqrt{3}}{2}$.

    (c) Calculate in radian mode: $\cos\frac{7\pi}{6} = -.8660254038$, which is equal to $-\cos\frac{\pi}{6} = -\frac{\sqrt{3}}{2}$.

87. Since $\sin\theta$ is positive in quadrant I and II, values for $\cot 315° = -\cot 45° = -\frac{1}{1} = -1$ can only be in these quadrants. In quadrant I, from the 30°-60° right triangle, $\sin 30° = \frac{1}{2}$, therefore 30° is one value. In quadrant II, use the reference angle 30° to find the other: $180° - 30° = 150°$. Therefore $\theta = 30°$ or $150°$.

89. Since $\tan\theta$ is negative in quadrant II and IV, values for θ can only be in these quadrants. From the 30°-60° right triangle, $\tan 60° = \sqrt{3}$, therefore 60° is the reference angle. In quadrant II, use the reference angle 60° to find the first value: $180° - 60° = 120°$. In quadrant IV, use the reference angle to find the other value: $360° - 60° = 300°$. Therefore, $\theta = 120°$ or $300°$.

91. Since $\cot\theta$ is negative in quadrant II and IV, values for θ can only be in these quadrants. From the 30° – 60° right triangle, $\cot 60° = \frac{\sqrt{3}}{3}$, therefore 60° is the reference angle. In quadrant II, use the reference angle 60° to find the first value: $360° - 60°$. In quadrant IV, use the reference angle 60° to find the other value: $360° - 60° = 300°$. Therefore, $\theta = 120°$ or $300°$

93. Since $\cos\theta$ is positive in quadrant I and IV, values for θ can only be in these quadrants. In quadrant I, we use the inverse trigonometric function (degree mode) of our calculator to find the angle: $\cos^{-1}.68716510 \Rightarrow \theta = 46.59388121°$. In quadrant IV, use the found reference angle from quadrant I to find $\theta: 360° - 46.59388121° = 313.4061188°$ Therefore, $\theta \approx 46.59388121°$ or $B = 90.00° - 61.00° \Rightarrow B = 29.00'$.

95. Since $\sin\theta$ is positive in quadrant I and II, values for θ can only be in these quadrants. In quadrant I, we use the inverse trigonometric function (degree mode) of our calculator to find the angle: $\sin^{-1}.41298643 \Rightarrow \theta = 24.39257624°$. In quadrant II, use the found reference angle from quadrant I to find $\theta: 24.39257624° = 155.6074238°$. Therefore, $\theta \approx 24.39257624$ or $155.6074238°$.

97. Since $\tan\theta$ is positive in quadrant I and III, values for θ can only be in these quadrants. In quadrant I, we use the inverse trigonometric function (degree mode) of our calculator to find the angle: $\tan^{-1}.876292035 \Rightarrow \theta = 41.24818261°$. In quadrant III, use the found reference angle from quadrant I to find $\theta: 180° + 41.24818261° = 221.2481826°$. Therefore, $\theta \approx 41.24818261°$ or $221.2481826°$.

99. Since $\tan\theta$ is positive in quadrant I and III, values for θ can only be in these quadrants. In quadrant I, we use the inverse trigonometric function (radian mode) of our calculator to find the angle: $\tan^{-1}.21264138 \Rightarrow \theta = .2095206607°$. In quadrant III, use the found reference angle from quadrant I to find $\theta: \pi + .2095206607 = 3.351113314$ radians. Therefore, $\theta \approx .2095206607$ or 3.351113314 radians.

101. Since $\cot\theta$ is positive in quadrant I and III, values for θ can only be in these quadrants. In quadrant I, we use the inverse trigonometric function (radian mode) of our calculator to find the angle: Since $\cot\theta = (\tan\theta)^{-1} \Rightarrow (\tan\theta)^{-1} - .29949853 \Rightarrow \tan\theta = (.29949853)^{-1} \Rightarrow \theta = \tan^{-1}(.29949853)^{-1} \Rightarrow \theta \approx 1.2799966$ radians. In quadrant III, use the found reference angle from quadrant I to find $\theta \approx 1.2799966$ radians. Therefore, $\theta \approx 1.27979966$ or 4.42139314 radians.

103. Using the point in the given example, $\sqrt{(x_1)^2+(y_1)^2}=r$ would yield: $r \approx 6.9032258$. This represents the distance from the point (x_1, y_1) to the origin.

104. Using the point in the given example and degree mode yields:
$$\tan^{-1}\left(\frac{y_1}{x_1}\right) = \tan^{-1}\left(\frac{5.9783689}{3.4516129}\right) \approx 59.9999° \approx 60°.$$

105. Using the point in the given example and degree mode yields:
$$\sin^{-1}\left(\frac{y_1}{r}\right) = \sin^{-1}\left(\frac{5.9783689}{6.9032258}\right) \approx 59.9999° \approx 60°.$$

106. Using the point in the given example and degree mode yields: $\cos^{-1}\left(\frac{x_1}{r}\right) = \cos^{-1}\left(\frac{3.4516129}{6.9032258}\right) \approx 60°$.

107. It is a measure (approximately 60°, for the example) of the angle formed by the positive x-axis and the ray $y = \sqrt{3}x,\ x \geq 0$.

108. …make a conjecture: The <u>slope</u> of a line passing through the origin is equal to the <u>tangent</u> of the angle it forms with the positive x-axis.

109. Solve for θ using the formula and given values: $400 = 5000(\sin\theta) \Rightarrow \sin\theta = \frac{400}{5000} \Rightarrow \theta = \sin^{-1}\frac{2}{25} \approx 4.6°$.

111. Solve for c_2 using the formula and given values:
$$\frac{3\times 10^8}{c_2} = \frac{\sin 46°}{\sin 31°} \Rightarrow c_2 = \frac{(3\times 10^8)\sin 31°}{\sin 46°} \approx 214{,}796{,}154 \approx 2\times 10^8 \text{ min/sec}.$$

113. Solve for θ using the formula and given values:
$$\frac{3\times 10^8}{1.5\times 10^8} = \frac{\sin 40°}{\sin\theta_2} \Rightarrow (3\times 10^8)\sin\theta_2 = (1.5\times 10^8)\sin 40° \Rightarrow \sin\theta_2 = \frac{(1.5\times 10^8)\sin 28°}{3\times 10^8} \Rightarrow$$
$$\theta_2 = \sin^{-1}\left(\frac{(1.5\times 10^8)\sin 40°}{3\times 10^8}\right) \Rightarrow \theta_2 \approx 18.747° \approx 19°.$$

115. Solve for using the formula and given values:
$$\frac{3\times 10^8}{2.254\times 10^8} = \frac{\sin 90°}{\sin\theta_2} \Rightarrow (3\times 10^8)\sin\theta_2 = (1.254\times 10^8)\sin 90° \Rightarrow \sin\theta_2 = \frac{(2.254\times 10^8)\sin 90°}{3\times 10^8} \Rightarrow$$
$$\theta_2 = \sin^{-1}\frac{(2.254\times 10^8)\sin 90°}{3\times 10^8} \Rightarrow \theta_2 \approx 48.706° \approx 48.7°.$$

117. (a) First change 55 and 30 mph to feet per second: $\frac{55\text{ mi}}{1\text{ hr}} \cdot \frac{5280\text{ ft}}{1\text{ mi}} \cdot \frac{1\text{ hr}}{3600\text{ sec}} = 80\frac{2}{3}$ ft/sec and

$\frac{30\text{ mi}}{1\text{ hr}} \cdot \frac{5280\text{ ft}}{1\text{ mi}} \cdot \frac{1\text{ hr}}{3600\text{ sec}} = 44$ ft/sec. Now solve for D using the formula, given, and found

values: $D = \dfrac{1.05\left(\left(80\frac{2}{3}\right)^2 - (44)^2\right)}{64.4(.4+.02+\sin 3.5°)} \approx 154.9303 \Rightarrow D \approx 155$ feet.

(b) Solve for *D* using the formula and given values:

$$D = \frac{1.05\left(\left(80\frac{2}{3}\right)^2 - (44)^2\right)}{64.4(.4 + .02 + \sin(-2°))} \approx 193.5313 \Rightarrow D \approx 194 \text{ feet}.$$

(c) As the grade decreases from uphill to downhill, the braking distance increases, which corresponds to driving experience.

8.7: Applications of Right Triangles

1. To find *B*: $B = 90° - 36°20' \Rightarrow B = 89°60' - 36°20' \Rightarrow B = 53°40'$

    To find *a*: $\sin A = \frac{a}{c} \Rightarrow \sin 36°20' = \frac{a}{964} \Rightarrow a = 964(\sin 36°20') \approx 571.1526 \Rightarrow a \approx 571$ m.

    To find *b*: $\cos A = \frac{b}{c} \Rightarrow \cos 36°20' = \frac{a}{964} \Rightarrow b = 964(\cos 36°20') \approx 776.5827 \Rightarrow b \approx 777$ m.

3. To find *M*: $M = 90° - 51.2° \Rightarrow M = 38.8°$.

    To find *n*: $\tan N = \frac{n}{m} \Rightarrow \tan 51.2° = \frac{n}{124} = n = 124(\tan 51.2°) \approx 154.2249 \Rightarrow n \approx 154$ m.

    To find *p*: $\cos N = \frac{n}{m} \Rightarrow \cos 51.2° = \frac{124}{p} \Rightarrow p = \frac{124}{\cos 51.2°} \approx 197.8922 \Rightarrow c \approx 198$ m.

5. To find *A*: $A = 90° - 42.0892° \Rightarrow A = 47.9108°$.

    To find *a*: $\tan B = \frac{b}{a} \Rightarrow a = \frac{b}{\tan B} = \frac{56.851}{\tan 42.0892°} \approx 62.942095 \Rightarrow a \approx 62.942$ cm.

    To find *c*: $\sin B = \frac{b}{c} \Rightarrow c = \frac{b}{\sin B} = \frac{56.851}{\sin 42.0892°} \approx 84.81594 \Rightarrow c \approx 84.816$ cm.

7. To find *A*: $\tan A = \frac{a}{b} \Rightarrow \tan A = \frac{7.1}{9.7} \Rightarrow A = \tan^{-1}\frac{7.1}{9.7} \Rightarrow A \approx 36.2026° \Rightarrow A \approx 36°$. To find *B*:

    $B = 90° - 36° \Rightarrow B = 54°$. To find *c*: $\sin A = \frac{a}{c} \Rightarrow \sin 36° = \frac{7.1}{c} \Rightarrow c = \frac{7.1}{\sin 36°} \approx 12.07924 \Rightarrow c \approx 12$ ft.

9. To find *A*: $\cos A = \frac{b}{c} \Rightarrow \cos A = \frac{7.3}{11} \Rightarrow A = \cos^{-1}\frac{7.3}{11} \Rightarrow A \approx 48.42220° \Rightarrow A \approx 48°$.

    To find *B*: $B = 90° - 48° \Rightarrow B = 42°$.

    To find *a*: $\sin A = \frac{a}{c} \Rightarrow \sin 48° = \frac{a}{11} \Rightarrow a = 11(\sin 48°) \approx 8.174593 \Rightarrow a \approx 8.2$ ft.

11. To find *B*: $B = 90.00° - 28.00° \Rightarrow B = 62.00°$.

    To find *a*: $\sin A = \frac{a}{c} \Rightarrow \sin 28.00° = \frac{a}{17.4} \Rightarrow a = 17.4(\sin 28.00°) \approx 8.1688 \Rightarrow a \approx 8.17$ ft.

    To find *b*: $\cos A = \frac{b}{c} \Rightarrow \cos 28.00° = \frac{b}{17.4} \Rightarrow b = 17.4(\cos 28.00°) \approx 15.3633 \Rightarrow b \approx 15.4$ ft.

13. To find A: $A = 90.00° - 73.00° \Rightarrow A = 17.00°$.

To find a: $\tan B = \dfrac{b}{a} \Rightarrow \tan 73.00° = \dfrac{128}{a} \Rightarrow a = \dfrac{128}{\tan 73.00°} \approx 39.1335 \Rightarrow a \approx 39.1$ in.

To find c: $\sin B = \dfrac{b}{c} \Rightarrow \sin 73.00° = \dfrac{128}{c} \Rightarrow c = \dfrac{128}{\sin 73.00°} \approx 133.849 \Rightarrow c \approx 134$ in.

15. To find c, use Pythagorean Theorem:

$c^2 = a^2 + b^2 \Rightarrow c^2 = (76.4)^2 + (39.3)^2 \Rightarrow c^2 = 7381.45 \Rightarrow c \approx 85.9154 \Rightarrow c \approx 85.9$ yd.

To find A: $\tan A = \dfrac{a}{b} \Rightarrow \tan A = \dfrac{76.4}{39.3} \Rightarrow A = \tan^{-1}\left(\dfrac{76.4}{39.3}\right) \approx 62.7788° \Rightarrow A \approx 62°46'44'' \Rightarrow A \approx 62°50'$.

To find B: $B = 90°00 - 62°50' \Rightarrow B = 89°60' - 62°50' \Rightarrow B = 27°10'$.

17. The other acute angle requires the least work to find, simply subtract the given angle from $90°$.

19. Because x and y are known, use tangent to find: $\tan\theta = \dfrac{y}{x} \Rightarrow \tan\theta = \dfrac{3.68}{4.6} \Rightarrow \theta = \tan^{-1}\left(\dfrac{3.68}{4.6}\right) \approx 38.6598°$.

21. Because AD and BC are parallel, angle DAB is congruent to angle ABC, as they are alternate interior angles of the transversal AB. (A theorem of elementary geometry assures us of this.)

23. It is measured clockwise from the north.

25. $\sin 43°50' = \dfrac{d}{13.5} \Rightarrow d = 13.5(\sin 43°50') \Rightarrow d \approx 9.34959996 \Rightarrow d \approx 9.35$ m.

27. $\tan 23.4° = \dfrac{5.75}{x} \Rightarrow x = \dfrac{5.75}{\tan 23.4°} \approx 13.2875 \Rightarrow x \approx 13.3$ ft.

29. First find the distance between the buildings, using the angle of depression and $h_1 = 30.0$ feet, since a point on the building horizontally across the street is, like the window, 30 feet from the ground. Find d:

$\tan 20.0 = \dfrac{30.0}{d} \Rightarrow d = \dfrac{30.0}{\tan 20.0°} \approx 82.424$. Now use the found distance and the angle elevation to find h_2 (the height from the horizontal point on the building to the top of the building):

$\tan 50° = \dfrac{h_2}{d} \Rightarrow \tan 50° = \dfrac{h_2}{82.424} \Rightarrow h_2 = 82.424(\tan 50°) \approx 98.229$. Finally, the height of the building is:

$h_1 + h_2 = 30 + 98.229 = 128.229 \approx 128$ feet.

31. First find the complementary angle to the angle of depression:

$\tan C = \dfrac{12.2}{5.93} \Rightarrow C = \tan^{-1}\left(\dfrac{12.02}{5.93}\right) \Rightarrow C \approx 63.74°$.

Therefore, the angle of depression is: $90° - 63.74° = 26.26° \approx 26.3°$ or $26°20'$.

33. To find A: $\tan A = \dfrac{a}{b} \Rightarrow \tan A = \dfrac{1.0837}{1.4923} \Rightarrow A = \tan^{-1}\dfrac{1.0837}{1.4923} \Rightarrow A \approx 35.9869° \Rightarrow A \approx 35.987°$ or $35°59'10''$. To find B: $B = 90.0° - 35.987° \Rightarrow B = 54.013°$ or $54°00'50''$.

35. Let be the base of the smaller right triangle, then: $\tan 21°10' = \dfrac{x}{135+y} \Rightarrow x = (135+y)\tan 21°10'$ and

$\tan 35°30' = \dfrac{x}{y} \Rightarrow x = y(\tan 35°30')$. Now $(135+y)\tan 21°10' = y(\tan 35°30') \Rightarrow$

$135(\tan 21°10') = y(\tan 35°30) - y(\tan 21°10') \Rightarrow 135(\tan 21°10') = y(\tan 35°30' - \tan 21°10') \Rightarrow$

$y = \dfrac{135(\tan 21°10')}{\tan 35°30' - \tan 21°10'} \Rightarrow y \approx 160.30258$. Use the small triangle to solve for x: $x = y(\tan 35°30') \Rightarrow$

$x = 160.30258(\tan 35°30') \Rightarrow x \approx 114.343$. The height of the pyramid is approximately: 114 feet.

37. Let $h=$ the height of the house and $x =$ the height of the antenna, then using the angles of elevation yields the

following equations: $\tan 18°10' = \dfrac{h}{28.0} \Rightarrow h = 28.0(\tan 18°10')$. and

$\tan 27°10' = \dfrac{h+x}{28.0} = h+x = 28.0(\tan 27°10')$. Using these equations we can use substitution for h and solve

for x: $28.0(\tan 18°10') + x = 28.0(\tan 27°10') \Rightarrow x = 28.0(\tan 27°10') - 28.0(\tan 18°10') \Rightarrow x \approx 5.18157$.

The height of the antenna is approximately 5.18 meters.

39. First solve for the hypotenuse of the top triangle: $\cos 30°50' = \dfrac{198.4}{c} \Rightarrow c = \dfrac{198.4}{\cos 30°50'} \Rightarrow c \approx 231.05719$.

Now use this value and the smaller angle of the bottom triangle $\cot 30° = \dfrac{3}{\sqrt{3}} = \dfrac{3\sqrt{3}}{3} = \sqrt{3}$ solve for x:

$\sin 21°30' = \dfrac{x}{c} \Rightarrow \sin 21°30' = \dfrac{x}{231.05719} \Rightarrow x = 231.05719(\sin 21°30') \Rightarrow x \approx 84.7$ m.

41. The angle between the two ships is $90°[180 - (28°10' + 61°50')]$; the first ship sails 96 miles (4×24) and

the second ship sails 112 miles (4×28). Using Pythagorean Theorem we can find c, the distance between

them: $c^2 = 96^2 + 112^2 \Rightarrow c^2 = 21,760 \Rightarrow c \approx 17.51$. The ships are approximately 148 miles apart.

43. From exercise 42, use angle $A = 53°40'$ and solve for d, the distance from point A to the transmitter:

$\sin A = \cos A$. . The distance is approximately 1.48 miles.

45. The angle at the top of the triangle is $90°((27° + (180° - 117°))$, therefore a right triangle is formed. Now

use Pythagorean Theorem to solve for x, the distance between starting and ending points:

$c^2 = 50^2 = 140^2 \Rightarrow c^2 = 22,100 \Rightarrow c \approx 148.66$. The distance is approximately 150 kilometers.

47. (a) A right triangle is formed, since the two acute angles at the bottom of the triangle add up to

$90°: [A(180° - 129°25') + B(39°25') = 90°]$. Now using angle $B = 39°25'$, of the triangle, solve for

distance AC, $\sin 39°25' = \dfrac{x}{15} \Rightarrow x = 15(\sin 39°35') \Rightarrow x \approx 9.524$ miles

(b) Use Pythagorean Theorem to find distance BC. $9.524^2 + b^2 = 15^2 \Rightarrow b = \sqrt{15^2 - 9.524^2} \Rightarrow b \approx 11.59$

49. Let the length of RS be x: $\tan 32°10' = \dfrac{x}{53.1} \Rightarrow x = 53.1(\tan 32°10') \Rightarrow x \approx 33.3957 \approx 33.4$ m.

51. First solve for h, the height of the searchlight beam: $\tan 30° = \dfrac{h}{1000} \Rightarrow h = 1000(\tan 30°) \Rightarrow h \approx 577.35$. The cloud ceiling is searchlight beam height plus observer height, therefore: $6 + 577.35 = 583.35 \approx 583$ feet.

53. (a) First solve for β and then for d, using the given formula and information:

$\beta \approx \dfrac{57.3S}{R} \Rightarrow \beta \approx \dfrac{57.3(336)}{600} \Rightarrow \beta \approx 32.088°$. Therefore: $d = 600\left(1 - \cos\left(\dfrac{32.088}{2}\right)°\right) \Rightarrow$

$d \approx 23.3702 \approx 23.4$ feet.

(b) First solve for β and then for d, using the given formula and information:

$\beta \approx \dfrac{57.3S}{R} \Rightarrow \beta \approx \dfrac{57.3(485)}{600} \Rightarrow \beta \approx 46.3175°$.

$d = 600\left(1 - \cos\left(\dfrac{46.3175}{2}\right)°\right) \Rightarrow d \approx 48.34877 \approx 48.3$ ft.

(c) The faster the speed, the more land that needs to be cleared on the inside of the curve.

55. (a) $\tan \theta = \dfrac{y}{x}$

(b) $\tan \theta = \dfrac{y}{x} \Rightarrow x(\tan \theta) = y \Rightarrow x = \dfrac{y}{\tan \theta}$

57. Find a: $\cos 60° = \dfrac{a}{24} \Rightarrow a = 24(\cos 60°) = 24\left(\dfrac{1}{2}\right) = 12$

Find b: $\sin 60° = \dfrac{b}{24} \Rightarrow b = 24(\sin 60°) = 24\left(\dfrac{\sqrt{3}}{2}\right) = 12\sqrt{3}$

Using $b = 12\sqrt{3}$, find c: $\sin 45° = \dfrac{12\sqrt{3}}{c} \Rightarrow c = \dfrac{12\sqrt{3}}{\cos 45°} = \dfrac{12\sqrt{3}}{\dfrac{\sqrt{2}}{2}} = 12\sqrt{3} \cdot \dfrac{2}{\sqrt{2}} \cdot \dfrac{\sqrt{2}}{\sqrt{2}} = 12\sqrt{6}$

Using $c = 12\sqrt{6}$, find d: $\sin 45° = \dfrac{d}{12\sqrt{6}} \Rightarrow d = 12\sqrt{6}(\sin 45°) = 12\sqrt{6}\left(\dfrac{\sqrt{2}}{2}\right) = 6\sqrt{12} = 6(2\sqrt{3}) = 12\sqrt{3}$.

59. Find a: $\sin 60° = \dfrac{7}{a} \Rightarrow a = \dfrac{7}{\sin 60°} = \dfrac{7}{\dfrac{\sqrt{3}}{2}} = 7 \cdot \dfrac{2}{\sqrt{3}} \cdot \dfrac{\sqrt{3}}{\sqrt{3}} = \dfrac{14\sqrt{3}}{3}$ Since the triangle is a $45° - 45°$ right triangle, $a = n$ and $n = \dfrac{14\sqrt{3}}{3}$

Using $a = \dfrac{14\sqrt{3}}{3}$, find m: $\cos 60° = \dfrac{m}{\frac{14\sqrt{3}}{3}} \Rightarrow m = \dfrac{14\sqrt{3}}{3}(\cos 60°) = \dfrac{14\sqrt{3}}{3} \cdot \dfrac{1}{2} = \dfrac{7\sqrt{3}}{3}$

Using $n = \dfrac{14\sqrt{3}}{3}$, find q: $\cos 45° = \dfrac{\frac{14\sqrt{3}}{3}}{q} \Rightarrow q = \dfrac{\frac{14\sqrt{3}}{3}}{\cos 45°} = \dfrac{\frac{14\sqrt{3}}{3}}{\frac{\sqrt{2}}{2}} = \dfrac{14\sqrt{3}}{3} \cdot \dfrac{2}{\sqrt{2}} \cdot \dfrac{\sqrt{2}}{\sqrt{2}} = \dfrac{28\sqrt{6}}{6} = \dfrac{14\sqrt{6}}{3}$

61. First, bisect the upper angle, which will also be the height (h) of the original triangle. Now solve for h using the smaller right triangle: $\sin 60° = \dfrac{h}{s} \Rightarrow h = s(\sin 60°) \Rightarrow h = \dfrac{s\sqrt{3}}{2}$. Finally find the area of the original triangle: $A = \dfrac{1}{2}bh = \dfrac{1}{2} \cdot s \cdot \dfrac{s\sqrt{3}}{2} \Rightarrow A = \dfrac{s^2\sqrt{3}}{4}$..

8.8 Harmonic Motion

1. (a) If $s(0) = 2$, then we can solve for a: $2 = \cos(w \cdot 0) \Rightarrow 2 = a(1) \Rightarrow a = 2$. Now, since the period is .5 seconds, $\dfrac{2\pi}{w} = \dfrac{1}{2} \Rightarrow w = 4\pi$. Thus $s(t) = a\cos(wt) \Rightarrow s(t) = 2\cos(4\pi t)$.

    (b) $s(1) = 2\cos(4\pi(1)) \Rightarrow s(1) = 2$. The weight is neither moving upward nor downward. At $t = 1$ the motion of the weight is changing from up to down. The calculator graph supports this.

3. (a) If $s(0) = -3$, then we can solve for a: $-3 = a\cos(w \cdot 0) \Rightarrow -3 = a(1) \Rightarrow a = -3$. Now, since the period is .8 seconds, $\dfrac{2\pi}{w} = \dfrac{8}{10} \Rightarrow 8w = 2.5\pi$. Thus $s(t) = a\cos(wt) \Rightarrow s(t) = -3\cos(2.5\pi t)$.

    (b) $s(1) = -3\cos(2.5\pi(1)) \Rightarrow s(1) = 0$. The spring is at its natural length one second after the weight is released. The weight is moving upward. The calculator graph supports this.

5. Using $F = 27.5$, note that $b = w = 2\pi(27.5) = 55\pi$, therefore $s(t) = a\cos(55\pi t)$. Now since $s(0) = .21$, we can solve for a: $.21 = a\cos(55\pi(0)) \Rightarrow .21 = a(1) \Rightarrow a = .21$. The equation is: $s(t) = .21\cos(55\pi t)$.
    See Figure 5.

7. Using $F = 110$ note that $b = w = 2\pi(55) = 110\pi$, therefore $s(t) = a\cos(110\pi t)$. Now since $s(0) = .14$, we can solve for a: $.14 = a\cos(110\pi(0)) \Rightarrow .14 = a(1) \Rightarrow a = .14$. The equation is: $s(t) = .14\cos(110\pi t)$.
    See Figure 7.

[0,0.05] by [-0.3,0.3]
Xscl = 0.01   Yscl = 0.1

[0,0.05] by [-0.3,0.3]
Xscl = 0.01   Yscl = 0.1

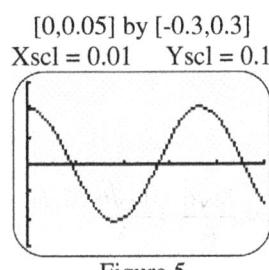

Figure 5

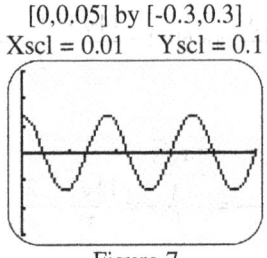

Figure 7

9. (a) Using the simple harmonic motion equation $s(t) = a\sin wt$ with $a = 2$ (radius 2) and $w = 2$ (2 radians/sec) yields the equation: $s(t) = 2\sin 2t$. Therefore, from this equation, the amplitude is $|a| = |2| = 2$, the period is $\frac{2\pi}{2} = \pi$, and the frequency is $\frac{w}{2\pi} = \frac{2}{2\pi} = \frac{1}{\pi}$.

(b) Using the simple harmonic motion equation $s(t) = a\sin wt$ with $a = 2$ (radius 2) and $w = 4$ (4 radians/sec) yields the equation: $s(t) = 2\sin 4t$. Therefore, from this equation, the amplitude is $|a| = |2| = 2$, the period is $\frac{2\pi}{4} = \frac{\pi}{2}$, and the frequency is $\frac{w}{2\pi} = \frac{4}{2\pi} = \frac{2}{\pi}$.

11. Using $P = 1$ and $P = 2\pi\sqrt{\frac{L}{32}}$ (from problem 10), we can solve for L:

$1 = 2\pi\sqrt{\frac{L}{32}} \Rightarrow \frac{1}{2\pi} = \sqrt{\frac{L}{32}} \Rightarrow 2\pi = \sqrt{\frac{32}{L}} \Rightarrow (2\pi)^2 = \frac{32}{L} \Rightarrow 4\pi^2 L = 32 \Rightarrow L = \frac{32}{4\pi^2} \Rightarrow L = \frac{8}{\pi^2}$

13. (a) Using the formula (from problem 12), $s(t) = a\sin\sqrt{\frac{k}{m}}t$, as the simple harmonic motion formula gives us $w = \sqrt{\frac{k}{m}}$, therefore $w = \sqrt{\frac{2}{1}} \Rightarrow w = \sqrt{2}$. With a spring stretch of $\frac{1}{2}$ foot the amplitude is: $\frac{1}{2}$; the period is: $\frac{2\pi}{\sqrt{2}} = \frac{2\sqrt{2}\pi}{2} = \sqrt{2}\pi$; and the frequency is: $\frac{w}{2\pi} = \frac{\sqrt{2}}{2\pi}$.

(b) Using the answers from part (a) and the simple harmonic motion formula $s(t) = a\sin wt$ yields: $s(t) = \frac{1}{2}\sin\sqrt{2}t$.

15. (a) From the equation, $a = -4$ and $w = 10$, therefore the maximum height is the amplitude $|-4| = 4$ in.

(b) From the equation, $a = -4$ and $w = 10$, therefore frequency $\frac{w}{2\pi} = \frac{10}{2\pi} = \frac{5}{\pi}$ cycles/second; and the period is: $\frac{2\pi}{w} = \frac{2\pi}{10} = \frac{\pi}{5}$ seconds.

(c) If $s(t) = 4$, solve $4 = -4\cos 10t \Rightarrow -1 = \cos 10t \Rightarrow 10t = \pi \Rightarrow t = \dfrac{\pi}{10}$. The weight first reaches its maximum height after $\dfrac{\pi}{10}$ seconds.

(d) $s(1.466) = -4\cos(10(1.466)) \approx 2$. After 1.466 seconds, the weight is about 2 inches above the equilibrium position.

17. (a) If the spring is pulled down 2 inches, then $a = -2$ Now use the given period to find w:

$\dfrac{2\pi}{w} = \dfrac{1}{3} \Rightarrow w = 6\pi$ Therefore the equation is $s(t) = -2\cos 6\pi t$

(b) The frequency is: $\dfrac{w}{2\pi} = \dfrac{6\pi}{2\pi} = 3$ cycles/second.

19. (a) From the equation the amplitude is $a = 2$, the spring is compressed 2 inches.

(b) From the equation $w = 2\pi$ therefore the frequency is $\dfrac{w}{2\pi} = \dfrac{2\pi}{2\pi} = 1$ cycle per second.

(c) Graph the equation on a calculator, using the capabilities of the calculator $D(t) = \dfrac{1}{e}$ inches when $t \approx 0.2053$ sec.

Reviewing Basic Concepts (Sections 8.5 - 8.8)

1. First find the value of r: $r = \sqrt{(-2)^2 + 5^2} \Rightarrow r = \sqrt{29}$ Now each of the following is:

$\sin\theta = \dfrac{y}{r} = \dfrac{5}{\sqrt{29}} = \dfrac{5\sqrt{29}}{29}$ $\cos\theta = \dfrac{x}{r} = \dfrac{-2}{\sqrt{29}} = -\dfrac{2\sqrt{29}}{29}$ $\tan\theta = \dfrac{y}{x} = \dfrac{5}{-2} = -\dfrac{5}{2}$

$\csc\theta = \dfrac{r}{y} = \dfrac{\sqrt{29}}{5}$ $\sec\theta = \dfrac{r}{x} = \dfrac{\sqrt{29}}{-2} = -\dfrac{\sqrt{29}}{2}$ $\cot\theta = \dfrac{x}{y} = \dfrac{-2}{5} = -\dfrac{2}{5}$

2. Using a calculator: $\sin 270° = -1$ $\cos 270° = 0$ $\tan 270°$ is undefined

$\csc 270° = -1$ $\sec 270°$ is undefined $\cot 270° = 0$

3. (a) Since $-1 \leq \cos\theta \leq 1$ for all values of θ, $\cos\theta = \dfrac{3}{2}$ is impossible.

(b) Since the range of $\tan\theta$ is: $-\infty < \tan\theta < \infty$, $\tan\theta = 300$, is possible.

(c) Since the range of $\csc\theta$ is: $\csc\theta \leq -1$ or $\csc\theta \geq 1$, $\sec\theta = 5$ is possible.

4. Since θ is in quadrant III, $\sin\theta = \dfrac{-2}{3} = -\dfrac{2}{3}$, $x = -2$ and $y = 3$ First find

$\cos\theta, \sin^2\theta + \cos^2\theta = 1: \left(-\dfrac{2}{3}\right)^2 + \cos^2\theta = 1 \Rightarrow \cos^2\theta = 1 - \dfrac{4}{9} \Rightarrow \cos^2\theta = \dfrac{5}{9} \Rightarrow \cos\theta = \pm\dfrac{\sqrt{5}}{3}$ Since θ is found

in quadrant III, $\cos\theta = -\dfrac{\sqrt{5}}{3}$ Find $\csc\theta$, $\csc\theta = \dfrac{1}{\sin\theta} \Rightarrow \csc\theta = -\dfrac{3}{2}$; find

$\sec\theta, \sec\theta = \dfrac{1}{\cos\theta} \Rightarrow \sec\theta = -\dfrac{3}{\sqrt{5}}$, therefore $\sec\theta = -\dfrac{3\sqrt{5}}{5}$; find

$\tan\theta, \tan\theta = \dfrac{\sin\theta}{\cos\theta} \Rightarrow -\dfrac{2}{3} \div -\dfrac{\sqrt{5}}{3} \Rightarrow \tan\theta = \dfrac{2}{\sqrt{5}}$, therefore $\tan\theta = \dfrac{2\sqrt{5}}{5}$; and

find $\cot\theta, \cot\theta = \dfrac{1}{\tan\theta} \Rightarrow \cot\theta = \dfrac{5}{2\sqrt{5}} = \dfrac{5\sqrt{5}}{10} \Rightarrow \cot\theta = \dfrac{\sqrt{5}}{2}$ The five Functions are:

$\cos\theta = -\dfrac{\sqrt{5}}{3}; \tan\theta = \dfrac{2\sqrt{5}}{5}; \cot\theta = \dfrac{\sqrt{5}}{2}; \sec\theta = -\dfrac{3\sqrt{5}}{5};$ and $\csc\theta = -\dfrac{3}{2}$

5. $\sin A = \dfrac{opp}{hyp} = \dfrac{18}{17}$ $\cos A = \dfrac{adj}{hyp} = \dfrac{15}{17}$ $\tan A = \dfrac{opp}{adj} = \dfrac{8}{15}$

   $\csc A = \dfrac{hpy}{opp} = \dfrac{17}{8}$ $\sec A = \dfrac{hyp}{adj} = \dfrac{17}{15}$ $\cot A = \dfrac{adj}{opp} = \dfrac{15}{8}$

6. By the $30° - 60°$ right triangle,

   $\sin 30° = \dfrac{1}{2}$ $\cos 30° = \dfrac{\sqrt{3}}{2}$ $\tan 30° = \dfrac{\sqrt{3}}{3}$

   $\csc 30° = \dfrac{2}{1} = 2$ $\sec 30° = \dfrac{2}{\sqrt{3}} = \dfrac{2\sqrt{3}}{3}$ $\cot 30° = \dfrac{3}{\sqrt{3}} = \dfrac{3\sqrt{3}}{3} = \sqrt{3}$

   By the $45° - 45°$ right triangle,

   $\sin 45° = \dfrac{\sqrt{2}}{2}$ $\cos 45° = \dfrac{\sqrt{2}}{2}$ $\tan 45° = \dfrac{\sqrt{2}}{\sqrt{2}} = 1$

   $\csc 45° = \dfrac{2}{\sqrt{2}} = \dfrac{2\sqrt{2}}{2} = \sqrt{2}$ $\sec 45° = \dfrac{2}{\sqrt{2}} = \dfrac{2\sqrt{2}}{\sqrt{2}} = \sqrt{2}$ $\cot 45° = \dfrac{\sqrt{2}}{\sqrt{2}} = 1$

   By the $30° - 60°$ right triangle,

   $\sin 60° = \dfrac{\sqrt{3}}{2}$ $\cos 60° = \dfrac{1}{2}$ $\tan 60° = \dfrac{\sqrt{3}}{1} = \sqrt{3}$

   $\csc 30° = \dfrac{2}{\sqrt{3}} = \dfrac{2\sqrt{3}}{3}$ $\sec 60° = \dfrac{2}{1} = 2$ $\cot 60° = \dfrac{1}{\sqrt{3}} = \dfrac{\sqrt{3}}{3}$

7. (a) $\sin 27° = \cos(90° - 27°) = \cos 63°$

   (b) $\tan\dfrac{\pi}{5} = \cot\left(\dfrac{\pi}{2} - \dfrac{\pi}{5}\right) = \cot\left(\dfrac{5\pi}{10} - \dfrac{2\pi}{10}\right) = \cot\dfrac{3\pi}{10}$

8. (a) If $\theta = 100°$ then $\theta° = 180° - 100° = 80°$

   (b) If $\theta = -365° = 720° - 365° = 355°$ then $\theta° = 360° - 355° = 5°$

   (c) If $\theta = \dfrac{8\pi}{3} - 2\pi = \dfrac{8\pi}{3} - \dfrac{6\pi}{3} = \dfrac{2\pi}{3}$ then $\theta° = \pi - \dfrac{2\pi}{3} = \dfrac{3\pi}{3} - \dfrac{2\pi}{3} = \dfrac{\pi}{3}$

9. First find the reference angle: $(360° - 315°) = 45°$ Using the $45° - 45°$ right triangle rules, for a $45°$ angle the hypotenuse $= \sqrt{2}$, the opposite side $= 1$, and the adjacent $= 1$ Since $\theta = 315°$ is in quadrant IV, y is negative and sine, tangent, cotangent, and cosecant are negative, therefore:

$$\sin 315° = -\sin 45° = -\frac{1}{\sqrt{2}} = -\frac{\sqrt{2}}{2} \qquad \csc 315° = -\csc 45° = -\frac{\sqrt{2}}{1} = -\sqrt{2}$$

$$\cos 315° = \cos 45° = \frac{1}{\sqrt{2}} = \frac{\sqrt{2}}{2} \qquad \sec 315° = \sec 45° = \frac{\sqrt{2}}{1} = \sqrt{2}$$

$$\tan 315° = -\tan 45° = -\frac{1}{1} = -1 \qquad \cot 315° = -\cot 45° = -\frac{1}{1} = -1$$

10. (a) Using the calculator, $\sin 46°30' \approx .725374371$

    (b) Using the calculator, $\tan(-100°) \approx 5.67128182$

    (c) Using the calculator, $\csc 4 = (\sin 4)^{-1} \approx -1.321348709$

11. Since $\tan \theta$ is negative in quadrant II and IV, values for θ can only be in these quadrants. From the $30° - 60°$ right triangle, $\tan 30° = \frac{\sqrt{3}}{3}$, therefore $30°$ is the reference angle. In quadrant II, use the reference angle $30°$ to find the first value: $180° - 30° = 150°$. In quadrant IV, use the reference angle to find the other value: $360° - 30° = 330°$. Therefore, $\theta = 150°$ or $330°$

12. Since $(2, -5)$, is positive in quadrant I and II, values for θ can only be in these quadrants. In quadrant I, we use the inverse trigonometric function (radian mode) of our calculator to find the angle: $\sin^{-1} .68163876 \Rightarrow \theta = .75$ In quadrant II, use the found reference angle from quadrant I to find $\theta : \pi - .75 \approx 2.391592654$ Therefore, $\theta \approx .75$ or 2.391592654

13. Let x be the base of the smaller right triangle and h the height of Mt. Kilimanjaro, then:

    $\tan 13.7° = \frac{h}{x} \Rightarrow x = \frac{h}{\tan 13.7°}$ and $\tan 10.4° = \frac{h}{x+5}$. Now substitute the second equation into the first

    equation: $\tan 10.4° = \dfrac{h}{\dfrac{h}{\tan 13.7°} + 5}$, now multiply by $\dfrac{\tan 13.7°}{\tan 13.7°}$ and solve for h:

    $\tan 10.4° = \dfrac{h}{\dfrac{h}{\tan 13.7°} + 5} \cdot \dfrac{\tan 13.7°}{\tan 13.7°} \Rightarrow \tan 10.4° = \dfrac{h(\tan 13.7°)}{h + 5(\tan 13.7°)} \Rightarrow$

    $\tan 10.4°(h + 5(\tan 13.7°)) = h(\tan 13.7°) \Rightarrow h(\tan 10.4°) + 5(\tan 13.7°)(\tan 10.4°) = h(\tan 13.7°) \Rightarrow$

    $h(\tan 10.4°) - h(\tan 13.7°) = -5(\tan 13.7°)(\tan 10.4°) \Rightarrow$

    $h(\tan 10.4° - \tan 13.7°) = -5(\tan 13.7°)(\tan 10.4°) \Rightarrow h = \dfrac{-5(\tan 13.7°)(\tan 10.4°)}{\tan 10.4° - \tan 13.7°} \Rightarrow h \approx 3.713588$ miles

Finally convert to feet: $h \approx \dfrac{3.713588 \text{ mi}}{1} \cdot \dfrac{5280 \text{ ft}}{1 \text{ mi}} \approx 19{,}607.7$

The mountain is approximately 19,600 feet high.

14. (a) From the equation, $a = -4$, therefore the amplitude is $|-4| = 4$ The maximum height is 4 inches.

    (b) Solve for t: $4 = -4\cos 8\pi t \Rightarrow -1 = \cos 8\pi t \Rightarrow 8\pi t = \pi \Rightarrow t = \dfrac{\pi}{8\pi} \Rightarrow t = \dfrac{1}{8}$ seconds.

    (c) The period is: $\dfrac{2\pi}{w} = \dfrac{2\pi}{8\pi} = \dfrac{1}{4}$; and the frequency is: $\dfrac{w}{2\pi} = \dfrac{8\pi}{2\pi} = 4$ cycles/second.

Chapter 8 Review

1. The smallest positive degree measure of the coterminal angle is: $-174° + 360° = 186°$.

2. All degree measure coterminal angles will be multiples of $360°$, therefore: $270° + n \cdot 360°$.

3. First find the radians per second: $\theta = \dfrac{320(2\pi)}{60} \Rightarrow \theta = \dfrac{32\pi}{3}$ radians per second. Now multiply by $\dfrac{2}{3}$ seconds and by $\dfrac{180}{\pi}$ to change to degrees: $\theta = \dfrac{32\pi}{3} \cdot \dfrac{2}{3} \cdot \dfrac{180}{\pi} \Rightarrow \theta = 1280°$.

4. First find degree rotated per second: $\theta = \dfrac{650(360°)}{60} \Rightarrow \theta = 3900°$. Now multiply by 2.4 seconds: $3900 \cdot 2.4 = 9360°$.

5. 1 radian $= 1 \cdot \dfrac{180}{\pi} = 57.3°$ therefore 1 radian $\approx 57.3° > 1°$.

6. (a) Change to degrees and determine the quadrant: $3 \cdot \dfrac{180}{\pi} = 171.9°$, therefore quadrant II.

    (b) Change to degrees and determine the quadrant: $4 \cdot \dfrac{180}{\pi} = 292.2°$, therefore quadrant III.

    (c) Change to degrees and determine the quadrant: $-2 \cdot \dfrac{180}{\pi} = 114.6°$, therefore quadrant III.

    (d) Change to degrees and determine the quadrant: $7 \cdot \dfrac{180}{\pi} = 401.1° - 360° = 41.1°$, therefore quadrant I.

7. $120° \cdot \dfrac{\pi}{180} = \dfrac{2\pi}{3}$

8. $800° \cdot \dfrac{\pi}{180} = \dfrac{40\pi}{9}$

9. $\dfrac{5\pi}{4} \cdot \dfrac{180}{\pi} = 225°$

10. $-\dfrac{6\pi}{5} \cdot \dfrac{\pi}{180} = -216°$

11. Using the arc length formula, 1 rotation has a length: $s = r\theta \Rightarrow s = 2(2\pi) \Rightarrow s = 4\pi$ inches. Then 20 minutes equals: $\dfrac{20}{60} \cdot 4\pi = \dfrac{4\pi}{3}$ inches.

12. Using the arc length formula, 1 rotation has a length: $s = r\theta \Rightarrow s = 2(2\pi) \Rightarrow s = 4\pi$ inches. Then 3 hours equals: $3 \cdot 4\pi = 12\pi$ inches.

13. Since arc length is found by the formula $s = r\theta$, the radius is: $s = 15.2 \cdot \dfrac{3\pi}{4} \Rightarrow s = 35.8$ cm.

14. Using the area of a sector formula $A = \dfrac{1}{2}r^2\theta$ yields: $A = \dfrac{1}{2}(28.69)^2\left(\dfrac{7\pi}{4}\right) \Rightarrow A \approx 2263$ in^2.

15. Because the central angle is very small, the arc length is approximately equal to the length of the inscribed chord. Using the arc length formula yields: $s = 2000\left(1 + \dfrac{10}{60}\right)\left(\dfrac{\pi}{180}\right) \approx 41$ yards.

16. Since arc length is found by the formula $s = r\theta$, the central angle is: $4 = 8\theta \Rightarrow \theta = \dfrac{4}{8} \Rightarrow \theta = \dfrac{1}{2}$ radians. Now using the area of a sector formula $A = \dfrac{1}{2}r^2\theta$ yields: $A = \dfrac{1}{2}(8)^2\left(\dfrac{1}{2}\right) \Rightarrow A = 16$ units^2.

17. From the properties 30°-60° of right triangles, an angle of $s = \dfrac{2\pi}{3}$ radians intersects the unit circle at the point $\left(-\dfrac{1}{2}, \dfrac{\sqrt{3}}{2}\right)$. Since $\cos s = x, \cos\dfrac{2\pi}{3} = -\dfrac{1}{2}$.

18. From the properties 30°-60° of right triangles, an angle of $s = -\dfrac{11\pi}{6}$ radians intersects the unit circle at the point $\left(\dfrac{\sqrt{3}}{2}, \dfrac{1}{2}\right)$. Since $\sin s = y, \sin\left(-\dfrac{11\pi}{6}\right) = \dfrac{1}{2}$.

19. First a coterminal angle: $4\pi - \dfrac{7\pi}{3} = \dfrac{5\pi}{3} \Rightarrow \theta' = -\dfrac{\pi}{3}$, From the properties of 30°-60° right triangles, an angle of $s = -\dfrac{\pi}{3}$ radians intersects the unit circle at $\left(\dfrac{1}{2}, -\dfrac{\sqrt{3}}{2}\right)$. Since $\tan s = \dfrac{y}{x}$, $\tan-\dfrac{\pi}{3} = -\dfrac{\sqrt{3}}{2} \cdot \dfrac{2}{1} = -\sqrt{3}$.

20. From the properties 45°-45° of right triangles, an angle of $s = \dfrac{5\pi}{4}$ radians intersects the unit circle at the point $\left(-\dfrac{\sqrt{2}}{2}, -\dfrac{\sqrt{2}}{2}\right)$. Since $\cot s = \dfrac{x}{y}, \cot\left(\dfrac{5\pi}{4}\right) = \dfrac{-\dfrac{\sqrt{2}}{2}}{-\dfrac{\sqrt{2}}{2}} = 1$.

21. First find θ: $\theta' = 2\pi - \dfrac{11\pi}{6} \Rightarrow \theta' = \dfrac{\pi}{6}$. From the properties of 30°-60° right triangles, an angle of $s = \dfrac{\pi}{6}$ radians intersects the unit circle at the point $\left(\dfrac{\sqrt{3}}{2}, \dfrac{1}{2}\right)$. Since $\csc s = \dfrac{1}{y}$, $\csc \dfrac{\pi}{6} = \dfrac{1}{\frac{1}{2}} = 2$

22. First a coterminal angle: $4\pi - 3\pi = \pi \Rightarrow \theta' = \pi$, an angle of $s = \pi$ radians intersects the unit circle at $(-1, 0)$. Since $\sec s = \dfrac{1}{x}$, $\sec 3\pi = \dfrac{1}{-1} = -1$.

23. Using the calculator (radian mode), $\cos(-.2443) \approx .97030688 \approx .9703$

24. Using the calculator (radian mode), $\cot 3.0543 = [\tan 3.0543]^{-1} \approx -11.426605 \approx -11.4266$.

25. From the properties of 30°-60° right triangles, an angle of $s = \dfrac{\pi}{3}$ radians intersects the unit circle at the point $\left(\dfrac{1}{2}, \dfrac{\sqrt{3}}{2}\right)$. Since $\cos s = \dfrac{1}{2} \Rightarrow s = \dfrac{\pi}{3}$

26. Using the calculator (radian mode), if $\sin s = .49244294$, then $s = \sin^{-1} .49244294 \approx .51489440 \approx .5149$

27. First find θ. Since this is a unit circle, $\sin \theta = y$, therefore $\sin \theta = -.5250622$ and $\theta = \sin^{-1} -.5250622 \Rightarrow \theta \approx -.5528$. Now with $r = 1$, use the arc length formula $s = |r\theta| \Rightarrow s \approx |(1)(-.5528)| \Rightarrow s \approx .5528$. The length of the shortest arc of the circle from $(1, 0)$ to $(.85106383, -.5250622)$ is .5528.

28. B, from the equation, the amplitude is 4 and the period is $\dfrac{2\pi}{2} = \pi$.

29. The amplitude is 2, the period is $\dfrac{2\pi}{(1)} = 2\pi$, and there is no vertical translation or phase shift. See Figure 29.

30. The amplitude (since a tangent function) is not applicable, the period is $\dfrac{\pi}{(3)}$, and there is no vertical translation or phase shift. See Figure 30.

31. The amplitude is $\dfrac{1}{2}$, the period is $\dfrac{2\pi}{(3)}$, and there is no vertical translation or phase shift. See Figure 31.

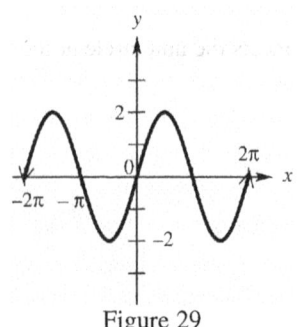
Figure 29

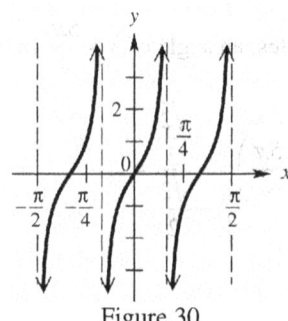
Figure 30

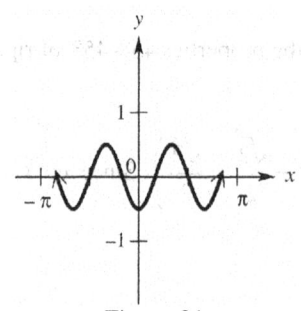
Figure 31

32. The amplitude is 2, the period is $\dfrac{2\pi}{(5)}$, and there is no vertical translation or phase shift. See Figure 32.

33. The amplitude is 2, the period is $\dfrac{2\pi}{\left(\frac{1}{4}\right)} = 8\pi$, the vertical shift is 1 unit upward, and there is no phase shift.

    See Figure 33.

34. The amplitude is $\dfrac{1}{4}$, the period is $\dfrac{2\pi}{\left(\frac{2}{3}\right)} = 3\pi$, the vertical shift is 3 units upward, and there is no phase shift.

    See Figure 34.

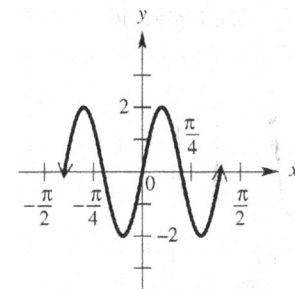
Figure 32

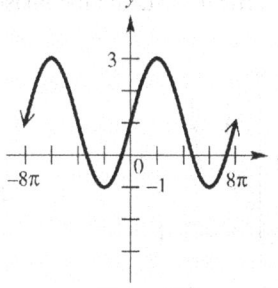
Figure 33

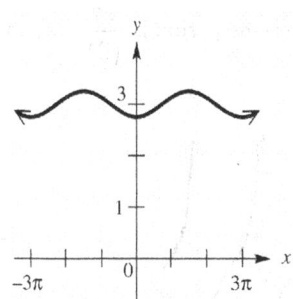
Figure 34

35. The amplitude is 3, the period is $\dfrac{2\pi}{(1)} = 2\pi$, there is no vertical shift, and the phase shift is $-\dfrac{\pi}{2}$.

    See Figure 35.

36. The amplitude is $|-1| = 1$, the period is $\dfrac{2\pi}{(1)} = 2\pi$, there is no vertical shift, and the phase shift is $\dfrac{3\pi}{4}$.

    See Figure 36.

37. Since $y = \dfrac{1}{2}\csc\left(2x - \dfrac{\pi}{4}\right) \Rightarrow y = \dfrac{1}{2}\csc 2\left(x - \dfrac{\pi}{8}\right)$ and the equation, the amplitude is not applicable (cosecant function), the period is $\dfrac{2\pi}{(2)} = \pi$, there is no vertical shift, and the phase shift is $\dfrac{\pi}{8}$. See Figure 37.

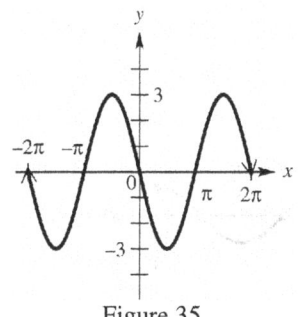
Figure 35

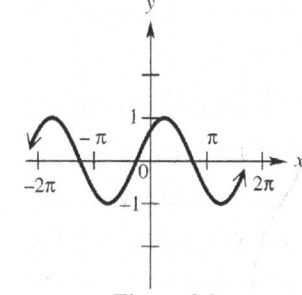
Figure 36

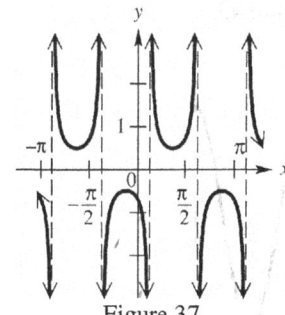
Figure 37

434   Chapter 8: The Unit Circle and the Functions of Trigonometry

38. There is no amplitude, the period is $\dfrac{\pi}{\left(\dfrac{1}{2}\right)} = 2\pi$, and there is no vertical translation or phase shift.

   See Figure 38.

39. There is no amplitude, the period is $\dfrac{2\pi}{(2)} = \pi$, and there is no vertical translation or phase shift. See Figure 39.

40. Since $y = \csc(2x - \pi) = \csc 2\left(x - \dfrac{\pi}{2}\right)$ and now from the equation, the amplitude is not applicable, (cosecant function) the period is $\dfrac{2\pi}{(2)} = \pi$, there is no vertical shift, and the phase shift is $\dfrac{\pi}{2}$. See Figure 40.

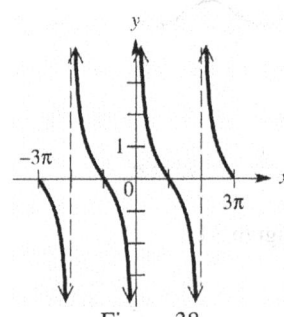
Figure 38

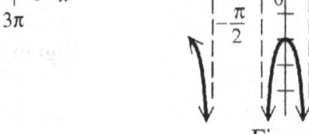
Figure 39

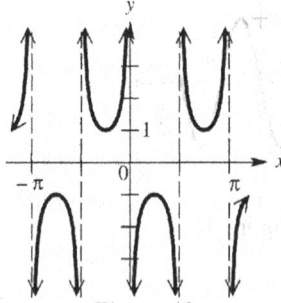
Figure 40

41. Graph a cosine function with an amplitude of 3 and a period of $\dfrac{2\pi}{(2)} = \pi$. See Figure 41.

42. Graph a cotangent function with a period of $\dfrac{\pi}{(3)}$, and passing through the points $\left(\dfrac{\pi}{6}, 0\right)$ (midpoint), $\left(\dfrac{\pi}{12}, 0\right)$, and $\left(\dfrac{\pi}{4}, -\dfrac{1}{2}\right)$. See Figure 42.

43. Graph a cosine function with amplitude 1, period $\dfrac{2\pi}{(1)} = 2\pi$, and phase shift $\dfrac{\pi}{4}$ units to the right.

   See Figure 43.

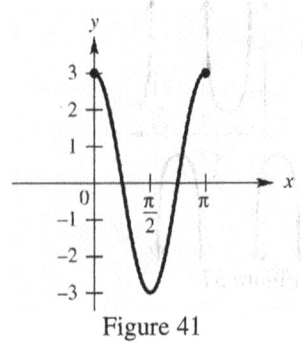
Figure 41

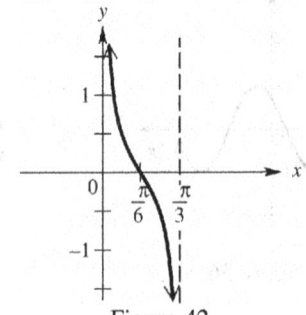
Figure 42

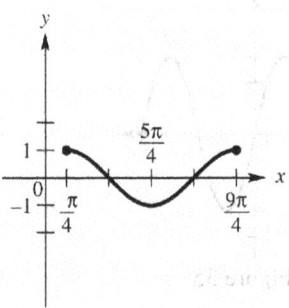
Figure 43

44. Graph a tangent function with a period of $\frac{\pi}{(1)} = \pi$, a phase shift $\frac{\pi}{2}$ units to the right, and passing through the points $\left(\frac{\pi}{2}, 0\right)$ (midpoint), $\left(\frac{\pi}{4}, -1\right)$, and $\left(\frac{3\pi}{4}, 1\right)$. See Figure 44.

45. Graph a cosine function with amplitude 2, period $\frac{2\pi}{(3)}$, and vertical translation 1 unit upward. See Figure 45.

46. Graph a sine function with a amplitude of $|-3| = 3$, a period of $\frac{2\pi}{(2)} = \pi$, and a vertical translation 1 unit downward. See Figure 80.

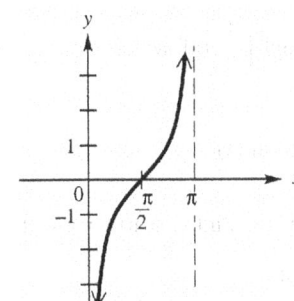
Figure 44

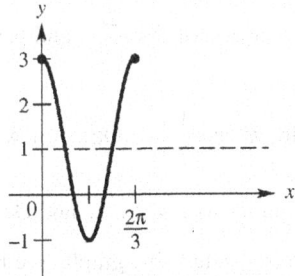
Figure 45

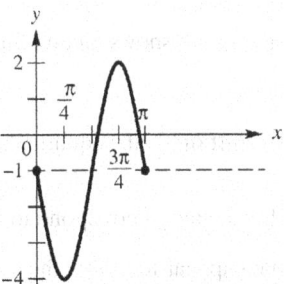
Figure 46

47. Since the period is π, the function is either $\tan x$ or $\cot x$. With an x-intercept $n\pi$, the function is tangent.

48. Since the period is 2π, the function is not $\tan x$ or $\cot x$. With the graph passing through $(0,0)$, the function is sine.

49. Since the period is 2π, the function is not $\tan x$ or $\cot x$. With the graph passing through $\left(\frac{\pi}{2}, 0\right)$, the function is cosine.

50. Since the period is 2π, the function is not $\tan x$ or $\cot x$. With the graph having the domain: $\{x | x \neq n\pi,$ where n is an integer$\}$ the function is cosecant.

51. Since the period is the function is either $\tan x$ or $\cot x$. With the graph decreasing over the interval $(0, \pi)$, the function is cotangent.

52. Since the period is 2π, the function is not $\tan x$ or $\cot x$. With the graph having asymptotes: $x = (2n+1)\frac{\pi}{2}$, where n is an integer, the function is secant.

53. Since the graph shows an amplitude of 3, a period of $\pi = \frac{2\pi}{(2)}$, and passes through $\left(\frac{\pi}{4}, 0\right)$ which means it has a phase shift of $\frac{\pi}{4}$, the equation is $y = 3\sin\left[2\left(x - \frac{\pi}{4}\right)\right]$. (Other answers are possible)

54. Since the graph shows an amplitude of 4, a period of $4\pi = \dfrac{2\pi}{\left(\frac{1}{2}\right)}$, and passes through $(0,0)$ which means it has no phase shift, the equation is $y = 4\sin\dfrac{1}{2}x$. (Other answers are possible)

55. Since the graph shows an amplitude of $\dfrac{1}{3}$, a period of $4\pi = \dfrac{2\pi}{\left(\frac{\pi}{2}\right)}$, and passes through $(0,0)$ which means it has no phase shift, the equation is $y = \dfrac{1}{3}\sin\dfrac{\pi}{2}x$. (Other answers are possible)

56. Since the graph shows an amplitude of π, a period of $2 = \dfrac{2\pi}{(\pi)}$, and passes through $\left(\dfrac{1}{2}, 0\right)$ which means it has a phase shift of $\dfrac{1}{2}$, the equation is $y = \pi\sin\left[\pi\left(x - \dfrac{1}{2}\right)\right]$. (Other answers are possible)

57. (a) Let January correspond to $x = 1$, Februrary to $x = 2,\ldots$, and December of the 2nd year to $x = 24$. The data appear to follow the pattern of a translated sine graph. See Figure 57a.

    (b) Using the model $f(x) = a\sin[b(x-d)] + c$, we can find the constants: The maximum average monthly temperature is 72° F, and the minimum is 22° F. Let the amplitude a be $\dfrac{72-22}{2} = \dfrac{50}{2}$, so $a = 25$. Since the period is $12 = \dfrac{2\pi}{b}$, $b = \dfrac{\pi}{6}$. The data are centered vertically around the line $y = \dfrac{75+25}{2} = 50$, therefore $c = 50$. The minimum temperature occurs in January. Thus, when $x = 1$, $b(x-d) = -\dfrac{\pi}{2}$ since the sine function is minimum at $-\dfrac{\pi}{2}$. Using this and solving for d yields: $\dfrac{\pi}{6}(1-d) = -\dfrac{\pi}{2} \Rightarrow d = 4$. Since the months before January are slightly colder than the months following January the value of d can be slightly adjusted to give a better visual fit, Trying $d = 4.2$ gives a better fit. Using these constant values yields the equation: $f(x) = 25\sin\left[\dfrac{\pi}{6}(x-4.2)\right] + 50$.

    (c) The constant values a controls the amplitude, b the period, c the vertical shift, and d the phase shift.

    (d) See Figure 57d. The function gives an excellent model.

    (e) The regression function gives $y = 25.77\sin(0.52x - 2.19) + 50.57$: see Figure 57e.

Section 8.R   437

[1,25] by [20,80]
Xscl = 5   Yscl = 10

[1,25] by [20,80]
Xscl = 5   Yscl = 10

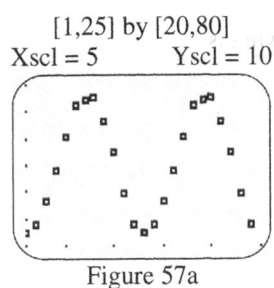
Figure 57a

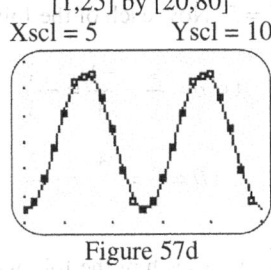
Figure 57d

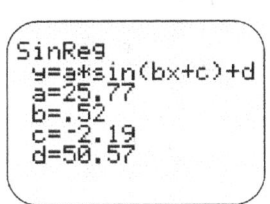
Figure 57e

58. (a) If the shorter leg of the right triangle has length $h_2 - h_1$, then $\cot\theta = \dfrac{d}{h_2 - h_1} \Rightarrow d = (h_2 - h_1)\cot\theta$.

(b) With the given values the equation is: $d = (55-5)\cot\theta \Rightarrow d = 50\cot\theta$. Since the period is π, and the graph wanted is for the interval $0 < \theta \leq \dfrac{\pi}{2}$, the graph will be the left half of a cotangent function. The asymptote is the line $\theta = 0$ and when $\theta = \dfrac{\pi}{4}, d = 50(1) = 50$. See Figure 58.

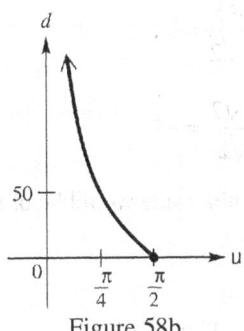
Figure 58b

59. First find the value of r: $r = \sqrt{(-3)^2 + (-3)^2} \Rightarrow r = \sqrt{18.} = 3\sqrt{2}$. Now each of the following is:

$\sin\theta = \dfrac{y}{r} = \dfrac{-3}{3\sqrt{2}} = -\dfrac{\sqrt{2}}{2}$ $\cos\theta = \dfrac{x}{r} = \dfrac{-3}{3\sqrt{2}} = -\dfrac{\sqrt{2}}{2}$ $\tan\theta = \dfrac{y}{x} = \dfrac{-3}{-3} = 1$

$\csc\theta = \dfrac{r}{y} = \dfrac{3\sqrt{2}}{-3} = -\sqrt{2}$ $\sec\theta = \dfrac{r}{x} = \dfrac{3\sqrt{2}}{-3} = -\sqrt{2}$ $\cot\theta = \dfrac{x}{y} = \dfrac{-3}{-3} = 1$

60. First find the value of r: $r = \sqrt{(1)^2 + (-\sqrt{3})^2} \Rightarrow r = \sqrt{4.} = 2$. Now each of the following is:

$\sin\theta = \dfrac{y}{r} = \dfrac{-\sqrt{3}}{2} = -\dfrac{\sqrt{3}}{2}$ $\cos\theta = \dfrac{x}{r} = \dfrac{1}{2}$ $\tan\theta = \dfrac{y}{x} = \dfrac{-\sqrt{3}}{1} = -\sqrt{3}$

$\csc\theta = \dfrac{r}{y} = \dfrac{2}{-\sqrt{3}} = -\dfrac{2\sqrt{3}}{3}$ $\sec\theta = \dfrac{r}{x} = \dfrac{2}{1} = 2$ $\cot\theta = \dfrac{x}{y} = \dfrac{1}{-\sqrt{3}} = -\dfrac{\sqrt{3}}{3}$

61. Using the calculator:

$\sin 180° = 0$ $\cos 180° = -1$ $\tan 180° = 0$

$\csc 180°$ is undefined $\sec 180° = -1$ $\cot 180°$ is undefined

62. First find the value of r: $r = \sqrt{(3)^2 + (-4)^2} \Rightarrow r = \sqrt{25} = 5$. Now each of the following is:

$\sin\theta = \dfrac{y}{r} = \dfrac{-4}{5} = -\dfrac{4}{5}$ $\qquad \cos\theta = \dfrac{x}{r} = \dfrac{3}{5}$ $\qquad \tan\theta = \dfrac{y}{x} = \dfrac{-4}{3} = -\dfrac{4}{3}$

$\csc\theta = \dfrac{r}{y} = \dfrac{5}{-4} = -\dfrac{5}{4}$ $\qquad \sec\theta = \dfrac{r}{x} = \dfrac{5}{3}$ $\qquad \cot\theta = \dfrac{x}{y} = \dfrac{3}{-4} = -\dfrac{3}{4}$

63. First find the value of r: $r = \sqrt{(9)^2 + (-2)^2} \Rightarrow r = \sqrt{85}$. Now each of the following is:

$\sin\theta = \dfrac{y}{r} = \dfrac{-2}{\sqrt{85}} = -\dfrac{2\sqrt{85}}{85}$ $\qquad \cos\theta = \dfrac{x}{r} = \dfrac{9}{\sqrt{85}} = \dfrac{9\sqrt{85}}{85}$ $\qquad \tan\theta = \dfrac{y}{x} = \dfrac{-2}{9} = -\dfrac{2}{9}$

$\csc\theta = \dfrac{r}{y} = \dfrac{\sqrt{85}}{-2} = -\dfrac{\sqrt{85}}{2}$ $\qquad \sec\theta = \dfrac{r}{x} = \dfrac{\sqrt{85}}{9}$ $\qquad \cot\theta = \dfrac{x}{y} = \dfrac{9}{-2} = -\dfrac{9}{2}$

64. First find the value of r: $r = \sqrt{(-2\sqrt{2})^2 + (2\sqrt{2})^2} \Rightarrow r = \sqrt{16.} = 4$. Now each of the following is:

$\sin\theta = \dfrac{y}{r} = \dfrac{2\sqrt{2}}{4} = \dfrac{\sqrt{2}}{2}$ $\qquad \cos\theta = \dfrac{x}{r} = \dfrac{-2\sqrt{2}}{4} = -\dfrac{\sqrt{2}}{2}$ $\qquad \tan\theta = \dfrac{y}{x} = \dfrac{2\sqrt{2}}{-2\sqrt{2}} = -1$

$\csc\theta = \dfrac{r}{y} = \dfrac{4}{2\sqrt{2}} = \sqrt{2}$ $\qquad \sec\theta = \dfrac{r}{x} = \dfrac{4}{-2\sqrt{2}} = -\sqrt{2}$ $\qquad \cot\theta = \dfrac{x}{y} = \dfrac{-2\sqrt{2}}{2\sqrt{2}} = -1$

65. If the terminal side of a quadrantal angle lies along the y-axis, a point on the terminal side would be of the form $(0, k)$ where k is a real number, $k \neq 0$

$\sin\theta = \dfrac{y}{r} = \dfrac{k}{r}$ $\qquad \cos\theta = \dfrac{x}{r} = \dfrac{0}{r} = 0$ $\qquad \tan\theta = \dfrac{y}{x} = \dfrac{k}{0}$ is undefined

$\csc\theta = \dfrac{r}{y} = \dfrac{r}{k}$ $\qquad \sec\theta = \dfrac{r}{x} = \dfrac{r}{0}$ is undefined $\qquad \cot\theta = \dfrac{x}{y} = \dfrac{0}{k} = 0$

66. Since the range of $\sec\theta$ is: $\sec\theta \leq -1$ or $\sec\theta \geq 1$, $\sec\theta = -\dfrac{2}{3}$ is impossible.

67. Since the range of $\tan\theta$ is: $-\infty \leq \tan\theta \leq \infty$, $\tan\theta = 1.4$ is possible.

68. Since $\sin\theta = \dfrac{\sqrt{3}}{5}$, $y = \sqrt{3}$ and $r = 5$. Now use Pythagorean Theorem to solve for x: $r^2 = x^2 + y^2 \Rightarrow$

    $25 = x^2 + 3 \Rightarrow x^2 = 22 \Rightarrow x = \pm\sqrt{22}$. Since $\cos\theta < 0$, $x = -\sqrt{22}$. Therefore,

$\sin\theta = \dfrac{\sqrt{3}}{5}$ $\qquad \cos\theta = \dfrac{x}{r} = \dfrac{-\sqrt{22}}{5} = -\dfrac{\sqrt{22}}{5}$ $\qquad \tan\theta = \dfrac{y}{x} = \dfrac{\sqrt{3}}{-\sqrt{22}} = -\dfrac{\sqrt{66}}{22}$

$\csc\theta = \dfrac{r}{y} = \dfrac{5}{\sqrt{3}} = \dfrac{5\sqrt{3}}{3}$ $\qquad \sec\theta = \dfrac{r}{x} = \dfrac{5}{-\sqrt{22}} = -\dfrac{5\sqrt{22}}{22}$ $\qquad \cot\theta = \dfrac{x}{y} = \dfrac{-\sqrt{22}}{\sqrt{3}} = -\dfrac{\sqrt{66}}{3}$

69. Since $\cos\theta = \dfrac{\sqrt{3}}{5}$, $x = -5$ and $r = 8$. Now use Pythagorean Theorem to solve for x:

    $r^2 = x^2 + y^2 \Rightarrow 64 = 25 + y^2 \Rightarrow y^2 = 39 \Rightarrow y = \pm\sqrt{39}$. Since θ is in quadrant III, $y = -\sqrt{39}$. Therefore,

$$\sin\theta = \frac{y}{r} = \frac{-\sqrt{39}}{8} = -\frac{\sqrt{39}}{8} \qquad \cos\theta = -\frac{5}{8} \qquad \tan\theta = \frac{y}{x} = \frac{-\sqrt{39}}{-5} = \frac{\sqrt{39}}{5}$$

$$\csc\theta = \frac{r}{y} = \frac{8}{-\sqrt{39}} = -\frac{8\sqrt{39}}{39} \qquad \sec\theta = \frac{r}{x} = \frac{8}{-5} = -\frac{8}{5} \qquad \cot\theta = \frac{x}{y} = \frac{-5}{-\sqrt{39}} = \frac{5\sqrt{39}}{39}$$

70. The sine function is negative in quadrant III and IV. The cosine function is positive in quadrants I and IV. Therefore, since $\sin\theta < 0$ and $\cos > 0$, θ must be in quadrant IV and in quadrant IV $\tan\theta$ is negative.

71. $\sin A = \frac{\text{opp}}{\text{hyp}} = \frac{40}{58} = \frac{20}{29} \qquad \cos A = \frac{\text{adj}}{\text{hyp}} = \frac{42}{58} = \frac{21}{29} \qquad \tan A = \frac{\text{opp}}{\text{adj}} = \frac{40}{42} = \frac{20}{21}$

$\csc A = \frac{\text{hyp}}{\text{opp}} = \frac{58}{40} = \frac{29}{20} \qquad \sec A = \frac{\text{hyp}}{\text{adj}} = \frac{58}{42} = \frac{29}{21} \qquad \cot A = \frac{\text{adj}}{\text{opp}} = \frac{42}{40} = \frac{21}{20}$

72. $\sin A = \frac{\text{opp}}{\text{hyp}} = \frac{60}{61} \qquad \cos A = \frac{\text{adj}}{\text{hyp}} = \frac{11}{61} \qquad \tan A = \frac{\text{opp}}{\text{adj}} = \frac{60}{11}$

$\csc A = \frac{\text{hyp}}{\text{opp}} = \frac{61}{60} \qquad \sec A = \frac{\text{hyp}}{\text{adj}} = \frac{61}{11} \qquad \cot A = \frac{\text{adj}}{\text{opp}} = \frac{11}{60}$

73. First find the reference angle: $(360° - 300°) = 60°$. Using the $30°$-$60°$ right triangle rules, for a $60°$ angle the hypotenuse = 2, the opposite side = $\sqrt{3}$ and the adjacent side=1. Since $\theta = 300°$ is in quadrant IV, y is negative and sine, tangent, cotangent, and cosecant are negative, therefore:

$$\sin 300° = -\sin 60° = -\frac{\sqrt{3}}{2} \qquad \csc 300° = -\csc 60° = -\frac{2}{\sqrt{3}} = -\frac{2\sqrt{3}}{3}$$

$$\cos 300° = \cos 60° = \frac{1}{2} \qquad \sec 300° = \sec 60° = \frac{2}{1} = 2$$

$$\tan 300° = -\tan 60° = -\frac{\sqrt{3}}{1} = -\sqrt{3} \qquad \cot 300° = -\cot 60° = -\frac{1}{\sqrt{3}} = -\frac{\sqrt{3}}{3}.$$

74. First find the reference angle: $-225°$ is coterminal with $-225° + 360° = 135°$ and the reference angle is: $360° - 135° = 45°$. Using the $45°$-$45°$ right triangle rules, for a $45°$ angle the hypotenuse = $\sqrt{2}$, the opposite side=1, and the adjacent=1. Since $\theta = -225°$ is in quadrant II, x is negative and cosine, tangent, cotangent, and secant are negative, therefore:

$$\sin(-225°) = \sin 45° = \frac{1}{\sqrt{2}} = \frac{\sqrt{2}}{2} \qquad \csc(-225°) = \csc 45° = \frac{\sqrt{2}}{1} = \sqrt{2}$$

$$\cos(-225°) = -\cos 45° = -\frac{1}{\sqrt{2}} = -\frac{\sqrt{2}}{2} \qquad \sec(-225°) = -\sec 45° = -\frac{\sqrt{2}}{1} = -\sqrt{2}$$

$$\tan(-225°) = -\tan 45° = -\frac{1}{1} = -1 \qquad \cot(-225°) = -\cot 45° = -\frac{1}{1} = -1$$

75. First find the reference angle: $-390°$ is co-terminal with $-390° + 720° = 330°$ and the reference angle is: $360° - 330° = 30°$. Using the $30° - 60°$ right triangle rules, for a $30°$ angle the hypotenuse = 2, the opposite

side=1, and the adjacent = $\sqrt{3}$. Since $\theta = -390°$ is in quadrant IV, y is negative and sine, tangent, cotangent, and cosecant are negative, therefore:

$\sin(-390°) = -\sin 30° = -\dfrac{1}{2}$ $\csc(-390°) = -\csc 30° = -\dfrac{20}{1} = -2$

$\cos(-390°) = \cos 30° = -\dfrac{\sqrt{3}}{2}$ $\sec(-390°) = \sec 30° = -\dfrac{2}{\sqrt{3}} = \dfrac{2\sqrt{3}}{3}$

$\tan(-390°) = -\tan 30° = -\dfrac{1}{\sqrt{3}} = -\dfrac{\sqrt{3}}{3}$ $\cot(-390°) = -\cot 30° = -\dfrac{\sqrt{3}}{1} = -\sqrt{3}$

76. $\sin 72°30' = \sin\left(72 + \dfrac{30}{60}\right)° = \sin 72° \approx .95371695$

77. $\sec 222°30' = \sec\left(222 + \dfrac{30}{60}\right)° = \sec 222.5° = (\cos 222.5°)^{-1} \approx -1.3563417$

78. $\cot 305.6° = (\tan 305.6°)^{-1} \approx -.7159268$

79. $\tan 11.7689° \approx .20834446$

80. If $\theta = 135°, \theta' = 45°$, if $\theta = 45°, \theta' = 45°$, if $\theta = 300°, \theta' = 60°$, and if $\theta = 140°, \theta' = 40°$. Of these reference angles, $40°$ is the only one which is not a special angle, so D, $\tan 140°$, is the only one which cannot be determined exactly.

81. $\theta = \sin^{-1}.82584121 \approx 55.673870° \approx 55.7°$

82. $\cot\theta = 1.1249386 \Rightarrow \dfrac{1}{\tan\theta} = 1.1249386 \Rightarrow \tan\theta = (1.1249386)^{-1} \Rightarrow \theta = \tan^{-1}(1.1249386)^{-1} \approx$
    $41.635092° \approx 41.6°$

83. To find B: $B = 90° - 58°30' \Rightarrow B = 89°60' - 58°30' \Rightarrow B = 31°30'$.

    To find a: $\sin A = \dfrac{a}{c} \Rightarrow \sin 58°30' = \dfrac{a}{748} \Rightarrow a = 748(\sin 58°30') \approx 637.7748 \Rightarrow a \approx 638$.

    To find b: $\cos A = \dfrac{b}{c} \Rightarrow \cos 58°30' = \dfrac{b}{748} \Rightarrow b = 748(\cos 58°30') \approx 390.8289 \Rightarrow b \approx 391$

84. To find B: $B = 90° - 39.72° \Rightarrow B = 50.28°$.

    To find a: $\tan A = \dfrac{a}{c} \Rightarrow \tan 39.72° = \dfrac{a}{38.97} \Rightarrow a = 38.97(\tan 39.72°) \approx 32.3765 \Rightarrow a \approx 32.38$

    To find c: $\cos A = \dfrac{b}{c} \Rightarrow \cos 39.72° = \dfrac{38.97}{c} \Rightarrow c = \dfrac{38.97}{\cos 39.72°} \approx 50.6646 \Rightarrow c \approx 50.66$

85. Draw a picture of these points (not shown). Since $344° - 254° = 90°$, points A, B, and C form a right triangle with angle C the right angle and angle. $B = 42°((254° - 180°) - 32°)$.

    Now set $d =$ the distance between point A and point B, now use the sine function to solve for d:

    $\sin 42° = \dfrac{780}{d} \Rightarrow d = \dfrac{780}{\sin 42°} \Rightarrow d \approx 1165.692$. The distance from A to B is approximately 1200 meters.

86. Draw a picture of these points (not shown). A right triangle is formed since the angle where the ship turns is $90°(35°+55°$ by alternate interior angles). Solve by Pythagorean theorem:

    $d^2 = 80^2 + 74^2 \Rightarrow d^2 = 11,876 \Rightarrow d \approx 108.97706$. The ship is approximately 110 km from the pier.

87. A right triangle is formed with a bottom angle of $36°(360°-324°)$, and the adjacent side to this $36°$ angle is 110 mph $(2\cdot 55)$. Let x be the distance between the cars and solve for x using cosine:

    $\cos 36° = \dfrac{110}{x} \Rightarrow x = \dfrac{110}{\cos 36°} \Rightarrow x \approx 135.96748$. The cars are approximately 140 miles apart.

88. Two right triangles are formed. Let x be the distance the boat travels, and y be the distance from shore at the second observation. First, solve for y using the larger right triangle: $\angle 1 = 27°$ (by alternate interior angles)

    $\Rightarrow \tan 27° = \dfrac{150}{x+y} \Rightarrow x+y = \dfrac{150}{\tan 27°} \Rightarrow y = \dfrac{150}{\tan 27°} - x$. Next, solve for y using the smaller right triangle:

    $<2 = 39°$ (by alternate interior angles) $\Rightarrow \tan 39° = \dfrac{150}{y} \Rightarrow y = \dfrac{150}{\tan 39°}$. Finally, since each equation equals

    y, set them equal to each other: $\dfrac{150}{\tan 27°} - x = \dfrac{150}{\tan 39°} \Rightarrow x = \dfrac{150}{\tan 27°} \Rightarrow x \approx 109.157$.

    The boat travels about 109 feet.

89. Let h = height of the tower, now use the tangent function to solve for h:

    $\tan 38°20' = \dfrac{h}{93.2} \Rightarrow h = 93.2 \tan 38°20' \approx 73.69300534 \Rightarrow h \approx 73.7$ feet.

90. The angle at the point on the ground is $29.5°$ (by geometry, alternate interior angles are equal). Now set h = height of the tower and use the tangent function to solve for h:

    $\tan 29.5° = \dfrac{h}{36.0} \Rightarrow h = 36.0 \tan 29.5° \Rightarrow h \approx 20.36782 \Rightarrow h \approx 20.4$ meters.

91. Let x be the length of the base of the smaller right triangle. First, solve for x using the larger triangle:

    $\tan 29° = \dfrac{h}{392+x} \Rightarrow 392+x = \dfrac{h}{\tan 29°} \Rightarrow x = \dfrac{h}{\tan 29°} - 392$. Next, solve for x using the smaller triangle:

    $\tan 49° = \dfrac{h}{x} \Rightarrow x = \dfrac{h}{\tan 49°}$. Finally, since each equation is equal to x, set them equal to each other:

    $\dfrac{h}{\tan 29°} - 392 = \dfrac{h}{\tan 49°} \Rightarrow \dfrac{h}{\tan 29°} - \dfrac{h}{\tan 49°} = 392 \Rightarrow h \tan 49° - h \tan 29° = 392 \tan 29° \tan 49° \Rightarrow$

    $h(\tan 49° - \tan 29°) = 392 \tan 29° \tan 49° \Rightarrow h = \dfrac{392 \tan 29° \tan 49°}{\tan 49° - \tan 29°} \Rightarrow h \approx 419.3585 \Rightarrow h \approx 419$.

92. (a) $\sin \theta = \dfrac{x_Q - x_P}{d} \Rightarrow x_Q = x_P + d \sin \theta$. Similarly, $\cos \theta = \dfrac{y_Q - y_P}{d} \Rightarrow y_Q = y_P + d \cos \theta$.

    (b) Using the given information yields: $y_Q = y_P + d \cos \theta \Rightarrow 337.95 + 193.86 \cos 17°19'22'' =$

    $337.95 + 193.86 \cos 17.3228° \Rightarrow y_Q \approx 523.02$ The coordinates of Q are $(181.34, 523.02)$.

93. From the equation, the amplitude is 4, the period is $\frac{2\pi}{(\pi)} = 2$, and the frequency is $\frac{(\pi)}{2\pi} = \frac{1}{2}$.

94. From the equation, the amplitude is 3, the period is $\frac{2\pi}{(2)} = \pi$, and the frequency is $\frac{(2)}{2\pi} = \frac{1}{\pi}$.

95. It represents the number of oscillations in one second. The position from the initial point after 1.5 seconds is given as $4\sin\left(\frac{3\pi}{2}\right) = -4 \Rightarrow 4$ inches below the initial point; after 2 seconds, $4\sin(2\pi) = 0 \Rightarrow$ at the intial point; after 3.25 seconds, $4\sin\left(\frac{13\pi}{4}\right) = -2\sqrt{2} \Rightarrow 2\sqrt{2}$ inches below the initial point.

96. The period is the time to complete one cycle. The amplitude is the maximum distance (on either side) from the initial point.

Chapter 8 Test:

1. The smallest positive degree measure of the coterminal angle is: $-157° + 360° = 203°$.

2. First find the revolutions per second: $\frac{450 \text{ rev}}{1 \text{ min}} \cdot \frac{1 \text{ min}}{60 \text{ sec}} = 7.5$ revolutions per second. Now find the degrees: $7.5(360°) = 2700°$. The point on the edge of the tire moves $2700°$ in one second.

3. (a) $120° \cdot \frac{\pi}{180} = \frac{2\pi}{3}$ radians.

    (b) $\frac{9\pi}{10} \cdot \frac{180}{\pi} = 162°$

4. (a) Since arc length is found by the formula $s = r\theta$, the central angle is: $200 = 150\theta \Rightarrow \theta = \frac{200}{150} \Rightarrow \theta = \frac{4}{3}$.

    (b) Using the area of a sector formula $A = \frac{1}{2}r^2\theta$ yields: $A = \frac{1}{2}(150)^2\left(\frac{4}{3}\right) \Rightarrow A = 15,000 \text{ km}^2$

5. Since $36° = 36 \cdot \frac{\pi}{180} = \frac{\pi}{5}$ radians and arc length is found by the formula $s = r\theta$, the arc length is: $s = 12\left(\frac{\pi}{5}\right) \Rightarrow s = \frac{12}{5}\pi \Rightarrow s \approx 7.54 \text{ in}$

6. From the equation, the amplitude is 2, the period is $\frac{2\pi}{(1)} = 2\pi$, the vertical translation is 1 unit downward, and the phase shift is π units to the left. See Figure 7.

7. From the equation, the amplitude is $|-1| = 1$ the period is $\frac{2\pi}{(2)} = \pi$, and there is no vertical translation or phase shift, and the graph is reflected across the x-axis. See Figure 18.

8. From the equation, the amplitude (since a tangent function) is not applicable, the period is $\frac{\pi}{(1)} = \pi$, and the phase shift is $\frac{\pi}{2}$ units to the right. See Figure 8.

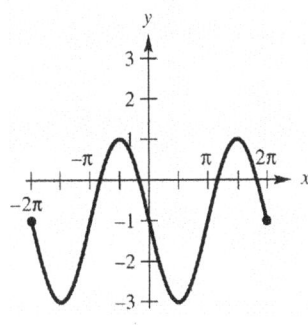

Figure 6

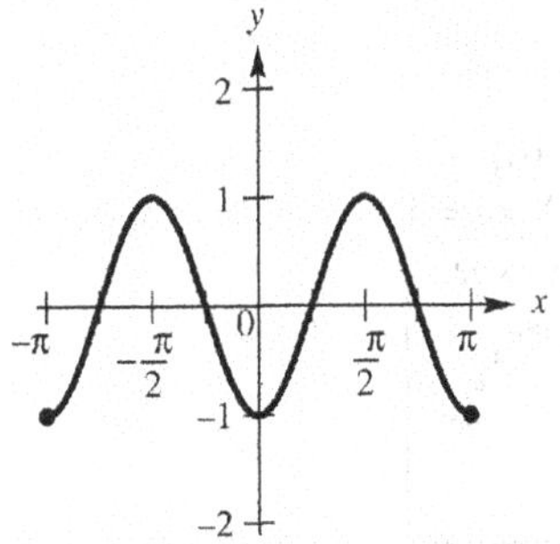

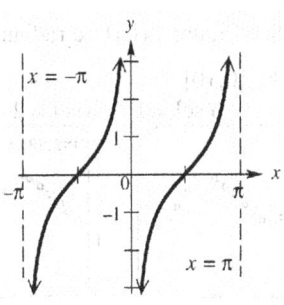

Figure 7

Figure 8

9. Graph the secant function with a period of 2π and shifted up 1 unit. See Figure 9.

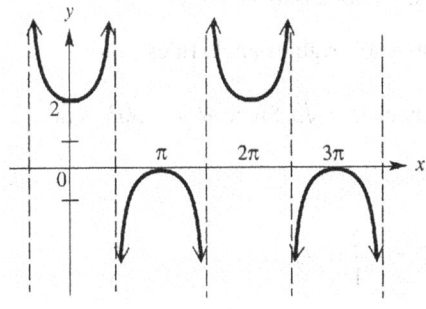

Figure 9

10. The graph has an amplitude of 2 therefore the value of a is 2. The graph repeats itself twice in the interval of 2π therefore the value of b is 2. The shape of the graph shows that we are graphing the sine function. Therefore, the equation of the graph is $y = 2\sin 2x$.

11. (a) Convert the times to decimals hours and enter the values in your calculator as described. Now make a scatterplot of the data on the calculator. See Figure 11a.

    (b) The minimum sunset time is 4:35 or 4.58; the maximum sunset time is 7:33 or 7.55. Using these values, the amplitude is $\frac{7.55 - 4.58}{2} = 1.48$ or 1:29. In the equation $y = a\sin b(x - d) + c$, the amplitude is a, therefore $a = 1.48$.

    (c) The times repeat every 12 months, so the period is $\frac{2\pi}{(12)} = \frac{\pi}{6} \approx .52$. Therefore $b \approx .52$.

    (d) We want the cycle to start with March 21, which corresponds to 3.68, therefore the phase shift is $\frac{2\pi}{(12)} = \frac{\pi}{6} d \approx 3.68$.

444 Chapter 8: The Unit Circle and the Functions of Trigonometry

(e) The vertical shift is the average of the maximum and minimum sunset times,

so $c = \dfrac{4.58 + 7.55}{2} = 6.065$. Therefore $c \approx 6.07$.

(f) Using $y = a\sin b(x - d) + c$ yields: $y = 1.48\sin[.52(x - 3.68)] + 6.07 \Rightarrow y = 1.48\sin(.52x - 1.91) + 6.07$.

See Figure 11f. (Use radian mode)

[0,25] by [0,10]   [0,25] by [0,10]
Xscl = 2   Yscl = 1   Xscl = 2   Yscl = 1

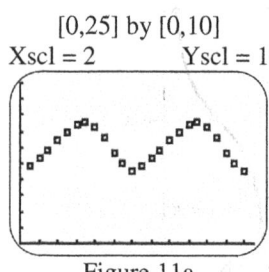
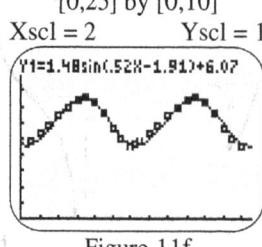

Figure 11a   Figure 11f

12. (a) The smallest positive degree measure of the coterminal angle is: $-150° + 360° = 210°$.

(b) First find the reference angle: $(210° - 180°) = 30°$. Using the $30°$-$60°$ right triangle rules, for a $30°$ angle the hypotenuse $= 2$, the opposite side $= 1$, and the adjacent $= \sqrt{3}$. Since $\theta = -150°$ is in quadrant III, both x and y are negative and the point is: $\left(-\sqrt{3}, -1\right)$.

(c) $\sin(-150°) = -\sin 30° = -\dfrac{1}{2}$ $\csc(-150°) = -\csc 30° = -\dfrac{2}{1} = -2$

$\cos(-150°) = -\cos 30° = -\dfrac{\sqrt{3}}{2}$ $\sec(-150°) = -\sec 30° = -\dfrac{2}{\sqrt{3}} = -\dfrac{2\sqrt{3}}{3}$

$\tan(-150°) = \tan 30° = \dfrac{1}{\sqrt{3}} = \dfrac{\sqrt{3}}{3}$ $\cot(-150°) = \cot 30° = \dfrac{\sqrt{3}}{1} = \sqrt{3}$

(d) $-150° = -\dfrac{150°}{1} \cdot \dfrac{\pi}{180°} = -\dfrac{5\pi}{6}$

13. If $\sin s = .82584121$, then $s = \sin^{-1}.82584121 \approx .97169234$.

14. If $\cos \theta < 0$, then θ is in quadrant II or III. If $\cot \theta > 0$, is in quadrant I or III. Therefore, θ terminates in quadrant III.

15. With the coordinate $(2, -5)$, we will have a radius of $r = \sqrt{(2)^2 + (-5)^2} = \sqrt{4 + 25} \Rightarrow r = \sqrt{29}$. Therefore:

$\sin \theta = \dfrac{y}{r} = \dfrac{-5}{\sqrt{29}} = -\dfrac{5\sqrt{29}}{29}$ $\cos \theta = \dfrac{x}{r} = \dfrac{2}{\sqrt{29}} = \dfrac{2\sqrt{29}}{29}$ $\tan \theta = \dfrac{y}{x} = \dfrac{-5}{2} = -\dfrac{5}{2}$.

16. Since $\cos \theta = \dfrac{4}{5}$, then $x = 4$ and $r = 5$. Now use the pythagorean theorem to find y

$5^2 = 4^2 + y^2 \Rightarrow 25 = 16 + y^2 \Rightarrow y^2 = 9 \Rightarrow y = \pm 3$. Since θ is in quadrant IV, $y = -3$.

Therefore: $\sin \theta = \dfrac{y}{r} = \dfrac{-3}{5} = -\dfrac{3}{5}$ $\tan \theta = \dfrac{y}{x} = \dfrac{-3}{4} = -\dfrac{3}{4}$

$$\csc\theta = \frac{r}{y} = \frac{5}{-3} = -\frac{5}{3} \qquad \sec\theta = \frac{r}{x} = \frac{5}{4} = \frac{5}{4} \qquad \cot\theta = \frac{x}{y} = \frac{4}{-3} = -\frac{4}{3}$$

17. Use knowledge of $(30°\text{-}60°)$ and $(45°\text{-}45°)$ right triangles to find each:

    To find w, use $\sin 30° = \frac{4}{w} \Rightarrow w = \frac{4}{\sin 30°} = \frac{4}{\frac{1}{2}} = 8$.

    To find x, use $\tan 45° = \frac{4}{x} \Rightarrow x = \frac{4}{\tan 45°} = \frac{4}{1} = 4$.

    To find y, use $\cos 30° = \frac{y}{w} = \frac{y}{8} \Rightarrow y = 8\cos 30° = 8 \cdot \frac{\sqrt{3}}{2} = 4\sqrt{3}$.

    To find z, use $\sin 45° = \frac{4}{z} \Rightarrow z = \frac{4}{\sin 45°} = \frac{4}{\frac{1}{\sqrt{2}}} = 4\sqrt{2}$.

18. First, $\cot(-750°)$ is coterminal with $(3 \cdot 360° - 750°) = \cot 330°$. Now find the reference angle: $\cot(360° - 330°) = \cot 30°$. Finally, since $\cot(-750°)$ is terminal in quadrant IV, we will find $-\cot 30°$ and using the $(30°-60°)$ right triangle: $-\cot 30° = -\sqrt{3}$.

19. (a) $\sin 78°21' = \sin\left(78 + \frac{21}{60}\right)° = \sin 78.35° \approx .97939940$

    (b) $\tan 11.7689° \approx .20834446$

    (c) $\sec 58.9041° = \frac{1}{\cos 58.9041°} = (\cos 58.9041°)^{-1} \approx 1.9362132$

20. To find B: $B = 90° - 58°30' \Rightarrow B = 89°60' - 58°30' \Rightarrow B = 31°30'$.

    To find a: $\sin A = \frac{a}{c} \Rightarrow \sin 58°30' = \frac{a}{748} \Rightarrow a = 748(\sin 58°30') \approx 637.7748 \Rightarrow a \approx 638$.

    To find b: $\cos A = \frac{b}{c} \Rightarrow \cos 58°30' = \frac{b}{748} \Rightarrow b = 748(\cos 58°30') \approx 390.8289 \Rightarrow b \approx 391$

21. Let x be the height of the flag pole. Now use the tangent function to solve for x:

    $\tan 32°10' = \frac{x}{24.7} \Rightarrow x = 24.7\tan 32°10' \approx 15.5$ feet.

22. Draw a picture of the ships travels (not shown). Angle ABX is $55°$ (using geometry—alternate interior angles are equal) and angle ABC is $55° + 35° = 90°$, therefore triangle ABC is a right triangle and we can use Pythagorean theorem to find AC: $AC^2 = 80^2 + 74^2 \Rightarrow AC = \sqrt{80^2 + 74^2} \approx 108.977 \Rightarrow AC \approx 110$ km.

23. Because the amplitude is $|-3| = 3$, the maximum height the weight rises above an equilibrium position of $y = 0$ is 3 inches.

24. If $s(t) = 3$, then $3 = -3\cos 2\pi t \Rightarrow -1 = \cos 2\pi t$. Since $\cos\theta = -1$ when $\theta = \pi$,

    then $2\pi t = \pi \Rightarrow 2t = 1 \Rightarrow t = \frac{1}{2}$. Therefore it reaches the maximum height at $\frac{1}{2}$ seconds.

Chapter 9: Trigonometric Identities and Equations

9.1: Trigonometric Identities

1. Since by the negative-number identities $\sin x = -\sin(-x)$, the function is: Odd.

3. Since by the negative-number identities $\tan x = -\tan(-x)$, the function is: Odd.

5. Since by the negative-number identities $\sec x = \sec(-x)$, the function is: Even.

7. By a negative-number identity, if $\cos(-\theta) = \cos\theta$, then $\cos(-4.38) = \cos 4.38$.

9. By a negative-number identity, if $\sin(-\theta) = -\sin\theta$, then $\sin(-0.5) = -\sin 0.5$.

11. By a negative-number identity, if $\tan(-\theta) = -\tan\theta$, then $\tan\left(-\dfrac{\pi}{7}\right) = -\tan\dfrac{\pi}{7}$.

13. By a quotient identity, $\dfrac{\cos x}{\sin x} = \cot x$, therefore B.

15. By a negative-number identity, $\cos(-x) = \cos x$, therefore E.

17. By a Pythagorean identity, $1 = \sin^2 x + \cos^2 x$, therefore A.

19. Using a Pythagorean identity and then a quotient identity, $\sec^2 x - 1 = \tan^2 x = \dfrac{\sin^2 x}{\cos^2 x}$, therefore A.

21. Using a Pythagorean identity, $1 + \sin^2 x = (\csc^2 x - \cot^2 x) + \sin^2 x$, therefore D.

23. The correct identity is $1 + \cot^2 x = \csc^2 x$; the function must have the argument "x" or θ, t, etc.

25. $\sin\theta$ in terms of $\cot\theta$: $\sin\theta = \dfrac{1}{\csc\theta} = \dfrac{1}{\pm\sqrt{1+\cot^2\theta}} = \pm\dfrac{\sqrt{1+\cot^2\theta}}{1+\cot^2\theta}$.

$P = 16k\left[1 - \sin^2(2\pi t)\right]$ in terms of $\sec\theta$:

$\sin\theta = \cos\theta \cdot \dfrac{\sin\theta}{\cos\theta} = \cos\theta \cdot \tan\theta = \dfrac{1}{\sec\theta} \cdot (\pm\sqrt{\sec^2\theta - 1}) = \pm\dfrac{\sqrt{\sec^2\theta - 1}}{\sec\theta}$.

27. $\tan\theta$ in terms of $\sin\theta$: $\tan\theta = \dfrac{\sin\theta}{\cos\theta} = \dfrac{\sin\theta}{\pm\sqrt{1-\sin^2\theta}} = \pm\dfrac{\sin\theta\sqrt{1-\sin^2\theta}}{1-\sin^2\theta}$.

$\tan\theta$ in terms of $\cos\theta$: $\tan\theta = \dfrac{\sin\theta}{\cos\theta} = \pm\dfrac{\sqrt{1-\cos^2\theta}}{\cos\theta}$.

$\tan\theta$ in terms of $\sec\theta$: $\tan\theta = \pm\sqrt{\sec^2\theta - 1}$.

$\tan\theta$ in terms of $\csc\theta$: $\tan\theta = \dfrac{1}{\cot\theta} = \dfrac{1}{\pm\sqrt{\csc^2\theta - 1}} = \pm\dfrac{\sqrt{\csc^2\theta - 1}}{\csc^2\theta - 1}$.

29. $\sec\theta$ in terms of $\sin\theta$: $\sec\theta = \dfrac{1}{\cos\theta} = \dfrac{1}{\pm\sqrt{1-\sin^2\theta}} = \pm\dfrac{\sqrt{1-\sin^2\theta}}{1-\sin^2\theta}$.

$\sec\theta$ in terms of $\tan\theta$: $\sec\theta = \pm\sqrt{\tan^2\theta + 1}$.

$\sec\theta$ in terms of $\cot\theta$: $\sec\theta = \pm\sqrt{\tan^2\theta+1} = \pm\sqrt{\dfrac{1}{\cot^2\theta}+1} = \pm\sqrt{\dfrac{1+\cot^2\theta}{\cot^2\theta}} = \pm\dfrac{\sqrt{1+\cot^2\theta}}{\cot\theta}$.

$\sec\theta$ in terms of $\csc\theta$: $\sec\theta = \dfrac{1}{\cos\theta} = \dfrac{1}{\pm\sqrt{1-\sin^2\theta}} = \dfrac{1}{\pm\sqrt{1-\dfrac{1}{\csc^2\theta}}} = \dfrac{1}{\pm\sqrt{\dfrac{\csc^2\theta-1}{\csc^2\theta}}} =$

$\dfrac{\pm\sqrt{\csc^2\theta}}{\sqrt{\csc^2\theta-1}} = \dfrac{\pm\csc\theta}{\sqrt{\csc^2\theta-1}} = \pm\dfrac{\csc\theta\sqrt{\csc^2\theta-1}}{\csc^2\theta-1}$.

31. $\tan\theta\cos\theta = \dfrac{\sin\theta}{\cos\theta}\cdot\dfrac{\cos\theta}{1} = \sin\theta$.

33. $\dfrac{\sin\beta\tan\beta}{\cos\beta} = \dfrac{\sin\beta}{\cos\beta}\cdot\tan\beta = \tan\beta\cdot\tan\beta = \tan^2\beta$.

35. $\sec^2 x - 1 = (\tan^2 x + 1) - 1 = \tan^2 x$.

37. $\dfrac{\sin^2 x}{\cos^2 x} + \sin x\csc x = \tan^2 x + \dfrac{\sin x}{1}\cdot\dfrac{1}{\sin x} = \tan^2 x + 1 = \sec^2 x$.

39. $\cot\theta\sin\theta = \dfrac{\cos\theta}{\sin\theta}\cdot\sin\theta = \cos\theta$.

41. $\cos\theta\csc\theta = \cos\theta\cdot\dfrac{1}{\sin\theta} = \dfrac{\cos\theta}{\sin\theta}$, which simplifies to $\cot\theta$.

43. $\dfrac{\cot^2\theta}{\csc^2\theta} = \dfrac{\dfrac{\cos^2\theta}{\sin^2\theta}}{\dfrac{1}{\sin^2\theta}} = \dfrac{\cos^2\theta}{\sin^2\theta}\cdot\dfrac{\sin^2\theta}{1} = \cos^2\theta$.

45. $\sin^2\theta + \cos^2\theta = 1 \Rightarrow 1 - \cos^2\theta = \sin^2\theta$

47. $\dfrac{1}{\sec^2\theta - 1} = \dfrac{1}{\dfrac{1}{\cos^2\theta}-1} = \dfrac{1}{\dfrac{1-\cos^2\theta}{\cos^2\theta}} = \dfrac{\cos^2\theta}{\sin^2\theta} = \cot^2\theta$.

49. $\sin^2\theta(\csc^2\theta - 1) = \sin^2\theta\cdot\cot^2\theta = \sin^2\theta\cdot\dfrac{\cos^2\theta}{\sin^2\theta} = \cos^2\theta$.

51. $(1-\cos\theta)(1+\sec\theta) = (1-\cos\theta)\left(1+\dfrac{1}{\cos}\right) = 1 + \dfrac{1}{\cos\theta} - \cos\theta - 1 = \dfrac{1}{\cos\theta} - \cos\theta$,

which simplifies to $\sec\theta - \cos\theta$.

53. It is in terms of sine and cosine, but simplifies to $\dfrac{\cos^2\theta - \sin^2\theta}{\sin\theta\cos\theta} = \dfrac{\cos^2\theta}{\sin\theta\cos\theta} - \dfrac{\sin^2\theta}{\sin\theta\cos\theta} =$

$\dfrac{\cos\theta}{\sin\theta} - \dfrac{\sin\theta}{\cos\theta} = \cot\theta - \tan\theta$.

55. $\sec\theta - \cos\theta = \dfrac{1}{\cos\theta} - \dfrac{\cos^2\theta}{\cos\theta} = \dfrac{1-\cos^2\theta}{\cos\theta} = \dfrac{\sin^2\theta}{\cos\theta}$.

57. $\sin\theta(\csc\theta - \sin\theta) = \sin\theta\left(\dfrac{1}{\sin\theta} - \sin\theta\right) = 1 - \sin^2\theta = \cos^2\theta.$

59. $\csc\theta\sec\theta\tan\theta = \dfrac{1}{\sin\theta}\dfrac{1}{\cos\theta}\dfrac{\sin\theta}{\cos\theta} = \dfrac{1}{\cos^2\theta} = \sec^2\theta.$

61. $\cot\theta + \dfrac{1}{\cot\theta} = \dfrac{\cos\theta}{\sin\theta} + \tan\theta = \dfrac{\cos\theta}{\sin\theta} + \dfrac{\sin\theta}{\cos\theta} = \dfrac{\cos^2\theta}{\sin\theta\cos\theta} + \dfrac{\sin^2\theta}{\sin\theta\cos\theta} = \dfrac{\sin^2\theta + \cos^2\theta}{\sin\theta\cos\theta} =$

    $\dfrac{1}{\sin\theta\cos\theta}$, or $\csc\theta\sec\theta.$

63. $\tan s(\cot s + \csc s) = \tan s\left(\dfrac{1}{\tan s} + \dfrac{1}{\sin s}\right) = 1 + \dfrac{\tan s}{\sin s} = 1 + \left(\dfrac{\sin s}{\cos s} \div \sin s\right) = 1 + \left(\dfrac{\sin s}{\cos s} \cdot \dfrac{1}{\sin s}\right) =$

    $1 + \dfrac{1}{\cos s} = 1 + \sec s.$

65. $\dfrac{1}{\csc^2\theta} + \dfrac{1}{\sec^2\theta} = \sin^2\theta + \cos^2\theta = 1.$

67. $\dfrac{\cos x}{\sec x} + \dfrac{\sin x}{\csc x} = \left(\dfrac{\cos x}{1} \div \dfrac{1}{\cos x}\right) + \left(\dfrac{\sin x}{1} \div \dfrac{1}{\sin x}\right) = \left(\dfrac{\cos x}{1} \cdot \dfrac{\cos x}{1}\right) + \left(\dfrac{\sin x}{1} \cdot \dfrac{\sin x}{1}\right) = \sin^2 x + \cos^2 x = 1.$

69. $(1 + \sin t)^2 + \cos^2 t = 1 + 2\sin t + \sin^2 t + \cos^2 t = 1 + 2\sin t + 1 = 2 + 2\sin t.$

71. $\dfrac{1}{1 + \cos x} - \dfrac{1}{1 - \cos x} = \dfrac{1(1 - \cos x)}{(1 + \cos x)(1 - \cos x)} - \dfrac{1(1 + \cos x)}{(1 + \cos x)(1 - \cos x)} = \dfrac{1 - \cos x - 1 - \cos x}{1 - \cos^2 x} =$

    $\dfrac{-2\cos x}{\sin^2 x} = -\dfrac{2\cos x}{\sin^2 x}$, or $-2\cot x \csc x.$

73. $\dfrac{\cot\theta}{\csc\theta} = \dfrac{\frac{\cos\theta}{\sin\theta}}{\frac{1}{\sin\theta}} = \dfrac{\cos\theta}{\sin\theta} \cdot \dfrac{\sin\theta}{1} = \dfrac{\cos\theta}{1} = \cos\theta.$

75. $\cos^2\theta(\tan^2\theta + 1) = \cos^2\theta(\sec^2\theta) = \cos^2\theta\left(\dfrac{1}{\cos^2\theta}\right) = 1.$

77. $\dfrac{\tan^2\gamma + 1}{\sec\gamma} = \dfrac{\sec^2\gamma}{\sec\gamma} = \sec\gamma.$

79. $\dfrac{1 - \sin^2\beta}{\cos\beta} = \dfrac{\cos^2\beta}{\cos\beta} = \cos\beta$

81. $\dfrac{1 - \cos x}{1 + \cos x} = \dfrac{1 - \cos x}{1 + \cos x} \cdot \dfrac{1 - \cos x}{1 - \cos x} = \dfrac{1 - 2\cos x + \cos^2 x}{1 - \cos^2 x} = \dfrac{1 - 2\cos x + \cos^2 x}{\sin^2 x}$. Work with the right side of the

    equation. $(\cot x - \csc x)^2 = \left(\dfrac{\cos x}{\sin x} - \dfrac{1}{\sin x}\right)^2 = \left(\dfrac{\cos x - 1}{\sin x}\right)^2 = \dfrac{\cos^2 x - 2\cos x - 1}{\sin^2 x}$. Therefore,

    $\dfrac{1 - \cos x}{1 + \cos x} = (\cot x - \csc x)^2.$

83. $\dfrac{\cot\alpha+1}{\cot\alpha-1} = \dfrac{\dfrac{\cos\alpha}{\sin\alpha}+1}{\dfrac{\cos\alpha}{\sin\alpha}-1} = \dfrac{\dfrac{\cos\alpha+\sin\alpha}{\sin\alpha}}{\dfrac{\cos\alpha-\sin\alpha}{\sin\alpha}} = \dfrac{\cos\alpha+\sin\alpha}{\cos\alpha-\sin\alpha} = \dfrac{\cos\alpha+\sin\alpha}{\cos\alpha-\sin\alpha} \cdot \dfrac{\dfrac{1}{\cos\alpha}}{\dfrac{1}{\cos\alpha}}$

$= \dfrac{\dfrac{\cos\alpha}{\cos\alpha}+\dfrac{\sin\alpha}{\cos\alpha}}{\dfrac{\cos\alpha}{\cos\alpha}-\dfrac{\sin\alpha}{\cos\alpha}} = \dfrac{1+\tan\alpha}{1-\tan\alpha}$.

85. $\sin^2\alpha + \tan^2\alpha + \cos^2\alpha = \sin^2\alpha + \cos^2\alpha + \tan^2\alpha = 1 + \tan^2\alpha = \sec^2\alpha$.

87. $\dfrac{\sin^2\gamma}{\cos\gamma} = \dfrac{1-\cos^2\gamma}{\cos\gamma} = \dfrac{1}{\cos\gamma} - \dfrac{\cos^2\gamma}{\cos\gamma} = \sec\gamma - \cos\gamma$.

89. $\dfrac{\cos\theta}{\sin\theta\cot\theta} = \dfrac{\cos\theta}{\sin\theta \cdot \frac{\cos\theta}{\sin\theta}} = \dfrac{\cos\theta}{\cos\theta} = 1$.

91. $\tan^2\gamma\sin^2\gamma = (\sec^2\gamma - 1)(1 - \cos^2\gamma) = \sec^2\gamma - \sec^2\gamma\cos^2\gamma - 1 + \cos^2\gamma =$

$\sec^2\gamma - 1 + \cos^2\gamma - \sec^2\gamma\cos^2\gamma = \tan^2\gamma + \cos^2\gamma - \dfrac{1}{\cos^2\gamma}\cdot\cos^2\gamma = \tan^2\gamma + \cos^2\gamma - 1$.

93. $\dfrac{(\sec\theta - \tan\theta)^2 + 1}{\sec\theta\csc\theta - \tan\theta\csc\theta} = \dfrac{\sec^2\theta - 2\sec\theta\tan\theta + \tan^2\theta + 1}{\csc\theta(\sec\theta - \tan\theta)} = \dfrac{\sec^2\theta - 2\sec\theta\tan\theta + \sec^2\theta}{\csc\theta(\sec\theta - \tan\theta)} =$

$\dfrac{2\sec^2\theta - 2\sec\theta\tan\theta}{\csc\theta(\sec\theta - \tan\theta)} = \dfrac{2\sec\theta(\sec\theta - \tan\theta)}{\csc\theta(\sec\theta - \tan\theta)} = \dfrac{2\sec\theta}{\csc\theta} = 2\left(\dfrac{1}{\cos\theta}\cdot\dfrac{\sin\theta}{1}\right) = 2\tan\theta$.

95. $\dfrac{1}{\tan\alpha - \sec\alpha} + \dfrac{1}{\tan\alpha + \sec\alpha} = \dfrac{(\tan\alpha + \sec\alpha) + (\tan\alpha - \sec\alpha)}{\tan^2\alpha - \sec^2\alpha} = \dfrac{2\tan\alpha}{\tan^2\alpha - (\tan^2\alpha + 1)} = \dfrac{2\tan\alpha}{-1} = -2\tan\alpha$.

97. $\sec^4 x - \sec^2 x = \sec^2 x(\sec^2 x - 1) = \sec^2 x \cdot \tan^2 x$. Simplify the right side of the equation.

$\tan^4 x + \tan^2 x = \tan^2 x(\tan^2 x + 1) = \tan^2 x \cdot \sec^2 x$. Therefore, $\sec^4 x - \sec^2 x = \tan^4 x + \tan^2 x$.

99. $\dfrac{\sec^4 s - \tan^4 s}{\sec^2 s + \tan^2 s} = \dfrac{(\sec^2 s - \tan^2 s)(\sec^2 s + \tan^2 s)}{\sec^2 s + \tan^2 s} = \sec^2 s - \tan^2 s$.

101. $\dfrac{\tan t - \cot t}{\tan t + \cot t} = \dfrac{\tan t - \dfrac{1}{\tan t}}{\tan t + \dfrac{1}{\tan t}} = \dfrac{\tan t - \dfrac{1}{\tan t}}{\tan t + \dfrac{1}{\tan t}} \cdot \dfrac{\tan t}{\tan t} = \dfrac{\tan^2 t - 1}{\tan^2 t + 1} = \dfrac{\tan^2 t - 1}{\sec^2 t}$

103. $\sin^2\alpha\sec^2\alpha + \sin^2\alpha\csc^2\alpha = \sin^2\alpha(\sec^2\alpha + \csc^2\alpha) = \sin^2\alpha\left(\dfrac{1}{\cos^2\alpha} + \dfrac{1}{\sin^2\alpha}\right) =$

$\tan^2\alpha + 1 = \sec^2\alpha$.

105. $\sec^2\theta - 2\sec\theta\tan\theta + \tan^2\theta = \dfrac{1}{\cos^2\theta} - 2\cdot\dfrac{1}{\cos\theta}\cdot\dfrac{\sin\theta}{\cos\theta} + \dfrac{\sin^2\theta}{\cos^2\theta} = \dfrac{1 - 2\sin\theta + \sin^2\theta}{\cos^2\theta}$

$= \dfrac{(1-\sin\theta)^2}{1-\sin^2\theta} = \dfrac{(1-\sin\theta)^2}{(1-\sin\theta)(1+\sin\theta)} = \dfrac{1-\sin\theta}{1+\sin\theta}.$

107. $\dfrac{1+\sin\theta}{1-\sin\theta} - \dfrac{1-\sin\theta}{1+\sin\theta} = \dfrac{(1+\sin\theta)(1+\sin\theta) - (1-\sin\theta)(1-\sin\theta)}{(1-\sin\theta)(1+\sin\theta)} = \dfrac{1+2\sin\theta+\sin^2\theta - 1 + 2\sin\theta - \sin^2\theta}{1-\sin^2\theta}$

$= \dfrac{4\sin\theta}{\cos^2\theta} = \dfrac{4\sin\theta}{\cos\theta}\cdot\dfrac{1}{\cos\theta} = 4\tan\theta\sec\theta.$

109. $(2\sin x + \cos x)^2 + (2\cos x - \sin x)^2 = (4\sin^2 x + 4\sin x\cos x + \cos^2 x) + (4\cos^2 x - 4\sin x\cos x + \sin^2 x) =$

$4(\sin^2 x + \cos^2 x) + (\cos^2 x + \sin^2 x) = 4 + 1 = 5.$

111. $\sec x - \cos x + \csc x - \sin x - \sin x\tan x = \dfrac{1}{\cos x} - \cos x + \dfrac{1}{\sin x} - \sin x - \sin x\left(\dfrac{\sin x}{\cos x}\right) =$

$\left(\dfrac{1}{\cos x} - \cos x\right) + \left(\dfrac{1}{\sin x} - \sin x\right) - \dfrac{\sin^2 x}{\cos x} = \dfrac{1-\cos^2 x}{\cos x} + \dfrac{1-\sin^2 x}{\sin x} - \dfrac{\sin^2 x}{\cos x} =$

$\left(\dfrac{1-\cos^2 x}{\cos x} - \dfrac{\sin^2 x}{\cos x}\right) + \dfrac{1-\sin^2 x}{\sin x} = \dfrac{1-\cos^2 x - \sin^2 x}{\cos x} + \dfrac{\cos^2 x}{\sin x} = \dfrac{1-(\cos^2 x + \sin^2 x)}{\cos x} + \dfrac{\cos^2 x}{\sin x} =$

$\dfrac{1-1}{\cos x} + \cos x\cdot\dfrac{\cos x}{\sin x} = \cos x\cot x.$

113. (a) Using an identity yields $I = k(1-\sin^2\theta)$.

(b) The function reaches its maximum value of k when $\cos^2\theta = 1$. This happens when $\theta = 0$.

115. (a) See Figure 115a. The total mechanical energy E is always 2. The spring has maximum potential energy when it is fully stretched but not moving. The spring has maximum kinetic energy when it is not stretched but is moving fastest.

(b) Let $Y_1 = P(t)$, $Y_2 = k(t)$, $Y_3 = E(t) = 2$ for all inputs; see Figure 115b. The spring is stretched the most (has the greatest potential energy) when $t = 0.25, 0.5, 0.75$, etc. At these times kinetic energy is 0.

(c) $E(t) = P(t) + k(t) = 2\cos^2(4\pi t) + 2\sin^2(4\pi t) = 2(\cos^2(4\pi t) + \sin^2(4\pi t)) = 2(1) = 2.$

[0,0.5] by [-1,3]
Xscl = 0.25   Yscl = 1

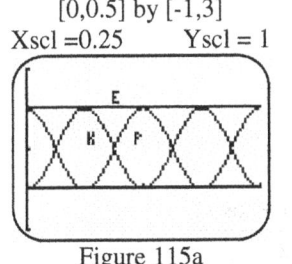

Figure 115a

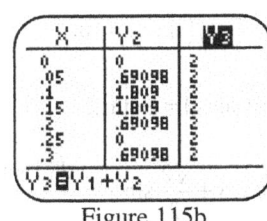

Figure 115b

452 CHAPTER 9 Trigonometric Identities and Equations

9.2: Sum and Difference Identities

1. By cosine of a sum, $\cos(x+y) = \cos x \cos y - \sin x \sin y$, therefore F.

3. By sine of a sum, $\sin(x+y) = \sin x \cos y + \cos x \sin y$, therefore C.

5. $\sin\dfrac{\pi}{12} = \sin\left(\dfrac{\pi}{3} - \dfrac{\pi}{4}\right) = \sin\dfrac{\pi}{3}\cos\dfrac{\pi}{4} - \cos\dfrac{\pi}{3}\sin\dfrac{\pi}{4} = \dfrac{\sqrt{3}}{2}\cdot\dfrac{\sqrt{2}}{2} - \dfrac{1}{2}\cdot\dfrac{\sqrt{2}}{2} = \dfrac{\sqrt{6}-\sqrt{2}}{4}$.

7. $\sin\left(-\dfrac{5\pi}{12}\right) = -\sin\left(\dfrac{5\pi}{12}\right) = -\sin\left(\dfrac{\pi}{6}+\dfrac{\pi}{4}\right) = -\left(\sin\dfrac{\pi}{6}\cos\dfrac{\pi}{4} + \cos\dfrac{\pi}{6}\sin\dfrac{\pi}{4}\right) =$
$-\left(\dfrac{1}{2}\cdot\dfrac{\sqrt{2}}{2} + \dfrac{\sqrt{3}}{2}\cdot\dfrac{\sqrt{2}}{2}\right) = \dfrac{-\sqrt{2}-\sqrt{6}}{4}$.

9. $\sin\dfrac{13\pi}{12} = \sin\left(\dfrac{5\pi}{4} - \dfrac{\pi}{6}\right) = \sin\dfrac{5\pi}{4}\cos\dfrac{\pi}{6} - \cos\dfrac{5\pi}{4}\sin\dfrac{\pi}{6} = \dfrac{-\sqrt{2}}{2}\cdot\dfrac{\sqrt{3}}{2} - \dfrac{-\sqrt{2}}{2}\cdot\dfrac{1}{2} = \dfrac{-\sqrt{6}+\sqrt{2}}{4}$.

11. $\cos 75° = \cos(45° + 30°) = \cos 45°\cos 30° - \sin 45°\sin 30° = \dfrac{\sqrt{2}}{2}\cdot\dfrac{\sqrt{3}}{2} - \dfrac{\sqrt{2}}{2}\cdot\dfrac{1}{2} = \dfrac{\sqrt{6}-\sqrt{2}}{4}$.

13. $\tan 105° = \tan(60° + 45°) = \dfrac{\tan 60° + \tan 45°}{1 - \tan 60°\tan 45°} = \dfrac{\sqrt{3}+1}{1-\sqrt{3}}\cdot\dfrac{1+\sqrt{3}}{1+\sqrt{3}} = \dfrac{2\sqrt{3}+4}{-2} = -\sqrt{3}-2$.

15. $\cos(-15°) = \cos 15° = \cos(60° - 45°) = \cos 60°\cos 45° + \sin 60°\sin 45° = \dfrac{1}{2}\cdot\dfrac{\sqrt{2}}{2} + \dfrac{\sqrt{3}}{2}\cdot\dfrac{\sqrt{2}}{2} = \dfrac{\sqrt{2}+\sqrt{6}}{4}$.

17. $\cos\dfrac{\pi}{3}\cos\dfrac{2\pi}{3} - \sin\dfrac{\pi}{3}\sin\dfrac{2\pi}{3} = \cos\left(\dfrac{\pi}{3}+\dfrac{2\pi}{3}\right) = \cos\pi = -1$.

19. $\sin 76°\cos 31° + \cos 76°\sin 31° = \sin(76° - 31°) = \sin 45° = \dfrac{\sqrt{2}}{2}$.

21. $\dfrac{\tan 80° + \tan 55°}{1 - \tan 80°\tan 55°} = \tan(80° + 55°) = \tan 135° = -1$.

23. $\sin(180° - x) = \sin 180°\cos x - \cos 180°\sin x = (0\cdot\cos x) - (-1)\sin x = 0 - (-\sin x) = \sin x$.

25. $\cos(180° + x) = \cos 180°\cos x - \sin 180°\sin x = (-1)\cos x - (0\cdot\sin x) = -\cos x$.

27. $\sin(x - 90°) = \sin x\cos 90° - \cos x\sin 90° = (\sin x \cdot 0) - (\cos x \cdot 1) = -\cos x$.

29. $\tan(180° - x) = \dfrac{\tan 180° - \tan x}{1 + \tan 180°\tan x} = \dfrac{0 - \tan x}{1 + (0\cdot\tan x)} = \dfrac{-\tan x}{1} = -\tan x$.

31. $\cos\left(\dfrac{\pi}{2} - x\right) = \cos\dfrac{\pi}{2}\cos x + \sin\dfrac{\pi}{2}\sin x = (0)(\cos x) + (1)(\sin x) = \sin x$.

33. $\cos\left(\dfrac{3\pi}{2} + x\right) = \cos\dfrac{3\pi}{2}\cos x - \sin\dfrac{3\pi}{2}\sin x = (0)(\cos x) - (-1)(\sin x) = \sin x$.

35. $\sin(\pi + x) = \sin\pi\cos x + \cos\pi\sin x = (0)(\cos x) + (-1)(\sin x) = -\sin x$.

37. $\cos(135° - x) = \cos 135°\cos x + \sin 135°\sin x = -\dfrac{\sqrt{2}}{2}\cdot\cos x + \dfrac{\sqrt{2}}{2}\sin x = \dfrac{\sqrt{2}(\sin x - \cos x)}{2}$.

39. $\tan(45° + x) = \dfrac{\tan 45° + \tan x}{1 - \tan 45° \tan x} = \dfrac{1 + \tan x}{1 - (1)\tan x} = \dfrac{1 + \tan x}{1 - \tan x}$.

41. $\tan(\pi - x) = \dfrac{\tan \pi - \tan x}{1 + \tan \pi \tan x} = \dfrac{0 - \tan x}{1 + (0)\tan x} = -\tan x$.

43. $\tan\left(\dfrac{5\pi}{4} - x\right) = \dfrac{\tan \dfrac{5\pi}{4} - \tan x}{1 + \tan \dfrac{5\pi}{4} \tan x} = \dfrac{1 - \tan x}{1 + \tan x}$.

45. $\cos(2\pi - x) = \cos 2\pi \cos x + \sin 2\pi \sin x = \cos x + 0 \cdot \sin x = \cos x$.

47. If $0 < A < \dfrac{\pi}{2}$ and $0 < B < \dfrac{\pi}{2}$, then A and B are both found in quadrant I. Next, using $\cos A = \dfrac{3}{5}$ and $\sin B = \dfrac{5}{13}$, find $\sin A$ and $\cos B$.

$\sin^2 A = 1 - \cos^2 A = 1 - \left(\dfrac{3}{5}\right)^2 = 1 - \dfrac{9}{25} = \dfrac{16}{25} \Rightarrow \sin A = \pm\sqrt{\dfrac{16}{25}} \Rightarrow \sin A = \dfrac{4}{5}$;

$\cos^2 B = 1 - \sin^2 B = 1 - \left(\dfrac{5}{13}\right)^2 = 1 - \left(\dfrac{25}{169}\right) = \dfrac{144}{169} \Rightarrow \cos B = \pm\sqrt{\dfrac{144}{169}} \Rightarrow \cos B = \dfrac{12}{13}$.

Now use $\cos A = \dfrac{3}{5}$, $\sin B = \dfrac{5}{13}$, $\sin A = \dfrac{4}{5}$, and $\cos B = \dfrac{12}{13}$ to find

(a) $\sin(A + B) = \sin A \cos B + \cos A \sin B = \dfrac{4}{5} \cdot \dfrac{12}{13} + \dfrac{3}{5} \cdot \dfrac{5}{13} = \dfrac{48 + 15}{65} \Rightarrow \sin(A + B) = \dfrac{63}{65}$.

(b) $\sin(A - B) = \sin A \cos B - \cos A \sin B = \dfrac{4}{5} \cdot \dfrac{12}{13} - \dfrac{3}{5} \cdot \dfrac{5}{13} = \dfrac{48 - 15}{65} \Rightarrow \sin(A - B) = \dfrac{33}{65}$.

(c) First find $\tan A$ and $\tan B$: $\tan A = \dfrac{\sin A}{\cos A} = \dfrac{\frac{4}{5}}{\frac{3}{5}} = \dfrac{4}{5} \cdot \dfrac{5}{3} = \dfrac{4}{3}$; $\tan B = \dfrac{\sin B}{\cos B} = \dfrac{\frac{5}{13}}{\frac{12}{13}} = \dfrac{5}{13} \cdot \dfrac{13}{12} = \dfrac{5}{12}$.

Now solve $\tan(A + B) = \dfrac{\tan A + \tan B}{1 - \tan A \tan B} = \dfrac{\frac{4}{3} + \frac{5}{12}}{1 - \frac{4}{3} \cdot \frac{5}{12}} \cdot \dfrac{36}{36} = \dfrac{48 + 15}{36 - 20} \Rightarrow \tan(A + B) = \dfrac{63}{16}$.

(d) $\tan(A - B) = \dfrac{\tan A - \tan B}{1 + \tan A \tan B} = \dfrac{\frac{4}{3} - \frac{5}{12}}{1 + \frac{4}{3} \cdot \frac{5}{12}} \cdot \dfrac{36}{36} = \dfrac{48 - 15}{36 + 20} \Rightarrow \tan(A - B) = \dfrac{33}{56}$.

(e) Since $\sin(A + B) > 0$ and $\tan(A + B) > 0$, $A + B$ is found in quadrant I.

(f) Since $\sin(A - B) > 0$ and $\tan(A - B) > 0$, $A - B$ is found in quadrant I.

49. If $\pi < A < \dfrac{3\pi}{2}$ and $\pi < B < \dfrac{3\pi}{2}$, then A and B are both found in quadrant III. Next, using $\cos A = -\dfrac{8}{17}$ and $\cos B = -\dfrac{3}{5}$, find $\sin A$ and $\sin B$.

$\sin^2 A = 1 - \cos^2 A = 1 - \left(-\dfrac{8}{17}\right)^2 = 1 - \dfrac{64}{289} = \dfrac{225}{289} \Rightarrow \sin A = \pm\sqrt{\dfrac{225}{289}} \Rightarrow \sin A = \pm\dfrac{15}{17}$.

454 CHAPTER 9 Trigonometric Identities and Equations

Since A is found in quadrant III, $\sin A = -\dfrac{15}{17}$.

$\sin^2 B = 1 - \cos^2 B = 1 - \left(-\dfrac{3}{5}\right)^2 = 1 - \dfrac{9}{25} = \dfrac{16}{25} \Rightarrow \sin B = \pm\sqrt{\dfrac{16}{25}} \Rightarrow \sin B = \pm\dfrac{4}{5}$. Since B is in quadrant III,

$\sin B = -\dfrac{4}{5}$. Now use $\cos A = -\dfrac{8}{17}$, $\cos B = -\dfrac{3}{5}$, $\sin A = -\dfrac{15}{17}$, and $\sin B = -\dfrac{4}{5}$ to find:

(a) $\sin(A+B) = \sin A \cos B + \cos A \sin B = \left(-\dfrac{15}{17}\right)\left(-\dfrac{3}{5}\right) + \left(-\dfrac{8}{17}\right)\left(-\dfrac{4}{5}\right) = \dfrac{45+32}{85} \Rightarrow \sin(A+B) = \dfrac{77}{85}$.

(b) $\sin(A-B) = \sin A \cos B - \cos A \sin B = \left(-\dfrac{15}{17}\right)\left(-\dfrac{3}{5}\right) - \left(-\dfrac{8}{17}\right)\left(-\dfrac{4}{5}\right) = \dfrac{45-32}{85} \Rightarrow \sin(A-B) = \dfrac{13}{85}$.

(c) First find $\tan A$ and $\tan B$.

$\tan A = \dfrac{\sin A}{\cos A} = \dfrac{-\frac{15}{17}}{-\frac{8}{17}} = \left(-\dfrac{15}{17}\right)\left(-\dfrac{17}{8}\right) = \dfrac{15}{8}$; $\tan B = \dfrac{\sin B}{\cos B} = \dfrac{-\frac{4}{5}}{-\frac{3}{5}} = \left(-\dfrac{4}{5}\right)\left(-\dfrac{5}{3}\right) = \dfrac{4}{3}$.

Now solve $\tan(A+B) = \dfrac{\tan A + \tan B}{1 - \tan A \tan B} = \dfrac{\frac{15}{8} + \frac{4}{3}}{1 - \frac{15}{8} \cdot \frac{4}{3}} \cdot \dfrac{24}{24} = \dfrac{45+32}{24-60} \Rightarrow \tan(A+B) = -\dfrac{77}{36}$.

(d) $\tan(A-B) = \dfrac{\tan A - \tan B}{1 + \tan A \tan B} = \dfrac{\frac{15}{8} - \frac{4}{3}}{1 + \frac{15}{8} \cdot \frac{4}{3}} \cdot \dfrac{24}{24} = \dfrac{45-32}{24+60} \Rightarrow \tan(A-B) = \dfrac{13}{84}$.

(e) Since $\sin(A+B) > 0$ and $\tan(A+B) < 0$, $A+B$ is found in quadrant II.

(f) Since $\sin(A-B) > 0$ and $\tan(A-B) > 0$, $A-B$ is found in quadrant I.

51. $\sin(x+x) = \sin(2x) = \sin x \cos x + \sin x \cos x = 2\sin x \cos x$.

53. $\sin(x+y) + \sin(x-y) = \sin x \cos y + \cos x \sin y + \sin x \cos y - \cos x \sin y = 2\sin x \cos y$.

55. $\dfrac{\cos(A-B)}{\cos A \sin B} = \dfrac{\cos A \cos B + \sin A \sin B}{\cos A \sin B} = \dfrac{\cos A \cos B}{\cos A \sin B} + \dfrac{\sin A \sin B}{\cos A \sin B} = \dfrac{\cos B}{\sin B} + \dfrac{\sin A}{\cos A} =$
$\cot B + \tan A = \tan A + \cot B$.

57. $\dfrac{\sin(A-B)}{\sin B} + \dfrac{\cos(A-B)}{\cos B} = \dfrac{\sin A \cos B - \cos A \sin B}{\sin B} + \dfrac{\cos A \cos B + \sin A \sin B}{\cos B} =$

$\dfrac{\sin A \cos^2 B + \sin A \sin^2 B}{\sin B \cos B} = \dfrac{\sin A (\cos^2 B + \sin^2 B)}{\sin B \cos B} = \dfrac{\sin A}{\sin B \cos B}$.

59. $\dfrac{\tan x - \tan y}{\tan x + \tan y} = \dfrac{\frac{\sin x}{\cos x} - \frac{\sin y}{\cos y}}{\frac{\sin x}{\cos x} + \frac{\sin y}{\cos y}} = \dfrac{\frac{\sin x \cos y - \cos x \sin y}{\cos x \cos y}}{\frac{\sin x \cos y + \cos x \sin y}{\cos x \cos y}} = \dfrac{\sin x \cos y - \cos x \sin y}{\sin x \cos y + \cos x \sin y} = \dfrac{\sin(x-y)}{\sin(x+y)}$.

61. Since there are 60 cycles per second, the number of cycles in 0.05 seconds is given by
(0.05 sec.)(60 cycles/sec.) = 3 cycles.

63. (a) $F = \dfrac{0.6(170)\sin(30°+90°)}{\sin 12°} \approx 424.8659171 \approx 425$ pounds.

(b) Using the sine of a sum identity yields $F = \dfrac{0.6W \sin(\theta+90°)}{\sin 12°} \Rightarrow$

$$F = \frac{0.6W}{\sin 12°}(\sin\theta\cos 90° + \cos\theta\sin 90°) \approx 2.8858W(\sin\theta(0) + \cos\theta(1)) \approx 2.9W\cos\theta.$$

(c) The function F is at a maximum when $\sin(\theta + 90°) = 1$. $\sin^{-1} 1 = \theta + 90° \Rightarrow 90° = \theta + 90° \Rightarrow \theta = 0°$.

65. (a) Using the given values, $P = \dfrac{a}{r}\cos\left[\dfrac{2\pi r}{\lambda} - ct\right] = \dfrac{0.4}{10}\cos\left[\dfrac{20\pi}{4.9} - 1026t\right]$. Graph this on $0 \le t \le 10$. See Figure 65a. At this distance, the pressure P is oscillating.

(b) Using the given values, $P = \dfrac{a}{r}\cos\left[\dfrac{2\pi r}{\lambda} - ct\right] = \dfrac{3}{r}\cos\left[\dfrac{2\pi r}{4.9} - 10,260\right]$. Graph this on $0 \le t \le 20$.

See Figure 65a. At this distance, the pressure P is oscillating. See Figure 65b. As the radius increases, the pressure P oscillates, and the amplitude decreases as r increases.

(c) If $r = n\lambda$, $P = \dfrac{a}{r}\cos\left[\dfrac{2\pi r}{\lambda} - ct\right] = \dfrac{a}{n\lambda}\cos\left[\dfrac{2\pi n\lambda}{\lambda} - ct\right] = \dfrac{a}{n\lambda}\cos[2\pi n - ct] =$

$\dfrac{a}{2n\lambda}[\cos(2\pi n)\cos(ct) + \sin(2\pi n)\sin(ct)] = \dfrac{a}{n\lambda}[(1)\cos(ct) + (0)\sin(ct)] = \dfrac{a}{n\lambda}\cos(ct).$

[0,0.05] by [-0.05,0.05]   [0,20] by [-2,2]

Xscl =0.01   Yscl = 1   Xscl = 1   Yscl = 1

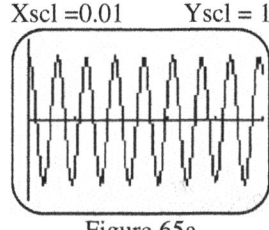

Figure 65a   Figure 65b

Reviewing Basic Concepts (Sections 9.1 – 9.2)

1. $\dfrac{\csc x}{\cot x} - \dfrac{\cot x}{\csc x} = \dfrac{1}{\cot x} \cdot \dfrac{\sin x}{\sin x} - \dfrac{\cos x}{\sin x} \cdot \dfrac{\sin x}{1} = \dfrac{1}{\cos x} - \cos x = \dfrac{1 - \cos^2 x}{\cos x} = \dfrac{\sin^2 x}{\cos x}.$

2. $\tan\left(-\dfrac{\pi}{12}\right) = \tan\left(\dfrac{\pi}{4} - \dfrac{\pi}{3}\right) = \dfrac{\tan\left(\frac{\pi}{4}\right) - \tan\left(\frac{\pi}{3}\right)}{1 + \tan\left(\frac{\pi}{4}\right)\tan\left(\frac{\pi}{3}\right)} = \dfrac{1 - \sqrt{3}}{1 + 1(\sqrt{3})} = \dfrac{1 - \sqrt{3}}{1 + \sqrt{3}} \cdot \dfrac{1 - \sqrt{3}}{1 - \sqrt{3}} = \dfrac{4 - 2\sqrt{3}}{-2}$ or $\sqrt{3} - 2$.

3. $\cos 18°\cos 108° + \sin 18°\sin 108° = \cos(18° - 108°) = \cos(-90°) = \cos 90° = 0.$

4. $\sin\left(x - \dfrac{\pi}{4}\right) = \sin x \cos\dfrac{\pi}{4} - \cos x \sin\dfrac{\pi}{4} = \sin x\left(\dfrac{\sqrt{2}}{2}\right) - \cos x\left(\dfrac{\sqrt{2}}{2}\right) = \dfrac{\sqrt{2}}{2}(\sin x - \cos x).$

5. If A is found in quadrant II and $\sin A = \dfrac{2}{3}$, then $y = 2$, $r = 3$, and, by the Pythagorean theorem,

    $x^2 + 2^2 = 3^2 \Rightarrow x^2 + 4 = 9 \Rightarrow x^2 = 5 \Rightarrow x = \pm\sqrt{5}$. Because A is found in quadrant II,

    $x = -\sqrt{5}$; therefore, $\sin A = \dfrac{2}{3}$, $\cos A = -\dfrac{\sqrt{5}}{3}$, and $\tan A = -\dfrac{2}{\sqrt{5}}$.

    If B is in quadrant III and $\cos B = -\dfrac{1}{2}$, then $x = -1$, $r = 2$, and, by the Pythagorean theorem,

    $(-1)^2 + y^2 = 2^2 \Rightarrow 1 + y^2 = 4 \Rightarrow y^2 = 3 \Rightarrow y = \pm\sqrt{3}$. Because B is found in quadrant III, $y = -\sqrt{3}$;

456 CHAPTER 9 Trigonometric Identities and Equations

therefore, $\sin B = -\frac{\sqrt{3}}{2}$, $\cos B = -\frac{1}{2}$, and $\tan B = \frac{\sqrt{3}}{1} = \sqrt{3}$. Use these values to find each compound

value. $\sin(A+B) = \sin A \cos B + \cos A \sin B = \frac{2}{3}\left(-\frac{1}{2}\right) + \left(-\frac{\sqrt{5}}{3}\right)\left(-\frac{\sqrt{3}}{2}\right) = -\frac{2}{6} + \frac{\sqrt{15}}{6} \Rightarrow$

$\sin(A+B) = \frac{-2+\sqrt{15}}{6}$.

$\cos(A-B) = \cos A \cos B + \sin A \sin B = \left(-\frac{\sqrt{5}}{3}\right)\left(-\frac{1}{2}\right) + \frac{2}{3}\left(-\frac{\sqrt{3}}{2}\right) = \frac{\sqrt{5}}{6} - \frac{2\sqrt{3}}{6} \Rightarrow$

$\cos(A-B) = \frac{\sqrt{5}-2\sqrt{3}}{6}$. $\tan(A-B) = \frac{\tan A - \tan B}{1+\tan A \tan B} = \frac{-\frac{2}{\sqrt{5}} - \sqrt{3}}{1+\left(-\frac{2}{\sqrt{5}}\right)\cdot(\sqrt{3})} \cdot \frac{\sqrt{5}}{\sqrt{5}} \Rightarrow \tan(A-B) = \frac{-2-\sqrt{15}}{\sqrt{5}-2\sqrt{3}}$.

6. $\csc^2\theta - \cot^2\theta = 1 + \cot^2\theta - \cot^2\theta = 1$.

7. $\frac{\sin t}{1-\cos t} = \frac{\sin t}{1-\cos t} \cdot \frac{1+\cos t}{1+\cos t} = \frac{\sin t(1+\cos t)}{1-\cos^2 t} = \frac{\sin t(1+\cos t)}{\sin^2 t} = \frac{1+\cos t}{\sin t}$.

8. $\frac{\cot A - \tan A}{\csc A \sec A} = \frac{\frac{\cos A}{\sin A} - \frac{\sin A}{\cos A}}{\frac{1}{\sin A} \cdot \frac{1}{\cos A}} \cdot \frac{\sin A \cos A}{\sin A \cos A} = \frac{\cos^2 A - \sin^2 A}{1} = \cos^2 A - \sin^2 A$.

9. $\frac{\sin(x-y)}{\sin x \sin y} = \frac{\sin x \cos y - \cos x \sin y}{\sin x \sin y} = \frac{\sin x \cos y}{\sin x \sin y} - \frac{\cos x \sin y}{\sin x \sin y} = \frac{\cos y}{\sin y} - \frac{\cos x}{\sin x} = \cot y - \cot x$.

10. $V = 20\sin\left(\frac{\pi t}{4} - \frac{\pi}{2}\right) = 20\left[\sin\frac{\pi t}{4}\cos\frac{\pi}{2} - \cos\frac{\pi t}{4}\sin\frac{\pi}{2}\right] = 20\left[\sin\frac{\pi t}{4}(0) - \cos\frac{\pi t}{4}(1)\right] = -20\cos\frac{\pi t}{4}$.

9.3: Further Identities

1. First find $\cos\theta$. If $\sin\theta = \frac{2}{5}$, then $\cos^2\theta = 1 - \sin^2\theta = 1 - \left(\frac{2}{5}\right)^2 = 1 - \frac{4}{25} \Rightarrow \cos\theta = \pm\frac{\sqrt{21}}{5}$, since for

   $\cos\theta < 0$, $\cos\theta = \frac{\sqrt{21}}{5}$. Now use $\sin\theta = \frac{2}{5}$ and $\cos\theta = -\frac{\sqrt{21}}{5}$ to find:

   (a) $\sin 2\theta = 2\sin\theta\cos\theta = 2\left(\frac{2}{5}\right)\left(-\frac{\sqrt{21}}{5}\right) = -\frac{4\sqrt{21}}{25}$.

   (b) $\cos 2\theta = \cos^2\theta - \sin^2\theta = \left(-\frac{\sqrt{21}}{5}\right)^2 - \left(\frac{2}{5}\right)^2 = \frac{21}{25} - \frac{4}{25} = \frac{17}{25}$.

3. First find $\sin\theta$ and $\cos\theta$. If $\tan\theta = 2$, then $\sec^2\theta = 1 + \tan^2\theta = 1 + 2^2 = 1 + 4 = 5 \Rightarrow \sec\theta = \pm\sqrt{5}$.

   Since $\cos\theta > 0$, and θ is in quadrant I, $\sec\theta = \sqrt{5}$. Now use this to find $\cos\theta$. $\cos\theta = \frac{1}{\sec\theta} = \frac{1}{\sqrt{5}} = \frac{\sqrt{5}}{5}$.

   Then use this to find $\sin x$. $\sin^2\theta = 1 - \cos^2\theta = 1 - \left(\frac{\sqrt{5}}{5}\right)^2 = 1 - \frac{5}{25} = \frac{20}{25} = \frac{4}{5} \Rightarrow \sin\theta = \pm\sqrt{\frac{4}{5}} = \pm\frac{2\sqrt{5}}{5}$.

$\sin\theta = \dfrac{2\sqrt{5}}{5}$ (θ is in quadrant I). Use $\sin x = \dfrac{2\sqrt{5}}{5}$ and $\cos x = \dfrac{\sqrt{5}}{5}$ to find:

(a) $\sin 2\theta = 2\sin\theta\cos\theta = 2\left(\dfrac{2\sqrt{5}}{5}\right)\left(\dfrac{\sqrt{5}}{5}\right) = \dfrac{20}{25} = \dfrac{4}{5}$.

(b) $\cos 2\theta = \cos^2\theta - \sin^2\theta = \left(\dfrac{\sqrt{5}}{5}\right)^2 - \left(\dfrac{2\sqrt{5}}{5}\right)^2 = \dfrac{5}{25} - \dfrac{20}{25} = -\dfrac{15}{25} = -\dfrac{3}{5}$.

5. First find $\cos\theta$. I $\sin\theta = -\dfrac{\sqrt{5}}{7}$, then $\cos^2\theta = 1 - \sin^2\theta = 1 - \left(-\dfrac{\sqrt{5}}{7}\right)^2 = 1 - \dfrac{5}{49} = \dfrac{44}{49} \Rightarrow$

$\cos\theta = \pm\sqrt{\dfrac{44}{49}} = \pm\dfrac{2\sqrt{11}}{7}$. Since $\cos\theta > 0$, $\cos\theta = \dfrac{2\sqrt{11}}{7}$. Now use $\sin\theta = -\dfrac{\sqrt{5}}{7}$ and $\cos\theta = \dfrac{2\sqrt{11}}{7}$ to find:

(a) $\sin 2\theta = 2\sin\theta\cos\theta = 2\left(-\dfrac{\sqrt{5}}{7}\right)\left(\dfrac{2\sqrt{11}}{7}\right) = -\dfrac{4\sqrt{55}}{49}$.

(b) $\cos 2\theta = 1 - 2\sin^2\theta = 1 - 2\left(-\dfrac{\sqrt{5}}{7}\right)^2 = 1 - 2\left(\dfrac{5}{49}\right) = \dfrac{39}{49}$.

7. $\cos^2 15° - \sin^2 15° = \cos[2(15°)] = \cos 30° = \dfrac{\sqrt{3}}{2}$.

9. $1 - 2\sin^2 15° = \cos[2(15°)] = \cos 30° = \dfrac{\sqrt{3}}{2}$.

11. $2\cos^2 67.5° - 1 = \cos[2(67.5°)] = \cos 135° = -\dfrac{\sqrt{2}}{2}$.

13. $\dfrac{\tan 51°}{1-\tan^2 51°} = \dfrac{1}{2}\cdot\dfrac{2\tan 51°}{1-\tan^2 51°} = \dfrac{1}{2}\tan[2\cdot 51°] = \dfrac{1}{2}\tan 102°$.

15. $\dfrac{1}{4} - \dfrac{1}{2}\sin^2 47.1° = \dfrac{1}{4}\left[4\left(\dfrac{1}{4} - \dfrac{1}{2}\sin^2 47.1°\right)\right] = \dfrac{1}{4}\left[1 - 2\sin^2 47.1°\right] = \dfrac{1}{4}\cos[2(47.1°)] = \dfrac{1}{4}\cos 94.2°$.

17. $4\sin 15°\cos 15° = 2\sin 2(15°) = 2\sin 30° = 2\cdot\dfrac{1}{2} = 1$.

19. When graphing the equation on the calculator, the graph looks like that of $\cos 2x$. Verify this result.

$\cos^4 x - \sin^4 x = (\cos^2 x - \sin^2 x)(\cos^2 x + \sin^2 x) = (\cos^2 x - \sin^2 x)(1) = \cos 2x$.

21. $\cos 3x = \cos(2x + x) = \cos 2x\cos x - \sin 2x\sin x = (2\cos^2 x - 1)\cos x - (2\sin x\cos x)\sin x =$

$2\cos^3 x - \cos x - 2\sin^2 x\cos x = 2\cos^3 x - \cos x - 2(1-\cos^2 x)\cos x =$

$2\cos^3 x - \cos x - 2\cos x + 2\cos^3 x = 4\cos^3 x - 3\cos x$.

The graph of each equation supports that they are equal.

458 CHAPTER 9 Trigonometric Identities and Equations

23. $\tan 4x = \tan 2(2x) = \dfrac{2\tan 2x}{1-\tan^2 2x} = \dfrac{2\left(\frac{2\tan x}{1-\tan^2 x}\right)}{1-\left(\frac{2\tan x}{1-\tan^2 x}\right)^2} \cdot \dfrac{\left(1-\tan^2 x\right)^2}{\left(1-\tan^2 x\right)^2} = \dfrac{4\tan x(1-\tan^2 x)}{(1-\tan^2 x)^2 - 4\tan^2 x} =$

$\dfrac{4\tan x - 4\tan^3 x}{1 - 2\tan^2 x + \tan^4 x - 4\tan^2 x} = \dfrac{4\tan x - 4\tan^3 x}{1 - 6\tan^2 x + \tan^4 x}$. The graph of each equation supports that they are equal.

25. Since $\sin\dfrac{\pi}{12}$ is found in quadrant I, the sine value will be positive; therefore:

$\sin\dfrac{\pi}{12} = \sin\left(\dfrac{\pi/6}{2}\right) = \sqrt{\dfrac{1-\cos\frac{\pi}{6}}{2}} = \sqrt{\dfrac{1-\frac{\sqrt{3}}{2}}{2} \cdot \dfrac{2}{2}} = \sqrt{\dfrac{2-\sqrt{3}}{4}} = \dfrac{\sqrt{2-\sqrt{3}}}{2}$.

27. $\tan\left(-\dfrac{\pi}{8}\right) = -\tan\left(\dfrac{\pi}{8}\right) = -\tan\left(\dfrac{\pi/4}{2}\right) = -\left(\dfrac{1-\cos\frac{\pi}{4}}{\sin\frac{\pi}{4}}\right) = -\dfrac{1-\frac{\sqrt{2}}{2}}{\frac{\sqrt{2}}{2}} \cdot \dfrac{2}{2} = -\dfrac{2-\sqrt{2}}{\sqrt{2}} \cdot \dfrac{\sqrt{2}}{\sqrt{2}} = -\dfrac{2\sqrt{2}-2}{2} = 1-\sqrt{2}$. An

Alternate method yields $-\sqrt{3-2\sqrt{2}}$.

29. Since $\sin 67.5°$ is found in quadrant I, the sine value will be positive, therefore:

$\sin 67.5° = \sin\left(\dfrac{135°}{2}\right) = \sqrt{\dfrac{1-\cos 135°}{2}} = \sqrt{\dfrac{1-\left(-\frac{\sqrt{2}}{2}\right)}{2} \cdot \dfrac{2}{2}} = \sqrt{\dfrac{2+\sqrt{2}}{4}} = \dfrac{\sqrt{2+\sqrt{2}}}{2}$.

31. If $\cos x = \dfrac{1}{4}$ and $0 < x < \dfrac{\pi}{2}$, then x is found in quadrant I. With x in quadrant I, the cosine value will be

positive; therefore: $\cos\dfrac{x}{2} = \sqrt{\dfrac{1+\cos x}{2}} = \sqrt{\dfrac{1+\frac{1}{4}}{2} \cdot \dfrac{4}{4}} = \sqrt{\dfrac{4+1}{8}} = \dfrac{\sqrt{5}}{\sqrt{8}} \cdot \dfrac{\sqrt{2}}{\sqrt{2}} = \dfrac{\sqrt{10}}{4}$.

33. If $\sin x = \dfrac{3}{5}$ and $\dfrac{\pi}{2} < x < \pi$, then x is found in quadrant II. With x in quadrant II, the cosine value will be

negative; therefore: $\cos x = -\sqrt{1-\sin^2 x} = -\sqrt{1-\dfrac{9}{25}} = -\sqrt{\dfrac{16}{25}} = -\dfrac{4}{5}$. Now use $\sin x = \dfrac{3}{5}$ and $\cos x = -\dfrac{4}{5}$ to

find $\tan\dfrac{x}{2}$. $\tan\dfrac{x}{2} = \dfrac{1-\cos\theta}{\sin\theta} = \dfrac{1-\left(-\frac{4}{5}\right)}{\frac{3}{5}} \cdot \dfrac{5}{5} = \dfrac{5+4}{3} = 3$.

35. If $\tan x = \dfrac{\sqrt{7}}{3}$ and $\pi < x < \dfrac{3\pi}{2}$, then x is found in quadrant III. With x in quadrant III, both sine and secant

values are negative; therefore: $\sec x = -\sqrt{1+\tan^2 x} = -\sqrt{1+\dfrac{7}{9}} = -\sqrt{\dfrac{16}{9}} = -\dfrac{4}{3}$. Therefore $\cos x = -\dfrac{3}{4}$, and

$\sin x = -\sqrt{1-\cos^2 x} = -\sqrt{1-\dfrac{9}{16}} = -\sqrt{\dfrac{7}{16}} = -\dfrac{\sqrt{7}}{4}$. Now use $\sin x = -\dfrac{\sqrt{7}}{4}$ and $\cos x = -\dfrac{3}{4}$ to find $\tan\dfrac{x}{2}$.

$\tan\dfrac{x}{2} = \dfrac{1-\cos x}{\sin x} = \dfrac{1-\left(-\frac{3}{4}\right)}{-\frac{\sqrt{7}}{4}} \cdot \dfrac{4}{4} = \dfrac{4+3}{-\sqrt{7}} \cdot \dfrac{\sqrt{7}}{\sqrt{7}} = \dfrac{7\sqrt{7}}{-7} = -\sqrt{7}$.

37. If $\tan x = 2$ and $0 < x < \dfrac{\pi}{2}$, then x is found in quadrant I. With x in quadrant I, then $\sec x > 0$.

$\sec^2 x = \tan^2 x + 1 \Rightarrow \sec^2 x = 2^2 + 1 = 5 \Rightarrow \sec x = \sqrt{5} \Rightarrow \cos x = \dfrac{1}{\sqrt{5}} = \dfrac{\sqrt{5}}{5}$. Since

$0 < x < \dfrac{\pi}{2} \Rightarrow 0 < \dfrac{x}{2} < \dfrac{\pi}{4} \Rightarrow \dfrac{x}{2}$ is in quadrant I and $\dfrac{x}{2} > 0$. $\sin \dfrac{x}{2} = \sqrt{\dfrac{1-\cos x}{2}} = \sqrt{\dfrac{1-\dfrac{\sqrt{5}}{5}}{2}} = \dfrac{\sqrt{50-10\sqrt{5}}}{10}$.

39. Since $\dfrac{\pi}{2} < x < \pi \Rightarrow \cos x < 0$. $\cos x = \sqrt{\dfrac{1+\cos 2x}{2}} \Rightarrow \sqrt{\dfrac{1+\left(-\dfrac{5}{12}\right)}{2}} = -\sqrt{\dfrac{7}{24}} = -\dfrac{\sqrt{42}}{12}$

41. (a) The function $\tan \dfrac{\pi}{2}$ is undefined, so it cannot be used.

   (b) $\tan\left(\dfrac{\pi}{2} + x\right) = \dfrac{\sin(\dfrac{\pi}{2} + x)}{\cos(\dfrac{\pi}{2} + x)}$.

   (c) $\tan\left(\dfrac{\pi}{2} + x\right) = \dfrac{\sin \dfrac{\pi}{2} \cos x + \cos \dfrac{\pi}{2} \sin x}{\cos \dfrac{\pi}{2} \cos x - \sin \dfrac{\pi}{2} \sin x} = \dfrac{1 \cdot \cos x + 0 \cdot \sin x}{0 \cdot \cos x - 1 \cdot \sin x} = \dfrac{\cos x}{-\sin x} = -\cot x$.

43. $\sqrt{\dfrac{1-\cos 40°}{2}} = \sin \dfrac{40°}{2} = \sin 20°$.

45. $\sqrt{\dfrac{1-\cos 147°}{1+\cos 147°}} = \tan \dfrac{147°}{2} = \tan 73.5°$.

47. $\dfrac{1-\cos 59.74°}{\sin 59.74°} = \tan \dfrac{59.74°}{2} = \tan 29.87°$.

49. $\dfrac{2\cos 2\alpha}{\sin 2\alpha} = \dfrac{2(\cos^2 \alpha - \sin^2 \alpha)}{2\sin \alpha \cos \alpha} = \dfrac{\cos^2 \alpha}{\sin \alpha \cos \alpha} - \dfrac{\sin^2 \alpha}{\sin \alpha \cos \alpha} = \dfrac{\cos \alpha}{\sin \alpha} - \dfrac{\sin \alpha}{\cos \alpha} = \cot \alpha - \tan \alpha$.

51. $\sec^2 \dfrac{x}{2} = \left(\dfrac{1}{\cos \dfrac{x}{2}}\right)^2 = \left(\pm \dfrac{1}{\sqrt{\dfrac{1+\cos x}{2}}}\right)^2 = \dfrac{1}{\dfrac{1+\cos x}{2}} = \dfrac{2}{1+\cos x}$.

53. Working the right side of the equation.

$\dfrac{2-\sec^2 \theta}{\sec^2 \theta} = \dfrac{2 - \dfrac{1}{\cos^2 \theta}}{\dfrac{1}{\cos^2 \theta}} = \dfrac{2 - \dfrac{1}{\cos^2 \theta}}{\dfrac{1}{\cos^2 \theta}} \cdot \dfrac{\cos^2 \theta}{\cos^2 \theta} = 2\cos^2 \theta - 1 = \cos 2\theta$.

55. If $\tan s + \cot s = \dfrac{\sin s}{\cos s} + \dfrac{\cos s}{\sin s} = \dfrac{\sin^2 s + \cos^2 s}{\sin s \cos s} = \dfrac{1}{\sin s \cos s}$, and if $2 \csc 2s = 2\left(\dfrac{1}{2\sin 2s}\right) = $

$2\left(\dfrac{1}{2\sin s \cos s}\right) = \dfrac{1}{\sin s \cos s}$, then $\tan s + \cot s = 2\csc 2s$.

57. Working the left side of the equation. $\sin^2 \frac{x}{2} = \left(\pm\sqrt{\frac{1-\cos x}{2}}\right)^2 = \frac{1-\cos x}{2}$.

Working the right side of the equation. $\dfrac{\tan x - \sin x}{2\tan x} = \dfrac{\dfrac{\sin x}{\cos x} - \sin x}{2 \cdot \dfrac{\sin x}{\cos x}} = \dfrac{\dfrac{\sin x}{\cos x} - \sin x}{2 \cdot \dfrac{\sin x}{\cos x}} \cdot \dfrac{\cos x}{\cos x} =$

$\dfrac{\sin x - \cos x \sin x}{2\sin x} = \dfrac{\sin x(1-\cos x)}{2\sin x} = \dfrac{1-\cos x}{2}$.

59. Working the right side of the equation.

$\dfrac{1-\tan^2 x}{1+\tan^2 x} = \dfrac{1-\dfrac{\sin^2 x}{\cos^2 x}}{1+\dfrac{\sin^2 x}{\cos^2 x}} = \dfrac{1-\dfrac{\sin^2 x}{\cos^2 x}}{1+\dfrac{\sin^2 x}{\cos^2 x}} \cdot \dfrac{\cos^2 x}{\cos^2 x} = \dfrac{\cos^2 x - \sin^2 x}{\cos^2 x + \sin^2 x} = \dfrac{\cos^2 x - \sin^2 x}{1} = \cos 2x$.

61. $\sin 2\alpha \cos 2\alpha = \sin 2\alpha(1-2\sin^2 \alpha) = \sin 2\alpha - 2\sin 2\alpha \sin^2 \alpha =$

    $\sin 2\alpha - 2(2\sin \alpha \cos \alpha)\sin^2 = \sin 2\alpha - 4\sin^3 \alpha \cos \alpha$.

63. $\sin 4\alpha = 2\sin 2\alpha \cos 2\alpha = 2(2\sin \alpha \cos \alpha)\cos 2\alpha = 4\sin \alpha \cos \alpha \cos 2\alpha$.

65. $2\sin 58° \cos 102° = 2\left[\dfrac{1}{2}[\sin(58°+102°)+\sin(58°-102°)]\right] = \sin 160° + \sin(-44°) = \sin 160° - \sin 44°$.

67. $2\cos 85° \sin 140° = \dfrac{1}{2}[2[\sin(85°+140°)-\sin(85°-140°)]] = \sin 225° - \sin(-55°) = \sin 225° + \sin 55°$.

69. $\cos 4x - \cos 2x = -2\sin\left(\dfrac{4x+2x}{2}\right)\sin\left(\dfrac{4x-2x}{2}\right) = -2\sin 3x \sin x$.

71. $\sin 25° + \sin(-48)° = 2\sin\left(\dfrac{25°+(-48°)}{2}\right)\cos\left(\dfrac{25°-(-48°)}{2}\right) = 2\sin(-11.5°)\cos 36.5° =$

    $-2\sin 11.5° \cos 36.5°$.

73. $\cos 4x + \cos 8x = 2\cos\left(\dfrac{4x+8x}{2}\right)\cos\left(\dfrac{4x-8x}{2}\right) = 2\cos 6x \cos(-2x) = 2\cos 6x \cos 2x$.

75. (a) Since R is the radius of the circle, the dashed line has length $R-b$, so $\cos\dfrac{\theta}{2} = \dfrac{R-b}{R}$.

    (b) $\tan\dfrac{\theta}{4} = \dfrac{1-\cos\frac{\theta}{2}}{\sin\frac{\theta}{2}} = \dfrac{1-\frac{R-b}{R}}{\frac{50}{R}} = \dfrac{R-(R-b)}{50} = \dfrac{b}{50}$.

    (c) If $b = 12$, then $\tan\dfrac{\theta}{4} = \dfrac{b}{50}$ yields $\tan\dfrac{\theta}{4} = \dfrac{12}{50}$. Now solve for θ.

    $\dfrac{\theta}{4} = \tan^{-1}\left(\dfrac{12}{50}\right) \Rightarrow \theta = 4\tan^{-1}\left(\dfrac{12}{50}\right) \approx 53.98° \Rightarrow \theta \approx 54°$.

77. (a) Graph $W = VI = [163\sin(120\pi t)][1.23\sin(120\pi t)] = 200.49\sin^2(120\pi t)$. See Figure 77.

    (b) The minimum wattage is 0 watts and occurs whenever $\sin(120\pi t) = 0$. The maximum wattage will occur when $\sin(120\pi t) = 1$. This would be $200.49(1) = 200.49$ watts.

(c) Use the identity, $\sin^2 A = \dfrac{1}{2}(1-\cos 2A)$.

$W = 200.49\sin^2(120\pi t) = 200.49\left[\dfrac{1}{2}(1-\cos(240\pi t))\right] = -100.245\cos(240\pi t) + 100.245$.

From this equation, $a = -100.245$, $w = 240\pi$, and $c = 100.245$.

(d) Graphing $(120\pi t)$ and $W = -100.245\cos(240\pi t) + 100.245$ in the same window shows that both equations have the same graph.

(e) Graph W and $y = 100.245$ together. The cosine (or sine) graph of $y = \tan x$ appears to be vertically centered about this line. An estimate for the average wattage consumed is 100.245 watts. The light bulb would be rated at about 100 watts.

[0,0.5] by [-1,6]
Xscl = 0.1   Yscl = 1

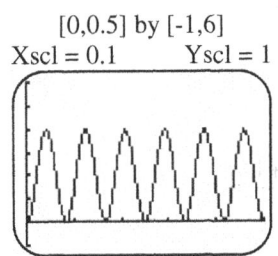

Figure 77

79. $\tan\theta + \cot\theta = \dfrac{\sin\theta}{\cos\theta} + \dfrac{\cos\theta}{\sin\theta} = \dfrac{\sin^2\theta}{\sin\theta\cos\theta} + \dfrac{\cos^2\theta}{\sin\theta\cos\theta} = \dfrac{\sin^2\theta + \cos^2\theta}{\sin\theta\cos\theta} =$

$\dfrac{1}{\sin\theta\cos\theta} = \dfrac{1}{\cos\theta}\cdot\dfrac{1}{\sin\theta} = \sec\theta\csc\theta$.

80. $\csc\theta\cos^2\theta + \sin\theta = \dfrac{1}{\sin\theta}\cdot\cos^2\theta + \sin\theta = \dfrac{\cos^2\theta}{\sin\theta} + \sin\theta = \dfrac{\cos^2\theta + \sin^2\theta}{\sin\theta} = \dfrac{1}{\sin\theta} = \csc\theta$.

81. $\tan\dfrac{x}{2} = \dfrac{1-\cos x}{\sin x} = \dfrac{1}{\sin x} - \dfrac{\cos x}{\sin x} = \csc x - \cot x$.

82. $\sec(\pi - x) = \dfrac{1}{\cos(\pi - x)} = \dfrac{1}{\cos\pi\cos x + \sin\pi\sin x} = \dfrac{1}{-1\cdot\cos x + 0\cdot\sin x} = \dfrac{1}{-\cos x} = -\sec x$.

83. $\dfrac{\sin t}{1+\cos t} = \tan\dfrac{t}{2} = \dfrac{1-\cos t}{\sin t}$.

84. $\dfrac{1-\sin t}{\cos t} = \dfrac{1}{\cos t} - \dfrac{\sin t}{\cos t} = \sec t - \tan t = (\sec t - \tan t)\cdot\dfrac{\sec t + \tan t}{\sec t + \tan t} = \dfrac{\sec^2 t - \tan^2 t}{\sec t + \tan t} = \dfrac{1}{\sec t + \tan t}$.

85. $\sin 2\theta = 2\sin\theta\cos\theta = 2\sin\theta\cos\theta\cdot\dfrac{\cos\theta}{\cos\theta} = \dfrac{2\sin\theta\cos^2\theta}{\cos\theta} = 2\cdot\dfrac{\sin\theta}{\cos\theta}\cdot\cos^2\theta = 2\tan\theta\cos^2\theta =$

$2\cdot\tan\theta\cdot\dfrac{1}{\sec^2\theta} = \dfrac{2\tan\theta}{\sec^2\theta} = \dfrac{2\tan\theta}{1+\tan^2\theta}$.

86. $\dfrac{2}{1+\cos x} - \tan^2\dfrac{x}{2} = \dfrac{2}{1-\cos x} - \dfrac{\sin^2\frac{x}{2}}{\cos^2\frac{x}{2}} = \dfrac{2}{1+\cos x} - \left(\sqrt{\dfrac{1-\cos x}{1+\cos x}}\right)^2 = \dfrac{2}{1+\cos x} - \dfrac{1-\cos x}{1+\cos x} = \dfrac{1+\cos x}{1+\cos x} = 1$.

87. $\cot\theta - \tan\theta = \dfrac{\cos\theta}{\sin\theta} - \dfrac{\sin\theta}{\cos\theta} = \dfrac{\cos^2\theta}{\sin\theta\cos\theta} - \dfrac{\sin^2\theta}{\sin\theta\cos\theta} = \dfrac{\cos^2\theta - \sin^2\theta}{\sin\theta\cos\theta} = \dfrac{\cos^2\theta - (1-\cos^2\theta)}{\sin\theta\cos\theta} = \dfrac{2\cos^2\theta - 1}{\sin\theta\cos\theta}.$

88. $1 - \tan^2\dfrac{\theta}{2} = 1 - \left(\sqrt{\dfrac{1-\cos\theta}{1+\cos\theta}}\right)^2 = 1 - \dfrac{1-\cos\theta}{1+\cos\theta} = \dfrac{1+\cos\theta}{1+\cos\theta} - \dfrac{1-\cos\theta}{1+\cos\theta} = \dfrac{2\cos\theta}{1+\cos\theta}.$

89. $\dfrac{\sin\theta + \tan\theta}{1 + \cos\theta} = \dfrac{\frac{\sin\theta}{1} + \frac{\sin\theta}{\cos\theta}}{1 + \cos\theta} = \dfrac{\frac{\cos\theta\sin\theta + \sin\theta}{\cos\theta}}{1+\cos\theta} = \dfrac{\frac{\sin\theta(\cos\theta+1)}{\cos\theta}}{1+\cos\theta} = \dfrac{\sin\theta}{\cos\theta} = \tan\theta.$

90. $\csc^4 x - \cot^4 x = (\csc^2\theta + \cot^2\theta)(\csc^2\theta - \cot^2\theta) = (\csc^2\theta + \cot^2\theta)(1 + \cot^2\theta - \cot^2\theta) =$

$(\csc^2\theta + \cot^2\theta)(1) = (\csc^2\theta + \cot^2\theta) = \dfrac{1}{\sin^2\theta} + \dfrac{\cos^2 x}{\sin^2 x} = \dfrac{1+\cos^2 x}{\sin x} = \dfrac{1+\cos^2 x}{1 - \cos^2 x}.$

91. $\dfrac{\tan^2 t + 1}{\tan t \csc^2 t} = \dfrac{\sec^2 t}{\tan t \csc^2 t} = \dfrac{\sec^2 t}{\csc^2 t} \cdot \dfrac{1}{\tan t} = (\tan^2 t) \cdot \dfrac{1}{\tan t} = \tan t.$

92. $\dfrac{\sin s}{1+\cos s} + \dfrac{1+\cos s}{\sin s} = \dfrac{\sin^2 s}{\sin s(1+\cos s)} + \dfrac{1 + 2\cos s + \cos^2 s}{\sin s(1+\cos s)} = \dfrac{\sin^2 s + \cos^2 s + 2\cos s + 1}{\sin s(1+\cos s)} =$

$\dfrac{1 + 2\cos s + 1}{\sin s(1+\cos s)} = \dfrac{2 + 2\cos s}{\sin s(1+\cos s)} = \dfrac{2(1+\cos s)}{\sin s(1+\cos s)} = \dfrac{2}{\sin s} = 2 \cdot \dfrac{1}{\sin s} = 2\csc s.$

93. $\tan 4\theta = \tan 2(2\theta) = \dfrac{2\tan 2\theta}{1 - \tan^2 2\theta} = \dfrac{2\tan 2\theta}{1 - (\sec^2\theta - 1)} = \dfrac{2\tan 2\theta}{2 - \sec^2\theta}.$

94. $\tan\left(\dfrac{x}{2} + \dfrac{\pi}{4}\right) = \dfrac{\tan\frac{x}{2} + \tan\frac{\pi}{4}}{1 - \tan\frac{x}{2}\tan\frac{\pi}{4}} = \dfrac{\frac{\sin x}{1+\cos x} + 1}{1 - \frac{\sin x}{1+\cos x}(1)} = \dfrac{\frac{\sin x + 1 + \cos x}{1+\cos x}}{\frac{1+\cos x - \sin x}{1+\cos x}} = \dfrac{1 + \cos x + \sin x}{1 + \cos x - \sin x} =$

$\dfrac{1+\cos x + \sin x}{1+\cos x - \sin x} \cdot \dfrac{\cos x}{\cos x} = \dfrac{\cos x + \cos^2 x + \cos x \sin x}{(1+\cos x - \sin x)\cos x} = \dfrac{\cos x + 1 - \sin^2 x + \cos x \sin x}{(1+\cos x - \sin x)\cos x} =$

$\dfrac{\cos x + (1+\sin x)(1-\sin x) + \cos x \sin x}{(1+\cos x - \sin x)\cos x} = \dfrac{\cos x(1+\sin x) + (1+\sin x)(1-\sin x)}{(1+\cos x - \sin x)\cos x} =$

$\dfrac{(1+\sin x)[\cos x + (1-\sin x)]}{(1+\cos x - \sin x)\cos x} = \dfrac{1+\sin x}{\cos x} = \dfrac{1}{\cos x} + \dfrac{\sin x}{\cos x} = \sec x + \tan x.$

95. $\dfrac{\cot s - \tan s}{\cos s + \sin s} = \dfrac{\frac{\cos s}{\sin s} - \frac{\sin s}{\cos s}}{\cos s + \sin s} = \dfrac{\frac{\cos s}{\sin s} - \frac{\sin s}{\cos s}}{\cos s + \sin s} \cdot \dfrac{\sin s \cos s}{\sin s \cos s} = \dfrac{\cos^2 s - \sin^2 s}{(\cos s + \sin s)\sin s \cos s} =$

$\dfrac{(\cos s + \sin s)(\cos s - \sin s)}{(\cos s + \sin s)\sin s \cos s} = \dfrac{\cos s - \sin s}{\sin s \cos s}$

96. $\dfrac{\tan\theta - \cot\theta}{\tan\theta + \cot\theta} = \dfrac{\frac{\sin\theta}{\cos\theta} - \frac{\cos\theta}{\sin\theta}}{\frac{\sin\theta}{\cos\theta} + \frac{\cos\theta}{\sin\theta}} = \dfrac{\frac{\sin\theta}{\cos\theta} - \frac{\cos\theta}{\sin\theta}}{\frac{\sin\theta}{\cos\theta} + \frac{\cos\theta}{\sin\theta}} \cdot \dfrac{\cos\theta\sin\theta}{\cos\theta\sin\theta} = \dfrac{\sin^2\theta - \cos^2\theta}{\sin^2\theta + \cos^2\theta} = \dfrac{\sin^2\theta - \cos^2\theta}{1} =$

$\sin^2\theta - \cos^2\theta = (1 - \cos^2\theta) - \cos^2\theta = 1 - 2\cos^2\theta$

Section 9.4   463

97. $\dfrac{\tan(x+y)-\tan y}{1+\tan(x+y)\tan y} = \dfrac{\dfrac{\tan x+\tan y}{1-\tan x\tan y}-\tan y}{1+\dfrac{\tan x+\tan y}{1-\tan x\tan y}\cdot\tan y} = \dfrac{\dfrac{\tan x+\tan y}{1-\tan x\tan y}-\tan y}{1+\dfrac{\tan x+\tan y}{1-\tan x\tan y}\cdot\tan y}\cdot\dfrac{1-\tan x\tan y}{1-\tan x\tan y} =$

$\dfrac{\tan x+\tan y-\tan y(1-\tan x\tan y)}{1-\tan x\tan y+(\tan x+\tan y)\tan y} = \dfrac{\tan x+\tan x\tan^2 y}{1-\tan x\tan y+\tan x\tan y+\tan^2 y} = \dfrac{\tan x(1+\tan^2 y)}{1+\tan^2 y} = \tan x$

98. $2\cos^2\dfrac{x}{2}\tan x = 2\left(\pm\sqrt{\dfrac{1+\cos x}{2}}\right)^2\cdot\dfrac{\sin x}{\cos x} = 2\cdot\dfrac{1+\cos x}{2}\cdot\dfrac{\sin x}{\cos x} = (1+\cos x)\cdot\dfrac{\sin x}{\cos x} =$

$\dfrac{\sin x}{\cos x}+\sin x = \tan x+\sin x$

99. $\dfrac{\cos^4 x-\sin^4 x}{\cos^2 x} = \dfrac{(\cos^2 x-\sin^2 x)(\cos^2 x+\sin^2 x)}{\cos^2 x} = \dfrac{\cos^2 x-\sin^2 x}{\cos^2 x} = \dfrac{\cos^2 x}{\cos^2 x}-\dfrac{\sin^2 x}{\cos^2 x} = 1-\tan^2 x$

100. $\dfrac{\csc t+1}{\csc t-1} = \dfrac{\dfrac{1}{\sin t}+1}{\dfrac{1}{\sin t}-1} = \dfrac{\dfrac{1}{\sin t}+1}{\dfrac{1}{\sin t}-1}\cdot\dfrac{\sin t}{\sin t} = \dfrac{1+\sin t}{1-\sin t} = \dfrac{1+\sin t}{1-\sin t}\cdot\dfrac{1+\sin t}{1+\sin t} = \dfrac{(1+\sin t)^2}{1-\sin^2 t} = \dfrac{(1+\sin t)^2}{\cos^2 t} =$

$\left(\dfrac{1+\sin t}{\cos t}\right)^2 = \left(\dfrac{1}{\cos t}+\dfrac{\sin t}{\cos t}\right)^2 = (\sec t+\tan t)^2$

101. $\dfrac{2(\sin x-\sin^3 x)}{\cos x} = \dfrac{2\sin x(1-\sin^2 x)}{\cos x} = \dfrac{2\sin x\cos^2 x}{\cos x} = 2\sin x\cos x = \sin 2x$

102. $\dfrac{1}{2}\cot\dfrac{x}{2}-\dfrac{1}{2}\tan\dfrac{x}{2} = \dfrac{1}{2}\cdot\dfrac{1}{\tan\dfrac{x}{2}}-\dfrac{1}{2}\tan\dfrac{x}{2} = \dfrac{1}{2}\cdot\dfrac{1}{\dfrac{\sin x}{1+\cos x}}-\dfrac{1}{2}\cdot\dfrac{1-\cos x}{\sin x} = \dfrac{1+\cos x}{2\sin x}-\dfrac{1-\cos x}{2\sin x} =$

$\dfrac{1+\cos x-(1-\cos x)}{2\sin x} = \dfrac{2\cos x}{2\sin x} = \dfrac{\cos x}{\sin x} = \cot x$

103. $\dfrac{\sin(x+y)}{\cos(x-y)} = \dfrac{\sin x\cos y+\cos x\sin y}{\cos x\cos y+\sin x\sin y} = \dfrac{\cos x\cos y+\cos x\sin y}{\cos x\cos y+\sin x\sin y}\cdot\dfrac{\dfrac{1}{\sin x\sin y}}{\dfrac{1}{\sin x\sin y}} = \dfrac{\dfrac{\cos y}{\sin y}+\dfrac{\cos x}{\sin x}}{\dfrac{\cos x\cos y}{\sin x\sin y}+1} =$

$\dfrac{\cot y+\cot x}{\cot x\cot y+1} = \dfrac{\cot x+\cot y}{1+\cot x\cot y}$.

104. $\dfrac{1}{\sec t-1}+\dfrac{1}{\sec t+1} = \dfrac{\sec t+1}{\sec^2 t-1}+\dfrac{\sec t-1}{\sec^2 t-1} = \dfrac{\sec t+1}{\tan^2 t}+\dfrac{\sec t-1}{\tan^2 t} = \dfrac{2\sec t}{\tan^2 t} = 2\sec t\cdot\dfrac{1}{\tan^2 t} =$

$2\sec t\cdot\cot^2 t = 2\cdot\dfrac{1}{\cos t}\cdot\dfrac{\cos^2 t}{\sin^2 t} = \dfrac{2\cos t}{\sin^2 t} = 2\cdot\dfrac{\cos t}{\sin t}\cdot\dfrac{1}{\sin t} = 2\cot t\csc t$.

9.4: The Inverse Circular Functions

1. one-to-one

3. $\cos y$

5. π

7. (a) The domain of $y = \sin^{-1} x$ is the range of $y = \sin x$, therefore the domain is: $[-1, 1]$

   (b) The range of $y = \sin^{-1} x$ is the domain of $y = \sin x$, therefore the range is: $\left[-\dfrac{\pi}{2}, \dfrac{\pi}{2}\right]$

   (c) For this function, as x increases, y increases. Therefore, it in an <u>increasing</u> function.

   (d) Arcsin (-2) is not defined since -2 is not in the domain.

9. (a) The domain of $y = \tan^{-1} x$ is the range of $y = \tan x$, therefore the domain is: $(-\infty, \infty)$

   (b) The range of $y = \tan^{-1} x$ is the domain of $y = \tan x$, therefore the range is: $\left(-\dfrac{\pi}{2}, \dfrac{\pi}{2}\right)$

   (c) For this function, as x increases, y increases. Therefore, it in an <u>increasing</u> function.

   (d) No, since the domain is $(-\infty, \infty)$ arctan x is defined for all numbers.

11. $y = \tan^{-1} 1 \Rightarrow 1 = \tan y \Rightarrow y = \dfrac{\pi}{4} \left(range: \left(-\dfrac{\pi}{2}, \dfrac{\pi}{2}\right)\right)$

13. $y = \cos^{-1}(-1) \Rightarrow -1 = \cos y \Rightarrow y = \pi \ (range: [0, \pi])$

15. $y = \sin^{-1}(-1) \Rightarrow -1 = \sin y \Rightarrow y = -\dfrac{\pi}{2} \left(range: \left[-\dfrac{\pi}{2}, \dfrac{\pi}{2}\right]\right)$

17. $y = \arctan 0 \Rightarrow 0 = \tan y \Rightarrow y = 0 \left(range: \left(-\dfrac{\pi}{2}, \dfrac{\pi}{2}\right)\right)$

19. $y = \arccos 0 \Rightarrow 0 = \cos y \Rightarrow y = \dfrac{\pi}{2} \ (range: [0, \pi])$

21. $y = \sin^{-1}\left(\dfrac{\sqrt{2}}{2}\right) \Rightarrow \dfrac{\sqrt{2}}{2} = \sin y \Rightarrow y = \dfrac{\pi}{4} \left(range: \left[-\dfrac{\pi}{2}, \dfrac{\pi}{2}\right]\right)$

23. $y = arc\cos\left(-\dfrac{\sqrt{3}}{2}\right) \Rightarrow -\dfrac{\sqrt{3}}{2} = \cos y \Rightarrow y = \dfrac{5\pi}{6} \ (range: [0, \pi])$

25. $y = \cot^{-1}(-1) \Rightarrow y = \tan^{-1}\left(\dfrac{1}{-1}\right) + \pi \Rightarrow y = \tan^{-1}(-1) + \pi \Rightarrow (-1 = \tan y) + \pi \Rightarrow$

    $y = -\dfrac{\pi}{4} + \pi \Rightarrow y = \dfrac{3\pi}{4} \ (range: (0, \pi))$.

27. $y = \csc^{-1}(-2) \Rightarrow y = \sin^{-1}\left(\dfrac{1}{-2}\right) \Rightarrow y = \sin^{-1}\left(-\dfrac{1}{2}\right) \Rightarrow -\dfrac{1}{2} = \sin y \Rightarrow y = -\dfrac{\pi}{6} \left(range: \left[-\dfrac{\pi}{2}, 0\right) \cup \left(0, \dfrac{\pi}{2}\right]\right)$

29. $y = arc\sec \dfrac{2\sqrt{3}}{3} \Rightarrow y = \cos^{-1}\left(\dfrac{1}{\frac{2\sqrt{3}}{3}}\right) \Rightarrow y = \cos^{-1}\left(\dfrac{3}{2\sqrt{3}}\right) \Rightarrow y = \cos^{-1}\dfrac{\sqrt{3}}{2} \Rightarrow$

    $\dfrac{\sqrt{3}}{2} = \cos y \Rightarrow y = \dfrac{\pi}{6} \left(range: \left[0, \dfrac{\pi}{2}\right) \cup \left(\dfrac{\pi}{2}, \pi\right]\right)$

31. $y = \tan^{-1}(\sqrt{3}) \Rightarrow \sqrt{3} = \tan y \Rightarrow y = \dfrac{\pi}{3}\ \left(range: \left(-\dfrac{\pi}{2}, \dfrac{\pi}{2}\right)\right)$

33. $y = \csc^{-1}(2) \Rightarrow y = \sin^{-1}\left(\dfrac{1}{2}\right) \Rightarrow \dfrac{1}{2} = \sin y \Rightarrow y = \dfrac{\pi}{6}\ \left(range: \left[-\dfrac{\pi}{2}, 0\right) \cup \left(0, \dfrac{\pi}{2}\right]\right)$

35. $\theta = \arctan(-1) \Rightarrow -1 = \tan\theta \Rightarrow \theta = -45°\ (range: (-90°, 90°))$

37. $\theta = \arcsin\left(-\dfrac{\sqrt{3}}{2}\right) \Rightarrow -\dfrac{\sqrt{3}}{2} = \sin\theta \Rightarrow \theta = -60°\ (range: [-90°, 90°])$

39. $\theta = \cot^{-1}\left(-\dfrac{\sqrt{3}}{3}\right) \Rightarrow \theta = \tan^{-1}\left(\dfrac{1}{-\frac{\sqrt{3}}{3}}\right) + 180° \Rightarrow \theta = \tan^{-1}\left(-\dfrac{3}{\sqrt{3}}\right) + 180° \Rightarrow$

$\theta = \tan^{-1}(-\sqrt{3}) + 180° \Rightarrow (-\sqrt{3} = \tan\theta) + 180° \Rightarrow \theta = -60° + 180° \Rightarrow \theta = 120°\ (range: (0°, 180°))$

41. $\theta = \csc^{-1}(-2) \Rightarrow \theta = \sin^{-1}\left(\dfrac{1}{-2}\right) \Rightarrow \theta = \sin^{-1}\left(-\dfrac{1}{2}\right) \Rightarrow \left(-\dfrac{1}{2} = \sin\theta\right) \Rightarrow \theta = -30°$

$(range: [90°, 0°) \cup (0°, 90°])$

43. $\theta = \sin^{-1}(2) \Rightarrow 2 = \sin\theta \Rightarrow \theta$ does not exist $(range\ of\ \sin\theta: [-1,1])$

45. $\theta = \sec^{-1}\left(-\dfrac{1}{2}\right) \Rightarrow \theta = \cos^{-1}(-2) \Rightarrow -2 = \cos\theta \Rightarrow \theta$ does not exist $(range\ of\ \cos\theta: [-1,1])$

47. $\theta = \sin^{-1}(-.13349122) \Rightarrow \theta \approx -7.6713835°$

49. $\theta = \arccos(-.39876459) \Rightarrow \theta \approx 113.500970°$

51. $\theta = \csc^{-1}(1.9422833) \Rightarrow \theta = \sin^{-1}\dfrac{1}{1.9422833} \Rightarrow \theta = \sin^{-1}(1.9422833)^{-1} \Rightarrow \theta \approx 30.987961°$

53. $y = \arctan 1.1111111 \Rightarrow y \approx 0.83798122$

55. $y = \cot^{-1}(-.92170128) \Rightarrow y = \left(\tan^{-1}\dfrac{1}{-.92170128}\right) + \pi \Rightarrow y = (\tan^{-1}(-.92170128)^{-1}) + \pi \Rightarrow$

$y \approx -.8261201193 + \pi \Rightarrow y \approx 2.315472534$

57. $y = \arcsin .92837781 \Rightarrow y \approx 1.1900238$

59. Graph $y = \cot^{-1} x$, see Figure 59

61. Graph $y = \sec^{-1} x$, see Figure 61.

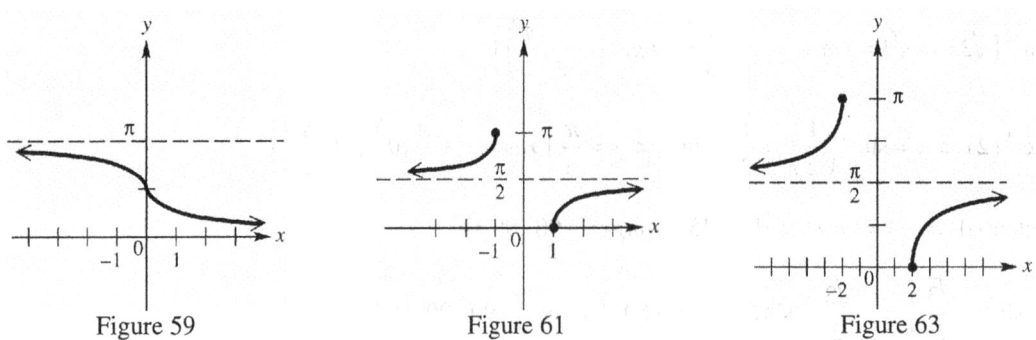

Figure 59   Figure 61   Figure 63

63. Graph $y = \text{arc}\sec\dfrac{1}{2}x$ $\left(\text{like the graph of } y = \sec^{-1} x, \text{with a domain}\left(-\infty, 2\right] \cup [2, \infty)\right)$ See Figure 63.

65. The domain of $y = \tan^{-1} x$ is $(-\infty, \infty)$ Therefore 1.003 is in this domain and $\tan^{-1} 1.003$ can be found.

67. Since $\sin(\sin^{-1} x) = x$ when $-1 < x < 1$, $\sin\left(\sin^{-1}\dfrac{1}{2}\right) = \dfrac{1}{2}$

69. First find $\sin\dfrac{4\pi}{3} = -\dfrac{\sqrt{3}}{2}$ now solve for $\sin^{-1}\left(-\dfrac{\sqrt{3}}{2}\right) \Rightarrow -\dfrac{\sqrt{3}}{2} = \sin\theta \Rightarrow \theta = -\dfrac{\pi}{3}$

71. First find $\cos\dfrac{3\pi}{2} = 0$ now solve for $\cos^{-1} 0 \Rightarrow 0 = \cos\theta \Rightarrow \theta = \dfrac{\pi}{2}$.

73. Since $\sin^2\dfrac{x}{2} = \left(\pm\sqrt{\dfrac{1-\cos x}{2}}\right)^2 = \dfrac{1-\cos x}{2}$ for all values of x $\tan(\tan^{-1} 5) = 5$

75. Since $\sec(\sec^{-1} x) = x$ when $x \leq -1$ or $x \geq 1$, $\sec(\sec^{-1} 2) = 2$.

77. First find $\tan\dfrac{5\pi}{6} = -\dfrac{1}{\sqrt{3}} = \dfrac{-\sqrt{3}}{3}$ now solve for $\tan^{-1}\left(\dfrac{-\sqrt{3}}{3}\right) \Rightarrow \dfrac{-\sqrt{3}}{3} = \tan\theta \Rightarrow \theta = -\dfrac{\pi}{6}$.

79. Since $\cos\theta = \dfrac{3}{4}$ is in quadrant I. Sketch and label a triangle in quadrant I $x = 3$ and $r = 4$. Now use Pythagorean Theorem to find y: $3^2 + y^2 = 4^2 \Rightarrow y^2 = 16 - 9 \Rightarrow y^2 = 7 \Rightarrow y = \sqrt{7}$. Therefore, $\tan\theta = \dfrac{\sqrt{7}}{3}$ and $\tan\left(\arccos\dfrac{3}{4}\right) = \dfrac{\sqrt{7}}{3}$.

81. Since $\tan\theta = -2$ then θ is in quadrant IV. Sketch and label a triangle in quadrant IV, with $x = 1$ and $y = -1$ Now use Pythagorean theorem to find r: $1^2 + (-2)^2 = r^2 \Rightarrow r^2 = 1 + 4 \Rightarrow r^2 = 5 \Rightarrow r = \sqrt{5}$ Therefore, $\cos\theta = \dfrac{1}{\sqrt{5}} = \dfrac{\sqrt{5}}{5}$ and $\cos(\tan^{-1}(-2)) = \dfrac{\sqrt{5}}{5}$.

83. Since $\tan\theta = \dfrac{12}{5}$ then θ is in quadrant I. Sketch and label a triangle in quadrant I, with $x = 5$ and $y = 12$ Use Pythagorean theorem to find r: $5^2 + 12^2 = r^2 \Rightarrow r^2 = 25 + 144 \Rightarrow r^2 = 169 \Rightarrow r = 13$ Now $\sin 2\theta = 2\sin\theta\cos\theta$ therefore, $\sin 2\theta = 2\left(\dfrac{12}{13}\right)\left(\dfrac{5}{13}\right) = \dfrac{120}{169}$ and $\sin\left(2\tan^{-1}\dfrac{12}{5}\right) = \dfrac{120}{169}$.

Copyright © 2015 Pearson Education, Inc

Section 9.4   467

85. Since $\tan\theta = \dfrac{4}{3}$, then θ is in quadrant I. Sketch and label a triangle in quadrant I, with $=\dfrac{\sqrt{u^2+5}}{u}$ and

$y = 4$. Use Pythagorean theorem to find r: $3^2 + 4^2 = r^2 \Rightarrow r^2 = 9+16 \Rightarrow r^2 = 25 \Rightarrow r = 5$. Now

$\cos 2\theta = \cos^2\theta - \sin^2\theta$, therefore, $\cos 2\theta = \left(\dfrac{3}{5}\right)^2 - \left(\dfrac{4}{5}\right)^2 = -\dfrac{7}{25}$ and $\cos\left(2\arctan\dfrac{4}{3}\right) = -\dfrac{7}{25}$.

87. Since $\cos\theta = \dfrac{1}{5}$, then θ is in quadrant I. Sketch and label a triangle in quadrant I, with $x = 1$ and $r = 5$.

Use Pythagorean theorem to find y: $1^2 + y^2 = 5^2 \Rightarrow y^2 = 25-1 \Rightarrow y^2 = 24 \Rightarrow y = \sqrt{24} = 2\sqrt{6}$. Now

$\sin 2\theta = 2\sin\theta\cos\theta$, therefore, $\sin 2\theta = 2\left(\dfrac{2\sqrt{6}}{5}\right)\left(\dfrac{1}{5}\right) = \dfrac{4\sqrt{6}}{25}$ and $\sin\left(2\cos^{-1}\dfrac{1}{5}\right) = \dfrac{4\sqrt{6}}{25}$.

89. Since $\sin\theta = \dfrac{3}{5}$, then θ is in quadrant I. Sketch and label a triangle in quadrant I, with $y = 3$ and $r = 5$.

Use Pythagorean theorem to find x: $x^2 + 3^2 = 5^2 \Rightarrow x^2 = 25-9 \Rightarrow x^2 = 16 \Rightarrow x = 4$. Since $\cos\beta = \dfrac{12}{13}$, then

β is in quadrant I. Use Pythagorean theorem to find y:

$12^2 + y^2 = 13^2 \Rightarrow y^2 = 169-144 \Rightarrow y^2 = 25 \Rightarrow y = 5$. Now $\cos(\theta - \beta) = \cos\theta\cos\beta + \sin\theta\sin\beta$, therefore,

$\cos(\theta + \beta) = \dfrac{4}{5}\cdot\dfrac{12}{13} + \dfrac{3}{5}\cdot\dfrac{5}{13} = \dfrac{48}{65} + \dfrac{15}{65} = \dfrac{63}{65}$ and $\cos\left(\sin^{-1}\dfrac{3}{5} - \cos^{-1}\dfrac{12}{13}\right) = \dfrac{63}{65}$

91. Use $\tan\theta = \dfrac{3}{4}$ and $\tan\beta = \dfrac{12}{5}$ in $\tan(\theta + \beta) = \dfrac{\tan\theta + \tan\beta}{1 - \tan\theta\tan\beta}$, therefore, $\tan x = -2 + \sqrt{2}$ and

$\tan\left(\tan^{-1}\dfrac{3}{4} + \tan^{-1}\dfrac{12}{5}\right) = \dfrac{\dfrac{3}{4} + \dfrac{12}{5}}{1 - \left(\dfrac{3}{4}\cdot\dfrac{12}{5}\right)} - \dfrac{63}{16}$

93. Since $\tan\theta = \dfrac{5}{12}$, then θ is in quadrant I. Sketch and label a triangle in quadrant I, with $x = 12$ and $y = 5$.

Use Pythagorean theorem to find r: $12^2 + 5^2 = r^2 \Rightarrow r^2 = 144+25 \Rightarrow r^2 = 169 \Rightarrow r = 13$. Since $\tan\beta = \dfrac{3}{4}$,

then β is in quadrant I. Sketch and label a triangle in quadrant I, with $x = 4$ and $y = 3$.

Use Pythagorean theorem to find y: $4^2 + 3^2 = r^2 \Rightarrow r^2 = 16+9 \Rightarrow r^2 = 25 \Rightarrow r = 5$.

Now $\cos(\theta - \beta) = \cos\theta\cos\beta + \sin\theta\sin\beta$, therefore, $\cos(\theta + \beta) = \dfrac{12}{13}\cdot\dfrac{4}{5} + \dfrac{5}{13}\cdot\dfrac{3}{5} = \dfrac{48}{65} + \dfrac{15}{65} = \dfrac{63}{65}$ and

$\cos\left(\tan^{-1}\dfrac{5}{12} - \tan^{-1}\dfrac{3}{4}\right) = \dfrac{63}{65}$

95. Since $\sin\theta = \dfrac{1}{2}$, then θ is in quadrant I. Sketch and label a triangle in quadrant I, with $y = 1$ and $r = 2$.

Use Pythagorean theorem to find x: $x^2 + 1^2 = 2^2 \Rightarrow x^2 = 4-1 \Rightarrow x^2 = 3 \Rightarrow x = \sqrt{3}$. Since $\tan\beta = (-3)$, then β is in quadrant IV. Sketch and label a triangle in quadrant IV, with $x = 1$ and $y = -3$. Use Pythagorean theorem to find r: $1^2 + (-3)^2 = r^2 \Rightarrow r^2 = 1+9 \Rightarrow r^2 = 10 \Rightarrow y = \sqrt{10}$. Now $\sin(\theta + \beta) = \sin\theta\cos\beta + \cos\theta\sin\beta$, therefore

$$\sin(\theta + \beta) = \frac{1}{2} \cdot \frac{1}{\sqrt{10}} + \frac{\sqrt{3}}{2} \cdot \frac{-3}{\sqrt{10}} = \frac{1}{2\sqrt{10}} + \frac{-3\sqrt{3}}{2\sqrt{10}} = \frac{\sqrt{10} - 3\sqrt{30}}{20} \text{ and } \sin\left(\sin^{-1}\frac{1}{2} - \tan^{-1}(-3)\right) = \frac{\sqrt{10} - 3\sqrt{30}}{20}$$

97. $\cos(\tan^{-1} 5) \approx 0.894427191$

99. $\tan(\arcsin .12251014) \approx 0.1234399811$

101. $\sec(\cos^{-1} u) = \dfrac{1}{\cos(\cos^{-1} u)} = \dfrac{1}{u}$

103. Since $\cos\theta = u$, then θ is in quadrant I. Sketch and label a triangle in quadrant I, with $x = u$ and $r = 1$.

   Use Pythagorean theorem to find y: $u^2 + y^2 = 1^2 \Rightarrow y^2 = 1 - u^2 \Rightarrow y = \sqrt{1-u^2}$.

   Now $\sin\theta = \dfrac{\sqrt{1-u^2}}{1} = \sqrt{1-u^2}$ and $\sin(\arccos u) = \sqrt{1-u^2}$.

105. Since $\sin\theta = u$, then θ is in quadrant I. Sketch and label a triangle in quadrant I, with $y = u$ and $r = 1$.

   Use Pythagorean theorem to find x: $x^2 + u^2 = 1^2 \Rightarrow x^2 = 1 - u^2 \Rightarrow x = \sqrt{1-u^2}$.

   Now $\cot\theta = \dfrac{\sqrt{1-u^2}}{u}$ and $\cot(\arcsin u) = \dfrac{\sqrt{1-u^2}}{u}$.

107. Since $\sec\theta = \dfrac{u}{2}$, then θ is in quadrant I. Sketch and label a triangle in quadrant I, $x = 2$ and $r = u$.

   Use Pythagorean theorem to find y: $2^2 + y^2 = u^2 \Rightarrow y^2 = u^2 - 4 \Rightarrow y = \sqrt{u^2 - 4}$.

   Now $\sin\theta = \dfrac{\sqrt{u^2-1}}{u}$ and $\sin\left(\sec^{-1}\dfrac{u}{2}\right) = \dfrac{\sqrt{u^2-4}}{u}$.

109. Since $\theta\dfrac{u}{\sqrt{u^2+2}}$, then θ is in quadrant I. Sketch and label a triangle in quadrant I. Use $\sqrt{u^2+2}$ and Pythagorean theorem to find x. $x^2 u^2 = \left(\sqrt{u^2+2}\right)^2 \Rightarrow x^2 = u^2 + 2 - u^2 \Rightarrow x^2 = 2 \Rightarrow x = \sqrt{2}$. Now

   $\tan\theta = \dfrac{u}{\sqrt{2}} = \dfrac{u\sqrt{2}}{2}$ and $\tan\left(\sin^{-1}\dfrac{u}{\sqrt{u^2+2}}\right) = \dfrac{u\sqrt{2}}{2}$.

111. Since $\cos\theta = \dfrac{\sqrt{4-u^2}}{u}$, then θ is in quadrant I. Sketch and label a triangle in quadrant I. Use $x = \sqrt{4-u^2}$

   and Pythagorean theorem to find r. $\left(\sqrt{4-u^2}\right)^2 + u^2 = r^2 \Rightarrow r^2 = 4 - u^2 + u^2 \Rightarrow r^2 = 4 \Rightarrow r = 2$. Now

   $\sec\theta = \dfrac{2}{\sqrt{4-u^2}} = \dfrac{2\sqrt{4-u^2}}{4-u^2}$ and $\sec\left(\text{arc}\cot\dfrac{\sqrt{4-u^2}}{u}\right) = \dfrac{2\sqrt{4-u^2}}{4-u^2}$.

113. (a) $\theta = \arcsin\left(\sqrt{\dfrac{v^2}{2v^2+64(0)}}\right) = arcsin\left(\sqrt{\dfrac{v^2}{2v^2}}\right) = arcsin\sqrt{\dfrac{1}{4}} = \arcsin\dfrac{1}{\sqrt{2}} = 45°$

(b) $\theta = \arcsin\left(\sqrt{\dfrac{v^2}{2v^2+64(6)}}\right) = arcsin\left(\sqrt{\dfrac{v^2}{2v^2+384}}\right)$. As $v \to \infty$, $\sqrt{\dfrac{v^2}{2v^2+384}} \to \sqrt{\dfrac{1}{2}}$, therefore

$\theta = \arcsin\sqrt{\dfrac{1}{2}} = \arcsin\dfrac{1}{\sqrt{2}} = 45°$. The equation of the asymptote is $\theta = 45° = \cos 45°, x = y$.

115. (a) For $3: \theta = \tan^{-1}\left(\dfrac{3(3)}{(3)^2+4}\right) = \tan^{-1}\dfrac{9}{13} \approx 34.70 \approx 35°$

(b) For $6: \theta = \tan^{-1}\left(\dfrac{3(6)}{(6)^2+4}\right) = \tan^{-1}\dfrac{18}{40} = \tan^{-1}\dfrac{9}{20} \approx 24.23 \approx 24°$

(c) For $9: \theta = \tan^{-1}\left(\dfrac{3(9)}{(9)^2+4}\right) = \tan^{-1}\dfrac{27}{85} \approx 17.62 \approx 18°$

(d) Sketch and label the two triangles formed above the sight line. From this sketch $(\theta + a) = \dfrac{3+1}{x} = \dfrac{4}{x}$

and $\tan a = \dfrac{1}{x}$. Now use these values in the tangent of a sum identity

$\tan(\theta + a) = \dfrac{\tan\theta + \tan a}{1-\tan\theta \tan a} : \dfrac{4}{x} = \dfrac{\tan\theta + \dfrac{1}{2}}{1-(\tan\theta)\left(\dfrac{1}{x}\right)} \Rightarrow \dfrac{4}{x} = \dfrac{x\tan\theta + 1}{x-\tan\theta} \Rightarrow 4(x-\tan\theta+1) =$

$4x - 4\tan\theta = x^2\tan\theta + x \Rightarrow 4x - x = x^2\tan\theta + 4\tan\theta \Rightarrow 3x = \tan\theta(x^2+4) \Rightarrow$

$\tan\theta = \dfrac{3x}{x^2+4} \Rightarrow \theta = \tan^{-1}\left(\dfrac{3x}{x^2+4}\right)$

(e) Graph $y_1 = \tan^{-1}\left(\dfrac{3x}{x^2+4}\right)$, Figure 115. The maximum value occurs when $x \approx 2$ feet.

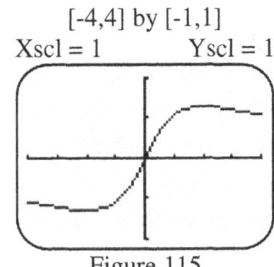

[-4,4] by [-1,1]
Xscl = 1   Yscl = 1

Figure 115

117. Let be the angle to the right of θ, and let β be the angle to the left of θ. Then $\beta + \theta + a = \pi$ and

$\theta = \pi - a - \beta$. Now from the picture $\tan a = \dfrac{150}{x}$, therefore $a = \tan^{-1}\left(\dfrac{105}{x}\right)$: and $\tan\beta = \dfrac{75}{100-x}$,

470   CHAPTER 9   Trigonometric Identities and Equations

therefore $\beta = \tan^{-1}\left(\dfrac{75}{100-x}\right)$. As a result: $\theta = \pi - \tan^{-1}\left(\dfrac{150}{x}\right) - \tan^{-1}\left(\dfrac{75}{100-x}\right) =$

$\pi - \arctan\left(\dfrac{150}{x}\right) - \arctan\left(\dfrac{75}{100-x}\right)$.

Reviewing Basic Concepts (Sections 9.3 - 9.4)

1. Since $\dfrac{\pi}{2} < x < \pi$ and $\cos 2x = -\dfrac{5}{12}$, x is found in quadrant II. Now solve for x:

   $\cos 2x = 1 - 2\sin^2 x \Rightarrow -\dfrac{5}{12} = 1 - 2\sin^2 x \Rightarrow 2\sin^2 x = \dfrac{17}{12} \Rightarrow \sin^2 x = \dfrac{17}{24} \Rightarrow \sin x = \dfrac{\sqrt{17}}{\sqrt{24}}$

   (positive because in quadrant II) $\Rightarrow \sin x = \dfrac{\sqrt{17}}{2\sqrt{6}} \cdot \dfrac{\sqrt{6}}{\sqrt{6}} \Rightarrow \sin x = \dfrac{\sqrt{102}}{12}$. Sketch and label a triangle in

   quadrant II, with $y = \sqrt{102}$ and $r = 12$. Now use Pythagorean theorem to find θ. Therefore, since x is in

   quadrant II, $\tan x = -\dfrac{\sqrt{102}}{\sqrt{42}} = -\dfrac{\sqrt{102}}{\sqrt{42}} \cdot \dfrac{\sqrt{42}}{\sqrt{42}} = -\dfrac{\sqrt{4284}}{42} = -\dfrac{6\sqrt{119}}{42} \Rightarrow \tan x = -\dfrac{\sqrt{119}}{7}$.

2. Since $\sin\theta = -\dfrac{1}{3}$ and θ is in quadrant III. Sketch and label a triangle in quadrant III, with $y = -1$ and $r = 3$.

   Now use pythagorean theorem to find x: $x^2 + (-1)^2 = 3^2 \Rightarrow x^2 = 9 - 1 \Rightarrow x^2 = 8 \Rightarrow x = \sqrt{8} = 2\sqrt{2}$,

   Since x is in quadrant III, $x = -2\sqrt{2}$. Therefore, $\cos\theta = -\dfrac{2\sqrt{2}}{3}$. Now find:

   $\sin 2\theta = 2\sin\theta\cos\theta = 2\left(-\dfrac{1}{2}\right)\left(-\dfrac{2\sqrt{2}}{3}\right) = \dfrac{4\sqrt{2}}{9}$;

   $\cos 2\theta = 2\cos^2\theta - 1 = 2\left(-\dfrac{2\sqrt{2}}{3}\right)^2 - 1 = 2\left(\dfrac{8}{9}\right) - 1 = \dfrac{7}{9}$: $\tan 2\theta = \dfrac{\sin 2\theta}{\cos 2\theta} = \dfrac{\dfrac{4\sqrt{2}}{9}}{\dfrac{7}{9}} = \dfrac{4\sqrt{2}}{7}$.

3. $\sin 75° = \sin\dfrac{150°}{2} = \sqrt{\dfrac{1-\cos 150°}{2}} = \sqrt{\dfrac{1-\left(-\dfrac{\sqrt{3}}{2}\right)}{2} \cdot \dfrac{2}{2}} = \dfrac{\sqrt{2+\sqrt{3}}}{2}$ or:

   $\sin 75° = \sin(30°+45°) = \sin 30°\cos 45° + \cos 30°\sin 45° = \dfrac{1}{2}\cdot\dfrac{\sqrt{2}}{2} + \dfrac{\sqrt{3}}{2}\cdot\dfrac{\sqrt{2}}{2} = \dfrac{\sqrt{2}}{4} + \dfrac{\sqrt{6}}{4} = \dfrac{\sqrt{2}+\sqrt{6}}{4}$

4. $2\sin 25°\cos 150° = 2\left[\dfrac{1}{2}\left[\sin(25°+150°) + \sin(25°-150°)\right]\right] = \sin 175° + \sin(-125°) = \sin 175° - \sin 125°$

Section 9.4   471

5. (a) If the left side equals $\sin^2\dfrac{x}{2} = \left(\pm\sqrt{\dfrac{1-\cos x}{2}}\right)^2 = \dfrac{1-\cos x}{2}$, and the right side equals:

$\dfrac{\tan x - \sin x}{2\tan x} = \dfrac{\frac{\sin x}{\cos x} - \sin x}{2\frac{\sin x}{\cos x}} = \dfrac{\frac{\sin x}{\cos x} - \sin x}{2\frac{\sin x}{\cos x}} \cdot \dfrac{\cos x}{\cos x} = \dfrac{\sin x - \sin x \cos x}{2\sin x} = \dfrac{\sin x(1-\cos x)}{2\sin x} = \dfrac{1-\cos x}{2}$, then

$\sin^2\dfrac{x}{2} = \dfrac{\tan x - \sin x}{2\tan x}$.

(b) If the left side equals: $\dfrac{\sin 2x}{2\sin x} = \dfrac{2\sin x\cos x}{2\sin x} = \cos x$, and the right side equals:

$\cos^2\dfrac{x}{2} - \sin^2\dfrac{x}{2} = \left(\pm\sqrt{\dfrac{1+\cos x}{2}}\right)^2 - \left(\pm\sqrt{\dfrac{1-\cos x}{2}}\right)^2 = \dfrac{1+\cos x}{2} - \dfrac{1-\cos x}{2} =$

$\dfrac{1+\cos x - (1-\cos x)}{2} = \dfrac{2\cos x}{2} = \cos x$, then $\dfrac{\sin 2x}{2\sin x} = \cos^2\dfrac{x}{2} - \sin^2\dfrac{x}{2}$.

6. (a) $y = \arccos\dfrac{\sqrt{3}}{2} \Rightarrow \dfrac{\sqrt{3}}{2} = \cos y \Rightarrow y = \dfrac{\pi}{6}$

(b) $y = \sin^{-1}\left(-\dfrac{\sqrt{2}}{2}\right) \Rightarrow -\dfrac{\sqrt{2}}{2} = \sin y \Rightarrow y = -\dfrac{\pi}{4}$

7. (a) $\theta = \arccos .5 \Rightarrow .5 = \cos\theta \Rightarrow \theta = 60°$

(b) $\theta = \cot^{-1}(-1) \Rightarrow -1 = \cot\theta \Rightarrow \theta = 135°$

8. Graph $y = 2\csc^{-1} x$ like the graph of $y = \csc^{-1} x$, with a range $2\left(-\dfrac{\pi}{2},\dfrac{\pi}{2}\right) = (-\pi,\pi)$, see Figure 8.

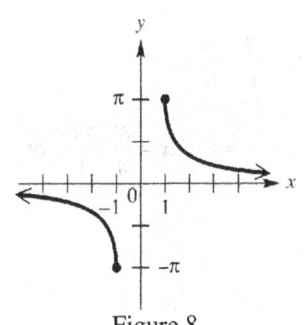

Figure 8

9. (a) Since $\sin\theta = -\dfrac{2}{3}$, then θ is in quadrant IV. Sketch and label a triangle in quadrant IV, with $y = -2$ and $r = 3$. Now use Pythagorean theorem to find $x: x^2 + (-2)^2 = 3^2 \Rightarrow x^2 = 9 - 4 \Rightarrow x^2 = 5 \Rightarrow x = \sqrt{5}$.

Therefore, $\cot\theta = \dfrac{\sqrt{5}}{-2} = -\dfrac{\sqrt{5}}{2}$ and $\cot\left(\arcsin\left(-\dfrac{2}{3}\right)\right) = -\dfrac{\sqrt{5}}{2}$.

(b) Since $\tan\theta = \dfrac{5}{12}$, then θ is in quadrant I. Sketch and label a triangle in quadrant I, with $x = 12$ and $y = 5$. Use Pythagorean theorem to find $r: 12^2 + 5^2 = r^2 = 144 + 25 \Rightarrow r^2 = 169 \Rightarrow r = 13$. Since

$\sin\beta = \dfrac{3}{5}$, then β is in quadrant I. Sketch and label a triangle in quadrant I, with $y = 3$ and $r = 5$. Use Pythagorean theorem to find $x: x^2 + 3^2 = 5^2 \Rightarrow r^2 = 25 - 9 \Rightarrow x^2 = 16 \Rightarrow x = 4$. Now $\cos(\theta - \beta) = \cos\theta\cos\beta + \sin\theta\sin\beta$, therefore, $\cos(\theta + \beta) = \dfrac{12}{13}\cdot\dfrac{4}{5} + \dfrac{5}{13}\cdot\dfrac{3}{5} = \dfrac{48}{65} + \dfrac{15}{65} = \dfrac{63}{65}$ and $\cos\left(\tan^{-1}\dfrac{5}{12} - \sin^{-1}\dfrac{3}{5}\right) = \dfrac{63}{65}$.

10. Since $\cot\theta = u$, then θ is in quadrant I. Sketch and label a triangle in quadrant I, with $x = u$ and $y = 1$. Use Pythagorean theorem to find $r: u^2 + 1^2 = r^2 \Rightarrow r^2 = u^2 + 1 \Rightarrow r = \sqrt{u^2 + 1}$. Now $\sin\theta = \dfrac{1}{\sqrt{u^2+1}} = \dfrac{1}{\sqrt{u^2+1}}\cdot\dfrac{\sqrt{u^2+1}}{\sqrt{u^2+1}} = \dfrac{\sqrt{u^2+1}}{u^2+1}$ and $\sin(\text{arccot } u) = \dfrac{\sqrt{u^2+1}}{u^2+1}$.

9.5: Trigonometric Equations and Inequalities (I)

1. $2\cos x + 1 = 0 \Rightarrow 2\cos x = -1 \Rightarrow \cos x = -\dfrac{1}{2} \Rightarrow x = \dfrac{2\pi}{3}, \dfrac{4\pi}{3}$. The solution set is $\left\{\dfrac{2\pi}{3}, \dfrac{4\pi}{3}\right\}$.

3. $5\sin x - 6 = 0 \Rightarrow 5\sin x = 6 \Rightarrow \sin x = \dfrac{6}{5} \Rightarrow x$ does not exist. The solution set is $\varnothing$.

5. $2\tan x + 1 = -1 \Rightarrow 2\tan x = -2 \Rightarrow \tan x = -1 \Rightarrow x = \dfrac{3\pi}{4}, \dfrac{7\pi}{4}$. The solution set is $\left\{\dfrac{3\pi}{4}, \dfrac{7\pi}{4}\right\}$.

7. $2\cos x + 5 = 6 \Rightarrow 2\cos x = 1 \Rightarrow \cos x = \dfrac{1}{2} \Rightarrow x = \dfrac{\pi}{3}, \dfrac{5\pi}{3}$. The solution set is $\left\{\dfrac{\pi}{3}, \dfrac{5\pi}{3}\right\}$.

9. $2\csc x + 4 = \csc x + 6 \Rightarrow \csc x = 2 \Rightarrow \sin x = \dfrac{1}{2} \Rightarrow x = \dfrac{\pi}{6}, \dfrac{5\pi}{6}$. The solution set is $\left\{\dfrac{\pi}{6}, \dfrac{5\pi}{6}\right\}$.

11. From the factored equation $(\cot x - 1)(\sqrt{3}\cot x + 1) = 0$, either $\cot x - 1 = 0 \Rightarrow \cot x = 1 \Rightarrow x = \dfrac{\pi}{4}, \dfrac{5\pi}{4}$, or $\sqrt{3}\cot x + 1 = 0 \Rightarrow \sqrt{3}\cot x = -1 \Rightarrow \cot x = -\dfrac{1}{\sqrt{3}} \Rightarrow \cot x = -\dfrac{\sqrt{3}}{3} \Rightarrow x = \dfrac{2\pi}{3}, \dfrac{5\pi}{3}$.

The solution set is $\left\{\dfrac{\pi}{4}, \dfrac{2\pi}{3}, \dfrac{5\pi}{4}, \dfrac{5\pi}{3}\right\}$.

13. First set the equation equal to zero and factor. $\cos x \cot x = \cos x \Rightarrow \cos x \cot x - \cos x = 0 \Rightarrow \cos x(\cot x - 1) = 0$. Now from this factored equation either $\cos x = 0 \Rightarrow x = \dfrac{\pi}{2}, \dfrac{3\pi}{2}$, or $\cot x - 1 = 0 \Rightarrow \cot x = 1 \Rightarrow x = \dfrac{\pi}{4}, \dfrac{5\pi}{4}$. The solution set is $\left\{\dfrac{\pi}{4}, \dfrac{\pi}{2}, \dfrac{5\pi}{4}, \dfrac{3\pi}{2}\right\}$.

15. First set the equation equal to zero and factor. $\sin^2 x - 2\sin x + 1 = 0 \Rightarrow (\sin x - 1)^2 = 0$. Now, from this factored equation, $\sin x - 1 = 0 \Rightarrow \sin x = 1 \Rightarrow x = \dfrac{\pi}{2}$. The solution set is $\left\{\dfrac{\pi}{2}\right\}$.

17. If $4(1+\sin x)(1-\sin x) = 3$, then $1-\sin^2 x = \dfrac{3}{4} \Rightarrow \cos^2 x = \dfrac{3}{4} \Rightarrow \cos x = \pm\dfrac{\sqrt{3}}{2} \Rightarrow x = \left\{\dfrac{\pi}{6}, \dfrac{5\pi}{6}, \dfrac{7\pi}{6}, \dfrac{11\pi}{6}\right\}$.

    The solution set is $\left\{\dfrac{\pi}{6}, \dfrac{5\pi}{6}, \dfrac{7\pi}{6}, \dfrac{11\pi}{6}\right\}$.

19. First set the equation equal to zero and factor. $\tan x + 1 = \sqrt{3} + \sqrt{3}\cot x \Rightarrow \tan x + 1 - \sqrt{3} - \dfrac{\sqrt{3}}{\tan x} = 0 \Rightarrow$

    $\tan^2 x + \tan(1-\sqrt{3}) - \sqrt{3} = 0 \Rightarrow (\tan x + 1)(\tan x - \sqrt{3}) = 0$. Now from this factored equation, either

    $\tan x + 1 = 0 \Rightarrow \tan x = -1 \Rightarrow x = \dfrac{3\pi}{4}, \dfrac{7\pi}{4}$, or $\tan x - \sqrt{3} = 0 \Rightarrow \tan x = \sqrt{3} \Rightarrow x = \dfrac{\pi}{3}, \dfrac{4\pi}{3}$.

    The solution set is $\left\{\dfrac{\pi}{3}, \dfrac{3\pi}{4}, \dfrac{4\pi}{3}, \dfrac{7\pi}{4}\right\}$.

21. First set the equation equal to zero and factor. $2\sin x - 1 = \csc x \Rightarrow 2\sin x - 1 - \dfrac{1}{\sin x} = 0 \Rightarrow$

    $2\sin^2 x - \sin x - 1 = 0 \Rightarrow (2\sin x + 1)(\sin x - 1) = 0$. From this factored equation, either

    $2\sin x + 1 = 0 \Rightarrow 2\sin x = -1 \Rightarrow \sin x = -\dfrac{1}{2} \Rightarrow x = \dfrac{7\pi}{6}, \dfrac{11\pi}{6}$, or $\sin x - 1 = 0 \Rightarrow \sin x = 1 \Rightarrow x = \dfrac{\pi}{2}$.

    The solution set is $\left\{x = \dfrac{\pi}{2}, \dfrac{7\pi}{6}, \dfrac{11\pi}{6}\right\}$.

23. $\cos^2 x - \sin^2 x = 1 \Rightarrow 1 - \sin^2 x - \sin^2 x = 1 \Rightarrow 1 - 2\sin^2 x = 1 \Rightarrow -2\sin^2 x = 0 \Rightarrow$

    $\sin^2 x = 0 \Rightarrow \sin x = 0 \Rightarrow x = 0, \pi$. The solution set is $\{0, \pi\}$.

25. (a) First simplify. $-2\cos x + 1 = 0 \Rightarrow -2\cos x = -1 \Rightarrow \cos x = \dfrac{1}{2}$. Now the reference angle is $\dfrac{\pi}{3}$ and x is

    found in quadrant I and IV; therefore, $f(x) = 0$ when $x = \dfrac{\pi}{3}, \dfrac{5\pi}{3}$.

    (b) Graph $y_1 = -2\cos x + 1$ on the calculator. From this graph, $f(x) > 0$ when the graph is above the x-

    axis; therefore, it is true for the interval $\left(\dfrac{\pi}{3}, \dfrac{5\pi}{3}\right)$.

    (c) Graph $y_1 = -2\cos x + 1$ on the calculator. From this graph, $f(x) < 0$ when the graph is below the x-

    axis; therefore, it is true for the interval $\left[0, \dfrac{\pi}{3}\right) \cup \left(\dfrac{5\pi}{3}, 2\pi\right)$.

27. (a) First simplify. $\tan^2 x - 3 = 0 \Rightarrow \tan^2 x = 3 \Rightarrow \tan x = \pm\sqrt{3}$. Now the reference angle is $\dfrac{\pi}{3}$ and x is found

    in all quadrants; therefore, $f(x) = 0$ when $x = \left\{\dfrac{\pi}{3}, \dfrac{2\pi}{3}, \dfrac{4\pi}{3}, \dfrac{5\pi}{3}\right\}$.

474   CHAPTER 9   Trigonometric Identities and Equations

(b) Graph $y_1 = \tan^2 x - 3$ on the calculator. From this graph, the asymptotes are $\frac{\pi}{2}$ and $\frac{3\pi}{2}$, and $f(x) > 0$ when the graph is above the x-axis; therefore, it is true for the interval $\left(\frac{\pi}{3}, \frac{\pi}{2}\right) \cup \left(\frac{\pi}{2}, \frac{2\pi}{3}\right) \cup \left(\frac{4\pi}{3}, \frac{3\pi}{2}\right) \cup \left(\frac{5\pi}{3}, 2\pi\right)$.

(c) Graph $y_1 = \tan^2 x - 3$ on the calculator. From this graph, $f(x) < 0$ when the graph is below the x-axis; therefore, it is true for the interval $\left[0, \frac{\pi}{3}\right) \cup \left(\frac{2\pi}{3}, \frac{4\pi}{3}\right) \cup \left(\frac{3\pi}{2}, \frac{5\pi}{3}\right)$.

29. (a) First, set the equation equal to zero, and factor. $2\cos^2 x - \sqrt{3}\cos x = 0 \Rightarrow \cos x\left(2\cos x - \sqrt{3}\right) = 0$. Now from this factored equation, either $\cos x = 0 \Rightarrow x = \frac{\pi}{2}, \frac{3\pi}{2}$, or $2\cos x - \sqrt{3} = 0 \Rightarrow$

$2\cos x = \sqrt{3} \Rightarrow \cos x = \frac{\sqrt{3}}{2}$; therefore, the reference angle is $\frac{\pi}{6}$. Since x is found in quadrant I and IV,

and $x = \frac{\pi}{6}, \frac{11\pi}{6}$, the solution for $f(x) = 0$ is true when $x = \left\{\frac{\pi}{6}, \frac{\pi}{2}, \frac{3\pi}{2}, \frac{11\pi}{6}\right\}$.

(b) Graph $y_1 = 2\cos^2 x - \sqrt{3}\cos x$ on the calculator. From this graph, $f(x) > 0$ when the graph is above the x-axis; therefore, it is true for the interval $\left(0, \frac{\pi}{6}\right) \cup \left(\frac{\pi}{2}, \frac{3\pi}{2}\right) \cup \left(\frac{11\pi}{6}, 2\pi\right)$.

(c) Graph $y_1 = 2\cos^2 x - \sqrt{3}\cos x$ on the calculator. From this graph, $f(x) < 0$ when the graph is below the x-axis; therefore, it is true for the interval $\left(\frac{\pi}{6}, \frac{\pi}{2}\right) \cup \left(\frac{3\pi}{2}, \frac{11\pi}{6}\right)$.

31. (a) First, set the equation equal to zero, and factor. $\sin^2 x \cos x - \cos x = 0 \Rightarrow \cos x\left(\sin^2 x - 1\right) = 0$.

Now, from this factored equation, either $\cos x = 0 \Rightarrow x = \frac{\pi}{2}, \frac{3\pi}{2}$, or $\sin^2 x - 1 = 0 \Rightarrow$

$\sin^2 x = 1 \Rightarrow \sin x = \pm 1 \Rightarrow x = \frac{\pi}{2}, \frac{3\pi}{2}$; therefore, $f(x) = 0$ when $x = \left\{\frac{\pi}{2}, \frac{3\pi}{2}\right\}$.

(b) Graph $y_1 = \sin^2 x \cos x - \cos x$ on the calculator. From this graph, $f(x) > 0$ when the graph is above the x-axis; therefore, it is true for the interval $\left(\frac{\pi}{2}, \frac{3\pi}{2}\right)$.

(c) Graph $y_1 = \sin^2 x \cos x - \cos x$ on the calculator. From this graph, $f(x) < 0$ when the graph is below the x-axis; therefore, it is true for the interval $\left[0, \frac{\pi}{2}\right) \cup \left(\frac{3\pi}{2}, 2\pi\right)$.

33. $\tan\theta + \cot\theta = 0 \Rightarrow \tan\theta + \frac{1}{\tan\theta} = 0 \Rightarrow \tan^2\theta + 1 = 0 \Rightarrow \tan^2\theta = -1 \Rightarrow \tan\theta$ does not exist, The solution set is $\varnothing$.

35. $2\tan^2\theta\sin\theta - \tan^2\theta = 0 \Rightarrow \tan^2\theta(2\sin\theta - 1) = 0 \Rightarrow \tan^2\theta = 0$ or $2\sin\theta - 1 = 0$;

$\tan^2\theta = 0 \Rightarrow \tan\theta = 0$ or $2\sin\theta - 1 = 0 \Rightarrow 2\sin\theta = 1 \Rightarrow \sin\theta = \frac{1}{2}$, Over the interval $[0°, 360°)$, the

equation $\tan\theta = 0$ has two solutions. These are $0°$ and $180°$. In the same interval, the equation $\sin\theta = \frac{1}{2}$

has two solutions, the angles in quadrants I and II that have a reference angle is $30°$. These are

$30°$ and $150°$. The solution set is $\{0°, 30°, 150°, 180°\}$.

37. $\sec^2\theta\tan\theta = 2\tan\theta \Rightarrow \sec^2\theta\tan\theta - 2\tan\theta = 0 \Rightarrow \tan\theta(\sec^2\theta - 2) = 0 \Rightarrow \tan\theta = 0$ or $\sec^2\theta - 2 = 0$;

$\sec^2\theta - 2 = 0 \Rightarrow \sec^2\theta = 2 \Rightarrow \sec\theta = \pm\sqrt{2}$, Over the interval $[0°, 360°)$, the equation $\tan\theta = 0$ has two

solutions. These are $0°$ and $180°$. In the same interval, the equation $\sec\theta = \sqrt{2}$ has two solutions, the

angles in quadrants I and IV that have a reference angle is $45°$. These are $45°$ and $315°$. The equation

$\sec\theta = -\sqrt{2}$ has two solutions, the angles in quadrants II and III that have a reference angle of $45°$. These

are $135°$ and $225°$ The solution set is $\{0°, 45°, 135°, 180°, 225°, 315°\}$.

39. $9\sin^2\theta - 6\sin\theta = 1 \Rightarrow 9\sin^2\theta - 6\sin\theta - 1 = 0$, Using the quadratic formula with $a = 9$, $b = -6$, and

$c = -1$. $\sin\theta = \dfrac{6 \pm \sqrt{36 - 4(9)(-1)}}{2(9)} = \dfrac{6 \pm \sqrt{36 + 36}}{18} = \dfrac{6 \pm \sqrt{72}}{18} = \dfrac{6 \pm 6\sqrt{2}}{18} = \dfrac{1 \pm \sqrt{2}}{3}$; The quadrant I

angle is $\sin^{-1}\left(\dfrac{1+\sqrt{2}}{3}\right) \approx 53.6°$. The quadrant II angle is approximately $180° - 53.6° = 126.4°$. The

other solution is $\sin^{-1}\left(\dfrac{1-\sqrt{2}}{3}\right) \approx -7.9°$. Since this angle is not in the interval $[0°, 360°)$ we will use the

reference angle $7.9°$ to find angles in Quadrant III and IV. The quadrant III angle is approximately

$180° + 7.9° = 187.9°$. The quadrant IV angle is approximately $360° - 7.9° = 352.1°$. The solution set is

$\{53.6°, 126.4°, 187.9°, 352.1°\}$.

41. $\tan^2\theta + 4\tan\theta + 2 = 0$, Using the quadratic formula with $a = 1$, $b = 4$, and $c = 2$.

$\tan\theta = \dfrac{-4 \pm \sqrt{16 - 4(1)(2)}}{2(1)} = \dfrac{-4 \pm \sqrt{16-8}}{2} = \dfrac{-4 \pm \sqrt{8}}{2} = \dfrac{-4 \pm 2\sqrt{2}}{2} = -2 \pm \sqrt{2}$; The quadrant II

angle is $\tan^{-1}(-2+\sqrt{2}) \approx -30.4°$. Since this angle is not in the interval $[0°, 360°)$ we will use the reference angle 30.4° to find angles in Quadrant II and IV. The quadrant II angle is approximately $180° - 30.4° = 149.6°$. The quadrant IV angle is approximately $360° - 30.4° = 329.6°$. The other solution is $\tan^{-1}(-2-\sqrt{2}) \approx -73.7°$. Since this angle is not in the interval $[0°, 360°)$ we will use the reference angle 73.7° to find angles in Quadrant II and IV. The quadrant II angle is approximately $180° - 73.7° = 106.3°$. The quadrant IV angle is approximately $360° - 73.7° = 286.3°$. The solution set is $\{106.3°, 149.6°, 286.3°, 329.6°\}$.

43. $\sin^2 \theta - 2\sin \theta + 3 = 0$, Using the quadratic formula with $a = 1$, $b = -2$, and $c = 3$

$$\sin \theta = \frac{2 \pm \sqrt{4 - 4(1)(3)}}{2(1)} = \frac{2 \pm \sqrt{4-12}}{2} = \frac{2 \pm \sqrt{-8}}{2} = \frac{2 \pm 2i\sqrt{2}}{2} = 1 \pm i\sqrt{2}$$; Since the result is not a real number, the equation has no real solutions. The solution set is the empty set.

45. $\cot \theta + 2\csc \theta = 3 \Rightarrow \dfrac{\cos \theta}{\sin \theta} + \dfrac{2}{\sin \theta} = 3 \Rightarrow \cos \theta + 2 = 3\sin \theta \Rightarrow (\cos \theta + 2)^2 = (3\sin \theta)^2 \Rightarrow$

$\cos^2 \theta + 4\cos \theta + 4 = 9\sin^2 \theta \Rightarrow \cos^2 \theta + 4\cos \theta + 4 = 9(1 - \cos^2 \theta) \Rightarrow$

$\cos^2 \theta + 4\cos \theta + 4 = 9 - 9\cos^2 \theta \Rightarrow 10\cos^2 \theta + 4\cos \theta - 5 = 0$

We use the quadratic formula with $a = 10$, $b = 4$, and $c = -5$.

$$\cos \theta = \frac{-4 \pm \sqrt{4^2 - 4(10)(-5)}}{2(10)} = \frac{-4 \pm \sqrt{16 + 200}}{20} = \frac{-4 \pm \sqrt{216}}{20} = \frac{-4 \pm 6\sqrt{6}}{20} = \frac{-2 \pm 3\sqrt{6}}{10}$$

Since $\cos \theta = \dfrac{-2 + 3\sqrt{6}}{10} > 0$ (and less than 1), we will obtain two angles. One angle will be in quadrant I and the other will be in quadrant IV. Using a calculator, if $\cos \theta = \dfrac{-2 + 3\sqrt{6}}{10} \approx 0.53484692$, the quadrant I angle will be approximately 57.7°. The quadrant IV angle will be approximately $360° - 57.7° = 302.3°$.

Since $\cos \theta = \dfrac{-2 - 3\sqrt{6}}{10} < 0$ (and greater than –1), we will obtain two angles. One angle will be in quadrant II and the other will be in quadrant III. Using a calculator, if $\cos \theta = \dfrac{-2 - 3\sqrt{6}}{10} \approx -0.93484692$, the quadrant II angle will be approximately 159.2°. The reference angle is $180° - 159.2° = 20.8°$. Thus, the quadrant III angle will be approximately $180° + 20.8° = 200.8°$. Since the solution was found by squaring both sides of an equation, we must check that each proposed solution is a solution of the original equation. 302.3° and 200.8° do not satisfy our original equation. Thus, they are not elements of the solution set.

Solution set: {57.7°, 159.2°}

47. $\tan^3 x = 3\tan x \Rightarrow \tan^3 - 3\tan x = 0$.

48. First factor. $\tan^3 x - 3\tan x = 0 \Rightarrow \tan x(\tan^2 x - 3) = 0$. Now, from this factored equation, either

$\tan x = 0 \Rightarrow x = 0, \pi$, or $\tan^2 x - 3 = 0 \Rightarrow \tan^2 x = 3 \Rightarrow \tan x = \pm\sqrt{3} \Rightarrow x = \frac{\pi}{3}, \frac{2\pi}{3}, \frac{4\pi}{3}, \frac{5\pi}{3}$; therefore, the

solution set is $\left\{0, \frac{\pi}{3}, \frac{2\pi}{3}, \pi, \frac{4\pi}{3}, \frac{5\pi}{3}\right\}$.

49. $\frac{\tan^2 x}{\tan x} = \frac{3\tan x}{\tan x} \Rightarrow \tan^2 x = 3 \Rightarrow \tan x = \pm\sqrt{3} \Rightarrow x = \frac{\pi}{3}, \frac{2\pi}{3}, \frac{4\pi}{3}, \frac{5\pi}{3}$.

50. The answers do not agree. The solutions 0 and π were lost when dividing by $\tan x$.

51. First, put the equation in quadratic form, and factor.

$3\sin^2 x - \sin x = 2 \Rightarrow 3\sin^2 x - \sin x - 2 = 0 \Rightarrow (3\sin x + 2)(\sin x - 1) = 0$. From this factored form, either

$3\sin x + 2 = 0 \Rightarrow 3\sin x = -2 \Rightarrow \sin x = -\frac{2}{3}$, or $\sin x - 1 = 0 \Rightarrow \sin x = 1$. Now find x:

(i) For $\sin x = 1$: $x = \sin^{-1}(1) \Rightarrow 1 = \sin x \Rightarrow x = \frac{\pi}{2}$.

(ii) For $\sin x = -\frac{2}{3}$: find the reference angle (calculate in radian mode). $\sin^{-1}\left(\frac{2}{3}\right) \approx 0.7297$.

Since x is in quadrants III and IV, $x = \pi + 0.7297 \approx 3.87$, and $x = 2\pi - 0.7297 \approx 5.55$; therefore, $f(x) = 0$,

when $x = \left\{\frac{\pi}{2}, 3.87, 5.55\right\}$.

53. First, put the equation in quadratic form, and factor by the quadratic formula.

$\tan x = \frac{-4 \pm \sqrt{(4)^2 - 4(1)(2)}}{2(1)} = \frac{-4 \pm \sqrt{8}}{2} = \frac{-4 \pm 2\sqrt{2}}{2} \Rightarrow \tan x = -2 \pm \sqrt{2}$. Now find x:

(i) For $\tan x = -2 + \sqrt{2}$, find the reference angle (calculate in radian mode). $\tan^{-1}(-2 + \sqrt{2}) \approx 0.5299$.

Since x is found in quadrants II and IV, $x = \pi - 0.5299 \approx 2.61$, and $x = 2\pi - 0.5299 \approx 5.75$.

(ii) For $\tan x = -2 - \sqrt{2}$, find the reference angle (calculate in radian mode). $\tan^{-1}(-2 - \sqrt{2}) \approx 1.2859$.

Since x is found in quadrants II and IV, $x = \pi - 1.2859 \approx 1.86$, and $x = 2\pi - 1.2859 \approx 5.00$.

Therefore, $f(x) = 0$ when $x = \{1.86, 2.61, 5.00, 5.75\}$.

55. First, set the equation equal to zero, and factor by the quadratic formula:

$2\cos^2 x + 2\cos x = 1 \Rightarrow 2\cos^2 x + 2\cos x - 1 = 0 \Rightarrow \cos x = \frac{-2 \pm \sqrt{(2)^2 - 4(2)(-1)}}{2(2)} =$

$\frac{-2 \pm \sqrt{12}}{4} = \frac{-2 \pm 2\sqrt{3}}{4} \Rightarrow \cos x = \frac{-1 \pm \sqrt{3}}{2}$. Now find x:

(i) For $x = \frac{-1 + \sqrt{3}}{2}$, find the reference angle (calculate in radian mode): $\cos^{-1}\left(\frac{-1 \pm \sqrt{3}}{2}\right) \approx 1.196$. Since x

is found in quadrants I and IV, $x \approx 1.20$, and $x = 2\pi - 1.196 = 5.09$.

478   CHAPTER 9   Trigonometric Identities and Equations

(ii) For $x = \dfrac{-1-\sqrt{3}}{2}$, find the reference angle (calculate in radian mode): $\cos^{-1}\left(\dfrac{-1-\sqrt{3}}{2}\right) = \varnothing$, because $\dfrac{-1-\sqrt{3}}{2}$ is outside the range of $\cos x$.

Therefore, $f(x) = 0$ when $x = \{1.20, 5.09\}$.

57. First, set the equation equal to zero, then use identities to put it into the quadratic form and factor.
$\sec^2\theta = 2\tan\theta + 4 \Rightarrow \tan^2\theta + 1 - 2\tan\theta - 4 = 0 \Rightarrow \tan^2\theta - 2\tan\theta - 3 = 0 \Rightarrow (\tan\theta - 3)(\tan\theta + 1) = 0$. From this factored form, either $\tan\theta - 3 = 0 \Rightarrow \tan\theta = 3$, or $\tan\theta + 1 = 0 \Rightarrow \tan\theta = -1$; therefore, $\tan x = -1, 3$.
Now find x:

(i) For $\tan x = 3$, find the reference angle (calculate in degree mode): $\cos^{-1} 3 \approx 71.57°$. Since x is found in quadrants I and III, $x \approx 71.57°$ and $x = 180° + 71.57° = 251.57°$.

(ii) For $\tan x = -1$, find the reference angle (calculate in degree mode): $\tan^{-1}(-1) = 45°$. Since x is found in quadrants II and IV, $x = 180° - 45° = 135°$, and $x = 360° - 45° = 315°$.

Therefore, $f(x) = 0$ when $x = \{71.6°, 135°, 251.6°, 315°\}$.

59. Use identities to get the equation in quadratic form, and factor by the quadratic formula:
$2\sin\theta = 1 - 2\cos\theta \Rightarrow (2\sin\theta)^2 = (1-2\cos\theta)^2 \Rightarrow 4\sin^2\theta = 1 - 4\cos\theta + 4\cos^2\theta \Rightarrow$
$4(1-\cos^2\theta) = 1 - 4\cos\theta + 4\cos^2\theta \Rightarrow 4 - 4\cos^2\theta = 1 - 4\cos\theta + 4\cos^2\theta \Rightarrow$
$0 = 8\cos^2\theta - 4\cos\theta - 3 \Rightarrow \cos\theta = \dfrac{4 \pm \sqrt{(-4)^2 - 4(8)(-3)}}{2(8)} = \dfrac{4 \pm \sqrt{112}}{16} = \dfrac{4 \pm 4\sqrt{7}}{16} \Rightarrow \cos\theta = \dfrac{1 \pm \sqrt{7}}{4}$.

Now find x:

(i) For $\cos x = \dfrac{1+\sqrt{7}}{4}$, find the reference angle (calculate in degree mode). $\cos\theta = \dfrac{1+\sqrt{7}}{4} \Rightarrow$
$\cos\theta \approx 0.91143783 \Rightarrow \theta = \cos^{-1} 0.91143783 \approx 24.30°$. Since x is found in quadrants I and IV, $x \approx 24.30°$, and $x = 360° - 24.30 = 335.70°$.

(ii) For $\cos\theta = \dfrac{1-\sqrt{7}}{4}$, find the reference angle (calculate in degree mode). $\cos\theta = \dfrac{1-\sqrt{7}}{4} \Rightarrow$
$\cos\theta \approx -0.41143783 \Rightarrow \theta = \cos^{-1}(-0.41143783) \approx 65.70°$. Since x is found in quadrants II and III, $x = 180° - 65.70° \approx 114.30°$, and $x = 180° + 65.70° \approx 245.70°$.

Finally, since the equation was square, we will need to check each solution.
Check $24.30°$. $2\sin 24.30° \approx 0.82$, and $1 - 2\cos 24.30° \approx -0.82$; this is not a solution.
Check $114.30°$. $2\sin 114.30° \approx 1.82$, and $1 - 2\cos 114.30° \approx 1.82$; this is a solution.
Check $245.70°$. $2\sin 245.70° \approx -1.82$, and $1 - 2\cos 114.30° \approx 1.82$; this is not a solution.
Check $335.70°$. $2\sin 335.70° \approx -0.82$, and $1 - 2\cos 335.70° \approx -0.82$; this is a solution.
Therefore, $f(x) = 0$ when $x = \{114.3°, 335.7°\}$.

61. $\cos\theta + 1 = 0 \Rightarrow \cos\theta = -1 \Rightarrow \theta = 180°$ in the interval $[0°, 360°)$. The solution set is $\{180° + 360°n,$ where n is any integer$\}$.

63. $3\csc x - 2\sqrt{3} = 0 \Rightarrow 3\csc x = 2\sqrt{3} \Rightarrow \csc x = \dfrac{2\sqrt{3}}{3} \Rightarrow x = \dfrac{\pi}{3}, \dfrac{2\pi}{3}$ in the interval $[0, 2\pi)$.

  The solution set is $\left\{\dfrac{\pi}{3} + 2n\pi, \dfrac{2\pi}{3} + 2n\pi, \text{ where } n \text{ is any integer}\right\}$.

65. $6\sin^2\theta + \sin\theta = 1 \Rightarrow 6\sin^2\theta + \sin\theta - 1 = 0 \Rightarrow (3\sin\theta - 1)(2\sin\theta + 1) = 0 \Rightarrow$
   $\sin\theta = \dfrac{1}{3} \Rightarrow \theta \approx 19.5°$ or $\theta \approx 180° - 19.5° = 160.5°$ or $\sin\theta = -\dfrac{1}{2} \Rightarrow \theta = 210°$ or $\theta = 330°$

  The solution set is $\{19.5° + 360°n, 160.5° + 360°n, 210° + 360°n, 330° + 360°n, \text{ where } n \text{ is any integer}\}$.

67. $2\cos^2 x + \cos x - 1 = 0 \Rightarrow (2\cos x - 1)(\cos x + 1) = 0 \Rightarrow 2\cos x - 1 = 0 \Rightarrow$
   $\cos x = \dfrac{1}{2}$ or $\cos x + 1 = 0 \Rightarrow \cos x = -1$, Over the interval $[0, 2\pi)$, the equation $\cos x = \dfrac{1}{2}$ has two

   solutions. The angles in quadrants I and IV that have a reference angle of $\dfrac{\pi}{3}$ are $\dfrac{\pi}{3}$ and $\dfrac{5\pi}{3}$. In the same

   interval, $\cos x = -1$ when the angle is π. Thus, the solution set is $\left\{\dfrac{\pi}{3} + 2n\pi, \pi + 2n\pi,\right.$

   and $\left.\dfrac{5\pi}{3} + 2n\pi, \text{ where } n \text{ is any integer}\right\}$.

69. $\sin\theta\cos\theta - \sin\theta = 0 \Rightarrow \sin\theta(\cos\theta - 1) = 0 \Rightarrow \sin\theta = 0 \Rightarrow \theta = 0°$ or $\theta = 180°$ or $\cos\theta = 1 \Rightarrow \theta = 0°$
   The solution set is $\{180°n, \text{ where } n \text{ is any integer}\}$.

71. $\sin x(3\sin x - 1) = 1 \Rightarrow 3\sin^2 x - \sin x - 1 = 0$, We use the quadratic formula with $a = 3$, $b = -1$, and $c = -1$.
   $\sin x = \dfrac{-(-1) \pm \sqrt{(-1)^2 - 4(3)(-1)}}{2(3)} = \dfrac{1 \pm \sqrt{1 + 12}}{6} = \dfrac{1 \pm \sqrt{13}}{6}$, Since $\sin x = \dfrac{1 + \sqrt{13}}{6} > 0$ (and less than 1), we

   will obtain two angles. One angle will be in quadrant I and the other will be in quadrant II. Using a calculator,

   if $\sin x = \dfrac{1 + \sqrt{13}}{6} \approx 0.76759188$, the quadrant I angle will be approximately 0.8751.

   The quadrant II angle will be approximately $\pi - 0.8751 \approx 2.2665$. Since $\sin x = \dfrac{1 - \sqrt{13}}{6} < 0$ (and greater than

   -1), we will obtain two angles. One angle will be in quadrant III and the other will be in quadrant IV. Using a

   calculator, if $\sin x = \dfrac{1 - \sqrt{13}}{6} \approx -0.43425855$, then $x \approx -0.4492$. Since this solution is not in the interval

   $[0, 2\pi)$, we must use it as a reference angle to find angles in the interval. Our reference angle will be 0.4492.

   The angle in quadrant III will be approximately $\pi + 0.4492 \approx 3.5908$. The angle in quadrant IV will be

   approximately $2\pi - 0.4492 \approx 5.8340$. Thus, the solution set is $\{0.8751 + 2n\pi, 2.2665 + 2n\pi, 3.5908 + 2n\pi,$

   and $5.8340 + 2n\pi$, where n is any integer$\}$.

480   CHAPTER 9   Trigonometric Identities and Equations

73. $5 + 5\tan^2\theta = 6\sec\theta \Rightarrow 5(1+\tan^2\theta) = 6\sec\theta \Rightarrow 5\sec^2\theta = 6\sec\theta \Rightarrow 5\sec^2\theta - 6\sec\theta = 0 \Rightarrow$

$\sec\theta(5\sec\theta - 6) = 0 \Rightarrow \sec\theta = 0$ or $5\sec\theta - 6 = 0 \Rightarrow \sec\theta = \dfrac{6}{5}$, $\sec\theta = 0$ is an impossible value since the

secant function must be either ≥ 1 or ≤ -1. Since $\sec\theta = \dfrac{6}{5} > 1$, we will obtain two angles. One angle will be in

quadrant I and the other will be in quadrant IV. Using a calculator, if $\sec\theta = \dfrac{6}{5} = 1.2$, the quadrant I angle will

be approximately 33.6°. The quadrant IV angle will be approximately $360° - 33.6° = 326.4°$. Thus, the solution set is { $33.6° + 360°n$ and $326.4° + 360°n$, where n is any integer }.

75. $\dfrac{2\tan\theta}{3-\tan^2\theta} = 1 \Rightarrow 2\tan\theta = 3 - \tan^2\theta \Rightarrow \tan^2\theta + 2\tan\theta - 3 = 0 \Rightarrow (\tan\theta - 1)(\tan\theta + 3) = 0 \Rightarrow$

$\tan\theta - 1 = 0 \Rightarrow \tan\theta = 1$ or $\tan\theta + 3 = 0 \Rightarrow \tan\theta = -3$, Over the interval [0°, 360°), the equation $\tan\theta = 1$ has two solutions 45° and 225°. Over the same interval, the equation $\tan\theta = -3$ has two solutions that are approximately $-71.6° + 180° = 108.4°$ and $-71.6° + 360° = 288.4°$.

Thus, the solutions are $45° + 360°n$, $108.4° + 360°n$, $225° + 360°n$ and $288.4° + 360°n$, where n is any integer. Since the period of the tangent function is 180°, the solution set can also be written as { $45° + 180°n$ and $108.4° + 180°n$, where n is any integer }.

77. The equation $2x - 1 = 0$ has one solution. The equation $2\sin x - 1 = 0$ has an infinite number of solutions because the sine function is periodic.

79. Graph $y = 2\sin x - 1 + 2\cos x$ (not shown). The x-intercepts are $\{1.99, 5.86\}$.

81. Graph $y = 2\cos^3 x + \sin x + 1$ (not shown). The x-intercepts are $\{2.68, 4.46, 4.71\}$.

83. Graph $y = \ln x - \cos x$ (not shown). The x-intercept is $\{1.30\}$.

85. (a) $14 = \dfrac{35}{3} + \dfrac{7}{3}\sin\dfrac{2x\pi}{365} \Rightarrow \dfrac{7}{3} = \dfrac{7}{3}\sin\dfrac{2x\pi}{365} \Rightarrow 1 = \sin\dfrac{2x\pi}{365} \Rightarrow \dfrac{2x\pi}{365} = \dfrac{\pi}{2} \Rightarrow 4\pi x = 365\pi \Rightarrow x \approx 91.25$.

Fourteen hours of daylight will occur approximately 91.3 days after March 21, or on June 20.

(b) The minimum will occur when $\sin\dfrac{2\pi x}{365} = -1$; therefore, $\dfrac{2\pi x}{365} = \dfrac{3\pi}{2} \Rightarrow 4\pi x = 1095\pi \Rightarrow x \approx 273.75$.

The minimum hours of daylight will occur approximately 273.8 days after March 21, December 19.

(c) $10 = \dfrac{35}{3} + \dfrac{7}{3}\sin\dfrac{2\pi x}{365} \Rightarrow 30 = 35 + 7\sin\dfrac{2\pi x}{365} \Rightarrow -\dfrac{5}{7} = \sin\dfrac{2\pi x}{365}$. Now, for $\sin\dfrac{2\pi x}{365}$, find the reference

angle (calculate in radian mode): $\dfrac{2\pi x}{365} = \sin^{-1}\dfrac{5}{7} \Rightarrow \dfrac{2\pi x}{365} \approx 0.7956$. Since $\sin\dfrac{2\pi x}{365} = -\dfrac{5}{7}$, $\dfrac{2\pi x}{365}$ is found

in quadrants III and IV, and $\dfrac{2\pi x}{365} \approx \pi + 0.7956 \Rightarrow \dfrac{2\pi x}{365} \approx 3.9372 \Rightarrow x \approx 228.7$, or

$\frac{2\pi x}{365} \approx 5.4876 \Rightarrow x \approx 318.8$. There will be about 10 hours of daylight twice, and they are approximately 228.7 days after March 21, or on Nov 4, and 318.8 days after March 21, or on Feb 2.

87. First, put the equation in quadratic form, and then factor by the quadratic formula:

$$0.342(80)\cos\theta + 2\cos^2\theta = \frac{16(80)^2}{(60)^2} \Rightarrow 27.36\cos\theta + 2\cos^2\theta = \frac{256}{9} \Rightarrow 2\cos^2\theta + 27.36\cos\theta - \frac{256}{9} = 0 \Rightarrow$$

$$\cos\theta = \frac{-27.36 \pm \sqrt{748.5696 - 4(2)\left(-\frac{256}{9}\right)}}{2(2)} = \frac{-27.36 \pm 31.243}{4}.$$ Therefore,

$$\cos\theta = \frac{-27.36 + 31.243}{4} = 0.97075, \text{ or } \cos\theta = \frac{-27.36 - 31.243}{4} = -14.65.$$

Since the range of $\cos\theta$ is $-1 < \cos\theta < 1$, the only solution is $\theta = \cos^{-1}0.97075 \approx 13.892° \approx 14°$.

89. Let $s(t) = \frac{2+\sqrt{3}}{2}$, and find $\sin t$. $\sin t + 2\cos t = \frac{2+\sqrt{3}}{2} \Rightarrow 2\sin t + 4\cos t = 2+\sqrt{3} \Rightarrow$

$4\cos t = (2+\sqrt{3}) - 2\sin t \Rightarrow (4\cos t)^2 = \left((2+\sqrt{3}) - 2\sin t\right)^2 \Rightarrow$

$16\cos^2 t = (7+4\sqrt{3}) - 4(2+\sqrt{3})\sin t + 4\sin^2 t \Rightarrow 16(1-\sin^2 t) = (7+4\sqrt{3}) - 4(2+\sqrt{3})\sin t + 4\sin^2 t \Rightarrow$

$0 = 20\sin^2 t - 4(2+\sqrt{3})\sin t + (-9+4\sqrt{3}) \Rightarrow 0 = (2\sin t - \sqrt{3})(10\sin t - 4 + 3\sqrt{3})$. Now, when

$2\sin t - \sqrt{3} = 0 \Rightarrow 2\sin t = \sqrt{3} \Rightarrow \sin t = \frac{\sqrt{3}}{2}$, and when

$10\sin t - 4 + 3\sqrt{3} = 0 \Rightarrow 10\sin t = 4 - 3\sqrt{3} \Rightarrow \sin t = \frac{4-3\sqrt{3}}{10}$.

To find a solution, choose $\sin t = \frac{\sqrt{3}}{2}$, which yields $t = \frac{\pi}{3}$.

9.6: Trigonometric Equations and Inequalities (II)

1. Dividing each by 2 yields $x = \frac{\pi}{3}, \pi, \frac{4\pi}{3}$.

3. Use identities to solve for x. $\sin\frac{x}{2} = \cos\frac{x}{2} \Rightarrow \left(\sin\frac{x}{2}\right)^2 = \left(\cos\frac{x}{2}\right)^2 \Rightarrow$

$\frac{1-\cos x}{2} = \frac{1+\cos x}{2} \Rightarrow 1-\cos x = 1+\cos x \Rightarrow -2\cos x = 0 \Rightarrow x = \frac{\pi}{2}, \frac{3\pi}{2}$. Since both sides of the equation

have been squared, we must check each solution. Check $x = \frac{\pi}{2}$. $\sin\frac{\left(\frac{\pi}{2}\right)}{2} = \sin\frac{\pi}{4} = \frac{\sqrt{2}}{2}$, and

$\cos\frac{\frac{\pi}{2}}{2} = \cos\frac{\pi}{4} = \frac{\sqrt{2}}{2}$; therefore, $x = \frac{\pi}{2}$ is a solution. Check $x = \frac{3\pi}{2}$. $\sin\frac{\left(\frac{3\pi}{2}\right)}{2} = \sin\frac{3\pi}{4} = \frac{\sqrt{2}}{2}$, and

$\cos\frac{\left(\frac{3\pi}{2}\right)}{4} = -\frac{\sqrt{2}}{2}$; therefore, $x = \frac{3\pi}{2}$ is not a solution. The solution is $x = \frac{\pi}{2}$.

482   CHAPTER 9   Trigonometric Identities and Equations

5. Use identities to solve for x. $\sin^2\left(\dfrac{x}{2}\right) - 1 = 0 \Rightarrow \left(\dfrac{\sqrt{1-\cos x}}{2}\right)^2 - 1 = 0 \Rightarrow \dfrac{1-\cos x}{2} - 1 = 0 \Rightarrow$

   $1 - \cos x - 2 = 0 \Rightarrow -\cos x = 1 \Rightarrow \cos x = -1 \Rightarrow x = \pi$.

7. Use identities to solve for x. $\sin 2x = 2\cos^2 x \Rightarrow 2\sin x \cos x = 2\cos^2 x \Rightarrow$

   $2\sin x \cos x - 2\cos^2 x = 0 \Rightarrow 2\cos x (\sin x - \cos x) = 0$. Now, either $2\cos x = 0 \Rightarrow \cos x = 0 \Rightarrow x = \dfrac{\pi}{2}, \dfrac{3\pi}{2}$,

   $\sin x - \cos x = 0 \Rightarrow \sin x = \cos x \Rightarrow x = \dfrac{\pi}{4}, \dfrac{5\pi}{4}$. Therefore, $x = \dfrac{\pi}{4}, \dfrac{\pi}{2}, \dfrac{5\pi}{4}, \dfrac{3\pi}{2}$.

9. Use identities to solve for x. $\cos x - 1 = \cos 2x \Rightarrow \cos x - 1 = 2\cos^2 x - 1 \Rightarrow \cos x - 2\cos^2 x = 0 \Rightarrow$

   $\cos x (1 - 2\cos x) = 0$. Now, either $\cos x = 0 \Rightarrow x = \dfrac{\pi}{2}, \dfrac{3\pi}{2}$, or $1 - 2\cos x = 0 \Rightarrow$

   $-2\cos x = -1 \Rightarrow \cos x = \dfrac{1}{2} \Rightarrow x = \dfrac{\pi}{3}, \dfrac{5\pi}{3}$. Therefore, $x = \dfrac{\pi}{3}, \dfrac{\pi}{2}, \dfrac{3\pi}{2}, \dfrac{5\pi}{3}$.

11. Use identities to solve for x: $\sin 2x - \cos x = 0 \Rightarrow 2\sin x \cos x - \cos x = 0 \Rightarrow \cos x (2\sin x - 1) = 0$.

    Now, either $\cos x = 0 \Rightarrow x = \dfrac{\pi}{2}, \dfrac{3\pi}{2}$ or $2\sin x - 1 = 0 \Rightarrow$

    $2\sin x = 1 \Rightarrow \sin x = \dfrac{1}{2} \Rightarrow x = \dfrac{\pi}{6}, \dfrac{5\pi}{6}$. Therefore, $x = \dfrac{\pi}{2}, \dfrac{\pi}{6}, \dfrac{5\pi}{6}, \dfrac{3\pi}{2}$.

13. (a) If the required interval for x is $0 \leq x < 2\pi$, then $0 \leq 2x < 4\pi$. Therefore, if $\cos 2x = \dfrac{\sqrt{3}}{2}$, then

    $2x = \dfrac{\pi}{6}, \dfrac{11\pi}{6}, \dfrac{13\pi}{6}, \dfrac{23\pi}{6}$. Now, dividing each solution by 2 (or multiplying by ½) yields

    $x = \dfrac{\pi}{12}, \dfrac{11\pi}{12}, \dfrac{13\pi}{12}, \dfrac{23\pi}{12}$.

    (b) Using a calculator, the graph of $\cos 2x = \dfrac{\sqrt{3}}{2}$ is above the graph of $y = \dfrac{\sqrt{3}}{2}$ for the interval:

    $\left[0, \dfrac{\pi}{12}\right) \cup \left(\dfrac{11\pi}{12}, \dfrac{13\pi}{12}\right) \cup \left(\dfrac{23\pi}{12}, 2\pi\right)$.

15. (a) If the required interval for x is $0 \leq x < 2\pi$, then $0 \leq 3x < 6\pi$. Therefore, if $\sin 3x = -1$, then

    $3x = \dfrac{3\pi}{2}, \dfrac{7\pi}{2}, \dfrac{11\pi}{2}$. Now, dividing each solution by 3 (or multiplying by ⅓) yields $x = \dfrac{\pi}{2}, \dfrac{7\pi}{6}, \dfrac{11\pi}{6}$.

    (b) Using a calculator, the graph of $\sin 3x = -1$ is never below the graph of $y = -1$; therefore,

    the interval is ∅.

17. (a) First, solve for $\cos 2x$. $\sqrt{2}\cos 2x = -1 \Rightarrow \cos 2x = -\dfrac{1}{\sqrt{2}}$. If the required interval for x is $0 \le x < 2\pi$, then $0 \le 2x < 4\pi$. Therefore, if $\cos 2x = -\dfrac{1}{\sqrt{2}}$, then $2x = \dfrac{3\pi}{4}, \dfrac{5\pi}{4}, \dfrac{11\pi}{4}, \dfrac{13\pi}{4}$. Now dividing each solution by 2 (or multiplying by $\frac{1}{2}$) yields $x = \dfrac{3\pi}{8}, \dfrac{5\pi}{8}, \dfrac{11\pi}{8}, \dfrac{13\pi}{8}$.

(b) Using a calculator, the graph of $\sqrt{2}\cos 2x = -1$ intersects or is below the graph of $y = -1$ for the interval: $\left[\dfrac{3\pi}{8}, \dfrac{5\pi}{8}\right] \cup \left[\dfrac{11\pi}{8}, \dfrac{13\pi}{8}\right]$.

19. (a) First solve for $\sin\dfrac{x}{2}$. $\sin\dfrac{x}{2} = \sqrt{2} - \sin\dfrac{x}{2} \Rightarrow 2\sin\dfrac{x}{2} = \sqrt{2} \Rightarrow \sin\dfrac{x}{2} = \dfrac{\sqrt{2}}{2}$. If the required interval for x is $0 \le x < 2\pi$, then $0 \le \dfrac{x}{2} < \pi$. Therefore, if $\sin\dfrac{x}{2} = \dfrac{\sqrt{2}}{2}$, then $\dfrac{x}{2} = \dfrac{\pi}{4}, \dfrac{3\pi}{4}$.

Now multiplying each solution by 2 yields $x = \dfrac{\pi}{2}, \dfrac{3\pi}{2}$.

(b) Using a calculator, the graph of $y = \sin\dfrac{x}{2}$ is above the graph of $y = \sqrt{2} - \sin\dfrac{x}{2}$ for the interval: $\left(\dfrac{\pi}{2}, \dfrac{3\pi}{2}\right)$.

21. $\sqrt{2}\sin 3x - 1 = 0 \Rightarrow \sqrt{2}\sin 3x = 1 \Rightarrow \sin 3x = \dfrac{1}{\sqrt{2}} \Rightarrow \sin 3x = \dfrac{\sqrt{2}}{2}$. In quadrant I and II, sine is positive. Thus,

$3x = \dfrac{\pi}{4} + 2n\pi, \dfrac{3\pi}{4} + 2n\pi \Rightarrow x = \dfrac{\pi}{12} + \dfrac{2n\pi}{3}, \dfrac{\pi}{4} + \dfrac{2n\pi}{3}$

Solution set: $\left\{\dfrac{\pi}{12} + \dfrac{2n\pi}{3}, \dfrac{\pi}{4} + \dfrac{2n\pi}{3}, \text{ where } n \text{ is any integer}\right\}$

23. $\cos\dfrac{\theta}{2} = 1 \Rightarrow \dfrac{\theta}{2} = 0° + 360°n \Rightarrow \theta = 720°n$. Solution set: $\{720°n, \text{ where } n \text{ is any integer}\}$

25. $2\sqrt{3}\sin\dfrac{x}{2} = 3 \Rightarrow \sin\dfrac{x}{2} = \dfrac{3}{2\sqrt{3}} \Rightarrow \sin\dfrac{x}{2} = \dfrac{3\sqrt{3}}{6} \Rightarrow \sin\dfrac{x}{2} = \dfrac{\sqrt{3}}{2}$

Since $0 \le \theta < 2\pi$, $0° \le \dfrac{x}{2} < \pi$. Thus, $\dfrac{x}{2} = \dfrac{\pi}{3} + 2n\pi, \dfrac{2\pi}{3} + 2n\pi \Rightarrow x = \dfrac{2\pi}{3} + 4n\pi, \dfrac{4\pi}{3} + 4n\pi$

Solution set: $\left\{\dfrac{2\pi}{3} + 4n\pi, \dfrac{4\pi}{3} + 4n\pi, \text{ where } n \text{ is any integer}\right\}$

27. $2\sin\theta = 2\cos 2\theta \Rightarrow \sin\theta = \cos 2\theta \Rightarrow \sin\theta = 1 - 2\sin^2\theta \Rightarrow 2\sin^2\theta + \sin\theta - 1 = 0 \Rightarrow$
$(2\sin\theta - 1)(\sin\theta + 1) = 0 \Rightarrow 2\sin\theta - 1 = 0 \text{ or } \sin\theta + 1 = 0$

Over the interval $[0°, 360°)$, we have $2\sin\theta - 1 = 0 \Rightarrow 2\sin\theta = 1 \Rightarrow \sin\theta = \dfrac{1}{2} \Rightarrow \theta = 30°$ or $150°$

$\sin\theta + 1 = 0 \Rightarrow \sin\theta = -1 \Rightarrow \theta = 270°$, Solution set: $\{30° + 360°n, 150° + 360°n,$
$270° + 360°n$, where n is any integer$\}$

29. $1 - \sin x = \cos 2x \Rightarrow 1 - \sin x = 1 - 2\sin^2 x \Rightarrow 2\sin^2 x - \sin x = 0 \Rightarrow \sin x(2\sin x - 1) = 0$

Over the interval $[0, 2\pi)$, we have $\sin x = 0 \Rightarrow x = 0$ or π.

$2\sin x - 1 = 0 \Rightarrow \sin x = \dfrac{1}{2} \Rightarrow x = \dfrac{\pi}{6}$ or $\dfrac{5\pi}{6}$

Solution set: $\left\{ n\pi, \dfrac{\pi}{6} + 2n\pi, \dfrac{5\pi}{6} + 2n\pi, \text{ where } n \text{ is any integer} \right\}$

31. $3\csc^2 \dfrac{x}{2} = 2\sec x \Rightarrow \dfrac{3}{\sin^2 \dfrac{x}{2}} = \dfrac{2}{\cos x} \Rightarrow \sin^2 \dfrac{x}{2} = \dfrac{3}{2}\cos x \Rightarrow \dfrac{1 - \cos x}{2} = \dfrac{3}{2}\cos x \Rightarrow$

$1 - \cos x = 3\cos x \Rightarrow 1 = 4\cos x \Rightarrow \dfrac{1}{4} = \cos x$

Over the interval $[0, 2\pi)$, we have $\cos x = \dfrac{1}{4} \Rightarrow x = 1.3181$ or $x = 4.9651$

Solution set: $\{1.3181 + 2n\pi, 4.9651 + 2n\pi, \text{ where } n \text{ is any integer}\}$

33. $2 - \sin 2\theta = 4\sin 2\theta \Rightarrow 2 = 5\sin 2\theta \Rightarrow \sin 2\theta = \dfrac{2}{5} \Rightarrow \sin 2\theta = 0.4$ Since $0 \le \theta < 360°$, $0° \le 2\theta < 720°$.

In quadrant I and II, sine is positive. $\sin 2\theta = 0.4 \Rightarrow 2\theta = 23.6°, 156.4°, 383.6°, 516.4°$

Thus, $\theta = 11.8°, 78.2°, 191.8°, 258.2°$.

Solution set: $\{11.8° + 360°n, 78.2° + 360°n, 191.8° + 360°n, 258.2° + 360°n, \text{ where } n \text{ is any integer}\}$ or

$\{11.8° + 180°n, 78.2° + 180°n, \text{ where } n \text{ is any integer}\}$

35. $2\cos^2 2\theta = 1 - \cos 2\theta \Rightarrow 2\cos^2 2\theta + \cos 2\theta - 1 = 0 \Rightarrow (2\cos 2\theta - 1)(\cos 2\theta + 1) = 0$

Since $0 \le \theta < 360° \Rightarrow 0° \le 2\theta < 720°$, we have $2\cos 2\theta - 1 = 0 \Rightarrow 2\cos 2\theta = 1 \Rightarrow \cos 2\theta = \dfrac{1}{2}$. Thus,

$2\theta = 60°, 300°, 420°, 660° \Rightarrow \theta = 30°, 150°, 210°, 330°$ or $\cos 2\theta + 1 = 0 \Rightarrow \cos 2\theta = -1$

$2\theta = 180°, 540° \Rightarrow \theta = 90°, 270°$

Solution set: $\{30° + 360°n, 90° + 360°n, 150° + 360°n, 210° + 360°n, 270° + 360°n,$

$330° + 360°n, \text{ where } n \text{ is any integer}\}$ or $\{30° + 180°n, 90° + 180°n, 150° + 180°n, \text{ where } n \text{ is any integer}\}$

37. Graph $y = \sin x + \sin 3x - \cos x$. Using the capabilities of the calculator, the x-intercepts are
0.262, 1.309, 1.571, 3.403, 4.451, and 4.712.

39. Graph $y = \cos 2x + \cos x$. Using the capabilities of the calculator, the x-intercepts are 1.047, 3.142, and 5.236.

41. Graph $y = \cos\dfrac{x}{2} - 2\sin 2x$. Using the capabilities of the calculator, the x-intercepts are 0.259, 1.372, 3.142, 4.911, and 6.024.

43. Since $1 + \tan^2 x = \sec^2 x$, we will express the equation in terms of secant. $\sec 2x + \tan 2x = 2 \Rightarrow$
$\tan 2x = 2 - \sec 2x \Rightarrow \tan^2 2x = 4 - 4\sec x + \sec^2 2x \Rightarrow \sec^2 2x - 1 = 4 - 4\sec x + \sec^2 2x \Rightarrow$
$0 = 5 - 4\sec 2x \Rightarrow \sec 2x = \dfrac{5}{4} \Rightarrow \dfrac{1}{\cos 2x} = \dfrac{5}{4} \Rightarrow \cos 2x = \dfrac{4}{5}$. Multiply the inequality $0 \leq x < 2\pi$ by 2 to find the interval for 2x is $[0, 4\pi)$. Using a calculator and the fact that cosine is positive in quadrants I and IV, we get $2x \approx 0.64350111, 5.6396842, 6.9266864, 11.922870..$ Dividing by 2
$x \approx 0.321750555, 2.819421, 3.463342, 5.961435$. Check answers for extraneous solutions:
$\sec(2(0.32175055)) + \tan(2(0.32175055)) = 2$, $\sec(2(3.463342)) + \tan(2(3.463342)) = 2$,
$\sec(2(5.961435)) + \tan(2(5.961435)) \neq 2$, $\sec(2(2.8198421)) + \tan(2(2.8198421)) \neq 2$
Therefore, $x \approx 0.32175055, 3.463342$.

45. Since $\sin^2 x + \cos^2 x = 1 \Rightarrow \cos^2 x = 1 - \sin^2 x$, we will use this as a substitution in the equation below.
$\cos 2x = 1 - \sin 2x \Rightarrow \cos^2 2x = 1 - 2\sin 2x + \sin^2 2x \Rightarrow 1 - \sin^2 2x = 1 - 2\sin 2x + \sin^2 2x \Rightarrow$
$2\sin^2 2x - 2\sin 2x = 0 \Rightarrow 2\sin 2x(\sin 2x - 1) = 0 \Rightarrow 2\sin 2x = 0 \text{ or } \sin 2x - 1 = 0$. Multiply the inequality $0 \leq x < 2\pi$ by 2 to find the interval for 2x is $[0, 4\pi)$. We know that $x = 0, \dfrac{\pi}{2}, \pi, 2\pi, \dfrac{5\pi}{2}$. Dividing by 2.
$x = 0, \dfrac{\pi}{4}, \dfrac{\pi}{2}, \pi, \dfrac{5\pi}{4}$. Check answers for extraneous solutions: $\cos(2 \cdot 0) = 1 - \sin(2 \cdot 0) \Rightarrow 1 = 1$,
$\cos\left(2 \cdot \dfrac{\pi}{4}\right) = 1 - \sin\left(2 \cdot \dfrac{\pi}{4}\right) \Rightarrow 0 = 0$, $\cos\left(2 \cdot \dfrac{\pi}{2}\right) = 1 - \sin\left(2 \cdot \dfrac{\pi}{2}\right) \Rightarrow -1 \neq 0$, $\cos(2 \cdot \pi) = 1 - \sin(2 \cdot \pi) \Rightarrow 1 = 1$,
$\cos\left(2 \cdot \dfrac{5\pi}{4}\right) = 1 - \sin\left(2 \cdot \dfrac{5\pi}{4}\right) \Rightarrow 0 = 0$. Therefore, $x = 0, \dfrac{\pi}{4}, \pi, \dfrac{5\pi}{4}$.

47. The function $\dfrac{\tan 2\theta}{2} \neq \tan \theta$, because the 2 in 2θ is not a factor of the numerator. It is a factor in the argument of the tangent function.

49. (a) If $e = 0$, then $0 = 20\sin\left(\dfrac{\pi t}{4} - \dfrac{\pi}{2}\right)$. Since $\arcsin 0 = 0$, we can solve the following equation for t.
$\dfrac{\pi t}{4} - \dfrac{\pi}{2} = 0 \Rightarrow \dfrac{\pi t}{4} = \dfrac{\pi}{2} \Rightarrow 2\pi t = 4\pi \Rightarrow t = 2$ seconds.

(b) If $e = 10\sqrt{3}$, then $10\sqrt{3} = 20\sin\left(\dfrac{\pi t}{4} - \dfrac{\pi}{2}\right) \Rightarrow \dfrac{\sqrt{3}}{2} = \sin\left(\dfrac{\pi t}{4} - \dfrac{\pi}{2}\right)$. Since $\arcsin\dfrac{\sqrt{3}}{2} = \dfrac{\pi}{2}$, we can solve the following equation for t. $\dfrac{\pi t}{4} - \dfrac{\pi}{2} = \dfrac{\pi}{3} \Rightarrow \dfrac{\pi t}{4} = \dfrac{\pi}{3} + \dfrac{\pi}{2} \Rightarrow \dfrac{\pi t}{4} = \dfrac{10\pi}{12} \Rightarrow 12\pi t = 40\pi \Rightarrow t = \dfrac{10}{3}$ seconds.

51. (a) For $x = t$, graph $P(t) = 0.004\sin\left(2\pi(261.63)t + \dfrac{\pi}{7}\right)$. See Figure 51.

(b) $0 = 0.004\sin\left[2\pi(261.63)t + \dfrac{\pi}{7}\right] \Rightarrow 0 = \sin(1643.87t + 0.45)$. Since

$\sin(1643.87t + 0.45) = 0$, $1643.87t + 0.45 = n\pi$, where n is an integer, and $t = \dfrac{n\pi - 0.45}{1643.87}$. If $n = 0$, then $t \approx -0.000274$. If $n = 1$, then $t \approx 0.00164$. If $n = 2$, then $t \approx 0.00355$. If $n = 3$, then $t \approx 0.00546$. The only solutions for $t \in [0, 0.005]$ are $t = 0.00164, 0.00355$.

(c) Graph $y = \sin(1643.87t + 0.45)$ on the calculator. The x-intercepts are $t \approx 0.00164$ and 0.00355; therefore, from the graph, $P < 0$ for the interval $(0.00164, 0.00355)$.

(d) The inequality $P < 0$ implies that there is a decrease in pressure, so an eardrum would be vibrating outward.

[0,0.005] by [-0.005,0.005]   [0.15,1.15] by [-0.01,0.01]   [0.15,1.15] by [-0.01,0.01]
Xscl = 0.001   Yscl = 1   Xscl =0.05   Yscl =0.01   Xscl =0.05   Yscl =0.01

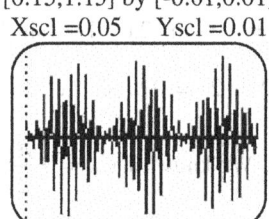
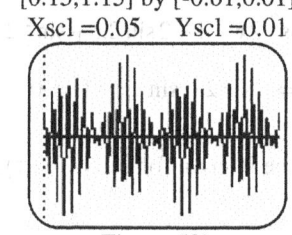

Figure 51   Figure 53a   Figure 53b

53. (a) For $x = t$, graph $P(t) = 0.005\sin 440\pi t + 0.005\sin 446\pi t$. See Figure 53a. There are 3 beats a second.

(b) For $x = t$, graph $P(t) = 0.005\sin 440\pi t + 0.005\sin 432\pi t$. See Figure 53b. There are 4 beats a second.

(c) The number of beats is equal to the absolute value of the difference in the frequencies of the two tones.

Reviewing Basic Concepts (Sections 9.5 - 9.6)

1. If the required interval for x is $0 \le x < 2\pi$, then $0 \le 2x < 4\pi$. Therefore, if $\cos 2x = \dfrac{\sqrt{3}}{2}$, then $2x = \dfrac{\pi}{6}, \dfrac{11\pi}{6}, \dfrac{13\pi}{6}, \dfrac{23\pi}{6}$. Now, dividing each solution by 2 (or multiplying by ½) yields $x = \dfrac{\pi}{12}, \dfrac{11\pi}{12}, \dfrac{13\pi}{12}, \dfrac{23\pi}{12}$.

2. First solve for $\sin x$. $2\sin x + 1 = 0 \Rightarrow 2\sin x = -1 \Rightarrow \sin x = -\dfrac{1}{2}$. If $\sin x = -\dfrac{1}{2}$, then $x = \dfrac{7\pi}{6}, \dfrac{11\pi}{6}$.

Section 9.6   487

3. Using the factored equation, either $\tan x - 1 = 0 \Rightarrow \tan x = 1 \Rightarrow x = \dfrac{\pi}{4}, \dfrac{5\pi}{4}, \ldots$ or

   $\cos x - 1 = 0 \Rightarrow \cos x = 1 \Rightarrow x = 0, 2\pi, \ldots$ Therefore, $x = 2n\pi, \dfrac{\pi}{4} + n\pi$ where n is any integer.

4. Solve for x. $2\cos^2 x = \sqrt{3}\cos x \Rightarrow 2\cos^2 x - \sqrt{3}\cos x = 0 \Rightarrow \cos x(2\cos x - \sqrt{3}) = 0$. Now, either

   $\cos x = 0 \Rightarrow x = \dfrac{\pi}{2}, \dfrac{3\pi}{2}, \ldots$ or $2\cos x - \sqrt{3} = 0 \Rightarrow 2\cos x = \sqrt{3} \Rightarrow \cos x = \dfrac{\sqrt{3}}{2} \Rightarrow x = \dfrac{\pi}{6}, \dfrac{11\pi}{6}, \ldots$ Therefore,

   $x = \dfrac{\pi}{6} + 2n\pi, \dfrac{\pi}{2} + n\pi, \dfrac{11\pi}{6} + 2n\pi$, where n is any integer.

5. First, set the equation equal to zero and factor by the quadratic formula.

   $3\cot^2 \theta - 3\cot \theta - 1 = 0 \Rightarrow \cot \theta = \dfrac{3 \pm \sqrt{(-3)^2 - 4(3)(-1)}}{2(3)} = \dfrac{3 \pm \sqrt{21}}{6}$. If $\cot \theta = \dfrac{3 \pm \sqrt{21}}{6}$, then

   $\tan \theta = \dfrac{6}{3 \pm \sqrt{21}}$. Now find θ.

   (i) For $\tan \theta = \dfrac{6}{3 + \sqrt{21}}$: Find the reference angle (calculate in degree mode). $\tan \theta = \dfrac{6}{3 + \sqrt{21}} \Rightarrow$

   $\tan \theta \approx 0.79128785 \Rightarrow \theta = \tan^{-1} 0.79128785 \approx 38.4°$. Since θ is found in quadrants I and III,

   $\theta \approx 38.4°$, and $\theta = 180° + 38.4 = 218.4°$.

   (ii) For $\tan \theta = \dfrac{6}{3 - \sqrt{21}}$: Find the reference angle (calculate in degree mode). $\tan \theta = \dfrac{6}{3 - \sqrt{21}} \Rightarrow$

   $\tan \theta \approx -3.79128785 \Rightarrow \theta = \tan^{-1}(-3.79128785) \approx 75.2°$. Since θ is found in quadrants II and IV,

   $\theta = 180° - 75.2° \approx 104.8°$, and $\theta = 360° - 75.2° \approx 284.8°$.

   Therefore, $\theta = 38.4°, 104.8°, 218.4°, 284.8°$.

6. First, factor by the quadratic formula. $4\cos^2 \theta + 4\cos \theta - 1 = 0 \Rightarrow$

   $\cos \theta = \dfrac{-4 \pm \sqrt{(4)^2 - 4(4)(-1)}}{2(4)} = \dfrac{-4 \pm \sqrt{32}}{8} = \dfrac{-4 \pm 4\sqrt{2}}{8} \Rightarrow \cos \theta = \dfrac{-1 \pm \sqrt{2}}{2}$. Now find x.

   (i) For $\cos \theta = \dfrac{-1 + \sqrt{2}}{2}$: find the reference angle (calculate in degree mode): $\cos \theta = \dfrac{-1 + \sqrt{2}}{2} \Rightarrow$

   $\cos \theta \approx 0.20710678 \Rightarrow \theta = \cos^{-1}(0.20710678) \approx 78.0°$. Since θ is found in quadrants I and IV,

   $\theta \approx 78.0°$, and $\theta = 360° - 78.0° = 282.0°$.

   (ii) For $\cos \theta = \dfrac{-1 - \sqrt{2}}{2}$, find the reference angle (calculate in degree mode). $\cos \theta = \dfrac{-1 - \sqrt{2}}{2} \Rightarrow$

   $\cos \theta \approx -1.207$. This value is outside the range of $\cos \theta$; therefore, $\emptyset$.

7. Use identities to solve for θ. $2\sin \theta - 1 = \csc \theta \Rightarrow 2\sin \theta - 1 = \dfrac{1}{\sin \theta} \Rightarrow 2\sin^2 \theta - \sin \theta = 1 \Rightarrow$

488 CHAPTER 9 Trigonometric Identities and Equations

$2\sin^2\theta - \sin\theta - 1 = 0 \Rightarrow (2\sin\theta + 1)(\sin\theta - 1) = 0$. Now, either $2\sin\theta + 1 = 0 \Rightarrow$

$2\sin\theta = -1 \Rightarrow \sin\theta = -\dfrac{1}{2} \Rightarrow \theta = 210°, 330°$, or $\sin\theta - 1 = 0 \Rightarrow \sin\theta = 1 \Rightarrow \theta = 90°$.

Therefore, $\theta = 90°, 210°, 330°$.

8. If $\sec^2\dfrac{\theta}{2} = 2$, then $\cos^2\dfrac{\theta}{2} = \dfrac{1}{2}$. If the required interval for θ is $0 \leq \theta < 360°$, then $0 \leq \dfrac{\theta}{2} < 180°$. If

$\cos\dfrac{\theta}{2} = \pm\dfrac{1}{\sqrt{2}} = \pm\dfrac{\sqrt{2}}{2}$, then $\dfrac{\theta}{2} = 45°, 135°$. Multiplying these solutions by 2 yields $\theta = 90°, 270°$.

9. Graph $y = x^2 + \sin x - x^3 - \cos x$. Using the capabilities of the calculator, the x-intercepts are

   $x \approx 0.68058878, 1.4158828$.

10. Graph $y_1 = x^3 - \cos^2 x$ and $y_2 = \dfrac{1}{2}x - 1$ in the same screen. Using the capabilities of the calculator, the

    intersection of these two graphs is $x \approx 0, 0.37600772$.

Chapter 9 Review Exercises

1. If $f(-x) = -f(x)$, then the function is an odd function, and (x, y) yields $(-x, -y)$. The following functions are odd: sine, tangent, cotangent, and cosecant.

2. If $f(-x) = f(x)$, then the function is an even function, and (x, y) yields $(-x, y)$. The following functions are even: cosine and secant.

3. Since cosine is an even function, $\cos(-x) = \cos x$, and $\cos(-3) = \cos 3$.

4. Since sine is an odd function, $\sin(-x) = -\sin x$, and $\sin(-3) = -\sin 3$.

5. Since tangent is an odd function, $\tan(-x) = -\tan x$, and $\tan(-3) = -\tan 3$.

6. Since secant is an even function $\sec(-x) = \sec x$, and $\sec(-3) = \sec 3$.

7. Since cosecant is an odd function, $\csc(-x) = -\csc x$, and $\csc(-3) = -\csc 3$.

8. Since cotangent is an odd function, $\cot(-x) = -\cot x$, and $\cot(-3) = -\cot 3$.

9. By reciprocal identity, $\sec x = \dfrac{1}{\cos x}$, therefore B.

10. By quotient identity, $\tan x = \dfrac{\sin x}{\cos x}$, therefore C.

11. By quotient identity, $\cot x = \dfrac{\cos x}{\sin x}$, therefore F.

12. By Pythagorean identity, $\tan^2 x + 1 = \sec^2 x = \dfrac{1}{\cos^2 x}$, therefore E.

13. By reciprocal identity, $\tan^2 x = \dfrac{1}{\cot^2 x}$, therefore D.

14. By reciprocal identity, $\csc x = \dfrac{1}{\sin x}$, therefore A.

15. $\dfrac{\cot\theta}{\sec\theta} = \dfrac{\frac{\cos\theta}{\sin\theta}}{\frac{1}{\cos\theta}} = \dfrac{\cos\theta}{\sin\theta}\cdot\dfrac{\cos\theta}{1} = \dfrac{\cos^2\theta}{\sin\theta}$.

16. $\tan^2\theta(1+\cot^2\theta) = \dfrac{\sin^2\theta}{\cos^2\theta}(\csc^2\theta) = \dfrac{\sin^2\theta}{\cos^2\theta}\left(\dfrac{1}{\sin^2\theta}\right) = \dfrac{1}{\cos^2\theta}$.

17. $\csc\theta + \cot\theta = \dfrac{1}{\sin\theta} + \dfrac{\cos\theta}{\sin\theta} = \dfrac{1+\cos\theta}{\sin\theta}$.

18. Since $x = \dfrac{3}{5}$, and x is in quadrant IV, $\sin x = -\sqrt{1-\cos^2 x}$; therefore,

    $\sin x = -\sqrt{1-\left(\dfrac{3}{5}\right)^2} = -\sqrt{1-\dfrac{9}{25}} = -\sqrt{\dfrac{16}{25}} = -\dfrac{4}{5}$. Now use these values to solve for

    $\tan x = \dfrac{\sin x}{\cos x} = \dfrac{-\frac{4}{5}}{\frac{3}{5}} = -\dfrac{4}{3}$, $\sec x = \dfrac{1}{\cos x} = \dfrac{5}{3}$, $\csc x = \dfrac{1}{\sin x} = -\dfrac{5}{4}$, $\cot x = -\dfrac{3}{4}$.

19. Since $x = -\dfrac{5}{4}$, and, since $\dfrac{\pi}{2} < x < \pi$, x is in quadrant II, $\sec x = -\sqrt{1+\tan^2 x} = -\sqrt{1+\dfrac{25}{16}} = -\sqrt{\dfrac{41}{16}} = -\dfrac{\sqrt{41}}{4}$.

    Now, use these to find the other functions.

    $\cos x = \dfrac{1}{\sec x} = -\dfrac{4}{\sqrt{41}} = -\dfrac{4\sqrt{41}}{41}$; $\cot x = \dfrac{1}{\tan x} = -\dfrac{4}{5}$; $\sin x = \sqrt{1-\cos^2 x} =$

    $\sqrt{1-\left(\dfrac{4\sqrt{41}}{41}\right)^2} = \sqrt{1-\dfrac{656}{1681}} = \sqrt{\dfrac{1025}{1681}} = \dfrac{5\sqrt{41}}{41}$; $\csc x = \dfrac{1}{\sin x} = \dfrac{41}{5\sqrt{41}}\cdot\dfrac{\sqrt{41}}{\sqrt{41}} = \dfrac{41\sqrt{41}}{5(41)} = \dfrac{\sqrt{41}}{5}$.

20. E, by a sum identity, $\cos 210° = \cos(150°+60°) = \cos 150°\cos 60° - \sin 150°\sin 60°$.

21. B, by a cofunctional identity, $\sin 35° = \cos(90°-35°) = \cos 55°$.

22. J, by a cofunctional identity, $\tan 35° = \tan(90°-(-35°)) = \cot 125°$.

23. A, by a negative number identity, $-\sin 35° = \sin(-35°)$.

24. I, by a negative number identity, $\cos 35° = \cos(-35°)$.

25. C, by a half-number identity, $\cos 75° = \cos\dfrac{150°}{2} = \sqrt{\dfrac{1+\cos 150°}{2}}$.

26. H, by a sum identity, $\sin 75° = \sin 15°\cos 60° + \cos 15°\sin 60°$.

27. D, by a double number identity, $\sin 300° = 2\sin 150°\cos 150°$.

28. G, by a double number identity, $\cos 300° = \cos(2\cdot 150°) = \cos^2 150° - \sin^2 150°$.

29. F, by a cofunctional identity, $\tan(-55°) = \cot(-35°)$.

30. $\sin^2 x - \sin^2 y = (1-\cos^2 x) - (1-\cos^2 y) = -\cos^2 x + \cos^2 y = \cos^2 y - \cos^2 x$.

31. $2\cos^3 x - \cos x = \cos x(2\cos^2 x - 1) = \dfrac{1}{\sec x}(\cos 2x) = \dfrac{\cos^2 x - \sin^2 x}{\sec x}$.

32. The right side of the equation equals $\dfrac{\sin 2x + \sin x}{\cos 2x - \cos x} = \dfrac{2\sin x\cos x + \sin x}{2\cos^2 x - 1 - \cos x} = \dfrac{\sin x(2\cos x + 1)}{(2\cos x + 1)(\cos x - 1)} = \dfrac{\sin x}{\cos x - 1}$.

    The left side of the equation equals $-\cot\dfrac{x}{2} = -\dfrac{1}{\tan\frac{x}{2}} = -\dfrac{1}{\frac{1-\cos x}{\sin x}} = \dfrac{-\sin x}{1-\cos x} = \dfrac{\sin x}{\cos x - 1}$. Since both sides of

    the equation equal the same expression, $-\cot\dfrac{x}{2} = \dfrac{\sin 2x + \sin x}{\cos 2x - \cos x}$.

33. The left side of the equation equals $\dfrac{\sin^2 x}{2 - 2\cos x} = \dfrac{1 - \cos^2 x}{2(1 - \cos x)} = \dfrac{(1-\cos x)(1+\cos x)}{2(1-\cos x)} = \dfrac{1 + \cos x}{2}$. The right

    side of the equation equals $\cos^2\dfrac{x}{2} = \left(\pm\sqrt{\dfrac{1+\cos x}{2}}\right)^2 = \dfrac{1+\cos x}{2}$. Since both sides of the equation equal the

    same expression, $\dfrac{\sin^2 x}{2 - 2\cos x} = \cos^2\dfrac{x}{2}$.

34. $\dfrac{\sin 2x}{\sin x} = \dfrac{2\sin x\cos x}{\sin x} = 2\cos x = \dfrac{2}{\sec x}$.

35. The right side of the equation equals $\cos A - \dfrac{\tan A}{\csc A} = \cos A - \dfrac{\frac{\sin A}{\cos A}}{\frac{1}{\sin A}} = \cos A - \dfrac{\sin^2 A}{\cos A} =$

    $\dfrac{\cos^2 A - \sin^2 A}{\cos A} = \dfrac{\cos 2A}{\cos A}$. The left side of the equation equals $2\cos A - \sec A = 2\cos A - \dfrac{1}{\cos A}$

    $= \dfrac{2\cos^2 A - 1}{\cos A} = \dfrac{\cos 2A}{\cos A}$. Since both sides of the equation equal the same expression,

    $2\cos A - \sec A = \cos A - \dfrac{\tan A}{\csc A}$.

36. $\dfrac{2\tan B}{\sin 2B} = \dfrac{\frac{2\sin B}{\cos B}}{2\sin B\cos B} = \dfrac{2\sin B}{\cos B} \cdot \dfrac{1}{2\sin B\cos B} = \dfrac{1}{\cos^2 B} = \sec^2 B$.

37. $2\tan\alpha\csc 2\alpha = \dfrac{2\sin\alpha}{\cos\alpha} \cdot \dfrac{1}{\sin 2\alpha} = \dfrac{2\sin\alpha}{\cos\alpha(2\sin\alpha\cos\alpha)} = \dfrac{1}{\cos^2\alpha} = \sec^2\alpha = 1 + \tan^2\alpha$.

38. $\cot\dfrac{t}{2} = \dfrac{1}{\tan\frac{t}{2}} = \dfrac{1}{\frac{1-\cos t}{\sin t}} = \dfrac{\sin t}{1 - \cos t}$.

39. $\dfrac{2\cot x}{\tan 2x} = \dfrac{2\cos x}{\sin x} + \dfrac{\sin 2x}{\cos 2x} = \dfrac{2\cos x}{\sin x} \cdot \dfrac{1 - 2\sin^2 x}{2\sin x\cos x} = \dfrac{1 - 2\sin^2 x}{\sin^2 x} = \dfrac{1}{\sin^2 x} - \dfrac{2\sin^2 x}{\sin^2 x} = \csc^2 x - 2$.

40. $\tan\theta\sin 2\theta = \dfrac{\sin\theta}{\cos\theta}(2\sin\theta\cos\theta) = 2\sin^2\theta = 2(1 - \cos^2\theta) = 2 - 2\cos^2\theta$.

41. $2\tan x\csc 2x - \tan^2 x = \tan x(2\csc 2x - \tan x) = \tan x\left(\dfrac{2}{\sin 2x} - \dfrac{\sin x}{\cos x}\right) =$

$$\tan x \left(\frac{2}{2\sin x \cos x} - \frac{\sin x}{\cos x} \right) = \tan x \left(\frac{2 - 2\sin^2 x}{2\sin x \cos x} \right) = \tan x \left(\frac{2(1-\sin^2 x)}{2\sin x \cos x} \right) =$$

$$\frac{\sin x}{\cos x} \cdot \left(\frac{\cos^2 x}{\sin x \cos x} \right) = \frac{\sin x}{\cos x} \cdot \frac{\cos x}{\sin x} = 1.$$

42. $y = \sin^{-1}\frac{\sqrt{2}}{2} \Rightarrow \frac{\sqrt{2}}{2} = \sin y \Rightarrow y = \frac{\pi}{4}.$ $\left(\text{range: } \left[-\frac{\pi}{2}, \frac{\pi}{2} \right] \right)$

43. $y = \arccos\left(-\frac{1}{2}\right) \Rightarrow -\frac{1}{2} = \cos y \Rightarrow y = \frac{2\pi}{3}.$ (range: $[0, \pi]$)

44. $y = \arctan\frac{\sqrt{3}}{3} \Rightarrow \frac{\sqrt{3}}{3} = \tan y \Rightarrow y = \frac{\pi}{6}.$ $\left(\text{range: } \left[-\frac{\pi}{2}, \frac{\pi}{2} \right] \right)$

45. $y = \sec^{-1}(-2) \Rightarrow y = \cos^{-1}\left(-\frac{1}{2}\right) \Rightarrow -\frac{1}{2} = \cos y \Rightarrow y = \frac{2\pi}{3}.$ $\left(\text{range: } \left[0, \frac{\pi}{2} \right) \cup \left(\frac{\pi}{2}, \pi \right] \right)$

46. $y = \text{arccsc}\frac{2\sqrt{3}}{3} \Rightarrow y = \arcsin\frac{3}{2\sqrt{3}} \Rightarrow y = \arcsin\frac{\sqrt{3}}{2} \Rightarrow \frac{\sqrt{3}}{2} = \sin y \Rightarrow y = \frac{\pi}{3}.$ $\left(\text{range: } \left[-\frac{\pi}{2}, 0 \right) \cup \left(0, \frac{\pi}{2} \right] \right)$

47. $y = \cot^{-1}(-1) \Rightarrow y = \tan^{-1}\left(\frac{1}{-1}\right) + \pi \Rightarrow y = \tan^{-1}(-1) + \pi \Rightarrow (-1 = \tan y) + \pi \Rightarrow$

$y = -\frac{\pi}{4} + \pi \Rightarrow y = \frac{3\pi}{4}.$ (range: $(0, \pi)$)

48. $\theta = \arccos\frac{1}{2} \Rightarrow \frac{1}{2} = \cos\theta \Rightarrow \theta = 60°.$ (range: $[0°, 180°]$)

49. $\theta = \arcsin\left(-\frac{\sqrt{3}}{2}\right) \Rightarrow -\frac{\sqrt{3}}{2} = \sin\theta \Rightarrow \theta = -60°.$ (range: $[-90°, 90°]$)

50. $\theta = \tan^{-1}(0) \Rightarrow 0 = \tan\theta \Rightarrow \theta = 0°.$ (range: $[-90°, 90°]$)

51. $\theta = \arcsin(-0.656059029) \Rightarrow \theta \approx -41°.$

52. $\theta = \arccos(0.7095707365) \Rightarrow \theta \approx 44.8°.$

53. $\theta = \arctan(-0.1227845609) \Rightarrow \theta \approx -7°.$

54. $\theta = \cot^{-1}(4.70463109) \Rightarrow \theta = \tan^{-1}\frac{1}{4.704630109} \Rightarrow \theta = \tan^{-1}(4.704630109)^{-1} \Rightarrow \theta \approx 12°.$

55. $\theta = \sec^{-1}(28.65370835) \Rightarrow \theta = \cos^{-1}\frac{1}{28.65370835} \Rightarrow \theta = \cos^{-1}(28.65370835)^{-1} \Rightarrow \theta \approx 88°.$

56. $\theta = \csc^{-1}(19.10732261) \Rightarrow \theta = \sin^{-1}\frac{1}{19.10732261} \Rightarrow \theta = \sin^{-1}(19.10732261)^{-1} \Rightarrow \theta \approx 3°.$

57. The value -3 is in the domain of the inverse tangent function but not in the domain of the inverse sine function.

58. The function $\cos x$ is defined for every real number, but $\arccos x$ is defined only on the interval $[-1,1]$. The function $\arccos(\cos x) = x$ only for x in the interval $[0,\pi]$.

59. Since $\sin(\sin^{-1} x) = x$ when $-1 < x < 1$, $\sin\left(\sin^{-1}\dfrac{1}{2}\right) = \dfrac{1}{2}$.

60. Since $\cos\theta = \dfrac{3}{4}$, θ is in quadrant I. Sketch and label a triangle in quadrant I, with $x = 3$ and $r = 4$. Now use the Pythagorean theorem to find y. $3^2 + y^2 = 4^2 \Rightarrow y^2 = 16 - 9 \Rightarrow y^2 = 7 \Rightarrow y = \sqrt{7}$.

    Therefore, $\sin\theta = \dfrac{\sqrt{7}}{4}$, and $\sin\left(\cos^{-1}\dfrac{3}{4}\right) = \dfrac{\sqrt{7}}{4}$.

61. Since $\tan\theta = \dfrac{3}{1}$, θ is in quadrant I. Sketch and label a triangle in quadrant I, with $x = 1$ and $y = 3$. Use the Pythagorean theorem to find r. $1^2 + 3^2 = r^2 \Rightarrow r^2 = 1 + 9 \Rightarrow r^2 = 10 \Rightarrow r = \sqrt{10}$.

    Therefore, $\cos\theta = \dfrac{1}{\sqrt{10}} = \dfrac{\sqrt{10}}{10}$, and $\cos(\arctan 3) = \dfrac{\sqrt{10}}{10}$.

62. Since $\theta = -\dfrac{1}{3}$, θ is in quadrant IV. Sketch and label a triangle in quadrant I, with $y = -1$ and $r = 3$. Use the Pythagorean theorem to find x. $x^2 + (-1)^2 = 3^2 \Rightarrow x^2 = 9 - 1 \Rightarrow x^2 = 8 \Rightarrow x = \sqrt{8} = 2\sqrt{2}$. Now,

    $\cos 2\theta = \cos^2\theta - \sin^2\theta$, thus $\cos 2\theta = \left(\dfrac{2\sqrt{2}}{3}\right)^2 - \left(-\dfrac{1}{3}\right)^2 = \dfrac{8}{9} - \dfrac{1}{9} = \dfrac{7}{9}$, and $\cos\left(2\sin^{-1}\dfrac{1}{3}\right) = \dfrac{7}{9}$;

    Finally, if $\cos\left(2\sin^{-1}\left(-\dfrac{1}{3}\right)\right) = \dfrac{7}{9}$, then $\sec\left(2\sin^{-1}\left(-\dfrac{1}{3}\right)\right) = \dfrac{9}{7}$.

63. Since $\cos\dfrac{3\pi}{2} = 0$, we can solve $\cos^{-1}(0) \Rightarrow 0 = \cos y \Rightarrow y = \dfrac{\pi}{2}$. Therefore, $\cos^{-1}\left(\cos\dfrac{3\pi}{2}\right) = \dfrac{\pi}{2}$.

64. Since $\sin\theta = \dfrac{3}{5}$, θ is in quadrant I. Sketch and label a triangle in quadrant I, with $y = 3$ and $r = 5$. Use the Pythagorean theorem to find x. $x^2 + 3^2 = 5^2 \Rightarrow x^2 = 25 - 9 \Rightarrow x^2 = 16 \Rightarrow x = 4$. Since $\cos\beta = \dfrac{5}{7}$, then β is in quadrant I. Sketch and label a triangle in quadrant I, with $x = 5$ and $r = 7$. Use the Pythagorean theorem to find y. $5^2 + y^2 = 7^2 \Rightarrow y^2 = 49 - 25 \Rightarrow y^2 = 24 \Rightarrow y = \sqrt{24} = 2\sqrt{6}$. Now use $\tan\theta = \dfrac{3}{4}$ and $\tan\beta = \dfrac{2\sqrt{6}}{5}$

    in $\tan(\theta+\beta) = \dfrac{\tan\theta + \tan\beta}{1 - \tan\theta\tan\beta}$; therefore, $\dfrac{\dfrac{3}{4} + \dfrac{2\sqrt{6}}{5}}{1 - \left(\dfrac{3}{4}\cdot\dfrac{2\sqrt{6}}{5}\right)} = \dfrac{\dfrac{3}{4} + \dfrac{2\sqrt{6}}{5}}{1 - \left(\dfrac{3}{4}\cdot\dfrac{2\sqrt{6}}{5}\right)} \cdot \dfrac{20}{20} = \dfrac{15 + 8\sqrt{6}}{20 - 6\sqrt{6}}$

    $= \dfrac{15 + 8\sqrt{6}}{20 - 6\sqrt{6}} \cdot \dfrac{20 + 6\sqrt{6}}{20 + 6\sqrt{6}} = \dfrac{588 + 250\sqrt{6}}{184} = \dfrac{294 + 125\sqrt{6}}{92}$. Therefore, $\tan\left(\sin^{-1}\dfrac{3}{5} + \cos^{-1}\dfrac{5}{7}\right) = \dfrac{294 + 125\sqrt{6}}{92}$.

65. Since $\theta = u$, θ is in quadrant I. Sketch and label a triangle in quadrant I, with $x = 1$ and $y = u$. Use the Pythagorean theorem to find r. $1^2 + u^2 = r^2 \Rightarrow r^2 = 1 + u^2 \Rightarrow r = \sqrt{u^2 + 1}$. Now $\sin\theta = \dfrac{u}{\sqrt{u^2+1}} = \dfrac{u\sqrt{u^2+1}}{u^2+1}$, and $\sin(\tan^{-1} u) = \dfrac{u\sqrt{u^2+1}}{u^2+1}$.

66. Since $\tan\theta = \dfrac{u}{\sqrt{1-u^2}}$, θ is in quadrant I. Sketch and label a triangle in quadrant I, $x = \sqrt{1-u^2}$ and $y = u$. Use the Pythagorean theorem to find r. $\left(\sqrt{1-u^2}\right)^2 + u^2 = r^2 \Rightarrow r^2 = 1 - u^2 + u^2 \Rightarrow r = 1$.

    Now $\cos\theta = \dfrac{\sqrt{1-u^2}}{1} = \sqrt{1-u^2}$, and $\cos\left(\arctan\dfrac{u}{\sqrt{1-u^2}}\right) = \sqrt{1-u^2}$.

67. Since $\cos\theta = \dfrac{u}{\sqrt{u^2+1}}$, θ is in quadrant I. Sketch and label a triangle in quadrant I, with $x = u$, and $r = \sqrt{u^2+1}$. Use the Pythagorean theorem to find y. $u^2 + y^2 = \left(\sqrt{u^2+1}\right)^2 \Rightarrow y^2 = u^2 + 1 - u^2 \Rightarrow y = 1$.

    Now $\tan\theta = \dfrac{1}{u}$ and $\tan(\arccos u) = \dfrac{1}{u}$.

68. $\sin^2 x = 1 \Rightarrow \sin x = \pm 1 \Rightarrow x = \dfrac{\pi}{2}, \dfrac{3\pi}{2}$. The solution set is $x = \left\{\dfrac{\pi}{2}, \dfrac{3\pi}{2}\right\}$.

69. $2\tan x - 1 = 0 \Rightarrow 2\tan x = 1 \Rightarrow \tan x = \dfrac{1}{2}$. Now, for $x = \dfrac{1}{2}$, find the reference angle (calculate in radian mode) $x = \tan^{-1}\left(\dfrac{1}{2}\right) \approx 0.463647609$. Since x is found in quadrants I and III, $x \approx 0.463647609$, and $x = \pi + 0.463647609 \approx 3.605240263$. The solution set is $x = \{0.463647609, 3.605240263\}$.

70. First, factor and solve for $\sin x$. $3\sin^2 x - 5\sin x + 2 = 0 \Rightarrow (3\sin x - 2)(\sin x - 1) = 0$. Now, either $3\sin x - 2 = 0 \Rightarrow 3\sin x = 2 \Rightarrow \sin x = \dfrac{2}{3}$, or $\sin x - 1 = 0 \Rightarrow \sin x = 1$. If $\sin x = \dfrac{2}{3}$, find the reference angle (calculate in radian mode) $x = \sin^{-1}\left(\dfrac{2}{3}\right) \approx 0.729726562$. Since x is found in quadrants I and II, $x \approx 0.729726562$, and $x = \pi - 0.729726562 \approx 2.411864997$. If $\sin x = 1$, then $x = \dfrac{\pi}{2}$. The solution is $x = 0.729726562, \dfrac{\pi}{2}, 2.411864997$.

71. Use identities to find $\tan x$. $\tan x = \cot x \Rightarrow \tan x = \dfrac{1}{\tan x} \Rightarrow \tan^2 x = 1 \Rightarrow \tan x = \pm 1$. If $\tan x = \pm 1$, then the solution is $x = \dfrac{\pi}{4}, \dfrac{3\pi}{4}, \dfrac{5\pi}{4}, \dfrac{7\pi}{4}$.

494 CHAPTER 9 Trigonometric Identities and Equations

72. First set equal to zero, factor, and solve for $\cot x$. $5\cot^2 x + 3\cot x = 2 \Rightarrow 5\cot^2 x + 3\cot x - 2 = 0 \Rightarrow$

    $(5\cot x - 2)(\cot x + 1) = 0$. Now, either $5\cot x - 2 = 0 \Rightarrow 5\cot x = 2 \Rightarrow \cot x = \dfrac{2}{5}$, or

    $\cot x + 1 = 0 \Rightarrow \cot x = -1$. If $\cot x = \dfrac{2}{5}$, then $\tan x = \dfrac{5}{2}$. Now find the reference angle in radian mode.

    $x = \tan^{-1}\left(\dfrac{5}{2}\right) \approx 1.19028995$. Since x is found in quadrants I and III, $x \approx 1.19028995$, and

    $x = \pi + 1.19028995 \approx 4.331882603$. If $\cot x = -1$, then $x = \dfrac{3\pi}{4}, \dfrac{7\pi}{4}$.

    The solutions are $x \approx 1.19028995, \dfrac{3\pi}{4}, 4.331882603, \dfrac{7\pi}{4}$.

73. Use identities to find $\cos x$. $\sec\dfrac{x}{2} = \cos\dfrac{x}{2} \Rightarrow \dfrac{1}{\cos\frac{x}{2}} = \cos\dfrac{x}{2} \Rightarrow 1 = \cos^2\dfrac{x}{2} \Rightarrow 1 = \left(\pm\sqrt{\dfrac{1+\cos x}{2}}\right)^2 \Rightarrow$

    $1 = \dfrac{1+\cos x}{2} \Rightarrow 2 = 1 + \cos x \Rightarrow \cos x = 1$. If $\cos x = 1$, then the solution is $x = 0$.

74. Use identities and factor. $\sin 2x = \cos 2x + 1 \Rightarrow \sin 2x - \cos 2x - 1 = 0 \Rightarrow$

    $2\sin x \cos x - (2\cos^2 x - 1) - 1 = 0 \Rightarrow 2\sin x \cos x - 2\cos^2 x = 0 \Rightarrow 2\cos x(\sin x - \cos x) = 0$. Now, either

    $2\cos x = 0 \Rightarrow \cos x = 0 \Rightarrow x = \dfrac{\pi}{2}, \dfrac{3\pi}{2}$, or $\sin x - \cos x = 0 \Rightarrow \sin x = \cos x \Rightarrow$

    $\cos^2 x = \sin^2 x \Rightarrow \cos^2 x = 1 - \cos^2 x \Rightarrow 2\cos^2 x = 1 \Rightarrow \cos^2 x = \dfrac{1}{2} \Rightarrow \cos x = \pm\dfrac{1}{\sqrt{2}} \Rightarrow x = \dfrac{\pi}{4}, \dfrac{3\pi}{4}, \dfrac{5\pi}{4}, \dfrac{7\pi}{4}$.

    Since we squared the equation to solve it, we need to check the second set of answers. The functions $\cos x$ and $\sin x$ have different signs in quadrants II and IV, so only $\dfrac{\pi}{4}$ and $\dfrac{5\pi}{4}$ will check.

    The solution is $x = \dfrac{\pi}{4}, \dfrac{3\pi}{4}, \dfrac{5\pi}{4}, \dfrac{7\pi}{4}$.

75. First solve for $\sin 2x$. $2\sin 2x = 1 \Rightarrow \sin 2x = \dfrac{1}{2}$. If the required interval for x is $0 \le x < 2\pi$, then

    $0 \le 2x < 4\pi$. Therefore, if $2x = \dfrac{1}{2}$, then $2x = \dfrac{\pi}{6}, \dfrac{5\pi}{6}, \dfrac{13\pi}{6}, \dfrac{17\pi}{6}$. Now, dividing each solution by 2

    (or multiplying by ½) yields $x = \dfrac{\pi}{12}, \dfrac{5\pi}{12}, \dfrac{13\pi}{12}, \dfrac{17\pi}{12}$.

76. Use identities and factor. $\sin 2x + \sin 4x = 0 \Rightarrow \sin 2x + 2\sin 2x \cos 2x = 0 \Rightarrow \sin 2x(1 + 2\cos 2x) = 0$. If the required interval for x is $0 \le x < 2\pi$, then $0 \le 2x < 4\pi$. Now, either $\sin 2x = 0 \Rightarrow 2x = 0, \pi, 2\pi, 3\pi$, or

$1+2\cos 2x = 0 \Rightarrow 2\cos 2x = -1 \Rightarrow 1+\cos 2x = -\frac{1}{2} \Rightarrow 2x = \frac{2\pi}{3}, \frac{4\pi}{3}, \frac{8\pi}{3}, \frac{10\pi}{3}$. Divide each solution by 2 (or multiply by ½) to get: $x = 0, \frac{\pi}{3}, \frac{\pi}{2}, \frac{2\pi}{3}, \pi, \frac{4\pi}{3}, \frac{3\pi}{2}, \frac{5\pi}{3}$.

77. Use identities and solve for x. $\cos x - \cos 2x = 2\cos x \Rightarrow -\cos x - (2\cos^2 x - 1) = 0 \Rightarrow$
$-\cos x - 2\cos^2 x + 1 = 0 \Rightarrow 2\cos^2 x + \cos x - 1 = 0 \Rightarrow (2\cos x - 1)(\cos x + 1) = 0$. Now, either
$2\cos x - 1 = 0 \Rightarrow 2\cos x = 1 \Rightarrow \cos x = \frac{1}{2} \Rightarrow x = \frac{\pi}{3}, \frac{5\pi}{3}$, or $\cos x + 1 = 0 \Rightarrow \cos x = -1 \Rightarrow x = \pi$.
The solution is $x = \frac{\pi}{3}, \pi, \frac{5\pi}{3}$.

78. If the required interval for x is $0 \le x < 2\pi$, then $0 \le 2x < 4\pi$. Therefore, if $\tan 2x = \sqrt{3}$, then
$2x = \frac{\pi}{3}, \frac{4\pi}{3}, \frac{7\pi}{3}, \frac{10\pi}{3}$. Now, dividing each solution by 2 (or multiplying by ½) yields $x = \frac{\pi}{6}, \frac{2\pi}{3}, \frac{7\pi}{6}, \frac{5\pi}{3}$.
Since we are looking for all solutions we can generalize the solution set as follows:
$\left\{\frac{\pi}{6} + n\pi, \frac{2\pi}{3} + n\pi, \text{ where } n \text{ is any integer}\right\}$

79. Factor to solve for $\cos\frac{x}{2}$. $\cos^2\frac{x}{2} - 2\cos\frac{x}{2} + 1 = 0 \Rightarrow \left(\cos\frac{x}{2} - 1\right)\left(\cos\frac{x}{2} - 1\right) = 0$. If the required interval for x is $0 \le x < 2\pi$, then $0 \le \frac{x}{2} < \pi$. If $\cos\frac{x}{2} - 1 = 0 \Rightarrow \cos\frac{x}{2} = 1 \Rightarrow \frac{x}{2} = 0$, then multiplying this by 2 yields the solution $x = 0$. Since we are looking for all solutions we can generalize the solution set as follows:
$\{2n\pi, \text{ where } n \text{ is any integer}\}$

80. Graph $y = \sin 2x - \cos 2x - 1$. From the calculator, the x intercepts are $\frac{\pi}{4}, \frac{\pi}{2}, \frac{5\pi}{4}, \frac{3\pi}{2}$.

   (a) For $\sin 2x > \cos 2x + 1$, the graph is above the x-axis for the interval $\left(\frac{\pi}{4}, \frac{\pi}{2}\right) \cup \left(\frac{5\pi}{4}, \frac{3\pi}{2}\right)$.

   (b) For $2x < \cos 2x + 1$, the graph is below the x-axis for the interval $\left[0, \frac{\pi}{4}\right) \cup \left(\frac{\pi}{2}, \frac{5\pi}{4}\right) \cup \left(\frac{3\pi}{2}, 2\pi\right)$.

81. (a) Let α be the angle to the left of θ, then $\tan\alpha = \frac{5}{x}$ and $\alpha = \arctan\frac{5}{x}$. Now,
$\tan(\alpha + \theta) = \frac{5+10}{x} \Rightarrow \alpha + \theta = \arctan\frac{15}{x} \Rightarrow \theta = \arctan\frac{15}{x} - \alpha \Rightarrow \theta = \arctan\frac{15}{x} - \arctan\frac{5}{x}$.

   (b) Graph $f(x) = \arctan\left(\frac{15}{x}\right) - \arctan\left(\frac{5}{x}\right)$. See Figure 81. The maximum occurs at $x \approx 8.6602567$.

[0,20] by [-1,1]   [0,0.01] by [-0.006,0.006]
Xscl = 1   Yscl = 1   Xscl = 0.001   Yscl = 0.001

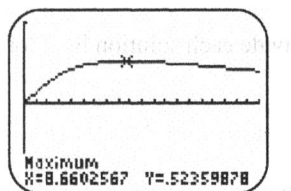

Figure 81

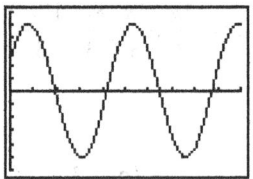

Figure 82

82. (a) Make sure your calculator is in radian mode. Let $A_1 = 0.0012$, $\phi_1 = 0.052$, $A_2 = 0.004$, and $\phi_2 = 0.61$.

$$A = \sqrt{(0.0012\cos.052 + 0.004\cos 0.61)^2 + (0.0012\sin 0.052 + 0.004\sin 0.61)^2} \approx 0.00506$$

$$\phi = \arctan\left(\frac{0.0012\sin 0.052 + 0.004\sin 0.61}{0.0012\cos 0.052 + 0.004\cos 0.61}\right) \approx 0.484$$

If $f = 220$, then $P = A\sin(2\pi ft + \phi)$ becomes $P = 0.00506\sin(440\pi t + 0.484)$.

(b) The two graphs are the same. See Figure 82.

83. $40 = 100\sin(2\pi \cdot 60)t \Rightarrow 0.4 = \sin 120\pi t \Rightarrow 120\pi t = \sin^{-1} 0.4 \Rightarrow t = \dfrac{\sin^{-1} 0.4}{120\pi} \Rightarrow t \approx 0.00109 \approx 0.001$ seconds.

84. $50 = 100\sin(2\pi \cdot 120)t \Rightarrow 0.5 = \sin 240\pi t \Rightarrow 240\pi t = \sin^{-1} 0.5 \Rightarrow t = \dfrac{\sin^{-1} 0.5}{240\pi} \Rightarrow t \approx 0.000694 \approx 0.0007$

seconds.

85. For $0.752 = \dfrac{\sin\theta_1}{\sin\theta_2}$, if $\theta_2 = 90°$, then $0.752 = \dfrac{\sin\theta_1}{\sin 90°} \Rightarrow 0.752 = \dfrac{\sin\theta_1}{1} \Rightarrow 0.752 = \sin\theta_1 \Rightarrow$

$\theta_1 = \sin^{-1} 0.752 \Rightarrow \theta_1 \approx 48.8°$.

86. If $\theta_1 > 48.8°$, then $\theta_2 > 90°$ and the light beam will stay completely under the water. The beam will be reflected at the surface of the water.

Chapter 9 Test

1. If $\sin y = -\dfrac{3}{5}$, and $\pi < y < \dfrac{3\pi}{2}$, then y is in quadrant III. Sketch and label a triangle in quadrant III, with $y = -3$ and $r = 5$. Use the Pythagorean theorem to find x.

$x^2 + (-3)^2 = 5^2 \Rightarrow x^2 = 25 - 9 \Rightarrow x^2 = 16 \Rightarrow x = \pm 4$. Because x is found in quadrant III, $x = -4$ Therefore, $\cos y = -\dfrac{4}{5}$. If $\cos x = -\dfrac{4}{5}$ and $\dfrac{\pi}{2} < x < \pi$, then x is in quadrant II. Sketch and label a triangle in quadrant II, with $x = -4$ and $r = 5$. Use the Pythagorean theorem to find y.

$(-4)^2 + y^2 = 5^2 \Rightarrow y^2 = 25 - 16 \Rightarrow y^2 = 9 \Rightarrow y = \pm 3$ Therefore, $\sin x = \dfrac{3}{5}$. Using these values,

$\sin(x+y) = \sin x \cos y + \cos x \sin y \Rightarrow \left(\dfrac{3}{5}\right)\left(-\dfrac{4}{5}\right) + \left(-\dfrac{4}{5}\right)\left(-\dfrac{3}{5}\right) = -\dfrac{12}{25} + \dfrac{12}{25} = 0.$

2. If $\sin y = -\dfrac{3}{5}$, and $\pi < y < \dfrac{3\pi}{2}$, then y is in quadrant III. Sketch and label a triangle in quadrant III, with $y = -3$ and $r = 5$. Use the Pythagorean theorem to find x.

   $x^2 + (-3)^2 = 5^2 \Rightarrow x^2 = 25 - 9 \Rightarrow x^2 = 16 \Rightarrow x = \pm 4$. Because x is found in quadrant III, $x = -4$. Therefore, $\cos y = -\dfrac{4}{5}$. If $\cos x = -\dfrac{4}{5}$ and $\dfrac{\pi}{2} < x < \pi$, then x is in quadrant II. Sketch and label a triangle in quadrant II, with $x = -4$ and $r = 5$. Use the Pythagorean theorem to find y.

   $(-4)^2 + y^2 = 5^2 \Rightarrow y^2 = 25 - 16 \Rightarrow y^2 = 9 \Rightarrow y = \pm 3$ Therefore, $\sin x = \dfrac{3}{5}$. Using these values,

   $\cos(x - y) = \cos x \cos y + \sin x \sin y \Rightarrow \left(-\dfrac{4}{5}\right)\left(-\dfrac{4}{5}\right) + \left(\dfrac{3}{5}\right)\left(-\dfrac{3}{5}\right) = \dfrac{16}{25} - \dfrac{9}{25} = \dfrac{7}{25}$.

3. If $\sin y = -\dfrac{3}{5}$, and $\pi < y < \dfrac{3\pi}{2}$, then y is in quadrant III. Sketch and label a triangle in quadrant III, with $y = -3$ and $r = 5$. Use the Pythagorean theorem to find x.

   $x^2 + (-3)^2 = 5^2 \Rightarrow x^2 = 25 - 9 \Rightarrow x^2 = 16 \Rightarrow x = \pm 4$. Because x is found in quadrant III, $x = -4$ Therefore, $\cos y = -\dfrac{4}{5}$. If $\cos x = -\dfrac{4}{5}$ and $\dfrac{\pi}{2} < x < \pi$, then x is in quadrant II. Using these values

   $\tan \dfrac{y}{2} = \dfrac{1 - \cos y}{\sin y} \Rightarrow \dfrac{1 - \left(-\dfrac{4}{5}\right)}{-\dfrac{3}{5}} = \dfrac{\dfrac{9}{5}}{-\dfrac{3}{5}} = -3$

4. If $\cos x = -\dfrac{4}{5}$ and $\dfrac{\pi}{2} < x < \pi$, then x is in quadrant II. Sketch and label a triangle in quadrant II, with $x = -4$ and $r = 5$. Use the Pythagorean theorem to find y.

   $(-4)^2 + y^2 = 5^2 \Rightarrow y^2 = 25 - 16 \Rightarrow y^2 = 9 \Rightarrow y = \pm 3$ Therefore, $\sin x = \dfrac{3}{5}$.

   Using these values $\cos 2x = 2\cos^2 x - 1 \Rightarrow 2\left(-\dfrac{4}{5}\right)^2 - 1 = \dfrac{32}{25} - \dfrac{25}{25} = \dfrac{7}{25}$.

5. $\tan^2 x - \sec^2 x = \dfrac{\sin^2 x}{\cos^2 x} - \dfrac{1}{\cos^2 x} = \dfrac{\sin^2 x - 1}{\cos^2 x} = -\dfrac{\cos^2 x}{\cos^2 x} = -1$.

6. Graph $y = \sec x - \sin x \tan x$ on the calculator. The graph looks like $\cos x$, so the identity is

   $\sec x - \sin x \tan x = \cos x$. Verify this: $\sec x - \sin x \tan x = \dfrac{1}{\cos x} - \dfrac{\sin x}{1} \cdot \dfrac{\sin x}{\cos x} = \dfrac{1 - \sin^2 x}{\cos x} = \dfrac{\cos^2 x}{\cos x} = \cos x$.

   Therefore, $\sec x - \sin x \tan x = \cos x$.

7. $\sec^2 B = \dfrac{1}{\cos^2 B} = \dfrac{1}{1 - \sin^2 B}$.

498   CHAPTER 9   Trigonometric Identities and Equations

8. $\dfrac{\cot A - \tan A}{\csc A \sec A} = \dfrac{\dfrac{\cos A}{\sin A} - \dfrac{\sin A}{\cos A}}{\dfrac{1}{\sin A} \cdot \dfrac{1}{\cos A}} = \dfrac{\cos^2 A - \sin^2 A}{\sin A \cos A} \cdot \dfrac{\sin A \cos A}{1} = \cos^2 A - \sin^2 A = \cos 2A.$

9. $\dfrac{\cos x + 1}{\sin x + \tan x} = \dfrac{\cos x + 1}{\sin x + \dfrac{\sin x}{\cos x}} = \dfrac{\cos x + 1}{\dfrac{\sin x \cos x + \sin x}{\cos x}} = \dfrac{\cos x (\cos x + 1)}{\sin x (\cos x + 1)} = \dfrac{\cos x}{\sin x} = \cot x.$

10. $\dfrac{\sec^2 x - 1}{1 + \tan^2 x} = \dfrac{\sec^2 x - 1}{\sec^2 x} = \dfrac{\sec^2 x}{\sec^2 x} - \dfrac{1}{\sec^2 x} = 1 - \cos^2 x = \sin^2 x.$

11. $\cos(270° - \theta) = \cos 270° \cos \theta + \sin 270° \sin \theta = 0 \cdot \cos \theta + (-1)\sin \theta = -\sin \theta.$

12. $\sin(\pi + \theta) = \sin \pi \cos \theta + \cos \pi \sin \theta = 0 \cdot \cos \theta + (-1)\sin \theta = -\sin \theta.$

13. (a) See Figure 13.

    (b) The domain is $[-1,1]$, the same as $f(x) = \sin^{-1} x$. The range is that of $f(x) = \sin^{-1} x$, multiplied by -2; therefore, it is $[-\pi, \pi]$.

    (c) The domain of $f(x) = -2\sin^{-1} x$ is $[-1,1]$, and 2 is not in this interval. (No number has sine value 2.)

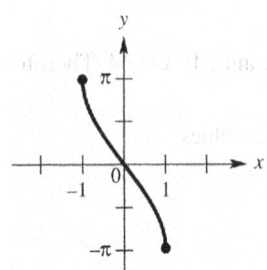

Figure 13

14. $y = \arccos\left(-\dfrac{1}{2}\right) \Rightarrow -\dfrac{1}{2} = \cos y \Rightarrow y = \dfrac{2\pi}{3}.$

15. $y = \tan^{-1}(0) \Rightarrow 0 = \tan y \Rightarrow y = 0.$

16. $y = \csc^{-1} \dfrac{2\sqrt{3}}{3} \Rightarrow \dfrac{2\sqrt{3}}{3} = \csc y \Rightarrow \sin y = \dfrac{3}{2\sqrt{3}} \Rightarrow \sin y = \dfrac{\sqrt{3}}{2} \Rightarrow y = \dfrac{\pi}{3}.$

17. Since $\sin\left(\dfrac{5\pi}{6}\right) = \dfrac{1}{2}$, $y = \sin^{-1}\left(\dfrac{1}{2}\right) \Rightarrow \dfrac{1}{2} = \sin y \Rightarrow y = \dfrac{\pi}{6}.$

18. Since $\sin \theta = \dfrac{2}{3}$, θ is in quadrant I. Sketch and label a triangle in quadrant I, with $y = 2$ and $r = 3$. Use the Pythagorean theorem to find x. $x^2 + 2^2 = 3^2 \Rightarrow x^2 = 9 - 4 \Rightarrow x^2 = 5 \Rightarrow x = \pm\sqrt{5}$. Therefore, $\cos \theta = \dfrac{\sqrt{5}}{3}$, and $\cos\left(\arcsin \dfrac{2}{3}\right) = \dfrac{\sqrt{5}}{3}.$

19. Since $\theta = \dfrac{1}{3}$, θ is in quadrant I. Sketch and label a triangle in quadrant I, with $x = 1$ and $r = 3$. Use the Pythagorean theorem to find y. $1^2 + y^2 = 3^2 \Rightarrow y^2 = 9 - 1 \Rightarrow y^2 = 8 \Rightarrow y = \pm\sqrt{8} = \pm 2\sqrt{2}.$

Now, $\sin 2\theta = 2\sin\theta\cos\theta$; therefore, $\sin 2\theta = 2\left(\dfrac{2\sqrt{2}}{3}\right)\left(\dfrac{1}{3}\right) = \dfrac{4\sqrt{2}}{9}$, and $\sin\left(2\cos^{-1}\dfrac{1}{3}\right) = \dfrac{4\sqrt{2}}{9}$.

20. $\sec(\cos^{-1} u) = \dfrac{1}{\cos(\cos^{-1} u)} = \dfrac{1}{u}$.

21. Since $\theta = \dfrac{u}{1}$, θ is in quadrant I. Sketch and label a triangle in quadrant I. Use $r = 1$, $y = u$, and the Pythagorean theorem to find x. $x^2 + u^2 = 1^2 \Rightarrow x^2 = 1 - u^2 \Rightarrow x = \sqrt{1-u^2}$. Now, $\tan\theta = \dfrac{u}{\sqrt{1-u^2}} = \dfrac{u\sqrt{1-u^2}}{1-u^2}$, and $\tan(\arcsin u) = \dfrac{u\sqrt{1-u^2}}{1-u^2}$.

22. Use identities to solve for θ. $\sin^2\theta = \cos^2\theta + 1 \Rightarrow 1 - \cos^2\theta = \cos^2\theta + 1 \Rightarrow 0 = 2\cos^2\theta \Rightarrow \cos\theta = 0 \Rightarrow \theta = \dfrac{\pi}{2}, \dfrac{3\pi}{2}$.

23. Use identities and factor. $\csc^2\theta - 2\cot\theta = 4 \Rightarrow 1 + \cot^2\theta - 2\cot\theta = 4 \Rightarrow \cot^2\theta - 2\cot\theta - 3 = 0 \Rightarrow (\cot\theta - 3)(\cot\theta + 1) = 0$. Now, either $\cot\theta - 3 = 0 \Rightarrow \cot\theta = 3$, or $\cot\theta + 1 = 0 \Rightarrow \cot\theta = -1$. If $\cot\theta = 3$, then $\tan\theta = \dfrac{1}{3} \Rightarrow \theta = \tan^{-1}\left(\dfrac{1}{3}\right)$. We find the reference angle in degree mode. $\tan^{-1}\left(\dfrac{1}{3}\right) \approx 18.4°$. Since θ is in quadrants I and III, $\theta \approx 18.4°$, and $\theta \approx 180° + 18.4° \approx 198.4°$. If $\cot\theta = -1 \Rightarrow \theta = 135°, 315°$, the solution set is $\theta \approx \{18.4°, 135°, 198.4°, 315°\}$.

24. Use identities and factor. $\cos x = \cos 2x \Rightarrow \cos x = 2\cos^2 x - 1 \Rightarrow 0 = 2\cos^2 x - \cos x - 1 \Rightarrow (2\cos x + 1)(\cos x - 1) = 0$. Now, either $2\cos x + 1 = 0 \Rightarrow 2\cos x = -1 \Rightarrow \cos x = -\dfrac{1}{2} \Rightarrow x = \dfrac{2\pi}{3}, \dfrac{4\pi}{3}$, or $\cos x - 1 = 0 \Rightarrow \cos x = 1 \Rightarrow x = 0$. Therefore, the solution set is $x = \left\{0, \dfrac{2\pi}{3}, \dfrac{4\pi}{3}\right\}$.

25. If the required interval for θ is $0° \leq \theta < 360°$, then $0° \leq \dfrac{\theta}{2} < 180°$.

    Now solve for $\dfrac{\theta}{2}$. $2\sqrt{3}\sin\dfrac{\theta}{2} = 3 \Rightarrow \sin\dfrac{\theta}{2} = \dfrac{3}{2\sqrt{3}} \Rightarrow \sin\dfrac{\theta}{2} = \dfrac{\sqrt{3}}{2} \Rightarrow \dfrac{\theta}{2} = 60°, 120°$. Finally, multiplying the solutions by 2 yields the solution $\theta = 120°, 240°$.

26. Graph $y = 2\sin x - 1$. Using the capabilities of the calculator, the x-intercepts are $\dfrac{\pi}{6}$ and $\dfrac{5\pi}{6}$. From the graph, $2\sin x - 1 \leq 0$, or the graph of the equation is below the x-axis for the interval $\left[0, \dfrac{\pi}{6}\right] \cup \left[\dfrac{5\pi}{6}, 2\pi\right)$.

27. (a) $2\sin x + 1 = 2 \Rightarrow 2\sin x = -1 \Rightarrow \sin x = -\dfrac{1}{2}$ then $x = \dfrac{7\pi}{6}, \dfrac{11\pi}{6}$. Since we are looking for all solutions we can generalize the solution set as follows: $\left\{\dfrac{7\pi}{6} + 2n\pi, \dfrac{11\pi}{6} + 2n\pi, \text{ where } n \text{ is any integer}\right\}$

(b) $\tan x + \sec x = 1 \Rightarrow \dfrac{\sin x}{\cos x} + \dfrac{1}{\cos x} = 1 \Rightarrow \sin x + 1 = \cos x \Rightarrow (\sin x + 1)^2 = \cos^2 x \Rightarrow$

$(\sin x + 1)^2 = 1 - \sin^2 x \Rightarrow \sin^2 x + 2\sin x + 1 = 1 - \sin^2 x \Rightarrow 2\sin^2 x + 2\sin x = 0 \Rightarrow \sin x(\sin x + 1) = 0 \Rightarrow$

$\sin x = 0$ or $\sin x = -1$. If $\sin x = -1$ then $\cos x = 0$ and $\sec x$ and $\tan x$ is undefined. If

$\sin x = 0$ then x is $0, \pi, 2\pi$. Since we are looking for all solutions we can generalize the solution set as

follows: $\{n\pi, \text{ where } n \text{ is any integer}\}$

(c) $\cos^2 x - \sin^2 x = \dfrac{1}{2} \Rightarrow (1 - \sin^2 x) - \sin^2 x = \dfrac{1}{2} \Rightarrow -2\sin^2 x = -\dfrac{1}{2} \Rightarrow \sin^2 x = \dfrac{1}{4} \Rightarrow \sin x = \pm\dfrac{1}{2}$ then

$x = \dfrac{\pi}{6}, \dfrac{5\pi}{6}, \dfrac{7\pi}{6}, \dfrac{11\pi}{6}$. Since we are looking for all solutions we can generalize the solution set as

follows: $\left\{\dfrac{\pi}{6} + n\pi, \dfrac{5\pi}{6} + n\pi \text{ where } n \text{ is any integer}\right\}$

28. (a) Since t will repeat every 12 months, the domain for 1 year will be $[0, 11]$. The function $T(x)$ is limited

by the range of cosine; at the minimum range of (-1), $50 + 50\cos(-1) = 0$, and at the maximum range

of (1), $50 + 50\cos(1) = 100$; therefore, the range of the function is $[0, 100]$ in hundreds.

(b) See Figure 28.

(c) From the graph, the maximum of 10,000 animals occurs at 0 or 12 months (July). The minimum of 0

animals occurs at 6 months (January).

(d) $T(3) = 50 + 50\cos\left(\dfrac{(3)\pi}{6}\right) = 50 + 50(0) = 50$ hundreds $= 5000$. There are 5000 animals at 3 months and

at 9 months. This is supported by the graph.

(e) $75 = 50 + 50\cos\left(\dfrac{\pi}{6}t\right) = 25 \Rightarrow 50\cos\left(\dfrac{\pi}{6}t\right) \Rightarrow \dfrac{1}{2} = \cos\left(\dfrac{\pi}{6}t\right) \Rightarrow \dfrac{\pi}{6}t = \dfrac{\pi}{3}$,

or $\dfrac{\pi}{6}t = \dfrac{5\pi}{3} \Rightarrow t = 2, 10$. At 2 months (September) and at 10 months (May), there will be 7500 animals.

(f) $T = 50 + 50\cos\left(\dfrac{\pi}{6}t\right) \Rightarrow T - 50 = 50\cos\left(\dfrac{\pi}{6}t\right) \Rightarrow \dfrac{T - 50}{50} = \cos\left(\dfrac{\pi}{6}t\right) \Rightarrow$

$\dfrac{\pi}{6}t = \arccos\left(\dfrac{T - 50}{50}\right) \Rightarrow t = \dfrac{6}{\pi}\arccos\left(\dfrac{T - 50}{50}\right)$.

[0,12] by [0,110]

Xscl = 1   Yscl = 10

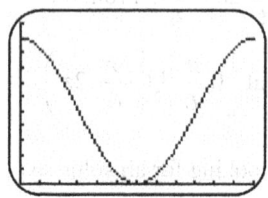

Figure 28

Chapter 10: Applications of Trigonometry and Vectors

10.1 The Law of Sines

1. The proportion shown in C is not valid because it cannot be written in the form of the Law of Sines.

3. The given information is AAS which does not result in the ambiguous case.

5. The given information is SSS which does not result in the ambiguous case.

7. The given information is SSA which results in the ambiguous case.

9. The given information is SSA which results in the ambiguous case.

11. Angle C has measure $180° - 60° - 75° = 45°$. Now, using the Law of Sines,

    $$\frac{a}{\sin 60°} = \frac{\sqrt{2}}{\sin 45°} \Rightarrow a = \frac{\sqrt{2}\sin 60°}{\sin 45°} \Rightarrow a = \frac{\sqrt{2} \cdot \frac{\sqrt{3}}{2}}{\frac{\sqrt{2}}{2}} \Rightarrow a = \frac{\frac{\sqrt{6}}{2}}{\frac{\sqrt{2}}{2}} \Rightarrow a = \frac{\sqrt{6}}{2} \cdot \frac{2}{\sqrt{2}} = \sqrt{3}.$$

13. Angle A has measure $180° - 120° - 15° = 45°$. Now, using the Law of Sines,

    $$\frac{a}{\sin 45°} = \frac{5}{\sin 120°} \Rightarrow a = \frac{5\sin 45°}{\sin 120°} \Rightarrow a = \frac{5 \cdot \frac{\sqrt{2}}{2}}{\frac{\sqrt{3}}{2}} \Rightarrow a = \frac{\frac{5\sqrt{6}}{2}}{\frac{3}{2}} \Rightarrow a = \frac{5\sqrt{6}}{3}.$$

15. Angle C has measure $180° - 37° - 48° = 95°$. Now, using the Law of Sines,

    $$\frac{a}{\sin 37°} = \frac{18}{\sin 95°} \Rightarrow a = \frac{18\sin 37°}{\sin 95°} \Rightarrow a \approx 10.87; \quad \frac{b}{\sin 48°} = \frac{18}{\sin 95°} \Rightarrow b = \frac{18\sin 48°}{\sin 95°} \Rightarrow b \approx 13.43.$$

    The solutions are $C = 95°$, $b \approx 13$ m, $a \approx 11$ m.

17. Angle B has measure $180° - 115.5° - 27.2° = 37.3°$. Now, using the Law of Sines,

    $$\frac{a}{\sin 27.2°} = \frac{76.0}{\sin 115.5°} \Rightarrow a = \frac{76.0\sin 27.2°}{\sin 115.5°} \Rightarrow a \approx 38.49;$$

    $$\frac{b}{\sin 37.3°} = \frac{76.0}{\sin 115.5°} \Rightarrow b = \frac{76.0\sin 37.3°}{\sin 115.5°} \Rightarrow b \approx 51.03. \text{ The solutions are } B = 37.3°, a \approx 38.5 \text{ ft}, b \approx 51.0 \text{ ft}.$$

19. Angle B has measure $180° - 37° - 95° = 48°$. Now, using the Law of Sines,

    $$\frac{a}{\sin 37°} = \frac{18}{\sin 95°} \Rightarrow a = \frac{18\sin 37°}{\sin 95°} \Rightarrow a \approx 10.87;$$

    $$\frac{b}{\sin 48°} = \frac{18}{\sin 95°} \Rightarrow b = \frac{18\sin 48°}{\sin 95°} \Rightarrow b \approx 13.43. \text{ The solutions are } B = 48°, a \approx 11 \text{ m}, b \approx 13 \text{ m}.$$

21. Angle A has measure $180° - 74.08° - 69.38° = 36.54°$. Now, using the Law of Sines,

    $$\frac{a}{\sin 36.54°} = \frac{45.38}{\sin 74.08°} \Rightarrow a = \frac{45.38\sin 36.54°}{\sin 74.08°} \Rightarrow a \approx 28.096;$$

    $$\frac{b}{\sin 69.38°} = \frac{45.38}{\sin 74.08°} \Rightarrow b = \frac{45.38\sin 69.38°}{\sin 74.08°} \Rightarrow b \approx 44.167.$$

    The solutions are $A = 36.54°$, $a \approx 28.10$ m, $b \approx 44.17$ m.

502   Chapter 10: Applications of Trigonometry and Vectors

23. Angle A has measure $180° - 38°40' - 91°40' = 49°40'$. Now, using the Law of Sines,

$$\frac{b}{\sin 38°40'} = \frac{19.7}{\sin 49°40'} \Rightarrow b = \frac{19.7 \sin 38°40'}{\sin 49°40'} \Rightarrow b \approx 16.146;$$

$$\frac{c}{\sin 91°40'} = \frac{19.7}{\sin 49°40'} \Rightarrow c = \frac{19.7 \sin 91°40'}{\sin 49°40'} \Rightarrow c \approx 25.832.$$

The solutions are $A = 49°40'$, $b \approx 16.1$ cm, $c \approx 25.8$ cm.

25. Angle C has measure $180° - 35.3° - 52.8° = 91.9°$. Now, using the Law of Sines,

$$\frac{a}{\sin 35.3°} = \frac{675}{\sin 52.8°} \Rightarrow a = \frac{675 \sin 35.3°}{\sin 52.8°} \Rightarrow a \approx 489.69;$$

$$\frac{c}{\sin 91.9°} = \frac{675}{\sin 52.8°} \Rightarrow c = \frac{675 \sin 91.9°}{\sin 52.8°} \Rightarrow c \approx 846.96.$$ The solutions are $C = 91.9°$, $a \approx 490$ ft, $c \approx 847$ ft.

27. Angle B has measure $180° - 39.70° - 30.35° = 109.95° \approx 110.0°$. Now, using the Law of Sines,

$$\frac{a}{\sin 39.70°} = \frac{39.74}{\sin 110.0°} \Rightarrow a = \frac{39.74 \sin 39.70°}{\sin 110.0°} \Rightarrow a \approx 27.01;$$

$$\frac{c}{\sin 30.35°} = \frac{39.74}{\sin 110.0°} \Rightarrow c = \frac{39.74 \sin 30.35°}{\sin 110.0°} \Rightarrow c \approx 21.37.$$

The solutions are $B = 110.0°$, $a \approx 27.01$ m, $c \approx 21.37$ m.

29. Angle A has measure $180° - 42.88° - 102.40° = 34.72°$. Now, using the Law of Sines,

$$\frac{a}{\sin 34.72°} = \frac{3974}{\sin 42.88°} \Rightarrow a = \frac{3974 \sin 34.72°}{\sin 42.88°} \Rightarrow a \approx 3326;$$

$$\frac{c}{\sin 102.40°} = \frac{3974}{\sin 42.88°} \Rightarrow c = \frac{3974 \sin 102.40°}{\sin 42.88°} \Rightarrow c \approx 5704.$$

The solutions are $A = 34.72°$, $a \approx 3326$ ft, $c \approx 5704$ ft.

31. Three given angles do not determine a unique triangle. Data set A does not determine a unique triangle.

33. (a) Consider the point (3, 0) which is on the x-axis and 4 units below the given point. If the length of the line segment is $4 < h < 5$, two triangles can be drawn. One triangle would intersect the x-axis to the left of (3, 0) and to the right of (0, 0), and the other would intersect the x-axis to the right of (3, 0).

    (b) A line segment with length $h = 4$ would form a single right triangle. Also, if $h \geq 5$, a single triangle would be formed with the line segment intersecting the positive x-axis to the right of (3, 0).

    (c) If $h < 4$, no triangle could be drawn because the line segment would not intersect the positive x-axis.

35. Using the Law of Sines, $\frac{\sin A}{31} = \frac{\sin 48°}{26} \Rightarrow \sin A = \frac{31 \sin 48°}{26} \Rightarrow A = \sin^{-1}\left(\frac{31 \sin 48°}{26}\right) \approx 62.4°$.

    Since $180° - 62.4° = 117.6°$ and $48° + 117.6° < 180°$, there are two triangles.

37. Using the Law of Sines, $\frac{\sin B}{61} = \frac{\sin 58°}{50} \Rightarrow \sin B = \frac{61 \sin 58°}{50} \Rightarrow B = \sin^{-1}\left(\frac{61 \sin 58°}{50}\right) \Rightarrow B \approx \sin^{-1}(1.03)$.

    Since 1.03 is not in the domain of the inverse sine function, no such angle exists.
    Thus no such triangle exists.

Section 10.1   503

39. Using the Law of Sines, $\dfrac{\sin B}{41.5} = \dfrac{\sin 29.7°}{27.2} \Rightarrow \sin B = \dfrac{41.5\sin 29.7°}{27.2} \Rightarrow B = \sin^{-1}\left(\dfrac{41.5\sin 29.7°}{27.2}\right)$

$\approx 49.1°$ or $180 - 49.1 = 130.9°$

If $B = 49.1$, $C = 180° - 29.7° - 49.1° = 101.2°$. If $B = 130.9°$, $C = 180° - 29.7° - 130.9° = 19.4°$.

The solutions are $B_1 = 49.1°$, $C_1 = 101.2°$ or $B_2 = 130.9°$, $C_2 = 19.4°$.

41. Using the Law of Sines,

$\dfrac{\sin A}{859} = \dfrac{\sin 74.3°}{783} \Rightarrow \sin A = \dfrac{859\sin 74.3°}{783} \Rightarrow A = \sin^{-1}\left(\dfrac{859\sin 74.3°}{783}\right) \Rightarrow A \approx \sin^{-1}(1.056)$. Since 1.056 is not

in the domain of the inverse sine function, no such angle exists. Thus no such triangle exists.

43. Using the Law of Sines, $\dfrac{\sin B}{5.432} = \dfrac{\sin 142.13°}{7.297} \Rightarrow \sin B$

$= \dfrac{5.432\sin 142.13°}{7.297} \Rightarrow B = \sin^{-1}\left(\dfrac{5.432\sin 142.13°}{7.297}\right) \approx 27.19°$ Since

$180° - 27.19° = 152.81$ and $142.13° + 152.81° > 180°$ there is only one triangle.

$C = 180° - 142.13° - 27.19° = 10.68°$. The solutions are . $B = 27.19°$, $c = 10.68°$.

45. Using the Law of Sines,

$\dfrac{\sin B}{8.14} = \dfrac{\sin 42.5°}{15.6} \Rightarrow \sin B = \dfrac{8.14\sin 42.5°}{15.6} \Rightarrow B = \sin^{-1}\left(\dfrac{8.14\sin 42.5°}{15.6}\right) \approx 20.6°$.

Since $180° - 42.5° - 20.6° = 159.4°$ and $42.5° + 159.4° > 180°$, there is one triangle.

$C = 180° - 42.5° - 20.6° = 116.9°$. $\dfrac{c}{\sin 116.9°} = \dfrac{15.6}{\sin 42.5°} \Rightarrow c = \dfrac{15.6\sin 116.9°}{\sin 42.5°} \approx 20.6$.

The solutions are $B = 20.6°$, $C = 116.9°$, $c = 20.6$ ft.

47. Using the Law of Sines,

$\dfrac{\sin C}{145} = \dfrac{\sin 72.2°}{78.3} \Rightarrow \sin C = \dfrac{145\sin 72.2°}{78.3} \Rightarrow C = \sin^{-1}\left(\dfrac{145\sin 72.2°}{78.3}\right) \approx c \approx \sin^{-1}(1.76)$.

Since 1.76 is not in the domain of the inverse sine function, no such angle exists.

Thus no such triangle exists.

49. Using the Law of Sines,

$\dfrac{\sin B}{11.8} = \dfrac{\sin 38°40'}{9.72} \Rightarrow \sin B = \dfrac{11.8\sin 38°40'}{9.72} \Rightarrow B = \sin^{-1}\left(\dfrac{11.8\sin 38°.40'}{9.72}\right) \approx 49°20'$. There are two angles:

$B_1 = 49°20'$ and $B_2 = 180 - 49°20' = 130°40$ (since $38°40' + 130°40' < 180°$)

$C_1 = 180° - 38°40' - 49°20' = 92°00'$ and $C_2 = 180° - 38°40' - 130°40' = 10°40'$

$\dfrac{c_1}{\sin 92°00'} = \dfrac{9.72}{\sin 38°40'} \Rightarrow c_1 = \dfrac{9.72\sin 92°00'}{\sin 38°40'} \approx 15.5$ $\dfrac{c_2}{\sin 10°40'} = \dfrac{9.72}{\sin 38°40'} \Rightarrow c_2 = \dfrac{9.72\sin 10°40'}{\sin 38°40'} \approx 2.88$.

The solutions are $B_1 = 49°20'$, $C_1 = 92°00'$, $c_1 = 15.5$ km or $B_2 = 130°40'$, $C_2 = 10°40'$, $c_2 = 2.88$ km

51. Using the Law of Sines,

    $\dfrac{\sin A}{7540} = \dfrac{\sin 32°50'}{5180} \Rightarrow \sin A = \dfrac{7540 \sin 32°50'}{5180} \Rightarrow A = \sin^{-1}\left(\dfrac{7540 \sin 32°50'}{5180}\right) \approx 52°10'.$

    There are two angles: $A_1 = 52°10'$ and $A_2 = 180° - 52°10' = 127°50'$ (since $32°50' + 127°50' < 180°$)

    $C_1 = 180° - 32°50' - 52°10' = 95°00'$ and $C_2 = 180° - 32°50' - 127°50' = 19°20'$

    $\dfrac{c_1}{\sin 95°00'} = \dfrac{5180}{\sin 32°50'} \Rightarrow c_1 = \dfrac{5180 \sin 95°00'}{\sin 32°50'} \approx 9520$

    $\dfrac{c_2}{\sin 19°20'} = \dfrac{5180}{\sin 32°50'} \Rightarrow c_2 = \dfrac{5180 \sin 19°20'}{\sin 32°50'} \approx 3160.$ The solutions are

    $A_1 = 52°10', C_1 = 95°00', c_1 = 9520$ cm or $A_2 = 127°50', C_2 = 19°20', c_2 = 3160$ cm.

53. The Pythagorean theorem only applies to right triangles.

55. If we are given only three sides, then any equation from the Law of Sines will contain two unknowns. At least one angle must be given.

57. Angle A has measure $180° = 112°10' - 15°20' = 52°20'$. Now, using the Law of Sines,

    $\dfrac{AB}{\sin 15°20'} = \dfrac{354}{\sin 52°30'} \Rightarrow AB = \dfrac{354 \sin 15°20'}{\sin 52°30'} \Rightarrow AB \approx 118$ m.

59. Triangle ABC has the following measurements:

    $A = 90° - 47.7° = 42.3°, B = 302.5° - 270° - 270° = 32.5°, C = 180° - 42.3° - 32.5° = 105.2°$ and $c = 3.46.$

    Now, using the Law of Sines, $\dfrac{b}{\sin 32.5°} = \dfrac{3.46}{\sin 105.2°} \Rightarrow b = \dfrac{3.46 \sin 32.5°}{\sin 105.2°} \Rightarrow b \approx 1.93$ mi.

61. Using the Law of Sines, $\dfrac{x}{\sin 54.8°} = \dfrac{12}{\sin 70.4°} \Rightarrow x = \dfrac{12 \sin 54.8°}{\sin 70.4°} \Rightarrow x \approx 10.4$ in.

63. Note that the distance between the centers of the small gear and middle-size gear is $2.7 + 1.6 = 4.3$ and the distance between the centers of the small gear and large gear is $3.6 + 1.6 = 5.2$. Use the Law of Sines to find the angle α on the large gear. $\dfrac{\sin \alpha}{4.3} = \dfrac{\sin 38°}{5.2} \Rightarrow \sin \alpha = \dfrac{4.3 \sin 38°}{5.2} \Rightarrow \alpha \approx \sin^{-1}\left(\dfrac{4.3 \sin 38°}{5.2}\right) \approx 30.6°.$

    It follows that $\theta = 180° - 38° - 30.6° = 111.4° \approx 111°$.

65. Let A, B, and C be the ship's initial position, new position, and position of the lighthouse, respectively. Triangle ABC has the following measurements:

    $A = 180° - 37° = 143°, B = 25°, C = 180° - 143° - 25° = 12°$, and $c = 2.5$.

    Now, using the Law of Sines, $\dfrac{a}{\sin 143°} = \dfrac{2.5}{\sin 12°} \Rightarrow a = \dfrac{2.5 \sin 143°}{\sin 12°} \Rightarrow a \approx 7.2$ mi and

    $\dfrac{b}{\sin 25°} = \dfrac{2.5}{\sin 12°} \Rightarrow a = \dfrac{2.5 \sin 25°}{\sin 12°} \Rightarrow a \approx 5.1$ mi.

67. Triangle ABC has the following measurements:

$A = 90° - 22.4° + 45° = 112.6°$, $B = 45° - 10.6° = 34.4°$,
$C = 180° - 112.6° - 34.4° = 33°$, $c = 25.5$

Now, using the Law of Sines, $\dfrac{b}{\sin 34.4°} = \dfrac{25.5}{\sin 33°} = \dfrac{25.5}{\sin 33°} \Rightarrow b = \dfrac{25.5 \sin 34.4°}{\sin 33°} \Rightarrow b \approx 26.5$ km.

69. Let R be the position of the rocket. Triangle T_1RT_2 has the following measurements:

    $T_1 = 28.1°$, $T_2 = 180° - 79.5° = 100.5°$, $R = 180° - 28.1° - 100.5° = 51.4°$, and $r = 1.73$.

    Now, using the Law of Sines, $\dfrac{t_2}{\sin 100.5°} = \dfrac{1.73}{\sin 51.4°} \Rightarrow t_2 = \dfrac{1.73 \sin 100.5°}{\sin 51.4°} \Rightarrow t_2 \approx 2.18$ km.

71. Use the Law of Sines to find angle W.

    $\dfrac{\sin W}{11.2} = \dfrac{\sin 25.5°}{28.6} \Rightarrow \sin W = \dfrac{11.2 \sin 25.5°}{28.6} \Rightarrow W = \sin^{-1}\left(\dfrac{11.2 \sin 25.5°}{28.6}\right) \approx 9.7°$.

    Thus, $P = 180° - 25.5° - 9.7° = 144.8°$. Now use the Law of Sines to find the required distance.

    $\dfrac{p}{\sin 144.8°} = \dfrac{11.2}{\sin 9.7°} \Rightarrow p = \dfrac{11.2 \sin 144.8°}{\sin 9.7°} \Rightarrow p \approx 38.3$ cm.

73. $\dfrac{\sin C}{2\sqrt{5}} = \dfrac{\sin 30°}{\sqrt{5}} \Rightarrow \sin C = \dfrac{2\sqrt{5} \sin 30°}{\sqrt{5}} = 1$. Thus $C = 90°$. This is a right triangle.

75. The longest side must be opposite the largest angle. Thus, B must be larger than A, which is impossible because A and B cannot both be obtuse.

77. Let B, M, and D be the positions of Bochum, the moon, and Donaueschingen, respectively. Triangle BMD has the following measurements:

    $B = 52.6997°$, $D = 180° - 52.7430° = 127.2570°$,
    $M = 180° - 52.6997° - 127.2570° = 0.433$, $m = 398$

    Now, using the Law of Sines, $\dfrac{d}{\sin 127.2570°} = \dfrac{398}{\sin 0433°} \Rightarrow a = \dfrac{398 \sin 127.2570°}{\sin .0433°} \Rightarrow a \approx 419,000$ km.

    This compares favorably to the actual value.

79. (a) Note: this solution utilizes the area formula introduced in section 10.2. First note that

    $\dfrac{R}{\sin C} = \dfrac{r}{\sin A} \Rightarrow r = \dfrac{R \sin A}{\sin C} \Rightarrow r = \dfrac{R \sin A}{\sin(A+B)}$. Substituting in the area formula gives

    $A = 10\left(\dfrac{1}{2} Rr \sin B\right) = 5R\left(\dfrac{R \sin A}{\sin(A+B)}\right) \sin B = \left[5\dfrac{\sin A \sin B}{\sin(A+B)} R^2\right]$.

    (b) $A = \left[5\dfrac{\sin 18° \sin 36°}{\sin(18° + 36°)} R^2\right] \approx 1.12257 R^2$.

    (c) (i) The stripe has height $10 \div 13 \approx .76923$ in. and area of $11.4(.76923) \approx 8.77$ in^2.

    (ii) The 50 stars have area $A = 50(1.12257)(.308)^2 \approx 5.32$ in^2.

    (iii) Red occupies the greatest area on the flag.

80. On the given interval, the graph is increasing.

81. If $B < A$, and $\sin B < \sin A$ because $y \sin x$ is increasing on $\left[0, \dfrac{\pi}{2}\right]$.

82. $\dfrac{b}{\sin B} = \dfrac{a}{\sin A} \Rightarrow b = \dfrac{a \sin B}{\sin A}$.

83. $b = \dfrac{a \sin B}{\sin A} = a \cdot \dfrac{\sin B}{\sin A}$. Since $\dfrac{\sin B}{\sin A} < 1, b = a \cdot \dfrac{\sin B}{\sin A} < a \cdot 1 = a$, so $b < a$.

84. If $B < A$, then $b < a$, but $b > a$ in triangle ABC

10.2 The Law of Cosines and Area Formulas

1. (a) Two sides and the included angle are given. This is form SAS.
   (b) SAS should be solved using the Law of Cosines.

3. (a) Two sides and a non-included angle are given. This is form SSA.
   (b) SSA should be solved using the Law of Sines.

5. (a) Two angles and the included side are given. This is form ASA.
   (b) ASA should be solved using the Law of Sines.

7. (a) Two angles and the included side are given. This is form ASA.
   (b) ASA should be solved using the Law of Sines

9. $a^2 = 3^2 + 8^2 - 2(3)(8)\cos 60° \Rightarrow a^2 = 73 - 48(.5) \Rightarrow a^2 = 73 - 24 \Rightarrow a^2 = 49 \Rightarrow a = 7$.

11. $1^2 = 1^2 + \left(\sqrt{3}\right)^2 - 2(1)\left(\sqrt{3}\right)\cos\theta \Rightarrow 1 = 4 - 2\sqrt{3}\cos\theta \Rightarrow \cos\theta = \dfrac{-3}{-2\sqrt{3}} \Rightarrow \cos\theta = \dfrac{\sqrt{3}}{2} \Rightarrow \theta = 30°$

13. Use the Law of Cosines to find a: $a^2 = 4^2 + 6^2 - 2(4)(6)\cos 61° \Rightarrow a = \sqrt{52 - 48\cos 61°} \approx 5.36$.

    Use the Law of Sines to find B: $\dfrac{\sin B}{4} = \dfrac{\sin 61°}{5.36} \Rightarrow \sin B = \dfrac{4\sin 61°}{5,36} \Rightarrow B = \sin^{-1}\left(\dfrac{4\sin 61°}{5.36}\right) \approx 40.7°$.

    Then $C = 180° - 61° - 40.7° = 78.3°$. The solutions are $a \approx 5.4, B \approx 40.7°, C \approx 78.3°$.

15. Use the Law of Cosines to find A: $4^2 = 8^2 + 10^2 - 2(8)(10)\cos A \Rightarrow A = \cos^{-1}\left(\dfrac{16 - 164}{-160}\right) \approx 22.33°$. Use the

    Law of Sines to find B: $\dfrac{\sin B}{10} = \dfrac{\sin 22.33°}{4} \Rightarrow \sin B = \dfrac{10\sin 22.33°}{4} \Rightarrow B = \sin^{-1}\left(\dfrac{10\sin 22.33°}{4}\right) \approx 71.8°$

    Since angle B is obtuse, $B = 180° - 71.8° = 108.2°$. The value of C is $180° - 22.3° - 108.2° = 49.5°$.
    The solutions are $A \approx 22.3°, B \approx 108.2°, C \approx 49.5°$.

17. Use the Law of Cosines to find A: $5^2 = 7^2 + 9^2 - 2(7)(9)\cos A \Rightarrow A = \cos^{-1}\left(\dfrac{25 - 130}{-126}\right) \approx 33.55°$. Use the Law

    of Sines to find B: $\dfrac{\sin B}{7} = \dfrac{\sin 33.55°}{5} \Rightarrow \sin B = \dfrac{7\sin 33.55°}{5} \Rightarrow B = \sin^{-1}\left(\dfrac{7\sin 33.55°}{5}\right) \approx 50.7°$. The value of

    C is $180° - 33.6° - 50.7° = 95.7°$ The solutions are $A \approx 33.6°, B \approx 50.7°, C \approx 95.7°$.

19. Use the Law of Cosines to find c:

$c^2 = 5.71^2 + 4.21^2 - 2(5.71)(4.21)\cos 28.3° \Rightarrow c = \sqrt{50.3282 - 48.0782\cos 28.3°} \approx 2.83$ Use the Law of Sines

to find A: $\dfrac{\sin A}{4.21} = \dfrac{\sin 28.3°}{28.3} \Rightarrow \sin A = \dfrac{4.21\sin 28.3°}{28.3} \Rightarrow A = \sin^{-1}\left(\dfrac{4.21\sin 28.3°}{28.3}\right) \approx 44.9°$.

Then $B = 180° - 28.3° - 44.9° = 106.8°$. The solutions are $c \approx 2.83$ in, $A \approx 44.9°$, $B \approx 106.8°$.

21. Use the Law of Cosines to find c:

$c^2 = 8.94^2 + 7.23^2 - 2(8.94)(7.23)\cos 45.6° \Rightarrow c = \sqrt{132.1965 - 129.274\cos 45.6°} \approx 6.46$

Use the Law of Sines to find A:

$\dfrac{\sin A}{7.23} = \dfrac{\sin 45.6°}{6.46} \Rightarrow \sin A = \dfrac{7.23\sin 45.6°}{6.46} \Rightarrow A = \sin^{-1}\left(\dfrac{7.23\sin 45.6°}{6.46}\right) \approx 53.1°$.

Then $B = 180° - 45.6° - 53.1° = 81.3°$. The solutions are $c \approx 6.46$ m, $A \approx 53.1°$, $B \approx 81.3°$.

23. Use the Law of Cosines to find A:

$9.3^2 = 5.7^2 + 8.2^2 - 2(5.7)(8.2)\cos A \Rightarrow A = \cos^{-1}\left(\dfrac{86.49 - 99.73}{-93.48}\right) \approx 81.86°$.

Use the Law of Sines to find B:

$\dfrac{\sin B}{5.7} = \dfrac{\sin 81.86°}{9.3} \Rightarrow \sin B = \dfrac{5.7\sin 81.86°}{9.3} \Rightarrow B = \sin^{-1}\left(\dfrac{5.7\sin 81.86°}{9.3}\right) \approx 37.35°$.

The value of C is $180° - 82° - 37° = 61°$. The solutions are $A \approx 82°$, $B \approx 37°$, $C \approx 61°$.

25. Use the Law of Cosines to find A:

$42.9^2 = 37.6^2 + 62.7^2 - 2(37.6)(62.7)\cos A \Rightarrow A = \cos^{-1}\left(\dfrac{1840.41 - 5345.05}{-4715.04}\right) \approx 41.99°$.

Use the Law of Sines to find B:

$\dfrac{\sin B}{37.6} = \dfrac{\sin 41.99°}{42.9} \Rightarrow \sin B = \dfrac{37.6\sin 41.99°}{42.9} \Rightarrow B = \sin^{-1}\left(\dfrac{37.6\sin 41.99°}{42.9}\right) \approx 35.90°$

$C \approx 180° - 42°00' - 35°50' = 102°10'$ The solutions are $A \approx 42°00', B \approx 35°50' C \approx 102°10'$.

27. Use the Law of Cosines to find A:

$965^2 = 1240^2 + 876^2 - 2(1240)(876)\cos A \Rightarrow A = \cos^{-1}\left(\dfrac{931,225 - 2,304,976}{-2,172,480}\right) \approx 50.78°$.

Use the Law of Sines to find B:

$\dfrac{\sin B}{876} = \dfrac{\sin 50.78°}{965} \Rightarrow \sin B = \dfrac{876\sin 50.78°}{965} \Rightarrow B = \sin^{-1}\left(\dfrac{876\sin 50.78°}{965}\right) \approx 44.69°$

$C \approx 180° - 50°50' - 44°40' = 80°30'$. The solutions are $A \approx 50°50'$, $B \approx 44°40'$ $C \approx 84°30'$.

29. Use the Law of Cosines to find a:

$a^2 = 143^2 + 89.6^2 - 2(143)(89.6)\cos 80°40 \Rightarrow a = \sqrt{28,477.16 - 25,625\cos 80°40'} \approx 155.95$.

Use the Law of Sines to find B:

$$\frac{\sin B}{143} = \frac{\sin 80°40'}{155.95} \Rightarrow \sin B = \frac{143\sin 80°40'}{155.95} \Rightarrow B = \sin^{-1}\left(\frac{143\sin 80°40'}{155.95}\right) \approx 64°50'$$

Then $C = 180° - 80°40' - 64°50' = 34°30'$ The solutions are $a \approx 156\,\text{cm}$, $B \approx 64°50'$, $C \approx 34°30'$.

31. Use the Law of Cosines to find b:

    $$b^2 = 8.919^2 + 6.427^2 - 2(8919)(6.427)\cos 74.80° \Rightarrow b = \sqrt{120.85489 - 114.644826\cos 74.80°} \approx 9.529.$$

    Use the Law of Sines to find A:

    $$\frac{\sin A}{8919} = \frac{\sin 74.80°}{9.529} \Rightarrow \sin A = \frac{8.919\sin 74.80°}{9.529} \Rightarrow A = \sin^{-1}\left(\frac{8919\sin 74.80°}{9.529}\right) \approx 64.59°.$$

    Then $C = 180° - 74.80° - 64.59° = 40.61°$. The solutions are $b \approx 9.529$ in, $A \approx 64.59°$, $C \approx 40.61°$.

33. Use the Law of Cosines to find a:

    $$a^2 = 6.28^2 + 12.2^2 - 2(6.28)(12.2)\cos 112.8° \Rightarrow a = \sqrt{188.2784 - 153.232\cos 112.8°} \approx 15.7.$$

    Use the Law of Sines to find B:

    $$\frac{\sin B}{6.28} = \frac{\sin 112.8°}{15.7} \Rightarrow \sin B = \frac{6.25\sin 112.8°}{15.7} \Rightarrow B = \sin^{-1}\left(\frac{6.28\sin 112.8°}{15.7}\right) \approx 21.6°.$$

    Then $C = 180° - 112.8° - 21.6° = 45.6°$. The solutions are $a \approx 15.7\,\text{m}$, $B \approx 21.6°$, $C \approx 45.6°$.

35. Use the Law of Cosines to find A: $3.0^2 = 5.0^2 + 6.0^2 - 2(5.0)(6.0)\cos A \Rightarrow A = \cos^{-1}\left(\frac{9-61}{-60}\right) \approx 30°$.

    Use the Law of Sines to find B: $\dfrac{\sin B}{5.0} = \dfrac{\sin 30°}{3.0} \Rightarrow \sin B = \dfrac{5.0\sin 30°}{3.0} \Rightarrow B = \sin^{-1}\left(\dfrac{5.0\sin 30°}{3.0}\right) \approx 56°$.

    The value of C is $180° - 30° - 56° = 94°$. The solutions are $A \approx 30°$, $B \approx 56°$, $C \approx 94°$.

37. Case 1. First use the triangle sum formula to find angle A: $179°60' - 50°52' - 28°37' = 101°30'$

    Use the Law of Sines: $\dfrac{59.49}{\sin 100°31'} = \dfrac{b}{\sin 50°52'} \Rightarrow \sin 100°31'b = 59.49\cdot\sin 50°52' \Rightarrow b = 46.93$

    $\dfrac{59.49}{\sin 100°31'} = \dfrac{c}{\sin 28°31'} \Rightarrow \sin 100°31'c = 59.49\cdot\sin 28°31' \Rightarrow c = 28.98$

39. Case 3. First use the Law of Cosines to find b:

    $$b^2 = (3.961)^2 + (5.308)^2 - 2(3.961)(5.308)\cos 58°12' = 21.7063 \Rightarrow b = 4.659$$

    Use the Law of Sines to find A: $\dfrac{3.961}{\sin A} = \dfrac{4.659}{\sin 58°12'} \Rightarrow 4.659\sin A = 3.961\cdot\sin 58°12' \Rightarrow A = 46°16'$

    Finally, use the triangle sum formula to find angle C: $179°60' - 46°16' - 58°12' = 75°32'$

41. Case 4. First use the Law of Cosines to find angle C.

    $$(65.88)^2 = (51.41)^2 + (37.29)^2 - 2(51.41)(37.29)\cos C \Rightarrow C = 94°35'$$

    Use the Law of Sines to find Angle A.

$$\frac{51.41}{\sin A} = \frac{65.88}{\sin 94°35'} \Rightarrow 65.88 \sin A = 51.41 \cdot \sin 94°35' \Rightarrow A = 51°04'$$

Finally, use the triangle sum formula to find angle B: $179°60' - 51°4' - 94°35' = 34°21'$

43. Case 2. Use the Law of Sines to find angle B:

$$\frac{7.031}{\sin 41°12'} = \frac{9.947}{\sin B} \Rightarrow 7.031 \sin B = 9.947 \cdot \sin 41°12 \Rightarrow B = 68°43'$$

There are two triangles $B_1 = 68°43'$ and $B_2 = 180 - 68°43' = 111°17'$. Since

$41°12' + 111°17' < 180°, C_1 = 180 - 41°12' - 68°43' = 70°05'$ and $C_2 = 180 - 41°12' - 111°17' = 27°31'$

Use the Law of Sines to find c_1 and c_2:

$$\frac{c_1}{\sin 70°05'} = \frac{7.031}{\sin 41°12'} \Rightarrow c_1 \sin 41°12' = 7.031 \cdot \sin 70°05' \Rightarrow c_1 = 10.04$$

$$\frac{c_2}{\sin 27°31'} = \frac{7.031}{\sin 41°12'} \Rightarrow c_2 \sin 41°12' = 7.031 \cdot \sin 27°31 \Rightarrow c_2 = 4.933$$

45. Case 2. Use the Law of Sines to find angle A:

$$\frac{34.22}{\sin 14°19'} = \frac{27.16}{\sin A} \Rightarrow 34.22 \sin A = 27.16 \cdot \sin 14°19' \Rightarrow A = 11°19'$$

There is one triangle since $180° - 11°19' + 14°19' > 180°$. Angle B $= 180° - 11°19' - 14°19' = 154°22'$

Use the Law of Sines to find b:

$$\frac{34.22}{\sin 14°19'} = \frac{b}{\sin 154°22'} \Rightarrow b \sin 14°19' = 34.22 \cdot \sin 154°22' \Rightarrow b = 59.87$$

47. Case 2. Use the Law of Sines to find angle A:

$$\frac{2634}{\sin A} = \frac{2220}{\sin 18°37'} \Rightarrow 2220 \sin A = 2634 \cdot \sin 18°37' \Rightarrow \sin A > 1..$$ There is no triangle that exists.

49. The absolute value of $\cos \theta$ will be greater than 1. The calculator will give an error message (or a complex number) when using the inverse cosine function.

51. Use the Law of Cosines to find c:

$$c^2 = 350^2 + 286^2 - 2(350)(286)\cos 46.3° \Rightarrow c = \sqrt{204,296 - 200,200\cos 46.3°} \approx 257 \text{ m}$$

53. Let the vertical line passing through airport C intersect the line from A to B at the point D. Now, using the right triangle CDB we can find the measure of angle B. The angle of this right triangle at position C is given by $180° - 128°40' = 51°20'$. Thus $B = 180° - 90° - 51°20' = 38°40'$. Use the Law of Cosines on ABC to find b: $b^2 = 450^2 + 359^2 - 2(450)(359)\cos 38°40' \Rightarrow d = \sqrt{331,323,100\cos 38°40'} \approx 281$ km

55. Let A, B, and C be the ship's initial position, new position and position of the rock, respectively. Triangle ABC has the following measurements:

$A = 90° - 45°20' = 44°40'$, $B = 308°40' - 270° = 38°40'$, $C = 180° - 44°40' - 38°40' = 96°40'°$, and

$c = 15.2$. Now, using the Law of Sines, $\dfrac{a}{\sin 44°40} = \dfrac{15.2}{\sin 96°40'} \Rightarrow a = \dfrac{15.2 \sin 44°40'}{\sin 96°40'} \Rightarrow a \approx 10.8$ mi.

57. Let A, B, and C be the positions of the airplane, battleship and submarine, respectively. Triangle ABC has the following measurements: $A = 24°10' - 17°30' = 6°40'$, $B = 17°30'$, $C = 180° - 6°40' - 70°30' = 155°50'°$, and $c = 5120$. Now, using the Law of Sines, $\dfrac{a}{\sin 6°40'} = \dfrac{5120}{\sin 155°50'} \Rightarrow a = \dfrac{5120 \sin 6°40'}{\sin 155°50'} \Rightarrow a \approx 1450$ ft

59. Use the Law of Cosines to find the distance d:
$d^2 = 10^2 + 10^2 - 2(10)(10)\cos 128° \Rightarrow d = \sqrt{200 - 200 \cos 128°} \approx 18$ ft.

61. Use the Law of Cosines to find the distance c: $c^2 = 3800^2 + 2900^2 - 2(3800)(2900)\cos 110° \Rightarrow$
$c = \sqrt{22{,}850{,}000 - 22{,}040{,}000 \cos 110°} \approx 5500$ m

63. The distances traveled by the sound are $3(344) = 1032$ m and $6(344) = 2064$ m. Use the Law of Cosines to find the distance d:
$d^2 = 1032^2 + 2064^2 - 2(1032)(2064)\cos 42.2° \Rightarrow d = \sqrt{5{,}325{,}120 - 4{,}260{,}096 \cos 42.2°} \approx 1473$ m

65. Use the Law of Cosines to find the angle of the triangle located at position A:
$9^2 = 17^2 + 21^2 - 2(17)(21)\cos A \Rightarrow A = \cos^{-1}\left(\dfrac{81 - 730}{-714}\right) \approx 25°$. The bearing is $325° + 25° = 350°$.

67. If the satellite travels one orbit in 2 hours, it is traveling at a rate of $360 \div 120 = 3°$ per minute. At 12:03 P.M. the angle formed at the center of Earth is $9°$. Noting that the sides of the triangle shown are 6400 km and $6400 + 1600 = 8000$ km, use the Law of Cosines to find the distance d:
$d^2 = 8000^2 + 6400^2 - 2(8000)(6400)\cos 9° \Rightarrow d = \sqrt{104{,}960{,}000 - 102{,}400{,}000 \cos 9°} \approx 2000$ km

69. Use the Law of Cosines to find angle θ
$57.8^2 = 25.9^2 + 32.5^2 - 2(25.9)(32.5)\cos \theta \Rightarrow \theta = \cos^{-1}\left(\dfrac{3340.84 - 1727.06}{-1683.5}\right) \approx 163.5°$.

71. Use the Law of Cosines to find x: $x^2 = 25^2 + 25^2 - 2(25)(25)\cos 52° \Rightarrow x = \sqrt{1250 - 1250 \cos 52°} \approx 22$ ft

73. Since A is obtuse, $90° < A < 180°$. The cosine of a quadrant II angle is negative.

74. In $a^2 = b^2 + c^2 - 2ab \cos A$, $\cos A$ is negative, so $a^2 = b^2 + c^2 +$ (a positive quantity). Thus, $a^2 > b^2 + c^2$.

75. $b^2 + c^2 > b^2$ and $b^2 + c^2 > c^2$. If $a^2 > b^2 + c^2$, then $a^2 > b^2$ and $a^2 > c^2$ from which $a > b$ and $a > c$ because a, b, and c are nonnegative.

76. Because A is obtuse, it is the largest angle, so the longest side should be a, not c.

77. $A = \dfrac{1}{2}(13.6)(10.1)\sin 42.5° \approx 46.4$ m^2

79. $s = \dfrac{1}{2}(12 + 16 + 25) = 26.5$; $A = \sqrt{26.5(26.5 - 12)(26.5 - 16)(26.5 - 25)} \approx 78$ m^2

Section 10.3   511

81. $s = \frac{1}{2}(76.3 + 109 + 98.8) = 142.05;\ A = \sqrt{142.05(142.05 - 76.3)(142.05 - 109)(142.05 - 98.8)} \approx 3650\ \text{ft}^2$

83. $s = \frac{1}{2}(25.4 + 38.2 + 19.8) = 41.7;\ A = \sqrt{41.7(41.7 - 25.4)(41.7 - 38.2)(41.7 - 19.8)} \approx 228\ \text{yd}^2$

85. $s = \frac{1}{2}(75 + 68 + 85) = 114;\ A = \sqrt{114(114 - 75)(114 - 68)(114 - 85)} \approx 2435\ \text{m}^2$ The number of cans needed is $2435 \div 75 \approx 32.5$ or 33 cans.

87. $A = \frac{1}{2}(15.2)(16.1)\sin 125° \approx 100\ \text{m}^2$

89. $s = \frac{1}{2}(9 + 10 + 17) = 18;\ A = \sqrt{18(18 - 9)(18 - 10)(18 - 17)} = 36\ \text{m}^2$ and $9 + 10 + 17 = 36$

91. (a) Using the law of sines, we have $\frac{\sin C}{c} = \frac{\sin A}{a} \Rightarrow \frac{\sin C}{15} = \frac{\sin 60°}{13} \Rightarrow \sin C = \frac{15 \sin 60°}{13} =$

    $\frac{15}{13} \cdot \frac{\sqrt{3}}{2} \approx 0.99926008$. There are two angles C between 0° and 180° that satisfy the condition. Since $\sin C \approx 0.99926008$, to the nearest tenth value of C is $C_1 = 87.8°$. Supplementary angles have the same sine value, so another possible value of C is $B_2 = 180° - 87.8° = 92.2°$.

    (b) By the law of cosines, we have $\cos C = \frac{a^2 + b^2 - c^2}{2ab} \Rightarrow \cos C = \frac{13^2 + 7^2 - 15^2}{2(13)(7)} =$

    $\frac{-7}{182} \approx -0.03846154 \Rightarrow C \approx 92.2°$

    (c) With the law of cosines, we are required to find the inverse cosine of a negative number; therefore; we know angle C is greater than 90°.

10.3 Vectors and their Applications

1. The vector pairs that have the same direction and length are **m** & **p** and **n** & **r**.

3. m = 2t, p = 2t, Or $t = \frac{1}{2}$m and $t = \frac{1}{2}$p; also m = 1p and n = 1r or p = 1m and r = 1n

5. See Figure 5.

7. See Figure 7.

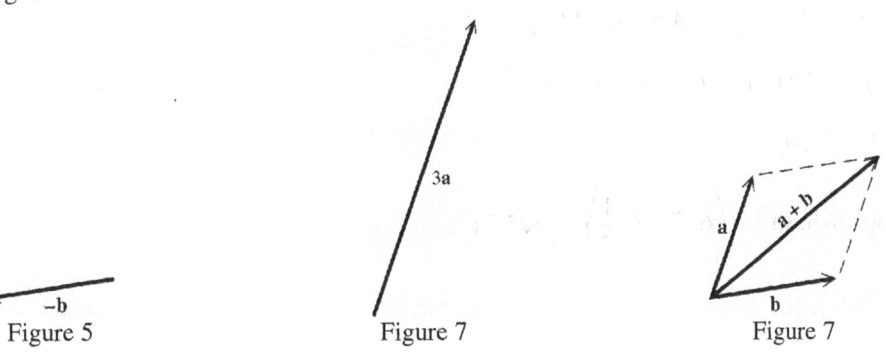

Figure 5   Figure 7   Figure 7

9. See Figure 9.

11. See Figure 11.

13. See Figure 13.

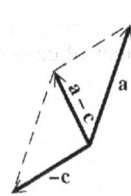
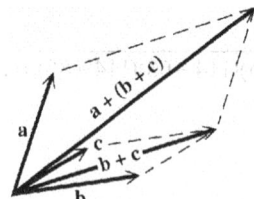

Figure 11 Figure 13

15. See Figure 15.

17. (a) $u + v = \langle -8,8 \rangle + \langle 4,8 \rangle = \langle -8+4, 8+8 \rangle = \langle -4, 16 \rangle$

    (b) $u - v = \langle -8,8 \rangle - \langle 4,8 \rangle = \langle -8-4, 8-8 \rangle = \langle -12, 0 \rangle$

    (c) $-u = -\langle -8,8 \rangle = \langle 8, -8 \rangle$

19. (a) $u + v = \langle 4,8 \rangle + \langle 4,-8 \rangle = \langle 4+4, 8+(-8) \rangle = \langle 8, 0 \rangle$

    (b) $u - v = \langle 4,8 \rangle - \langle 4,-8 \rangle = \langle 4-4, 8-(-8) \rangle = \langle 0, 16 \rangle$

    (c) $-u = -\langle 4,8 \rangle = \langle -4, -8 \rangle$

21. (a) $u + v = \langle -8,4 \rangle + \langle 8,8 \rangle = \langle -8+8, 4+8 \rangle = \langle 0, 12 \rangle$

    (b) $u - v = \langle -8,4 \rangle - \langle 8,8 \rangle = \langle -8-8, 4-8 \rangle = \langle -16, -4 \rangle$

    (c) $-u = -\langle -8,4 \rangle = \langle 8, -4 \rangle$

23. (a) $2u = 2(2i) = 4i$

    (b) $2u + 3v = 2(2i) + 3(i+j) = 4i + 3i + 3j = 7i + 3j$

    (c) $v - 3u = i + j - 3(2i) = i + j - 6i = -5i + j$

25. (a) $2u = 2\langle -1,2 \rangle = \langle -2, 4 \rangle$

    (b) $2u + 3v = 2\langle -1,2 \rangle + 3\langle 3,0 \rangle = \langle -2,4 \rangle + \langle 9,0 \rangle = \langle -2+9, 4+0 \rangle = \langle 7, 4 \rangle$

    (c) $v - 3u = \langle 3,0 \rangle - 3\langle -1,2 \rangle = \langle 3,0 \rangle + \langle 3,-6 \rangle = \langle 3+3, 0+(-6) \rangle = \langle 6, -6 \rangle$

27. $u + v = \langle -2,5 \rangle + \langle 4,3 \rangle = \langle -2+4, 5+3 \rangle = \langle 2, 8 \rangle$

29. $v - u = \langle 4,3 \rangle - \langle -2,5 \rangle = \langle 4-(-2), 3-5 \rangle = \langle 6, -2 \rangle$

31. $-5v = -5\langle 4,3 \rangle = \langle -20, -15 \rangle$

33. $v = \langle 6\cos 30°, 6\sin 30° \rangle = \left\langle 6 \cdot \frac{\sqrt{3}}{2}, 6 \cdot \frac{1}{2} \right\rangle = \langle 3\sqrt{3}, 3 \rangle$

35. $v = \langle 9\cos 225°, 9\sin 225°\rangle = \left\langle 9\cdot\left(-\frac{\sqrt{2}}{2}\right), 9\cdot\left(-\frac{\sqrt{2}}{2}\right)\right\rangle = \left\langle -\frac{9\sqrt{2}}{2}, -\frac{9\sqrt{2}}{2}\right\rangle$

37. $v = \langle 4\cos 40°, 4\sin 40°\rangle \approx \langle 3.06, 2.57\rangle$

39. $v = \langle 5\cos(-35°), 5\sin(-35°)\rangle \approx \langle 4.10, -2.87\rangle$

41. The adjacent angle in the parallelogram is supplementary to 40°, thus it has measure 140°.
    $|v|^2 = 40^2 + 60^2 - 2(40)(60)\cos 140° \approx 8877.0133 \Rightarrow |v| = \sqrt{8877.0133} \approx 94.2$ lb

43. The adjacent angle in the parallelogram is supplementary to 110°, thus it has measure 70°.
    $|v|^2 = 15^2 + 25^2 - 2(15)(25)\cos 70° \approx 593.4849 \Rightarrow |v| = \sqrt{593.4849} \approx 24.4$ lb

45. $\langle -5, 8\rangle = -5\mathbf{i} + 8\mathbf{j}$

47. $\langle 2, 0\rangle = 2\mathbf{i} + 0\mathbf{j} = 2\mathbf{i}$

49. $(8\cos 45°)\mathbf{i} + (8\sin 45°)\mathbf{j} = \left(8\cdot\frac{\sqrt{2}}{2}\right)\mathbf{i} + \left(8\cdot\frac{\sqrt{2}}{2}\right)\mathbf{j} = 4\sqrt{2}\mathbf{i} + 4\sqrt{2}\mathbf{j}$

51. $(.6\cos 115°)\mathbf{i} + (.6\sin 115°)\mathbf{j} = -.25\mathbf{i} + .54\mathbf{j}$

53. $|\langle 1,1\rangle| = \sqrt{1^2 + 1^2} = \sqrt{1+1} = \sqrt{2}$; direction angle: $\tan^{-1}(1) = 45°$

55. $|\langle 8\sqrt{2}, -8\sqrt{2}\rangle| = \sqrt{(8\sqrt{2})^2 + (-8\sqrt{2})^2} = \sqrt{128+128} = \sqrt{256} = 16$; direction angle: $\tan^{-1}\left(\frac{-8\sqrt{2}}{8\sqrt{2}}\right) = 315°$

57. $|\langle 15, -8\rangle| = \sqrt{15^2 + (-8)^2} = \sqrt{225+64} = \sqrt{289} = 17$; direction angle: $\tan^{-1}\left(\frac{-8}{15}\right) = 331.9°$

59. $|\langle -6, 0\rangle| = \sqrt{(-6)^2 + 0^2} = \sqrt{36+0} = \sqrt{36} = 6$; direction angle: $\tan^{-1}\left(\frac{0}{-6}\right) = 180°$

61. $\langle 6, -1\rangle \cdot \langle 2, 5\rangle = (6)(2) + (-1)(5) = 12 - 5 = 7$

63. $\langle 2, -3\rangle \cdot \langle 6, 5\rangle = (2)(6) + (-3)(5) = 12 - 15 = -3$

65. $4\mathbf{i} \cdot (5\mathbf{i} - 9\mathbf{j}) = (4)(5) + (0)(-9) = 20 + 0 = 20$

67. $\cos\theta = \frac{\mathbf{u}\cdot\mathbf{v}}{|\mathbf{u}||\mathbf{v}|} = \frac{\langle 2,1\rangle\cdot\langle -3,1\rangle}{|\langle 2,1\rangle||\langle -3,1\rangle|} = \frac{(2)(-3)+(1)(1)}{\sqrt{4+1}\sqrt{9+1}} = \frac{-5}{\sqrt{5}\sqrt{10}} = \frac{-5}{\sqrt{50}} = \frac{-5}{5\sqrt{2}} = -\frac{1}{\sqrt{2}} \Rightarrow \theta = \cos^{-1}\left(-\frac{1}{\sqrt{2}}\right) = 135°$

69. $\cos\theta = \frac{\mathbf{u}\cdot\mathbf{v}}{|\mathbf{u}||\mathbf{v}|} = \frac{\langle 1,2\rangle\cdot\langle -6,3\rangle}{|\langle 1,2\rangle||\langle -6,3\rangle|} = \frac{(1)(-6)+(2)(3)}{\sqrt{1+4}\sqrt{36+9}} = \frac{0}{\sqrt{5}\sqrt{45}} = 0 \Rightarrow \theta = \cos^{-1} 0 = 90°$

71. $\cos\theta = \frac{\mathbf{u}\cdot\mathbf{v}}{|\mathbf{u}||\mathbf{v}|} = \frac{(\mathbf{i}+7\mathbf{j})\cdot(\mathbf{i}+\mathbf{j})}{|\mathbf{i}+7\mathbf{j}||\mathbf{i}+\mathbf{j}|} = \frac{(1)(1)+(7)(1)}{\sqrt{1+49}\sqrt{1+1}} = \frac{8}{\sqrt{50}\sqrt{2}} = \frac{8}{\sqrt{100}} = \frac{8}{10} = \frac{4}{5} \Rightarrow \theta = \cos^{-1}\left(\frac{4}{5}\right) \approx 36.87°$

73. $\cos\theta = \frac{\mathbf{u}\cdot\mathbf{v}}{|\mathbf{u}||\mathbf{v}|} = \frac{(\mathbf{i}+\mathbf{j})\cdot(3\mathbf{i}+4\mathbf{j})}{|\mathbf{i}+\mathbf{j}||3\mathbf{i}+4\mathbf{j}|} = \frac{(1)(3)+(1)(4)}{\sqrt{1+1}\sqrt{9+16}} = \frac{7}{5\sqrt{2}} = \frac{7\sqrt{2}}{10} \Rightarrow \theta = \cos^{-1}\left(\frac{7\sqrt{2}}{10}\right) \approx 8.13°$

514 Chapter 10: Applications of Trigonometry and Vectors

75. $(3\mathbf{u})\cdot\mathbf{v} = 3\langle -2,1\rangle \cdot \langle 3,4\rangle = \langle -6,3\rangle \cdot \langle 3,4\rangle = (-6)(3)+(3)(4) = -18+12 = -6$

77. $\mathbf{u}\cdot\mathbf{v}-\mathbf{u}\cdot\mathbf{w} = \langle -2,1\rangle \cdot \langle 3,4\rangle - \langle -2,1\rangle \cdot \langle -5,12\rangle = \left[(-2)(3)+(1)(4)\right]\left[(-2)(-5)+(1)(12)\right] = -24$

79. $\langle 1,2\rangle \cdot \langle -6,3\rangle = (1)(-6)+(2)(3) = -6+6 = 0 \Rightarrow$ orthogonal

81. $\langle 1,0\rangle \cdot \langle \sqrt{2},0\rangle = (1)(\sqrt{2})+(0)(0) = \sqrt{2}+0 = \sqrt{2} \Rightarrow$ not orthogonal

83. $(\sqrt{5}\mathbf{i}-2\mathbf{j})\cdot(-5\mathbf{i}+2\sqrt{5}\mathbf{j}) = (\sqrt{5})(-5)+(-2)(2\sqrt{5}) = -5\sqrt{5}-4\sqrt{5} = -9\sqrt{5} \Rightarrow$ not orthogonal

85. By completing the parallelogram with the resultant vector as the diagonal, the triangle formed by two sides of the parallelogram and the resultant has a side of measure 176 and angles with the following measures: $41°10', 78°50'-41°10' = 37°40',$ and $180°-41°10'-37°40' = 101°10'.$ Using the Law of Sines,

$$\frac{F_2}{\sin 41°10'} = \frac{176}{\sin 37°40'} \Rightarrow F_2 = \frac{176\sin 41°10'}{\sin 37°40'} \approx 190\,\text{lb}$$

$$\frac{R}{\sin 101°10'} = \frac{176}{\sin 37°40'} \Rightarrow F_2 = \frac{176\sin 101°10'}{\sin 37°40'} \approx 283\,\text{lb}$$

87. $\theta = \sin^{-1}\left(\dfrac{25}{80}\right) \approx 18°$

89. $\sin 2.3° = \dfrac{F}{60} \Rightarrow F = 60\sin 2.3° \approx 2.4$ tons

91. $\theta = \sin^{-1}\left(\dfrac{18}{60}\right) \approx 17.5°$

93. The weight of the crate is $\sin 46°20' = \dfrac{F}{89.6} \Rightarrow F = 89.6\sin 46°20' \approx 64.8\,\text{lb}$.

The tension on the other rope is $\cos 46°20' = \dfrac{F}{89.6} \Rightarrow F = 89.6\cos 46°20' \approx 61.9\,\text{lb}$.

95. Let A, B, and C be the ship's initial position, turning position, and final position, respectively. Triangle ABC has the following measurements: $B = 90°+34.0° = 124.0°, a = 4.6,$ and $c = 10.4$.

Now, $b^2 = 10.4^2 + 4.6^2 - 2(10.4)(4.6)\cos 124.0° \Rightarrow b = \sqrt{129.32-95.68\cos 124.0°} \approx 13.5$ mi

$\dfrac{\sin A}{4.6} = \dfrac{\sin 124.0°}{13.5} \Rightarrow \sin A = \dfrac{4.6\sin 124.0°}{13.5} \Rightarrow A = \sin^{-1}\left(\dfrac{4.6\sin 124.0°}{13.5}\right) \approx 16.4°$.

The ship is 13.5 miles from its starting point on a bearing of $34.0°+16.4° = 50.4°$.

97. Let A, B, and C be the ship's initial position, turning position, and final position, respectively. Triangle ABC has the following measurements:

$B = 360°-\left[317°-(189°-180°)\right] = 52°, a = 47.8,$ and $c = 18.5$

Now, $b^2 = 47.8^2 + 18.5^2 - 2(47.8)(18.5)\cos 52° \Rightarrow b = \sqrt{2627.09-1768.6\cos 52°} \approx 39.2$ mi

Copyright © 2015 Pearson Education, Inc

99. The speed of the boat in still water, 20, is the hypotenuse of a right triangle with the shorter leg representing the speed of the current and the longer leg representing the actual speed of the boat. The smallest angle of the right triangle is $90° - 80° = 10°$. The actual speed of the boat is $20\cos 10° \approx 19.7$ mph. The speed of the current is $20\sin 10° \approx 3.5$ mph.

101. If the wind is from the direction of $114°$, the bearing of the wind is $114° + 180° = 294°$. The angle between the wind and the flight of the jet is $(360° - 294°) + [180° - (360° - 223°)] = 119°$. If b is the missing side of the triangle, $b^2 = 450^2 + 39^2 - 2(450)(39)\cos 119° \Rightarrow b = \sqrt{204,021 - 35,100\cos 119°} \approx 470$ mph. Then $\dfrac{\sin A}{39} = \dfrac{\sin 119°}{470} \Rightarrow \sin A = \dfrac{39\sin 119°}{470} \Rightarrow A = \sin^{-1}\left(\dfrac{39\sin 119°}{470}\right) \approx 4.2°$. The ground speed of the jet is 470 mph, and the bearing is $233° + 4.2° = 237°$.

103. The triangle formed is a right triangle with one leg representing the wind speed of 42 mph, the hypotenuse representing airspeed, and the other leg representing the groundspeed. The angle between the airspeed and groundspeed is $90° - 74.9° = 15.1°$. Let g represent the hypotenuse and let a represent the unknown leg. The groundspeed is given by $\sin 15.1° = \dfrac{42}{g} \Rightarrow g = \dfrac{42}{\sin 15.1°} \approx 161$ mph. The airspeed is given by $\tan 15.1° = \dfrac{42}{a} \Rightarrow g = \dfrac{42}{\tan 15.1°} \approx 156$ mph.

105. Let A, B, and C represent the angle between the flight path and the desired bearing, the angle between the wind vector and the original flight path, and the angle between the wind vector and the desired bearing. Triangle ABC has the following measurements: $C = 64°30'$, $a = 35$, and $c = 190$. Using the Law of Sines, $\dfrac{\sin A}{35} = \dfrac{\sin 91.3°}{190} \Rightarrow \sin A = \dfrac{35\sin 64°30'}{190} \Rightarrow A = \sin^{-1}\left(\dfrac{35\sin 64°30'}{190}\right) \approx 9°30'$.

So $B = 180° - 9°30' - 64°30' = 106°$. Use the Law of Sines to find b:

$\dfrac{b}{\sin 106°} = \dfrac{190}{\sin 64°30'} \Rightarrow b = \dfrac{190\sin 106°}{\sin 64°30'} \approx 202$ mph. The bearing is $r = \dfrac{3}{1+\cos\theta} \Rightarrow 64\ 64°30' + 9°30' = 74°$ and the ground speed is 202 mph.

107. Let A, B, and C represent the angle between the required flight path and due north, the angle between the wind vector and due north, and the angle between the wind vector and the required flight path, respectively. Triangle ABC has the following measurements: $C = 360° - 328° = 32°$, $a = 11$, and $c = 400 \div 2.5 = 160$

Using the Law of Sines, $\dfrac{\sin A}{11} = \dfrac{\sin 32°}{160} \Rightarrow \sin A = \dfrac{11\sin 32°}{160} \Rightarrow A = \sin^{-1}\left(\dfrac{11\sin 32°}{160}\right) \approx 2°$

So $B = 180° - 2° - 32° = 146°$. Use the Law of Sines to find b:

$\dfrac{b}{\sin 146°} = \dfrac{160}{\sin 32°} \Rightarrow b = \dfrac{160\sin 146°}{\sin 32°} \approx 170$ mph.

The bearing is $360° - 2° = 358°$ and the ground speed is 170 mph.

516   Chapter 10: Applications of Trigonometry and Vectors

109. If the wind is from the direction of 245°, the bearing of the wind is $245° - 180° = 65°$. The angle between the wind and the flight of the plane is $65° + (180° + 174°) = 71°$. If b is the missing side of the triangle,

$b^2 = 240^2 + 30^2 - 2(240)(30)\cos 71° \Rightarrow b = \sqrt{58500 - 14400\cos 71°} \approx 230$ km per hr.

Then, $\dfrac{\sin A}{30} = \dfrac{\sin 71°}{230} \Rightarrow \sin A = \dfrac{30\sin 71°}{230} \Rightarrow A = \sin^{-1}\left(\dfrac{30\sin 71°}{230}\right) \approx 7°$.

The ground speed is 230 km per hr and the bearing is $174° - 7° = 167°$.

111. (a) $|\mathbf{R}| = \sqrt{1^2 + (-2)^2} = \sqrt{5} \approx 2.2;\ |\mathbf{A}| = \sqrt{.5^2 + 1^2} = \sqrt{1.25} \approx 1.1$ About 2.2 inches of rain fell. The area of the opening is about 1.1 in^2.

(b) $V = |\mathbf{R} \cdot \mathbf{A}| = |(1)(.5) + (-2)(1)| = |-1.5| = 1.5$; The volume of rain was 1.5 in^3.

(c) To collect the maximum amount of rain, $\mathbf{R}$ and $\mathbf{A}$ should be parallel and point in opposite directions.

Reviewing Basic Concepts (Sections 10.1—10.3)

1. Angle B has measure $180° - 44° - 62° = 74°$. Now, using the Law of Sines,

$\dfrac{c}{\sin 62°} = \dfrac{12}{\sin 44°} \Rightarrow \dfrac{12\sin 62°}{\sin 44°} \Rightarrow c \approx 15.3;\ \dfrac{b}{\sin 74°} = \dfrac{12}{\sin 44°} \Rightarrow b = \dfrac{12\sin 74°}{\sin 44°} \Rightarrow b \approx 16.6$. The solutions are

$B = 74°,\ b \approx 16.6,\ c = 15.3$.

2. There are two solutions. Using the Law of Sines,

$\dfrac{\sin B}{8} = \dfrac{\sin 32°}{6} \Rightarrow \sin B = \dfrac{8\sin 32°}{6} \Rightarrow B = \sin^{-1}\left(\dfrac{8\sin 32°}{6}\right) \approx 45.0°$. There are two angles: $B_1 = 45.0°$ and

$B_2 = 180° - 45.0° = 135.0°$ (since $32° + 135.0° < 180°$). $c_1 = 180° - 32° - 45.0° = 103°$ and

$c_2 = 180° - 32° - 135° = 13°$ $\dfrac{c_1}{\sin 103°} = \dfrac{6}{\sin 32°} \Rightarrow c_1 = \dfrac{6\sin 103°}{\sin 32°} \approx 11.0$

$\dfrac{c_2}{\sin 13°} = \dfrac{6}{\sin 32°} \Rightarrow c_2 = \dfrac{6\sin 13°}{\sin 32°} \approx 2.5$

The solutions are $B_1 = 45.0°, c_1 = 103°, c_1 = 11.0$ or $B_2 = 135.0°, c_2 = 13°, c_2 = 2.5$.

3. Using the Law of Sines, $\dfrac{\sin A}{7} = \dfrac{\sin 41°}{12} \Rightarrow \sin A = \dfrac{7\sin 41°}{12} \Rightarrow A = \sin^{-1}\left(\dfrac{7\sin 41°}{12}\right) \approx 22.5°$. Since

$180° - 22.5° = 157.5°$ and $41° + 157.5° > 180°$, there is one triangle.

$B = 180° - 41° - 22.5° = 116.5°\cdot \dfrac{b}{\sin 116.5°} = \dfrac{12}{\sin 41°} \Rightarrow b = \dfrac{12\sin 116.5°}{\sin 41°} \approx 16.4$. The solutions are

$A = 22.5°, B = 116.5°, b = 16.4$.

4. (a) Use the Law of Cosines to find b:

$b^2 = 8.1^2 + 8.3^2 - 2(8.1)(8.3)\cos 51° \Rightarrow b = \sqrt{134.5 - 134.46\cos 51°} \approx 7.063$

Use the Law of Sines: $\dfrac{\sin A}{8.1} = \dfrac{\sin 51°}{7.063} \Rightarrow \sin A = \dfrac{8.1\sin 51°}{7.063} \Rightarrow A = \sin^{-1}\left(\dfrac{8.1\sin 51°}{7.063}\right) \approx 63.0°$

Then $C = 180° - 51° - 63.0° = 66.0°$. The solutions are $b \approx 7.1$, $A \approx 63.0°$, $C \approx 66.0°$.

(b) Use the Law of Cosines to find A: $14^2 = 8^2 + 9^2 - 2(8)(9)\cos A \Rightarrow A = \cos^{-1}\left(\dfrac{196-145}{-144}\right) \approx 110.7°$

Use the Law of Sines to find B:

$\dfrac{\sin B}{9} = \dfrac{\sin 110.7°}{14} \Rightarrow \sin B = \dfrac{9\sin 110.7°}{14} \Rightarrow B = \sin^{-1}\left(\dfrac{9\sin 110.7°}{14}\right) \approx 37.0°$.

The value of C is $180° - 110.7° - 37.0° = 32.3°$. The solutions are $A \approx 110.7°$, $B \approx 37.0°$, $C \approx 32.3°$.

5. $A = \dfrac{1}{2}(4.5)(5.2)\sin 55° \approx 9.6$

6. $s = \dfrac{1}{2}(6+7+9) = 11; A = \sqrt{11(11-6)(11-7)(11-9)} \approx 21$

7. (a) $2\mathbf{v}+\mathbf{u} = 2(2\mathbf{i}-\mathbf{j})+(-3\mathbf{i}+2\mathbf{j}) = 4\mathbf{i}-2\mathbf{j}+(-3\mathbf{i}+2\mathbf{j}) = (4\mathbf{i}-3\mathbf{i})+(-2\mathbf{j}+2\mathbf{j}) = \mathbf{i}$

   (b) $2\mathbf{v} = 2(2\mathbf{i}-\mathbf{j}) = 4\mathbf{i}-2\mathbf{j}$

   (c) $\mathbf{v}-3\mathbf{u} = (2\mathbf{i}-\mathbf{j})-3(-3\mathbf{i}+2\mathbf{j}) = 2\mathbf{i}-\mathbf{j}+9\mathbf{i}-6\mathbf{j}) = (2\mathbf{i}+9\mathbf{i})+(-\mathbf{j}-6\mathbf{j}) = 11\mathbf{i}-7\mathbf{j}$

8. $\langle 3,-2\rangle \cdot \langle -1,3\rangle = (3)(-1)+(-2)(3) = -3-6 = -9$

   $\cos\theta = \dfrac{\mathbf{u}\cdot\mathbf{v}}{|\mathbf{u}||\mathbf{v}|} = \dfrac{-9}{\sqrt{9+4}\sqrt{1+9}} = \dfrac{-9}{\sqrt{13}\sqrt{10}} = \dfrac{-9}{\sqrt{130}} \Rightarrow \theta = \cos^{-1}\left(-\dfrac{9}{\sqrt{130}}\right) \approx 142.1°$

9. The adjacent angle in the parallelogram is supplementary to $52°$, thus it has measure $128°$.

   $|\mathbf{v}|^2 = 100^2+130^2-2(100)(130)\cos 128° \approx 42{,}907.19836 \Rightarrow |\mathbf{v}| = \sqrt{42{,}907.19836} \approx 207$ lb

10. Angle B is supplementary to $52°$ and has measure $180°-57° = 123°$. The other angle of the triangle, C, has measure $180°-52°-123° = 5°$. Using the Law of Sines, $\dfrac{a}{\sin 52°} = \dfrac{950}{\sin 5°} \Rightarrow a = \dfrac{950\sin 52°}{\sin 5°} \Rightarrow a \approx 8589$. If a vertical line from the plane to the ground intersects the ground at D, then triangle CBD is a right triangle.

    Thus, $\sin 57° = \dfrac{h}{8589} \Rightarrow h = 8589\sin 57° \approx 7200$ ft.

10.4 Trigonometric (Polar) Form of Complex Numbers

1. The modulus of a complex number represents the magnitude (length) of the vector representing it in the complex plane.

3. See Figure 3.

5. See Figure 5.

518   Chapter 10: Applications of Trigonometry and Vectors

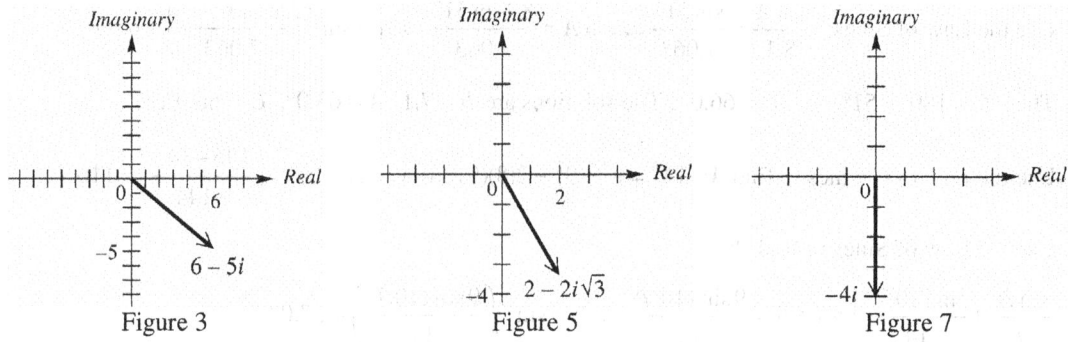

Figure 3   Figure 5   Figure 7

7. See Figure 7.

9. See Figure 9.

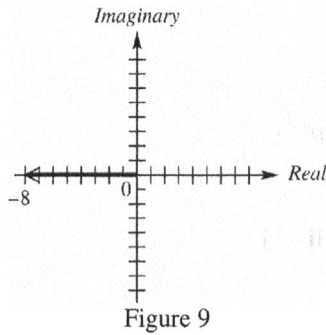

Figure 9   Figure 10

11. Since the vector has terminal point $(1, -4),$ the rectangular form is $1 - 4i$.

13. The imaginary part must be 0.

15. $a = 0$

17. $(4 - 3i) + (-1 + 2i) = (4 - 1) + (-3 + 2)i = 3 - i$

19. $(-3 + 0i) + (0 + 3i) = (-3 + 0) + (0 + 3)i = -3 + 3i$

21. $(2 + 6i) + (0 - 2i) = (2 + 0) + (6 - 2)i = 2 + 4i$

23. $(4 - 2i) + (5 + 0i) = (4 + 5) + (-2 + 0)i = 9 - 2i$

25. $r = \sqrt{1^2 + 1^2} = \sqrt{2}$

27. $r = \sqrt{12^2 + (-5)^2} = \sqrt{169} = 13$

29. $r = \sqrt{(-6)^2 + 0^2} = \sqrt{36} = 6$

31. $r = \sqrt{2^2 + (-3)^2} = \sqrt{13}$

33. $2(\cos 45° + i \sin 45°) = 2\left(\dfrac{\sqrt{2}}{2} + i\dfrac{\sqrt{2}}{2}\right) = \sqrt{2} + i\sqrt{2}$

35. $10 \text{ cis } 90° = 10(\cos 90° + i \sin 90°) = 10(0 + 1i) = 10i$

Section 10.4   519

37. $4(\cos 240° - i\sin 240°) = 4\left(-\dfrac{1}{2} - i\dfrac{\sqrt{3}}{2}\right) = -2 - 2i\sqrt{3}$

39. $\left(\cos\dfrac{\pi}{6} + i\sin\dfrac{\pi}{6}\right) = \left(\dfrac{\sqrt{3}}{2} + i\dfrac{1}{2}\right) = \dfrac{\sqrt{3}}{2} + \dfrac{1}{2}i$

41. $5\operatorname{cis}\left(-\dfrac{\pi}{6}\right) = 5\left[\cos\left(-\dfrac{\pi}{6}\right) + i\sin\left(-\dfrac{\pi}{6}\right)\right] = 5\left(\dfrac{\sqrt{3}}{2} - i\dfrac{1}{2}\right) = \dfrac{5\sqrt{3}}{2} - \dfrac{5}{2}i$

43. $\sqrt{2}\operatorname{cis}\pi = \sqrt{2}(\cos\pi + i\sin\pi) = \sqrt{2}(-1 - 0i) = -\sqrt{2}$

45. $r = \sqrt{3^2 + (-3)^2} = \sqrt{18} = 3\sqrt{2}; \tan\theta = \dfrac{y}{x} \Rightarrow \tan\theta = \dfrac{-3}{3} \Rightarrow \tan\theta = -1 \Rightarrow \theta = \tan^{-1}(-1) = -45°$ Since θ is in

   quadrant IV and $0° \le \theta \le 360°$, $\theta = 36 - 45 = 315°$. Therefore $3 - 3i = 3\sqrt{2}\left[\cos(315°) + i\sin(315°)\right]$.

47. $r = \sqrt{1^2 + (\sqrt{3})^2} = \sqrt{4} = 2; \tan\theta = \dfrac{y}{x} \Rightarrow \tan\theta = \dfrac{\sqrt{3}}{1} \Rightarrow \tan\theta = \sqrt{3} \Rightarrow \theta = \tan^{-1}(\sqrt{3}) = 60°$

   Since θ is in quadrant I, $\theta = 60°$. Therefore $1 + i\sqrt{3} = 2(\cos 60° + i\sin 60°)$.

49. $r = \sqrt{0^2 + (-2)^2} = \sqrt{4} = 2; \tan\theta = \dfrac{y}{x} \Rightarrow \tan\theta = \dfrac{-2}{0} \Rightarrow \tan\theta$ is undefined $\Rightarrow \theta = 90°$. Since θ is on the

   negative y-axis and $0° \le \theta \le 360°$, $\theta = 90° + 180° = 270°$. Therefore $-2i = 2\left[\cos(270°) + i\sin(270°)\right]$.

51. $r = \sqrt{(4\sqrt{3})^2 + 4^2} = \sqrt{64} = 8; \tan\theta = \dfrac{y}{x} \Rightarrow \tan\theta = \dfrac{1}{\sqrt{3}} \Rightarrow \tan\theta = \dfrac{1}{\sqrt{3}} \Rightarrow \theta = \tan^{-1}\left(\dfrac{1}{\sqrt{3}}\right) = \dfrac{\pi}{6}$.

   Since θ is in quadrant I and $0 \le \theta \le 2\pi$, $\theta = \dfrac{\pi}{6}$. Therefore $4\sqrt{3} + 4i = 8\left(\cos\dfrac{\pi}{6} + i\sin\dfrac{\pi}{6}\right)$.

53. $r = \sqrt{(-\sqrt{2})^2 + (\sqrt{2})^2} = \sqrt{4} = 2; \tan\theta = \dfrac{y}{x} \Rightarrow \tan\theta = -\dfrac{\sqrt{2}}{\sqrt{2}} \Rightarrow \tan\theta = -1 \Rightarrow \theta = \tan^{-1}(-1) = -\dfrac{\pi}{4}$

   Since θ is in quadrant II and $0 \le \theta \le 2\pi$, $\theta = -\dfrac{\pi}{4} + \pi = \dfrac{3\pi}{4}$. Therefore $-\sqrt{2} + i\sqrt{2} = 2\left(\cos\dfrac{3\pi}{4} + i\sin\dfrac{3\pi}{4}\right)$.

55. $r = \sqrt{(-4)^2 \, 0^2} = \sqrt{16} = 4; \tan\theta = \dfrac{y}{x} \Rightarrow \tan\theta = \dfrac{0}{-4} \Rightarrow \tan\theta = 0 \Rightarrow \theta = \tan^{-1}(0) = 0$

   Since θ is on the negative x-axis and $0 \le \theta \le 2\pi$, $\theta = 0 + \pi = \pi$. Therefore $-4 = 4(\cos\pi + i\sin\pi)$.

57. $[3(\cos 60° + i\sin 60°)][2(\cos 90° + i\sin 90°)] = (3 \cdot 2)[\cos(60° + 90°) + i\sin(60° + 90°)]$

   $= 6(\cos 150° + i\sin 150°) = 6\left(-\dfrac{\sqrt{3}}{2} + \dfrac{1}{2}i\right) = -3\sqrt{3} + 3i$

59. $[2(\cos 45° + i\sin 45°)][2(\cos 225° + i\sin 225°)] = (2 \cdot 2)[\cos(45° + 225°) + i\sin(45° + 225°)]$

   $= 4(\cos 270° + i\sin 270°) = 4(0 - 1i) = -4i$

61. $\left[5\operatorname{cis}\dfrac{\pi}{2}\right]\left[3\operatorname{cis}\dfrac{\pi}{2}\right] = \left[5\left(\cos\dfrac{\pi}{2}+i\sin\dfrac{\pi}{2}\right)\right]\left[3\left(\cos\dfrac{\pi}{4}+i\sin\dfrac{\pi}{4}\right)\right]$

$= (5\cdot 3)\left[\cos\left(\dfrac{\pi}{2}+\dfrac{\pi}{4}\right)+i\sin\left(\dfrac{\pi}{2}+\dfrac{\pi}{4}\right)\right] = 15\left(\cos\dfrac{3\pi}{4}+i\sin\dfrac{3\pi}{4}\right) = 15\left(-\dfrac{\sqrt{2}}{2}+\dfrac{\sqrt{2}}{2}i\right) = -\dfrac{15\sqrt{2}}{2}+\dfrac{15\sqrt{2}}{2}i$

63. $\left(\sqrt{3}\operatorname{cis}\dfrac{\pi}{4}\right)\left(\sqrt{3}\operatorname{cis}\dfrac{5\pi}{4}\right) = \left[\sqrt{3}\left(\cos\dfrac{\pi}{4}+i\sin\dfrac{\pi}{4}\right)\right]\left[\sqrt{3}\left(\cos\dfrac{5\pi}{4}+i\sin\dfrac{5\pi}{4}\right)\right]$

$= (\sqrt{3}\cdot\sqrt{3})\left[\cos\left(\dfrac{\pi}{4}+\dfrac{5\pi}{4}\right)+i\sin\left(\dfrac{\pi}{4}+\dfrac{5\pi}{4}\right)\right] = 3\left(\cos\dfrac{3\pi}{2}+i\sin\dfrac{3\pi}{2}\right) = 3(0+1i) = -3i$

65. $\dfrac{4(\cos 120°+i\sin 120°)}{2(\cos 150°+i\sin 150°)} = \dfrac{4}{2}[\cos(120°-150°)+i\sin(120°-150°)]$

$= 2[\cos(-30°)+i\sin(-30°)] = 2\left(\dfrac{\sqrt{3}}{2}-\dfrac{1}{2}i\right) = \sqrt{3}-i$

67. $\dfrac{10(\cos\frac{5\pi}{4}+i\sin\frac{5\pi}{4})}{5(\cos\frac{\pi}{4}+i\sin\frac{\pi}{4})} = \dfrac{10}{5}\left[\cos(\dfrac{5\pi}{4}-\dfrac{\pi}{4})+i\sin(\dfrac{5\pi}{4}-\dfrac{\pi}{4})\right] = 2(\cos\pi+i\sin\pi) = 2(-1-0i) = -2$

69. $\dfrac{3\operatorname{cis}\frac{61\pi}{36}}{9\operatorname{cis}\frac{13\pi}{36}} = \dfrac{3(\cos\frac{61\pi}{36}+i\sin\frac{61\pi}{36})}{9(\cos\frac{13\pi}{36}+i\sin\frac{13\pi}{36})} = \dfrac{3}{9}[\cos(\dfrac{61\pi}{36}-\dfrac{13\pi}{36})+i\sin(\dfrac{61\pi}{36}-\dfrac{13\pi}{36})] =$

$\dfrac{1}{3}\left(\cos\dfrac{4\pi}{3}+\sin\dfrac{4\pi}{3}\right) = \dfrac{1}{3}\left(-\dfrac{1}{2}-\dfrac{\sqrt{3}}{2}i\right) = -\dfrac{1}{6}-\dfrac{\sqrt{3}}{6}i$

71. $\dfrac{8}{\sqrt{3}+i}$ numerator: $8 = 8+0i$ and $r = \sqrt{8^2+0^2} = 8$ $\theta = 0°$ since $\cos 0° = 1$ and $\sin 0° = 0$, so $8 =$

8 cis 0°; denominator: $\sqrt{3}+i$ and $r = \sqrt{(\sqrt{3})^2+1^2} = \sqrt{3+1} = \sqrt{4} = 2$; $\tan\theta = \dfrac{1}{\sqrt{3}} = \dfrac{\sqrt{3}}{3}$

Since x and y are both positive, θ is in quadrant I, so $\theta = 30°$. Thus $\sqrt{3}+i = 2\operatorname{cis} 30°$.

$\dfrac{8}{\sqrt{3}+i} = \dfrac{8\operatorname{cis} 0°}{2\operatorname{cis} 30°} = \dfrac{8}{2}\operatorname{cis}(0-30°) = 4[\cos(-30°)+i\sin(-30°)] = 4\left(\dfrac{\sqrt{3}}{2}-\dfrac{1}{2}i\right) = 2\sqrt{3}-2i$

73. $\dfrac{-i}{1+i}$ numerator: $-i = 0-i$ and $r = \sqrt{0^2+(-1)^2} = \sqrt{0+1} = \sqrt{1} = 1$, $\theta = 270°$ since $\cos 270° = 0$ and

$\sin 270° = -1$, so $-i = 1\operatorname{cis} 270°$.; denominator: $1+i$ $r = \sqrt{1^2+1^2} = \sqrt{1+1} = \sqrt{2}$ and $\tan\theta = \dfrac{y}{x} = \dfrac{1}{1} = 1$

Since x and y are both positive, θ is in quadrant I, so $\theta = 45°$. Thus, $1+i = \sqrt{2}\operatorname{cis} 45°$

$\dfrac{-i}{1+i} = \dfrac{\operatorname{cis} 270°}{\sqrt{2}\operatorname{cis} 45°} = \dfrac{1}{\sqrt{2}}\operatorname{cis}(270°-45°) = \dfrac{\sqrt{2}}{2}\operatorname{cis} 225° = \dfrac{\sqrt{2}}{2}(\cos 225°+i\sin 225°) =$

$$\frac{\sqrt{2}}{2}\left(-\frac{\sqrt{2}}{2}-i\cdot\frac{\sqrt{2}}{2}\right)=-\frac{1}{2}-\frac{1}{2}i$$

75. $\frac{2\sqrt{6}-2i\sqrt{2}}{\sqrt{2}-i\sqrt{6}}$ numerator: $2\sqrt{6}-2i\sqrt{2}$ and $r=\sqrt{\left(2\sqrt{6}\right)^2+\left(-2\sqrt{2}\right)^2}=\sqrt{24+8}=\sqrt{32}=4\sqrt{2}$

$\tan\theta=\frac{-2\sqrt{2}}{2\sqrt{6}}=-\frac{1}{\sqrt{3}}=-\frac{\sqrt{3}}{3}$. Since x is positive and y is negative, θ is in quadrant IV, so $\theta=-30°$.

Thus, $2\sqrt{6}-2i\sqrt{2}=4\sqrt{2}\operatorname{cis}(-30°)$. denominator: $\sqrt{2}-i\sqrt{6}$ and

$r=\sqrt{\left(\sqrt{2}\right)^2+\left(-\sqrt{6}\right)^2}=\sqrt{2+6}=\sqrt{8}=2\sqrt{2}$, $\tan\theta=\frac{-\sqrt{6}}{\sqrt{2}}=-\sqrt{3}$

Since x is positive and y is negative, θ is in quadrant IV, so $\theta=-60°$. Thus, $\sqrt{2}-i\sqrt{6}=2\sqrt{2}\operatorname{cis}(-60°)$

$\frac{2\sqrt{6}-2i\sqrt{2}}{\sqrt{2}-i\sqrt{6}}=\frac{4\sqrt{2}\operatorname{cis}(-30°)}{2\sqrt{2}\operatorname{cis}(-60°)}=\frac{4\sqrt{2}}{2\sqrt{2}}\operatorname{cis}\left[-30°-(-60°)\right]=2\operatorname{cis}30°=2(\cos 30°+i\sin 30°)=$

$2\left(\frac{\sqrt{3}}{2}+i\frac{1}{2}\right)=\sqrt{3}+i$

77. (a) $|a+bi|=\sqrt{a^2+b^2}$ and $|a-bi|=\sqrt{a^2+(-b^2)}=\sqrt{a^2+b^2}$

   (b) $Z_1^2-1=(a+bi)^2-1=a^2+2abi-b^2-1=a^2-b^2-1+2abi$

   $Z_2^2-1=(a-bi)^2-1=a^2-2abi-b^2-1=a^2-b^2-1-2abi$

   (c) If $z_1=a+bi$ and $z_2=a-bi$, then z_1^2-1 and z_2^2-1 are also conjugates with the same modulus.

   Therefore, if z_1 is in the Julia set, so is z_2. Thus (a,b) in the Julia set implies $(a,-b)$ is also in the set.

   (d) Yes, see part (e) below.

   (e) $z_1^2-1=(a+bi)^2-1=a^2+2abi-b^2-1=a^2-b^2-1+2abi$

   $z_2^2-1=(-a+bi)^2-1=a^2-2abi-b^2-1=a^2-b^2-1-2abi$. If $z_1=a+bi$ and

   $z_2=-a+bi$, then z_1^2-1 and z_2^2-1 are also conjugates with the same modulus.

   Therefore, if z_1 is in the Julia set, so is z_2. Thus (a,b) in the Julia set implies $(a,-b)$ is also in the set.

79. First find the trigonometric form of $Z=6+3i$: $r=\sqrt{6^2+3^2}=\sqrt{45}\approx 6.71$;

$\tan\theta=\frac{3}{6}\Rightarrow\tan\theta=\frac{1}{2}\Rightarrow\theta\tan^{-1}\frac{1}{2}\Rightarrow\theta\approx 26.6°$. Therefore $Z\approx 6.71(\cos 26.6°+i\sin 26.6°)$.

$I=\frac{E}{Z}=\frac{8(\cos 20°+i\sin 20°)}{6.71(\cos 26.57°+i\sin 26.57°)}=\frac{8}{6.71}[\cos(20°-26.57°)+i\sin(20°-26.57°)]\approx 1.18-.14i$

81. Noting that $Z=\dfrac{1}{\dfrac{1}{Z_1}+\dfrac{1}{Z_2}}=\dfrac{1}{\dfrac{Z_2+Z_1}{Z_1Z_2}}=\dfrac{Z_1Z_2}{Z_1+Z_2}$, we find the following:

First find the trigonometric form of $Z_1 = 50+25i$: $r = \sqrt{50^2 + 25^2} = \sqrt{3125}$;

$\tan\theta = \dfrac{25}{50} \Rightarrow = \tan^{-1}\dfrac{1}{2} \Rightarrow \theta \approx 25.565°$. The value is $\sqrt{3125}(\cos 26.565° + i\sin 26.565°)$.

Next find the trigonometric form of $Z_2 = 60+20i$: $r = \sqrt{60^2 + 20^2} = \sqrt{4000}$;

$\tan\theta = \dfrac{20}{60} \Rightarrow\Rightarrow \theta = \tan^{-1}\dfrac{1}{3} \Rightarrow \theta \approx 18.435°$. The value is $\sqrt{4000}(\cos 18.435° + i\sin 18.435°)$. Finally find

the trigonometric form of $Z_1 + Z_2 = 110+45i$: $r = \sqrt{110^2 + 45^2} = \sqrt{14,125}$;

$\tan\theta = \dfrac{45}{110} \Rightarrow\Rightarrow \theta = \tan^{-1}\dfrac{9}{22} \Rightarrow \theta \approx 22.249°$. The value is $\sqrt{14,125}(\cos 22.249° + i\sin 22.249°)$.

$$Z = \dfrac{[\sqrt{3125}(\cos 26.565° + i\sin 26.565°)][\sqrt{4000}(\cos 18.435° + i\sin 18.435°)]}{\sqrt{14,125}(\cos 22.249° + i\sin 22.249°)} =$$

$$\dfrac{\sqrt{3125} \cdot \sqrt{4000}}{\sqrt{14,125}}[(\cos(26.565° + 18.435° - 22.249°)) + i\sin(26.565° + 18.435° - 22.249°)] \approx 27.43 + 11.5i$$

83. To square a complex number in trigonometric form, square the modulus r and double the argument θ.

85. (a) If the real part equals 0, then $\cos\theta = 0 \Rightarrow \theta = \dfrac{\pi}{2}$.

    (b) If the imaginary part equals 0, then $\sin\theta = 0 \Rightarrow \theta = \pi$.

10.5 Powers and Roots of Complex Numbers

1. $[3(\cos 30° + i\sin 30°)]^3 = 3^3[\cos(3 \cdot 30°) + i\sin(3 \cdot 30°)] = 27(\cos 90° + i\sin 90°) = 27(0 + 1i) = 27i$

3. $\left(\cos\dfrac{\pi}{4} + i\sin\dfrac{\pi}{4}\right)^8 = \cos\left(8 \cdot \dfrac{\pi}{4}\right) + i\sin\left(8 \cdot \dfrac{\pi}{4}\right) = \cos 2\pi + i\sin 2\pi = 1 + 0i = 1$

5. $\left[2\left(\cos\dfrac{2\pi}{3} + i\sin\dfrac{2\pi}{3}\right)\right]^3 = 2^3\left[\cos\left(3 \cdot \dfrac{2\pi}{3}\right) + i\sin\left(3 \cdot \dfrac{2\pi}{3}\right)\right] = 8(\cos 2\pi + i\sin 2\pi) = 8(1 + 0i) = 8$

7. $[3cis100°]^3 = [3(\cos 100° + i\sin 100°)]^3 = 3^3[\cos(3 \cdot 100°) + i\sin(3 \cdot 100°)] =$

   $27(\cos 300° + i\sin 300°) = 27\left(\dfrac{1}{2} - \dfrac{\sqrt{3}}{2}i\right) = \dfrac{27}{2} - \dfrac{27\sqrt{3}}{2}i$

9. First find the trigonometric form of $\sqrt{3} + i$; $r = \sqrt{(\sqrt{3})^2 + 1^2} = \sqrt{4} = 2$;

   $\tan\theta = \dfrac{y}{x} \Rightarrow \tan\theta = \dfrac{1}{\sqrt{3}} \Rightarrow\Rightarrow \theta = \tan^{-1}\dfrac{1}{\sqrt{3}} = 30°$ $\sqrt{3} + i = 2(\cos 30° + i\sin 30°)$.

   $(\sqrt{3} + i)^3 = [2(\cos 30° + i\sin 30°)]^3 = 2^3[\cos(3 \cdot 30°) + i\sin(3 \cdot 30°)] = 8(\cos 90° + i\sin 90°) + 8(0 + 1i) = 8i$

11. First find the trigonometric form of $1 + i\sqrt{3}$; $r = \sqrt{1^2 + (\sqrt{3})^2} = \sqrt{4} = 2$;

$\tan\theta = \dfrac{y}{x} \Rightarrow \tan\theta = \dfrac{\sqrt{3}}{1} \Rightarrow \Rightarrow \theta = \tan^{-1}\sqrt{3} = 60°$. Therefore

$1+i\sqrt{3} = 2(\cos 60° + i\sin 60°)$. $(1+i\sqrt{3})^4 = [2(\cos 60° + i\sin 60°)]^4 = 2^4[\cos(4\cdot 60°) + i\sin(4\cdot 60°)] =$

$16(\cos 240° + i\sin 240°) = 16\left(-\dfrac{1}{2} - \dfrac{\sqrt{3}}{2}i\right) = -8 - 8i\sqrt{3}$

13. First find the trigonometric form of $-\dfrac{\sqrt{2}}{2} + \dfrac{\sqrt{2}}{2}i$; $r = \sqrt{\left(-\dfrac{\sqrt{2}}{2}\right)^2 + \left(\dfrac{\sqrt{2}}{2}\right)^2} = \sqrt{1} = 1$;

$\tan\theta = \dfrac{y}{x} \Rightarrow \tan\theta = \left[\dfrac{\sqrt{2}}{2} \div \left(-\dfrac{\sqrt{2}}{2}\right)\right] \Rightarrow \tan\theta = -1 \Rightarrow \theta = \tan^{-1} 1 = -45°$. Since θ is in quadrant II,

$\theta = -45° + 180° = 135°$. Therefore $-\dfrac{\sqrt{2}}{2} + \dfrac{\sqrt{2}}{2}i = \cos 135° + i\sin 135°$.

$\left(-\dfrac{\sqrt{2}}{2} + \dfrac{\sqrt{2}}{2}i\right)^4 = (\cos 135° + i\sin 135°)^4 = \cos(4.135°) + i\sin(4.135°) = \cos 540° + i\sin 540° = -1$

15. First find the trigonometric form of $1-i$; $r = \sqrt{1^2 + (-1)^2} = \sqrt{2}$;

$\tan\theta = \dfrac{y}{x} \Rightarrow \tan\theta = \dfrac{-1}{1} \Rightarrow \Rightarrow \theta = \tan^{-1}(-1) = -45°$. Therefore $1-i = \sqrt{2}[\cos(-45°) + i\sin(-45°)]$.

$(1-i)^6 = [\sqrt{2}(\cos(-45°) + i\sin(-45°))]^6 = (\sqrt{2})^6\{\cos[6.(-45°)] + i\sin[6.(-45°)]\}$

$= 8[\cos(-270°) + i\sin(-270°)] = 8(0 + 1i) = 8i$

17. First find the trigonometric form of $-2-2i$; $r = \sqrt{(-2)^2 + (-2)^2} = \sqrt{8} = 2\sqrt{2}$;

$\tan\theta = \dfrac{y}{x} \Rightarrow \tan\theta = \dfrac{-2}{-2} \Rightarrow \Rightarrow \theta = \tan^{-1} 1 = 225°$. Therefore, $-2-2i = 2\sqrt{2}(\cos 225° + i\sin 225°)$.

$(-2-2i)^5 = [2\sqrt{2}(\cos 225° + i\sin 225°)]^5 = (2\sqrt{2})^5[\cos(5.225°) + i\sin(5.225°)] =$

$128\sqrt{2}(\cos 1125° + i\sin 1125°) = 128\sqrt{2}\left(\dfrac{\sqrt{2}}{2} + \dfrac{\sqrt{2}}{2}i\right) = 128 + 128i$

19. Note that $1 = (\cos 0° + i\sin 0°)$. Here $r = 1$, so $\sqrt[3]{r} = 1$, $n = 3$, and $k = 0, 1,$ or 2. $\alpha = \dfrac{0° + 360°\cdot k}{3}$: For

$k = 0, \alpha = 0°$. For $k = 1, \alpha = 120°$. For $k = 2, \alpha = 240°$. The cube roots are

$\cos 0° + i\sin 0°, \cos 120° + i\sin 120°,$ and $\cos 240° + i\sin 240°$. See Figure 19.

21. Here $r = 8$ so $\sqrt[3]{r} = 2$, $n = 3$, and $k = 0, 1,$ or 2. $\alpha = \dfrac{60° + 360°\cdot k}{3}$: For $k = 0, \alpha = 20°$. For

$k = 1, \alpha = 140°$. For $k = 2, \alpha = 260°$. The cube roots are $2(\cos 20° + i\sin 20°), 2(\cos 140° + i\sin 140°),$ and

$2(\cos 260° + i\sin 260°)$. See Figure 21.

524 Chapter 10: Applications of Trigonometry and Vectors

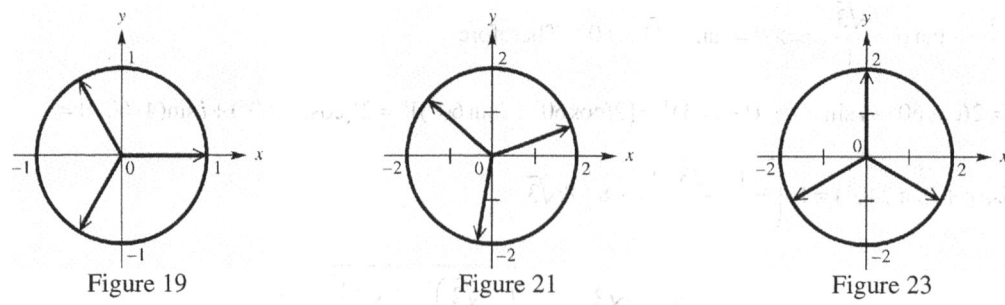

Figure 19 Figure 21 Figure 23

23. Note that $-8i = 8(\cos 270° + i \sin 270°)$. Here $r = 8$, so $\sqrt[3]{r} = 2$, $n = 3$, and $k = 0, 1,$ or 2. For

$\alpha = \dfrac{270° + 360° \cdot k}{3}$: For $k = 0$, $\alpha = 90°$. For $k = 1, \alpha = 210°$. For $k = 2$, $\alpha = 330°$. The cube roots

are $2(\cos 90° + i \sin 90°)$, $2(\cos 210° + i \sin 210°)$, and $2(\cos 330° + i \sin 330°)$. See Figure 23.

25. Note that $-64 = 64(\cos 180° + i \sin 180°)$. Here $r = 64$, so $\sqrt[3]{r} = 4$, $n = 3$, and $k = 0, 1,$ or 2.

$\alpha = \dfrac{180° + 360° \cdot k}{3}$: For $k = 0$, $\alpha = 60°$. For $k = 1$, $\alpha = 180°$. For $k = 2$, $\alpha = 300°$. The cube roots are

$4(\cos 60° + i \sin 60°), 4(\cos 180° + i \sin 180°)$, and $4(\cos 300° + i \sin 300°)$. See Figure 25.

27. Note that $1 + i\sqrt{3} = 2(\cos 60° + i \sin 60°)$. Here $r = 2$, so $\sqrt[3]{r} = \sqrt[3]{2}$, $n = 3$, and $k = 0, 1,$ or 2.

$\alpha = \dfrac{60° + 360° \cdot k}{3}$: For $k = 0$, $\alpha = 20°$. For $k = 1$, $\alpha = 140°$. For $k = 2$, $\alpha = 260°$. The cube roots are

$\sqrt[3]{2}(\cos 20° + i \sin 20°), \sqrt[3]{2}(\cos 140° + i \sin 140°)$, and $\sqrt[3]{2}(\cos 260° + i \sin 260°)$. See Figure 27.

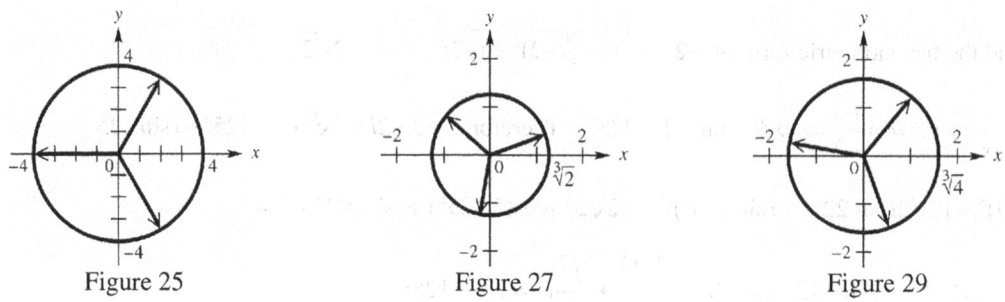

Figure 25 Figure 27 Figure 29

29. Note that $-2\sqrt{3} + 2i = 4(\cos 150° + i \sin 150°)$. Here $r = 4$, so $\sqrt[3]{r} = \sqrt[3]{4}$, $n = 3$, and

$k = 0, 1, 2$. $\alpha = \dfrac{150° + 360° \cdot k}{3}$: For $k = 0$, $\alpha = 50°$. For $k = 1$, $\alpha = 170°$. For $k = 2$, $\alpha = 290°$. The cube

roots are $\sqrt[3]{4}(\cos 50° + i \sin 50°)$, $\sqrt[3]{4}(\cos 170° + i \sin 170°)$, and $\sqrt[3]{4}(\cos 290° + i \sin 290°)$. See Figure 29.

31. The complex number is $4(\cos 120° + i \sin 120°)$. $r = 4$, so $\sqrt{r} = 2$, $n = 2$, and $k = 0$ or 1.

$\alpha = \dfrac{120° + 360° \cdot k}{2}$: For $k = 0$, $\alpha = 60°$. For $k = 1$, $\alpha = 240°$. The square roots are

$2(\cos 60° + i \sin 60°) = 1 + i\sqrt{3}$ and $2(\cos 240° + i \sin 240°) = -1 - i\sqrt{3}$.

Copyright © 2015 Pearson Education, Inc

33. The complex number is $\cos 180° + i\sin 180°$ Here $r = 1$ so, $\sqrt[3]{r} = 1$, $n = 3$, and

$k = 0, 1,$ or 2. $\alpha = \dfrac{180° + 360° \cdot k}{3}$: For $k = 0$, $\alpha = 60°$. For $k = 1$, $\alpha = 180°$. For $k = 2$, $\alpha = 300°$. The

cube roots are $\cos 60° + i\sin 60° = \dfrac{1}{2} + \dfrac{\sqrt{3}}{2}i$, $\cos 180° + i\sin 180° = -1$, and $\cos 300° + i\sin 300° = \dfrac{1}{2} - \dfrac{\sqrt{3}}{2}i$.

35. Note that $i = \cos 90° + i\sin 90°$. Here $r = 1$, so $\sqrt{r} = 1$, $n = 2$, and $k = 0$ or 1. $\alpha = \dfrac{90° + 360° \cdot k}{2}$:

For $k = 0$, $\alpha = 45°$. For $k = 1$, $\alpha = 225°$. The square roots are $\cos 45° + i\sin 45° = \dfrac{\sqrt{2}}{2} + \dfrac{\sqrt{2}}{2}i$

and $\cos 225° + i\sin 225° = -\dfrac{\sqrt{2}}{2} - \dfrac{\sqrt{2}}{2}i$.

37. Note that $64i = 64(\cos 90° + i\sin 90°)$. Here $r = 64$, So $\sqrt[3]{r} = 4$, $n = 3$, and

$k = 0, 1,$ or 2. $\alpha = \dfrac{90° + 360° \cdot k}{3}$: For $k = 0$, $\alpha = 30°$. For $k = 1$, $\alpha = 150°$. For $k = 2$, $\alpha = 270°$. The cube

roots are $4(\cos 30° + i\sin 30°) = 2\sqrt{3} + 2i$, $4(\cos 150° + i\sin 150°) = -2\sqrt{3} + 2i$ and

$4(\cos 270° + i\sin 270°) = -4i$.

39. Note that $81 = 81(\cos 0° + i\sin 0°)$. Here $r = 81$, so $\sqrt[4]{r} = 3$, $n = 4$, and $k = 0, 1, 2,$ or 3. $\alpha = \dfrac{0° + 360° \cdot k}{4}$:

For $k = 0$, $\alpha = 0°$. For $k = 1$, $\alpha = 90°$. For $k = 2$, $\alpha = 180°$. For $k = 3$, $\alpha = 270°$. The fourth roots

are $3(\cos 0° + i\sin 0°) = 3$, $3(\cos 90° + i\sin 90°) = 3i$, $3(\cos 180° + i\sin 180°) = -3$, and

$3(\cos 270° + i\sin 270°) = -3i$.

41. (a) Note that $1 = \cos 0° + i\sin 0°$. Here $r = 1$, so $\sqrt[4]{r} = 1$, $n = 4$, and $k = 0, 1, 2,$ or 3 $\alpha = \dfrac{0° + 360°k}{4}$:

For $k = 0$, $\alpha = 0°$. For $k = 1$, $\alpha = 90°$. For $k = 2$, $\alpha = 180°$. For $k = 3$, $\alpha = 270°$. The fourth roots are

$\cos 0° + i\sin 0° = 1$, $\cos 90° + i\sin 90° = i$ $\cos 180° + i\sin 180° = -1$ and $\cos 270° + i\sin 270° = -i$.

See Figure 41a.

(b) Note that $1 = \cos 0° + i\sin 0°$. Here $r = 1$, so $\sqrt[6]{r} = 1$, $n = 6$, and $k = 0, 1, 2, 3, 4$ or 5. $\alpha = \dfrac{0° + 360° \cdot k}{6}$:

For $k = 0$, $\alpha = 0°$. For $k = 1$, $\alpha = 60°$. For $k = 2$, $\alpha = 120°$. For $k = 3$, $\alpha = 180°$. For $k = 4$, $\alpha = 240°$.

For $k = 5$, $\alpha = 300°$. The sixth roots are

$\cos 0° + i\sin 0° = 1$, $\cos 60° + i\sin 60° = \dfrac{1}{2} + \dfrac{\sqrt{3}}{2}i$, $\cos 120° + i\sin 120° = -\dfrac{1}{2} + \dfrac{\sqrt{3}}{2}i$,

$\cos 180° + i\sin 180° = -1$, $\cos 240° + i\sin 240° = -\dfrac{1}{2} - \dfrac{\sqrt{3}}{2}i$ $\cos 300° + i\sin 300° = \dfrac{1}{2} - \dfrac{\sqrt{3}}{2}i$.

See Figure 41b

526 Chapter 10: Applications of Trigonometry and Vectors

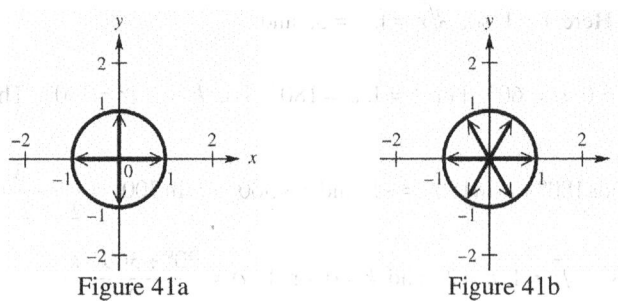

Figure 41a   Figure 41b

43. The argument for a positive real number is $\theta = 0°$. By the nth root theorem with $k = 0$, $\alpha = 0°$. Thus, one nth root has an argument of $0°$ and it must be real.

45. $x^3 + 8 = (x+2)(x^2 - 2x + 4)$

46. $x + 2 = 0 \Rightarrow x = -2$

47. $x^2 - 2x + 4 = 0 \Rightarrow x^2 - 2x + 1 = -4 + 1 \Rightarrow (x-1)^2 = -3 \Rightarrow x - 1 = \pm\sqrt{-3} \Rightarrow x = 1 \pm i\sqrt{3}$

48. Note that $8(\cos 180° + i \sin 180°)$. Here $r = 8$, so $\sqrt[3]{r} = 2$, $n = 3$, and $k = 0, 1,$ or 2. $\alpha = \dfrac{180° + 360° \cdot k}{3}$: For $k = 0$, $\alpha = 60°$. For $k = 1$, $\alpha = 180°$. For $k = 2$, $\alpha = 300°$. The cube roots are

    $2(\cos 60° + i \sin 60°), 2(\cos 180° + i \sin 180°),$ and $2(\cos 300° + i \sin 300°)$

49. $2(\cos 60° + i \sin 60°) = 1 + i\sqrt{3}, 2(\cos 180° + i \sin 180°) = -2$, and $2(\cos 300° + i \sin 300°) = 1 - i\sqrt{3}$.

50. The results are the same.

51. $x^4 + 1 = 0 \Rightarrow x^4 = -1$. Find the fourth roots of -1. Note that $-1 = \cos 180° + i \sin 180°$. Here $r = 1$, so

    $\sqrt[4]{r} = 1$, $n = 4$, and $k = 0, 1, 2,$ or 3 $\alpha = \dfrac{180° + 360° \cdot k}{4}$: For $k = 0$, $\alpha = 45°$. For $k = 1$, $\alpha = 135°$. For $k = 2$, $\alpha = 225°$. For $k = 3$, $\alpha = 315°$. The fourth roots are

    $\cos 45° + i \sin 45°, \cos 135° + i \sin 135°, \cos 225° + i \sin 225°,$ and $\cos 315° + i \sin 315°$.

53. $x^5 - i = 0 \Rightarrow x^5 = i$. Find the fifth roots of i. Note that $i = \cos 90° + i \sin 90°$. Here $r = 1$, so

    $\sqrt[5]{r} = 1$, $n = 5$, and $k = 0, 1, 2, 3,$ or 4. $\alpha = \dfrac{90° + 360° \cdot k}{5}$: For $k = 0$, $\alpha = 18°$. For $k = 1$, $\alpha = 90°$. For $k = 2$, $\alpha = 162°$. For $k = 3$, $\alpha = 234°$. For $k = 4$, $\alpha = 306°$. The fifth roots are

    $\cos 18° + i \sin 18°, \cos 90° + i \sin 90°, \cos 162° + i \sin 162°, \cos 234° + i \sin 234°,$ and $\cos 306° + i \sin 306°$.

55. $x^3 + 1 = 0 \Rightarrow x^3 = -1$. Find the cube roots of -1. Note that $-1 = \cos 180° + i \sin 180°$. Here $r = 1$, so

    $\sqrt[3]{r} = 1$, $n = 3$, and $k = 0, 1,$ or 2. $\alpha = \dfrac{180° + 360° \cdot k}{3}$: For $k = 0$, $\alpha = 60°$. For $k = 1$, $\alpha = 180°$. For $k = 2$, $\alpha = 300°$. The fourth roots are $\cos 60° + i \sin 60°, \cos 180° + i \sin 180°,$ and $\cos 300° + i \sin 300°$.

57. $x^3 - 8 = 0 \Rightarrow x^3 = 8$. Find the cube roots of 8. Note that $8 = 8(\cos 0° + i \sin 0°)$. Here $r = 8$, so $\sqrt[n]{r} = 2$, $n = 3$, and $k = 0, 1$, or 2. $\alpha = \dfrac{0° + 360° \cdot k}{3}$. For $k = 0$, $\alpha = 0°$. For $k = 1$, $\alpha = 120°$. For $k = 2$, $\alpha = 240°$. The cube roots are $2(\cos 0° + i \sin 0°)$, $2(\cos 120° + i \sin 120°)$, and $2(\cos 240° + i \sin 240°)$.

59. (a) Using a calculator yields: $f(z_1) = \dfrac{2(i)^3 + 1}{3(i)^2} = -\dfrac{1}{3} + \dfrac{2}{3}i$; $f(z_2) = \dfrac{2(\frac{1}{3} + \frac{2}{3}i)^3 + 1}{3(-\frac{1}{3} + \frac{2}{3}i)^2} = -\dfrac{131}{225} + \dfrac{208}{225}i$

The value is approaching w_2 and the pixel should be colored blue.

(b) Using a calculator yields:

$f(z_1) = \dfrac{2(2+i)^3 + 1}{3(2+i)^2} = -\dfrac{103}{75} + \dfrac{46}{75}i$; $f(z_2) = \dfrac{2(\frac{103}{75} + \frac{46}{75}i)^3 + 1}{3(-\frac{103}{75} + \frac{46}{75}i)^2} \approx 1.01 + .23i$

The value is approaching w_2 and the pixel should be colored red.

(c) Using a calculator yields: $f(z_1) = \dfrac{2(-1-i)^3 + 1}{3(-1-i)^2} = -\dfrac{2}{3} - \dfrac{5}{6}i$; $f(z_2) = \dfrac{2(-\frac{2}{3} - \frac{5}{6}i)^3 + 1}{3(-\frac{2}{3} + \frac{5}{6}i)^2} \approx -.51 - .84i$

The value is approaching w_3 and the pixel should be colored yellow.

Reviewing Basic Concepts (Sections 10.4 and 10.5)

1. $2(\cos 60° + i \sin 60°) = 2\left(\dfrac{1}{2} + \dfrac{\sqrt{3}}{2}\right) = 1 + i\sqrt{3}$.

2. $|3 - 4i| = \sqrt{3^2 + (-4)^2} = \sqrt{25} = 5$

3. $r = \sqrt{(-\sqrt{2})^2 + (\sqrt{2})^2} = \sqrt{4} = 2$; $\tan \theta = \dfrac{y}{x} \Rightarrow \tan \theta = \dfrac{\sqrt{2}}{-\sqrt{2}} \Rightarrow \tan \theta = -1 \Rightarrow \theta = \tan^{-1}(-1) = -45°$

Since θ is in quadrant II, $\theta = -45° + 180° = 135°$. Therefore $-\sqrt{2} + i\sqrt{2} = 2(\cos 135° + i \sin 135°)$.

4. $[4(\cos 135° + i \sin 135°)][2(\cos 45° + i \sin 45°)] = (4 \cdot 2)[\cos(135° + 45°) + i \sin(135° + 45°)]$

$= 8(\cos 180° + i \sin 180°) = 8(-1 + 0i) = -8$

5. $\dfrac{4(\cos 135° + i \sin 135°)}{2(\cos 45° + i \sin 45°)} = \dfrac{4}{2}[\cos(135° - 45°) + i \sin(135° - 45°)] = 2(\cos 90° + i \sin 45°) = 2(0 + i) = 2i$

6. $[4 \text{cis} 17°]^3 = [4(\cos 17° + i \sin 17°)]^3 = 4^3[\cos(3 \cdot 17°) + i \sin(3 \cdot 17°)] = 64(\cos 51° + i \sin 51°) = 64 \text{cis} 51°$

7. First find the trigonometric form of $2 - 2i$; $r = \sqrt{2^2 + 2^2} = \sqrt{8} = 2\sqrt{2}$;

$\tan \theta = \dfrac{y}{x} \Rightarrow \tan \theta = \dfrac{-2}{2} \Rightarrow \Rightarrow \theta = \tan^{-1}(-1) = -45°$. Therefore $2 - 2i = 2\sqrt{2};[\cos(-45°) + i \sin(-45°)]$.

$(2 - 2i) = \{2\sqrt{2};[\cos(-45°) + i \sin(-45°)]\}^4 = (2\sqrt{2})^4 \{\cos[4 \cdot (-45°)] + i \sin[4 \cdot (-45°)]\}$

528 Chapter 10: Applications of Trigonometry and Vectors

$$= 64\left[\cos(-180°) + i\sin(180°)\right] = 64(-1 + 0i) = -64$$

8. Note that $-64 = 64(\cos 180° + i \sin 180°)$. Here $r = 64$, so $\sqrt[3]{r} = 4$, $n = 3$, and $k = 0, 1,$ or 2.

   $\alpha = \dfrac{180° + 360° \cdot k}{3}$: For $k = 0$, $\alpha = 60°$. For $k = 1$, $\alpha = 180°$. For $k = 2$, $\alpha = 300°$. The cube roots are $4(\cos 60° + i \sin 60°) = 2 + 2i\sqrt{3}$, $4(\cos 180° + i \sin 180°) = -4$, and $4(\cos 300° + i \sin 300°) = 2 - 2i\sqrt{3}$.

9. Note that $2i = 2(\cos 90° + i \sin 90°)$. Here $r = 2$, so $\sqrt{r} = \sqrt{2}$, $n = 2$, and $k = 0$ or $\alpha = \dfrac{90° + 360° \cdot k}{2}$:

   For $k = 0$, $\alpha = 45°$. For $k = 1$, $\alpha = 225°$. The square roots are $\sqrt{2}(\cos 45° + i \sin 45°) = 1 + i$ and $\sqrt{2}(\cos 225° + i \sin 225°) = -1 - i$.

10. Find the cube roots of -1. Note that $-1 = \cos 180° + i \sin 180°$. Here $r = 1$, so $\sqrt[3]{r} = 1$, $n = 3$, and $k = 0, 1,$ or 2. $\alpha = \dfrac{180° + 360° \cdot k}{3}$: For $k = 0$, $\alpha = 60°$. For $k = 1$, $\alpha = 180°$. For $k = 2$, $\alpha = 300°$. The cube roots are $\cos 60° + i \sin 60°$, $\cos 180° + i \sin 180°$, and $\cos 300° + i \sin 300°$.

10.6 Polar Equations and Graphs

1. (a) The point is in quadrant II.
   (b) The point is in quadrant I.
   (c) The point is in quadrant IV.
   (d) The point is in quadrant III.

3. See Figure 3-13. Two other forms are $(1, 45° + 360°) = (1, 405°)$ or $(-1, 45° + 180°) = (-1, 225°)$.

5. See Figure 3-13. Two other forms are $(-2, 135° + 360°) = (-2, 495°)$ or $(2, 135° + 180°) = (2, 315°)$.

7. See Figure 3-13. Two other forms are $(5, -60° + 360°) = (5, 300°)$ or $(-5, -60° + 180°) = (-5, 120°)$.

9. See Figure 3-13. Two other forms are $(-3, -210° + 360°) = (-3, 150°)$ or $(3, -210° + 180°) = (3, -30°)$.

11. See Figure 3-13. Two other forms are $\left(3, \dfrac{5\pi}{3} + 2\pi\right) = \left(3, \dfrac{11\pi}{3}\right)$ or $\left(-3, \dfrac{5\pi}{3} - \pi\right) = \left(-3, \dfrac{2\pi}{3}\right)$.

13. See Figure 3-13. Two other forms are $(2, 0 + \pi) = (2, \pi)$ or $(-2, 0 + 2\pi) = (-2, 2\pi)$.

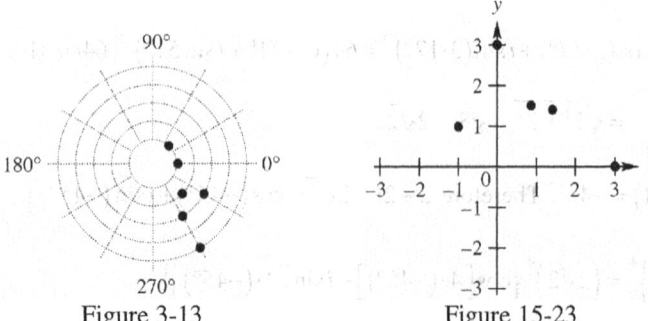

Figure 3-13 Figure 15-23

15. See Figure 15-23. $r = \sqrt{(-1)^2 + 1^2} = \sqrt{2}$; $\theta = \tan^{-1}\left(\dfrac{1}{-1}\right) = -45°$. Since the point is in QII, $\left(\sqrt{2}, 135°\right)$. Two forms are $\left(\sqrt{2}, 135°\right)$ and $\left(-\sqrt{2}, 315°\right)$.

17. See Figure 15-23. $r = \sqrt{0^2 + 3^2} = 3$; $\theta = \tan^{-1}\left(\dfrac{3}{0}\right) \Rightarrow$ undefined $\Rightarrow \theta = 90°$ (positive y-axis). Two forms are $(3, 90°)$ and $(-3, 270°)$.

19. See Figure 15-23. $r = \sqrt{\left(\sqrt{2}\right)^2 + \left(\sqrt{2}\right)^2} = 2$; $\theta = \tan^{-1}\left(\dfrac{\sqrt{2}}{\sqrt{2}}\right) = 45°$. Two forms are $(2, 4.5°)$. and $(-2, 225°)$.

21. See Figure 15-23. $r = \sqrt{\left(\dfrac{\sqrt{3}}{2}\right)^2 + \left(\dfrac{3}{2}\right)^2} = \sqrt{3}$; $\theta = \tan^{-1}\left(\dfrac{3}{2} \div \dfrac{\sqrt{3}}{2}\right) = 60°$. Two forms are $\left(\sqrt{3}, 60°\right)$ and $\left(-\sqrt{3}, 240°\right)$.

23. See Figure 15-23. $r = \sqrt{3^2 + 0^2} = 3$; $\theta = \tan^{-1}\left(\dfrac{0}{3}\right) = 0°$ (positive x-axis). Two forms are $(3, 0°)$ and $(-3, 180°)$.

25. $x - y = 4 \Rightarrow r\cos\theta - r\sin\theta = 4 \Rightarrow r(\cos\theta - \sin\theta) = 4 \Rightarrow r = \dfrac{4}{\cos\theta - \sin\theta}$. See Figure 25.

27. $x^2 + y^2 = 16 \Rightarrow (r\cos\theta)^2 - (r\sin\theta)^2 = 16 \Rightarrow r^2\left(\cos^2\theta + \sin^2\theta\right) = 16 \Rightarrow r = 4, r = -4$. See Figure 27.

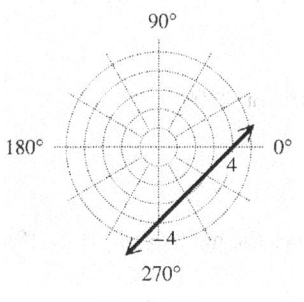
Figure 25

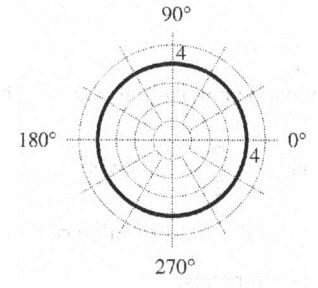
Figure 27

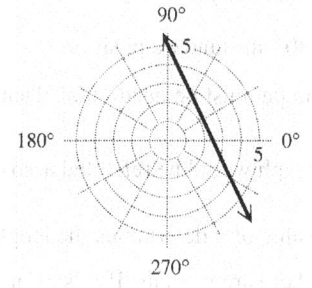
Figure 29

29. $2x + y = 5 \Rightarrow 2r\cos\theta + r\sin\theta = 5 \Rightarrow r(2\cos\theta + \sin\theta) = 5 \Rightarrow r = \dfrac{5}{2\cos\theta + \sin\theta}$. See Figure 29.

31. This is a circle of radius 3. Graph C.

33. This is a rose with four petals. Graph A.

35. The graph is a cardioid. See Figure 35.

37. The graph is a limaçon. See Figure 37.

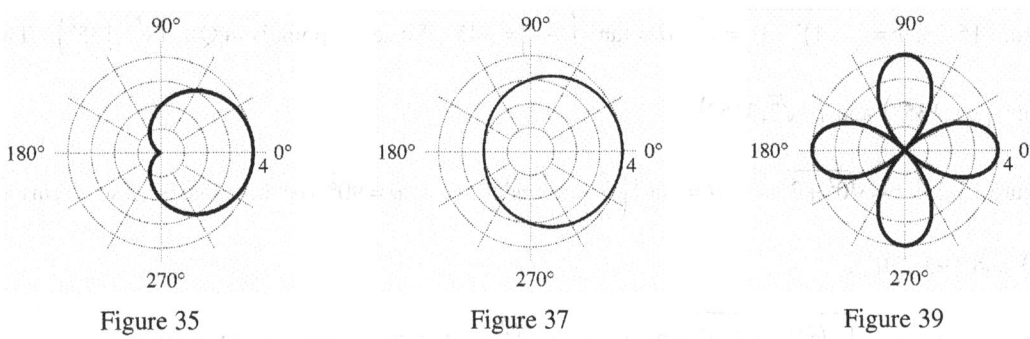

Figure 35   Figure 37   Figure 39

39. The graph is a four-leaved rose. See Figure 39.

41. The graph is a lemniscate. See Figure 41.

43. The graph is a cardioid. See Figure 43

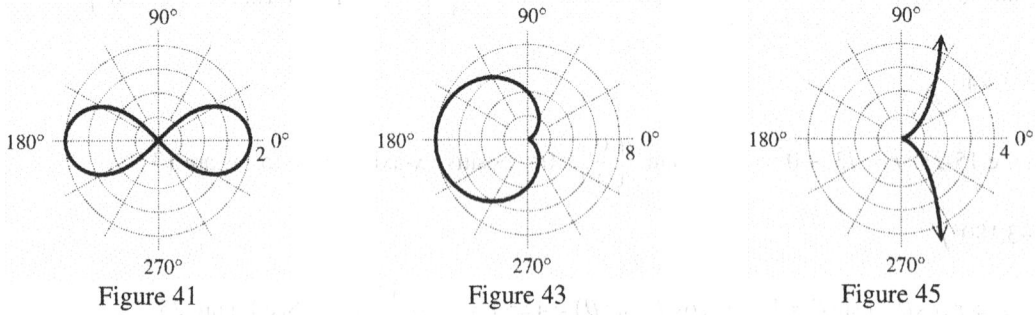

Figure 41   Figure 43   Figure 45

45. The graph is a cissoid. See Figure 45.

47. To graph $(r, \theta), r < 0,$ you could locate θ, add $180°$ to it, and move $|r|$ units along the terminal ray of $\theta + 180°$ in standard position.

49. The angle must be quadrantal. That is, it must be coterminal with $0°, 90°, 180°,$ or $270°$.

51. The graph would be reflected across the line $\theta = \dfrac{\pi}{2}$ (the y-axis).

53. The value of a determines the length of the petals, and the value of n determines the number of petals. If n is odd, there are n petals. If n is even, there are $2n$ petals.

55. $r = 2\sin\theta \Rightarrow r^2 = 2r\sin\theta \Rightarrow x^2 + y^2 = 2y \Rightarrow x^2 + y^2 - 2y + 1 = 1 \Rightarrow x^2 + (y-1)^2 = 1.$ See Figure 55.

57. $r = \dfrac{2}{1-\cos\theta} \Rightarrow r - r\cos\theta = 2 \Rightarrow \sqrt{x^2+y^2} - x - 2 \Rightarrow \sqrt{x^2+y^2} = x+2 \Rightarrow x^2 + y^2 = (x+2)^2$

$\Rightarrow x^2 + y^2 = x^2 + 4x + 4 \Rightarrow y^2 = 4x + 4 \Rightarrow y^2 = 4(x+1).$ See Figure 57.

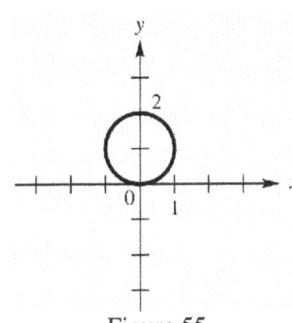

Figure 55

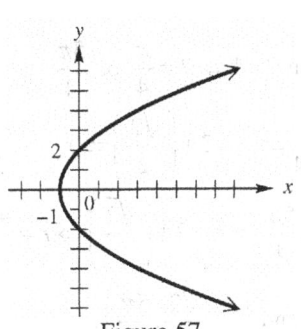

Figure 57

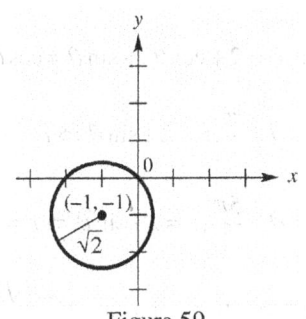

Figure 59

59. $r = -2\cos\theta - 2\sin\theta \Rightarrow r^2 = -2r\cos\theta - 2r\sin\theta \Rightarrow x^2 + y^2 = -2x - 2y \Rightarrow x^2 + y^2 + 2x + 2y = 0 \Rightarrow$
$x^2 + 2x + 1 + y^2 + 2y + 1 = 2 \Rightarrow (x+1)^2 + (y+1)^2 = 2$. See Figure 59.

61. $r = 2\sec\theta \Rightarrow r = \dfrac{2}{\cos\theta} = 2 \Rightarrow x = 2$. See Figure 61.

63. $r = \dfrac{2}{\cos\theta + \sin\theta} \Rightarrow r\cos\theta + r\sin\theta = 2 \Rightarrow x + y = 2$. See Figure 63.

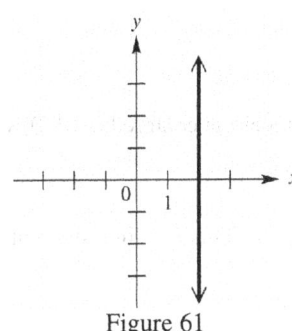

Figure 61

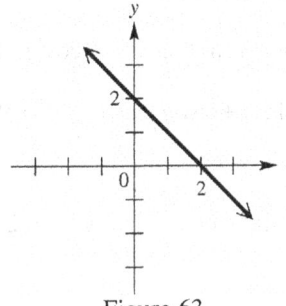

Figure 63

Figure 63

65. See Figure 65.

67. See Figure 67.

[-15,15] by [-15,15]
Xscl = 1   Yscl = 1

[-20,20] by [-20,20]
Xscl = 1   Yscl = 5

[-2.4,2.4] by [-1.6,1.6]
Xscl = 0.2   Yscl = 0.1

[-60,60] by [-40,40]
Xscl = 10   Yscl = 10

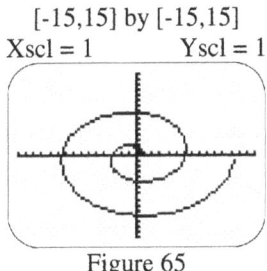

Figure 65

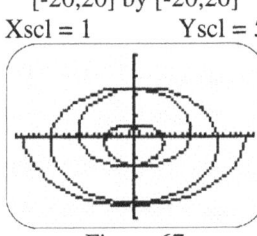

Figure 67

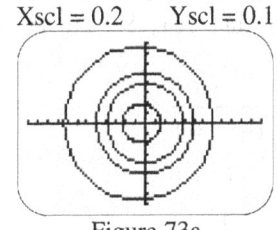

Figure 73a

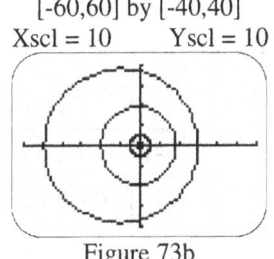

Figure 73b

69. $4\sin\theta = 1 + 2\sin\theta \Rightarrow 2\sin\theta = 1 \Rightarrow \sin\theta = \dfrac{1}{2} \Rightarrow \theta = \sin^{-1}\dfrac{1}{2} \Rightarrow \theta = \dfrac{\pi}{6}$ or $\dfrac{5\pi}{6}$ Then
$r = 4\sin\theta \Rightarrow r = 4\sin\dfrac{\pi}{6} \Rightarrow r = 4\left(\dfrac{1}{2}\right) \Rightarrow r = 2.$. The intersection points are $\left(2, \dfrac{\pi}{6}\right)$ and $\left(2, \dfrac{5\pi}{6}\right)$.

71. $2+\sin\theta = 2+\cos\theta \Rightarrow \sin\theta = \cos\theta \Rightarrow \tan\theta = 1 \Rightarrow \theta = \dfrac{\pi}{4}$ or $\dfrac{5\pi}{4}$.

   When $\theta = \dfrac{\pi}{4}, r = 2+\sin\theta \Rightarrow r = 2+\sin\dfrac{\pi}{4} \Rightarrow r = 2+\left(\dfrac{\sqrt{2}}{2}\right) \Rightarrow r = \dfrac{4+\sqrt{2}}{2}$.

   When $\theta = \dfrac{5\pi}{4}, r = 2+\sin\theta \Rightarrow r = 2+\sin\dfrac{5\pi}{4} \Rightarrow r = 2+\left(\dfrac{\sqrt{2}}{2}\right) \Rightarrow r = \dfrac{4-\sqrt{2}}{2}$.

   The intersection points are $\left(\dfrac{4+\sqrt{2}}{2}, \dfrac{\pi}{4}\right)$ and $\left(\dfrac{4-\sqrt{2}}{2}, \dfrac{5\pi}{4}\right)$.

73. (a) See Figure 73a.

   (b) See Figure 73b. Earth is closest to the sun.

   (c) By graphing the orbits of Neptune and Pluto (not shown), we see that Pluto is not always farthest from the sun.

10.7 More Parametric Equations

1. At $t = 2$, $x = 3(2)+6 = 12$ and $y = -2(2)+4 = 0$. The correct choice is C.

3. At $t = 5$, $x = 5$ and $y = 5^2 = 25$. The correct choice is A.

5. Note that $x = 3\sin t \sin \Rightarrow x^2 = 9\sin^2$ and $y = 3\cos t \Rightarrow y^2 = 9\cos^2 t$. Thus

   $x^2 + y^2 = 9\sin^2 t + 9\cos^2 t \Rightarrow x^2 + y^2 = 9(\sin^2 t + \cos^2 t) \Rightarrow x^2 + y^2 = 9$. This is a circle centered at (0, 0) with radius 3.

7. Here $y+x = 2\sin^2 t + 2\cos^2 t \Rightarrow y+x = 2(\sin^2 t + \cos^2 t) \Rightarrow y+x = 2 \Rightarrow y = 2-x$. This is a line segment connecting the points (2, 0) and (0, 2).

9. Note that $x = 3\tan t \Rightarrow x^2 = 9\tan^2 t$ and $y = 2\sec t \Rightarrow y^2 = 4\sec^2 t$. Thus

   $9y^2 - 4x^2 = 36\sec^2 t - 36\tan^2 t \Rightarrow \dfrac{9y^2}{36} - \dfrac{4x^2}{36} = \sec^2 t - \tan^2 t \Rightarrow \dfrac{y^2}{4} - \dfrac{x^2}{9} = 1$. This is the upper branch of a hyperbola.

11. (a) $x = t+2$, $y = t^2$, for t in $[-1, 1]$ See Figure 11.

t	$x = t+2$	$y = t^2$
-1	$-1+2 = 1$	$(-1)^2 = 1$
0	$0+2 = 2$	$0^2 = 0$
1	$1+2 = 3$	$1^2 = 1$

    (b) $x - 2 = t$, therefore $y = (x-2)^2$ or $y = x^2 - 4x + 4$. Since t is in $[-1, 1]$, x is in $[-1+2, 1+2]$ or $[1, 3]$.

13. (a) $x = \sqrt{t}$, $y = 3t-4$, for t in $[0, 4]$. See Figure 13.

t	$x = \sqrt{t}$	$y = 3t - 4$
0	$\sqrt{0} = 0$	$3(0) - 4 = -4$
1	$\sqrt{1} = 1$	$3(1) - 4 = -1$
2	$\sqrt{2} \approx 1.4$	$3(2) - 4 = 2$
3	$\sqrt{3} \approx 1.7$	$3(3) - 4 = 5$
4	$\sqrt{4} = 2$	$3(4) - 4 = 8$

(b) $x = \sqrt{t}$, $y = 3t - 4$ Since $x = \sqrt{t} \Rightarrow x^2 = t$, we have $y = 3x^2 - 4$. Since t is in $[0, 4]$, x is in $[\sqrt{0}, \sqrt{4}]$ or $[0, 2]$.

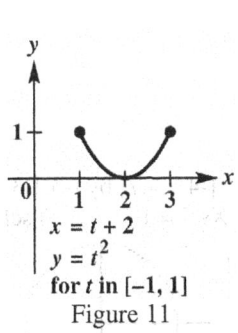
$x = t + 2$
$y = t^2$
for t in $[-1, 1]$
Figure 11

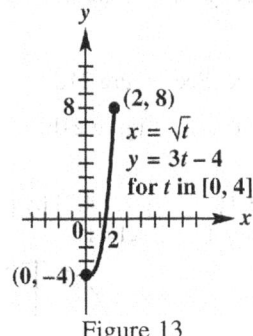
$x = \sqrt{t}$
$y = 3t - 4$
for t in $[0, 4]$
Figure 13

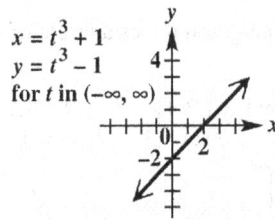
$x = t^3 + 1$
$y = t^3 - 1$
for t in $(-\infty, \infty)$
Figure 15

15. (a) $x = t^3 + 1$, $y = t^3 - 1$, for t in $(-\infty, \infty)$. See Figure 15.

t	$x = t^3 + 1$	$y = t^3 - 1$
-2	$(-2)^3 + 1 = -7$	$(-2)^3 - 1 = -9$
-1	$(-1)^3 + 1 = 0$	$(-1)^3 - 1 = -2$
0	$0^3 + 1 = 1$	$0^3 - 1 = -1$
1	$1^3 + 1 = 2$	$1^3 - 1 = 0$
2	$2^3 + 1 = 9$	$2^3 - 1 = 7$
3	$3^3 + 1 = 28$	$3^3 - 1 = 26$

(b) Since $x = t^3 + 1$, we have $x - 1 = t^3$. Since $y = t^3 - 1$, we have $y = (x - 1) - 1 = x - 2$. Since t is in $(-\infty, \infty)$, x is in $(-\infty, \infty)$.

17. (a) $x = t + 2$, $y = \dfrac{1}{t + 2}$, for $t \neq 2$ .. See Figure 17.

(b) Since $x = t + 2$ and $y = \dfrac{1}{t + 2}$, we have $y = \dfrac{1}{x}$. Since $t \neq -2$, $x \neq -2 + 2$, $x \neq 0$. Therefore, x is in $(-\infty, 0) \cup (0, \infty)$.

534 Chapter 10: Applications of Trigonometry and Vectors

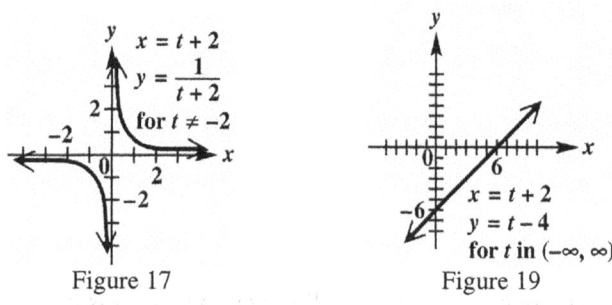

Figure 17   Figure 19

19. (a) $x = t + 2, y = t - 4,$ for t in $(-\infty, \infty)$. See Figure 19.

   (b) Since $x = t + 2$, we have $t = x - 2$. Since $y = t - 4$, we have $y = (x - 2) - 4 = x - 6$. Since t is in $(-\infty, \infty)$, x is in $(-\infty, \infty)$.

21. (a) The graph traces a circle of radius 3 once. See Figure 21a.

   (b) The graph traces a circle of radius 3 twice. See Figure 21b.

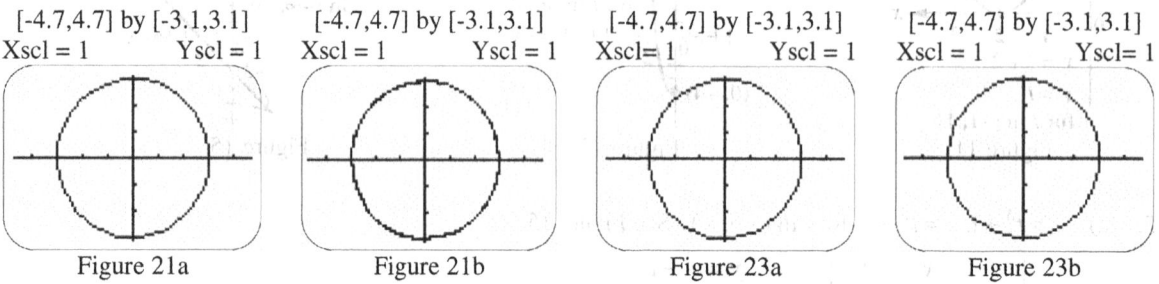

Figure 21a   Figure 21b   Figure 23a   Figure 23b

23. (a) The graph traces a circle of radius 3 once counterclockwise starting at (3, 0). See Figure 23a.

   (b) The graph traces a circle of radius 3 once clockwise starting at (0, 3). See Figure 23b.

25. $xy = \sin t \csc t \Rightarrow xy = 1 \Rightarrow y = \dfrac{1}{x}$. For t in the interval $(0, \pi), x = \sin t$ takes on the values in $(0, 1)$.

   See Figure 25.

27. $x = 2 + \sin t \Rightarrow x - 2 = \sin t \Rightarrow (x-2)^2 = \sin^2 t$ and $y = 1 + \cos t \Rightarrow y - 1 = \cos t \Rightarrow (y-1)^2 = \cos^2 t.$

   Thus $(x-2)^2 + (y-1)^2 = \sin^2 t + \cos^2 t \Rightarrow (x-2)^2 + (y-1)^2 = 1$. For

   in the interval $[0, 2\pi], x = 2 + \sin t$ takes on values in $[1, 3]$. See Figure 27.

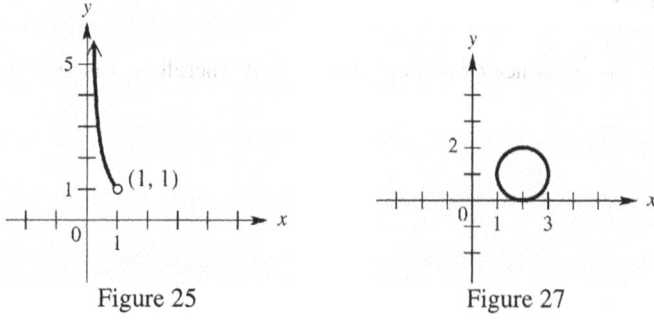

Figure 25   Figure 27

29. See Figure 29.

Section 10.7   535

31. See Figure 31.

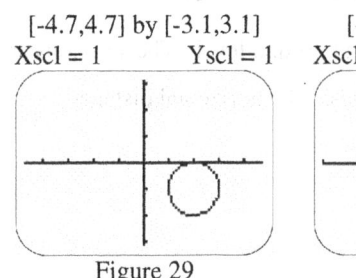
[-4.7,4.7] by [-3.1,3.1]
Xscl = 1   Yscl = 1
Figure 29

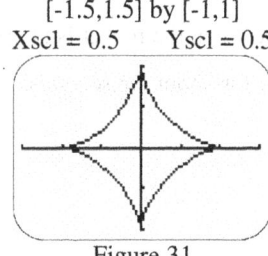
[-1.5,1.5] by [-1,1]
Xscl = 0.5   Yscl = 0.5
Figure 31

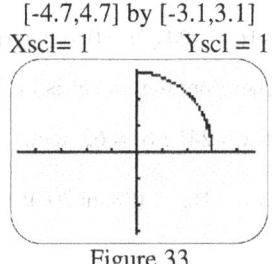
[-4.7,4.7] by [-3.1,3.1]
Xscl= 1   Yscl = 1
Figure 33

33. See Figure 33.

35. See Figure 35.

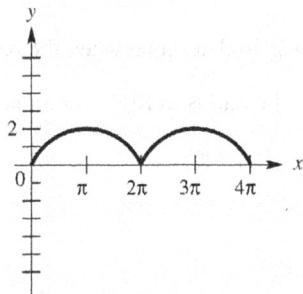

Figure 35

37. The letter graphed is F. See Figure 37.

39. The letter graphed is D. See Figure 39.

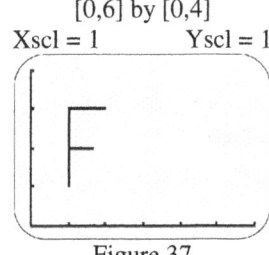
[0,6] by [0,4]
Xscl = 1   Yscl = 1
Figure 37

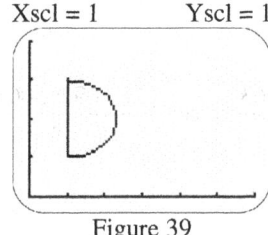
[0,6] by [0,4]
Xscl = 1   Yscl = 1
Figure 39

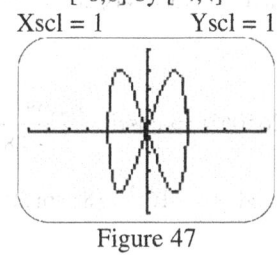
[-6,6] by [-4,4]
Xscl = 1   Yscl = 1
Figure 47

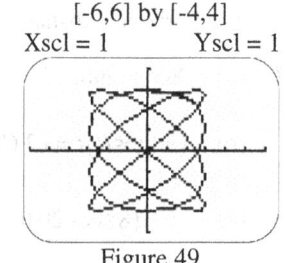
[-6,6] by [-4,4]
Xscl = 1   Yscl = 1
Figure 49

41. Answers may vary. One possibility is: $x_1 = 0, y_1 = 2t, x_2 = t, y_2 = 0$ for $0 \le t \le 1$.

43. Answers may vary. One possibility is: $x_1 = \sin t, y_1 = \cos t, x_2 = 0, y_2 = t - 2$ for $0 \le t \le \pi$.

45. Answers may vary.

47. See Figure 47.

49. See Figure 49.

51. (a) $x = (48\cos 60°)t \Rightarrow x = 48\left(\dfrac{1}{2}\right)t \Rightarrow x = 24t$

$y = (48\sin 60°)t - 16t^2 + 0 \Rightarrow y = 48\left(\dfrac{\sqrt{3}}{2}\right)t - 16t^2 \Rightarrow y = -16t^2 + 24\sqrt{3}t$

536 Chapter 10: Applications of Trigonometry and Vectors

(b) $x = 24t \Rightarrow t = \dfrac{x}{24}$, thus $y = -16t^2 + 24\sqrt{3}t \Rightarrow y = -16\left(\dfrac{x}{24}\right)^2 + 24\sqrt{3}\left(\dfrac{x}{24}\right) \Rightarrow y = -\dfrac{1}{36}x^2 + \sqrt{3}x$

(c) Solve the equation $-16t^2 + 24\sqrt{3}t = 0$ to determine when the rocket is at ground level. The solutions are 0 and 2.6 seconds. Therefore the rocket is in flight for about 2.6 seconds. The horizontal distance traveled is $x = 24t \Rightarrow x = 24(2.6) \approx 62$ feet.

53. (a) $x = (88\cos 20°)t$, $y = -16t^2 + (88\sin 20°)t + 2$,

(b) $x = (88\cos 20°)t \Rightarrow t = \dfrac{x}{88\cos 20°}$, thus

$y = 2 - 16\left(\dfrac{x}{88\cos 20°}\right)^2 + (88\sin 20°)\left(\dfrac{x}{88\cos 20°}\right) \Rightarrow y = 2 - \dfrac{x^2}{484\cos^2 20°} + (\tan 20°)x$

(c) Use the quadratic formula to solve the equation $y = -16t^2 + (88\sin 20°)t + 2$ to determine when the ball is at ground level. The solutions are $-.064$ and 1.945 seconds. Therefore the ball is in flight for about 1.9 seconds. The horizontal distance traveled is $x = (88\cos 20°)(1.945) \approx 161$ feet.

55. $x = (88\cos 45°)t = x = 88\left(\dfrac{\sqrt{2}}{2}\right)t \Rightarrow x = 44\sqrt{2}t$

$y = (88\cos 45°)t - 2.66t^2 + 0 \Rightarrow y = 88\left(\dfrac{\sqrt{2}}{2}\right)t - 2.66t^2 \Rightarrow -2.66t^2 + 44\sqrt{2}t$. Solve the equation $-2.66t^2 + 44\sqrt{2}t = 0$ to determine when the ball is at ground level. The solutions are 0 and 23.393 seconds. The horizontal distance traveled is $x = 44\sqrt{2}t \Rightarrow x = 24\sqrt{2}(23.393) \approx 1456$ feet.

57. (a) See Figure 57.

(b) $(88\cos\theta)t = 82.69265063t \Rightarrow \cos\theta = \dfrac{82.69265063}{88} \Rightarrow \cos^{-1}\left(\dfrac{82.69265063}{88}\right) \approx 20.0°$

(c) $x = (88\cos 20.0°)t$ and $y = -16t^2 + (88\sin 20.0°)t$

[0,200] by [0,30]
Xscl = 50   Yscl = 10

[-6,6] by [-4,4]
Xscl = 1   Yscl = 1

[-3,3] by [-3,3]
Xscl = 1   Yscl = 1

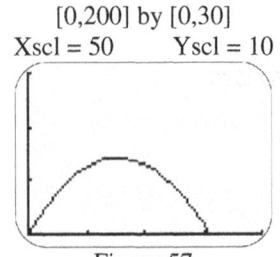
Figure 57

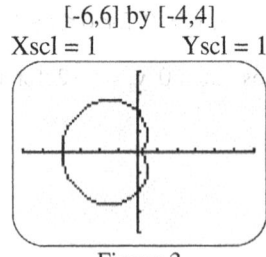
Figure 3

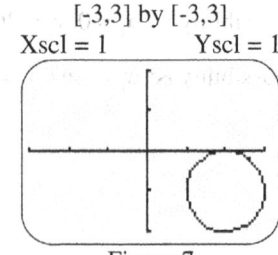
Figure 7

59. Since $x = r\cos\theta$ and $y = r\sin\theta$, by substitution, $x = a\theta\cos\theta$ and $y = a\theta\sin\theta$ for θ in $(-\infty, \infty)$

Reviewing Basic Concepts (Sections 10.6 and 10.7)

1. The point is in quadrant IV.

2. $r = \sqrt{(-2)^2 + 2^2} = \sqrt{8} = 2\sqrt{2}$; $\theta = \tan^{-1}\left(\dfrac{2}{-2}\right) = -45°$. Since the point is in QII $\theta = 135°$. Two forms are $\left(2\sqrt{2}, 135°\right)$ and $\left(-2\sqrt{2}, -45°\right)$.

3. The graph is a cardioid. See Figure 3

4. $r = 2\cos\theta \Rightarrow r^2 = 2r\cos\theta \Rightarrow x^2 + y^2 = 2x \Rightarrow x^2 - 2x + 1 + y^2 = 1 \Rightarrow (x-1)^2 + y^2 = 1$

5. $x + y = 6 \Rightarrow r\cos\theta + r\sin\theta = 6 \Rightarrow r(\cos\theta + \sin\theta) = 6 \Rightarrow r = \dfrac{6}{\cos\theta + \sin\theta}$

6. Note that $x = 2\cos t \Rightarrow x^2 = 4\cos^2 t$ and $y = 4\sin t \Rightarrow y^2 = 16\sin^2 t$. Thus

$4x^2 + y^2 = 16\cos^2 t + 16\sin^2 t \Rightarrow 4x^2 + y^2 = 16(\cos^2 t + \sin^2 t) \Rightarrow 4x^2 + y^2 = 16 \Rightarrow \dfrac{x^2}{4} + \dfrac{y^2}{16} = 1$.

7. See Figure 7.

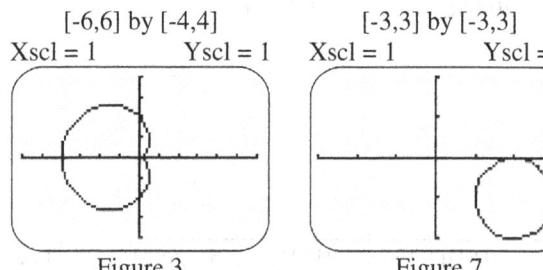

Figure 3   Figure 7

8. $x = (88\cos 45°)t \Rightarrow x = 88\left(\dfrac{\sqrt{2}}{2}\right)t \Rightarrow x = 44\sqrt{2}\,t$

$y = (88\cos 45°)t - 16t^2 + 50 \Rightarrow y = 88\left(\dfrac{\sqrt{2}}{2}\right)t - 16t^2 + 50 \Rightarrow y = 50 - 16t^2 + 88\sqrt{2}\,t$. Use the quadratic formula to solve the equation $50 - 16t^2 + 44\sqrt{2}\,t = 0$ to determine when the ball is at ground level. The solutions are $-.683$ and 4.5725 seconds. The horizontal distance traveled is $x = 44\sqrt{2}(4.5725) \approx 285$ feet.

Chapter 10 Review

1. Using the Law of Sines, $\dfrac{b}{\sin 39°30'} = \dfrac{96.3}{\sin 74°10'} \Rightarrow b = \dfrac{96.3\sin 39°30'}{\sin 74°10'} \Rightarrow b \approx 63.7$ m.

2. Using the Law of Sines, $\dfrac{b}{\sin 25.0°} = \dfrac{165}{\sin 100.2°} \Rightarrow b = \dfrac{165\sin 25.0°}{\sin 100.2°} \Rightarrow b \approx 70.9$ m.

3. Using the Law of Cosines,

$86.14^2 = 253.2^2 + 241.9^2 - 2(253.2)(241.9)\cos A \Rightarrow A = \cos^{-1}\left(\dfrac{7420.0996 - 122,625.85}{-122,498.16}\right) \approx 19.87°$

4. Using the Law of Cosines,

538   Chapter 10: Applications of Trigonometry and Vectors

$19.7^2 = 14.8^2 + 31.8^2 - 2(14.8)(31.8)\cos B \Rightarrow B = \cos^{-1}\left(\dfrac{388.09 - 1230.28}{-941.28}\right) \approx 26.5°$.

5. Using the Law of Sines,
$\dfrac{\sin B}{69.8} = \dfrac{\sin 129°40'}{127} \Rightarrow \sin B = \dfrac{69.8 \sin 129°40'}{127} \Rightarrow B = \sin^{-1}\left(\dfrac{69.8 \sin 129°40'}{127}\right) \approx 25°00'$.

6. Using the Law of Sines,
$\dfrac{\sin A}{340} = \dfrac{\sin 39°50'}{268} \Rightarrow \sin A = \dfrac{340 \sin 39°50'}{268} \Rightarrow A = \sin^{-1}\left(\dfrac{340 \sin 39°50'}{268}\right) \approx 54°20'$.

Since $180° - 54°20' = 125°40'$ and $39°50' + 125°40' < 180°$, the other possible angle is . $180° - 54°20' = 125°40'$

7. Using the Law of Cosines,
$b^2 = 127^2 + 69.8^2 - 2(127)(69.8)\cos 120.7° \Rightarrow b = \sqrt{21,001.04 - 17,729 \cos 120.7°} \approx 173$ ft.

8. Using the Law of Cosines,
$a^2 = 184^2 + 192^2 - 2(184)(192)\cos 46.2° \Rightarrow a = \sqrt{70,720 - 70,656 \cos 46.2°} \approx 148$ cm

9. $A = \dfrac{1}{2}(840.6)(715.9)\sin(149.3°) \approx 153600 \text{ m}^2$.

10. $A = \dfrac{1}{2}(6.90)(10.2)\sin 35°10' \approx 20.3 \text{ ft}^2$

11. $s = \dfrac{1}{2}(.913 + .816 + .582) = 1.1555$; $A = \sqrt{1.1555(1.1555 - .913)(1.1555 - .816)(1.1555 - .582)} \approx .234 \text{ km}^2$

12. $s = \dfrac{1}{2}(43 + 32 + 51) = 63$; $A = \sqrt{63(63 - 43)(63 - 32)(63 - 51)} \approx 680 \text{ m}^2$

13. First note that $C = 180° - 47°20' - 24°50' = 107°50'$. Now, using the Law of Sines,
$\dfrac{a}{\sin 24°50'} = \dfrac{8.4}{\sin 107°50'} \Rightarrow a = \dfrac{8.4 \sin 24°50'}{\sin 107°50'} \Rightarrow a \approx 3.71$ mi. If a perpendicular line segment joining C to the the ground intersects the ground at D, we can use right triangle BDC to find the distance d to the balloon:
$\sin 47°20' = \dfrac{d}{3.71} \Rightarrow d = 3.71 \sin 47°20' \approx 2.7$ mi.

14. Triangle XYZ has the following measurements: $X = 48°, Z = 36°, Y = 180° - 48° - 36° = 96°$, and $y = 10$.
Using the Law of Sines, $\dfrac{x}{\sin 48°} = \dfrac{10}{\sin 96°} \Rightarrow x = \dfrac{10 \sin 48°}{\sin 96°} \Rightarrow x \approx 7$ km.

15. Let C represent the position of the illegal transmitter. Triangle ABC has the following measurements:
$A = 90° - 48° = 42°, B = 302° - 270° = 32°, C = 180° - 42° - 32° = 160°$, and $c = 3.46$. Using the Law of Sines, $\dfrac{b}{\sin 32°} = \dfrac{3.46}{\sin 106°} \Rightarrow b = \dfrac{3.46 \sin 32°}{\sin 106°} \Rightarrow b \approx 1.91$ mi.

16. First note that $A = 180° - 58.4° - 27.9° = 93.7°$. Now, using the Law of Sines,

$$\frac{c}{\sin 27.9°} = \frac{125}{\sin 93.7°} \Rightarrow c = \frac{125\sin 27.9°}{\sin 93.7°} \Rightarrow c \approx 58.6 \text{ ft.}$$

17. Let A, B, and C represent the lower end of the brace, the lower end of the pole, and the upper end of the pole, respectively. Then $A = 180° - 115° - 22° = 43°, B = 115°, C = 22°$, and $a = 8.0$.

    Using the Law of Cosines, $\frac{b}{\sin 115°} = \frac{8.0}{\sin 43°} \Rightarrow b = \frac{8.0\sin 115°}{\sin 43°} \Rightarrow b \approx 11 \text{ ft.}$

18. Using the Law of Cosines,
    $c^2 = 15^2 + 12.2^2 - 2(15)(12.2)\cos 70.3° \Rightarrow c = \sqrt{373/.84 - 366\cos 70.3°} \approx 15.8 \text{ ft.}$

19. Using the Law of Cosines, $150^2 = 102^2 + 135^2 - 2(102)(135)\cos C \Rightarrow \cos^{-1}\left(\frac{22,500 - 28,629}{-27,540}\right) \approx 77.1°$.

20. This in not an ambiguous case because we are not given SSA.

21. This triangle cannot exist because a+b=c.

22. (a) If A and B lie on a horizontal line with C positioned above the line, then C lies $10\sin 30° = 5$ units above the line. Thus there will be exactly one value if b = 5 or if $b \geq 10$.

    (b) There will be two possible values if $5 < b < 10$.

    (c) There will be no value if $b < 5$.

23. If $C = 90°$, the value of $2ab\cos\theta$ is 0. The Law of Cosines becomes the Pythagorean theorem.

24. If the cosine value is positive, the angle is acute. If the cosine value is negative, the angle is obtuse.

25. See Figure 25.

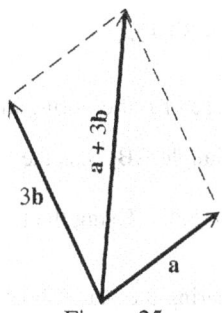

Figure 25

26. $|\langle 21, -20 \rangle| = \sqrt{21^2 + (-20)^2} = \sqrt{441 + 400} = \sqrt{841} = 29$; direction angle: $\tan^{-1}\left(\frac{-20}{21}\right) \approx 316.4°$.

27. $|\langle -9, 12 \rangle| = \sqrt{(-9)^2 + 12^2} = \sqrt{81 + 144} = \sqrt{225} = 15$; direction angle: $\tan^{-1}\left(\frac{12}{-9}\right) \approx 126.9°$.

28. $\langle 50\cos 45°, 50\sin 45° \rangle = \left\langle 50 \cdot \frac{\sqrt{2}}{2}, 50 \cdot \frac{\sqrt{2}}{2} \right\rangle = \langle 25\sqrt{2}, 25\sqrt{2} \rangle$.

29. $\langle 69.2\cos 75°, 69.2\sin 75° \rangle \approx \langle 17.9, 66.8 \rangle$.

30. $\langle 964\cos 154°20', 964\sin 154°20' \rangle \approx \langle -869, 418 \rangle$.

540　Chapter 10: Applications of Trigonometry and Vectors

31. (a) $\langle 6,2 \rangle \cdot \langle 3,-2 \rangle = (6)(3)+(2)(-2) = 18-4 = 14$.

   (b) $\cos\theta = \dfrac{u \cdot v}{|u||v|} = \dfrac{\langle 6,2 \rangle \cdot \langle 3,-2 \rangle}{|\langle 6,2 \rangle||\langle 3,-2 \rangle|} = \dfrac{(6)(3)+(2)(-2)}{\sqrt{36+4}\sqrt{9+4}} = \dfrac{14}{\sqrt{40}\sqrt{13}} = \dfrac{14}{\sqrt{520}} \Rightarrow$

   $\theta = \cos^{-1}\left(\dfrac{14}{\sqrt{520}}\right) = 52.13°$.

32. (a) $\langle 2\sqrt{3},2 \rangle \cdot \langle 5,5\sqrt{3} \rangle = (2\sqrt{3})(5)+(2)(5\sqrt{3}) = 10\sqrt{3}+10\sqrt{3} = 10\sqrt{3}+10\sqrt{3} = 20\sqrt{3}$.

   (b) $\cos\theta = \dfrac{u \cdot v}{|u||v|} = \dfrac{\langle 2\sqrt{3},2 \rangle \cdot \langle 5,5\sqrt{3} \rangle}{|\langle 2\sqrt{3},2 \rangle||\langle 5m5\sqrt{3} \rangle|} = \dfrac{(2\sqrt{3})(5)+(2)(5\sqrt{3})}{\sqrt{12+4}\sqrt{25+75}} = \dfrac{20\sqrt{3}}{\sqrt{16}\sqrt{100}} = \dfrac{20\sqrt{3}}{40} = \dfrac{\sqrt{3}}{2} \Rightarrow$

   $\theta = \cos^{-1}\left(\dfrac{\sqrt{3}}{2}\right) = 30°$.

33. The vectors are orthogonal because $u \cdot v = \langle 5,-1 \rangle \cdot \langle -2,-10 \rangle = (5)(-2)+(-1)(-10) = -10+10 = 0$.

34. The adjacent angle in the parallelogram is supplementary to $10°+15° = 25°$, thus it has measure $155°$.
    $|v|^2 = 12^2 + 18^2 - 2(12)(18)\cos 155° \approx 859.524964 \Rightarrow |v| = \sqrt{859.524964} \approx 29$ lb.

35. The adjacent angle in the parallelogram is supplementary to $45°$, thus it has measure $135°$.
    $|v|^2 = 1000^2 + 2000^2 - 2(1000)(2000)\cos 135° \approx 7,828,427.125 \Rightarrow |v| = \sqrt{7,828,427.125} \approx 2798$ The
    resultant is about 2800 newtons. The required angle can be found using the Law of Cosines:
    $2000^2 = 1000^2 + 2798^2 - 2(1000)(2798)\cos A \Rightarrow \cos^{-1}\left(\dfrac{4,000,000-8,828,804}{-5,596,000}\right) \approx 30.4°$.

36. Let A represent the plan's initial position. Let B represent the point at which the vector representing the desired flight path $(310°$ bearing$)$ intersects the vector representing the wind. Triangle ABC has the following measurements: $C = (360°-310°)+(121°-180°) = 82°$, $a = 37$, and $c = 520$. Using the Law of Sines, $\dfrac{\sin A}{37} = \dfrac{\sin 82°}{520} \Rightarrow \sin A = \dfrac{37\sin 82°}{520} \Rightarrow A = \sin^{-1}\dfrac{(37\sin 82°)}{520} \approx 4°$. The bearing the plane should take is $310°-4° = 306°$. Noting that $B = 180°-82°-4° = 94°$, $\dfrac{b}{\sin 94°} = \dfrac{520}{\sin 82°} \Rightarrow b = \dfrac{520\sin 94°}{\sin 82°} \Rightarrow b \approx 524$.
    The plane's actual speed is about 524 mph.

37. The angle between the current and the due north swim path is $180°-12° = 168°$. If b is the missing side of the triangle, $b^2 = 3.2^2 + 5.1^2 - 2(3.2)(5.1)\cos 168° \Rightarrow b = \sqrt{36.25-32.64\cos 168°} \approx 8.3$ mph. Then
    $\dfrac{\sin A}{5.1} = \dfrac{\sin 168°}{8.3} \Rightarrow \sin A = \dfrac{5.1\sin 168°}{8.3} \Rightarrow A = \sin^{-1}\left(\dfrac{5.1\sin 168°}{8.3}\right) \approx 7°20'$. The swimmer's actual speed is 8.3 mph, and the resulting bearing is $7°20'$.

38. (a) The speed of the wind is $|v| = \sqrt{6^2+8^2} = \sqrt{36+64} = \sqrt{100} = 10$ mph.

(b) $3\mathbf{v} = 3(6\mathbf{i} + 8\mathbf{j}) = 18\mathbf{i} + 24\mathbf{j}$; This represents a 30 mph wind in the direction of v.

(c) **u** represents a southeast wind with speed $|\mathbf{u}| = \sqrt{(-8)^2 + 8^2} = \sqrt{64+64} = \sqrt{128} \approx 11.3$ mph.

39. See Figure 39.
40. See Figure 40.

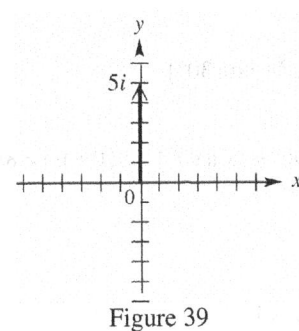
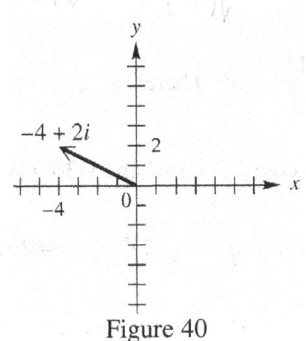

Figure 39   Figure 40

41. $(7+3i)+(-2+i) = (7+(-2))+(3+1)i = 5+4i$.

42. $(2-4i)+(5+i) = (2+5)+(-4+1)i = 7-3i$.

43. $r = \sqrt{(-2)^2 + 2^2} = \sqrt{8} = 2\sqrt{2}$; $\tan\theta = \dfrac{2}{-2} \Rightarrow \tan\theta = -1 \Rightarrow \theta = \tan^{-1}(-1) = -45°$. Since θ is in quadrant II, $\theta = -45° + 180° = 135°$. Therefore $-2+2i = 2\sqrt{2}\,\text{cis}\,135°$.

44. $3(\cos 90° + i\sin 90°) = 3(0+1i) = 3i$.

45. $2\text{cis}\,225° = 2(\cos 225° + i\sin 225°) = 2\left(-\dfrac{\sqrt{2}}{2} - \dfrac{\sqrt{2}}{2}i\right) = -\sqrt{2} - \sqrt{2}i$.

46. $r = \sqrt{(-4)^2 + (4\sqrt{3})^2} = \sqrt{64} = 8$; $\tan\theta = \dfrac{4\sqrt{3}}{-4} \Rightarrow \theta = -60°$. Since θ is in quadrant II, $\theta = -60° + 180° = 120°$. Therefore $-4 + 4i\sqrt{3} = 8\,\text{cis}\,120°$.

47. $[5(\cos 90° + i\sin 90°)][6(\cos 180° + i\sin 180°)] = (5 \cdot 6)[\cos(90°+180°) + i\sin(90°+180°)]$
$= 30(\cos 270° + i\sin 270°) = 30(0-i) = -30i$.

48. $(3\text{cis}\,135°)(2\text{cis}\,105°) = [3(\cos 135° + i\sin 135°)][2(\cos 105° + i\sin 105°)]$
$= (3 \cdot 2)[\cos(135°+105°) + i\sin(135°+105°)] = 6(\cos 240° + i\sin 240°) = 6\left(-\dfrac{1}{2} - \dfrac{\sqrt{3}}{2}i\right) = -3 - 3\sqrt{3}i$.

49. $\dfrac{2(\cos 60° + i\sin 60°)}{8(\cos 300° + i\sin 300°)} = \dfrac{2}{8}[\cos(60°-300°) + i\sin(60°-300°)]$

$\dfrac{1}{4}[\cos(-240°) + i\sin(-240°)] = \dfrac{1}{4}\left(-\dfrac{1}{2} + \dfrac{\sqrt{3}}{2}i\right) = -\dfrac{1}{8} + \dfrac{\sqrt{3}}{8}i$.

542   Chapter 10: Applications of Trigonometry and Vectors

50. $\dfrac{4\operatorname{cis}270°}{2\operatorname{cis}90°} = \dfrac{4(\cos 270° + i\sin 270°)}{2(\cos 90°) + i\sin 90°} = \dfrac{4}{2}\left[\cos(270° - 90°) + i\sin(270° - 90°)\right]$

$= 2(\cos 180° + i\sin 180°) = 2(-1 + 0i) = -2.$

51. First find the trigonometric form of $\sqrt{3} + i$; $r = \sqrt{\left(\sqrt{3}\right)^2 + 1^2} = \sqrt{4} = 2$;

$\tan\theta = \dfrac{y}{x} \Rightarrow \tan\theta = \dfrac{1}{\sqrt{3}} \Rightarrow \theta = \tan^{-1}\dfrac{1}{\sqrt{3}} = 30°$. Therefore $\sqrt{3} + i = 2(\cos 30° + i\sin 30°)$

$\left(\sqrt{3} + i\right)^3 = \left[2(\cos 30° + i\sin 30°)\right]^3 = 2^3\left[\cos(3\cdot 30°) + i\sin(3\cdot 30°)\right] = 8(\cos 90° + i\sin 90°) = 8(0 + 1i) = 8i.$

52. First find the trigonometric form of $2 - 2i$; $r = \sqrt{2^2 + (-2)^2} = \sqrt{8} = 2\sqrt{2}$;

$\tan\theta = \dfrac{y}{x} \Rightarrow \tan\theta = \dfrac{-2}{2} \Rightarrow \theta = \tan^{-1}(-1) = 315°$. Therefore $2 - 2i = 2\sqrt{2}(\cos 315° + i\sin 315°)$.

$(2 - 2i)^5 = \left[2\sqrt{2}(\cos 315° + i\sin 315°)\right]^5 = \left(2\sqrt{2}\right)^5\left[\cos(5\cdot 315°) + i\sin(5\cdot 315)\right] =$

$128\sqrt{2}(\cos 1575° + i\sin 1575°) = 128\sqrt{2}\left(-\dfrac{\sqrt{2}}{2} + \dfrac{\sqrt{2}}{2}i\right) = -128 + 128i$

53. $(\cos 100° + i\sin 100°)^6 = \cos(6\cdot 100°) + i\sin(6\cdot 100°) = \cos 600° + i\sin 600° = -\dfrac{1}{2} - \dfrac{\sqrt{3}}{2}i.$

54. $(\operatorname{cis}20°)^3 = (\cos 20° + i\sin 20°)^3 = \cos(3\cdot 20°) + i\sin(3\cdot 20°) = \cos 60° + i\sin 60° = \dfrac{1}{2} + \dfrac{\sqrt{3}}{2}i$

55. Note that $-27i = 27(\cos 270° + i\sin 270°)$. Here $r = 27$, so $\sqrt[3]{r} = 3$, $n = 3$ and $k = 0, 1,$ or 2.

$\alpha = \dfrac{270° + 360°\cdot k}{3}$: For $k = 0$, $\alpha = 90°$. For $k = 1$, $\alpha = 210°$. For $k = 2$, $\alpha = 330°$. The cube roots are

$3\operatorname{cis}90°$, $3\operatorname{cis}210°$, and $3\operatorname{cis}330°$. See Figure 55.

56. Note that $16i = 16(\cos 90° + i\sin 90°)$. Here $r = 16$ so $\sqrt[4]{r} = 2$, $n = 4$ and $k = 0, 1, 2,$ or 3.

$\alpha = \dfrac{90° + 360°\cdot k}{4}$: For $k = 0$, $\alpha = 22.5°$. For $k = 1$, $\alpha = 112.5°$. For $k = 2$, $\alpha = 202.5°$. For

$k = 3$, $\alpha = 292.5°$. The fourth roots are $2\operatorname{cis}22.5°$, $2\operatorname{cis}112.5°$, $2\operatorname{cis}202.5°$, and $2\operatorname{cis}292.5°$. See Figure 56.

57. Note that $32 = 32(\cos 0° + i\sin 0°)$.

Here $r = 32$ so $\sqrt[5]{r} = 2$, $n = 5$ and $k = 0.1.2.3.$or 4. $\alpha = \dfrac{0° + 360\cdot k}{5}$: For $k = 0$, $\alpha = 0°$.

For $k = 1$, $\alpha = 72°$. For $k = 2$, $\alpha = 144°$. For $k = 3, \alpha = 216°$. For $k = 4$, $\alpha = 288°$. The fifth roots are

$2\operatorname{cis}0°$, $2\operatorname{cis}72°$, $2\operatorname{cis}144°$, $2\operatorname{cis}216°$, and $2\operatorname{cis}288°$. See Figure 57.

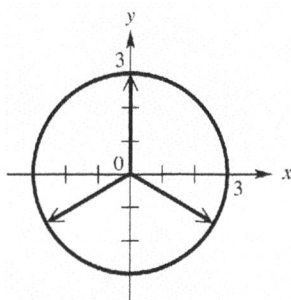
Figure 55

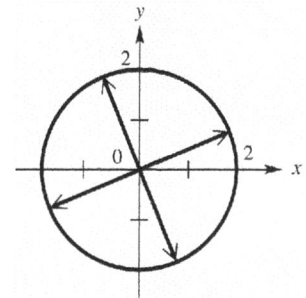
Figure 56

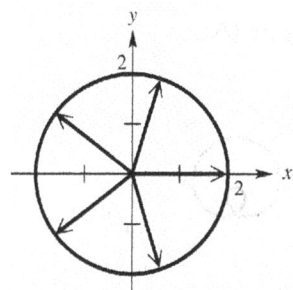
Figure 57

58. $x^4 + i = 0 \Rightarrow x^4 = -i$. Find the fourth roots of $-i$. Note that $-i = \cos 270° + i \sin 270°$.

    Here $r = 1$ so $\sqrt[4]{r} = 1$, $n = 4$ and $k = 0, 1, 2$, or 3. $\alpha = \dfrac{270° + 360° \cdot k}{4}$: For $k = 0$, $\alpha = 67.5°$.

    For $k = 1$, $\alpha = 157.5°$. For $k = 2$, $\alpha = 247.5°$. For $k = 3$, $\alpha = 337.5°$. The four roots are

    cis 67.5°, cis 157.7°, cis 247.5°, and cis 337.5°.

59. $x = r \cos \theta = 12 \cos 225 = 12 \left(-\dfrac{\sqrt{2}}{2} \right) = -6\sqrt{2}$; $y = r \sin \theta = 12 \sin 225° = 12 \left(-\dfrac{\sqrt{2}}{2} \right) = -6\sqrt{2}$

    The rectangular coordinates are $\left(-6\sqrt{2}, -6\sqrt{2} \right)$.

60. $x = r \cos \theta = -8 \cos \left(-\dfrac{\pi}{3} \right) = -8 \left(\dfrac{1}{2} \right) = -4$; $y = r \sin \theta = -8 \sin \left(-\dfrac{\pi}{3} \right) = -8 \left(-\dfrac{\sqrt{3}}{2} \right) = 4\sqrt{3}$

    The rectangular coordinates are $\left(-4, 4\sqrt{3} \right)$.

61. $r = \sqrt{(-6)^2 + 6^2} = \sqrt{72} = 6\sqrt{2}$; $\theta = \tan^{-1} \left(\dfrac{6}{-6} \right) = -45°$. Since the point is in QII, $\theta = 135°$.

    One possible form is $\left(6\sqrt{2}, 135° \right)$.

62. $r = \sqrt{0^2 + (-5)^2} = 5$; $\theta = \tan^{-1} \left(\dfrac{-5}{0} \right) \Rightarrow$ undefined $\Rightarrow \theta = 270°$ (negative y-axis).

    One possible form is $(5, 270°)$.

63. See Figure 63.
64. See Figure 64.
65. See Figure 65.

[-6,6] by [-4,4]
Xscl = 1   Yscl = 1

[-6,6] by [-4,4]
Xscl = 1   Yscl = 1

[-6,6] by [-4,4]
Xscl = 1   Yscl = 1

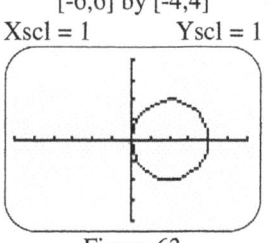
Figure 63

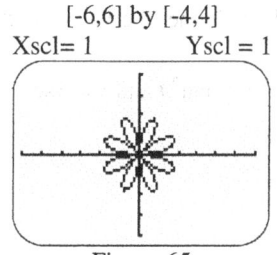
Figure 64   Figure 65

66. See Figure 66.

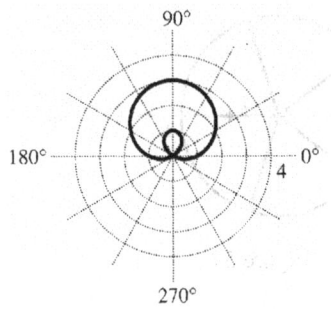

Figure 66

67. $r = \dfrac{3}{1+\cos\theta} \Rightarrow r + r\cos\theta = 3 + \sqrt{x^2+y^2} + x = 3 \Rightarrow \sqrt{x^2+y^2} = 3-x \Rightarrow x^2+y^2 = (3-x)^2 \Rightarrow x^2+y^2$

$= 9 - 6x + x^2 \Rightarrow y^2 = -6x + 9 \Rightarrow y^2 = -6\left(x - \dfrac{3}{2}\right)$

68. $r = \dfrac{4}{2\sin\theta - \cos\theta} \Rightarrow 2r\sin\theta - r\cos\theta = 4 \Rightarrow 2y - x = 4$

69. $r = \sin\theta + \cos\theta \Rightarrow r^2 = r\sin\theta + r\cos\theta \Rightarrow x^2 + y^2 = y + x \Rightarrow x^2 + y^2 - x - y = 0 \Rightarrow$

$x^2 - x + \dfrac{1}{4} + y^2 - y + \dfrac{1}{4} = \dfrac{1}{4} + \dfrac{1}{4} \Rightarrow \left(x - \dfrac{1}{2}\right)^2 + \left(y - \dfrac{1}{2}\right)^2 = \dfrac{1}{2}$

70. $r = 2 \Rightarrow r^2 = 4 \Rightarrow x^2 + y^2 = 4$

71. $x = -3 \Rightarrow r\cos\theta = -3 \Rightarrow r = \dfrac{-3}{\cos\theta} \Rightarrow r = -\dfrac{3}{\cos\theta}$

72. $y = x \Rightarrow r\sin\theta = r\cos\theta \Rightarrow \dfrac{r\sin\theta}{r\cos\theta} = 1 \Rightarrow \tan\theta = 1$

73. $y = x^2 \Rightarrow r\sin\theta = r^2\cos^2\theta \Rightarrow \dfrac{r\sin\theta}{r\cos^2\theta} = r \Rightarrow r = \tan\theta \cdot \dfrac{1}{\cos\theta} \Rightarrow r = \dfrac{\tan\theta}{\cos\theta}$

74. $x = y^2 \Rightarrow r\cos\theta = r^2\sin^2\theta \Rightarrow \dfrac{r\cos\theta}{r\sin^2\theta} = r \Rightarrow r = \cot\theta \cdot \dfrac{1}{\sin\theta} \Rightarrow r = \dfrac{\cot\theta}{\sin\theta}$

75. Note that $x = \cos 2t \Rightarrow x = \cos^2 t - \sin^2 t$ and $y = \sin t \Rightarrow y^2 = \sin^2 t$. Thus

$x + 2y^2 = \cos^2 t - \sin^2 t + 2\sin^2 t \Rightarrow x + 2y^2 = \cos^2 t + \sin^2 t \Rightarrow x + 2y^2 = 1 \Rightarrow 2y^2 + x - 1 = 0$. This can also be

written $y^2 = -\dfrac{1}{2}(x-1)$. For t in the interval $(-\pi, \pi)$, $x = \cos 2t$ takes on the values in. $[-1, 1]$.

76. Note that $x = 5\tan t \Rightarrow x^2 = 25\tan^2 t$ and $y = 3\sec t \Rightarrow y^2 = 9\sec^2 t$.

Thus $25y^2 - 9x^2 = 225\sec^2 t - 225\tan^2 t \Rightarrow \dfrac{25y^2}{225} - \dfrac{9x^2}{225} = \sec^2 t - \tan^2 t \Rightarrow \dfrac{y^2}{9} - \dfrac{x^2}{25} = 1$. This can also be written $y = 3\sqrt{1 + \dfrac{x^2}{25}}$. For t in the interval $\left(-\dfrac{\pi}{2}, \dfrac{\pi}{2}\right)$, $x = 5$ takes on the values in $(-\infty, \infty)$.

77. See Figure 77.

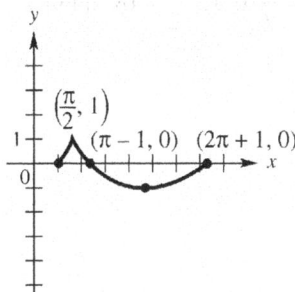

Figure 77

78. $x = (118\cos 27°)t;\ y = (118\sin 27°)t - 16t^2 + 3.2 \Rightarrow y = 3.2 - 16t^2 + (118\sin 27°)t$

Use the quadratic formula to solve the equation $y = 3.2 - 16t^2 + (118\sin 27°)t = 0$ to determine when the ball is at ground level. The solutions are $-.059$ and 3.4069 seconds. The horizontal distance traveled is $x = (1118\cos 27°)(3.4069) \approx 360$ feet.

Chapter 10 Test

1. Find C, given $A = 25.2°$, $a = 6.92$ yd, $b = 4.82$ yd.

   Use the law of sines to first find the measure of angle B.

   $\dfrac{\sin 25.2°}{6.92} = \dfrac{\sin B}{4.82} \Rightarrow \sin B = \dfrac{4.82 \sin 25.2°}{6.92} \Rightarrow B = \sin^{-1}\left(\dfrac{4.82 \sin 25.2°}{6.92}\right) \approx 17.3°$

   Use the fact that the angles of a triangle sum to $180°$ to find the measure of angle C.
   $C = 180° - A - B = 180° - 25.2° - 17.3° = 137.5°$

2. Find c, given $C = 118°$, $b = 131$ km, $a = 75.0$ km.

   Using the law of cosines to find the length of c.

   $c^2 = a^2 + b^2 - 2ab\cos C \Rightarrow c^2 = 75.0^2 + 131^2 - 2(75.0)(131)\cos 118° \approx 32011.12 \Rightarrow c \approx 178.9$ km

   c is approximately 179 km. (rounded to two significant digits)

3. Find B, given $a = 17.3$ ft, $b = 22.6$ ft, $c = 29.8$ ft.

   Using the law of cosines, find the measure of angle B.

   $b^2 = a^2 + c^2 - 2ac\cos B \Rightarrow \cos B = \dfrac{a^2 + c^2 - b^2}{2ac} = \dfrac{17.3^2 + 29.8^2 - 22.6^2}{2(17.3)(29.8)} \approx 0.65617605 \Rightarrow B \approx 49.0°$

546   Chapter 10: Applications of Trigonometry and Vectors

4. $a = 14, b = 30, c = 40$ We can use Heron's formula to find the area.

   $s = \frac{1}{2}(a+b+c) = \frac{1}{2}(14+30+40) = 42$

   $\mathcal{A} = \sqrt{s(s-a)(s-b)(s-c)} = \sqrt{42(42-14)(42-30)(42-40)} = \sqrt{42 \cdot 28 \cdot 12 \cdot 2} = \sqrt{28,224} = 168$ sq units

5. This is SAS, so we can use the formula $\mathcal{A} = \frac{1}{2}zy\sin X$. $\mathcal{A} = \frac{1}{2} \cdot 6 \cdot 12 \sin 30° = \frac{1}{2} \cdot 6 \cdot 12 \cdot \frac{1}{2} = 18$ sq units

6. Since $B > 90°$, b must be the longest side of the triangle.

   (a) $b > 10$

   (b) none

   (c) $b \le 10$

7. $A = 60°, b = 30$ m, $c = 45$ m   This is SAS, so use the law of cosines to find a:

   $a^2 = b^2 + c^2 - 2bc\cos A \Rightarrow a^2 = 30^2 + 45^2 - 2 \cdot 30 \cdot 45 \cos 60° = 1575 \Rightarrow a = 15\sqrt{7} \approx 40$ m

   Now use the law of sines to find B: $\frac{\sin B}{b} = \frac{\sin A}{a} \Rightarrow \frac{\sin B}{30} = \frac{\sin 60°}{15\sqrt{7}} \Rightarrow \sin B = \frac{30\sin 60°}{15\sqrt{7}} \Rightarrow B \approx 41°$

   $C = 180° - A - B = 180° - 60° - 41° = 79°$

8. $b = 1075$ in., $c = 785$ in., $C = 38°30'$ We can use the law of sines.

   $\frac{\sin B}{b} = \frac{\sin C}{c} \Rightarrow \frac{\sin B}{1075} = \frac{\sin 38°30'}{785} \Rightarrow \sin B = \frac{1075 \sin 38°30'}{785} \Rightarrow B_1 \approx 58.5° = 58°30'$ or

   $B_2 = 180° - 58°30' = 121°30'$

   Solving separately for triangles A_1B_1C and A_2B_2C, we have the following.

   A_1B_1C: $A_1 = 180° - B_1 - C = 180° - 58°30' - 38°30' = 83°00'$

   $\frac{a_1}{\sin A_1} = \frac{b}{\sin B_1} \Rightarrow \frac{a_1}{\sin 83°} = \frac{1075}{\sin 58°30'} \Rightarrow a_1 = \frac{1075 \sin 83°}{\sin 58°30'} \approx 1250$ in. (three significant digits) A_2B_2C:

   $A_2 = 180° - B_2 - C = 180° - 121°30' - 38°30' = 20°00'$

   $\frac{a_2}{\sin A_2} = \frac{b}{\sin B_2} \Rightarrow \frac{a_2}{\sin 20°} = \frac{1075}{\sin 121°30'} \Rightarrow a_2 = \frac{1075 \sin 20°}{\sin 121°30'} \approx 431$ in. (rounded to three significant digits)

9. magnitude: $|\mathbf{v}| = \sqrt{(-6)^2 + 8^2} = \sqrt{36+64} = \sqrt{100} = 10$

   angle: $\tan\theta = \frac{y}{x} \Rightarrow \tan\theta = \frac{8}{-6} = -\frac{4}{3} \approx -1.33333333 \Rightarrow \theta \approx -53.1° \Rightarrow \theta = -53.1° + 180° = 126.9°$

   (θ lies in quadrant II) The magnitude $|\mathbf{v}|$ is 10 and $\theta = 126.9°$.

10. (a) $\mathbf{u} + \mathbf{v} = \langle -1, 3 \rangle + \langle 2, -6 \rangle = \langle -1+2, 3+(-6) \rangle = \langle 1, -3 \rangle$

(b) $-3\mathbf{v} = -3\langle 2, -6 \rangle = \langle -3 \cdot 2, -3(-6) \rangle = \langle -6, 18 \rangle$

(c) $\mathbf{u} \cdot \mathbf{v} = \langle -1, 3 \rangle \cdot \langle 2, -6 \rangle = -1(2) + 3(-6) = -2 - 18 = -20$

(d) $|\mathbf{u}| = \sqrt{(-1)^2 + 3^2} = \sqrt{1+9} = \sqrt{10}$

11. $\mathbf{u} \cdot \mathbf{v} = \langle 4, 3 \rangle \cdot \langle 1, 5 \rangle = 4(1) + 3(5) = 19$, $|\mathbf{u}| = \sqrt{4^2 + 3^2} = \sqrt{25} = 5$, $|\mathbf{v}| = \sqrt{1^2 + 5^2} = \sqrt{26}$

$\cos\theta = \dfrac{\mathbf{u}\cdot\mathbf{v}}{|\mathbf{u}||\mathbf{v}|} \Rightarrow \cos\theta = \dfrac{19}{5\sqrt{26}} \Rightarrow \theta = \cos^{-1}\left(\dfrac{19}{5\sqrt{26}}\right) \approx 41.8°$

12. Given $A = 45°, B = 30°$ and $AB = 4.2$ mi, first find the measure of angle C.

$C = 180° - 45° - 30° = 105°$

Use this information and the law of sines to find AC. $\dfrac{AC}{\sin 45°} = \dfrac{4.2}{\sin 105°} \Rightarrow$

$AC = \dfrac{4.2\sin 45°}{\sin 105°} \approx 3.075$ mi   Drop a perpendicular line from C to segment AB.

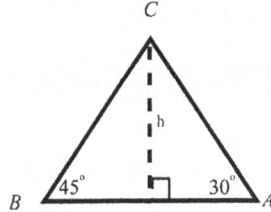

Thus, $\sin 30° = \dfrac{h}{3.075} \Rightarrow h \approx 3.075\sin 30° \approx 1.5$ mi. The balloon is 2.7 miles off the ground.

13. horizontal: $x = |\mathbf{v}|\cos\theta = 569\cos 127.5° \approx -346$ and vertical: $y = |\mathbf{v}|\sin\theta = 569\sin 127.5° \approx 451$

The vector is $\langle -346, 451 \rangle$.

14. Consider the figure below.

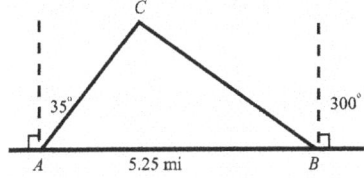

Since the bearing is 35° from A, angle A in ABC must be 90° − 35° = 55°. Since the bearing is 300° from B, angle B in ABC must be 300° − 270° = 30°. The angles of a triangle sum to 180°, so $C = 180° - A - B = 180° - 55° - 30° = 95°$. Using the law of sines, we have the distance from A to the transmitter is 2.64 miles. (rounded to two significant digits)

548 Chapter 10: Applications of Trigonometry and Vectors

15. Since $m\angle DAC = 8.0°$, $m\angle CAB = 90° - 8.0° = 82.0°$. $m\angle B = 66°$, so $m\angle C = 180° - 82° - 66° = 32°$. Now use the law of sines to find AC: $\dfrac{AC}{\sin B} = \dfrac{AB}{\sin C} \Rightarrow \dfrac{AC}{\sin 66°} = \dfrac{8.0}{\sin 32°} \Rightarrow AC = \dfrac{8.0 \sin 66°}{\sin 32°} \approx 13.8 \approx 14$ m

16. AX is the airspeed vector. Since the plane is flying 630 miles due north in 3 hours, the ground speed is 210 mph. The measure of angle ACX is $180° - 42° = 138°$.

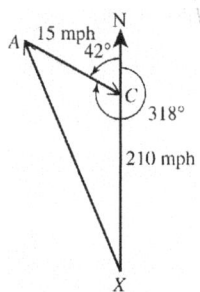

$\left|\overrightarrow{AX}\right|^2 = 15^2 + 210^2 - 2(15)(210)\cos 138° = 49006.8124 \Rightarrow \left|\overrightarrow{AX}\right| \approx 221.3748 \approx 220$ mph (two significant digits). Using the law of sines to find the measure of angle X, we have

$\dfrac{\sin X}{15} = \dfrac{\sin 138°}{220} \Rightarrow \sin X = \dfrac{15\sin 138°}{220} \Rightarrow X = \sin^{-1}\left(\dfrac{15\sin 138°}{220}\right) \approx 2.6°$

The plane's bearing is $360° - 2.6° = 357.4° \approx 357°$.

17. $\left|\overrightarrow{AC}\right| = 16.0$ lb; $\left|\overrightarrow{BA}\right| = 50.0$ lb

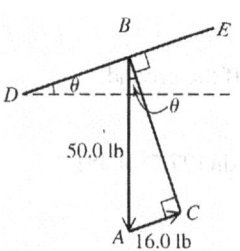

$\sin\theta = \dfrac{16.0}{50.0} \Rightarrow \theta = \sin^{-1}\left(\dfrac{16.0}{50.0}\right) \approx 18.7°$

18. $w + z = (2 - 4i) + (5 + i) = 7 - 3i$

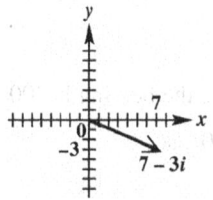

19. (a) $i^{15} = i^{12+3} = i^{12} \cdot i^3 = \left(i^4\right)^3 \cdot i^3 = 1(-i) = -i$

Copyright © 2015 Pearson Education, Inc

(b) $(1+i)^2 = (1+i)(1+i) = 1+i+i+i^2 = 1+2i+(-1) = 2i$

20. (a) $3i \Rightarrow r = \sqrt{0^2 + 3^2} = \sqrt{0+9} = \sqrt{9} = 3$

    The point $(0,3)$ is on the positive y-axis, so, $\theta = 90°$. Thus, $3i = 3(\cos 90° + i\sin 90°)$.

    (b) $1+2i \Rightarrow r = \sqrt{1^2 + 2^2} = \sqrt{1+4} = \sqrt{5}$

    Since θ is in quadrant I, $\theta = \tan^{-1}\left(\frac{2}{1}\right) = \tan^{-1} 2 \approx 63.43°$. Thus, $1+2i = \sqrt{5}(\cos 63.43° + i\sin 63.43°)$.

    (c) $-1-\sqrt{3}i \Rightarrow r = \sqrt{(-1)^2 + (-\sqrt{3})^2} = \sqrt{1+3} = \sqrt{4} = 2$ Since θ is in quadrant III,

    $\theta = \tan^{-1}\left(\frac{-\sqrt{3}}{-1}\right) = \tan^{-1}\sqrt{3} = 240°$. Thus, $-1-\sqrt{3}i = 2(\cos 240° + i\sin 240°)$

21. (a) $3(\cos 30° + i\sin 30°) = 3\left(\frac{\sqrt{3}}{2} + \frac{1}{2}i\right) = \frac{3\sqrt{3}}{2} + \frac{3}{2}i$

    (b) $4 \text{ cis } 40° \approx 3.06 + 2.57i$

    (c) $3(\cos 90° + i\sin 90°) = 3(0 + 1 \cdot i) = 0 + 3i = 3i$

22. (a) $wz = 8 \cdot 2\left[\cos(40° + 10°) + i\sin(40° + 10°)\right] = 16(\cos 50° + i\sin 50°)$

    (b) $\frac{w}{z} = \frac{8}{2}\left[\cos(40° - 10°) + i\sin(40° - 10°)\right] = 4(\cos 30° + i\sin 30°) = 4\left(\frac{\sqrt{3}}{2} + \frac{1}{2}i\right) = 2\sqrt{3} + 2i$

    (c) $z^3 = \left[2(\cos 10° + i\sin 10°)\right]^3 = 2^3(\cos 3 \cdot 10° + i\sin 3 \cdot 10°) = 8(\cos 30° + i\sin 30°) =$

    $8\left(\frac{\sqrt{3}}{2} + \frac{1}{2}i\right) = 4\sqrt{3} + 4i$

23. Since $r^4(\cos 4\alpha + i\sin 4\alpha) = 16(\cos 270° + i\sin 270°)$, then we have $r^4 = 16 \Rightarrow r = 2$ and

    $4\alpha = 270° + 360° \cdot k \Rightarrow \alpha = \frac{270° + 360° \cdot k}{4} = 67.5° + 90° \cdot k$, k any integer. If $k = 0$, then $\alpha = 67.5°$.

    If $k = 1$, then $\alpha = 157.5°$, If $k = 2$, then $\alpha = 247.5°$., If $k = 3$, then $\alpha = 337.5°$.

    The fourth roots of $-16i$ are $2(\cos 67.5° + i\sin 67.5)$, $2(\cos 157.5° + i\sin 157.5°)$, $2(\cos 247.5° + i\sin 247.5°)$,

    and $2(\cos 337.5° + i\sin 337.5°)$.

24. Answers may vary.

550 Chapter 10: Applications of Trigonometry and Vectors

(a) $(0, 5) \Rightarrow r = \sqrt{0^2 + 5^2} = \sqrt{0+25} = \sqrt{25} = 5$

The point $(0, 5)$ is on the positive y-axis. Thus, $\theta = 90°$. One possibility is $(5, 90°)$. Alternatively, if $\theta = 90° - 360° = -270°$, a second possibility is $(5, -270°)$.

(b) $(-2, -2) \Rightarrow r = \sqrt{(-2)^2 + (-2)^2} = \sqrt{4+4} = \sqrt{8} = 2\sqrt{2}$

Since θ is in quadrant III, $\theta = \tan^{-1}\left(\dfrac{-2}{-2}\right) = \tan^{-1} 1 = 225°$. One possibility is $\left(2\sqrt{2}, 225°\right)$.

Alternatively, if $\theta = 225° - 360° = -135°$, a second possibility is $\left(2\sqrt{2}, -135°\right)$.

25. (a) $(3, 315°) \Rightarrow x = r\cos\theta \Rightarrow x = 3\cos 315° = 3 \cdot \dfrac{\sqrt{2}}{2} = \dfrac{3\sqrt{2}}{2}$ and $y = r\sin\theta \Rightarrow$

$y = 3\sin 315° = 3\left(-\dfrac{\sqrt{2}}{2}\right) = \dfrac{-3\sqrt{2}}{2}$ The rectangular coordinates are $\left(\dfrac{3\sqrt{2}}{2}, \dfrac{-3\sqrt{2}}{2}\right)$.

(b) $(-4, 90°) \Rightarrow x = r\cos\theta \Rightarrow x = -4\cos 90° = 0$ and $y = r\sin\theta \Rightarrow y = -4\sin 90° = -4$

The rectangular coordinates are $(0, -4)$.

26. $r = 1 - \cos\theta$ is a cardioid.

θ	0°	30°	45°	60°	90°	135°
$r = 1 - \cos\theta$	0	0.1	0.3	0.5	1	1.7
θ	180°	225°	270°	315°	360°	
$r = 1 - \cos\theta$	2	1.7	1	0.3	0	

90°

180° 0°

270°
$r = 1 - \cos\theta$

27. $r = 3\cos 3\theta$ is a three-leaved rose.

θ	0°	30°	45°	60°	90°	120°	135°	150°	180°
$r = 3\cos 3\theta$	3	0	−2.1	−3	0	3	2.1	0	−3

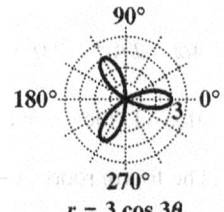

270°
$r = 3 \cos 3\theta$

Graph is retraced in the interval (180°, 360°).

28. (a) Since $r = \dfrac{4}{2\sin\theta - \cos\theta} = \dfrac{4}{-1\cdot\cos\theta + 2\sin\theta}$, we can use the general form for the polar equation of a line, $r = \dfrac{c}{a\cos\theta + b\sin\theta}$, with $a = -1$, $b = 2$, and $c = 4$, we have $-x + 2y = 4$ or $x - 2y = -4$. The graph is a line with intercepts $(-4, 0)$ and $(0, 2)$. See Figure 28a

(b) $r = 6$ represents the equation of a circle centered at the origin with radius 6, namely $x^2 + y^2 = 36$. See Figure 28b.

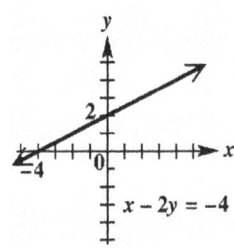

Figure 28a

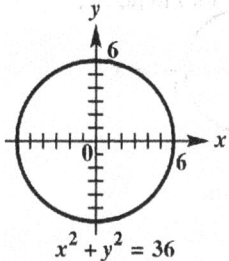

Figure 28b

29. $x = 2t - 1$, $y = t^2$ for t in $[-2, 3]$ See Figure 29.

t	x	Y
-2	-5	4
-1	-3	1
0	-1	0
1	1	1
2	3	4
3	5	9

Since $x = 2t - 1 \Rightarrow t = \dfrac{x+1}{2}$ and $y = t^2$, we have $y = \left(\dfrac{x+1}{2}\right)^2 = \dfrac{1}{4}(x+1)^2$, where x is in $[-5, 5]$

30. $x = 2\cos 2t$, $y = 2\sin 2t$ for t in $[0, 2\pi]$. See Figure 30.

T	0	$\frac{\pi}{8}$	$\frac{\pi}{4}$	$\frac{3\pi}{8}$	$\frac{\pi}{2}$	$\frac{5\pi}{8}$
X	2	$\sqrt{2}$	0	$-\sqrt{2}$	-2	$-\sqrt{2}$
Y	0	$\sqrt{2}$	2	$\sqrt{2}$	0	$-\sqrt{2}$

T	$\frac{3\pi}{4}$	π	$\frac{5\pi}{4}$	$\frac{3\pi}{2}$	$\frac{7\pi}{4}$	2π
X	0	2	0	-2	0	2
Y	-2	0	2	0	-2	0

Since $x = 2\cos 2t \Rightarrow \cos 2t = \dfrac{x}{2}$, $y = 2\sin 2t \Rightarrow \sin 2t = \dfrac{y}{2}$, and $\cos^2(2t) + \sin^2(2t) = 1$, we have

$$\left(\dfrac{x}{2}\right)^2 + \left(\dfrac{y}{2}\right)^2 = 1 \Rightarrow \dfrac{x^2}{4} + \dfrac{y^2}{4} = 1 \Rightarrow x^2 + y^2 = 4, \text{ where } x \text{ is in } [-1, 1].$$

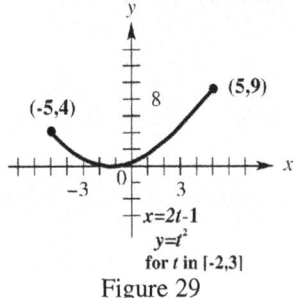

Figure 29

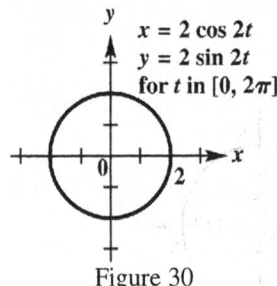

Figure 30

Chapter 11: Further Topics in Algebra

11.1: Sequences and Series

1. $a_1 = 4(1) + 10 = 14$; $a_2 = 4(2) + 10 = 18$; $a_3 = 4(3) + 10 = 22$; $a_4 = 4(4) + 10 = 26$; $a_5 = 4(5) + 10 = 30$

   The first five terms of the sequence are 14, 18, 22, 26, and 30.

3. $a_1 = 2^{1-1} = 2^0 = 1$; $a_2 = 2^{2-1} = 2^1 = 2$; $a_3 = 2^{3-1} = 2^2 = 4$; $a_4 = 2^{4-1} = 2^3 = 8$; $a_5 = 2^{5-1} = 2^4 = 16$

   The first five terms of the sequence are 1, 2, 4, 8, and 16.

5. $a_1 = \left(\frac{1}{3}\right)^1 (1-1) = \left(\frac{1}{3}\right)(0) = 0$; $a_2 = \left(\frac{1}{3}\right)^2 (2-1) = \left(\frac{1}{9}\right)(1) = \frac{1}{9}$;

   $a_3 = \left(\frac{1}{3}\right)^3 (3-1) = \left(\frac{1}{27}\right)(2) = \frac{2}{27}$; $a_4 = \left(\frac{1}{3}\right)^4 (4-1) = \left(\frac{1}{81}\right)(3) = \frac{1}{27}$; $a_5 = \left(\frac{1}{3}\right)^5 (5-1) = \left(\frac{1}{243}\right)(4) = \frac{4}{243}$

   The first five terms of the sequence are $0, \frac{1}{9}, \frac{2}{27}, \frac{1}{27}$, and $\frac{4}{243}$.

7. $a_1 = (-1)^1 [(2)(1)] = -2$; $a_2 = (-1)^2 [(2)(2)] = 4$; $a_3 = (-1)^3 [(2)(3)] = -6$;

   $a_4 = (-1)^4 [(2)(4)] = 8$; $a_5 = (-1)^5 [(2)(5)] = -10$

   The first five terms of the sequence are $-2, 4, -6, 8$, and -10.

9. $a_1 = \frac{4(1)-1}{1^2+2} = \frac{3}{3} = 1$; $a_2 = \frac{4(2)-1}{2^2+2} = \frac{7}{6}$; $a_3 = \frac{4(3)-1}{3^2+2} = \frac{11}{11} = 1$;

   $a_4 = \frac{4(4)-1}{4^2+2} = \frac{15}{3} = \frac{5}{6}$; $a_5 = \frac{4(5)-1}{5^2+2} = \frac{19}{27}$ The first five terms of the sequence are $1, \frac{7}{6}, 1, \frac{5}{6}$, and $\frac{19}{27}$.

11. The terms of a sequence are numbered according to their position in the sequence; a_1 is the first term, a_2 is the second term, etc. So a_n will be the nth term in the sequence for any positive integer value of n.

13. The sequence has 7 terms; it is finite.

15. The sequence has 4 terms; it is finite.

17. The sequence has no last term; it is infinite.

19. The sequence is defined for integer values of n from 1 through 10; it is finite.

21. $a_1 = -2$; $a_2 = a_1 + 3 = -2 + 3 = 1$; $a_3 = a_2 + 3 = 1 + 3 = 4$; $a_4 = a_3 + 3 = 4 + 3 = 7$

    The first four terms of the sequence are $-2, 1, 4$, and 7.

23. $a_1 = 1$; $a_2 = 1$; $a_3 = a_2 + a_1 = 1 + 1 = 2$; $a_4 = a_3 + a_2 = 2 + 1 = 3$.

    The first four terms of the sequence are 1, 1, 2, and 3.

25. $a_1 = 5$; $a_2 = 3(2) + 3a_1 = 6 + 3(5) = 21$; $a_3 = 3(3) + 3a_2 = 9 + 3(21) = 72$;
    $a_4 = 3(4) + 3a_3 = 12 + 3(72) = 228$.

    The first four terms of the sequence are 5, 21, 72, and 228.

27. $a_1 = 2$; $a_2 = 3$; $a_3 = a_2 \cdot a_1 = 3(2) = 6$; $a_4 = a_3 \cdot a_2 = 6(3) = 18$

The first four terms of the sequence are 2, 3, 6, and 18.

29. $\sum_{i=1}^{5} (2i+1) = 3+5+7+9+11 = 35$

31. $\sum_{j=1}^{4} \frac{1}{j} = \frac{1}{1}+\frac{1}{2}+\frac{1}{3}+\frac{1}{4} = \frac{25}{12}$

33. $\sum_{i=1}^{4} i^i = 1^1 + 2^2 + 3^3 + 4^4 = 288$

35. $\sum_{k=1}^{6} (-1)^k \cdot k = (-1)^1(1) + (-1)^2(2) + (-1)^3(3) + (-1)^4(4) + (-1)^5(5) + (-1)^6(6) = 3$

37. $\sum_{i=2}^{5} (6-3i) = (6-6) + (6-9) + (6-12) + (6-15) = -18$

39. $\sum_{i=-2}^{3} 2(3)^i = 2(3)^{-2} + 2(3)^{-1} + 2(3)^0 + 2(3)^1 + 2(3)^2 + 2(3)^3 = \frac{728}{9}$

41. $\sum_{i=-1}^{5} (i^2 - 2i) = \left[(-1)^2 - 2(-1)\right] + \left[0^2 - 2(0)\right] + \left[1^2 - 2(1)\right] + \left[2^2 - 2(2)\right] + \left[3^2 - 2(3)\right] +$

$\left[4^2 - 2(4)\right] + \left[5^2 - 2(5)\right] = 28$

43. $\sum_{i=1}^{5} (3^i - 4) = (3^1 - 4) + (3^2 - 4) + (3^3 - 4) + (3^4 - 4) + (3^5 - 4) = 343$

45. $\sum_{i=1}^{5} x_i = (-2) + (-1) + (0) + (1) + (2) = -2 - 1 + 0 + 1 + 2$

47. $\sum_{i=1}^{5} (2x_i + 3) = [2(-2)+3] + [2(-1)+3] + [2(0)+3] + [2(1)+3] + [2(2)+3] = -1+1+3+5+7$

49. $\sum_{i=1}^{3} (3x_i - x_i^2) = \left[3(-2) - (-2)^2\right] + \left[3(-1) - (-1)^2\right] + \left[3(0) - (0)^2\right] = -10 - 4 + 0$

51. $\sum_{i=2}^{5} \frac{x_i + 1}{x_i + 2} = \frac{-1+1}{-1+2} + \frac{0+1}{0+2} + \frac{1+1}{1+2} + \frac{2+1}{2+2} = 0 + \frac{1}{2} + \frac{2}{3} + \frac{3}{4}$

53. $\sum_{i=1}^{4} f(x_i)\Delta x = [4(0)-7](0.5) + [4(2)-7](0.5) + [4(4)-7](0.5) + [4(6)-7](0.5) = -0.35 + 0.5 + 4.5 + 8.5$

55. $\sum_{i=1}^{4} f(x_i)\Delta x = \left[2(0)^2\right](0.5) + \left[2(2)^2\right](0.5) + \left[2(4)^2\right](0.5) + \left[2(6)^2\right](0.5) = 0 + 4 + 16 + 36$

57. $\sum_{i=1}^{4} f(x_i)\Delta x = \left(\frac{-2}{0+1}\right)(0.5) + \left(\frac{-2}{2+1}\right)(0.5) + \left(\frac{-2}{4+1}\right)(0.5) + \left(\frac{-2}{6+1}\right)(0.5) = -1 - \frac{1}{3} - \frac{1}{5} - \frac{1}{7}$

59. $\sum_{i=1}^{100} 6 = (100)(6) = 600$

61. $\sum_{i=1}^{15} i^2 = \frac{(15)(15+1)[2(15)+1]}{6} = 1240$

63. $\sum_{i=1}^{5}(5i+3) = 5\left[\frac{(5)(5+1)}{2}\right] + 5(3) = 90$

65. $\sum_{i=1}^{5}(4i^2 - 2i + 6) = 4\left[\frac{(5)(5+1)[2(5)+1]}{6}\right] - 2\left[\frac{5(5+1)}{2}\right] + 5(6) = 220$

67. $\sum_{i=1}^{4}(3i^3 + 2i - 4) = 3\left[\frac{4^2(4+1)^2}{4}\right] + 2\left[\frac{(4)(4+1)}{2}\right] + 4(-4) = 304$

69. $\sum_{i=1}^{60}(i^3 - 2i^2) = \frac{60^2(60+1)^2}{4} - 2\left[\frac{(60)(60+1)[2(60)+1]}{6}\right] = 3,201,280$

71. $\sum_{i=1}^{77}(i^2 + 52i + 672) = \left[\frac{(77)(77+1)[2(77)+1]}{6}\right] + 52\left[\frac{77(77+1)}{2}\right] + 77(672) = 363,055$

73. A single fraction in the sum $\frac{2}{5(1)} + \frac{2}{5(2)} + \frac{2}{5(3)} + ... + \frac{2}{5(100)}$ can be shown as $\frac{2}{5(i)}$ where i begins at 1 and ends at 100. This sum can be shown as $\sum_{i=1}^{100} \frac{2}{5i}$.

75. A single fraction in the sum $1 + \frac{1}{2} + \frac{1}{3} + \frac{1}{4} + ... + \frac{1}{9}$ can be shown as $\frac{1}{i}$ where i begins at 1 and ends at 9. This sum can be shown as $\sum_{i=1}^{9} \frac{1}{i}$.

77. The graphing calculator graph of the first ten terms of this sequence is shown in Figure 77. From this graph, the terms of the sequence appear to converge to the value $\frac{1}{2}$ which, in fact, they do.

79. The graphing calculator graph of the first ten terms of this sequence is shown in Figure 79. From this graph, the terms of the sequence appear to diverge and, in fact, they do.

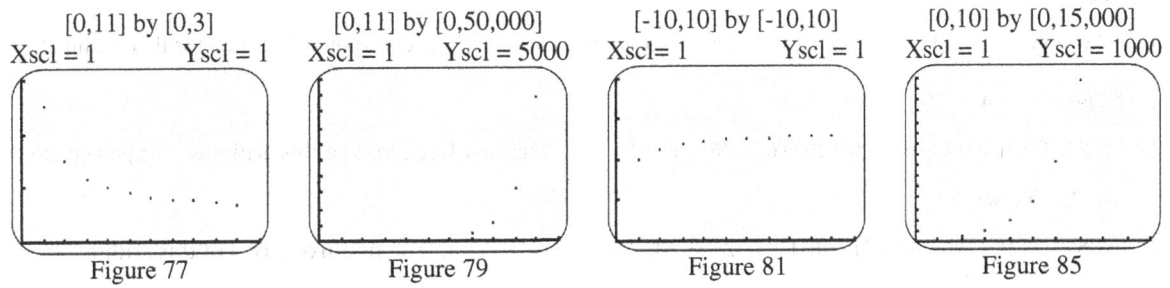

[0,11] by [0,3] Xscl = 1 Yscl = 1   Figure 77
[0,11] by [0,50,000] Xscl = 1 Yscl = 5000   Figure 79
[-10,10] by [-10,10] Xscl= 1 Yscl = 1   Figure 81
[0,10] by [0,15,000] Xscl = 1 Yscl = 1000   Figure 85

81. The graphing calculator graph of the first ten terms of this sequence is shown in Figure 81. From this graph, the terms of the sequence appear to converge to the value somewhat greater than 2.5. In fact, they converge to $e \approx 2.71828$.

83. The sum of the first six terms of the series is

$$\frac{1}{1^4}+\frac{1}{2^4}+\frac{1}{3^4}+\frac{1}{4^4}+\frac{1}{5^4}+\frac{1}{6^4}=1+\frac{1}{16}+\frac{1}{81}+\frac{1}{256}+\frac{1}{625}+\frac{1}{1296} \approx 1.081123534 \Rightarrow$$

$$\frac{\pi^4}{90} \approx 1.081123534 \Rightarrow \pi^4 \approx 97.30111806 \Rightarrow \pi \approx 3.140721718.$$

This approximation of π is accurate to three decimal places when rounded to 3.141.

85. (a) The number of bacteria doubles every 40 minutes, so $N_{j+1} = 2N_j$ for $j \geq 1$.

(b) Two hours = 120 minutes $\Rightarrow 120 = 40(j-1) \Rightarrow 3 = j-1 \Rightarrow j = 4$.

$N_1 = 230; N_2 = 2(230) = 460; N_3 = 2(460) = 920; N_4 = 2(920) = 1840$. If there are initially 230 bacteria, then there will be 1840 bacteria after two hours.

(c) The graph of the first seven terms of this sequence is shown in Figure 85.

(d) From the graph, the growth rate is seen to be very rapid. Doubling the number of bacteria at equal intervals of time produces an exponential growth rate.

87. (a) $1+1+\frac{1^2}{2!}+\frac{1^3}{3!}+\frac{1^4}{4!}+\frac{1^5}{5!}+\frac{1^6}{6!}+\frac{1^7}{7!} \approx 2.718254$; $e \approx 2.718282$. Eight terms of the series gives an estimate that matches to four decimal places.

(b) $1+(-1)+\frac{(-1)^2}{2!}+\frac{(-1)^3}{3!}+\frac{(-1)^4}{4!}+\frac{(-1)^5}{5!}+\frac{(-1)^6}{6!}+\frac{(-1)^7}{7!} \approx 0.367857$; $e \approx 0.367879$. Eight terms of the series gives an estimate that matches to four decimal places.

(c) $1+\frac{1}{2}+\frac{\left(\frac{1}{2}\right)^2}{2!}+\frac{\left(\frac{1}{2}\right)^3}{3!}+\frac{\left(\frac{1}{2}\right)^4}{4!}+\frac{\left(\frac{1}{2}\right)^5}{5!}+\frac{\left(\frac{1}{2}\right)^6}{6!}+\frac{\left(\frac{1}{2}\right)^7}{7!} \approx 1.648721$; $\sqrt{e} = e^{1/2} \approx 1.648721$. Eight terms of the series gives an estimate that matches to six decimal places.

11.2: Arithmetic Sequences and Series

1. $5-2=3$; $8-5=3$; $11-8=3$. The common difference for this arithmetic sequence is 3.

3. $-2-3=-5$; $-7-(-2)=-5$; $-12-(-7)=-5$. The common difference for this arithmetic sequence is -5.

5. $(2x+5y)-(x+3y)=x+2y$; $(3x+7y)-(2x+5y)=x+2y$. The common difference for this arithmetic sequence is $x+2y$.

7. 8; $8+6=14$; $14+6=20$; $20+6=26$; $26+6=32$. The first five terms of this arithmetic sequence are 8, 14, 20, 26, and 32.

9. 5; $5+(-2)=3$; $3+(-2)=1$; $1+(-2)=-1$; $(-1)+(-2)=-3$. The first five terms of this arithmetic sequence 5, 3, 1, -1, and -3.

11. $a_3 = 10$; $a_1 = 10-2(-2) = 14$; $a_2 = 10-(-2) = 12$; $a_4 = 10+(-2) = 8$; $a_5 = 8+(-2) = 6$. The first five terms of this arithmetic sequence are 14, 12, 10, 8, and 6.

13. $a_8 = 5 + (8-1)(2) = 19$; $a_n = 5 + (n-1)(2) = 2n + 3$. The eighth term of the sequence is 19. The nth term of the sequence is $2n + 3$.

14. $a_8 = -3 + (8-1)(-4) = -31$; $a_n = -3 + (n-1)(-4) = -4n + 1$ The eighth term of the sequence is -31 The nth term of the sequence is $-4n + 1$.

15. $a_3 = 2$; $d = 1 \Rightarrow a_1 = 2 - 2(1) = 0$; $a_8 = 0 + (8-1)(1) = 7$; $a_n = 0 + (n-1)(1)$. The eighth term of the sequence is 7. The nth term of the sequence is $n - 1$.

17. $a_1 = 8$; $a_6 = 6 \Rightarrow d = 6 - 8 = -2$; $a_8 = 8 + (8-1)(-2) = -6$; $a_n = 8 + (n-1)(-2) = -2n + 10$. The eighth term of the sequence is -6. The nth term of the sequence is $-2n + 10$.

19. $a_{10} = 6$; $a_{12} = 15 \Rightarrow 2d = 15 - 6 = 9$; $d = 4.5$; $a_1 = 6 - (9)(4.5) = -3.45$;
$a_8 = -34.5 + (8-1)(4.5) = -3$; $a_n = -34.5 + (n-1)(4.5) = 4.5n - 39$. The eighth term of the sequence is -3 The nth term of the sequence is $4.5n - 39$.

21. $a_1 = x$; $a_2 = x + 3 \Rightarrow d = (x+3) - x = 3$; $a_8 = x + (8-1)(3) = x + 21$; $a_n = x + (n-1)(3) = x + 3n - 3$. The eighth term of the sequence is $x + 21$. The nth term of the sequence is $x + 3n - 3$.

23. $a_3 = \pi + 2\sqrt{e}$; $a_4 = \pi + 3\sqrt{e} \Rightarrow d = (\pi + 3\sqrt{3}) - (\pi + 2\sqrt{e}) \Rightarrow a_1 = \pi$. $a_8 = \pi + 7\sqrt{e}$ $a_n = \pi + (n-1)\sqrt{e}$
The eighth term is $\pi + 7\sqrt{e}$ and the nth term is $\pi + (n-1)\sqrt{e}$.

25. $a_5 = 27$; $a_{15} = 87 \Rightarrow 87 = 27 + 10d \Rightarrow 10d = 60 \Rightarrow d = 6$; $27 = a_1 + (5-1)(6) \Rightarrow a_1 = 27 - 24 = 3$. The first term of the sequence is 3.

27. $a_5 = -3$; $a_{18} = -29 \Rightarrow -29 = -3 + 13d \Rightarrow 13d = -26 \Rightarrow d = -2$;
$-29 = a_1 + (18-1)(-2) \Rightarrow a_1 = -29 + 34 = 5$. The first term of the sequence is 5.

29. $S_3 = 75$; $a_3 = 22 \Rightarrow 75 = \frac{3}{2}[a_1 + (22)] \Rightarrow a_1 = 50 - 22 \Rightarrow a_1 = 28$. The first term of the sequence is 28.

31. $S_{16} = -160$; $a_{16} = -25 \Rightarrow -160 = \frac{16}{2}[a_1 + (-25)] \Rightarrow 8a_1 = -160 + 200 \Rightarrow a_1 = 5$. The first term of the sequence is 5.

33. $a_8 = -160$; $d = 3 \Rightarrow a_{10} = 8 + (10-1)(3) = 35 \Rightarrow S_{10} = \frac{10}{2}(8 + 35) = 215$. The sum of the first ten terms of the sequence is 215.

35. $a_3 = 5$; $a_4 = 8 \Rightarrow d = 8 - 5 = 3 \Rightarrow 5 = a_1 + (3-1)(3) \Rightarrow a_1 = -1 \Rightarrow a_{10} = -1 + (10-1)(3) = 26 \Rightarrow$
$S_{10} = \frac{10}{2}(-1 + 26) = 125$. The sum of the first ten terms of the sequence is 125.

37. $a_1 = 5$; $d = 9 - 5 = 4 \Rightarrow a_{10} = 5 + (10-1)(4) = 41 \Rightarrow S_{10} = \frac{10}{2}(5 + 41) = 230$. The sum of the first ten terms of the sequence is 230.

39. $a_1 = 10$; $a_{10} = 5.5 \Rightarrow S_{10} = \dfrac{10}{2}(10+55) = 77.5$. The sum of the first ten terms of the sequence is 77.5.

41. $S_{20} = 1090$; $a_{20} = 102 \Rightarrow 1090 = \dfrac{20}{2}(a_1 + 102) \Rightarrow 109 = a_1 + 102 \Rightarrow a_1 = 7 \Rightarrow 102 = 7 + (20-1)d \Rightarrow$

    $19d = 95 \Rightarrow d = 5$. The first term of the sequence is 7 and the common difference is 5.

43. $S_{12} = -108$; $a_{12} = -19 \Rightarrow -108 = \dfrac{12}{2}[a_1 + (-19)] \Rightarrow 6a_1 = -108 + 114 = 6 \Rightarrow$

    $a_1 = 1 \Rightarrow -19 = 1 + (12-1)d \Rightarrow 11d = -20 \Rightarrow d = -\dfrac{20}{11}$. The first term of the sequence is 1 and the

    common difference is $-\dfrac{20}{11}$.

45. From the graph, $a_1 = -2, a_2 = -1 \Rightarrow d = -1 - (-2) = 1 \Rightarrow a_n = -2 + (n-1) = n - 3$. Also from the graph,

    $D: \{1,2,3,4,5,6\}$; $R: \{-2,-1,0,1,2,3\}$. The nth term of the sequence is $n - 3$. The domain of the sequence

    is the set $\{1,2,3,4,5,6\}$ and the range of the sequence is set $\{-2,-1,0,1,2,3\}$.

47. From the graph, $a_1 = 2.5$, $a_2 = 2 \Rightarrow d = 2 - 2.5 = -0.5 \Rightarrow a_n = 2.5 + (n-1)(-0.5) = -0.5n + 3$. Also from

    the graph, $D: \{1,2,3,4,5,6\}$; $R: \{0.5,1,1.5,2,2.5\}$. The nth term of the sequence is $-0.5n + 3$. The domain of

    the sequence is the set $\{1,2,3,4,5,6\}$ and the range of the sequence is set $\{0.5,1,1.5,2,2.5\}$.

49. From the graph, $a_1 = 10$, $a_2 = -10 \Rightarrow d = -10 - 10 = -20 \Rightarrow a_n = 10 + (n-1)(-20) = -20n + 30$. Also

    from the graph, $D: \{1,2,3,4,5\}$; $R: \{-70,-50,-30,-10,10\}$. The nth term of the sequence is $-20n + 30$.

    The domain of the sequence is the set $\{1,2,3,4,5\}$ and the range of the sequence is set

    $\{-70,-50,-30,-10,10\}$.

51. $a_1 = 3$, $a_8 = 17$; $3+5+7+9+11+13+15+17 = S_8 = \dfrac{8}{2}(3+17) = 80$. The sum of the series is 80.

53. $a_1 = 1$; $a_{50} = 50$; $1+2+3+4+\cdots+50 = S_{50} = \dfrac{50}{2}(1+50) = 1275$. The sum of the series is 1275.

55. $a_1 = -7$; $d = -4 - (-7) = 3$; $101 = -7 + (n-1)(3) \Rightarrow 3n = 111 \Rightarrow n = 37$;

    $-7 + (-4) + (-1) + 2 + 5 + \ldots + 98 + 101 = S_{37} = \dfrac{37}{2}(-7 + 101) = 1739$. The sum of the series is 1739.

57. $a_1 = 5(1) = 5$; $a_{40} = 5(40) = 200$; $S_{40} = \dfrac{40}{20}(5+200) = 4100$. The sum of the series is 4100.

59. $a_1 = 1+4 = 5$; $a_3 = 3+4 = 7$; $\sum\limits_{i=1}^{3}(i+4) = S_3 = \dfrac{3}{2}(5+7) = 18$. The sum is 18.

61. $a_1 = 2(1)+3 = 5$; $a_{10} = 2(10)+3 = 23$; $\sum\limits_{j=1}^{10}(2j+3) = S_{10} = \dfrac{10}{2}(5+23) = 140$. The sum is 140.

63. $a_1 = -5 - 8(1) = -13$; $a_{12} = -5 - 8(12) = -101$; $\sum_{i=1}^{12}(-5-8i) = S_{12} = \frac{12}{2}[-13+(-101)] = -684$.

The sum is -684.

65. $a_1 = 1$; $a_{1000} = 1000$; $\sum_{i=1}^{1000} i = S_{1000} = \frac{1000}{2}(1+1000) = 500,500$. The sum is $500,500$.

67. $a_n = 4.2n + 9.73$. Using the sequence feature of a graphing calculator, we obtain $s_{10} = 328.3$.

69. $a_n = \sqrt{8}n + \sqrt{3}$. Using the sequence feature of a graphing calculator, we obtain $s_{10} = 172.884$.

71. $a_1 = 51$; $d = 1$; $71 = 51 + (n-1)(1) \Rightarrow n = 71 - 50 = 21$; $\sum_{i=51}^{71} i = s_{21} = \frac{21}{2}(51+71) = 1281$. The sum of all the integers from 51 to 71 is 1281.

73. $a_1 = 1$; $a_{12} = 12$; $s_{12} = \frac{12}{2}(1+12) = 78$; chimes per 24 hours $= 2(78) = 156$. Chimes per 30 days $= (30)(156) = 4680$. The clock will chime 4680 times in a month of 30 days.

75. $a_1 = 49,000$, $d = 580$, $n = 11$; $a_{11} = 49,000 + (11-1)(580) = 54,800$. The population five years from now will be 54,800.

77. $a_1 = 18$; $a_{31} = 28$; $s_{31} = \frac{31}{2}(18+28) = 713$. A total of 713 inches of material will be needed.

79. (a) $a_1 = 98.2$, $a_3 = 109.8 \Rightarrow 109.8 = 98.2 + (3-1)d \Rightarrow 2d = 11.6 \Rightarrow d = 5.8$. The common difference of the arithmetic sequence describing the child's height would be 5.8 centimeters.

(b) $a_6 = 98.2 + (6-1)(5.8) = 127.2$. We would expect the child's height to be 127.2 centimeters at age 8.

81. $d_{n+1} - d_n = (a_{n+1} + c \cdot b_{n+1}) - (a_n + c \cdot b_n) = (a_{n+1} - a_n) + c(b_{n+1} - b_n) = j + ck$, where j is the common difference for the sequence $a_1, a_2, a_3, \ldots$ and k is the common difference for the sequence $b_1, b_2, b_3, \ldots$ Thus, since $d_{n+1} - d_n$ is a constant, $d_1, d_2, d_3, \ldots$ is also an arithmetic sequence.

11.3: Geometric Sequences and Series

1. $a_1 = \frac{5}{3}$; $a_2 = \left(\frac{5}{3}\right)(3) = 5$; $a_3 = (5)(3) = 15$; $a_4 = (15)(3) = 45$. The first four terms of the sequence are

$\frac{5}{3}, 5, 15, 45$.

3. $a_4 = 5$, $a_5 = 10 \Rightarrow r = \frac{10}{5} = 2$; $a_3 = \frac{5}{2}$; $a_2 = \frac{\frac{5}{2}}{2} = \frac{5}{4}$; $a_1 = \frac{\frac{5}{4}}{2} = \frac{5}{8}$. The first five terms of the sequence are

$\frac{5}{8}, \frac{5}{4}, \frac{5}{2}, 5, 10$.

5. $a_5 = 5(-2)^{5-1} = (5)(16) = 80$; $a_n = 5(-2)^{n-1}$. The fifth term of the sequence is 80 and the nth term of the sequence is $5(-2)^{n-1}$.

7. $a_2 = -4, r = -3 \Rightarrow a_1 = \dfrac{4}{3}$; $a_5 = \left(\dfrac{4}{3}\right)(-3)^{5-1} = 108$; $a_n = \left(\dfrac{4}{3}\right)(-3)^{n-1}$. The fifth term of the sequence is 108 and the nth term of the sequence is $\left(\dfrac{4}{3}\right)(-3)^{n-1}$.

9. $a_4 = 243, r = -3 \Rightarrow a_1 = \dfrac{243}{(-3)^{4-1}} = -9$; $a_5 = (-9)(-3)^{5-1} = -729$; $a_n = (-9)(-3)^{n-1}$. The fifth term of the sequence is -729 and the nth term of the sequence is $(-9)(-3)^{n-1}$.

11. $r = \dfrac{-12}{-4} = \dfrac{-36}{-12} = \dfrac{-108}{-36} = 3$; $a_5 = (-4)(3)^{5-1} = -324$; $a_n = (-4)(3)^{n-1}$. The fifth term of the sequence is -324 and the nth term of the sequence is $(-4)(3)^{n-1}$.

13. $r = \dfrac{2}{\frac{4}{5}} = \dfrac{5}{2} = \dfrac{\frac{25}{2}}{5} = \dfrac{5}{2}$; $a_5 = \left(\dfrac{4}{5}\right)\left(\dfrac{5}{2}\right)^{5-1} = \dfrac{125}{4}$; $a_n = \left(\dfrac{4}{5}\right)\left(\dfrac{5}{2}\right)^{n-1}$. The fifth term of the sequence is $\dfrac{125}{4}$ and the nth term of the sequence is $\left(\dfrac{4}{5}\right)\left(\dfrac{5}{2}\right)^{n-1}$.

15. $r = \dfrac{-5}{10} = \dfrac{\frac{5}{2}}{-5} = \dfrac{-\frac{5}{4}}{\frac{5}{2}} = -\dfrac{1}{2}$; $a_5 = (10)\left(-\dfrac{1}{2}\right)^{5-1} = \dfrac{5}{8}$; $a_n = 10\left(-\dfrac{1}{2}\right)^{n-1}$. The fifth term of the sequence is $\dfrac{5}{8}$ and the nth term of the sequence is $10\left(-\dfrac{1}{2}\right)^{n-1}$.

17. $a_3 = 5, a_8 = \dfrac{1}{625} \Rightarrow r^{7-2} = \dfrac{\frac{1}{625}}{5} = \dfrac{1}{3125} \Rightarrow r = \dfrac{1}{5}$; $a_1 = \dfrac{5}{\left(\frac{1}{5}\right)^2} = 125$. The first term of the sequence is 125 and the common ratio is $\dfrac{1}{5}$.

19. $a_4 = -\dfrac{1}{4}, a_9 = -\dfrac{1}{128} \Rightarrow r^{8-3} = \dfrac{-\frac{1}{128}}{-\frac{1}{4}} = \dfrac{1}{32} \Rightarrow r = \dfrac{1}{2}$; $a_1 = \dfrac{-\frac{1}{4}}{\left(\frac{1}{2}\right)^3} = -2$. The first term of the sequence is -2 and the common ratio is $\dfrac{1}{2}$.

21. $r = \dfrac{8}{2} = \dfrac{32}{8} = \dfrac{128}{32} = 4$; $S_5 = \dfrac{2(1-4^5)}{1-4} = 682$. The sum of the first five terms of the sequence is 682.

23. $r = \dfrac{-9}{18} = \dfrac{\frac{9}{2}}{-9} = \dfrac{-\frac{9}{4}}{\frac{9}{2}} = -\dfrac{1}{2}$; $S_5 = \dfrac{18\left[1-\left(-\frac{1}{2}\right)^5\right]}{1-\left(-\frac{1}{2}\right)} = \dfrac{99}{8}$. The sum of the first five terms of the sequence is $\dfrac{99}{8}$.

25. $S_5 = \dfrac{(8.423)\left[1-(2.859)^5\right]}{1-2.859} \approx 860.95$. Rounded to the nearest hundredth, the sum of the first five terms of the sequence is 860.95.

27. $a_1 = 3$; $r = 3$; $S_5 = \dfrac{3(1-3^5)}{1-3} = 363$. The sum is 363.

29. $a_1 = (48)\left(\dfrac{1}{2}\right) = 24$; $r = \dfrac{1}{2}$; $S_6 = \dfrac{24\left[1-\left(\frac{1}{2}\right)^6\right]}{1-\frac{1}{2}} = \dfrac{189}{4}$. The sum is $\dfrac{189}{4}$.

31. $a_1 = (-2)^4 = 16$; $r = 2$; $n = 10-3 = 7$; $S_7 = \dfrac{16\left(1-(-2)^7\right)}{1-(-2)} = 688$. The sum is 688.

33. $a_1 = -2$; $r = 2$; $S_8 = \dfrac{(-2)\left[1-(2)^8\right]}{1-(2)} = -510$, In this case the index begins at 2 so we will subtract the value of a_1 from the sum. $-510-(-2) = -508$. The sum is -508.

35. $a_1 = 5$; $r = 2$; $S_6 = \dfrac{(5)\left[1-(2)^6\right]}{1-(2)} = 315$. The sum is 315.

37. $a_1 = -1$; $r = \dfrac{1}{2}$; $S_4 = \dfrac{(-1)\left[1-\left(\frac{1}{2}\right)^4\right]}{1-\left(\frac{1}{2}\right)} = \dfrac{-\frac{15}{16}}{\frac{1}{2}} = -\dfrac{15}{8}$, The sum is $-\dfrac{15}{8}$.

39. The sum of the terms of an infinite geometric sequence exists if the absolute value of the common ratio is less than 1.

41. $a_1 = 0.8$, $r = 0.1 \Rightarrow S_\infty = \dfrac{0.8}{1-0.1} = \dfrac{8}{9}$. The sum of the geometric series is $\dfrac{8}{9}$.

43. $a_1 = 0.45$, $r = 0.01 \Rightarrow S_\infty = \dfrac{0.45}{1-0.01} = \dfrac{5}{11}$. The sum of the geometric series is $\dfrac{5}{11}$.

45. $a_1 = 0.378$, $r = 0.001 \Rightarrow S_\infty = \dfrac{0.378}{1-0.001} = \dfrac{14}{37}$. The sum of the geometric series is $\dfrac{14}{37}$.

47. $r = \dfrac{24}{12} = \dfrac{48}{24} = \dfrac{96}{48} = 2$; $|r| > 1 \Rightarrow$ the sum will not converge. Because the common ratio, 2, is greater than 1, the sum of the terms of the geometric sequence does not converge.

49. $r = \dfrac{-24}{-48} = \dfrac{-12}{-24} = \dfrac{-6}{-12} = \dfrac{1}{2}; |r| < 1 \Rightarrow$ the sum would converge. The common ratio is $\dfrac{1}{2}$ and the sum of

the terms of the geometric sequence would converge.

51. $r = \dfrac{2}{16} = \dfrac{\frac{1}{4}}{2} = \dfrac{\frac{1}{32}}{\frac{1}{4}} = \dfrac{1}{8}; S_\infty = \dfrac{16}{1-\frac{1}{8}} = \dfrac{128}{7}$. The sum is $\dfrac{128}{7}$.

53. $r = \dfrac{10}{100} = \dfrac{1}{10}; S_\infty = \dfrac{100}{1-\frac{1}{10}} = \dfrac{1000}{9}$. The sum is $\dfrac{1000}{9}$.

55. $r = \dfrac{\frac{2}{3}}{\frac{4}{3}} = \dfrac{\frac{1}{3}}{\frac{2}{3}} = \dfrac{1}{2}; S_\infty = \dfrac{\frac{4}{3}}{1-\frac{1}{2}} = \dfrac{8}{3}$. The sum is $\dfrac{8}{3}$.

57. $a_1 = 3, r = \dfrac{1}{4} \Rightarrow S_\infty = \dfrac{3}{1-\frac{1}{4}} = 4$. The sum is 4.

59. $a_1 = 0.3, r = 0.3 \Rightarrow S_\infty = \dfrac{0.3}{1-0.3} = \dfrac{3}{7}$. The sum is $\dfrac{3}{7}$.

61. Since $5^{-k} = \left(\dfrac{1}{5}\right)^k$ we have $a_1 = \dfrac{1}{5}, r = \dfrac{1}{5} \Rightarrow S_\infty = \dfrac{\frac{1}{5}}{1-\frac{1}{5}} = \dfrac{1}{4}$. The sum is $\dfrac{1}{4}$.

63. $a_1 = \dfrac{1}{5}, r = -\dfrac{1}{2} \Rightarrow S_\infty = \dfrac{\frac{1}{5}}{1-\left(-\frac{1}{2}\right)} = \dfrac{2}{15}$. The sum is $\dfrac{2}{15}$.

65. See Figure 65. Rounded to the nearest thousandth, the sum is -97.739.

67. See Figure 67. Rounded to the nearest thousandth, the sum is 0.212.

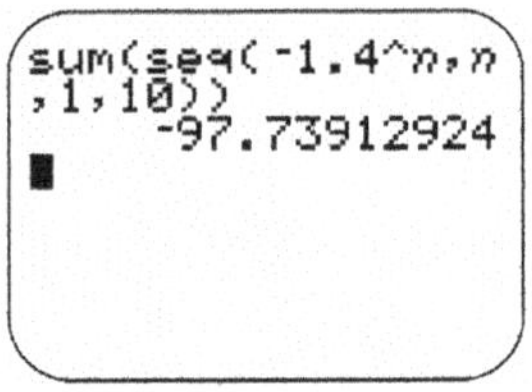

```
sum(seq(-1.4^n,n
,1,10))
       -97.73912924
■
```

```
sum(seq(2(.4)^n,
n,3,8))
        .21245952
```

Figure 65 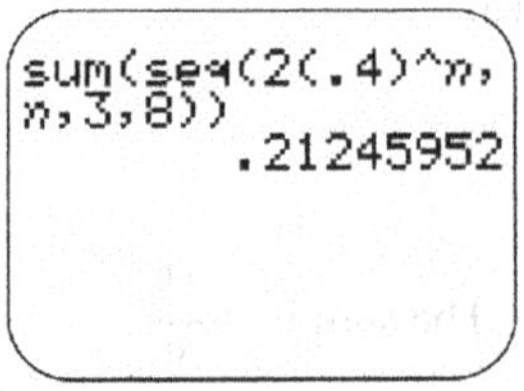   Figure 67

69. $S = 1000\left[\dfrac{(1+0.04)^9 - 1}{0.04}\right] \approx 10{,}582.80$. Rounded to the nearest penny, the future value of the annuity is

$\$10{,}582.80$.

71. $S = 2430\left[\dfrac{(1+0.025)^{10}}{0.025}\right] \approx 27{,}244.22$. Rounded to the nearest penny, the future value of the annuity is

$\$27{,}224.22$.

73. (a) $a_1 = 1276(0.916)^1 \approx 1169; r = 0.916$. Rounded to the nearest whole number, the first term of the sequence is 1169. The common ratio is 0.916.

(b) $a_{10} = 1276(0.916)^{10} \approx 531; a_{20} = 1276(0.916)^{20} \approx 221$. Rounded to the nearest whole number, the tenth term of the sequence is 531 and the twentieth term of the sequence is 221. This means that a person 10 years from retirement should have saved 531% of his or her annual income and a person 20 years from retirement should have saved 221% of his or her annual income.

75. (a) $a_2 = 2a_1; a_3 = 2a_2 = 4a_1; \ldots a_n = a_1(20)^{n-1}$. The nth term of the geometric series is $a_1(2)^{n-1}$.

(b) $a_1 = 100; a_n > 1,000,000 \Rightarrow (2)^{n-1} > 10,000 \Rightarrow n-1 > \dfrac{4}{\log(2)} \Rightarrow n > 14.25 = 15$.

(c) $n = 4$ time $= (15-1)40$ minutes $= 560$ minutes $= 9$ hours 20 minutes. After 9 hours and 20 minutes, the number of bacteria will exceed one million.

77. $a_1 = 0.8, r = 0.8 \Rightarrow a_9 = (0.8)(0.8)^{9-1} \approx 0.134 = 13.4\%$. After nine drainings and replacements with water, the strength of the mixture will be approximately 13.4%.

79. $a_1 = (100,000)(1-0.2) = 80,000; r = 0.8 \Rightarrow a_6 = 80,000(0.8)^{6-1} = 26,214.40\ldots$ The value of the machine at the end of six years will be $26,214.40.

81. $a_1 = 100, r = 1.5 \Rightarrow a_n = 100(1.5)^{n-1}; a_4 = 100(1.5)^{4-1} = 337.5$ In the fourth generation there will be about 338 flies.

83. $a_1 = 40, r = 0.8 \Rightarrow S_\infty = \dfrac{40}{1-0.8} = 200$. The total length of arc through which the pendulum will swing is 200 centimeters.

85. $a_1 = 2, r = 2 \Rightarrow S_5 = \dfrac{2(1-2^5)}{1-2} = 62; S_{10} = \dfrac{2(1-2^{10})}{1-2} = 2046$. Going back 5 generations, a person has 62 ancestors and going back 10 generations, a person has 2046 ancestors

87. Option 1: Arithmetic sequences with $a_1 = 5000$ and $d = 10,000 \Rightarrow$

$S_{30} = \dfrac{30}{2}[2(5000) + (30-1)(10,000)] = 4,500,000$.

Option 2: Geometric sequences with $a_1 = 0.01$ and $r = 2 \Rightarrow S_{30} = \dfrac{0.01(1-2^{30})}{1-2} = 10,737,418.23$.

Option 1 pays a total of $4,500,000 while Option 2 pays a total of $10,737,418.23. Choose Option 2.

89. $a_1 = 2, r = \dfrac{1}{2} \Rightarrow a_8 = 2\left(\dfrac{1}{2}\right)^{8-1} = \dfrac{1}{64}$. The eighth such triangle will have sides of length $\dfrac{1}{64}$.

Reviewing Basic Concepts (Sections 11.1—11.3)

1. $a_1 = (-1)^{1-1}(4 \cdot 1) = 4; a_2 = (-1)^{2-1}(4 \cdot 2) = -8; a_3 = (-1)^{3-1}(4 \cdot 3) = 12; a_4 = (-1)^{4-1}(4 \cdot 4);$

$a_5 = (-1)^{5-1}(4 \cdot 5) = 20$. The first five terms of the sequence are $4, -8, 12, -16, 20$.

2. $a_1 = 3 \cdot 1 + 1 = 4$; $a_5 = 3 \cdot 5 + 1 = 16$; $s_5 = \frac{5}{2}(4+16) = 50$. The series sum is 50.

3. From Figure 3, it can be seen that as n increases, the terms of the sequence converge to 1.

[0,11] by [-2,2]
Xscl = 1   Yscl = 1

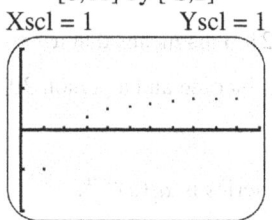

Figure 3

4. $a_1 = 8, d = -2 \Rightarrow a_2 = 8 - 2 = -6, a_3 = 6 - 2 = 4, a_4 = 4 - 2 = 2, a_5 = 2 - 2 = 0$. The first five terms of the sequence are 8, 6, 4, 2, 0.

5. $a_5 = 5, a_8 = 17 \Rightarrow 3d = 17 - 5 \Rightarrow d = 4 \Rightarrow a_1 = 5 - 4 \cdot 4 = -11$. The first term of the sequence is -11.

6. $a_{10} = 2 + 5(10-1) = 47$; $S_{10} = \frac{10}{2}(2+47) = 245$. The sum of the first ten terms of the sequence is 245.

7. $a_3 = (-2)(-3)^{3-1} = -18$; $a_n = (-2)(-3)^{n-1}$. The third term of the sequence is -18 and the nth term of the sequence is $(-2)(-3)^{n-1}$.

8. $r = \frac{3}{5} = \frac{\frac{9}{5}}{3} = \frac{3}{5}$; $\frac{244}{625} = 5\left(\frac{3}{5}\right)^{n-1} \Rightarrow \left(\frac{3}{5}\right)^{n-1} = \frac{243}{3125} \Rightarrow n - 1 = 5 \Rightarrow n = 6$.

$S_6 = \frac{5\left[1-\left(\frac{3}{5}\right)^6\right]}{1-\frac{3}{5}} = \frac{7448}{625}$. The series is geometric with common ratio $\frac{3}{5}$. The series sum is $\frac{7448}{625}$.

9. $a_1 = 3\left(\frac{2}{3}\right) = 2$. $S_\infty = \frac{2}{1-\frac{2}{3}} = 6$. The series sum is 6.

10. $S = 500\left[\frac{(1+0.035)^{13}-1}{0.035}\right] \approx 8056.52$. Rounded to the nearest penny, the future value of the annuity is $8,056.52.

11.4: Counting Theory

1. $4! = 4 \cdot 3 \cdot 2 \cdot 1 = 24$

3. $(4-2)! = 2! = 2 \cdot 1 = 2$

5. $\frac{6!}{5!} = \frac{6 \cdot 5 \cdot 4 \cdot 3 \cdot 2 \cdot 1}{5 \cdot 4 \cdot 3 \cdot 2 \cdot 1} = 6$

7. $\frac{8!}{6!} = \frac{8 \cdot 7 \cdot 6 \cdot 5 \cdot 4 \cdot 3 \cdot 2 \cdot 1}{6 \cdot 5 \cdot 4 \cdot 3 \cdot 2 \cdot 1} = 8 \cdot 7 = 56$

9. $3! \cdot 4 = 3 \cdot 2 \cdot 1 \cdot (4) = 24$

11. Divide the common factor $6 \cdot 5 \cdot 4 \cdot 3 \cdot 2 \cdot 1$ from both the numerator and denominator to begin. Then multiply the factors 7 and 8 which remain in the denominator to obtain 56.

13. $P(7,7) = \dfrac{7!}{(7-7)!} = \dfrac{7!}{0!} = 7 \cdot 6 \cdot 5 \cdot 4 \cdot 3 \cdot 2 \cdot 1 = 5040$. The value of $P(7,7)$ is 50,400

15. $P(9,2) = \dfrac{9!}{(9-2)!} = \dfrac{9!}{7!} = 9 \cdot 8 = 72$. The value of $P(9,2)$ is 72.

17. $P(5,1) = \dfrac{5!}{(5-1)!} = \dfrac{5!}{4!} = 5$. The value of $P(5,4)$ is 5.

19. $C(4,2) = \dfrac{4!}{(4-2)!2!} = \dfrac{4!}{2!2!} = \dfrac{4 \cdot 3}{2 \cdot 1} = 6$. The value of $C(4,2)$ is 6.

21. $C(6,0) = \dfrac{6!}{(6-0)!0!} = \dfrac{6!}{6!} = 1$. The value of $C(6,0)$ is 1.

23. $C(12,4) = \dfrac{12!}{(12-4)!4!} = \dfrac{12!}{8!4!} = \dfrac{12 \cdot 11 \cdot 10 \cdot 9}{4 \cdot 3 \cdot 2 \cdot 1} = 495$. The value of $C(12,4)$ is 495.

25. $_{20}P_5 = 20\ _nP_r\ 5 = 1,860,480$ The value of $_{20}P_5$ is $1,860,480$

27. $_{15}P_8 = 15\ _nP_r\ 8 = 259,459,200$. The value of $_{15}P_8$ is $259,459,200$.

29. $_{20}C_5 = 20\ _nC_r\ 5 = 15,504$. The value of $_{20}C_5$ is $15,504$.

31. $_{15}C_8 = 15\ _nC_r\ 8 = 6435$. The value of $_{15}C_8$ is 6435.

33. (a) A telephone number involves a permutation of digits because order matters.

　　(b) A social security number involves a permutation of digits because order matters.

　　(c) A hand of cards in poker involves a combination of cards because order does not matter.

　　(d) A committee of politicians involves a combination of persons because order does not matter.

　　(e) The "combination" on a combination lock involves a permutation of numbers because order matters.

　　(f) A lottery choice of six numbers where the order does not matter involves a combination of numbers.

　　(g) An automobile license plate involves a permutation of characters because order matters.

35. $5 \times 3 \times 2 = 30$. 30 different types of homes are available.

37. (a) $2 \times 25 \times 24 \times 23 = 27,600$. 27,600 radio station calls can be made.

　　(b) $2 \times 26 \times 26 \times 26 = 35,152$. 35,152 radio station calls can be made.

　　(c) $2 \times 24 \times 24 \times 1 = 1104$. 1104 radio station calls can be made.

39. $3 \times 5 = 15$. 15 first and middle name combinations are possible.

41. (a) $26 \times 26 \times 26 \times 10 \times 10 \times 10 = 17,576,000$. 17,576,000 different license plates are possible.

　　(b) $10 \times 10 \times 10 \times 26 \times 26 \times 26 = 17,576,000$. 17,576,000 additional plates are possible.

　　(c) $26 \times 10 \times 10 \times 10 \times 26 \times 26 \times 26 = 456,976,000$. The new scheme provides 456,976,000 plates.

43. $_6P_6 = 720$. 720 arrangements of the people are possible.

45. $_6P_3 = 120$. 120 course schedules are possible.

47. $_{15}P_3 = 2730$. 2730 slates of 3 officers are possible.

49. $_5P_5 = 120$; $_{10}P_5 = 30,240$. With 5 players, 120 assignments are possible and with 10 players, 30,240 assignments are possible.

51. $_{30}P_4 = 27,405$. 27,405 different groups are possible.

53. $_6C_3 = 20$. 20 different garnished hamburgers are possible.

55. $_{15}C_2 = 105$; $_{15}C_4 = 1365$. 105 samples of 2 may be drawn and 1365 samples of 4 may be drawn.

57. $_8C_2 = 28$. 28 samples of 2 may be drawn where both marbles are blue.

59. (a) $_9C_3 = 84$. 84 delegations are possible.

   (b) $_5C_3 = 10$. 10 delegations could have all liberals.

   (c) $(_5C_2)(_4C_1) = (10)(4) = 40$. 40 delegations could have 2 liberals and 1 conservative.

   (d) $_8C_2 = 28$. 28 delegations are possible that include the mayor.

61. $_8P_4 = 1680$. 1680 course schedules are possible.

63. $_6C_4 = 15$. 15 different soups can be made.

65. $_{12}P_{11} = 479,001,600$. 479,001,600 different seatings are possible.

67. (a) $_8C_5 = 56$. 56 committees of all men may be chosen.

   (b) $_{11}C_5 = 462$. 462 committees of all women may be chosen.

   (c) $(_8C_3)(_{11}C_2) = (56)(55) = 3080$. 3080 committees of 3 men and 2 women may be chosen.

   (d) $(_8C_5)(_{11}C_0) + (_8C_4)(_{11}C_1) + (_8C_3)(_{11}C_2) + (_8C_2)(_{11}C_3) =$
   $(56)(1) + (70)(11) + (56)(55) + (28)(165) = 8526$. 8526 committees with no more than 3 women are possible.

69. $2^{12} = 4096$. 4096 codes are possible.

71. $(10 \times 10 \times 10)(10 \times 10 \times 10) = 1,000,000$. 1,000,000 different combinations are possible.

73. Circular ring $\Rightarrow$ 1 key to start; then, $_3P_3 = 6$ ways to add the remaining 3. The keys can be put on in 6 distinguishable ways.

75. $P(n, n-1) = \dfrac{n!}{[n-(n-1)]!} = \dfrac{n!}{1!} = n!$; $P(n,n) = \dfrac{n!}{(n-n)!} = \dfrac{n!}{0!} = n!$. Thus, $P(n, n-1) = P(n,n)$.

77. $P(n,0) = \dfrac{n!}{(n-0)!} = \dfrac{n!}{n!} = 1$. Thus, $P(n,0) = 1$.

79. $C(n,0) = \dfrac{n!}{(n-0)!0!} = \dfrac{n!}{n!} = 1$. Thus, $C(n,0) = 1$.

81. $C(n, n-1) = \dfrac{n!}{[n-(n-1)]!(n-1)!} = \dfrac{n!}{1!(n-1)!} = \dfrac{n(n-1)!}{(n-1)!} = n.$ Thus, $C(n, n-1) = n.$

11.5: The Binomial Theorem

1. $\dfrac{6!}{3!3!} = \dfrac{6 \cdot 5 \cdot 4 \cdot 3 \cdot 2 \cdot 1}{3 \cdot 2 \cdot 1 \cdot 3 \cdot 2 \cdot 1} = 20$ The expression is equal to 20.

3. $\dfrac{7!}{3!4!} = \dfrac{7 \cdot 6 \cdot 5 \cdot 4 \cdot 3 \cdot 2 \cdot 1}{3 \cdot 2 \cdot 1 \cdot 4 \cdot 3 \cdot 2 \cdot 1} = 35.$ The expression is equal to 35.

5. $\binom{8}{3} = C(8,3) = \dfrac{8!}{(8-3)!3!} = \dfrac{8!}{5!3!} = 56$ The expression is equal to 56.

7. $\binom{10}{8} = C(10,8) = \dfrac{10!}{(10-8)!10!} = \dfrac{10!}{2!10!} = 45.$ The expression is equal to 45.

9. $\binom{13}{13} = C(13,13) = \dfrac{13!}{(13-13)!13!} = \dfrac{13!}{13!} = 1.$ The expression is equal to 1. 11.

$\binom{8}{3} = C(8,3) = \dfrac{8!}{(8-3)!3!} = \dfrac{8!}{5!3!} = 56.$ The expression is equal to 56.

13. $\binom{100}{2} = C(100,2) = \dfrac{100!}{(100-2)!2!} = \dfrac{100!}{98!2!} = 4950.$ The expression is equal to 4950.

15. $\binom{5}{0} = C(5,0) = \dfrac{5!}{(5-0)!0!} = \dfrac{5!}{5!} = 1.$ The expression is equal to 1.

17. $\binom{n}{n-1} = \dfrac{n!}{(n-1)!(n-(n-1))!} = \dfrac{n!}{(n-1)!(1)!} = \dfrac{n(n-1)!}{(n-1)!} = n.$ The expression is equal to n.

19. The expansion of $(x+y)^8$ has a term where x is raised to each of the following powers: 8, 7, 6, 5, 4, 3, 2, 1, and 0. Thus, there are 9 terms.

21. $(2x)^4 = 16x^4 ; (3y)^4 = 81y^4.$ In the expansion of $(2x)^4$, $16x^4$ is the first term and $81y^4$ is the last term.

23. The binomial expansion for $(x+y)^6$ is given by:

$(x+y)^6 = \binom{6}{0}x^6 + \binom{6}{1}x^5 y + \binom{6}{2}x^4 y^2 + \binom{6}{3}x^3 y^3 + \binom{6}{4}x^2 y^4 + \binom{6}{5}xy^5 + \binom{6}{6}y^6 =$

$x^6 + 6x^5 y + 15x^4 y^2 + 20x^3 y^3 + 15x^2 y^4 + 6xy^5 + y^6.$

25. The binomial expansion for $(p-q)^5$ is given by:

$(p-q)^5 = \binom{5}{0}p^5 + \binom{5}{1}p^4(-q) + \binom{5}{2}p^3(-q)^2 + \binom{5}{3}p^2(-q)^3 + \binom{5}{4}p(-q)^4 + \binom{5}{5}(-q)^5 =$

$p^5 - 5p^4 q + 10p^3 q^2 - 10p^2 q^3 + 5pq^4 - q^5.$

27. The binomial expansion for $(r^2+s)^5$ is given by:

$$(r^2+s)^5 = \binom{5}{0}(r^2)^5 + \binom{5}{1}(r^2)^4 s + \binom{5}{2}(r^2)^3 s^2 + \binom{5}{3}(r^2)^2 s^3 + \binom{5}{4}(r^2)s^4 + \binom{5}{5}s^5 =$$

$$r^{10} + 5r^8 s + 10r^6 s^2 + 10r^4 s^3 + 5r^2 s^4 + s^5.$$

29. The binomial expansion for $(p+2q)^4$ is given by:

$$(p+2q)^4 = \binom{4}{0}p^4 + \binom{4}{1}p^3(2q) + \binom{4}{2}p^2(2q)^2 + \binom{4}{3}p(2q)^3 + \binom{4}{4}(2q)^4 =$$

$$p^4 + 8p^3 q + 24p^2 q^2 + 32pq^3 + 16q^4.$$

31. The binomial expansion for $(7p+2q)^4$ is given by:

$$(7p+2q)^4 = \binom{4}{0}(7p)^4 + \binom{4}{1}(7p)^3(2q) + \binom{4}{2}(7p)^2(2q)^2 + \binom{4}{3}(7p)(2q)^3 + \binom{4}{4}(2q)^4 =$$

$$2401p^4 + 2744p^3 q + 1176p^2 q^2 + 224pq^3 + 16q^4.$$

33. The binomial expansion for $(3x-2y)^6$ is given by:

$$(3x-2y)^6 = \binom{6}{0}(3x)^6 + \binom{6}{1}(3x)^5(-2y) + \binom{6}{2}(3x)^4(-2y)^2 + \binom{6}{3}(3x)^3(-2y)^3 + \binom{6}{4}(3x)^2(-2y)^4 +$$

$$\binom{6}{5}(3x)(-2y)^5 + \binom{6}{6}(-2y)^6 = 729x^6 - 2916x^5 y + 4860x^4 y^2 - 4320x^3 y^3 + 2160x^2 y^4 - 576xy^5 + 64y^6.$$

35. The binomial expansion for $\left(\dfrac{m}{2}-1\right)^6$ is given by:

$$\left(\dfrac{m}{2}-1\right)^6 = \binom{6}{0}\left(\dfrac{m}{2}\right)^6 + \binom{6}{1}\left(\dfrac{m}{2}\right)^5(-1) + \binom{6}{2}\left(\dfrac{m}{2}\right)^4(-1)^2 + \binom{6}{3}\left(\dfrac{m}{2}\right)^3(-1)^3 + \binom{6}{4}\left(\dfrac{m}{2}\right)^2(-1)^4 +$$

$$\binom{6}{5}\left(\dfrac{m}{2}\right)(-1)^5 + \binom{6}{6}(-1)^6 = \dfrac{m^6}{64} - \dfrac{3m^5}{16} + \dfrac{15m^4}{16} - \dfrac{5m^3}{2} + \dfrac{15m^2}{4} - 3m + 1.$$

37. The binomial expansion for $\left(\sqrt{2}r + \dfrac{1}{m}\right)^4$ is given by:

$$\left(\sqrt{2}r + \dfrac{1}{m}\right)^4 = \binom{4}{0}(\sqrt{2}r)^4 + \binom{4}{1}(\sqrt{2}r)^3\left(\dfrac{1}{m}\right) + \binom{4}{2}(\sqrt{2}r)^2\left(\dfrac{1}{m}\right)^2 + \binom{4}{3}(\sqrt{2}r)\left(\dfrac{1}{m}\right)^3 + \binom{4}{4}\left(\dfrac{1}{m}\right)^4 =$$

$$4r^4 + \dfrac{8\sqrt{2}r^3}{m} + \dfrac{4\sqrt{2}r^2}{m^2} + \dfrac{4\sqrt{2}r}{m^3} + \dfrac{1}{m^4}.$$

39. $\binom{8}{5}(4h)^3(-j)^5 = -3584h^3 j^5$ The sixth term of the binomial expansion of $(4h-j)^8$ is $-3584n^3 j^5$.

41. $\binom{22}{14}(a^2)(b^{14}) = 319,770a^{16}b^{14}$ The fifteenth term of the binomial expansion of $(a^2+b)^{22}$ is

    $319,770a^{16}b^{14}$.

43. $\binom{20}{14}(x)^6(-y^3)^{14} = 38,760x^6y^{42}$ The fifteenth term of the binomial expansion of $(x-y^3)^{20}$ is

    $38,760x^6y^{42}$.

45. $\binom{8}{4}(3x^7)(2y^3)^4 = 90,720x^{28}y^{12}$ The middle term of the binomial expansion of $(3x^7+2y^3)^8$ is the fifth

    term which is $90,720x^{28}y^{12}$.

47. $n-4=7$ and $n-7=4 \Rightarrow n=11$. The coefficients of the fifth and eighth terms in the expansion of

    $(x+y)^n$ are the same for n=11.

49. $10! = 3,628,800$; $\sqrt{2\pi(10)}(10^{10})(e^{-10}) \approx 3,598,695.619$. The exact value of 10! is 3,628,800 and the

    Stirling's formula approximation of 10! is about 3,598,695.619.

50. $\dfrac{3,628,800 - 3,598,695.619}{3,628,800} \approx 0.00830 = 0.830\%$. The percentage error in the Stirling's formula

    approximation of 10! is about 0.830%.

51. $12! = 479,001,600$; $\sqrt{2\pi(12)}(12^{12})(e^{-12}) \approx 475,687,486.5$;

    $\dfrac{479,001,600 - 475,687,486.5}{479,001,600} \approx 0.00692 = 0.692\%$. The exact value of 12! is 479,001,600 and the

    Stirling's formula approximation of 12! is about 475,687,486.5 which has a percent error of about 0.692%.

52. $13! = 6,227,020,800$; $\sqrt{2\pi(13)}(13^{13})(e^{-13}) \approx 6,187,239,475$;

    $\dfrac{6,227,020,800 - 6,187,239,475}{6,227,020,800} \approx 0.00639 = 0.639\%$. The exact value of 13! Is 6,227,020,800 and the

    Stirling's formula approximation of 13! is about 6,187,239,475 which has a percent error of about 0.639%.
    Based on this series of exercises, it appears that the percent error in the Stirling's formula approximation of
    n! decreases as n increases.

53. $(1.02)^{-3} = (1+0.02)^{-3} \approx 1 + (-3)(0.02) + \dfrac{(-3)(-3-1)}{2!}(0.02)^2 +$

    $\dfrac{(-3)(-3-1)(-3-2)}{3!}(0.02)^3 \approx 0.942$. To the nearest thousandth, $(1.02)^{-3}$ is 0.942.

55. $(1.01)^{3/2} = (1+0.01)^{3/2} \approx 1 + \left(\frac{3}{2}\right)(0.01) + \frac{\left(\frac{3}{2}\right)\left(\frac{3}{2}-1\right)}{2!}(0.01)^2 + \frac{\left(\frac{3}{2}\right)\left(\frac{3}{2}-2\right)}{3!}(0.01)^3 \approx 1.015$. To the nearest thousandth, $(1.01)^{3/2}$ is 1.015.

Reviewing Basic Concepts (Sections 11.4 and 11.5)

1. $4! = 24$. There are 24 different arrangements.

2. $P(7,3) = \frac{7!}{(7-3)!} = \frac{7!}{4!} = 210$.

3. $C(10,4) = \frac{10!}{(10-4)!4!} = \frac{10!}{6!4!} = 210$

4. $_6C_2 \cdot _5C_2 \cdot _3C_1 = 450$. There are 450 different arrangements for this basketball team.

5. $9 \cdot 4 \cdot 2 = 72$. There are 72 different homes available.

6. To expand $(x+y)^n$ use row $n+1$ of Pascal's Triangle.

7. Given $(a+2b)^4$. We will let $x = a$ and $y = 2b$ in the binomial theorem. Using the 5th row of Pascal's Triangle we find the coefficients 1,4,6,4,1
$\Rightarrow (a+2b)^4 = (a)^4 + 4(a)^3(2b) + 6(a)^2(2b)^2 + 4(a)(2b)^3 + (2b)^4$

8. $\binom{6}{2}(x)^4(-2y)^2 = 60x^4y^2$. The third term of the binomial $(x-2y)^6$ is $60x^4y^2$.

11.6: Mathematical Induction

1. The domain of the variable must be all positive integers (natural numbers).

3. Since $2^1 = 2(1)$ and $2^2 = 2(2)$, the statement is not true for $n = 1$ and $n = 2$.

5. $3+6+9+\cdots+3n = \frac{3n(n+1)}{2}$

   (i) Show that the statement is true for $n = 1$: $3(1) = \frac{3(1)(2)}{2} \Rightarrow 3 = 3$.

   (ii) Assume that S_k is true: $3+6+9+\cdots+3k = \frac{3k(k+1)}{2}$. Show that S_{k+1} is true: $3+6+\cdots+3(k+1) = \frac{3(k+1)(k+2)}{2}$. Add $3(k+1)$ to each side of

   S_k: $3+6+9+\cdots+3k+3(k+1) = \frac{3k(k+1)}{2}+3(k+1) = \frac{3k(k+1)+6(k+1)}{2} = \frac{(k+1)(3k+6)}{2} = \frac{3(k+1)(k+2)}{2}$.

Since S_k implies S_{k+1}, the statement is true for every positive integer n.

7. $5+10+15+\cdots+5n = \dfrac{5n(n+1)}{2}$

    (i) Show that the statement is true for $n=1$: $5(1) = \dfrac{5(1)(2)}{2} \Rightarrow 5 = 5$.

    (ii) Assume that S_k is true: $5+10+15+\cdots+5k = \dfrac{5k(k+1)}{2}$. Show that S_{k+1} is true:

    $5+10+\cdots+5(k+1) = \dfrac{5(k+1)(k+2)}{2}$. Add $5(k+1)$ to each side of S_k:

    $5+10+15+\cdots+5k+5(k+1) = \dfrac{5k(k+1)}{2}+5(k+1) =$

    $\dfrac{5k(k+1)+10(k+1)}{2} = \dfrac{(k+1)(5k+10)}{2} = \dfrac{5(k+1)(k+2)}{2}$.

    Since S_k implies S_{k+1}, the statement is true for every positive integer n.

9. $3+3^2+3^3+\cdots+3^n = \dfrac{3(3^n-1)}{2}$

    (i) Show that the statement is true for $n=1$: $3^1 = \dfrac{3(3^1-1)}{2} \Rightarrow 3 = 3$.

    (ii) Assume that S_k is true: $3+3^2+3^3+\cdots+3^k = \dfrac{3(3^k-1)}{2}$. Show that S_{k+1} is true:

    $3+3^2+3^3+\cdots+3^{k+1} = \dfrac{3(3^{k+1}-1)}{2}$ Add 3^{k+1} to each side of S_k:

    $3+3^2+3^3+\cdots 3^k + 3^{k+1} = \dfrac{3(3^k-1)}{2} + 3^{k+1} = \dfrac{3(3^k-1)+2(3^{k+1})}{2} =$

    $\dfrac{3^{k+1}-3+2(3^{k+1})}{2} = \dfrac{3(3^{k+1})-3}{2} = \dfrac{3(3^{k+1}-1)}{2}$

    Since S_k implies S_{k+1}, the statement is true for every positive integer n.

11. $1^3+2^3+3^3+\cdots+n^3 = \dfrac{n^2(n+1)^2}{4}$

    (i) Show that the statement is true for $n=1$: $1^3 = \dfrac{1^2(1+1)^2}{4} \Rightarrow 1 = 1$.

    (ii) Assume that S_k is true: $1^3+2^3+3^3+\cdots+k^3 = \dfrac{k^2(k+1)^2}{4}$. Show that S_{k+1} is true:

    $1^3+2^3+3^3+\cdots+(k+1)^3 = \dfrac{(k+1)^2(k+2)^2}{4}$. Add $(k+1)^3$ to each side of

S_k: $1^3 + 2^3 + 3^3 + \cdots + k^3 + (k+1)^3 = \dfrac{k^2(k+1)^2}{4} + (k+1)^3 =$

$\dfrac{k^2(k+1)^2 + 4(k+1)^3}{4} = \dfrac{(k+1)^2(k^2+4k+4)}{4} = \dfrac{(k+1)^2(k+2)^2}{4}$

Since S_k implies S_{k+1}, the statement is true for every positive integer n.

13. $\dfrac{1}{1\cdot 2} + \dfrac{1}{2\cdot 3} + \cdots + \dfrac{1}{n(n+1)} = \dfrac{n}{n+1}$

   (i) Show that the statement is true for $n = 1$: $\dfrac{1}{1(1+1)} = \dfrac{1}{1+1} \Rightarrow \dfrac{1}{2} = \dfrac{1}{2}$.

   (ii) Assume that S_k is true: $\dfrac{1}{1\cdot 2} + \dfrac{1}{2\cdot 3} + \cdots + \dfrac{1}{k(k+1)} = \dfrac{k}{k+1}$. Show that S_{k+1} is true:

   $\dfrac{1}{1\cdot 2} + \dfrac{1}{2\cdot 3} + \cdots + \dfrac{1}{(k+1)(k+2)} = \dfrac{k+1}{k+2}$. Add $\dfrac{1}{(k+1)(k+2)}$ to each side of

   S_k: $\dfrac{1}{1\cdot 2} + \dfrac{1}{2\cdot 3} + \cdots + \dfrac{1}{(k+1)(k+2)} = \dfrac{k}{k+1} + \dfrac{1}{(k+1)(k+2)} =$

   $\dfrac{k(k+2)+1}{(k+1)(k+2)} = \dfrac{k^2+2k+1}{(k+1)(k+2)} = \dfrac{(k+1)(k+1)}{(k+1)(k+2)} = \dfrac{k+1}{(k+2)}$.

   Since S_k implies S_{k+1}, the statement is true for every positive integer n.

15. $\dfrac{4}{5} + \dfrac{4}{5^2} + \dfrac{4}{5^3} + \cdots + \dfrac{4}{5^n} = 1 - \dfrac{1}{5^n}$

   (i) Show that the statement is true for $n = 1$: $\dfrac{4}{5^1} = 1 - \dfrac{1}{5^1} \Rightarrow \dfrac{4}{5} = \dfrac{4}{5}$.

   (ii) Assume that S_k is true: $\dfrac{4}{5} + \dfrac{4}{5^2} + \dfrac{4}{5^3} + \cdots + \dfrac{4}{5^k} = 1 - \dfrac{1}{5^k}$.

   Show that S_{k+1} is true: $\dfrac{4}{5} + \dfrac{4}{5^2} + \cdots + \dfrac{4}{5^{k+1}} = 1 - \dfrac{1}{5^{k+1}}$. Add $\dfrac{4}{5^{k+1}}$ to each side of S_k:

   $\dfrac{4}{5} + \dfrac{4}{5^2} + \dfrac{4}{5^3} + \cdots + \dfrac{4}{5^k} + \dfrac{4}{5^{k+1}} = 1 - \dfrac{1}{5^k} + \dfrac{4}{5^{k+1}} = 1 - \dfrac{1}{5^k} \cdot \dfrac{5}{5} + \dfrac{4}{5^{k+1}} = 1 - \dfrac{5}{5^{k+1}} + \dfrac{4}{5^{k+1}} = 1 - \dfrac{1}{5^{k+1}}$.

   Since S_k implies S_{k+1}, the statement is true for every positive integer n.

17. $\dfrac{1}{1\cdot 4} + \dfrac{1}{4\cdot 7} + \cdots + \dfrac{1}{(3n-2)(3n+1)} = \dfrac{n}{3n+1}$

   (i) Show that the statement is true for $n = 1$: $\dfrac{1}{1\cdot 4} = \dfrac{1}{3(1)+1} \Rightarrow \dfrac{1}{4} = \dfrac{1}{4}$.

   (ii) Assume that S_k is true: $\dfrac{1}{1\cdot 4} + \cdots + \dfrac{1}{(3k-2)(3k+1)} = \dfrac{k}{3k+1}$.

Show that S_{k+1} is true: $\dfrac{1}{1\cdot 4}+\cdots+\dfrac{1}{[3(k+1)-2][3(k+1)+1]}=\dfrac{k+1}{3(k+1)+1}$. Add

$\dfrac{1}{[3(k+1)-2][3(k+1)+1]}$ to each side of S_k: $\dfrac{1}{1\cdot 4}+\cdots+\dfrac{1}{[3(k+1)-2][3(k+1)+1]}=$

$\dfrac{k}{3k+1}+\dfrac{1}{[3(k+1)-2][3(k+1)+1]}=\dfrac{k}{3k+1}+\dfrac{1}{(3k+1)(3k+4)}=\dfrac{k(3k+4)+1}{(3k+1)(3k+4)}=$

$\dfrac{3k^2+4k+1}{(3k+1)(3k+4)}=\dfrac{(3k+1)(k+1)}{(3k+1)(3k+4)}=\dfrac{k+1}{3k+4}=\dfrac{k+1}{3(k+1)+1}$.

Since S_k implies S_{k+1}, the statement is true for every positive integer n.

19. When $n=1$, $3^1<6(1)\Rightarrow 3<6$. When $n=2$, $3^2<6(2)\Rightarrow 9<12$. When $n=3$, $3^3>6(3)\Rightarrow 27>18$. For

all $n\geq 3$, $3^n>6n$. The only values are 1 and 2.

21. When $n=1$, $2^1>1^2\Rightarrow 2>1$. When $n=2$, $2^2=2^2\Rightarrow 4=4$. When $n=3$, $2^3<3^2\Rightarrow 8<9$. When

$n=4$, $2^4=4^2\Rightarrow 16=16$. For all $n\geq 5$, $2^n>n^2$. The only values are 2, 3, and 4.

23. $(a^m)^n=a^{mn}$

    (i) Show that the statement is true for $n=1$: $(a^m)^1=a^{m\cdot 1}\Rightarrow a^m=a^m$.

    (ii) Assume that S_k is true: $(a^m)^k=a^{mk}$.

    Show that S_{k+1} is true: $(a^m)^{k+1}=a^{m(k+1)}$.

    Multiply each side of S_k by a^m: $(a^m)^k\cdot(a^m)^1=a^{mk}\cdot a^m\Rightarrow(a^m)^{k+1}=a^{mk+m}\Rightarrow$

    $(a^m)^{k+1}=a^{m(k+1)}$.

Since S_k implies S_{k+1}, the statement is true for every positive integer n.

25. $2^n>2n$, if $n\geq 3$

    (i) Show that the statement is true for $n=3$: $2^3>2(3)\Rightarrow 8>6$.

    (ii) Assume that S_k is true: $2^k>2k$.

Show that S_{k+1} is true: $2^{k+1}>2(k+1)$. Multiply each side of S_k by 2:

$2^k\cdot 2>2k\cdot 2\Rightarrow 2^{k+1}>2(2k)$. Because $2k>k+1$ for all $k>1$, we have $2(2k)>2(k+1)$; therefore,

$2^{k+1}>2(k+1)$.

Since S_k implies S_{k+1}, the statement is true for every positive integer $n\geq 3$.

27. $a^n>1$, if $a>1$

    (i) Show that the statement is true for $n=1$: $a^1>1\Rightarrow a>1$, which is true by the given restriction.

574 CHAPTER 11 Further Topics in Algebra

(ii) Assume that S_k is true: $a^k > 1$. Show that S_{k+1} is true: $a^{k+1} > 1$.

Multiply each side of S_k by a: $a^k \cdot a > 1 \cdot a \Rightarrow a^{k+1} > a$. Because $a > 1$, we may substitute 1 for a in the expression. That is, $a^{k+1} > 1$.

Since S_k implies S_{k+1}, the statement is true for every positive integer n.

29. $a^n < a^{n-1}$, if $0 < a < 1$

(i) Show that the statement is true for $n = 1$: $a^1 < a^0 \Rightarrow a < 1$, which is true by the given restriction.

(ii) Assume that S_k is true: $a^k < a^{k-1}$. Show that S_{k+1} is true: $a^{k+1} < a^k$.

Multiply each side of S_k by a: $a^k \cdot a < a^{k-1} \cdot a \Rightarrow a^{k+1} < a^k$.

Since S_k implies S_{k+1}, the statement is true for every positive integer n.

31. $n! > 2^n$, if $n \geq 4$

(i) Show that the statement is true for $n = 4$: $4! > 2^4 \Rightarrow 24 > 16$.

(ii) Assume that S_k is true: $k! > 2^k$. Show that S_{k+1} is true: $(k+1)! > 2^{k+1}$.

Multiply each side of S_k by $k+1$: $(k+1)k! > 2^k(k+1) \Rightarrow (k+1)! > 2^k(k+1)$.

Because $(k+1) > 2$ for all $k \geq 4$, we may substitute 2 for $(k+1)$ in the expression.

That is, $(k+1)! > 2^k(2)$ or $(k+1)! > 2^{k+1}$.

Since S_k implies S_{k+1}, the statement is true for every positive integer $n \geq 4$.

33. The number of handshakes is $\dfrac{n^2 - n}{2}$ if $n \geq 2$.

(i) Show that the statement is true for $n = 2$. The number of handshakes for 2 people is $\dfrac{2^2 - 2}{2} = \dfrac{2}{2} = 1$, which is true.

(ii) Assume that S_k is true: the number of handshakes for k people is $\dfrac{k^2 - k}{2}$.

Show that S_{k+1} is true: the number of handshakes for $k+1$ people is

$\dfrac{(k+1)^2 - (k+1)}{2} = \dfrac{k^2 + 2k + 1 - k - 1}{2} = \dfrac{k^2 + k}{2}$. When a person joins a group of k people, each person must shake hands with the new person. Since there are a total of k people that will shake hands with the new person, the total number of handshakes for $k+1$ people is

$\dfrac{k^2 - k}{2} + k = \dfrac{k^2 - k + 2k}{2} = \dfrac{k^2 + k}{2}$.

Since S_k implies S_{k+1}, the statement is true for every positive integer $n \geq 2$.

35. The first figure has perimeter $P = 3$. When a new figure is generated, each side of the previous figure increases in length by a factor of $\frac{4}{3}$. Thus, the second figure has perimeter $P = 3\left(\frac{4}{3}\right)$, the third figure has perimeter $P = 3\left(\frac{4}{3}\right)^2$, and so on. In general, the nth figure has perimeter $P = 3\left(\frac{4}{3}\right)^{n-1}$.

37. With 1 ring, 1 move is required. With 2 rings, 3 moves are required. Note that $3 = 2+1$. With 3 rings, 7 moves are required. Note that $7 = 2^2 + 2 + 1$. With n rings, $2^{n-1} + 2^{n-2} + \cdots + 2^1 + 1 = 2^n - 1$ moves are required.

    (i) Show that the statement is true for $n = 1$. The number of moves for 1 ring is $2^1 - 1 = 1$, which is true.

    (ii) Assume that S_k is true: the number of moves for k rings is $2^k - 1$. Show that S_{k+1} is true: the number of moves for $k+1$ rings is $2^{k+1} - 1$. Assume $k+1$ rings are on the first peg. Since S_k is true, the top k rings can be moved to the second peg in $2^k - 1$ moves. Now move the bottom ring to the third peg. Since S_k is true, move the k rings from the second peg on top of the ring on the third peg in $2^k - 1$ moves. The total number of moves is $\left(2^k - 1\right) + 1 + \left(2^k - 1\right) = 2 \cdot 2^k - 1 = 2^{k+1} - 1$.

    Since S_k implies S_{k+1}, the statement is true for every positive integer n.

11.7: Probability

1. Since the coin has a head on each side, the sample space is $S = \{H\}$.

3. Since each of the three coins can be either heads or tails, the sample space is
$$S = \{(H,H,H),(H,H,T),(H,T,H),(H,T,T),(T,H,H),(T,H,T),(T,T,H),(T,T,T)\}.$$

5. On each spin, the spinner may land on 1, 2, or 3. The sample space is
$$S = \{(1,1),(1,2),(1,3),(2,1),(2,2),(2,3),(3,1),(3,2),(3,3)\}.$$

7. (a) The event $E_1 = \{H\}$. The probability of the event, $P(E_1) = 1$.

    (b) The event $E_2 = \emptyset$. The probability of the event, $P(E_2) = 0$.

9. (a) The event $E_1 = \{(1,1),(2,2),(3,3)\}$. The probability of the event, $P(E_1) = \frac{3}{9} = \frac{1}{3}$.

    (b) The event $E_2 = \{(1,1),(1,3),(2,1),(2,3),(3,1)(3,3)\}$. The probability of the event, $P(E_2) = \frac{6}{9} = \frac{2}{3}$.

    (c) The event $E_3 = \{(2,1),(2,3)\}$. The probability of the event, $P(E_3) = \frac{2}{9}$.

11. All probability values must be greater than or equal to 0 and less than or equal to 1. Since $\frac{6}{5} > 1$, it cannot be a probability.

13. (a) The probability of drawing a yellow marble is $P(\text{yellow}) = \frac{3}{15} = \frac{1}{5}$.

    (b) The probability of drawing a black marble is $P(\text{black}) = \frac{0}{15} = 0$.

    (c) The probability of drawing a yellow or white marble is $P(\text{yellow} \cup \text{white}) = \frac{3+4}{15} = \frac{7}{15}$.

    (d) $P(\text{yellow}) = \frac{1}{5}$; $P(\text{not yellow}) = \frac{4}{5}$. The odds in favor of drawing a yellow marble are $\frac{\frac{1}{5}}{\frac{4}{5}} = \frac{1}{4}$ or 1 to 4.

    (e) $P(\text{blue}) = \frac{8}{15}$; $P(\text{not blue}) = \frac{7}{15}$. The odds against drawing a blue marble are $\frac{\frac{7}{15}}{\frac{8}{15}} = \frac{7}{8}$ or 7 to 8.

15. $P(\text{sum is }5) = \frac{2}{10} = \frac{1}{5}$; $P(\text{sum is not }5) = \frac{8}{10} = \frac{4}{5}$. The odds in favor of the sum being 5 are $\frac{\frac{1}{5}}{\frac{4}{5}} = \frac{1}{4}$ or 1 to 4.

17. Odds in favor of candidate are 3 to 2 $\Rightarrow P(\text{lose}) = \frac{2}{3+2} = \frac{2}{5}$. The probability the candidate will lose is $\frac{2}{5}$.

19. (a) The probability of an uncle or brother arriving first is $P(\text{uncle} \cup \text{brother}) = \frac{2+3}{10} = \frac{5}{10} = \frac{1}{2}$.

    (b) The probability of a brother or cousin arriving first is $P(\text{brother} \cup \text{cousin}) = \frac{3+4}{10} = \frac{7}{10}$.

    (c) The probability of a brother or her mother arriving first is $P(\text{brother} \cup \text{mother}) = \frac{3+1}{10} = \frac{4}{10} = \frac{2}{5}$.

21. (a) $P(E) = -0.1$ matches with statement F, the event is impossible, because a probability value cannot be negative.

    (b) $P(E) = 0.01$ matches with statement D, the event is very unlikely to occur, because the probability value is relatively low.

    (c) $P(E) = 1$ matches with statement A, the event is certain to occur.

    (d) $P(E) = 2$ matches with statement F, the probability cannot occur, because a probability value cannot be greater than 1.

    (e) $P(E) = 0.99$ matches with statement C, the event is very likely to occur, because the probability value is relatively high.

(f) $P(E) = 0$ matches with statement B, the event is impossible.

(g) $P(E) = 0.5$ matches with statement E, the event is just as likely to occur as not occur.

23. (a) The probability that a randomly selected patient will need a kidney or a heart transplant is

$P(\text{kidney} \cup \text{heart}) = \dfrac{35,025 + 3774}{51,277} \approx 0.76.$

(b) The probability that a randomly selected patient will need neither a kidney nor a heart transplant is
$P(\text{not kidney} \cap \text{not heart}) = P'(\text{kidney} \cup \text{heart}) \approx 1 - 0.76 \approx 0.24.$

25. (a) $P(\text{less than } \$20) = 0.25 + 0.37 = 0.62$. The probability of a purchase that is less then $20 is 0.62.

(b) $P(\$40 \text{ or more}) = 0.09 + 0.07 + 0.08 + 0.03 = 0.27$. The probability of a purchase that is $40 or more is 0.27.

(c) $P(\text{more than } \$99.99) = 0.08 + 0.03 = 0.11$. The probability of a purchase that is more than $99.99 is 0.11.

(d) $P(\text{less than } \$100) = 1 - 0.11 = 0.89$. The probability of a purchase that is less than $100 is 0.89.

27. Number of picks with all cards correct except the heart $= 12$.
Number of picks with all cards correct except the club $= 12$.
Number of picks with all cards correct except the diamond $= 12$.
Number of picks with all cards correct except the spade $= 12$. Total number of picks with all cards correct but one $= 48$. $P(\text{all cards correct but one}) = \dfrac{48}{28,561} \approx 0.001681$. The probability of getting three of the four selections correct is $\dfrac{48}{28,561}$ or approximately 0.001681.

29. (a) $P(\text{male selected}) = 1 - 0.28 = 0.72$. The probability that a male worker is selected is 0.72.

(b) $P(5 \text{ years or less}) = 1 - 0.3 = 0.7$. The probability that a worker is selected who has worked for the company 5 years or less is 0.7.

(c) $P(\text{contribute} \cup \text{female}) = P(\text{contribute}) + P(\text{female}) - P(\text{contribute} \cap \text{female})$
$= 0.65 + 0.28 - \dfrac{0.28}{2} = 0.79$. The probability that a worker is selected who contributes to the retirement plan or is female is 0.79.

31. There are $5^2 = 32$ possible outcomes, each with probability $\dfrac{1}{32}$. $\binom{5}{2} = 10$ outcomes with 2 girls (and 3 boys)

$\Rightarrow P(2 \text{ girls and } 3 \text{ boys}) = 10\left(\dfrac{1}{32}\right) = \dfrac{5}{16} = 0.3125$. The probability of having exactly 2 girls and 3 boys is $\dfrac{5}{16} = 0.3125$.

578   CHAPTER 11   Further Topics in Algebra

33. $\binom{5}{0} = 1$ outcome has no girls $\Rightarrow P(\text{no girls}) = 1\left(\frac{1}{32}\right) = \frac{1}{32} = 0.03125.$

   The probability of having no girls is $\frac{1}{32} = 0.03125.$

35. $\binom{5}{5} + \binom{5}{4} + \binom{5}{3} = 1 + 5 + 10 = 16$ outcomes have at least 3 boys $\Rightarrow P(\text{at least 3 boys}) = 16\left(\frac{1}{32}\right) = \frac{1}{2} = 0.5.$

   The probability of having at least 3 boys is $\frac{1}{2} = 0.5.$

37. $P(1 \text{ student smokes less than 10 per day}) = 0.45 + 0.24 = 0.69.$ $P(4 \text{ of 10 smoke less than 10 per day}) =$

   $\binom{10}{4}(0.69)^4(1-0.69)^6 \approx 0.042246.$ The probability that 4 of 10 students selected at random smoked less than 10 cigarettes per day is approximately 0.042246.

39. $P(1 \text{ student smokes between 1 and 19 per day}) = 0.023831.$

   $P(\text{fewer than 2 smoke between 1 and 19 per day}) =$

   $P(0 \text{ smoke between 1 and 19 per day}) + P(1 \text{ smokes between 1 and 19 per day}) =$

   $= \binom{10}{0}(0.44)^0(1-0.44)^{10} + \binom{10}{1}(0.44)^1(1-0.44)^9 \approx 0.026864.$ The probability that fewer than 2 of 10 students selected at random smoked between 1 and 19 cigarettes per day is approximately 0.026864.

41. $P(\text{exactly 12 ones}) = \binom{12}{12}\left(\frac{1}{6}\right)^{12}\left(\frac{5}{6}\right)^0 = \frac{1}{6^{12}} \approx 4.6 \times 10^{-10}.$ The probability of rolling exactly 12 ones is $\frac{1}{6^{12}} \approx 4.6 \times 10^{-10}.$

43. $P(\text{no more than 3 ones}) = P(0 \text{ ones}) + P(1 \text{ ones}) + P(2 \text{ ones}) + P(3 \text{ ones}) =$

   $\binom{12}{0}\left(\frac{1}{6}\right)^0\left(\frac{5}{6}\right)^{12} + \binom{12}{1}\left(\frac{1}{6}\right)^1\left(\frac{5}{6}\right)^{11} + \binom{12}{2}\left(\frac{1}{6}\right)^2\left(\frac{5}{6}\right)^{10} + \binom{12}{3}\left(\frac{1}{6}\right)^3\left(\frac{5}{6}\right)^9 \approx 0.875.$ The probability of rolling no more than 3 ones is approximately 0.875.

45. $P(\text{fewer than 4}) = P(1) + P(2 \text{ or } 3) = 0.2 + 0.29 = 0.49.$ The probability that a randomly selected student applied to fewer than 4 colleges is 0.49.

47. $P(\text{more than 3}) = P(4\text{-}6) + P(7 \text{ or more}) = 0.37 + 0.14 = 0.51.$ The probability that a randomly selected student applied to more than 3 colleges is 0.51.

49. (a) $P(5 \text{ of 53 are color blind}) = \binom{53}{5}(0.042)^5(1-0.042)^{48} \approx 0.047822.$ The probability that exactly 5 of 53 men are color blind is approximately 0.047822.

(b) $P(\text{no more than } 5) = P(0) + P(1) + P(2) + P(3) + P(4) + P(5) =$

$\binom{53}{0}(0.042)^0(1-0.42)^{53} + \binom{53}{1}(0.042)^1(1-0.042)^{52} + \binom{53}{2}(0.042)^2(1-0.042)^{51} +$

$\binom{53}{3}(0.042)^3(1-0.042)^{50} + \binom{53}{4}(0.042)^4(1-0.042)^{49} + \binom{53}{5}(0.042)^5(1-0.042)^{48} \approx 0.976710.$

The probability that no more than 5 of 53 men are color blind is approximately 0.976710.

(c) $P(\text{none are color blind}) = \binom{53}{0}(0.042)^0(1-0.042)^{53} \approx 0.102890.$

$P(\text{at least 1 color blind}) = 1 - P(\text{none are color blind}) \approx 0.897110.$

The probability that at least 1 man of 53 men is color blind is approximately 0.897110.

51. (a) $I = 2, S = 4, p = 0.1 \Rightarrow q(1-p)^I = (1-0.1)^2 = 0.81..$

$P(\text{3 not becoming infected}) = \binom{4}{3}(0.81)^3(1-0.81)^{4-3} \approx 0.404 = 40.4\%.$ The probability of 3 family members not becoming infected is approximately 40.4%.

(b) $I = 2, S = 4, p = 0.5 \Rightarrow q = (1-p)^I = (1-0.5)^2 = 0.25.$

$P(\text{3 not becoming infected}) = \binom{4}{3}(0.25)^3(1-0.25)^{4-3} \approx 4.7\%.$ The probability of 3 family members not becoming infected is approximately 4.7%.

(c) $I = 1, S = 9, p = 0.5 \Rightarrow q = (1-p)^I = (1-0.5)^1 = 0.5.$

$P(\text{0 not becoming infected}) = \binom{9}{0}(0.5)^0(1-0.5)^{9-0} \approx 0.002$

The probability that all of the other family members becoming sick is approximately 0.2%. Thus, it is unlikely that everyone in a large family would become sick even though the disease is highly infectious.

Reviewing Basic Concepts (Sections 11.6 and 11.7)

1. $4 + 8 + 12 + 16 + \cdots + 4n = 2n(n+1).$

   (i) Show that the statement is true for $n = 1$: $4(1) = 2(1)(1+1) \Rightarrow 4 = 4.$

   (ii) Assume that S_k is true: $4 + 8 + 12 + 16 + \cdots + 4k = 2k(k+1).$ Show that S_{k+1} is true:

   $4 + 8 + 12 + 16 + \cdots + 4(k+1) = 2(k+1)(k+2).$ Add $4(k+1)$ to each side of S_k:

   $4 + 8 + 12 + 16 + \cdots + 4k + 4(k+1) = 2k(k+1) + 4(k+1).$

   $= 2k^2 + 2k + 4k + 4 = 2k^2 + 6k + 4 = 2(k^2 + 3k + 2) = 2(k+1)(k+2).$

   Since S_k implies S_{k+1}, the statement is true for every positive integer n.

2. $n^2 \leq 2^n$, if $n \geq 4$

(i) Show that the statement is true for $n = 4$: $4^2 \leq 2^4 \Rightarrow 16 \leq 16$.

(ii) Assume that S_k is true: $k^2 \leq 2^k$. Show that S_{k+1} is true: $(k+1)^2 \leq 2^{(k+1)}$.

Multiply each side of S_k by 2: $k^2 \cdot 2 \leq 2^k \cdot 2 \Rightarrow 2k^2 \leq 2^{k+1}$.

Because $(k+1)^2 < 2k^2$ for all $k \geq 4$, we may substitute $(k+1)^2$ for $2k^2$ in the expression.

That is, $(k+1)^2 \leq 2^{k+1}$.

Since S_k implies S_{k+1}, the statement is true for every positive integer $n \geq 4$.

3. The sample space S for tossing a coin twice is $S = \{(H,H),(H,T),(T,H),(T,T)\}$.

4. 36 possible outcomes, each with probability $\dfrac{1}{36}$. 2 outcomes yield 11, $\{(5,6),(6,5)\}$.

Therefore, $1^3 = 1; 1^2(2(1)^2 - 1) = 1(2-1) = 1$; The probability of rolling a sum of 11 is $\dfrac{2}{36} = \dfrac{1}{18}$.

5. $\binom{4}{4} = 1$ way of drawing 4 aces; $\binom{4}{1} = 4$ ways of drawing 1 queen; $\binom{52}{5} = 2{,}598{,}960$ ways of drawing 5 cards. P (4 aces and 1 queen) $= \dfrac{1 \times 4}{2{,}598{,}960} \approx 0.0000015$. The probability of drawing 4 aces and 1 queen is approximately 0.0000015.

6. From number 5, the probability of drawing 4 aces and 1 queen is given by $\dfrac{4}{2{,}598{,}960}$. Therefore, the probability of not drawing 4 aces and 1 queen is given by $1 - \dfrac{4}{2{,}598{,}960} = \dfrac{2{,}598{,}956}{2{,}598{,}960} \approx 0.9999985$.

7. P (rain) $= \dfrac{3}{3+7} = \dfrac{3}{10}$. The probability of rain is $\dfrac{3}{10}$.

8. P (female) $= \dfrac{2.81 - 1.45}{2.81} \approx 0.484$. The probability that a randomly selected graduate is female is approximately 0.484.

Chapter 11 Review Exercises

1. $a_1 = \dfrac{1}{1+1} = \dfrac{1}{2}$; $a_2 = \dfrac{2}{2+1} = \dfrac{2}{3}$; $a_3 = \dfrac{3}{3+1} = \dfrac{3}{4}$; $a_4 = \dfrac{4}{4+1} = \dfrac{4}{5}$; $a_5 = \dfrac{5}{5+1} = \dfrac{5}{6}$. The first five terms of the sequence are $\dfrac{1}{2}, \dfrac{2}{3}, \dfrac{3}{4}, \dfrac{4}{5},$ and $\dfrac{5}{6}$. The sequence is neither arithmetic nor geometric.

2. $a_1 = (-2)^1 = -2$; $a_2 = (-2)^2 = 4$; $a_3 = (-2)^3 = -8$; $a_4 = (-2)^4 = 16$; $a_5 = (-2)^5 = -32$. The first five terms of the sequence are –2, 4, –8, 16, and –32. The sequence is geometric with common ratio –2.

3. $a_1 = 2(1+3) = 8; a_2 = 2(2+3) = 10; a_3 = 2(3+3) = 12; a_4 = 2(4+3) = 14; a_5 = 2(5+3) = 16$. The first five terms of the sequence are 8, 10, 12, 14, and 16. The sequence is arithmetic with common difference 2.

4. $a_1 = 1(1+1) = 2; a_2 = 2(2+1) = 6; a_3 = 3(3+1) = 12; a_4 = 4(4+1) = 20; a_5 = 5(5+1) = 30$. The first five terms of the sequence are 2, 6, 12, 20, and 30. The sequence is neither arithmetic nor geometric.

5. $a_1 = 5; a_2 = 5-3 = 2; a_3 = 2-3 = -1; a_4 = -1-3 = -4; a_5 = -4-3 = -7$. The first five terms of the sequence are 5, 2, –1, –4, and –7. The sequence is arithmetic with common difference –3.

6. $a_1 = \left(\frac{1}{5}\right)^{1-1}; a_2 = \left(\frac{1}{5}\right)^{2-1}; a_3 = \left(\frac{1}{5}\right)^{3-1}; a_4 = \left(\frac{1}{5}\right)^{4-1}; a_5 = \left(\frac{1}{5}\right)^{5-1}$. The first five terms of the sequence are, $1, \frac{1}{5}, \frac{1}{25}, \frac{1}{125}, \frac{1}{625}$. The sequence is geometric with common ratio $\frac{1}{5}$.

7. $a_2 = 10, d = -2 \Rightarrow a_1 = 10+2 = 12; a_3 = 10-2 = 8; a_4 = 8-2 = 6; a_5 = 6-2 = 4$. The first five terms of the sequence are 12, 10, 8, 6, and 4.

8. $a_3 = \pi, a_4 = 1 \Rightarrow d = 1 - \pi \Rightarrow a_2 = \pi - (1-\pi) = 2\pi - 1; a_1 = 2\pi - 1 - (1-\pi) = 3\pi - 2;$
$a_5 = 1 + (1-\pi) = -\pi + 2$. The first five terms of the sequence are $3\pi - 2, 2\pi - 1, \pi, 1,$ and $-\pi + 2$.

9. $a_1 = 6, r = 2 \Rightarrow a_2 = 6 \cdot 2 = 12; a_3 = 12 \cdot 2 = 24; a_4 = 24 \cdot 2 = 48; a_5 = 48 \cdot 2 = 96$. The first five terms of the sequence are 6, 12, 24, 48, and 96.

10. $a_1 = -5, a_2 = -1 \Rightarrow r = \frac{1}{5} \Rightarrow a_3 = (-1)\left(\frac{1}{5}\right) = -\frac{1}{5}; a_4 = \left(\frac{-1}{5}\right)\left(\frac{1}{5}\right) = -\frac{1}{25}; a_5 = \left(-\frac{1}{25}\right)\left(\frac{1}{5}\right) = -\frac{1}{125}$. The first five terms of the sequence are $-5, -1, -\frac{1}{5}, -\frac{1}{25}, -\frac{1}{125}$.

11. $a_5 = -3, a_{15} = 17 \Rightarrow 17 = -3 + 10d \Rightarrow d = 2 \Rightarrow -3 = a_1 + 4 \cdot 2 \Rightarrow a_1 = -11 \Rightarrow$
$a_n = -11 + 2(n-1) = 2n - 13$. The first term of the sequence is –11 and the nth term of the sequence is given by $a_n = 2n - 13$.

12. $a_1 = -8, a_7 = -\frac{1}{8} \Rightarrow -\frac{1}{8} = (-8)r^6 \Rightarrow r^6 = \frac{1}{64} \Rightarrow r = \pm\frac{1}{2}$. Therefore, $a_4 = (-8)\left(\frac{1}{2}\right)^3 = -1$ and
$a_n = (-8)\left(\frac{1}{2}\right)^{n-1} = -\left(\frac{1}{2}\right)^{n-4}$ or $a_4 = (-8)\left(-\frac{1}{2}\right)^3 = 1$ and $a_n = (-8)\left(-\frac{1}{2}\right)^{n-1} = -\left(-\frac{1}{2}\right)^{n-4}$. Either the common ratio is $\frac{1}{2}$ and the fourth term of the sequence is –1 and the nth term of the sequence is given by
$a_n = (-8)\left(\frac{1}{2}\right)^{n-1} = -\left(\frac{1}{2}\right)^{n-4}$ or the common ratio is $-\frac{1}{2}$ and the fourth term of the sequence is 1 and the
n^{th} term of the sequence is given by $a_n = (-8)\left(-\frac{1}{2}\right)^{n-1} = -\left(-\frac{1}{2}\right)^{n-4}$.

582 CHAPTER 11 Further Topics in Algebra

13. $a_1 = 6, d = 2 \Rightarrow a_8 = 6 + (8-1)(2) = 20$. The eighth term of the sequence is 20.

14. $a_1 = 6x-9, a_2 = 5x+1 \Rightarrow d = (5x+1)-(6x-9) = -x+10 \Rightarrow a_8 = (6x-9)+(8-1)(-x+10) = -x+61$.

    The eighth term of the sequence is $-x+61$.

15. $a_1 = 2, d = 3 \Rightarrow a_{12} = 2+(12-1)(3) = 35 \Rightarrow S_{12} = \frac{12}{2}(2+35) = 222$. The sum of the first twelve terms of

    the sequence is 222.

16. $a_2 = 6, d = 10 \Rightarrow a_1 = 6-10 = -4 \Rightarrow a_{12} = -4+(12-1)(10) = 106 \Rightarrow S_{12} = \frac{12}{2}(-4+106) = 612$. The

    sum of the first twelve terms of the sequence is 612.

17. $a_1 = -2, r = 3 \Rightarrow a_5 = (-2)(3)^{5-1} = -162$. The fifth term of the sequence is -162.

18. $a_3 = 4, r = \frac{1}{5} \Rightarrow a_1 = \frac{4}{\left(\frac{1}{5}\right)^2} = 100 \Rightarrow a_5 = (100)\left(\frac{1}{5}\right)^{5-1} = \frac{100}{625} = \frac{4}{25}$. The fifth term of the sequence is $\frac{4}{25}$.

19. $a_1 = 3, r = 2 \Rightarrow S_4 = \frac{3(1-2^4)}{1-2} = 45$. The sum of the first four terms of the sequence is 45.

20. $a_1 = \frac{3}{4}, a_2 = -\frac{1}{2}, a_3 = \frac{1}{3} \Rightarrow r = -\frac{2}{3} \Rightarrow S_4 = \frac{\frac{3}{4}(1-(-\frac{2}{3})^4)}{1-(-\frac{2}{3})} = \frac{13}{36}$. The sum of the first four terms is $\frac{13}{36}$.

21. $S = 2000\left[\frac{(1+0.03)^5 - 1}{0.03}\right] = 10,618.27$. The future value of the annuity is \$10,618.27.

22. $a_1 = 6, r = 0.9$; therefore $a_n = 6(0.9)^{n-1}$

23. $a_1 = (-1)^{1-1} = 1; r = -1; \sum_{i=1}^{7}(-1)^{i-1} = S_7 = \frac{1\left[1-(-1)^7\right]}{1-(-1)} = \frac{1(2)}{2} = 1$. The value of the sum is 1.

24. $\sum_{i=1}^{5}(i^2+i) = \sum_{i=1}^{5}i^2 + \sum_{i=1}^{5}i = \frac{5(5+1)(2\cdot 5+1)}{6} + \frac{5(5+1)}{2} = 55+15 = 70$. The value of the sum is 70.

25. $\sum_{i=1}^{4}\frac{i+1}{i} = \frac{2}{1}+\frac{3}{2}+\frac{4}{3}+\frac{5}{4} = \frac{73}{12}$. The value of the sum is $\frac{73}{12}$.

26. $a_1 = 3(1)-4 = -1; a_{10} = 3(10)-4 = 26; \sum_{j=1}^{10}(3j-4) = S_{10} = \frac{10}{2}(-1+26) = 125$.

    The value of the sum is 125.

27. $\sum_{j=1}^{2500} j = \frac{2500(2500+1)}{2} = 3,126,250$. The value of the sum is 3,126,250.

28. $a_1 = 4\cdot 2^1 = 8; r = 2; \sum_{i=1}^{5} 4\cdot 2^i = S_5 = \frac{8(1-2^5)}{1-2} = 248$. The value of the sum is 248.

29. $a_1 = \left(\frac{4}{7}\right)^1 = \frac{4}{7}; r = \frac{4}{7}; \sum_{i=1}^{\infty}\left(\frac{4}{7}\right)^i = S_\infty = \frac{\frac{4}{7}}{1-\frac{4}{7}} = \frac{4}{3}$. The value of the sum is $\frac{4}{3}$.

30. $r = \frac{6}{5} \Rightarrow |r| \geq 1 \Rightarrow \sum_{i=1}^{\infty} -2\left(\frac{6}{5}\right)^i$ does not exist.

31. $a_1 = 24, a_2 = 8, a_3 = \frac{8}{3}, a_4 = \frac{8}{9} \Rightarrow r = \frac{1}{3} \Rightarrow S_\infty = \frac{24}{1-\frac{1}{3}} = 36$. The value of the sum is 36.

32. $a_1 = -\frac{3}{4}, a_2 = \frac{1}{2}, a_3 = -\frac{1}{3}, a_4 = \frac{2}{9} \Rightarrow r = -\frac{2}{3} \Rightarrow S_\infty = \frac{-\frac{3}{4}}{1-\left(-\frac{2}{3}\right)} = -\frac{9}{20}$. The value of the sum is $-\frac{9}{20}$.

33. $a_1 = \frac{1}{12}, a_2 = \frac{1}{6}, a_3 = \frac{1}{3}, a_4 = \frac{2}{3} \Rightarrow r = 2 \Rightarrow |r| \geq 1 \Rightarrow S_\infty$ diverges. The value of the sum diverges and does not exist.

34. $a_1 = 0.9, a_2 = 0.09, a_3 = 0.009, a_4 = 0.0009 \Rightarrow r = \frac{1}{10} \Rightarrow S_\infty = \frac{0.9}{1-\frac{1}{10}} = 1$. The value of the sum is 1.

35. $\sum_{i=1}^{4}(x_i^2 - 6) = \sum_{i=1}^{4}x_i^2 - \sum_{i=1}^{4}6 = \sum_{i=1}^{4}(x_i+1)^2 - 24 = \frac{3(3+1)(2\cdot 3+1)}{6} - 24 = -10$. The value of the sum is -10.

36. $\sum_{i=1}^{6} f(x_i)\Delta x = (0-2)^3(0.1) + (1-2)^3(0.1) + (2-2)^3(0.1) + (3-2)^3(0.1) +$

    $(4-2)^3(0.1) + (5-2)^3(0.1) = 2.7$. The value of the sum is 2.7.

37. $a_1 = 4, a_2 = -1, a_3 = -6 \Rightarrow d = -5 \Rightarrow a_n = 4 - 5(n-1) = -5n + 9$.

    $a_n = -66 = -5n + 9 \Rightarrow n = 15 \Rightarrow 4 - 1 - 6 - \ldots - 66 = \sum_{i=1}^{15}(-5i+9)$.

    The sum may be written as $\sum_{i=1}^{15}(-5i+9)$.

38. $a_1 = 10, a_2 = 14, a_3 = 18 \Rightarrow d = 4 \Rightarrow a_n = 10 + 4(n-1) = 4n + 6$..

    $a_n = 86 = 4n + 6 \Rightarrow n = 20 \Rightarrow 10 + 14 + 18 + \ldots + 86 = \sum_{i=1}^{20}(4i+6)$. The sum may be written as $\sum_{i=1}^{20}(4i+6)$.

39. $a_1 = 4, a_2 = 12, a_3 = 36 \Rightarrow r = 3 \Rightarrow a_n 4(3)^{n-1}$. $a_n = 972 = 4(3)^{n-1} \Rightarrow$

    $n - 1 = 5 \Rightarrow n = 6 \Rightarrow 4 + 12 + 36 + \ldots + 972 = \sum_{i=1}^{6}4(3)^{n-1}$. The sum may be written as $\sum_{i=1}^{6}4(3)^{n-1}$.

40. $a_n = \frac{n}{n+1}$ for $5 \leq n \leq 12$; $\frac{5}{6} + \frac{6}{7} + \frac{7}{8} + \ldots + \frac{12}{13} = \sum_{i=5}^{12}\frac{i}{i+1}$. The sum may be written as $\sum_{i=5}^{12}\frac{i}{i+1}$.

41. $9! = 362{,}880$. The value of $9!$ is $362{,}880$.

42. $P(9,2) = {}_9P_r 2 = 72$. The value of $P(9,2)$ is 72.

43. $P(6,0) = {}_6P_r 0 = 1$. The value of $P(6,0)$ is 1.

584   CHAPTER 11   Further Topics in Algebra

44. $C(10,5) = 10_n C_r 5 = 252$. The value of $C(10,5)$ is 252.

45. $\binom{8}{3} = 8_n C_r 3 = 56$. The value of $\binom{8}{3}$ is 56.

46. Order is significant in the digits of a student identification number. Thus, such a number is an example of a permutation.

47. $(x+2y)^4 = \binom{4}{0}x^4(2y)^0 + \binom{4}{1}x^3(2y)^1 + \binom{4}{2}x^2(2y)^2 + \binom{4}{3}x^1(2y)^3 + \binom{4}{4}x^0(2y)^4 =$

$x^4 + 8x^3y + 24x^2y^2 + 32xy^3 + 16y^4$. The binomial expansion of $(x+2y)^4$ is

$x^4 + 8x^3y + 24x^2y^2 + 32xy^3 + 16y^4$.

48. $(3z-5w)^3 = \binom{3}{0}(3z)^3(-5w)^0 + \binom{3}{1}(3z)^2(-5w)^1 + \binom{3}{2}(3z)^1(-5w)^2 + \binom{3}{3}(3z)^0(-5w)^3 = \backslash$

$27z^3 - 135z^2w + 225zw^2 - 125w^3$. The binomial expansion of $(3z-5w)^3$ is

$27z^3 - 135z^2w + 225zw^2 - 125w^3$.

49. $\left(3\sqrt{x} - \dfrac{1}{\sqrt{x}}\right)^5 = \binom{5}{0}(3x^{1/2})^5(-x^{-1/2})^0 + \binom{5}{1}(3x^{1/2})^4(-x^{-1/2})^1 + \binom{5}{2}(3x^{1/2})^3(-x^{-1/2})^2 +$

$\binom{5}{3}(3x^{1/2})^2(-x^{-1/2})^3 + \binom{5}{4}(3x^{1/2})^1(-x^{-1/2})^4 + \binom{5}{5}(3x^{1/2})^0(-x^{-1/2})^5 =$

$243x^{5/2} - 405x^{3/2} + 270x^{1/2} - 90x^{-1/2} + 15x^{-3/2} - x^{-5/2}$. The binomial expansion of $\left(3\sqrt{x} - \dfrac{1}{\sqrt{x}}\right)^5$ is

$243x^{5/2} - 405x^{3/2} + 270x^{1/2} - 90x^{-1/2} + 15x^{-3/2} - x^{-5/2}$.

50. $(m^3 - m^{-2})^4 = \binom{4}{0}(m^3)^4(-m^{-2})^0 + \binom{4}{1}(m^3)^3(-m^{-2})^1 + \binom{4}{2}(m^3)^2(-m^{-2})^2 +$

$\binom{4}{3}(m^3)^1(-m^{-2})^3 + \binom{4}{4}(m^3)^0(-m^{-2})^4 = m^{12} - 4m^7 + 6m^2 - 4m^{-3} + m^{-8}$. The binomial expansion of

$(m^3 - m^{-2})^4$ is $m^{12} - 4m^7 + 6m^2 - 4m^{-3} + m^{-8}$.

51. $\binom{8}{5}(4x)^3(-y)^5 = -3584x^3y^5$. The sixth term of $(4x-y)^8$ is $-3584x^3y^5$.

52. $\binom{14}{6}(m)^8(-3n)^6 = 2,189,187m^8n^6$. The seventh term of $(m-3n)^{14}$ is $2,189,187 \, m^8n^6$.

53. $(x+2)^{12} = \binom{12}{0}(x)^{12}(2)^0 + \binom{12}{1}(x)^{11}(2)^1 + \binom{12}{2}(x)^{10}(2)^2 +$

$\binom{12}{3}(x)^9(2)^3 + \ldots = x^{12} + 24x^{11} + 264x^{10} + 1760x^9 + \ldots$. The first four terms of $(x+12)^{12}$ are

$x^{12} + 24x^{11} + 264x^{10} + 1760x^9$.

54. $(2a+5b)^{16} = \ldots + \binom{16}{14}(2a)^2(5b)^{14} + \binom{16}{15}(2a)^1(5b)^{15} + \binom{16}{16}(2a)^0(5b)^{16} =$

    $\ldots + 480 \cdot 5^{14}a^2b^{14} + 32 \cdot 5^{15}ab^{15} + 5^{16}b^{16}$. The last three terms of $(2a+5b)^{16}$ are

    $480 \cdot 5^{14}a^2b^{14} + 32 \cdot 5^{15}ab^{15} + 5^{16}b^{16}$.

55. Statements which are defined on the natural numbers; that is, statements which have the natural numbers as their domain, are proved by mathematical induction. An example is $\sum_{i=1}^{n} i = \frac{n(n+1)}{2}$.

56. A proof by mathematical induction consists of two steps. First, show that the statement is true for $n=1$. Then show that if the statement is true for $n=k$, it must follow that the statement is also true for $n=k+1$.

57. Prove $1+3+5+7+\ldots+(2n-1) = n^2$.

    Step 1: $1 = 1^2 \Rightarrow 1+3+5+7+\ldots+(2n-1) = n^2$ for $n=1$.

    Step 2: Assume $1+3+5+7+\ldots+(2k-1) = k^2$, then

    $1+3+5+7+\ldots+(2k-1)+(2k+1) = k^2+2k+1 \Rightarrow 1+3+5+7+\ldots+(2k-1)+(2(k+1)-1) = (k+1)^2$.

    Thus, if $1+3+5+7+\ldots+(2n-1) = n^2$ for $n=k$, then it must follow that

    $1+3+5+7+\ldots+(2n-1) = n^2$ for $n=k+1$ also.

58. Prove $2+6+10+14+\ldots+(4n-2) = 2n^2$.

    Step 1: $2 = 2(1)^2 \Rightarrow 2+6+10+14+\ldots+(4n-2) = 2n^2$ for n = 1.

    Step 2: Assume $2+6+10+14+\ldots+(4k-2) = 2k^2$, then

    $2+6+10+14+\ldots+(4k-2)+(4k+2) = 2k^2+4k+2 \Rightarrow$

    $2+6+10+14+\ldots+(4k-2)+(4(k+1)-1) = 2(k+1)^2$. Thus if $2+6+10+14+\ldots+(4n-2) = 2n^2$ for

    $n=k$, then it must follow that $2+6+10+14+\ldots+(4n-2) = 2n^2$ for $n=k+1$ also.

59. Prove $2+2^2+2^3+\ldots+2^n = 2(2^n-1)$.

    Step 1: $2 = 2(2^1-1) \Rightarrow 2+2^2+2^3+\ldots+2^n = 2(2^n-1)$ for $n=1$.

    Step 2: Assume $2+2^2+2^3+\ldots+2^k = 2(2^k-1)$, then

    $2+2^2+2^3+\ldots+2^k+2^{k+1} = 2(2^k-1)+2^{k+1} = 2^{k+1}-2+2^{k+1} = 2(2^{k+1}-1)$ Thus, if

$2+2^2+2^3+...+2^n = 2(2^n-1)$ for $n = k$, then it must follow that $2+2^2+2^3+...+2^n = 2(2^n-1)$ for $n = k+1$ also.

60. Prove $1^3+3^3+5^3+...+(2n-1)^2 = n^2(2n^2-1)$.

    Step 1: $1^3 = 1; 1^2(2(1)^2-1) = 1(2-1) = 1$, so $1^3+3^3+5^3+...+(2n-1)^3 = n^2(2n^2-1)$ for n = 1.

    Step 2: Assume $1^3+3^3+5^3+...+(2k-1)^3 = k^2(2k^2-1)$. Then,

    $1^3+3^3+5^3+...+(2k-1)^3+(2k+1)^3 = k^2(2k^2-1)+(2k=1)^3$. Then

    $1^3+3^3+5^3+...+(2k-1)^3+(2(k+1)-1)^3 = 2k^4+8k^3+11k^2+6k+1 =$

    $(k^2+2k+1)(2k^2+4k+1) = (k+1)^2(2(k+1)^2-1)$. Thus, if $1^3+3^3+5^3+...+(2n-1)^3 = n^2(2n^2-1)$ for

    $n = k$, then it must follow that $1^3+3^3+5^3+...+(2n-1)^3 = n^2(2n^2-1)$ for $n = k+1$ also.

61. $2 \times 4 \times 3 \times 2 = 48$. The number of wedding arrangements possible is 48.

62. $5 \times 3 \times 6 = 90$. The number of available couches is 90.

63. $_4P_r4 = 24$. The jobs can be assigned in 24 different ways.

64. (a) $\binom{6}{3} = 20$. The number of different delegations possible is 20.

    (b) $\binom{5}{2} = 10$. If the president must attend, 10 different delegations are possible.

65. $_9P_r3 = 504$. There are 504 different ways the winners could be determined.

66. $26 \times 10 \times 10 \times 10 \times 26 \times 26 \times 26 = 456,976,000$. The number of possible different license plates is 456,976,000.

67. (a) P(green) = $\frac{4}{15}$. The probability of drawing a green marble is $\frac{4}{15}$.

    (b) P(not black) = $\frac{4+6}{15} = \frac{10}{15} = \frac{2}{3}$. The probability of drawing a marble that is not black is $\frac{2}{3}$.

    (c) P(blue) = $\frac{0}{15} = 0$. The probability of drawing a green blue is 0.

68. (a) P(green) = $\frac{4}{15} \Rightarrow \frac{4}{15-4} = \frac{4}{11}$. The odds in favor of drawing a green marble are 4 to 11.

    (b) P(not white) = $\frac{4+5}{15} = \frac{9}{15} = \frac{3}{5} \Rightarrow \frac{3}{5-3} = \frac{3}{2}$. The odds against drawing a white marble are 3 to 2.

    (c) From (b), the odds in favor of drawing a marble that is not white are 3 to 2.

69. P(black king) = $\frac{2}{52} = \frac{1}{26}$. The probability of drawing a black king is $\frac{1}{26}$.

70. P(face or ace) = $\frac{16}{52} = \frac{4}{13}$. The probability of drawing a face card or an ace is $\frac{4}{13}$.

71. $P(\text{ace} \cup \text{diamond}) = P(\text{ace}) + P(\text{diamond}) - P(\text{ace} \cap \text{diamond}) = \frac{4}{52} + \frac{13}{52} - \frac{1}{52} = \frac{16}{52} = \frac{4}{13}$. The probability of drawing an ace or a diamond is $\frac{4}{13}$.

72. $P(\text{not a diamond}) = 1 - P(\text{diamond}) = 1 - \frac{1}{4} = \frac{3}{4}$.

    The probability of drawing a card that is not a diamond is $\frac{3}{4}$.

73. $P(\text{no more than 3}) = 1 - [P(4) + P(5)] = 1 - (0.08 + 0.06) = 0.86$. The probability that no more than 3 filters are defective is 0.86.

74. $P(\text{at least 2}) = 1 - [P(0) + P(1)] = 1 - (0.31 + 0.25) = 0.44$. The probability that at least 2 filters are defective is 0.44.

75. $P(\text{more than 5}) = 0$. Only 5 filters were selected, so it is not possible for more than 5 to be defective. Note that, from the probabilities in the table, $P(0) + P(1) + P(2) + P(3) + P(4) + P(5) = 1$.

76. $\binom{12}{2}\left(\frac{1}{6}\right)^2\left(\frac{5}{6}\right)^{10} \approx 0.296$. The probability that exactly 2 of 12 rolls results in a 5 is approximately 0.296.

77. $\binom{10}{4}\left(\frac{1}{2}\right)^4\left(\frac{1}{2}\right)^6 \approx 0.205$. The probability that exactly 4 of 10 coins tossed result in a tail is approximately 0.205.

78. (a) $P(\text{conservation}) = \frac{56.51}{282.2} \approx 0.2002$. The probability that a randomly selected student is in the conservative group is approximately 0.2002.

    (b) $P(\text{far left or far right}) = \frac{7.06 + 3.673}{282.2} \approx 0.0380$. The probability that a randomly selected student is on the far left or the far right is approximately 0.0380.

    (c) $P(\text{not middle of road}) = 1 - P(\text{middle of road}) = 1 - \frac{143.5}{282.2} \approx 0.4915$. The probability that a randomly selected student is not middle of the road is approximately 0.4915.

Chapter 11 Test

1. (a) $a_1 = (-1)^1(1+2) = -3$; $a_2 = (-1)^2(2+2) = 4$; $a_3 = (-1)^3(3+2) = -5$;

    $a_4 = (-1)^4(4+2) = 6$; $a_5 = (-1)^5(5+2) = -7$. The first five terms of the sequence are -3, 4, -5, 6, and -7. The sequence is neither arithmetic nor geometric.

(b) $a_1 = (-3)\left(\dfrac{1}{2}\right)^1 = -\dfrac{3}{2}$; $a_2 = (-3)\left(\dfrac{1}{2}\right)^2 = -\dfrac{3}{4}$; $a_3 = (-3)\left(\dfrac{1}{2}\right)^3 = -\dfrac{3}{8}$;

$a_4 = (-3)\left(\dfrac{1}{2}\right)^4 = -\dfrac{3}{16}$; $a_5 = (-3)\left(\dfrac{1}{2}\right)^5 = -\dfrac{3}{32}$. The first five terms of the sequence are

$-\dfrac{3}{2}, -\dfrac{3}{4}, -\dfrac{3}{8}, -\dfrac{3}{16}$, and $-\dfrac{3}{32}$. The sequence is geometric with common ratio $\dfrac{1}{2}$.

(c) $a_1 = 2$; $a_2 = 3$; $a_3 = 3 + 2(2) = 7$; $a_4 = 7 + 2(3) = 13$; $a_5 = 13 + 2(7) = 27$. The first five terms of the sequence are 2, 3, 7, 13, and 27. The sequence is neither arithmetic nor geometric.

2. (a) $a_1 = 1$, $a_3 = 25 \Rightarrow 25 = 1 + (3-1)d \Rightarrow 2d = 24 \Rightarrow d = 12 \Rightarrow a_5 = 1 + (5-1)(12) = 49$. The fifth term of the sequence is 49.

(b) $a_1 = 81, r = -\dfrac{2}{3} \Rightarrow a_5 = 81\left(-\dfrac{2}{3}\right)^{5-1} = 16$. The fifth term of the sequence is 16

3. (a) $a_1 = -43, d = 12 \Rightarrow a_{10} = -43 + 12(10-1) = 65 \Rightarrow S_{10} = \dfrac{10}{2}(-43 + 65) = 110$. The sum of the first ten terms of the sequence is 110.

(b) $a_1 = 5, r = -2 \Rightarrow S_{10} = \dfrac{5(1-(-2)^{10})}{1-(-2)} = -1705$.

The sum of the first ten terms of the sequence is -1705.

4. (a) $a_1 = 5(1) + 2 = 7$; $a_{30} = 5(30) + 2 = 152$; $d = 5 \Rightarrow \sum_{i=1}^{30}(5i+2) = S_{30} = \dfrac{30}{2}(7 + 152) = 2385$. The value of the sum is 2385.

(b) $a_1 = (-3)(2)^1 = -6; r = 2 \Rightarrow \sum_{i=1}^{5}(-3 \cdot 2^i) = \dfrac{-6(1-(2)^5)}{1-2} = -186$. The value of the sum is -186.

(c) $r = 2 \Rightarrow |r| \geq 1 \Rightarrow \sum_{i=1}^{\infty}(2^i) \cdot 4$ does not exist. The value of the sum diverges and does not exist.

(d) $a_1 = 54\left(\dfrac{2}{9}\right)^1 = 12; r = \dfrac{2}{9} \Rightarrow \sum_{i=1}^{\infty} 54\left(\dfrac{2}{9}\right)^i = S_\infty = \dfrac{12}{1-\dfrac{2}{9}} = \dfrac{108}{7}$. The value of the sum is $\dfrac{108}{7}$.

5. (a) $10 {_nC_r} 2 = 45$. The value of $10 {_nC_r} 2 = 45$.

(b) $\binom{7}{3} = 7 {_nC_r} 3 = 35$. The value of $\binom{7}{3}$ is 35.

(c) $7! = 5040$. The value of $7!$ is 5040.

(d) $P(11, 3) = 11 {_nP_r} 3 = 990$. The value of $P(11, 3)$ is 990.

6. (a) $(2x-3y)^4 = \binom{4}{0}(2x)^4(-3y)^0 + \binom{4}{1}(2x)^3(-3y)^1 + \binom{4}{2}(2x)^2(-3y)^2 +$

$\binom{4}{3}(2x)^1(-3y)^3 + \binom{4}{4}(2x)^0(-3y)^4 = 16x^4 - 96x^3y + 216x^2y^2 - 216xy^3 + 81y^4.$

The binomial expansion of $(2x-3y)^4$ is $16x^4 - 96x^3y + 216x^2y^2 - 216xy^3 + 81y^4$.

(b) $\binom{6}{2}(w)^4(-2y)^2 = 60w^4y^2$. The third term of the expansion of $(w-2y)^6 = 60w^4y^2$.

7. Prove $8+14+20+26+...+(6n+2) = 3n^2+5n$.

Step 1: $3(1)^2 + 5(1) = 8 \Rightarrow 8+14+20+26+...+(6n+2) = 3n^2+5n$ for $n=1$.

Step 2: Assume $8+14+20+26+...+(6k+2) = 3k^2+5k$, then

$8+14+20+26+...+(6k+2)+(6k+8) = 3k^2+5k+6k+8 \Rightarrow$

$8+14+20+26+...+(6k+2)+[6(k+1)+2] = 3k^2+11k+8 =$

$3k^2+6k+3+5k+5 = 3(k+1)^2+5(k+1)$. Thus, if $8+14+20+26+...+(6n+2) = 3n^2+5n$ for

$n=k$, then it must follow that $8+14+20+26+...+(6n+2) = 3n^2+5n$ for $n=k+1$ also.

8. $4 \times 3 \times 2 = 24$. 24 different types of shoes can be made.

9. $20_nP_r3 = 6840$. The three offices can be filled in 6840 different ways.

10. $\binom{8}{2}\binom{12}{3} = 28 \cdot 220 = 6160$. Two men and three women can be chosen in 6160 different ways.

11. (a) $P(\text{red } 3) = \frac{2}{52} = \frac{1}{26}$. The probability of drawing a red three is $\frac{1}{26}$.

(b) $4 \times 3 = 12$ cards are face cards $\Rightarrow 52-12 = 40$ cards are not face cards $\Rightarrow P(\text{not a face card}) =$

$\frac{40}{52} = \frac{10}{13}$. The probability of drawing a card that is not a face card is $\frac{10}{13}$.

(c) $P(\text{king} \cup \text{spade}) = P(\text{king}) + P(\text{spade}) - P(\text{king} \cap \text{spade}) = \frac{4}{52} + \frac{13}{52} - \frac{1}{52} = \frac{16}{52} = \frac{4}{13}$.

(d) $P(\text{facecard}) = \frac{12}{52} = \frac{3}{13} \Rightarrow \frac{3}{13-3} = \frac{3}{10}$. The odds in favor of drawing a face card are 3 to 10.

12. (a) $\binom{8}{3}\left(\frac{1}{6}\right)^3\left(\frac{5}{6}\right)^5 \approx 0.104$. The probability that exactly 3 of 8 rolls will result in a 4 is approximately 0.104.

(b) $\binom{8}{8}\left(\frac{1}{6}\right)^8\left(\frac{5}{6}\right)^0 \approx 0.000000595$. The probability that all 8 of 8 rolls will result in a 6 is approximately 0.000000595.

Chapter 12: Limits, Derivatives, and Definite Integrals

12.1: An Introduction to Limits

1. The statement is false. Consider the following function: $f(x) = \begin{cases} x & \text{if } x \neq 0 \\ 2 & \text{if } x = 0 \end{cases}$

   For this function, $\lim_{x \to 0} f(x) = 0 \neq 2 = f(0)$.

3. The statement is false. Consider the following function: $f(x) = \begin{cases} x+4 & \text{for } x \neq 1 \\ \text{undefined} & \text{for } x = 1 \end{cases}$

   For this function, $\lim_{x \to 1} f(x) = 5$, but $x = 1$ is not in the domain of $f(x)$. For $\lim_{x \to a} f(x)$ to exist, values of x arbitrarily near a must be in the domain of $f(x)$ but $x = a$ need not be in the domain of $f(x)$.

5. The statement is true. If $y_1 = 5/x$ then there must be some value of x near a where
   $|f(x) - (-5)| \leq .001 \Rightarrow -5.001 \leq f(x) \leq -4.999$.

7. From the graph, $\lim_{x \to 3} f(x) = 2.5$.

9. From the graph, as x approaches 2, $|F(x)|$ becomes arbitrarily large. Therefore, $\lim_{x \to 2} f(x)$ does not exist.

11. From the graph, $\lim_{x \to 0} f(x) = 0$.

13. From the graph, as x approaches 1 from the left, $f(x)$ approaches 1.5, but as x approaches 1 from the right, $f(x)$ approaches 3. Thus, $\lim_{x \to 1} f(x)$ does not exist.

15. From the graph, $\lim_{x \to 3} g(x) = 2$.

17. From the graph, as x approaches .5, $h(x)$ has infinitely many oscillations between the values of $y = 0$ and $y = 2$. Thus, $\lim_{x \to 0.5} h(x)$ does not exist.

19. From the table of values, it appears that $\lim_{x \to 1} f(x) = 2$.

21. The completed table is shown in Figure 21. From the table, $\lim_{x \to 1} f(x) = 1$.

(x)	.9	.99	.999	1.001	1.01	1.1
$f(x)$	1.02	1.0002	1.000002	1.000002	1.0002	1.02

    Figure 21

23. The completed table is shown in Figure 23. From the table, $\lim_{x \to 2} f(x) = 10$.

x	1.9	1.99	1.999	2.001	2.01	2.1
$f(x)$	9.41	9.9401	9.994	10.006	10.0601	10.61

    Figure 23

25. The completed table is shown in Figure 25. From the table, as x approaches 1 from the left, $f(x)$ goes to large positive values, but as x approaches 1 from the right, $f(x)$ goes to large negative values. Thus, $\lim_{x \to 1} f(x)$ does not exist.

x	.9	.99	.999	1.001	1.01	1.1
$f(x)$	10.5132	100.501	1000.5	−999.5	−99.5012	−9.51191

Figure 25

27. The completed table is shown in Figure 27. From the table, $\lim_{x \to 0} f(x) = 2$.

x	−.1	−.01	−.001	.001	.01	.1
$f(x)$	1.987	1.99987	1.9999987	1.9999987	1.99987	1.987

Figure 27

29. Graphing $y_1 = \text{abs}(2x-4)$ in the window $0 \le x \le 10$, $0 \le y \le 10$ (not shown), it can be seen that $\lim_{x \to 5} |2x-4| = 6$.

31. Graphing $y_1 = (x^2 - 3x - 10)/(x-5)$ in the window $0 \le x \le 10$, $0 \le y \le 10$ (not shown), it can be seen that even though $\dfrac{x^2 - 3x - 10}{x-5}$ does not exist at $x = 5$, $\lim_{x \to 5} \dfrac{x^2 - 3x - 10}{x-5} = 7$.

33. Graphing $y_1 = (x^2 + 2)/(x+2)$ in the window $-4 \le x \le 0$, $-100 \le y \le 100$ (not shown), it can be seen that $\dfrac{x^2 + 2}{x+2}$ goes to unbounded negative values as x approaches -2 from the left and unbounded positive values as x approaches -2 from the right. Thus $\lim_{x \to -2} \dfrac{x^2 + 2}{x+2}$ does not exist.

35. Graphing $y_1 = (x^2 - x - 2)/(x-2)$ in the window $0 \le x \le 4$, $0 \le y \le 6$ (not shown), it can be seen that even though $\dfrac{x^2 - x - 2}{x-2}$ does not exist at $x = 2$, $\lim_{x \to 2} \dfrac{x^2 - x - 2}{x-2} = 3$.

37. Graphing $y_1 = x + 7$ for $(x \le 3)$ and $y_2 = 5x - 5$ for in the window $0 \le x \le 6$, $0 \le y \le 20$ (not shown), it can be seen that $\lim_{x \to 3} f(x) = 10$.

39. Graphing $y_1 = x^2 - 3$ for $(x < 2)$ and $y_2 = 5 - x^2$ for $(x > 2)$ in the window $1 \le x \le 3$, $.5 \le y \le 1.5$ (not shown), it can be seen that even though $f(x)$ does not exist at $x = 2$, $\lim_{x \to 2} f(x) = 1$.

41. Graphing $y_1 = e^x$ for $(x \le 1)$, $y_2 = \sqrt{x}$ for $(x > 1)$ and $y_3 = e^1$ in the window $0 \le x \le 2$, $0 \le y \le 4$ (not shown), it can be seen that $f(x)$ goes to e as x approaches 1 from the left and $f(x)$ approaches 1 as x approaches 1 from the right. Thus $\lim_{x \to 1} f(x)$ does not exist.

43. Graphing $y_1 = (x^3)/(x - \sin x)$ in the window $-1 \leq x \leq 1, 5 \leq y \leq 7$ (not shown), it can be seen that even though $\dfrac{x^3}{x - \sin x}$ does not exist at $x = 0$, $\lim\limits_{x \to 0} \dfrac{x^3}{x - \sin x} = 6$

45. Graphing $y_1 = (\cos x - 1)/x$ in the window $-1 \leq x \leq 1, 0 \leq y \leq 1$ (not shown), it can be seen that even though $\dfrac{\cos x - 1}{x}$ does not exist at $x = 0$, $\lim\limits_{x \to 0} \dfrac{\cos x - 1}{x} = 0$.

47. Graphing $y_1 = (e^{2x} - 1)/(e^x - 1)$ in the window $-1 \leq x \leq 1, 0 \leq y \leq 4$ (not shown), it can be seen that even though $\dfrac{e^{2x} - 1}{e^x - 1}$ does not exist at $x = 0$, $\lim\limits_{x \to 0} \dfrac{e^{2x} - 1}{e^x - 1} = 2$.

49. Graphing $y_1 = (\ln x^2)/(\ln x)$ in the window $0 \leq x \leq 2, 0 \leq y \leq 4$ (not shown), it can be seen that even though $\dfrac{\ln x^2}{\ln x}$ does not exist at $x = 1$, $\lim\limits_{x \to 1} \dfrac{\ln x^2}{\ln x} = 2$.

51. Graphing $y_1 = x \sin x$ in the window $-1 \leq x \leq 1, -1 \leq y \leq 1$ (not shown), it can be seen that $\lim\limits_{x \to 0} x \sin x = 0$.

53. Graphing $y_1 = \tan(1/x)$ in the window $-2 \leq x \leq 2, -1 \leq y \leq 1$ (not shown), it can be seen that the graph approaches infinity as x approaches 0. Thus $\lim\limits_{x \to 0} \tan \dfrac{1}{x}$ does not exist.

12.2: Techniques for Calculating Limits

1. $\lim\limits_{x \to 4}[f(x) - g(x)] = \lim\limits_{x \to 4} f(x) - \lim\limits_{x \to 4} g(x) = 16 - 8 = 8$. Thus, the limit is 8.

3. Since $\lim\limits_{x \to 4} g(x) = 8 \neq 0$, $\lim\limits_{x \to 4} \dfrac{f(x)}{g(x)} = \dfrac{\lim\limits_{x \to 4} f(x)}{\lim\limits_{x \to 4} g(x)} = \dfrac{16}{8} = 2$. Thus, the limit is 2.

5. Since $\lim\limits_{x \to 4} f(x) = 16 \geq 0$, $\lim\limits_{x \to 4} \sqrt{f(x)} = \left[\lim\limits_{x \to 4} f(x)\right]^{1/2} = (16)^{1/2} = 4$. Thus, the limit is 4.

7. $\lim\limits_{x \to 4} 2^{g(x)} = 2^{\lim\limits_{x \to 4} g(x)} = 2^8 = 256$. Thus, the limit is 256.

9. Since $\lim\limits_{x \to 4} g(x) = 8 \neq 0$, $\lim\limits_{x \to 4} \dfrac{f(x) + g(x)}{2g(x)} = \dfrac{\lim\limits_{x \to 4} f(x) + \lim\limits_{x \to 4} g(x)}{2 \cdot \lim\limits_{x \to 4} g(x)} = \dfrac{16 + 8}{2 \cdot 8} = \dfrac{3}{2}$. Thus, the limit is $\dfrac{3}{2}$.

11. $\lim\limits_{x \to -3} 7 = 7$. The limit is 7.

13. $\lim\limits_{x \to \pi} x = \pi$. The limit is π.

15. $\lim\limits_{x \to 3} 4x^2 = 4(3)^2 = 36$. The limit is 36.

17. $\lim\limits_{x \to -1} 4x^3 = 4(-1)^3 = -4$. The limit is -4.

19. $\lim\limits_{x \to 2}(x^3 + 4x^2 - 5) = (2)^3 + 4(2)^2 - 5 = 19$. The limit is 19.

21. $\lim\limits_{x \to -1} \dfrac{2x+3}{3x+4} = \dfrac{2(-1)+3}{3(-1)+4} = 1$. The limit is 1.

23. $\lim\limits_{x \to 3} \dfrac{x^2-9}{x-3} = \lim\limits_{x \to 3} \dfrac{(x+3)(x-3)}{x-3} = \lim\limits_{x \to 3}(x+3) = 6$. The limit is 6.

25. $\lim\limits_{x \to -2} \dfrac{x^2-x-6}{x+2} = \lim\limits_{x \to -2} \dfrac{(x-3)(x+2)}{x+2} = \lim\limits_{x \to -2}(x-3) = -5$. The limit is -5.

27. $\lim\limits_{x \to 1} \dfrac{x^2+x-2}{x-1} = \lim\limits_{x \to 1} \dfrac{(x+2)(x-1)}{x-1} = \lim\limits_{x \to 1}(x+2) = 3$. The limit is 3.

29. $\lim\limits_{x \to 1} \dfrac{(x-1)^2}{x^2+x-2} = \lim\limits_{x \to 1} \dfrac{(x-1)(x-1)}{(x-1)(x+2)} = \lim\limits_{x \to 1} \dfrac{x-1}{x+2} = \dfrac{0}{3} = 0$. The limit is 0.

31. $\lim\limits_{x \to 2} \dfrac{x^3-8}{x^4-16} = \lim\limits_{x \to 2} \dfrac{(x-2)(x^2+2x+4)}{(x-2)(x+2)(x^2+4)} = \lim\limits_{x \to 2} \dfrac{x^2+2x+4}{(x+2)(x^2+4)} = \dfrac{12}{32} = \dfrac{3}{8}$. The limit is $\dfrac{3}{8}$.

33. $\lim\limits_{x \to 4} \dfrac{x-4}{\sqrt{x}-2} = \lim\limits_{x \to 4} \dfrac{(\sqrt{x}-2)(\sqrt{x}+2)}{(\sqrt{x}-2)} = \lim\limits_{x \to 4}(\sqrt{x}+2) = 4$. The limit is 4.

35. $\lim\limits_{x \to 3} \sqrt{6x-2} = \sqrt{6(3)-2} = 4$. The limit is 4.

37. $\lim\limits_{x \to 1} 9^{1/(x+1)} = 9^{1/(1+1)} = 3$. The limit is 3.

39. $\lim\limits_{x \to 5}[\log_3(2x-1)] = \log_3(2(5)-1) = 2$. The limit is 2.

41. $\lim\limits_{x \to 1}[\sqrt{x}(1+x)] = \sqrt{1}(1+1) = 2$. The limit is 2.

43. $\lim\limits_{x \to 3} \dfrac{\sqrt{x+1}}{\log_2(5x+1)} = \dfrac{\sqrt{3+1}}{\log_2(5(3)+1)} = \dfrac{2}{4} = \dfrac{1}{2}$. The limit is $\dfrac{1}{2}$.

45. $\sqrt{-1}$ does not exist and $\sqrt{x}$ does not exist for values of x near -1. Thus, $\lim\limits_{x \to -1} \sqrt{x}$ does not exist.

47. $\lim\limits_{x \to 0} \dfrac{\sin x - 3x}{x} = \lim\limits_{x \to 0} \dfrac{\sin x}{x} - 3\lim\limits_{x \to 0} \dfrac{x}{x} = 1 - 3(1) = -2$. The limit is -2.

49. $\lim\limits_{x \to 0}(x \cot x) = \lim\limits_{x \to 0}\left(x \dfrac{\cos x}{\sin x}\right) = \dfrac{1}{\lim\limits_{x \to 0} \dfrac{\sin x}{x}} \cdot \lim\limits_{x \to 0} \cos x = 1 \cdot 1 = 1$. The limit is 1.

51. $\dfrac{\cos x - 1}{3x} = \dfrac{\cos x - 1}{3x} \cdot \dfrac{\cos x + 1}{\cos x + 1} = \dfrac{\cos^2 x - 1}{3x(\cos x + 1)} = \dfrac{-\sin^2 x}{3x(\cos x + 1)} = -\dfrac{1}{3}(\sin x)\left(\dfrac{\sin x}{x}\right)\left(\dfrac{1}{\cos x + 1}\right)$.

Thus, $\lim\limits_{x \to 0} \dfrac{\cos x - 1}{3x} = \lim\limits_{x \to 0}\left[-\dfrac{1}{3}(\sin x)\left(\dfrac{\sin x}{x}\right)\left(\dfrac{1}{\cos x + 1}\right)\right] = -\dfrac{1}{3}(0)(1)\left(\dfrac{1}{2}\right) = 0$. The limit is 0.

53. As the angle x approaches 0, the length of the line segment AB approaches 0 and the length of the line segment OB approaches 1 (the radius of the unit circle). Thus, $\lim\limits_{x \to 0} \sin x = 0$ and $\lim\limits_{x \to 0} \cos x = 1$.

54. The area of triangle $OAB = \dfrac{1}{2}(AB)(OB) = \dfrac{1}{2}\sin x \cos x$.

55. The area of triangle $OCD = \frac{1}{2}(1)(CD) = \frac{1}{2}\tan x$.

56. The area of sector $OAD = \pi(1)^2\left(\frac{x}{2\pi}\right) = \frac{x}{2}$. From the figure, we see that area of triangle $OAB <$ area of sector $OAD <$ area of triangle OCD. Thus, $\frac{1}{2}\sin x\cos x < \frac{1}{2}x < \frac{1}{2}\frac{\sin x}{\cos x} \Rightarrow \cos x < \frac{x}{\sin x} < \frac{1}{\cos x}$. Thus, $\frac{1}{\cos x} > \frac{\sin x}{x} > \cos x$ or $\cos x < \frac{\sin x}{x} < \frac{1}{\cos x}$.

57. From the inequality $\cos x < \frac{\sin x}{x} < \frac{1}{\cos x}$ we see that, as x approaches 0, the values of $\frac{\sin x}{x}$ are between the values of two other functions, both of which go to 1. Thus, $\lim_{x\to 0}\frac{\sin x}{x} = 1$.

58. $\frac{1-\cos x}{x} = \frac{1-\cos x}{x} \cdot \frac{1+\cos x}{1+\cos x} = \frac{1-\cos^2 x}{x(1+\cos x)} = \frac{\sin^2 x}{x(1+\cos x)} = (\sin x)\left(\frac{\sin x}{x}\right)\left(\frac{1}{1+\cos x}\right)$.

Thus, $\lim_{x\to 0}\frac{1-\cos x}{x} = \lim_{x\to 0}\left[(\sin x)\left(\frac{\sin x}{x}\right)\left(\frac{1}{1+\cos x}\right)\right] = (0)(1)\left(\frac{1}{2}\right) = 0$. The limit is 0.

12.3: One-Sided Limits; Limits Involving Infinity

1. (a) Since $f(x) = 4$ for $x > 2$, $\lim_{x\to 2^+} f(x) = 4$.

    (b) Since $f(x) = x$ for $x < 2$, $\lim_{x\to 2^-} f(x) = 2$.

3. (a) As shown in the graph of $f(x) = \frac{x}{5(3-x)^3}$, $\lim_{x\to 3^+} f(x) = -\infty$.

    (b) As shown in the same graph, $\lim_{x\to 3^-} f(x) = \infty$.

5. (a) As shown in the graph of $f(x) = \frac{x}{(x+1)^2}$, $\lim_{x\to -1^+} f(x) = -\infty$.

    (b) As shown in the same graph, $\lim_{x\to -1^-} f(x) = -\infty$.

7. Since $3x - 5$ is continuous at $x = 5$, $\lim_{x\to 5^+}(3x-5) = 3(5) - 5 = 10$.

9. Since 100 is continuous at $x = 7$, $\lim_{x\to 7^-} 100 = 100$

11. Since $\sqrt{x+3}$ does not exist for $x < -3$, $\lim_{x\to -3^-}\sqrt{x+3}$ does not exist.

13. Since $\frac{|x|}{x} = -1$ for $x < 0$, $\lim_{x\to 0^-}\frac{|x|}{x} = -1$.

15. Since $\frac{|x+3|}{x+3} = -1$ for $x < -3$, $\lim_{x\to -3^-}\frac{|x+3|}{x+3} = -1$.

17. As shown in the graph of $2 + e^{-x}$, $\lim_{x\to\infty}(2+e^{-x}) = 2$.

19. As shown in the graph of $x+\dfrac{1}{x}$, $\displaystyle\lim_{x\to\infty}\left(x+\dfrac{1}{x}\right)=\infty$.

21. Graphing $y_1 = x\cdot\sin(1/x^2)$ in the window $0\le x\le 100$, $-1\le y\le 1$ (not shown), it can be seen that
$$\lim_{x\to\infty}\left(x\sin\dfrac{1}{x^2}\right)=0.$$

23. Graphing $y_1 = x-\sqrt{(x^2+5)}$ in the window $0\le x\le 100$, $-1\le y\le 1$ (not shown), it can be seen that
$$\lim_{x\to\infty}(x-\sqrt{x^2+5})=0.$$

25. Graphing $y_1 = \tan^{-1}\left(\dfrac{x}{x-1}\right)$ in the window $-100\le x\le 100$, $-\dfrac{\pi}{2}\le y\le\dfrac{\pi}{2}$ (not shown), it can be seen that $y=\dfrac{\pi}{4}$ is a horizontal asymptote both when $x\to\infty$ and when $x\to -\infty$. Changing the window to $0\le x\le 2$, $-\pi\le y\le \pi$, shows that $x=1$ is not a vertical asymptote.

27. Graphing $y_1 = 5-e^{-x}$ in the window $-10\le x\le 10$, $-10\le y\le 10$ (not shown), it can be seen that $y=5$ is a horizontal asymptote as $x\to\infty$.

29. (a) Since $f(x)=x-1$ if $x>2$, $\displaystyle\lim_{x\to 2^+}f(x)=2-1=1$.

    (b) Since $f(x)=7x$ if $x\le 2$, $\displaystyle\lim_{x\to 2^-}f(x)=7(2)=14$.

31. (a) Graphing $y_1 = x/(4-x)^3$ in the window $0\le x\le 8$, $-50\le y\le 50$ (not shown), shows that
$$\lim_{x\to 4^+}f(x)=-\infty.$$

    (b) The same graph shows that $\displaystyle\lim_{x\to 4^-}f(x)=\infty$.

33. (a) Graphing $y_1 = x/(x+3)^3$ in the window $-6\le x\le 0$, $-50\le y\le 50$ (not shown), shows that
$$\lim_{x\to -3^+}f(x)=-\infty.$$

    (b) The same graph shows that $\displaystyle\lim_{x\to -3^-}f(x)=\infty$.

35. $\displaystyle\lim_{x\to\infty}\dfrac{5x}{3x-1}=\lim_{x\to\infty}\dfrac{5}{3-\dfrac{1}{x}}=\dfrac{5}{3}$. The limit is $\dfrac{5}{3}$.

37. $\displaystyle\lim_{x\to -\infty}\dfrac{8x+2}{2x-5}=\lim_{x\to -\infty}\dfrac{8+\dfrac{2}{x}}{2-\dfrac{5}{x}}=\dfrac{8}{2}=4$. The limit is 4.

39. $\displaystyle\lim_{x\to\infty}\dfrac{x^2+2x-5}{3x^2+2}=\lim_{x\to\infty}\dfrac{1+\dfrac{2}{x}-\dfrac{5}{x^2}}{3+\dfrac{2}{x^2}}=\dfrac{1}{3}$. The limit is $\dfrac{1}{3}$.

41. $\lim_{x \to -\infty} \frac{5x + 8x^2}{3 + 2x^2} = \lim_{x \to -\infty} \frac{\frac{5}{x} + 8}{\frac{3}{x^2} + 2} = \frac{8}{2} = 4$. The limit is 4.

43. $\lim_{x \to \infty} \frac{1 - 7x^3}{x^2 + 7x^3} = \lim_{x \to \infty} \frac{\frac{1}{x^3} - 7}{\frac{1}{x} + 7} = \frac{-7}{7} = -1$. The limit is -1.

45. $\lim_{x \to \infty} \frac{-4x^4 - x^2 + 8}{6x^4 - 5x} = \lim_{x \to \infty} \frac{-4 - \frac{1}{x^2} + \frac{8}{x^4}}{6 - \frac{5}{x^3}} = -\frac{4}{6} = -\frac{2}{3}$. The limit is $-\frac{2}{3}$.

47. $\lim_{x \to \infty} \frac{2x^2 - 1}{3x^4 + 2} = \lim_{x \to \infty} \frac{\frac{2}{x^2} - \frac{1}{x^4}}{3 + \frac{2}{x^4}} = \frac{0}{3} = 0$. The limit is 0.

49. $\lim_{x \to \infty} \frac{x^4 - x^3 - 3x}{7x^2 + 9} = \lim_{x \to \infty} \frac{x^2 - x - \frac{3}{x}}{7 + \frac{9}{x^2}} = \infty$. The limit is ∞.

51. $\lim_{x \to -\infty} \frac{2x - 3x^3}{4x^3 + x} = \lim_{x \to -\infty} \frac{\frac{2x}{x^3} - \frac{3x^3}{x^3}}{\frac{4x^3}{x^3} + \frac{x}{x^3}} = \frac{-3}{4}$. The limit is $-\frac{3}{4}$.

53. The function $f(x) = \frac{1}{x - 5}$ has the properties that $\lim_{x \to 5^+} f(x) = \infty$ and $\lim_{x \to 5^-} f(x) = -\infty$

55. The function $f(x) = -x^3$ has the properties that $f(x)$ is a polynomial and $\lim_{x \to \infty} f(x) = -\infty$.

57. The function $f(x) = 2x$ and $g(x) = x$ have the properties that $\lim_{x \to \infty} f(x) = \infty$, $\lim_{x \to \infty} g(x) = \infty$, and $\lim_{x \to \infty} [f(x) - g(x)] = \infty$.

59. The functions $f(x) = \frac{1}{x}$ and $g(x) = x^2$ have the properties that $\lim_{x \to \infty} f(x) = 0$, $\lim_{x \to \infty} g(x) = \infty$, and $\lim_{x \to \infty} [f(x) \cdot g(x)] = \infty$.

61. If the graph of $y = f(x)$ has oblique asymptote $y = \frac{1}{2}x + 3$, then $\lim_{x \to \infty} f(x) = \infty$.

63. (a) Graphing $y_1 = xe^{-x}$ in the window $0 \le x \le 10$, $-.1 \le y \le .5$ (not shown), shows that $\lim_{x \to \infty}(xe^{-x}) = 0$.

    (b) Graphing $y_1 = x^2 e^{-x}$ in the window $0 \le x \le 20$, $-.1 \le y \le .7$ (not shown), shows c) that $\lim_{x \to \infty}(x^2 e^{-x}) = 0$.

    (c) Graphing $y_1 = x^{10} e^{-x}$ in the window $0 \le x \le 25$, $0 \le y \le 500,000$ (not shown), shows that

    $\lim_{x \to \infty}(x^{10} e^{-x}) = 0$. It would seem that $\lim_{x \to \infty}(x^n e^{-x}) = 0$ for any positive integer n.

598   Chapter 12 Limits, Derivatives, and Definite Integrals

65. From the graph in the figure $\lim_{t \to 1^-} f(t)$ is the quantity of the drug in the body just prior to the second injection and $\lim_{t \to 1^+} f(t)$ is the quantity of the drug in the body immediately after the second injection.

67. $\lim_{t \to \infty} p(t) = 12$. The limit is $12. This limit represents the long term ultimate price for the commodity.

69. $f(x) = a_n x^n + a_{n-1} x^{n-1} + \cdots + a_1 x + a_0 = a_n x^n \left(1 + \frac{a_{n-1}}{a_n} \cdot \frac{1}{x} + \frac{a_{n-2}}{a_n} \cdot \frac{1}{x^2} + \cdots + \frac{a_1}{a_n} \cdot \frac{1}{x^{n-1}} + \frac{a_0}{a_n} \cdot \frac{1}{x^n}\right)$

70. $\lim_{x \to \infty} f(x) = \left[\lim_{x \to \infty}(a_n x^n)\right] \cdot \left[\lim_{x \to \infty}\left(1 + \frac{a_{n-1}}{a_n} \cdot \frac{1}{x} + \cdots + \frac{a_0}{a_n} \cdot \frac{1}{x^n}\right)\right] = \left[a_n \lim_{x \to \infty} x^n\right] \cdot [1] = a_n \lim_{x \to \infty} x^n$

$\lim_{x \to -\infty} f(x) = \left[\lim_{x \to -\infty}(a_n x^n)\right] \cdot \left[\lim_{x \to -\infty}\left(1 + \frac{a_{n-1}}{a_n} \cdot \frac{1}{x} + \cdots + \frac{a_0}{a_n} \cdot \frac{1}{x^n}\right)\right] = \left[a_n \lim_{x \to -\infty} x^n\right] \cdot [1] = a_n \lim_{x \to -\infty} x^n$

71. Since $\lim_{x \to \infty} f(x) = a_n \lim_{x \to \infty} x^n$ and $\lim_{x \to -\infty} f(x) = a_n \lim_{x \to -\infty} x^n$,

   (a) if a_n is positive and n is even, then $\lim_{x \to \infty} f(x) = \infty$ and $\lim_{x \to -\infty} f(x) = \infty$.

   (b) if a_n is negative and n is even, then $\lim_{x \to \infty} f(x) = -\infty$ and $\lim_{x \to -\infty} f(x) = -\infty$.

   (c) if a_n is positive and n is odd, then $\lim_{x \to \infty} f(x) = \infty$ and $\lim_{x \to -\infty} f(x) = -\infty$.

   (d) if a_n is negative and n is odd, then $\lim_{x \to \infty} f(x) = -\infty$ and $\lim_{x \to -\infty} f(x) = \infty$.

72. (a) ∪   (b) ∩   (c) ⌣   (d) ⌢

Reviewing Basic Concepts (Sections 12.1—12.3)

1. (a) Based on the intercept shown in the graph, $f(x) = \frac{2}{3}x + 1$, $\lim_{x \to 3} f(x) = \frac{2}{3}(3) + 1 = 3$. The limit is 3.

   (b) Even though $F(x)$ is not defined at $x = 2$, the graph shows that $\lim_{x \to 2} f(x) = 4$. The limit is 4.

   (c) Even though $f(x)$ is not defined at $x = 0$, the graph shows that $\lim_{x \to 0} f(x) = 0$. The limit is 0.

   (d) The graph shows that $\lim_{x \to 3} g(x) = 2$. The limit is 2.

2. (a) The graph shows that $\lim_{x \to -2^-} f(x) = -1$ and that $\lim_{x \to -2^+} f(x) = -\frac{1}{2}$ and that $\lim_{x \to -2} f(x)$ does not exist.

   (b) The graph shows that $\lim_{x \to -1^-} f(x) = -\frac{1}{2}$ and that $\lim_{x \to -1^+} f(x) = -\frac{1}{2}$ and that $\lim_{x \to -1} f(x) = -\frac{1}{2}$.

3. (a) The graph shows that $\lim_{x \to 1^-} f(x) = 1$ and that $\lim_{x \to 1^+} f(x) = 1$ and, even though $f(1) = 2$, $\lim_{x \to 1} f(x) = 1$.

   (b) The graph shows that $\lim_{x \to 2^-} f(x) = 0$ and that $\lim_{x \to 2^+} f(x) = 0$ and that $\lim_{x \to 2} f(x) = 0$

4. (a) The graph shows that $\lim_{x \to \infty} f(x) = 3$. The limit is 3.

   (b) The graph shows that $\lim_{x \to -\infty} g(x) = \infty$. The limit is ∞ (or does not exist).

5. The completed table is shown in Figure 5. From the table of values, $\lim_{x \to 4} \frac{\sqrt{x}-2}{x-4} = \frac{1}{4}$.

x	3.9	3.99	3.999	4.001	4.01	4.1
f(x)	.251582	.250156	.250015	.249984	.249844	.248457

Figure 5

6. (a) $\lim_{x \to 8}[f(x) - g(x)] = \lim_{x \to 8} f(x) - \lim_{x \to 8} g(x) = 32 - 4 = 28$. The limit is 28.

   (b) $\lim_{x \to 8}[g(x) \cdot f(x)] = \left[\lim_{x \to 8} g(x)\right] \cdot \left[\lim_{x \to 8} f(x)\right] = 4 \cdot 32 = 128$. The limit is 128.

   (c) $\lim_{x \to 8} \frac{f(x)}{g(x)} = \frac{\lim_{x \to 8} f(x)}{\lim_{x \to 8} g(x)} = \frac{32}{4} = 8$. The limit is 8.

   (d) $\lim_{x \to 8}[\log_2 f(x)] = \log_2\left[\lim_{x \to 8} f(x)\right] = \log_2(32) = 5$. The limit is 5.

   (e) $\lim_{x \to 8} \sqrt{f(x)} = \sqrt{\lim_{x \to 8} f(x)} = \sqrt{32} = 4\sqrt{2}$. The limit is $4\sqrt{2}$.

   (f). $\lim_{x \to 8} = \sqrt[3]{g(x)} = \sqrt[3]{\lim_{x \to 8} g(x)} = \sqrt[3]{4}$. The limit is $\sqrt[3]{4}$.

   (g) $\lim_{x \to 8} 2^{g(x)} = 2^{\lim_{x \to 8} g(x)} = 2^4 = 16$. Thus, the limit is 16.

   (h) $\lim_{x \to 8}[1 + f(x)]^2 = \left[1 + \lim_{x \to 8} f(x)\right]^2 = [1 + 32]^2 = 1089$. The limit is 1089.

   (i) $\lim_{x \to 8^-} \frac{f(x) - g(x)}{4g(x)} = \frac{\lim_{x \to 8^-} f(x) - \lim_{x \to 8^-} g(x)}{4 \lim_{x \to 8^-} g(x)} = \frac{32 - 4}{4(4)} = \frac{7}{4}$. The limit is $\frac{7}{4}$.

   (j) $\lim_{x \to 8^+} \frac{2g(x) + 3}{1 + f(x)} = \frac{2 \lim_{x \to 8^+} g(x) + 3}{1 + \lim_{x \to 8^+} f(x)} = \frac{2(4) + 3}{1 + 32} = \frac{1}{3}$. The limit is $\frac{1}{3}$.

   (k) $\lim_{x \to 8^+}[f(x) + g(x)]^2 = \left[\lim_{x \to 8^+} f(x) + \lim_{x \to 8^+} g(x)\right]^2 = [32 + 4]^2 = 1296$

   (l) $\lim_{x \to 8^-}[\log_6(f(x) + g(x))] = \log_6\left[\lim_{x \to 8^-} f(x) + \lim_{x \to 8^-} g(x)\right] = \log_6(36) = 2$

7. $\lim_{x \to 3} \frac{x^2 - 9}{x - 3} = \lim_{x \to 3} \frac{(x+3)(x-3)}{x-3} = 6$. Even though $\frac{x^2-9}{x-3}$ does not exist at $x = 3$, the limit is 6.

8. $\lim_{x \to \infty} \frac{2x^2 - 1}{3x^4 + 5} = \lim_{x \to \infty} \frac{\frac{2}{x^2} - \frac{1}{x^4}}{3 + \frac{5}{x^4}} = \frac{0}{3} = 0$. The limit is 0.

9. $\lim_{x \to -\infty} \frac{2x^3 - x + 3}{6x^3 + 4x - 9} = \lim_{x \to -\infty} \frac{2 - \frac{1}{x^2} + \frac{3}{x^3}}{6 + \frac{4}{x^2} - \frac{9}{x^3}} = \frac{2}{6} = \frac{1}{3}$. The limit is $\frac{1}{3}$.

600   Chapter 12 Limits, Derivatives, and Definite Integrals

10. $\lim\limits_{x\to 4^-} f(x) = \lim\limits_{x\to 4^-}(x+2) = 6$ and $\lim\limits_{x\to 4^+} f(x) = \lim\limits_{x\to 4^+}(x^2-6) = 10$. Therefore $\lim\limits_{x\to 4} f(x)$ does not exist.

12. 4: Tangent Lines and Derivatives

1. The tangent line passes through the points $(5,3)$ and $(6,5)$ and has slope $m = \dfrac{5-3}{6-5} = 2$.

3. The tangent line passes through the points $(-2,2)$ and $(3,3)$ and has slope $m = \dfrac{3-2}{3-(-2)} = \dfrac{1}{5}$.

5. $m = \lim\limits_{x\to 4}\dfrac{x^2-4^2}{x-4} = \lim\limits_{x\to 4}\dfrac{(x+4)(x-4)}{x-4} = 8$. The slope of the tangent line is 8.

7. $m = \lim\limits_{x\to -2}\dfrac{\left(-4x^2+11x\right) - \left[-4(-2)^2+11(-2)\right]}{x-(-2)} = \lim\limits_{x\to -2}\dfrac{-4x^2+11x+38}{x+2} = \lim\limits_{x\to -2}\dfrac{(-4x+19)(x+2)}{x+2} = 27$

   The slope of the tangent line is 27.

9. $m = \lim\limits_{x\to 4}\dfrac{\left(-\frac{2}{x}\right)-\left(-\frac{2}{4}\right)}{x-4} = \lim\limits_{x\to 4}\dfrac{-\frac{2}{x}+\frac{1}{2}}{x-4} = \lim\limits_{x\to 4}\dfrac{\frac{x-4}{2x}}{x-4} = \dfrac{1}{8}$. The slope of the tangent line is $\dfrac{1}{8}$.

11. $m = \lim\limits_{x\to 1}\dfrac{-3\sqrt{x}+3\sqrt{1}}{x-1} = \lim\limits_{x\to 1}\dfrac{-3(\sqrt{x}-1)}{(\sqrt{x}-1)(\sqrt{x}+1)} = -\dfrac{3}{2}$. The slope of the tangent line is $-\dfrac{3}{2}$.

13. $m = \lim\limits_{x\to 1}\dfrac{2x^3-2(1)^3}{x-1} = \lim\limits_{x\to 1}\dfrac{2(x^3-1)}{x-1} = \lim\limits_{x\to 1}\dfrac{2(x-1)(x^2+x+1)}{x-1} = 6$. The slope of the tangent line is 6.

15. $m = \lim\limits_{x\to -1}\dfrac{\left(4-x^2\right)-\left[4-(-1)^2\right]}{x-(-1)} = \lim\limits_{x\to -1}\dfrac{1-x^2}{x+1} = \lim\limits_{x\to -1}\dfrac{-(x+1)(x-1)}{x+1} = 2$.

   The slope of the tangent line is 2.

17. $m = \lim\limits_{x\to 3}\dfrac{\left(x^2+2x\right)-\left[3^2+2(3)\right]}{x-3} = \lim\limits_{x\to 3}\dfrac{x^2+2x-15}{x-3} = \lim\limits_{x\to 3}\dfrac{(x+5)(x-3)}{x-3} = 8$.

   $f(3) = 15$; $y - 15 = 8(x-3) = 8x - 24$. The tangent line is $y = 8x - 9$. Graphing $y_1 = x^2 + 2x$ and $y_2 = 8x - 9$ in the window $0 \le x \le 6$, $0 \le y \le 50$ (not shown), shows this result.

19. $m = \lim\limits_{x\to 2}\dfrac{\frac{5}{x}-\frac{5}{2}}{x-2} = \lim\limits_{x\to 2}\dfrac{\frac{-5(x-2)}{2x}}{x-2} = -\dfrac{5}{4}$. $f(2) = \dfrac{5}{2}$; $y - \dfrac{5}{2} = -\dfrac{5}{4}(x-2) = -\dfrac{5}{4}x + \dfrac{5}{2}$. The tangent line is

   $y = -\dfrac{5}{4}x + 5$. Graphing $y_1 = 5/x$ and $y_2 = -(5/4)x + 5$ in the window

   $0 \le x \le 4$, $0 \le y \le 10$ (not shown), shows this result.

21. $m = \lim\limits_{x \to 9} \dfrac{4\sqrt{x} - 4\sqrt{9}}{x-9} = \lim\limits_{x \to 9} \dfrac{4(\sqrt{x}-3)}{(\sqrt{x}-3)(\sqrt{x}+3)} = \dfrac{2}{3}$. $f(9) = 12$; $y - 12 = \dfrac{2}{3}(x-9) = \dfrac{2}{3}x - 6$. The tangent line is $y = \dfrac{2}{3}x + 6$. Graphing $y_1 = 4\sqrt{x}$ and $y_2 = (2/3)x + 6$ in the window $0 \le x \le 18, 0 \le y \le 20$ (not shown), shows this result.

23. Graphing $y_1 = 5$, we see that the graph of $f(x)$ is a horizontal line which never changes. Thus, the rate of change of $f(x)$ is 0 everywhere and $f'(2) = 0$.

25. Graphing $y_1 = -x$, we see that the graph of $f(x)$ is a straight line with slope $m = -1$. Thus, the rate of change of $f(x)$ is -1 everywhere and $f'(2) = -1$.

27. On a TI-86, nDer$(e^x, x, 0) = 1.00000016667$. Thus, we conclude that $f'(0)$ is 1.

29. On a TI-86, nDer$(10x/(1+.25x^2), x, 2) = 6.25$ E^{-7}. Thus, we conclude that $f'(2)$ is 0.

31. On a TI-86, nDer$(x\cos x, x, \pi/4) = .151746152925$. Thus, we conclude that $f'\left(\dfrac{\pi}{4}\right)$ is approximately .1517.

33. From the figure, the tangent line at (0, 1) has slope $m = \dfrac{1}{3}$. Thus, $f'(0)$ is $\dfrac{1}{3}$

35. Using the first two secant line equations, we get $f(a) = 2.03a - .53$ and $f(a) = 2.02a - .52$. Solving this simultaneously, we get $a = 1$ and $f(a) = 1.5$. The slope of the tangent line is the limit of the slopes of the secant lines as $x \to a$ and, from the figure, this limit appears to be 2. Thus $f'(a)$ is 2.

37. $s'(3) = \lim\limits_{t \to 3} \dfrac{9t^2 - 9(3)^2}{t-3} = \lim\limits_{t \to 3} \dfrac{9(t+3)(t-3)}{t-3} = 9(6) = 54$. The car's velocity when $t = 3$ seconds is 54 f feet/second.

39. $s'(3) = \lim\limits_{t \to 3} \dfrac{(3t^3 - t^2) - [3(3)^3 - (3)^2]}{t-3} = \lim\limits_{t \to 3} \dfrac{3t^3 - t^2 - 72}{t-3} = \lim\limits_{t \to 3} \dfrac{(t-3)(3t^2 + 8t + 24)}{t-3} =$
$3(3)^2 + 8(3) + 24 = 75$. The car's velocity when $t = 3$ seconds is approximately 75 feet/second.

41. $f'(a) = \lim\limits_{x \to a} \dfrac{x^2 - a^2}{x-a} = \lim\limits_{x \to a} \dfrac{(x-a)(x+a)}{x-a} = \lim\limits_{x \to a}(x+a) = 2a$

43. $f'(a) = \lim\limits_{x \to a} \dfrac{(3x-1) - (3a-1)}{x-a} = \lim\limits_{x \to a} \dfrac{3(x-a)}{x-a} = \lim\limits_{x \to a} 3 = 3$

45. $f'(a) = \lim\limits_{x \to a} \dfrac{(4x - x^2) - (4a - a^2)}{x-a} = \lim\limits_{x \to a} \dfrac{4x - 4a + a^2 - x^2}{x-a} = \lim\limits_{x \to a} \dfrac{(x-a)(4-a-x)}{x-a} = 4 - 2a$

47. $f'(a) = \lim\limits_{x \to a} \dfrac{\sqrt{x}-\sqrt{a}}{x-a} = \lim\limits_{x \to a} \dfrac{\sqrt{x}-\sqrt{a}}{\left(\sqrt{x}-\sqrt{a}\right)\left(\sqrt{x}+\sqrt{a}\right)} = \lim\limits_{x \to a} \dfrac{1}{\sqrt{x}+\sqrt{a}} = \dfrac{1}{2\sqrt{a}}$

49. $f'(x) = \lim\limits_{h \to 0} \dfrac{\left(-(x+h)^2 + 4(x+h)\right) - \left(-x^2 + 4x\right)}{h} = \lim\limits_{h \to 0} \dfrac{-x^2 - 2xh + h^2 + 4x + 4h + x^2 - 4x}{h} =$

    $\lim\limits_{h \to 0} \dfrac{-2xh + h^2 + 4h}{h} = \lim\limits_{h \to 0} -2x + h + 4 = -2x + 4$

51. $f'(x) = \lim\limits_{h \to 0} \dfrac{\left(2(x+h)^2 - (x+h)\right) - \left(2x^2 - x\right)}{h} = \lim\limits_{h \to 0} \dfrac{2x^2 + 4xh + 2h^2 - x - h - 2x^2 + x}{h} =$

    $\lim\limits_{h \to 0} \dfrac{4xh + 2h^2 - h}{h} = \lim\limits_{h \to 0} 4x + 2h - 1 = 4x - 1$

53. $f'(x) = \lim\limits_{h \to 0} \dfrac{\left(2(x+h)^2 - (x+h) + 1\right) - \left(2x^2 - x + 1\right)}{h} = \lim\limits_{h \to 0} \dfrac{2x^2 + 4xh + 2h^2 - x - h + 1 - 2x^2 + x - 1}{h} =$

    $\lim\limits_{h \to 0} \dfrac{4xh + 2h^2 - h}{h} = \lim\limits_{h \to 0} 4x + 2h - 1 = 4x - 1$

55. $f'(x) = \lim\limits_{h \to 0} \dfrac{\left((x+h)^3\right) - \left(x^3\right)}{h} = \lim\limits_{h \to 0} \dfrac{x^3 + 3x^2h + 3xh^2 + h^3 - x^3}{h} =$

    $\lim\limits_{h \to 0} \dfrac{3x^2h + 3xh^2 + h^3}{h} = \lim\limits_{h \to 0} 3x^2 + 3xh + h^2 = 3x^2$

57. The tangent line when $t = 6$ years passes through the points $(6, 5)$ and $(2, 2)$ and, therefore, has slope

    $m = \dfrac{5-2}{6-2} = \dfrac{3}{4}$. The interest rates were rising at a rate of $\dfrac{3}{4}\%$ per year on January 1, 2006.

59. $W'(4) = \lim\limits_{t \to 4} \dfrac{.1t^2 - .1(4)^2}{t-4} = \lim\limits_{t \to 4} \dfrac{.1(t-4)(t+4)}{t-4} = .8$. The tumor is growing at a rate of .8 grams/week when

    $t = 4$ weeks.

61. (a) $20 = t^2 + t \Rightarrow t^2 + t - 20 = 0 \Rightarrow (t+5)(t-4) = 0 \Rightarrow t = -5$ or $t = 4$ The helicopter will reach a height of 20 feet in 4 seconds.

    (b) $s'(4) = \lim\limits_{t \to 4} \dfrac{\left(t^2 + t\right) - \left[4^2 + 4\right]}{t-4} = \lim\limits_{t \to 4} \dfrac{t^2 + t - 20}{t-4} = \lim\limits_{t \to 4} \dfrac{(t+5)(t-4)}{t-4} = 9$. The velocity of the helicopter when it is 20 feet above the ground will be 9 feet/second.

63. $R'(1000) = \lim\limits_{x \to 1000} \dfrac{\left(10x - .002x^2\right) - \left[10(1000) - .002(1000)^2\right]}{x - 1000} = \lim\limits_{x \to 1000} \dfrac{-.002x^2 + 10x - 8000}{x - 1000} =$

    $\lim\limits_{x \to 1000} \dfrac{(x - 1000)(-.002x + 8)}{x - 1000} = 6$. The marginal revenue at $x = 1000$ is $6000 per unit.

65. Graph $y_1 = 100,000/\left(1+9.134(0.8)^x\right)$ in the window $0 \le x \le 32$, $0 \le y \le 100,000$ to obtain the graph shown in Figure 65. $\text{nDer}(y_1, x, 8) = 5331.9986515$. Thus, we conclude that the rumor is spreading by about 5332 people per day when $x = 8$ days.

[0,32] by [0,100,000]
Xscl = 6   Yscl = 10000

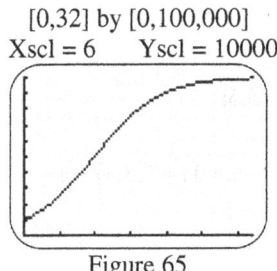

Figure 65

12.5: Area and the Definite Integral

1. (a) $f(x_1) = 2(0)+1 = 1; f(x_2) = 2(2)+1 = 5; f(x_3) = 2(4)+1 = 9; f(x_4) = 2(6)+1 = 13;$

   $\sum_{i=1}^{4} f(x_i) \Delta x = 1(2) + 5(2) + 9(2) + 13(2) = 56$. The sum is 56.

   (b) $\int_0^8 (2x+1) dx$ is the definite integral approximated by the sum in part (a).

3. (a) $x_1 = 1; x_2 = 2; x_3 = 3; x_4 = 4;$

   $f(x_1) = 3(1)+2 = 5; f(x_2) = 3(2)+2 = 8; f(x_3) = 3(3)+2 = 11; f(x_4) = 3(4)+2 = 14;$

   $\sum_{i=1}^{4} f(x_i) \Delta x = 5(1) + 8(1) + 11(1) + 14(1) = 38$. Using left endpoints, the area is approximately 38.

   (b) $x_1 = 2; x_2 = 3; x_3 = 4; x_4 = 5;$

   $f(x_1) = 3(2)+2 = 8; f(x_2) = 3(3)+2 = 11; f(x_3) = 3(4)+2 = 14; f(x_4) = 3(5)+2 = 17;$

   $\sum_{i=1}^{4} f(x_i) \Delta x = 8(1) + 11(1) + 14(1) + 17(1) = 50$. Using right endpoints, the area is approximately 50.

   (c) $\dfrac{38+50}{2} = 44$. Averaging the answers to (a) and (b), the area is approximately 44.

   (d) $x_1 = 1.5; x_2 = 2.5; x_3 = 3.5; x_4 = 4.5; f(x_1) = 3(1.5)+2 = 6.5; f(x_2) = 3(2.5)+2 = 9.5;$

   $f(x_3) = 3(3.5)+2 = 12.5; f(x_4) = 3(4.5)+2 = 15.5;$

   $\sum_{i=1}^{4} f(x_i) \Delta x = 6.5(1) + 9.5(1) + 12.5(1) + 15.5(1) = 44$. Using midpoints, the area is approximately 44.

5. (a) $x = 0; x_2 = 1; x_3 = 2; x_4 = 3;$

   $f(x_1) = 0+2 = 2; f(x_2) = 1+2 = 3; f(x_3) = 2+2 = 4; f(x_4) = 3+2 = 5;$

   $\sum_{i=1}^{4} f(x_i) \Delta x = 2(1) + 3(1) + 4(1) + 5(1) = 14$. Using left endpoints, the area is approximately 14.

(b) $x_1 = 1; x_2 = 2; x_3 = 3; x_4 = 4;$

$f(x_1) = 1+2 = 3; f(x_2) = 2+2 = 4; f(x_3) = 3+2 = 5; f(x_4) = 4+2 = 6;$

$\sum_{i=1}^{4} f(x_i)\Delta x = 3(1)+4(1)+5(1)+6(1) = 18$. Using right endpoints, the area is approximately 18.

(c) $\dfrac{14+18}{2} = 16$. Averaging the answers to (a) and (b), the area is approximately 16.

(d) $x_1 = 0.5; x_2 = 1.5; x_3 = 2.5; x_4 = 3.5; f(x_1) = .5+2 = 2.5; f(x_2) = 1.5+2 = 3.5;$

$f(x_3) = 2.5+2 = 4.5; f(x_4) = 3.5+2 = 5.5; \sum_{i=1}^{4} f(x_i)\Delta x = 2.5(1)+3.5(1)+4.5(1)+5.5(1) = 16.$

Using midpoints, the area is approximately 16.

7. (a) $x_1 = 1; x_2 = 2; x_3 = 3; x_4 = 4\ f(x_1) = 1^2 = 1; f(x_2) = 2^2 = 4; f(x_3) = 3^2 = 9; f(x_4) = 4^2 = 16;$

$\sum_{i=1}^{4} f(x_i)\Delta x = 1(1)+4(1)+9(1)+16(1) = 30$. Using left endpoints, the area is approximately 30.

(b) $x_1 = 2; x_2 = 3; x_3 = 4; x_4 = 5; f(x_1) = 2^2 = 4; f(x_2) = 3^2 = 9; f(x_3) = 4^2 = 16; f(x_4) = 5^2 = 25;$

$\sum_{i=1}^{4} f(x_i)\Delta x = 4(1)+9(1)+16(1)+25(1) = 54$. Using right endpoints, the area is approximately 54.

(c) $\dfrac{30+54}{2} = 42$ Averaging the answers to (a) and (b), the area is approximately 42.

(d) $x_1 = 1.5; x_2 = 2.5; x_3 = 3.5; x_4 = 4.5; f(x_1) = (1.5)^2 = 2.25; f(x_2) = (2.5)^2 = 6.25;$

$f(x_3) = (3.5)^2 = 12.25; f(x_4) = (4.5)^2 = 20.25;$

$\sum_{i=1}^{4} f(x_i)\Delta x = 2.25(1)+6.25(1)+12.25(1)+20.25(1) = 41$

Using midpoints, the area is approximately 41.

9 (a) $x_1 = 0; x_2 = 1; x_3 = 2; x_4 = 3;$

$f(x_1) = e^0 - 1 = 0; f(x_2) = e^1 - 1 \approx 1.718; f(x_3) = e^2 - 1 \approx 6.389; f(x_4) = e^3 - 1 \approx 19.086;$

$\sum_{i=1}^{4} f(x_i)\Delta x = 0(1)+1.718(1)+6.389(1)+19.086(1) \approx 27.19.$

Using left endpoints, the area is approximately 27.19.

(b) $x_1 = 1; x_2 = 2; x_3 = 3; x_4 = 4;$

$f(x_1) = e^1 - 1 \approx 1.718; f(x_2) = e^2 - 1 \approx 6.389; f(x_3) = e^3 - 1 \approx 19.086; f(x_4) = e^4 - 1 \approx 53.598;$

$\sum_{i=1}^{4} f(x_i)\Delta x = 1.718(1)+6.389(1)+19.086(1)+53.598(1) \approx 80.79.$

Using right endpoints, the area is approximately 80.79.

(c) $\dfrac{27.19+80.79}{2} = 53.99$. Averaging the answers to (a) and (b), the area is approximately 53.99.

(d) $x_1 = .5;\ x_2 = 1.5;\ x_3 = 2.5;\ x_4 = 3.5;\ f(x_1) = e^{.5} - 1 \approx .649;\ f(x_2) = e^{1.5} - 1 \approx 3.482;$

$f(x_3) = e^{2.5} - 1 \approx 11.182;\ f(x_4) = e^{3.5} - 1 \approx 32.115;$

$\sum\limits_{i=1}^{4} f(x_i)\Delta x = .649(1) + 3.482(1) + 11.182(1) + 32.115(1) \approx 47.43$.

Using midpoints, the area is approximately 47.43.

11. (a) $x_1 = 1;\ x_2 = 2;\ x_3 = 3;\ x_4 = 4;\ f(x_1) = \dfrac{1}{1} = 1;\ f(x_2) = \dfrac{1}{2};\ f(x_3) = \dfrac{1}{3};\ f(x_4) = \dfrac{1}{4};$

$\sum\limits_{i=1}^{4} f(x_i)\Delta x = (1)(1) + \left(\dfrac{1}{2}\right)(1) + \left(\dfrac{1}{3}\right)(1) + \left(\dfrac{1}{4}\right)(1) \approx \dfrac{25}{12}$.

Using left endpoints, the area is approximately $\dfrac{25}{12}$.

(b) $x_1 = 2;\ x_2 = 3;\ x_3 = 4;\ x_4 = 5;\ f(x_1) = \dfrac{1}{2};\ f(x_2) = \dfrac{1}{3};\ f(x_3) = \dfrac{1}{4};\ f(x_4) = \dfrac{1}{5};$

$\sum\limits_{i=1}^{4} f(x_i)\Delta x = \left(\dfrac{1}{2}\right)(1) + \left(\dfrac{1}{3}\right)(1) + \left(\dfrac{1}{4}\right)(1) + \left(\dfrac{1}{5}\right)(1) \approx \dfrac{77}{66}$.

Using right endpoints, the area is approximately $\dfrac{77}{60}$.

(c) $\dfrac{\frac{25}{12} + \frac{77}{60}}{2} = \dfrac{101}{60}$ Averaging the answers to (a) and (b), the area is approximately $\dfrac{101}{60}$.

(d) $x_1 = 1.5;\ x_2 = 2.5;\ x_3 = 3.5;\ x_4 = 4.5;\ f(x_1) = \dfrac{1}{1.5} = \dfrac{2}{3};\ f(x_2) = \dfrac{1}{2.5} = \dfrac{2}{5};$

$f(x_3) = \dfrac{1}{3.5} = \dfrac{2}{7};\ f(x_4) = \dfrac{1}{4.5} = \dfrac{2}{9};\ \sum\limits_{i=1}^{4} f(x_i)\Delta x = \left(\dfrac{2}{3}\right)(1) + \left(\dfrac{2}{5}\right)(1) + \left(\dfrac{2}{7}\right)(1) + \left(\dfrac{2}{9}\right)(1) \approx \dfrac{496}{315}$.

Using midpoints, the area is approximately $\dfrac{496}{315}$.

13. (a) $x_1 = .5;\ x_2 = 1.5;\ x_3 = 2.5;\ x_4 = 3.5;\ f(x_1) = \dfrac{.5}{2} = \dfrac{1}{4};\ f(x_2) = \dfrac{1.5}{2} = \dfrac{3}{4};$

$f(x_3) = \dfrac{2.5}{2} = \dfrac{5}{4};\ f(x_4) = \dfrac{3.5}{2} = \dfrac{7}{4};\ \sum\limits_{i=1}^{4} f(x_i)\Delta x = \left(\dfrac{1}{4}\right)(1) + \left(\dfrac{3}{4}\right)(1) + \left(\dfrac{5}{4}\right)(1) + \left(\dfrac{7}{4}\right)(1) = \dfrac{16}{4} = 4$.

Using midpoints, the area is approximately 4.

(b) Triangle base $= 4 - 0 = 4$; Triangle height $= \dfrac{4}{2} = 2$; Triangle area $= \dfrac{1}{2}(4)(2) = 4$. Using the formula

for the area of a triangle, the area is 4.

15. (a) Triangle base $= 4$; Triangle height $= 2$; Triangle area $= \frac{1}{2}(4)(2) = 4$. Using the formula for the area of a triangle, the area is 4.

    (b) First triangle base $= 3$; First triangle height $= 3$; First triangle area $= \frac{1}{2}(3)(3) = \frac{9}{2}$. Second triangle base $= 1$; Second triangle height $= 1$; Second triangle area $= \frac{1}{2}(1)(1) = \frac{1}{2}$. Using the formula for the area of a triangle, the area is $\frac{9}{2} + \frac{1}{2} = 5$.

    (c) Triangle base $= 4$; Triangle height $= 4$; Triangle area $= \frac{1}{2}(4)(4) = 8$. Using the formula for the area of a triangle, the area is 8.

    (d) The graph is a semi-circle with radius 2. Semi-Circle area $= \frac{1}{2}\pi r^2 = \frac{1}{2}\pi(2)^2 = 2\pi$.

17. $\sqrt{16-x^2}$ for $-4 \leq x \leq 0$ is a quarter circle with center $(0,0)$ and radius 4. Area of quarter circle $= \left(\frac{1}{4}\right)(\pi)(4)^2 = 4\pi$. The area is 4π.

19. $(1+2x)$ for $2 \leq x \leq 5$ is a (sideways) trapezoid with height $= 3$, first base $= 11$, second base $= 5$. Area of trapezoid $= \left(\frac{1}{2}\right)(11+5)(3) = 24$. The area is 24

21. $(2x-1)$ for $1 \leq x \leq 4$ is a (sideways) trapezoid with height $= 3$, first base $= 1$, second base $= 7$. Area of trapezoid $= \left(\frac{1}{2}\right)(1+7)(3) = 12$. The area is 12

Reviewing Basic Concepts (Sections 12.4 and 12.5)

1. The tangent line passes through the points $(-3, 4)$ and $(0, 1.5)$ and has slope $m = \frac{4-1.5}{-3-0} = -\frac{5}{6}$.

2. The tangent line passes through the points $(2,1)$ and $(0, -3)$ and has slope $m = \frac{-3-1}{0-2} = \frac{-4}{-2} = 2$.

3. The tangent line is a horizontal line and has slope $m = 0$.

4. The tangent line is a vertical line and its slope does not exist.

5. $\lim\limits_{x \to 1800} R(x) = \lim\limits_{x \to 1800} \frac{(-.0012x^2 + 3x) - \left[-.0012(1800)^2 + 3(1800)\right]}{x - 1800} = \lim\limits_{x \to 1800} \frac{-.0012x^2 + 3x + -1512}{x - 1800} =$
   $= \lim\limits_{x \to 1800} \frac{(x-1800)(-.0012x + .84)}{x - 1800} = -1.32$

   The marginal revenue when producing 1800 units is $-\$1.32$ per unit.

6. $\lim\limits_{x\to -1} f(x) = \lim\limits_{x\to -1} \dfrac{(6-x^2)-(6-(-1)^2)}{x--1} = \lim\limits_{x\to -1} \dfrac{1-x^2}{x+1} = \lim\limits_{x\to -1} \dfrac{(1-x)(1+x)}{x+1} = 2$. The slope of the tangent line is $m = 2$. $f(-1) = 6-(-1)^2 = 5 \Rightarrow$ the tangent line passes through $(-1, 5)$.

    $y - 5 = 2(x-(-1)) = 2x+2$. The equation of the tangent line is $y = 2x + 7$.

7. $f'(9) = \lim\limits_{x\to 9} \dfrac{(\sqrt{x}+2)-(\sqrt{9}+2)}{x-9} = \lim\limits_{x\to 9} \dfrac{\sqrt{x}-3}{(\sqrt{x}-3)(\sqrt{x}+3)} = \dfrac{1}{6}$. $f'(9)$ is $\dfrac{1}{6}$.

8. $x_1 = .5; x_2 = 1.5; x_3 = 2.5; x_4 = 3.5; x_5 = 4.5; f(x_1) = (.5)^2 = .25; f(x_2) = (1.5)^2 = 2.25;$

    $f(x_3) = (2.5)^2 = 6.25; f(x_4) = (3.5)^2 = 12.25; f(x_5) = (4.5)^2 = 20.25$

    $\lim\limits_{x\to 0^-} f(x) = \lim\limits_{x\to 0^-} \sum\limits_{i=1}^{5} f(x_i)\Delta x = (.25)(1)+(2.25)(1)+(6.25)(1)+(12.25)(1)+(20.25)(1) = 41.25$.

    The area is approximately 41.25.

9. Triangle base $= 8$. Triangle height $= 8$. Triangle area $= \dfrac{1}{2}(8)(8) = 32$. Using the formula for the area of a triangle, the area is 32.

10. $\sqrt{9-x^2}$ for $0 \leq x \leq 3$ is a quarter circle with center $(0, 0)$ and radius 3. Area of quarter circle $= \left(\dfrac{1}{4}\right)(\pi)(3)^2 = \dfrac{9\pi}{4}$. The area is $\dfrac{9\pi}{4}$.

Chapter 12 Review Exercises

1. (a) From the graph, $\lim\limits_{x\to 1^-} f(x) = 2$.

    (b) From the graph, $\lim\limits_{x\to 1^+} f(x) = 2$.

    (c) From the graph, $\lim\limits_{x\to 1} f(x) = 2$.

2. (a) From the graph, $\lim\limits_{x\to -1^-} f(x) = -2$.

    (b) From the graph, $\lim\limits_{x\to -1^+} f(x) = 2$.

    (c) From the graph, $\lim\limits_{x\to -1} f(x)$ does not exist.

3. (a) From the graph, $\lim\limits_{x\to 4^-} f(x) = \infty$.

    (b) From the graph, $\lim\limits_{x\to 4^+} f(x) = -\infty$.

    (c) From the graph, $\lim\limits_{x\to 4} f(x)$ does not exist.

4. (a) From the graph, $\lim\limits_{x\to \infty} f(x) = -3$.

(b) From the graph, $\lim\limits_{x \to 0^-} f(x) = -3$.

(c) From the graph, $\lim\limits_{x \to 0^+} f(x) = -3$.

5. $\lim\limits_{x \to 1}(2x^2 - 3x) = 2(1)^2 - 3(1) = -1$. The limit is -1.

6. $\lim\limits_{x \to -1}(x - x^3) = (-1) - (-1)^3 = 0$. The limit is 0.

7. $\lim\limits_{x \to 2}\dfrac{3x+4}{x+3} = \dfrac{3(2)+4}{2+3} = 2$. The limit is 2.

8. $\lim\limits_{x \to 4}\dfrac{x-4}{x^3+5x} = \dfrac{4-4}{4^3+5(4)} = \dfrac{0}{84} = 0$. The limit is 0.

9. $\lim\limits_{x \to -1}\sqrt{5x+21} = \sqrt{5(-1)+21} = 4$. The limit is 4.

10. $\lim\limits_{x \to 2} 27^{(3-x)/(1+x)} = 27^{(3-2)/(1+2)} = 3$. The limit is 3.

11. $\lim\limits_{x \to 1}[\log_2(5x+3)] = \log_2(5(1)+3) = 3$. The limit is 3.

12. $\lim\limits_{x \to -3}(5-9x)^{2/5} = (5-9(-3))^{2/5} = 4$. The limit is 4.

13. $\lim\limits_{x \to 5}\dfrac{2x-10}{5-x} = \lim\limits_{x \to 5}\dfrac{-2(5-x)}{5-x} = -2$. The limit is -2.

14. $\lim\limits_{x \to 6}\dfrac{x^2-36}{x-6} = \lim\limits_{x \to 6}\dfrac{(x-6)(x+6)}{x-6} = 12$. The limit is 12.

15. $\lim\limits_{x \to -3}\dfrac{x^2+2x-3}{x+3} = \lim\limits_{x \to -3}\dfrac{(x+3)(x-1)}{x+3} = -4$. The limit is -4.

16. $\lim\limits_{x \to 1}\dfrac{x^2-2x+1}{x-1} = \lim\limits_{x \to 1}\dfrac{(x-1)(x-1)}{x-1} = 0$. The limit is 0.

17. $\lim\limits_{x \to 2}\dfrac{x^2-x-2}{x^2-5x+6} = \lim\limits_{x \to 2}\dfrac{(x-2)(x+1)}{(x-2)(x-3)} = \dfrac{3}{-1} = -3$. The limit is -3.

18. $\lim\limits_{x \to -2}\dfrac{x^3+3x^2+2x}{x^2+2x} = \lim\limits_{x \to -2}\dfrac{x(x+2)(x+1)}{x(x+2)} = -1$. The limits is -1.

19. $\lim\limits_{x \to 1}\dfrac{x^2+x}{x-1} = \lim\limits_{x \to 1}\dfrac{x(x+1)}{x-1} = \infty$. The limit does not exist.

20. $\lim\limits_{x \to 0}\dfrac{x^2+1}{x} = \infty$. The limit does not exist.

21. $\lim\limits_{x \to 0}\dfrac{\sin x}{3x} = \dfrac{1}{3}\lim\limits_{x \to 0}\dfrac{\sin x}{x} = \dfrac{1}{3}(1) = \dfrac{1}{3}$. The limit is $\dfrac{1}{3}$.

22. Graphing $y_1 = (\sin(1/x))/x$ in the window $-.5 \leq x \leq .5, -20 \leq y \leq 20$ (not shown), it can be seen that

$\dfrac{\sin \frac{1}{x}}{x}$ oscillates wildly as $x \to 0$ Thus, $\lim\limits_{x \to 0} \dfrac{\sin \frac{1}{x}}{x}$ does not exist.

23. Graphing $y_1 = (x\cos x - 1)/x^2$ in the window $-.5 \leq x \leq .5, -100 \leq y \leq 0$ (not shown), it can be seen that

$\lim\limits_{x \to 0} \dfrac{x\cos x - 1}{x^2} = -\infty$ The limits is $-\infty$.

24. $\lim\limits_{x \to 0} \dfrac{\tan x}{2x} = \lim\limits_{x \to 0} \left(\dfrac{\sin x}{\cos x}\right)\left(\dfrac{1}{2x}\right) = \dfrac{1}{2}\lim\limits_{x \to 0}\left(\dfrac{\sin x}{x}\right)\left(\dfrac{1}{\cos x}\right) = \left(\dfrac{1}{2}\right)(1) = \dfrac{1}{2}$. The limit is $\dfrac{1}{2}$.

25. $\lim\limits_{x \to 2^-} f(x) = \lim\limits_{x \to 2^-} (3x - 1) = 5$; $\lim\limits_{x \to 2^+} f(x) = \lim\limits_{x \to 2^+} (x + 3) = 5$; Thus, $\lim\limits_{x \to 2} f(x) = 5$. The limit is 5.

26. $\lim\limits_{x \to 1^-} f(x) = \lim\limits_{x \to 1^-} x^2 = 1$; $\lim\limits_{x \to 1^+} f(x) = \lim\limits_{x \to 1^+} (3x - 2) = 1$; Thus, even though $f(1) = 5$, $\lim\limits_{x \to 1} f(x) = 1$.

The limit is 1.

27. $\lim\limits_{x \to 2^-} f(x) = \lim\limits_{x \to 2^-} (x^2 - 1) = 3$. The limit is 3.

28. $\lim\limits_{x \to 0^+} f(x) = \lim\limits_{x \to 0^+} \sqrt{x} = 0$. The limit is 0.

29. $\lim\limits_{x \to 0^-} f(x) = \lim\limits_{x \to 0^-} \ln(-x) = \lim\limits_{x \to 0^+} \ln(x) = -\infty$. The limit is $-\infty$.

30. $\lim\limits_{x \to 0^-} f(x) = \lim\limits_{x \to 0^-} \left(\dfrac{\sin x}{x}\right) = 1$. The limit is 1.

31. $\lim\limits_{x \to 3^+} (\pi - 1) = \pi - 1$. The limit is $\pi - 1$.

32. $\lim\limits_{x \to -2^-} f(x) = \lim\limits_{x \to -2^-} -5x^3 = -5(-2)^3 = 40$. The limit is 40.

33. Graphing $y_1 = 1/(x - 7)$ in the window $6.5 \leq x \leq 7.5, -100 \leq y \leq 100$ (not shown), shows that

$\lim\limits_{x \to 7^-} \dfrac{1}{x - 7} = -\infty$. The limit is $-\infty$.

34. $x \to -2^+ \Rightarrow x \geq -2 \Rightarrow x + 2 \geq 0 \Rightarrow \lim\limits_{x \to -2^+} \sqrt{x + 2} = \sqrt{-2 + 2} = 0$. The limit is 0.

35. $x \to 1^+ \Rightarrow x \geq 1 \Rightarrow 1 - x \leq 0 \Rightarrow \lim\limits_{x \to 1^+} \sqrt{1 - x}$ does not exist. The limit does not exist.

36. $\lim\limits_{x \to 2^-} (3x - 1) = 3(2) - 1 = 5$. The limit is 5.

37. $\lim\limits_{x \to 1^-} \dfrac{|x - 1|}{x - 1} = \lim\limits_{x \to 1^-} (-1) = -1$. The limit is -1.

38. $\lim\limits_{x \to 2^+} \dfrac{x + 2}{|x + 2|} = \lim\limits_{x \to -2^+} (1) = 1$. The limit is 1.

39. Graphing $y_1 = x/(x-4)^2$ in the window $3.5 \leq x \leq 4.5, 0 \leq y \leq 1000$ (not shown), shows that

$$\lim_{x \to 4^+} \frac{x}{(x-4)^2} = \infty.$$ The limit is ∞.

40. Graphing $y_1 = x/(x-4)^2$ in the window $3.5 \leq x \leq 4.5, 0 \leq y \leq 1000$ (not shown), shows that

$$\lim_{x \to 4^-} \frac{x}{(x-4)^2} = \infty.$$ The limit is ∞.

41. Graphing $y_1 = x^2/(x-1)^3$ in the window $.75 \leq x \leq 1.25, -10,000 \leq y \leq 10,000$ (not shown), shows that

$$\lim_{x \to 1^+} \frac{x^2}{(x-1)^3} = \infty.$$ The limit is ∞.

42. Graphing $y_1 = x^2/(x-1)^3$ in the window $.75 \leq x \leq 1.25, -10,000 \leq y \leq 10,000$ (not shown), shows that

$$\lim_{x \to 1^-} \frac{x^2}{(x-1)^3} = -\infty.$$ The limit is $-\infty$.

43. $\lim\limits_{x \to \infty} \dfrac{5x+1}{2x-7} = \lim\limits_{x \to \infty} \dfrac{5+\frac{1}{x}}{2-\frac{7}{x}} = \dfrac{5}{2}$. The limit is $\dfrac{5}{2}$.

44. $\lim\limits_{x \to \infty} \dfrac{4x^2 - 5x}{2x^2} = \lim\limits_{x \to \infty} \dfrac{4 - \frac{5}{x}}{2} = \dfrac{4}{2} = 2$. The limit is 2.

45. $\lim\limits_{x \to -\infty} \dfrac{x^3 + 1}{x^2 - 1} = \lim\limits_{x \to -\infty} \dfrac{x + \frac{1}{x^2}}{1 + \frac{1}{x^2}} = -\infty$. The limit is $-\infty$.

46. $\lim\limits_{x \to -\infty} \dfrac{x^4 + x + 1}{x^5 - 2} = \lim\limits_{x \to -\infty} \dfrac{\frac{1}{x} + \frac{1}{x^4} + \frac{1}{x^5}}{1 + \frac{2}{x^5}} = \dfrac{0}{1} = 0$. The limit is 0.

47. $\lim\limits_{x \to \infty} \left(5 + \dfrac{x}{1+x^2}\right) = 5 + \lim\limits_{x \to \infty} \left(\dfrac{\frac{1}{x}}{\frac{1}{x^2}+1}\right) = 5 + 0 = 5$. The limit is 5.

48. $\lim\limits_{x \to \infty} \left(e^{-2x} + 7\right) = \lim\limits_{x \to \infty} e^{-2x} + 7 = 0 + 7 = 7$. This limit is 7.

49. $\lim\limits_{x \to \infty} \left(2 - \dfrac{3}{1-e^{-x}}\right) = 2 - \dfrac{3}{1 - \lim\limits_{x \to \infty} e^{-x}} = 2 - 3 = -1$. The limit is -1.

50. $\lim\limits_{x \to \infty} \left(\dfrac{5}{1+2^{-x}} - 3\right) = \dfrac{5}{1 - \lim\limits_{x \to \infty} 2^{-x}} - 3 = 5 - 3 = 2$. The limit is 2.

51. $\lim\limits_{x \to \infty} f(t) = 70 + 110 \lim\limits_{x \to \infty} e^{-.25t} = 70$ In the time, the coffee ultimately cools to $70°$.

52. The functions $f(x) = x^2$ and $g(x) = x$ have the properties that $\lim_{x \to \infty} f(x) = \infty$, $\lim_{x \to \infty} g(x) = \infty$, and $\lim_{x \to \infty} \frac{f(x)}{g(x)} = \infty$.

53. The functions $f(x) = \frac{1}{x-2}$ and $g(x) = -\frac{1}{x-2}$ have the properties that neither $\lim_{x \to 2} f(x)$ nor $\lim_{x \to 2} g(x)$ exists, but $\lim_{x \to 2} [f(x) + g(x)] = 0$ does exists.

54. $m = \lim_{x \to 3} \frac{(1+x^2)-(1+3^2)}{x-3} = \lim_{x \to 3} \frac{x^2-9}{x-3} = \lim_{x \to 3} \frac{(x-3)(x+3)}{x-3} = 6$. The slope of the tangent line to $f(x)$ at $x = 3$ is 6.

55. $m = \lim_{x \to 1} \frac{\frac{3}{x} - \frac{3}{1}}{x-1} = \lim_{x \to 1} \frac{\frac{3-3x}{x}}{x-1} = \lim_{x \to 1} \frac{\frac{-3(x-1)}{x}}{x-1} = -3$. The slope of the tangent line to $f(x)$ at $x = 1$ is -3.

56. $m = \lim_{x \to 2} \frac{\frac{4}{x} - \frac{4}{2}}{x-2} = \lim_{x \to 2} \frac{\frac{-2(x-2)}{x}}{x-2} = -1$ $f(2) = \frac{4}{2} = 2$; $y - 2 = -1(x-2) = -x+2$. The equation of the tangent line is $y = -x + 4$. Graphing $y_1 = 4/x$ and $y_2 = -x + 4$ in the window $0 \le x \le 4, 0 \le y \le 10$ (not shown), shows this to be so.

57. $m = \lim_{x \to 2} \frac{(x^2-x)-(2^2-2)}{x-2} = \lim_{x \to 2} \frac{x^2-x-2}{x-2} = \lim_{x \to 2} \frac{(x-2)(x+1)}{x-2} = 3$. $f(2) = 2^2 - 2 = 2$; $y - 2 = 3(x-2) = 3x - 6$. The equation of the tangent line is $y = 3x - 4$. Graphing $y_1 = x^2 - x$ and $y_2 = 3x - 4$ in the window $0 \le x \le 4, -5 \le y \le 10$ (not shown), shows this to be so.

58. $\lim_{x \to 4} \frac{\sqrt{x}-2}{x-4}$ will be the slope of the tangent line to $f(x) = \sqrt{x}$ at the point $(4, 2)$ From the figure, this slope is .25. Thus, $\lim_{x \to 4} \frac{\sqrt{x}-2}{x-4} = .25$.

59. $f'\left(\frac{\pi}{2}\right)$ will be the slope of the tangent line to $f(x) = \sin x$ at the point $\left(\frac{\pi}{2}, 1\right)$ From the figure, this slope is 0. Thus, $f'\left(\frac{\pi}{2}\right) = 0$.

60. nDeriv $(x \sin x, x, \pi) = -3.14159212999 \approx -\pi$. The value of $f'(\pi)$ is $-\pi$.

61. nDeriv $(e^x, x, 0) = 1.00000016667 \approx 1$. The value of $f'(0)$ is 1.

62. The tangent line passes through the points (40, 150) and (80, 400). Thus, the slope of the tangent line is

$m = \frac{400 - 150}{80 - 40} = 6.25$. The average farm size was increasing by 6.25 acres per year on January 1, 1950.

63. $S(t) = -16t^2 + 100t + 4$;

$$S'(3) = \lim_{t \to 3} \frac{\left(-16t^2 + 100t + 4\right) - \left[-16(3)^2 + 100(3) + 4\right]}{t-3} = \lim_{t \to 3} \frac{-16t^2 + 100t - 156}{t-3} =$$

$$\lim_{t \to 3} \frac{(t-3)(-16t+52)}{t-3} = 4$$ The velocity of the ball when $t = 3$ seconds is 4 feet per second.

64. $\text{nDeriv}\left(.006x^3 - .7x^2 + 32x + 250, x, 72\right) = 24.512$. The marginal cost at $x = 72$ units is \$2451.20 per unit.

65. $f(x_1) = 3(-1) + 1 = -2$; $f(x_2) = 3(0) + 1 = 1$; $f(x_3) = 3(1) + 1 = 4$; $f(x_4) = 3(2) + 1 = 7$;

$f(x_5) = 3(3) + 1 = 10$; $\sum_{i=1}^{5} f(x_i) \Delta x = (-2)(1) + (1)(1) + (4)(1) + (7)(1) + (10)(1) = 20$. The sum is 20.

66. $\int_0^3 f(x) dx$ = area of a trapezoid. Height of the trapezoid $= 3$, first base of the trapezoid $= 2$ second base of the trapezoid $= 1$, area of the trapezoid $= \left(\frac{1}{2}\right)(3)(2+1) = \frac{9}{2}$. Thus, the value of $\int_0^3 f(x) dx$ is $\frac{9}{2} = 4.5$.

67. $x_1 = 0$; $x_2 = 1$; $x_3 = 2$; $x_4 = 3$; $f(x_1) = 2(0) + 3 = 3$; $f(x_2) = 2(1) + 3 = 5$;

$f(x_3) = 2(2)3 = 7$; $f(x_4) = 2(3) + 3 = 9$; $\sum_{i=1}^{4} f(x_i)\Delta x = 3(1) + 5(1) + 7(1) + 9(1) = 24$.

The area is approximately 24.

68. Height of the trapezoid $=4$, first base of the trapezoid $=2(4)+3=11$, second base of the trapezoid $= 2(0) + 3 = 3$, area of the trapezoid $= \left(\frac{1}{2}\right)(4)(11+3) = 28$. The area is 28, which is 4 greater than the approximation in exercise 67. We also conclude that the value of $\int_0^4 (2x+3) dx$ is 28.

69. Height of the triangle $= 5$, and the base of the triangle $= 5$. Thus, the area of the triangle $= \left(\frac{1}{2}\right)(5)(5) = \frac{25}{2} = 12.5$ Thus, we conclude that the value of $\int_0^5 (5-x) dx$ is 12.5.

70. $\sqrt{1-x^2}$ for $0 \leq x \leq 1$ is a quarter of a circle centered at (0, 0) with radius 1. The area of the quarter circle is $\left(\frac{1}{4}\right)(\pi)(1)^2 = \frac{\pi}{4}$. Thus, we conclude that the value of $\int_0^1 \sqrt{1-x^2} dx$ is $\frac{\pi}{4}$.

Chapter 12 Test

1. From the graph, we see that $\lim_{x \to 4^-} f(x)$ is 5.

2. From the graph, we see that $\lim_{x \to \infty} f(x)$ is 0.

3. (a) From the graph, we see that $\lim_{x \to 3^+} f(x)$ is ∞.

(b) From the graph, we see that $\lim\limits_{x \to 3^-} f(x)$ is 4.

4. $\lim\limits_{x \to 1} \dfrac{x^2 + x + 1}{x^2 + 1} = \dfrac{1^2 + 1 + 1}{1^2 + 1} = \dfrac{3}{2}$ The limit is $\dfrac{3}{2}$.

5. $\lim\limits_{x \to -2} \dfrac{x^2 + 2x}{x + 2} = \lim\limits_{x \to -2} \dfrac{x(x+2)}{x+2} = -2$. The limit is -2.

6. $\lim\limits_{x \to 3} \dfrac{x^2 - 6x + 9}{x - 3} = \lim\limits_{x \to 3} \dfrac{(x-3)(x-3)}{x-3} = 0$. The limit is 0.

7. $\lim\limits_{x \to 2} \dfrac{x^2 + x - 6}{x^2 - 4} = \lim\limits_{x \to 2} \dfrac{(x-2)(x+3)}{(x-2)(x+2)} = \dfrac{5}{4}$. The limit is $\dfrac{5}{4}$.

8. $\lim\limits_{x \to 3} \sqrt{x^2 + 7} = \sqrt{3^2 + 7} = 4$. The limit is 4.

9. $\lim\limits_{x \to \infty} \dfrac{2x^2 - 3}{5x^2 + x + 1} = \lim\limits_{x \to \infty} \dfrac{2 - \frac{3}{x^2}}{5 + \frac{1}{x} + \frac{1}{x^2}} = \dfrac{2}{5}$. The limit is $\dfrac{2}{5}$.

10. $\lim\limits_{x \to -\infty} \dfrac{3x - 4}{4x - 3} = \lim\limits_{x \to -\infty} \dfrac{3 - \frac{4}{x}}{4 - \frac{3}{x}} = \dfrac{3}{4}$. The limit is $\dfrac{3}{4}$.

11. $\lim\limits_{x \to 0} \dfrac{\sin x}{x \cos x} = \left(\lim\limits_{x \to 0} \dfrac{\sin x}{x} \right)\left(\lim\limits_{x \to 0} \dfrac{1}{\cos x} \right) = (1)(1) = 1$. The limit is 1.

12. $\lim\limits_{x \to 0} \dfrac{x^2 - 10}{x^3 + 1} = \dfrac{0^2 - 10}{0^3 + 1} = -10$. The limit is -10.

13. $\lim\limits_{x \to 1^+} f(x) = \lim\limits_{x \to 1^+} (1 - 2x^2) = 1 - 2(1)^2 = -1$ The limit is -1.

14. $\lim\limits_{x \to 4^+} 55 = 55$. The limit is 55.

15. $\lim\limits_{x \to 3^-} (4x^2 - 3x) = 4(3)^2 - 3(3) = 27$. The limit is 27.

16. For $x > 2$, $2 - x < 0$. Thus, $\lim\limits_{x \to 2^+} \sqrt{2 - x}$ does not exist.

17. $\lim\limits_{x \to 3^-} \dfrac{|3 - x|}{3 - x} = 1$. The limit is 1.

18. For $x > -1$, $x + 1 > 0$. Thus, $\lim\limits_{x \to -1^+} \sqrt{x+1} = \sqrt{-1+1} = 0$. The limit is 0.

19. Since we are looking at evaluating the limit as x approaches from the right, we will evaluate the function when $x > 1$. $\lim\limits_{x \to 1^+} f(x) = 1 - 2(1)^2 = 1 - 2 = -1$.

20. Evaluate the limit as x approaches from both the left and the right.

$$\lim_{x \to 3^+} f(x) = 3(3) - 1 = 9 - 1 = 8, \quad \lim_{x \to 3^-} f(x) = 2(3) + 1 = 6 + 1 = 7$$

Since the limit as x approaches 3 from the left is not equal to the limit as x approaches from the right, the limit as x approaches 3 of $f(x)$ does not exist.

21. $m = \lim_{x \to 1} \dfrac{(2x^2 - 1) - (2(1)^2 - 1)}{x - 1} = \lim_{x \to 1} \dfrac{2x^2 - 2}{x - 1} = \lim_{x \to 1} \dfrac{2(x-1)(x+1)}{x-1} = 4$. The slope is 4.

22. $m = \lim_{x \to 1} \dfrac{\frac{-3}{x} - \left(\frac{-3}{1}\right)}{x - 1} = \lim_{x \to 1} \dfrac{\frac{3(x-1)}{x}}{x - 1} = 3$. $y + 3 = 3(x - 1) = 3x - 3$. The equation of the tangent line is $y = 3x - 6$.

23. $\text{nDeriv}\left((1 + e^x)/x, x, 4\right) = 10.174654336$. $f'(4)$ is approximately 10.1747.

24. The tangent line passes through the points $(14, .80)$ and $(22, 0)$. Thus, the slope of the tangent line is

    $m = \dfrac{0 - .8}{22 - 14} = -.1$ At $t = 14$ years, the cobalt is disintegrating at a rate of $\dfrac{1}{10}$ gram per year.

25. The graph of $y_1 = 4{,}000\left(1 - e^{-.25x}\right)$ in the window $0 \le x \le 36$, $0 \le y \le 45{,}000$ is shown in Figure 25.

    $\text{nDeriv}\left(40{,}000\left(1 - e^{-.25x}\right), x, 3\right) \approx 4723.67$. When $t = 3$ days, the information is spreading at a rate of approximately 4724 persons per day.

[0,36] by [0,45,000]
Xscl = 6   Yscl = 10000

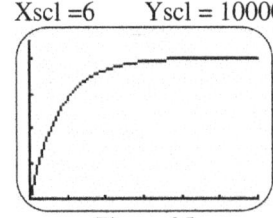

Figure 25

26. $x_1 = .5$; $x_2 = 1.5$; $x_3 = 2.5$; $x_4 = 3.5$; $f(x_1) = (.5)^2 = .25$; $f(x_2) = (1.5)^2 = 2.25$; $f(x_3) = (2.5)^2 = 6.25$;

    $f(x_4) = (3.5)^2 = 12.25$; $\sum_{i=1}^{4} f(x_i) \Delta x = (.25)(1) + (2.25)(1) + (6.25)(1) + (12.25)(1) = 21$. The area is approximately 21.

27. Height of the triangle is 6 and the base of the triangle is 6.

    Thus, the area of the triangle is $\left(\dfrac{1}{2}\right)(6)(6) = \dfrac{36}{2} = 18$. We conclude that the value of $\int_0^6 (6 - x)\,dx$ is 18.

28. $\int_{-2}^{2} \sqrt{4 - x^2}$ is equivalent to finding the area of the semi circle centered at the origin with a radius of 2.

    $A = \dfrac{1}{2}\pi(2)^2 = 2\pi$

Chapter R: Reference: Basic Algebraic Concepts

R.1: Review of Exponents and Polynomials

1. $(-4)^3 \cdot (-4)^2 = (-4)^{3+2} = (-4)^5$

3. $2^0 = 1$

5. $(5m)^0 = 1$, if $m \neq 0$

7. $(2^2)^5 = 2^{2 \cdot 5} = 2^{10}$

9. $(2x^5 y^4)^3 = 2^3 (x^5)^3 (y^4)^3 = 2^3 x^{15} y^{12}$ or $8x^{15} y^{12}$

11. $-\left(\dfrac{p^4}{q}\right)^2 = -\left(\dfrac{p^{4 \cdot 2}}{q^2}\right) = -\dfrac{p^8}{q^2}$

13. $-5x^{11}$ is a polynomial. It is a monomial since it has one term. It has degree 11 since 11 is the highest exponent.

15. $18p^5 q + 6pq$ is a polynomial. It is a binomial since it has two terms. It has degree 6 since 6 is the sum of the exponents in the term $18p^5 q$. (The term $6pq$ has degree 2.)

17. $\sqrt{2}x^2 + \sqrt{3}x^6$ is a polynomial. It is a binomial since it has two terms. It has degree 6 since 6 is the highest exponent.

19. $\dfrac{1}{3}r^2 s^2 - \dfrac{3}{5}r^4 s^2 + rs^3$ is a polynomial. It is a trinomial since it has three terms. It has degree 6 since 6 is the sum of the exponents in the term $-\dfrac{3}{5}r^4 s^2$. (The other terms have degree 4.)

21. $-5\sqrt{z} + 2\sqrt{z^3} - 5\sqrt{z^5} = -5z^{1/2} + 2z^{3/2} - 5z^{5/2}$ is not a polynomial since the exponents are not integers.

23. $(4m^3 - 3m^2 + 5) + (-3m^3 - m^2 + 5) = (4m^3 - 3m^3) + (-3m^2 - m^2) + (5 + 5) = m^3 - 4m^2 + 10$

25. $(8p^2 - 5p) - (3p^2 - 2p + 4) = 8p^2 - 5p - 3p^2 + 2p - 4 = 5p^2 - 3p - 4$

27. $-(8x^3 + x - 3) + (2x^3 + x^2) - (4x^2 + 3x - 1) = -8x^3 - x + 3 + 2x^3 + x^2 - 4x^2 - 3x + 1 = -6x^3 - 3x^2 - 4x + 4$

29. $(5m - 6)(3m + 4) = 5m \cdot 3m + 5m \cdot 4 - 6 \cdot 3m - 6 \cdot 4 = 15m^2 + 20m - 18m - 24 = 15m^2 + 2m - 24$

31. $\left(2m - \dfrac{1}{4}\right)\left(3m + \dfrac{1}{2}\right) = 2m \cdot 3m + 2m \cdot \dfrac{1}{2} - \dfrac{1}{4} \cdot 3m - \dfrac{1}{4} \cdot \dfrac{1}{2} = 6m^2 + m - \dfrac{3}{4}m - \dfrac{1}{8} = 6m^2 + \dfrac{1}{4}m - \dfrac{1}{8}$

33. $2b^3(b^2 - 4b + 3) = 2b^3 \cdot b^2 + 2b^3 \cdot (-4b) + 2b^3 \cdot 3 = 2b^5 - 8b^4 + 6b^3$

35. $(m - n + k)(m + 2n - 3k) = m^2 + 2mn - 3km - mn - 2n^2 + 3kn + km + 2kn - 3k^2 = m^2 + mn - 2km - 2n^2 + 5kn - 3k^2$

37. To find the square of a binomial, find the sum of the square of the first term, twice the product of the two terms, and the square of the last term.

616   Chapter R: Reference: Basic Algebraic Concepts

39. $(2m+3)(2m-3) = (2m)^2 - (3)^2 = 4m^2 - 9$

41. $(4m+2n)^2 = (4m)^2 + 2(4m)(2n) + (2n)^2 = 16m^2 + 16mn + 4n^2$

43. $(5r+3t^2)^2 = (5r)^2 + 2(5r)(3t^2) + (3t^2)^2 = 25r^2 + 30rt^2 + 9t^4$

45. $[(2p-3)+q]^2 = (2p-3)^2 + 2(2p-3)(q) + (q)^2 = [(2p)^2 - 2(2p)(3) + 3^2] + 4pq - 6q + q^2 =$
    $4p^2 - 12p + 9 + 4pq - 6q + q^2$

47. $[(3q+5)-p][(3q+5)+p] = (3q+5)^2 - (p)^2 = [(3q)^2 + 2(3q)(5) + (5)^2] - p^2 = 9q^2 + 30q + 25 - p^2$

49. $[(3a+b)-1]^2 = (3a+b)^2 - 2(3a+b)(1) + (-1)^2 = [(3a)^2 + 2(3a)(b) + (b)^2] - 6a - 2b + 1 =$
    $9a^2 + 6ab + b^2 - 6a - 2b + 1$

51. $(6p+5q)(3p-7q) = (6p)(3p) + (6p)(-7q) + (5q)(3p) + (5q)(-7q) = 18p^2 - 42pq + 15pq - 35q^2 =$
    $18p^2 - 27pq - 35q^2$

53. $(p^3 - 4p^2 + p) - (3p^2 + 2p + 7) = p^3 - 4p^2 + p - 3p^2 - 2p - 7 = p^3 - 7p^2 - p - 7$

55. $y(4x+3y)(4x-3y) = y[(4x)^2 - (3y)^2] = y[16x^2 - 9y^2] = 16x^2y - 9y^3$

57. $(2z+y)(3z-4y) = (2z)(3z) + (2z)(-4y) + (y)(3z) + (y)(-4y) = 6z^2 - 8yz + 3yz - 4y^2 = 6x^2 - 5yz - 4y^2$

59. $(3p+5)^2 = (3p)^2 + 2(3p)(5) + 5^2 = 9p^2 + 30p + 25$

61. $p(4p-6) + 2(3p-8) = 4p^2 - 6p + 6p - 16 = 4p^2 - 16$

63. $-y(y^2 - 4) + 6y^2(2y - 3) = -y^3 + 4y + 12y^3 - 18y^2 = 11y^3 - 18y^2 + 4y$

R.2: Review of Factoring

1. (a) $(x+5y)^2 = x^2 + 10xy + 25y^2$; B

    (b) $(x-5y)^2 = x^2 - 10xy + 25y^2$; C

    (c) $(x+5y)(x-5y) = x^2 - 25y^2$; A

    (d) $(5y+x)(5y-x) = 25y^2 - x^2$; D

3. $4k^2m^3 + 8k^4m^3 - 12k^2m^4 = 4k^2m^3(1 + 2k^2 - 3m)$

5. $2(a+b) + 4m(a+b) = (a+b)(2+4m) = 2(a+b)(1+2m)$

7. $(2y-3)(y+2) + (y+5)(y+2) = (y+2)(2y-3+y+5) = (y+2)(3y+2)$

9. $(5r-6)(r+3) - (2r-1)(r+3) = (r+3)(5r-6-(2r-1)) = (r+3)(3r-5)$

11. $2(m-1)-3(m-1)^2+2(m-1)^3 = (m-1)\left(2-3(m-1)+2(m-1)^2\right) =$
    $(m-1)\left(2-3m+3+2\left(m^2-2m+1\right)\right) = (m-1)\left(5-3m+2m^2-4m+2\right) = (m-1)\left(2m^2-7m+7\right)$

13. $6st+9t-10s-15 = 3t(2s+3)-5(2s+3) = (2s+3)(3t-5)$

15. $10x^2-12y+15x-8xy = 10x^2+15x-8xy-12y = 5x(2x+3)-4y(2x+3) = (2x+3)(5x-4y)$

17. $t^3+2t^2-3t-6 = t^2(t+2)-3(t+2) = (t+2)\left(t^2-3\right)$

19. $(8a-3)(2a-5) = \left[-1(-8a+3)\right]\left[-1(-2a+5)\right] = (3-8a)(5-2a)$; Both are correct.

21. $8h^2-24h-320 = 8\left(h^2-3h-40\right) = 8(h-8)(h+5)$

23. $9y^4-54y^3+45y^2 = 9y^2\left(y^2-6y+5\right) = 9y^2(y-1)(y-5)$

25. $14m^2+11mr-15r^2 = (7m-5r)(2m+3r)$

27. $12s^2+11st-5t^2 = (3s-t)(4s+5t)$

29. $30a^2+am-m^2 = (5a+m)(6a-m)$

31. $18x^5+15x^4z-75x^3z^2 = 3x^3\left(6x^2+5xz-25z^2\right) = 3x^3(2x+5z)(3x-5z)$

33. $16p^2-40p+25 = (4p-5)^2$

35. $20p^2-100pq+125q^2 = 5\left(4p^2-20pq+25q^2\right) = 5(2p-5q)^2$

37. $9m^2n^2-12mn+4 = (3mn-2)^2$

39. $(2p+q)^2-10(2p+q)+25 = \left((2p+q)-5\right)\left((2p+q)-5\right) = (2p+q-5)^2$

41. $9a^2-16 = (3a+4)(3a-4)$

43. $25s^4-9t^2 = \left(5s^2+3t\right)\left(5s^2-3t\right)$

45. $(a+b)^2-16 = (a+b+4)(a+b-4)$

47. $p^4-625 = \left(p^2+25\right)\left(p^2-25\right) = \left(p^2+25\right)(p+5)(p-5)$

49. $x^4-1 = \left(x^2+1\right)\left(x^2-1\right) = \left(x^2+1\right)(x+1)(x-1)$; B

51. $8-a^3 = 2^3-a^3 = (2-a)\left(4+2a+a^2\right)$

53. $125x^3-27 = (5x)^3-3^3 = (5x-3)\left(25x^2+15x+9\right)$

55. $27y^9+125z^6 = \left(3y^3\right)^3+\left(5z^2\right)^3 = \left(3y^3+5z^2\right)\left(9y^6-15y^3z^2+25z^4\right)$

57. $(r+6)^3-216 = (r+6)^3-6^3 = (r+6-6)\left((r+6)^2+6(r+6)+36\right) =$
    $r\left(r^2+12r+36+6r+36+36\right) = r\left(r^2+18r+108\right)$

59. $27-(m+2n)^3 = 3^3 -(m+2n)^3 = (3-(m+2n))(9+3(m+2n)+(m+2n)^2)$

$(3-m-2n)(9+3m+6n+m^2+4mn+4n^2)$

61. $3a^4+14a^2-5$; Let $u=a^2 \Rightarrow 3u^2+14u-5=(3u-1)(u+5)$. Then $a^2=u \Rightarrow (3a^2-1)(a^2+5)$ was not substituted back in for u.

63. a^4-2a^2-48; Let $u=a^2 \Rightarrow u^2-2u-48=(u-8)(u+6)$. Then $a^2=u \Rightarrow (a^2-8)(a^2+6)$.

65. $6(4z-3)^2+7(4z-3)-3$; Let $u=4z-3 \Rightarrow 6u^2+7u-3=(3u-1)(2u+3)$. Then

$4z-3=u \Rightarrow (3(4z-3)-1)(2(4z-3)+3) = (12z-10)(8z-3) = 2(6z-5)(8z-3)$.

67. $20(4-p)^2-3(4-p)-2$; Let $u=4-p \Rightarrow 20u^2-3u-2=(5u-2)(4u+1)$. Then

$4-p=u \Rightarrow (5(4-p)-2)(4(4-p)+1) = (18-5p)(17-4p)$.

69. $4b^2+4bc+c^2-16 = (4b^2+4b+c^2)-16 = (2b+c)^2-16 = (2b+c+4)(2b+c-4)$.

71. $x^2+xy-5y-5y = x(x+y)-5(x+y) = (x+y)(x-5)$

73. $p^4(m-2n)+q(m-2n) = (m-2n)(p^4+q)$

75. $4z^2+28z+49 = (2z+7)^2$

77. $1000x^3+343y^3 = (10x)^3+7(y)^3 = (10x+7y)(100x^2-70xy+49y^2)$

79. $125m^6-216 = (5m^2)^3-6^3 = (5m^2-6)(25m^4+30m^2+36)$

81. $12m^2+16mn-35n^2 = (6m-7n)(2m+5n)$

83. $4p^2+3p-1 = (4p-1)(p+1)$

85. $144z^2+121$ does not factor, it is prime.

87. $(4t+5)^2+16(4t+5)+64$; Let $u=4t+5 \Rightarrow u^2+16u+64 = (u+8)^2$ Then

$4t+5=u \Rightarrow (4t+5+8)^2 = (4t+13)^2$

R.3: Review of Rational Expressions

1. $\dfrac{x-2}{x+6}$; $x+6=0, \{x \mid x \neq -6\}$

3. $\dfrac{2x}{5x-3}$; $5x-3=0, \left\{x \mid x \neq \dfrac{3}{5}\right\}$

5. $\dfrac{-8}{x^2+1}$; No restrictions since $x^2+1 > 0$. Domain: $(-\infty, \infty)$

7. $\dfrac{3x+7}{(4x+2)(x-1)}$; $4x+2=0 \Rightarrow 4x=-2 \Rightarrow x=-\dfrac{2}{4}=-\dfrac{1}{2}$ and $x-1=0 \Rightarrow x=1$; $\left\{x \mid x \neq -\dfrac{1}{2}, 1\right\}$

9. $\dfrac{25p^3}{10p^2} = \dfrac{5p^2(5p)}{5p^2(2)} = \dfrac{5p}{2}$

11. $\dfrac{8k+16}{9k+18} = \dfrac{8(k+2)}{9(k+2)} = \dfrac{8}{9}$

13. $\dfrac{3(t+5)}{(t+5)(t-3)} = \dfrac{3}{t-3}$

15. $\dfrac{8x^2+16x}{4x^2} = \dfrac{8x(x+2)}{4x^2} = \dfrac{2(x+2)}{x} = \dfrac{2x+4}{x}$

17. $\dfrac{m^2-4m+4}{m^2+m-6} = \dfrac{(m-2)^2}{(m-2)(m+3)} = \dfrac{m-2}{m+3}$

19. $\dfrac{8m^2+6m-9}{16m^2-9} = \dfrac{(4m-3)(2m+3)}{(4m-3)(4m+3)} = \dfrac{2m+3}{4m+3}$

21. $\dfrac{15p^3}{9p^2} \div \dfrac{6p}{10p^2} = \dfrac{15p^3}{9p^2} \cdot \dfrac{10p^2}{6p} = \dfrac{25p^2}{9}$

23. $\dfrac{2k+8}{6} \div \dfrac{3k+12}{2} = \dfrac{2(k+4)}{6} \times \dfrac{2}{3(k+4)} = \dfrac{2}{9}$

25. $\dfrac{x^2+x}{5} \cdot \dfrac{25}{xy+y} = \dfrac{x(x+1)}{5} \cdot \dfrac{25}{y(x+1)} = \dfrac{5x}{y}$

27. $\dfrac{4a+12}{2a-10} \div \dfrac{a^2-9}{a^2-a-20} = \dfrac{4(a+3)}{2(a-5)} \cdot \dfrac{(a+4)(a-5)}{(a-3)(a+3)} = \dfrac{2(a+4)}{a-3}$

29. $\dfrac{p^2-p-12}{p^2-2p-15} \cdot \dfrac{p^2-9p+20}{p^2-8p+16} = \dfrac{(p-4)(p+3)}{(p+3)(p-5)} \cdot \dfrac{(p-5)(p-4)}{(p-4)(p-4)} = 1$

31. $\dfrac{m^2+3m+2}{m^2+5m+4} \div \dfrac{m^2+5m+6}{m^2+10m+24} = \dfrac{(m+2)(m+1)}{(m+4)(m+1)} \cdot \dfrac{(m+4)(m+6)}{(m+3)(m+2)} = \dfrac{m+6}{m+3}$

33. $\dfrac{2m^2-5m-12}{m^2-10m+24} \div \dfrac{4m^2-9}{m^2-9m+18} = \dfrac{(2m+3)(m-4)}{(m-4)(m-6)} \cdot \dfrac{(m-3)(m-6)}{(2m+3)(2m-3)} = \dfrac{m-3}{2m-3}$

35. $\dfrac{x^3+y^3}{x^2-y^2} \cdot \dfrac{x+y}{x^2-xy+y^2} = \dfrac{(x+y)(x^2-xy+y^2)}{(x+y)(x-y)} \cdot \dfrac{x+y}{x^2-xy+y^2} = \dfrac{x+y}{x-y}$

37. $\dfrac{x^3+y^3}{x^3-y^3} \cdot \dfrac{x^2-y^2}{x^2+2xy+y^2} = \dfrac{(x+y)(x^2-xy+y^2)}{(x-y)(x^2+xy+y^2)} \cdot \dfrac{(x-y)(x+y)}{(x+y)(x+y)} = \dfrac{x^2-xy+y^2}{x^2+xy+y^2}$

39. A: $\dfrac{x-4}{x+4} \neq -1$, B: $\dfrac{-x-4}{x+4} = \dfrac{-1(x+4)}{x+4} = -1$, C: $\dfrac{x-4}{4-x} = \dfrac{x-4}{-1(x-4)} = -1$, D: $\dfrac{x-4}{-x-4} = \dfrac{x-4}{-1(x+4)} \neq -1$

41. $\dfrac{3}{2k}+\dfrac{5}{3k}=\dfrac{9}{6k}+\dfrac{10}{6k}=\dfrac{19}{6k}$

43. $\dfrac{a+1}{2}-\dfrac{a-1}{2}=\dfrac{a+1-(a-1)}{2}=\dfrac{2}{2}=1$

45. $\dfrac{3}{p}+\dfrac{1}{2}=\dfrac{6}{2p}+\dfrac{p}{2p}=\dfrac{6+p}{2p}$

47. $\dfrac{1}{6m}+\dfrac{2}{5m}+\dfrac{4}{m}=\dfrac{5(1)+6(2)+30(4)}{30m}=\dfrac{5+12+120}{30m}=\dfrac{137}{30m}$

49. $\dfrac{1}{a+1}-\dfrac{1}{a-1}=\dfrac{a-1-(a+1)}{(a+1)(a-1)}=\dfrac{-2}{(a+1)(a-1)}$

51. $\dfrac{m+1}{m-1}+\dfrac{m-1}{m+1}=\dfrac{(m+1)^2+(m-1)^2}{(m-1)(m+1)}=\dfrac{m^2+2m+1+m^2-2m+1}{(m-1)(m+1)}=\dfrac{2m^2+2}{(m-1)(m+1)}$

53. $\dfrac{3}{a-2}-\dfrac{1}{2-a}=\dfrac{3}{a-2}-\dfrac{-1}{a-2}=\dfrac{3+1}{a-2}=\dfrac{4}{a-2}$ or $\dfrac{-4}{2-a}$

55. $\dfrac{x+y}{2x-y}-\dfrac{2x}{y-2x}=\dfrac{x+y}{2x-y}-\dfrac{-2x}{2x-y}=\dfrac{x+y+2x}{2x-y}=\dfrac{3x+y}{2x-y}$ or $\dfrac{-3x-y}{y-2x}$

57. $\dfrac{1}{a^2-5a+6}-\dfrac{1}{a^2-4}=\dfrac{1}{(a-2)(a-3)}-\dfrac{1}{(a-2)(a+2)}=\dfrac{1(a+2)-1(a-3)}{(a-2)(a-3)(a+2)}=$

$\dfrac{a+2-a+3}{(a-2)(a-3)(a+2)}=\dfrac{5}{(a-2)(a-3)(a+2)}$

59. $\dfrac{1}{x^2+x-12}-\dfrac{1}{x^2-7x+12}+\dfrac{1}{x^2-16}=\dfrac{1}{(x+4)(x-3)}-\dfrac{1}{(x-3)(x-4)}+\dfrac{1}{(x-4)(x+4)}=$

$\dfrac{1(x-4)-1(x+4)+1(x-3)}{(x+4)(x-3)(x-4)}=\dfrac{x-4-x-4+x-3}{(x+4)(x-3)(x-4)}=\dfrac{x-11}{(x+4)(x-3)(x-4)}$

61. $\dfrac{3a}{a^2+5a-6}-\dfrac{2a}{a^2+7a+6}=\dfrac{3a}{(a+6)(a-1)}-\dfrac{2a}{(a+6)(a+1)}=\dfrac{3a(a+1)-2a(a-1)}{(a+6)(a-1)(a+1)}=$

$\dfrac{3a^2+3a-2a^2+2a}{(a+6)(a-1)(a+1)}=\dfrac{a^2+5a}{(a+6)(a-1)(a+1)}$

63. $\dfrac{1+\frac{1}{x}}{1-\frac{1}{x}}=\dfrac{x(1+\frac{1}{x})}{x(1-\frac{1}{x})}=\dfrac{x+1}{x-1}$

65. $\dfrac{\frac{1}{x+1}-\frac{1}{x}}{\frac{1}{x}}=\dfrac{x(x+1)(\frac{1}{x+1}-\frac{1}{x})}{x(x+1)(\frac{1}{x})}=\dfrac{x-(x+1)}{x+1}=\dfrac{-1}{x+1}$

67. $\dfrac{1+\frac{1}{1-b}}{1-\frac{1}{1+b}}=\dfrac{(1-b)(1+b)(1+\frac{1}{1-b})}{(1-b)(1+b)(1-\frac{1}{1+b})}=\dfrac{(1-b)(1+b)+(1+b)}{(1-b)(1-b)-(1-b)}=\dfrac{1-b^2+1+b}{1-b^2-1+b}=\dfrac{-b^2+b+2}{-b^2+b}=\dfrac{(2-b)(1+b)}{b(1-b)}$

69. $\dfrac{m - \frac{1}{m^2-4}}{\frac{1}{m+2}} = \dfrac{(m^2-4)\left(m - \frac{1}{m^2-4}\right)}{(m^2-4)\left(\frac{1}{m+2}\right)} = \dfrac{m(m^2-4)-1}{m-2} = \dfrac{m^3 - 4m - 1}{m-2}$

R.4: Review of Negative and Rational Exponents

1. $\left(\dfrac{4}{9}\right)^{3/2} = \left[\left(\dfrac{4}{9}\right)^{1/2}\right]^3 = \left(\dfrac{2}{3}\right)^3 = \dfrac{2^3}{3^3} = \dfrac{8}{27}$; E

3. $-\left(\dfrac{9}{4}\right)^{3/2} = -\left[\left(\dfrac{9}{4}\right)^{1/2}\right]^3 = -\left(\dfrac{3}{2}\right)^3 = -\dfrac{3^3}{2^3} = -\dfrac{27}{8}$; F

5. $\left(\dfrac{8}{27}\right)^{2/3} = \left[\left(\dfrac{8}{27}\right)^{1/3}\right]^2 = \left(\dfrac{2}{3}\right)^2 = \dfrac{2^2}{3^2} = \dfrac{4}{9}$; D

7. $-\left(\dfrac{27}{8}\right)^{2/3} = -\left[\left(\dfrac{27}{8}\right)^{1/3}\right]^2 = -\left(\dfrac{3}{2}\right)^2 = -\dfrac{3^2}{2^2} = -\dfrac{9}{4}$; B

9. $(-4)^{-3} = \left(-\dfrac{1}{4}\right)^3 = -\dfrac{1}{64}$

11. $\left(\dfrac{1}{2}\right)^{-3} = 2^3 = 8$

13. $-4^{1/2} = -(4^{1/2}) = -2$

15. $8^{2/3} = (8^{1/3})^2 = 2^2 = 4$

17. $27^{-2/3} = \left[\left(\dfrac{1}{27}\right)^{1/3}\right]^2 = \left(\dfrac{1}{3}\right)^2 = \dfrac{1}{9}$

19. $\left(\dfrac{27}{64}\right)^{-4/3} = \left[\left(\dfrac{64}{27}\right)^{1/3}\right]^4 = \left(\dfrac{4}{3}\right)^4 = \dfrac{256}{81}$

21. $(16p^4)^{1/2} = 4p^2$

23. $(27x^6)^{2/3} = [(27x^6)^{1/3}]^2 = (3x^2)^2 = 9x^4$

25. $2^{-3} \cdot 2^{-4} = 2^{-7} = \dfrac{1}{2^7}$

27. $27^{-2} \cdot 27^{-1} = 27^{-3} = \dfrac{1}{27^3}$

29. $\dfrac{4^{-2} \cdot 4^{-1}}{4^{-3}} = 4^{(-2+(-1)-(-3))} = 4^0 = 1$

31. $(m^{2/3})(m^{5/3}) = m^{(2/3+5/3)} = m^{7/3}$

33. $(1+n)^{1/2}(1+n)^{3/4} = (1+n)^{(2/4+3/4)} = (1+n)^{5/4}$

35. $(2y^{3/4}z)(3y^{-2}z^{-1/3}) = 6y^{(3/4-8/4)}z^{(1-1/3)} = 6y^{-5/4}z^{2/3} = \dfrac{6z^{2/3}}{y^{5/4}}$

37. $(4a^{-2}b^7)^{1/2} \cdot (2a^{1/4}b^3)^5 = (2a^{-1}b^{7/2})(2^5 a^{5/4}b^{15}) = 2^6 a^{(-1+5/4)}b^{(7/2+30/2)} = 2^6 a^{1/4}b^{37/2}$

39. $\left(\dfrac{r^{-2}}{s^{-5}}\right)^{-3} = \dfrac{r^6}{s^{15}}$

41. $\left(\dfrac{-a}{b^{-3}}\right)^{-1} = \left(\dfrac{b^{-3}}{-a}\right) = \dfrac{-1}{ab^3}$

43. $\dfrac{12^{5/4} \cdot y^{-2}}{12^{-1} y^{-3}} = 12^{(5/3-(-1))} y^{(-2-(-3))} = 12^{9/4} y$

45. $\dfrac{8p^{-3}(4p^2)^{-2}}{p^{-5}} = \dfrac{8p^5}{p^3(4p^2)^2} = \dfrac{8p^5}{16p^7} = \dfrac{1}{2p^2}$

47. $\dfrac{m^{7/3} n^{-2/5} p^{3/8}}{m^{-2/3} n^{3/5} p^{-5/8}} = m^{(7/3+2/3)} n^{(-2/5-3/5)} p^{(3/8+5/8)} = m^3 n^{-1} p^1 = \dfrac{m^3 p}{n}$

49. $\dfrac{-4a^{-1}a^{2/3}}{a^{-2}} = -4a^{(-3/3+2/3+6/3)} = -4a^{5/3}$

51. $\dfrac{(k+5)^{1/2}(k+5)^{-1/4}}{(k+5)^{3/4}} = (k+5)^{(1/2-1/4-3/4)} = (k+5)^{-1/2} = \dfrac{1}{(k+5)^{1/2}}$

53. $y^{5/8}(y^{3/8} - 10y^{11/8}) = y^{(5/8+3/8)} - 10y^{(5/8+11/8)} = y - 10y^2$

55. $-4k(k^{7/3} - 6k^{1/3}) = -4k^{(1+7/3)} + 24k^{(1+1/3)} = -4k^{10/3} + 24k^{4/3}$

57. $(x + x^{1/2})(x - x^{1/2}) = x^2 - x^{(1+1/2)} + x^{(1+1/2)} - x^{(1/2+1/2)} = x^2 - x$

59. $(r^{1/2} - r^{-1/2})^2 = (r^{1/2})^2 - 2(r^{1/2})(r^{-1/2}) + (r^{-1/2})^2 = r - 2r^0 + r^{-1} = r - 2 + \dfrac{1}{r}$

61. $4k^{-1} + k^{-2} = 4k^1 \cdot k^{-2} + k^{-2} = k^{-2}(4k + 1)$

63. $9z^{-1/2} + 2z^{1/2} = 9z^{-1/2} + 2z^{-1/2} \cdot z^{2/2} = z^{-1/2}(9 + 2z)$

65. $p^{-3/4} - 2p^{-7/4} = p^{-7/4} \cdot p^{4/4} - 2p^{-7/4} = p^{-7/4}(p - 2)$

67. $(p+4)^{-3/2} + (p+4)^{-1/2} + (p+4)^{1/2} = (p+4)^{-3/2}(1 + (p+4) + (p+4)^2) =$

    $(p+4)^{-3/2}(1 + p + 4 + p^2 + 8p + 16) = (p+4)^{-3/2}(p^2 + 9p + 21)$

R.5: Review of Radicals

1. $(-3x)^{1/3} = \sqrt[3]{-3x}$; F

3. $(-3x)^{-1/3} = \dfrac{1}{(-3x)^{1/3}} = \dfrac{1}{\sqrt[3]{-3x}}$; H

5. $(3x)^{1/3} = \sqrt[3]{3x}$; G

7. $(3x)^{-1/3} = \dfrac{1}{(3x)^{1/3}} = \dfrac{1}{\sqrt[3]{3x}}$; C

9. $(-m)^{2/3} = \sqrt[3]{(-m)^2}$ or $(\sqrt[3]{-m})^2$

11. $(2m+p)^{2/3} = \sqrt[3]{(2m+p)^2}$ or $(\sqrt[3]{(2m+p)})^2$

13. $\sqrt[5]{k^2} = k^{2/5}$

15. $-3\sqrt{5p^3} = -3(5p^3)^{1/2} = -3 \cdot 5^{1/2} p^{3/2}$

17. A: $\sqrt{ab} = \sqrt{a} \cdot \sqrt{b}$ is true for $a > 0, b > 0$.

19. $\sqrt{9ax^2} = 3x\sqrt{a}$ is true for all $x \geq 0$.

21. $\sqrt[3]{125} = \sqrt[3]{5^3} = 5$

23. $\sqrt[5]{-3125} = \sqrt[5]{(-5)^5} = -5$

25. $\sqrt{50} = \sqrt{25 \cdot 2} = 5\sqrt{2}$

27. $\sqrt[3]{81} = \sqrt[3]{3^4} = 3\sqrt[3]{3}$

29. $-\sqrt[4]{32} = -\sqrt[4]{2^5} = -2\sqrt[4]{2}$

31. $-\sqrt{\dfrac{9}{5}} = -\dfrac{\sqrt{9}}{\sqrt{5}} \cdot \dfrac{\sqrt{5}}{\sqrt{5}} = -\dfrac{3\sqrt{5}}{5}$

33. $-\sqrt[3]{\dfrac{4}{5}} = -\dfrac{\sqrt[3]{4}}{\sqrt[3]{5}} \cdot \dfrac{\sqrt[3]{5^2}}{\sqrt[3]{5^2}} = -\dfrac{\sqrt[3]{100}}{5}$

35. $\sqrt[3]{16(-2)^4(2)^8} = \sqrt[3]{(2)^4(-2)^4(2)^8} = \sqrt[3]{(2)^{12}(-2)^4} = 2^4(-2)\sqrt[3]{-2} = -32\sqrt[3]{-2}$ or $32\sqrt[3]{2}$

37. $\sqrt{8x^5 z^8} = \sqrt{2^3 x^5 z^8} = 2x^2 z^4 \sqrt{2x}$

39. $\sqrt[3]{16z^5 x^8 y^4} = \sqrt[3]{2^4 z^5 x^8 y^4} = 2zx^2 y \sqrt[3]{2z^2 x^2 y}$

41. $\sqrt[4]{m^2 n^7 p^8} = np^2 \sqrt[4]{m^2 n^3}$

43. $\sqrt[4]{x^4 + y^4}$ cannot be simplified.

45. $\sqrt{\dfrac{2}{3x}} = \dfrac{\sqrt{2}}{\sqrt{3x}} \cdot \dfrac{\sqrt{3x}}{\sqrt{3x}} = \dfrac{\sqrt{6x}}{3x}$

47. $\sqrt{\dfrac{x^5 y^3}{z^2}} = \dfrac{\sqrt{x^5 y^3}}{\sqrt{z^2}} = \dfrac{x^2 y \sqrt{xy}}{z}$

49. $\sqrt[3]{\dfrac{8}{x^2}} = \dfrac{\sqrt[3]{2^3}}{\sqrt[3]{x^2}} \cdot \dfrac{\sqrt[3]{x}}{\sqrt[3]{x}} = \dfrac{2\sqrt[3]{x}}{x}$

51. $\sqrt[4]{\dfrac{g^3h^5}{9r^6}} = \dfrac{\sqrt[4]{g^3h^5}}{\sqrt[4]{3^2r^6}} = \dfrac{h\sqrt[4]{g^3h}}{r\sqrt[4]{3^2r^2}} \cdot \dfrac{\sqrt[4]{3^2r^2}}{\sqrt[4]{3^2r^2}} = \dfrac{h\sqrt[4]{9g^3hr^2}}{3r^2}$

53. $\dfrac{\sqrt[3]{mn} \cdot \sqrt[3]{m^2}}{\sqrt[3]{n^2}} \cdot \dfrac{\sqrt[3]{n}}{\sqrt[3]{n}} = \dfrac{\sqrt[3]{m^3n^2}}{n} = \dfrac{m\sqrt[3]{n^2}}{n}$

55. $\dfrac{\sqrt[4]{32x^5y} \cdot \sqrt[4]{2xy^4}}{\sqrt[4]{4x^3y^2}} = \dfrac{\sqrt[4]{2^6x^6y^5}}{\sqrt[4]{2^2x^3y^2}} \cdot \dfrac{\sqrt[4]{2^2xy^2}}{\sqrt[4]{2^2xy^2}} = \dfrac{\sqrt[4]{2^8x^7y^7}}{2xy} = \dfrac{4x\sqrt[4]{x^3y^3}}{2xy} = 2\sqrt[4]{x^3y^3}$

57. $\sqrt[3]{\sqrt{4}} = \sqrt[3]{2}$

59. $\sqrt[6]{\sqrt[3]{x}} = (x^{1/3})^{1/6} = x^{1/18} = \sqrt[18]{x}$

61. $4\sqrt{3} - 5\sqrt{12} + 3\sqrt{75} = 4\sqrt{3} - 5(2\sqrt{3}) + 3(5\sqrt{3}) = 4\sqrt{3} - 10\sqrt{3} + 15\sqrt{3} = 9\sqrt{3}$

63. $3\sqrt{28p} - 4\sqrt{63p} + \sqrt{112p} = 3(2\sqrt{7p}) - 4(3\sqrt{7p}) + 4\sqrt{7p} = 6\sqrt{7p} - 12\sqrt{7p} + 4\sqrt{7p} = -2\sqrt{7p}$

65. $2\sqrt[3]{3} + 4\sqrt[3]{24} - \sqrt[3]{81} = 2\sqrt[3]{3} + 4(2\sqrt[3]{3}) - 3\sqrt[3]{3} = 2\sqrt[3]{3} + 8\sqrt[3]{3} - 3\sqrt[3]{3} = 7\sqrt[3]{3}$

67. $\dfrac{1}{\sqrt{3}} - \dfrac{2}{\sqrt{12}} + 2\sqrt{3} = \dfrac{1}{\sqrt{3}} \cdot \dfrac{\sqrt{3}}{\sqrt{3}} - \dfrac{2}{2\sqrt{3}} \cdot \dfrac{\sqrt{3}}{\sqrt{3}} + 2\sqrt{3} = \dfrac{\sqrt{3}}{3} - \dfrac{2\sqrt{3}}{6} + 2\sqrt{3} = \dfrac{2\sqrt{3} - 2\sqrt{3} + 12\sqrt{3}}{6} = \dfrac{12\sqrt{3}}{6} = 2\sqrt{3}$

69. $\dfrac{5}{\sqrt[3]{2}} - \dfrac{2}{\sqrt[3]{16}} + \dfrac{1}{\sqrt[3]{54}} = \dfrac{5}{\sqrt[3]{2}} \cdot \dfrac{\sqrt[3]{4}}{\sqrt[3]{4}} - \dfrac{2}{\sqrt[3]{16}} \cdot \dfrac{\sqrt[3]{4}}{\sqrt[3]{4}} + \dfrac{1}{\sqrt[3]{54}} \cdot \dfrac{\sqrt[3]{4}}{\sqrt[3]{4}} = \dfrac{5\sqrt[3]{4}}{2} - \dfrac{\sqrt[3]{4}}{2} + \dfrac{\sqrt[3]{4}}{6} = \dfrac{15\sqrt[3]{4} - 3\sqrt[3]{4} + \sqrt[3]{4}}{6} = \dfrac{13\sqrt[3]{4}}{6}$

71. $(\sqrt{2}+3)(\sqrt{2}-3) = (\sqrt{2})^2 - 3^2 = 2 - 9 = -7$

73. $(\sqrt[3]{11} - 1)(\sqrt[3]{11^2} + \sqrt[3]{11} + 1) = \sqrt[3]{11} \cdot \sqrt[3]{11^2} + \sqrt[3]{11} \cdot \sqrt[3]{11} + \sqrt[3]{11} \cdot 1 - \sqrt[3]{11^2} - \sqrt[3]{11} - 1 =$
$11 + \sqrt[3]{11^2} + \sqrt[3]{11} - \sqrt[3]{11^2} - \sqrt[3]{11} - 1 = 11 - 1 = 10$

75. $(\sqrt{3} + \sqrt{8})^2 = (\sqrt{3})^2 + 2\sqrt{3} \cdot \sqrt{8} + (\sqrt{8})^2 = 3 + 2\sqrt{24} + 8 = 11 + 2(2\sqrt{6}) = 11 + 4\sqrt{6}$

77. $(3\sqrt{2} + \sqrt{3})(2\sqrt{3} - \sqrt{2}) = 3\sqrt{2} \cdot 2\sqrt{3} + 3\sqrt{2}(-\sqrt{2}) + \sqrt{3} \cdot 2\sqrt{3} + \sqrt{3}(-\sqrt{2}) = 6\sqrt{6} - 6 + 6 - \sqrt{6} = 5\sqrt{6}$

79. $\dfrac{8}{\sqrt{5}} = \dfrac{8}{\sqrt{5}} \cdot \dfrac{\sqrt{5}}{\sqrt{5}} = \dfrac{8\sqrt{5}}{5}$

81. $\dfrac{6}{\sqrt[3]{x^2}} = \dfrac{6}{\sqrt[3]{x^2}} \cdot \dfrac{\sqrt[3]{x}}{\sqrt[3]{x}} = \dfrac{6\sqrt[3]{x}}{x}$

83. $\dfrac{\sqrt{3}}{\sqrt{5} + \sqrt{3}} \cdot \dfrac{\sqrt{5} - \sqrt{3}}{\sqrt{5} - \sqrt{3}} = \dfrac{\sqrt{3} \cdot \sqrt{5} - \sqrt{3} \cdot \sqrt{3}}{(\sqrt{5})^2 - (\sqrt{3})^2} = \dfrac{\sqrt{15} - 3}{5 - 3} = \dfrac{\sqrt{15} - 3}{2}$

85. $\dfrac{1 + \sqrt{3}}{3\sqrt{5} + 2\sqrt{3}} \cdot \dfrac{3\sqrt{5} - 2\sqrt{3}}{3\sqrt{5} - 2\sqrt{3}} = \dfrac{3\sqrt{5} - 2\sqrt{3} + \sqrt{3} \cdot 3\sqrt{5} - 2(\sqrt{3})^2}{(3\sqrt{5})^2 - (2\sqrt{3})^2} = \dfrac{3\sqrt{5} - 2\sqrt{3} + 3\sqrt{15} - 6}{45 - 12} = \dfrac{3\sqrt{5} - 2\sqrt{3} + 3\sqrt{15} - 6}{33}$

87. $\dfrac{p}{\sqrt{p} + 2} \cdot \dfrac{\sqrt{p} - 2}{\sqrt{p} - 2} = \dfrac{p\sqrt{p} - 2p}{(\sqrt{p})^2 - (2)^2} = \dfrac{p(\sqrt{p} - 2)}{p - 4}$

89. $\dfrac{a}{\sqrt{a+b}-1} \cdot \dfrac{\sqrt{a+b}+1}{\sqrt{a+b}+1} = \dfrac{a(\sqrt{a+b}+1)}{(\sqrt{a+b})^2 - (1)^2} = \dfrac{a(\sqrt{a+b}+1)}{a+b-1}$

Chapter R-Test

1. (a) $(-3)^4 \cdot (-3)^5 = (-3)^{4+5} = (-3)^9$

   (b) $(2x^3 y)^2 = 2^2 (x^3)^2 y^2 = 4x^6 y^2$

   (c) $(-5z)^0 = 1$

   (d) $\left(-\dfrac{4}{5}\right)^2 = \dfrac{4^2}{5^2}$

   (e) $-\left(\dfrac{m^2}{p}\right)^3 = -\dfrac{m^6}{p^3}$

2. (a) $(x^2 - 3x + 2) - (x - 4x^2) + 3x(2x+1) = (x^2 - 3x + 2) - (x - 4x^2) + 6x^2 + 3x =$

   $x^2 - 3x + 2 - x + 4x^2 + 6x^2 + 3x = 11x^2 - x + 2$

   (b) $(6r-5)^2 = (6r-5)(6r-5) = 36r^2 - 60r + 25$

   (c) $(u+2)(3u^2 - u + 4) = 3u^3 - u^2 + 4u + 6u^2 - 2u + 8 = 3u^3 + 5u^2 + 2u + 8$

   (d) $(4x-5)(4x+5) = 16x^2 - 25$

   (e) $[(5p-1)+4]^2 = [5p+3]^2 = (5p+3)(5p+3) = 25p^2 + 30p + 9$

3. (a) $6x^2 - 17x + 7 = (3x-7)(2x-1)$

   (b) $x^4 - 16 = (x^2)^2 - 4^2 = (x^2 - 4)(x^2 + 4) = (x-2)(x+2)(x^2+4)$

   (c) $z^2 - 6zk - 16k^2 = (z+2k)(z-8k)$

   (d) $x^3 y^2 - 9x^3 - 8y^2 + 72 = x^3(y^2 - 9) - 8(y^2 - 9) = (y^2 - 9)(x^3 - 8) =$

   $(x-2)(x^2 + 2x + 4)(y+3)(y-3)$

4. (a) $\dfrac{16x^3}{4x^5} = \dfrac{4}{x^2}; \{x \mid x \neq 0\}$

   (b) $\dfrac{1+k}{k^2 - 1} = \dfrac{1+k}{(k+1)(k-1)} = \dfrac{1}{k-1}; \{k \mid k \neq -1, 1\}$

626 Chapter R: Reference: Basic Algebraic Concepts

(c) $\dfrac{x^2+x-2}{x^2+5x+6} = \dfrac{(x+2)(x-1)}{(x+2)(x+3)} = \dfrac{x-1}{x+3}; \{x \mid x \neq -3, -2\}$

5. (a) $\dfrac{5x^2-9x-2}{30x^3+6x^2} \cdot \dfrac{2x^8+6x^7+4x^6}{x^4-3x^2-4} = \dfrac{(5x+1)(x-2)}{6x^2(5x+1)} \cdot \dfrac{2x^6(x+2)(x+1)}{(x+2)(x-2)(x^2+1)} = \dfrac{x^4(x+1)}{3(x^2+1)}$

(b) $\dfrac{x}{x^2+3x+2} + \dfrac{2x}{2x^2-x-3} = \dfrac{x}{(x+2)(x+1)} + \dfrac{2x}{(2x-3)(x+1)} = \dfrac{x(2x-3)+2x(x+2)}{(2x-3)(x+2)(x+1)} =$

$\dfrac{4x^2+x}{(2x-3)(x+2)(x+1)} = \dfrac{x(4x+1)}{(2x-3)(x+2)(x+1)}$

(c) $\dfrac{a+b}{2a-3} - \dfrac{a-b}{3-2a} = \dfrac{a+b}{2a-3} + \dfrac{a-b}{2a-3} = \dfrac{2a}{2a-3} = \dfrac{-2a}{3-2a}$

(d) $\dfrac{g-\frac{2}{g}}{g-\frac{4}{g}} = \dfrac{g^2-2}{g^2-4} = \dfrac{g^2-2}{(g-2)(g+2)}$

6. (a) $(-7)^{-2} = \dfrac{1}{(-7)^2} = \dfrac{1}{49}$

(b) $(16x^8)^{3/4} = 16^{3/4}(x^8)^{3/4} = 8x^6$

(c) $\left(\dfrac{64}{27}\right)^{-2/3} = \left(\dfrac{27}{64}\right)^{2/3} = \dfrac{9}{16}$

7. (a) $\dfrac{5^{-3} \cdot 5^{-1}}{5^{-2}} = \dfrac{5^{-4}}{5^{-2}} = 5^{-2} = \dfrac{1}{5^2}$

(b) $(x+2)^{-1/5}(x+2)^{-7/10} = (x+2)^{-9/10} = \dfrac{1}{(x+2)^{9/10}}$

(c) $(m^{-1}n^{1/2})^4(4m^3n^{-2})^{-1/2} = \left(m^{-4}n^2 \dfrac{1}{2}m^{-3/2}n\right) = \dfrac{n^3}{2m^{11/2}}$

8. (a) $\sqrt[4]{16} = 2$

(b) $\sqrt[3]{\dfrac{2}{3}} = \dfrac{\sqrt[3]{2}}{\sqrt[3]{3}} = \dfrac{\sqrt[3]{2 \cdot 9}}{\sqrt[3]{3 \cdot 9}} = \dfrac{\sqrt[3]{18}}{3}$

(c) $\sqrt{18x^5y^8} = \sqrt{9x^4y^8}\sqrt{2x} = 3x^2y^4\sqrt{2x}$

(d) $\dfrac{\sqrt[4]{pq} \cdot \sqrt[4]{q^2}}{\sqrt[4]{p^3}} = \sqrt[4]{\dfrac{pq^3}{p^3}} = \sqrt[4]{\dfrac{q^3}{p^2}} = \dfrac{\sqrt[4]{p^2q^3}}{p}$

9. (a) $\sqrt{32x} + \sqrt{2x} - \sqrt{18x} = 4\sqrt{2x} + \sqrt{2x} - 3\sqrt{2x} = 2\sqrt{2x}$

(b) $\left(\sqrt[3]{2}+4\right)\left(\sqrt[3]{4}+1\right)=\sqrt[3]{8}+\sqrt[3]{2}+4\sqrt[3]{4}+4=6+\sqrt[3]{2}+4\sqrt[3]{4}$

(c) $\left(\sqrt{x}-\sqrt{y}\right)\left(\sqrt{x}+\sqrt{y}\right)=x-\sqrt{xy}+\sqrt{xy}-y=x-y$

10. $\dfrac{14}{\sqrt{11}-\sqrt{7}}=\dfrac{14}{\sqrt{11}-\sqrt{7}}\cdot\dfrac{\sqrt{11}+\sqrt{7}}{\sqrt{11}+\sqrt{7}}=\dfrac{14\left(\sqrt{11}+\sqrt{7}\right)}{11-7}=\dfrac{7\left(\sqrt{11}+\sqrt{7}\right)}{2}$

Appendix B: Vectors in Space

1. The plane determined by the x-axis and the z-axis is called the xz-plane.

3. The component form of the position vector with terminal point $(5, 3, -2)$ is $(5, 3, -2)$.

5. $d = \sqrt{(2-0)^2 + (-2-0)^2 + (5-0)^2} = \sqrt{4+4+25} = \sqrt{33}$

7. $d = \sqrt{(8-10)^2 + (3-15)^2 + (-4-9)^2} = \sqrt{4+144+169} = \sqrt{317}$

9. $d = \sqrt{(5-20)^2 + (5-25)^2 + (6-16)^2} = \sqrt{225+400+100} = \sqrt{725} = 5\sqrt{29}$

11. $PQ = \langle (2-0), (-2-0), (5-0) \rangle = \langle 2, -2, 5 \rangle; 2i - 2j + 5k$

13. $PQ = \langle (8-10), (3-15), (-4-0) \rangle = \langle -2, -12, -4 \rangle; -2i - 12j - 4k$

15. $PQ = \langle (5-20), (5-25), (16-6) \rangle = \langle -15, -20, 10 \rangle; -15i - 20j + 10k$

17. $QP = \langle (0-2), (0-(-2)), (0-5) \rangle = \langle -2, 2, -5 \rangle$; **QP** is the opposite of **PQ**. That is **QP = -PQ**.

19. $u - w = (2-4)i + (4-(-3))j + (7-(-6))k = -2i + 7j + 13k$

21. $4u + 5v = [4(2) + 5(-3)]i + [4(4) + 5(5)]j + [4(7) + 5(2)]k = -7i + 41j + 38k$

23. $|\mathbf{u}| = \sqrt{2^2 + 4^2 + 7^2} = \sqrt{69}$

25. $w + u = (4+2)i + (-(-3)+4)j + ((-6)+7)k = 6i + j + k \Rightarrow |w+u| = \sqrt{6^2 + 1^2 + 1^2} = \sqrt{38}$

27. $v \cdot w = (-3)(4) + (5)(-3) + (2)(-6) = -39$

29. $v \cdot v = (-3)(-3) + (5)(5) + (2)(2) = 38$

31. Let $v = \langle 2, -2, 0 \rangle$ and $w = \langle 5, -2, -1 \rangle$. The dot product is $v \cdot w = (2)(5) + (-2)(-2) + (0)(-1) = 14$. The required magnitudes are $|v| = \sqrt{2^2 + (-2)^2 + 0^2} = \sqrt{8}$ and $|w| = \sqrt{5^2 + (-2)^2 + (-1)^2} = \sqrt{30}$.

    $\cos\theta = \dfrac{v \cdot w}{|v||w|} \Rightarrow \cos\theta = \dfrac{14}{\sqrt{8}\sqrt{30}} \Rightarrow \theta = \cos^{-1}\dfrac{14}{(\sqrt{8}\sqrt{30})} \approx 25.4°$

33. Let $\mathbf{v} = \langle 6, 0, 0 \rangle$ and $\mathbf{w} = \langle 8, 3, -4 \rangle$. The dot product is $v \cdot w = (6)(8) + (0)(3) + (0)(-4) = 48$. The required magnitudes are $|\mathbf{v}| = \sqrt{6^2 + 0^2 + 0^2} = 6$ and $|\mathbf{w}| = \sqrt{8^2 + 3^2 + (-4)^2} = \sqrt{89}$.

    $\cos\theta = \dfrac{v \cdot w}{|v||w|} \Rightarrow \cos\theta = \dfrac{48}{6\sqrt{89}} \Rightarrow \theta = \cos^{-1}\left(\dfrac{48}{6\sqrt{89}}\right) \approx 32.0°$

35. Let $\mathbf{v} = \langle 1, 0, 0 \rangle$ and $\mathbf{w} = \langle 0, 1, 0 \rangle$. The dot product is $v \cdot w = (-1)(0) + (0)(1) + (0)(0) = 0$. The required magnitudes are $|v| = \sqrt{1^2 + 0^2 + 0^2} = 1$ and $|w| = \sqrt{0^2 + 1^2 + 0^2} = 1$.

630 Appendix

$$\cos\theta = \frac{v \cdot w}{|v||w|} \Rightarrow \cos\theta = \frac{0}{1(1)} \Rightarrow \theta = \cos^{-1}0 = 90°$$

37. $|u| = \sqrt{2^2 + 4^2 + 7^2} = \sqrt{69}; \cos\alpha = \frac{a}{|u|} = \frac{2}{\sqrt{69}} \Rightarrow \alpha = \cos^{-1}\left(\frac{2}{\sqrt{69}}\right) \approx 76.1°$

$\cos\beta = \frac{b}{|u|} = \frac{4}{\sqrt{69}} \Rightarrow \beta = \cos^{-1}\left(\frac{4}{\sqrt{69}}\right) \approx 61.2°; \cos\gamma = \frac{c}{|u|} = \frac{7}{\sqrt{69}} \Rightarrow \gamma = \cos^{-1}\left(\frac{7}{\sqrt{69}}\right) \approx 32.6°$

39. $|w| = \sqrt{4^2 + (-3)^2 + (-6)^2} = \sqrt{61}; \cos\alpha = \frac{a}{|w|} = \frac{4}{\sqrt{61}} \Rightarrow \alpha = \cos^{-1}\left(\frac{4}{\sqrt{61}}\right) \approx 59.2°$

$\cos\beta = \frac{b}{|w|} = \frac{-3}{\sqrt{61}} \Rightarrow \beta = \cos^{-1}\left(\frac{-3}{\sqrt{61}}\right) \approx 112.6°; \cos\gamma = \frac{c}{|w|} = \frac{-6}{\sqrt{61}} \Rightarrow \gamma = \cos^{-1}\left(\frac{-6}{\sqrt{61}}\right) \approx 140.2°$

41. Here $\cos\alpha = \cos 45° = \frac{\sqrt{2}}{2}$ and $\cos\beta = \cos 120° = -\frac{1}{2}$. Since $\cos^2\alpha + \cos^2\beta + \cos^2\gamma = 1$,

$\cos^2\gamma = 1 - \cos^2\alpha - \cos^2\beta = 1 - \frac{1}{2} - \frac{1}{4} = \frac{1}{4} \Rightarrow \cos\gamma = \frac{1}{2} \Rightarrow \gamma = \cos^{-1}\frac{1}{2} = 60°$

43. Two vectors are parallel if the position vector for one is a scalar multiple of the position vector of the other.

45. $\mathbf{PQ} = \langle(1-0),(3-0),(2-0)\rangle = \langle 1,3,2\rangle; \mathbf{F \cdot PQ} = (2)(1) + (0)(3) + (5)(2) = 12$ work units

47. $\mathbf{PQ} = \langle(5-2),(7-(-1)),(8-2)\rangle = \langle 3,8,6\rangle; \mathbf{F \cdot PQ} = (1)(3) + (2)(8) + (-1)(6) = 13$ work units

49. $\cos^2\alpha + \cos^2\beta + \cos^2\gamma = \left(\frac{a}{|\mathbf{v}|}\right)^2 + \left(\frac{b}{|\mathbf{v}|}\right)^2 + \left(\frac{c}{|\mathbf{v}|}\right)^2 = \frac{a^2}{|\mathbf{v}|^2} + \frac{b^2}{|\mathbf{v}|^2} + \frac{c^2}{|\mathbf{v}|^2} =$

$\frac{a^2}{(\sqrt{a^2+b^2+c^2})^2} + \frac{b^2}{(\sqrt{a^2+b^2+c^2})^2} + \frac{c^2}{(\sqrt{a^2+b^2+c^2})^2} = \frac{a^2+b^2+c^2}{a^2+b^2+c^2} = 1$

Appendix C: Polar Form of Conic Sections

1. Only the calculator graph is shown here. See Figure 1.
3. Only the calculator graph is shown here. See Figure 3.

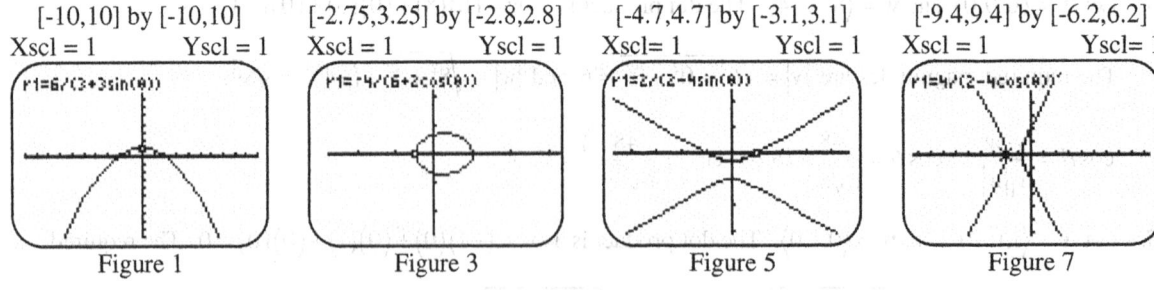

Figure 1   Figure 3   Figure 5   Figure 7

5. Only the calculator graph is shown here. See Figure 5.
7. Only the calculator graph is shown here. See Figure 7.

Appendix C   631

9. Only the calculator graph is shown here. See Figure 9.

11. Only the calculator graph is shown here. See Figure 11.

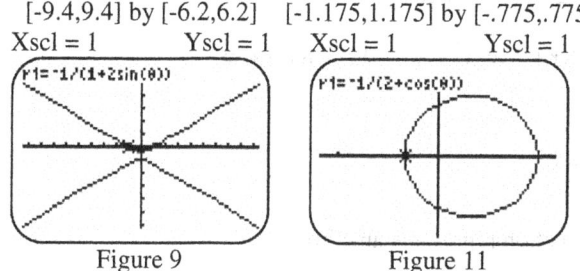

[-9.4,9.4] by [-6.2,6.2]   [-1.175,1.175] by [-.775,.775]
Xscl = 1   Yscl = 1   Xscl = 1   Yscl = 1

Figure 9   Figure 11

13. The conic is a parabola, so $e = 1$. Since the vertical directrix is 3 units to the right of the pole, the equation is of the form $r = \dfrac{ep}{1 + e\cos\theta}$ with $p = 3$. The equation for this parabola is $r = \dfrac{3}{1 + \cos\theta}$.

15. The conic is a parabola, so $e = 1$. Since the horizontal directrix is 5 units below the pole, the equation is of the form $r = \dfrac{ep}{1 - e\sin\theta}$ with $p = 5$. The equation for this parabola is $r = \dfrac{5}{1 - \sin\theta}$.

17. Since the vertical directrix is 5 units to the right of the pole, the equation is of the form $r = \dfrac{ep}{1 + e\cos\theta}$ with $p = 5$. Since $e = \dfrac{4}{5} < 1$, the conic is an ellipse with equation

$$r = \dfrac{\left(\frac{4}{5}\right)5}{1 + \frac{4}{5}\cos\theta} \Rightarrow r = \dfrac{4}{1 + \frac{4}{5}\cos\theta} \Rightarrow r = \dfrac{4}{1 + \frac{4}{5}\cos\theta} \cdot \dfrac{5}{5} \Rightarrow r = \dfrac{20}{5 + 4\cos\theta}.$$

19. Since the horizontal directrix is 8 units below the pole, the equation is of the form $r = \dfrac{ep}{1 - e\sin\theta}$ with $p = 8$. Since $e = \dfrac{5}{4} > 1$, the conic is an hyperbola with equation

$$r = \dfrac{\left(\frac{5}{4}\right)8}{1 - \frac{5}{4}\sin\theta} \Rightarrow r = \dfrac{10}{1 - \frac{5}{4}\sin\theta} \Rightarrow r = \dfrac{10}{1 - \frac{5}{4}\sin\theta} \cdot \dfrac{4}{4} \Rightarrow r = \dfrac{40}{4 - 5\sin\theta}.$$

21. $r = \dfrac{6}{3 - \cos\theta} \cdot \dfrac{\frac{1}{3}}{\frac{1}{3}} = \dfrac{2}{1 - \frac{1}{3}\cos\theta}$. Since $e = \dfrac{1}{3} < 1$, this equation represents an ellipse.

$r = \dfrac{6}{3 - \cos\theta} \Rightarrow r(3 - \cos\theta) = 6 \Rightarrow 3r - r\cos\theta = 6 \Rightarrow 3r = r\cos\theta + 6 \Rightarrow (3r)^2 = (r\cos\theta + 6)^2 \Rightarrow$
$(3r)^2 = (x + 6)^2 \Rightarrow 9r^2 = x^2 + 12x + 36 \Rightarrow 9(x^2 + y^2) = x^2 + 12x + 36 \Rightarrow 8x^2 + 9y^2 - 12x - 36 = 0$

The rectangle form of the equation is $8x^2 + 9y^2 - 12x - 36 = 0$.

23. $r = \dfrac{-2}{1+2\cos\theta}$; Since $e = 2 > 1$, this equation represents a hyperbola

$r = \dfrac{-2}{1+2\cos\theta} \Rightarrow r(1+2\cos\theta) = -2 \Rightarrow r + 2r\cos\theta = -2 \Rightarrow r = -2r\cos\theta - 2 \Rightarrow$

$r^2 = (-2r\cos\theta - 2)^2 \Rightarrow r^2 = (-2x - 2)^2 \Rightarrow r^2 = 4x^2 + 8x + 4 \Rightarrow x^2 + y^2 = 4x^2 + 8x + 4 \Rightarrow$

$3x^2 - y^2 + 8x + 4 = 0$;

The rectangular form of equation is $3x^2 - y^2 + 8x + 4 = 0$.

25. $r = \dfrac{-6}{4+2\sin\theta} \cdot \dfrac{\frac{1}{4}}{\frac{1}{4}} = \dfrac{-\frac{3}{2}}{1+\frac{1}{2}\sin\theta}$; Since $e = \dfrac{1}{2} < 1$, this equation represents an ellipse.

$r = \dfrac{-6}{4+2\sin\theta} \Rightarrow r(4+2\sin\theta) = -6 \Rightarrow 4r + 2r\sin\theta = -6 \Rightarrow 4r = -2r\sin\theta - 6 \Rightarrow$

$(4r)^2 = (-2r\sin\theta - 6)^2 \Rightarrow (4r)^2 = (-2y - 6)^2 \Rightarrow 16r^2 = 4y^2 + 24y + 36 \Rightarrow$

$16(x^2 + y^2) = 4y^2 + 24y + 36 = 0 \Rightarrow 16x^2 + 12y^2 - 24y - 36 = 0 \Rightarrow 4x^2 + 3y^2 - 6y - 9 = 0$

The rectangular form of equation is $4x^2 + 3y^2 - 6y - 9 = 0$.

27. $r = \dfrac{10}{2-2\sin\theta} \cdot \dfrac{\frac{1}{2}}{\frac{1}{2}} = \dfrac{5}{1-\sin\theta}$; Since $e = 1$, this equation represents a parabola.

$r = \dfrac{10}{2-2\sin\theta} \Rightarrow r(2-2\sin\theta) = 10 \Rightarrow 2r - 2r\sin\theta = 10 \Rightarrow 2r = 2r\sin\theta + 10 \Rightarrow$

$(2r)^2 = (2r\sin\theta + 10)^2 \Rightarrow (2r)^2 = (2y + 10)^2 \Rightarrow 4r^2 = 4y^2 + 40y + 100 \Rightarrow$

$4(x^2 + y^2) = 4y^2 + 40y + 100 = 0 \Rightarrow 4x^2 - 40y - 100 = 0 \Rightarrow x^2 - 10y - 25 = 0$

The rectangular form of equation is $x^2 - 10y - 25 = 0$.

Appendix D: Rotation of Axes

1. $4x^2 + 3y^2 + 2xy - 5x = 8 \Rightarrow B^2 - 4AC = 2^2 - 4(4)(3) = 4 - 48 < 0$. Circle, ellipse, or a point.

3. $2x^2 + 3xy - 4y^2 = 0 \Rightarrow B^2 - 4AC = 3^2 - 4(2)(-4) = 9 + 32 > 0$. Hyperbola or 2 intersecting lines.

5. $4x^2 + 4xy + y^2 + 15 = 0 \Rightarrow B^2 - 4AC = 4^2 - 4(4)(1) = 16 - 16 = 0$. Parabola, one line, or 2 parallel lines.

7. $2x^2 + \sqrt{3}xy + y^2 + x = 5 \Rightarrow \cot 2\theta = \dfrac{A-C}{B} = \dfrac{2-1}{\sqrt{3}} \Rightarrow \cot 2\theta = \dfrac{1}{\sqrt{3}} \Rightarrow 2\theta = 60° \Rightarrow \theta = 30°$

9. $3x^2 + \sqrt{3}xy + 4y^2 + 2x - 3y = 12 \Rightarrow \cot 2\theta = \dfrac{A-C}{B} = \dfrac{3-4}{\sqrt{3}} \Rightarrow \cot 2\theta = -\dfrac{1}{\sqrt{3}} \Rightarrow 2\theta = 120° \Rightarrow \theta = 60°$

11. $x^2 - 4xy + 5y^2 = 18 \Rightarrow \cot 2\theta = \dfrac{A-C}{B} = \dfrac{1-5}{-4} = 1 \Rightarrow \cot 2\theta = 1 \Rightarrow 2\theta = 45° \Rightarrow \theta = 22.5°$

13. $x^2 - xy + y^2 = 6$ [1]; $\theta = 45°$; $x = x'\cos\theta - y'\sin\theta = \dfrac{\sqrt{2}}{2}x' - \dfrac{\sqrt{2}}{2}y'$ [2]; $y = x'\sin\theta + y'\cos\theta = \dfrac{\sqrt{2}}{2}x' + \dfrac{\sqrt{2}}{2}y'$ [3].

Substitute [2] and [3] in [1].

$\left(\dfrac{\sqrt{2}}{2}x' - \dfrac{\sqrt{2}}{2}y'\right)^2 - \left(\dfrac{\sqrt{2}}{2}x' - \dfrac{\sqrt{2}}{2}y'\right)\left(\dfrac{\sqrt{2}}{2}x' + \dfrac{\sqrt{2}}{2}y'\right) + \left(\dfrac{\sqrt{2}}{2}x' + \dfrac{\sqrt{2}}{2}y'\right)^2 = 6 \Rightarrow$

See Figure 13.

$\dfrac{1}{2}x'^2 - x'y' + \dfrac{1}{2}y'^2 - \dfrac{1}{2}x'^2 + \dfrac{1}{2}y'^2 + \dfrac{1}{2}x'^2 + x'y' + \dfrac{1}{2}y'^2 = 6 \Rightarrow \dfrac{1}{2}x'^2 + \dfrac{3}{2}y'^2 = 6 \Rightarrow \dfrac{x'^2}{12} + \dfrac{y'^2}{4} = 1.$

15. $8x^2 - 4xy + 5y^2 = 36 [1]; \sin\theta = \dfrac{2}{\sqrt{5}}, y = 2, r = \sqrt{5}, x = \sqrt{5-4} = 1 \Rightarrow \cos\theta = \dfrac{1}{\sqrt{5}};$

$x = x'\cos\theta - y'\sin\theta = \dfrac{1}{\sqrt{5}}x' - \dfrac{2}{\sqrt{5}}y' [2]; y = x'\sin\theta + y'\cos\theta = \dfrac{2}{\sqrt{5}}x' + \dfrac{1}{\sqrt{5}}y' [3].$

Substitute [2] and [3] in [1].

$8\left(\dfrac{1}{\sqrt{5}}x' - \dfrac{2}{\sqrt{5}}y'\right)^2 - 4\left(\dfrac{1}{\sqrt{5}}x' - \dfrac{2}{\sqrt{5}}y'\right)\left(\dfrac{2}{\sqrt{5}}x' + \dfrac{1}{\sqrt{5}}y'\right) + 5\left(\dfrac{2}{\sqrt{5}}x' + \dfrac{1}{\sqrt{5}}y'\right)^2 = 36 \Rightarrow$

$8\left(\dfrac{1}{5}x'^2 - \dfrac{4}{5}x'y' + \dfrac{4}{5}y'^2\right) - 4\left(\dfrac{2}{5}x'^2 - \dfrac{3}{5}x'y' - \dfrac{2}{5}y'^2\right) 5\left(\dfrac{4}{5}x'^2 + \dfrac{4}{5}x'y' + \dfrac{1}{5}y'^2\right) = 36 \Rightarrow$

See Figure 15.

$\dfrac{8}{5}x'^2 - \dfrac{32}{5}x'y' + \dfrac{32}{5}y'^2 - \dfrac{8}{5}x'^2 + \dfrac{12}{5}x'y' + \dfrac{8}{5}y'^2 + 4x'^2 + 4x'y' + y'^2 = 36 \Rightarrow 4x'^2 + 9y'^2 = 36 \Rightarrow$

$\dfrac{x'^2}{9} + \dfrac{y'^2}{4} = 1.$

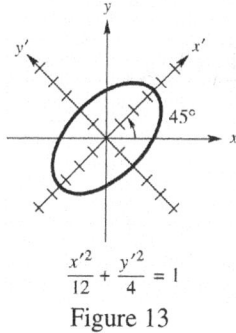
$\dfrac{x'^2}{12} + \dfrac{y'^2}{4} = 1$
Figure 13

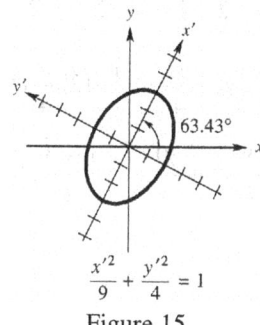
$\dfrac{x'^2}{9} + \dfrac{y'^2}{4} = 1$
Figure 15

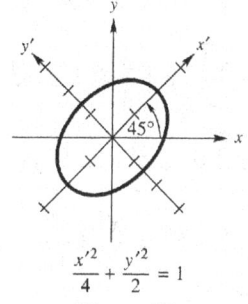
$\dfrac{x'^2}{4} + \dfrac{y'^2}{2} = 1$
Figure 17

17. $3x^2 - 2xy + 3y^2 = 8 [1]; \cot 2\theta = \dfrac{A-C}{B} = \dfrac{3-3}{-2} = 0 \Rightarrow 2\theta = 90° \Rightarrow \theta = 45°;$

$x = x'\cos\theta - y'\sin\theta = \dfrac{\sqrt{2}}{2}x' - \dfrac{\sqrt{2}}{2}y' [2]; y = x'\sin\theta + y'\cos\theta = \dfrac{\sqrt{2}}{2}x' + \dfrac{\sqrt{2}}{2}y' [3].$

Substitute [2] and [3] in [1].

$3\left(\dfrac{\sqrt{2}}{2}x' - \dfrac{\sqrt{2}}{2}y'\right)^2 - 2\left(\dfrac{\sqrt{2}}{2}x' - \dfrac{\sqrt{2}}{2}y'\right)\left(\dfrac{\sqrt{2}}{2}x' + \dfrac{\sqrt{2}}{2}y'\right) + 3\left(\dfrac{\sqrt{2}}{2}x' + \dfrac{\sqrt{2}}{2}y'\right)^2 = 8 \Rightarrow$

$3\left(\dfrac{1}{2}x'^2 - x'y' + \dfrac{1}{2}y'^2\right) - 2\left(\dfrac{1}{2}x'^2 - \dfrac{1}{2}y'^2\right) + 3\left(\dfrac{1}{2}x'^2 + x'y' + \dfrac{1}{2}y'^2\right) = 8 \Rightarrow$

$\dfrac{3}{2}x'^2 - 3x'y' + \dfrac{3}{2}y'^2 - x'^2 + y'^2 + \dfrac{3}{2}x'^2 + 3x'y' + \dfrac{3}{2}y'^2 = 8 \Rightarrow 2x'^2 + 4y'^2 = 8 \Rightarrow \dfrac{x'^2}{4} + \dfrac{y'^2}{2} = 1$

See Figure 17.

19. $x^2 - 4xy + y^2 = -5$ [1]; $\cot 2\theta = \dfrac{A-C}{B} = \dfrac{1-1}{-4} = 0 \Rightarrow 2\theta = 90° \Rightarrow \theta = 45°$;

$x = x'\cos\theta - y'\sin\theta = \dfrac{\sqrt{2}}{2}x' - \dfrac{\sqrt{2}}{2}y'$ [2]; $y = x'\sin\theta + y'\cos\theta = \dfrac{\sqrt{2}}{2}x' + \dfrac{\sqrt{2}}{2}y'$ [3].

Substitute [2] and 3 in [1].

$\left(\dfrac{\sqrt{2}}{2}x' - \dfrac{\sqrt{2}}{2}y'\right)^2 - 4\left(\dfrac{\sqrt{2}}{2}x' - \dfrac{\sqrt{2}}{2}y'\right)\left(\dfrac{\sqrt{2}}{2}x' + \dfrac{\sqrt{2}}{2}y'\right) + \left(\dfrac{\sqrt{2}}{2}x' + \dfrac{\sqrt{2}}{2}y'\right)^2 = -5 \Rightarrow$

$\dfrac{1}{2}x'^2 - x'y' + \dfrac{1}{2}y'^2 - 4\left(\dfrac{1}{2}x'^2 - \dfrac{1}{2}y'^2\right) + \dfrac{1}{2}x'^2 + x'y' + \dfrac{1}{2}y'^2 = -5 \Rightarrow$

$\dfrac{1}{2}x'^2 - x'y' + \dfrac{1}{2}y'^2 - 2x'^2 + 2y'^2 + \dfrac{1}{2}x'^2 + x'y' + \dfrac{1}{2}y'^2 = -5 \Rightarrow -x'^2 + 3y'^2 = -5 \Rightarrow \dfrac{x'^2}{5} - \dfrac{3y'^2}{5} = 1.$

See Figure 19.

21. $7x^2 + 6\sqrt{3}xy + 13y^2 = 64$ [1]; $\cot 2\theta = \dfrac{A-C}{B} = \dfrac{7-13}{6\sqrt{3}} = \dfrac{-6}{6\sqrt{3}} = -\dfrac{1}{\sqrt{3}} \Rightarrow 2\theta = 120° \Rightarrow \theta = 60°$;

$x = x'\cos\theta - y'\sin\theta = \dfrac{1}{2}x' - \dfrac{\sqrt{3}}{2}y'$ [2]; $y = x'\sin\theta + y'\cos\theta = \dfrac{\sqrt{3}}{2}x' + \dfrac{1}{2}y'$ [3].

Substitute [2] and 3 in [1].

$7\left(\dfrac{1}{2}x' - \dfrac{\sqrt{3}}{2}y'\right)^2 + 6\sqrt{3}\left(\dfrac{1}{2}x' - \dfrac{\sqrt{3}}{2}y'\right)\left(\dfrac{\sqrt{3}}{2}x' + \dfrac{1}{2}y'\right) + 13\left(\dfrac{\sqrt{3}}{2}x' + \dfrac{1}{2}y'\right)^2 = 64 \Rightarrow$

$7\left(\dfrac{1}{4}x'^2 - \dfrac{\sqrt{3}}{2}x'y' + \dfrac{3}{4}y'^2\right) + 6\sqrt{3}\left(\dfrac{\sqrt{3}}{4}x'^2 - \dfrac{1}{2}x'y' - \dfrac{\sqrt{3}}{4}y'^2\right) + 13\left(\dfrac{3}{4}x'^2 + \dfrac{\sqrt{3}}{2}x'y' + \dfrac{1}{4}y'^2\right) = 64 \Rightarrow$

$\dfrac{7}{4}x'^2 - \dfrac{7\sqrt{3}}{2}x'y' + \dfrac{21}{4}y'^2 + \dfrac{18}{4}x'^2 - \dfrac{6\sqrt{3}}{2}x'y' - \dfrac{18}{4}y'^2 + \dfrac{39}{4}x'^2 + \dfrac{13\sqrt{3}}{2}x'y' + \dfrac{13}{4}y' = 64 \Rightarrow$

$16x'^2 + 4y'^2 = 64 \Rightarrow \dfrac{x'^2}{4} + \dfrac{y'^2}{16} = 1.$

See Figure 21.

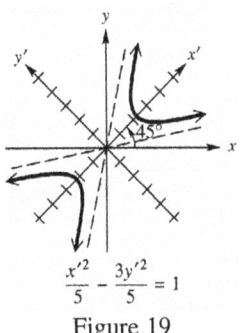
$\dfrac{x'^2}{5} - \dfrac{3y'^2}{5} = 1$
Figure 19

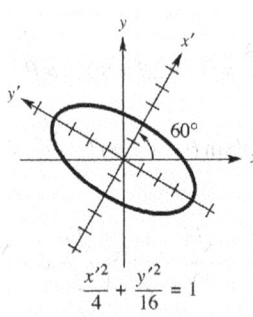
$\dfrac{x'^2}{4} + \dfrac{y'^2}{16} = 1$
Figure 21

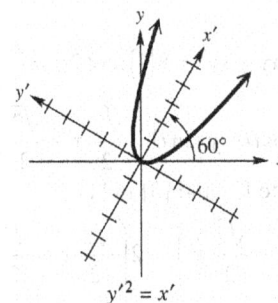
$y'^2 = x'$
Figure 23

23. $3x^2 - 2\sqrt{3}xy + y^2 - 2x - 2\sqrt{3}y = 0$ [1]; $\cot 2\theta = \dfrac{A-C}{B} = \dfrac{3-1}{-2\sqrt{3}} = -\dfrac{1}{\sqrt{3}} \Rightarrow 2\theta = 120° \Rightarrow$

$\theta = 60°$; $x = x'\cos\theta - y'\sin\theta = \dfrac{1}{2}x' - \dfrac{\sqrt{3}}{2}y'$ [2]; $y = x'\sin\theta + y'\cos\theta = \dfrac{\sqrt{3}}{2}x' + \dfrac{1}{2}y'$ [3].

Substitute [2] and 3 in [1].

$$3\left(\frac{1}{2}x' - \frac{\sqrt{3}}{2}y'\right)^2 - 2\sqrt{3}\left(\frac{1}{2}x' - \frac{\sqrt{3}}{2}y'\right)\left(\frac{\sqrt{3}}{2}x' + \frac{1}{2}y'\right) +$$

$$\left(\frac{\sqrt{3}}{2}x' + \frac{1}{2}y'\right)^2 - 2\left(\frac{1}{2}x' - \frac{\sqrt{3}}{2}y'\right) - 2\sqrt{3}\left(\frac{\sqrt{3}}{2}x' + \frac{1}{2}y'\right) = 0 \Rightarrow 3\left(\frac{1}{4}x'^2 - \frac{\sqrt{3}}{2}x'y' + \frac{3}{4}y'^2\right) -$$

$$2\sqrt{3}\left(\frac{\sqrt{3}}{4}x'^2 - \frac{1}{2}x'y' - \frac{\sqrt{3}}{4}y'^2\right) + \left(\frac{3}{4}x'^2 + \frac{\sqrt{3}}{2}x'y' + \frac{1}{4}y'^2\right) - x' + \sqrt{3}y' - 3x - \sqrt{3}y' = 0 \Rightarrow$$

$$\frac{4}{3}x'^2 - \frac{3\sqrt{3}}{2}x'y' + \frac{9}{4}y'^2 - \frac{3}{2}x'^2 + \sqrt{3}x'y' + \frac{3}{2}y'^2 + \frac{3}{4}x'^2 + \frac{\sqrt{3}}{2}x'y' + \frac{1}{4}y'^2 - 4x = 0 \Rightarrow$$

$$4y'^2 - 4x' = 0 \Rightarrow 4y'^2 = 4x' \Rightarrow y'^2 = x'.$$

See Figure 23.

25. $x^2 + 3xy + y^2 - 5\sqrt{2}y = 15$ [1]; $\cot 2\theta = \dfrac{A-C}{B} = \dfrac{1-1}{3} = 0 \Rightarrow 2\theta = 90° \Rightarrow \theta = 45°$;

$x = x'\cos\theta - y'\sin\theta = \dfrac{\sqrt{2}}{2}x' - \dfrac{\sqrt{2}}{2}y'$ [2]; $y = x'\sin\theta + y'\cos\theta = \dfrac{\sqrt{2}}{2}x' + \dfrac{\sqrt{2}}{2}y'$ [3].

Substitute [2] and [3] in [1].

$$\left(\frac{\sqrt{2}}{2}x' - \frac{\sqrt{2}}{2}y'\right)^2 + 3\left(\frac{\sqrt{2}}{2}x' - \frac{\sqrt{2}}{2}y'\right)\left(\frac{\sqrt{2}}{2}x' + \frac{\sqrt{2}}{2}y'\right) +$$

$$\left(\frac{\sqrt{2}}{2}x' + \frac{\sqrt{2}}{2}y'\right)^2 - 5\sqrt{2}\left(\frac{\sqrt{2}}{2}x' + \frac{\sqrt{2}}{2}y'\right) = 15 \Rightarrow$$

$$\frac{1}{2}x'^2 - x'y' + \frac{1}{2}y'^2 + 3\left(\frac{1}{2}x'^2 - \frac{1}{2}y'^2\right) + \frac{1}{2}x'^2 + x'y' + \frac{1}{2}y'^2 - 5x' - 5y' = 15 \Rightarrow$$

$$\frac{1}{2}x'^2 - x'y' + \frac{1}{2}y'^2 + \frac{3}{2}x'^2 - \frac{3}{2}y'^2 + \frac{1}{2}x'^2 + x'y' + \frac{1}{2}y'^2 - 5x' - 5y' = 15 \Rightarrow$$

$$\frac{5}{2}x'^2 - \frac{1}{2}y'^2 - 5x' - 5y' = 15 \Rightarrow 5x'^2 - 10x' - y'^2 - 10y' = 30 \Rightarrow$$

$$5(x'^2 - 2x' + 1) - (y'^2 + 10y' + 25) = 30 + 5 - 25 \Rightarrow 5(x'-1)^2 - (y'+5)^2 = 10 \Rightarrow$$

$$\frac{(x'-1)^2}{2} - \frac{(y'+5)^2}{10} = 1.$$

See Figure 25.

The graph of the equation is a hyperbola with its center at (1, −5). By translating the axes of the $x'y'$ −system down 5 units and right 1 unit, we get an $x''y''$ −coordinate system, in which the hyperbola is centered at the origin. Thus $\dfrac{x''^2}{2} - \dfrac{y''^2}{10} = 1$.

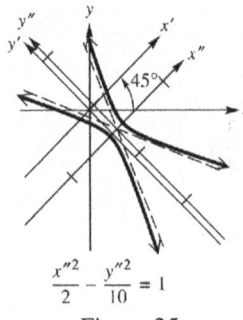

y″
y′
y
x′
x″
45°
x
$\frac{x''^2}{2} - \frac{y''^2}{10} = 1$

Figure 25

y″
y′
y
x″
x′
26.57°
x
$x''^2 \approx -8.94y''$

Figure 27

27. $4x^2 + 4xy + y^2 - 24x + 38y - 19 = 0[1]; \cot 2\theta = \frac{A-C}{B} = \frac{4-1}{4} = \frac{3}{4} \Rightarrow 2\theta \approx 53.13^\circ \Rightarrow \theta \approx 26.57^\circ$. For

$2\theta; x = 3, y = 4, r = \sqrt{3^2 + 4^2} = 5 \Rightarrow \cos 2\theta = \frac{3}{5}$.

$\sin\theta = \sqrt{\frac{1-\cos 2\theta}{2}} = \sqrt{\frac{1-\frac{3}{5}}{2}} = \sqrt{\frac{2}{10}} = \frac{\sqrt{5}}{5}; \cos\theta = \sqrt{\frac{1+\cos 2\theta}{2}} = \sqrt{\frac{1+\frac{3}{5}}{2}} = \sqrt{\frac{8}{10}} = \frac{2\sqrt{5}}{5}$;

$x = x'\cos\theta - y'\sin\theta = \frac{2\sqrt{5}}{5}x' - \frac{\sqrt{5}}{5}y'[2]; y = x'\sin\theta + y'\cos\theta = \frac{\sqrt{5}}{5}x' + \frac{2\sqrt{5}}{5}y'[3]$.

Substitute [2] and [3] in [1]. $4\left(\frac{2\sqrt{5}}{5}x' - \frac{\sqrt{5}}{5}y'\right)^2 + 4\left(\frac{2\sqrt{5}}{5}x' - \frac{\sqrt{5}}{5}y'\right)\left(\frac{\sqrt{5}}{5}x' + \frac{2\sqrt{5}}{5}y'\right) +$

$\left(\frac{\sqrt{5}}{5}x' + \frac{2\sqrt{5}}{5}y'\right)^2 - 24\left(\frac{2\sqrt{5}}{5}x' - \frac{\sqrt{5}}{5}y'\right)^2 + 38\left(\frac{\sqrt{5}}{5}x' + \frac{2\sqrt{5}}{5}y'\right)^2 = 19 \Rightarrow$

$4\left(\frac{4}{5}x'^2 - \frac{4}{5}x'y' + \frac{1}{5}y'^2\right) + 4\left(\frac{2}{5}x'^2 + \frac{3}{5}x'y' - \frac{1}{5}y'^2\right) + \left(\frac{1}{5}x'^2 + \frac{4}{5}x'y' + \frac{4}{5}y'^2\right) - \frac{48\sqrt{5}}{5}x' + \frac{25\sqrt{5}}{5}y' +$

$\frac{38\sqrt{5}}{5}x' + \frac{76\sqrt{5}}{5}y' = 19 \Rightarrow 5x'^2 - 2\sqrt{5}x' + 20\sqrt{5}y' = 19 \Rightarrow$

$5\left(x'^2 - \frac{2\sqrt{5}}{5}x' + \frac{1}{5}\right) + 20\sqrt{5}y' = 19 + 1 \Rightarrow 5\left(x' - \frac{\sqrt{5}}{5}\right)^2 = 20 - 20\sqrt{5}y \Rightarrow$

$\left(x' - \frac{\sqrt{5}}{5}\right)^2 = 4 - 4\sqrt{5}y' \Rightarrow \left(x' - \frac{\sqrt{5}}{5}\right)^2 = -4\sqrt{5}\left(y' - \frac{\sqrt{5}}{5}\right)$.

See Figure 27.

29. $16x^2 + 24xy + 9y^2 - 130x + 90y = 0[1]; \cot 2\theta = \frac{A-C}{B} = \frac{16-9}{24} = -\frac{7}{24} \Rightarrow$

$2\theta \approx 73.74° \Rightarrow \theta \approx 36.87°$. For $2\theta; x = 7, y = 24, r = \sqrt{7^2 + 24^2} = 25 \Rightarrow \cos 2\theta = \frac{7}{25}$.

$\sin\theta = \sqrt{\frac{1-\cos 2\theta}{2}} = \sqrt{\frac{1-\frac{7}{25}}{2}} = \sqrt{\frac{18}{50}} = \frac{3}{5}; \cos\theta = \sqrt{\frac{1+\cos 2\theta}{2}} = \sqrt{\frac{1+\frac{7}{25}}{2}} = \sqrt{\frac{32}{50}} = \frac{4}{5}$;

$x = x'\cos\theta - y'\sin\theta = \frac{4}{5}x' - \frac{3}{5}y'[2]; y = x'\sin\theta + y'\cos\theta = \frac{3}{5}x' + \frac{4}{5}y'[3]$.

Substitute [2] and [3] in [1].

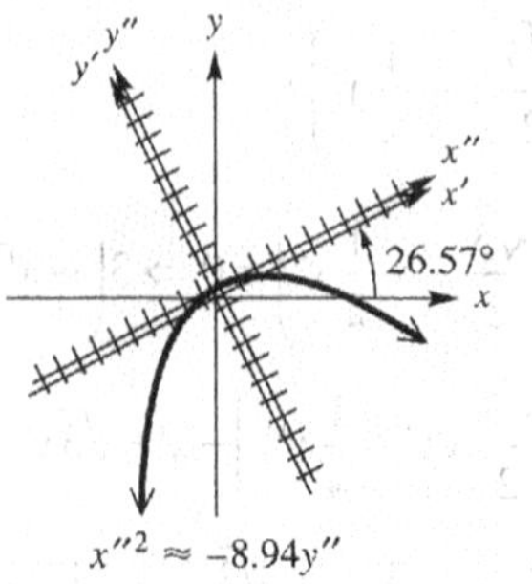

$$16\left(\frac{4}{5}x'-\frac{3}{5}y'\right)^2+24\left(\frac{4}{5}x'-\frac{3}{5}y'\right)\left(\frac{3}{5}x'+\frac{4}{5}y'\right)+$$

$$9\left(\frac{3}{5}x'+\frac{4}{5}y'\right)^2-130\left(\frac{4}{5}x'-\frac{3}{5}y'\right)+90\left(\frac{3}{5}x'+\frac{4}{5}y'\right)=0 \Rightarrow$$

$$16\left(\frac{16}{25}x'^2-\frac{24}{25}x'y'+\frac{9}{25}y'^2\right)+24\left(\frac{12}{25}x'^2+\frac{7}{25}x'y'-\frac{12}{25}y'^2\right)+9\left(\frac{9}{25}x'^2+\frac{24}{25}x'y'+\frac{16}{25}y'^2\right)-$$

$$104x'+78y'+54x'+72y'=0 \Rightarrow \frac{256}{25}x'^2-\frac{384}{25}x'y'+\frac{144}{25}y'^2+\frac{288}{25}x'^2+\frac{168}{25}x'y'-\frac{288}{25}y'^2+$$

$$\frac{81}{25}x'^2+\frac{216}{25}x'y'+\frac{144}{25}y'^2-50x'+150y'=0 \Rightarrow 25x'^2-50x'+150y'=0 \Rightarrow$$

$$25(x'^2-2x'+1)=-150y'+25 \Rightarrow 25(x'-1)^2=-150\left(y'-\frac{1}{6}\right) \Rightarrow (x'-1)^2=-6\left(y'-\frac{1}{6}\right).$$

See Figure 29. The graph of the equation is a parabola with its vertex at $\left(1,\frac{1}{6}\right)$. By translating the axes of the $x'y'$–system up $\frac{1}{6}$ units and right 1 unit, we get an $x''y''$–coordinate system, in which the parabola is centered at the origin. Thus $x''^2=-6y''$.

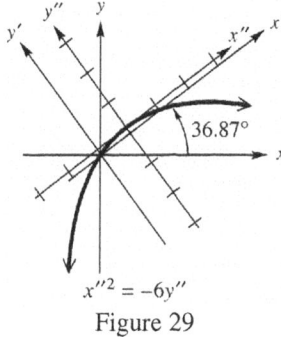

$x''^2 = -6y''$
Figure 29

31. If $B=0$, cot 2θ is undefined, and the graph may be translated but not rotated.

32. If $A=C$, then $A-C=0$, cot $2\theta=0, 2\theta=90°$ and $\theta=45°$.

Join Our Online Discussion Group:

Managed Care Exchange

The **Managed Care Exchange Discussion Group** serves executives and professionals working in health and managed care organizations. The group is sponsored by the Managed Care Information Center. (MCIC)

The group is dedicated to providing members with professional information sharing; opportunities for networking and offering opinion and commentary; and connections to other resources. There is no cost to join.

The members of the online managed care community include managed care and healthcare industry executives and decision makers, consultants, pharmaceutical executives and executives from companies providing goods and services to the industry.

The mission of the **Managed Care Exchange Discussion Group** is to provide members with useful information for decision-making through a variety of means. Discussion open only to professionals and managed care-related postings of professional interest.

You are encouraged to participate in this management-level group.

To Join Go To:

http://groups.yahoo.com/group/ManagedCareExchange

Or Complete This Form and Fax it Toll-Free to (888)329-6242:

Name_____
Title_____
Organization_____
Organization Type_____
Address_____
City_____ State_____ Zipcode_____
Phone_____ Fax_____
E-mail_____
Web Address_____

Order Code: DMC7AD07

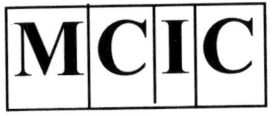

Managed Care InformationCenter
The Executive Report on Managed Care
P.O. Box 456, Allenwood, NJ 08720
Call Toll-Free 1-800-516-4343 or FAX 1-888-329-6242
www.themcic.com   www.healthresourcesonline.com

FREE Weekly E-Mail Newsletter

Sign Up Form

☐ **YES!** Sign me up for Wellness Junction's FREE weekly e-mail newsletter, *"Wellness Junction Professional Weekly Update,"* the twice-a-month briefing providing valuable management tips and program planning ideas. I understand I am under no obligation and can cancel my subscription at any time. To sign up for the FREE *"Wellness Junction Professional Weekly Update,"* fill out this form and fax it back toll-free to (888) 329-6242 or e-mail your request to be added afidalgo@themcic.com.

Name_____
Title_____
Organization_____
Organization Type_____
Address_____
City_____ State_____ Zipcode_____
Phone_____ Fax_____
E-mail_____
Web Address_____

Please share this Sign Up Form with your Director of Health Promotion/Education

FAX BACK TOLL-FREE: (888) 329-6242

Order No. DMC7AD07

Join our Wellness Manager discussion group
at: www.wellnessjunction.com/forum/

This is the place where you can post questions, share stories and search for answers to your health and wellness questions. Whether you have concerns about getting a wellness initiative started, or are looking for information on specific issues such as smoking cessation and nutrition, users can tap into a worldwide community of everyday people and professionals.

Keeping up on the latest wellness-related issues used to involve lengthy reviews of professional literature, poring over stacks of magazines and journals and time-consuming searches of overwhelming amounts of data on the Internet. Now there's...

── www.WellnessJunction.com ──

"Where the Health and Wellness Needs of Consumers and Professionals Meet"

Whether you're looking for return on investment statistics to prove your program's worth, profiles of successful worksite programs or a bookstore of professional resources, Wellness Junction is the place busy professionals can go to find answers to their daily dilemmas. You'll get tons of management tips and insights — and your program participants can find information about a range of such wellness-related issues as diet and nutrition, fitness and smoking cessation.

Visit the Wellness Junction web site today at **www.wellnessjunction.com** and see all we have to offer!

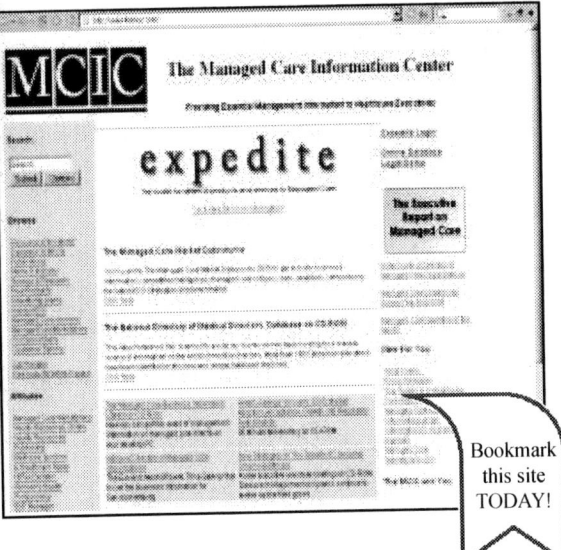

Find the Latest News on Managed Care in one easy stop...

www.themcic.com

From top headline news to managed care market developments, free special reports, and new products and services that can help you get the job done this is the one managed care website that links you to the entire world of managed care. Continuously updated to bring you the latest breaking news.

Bookmark this site TODAY!

"Turning Healthcare Data Into Knowledge"

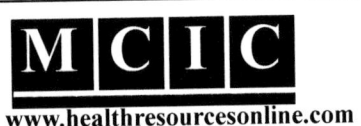
www.healthresourcesonline.com

Managed Care Information Center
PO Box 559
Allenwood, NJ 08720

Call Toll-Free 1-888-THE-MCIC (1-888-843-6242)

FREE Weekly E-Mail Newsletter

• • • • • • • • • • • • • • • Sign Up Form • • • • • • • • • • • • • • •

☐ **YES!** Sign me up for The Managed Care Information Center's free weekly e-mail newsletter, "Managed Care Weekly Watch", the weekly, capsulated managed care briefing on industry activities. I understand I am under no obligation and can cancel my subscription at any time. To sign up for the FREE Managed Care Weekly Watch, fill out this form and fax it back toll-free to (888) 329-6242, e-mail: addmcww@themcic.com, or sign up online at: www.themcic.com/mcww.htm

Name _____
Title _____
Organization _____
Address _____
City _____ State _____ Zip _____
Phone ( ) _____ Fax ( ) _____
E-Mail _____
Type of service provided by your organization _____
Web site _____

FAX BACK TOLL-FREE: (888) 329-6242

Order Code:
DMC7AD07

FREE Weekly E-Mail Newsletter

Sign Up Form

☐ **YES!** Sign me up for Health Resource Publishing's free weekly e-mail newsletter, "Healthcare Industry Weekly Watch," the weekly, capsulated healthcare briefing on industry activities. I understand I am under no obligation and can cancel my subscription at any time. To sign up for the FREE Healthcare Industry Weekly Watch, fill out this form and fax it back toll-free to (888) 329-6242 or sign up online at: www.healthresourcesonline.com/freenews.htm

Order Code: DMC7AD07

Name _____

Title _____

Organization _____

Address _____

City _____ State _____ Zip Code _____

Phone (____) _____ Fax (____) _____

E-Mail _____

Web Address _____

Type of service provided by your organization _____

www.healthrespubs.com

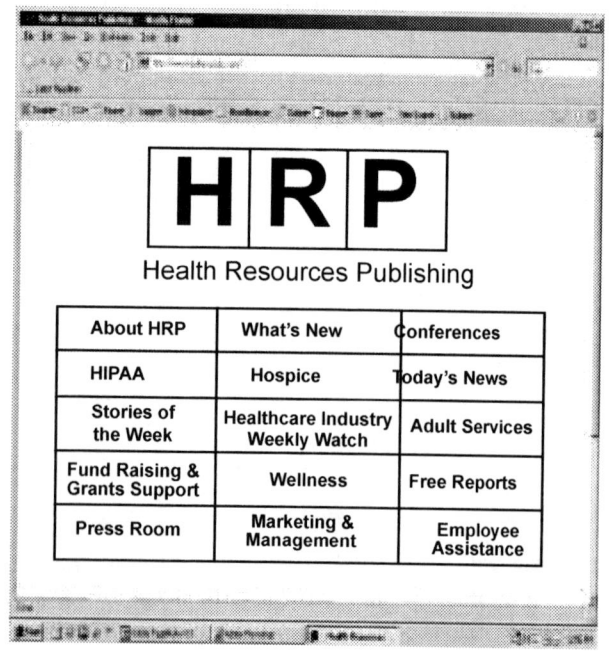

Healthrespubs.com contains information for healthcare professionals from an array of disciplines, including fund raising and grant development, hospice, adult day services, senior services, management, marketing, long-term care administration, wellness and health promotion, and employee assistance program professionals. To foster networking, the site contains forums where visitors can post questions about their most pressing professional needs and concerns. Presented by Health Resources Publishing, the site is updated regularly with useful information for these executives.

| H R P | **Health Resources Publishing**
PO Box 456
Allenwood, NJ 08720 | **Call Toll-Free**
1-800-516-4343 |

Index VIII: Personnel

Zercher, Stephanie
Broadspire Inc — Page 105
Zibes, Zloria
Blue Cross of Puerto Rico/
La Cruz Azul de Puerto Rico — Page 377
Ziesmer, Linda
M-Care Inc — Page 225
Zilligen, Kathy
UnitedHealthcare of
the Midwest Inc — Page 251
Zimmer, Kirk I
DakotaCare — Page 387
Zimmerman, Deborah, MD
Mercy Health Plans of Missouri Inc — Page 249
Zimmerman, Kay
Advantage Health Solutions Inc — Page 157
Zimmerman, Kenneth B
Arkansas Community Care Inc — Page 26
Zimmerman, Natalie
Berkshire Health Partners/Medicus
Resource Management — Page 357
Zingsheim, Jennifer
Catalina Behavioral
Health Services Inc — Page 13
Ziogas, Mike
Aetna Inc - Dental Plan of TX — Page 403
Zlotnick-Hale, Susan
Premier Hlth Ntwrks of AL LLC — Page 6
Zoccoli, Zeke
Horizon Behavioral Services — Page 417
Zoeller, Curt
HealthEOS by MultiPlan — Page 466
Zomermaand, Randall D
WellCare Health Plans Inc -
Corporate Headquarters — Page 124
Zoretic, Richard C
AmeriGroup Corporation — Page 442
Zorn, Christian
Scan Health Plan — Page 68
Zriny, Jeff
Security Health Plan of WI Inc — Page 469
Zubretsky, Joseph M
Aetna Inc - Arkansas — Page 25
Aetna Inc - Dental Care of CA — Page 32
Aetna Inc — Page 87
Aetna Inc - Corp Hdqrtrs — Page 87
Aetna Inc - Altamonte Springs — Page 99
Aetna Inc - Florida — Page 100
Aetna Inc - Jacksonville — Page 100
Aetna Inc - Plantation — Page 100
Aetna Health of Illinois Inc — Page 143
Aetna Inc - Louisiana — Page 189
Aetna Inc - Maryland — Page 199
Aetna Inc - Michigan — Page 217
Aetna Inc - Missouri — Page 243
Aetna Inc - Nevada — Page 259
Aetna Inc - New Jersey — Page 267
Aetna Inc - New York — Page 283
Aetna Inc of the Carolinas — Page 309
Aetna Inc - Ohio — Page 319
Aetna Inc - Oklahoma — Page 339
Aetna Inc - Tulsa — Page 339
Aetna Inc - Corp Hdqrtrs — Page 355
Aetna Inc - Pennsylvania — Page 355
Aetna Inc - Pennsylvania — Page 355
Aetna Inc - Pennsylvania Rgn — Page 356
Aetna Inc - Tennessee — Page 391
Aetna Inc - Dental Plan of TX — Page 403
Aetna Inc - Houston — Page 403
Aetna Health Plans
of Mid-Atlantic — Page 441
Aetna Inc - Virginia — Page 441
Aetna Health Inc - Colorado — Page 77
Zucker, Hymin, MD
Metcare Health Plans Inc — Page 116
Zurblis, Eileen
Hines & Associates Inc — Page 150

Zvelke, Bill
Delta Dental Ins Co - GA — Page 131
Zweig, Neal
CIGNA Healthcare of NH — Page 265
Zybelman, Jay
Primary Provider Management
Company Inc — Page 64

Index VIII: Personnel

Woods, Rick
Group Health Options Inc — Page 452
Group Health Cooperative — Page 451
Woodson, Tonya
Virginia Premier Hlth Plans Inc — Page 447
Woodworth, Judy
Humana Medical Plan - Central Florida — Page 113
Woolf, Allen, MD
CIGNA HealthCare - Corporate Headquarters — Page 360
Intracorp — Page 367
Woolley, Mary
Cariten Healthcare — Page 393
PHP Companies Inc — Page 397
Wooten, Lewis
Health Plus of Louisiana Inc — Page 191
Worcester, Ghita
Ucare Minnesota — Page 238
Worek, Margaret
Gateway Health Plan Inc — Page 362
Worobow, Robert
Trustmark Insurance Company — Page 153
Worthen, Jason
Molina HealthCare of Utah Inc — Page 435
Woys, James
Health Net Inc - Corp Hdqrtrs — Page 49
Wozniak, Richard, MD
Penn Highlands Health Plan — Page 370
Wray, Linton, MD
CareFirst BlueChoice Inc — Page 97
Wright, Daniel
United Concordia Co Inc - AL — Page 6
United Concordia Co Inc - AZ — Page 21
United Concordia Co Inc - CA — Page 72
United Concordia Co Inc - FL — Page 121
United Concordia Co Inc - IL — Page 154
United Concordia Co Inc - MD — Page 206
United Concordia Co Inc - MI — Page 231
United Concordia Co Inc - MO — Page 251
United Concordia Co Inc - NM — Page 282
United Concordia Co Inc - NY — Page 306
United Concordia Co Inc - Corporate Headquarters — Page 373
United Concordia Co Inc - PA — Page 374
United Concordia Co Inc - PA Central — Page 374
United Concordia Co Inc - TX — Page 429
United Concordia Co Inc - VA — Page 446
United Concordia Co Inc - WA — Page 457
Wright, Elease E
Aetna Inc — Page 87
Aetna Inc - New York — Page 283
Aetna Inc of the Carolinas — Page 309
Aetna Inc - Pennsylvania — Page 355
Aetna Inc - Tennessee — Page 391
Wright, Eric
Mutual Assurance Administrators Inc — Page 342
Wright, Jacqueline
Santa Barbara Regional Health Authority — Page 67
Wright, Jonathan
PHP Companies Inc — Page 397
Wright, Kelly
Preferred Provider Organization of Michigan (PPOM) — Page 229
Wright, Lorenzo
Renaissance Health Sys Inc — Page 119
Wright, Nancy
OSF Health Plans — Page 151
Wright, Philip D
Health Plan of the Upper Ohio Valley — Page 327
Health Plan, The Hometown Region — Page 327
Wright, Philip, MD
Physicians Health Plan of Northern Indiana — Page 164

Wristen, Edward L
First Health — California — Page 46
Wroth, Renee
Health New England — Page 212
Wynkoop, Paul
PacificSource Health Plans — Page 350

X

Xie, Frank
Family Choice Health Alliance — Page 272

Y

Yacos, Nadine
Preferred Health Professionals — Page 180
Yaeger, Lisa
Healthplex Inc — Page 296
Yalowitz, David, MD
Bravo Health Inc — Page 200
Bravo Health Pennsylvania Inc — Page 358
Yamaykina, Anna
Northeast Pharmacy Srvc Corp — Page 490
Yambert, Jay, A MD, FACP, FACEP
CIMRO Quality Healthcare Solutions — Page 144
Yancey, Betty
Coastal Healthcare Administrators — Page 41
Yanchak, Adam
Ohio Health Choice — Page 332
Yang, Anna, PharmD
Alameda Alliance for Health — Page 33
Yanuk, Michael, MD
Quality Health Plan Inc — Page 119
Yates, Alan, MD
Stanislaus Medical Society — Page 70
Yates, Libba
Viva Health Inc — Page 7
Yates, Steven
Windsor Health Plan of TN Inc — Page 401
Yearwood, Lynn
HealthLink Inc - Corp Hdqrtrs — Page 249
Yee, David
Capitol Administrators — Page 38
Yee, Don
Vision Service Plan of Arizona — Page 22
Yelorda, Peter K
BCBS of Kansas City — Page 244
Yoder, David, PharmD, MBA
Bravo Health Pennsylvania Inc — Page 358
Yoder, Eric MD, MBA
AmeriGroup Texas Inc — Page 404
Yong, Eben
Health Plan of San Mateo — Page 50
Yordy, Matt S
Prime Therapeutics — Page 493
York, Billie
American WholeHealth Networks Inc — Page 442
York, Rebecca
Superior Dental Care Alliance — Page 335
Yost, R David
Amerisource Bergen Performance Plus Network - West — Page 480
Yost, Tina
Humana Health Care Plans of Houston — Page 418
Young, Albert, MD
UHP Healthcare — Page 71
Young, Ann
Dental Care Plus Inc — Page 324

Young, Ann
Dental Care Plus Inc — Page 324
Young, Bill
Blue Cross Blue Shield of TN — Page 392
Blue Cross Blue Shield of TN - Memphis — Page 393
Young, Charles N
Delta Dental Plan of Tennessee — Page 394
Young, Dennis, MD
UnitedHealthcare of Florida Inc — Page 121
Young, Gerald
National Capital PPO — Page 444
Young, Jeffrey, MD
Arise Health Plan — Page 461
Young, John T
Managed Health Services Indiana Inc — Page 163
Young, Leslie
XL Health — Page 207
Young, Margaret, RN, BSN, MBA
Molina Healthcare of Texas Inc — Page 421
Young, Michael, CPA
Molina Healthcare of Texas Inc — Page 421
Young, Thomas
Aetna Inc - Pennsylvania — Page 355
Young, Wes
Health Management Network Inc — Page 16
Young, Ze'ev, MD
First Choice Health Network — Page 451
Youso, Steven
Security Health Plan of WI Inc — Page 469
Yucht, Gerry, MD
Medcore Health Plan — Page 58
Yung, Patrick
Connecticare Inc — Page 89
Yust, Greg
Sagamore Health Network Inc — Page 164

Z

Zaback, David
National Health Plan — Page 302
Zaferos, Bill
Anthem BCBS of Wisconsin — Page 461
Zaftoupil, Stacy
Delta Dental Plan of Wyoming — Page 473
Zagorski, Pam
Health New England — Page 212
Zakrzewski, Devin
Texas True Choice — Page 428
Zaldivar, Nieves M, MD
D C Chartered Health Plan Inc — Page 97
Zaldivar, Sergio
CareMore Health Plan — Page 38
Zambino, Sondra
Dentistat (Insurance Dentists of America) — Page 45
Zane, Linda
Physical Therapy Provider Network — Page 117
Zanoni, Lawrence J
Group Health Cooperative South Central Wisconsin — Page 464
Zarza-Garrido, Joann
Molina Healthcare Inc - CA — Page 59
Zastrow, Allan W
Keokuk Area Hospital Organized Delivery System Inc — Page 171
Zeitenberg, Lynn
Mental Health Consultants Inc — Page 369
Zelkind, Sharon
Healthplex Inc — Page 296
Zeppetello, Angela
SCHC Total Care Inc — Page 305

Index VIII: Personnel

Williams, Wayne, COO
Atlantic Integrated Health Inc — Page 309
Williamson, Jane, RN
HealthSmart Preferred Care — Page 416
Williamson, Vicki
Great-West Healthcare of PA — Page 363
Willingham, Edna
Memphis Managed Care Corp — Page 397
Willingham, Ellen
Pacific Union Dental Inc — Page 63
Nevada Pacific Dental — Page 262
Willis, Kerry A, MD
Atlantic Integrated Health Inc — Page 309
Willis, Richard
Humana Health Plan of Austin — Page 419
Willoughby, Brenda
NAMCI — Page 6
Premier Hlth Networks of AL LLC — Page 6
Wills, Charles
Berkshire Health Partners/Medicus Resource Management — Page 357
Wills, Jennifer
Humana Hlth Care Plans of AZ — Page 17
Wilson, Brian
Zurich Services Corporation — Page 155
Wilson, Chris P
ValueOptions - Corp Hdqrtrs — Page 447
Wilson, Clint
Mutual Assurance Administrators Inc — Page 342
Wilson, Deborah
Preferred Provider Organization of Michigan (PPOM) — Page 229
Wilson, Deborah
AmeriGroup District of Columbia — Page 97
Wilson, Dennis
Lovelace Health Plan — Page 280
Wilson, Doug
Mountain Medical Affiliates — Page 83
Wilson, Ellen G
Excellus BlueCross BlueShield, Central New York Region — Page 291
Wilson, J Bradley
BCBS of North Carolina — Page 310
BCBS of North Carolina — Page 481
Wilson, Jennifer
Blue Cross Blue Shield of MS — Page 241
Wilson, Judith
Acumentra Health — Page 345
Wilson, Keith, MD
Talbert Health Plan — Page 70
Talbert Health Plan — Page 70
Wilson, Kern
Gulf Health Plans PPO Inc — Page 4
Wilson, Lance
Assurant Health - Corp Hdqrtrs — Page 462
Wilson, Lawrence, MD
Blue Cross Blue Shield of NM — Page 279
HMO New Mexico Inc — Page 280
Wilson, Linda
Mutual Assurance Administrators Inc — Page 342
Wilson, Lonny
Pharmacy Providers of OK — Page 492
Wilson, M Haley
Qca Health Plan Inc — Page 28
Wilson, Michael
Texas True Choice — Page 428
Wilson, Mike
Fidelio Insurance Company — Page 362
Wilson, Teresa
Center Care — Page 184
Wimmer, Judith, RN
New York Presbyterian Community Health Plan — Page 302
Winderman, Jonathan
Intracorp — Page 367

Windfeldt, Ty
Hometown Health Plan — Page 260
Wing, Deborah
CIGNA Healthcare of NH — Page 265
Wingaurd, Susan
Atrio Health Plans Inc — Page 345
Winger, Curtis L
Mid-Atlantic Managed Care Org of Pennsylvania Inc — Page 369
Winkler, Walter H
Keokuk Area Hospital Organized Delivery System Inc — Page 171
Winn, Daniel, MD
CareFirst Blue Cross Blue Shield — Page 200
Winner, Mark
American Healthcare Alliance — Page 243
Winskas, Robin
Health Net of Arizona — Page 17
Health Alliance Medical Plans - Corporate Headquarters — Page 149
Winslett, Claudia
WelBorn Health Plans — Page 167
Winston, Taylor
San Francisco Health Plan — Page 66
Wintermeyer, Dorane
Blue Cross Blue Shield of NM — Page 279
Winzer, Kimulet
Care 1st Health Plan AZ Inc — Page 13
Wipperfurth, Rich
Innoviant Inc — Page 487
Wisdom, Keith
UnitedHealthcare of the Heartland States — Page 182
Wise, Greg, MD
Mount Carmel Health Plan — Page 331
Wise, Michael R
Connecticare Inc — Page 89
Wise, Mike
Delta Dental of Virginia — Page 443
Wise, Steve
MedSolutions — Page 396
Witkowski, Joseph
PPO USA Inc — Page 250
Witt, Bruce
Preferred Health Systems — Page 180
Witte, Barbara
Group Health Plan Inc — Page 248
Witte, Barbara A
Coventry Health Care of NE Inc — Page 255
Wittenauer, Douglas
Pharmacy Data Mngmnt Inc — Page 492
Witter, Dana
Vision Insurance Plan of America Inc - Corp Headquarters — Page 471
Wittman, Joyce
Individualized Care Mngmnt Inc — Page 162
Witty, Karey L CPA
Managed Health Services Insurance Corporation — Page 467
Wofford, John
1st Medical Network — Page 127
Wohlman, Doug
Williamette Dental Group PC — Page 352
Wojtaszek, Ronald
Santa Clara Family Health Plan — Page 67
Wolf, Dale B
First Health Group Corp — Page 147
Coventry Health Care Inc — Corporate Headquarters — Page 201
Cambridge Life Ins Co — Page 516
First Health Rx — Page 485
Coventry Healthcare — Page 394
Wolf, David D
CareFirst BlueChoice Inc — Page 97
CareFirst BCBS — Page 200
Delmarva Health Care Plan Inc — Page 202
Wolf, Jodi
Davis Vision — Page 288

Wolfe, Dennis
Berkshire Health Partners/Medicus Resource Management — Page 357
Wolff, Sherman M
Blue Cross Blue Shield of IL — Page 144
Blue Cross Blue Shield of Texas — HMO Blue - Midwest TX — Page 406
Wolgemuth, Sherry
Preferred Health Care — Page 370
Wolin, Leon
Union Health Service Inc — Page 154
Wolk, Larry, MD
HMS Colorado Inc — Page 82
Sloan's Lake Preferred Health Networks — Page 85
Wolk, Lawrence, MD
CIGNA Healthcare of Colorado — Page 79
Woll, Douglas R, MD
Blue Care Network of Michigan — Page 217
Woloszynski, Jay
Health Net Inc - Northeast Corporate Headquarters — Page 91
Wolson, Richard
Aetna Health of Illinois Inc — Page 143
Wong, Adrian
Chinese Community Hlth Plan — Page 39
Wong, Edward
Premera BCBS of Alaska — Page 9
LifeWise Health Plan of WA — Page 453
Premera - Corp Hdqrtrs — Page 454
Premera Blue Cross - Eastern — Page 454
Premera Blue Cross - Western — Page 454
Wong, Frank, MD
Managed HealthCare Northwest Inc — Page 348
Wong, Gloria
New York State Catholic Health Plan Inc — Page 303
Wong, Irene
SHPS Inc — Page 186
Wong, Josie, RN
Care 1st Health Plan — Page 38
Wong, Michael, WC
Hawaii Medical Services Association - BC/BS of Hawaii — Page 137
Wong, SR
Care 1st Health Plan — Page 38
Wong, Sue
On Lok Senior Health Services — Page 60
On Lok Senior Health Services — Page 512
Wong, Winston, PharmD
CareFirst BlueChoice Inc — Page 97
CareFirst BCBS — Page 200
Delmarva Health Care Plan Inc — Page 202
Woo, Herbert
Care 1st Health Plan — Page 38
Wood, Alan
Humana Health Plans of GA — Page 132
Wood, John
Comprehensive Health Group — Page 129
Wood, Ron
CompBenefits Corporation - Corporate Headquarters — Page 129
Woodall, Gilbert, Jr, MD
Prime Health Services Inc — Page 398
Woodall, John
KPS Health Plans — Page 452
Woodard, Bob
Kern Family Health Care — Page 55
Woodley, Michael, RPh
WellDyne Rx — Page 497
Woodriffe, Ramona, MD
Evercare Select — Page 15
Woods, Rick
KPS Health Plans — Page 452
Group Health Cooperative — Page 141
Group Health Cooperative of Puget Sound — Page 452

Index VIII: Personnel

White, Gary
American National Ins Co — Page 405
White, Heather C
Dental Bnft Providers of CA Inc — Page 45
White, Jan
Mutual Assurance
Administrators Inc — Page 342
White, Jayson R
New York State Catholic
Health Plan Inc — Page 303
White, Lorie
HealthLink Inc - Corp Hdqrtrs — Page 249
White, Mark
Arkansas Blue Cross/Blue Shield
a Mutual Insurance Company — Page 25
White, Michael
Delta Dental Plan of Illinois — Page 145
White, Michael, DDS
Dental Care of America Ltd — Page 146
White, Patty
Provider Ntwrks of America Inc — Page 424
White, Prowess
UnitedHealthcare of Texas Inc -
Houston — Page 429
White, Robert
MD-Individual Practice Association Inc
(MD IPA) — Page 204
Mid Atlantic Medical Services Inc
(MAMSI)- Corp Headquarters — Page 204
OneNet PPO — Page 205
White, Robert P
American Specialty
Health Plans Inc — Page 33
White, Sandra L, MD
Blue Cross Blue Shield of GA — Page 128
White, Stephen
Delta Dental Plans Association — Page 146
White, Steven A
Great-West Healthcare of FL — Page 111
Great-West Healthcare of GA — Page 131
Great-West Healthcare of NC — Page 313
White, Winona
Kaiser Permanente Health Plan — Page 137
Whiteford, Gary
Univera Community Health — Page 307
Whites, Bruce
Preferred Health Care — Page 370
Whitesel, Karen
United Concordia Co Inc - CA — Page 72
United Concordia Co Inc -
Corporate Headquarters — Page 373
Whiting, Kent
Deseret Healthcare — Page 434
Whitley, Kim R, MBA
Samaritan Health Plans Inc — Page 352
Whitley, Michael
Providence Health System — Page 514
Whitmer, Richard E
Blue Preferred Plan-Blue Cross/Blue Shield
Michigan — Page 519
Whittlesey, Dee, MD
Blue Cross Blue Shield of Texas —
Corporate Headquarters — Page 406
Blue Cross Blue Shield of Texas —
HMO Blue - Southeast — Page 407
Blue Cross Blue Shield of Texas — HMO
Blue - West — Page 407
Wiatrek, Karen
Community First Hlth Plans Inc — Page 410
Wichmann, David S
Dental Bnft Providers of CA Inc — Page 45
Wicks, Cynthia
Capital District Physicians
Health Plan — Page 286
Wiechers, David O, MD, MS, MBA
UnitedHealthcare of Illinois Inc — Page 154
Wiedenman, Charlotte, DMD
Delta Dental Insu Co - AL — Page 4

Wiesendanger, John C
West Virginia Medical Institute — Page 460
Wiewora, Ronald, MD
Healthy Palm Beaches Inc — Page 112
Wiffler, Thomas P
UnitedHealthcare of IL Inc — Page 154
Wiggins, Steven K
Blue Cross Blue Shield of SC -
Corporate Hqtrs — Page 383
Wightman, Deborah M
Aetna Inc - Georgia — Page 127
Aetna Inc - Maine — Page 195
Wilbanks, C Shane
CorpHealth Inc — Page 412
Wilber, Don, MD
Global Health Inc — Page 341
Wilbert, Jill
Lifetime Healthcare Companies, The -
Corporate Headquarters — Page 298
Wilcox, Bob
Iowa Health Solutions — Page 171
Wilcox, David, MD
Preferred One — Page 93
Wilcoxon, Samuel R
Fidelis SecureCare of MI Inc — Page 221
Wild, Barbara
Winhealth Partners — Page 473
Wild, Trei
Safeguard Health Plans Inc — Page 424
Wildenberg, Bob
Group Health Cooperative
of Eau Claire — Page 465
Wilder, Barbara, MBA
MDwise — Page 163
Wilhelm, Felicia, RN
Prairie States Enterprises Inc — Page 152
Wilhelmy, Cynthian, MD
Ventura County Health Care Plan — Page 73
Wilk, Joel, MD
Forte Managed Care — Page 414
Wilkerson, Leonard A, DO
UnitedHealthcare of NC Inc — Page 315
Wilkerson, Scott
Physicians Health Plan
of Mid-Michigan — Page 228
Wilkinson, Bruce
Providence Health Plans — Page 351
Wilkosz, Diane
HealthEase of Florida Inc — Page 111
WellCare of New York — Page 307
Will, Theodore O, MPA
IPRO — Page 298
Willard, Teresa
Geisinger Health Plan — Page 363
Willcoxon, Samuel R
Fidelis SeniorCare Inc — Page 147
Fidelis SecureCare of MI Inc — Page 221
Fidelis SecureCare of NC — Page 312
Fidelis SecureCare of Texas — Page 413
Willey, Charles J, MD
Essence Inc — Page 246
William-Lindgren, Suanne
Martins Point Health Care — Page 196
Williams, Amy
Managed Health Services
Indiana Inc — Page 163
Williams, Barbara
Careington International -
The Dental Network — Page 408
Williams, Christine
Western Health Advantage — Page 75
Williams, Craig
SCHC Total Care Inc — Page 305
Williams, Deborah
Dental Care Plus Inc — Page 324
Williams, Doyle, DDS
Denta Quest Mid-Atlantic Inc — Page 202
Denta Quest Ventures Inc — Page 211
Doral Dental USA — Page 464

Williams, Holly
Superior HealthPlan Inc — Page 426
Williams, Jim L
Oklahoma Foundation for
Medical Quality — Page 342
Williams, Laura
Community Health Plan — Page 42
Williams, Lauren
Connecticare Inc — Page 89
Williams, Lisa
Kansas Foundation Mdcl Care — Page 179
Williams, Lisa
Group Health Plan Inc — Page 248
Williams, Marinan
Legacy Health Solutions Inc — Page 420
Scott & White Health Plan — Page 424
Williams, Mark
Epoch Group LC, The — Page 178
Williams, Micael, Esq
San Joaquin Foundation PPO — Page 67
Williams, Myra L
Hawaii Medical Services Association - BC/
BS of Hawaii — Page 137
Williams, Ronald A
Aetna Inc - Arizona — Page 11
Aetna Inc - Arkansas — Page 25
Aetna Health of California Inc — Page 31
Aetna Inc - Dental Care of CA — Page 32
Aetna Health Inc - Colorado — Page 77
Aetna Inc - Connecticut — Page 87
Aetna Inc - Corp Hdqrtrs — Page 87
Aetna Inc Life Insurance Co — Page 87
Aetna Inc - Altamonte Springs — Page 99
Aetna Inc - Florida — Page 100
Aetna Inc - Jacksonville — Page 100
Aetna Inc - Plantation — Page 100
Aetna Inc - Georgia — Page 127
Aetna Health of Illinois Inc — Page 143
Aetna Inc - Louisiana — Page 189
Aetna Inc - Maine — Page 195
Aetna Inc - Maryland — Page 199
Aetna Inc - Massachusetts — Page 209
Aetna Inc - Michigan — Page 217
Aetna Inc - Missouri — Page 243
Aetna Inc - Nevada — Page 259
Aetna Dental Inc - New Jersey — Page 267
Aetna Inc - New Jersey — Page 267
Aetna Inc - New Jersey — Page 267
Aetna Inc - New York — Page 283
Aetna Inc - New York — Page 283
Aetna Inc of the Carolinas — Page 309
Aetna Inc - Ohio — Page 319
Aetna Inc - Oklahoma — Page 339
Aetna Inc - Tulsa — Page 339
Aetna Inc - Corp Hdqrtrs — Page 355
Aetna Inc - Pennsylvania — Page 355
Aetna Inc - Pennsylvania — Page 355
Aetna Inc - Pennsylvania Rgn — Page 356
Aetna Inc - Tennessee — Page 391
Aetna Inc - Tennessee — Page 391
Aetna Inc - Dental Plan of TX — Page 403
Aetna Inc - Houston — Page 403
Aetna Hlth Plans of Mid-Atlantic — Page 441
Aetna Inc - Virginia — Page 441
Aetna Inc - Washington — Page 449
Aetna Life Insurance Company — Page 516
Williams, Sharon
HFN Inc — Page 150
Williams, Shelly
Utah Public Employees
Health Program — Page 438
Williams, Thomas R
Aetna Health of California Inc — Page 31
Aetna Inc - Dental Care of CA — Page 32
Aetna Inc - Nevada — Page 259
Williams, Vince
Golden West Dental & Vision — Page 47

Index VIII: Personnel

Waters, Wes
UnitedHealthcare of TN Inc — Page 401
Watkins, Anne
Kern Family Health Care — Page 55
Watkins, Kenneth L
PacifiCare Behavioral Health — Page 61
Watkins, Letitia E
Viva Health Inc — Page 7
Watkins, Reg
All Florida PPO Inc — Page 101
All Florida PPO Inc — Page 101
Watrin, Elizabeth A
HMO New Mexico Inc — Page 280
Blue Cross Blue Shield of NM — Page 279
Watson, Anthony L
Connecticare Inc — Page 89
Connecticare of MN Inc — Page 210
Connecticare of NY — Page 288
EmblemHealth Inc — Page 290
HIP Health Plan of New York — Page 296
Watson, Esther, RN
Wellpath Select Inc — Page 315
Watson, Mary, MD
Community First Hlth Plans Inc — Page 410
Watson, Robert W
Allianz Life Insurance Company of North America — Page 233
Watson, Ron
Bucks County Physician Hospital Alliance — Page 358
Waugh, Sam
Humana Health Care Plans of Dallas — Page 417
Waxman, Albert, PhD
CareGuide — Page 105
Waymire, Sharin Danell
Puget Sound Health Partners — Page 455
Weafer, Patricia
Capital District Physicians Health Plan — Page 286
Wearing, Allen
Group Health Cooperative South Central Wisconsin — Page 464
Weaver, Lisa, MD
Humana Inc - Tennessee — Page 396
Humana WI Hlth Org Inc — Page 466
Weaver, Vicki
Cariten Healthcare — Page 393
PHP Companies Inc — Page 397
Webb, Deborah
Utah Public Employees Health Program — Page 438
Webb, Jane
Health Plan, The Hometown Region — Page 327
Webb, Larry
Athens Area Health Plan Select Inc — Page 127
Webb, Michael
Premier Pharmacy Plan — Page 493
Webb-Bowen, Ken
Preferred Health Plan Inc — Page 350
Weber, Chuck
CareMore Health Plan — Page 38
Weber, Darcee
Preferred One — Page 237
Weber, Kris
Sagamore Health Network Inc — Page 164
Weber, Ralph, MD
Blue Cross Blue Shield of KS — Page 177
Weber, Tim
Wellmark BCBS of Iowa — Page 174
Wellmark Inc — Corp Hdqrtrs — Page 175
Wellmark Health Plan of IA Inc — Page 175
Webster, Deborah
Altius Health Plans — Page 433
Wedin, Jeff
UnitedHealthcare of Alabama — Page 7
UnitedHealthcare of Louisiana — Page 193

Weeks, Cynthia G
Employers Dental Services Inc — Page 15
Wehier, Helge
Bayer Corporation Pharmaceutical Division — Page 481
Wehr, Ann, MD
Molina Healthcare of NM — Page 281
Wehr, Richard, CLU
Preferred Care Incorporated — Page 370
Weigle, Catherine
Neighborhood Hlth Providers — Page 302
Weigum, Eileen
Community First Hlth Plans Inc — Page 410
Weikel, David
Coordinated Health Systems — Page 361
Weimann, Fred
Suffolk Health Plan — Page 305
Weinberg, Rick
HealthPlus Inc — Page 296
Weinberg, Ted
Avera Health Plans Inc — Page 387
Weinberger, Dick
USA Managed Care Org — Page 22
Weiner, Scott
Health Net Hlth Plan of OR Inc — Page 346
Weingarten, Allan
Great-West Healthcare of AZ — Page 16
Weingarten, Jorge, MD
Care 1st Health Plan — Page 38
Weinper, Michael, MPH, PT
PTPN - Corporate Headquarters — Page 65
Weinschenk, Sherry
Healthy Palm Beaches Inc — Page 112
Weinstein, Audrey
Block Vision of Texas Inc — Page 405
Weinstein, Matthew
Community Behavioral Healthcare Cooperative of Pennsylvania — Page 361
Weinstein, Michael
AIDS Healthcare Foundation — Page 32
Weis, Marci, RN, MPH, CCM, CPUM
Qualis Health — Page 455
Weiser, Robert
Carolinas Center for Medical Excellence, The — Page 310
Weiss, Carl Jr, MD
Coordinated Health Systems — Page 361
Weiss, Clay
Alliance Regional Hlth Ntwrk — Page 404
Weiss, Jack, MD
Sun Health Medisun — Page 20
Weiss, James D
Aetna Inc - Washington — Page 449
Weiss, Mary
Humana Health Care Plans of Corpus Christi — Page 417
Humana Health Care Plans of San Antonio/Austin — Page 418
Weiss, Peter, MD
Health First Health Plans Inc — Page 111
Weisz, Jeffrey A, MD
Kaiser Foundation Health Plan of Southern California — Page 54
Welborn, Lynn
Blue Cross Blue Shield of GA — Page 128
Welch, Suzy
First Choice of the Midwest Inc — Page 388
Welch, Terri RN
New York Presbyterian Community Health Plan — Page 302
Welle-Powell, Debbie, CMPE
Exempla Healthcare LLC — Page 81
Wells, Brian
Missouri Care — Page 250
CIGNA Healthcare of NH — Page 265
Wells, Kevin
CareSource — Page 321

Wells, Mark
BeneScript Services Inc — Page 481
Wells, Scott
Sante Community Physicians — Page 67
Welters, Anthony
AmeriChoice of New York — Page 284
Wende, Joseph, MD
Davis Vision — Page 288
Wendt, Douglas R
Combined Insurance Company of America — Page 145
Wendt, Linda
Group Health Cooperative of Eau Claire — Page 465
Wenk, Philip, DDS
Delta Dental Plan of TN — Page 394
Wenners, Douglas
Anthem BCBS of Maine — Page 195
Wentworth, Katherine, JD
MDwise — Page 163
Wernsing, Donald, MD
Americhoice of New Jersey — Page 268
Wesley, Susan
UnitedHealthcare of WI Inc — Page 470
West, Malcolm R
Community Behavioral Healthcare Cooperative of Pennsylvania — Page 361
Westerman, Chris
Health Mngmnt Ntwrk Inc — Page 16
Westerman, George, MD
Behavioral Hlthcre Options Inc — Page 259
Westfall, Laurie
Blue Care Network of Michigan — Page 217
Care Choices HMO — Page 218
Westin, George, MD
Medcore Health Plan — Page 58
Westley, Randy
Abri Health Plan Inc — Page 461
Wexler, Eric
Great Lakes Health Plan — Page 222
Whalen, Joseph, MD
KHS a KMG America Co — Page 385
Whaley, Carla
Humana Health Plan - KY — Page 185
Whaley, Linda
Healthcare USA of Missouri LLC — Page 248
Whalley, John W
PacifiCare Dental & Vision — Page 61
Whalley, Nancy, BSN, MPA, CMAC
Action Hlth Care Mngmnt Srvcs — Page 11
Whamond, Don
Care-Plus Dental Plans Inc — Page 462
Wheat, Rich
Integrated Health Plan Inc — Page 115
Wheaton, Angela
Martins Point Health Care — Page 196
Wheeler, George
Coventry Health Care of KS - Wichita — Page 178
Coventry Hlth Care of KS Inc — Page 245
Wheeler, Jeffrey, MD, JD
Kansas Foundation Mdcl Care — Page 179
Wheelock, Ann
Columbia United Providers — Page 449
Whisman, Bill
Southeastern Indiana Health Organization — Page 166
Whitcomb, Ronald
Delta Dental Plan of Kansas — Page 178
White Crane, Angela
Comprehensive Behavioral Care Inc — Page 108
White, Brenda
Neighborhood Hlth Plan of RI — Page 380
White, Carolyn
Optimum HealthCare Inc — Page 117
White, Dale
MultiPlan Inc - Corp Hdqrtrs — Page 300

Index VIII: Personnel

Wachsman, Abraham
Atlantis Health Plan — Page 285
Wachtelhausen, Roberta
Meritain Health Inc — Page 299
Waddell, Deborah
Citrus Health Care Inc — Page 108
Wade, Michael
Serve You Custom
Prescription Management — Page 495
Wadle, Charles, DO
Magellan Behavioral
Care of IA Inc — Page 171
Waechter, Joachim
ScripNet — Page 494
Waegelein, Robert A
American Pioneer
Health Plans Inc — Page 101
American Progressive Life
& Health of New York — Page 501
Wagnar, Mark
Empire BCBS — Page 290
Wagner, Barry
Av-Med Health Plan - Tampa — Page 103
Wagner, Jean
University Family Care
Health Plan — Page 22
Wagner, John
Regence Blue Shield — Page 456
Wagner, Peggy
Horizon Behavioral Services — Page 112
Wagner, Sylvia R
Assurant Employee Benefits-AL — Page 3
Assurant Employee Benefits-AZ — Page 12
Assurant Employee Benefits-CA — Page 35
Assurant Employee Benefits-CO — Page 78
Assurant Employee Benefits-FL — Page 102
Assurant Employee Benefits-GA — Page 127
Assurant Employee Benefits-IL — Page 143
Assurant Employee Benefits-IN — Page 158
Assurant Employee Benefits-MI — Page 217
Assurant Employee Benefits -
Corporate Office — Page 244
Assurant Employee Benefits-NM — Page 279
Assurant Employee Benefits-NY — Page 285
Assurant Employee Benefits-NC — Page 309
Assurant Employee Benefits-PA — Page 357
Assurant Employee Benefits-TN — Page 392
Assurant Employee Benefits-TX — Page 429
Assurant Employee Benefits-WA — Page 449
Wagner, Yvon
Eyexam of California Inc — Page 46
Waibel, Robert
UnitedHealthcare of Arkansas — Page 28
Waite, Douglas D
Seton Health Plan — Page 425
Walbillig, Cathy
Evercare Select — Page 15
Walburn, Ed
AmeriGroup DC — Page 97
Walcott, Myles
Behavioral Health Systems Inc — Page 3
Waldo, Laura
Humana Inc - Indiana — Page 161
Waldron, Angela
Avesis Inc — Page 12
Waldron, Dave
American WholeHealth
Networks Inc — Page 442
Wales, Dirk O, MD
HealthSpring Inc-Tennessee — Page 395
HealthSpring Inc-Corp Hdqrtrs — Page 395
Walheim, Jon, MD
Bucks County Physician
Hospital Alliance — Page 358
Walker, Arthur, DC
Complementary Hlthcare Plans — Page 345
Walker, Bob
Delta Dental Plan of Wisconsin — Page 463

Walker, Janice, RN, CPHQ
Beech Street Corporation —
Corporate Headquarters — Page 36
Walker, Karen, RN
Fidelis SecureCare of NC — Page 312
Walker, Linda
HCH Administration — Page 148
Walker, Michelle L
HealthLink Inc - Corp Hdqrtrs — Page 249
Walko, Jeff
Anthem BCBS of Virginia Inc — Page 442
Wall, Bruce, MD
OhioHealth Group — Page 332
Wall, Eric M, MD, MPH
LifeWise Health Plan of OR — Page 348
Wall, Juli
Allianz Life Insurance Company
of North America — Page 233
Wall, Robert E
Blue Cross Blue Shield of FL
Health Options Inc — Page 104
Wallace, C Wayne
Blue Cross Blue Shield of OK — Page 339
Wallace, Jama, PharmD
WelBorn Health Plans — Page 167
Wallace, Jim, RPh
AmeriScript Inc — Page 479
Wallace, Wayne
Bluelincs HMO — Page 340
Wallace, William J
Blue Cross Blue Shield of KS — Page 177
Wallbank, Nigel
Strategic Health
Development Corporation — Page 119
Wallen, Robert
Great-West Healthcare of AZ — Page 16
Wallendjack, John C, MD
HealthAmerica Pennsylvania Inc -
Central Region — Page 364
HealthAmerica Pennsylvania Inc -
Eastern Region — Page 365
Waller, Jim
Nationwide Better Health — Page 204
Walli, Steve C
UnitedHealthcare of the
Midwest Inc — Page 251
Wallis, Robert, MD
Memorial Hermann
Health Network Providers — Page 420
Wallner, Mark P
Vision Insurance Plan of America Inc -
Corp Headquarters — Page 471
Walls, Phil, RPh
MyMatrixx — Page 489
Wallstrom, Nicole
Ameritas Mngd Dental Plan Inc — Page 34
Walsh, Andrea
HealthPartners Inc — Page 236
HealthPartners — Page 486
Walsh, Colleen
UMPC Health Plan Univ of
Pittsburgh Medical Center — Page 374
Walsh, Glenn
UnitedHealthcare of Arkansas — Page 28
Walsh, James P
Hawaii Medical Services Association -
BC/BS of Hawaii — Page 137
Walsh, Michael F
Delta Dental Plan of MN — Page 235
Walsh, Michael F
Delta Dental of Nebraska — Page 256
Delta Dental Plan of MN — Page 235
Walsh, Nancy
Humana Health Plan - KY — Page 185
Walsh, Robyn S
Aetna Inc - Corp Hdqrtrs — Page 87
Aetna Inc - Corp Hdqrtrs — Page 355
Aetna Inc - Pennsylvania — Page 355

Walter, Courtney B
HealthLink of Arkansas Inc — Page 27
HealthLink Inc — Page 248
HealthLink Inc - Corp Hdqrtrs — Page 249
Walters, Laurel
Rocky Mountain Health Plans — Page 84
Rocky Mountain HealthCare Options Inc
dba Healthcare Options — Page 84
Walton, Aaron A
Highmark Inc — Page 366
Walton, Cheryl, RN
Care 1st Health Plan AZ Inc — Page 13
Wamble-King, Sharon
Blue Cross Blue Shield of Florida/
Health Options Inc — Page 104
Wanchik, Nancy
Molina Healthcare of MI Inc — Page 227
Wander, Frank
Guardian Life Insurance Co
of America — Page 294
Wang, James, MD
CIGNA Healthcare of CA — Page 41
Wanger, Jeff
Contra Costa Health Plan — Page 43
Wann, Paul
HCH Administration — Page 148
Wanovich, Robert
Highmark Inc — Page 366
Warburton, R Paul
Regence BCBS of Utah — Page 436
Regence Healthwise — Page 436
Regence Valucare — Page 436
Ward, Butch
Independence Blue Cross — Page 366
Keystone Health Plan East Inc — Page 368
Ward, Gary
Lifetime Healthcare Companies, The -
Corporate Headquarters — Page 298
Ward, John
Maxor Plus — Page 488
Ward, Lisa
Delta Dental Plan of Kansas — Page 178
Ward, Matthew P
Partners Rx Management LLC — Page 491
Warner, Jeffrey E
Doral Dental USA — Page 464
Warner, Mark
Integra Group — Page 329
Warner, Tracy
Washington Dental Service — Page 457
Warren, Ann
Community Health Group — Page 41
Warren, Karen
Molina HealthCare of Utah Inc — Page 435
Warren, Kevin
Texas Medical Foundation
Health Quality Institute — Page 427
Warren, Lonny D
Winhealth Partners — Page 473
Warren, Patricia
AmeriGroup New Jersey Inc — Page 268
Warren, Robert
Aetna Inc - Oklahoma — Page 339
Warrington, J Marc, DMD
Assurant Employee Bnfts - NM — Page 279
Wasden, Phil
CIGNA Healthcare of Florida — Page 107
Washburn, Steve
Great Lakes Health Plan — Page 222
Washington, Adrienne
Kaiser Foundation Health
Plan of Georgia — Page 132
Wassom, Rhonda
Priority Health — Page 230
Wasson, Beth A
Winhealth Partners — Page 473
Waterman, Beth
HealthPartners Inc — Page 236

Index VIII: Personnel

V

Vaccaro, Jerome V, MD
PacifiCare Behavioral Health   Page 61
APS Healthcare Inc   Page 199
Vagas, Monica
American Specialty
Health Plans Inc   Page 33
Vagts, Joyce
Connecticare Inc   Page 89
Vail, Cheron
Regence BCBS of Oregon   Page 351
Vail, Cheron R
Regence Group, The —
Corporate Headquarters   Page 351
Valdes, Petra
Medical Card System   Page 377
Valdez, Josh
Blue Cross of California   Page 34
Valdimer, Leigh
CareIQ   Page 106
Valenti, John, DDS
Golden Dental Plans Inc   Page 221
Valentine, Joyce
Union Health Service Inc   Page 154
Valentine, Theresa E
UlliCare   Page 98
Union Labor Life Insurance Co   Page 276
Valenzuela, Susana P
Employers Dental Services Inc   Page 15
Valerio, David A, Esq
American Health Care   Page 480
Valesey, Janice
Vista Hlthplan of South FL Inc   Page 123
Valine, Roger
Vision Service Plan of Arizona   Page 22
Valiulis, Carl
Hines & Associates Inc   Page 150
Valosin, Jose
AmeriGroup Florida Inc   Page 101
Van Aken, Stefanie
Managed Care Consultants   Page 261
Van Amber, Alan
Navitus Health Solutions   Page 490
Van Amerongen, Derek, MD, MS
ChoiceCare/Humana   Page 322
Humana Hlth Plan of OH Inc   Page 328
Van Brunt, Walter
Delta Dental Plan of NJ   Page 271
Van Duren, Michael, MD
San Francisco Health Plan   Page 66
Van Etten, Ann
Affinity Health Plan Inc   Page 283
Van Faasen, William C
Blue Cross Blue Shield of MA   Page 209
Van Gieson, William
University Health Plans Inc   Page 277
Van Gilmore, Donald
AmeriGroup Florida Inc   Page 101
Van Ribbink, Steve
Hawaii Medical Services Association -
BC/BS of Hawaii   Page 137
Van Roekel, Nathan
Avera Health Plans Inc   Page 387
Van Trease, Sandra
Unicare Health Plans
of the Midwest Inc   Page 153
Unicare Health Plans
of the Midwest Inc   Page 521
Van Vessem, Nancy, MD
Capital Health Plan   Page 105
Van Wyk, Sharon
GenWorth Life & Hlth Ins Co   Page 90
VanAssendelft, Maryelle, RN
Fidelis SecureCare of Texas   Page 413
VanCleave, Ken
Ameritas Mngd Dental Plan Inc   Page 34
VanEck, Bob
Priority Health   Page 230

Vana, Mark
Trustmark Insurance Company   Page 153
Vanasdale, Sallie A
CIGNA Health Plan of Utah Inc   Page 433
Vander Kolk, Keith
Iowa Foundation for Medical Care/
Encompass   Page 170
Vanderlaan, Burton, MD
Aetna Health of Illinois Inc   Page 143
Aetna Inc - Missouri   Page 243
Vandever, Carla
Utah Public Employees
Health Program   Page 438
Vanyo, Darrell
Blue Cross Blue Shield of ND   Page 317
Vardaro, Richard
Visioncare of California   Page 75
Vargas, Karen
Coventry Hlth Care Inc - DE Inc   Page 96
Vargas, Peter
Neighborhood Hlth Plan of RI   Page 380
Vastardis, Anthony G
Care-Plus Dental Plans Inc   Page 462
Vaturi, Shani, MD
Mercer First Choice   Page 369
Vaughan, Stan
Community Health Plan   Page 245
Vavrina, Robert T
Blue Cross Blue Shield of NC   Page 310
Vayer, Julie
CIGNA Behavioral Health Inc -
Corporate Headquarters   Page 234
CIGNA Behavioral Health Inc   Page 88
Vecchioni, Sharon
CareFirst BCBS   Page 200
Vega, Jody
National Dntl Consultants Inc   Page 301
Velarde, Jeannette
Lovelace Health Plan   Page 280
Velazquez, Ralph, MD
OSF Health Plans   Page 151
Vele, Janice, MD
Managed Health Services
Insurance Corporation   Page 467
Veltri, Gregg
Denver Health Medical Plan Inc   Page 80
Vennari, Joe
Bluegrass Family Health Inc   Page 183
Ver Hulst, Jay R
Care Network   Page 359
Selectcare Access Corporation   Page 371
Vercillo, Arthur, MD
Excellus BlueCross BlueShield,
Central New York Region   Page 291
Verroca, Andrea
SummaCare Inc   Page 334
Verros, Kathy
HealthPlus of Michigan   Page 224
Verso, Maria A, MD
Arizona Foundation for
Medical Care   Page 11
Vibbert, Spencer
IPRO   Page 298
Vickery, Peggy
Select Health of SC   Page 385
Vidrick, Frank
Forte Managed Care   Page 414
Vieira, John
Human Affairs International
of California   Page 52
Vienne, Richard P, Jr, DO
Univera Community Health   Page 307
Vieth, George W, Jr
Landmark Healthcare Inc   Page 56
Vigil, Karen
Medica Health Plans   Page 506
Villa, Sonia
Superior HealthPlan Inc   Page 426
Villabba, Pedro
HIP Health Plan of New York   Page 296
Villano, JoAnn
Preferred One   Page 93

Villanveva, Rosella
Strategic Health
Development Corporation   Page 119
Villegan, Kim, OD
Eyexam of California Inc   Page 46
Vincent, Sandra
Care 1st Health Plan AZ Inc   Page 13
Vincenti, Claude
SummaCare Inc   Page 334
Vis, David
IBA Health Plans   Page 225
Physicians Health Plan
of Mid-Michigan   Page 228
Visaya, Teresita
National Health Plan   Page 302
Visuri, Jeanne
HealthPlus of Michigan   Page 224
Vitale, Paul
Elder Service Plan of the
Cambridge Health Alliance   Page 510
Viteri, Mario
Vision Plan of America   Page 75
Vitkauskas, Wendy
Fallon Community H
ealth Plan Inc   Page 211
Vivaldo, Flora
Human Affairs International
of California   Page 52
Voelsch, Linda
Complementary Hlthcare Plans   Page 345
Voigt, Delores
Healthnow   Page 395
Voisey, Ryan
Group Health Plan Inc   Page 248
Voit, Bennett O
Primary Provider Mngmnt Co Inc   Page 64
Volberg, Keith
Unison Health Plan -
Corporate Headquarters   Page 372
Volin, Barry
Elderplan Inc   Page 289
Volk, Kim
Delta Dental Plans Association   Page 146
Volkmar, Keith A
Lifetime Healthcare Companies, The -
Corporate Headquarters   Page 298
Volkover, John
Alameda Alliance for Health   Page 33
Volpe, Ralph
Blue Cross Blue Shield of
Western New York   Page 285
von Ebers, Paul
Excellus BCBS   Page 290
Excellus BCBS Rochester Area   Page 292
Lifetime Healthcare Companies, The -
Corporate Headquarters   Page 298
Von Hassel, Shawn
GenWorth Life & Health Ins Co   Page 90
VonFange, Steve
Blue Cross Blue Shield of SC -
Corporate Hqtrs   Page 383
VonderBrink, Tom
Ohio State University Managed
Health Care Systems Inc   Page 332
Vossmeyer, Mike, MD
ChoiceCare/Humana   Page 322
Voxakis, Angelo C, PD
Epic Pharmacy Network Inc   Page 484
Vroman, Tim
Cypress Care   Page 483
Vukmer, Daniel, Esq
UMPC Health Plan Univ of
Pittsburgh Medical Center   Page 374

W

Wachowiak, Victoria
UnitedHealthcare of Georgia   Page 134

Index VIII: Personnel

Tipton, Norman
SummaCare Inc — Page 334
Tirao, Pam
KPS Health Plans — Page 452
Tobin, Clara
Medical Review Institute - Corporate Headquarters — Page 435
Tobin, Jill
Amerigroup New York, LLC — Page 284
Touchstone Health HMO Inc — Page 305
Tobin, John
Argus Health System Inc — Page 480
Todd, Larry CPA
Arkansas Foundation for Medical Care — Page 26
Todd, Richard W
CommunityCare Managed Healthcare Plans of OK Inc — Page 340
CommunityCare Managed Healthcare Plans of OK Inc — Page 483
Tokar, Leo
Kaiser Foundation Health Plan of Colorado — Page 83
Toler, Wendy
Optimum Choice Inc — Page 205
Tolleson, Sidney
Coastal Healthcare Admnstrtrs — Page 41
Tom, Martin
Legacy Health Solutions Inc — Page 420
Tomey, Lori
Encore Health Network — Page 160
Tomlinson, Joseph C, DMD
Ndc-West Inc dba NADENT — Page 83
Tomlinson, Sandra
Highmark Inc — Page 366
Toohey, Thomas
One Call Medical Inc — Page 275
Toomey, David
CIGNA Healthcare of LA — Page 190
CIGNA Healthcare of North TX — Page 409
Toon, Tom
Delta Dental Ins Co - GA — Page 131
Torbeck, Terence P, MD
CareSource — Page 321
Torgenrud, Terry W, MD
Regence Blue Shield — Page 456
Torkelson, Richard E, MD
Winhealth Partners — Page 473
Torosian, Janice
Health Plan of Michigan — Page 224
Torres, Ann
Behavioral Healthcare Inc — Page 78
Torres, Cindy
Medical Care Referral Group — Page 420
Torres, Janneth
Atlantis Health Plan — Page 285
Torres, Jose A, MD
Physicians United Plan Inc — Page 118
Torres, Tony
Preferred Podiatry Group — Page 152
Toth, Imre, MD
CIGNA Healthcare of MA — Page 210
Tournoux, MaryAnn
Health Alliance Medical Plans - Corporate Headquarters — Page 149
Touslee, Ma'ata
Family Health Partners — Page 247
Towne, Cynthia, RN, BSN, CCM
Action Health Care Management Services — Page 11
Tracy, William C
UnitedHealthcare of the Heartland States — Page 182
UnitedHealthcare of the Midlands Inc — Page 257
Traczyk, Richard J, DPM
Preferred Podiatrists of OK — Page 342
Tran, Anna
Care 1st Health Plan — Page 38
Tran, Lili, MHA
Lakewood Health Plan Inc — Page 56

Tran, Tom
Blue Cross Blue Shield of Texas — Corporate Headquarters — Page 406
Traylor, Thomas
BMC HealthNet Plan — Page 209
Traynor, Mark
Ucare Minnesota — Page 238
Treadwell, Randall, MD
HealthSmart Preferred Care — Page 416
Trebino, Patricia
Tufts Health Plan — Page 216
Tredway, Al
Coventry Hlth Care Inc - LA — Page 190
Trembulak, Frank
Geisinger Health Plan — Page 363
Tretheway, Barb
HealthPartners Inc — Page 236
HealthPartners — Page 486
Trifone, John
Blue Cross Blue Shield of VT — Page 439
Vermont Hlth Plans (Blue Care) — Page 439
Trimble, Joan
Community First Hlth Plans Inc — Page 410
Trinchitella, Yvonne, RN
Humana Health Care Plans of Houston — Page 418
Triplett, Stefanie L
SW Preferred Dental Org — Page 20
Trlica, Cathy
Humana Health Care Plans of San Antonio/Austin — Page 418
Tromans, Marilyn T
BCBS of Kansas City — Page 244
Good Health HMO Inc — Page 247
Trombley, Amy
Health New England — Page 212
Trout, Deborah, PhD
Magellan Health Services Inc — Page 91
Trowbridge, Lee E
BCBS of Nebraska — Page 255
Truess, James W
AmeriGroup Corporation — Page 442
AmeriGroup Tennessee Inc — Page 391
Amerigroup Ohio Inc — Page 319
Truett, Angela
El Paso First Health Plans Inc — Page 413
Truitt, Gary R, ESQ
Highmark Inc — Page 366
Truitt, Lisa
AmeriGroup DC — Page 97
Trujillo, Alfonso
HMO New Mexico Inc — Page 280
Tsang, Steve
Chinese Community Health Plan — Page 39
Tsang, Wellman, MD
On Lok Senior Health Services — Page 60
Tucker, Cecily
Sanford Health Plan — Page 388
Tucker, JC
Chinese Community Health Plan — Page 39
Tucker, Mark, MD
Midwest Health Plan — Page 226
Tufano, Paul A
Independence Blue Cross — Page 366
Tull, Debra
Landmark Healthcare Inc — Page 56
Tuller, Ed
Care Choices HMO — Page 218
Tullman, Glen E
Allscripts Pharmaceuticals Inc — Page 479
Tulloch, Mark A
HealthSpring Inc-Tennessee — Page 395
HealthSpring Inc-Corp Hdqrtrs — Page 395
Tunney, Penny
LA Care Health Plan — Page 55
Turcu, Shelley
Great Lakes Health Plan — Page 222
Turek, Lori
Arise Health Plan — Page 461
Tures, John F, MD
El Paso First Health Plans Inc — Page 413

Turner, Amy
Aetna Hlth Plans of Mid-Atlantic — Page 441
Aetna Inc - Virginia — Page 441
Turner, Christine
Puget Sound Health Partners — Page 455
Turner, Jim
Humana Health Plan - KY — Page 185
Turner, Scott
Aids Healthcare Foundation — Page 32
Turpin, Michael A
Oxford Health Plans-CT — Page 91
Oxford Health Plans Inc — Corporate Headquarters — Page 92
Oxford Health Plans of NJ Inc — Page 275
UnitedHealthcare of NY Metropolitan — Page 306
Tuttle, Tamara
Ohio State University Managed Health Care Systems Inc — Page 332
Tye, Pattie D
Humana Health Care Plans of Houston — Page 418
Tyler, Susan M
HMO Health Ohio (Cleveland) — Page 328
Medical Mutual of Ohio — Page 330
Tylus, Kevin
CIGNA Dental Health of OH Inc — Page 322
Tysell, Jim, MD
Contra Costa Health Plan — Page 43
Tyson, Diane
United Concordia Co Inc - FL — Page 121

U

Udvaryhalyi, Steven, MD
Independence Blue Cross — Page 366
Keystone Health Plan East Inc — Page 368
Ueoka, Jamie
Care 1st Health Plan — Page 38
Ukani, Ahmed
CIGNA Dental Health of CA Inc — Page 40
Ulibarri, Frank
UnitedHealthcare of Alabama — Page 7
UnitedHealthcare of Louisiana — Page 193
Ullian, Elaine
BMC HealthNet Plan — Page 209
Ullman, Richard O
NPAX Inc — Page 490
Ulrich, Michael
Physicians Foundation for Medical Care — Page 64
Uma, Chet
Health Plan of San Joaquin, The — Page 50
Inland Empire Health Plan — Page 52
Umland, Mike
Preferred One — Page 237
Underwood, Dave
Health Plus — Page 150
Ungerlieder, Alex
Anthem BCBS of Connecticut — Page 88
Ungs, Matt
Wellpath Select Inc — Page 315
Unhjem, Michael B
BCBS of North Dakota — Page 317
Unruh, David
Winhealth Partners — Page 473
Urbani, Lynne A
Blue Cross Blue Shield of RI — Page 379
Urbanski, Susan
CIGNA Behavioral Health Inc — Page 40
Urbina, Patty
Community Health Group — Page 41
Urick, Paul
Independence Blue Cross — Page 366
Utley, Jim, MD
Coventry Health Care of KS Inc — Page 245

Index VIII: Personnel

Tanzer, Tobi
HealthPartners Inc — Page 236
Tapp, Kathy
Carolinas Center for
Medical Excellence, The — Page 310
Tarantino, Laura F, CPA
APS Healthcare Inc — Page 199
Tasinga, Martha, MD
Orange Prevention &
Treatment Integrated — Page 60
Tate, Bruce
Health First Health Plans Inc — Page 111
Tawney, Kim
Nationwide Better Health — Page 204
Taylor, Darren C
Good Health HMO Inc — Page 247
Taylor, Douglas A
WellDyne Rx — Page 497
Taylor, Geoffrey E
Lifetime Healthcare Companies, The -
Corporate Headquarters — Page 298
Taylor, James
OraQuest Dental Plans — Page 421
Taylor, Kay
Exempla Healthcare LLC — Page 81
Taylor, Larry
Hygeia Corporation — Page 114
Taylor, Laura
Dental Care Plus Inc — Page 324
Taylor, Mary
Vision Health Mngmnt Systems — Page 155
Taylor, Michael
UMPC Health Plan Univ of
Pittsburgh Medical Center — Page 374
Taylor, Sheila
AmeriGroup DC — Page 97
Taylor, Troy
M Plan Inc — Page 163
Taylor, Viston
Alexian Brothers
Health Systems Inc — Page 507
Teachout, Michael W
Coventry Health Care Inc - IA — Page 169
Teal, Jan
Advantage Health Solutions Inc — Page 157
Tearcy, John
United Concordia Co Inc - FL — Page 121
Tegenu, Mesfin, MS, RPh
PerformRx — Page 492
Tempeny, Linda
Univera Community Health — Page 307
Temperly, Tim
Network Health Plan WI — Page 468
Temple, Carolyn J
Kern Foundation/
Preferred Provider Organization — Page 55
Temple, Thomas R, RPh, MS
Iowa Pharmacists Association — Page 487
Ten Pas, Bill
ODS Health Plan — Page 349
Tenery, Joanne
Parkland Community
Health Plan Inc — Page 422
Tenorio, Susan, RN
Inter Valley Health Plan Inc — Page 53
Tepper, Dave
Global Medical Management — Page 110
Termini, John
American Healthcare Alliance — Page 243
Terrill, Jeff
CIGNA Healthcare of Arizona — Page 14
Terrill, Sonny
Signature Health Alliance — Page 398
Terrin, Tanna
Altius Health Plans — Page 433
Terry, David L, Jr
HealthSpring Inc - Tennessee — Page 395
HealthSpring Inc-Corp Hdqrtrs — Page 395
Terry, Donna
Pima Health Plan — Page 19

Terry, Fred
Mercycare Health Plan Inc — Page 468
Thames, Bill
Southwest Health Alliance
(SHALLC) — Page 425
Thames-Conley, Charmaine
Citrus Health Care Inc — Page 108
Thanert, Shawn
Humana Medical Plan Inc — Page 114
Tharp, Tommy L
Integrated Health Plan Inc — Page 115
Theado, Janet
Integra Group — Page 329
Thibdeau, Michael, CPA
Davis Vision — Page 288
Thielking, Patti
Sagamore Health Network Inc — Page 164
Thielking, Patti
Sagamore Health Network Inc — Page 164
Thiemann, Kendall
PacifiCare of Oregon — Page 350
Thierer, Mark A
SXC Health Solutions Inc — Page 495
Thode, Mary Ann
Kaiser Foundation Health
Plan of Northern California — Page 54
Thomas, Beverly
Kaiser Foundation Health
Plan of Georgia — Page 132
Thomas, David
New York State Catholic
Health Plan Inc — Page 303
Thomas, David, Esq
Unison Health Plan -
Corporate Headquarters — Page 372
Thomas, David W
Unison Health Plan of TN — Page 399
Thomas, J Grover, Jr
Trustmark Insurance Company — Page 153
Thomas, Jarrel
Memphis Managed Care Corp — Page 397
Thomas, Jesse
Molina Healthcare of MI Inc — Page 227
Thomas, Johnna
Arkansas Managed Care Org — Page 26
Thomas, Lamonte
CIGNA Healthcare of Virginia Inc -
Richmond — Page 443
Thomas, Lynn
Sanford Health Plan — Page 388
Thomas, Marshall, MD
Colorado Access — Page 79
Thomas, Rachel T
Optima Health Plan Inc — Page 445
Thomas, Ray
Davis Vision — Page 288
Thomas, Stefanie
Denver Health Medical Plan Inc — Page 80
Thomas, Terrina
Optima Health Plan Inc — Page 445
Thomas, William
PerfectHealth Ins Co — Page 304
Thomas-Brown, Marianne, RN
Molina Healthcare of MI Inc — Page 227
Thomashaver, Robin
Partnercare Health Plan Inc — Page 117
Thomason, Ed
Preferred Health Alliance — Page 6
Thomason, Kristi
CIGNA Healthcare of Arizona — Page 14
Thompson, Betsy, MD
Colorado Choice Health Plan/
San Luis Valley HMO Inc — Page 79
Thompson, Beverly, MD
Community Care Plus — Page 249
Thompson, Bryan
Em Risk Management,
A POMCO Company — Page 290
Thompson, Cathy
Humana Wisconsin
Health Organization Inc — Page 466

Thompson, Greg
UnitedHealthcare of
the Heartland States — Page 182
Thompson, Joaquin
BCBS of Georgia — Page 128
Thompson, Kim
Spectera Vision Inc - Indiana — Page 166
Thompson, Kris
Community Health Plan of WA — Page 450
Thompson, Kurt B
Oxford Health Plans of NY Inc — Page 303
Thompson, Robert H
Monroe Plan for
Medical Care, The — Page 300
Thompson, Scott
Primecare Medical Network Inc — Page 65
Thompson, Thomas
OhioHealth Group — Page 332
Thorbin, Patricia
Citrus Health Care Inc — Page 108
Thornberry, Brian
Pacific Health Alliance — Page 62
Thorne, Curt
MedSolutions — Page 396
Thorne, Donna
Blue Cross Blue Shield of SC -
Corporate Hqtrs — Page 383
Thorne, Jim
Anthem BCBS of Colorado — Page 77
Rocky Mountain Hospital & Medical
Services Inc — Page 85
Thorson, Rhonda
Group Health Cooperative
of Eau Claire — Page 465
Thrailkill, Julie
North Dakota Hlth Care Review — Page 318
Tiano, Linda
Health Net Inc - Corp Hdqrtrs — Page 49
Tice, Carrie
Santa Clara Family Health Plan — Page 67
Tidwell, Cindy
Secure Hlth Plans of GA LLC — Page 133
Tikker, Blair
HMS Colorado Inc — Page 82
Sloan's Lake Preferred
Health Networks — Page 85
Tildon, Maria
CareFirst BlueChoice Inc — Page 97
CareFirst BCBS — Page 200
Delmarva Hlth Care Plan Inc — Page 202
Tilford, David
Medica Health Plans — Page 236
Medica Health Plans — Page 518
Medica Health Plans — Page 506
Medica Health Plans of WI — Page 518
Tillery, Robert, DDS
Dental Health Services — Page 45
Dental Health Services Inc — Page 450
Tilley, Maggie
Colorado Health Networks LLC -
ValueOptions — Page 80
Tilly, Ken
Contra Costa Health Plan — Page 43
Tilow, Brian
TriHealth Senior Link — Page 515
Timmermans, Rebecca
South Central Preferred — Page 372
Timms, Dennis
Bluelincs HMO — Page 340
Timonere, Ron
Aetna Inc - Plantation — Page 100
Tindall, Jeffrey
CIGNA Healthcare of Virginia Inc -
Richmond — Page 443
Tindall, Julie
Abri Health Plan Inc — Page 461
Tingue, Dave
Horizon Behavioral Services — Page 112
Tipton, Meredith
Anthem BCBS of Maine — Page 195

Index VIII: Personnel

Strickland, John, BS, MCSE
Health Design Plus — Page 327
Strohmenger, Thomas
Aetna Inc - Pennsylvania — Page 355
Strollo, Mark
Keystone Health Plan East Inc — Page 368
Strombom, Elizabeth
Humana Medical Plan -
Central Florida — Page 113
Strother, Jack G
Regence Group, The —
Corporate Headquarters — Page 351
Strunk, Deana
LifeWise Health Plan of OR — Page 348
Stryker-Smit, Johanna
Pima Health Plan — Page 19
Stuart-Middleton, Deborah
On Lok Senior Health Services — Page 60
Stuckey, Dan, MD
PacifiCare of Texas - Houston — Page 422
Stuckey, Scott
Ameritas Managed Dental Plan Inc — Page 34
Stucky, Paul
Epoch Group LC, The — Page 178
Studebaker, Mark, MD
Aetna Inc - Ohio — Page 319
Stueve, Jo
Family Health Partners — Page 247
Stults, Evan
Qualis Health — Page 455
Stumpfel, James
Best Health Plans — Page 36
Stutes, Ronald
JPS Benefits — Page 419
Suarez, Debra
Evolutions Healthcare Sys Inc — Page 109
Suarez, Kim
Priority Health — Page 230
SubLaban, Grace
Jackson Memorial Health Plan — Page 115
Suchoski, Ken
Blue Cross of Northeastern PA — Page 358
Suchy, Bruce E
Pioneer Management Systems — Page 215
Suckow, Milisa
Community Health Plan — Page 245
Sucoloski, Mark
National Capital PPO — Page 444
Sud, Susdey
Galaxy Health Network — Page 414
Sudderth, Gregory
Blue Preferred Plan-BCBS MI — Page 218
Suenram, Roberta
Preferred Health Professionals — Page 180
Sugarman, Jonathan, MD, MPH
Qualis Health — Page 455
Suggs, Kim
Novasys Health Network — Page 28
Suleski, Carol
Elder Service Plan of the
North Shore — Page 510
Suleski, Jim
Delta Dental Plan of NJ — Page 271
Sullivan, Brett
ACN Group — Page 233
Sullivan, Jacquelyn
Physicians Foundation for
Medical Care — Page 64
Sullivan, Janet, MD
Hudson Health Plan — Page 297
Sullivan, Joseph M
New York State Catholic
Health Plan Inc — Page 303
Sullivan, Thomas
UnitedHealthcare of Ohio Inc-
Cleveland — Page 336
Sullivan, William
Oxford Health Plans of NY Inc — Page 303

Sumfest, Jill M, MD
Humana Medical Plan Inc — Page 114
Preferred Health Systems — Page 180
Summers, David
Virginia Premier Hlth Plans Inc — Page 447
Sumner, Pat, RN
Phoebe Health Partners — Page 133
Sun, Cary, DDS
CIGNA Dental Health of CA Inc — Page 40
Sun, Dan
LA Care Health Plan — Page 55
Sun, Eugene, MD
HealthAmerica Pennsylvania Inc -
NorthWest — Page 365
HealthAmerica Pennsylvania Inc -
Western Region — Page 365
Suris, Heather
MagnaCare — Page 298
Surman, Tom
Vantage PPO — Page 375
Sutherland, E J
Coordinated Health Plan — Page 379
Sutherland, Everett J
Blue Cross Blue Shield of RI — Page 379
Sutherland, Russ
Capitol Administrators — Page 38
Sutton, Cynthia
Legacy Health Solutions Inc — Page 420
Sutton, Terry, MD
Blue Cross Blue Shield of Texas —
HMO Blue - Southeast — Page 407
Swackhamer, Roy
Scan Health Plan — Page 68
Swain, Eric
UnitedHealthcare of
New England Inc — Page 381
Swaine, Bruce
Crawford and Co -
Corporate Headquarters — Page 130
Swanson, Michael
United Behavioral Health (UBH) — Page 71
Swanson, Sheryl, MBA
Community Behavioral Healthcare
Cooperative of Pennsylvania — Page 361
Swanson, Steve
Regence Blue Shield — Page 456
Swanson-Pico, Kelli
Interplan Health Group — Page 53
Superien Health Network Inc — Page 335
Swartz, Scott N
Mountain State BCBS — Page 460
Swartzbaugh, Tom
Vision Service Plan — Page 86
Sweda, Stewart
Careington International -
The Dental Network — Page 408
Sweeney, Mary Ellen
Santa Clara Family Health Plan — Page 67
Sweeris, Chuck
Blue Shield of California — Page 36
Sweetsler, Mark
AmeriHealth Ins Co — Page 95
Swenson, Nancy
Union Health Service Inc — Page 154
Swenson, Rich
HealthPlus of Michigan — Page 224
Swingle, Christine
Freedom Health Inc — Page 110
Sydell, Gerald A, DDS
Delta Dental Plan of NJ — Page 271
Sylvestro, Ann
Horizon BCBS of NJ — Page 273
Sylvies, Alicia
Utah Public Employees
Health Program — Page 438
Syoen, Sue Ann, RPh
4D Pharmacy
Management Systems Inc — Page 479

Syracuse, Jill
Independent Health Assoc Inc — Page 297
Szelis, Denise
Physicians Health Plan
of Northern Indiana — Page 164
Szilagyi, Peter, MD, MPH
Monroe Plan for
Medical Care, The — Page 300
Szumski, Ron
Molina Healthcare of MI Inc — Page 227
Szuto, Peter
Center for Elders Independence — Page 508
Szydlowski, Veronica
Mount Carmel Health Plan — Page 331

T

Tabak, Mark
Private Hlthcare Systems-CA — Page 65
Private Hlthcare Systems-GA — Page 133
Private Hlthcare Systems--IL — Page 153
Private Hlthcare Systems-
Corporate Headquarters — Page 215
Private Hlthcare Systems-MO — Page 251
MultiPlan Inc - Corp Hdqrtrs — Page 300
Private Hlthcare Systems-TX — Page 423
Private Hlthcare Systems-WA — Page 455
Tabakin, Scott
Bravo Health Mid-Atlantic Inc — Page 200
Bravo Health Pennsylvania Inc — Page 358
Bravo Health Texas Inc — Page 407
Tabela, Frank
Neighborhood Hlth Plan of RI — Page 380
Tabor, Thomas R
Highmark Inc — Page 366
Tabor, Ty
KPS Health Plans — Page 452
Taddeo, Michael
HMO Health Ohio (Cleveland) — Page 328
Medical Mutual of Ohio — Page 330
SuperMed Network — Page 334
Tafel, Jill
Humana Inc-Grand Rapids MI — Page 225
Taitano, Maria D R
Staywell Insurance Guam Inc — Page 135
Taitano, Taling M, CPA, CGFM
Staywell Insurance Guam Inc — Page 135
Takiki, Kazu, DDS
CIGNA Dental Health of Colorado — Page 78
Takkar, Preet
SmileCare/
Community Dental Services — Page 69
Talb, Eric
Humana Health Care Plans
of Dallas — Page 417
Taliafenno, Janae
CorpHealth Inc — Page 412
Tallent, John
Medical Associates Hlth Plans — Page 172
Tallent, Robert
OneNet PPO — Page 205
Tamayo, Jonathan
Community Health Group — Page 41
Tamborini, Ray
One Call Medical Inc — Page 275
Tanaka, Eric M
Regencecare — Page 456
Tankersley, Dwane
Novasys Health Network — Page 28
Tannos, Paul, CPA
Community Health Choice Inc — Page 410
Tanquary, Patricia
Contra Costa Health Plan — Page 43

Index VIII: Personnel

Stedman, Matt
Humana Health Care Plans
of San Antonio/Austin   Page 418
Steel, Patrick F
Delta Dental Plan of CA   Page 44
Steele, David, MD
Humana Hlth Care Plans of IL   Page 151
Steele, Patrick S
Delta Dental Ins Co - Nevada   Page 259
Delta Dental of Pennsylvania   Page 361
Delta Dental Plan Inc - Utah   Page 434
Steely, Sharon
Health Plan of San Joaquin, The   Page 50
Steere, Richard W
Vision Service Plan of Arizona   Page 22
Vision Service Plan   Page 75
Vision Service Plan   Page 86
Steffes, Craig
Anthem BCBS of Wisconsin   Page 461
Stegamen, Dale, MD
HealthLink of Arkansas Inc   Page 27
Stein, Steven, MD
Great Lakes Health Plan   Page 222
Steinberg, Gregory, MD
Active Health Management   Page 441
Steinbrecher-Loera, Carolyn
Regence Blue Shield of Idaho   Page 142
Steiner, Kathy
University Family Care Hlth Plan   Page 22
Steingerwalt, Eric
New England Financial -
Corporate Headquarters   Page 214
Stelben, John J
Coventry Health Care Inc —
Corporate Headquarters   Page 201
Stellmon, John
Regence Blue Shield of Idaho   Page 142
Stemple, Charles, MD
UnitedHealthcare of Ohio Inc-
Cleveland   Page 336
Stengel, Art
HealthLink Inc - Corp Hdqrtrs   Page 249
Stepec, Tom
Antares Mngmnt Solutions   Page 319
Stephen, Jane
Blue Cross Blue Shield of WY   Page 473
Stephens, Deborah L
Behavioral Health Systems Inc   Page 3
Stephens, Mark, PharmD
Memphis Managed Care Corp   Page 397
Stephens, Rosalyn
AmeriGroup DC   Page 97
Stephenson, George, II
Kern Foundation/
Preferred Provider Organization   Page 55
Stephenson, Lori, RN
Rocky Mountain Health Plans   Page 84
Steranka, Sarah D
American Hlthcre Group Inc   Page 356
Sterling, Jeff
El Paso First Health Plans Inc   Page 413
Stern, Kyle
Spectera Vision Inc - Indiana   Page 166
Stern, Peter
Kansas Pharmacy Service Corp   Page 487
Sternbergh, John
BCBS of North Carolina   Page 310
Sterns, George
Atlantic Integrated Health Inc   Page 309
Sterns, Melissa
Community Health Group   Page 41
Stetson, Paul
Medcost LLC   Page 313
Stevans, Joel, DC
Landmark Healthcare Inc   Page 56
Stevener, Evelyn
Kansas Fndtn Medical Care   Page 179

Stevens, John
Behavioral Healthcare Inc   Page 78
Stevens, Kenneth
Sun Health Medisun   Page 20
Stevens, Lisa
Flora Health Network   Page 325
Stevens, Ronald S, MBA
Samaritan Health Plans Inc   Page 352
Stevens, Sheila
Medcore Health Plan   Page 58
Stevenson, Gretchen
United Concordia Co Inc - TX   Page 429
Stevenson, James
HCH Administration   Page 148
Steward, Tracy
PacifiCare of Arizona   Page 19
Steward-Alexander, Victoria
Alexian Brothers
Community Services   Page 507
Stewart, Alan
CompBenefits   Page 410
Stewart, Charles D
Aetna Inc - Arizona   Page 11
Stewart, Debbie
KPS Health Plans   Page 452
Stewart, Donna
Nationwide Better Health   Page 204
Stewart, Eric
Humana Health Plan -
Jacksonville   Page 113
Stewart, Hal
Kern Family Health Care   Page 55
Stewart, Joanne
Orange County PPO   Page 61
Stewart, Judy
Physicians Health Plan of
Mid-Michigan   Page 228
Stewart, Marilyn, RN
Deseret Healthcare   Page 434
Stewart, Michael E
Colorado Choice Health Plan/
San Luis Valley HMO Inc   Page 79
Stewart, Shelly
Managed Hlth Services IN Inc   Page 163
Stewert, Tim
Comprehensive Health Group   Page 129
Stidham, Donna
AIDS Healthcare Foundation   Page 32
Stiefel, Maria
Connecticare Inc   Page 89
Stiefel, Melba
UTMB Health Plans Inc   Page 431
Stiff, Jacqueline E, MD
UnitedHealthcare of Colorado   Page 85
Stiller, Rod
Blue Cross of Idaho   Page 141
Stillwagon, Troy
Scott & White Health Plan   Page 424
Stilwell, Lisa
CIGNA Healthcare of Arizona   Page 14
Stinton, Roger
Great-West Healthcare of AZ   Page 16
Stirewalt, Charles, DMD
Newport Dental Plan   Page 60
Stith, Randy
Behavioral Healthcare Inc   Page 78
Stobbe, Greg
Dental Network of America   Page 146
Stock, Michael E
QCA Health Plan Inc   Page 28
Stocker, Judy
Avesis Inc   Page 12
Stoddard, Paul
Blue Cross Blue Shield of
Western New York   Page 285
Stokey, Joan
ppoNEXT   Page 423
Stoll, Christine
Unicare Health Plans
of the Midwest Inc   Page 153

Stoll, Steve
Delta Dental Plan of NJ   Page 271
Stollenwerk Petrulis, Alice, MD
Ohio Kepro Inc   Page 332
Stoller, Michael B
Hawaii Medical Services Association -
BC/BS of Hawaii   Page 137
Stoltz, Tammy
Health Net of Arizona   Page 17
Stom, Mary K, MD
Health Partners   Page 364
Stone, Betsy
Blue Shield of California   Page 36
Stone, Elaine
Private Healthcare Systems -
Corporate Headquarters   Page 215
Stone, Julie
First Plan of Minnesota   Page 235
First Plan of Minnesota   Page 505
Stone, W Clement
Combined Ins Co of America   Page 145
Stone, W Randy, MBA
LA Care Health Plan   Page 55
Stoneback, Keith
SHPS Inc   Page 186
Stoner, Andrew
M Plan Inc   Page 163
Stoner, Kenneth, DDS
Dominion Dental Services -
Corporate Headquarters   Page 444
Stoner, Patrick
OraQuest Dental Plans   Page 421
Stopper, James
Central Susquehanna
Healthcare Providers   Page 359
Storbakken, Norman
Delta Dental Plan of MN   Page 235
Storey, Donald, MD
Aetna Inc - Washington   Page 449
Storms, Susy
Nevada Pacific Dental   Page 262
Storrer, Scott A
CIGNA Healthcare of CT   Page 89
Stout, Julia
Legacy Health Solutions Inc   Page 420
Stout, Renee
Capitol Administrators   Page 38
Stovall, Dorrence B
Prime Health Services Inc   Page 398
Stover, James
University Family Care Hlth Plan   Page 22
Stowers, Phil
Arkansas Managed Care Org   Page 26
Straley, Hugh, MD
Group Health Cooperative   Page 141
Group Health Cooperative   Page 451
Group Health Cooperative
of Puget Sound   Page 452
Group Health Options Inc   Page 452
Straley, Peter F
Health New England   Page 212
Strand, David R
Medica Health Plans   Page 506
Strange, Kyle, LCSW
Behavioral Health Systems Inc   Page 3
Strangle, Nancy
Trustmark Insurance Company   Page 153
Strassberg, Leslie
HIP Health Plan of New York   Page 296
Straus, Daniel E
Aveta Inc   Page 270
Strautman, Kate
Vista Hlthplan of South FL Inc   Page 123
Streator, Scott
Ohio State University Managed
Health Care Systems Inc   Page 332
Strebig, James, MD
Orange County PPO   Page 61

Index VIII: Personnel

Solomon, Paul, MD
UnitedHealthcare of Texas Inc —
Dallas — Page 430
Soltesz, Lucille
Metcare Health Plans Inc — Page 116
Vista Hlthplan of South FL Inc — Page 123
Soman, Michael, MD
Group Health Cooperative
of Puget Sound — Page 452
Somers, Carola
University of PA, Trustees — Page 512
Somerville, Terry
Priority Health — Page 230
Sommer, Steve
MedScript — Page 488
Sommers, Jack, MD
CommunityCare Managed Healthcare
Plans of Oklahoma Inc — Page 340
CommunityCare Managed Healthcare
Plans of Oklahoma Inc — Page 483
Sondgeroth, Mary Dorothea
PhysiciansPlus & St Dominic Health
Maintenance Organization — Page 242
Soonthornsima, Worachote 'Ob'
BCBS of Louisiana Inc — Page 189
HMO Louisiana Inc — Page 191
Sorenson, Dan, MD
ConnectCare — Page 219
Sorkin, Hardy, MD
Signature Health Alliance — Page 398
Soroka, Dina
Centercare Inc — Page 287
Fidelis Care New York — Page 293
New York State Catholic
Health Plan Inc — Page 303
Sorrell, Carol, RN
Kern Family Health Care — Page 55
Sorrow, John W
CIGNA Healthcare of TN Inc — Page 394
Sosinski, James
Dental Group of New Jersey — Page 271
Soto Rojas, Ultra
Humana Inc/PCA - Puerto Rico — Page 377
Sotunde, Tunde, MD
UnitedHealthcare of Arkansas — Page 28
Soucheray, Philip
UnitedHealth Group —
Corporate Headquarters — Page 238
Southam, Arthur M, MD
Kaiser Permanente - Kaiser Foundation
Health Plan, Inc — Page 54
Kaiser Foundation Health
Plan of Ohio — Page 329
Southwell, David N
Wellmark BCBS of Iowa — Page 174
Wellmark Inc — Corp Hdqrtrs — Page 175
Wellmark Health Plan of IA Inc — Page 175
Southworth, Judith K
Virginia Health Network — Page 447
Soutor, Stefany
Delta Dental Plans Association — Page 146
Sowards, Farley
Molina HealthCare of Utah Inc — Page 435
Sowards, Vince
4MOST Health Network — Page 459
Sowers, Charles M
Health Net of Arizona — Page 17
Spadani, Ned
Community Medical Alliance — Page 210
Spafford, Kent
One Call Medical Inc — Page 275
Spafford, Kent
One Call Medical Inc — Page 275
Spain, R Dennis, DDS
Nevada Pacific Dental — Page 262
Spalding, George E, CPA
Comprehensive Health Group — Page 129

Sparkman, Annette
CBCA Care Management Inc — Page 408
Sparks, Allison
Pacific Health Alliance — Page 62
Sparks, Carol
Horizon Behavioral Services — Page 112
Sparks, Kevin P
BCBS of Kansas City — Page 244
Good Health HMO Inc — Page 247
Spear, Ken, MD
SelectHealth Network — Page 165
Spears, Tressa
Community Health Network
of Connecticut Inc — Page 89
Spector-Piotti, Karen
Family Choice Health Alliance — Page 272
Spence, David, MBA
Dedicated Dental Systems — Page 43
Spence, Glen A
CareGuide — Page 105
Spencer, Deborah
Care Choices HMO — Page 218
Spencer, Eric
Easy Choice Health Plan Inc — Page 46
Spencer, Kevin
OmniCare, A Coventry
Health Plan — Page 228
Spencer, Nancy
Delta Dental Plan of SC — Page 384
Sperandio, Stephen J
Delta Dental of Rhode Island — Page 380
Altus Dental Ins Co Inc — Page 379
Spiewak, Bruce
Care-Plus Dental Plans Inc — Page 462
Spillane, Timothy J
AmeriGroup Corporation — Page 442
Spinazola, Pam
Connecticare Inc — Page 89
Connecticare of MA Inc — Page 210
Connecticare of NY — Page 288
Spindler, Jayne
Gundersen Lutheran
Health Plan Inc — Page 465
Spitzig, Kevin
American Republic Ins Co — Page 169
Spogan, Daniel, MD
Universal Health Network -
Corporate Headquarters — Page 264
Sponer, Dennis M
ScripNet — Page 494
Sponer, Jennifer
ScripNet — Page 494
Sponsler, Linda
BCBS of Oklahoma — Page 339
Spoon, John, RPh
Aetna Inc - Tulsa — Page 339
Spooner, Tim
AmeriGroup DC — Page 97
Sporel, Heidi R
Masspro Inc — Page 213
Sprague, Charles W
Fiserv Inc — Page 464
Sprecher, Lon
Dean Health Plan — Page 463
Spring, Mitch
EyeMed Vision Care LLC — Page 325
Squarrell Shablin, Karen
AmeriGroup DC — Page 97
Squilanti, Todd
Meritain Health Inc — Page 299
St Clair, Rod, MD
Primecare Medical Network Inc — Page 65
St Hilare, Gary D
Keystone Health Plan Central — Page 367
Capital Blue Cross — Page 359
Stabelfeldt, Marty
American WholeHealth
Networks Inc — Page 442

Stablefeld, Susan
EBC — Page 464
Stacke, Mary
Delta Dental Plan of Minnesota — Page 235
Stackhouse, James, MD
Atlantic Integrated Health Inc — Page 309
Stacy, Cheryl
APS Healthcare Northwest Inc — Page 253
Stahl, Jeffrey, MD
Iowa Foundation for Medical Care/
Encompass — Page 170
Staker, Larry, MD
Deseret Healthcare — Page 434
Stala, Maria
SCHC Total Care Inc — Page 305
Stalker, Nancy
Blue Shield of California — Page 36
Stallings, Robert
Humana Health Benefit Plan
of Louisiana — Page 191
Stam, Pete
Assurant Employee Bnfts-NC — Page 309
Stambaugh, Elizabeth A
Employers Dental Services Inc — Page 15
Stamm, Joseph B
NYCHSRO/MedReview Inc — Page 303
Stanislaw, Sherry
Scan Health Plan — Page 68
Stanley, David A
University Health Care Inc -
Passport Health Plan — Page 187
Stanley, Donna Marie
Oxford Health Plans Inc —
Corporate Headquarters — Page 92
Stanley, Jeff
Care Network — Page 359
Stanley, Kathy
HMO New Mexico Inc — Page 280
Stanley, Lorena Jean
AmeriGroup Tennessee Inc — Page 391
Stanley, Margaret
Regence Blue Shield — Page 456
Stanley, Terri, RN, MPA
Partnership HealthPlan of CA — Page 64
Stanos, Steven P, Jr, DO
MyMatrixx — Page 489
Stanyer, Brent
Premera Blue Cross - Eastern — Page 454
Stapley, Michael J
Deseret Healthcare — Page 434
Starck, Daniel J
Corvel Corporation — Page 43
Corvel Corporation — Page 324
Stark, Charles R
Group Health Plan Inc — Page 248
Stark, Linda, MD
Health Plan,
The Hometown Region — Page 327
Starks-Jenkins, Nancy
HealthPlus of Michigan — Page 224
Starn, Kenneth J
S V S Visions Inc — Page 231
Starr, Harriet, MD
Nychsro/MedReview Inc — Page 303
Starr, Maureen
Interplan Health Group — Page 53
Superien Health Network Inc — Page 335
Statner, Mike
20/20 Eyecare Plan Inc — Page 99
Staudenmeier, Paul
Bravo Health Inc — Page 200
Stearns, Laura O
Delta Dental Plan of Ohio Inc — Page 324
Steber, John H
HIP Health Plan of New York — Page 296
Steckbeck, Marie
Colorado Access — Page 79

Index VIII: Personnel

Slawter, Todd
Aetna Inc - Plantation — Page 100
Slepin, Robert
WellCare of New York — Page 307
Sleszar, Thomas, DDS, MS
Delta Dental Plan of Ohio Inc — Page 324
Slick, Barbara, RN
Saint Mary's HealthFirst — Page 263
Slifka, Danielle
Wellmark BCBS of SD — Page 389
Slinger, Randy, MD
ChoiceCare/Humana — Page 322
Sloan, Cullen, CPA
Innoviant Inc — Page 487
Sloan, Mary Anne
Arnett Health Plans — Page 157
Sloan, Thom
Texas Medical Foundation
Health Quality Institute — Page 427
Slone, Carl J
Anthem BCBS of Virginia Inc — Page 442
Slotky, Barry, MD
CIMRO Quality
Healthcare Solutions — Page 144
Slowik, Donald J
Independent Care Health Plan — Page 467
Slubowski, James S
Priority Health — Page 230
Sluka, Joseph
Western Health — Page 389
Slusser, Eric R
Centene Corporation — Page 244
Slutsky, Alan, DMD
Dedicated Dental Systems — Page 43
Small, Eric
Community Clinical Services — Page 196
Smallie, Don, DC
Basic Chiropractic Hlth Plan Inc — Page 35
Smart, Deborah, MD
Trustmark Insurance Company — Page 153
Smart, Ellen
Care 1st Health Plan — Page 38
Smart, Rob
CIGNA Healthcare of Virginia Inc -
Richmond — Page 443
Smart, Shelli
Mutual Assurance
Administrators Inc — Page 342
Smart, Zina
Western Dental Services — Page 75
Smeltzer, Phil
BCBS of Western New York — Page 285
Smethers, Gary D, MD
Blue Cross Blue Shield of AZ — Page 12
Smiley, Bruce
Indiana Health Network — Page 161
Smit, Alan
LifeWise Health Plan of WA — Page 453
Premera Blue Cross - Eastern — Page 454
Smith, Anita M
Capital Blue Cross — Page 359
Keystone Health Plan Central — Page 367
Smith, Ann
Galaxy Health Network — Page 414
Smith, Bob
Arizona Foundation for
Medical Care — Page 11
Smith, Chris
HealthLink Inc - Corp Hdqrtrs — Page 249
Smith, Clarence, MD
Jackson Memorial Health Plan — Page 115
Smith, Craig, MD, MBA
Children's Community
Health Plan Inc — Page 462
Smith, D Wesley, MD
Alabama Quality
Assurance Foundation — Page 3
Smith, David
MedSolutions — Page 396

Smith, David R
EHP Inc — Page 362
Smith, Dawn
PersonalCare Ins of IL Inc — Page 151
Smith, Dennis H
Upper Peninsula Health Plan — Page 232
Smith, Dewitt M
HIP Health Plan of New York — Page 296
Smith, Donald E
Regence BCBS of Utah — Page 436
Regence Healthwise — Page 436
Smith, Donna
USA Managed Care Organization — Page 22
Smith, Doug
Martins Point Health Care — Page 196
Smith, Gail
MetroPlus Health Plan — Page 300
Smith, Gayle
Ohio Kepro Inc — Page 332
Smith, George, MD
Humana Health Care Plans of
San Antonio/Austin — Page 418
Smith, Gerry
Scriptrax — Page 495
Smith, Graham
Care Choices HMO — Page 218
Smith, Gregory K
Mountain State BCBS — Page 460
Smith, Howard
HealthPlus Inc — Page 296
Smith, Jack
Humana Health Care Plans
of Houston — Page 418
Smith, Jack A
Medco Health Solutions Inc — Page 488
Smith, Jackee
Co/OP Optical Services Inc — Page 219
Smith, Jackee
CO/OP Optical Services Inc — Page 219
Smith, James R
Excellus BCBS, Central
New York Region — Page 291
Smith, Jodi
ProviDRs Care Network — Page 181
Smith, Joseph
Arkansas Blue Cross/Blue Shield
a Mutual Insurance Company — Page 25
Smith, Karen
Presbyterian Health Plan — Page 281
Smith, Kevin, MD
Molina Healthcare of Ohio Inc — Page 330
Smith, Marsha
Evercare Select — Page 15
Smith, Martin
Global Medical Management — Page 110
Smith, Melissa
Preferred Mental Hlth Mngmnt — Page 180
Smith, Mike
Anthem BCBS of Ohio — Page 320
Smith, Patsy
Alliance Regional Hlth Ntwrk — Page 404
Smith, Ron
Renaissance Hlth Systems Inc — Page 119
Smith, Ron, MD
BCBS of North Carolina — Page 481
Smith, Roy D, DDS
Newport Dental Plan — Page 60
Smith, Russell P
Aetna Inc - Arizona — Page 11
Smith, Sandra
HMO Louisiana Inc — Page 191
Smith, Scott, MD
First Health — California — Page 46
Smith, Scott Sr
Coalition America Inc — Page 129
Smith, Sean
Coalition America Inc — Page 129
Smith, Sharon
Health Care Excel Inc — Page 160

Smith, Steve, RPh
Maxor Plus — Page 488
Smith, Susan
American Specialty
Health Plans Inc — Page 33
Smith, Tamara A
D C Chartered Health Plan Inc — Page 97
Smith, Thomas P
PacifiCare of Nevada — Page 263
Smith, Troy
Hometown Health Plan — Page 260
Smith, William
Bucks County Physician
Hospital Alliance — Page 358
Smith, William
South Central Preferred — Page 372
Smith, William P
Blue Preferred Plan-BCBS
Michigan — Page 218
Smith-Clem, Delores
El Paso First Health Plans Inc — Page 413
Smith-Hagman, Karen
Catalina Behavioral
Health Services Inc — Page 13
Smithson, Tammy
Americas PPO — Page 233
Smock, Nick
PBA Health — Page 491
Smoot, Karen
Blue Cross Blue Shield of NM — Page 279
HMO New Mexico Inc — Page 280
Snead, Thomas G, Jr
Anthem BCBS of Virginia Inc — Page 442
Snell, Chris
Evercare Select — Page 15
Snider, Mary
UnitedHealthcare of NC Inc — Page 315
Snider, Steve
Citrus Health Care Inc — Page 108
Snidersich, Gloria
HealthPlus of Michigan — Page 224
Snook O'Riva, Teresa
Contra Costa Health Plan — Page 43
Snow, David B, Jr
Medco Health Solutions Inc — Page 275
Medco Health Solutions Inc — Page 488
Snyder, Jeff
Hometown Health Plan — Page 260
Snyder, Kristin
Kaiser Foundation Health Plan
of Colorado — Page 83
Snyder, Samantha
CIGNA Dental Health of KS Inc — Page 177
CIGNA Dental Health of MD Inc — Page 201
Sobel, Lila, RN
Geisinger Health Plan — Page 363
Soberg, Elizabeth K
PacifiCare of Colorado — Page 84
UnitedHealthcare of Colorado — Page 85
Sobocinski, Vincent J
CIGNA Healthcare of PA — Page 360
Soczynski, Paul F
Community Care Hlth Plan Inc — Page 521
Soistman, Francis S Jr
Coventry Health Care Inc —
Corporate Headquarters — Page 201
Sokolow, Alan, MD
Blue Shield of California — Page 36
Sola, Marcus
Holman Group, The — Page 51
Soler, Morris
American National Ins Co — Page 405
Solma, Margaret
Avera Health Plans Inc — Page 387
Soloman, Carol
McLaren Health Plan — Page 226
Solomon, Carol A
Tenet Choices Inc — Page 192

Index VIII: Personnel

Shiflett, Jason
Mutual Assurance Admin Inc   Page 342
Shih, Anthony
IPRO   Page 298
Shilling, Terry S
Humana Health Benefit Plan
of Louisiana   Page 191
Humana Health Benefit Plan
of Louisiana   Page 517
Shin, Amy
On Lok Senior Health Services   Page 60
Shinto, Richard
Primecare Medical Network Inc   Page 65
Shipley, Kurt
Blue Cross Blue Shield of NM   Page 279
HMO New Mexico Inc   Page 280
Shipley, Marion
Innovative Care Management   Page 347
Shipp, Charles Brian
AmeriGroup Tennessee Inc   Page 391
Shiraishi, Allan
Scan Health Plan   Page 68
Shirley, Michael, MD
Sagamore Health Network Inc   Page 164
Shjerven, Tom
ValueOptions - Corp Hdqrtrs   Page 447
Shoaf, Kirby
Community Care Org Inc   Page 509
Community Care Hlth Plan Inc   Page 521
Shonk, Richard
UnitedHealthcare of SW Ohio Inc-
Dayton/Cincinnati   Page 337
Shonkoff, Fredi
Blue Cross Blue Shield of MA   Page 209
Shoop, Stephen E
Behavioral Hlthcare Options Inc   Page 259
Shoptaw, Robert L
Arkansas Blue Cross/Blue Shield
a Mutual Insurance Company   Page 25
Shore, Howard
Catalina Behavioral
Health Services Inc   Page 13
Short, Steve
Health Advantage   Page 27
Shorter, Gary C
4MOST Health Network   Page 459
Showalter, Kathryn
Medcost LLC   Page 313
Showalter, Michael
CIGNA Healthcare of CT   Page 89
Shrader, Will
Blue Cross Blue Shield of SC -
Corporate Hqtrs   Page 383
Shreck, Robert W, MD FAAP
Healthinsight   Page 435
Shriver, Ric
Horizon Behavioral Services   Page 112
Shulaiba, Refaat
Midwest Health Plan   Page 226
Shuler, Robin L, CPA, MBA
Qualis Health   Page 455
Shullick, Karen
CIGNA Healthcare of OH Inc   Page 323
Shulman, Steven J
Magellan Health Services Inc   Page 91
Magellan Health Services   Page 132
Magellan Behavioral Health   Page 274
Shuman, Bill
Flora Health Network   Page 325
Sidon, Ken
Antares Mngmnt Solutions   Page 319
Sidon, Kenneth
Medical Mutual of Ohio   Page 330
Sieber, Jack
Excellus BCBS   Page 290
Siegel, Jodi RN
Fidelis SecureCare of MI Inc   Page 221

Siegel, Michael MD
Molina Healthcare Inc -
Corporate Headquarters   Page 59
Sieman, Gary
HealthLink Inc   Page 248
HealthLink Inc -
Corporate Headquarters   Page 249
Sienik, Suzanne C
Concentra Inc   Page 144
Sigel, Deena
Care 1st Health Plan AZ Inc   Page 13
Sihkin, Daniel, RPh
Humana Medical Plan Inc   Page 114
Sikka, Anju, MD
Health Net - New Jersey   Page 272
Health Net - New York   Page 295
Silberstein, Charles, MD
National Dental Consultants Inc   Page 301
Silberstein, David
Ndc-West Inc dba NADENT   Page 83
National Dental Consultants Inc   Page 301
Silberstein, Nina
NDC-West Inc dba NADENT   Page 83
Silberstein, Nina
National Dntl Consultants Inc   Page 301
Silva, Pam
Grand Valley Health Plan   Page 221
Silverman, Bruce
Delta Dental Plan of NJ   Page 271
Silverstein, Jay
UnitedHealth Group —
Corporate Headquarters   Page 238
Simmer, Thomas L, MD
Blue Preferred Plan-BBCBS -
Michigan   Page 218
Simmon, Victoria, RN
Saint Mary's HealthFirst   Page 263
Simmons, Rick
Health Net Inc -
Corporate Headquarters   Page 49
Simon, Avrum, MD
Zurich Services Corporation   Page 155
Simon, Lois
Commonwealth Care
Alliance Inc   Page 505
Simone, Michael
New York Presbyterian
Community Health Plan   Page 302
Simonitsch, Kirsten
Premera BCBS of Alaska   Page 9
Premera - Corp Hdqrtrs   Page 454
Premera Blue Cross - Western   Page 454
Simpson, Charles A, DC
Complementary Hlthcare Plans   Page 345
Simpson, Christy
Utah Public Employees
Health Program   Page 438
Simpson, Edward, Jr
Florida Health Care Plan Inc   Page 109
Simpson, Jeanne
Kern Foundation/
Preferred Provider Organization   Page 55
Simpson, Kevin
Delta Dental Plan of NC   Page 312
Simpson, Mark
Great-West Hlthcare of Maine   Page 196
Simpson, Patricia
Delaware Physicians Care Inc   Page 521
Simpson, Ross J, Jr, MD
Carolinas Center for
Medical Excellence, The   Page 310
Simpson, Scott, MD
Humana Health Plan of Austin   Page 419
Simunza, Craig
Dental Network of America   Page 146
Sinclair, Brenda
Humana Health Care Plans
of Kansas & Missouri   Page 179

Sinclair, Christopher A
Cambridge Managed
Care Services   Page 38
Sing Loo, Lawrence Wing
Puget Sound Health Partners   Page 455
Singer, Ben
PacifiCare Health Systems-
Corporate Headquarters   Page 62
Singer, Eric
Immediate Pharmaceutical
Services Inc   Page 486
Singer, Steven
Blue Cross Blue Shield of FL
& Health Options Inc   Page 104
Singh, Randit
San Joaquin Foundation PPO   Page 67
Singletary, Carol
Behavioral Health Systems Inc   Page 3
Singleton, Mark E
Union Labor Life Insurance Co   Page 276
Sipski, M Leonide
CHN Solutions   Page 270
Siren, Pamela
Community Medical Alliance   Page 210
Neighborhood Health Plan   Page 214
Sirera, John
Preferred One   Page 93
WellCare Health Plans Inc -
Corporate Headquarters   Page 124
Sirois, Don
Anthem BCBS of Maine   Page 195
Sisco-Creed, Shirley, RN
ProviDRs Care Network   Page 181
Situ, Jamie
Pacific IPA   Page 63
Sivak, Christopher G, MD
Buckeye Community
Health Plan Inc   Page 321
Sivertsen, Darren
Health Plan of Nevada Inc   Page 260
Sivigliano, Denise
Mutual Assurance
Administrators Inc   Page 342
Sivori, Joseph
SmileCare/
Community Dental Services   Page 69
Sizemore, Kim
PPO Oklahoma Inc   Page 341
Skillern, Gwendoyln
CareFirst BCBS   Page 200
Skinner, David
GroupLink Inc   Page 160
Skinner, Robert
Presbyterian Health Plan   Page 281
Skinner, Roger W
GroupLink Inc   Page 160
Skipper, Ron, MD
Heart of America Health Plan   Page 317
Skolozdra, Michael
Connecticare Inc   Page 89
Skourtes, Eugene C
Williamette Dental Group PC   Page 352
Williamette Dental of WA Inc   Page 457
Skrocki, Ronald
Genex Services   Page 363
Slabosky, Alex
M Plan Inc   Page 163
Encore Health Network   Page 160
Slack, Steven
Pacific Health Alliance   Page 62
Slagle, Ydsia
Optima Health Plan Inc   Page 445
Slater, Chuck
Anthem BCBS of Ohio   Page 320
Slaughter, Richard, MD
Geisinger Health Plan   Page 363
Slavin, William, DDS
Managed Dental Care   Page 57

Index VIII: Personnel

Sell, Steven
Managed Health Network — Page 57
Sellers, Ken
Blue Cross Blue Shield of FL & Health Options Inc — Page 104
Sellers, M Edward
BlueChoice Hlth Plan of SC Inc — Page 383
BCBS of South Carolina - Corporate Hqtrs — Page 383
Sellers, Mary
Qualis Health — Page 455
Sellner, William
Sun Health Medisun — Page 20
Seltenheim, Jon
United Concordia Co Inc - AL — Page 6
United Concordia Co Inc - CA — Page 72
United Concordia Company Inc - Corporate Headquarters — Page 373
Selva, Manuel, MD
UnitedHealthcare of South FL — Page 122
Semands Suttles, Denise
Global Health Inc — Page 341
Sementi, Darcy
PersonalCare Ins of IL Inc — Page 151
Semingson, Bruce A, RPh
United Drugs — Page 496
Semkiw, Cindy
Jaimini Health Inc — Page 53
Sendlewski, Susan
Amerihealth Ins Co - NJ North — Page 269
Amerihealth Ins Co - NJ South — Page 269
Sengewalt, J Mark
Mountain State BCBS — Page 460
Senne, Jerry
Health First Health Plans Inc — Page 111
Senter, Pat
Unity Health Insurance — Page 470
Senterfitt, Colleen
New West Health Plan — Page 254
Sequra, Ernesto
Mercy Health Plans of MO Inc — Page 249
Serenelli, Christine
SunRx Inc — Page 495
Serini, Paul A, Esq
XL Health — Page 207
Serio, Angelo
Maxor Plus — Page 488
Sessoms, Vickie L
Health Partners — Page 364
Sevcik, Joseph A
Assurant Employee Benefits-AL — Page 3
Assurant Employee Benefits-AZ — Page 12
Assurant Employee Benefits-CA — Page 35
Assurant Employee Benefits-CO — Page 78
Assurant Employee Benefits-FL — Page 102
Assurant Employee Benefits-GA — Page 127
Assurant Employee Benefits-IL — Page 143
Assurant Employee Benefits-IN — Page 158
Assurant Employee Benefits-MI — Page 217
Assurant Employee Benefits - Corporate Office — Page 244
Assurant Employee Benefits-NM — Page 279
Assurant Employee Benefits-NY — Page 285
Assurant Employee Benefits-NC — Page 309
Assurant Employee Benefits-PA — Page 357
Assurant Employee Benefits-TN — Page 392
Assurant Employee Benefits-TX — Page 429
Assurant Employee Benefits-WA — Page 449
Severson, DuWayne
Mercycare Health Plan Inc — Page 468
Sewall, John
Blue Cross Blue Shield of MS — Page 241
Sewell, Gary
Medical Associates Hlth Plans — Page 172
Sewell, Jamie
Complementary Hlthcare Plans — Page 345
Seyerle, Jo Ellen
Humana Inc - Tennessee — Page 396

Shackleton, Robert, MD
Tenet Choices Inc — Page 192
Shadle, Dan
Galaxy Health Network — Page 414
Shadron, Jacqueline
Humana Health Care Plans of Corpus Christi — Page 417
Shafa, Mehrdad, MD
Maricopa Health Plan — Page 18
Shafer, Debbie
Partnership HealthPlan of CA — Page 64
Shaff, Karen E
Principal Life Ins Co — Page 172
Shaffer, Dave
Kern Family Health Care — Page 55
Shaffer, Ian A, MD
Managed Health Network — Page 57
Shaffer, Kathy
Sentinel Management Services - Corporate Headquarters — Page 372
Shaffer, Matthew M
Wellmark Inc — Corp Hdqrtrs — Page 175
Shah, Mansoor, MD
Lakewood Health Plan Inc — Page 56
Shah, Rupesh
Preferred One — Page 93
WellCare HMO Inc — Page 124
WellCare Health Plans Inc - Corporate Headquarters — Page 124
HealthEase of Florida Inc — Page 111
Shah, Sanjiv
MetroPlus Health Plan — Page 300
Shalowitz, Joel, MD
Delphi Card R — Page 145
Shanahan, Brian
Medical Mutual of Ohio — Page 330
Shandley, Audrey
Community Health Plan — Page 245
Shane, Paul J, Jr
Galaxy Health Network — Page 414
Shannon, Colleen
Pearle Vision Managed Care - HMO of Texas Inc — Page 423
Shapiro, Lee
Allscripts Pharmaceuticals Inc — Page 479
Shapiro, Sheila
Blue Cross Blue Shield of MT — Page 253
Shapiro, Sheila K, BS, MBA
Molina Healthcare Inc - Corporate Headquarters — Page 59
Shapley, Brian
Preferred Care — Page 304
Shappet, Aspasia
Medical Eye Services Inc — Page 58
Sharbatz, Kim
Health Care Exchange Limited Company — Page 223
Sharenow, Joel
Midwestern Dental Plans Inc — Page 226
Sharet, Melody
Global Medical Management — Page 110
Sharp, Brandon
Prime Health Services Inc — Page 398
Sharp, Brian A, MEd, CCM, CDMS
Prime Health Services Inc — Page 398
Shashati, Nick, OD
Visioncare of California — Page 75
Shaw, Carol
United Behavioral Health (UBH) — Page 71
Shaw, Robert, MD
UnitedHealthcare of Florida Inc — Page 122
Shea, Marcia
UnitedHealthcare of Texas Inc - Houston — Page 429
Shearer, Jacquelyn
Managed Hlth Services IN Inc — Page 163
Shearer, Lindsay
CIGNA Healthcare — Page 439

Sheehan, Dan
New England Financial - Corporate Headquarters — Page 214
Sheehan, Kathy
Southern Health Services Inc — Page 445
Sheehy, Joseph, MD
Southeastern Indiana Health Organization — Page 166
Sheehy, Robert J
UnitedHealthcare Services Co of the River Valley Inc — Page 154
UnitedHealthcare Services Co of the River Valley Inc — Page 172
UnitedHealthcare Services Co of the River Valley Inc — Page 173
UnitedHealthcare Services Co of the River Valley Inc — Page 174
UnitedHealthcare Services Co of the River Valley Inc — Page 400
Sheehy, Thomas J, Jr
IPRO — Page 298
Sheesley, Phil
Universal Health Care Inc — Page 122
Shehab, Phyllis
Care Network — Page 359
Selectcare Access Corp — Page 371
Sheldon, Kenneth M
National Pacific Dental — Page 421
Shellabarger, Scott
Novasys Health Network — Page 28
Shelton, Carol
Lovelace Health Plan — Page 280
Shelton, Jim
Indiana Health Network — Page 161
Shelton, Lesley
Humana Medical Plan Inc — Page 114
Shematek, Jon, MD
CareFirst BlueChoice Inc — Page 97
CareFirst BCBS — Page 200
Delmarva Hlth Care Plan Inc — Page 202
CareFirst BCBS — Page 481
Shen, Lili
Pacific IPA — Page 63
Shepard, Darcy
WellCare of New York — Page 307
Shepard, Robert M, MD
New West Health Plan — Page 254
Shepherd, W Hal
Preferred Health Alliance — Page 6
Shepperd, James
Innovative Care Management — Page 347
Sheridan, Joseph, DO
Unison Health Plan of PA — Page 373
Sheridan, Susan
CIGNA Behavioral Health Inc - Corporate Headquarters — Page 234
Sherif, Cindy
Horizon Behavioral Services — Page 112
Sherma, Sally
WellPoint NextRX — Page 497
Sherman, Amy
Health Care Exchange Limited Company — Page 223
Sherman, Jennifer
Coreview — Page 235
Shermer, Barry
Windsor Health Plan of TN Inc — Page 401
Sherwin, David A, CPA
Quality Health Plan Inc — Page 119
Shiba, David, MD
Stanislaus Medical Society — Page 70
Shields, Brian
Aetna Inc of the Carolinas — Page 309
Shields, Guy
Landmark Healthcare Inc — Page 56
Shields, Jack
UnitedHealthcare of NC Inc — Page 315
Shields, John
Williamette Dental Group PC — Page 352
Williamette Dental of WA Inc — Page 457

Index VIII: Personnel

Schneider, Dan
Parkview Signature Care — Page 164
Schneider, George, CPA, CMCP
Mercy Health Plans of MO Inc — Page 249
Schneider, Rachel
Optima Health Plan Inc — Page 445
Schnitzer, Mary
CHN MCO — Page 322
Schoellkopf, Nancy
Blue Cross Blue Shield
of Western New York — Page 285
Schoenbaum, John
Blue Cross Blue Shield
of Massachusetts — Page 209
Schoeplein, Kevin D
OSF Health Plans — Page 151
Schofield, Carolyn
Excellus BCBS — Page 290
Schofield, Linda
Preferred One — Page 93
Scholten, Gary P
Principal Life Insurance Co — Page 172
Schooley, Edwin, DDS, MHA
Delta Dental of Iowa — Page 169
Schotz, Michael D
Interplan Health Group — Page 53
Interplan Health Group -
Corporate Headquarters — Page 91
Superien Health Network Inc — Page 335
Interplan Health Group — Page 419
Schouweiler, Steven H
American National Ins Co — Page 405
Schrader, Michael
Santa Barbara Regional
Health Authority — Page 67
Schreck, Ronda
Keokuk Area Hospital
Organized Delivery System Inc — Page 171
Schreiber, Joy K
Block Vision of Texas Inc — Page 405
Schreiber, Richard
HMO California — Page 51
Schreier, Russell
Colorado Dental Service Inc,
dba: Delta Dental Plan of CO — Page 80
Schrock, Jon, MD
EHP Inc — Page 362
Schroeder, Gordon L
Fiserv Inc — Page 464
Schroeder, Wanda
20/20 Eyecare Plan Inc — Page 99
Schryver, Tim
Unicare Health Plans
of the Midwest Inc — Page 153
Unicare Health Plans
of the Midwest Inc — Page 521
Schub, Craig S
HealthSpring Inc - Tennessee — Page 395
Schubach, Stephen
Standard Optical — Page 437
Schuback, Aaron
Standard Optical — Page 437
Schuetz, Linda
CIGNA Healthcare of NH — Page 265
Schukman, Jay, MD
Anthem BCBS of Virginia Inc — Page 442
Schuler, Stephen T, DMD
Dental Care Plus Inc — Page 324
Schultz Clubbs, Amy
Molina Healthcare of Ohio Inc — Page 330
Schultz, Brent
Memorial Hermann Health
Network Providers — Page 420
Schultz, Carl
Mercy Health Plans of MO Inc — Page 249
Schultz, Eric H
Fallon Community Hlth Plan Inc — Page 211
Fallon Community Hlth Plan — Page 514

Schultz, Jennifer
Saint Mary's HealthFirst — Page 263
Schultz, Timothy J, MBA, CPA, M
Primaris — Page 250
Schultz-Evans, Jill
Dental Benefit Providers Inc — Page 202
Schum, Rick
Blue Cross Blue Shield of WY — Page 473
Schumacher, Laura
Corvel Corporation — Page 169
Schumacher, Tamara
Iba Health Plans — Page 225
Schuman, Dennis, MD
Saint Mary's HealthFirst — Page 263
Schumann, Scott
Great Lakes Health Plan — Page 222
Schurmann, Theresa
HealthPlus of Michigan — Page 224
Schuyler, Bradley
Avante Behavioral Health Plan — Page 35
Schwaazenburg, Lynn
UnitedHealthcare of Texas Inc -
Houston — Page 429
Schwab, Jeff
Dominion Dental Services -
Corporate Headquarters — Page 444
Schwab, Maryan
Community Health Plan of WA — Page 450
Schwab, Michael
Nd Pharmacy Service Corp — Page 490
Schwab, Timothy, MD
Scan Health Plan — Page 68
Schwartz, Milton, MD
Aetna Health of California Inc — Page 31
Aetna Inc - Dental Care of CA — Page 32
Schwartz, Steven P
Allscripts Pharmaceuticals Inc — Page 479
Schwarz, Jon
UnitedHealthcare of Florida Inc — Page 121
Schweppe, Richard
Corvel Corporation — Page 43
Sciammacco, Ann Marie
Fallon Community Hlth Plan Inc — Page 211
Scjeel, Jim
CIGNA Behavioral Health Inc — Page 40
Scoggins, Alan
Texas True Choice — Page 428
Scoon, Davey
Tufts Health Plan — Page 216
Scoones, Laura
New York State Catholic
Health Plan Inc — Page 303
Scott, Angela
New York Presbyterian
Community Health Plan — Page 302
Scott, Cory
Coventry Hlth Care Inc-GA Inc — Page 130
SouthCare/Hlthcare Preferred — Page 134
Coventry Health Care Inc —
Carolinas — Page 311
Scott, Dan
Berkshire Health Partners/Medicus
Resource Management — Page 357
Scott, Denise
Unipsych Systems — Page 120
Scott, Garland G, III
UnitedHealthcare of Arkansas — Page 28
UnitedHealthcare of TN Inc — Page 401
Scott, Gregory W
PacifiCare Health Systems-
Corporate Headquarters — Page 62
PacifiCare of California — Page 62
Pacificare Life & Health
Insurance Company — Page 63
APS Healthcare Inc — Page 199
Pacificare Life & Health
Insurance Company — Page 519

Scott, Jan
Texas Childrens Health Plan — Page 426
Scott, Kirby
Delta Dental Plan of SD — Page 387
Scott, Mary
Preferred Health Systems — Page 180
Scott, Peggy
BCBS of Louisiana Inc — Page 189
Scott, Robert, MD
Sentinel Management Services -
Corporate Headquarters — Page 372
Summit Health Plan Inc — Page 120
Scott, Steve
Vision Service Plan — Page 75
Vision Service Plan — Page 86
Scott, Steven M, MD
Vista Health Plan Inc — Page 123
Vista Hlthplan of South FL Inc — Page 123
Scott, Tameria
USA Managed Care Org — Page 22
Scott, Torje, RN
Humana Health Plan of Austin — Page 419
Scott, Tracey
Great-West Healthcare of Texas -
Dallas — Page 415
Scott, Weston P
Humana Health Care Plans
of Corpus Christi — Page 417
Scrase, David R, MD
Presbyterian Health Plan — Page 281
Scub, Craig S
HealthSpring Inc-Corp Hdqrtrs — Page 395
Scully, Robert, MD
Health Alliance Medical Plans -
Corporate Headquarters — Page 149
Seabert, Pat
Care 1st Health Plan AZ Inc — Page 13
Seabrooks, Norm
Aetna Inc - Washington — Page 449
Sebastian, Dennis
Gateway Health Plan Inc — Page 362
Sedlak, Cheryl
Vantage PPO — Page 375
Sedmark, Pamela
CareSource — Page 321
Sedqwick, Casper F
Excellus BlueCross BlueShield,
Central New York Region — Page 291
Seebolt, Andrew
South Central Preferred — Page 372
Sehring, Robert C
OSF Health Plans — Page 151
Seibel, John, MD
New Mexico Medical
Review Association — Page 281
Seibert, Cheryl
Preferred Health Systems — Page 180
Seidenfeld, John J, MD
Anthem Blue Cross Blue Shield
of Missouri — Page 243
HealthLink Inc — Page 248
HealthLink Inc -
Corporate Headquarters — Page 249
Seidman, Richard, MD
LA Care Health Plan — Page 55
Seifert, Randy
Santa Barbara Regional
Health Authority — Page 67
Seitzman, Sharon
QualCare Inc — Page 276
Selberg, Jeffrey D
Exempla Healthcare LLC — Page 81
Seleski, Dorothy
LA Care Health Plan — Page 55
Self, David
Primary Health Plan — Page 142
Seligman, Terry
Navitus Health Solutions — Page 490

Index VIII: Personnel

Sanders, Janet
Kern Family Health Care — Page 55
Sanders, Paige
Spectera Vision Srvcs of Ca Inc — Page 69
Sandoval, Lisa CPA
Colorado Choice Health Plan/
San Luis Valley HMO Inc — Page 79
Sandridge, Mary
Carelink Health Plans — Page 459
Sanfilippo, Fred, MD, PhD
Ohio State University Managed
Health Care Systems Inc — Page 332
Sanghui, Sujata
PacificSource Health Plans — Page 350
Sanjak, Amer
Molina Healthcare of MI Inc — Page 227
Sannes, Randall
UnitedHealthcare of WI Inc — Page 470
SantaCroce, Mark
RxAmerica LLC — Page 494
Santana, Kelli
CIGNA Healthcare of California — Page 41
Santelli, Lisa
Excellus BCBS, Central NY
Southern Tier — Page 291
Santiago, Carlos
Medical Card System — Page 377
Santiago, Mark
Hudson Health Plan — Page 297
Santoyo, Julian
Primecare Medical Network Inc — Page 65
Santry, Barbara
Primary Health Plan — Page 142
Saperstein, Arnold, MD
MetroPlus Health Plan — Page 300
Sarafian, Araksi H
HIP Health Plan of New York — Page 296
Sarbora, Russell
Community Health Plan of WA — Page 450
Sarcheck, James, DDS
Great Expressions
Dental Centers — Page 222
Sardegna, Carl
Nationwide Better Health — Page 204
Sarik, Patricia
Valley Preferred — Page 375
Sarli, Gail
MDNY Healthcare Inc — Page 299
Sarran, Scott, MD
Fidelis SeniorCare Inc — Page 147
Sarria, Dan
Preferred Therapy Providers of America -
Corp Headquarters — Page 19
Sarvello, Francesca
Molina HealthCare of Utah Inc — Page 435
Sasser, E Rhone
Blue Cross Blue Shield of NC — Page 310
Sassi, Brian A
Blue Cross of California — Page 34
Blue Cross of California — Page 517
Sates, Dennis
Safeguard Health Plans Inc — Page 424
Sattenspiel, John, MD
Lane Oregon Health Plans — Page 347
Sauby, Eric
UnitedHealthcare of FL Inc — Page 121
Saudek, Karen
Blue Cross Blue Shield of VT — Page 439
Vermont Hlth Plans (Blue Care) — Page 439
Sauer, Paula M
Medical Mutual of Ohio — Page 330
Saunders, Mary Ann
Health Plan,
The Hometown Region — Page 327
Savage, Larry
ChoiceCare/Humana — Page 322
Humana Health Plan of OH Inc — Page 328

Savenko, Kathy
OhioHealth Group — Page 332
Savers, Robert
Coordinated Health Systems — Page 361
Savin, Bruce A, OD
Vision Care Network — Page 471
Savin, Dale
Vision Care Network — Page 471
Savrin, Ronald A
Ohio Kepro Inc — Page 332
Sawchak, Bill
UMPC Health Plan Univ of
Pittsburgh Medical Center — Page 374
Sax, Richard, MD
Orange Prevention &
Treatment Integrated — Page 60
Saxton, Kim
Community Choice Michigan — Page 219
Sayer, Linda S
Advantica Eyecare Inc — Page 99
Scammon, James
CIGNA Healthcare of NH — Page 265
Scanavino, David
MMM Healthcare Inc — Page 378
Scanlon, Edward, MD
Network Health Plan WI — Page 468
Scantland, D Alan
MemberHealth Inc — Page 489
Scapellati, Mark
Community Health Network
of Connecticut Inc — Page 89
Scarbrough, Michael
Memphis Managed Care Corp — Page 397
Scarcelli, Betsy
Keystone Mercy Health Plan — Page 368
Scasny, Ron
Abri Health Plan Inc — Page 461
Scavo, Amy
Aetna Health of Illinois Inc — Page 143
Scelletar, Robert, MD
AmeriChoice of New York — Page 284
Schacht, Karla J
Assurant Employee Benefits-AL — Page 3
Assurant Employee Benefits-AZ — Page 12
Assurant Employee Benefits-CA — Page 35
Assurant Employee Benefits-CO — Page 78
Assurant Employee Benefits-FL — Page 102
Assurant Employee Benefits-GA — Page 127
Assurant Employee Benefits-IL — Page 143
Assurant Employee Benefits-IN — Page 158
Assurant Employee Benefits-MI — Page 217
Assurant Employee Benefits -
Corporate Office — Page 244
Assurant Employee Benefits-NM — Page 279
Assurant Employee Benefits-NY — Page 285
Assurant Employee Benefits-NC — Page 309
Assurant Employee Benefits-PA — Page 357
Assurant Employee Benefits-TN — Page 392
Assurant Employee Benefits-TX — Page 429
Assurant Employee Benefits-WA — Page 449
Schaefer, Sue
South Dakota
Pharmacist Association — Page 495
Schaen, Laurie A
American Progressive Life &
Insurance Company — Page 520
Schaffer, David
Medical Card System — Page 377
Schaffer, W Allen
CIGNA Healthcare of TX Inc — Page 409
Schaffner, Linda
Keokuk Area Hospital
Organized Delivery System Inc — Page 171
Schaich, Robert L
Sierra Health Services Inc-
Corporate Headquarters — Page 264
Health Plan of Nevada Inc — Page 260
Schambacher, Lisa
Parkview Signature Care — Page 164

Schandel, David
Florida Health Care Plan Inc — Page 109
Schandley, Audrey
Community Health Plan — Page 245
Schatz, Brian
Medical Associates Hlth Plans — Page 172
Schauer, Raymond
Mercer First Choice — Page 369
Schechtman, Jay, MD
HealthFirst Inc — Page 295
Scheff, Albert, MD
Med-Valu Inc — Page 329
Scheff, Jonathan H, MD
Health Net Inc - Corp Hdqrtrs — Page 49
Schell, Mike
Medical Eye Services Inc — Page 58
Schellhorn, Charles W
Argus Health System Inc — Page 480
Schenk, Sue
UnitedHealthcare & Mid Atlantic Medical
Services Inc — Page 206
Schenken, Penny
Health Plan of San Joaquin, The — Page 50
Scherer, Chris A
Great Lakes Health Plan — Page 222
Scherer, Jerry D
Blue Cross Blue Shield of OK — Page 339
Bluelincs HMO — Page 340
Scherer, Kurt
Cox Health Plans — Page 246
Schexnayder, Todd
BCBS of LA Inc — Page 189
Schiavo, Toni
Health Net Inc - Corp Hdqrtrs — Page 49
Health Net of California — Page 49
Schiess, Jack
Regence BCBS of Utah — Page 436
Schiesser, Heath
Preferred One — Page 93
HealthEase of Florida Inc — Page 111
WellCare HMO Inc — Page 124
WellCare Health Plans Inc -
Corporate Headquarters — Page 124
Harmony Health Plan — Page 148
WellCare of New York — Page 307
Schievelbein, Karen
Dental Benefit Prvidrs of CA Inc — Page 45
United Behavioral Health (UBH) — Page 71
Dental Benefit Providers Inc — Page 202
United Behavioral Health — Page 373
Schiffman, Debbie
Unity Health Insurance — Page 470
Schimmelbusch, Diane
Evercare of Texas LLC — Page 413
Schindler, Eric L
Blue Cross Blue Shield of MT — Page 253
Schirmer, Daniel
Denver Health Medical Plan Inc — Page 80
Schlottman, James E
Humana Health Benefit Plan
of Louisiana — Page 191
Humana Health Benefit Plan
of Louisiana — Page 517
Schmelzer, Dean C
Fiserv Inc — Page 464
Schmidt, Bradley E
Newport Dental Plan — Page 60
Schmidt, Christopher
DentCare Delivery Systems Inc — Page 289
Healthplex Inc — Page 296
Schmidt, Dave
Scan Health Plan — Page 68
Scan Health Plan — Page 502
Schmidt, Kurt W
Care-Plus Dental Plans Inc — Page 462
Schmitz, Ferdie
ParadigmHealth — Page 276

Index VIII: Personnel

Rowland, Lisa
Humana Health Care Plans
of Houston — Page 418
Roy, Bernie
Florida Health Partners Inc — Page 110
Roy, Denis J
Wellmark BCBS of Iowa — Page 174
Wellmark Inc —
Corporate Headquarters — Page 175
Wellmark Hlth Plan of IA Inc — Page 175
Wellmark BCBS of SD — Page 389
Roy-Czyzowski, Connie M
Delta Dental Plan of NH — Page 265
Royal, Nancy
Humana Health Care Plans
of Houston — Page 418
Roybal, Ray
Catalina Behavioral
Health Services Inc — Page 13
Royer, Richard A
Primaris — Page 250
Rozga, Sandy
Independent Care Health Plan — Page 467
Ruadez, Roberto
Olympus Managed
Health Care Inc — Page 117
Rubin, Ben, MD
Family Health Partners — Page 247
Rubin, Valerie
Av-Med Health Plan-Gainesville Page 102
Av-Med Health Plan-Miami — Page 103
Av-Med Health Plan-Orlando — Page 103
Rubino, Mark, RPh, MHA
Aetna Inc - Pennsylvania — Page 355
Rubino, Richard J, CPA
Medco Health Solutions Inc — Page 488
Rubino, Tami
Coventry Health Care Inc — IA — Page 169
Ruchman, Mark, MD
Opticare Managed Vision — Page 314
AECC Total Vision Health
Plan of Texas Inc — Page 403
Rudell, Jeff
Epoch Group LC, The — Page 178
Rudisill, Greg
EyeMed Vision Care LLC — Page 325
Ruecker, Rita
Western Health Advantage — Page 75
Ruflin, Anne
Excellus BCBS — Page 290
Ruiz, Ron MD
CIGNA Healthcare of Arizona — Page 14
Rule Sandler, Susan
Western Dental Services — Page 75
Rummelhoff, Monica
Global Medical Management — Page 110
Rumper, Pat
Great-West Healthcare of AZ — Page 16
Rundle, Mark
Hines & Associates Inc — Page 150
Runnoe, Philip
DeltaCare USA — Page 44
Rupp, Tammy
Care Choices HMO — Page 218
Rush, John, MD
PacifiCare of Colorado — Page 84
Rushnell, Christi
Health First Health Plans Inc — Page 111
Russell, Dolores
Managed HealthCare
Northwest Inc — Page 348
Russell, Elizabeth
Scan Health Plan — Page 68
Russell, Michelle
NAMCI — Page 6
Premier Hlth Ntwrks of AL LLC — Page 6
Russo, Joan
Great-West Hlthcare - NJ — Page 272
Great-West Hlthcare of NY — Page 294

Russo, Pam
United Behavioral Health (UBH) — Page 71
Russo, Pat
Anthem BCBS of Virginia Inc — Page 442
Ruszczyk, Mark
Excellus BCBS, Utica Region — Page 292
Rutelberg, Jack
Florida Pace Centers Inc — Page 511
Ruth, Kevin J
Dental Benefit Providers of CA Inc Page 45
Rutherford, Carla
Delta Dental Plan of Arkansas — Page 26
Ruthven, Courtney, PhD
Preferred Mental Health
Management — Page 180
Rutkowski, Barbara, EdD, MN
SelectHealth Network — Page 165
Rutledge, Valinda
St Francis Optimum
Health Network — Page 385
Ruttenberg, Valerie
Prime Therapeutics — Page 493
Ruzas, Laura
Group Health Plan Inc — Page 248
Ryan, Chris
SHPS Inc — Page 186
Ryan, Cindy
Aetna Inc - Arizona — Page 11
Aetna Inc - Dental Care of CA — Page 32
Ryan, Kathy
Health Advantage — Page 27
Ryan, Thomas M
Caremark/CVS - Arizona — Page 482
CVS/Caremark -
Corporate Headquarters — Page 483
Caremark/CVS - Tennessee — Page 482
Caremark/CVS - Illinois — Page 482
Ryba, Rhonda
Presbyterian Health Plan — Page 281
Rybak, Tina
Arise Health Plan — Page 461
Ryce, Patrick, MD
Blue Cross Blue Shield of AL — Page 3
Ryder, Judi
Vista Hlthplan of South FL Inc — Page 123
Rye, Matt
UnitedHealthcare of SW Ohio Inc-
Dayton/Cincinnati — Page 337
Rygiel, Chuck
Blue Cross Blue Shield of OK — Page 339
Rykaczeski, Robert
HFN Inc — Page 150
Rzewnicki, Robert, MD
HMO Health Ohio (Cleveland) — Page 328
Medical Mutual of Ohio — Page 330
SuperMed Network — Page 334

S

Saalwaechter, John, MD
HealthPlus of Michigan — Page 224
Sabir, Jenna
Vision Insurance Plan of America Inc -
Corp Headquarters — Page 471
Sabo, Robert J
Metcare Health Plans Inc — Page 116
Sabochek, Mike
Script Care Inc — Page 425
Sack, Kenneth
Pharmacy Services Group — Page 492
Sadanandan, Subash
Paragon Biomedical Inc — Page 491
Sadler, JoAnn
Integrated Health Plan Inc — Page 115

Sadler, Robin
Kaiser Foundation Health Plan
of Colorado — Page 83
Sadtler, John
Humana Inc - Indiana — Page 161
Saffer, Mark B, DPM
Midwest Health Plan — Page 226
Safo, Doris
Metropolitan Health Plan — Page 237
Safran, Bruce H
DentCare Delivery Systems Inc — Page 289
Healthplex Inc — Page 296
Sahin, Mete
Dental Benefit Providers Inc — Page 202
Sahney, Vinod K, PhD
Blue Cross Blue Shield of MA — Page 209
Said, Conception, RN
Community Health Plan — Page 42
Sakovits, Steve
HealthFirst Inc — Page 295
Salazar, Arnold
Colorado Health Networks LLC -
ValueOptions — Page 80
Salinas, Jacob
Cox Health Plans — Page 246
Salkowe, Jerry
MVP Health Plan Inc — Page 301
Salm, Gordon W
Health Alliance Medical Plans - Corporate
Headquarters — Page 149
Salter, Brenda, MD
Medwatch LLC — Page 116
Saltzgaber, Lee, G MD, MPH, CPE
Staywell Insurance Guam Inc — Page 135
Sammis, Elizabeth
MD-Individual Practice Association Inc
(MD IPA) — Page 204
Mid Atlantic Medical Services Inc
(MAMSI)- Corp Headquarters — Page 204
Optimum Choice Inc — Page 205
OneNet PPO — Page 205
Sams, Cassandra
UHP Healthcare — Page 71
Samuels, Harold
JPS Benefits — Page 419
Samuels, Julie
HMO Louisiana Inc — Page 191
SanFilippo, Joe
Nationwide Health Plans — Page 331
Sanabria, Farrah, PHR
Quality Health Plan Inc — Page 119
Sanborn, Douglas, Esq
Delta Dental Plan of NJ — Page 271
Sanborn, Rebecca
Group Health Plan Inc — Page 248
Sanchez, Alejandro, RN, BSN, CC
Olympus Managed Health
Care Inc — Page 117
Sanchez, Annette
Crawford and Co -
Corporate Headquarters — Page 130
Sanchez, Egal
Community Choice Health Plan of
Westchester Inc — Page 287
Sanchez, Ester
Inland Empire Foundation
for Medical Care — Page 52
Sanchez, Melvin
Medical Card System — Page 377
Sanchez, Richard L
Advantica Eyecare Inc — Page 99
Sanchez, Richard, MD
Group Health Plan Inc — Page 248
Sanders, Cindy
Blue Cross Blue Shield of GA — Page 128
Sanders, James
OraQuest Dental Plans — Page 421

Index VIII: Personnel

Rodriguez, Roger
Preferred Care Partners Inc — Page 118
Roe, Jeff
LifeWise Health Plan of WA — Page 453
Roeding, Janine
Total Script — Page 496
Roehm, John
Health Partners — Page 364
Roehrick, Charles
Prime Therapeutics — Page 493
Roge, Rich
PacifiCare of California — Page 62
Pacificare Life & Hlth Ins Co — Page 63
Rogers, Carol
Delphi Card R — Page 145
Rogers, David
Independent Health Assoc Inc — Page 297
Rogers, Dennis
PacificSource Health Plans — Page 350
Rogers, Emily
ECCA - Managed Vision Care Inc -
Corporate Headquarters — Page 413
Rogers, Gary
Delta Dental Plan of WI — Page 463
Rogers, James T, MD
Primaris — Page 250
Rogers, Joseph
Jackson Memorial Health Plan — Page 115
Rogers, Kenyata J
OmniCare, A Cvntry Hlth Plan — Page 228
Rogers, Nancy
Guardian Life Insurance
Company of America — Page 294
Rogers, Phyllis L
Delta Dental Plan of Arkansas — Page 26
Rogers, Richard
Connecticare Inc — Page 89
Connecticare of NY — Page 288
Rogers, Richard
Connecticare of MA Inc — Page 210
Rogier, Steve
EyeMed Vision Care LLC — Page 325
Rogissart, Dennis
Molina Healthcare of MI Inc — Page 227
Rohan, Karen S
CIGNA Dental Health
Plan of AZ Inc — Page 14
CIGNA Dental Health of CO — Page 78
CIGNA Dental Health of DE Inc — Page 95
CIGNA Dental Health Inc -
Corporate Headquarters — Page 106
CIGNA Dental Health of FL — Page 107
CIGNA Dental Health of KS Inc — Page 177
CIGNA Dental Health of MD Inc — Page 201
CIGNA Dental Health of NJ Inc — Page 270
CIGNA Dental Health of NC Inc — Page 310
CIGNA Dental Health of OH Inc — Page 322
CIGNA Dental Health of TX Inc — Page 409
CIGNA Dental Health of PA Inc — Page 360
Rohfritch, Jack
University Health Plans Inc — Page 277
Rohr, Jan
Rocky Mountain Health Plans — Page 84
Rocky Mountain HealthCare Options Inc
dba Healthcare Options — Page 84
Rolando, Jean
RxAmerica LLC — Page 494
Rolff, Christi
Sante Community Physicians — Page 67
Rollins, Darren
Medical Review Institute -
Corporate Headquarters — Page 435
Rollins, Jeff
Medical Review Institute -
Corporate Headquarters — Page 435
Rollinson, Jane
UnitedHealthcare of NC Inc — Page 315
Rollinson, Jane E
Touchstone Health HMO Inc — Page 305

Rollman, Roger
UnitedHealthcare of AL — Page 7
UnitedHealthcare of FL Inc — Page 122
UnitedHealthcare of GA — Page 134
UnitedHealthcare of LA — Page 193
UnitedHealthcare of NC Inc — Page 315
Rollow, Arthur B
Viva Health Inc — Page 7
Rolston, Richard, MD, FAAP
Prevea Health Network — Page 469
Roman, Pablo
Aids Healthcare Foundation — Page 32
Romanchok, Mary
Interplan Health Group — Page 53
Superien Health Network Inc — Page 335
AmeriScript Inc — Page 479
Romania, Matt, RN
Central Susquehanna
Healthcare Providers — Page 359
Romano, Michael, MD
Midlands Choice Inc — Page 256
Romansky, Eileen
Interplan Health Group — Page 53
Interplan Health Group -
Corporate Headquarters — Page 91
Superien Health Network Inc — Page 335
Interplan Health Group — Page 419
Romberger, Wesley, MD
Health Management Network Inc — Page 16
Ron, Aran, MD
GHI HMO Select Inc — Page 293
Rooney, William R, MD
Coventry Health Care of KS -
Wichita — Page 178
Roos, John T
BCBS of North Carolina — Page 310
BCBS of North Carolina — Page 481
Roosevelt, James, Jr
Tufts Health Plan — Page 216
Root, Leon A, Jr
AmeriGroup New Jersey Inc — Page 268
AmeriGroup Corporation — Page 442
Roper, Libby
Coalition America Inc — Page 129
Roqueta, Barbara
Renaissance Hlth Systems Inc — Page 119
Rosa, Thomas J, ABOC
Davis Vision — Page 288
Rose, Brian
Preferred Health Systems — Page 180
Preferred Health Systems — Page 180
Rose, Melissa, MBA
Magellan Health Services Inc — Page 91
Rose, Trevor, MD, MS, MMM
Quality Health Plan Inc — Page 119
Rosebrock, Carol
Blue Cross of Idaho — Page 141
Rosebrook, Steve
Kansas Foundation Mdcl Care — Page 179
Rosell, Jan
ProviDRs Care Network — Page 181
Rosen, Richard, MD
Aetna Inc - Pennsylvania — Page 355
Rosenbaum, Martin
Great-West Healthcare - Corp — Page 81
Rosenbaum, Stanley
BioScrip Inc — Page 481
Rosenberg, Alan
Unicare Health Plans of the
Midwest Inc — Page 153
Rosenblatt, Elaine
Unity Health Insurance — Page 470
Rosenbloom, Robert, Esq
Nychsro/MedReview Inc — Page 303
Rosenfeld, David
Aetna Inc - Arkansas — Page 25
Rosenhan, Debbie
Altius Health Plans — Page 433

Rosenhoch, Valerie J
Univera Healthcare of
Western New York — Page 307
Rosenthal, Daniel
UnitedHealthcare of South FL — Page 122
Rosenthal, Robert, DDS
Delta Dental Plan of NC — Page 312
Roset, Bob
Health Plan,
The Hometown Region — Page 327
Health Plan of the
Upper Ohio Valley — Page 327
Rosetti, Denise
Preferred Care Incorporated — Page 370
Rosnick, Michael, MD
MD-Individual Practice Association Inc
(MD IPA) — Page 204
Mid Atlantic Medical Services Inc
(MAMSI)- Corp Headquarters — Page 204
OneNet PPO — Page 205
Ross, Bonnie
Finger Lakes Community
Care Network — Page 293
Ross, Gail
Blue Care Network of Michigan — Page 217
Ross, Jan
Delta Dental Plan of Illinois — Page 145
Ross, Kelly
CommunityCare Managed Healthcare
Plans of Oklahoma Inc — Page 340
Ross, Michael, RN
Total Health Choice Inc — Page 120
Ross, Susan
Health Net Inc - Northeast
Corporate Headquarters — Page 91
Ross, Wendy
Group Health Cooperative
of Eau Claire — Page 465
Ross, William T
South Bay Independent
Physicians Medical Group Inc — Page 69
Rosse, Claire B
Nationwide Better Health — Page 204
Rossi, Sheila
Finger Lakes Community
Care Network — Page 293
Rossy, Miguel
Texas Community Care — Page 427
Rothbart, Marc E
Southeastern Indiana
Health Organization — Page 166
Rothenberg, Nancy
PTPN - Corporate Headquarters — Page 65
Rothman, Janet
Elderplan Inc — Page 289
Rothrock, Kirk
Texas Dental Plan — Page 427
Rothrock, Kirk E
HealthAmerica PA Inc -
Central Region — Page 364
HealthAmerica PA Inc -
Eastern Region — Page 365
HealthAmerica PA Inc -
NorthWest — Page 365
HealthAmerica PA Inc -
Western Region — Page 365
Rothstein, Randy
Capital District Physicians
Health Plan — Page 286
Roughen, Dave
Unity Health Insurance — Page 470
Routh, Charles, MD
Select Circle Health Plan — Page 165
Rovira, Awilda
Medical Card System — Page 377
Rowan, Michael
UHP Healthcare — Page 71
Rowland, Lisa
Aetna Inc - Houston — Page 403

Index VIII: Personnel

Rice, Jean
Action Health Care
Management Services — Page 11
Rice, Jon, MD
Blue Cross Blue Shield of ND — Page 317
Rice, Lonell D
Delta Dental Plan of IN Inc — Page 159
Delta Dental Plan of MI Inc — Page 220
Delta Dental Plan of OH Inc — Page 324
Rice, Michael
Atlantic Integrated Health Inc — Page 309
Rice, Tom
United Concordia Co Inc - MI — Page 231
Rice, Vivian, RN
Indiana Pro Health Network — Page 162
Rice, William
Community Health Group — Page 41
Ricevuto, Charles
Neighborhood Hlth Partnership — Page 116
Richard, David M
Fara Healthcare Management — Page 190
Richard, Martha
M-Care Inc — Page 225
Richards, Beth
Doral Dental USA — Page 464
Richards, Judy
PacifiCare Health Systems-
Corporate Headquarters — Page 62
Richards, Karl
Dean Health Plan — Page 463
Richards, Patricia Roe
Paramount Care of Michigan — Page 228
Richardson, Bob
Healthplex Inc — Page 296
Richardson, Jan
Preferred Care — Page 304
Richardson, Jodie
Humana Health Plan of Austin — Page 419
Richardson, Mark
Mount Carmel Health Plan — Page 331
Richardson, Scott
Humana Medical Plan Inc — Page 114
Richey, Becky
Sagamore Health Network Inc — Page 164
Richey, Carol
Health Net - Connecticut — Page 90
Health Net - New Jersey — Page 272
Richie, Carl, MD
Community Choice Health Plan of
Westchester Inc — Page 287
Richter, Shelley
Humana Health Plan - KY — Page 185
Rickenbach, Nancy
Puget Sound Health Partners — Page 455
Ricks, Luanne
Employee Benefit
Management Services Inc — Page 253
Ricks-Hawkins, Pam
Community Health Plan — Page 42
Ridao, Richard, MD
University Health Alliance — Page 138
Riddick, Charles
Carolinas Center for
Medical Excellence, The — Page 310
Ridge, Tiffany
Select Circle Health Plan — Page 165
Ried, R Scott
HCH Administration — Page 148
Riegner, Robin J RN
Berkshire Health Partners/Medicus
Resource Management — Page 357
Riemann, Gunner, MD
Bayer Corporation
Pharmaceutical Division — Page 481
Ries, Andrea, MD
Medical Associates Hlth Plans — Page 172
Rifaat, Hassan, MD
Humana Hlth Care Plans of IL — Page 151

Riggan, Yvonne
Hometown Health Plan — Page 260
Riggs, Elaine
American Dental Examiners — Page 284
Rigoletto, Diane
Alameda Alliance for Health — Page 33
Rigsby, Michael, MD
Yale University Health Plan — Page 93
Rim, Tom
Bravo Health Inc — Page 200
Riordan, James R
Wisconsin Physician
Services Insurance Company — Page 471
Rios, Ramon
Citrus Health Care Inc — Page 108
Ripepi, Frank
Kern Family Health Care — Page 55
Ripley, Robert C
Initial Group Inc, The — Page 396
Rish, Dale
Blue Cross Blue Shield of SC -
Corporate Hqtrs — Page 383
Rishell, Mark A
HmoLouisiana Inc — Page 191
Ritchie, Rayman
Community Choice Health Plan of
Westchester Inc — Page 287
Ritter, Kel
Affinity Health Plan Inc — Page 283
Ritz, Charles
Humana Hlth Care Plans of AZ — Page 17
Humana Health Care Plans
of Lexington — Page 185
Rivas, Lordes
Atlantic Dental Inc — Page 102
Rivas, Socotto
Triple-S Inc — Page 378
Rivera, Angel
Medical Card System — Page 377
Rivero, Lupe
Horizon Behavioral Services — Page 112
Rivers, Richard F
Great-West Hlthcre of VA Inc — Page 444
Great-West Healthcare - Corp — Page 81
Rizzuto, Phillip
DentCare Delivery Systems Inc — Page 289
Rizzuto, Phillip
Healthplex Inc — Page 296
Robak, Kim M
Fiserv Inc — Page 464
Robbins, Barry
Cariten Healthcare — Page 393
PHP Companies Inc — Page 397
Robbins, Chris
Arxcel Inc — Page 480
Robbins, Marv MD
Behavioral Healthcare Inc — Page 78
Roberts Simmons, Jacqueline, MD
University Health Care Inc -
Passport Health Plan — Page 187
Roberts, Ann H BSN
Individualized Care Mngmnt Inc — Page 162
Roberts, John S
Assurant Employee Benefits-AL — Page 3
Assurant Employee Benefits-AZ — Page 12
Assurant Employee Benefits-CA — Page 35
Assurant Employee Benefits-CO — Page 78
Assurant Employee Benefits-FL — Page 102
Assurant Employee Benefits-GA — Page 127
Assurant Employee Benefits-IL — Page 143
Assurant Employee Benefits-IN — Page 158
Assurant Employee Benefits-MI — Page 217
Assurant Employee Benefits -
Corporate Office — Page 244
Assurant Employee Benefits-NM — Page 279
Assurant Employee Benefits-NY — Page 285
Assurant Employee Benefits-NC — Page 309
Assurant Employee Benefits-PA — Page 357
Assurant Employee Benefits-TN — Page 392
Assurant Employee Benefits-TX — Page 429
Assurant Employee Benefits-WA — Page 449

Roberts, Kim
Valley Health Plan
Santa Clara County — Page 72
Roberts, Lisa
Eyexam of California Inc — Page 46
Roberts, Peter W
Wellmark Inc — Corp Hdqrtrs — Page 175
Roberts, Roger
Dencap Dental Plans — Page 220
Roberts, Stephanie
Health Plus of Louisiana Inc — Page 191
Roberts, Todd
Jackson Memorial Health Plan — Page 115
Robertson, Dwight, MD
Coventry Healthcare — Page 394
Robertson, Jeffrey A, MD
Regence Group, The —
Corporate Headquarters — Page 351
Regence Blue Shield — Page 456
Regencecare — Page 456
Robidon, Rob
Cooks Childrens Health Plan — Page 411
Robins, Jim
United Concordia Co Inc - AL — Page 6
United Concordia Co Inc - AZ — Page 21
United Concordia Co Inc - FL — Page 121
United Concordia Co Inc - MO — Page 251
United Concordia Co Inc - NM — Page 282
United Concordia Co Inc - TX — Page 429
United Concordia Co Inc - VA — Page 446
Robinson, Betsy
Intracorp — Page 367
Robinson, Harlon
United Concordia Co Inc - AZ — Page 21
United Concordia Co Inc - CA — Page 72
United Concordia Co Inc -
Corporate Headquarters — Page 373
Robinson, Jennifer
Arizona Foundation for
Medical Care — Page 11
Robinson, Katisha
Molina Healthcare of MI Inc — Page 227
Robinson, Kenneth L, Jr, Esq
Delta Dental Plan of NH — Page 265
Robinson, Marilyn
Healthnow — Page 395
Robinson, Mark
SummaCare Inc — Page 334
Robinson, Ron
Health Plan of San Mateo — Page 50
Robinson, Tamera K, CPA
Delta Dental Plan of Illinois — Page 145
Delta Dental of Iowa — Page 169
Robinson, Virgil
HMO Louisiana Inc — Page 191
Robinson-Beale, Rhonda, MD
CIGNA Behavioral Health Inc — Page 408
Robles, Milagros
National Dntl Consultants Inc — Page 301
Roche, Mark
Alameda Alliance for Health — Page 33
Rock, Rick
Sun Health Medisun — Page 20
Rockowitz, Steven, PsyD
ValueOptions of California Inc — Page 72
Rodgers, Brian
ConnectCare — Page 219
ConnectCare — Page 219
Rodgers, John
Independent Health Assoc Inc — Page 297
Rodriguez, Ada
HealthPlus Inc — Page 296
Rodriguez, Alex R, MD
Magellan Health Services Inc — Page 91
Rodriguez, Diane
Lakewood Health Plan Inc — Page 56
Rodriguez, Jimmy
Legacy Health Solutions Inc — Page 420

Index VIII: Personnel

Rai, Ashok, MD
Prevea Health Network — Page 469
Rainer, Sam
Vantage Health Plan Inc — Page 193
Rainey, Richard, MD
Regence Blue Shield of Idaho — Page 142
Rajan, Samuel, RPh
MemberHealth Inc — Page 489
Ralston, LeNore
Colorado Access — Page 79
Ram, Rakesh
Access Dental Services — Page 31
Ramakrishnan, Suresh
XL Health — Page 207
Rambo, Larry
Humana Wisconsin Health Organization Inc — Page 466
Ramer, Henry
Delta Dental Plan of TN — Page 394
Ramey, Catherine
Md-Individual Practice Association Inc (MD IPA) — Page 204
Ramicez, Adrian
Partnercare Health Plan Inc — Page 117
Ramos, Julie
Vision Service Plan — Page 75
Ramseier, Mike
Anthem BCBS of Colorado — Page 77
Ramsey, Dan
Prevea Health Network — Page 469
Ramsey, Garry
Bluegrass Family Health Inc — Page 183
Ramsey, Stephanie
Health Net of Arizona — Page 17
Randol, Tim
Preferred Health Professionals — Page 180
Randolph, John C
Paramount Care of Michigan — Page 228
Paramount Health Care Plan — Page 333
Randolph, Kerry, MD
Cox Health Plans — Page 246
Rangala, Thankam
Community Medical Alliance — Page 210
Neighborhood Health Plan — Page 214
Rank, Brian, MD
HealthPartners Inc — Page 236
HealthPartners — Page 486
Rankin, Jim
Management Sciences for Hlth — Page 488
Ransdell, Sheila
Delta Dental Plan Inc - Utah — Page 434
Rao, Shankar
PacifiCare Dental & Vision — Page 61
Rashid, Michael A
Keystone Mercy Health Plan — Page 368
Rath, Lorie
Prairie States Enterprises Inc — Page 152
Rausch, Jay
Dominion Dental Services - Corporate Headquarters — Page 444
Ravin, Richard
Combined Insurance Company of America — Page 145
Rawlinson, Dorien
Rocky Mountain Health Plans — Page 84
Ray, Brenda
Healthnow — Page 395
Raymond, Jane
Humana Inc - Tennessee — Page 396
Raymond, Nancy
Health Plan of San Joaquin, The — Page 50
Razo, Susana
Santa Clara Family Health Plan — Page 67
Reamer, Michael
Avesis Inc — Page 12
Reavis, Jay
Delta Dental Plan of TN — Page 394

Reay, Bill
Physicians Plus Ins Corp — Page 469
Redd, Judith B, MS
JPS Benefits — Page 419
Redfield, Betsy
Santa Barbara Regional Health Authority — Page 67
Redfield, David L
CorpHealth Inc — Page 412
Redlin, Kenneth, MD
APS Healthcare Midwest Inc — Page 461
Redmond, James
Excellus BCBS, Rochester Area — Page 292
Redmond, Lynn
Denta Quest Mid-Atlantic Inc — Page 202
Reed, Gena H
Paragon Biomedical Inc — Page 491
Reed, James
Excellus BCBS, Central NY Southern Tier — Page 291
Reed, Jeff
Excellus BCBS, Central New York Region — Page 291
Reed, JoAnn
Medco Health Solutions Inc — Page 275
Reed, John, MD
American WholeHealth Networks Inc — Page 442
Reed, Judith
Preferred Dental Ntwrk (PDN) — Page 215
Reed, Ron
Deseret Healthcare — Page 434
Reedy, Dan
Co/OP Optical Services Inc — Page 219
Reef, Christopher
WelBorn Health Plans — Page 167
Reeme, Peter, PharmD
ChoiceCare/Humana — Page 322
Reeves, Debbie
Delta Dental Ins Co - AL — Page 4
Delta Dental Ins Co - GA — Page 131
Reeves, Jennifer
Great-West Healthcare of TX - Dallas — Page 415
Reeves, Stacie
Kern Family Health Care — Page 55
Reeves, Vanessa
Jackson Memorial Health Plan — Page 115
Regotti, Ginger
Capitol Administrators — Page 38
Reichardt, Mary
Great-West Healthcare of TX - Dallas — Page 415
Reid, Allan L, DMD
Health Resources Inc — Page 161
Reid, James
Aetna Inc - New York — Page 283
Reid, LaZandra
OmniCare, A Cvntry Hlth Plan — Page 228
Reid, Rohan
Delta Dental Plan of California — Page 44
Reidell, Kris
MDNY Healthcare Inc — Page 299
Reikes, Jim
Physicians Foundation for Medical Care — Page 64
Reilley, Lee
Coventry Health Care Inc — LA — Page 190
Reimer, Renee
Presbyterian Health Plan — Page 281
Reimer, Tom
Arise Health Plan — Page 461
Reimers, Todd
Ameritas Mngd Dental Plan Inc — Page 34
Reinert, Pam, RN
Blue Care Network of MI — Page 217

Reinhardt, Glenn
UnitedHealthcare of WI Inc — Page 470
Reinhart, Larry
Elderhaus Inc — Page 510
Reis, Peter
Aids Healthcare Foundation — Page 32
Reisman, Lonny, MD
Active Health Management — Page 441
Reiswig, Robert, RPh
South Dakota Pharmacist Association — Page 495
Reitan, Colleen
BCBS of Minnesota — Page 234
BCBS of Minnesota — Page 505
Reitz, Mike
BCBS of Louisiana Inc — Page 189
Rekart, Tom
Spectera Vision Inc - Indiana — Page 166
Remillard, Dave
North Dakota Hlth Care Review — Page 318
Renaudin, George, II
Humana Health Benefit Plan of Louisiana — Page 191
Renfro, Charley
Dental Network of America — Page 146
Renollet, Charlene
QualCare Inc — Page 276
Renson, Maureen
Preferred Care Incorporated — Page 370
Renwick-Espinosa, Kate
Vision Service Plan — Page 75e
Vision Service Plan — Page 86
Replogle, Dennis
Broadspire Inc — Page 105
Ressel, Randy
HealthLink Inc - Corp Hdqrtrs — Page 249
Revels, David
Great-West Healthcare of TX - Dallas — Page 415
Revill, Lawrence
UTMB Health Plans Inc — Page 431
Reyes, David
Total Long Term Care — Page 515
Reyes, Mario
Community Health Plan — Page 42
Reynolds, Aaron
Medica Health Plans — Page 236
Medica Health Plans — Page 518
Reynolds, Dave
Humana Hlth Care Plans of IL — Page 151
Reynolds, David
Capitol Administrators — Page 38
Reynolds, David
Coventry Hlth Care of KS Inc — Page 245
Reynolds, Dorothy
ECCA - Managed Vision Care Inc - Corporate Headquarters — Page 413
Reynolds, Douglas
Allianz Life Insurance Company of North America — Page 233
Reynolds, Gloria
Virginia Premier Hlth Plans Inc — Page 447
Reynolds, Linda
Health Plan of San Joaquin, The — Page 50
Reynolds, Mark
Neighborhood Health Plan of Rhode Island — Page 380
Rheinberger, Paul
Horizon Health PPO — Page 261
Managed Care Consultants — Page 261
Rhoads, Mike
BCBS of Oklahoma — Page 339
Rhye, Sam
Anthem BCBS of Virginia Inc — Page 442
Riabov, Darelle
Blue Cross Blue Shield of DE — Page 95
Rice, Earle
CommunityCare Managed Healthcare Plans of Oklahoma Inc — Page 340
CommunityCare Managed Healthcare Plans of Oklahoma Inc — Page 483

Index VIII: Personnel

Poole, Anita L
CorpHealth Inc — Page 412
Poole, Steve
St Francis Optimum
Health Network — Page 385
Pope, G Phillip
Blue Cross Blue Shield of AL — Page 3
Popejoy, David L
Chiropractic Arizona Network Inc — Page 13
SW Preferred Dental Organization — Page 20
Popiel, Richard G, MD
Horizon BCBS of NJ — Page 273
Horizon Hlthcare Services Inc — Page 274
Popovich, Karen
Select Circle Health Plan — Page 165
Popp, Kurt
Unity Health Insurance — Page 470
Port, Ron
Community Care Plus — Page 249
Porter, Monica
Gateway Health Plan Inc — Page 362
Portocarrero, Rolondo
HealthPlus Inc — Page 296
Portune, Richard W, DDS
Superior Dental Care Alliance — Page 335
Posey, Pat
Santa Clara Family Health Plan — Page 67
Posner, Barry A
BioScrip Inc — Page 481
Posner, Robert, MD
Catalina Behavioral
Health Services Inc — Page 13
Post, J'Anna
Northwest Rehab Alliance — Page 349
Post, Linda L, MD
Unison Health Plan of Ohio Inc — Page 336
Potere, Marcia M
Renaissance Health Sys Inc — Page 119
Potisuk, Cathy
CareSource — Page 321
Potochnik, Wendy
UnitedHealthcare of WI Inc — Page 470
Potts, Sylvia
Hines & Associates Inc — Page 150
Poulos, Sharon
Optima Health Plan Inc — Page 445
Powell, Greg
Humana Health Plans of GA — Page 132
Powell, Marshall
Arnett Health Plans — Page 157
Powell, Michelle
Select Health of SC — Page 385
Powell, Tim
Texas True Choice — Page 428
Powell-Wick, Lynette
Community Choice Health Plan of
Westchester Inc — Page 287
Powers, Donald A
PacifiCare of Colorado — Page 84
UnitedHealthcare of Colorado — Page 85
Powers, Faith
Bluegrass Family Health Inc — Page 183
Powers, Rich
Humana Inc - Colorado — Page 82
Pozo, Justo L
Preferred Care Partners Inc — Page 118
Prack, Lyda E
XL Health — Page 207
Preisig, Christina
Zurich Services Corporation — Page 155
Preizler, Marty
Physicians Plus Ins Corp — Page 469
Prenderast, Victoria
Signature Health Alliance — Page 398
Press, Thomas E
Midlands Choice Inc — Page 256
Preston, Gregory, MD
Cooks Childrens Health Plan — Page 411

Preston, Harold E, Jr
Carelink Health Plans — Page 459
Preston, Randall
Delphi Card R — Page 145
Prevallet, Bart
Alabama Quality
Assurance Foundation — Page 3
Price, Betsy MD
San Francisco Health Plan — Page 66
Price, Don
Vision Service Plan of Arizona — Page 22
Vision Service Plan — Page 75
Vision Service Plan — Page 86
Price, Greg
Valley Health Plan
Santa Clara County — Page 72
Price, Joseph V
Advantica Eyecare Inc — Page 99
Price, Stew
Unity Health Insurance — Page 470
Prickman, Linda
Vista Hlthplan of South FL Inc — Page 123
Pricknell, Charles
Regence Blue Shield — Page 456
Princivalle, Karin
Medco Health Solutions Inc — Page 488
Printy, Edward T, CPA
Partners Rx Management LLC — Page 491
Pritz, Ernie
Preferred Medical Plan Inc — Page 118
Proctor, Jim
Memphis Managed Care Corp — Page 397
Pronk, Nico, PhD
HealthPartners Inc — Page 236
Provencher, Kenneth
PacificSource Health Plans — Page 350
Provenzano, Nancy
CHN Solutions — Page 270
Provjansky, Jed
Pioneer Management Systems — Page 215
Prows, Ralph, MD
Regence BCBS of Oregon — Page 351
Prue, John
Humana Health Care Plans of
Kansas & Missouri — Page 179
Prunty, Brenda
American Dental Examiners — Page 284
Pryor, Concetta A
MDNY Healthcare Inc — Page 299
Pryor, Ray
Humana Military Service Inc — Page 186
Przybilla, Jim
Primewest Health System — Page 506
Ptacek, Scott
Bravo Health Mid-Atlantic Inc — Page 200
Bravo Health Pennsylvania Inc — Page 358
Bravo Health Texas Inc — Page 407
Pudeman, Missy
Northeast Health Direct LLC — Page 92
Pudimott, Missy
CHN Solutions — Page 270
Puente, Kenneth M
AmeriGroup Maryland Inc — Page 199
Pugh, Dick
Community Health Plan — Page 245
Pujals, Manuela
Global Medical Management — Page 110
Pullom, Joyce
Behavioral Health Systems Inc — Page 3
Purcell, James E, Esq
Coordinated Health Plan — Page 379
BCBS of Rhode Island — Page 379
Pures, Robert J
Horizon BCBS of NJ — Page 273
Purk, Gary
RxAmerica LLC — Page 494
Pusateri, Jim
BCBS of Nebraska — Page 255

Pushin, Maya
Vision Plan of America — Page 75
Putiak, Mike
Tenet Choices Inc — Page 192
Putman, Shawn, MD
Opticare Managed Vision — Page 314
Putnam, Harold
Community Medical Alliance — Page 210
Neighborhood Health Plan — Page 214
Putnam, Sheri M
Bucks County Physician
Hospital Alliance — Page 358
Putt, Lisa
BCBS of Oklahoma — Page 339
Bluelincs HMO — Page 340
Pyle, David
Managed HealthCare
Northwest Inc — Page 348
Pyle, Kristina
First Choice of the Midwest Inc — Page 388

Q

Qualley, Thomas
Geisinger Health Plan — Page 363
Quan, Kelvin
San Francisco Health Plan — Page 66
Quarles, Travonya
Berkshire Health Partners/Medicus
Resource Management — Page 357
Queen, Pam
JP Farley Corp — Page 329
Quinlivan, Keith
Orange Prevention &
Treatment Integrated — Page 60
Quinn, Jennifer
Capital District
Physicians Health Plan — Page 286
Quinn, Peter
First Health Services Corp — Page 485
Quinones, Lourdes
Kaiser Foundation Health
Plan of Georgia — Page 132
Quiriconi, Frank
PhysiciansPlus & St Dominic Health
Maintenance Organization — Page 242
Quirk, Jack
Anthem BCBS of Maine — Page 195
Quirk, Thomas
UnitedHealthcare of Texas Inc —
Dallas — Page 430

R

Rabinowitz, Barbra
CBCA Care Management Inc — Page 408
Radigan, Joseph P
Hygeia Corporation — Page 114
Radine, Gary D
Delta Dental Plan of California — Page 44
Delta Dental of Pennsylvania — Page 361
Delta Dental Plan Inc - Utah — Page 434
Radner, Marc
Scan Health Plan — Page 68
Raffio, Thomas, FLMI
Delta Dental Plan of NH — Page 265
Raghavan, Anand
Great-West Healthcare of CA -
Southern — Page 48
Rahm, Janice
Meritain Health Inc — Page 299

Index VIII: Personnel

Petersen, Andee
Kaiser Foundation Health Plan -
Mid Atlantic States — Page 203
Petersen, Christine A, MD
Health Plan of Nevada Inc — Page 260
Petersen, Todd
PersonalCare Ins of IL Inc — Page 151
Peterson, Amanda, RPh
Envision Pharmaceutical
Services Inc — Page 484
Peterson, Bruce
Em Risk Management,
A POMCO Company — Page 290
Peterson, David, BS
CIGNA Behavioral Health Inc — Page 88
CIGNA Behavioral Health Inc -
Corporate Headquarters — Page 234
Peterson, Donald J, DDS
Total Dental Administrators
Health Plan — Page 21
Peterson, Leland
Sun Health Medisun — Page 20
Peterson, Lyndon T
Wellmark BCBS of SD — Page 389
Peterson, Mary Dale
Driscoll Children's Health Plan — Page 412
Peterson, Sandra
Network Health Plan WI — Page 468
Peterson, Timothy
Blue Cross Blue Shield of MN — Page 505
Peterson, Timothy J
Pima Health Plan — Page 19
Peterson, Tom
American Republic Ins Co — Page 169
Peterson-Smith, Debra
1st Medical Network — Page 127
Peach State Health Plan — Page 133
Petit, Lynn
Health Net Hlth Plan of OR Inc — Page 346
Petrella, Russell
Magellan Behavioral
Care of IA Inc — Page 171
Petrella, Russell C, PhD
Magellan Health Services Inc — Page 91
Magellan Health Services — Page 132
Premier Behavioral
Systems of TN LLC — Page 398
Tennessee Behavioral Hlth Inc — Page 399
Petrin, Thomas, MD
Indiana Pro Health Network — Page 162
Petroff, Thomas, DO
McLaren Health Plan — Page 226
Petroski, Alan, PhD
Community Behavioral Healthcare
Cooperative of Pennsylvania — Page 361
Petrovic, Jelka
Care Choices HMO — Page 218
Petrulis, Alice Stollenwerk, MD
KEPRO — Page 367
Petruzelli, Steve
Williamette Dental Group PC — Page 352
Williamette Dental of WA Inc — Page 457
Pettis, Sean
Lovelace Health Plan — Page 280
Pezzullo, Angelo
Delta Dental of Rhode Island — Page 380
Pflughoeft, Michael
Doral Dental USA — Page 464
Pham, Michael
Spectera Vision Inc - Indiana — Page 166
Spectera Vision Inc -
Corporate Headquarters — Page 206
Phanstiel, Howard G
PacifiCare Health Systems-
Corporate Headquarters — Page 62
PacifiCare of California — Page 62
Pacificare Life & Hlth Ins Co — Page 63
Pacificare Life & Hlth Ins Co — Page 519
Phelps, Charis, CPCS
Phoebe Health Partners — Page 133

Phelps, Chet
Colorado Health Networks LLC -
ValueOptions — Page 80
Phenow, Kenneth J, MD, MPH
CIGNA Healthcare of North TX — Page 409
Pheqley, Julie
Indiana Pro Health Network — Page 162
Phillip, Clark
Select Health of SC — Page 385
Phillips, Deborah
Priority Health — Page 230
Phillips, Patricia
HealthEOS by MultiPlan — Page 466
Philpott, Paul M
Connecticare Inc — Page 89
Connecticare of NY — Page 288
Piacentini, Karen
Aetna Inc - Pennsylvania — Page 355
Pica, Michael
University Health Plans Inc — Page 277
Piccioni, Lori
Alignis Inc — Page 268
Pickerman, Linda
Lutheran Preferred/
Three Rivers Preferred — Page 162
Piefer, Gary, MD
Seton Health Plan — Page 425
Pierre, John
Regence Blue Shield — Page 456
Pifalo, W Bradley, MD
Highmark Inc — Page 366
Pifer, Donald
Carolina Care Plan Inc — Page 383
Piggee, Charlotte
Community Health Plan — Page 42
Pighin, Shelly
Contra Costa Health Plan — Page 43
Pijor, Dennis
CHN MCO — Page 322
Pike, Edward
GenWorth Life & Hlth Ins Co — Page 90
Pileggi, Gale S, MBA
JPS Benefits — Page 419
Pilgrim, Gloria
OneNet PPO — Page 205
Pillari, George D
CBCA Care Management Inc — Page 408
Pilous, Betty, RN, MHSA, CPHQ
Ohio KEPRO Inc — Page 332
Pinkney, Mary
Denver Health Medical Plan Inc — Page 80
Pinn, Melvin T Jr, MD
Virginia Premier Hlth Plans Inc — Page 447
Pinnas, Susan Knapp
CIGNA Healthcare of Florida — Page 107
Pinzotto, Vince
United Concordia Co Inc - PA — Page 374
United Concordia Co Inc - PA -
Central — Page 374
Piotti, Karen
Family Choice Health Alliance — Page 272
Piper, Brian
Global Medical Management — Page 110
Pippin, Angela
Physicians Health Plan
of Northern Indiana — Page 164
Pirozzi, Cindy
Raytel Imaging Network — Page 371
Pitera, Raymond D
Health Plan of Michigan — Page 224
Pitman, Larry W
Kansas Fndtn Medical Care — Page 179
Pitoscia, Jennifer
Prime Health Services Inc — Page 398
Pitsenberger, William
Blue Cross Blue Shield of KS — Page 177
Pittman, Austin
PacifiCare of Oklahoma Inc/
Secure Horizons — Page 342
PacifiCare of Texas Inc — Page 422

Pittman, Denice
Humana Health Care
Plans of Houston — Page 418
Pittman, Lane
CIGNA Healthcare of Arizona — Page 14
Pittman, Shelley
Blue Cross Blue Shield of KS — Page 177
Pitts, Charles C
CIGNA Healthcare of NC — Page 311
CIGNA Healthcare of SC — Page 384
Pizzelanti, Janet
AmeriGroup New Jersey Inc — Page 268
Pizzini, Denise
New West Health Plan — Page 254
Plagge, Jeff
Delta Dental of Iowa — Page 169
Planchunas, Sharon
ScripNet — Page 494
Plaster, Linda J
Integrated Health Plan Inc — Page 115
Platt, Marcy
Managed Care Consultants — Page 261
Platt, Ronald, MD
Vista Health Plan Inc — Page 123
Plocher, David, MD
Blue Cross Blue Shield of MN — Page 234
Ploskonka, Len
MemberHealth Inc — Page 489
Plowman, Rebekah N
Individualized Care Mngmnt Inc — Page 162
Pluto, Victor J
PacifiCare of Oklahoma Inc/
Secure Horizons — Page 342
PacifiCare of Texas - Houston — Page 422
PacifiCare of Texas Inc — Page 422
Pocock, Rob
Priority Health — Page 230
Pointon, Karen
CareFirst BCNS — Page 200
Pointon, Meg
HealthPlus of Michigan — Page 224
Polan, Linda
Maricopa Health Plan — Page 18
Polasik, Connie
Arise Health Plan — Page 461
Polenske, Kathy
Interplan Health Group — Page 53
Superien Health Network Inc — Page 335
Polese, Anne
Active Health Management — Page 441
Politakis, Jean
Fallon Community Hlth Plan Inc — Page 211
Pollack, David
Neighborhood Hlth Partnership — Page 116
Pollock, Steven
Doral Dental USA — Page 464
Polter, Jeff
4D Pharmacy Management
Systems Inc — Page 479
Pomerantz, Jay I, MD, MMM, FACP
BCBS of Western New York — Page 285
Central New York East
HealthNow New York Inc — Page 287
Central New York West
HealthNow New York Inc — Page 287
HealthNow New York Inc — Page 295
BlueShield of Northeastern NY — Page 286
Pomfry, Robert W
Em Risk Management,
A POMCO Company — Page 290
Poniatowski, John
CIGNA Healthcare of CT — Page 89
Ponski, Jennifer
Advantage Health Solutions Inc — Page 157
Pontius, Greg
Bravo Health Inc — Page 200
Bravo Health PA Inc — Page 358

Index VIII: Personnel

Parks, Jess
DaVita VillageHealth of MI Inc   Page 220
Parks, Jess
Aveta Inc   Page 270
Parlette, Allita
Mountain Medical Affiliates   Page 83
Parra, Gabriel
Presbyterian Health Plan   Page 281
Parrish, B J
Med-Comp USA   Page 192
Parrish, Linda
Utah Public Employees
Health Program   Page 438
Parrott, James S
Virginia Premier Hlth Plans Inc   Page 447
Parton, Gerald
Tenet Choices Inc   Page 192
Parton, Ron, MD
Physicians Plus Ins Corp   Page 469
Parysek, Ginger E
Lifetime Healthcare Companies, The -
Corporate Headquarters   Page 298
Pascoe, Joy
UnitedHealthcare of Ohio Inc-
Cleveland   Page 336
Paskell, Mary
Compsych Behavioral Health   Page 145
Paskowski, Robert
Arnett Health Plans   Page 157
Paslidis, Nick J MD, PhD, MHCM
Arkansas Foundation
for Medical Care   Page 26
Passantino, Philip
MetroPlus Health Plan   Page 300
Patalano, Frank
Zurich Services Corporation   Page 155
Patalano, Kirsten L
Scripps Clinic Health
Plan Services Inc   Page 68
Patel, Deepak, MD
WellCare of New York   Page 307
Patel, Jayant, MD
Citrus Health Care Inc   Page 108
Patel, Kirit, MD
Medcore Health Plan   Page 58
Patel, Minal
Rayant Insurance Co of NY   Page 304
Patel, Nilesh
Pacific Union Dental Inc   Page 63
Patel, Rash
Americhoice of New Jersey   Page 268
Patric, John, MD
Blue Cross Blue Shield of TN   Page 392
Patrnchak, Joseph
Blue Cross Blue Shield of MA   Page 209
Pattarozzi, Edward
Dean Health Plan   Page 463
Patten, Doug, MD
1st Medical Network   Page 127
Patterson, Chris
CareGuide   Page 105
Patterson, Jamie
Memphis Managed Care Corp   Page 397
Patterson, Jill
Allianz Life Insurance Company
of North America   Page 233
Patterson, Laura
Medcost LLC   Page 313
Patterson, Terry
Nychsro/MedReview Inc   Page 303
Patterson, William M, MD
Behavioral Health Systems Inc   Page 3
Patti, Paul
Comprehensive Behavioral
Care Inc   Page 108
Patton, Mark
ParadigmHealth   Page 276

Patton, Robert K
FirstSight Vision Services Inc   Page 47
Patton, Sherry
Preferred Health Professionals   Page 180
Paul, James M
UlliCare   Page 98
Union Labor Life Insurance Co   Page 276
Paul, Kate
Colorado Dental Service Inc,
dba: Delta Dental Plan of CO   Page 80
Paul, Wayne
United Concordia Co Inc - MD   Page 206
Paulakuhn, Judy
Interactive Medical Systems   Page 313
Paules, Chris
United Behavioral Health   Page 373
Paulson, Sidney C
SelectHealth   Page 437
Paulus, Sharon
Sagamore Health Network Inc   Page 164
Paustian, Dale
Davis Vision   Page 288
Pautz, Edward
Group Health Cooperative
South Central Wisconsin   Page 464
Pavlek, Janie
Health Plan,
The Hometown Region   Page 327
Pavlicek, Stephen E
American National Ins Co   Page 405
Pawlyshyn, John
Santa Clara Family Health Plan   Page 67
Paynter, Lois
Saint Mary's HealthFirst   Page 263
Paz, George
Express Scripts Inc -
Corporate Headquarters   Page 484
Express Scripts Inc - MN   Page 484
Express Scripts Inc - NJ   Page 484
Express Scripts Inc - PA   Page 484
Pe Quilino, Nancy
CIGNA Dental Health of CA Inc   Page 40
Pearl, Lisa
Great-West Healthcare of CA -
Southern   Page 48
Pearl, Robert M, MD
Kaiser Foundation Health
Plan of Northern California   Page 54
Pearlman, Stacey
American Healthguard Corp   Page 33
Pearson, Doug
Sagamore Health Network Inc   Page 164
Peatross, Paul
Best Health Plans   Page 36
Peck, Charles A, MD
Aetna Inc Life Insurance Co   Page 87
Aetna Inc - Massachusetts   Page 209
Aetna Inc - Tennessee   Page 391
Peck, Laurie
Med-Valu Inc   Page 329
Pecoraro, David
Exempla Healthcare LLC   Page 81
Pederson, Karen
Valley Baptist Insurance Co   Page 431
Pegler, Lori
Signature Health Alliance   Page 398
Pelezo, Tony, MD
Mdwise   Page 163
Pels-Beck, Leslie
Sharp Health Plan   Page 68
Peltz, Leslie
Acumentra Health   Page 345
Pelyso, Lisa
Value Health Care   Page 277
Pena, Bobby
Aetna Inc - Arizona   Page 11
Pence, Gregory S
Managed Health Network   Page 57

Pence, Terry, RPh
Select Circle Health Plan   Page 165
Pendergast, Kevin
American Republic Ins Co   Page 169
Pendrak, Robert F, MD
American College of
Medical Quality   Page 199
Penney, Steven
Trustmark Insurance Co   Page 153
Pennington, James M
ppoNEXT   Page 423
Pennington, Jim
Health Care Evaluation   Page 48
Penrose, John
ParadigmHealth   Page 276
Perdomo, Marianella
Partners National Health
Plans of North Carolina Inc   Page 314
Perez, Martin
Medica Healthcare Plans Inc   Page 116
Pericone, Nancy L
Bucks County Physician
Hospital Alliance   Page 358
Perkins, Denise
Qualis Health   Page 455
Perkins, Duane
Zurich Services Corporation   Page 155
Perkins, Greg
Aids Healthcare Foundation   Page 32
Perkins, Sharon
El Paso First Health Plans Inc   Page 413
Perkins, Stephen, MD
Vermont Hlth Plans (Blue Care)   Page 439
Perlstein, John
CIGNA HealthCare —
Corporate Headquarters   Page 360
Pernell, Gary, DDS
Dental Health Services Inc   Page 45
Dental Health Services   Page 450
Pernell, Godfrey, DDS
Dental Health Services Inc   Page 450
Perrine, Anita, RN
Kern Family Health Care   Page 55
Perrone, Ronald, MD, MBA
MDNY Healthcare Inc   Page 299
Perroni, Jospeh
Altus Dental Ins Co Inc   Page 379
Perry, Adele
CareSource   Page 321
Perry, Bruce, MD, MPH
Kaiser Foundation Health
Plan of Georgia   Page 132
Perry, J Thomas
Delta Dental Plan of TN   Page 394
Perry, Jeff
Antares Management Solutions   Page 319
Perry, Vicki
Advantage Health Solutions Inc   Page 157
Pesano, Ted
United Concordia Co Inc - AL   Page 6
United Concordia Co Inc - FL   Page 121
United Concordia Co Inc - MI   Page 231
United Concordia Co Inc - MO   Page 251
United Concordia Co Inc - NM   Page 282
United Concordia Co Inc - NY   Page 306
United Concordia Co Inc - VA   Page 446
Pesetski, Eric Joel, MD
Tenet Choices Inc   Page 192
Pesko, Larry
Lovelace Health Plan   Page 280
Pete, Kevin
Aultcare   Page 320
Peters, Evan
CIGNA Healthcare of
Kansas/Missouri   Page 177
Peters, Sue
Aetna Inc - Pennsylvania   Page 355

Index VIII: Personnel

Oram, Mary
Northeast Pharmacy Srvc Corp   Page 490
Orchard, Kim, RPh
Group Health Cooperative   Page 141
Group Health Cooperative   Page 451
Ord, Steven
PacificSource Health Plans   Page 350
Ordner, Justine
Health Mngmnt Network Inc   Page 16
Ordway, Jody
Managed HealthCare
Northwest Inc   Page 348
Origer, Deborah L
Great-West Healthcare of MA   Page 212
Orland, Burton
Aveta Inc   Page 270
Orman, Morton, MD
Keystone Health Plan Central   Page 367
Orr, Rita
UMPC Health Plan Univ of
Pittsburgh Medical Center   Page 374
Orsbon, Nance
Delta Dental Plan of SD   Page 387
Orta, Francine
Total Health Choice Inc   Page 120
Orth, Cindy
Columbia United Providers   Page 449
Ortiz, Glenda
Strategic Health
Development Corporation   Page 119
Orvosh, Dennis
Great-West Healthcare of
Washington Inc   Page 451
Osband, Gerald E, MD
SHPS Healthcare Services   Page 20
SHPS Inc   Page 186
Osborn, Carl
Health Care Excel Inc   Page 160
Osborne, Mary Lou
HealthAmerica Pennsylvania Inc -
NorthWest   Page 365
Osbrink, Raymond, MD
Safeguard Health Enterprises Inc   Page 66
Osenar, Peter R
Emerald Hlth Network Inc, The   Page 325
Interplan Health Group -
Corporate Headquarters   Page 91
Osgood, Kenneth, MD
NevadaCare Inc   Page 262
Osgood, Teena
Fallon Community Hlth Plan Inc   Page 211
Oshensky, Janis
Delta Dental Plans Association   Page 146
Osheroff, William J, MD
Hawaii Medical Services Association -
BC/BS of Hawaii   Page 137
Osika, Andy
EHP Inc   Page 362
Osmanski-Harmon, Julie
Horizon Behavioral Services   Page 112
Osowski, Hank
Scan Health Plan   Page 68
Oster, Claude, DO
National Foot Care Program Inc   Page 227
Osterman, Nicholas
CIGNA Behavioral Health Inc   Page 40
Ostrander, Robert, MD
Finger Lakes Community
Care Network   Page 293
Ostrov, Michael
Group Health Cooperative
South Central Wisconsin   Page 464
Ostrowski, Lynn
Health New England   Page 212
Oswald, D Duane
Avante Behavioral Health Plan   Page 35
Oswald, Ed
Community Care Plus   Page 249

Oswald, Jeremy
Avante Behavioral Health Plan   Page 35
Otis, Tiffany
Preferred Provider Organization of
Michigan (PPOM)   Page 229
Outsen, Jalyn
Utah Public Employees
Health Program   Page 438
Outten, Cornelia
Interplan Health Group   Page 53
Superien Health Network Inc   Page 335
Overgaard, Wade
Kaiser Foundation Health
Plan of Colorado   Page 83
Overstreet, Julia, CPA
CIMRO Quality
Healthcare Solutions   Page 144
Owen, Carole
Bluegrass Family Health Inc   Page 183
Owen, Wanda
Medcost LLC   Page 313
Owens, Amy
Community Health Plan   Page 245
Owens, Curtis
UHP Healthcare   Page 71
Owens, Odell, MD
UnitedHealthcare of Ohio Inc-
Cleveland   Page 336
Owerbach, Joel, PharmD
Excellus BlueCross BlueShield,
Rochester Area   Page 292
Lifetime Healthcare Companies, The -
Corporate Headquarters   Page 298
Owings, Lorena, RN
Ohio State University Managed
Health Care Systems Inc   Page 332

P

Pachnik, Randy, DPM
Preferred Podiatry Group   Page 152
Pack, Ronald E, CLU
Mid-Atlantic Managed Care Org
of Pennsylvania Inc   Page 369
Padgett, Claude, DDS
United Concordia Co Inc - AZ   Page 21
Pagan, Richard
Pacific IPA   Page 63
Page, Brenda
Evercare Select   Page 15
Page, Jim
KPS Health Plans   Page 452
Page, Nick, PharmD
PBM Plus Inc   Page 491
Pagidipati, Daviah
Freedom Health Inc   Page 110
Pagliaro, Brian P
Tufts Health Plan   Page 216
Paine, Charles
Security Health Plan of WI Inc   Page 469
Painter, Lisa A
4MOST Health Network   Page 459
Pajil Battle, Maria
Keystone Mercy Health Plan   Page 368
Pak, Mary
Unity Health Insurance   Page 470
Palacios, Connie
Mega Life & Health Ins Co   Page 420
Palardy, Robert B, CPA
Masspro Inc   Page 213
Palenske, Fredrick D
BCBS of Kansas   Page 177
Palish, Sherri
Crawford and Co-Corp Hdqrtrs   Page 130

Palla, Barbara, MD
Central Coast Alliance for Hlth   Page 39
Palmateer, Michael
GHI HMO Select Inc   Page 293
Palmer, Bruce
Physicians Health Plan
of Northern Indiana   Page 164
Palmer, Cynthia
Colorado Choice Health Plan/
San Luis Valley HMO Inc   Page 79
Palmer, Paul H
Health Plan of Nevada Inc   Page 260
Palmer, Robert
Dean Health Plan   Page 463
Palmer, Robert
Navitus Health Solutions   Page 490
Palmer, Roland
Grand Valley Health Plan   Page 221
Palmer, William
CIGNA Behavioral Health Inc   Page 40
Palmier, Catherine L, MD
UnitedHealthcare of Georgia   Page 134
Panatera, Larry
Kaiser Foundation Health Plan
of Georgia   Page 132
Panfil, Ray
Preferred Hlth Professionals   Page 180
Pankau, David S
Blue Cross Blue Shield of SC -
Corporate Hqtrs   Page 383
Papa, Joseph
Neighborhood Hlth Partnership   Page 116
Papa, Tony J
Health Plus of Louisiana Inc   Page 191
Paplham, Lawrence J
Community Care Hlth Plan Inc   Page 521
Paquin, Daniel
CareSource   Page 321
Parades, Eddie
Fidelis SecureCare of Texas   Page 413
Pardes, Marion
Americhoice of New Jersey   Page 268
AmeriChoice of New York   Page 284
Pardi, Cherie
HealthChoice of Alabama   Page 4
Parietti, Dan
WellCare of New York   Page 307
WellCare Health Plans Inc -
Corporate Headquarters   Page 124
Parikh, Rajendra, MD
Community Care Plus   Page 249
Parisi, Don
CareGuide   Page 105
Park, Jason
Liberty Dental Plan of CA   Page 56
Park, Jeffrey
SXC Health Solutions Inc   Page 495
Parker, Angela
Bluegrass Family Health Inc   Page 183
Parker, Charles
Masspro Inc   Page 213
Parker, Francine
Health Alliance Plan   Page 223
Parker, Jerry
MedImpact Healthcare Sys Inc   Page 488
Parker, Maureen
Citrus Health Care Inc   Page 108
Parker, R Lance, PhD
Preferred Mental Hlth Mngmnt   Page 180
Parker, Tricia
First Choice of the Midwest Inc   Page 388
Parker, Trisha
GroupLink Inc   Page 160
Parkes, Carla
HealthPlus of Michigan   Page 224
Parkington, Sandra
Sharp Health Plan   Page 68

Index VIII: Personnel

Noonan Harnsberger, Helen
Providence Health Plans — Page 351
Noonan, Helen
UnitedHealthcare of NY Inc — Page 306
Norman, Frank C, Jr
Active Health Management — Page 441
Norman, Karol H, PHR
Southern Health Services Inc — Page 445
Norris, Cyndi
Mutual Assurance Administrators Inc — Page 342
Norris, Latricia
CIGNA Healthcare of Virginia Inc - Richmond — Page 443
North, Mike
DakotaCare — Page 387
Norton, Deborah A
Harvard Pilgrim Health Care - Corporate Headquarters — Page 212
Norwood, Felicia
Aetna Inc - Pennsylvania — Page 355
Aetna Inc - Pennsylvania Region — Page 356
Norwood, Felicia F
Active Health Management — Page 441
Norwood, Verdis
Interplan Health Group — Page 53
Superien Health Network Inc — Page 335
Nostrand, Charles
Health Net Inc - Northeast Corporate Headquarters — Page 91
Novak, Johanna
Physicians Health Plan of Mid-Michigan — Page 228
Novak, Margaret
Health Net of Arizona — Page 17
Novelli, Bob
Blue Shield of California — Page 36
Novick, Nancy
Phoenix Health Plan - Community Connection — Page 19
Novoa, Gabriel, MD
Preferred Medical Plan Inc — Page 118
Nuckols, Steve
Atlantic Integrated Health Inc — Page 309
Nueheisel, Dana
ACN Group — Page 233
Nussbaum, Samuel R, MD
WellPoint Inc - Corp Hdqrtrs — Page 167
Anthem BCBS of Ohio — Page 320
Nutter, Hal
SmileCare/ Community Dental Services — Page 69

O

O'Brian, Dan
Americhoice of PA Inc — Page 356
O'Brien, Anne Marie
UnitedHealthcare of NY Inc — Page 306
O'Brien, Carol A
Paragon Biomedical Inc — Page 491
O'Brien, Cyndle
Inter Valley Health Plan Inc — Page 53
O'Brien, David
Med-Valu Inc — Page 329
O'Brien, David
Highmark Inc — Page 366
O'Brien, Karen
Superior Vision Services Inc — Page 70
O'Brien, Lawrence
Saint Mary's HealthFirst — Page 263
O'Connell, Peg
Carolinas Center for Medical Excellence, The — Page 310
O'Connor, Kim
Vista Health Plan Inc — Page 123
Vista Hlthplan of South FL Inc — Page 123

O'Connor, Michael
Davis Vision — Page 288
O'Connor, Patrick F
Health Care Service Corp - Corporate Headquarters — Page 149
O'Connor, Richard
Iowa Health Solutions — Page 171
O'Connor, Sharon
Corvel Corporation — Page 43
Corvel Corporation — Page 159
Corvel Corporation — Page 169
Corvel Corporation — Page 324
O'Dell, Stephen T
Molina Healthcare Inc - CA — Page 59
O'Donnell, Amy
Molina Healthcare of MI Inc — Page 227
O'Donnell, Anita, RN
Med-Valu Inc — Page 329
O'Donnell, William
Great-West Healthcare of PA — Page 363
Great-West Hlthcare of VA Inc — Page 444
O'Farrell, Kathy
Encore Health Network — Page 160
M Plan Inc — Page 163
O'Gorman, Scott
Denta Quest Mid-Atlantic Inc — Page 202
Denta Quest Ventures Inc — Page 211
Neighborhood Health Plan of Rhode Island — Page 380
O'Grady, Brian G
BlueShield of Northeastern NY — Page 286
O'Keefe, Eileen
Mit Health Plan — Page 214
O'Keefe, Kevin
Lifetime Healthcare Companies, The - Corporate Headquarters — Page 298
O'Keefe, Mary A
Principal Life Ins Co — Page 172
O'Keefe, Michael
Central Susquehanna Healthcare Providers — Page 359
O'Malley, Michael
AIDS Healthcare Foundation — Page 32
O'Mara, Ed
Innovative Care Management — Page 347
O'Neal, Sandra
Florida Health Care Plan Inc — Page 109
O'Neil, Laurence G
Kaiser Foundation Health Plan of Southern California — Page 54
O'Neil-White, Alphonso
BCBS of Western New York — Page 285
HealthNow New York Inc — Page 295
O'Neill, Mark
Mountain Medical Affiliates — Page 83
Preferred Provider Organization of Michigan (PPOM) — Page 229
O'Shea Auen, Eileen, MBA
APS Healthcare Northwest Inc — Page 253
O'Sullivan, Patrick
Arkansas BCBS a Mutual Insurance Company — Page 25
O'Sullivan, Terence M
UlliCare — Page 98
UlliCare — Page 98
Oaks, Joseph
HealthChoice of Alabama — Page 4
Oatko, Rita
Sharp Health Plan — Page 68
Obon, John A
Blue Cross Blue Shield of IL — Page 144
Health Care Service Corporation - Corporate Headquarters — Page 149
HMO Illinois — Page 150
Odabashian, Julie
Intergroup Services Corp — Page 367

Oddo, Angel
HealthAmerica PA Inc - Western Region — Page 365
Odzer, Randall, CPA, MBA
CIGNA Behavioral Health Inc — Page 408
Oestriech, Kathy
University Family Care Hlth Plan — Page 22
Oetgen, Suzanne
Hometown Health Plan — Page 260
Ogilvie, Steven
HealthEase of Florida Inc — Page 111
Ogle, Jan, RN
CIGNA Healthcare of California — Page 41
Oglei, April, RN, MS
CIMRO Quality Healthcare Solutions — Page 144
Oh, Julee
Health Net - Connecticut — Page 90
Health Net - New Jersey — Page 272
Health Net - New York — Page 295
Ohman, Dan L
UnitedHealthcare of Georgia — Page 134
Ohmann, Kathy
HealthPartners Inc — Page 236
Ohton, Elizabeth
Care 1st Health Plan AZ Inc — Page 13
Oishi, Ken, BA
MPRO — Page 227
Ojard, Nancy
First Plan of Minnesota — Page 235
Ojeda, Alonso R, MD
Inland Empire Foundation for Medical Care — Page 52
Olague, Dolores
Care 1st Health Plan — Page 38
Olaka, Dave
Carolina Care Plan Inc — Page 383
Olig, Cameron
Prime Therapeutics — Page 493
Oliker, David W
MVP Health Plan of NH — Page 266
MVP Health Plan Inc — Page 301
Preferred Care — Page 304
Oliva, Lucy
MDNY Healthcare Inc — Page 299
Oliverez, Edward J, MD
California Benefits Dental Plan — Page 37
Oliveri, Maria
HealthFirst Inc — Page 295
Olsen, G Kirk
Molina HealthCare of Utah Inc — Page 435
Olson, David W
Health Net Inc - Corp Hdqrtrs — Page 49
Olson, Fred, MD
Blue Cross Blue Shield of MT — Page 253
Olson, Jeff
UnitedHealthcare of Florida Inc — Page 121
Olson, LeAnn
Community Hlth Ntwrk of CT Inc — Page 89
Olson, Michael
Fortified Provider Network Inc — Page 15
Olson, Patricia
Avera Health Plans Inc — Page 387
Onda, Ron
United Concordia Co Inc - NM — Page 282
United Concordia Co Inc - VA — Page 446
Onks, Claire
Forte Managed Care — Page 414
Onorati, Annette C
Preferred Care Partners Inc — Page 118
Ontiveros, Cathy
NAMCI — Page 6
Premier Hlth Networks of AL LLC — Page 6
Oprzadek, Tim
Health Plan, The Hometown Region — Page 327
Opstad, Elodie
Iowa Foundation for Medical Care/ Encompass — Page 170

Index VIII: Personnel

Napier, Donald P
Em Risk Management,
A POMCO Company — Page 290

Napier, Mark
UnitedHealthcare of IL Inc — Page 154

Narowitz, Randy A
Total Health Care Inc — Page 231

Narula, Mohander, DDS
Jaimini Health Inc — Page 53

Nash, Bruce, MD, MBA
Capital District Physicians
Health Plan — Page 286

Nasi, Brian A.
South Country Health Alliance — Page 507

Nasir, Musa, MD
Pacific IPA — Page 63

Nauman, Laura
West Virginia Medical Institute — Page 460

Navarra, Linda
Capital District Physicians
Health Plan — Page 286

Navarro, D Scott, DDS
Delta Dental Plan of NJ — Page 271

Navarro, Rubin
Omnicare Of South Florida — Page 490

Neal, Steve
Health Plan of the
Upper Ohio Valley — Page 327
Health Plan,
The Hometown Region — Page 327

Nee, Chris
UHP Healthcare — Page 71

Needleman, Phillip
Vision Plan of America — Page 75

Needleman, Stuart, OD
Vision Plan of America — Page 75

Neely, Marc
Great-West Healthcare - Corp — Page 81

Neer, David, MD, JD
Lakewood Health Plan Inc — Page 56

Neese, Stan
UnitedHealthcare of MS Inc — Page 242

Neff, Paul E
Genex Services — Page 363

Negron, David
Davis Vision — Page 288

Neibert, Juanita
Complementary Hlthcre Plans — Page 345

Neidorff, Michael F
Centene Corporation — Page 244

Neilson, Barbara
Regence Valucare — Page 436

Nelsen, Nancy
Beech Street Corporation —
Corporate Headquarters — Page 36

Nelson, Andrea
Great-West Healthcare of TX -
Dallas — Page 415

Nelson, Andrew
National Foot Care Prgrm Inc — Page 227

Nelson, Casey
Community Health Plan — Page 245

Nelson, Jennifer
Maricopa Health Plan — Page 18

Nelson, Jim
Humana Wisconsin
Health Organization Inc — Page 466

Nelson, Kevin
Hudson Health Plan — Page 297

Nelson, Laura
Aids Healthcare Foundation — Page 32

Nelson, Michael, DO
Coventry Health Care of NE Inc — Page 255

Nelson, Russell
Altius Health Plans — Page 433

Nelson, Sandy J
Wellmark BCBS of Iowa — Page 174
Wellmark Inc — Corp Hdqrtrs — Page 175
Wellmark BCBS of SD — Page 389
Wellmark Health Plan of IA Inc — Page 175

Nelson, Steve
Health Net Inc - Corp Hdqrtrs — Page 49

Nelson, Sue
Presbyterian Health Plan — Page 281
Anthem BCBS of Nevada — Page 259
Presbyterian Health Plan — Page 281

Nelson, William L, MD
Hines & Associates Inc — Page 150

Nemec, John
Health Tradition Health Plans — Page 466

Nemecek, Doug, MD
CIGNA Behavioral Health Inc — Page 88
CIGNA Behavioral Health Inc -
Corporate Headquarters — Page 234

Nemeth, Joseph
Mercycare Health Plan Inc — Page 468

Nemmers, Jo Ann
Coventry Health Care Inc — IA — Page 169

Nenni, Angie
Delta Dental Plan of KY Inc — Page 184

Nesbit, Lamar
PhysiciansPlus/St Dominic Health
Maintenance Organization — Page 242

Nesbit-Fisher, Sue
Iowa Foundation for Medical Care/
Encompass — Page 170

Nesbitt, Stephen, DO
UniCare Health Plans of TX Inc — Page 428

Neshat, Amir, DDS
Liberty Dental Plan of CA — Page 56

Netoskie, Mark, MD
Humana Health Care
Plans of Dallas — Page 417

Nettles, Rene, RN, CCM
Spectrum Review Services Inc — Page 426

Nettleton, Kim
Community Health Choice Inc — Page 410

Neuner, Richard P
Blue Cross Blue Shield of MN — Page 234

Neupauer, Vicki RN
Humana Medical Plan -
Central Florida — Page 113

Neuville, Eric
Anthem BCBS of Ohio — Page 320

Neuweiler, Diane
Ppnm's Mastercare Network — Page 263

Nevanen, Cathy
First Plan of Minnesota — Page 235

Nevins, Maggie
Delta Dental Plan of NM — Page 279

Nevins, Nancy
LifeWise Hlth Plan of OR — Page 348

Nevins, Tesa
Virginia Premier Hlth Plans Inc — Page 447

Newberry, Mitchel
El Paso First Health Plans Inc — Page 413

Newell, Anthony, MD
Peach State Health Plan — Page 133

Newman, Christy
Cariten Healthcare — Page 393
PHP Companies Inc — Page 397

Newman, Ken
Horizon Behavioral Services — Page 112
Horizon Behavioral Services — Page 417

Newman, Stephen L, MD
Tenet Choices Inc — Page 192

Newmeyer, Ed
Mercer First Choice — Page 369

Newsom, Larry J
Health Care Service Corporation -
Corporate Headquarters — Page 149

Newsome, Rick
Kaiser Foundation Health
Plan of Colorado — Page 83

Newsum, Benjamin
Health Management Network Inc — Page 16

Newton, Dean
Delta Dental Plan of Kansas — Page 178

Newton, Earl W
Racine Dental Group SC — Page 469

Newton, Linda H
Blue Cross Blue Shield
of Rhode Island — Page 379

Neyer, Tim
HealthLink Inc - Corp Hdqrtrs — Page 249

Nguyen, Anh, OD
FirstSight Vision Services Inc — Page 47

Nguyen, Michelle
CIGNA Dental Health of CA Inc — Page 40

Nguyen, Son
UnitedHealthcare of Texas Inc -
Houston — Page 429

Nguyen, Tricia MD
Humana Inc - Indiana — Page 161

Niceley, Christopher J
Denta Quest Mid-Atlantic Inc — Page 202

Nichol, Dan, MD
CIGNA Healthcare of
New York and New Jersey — Page 270

Nichols, Gaye
Universal Health Network -
Corporate Headquarters — Page 264

Nichols, Sandra
Americhoice of PA Inc — Page 356

Nicholson, Frank E
BCBS of Illinois — Page 144
HMO Illinois — Page 150
Health Care Service Corporation -
Corporate Headquarters — Page 149

Nicholson, Joe, MD
Bluelincs HMO — Page 340

Nicholson, Sherrie
Health Care Excel Inc — Page 160

Nicholson, Thomas
DakotaCare — Page 387

Nicknish, Mike
HAS Premier Providers Inc — Page 415

Niebling, Tammy
Health Net of Arizona — Page 17

Niederberger, Jane
Anthem BCBS of Indiana — Page 157

Niegel, Chad
Marion Polk Community
Health Plan Advantage — Page 349

Niehaus, William
Humana Health Plan - KY — Page 185

Nienow, Patricia
HealthEOS by MultiPlan — Page 466

Nieukirk, Mary Anne
OSF Health Plans — Page 151

Nightingdale, Gary
Mental Health Consultants Inc — Page 369

Niles, Chad
BCBS of North Dakota — Page 317

Nissenson, Allen, MD, FACP
DaVita VillageHealth of MI Inc — Page 220

Nittle, Terry
Humana Health Care
Plans of Arizona — Page 17

Noble, Ann
QualCare Inc — Page 276

Nobles, Jennifer
Vision Service Plan — Page 86

Noel, Mike
Scan Health Plan — Page 68

Nolan, Robert
Oxford Health Plans of NY Inc — Page 303

Nolan, Robert J
Aetna Inc - New York — Page 283

Nolan, Timothy E
Coventry Hlth Care Inc — DE Inc — Page 96

Noland, Tom
Humana Insurance Co - AL — Page 5
Humana Inc - DC — Page 98
Humana Inc - ND — Page 317
Humana Inc - CO — Page 82

Index VIII: Personnel

Mowreader, Diane
Columbia United Providers — Page 449
Moya, Angie
Catalina Behavioral
Health Services Inc — Page 13
Moya, Steve
Humana Inc — Page 486
Moya, Steven O
Humana Insurance Co - AL — Page 5
Humana Inc - CO — Page 82
Humana Inc - DC — Page 98
Humana Inc - Corp Hdqrtrs — Page 185
Humana Inc - MD — Page 203
Humana Inc - NM — Page 280
Humana Inc - ND — Page 317
Humana Health Care Plans
of Corpus Christi — Page 417
Humana Inc - UT — Page 435
Moyes, Karen, MD
Santa Barbara Regional
Health Authority — Page 67
Mozden, Annterese
CIGNA Healthcare of NH — Page 265
Mroue, Carol
Care Choices HMO — Page 218
Muchnicki, Michael A
Touchstone Health HMO Inc — Page 305
Mudra, Karl
Delta Dental Plan of MO — Page 246
Mueller, Susan, MD
Aetna Inc - Houston — Page 403
Muench, Paul
Molina HealthCare of UT Inc — Page 435
Mulcahy, Barbara
HMS Colorado Inc — Page 82
Sloan's Lake Preferred
Health Networks — Page 85
Mulichak, Lori
Buckeye Community
Health Plan Inc — Page 321
Mulland, Thomas, CPA
Spectrum Vision Systems Inc — Page 181
Mullaney, Joseph E, III, Esq
Masspro Inc — Page 213
Mullen, Ed
Broadspire Inc — Page 105
Mullen, Orie
Humana Military Service Inc — Page 186
Muller, Cecelia
United Concordia Co Inc - FL — Page 121
Muller, Debra
Avera Health Plans Inc — Page 387
Muller, Roger, MD
UnitedHealthcare of Washington — Page 457
Muller, Sheila
Blue Shield of California — Page 36
Muller, Wayne F
Superior Vision Services Inc — Page 70
Mulligan, Terri
National Foot Care Program Inc — Page 227
Mullins, Anita
Molina Healthcare of New Mexico — Page 281
Mullins, Larry A, DHA
Intercommunity Health Network — Page 347
Samaritan Health Plans Inc — Page 352
Samaritan Health Plans Inc — Page 352
Mullins, Micah
UHP Healthcare — Page 71
Fiserv Inc — Page 464
Mummery, Ray, MD
Dimension Health (PPO) — Page 109
Mundy, Claudia
Alameda Alliance for Health — Page 33
Mundy, Nancy
Coventry Health Care Inc — IA — Page 169
Mundy, Troy
United Concordia Co Inc - WA — Page 457

Muney, Alan M, MD, MHA
Oxford Health Plans Inc —
Corporate Headquarters — Page 92
Oxford Health Plans-CT — Page 91
Oxford Health Plans of NJ Inc — Page 275
Oxford Health Plans of NY Inc — Page 303
Muney, John
Atlantis Health Plan — Page 285
Munir, Naim, MD
Rayant Insurance Co of NY — Page 304
Munoz, Carlos A, MD
Medical Card System — Page 377
Munoz, Juan
Preferred Medical Plan Inc — Page 118
Munoz, Perfecto
Health Plan of San Joaquin, The — Page 50
Munroe, Sharon
Metcare Health Plans Inc — Page 116
Munshower, Ernest C
Spectrum Review Services Inc — Page 426
Spectrum Review Services Inc — Page 426
Munson, Russell J, MD
Anthem BCBS of Connecticut — Page 88
Murabito, John
CIGNA HealthCare —
Corporate Headquarters — Page 360
Murabito, John
CIGNA Healthcare of TX Inc — Page 409
Murar, Thomas
Molina Healthcare of MI Inc — Page 227
Murdock, Jake
Deseret Healthcare — Page 434
Murillo, Sharon
Serve You Custom
Prescription Management — Page 495
Murnane, Jane
New York Presbyterian
Community Health Plan — Page 302
Muro, JP
Sante Community Physicians — Page 67
Murphy, Don
Medical Review Institute -
Corporate Headquarters — Page 435
Murphy, Eileen
OhioHealth Group — Page 332
Murphy, Jeff
Aetna Health of Illinois Inc — Page 143
Murphy, Le'Dice
Community Choice Health Plan of
Westchester Inc — Page 287
Murphy, Louise
Aetna Behavioral Health - Utah Care
Management Center — Page 433
Murphy, Michael G
Mercy Health Plans of MO Inc — Page 249
Murphy, Susan
CIGNA Healthcare of NH — Page 265
Murray, Charles
University Health Alliance — Page 138
Murray, Doug
PerfectHealth Insurance Co — Page 304
Murray, James E
Humana Insurance Co - AL — Page 5
Humana Inc - CO — Page 82
Humana Inc - DC — Page 98
Humana Inc - Corp Hdqrtrs — Page 185
Humana Inc - MD — Page 203
Humana Inc - ND — Page 317
Humana Health Care Plans
of Corpus Christi — Page 417
Humana Inc - UT — Page 435
Humana Inc - Corp Hdqrtrs — Page 486
Murray, Michael
Blue Cross Blue Shield of MN — Page 234
Murrillo, Diane
Alliance Regional Hlth Ntwrk — Page 404
Muscatello, Todd
Excellus BlueCross BlueShield,
Rochester Area — Page 292

Musial, Brian
Advantage Hlth Solutions Inc — Page 157
Musial, Scott
IBA Health Plans — Page 225
Muskat, Denis
RxAmerica LLC — Page 494
Musser, Josephine W
Wisconsin Physician Services
Insurance Company — Page 471
Musser, Karen
Elder Care Health Plan Inc — Page 522
Musunuri, Sanjoy
Humana Hlth Care Plans of IL — Page 151
Muszynski, Thomas
Care Resources Inc — Page 508
Mutchler, Helen
Nychsro/MedReview Inc — Page 303
Muzzy, Tammy
Health First Health Plans Inc — Page 111
Myers, Cindy, MA, LPC, CHCQM
Behavioral Health Systems Inc — Page 3
Myers, Jack A
Blue Cross of Idaho — Page 141
True Blue — Page 142
Myers, Jeremy
Opticare Managed Vision — Page 314
Myers, Liana
Aetna Health of California Inc — Page 31
Aetna Inc - Dental Care of CA — Page 32
Myers, Robert
Dean Health Plan — Page 463
Myers, Tim
Oxford Health Plans-CT — Page 91
Myers, Wendy, MD
Florida Health Care Plan Inc — Page 109

N

Nabors, Dennis, DDS
Dental Care Plus Inc — Page 324
Nace, Josh
Dental Health Services — Page 45
Dental Health Services Inc — Page 450
Nadeau, Mark
Delta Dental Plan of NJ — Page 271
Naffaly, Robert
Blue Preferred Plan-BCBS MI — Page 519
Nageotte, Noreen
CIGNA Healthcare of OH Inc — Page 323
Nagle, Joseph A
Altus Dental Ins Co Inc — Page 379
Delta Dental of Rhode Island — Page 380
Nagle, Kevin M
Envision Pharmaceutical
Services Inc — Page 484
Nagy, Mary Ann
CHN Solutions — Page 270
Naimpally, Sobha, MD
Community Health Plan — Page 42
Nair, Mohandas
Regence Group, The —
Corporate Headquarters — Page 351
Nall, Larry
UnitedHealthcare of TN Inc — Page 401
Nameth, Michael A, RPh, MBA
HealthLink Inc — Page 248
Nangreave, Richard
Excellus BCBS — Page 290
Excellus BCBS,
Rochester Area — Page 292
Nankin, Gerald, OD
Vision Plan of America — Page 75
Napier, Annette
Vantage Health Plan Inc — Page 193

Index VIII: Personnel

Moeller-Roy, Nance
CIGNA Behavioral Health Inc -
Corporate Headquarters — Page 234
Moessner, Deborah W
Anthem BCBS of Kentucky
(HMO Kentucky) — Page 183
Moffa-Sipio, Felicia
Devon Health Services Inc — Page 361
Mohoney, Mike
Physicians Plus
Insurance Corporation — Page 469
Mohoric, Peggy RN
Blue Cross Blue Shield of NM — Page 279
HMO New Mexico Inc — Page 280
Mohr, Audrey
UnitedHealthcare of Texas Inc -
Houston — Page 429
Mohr, Joseph N
HDN PPO — Page 149
Moksnes, Mark
Delta Dental Plan of MN — Page 235
Molchan, Paul, MD
Regence BCBS of Utah — Page 436
Regence Healthwise — Page 436
Regence Valucare — Page 436
Molina, J Mario, MD
Molina Healthcare Inc — Page 489
Molina, John C, JD
Molina Healthcare Inc -
Corporate Headquarters — Page 59
Molina Healthcare Inc - CA — Page 59
Molina Healthcare Inc — Page 489
Molina, Joseph M, MD
Molina Healthcare Inc -
Corporate Headquarters — Page 59
Molina Healthcare Inc - CA — Page 59
Molina Healthcare of MI Inc — Page 227
Molina Healthcare of NM — Page 281
Molina Healthcare of TX Inc — Page 421
Molina HealthCare of UT Inc — Page 435
Molina HealthCare of WA Inc — Page 453
Monaco, Patricia
Northeast Pharmacy Srvc Corp — Page 490
Monahan, Frank A
CIGNA Healthcare of
Kansas/Missouri — Page 177
CIGNA Healthcare of St Louis — Page 245
Monen, Floyd
Northwest Pharmacy Services — Page 490
Monez, Sue
Partnership HealthPlan of CA — Page 64
Monfifetto, Ernest
AmeriChoice of New York — Page 284
Mongeon, Laura P
Univera Community Health — Page 307
Monnihan, Kay
Pioneer Management Systems — Page 215
Monroe, Brent
Interactive Medical Systems — Page 313
Monsen, Brian
Molina HealthCare of Utah Inc — Page 435
Montag, Jeff
Humana Hlth Care Plans of AZ — Page 17
Monte, John
Fallon Community Hlth Plan Inc — Page 211
Montepare, Carole
Capital District Physicians
Health Plan — Page 286
Montesino, Arlene
Preferred Care Partners Inc — Page 118
Montgomery, Carol
Mutual Assurance
Administrators Inc — Page 342
Montgomery, Harold
Pro-Care Health Plan — Page 230
Monti-Markowski, Diane, DMD
Delta Dental of Rhode Island — Page 380
Montjoy, George Rea
Mississippi Select Health Care — Page 241

Moody, Dennis, MBA
Magellan Health Services Inc — Page 91
Magellan Health Services — Page 132
Moody, Michael, MD
Arkansas Foundation for
Medical Care — Page 26
Moody, Robers
Community Health Plan — Page 42
Moody, Robert L
American National
Insurance Company — Page 405
Mooney, Kerry, ACSW
ValueOptions - Corp Hdqrtrs — Page 447
Moore, Allen
Delta Dental Plan of Arkansas — Page 26
Moore, Charles A
Community Health Choice Inc — Page 410
Moore, Dan
Forte Managed Care — Page 414
Moore, David, MD
Florida Health Partners Inc — Page 110
Moore, Donna O
Independence Blue Cross — Page 366
Moore, Ginny, MD
AmeriGroup Maryland Inc — Page 199
Moore, Kathy
American WholeHealth
Networks Inc — Page 442
Moore, Laura N, MPA
Masspro Inc — Page 213
Moore, Ned
Metropolitan Health Plan — Page 237
Moore, Stephen
PTPN - Corporate Headquarters — Page 65
Moore, Susie
Arkansas Foundation for
Medical Care — Page 26
Moore, Timothy J, MD, MS
Health Net - Connecticut — Page 90
Moorthy, Sachidananda, MD
Paragon Biomedical Inc — Page 491
Moran, Maureen
Northeast Health Direct LLC — Page 92
Moran, Rhonda
Corvel Corporation — Page 159
Morand, Mary Ann
ProviDRs Care Network — Page 181
Morano, Carmine
PerfectHealth Insurance Co — Page 304
Morgan, Gary
Kaiser Foundation Health Plan
Northwest — Page 347
Morgan, John, Jr
Midwestern Dental Plans Inc — Page 226
Morgan, Peter
Group Health Cooperative
of Puget Sound — Page 452
Morgan, Sue
IBA Health Plans — Page 225
Morgan, Thomas B
SelectHealth — Page 437
Morgan, Victor
ConnectCare — Page 219
Morin, Jeff
Medical Network Inc — Page 197
Moroney, Patrick
National Medical Health Card Systems -
Corporate Headquarter — Page 489
Morphew, Wendy
Aetna Health of Illinois Inc — Page 143
Morrell, Adrienne
Health Net Inc - Corp Hdqrtrs — Page 49
Morris, Carol
Anthem BCBS of Maine — Page 195
Morris, Carole
Community Choice Health
Plan of Westchester Inc — Page 287

Morris, Charles J, MD
UnitedHealthcare of Texas Inc -
Houston — Page 429
Morris, Harold
Community Choice Health Plan of
Westchester Inc — Page 287
Morris, Ken
CO/OP Optical Services Inc — Page 219
Morris, M Shawn
Signature Health Alliance — Page 398
Morris, Mark
Health New England — Page 212
Morris, Michael E
Aetna Inc - Maine — Page 195
Morris, Pamela
Community Choice Michigan — Page 219
Morris, Pamela B
CareSource — Page 321
Morris, Regina
Neighborhood Health Providers — Page 302
Morris, Sandra, MD
FirstCarolinaCare — Page 312
Morris, Shawn
HealthSpring Inc - Tennessee — Page 395
Morris, Susan
Delta Dental Plans Association — Page 146
Morris, Tracy
Primary Health Plan — Page 142
Morrison, JoAnn
Mountain State BCBS — Page 460
Morrison, Sheila R
Elder Service Plan of
Harbor Health Services Inc — Page 510
Morrone, Michael A
CHN Solutions — Page 270
Morrone, Rick
Health Care Exchange
Limited Company — Page 223
Morrow, Michael
BCBS of Minnesota — Page 234
Morrow, Robin
Health Plan of San Joaquin, The — Page 50
Morrow, Thomas, MD
Great-West Healthcare of FL — Page 111
Morse, David B
Delta Dental Plan of MN — Page 235
Morton, Rob
Secure Hlth Plans of GA LLC — Page 133
Morton, Ron, MD
MDX Hawaii — Page 138
Mosbacher, Michael
Vantage PPO — Page 375
Moscheo, Richard
Capital District Physicians
Health Plan — Page 286
Moscovic, David
Basic Chiropractic Hlth Plan Inc — Page 35
Moser, Brandon
Unison Health Plan -
Corporate Headquarters — Page 372
Moser, Mark H
Paramount Care of Michigan — Page 228
Paramount Health Care Plan — Page 333
Moses, John P
Blue Cross of Northeastern PA — Page 358
Moss, Debra L MD, MBA
MPRO — Page 227
Moss, Paul
Lutheran Preferred/
Three Rivers Preferred — Page 162
Motter, Jason
CIGNA Healthcare of North TX — Page 409
Mount, Edward
Blue Cross Blue Shield of TX —
HMO Blue - Southeast — Page 407
Moussavi, Mehdi
Dental Health Services Inc — Page 450

Index VIII: Personnel

Merson, James L, MD
Inland Empire Foundation
for Medical Care — Page 52
Merson, Michael R
CareFirst BlueChoice Inc — Page 97
CareFirst BCBS — Page 200
Delmarva Health Care Plan Inc — Page 202
CareFirst BCBS — Page 481
Mertel, Mark V
Partners Rx Management LLC — Page 491
Mertz, Laura
Valley Preferred — Page 375
Merz, Marcus
Preferred One — Page 237
Mesoras, Michael
Aetna Inc - Pennsylvania — Page 355
Metnick, Joyce
UMPC Health Plan Univ of
Pittsburgh Medical Center — Page 374
Metz, Gaylon
Group Health Cooperative
South Central Wisconsin — Page 464
Metz, Peter, MD
Humana Health Care
Plans of Arizona — Page 17
Metz, R Douglas, DC
American Specialty
Health Plans Inc — Page 33
Metzdorf, Kelly
CIGNA Healthcare of North TX — Page 409
Meuttenmuller, Paul
Essence Inc — Page 246
Meyer, Ann, RN, MBA
Active Health Management — Page 441
Meyer, Brian
DakotaCare — Page 387
Meyer, Carrie
Independent Health
Association Inc — Page 297
Meyer, Gregg S, MD, MSC
Masspro Inc — Page 213
Meyer, Mike
SXC Health Solutions Inc — Page 495
Meyers, James
HealthEOS by MultiPlan — Page 466
Meyers, Robert, MD
Atlantic Integrated Health Inc — Page 309
Meyers-Alessi, Lisa
Blue Cross Blue Shield
of Western New York — Page 285
Meyerson, Tamara
Preferred Medical Plan Inc — Page 118
Michaels, Melanie
Preferred Podiatry Group — Page 152
Michaelson, Marco, MD
Fidelis Care New York — Page 293
New York State Catholic
Health Plan Inc — Page 303
Michel, Richard E
Ventura County
Foundation for Medical Care — Page 73
Michelin, Nasry
Amerigroup New York, LLC — Page 284
Michelson, Dan
Allscripts Pharmaceuticals Inc — Page 479
Mickle, Byron
Navitus Health Solutions — Page 490
Mickle, William
Prescription Solutions — Page 493
Middleton, Darrell E
Blue Preferred Plan-BCBS
Michigan — Page 218
Middleton, Frank, III, MD
Phoebe Health Partners — Page 133
Midlikowski, Gail
Unity Health Insurance — Page 470
Mielke, John
Prime Therapeutics — Page 493

Miersch, Edward R
SunRx Inc — Page 495
Mihalik, Chuck
M Plan Inc — Page 163
Mikan, G Mike
Ovations Pharmacy Solutions — Page 490
Mikan, George L
UnitedHealthcare & Mid
Atlantic Medical Services Inc — Page 206
Mikrut, Paula, MD
Health Net of Arizona — Page 17
Mikula, Martin
Southwest Health Alliance
(SHALLC) — Page 425
Milazzo, Al
Health Net Inc - Northeast
Corporate Headquarters — Page 91
Miles, Vincent MD
Winhealth Partners — Page 473
Milich, David
UnitedHealthcare of the
Midwest Inc — Page 251
Miller, Cari
PRONJ, The Healthcare Quality
Improvement Org of NJ — Page 276
Miller, David
Humana Health Care Plans of
Kansas & Missouri — Page 179
Miller, Dawn
New Mexico Medical
Review Association — Page 281
Miller, Deborah
Scan Health Plan — Page 68
Miller, Epsy
ECCA - Managed Vision Care Inc -
Corporate Headquarters — Page 413
Miller, Howard
Assurant Health -
Corporate Headquarters — Page 462
Miller, Jim
Hometown Health Plan — Page 260
Miller, Kathy
CHN MCO — Page 322
Miller, Larry D
Mennonite Mutual
Aid Association — Page 519
Miller, Mike
Initial Group Inc, The — Page 396
Miller, Oliver C
Univera Community Health — Page 307
Miller, Pam, RN
Select Circle Health Plan — Page 165
Miller, Paul R, CPA
Prescription Solutions — Page 493
Miller, Rick DO
Avera Health Plans Inc — Page 387
Miller, Ruth
Delta Dental Ins Co - AL — Page 4
Delta Dental Ins Co - GA — Page 131
Miller, Sallie
PersonalCare Ins of IL Inc — Page 151
Miller, Sharon
EM Risk Management,
A POMCO Company — Page 290
Miller, Susan
Primary Health Plan — Page 142
Miller, Tara
Family Health Partners — Page 247
Miller, Terry
Iowa Foundation for Medical Care/
Encompass — Page 170
Miller, Timothy
First Plan of Minnesota — Page 235
First Plan of Minnesota — Page 505
Miller, Vicki
Best Health Plans — Page 36
Miller, William F
S V S Visions Inc — Page 231

Milliner, Roger
MetroPlus Health Plan — Page 300
Mills, Randy
Southeastern Indiana
Health Organization — Page 166
Milner, Roger
Preferred Health Care — Page 370
Milnes, William R, Jr
Blue Cross Blue Shield of VT — Page 439
Vermont Hlth Plans (Blue Care) — Page 439
Milo, Yori
Premera BCBS of Alaska — Page 9
LifeWise Health Plan of WA — Page 453
Premera - Corp Hdqrtrs — Page 454
Premera Blue Cross - Eastern — Page 454
Premera Blue Cross - Western — Page 454
Miloni, Donald L
Alpha Dental Plan of Colorado — Page 77
Mims, Pamela
Florida Health Care Plan Inc — Page 109
Mincy, Bill, RPh
Pharmacy Providers
Services Corp — Page 492
Miner, Mathew
Suffolk Health Plan — Page 305
Ming, Bart
Humana Health Care Plans
of Corpus Christi — Page 417
Minier, William, MD
Blue Cross Blue Shield of NE — Page 255
Minksy, Joseph
Western Dental Services — Page 75
Minsloff, Mark
Arise Health Plan — Page 461
Mintz, Adam
AmeriGroup New Jersey Inc — Page 268
Mirsky, Bob, MD
Gateway Health Plan Inc — Page 362
Misech, Evelyn
Mdx Hawaii — Page 138
Mitchell, Aurora B
UTMB Health Plans Inc — Page 431
Mitchell, Bruce
CompBenefits — Page 410
Texas Dental Plan — Page 427
Mitchell, Jon, FACHE
Acumentra Health — Page 345
Mitchell, Joseph
Mississippi Select Health Care — Page 241
Mitchell, Karen
CompBenefits Corporation -
Corporate Headquarters — Page 129
Mitchell, Kim
Center Care — Page 184
Mitchell, Mike
RxPlus Pharmacies Inc — Page 494
Mitchell, Rick
Maricopa Health Plan — Page 18
Mitchell, Tracy
Arizona Foundation for
Medical Care — Page 11
Mitchell-Yon, Carol
Pharmacy Providers
Services Corp — Page 492
Mitten, Anthony D
Arizona Foundation for
Medical Care — Page 11
Mizell, Gary M
Aetna Inc - Arizona — Page 11
Mlsna, Michael, MD
Upper Peninsula Health Plan — Page 232
Mock, Kathleen
Blue Cross Blue Shield of MN — Page 234
Moebus, Janis
SHPS Inc — Page 186
Moeller, Rob
JP Farley Corp — Page 329

Index VIII: Personnel

McGurgan, Kevin J
Excellus BCBS, Central NY
Southern Tier — Page 291
McHale, Marigene
Opticare Managed Vision — Page 314
McHugh, Joseph M
LDI Pharmacy
Benefit Management — Page 487
McHugh, William
AmeriGroup Florida Inc — Page 101
McHugh, William
Independent
Health Association Inc — Page 297
McInerny, Linda, MD
Health Plans Inc — Page 213
McIntire, Joe
OSF Health Plans — Page 151
McIntire, Pamala
Florida Health Care Plan Inc — Page 109
McIntosh, Cynthia
Alabama Quality
Assurance Foundation — Page 3
McIntyre, Brett
APS Healthcare Inc — Page 199
APS Healthcare Northwest Inc — Page 253
APS Healthcare Midwest Inc — Page 461
McKay, Alan
Central Coast Alliance for Hlth — Page 39
McKay, Neil
Allianz Life Insurance Company
of North America — Page 233
McKelvey, William G
Preferred Dental Network (PDN) — Page 215
McKenna, Denise
Blue Cross Blue Shield of MN — Page 234
McKenna, Rick
Berkley Administrators — Page 88
McKim, Mike
Preferred One — Page 237
McKinley, Lawrence
United Concordia Co Inc - CA — Page 72
United Concordia Co Inc -
Corporate Headquarters — Page 373
McKinney, Ann
Lovelace Health Plan — Page 280
McLaughlin, Joseph
Intergroup Services Corp — Page 367
McLaughlin, Maureen
Group Health Cooperative — Page 141
Group Health Cooperative — Page 451
Group Health Cooperative of
Puget Sound — Page 452
Group Health Options Inc — Page 452
McLean, Alexander H
University Health Plans Inc — Page 277
McLean, Gionne
Humana Health Benefit
Plan of Louisiana — Page 191
McLeod, CJ
Oregon Dealthan — Page 349
McMahon, John W, Sr, MD
Mountain Pacific Quality
Health Foundation — Page 254
McMahon, Patrick
Virginia Premier Hlth Plans Inc — Page 447
McMillan, Sheila E
Evercare of Texas LLC — Page 413
McMillen, Jay, MD
Community Health Plan — Page 245
McMorran, Nancy
Delta Dental Plan of Minnesota — Page 235
McMurphy, Patrick
Preferred Mental Health
Management — Page 180
McMurray, Maurice E
Health Alliance Plan — Page 223
McNair, Greg
Tennessee Healthcare LLC — Page 399

McNair, Pamela
New York State Catholic
Health Plan Inc — Page 303
McNally, Thomas
Dental Network of America — Page 146
McNamara, Kathy
First Plan of Minnesota — Page 235
McNamara, Kevin
Signature Health Alliance — Page 398
McNamara, Kevin M
HealthSpring Inc - Tennessee — Page 395
HealthSpring Inc -
Corporate Headquarters — Page 395
McNamara, Timothy M
Univera Healthcare of
Western New York — Page 307
McNamus, Kim
Community Health Plan — Page 245
McNatt, Rick
Evercare Health Plans — Page 502
McNaughton, Jim
Aetna Inc - Oklahoma — Page 339
McNeill, Dana
Wellmark Inc — Corp Hdqrtrs — Page 175
McPherson, Jamie
Virginia Premier Hlth Plans Inc — Page 447
McQuarrie, Howard G, MD
Utah Public Employees
Health Program — Page 438
McRee, Keith
Vantage Health Plan Inc — Page 193
McSorley, John
QualCare Inc — Page 276
McSorley, Mary
Americhoice of PA Inc — Page 356
McWaters, Jeffrey L
AmeriGroup Corporation — Page 442
Amerigroup Ohio Inc — Page 319
McWilliams, Kathy L
Pacific Visioncare WA Inc — Page 453
McWilliams, Mary O
Asuris Northwest Health — Page 449
Regencecare — Page 456
Regence Blue Shield — Page 456
Regence Blue Shield — Page 456
Regencecare — Page 456
Mckinnon, John
Northwest Rehab Alliance — Page 349
Mead, Robert M
Aetna Inc - Corp Hdqrtrs — Page 87
Aetna Inc - New Jersey — Page 267
Meade, Peter
Blue Cross Blue Shield of MA — Page 209
Meador, Sue
Capitol Administrators — Page 38
Means, Aaron A.
ppoNEXT — Page 423
Mearnic, Cynthia
CO/OP Optical Services Inc — Page 219
Mechling, William C
Central Benefits Mutual
Insurance Company — Page 321
Medack, Ruth, MD
Acumentra Health — Page 345
Medici, Christopher J
Coordinated Health Plan — Page 379
Blue Cross Blue Shield
of Rhode Island — Page 379
Medley, Sara
Mountain Pacific Quality
Health Foundation — Page 254
Medwid, Mike
Nationwide Health Plans — Page 331
Meehan, Carson
Carolina Care Plan Inc — Page 383
Humana Medical Plan -
Central Florida — Page 113
Humana Medical Plan -
Daytona — Page 113

Meek, Todd
Iowa Health Solutions — Page 171
Meguess, Christopher
PACE Greater New Orleans — Page 513
Meholic, Steven C
Aetna Pharmacy Management -
Corporate Headquarters — Page 479
Mehra, Rahul, MD
Unipsych Systems — Page 120
Mehra, Victor
Hygeia Corporation — Page 114
Mehrotra, Rishabh
SHPS Inc — Page 186
Mei Ko, Sin
Neighborhood Health Plan
of Rhode Island — Page 380
Meisel, Stephen B, MD
MedFocus Radiology Network — Page 58
Mejia, Gisela
KPS Health Plans — Page 452
Melani, Kenneth R, MD
Highmark Inc — Page 366
Melani, Kenneth R MD
Highmark Inc — Page 366
Keystone Health Plan West Inc — Page 368
Mele, Mario
Fidelio Insurance Company — Page 362
Meledez, Jose G
Medical Card System — Page 377
Meleski, Matthew
Southern Health Services Inc — Page 445
Mellentine, David
Primecare Medical Network Inc — Page 65
Melton, Jack, MD
APS Healthcare Midwest Inc — Page 461
Memmott, Daniel
Healthinsight — Page 435
Mendelson, Jackie
Aids Healthcare Foundation — Page 32
Mendis, Paul, MD
Community Medical Alliance — Page 210
Neighborhood Health Plan — Page 214
Mendrygal, Matthew A, CPA
HealthPlus of Michigan — Page 224
Meng, Max
Affinity Health Plan Inc — Page 283
Mengert, Steve
MedSolutions — Page 396
Meoli, Angie
Coventry Health Care Inc — LA — Page 190
Mera, Csaba
ODS Health Plan — Page 349
Mercier, Jill
Southern Health Services Inc — Page 445
Mercklein, Thomas
WellCare of New York — Page 307
Merkel, Chip
United Concordia Co Inc - CA — Page 72
United Concordia Co Inc -
Corporate Headquarters — Page 373
Merkel-Liberatore, Karen
Blue Cross Blue Shield of
Western New York — Page 285
Merkin, Richard
Heritage Provider Network Inc — Page 50
Merlino, Chuck
New York Presbyterian
Community Health Plan — Page 302
Merlo, Kristin
Washington Dental Service — Page 457
Merrill, Kathleen
West Virginia Medical Institute — Page 460
Merrill, Kay
Health Net of California — Page 49
Merriott, Debbie
Chiropractic Arizona Ntwrk Inc — Page 13
Merrow, Walter
Blue Cross Blue Shield of VT — Page 439
Vermont Hlth Plans (Blue Care) — Page 439

Index VIII: Personnel

Humana Health Care Plans
of San Antonio/Austin   Page 418
Humana Health Plan of Austin   Page 419
Humana Inc - UT   Page 435
Humana Inc - WY   Page 473
Humana Inc   Page 486
Humana Health Plan - KY   Page 517
Humana Ins Co of New York   Page 518

McCann, Doug
Aetna Inc - Oklahoma   Page 339

McCarey, Katie
UnitedHealthcare of Florida Inc Page 122

McCarthy, Brian M
Masspro Inc   Page 213

McCarthy, Chris
Golden West Dental & Vision   Page 47

McCarthy, Jeanne
CIGNA Healthcare - Cincinnati Page 323

McCarthy, Margaret
Aetna Inc - Corp Hdqrtrs   Page 87
Aetna Inc - New Jersey   Page 267
Aetna Inc of the Carolinas   Page 309
Aetna Inc - Pennsylvania   Page 355

McCartney, Terry
Blue Cross Blue Shield of AL   Page 3

McCarty, John
SHPS Inc   Page 186

McCaskey, Raymond F
Blue Cross Blue Shield of IL   Page 144
HMO Illinois   Page 150
Health Care Service Corporation -
Corporate Headquarters   Page 149
Blue Cross Blue Shield of NM   Page 279
HMO New Mexico Inc   Page 280
Blue Cross and Blue Shield of IL
Pharmacy Programs   Page 481

McCaughey, Tracy
Neighborhood Health Plan
of Rhode Island   Page 380

McClain, Barbara
Lifetime Healthcare Companies, The -
Corporate Headquarters   Page 298

McClain, Dave
Wellpath Select Inc   Page 315

McClanathan, Ann
PacifiCare Behavioral Health   Page 61

McClellan, Hassell
Denta Quest Ventures Inc   Page 211

McClerkin, Hayes C
Arkansas Blue Cross/Blue Shield
a Mutual Insurance Company   Page 25

McCloud, Scott
Corvel Corporation   Page 43
Corvel Corporation   Page 159
Corvel Corporation   Page 324

McClure, Nancy
HealthPartners Inc   Page 236

McClurg, Jack
HealthTrans LLC   Page 486

McCluskey, Mary T, MD
Aetna Inc - Maine   Page 195

McComas, John E
AlohaCare   Page 137

McCombs, Marc
West Virginia Medical Institute Page 460

McConnell, Wendy
Parkview Signature Care   Page 164

McCord, Robert
PerfectHealth Ins Co   Page 304

McCormack, Joseph
Immediate Pharmaceutical
Services Inc   Page 486

McCormick, Tom
APS Healthcare Midwest Inc   Page 461

McCosh, Alec, PhD
Behavioral Hlthcre Options Inc Page 259

McCowan, Steven
UnitedHealthcare of Kentucky   Page 186

McCoy, Molly
Colorado Access   Page 79

McCoy, Sarah
Dental Care Plus Inc   Page 324

McCrann, Kelly
PacifiCare Dental & Vision   Page 61

McCray, Joseph W, Jr, OD
Vision Health Mngmnt Sys   Page 155

McCrory, Tina
Colorado Health Networks LLC -
ValueOptions   Page 80

McCroskey, Barbara
Blue Cross Blue Shield of
Western New York   Page 285

McCrossen, Michael P
Med-Comp USA   Page 192

McCullough, Andrew R
Kaiser Foundation Health Plan
Northwest   Page 347

McCullum, Philip
United Concordia Co Inc - MO   Page 251

McCurry, Peggy
Cariten Healthcare   Page 393
PHP Companies Inc   Page 397

McCusker, Owen
Health Plan for Community
Living Inc   Page 522

McCutcheon, Pat
MedFocus Radiology Network   Page 58

McDade, Jean
Citrus Health Care Inc   Page 108

McDaniel, Debora A
CIGNA Healthcare of St Louis   Page 245

McDaniel, Donna
Mercy Health Plans of MO Inc   Page 249

McDaniel, Jeff
Nationwide Health Plans   Page 331

McDannold, Roger
First Plan of Minnesota   Page 235

McDermott, John
Highmark Inc   Page 366

McDonald, Donna C
Excellus BCBS   Page 290

McDonald, Janice
Northeast Health Direct LLC   Page 92

McDonald, Michael
Optimum HealthCare Inc   Page 117

McDonald, Vicki
Health Net of California   Page 49

McDonough, Dave
Trustmark Insurance Company   Page 153

McDonough, Thomas P
Coventry Health Care Inc —
Corporate Headquarters   Page 201

McDow, Anne
Geisinger Health Plan   Page 363

McDowell, David C
Excellus BCBS   Page 290
Lifetime Healthcare Companies, The -
Corporate Headquarters   Page 298
Univera Healthcare of
Western New York   Page 307

McDowell, Dennis
Great-West Healthcare of Texas -
Houston   Page 415

McDowell, John, RPh, MBA
Quality Health Plan Inc   Page 119

McDuffie, Scott
Viva Health Inc   Page 7

McElroy, Tom
Tennessee Healthcare LLC   Page 399

McEntee, Toni
Sanford Health Plan   Page 388

McFadden, John
Select Health of SC   Page 385

McFall, Tim
Aetna Inc - Oklahoma   Page 339

McFarland, Greg
Horizon Health PPO   Page 261
Managed Care Consultants   Page 261

McFarland, Kay
Alpha Dental Plan of Colorado Page 77

McFarland, Patti
Central Coast Alliance for Hlth Page 39

McFarlane, Don
Corvel Corporation   Page 43
Corvel Corporation   Page 159
Corvel Corporation   Page 324

McFarlane, Lawrence G, MD
Security Health Plan of WI Inc Page 469

McFeetors, Raymond L
Great-West Healthcare of California -
Southern   Page 48
Great West Life Annuity Ins Co Page 81
Great-West Healthcare - Corp   Page 81
Great-West Healthcare of CO   Page 81
Great-West Healthcare of IL   Page 148
Great-West Healthcare
of Kansas/Missouri   Page 179
Great-West Healthcare of ME   Page 196
Great-West Healthcare of MI   Page 223
Great-West Healthcare of MN   Page 236
Great-West Healthcare of NY   Page 294
Great-West Healthcare of NC   Page 313
Great-West Healthcare of OH   Page 326
Great-West Healthcare of TX -
Houston   Page 415

McGarry, Peter
Health Plan of CareOregon Inc Page 346

McGee, Judi
Primecare Medical Network Inc Page 65

McGeehan, Thomas
UniCare Health Plans of TX Inc Page 428

McGillen, Linda
Blue Cross Blue Shield of MT   Page 253

McGinnity, Mike
Innoviant Inc   Page 487

McGlynn, Mitchell E
Dominion Dental Services - Corporate
Headquarters   Page 444

McGovern, Kevin
Fallon Community Hlth Plan Inc Page 211

McGovern, Patrick
Preferred Care Incorporated   Page 370

McGowan, Daniel T
HIP Health Plan of New York   Page 296

McGowan, Katherine
Physicians Plus
Insurance Corporation   Page 469

McGrath, Katherine
BMC HealthNet Plan   Page 209

McGrath, Nicole
Medcore Health Plan   Page 58

McGriff, Sandra
OmniCare, A Coventry
Health Plan   Page 228

McGrory, Ken
RxAmerica LLC   Page 494

McGuinness, John
Great-West Healthcare of TX -
Dallas   Page 415

McGuinness, Sean
Center Care   Page 184

McGuire, Andy, MD
American Republic
Insurance Company   Page 169

McGuire, Erika
ProviDRs Care Network   Page 181

McGuire, Kathy
Independent Living for Seniors Page 511

McGuire, Kenneth
Delta Dental of Oklahoma   Page 340

McGuire, Marilee
Community Health Plan of WA   Page 450

McGuire, Nora K
HealthNow New York Inc   Page 295

Index VIII: Personnel

Martin, Peter
Humana Medical Plan Inc — Page 114
Martin, Steven R
Mennonite Mutual Aid Assoc — Page 519
Martin, Steven S
Blue Cross Blue Shield of NE — Page 255
Martin, Veronica
Humana Inc - Indiana — Page 161
Martinez, Belinda
Delta Dental Ins Co - AL — Page 4
Martinez, Carlos A
Total Health Choice Inc — Page 120
Martinez, Cesar D
D C Chartered Health Plan Inc — Page 97
WellCare Health Plans Inc -
Corporate Headquarters — Page 124
Martinez, Estela
Orange Prevention &
Treatment Integrated — Page 60
Martinez, Heather
Dedicated Dental Systems — Page 43
Martinez, Mark
LA Care Health Plan — Page 55
Martinez, Roberto, MD
Capital District Physicians
Health Plan — Page 286
Martinez, Sandra
Jaimini Health Inc — Page 53
Jaimini Health Inc — Page 53
Martinez, Terry
Humana Medical Plan Inc — Page 114
Martinez, Thomas
Community Choice Health Plan of
Westchester Inc — Page 287
Martins-Lopes, Maria, MD
GHI HMO Select Inc — Page 293
Martorelli, Jack
HealthLink Inc - Corp Hdqrtrs — Page 249
Martz, William, MD
University Family Care
Health Plan — Page 22
Marusin, Mark A
Great-West Healthcare of CO — Page 81
Marwede, Lee
Americas PPO — Page 233
Masciandaro, Mario
DentCare Delivery Systems Inc — Page 289
Masin, Jerry
One Call Medical Inc — Page 275
Maslen, Loy, RNC, MSN, NNP
Qualis Health — Page 455
Maslowski, Marie
UCARE Minnesota — Page 238
Mason, Christopher R, ESQ
New York Compensation
Managers Inc — Page 302
Mason, Mary Anne
American WholeHealth
Networks Inc — Page 442
Mason, Mary V, MD
Centene Corporation — Page 244
Mason, Peg
Iowa Foundation for Medical Care/
Encompass — Page 170
Mason, Sanford, DPM
Preferred Podiatry Group — Page 152
Massey, Mikki
Family Health Partners — Page 247
Master, Robert J, MD
Commonwealth Care
Alliance Inc — Page 505
Masterson, Robert
Coventry Hlth Care of NE Inc — Page 255
Matalon, Reuben, MD
UTMB Health Plans Inc — Page 431
Mateja, Anna
Texas Childrens Health Plan — Page 426

Matera, Andrew, MD
Missouri Care — Page 250
Matheis, Dennis
Anthem BCBS of Missouri — Page 243
Mathews, Christopher, MD
Community Health Plan of WA — Page 450
Mathews, Jeremy
WelBorn Health Plans — Page 167
Mathews, Randy
CIGNA Healthcare of California — Page 41
Mathias, Raub
Community Health Plan — Page 42
Mathieu, Dave
Health Plan of the
Upper Ohio Valley — Page 327
Mathuny, Robert
SmileCare/Community
Dental Services — Page 69
Matsumoto, Kerry
PacifiCare Behavioral Health — Page 61
Matsuoka, Marlene
Great-West Healthcare of
California - Northern — Page 48
Matthew, Richard L
Preferred Care Incorporated — Page 370
Matthews, Caroline S
Anthem BCBS of Nevada — Page 259
WellPoint Inc - Corp Hdqrtrs — Page 167
Matthews, Norman S, Jr
Hawaii Medical Services Association -
BC/BS of Hawaii — Page 137
Matthews, Robert
KHS a KMG America Company — Page 385
Mattola, Michael
MetroPlus Health Plan — Page 300
Maturi, Richard
Premera BCBS of Alaska — Page 9
Premera - Corpe Hdqrtrs — Page 454
Premera Blue Cross - Eastern — Page 454
Premera Blue Cross - Western — Page 454
Matzner, Gary C
Hygeia Corporation — Page 114
Maura, Erin
Med-Comp USA — Page 192
Maury, Albert
Leon Medical Centers
Health Plan Inc — Page 115
Mauthe, Deb
Prevea Health Network — Page 469
Mauzy, Larry
MD-Individual Practice Association Inc
(MD IPA) — Page 204
Mauzy, Larry
Mid Atlantic Medical Services Inc
(MAMSI)- Corp Headquarters — Page 204
Maxcy, Steven
Medical Network Inc — Page 197
Maxwell, Jamey
PersonalCare Ins of IL Inc — Page 151
Maxwell, Melanie
CommunityCare Managed Healthcare
Plans of Oklahoma Inc — Page 340
CommunityCare Managed Healthcare
Plans of Oklahoma Inc — Page 483
Maxwell, Paul
Humana Health Care
Plans of IL — Page 151
Maxwell, Rae Ann
UMPC Health Plan Univ of
Pittsburgh Medical Center — Page 374
May, Fred, MD
Blue Cross Blue Shield of MI — Page 241
Mayer, Holly
Buckeye Community
Health Plan Inc — Page 321
Mayer, Katherine
American Specialty
Health Plans Inc — Page 33

Mayhew, Karin B
Health Net Inc - Corp Hdqrtrs — Page 49
Maynard, Elizabeth
Kern Foundation/
Preferred Provider Organization — Page 55
Maynard, Jody
Vantage Health Plan Inc — Page 193
Maynard, Michael
Delta Dental Plan of NM — Page 279
Maynard, Virginia
Aetna Behavioral Health -
Utah Care Management Center — Page 433
Mays, Todd
PacifiCare of Nevada — Page 263
Mazza, Bill
Av-Med Health Plan - Tampa — Page 103
Mazzola Spivey, Mary
BlueChoice Hlth Plan of SC Inc — Page 383
McGowan, David T
EmblemHealth Inc — Page 290
Mc Mullin, Bart, MD
Regence BCBS of Oregon — Page 351
Mc Murren, Mitchell
Total Health Care Inc — Page 231
McAllister, Sandra
CIGNA Healthcare — Page 439
McAndrew, Cheryl
MDNY Healthcare Inc — Page 299
McArdle, Michael, MD
Physicians Health Plan of
Northern Indiana — Page 164
McAulifee, Mark
Martins Point Health Care — Page 196
McCaffrey, Frank
Humana Health Care
Plans of Dallas — Page 417
McCaffrey, Maura
Health New England — Page 212
McCain, Donald
Inter Valley Health Plan Inc — Page 53
McCallister, Ben D, MD
BCBS of Kansas City — Page 244
Good Health HMO Inc — Page 247
McCallister, Ed
UMPC Health Plan Univ of
Pittsburgh Medical Center — Page 374
McCallister, Michael B
Humana Insurance Co - AL — Page 5
Humana Inc - AR — Page 27
Humana Inc - CO — Page 82
Humana Inc - DC — Page 98
Humana Inc - IA — Page 170
Humana Inc - GA — Page 132
Humana Inc - IN — Page 161
Humana Inc - IA — Page 170
Humana Health Care Plans
of Kansas & Missouri — Page 179
CHA Health - Humana — Page 184
Humana Inc -
Corporate Headquarters — Page 185
Humana Health Care Plans
of Lexington — Page 185
Humana Inc - MD — Page 203
Humana Inc - Grand Rapids
Michigan — Page 225
Humana Inc - MS — Page 241
Humana Inc - NE — Page 256
Humana Inc - NM — Page 280
Humana Inc - NC — Page 313
Humana Inc - ND — Page 317
Humana Health Plan of OH Inc — Page 328
Humana Inc - OK — Page 341
Humana Inc - SC — Page 384
Humana Inc - SD — Page 388
Humana Inc - TN — Page 396
Humana Health Care Plans
of Corpus Christi — Page 417

Index VIII: Personnel

Mahaney, Phil, MD
Atlantic Integrated Health Inc — Page 309
Mahar, Peter J, MD
CIGNA Healthcare of NH — Page 265
Maher, Dan
Nevada Pacific Dental — Page 262
Mahler, Mark, MD, MBA
Unison Health Plan - Corporate Headquarters — Page 372
Mahony, Patricia
SmileCare/Community Dental Services — Page 69
Mailloux, Kirsten
Employee Benefit Management Services Inc — Page 253
Maisel, Garry
Western Health Advantage — Page 75
Majerik, Michael
Magellan Health Services Inc — Page 91
Malboeuf, Roland
Pioneer Management Systems — Page 215
Malek, Pierre M, MD
Great-West Healthcare of CO — Page 81
Maleri, Carl
Preferred Care — Page 304
Malko, Elizabeth, MD
Anthem BCBS of NH — Page 265
Mallard, Leonard
Citrus Health Care Inc — Page 108
Mallatt, Kathy Ann
Coventry Health Care of Nebraska Inc — Page 255
Mallicoat, Jerry
Anthem BCBS of Indiana — Page 157
Malloy, Marc
Coventry Hlth Care Inc -GA Inc — Page 130
SouthCare/Hlthcre Preferred — Page 134
Maloney, Marie
BMC HealthNet Plan — Page 209
Maloney, Sheila
Santa Clara Family Health Plan — Page 67
Maltz, Allen
Blue Cross Blue Shield of MA — Page 209
Malvick, Steve
Williamette Dental of WA Inc — Page 457
Manchandia, Mahesh
Jaimini Health Inc — Page 53
Mancini, Kathie
Molina Healthcare of Ohio Inc — Page 330
Mancini-Peare, Lisa
Fallon Community Hlth Plan Inc — Page 211
Manders, Matt
CIGNA HealthCare — Corporate Headquarters — Page 360
Maness, Dianne
San Joaquin Foundation PPO — Page 67
Manheim, Joseph
Interplan Health Group — Page 53
Superien Health Network Inc — Page 335
Manley, Thomas
Texas Medical Foundation Health Quality Institute — Page 427
ManleyGamel, Tom
Texas Medical Foundation Health Quality Institute — Page 427
Manlove, Celia
AmeriGroup Texas Inc — Page 404
Mann, Robert, MD
Cooks Childrens Health Plan — Page 411
Mann, Susan
Encore Health Network — Page 160
Mann, Todd DPM
Preferred Podiatry Group — Page 152
Mannen, Dan L, OD
Vision Service Plan — Page 86
Manning, Allison
Americhoice of New Jersey — Page 268
Manning, Deborah
Fidelis SecureCare of Texas — Page 413

Manning, Dennis J, CLU, CHFC
Guardian Life Insurance Co of America — Page 294
Manning, Karen
Secure Health Plans of GA LLC — Page 133
Manning, Kim
Baptist Health Services Group — Page 392
Mansheim, Bernard J, MD
Coventry Health Care Inc — Corporate Headquarters — Page 201
Manson, Rick
Medica Health Plans — Page 236
Mantegia, Frank, DDS
Atlantic Dental Inc — Page 102
Mapnet, Bryan
Crawford and Co - Corporate Headquarters — Page 130
Maquiren, Janet
Blue Care Network of MI — Page 217
Marbut, Cliff, MD
HealthPlus Inc — Page 296
March, Cabrini T, MD
March Vision Care Inc — Page 58
March, Glenville A, Jr, MD
March Vision Care Inc — Page 58
Marchand, Pamella J
Complementary Hlthcre Plans — Page 345
Marchant, Paul
New West Health Plan — Page 254
Marchany, Zoraida
Blue Cross of Puerto Rico/ La Cruz Azul de Puerto Rico — Page 377
Marchese, Denise, RN
Affinity Health Plan Inc — Page 283
Marchetti, Paul
UnitedHealthcare of NY Inc — Page 306
Marciano, Nick, MD
Primary Provider Management Company Inc — Page 64
Marciniak, Steven
Care Choices HMO — Page 218
Marco, Judith
SummaCare Inc — Page 334
Marcoux, Sara
Delta Dental Plan of California — Page 44
Marcuccilli, Brinke
Trustmark Insurance Company — Page 153
Marcum, Sharon
CorpHealth Inc — Page 412
Marenger, Abby RN
Humana Medical Plan - Central Florida — Page 113
Margolies, Martin P
PRONJ, The Healthcare Quality Improvement Org of NJ — Page 276
Margolin, Leslie A
Kaiser Permanente - Kaiser Foundation Health Plan, Inc — Page 54
Margulis, Heidi S
Humana Inc - Corp Hdqrtrs — Page 185
Mariencheck, Jenifer L RN CCM
Windsor Health Plan of TN Inc — Page 401
Marier, Carl
Inland Empire Health Plan — Page 52
Marino, Catherine, MD, FACP, FACR
MagnaCare — Page 298
Marino, Robert A
Horizon BCBS of NJ — Page 273
Marino, William J
Horizon BCBS of NJ — Page 273
Horizon Hlthcre Services Inc — Page 274
Marjar, Kathy
UnitedHealthcare of Florida Inc — Page 122
Mark, Joseph D
Aveta Inc — Page 270
Markello, Sam, PhD
Kansas Foundation Mdcl Care — Page 179
Markle, Nancy
SummaCare Inc — Page 334

Marks, Richard
KPS Health Plans — Page 452
Marks, Steven, MD
PacificSource Health Plans — Page 350
Markson, Deborah
Denver Health Medical Plan Inc — Page 80
Markus, Rick
Beech Street Corporation — Corporate Headquarters — Page 36
Marlon, Anthony M, MD
Sierra Health Services Inc- Corporate Headquarters — Page 264
Maroney, Dawn C
CareMore Health Plan — Page 38
Marootian, Beth
Neighborhood Health Plan of Rhode Island — Page 380
Marquardt, Cynthia
Kaiser Foundation Health Plan - Mid Atlantic States — Page 203
Marquardt, Jeff
Arise Health Plan — Page 461
Marquardt, Kent
Premera BCBS of Alaska — Page 9
LifeWise Health Plan of OR — Page 348
LifeWise Health Plan of WA — Page 453
Premera - Corp Hdqrtrs — Page 454
Premera Blue Cross - Eastern — Page 454
Premera Blue Cross - Western — Page 454
Marques, Clarissa C, PhD
Magellan Health Services — Page 132
Marquez, Keith
MyMatrixx — Page 489
Marquez, Lorenzo
CommunityCare Managed Healthcare Plans of Oklahoma Inc — Page 340
CommunityCare Managed Healthcare Plans of Oklahoma Inc — Page 483
Marra, Carlene
Humana Health Care Plans of Kansas & Missouri — Page 179
Marraffino, Cyndi
Lane Oregon Health Plans — Page 347
Marrero, Juan
Opticare Managed Vision — Page 314
AECC Total Vision Health Plan of Texas Inc — Page 403
Marroquin, Paula
Vision Plan of America — Page 75
Marshall, William, MD
OSF Health Plans — Page 151
Marsola, David, RPH
CIGNA Healthcare - Cincinnati — Page 323
Martel, Thomas
CIGNA Healthcare of Virginia Inc - Richmond — Page 443
CIGNA Healthcare of Mid-Atlantic Inc — Page 201
Martie, John
Anthem BCBS of Colorado — Page 77
Rocky Mountain Hospital & Medical Services Inc — Page 85
Martin, Craig
United Concordia Co Inc - TX — Page 429
Martin, Elizabeth
Excellus BCBS, Central New York Region — Page 291
Martin, JoAnn
Ameritas Group Dental — Page 255
Martin, John
Physicians Plus Insurance Corporation — Page 469
Martin, Kay
Fara Healthcare Management — Page 190
Martin, Marcia
Gateway Health Plan Inc — Page 362
Martin, Pam
Delta Dental Plan of Missouri — Page 246

Index VIII: Personnel

Lucey, Kate
CIGNA Healthcare of NH — Page 265
Lucht, Jeffrey
Aetna Health Plans of
Mid-Atlantic — Page 441
Lucia, Frank
CIGNA Dental Health of CO — Page 78
CIGNA Dental Health of DE Inc — Page 95
Lucier, Paula
Abri Health Plan Inc — Page 461
Lucy, Edward A.
HIP Health Plan of New York — Page 296
Ludington, Cory
Community Hlth Ntwrk of CT Inc — Page 89
Ludka, Debbie
Navitus Health Solutions — Page 490
Ludlum, Beverly
Unison Health Plan of TN — Page 399
Ludwig, Eric C
Interactive Medical Systems — Page 313
Lufrano, Robert I, MD
Blue Cross Blue Shield of FL &
Health Options Inc — Page 104
Lugo, Rosemarie
Community Health Plan — Page 42
Lukenda, Richard J, DMD
Dental Group of New Jersey — Page 271
Lukenda, Susan
Dental Group of New Jersey — Page 271
Lukens, Kay
Preferred Chiropractic Care, PA — Page 179
Lulla, Naren
MagnaCare — Page 298
Lum, Andrew, MD
Kaiser Foundation Health
Plan Northwest — Page 347
Luman, Bob
Delta Dental Ins Co - GA — Page 131
Lumpkins, John E.
CompBenefits — Page 410
Lun, Allison
San Francisco Health Plan — Page 66
Luna, Armando
Blue Cross Blue Shield of FL &
Health Options Inc — Page 104
Lundien, Keith
Southwest Health Alliance
(SHALLC) — Page 425
Lusk, Jerry
Blue Cross Blue Shield of MT — Page 253
Luskin, Barbara
Grand Valley Health Plan — Page 221
Lustick, Martin, MD
Excellus BlueCross BlueShield,
Rochester Area — Page 292
Lifetime Healthcare Companies, The -
Corporate Headquarters — Page 298
Luter, Larry J, MD, FAAFP
Meritain Health Inc — Page 299
Meritain Health — Page 330
Luther, Dr John, MD
Dentistat (Insurance
Dentists of America) — Page 45
Lutz, Kathleen J
Integra Group — Page 329
Lutz, Lincoln
Kroger Prescription Plans — Page 487
Luzzatti, Renzo
Us-Rx Care — Page 496
Lyman, Cheryl
Universal Health Network -
Corporate Headquarters — Page 264
Lynaugh, Kathleen
UnitedHealthcare of Oregon — Page 352
Lynch, James R
Vision Service Plan — Page 75
Lynch, Richard D
Anthem BCBS of Maine — Page 195

Anthem BCBS of NH — Page 265
Lynch, Robert
Vision Service Plan — Page 86
Lynch, Stephen
Health Net Inc - Corp Hdqrtrs — Page 49
Health Net of California — Page 49
Health Net Hlth Plan of OR Inc — Page 346
Lynn, Robert E
Doral Dental USA — Page 464
Lynne, Donna
Kaiser Foundation Health
Plan of Colorado — Page 83
Lyon, Judith
Medavant National
Preferred Provider Network — Page 299
Lyons, Daniel, MD
Independence Blue Cross — Page 366
Lyons, Lisa
UnitedHealthcare of Arkansas — Page 28
Lyski, James
CIGNA HealthCare —
Corporate Headquarters — Page 360
CIGNA Healthcare of TX Inc — Page 409

M

Ma, Patricia
Denta Quest Ventures Inc — Page 211
MaGill, Julie
Great-West Healthcare of Texas -
Dallas — Page 415
Maar, Mary
Lifetime Healthcare Companies, The -
Corporate Headquarters — Page 298
Maas, Diane
Community Health Alliance — Page 159
Maassen, Martin J, MD
Individualized Care
Management Inc — Page 162
Maassen, Mimi
Atlantic Integrated Health Inc — Page 309
MacDonald, Gregg
UnitedHealthcare of Florida Inc — Page 121
MacDonald, Jan, RN
Care Network — Page 359
MacDonald, Steven
MyMatrixx — Page 489
MacDonald, Stuart
Community Hlth Ntwrk of CT Inc — Page 89
MacEwan, Pam
Group Health Cooperative — Page 141
Group Health Cooperative — Page 451
Group Health Cooperative of
Puget Sound — Page 452
MacEwen, Scott
KHS a KMG America Company — Page 385
MacGillivray, Colin A
Delta Dental of Rhode Island — Page 380
Altus Dental Ins Co Inc — Page 379
MacKinnon, Elinor
Blue Shield of California — Page 36
MacKinnon, Matthew
Preferred Care — Page 304
MacLean, Tom, MD
BCBS of New Mexico — Page 279
Macbeth, Charlotte, JD
MDwise — Page 163
Macedo, Amrish
Alignis Inc — Page 268
Macfie, Sam
Secure Health Plans of GA LLC — Page 133
Mach, John
UnitedHealthcare of MA — Page 216
Mach, John R, Jr, MD
Evercare of Texas LLC — Page 413

Macheledt, Cheryl
First Plan of Minnesota — Page 235
Machtan, Kenneth
Group Health Cooperative
South Central Wisconsin — Page 464
Mack, David J
Lifetime Healthcare Companies, The -
Corporate Headquarters — Page 298
Mackail, Christopher E
Md-Individual Practice Association Inc
(MD IPA) — Page 204
Mackenzie, Laurinda
Spectera Vision Inc - Indiana — Page 166
Mackenzie, Ranald, OD
Henry Ford OptimEyes — Page 224
Mackler, Robert
Pacific Health Alliance — Page 62
Macko, William
WelBorn Health Plans — Page 167
Mackrell, James
Aetna Hlth Plans of Mid-Atlantic — Page 441
Aetna Inc - Virginia — Page 441
Madaus, James, OD
S V S Visions Inc — Page 231
Madden, Kathleen
Connecticare Inc — Page 89
Madden, Machelle
Liberty Dental Plan of CA — Page 56
Maddox, Lisa
Galaxy Health Network — Page 414
Madeaux, Judy
Yale University Health Plan — Page 93
Madeja, Peter C
GENEX Services — Page 363
Madill, Fred O
Unison Health Plan of TN — Page 399
Madill, Fred O
Unison Health Plan -
Corporate Headquarters — Page 372
Madison, Babette L
Mid-Atlantic Managed Care
Organization of PA Inc — Page 369
Madrid, Diane
Molina Healthcare of NM — Page 281
Mae, Willie
Community Medical Alliance — Page 210
Maesaka, Clifford T, Jr, DDS
Delta Dental Plan of KY Inc — Page 184
Maeyher, Phyllis
American Specialty
Health Plans Inc — Page 33
Mageau, Kim
Prime Therapeutics — Page 493
Maggio, Frank A, DDS
Delta Dental Plan of Illinois — Page 145
Magill, Julie
Great-West Healthcare of Texas -
Austin — Page 414
Magill, Martin A
National Medical Health Card Systems -
Corporate Headquarter — Page 489
Maginnis, John
BCBS of LA Inc — Page 189
HMO Louisiana Inc — Page 191
Magnuson, Richard
Group Health Cooperative — Page 141
Group Health Cooperative — Page 451
Group Health Cooperative of
Puget Sound — Page 452
Group Health Options Inc — Page 452
Maguire, Sharon
Health Net of California — Page 49
Magusin, Barbara
Premera BCBS of Alaska — Page 9
Premera - Corp Hdqrtrs — Page 454
Premera Blue Cross - Eastern — Page 454
Premera Blue Cross - Western — Page 454

Copyright MCIC -- The National Directory of Managed Care Organizations, Seventh Edition

Index VIII: Personnel

Linder, Jerry
Community Care Plus — Page 249
Linder, Michael J
Blue Cross Blue Shield of AZ — Page 12
Linderman, Pamela
Ventura County Hlth Care Plan — Page 73
Lindgren, Charles
Dimension Health (PPO) — Page 109
Lindlahr, Tara
Avante Behavioral Health Plan — Page 35
Lindley, Andrew
Employee Benefit Management Services Inc — Page 253
Lindquist, Brent
Avante Behavioral Health Plan — Page 35
Lindquist, Tom
UnitedHealthcare of MI Inc — Page 242
Lindsay, Jane
Blue Cross of Idaho — Page 141
Lindsey, James R
California Dental Network Inc — Page 37
Ling Antoire, Wer
Pacific IPA — Page 63
Lingenfelter, John, MD
Evercare Select — Page 15
Lining, Jodi
MDX Hawaii — Page 138
Link, Barbara
Health Management Ntwrk Inc — Page 16
Linkogle, Dorian
Aetna Health of California Inc — Page 31
Aetna Inc - Dental Care of CA — Page 32
Linsin, Catherine PhD
Mercy Health Plans of MO Inc — Page 249
Lipinski, Denise
Hometown Health Plan — Page 260
Lipomi, Jack D
Penn Highlands Health Plan — Page 370
Liponis, Lisa
Medical Network Inc — Page 197
Lippai, Steve
Combined Insurance Company of America — Page 145
Lippai, Steven E FSA
Sterling Life Insurance Co — Page 520
Lippert, Cheryl
UnitedHealthcare of Louisiana — Page 193
List, Samm M
South Bay Independent Physicians Medical Group Inc — Page 69
Liston, Tom
Humana Insurance Co - AL — Page 5
Humana Inc - Co — Page 82
Humana Inc - DC — Page 98
Humana Inc - ND — Page 317
Little, John M, MD
Blue Cross Blue Shield of SC - Corporate Hqtrs — Page 383
Little, Joyce F
Colorado Choice Health Plan/ San Luis Valley HMO Inc — Page 79
Littleton, Bruno
Humana Health Plan - Jacksonville — Page 113
Littleton, Lynn
ppoNEXT — Page 423
Livermore, Duke
Blue Cross Blue Shield of Florida & Health Options Inc — Page 104
LoBasso, Tony
Community First Hlth Plans Inc — Page 410
Lobe, Michelle
Encore Health Network — Page 160
Locke, Julie
AmeriGroup Maryland Inc — Page 199
Locke, Sandy
Mutual Assurance Administrators Inc — Page 342
Loder, Sandra
Clear Choice Health Plans — Page 345

Loepp, Daniel J
Blue Preferred Plan-BCBS MI — Page 218
Loerch, Bob
Pearle Vision Managed Care - HMO of Texas Inc — Page 423
Loft, Richard S, MD
Ventura County Foundation for Medical Care — Page 73
Lohcamp, Doug
BCBS of New Mexico — Page 279
HMO New Mexico Inc — Page 280
Loi, Liang Lee
NevadaCare Inc — Page 262
Lollar, Keith
GroupLink Inc — Page 160
Lollar, Ketrina
GroupLink Inc — Page 160
Lomba, Susan
Community First Hlth Plans Inc — Page 410
Lon, Robyn, Dr
PharmAvail Benefit Management Company — Page 492
London, Alan, MD
CHN MCO — Page 322
London, Robert, MD
Anthem BCBS of Colorado — Page 77
Rocky Mountain Hospital & Medical Services Inc — Page 85
Londow, Kathy
Memphis Managed Care Corp — Page 397
Long, JoAnne
Regence Blue Shield — Page 456
Long, Laura, MD
BlueChoice Health Plan of SC Inc — Page 383
Long, Marshall
Crawford and Co - Corporate Headquarters — Page 130
Longalong-Coz, Erlinda
Renaissance Hlth Systems Inc — Page 119
Longendyke, Robert
Medica Health Plans — Page 236
Longtin, Sandie
PacificSource Health Plans — Page 350
Lonsdale, Winston
Av-Med Health Plan - Gainesville — Page 102
Av-Med Health Plan - Jacksonville — Page 102
Av-Med Health Plan - Miami — Page 103
Av-Med Health Plan - Orlando — Page 103
Av-Med Health Plan - Tampa — Page 103
Looney, C Evans
Humana Inc - Tennessee — Page 396
Loos, Richard
Chinese Community Hlth Plan — Page 39
Loper, David
HAS Premier Providers Inc — Page 415
Lopez De Choudens, Gerald
Medical Card System — Page 377
Lopez, Cheryl
Lovelace Health Plan — Page 280
Lopez, John
Lakewood Health Plan Inc — Page 56
Lopez, Julia
Triple-S Inc — Page 378
Lopez, Nilda
Medica Healthcare Plans Inc — Page 116
Lopez-Fernandez, Orlando, MD
Preferred Care Partners Inc — Page 118
Lopilato, David M
Olympus Managed Health Care Inc — Page 117
Lord, Jonathan T, MD
Humana Insurance Co - AL — Page 5
Humana Inc - AR — Page 27
Humana Inc - CO — Page 82

Humana Inc - DC — Page 98
Humana Inc - IA — Page 170
Humana Inc - Corp Hdqrtrs — Page 185
Humana Inc - MD — Page 203
Humana Inc - Grand Rapids, MI — Page 225
Humana Inc - MS — Page 241
Humana Inc - NE — Page 256
Humana Inc - NM — Page 280
Humana Inc - ND — Page 317
Humana Inc - OK — Page 341
Humana Inc - SC — Page 384
Humana Inc - SD — Page 388
Humana Inc - UT — Page 435
Humana Inc - WY — Page 473
Lorda, Pat
Southwest Health Alliance (SHALLC) — Page 425
Lorentz, William B, Jr, MD
Medcost LLC — Page 313
Lorenz, Bruce
Molina Healthcare of NM — Page 281
Lorenzen, Steve
Blue Cross Blue Shield of NE — Page 255
Lorge, Vicki
Arise Health Plan — Page 461
Lott, Jim
LA Care Health Plan — Page 55
Loudermilk, Kerry
Phoebe Health Partners — Page 133
Lounsbery, Christine, PharmD
DakotaCare — Page 387
Louro, Judith
Contra Costa Health Plan — Page 43
Lovata, Debbie, RN
Texas Medical Foundation Health Quality Institute — Page 427
Lovato, Lou
Blue Shield of California — Page 36
Love, Vincent J
Alignis Inc — Page 268
Lovelace, John
UMPC Health Plan Univ of Pittsburgh Medical Center — Page 374
Low, William W
Medical Review Institute - Corporate Headquarters — Page 435
Lowe, Art
Bluegrass Family Health Inc — Page 183
Lower, Kathy
Anthem BCBS of Kentucky (HMO Kentucky) — Page 183
Lowery-Born, Bebo
Blue Cross Blue Shield of KS — Page 177
Lown, Ryan
Pueblo Health Care — Page 84
Lowry, Jeffrey K
Univera Healthcare of Western New York — Page 307
Lowry, Robert
Neighborhood Health Providers — Page 302
Loy, Bryan, MD
Humana Health Care Plans of Lexington — Page 185
Humana Health Plan - KY — Page 185
Lubben, David J
UnitedHealth Group — Corporate Headquarters — Page 238
Lubbers, Serena
ProviDRs Care Network — Page 181
Luben, William J
American WholeHealth Networks Inc — Page 442
Lubitz, Mitch
Humana Inc - South Carolina — Page 384
Lucci, Barbara
Safeguard Hlth Enterprises Inc — Page 66
Luce, David B, MD
Wisconsin Physician Services Insurance Company — Page 471

Index VIII: Personnel

Lawhead, Jean
Colorado Dental Service Inc,
dba: Delta Dental Plan of CO — Page 80
Lawrence, Joseph
Managed Care Consultants — Page 261
Lawrence, Melissa
Aetna Inc - Tulsa — Page 339
Lawrence, Ron
Blue Cross Blue Shield of GA — Page 128
Lawrence, Shawna
Preferred Therapy Providers of America -
Corp Headquarters — Page 19
Lawreno, Joseph
Horizon Health PPO — Page 261
Lawrenz, Donald R
Best Health Plans — Page 36
Layland, David, MD
AmeriGroup Texas Inc — Page 404
Layman, Katrina, RN
Carelink Health Plans — Page 459
Le Meir, Sherrie
Blue Cross Blue Shield of AL — Page 3
LeDuc, Gary
ACN Group — Page 233
LeForge, Gary
ConnectCare — Page 219
LeMar, Jerry, DO
Coventry Hlth Care Inc — IA — Page 169
Leach, Charles W, MBA
Health Design Plus — Page 327
Leaf, Robert
American Dental Examiners — Page 284
Learner, Rebecca
Scan Health Plan — Page 68
Leary, Edward, MD
Humana Hlth Care Plans of IL — Page 151
Leary, Mary
Medical Associates Hlth Plans — Page 172
Leber, Jeff
BCBS of Mississippi — Page 241
Lechner, David
LifeWise Health Plan of OR — Page 348
Lederberg, Michele B
Blue Cross Blue Shield of
Rhode Island — Page 379
Lederman, Janet
Grand Valley Health Plan — Page 221
Lee, Chad
University Health Alliance — Page 138
Lee, Christine V, PharmD, CLS
American Health Care — Page 480
Lee, David
SHPS Inc — Page 186
Lee, Douglas A
BioScrip Inc — Page 481
Lee, Frank
Contra Costa Health Plan — Page 43
Lee, Grover C, Pharm D, BCMCM
American Health Care — Page 480
Lee, Howard KF
University Health Alliance — Page 138
Lee, Kathy
Scott & White Health Plan — Page 424
Lee, Laurel A MSPH
Molina HealthCare of WA Inc — Page 453
Lee, Linda
Orange Prevention &
Treatment Integrated — Page 60
Lee, Sherri E, CPA
AmeriGroup Corporation — Page 442
Lee, Steve, MD
Humana Medical Plan -
Central Florida — Page 113
Humana Medical Plan -
Daytona — Page 113
Lee, Wayne, MD
Global Medical Management — Page 110
Lee, Yolanda
Chinese Community Health Plan — Page 39

Lee-McCord, Jackie
Sagamore Health Network Inc — Page 164
Lefko, Bruce
HealthEOS by MultiPlan — Page 466
Lefler, Mark, MD
1st Medical Network — Page 127
Leftwich, Inda
Strategic Health
Development Corporation — Page 119
Lehman, Brian
Ohio State University Managed
Health Care Systems Inc — Page 332
Lehr, William
Capital Blue Cross — Page 359
Keystone Health Plan Central — Page 367
Lehrer, Randee
CIGNA Dental Health of NC Inc — Page 310
Leichtle, Robert A
BCBS of South Carolina -
Corporate Hqtrs — Page 383
Leider, Harry L, MD
XL Health — Page 207
Leihbacher, Carloyn
Hudson Health Plan — Page 297
Lemoine, Jean Claude, MD
Atlantis Health Plan — Page 285
Lemonds, Jeannine
HealthPlus of Michigan — Page 224
Lemons, Susan
SHPS Inc — Page 186
Lenahan, Michael G
Active Health Management — Page 441
Lendino, Angelo
Dental Care of America Ltd — Page 146
Lenhart, Jack, RN
Valley Preferred — Page 375
Lent, Ellen
Contra Costa Health Plan — Page 43
Lentine, Anthony
Golden Dental Plans Inc — Page 221
Lentine, Joseph S
Golden Dental Plans Inc — Page 221
Lentine, Joseph T
Dencap Dental Plans — Page 220
Lentine, Sam
Golden Dental Plans Inc — Page 221
Lentz, Loran
Navitus Health Solutions — Page 490
Lenza, Robert
Anthem BCBS of NH — Page 265
Leon, Benjamin, Jr
Leon Medical Centers
Health Plan Inc — Page 115
Leonard, Dennis
Denta Quest Mid-Atlantic Inc — Page 202
Denta Quest Ventures Inc — Page 211
Leonard, Karen
CIGNA Healthcare of NH — Page 265
Leone, Nancy, RN
Medwatch LLC — Page 116
Leopold, Larry
Washington Dental Service — Page 457
Lepore, Michele
BMC HealthNet Plan — Page 209
Lerer, Rene, MD
Magellan Health Services Inc — Page 91
Magellan Health Services — Page 132
Magellan Behavioral Health — Page 274
Magellan Behavioral Health — Page 274
Lerner, Ken
Blue Cross Blue Shield of NC — Page 310
Lesley, Craig
Physicians Health Plan of
Mid-Michigan — Page 228
Lesley, E Craig
Delta Dental Plan of Ohio Inc — Page 324
Lesnewski, Judy
PPO Oklahoma Inc — Page 341

Lessin, Leeba
CareMore Health Plan — Page 38
Lessner, Wanda
CareFirst BCBS — Page 200
Lettko, John G
Medavant National
Preferred Provider Network — Page 299
Leuchars, Elaine
Vision Service Plan — Page 75
Vision Service Plan — Page 86
Levicki, George A, DDS
Delta Dental of Virginia — Page 443
Levin, Howard, OD
Block Vision of Texas Inc — Page 405
Levin, Julie
Hudson Health Plan — Page 297
Levine, Barry
Pequot Pharmaceutical Ntwrk — Page 491
Levine, Chuck
Group Health Options Inc — Page 452
Levine, Gary
Mercy Health Plans of MO Inc — Page 249
Levine, Hal DO
ValueOptions - Corp Hdqrtrs — Page 447
Levine, Susan
Behavioral Health Systems Inc — Page 3
Levinson, Anthony
Coalition America Inc — Page 129
Lewis, Catherine
MedFocus Radiology Network — Page 58
Lewis, David
Deseret Healthcare — Page 434
Lewis, Kenneth J
FirstCarolinaCare — Page 312
Lewis, Kim
UnitedHealthcare of Alabama — Page 7
UnitedHealthcare of Louisiana — Page 193
Lewis, Linda, MD
Innovative Care Management — Page 347
Lewis, Nam
Great-West Healthcare of OR — Page 346
Lewis, Steve
Health First Health Plans Inc — Page 111
Lewis, T David
UnitedHealthcare of MI Inc — Page 242
Lewis-Clapper, Caskie, MS
Magellan Health Services Inc — Page 91
Magellan Health Services — Page 132
Magellan Behavioral Health — Page 274
Leyden, Thomas, BA
MPRO — Page 227
Li, Grace, MHA
On Lok Senior Health Services — Page 60
Liang, Louise, MD
Kaiser Permanente - Kaiser
Foundation Health Plan, Inc — Page 54
Libby, Charlene
Nevada Prfrrd Professionals — Page 262
Liberato, Christine
Sun Health Medisun — Page 20
Liburdi, Matthew
Mercer First Choice — Page 369
Lider, Jerry
Community Care Plus — Page 249
Light, Leao
Health Management Network Inc — Page 16
Lihott, Karem
Physicians Health Plan of
Northern Indiana — Page 164
Lilly, John P MD
4MOST Health Network — Page 459
Limoreaux, William
Health Net - New Jersey — Page 272
Lindbion, Peter
Pacific IPA — Page 63
Linde, Michael
Med-Valu Inc — Page 329
Linden, Karen
Beech Street Corporation —
Corporate Headquarters — Page 36

Index VIII: Personnel

Kupfer, Charles
Medical Eye Services Inc — Page 58
Kurek, Tim
Wellpath Select Inc — Page 315
Kuretich, Kathleen
Newport Dental Plan — Page 60
Kurian, Jaya
Heritage Provider Network Inc — Page 50
Kurpiel, Tom
UnitedHealthcare of South FL — Page 122
Kutner, David
American Healthguard Corp — Page 33
Kutz, George
Geisinger Health Plan — Page 363
Kwavnick, Myer
Vista Hlthplan of South FL Inc — Page 123
Kyle, Frank
Altius Health Plans — Page 433
Kynsz, Janet, MD
Great Expressions
Dental Centers — Page 222
Kynsz, Walter, Jr, MD
Great Expressions
Dental Centers — Page 222

L

La Haye, Jim
Prevea Health Network — Page 469
LaBarga, Maria, MD
CarePlus Health Plans Inc — Page 106
LaBresh, Kenneth A, MD, FAHA
Masspro Inc — Page 213
LaCombe, Philip M
Health New England — Page 212
LaFrance, Jason, MA
Community Behavioral Healthcare
Cooperative of Pennsylvania — Page 361
LaGere-Litsch, Tracie
Oklahoma Foundation for
Medical Quality — Page 342
LaGralious, Thomas
South Bay Independent
Physicians Medical Group Inc — Page 69
LaGreca, Celann
Blue Cross Blue Shield of NE — Page 255
LaHousse, Carolyn
Review Works — Page 230
LaMagna, Kathy
Vista Healthplan of South FL Inc — Page 123
LaMere, Hannah
Metropolitan Health Plan — Page 237
LaTourette, Charlie
Oregon Dealthan — Page 349
Labby, David, MD
Health Plan of CareOregon Inc — Page 346
Lach, Maureen
Citrus Health Care Inc — Page 108
Lachman, Barry, MD
Parkland Community
Health Plan Inc — Page 422
Lad, Rajnikant, MD
Community Behavioral Healthcare
Cooperative of Pennsylvania — Page 361
Laderman, Andy
Safeguard Health Plans Inc — Page 424
Ladig, Curtis R
Delta Dental Plan of KY Inc — Page 184
Lagorio, Lora
Medcore Health Plan — Page 58
Lahr, John, MD
EyeMed Vision Care LLC — Page 325
Lahti, Alan
Humana Health Plan of Austin — Page 419
Laiben, Gregg R, MD
Primaris — Page 250

Lail, Neal
Fidelis SecureCare of NC — Page 312
Laird, Brend
Delta Dental Plan of MI Inc — Page 220
Laird, Gina
HmoLouisiana Inc — Page 191
Lake, Betty
ACN Group — Page 233
Lally, Joseph
Delta Dental Plan of MN — Page 235
Lam, Troy
Alameda Alliance for Health — Page 33
Lambdin, Paul
Health Net Inc - Northeast
Corporate Headquarters — Page 91
Lambert, Paul
Delta Dental Ins Co - AL — Page 4
Lambrukos, William H
Delta Dental Plan of NH — Page 265
Lamendola, Damien
WellDyne Rx — Page 497
Lamirault, Ingrid
Alameda Alliance for Health — Page 33
Lamkin, Jim
Community Care Plus — Page 249
Lammie, Scott
UMPC Health Plan Univ of
Pittsburgh Medical Center — Page 374
Lammons, Nicole
Provider Ntwrks of America Inc — Page 424
Lamoreaux, Leon D
Priority Health — Page 230
Excellus BlueCross BlueShield — Page 290
Lamoreaux, William
Health Net Inc - Northeast
Corporate Headquarters — Page 91
Health Net - New York — Page 295
Lanava, Tom, MD
Partners National Health
Plans of North Carolina Inc — Page 314
Lancaster, Kathy
Kaiser Foundation Health
Plan of Southern California — Page 54
Kaiser Foundation Health
Plan of Ohio — Page 329
Land, Kenneth
Managed Care Consultants — Page 261
Landin, Lindie
Delta Dental Plan of WI — Page 463
Landis, Robert
Comprehensive Bhvrl Care Inc — Page 108
Landkamer, Steve
Partnership Health Plan Inc — Page 522
Landry, Joann
Community Medical Alliance — Page 210
Neighborhood Health Plan — Page 214
Lane, Mark
Centercare Inc — Page 287
Lane, Mark L
Fidelis Care New York — Page 293
New York State Catholic
Health Plan Inc — Page 303
Lang, James, PharmD
Blue Care Network of MI — Page 217
Langenus, John
First Health Group Corp — Page 147
Langer, Donald
AmeriChoice of New York — Page 284
Langlois, Darrel
BCBS of Louisiana Inc — Page 189
HMO Louisiana Inc — Page 191
Lanoon, Allan R
Hawaii Medical Services Association -
BC/BS of Hawaii — Page 137
Lantos, Phyllis
New York Presbyterian
Community Health Plan — Page 302

Lapetina, Antoinette
PerfectHealth Ins Co — Page 304
Lapp, Roger
Scan Health Plan — Page 68
Laraway, Dennis L
Scott & White Health Plan — Page 424
Larimore, Rhonda
UMPC Health Plan Univ of
Pittsburgh Medical Center — Page 374
Larkin, Betty
Jackson Memorial Health Plan — Page 115
Larossi, Corte
Coalition America Inc — Page 129
Larsen, Chris
Regence Blue Shield of Idaho — Page 142
Larson, Beverly, RN
Health Tradition Health Plans — Page 466
Larson, Jan, RN
Managed Health Services
Insurance Corporation — Page 467
Larson, Michael
Iowa Foundation for
Medical Care/Encompass — Page 170
Larson, Milt
First Plan of Minnesota — Page 235
Larson, Nicki
Employee Benefit
Management Services Inc — Page 253
Larson, Steven B
AmeriGroup Maryland Inc — Page 199
Larson, Steven E MD
Inland Empire
Foundation for Medical Care — Page 52
Laspina, Laurie
United Concordia Co Inc - CA — Page 72
Lathrop-Warriner, Laura
Community Health Plan — Page 42
Latimer, Scott, MD
Humana Medical Plan -
Central Florida — Page 113
Humana Mdcl Plan - Daytona — Page 113
Latkowski, Anglea
Community Health Alliance — Page 159
Lattig, John
Aetna Health of California Inc — Page 31
Latts, Lisa, MD
Anthem BCBS of Colorado — Page 77
Rocky Mountain Hospital &
Medical Services Inc — Page 85
Laudeman, Lisa A, CPAM, CCAM
Blue Ridge Health Network — Page 357
Laudenslager, Debbie
KPS Health Plans — Page 452
Laufenburger, Mike
Safeguard Health Plans Inc — Page 424
Safeguard Hlth Enterprises Inc — Page 66
Lauzon, Thomas
Health Plan of Michigan — Page 224
Lavelle, J Stewart
Coventry Health Care Inc —
Corporate Headquarters — Page 201
Lavely, David
AECC Total Vision Health
Plan of Texas Inc — Page 403
Opticare Managed Vision — Page 314
Lavia, Denny
Unicare Health Plans of
the Midwest Inc — Page 153
Lavine, Faith
Preferred Provider Organization of
Michigan (PPOM) — Page 229
Lavoie, Raymond J, Jr
Neighborhood Health Plan
of Rhode Island — Page 380
Law, Cindy
Dental Care Plus Inc — Page 324

Index VIII: Personnel

Koch, Connie
UMPC Health Plan Univ of
Pittsburgh Medical Center — Page 374
Koch, Jeff
OSF Health Plans — Page 151
Koch, Robert
Preferred Care Incorporated — Page 370
Kodora, Richard, MBA
APS Healthcare Inc — Page 199
APS Healthcare Northwest Inc — Page 253
Koehler, Dawn
Great Lakes Health Plan — Page 222
Koehler, Michael J
UnitedHealthcare of Texas Inc -
Houston — Page 429
Koehn, Gregg
Oklahoma Foundation for
Medical Quality — Page 342
Koeling, Pat
AtlantiCare Health Plans Inc — Page 269
Koening, Teresa, MD
SummaCare Inc — Page 334
Kofsky, Lisa
Neighborhood Hlth Partnership — Page 116
Kogan, Allan, MD
Great-West Healthcare of Texas -
Austin — Page 414
Great-West Healthcare of Texas -
Dallas — Page 415
Great-West Healthcare of Texas -
Houston — Page 415
Koh, Rachel
Community Health Plan of WA — Page 450
Kohl, Rebecca
Presbyterian Health Plan — Page 281
Kohler, Nancy
KEPRO — Page 367
Kohn, Judy A
HIP Health Plan of New York — Page 296
Kohn, Patricia
Interplan Health Group — Page 419
Kohut, Mary Kay
KEPRO — Page 367
Koizumi, Noreen
Community Health Group — Page 41
Kokoszka, Margaret
HealthPlus of Michigan — Page 224
Kolb, David
HFN Inc — Page 150
Kole-James, Augustine, MD
Pro-Care Health Plan — Page 230
Kollefrath, Dan
Physicians United Plan Inc — Page 118
Kolodgy, Robert James
Paramount Care of Michigan — Page 228
Kolowrat, Jean M
Wisconsin Physician
Services Insurance Company — Page 471
Konigsberg, Alvin
National Health Plan — Page 302
Konzen, Mike
Group Health Cooperative
of Eau Claire — Page 465
Koo, Doug
CBCA Care Management Inc — Page 408
Koransky, Alan
Best Health Plans — Page 36
Kordish, Roberta, RN, MSN
Health Design Plus — Page 327
Korenek, Becky
UniCare Health Plans of TX Inc — Page 428
Korpal, Gail
Phoebe Health Partners — Page 133
Kosak, Traci
Neighborhood Hlth Providers — Page 302
Kosecoff, Jacqueline, PhD
PacifiCare Health Systems-
Corporate Headquarters — Page 62

Kosior, Robert A
Health New England — Page 212
Kosloff, Tom
ACN Group — Page 233
Kota, Bob
Health Plan,
The Hometown Region — Page 327
Kotcamp, Wendy D
Excellus BCBS, Central
New York Region — Page 291
Kotecki, John
Dentistat (Insurance
Dentists of America) — Page 45
Kotin, Anthony M, MD
Magellan Health Services Inc — Page 91
Magellan Health Services — Page 132
Magellan Behavioral Health — Page 274
Kotonias-Ray, Carol
PacifiCare of Oregon — Page 350
Kottooor, Anil
WellCare Health Plans Inc -
Corporate Headquarters — Page 124
Kottoor, Anil
Preferred One — Page 93
Koumaras, George
Aetna Inc - Corp Hdqrtrs — Page 87
Aetna Inc Life Insurance Co — Page 87
Koury, David
Health Net of California — Page 49
Kovaleski, Kerry, CPUM
Arizona Foundation for
Medical Care — Page 11
Kovel, Scott
BCBS of Western New York — Page 285
Kowalski, Robert
Parkland Community
Health Plan Inc — Page 422
Kowamura, Marilyn
Kaiser Foundation Health Plan - Mid
Atlantic States — Page 203
Kowitz, M Donald
Saint Mary's HealthFirst — Page 263
Kozal, Ann
Grand Valley Health Plan — Page 221
Koziara, Michael R
Care Choices HMO — Page 218
Koziej, Marcin, MD
Paragon Biomedical Inc — Page 491
Kozman, Melissa, BA
Health Design Plus — Page 327
Kracik, Jay
Preferred Podiatry Group — Page 152
Kraemer, Karen
HealthPartners Inc — Page 236
Krafka, Thomas, MD
DakotaCare — Page 387
Kraft, Judy RN, MSN
Driscoll Children's Hlth Plan — Page 412
Krainert, John
Partnership HealthPlan of CA — Page 64
Kramer, Debbie
Assurant Health - Corp Hdqrtrs — Page 462
Kramer, James
Neighborhood Health Providers — Page 302
Krause, John
Care-Plus Dental Plans Inc — Page 462
Kraymer, Lisa
Santa Clara Family Health Plan — Page 67
Krebens, Sara
Sutter Senior Care — Page 515
Krebs, David M
Humana Inc/PCA - Puerto Rico — Page 377
Humana Inc/PCA - Puerto Rico — Page 518
Krebs, Rose
Health Net of Arizona — Page 17
Kremer, Adi
Health Plan of San Joaquin, The — Page 50

Krenek, Bryant H, Jr
Healthcare Partners of
East Texas Inc — Page 416
Krentzlin, Paul, MD, MBA
Horizon BCBS of NJ — Page 273
Krigstein, Alan
Keystone Mercy Health Plan — Page 368
Kring, Gerald W
Horizon Health PPO — Page 261
Managed Care Consultants — Page 261
Krisologo-Elliott, Cris
KPS Health Plans — Page 452
Kroft, Jim
Nevada Prfrrd Professionals — Page 262
Universal Health Network -
Corporate Headquarters — Page 264
Kropp, Robert, MD
CIGNA Healthcare of Florida — Page 107
Krovisky, Mary Beth
Aetna Inc - Pennsylvania — Page 355
Kruger, Daniel A
Sierra Health Services Inc-
Corporate Headquarters — Page 264
Krugman, Mark E
Orange County PPO — Page 61
Krumholz, Alan, MD
Health Tradition Health Plans — Page 466
Krupa, David
Blue Cross Blue Shield of VT — Page 439
Vermont Hlth Plans (Blue Care) — Page 439
Kruse, Lowell
Community Health Plan — Page 245
Krysh, Josesph C
Medical Mutual of Ohio — Page 330
Krystopolski, Ruth
Sanford Health Plan of MN — Page 238
Sanford Health Plan — Page 388
Kubel, Judy Y
Managed Health Network — Page 57
Kuckarni, Tammaji, MD
Harmony Health Plan — Page 148
Kudgis, Leonard
Horizon NJ Health — Page 274
Kudla, Keith
WellCare Health Plans Inc -
Corporate Headquarters — Page 124
Harmony Health Plan — Page 148
Kuester, Cynthia A
Health Resources Inc — Page 161
Kuhn, Jeffrey Craig
Paramount Care of Michigan — Page 228
Kujawa, Kevin
American Specialty
Health Plans Inc — Page 33
Kulbick, Robert
Cypress Care — Page 483
Kulich, Roman T
Molina Healthcare of MI Inc — Page 227
Kulka, Don
Great Expressions
Dental Centers — Page 222
Kummer, Randy
Physicians Health Plan of
Northern Indiana — Page 164
Kumpula, Dale
Trustmark Insurance Company — Page 153
Kunder, Celissa
Unipsych Systems — Page 120
Kunes, Steven M
Health Tradition Health Plans — Page 466
Kunkle, Jeffrey A
Athens Area Health
Plan Select Inc — Page 127
Kunkle, John
Nationwide Better Health — Page 204
Kunz, Eileen, MPH
On Lok Senior Health Services — Page 512
Kunz, Heidi
Blue Shield of California — Page 36

Index VIII: Personnel

Kile, Gregory
Valley Preferred — Page 375
Kiley, Catherine
Fidelis SecureCare of MI Inc — Page 221
Kilgore, Margaret
Coventry Health Care of KS Inc — Page 245
Killeen, Patrick
Gundersen Lutheran
Health Plan Inc — Page 465
Killilea, Terry
Regence Valucare — Page 436
Killingsworth, Cleve L
Blue Cross Blue Shield of MA — Page 209
Kimaitas, Tracy
SummaCare Inc — Page 334
Kime, Stuart
MyMatrixx — Page 489
Kimrey, Tom
Dental Network of America — Page 146
Kincaid, Catharine
Molina Healthcare of NM — Page 281
Kincheloe, Earl, DDS
Delta Dental Plan of WY — Page 473
Kindred, Kim
Provider Networks of America Inc — Page 424
King, Al
Memphis Managed Care Corp — Page 397
King, Alice
Affinity Health Plan Inc — Page 283
King, Allan F
IPRO — Page 298
King, Amy
Complementary Hlthcare Plans — Page 345
King, Carl
Aetna Inc - Altamonte Springs — Page 99
Aetna Inc - Florida — Page 100
Aetna Inc - Jacksonville — Page 100
Aetna Inc - Plantation — Page 100
Aetna Inc - Houston — Page 403
King, Clarence C, III
Aetna Inc - Georgia — Page 127
King, David
WellDyne Rx — Page 497
King, Ethelle
CO/OP Optical Services Inc — Page 219
King, Jennifer
Humana Health Care
Plans of Dallas — Page 417
Humana Health Plan of Austin — Page 419
King, Ray, MD
Physicians Health Plan
of South Michigan — Page 229
King, Richard
Blue Cross Blue Shield of AL — Page 3
King, Ronald F
Blue Cross Blue Shield of OK — Page 339
Bluelincs HMO — Page 340
King, Tim
Great-West Healthcare of GA — Page 131
Kingsdale, Jon M, PhD
Tufts Health Plan — Page 216
Kinkelaar, Judy, RN, BSN
CIMRO Quality
Healthcare Solutions — Page 144
Kinn, Grant
RxPlus Pharmacies Inc — Page 494
Kinney, James T
Dms Dental Plan — Page 380
Kinney, Karen
Provider Ntwrks of America Inc — Page 424
Kinney, Linda S
Dms Dental Plan — Page 380
Kiraly, Thomas E
Concentra Inc — Page 411
Kircher, Debra A
Health Partners — Page 364
Kirdzik, Jamie
Northeast Health Direct LLC — Page 92

Kirges, Jenny
PacifiCare of Arizona — Page 19
Kirk, Cliff
Blue Cross Blue Shield of WY — Page 473
Kirk, Gary M, MD
Community Choice Michigan — Page 219
Kirk, Jennifer
Managed HealthCare
Northwest Inc — Page 348
Kirk, Troy
PacificSource Health Plans — Page 350
Kirkendall, Richard, PhD
Inter Valley Health Plan Inc — Page 53
Kirkland, Jennifer, RN, BS, CPH
CIMRO Quality
Healthcare Solutions — Page 144
Kirkman, Brett
HealthLink of Arkansas Inc — Page 27
Mercy Health Plans of MO Inc — Page 249
Kirkwood, Jonna
1st Medical Network — Page 127
Peach State Health Plan — Page 133
Kish, Angela S
Doral Dental USA — Page 464
Kissner, Larry J
UnitedHealthcare of Kentucky — Page 186
Kite, Carl J, MD
Health Plan,
The Hometown Region — Page 327
Kitson, Bonnie
Group Health Plan Inc — Page 248
Kittrell, Christine
Capital District Physicians
Health Plan — Page 286
Kivimaki, Kim
Ohio State University Managed
Health Care Systems Inc — Page 332
Klammer, Tom
Landmark Healthcare Inc — Page 56
Klarner, Susan
SmileCare/Community
Dental Services — Page 69
Klassen, Richard
Delta Dental Plan of Missouri — Page 246
Kleaver, Elwood
Primary Health Plan — Page 142
Kleefisch, Boyd
New Mexico Medical
Review Association — Page 281
Kleese, Kathy
HealthAmerica Pennsylvania Inc -
Eastern Region — Page 365
Klein, David H, MD
Excellus BCBS — Page 290
Excellus BCBS,
Central NY Southern Tier — Page 291
Excellus BCBS,
Central New York Region — Page 291
Excellus BCBS, Rochester Area — Page 292
Excellus BCBS, Utica Region — Page 292
Lifetime Healthcare Companies,
The - Corporate Headquarters — Page 298
Univera Healthcare of
Western New York — Page 307
Lifetime Healthcare Companies, The -
Corporate Headquarters — Page 298
Klein, Garner, MD
Valley Baptist Insurance Co — Page 431
Klein, Gary
Florida Health Care Plan Inc — Page 109
Klein, Judy
IBA Health Plans — Page 225
Vision Service Plan — Page 75
Kleinberg, Nate
United Concordia Company Inc -
Alabama — Page 6
United Concordia Company Inc -
Arizona — Page 21

Kleinfeldt, Mary Jo
Blue Cross of Idaho — Page 141
Kleman, Laurie
Aetna Inc - New Jersey — Page 267
Klenk, Scott
Capital District Physicians
Health Plan — Page 286
Kleppe, Roger W
Blue Cross Blue Shield of MN — Page 234
Klepper, Kenneth O
Medco Health Solutions Inc — Page 275
Medco Health Solutions Inc — Page 488
Klich, Richard, DMD
United Concordia Co Inc - AL — Page 6
United Concordia Co Inc - AZ — Page 21
United Concordia Co Inc - CA — Page 72
United Concordia Co Inc - FL — Page 121
United Concordia Co Inc - IL — Page 154
United Concordia Co Inc - MD — Page 206
United Concordia Co Inc - MI — Page 231
United Concordia Co Inc - MO — Page 251
United Concordia Co Inc - NM — Page 282
United Concordia Co Inc - NY — Page 306
United Concordia Co Inc -
Corporate Headquarters — Page 373
United Concordia Co Inc - PA — Page 374
United Concordia Co Inc - PA
Central — Page 374
United Concordia Co Inc - TX — Page 429
United Concordia Co Inc - VA — Page 446
United Concordia Co Inc - WA — Page 457
Klima, Cliff
LifeWise Health Plan of Arizona — Page 17
Klimansky, Mike
Mercy Care Plan — Page 18
Kline, Gretchen
Great-West Healthcare of MI — Page 223
Klingensmith, James M, ScD
Highmark Inc — Page 366
Klinkner, John
American Republic
Insurance Company — Page 169
Klister, Steve
Dental Network of America — Page 146
Klock, David R, MD
CompBenefits Corporation -
Corporate Headquarters — Page 129
Kloss, John G
MemberHealth Inc — Page 489
Klotz, Nancy, MD
Centercare Inc — Page 287
Kluge, Susan A
Blue Care Network of MI — Page 217
Knackstedt, Christopher M
Great-West Healthcare of AZ — Page 16
Great-West Healthcare -
Corporate — Page 81
Knellinger, Mike
CareSource — Page 321
Kniess, April
Williamette Dental Group PC — Page 352
Knight, Alferd, MD
Scott & White Health Plan — Page 424
Knight, Jeff
Health Plan of the
Upper Ohio Valley — Page 327
Health Plan,
The Hometown Region — Page 327
Knight, Terry
Viva Health Inc — Page 7
Knighton, Larry D
Health Plus of Louisiana Inc — Page 191
Knox, Jeff
Mutual Assurance
Administrators Inc — Page 342
Knudsen, Eric
Fara Healthcare Management — Page 190
Knutson, Deb
Medica Health Plans — Page 236

Index VIII: Personnel

Kaplan, Paul, MD
Blue Cross Blue Shield of DE — Page 95
Kaplan, Rick
Health Net Inc - Northeast
Corporate Headquarters — Page 91
Karas, Richard
Delta Dental Plan of IN Inc — Page 159
Delta Dental Plan of OH Inc — Page 324
Delta Dental Plan of MI Inc — Page 220
Karjala, Kenneth
Orange County PPO — Page 61
Karl, Jim
Community Health
Network of CT Inc — Page 89
Karlson, Susan
Mercy Care Plan — Page 18
Karpinski, Judy
Health Plan,
The Hometown Region — Page 327
Kasabian, Carolyn
Community Clinical Services — Page 196
Kasitz, Todd
Preferred Health Systems — Page 180
Kasle, Dan
Elderplan Inc - SHMO — Page 289
Kasper, Mike
Humana Health Care
Plans of Illinois — Page 151
Kassem, Amin
SHPS Inc — Page 186
Kassner, Diane
Outlook Vision Services — Page 18
Kastelitz, Rod
Employee Benefit
Management Services Inc — Page 253
Kastner, Richard J
BCBS of Kansas City — Page 244
Kates, Peter B
Univera Healthcare of
Western New York — Page 307
Katulic, Joseph
M-Care Inc — Page 225
Katz, Amy
Fidelis SecureCare of MI Inc — Page 221
Katz, Barry I, RPh
Envision Pharmaceutical
Services Inc — Page 484
Katz, Leah
Connecticare Inc — Page 89
Katz, Mitchell, MD
San Francisco Health Plan — Page 66
Katz, Richard, PT
Northwest Rehab Alliance — Page 349
Kaufman, Joseph A, MD
Sierra Health Services Inc-
Corporate Headquarters — Page 264
Kaufmann, Michael
Delta Dental Plan of California — Page 44
Kaukas, John
Community Health Network
of Connecticut Inc — Page 89
Kawaguchi, Sharon
On Lok Senior Health Services — Page 60
Kawate, Chris
Community Health Plan — Page 42
Kaye, Mitchel PT
PTPN - Corporate Headquarters — Page 65
Kaye, Tom, RPh
Bluelincs HMO — Page 340
Kearney, Jessice
Bluegrass Family Health Inc — Page 183
Kearns, James
Medavant National
Preferred Provider Network — Page 299
Keating, Ken
Safeguard Hlth Enterprises Inc — Page 66
Keck, Kevin, MD
Providence Health Plans — Page 351

Keegan, Albert F, MD
NYCHSRO/MedReview Inc — Page 303
Keeley, Larry
Opticare Managed Vision — Page 314
Keester, Don
Providence Health System-OR — Page 513
Keffer, Mark, MD
UnitedHealthcare of South FL — Page 122
Kehl, Thomas, MD
Coastal Hlthcare Administrators — Page 41
Kehoe, Patty
NM Medical Review Assoc — Page 281
Kehres, Deborah
South Central Preferred — Page 372
Keiler, Susan
Community Clinical Services — Page 196
Keim, Scott
PacifiCare of Colorado — Page 84
Keiserman, Wayne, MD
Managed Health Services
Insurance Corporation — Page 467
Keitel, Cindy
Health Net of California — Page 49
Keith, Barbara
AZ Foundation for Medical Care — Page 11
Kelch, Robert P MD
M-Care Inc — Page 225
Kellenberger, Debbie
Inland Empire Foundation for
Medical Care — Page 52
Keller, Larry
Central Health Plan of CA Inc — Page 39
Ventura County Hlth Care Plan — Page 73
Keller, Reed
SHPS Inc — Page 186
Kellogg, Terry
Blue Cross Blue Shield of AL — Page 3
Kelly, Barbara
Blue Cross Blue Shield of SC -
Corporate Hqtrs — Page 383
Kelly, Dan
Mid-Atlantic Managed Care Org of
Pennsylvania Inc — Page 369
Kelly, Jennifer
ECCA - Managed Vision Care Inc -
Corporate Headquarters — Page 413
Kelly, Kathy
Keystone Health Plan Central — Page 367
Kelly, Sylvia
Community Hlth Ntwrk of CT Inc — Page 89
Kelly, William
Employees Benefit Systems — Page 170
Kelman, Barbara
Affinity Health Plan Inc — Page 283
Kelso, David
Aetna Inc - Pennsylvania — Page 355
Kelso, Harry, Jr, MD
American National
Insurance Company — Page 405
Kendall, Edie, DDS
Careington International -
The Dental Network — Page 408
Kendall, Kathy
McLaren Health Plan — Page 226
Kendall, Paula
Aetna Inc - Altamonte Springs — Page 99
Kendall, Ralph, PharmD
Healthesystems — Page 486
Kening, Larry
Zurich Services Corporation — Page 155
Kennard, Betty
Health First Health Plans Inc — Page 111
Kennedy, Bryan
Ohio Health Choice — Page 332
Kennedy, James J, Jr
UlliCare — Page 98
Union Labor Life Insurance Co — Page 276

Kennedy, Janna
SummaCare Inc — Page 334
Kennedy, John W
BCBS of Kansas City — Page 244
Good Health HMO Inc — Page 247
Kennedy, Michael
Evercare Select — Page 15
Kennedy, Thomas F
Regence Group, The —
Corporate Headquarters — Page 351
Regence BCBS of Oregon — Page 351
Kennedy-Scott, Patricia
Kaiser Foundation
Health Plan of Ohio — Page 329
Kenny, Carolyn
Kaiser Foundation
Health Plan of Georgia — Page 132
Kenslea, Ged
AIDS Healthcare Foundation — Page 32
Keohane, John D
GENEX Services — Page 363
Keough, Kim
Coordinated Health Plan — Page 379
Kerby, James, MD
Grand Valley Health Plan — Page 221
Kerlin, Mary
Partnership HealthPlan of CA — Page 64
Kern, Sue
Group Health Cooperative
of Eau Claire — Page 465
Kerr, Thomas W
Highmark Inc — Page 366
Kerr, William MD
WellCare Health Plans Inc -
Corporate Headquarters — Page 124
Kerrigan, Brendan
Oxford Health Plans-CT — Page 91
Kessel, Stacy
Community Health Plan of WA — Page 450
First Choice Health Network — Page 451
Kessler, Allen A, CPA
Midwest Health Plan — Page 226
Kessler, James S
Health New England — Page 212
Kessler, Ken, MD
APS Healthcare Northwest Inc — Page 253
Ketner, William D
Medcost LLC — Page 313
Kettyle, William, MD
MIT Health Plan — Page 214
Khalil, Adnane
Medavant National
Preferred Provider Network — Page 299
Khan, Nazeer H, MD
Quality Health Plan Inc — Page 119
Khan, Rashid
Coreview — Page 235
Khan, Sabiha
Quality Health Plan Inc — Page 119
Khan, Sianam
UHP Healthcare — Page 71
Khatib, Chaker
Americas PPO — Page 233
HCH Administration — Page 148
Kibbe, David
IBA Health Plans — Page 225
New West Health Plan — Page 254
Kiernan, Cathy
Delta Dental Plan of Ohio Inc — Page 324
Kieser, Brian
El Paso First Health Plans Inc — Page 413
Kight, Charles L
Community First Hlth Plans Inc — Page 410
Kilcher, Lisa
CIGNA Healthcare of Ohio Inc — Page 323
Kilcullin, Tracy, Esq
Intracorp — Page 367

Index VIII: Personnel

Jonas, Cecio, MD
Pro-Care Health Plan — Page 230
Jones, Barbara G
Keystone Mercy Health Plan — Page 368
Jones, Brooks
Care 1st Health Plan — Page 38
Jones, Christine
Preferred Health Systems — Page 180
Jones, David A, Jr
Humana Insurance Co - AL — Page 5
Humana Inc - AR — Page 27
Humana Hlth Care Plans of AZ — Page 17
Humana Inc - CO — Page 82
Humana Inc - DC — Page 98
Humana Health Plan - Jacksonville — Page 113
Humana Medical Plan - Central Florida — Page 113
Humana Medical Plan - Daytona — Page 113
Humana Medical Plan Inc — Page 114
Humana Health Plans of GA — Page 132
Humana Hlth Care Plans of IL — Page 151
Humana Inc - IN — Page 161
Humana Inc - IA — Page 170
Humana Health Care Plans of Kansas & Missouri — Page 179
CHA Health - Humana — Page 184
Humana Inc - Corporate Headquarters — Page 185
Humana Health Plan - Kentucky — Page 185
Humana Health Care Plans of Lexington — Page 185
Humana Military Service Inc — Page 186
Humana Hlth Benefit Plan of LA — Page 191
Humana Inc - MD — Page 203
Humana Inc - Grand Rapids MI — Page 225
Humana Inc - MS — Page 241
Humana Inc - NE — Page 256
Humana Inc - NM — Page 280
Humana Inc - NC — Page 313
Humana Inc - ND — Page 317
Humana Health Plan of OH Inc — Page 328
Humana Inc - OK — Page 341
Humana Inc - SC — Page 384
Humana Inc - SD — Page 388
Humana Inc - TN — Page 396
Humana Health Care Plans of Corpus Christi — Page 417
Humana Health Care Plans of Dallas — Page 417
Humana Health Care Plans of Houston — Page 418
Humana Health Care Plans of San Antonio/Austin — Page 418
Humana Health Plan of Austin — Page 419
Humana Inc - UT — Page 435
Humana WI Health Org Inc — Page 466
Humana Inc - Wyoming — Page 473
Humana Inc — Page 486
Humana Health Care Plans of San Antonio/Austin — Page 418
Humana Health Plan of Austin — Page 419
Jones, Elliott
Blue Cross Blue Shield of Texas — HMO Blue - Southeast — Page 407
Jones, Hugh A
Health Net of California — Page 49
Jones, Jacqueline
Peach State Health Plan — Page 133
Jones, James, MD
CareGuide — Page 105
Jones, Jan
Grand Valley Health Plan — Page 221
Jones, Jeri
UnitedHealthcare of Colorado — Page 85
Jones, Jetta
Bluegrass Family Health Inc — Page 183

Jones, John D, RPh, JD
Prescription Solutions — Page 493
Jones, Karen
HealthLink Inc - Corp Hdqrtrs — Page 249
Jones, Kori
Best Health Plans — Page 36
Jones, Larry, MD
Hlthcare USA of Missouri LLC — Page 248
Jones, Latasha
Memphis Managed Care Corp — Page 397
Jones, Marcie
Upper Peninsula Health Plan — Page 232
Jones, Mark
Texas True Choice — Page 428
Jones, Michael
Memphis Managed Care Corp — Page 397
Jones, Michael
Alabama Quality Assurance Foundation — Page 3
Jones, Michael, MBA
CIGNA Behavioral Health Inc — Page 408
Jones, Patrick G, MD
Vantage Health Plan Inc — Page 193
Jones, Rich, RN
DakotaCare — Page 387
Jones, Richard
Aetna Inc - Nevada — Page 259
Jones, Robert E
Blue Ridge Health Network — Page 357
Jones, Scott
Delta Dental Plan of SD — Page 387
Jones, Sheila
Care 1st Health Plan AZ Inc — Page 13
Jones, Stacey
Aetna Health of Illinois Inc — Page 143
Jones, Stephanie
Vista Hlthplan of South FL Inc — Page 123
Jones, Steve
Encore Health Network — Page 160
Jones, Tammy
Kaiser Foundation Health Plan of Georgia — Page 132
Jones, WH
Med-Comp USA — Page 192
Jones, William
Grand Valley Health Plan — Page 221
Jones, Willis E, III
Windsor Health Plan of TN Inc — Page 401
Jordan, Mary, RN
Health Plan of San Joaquin, The — Page 50
Josephs, Scott T, MD
CIGNA Healthcare of NC Inc — Page 311
Joshi, Ramesh
Union Health Service Inc — Page 154
Joswick, Lois
Delta Dental Plan of WI — Page 463
Joy, James J
Blue Cross Blue Shield of RI — Page 379
Coordinated Health Plan — Page 379
Joyce, Drew A
Southern Health Services Inc — Page 445
Joyce, Kevin
QualCare Inc — Page 276
Joyner, David
Blue Shield of California — Page 36
Jubert, Rose
Pueblo Health Care — Page 84
Julia, Julio F
MMM Healthcare Inc — Page 378
Jurena, Jerry
Heart of America Health Plan — Page 317
Jurevic, Jon
Oregon Dealthan — Page 349
Justice, Shelly
HMS Colorado Inc — Page 82
Sloan's Lake Preferred Health Networks — Page 85

Justice, William
Vantage Health Plan Inc — Page 193

K

Kabarsky, Kay
DeltaCare USA — Page 44
Kack, Kyla
Managed Health Services Insurance Corporation — Page 467
Kaden, William S, MD
Masspro Inc — Page 213
Kadja, Judy
Ohio State University Managed Health Care Systems Inc — Page 332
Kaehler, Mary
Pima Health Plan — Page 19
Kahen, Parvis
Honored Citizen's Choice Health Plan — Page 51
Kahn, Howard A
LA Care Health Plan — Page 55
Kaiser, Angela
Metropolitan Health Plan — Page 237
Kaiser, Kelley C, MPH
Samaritan Health Plans Inc — Page 352
Kakuno, Jeff
Mdx Hawaii — Page 138
Kalahiki, Linda
University Health Alliance — Page 138
Kaldenbaugh, Henry, MD
Evercare Select — Page 15
Kalor, Ali
WelBorn Health Plans — Page 167
Kalustian, Lisa
Health Net of California — Page 49
Kam, Sam
Central Health Plan of CA Inc — Page 39
Kamil, Ivan Jeffrey
Blue Cross of California — Page 34
Kan, Bruce
MDX Hawaii — Page 138
Kanard, Michael
Kaiser Foundation Health Plan Northwest — Page 347
Kandalaft, Kevin
Lovelace Health Plan — Page 280
Kane, Barbara, MSN, BSN, CCM
Corporate Care Mngmnt Inc — Page 288
Kane, Edward
Guardian Life Ins Co of America — Page 294
Kane, Martin, MD
Healthplex Inc — Page 296
Kane, Suzanne M
MedSolutions — Page 396
Kane, William J
Innovative Care Management — Page 347
Kang, Jeffery, MD
CIGNA Healthcare of CT — Page 89
Kania, Cathy
GHI HMO Select Inc — Page 293
Kanter, Gene
Carelink Health Plans — Page 459
Kanwal, Neeraj, MD
Paramount Care of Michigan — Page 228
Paramount Health Care Plan — Page 333
Paramount Advantage — Page 333
Kapic, Maja
Liberty Dental Plan of CA — Page 56
Kaplan, David
Fidelis SecureCare of NC — Page 312
Kaplan, Jonathan S, MD
Excellus BlueCross BlueShield — Page 290
Kaplan, Leon
CareFirst BlueChoice Inc — Page 97
CareFirst BCBS — Page 200
Delmarva Health Care Plan Inc — Page 202

Index VIII: Personnel

Delta Dental Plan of MI Inc	Page 220
Delta Dental Plan of OH Inc	Page 324

Jacobson, Kathy
UnitedHealthcare of Arkansas — Page 28

Jacobson, Robert
Compsych Behavioral Health — Page 145

Jacobson, Stephen W
Olympus Mngd Hlth Care Inc — Page 117

Jacobson, Trish
Inter Valley Health Plan Inc — Page 53

Jaegar, Michael, MD
Anthem BCBS of Wisconsin — Page 461

Jaeger, Mary Ann
Heart of America Health Plan — Page 317

Jaffe, John, MD
Valley Preferred — Page 375

Jaffe, Roger
APS Healthcare Inc — Page 199

Jaillette, Debbie
KHS a KMG America Company — Page 385

Jakubowski, Stanley S
Genex Services — Page 363

Jamal, Asif
Jackson Memorial Health Plan — Page 115

James, Don
Beech Street Corporation — Corporate Headquarters — Page 36

James, Jackie L
Horizon Behavioral Services — Page 112
Horizon Behavioral Services — Page 417

Jamieson, Elizabeth
Ohio Health Choice — Page 332

Jamison, Patricia
Vista Health Plan Inc — Page 123

Jamison, Scott
DakotaCare — Page 387

Jan, Janet
Care 1st Health Plan — Page 38

Janczak, Linda
Finger Lakes Community Care Network — Page 293

Jani, David
Geisinger Health Plan — Page 363

Janicak, Steve
MedSolutions — Page 396

Jansen, Steve
Mercy Health Plans of MO Inc — Page 249

Jaques, Douglas
Scan Health Plan — Page 68

Jaramillo, Robert
Altius Health Plans — Page 433

Jarboe, David
CarePlus Health Plans Inc — Page 106

Jarmon, Margaret
Atlantic Integrated Health Inc — Page 309

Jarv, Karen
Medavant National Preferred Provider Network — Page 299

Javier-Obinger, Sonia
Neighborhood Health Plan — Page 214

Jaycox, Tracey
Flora Health Network — Page 325

Jazo-Bajet, Martha, RN, MPH
Community Health Group — Page 41

Jedynak-Bell, Corinne E, DO
Puget Sound Health Partners — Page 455

Jefferson, Amanda
American Pharmacy Services Corporation — Page 183

Jeffries, Faye RN
Geisinger Health Plan — Page 363

Jehle, Christopher A
Total Dental Administrators Health Plan — Page 21

Jenkins, Craig
Healthy Palm Beaches Inc — Page 112

Jenkins, Harry
American Pioneer Health Plans Inc — Page 101

Jenkins, Mary Beth
UMPC Health Plan Univ of Pittsburgh Medical Center — Page 374

Jenkins, Mary, Pharm D, MS
Innoviant Inc — Page 487

Jenkins, Nancy
HealthPlus of Michigan — Page 224

Jenkins, Shiela
Network Health Plan Wisconsin — Page 468

Jenkins, Steven
Memphis Managed Care Corp — Page 397

Jennings, Donna
Coventry Health Care of Nebraska Inc — Page 255

Jennings, Lane, MD
Volusia Health Network — Page 124

Jennings, Michele
Interplan Health Group — Page 419

Jennings, Tanya
Upper Peninsula Health Plan — Page 232

Jennings, Tim
Optima Health Plan Inc — Page 445

Jensen, Jeffrey L, CPA
Utah Public Employees Health Program — Page 438

Jensen, Kenneth R
Fiserv Inc — Page 464

Jensen, William F
Independent Care Health Plan — Page 467

Jernigan, J Michael
Select Health of South Carolina — Page 385

Jerominski, Patricia M
Independent Care Health Plan — Page 467

Jesse, Sandra L
Blue Cross Blue Shield of MA — Page 209

Jesserer, William
Aetna Inc - Pennsylvania — Page 355

Jewell, Deb
CHN MCO — Page 322

Jewett, Jan
United Concordia Company Inc - California — Page 72
United Concordia Company Inc - Corporate Headquarters — Page 373

Jewett, Stephen
Connecticare Inc — Page 89

Jhaveri, Vishu, MD
Nationwide Better Health — Page 204

Murray, Jim
Humana Inc - New Mexico — Page 280

Jimenez, Martin
Community First Hlth Plans Inc — Page 410

Jimenez, Peter
CarePlus Health Plans Inc — Page 106

Joaquin, Jackie
Midlands Choice Inc — Page 256

Joe, David
Western Dental Services — Page 75

Joehl-Colling, Jane, Esq
MemberHealth Inc — Page 489

Johnes, Ed
Evolutions Hlthcre Sys Inc — Page 109

Johnson, Amy
Great-West Healthcare of ME — Page 196

Johnson, B Randy
AmeriGroup Texas Inc — Page 404

Johnson, Barbara
Security Health Plan of WI Inc — Page 469
Mercycare Health Plan Inc — Page 468

Johnson, Carlene
Primaris — Page 250

Johnson, Carolyn
Best Health Plans — Page 36

Johnson, Cheryl
Vision Service Plan — Page 75

Johnson, Dave, MD
Parkview Signature Care — Page 164

Johnson, David R
Metropolitan Health Plan — Page 237
Metropolitan Health Plan — Page 506

Johnson, David T
UnitedHealthcare of Arkansas — Page 28

Johnson, Eam
Atrio Health Plans Inc — Page 345

Johnson, Glen R
Community Health Choice Inc — Page 410

Johnson, J D
American National Ins Co — Page 405

Johnson, Jana
Medica Health Plans — Page 236
Medica Health Plans — Page 518

Johnson, Jeffrey
Vermont Hlth Plans (Blue Care) — Page 439

Johnson, John
Health Tradition Health Plans — Page 466

Johnson, John
Humana Inc - Indiana — Page 161

Johnson, Karen
Delta Dental Plan of WI — Page 463

Johnson, L Gray, Jr
Optimum Choice Inc — Page 205

Johnson, Linda
Medical Mutual of Ohio — Page 330

Johnson, Mark
Independent Health Assoc Inc — Page 297

Johnson, Mark
Zurich Services Corporation — Page 155

Johnson, Mary Jane, RN, MBA
Comprehensive Behavioral Care Inc — Page 108

Johnson, Michelle
Vista Health Plan Inc — Page 123
Vista Hlthplan of South FF Inc — Page 123

Johnson, Owen, MD
UnitedHealthcare of Ohio Inc — Page 336

Johnson, Pat
UHP Healthcare — Page 71

Johnson, Paula
Upper Peninsula Health Plan — Page 232

Johnson, Randy
BCBS of North Dakota — Page 317

Johnson, Robert
InStil Health Insurance Co — Page 518

Johnson, Robert L, OD, MS
Vision Health Mngmnt Systems — Page 155

Johnson, Ronald
Outlook Vision Services — Page 18

Johnson, Terry, MD
Superior HealthPlan Inc — Page 426

Johnson, Twild R
Security Health Plan of WI Inc — Page 469

Johnson, Vicki Lee
Physicians Health Plan of Northern Indiana — Page 164

Johnson-Mills, Rita
Managed Hlth Services IN Inc — Page 163

Johnston, Jennifer
Health Plan, The Hometown Region — Page 327

Johnston, L McTyeire, MD
Neighborhood Health Plan of Rhode Island — Page 380

Johnston, Robert
Regence BCBS of Utah — Page 436

Johnston, Steve
Healthcare Partners of East Texas Inc — Page 416

Joiner, Ronald V
D C Chartered Health Plan Inc — Page 97

Jollie, Bill
Physicians Plus Ins Corp — Page 469

Jolly, Mark
ECCA - Managed Vision Care Inc - Corporate Headquarters — Page 413

Jolly, Nicki
Prime Health Services Inc — Page 398

Index VIII: Personnel

Hueben, Craig
AmeriChoice of New York — Page 284
Huerta, Sharon
Molina Healthcare of NM — Page 281
Huether, Jamie
HealthLink Inc - Corporate Headquarters — Page 249
Huey, Lynne
Optimum HealthCare Inc — Page 117
Huey, Rodney I, MD
BCBS of Oklahoma — Page 339
Bluelincs HMO — Page 340
Huff, Dale D
Coordinated Health Plan — Page 379
Huffer, Michael
Argus Health System Inc — Page 480
Huffman, Vicki
Gateway Health Plan Inc — Page 362
Hufford, Don MD
Western Health Advantage — Page 75
Hughes, Paul A,, ESQ
Emerald Hlth Network Inc, The — Page 325
Hulen, Debbie
Md-Individual Practice Association Inc (MD IPA) — Page 204
Optimum Choice Inc — Page 205
Hulin, Colin
Tenet Choices Inc — Page 192
Hull, Leigh
Mountain Medical Affiliates — Page 83
Hullett, Joseph MD
ValueOptions of California Inc — Page 72
Humbert, Ernest E
Molina Healthcare of Ohio Inc — Page 330
Hummel, Cynthia C
Excellus BlueCross BlueShield, Utica Region — Page 292
Hummel, Linda T
Humana Health Care Plans of Corpus Christi — Page 417
Humana Health Care Plans of San Antonio/Austin — Page 418
Humphrey, Bob
UnitedHealthcare of Louisiana — Page 193
Humphries, O Guy, DDS
Nevada Pacific Dental — Page 262
Hundley, Charley
Blue Cross Blue Shield of ND — Page 317
Hung, Amy
Pacific IPA — Page 63
Hungness, Kathy
Primewest Health System — Page 506
Hunsaker, David
APS Healthcare Inc — Page 199
APS Healthcare Northwest Inc — Page 253
Hunsinger, Lance
Cariten Healthcare — Page 393
PHP Companies Inc — Page 397
Hunt, Ann
First Commonwealth — Page 147
Hunt, Doris
Cooks Childrens Health Plan — Page 411
Hunt, Joseph J
Union Labor Life Insurance Co — Page 276
Hunt, Sue
Blue Cross Blue Shield of Texas — Corporate Headquarters — Page 406
Hunter, Bob
Doral Dental USA — Page 464
Hunter, Regina
Aetna Inc - Houston — Page 403
Hunziker, Bryan BS, MS
Prime Health Services Inc — Page 398
Hupman, Raedina
Preferred Health Systems — Page 180
Hurban, Alesia, RN, CCM, MSC
Corporate Care Management Inc — Page 288

Hurd, Herman E, MD
Delta Dental Plan of Arkansas — Page 26
Hurlburt, Ward B, MD, MBA
Molina HealthCare of WA Inc — Page 453
Hurley, Barbara, RN
Affinity Health Plan Inc — Page 283
Hurst, David
Health Plan of San Joaquin, The — Page 50
Hurst, Keith
Community Health Plan of WA — Page 450
Hurt, John
Neighborhood Hlth Partnership — Page 116
Husband, Monica
Care 1st Health Plan AZ Inc — Page 13
Huschie, Patricia
Neighborhood Health Plan of Rhode Island — Page 380
Huschka, Angela
New West Health Plan — Page 254
Huss, C Eric
Gateway Health Plan Inc — Page 362
Hussey, Tim
EBC — Page 464
Husted, Kevin
Preferred Care — Page 304
Hutchins, Diane
Peach State Health Plan — Page 133
Hutchins, Gary
1st Medical Network — Page 127
Hutchins, Leigh
Primecare Medical Network Inc — Page 65
Hutchinson, Donn
Delta Dental of Iowa — Page 169
Hutchinson, Sherrie
Florida Health Care Plan Inc — Page 109
Hutchison, John
Regence BCBS of Oregon — Page 351
Hutchson, Louis, Jr
HealthTrans LLC — Page 486
Hutt, Edward D, MD, MBA
Carolina Care Plan Inc — Page 383
Huyghue, Bruce
PacifiCare of Nevada — Page 263
Hyatt, Ronnie
St Francis Optimum Health Network — Page 385
Hynek, James
Coventry Hlth Care Inc-DE Inc — Page 96
Hyre, Barbara
Nationwide Health Plans — Page 331

I

Ianniello, Cara
CHN Solutions — Page 270
Iazarovic, Jacob, MD
Broadspire Inc — Page 105
Ibanuz, Grace, RN
Community Health Plan — Page 42
Ideson, D Scott
Regence BCBS of Utah — Page 436
Ideson, D Scott
Regence Healthwise — Page 436
Imai, Kent, MD
Valley Health Plan Santa Clara County — Page 72
Imes, Bettina
Superior Dental Care Alliance — Page 335
Immel, Deborah, RN
Care Network — Page 359
Infante, Nelia
CIGNA Behavioral Health Inc — Page 88
CIGNA Behavioral Health Inc - Corporate Headquarters — Page 234

Ingala, Robert J
Neighborhood Health Plan — Page 214
Inge, Ron, DDS
Washington Dental Service — Page 457
Ingrum, Jeffrey C, MD
Health Alliance Medical Plans - Corporate Headquarters — Page 149
Intfen, Joseph
Preferred Health Professionals — Page 180
Ireland, Jeff
New West Health Plan — Page 254
Irizarry, Vincente J Leon, CPA
Triple-S Inc — Page 378
Irwin, Mark
Pennsylvania PACE Inc — Page 514
Isaac, Sharon
UHP Healthcare — Page 71
Isaacs, Jason, BS
Primaris — Page 250
Isaacs, Steven, K LLIF
CompBenefits — Page 410
Isham, George, MD
HealthPartners Inc — Page 236
HealthPartners — Page 486
Ishibashi, Tammy
Nevada Pacific Dental — Page 262
Itzchaki, Raija
Global Medical Management — Page 110
Ivan, Cynthia
Health Net of Arizona — Page 17
Ivey, Sheri
Humana Medical Plan Inc — Page 114
Iwanaga, Jim
ppoNEXT — Page 423

J

Jackson, Laura
Wellmark BCBS of Iowa — Page 174
Wellmark Inc — Corp Hdqtrs — Page 175
Wellmark Health Plan of IA Inc — Page 175
Wellmark BCBS of SD — Page 389
Wellmark Health Plan of IA Inc — Page 175
Jackson, Marianne
Blue Shield of California — Page 36
Jackson, Micki
Horizon BCBS of NJ — Page 273
Jackson, Morgan
OhioHealth Group — Page 332
Jackson, Paul
PacifiCare of Colorado — Page 84
Jackson, Phil
Providence Health Plans — Page 351
Jackson, Rick
MDX Hawaii — Page 138
Jaco, Dan, MA, MSPH
New Mexico Medical Review Association — Page 281
Jacobi, Jeff
Blue Cross Blue Shield of Texas — HMO Blue - Midwest TX — Page 406
Jacobs, Annette
Mit Health Plan — Page 214
Jacobs, Beverly
Contra Costa Health Plan — Page 43
Jacobs, Gary M
American Pioneer Health Plans Inc — Page 101
Jacobs, John L
Hawaii Medical Services Association - BC/BS of Hawaii — Page 137
Jacobson, Brae D, MD
CorpHealth Inc — Page 412
Jacobson, Jed J, DDS, MPH
Delta Dental Plan of IN Inc — Page 159

Index VIII: Personnel

Hohing, Laura
Assurant Health -
Corporate Headquarters — Page 462
Hoidal, David
Viva Health Inc — Page 7
Holcombe, Jerry
Delta Dental Plan of California — Page 44
Holden, Bissy
Florida Health Care Plan Inc — Page 109
Holden, Stephen
Pearle Vision Managed Care -
HMO of Texas Inc — Page 423
Holder, Diane P
UMPC Health Plan Univ of
Pittsburgh Medical Center — Page 374
Holgerson, Kris
Williamette Dental Group PC — Page 352
Williamette Dental of WA Inc — Page 457
Holladay, Allen
Evergreen Medical Group LLC — Page 131
Holland, Vicki
Crawford and Co -
Corporate Headquarters — Page 130
Hollifield, Mark
Prescription Management
Services Inc — Page 493
Hollifield, Mark
Tmesys — Page 496
Hollinger, Stacy
Galaxy Health Network — Page 414
Hollingsworth, Karen
Blue Cross Blue Shield of NE — Page 255
Holloway, Joshua, MD
D C Chartered Health Plan Inc — Page 97
Holman, Steven C
Selectcare of Texas LLC — Page 521
Heritage Health Systems Inc — Page 416
Holmberg, David
ECCA - Managed Vision Care Inc -
Corporate Headquarters — Page 413
Holmes, Ava
Lakewood Health Plan Inc — Page 56
Holmes, Barbara
Parkland Community
Health Plan Inc — Page 422
Holmes, Susan
Alabama Quality
Assurance Foundation — Page 3
Holmon, Linda
Holman Group, The — Page 51
Holmon, Ron
Holman Group, The — Page 51
Holmstrom, Jeff, MD
Anthem BCBS of Maine — Page 195
Holsenbeck, Stephen, MD
Colorado Health Networks LLC -
ValueOptions — Page 80
Holt, Albert
ParadigmHealth — Page 276
Holt, Jamie
UnitedHealthcare of Georgia — Page 134
Holt, Timothy A
Aetna Inc - Georgia — Page 127
Holt-Darcy, Lenore
Unicare Health Plans of the
Midwest Inc — Page 153
Holtz, Julie
Behavioral Healthcare Inc — Page 78
Holtzman, Roberta, MBA
Molina Healthcare Inc - CA — Page 59
Holvey, Michael C, Jr
Univera Community Health — Page 307
Holzhauer, Robert J, MD, MBA
Univera Healthcare of
Western New York — Page 307
Hom, Jim
Combined Insurance
Company of America — Page 145
Hom, John, DDS
Dental Health Services Inc — Page 450

Homeister, John
National Foot Care Prgrm Inc — Page 227
Hondel, Richard J
Molina Healthcare Inc - CA — Page 59
Honeycott, Bruce
Blue Cross Blue Shield of SC -
Corporate Hqtrs — Page 383
Hood, Bob
Midlands Choice Inc — Page 256
Hood, Brenton
Metcare Health Plans Inc — Page 116
Hood, Hugh, MD
Healthspring of Alabama Inc — Page 5
Hooker, Dennis
Blue Cross Blue Shield of IL — Page 144
HMO Illinois — Page 150
Hooker, Steven L
Regence BCBS of Oregon — Page 351
Regence Group, The —
Corporate Headquarters — Page 351
Hooley, Jim
Community Medical Alliance — Page 210
Hoops, Alan
CareMore Health Plan — Page 38
Hoorwitz, Sheila
Capital District Physicians
Health Plan — Page 286
Hooven, Eileen
University Health Plans Inc — Page 277
Hoover, Mary
Nevada Prfrrd Professionals — Page 262
Hoover, Mary
Universal Health Network -
Corporate Headquarters — Page 264
Hoover, Robert
Independent Health
Association Inc — Page 297
Hooyenga, Judith
Priority Health — Page 230
Hopkins, Jeannette
Med-Valu Inc — Page 329
Hopkins, John P, RPh
Rocky Mountain Health Plans — Page 84
Rocky Mountain HealthCare Options Inc
dba Healthcare Options — Page 84
Hopper, Ken, MD
CorpHealth Inc — Page 412
Hopsicker, James
MVP Health Plan Inc — Page 301
Horn, Debra Rose
UMPC Health Plan Univ of
Pittsburgh Medical Center — Page 374
Horn, Jack
Partnership HealthPlan of CA — Page 64
Horn, Kathy
Excellus BlueCross BlueShield, Utica
Region — Page 292
Horn, Kimberly K
Priority Health — Page 230
Horozaniecki, Joseph C, MD
Metropolitan Health Plan — Page 237
Horstmann, Nancy
CommunityCare Managed Healthcare
Plans of Oklahoma Inc — Page 340
CommunityCare Managed Healthcare
Plans of Oklahoma Inc — Page 483
Hostetler, Nancy E
Delta Dental Plan of IN Inc — Page 159
Delta Dental Plan of MI Inc — Page 220
Delta Dental Plan of OH Inc — Page 324
Houghton, Jacki
California Dental Network Inc — Page 37
Houlihan, Richard P, Esq
Fallon Community Hlth Plan Inc — Page 211
House, Anthony
Community Behavioral Healthcare
Cooperative of Pennsylvania — Page 361
House, Margaret, LVP, CPHQ
Orange County PPO — Page 61
Houser, Cynthia
Preferred Health Systems — Page 180

Houser, Matt, RPh
CIGNA Healthcare of Ohio Inc — Page 323
Houy, William
Delphi Card R — Page 145
Hovagimian, Deb
Health Plans Inc — Page 213
Hovencamp, Dean
Aetna Inc - Arkansas — Page 25
Hoverman, Ken L
UnitedHealthcare of Florida Inc — Page 122
Hovila, Gary
UnitedHealthcare of WI Inc — Page 470
Howard, Phyllis
Value Health Care — Page 277
Howard, Randy, MD
Anthem BCBS of Indiana — Page 157
Howatt, James W, MD
Molina Healthcare Inc -
Corporate Headquarters — Page 59
Molina Healthcare Inc — Page 489
Howe, Roger K MD, MMM
Qca Health Plan Inc — Page 28
Howe, Sharon
LifeWise Health Plan of Oregon — Page 348
Howell, Curt
UnitedHealthcare of Utah — Page 437
Howell, Scott, MD
Aids Healthcare Foundation — Page 32
Howell, Wendy
Innovative Care Management — Page 347
Howes, David H, MD
Martins Point Health Care — Page 196
Howry, Cyndy
Zurich Services Corporation — Page 155
Howze, Ken
AmeriGroup District of Columbia — Page 97
Hoy, Janet
Sharp Health Plan — Page 68
Hoyt, Debra
Connecticare of NY — Page 288
Hrobowchec, Carol
Valley Baptist Insurance Co — Page 431
Hromadka, Donnie
Humana Health Plan of Austin — Page 419
Hronek, Mike
Primary Health Plan — Page 142
Hrr, Paula M
Nationwide Better Health — Page 204
Hubbard, AJ
Humana Health Plan - KY — Page 185
Hubbard, Linda
Lovelace Health Plan — Page 280
Hubbell, Connie
Kansas Fndtn Medical Care — Page 179
Hubbell, Greg
Alternative Care Mngmnt Sys — Page 319
Huber, Jack
Community Health Network
of Connecticut Inc — Page 89
Hubler, Kurt
Orange Prevention &
Treatment Integrated — Page 60
Huckle, Tim
Blue Cross Blue Shield of ND — Page 317
Hudak, Jim
United Behavioral Health (UBH) — Page 71
United Behavioral Health — Page 373
Hudkins, Garrison
Great-West Healthcare of NY — Page 294
Hudson, Joyce
Deaconess Health Plans — Page 159
Hudson, Lori
KPS Health Plans — Page 452
Hudson, Mark
UCARE Minnesota — Page 238
UCARE of Minnesota — Page 505
UCARE of Minnesota — Page 507

Index VIII: Personnel

Hernandez, Madeline, CPA
Medical Card System — Page 377
Hernandez, Rhea
UTMB Health Plans Inc — Page 431
Herndon, Larry
Utah Public Employees
Health Program — Page 438
Herndon, Robert
UnitedHealthcare of Texas Inc -
San Antonio — Page 430
Herr, David S, MD, FAAP
Rocky Mountain Health Plans — Page 84
Rocky Mountain HlthCare Options Inc
dba Healthcare Options — Page 84
Herrera, Kristy
Evergreen Medical Group LLC — Page 131
Herrera, Teresa
Inland Empire Foundation
for Medical Care — Page 52
Herrin, Tom, MD
PhysiciansPlus & St Dominic — Page 242
Herron, George, MD
Medcore Health Plan — Page 58
Herron, Judith
CIGNA Dental Health of NC Inc — Page 310
CIGNA Dental Health of OH Inc — Page 322
Texas Dental Plan — Page 427
Hershberger, Michael
American Healthguard Corp — Page 33
Hert, Myrna
Strategic Health
Development Corporation — Page 119
Hervy, Patrick MBA
XL Health — Page 207
Hess, Carolyn
Healthcare Partners of
East Texas Inc — Page 416
Hess, Kimberly
Superior Vision Services Inc — Page 70
Hesson, Patty
UnitedHealthcare of Florida Inc — Page 122
Hester, Bambi
Scott & White Health Plan — Page 424
Hettrick, Robert
Sentinel Management Services -
Corporate Headquarters — Page 372
Heuer, Max
Arkansas Blue Cross/Blue Shield
a Mutual Insurance Company — Page 25
Heuser, George, MD
Optima Health Plan Inc — Page 445
Heyl, Ross D
First Choice Health Network — Page 451
Heyman, Dick
CHN Solutions — Page 270
Hiam, Robert P
Hawaii Medical Services Association -
BC/BS of Hawaii — Page 137
Hice, Diane
Presbyterian Health Plan — Page 281
Hickey, James W CHE
Great-West Healthcare of NC — Page 313
Hickey, Jim
Unicare Life and Hlth Ins Co Inc — Page 428
Hickey, Jim
Humana Health Care Plans of
Houston — Page 418
Hickey, Mary
Coordinated Health Plan — Page 379
Hickie, Mary
Sun Health Medisun — Page 20
Hicks, Deborah
Harvard Pilgrim Health Care -
Corporate Headquarters — Page 212
Hicks, Matt
Mercycare Health Plan Inc — Page 468
Hieber, Klaus A, RPh
PBM Plus Inc — Page 491

Higashida, Neil, PharmD
Health Net of California — Page 49
Higbee, John R
Av-Med Health Plan -
Gainesville — Page 102
Av-Med Health Plan -
Jacksonville — Page 102
Av-Med Health Plan - Miami — Page 103
Av-Med Health Plan - Orlando — Page 103
Av-Med Health Plan - Tampa — Page 103
Hightower, Gina
UTMB Health Plans Inc — Page 431
Hilbert, J Andy
Tufts Health Plan — Page 216
Hilferty, Daniel J
Keystone Mercy Health Plan — Page 368
Keystone Mercy Health Plan — Page 368
Hill, Barbara B
ValueOptions of Texas Inc — Page 431
ValueOptions -
Corporate Headquarters — Page 447
Hill, Bruce
HealthPlus of Michigan — Page 224
Hill, Catherine
Ppoplus LLC — Page 192
Hill, Kevin N
Excellus BlueCrossBlueShield — Page 290
Lifetime Healthcare Companies, The -
Corporate Headquarters — Page 298
Hill, Mike
Evergreen Medical Group LLC — Page 131
Hill, Robert
Dedicated Dental Systems — Page 43
Hill, Stacey
UAHC Health Plan of TN — Page 399
Hill, Teresa
UnitedHealthcare of Arkansas — Page 28
Hill, Virginia
IPRO — Page 298
Hillard, Mark
University Family Care Hlth Plan — Page 22
Hillebert, Jaxene
Preferred Therapy Providers of America -
Corp Headquarters — Page 19
Hillman, Robert
Medical Network Inc — Page 197
Hillman, Robert W
Anthem BCBS of Indiana — Page 157
Hillyer, Richard
Has Premier Providers Inc — Page 415
Hilst, Kevin
Pearle Vision Managed Care -
HMO of Texas Inc — Page 423
Hilton, Gordon R
Hawaii Medical Services Association -
BC/BS of Hawaii — Page 137
Hilton, March
Employee Hlth Ins Mngmnt Inc — Page 483
Hilycord, Angela
Southeastern Indiana
Health Organization — Page 166
Hilzinger, Kurt J
Amerisource Bergen
Performance Plus Network - West — Page 480
Hinckley, Robert
Capital District Physicians
Health Plan — Page 286
Hiner, Nick
Health Net of Arizona — Page 17
Hines, Judith
Hines & Associates Inc — Page 150
Hines, Linda
Virginia Premier Hlth Plans Inc — Page 447
Hinkle, Allen J MD
Tufts Health Plan — Page 216
Hinkle, Gary
Advantage Health Solutions Inc — Page 157
Hinton, James H
Presbyterian Health Plan — Page 281

Hipwell, Art
Humana Insurance Co - AL — Page 5
Humana Inc - CO — Page 82
Humana Inc - DC — Page 98
Humana Inc - ND — Page 317
Hird, Andrea
First Health — California — Page 46
Hirsch, Thomas J, MD
Dean Health Plan — Page 463
Hirsh, Alan, MD
Health Design Plus — Page 327
Hiza, Douglas, MD
First Plan of Minnesota — Page 235
Hjerpe, Fred, MD
For Eyes Vision Plan Inc — Page 47
Ho, Sam N, MD
PacifiCare Health Systems-
Corporate Headquarters — Page 62
PacifiCare of California — Page 62
Pacificare Life & Health
Insurance Company — Page 63
PacifiCare of Nevada — Page 263
Hobbs, Cary D
Centene Corporation — Page 244
Hobbs, Sherry
Ameritas Mngd Dental Plan Inc — Page 34
Hobgood, Mark
Healthcare Partners of
East Texas Inc — Page 416
Hochstetler, Mark A, MD
Encore Health Network — Page 160
Hockenson, Susan
Behavioral Hlthcare Options Inc — Page 259
Hockett, Bill
ODS Health Plan — Page 349
Hockmuth, Robert, MD
CIGNA Healthcare of Maine Inc — Page 195
Hodge, Grace, RN
Humana Medical Plan - Daytona — Page 113
Hodge, Jerry, RPh
Maxor Plus — Page 488
Hodges, Debbie
Health Plans Inc — Page 213
Hodgin, Ace M, MD
Bravo Health Mid-Atlantic Inc — Page 200
Bravo Health Texas Inc — Page 407
Bravo Health Inc — Page 200
Bravo Health Mid-Atlantic Inc — Page 517
Hodgkins, Robert C Jr
Dental Care Plus Inc — Page 324
Hoeflinger, Erin
Anthem BCBS of Maine — Page 195
Hoernis, Pamela CPA
Texas Medical Foundation
Health Quality Institute — Page 427
Hoernke, Daniel
Humana Hlth Care Plans of AZ — Page 17
Hofflander, John
Preferred One — Page 237
Hoffman, Joseph H
Central Benefits Mutual
Insurance Company — Page 321
Hoffman, Susan, RN
Humana Medical Plan Inc — Page 114
Hoffmann, Bruce, DC
ACN Group — Page 233
Hoffmann, Julie
Medical Associates Clinic
Health Plan of WI — Page 467
Hofkes, Steven
Group Health Cooperative
of Eau Claire — Page 465
Hofman, Allison
QualCare Inc — Page 276
Hogan, John M
Capital Health Plan — Page 105
Hogan, Kathryn
Lakewood Health Plan Inc — Page 56

Index VIII: Personnel

Haugen, Rich, CPA
North Dakota Hlth Care Review Page 318
Haughton, ELizabeth, JD
Primecare Medical Network Inc Page 65
Hauptman, Mark D
Mega Life & Health
Insurance Company Page 420
Hauser, Martin
CHN MCO Page 322
SummaCare Inc Page 334
Hauser, William E, Jr, MD
Aetna Inc - Georgia Page 127
Hauteman, Wendy
EyeMed Vision Care LLC Page 325
Havard, Jerry
Maxor Plus Page 488
Havel, Thomas, MD
Concern: Employee
Assistance Program Page 42
Havill, Mark
Paragon Biomedical Inc Page 491
Havlicek, Karen
Aetna Inc - Dental Care of CA Page 32
Hawkins, Gregory A
M-Care Inc Page 225
Hawkins, Greogry, CPA
Priority Health Page 230
Hawkins, Michael MD
UnitedHealthcare of Texas Inc -
San Antonio Page 430
Hayburn, Renee
Health Net Hlth Plan of OR Inc Page 346
Haydel, Augustavia JD
LA Care Health Plan Page 55
Hayden, Gerard M JR
Medavant National
Preferred Provider Network Page 299
Hayden-Cook, Melissa
Sharp Health Plan Page 68
Hayek, Andrew
DaVita VillageHealth of MI Inc Page 220
Hayes, Darin
HealthAmerica Pennsylvania Inc -
Western Region Page 365
HealthAmerica Pennsylvania Inc -
NorthWest Page 365
Hayes, Jerry
Rocky Mountain Health Plans Page 84
Hayes, Lori
Dominion Dental Services -
Corporate Headquarters Page 444
Haygood, Lori
Health Net of Arizona Page 17
Haygood, Rhonda
Vantage Health Plan Inc Page 193
Haynes, Benjamin K
CIGNA Dental Health of CO Page 78
CIGNA Dental Health of DE Inc Page 95
Haynes, David
Delta Dental Plan of Missouri Page 246
Haynes, Jay, MD
JPS Benefits Page 419
Haynes, Jean
BMC HealthNet Plan Page 209
Haynes, Kelly
Mutual Assurance
Administrators Inc Page 342
Haynes, Ted
Blue Cross Blue Shield of Texas —
Corporate Headquarters Page 406
Hays, Bonnie
Metropolitan Health Plan Page 237
Hays, Cheryl
Oklahoma Foundation for
Medical Quality Page 342
Haytaian, Peter D Esq
AmeriGroup New Jersey Inc Page 268
Hayward, Doug
WellCare Health Plans Inc -
Corporate Headquarters Page 124

Hazelip, Tina
Deaconess Health Plans Page 159
Deaconess Health Plans Page 159
Hazen, Wynn
Physicians Health Plan of
South Michigan Page 229
Hazlewood, Hugh
Liberty Dental Plan of CA Page 56
Hazlewood, Marsha
Liberty Dental Plan of CA Page 56
Head, Janice L
Kaiser Permanente Health Plan Page 137
Headley, Patricia
MPRO Page 227
Healey, Eileen
Medavant National
Preferred Provider Network Page 299
Heaps, Collette
Altius Health Plans Page 433
Hearell, John
Mega Life & Health
Insurance Company Page 420
Heavens, Teresa L
Health Partners Page 364
Hebert, Mundy
Forte Managed Care Page 414
Hebner, Tom
LifeWise Health Plan of OR Page 348
Heckenlaible, Mick
Delta Dental Plan of SD Page 387
Hedlund, Janet
Sagamore Health Network Inc Page 164
Hedstrom, David, DDS
Delta Dental Plan of NH Page 265
Hedstrom, Nancy
CIGNA Behavioral Health Inc Page 88
CIGNA Behavioral Health Inc -
Corporate Headquarters Page 234
Heffernan, Regina
Keystone Mercy Health Plan Page 368
Hefner, Jaunell
Managed Health Network Page 57
Hegschweiler, Kurt DC
American Spclty Hlth Plans Inc Page 33
Hegstad, Rich
HMS Colorado Inc Page 82
Sloan's Lake Preferred
Health Networks Page 85
Heidelman, Joseph T
FirstSight Vision Services Inc Page 47
Hein, David
Complementary Hlthcare Plans Page 345
Heine, Kevin
Aetna Inc - Pennsylvania Page 355
Heinz, Scott
Saint Mary's HealthFirst Page 263
Hekman, Steve
Grand Valley Health Plan Page 221
Held, Arthur
APS Healthcare Northwest Inc Page 253
APS Healthcare Midwest Inc Page 461
Helenius, Beth
Fallon Community Hlth Plan Inc Page 211
Helling, Cindy
Select Health of SC Page 385
Hembrick, Monica
Coalition America Inc Page 129
Hemeon, Frank
Kaiser Foundation Health
Plan Northwest Page 347
Hemingway Hall, Patricia A
Health Care Service Corporation -
Corporate Headquarters Page 149
Hemmer, Laura
Dental Care Plus Inc Page 324
Hemmingsen-Souza, Lori RN
Superior Vision Services Inc Page 70

Hemsley, Stephen J
Ovations Pharmacy Solutions Page 490
UnitedHealth Group —
Corporate Headquarters Page 238
United Healthcare Ins Co Page 519
Henchey, Chris
MVP Health Plan of NH Page 266
Henderson, David
GHI HMO Select Inc Page 293
Henderson, Elizabeth, DDS
California Dental Network Inc Page 37
Henderson, Jeff
LeaderNET/Leader Drug Stores —
Cardinal Health Inc Page 487
Henderson, Lisa
Beech Street Corporation —
Corporate Headquarters Page 36
Hendrick, Jeremy
Careington International -
The Dental Network Page 408
Hendrikson, Kay
Metropolitan Health Plan Page 237
Henneman, Phil
Parkview Signature Care Page 164
Hennes, David, MD
KPS Health Plans Page 452
Henningsen, Rod
Alpha Dental Plan of Colorado Page 77
Henrickson, Robert
New England Financial - Corporate
Headquarters Page 214
Henriksen, Rich
Americas PPO Page 233
Henry, Dave
New West Health Plan Page 254
Henry, Debra M
Blue Cross of Idaho Page 141
Henry, Elizabeth
CIGNA Healthcare of Connecticut Page 89
Henry, Robert
Yale University Health Plan Page 93
Hensley, Murphy J
UnitedHealthcare of Washington Page 457
Hentschel, Bruce R
Employers Dental Services Inc Page 15
Herbert, Michael
Delta Dental Plan of Kansas Page 178
Delta Dental Plan of Kansas Page 178
Herbert, Michael E
Connecticare Inc Page 89
Connecticare of NY Page 288
Connecticare of MA Inc Page 210
Herdman, Bruce, MBA, PhD
Keystone Mercy Health Plan Page 368
Herduin, Robert
Preferred Health Professionals Page 180
Herman, Joan E
WellPoint Inc - Corp Hdqrtrs Page 167
Herman, Michael
Coventry Hlth Care Inc-DE Inc Page 96
Herman, Roberta, MD
Harvard Pilgrim Health Care -
Corporate Headquarters Page 212
Herman, Scott
Humana Health Care Plans of
Houston Page 418
Herman, Ted
Hudson Health Plan Page 297
Hermann, Karen
Sentinel Management Services -
Corporate Headquarters Page 372
Hermniz, Nancy
Neighborhood Health Plan of
Rhode Island Page 380
Hernandez, Ismael
Select Health of South Carolina Page 385
Hernandez, Linda
Primary Provider Mngmnt Co Inc Page 64

Index VIII: Personnel

Texas Dental Plan — Page 427
Hammergren, John
McKesson Pharmacy
Provider Network — Page 488
Hammond, J D, PharmD
American Pharmacy
Services Corporation — Page 183
Hamnick, Martha
United Concordia Company Inc -
Maryland — Page 206
Hamrick, Gary
West Virginia Medical Institute — Page 460
Hamslay, Lisa, RN
Phoebe Health Partners — Page 133
Hanaway, Edward
CIGNA Healthcare of TN Inc — Page 394
Hancovsky, Jim
Unison Health Plan of TN — Page 399
Handa, Angela
Health First Health Plans Inc — Page 111
Handel, Paul, MD
Health Care Service Corporation -
Corporate Headquarters — Page 149
Blue Cross Blue Shield of Texas —
Corporate Headquarters — Page 406
Blue Cross Blue Shield of Texas —
HMO Blue - Midwest TX — Page 406
Blue Cross Blue Shield of Texas —
HMO Blue - West — Page 407
Handelman, Warren
MultiPlan Inc - Corp Hdqrtrs — Page 300
Private Hlthcr Systems Inc — Page 455
Handkins, Shelly
Providence Health Plans — Page 351
Hanford, Patrick, MD
Texas Medical Foundation
Health Quality Institute — Page 427
Hanks, Christopher B
HealthTrans LLC — Page 486
Hanks, Rick
Utah Public Employees
Health Program — Page 438
Hanna, Cathy
American Pharmacy
Services Corporation — Page 183
Hanna, Gabriel J
D C Chartered Health Plan Inc — Page 97
Hanna, George B
Wellmark Inc —
Corporate Headquarters — Page 175
Hannah, Paulette
Concern: Employee
Assistance Program — Page 42
Hannigan-Farley, Patricia, PhD
JP Farley Corp — Page 329
Hannon, Richard M
Blue Cross Blue Shield of AZ — Page 12
Hansen, Ann
Great Lakes Medical Review — Page 326
Hansen, Bonnie
Altius Health Plans — Page 433
Hansen, David
PacifiCare of Oregon — Page 350
Hansen, Gunnar
Clear Choice Health Plans — Page 345
Hansen, Jennie Chin
On Lok Senior Health Services — Page 512
Hansen, R.Scott
Utah Public Employees
Health Program — Page 438
Hanson, Mike
UnitedHealthcare of Florida Inc — Page 122
Hanson, Suzy
Cariten Healthcare — Page 393
PHP Companies Inc — Page 397
Hanway, H Edward
CIGNA Healthcare of AZ — Page 14
CIGNA Healthcare of CT — Page 89

CIGNA Healthcare of IL Inc — Page 144
CIGNA Dental Health of MD Inc — Page 201
CIGNA Healthcare of NC Inc — Page 311
CIGNA Healthcare - Cincinnati — Page 323
CIGNA HealthCare —
Corporate Headquarters — Page 360
CIGNA Dental Health of PA Inc — Page 360
CIGNA Healthcare of TN — Page 393
CIGNA Healthcare of TX Inc — Page 409
Haraway, Mark
Denta Quest Ventures Inc — Page 211
Harbert, Lynn
Delta Dental Plan of Arkansas — Page 26
Harder, Ralph, MD
Community Clinical Services — Page 196
Hardesty, Cliff
PacifiCare of Arizona — Page 19
PacifiCare of Colorado — Page 84
Hardin, Dianna R
4MOST Health Network — Page 459
Harding, Cynthia M, APR
Kaiser Foundation Health
Plan of Southern California — Page 54
Harding, John, MD
Corporate Care Mngmnt Inc — Page 288
Hardwick, Debi
Coastal Hlthcare Administrators — Page 41
Hare, James MD
UnitedHealthcare of WI Inc — Page 470
Haring, Carissa
McLaren Health Plan — Page 226
Harless, Jim
Antares Management Solutions — Page 319
Harman, Charles E
Blue Cross Blue Shield of GA — Page 128
Harmer, MaryAnne
Regence BCBS — Page 351
Harp, Joan
BCBS of Tennessee — Page 392
BCBS of Tennessee - Memphis — Page 393
Harper, Candy
WelBorn Health Plans — Page 167
Harper, Jennifer, MD
CIGNA Healthcare - Cincinnati — Page 323
Harrell, Traci
Superior Dental Care Alliance — Page 335
Harriger, Craig MBA, JD
Magellan Health Services Inc — Page 91
Harrington, Eric
HMO Louisiana Inc — Page 191
BCBS of Louisiana Inc — Page 189
Harrington, Judy B
Health Partners — Page 364
Harris, Cheryl
Wellpath Select Inc — Page 315
Harris, Eddie
Blue Cross Blue Shield of AL — Page 3
Harris, Edwin J
Delta Dental Plan of NM — Page 279
Harris, Meghan
Ohio Kepro Inc — Page 332
Harris, Ryan
MetroPlus Health Plan — Page 300
Harris, Shawn
MedFocus Radiology Network — Page 58
Harris, Stephen
UAHC Health Plan of TN — Page 399
Harrison, Dorothy, PhD
Horizon Behavioral Services — Page 417
Horizon Behavioral Services — Page 112
Harrison, Larry
Managed Hlth Services IN Inc — Page 163
Harrison, Larry J
Scripps Clinic Health
Plan Services Inc — Page 68
Harrison, Linda
Health Net Hlth Plan of OR Inc — Page 346
Harrison, Richard
Contra Costa Health Plan — Page 43

Harrold, Jason
Opticare Managed Vision — Page 314
AECC Total Vision Health
Plan of Texas Inc — Page 403
Harrop, Donald E, MD
KePRO — Page 367
Harston, Dennis T, MD, MBA
Altius Health Plans — Page 433
Hart, Erin
American Hlthcare Group Inc — Page 356
Hart, Laura
Secure Hlth Plans of GA LLC — Page 133
Hart, Marcy
Arnett Health Plans — Page 157
Hart, Ned
Parkview Signature Care — Page 164
Hart, Roland, MD
San Joaquin Foundation PPO — Page 67
Hart, Steve
Nationwide Better Health — Page 204
Harte, Helen
Community Health Plan of WA — Page 450
Hartert, James E, MD, MS, FACP
Prime Therapeutics — Page 493
Hartz, Leo
Blue Cross of Northeastern PA — Page 358
Hartzell, Ed
Antares Management Solutions — Page 319
Harvill, Mark
Paragon Biomedical Inc — Page 491
Haslam, Christine
Aetna Inc - Maine — Page 195
Hassan, Pamela
Centercare Inc — Page 287
Hassel, Mike
SelectHealth Network — Page 165
Hassen, Pamela
New York State Catholic
Health Plan Inc — Page 303
Hastings, Thomas, MD
Essence Inc — Page 246
Hastreiter, Richard, DDS
Delta Dental Plan of Minnesota — Page 235
Hatcher-Sneed, Karen
Pequot Pharmaceutical Network — Page 491
Hatfield, Fred
Aetna Health of California Inc — Page 31
Hatfield, Laura, RN
Humana Hlth Care Plans of IL — Page 151
Hatfield, Susan
Nationwide Health Plans — Page 331
Hathcock, Bonnie C
Humana Insurance Co - AL — Page 5
Humana Inc - AR — Page 27
Humana Inc - CO — Page 82
Humana Inc - DC — Page 98
Humana Inc - Indiana — Page 161
Humana Inc - IA — Page 170
Humana Inc -
Corporate Headquarters — Page 185
Humana Inc - MD — Page 203
Humana Inc - MI — Page 241
Humana Inc - NE — Page 256
Humana Inc - NM — Page 280
Humana Inc - NC — Page 313
Humana Inc - ND — Page 317
Humana Health Plan of OH Inc — Page 328
Humana Inc - OK — Page 341
Humana Inc - SC — Page 384
Humana Inc - SD — Page 388
Humana Inc - TN — Page 396
Humana Health Care Plans
of Corpus Christi — Page 417
Humana Inc - UT — Page 435
Humana Inc - Wyoming — Page 473
Humana Inc — Page 486
Hau, Kilo
UnitedHealthcare of Arkansas — Page 28

Index VIII: Personnel

Guardia, Angela
Pharmacy Providers
Services Corp — Page 492
Guarneschelli, N Timothy
HealthAmerica Pennsylvania Inc -
NorthWest — Page 365
HealthAmerica Pennsylvania Inc -
Central Region — Page 364
HealthAmerica Pennsylvania Inc -
Eastern Region — Page 365
Guenther, Bret W, CEBS
Dentistat (Insurance
Dentists of America) — Page 45
Guertin, Lisa M
Anthem BCBS of NH — Page 265
Guertin, Shawn M
First Health Group Corp — Page 147
Coventry Health Care Inc —
Corporate Headquarters — Page 201
Guerue, Chris
Galaxy Health Network — Page 414
Guethon, Josa A, MD, MBA
Metcare Health Plans Inc — Page 116
Guillama, Noel J
Renaissance Hlth Systems Inc — Page 119
Guillama, Susan D
Renaissance Health Systems Inc — Page 119
Guinn, Joe
PacifiCare of Texas Inc — Page 422
Gularte, Marla
Concern: Employee
Assistance Program — Page 42
Gulau, Jere
Evolutions Hlthcare Sys Inc — Page 109
Gurber, Tara Dowd
Health Care Service Corporation -
Corporate Headquarters — Page 149
Gurk, Peter, MD
Bluegrass Family Health Inc — Page 183
Gustafson, Greg A
Upper Peninsula Health Plan — Page 232
Gustavel, Jack
Blue Cross of Idaho — Page 141
Gustin, Karen
Ameritas Group Dental — Page 255
Gustrand, Paul
Dental Benefit Providers Inc — Page 202
Guthrie, Cindy
PersonalCare Insurance of IL Inc — Page 151
Gutierrez, Patricia
Primecare Medical Network Inc — Page 65
Gutierrez, Victor, MD
Humana Inc/PCA - Puerto Rico — Page 377
Humana Inc/PCA - Puerto Rico — Page 518
Gutman, Steve
CareGuide — Page 105
Gutzmore, Jennifer M, MD
Health Net of California — Page 49
Guzman, Cynthia, CPA
Lakewood Health Plan Inc — Page 56
Gyton, Mike
Unicare Health Plans of the
Midwest Inc — Page 153

H

Haaland, Doug
Cariten Healthcare — Page 393
PHP Companies Inc — Page 397
Haarala, Karen
Delta Dental Plan of Minnesota — Page 235
Haas, David R, MD
Opticare Managed Vision — Page 314

Haas, Jeffrey
Aetna Inc - Washington — Page 449
Haas, Marci B
MDNY Healthcare Inc — Page 299
MDNY Healthcare Inc — Page 299
Haas, Michelle I
CIGNA Dental Health Inc -
Corporate Headquarters — Page 106
CIGNA Dental Health of FL — Page 107
CIGNA Dental Health of NC Inc — Page 310
CIGNA Dental Health of OH Inc — Page 322
CIGNA Dental Health of TX Inc — Page 409
Haas, Terrance P
Amerisource Bergen
Performance Plus Network - West — Page 480
Haaz, Edward J
Mental Health Consultants Inc — Page 369
Haban, Gregory, MD
Aultcare — Page 320
Primetime Medical Health Plan — Page 333
Habowski, Sandra
Health Net of Arizona — Page 17
Hackworth, John
Health Plan of San Joaquin, The — Page 50
Haden, Eric
Inland Empire Health Plan — Page 52
Hadley, Michael
Healthnow — Page 395
Haessler, Greg, MD
Principal Life Insurance Company — Page 172
Hafer, Roderick J, PhD
APS Healthcare Inc — Page 199
APS Healthcare Northwest Inc — Page 253
Haffner, Richard J, DDS
Delta Dental Plan of Missouri — Page 246
Delta Dental Plan of SC — Page 384
Hafford, Juliet
Flora Health Network — Page 325
Hagan, Lynn Datsko
American Hlthcare Group Inc — Page 356
Hagan, Robert E, Jr, CPA
American Hlthcare Group Inc — Page 356
Hagan, Thomas
ParadigmHealth — Page 276
Hagen, Joyce S
University Health Care Inc -
Passport Health Plan — Page 187
Hager, Chad
Heart of America Health Plan — Page 317
Hagert, Michael
First Choice of the Midwest Inc — Page 388
Haggett, William F
Amerihealth Ins Co - NJ North — Page 269
Amerihealth Ins Co - NJ South — Page 269
Haglund, Jacqueline
BCBS of Oklahoma — Page 339
Bluelincs HMO — Page 340
Hague, Richard DMD
Liberty Dental Plan of California — Page 56
Haigler, Steven
CIGNA Healthcare of Florida — Page 107
Hailey, James R
Coventry Health Care Inc —
Corporate Headquarters — Page 201
Haines, Rick L
Aultcare — Page 320
Primetime Medical Health Plan — Page 333
Haincy, Jenny, RN
Family Health Partners — Page 247
Hairston, Don
Citrus Health Care Inc — Page 108
Hakanson, Tim
Trustmark Insurance Company — Page 153
Hale, Kathy
Healthcare Partners of
East Texas Inc — Page 416
Hale, Richard
BCBS of Mississippi — Page 241

Hale, Rick
HMS Colorado Inc — Page 82
Sloan's Lake Preferred
Health Networks — Page 85
Hale, William E
Beech Street Corporation — Corporate
Headquarters — Page 36
Hall, David T
Dental Benefit Prvdrs of CA Inc — Page 45
Hall, Dr A Edward
Delta Dental Plan of Kansas — Page 178
Hall, Jeffrey
Express Scripts Inc - MN — Page 484
Express Scripts Inc -
Corporate Headquarters — Page 484
Express Scripts Inc - NJ — Page 484
Express Scripts Inc - PA — Page 484
Hall, Kerry
Delta Dental Plan of Wyoming — Page 473
Hall, Miles, DDS
CIGNA Dental Health of NC Inc — Page 310
CIGNA Dental Health of OH Inc — Page 322
Hallam, Bernadette
Senior Care Connection Inc — Page 509
Hallam, Cynthia
HmoLouisiana Inc — Page 191
Hallberg, Charles E, JD
MemberHealth Inc — Page 489
Hallet, Susan
Great-West Healthcare of
California - Northern — Page 48
Halley, Melissa
Vantage Health Plan Inc — Page 193
Hallock, Kristine M
Innovative Care Management — Page 347
Halow, Joseph
Medical Care Referral Group — Page 420
Halow, Lorri
Medical Care Referral Group — Page 420
Halpert, Andy MD
Blue Shield of California — Page 36
Halseth, Marilyn
Ucare Minnesota — Page 238
Halvorsen, George C
Kaiser Foundation Health Plan of
Northern California — Page 54
Kaiser Foundation Health
Plan of Southern California — Page 54
Kaiser Permanente - Kaiser
Foundation Health Plan, Inc — Page 54
Kaiser Foundation Health
Plan of Colorado — Page 83
Hamblin, Greg BS, CPA
Molina Healthcare Inc - CA — Page 59
Hambrick, Harold
UHP Healthcare — Page 71
Hamilton, Janet
Columbia United Providers — Page 449
Hamilton, Melissa
CorpHealth Inc — Page 412
Hamilton, Roderick
Hygeia Corporation — Page 114
Hamilton, Stuart A, MD
Select Health of South Carolina — Page 385
Hamilton, Tyrette
Safeguard Hlth Enterprises Inc — Page 66
Hamm, Don
Assurant Health -
Corporate Headquarters — Page 462
Hamm, Kenneth
First Choice Health Network — Page 451
Hammant, Bridgette
Fara Healthcare Management — Page 190
Hammer, Kenneth J, DDS, MBA
CompBenefits Corporation -
Corporate Headquarters — Page 129
CompBenefits — Page 410

Index VIII: Personnel

Gray, Donnie
Broadspire Inc — Page 105
Gray, James, MD
Brazos Valley Health Network — Page 408
Gray, Kimberly S, Esq CIPP
Highmark Inc — Page 366
Gray, Lisa
Great Lakes Health Plan — Page 222
Gray, Rhesa
CorpHealth Inc — Page 412
Gray, Walter
Care 1st Health Plan — Page 38
Graye, Mitchell
Great-West Healthcare of CO — Page 81
Great-West Healthcare of IL — Page 148
Great-West Healthcare of Kansas/Missouri — Page 179
Great West Life Annuity Insurance Co — Page 81
Grden, Nancy L
AmeriGroup Corporation — Page 442
Greaves, Roger F
Health Net Inc - Corp Hdqrtrs — Page 49
Grebow, Edward
UlliCare — Page 98
Greczyn, Robert J, Jr
BCBS of North Carolina — Page 310
BCBS of North Carolina — Page 481
Green, Christopher
Brazos Valley Health Network — Page 408
Green, Dolores L
Inland Empire Foundation for Medical Care — Page 52
Green, Lee
Scott & White Health Plan — Page 424
Green, Lee B
Unicare Health Plans of the Midwest Inc — Page 153
Green, Taira
Family Health Partners — Page 247
Green, Theodore T
UlliCare — Page 98
Green, W Bradley
Healthspring of Alabama Inc — Page 5
Green, Warren
One Call Medical Inc — Page 275
Green-EL, Diane, MD
SCHC Total Care Inc — Page 305
Greena, Karen M
Delta Dental Plan of Indiana Inc — Page 159
Greenberg, Allan I
Aetna Inc - Missouri — Page 243
Aetna Health Inc - Colorado — Page 77
Greenberg, Ann
Lovelace Health Plan — Page 280
Greenberg, Helen
Great-West Healthcare - NJ — Page 272
Greene, Judith
Community Health Network of Connecticut Inc — Page 89
Greene, Thomas E
Medical Mutual of Ohio — Page 330
Greenfield, Craig B
MagnaCare — Page 298
Greenhouse, Kara
Dominion Dental Services - Corporate Headquarters — Page 444
Greenman, Jack
Vista Health Plan Inc — Page 123
Vista Hlthplan of South FL Inc — Page 123
Greensberg, Marsha
Altius Health Plans — Page 433
Greenwalt, Pamela
UlliCare — Page 98
Greenway, Claudette RN
Oklahoma Foundation for Medical Quality — Page 342

Greenwood, Jim
Concentra Inc — Page 411
Greenwood, Marilyn
Pioneer Management Systems — Page 215
Greer, Len
Active Health Management — Page 441
Greeson, Dean, MD
Great-West Healthcare of GA — Page 131
Gregg, Vicky
BCBS of TN — Page 392
Gregg, Vicky
BCBS of Tennessee - Memphis — Page 393
Gregoire, Daniel N
Oxford Health Plans Inc — Corporate Headquarters — Page 92
Oxford Health Plans of NY, Inc — Page 303
Gregoire, John
South Country Health Alliance — Page 507
Gregory, Beth, PhD
Behavioral Health Systems Inc — Page 3
Gregory, Glen
American LIFECARE - Mississippi - PHCS — Page 241
Gregory, Steve
BCBS of Mississippi — Page 241
Gress, Elaine
Mega Life & Health Ins Co — Page 420
Grezcyn, Robert
Partners National Health Plans of North Carolina Inc — Page 314
Gries, Tanna
Avera Health Plans Inc — Page 387
Griffin, Brian T
Medco Health Solutions Inc — Page 488
Griffin, Cynthia
Humana Health Plan - Jacksonville — Page 113
Griffin, Susan
Great-West Healthcare of FL — Page 111
Griffin, Susan
Concordia Care — Page 509
Griffin, Thomas
Great-West Healthcare of ME — Page 196
Griffin, William
Baptist Health Services Group — Page 392
Griffith, David T
Excellus BlueCross BlueShield, Utica Region — Page 292
Griffith, Jacque
Care 1st Health Plan AZ Inc — Page 13
Griffith, Julie
Physicians Health Plan of Mid-Michigan — Page 228
Griffiths, Linda
CIGNA Healthcare of MA — Page 210
Griggs, Johnny D
UHP Healthcare — Page 71
Griggs, Roland, MD
Care Network — Page 359
Griggs, Stephanie W
Community Care Health Plan Inc — Page 521
Grigson, John
Cooks Childrens Health Plan — Page 411
Grimes, Alan, MD
UnitedHealthcare of Kentucky — Page 186
Grimes, Sandra
Ventura County Foundation for Medical Care — Page 73
Grimm, Michelle
UnitedHealthcare of the Midwest Inc — Page 251
Grimm, William
Magellan Bhvrl Care of IA Inc — Page 171
Grimm, William R
Premier Bhvrl Systems of TN LLC — Page 398
Grimshaw, Thomas
Exempla Healthcare LLC — Page 81
Griswell, J Barry
Principal Life Insurance Co — Page 172

Griswold, Roger
UnitedHealthcare of Ohio Inc- Cleveland — Page 336
Groban, Mark D, MD
OneNet PPO — Page 205
MD-Individual Practice Association Inc (MD IPA) — Page 204
Mid Atlantic Medical Services Inc (MAMSI)- Corp Headquarters — Page 204
Optimum Choice Inc — Page 205
Groce, Joel
Medcost LLC — Page 313
Grodus, Michael G
McLaren Health Plan — Page 226
Groffman, Aaron
CIGNA Dental Health of CA Inc — Page 40
CIGNA Dental Health of CO — Page 78
CIGNA Dental Health of DE Inc — Page 95
CIGNA Dental Health Inc - Corporate Headquarters — Page 106
CIGNA Dental Health of FL — Page 107
Grohskopf, Dean
Mountain Medical Affiliates — Page 83
HMS Colorado Inc — Page 82
Sloan's Lake Preferred Health Networks — Page 85
Groover, Linda
HealthTrans LLC — Page 486
Groover, Ron
KHS a KMG America Company — Page 385
Groover, Steve
HealthTrans LLC — Page 486
Grosand, Paul
Spectera Vision Inc - Corporate Headquarters — Page 206
Gross, Barry L, MD
Virginia Health Network — Page 447
Gross, Brenda
Priority Health — Page 230
Gross, Sharon
Phoebe Health Partners — Page 133
Grossman, Elliot
Eyexam of California Inc — Page 46
Grossman, Robert, MD
Health Net - New Jersey — Page 272
Grossman, Robert, MD
BCBS of North Dakota — Page 317
Grote, Gretchen
Strategic Health Development Corporation — Page 119
Groutt, Barbara, MSA
North Dakota Hlth Care Review — Page 318
Grove, Andrew
Humana Health Care Plans of Corpus Christi — Page 417
Humana Health Care Plans of San Antonio/Austin — Page 418
Grove, Chris
Mountain Pacific Quality Health Foundation — Page 254
Grove, Jane
South Central Preferred — Page 372
Grover, Mike
Health Plus — Page 150
Grubbs, Walter
Vision Service Plan of Arizona — Page 22
Gruber, Lynn
CIGNA Healthcare of Ohio Inc — Page 323
Gruenbaum, Samuel
Western Dental Services — Page 75
Grujich, Nick J
HealthExtras Inc — Page 485
Catalyst Rx, A Healthextras Co — Page 482
Grundy, Gordon W, MD
Aetna Inc - Massachusetts — Page 209
Aetna Inc - New York — Page 283
Grussi, Katherine
Anthem BCBS of Connecticut — Page 88

Index VIII: Personnel

Glover, Paul W
Interplan Health Group — Page 53
Interplan Health Group -
Corporate Headquarters — Page 91
Superien Health Network Inc — Page 335
Interplan Health Group — Page 419
AmeriScript Inc — Page 479
Glover, Paul W, III
Emerald Hlth Network Inc, The — Page 325
Glover, Wendy
Superior Dental Care Alliance — Page 335
Glover, Zina
Alameda Alliance for Health — Page 33
Gnisci, Frank J
Hygeia Corporation — Page 114
Goddard, Kevin
Blue Cross Blue Shield of VT — Page 439
Godin, Gary
CIGNA Healthcare of
Kansas/Missouri — Page 177
Godley, Pat
Contra Costa Health Plan — Page 43
Godwin, Rachel
Care Choices HMO — Page 218
Great Lakes Health Plan — Page 222
Goff, Susan A
Md-Individual Practice
Association Inc (MD IPA) — Page 204
Mid Atlantic Medical Services Inc
(MAMSI)- Corp Headquarters — Page 204
Optimum Choice Inc — Page 205
Goheen, Charles
Fallon Community Hlth Plan Inc — Page 211
Goheen, Lezli
Health Net Hlth Plan of OR Inc — Page 346
Gohlke, Robert, DDS
National Pacific Dental — Page 421
Gold, Clifford D
Wellmark BCBS of Iowa — Page 174
Wellmark Inc — Corp Hdqrtrs — Page 175
Gold, Mari S
MetroPlus Health Plan — Page 300
Gold, Michael A
Hawaii Medical Services Association -
BC/BS of Hawaii — Page 137
Goldberg, Steve
Blue Care Network of MI — Page 217
Goldberg, Steven, MD
Excellus BlueCross BlueShield,
Central NY Southern Tier — Page 291
Golden, William
UnitedHealthcare of New York
Metropolitan — Page 306
Oxford Health Plans of NY, Inc — Page 303
Goldin, Donna
Great-West Healthcare - Corp — Page 81
Great-West Healthcare of
Kansas/Missouri — Page 179
Great-West Healthcare of NC — Page 313
Great-West Healthcare of OH — Page 326
Goldman, Carol E
Centene Corporation — Page 244
Goldman-Wilkinson, Roberta
Community Medical Alliance — Page 210
Neighborhood Health Plan — Page 214
Goldstein, Alan, MD
HealthChoice of Alabama — Page 4
Goldstein, Allan MD
Amerihealth Ins - Co-NJ North — Page 269
Amerihealth Ins Co - NJ South — Page 269
Goldstein, Gary, MD
Humana Health Care Plans of
Dallas — Page 417
Humana Health Care Plans of
Houston — Page 418
Humana Health Plan of
Austin — Page 419
Goldstein, George S, PhD
Molina Healthcare of MI Inc — Page 227

Molina HealthCare of UT Inc — Page 435
Molina Healthcare Inc-CA — Page 59
Goldstone, Michael, MD
North Dakota Hlth Care Review — Page 318
Golemi, Glen J
UnitedHealthcare of Alabama — Page 7
UnitedHealthcare of Louisiana — Page 193
Golinkoff, Michael, MD
United Behavioral Health — Page 373
Golonski, Dave
Health Net of California — Page 49
Goltz, David
Fidelis SeniorCare Inc — Page 147
Gonis, John G, MD
Care-Plus Dental Plans Inc — Page 462
Gonzalez, Maria
Community First Health Plans Inc — Page 410
Gonzalez, Mary Helen
Community First Health Plans Inc — Page 410
Gonzalez, Virgilina
MetroPlus Health Plan — Page 300
Good, Laurie, RN
Fidelis SecureCare of MI Inc — Page 221
Goode, Steve
4D Pharmacy Management
Systems Inc — Page 479
Goodman, Bruce J
Humana Insurance Co - AL — Page 5
Humana Inc - AR — Page 27
Humana Inc - CO — Page 82
Humana Inc - DC — Page 98
Humana Inc - IA — Page 170
Humana Inc- IN — Page 161
Humana Inc -
Corporate Headquarters — Page 185
Humana Inc - MD — Page 203
Humana Inc - MI — Page 241
Humana Inc - NE — Page 256
Humana Inc - NM — Page 280
Humana Inc - NC — Page 313
Humana Inc - ND — Page 317
Humana Health Plan of OH Inc — Page 328
Humana Inc - OK — Page 341
Humana Inc - SD — Page 388
Humana Inc - TN — Page 396
Humana Health Care Plans
of Corpus Christi — Page 417
Humana Inc - UT — Page 435
Humana Inc - Wyoming — Page 473
Goodman, Kim
American College of Medical
Quality — Page 199
Goodman, Princess
Dominion Dental Services -
Corporate Headquarters — Page 444
Gootee, Robert
ODS Health Plan — Page 349
ODS Health Plan — Page 349
Gorczycd, Ed
Comprehensive Behavioral
Care Inc — Page 108
Gordan, Neil MD
Nationwide Better Health — Page 204
Gordon, Mark, CPA
Behavioral Health Systems Inc — Page 3
Gore, Christina, DDS
Delta Dental Plan of Kansas — Page 178
Gore, James L
Virginia Health Network — Page 447
Gore, John, MD
Landmark Healthcare Inc — Page 56
Gorecki, Chris
CIGNA Healthcare of Arizona — Page 14
Goren, Richard, DDS
Managed Dental Care — Page 57
First Commonwealth — Page 147
Gorlitz, Vicki
Great Expressions
Dental Centers — Page 222

Gorman, John H
BCBS of Rhode Island — Page 379
Gorman, Preston
Bluegrass Family Health Inc — Page 183
Gorton, Christopher, MD, MHSA
APS Healthcare Inc — Page 199
Gosnell, Deborah
Aetna Inc - Arkansas — Page 25
Gosnell, Ross
Delta Dental Plan of Illinois — Page 145
Goss, Laurie
Denver Health Medical Plan Inc — Page 80
Gosser, Bruce
HealthLink of Arkansas Inc — Page 27
Gotcher, Patrick D
CorpHealth Inc — Page 412
Gotkin, Trina
Denta Quest Mid-Atlantic Inc — Page 202
Gougler, Matt
Health Net Hlth Plan of OR Inc — Page 346
Gould, R Max
Aetna Health of Illinois Inc — Page 143
Gowdey, Craig
Washington Dental Service — Page 457
Gozon, Richard C
Amerisource Bergen Performance
Plus Network - Corporate — Page 480
Grabara, Kelly
Group Health Cooperative
of Eau Claire — Page 465
Grabow, Rhonda
Innoviant Inc — Page 487
Grady, Kara
Crawford and Co-Corp Hdqrtrs — Page 130
Graff, Sean
USA Managed Care Org — Page 22
Graham, Judy
OneNet PPO — Page 205
Md-Individual Practice Association Inc
(MD IPA) — Page 204
Mid Atlantic Medical Services Inc
(MAMSI)- Corp Headquarters — Page 204
Optimum Choice Inc — Page 205
Gran, Sid
Delta Dental Plan of SD — Page 387
Grandfield, Steve
BCBS of Nebraska — Page 255
Grangaard, Jean
Americas PPO — Page 233
Grant, Janet
CareSource — Page 321
Grantham, Sylvia
UHP Healthcare — Page 71
Granzier, Mark
Aetna Inc - Maine — Page 195
Grassy, Richard G, MD
PersonalCare Ins of IL Inc — Page 151
Gratton, Patricia
PACE Vermont Inc — Page 513
Gratton, Robert
Great West Life Annuity Ins Co — Page 81
Graves, Edward
UnitedHealthcare of the
Midwest Inc — Page 251
Graves, Lon MD
Kern Family Health Care — Page 55
Graves, Tania
CIGNA Healthcare of Arizona — Page 14
Graves, Tom
Coventry Health Care Inc — LA — Page 190
Gravette, Jim
PacificSource Health Plans — Page 350
Gray, Anita
Md-Individual Practice Association Inc
(MD IPA) — Page 204
Gray, Deanna H
Coventry Health Care Inc- IA — Page 169
Coventry Health Care of NE Inc — Page 255

Index VIII: Personnel

Gedwed, William J
Mega Life & Hlth Ins Company Page 420
Chesapeake Life Insurance Co Page 517

Gee, Karen
Primecare Medical Network Inc Page 65

Geiwitz, Paul
Preferred One Page 237

Geller, Roberta, RN, Esq
Community Health Network
of Connecticut Inc Page 89

Gellert, Jay M
Health Net Inc - Corp Hdqrtrs Page 49
Health Net - New York Page 295
Health Net - Connecticut Page 90

Gelpi, Leslie A
Unison Health Plan of TN Page 399
Unison Health Plan of OH Inc Page 336
Unison Health Plan -
Corporate Headquarters Page 372

Gelzer, Andrea, MD
BMC HealthNet Plan Page 209

Genecin, Paul, MD
Yale University Health Plan Page 93

Gentile, David R
BCBS of Kansas City Page 244

Gentile, Douglas A, MD, MBA
Allscripts Pharmaceuticals Inc Page 479

Gentile, Jane
Preferred Care Page 304

Gentry, Kevin
PTPN - Corporate Headquarters Page 65

Geoghan, Karen
Maricopa Health Plan Page 18
University Family Care Hlth Plan Page 22

George, David A
Cypress Care Page 483

George, Don
BCBS Shield of Vermont Page 439

George, Elizabeth, JD
CIGNA Behavioral Health Inc Page 408

George, John A
Intergroup Services Corp Page 367

George, Tim
M-Care Inc Page 225

George, William S
Health Partners Page 364

Georgopoulous, Larry
Presbyterian Health Plan Page 281

Georgy, Tina RN, MS
CIMRO Qlity Hlthcre Solutions Page 144

Gerace, James
USA Managed Care Org Page 22

Geraci, Danla
Aetna Inc - Louisiana Page 189

Geraghty, Patrick J
Horizon BCBS of NJ Page 273

Gerbo, Christine
Santa Clara Family Health Plan Page 67

Gerdas, John R, MD, FACOG
Spectrum Review Services Inc Page 426

Gericke, Kris PharmD
Orange Prevention &
Treatment Integrated Page 60

Germain, Carrie RPh
HealthPlus of Michigan Page 224

Germano, Emanuel F
Aetna Inc Life Insurance Co Page 87
Aetna Inc - Massachusetts Page 209

Gerrard, Allison
Us Script Inc Page 496

Gersie, Michael H
Principal Life Insurance Co Page 172

Gerstein, Richard
MultiPlan Inc - Corp Hdqrtrs Page 300
Private Hlthcare Systems-WA Page 455

Gesaman, Greg
Iowa Foundation for Medical Care/
Encompass Page 170

Gevens, Teresa
DakotaCare Page 387
DakotaCare Page 387

Geyer-Sylvia, Zelda
M-Care Inc Page 225
M-Care Inc Page 225

Giammona, Mary, MD
Health Plan of San Mateo Page 50

Giancursio, Donald J
Health Plan of Nevada Inc Page 260
Sierra Health Services Inc-
Corporate Headquarters Page 264

Giannotti, Jennifer
Windsor Health Plan of TN Inc Page 401

Giardina, Frank
Spectera Vision Services of
California Inc Page 69

Giardino, Angelo MD
Texas Childrens Health Plan Page 426

Gibboney, Liz
Partnership HealthPlan of CA Page 64

Gibford, Pat
Clear Choice Health Plans Page 345

Giblien, John
Blue Cross Blue Shield of TN Page 392

Gibson, Dale, DDS
Delta Dental Plan of SD Page 387

Giddings, Cindy
CommunityCare Managed Healthcare
Plans of Oklahoma Inc Page 340

Gies, Kathy
CIGNA Healthcare of California Page 41

Gies, Mary Ellen
Great Lakes Health Plan Page 222

Gifford, Joe, MD
Asuris Northwest Health Page 449

Gijsbers, Gary
Molina Healthcare of NM Page 281

Gil, Eladio
Preferred Care Partners Inc Page 118

Gilbert, Brad, MD
Inland Empire Health Plan Page 52

Gilbert, Jay M
Physicians Health Plan of
Northern Indiana Page 164

Gilbert, Joy
Health First Health Plans Inc Page 111

Gilbert, Mary Kay
CompBenefits Corporation -
Corporate Headquarters Page 129
CompBenefits Page 410
Texas Dental Plan Page 427

Gilbert, Mike
Prevea Health Network Page 469

Gilbody, Karl, RN
Orange County PPO Page 61

Giles, Randy
UnitedHealthcare of Texas Inc -
Houston Page 429

Gilfillan, Richard, MD
Geisinger Health Plan Page 363

Gilham, Charles
Mercy Health Plans of MO Inc Page 249

Gilkin, Bob
Coventry Hlth Care Inc-DE Inc Page 96
HealthAmerica Pennsylvania Inc -
Western Region Page 365
Carelink Health Plans Page 459
Carelink Health Plans Page 459

Gill, James F, Esq
GHI HMO Select Inc Page 293

Gillepsie, John, MD
Independent Health Assoc Inc Page 297

Gillert, Jay M
Health Net Inc - Northeast
Corporate Headquarters Page 91

Gillespie, Pat
Cariten Healthcare Page 393
PHP Companies Inc Page 397

Gilliland, Rob
Florida Health Care Plan Inc Page 109

Gilster, Mark
Sterling Life Insurance Co Page 501

Gimarelli, James R, Jr
UDC Ohio Inc Page 335

Gimbel, Marlin W
Pacific Visioncare WAInc Page 453

Gimble, Anna
UnitedHealthcare of Utah Page 437

Ginsberg, J Lawrence, MD
Central Susquehanna
Healthcare Providers Page 359
UnitedHealthcare of the
Midwest Inc Page 251

Girgenti, Anthony
Avesis Inc Page 12

Girolami, Sabrina RN, BSN
Geisinger Health Plan Page 363

Girten, Julie, RN
WelBorn Health Plans Page 167

Gist, JoAnna
Arkansas Managed Care Org Page 26

Giunta, Kavoi
Coventry Health Care of KS Inc Page 245

Gladden, John
Delta Dental of Oklahoma Page 340

Gladitsch, Peter
Health Net Inc - Northeast
Corporate Headquarters Page 91

Gladkov, Alexander, DDS
Affinity Dental Health Plans Page 32

Glas, Bob
Managed Health Network Page 57

Glaser, Daniel E
BCBS of North Carolina Page 310
BCBS North Carolina Page 481

Glass, Andrew MD
Health Net Hlth Plan of OR Inc Page 346

Glass, Sharon
Humana Mdicl Plan - Daytona Page 113

Glassbrenner, Mary J
Group Health Cooperative
of Eau Claire Page 465

Glasscock, Larry C
HealthLink Inc Page 248
Anthem BCBS of CO Page 77
WellPoint Inc - Corp Hdqrtrs Page 167
Anthem BCBS of Maine Page 195
Anthem BCBS of Nevada Page 259
Rocky Mountain Hospital &
Medical Services Inc Page 85

Glasscock, Larry C
WellPoint NextRX Page 497

Glasser, Michael, MD
CIGNA Behavioral Health Inc Page 40

Glassford, John
Novasys Health Network Page 28

Glatt, David J, MD
North Dakota Hlth Care Review Page 318

Glauser, David
Educators Health Care Page 434

Glavey, Patrick
Preferred Care Page 304

Glazer, Leslie
Dimension Health (PPO) Page 109

Gleit, Larry
CIGNA Behavioral Health Inc Page 408

Glenn, Gordon S
SXC Health Solutions Inc Page 495

Glenney, Karen
Community First Hlth Plans Inc Page 410

Glennon, Patty
Delta Dental Plan of WI Page 463

Glossy, Bernard
Delta Dental Plan of Arizona Inc Page 14

Glouner, Tanya
Berkshire Health Partners/Medicus
Resource Management Page 357

Index VIII: Personnel

Frost, Lynne
HealthLink Inc - Corp Hdqrtrs — Page 249
Frucella, Maureen
Preferred Hlthcare System Inc — Page 371
Fry, Robert S, Jr
CIGNA Healthcare of IL Inc — Page 144
Fuentes, Hector M
Medical Card System — Page 377
Fuerish, Sandy
Primary Provider
Management Company Inc — Page 64
Fugate, Hollace
CommunityCare Managed Healthcare
Plans of Oklahoma Inc — Page 340
Fuhrman, James
Pacific Union Dental Inc — Page 63
Spectera Vision Inc - Indiana — Page 166
Nevada Pacific Dental — Page 262
Fulkerson, Cathy
SelectHealth Network — Page 165
Fuller, Christy
Mountain Pacific Quality
Health Foundation — Page 254
Fullmer, Jane
Superior Dental Care Alliance — Page 335
Fullwood, Michael D, Esq
Hip Health Plan of New York — Page 296
Furey, Vincent, Jr
Medical Network Inc — Page 197
Furman, Donald S, MD, MBA
CareMore Health Plan — Page 38
Fusco, Robert, MD
United Behavioral Health (UBH) — Page 71
United Behavioral Health — Page 373

G

Gaal, Steve P III
Delta Dental Plan of Missouri — Page 246
Delta Dental Plan of SC — Page 384
Gabbard, Jennifer
UTMB Health Plans Inc — Page 431
Gabbert, John R
Great West Life Annuity
Insurance Co — Page 81
Great-West Healthcare -
Corporate — Page 81
Great-West Healthcare of
Kansas/Missouri — Page 179
Great-West Healthcare of NC — Page 313
Great-West Healthcare of OH — Page 326
Great-West Healthcare of OH — Page 326
Gabel, Larry, CPA
Davis Vision — Page 288
Gadola, Bob
Preferred One — Page 237
Gadsby, Laura R
Sentara Life Care Corp Inc — Page 514
Gaebel, John, DDS
Nevada Pacific Dental — Page 262
Pacific Union Dental Inc — Page 63
Gaffney, Paulette
Total Dental Administrators
Health Plan — Page 21
Gaglioti, Joseph
Pearle Vision Managed Care -
HMO of Texas Inc — Page 423
Gagne, Mark
CIGNA Healthcare — Page 439
Galanate, Dominic, MD
Preferred Care — Page 304
Galano, Rolando I
Educators Health Care — Page 434
Galbraith, George
Gateway Health Plan Inc — Page 362

Galbraith, Polly M, MD
Assurant Employee Benefits-AL — Page 3
Assurant Employee Benefits-AZ — Page 12
Assurant Employee Benefits-CA — Page 35
Assurant Employee Benefits-CO — Page 78
Assurant Employee Benefits-FL — Page 102
Assurant Employee Benefits-GA — Page 127
Assurant Employee Benefits-IL — Page 143
Assurant Employee Benefits-IN — Page 158
Assurant Employee Benefits-MI — Page 217
Assurant Employee Benefits -
Corporate Office — Page 244
Assurant Employee Benefits-NM — Page 279
Assurant Employee Benefits-NY — Page 285
Assurant Employee Benefits-NC — Page 309
Assurant Employee Benefits-PA — Page 357
Assurant Employee Benefits-TN — Page 392
Assurant Employee Benefits-TX — Page 429
Assurant Employee Benefits-WA — Page 449
Galinko, Neal, MD
UnitedHealthcare of
New England Inc — Page 381
Gallagher, Daniel
Unison Health Plan of SC Inc — Page 386
Gallagher, Michael
Av-Med Health Plan -
Gainesville — Page 102
Av-Med Health Plan -
Jacksonville — Page 102
Av-Med Health Plan - Miami — Page 103
Av-Med Health Plan - Orlando — Page 103
Av-Med Health Plan - Tampa — Page 103
Gallitano, Frances
Denta Quest Ventures Inc — Page 211
Gamache, Alanda
GenWorth Life & Health Ins Co — Page 90
Ganc, Cyndie
Coventry Health Care Inc-DE Inc — Page 96
Gandhi, Jay, PharmD, CDM
Fidelis SeniorCare Inc — Page 147
Gann, Merry
Strategic Health
Development Corporation — Page 119
Gannaway, Gary R
First Choice Health Network — Page 451
Ganoni, Sandy
Humana Wisconsin
Health Organization Inc — Page 466
Gantos, Russell P Jr
Community First Hlth Plans Inc — Page 410
Selectcare of Texas LLC — Page 521
Ganz, Mark B
Regence Blue Shield of Idaho — Page 142
Regence BCBS of Oregon — Page 351
Regence Group, The -
Corporate Headquarters — Page 351
Regence Valucare — Page 436
Asuris Northwest Health — Page 449
RegenceRx — Page 493
Garber, Judy, RN
Medwatch LLC — Page 116
Garboden, Steve
Mennonite Mutual Aid Assoc — Page 519
Garcia Romain, Oscar
Blue Cross of Puerto Rico/
La Cruz Azul de Puerto Rico — Page 377
Garcia, Daniel P
Kaiser Permanente - Kaiser
Foundation Health Plan, Inc — Page 54
Garcia, Joseph A
Community Health Group — Page 41
Garcia, Mary Alice
Molina Healthcare of NM — Page 281
Garcia, Melinda
Alameda Alliance for Health — Page 33
Garcia, Nancy
Preferred Medical Plan Inc — Page 118
Garcia, Stevan
UnitedHealthcare of Ohio Inc — Page 336

Garcia, Tida
Care 1st Health Plan Arizona Inc — Page 13
Gardner, Peter
Texas HealthSpring I LLC — Page 427
Gardynik, John, PharmD, MBA
RxAmerica LLC — Page 494
Garland, Patrick
Centercare Inc — Page 287
Garner, Dick
American Republic Ins Co — Page 169
Garner, Fredric, MD
National Capital PPO — Page 444
Garnes, Elizabeth
Union Health Service Inc — Page 154
Garrett, Barb
Community Health Alliance — Page 159
Garrett, Debbie
Scott & White Health Plan — Page 424
Garrett, Michael B, MS, CCM
Qualis Health — Page 455
Garrett, Sharon
Pacificare Life & Health
Insurance Company — Page 63
Garrett, Terry
Anthem BCBS of Maine — Page 195
Garrett, W Joe
Union Health Service Inc — Page 154
Garrison, Frank
Blue Care Network of MI — Page 217
Garrison, Kerri
BCBS of Western New York — Page 285
Garrison, Lynne
BCBS of North Carolina — Page 310
Gartner, Darcy
Vista Healthplan of
South Florida Inc — Page 123
Vista Health Plan Inc — Page 123
Garvanian, Kelli
Trustmark Insurance Company — Page 153
Garvey, Thomas E
Immediate Pharmaceutical
Services Inc — Page 486
Garvey, Tom
CIGNA Healthcare of CT — Page 89
CIGNA Healthcare of
New York and New Jersey — Page 270
Gasbarro, Eric
BCBS of Rhode Island — Page 379
Gaskill, Jerry
Humana Health Care Plans of
Kansas & Missouri — Page 179
Gasque, Damon
UlliCare — Page 98
Union Labor Life Insurance Co — Page 276
Gates, Dennis
Safeguard Hlth Enterprises Inc — Page 66
Gaucher, Ellen
Wellmark Inc-Corp Hdqrtrs — Page 175
Gaulstrand, Paul
Spectera Vision Inc - Indiana — Page 166
Gauper, Larry
BCBS of North Dakota — Page 317
Gauthier, Guy S
Priority Health — Page 230
Gauthier, Kathleen
Connecticare Inc — Page 89
Gaven, Steve
Has Premier Providers Inc — Page 415
Gavinski, Mary Parish, MD
Community Care Hlth Plan Inc — Page 521
Gavras, Debi
Healthy Palm Beaches Inc — Page 112
Gavras, Jonathan B, MD
Blue Cross Blue Shield of FL/
Health Options Inc — Page 104
Gedman, Bill
UMPC Health Plan Univ of
Pittsburgh Medical Center — Page 374

Index VIII: Personnel

Forrest, Patrick
Care Network   Page 359
Selectcare Access Corp   Page 371
Forsberg, Marilee
HealthPartners Inc   Page 236
Forsell, Annette
First Plan of Minnesota   Page 235
Forshee, James, MD
Molina Healthcare of MI Inc   Page 227
Forsyth, John D
Wellmark BCBS of Iowa   Page 174
Forsyth, John D
Wellmark Inc — Corp Hdqrtrs   Page 175
Forsyth, John D
Wellmark BCBS Shield of SD   Page 389
Forsyth, John D
Wellmark Health Plan of Iowa Inc Page 175
Fortini, John L
Assurant Employee Benefits-AL   Page 3
Assurant Employee Benefits-AZ   Page 12
Assurant Employee Benefits-CA   Page 35
Assurant Employee Benefits-CO   Page 78
Assurant Employee Benefits-FL   Page 102
Assurant Employee Benefits-GA   Page 127
Assurant Employee Benefits-IL   Page 143
Assurant Employee Benefits-IN   Page 158
Assurant Employee Benefits-MI   Page 217
Assurant Employee Benefits -
Corporate Office   Page 244
Assurant Employee Benefits-NM   Page 279
Assurant Employee Benefits-NY   Page 285
Assurant Employee Benefits-NC   Page 309
Assurant Employee Benefits-PA   Page 357
Assurant Employee Benefits-TN   Page 392
Assurant Employee Benefits-TX   Page 429
Assurant Employee Benefits-WA   Page 449
Fortner, Scott
Central Coast Alliance for Hlth Page 39
Fosjord, Vikki
Employee Benefit
Management Services Inc   Page 253
Foss, Robert
Mid Atlantic Medical Services Inc
(MAMSI)- Corp Headquarters   Page 204
Foss, Robert
Optimum Choice Inc   Page 205
Foster, Kelly
Community Health Alliance   Page 159
Foster, Martin G
Blue Cross Blue Shield of Texas —
Corporate Headquarters   Page 406
Blue Cross Blue Shield of Texas —
HMO Blue - Midwest TX   Page 406
Blue Cross Blue Shield of Texas —
HMO Blue - Southeast   Page 407
Blue Cross Blue Shield of Texas —
HMO Blue - West   Page 407
UnitedHealthcare of Texas Inc —
Dallas   Page 430
Foster, Noe
AlohaCare   Page 137
Foster, Scott
Peach State Health Plan   Page 133
Fouts, Terry L, MD
Great West Life Annuity
Insurance Co   Page 81
Great-West Healthcare -
Corporate   Page 81
Great-West Healthcare of IL   Page 148
Great-West Healthcare of
Kansas/Missouri   Page 179
Great-West Healthcare of Ohio   Page 326
Great-West Healthcare of Ohio   Page 326
Fowell, Ron
Center Care   Page 184
Fowler, Steve
Healthy Palm Beaches Inc   Page 112
Fox, Clement, MD
Health Advantage   Page 27

Fox, Don
Bravo Health Pennsylvania Inc   Page 358
Fox, Richard E
Unity Dental Health Services   Page 277
Francey, David
New York Compensation
Managers Inc   Page 302
Francis, Matt
Health Net of Arizona   Page 17
Franey, David, MD
Care 1st Health Plan AZ Inc   Page 13
Frank, Carole, RN
Optimum HealthCare Inc   Page 117
Frank, Leslie
Medica Health Plans   Page 236
Frank, Lisa
University Family Care
Health Plan   Page 22
Frank, Michael
Blue Cross Blue Shield of MT   Page 253
Franke, Donald A
Great-West Healthcare of IL   Page 148
Franklin, Andrew
Oregon Dealthan   Page 349
Frantz, James M
Health Plus of Louisiana Inc   Page 191
Franzoi, R.J.
Aetna Inc - Virginia   Page 441
Frasier, Jean S
San Francisco Health Plan   Page 66
Frawley, Patrick J, Rev
Centercare Inc   Page 287
Fidelis Care New York   Page 293
New York State Catholic
Health Plan Inc   Page 303
Frazier, Lynne
APS Healthcare Inc   Page 199
Frederick, David
NAMCI   Page 6
Premier Health Networks
of Alabama LLC   Page 6
Frederickson, Paula
Partnership HealthPlan of CA   Page 64
Fredrick, John, MD
Preferred One   Page 237
Fredrickson, Richard L
Buckeye Community
Health Plan Inc   Page 321
Freeman, Barbara, MD, FAAFP
Strategic Health
Development Corporation   Page 119
Freeman, Jennifer L, CPA
Molina HealthCare of WA Inc   Page 453
Freeman, Joanna
Superior Vision Services Inc   Page 70
Freeman, Keenan B
Southwest Health Alliance
(SHALLC)   Page 425
Freeman, Nancy E
Arkansas Community Care Inc   Page 26
Freeman, Robert
Santa Barbara Regional
Health Authority   Page 67
Frelick, Stephanie
Anthem BCBS of Wisconsin   Page 461
Fremion, Beth
Lutheran Preferred/
Three Rivers Preferred   Page 162
French, Judy
CIGNA Healthcare of Virginia Inc -
Richmond   Page 443
French, R Scott, MD
Regence Blue Shield   Page 456
Frenkel, Jillian M
Humana Health Plans of GA   Page 132
Frey, Jeannette
Fallon Community Hlth Plan Inc   Page 211

Frey, John P
CIGNA Dental Health of TX Inc   Page 409
Freysinger, Edward
Exempla Healthcare LLC   Page 81
Friberg, Kristina
UnitedHealthcare of Arkansas   Page 28
Fricchione, James M
MDNY Healthcare Inc   Page 299
Frick, Joseph A
Independence Blue Cross   Page 366
Keystone Health Plan East Inc   Page 368
Fridell, Cathy
OneNet PPO   Page 205
Fried, William, MD
Aetna Inc - New Jersey   Page 267
Aetna Hlth Plans of Mid-Atlantic Page 441
Aetna Inc - Virginia   Page 441
Friedley, Pat
Behavioral Health Systems Inc   Page 3
Friedman, David, MD
Chiropractic Arizona Network Inc Page 13
Friedman, Michelle
MedFocus Radiology Network   Page 58
Friedman, Neal
South Central Preferred   Page 372
Friedman, Richard H
BioScrip Inc   Page 481
Friedman, Robert, MD
Primary Health Plan   Page 142
Friedman, Scott W
BioScrip Inc   Page 481
Friedman, Yrena
Aetna Inc - Arizona   Page 11
Aetna Health of California Inc   Page 31
Friedrich, Jamie, MS
Innoviant Inc   Page 487
Friedrichs, Robert
UnitedHealthcare of Georgia   Page 134
Fries, John
Neighborhood Hlth Partnership   Page 116
Friscan, Bernice
United Behavioral Health (UBH)   Page 71
Frisch, Delphia B
Genex Services   Page 363
Friscino, Deborah
Mit Health Plan   Page 214
Fritch, Herb
Signature Health Alliance   Page 398
Fritch, Herbert A
Healthspring of Alabama Inc   Page 5
HealthSpring Inc - Tennessee   Page 395
HealthSpring Inc - Corp Hdqrtrs Page 395
Fritch, Vikki
MyMatrixx   Page 489
Fritz, Chris
Scripps Clinic Health
Plan Services Inc   Page 68
Fritz, Edward L, DDS
Health Resources Inc   Page 161
Fritz, James S
Bluegrass Family Health Inc   Page 183
Fritz, Richard A
Delta Dental of Rhode Island   Page 380
Altus Dental Insurance Co Inc   Page 379
Frock, Thomas
HMO New Mexico Inc   Page 280
Frock, Tom
Blue Cross Blue Shield of NM   Page 279
Frock, Tom
HMO New Mexico Inc   Page 280
Froeschle, Leslie, PHR
Texas Medical Foundation
Health Quality Institute   Page 427
Fronczek, Jodi
Dental Care Plus Inc   Page 324
Frost, Dena
PTPN - Corporate Headquarters   Page 65

Index VIII: Personnel

Fiebert, Ira
Physical Therapy Prvdr Ntwrk   Page 117
Fiedler, Alice
Atlantic Integrated Health Inc   Page 309
Fiegel, Susan
Anthem BCBS of Wisconsin   Page 461
Field, Robert W
Partners Rx Management LLC   Page 491
Fielder, Jay
Humana Health Benefit
Plan of Louisiana   Page 191
Fieldler, Justin
GHI HMO Select Inc   Page 293
Fields, Candia
CommunityCare Managed Healthcare
Plans of Oklahoma Inc   Page 340
Fields, Cherie
LA Care Health Plan   Page 55
Fields, David W
HealthLink Inc   Page 248
HealthLink Inc - Corp Hdqrtrs   Page 249
UniCare Health Plans of TX Inc   Page 428
Unicare Health Plans of the
Midwest Inc   Page 521
Fife, Carol
Med-Comp USA   Page 192
Figenshu, Bill
Western Health Advantage   Page 75
Figge, James, MD
Capital District Physicians
Health Plan   Page 286
Fikes, Francis, BA
Health Design Plus   Page 327
Film, George
Primetime Medical Hlth Plan   Page 333
Finkelstein, Loren
Great-West Healthcare of
California - Southern   Page 48
Finley, Deborah K, MPA
Primaris   Page 250
Finnegan, Geriann, RN, MSA
Health Plan of Michigan   Page 224
Finnegan, Paul
GenWorth Life & Hlth Ins Co   Page 90
Finnel, Debra A
Metcare Health Plans Inc   Page 116
Finnerty, Michael
American Specialty
Health Plans Inc   Page 33
Finora, Rosemary
APS Healthcare Midwest Inc   Page 461
Finter, Cynthia
Kaiser Foundation Health
Plan Northwest   Page 347
Finuf, Bob
Family Health Partners   Page 247
Fischer, Donald, MD
Highmark Inc   Page 366
Fischer, John A
4MOST Health Network   Page 459
Fish, Leslie, PharmD
Fallon Community Health Plan Inc   Page 211
Fishbein, Daniel, MD
Aetna Inc - Maine   Page 195
Fisher, Andrea
Devon Health Services Inc   Page 361
Fisher, Bruce, MD
QualCare Inc   Page 276
Fisher, Mark
Fallon Community Health Plan Inc   Page 211
Fisher, Marsha
ProviDRs Care Network   Page 181
Fisher, Roman G, MS, LLM
Metcare Health Plans Inc   Page 116
Fisher-Gable, Hazel
Delta Dental Plan of Illinois   Page 145
Fisk, Suzanne
Arnett Health Plans   Page 157

Fitzgerald, Desmond
Garden State Pharmacy
Owners Provider Services   Page 485
Fitzgerald, Eleanor
SCHC Total Care Inc   Page 305
Fitzgerald, James P
Masspro Inc   Page 213
Fitzgerald, Judy
Capital District Physicians
Health Plan   Page 286
Fitzwater, Ron
Pharmacy Association, The   Page 492
Fitzwater, Travis
Pharmacy Association, The   Page 492
Fjelstad, Dani
Delta Dental Plan of Minnesota   Page 235
Flachbart, Raymond
Blue Cross of Idaho   Page 141
True Blue   Page 142
Flanagan, Patrick
Eye Care of Wisconsin Inc   Page 464
Flanegin, Jeff
Raytel Imaging Network   Page 371
Flannery, Guy, CPA
Great Expressions
Dental Centers   Page 222
Flatt, Andy
Signature Health Alliance   Page 398
Flebotte, Laurel A
CIGNA Dental Health of CA Inc   Page 40
CIGNA Dental Health of CO   Page 78
CIGNA Dental Health of DE Inc   Page 95
CIGNA Dental Health Inc -
Corporation Headquarters   Page 106
CIGNA Dental Health of FL   Page 107
CIGNA Dental Health of KS Inc   Page 177
CIGNA Dental Health of MD Inc   Page 201
CIGNA Dental Health of NC Inc   Page 310
CIGNA Dental Health of OH Inc   Page 322
Fleishman, Tom
Health Net of California   Page 49
Fleming, Beth
Health First Health Plans Inc   Page 111
Fleming, Jamie, RN
Blue Care Network of Michigan   Page 217
Fleming, Jerry C
Kaiser Permanente - Kaiser Foundation
Health Plan, Inc   Page 54
Fleming, John
Crawford and Co-Corp Hdqrtrs   Page 130
Fleming, Katie
Health First Health Plans Inc   Page 111
Fleszar, George
Aetna Inc - Pennsylvania   Page 355
Fleszar, Thomas J, DDS, MS
Delta Dental Plan of IN Inc   Page 159
Delta Dental Plan of MI Inc   Page 220
Delta Dental Plan of OH Inc   Page 324
Fletcher, Alan
HealthPartners Inc   Page 236
Fletcher, Gary Hall
Amerigroup Ohio Inc   Page 319
Fletcher, Melvyn
Blue Cross Blue Shield of
Florida & Health Options Inc   Page 104
Flinn, Sandra, RN
Cooks Childrens Health Plan   Page 411
Flood, Marc
Em Risk Management,
A POMCO Company   Page 290
Flora, Devonna
Virginia Health Network   Page 447
Flores, Robin
Freedom Health Inc   Page 110
Flores-Witte, Amanda
Alameda Alliance for Health   Page 33
Flowers, Eric A, MBA
Ramsell Holding Corporation   Page 493

Flowers, Sandra
Arizona Foundation for
Medical Care   Page 11
Floyd, Charles E, CEBS
Delta Dental Plan of Ohio Inc   Page 324
Delta Dental Plan of MI Inc   Page 220
Delta Dental Plan of IN Inc   Page 159
Delta Dental Plan of MI Inc   Page 220
Floyd, Paul J
CorpHealth Inc   Page 412
Flunker, Bruce
EBC   Page 464
Flynn, Peter
Corvel Corporation   Page 43
Fody, Kenneth W
Independence Blue Cross   Page 366
Fogel, Baruch
Arta Medicare Health Plan Inc   Page 34
Fogarty, W Thomas, MD
Concentra Inc   Page 411
Foley, David
Memorial Hermann
Health Network Providers   Page 420
Foley, John
UnitedHealthcare of WI Inc   Page 470
Foley, Patrick M
Allianz Life Insurance
Company of North America   Page 233
Foley, Susie, RN, MSN
Lakewood Health Plan Inc   Page 56
Folick, Jeff
Bravo Health Mid-Atlantic Inc   Page 200
Bravo Health Pennsylvania Inc   Page 358
Bravo Health Texas Inc   Page 407
Bravo Health Inc   Page 200
Bravo Health Mid-Atlantic Inc   Page 517
Follmer, Cindy
UnitedHealthcare of Georgia   Page 134
Foltin, Jean, RN
Fidelis SeniorCare Inc   Page 147
Fones, John Mark
Center Care   Page 184
Fookes, Melissa
Integra Group   Page 329
Foos, John G
Independence Blue Cross   Page 366
Keystone Health Plan East Inc   Page 368
Foote, Don
American LIFECARE -
Mississippi - PHCS   Page 241
Forbes, Brian
Aetna Inc - Tulsa   Page 339
Ford, Amos
Delta Dental Plan of Ohio Inc   Page 324
Ford, Cory
Anthem BCBS of Wisconsin   Page 461
Ford, David
Health Plan of CareOregon Inc   Page 346
Ford, Milam
HmoLouisiana Inc   Page 191
Ford, Stephen, MD
PerfectHealth Insurance Co   Page 304
Foreman, Roger L
BCBS of Kansas City   Page 244
Foreman, Roger L
Good Health HMO Inc   Page 247
Foresame, Michael
CIGNA Healthcare of SC   Page 384
Forestieri, Teri
Delta Dental Plan of CA   Page 44
Fornadel, Richard M, MD
CIGNA Healthcare of
Mid-Atlantic Inc   Page 201
Fornadel, Rick, MD
Aetna Inc - Maryland   Page 199
Forney, David L
Western Dental Services   Page 75

Index VIII: Personnel

Evans, Patricia, CPA
Kansas Foundation Medical Care Page 179
Evelyn, Scott
CIGNA Healthcare of Georgia Page 128
Everetez, Juanita, MD
Nychsro/MedReview Inc Page 303
Everett, Junetta
Delta Dental Plan of Kansas Page 178
Ezell, DeWitt, Jr
Blue Cross Blue Shield of TN Page 392
Blue Cross Blue Shield of TN - Memphis Page 393

F

Fabrizio, John
Maxor Plus Page 488
Fad, P Scott
Coventry Hlth Care Inc - DE Inc Page 96
Fagan, Janice
Great-West Healthcare of Texas - Austin Page 414
Unicare Life and Health Insurance Co Inc Page 428
Fahey, Ronald, CPA
Medical Associates Hlth Plans Page 172
Medical Associates Clinic Health Plan of WI Page 467
Fahy, Kevin
Avera Health Plans Inc Page 387
Faine, Nora, MD
Sharp Health Plan Page 68
Fairchild, Philip
Select Health of SC Page 385
Fairweather, Leslie
Comprehensive Behavioral Care Inc Page 108
Fakurnejad, Adeebeh
Contra Costa Health Plan Page 43
Falcone, Charles
Devon Health Services Inc Page 361
Fallon, John, A MD, MBA, FACP
Blue Cross Blue Shield of MA Page 209
Fallon, Robert
Commonwealth Care Alliance Inc Page 505
Fanning, Chris
Southern Health Services Inc Page 445
Farah, Thomas M
HealthExtras Inc Page 485
Farkus, Darrell
Oxford Health Plans of NJ Inc Page 275
Farley, James P
Jp Farley Corp Page 329
Farnan, Lisa
Blue Shield of California Page 36
Farnsley, John
HealthSmart Preferred Care Page 416
Farrar, Bob
Hometown Health Plan Page 260
Farrell, Barbara
Bluegrass Family Health Inc Page 183
Farrell, T Mark
Intracorp Page 367
Farrell, Lisa
Presbyterian Health Plan Page 281
Farrell, Paul
Coventry Health Care Inc — Georgia Inc Page 130
SouthCare/Hlthcare Preferred Page 134
Farrell, Robert G, Jr
S V S Visions Inc Page 231
Farrell, Stephen J
UnitedHealthcare of New England Inc Page 381
Farrow, Peter
Group Health Cooperative of Eau Claire Page 465

Farry, Bill
Orange Prevention & Treatment Integrated Page 60
Fasano, Philip
Kaiser Foundation Health Plan of Southern California Page 54
Kaiser Permanente - Kaiser Foundation Health Plan, Inc Page 54
Fast, Patti
Health Plan, The Hometown Region Page 327
Faulk, Janice
Great-West Healthcare of Texas - Dallas Page 415
Faulk, Kathleen
Lifetime Healthcare Companies, The - Corporate Headquarters Page 298
Faulk, Robert
Mendocino and Lake Counties Foundation for Medical Care Page 59
Faust-Thomas, Brenda
National Capital PPO Page 444
Fava, Ron
UnitedHealthcare of FL Inc Page 121
Fay, Mike
Wellmark BCBS of Iowa Page 174
Wellmark Hlth Plan of Iowa Inc Page 175
Wellmark Inc — Corp Hdqrtrs Page 175
Fazio, Charles, MD
Medica Health Plans Page 236
Feaver, Ed
PacifiCare of California Page 62
Pacificare Life & Health Insurance Company Page 63
Feaver, Edward M, PharmD
Prescription Solutions Page 493
Feay, Suzanne RN
Superior HealthPlan Inc Page 426
Fedderly, Michele
Ucare Minnesota Page 238
Federico, John, MD
Community Health Network of Connecticut Inc Page 89
Feeney, Carol, RN
Affinity Health Plan Inc Page 283
Feingold, Glenn
Managed Care of North America Inc Page 115
Feingold, Orrin D, CFA
MagnaCare Page 298
Feldman, Eileen
Family Choice Health Alliance Page 272
Feldman, Eli S
Elderplan Inc Page 289
Elderplan Inc - SHMO Page 289
Feldman, Gary
Delta Dental Plan of AZ Inc Page 14
Feldman, James, DDS
Dencap Dental Plans Page 220
Feldman, Karen, DDS
Golden West Dental & Vision Page 47
Feldman, Nancy
UCARE of Minnesota Page 238
UCARE of Minnesota Page 505
UCARE of Minnesota Page 507
Feldman, Saul, MD
United Behavioral Health (UBH) Page 71
United Behavioral Health Page 373
Feldman, Victor
ACN Group Page 233
Feldstein, Jay, DO
Keystone Mercy Health Plan Page 368
Felice, Ginny
Elder Service Plan of East Boston Health Center Page 510
Felix, Joseph
Valley Preferred Page 375

Felix, Zule Ka
Family Choice Health Alliance Page 272
Feller, Marcy
MultiPlan Inc - Corp Hdqrtrs Page 300
Fellin, Eugene J, DO
Berkshire Health Partners/Medicus Resource Management Page 357
Felsted, Steve
Deseret Healthcare Page 434
Fenn, Scott
Memorial Hermann Health Network Providers Page 420
Fennell, Barbara
Delta Dental of Oklahoma Page 340
Fennell, Emile
Texas Medical Foundation Health Quality Institute Page 427
Fennell, Kathleen
Delta Dental Plan of NJ Page 271
Fenster, Dennis
Preferred One Page 237
Fenton, Leticia
CIGNA Behavioral Health Inc Page 40
Fenton, Michael
Dental Health Services Page 45
Ferdinandtsen, G Richard
American National Insurance Company Page 405
Ferguson, Bill
BlueChoice Health Plan of South Carolina Inc Page 383
Ferguson, Karin, RN
Southern Health Services Inc Page 445
Ferguson, Sally
Corvel Corporation Page 159
Ferkan, John
Jackson Memorial Health Plan Page 115
Fermin, Mariella
Amerigroup New York, LLC Page 284
Fernandez, Jeffrey
Humana Health Benefit Plan of Louisiana Page 191
Fernandez, Miguel
Humana Health Plan - Jacksonville Page 113
Ferrante, Michael
MultiPlan Inc - Corp Hdqrtrs Page 300
Private Healthcare Systems-WA Page 455
Ferraro, Stephen
Galaxy Health Network Page 414
Ferree, Fred
Alabama Quality Assurance Foundation Page 3
Ferrier, Tim
Gundersen Lutheran Health Plan Inc Page 465
Ferrin, Tanna
Altius Health Plans Page 433
Ferro, Gerard J
SunRx Inc Page 495
Ferro, Margo
Fallon Community Hlth Plan Inc Page 211
Feruck, Dan
Humana Health Plans of GA Page 132
Fessler, Thomas
Vision Service Plan Page 75
Fetterolf, Donald E, MD
American College of Medical Quality Page 199
Feuerman, Jason
Bravo Health Inc Page 200
Feyen, Patrick
Bravo Health Texas Inc Page 407
Fianu, Peter
Meritain Health Inc Page 299
Fickling, William A, Jr
Beech Street Corporation — Corporate Headquarters Page 36

Index VIII: Personnel

Edge, Dan
Dean Health Plan — Page 463
Edley, Richard S, PhD
Community Behavioral Healthcare Cooperative of Pennsylvania — Page 361
Edmonds, Daryl W
CIGNA Healthcare of Colorado — Page 79
CIGNA Health Plan of Utah Inc — Page 433
Edmonson, Robert
On Lok Senior Health Services — Page 60
Edwards, Benjamin
CO/OP Optical Services Inc — Page 219
Edwards, Bruce
CareFirst BC/BS — Page 200
Edwards, Dave
Metropolitan Health Plan — Page 237
Metropolitan Health Plan — Page 506
Edwards, Janet
UnitedHealthcare of WI Inc — Page 470
Edwards, Kathy
Select Circle Health Plan — Page 165
Edwards, Kevin
Humana Health Care Plans of Kansas & Missouri — Page 179
Edwards, Z Colette, MD
CIGNA Healthcare of Ohio Inc — Page 323
CIGNA Healthcare of Ohio Inc — Page 323
CIGNA Healthcare of VA Inc - Richmond — Page 443
CIGNA Healthcare of Mid-Atlantic Inc — Page 201
Eftekhari, Amir
Americas PPO — Page 233
Eftekhari, Nazie
Americas PPO — Page 233
Efusy, Brian
Total Health Care Inc — Page 231
Egan, Dan
Care-Plus Dental Plans Inc — Page 462
Egan, Robert D
Tufts Health Plan — Page 216
Egbert, Michael
Molina HealthCare of Utah Inc — Page 435
Eggert, Mark W
Centene Corporation — Page 244
Ehrenreich, Judy
PacifiCare Health Systems-Corporate Headquarters — Page 62
Eiesland, Susie
First Choice of the Midwest Inc — Page 388
Eigel, Linda
Humana Health Care Plans of San Antonio/Austin — Page 418
Eiler, Roger
CHN Solutions — Page 270
Einboden, Allan
Scott & White Health Plan — Page 424
Eisenberg, Jerry
QualCare Inc — Page 276
El-Azma, Majd
LifeWise Health Plan of OR — Page 348
El-Tawil, Mark
Health Net Inc - Corp Hdqrtrs — Page 49
Elder, Renwcyk
WellPoint NextRX — Page 497
Eldred, James
ChoiceCare/Humana — Page 322
Eldredge, Debbie
Pacific Visioncare WA Inc — Page 453
Elkins, Alan M. MD
Magellan Health Services — Page 132
Eller, Kim
Tenet Choices Inc — Page 192
Ellerbrock, Suzanne
Quincy Hlth Care Mngmnt Inc — Page 153
Ellerman, Brad
Behavioral Hlthcare Options Inc — Page 259

Ellerman, Steve
One Call Medical Inc — Page 275
Ellertson, Chris
Health Net Hlth Plan of OR Inc — Page 346
Ellex, Tina
Coalition America Inc — Page 129
Ellington, Hayley
CorpHealth Inc — Page 412
Elliot, David
Baptist Health Services Group — Page 392
Elliot, Tom
UnitedHealthcare of Colorado — Page 85
Elliott, Eric
CIGNA Pharmacy Management — Page 483
Elliott, Karen Louise
LA Care Health Plan — Page 55
Elliott, Robert B
Delta Dental Insurance Company - Nevada — Page 259
Delta Dental Insurance Company - Texas — Page 412
DeltaCare USA — Page 44
Delta Dental of Florida — Page 108
Delta Dental Insurance Company - Georgia — Page 131
Alpha Dental Programs Inc — Page 404
Ellis, Gary
Managed Pharmacy Care — Page 488
Ellis, John, MD
M Plan Inc — Page 163
Ellis, Lyndle
Bluelincs HMO — Page 340
BCBS of Oklahoma — Page 339
Ellis, Susan, RN
Mdx Hawaii — Page 138
Ellison, Amy
Delta Dental Plan of Kansas — Page 178
Elloway, Doug
Pacific Union Dental Inc — Page 63
Ellsworth, Scott G
Excellus BCBS, Rochester Area — Page 292
Elrod, Buster
Carolina Care Plan Inc — Page 383
Elrod, James K
Health Plus of Louisiana Inc — Page 191
Elsas, Robert
Davis Vision — Page 288
Elsea, Barbara
Santa Clara Family Health Plan — Page 67
Elson'Dew, Craig
Alameda Alliance for Health — Page 33
Elston, Michael P, MD
Western Health — Page 389
Elton, David DC
ACN Group — Page 233
Emerson, Jeff D
Magellan Health Services — Page 132
Magellan Health Services Inc — Page 91
Magellan Behavioral Health — Page 274
Emerson, Jeff D
ValueOptions - Corp Hdqrtrs — Page 447
Emery, Charles C, Jr
Horizon Hlthcare Services Inc — Page 274
Emery, Gene
Delta Dental Plan of NH — Page 265
Eng, Catherine, MD
On Lok Senior Health Services — Page 60
Engelman, Rebecca
Select Health of South Carolina — Page 385
England, Greg
Physicians Health Plan of Mid-Michigan — Page 228
England, Patricia
KHS a KMG America Company — Page 385
English, Debra
Arnett Health Plans — Page 157
English, George H, Jr
Blue Cross Blue Shield of DE — Page 95

English, Robert L
Blue Cross Blue Shield of Texas — HMO Blue - West — Page 407
Enigl, Debbie
Landmark Healthcare Inc — Page 56
Enos, Deborah
Neighborhood Health Plan — Page 214
Community Medical Alliance — Page 210
Enos, Scott
UnitedHealthcare of New England Inc — Page 381
Enright, Sherri
BCBS of Kansas City — Page 244
Epperson, Denise, RN
Saint Mary's HealthFirst — Page 263
Epstein, Robert S, MD, MS
Medco Health Solutions Inc — Page 275
Medco Health Solutions Inc — Page 488
Epstein, Tom
Blue Shield of California — Page 36
Eranch, Mary Jane, RN
Humana Medical Plan - Daytona — Page 113
Erickson, Gary
Partnership HealthPlan of CA — Page 64
Erickson, Kecia
ACN Group — Page 233
Ericson, Wade
DakotaCare — Page 387
Erlandson, Patrick
UnitedHealth Group - Corporate Headquarters — Page 238
Erlandson, Patrick
United Hlthcare Insurance Co — Page 519
Erney, Connie
HealthAmerica Pennsylvania Inc - Central Region — Page 364
Espinola, Nick
Valley Baptist Ins Company — Page 431
Esposito, Bob
ValueOptions of Texas Inc — Page 431
ValueOptions - Corp Hdqrtrs — Page 447
Esser, Deb, MD
UnitedHealthcare of the Midlands Inc — Page 257
Estep, Joan
Med-Valu Inc — Page 329
Estrella, Elisa
Community Health Plan — Page 42
Ethinger, Robert
MetroPlus Health Plan — Page 300
Ethridge, Larry
BeneScript Services Inc — Page 481
Eu, James K OD, PhD
Vision First Eye Care Inc — Page 73
Eull, Mary Ann
Bravo Health Mid-Atlantic Inc — Page 200
Bravo Health Mid-Atlantic Inc — Page 517
Eutledge, John
Wellpath Select Inc — Page 315
Evancho, John
OSF Health Plans — Page 151
Evans, Cornelius D
American LIFECARE - Mississippi - PHCS — Page 241
Evans, Dan CIU
LifeWise Health Plan of AZ — Page 17
Evans, David
Geisinger Health Plan — Page 363
Evans, Gary
ppoNEXT — Page 423
Evans, Joseph, MD
PPNM's Mastercare Network — Page 263
Evans, Kathy
Florida Health Care Plan Inc — Page 109
Evans, Marlene
Priority Health — Page 230
Evans, Nancy
PPNMs Mastercare Network — Page 263

Index VIII: Personnel

DuFresne, J Stevens
Optimum Choice Inc — Page 205
Dubbs, Allison
Dental Care Plus Inc — Page 324
Dubeck, Frank, MD
Excellus BlueCross BlueShield,
Utica Region — Page 292
Dubman, Robert, MD
Unity Dental Health Services — Page 277
Dubuc, Louis R
Fara Healthcare Management — Page 190
Duda, Emil D
Excellus BlueCross BlueShield — Page 290
Excellus BlueCross BlueShield,
Central NY Southern Tier — Page 291
Excellus BlueCross BlueShield,
Central New York Region — Page 291
Excellus BlueCross BlueShield,
Rochester Area — Page 292
Excellus BlueCross BlueShield,
Utica Region — Page 292
Lifetime Healthcare Companies,
The - Corp Headquarters — Page 298
Univera Healthcare of
Western New York — Page 307
Dudash, Steve
Delta Dental Plan of NC — Page 312
Dudley, G Martin
Intergroup Services Corporation — Page 367
Dudley, Gregory
Intergroup Services Corporation — Page 367
Dudley, Michael
Optima Health Plan Inc — Page 445
Duer, Linda
Primary Health Plan — Page 142
Duerr, Jeannette
Spectera Vision Inc - Indiana — Page 166
Spectera Vision Inc -
Corporate Headquarters — Page 206
Duford, Don
One Call Medical Inc — Page 275
Dugan, Chris
Anthem Blue Cross/Blue Shield
of New Hampshire — Page 265
Dugan, Dr
Pacific Union Dental Inc — Page 63
Dugan, Karen
Priority Health — Page 230
Dugan, Nicolle
Strategic Health
Development Corporation — Page 119
Duggin, Thelma
AmeriChoice of New York — Page 284
Duke, Derrick A.
Mega Life & Health
Insurance Company — Page 420
Dukes, R W, MD
Primary Provider
Management Company Inc — Page 64
Dulik, Edward
Aetna Health of Illinois Inc — Page 143
Dulik, Edward
Aetna Inc - Ohio — Page 319
Dulsky, Mark G
Blue Cross Blue Shield of KS — Page 177
Dunaway, George
CompBenefits Corporation -
Corporate Headquarters — Page 129
CompBenefits — Page 410
Texas Dental Plan — Page 427
Cypress Care — Page 483
Dunaway, Suzie
Family Health Partners — Page 247
Duncan, Patrick
Rocky Mountain Health Plans — Page 84
Rocky Mountain HealthCare Options Inc
dba Healthcare Options — Page 84

Duncan, Peter G
Blue Shield of California — Page 36
Duncan, Salli, RN
CareSource — Page 321
Duncan, Sharon
Geisinger Health Plan — Page 363
Dunlap, Robert
Fidelis SecureCare of NC — Page 312
Dunlop, Richard
UnitedHealthcare of Ohio Inc — Page 336
Dunn, E Paul Jr
AmeriGroup New Jersey Inc — Page 268
ValueOptions - Corp Hdqrtrs — Page 447
Dunn, Jodi
Nationwide Better Health — Page 204
Dunn, Paul
ValueOptions of Texas Inc — Page 431
Dunning, Jayna
Corvel Corporation — Page 159
Duran, Sally
OneNet PPO — Page 205
Md-Individual Practice
Association (MD IPA) — Page 204
Mid Atlantic Medical Services Inc
(MAMSI)- Corp Hdqrtrs — Page 204
Duran, Sally
Optimum Choice Inc — Page 205
Durand, Pierre, DPA
Ventura County Hlth Care Plan — Page 73
Durante, Robert
Elder Service Plan
of the North Shore — Page 510
Dury, Kathy
Eyexam of California Inc — Page 46
Dusenbury, Brenda
Spectrum Review Services Inc — Page 426
Dutcher, JoAnne
Citrus Health Care Inc — Page 108
Duvall, Judith Ann, OSF
OSF Health Plans — Page 151
Duvall, Steve
Has Premier Providers Inc — Page 415
Dvorak, Vera C, MD
UnitedHealthcare & Mid Atlantic
Medical Services Inc — Page 206
Dworak, Jerry
True Blue — Page 142
Dworsky, Dan, MD
Scripps Clinic Health
Plan Services Inc — Page 68
Dwyer, James D
Washington Dental Service — Page 457
Dwyer, Thomas
Atlantis Health Plan — Page 285
Dyer, Gary M
Blue Cross of Idaho — Page 141
Dyer, Gary M
True Blue — Page 142
Dyer, James D
Summerline Life &
Health Insurance Company — Page 138
Dyer, James D
Iowa Health Solutions — Page 171
Summerline Life &
Health Insurance Company — Page 138
Summerlin Life &
Health Insurance Company — Page 264
Dyer, Mark
Health Management Network Inc — Page 16
Dziedzicki, Ron
CIGNA Healthcare - Cincinnati — Page 323
Dzuryachko, Thomas A
United Concordia Company Inc -
California — Page 72

Dzuryachko, Thomas A
United Concordia Company Inc -
Corporate Headquarters — Page 373
United Concordia Company Inc -
Alabama — Page 6
United Concordia Company Inc -
Arizona — Page 21
United Concordia Company Inc -
Florida — Page 121
United Concordia Company Inc -
Illinois — Page 154
United Concordia Company Inc -
Maryland — Page 206
United Concordia Company Inc -
Michigan — Page 231
United Concordia Company Inc -
Missouri — Page 251
United Concordia Company Inc -
New Mexico — Page 282
United Concordia Company Inc -
New York — Page 306
United Concordia Company Inc -
Pennsylvania — Page 374
United Concordia Company Inc -
Pennsylvania - Central — Page 374
United Concordia Company Inc -
Texas — Page 429
United Concordia Company Inc -
Virginia — Page 446
United Concordia Company Inc -
Washington — Page 457

E

Eardley, Jennifer
Fallon Community Health Plan Inc — Page 211
Earl, Ann
Medica Health Plans — Page 236
Earley, J Fred, II
Mountain State BCBS — Page 460
Earley, Michael M
Metcare Health Plans Inc — Page 116
Early, Thomas
HealthPlus Inc — Page 296
East, Jeffrey
Masspro Inc — Page 213
Easterling, Alice
Care Choices HMO — Page 218
Eaton, Emily
Fallon Community Health Plan Inc — Page 211
Ebbib, Allan, MD
Health Plan of Nevada Inc — Page 260
Ebeling, Brian, MD
Americas PPO — Page 233
Ebert, Thomas H, MD
Health New England — Page 212
Eck, Cathy
CIGNA Healthcare - Cincinnati — Page 323
CIGNA Healthcare of Ohio Inc — Page 323
Eckbert, William, MD
Horizon Behavioral Services — Page 112
Horizon Behavioral Services — Page 417
Eckert, Christina
South Central Preferred — Page 372
Eckert, Karen
Lifetime Healthcare Companies, The -
Corporate Headquarters — Page 298
Eckstein, Michael
Health Tradition Health Plans — Page 466
Eder, Dennis
Scan Health Plan — Page 68
Scan Health Plan — Page 502
Scan Health Plan — Page 502

Index VIII: Personnel

Dillon, Donald F
Fiserv Inc — Page 464
Dillon, Jeff
OSF Health Plans — Page 151
Dines, Keith
Sun Health Medisun — Page 20
Dinkel, Suzanne
Golden Dental Plans Inc — Page 221
Dino, Leonard S, Jr, Pharm D
LDI Pharmacy Benefit Mngmnt — Page 487
Discher, Joan
Magellan Bhvrl Care of IA Inc — Page 171
Dishman, Pam
Delta Dental Plan of TN — Page 394
Dishneau, Shannon
Great-West Healthcare of MI — Page 223
Disser, Evan J
Spectrum Vision Systems Inc — Page 181
Disser, Hollace M
Spectrum Vision Systems Inc — Page 181
Disser, Paul
Spectrum Vision Systems Inc — Page 181
Ditman, Steven L
Interplan Health Group — Page 53
Interplan Health Group -
Corporate Headquarters — Page 91
Emerald Health Ntwrk Inc, The — Page 325
Superien Health Network Inc — Page 335
Interplan Health Group — Page 419
AmeriScript Inc — Page 479
Divinty, Shirley
Aetna Inc - Louisiana — Page 189
Dixon, Glenn
CBCA Care Management Inc — Page 408
Dixon, Keith, PhD
CIGNA Behavioral Health Inc — Page 88
CIGNA Behavioral Health Inc -
Corporate Headquarters — Page 234
CIGNA Behavioral Health Inc — Page 408
Dixon, Mark G
Connecticare Inc — Page 89
Connecticare of NY — Page 288
Connecticare of MA Inc — Page 210
Colorado Health Networks LLC -
ValueOptions — Page 80
Djordjevic, Nancy
AmeriGroup District of Columbia — Page 97
Dlugos, Michael
Interplan Health Group — Page 53
Superien Health Network Inc — Page 335
Dobbins-Wolfe, Tami
Carelink Health Plans — Page 459
Dobson, Karen
Blue Cross Blue Shield of WY — Page 473
Dobson, Ron
Humana Health Plan -
Jacksonville — Page 113
Dodge, Patrick
Atlantis Health Plan — Page 285
Doerr, R Chris
Blue Cross Blue Shield of FL
& Health Options Inc — Page 104
Dolatowski, Tom
Delta Dental Plans Association — Page 146
Dominguez, Mary
El Paso First Health Plans Inc — Page 413
Domintz, Jack, MD
Health Plus — Page 150
Donahue, Kevin
HealthTrans LLC — Page 486
Donahue, RT
ACN Group — Page 233
Donahue, Russ
Community Clinical Services — Page 196

Donigan, Heyward
Premera BCBS of AK — Page 9
LifeWise Health Plan of WA — Page 453
Premera - Corp Headquarters — Page 454
Premera Blue Cross - Eastern — Page 454
Premera Blue Cross - Western — Page 454
Donohue, Fay
Denta Quest Ventures Inc — Page 211
Donovan, Charles
HealthTrans LLC — Page 486
Donovan, Creighton
Evercare Select — Page 15
Donovan, LeAnn
M Plan Inc — Page 163
Donovan, Michael P
HealthExtras Inc — Page 485
Donovan, Raymond
Athens Area Health Plan
Select Inc — Page 127
Donze, Michael
Anthem BC BS of MO — Page 243
Doolen, Erick
PacificSource Health Plans — Page 350
Dooley, Donna
Pequot Pharmaceutical Ntwrk — Page 491
Dooley, Judy
Texas Medical Foundation
Health Quality Institute — Page 427
Dopps, Brad
Preferred Chiropractic Care PA — Page 179
Dopps, Mark
Preferred Chiropractic Care PA — Page 179
Doran, Gail
Physicians Health Plan of
Northern Indiana — Page 164
Dorfman, Nancy
Excellus BlueCross BlueShield,
Central NY Southern Tier — Page 291
Doris, Teresa
American Pharmacy Services
Corporation — Page 183
Dorma-O'Donnell, Margie RN
Cooks Childrens Health Plan — Page 411
Dorman-Rodriguez, Deborah
Health Care Service Corporation -
Corporate Headquarters — Page 149
BC BS of NM — Page 279
Dorney, William P, DC
Alignis Inc — Page 268
Dornig, Kara
United Behavioral Health (UBH) — Page 71
Anthem BC BS of CT — Page 88
Anthem BC BS of OH — Page 320
Dorrell, John
HMO Health Ohio (Cleveland) — Page 328
SuperMed Network — Page 334
Medical Mutual of Ohio — Page 330
Dorris, Robert T, Jr
Robert T Dorris Associates — Page 66
Doty, Dreux
Midland Care Connection — Page 512
Double, Mary Hagan
American Healthcare
Group INC — Page 356
Dougher, Joseph
KEPRO — Page 367
Dovi, Sebastion F, MD
University Health Plans Inc — Page 277
Dowd, Terrence C, Jr
Em Risk Management,
A POMCO Company — Page 290
Dowell, Stephanie
UAHC Health Plan of TN — Page 399
Downey, Ellen
Care Choices HMO — Page 218
Downey, Robin
Aetna Inc - Pennsylvania — Page 355

Downs, Barbara RN
Capital District
Physicians Health Plan — Page 286
Doyle, Anne
Fallon Community
Health Plan Inc — Page 211
Doyle, John
Dental Network of America — Page 146
Doyle, John G, Jr
Excellus BlueCross BlueShield — Page 290
Excellus BlueCross BlueShield,
Rochester Area — Page 292
Lifetime Healthcare Companies, The -
Corporate Headquarters — Page 298
Univera Healthcare of
Western New York — Page 307
Doyle, Patricia L
Dominion Dental Services -
Corporate Headquarters — Page 444
Dozoretz, Ronald I, MD
ValueOptions of Texas Inc — Page 431
ValueOptions -
Corporate Headquarters — Page 447
Drabelle, Tom
PersonalCare Ins of IL Inc — Page 151
Drabik, Ronald C
Horizon Behavioral Services — Page 112
Drablos, Craig
Humana Health Plan -
Jacksonville — Page 113
Humana Medical Plan -
Central Florida — Page 113
Humana Medical Plan -
Daytona — Page 113
Humana Medical Plan Inc — Page 114
Dragalin, Dan J, MD
HIP Health Plan of New York — Page 296
Dragila, Tim CPA
Acumentra Health — Page 345
Drake, Bonnie
Humana Health Care
Plans of Houston — Page 418
Drake, Howard
Innoviant Inc — Page 487
Dreibelbis, Dawn, RN
Berkshire Health Partners/Medicus
Resource Management — Page 357
Drennen, Mark
PACE Greater New Orleans — Page 513
Drew, Greg, RPh
Rite Aid Health Solutions — Page 494
Dreyfus, Andrew
Blue Cross Blue Shield of MA — Page 209
Dreyling, Scott
ACN Group — Page 233
Drinkwater, Deborah
LifeWise Health Plan of AZ — Page 17
Driscoll, Jackie
HMS Colorado Inc — Page 82
Sloan's Lake Preferred
Health Networks — Page 85
Drivedi, Jadeep
Elder Service Plan of
Harbor Health Services Inc — Page 510
Drohan, Mariann
GHI HMO Select Inc — Page 293
Dropski, Richard
Community Medical Alliance — Page 210
Druby, Thomas
Blue Cross of Northeastern PA — Page 358
Drucker, Alan, MD
Avante Behavioral Health Plan — Page 35
Drvenkar, Rita
CHN MCO — Page 322
DuCharme, James
Capital District
Physicians Health Plan — Page 286

Index VIII: Personnel

DeShambo, Cheryl
Serve You Custom
Prescription Management   Page 495
DeSmet, John
ACN Group   Page 233
DeTurk, Nanette P
Highmark Inc   Page 366
DeVaney, Tom
Health Plan of CareOregon Inc   Page 346
DeVay, Kathe
Unity Health Insurance   Page 470
DeVeydt, Wayne S
Blue Cross of California   Page 34
WellPoint Inc - Corp Hdqrtrs   Page 167
Anthem BC BS of MO   Page 243
UniCare Health Plans of TX Inc   Page 428
Unicare Life and
Health Insurance Co Inc   Page 428
DeVille, Greg
Beech Street Corporation —
Corporate Headquarters   Page 36
DeVries, George T III
American Spclty Hlth Plans Inc   Page 33
DeVyet, Wayne
Anthem BC BS OF IN   Page 157
DeWeese, Timothy
Delta Dental Plan of Ohio Inc   Page 324
DeWitt, Jackie
Humana Inc - Colorado   Page 82
Deacon, Whit
Blue Cross Blue Shield of TN
- Memphis   Page 393
Deadrick, Carol
Assurant Employee Benefits -
Michigan   Page 217
Deal, David
Blue Cross Blue Shield of TN -
Memphis   Page 393
Deal, Judy M
Safeguard Hlth Enterprises Inc   Page 66
Dean, Mary
Great-West Healthcare of Texas -
Austin   Page 414
Dean, Pam
Lakewood Health Plan Inc   Page 56
Dean, Val
MMM Healthcare Inc   Page 378
Debriae, Carrie
KPS Health Plans   Page 452
Decker, Chad
Health Resources Inc   Page 161
Decker, Dave
Evercare Select   Page 15
Dedrick, Matt
Unity Health Insurance   Page 470
Deelsnyder, Christopher
ACS Government
Healthcare Solutions   Page 479
Defazio, Randy
CHN Solutions   Page 270
Deguio, Patti, RN
Humana Health Plan -
Jacksonville   Page 113
Dehis Cornell, Lois
Tufts Health Plan   Page 216
Deitch, Jeffrey, DO
MPRO   Page 227
Deitch, Jennifer
Health Design Plus   Page 327
Delahongra, Arturo
Triple-S Inc   Page 378
Delaney, Dave
Kaiser Permanente Health Plan   Page 137
Delaney, David
Indiana Pro Health Network   Page 162
Delatorre, Aurora
Ndc-West Inc dba NADENT   Page 83
Delgado, Abraham, MD, FACP
Texas Medical Foundation Health Quality
Institute   Page 427

Dellacorte, Robert N
UnitedHealthcare of
New England Inc   Page 381
Dellavecchia, Ted
CareFirst BCBS   Page 200
Delmarva Health Care Plan Inc   Page 202
CareFirst BCBS   Page 481
Delz, Gary
United Concordia Co Inc - TX   Page 429
Demaio, Barbara
CIGNA Dental Health of KS Inc   Page 177
Demartini, Gretchen
HealthEase of Florida Inc   Page 111
WellCare Health Plans Inc -
Corporate Headquarters   Page 124
WellCare of New York   Page 307
Demers, John
GHI HMO Select Inc   Page 293
Demilio, Mark S
Magellan Health Services   Page 132
Magellan Health Services Inc   Page 91
Demosthenes, James
CIGNA Healthcare of ME Inc   Page 195
Denes, Steven
Atlantis Health Plan   Page 285
Dengler, Stephen R
HealthAmerica Pennsylvania Inc -
NorthWest   Page 365
HealthAmerica Pennsylvania Inc -
Western Region   Page 365
HealthAmerica Pennsylvania Inc -
Central Region   Page 364
HealthAmerica Pennsylvania Inc -
Eastern Region   Page 365
Denham, Linda
EyeMed Vision Care LLC   Page 325
Denney, Renessa
Atlantic Integrated Health Inc   Page 309
Denning, Carl
Mutual Assurance
Administrators Inc   Page 342
Denning-Bell, Larecia
Center Care   Page 184
Dennis, Lyman
Partnership HealthPlan of CA   Page 64
Dennis, Marisa
Mount Carmel Health Plan   Page 331
Dennis, Patricia
Medica Health Plans   Page 236
Dennison, Robert E, DMD
Delta Dental Plan of Illinois   Page 145
Denny, James J
ECCA - Managed Vision Care Inc -
Corporate Headquarters   Page 413
Dent, Darnell
Community Health Plan of WA   Page 450
Dent, Sue
XL Health   Page 207
Dentone, Stephen, MD
Visioncare of California   Page 75
Depace, Gerry
National Dental Consultants Inc   Page 301
Derback, Glen R
Great West Life
Annuity Insurance Co   Page 81
Derdzinski, Mike
UnitedHealthcare of WI Inc   Page 470
Desai, Akshay, MD
Universal Health Care Inc   Page 122
Deters, Beth
Deaconess Health Plans   Page 159
Detrick, Mary Ellen
HealthLink Inc - Corp Hdqrtrs   Page 249
Deus, Frank N, MD
Tenet Choices Inc   Page 192

Devou, Gregory A
CareFirst BlueChoice Inc   Page 97
CareFirst BCBS   Page 200
Delmarva Health Care Plan Inc   Page 202
CareFirst BCBS   Page 481
Deyling, James
Blue Cross Blue Shield of SC -
Corporate Hqtrs   Page 383
Di Salvo, George
Kaiser Foundation Health
Plan of Northern California   Page 54
DiBella, Kenneth
CBCA Care Management Inc   Page 408
CBCA   Page 483
DiCandilo, Michael D
Amerisource Bergen Performance
Plus Network - West   Page 480
DiGiandomenico, Liz
Eyexam of California Inc   Page 46
EyeMed Vision Care LLC   Page 325
DiGiovanni, Frank
Hudson Health Plan   Page 297
DiLeva, Lisa M
South Bay Independent
Physicians Medical Group Inc   Page 69
DiLorio, Emil MD
Coordinated Health Systems   Page 361
DiMartini, Gretchen
WellCare HMO Inc   Page 124
DiMura, Vincent, CPA
Meritain Health Inc   Page 299
Meritain Health   Page 330
DiPaula, John
SCHC Total Care Inc   Page 305
DiTirro, Frank, PhD, MD, FCCP
BC BS of Kansas City   Page 244
Good Health HMO Inc   Page 247
Diamond, Stuart
National Medical Health Card Systems -
Corporate Headquarter   Page 489
Diaz, Felipe, MD
SCHC Total Care Inc   Page 305
Diaz, Norma A
Community Health Group   Page 41
Dice, Mary
Behavioral Healthcare Inc   Page 78
Dichter, Debby
Mental Health Consultants Inc   Page 369
Dick, Tom
CO/OP Optical Services Inc   Page 219
Dickerson, James
BC BS of Western New York   Page 285
HealthNow New York Inc   Page 295
Dickerson, Susan
Community First Hlth Plans Inc   Page 410
Dickes, Robert
Landmark Healthcare Inc   Page 56
Dickey, Gina
Superior Vision Services Inc   Page 70
Dickhart, Russell
Aetna Inc - New Jersey   Page 267
Dickman, Timothy F
Prime Therapeutics   Page 493
Dickstein, Paul
HealthFirst Inc   Page 295
Diehs, Creta
Dimension Health (PPO)   Page 109
Diemert, Roger, MD
Humana Health Care
Plans of Kansas & Missouri   Page 179
Dietch, Jen
Superien Health Network Inc   Page 335
Dietsch, Linda
Maryland Care Inc   Page 521
Dilday, Gwyn
CIGNA Healthcare of CA   Page 41
CIGNA Health Plan of UT Inc   Page 433

Index VIII: Personnel

D'Apolito, Joseph
PerfectHealth Insurance Co — Page 304
D'Arcy, Colin P
Humana Medical Plan Inc — Page 114
Dabiri, Norman, DDS
Union Health Service Inc — Page 154
Dachille, Susan
UMPC Health Plan Univ of Pittsburgh Medical Center — Page 374
Daddairo, Donald
Health Partners — Page 364
Daffron, Mitzi
Health Care Excel Inc — Page 160
Daigle, Danis
Blue Cross Blue Shield - LA Inc — Page 189
Dailey, Karen
Parkview Signature Care — Page 164
Dailey, Lois
University Health Care Inc - Passport Health Plan — Page 187
Dalessio, James P
Horizon NJ Health — Page 274
University Health Plans Inc — Page 277
Daley, Laura
Medical Review Institute - Corporate Headquarters — Page 435
Dallafior, Kenneth R
Blue Preferred Plan- BC BS Michigan — Page 218
Daly Lauenstein, Teri
Community Health Plan — Page 42
Daly, Dennis, MD
Em Risk Management, A POMCO Company — Page 290
Daly, Marilyn
Neighborhood Health Plan — Page 214
Dameron, Emery
UnitedHealthcare of Oregon — Page 352
Dameron, Gene
Evercare Select — Page 15
Damico, Gail
Blue Cross Blue Shield of AZ — Page 12
Dammon, John
Humana Health Plans of GA — Page 132
Humana Inc - South Carolina — Page 384
Dammrose, Douglas, MD
Blue Cross of Idaho — Page 141
True Blue — Page 142
Danforth, Patricia
Nevada Prefrrd Professionals — Page 262
Dang, Long, MD
Molina Healthcare Inc - CA — Page 59
Daniel, Patty
HmoLouisiana Inc — Page 191
Daniels, Andrew R
Concentra Inc — Page 411
Daniels, Cheryl
Community Health Plan — Page 245
Daniels, Heather
CIGNA Behavioral Health Inc — Page 88
Daniels, Joni S
Qca Health Plan Inc — Page 28
Danielson, Russ
Providence Health Plans — Page 351
Dannels, Linda
PacifiCare Health Systems- Corporate Headquarters — Page 62
Dannenbaum, Steve
Catalina Behavioral Health Services Inc — Page 13
Danz, Kris
EHP Inc — Page 362
Darnley, Patricia J
Centene Corporation — Page 244
Darr, Katie
Henry Ford OptimEyes — Page 224
Darrell, Christopher G
Genex Services — Page 363

Daubert, Scott, PhD
Community Behavioral Healthcare Cooperative of Pennsylvania — Page 361
Daun, Lowell
Delta Dental Plan of CA — Page 44
Dauner, Beth
Preferred Chiropractic Care PA — Page 179
Dauner, Marlon R
Preferred Health Systems — Page 180
Davenport, Becky
Kern Family Health Care — Page 55
Davenport, Cathie
Nevada Pacific Dental — Page 262
Davenport, Terry Jones
Select Health of SC — Page 385
Davidson, Joel, MD
Horizon Health PPO — Page 261
Managed Care Consultants — Page 261
Davidson, Revathi A
Presbyterian Health Plan — Page 281
Davies, Dyke
Delta Dental of Virginia — Page 443
Davies, Matthew M
UnitedHealthcare of FL Inc — Page 121
Davis, Addie
Vision Health Mngmnt Sys — Page 155
Davis, Barbara
Oxford Health Plans of NY, Inc — Page 303
Davis, Barry, OD
Block Vision of Texas Inc — Page 405
Davis, Benton
UnitedHealthcare of AZ Inc — Page 21
Davis, Camilla Q
Fara Healthcare Management — Page 190
Davis, Clarence, MD
Memphis Managed Care Corp — Page 397
Davis, Cosby M, III
Southern Health Services Inc — Page 445
Carelink Health Plans — Page 459
Davis, Cynthia
CIGNA Healthcare of KS/MO — Page 177
Davis, Dan
Suburban Health Organization — Page 166
Davis, Denise, RN
Medwatch LLC — Page 116
Davis, Donald, Jr
Health Alliance Plan — Page 223
Davis, Duane E, MD
Geisinger Health Plan — Page 363
Davis, Grover
Crawford and Co - Corporate Headquarters — Page 130
Davis, Howard E
HMO California — Page 51
Davis, James P
Delta Dental Plan of AZ Inc — Page 14
Davis, Jay D
HMO California — Page 51
Davis, Jeffrey V
HMO California — Page 51
Davis, Jeffrey W
Premera BC BS of AK — Page 9
Davis, Judith M
BC BS of South Carolina - Corporate Hqtrs — Page 383
Davis, Karen
Ventura County Hlth Cre Plan — Page 73
Davis, Ken, MD
PacifiCare of Arizona — Page 19
Davis, Kevin
Coventry Hlth Care Inc - DE Inc — Page 96
Davis, Lynda
Med-Valu Inc — Page 329
Davis, Michael
Dominion Dental Services - Corporate Headquarters — Page 444
Davis, Nancy P
Harvard Pilgrim Health Care - Corporate Headquarters — Page 212

Davis, Patrisha L
Coventry Health Care Inc — Corporate Headquarters — Page 201
Davis, Philip M
Wellmark BC BS of SD — Page 389
Davis, Phillip G
Health Net Inc - Corporate Headquarters — Page 49
Davis, Robert
Healthspring of Alabama Inc — Page 5
Davis, Ronald A
Olympus Managed Hlth Cre Inc — Page 117
Davis, Stepanie K
Excellus BC BS, Utica Region — Page 292
Excellus BC BS, Central NY Southern Tier — Page 291
Davis, Teresa
Great-West Hlthcare of WA Inc — Page 451
Davis, Thomas A
Coventry Hlth Care Inc- GA Inc — Page 130
SouthCare/Hlthcare Preferred — Page 134
Davis, Thomas, MD
Humana Hlth Care Plans of AZ — Page 17
Davis, William J
Allscripts Pharmaceuticals Inc — Page 479
Davis, William, RPh
Immediate Pharmaceutical Services Inc — Page 486
Davydov, Liya
Fidelis Care New York — Page 293
New York State Catholic Health Plan Inc — Page 303
Dawes, Deborah
Rocky Mountain Health Plans — Page 84
Day, Peter A
Alignis Inc — Page 268
Day, Stephen C
Delta Dental Plan of KY Inc — Page 184
Daza, Marilou
Health Delivery Mngmnt LLC — Page 485
de la Rocha, Castulo
AltaMed Health Services Corporation — Page 507
De Soto, Mateo, MD
Sante Community Physicians — Page 67
DeAnnuntis, Liza, MD
Paragon Biomedical Inc — Page 491
DeBold, Cheryl
Humana Hlth Benefit Plan of LA — Page 191
DeCorte, Ted
Nevada Pacific Dental — Page 262
DeGrace, Margie
Meritain Health Inc — Page 299
DeGroat, James S
El Paso First Health Plans Inc — Page 413
DeGroote, Anna
Health Net of California — Page 49
DeLaine, Brenna, MD
Unison Health Plan of SC Inc — Page 386
DeLong, Beattie
Fidelis SeniorCare Inc — Page 147
DeMartini, Gretchen
Preferred One — Page 93
DeMovick, Harvey C, Jr
Coventry Health Care Inc — Corporate Headquarters — Page 201
DePasquale, Ed
Penn Highlands Health Plan — Page 370
DePuch, Felicia
Care 1st Health Plan — Page 38
deRanitz, Mary
Ucare Minnesota — Page 238
DeRitis, Lisa
Cambridge Mngd Cre Srvcs — Page 38
DeRosa, Christopher
CIGNA Healthcare of California — Page 41
DeRosa, John
OneNet PPO — Page 205
DeRouin, Steve
Health Management Ntwrk Inc — Page 16

Index VIII: Personnel

Courchaine, Dolph
M-Care Inc — Page 225
Course, Steve
Best Health Plans — Page 36
Coussoule, Nick
Crawford and Co -
Corporate Headquarters — Page 130
Covert, Kim D
Coventry Health Care of KS Inc — Page 245
Cowart, Ruben P, DDS
SCHC Total Care Inc — Page 305
Cowyer, David, MD
Preferred Hlthcare System Inc — Page 371
Cox, Belinda, RN, CPHP
Carolina Care Plan Inc — Page 383
Cox, Ralph W, ESQ
Excellus BlueCross BlueShield — Page 290
Excellus BlueCross BlueShield,
Rochester Area — Page 292
Cox, Ralph, Jr, MD
Beech Street Corporation —
Corporate Headquarters — Page 36
Cox, Steve
Health Plan of San Joaquin, The — Page 50
Cox, Susan E
Dental Benefit Providers Inc — Page 202
Spectera Vision Inc -
Corporate Headquarters — Page 206
Coyle, Danny
Valley Baptist Insurance Co — Page 431
Coyle, Keely
Avante Behavioral Health Plan — Page 35
Craig, Kay
Ventura County Foundation for
Medical Care — Page 73
Craig, Mary
Gateway Health Plan Inc — Page 362
Crammond, Stefanie J
Block Vision of Texas Inc — Page 405
Crampton, Kathleen R
Managed Health Services
Insurance Corporation — Page 467
Crandel, Cindy
Iba Health Plans — Page 225
Crandel, Michael, MD
Sanford Health Plan — Page 388
Cranford, Allen K
Evolutions Healthcare
Systems Inc — Page 109
Crawford, Michelle
Aetna Inc - Tulsa — Page 339
Crawford, Thomas W
Crawford and Co -
Corporate Headquarters — Page 130
Creager, Dick, MD
Medical Review Institute -
Corporate Headquarters — Page 435
Creamer, Jodie
CorpHealth Inc — Page 412
Creticos, Angelo P, MD
Union Health Service Inc — Page 154
Crider, Annetta
Behavioral Hlthcre Options Inc — Page 259
Crilly, Tim J
Blue Cross Blue Shield of WY — Page 473
Crim, Fred
Cambridge Managed
Care Services — Page 38
Crisp, Sherry L
Delta Dental Plan of IN Inc — Page 159
Delta Dental Plan of MI Inc — Page 220
Delta Dental Plan of OH Inc — Page 324
Cristea, Cris
Community Care Plus — Page 249
Crocker, Robert, MD
American Spclty Hlth Plans Inc — Page 33
Cromie, William J, MD, MBA
Capital District
Physicians Health Plan — Page 286

Cromwell, Adrienne
Integrated Health Plan Inc — Page 115
Cronister, Kevin
Kansas Fndtn Medical Care — Page 179
Crooks, Andrew D
CIGNA Healthcare of Florida — Page 107
Cropp, Michael, MD
Independent Health Assoc Inc — Page 297
Crosby, David
HealthPlus of Michigan — Page 224
Crosby, Lynette
Delta Dental Plan of California — Page 44
Cross, Laurie
Community Behavioral Healthcare
Cooperative of Pennsylvania — Page 361
Crosson, Francis J, MD
Kaiser Permanente - Kaiser
Foundation Health Plan, Inc — Page 54
Crouch, Jeff
Blue Cross of Idaho — Page 141
Crouser, Lisa
Pioneer Management Systems — Page 215
Crow, Catherine R
Newport Dental Plan — Page 60
Crow, Lisa
Community First Hlth Plans Inc — Page 410
Crow, Margie
Blue Cross Blue Shield of NM — Page 279
Crow, Randall
Qca Health Plan Inc — Page 28
Crowder, Phil
Anthem BC BS of Virginia Inc — Page 442
Crowley, Chris
Mountain Medical Affiliates — Page 83
Crowley, Christopher
Preferred Provider Organization of
Michigan (PPOM) — Page 229
Crowley, Christopher
Flora Health Network — Page 325
Crowley, Daniel D
SmileCare/Community
Dental Services — Page 69
Delta Dental Plan of California — Page 44
Crowley, Dennis W
Serve You Custom
Prescription Management — Page 495
Crowley, John
CIGNA Healthcare of Virginia Inc -
Richmond — Page 443
Crowley, Maureen, MD, MPH
Suffolk Health Plan — Page 305
Crowner, Matther
Mid-Atlantic Managed Care
Organization of PA Inc — Page 369
Crowsell, Thomas A
Tufts Health Plan — Page 216
Crum, John MD
Humana Military Service Inc — Page 186
Crusse, John
Humana Inc - Grand Rapids MI — Page 225
Cuchel, Stephen, MD
Healthplex Inc — Page 296
DentCare Delivery Systems Inc — Page 289
Cuda, John
MetroPlus Health Plan — Page 300
Cuddaback, Brian
CIGNA Healthcare of CT — Page 89
Cueny, Douglas G
Av-Med Hlth Plan - Gainesville — Page 102
Av-Med Hlth Plan - Jacksonville — Page 102
Av-Med Hlth Plan - Miami — Page 103
Av-Med Hlth Plan - Orlando — Page 103
Av-Med Hlth Plan - Tampa — Page 103
Cuevas, Vicky
Health Net of California — Page 49
Cukierman, Mark, MD
QualCare Inc — Page 276

Culberson, Lynne
Dental Network of America — Page 146
Culhane, Thomas, MD
Columbia United Providers — Page 449
Cull, John G
Allscripts Pharmaceuticals Inc — Page 479
Cullen, Caron
Affinity Health Plan Inc — Page 283
Cullen, Mary Ann
Corvel Corporation — Page 169
Culp, Ann
Medcost LLC — Page 313
Culyba, Michael, MD
UMPC Health Plan Univ of
Pittsburgh Medical Center — Page 374
Cummings, Andrew M
Tennessee Behavioral Hlth Inc — Page 399
Cummings, Kelly
Fallon Community Hlth Plan Inc — Page 211
Cummings, Scott
Care 1st Health Plan AZ Inc — Page 13
Cummins, Charles, MD
ECCA - Managed Vision Care Inc -
Corporate Headquarters — Page 413
Cunningham, Kim
Orange Prevention &
Treatment Integrated — Page 60
Cunningham, Maureen MHA RN CCM
Coventry Health Care Inc-DE Inc — Page 96
Cunningham, R Joseph, MD
BC BS of Oklahoma — Page 339
Curran, Pat
Nationwide Better Health — Page 204
Curran, Rick
Blue Cross Blue Shield of FL/
Health Options Inc — Page 104
Currie, Jay
Iowa Pharmacists Association — Page 487
Currier, Cecile
Concern: Employee
Assistance Program — Page 42
Curry, Donald M
CIGNA Healthcare of ME Inc — Page 195
CIGNA Healthcare of MA — Page 210
CIGNA Healthcare of NH — Page 265
CIGNA Healthcare — Page 439
Curtin, Kathleen
Excellus BC BS — Page 290
Curtis, Arda
Comprehensive Bhvrl Care Inc — Page 108
Curtis, Patricia
Optima Health Plan Inc — Page 445
Cusatis, James
Susquehanna Health Care — Page 372
Cusatis, William
Susquehanna Health Care — Page 372
Custer, Tim DDS
Dental Network of America — Page 146
Cutsinger, Jennifer
Southeastern Indiana Hlth Org — Page 166
Cuva, Tony
Intracorp — Page 367
Cyndi, Mincy
Pharmacy Providers Srvcs Corp — Page 492
Czelada, Laura L, CPA
Delta Dental Plan of IN Inc — Page 159
Delta Dental Plan of MI Inc — Page 220
Delta Dental Plan of OH Inc — Page 324

D

D'Allesandro, Sylvia
HealthPlus Inc — Page 296
D'Antonio, Frank
Group Health Plan Inc — Page 248

Index VIII: Personnel

Cole, Jeff, MD
Athens Area Health Plan
Select Inc — Page 127
Cole, Terry, CPA
MDwise — Page 163
Coleman, Dorothy
UnitedHealthcare of SW
Ohio Inc-Dayton/Cincinnati — Page 337
Coleman, M Ruth, RN, MA
Health Design Plus — Page 327
Coley, Dawn
Pequot Pharmaceutical Ntwrk — Page 491
Colgan, Thomas J
Delta Dental Plan of Illinois — Page 145
Colin, Wendy, MD
Preferred Care — Page 304
Collake, Jeff
Cariten Healthcare — Page 393
PHP Companies Inc — Page 397
Collazo, Theresa
AmeriGroup Corporation — Page 442
Colles, Cheryl
CIGNA Healthcare - Cincinnati — Page 323
CIGNA Healthcare of Ohio Inc — Page 323
Collier, James
UnitedHealthcare of Arkansas — Page 28
Collier, John
Delta Dental Plan of TN — Page 394
Colligan, Tim
SummaCare Inc — Page 334
Collingflower, Michael A.
Mega Life & Health
Insurance Company — Page 420
Collins, Dennis, MD
Santa Clara Family Health Plan — Page 67
Collins, Joseph, MD
Health First Health Plans Inc — Page 111
Collins, Linda
UnitedHealthcare of AZ Inc — Page 21
Collins, Paul
Behavioral Health Systems Inc — Page 3
Coltabaugh, Jeffery P
Preferred Hlthcr System Inc — Page 371
Colvin, Carolyn W
AmeriGroup DC — Page 97
Combs, Thomas
MVP Health Plan Inc — Page 301
Combs, Thomas J
Preferred Care — Page 304
Comeaux, Lynn
Humana Health Benefit
Plan of Louisiana — Page 191
Humana Health Benefit
Plan of Louisiana — Page 517
Comerford, Bill
Humana Health Care Plans
of Dallas — Page 417
Comrie, Daniel J
PacifiCare of Oklahoma Inc/
Secure Horizons — Page 342
PacifiCare of Texas - Houston — Page 422
PacifiCare of Texas Inc — Page 422
Concaugh, Daniel
Fallon Community Hlth Plan Inc — Page 211
Conde, Juan
CIGNA HealthCare —
Corporate Headquarters — Page 360
Condon, Bill
Humana Medical Plan Inc — Page 114
Conlin, Marci
Beech Street Corporation —
Corporate Headquarters — Page 36
Conlin, Paul
Oxford Health Plans-Connecticut — Page 91
Conner, Bill
Vision Service Plan — Page 75
Connington, Mary Ellen
New York State
Catholic Health Plan Inc — Page 303

Connolly, Jeff
Flora Health Network — Page 325
Connolly, Karen W, RN
Total Health Care Inc — Page 231
Connolly, Monye
Blue Cross Blue Shield of GA — Page 128
Connor, Renee
EHP Inc — Page 362
Connors, Janice
Mountain Pacific Quality
Health Foundation — Page 254
Consiglio, Denise
Preferred One — Page 93
Console, Rita
Evercare Select — Page 15
Constantine, Timothy J
Blue Cross Blue Shield of DE — Page 95
Conte, George
Priority Health — Page 230
Conte, Susan
Capital Health Plan — Page 105
Conti, Stacy
Intracorp — Page 367
Conway, Michael
Combined Insurance
Company of America — Page 145
Cook, Anthony A MBA, MS
Dental Care Plus Inc — Page 324
Cook, Barbara
LA Care Health Plan — Page 55
Cook, Bethany
Prime Health Services Inc — Page 398
Cook, Bonnie
Health Plan of the
Upper Ohio Valley — Page 327
Health Plan, The
Hometown Region — Page 327
Cook, Connie
Opticare Managed Vision — Page 314
Cook, David, MD
Indiana Health Network — Page 161
Cook, Jeffrey
UnitedHealthcare of Texas Inc -
San Antonio — Page 430
Cook, Joyce, RN, CHCM, CLNC
ConnectCare — Page 219
Cook, Larry N, MD
University Health Care Inc -
Passport Health Plan — Page 187
Cook, Peter
Assurant Employee Bnfits-NC — Page 309
Cook, Stephanie, DO
Ohio State University Managed
Health Care Systems Inc — Page 332
Coombs, Ed, CPA
New York Compensation
Managers Inc — Page 302
Cooner, Danny
Behavioral Health Systems Inc — Page 3
Cooney, Christopher W
Magellan Behavioral Health — Page 274
Cooney, Kathy
HealthPartners Inc — Pages 236, 486, 506
Cooper, Douglas, MD
Vision Service Plan — Page 75
Cooper, Linda
Aetna Hlth Plns of Mid-Atlantic — Page 441
Aetna Inc - Virginia — Page 441
Cooper, Michael, RN, MN
Acumentra Health — Page 345
Cooper, Richard
Arkansas Blue Cross/Blue Shield
a Mutual Insurance Company — Page 25
Health Advantage — Page 27
Cooper, Sunny
LA Care Health Plan — Page 55
Cooper, Wayne, DPM
Preferred Podiatry Group — Page 152

Coors, Margaret
Horizon BC BS of NJ — Page 273
Coplin, Terry W
Lane Oregon Health Plans — Page 347
Coppola, Robert C
20/20 Eyecare Plan Inc — Page 99
Corba, Bill
Kaiser Permanente Hlth Plan — Page 137
Corbett, Debra
MetroPlus Health Plan — Page 300
Corbett, Rick P
Superior Vision Services Inc — Page 70
Corcoran, Mark T
Carolina Care Plan Inc — Page 383
Cordani, David M
CIGNA HealthCare —
Corporate Headquarters — Page 360
CIGNA Healthcare of TX Inc — Page 409
Cordes, Paul
Health Management Network Inc — Page 16
Corgin, Andrew C
Blue Cross Blue Shield of KS — Page 177
Corley, William E
Indiana Pro Health Network — Page 162
Cormany, Doug
Preferred Care Partners Inc — Page 118
Cornell, Lois Dehls
Tufts Health Plan — Page 216
Coronado, Raul, MD
Neighborhood Health Providers — Page 302
Corr, Daryl
Healthsystems — Page 486
Corrado, Ann
Delta Dental of Rhode Island — Page 380
Correa, Norberto
El Paso First Health Plans Inc — Page 413
Corrigan, Ann E
Humana Health Benefit
Plan of Louisiana — Page 191
Cortez, Christian
UDC Dental California Inc — Page 71
Cortez, Kathy
Fidelis SeniorCare Inc — Page 147
Cortez, Larry, MD
Humana Health Benefit Plan of Louisiana
Page 191
Cory, Patrick, PharmD
Unity Health Insurance — Page 470
Cosler, Ed
American Healthcare Alliance — Page 243
Coss, Lance
Healthinsight — Page 435
Costa, Laura
Vision Service Plan — Page 75
Costello, Gwen
Rocky Mountain Health Plans — Page 84
Costello, Jeff
Community Health Alliance — Page 159
Costello, Rita
CareFirst BC BS — Page 200
Cotton, David B, MD
Health Plan of Michigan — Page 224
Cotton, Sheryl L
Health Plan of Michigan — Page 224
Couch, Beth
NAMCI — Page 6
Premier Hlth Ntwrks of AL LLC — Page 6
Coughlin, Thomas S
Excellus BlueCross BlueShield,
Central NY Southern Tier — Page 291
Coulter, Steven, MD
Blue Cross Blue Shield of TN -
Memphis — Page 393
Counts, Alice
CIGNA Healthcare of VA Inc -
Richmond — Page 443
Countsms, Stacey
Community Health Plan — Page 245

Index VIII: Personnel

Christopher, Laurie
Acumentra Health — Page 345
Christy, Denise
Humana Inc - Grand Rapids MI — Page 225
Christy, Paul A
Physicians United Plan Inc — Page 118
Christy, Susan
Missouri Care — Page 250
Chu, Benjamin, MD
Kaiser Foundation Health Plan
of Southern California — Page 54
Chu, Lisa
First Health Network — Page 46
Chuong, Edwin
Central Health Plan of CA Inc — Page 39
Church, C Franklin, MD
Optimum Choice of the
Carolina Inc — Page 205
Church, Patty
Regence BS BS of OR — Page 351
Churchill, Carol A, MD
AmeriGroup Tennessee Inc — Page 391
Ciaccio, Elizabeth, RN, MBA
Orange County PPO — Page 61
Cianciolo, Kirk, DO
Av-Med Health Plan - Tampa — Page 103
Cianfrocco, Heather
Unison Health Plan -
Corporate Headquarters — Page 37
Unison Health Plan of TN — Page 399
Ciarocchi, Michael
Aetna Inc - Houston — Page 403
Cichon, Kristen
Grand Valley Health Plan — Page 221
Cierpka, Lisa, RN, BSN
Quality Health Plan Inc — Page 119
Cierzan, Karen
CIGNA Behavioral Health Inc -
Corporate Headquarters — Page 234
Cieszkowski, Colleen, RN, MA
MPRO — Page 227
Cinquegrana, Robert L, CPA
XL Health — Page 207
Citrin, Richard S, PhD, MBA
UPMC Health Plan Univ of
Pittsburgh Medical Center — Page 374
Ciullo, Rose Ungaro
KEPRO — Page 367
Civera, Edward S
HealthExtras Inc — Page 485
Claassen, Mel
Mennonite Mutual Aid Assoc — Page 519
Cladouhos, Sherry L
Blue Cross Blue Shield of MT — Page 253
Clancey, Cathy
Hudson Health Plan — Page 297
Clancy, Ann
CIGNA Healthcare of Arizona — Page 14
Clancy, Mike
Southeastern IN Health Org — Page 166
Clanton, Craig, MD
Scott & White Health Plan — Page 424
Clanton, Ken, MD
Pearle Vision Managed Care - HMO of
Texas Inc — Page 423
Clapp, Kent W
HMO Health Ohio (Cleveland) — Page 328
Medical Mutual of Ohio — Page 330
SuperMed Network — Page 334
Clark Stanley, Janet
UDC Dental California Inc — Page 71
Clark, Bob
Family Health Partners — Page 247
Clark, Bobby
HealthSmart Preferred Care — Page 416
Clark, Casey
New West Health Plan — Page 254

Clark, Cathi
American Pharmacy
Services Corporation — Pages 183, 480
Clark, Christian
Integrated Health Plan Inc — Page 115
Clark, George
Devon Health Services Inc — Page 361
Clark, Greg
Preferred Health Plan Inc — Page 350
Clark, Jenny
Evercare Select — Page 15
Clark, Karen L
Horizon NJ Health — Page 274
Clark, Kerry
LeaderNET/Leader Drug Stores —
Cardinal Health Inc — Page 487
Clark, Lucia
Delta Dental Plans Association — Page 146
Clark, Michael
Delta Dental Plan of Kansas — Page 178
Clark, Michael E
PacifiCare of Nevada — Page 263
Clark, Michael W
Restat — Page 494
Clark, Robin
Aultcare — Page 320
Clark, Scott
Signature Health Alliance — Page 398
Clark, Scott E
Total Dental Administrators
Health Plan — Page 21
Clark, Sherree
NAMCI — Page 6
Premier Health Networks
of Alabama LLC — Page 6
Clark, Valerie A
California Benefits Dental Plan — Page 37
Clarke, James N, RPh, MS
Molina Healthcare of MI Inc — Page 227
Clary, Janet
Kern Foundation/
Preferred Provider Organization — Page 55
Clason, Roy, Jr
Aetna Inc - Corp Headquarters — Page 87
Aetna Inc Life Insurance Co — Page 87
Claudio, Cecilia
Anthem BCI BS of OH — Page 320
Clawson, Byron
Regence BC BS of Utah — Page 436
Regence Healthwise — Page 436
Clay, Brett
Altius Health Plans — Page 433
Clay, Peter
Coventry Health Care Inc —
Corporate Headquarters — Page 201
Clayton, Dawn
BC BS of Louisiana Inc — Page 189
Clement, Jeanne, RN, MPH
ParadigmHealth — Page 276
Clements, Anne
AmeriGroup DC — Page 97
Clements, Janice
PACE Vermont Inc — Page 513
Clemons, V Gordon
Corvel Corporation — Page 43
Corvel Corporation — Page 159
Corvel Corporation — Page 169
Corvel Corporation — Page 324
Cleven, Steven, MD
Holman Group, The — Page 51
Cliett, Charles
Community First Hlth Plans Inc — Page 410
Clinkscales, Douglas
Denver Health Medical Plan Inc — Page 80
Clinqueonce, Carmelo, MBA
Carolina Pharmacy Network — Page 482
Closson, Tim
Great-West Healthcare
of California - Southern — Page 48

Clothier, Brad
Preferred Health Systems — Page 180
Clough, Dee Dee
Beech Street Corporation —
Corporate Headquarters — Page 36
Clough-Gitchell, Deborah, RN C
Corporate Care Mngmnt Inc — Page 288
Cloyd, Michael, MD
Behavioral Health Systems Inc — Page 3
Coakley, Susan
BMC HealthNet Plan — Page 209
Coats, Bard H, MD
PacifiCare of Nevada — Page 263
Coberly, Sandi
Outlook Vision Services — Page 18
Cobern, Marvin C
Landmark Healthcare Inc — Page 56
Coburn, Nancy
Neighborhood Health Plan of RI — Page 380
Cochran, James
South Central Preferred — Page 372
Cochran, John H, Jr, MD
Kaiser Foundation Health Plan
of Colorado — Page 83
Cochran, Patricia C
Vision Service Plan of Arizona — Page 22
Vision Service Plan — Page 75
Vision Service Plan — Page 86
Coe, Susan
Bravo Health Inc — Page 200
Coenson, Craig, MD
CIGNA Behavioral Health Inc -
Corporate Headquarters — Page 234
Coffield, Patty
Carelink Health Plans — Page 459
Cogar, Mary
Cariten Healthcare — Page 393
PHP Companies Inc — Page 397
Cohen, Barry, MD
AmeriGroup DC — Page 97
Cohen, Bernie, MD
Coventry Health Care Inc —
Georgia Inc — Page 130
SouthCare/Hlthcre Preferred — Page 134
Cohen, Dale
ACN Group of California -
Western Region — Page 31
Cohen, Debra B
Capital Blue Cross — Page 359
Cohen, Donald C
Renaissance Hlth Systems Inc — Page 119
Cohen, Fred
Independent Hlth Assoc Inc — Page 297
Cohen, Julian
United Behavioral Health (UBH) — Page 71
Cohen, Michael, MD
Interplan Health Group — Page 53
Superien Health Network Inc — Page 335
Cohen, Robb A, MBA
XL Health — Page 207
Cohen, Steven, MD
Preferred Care — Page 304
Cohn, Alan S
Avesis Inc — Page 12
Coil, Gerald V
HealthSpring Inc - Tennessee — Page 395
HealthSpring Inc -
Corporate Headquarters — Page 395
Colbert, Ramona
Dental Associates of Torrance — Page 45
Cole, David L
Lane Oregon Health Plans — Page 347
Cole, Gary M
Humana Health Care Plans
of Dallas — Page 417
Cole, Jacque, RN
DakotaCare — Page 387

Index VIII: Personnel

Cassidy, Monique, MA
Masspro Inc — Page 213
Castellano, Louis, CPA
Health Design Plus — Page 327
Caster, Jean
Mdwise — Page 163
Castiglia, John L, MD
Premera BC BS of Alaska — Page 9
LifeWise Health Plan of WA — Page 453
Premera - Corp Headquarters — Page 454
Premera Blue Cross - Eastern — Page 454
Premera Blue Cross - Western — Page 454
Castiglia, Joseph J
Blue Cross Blue Shield
of Western New York — Page 285
HealthNow New York Inc — Page 295
Castillo, Abie
Community Health Plan of WA — Page 450
Castillo, Rosemary
Bienvivir Senior Health Srvcs — Page 508
Castro, Michael J
Delta Dental Plan of California — Page 44
Delta Dental of Pennsylvania — Page 361
Delta Dental Plan Inc - Utah — Page 434
Castro, Stephen
ACN Group of California -
Western Region — Page 31
Caswell, William B
Kaiser Foundation Health Plan
of Southern California — Page 54
Catalan, John
Aetna Inc — Page 87
Aetna Inc - New York — Page 283
Catalano, Charles
CIGNA Healthcare of
New York and New Jersey — Page 270
Cataldo, Jeanette M
Basic Chiropractic Hlth Plan Inc — Page 35
ChiroSource -
Corporate Headquarters — Page 40
Cataldo, Ron S, Jr, DC
Basic Chiropractic Hlth Plan Inc — Page 35
ChiroSource -
Corporate Headquarters — Page 40
Cataldo, Todd
Basic Chiropractic Hlth Pln Inc — Page 35
ChiroSource -
Corporate Headquarters — Page 40
Cate, Virginia
CIGNA Healthcare of NH — Page 265
Catino, Annette
QualCare Inc — Page 276
Catol, Rose Anne
QCA Health Plan Inc — Page 28
Catron, Tim
JP Farley Corp — Page 329
Catt, Kimberly, RN
Deaconess Health Plans — Page 159
Caughlin, Beth, RN
McLaren Health Plan — Page 226
Cavalier, Kevin
SummaCare Inc — Page 334
Cavalieri, Stephen L, MD
Southern Health Services Inc — Page 445
Cavanagh, Mary Ann
Vision Service Plan — Page 75
Cavavlier, Kevin
SummaCare Inc — Page 334
Cavender, Lenny
Advantage Health Solutions Inc — Page 157
Cecero, David M
JPS Benefits — Page 419
Celli, Pat
Americhoice of New Jersey — Page 268
Cerio, Robyn
UnitedHealthcare of
Florida Inc — Pages 121, 122

Cerrito, Diana
CIGNA Healthcare of AZ — Page 14
Cerven, Ted
Dental Network of America — Page 146
Cesare, Denise S
Blue Cross of Northeastern PA — Page 358
Cetiro, Robert
Hope Resources Providers (HRP) — Page 273
Chaddick, John
Scott & White Health Plan — Page 424
Chadee, Floyd F
Assurant Employee Benefits-AL — Page 3
Assurant Employee Benefits-AZ — Page 12
Assurant Employee Benefits-CA — Page 35
Assurant Employee Benefits-CO — Page 78
Assurant Employee Benefits-FL — Page 102
Assurant Employee Benefits-GA — Page 127
Assurant Employee Benefits-IL — Page 143
Assurant Employee Benefits-IN — Page 158
Assurant Employee Benefits-MI — Page 217
Assurant Employee Benefits -
Corporate Office — Page 244
Assurant Employee Benefits-NM — Page 279
Assurant Employee Benefits-NY — Page 285
Assurant Employee Benefits-NC — Page 309
Assurant Employee Benefits-PA — Page 357
Assurant Employee Benefits-TN — Page 392
Assurant Employee Benefits-TX — Page 429
Assurant Employee Benefits-WA — Page 449
Chaffee, Hamilton
Interplan Health Group — Page 53
Interplan Health Group -
Corporate Headquarters — Page 91
Superien Health Network Inc — Page 335
Interplan Health Group — Page 419
Chaifetz, Richard, PhD
Compsych Behavioral Health — Page 145
Chaitkin, Paul, DDS
First Commonwealth — Page 147
Challener, Ken, MD
Vantage PPO — Page 375
Chambers, Carla
Blue Care Network of MI — Page 217
Chambers, Richard
Orange Prevention &
Treatment Integrated — Page 60
Chamorro, Cheryl
CIGNA Healthcare of KS/MI — Page 177
CIGNA Healthcare of St Louis — Page 245
Chan, Florance
Contra Costa Health Plan — Page 43
Chandler, Jody
Blue Cross Blue Shield of AZ — Page 12
Chandra, Kathleen
National Capital PPO — Page 444
Chaney, G Mark
CareFirst BlueChoice Inc — Page 97
CareFirst BC BS — Page 200
Delmarva Health Care Plan Inc — Page 202
CareFirst BC BS — Page 481
Chaney, Jared P
HMO Health Ohio (Cleveland) — Page 328
Medical Mutual of Ohio — Page 330
SuperMed Network — Page 334
Chapin, Georganne
Hudson Health Plan — Page 297
Chapman, Carole
Preferred Care Incorporated — Page 370
Chard, Douglas
Medcore Health Plan — Page 58
Charlier, Brian
Prevea Health Network — Page 469
Charlton, Greg
Regence Blue Shield of Idaho — Page 142
Charlton, Sharon
Lovelace Health Plan — Page 280
Chase, Barbara, MD
Masspro Inc — Page 213

Chatfield, Jim
National Foot Care Prgm Inc — Page 227
Chauncey, Peter
Wellpath Select Inc — Page 315
Chavanu, Patrick
Intracorp — Page 367
Chavey, Francisca
Community Health Group — Page 41
Checkett, Donna
Missouri Care — Page 250
Chee, Michael
Blue Cross of California — Page 34
Cheek, Liz
Delta Dental Plan of TN — Page 394
Chejanovski, Arlene
CareIQ — Page 106
Chen, Arthur, MD
Alameda Alliance for Health — Page 33
Chen, Bill
Inter Valley Health Plan Inc — Page 53
Chenell, Sherry
Innovative Care Management — Page 347
Chenette, Dwight
Healthy Palm Beaches Inc — Page 112
Cheney, Chris
Sante Community Physicians — Page 67
Cheng, Wei-Tih, PhD
Aetna Inc - Tennessee — Page 391
Chenoweth, Joni
Qualis Health — Page 455
Chernis, Bob
Central Coast Alliance for Hlth — Page 39
Chesrown, Karen A
Blue Cross Blue Shield of IL — Page 144
HMO Illinois — Page 150
Chester, Mike
Arise Health Plan — Page 461
Chilcote, Alana
Amarillo Multi Service
Center for the Aging Inc — Page 508
Childs, Lynn
Community Health
Network of Connecticut Inc — Page 89
Chin, Stephen
Sharp Health Plan — Page 68
Chin, Yuen
Williamette Dental Group PC — Page 352
Williamette Dental of WA Inc — Page 457
Chin-Wardwell, Eleanor
Affinity Health Plan Inc — Page 283
Chipperfield, Michael
Primary Provider
Management Company Inc — Page 64
Chism, Terry
Ucare Minnesota — Page 238
Chiu, Thomas, MD
Pacific IPA — Page 63
Choate, Eddie A
Delta Dental Plan of Arkansas — Page 26
Chodroff, Charles, MD
South Central Preferred — Page 372
Chomiuk, Ron
Wal-Mart Stores Pharmacy Div — Page 496
Chong, Dennis, MD
CIGNA Health Plan of Utah Inc — Page 433
Chow, Edward, MD
Chinese Community Health Plan — Page 39
Christel, Karen
Arise Health Plan — Page 461
Christensen, Barb
Providence Health Plans — Page 351
Christensen, Donald E, MD
ValueOptions of Texas Inc — Page 431
Christiansen, Donna
Qualis Health — Page 455
Christopher, Adam
Med-Comp USA — Page 192

Index VIII: Personnel

Calomeni, Carolyn
Ucare Minnesota — Page 238
Calos, Chris
Humana Inc/PCA - Puerto Rico — Page 377
Cammisa, Chris, MD
Partnership HealthPlan of CA — Page 64
Campbell, Colleen
PacifiCare of Colorado — Page 84
Campbell, Jerry
Group Health Cooperative
of Puget Sound — Page 452
Group Health Options Inc — Page 452
Campbell, John W
Horizon BC BS of NJ — Page 273
Campbell, Juan
Health New England — Page 212
Campbell, Karen
Itasca Medical Care — Page 506
Campbell, Lee, MD
Humana Medical Plan - Daytona — Page 113
Campbell, Mark, Pharm D
Innoviant Inc — Page 487
Campbell, Stuart K
Anthem BC BS of Missouri — Page 243
Anthem BC BS of Wisconsin — Page 461
Campbell-Wisley, Mary Lee
Univera Healthcare of
Western New York — Page 307
Campos, Alena
Leon Medical Centers
Health Plan Inc — Page 115
Canacan, Colleen
United Behavioral Health — Page 373
Canavan, Neil T
Keystone Health Plan East Inc — Page 368
Cannella, Gregg, MD
Aetna Inc - Tennessee — Page 391
Cannizzaro, Joe
Dental Health Services Inc — Page 450
Cannon, Doug
Viva Health Inc — Page 7
Cannon, Mike D
Blue Cross of Idaho — Page 141
True Blue — Page 142
Canova, Jacob L
Meritain Health Inc — Pages 299, 330
Canterbury, Norman
Arkansas BC BS
a Mutual Insurance Company — Page 25
Health Advantage — Page 27
Cantrell, Dawn
BC BS of LA Inc — Page 189
HMO Louisiana Inc — Page 191
Cantu, Dubie
Humana Health Plan of Austin — Page 419
Caolo, Michael
American Preferred
Provider Organization INC — Page 405
Capaldo, Lynn
Blue Cross Blue Shield of
Florida & Health Options Inc — Page 104
Capezza, Joseph C, CPA
Health Net Inc -
Corporate Headquarters — Page 49
Capo, Zaydee
Global Medical Management — Page 110
Caponi, Vincent
Advantage Health Solutions Inc — Page 157
Caporello, Ed
CIGNA Healthcare of NH — Page 265
Capozzi, Vincent
Harvard Pilgrim Health Care -
Corporate Headquarters — Page 212
Cappel, Lawrence W, PhD
Pacific Health Alliance — Page 62
Cappel, Tim
Humana Health Plan of OH Inc — Page 328
Carales, Rene
Safeguard Health Plans Inc — Page 424

Cardamone, Thea
GenWorth Life &
Health Insurance Co — Page 90
Cardona, Alexis
APS Healthcare Inc — Page 199
Carendi, Jan
Allianz Life Insurance
Company of North America — Page 233
Carillo, J Emilio, MD
New York Presbyterian
Community Health Plan — Page 302
Carl Papp, Carl
Initial Group Inc, The — Page 396
Carley, Mark J
Great-West Healthcare of CO — Page 81
Carlin, Sharon A
UCARE of Minnesota — Page 238
UCARE of Minnesota — Page 505
UCARE of Minnesota — Page 507
Carlisle, Scott
Alliance Regional Hlth Network — Page 404
Carlisle, Sylvia, MD
Health Plan of San Joaquin, The — Page 50
Carllson, Richard E
Mutual Assurance Admns Inc — Page 342
Carlomusto, Joseph ABOC, FNAO
Davis Vision — Page 288
Carlson, Anthony
Anthem BC BS of Colorado — Page 77
Rocky Mountain Hospital &
Medical Services Inc — Page 85
Carlson, Carroll
Group Health Cooperative
of Eau Claire — Page 465
Carlson, James G
AmeriGroup Corporation — Page 442
AmeriGroup Florida Inc — Page 101
Carlson, Jeanne H
Blue Care Network of MI — Page 217
Carlson, Lisa
Sanford Health Plan — Page 388
Carlton, Cindy
Humana Health Plan -
Jacksonville — Page 113
Carlton, Pam
Preferred Therapy Providers of America -
Corp Headquarters — Page 19
Carmichael, Julie
Suburban Health Organization — Page 166
Carmona, James
Affinity Health Plan Inc — Page 283
Carmona, Laura
HMO California — Page 51
Carney, James J, MD
BC BS of Louisiana Inc — Page 189
HMO Louisiana Inc — Page 191
Carney, Patricia
Parkland Community
Health Plan Inc — Page 422
Carney, Philip S, MD
Kaiser Foundation Health Plan -
Mid Atlantic States — Page 203
Carney, Timothy W
Delta Dental Plan of Arkansas — Page 26
Carovello, Victoria
San Francisco Health Plan — Page 66
Carpenter, Steve
CBCA Care Management Inc — Page 408
Carpenter, Theodore M, Jr
Heritage Health Systems Inc — Page 416
Selectcare of Texas LLC — Page 521
Carpenter, Tim CPA
Virginia Premier Hlth Plans Inc — Page 447
Carr, Cherry
Secure Health Plans of GA LLC — Page 133
Carrasco, Angie
Medical Care Referral Group — Page 420
Carrico, Laura
Physicians Health Plan of
Northern Indiana — Page 164

Carril, Doris
Hudson Health Plan — Page 297
Carrillo, Veronique
El Paso First Health Plans Inc — Page 413
Carroll, Bob
CIGNA Healthcare of AZ — Page 14
Carroll, Charles
Driscoll Children's Health Plan — Page 412
Carroll, Chuck
Molina Healthcare of Texas Inc — Page 421
Carroll, Deidre
AmeriGroup District of Columbia — Page 97
Carroll, Jean
Volusia Health Network — Page 124
Carroll, Milton
Health Care Service Corporation -
Corporate Headquarters — Page 149
Carroll, Nicole
Davis Vision — Page 288
Carter, Hodge, CHE
Mercy of Iowa City Regional PHO -
Priority Health Network — Page 172
Carter, Paul
Health Management Network Inc — Page 16
NevadaCare Inc — Page 262
Iowa Health Solutions — Page 171
Carter, Philip
Blue Cross Blue Shield of DE — Page 95
Carter, Trudi, MD
Orange Prevention &
Treatment Integrated — Page 60
Cartwright, Kathy
UnitedHealthcare of TN Inc — Page 401
Caruana, Carm
Independent Health
Association Inc — Page 297
Carufel, David
ACN Group — Page 233
Caruncho, Jospeh
Preferred Care Partners Inc — Page 118
Casady, Beth
Upper Peninsula Health Plan — Page 232
Casalino, Marie, MD
Amerigroup New York, LLC — Page 284
Casberg, Jeffrey
Connecticare Inc — Page 89
Connecticare of MA Inc — Page 210
Connecticare of NY — Page 288
Cascino, Jeff
Coordinated Health Systems — Page 361
Casey, Stephen R
California Dental Network Inc — Page 37
Cash, Bruce
Coventry Health Care of Kansas -
Wichita — Page 178
Carelink Health Plans — Page 459
Cashin, Patrick
Eye Care of Wisconsin Inc — Page 464
Cashman, Christopher
Independence Blue Cross — Page 366
Casler, Laurie
Integrated Health Plan Inc — Page 115
Casper, Steven
MedFocus Radiology Network — Page 58
Cassady, Margaret M Esq
Excellus BlueCross BlueShield,
Central New York Region — Page 291
Excellus BlueCross BlueShield,
Utica Region — Page 292
Cassano, Scott G
Health Plan of Nevada Inc — Page 260
Sierra Health Services Inc-Corporate
Headquarters — Page 264
Cassetta, Toni
MetroPlus Health Plan — Page 300
Cassidy, James E
Community Clinical Services — Page 196

Index VIII: Personnel

Bunker, Jonathan W
Health Plan of Nevada Inc   Page 260
Sierra Health Services Inc-
Corporate Headquarters   Page 264
Bunkley, Mike
MyMatrixx   Page 489
Burcham, Michael
ParadigmHealth   Page 276
Burchuk, Robert, MD
PacifiCare Behavioral Health   Page 61
Burge, Warren
Preferred Health Systems   Page 180
Burgess, Howard
Physicians Health Plan of
Mid-Michigan   Page 228
Burgess, Trixy
Sanford Health Plan   Page 388
Burggraff, Lori
UnitedHealthcare of Texas Inc -
Houston   Page 429
Burgos, Gilbert, MD
Care Choices HMO   Page 218
Burke, James
Private Healthcare Systems -
Corporate Headquarters   Page 215
Burke, John
HealthFirst Inc   Page 295
Burke, Melissa
Careington International - The Dental
Network   Page 408
Burke, Richard P
Fallon Community Hlth Pln Inc   Page 211
Burke, Richard T
UnitedHealthcare of AZ Inc   Page 21
UnitedHealthcare of AR   Page 28
UnitedHealthcare of CO   Page 85
UnitedHealthcare of FL Inc   Page 121
UnitedHealthcare of FL Inc   Page 122
UnitedHealthcare of South FL   Page 122
UnitedHealthcare of GA   Page 134
UnitedHealthcare Services
Co of the River Valley Inc   Page 154
UnitedHealthcare of Illinois Inc   Page 154
UnitedHealthcare Services
Co of the River Valley Inc   Page 172
UnitedHealthcare Services
Co of the River Valley Inc   Page 173
UnitedHealthcare of the
Heartland States   Page 182
UnitedHealthcare of KY   Page 186
UnitedHealthcare of LA   Page 193
UnitedHealthcare & Mid Atlantic
Medical Services Inc   Page 206
UnitedHealth Group —
Corporate Headquarters   Page 238
UnitedHealthcare of MI Inc   Page 242
UnitedHealthcare of the
Midwest Inc   Page 251
UnitedHealthcare of the
Midlands Inc   Page 257
UnitedHealthcare of NY Inc   Page 306
UnitedHealthcare of
New York Metropolitan   Page 306
UnitedHealthcare of NC Inc   Page 315
UnitedHealthcare of OH Inc-
Cleveland   Page 336
UnitedHealthcare of SW OH Inc-
Dayton/Cincinnati   Page 337
UnitedHealthcare of OR   Page 352
UnitedHealthcare of
New England Inc   Page 381
UnitedHealthcare Services
Co of the River Valley Inc   Page 400
UnitedHealthcare of TN Inc   Page 401
UnitedHealthcare of TX Inc -
Houston   Page 429
UnitedHealthcare of TX Inc -
San Antonio   Page 430

UnitedHealthcare of TX Inc —
Dallas   Page 430
UnitedHealthcare of VA   Page 446
UnitedHealthcare of WI Inc   Page 470
UnitedHealthcare Services
Co of the River Valley Inc   Page 173
Burke, Shawn
Coventry Health Care of KS Inc   Page 245
Burkett, Charles, MD
Volusia Health Network   Page 124
Burkett, Kristen
Exempla Healthcare LLC   Page 81
Burkhart, Eddie
NevadaCare Inc   Page 262
Burley, Brian
Aultcare   Page 320
Burlock, Samuel
Blue Ridge Health Network   Page 357
Burn, Greg
Blue Cross Blue Shield of OK   Page 339
Burnaugh, Bob
Employee Benefit
Management Services Inc   Page 253
Burnett, Ann
BlueChoice Hlth Plan of SC Inc   Page 383
Burnett, Janet
WelBorn Health Plans   Page 167
Burnette, Peg
Denver Health Medical Plan Inc   Page 80
Burnette, Ron
Pharmacy Providers
Services Corp   Page 492
Burnham, Heather
Corvel Corporation   Page 43
Burns, Nancy
Southeastern Indiana
Health Organization   Page 166
Burns, Susan, BA
MPRO   Page 227
Burnside, Terry
Medicap Pharmacies Inc   Page 489
Burrell, Chester
CareFirst BlueChoice Inc   Page 97
CareFirst BC BS   Page 200
Delmarva Health Care Plan Inc   Page 202
CareFirst BC BS   Page 481
Burris, Bonita
HMS Colorado Inc   Page 82
Sloan's Lake Preferred
Health Networks   Page 85
Bursac, Radovan
Unity Health Insurance   Page 470
Burton, James
Block Vision of Texas Inc   Page 405
Burzynski, Mark
Blue Cross Blue Shield of MT   Page 253
Busack, Gary
Coventry Health Care Inc _ IA   Page 169
Busby, Tom
Educators Health Care   Page 434
Busch, Charles E
Beech Street Corporation —
Corporate Headquarters   Page 36
PpoNEXT   Page 423
Busek, Rhonda
Lane Oregon Health Plans   Page 347
Bushardt, Keith G
Blue Cross Blue Shield of NE   Page 255
Bushnell, Ian, MD
Southern Health Services Inc   Page 445
Bussey, Larry
Medica Health Plans   Page 236
Butcher, Jeff
Hometown Health Plan   Page 260
Butera, Jody
University Family Care Hlth Plan   Page 22
Butler, Christopher D
Independence Blue Cross   Page 366
Keystone Health Plan East Inc   Page 368

Butler, Chuck
Blue Cross Blue Shield of MT   Page 253
Butler, Leona M
Santa Clara Family Health Plan   Page 67
Butler, Vince
Medwatch LLC   Page 116
Butora, Joseph
Keystone Health Plan Central   Page 367
Butts, Wayne
Western Dental Services   Page 75
Byers, Marnie
Priority Health   Page 230
Bymark, Lori, MSIA
Partners Rx Management LLC   Page 491
Byrd, Karen
MedFocus Radiology Network   Page 58
Byrd, Rosemarie
M Plan Inc   Page 163
Byrd, Thomas R
Anthem BC BS of VA Inc   Page 442
WellPoint Inc -
Corporate Headquarters   Page 167
Byrne, James J, MD
Priority Health   Page 230

C

Cabrera, Marcio
Atlantic Dental Inc   Page 102
Cabrera, Patricia
Central Benefits Mutual
Insurance Company   Page 321
Cadger, Michael
Peach State Health Plan   Page 133
Cadoret, Judy
Integrated Health Plan Inc   Page 115
Cagle, Mary Jo, MD
St Francis Optimum
Health Network   Page 385
Cahill, Maureen
Ohio State University Managed
Health Care Systems Inc   Page 332
Cahill, Patrick T
Delta Dental Plan of IN Inc   Page 159
Delta Dental Plan of MI Inc   Page 220
Delta Dental Plan of OH Inc   Page 324
Cain, Susan
WellDyne Rx   Page 497
Cairo, Karen
Nationwide Health Plans   Page 331
Calabrese, Steven
Health Net - New Jersey   Page 272
Health Net - New York   Page 295
Health Net Inc - Northeast
Corporate Headquarters   Page 91
Calarco, Christine
Meritain Health Inc   Page 299
Calder, Jen
Mount Carmel Health Plan   Page 331
Calhoun-Davis, Gloria, LVN
Lakewood Health Plan Inc   Page 56
Call, David D
Deseret Healthcare   Page 434
Call, Gary, MD
Molina HealthCare of Utah Inc   Page 435
Callaghan, Karron
Delta Dental Plans Association   Page 146
Callahan, Charles, RPh, CDM
PharmAvail Benefit
Management Company   Page 492
Callahan, Kevin J
Newport Dental Plan   Page 60
Callenberger, Douglas
HealthAmerica Pennsylvania Inc -
Eastern Region   Page 365

Index VIII: Personnel

Broadhead, Stephen Y, CPA
Utah Public Employees
Health Program — Page 438
Broatch, Robert E
Guardian Life Insurance
Co of America — Page 294
Brockey, Alicia
CIGNA Healthcare of Arizona — Page 14
Brocksome, Steve
Blue Cross of Idaho — Page 141
True Blue — Page 142
Broda, Mindy, DDS
Delta Dental Insurance Company -
Georgia — Page 131
Brodeur, Michael
Aetna Specialty Pharmacy — Page 479
Brodie, Bridget
American College of
Medical Quality — Page 199
Brody, David, MD
Denver Health Medical Plan Inc — Page 80
Broeren, Marcia
Network Health Plan WI — Page 468
Bromley, Debbi
Genex Services — Page 363
Brooks, Gary N
Vision Service Plan of Arizona — Page 22
Vision Service Plan — Page 75
Vision Service Plan — Page 86
Brooks, Mike
Humana Health Plan of OH Inc — Page 328
Brophy, J Paul
CIGNA Healthcare of OH Inc — Page 323
Brophy, Paul
UnitedHealthcare of SW OH Inc-
Dayton/Cincinnati — Page 337
Brower, Dwight
Blue Cross Blue Shield of LA Inc — Page 189
HMO Louisiana Inc — Page 191
Brown, Amy
Advantage Health Solutions Inc — Page 157
Brown, Anne
Individualized Care
Management Inc — Page 162
Brown, Beverly
Cariten Healthcare — Page 393
PHP Companies Inc — Page 397
Brown, Brent
Anthem BC BS of Colorado — Page 77
Brown, Brent
Rocky Mountain Hospital
& Medical Services Inc — Page 85
Brown, Charles T
Aetna Inc - Oklahoma — Page 339
Aetna Inc - Tulsa — Page 339
Aetna Inc - Dental Plan of Texas — Page 403
Brown, Constance
Encore Health Network — Page 160
M Plan Inc — Page 163
Brown, Dale
CareGuide — Page 105
MedImpact Hlthcr Sys Inc — Page 488
Brown, Deanna
Spectera Vision Srvcs of CA Inc — Page 69
Brown, Dennis
Delta Dental Plan of WI — Page 463
Brown, Dewey
Coventry Health Care Inc —
Carolinas — Page 311
Wellpath Select Inc — Page 315
Brown, Douglas
Blue Cross Blue Shield of GA — Page 128
Brown, Frederick
CarePlus Health Plans Inc — Page 106
Brown, Frederick G, MD
KePRO — Page 367
Brown, James M
Blue Cross Blue Shield of AL — Page 3

Brown, Jim
Presbyterian Health Plan — Page 281
Brown, Jim, RPh
Script Care Inc — Page 425
Script Care Inc - Texas — Page 494
Brown, Kathy
El Paso First Health Plans Inc — Page 413
Brown, Kenneth
AmeriGroup Maryland Inc — Page 199
Brown, Michael
HealthPlus Inc — Page 296
Brown, Neal
Aetna Inc - Pennsylvania — Page 355
Brown, Randy L
WellPoint Inc -
Corporate Headquarters — Page 167
Brown, Rick
Newport Dental Plan — Page 60
Brown, Robin
Health Net of California — Page 49
Brown, Sandra, MD
Community Health Alliance — Page 159
Brown, Sandy
Health Plus of Louisiana Inc — Page 191
Brown, Tammy
4MOST Health Network — Page 459
Brown, Tom
ValueOptions -
Corporate Headquarters — Page 447
Brown-Stevenson, Tina
Aetna Inc - Pennsylvania — Page 355
Browning, Francis L
Qca Health Plan Inc — Page 28
Browning, Mike, MBA, CPA
SelectHealth Network — Page 165
Brubaker, Laurie
Aetna Inc - Houston — Page 403
Brubaker, Lisa
Preferred Care — Page 304
Brubaker, Mary Jane
ProNJ, The Healthcare Quality Improve-
ment Organization of NJ — Page 276
Bruce, Bill
Devon Health Services Inc — Page 361
Bruce-Nichols, Sandra D, MD
AmeriGroup Maryland Inc — Page 199
Brumbaugh, Brian
Preferred Hlthcr System Inc — Page 371
Brunetti, Louis
MedImpact Hlthcr Sys Inc — Page 488
Bruno, Anthony
Community Health Network
of Connecticut Inc — Page 89
Bruno, Richard
Inland Empire Health Plan — Page 52
Bruns, Dennis, CPA
Primary Health Plan — Page 142
Brunstad, John
Group Health Cooperative
of Eau Claire — Page 465
Bruntgen, Patti
Delta Dental Plan of Minnesota — Page 235
Bruzek, Rick
HealthPartners Inc — Page 236
Bryant, Gary W, CPA
American Pioneer Health
Plans Inc — Page 101
Bryant, James
Humana Inc - Indiana — Page 161
Bryant, Oscar
Delta Dental of Virginia — Page 443
Bryant, Ruth Ann
Alabama Quality
Assurance Foundation — Page 3
Bryant, Sharon
Columbia United Providers — Page 449
Bryant, Vicki
Concentra Inc — Page 411

Bubach, Richard, MSA
North Dakota Hlth Cre Review — Page 318
Buccheri, Jim
Connecticare Inc — Page 89
Bucher, George
Coventry Health Care Inc — LA — Page 190
Buchert, Greg, MD
Orange Prevention &
Treatment Integrated — Page 60
Buck, Eric E
Preferred Health Care — Page 370
Buck, Ernest, MD
Driscoll Children's Health Plan — Page 412
Buck, John
Medica Health Plans — Page 236
Buck, Rick
Keystone Mercy Health Plan — Page 368
PerformRx — Page 492
Buckley, David
Colorado Choice Health Plan/
San Luis Valley HMO Inc — Page 79
Buckwold, Frederick, MD
Evercare of Texas LLC — Page 413
Budd, Robert
Delta Dental Insurance Company -
Georgia — Page 131
Alpha Dental Programs Inc — Page 404
Budnick, John
Active Health Management — Page 441
Buehrle, Charmaane
Nevada Prfrrd Professionals — Page 262
Universal Health Network -
Corporate Headquarters — Page 264
Buffa, Jan L, PhD, MBA
Marion Polk Community
Health Plan Advantage — Page 349
Buffington, Jody
Magellan Health Services — Page 132
Bugajski, Steve
Unison Health Plan -
Corporate Headquarters — Page 372
Unison Health Plan of TN — Page 399
Buggle, Janet
QualCare Inc — Page 276
Buitkus, Kastytis, MD
Review Works — Page 230
Bujak, Denise A
Blue Cross Blue Shield of IL — Page 144
Health Care Service Corporation -
Corporate Headquarters — Page 149
Blue Cross Blue Shield of TX —
Corporate Headquarters — Page 406
Buka, Chris
Great-West Healthcare of GA — Page 131
Bukovinsky, Richard
Meritain Health — Page 330
Bulkley, Benjamin
Allscripts Pharmaceuticals Inc — Page 479
Bullard, Richard, RPh
Partners Rx Management LLC — Page 491
Bullard, Stacy
Elderhaus Inc — Page 510
Bullen, Bruce M
Harvard Pilgrim Health Care -
Corporate Headquarters — Page 212
Bulloch, Karen
Partnership Health Plan Inc — Page 522
Bullock, Ralph T
Anthem BC BS of VA Inc — Page 442
Bultemeier, Dale
Physicians Health Plan of
Northern Indiana — Page 164
Bumbard, Joycea
Healthcare Partners of
East Texas Inc — Page 416
Bumeter, Cindy
Health Plus — Page 150
Buncher, James E
Safeguard Hlth Plns Inc — Pages 119, 424

Index VIII: Personnel

Bowers, Krista
Health Net - Connecticut — Page 90
Health Net Inc - Northeast
Corporate Headquarters — Page 91
Bowers, Lee
Humana Health Plan -
Jacksonville — Page 113
Bowers, Lynn, MD
Suburban Health Organization — Page 166
Bowers, Scott A
Unison Health Plan of Ohio Inc — Page 336
Bowlenbaugh, Scott
Aetna Inc - Tennessee — Page 391
Bowles, Charles, Jr, MD
D C Chartered Health Plan Inc — Page 97
Bowling, Elaine
Santa Barbara Regional
Health Authority — Page 67
Bowling, Rita, RN MSN MBA CPHQ
Ohio Kepro Inc — Page 332
Bowlus, Brad
PacifiCare Health Systems-
Corporate Headquarters — Page 62
Bowser, Tom
Blue Cross Blue Shield of
Kansas City — Page 244
Good Health HMO Inc — Page 247
Boxer, Mark L
WellPoint Inc -
Corporate Headquarters — Page 167
Anthem Insurance Co Inc — Page 516
Boyce-Smith, Gifford, MD
Blue Shield of California — Page 36
Boyd, Jeff
Oxford Health Plans-CT — Page 91
Boyd, Laura
Community Health Plan of WA — Page 450
Boyd, Lynn
South Central Preferred — Page 372
Boyd, Thomas A
Blue Cross Blue Shield of RI — Page 379
Boyd, Todd
Assurant Employee Benefits-AZ — Page 12
Assurant Employee Benefits-CA — Page 35
Assurant Employee Benefits-CO — Page 78
Assurant Employee Benefits-FL — Page 102
Assurant Employee Benefits-GA — Page 127
Assurant Employee Benefits-IL — Page 143
Assurant Employee Benefits-IN — Page 158
Assurant Employee Benefits-MI — Page 217
Assurant Employee Benefits -
Corporate Office — Page 244
Assurant Employee Benefits-NM — Page 279
Assurant Employee Benefits-NY — Page 285
Assurant Employee Benefits-NC — Page 309
Assurant Employee Benefits-PA — Page 357
Assurant Employee Benefits-TN — Page 392
Assurant Employee Benefits-TX — Page 429
Assurant Employee Benefits-WA — Page 449
Boyer, Guy
Blue Cross Blue Shield of VT — Page 439
Boyer, Julie
HealthPlus of Michigan — Page 224
Boyer, Spencer
Bluegrass Family Health Inc — Page 183
Boyle, Judy
Independent Health
Association Inc — Page 297
Boyle, Kathy, RN
HMO New Mexico Inc — Page 280
Bracciodieta, William P, MD
Health Net of California — Page 49
Health Net Health Plan
of Oregon Inc — Page 346
Brace, Aaron
UnitedHealthcare of Alabama — Page 7
UnitedHealthcare of Louisiana — Page 193
Bracikowski, James, MD, FACP
Windsor Health Plan of TN Inc — Page 401

Brackett, Roger
GroupLink Inc — Page 160
Braden, Stephen
1st Medical Network — Page 127
Bradford, William
Denta Quest Ventures Inc — Page 211
Bradley, Clare B, MD, MPH
IPRO — Page 298
Bradley, Don W, MD MHS-CL
Blue Cross
Blue Shield of NC — Pages 310, 481
Bradley, Kerry
EyeMed Vision Care LLC — Page 325
Bradman, Leo, PsyD
Unipsych Systems — Page 120
Brady, Dan
Florida Pace Centers Inc — Page 511
Brady, Rupert
Fidelis Care New York — Page 293
Brainerd, Mary
HealthPartners Inc — Pages 236, 486, 506
Braly, Angela F
Anthem Blue Cross
Blue Shield of Colorado — Page 77
WellPoint Inc -
Corporate Headquarters — Page 167
Anthem Blue Cross
Blue Shield of Nevada — Page 259
Anthem Blue Cross
Blue Shield of Ohio — Page 320
Anthem Blue Cross and
Blue Shield of Ohio — Page 320
Rocky Mountain Hospital
& Medical Services Inc — Page 85
Anthem Blue Cross
Blue Shield of Maine — Page 195
WellPoint NextRx — Page 497
Bramstenner, Tamara
Delta Dental Plan of Idaho — Page 141
Branch, Derrick
Union Health Service Inc — Page 154
Branchini, Frank J
GHI HMO Select Inc — Page 293
EmblemHealth Inc — Page 290
Brander, Christy
Beech Street Corporation —
Corporate Headquarters — Page 36
Brandt, Mike
Health Net of California — Page 49
Branham, Stacy, MD
Viva Health Inc — Page 7
Brannigan, Matthew T
Blue Cross Blue Shield of RI — Page 379
Coordinated Health Plan — Page 379
Branstetter, Phil
Inland Empire Health Plan — Page 52
Brantley, Viviana
BeneScript Services Inc — Page 481
Brantner, Linda
Delta Dental Plan of Kansas — Page 178
Brash-Sorensen, Charlene
Universal Health Care Inc — Page 122
Brauer, Keith
Aveta Inc — Page 270
Braun, Janet, RN
Health Plan of San Joaquin, The — Page 50
Braun, Stephen
KPS Health Plans — Page 452
Braverman, Howard J, OD
CompBenefits — Page 410
Bravo, Edith
Dental Health Services Inc — Page 450
Brazier, Bruce
KPS Health Plans — Page 452
Breard, Mike W
Vantage Health Plan Inc — Page 193
Brecher, Randy A
Pacific Union Dental Inc — Page 63

Nevada Pacific Dental — Page 262
National Pacific Dental — Page 421
Brede, Rhonda
Evercare Select — Page 15
Brehm, John G, MD, FACP
West Virginia Medical Institute — Page 460
Breidenstein, Stacy
CareFirst BC/BS — Page 200
Breitbach, Lynn
Hines & Associates Inc — Page 150
Brendzel, Ronald I
Safeguard Hlth Enterprises Inc — Page 66
Breneman, Brian
New England Financial -
Corporate Headquarters — Page 214
Brennan, Laura
PacificSource Health Plans — Page 350
Brennan, Troyen A, MD
Aetna Inc - Corp Headquarters — Page 87
Aetna Inc of the Carolinas — Page 309
Aetna Inc - Corp Headquarters — Page 355
Aetna Inc - Pennsylvania — Page 355
Aetna Inc - PA Region — Page 356
Aetna Inc - Tennessee — Page 391
Bresler, Catherine
Trustmark Insurance Company — Page 153
Bretz, Virgil
Hygeia Corporation — Page 114
Breuer, David
Blue Cross Blue Shield of ND — Page 317
Brian, Michael
Great-West Healthcare of MA — Page 212
Brick, Errol D
HMO Health Ohio (Cleveland) — Page 328
Medical Mutual of Ohio — Page 330
SuperMed Network — Page 334
Bricker, Frederick
UnitedHealthcare of Texas Inc -
Houston — Page 429
Bridges, David Frank
Health Advantage — Page 27
Bridges, Derek
Golden West Dental & Vision — Page 47
Briedenbach, William
Health Plans Inc — Page 213
Brigden, Cathy
SCHC Total Care Inc — Page 305
Briggs, Marc R
Sierra Health Services Inc-
Corporate Headquarters — Page 264
Briggs, Patricia Cecilia
Puget Sound Health Partners — Page 455
Brill, Joel, MD
Action Health Care
Management Services — Page 11
Brill, Martin J
Health Partners — Page 364
Brill, Marty
Amerihealth Insurance Company -
NJ North — Page 269
Amerihealth Insurance Company -
NJ South — Page 269
Bringardner, Jeff
Humana Health Care Plans of
Lexington — Page 185
Brinkley, Cary
Allianz Life Insurance
Company of North America — Page 233
Britt, Judy
Hometown Health Plan — Page 260
Brittain, James W
Virginia Health Network — Page 447
Brittain, John S
Aveta Inc — Page 270
Brizendine, Kevin
Saint Mary's HealthFirst — Page 263
Broader, Michael
SCHC Total Care Inc — Page 305

Index VIII: Personnel

Humana Inc - IA — Page 170
Humana Inc - Corporate Headquarters — Page 185
Humana Inc - MD — Page 203
Humana Inc - MI — Page 241
Humana Inc - NE — Page 256
Humana Inc - NM — Page 280
Humana Inc - NC — Page 313
Humana Inc - ND — Page 317
Humana Health Plan of OH Inc — Page 328
Humana Inc - OK — Page 341
Humana Inc - SC — Page 384
Humana Inc - SD — Page 388
Humana Inc - TN — Page 396
Humana Health Care Plans of Corpus Christi — Page 417
Humana Inc - UT — Page 435
Humana Inc - Wyoming — Page 473
Humana Inc — Page 486

Blomberg, Dan
Blue Cross Blue Shield of TN — Page 392
Blue Cross Blue Shield of TN - Memphis — Page 393

Bloom, Alan
UHP Healthcare — Page 71

Bloom, Celia
Coventry Health Care Inc — Delaware Inc — Page 96

Bloschichak, Andrew, MD
Keystone Health Plan West Inc — Page 368

Blount, Jospeh L, MD
OmniCare, A Coventry Health Plan — Page 228

Bluestein, Paul A MD
Connecticare Inc — Page 89
Connecticare of NY — Page 288
Connecticare of MA Inc — Page 210

Bluestone, Daniel, MD
Sante Community Physicians — Page 67

Bluestone, Maura
Affinity Health Plan Inc — Page 283

Blume, Lisa
Humana Health Benefit Plan of Louisiana — Pages 191, 517

Boals, Richard
Blue Cross Blue Shield of AZ — Page 12

Bock, Kelly
Great-West Healthcare of FL — Page 111

Bodaken, Bruce G
Blue Shield of California — Page 36

Bode, Edwin
Healthnow — Page 395

Bode, Tim
Americas PPO — Page 233

Bodgewiecz, George C
Great West Life Annuity Insurance Co — Page 81

Boehm, Jonathan
Argus Health System Inc — Page 480

Boehning, Kathy
Behavioral Healthcare Options Inc — Page 259

Boeing, Donna
Anthem Blue Cross Blue Shield of Colorado — Page 77
Rocky Mountain Hospital & Medical Services Inc — Page 85

Boetcher, Nancy
Health Management Network Inc — Page 16

Bogdewiecz, George C
Great-West Healthcare of Kansas/Missouri — Page 179

Boggus, Terrie
Physicians Health Plan of Mid-Michigan — Page 228

Bogle, George
USA Managed Care Org — Page 22

Bogle, Mike
USA Managed Care Org — Page 22

Bogossian, Gail
Connecticare Inc — Page 89

Bohlmann, Pamela
Santa Clara Family Health Plan — Page 67

Bohner, Scott
KEPRO — Page 367

Boisette, Serge
Jackson Memorial Health Plan — Page 115

Boland Docimo, Ann, MD
UPMC Health Plan Univ of Pittsburgh Medical Center — Page 374

Bolding, Ronald
Inter Valley Health Plan Inc — Page 53

Bolen, Joe
Blue Cross Blue Shield of AL — Page 3

Boles, Christopher D
PacifiCare Dental & Vision — Page 61

Bolic, Walter
Delta Dental Plan of NM — Page 279

Bolovrelchi, Cindy
CompBenefits Corporation - Corporate Headquarters — Page 129

Bolster, Jennifer
SCHC Total Care Inc — Page 305

Bolton, Mary Beth, MD
Health Alliance Plan — Page 223

Bolton, Roger
Aetna Inc of the Carolinas — Page 309

Bolyog, Candee
Managed Dental Care — Page 57

Bolz, Terry
Unity Health Insurance — Page 470

Bonaparte, Philip M, MD
Horizon NJ Health — Page 274

Bond, Janis RN, CMCN
ConnectCare — Page 219

Bond, Jeffrey C
Cox Health Plans — Page 246

Bond, Rosemary
Preferred Care — Page 304

Bonde, Toni
Hudson Health Plan — Page 297

Bonner, Mary Claire
Aetna Inc — Page 87
Aetna Inc - Pennsylvania — Page 355

Booher, Scott
Medica Health Plans — Page 236

Bookhardt, Dawn
Denver Health Medical Plan Inc — Page 80

Booma, Stephen J
Blue Cross Blue Shield of MA — Page 209

Boone, Merrill
Kaiser Foundation Health Plan of Georgia — Page 132

Booth, Randy
Utah Public Employees Health Program — Page 438

Boothe, James O
HealthFirst Inc — Page 295

Boozer, Sandra
Blue Care Network of MI — Page 217

Bopp, George
NYCHSRO/MedReview Inc — Page 303

Borden, Jay
Prairie States Enterprises Inc — Page 152

Borders, Phyllis
Physicians Health Plan of Northern Indiana — Page 164

Bordreaux, Gail K
HMO Illinois — Page 150

Borgstrom, Ned Jr
Exempla Healthcare LLC — Page 81

Born, Chris
Texas Childrens Health Plan — Page 426

Borrell, Judy M
American Progressive Life & Health of New York — Page 501

Borsand, Gerald C, RPh
4D Pharmacy Management Systems Inc — Page 479

Borsand, Jonathan D
4D Pharmacy Management Systems Inc — Page 479

Borup, Lynn
Colorado Choice Health Plan/San Luis Valley HMO Inc — Page 79

Bory, Steven
Neighborhood Health Providers — Page 302

Boscio, Raymond M
Rayant Insurance Company of New York — Page 304

Bossi, Anne E
Union Labor Life Insurance Co — Page 276

Boston, Trina
Individualized Care Management Inc — Page 162

Boswell, Allen
Encore Health Network — Page 160

Botticelli, Max G, MD
University Health Alliance — Page 138

Bottitta, Louis
Valley Preferred — Page 375

Bottrill, Lorry
Health Net of Arizona — Page 17

Boucher, David
Blue Cross Blue Shield of SC - Corporate Hqtrs — Page 383

Bouharoun, Khalil
D C Chartered Health Plan Inc — Page 97

Boulis, Paul S
Blue Cross and Blue Shield of IL Pharmacy Programs — Page 481
Blue Cross Blue Shield of IL — Page 144

Boullion, Michelle
Fara Healthcare Management — Page 190

Bourbeau, Michael D
Delta Dental Plan of NH — Page 265

Bourdon, David, MBA
CIGNA Behavioral Health Inc — Page 88
CIGNA Behavioral Health Inc - Corporate Headquarters — Page 234

Bourgvignon, Ramona
Community Medical Alliance — Page 210

Bourquin, Judy
Indiana Pro Health Network — Page 162

Boutin, Jeannine
Action Health Care Management Services — Page 11

Bouton, Charles
Fallon Community Hlth Pln Inc — Page 211

Bouvette, Ralph E, RPA, PhD, JD
American Pharmacy Services Corporation — Page 183
American Pharmacy Services Corp — Page 480

Bouvier, Chris
KEPRO — Page 367
Amerigroup New York, LLC — Page 284

Bove, Frank
Atlantis Health Plan — Page 285

Bovine, Sarah
SHPS Inc — Page 186

Bowen, Amy
Geisinger Health Plan — Page 363

Bowen, Kenneth W, Jr
QCA Health Plan Inc — Page 28

Bowen, Mark J
Assurant Employee Benefits-PA — Page 357

Bowers, Christopher D
Superior HealthPlan Inc — Page 426

Bowers, Christopher D
Centene Corporation — Page 244

Bowers, David, MD
Preferred Health Care — Page 370

Index VIII: Personnel

Berkel, Susan L
PacifiCare of Oregon — Page 350
UnitedHealthcare of WA — Page 457
Berkowitz, Kenneth
Blue Cross Blue Shield of
Florida & Health Options Inc — Page 104
Berman, Eric, MD
AmeriGroup New Jersey Inc — Page 268
Berman, Jim
UnitedHealthcare of Colorado — Page 85
Berman, Neil E
Humana Medical Plan Inc — Page 114
Bermel, Margaret
Suffolk Health Plan — Page 305
Bernadett, Martha, MD
Molina Healthcare Inc -
Corporate Headquarters — Page 59
Bernal, Rose
Care 1st Health Plan AZ Inc — Page 13
Bernard-Shaw, Cheryle, JD
On Lok Senior Health Services — Page 60
Bernath, Robert, CPA
Jp Farley Corp — Page 329
Bernhardt, Peggy
UnitedHealth Group —
Corporate Headquarters — Page 238
Bernstein, Michael
Anthem Blue Cross
Blue Shield of Wisconsin — Page 461
Bero, Marvin
Preferred Podiatry Group — Page 152
Berrier, Frank J, Jr, PhD
Spectrum Review Services Inc — Page 426
Berry, Elyse
HealthPlus of Michigan — Page 224
Berry, Gery J
HmoLouisiana Inc — Page 191
Berry, Jack, MD
HealthPlus of Michigan — Page 224
Berry, Laurie
ACN Group — Page 233
Berry, Melody
OSF Health Plans — Page 151
Berry, Ronald
Health Alliance Plan — Page 223
Berryman, Patrick M
Epic Pharmacy Network Inc — Page 484
Berthiaume, John T, MD
Hawaii Medical Services Association -
BC/BS of Hawaii — Page 137
Bertolini, Mark T
Aetna Inc - Arizona — Page 11
Aetna Inc - Maryland — Page 199
Aetna Inc - Michigan — Page 217
Aetna Inc - New Jersey — Page 267
Aetna Inc - New York — Page 283
Aetna Inc of the Carolinas — Page 309
Aetna Inc - Corp Headquarters — Page 87
Aetna Inc - Corp Headquarters — Page 355
Aetna Inc - Pennsylvania — Page 355
Aetna Inc - Tennessee — Page 391
Aetna Health Plans
of Mid-Atlantic — Page 441
Aetna Inc - Virginia — Page 441
Bertonellit, Mindi
Capitol Administrators — Page 38
Berube, Paul
BeneScript Services Inc — Page 481
Berwick, Tracy
Careington International -
The Dental Network — Page 408
Best, Marc
New West Health Plan — Page 254
Beste, Pete
Navitus Health Solutions — Page 490
Bevil, Stacey
Memorial Hermann
Health Network Providers — Page 420

Bhatia, Arun
MagnaCare — Page 298
Bhojwani, Gary C
Allianz Life Insurance
Company of North America — Page 233
Biats, Steve
CIGNA Healthcare - Cincinnati — Page 323
CIGNA Healthcare of Ohio Inc — Page 323
Bickford, Robert, MBA
Community Behavioral
Healthcare Cooperative of PA — Page 361
Bicknell, Patrick F
Health Plus of Louisiana Inc — Page 191
Biedes, Phyllis
Maricopa Health Plan — Page 18
Biehn, Doug
Blue Shield of California — Page 36
Biglin, Helen T
Delta Dental Plan of NH — Page 265
Bigney, Dawn, BSN RN CCM CLCP
Corporate Care Mngmnt Inc — Page 288
Bikoff, Morris, DDS
SW Preferred Dental Org — Page 20
Bildstein, Megan
Great Expressions
Dental Centers — Page 222
Billard, William T
Delta Dental Plan of IN Inc — Page 159
Delta Dental Plan of MI Inc — Page 220
Delta Dental Plan of OH Inc — Page 324
Billerbeck, Robert, MD
Humana Health Care
Plans of Arizona — Page 17
Bilt, Steven C
Newport Dental Plan — Page 60
Bindschadler, Darryl D, MD
Blue Cross Blue Shield of WY — Page 473
Bingaman, Gary
Golden Dental Plans Inc — Page 221
Binley, Malissa, PhD
Carolina Care Plan Inc — Page 383
Binn, Martha
Health Tradition Health Plans — Page 466
Birch, Bryan D
Medco Health Solutions Inc — Page 488
Birch, Pamela
Combined Insurance
Company of America — Page 145
Bird, A David
CIGNA Healthcare of St Louis — Page 245
Bird, Jon
Beech Street Corporation —
Corporate Headquarters — Page 36
Birdsong, Carl, RPh
Maxor Plus — Page 488
Birnbawn, Howard
Hudson Health Plan — Page 297
Bischoff, Kevin
Regence Blue Cross
Blue Shield of Utah — Page 436
Bishoff, Suzanne
Interactive Medical Systems — Page 313
Bishop, Stephen T
Community First Hlth Plans Inc — Page 410
Bishop, Steven
Humana Health Care Plans
of Corpus Christi — Page 417
Bitter, Anita
Optimum Choice Inc — Page 205
Bittner, Clay
UnitedHealthcare of Arkansas — Page 28
Bixenmann, Helen
Sun Health Medisun — Page 20
Bjerre, Claudia
Healthcare USA of MI LLC — Page 248
Group Health Plan Inc — Page 248
Bjorum, John S
First Plan of Minnesota — Pages 235, 505

Bjostad, Teri, MD
Preferred Mental
Health Management — Page 180
Black, Baeteena, RPh
Tennessee Pharmacist Assoc — Page 495
Black, Glenn
Henry Ford Health System — Page 508
Black, Steven H
Oxford Health Plans-CT — Page 91
Oxford Health Plans Inc —
Corporate Headquarters — Page 92
Oxford Health Plans of NY, Inc — Page 303
Blackburn, John
Center Care — Page 184
Blackett, Melrose, MD
UAHC Health Plan of Tennessee — Page 399
Blackshear, Murray
Texas HealthSpring I LLC — Page 427
Blackwood, Michael
Gateway Health Plan Inc — Page 362
Blain, Kathy
PacificSource Health Plans — Page 350
Blair, David T
HealthExtras Inc — Page 485
Catalyst Rx,
A Healthextras Company — Page 482
Blake, John
Humana Health Benefit
Plan of Louisiana — Page 191
Blakely, Richard, MD
Memorial Hermann
Health Network Providers — Page 420
Blancas, Gilbert
El Paso First Health Plans Inc — Page 413
Blaney, Dan
Genex Services — Page 363
Blaney, Dina
Community Health
Network of Connecticut Inc — Page 89
Blanford, Joseph
Aetna Inc - Arkansas — Page 25
Aetna Inc - Louisiana — Page 189
Blank, John P, MD
Unison Health Plan of PA — Page 373
Unison Health Plan of OH Inc — Page 336
Unison Health Plan -
Corporate Headquarters — Page 372
Unison Health Plan of TN — Page 399
Blank, William
Paragon Biomedical Inc — Page 491
Blankenship, Arin
Humana Inc - Grand Rapids MI — Page 225
Blaser, Lon, DO
Group Health Cooperative
of Eau Claire — Page 465
Blasko, Kristin
APS Healthcare Northwest Inc — Page 253
Blaxton, Sharon
Evergreen Medical Group LLC — Page 131
Blaylock, Stanley B
Walgreens Health Initiatives — Page 496
Blevins, Shirley J
Unison Health Plan -
Corporate Headquarters — Page 372
Unison Health Plan of TN — Page 399
Blickman, Fred
Hip Health Plan of New York — Page 296
Bliss, Patti, RN
ChoiceCare/Humana — Page 322
Block, Martin, MD
Mercy Care Plan — Page 18
Bloedorn, David
Network Health Plan WI — Page 468
Bloem, James H
Humana Insurance Co - AL — Page 5
Humana Inc - AR — Page 27
Humana Inc - CO — Page 82
Humana Inc - DC — Page 98

Index VIII: Personnel

Baum, J Robert
Highmark Inc — Page 366
Baum, Lisa
Capital District
Physicians Health Plan — Page 286
Baum, Paul
Group Health Cooperative
South Central Wisconsin — Page 464
Bauman, Brent
Partnership Health Plan Inc — Page 522
Bavier, Charles
First Script Network Services — Page 485
Bawel, Terry
Health Resources Inc — Page 161
Baxter, Christie
Athens Area Health Plan Select Inc — Page 127
Bayer, Gregory A, PhD
United Behavioral Health (UBH) — Page 71
Bayer, Sue
McLaren Health Plan — Page 226
Bayer, Terry BS, MPH, JD
Molina Healthcare Inc -
Corporate Headquarters — Pages 59, 489
Bea, Javon
Mercycare Health Plan Inc — Page 468
Beach, Bill
Crawford and Co -
Corporate Headquarters — Page 130
Beach, Jason S
Central Susquehanna
Healthcare Providers — Page 359
Beach, Pamela
United Behavioral Health (UBH) — Page 71
Beadle, Zena
Unipsych Systems — Page 120
Beal, Dennis N
American Specialty
Health Plans Inc — Page 33
Beane, Susan J, MD
Affinity Health Plan Inc — Page 283
Beaodin Klein, Shannon
HealthPartners Inc — Page 236
Beard, Patricia
OmniCare,
A Coventry Health Plan — Page 228
Beard, Sandy
CareFirst Blue Cross Blue Shield — Page 200
Beardall, Robert W, MD
Exempla Healthcare LLC — Page 81
Beardmore, Jeffrey, MD
Arnett Health Plans — Page 157
Beaty, Sonja
Texas Childrens Health Plan — Page 426
Beauchaine, David
Healthspring of Alabama Inc — Page 5
Beauchamp, Christy
Preferred Therapy Providers of America -
Corp Headquarters — Page 19
Beauchamp, Karen
Oregon Dealthan — Page 349
Beauchamp, Robert, MD
UnitedHealthcare of Arizona Inc — Page 21
UnitedHealthcare of Utah — Page 437
Beaudoin, Harry
UnitedHealthcare of AL — Page 7
UnitedHealthcare of LA — Page 193
Beaumont, Nancy
Avera Health Plans Inc — Page 387
Bechtol, Allison
LifeWise Health Plan of OR — Page 348
Beck, Dave
Community Health Plan — Page 42
Beck, Jim
SHPS Healthcare Services — Page 20
SHPS Inc — Page 186
Beck, Joann
Aetna Inc - Houston — Page 403

Beck, John
Care Network — Page 359
Beck, John G
Unison Health Plan -
Corporate Headquarters — Page 372
Unison Health Plan of TN — Page 399
Becker, Denise
GHI HMO Select Inc — Page 293
Becker, George H
PacifiCare of Oklahoma Inc/
Secure Horizons — Page 342
PacifiCare of Texas Inc — Page 422
PacifiCare of Texas - Houston — Page 422
Beckies, Valerie, MD
Aetna Inc - Plantation — Page 100
Beckman, Linda
Health Plus — Page 150
Beckman, Richard
Great Expressions
Dental Centers — Page 222
Beckwith, G Nicholas, III
UPMC Health Plan Univ of Pittsburgh
Medical Center — Page 374
Becque, Kathie
Humana Health Plan of Austin — Page 419
Bedrin, Linda
Memphis Managed Care Corp — Page 397
Bedrossian, Phillip, MD
Mercycare Health Plan Inc — Page 468
Beeman, Charles, PharmD
Managed Pharmacy Care — Page 488
Begley, Kate
Aetna Inc - Houston — Page 403
Behrani, Neda
Superior Dental Care Alliance — Page 335
Behremand, Ferial
PacifiCare Health Systems-
Corporate Headquarters — Page 62
Behrens, Patricia L
AmeriGroup Texas Inc — Page 404
Behrman, Jaudon, MD
Bluegrass Family Health Inc — Page 183
Behuniak, Darren M
Devon Health Services Inc — Page 361
Beigian, Koorosh
Combined Insurance
Company of America — Page 145
Beisenstein, William C
Wisconsin Physician
Services Insurance Company — Page 471
Beitel, Rem
CommunityCare Managed Healthcare
Plans of OK Inc — Pages 340, 483
Beland, Rich
Active Health Management — Page 441
Belek, Marilynn G, DMD
Delta Dental Plan of California — Page 44
Belemjian, Glenn
UnitedHealthcare of Arkansas — Page 28
Belfield, Tricia
Americas PPO — Page 233
Bell, Christy W
Horizon Blue Cross/
Blue Shield of NJ — Page 273
Bell, Donna
Aetna Inc - Pennsylvania — Page 355
Bell, Jill Joseph
University Health Care Inc -
Passport Health Plan — Page 187
Bell, John, MD
Global Health Inc — Page 341
Bell, Michael
CIGNA Healthcare of
New York and New Jersey — Page 270
CIGNA Healthcare of Texas Inc — Page 409
CIGNA HealthCare —
Corporate Headquarters — Page 360
Bell, Reed A
Fara Healthcare Management — Page 190

BellaVecchia, Theodore
CareFirst BlueChoice Inc — Page 97
Bellah, Ann
Pueblo Health Care — Page 84
Belle, Diane
Delta Dental Plan of NJ — Page 271
Belleck, Marilyn
Delta Dental Insurance Company -
Nevada — Page 259
Bellinger, Susan
MultiPlan Inc -
Corporate Headquarters — Page 300
Belliveau, Carole
Medical Network Inc — Page 197
Bellofatto, Susan
Horizon Behavioral Services — Page 112
Beltch, Robert
Health Net of California — Page 49
Belton, Paul
Sharp Health Plan — Page 68
Bendel, Kerry
Medica Health Plans — Page 236
Bender, Karen
Unity Health Insurance — Page 470
Benigar, Sandy
UTMB Health Plans Inc — Page 431
Benita, Michael
Fallon Community Hlth Plan Inc — Page 211
Benitez, Abraham
Community Choice Health Plan of
Westchester Inc — Page 287
Benjamin, Georganne
Regence Blue Shield of Idaho — Page 142
Benn, John
UnitedHealthcare of Arizona Inc — Page 21
Bennett, John D, MD
Capital District Physicians
Health Plan — Page 286
Bennett, Marc H
Healthinsight — Page 435
Benson, Charles
Co/OP Optical Services Inc — Page 219
Benson, Tom
Corvel Corporation — Pages 43, 159, 324
Benteler, Joanne
KEPRO — Page 367
Bentrup, Barbara C
UnitedHealthcare of the
Midwest Inc — Page 251
Bentz Seal, Joni
Ohio State University
Managed Health Care
Systems Inc — Page 332
Berardo, Joseph, Jr
MagnaCare — Page 298
Berg, Charles G
Preferred One — Page 93
HealthEase of Florida Inc — Page 111
WellCare HMO Inc — Page 124
WellCare Health Plans Inc -
Corporate Headquarters — Page 124
WellCare of New York — Page 307
Bergdall, Thomas W, Esq
HealthFirst Inc — Page 295
Berge, Leanne
Harvard Pilgrim Health Care - Corporate
Headquarters — Page 212
Bergen, Eric L
UnitedHealth Group —
Corporate Headquarters — Page 238
Berger, Gregory, MD
Health Plan of Michigan — Page 224
Berger, Ivan, DDS, MAGD
SmileCare/Community
Dental Services — Page 69
Bergh, Wendy
Group Health Cooperative
of Eau Claire — Page 465

Index VIII: Personnel

Balcom, Clark
Pba Health — Page 491

Baldino, Micki
Blue Cross Blue Shield of NE — Page 255

Baldwin, James G Jr, MD
Select Health of SC — Page 385

Baldwin, K Rone
GenWorth Life & Health Ins Co — Page 90

Baldwin, Stanley F
AmeriGroup Corporation — Page 442

Balko, Alex
Elderplan Inc - SHMO — Page 289

Ballerdine, Lorie
Health Net of California — Page 49

Ballman, Gary
Delta Dental Plan of Minnesota — Page 235

Baltar, Marlene
Aetna Inc - Georgia — Page 127

Balthasar, Norman J
Fiserv Inc — Page 464

Balthaser, Harvey, MD
Humana Health Care Plans of Houston — Page 418

Bandini, Beverly
Health Net of California — Page 49

Banks, Mark W MD
Blue Cross Blue Shield of MInnesota — Pages 234, 505

Bannen, William, MD
Anthem Blue Cross Blue Shield of Nevada — Page 259
HMO Nevada — Page 260

Banner, Rio, MD
AlohaCare — Page 137

Baptiste, Arnie
Hawaii Management Alliance Association — Page 137

Baquiran, Delia, RN
Atlantis Health Plan — Page 285

Baraket, Doug
American Republic Insurance Company — Page 169

Barasch, Richard A
American Pioneer Health Plans Inc — Page 101

Barasch, Richard A
American Progressive Life & Health of New York — Page 501

Barasch, Richard A
Marquette National Life Insurance Company — Page 520

Barasch, Richard A
Pyramid Life Insurance Co — Page 520

Barbanell, Linda
Vista Healthplan of South Florida Inc — Page 123

Barber, Kristen
Nationwide Better Health — Page 204

Barbera, Thomas P
Md-Individual Practice Association Inc (MD IPA) — Page 204
Mid Atlantic Medical Services Inc (MAMSI)- Corp Headquarters — Page 204
Optimum Choice Inc — Page 205
OneNet PPO — Page 205
Optimum Choice of the Carolina Inc — Page 205
UnitedHealthcare & Mid Atlantic Medical Services Inc — Page 206

Barco, Daniel, MD
Coventry Health Care Inc — Carolinas — Page 311
Wellpath Select Inc — Page 315

Barden, J Gentry
HealthSpring Inc - Tennessee — Page 395

Bare, James W, Jr
Florida Health Care Plan Inc — Page 109

Barger, John
Humana Medical Plan - Central Florida — Page 113

Barger, Shawn
Av-Med Health Plan - Gainesville — Page 102
Av-Med Health Plan - Jacksonville — Page 102
Av-Med Health Plan - Miami — Page 103
Av-Med Health Plan - Orlando — Page 103
Av-Med Health Plan - Tampa — Page 103

Barker, Curt
Health Management Network Inc — Page 16

Barker, David
Southeastern Indiana Health Organization — Page 166

Barker, Pat
Exempla Healthcare LLC — Page 81

Barlow, HR Brereton
Premera Blue Cross Blue Shield of Alaska — Page 9

Barlow, HR Brereton
Premera - Corp Headquarters — Page 454
Premera Blue Cross - Eastern — Page 454
Premera Blue Cross - Western — Page 454

Barlow, Stephen L, MD
SelectHealth — Page 437

Barnard, Mark
Horizon Blue Cross/ Blue Shield of NJ — Page 273

Barnes, Arthur
Hip Health Plan of New York — Page 296

Barnes, Dawn
Evercare Select — Page 15

Barnes, Linda
Nevada Preferred Professionals — Page 262
Universal Health Network - Corporate Headquarters — Page 264

Barnes, Mary
Inland Empire Foundation for Medical Care — Page 52

Barnett, Charles J
Seton Health Plan — Page 425

Barnette, Kevin
Medcost LLC — Page 313

Barnhart, Karla
Lutheran Preferred/ Three Rivers Preferred — Page 162

Barnhart, Keith
Suburban Health Organization — Page 166

Barone, Charles, II, MD
MPRO — Page 227

Barr, William C, MA
Magellan Health Services Inc — Page 91

Barr, William C, MA
Regence Group, The — Corporate Headquarters — Page 351

Barresi, Gina
Berkley Administrators — Page 88

Barrett, James A, DMD
Assurant Employee Benefits-AL — Page 3
Assurant Employee Benefits-AZ — Page 12
Assurant Employee Benefits-CA — Page 35
Assurant Employee Benefits-CO — Page 78
Assurant Employee Benefits-FL — Page 102
Assurant Employee Benefits-GA — Page 127
Assurant Employee Benefits-IL — Page 143
Assurant Employee Benefits-IN — Page 158
Assurant Employee Benefits-MI — Page 217
Assurant Employee Benefits - Corporate Office — Page 244
Assurant Employee Benefits-NM — Page 279
Assurant Employee Benefits-NY — Page 285
Assurant Employee Benefits-NC — Page 309
Assurant Employee Benefits-PA — Page 357
Assurant Employee Benefits-TN — Page 392
Assurant Employee Benefits-TX — Page 429
Assurant Employee Benefits-WA — Page 449

Barrett, William A, DC
Chirocare of Minnesota — Page 234

Barringer, Karen
Gateway Health Plan Inc — Page 362

Barrington, Christina
Health Alliance Medical Plans - Corporate Headquarters — Page 149

Barry, Gery J
Blue Cross Blue Shield of Louisiana Inc — Page 189

Barry, Michelle
Keystone Health Plan East Inc — Page 368

Barth, Anthony
Delta Dental Plan of California — Page 44

Barth, Tony
Delta Dental Insurance Company - Alabama — Page 4

Bartholomew, Ginger
Susquehanna Health Care — Page 372

Bartholomew, Lydia, MD
Qualis Health — Page 455

Bartlett, Karen
Premera Blue Cross Blue Shield of Alaska — Page 9
LifeWise Health Plan of WA — Page 453
Premera - Corporate Hdqrtrs — Page 454
Premera Blue Cross - Eastern — Page 454
Premera Blue Cross - Western — Page 454

Bartlett, Marilyn
Employee Benefit Management Services Inc — Page 253

Bartlett, Mark R
Blue Preferred Plan-Blue Cross/ Blue Shield MI — Pages 218, 519

Bartlett, Robert
Review Works — Page 230

Bartone, Dominic
American Pharmacy Services Corporation — Page 183

Bartsch, Richard L
UnitedHealthcare Services Company of the River Valley Inc — Page 400

Bartsen, Richard, MD
UnitedHealthcare Services Company of the River Valley Inc — Page 400

Basacci, Cathy
Independent Health Assoc Inc — Page 297

Basco, Michael, MD
Molina Healthcare of Texas Inc — Page 421

Bascombe, Eileen
Horizon Behavioral Services — Page 112

Baskins, Judy
Palmetto SeniorCare — Page 513

Basoco, Soledad
El Paso First Health Plans Inc — Page 413

Bass, Sabin
Capital Health Plan — Page 105

Bassett, Paula
Parkland Community Health Plan Inc — Page 422

Batay, Dennis, MD
Fallon Community Hlth Plan Inc — Page 211

Batchlor, Elaine, MD
LA Care Health Plan — Page 55

Bateman, Kim MD
Healthinsight — Page 435

Bates, Debra
UnitedHealthcare of Arkansas — Page 28

Bates, Robin O
Avera Health Plans Inc — Page 387

Bathke, William T
Wisconsin Physician Services Insurance Company — Page 471

Battani, Lorenzo
American Republic Insurance Company — Page 169

Battista, Jeanette
Delta Dental Plan of Illinois — Page 145

Index VIII: Personnel

Armstrong, Richard M
Blue Cross of Idaho — Page 141
Armstrong, Scott
Group Health Cooperative — Page 141
Group Health Cooperative — Page 451
Group Health Cooperative of Puget Sound — Page 452
Group Health Options Inc — Page 452
Armstrong, Vicki
South Central Preferred — Page 372
Armstrong, Wayne
Argus Health System Inc — Page 480
Arneson, Linda
Colorado Dental Service Inc, DBA: Delta Dental Plan of CO — Page 80
Arnim, Jeff
Dental Health Services Inc — Page 450
Arnold, John
CompBenefits Corporation - Corporate Headquarters — Page 129
Arnold, Roy, MD
WelBorn Health Plans — Page 167
Arnold-Miller, Erica, MBA
Colorado Health Networks LLC - ValueOptions — Page 80
Arnone, Wendy
UnitedHealthcare of WI Inc — Page 470
Aronovitch, Stan
Mercy Care Plan — Page 18
Aronson Prohofsky, Jodi, PhD
CIGNA Behavioral Health Inc — Page 88
CIGNA Behavioral Health Inc - Corporate Headquarters — Page 234
CIGNA Behavioral Health Inc — Page 408
Arrington, Robyn J Jr, MD
Total Health Choice Inc — Page 120
Total Health Care Inc — Page 231
Arritola, Madeleine
Humana Medical Plan Inc — Page 114
Arroyo, Ivonne
Medical Card System — Page 377
Arth, Lawrence J
Ameritas Group Dental — Page 255
Arthur, Megan M, JD
Magellan Health Services Inc — Page 91
Asao, Duane, Pharm D
Community Health Plan — Page 42
Ascenzo, Carl
Blue Cross Blue Shield of MA — Page 209
Ascher, Erin
Prime Therapeutics — Page 493
Ash, Sharon, MD
Secure Health Plans of GA LLC — Page 133
Ash-Jackson, Linda, MD
Hometown Health Plan — Page 260
Ashanin, Lydia
Blue Cross Blue Shield of NM — Page 279
Asher, Chris
Southeastern Indiana Health Organization — Page 166
Asher, Drew
Coventry Health Care Inc — Corporate Headquarters — Page 201
Ashkenaz, Peter
Evercare of Texas LLC — Page 413
Assadi, Nadia
CIGNA Healthcare of Virginia Inc - Richmond — Page 443
Astorga, Tony, CPA
Blue Cross Blue Shield of AZ — Page 12
Ater, Candus
Scott & White Health Plan — Page 424
Atkins, C Richard, DDS
Blue Cross Blue Shield of Louisiana Inc — Page 189

Atkins, Nancy
Bluegrass Family Health Inc — Page 183
Atkins, Ruth
University Health Care Inc - Passport Health Plan — Page 187
Atkins, Sue M, RHR
Southern Health Services Inc — Page 445
Atkinson, Brian
Devon Health Services Inc — Page 361
Atkinson, Mary
CIGNA Healthcare of Florida — Page 107
Attalla, Yvonne
QualCare Inc — Page 276
Aubrey, Rob
Athens Area Health Plan Select Inc — Page 127
Auen, Eileen, MD
APS Healthcare Midwest Inc — Page 461
Aug, Matthew
Cox Health Plans — Page 246
Aukerman, Glen, MD
Ohio State University Managed Health Care Systems Inc — Page 332
Ault, Jennifer
Health Plan, The Hometown Region — Page 327
Aurich, Lee Durham
Aetna Inc - Washington — Page 449
Austin, Jeanell
National Capital PPO — Page 444
Austin, John H, MD
Coventry Health Care Inc — Corporate Headquarters — Page 201
Austin, John H, MD
Arkansas Community Care Inc — Page 26
Austin, Mark
Blue Cross Blue Shield of TN — Page 392
Blue Cross Blue Shield of TN - Memphis — Page 393
Avelar, Marta
Santa Clara Family Health Plan — Page 67
Averill, Scott W
Health Alliance Plan — Page 223
MVP Health Plan Inc — Page 301
Avery, Alan
Medical Associates Clinic Health Plan of WI — Page 467
Medical Associates Health Plans — Page 172
Avey, Steven G
Partners Rx Management LLC — Page 491
Ayers, Skip, DDS
Dental Health Services — Page 45
Azzolina, David S
MemberHealth Inc — Page 489

B

Baackes, John
Senior Whole Health LLC — Page 505
Baca, Mari
Health Plan of San Mateo — Page 50
Bachmann, Anita
UnitedHealthcare of NC — Page 315
Baeten, Bill
Arise Health Plan — Page 461
Baetz, Joan
Cambridge Managed Care Services — Page 38
Bagby, David
New Mexico Medical Review Association — Page 281
Bagby, Rhonda
Humana Health Plan - Jacksonville — Page 113

Bagby, Rhonda
Humana Health Benefit Plan of Louisiana — Page 191
Bagnall, Dana
Vision Insurance Plan of America Inc - Corp Headquarters — Page 471
Bahe, Tim
Parkland Community Health Plan Inc — Page 422
Bahr, Michael
Altius Health Plans — Page 433
Bahrke, Linda
Community Health Plan — Page 245
Bahy, Ryan
Sanford Health Plan — Page 388
Bailey, Bary, CSO
PacifiCare Health Systems- Corporate Headquarters — Page 62
Bailey, Chad
Indiana Pro Health Network — Page 162
Bailey, Jim
Health Advantage — Page 27
Bailey, Mark
VIA Christi HOPE Inc — Page 516
Bailey, Michael D
Windsor Health Plan of TN Inc — Page 401
Bailey, S Graham
Blue Cross Blue Shield of KS — Page 177
Baine, Gary
Metcare Health Plans Inc — Page 116
Baines, Barry, MD
Ucare Minnesota — Page 238
Baker, Andrew
Family Choice Health Alliance — Page 272
Baker, Brendan
PacifiCare of Arizona — Page 19
Baker, Charles F
Harvard Pilgrim Health Care - Corporate Headquarters — Page 212
Baker, Dan
Jaimini Health Inc — Page 53
Baker, David
Humana Military Service Inc — Page 186
Baker, Gary Charles
UnitedHealthcare of Arkansas — Page 28
Baker, John
AmeriScript Inc — Page 479
Baker, Karen
Cooks Childrens Health Plan — Page 411
Baker, Laila, MD
Access Dental Services — Page 31
Baker, Linda
Managed Health Srvcs IN Inc — Page 163
Baker, Linda
Health Net Hlth Pln of OR Inc — Page 346
Baker, Linn
Utah Public Employees Health Program — Page 438
Baker, Michael G
CorpHealth Inc — Page 412
Baker, Stephen
Safeguard Hlth Enterprises Inc — Page 66
Safeguard Health Plans Inc — Page 424
Baker, Tracy H
Coventry Health Care Inc — Carolinas — Page 311
Wellpath Select Inc — Page 315
Baker, William
Superior HealthPlan Inc — Page 426
Bakshi, Sharon, PharmD
Scan Health Plan — Page 68
Bal, Rajeev
Assurant Health - Corporate Headquarters — Page 462
Balboni, Jill
Delta Dental Insurance Company - Georgia — Page 131

Index VIII: Personnel

Alperstein, Joel
Avesis Inc ..... Page 12
Alrich, Christine L
Blue Cross Blue Shield of
Delaware ..... Page 95
Alston, Cynthia, MD
CIGNA Healthcare of Illinois Inc ..... Page 144
Alt, Edward, MD
Medical Associates
Health Plans ..... Pages 172, 467
Althaus, Jennifer
Managed Dental Care ..... Page 57
Altizer, Chutamar
CIGNA Healthcare of
North Carolina ..... Page 311
Altman, Donald S, DDS
Employers Dental Services Inc ..... Page 15
Altman, Maya
Health Plan of San Mateo ..... Page 50
Altstadt, Rick
M Plan Inc ..... Page 163
Alvarado, Arcilio
Blue Cross of Puerto Rico/
La Cruz Azul de Puerto Rico ..... Page 377
Alvarenga, Monica
Health Net of California ..... Page 49
Alverez, Tony
CarePlus Health Plans Inc ..... Page 106
Alvin, William R
Care Choices HMO ..... Page 218
Amacker, Larry B, MD
UnitedHealthcare of Alabama ..... Page 7
UnitedHealthcare of Louisiana ..... Page 193
UnitedHealthcare of
Mississippi Inc ..... Page 242
Amaro, Rafael, MD
Community Health Group ..... Page 41
Amato, Peter, MD
Berkley Administrators ..... Page 88
Amaya, Sandra
El Paso First Health Plans Inc ..... Page 413
Ambrose, Nalini
OSF Health Plans ..... Page 151
Ambrose, Sandra
Deaconess Health Plans ..... Page 159
Ambrosia, Renee
Preferred One ..... Page 237
Amburn, Linda
Blue Cross Blue Shield of NM ..... Page 279
Amendola, Louis J
Western Dental Services ..... Page 75
Ammons, Mark
Primary Health Plan ..... Page 142
Amodio, Danielle
Renaissance Health Systems Inc ..... Page 119
Amundson, Paul, MD
DakotaCare ..... Page 387
Anand, Sury, MD
Atlantis Health Plan ..... Page 285
Anania, Andrea
CIGNA Healthcare of Texas Inc ..... Page 409
Ancell, Brian
Premera Blue Cross
Blue Shield of Alaska ..... Page 9
Premera - Corp Headquarters ..... Page 454
Anderson, Bill
Health First Health Plans Inc ..... Page 111
Anderson, Calvin
Blue Cross Blue Shield of Tennessee - Memphis ..... Page 393
Anderson, Carol, RN
Community Health Group ..... Page 41
Anderson, Darleen
Optima Health Plan Inc ..... Page 445
Anderson, David W
Health Net - Connecticut ..... Page 90
Health Net Inc - Northeast Corporate Headquarters ..... Page 91

Health Net - New Jersey ..... Page 272
Health Net - New York ..... Page 295
Health Net of California ..... Page 49
Anderson, Diane
20/20 Eyecare Plan Inc ..... Page 99
Anderson, Doris
Blue Cross Blue Shield of GA ..... Page 128
Anderson, Dorothy
San Joaquin Foundation PPO ..... Page 67
Anderson, Ellen, RN
Midwest Health Plan ..... Page 226
Anderson, Gary
San Joaquin Foundation PPO ..... Page 67
Anderson, James
PRONJ, The Healthcare Quality Improvement Organization of NJ ..... Page 276
Anderson, Jeremy, BA, MBA, MCS
CIMRO Quality
Healthcare Solutions ..... Page 144
Anderson, Jim
Olympus Managed Health
Care Inc ..... Page 117
Anderson, Jon
Sagamore Health Network Inc ..... Page 164
Anderson, Lani
Altius Health Plans ..... Page 433
Anderson, Larry
ValueOptions - Corp Hdqrtrs ..... Page 447
Anderson, Mark
Delta Dental Plan of Arizona Inc ..... Page 14
Anderson, Max, DDS
Delta Dental Plans Association ..... Page 146
Anderson, Maxwell, DDS
Colorado Dental Service Inc, DBA: Delta Dental Plan of CO ..... Page 80
Anderson, Randa Stice
Humana Health Care Plans of
Kansas & Missouri ..... Page 179
Anderson, Richard C
Wellmark Blue Cross & Blue Shield of
South Dakota ..... Page 389
Anderson, Rick D, OD
Vision Care Network ..... Page 471
Anderson, Robert, DDS
Jaimini Health Inc ..... Page 53
Anderson, Roland, MD
Novasys Health Network ..... Page 28
Interplan Health Group ..... Page 419
Anderson, Ron J, MD
Parkland Community
Health Plan Inc ..... Page 422
Anderson, Stacy
American College of
Medical Quality ..... Page 199
Andrakowicz, Stanley J
Western Dental Services ..... Page 75
Andreini-Arnold, Patti
Medica Health Plans ..... Page 506
Andreshak, Mike
Preferred Provider Organization of
Michigan (PPOM) ..... Page 229
Andretta, Dean
Marion Polk Community Health Plan
Advantage ..... Page 349
Andrew, Bob
Wisconsin Physician Services
Insurance Company ..... Page 471
Andrews, Cheryl
Maricopa Health Plan ..... Page 18
Andrews, Darlene
Blue Cross Blue Shield of GA ..... Page 128
Andrews, George, MD
Cariten Healthcare ..... Page 393
PHP Companies Inc ..... Page 397
Andrews, George, MD
CIGNA Healthcare of Florida ..... Page 107
Andrews, Leslie H
Humana Inc - Colorado ..... Page 82
Andrews, Mark L, ESQ
Molina Healthcare Inc - CA ..... Page 59

Andringa, Dale J, MD
Wellmark Blue Cross
Blue Shield of Iowa ..... Page 174
Wellmark Inc — Corp Hdqrtrs ..... Page 175
Wellmark Blue Cross &
Blue Shield of South Dakota ..... Page 389
Wellmark Health Plan of IA Inc ..... Page 175
Andron, Kelly
Healthplex Inc ..... Page 296
Angellis, Dennis, MD
Presbyterian Health Plan ..... Page 281
Ansari, Nazir
Hometown Health Plan ..... Page 260
Ansert, Art
Memphis Managed Care Corp ..... Page 397
Anthony, Robert A, DDS
Delta Dental Plan of IN Inc ..... Page 159
Delta Dental Plan of MI Inc ..... Page 220
Antihik, Jeffrey
UnitedHealthcare of Florida Inc ..... Page 122
Antonello, William
CIGNA Healthcare of Florida ..... Page 107
Antun, Mayda, MD
Neighborhood Health
Partnership ..... Page 116
Anzalmo, John
Horizon Behavioral Services ..... Page 112
Apland, Babette
HealthPartners Inc ..... Pages 236
Aponte, Pedro
Medical Card System ..... Page 377
Apostle, Paul B
Antares Management Solutions ..... Page 319
Medical Mutual of Ohio ..... Page 330
Aracich, Dick
Delta Dental Insurance Company -
Alabama ..... Page 4
Aracich, Dick
Delta Dental Insurance Company -
Georgia ..... Page 131
Arasi, Deb
20/20 Eyecare Plan Inc ..... Page 99
Arca, Albert
Preferred Medical Plan Inc ..... Page 118
Archer, David
Healthnow ..... Page 395
Archer, Richard
Employees Benefit Systems ..... Page 170
Archer, Todd
Mutual Assurance
Administrators Inc ..... Page 342
Arfin, Ronald
Neighborhood Health Providers ..... Page 302
Argwin, Juliette
CIGNA Healthcare of California ..... Page 41
Arkin, Steve
Physicians United Plan Inc ..... Page 118
Armacost, Karen RNC
Johns Hopkins
Health System Inc ..... Page 511
Armao, Anne
SummaCare Inc ..... Page 334
Armijo, Al
HMS Colorado Inc ..... Page 82
Sloan's Lake
Preferred Health Networks ..... Page 85
Armijo, Kathy
Total Dental Administrators
Health Plan ..... Page 21
Armstead, Rodney C, MD
Family Choice Health Alliance ..... Page 272
Armstron, Richard M
Blue Cross of Idaho ..... Page 141
Armstrong, Jim
Mount Carmel Health Plan ..... Page 331
Armstrong, Mary
Humana Health Benefit
Plan of Louisiana ..... Page 191

Index VIII: Personnel

Aalbregtse, Karen
Volusia Health Network   Page 124
Aardsma, Wayne
Aveta Health Illinois Inc   Page 143
Aaronson, Daniel
Excellus BlueCross BlueShield   Page 290
Abbas, Mohammed
Valley Baptist
Insurance Company   Page 431
Abbaszadeh, Reza, DDS
Access Dental Services   Page 31
Abbaszadeh, Terri
Access Dental Services   Page 31
Abboa-Offei, Abenaa
Affinity Health Plan Inc   Page 283
Abbott, Mary, MD
Community Health Plan   Page 42
Abbott, Michael E
American Republic Insurance Company
Page 169
Abernethy, David
Hip Health Plan of New York   Page 296
Aberson, Dan
DakotaCare   Page 387
Abner, LaShaundia
Humana Inc -
Grand Rapids Michigan   Page 225
Abramson, Alan
HealthPartners Inc   Page 236
Abulencra, Penny
Independent Living Services
of Central New York   Page 512
Abutin, Ceaser
Lakewood Health Plan Inc   Page 56
Accardi, Paul T
MDNY Healthcare Inc   Page 299
Acevedo, Caridad S, RN, BSN,
Olympus Managed
Health Care Inc   Page 117
Acevedo, Enrique
Medica Healthcare Plans Inc   Page 116
Achillare, Vince
Amerigroup New York, LLC   Page 284
Acholonu, Lincoln
CIGNA Healthcare of California   Page 41
Acker, Kenneth
Standard Optical   Page 437
Ackermen, Glen, MD
Nationwide Health Plans   Page 331
Acosta, Jamie
ECCA - Managed Vision Care Inc -
Corporate Headquarters   Page 413
Adamo, Amy
SmileCare/Community Dental Services
Page 69
Adams, Chuck
Complementary
Healthcare Plans   Page 345
Adams, David
HealthSmart Preferred Care   Page 416
Adams, John, MD
HMO California   Page 51
Adams, Larry
United Concordia Company Inc -
New Mexico   Page 282
Adams, Michael R, ACSW
Behavioral Healthcare
Options Inc   Page 259
Adamson, James, MD
Arkansas Blue Cross/Blue Shield
a Mutual Insurance Company   Page 25

Adank, Kari
Gundersen Lutheran
Health Plan Inc   Page 465
Addiego, Joseph, MD
Prescription Solutions   Page 493
Adeleye, Anthony, MD
Pro-Care Health Plan   Page 230
Adetola, Angela
MetroPlus Health Plan   Page 300
Adkins, Gary W
Windsor Health Plan of
Tennessee Inc   Page 401
Adkins, L Aaron
UnitedHealthcare of SW Ohio
Inc-Dayton/Cincinnati   Page 337
Adkison, Mark, A
National Medical Health Card Systems -
Corporate Headquarter   Page 489
Adler, Laura
Healthnow   Page 395
Adye, Candace
SelectHealth Network   Page 165
Aebischer, Scott
HealthPartners Inc   Page 236
Aguas, Stacy, RN, MBA
Acumentra Health   Page 345
Aguilar, Ronald
Denver Health Medical Plan Inc   Page 80
Aguirre, Kathy
Vista Health Plan Inc   Page 123
Vista Healthplan of
South Florida Inc   Page 123
Ahlskog, Dale C
Molina HealthCare of
Washington Inc   Page 453
Aizen, Lance
Rite Aid Health Solutions   Page 494
Akaski, Ronald, MD
Pacific IPA   Page 63
Akenberger, Gary
Paramount Advantage   Page 333
Paramount Health Care Plan   Page 333
Akers, Jeff
Complementary
Healthcare Plans   Page 345
Akers, William
Group Health Cooperative   Page 451
Akosa, Anthony, MD
Advantage Health Solutions Inc   Page 157
Album, Jeffrey
Delta Dental Insurance
Company - Alabama   Page 4
Delta Dental Plan of California   Page 44
DeltaCare USA   Page 44
Delta Dental Insurance
Company - Georgia   Page 131
Delta Dental Insurance
Company - Nevada   Page 259
Alcorn, Andrew
Block Vision of Texas Inc   Page 405
Aldrich, Susan
Comprehensive Care
Management Corp   Page 509
Aldridge, Marcia
Community Care Plus   Page 249
Alexander, Brenda Deann
UDC Dental California Inc   Page 71
Alexander, Brenda K
4MOST Health Network   Page 459
Alexander, Jerri
Humana Health Benefit Plan
of Louisiana   Page 191
Alexander, S Tyrone
Highmark Inc   Page 366
Alfano, Michele D
ValueOptions of Texas Inc   Page 431
ValueOptions - Corp Hqrtrs   Page 447

Alfieri, Richard A
IPRO   Page 298
Alford, Steve
Coalition America Inc   Page 129
Alfred, Doug
Mount Carmel Health Plan   Page 331
Algate, Lyle E
Total Health Choice Inc   Page 120
Total Health Care Inc   Page 231
Alison, Lani
HealthFirst Inc   Page 295
Alkin, Frank
University Health Plans Inc   Page 277
All, Matthew D
Blue Cross Blue Shield of Kansas Page 177
Allan, Kenneth, MD
Health Plan, The Hometown Region   Page 327
Allari, Don, MD
Physicians Foundation for Medical Care
Page 64
Allen, Beverly A
OmniCare,
A Coventry Health Plan   Page 228
Allen, Calvin
HealthPartners Inc   Page 236
Allen, Christine
Life at Home LLC   Page 512
Allen, Dennis, MD
MVP Health Plan Inc   Page 301
Allen, Flora
Lifetime Healthcare Companies, The -
Corporate Headquarters   Page 298
Allen, Gary, DMD
Williamette Dental Group PC   Page 352
Williamette Dental of
Washington Inc   Page 457
Allen, Greg
Texas HealthSpring I LLC   Page 427
Allen, Greg
Signature Health Alliance   Page 398
Allen, Gregg, MD
MedSolutions   Page 396
Allen, Jene
Care Choices HMO   Page 218
Allen, Kenneth, MD
Health Plan of the
Upper Ohio Valley   Page 327
Allen, Libby
Dental Care Plus Inc   Page 324
Allen, Lynn
Molina Healthcare of
New Mexico   Page 281
Allen, Robert, MD
Great-West Healthcare of
Washington Inc   Page 451
Allen, Robin
Anthem Blue Cross
Blue Shield of Maine   Page 195
Allen, Sharon
Arkansas Blue Cross/Blue Shield
a Mutual Insurance Company   Page 25
Allenbach, Karen
Mount Carmel Health Plan   Page 331
Allenburg, Thomas J, DC
ACN Group   Page 233
Allgood, John
Community Care of San Diego   Page 514
Allison, Carey C, MD
Health Plus of Louisiana Inc   Page 191
Allman, Alice
Sante Community Physicians   Page 67
Allocco, Andrew
Blue Cross of California   Page 34
Almquist, Stacia N
UDC Ohio Inc   Page 335
Alonge, Gerald
Vantage PPO   Page 375

Index VIII

Personnel

Index VII: Miscellaneous Organizations

RxAmerica LLC
Salt Lake City, UT — Page 494
RxPlus Pharmacies Inc
Wheat Ridge, CO — Page 494

S

Scan Health Plan
Long Beach, CA — Page 502
ScripNet
Las Vegas, NV — Page 494
Script Care Inc - Texas
Beaumont, TX — Page 494
Scriptrax
Winston-Salem, NC — Page 495
Selectcare of Texas LLC
Houston, TX — Page 521
Senior Care Connection Inc
Schenectady, NY — Page 509
Senior Whole Health LLC
Cambridge, MA — Page 505
Sentara Life Care Corporation Inc
Virginia Beach, VA — Page 514
Serve You Custom Prescription Management
Milwaukee, WI — Page 495
South Country Health Alliance
Owatonna, MN — Page 507
South Dakota Pharmacist Association
Pierre, SD — Page 495
St Agnes Medical Center
Philadelphia, PA — Page 511
Sterling Life Insurance Company
Bellingham, WA — Page 520
Sterling Life Insurance Company
Bellingham, WA — Page 501
SunRx Inc
Mount Laurel, NJ — Page 495
Sutter Senior Care
Sacramento, CA — Page 515
SXC Health Solutions Inc
Lisle, IL — Page 495

T

Tennessee Pharmacist Association
Nashville, TN — Page 495
Tmesys
Tampa, FL — Page 496
Total Community Care
Albuquerque, NM — Page 515
Total Long Term Care
Denver, CO — Page 515
Total Script
Broomfield, CO — Page 496
TriHealth Senior Link
Cincinnati, OH — Page 515

U

UCARE of Minnesota
Minneapolis, MN — Page 505
Minneapolis, MN — Page 507
Unicare Health Plans of the Midwest Inc
Chicago, IL — Page 521
United Drugs
Phoenix, AZ — Page 496

United Healthcare Insurance Company
Minnetonka, MN — Page 519
Minnetonka, MN — Page 501
UnitedHealthcare Insurance Company of New York
Minnetonka, MN — Page 519
University of Pennsylvania, Trustees
Philadelphia, PA — Page 512
Uphams Corner Health Committee Inc
Boston, MA — Page 515
US Script Inc
Fresno, CA — Page 496
US-Rx Care
Jersey City, NJ — Page 496

V

VIA Christi HOPE Inc
Wichita, KS — Page 516

W

Wal-Mart Stores Pharmacy Div
Bentonville, AR — Page 496
Walgreens Health Initiatives
Deerfield, IL — Page 496
WellDyne Rx
Centennial, CO — Page 497
WellPoint NextRX
West Hills, CA — Page 497
Mason, OH — Page 497

Index VII: Miscellaneous Organizations

Healthesystems
Tampa, FL — Page 486
Henry Ford Health System
Detroit, MI — Page 508
Humana Health Benefit Plan of Louisiana
Metairie, LA — Page 517
Humana Health Plan - Kentucky
DePere, WI — Page 517
Humana Inc
Louisville, KY — Page 486
Humana Inc/PCA - Puerto Rico
San Juan, PR — Page 518
Humana Insurance Company of New York
Louisville, KY — Page 518

I

Immediate Pharmaceutical Services Inc
Avon Lake, OH — Page 486
InStil Health Insurance Company
Columbia, SC — Page 518
Independent Living Services of Central New York
N Syracuse, NY — Page 512
Independent Living for Seniors
Rochester, NY — Page 511
Innoviant Inc
Wausau, WI — Page 487
Iowa Pharmacists Association
Des Moines, IA — Page 487
Itasca Medical Care
Grand Rapids, MN — Page 506

J

Johns Hopkins Health System Inc
Baltimore, MD — Page 511

K

Kansas Pharmacy Service Corporation
Topeka, KS — Page 487
Kroger Prescription Plans
Cincinnati, OH — Page 487

L

LDI Pharmacy Benefit Management
St Louis, MO — Page 487
LeaderNET/Leader Drug Stores — Cardinal Health Inc
Dublin, OH — Page 487
LIFE - Pittsburgh Inc
Pittsburgh, PA — Page 511
Life at Home LLC
Kennett Square, PA — Page 512

M

Managed Pharmacy Care
Lake Arrowhead, CA — Page 488

Management Sciences for Health
Arlington, VA — Page 488
Marquette National Life Insurance Company
Lake Mary, FL — Page 520
Maryland Care Inc
Linthicum, MD — Page 521
Maxor Plus
Amarillo, TX — Page 488
McKesson Pharmacy Provider Network
San Francisco, CA — Page 488
MedImpact Healthcare Systems Inc
San Diego, CA — Page 488
MedScript
Earth City, MO — Page 488
Medco Health Solutions Inc
Franklin Lakes, NJ — Page 488
Medica Health Plans
Minnetonka, MN — Page 518
Medica Health Plans
Minnetonka, MN — Page 506
Medica Health Plans of Wisconsin
Minnetonka, MN — Page 518
Medicap Pharmacies Inc
West Des Moines, IA — Page 489
MemberHealth Inc
Solon, OH — Page 489
Mennonite Mutual Aid Association
Goshen, IN — Page 519
Metropolitan Health Plan
Minneapolis, MN — Page 506
Midland Care Connection
Topeka, KS — Page 512
Molina Healthcare Inc
Long Beach, CA — Page 489
MyMatrixx
Tampa, FL — Page 489

N

National Medical Health Card Systems - Corporate Headquarter
Port Washington, NY — Page 489
Navitus Health Solutions
Madison, WI — Page 490
ND Pharmacy Service Corp
Bismarck, ND — Page 490
Northeast Pharmacy Service Corp
Framingham, MA — Page 490
Northwest Pharmacy Services
Puyallup, WA — Page 490
NPAX Inc
Clifton, NJ — Page 490

O

Omnicare Of South Florida
Weston, FL — Page 490
On Lok Senior Health Services
San Francisco, CA — Page 512
Ovations Pharmacy Solutions
Minnetonka, MN — Page 490

P

Pace Greater New Orleans
New Orleans, LA — Page 513
Pace Organization of Rhode Island
Providence, RI — Page 513

Pace Vermont Inc
Colchester, VT — Page 513
Pacificare Life & Health Insurance Company
Cypress, CA — Page 519
Palmetto SeniorCare
Columbia, SC — Page 513
Paragon Biomedical Inc
Irvine, CA — Page 491
Partners Rx Management LLC
Scottsdale, AZ — Page 491
Partnership Health Plan Inc
Eau Claire, WI — Page 522
PBA Health
Kansas City, MO — Page 491
Pbm Plus Inc
Milford, OH — Page 491
Pennsylvania Life Insurance Company
Houston, TX — Page 501
Pennsylvania PACE Inc
Johnstown, PA — Page 514
Pequot Pharmaceutical Network
Mashantucket, CT — Page 491
PerformRx
Philadelphia, PA — Page 492
PharmAvail Benefit Management Company
Woodstock, GA — Page 492
Pharmacy Association, The
Jefferson City, MO — Page 492
Pharmacy Data Management Inc
Boardman, OH — Page 492
Pharmacy Providers Services Corp
Tallahassee, FL — Page 492
Pharmacy Providers of Oklahoma
Oklahoma City, OK — Page 492
Pharmacy Services Group
Fort Lauderdale, FL — Page 492
Pittsburgh Care Partnership Inc
Pittsburgh, PA — Page 509
Premier Pharmacy Plan
Spartanburg, SC — Page 493
Prescription Management Services Inc
Tampa, FL — Page 493
Prescription Solutions
Irvine, CA — Page 493
Prime Therapeutics
Eagan, MN — Page 493
Primewest Health System
Minneapolis, MN — Page 506
Providence Health System
Seattle, WA — Page 514
Providence Health System - Oregon
Portland, OR — Page 513
Pyramid Life Insurance Company
Lake Mary, FL — Page 520

Q

QCC Insurance Company
Philadelphia, PA — Page 520

R

Ramsell Holding Corporation
Oakland, CA — Page 493
RegenceRx
Portland, OR — Page 493
Restat
West Bend, WI — Page 494
Rite Aid Health Solutions
Camp Hill, PA — Page 494

Index VII: Miscellaneous Organizations

4D Pharmacy Management Systems Inc
Troy, MI — Page 479

A

ACS Government Healthcare Solutions
Atlanta, GA — Page 479
Aetna Life Insurance Company
Hartford, CT — Page 516
Aetna Pharmacy Management - Corporate Headquarters
Hartford, CT — Page 479
Aetna Specialty Pharmacy
Alpharetta, GA — Page 479
Alexian Brothers Community Services
St Louis, MO — Page 507
Alexian Brothers Health Systems Inc
Chattanooga, TN — Page 507
Allscripts Pharmaceuticals Inc
Chicago, IL — Page 479
AltaMed Health Services Corporation
Los Angeles, CA — Page 507
Amarillo Multi Service Center for the Aging Inc
Amarillo, TX — Page 508
AmeriScript Inc
Stow, OH — Page 479
American Health Care
Rocklin, CA — Page 480
American Pharmacy Services Corp
Frankfort, KY — Page 480
American Progressive Life & Health of New York
Rye Brook, NY — Page 501
American Progressive Life & Insurance Company
Rye Brook, NY — Page 520
Amerisource Bergen Performance Plus Network - Corporate
Chesterbrook, PA — Page 480
Amerisource Bergen Performance Plus Network - West
Orange, CA — Page 480
Anthem Insurance Companies Inc
Cincinnati, OH — Page 516
Argus Health System Inc
Kansas City, MO — Page 480
Arxcel Inc
Williamsville, NY — Page 480
Avalon Insurance Company
Harrisburg, PA — Page 516

B

Bayer Corporation Pharmaceutical Division
West Haven, CT — Page 481
BeneScript Services Inc
Norcross, GA — Page 481
Bienvivir Senior Health Services
El Paso, TX — Page 508
BioScrip Inc
Elmsford, NY — Page 481
Blue Cross & Blue Shield of North Carolina
Durham, NC — Page 481
Blue Cross Blue Shield of Minnesota
St Paul, MN — Page 505
Blue Cross and Blue Shield of IL Pharmacy Programs
Chicago, IL — Page 481
Blue Cross of California
Woodland Hills, CA — Page 517
Blue Preferred Plan-Blue Cross/Blue Shield Michigan
Detroit, MI — Page 519
Bravo Health Mid-Atlantic Inc
Baltimore, MD — Page 517

C

Cambridge Life Insurance Company
Downers Grove, IL — Page 516
Care Resources Inc
Grand Rapids, MI — Page 508
CareFirst Blue Cross Blue Shield
Owings Mills, MD — Page 481
Caremark/CVS - Arizona
Scottsdale, AZ — Page 482
Caremark/CVS - Illinois
Northbrook, IL — Page 482
Caremark/CVS - Tennessee
Nashville, TN — Page 482
Caremark/CVS - Texas
Irving, TX — Page 482
Carolina Pharmacy Network
Columbia, SC — Page 482
Catalyst Rx, A Healthextras Company
Las Vegas, NV — Page 482
Catalyst Rx, A Healthextras Company
Rockville, MD — Page 482
CBCA
East Haven, CT — Page 483
Center for Elders Independence
Oakland, CA — Page 508
Chesapeake Life Insurance Company
North Richland Hills, TX — Page 517
CIGNA Pharmacy Management
Hartford, CT — Page 483
Commonwealth Care Alliance Inc
Boston, MA — Page 505
Community Care Health Plan Inc
Milwaukee, WI — Page 521
Community Care Organization Inc
Milwaukee, WI — Page 509
Community Care of San Diego
San Diego, CA — Page 514
CommunityCare Managed Healthcare Plans of Oklahoma Inc
Tulsa, OK — Page 483
Comprehensive Care Management Corp
Bronx, NY — Page 509
Concordia Care
Cleveland Heights, OH — Page 509
CVS/Caremark - Corporate Headquarters
Lincoln, RI — Page 483
Cypress Care
Duluth, GA — Page 483

D

Delaware Physicians Care Inc
Newark, DE — Page 521

E

Elder Care Health Plan Inc
Madison, WI — Page 522
Elder Service Plan of East Boston Health Center
East Boston, MA — Page 510
Elder Service Plan of Harbor Health Services Inc
Dorchester, MA — Page 510
Elder Service Plan of the Cambridge Health Alliance
Cambridge, MA — Page 510
Elder Service Plan of the North Shore
Lynn, MA — Page 510
Elderhaus Inc
Wilmington, NC — Page 510
Employee Health Insurance Management Inc
Southfield, MI — Page 483
Envision Pharmaceutical Services Inc
Twinsburg, OH — Page 484
Epic Pharmacy Network Inc
Mechanicsville, VA — Page 484
Evercare Health Plans
Norcross, GA — Page 502
Express Scripts Inc - Corporate Headquarters
St Louis, MO — Page 484
Express Scripts Inc - Minnesota
Bloomington, MN — Page 484
Express Scripts Inc - New Jersey
East Hanover, NJ — Page 484
Express Scripts Inc - Pennsylvania
Horsham, PA — Page 484

F

Fallon Community Health Plan
Worchester, MA — Page 514
First Health Rx
Downers Grove, IL — Page 485
First Health Services Corp
Glen Allen, VA — Page 485
First Plan of Minnesota
Two Harbors, MN — Page 505
First Script Network Services
Tucson, AZ — Page 485
Florida Pace Centers Inc
Miami, FL — Page 511

G

Garden State Pharmacy Owners Provider Services
Hamilton, NJ — Page 485

H

Health Delivery Management LLC
Chicago, IL — Page 485
Health Plan for Community Living Inc
Madison, WI — Page 522
HealthExtras Inc
Rockville, MD — Page 485
HealthPartners
Bloomington, MN — Page 486
HealthPartners Inc
Bloomington, MN — Page 506
HealthTrans LLC
Greenwood Village, CO — Page 486

Index VII

Miscellaneous Organizations

Index VI: Point of Service Organizations

Wellmark Health Plan of Iowa Inc
Des Moines, IA — Page 175
**Wellmark Inc —
Corporate Headquarters**
Des Moines, IA — Page 175
Wellpath Select Inc
Morrisville, NC — Page 315
WINHealth Partners
Cheyenne, WY — Page 473
**Wisconsin Physician Services
Insurance Company**
Madison, WI — Page 471

Index VI: Point of Service Organizations

Secure Health Plans of Georgia LLC
Macon, GA Page 133
SelectHealth
Salt Lake City, UT Page 437
Sierra Health Services Inc-
Corporate Headquarters
Las Vegas, NV Page 264
South Bay Independent Physicians
Medical Group Inc
Torrance, CA Page 69
Southeastern Indiana Health
Organization
Columbus, IN Page 166
Southern Health Services Inc
Charlottesville, VA Page 445
Southern Health Services Inc
Richmond, VA Page 445
Spectrum Vision Systems Inc
Overland Park, KS Page 181
Summacare Inc
Akron, OH Page 334
Summerlin Life & Health Insurance
Company
Las Vegas, NV Page 264

T

Tufts Health Plan
Watertown, MA Page 216

U

Unicare Health Plans of the
Midwest Inc
Chicago, IL Page 153
United Behavioral Health
Philadelphia, PA Page 373
United Behavioral Health (UBH)
San Francisco, CA Page 71
United Concordia Company Inc -
Alabama
Birmingham, AL Page 6
United Concordia Company Inc -
Arizona
Phoenix, AZ Page 21
United Concordia Company Inc -
California
Woodland Hills, CA Page 72
United Concordia Company Inc -
Corporate Headquarters
Harrisburg, PA Page 373
United Concordia Company Inc - Florida
Tampa, FL Page 121
United Concordia Company Inc -
Maryland
Hunt Valley, MD Page 206
United Concordia Company Inc -
Michigan
Troy, MI Page 231
United Concordia Company Inc -
Missouri
Chesterfield, MO Page 251
United Concordia Company Inc - New
Mexico
Albuquerque, NM Page 282
United Concordia Company Inc - New
York
Plainview, NY Page 306
United Concordia Company Inc -
Pennsylvania
Pittsburgh, PA Page 374

United Concordia Company Inc -
Pennsylvania - Central
Harrisburg, PA Page 374
United Concordia Company Inc - Texas
Dallas, TX Page 429
United Concordia Company Inc -
Virginia
Glen Allen, VA Page 446
United Concordia Company Inc -
Washington
Seattle, WA Page 457
UnitedHealth Group—
Corporate Headquarters
Minnetonka, MN Page 238
UnitedHealthcare & Mid Atlantic
Medical Services Inc
Rockville, MD Page 206
UnitedHealthcare of Alabama
Birmingham, AL Page 7
UnitedHealthcare of Arizona Inc
Phoenix, AZ Page 21
UnitedHealthcare of Arkansas
Little Rock, AR Page 28
UnitedHealthcare of Colorado
Centennial, CO Page 85
UnitedHealthcare of Florida Inc
Maitland, FL Page 121
UnitedHealthcare of Florida Inc
Tampa, FL Page 122
UnitedHealthcare of Georgia
Norcross, GA Page 134
UnitedHealthcare of Illinois Inc
Chicago, IL Page 154
UnitedHealthcare of Kentucky
Lexington, KY Page 186
UnitedHealthcare of Louisiana
Metairie, LA Page 193
UnitedHealthcare of Mississippi Inc
Ridgeland, MS Page 242
UnitedHealthcare of New England Inc
Warwick, RI Page 381
UnitedHealthcare of New York Inc
East Syracuse, NY Page 306
UnitedHealthcare of New York
Metropolitan
New York, NY Page 306
UnitedHealthcare of Ohio Inc-Cleveland
Cleveland, OH Page 336
UnitedHealthcare of Oregon
Long Beach, CA Page 352
UnitedHealthcare of SW Ohio Inc-
Dayton/Cincinnati
Westchester, OH Page 337
UnitedHealthcare of South Florida
Sunrise, FL Page 122
UnitedHealthcare of Tennessee Inc
Brentwood, TN Page 401
UnitedHealthcare of Texas Inc -
Houston
Houston, TX Page 429
UnitedHealthcare of Texas Inc -
San Antonio
San Antonio, TX Page 430
UnitedHealthcare of Texas Inc — Dallas
Plano, TX Page 430
UnitedHealthcare of Utah
Salt Lake City, UT Page 437
UnitedHealthcare of Virginia
Richmond, VA Page 446
UnitedHealthcare of Washington
Mercer Island, WA Page 457
UnitedHealthcare of Wisconsin Inc
Milwaukee, WI Page 470
UnitedHealthcare of the Heartland
States
Overland Park, KS Page 182

UnitedHealthcare of the Midlands Inc
Omaha, NE Page 257
UnitedHealthcare of the Midwest Inc
Maryland Heights, MO Page 251
UnitedHealthcare Services Company of
the River Valley Inc
Peoria, IL Page 154
UnitedHealthcare Services Company of
the River Valley Inc
Moline, IL Page 154
UnitedHealthcare Services Company of
the River Valley Inc
Bettendorf, IA Page 172
UnitedHealthcare Services Company of
the River Valley Inc
Chattanooga, TN Page 400
UnitedHealthcare Services Company of
the River Valley Inc
Dubuque, IA Page 173
UnitedHealthcare Services Company of
the River Valley Inc
Kingsport, TN Page 400
UnitedHealthcare Services Company of
the River Valley Inc
Knoxville, TN Page 400
UnitedHealthcare Services Company of
the River Valley Inc
Marion, IA Page 173
UnitedHealthcare Services Company of
the River Valley Inc
Urbandale, IA Page 173
UnitedHealthcare Services Company of
the River Valley Inc
Waterloo, IA Page 174
Unity Health Insurance
Sauk City, WI Page 470
Univera Healthcare of Western New
York
Buffalo, NY Page 307
University Health Plans Inc
Newark, NJ Page 277
UPMC Health Plan University of
Pittsburgh Medical Center
Pittsburgh, PA Page 374

V

Valley Baptist Insurance Company
Harlingen, TX Page 431
ValueOptions - Corporate Headquarters
Norfolk, VA Page 447
Vermont Health Plans (Blue Care)
Montpelier, VT Page 439
Virginia Health Network
Richmond, VA Page 447
Virginia Premier Health Plans Inc
Richmond, VA Page 447
Vista Health Plan Inc
Hollywood, FL Page 123
Vista Healthplan of South Florida Inc
Sunrise, FL Page 123

W

WelBorn Health Plans
Evansville, IN Page 167
WellPoint Inc -
Corporate Headquarters
Indianapolis, IN Page 167
Wellmark Blue Cross Blue Shield of
Iowa
Des Moines, IA Page 174

Index VI: Point of Service Organizations

Lovelace Health Plan
Albuquerque, NM — Page 280
**Lutheran Preferred/
Three Rivers Preferred**
Ft Wayne, IN — Page 162

M

M Plan Inc
Indianapolis, IN — Page 163
M-Care Inc
Ann Arbor, MI — Page 225
Magellan Health Services
Macon, GA — Page 132
Magellan Health Services Inc
Avon, CT — Page 91
MagnaCare
Garden City, NY — Page 298
Managed Care Consultants
Henderson, NV — Page 261
Managed Health Network
Point Richmond, CA — Page 57
MDNY Healthcare Inc
Melville, NY — Page 299
Medica Health Plans
Minnetonka, MN — Page 236
Medical Associates Health Plans
Dubuque, IA — Page 172
Medical Card System
Hato Rey, PR — Page 377
Medical Care Referral Group
El Paso, TX — Page 420
Medical Mutual of Ohio
Cleveland, OH — Page 330
Medical Network Inc
Portland, ME — Page 197
Mercy Health Plans of Missouri Inc
Chesterfield, MO — Page 249
Mercycare Health Plan Inc
Janesville, WI — Page 468
Meritain Health Inc
Amherst, NY — Page 299
**Mid Atlantic Medical Services Inc
(MAMSI)- Corp Headquarters**
Rockville, MD — Page 204
Mississippi Select Health Care
Gulfport, MS — Page 241
Molina Healthcare of New Mexico
Albuquerque, NM — Page 281
Molina Healthcare of Washington Inc
Bothell, WA — Page 453
Mountain State Blue Cross Blue Shield
Parkersburg, WV — Page 460
MVP Health Plan Inc
Schenectady, NY — Page 301

N

National Health Plan
New York, NY — Page 302
Nationwide Health Plans
Columbus, OH — Page 331
Neighborhood Health Partnership
Miami, FL — Page 116
Network Health Plan Wisconsin
Menasha, WI — Page 468
Nevada Pacific Dental
Las Vegas, NV — Page 262
New West Health Services
Helena, MT — Page 254

O

ODS Health Plan
Portland, OR — Page 349
Ohio Health Choice
Akron, OH — Page 332
OmniCare, A Coventry Health Plan
Detroit, MI — Page 228
Optima Health Plan Inc
Virginia Beach, VA — Page 445
OSF Health Plans
Peoria, IL — Page 151
**Oxford Health Plans Inc —
Corporate Headquarters**
Trumbell, CT — Page 92
Oxford Health Plans of New Jersey Inc
Iselin, NJ — Page 275
Oxford Health Plans of New York, Inc
New York, NY — Page 303
Oxford Health Plans-Connecticut
Trumbell, CT — Page 91

P

PacifiCare Behavioral Health
Santa Ana, CA — Page 61
**PacifiCare Health Systems-
Corporate Headquarters**
Santa Ana, CA — Page 62
PacifiCare of Arizona
Phoenix, AZ — Page 19
PacifiCare of California
Cypress, CA — Page 62
**PacifiCare of Colorado/United
Healthcare**
Greenwood Village, CO — Page 84
PacifiCare of Nevada
Las Vegas, NV — Page 263
PacifiCare of Oregon
Lake Oswego, OR — Page 350
PacifiCare of Texas - Houston
Houston, TX — Page 422
PacifiCare of Texas Inc
Dallas, TX — Page 422
Paramount Health Care Plan
Maumee, OH — Page 333
**Partners National Health Plans of
North Carolina Inc**
Winston-Salem, NC — Page 314
Penn Highlands Health Plan
Johnstown, PA — Page 370
PersonalCare Insurance of Illinois Inc
Champaign, IL — Page 151
PHP Companies Inc
Knoxville, TN — Page 397
**Physicians Health Plan of Mid-
Michigan**
Lansing, MI — Page 228
**Physicians Health Plan of Northern
Indiana**
Ft Wayne, IN — Page 164
**Physicians Health Plan of South
Michigan**
Jackson, MI — Page 229
Preferred Care
Rochester, NY — Page 304
Preferred Health Systems
Wichita, KS — Page 180
Premera - Corporate Headquarters
Mountlake Terrace, WA — Page 454
Premera Blue Cross - Eastern
Spokane, WA — Page 454
Premera Blue Cross - Western
Mountlake Terrace, WA — Page 454
Presbyterian Health Plan
Alburquerque, NM — Page 281
Primary Health Plan
Boise, ID — Page 142
Primecare Medical Network Inc
Ontario, CA — Page 65
Priority Health
Grand Rapids, MI — Page 230
**Private Healthcare Systems -
California**
Irvine, CA — Page 65
**Private Healthcare Systems -
Corporate Headquarters**
Waltham, MA — Page 215
Private Healthcare Systems - Georgia
Atlanta, GA — Page 133
Private Healthcare Systems - Illinois
Rosemont, IL — Page 153
Private Healthcare Systems - Missouri
Kansas City, MO — Page 251
Private Healthcare Systems - Texas
Dallas, TX — Page 423
**Private Healthcare Systems -
Washington**
Bothell, WA — Page 455
ProviDRs Care Network
Wichita, KS — Page 181
Providence Health Plans
Beaverton, OR — Page 351

Q

QCA Health Plan Inc
Little Rock, AR — Page 28
QualCare Inc
Piscataway, NJ — Page 276
Quincy Health Care Management Inc
Quincy, IL — Page 153

R

**Regence Blue Cross Blue Shield of
Oregon**
Portland, OR — Page 351
Regence Blue Shield
Burlington, WA — Page 456
Regence Blue Shield
Seattle, WA — Page 456
Regence Blue Shield of Idaho
Lewiston, ID — Page 142
Rocky Mountain Health Plans
Grand Junction, CO — Page 84
**Rocky Mountain Hosital &
Medical Services Inc**
Denver, CO — Page 85

S

Saint Mary's HealthFirst
Reno, NV — Page 263
Sante Community Physicians
Fresno, CA — Page 67
Scott & White Health Plan
Temple, TX — Page 424

Index VI: Point of Service Organizations

GHI HMO Select Inc
New York, NY — Page 293
Great West Life Annuity Insurance Co
Greenwood Village, CO — Page 81
Great-West Healthcare - Corporate
Greenwood Village, CO — Page 81
Great-West Healthcare - New Jersey
Piscataway, NJ — Page 272
Great-West Healthcare of Arizona
Scottsdale, AZ — Page 16
Great-West Healthcare of California - North
Pleasant Hill, CA — Page 48
Great-West Healthcare of Colorado
Greenwood Village, CO — Page 81
Great-West Healthcare of Florida
Tampa, FL — Page 111
Great-West Healthcare of Georgia
Atlanta, GA — Page 131
Great-West Healthcare of Michigan
Southfield, MI — Page 223
Great-West Healthcare of North Carolina
Charlotte, NC — Page 313
Great-West Healthcare of Ohio
North Olmstead, OH — Page 326
Great-West Healthcare of Oregon
Portland, OR — Page 346
Great-West Healthcare of Pennsylvania
Media, PA — Page 363
Great-West Healthcare of Texas - Austin
Austin, TX — Page 414
Great-West Healthcare of Texas - Dallas
Dallas, TX — Page 415
Great-West Healthcare of Washington Inc
Bellevue, WA — Page 451
Group Health Cooperative
Coeur D'Alene, ID — Page 141
Group Health Cooperative
Spokane, WA — Page 451
Group Health Cooperative of Puget Sound
Seattle, WA — Page 452
Group Health Options Inc
Seattle, WA — Page 452
Group Health Plan Inc
Earth City, MO — Page 248
GroupLink Inc
Indianapolis, IN — Page 160
Guardian Life Insurance Co of America
New York, NY — Page 294
Gundersen Lutheran Health Plan Inc
La Crosse, WI — Page 465

H

Harvard Pilgrim Health Care - Corporate Headquarters
Wellesley, MA — Page 212
Hawaii Medical Services Association - BC/BS of Hawaii
Honolulu, HI — Page 137
Health Alliance Medical Plans - Corporate Headquarters
Urbana, IL — Page 149
Health Alliance Plan of Michigan
Detroit, MI — Page 223
Health Care Exchange Limited Company
Southfield, MI — Page 223

Health Care Service Corporation - Corporate Headquarters
Chicago, IL — Page 149
Health First Health Plans Inc
Rockledge, FL — Page 111
Health Net - Connecticut
Shelton, CT — Page 90
Health Net - New Jersey
Neptune, NJ — Page 272
Health Net - New York
White Plains, NY — Page 295
Health Net Health Plan of Oregon Inc
Tigard, OR — Page 346
Health Net Inc - Corporate Headquarters
Woodland Hills, CA — Page 49
Health Net Inc - Northeast Corporate Headquarters
Shelton, CT — Page 91
Health Net of Arizona
Tucson, AZ — Page 17
Health Net of California
Woodland Hills, CA — Page 49
Health New England
Springfield, MA — Page 212
Health Plan of Nevada Inc
Las Vegas, NV — Page 260
Health Plan, The/Hometown Region
Massillon, OH — Page 327
Health Plus
Peoria, IL — Page 150
Health Plus of Louisiana Inc
Shreveport, LA — Page 191
Health Tradition Health Plans
Onalaska, WI — Page 466
HealthAmerica Pennsylvania Inc - Central Region
Harrisburg, PA — Page 364
HealthAmerica Pennsylvania Inc - Eastern Region
Plymouth Meeting, PA — Page 365
HealthAmerica Pennsylvania Inc - Nortwestern
Erie, PA — Page 365
HealthAmerica Pennsylvania Inc - Western Region
Pittsburgh, PA — Page 365
HealthLink Inc
St Louis, MO — Page 248
HealthLink Inc - Corporate Headquarters
St Louis, MO — Page 249
HealthNow New York Inc
Buffalo, NY — Page 295
HealthPlus of Michigan
Flint, MI — Page 224
HealthSmart Preferred Care
Lubbock, TX — Page 416
HealthSpring Inc - Corporate Headquarters
Franklin, TN — Page 395
HealthSpring Inc - Tennessee
Nashville, TN — Page 395
Healthplex Inc
Uniondale, NY — Page 296
Highmark Inc
Pittsburgh, PA — Page 366
HIP Health Plan of New York
New York, NY — Page 296
HMO California
Signal Hill, CA — Page 51
HMO Louisiana Inc
Baton Rouge, LA — Page 191
HMO New Mexico Inc
Albuquerque, NM — Page 280
Horizon Blue Cross/Blue Shield of NJ
Newark, NJ — Page 273

Horizon Healthcare Services Inc
Newark, NJ — Page 274
Humana Health Benefit Plan of Louisiana
Metairie, LA — Page 191
Humana Health Care Plans of Arizona
Phoenix, AZ — Page 17
Humana Health Care Plans of Illinois
Chicago, IL — Page 151
Humana Health Care Plans of Kansas & Missouri
Overland Park, KS — Page 179
Humana Health Care Plans of Lexington
Lexington, KY — Page 185
Humana Health Care Plans of San Antonio/Austin
San Antonio, TX — Page 418
Humana Health Plan - Jacksonville
Jacksonville, FL — Page 113
Humana Health Plan - Kentucky
Louisville, KY — Page 185
Humana Health Plan of Ohio Inc
Cincinnati, OH — Page 328
Humana Health Plans of Georgia
Atlanta, GA — Page 132
Humana Inc - Arkansas
Louisville, KY — Page 27
Humana Inc - Corporate Headquarters
Louisville, KY — Page 185
Humana Military Service Inc
Louisville, KY — Page 186

I

Independence Blue Cross
Philadelphia, PA — Page 366
Independent Health Association Inc
Buffalo, NY — Page 297
Initial Group Inc, The
Nashville, TN — Page 396
Iowa Foundation for Medical Care/Encompass
West Des Moines, IA — Page 170

K

Kaiser Foundation Health Plan - Mid Atlantic States
Rockville, MD — Page 203
Kaiser Foundation Health Plan of Georgia
Atlanta, GA — Page 132
Kaiser Foundation Health Plan of Ohio
Cleveland, OH — Page 329
Keystone Health Plan East Inc
Philadelphia, PA — Page 368
Keystone Health Plan West Inc
Pittsburgh, PA — Page 368

L

Lakewood Health Plan Inc
Lakewood, CA — Page 56
Landmark Healthcare Inc
Sacramento, CA — Page 56
Lifetime Healthcare Companies, The - Corporate Headquarters
Rochester, NY — Page 298

Index VI: Point of Service Organizations

C

Capital Blue Cross
Harrisburg, PA   Page 359
Capital District Physicians Health Plan
Albany, NY   Page 286
Capitol Administrators
Rancho Cordova, CA   Page 38
CareFirst Blue Cross Blue Shield
Owings Mills, MD   Page 200
CareFirst BlueChoice Inc
Washington, DC   Page 97
Carelink Health Plans
Wheeling, WV   Page 459
Carelink Health Plans
Charleston, WV   Page 459
Cariten Healthcare
Knoxville, TN   Page 393
Carolina Care Plan Inc
Columbia, SC   Page 383
Catalina Behavioral Health Services Inc
Mesa, AZ   Page 13
Center Care
Bowling Green, KY   Page 184
Central New York East HealthNow New York Inc
East Syracuse, NY   Page 287
Central New York West HealthNow New York Inc
Rochester, NY   Page 287
Cha Health - Humana
Lexington, KY   Page 184
ChiroSource - Corporate Headquarters
Concord, CA   Page 40
CHN MCO
Independence, OH   Page 322
ChoiceCare/Humana
Cincinnati, OH   Page 322
CIGNA Health Plan of Utah Inc
Salt Lake City, UT   Page 433
CIGNA HealthCare — Corporate Headquarters
Philadelphia, PA   Page 360
CIGNA Healthcare
Burlington, VT   Page 439
CIGNA Healthcare - Cincinnati
Cincinnati, OH   Page 323
CIGNA Healthcare of Arizona
Phoenix, AZ   Page 14
CIGNA Healthcare of California
Glendale, CA   Page 41
CIGNA Healthcare of Colorado
Denver, CO   Page 79
CIGNA Healthcare of Connecticut
Hartford, CT   Page 89
CIGNA Healthcare of Florida
Tampa, FL   Page 107
CIGNA Healthcare of Florida
Sunrise, FL   Page 107
CIGNA Healthcare of Georgia
Atlanta, GA   Page 128
CIGNA Healthcare of Illinois Inc
Chicago, IL   Page 144
CIGNA Healthcare of Indiana
Indianapolis, IN   Page 158
CIGNA Healthcare of Kansas/Missouri
Overland Park, KS   Page 177
CIGNA Healthcare of Maine Inc
Falmouth, ME   Page 195
CIGNA Healthcare of Massachusetts
Newton, MA   Page 210
CIGNA Healthcare of New Hampshire
Hooksett, NH   Page 265

CIGNA Healthcare of New York and New Jersey
Jersey City, NJ   Page 270
CIGNA Healthcare of North Carolina
Raleigh, NC   Page 311
CIGNA Healthcare of North Carolina Inc
Charlotte, NC   Page 311
CIGNA Healthcare of Ohio Inc
Cleveland, OH   Page 323
CIGNA Healthcare of Ohio Inc
Columbus, OH   Page 323
CIGNA Healthcare of PA
Blue Bell, PA   Page 360
CIGNA Healthcare of St Louis
St Louis, MO   Page 245
CIGNA Healthcare of Tennessee
Memphis, TN   Page 393
CIGNA Healthcare of Tennessee Inc
Franklin, TN   Page 394
CIGNA Healthcare of Virginia Inc - Richmond
Richmond, VA   Page 443
Colorado Dental Service Inc, dba: Delta Dental Plan of CO
Denver, CO   Page 80
Community Health Plan
St Joseph, MO   Page 245
CommunityCare Managed Healthcare Plans of Oklahoma Inc
Tulsa, OK   Page 340
ConnectCare
Midland, MI   Page 219
Connecticare Inc
Farmington, CT   Page 89
Connecticare of Massachusetts Inc
Farmington, CT   Page 210
Coordinated Health Plan
Providence, RI   Page 379
Coventry Health Care Inc — Carolinas
Charlotte, NC   Page 311
Coventry Health Care Inc — Corporate Headquarters
Bethesda, MD   Page 201
Coventry Health Care Inc — Delaware Inc
Wilmington, DE   Page 96
Coventry Health Care Inc — Georgia Inc
Atlanta, GA   Page 130
Coventry Health Care Inc — Iowa
Urbandale, IA   Page 169
Coventry Health Care Inc — Louisiana
Metairie, LA   Page 190
Coventry Health Care of Kansas - Wichita
Wichita, KS   Page 178
Coventry Health Care of Kansas Inc
Kansas City, MO   Page 245
Coventry Health Care of Nebraska Inc
Omaha, NE   Page 255
Cox Health Plans
Springfield, MO   Page 246

D

DakotaCare
Sioux Falls, SD   Page 387
Dean Health Plan
Madison, WI   Page 463
Delmarva Health Care Plan Inc
Easton, MD   Page 202
Delphi Card R
Fox River Grove, IL   Page 145

Delta Dental Plan of California
San Francisco, CA   Page 44
Delta Dental Plan of Illinois
Lisle, IL   Page 145
Delta Dental Plan of Indiana Inc
Indianapolis, IN   Page 159
Delta Dental Plan of Michigan Inc
Okemos, MI   Page 220
Delta Dental Plan of Minnesota
Eagan, MN   Page 235
Delta Dental Plan of Missouri
St Louis, MO   Page 246
Delta Dental Plan of New Jersey
Parsippany, NJ   Page 271
Delta Dental Plan of Ohio Inc
Westerville, OH   Page 324
Delta Dental Plan of Tennessee
Nashville, TN   Page 394
Delta Dental Plan of Wisconsin
Racine, WI   Page 463
Delta Dental Plans Association
Oak Brook Village, IL   Page 146
Delta Dental of Virginia
Roanoke, VA   Page 443
DeltaCare USA
Cerritos, CA   Page 44
DentCare Delivery Systems Inc
Uniondale, NY   Page 289
Dental Benefit Providers Inc
Rockville, MD   Page 202

E

Empire Blue Cross Blue Shield
New York, NY   Page 290
Employee Benefit Management Services Inc
Billings, MT   Page 253
Employee Benefits Corporation
Middletown, WI   Page 464
Evergreen Medical Group LLC
Columbus, GA   Page 131
Excellus BlueCross BlueShield
Rochester, NY   Page 290
Excellus BlueCross BlueShield, Utica Region
Utica, NY   Page 292

F

Fallon Community Health Plan Inc
Worcester, MA   Page 211
Fara Healthcare Management
Mandeville, LA   Page 190
First Health Network
San Diego, CA   Page 46
First Plan of Minnesota
Duluth, MN   Page 235
Flora Health Network
Cleveland, OH   Page 325
Florida Health Care Plan Inc
Holly Hill, FL   Page 109

G

Geisinger Health Plan
Danville, PA   Page 363

Index VI: Point of Service Organizations

A

Advantage Health Solutions Inc
Indianapolis, IN   Page 157
Aetna Health Inc
Houston, TX   Page 403
Aetna Health Inc - Colorado
Greenwood Village, CO   Page 77
Aetna Health Plans of Mid-Atlantic
Falls Church, VA   Page 441
Aetna Health of California Inc
Walnut Creek, CA   Page 31
Aetna Health of Illinois Inc
Chicago, IL   Page 143
Aetna Inc
Norwalk, CT   Page 87
Aetna Inc - Altamonte Springs
Altamonte Springs, FL   Page 99
Aetna Inc - Arizona
Phoenix, AZ   Page 11
Aetna Inc - Arkansas
Metairie, LA   Page 25
Aetna Inc - Arkansas
Little Rock, AR   Page 25
Aetna Inc - Corporate Headquarters
Hartford, CT   Page 87
Aetna Inc - Corporate Headquarters
Blue Bell, PA   Page 355
Aetna Inc - Florida
Tampa, FL   Page 100
Aetna Inc - Georgia
Alpheretta, GA   Page 127
Aetna Inc - Jacksonville
Jacksonville, FL   Page 100
Aetna Inc - Louisiana
Metairie, LA   Page 189
Aetna Inc - Maine
Portland, ME   Page 195
Aetna Inc - Maryland
Linthicum, MD   Page 199
Aetna Inc - Michigan
Southfield, MI   Page 217
Aetna Inc - Missouri
Chesterfield, MO   Page 243
Aetna Inc - New Jersey
Mt Laurel, NJ   Page 267
Aetna Inc - New Jersey
Fairfield, NJ   Page 267
Aetna Inc - Ohio
Richfield, OH   Page 319
Aetna Inc - Oklahoma
Oklahoma City, OK   Page 339
Aetna Inc - Pennsylvania
Pittsburgh, PA   Page 355
Aetna Inc - Pennsylvania
King of Prussia, PA   Page 355
Aetna Inc - Pennsylvania Region
Blue Bell, PA   Page 356
Aetna Inc - Plantation
Plantation, FL   Page 100
Aetna Inc - Tennessee
Memphis, TN   Page 391
Aetna Inc - Tennessee
Nashville, TN   Page 391
Aetna Inc - Tulsa
Tulsa, OK   Page 339
Aetna Inc of New England
Middletown, CT   Page 87
Aetna Inc of the Carolinas
Charlotte, NC   Page 309
Alignis Inc
Paramus, NJ   Page 268
Altius Health Plans
South Jordan, UT   Page 433

AmeriGroup Florida Inc
Tampa, FL   Page 101
AmeriHealth Insurance Company
Wilmington, DE   Page 95
American LIFECARE - Louisiana
New Orleans, LA   Page 189
American Specialty Health Plans Inc
San Diego, CA   Page 33
Americas PPO
Bloomington, MN   Page 233
Amerihealth Insurance Company - NJ North
Iselin, NJ   Page 269
Amerihealth Insurance Company - NJ South
Mt Laurel, NJ   Page 269
Anthem Blue Cross
Woodland Hills, CA   Page 34
Anthem Blue Cross Blue Shield of Colorado
Denver, CO   Page 77
Anthem Blue Cross Blue Shield of Maine
South Portland, ME   Page 195
Anthem Blue Cross Blue Shield of Missouri
St Louis, MO   Page 243
Anthem Blue Cross Blue Shield of Virginia Inc
Richmond, VA   Page 442
Anthem Blue Cross and Blue Shield of Kentucky (HMO Kentucky)
Louisville, KY   Page 183
Anthem Blue Cross and Blue Shield of Ohio
Cincinnati, OH   Page 320
Anthem Blue Cross/Blue Shield of Indiana
Indianapolis, IN   Page 157
Anthem Blue Cross/Blue Shield of New Hampshire
Manchester, NH   Page 265
Anthem Health Plan Inc dba: Anthem Blue Cross Blue Shield CT
North Haven, CT   Page 88
APS Healthcare Northwest Inc
Missoula, MT   Page 253
Arise Health Plan
Green Bay, WI   Page 461
Arizona Foundation for Medical Care
Phoenix, AZ   Page 11
Arkansas Blue Cross/Blue Shield a Mutual Insurance Company
Little Rock, AR   Page 25
Arnett Health Plans
Lafayette, IN   Page 157
Assurant Employee Benefits - New Mexico
Albuquerque, NM   Page 279
Athens Area Health Plan Select Inc
Athens, GA   Page 127
Atlantis Health Plan
New York, NY   Page 285
Av-Med Health Plan - Jacksonville
Jacksonville, FL   Page 102
Av-Med Health Plan - Miami
Miami, FL   Page 103
Av-Med Health Plan - Orlando
Maitland, FL   Page 103
Av-Med Health Plan - Tampa
Tampa, FL   Page 103
Avera Health Plans Inc
Sioux Falls, SD   Page 387

B

Baptist Health Services Group
Memphis, TN   Page 392
Behavioral Healthcare Options Inc
Las Vegas, NV   Page 259
Blue Cross Blue Shield of Alabama
Birmingham, AL   Page 3
Blue Cross Blue Shield of Delaware
Wilmington, DE   Page 95
Blue Cross Blue Shield of Florida & Health Options Inc
Miami, FL   Page 104
Blue Cross Blue Shield of Florida/Health Options Inc
Jacksonville, FL   Page 104
Blue Cross Blue Shield of Illinois
Chicago, IL   Page 144
Blue Cross Blue Shield of Louisiana Inc
Baton Rouge, LA   Page 189
Blue Cross Blue Shield of Massachusetts
Boston, MA   Page 209
Blue Cross Blue Shield of Minnesota
St Paul, MN   Page 234
Blue Cross Blue Shield of Mississippi
Jackson, MS   Page 241
Blue Cross Blue Shield of Montana
Helena, MT   Page 253
Blue Cross Blue Shield of Nebraska
Omaha, NE   Page 255
Blue Cross Blue Shield of New Mexico
Albuquerque, NM   Page 279
Blue Cross Blue Shield of North Carolina
Durham, NC   Page 310
Blue Cross Blue Shield of South Carolina - Corporate Hqtrs
Columbia, SC   Page 383
Blue Cross Blue Shield of Tennessee
Chattanooga, TN   Page 392
Blue Cross Blue Shield of Tennessee - Memphis
Memphis, TN   Page 393
Blue Cross Blue Shield of Texas — Corporate Headquarters
Richardson, TX   Page 406
Blue Cross Blue Shield of Texas — HMO Blue - Southeast
Houston, TX   Page 407
Blue Cross Blue Shield of Texas — HMO Blue - West
El Paso, TX   Page 407
Blue Cross Blue Shield of Vermont
Berlin, VT   Page 439
Blue Cross Blue Shield of Western New York
Buffalo, NY   Page 285
Blue Cross of Idaho
Meridian, ID   Page 141
Blue Shield of California
San Francisco, CA   Page 36
BlueChoice Health Plan of South Carolina Inc
Columbia, SC   Page 383
BlueCross of Northeastern Pennsylvania
Wilkes-Barre, PA   Page 358
BlueShield of Northeastern New York
Latham, NY   Page 286
Bluegrass Family Health Inc
Lexington, KY   Page 183

Index VI

Point of Service Organizations

Index V: Specialty PPOs

United Concordia Company Inc - California
Woodland Hills, CA — Page 72

United Concordia Company Inc - Corporate Headquarters
Harrisburg, PA — Page 373

United Concordia Company Inc - Florida
Tampa, FL — Page 121

United Concordia Company Inc - Illinois
Chicago, IL — Page 154

United Concordia Company Inc - Maryland
Hunt Valley, MD — Page 206

United Concordia Company Inc - Michigan
Troy, MI — Page 231

United Concordia Company Inc - Missouri
Chesterfield, MO — Page 251

United Concordia Company Inc - New Mexico
Albuquerque, NM — Page 282

United Concordia Company Inc - New York
Plainview, NY — Page 306

United Concordia Company Inc - Pennsylvania
Pittsburgh, PA — Page 374

United Concordia Company Inc - Pennsylvania - Central
Harrisburg, PA — Page 374

United Concordia Company Inc - Texas
Dallas, TX — Page 429

United Concordia Company Inc - Virginia
Glen Allen, VA — Page 446

United Concordia Company Inc - Washington
Seattle, WA — Page 457

Unity Dental Health Services
Lyndhurst, NJ — Page 277

Valley Preferred
Allentown, PA — Page 375

ValueOptions - Corporate Headquarters
Norfolk, VA — Page 447

Ventura County Foundation for Medical Care
Camarillo, CA — Page 73

Vision Health Management Systems
Chicago, IL — Page 155

Vision Plan of America
Los Angeles, CA — Page 75

Vision Service Plan
Rancho Cordova, CA — Page 75

Vision Service Plan
Denver, CO — Page 86

Washington Dental Service
Seattle, WA — Page 457

Index V: Specialty PPOs

Employee Benefit Management Services Inc
Billings, MT — Page 253
Eye Care of Wisconsin Inc
Milwaukee, WI — Page 464
EyeMed Vision Care LLC
Mason, OH — Page 325

F

Fidelio Insurance Company
Glenside, PA — Page 362
First Choice Health Network
Seattle, WA — Page 451
First Commonwealth
Chicago, IL — Page 147

G

GENEX Services
Wayne, PA — Page 363
Global Medical Management
Davie, FL — Page 110
Golden West Dental & Vision
Camarillo, CA — Page 47
Great Expressions Dental Centers
Bloomfield Hills, MI — Page 222
GroupLink Inc
Indianapolis, IN — Page 160

H

Health Care Exchange Limited Company
Southfield, MI — Page 223
HealthLink Inc - Corporate Headquarters
St Louis, MO — Page 249
Healthplex Inc
Uniondale, NY — Page 296
Henry Ford OptimEyes
Madison Heights, MI — Page 224
Horizon Behavioral Services
Lake Mary, FL — Page 112
Horizon Behavioral Services
Lewisville, TX — Page 417
Humana Inc - Corporate Headquarters
Louisville, KY — Page 185

I

Iowa Foundation for Medical Care/Encompass
West Des Moines, IA — Page 170

L

Landmark Healthcare Inc
Sacramento, CA — Page 56

M

Magellan Behavioral Health
Parsippany, NJ — Page 274
Magellan Health Services
Macon, GA — Page 132
Managed Health Network
Point Richmond, CA — Page 57
Managed HealthCare Northwest Inc
Portland, OR — Page 348
Med-Comp USA
Metairie, LA — Page 192
MedSolutions
Franklin, TN — Page 396
Medco Health Solutions Inc
Franklin Lakes, NJ — Page 275
Medfocus Radiology Network
Santa Monica, CA — Page 58
Medical Card System
Hato Rey, PR — Page 377
Medical Eye Services Inc
Santa Ana, CA — Page 58
Mental Health Consultants Inc
Jamison, PA — Page 369

N

National Dental Consultants Inc
Islip, NY — Page 301
National Foot Care Program Inc
Lathrup Village, MI — Page 227
Nevada Preferred Professionals
Las Vegas, NV — Page 262
New York State Catholic Health Plan Inc
Rego Park, NY — Page 303
Newport Dental Plan
Santa Ana, CA — Page 60
Northwest Rehab Alliance
Portland, OR — Page 349

O

One Call Medical Inc
Parsippany, NJ — Page 275
Outlook Vision Services
Mesa, AZ — Page 18

P

PacifiCare Behavioral Health
Santa Ana, CA — Page 61
PacifiCare Dental & Vision
Santa Ana, CA — Page 61
PacifiCare of Colorado/United Healthcare
Greenwood Village, CO — Page 84
Pacific Union Dental Inc
Concord, CA — Page 63
Pacific Visioncare Washington Inc
Chehalis, WA — Page 453
Physical Therapy Provider Network
Delray Beach, FL — Page 117
PPNM's Mastercare Network
Sparks, NV — Page 263

Preferred Chiropractic Care Inc
Wichita, KS — Page 179
Preferred Dental Network (PDN)
Quincy, MA — Page 215
Preferred Mental Health Management
Wichita, KS — Page 180
Preferred Podiatry Group
Northbrook, IL — Page 152
Preferred Therapy Providers of America - Corp Headquarters
Phoenix, AZ — Page 19
PTPN - Corporate Headquarters
Calabasas, CA — Page 65

R

Racine Dental Group SC
Racine, WI — Page 469
Raytel Imaging Network
Collegeville, PA — Page 371
Renaissance Health Systems Inc
Wellington, FL — Page 119

S

Safeguard Health Enterprises Inc
Aliso Viejo, CA — Page 66
Safeguard Health Plans Inc
Ft Lauderdale, FL — Page 119
Script Care Inc
Beaumont, TX — Page 425
SecureCare Dental
Phoenix, AZ — Page 20
SmileCare/Community Dental Services
Santa Ana, CA — Page 69
Spectrum Vision Systems Inc
Overland Park, KS — Page 181
Superior Vision Services Inc
Laguna Hills, CA — Page 70
Susquehanna Health Care
Berwick, PA — Page 372

T

Texas Dental Plan
San Antonio, TX — Page 427
Total Dental Administrators Health Plan
Phoenix, AZ — Page 21

U

Union Labor Life Insurance Co
Mount Laurel, NJ — Page 276
Unipsych Systems
Hollywood, FL — Page 120
United Behavioral Health
Philadelphia, PA — Page 373
United Behavioral Health (UBH)
San Francisco, CA — Page 71
United Concordia Company Inc - Alabama
Birmingham, AL — Page 6
United Concordia Company Inc - Arizona
Phoenix, AZ — Page 21

Index V: Specialty PPOs

20/20 Eyecare Plan Inc
Ft Lauderdale, FL   Page 99

A

Access Dental Services
Sacramento, CA   Page 31
ACN Group
Golden Valley, MN   Page 233
ACN Group of California - Western Region
San Diego, CA   Page 31
Advantica Eyecare Inc
Clearwater, FL   Page 99
Aetna Behavioral Health - Utah Care Management Center
Sandy, UT   Page 433
Aetna Dental Inc - New Jersey
Fairfield, NJ   Page 267
Aetna Inc - Dental Plan of Texas
Dallas, TX   Page 403
Alignis Inc
Paramus, NJ   Page 268
Alpha Dental Plan of Colorado
Denver, CO   Page 77
American Pharmacy Services Corporation
Frankfort, KY   Page 183
American Specialty Health Plans Inc
San Diego, CA   Page 33
American WholeHealth Networks Inc
Sterling, VA   Page 442
Americas PPO
Bloomington, MN   Page 233
Ameritas Group Dental
Lincoln, NE   Page 255
APS Healthcare Inc
Silver Springs, MD   Page 199
APS Healthcare Midwest Inc
Brookfield, WI   Page 461
APS Healthcare Northwest Inc
Missoula, MT   Page 253
Assurant Employee Benefits - New Mexico
Albuquerque, NM   Page 279
Assurant Employee Benefits - North Carolina
Raleigh, NC   Page 309
Avante Behavioral Health Plan
Fresno, CA   Page 35
Avesis Inc
Phoenix, AZ   Page 12

B

Behavioral Health Systems Inc
Birmingham, AL   Page 3
Behavioral Healthcare Options Inc
Las Vegas, NV   Page 259
Berkley Administrators of Connecticut Inc
Farmington, CT   Page 88
Blue Cross Blue Shield of Florida/Health Options Inc
Jacksonville, FL   Page 104
Blue Cross Blue Shield of Tennessee
Chattanooga, TN   Page 392

C

Capitol Administrators
Rancho Cordova, CA   Page 38
CareIQ
Miramar, FL   Page 106
Careington International - The Dental Network
Frisco, TX   Page 408
Catalina Behavioral Health Services Inc
Mesa, AZ   Page 13
ChiroSource - Corporate Headquarters
Concord, CA   Page 40
Chirocare of Minnesota INC
Shoreview, MN   Page 234
Chiropractic Arizona Network Inc
Phoenix, AZ   Page 13
CIGNA Behavioral Health Inc - Corporate Headquarters
Eden Prairie, MN   Page 234
CIGNA Dental Health of Colorado
Sunrise, FL   Page 78
CIGNA Dental Health of New Jersey Inc
Sunrise, FL   Page 270
CIGNA Healthcare
Burlington, VT   Page 439
Coalition America Inc
Atlanta, GA   Page 129
Colorado Dental Service Inc, dba: Delta Dental Plan of CO
Denver, CO   Page 80
Community Behavioral Healthcare Cooperative of Pennsylvania
Harrisburg, PA   Page 361
CompBenefits Corporation - Corporate Headquarters
Roswell, GA   Page 129
Complementary Healthcare Plans
Beaverton, OR   Page 345
Comprehensive Health Group
Duluth, GA   Page 129
Compsych Behavioral Health
Chicago, IL   Page 145
CorpHealth Inc
Fort Worth, TX   Page 412
Corvel Corporation
Toledo, OH   Page 324
Coventry Health Care Inc — Iowa
Urbandale, IA   Page 169

D

Davis Vision
Plainview, NY   Page 288
Delphi Card R
Fox River Grove, IL   Page 145
Delta Dental Insurance Company - Alabama
Birmingham, AL   Page 4
Delta Dental Insurance Company - Georgia
Alpharetta, GA   Page 131
Delta Dental Insurance Company - Nevada
Las Vegas, NV   Page 259
Delta Dental Insurance Company - Texas
Irving, TX   Page 412
Delta Dental Plan of Arizona Inc
Phoenix, AZ   Page 14
Delta Dental Plan of Arkansas
Sherwood, AR   Page 26
Delta Dental Plan of California
San Francisco, CA   Page 44
Delta Dental Plan of Idaho
Boise, ID   Page 141
Delta Dental Plan of Illinois
Lisle, IL   Page 145
Delta Dental Plan of Indiana Inc
Indianapolis, IN   Page 159
Delta Dental Plan of Kansas
Wichita, KS   Page 178
Delta Dental Plan of Kentucky Inc
Louisville, KY   Page 184
Delta Dental Plan of Michigan Inc
Okemos, MI   Page 220
Delta Dental Plan of Minnesota
Eagan, MN   Page 235
Delta Dental Plan of Missouri
St Louis, MO   Page 246
Delta Dental Plan of New Hampshire
Concord, NH   Page 265
Delta Dental Plan of New Jersey
Parsippany, NJ   Page 271
Delta Dental Plan of Ohio Inc
Westerville, OH   Page 324
Delta Dental Plan of South Dakota
Pierre, SD   Page 387
Delta Dental Plan of Tennessee
Nashville, TN   Page 394
Delta Dental Plan of Wisconsin
Racine, WI   Page 463
Delta Dental Plans Association
Oak Brook Village, IL   Page 146
Delta Dental of Florida
Maitland, FL   Page 108
Delta Dental of Iowa
Ankeny, IA   Page 169
Delta Dental of Nebraska
Omaha, NE   Page 256
Delta Dental of Virginia
Roanoke, VA   Page 443
DentCare Delivery Systems Inc
Uniondale, NY   Page 289
Denta Quest Mid-Atlantic Inc
Calverton, MD   Page 202
Denta Quest Ventures Inc
Boston, MA   Page 211
Dental Benefit Providers Inc
Rockville, MD   Page 202
Dental Benefit Providers of CA Inc
San Francisco, CA   Page 45
Dental Care of America Ltd
Buffalo Grove, IL   Page 146
Dental Group of New Jersey
Linden, NJ   Page 271
Dental Health Services
Long Beach, CA   Page 45
Dental Health Services Inc
Seattle, WA   Page 450
Dental Network of America
Oakbrook Terrace, IL   Page 146
Dentistat (Insurance Dentists of America)
Saratoga, CA   Page 45

E

ECCA - Managed Vision Care Inc - Corporate Headquarters
San Antonio, TX   Page 413
EM Risk Management, A POMCO Company
Endicott, NY   Page 290

Index V

Specialty PPOs

Index IV: Specialty HMOs

Pearle Vision Managed Care - HMO of Texas Inc
Dallas, TX   Page 423
Preferred Podiatrists of Oklahoma
Bethany, OK   Page 342
Premier Behavioral Systems of Tennessee LLC
Nashville, TN   Page 398

R

Racine Dental Group SC
Racine, WI   Page 469
Robert T Dorris Associates
Westlake Village, CA   Page 66

S

S V S Visions Inc
Mt Clemens, MI   Page 231
Safeguard Health Enterprises Inc
Aliso Viejo, CA   Page 66
Safeguard Health Plans Inc
Ft Lauderdale, FL   Page 119
Safeguard Health Plans Inc
Dallas, TX   Page 424
SCHC Total Care Inc
Syracuse, NY   Page 305
SmileCare/Community Dental Services
Santa Ana, CA   Page 69
Spectera Vision Inc - Corporate Headquarters
Baltimore, MD   Page 206
Spectera Vision Inc - Indiana
Indianapolis, IN   Page 166
Spectera Vision Services of California Inc
Culver City, CA   Page 69
Standard Optical
Salt Lake City, UT   Page 437
Superior Dental Care Alliance
Dayton, OH   Page 335

T

Tennessee Behavioral Health Inc
Nashville, TN   Page 399
Total Dental Administrators Health Plan
Phoenix, AZ   Page 21

U

UDC Dental California Inc
San Diego, CA   Page 71
UDC Ohio Inc
Cincinnati, OH   Page 335
United Behavioral Health (UBH)
San Francisco, CA   Page 71
United Concordia Company Inc - Alabama
Birmingham, AL   Page 6
United Concordia Company Inc - Arizona
Phoenix, AZ   Page 21
United Concordia Company Inc - California
Woodland Hills, CA   Page 72
United Concordia Company Inc - Corporate Headquarters
Harrisburg, PA   Page 373
United Concordia Company Inc - Florida
Tampa, FL   Page 121
United Concordia Company Inc - Illinois
Chicago, IL   Page 154
United Concordia Company Inc - Maryland
Hunt Valley, MD   Page 206
United Concordia Company Inc - Michigan
Troy, MI   Page 231
United Concordia Company Inc - Missouri
Chesterfield, MO   Page 251
United Concordia Company Inc - New Mexico
Albuquerque, NM   Page 282
United Concordia Company Inc - New York
Plainview, NY   Page 306
United Concordia Company Inc - Pennsylvania
Pittsburgh, PA   Page 374
United Concordia Company Inc - Pennsylvania - Central
Harrisburg, PA   Page 374
United Concordia Company Inc - Texas
Dallas, TX   Page 429
United Concordia Company Inc - Virginia
Glen Allen, VA   Page 446
United Concordia Company Inc - Washington
Seattle, WA   Page 457
United Dental Care of Texas Inc - Assurant Employee Benefits
Addison, TX   Page 429
UnitedHealthcare of the Midlands Inc
Omaha, NE   Page 257
Unity Dental Health Services
Lyndhurst, NJ   Page 277

V

ValueOptions of California Inc
Cypress, CA   Page 72
ValueOptions of Texas Inc
Coppell, TX   Page 431
Vision Care Network
Racine, WI   Page 471
Vision First Eye Care Inc
San Jose, CA   Page 73
Vision Insurance Plan of America Inc - Corp Headquarters
Milwaukee, WI   Page 471
Vision Plan of America
Los Angeles, CA   Page 75
Vision Service Plan
Rancho Cordova, CA   Page 75
Vision Service Plan of Arizona
Phoenix, AZ   Page 22
Visioncare of California
San Diego, CA   Page 75

W

Western Dental Services
Orange, CA   Page 75

Williamette Dental Group PC
Hillsboro, OR   Page 352
Williamette Dental of Washington Inc
Hillsboro, OR   Page 457

Index IV: Specialty HMOs

Delta Dental Plan of Minnesota
Eagan, MN — Page 235
Delta Dental Plan of Missouri
St Louis, MO — Page 246
Delta Dental Plan of New Hampshire
Concord, NH — Page 265
Delta Dental Plan of New Jersey
Parsippany, NJ — Page 271
Delta Dental Plan of New Mexico
Albuquerque, NM — Page 279
Delta Dental Plan of North Carolina
Raleigh, NC — Page 312
Delta Dental Plan of Ohio Inc
Westerville, OH — Page 324
Delta Dental Plan of Puerto Rico
Santruce, PR — Page 377
Delta Dental Plan of South Carolina
Columbia, SC — Page 384
Delta Dental Plan of Wisconsin
Racine, WI — Page 463
Delta Dental Plan of Wyoming
Cheyenne, WY — Page 473
Delta Dental Plans Association
Oak Brook Village, IL — Page 146
Delta Dental of Florida
Maitland, FL — Page 108
Delta Dental of Nebraska
Omaha, NE — Page 256
Delta Dental of Oklahoma
Oklahoma City, OK — Page 340
Delta Dental of Pennsylvania
Mechanicsburg, PA — Page 361
Delta Dental of Rhode Island
Providence, RI — Page 380
Delta Dental of Virginia
Roanoke, VA — Page 443
DeltaCare USA
Cerritos, CA — Page 44
Dencap Dental Plans
Detroit, MI — Page 220
DentCare Delivery Systems Inc
Uniondale, NY — Page 289
Denta Quest Mid-Atlantic Inc
Calverton, MD — Page 202
Denta Quest Ventures Inc
Boston, MA — Page 211
Dental Benefit Providers Inc
Rockville, MD — Page 202
Dental Benefit Providers of CA Inc
San Francisco, CA — Page 45
Dental Health Services
Long Beach, CA — Page 45
Dental Health Services Inc
Seattle, WA — Page 450
Dental Network of America
Oakbrook Terrace, IL — Page 146
Dms Dental Plan
Warwick, RI — Page 380
Dominion Dental Services - Corporate Headquarters
Alexandria, VA — Page 444
Doral Dental USA
Mequon, WI — Page 464

E

Elderplan Inc
Brooklyn, NY — Page 289
Employers Dental Services Inc
Tucson, AZ — Page 15
Eye Care of Wisconsin Inc
Milwaukee, WI — Page 464
Eyexam of California Inc
Mission Viejo, CA — Page 46

F

First Commonwealth
Chicago, IL — Page 147
FirstSight Vision Services Inc
Upland, CA — Page 47
Florida Health Partners Inc
Tampa, FL — Page 110
For Eyes Vision Plan Inc
Berkeley, CA — Page 47

G

Golden Dental Plans Inc
Warren, MI — Page 221
Golden West Dental & Vision
Camarillo, CA — Page 47
Great Expressions Dental Centers
Bloomfield Hills, MI — Page 222

H

Health Resources Inc
Evansville, IN — Page 161
Healthplex Inc
Uniondale, NY — Page 296
Holman Group, The
Northridge, CA — Page 51
Horizon Behavioral Services
Lewisville, TX — Page 417
Horizon Healthcare Dental Inc
Newark, NJ — Page 273
Human Affairs International of California
El Segundo, CA — Page 52
Humana Health Care Plans of Arizona
Phoenix, AZ — Page 17
Humana Inc - Arkansas
Louisville, KY — Page 27
Humana Inc - Colorado
Englewood, CO — Page 82
Humana Inc - Corporate Headquarters
Louisville, KY — Page 185

I

Iowa Health Solutions
Rock Island, IL — Page 171

J

Jaimini Health Inc
Rancho Cucamonga, CA — Page 53
JPS Benefits
Fort Worth, TX — Page 419

K

Keystone Health Plan East Inc
Philadelphia, PA — Page 368

L

Landmark Healthcare Inc
Sacramento, CA — Page 56
Liberty Dental Plan of California
Irvine, CA — Page 56

M

Magellan Behavioral Care of Iowa Inc
West Des Moines, IA — Page 171
Magellan Health Services
Macon, GA — Page 132
Managed Care of North America Inc
Ft Lauderdale, FL — Page 115
Managed Dental Care
Woodland Hills, CA — Page 57
Managed Health Network
Point Richmond, CA — Page 57
Managed Health Services Indiana Inc
Indianapolis, IN — Page 163
Medical Eye Services Inc
Santa Ana, CA — Page 58
Meritain Health
Cleveland, OH — Page 330
Midwestern Dental Plans Inc
Dearborn, MI — Page 226

N

National Pacific Dental
Houston, TX — Page 421
Neighborhood Health Providers
New York, NY — Page 302
Nevada Pacific Dental
Las Vegas, NV — Page 262
New York Compensation Managers Inc
Syracuse, NY — Page 302
New York State Catholic Health Plan Inc
Rego Park, NY — Page 303
Newport Dental Plan
Santa Ana, CA — Page 60

O

On Lok Senior Health Services
San Francisco, CA — Page 60
Opticare Managed Vision
Rocky Mount, NC — Page 314
OraQuest Dental Plans
Sugarland, TX — Page 421

P

PacifiCare Behavioral Health
Santa Ana, CA — Page 61
PacifiCare Dental & Vision
Santa Ana, CA — Page 61
PacifiCare of Colorado/United Healthcare
Greenwood Village, CO — Page 84
Pacific Union Dental Inc
Concord, CA — Page 63

Index IV: Specialty HMOs

20/20 Eyecare Plan Inc
Ft Lauderdale, FL — Page 99

A

Access Dental Services
Sacramento, CA — Page 31
ACN Group
Golden Valley, MN — Page 233
ACN Group of California - Western Region
San Diego, CA — Page 31
Advantica Eyecare Inc
Clearwater, FL — Page 99
AECC Total Vision Health Plan of Texas Inc
Dallas, TX — Page 403
Aetna Dental Inc - New Jersey
Fairfield, NJ — Page 267
Aetna Inc - Dental Care of California
Thousand Oaks, CA — Page 32
Aetna Inc - Dental Plan of Texas
Dallas, TX — Page 403
Affinity Dental Health Plans
Culver City, CA — Page 32
Aids Healthcare Foundation
Los Angeles, CA — Page 32
Alignis Inc
Paramus, NJ — Page 268
Alpha Dental Programs Inc
Flower Mound, TX — Page 404
Altus Dental Insurance Company Inc
Providence, RI — Page 379
American Healthguard Corporation
Arcadia, CA — Page 33
American Specialty Health Plans Inc
San Diego, CA — Page 33
American WholeHealth Networks Inc
Sterling, VA — Page 442
Ameritas Managed Dental Plan Inc
Costa Mesa, CA — Page 34
Anthem Blue Cross Blue Shield of Wisconsin
Milwaukee, WI — Page 461
APS Healthcare Inc
Silver Springs, MD — Page 199
APS Healthcare Midwest Inc
Brookfield, WI — Page 461
APS Healthcare Northwest Inc
Missoula, MT — Page 253
Assurant Employee Benefits - Alabama
Birmingham, AL — Page 3
Assurant Employee Benefits - Arizona
Phoenix, AZ — Page 12
Assurant Employee Benefits - California
San Diego, CA — Page 35
Assurant Employee Benefits - Colorado
Greenwood Village, CO — Page 78
Assurant Employee Benefits - Corporate Office
Kansas City, MO — Page 244
Assurant Employee Benefits - Florida
Tampa, FL — Page 102
Assurant Employee Benefits - Georgia
Atlanta, GA — Page 127
Assurant Employee Benefits - Illinois
Oakbrook Terrace, IL — Page 143
Assurant Employee Benefits - Indiana
Mooresville, IN — Page 158
Assurant Employee Benefits - Michigan
Troy, MI — Page 217
Assurant Employee Benefits - New Mexico
Albuquerque, NM — Page 279
Assurant Employee Benefits - New York
New York, NY — Page 285
Assurant Employee Benefits - North Carolina
Raleigh, NC — Page 309
Assurant Employee Benefits - Pennsylvania
Radnor, PA — Page 357
Assurant Employee Benefits - Tennessee
Nashville, TN — Page 392
Assurant Employee Benefits - Washington
Seattle, WA — Page 449
Atlantic Dental Inc
Coral Gables, FL — Page 102
Avante Behavioral Health Plan
Fresno, CA — Page 35
Avesis Inc
Phoenix, AZ — Page 12

B

Basic Chiropractic Health Plan Inc
Stockton, CA — Page 35
Behavioral Healthcare Inc
Centennial, CO — Page 78
Behavioral Healthcare Options Inc
Las Vegas, NV — Page 259
Block Vision of Texas Inc
Dallas, TX — Page 405
Blue Cross Blue Shield of Florida/ Health Options Inc
Jacksonville, FL — Page 104

C

California Benefits Dental Plan
Santa Ana, CA — Page 37
California Dental Network Inc
Santa Ana, CA — Page 37
Care-Plus Dental Plans Inc
Wauwatosa, WI — Page 462
CareGuide
Coral Springs, FL — Page 105
Catalina Behavioral Health Services Inc
Mesa, AZ — Page 13
ChiroSource - Corporate Headquarters
Concord, CA — Page 40
CIGNA Behavioral Health Inc
Glendale, CA — Page 40
CIGNA Behavioral Health Inc
Hartford, CT — Page 88
CIGNA Behavioral Health Inc
Irving, TX — Page 408
CIGNA Behavioral Health Inc - Corporate Headquarters
Eden Prairie, MN — Page 234
CIGNA Dental Health Inc - Corporation Headquarters
Sunrise, FL — Page 106
CIGNA Dental Health Plan of Arizona Inc
Sunrise, FL — Page 14
CIGNA Dental Health of California Inc
Glendale, CA — Page 40
CIGNA Dental Health of Colorado
Sunrise, FL — Page 78
CIGNA Dental Health of Delaware Inc
Sunrise, FL — Page 95
CIGNA Dental Health of Florida
Sunrise, FL — Page 107
CIGNA Dental Health of Kansas Inc
Sunrise, FL — Page 177
CIGNA Dental Health of Maryland Inc
Sunrise, FL — Page 201
CIGNA Dental Health of North Carolina Inc
Sunrise, FL — Page 310
CIGNA Dental Health of Ohio Inc
Sunrise, FL — Page 322
CIGNA Dental Health of Pennsylvania Inc
Sunrise, FL — Page 360
CIGNA Dental Health of Texas Inc
Irving, TX — Page 409
CIGNA Dental Health of Virginia Inc
Sunrise, FL — Page 443
CO/OP Optical Services Inc
Detroit, MI — Page 219
Colorado Dental Service Inc, dba: Delta Dental Plan of CO
Denver, CO — Page 80
Colorado Health Networks LLC
Colorado Springs, CO — Page 80
Community Medical Alliance
Boston, MA — Page 210
CompBenefits - Denticare Inc
Houston, TX — Page 410
CompBenefits Corporation - Corporate Headquarters
Roswell, GA — Page 129
Comprehensive Behavioral Care Inc
Tampa, FL — Page 108
Concern: Employee Assistance Program
Mountain View, CA — Page 42
CorpHealth Inc
Fort Worth, TX — Page 412
Coventry Health Care Inc — Iowa
Urbandale, IA — Page 169

D

Dedicated Dental Systems
Bakersfield, CA — Page 43
Delta Dental Insurance Company - Georgia
Alpharetta, GA — Page 131
Delta Dental Insurance Company - Nevada
Las Vegas, NV — Page 259
Delta Dental Insurance Company - Texas
Irving, TX — Page 412
Delta Dental Plan Inc - Utah
Salt Lake City, UT — Page 434
Delta Dental Plan of Arizona Inc
Phoenix, AZ — Page 14
Delta Dental Plan of Arkansas
Sherwood, AR — Page 26
Delta Dental Plan of California
San Francisco, CA — Page 44
Delta Dental Plan of Idaho
Boise, ID — Page 141
Delta Dental Plan of Illinois
Lisle, IL — Page 145
Delta Dental Plan of Indiana Inc
Indianapolis, IN — Page 159
Delta Dental Plan of Kansas
Wichita, KS — Page 178
Delta Dental Plan of Kentucky Inc
Louisville, KY — Page 184
Delta Dental Plan of Michigan Inc
Okemos, MI — Page 220

Index IV

Specialty HMOs

Index III: Preferred Provider Organizations

Wellmark Blue Cross & Blue Shield of South Dakota
Sioux Falls, SD — Page 389

Wellmark Blue Cross Blue Shield of Iowa
Des Moines, IA — Page 174

**Wellmark Inc —
Corporate Headquarters**
Des Moines, IA — Page 175

Wellpath Select Inc
Morrisville, NC — Page 315

Wisconsin Physician Services Insurance Company
Madison, WI — Page 471

Index III: Preferred Provider Organizations

Regence Blue Cross Blue Shield of Utah
Salt Lake City, UT — Page 436
Regence Blue Shield
Burlington, WA — Page 456
Regence Blue Shield
Seattle, WA — Page 456
Regence Group, The — Corporate Headquarters
Portland, OR — Page 351
Regence Valucare
Salt Lake City, UT — Page 436
Rocky Mountain HealthCare Options Inc dba Healthcare Options
Grand Junction, CO — Page 84
Rocky Mountain Hosital & Medical Services Inc
Denver, CO — Page 85

S

Sagamore Health Network Inc
Carmel, IN — Page 164
Saint Mary's HealthFirst
Reno, NV — Page 263
San Joaquin Foundation PPO
Murphys, CA — Page 67
Secure Health Plans of Georgia LLC
Macon, GA — Page 133
SecureCare Dental
Phoenix, AZ — Page 20
Select Circle Health Plan
Muncie, IN — Page 165
SelectHealth
Salt Lake City, UT — Page 437
SelectHealth Network
Evansville, IN — Page 165
Selectcare Access Corporation
Pittsburgh, PA — Page 371
Sierra Health Services Inc-Corporate Headquarters
Las Vegas, NV — Page 264
Signature Health Alliance
Nashville, TN — Page 398
Sloan's Lake Preferred Health Networks
Greenwood Village, CO — Page 85
South Bay Independent Physicians Medical Group Inc
Torrance, CA — Page 69
South Central Preferred
York, PA — Page 372
Southcare/Healthcare Preferred
Atlanta, GA — Page 134
Southeastern Indiana Health Organization
Columbus, IN — Page 166
Southern Health Services Inc
Charlottesville, VA — Page 445
Southwest Health Alliance (SHALLC)
Austin, TX — Page 425
St Francis Optimum Health Network
Greenville, SC — Page 385
Stanislaus Medical Society
Modesto, CA — Page 70
Staywell Insurance Guam Inc
Hagatna, GU — Page 135
Summacare Inc
Akron, OH — Page 334
Summerlin Life & Health Insurance Company
Las Vegas, NV — Page 264
Summerline Life & Health Insurance Company
Honolulu, HI — Page 138

SuperMed Network
Cleveland, OH — Page 334
Superien Health Network Inc
Stow, OH — Page 335
Susquehanna Health Care
Berwick, PA — Page 372

T

Tenet Choices Inc
Metaire, LA — Page 192
Tennessee Healthcare LLC
Brentwood, TN — Page 399
Texas True Choice
Plano, TX — Page 428
Triple-S Inc
San Juan, PR — Page 378
Trustmark Insurance Company
Lake Forest, IL — Page 153
Tufts Health Plan
Watertown, MA — Page 216

U

Unicare Health Plans of the Midwest Inc
Chicago, IL — Page 153
Unicare Life and Health Insurance Co Inc
Houston, TX — Page 428
United Behavioral Health
Philadelphia, PA — Page 373
UnitedHealth Group — Corporate Headquarters
Minnetonka, MN — Page 238
UnitedHealthcare & Mid Atlantic Medical Services Inc
Rockville, MD — Page 206
UnitedHealthcare Services Company of the River Valley Inc
Peoria, IL — Page 154
UnitedHealthcare Services Company of the River Valley Inc
Moline, IL — Page 154
UnitedHealthcare of Alabama
Birmingham, AL — Page 7
UnitedHealthcare of Arizona Inc
Phoenix, AZ — Page 21
UnitedHealthcare of Arkansas
Little Rock, AR — Page 28
UnitedHealthcare of Colorado
Centennial, CO — Page 85
UnitedHealthcare of Florida Inc
Jacksonville, FL — Page 121
UnitedHealthcare of Florida Inc
Maitland, FL — Page 121
UnitedHealthcare of Florida Inc
Tampa, FL — Page 122
UnitedHealthcare of Georgia
Norcross, GA — Page 134
UnitedHealthcare of Illinois Inc
Chicago, IL — Page 154
UnitedHealthcare of Kentucky
Lexington, KY — Page 186
UnitedHealthcare of Louisiana
Metairie, LA — Page 193
UnitedHealthcare of Massachusetts
Waltham, MA — Page 216
UnitedHealthcare of Mississippi Inc
Ridgeland, MS — Page 242
UnitedHealthcare of New England Inc
Warwick, RI — Page 381
UnitedHealthcare of New York Metropolitan
New York, NY — Page 306

UnitedHealthcare of Ohio Inc
Westerville, OH — Page 336
UnitedHealthcare of Ohio Inc-Cleveland
Cleveland, OH — Page 336
UnitedHealthcare of Oregon
Long Beach, CA — Page 352
UnitedHealthcare of SW Ohio Inc-Dayton/Cincinnati
Westchester, OH — Page 337
UnitedHealthcare of South Florida
Sunrise, FL — Page 122
UnitedHealthcare of Tennessee Inc
Brentwood, TN — Page 401
UnitedHealthcare of Texas Inc - Houston
Houston, TX — Page 429
UnitedHealthcare of Texas Inc - San Antonio
San Antonio, TX — Page 430
UnitedHealthcare of Texas Inc — Dallas
Plano, TX — Page 430
UnitedHealthcare of Utah
Salt Lake City, UT — Page 437
UnitedHealthcare of Virginia
Richmond, VA — Page 446
UnitedHealthcare of Wisconsin Inc
Milwaukee, WI — Page 470
UnitedHealthcare of the Heartland States
Overland Park, KS — Page 182
UnitedHealthcare of the Midlands Inc
Omaha, NE — Page 257
Unity Health Insurance
Sauk City, WI — Page 470
Univera Healthcare of Western New York
Buffalo, NY — Page 307
Universal Health Network - Corporate Headquarters
Reno, NV — Page 264
University Health Alliance
Honolulu, HI — Page 138
University Health Plans Inc
Newark, NJ — Page 277
USA Managed Care Organization
Phoenix, AZ — Page 22
Utah Public Employees Health Program
Salt Lake City, UT — Page 438

V

Valley Preferred
Allentown, PA — Page 375
Vantage Health Plan Inc
Monroe, LA — Page 193
Vantage PPO
Meadville, PA — Page 375
Ventura County Foundation for Medical Care
Camarillo, CA — Page 73
Virginia Health Network
Richmond, VA — Page 447
Vista Health Plan Inc
Hollywood, FL — Page 123
Vista Healthplan of South Florida Inc
Sunrise, FL — Page 123
Volusia Health Network
Holly Hill, FL — Page 124

W

WellPoint Inc - Corporate Headquarters
Indianapolis, IN — Page 167

Index III: Preferred Provider Organizations

Mercy of Iowa City Regional PHO - Priority Health Network
Iowa City, IA — Page 172
Meritain Health Inc
Amherst, NY — Page 299
Mid Atlantic Medical Services Inc (MAMSI)- Corp Headquarters
Rockville, MD — Page 204
Mid-Atlantic Managed Care Organization of Pennsylvania Inc
Gettysburg, PA — Page 369
Midlands Choice Inc
Omaha, NE — Page 256
Mountain Medical Affiliates
Greenwood Village, CO — Page 83
Mountain State Blue Cross Blue Shield
Parkersburg, WV — Page 460
MultiPlan Inc - Corporate Headquarters
New York, NY — Page 300
MVP Health Plan Inc
Schenectady, NY — Page 301
MVP Health Plan of New Hampshire
Bedford, NH — Page 266

N

NAMCI
Huntsville, AL — Page 6
National Capital PPO
Springfield, VA — Page 444
National Health Plan
New York, NY — Page 302
Nationwide Health Plans
Columbus, OH — Page 331
Network Health Plan Wisconsin
Menasha, WI — Page 468
Nevada Preferred Professionals
Las Vegas, NV — Page 262
New England Financial - Corporate Headquarters
Boston, MA — Page 214
New West Health Services
Helena, MT — Page 254
Northeast Health Direct LLC
Marlborough, CT — Page 92
Novasys Health Network
Little Rock, AR — Page 28

O

ODS Health Plan
Portland, OR — Page 349
Ohio Health Choice
Akron, OH — Page 332
Ohio State University Managed Health Care Systems Inc
Columbus, OH — Page 332
OhioHealth Group
Columbus, OH — Page 332
Olympus Managed Health Care Inc
Miami, FL — Page 117
OneNet PPO
Rockville, MD — Page 205
Optima Health Plan Inc
Virginia Beach, VA — Page 445
Orange County PPO
Orange, CA — Page 61
OSF Health Plans
Peoria, IL — Page 151

Oxford Health Plans Inc — Corporate Headquarters
Trumbell, CT — Page 92
Oxford Health Plans of New Jersey Inc
Iselin, NJ — Page 275
Oxford Health Plans of New York, Inc
New York, NY — Page 303

P

PacifiCare Health Systems- Corporate Headquarters
Santa Ana, CA — Page 62
PacifiCare of California
Cypress, CA — Page 62
PacifiCare of Colorado/ United Healthcare
Greenwood Village, CO — Page 84
PacifiCare of Nevada
Las Vegas, NV — Page 263
PacifiCare of Oregon
Lake Oswego, OR — Page 350
PacifiCare of Texas Inc
Dallas, TX — Page 422
Pacific Health Alliance
Burlingame, CA — Page 62
PacificSource Health Plans
Springfield, OR — Page 350
Paramount Health Care Plan
Maumee, OH — Page 333
Parkview Signature Care
Ft Wayne, IN — Page 164
Partners National Health Plans of North Carolina Inc
Winston-Salem, NC — Page 314
Penn Highlands Health Plan
Johnstown, PA — Page 370
PerfectHealth Insurance Company
Staten Island, NY — Page 304
PersonalCare Insurance of Illinois Inc
Champaign, IL — Page 151
Phoebe Health Partners
Albany, GA — Page 133
PHP Companies Inc
Knoxville, TN — Page 397
Physicians Foundation for Medical Care
San Jose, CA — Page 64
Physicians Health Plan of South Michigan
Jackson, MI — Page 229
Pioneer Health - The PPO
West Springfield, MA — Page 215
PPO USA Inc
Lee's Summit, MO — Page 250
ppoNEXT
Dallas, TX — Page 423
Ppoplus LLC
New Orleans, LA — Page 192
Preferred Care
Rochester, NY — Page 304
Preferred Care Incorporated
Ft Washington, PA — Page 370
Preferred Chiropractic Care Inc
Wichita, KS — Page 179
Preferred Health Care
Lancaster, PA — Page 370
Preferred Health Plan Inc
Klamath Falls, OR — Page 350
Preferred Health Professionals
Overland Park, KS — Page 180
Preferred Health Systems
Wichita, KS — Page 180
Preferred Healthcare System Inc
Altoona, PA — Page 371

Preferred One
Golden Valley, MN — Page 237
Preferred Provider Organization of Michigan (PPOM)
Southfield, MI — Page 229
Premera - Corporate Headquarters
Mountlake Terrace, WA — Page 454
Premera Blue Cross - Eastern
Spokane, WA — Page 454
Premera Blue Cross - Western
Mountlake Terrace, WA — Page 454
Premera Blue Cross Blue Shield of Alaska
Anchorage, AK — Page 9
Premier Health Networks of Alabama LLC
Huntsville, AL — Page 6
Presbyterian Health Plan
Alburquerque, NM — Page 281
Prevea Health Network
Green Bay, WI — Page 469
Primary Health Plan
Boise, ID — Page 142
Primary Provider Management Company Inc
San Diego, CA — Page 64
Prime Health Services Inc
Brentwood, TN — Page 398
Principal Life Insurance Company
West Des Moines, IA — Page 172
Priority Health
Grand Rapids, MI — Page 230
Private Healthcare Systems - California
Irvine, CA — Page 65
Private Healthcare Systems - Corporate Headquarters
Waltham, MA — Page 215
Private Healthcare Systems - Georgia
Atlanta, GA — Page 133
Private Healthcare Systems - Illinois
Rosemont, IL — Page 153
Private Healthcare Systems - Missouri
Kansas City, MO — Page 251
Private Healthcare Systems - Texas
Dallas, TX — Page 423
Private Healthcare Systems - Washington
Bothell, WA — Page 455
ProviDRs Care Network
Wichita, KS — Page 181
Providence Health Plans
Beaverton, OR — Page 351
Provider Networks of America Inc
Arlington, TX — Page 424
Pueblo Health Care
Pueblo, CO — Page 84

Q

QualCare Inc
Piscataway, NJ — Page 276
Quincy Health Care Management Inc
Quincy, IL — Page 153

R

Regence Blue Cross Blue Shield of Oregon
Portland, OR — Page 351

Index III: Preferred Provider Organizations

HealthSpring Inc - Tennessee
Nashville, TN — Page 395
Healthcare Partners of East Texas Inc
Longview, TX — Page 416
Healthnow
Memphis, TN — Page 395
HFN Inc
Oak Brook, IL — Page 150
Highmark Inc
Pittsburgh, PA — Page 366
HIP Health Plan of New York
New York, NY — Page 296
HMO Louisiana Inc
Baton Rouge, LA — Page 191
HMS Colorado Inc
Greenwood Village, CO — Page 82
Hometown Health Plan
Reno, NV — Page 260
Horizon Blue Cross/Blue Shield of NJ
Newark, NJ — Page 273
Horizon Health PPO
Henderson, NV — Page 261
Horizon Healthcare Services Inc
Newark, NJ — Page 274
Humana Health Care Plans of Arizona
Phoenix, AZ — Page 17
Humana Health Care Plans of Corpus Christi
Corpus Christi, TX — Page 417
Humana Health Care Plans of Dallas
Dallas, TX — Page 417
Humana Health Care Plans of Houston
Houston, TX — Page 418
Humana Health Care Plans of Illinois
Chicago, IL — Page 151
Humana Health Care Plans of Kansas & Missouri
Overland Park, KS — Page 179
Humana Health Care Plans of Lexington
Lexington, KY — Page 185
Humana Health Care Plans of San Antonio/Austin
San Antonio, TX — Page 418
Humana Health Plan - Jacksonville
Jacksonville, FL — Page 113
Humana Health Plan - Kentucky
Louisville, KY — Page 185
Humana Health Plan of Austin
Austin, TX — Page 419
Humana Health Plan of Ohio Inc
Cincinnati, OH — Page 328
Humana Health Plans of Georgia
Atlanta, GA — Page 132
Humana Inc - Arkansas
Louisville, KY — Page 27
Humana Inc - Colorado
Englewood, CO — Page 82
Humana Inc - Corporate Headquarters
Louisville, KY — Page 185
Humana Inc - District of Columbia
Louisville, KY — Page 98
Humana Inc - Grand Rapids Michigan
Grand Rapids, MI — Page 225
Humana Inc - Indiana
Indianapolis, IN — Page 161
Humana Inc - Iowa
Louisville, KY — Page 170
Humana Inc - Maryland
Louisville, KY — Page 203
Humana Inc - Mississippi
Louisville, KY — Page 241
Humana Inc - Nebraska
Louisville, KY — Page 256
Humana Inc - New Mexico
Louisville, KY — Page 280

Humana Inc - North Carolina
Charlotte, NC — Page 313
Humana Inc - North Dakota
Louisville, KY — Page 317
Humana Inc - Oklahoma
Louisville, KY — Page 341
Humana Inc - South Carolina
Louisville, KY — Page 384
Humana Inc - South Dakota
Louisville, KY — Page 388
Humana Inc - Tennessee
Memphis, TN — Page 396
Humana Inc - Utah
Louisville, KY — Page 435
Humana Inc - Wyoming
Laramie, WY — Page 473
Humana Inc/PCA - Puerto Rico
San Juan, PR — Page 377
Humana Insurance Co - Alabama
DePere, AL — Page 5
Humana Medical Plan - Daytona
Daytona Beach, FL — Page 113
Humana Military Service Inc
Louisville, KY — Page 186
Hygeia Corporation
Miami Lakes, FL — Page 114

I

IBA Health Plans
Kalamazoo, MI — Page 225
Independence Blue Cross
Philadelphia, PA — Page 366
Independent Health Association Inc
Buffalo, NY — Page 297
Indiana Health Network
Indianapolis, IN — Page 161
Indiana Pro Health Network
Indianapolis, IN — Page 162
Individualized Care Management Inc
Lafayette, IN — Page 162
Initial Group Inc, The
Nashville, TN — Page 396
Inland Empire Foundation for Medical Care
Riverside, CA — Page 52
Integra Group
Cincinnati, OH — Page 329
Integrated Health Plan Inc
St Petersburg, FL — Page 115
Intergroup Services Corporation
Malvern, PA — Page 367
Interplan Health Group
Stockton, CA — Page 53
Interplan Health Group
Arlington, TX — Page 419
Interplan Health Group - Corporate Headquarters
Farmington, CT — Page 91
Iowa Foundation for Medical Care/ Encompass
West Des Moines, IA — Page 170

K

Kern Foundation/Preferred Provider Organization
Bakersfield, CA — Page 55

Keystone Health Plan East Inc
Philadelphia, PA — Page 368
KHS a KMG America Company
Lancaster, SC — Page 385
KPS Health Plans
Bremerton, WA — Page 452

L

Lakewood Health Plan Inc
Lakewood, CA — Page 56
Legacy Health Plan Inc
San Angelo, TX — Page 420
LifeWise Health Plan of Arizona
Scottsdale, AZ — Page 17
LifeWise Health Plan of Oregon
Portland, OR — Page 348
LifeWise Health Plan of Washington
Mountlake Terrace, WA — Page 453
Lifetime Healthcare Companies, The - Corporate Headquarters
Rochester, NY — Page 298
Lovelace Health Plan
Albuquerque, NM — Page 280
Lutheran Preferred/Three Rivers Preferred
Ft Wayne, IN — Page 162

M

M Plan Inc
Indianapolis, IN — Page 163
M-Care Inc
Ann Arbor, MI — Page 225
MagnaCare
Garden City, NY — Page 298
Managed Care Consultants
Henderson, NV — Page 261
Managed HealthCare Northwest Inc
Portland, OR — Page 348
Martins Point Health Care
Portland, ME — Page 196
MD-Individual Practice Association Inc (MD IPA)
Rockville, MD — Page 204
MedAvant National Preferred Provider Network
Middletown, NY — Page 299
Medcost LLC
Winston-Salem, NC — Page 313
Medica Health Plans
Minnetonka, MN — Page 236
Medical Card System
Hato Rey, PR — Page 377
Medical Care Referral Group
El Paso, TX — Page 420
Medical Eye Services Inc
Santa Ana, CA — Page 58
Medical Mutual of Ohio
Cleveland, OH — Page 330
Medical Network Inc
Portland, ME — Page 197
Mega Life & Health Insurance Company
North Richland Hills, TX — Page 420
Mendocino and Lake Counties Foundation for Medical Care
Ukiah, CA — Page 59
Mercer First Choice
Sharon, PA — Page 369
Mercy Health Plans of Missouri Inc
Chesterfield, MO — Page 249

Index III: Preferred Provider Organizations

E

Ehp Inc
Lancaster, PA — Page 362
EM Risk Management, A POMCO Company
Endicott, NY — Page 290
EmblemHealth Inc
New York, NY — Page 290
Emerald Health Network Inc, The
Cleveland, OH — Page 325
Empire Blue Cross Blue Shield
New York, NY — Page 290
Employee Benefits Corporation
Middletown, WI — Page 464
Encore Health Network
Indianapolis, IN — Page 160
Evergreen Medical Group LLC
Columbus, GA — Page 131
Evolutions Healthcare Systems Inc
New Port Richey, FL — Page 109
Excellus BlueCross BlueShield
Rochester, NY — Page 290
Excellus BlueCross BlueShield, Rochester Region
Rochester, NY — Page 292
Exempla Healthcare LLC
Denver, CO — Page 81

F

Fallon Community Health Plan Inc
Worcester, MA — Page 211
Family Choice Health Alliance
Hackensack, NJ — Page 272
Fara Healthcare Management
Mandeville, LA — Page 190
Finger Lakes Community Care Network
Canandaigua, NY — Page 293
First Choice Health Network
Seattle, WA — Page 451
First Choice of the Midwest Inc
Sioux Falls, SD — Page 388
First Health — California
W Sacramento, CA — Page 46
First Health Group Corp
Downers Grove, IL — Page 147
First Health Network
San Diego, CA — Page 46
First Health Network (PPO Oklahoma Inc)
Oklahoma City, OK — Page 341
Flora Health Network
Cleveland, OH — Page 325
Forte Managed Care
Austin, TX — Page 414
Fortified Provider Network Inc
Scottsdale, AZ — Page 15

G

Galaxy Health Network
Arlington, TX — Page 414
Geisinger Health Plan
Danville, PA — Page 363
GenWorth Life & Health Insurance Co
Windsor, CT — Page 90
Good Health HMO Inc
Kansas City, MO — Page 247
Great West Life Annuity Insurance Co
Greenwood Village, CO — Page 81
Great-West Healthcare - Corporate
Greenwood Village, CO — Page 81
Great-West Healthcare - New Jersey
Piscataway, NJ — Page 272
Great-West Healthcare of Arizona
Scottsdale, AZ — Page 16
Great-West Healthcare of California
Glendale, CA — Page 48
Great-West Healthcare of California - North
Pleasant Hill, CA — Page 48
Great-West Healthcare of Colorado
Greenwood Village, CO — Page 81
Great-West Healthcare of Florida
Tampa, FL — Page 111
Great-West Healthcare of Georgia
Atlanta, GA — Page 131
Great-West Healthcare of Illinois
Rosemont, IL — Page 148
Great-West Healthcare of Kansas/Missouri
Overland Park, KS — Page 179
Great-West Healthcare of Maine
S Portland, ME — Page 196
Great-West Healthcare of Massachusetts
Waltham, MA — Page 212
Great-West Healthcare of Michigan
Southfield, MI — Page 223
Great-West Healthcare of New York
White Plains, NY — Page 294
Great-West Healthcare of North Carolina
Charlotte, NC — Page 313
Great-West Healthcare of Ohio
Columbus, OH — Page 326
Great-West Healthcare of Ohio
North Olmstead, OH — Page 326
Great-West Healthcare of Oregon
Portland, OR — Page 346
Great-West Healthcare of Pennsylvania
Media, PA — Page 363
Great-West Healthcare of Texas - Austin
Austin, TX — Page 414
Great-West Healthcare of Texas - Dallas
Dallas, TX — Page 415
Great-West Healthcare of Washington Inc
Bellevue, WA — Page 451
Group Health Plan Inc
Earth City, MO — Page 248
GroupLink Inc
Indianapolis, IN — Page 160
Guardian Life Insurance Co of America
New York, NY — Page 294
Gulf Health Plans PPO Inc
Mobile, AL — Page 4

H

Harvard Pilgrim Health Care - Corporate Headquarters
Wellesley, MA — Page 212
Hawaii Management Alliance Association
Honolulu, HI — Page 137
Hawaii Medical Services Association - BC/BS of Hawaii
Honolulu, HI — Page 137
HDN PPO
Wilmette, IL — Page 149
Health Alliance Medical Plans - Corporate Headquarters
Urbana, IL — Page 149
Health Alliance Plan of Michigan
Detroit, MI — Page 223
Health Care Exchange Limited Company
Southfield, MI — Page 223
Health Care Service Corporation - Corporate Headquarters
Chicago, IL — Page 149
Health Design Plus
Hudson, OH — Page 327
Health Management Network Inc
Tempe, AZ — Page 16
Health Net - Connecticut
Shelton, CT — Page 90
Health Net Health Plan of Oregon Inc
Tigard, OR — Page 346
Health Net Inc - Corporate Headquarters
Woodland Hills, CA — Page 49
Health Net Inc - Northeast Corporate Headquarters
Shelton, CT — Page 91
Health Net of Arizona
Tucson, AZ — Page 17
Health Net of California
Woodland Hills, CA — Page 49
Health New England
Springfield, MA — Page 212
Health Plan, The/Hometown Region
Massillon, OH — Page 327
Health Plans Inc
Westborough, MA — Page 213
Health Plus
Peoria, IL — Page 150
Health Resources Inc
Evansville, IN — Page 161
HealthAmerica Pennsylvania Inc - Central Region
Harrisburg, PA — Page 364
HealthAmerica Pennsylvania Inc - Eastern Region
Plymouth Meeting, PA — Page 365
HealthAmerica Pennsylvania Inc - Nortwestern
Erie, PA — Page 365
HealthAmerica Pennsylvania Inc - Western Region
Pittsburgh, PA — Page 365
HealthCare Value Management Inc
Norwood, MA — Page 213
HealthChoice of Alabama
Birmingham, AL — Page 4
HealthEOS by MultiPlan
Brookfield, WI — Page 466
HealthFirst Inc
New York, NY — Page 295
HealthLink Inc
St Louis, MO — Page 248
HealthLink Inc - Corporate Headquarters
St Louis, MO — Page 249
HealthLink of Arkansas Inc
North Little Rock, AR — Page 27
HealthNow New York Inc
Buffalo, NY — Page 295
HealthPartners Inc
Bloomington, MN — Page 236
HealthSmart Preferred Care
Lubbock, TX — Page 416
HealthSpring Inc - Corporate Headquarters
Franklin, TN — Page 395

Index III: Preferred Provider Organizations

Blue Cross Blue Shield of South Carolina - Corporate Hqtrs
Columbia, SC — Page 383

Blue Cross Blue Shield of Tennessee
Chattanooga, TN — Page 392

Blue Cross Blue Shield of Tennessee - Memphis
Memphis, TN — Page 393

Blue Cross Blue Shield of Texas — Corporate Headquarters
Richardson, TX — Page 406

Blue Cross Blue Shield of Texas — HMO Blue - Midwest TX
Austin, TX — Page 406

Blue Cross Blue Shield of Texas — HMO Blue - Southeast
Houston, TX — Page 407

Blue Cross Blue Shield of Texas — HMO Blue - West
El Paso, TX — Page 407

Blue Cross Blue Shield of Vermont
Berlin, VT — Page 439

Blue Cross Blue Shield of Western New York
Buffalo, NY — Page 285

Blue Cross Blue Shield of Wyoming
Cheyenne, WY — Page 473

Blue Cross of Idaho
Meridian, ID — Page 141

Blue Preferred Plan-Blue Cross/Blue Shield Michigan
Detroit, MI — Page 218

Blue Ridge Health Network
Pottsville, PA — Page 357

Blue Shield of California
San Francisco, CA — Page 36

BlueChoice Health Plan of South Carolina Inc
Columbia, SC — Page 383

BlueCross of Northeastern Pennsylvania
Wilkes-Barre, PA — Page 358

BlueShield of Northeastern New York
Latham, NY — Page 286

Bluegrass Family Health Inc
Lexington, KY — Page 183

Brazos Valley Health Network
Waco, TX — Page 408

Broadspire Inc
Plantation, FL — Page 105

Bucks County Physician Hospital Alliance
Doylestown, PA — Page 358

C

Capital Blue Cross
Harrisburg, PA — Page 359

Capital District Physicians Health Plan
Albany, NY — Page 286

Capitol Administrators
Rancho Cordova, CA — Page 38

Care Choices
Farmington Hills, MI — Page 218

CareIQ
Miramar, FL — Page 106

Carelink Health Plans
Wheeling, WV — Page 459

Carelink Health Plans
Charleston, WV — Page 459

Cariten Healthcare
Knoxville, TN — Page 393

Center Care
Bowling Green, KY — Page 184

Central Benefits Mutual Insurance Company
Columbus, OH — Page 321

Central New York East HealthNow New York Inc
East Syracuse, NY — Page 287

Central New York West HealthNow New York Inc
Rochester, NY — Page 287

Central Susquehanna Healthcare Providers
Lewisburg, PA — Page 359

ChiroSource - Corporate Headquarters
Concord, CA — Page 40

CHN Solutions
Hamilton, OH — Page 270

ChoiceCare/Humana
Cincinnati, OH — Page 322

CIGNA Health Plan of Utah Inc
Salt Lake City, UT — Page 433

CIGNA HealthCare — Corporate Headquarters
Philadelphia, PA — Page 360

CIGNA Healthcare
Burlington, VT — Page 439

CIGNA Healthcare - Cincinnati
Cincinnati, OH — Page 323

CIGNA Healthcare of Arizona
Phoenix, AZ — Page 14

CIGNA Healthcare of Colorado
Denver, CO — Page 79

CIGNA Healthcare of Connecticut
Hartford, CT — Page 89

CIGNA Healthcare of Florida
Tampa, FL — Page 107

CIGNA Healthcare of Florida
Sunrise, FL — Page 107

CIGNA Healthcare of Georgia
Atlanta, GA — Page 128

CIGNA Healthcare of Indiana
Indianapolis, IN — Page 158

CIGNA Healthcare of Kansas/Missouri
Overland Park, KS — Page 177

CIGNA Healthcare of Louisiana
Houston, TX — Page 190

CIGNA Healthcare of Maine Inc
Falmouth, ME — Page 195

CIGNA Healthcare of Massachusetts
Newton, MA — Page 210

CIGNA Healthcare of New Hampshire
Hooksett, NH — Page 265

CIGNA Healthcare of New York and New Jersey
Jersey City, NJ — Page 270

CIGNA Healthcare of North Carolina Inc
Charlotte, NC — Page 311

CIGNA Healthcare of North Texas
Irving, TX — Page 409

CIGNA Healthcare of Ohio Inc
Cleveland, OH — Page 323

CIGNA Healthcare of Ohio Inc
Columbus, OH — Page 323

CIGNA Healthcare of PA
Blue Bell, PA — Page 360

CIGNA Healthcare of St Louis
St Louis, MO — Page 245

CIGNA Healthcare of Tennessee
Memphis, TN — Page 393

CIGNA Healthcare of Texas Inc
Houston, TX — Page 409

CIGNA Healthcare of Virginia Inc - Richmond
Richmond, VA — Page 443

Coalition America Inc
Atlanta, GA — Page 129

Coastal Healthcare Administrators
Salinas, CA — Page 41

Community Health Alliance
South Bend, IN — Page 159

Community Health Plan
St Joseph, MO — Page 245

CommunityCare Managed Healthcare Plans of Oklahoma Inc
Tulsa, OK — Page 340

Complementary Healthcare Plans
Beaverton, OR — Page 345

Concentra Operating Corporation
Addison, TX — Page 411

ConnectCare
Midland, MI — Page 219

Connecticare Inc
Farmington, CT — Page 89

Connecticare of Massachusetts Inc
Farmington, CT — Page 210

Coordinated Health Plan
Providence, RI — Page 379

Coordinated Health Systems
Bethlehem, PA — Page 361

Corvel Corporation
Irvine, CA — Page 43

Corvel Corporation
Indianapolis, IN — Page 159

Corvel Corporation
West Des Moines, IA — Page 169

Coventry Health Care
Franklin, TN — Page 394

Coventry Health Care Inc — Carolinas
Charlotte, NC — Page 311

Coventry Health Care Inc — Corporate Headquarters
Bethesda, MD — Page 201

Coventry Health Care Inc — Delaware Inc
Wilmington, DE — Page 96

Coventry Health Care Inc — Georgia Inc
Atlanta, GA — Page 130

Coventry Health Care Inc — Iowa
Urbandale, IA — Page 169

Coventry Health Care Inc — Louisiana
Metairie, LA — Page 190

Coventry Health Care of Kansas - Wichita
Wichita, KS — Page 178

Coventry Health Care of Kansas Inc
Kansas City, MO — Page 245

Coventry Health Care of Nebraska Inc
Omaha, NE — Page 255

Cox Health Plans
Springfield, MO — Page 246

D

Deaconess Health Plans
Evansville, IN — Page 159

Dean Health Plan
Madison, WI — Page 463

Delta Dental Plan of Minnesota
Eagan, MN — Page 235

Delta Dental Plan of Tennessee
Nashville, TN — Page 394

Deseret Healthcare
Salt Lake City, UT — Page 434

Devon Health Services Inc
King of Prussia, PA — Page 361

Dimension Health (PPO)
Miami Lakes, FL — Page 109

DMC Care
Detroit, MI — Page 22

Index III: Preferred Provider Organizations

1st Medical Network
Atlanta, GA — Page 127
4MOST Health Network
Charleston, WV — Page 459

A

ACN Group
Golden Valley, MN — Page 233
ACN Group of California - Western Region
San Diego, CA — Page 31
Aetna Health Inc
Houston, TX — Page 403
Aetna Health Inc - Colorado
Greenwood Village, CO — Page 77
Aetna Health Plans of Mid-Atlantic
Falls Church, VA — Page 441
Aetna Health of California Inc
Walnut Creek, CA — Page 31
Aetna Health of Illinois Inc
Chicago, IL — Page 143
Aetna Inc
Norwalk, CT — Page 87
Aetna Inc - Arizona
Phoenix, AZ — Page 11
Aetna Inc - Arkansas
Metairie, LA — Page 25
Aetna Inc - Arkansas
Little Rock, AR — Page 25
Aetna Inc - Corporate Headquarters
Hartford, CT — Page 87
Aetna Inc - Corporate Headquarters
Blue Bell, PA — Page 355
Aetna Inc - Florida
Tampa, FL — Page 100
Aetna Inc - Georgia
Alpheretta, GA — Page 127
Aetna Inc - Jacksonville
Jacksonville, FL — Page 100
Aetna Inc - Maine
Portland, ME — Page 195
Aetna Inc - Maryland
Linthicum, MD — Page 199
Aetna Inc - Missouri
Chesterfield, MO — Page 243
Aetna Inc - New Jersey
Mt Laurel, NJ — Page 267
Aetna Inc - New Jersey
Fairfield, NJ — Page 267
Aetna Inc - New York
Uniondale, NY — Page 283
Aetna Inc - Pennsylvania
Pittsburgh, PA — Page 355
Aetna Inc - Pennsylvania
King of Prussia, PA — Page 355
Aetna Inc - Pennsylvania Region
Blue Bell, PA — Page 356
Aetna Inc - Plantation
Plantation, FL — Page 100
Aetna Inc - Tennessee
Nashville, TN — Page 391
Aetna Inc - Tulsa
Tulsa, OK — Page 339
Aetna Inc - Virginia
Richmond, VA — Page 441
Aetna Inc - Washington
Seattle, WA — Page 449
Aetna Inc of New England
Middletown, CT — Page 87
Aetna Inc of the Carolinas
Charlotte, NC — Page 309
All Florida PPO Inc
Pompano Beach, FL — Page 101

Alliance Regional Health Network
Amarillo, TX — Page 404
Allianz Life Insurance Company of North America
Minneapolis, MN — Page 233
Altius Health Plans
South Jordan, UT — Page 433
AmeriHealth Insurance Company
Wilmington, DE — Page 95
American Healthcare Alliance
Kansas City, MO — Page 243
American Healthcare Group INC
Pittsburgh, PA — Page 356
American LIFECARE - Louisiana
New Orleans, LA — Page 189
American LIFECARE - Mississippi
Jackson, MS — Page 241
American National Insurance Company
Galveston, TX — Page 405
American Preferred Provider Organization LLC
Irving, TX — Page 405
American Republic Insurance Company
Des Moines, IA — Page 169
Americas PPO
Bloomington, MN — Page 233
Amerihealth Insurance Company - NJ North
Iselin, NJ — Page 269
Amerihealth Insurance Company - NJ South
Mt Laurel, NJ — Page 269
Anthem Blue Cross
Woodland Hills, CA — Page 34
Anthem Blue Cross Blue Shield of Colorado
Denver, CO — Page 77
Anthem Blue Cross Blue Shield of Maine
South Portland, ME — Page 195
Anthem Blue Cross Blue Shield of Missouri
St Louis, MO — Page 243
Anthem Blue Cross Blue Shield of Nevada
Reno, NV — Page 259
Anthem Blue Cross Blue Shield of Ohio
Mason, OH — Page 320
Anthem Blue Cross Blue Shield of Virginia Inc
Richmond, VA — Page 442
Anthem Blue Cross Blue Shield of Wisconsin
Milwaukee, WI — Page 461
Anthem Blue Cross and Blue Shield of Kentucky (HMO Kentucky)
Louisville, KY — Page 183
Anthem Blue Cross and Blue Shield of Ohio
Cincinnati, OH — Page 320
Anthem Blue Cross/Blue Shield of Indiana
Indianapolis, IN — Page 157
Anthem Blue Cross/Blue Shield of New Hampshire
Manchester, NH — Page 265
Anthem Health Plan Inc dba: Anthem Blue Cross Blue Shield CT
North Haven, CT — Page 88
Arise Health Plan
Green Bay, WI — Page 461
Arizona Foundation for Medical Care
Phoenix, AZ — Page 11
Arkansas Blue Cross/Blue Shield a Mutual Insurance Company
Little Rock, AR — Page 25

Arkansas Managed Care Organization
Little Rock, AR — Page 26
Assurant Employee Benefits - Michigan
Troy, MI — Page 217
Assurant Health - Corporate Headquarters
Milwaukee, WI — Page 462
Asuris Northwest Health
Spokane, WA — Page 449
AtlantiCare Health Plans Inc
Hammonton, NJ — Page 269
Atlantic Integrated Health Inc
New Bern, NC — Page 309
Aultcare
Canton, OH — Page 320
Av-Med Health Plan - Jacksonville
Jacksonville, FL — Page 102
Av-Med Health Plan - Orlando
Maitland, FL — Page 103

B

Baptist Health Services Group
Memphis, TN — Page 392
Beech Street Corporation — Corporate Headquarters
Lake Forest, CA — Page 36
Berkshire Health Partners/Medicus Resource Management
Wyomissing, PA — Page 357
Best Health Plans
Irvine, CA — Page 36
Blue Cross Blue Shield of Alabama
Birmingham, AL — Page 3
Blue Cross Blue Shield of Arizona
Phoenix, AZ — Page 12
Blue Cross Blue Shield of Delaware
Wilmington, DE — Page 95
Blue Cross Blue Shield of Florida & Health Options Inc
Miami, FL — Page 104
Blue Cross Blue Shield of Florida/ Health Options Inc
Jacksonville, FL — Page 104
Blue Cross Blue Shield of Georgia
Atlanta, GA — Page 128
Blue Cross Blue Shield of Illinois
Chicago, IL — Page 144
Blue Cross Blue Shield of Kansas
Topeka, KS — Page 177
Blue Cross Blue Shield of Kansas City
Kansas City, MO — Page 244
Blue Cross Blue Shield of Louisiana Inc
Baton Rouge, LA — Page 189
Blue Cross Blue Shield of Massachusetts
Boston, MA — Page 209
Blue Cross Blue Shield of Minnesota
St Paul, MN — Page 234
Blue Cross Blue Shield of Mississippi
Jackson, MS — Page 241
Blue Cross Blue Shield of Nebraska
Omaha, NE — Page 255
Blue Cross Blue Shield of New Mexico
Albuquerque, NM — Page 279
Blue Cross Blue Shield of North Carolina
Durham, NC — Page 310
Blue Cross Blue Shield of Oklahoma
Tulsa, OK — Page 339
Blue Cross Blue Shield of Rhode Island
Providence, RI — Page 379

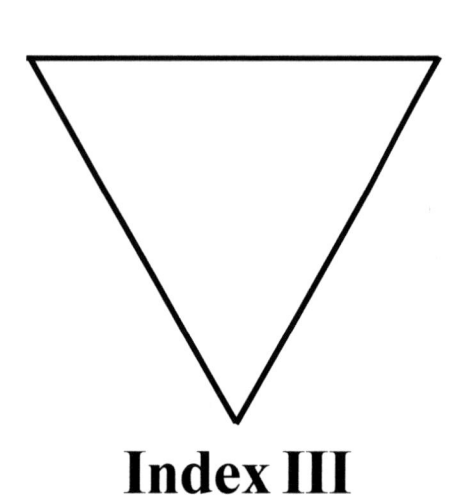

Index III

Preferred Provider Organizations

Index II: Health Maintenance Organizations

**Unison Health Plan -
Corporate Headquarters**
Pittsburgh, PA Page 372
Unison Health Plan of Ohio Inc
Cleveland, OH Page 336
Unison Health Plan of Pennsylvania
Pittsburgh, PA Page 373
**Unison Health Plan of
South Carolina Inc**
Columbia, SC Page 386
Unison Health Plan of Tennessee
Memphis, TN Page 399
**UnitedHealth Group—
Corporate Headquarters**
Minnetonka, MN Page 238
**UnitedHealthcare & Mid Atlantic
Medical Services Inc**
Rockville, MD Page 206
**UnitedHealthcare Services Company of
the River Valley Inc**
Peoria, IL Page 154
**UnitedHealthcare Services Company of
the River Valley Inc**
Moline, IL Page 154
**UnitedHealthcare Services Company of
the River Valley Inc**
Bettendorf, IA Page 172
**UnitedHealthcare Services Company of
the River Valley Inc**
Dubuque, IA Page 173
**UnitedHealthcare Services Company of
the River Valley Inc**
Urbandale, IA Page 173
**UnitedHealthcare Services Company of
the River Valley Inc**
Waterloo, IA Page 174
**UnitedHealthcare Services Company of
the River Valley Inc**
Marion, IA Page 173
**UnitedHealthcare Services Company of
the River Valley Inc**
Kingsport, TN Page 400
**UnitedHealthcare Services Company of
the River Valley Inc**
Knoxville, TN Page 400
**UnitedHealthcare Services Company of
the River Valley Inc**
Chattanooga, TN Page 400
UnitedHealthcare of Alabama
Birmingham, AL Page 7
UnitedHealthcare of Arizona Inc
Phoenix, AZ Page 21
UnitedHealthcare of Arkansas
Little Rock, AR Page 28
UnitedHealthcare of Colorado
Centennial, CO Page 85
UnitedHealthcare of Florida Inc
Jacksonville, FL Page 121
UnitedHealthcare of Florida Inc
Maitland, FL Page 121
UnitedHealthcare of Florida Inc
Tampa, FL Page 122
UnitedHealthcare of Georgia
Norcross, GA Page 134
UnitedHealthcare of Illinois Inc
Chicago, IL Page 154
UnitedHealthcare of Kentucky
Lexington, KY Page 186
UnitedHealthcare of Louisiana
Metairie, LA Page 193
UnitedHealthcare of Massachusetts
Waltham, MA Page 216
UnitedHealthcare of Mississippi Inc
Ridgeland, MS Page 242
UnitedHealthcare of New England Inc
Warwick, RI Page 381
UnitedHealthcare of New York Inc
East Syracuse, NY Page 306

**UnitedHealthcare of New York
Metropolitan**
New York, NY Page 306
UnitedHealthcare of North Carolina Inc
Greensboro, NC Page 315
UnitedHealthcare of Ohio Inc
Westerville, OH Page 336
UnitedHealthcare of Ohio Inc-Cleveland
Cleveland, OH Page 336
UnitedHealthcare of Oregon
Long Beach, CA Page 352
**UnitedHealthcare of SW Ohio Inc-
Dayton/Cincinnati**
Westchester, OH Page 337
UnitedHealthcare of South Florida
Sunrise, FL Page 122
UnitedHealthcare of Tennessee Inc
Brentwood, TN Page 401
**UnitedHealthcare of Texas Inc -
Houston**
Houston, TX Page 429
**UnitedHealthcare of Texas Inc - San
Antonio**
San Antonio, TX Page 430
UnitedHealthcare of Texas Inc — Dallas
Plano, TX Page 430
UnitedHealthcare of Utah
Salt Lake City, UT Page 437
UnitedHealthcare of Virginia
Richmond, VA Page 446
UnitedHealthcare of Washington
Mercer Island, WA Page 457
UnitedHealthcare of Wisconsin Inc
Milwaukee, WI Page 470
**UnitedHealthcare of the Heartland
States**
Overland Park, KS Page 182
UnitedHealthcare of the Midlands Inc
Omaha, NE Page 257
UnitedHealthcare of the Midwest Inc
Maryland Heights, MO Page 251
Unity Health Insurance
Sauk City, WI Page 470
Univera Community Health
Buffalo, NY Page 307
**Univera Healthcare of Western New
York**
Buffalo, NY Page 307
Universal Health Care Inc
St Petersburg, FL Page 122
University Family Care Health Plan
Tucson, AZ Page 22
**University Health Care Inc - Passport
Health Plan**
Louisville, KY Page 187
University Health Plans Inc
Newark, NJ Page 277
**UPMC Health Plan Univ of Pittsburgh
Medical Center**
Pittsburgh, PA Page 374
Upper Peninsula Health Plan
Marquette, MI Page 232
UTMB Health Plans Inc
Galveston, TX Page 431

V

Valley Baptist Insurance Company
Harlingen, TX Page 431
Valley Health Plan Santa Clara County
San Jose, CA Page 72
Vantage Health Plan Inc
Monroe, LA Page 193
Ventura County Health Care Plan
Ventura, CA Page 73

Vermont Health Plans (Blue Care)
Montpelier, VT Page 439
Virginia Premier Health Plans Inc
Richmond, VA Page 447
Vista Health Plan Inc
Hollywood, FL Page 123
Vista Healthplan of South Florida Inc
Sunrise, FL Page 123
Viva Health Inc
Birmingham, AL Page 7

W

WelBorn Health Plans
Evansville, IN Page 167
WellCare HMO Inc
Tampa, FL Page 124
**WellCare Health Plans Inc -
Corporate Headquarters**
Tampa, FL Page 124
WellCare of New York
Poughkeepsie, NY Page 307
**WellPoint Inc - Corporate
Headquarters**
Indianapolis, IN Page 167
**Wellmark Blue Cross Blue Shield of
Iowa**
Des Moines, IA Page 174
Wellmark Health Plan of Iowa Inc
Des Moines, IA Page 175
**Wellmark Inc—
Corporate Headquarters**
Des Moines, IA Page 175
Wellpath Select Inc
Morrisville, NC Page 315
Western Health Advantage
Sacramento, CA Page 75
WINHealth Partners
Cheyenne, WY Page 473
Windsor Health Plan of Tennessee Inc
Brentwood, TN Page 401
**Wisconsin Physician Services
Insurance Company**
Madison, WI Page 471

X

XL Health
Baltimore, MD Page 207

Y

Yale University Health Plan
New Haven, CT Page 93

Index II: Health Maintenance Organizations

Pacificare Life & Health Insurance Company
Cypress, CA — Page 63
Paramount Advantage
Maumee, OH — Page 333
Paramount Care of Michigan
Dundee, MI — Page 228
Paramount Health Care Plan
Maumee, OH — Page 333
Parkland Community Health Plan Inc
Dallas, TX — Page 422
Partnercare Health Plan Inc
Tampa, FL — Page 117
Partners National Health Plans of North Carolina Inc
Winston-Salem, NC — Page 314
Partnership HealthPlan of California
Fairfield City, CA — Page 64
Peach State Health Plan
Smyrna, GA — Page 133
PersonalCare Insurance of Illinois Inc
Champaign, IL — Page 151
Phoenix Health Plan - Community Connection
Phoenix, AZ — Page 19
Php Companies Inc
Knoxville, TN — Page 397
Physicians Health Plan of Mid-Michigan
Lansing, MI — Page 228
Physicians Health Plan of Northern Indiana
Ft Wayne, IN — Page 164
Physicians Health Plan of South Michigan
Jackson, MI — Page 229
Physicians Plus Insurance Corporation
Madison, WI — Page 469
Physicians United Plan Inc
Orlando, FL — Page 118
PhysiciansPlus Baptist St Dominic Inc
Jackson, MS — Page 242
Pima Health Plan
Tucson, AZ — Page 19
Preferred Care
Rochester, NY — Page 304
Preferred Care Partners Inc
Miami, FL — Page 118
Preferred Health Systems
Wichita, KS — Page 180
Preferred Medical Plan Inc
Coral Gables, FL — Page 118
Preferred One
North Haven, CT — Page 93
Preferred One
Golden Valley, MN — Page 237
Preferred Plus of Kansas Inc
Wichita, KS — Page 181
Premera - Corporate Headquarters
Mountlake Terrace, WA — Page 454
Premera Blue Cross - Eastern
Spokane, WA — Page 454
Premera Blue Cross - Western
Mountlake Terrace, WA — Page 454
Premera Blue Cross Blue Shield of Alaska
Anchorage, AK — Page 9
Presbyterian Health Plan
Alburquerque, NM — Page 281
Primary Health Plan
Boise, ID — Page 142
Primecare Medical Network Inc
Ontario, CA — Page 65
Primetime Medical Health Plan
Canton, OH — Page 333
Priority Health
Grand Rapids, MI — Page 230

Pro-Care Health Plan
Detroit, MI — Page 230
Providence Health Plans
Beaverton, OR — Page 351
Puget Sound Health Partners
Lakewood, WA — Page 455

Q

QCA Health Plan Inc
Little Rock, AR — Page 28
QualCare Inc
Piscataway, NJ — Page 276
Quality Health Plan Inc
Holiday, FL — Page 119

R

Rayant Insurance Company of New York
New York, NY — Page 304
Regence Blue Cross Blue Shield of Oregon
Portland, OR — Page 351
Regence Blue Cross Blue Shield of Utah
Salt Lake City, UT — Page 436
Regence Blue Shield
Seattle, WA — Page 456
Regence Group, The — Corporate Headquarters
Portland, OR — Page 351
Regence Healthwise
Salt Lake City, UT — Page 436
Regence Valucare
Salt Lake City, UT — Page 436
Regencecare
Seattle, WA — Page 456
Rocky Mountain Health Plans
Grand Junction, CO — Page 84
Rocky Mountain Hosital & Medical Services Inc
Denver, CO — Page 85

S

Saint Mary's HealthFirst
Reno, NV — Page 263
Samaritan Health Plans Inc
Corvallis, OR — Page 352
San Francisco Health Plan
San Francisco, CA — Page 66
Sanford Health Plan
Sioux Falls, SD — Page 388
Sanford Health Plan of Minnesota
Sioux Falls, SD — Page 238
Santa Barbara Regional Health Authority
Goleta, CA — Page 67
Santa Clara Family Health Plan
Campbell, CA — Page 67
Sante Community Physicians
Fresno, CA — Page 67
Scan Health Plan
Long Beach, CA — Page 68
Scott & White Health Plan
Temple, TX — Page 424
Scripps Clinic Health Plan Services Inc
San Diego, CA — Page 68

Security Health Plan of Wisconsin Inc
Marshfield, WI — Page 469
Select Health of South Carolina
North Charleston, SC — Page 385
SelectHealth
Salt Lake City, UT — Page 437
Seton Health Plan
Austin, TX — Page 425
Sharp Health Plan
San Diego, CA — Page 68
Sierra Health Services Inc- Corporate Headquarters
Las Vegas, NV — Page 264
Southeastern Indiana Health Organization
Columbus, IN — Page 166
Southern Health Services Inc
Charlottesville, VA — Page 445
Southern Health Services Inc
Richmond, VA — Page 445
Southwest Health Alliance (SHALLC)
Austin, TX — Page 425
Suburban Health Organization
Indianapolis, IN — Page 167
Suffolk Health Plan
Hauppauge, NY — Page 305
Summacare Inc
Akron, OH — Page 334
Summit Health Plan Inc
Hollywood, FL — Page 120
Sun Health Medisun
Sun City, AZ — Page 20
SuperMed Network
Cleveland, OH — Page 334
Superior HealthPlan Inc
Austin, TX — Page 426
Talbert Health Plan
Costa Mesa, CA — Page 70
Tenet Choices Inc
Metaire, LA — Page 192
Texas Childrens Health Plan
Houston, TX — Page 426
Texas Community Care
El Paso, TX — Page 427
Texas HealthSpring I LLC
Houston, TX — Page 427
Total Health Care Inc
Detroit, MI — Page 231
Total Health Choice Inc
Miami, FL — Page 120
Touchstone Health HMO Inc
New York, NY — Page 305
Triple-S Inc
San Juan, PR — Page 378
True Blue
Meridian, ID — Page 142
Tufts Health Plan
Watertown, MA — Page 216

U

UAHC Health Plan of Tennessee
Memphis, TN — Page 399
Ucare Minnesota
Minneapolis, MN — Page 238
UHP Healthcare
Los Angeles, CA — Page 71
UniCare Health Plans of TX Inc
Houston, TX — Page 428
Unicare Health Plans of the Midwest Inc
Chicago, IL — Page 153
Union Health Service Inc
Chicago, IL — Page 154

Index II: Health Maintenance Organizations

Kaiser Foundation Health Plan of Southern California
Pasadena, CA — Page 54

Kaiser Permanente - Kaiser Foundation Health Plan, Inc
Oakland, CA — Page 54

Kaiser Permanente Health Plan
Honolulu, HI — Page 137

Keokuk Area Hospital Organized Delivery System Inc
Keokuk, IA — Page 171

Kern Family Health Care
Bakersfield, CA — Page 55

Keystone Health Plan Central
Harrisburg, PA — Page 367

Keystone Health Plan East Inc
Philadelphia, PA — Page 368

Keystone Health Plan West Inc
Pittsburgh, PA — Page 368

Keystone Mercy Health Plan
Philadelphia, PA — Page 368

KPS Health Plans
Bremerton, WA — Page 452

L

LA Care Health Plan
Los Angeles, CA — Page 55

Lakewood Health Plan Inc
Lakewood, CA — Page 56

Lane Oregon Health Plans
Eugene, OR — Page 347

Legacy Health Plan Inc
San Angelo, TX — Page 420

Leon Medical Centers Health Plan Inc
Miami, FL — Page 115

Lifetime Healthcare Companies, The - Corporate Headquarters
Rochester, NY — Page 298

Lovelace Health Plan
Albuquerque, NM — Page 280

M

M Plan Inc
Indianapolis, IN — Page 163

M-Care Inc
Ann Arbor, MI — Page 225

MagnaCare
Garden City, NY — Page 298

Managed Health Services Indiana Inc
Indianapolis, IN — Page 163

Managed Health Services Insurance Corporation
West Allis, WI — Page 467

March Vision Care Inc
Los Angeles, CA — Page 58

Maricopa Health Plan
Phoenix, AZ — Page 18

Marion Polk Community Health Plan Advantage
Salem, OR — Page 349

Martins Point Health Care
Portland, ME — Page 196

McLaren Health Plan
Flint, MI — Page 226

MD-Individual Practice Association Inc (MD IPA)
Rockville, MD — Page 204

MDNY Healthcare Inc
Melville, NY — Page 299

MDWise
Indianapolis, IN — Page 163

Medcore Health Plan
Stockton, CA — Page 58

Medica Health Plans
Minnetonka, MN — Page 236

Medica Healthcare Plans Inc
Coral Gables, FL — Page 116

Medical Associates Clinic Health Plan of WI
Dubuque, IA — Page 467

Medical Associates Health Plans
Dubuque, IA — Page 172

Medical Card System
Hato Rey, PR — Page 377

Medical Mutual of Ohio
Cleveland, OH — Page 330

Memphis Managed Care Corp
Memphis, TN — Page 397

Mercy Care Plan
Phoenix, AZ — Page 18

Mercy CarePlus
St Louis, MO — Page 249

Mercy Health Plans of Missouri Inc
Chesterfield, MO — Page 249

Mercycare Health Plan Inc
Janesville, WI — Page 468

Metcare Health Plans Inc
West Palm Beach, FL — Page 116

MetroPlus Health Plan
New York, NY — Page 300

Metropolitan Health Plan
Minneapolis, MN — Page 237

Mid Atlantic Medical Services Inc (MAMSI)- Corp Headquarters
Rockville, MD — Page 204

Midwest Health Plan
Dearborn, MI — Page 226

Missouri Care
Columbia, MO — Page 250

MIT Health Plan
Cambridge, MA — Page 214

MMM Healthcare Inc
San Juan, PR — Page 378

Molina Healthcare Inc - Corporate Headquarters
Long Beach, CA — Page 59

Molina Healthcare Inc of California
Long Beach, CA — Page 59

Molina Healthcare of Michigan Inc
Troy, MI — Page 227

Molina Healthcare of New Mexico
Albuquerque, NM — Page 281

Molina Healthcare of Ohio Inc
Columbus, OH — Page 330

Molina Healthcare of Texas Inc
Houston, TX — Page 421

Molina Healthcare of Utah Inc
Midvale, UT — Page 435

Molina Healthcare of Washington Inc
Bothell, WA — Page 453

Monroe Plan for Medical Care, The
Rochester, NY — Page 300

Mount Carmel Health Plan
Columbus, OH — Page 331

MVP Health Plan Inc
Schenectady, NY — Page 301

MVP Health Plan of New Hampshire
Bedford, NH — Page 266

N

Nationwide Health Plans
Columbus, OH — Page 331

Neighborhood Health Partnership
Miami, FL — Page 116

Neighborhood Health Plan
Boston, MA — Page 214

Neighborhood Health Plan of Rhode Island
Providence, RI — Page 380

Network Health Plan Wisconsin
Menasha, WI — Page 468

NevadaCare Inc
Las Vegas, NV — Page 262

New West Health Services
Helena, MT — Page 254

New York Presbyterian Community Health Plan
New York, NY — Page 302

O

OmniCare, A Coventry Health Plan
Detroit, MI — Page 228

Optima Health Plan Inc
Virginia Beach, VA — Page 445

Optimum Choice Inc
Rockville, MD — Page 205

Optimum Choice of the Carolina Inc
Rockville, MD — Page 205

Optimum HealthCare Inc
Spring Hill, FL — Page 117

Orange County Health Authority
Orange, CA — Page 60

OSF Health Plans
Peoria, IL — Page 151

Oxford Health Plans Inc — Corporate Headquarters
Trumbell, CT — Page 92

Oxford Health Plans of New Jersey Inc
Iselin, NJ — Page 275

Oxford Health Plans of New York, Inc
New York, NY — Page 303

Oxford Health Plans-Connecticut
Trumbell, CT — Page 91

P

PacifiCare Health Systems- Corporate Headquarters
Santa Ana, CA — Page 62

PacifiCare of Arizona
Phoenix, AZ — Page 19

PacifiCare of California
Cypress, CA — Page 62

PacifiCare of Colorado/ United Healthcare
Greenwood Village, CO — Page 84

PacifiCare of Nevada
Las Vegas, NV — Page 263

PacifiCare of Oklahoma Inc/Secure Horizons
Tulsa, OK — Page 342

PacifiCare of Oregon
Lake Oswego, OR — Page 350

PacifiCare of Texas - Houston
Houston, TX — Page 422

PacifiCare of Texas Inc
Dallas, TX — Page 422

Pacific IPA
El Monte, CA — Page 63

PacificSource Health Plans
Springfield, OR — Page 350

Index II: Health Maintenance Organizations

Health Care Service Corporation -
Corporate Headquarters
Chicago, IL   Page 149
Health Choice Arizona
Tempe, AZ   Page 16
Health First Health Plans Inc
Rockledge, FL   Page 111
Health Net - Connecticut
Shelton, CT   Page 90
Health Net - New Jersey
Neptune, NJ   Page 272
Health Net - New York
White Plains, NY   Page 295
Health Net Health Plan of Oregon Inc
Tigard, OR   Page 346
**Health Net Inc -
Corporate Headquarters**
Woodland Hills, CA   Page 49
**Health Net Inc - Northeast
Corporate Headquarters**
Shelton, CT   Page 91
Health Net of Arizona
Tucson, AZ   Page 17
Health Net of California
Woodland Hills, CA   Page 49
Health New England
Springfield, MA   Page 212
Health Partners
Philadelphia, PA   Page 364
Health Plan of CareOregon Inc
Portland, OR   Page 346
Health Plan of Michigan
Southfield, MI   Page 224
Health Plan of Nevada Inc
Las Vegas, NV   Page 260
Health Plan of San Joaquin, The
French Camp, CA   Page 50
Health Plan of San Mateo
San Francisco, CA   Page 50
Health Plan of the Upper Ohio Valley
St Clairsville, OH   Page 327
Health Plan, The/Hometown Region
Massillon, OH   Page 327
Health Plus of Louisiana Inc
Shreveport, LA   Page 191
Health Tradition Health Plans
Onalaska, WI   Page 466
**HealthAmerica Pennsylvania Inc -
Central Region**
Harrisburg, PA   Page 364
**HealthAmerica Pennsylvania Inc -
Eastern Region**
Plymouth Meeting, PA   Page 365
**HealthAmerica Pennsylvania Inc -
Nortwestern**
Erie, PA   Page 365
**HealthAmerica Pennsylvania Inc -
Western Region**
Pittsburgh, PA   Page 365
HealthCare USA of Missouri LLC
St Louis, MO   Page 248
HealthEase of Florida Inc
Tampa, FL   Page 111
HealthFirst Inc
New York, NY   Page 295
HealthLink Inc
St Louis, MO   Page 248
**HealthLink Inc -
Corporate Headquarters**
St Louis, MO   Page 249
HealthLink of Arkansas Inc
North Little Rock, AR   Page 27
HealthNow New York Inc
Buffalo, NY   Page 295
HealthPartners Inc
Bloomington, MN   Page 236
HealthPlus of Michigan
Flint, MI   Page 224

**HealthSpring Inc - Corporate Head-
quarters**
Franklin, TN   Page 395
HealthSpring Inc - Tennessee
Nashville, TN   Page 395
Healthnow
Memphis, TN   Page 395
Healthplus Inc
Brooklyn, NY   Page 296
Healthspring of Alabama Inc
Birmingham, AL   Page 5
Healthsun Health Plans Inc
Miami, FL   Page 112
Healthy Palm Beaches Inc
West Palm Beach, FL   Page 112
Heart of America Health Plan
Rugby, ND   Page 317
Heritage Health Systems Inc
Houston, TX   Page 416
Heritage Provider Network Inc
Northridge, CA   Page 50
Highmark Inc
Pittsburgh, PA   Page 366
HIP Health Plan of New York
New York, NY   Page 296
HMO California
Signal Hill, CA   Page 51
HMO Health Ohio (Cleveland)
Cleveland, OH   Page 328
HMO Illinois
Chicago, IL   Page 150
HMO Louisiana Inc
Baton Rouge, LA   Page 191
HMO Nevada
Las Vegas, NV   Page 260
HMO New Mexico Inc
Albuquerque, NM   Page 280
Hometown Health Plan
Reno, NV   Page 260
Honored Citizen's Choice Health Plan
Beverly Hills, CA   Page 51
Horizon Blue Cross/Blue Shield of NJ
Newark, NJ   Page 273
Horizon Healthcare Services Inc
Newark, NJ   Page 274
Horizon NJ Health
Trenton, NJ   Page 274
Hudson Health Plan
Tarrytown, NY   Page 297
**Humana Health Benefit Plan of
Louisiana**
Metairie, LA   Page 191
Humana Health Care Plans of Arizona
Phoenix, AZ   Page 17
**Humana Health Care Plans of Corpus
Christi**
Corpus Christi, TX   Page 417
Humana Health Care Plans of Houston
Houston, TX   Page 418
Humana Health Care Plans of Illinois
Chicago, IL   Page 151
**Humana Health Care Plans of Kansas
& Missouri**
Overland Park, KS   Page 179
**Humana Health Care Plans of
Lexington**
Lexington, KY   Page 185
**Humana Health Care Plans of San
Antonio/Austin**
San Antonio, TX   Page 418
Humana Health Plan - Jacksonville
Jacksonville, FL   Page 113
Humana Health Plan - Kentucky
Louisville, KY   Page 185
Humana Health Plan of Austin
Austin, TX   Page 419
Humana Health Plan of Ohio Inc
Cincinnati, OH   Page 328

Humana Health Plans of Georgia
Atlanta, GA   Page 132
Humana Inc - Corporate Headquarters
Louisville, KY   Page 185
Humana Inc - Indiana
Indianapolis, IN   Page 161
Humana Inc - North Carolina
Charlotte, NC   Page 313
Humana Inc - Oklahoma
Louisville, KY   Page 341
Humana Inc/PCA - Puerto Rico
San Juan, PR   Page 377
Humana Medical Plan - Central Florida
Tampa, FL   Page 113
Humana Medical Plan - Daytona
Daytona Beach, FL   Page 113
Humana Medical Plan Inc
Miramar, FL   Page 114
Humana Military Service Inc
Louisville, KY   Page 186
**Humana Wisconsin Health
Organization Inc**
Waukesha, WI   Page 466

I

IBA Health Plans
Kalamazoo, MI   Page 225
Independence Blue Cross
Philadelphia, PA   Page 366
Independent Care Health Plan
Milwaukee, WI   Page 467
Independent Health Association Inc
Buffalo, NY   Page 297
Indiana Pro Health Network
Indianapolis, IN   Page 162
Inland Empire Health Plan
San Bernardino, CA   Page 52
Inter Valley Health Plan Inc
Pomona, CA   Page 53
Intercommunity Health Network
Corvallis, OR   Page 347
Iowa Health Solutions
Rock Island, IL   Page 171

J

Jackson Memorial Health Plan
Miami, FL   Page 115

K

**Kaiser Foundation Health Plan - Mid
Atlantic States**
Rockville, MD   Page 203
**Kaiser Foundation Health Plan North-
west**
Portland, OR   Page 347
**Kaiser Foundation Health Plan of
Colorado**
Denver, CO   Page 83
**Kaiser Foundation Health Plan of
Georgia**
Atlanta, GA   Page 132
**Kaiser Foundation Health Plan of
Northern California**
Oakland, CA   Page 54
Kaiser Foundation Health Plan of Ohio
Cleveland, OH   Page 329

Index II: Health Maintenance Organizations

Connecticare Inc
Farmington, CT — Page 89
Connecticare of Massachusetts Inc
Farmington, CT — Page 210
Connecticare of NY
Tarrytown, NY — Page 288
Contra Costa Health Plan
Martinez, CA — Page 43
Cooks Childrens Health Plan
Fort Worth, TX — Page 411
Coordinated Health Plan
Providence, RI — Page 379
Coordinated Health Systems
Bethlehem, PA — Page 361
Coventry Health Care Inc — Carolinas
Charlotte, NC — Page 311
Coventry Health Care Inc — Corporate Headquarters
Bethesda, MD — Page 201
Coventry Health Care Inc — Delaware Inc
Wilmington, DE — Page 96
Coventry Health Care Inc — Georgia Inc
Atlanta, GA — Page 130
Coventry Health Care Inc — Iowa
Urbandale, IA — Page 169
Coventry Health Care Inc — Louisiana
Metairie, LA — Page 190
Coventry Health Care of Kansas - Wichita
Wichita, KS — Page 178
Coventry Health Care of Kansas Inc
Kansas City, MO — Page 245
Coventry Health Care of Nebraska Inc
Omaha, NE — Page 255
Cox Health Plans
Springfield, MO — Page 246

D

D C Chartered Health Plan Inc
Washington, DC — Page 97
DaVita VillageHealth of Michigan Inc
Brighton, MI — Page 220
DakotaCare
Sioux Falls, SD — Page 387
Dean Health Plan
Madison, WI — Page 463
Delmarva Health Care Plan Inc
Easton, MD — Page 202
Dental Care Plus Inc
Cincinnati, OH — Page 324
Denver Health Medical Plan Inc
Denver, CO — Page 80
Deseret Healthcare
Salt Lake City, UT — Page 434
Driscoll Children's Health Plan
Corpus Christi, TX — Page 412

E

Easy Choice Health Plan Inc
Newport Beach, CA — Page 46
Educators Health Care
Murray, UT — Page 434
El Paso First Health Plans Inc
El Paso, TX — Page 413
Elderplan Inc - SHMO
Brooklyn, NY — Page 289
EmblemHealth Inc
New York, NY — Page 290
Empire Blue Cross Blue Shield
New York, NY — Page 290
Essence Inc
St Louis, MO — Page 246
Evercare Select
Phoenix, AZ — Page 15
Evercare of Texas LLC
Houston, TX — Page 413
Evergreen Medical Group LLC
Columbus, GA — Page 131
Excellus BlueCross BlueShield
Rochester, NY — Page 290
Excellus BlueCross BlueShield, Central NY Southern Tier
Syracuse, NY — Page 291
Excellus BlueCross BlueShield, Central New York Region
Syracuse, NY — Page 291
Excellus BlueCross BlueShield, Rochester Region
Rochester, NY — Page 292
Excellus BlueCross BlueShield, Utica Region
Utica, NY — Page 292

F

Fallon Community Health Plan Inc
Worcester, MA — Page 211
Family Health Partners
Kansas City, MO — Page 247
Fidelis Care New York
Rego Park, NY — Page 293
Fidelis SecureCare of Michigan Inc
Livonia, MI — Page 221
Fidelis SecureCare of North Carolina
Charlotte, NC — Page 312
Fidelis SeniorCare Inc
Schaumburg, IL — Page 147
First Medical Health Plan of Florida
Miami, FL — Page 109
First Plan of Minnesota
Duluth, MN — Page 235
FirstCarolinaCare
Pinehurst, NC — Page 312
Florida Health Care Plan Inc
Holly Hill, FL — Page 109
Freedom Health Inc
St Petersburg, FL — Page 110

G

Gateway Health Plan Inc
Pittsburgh, PA — Page 362
Geisinger Health Plan
Danville, PA — Page 363
GHI HMO Select Inc
New York, NY — Page 293
Global Health Inc
Oklahoma City, OK — Page 341
Good Health HMO Inc
Kansas City, MO — Page 247
Grand Valley Health Plan
Grand Rapids, MI — Page 221
Great Lakes Health Plan
Southfield, MI — Page 222
Great West Life Annuity Insurance Co
Greenwood Village, CO — Page 81
Great-West Healthcare - Corporate
Greenwood Village, CO — Page 81
Great-West Healthcare of Arizona
Scottsdale, AZ — Page 16
Great-West Healthcare of California
Glendale, CA — Page 48
Great-West Healthcare of California - North
Pleasant Hill, CA — Page 48
Great-West Healthcare of Colorado
Greenwood Village, CO — Page 81
Great-West Healthcare of Florida
Tampa, FL — Page 111
Great-West Healthcare of Georgia
Atlanta, GA — Page 131
Great-West Healthcare of Illinois
Rosemont, IL — Page 148
Great-West Healthcare of Kansas/Missouri
Overland Park, KS — Page 179
Great-West Healthcare of Michigan
Southfield, MI — Page 223
Great-West Healthcare of Minnesota
Eden Prairie, MN — Page 236
Great-West Healthcare of New York
New York, NY — Page 294
Great-West Healthcare of Ohio
Columbus, OH — Page 326
Great-West Healthcare of Ohio
North Olmstead, OH — Page 326
Great-West Healthcare of Pennsylvania
Media, PA — Page 363
Great-West Healthcare of Texas - Austin
Austin, TX — Page 414
Great-West Healthcare of Texas - Dallas
Dallas, TX — Page 415
Great-West Healthcare of Texas - Houston
Houston, TX — Page 415
Great-West Healthcare of Virginia Inc
Falls Church, VA — Page 444
Group Health Cooperative
Coeur D'Alene, ID — Page 141
Group Health Cooperative
Spokane, WA — Page 451
Group Health Cooperative South Central Wisconsin
Madison, WI — Page 464
Group Health Cooperative of Eau Claire
Altoona, WI — Page 465
Group Health Cooperative of Puget Sound
Seattle, WA — Page 452
Group Health Plan Inc
Earth City, MO — Page 248
Guardian Life Insurance Co of America
New York, NY — Page 294
Gundersen Lutheran Health Plan Inc
La Crosse, WI — Page 465

H

Harmony Health Plan
Chicago, IL — Page 148
Harvard Pilgrim Health Care - Corporate Headquarters
Wellesley, MA — Page 212
Hawaii Medical Services Association - BC/BS of Hawaii
Honolulu, HI — Page 137
Health Advantage
Little Rock, AR — Page 27
Health Alliance Medical Plans - Corporate Headquarters
Urbana, IL — Page 149
Health Alliance Plan of Michigan
Detroit, MI — Page 223

Index II: Health Maintenance Organizations

Blue Cross Blue Shield of Nebraska
Omaha, NE — Page 255
Blue Cross Blue Shield of New Mexico
Albuquerque, NM — Page 279
Blue Cross Blue Shield of North Dakota
Fargo, ND — Page 317
Blue Cross Blue Shield of Oklahoma
Tulsa, OK — Page 339
Blue Cross Blue Shield of Rhode Island
Providence, RI — Page 379
Blue Cross Blue Shield of South Carolina - Corporate Hqtrs
Columbia, SC — Page 383
Blue Cross Blue Shield of Tennessee
Chattanooga, TN — Page 392
Blue Cross Blue Shield of Tennessee - Memphis
Memphis, TN — Page 393
Blue Cross Blue Shield of Texas — Corporate Headquarters
Richardson, TX — Page 406
Blue Cross Blue Shield of Texas — HMO Blue - Midwest TX
Austin, TX — Page 406
Blue Cross Blue Shield of Texas — HMO Blue - Southeast
Houston, TX — Page 407
Blue Cross Blue Shield of Texas — HMO Blue - West
El Paso, TX — Page 407
Blue Cross Blue Shield of Vermont
Berlin, VT — Page 439
Blue Cross Blue Shield of Western New York
Buffalo, NY — Page 285
Blue Cross Blue Shield of Wyoming
Cheyenne, WY — Page 473
Blue Cross of Puerto Rico/La Cruz Azul de Puerto Rico
San Juan, PR — Page 377
Blue Shield of California
San Francisco, CA — Page 36
BlueChoice Health Plan of South Carolina Inc
Columbia, SC — Page 383
BlueCross of Northeastern Pennsylvania
Wilkes-Barre, PA — Page 358
BlueShield of Northeastern New York
Latham, NY — Page 286
Bluegrass Family Health Inc
Lexington, KY — Page 183
Bluelincs HMO
Tulsa, OK — Page 340
BMC HealthNet Plan
Boston, MA — Page 209
Bravo Health Inc
Baltimore, MD — Page 200
Bravo Health Mid-Atlantic Inc
Baltimore, MD — Page 200
Bravo Health Pennsylvania Inc
Philadelphia, PA — Page 358
Bravo Health Texas Inc
San Antonio, TX — Page 407
Buckeye Community Health Plan Inc
Columbus, OH — Page 321

C

Capital Blue Cross
Harrisburg, PA — Page 359
Capital District Physicians Health Plan
Albany, NY — Page 286

Capital Health Plan
Tallahassee, FL — Page 105
Care 1st Health Plan
Alhambra, CA — Page 38
Care 1st Health Plan Arizona Inc
Phoenix, AZ — Page 13
Care Choices
Farmington Hills, MI — Page 218
CareFirst Blue Cross Blue Shield
Owings Mills, MD — Page 200
CareFirst BlueChoice Inc
Washington, DC — Page 97
CareMore Health Plan
Cerritos, CA — Page 38
CarePlus Health Plans Inc
Coral Gables, FL — Page 106
CareSource
Dayton, OH — Page 321
Carelink Health Plans
Wheeling, WV — Page 459
Carelink Health Plans
Charleston, WV — Page 459
Cariten Healthcare
Knoxville, TN — Page 393
Carolina Care Plan Inc
Columbia, SC — Page 383
Centene Corporation
St Louis, MO — Page 244
Centercare Inc
Rego Park, NY — Page 287
Central Coast Alliance for Health
Scotts Valley, CA — Page 39
Central Health Plan of California Inc
Covina, CA — Page 39
Central New York East HealthNow New York Inc
East Syracuse, NY — Page 287
Central New York West HealthNow New York Inc
Rochester, NY — Page 287
CHA Health - Humana
Lexington, KY — Page 184
Children's Community Health Plan Inc
Madison, WI — Page 462
Chinese Community Health Plan
San Francisco, CA — Page 39
CHN MCO
Independence, OH — Page 322
ChoiceCare/Humana
Cincinnati, OH — Page 322
CIGNA Health Plan of Utah Inc
Salt Lake City, UT — Page 433
CIGNA HealthCare — Corporate Headquarters
Philadelphia, PA — Page 360
CIGNA Healthcare
Burlington, VT — Page 439
CIGNA Healthcare - Cincinnati
Cincinnati, OH — Page 323
CIGNA Healthcare of Arizona
Phoenix, AZ — Page 14
CIGNA Healthcare of California
Glendale, CA — Page 41
CIGNA Healthcare of Colorado
Denver, CO — Page 79
CIGNA Healthcare of Connecticut
Hartford, CT — Page 89
CIGNA Healthcare of Florida
Tampa, FL — Page 107
CIGNA Healthcare of Florida
Sunrise, FL — Page 107
CIGNA Healthcare of Georgia
Atlanta, GA — Page 128
CIGNA Healthcare of Illinois Inc
Chicago, IL — Page 144
CIGNA Healthcare of Indiana
Indianapolis, IN — Page 158

CIGNA Healthcare of Kansas/Missouri
Overland Park, KS — Page 177
CIGNA Healthcare of Maine Inc
Falmouth, ME — Page 195
CIGNA Healthcare of Massachusetts
Newton, MA — Page 210
CIGNA Healthcare of Mid-Atlantic Inc
Columbia, MD — Page 201
CIGNA Healthcare of New Hampshire
Hooksett, NH — Page 265
CIGNA Healthcare of New York and New Jersey
Jersey City, NJ — Page 270
CIGNA Healthcare of North Carolina
Raleigh, NC — Page 311
CIGNA Healthcare of North Carolina Inc
Charlotte, NC — Page 311
CIGNA Healthcare of North Texas
Irving, TX — Page 409
CIGNA Healthcare of Ohio Inc
Cleveland, OH — Page 323
CIGNA Healthcare of PA
Blue Bell, PA — Page 360
CIGNA Healthcare of South Carolina
Greenville, SC — Page 384
CIGNA Healthcare of St Louis
St Louis, MO — Page 245
CIGNA Healthcare of Tennessee
Memphis, TN — Page 393
CIGNA Healthcare of Tennessee Inc
Franklin, TN — Page 394
CIGNA Healthcare of Texas Inc
Houston, TX — Page 409
CIGNA Healthcare of Virginia Inc - Richmond
Richmond, VA — Page 443
Citrus Health Care Inc
Tampa, FL — Page 108
Clear Choice Health Plans
Bend, OR — Page 345
Colorado Access
Denver, CO — Page 79
Colorado Choice Health Plana/San Luis Valley HMO Inc
Alamosa, CO — Page 79
Columbia United Providers
Vancouver, WA — Page 449
Combined Insurance Company of America
Glenview, IL — Page 145
Community Choice Health Plan of Westchester Inc
Yonkers, NY — Page 287
Community Choice Michigan
Okemos, MI — Page 219
Community Clinical Services
Lewiston, ME — Page 196
Community First Health Plans Inc
San Antonio, TX — Page 410
Community Health Choice Inc
Houston, TX — Page 410
Community Health Group
Chula Vista, CA — Page 41
Community Health Network of Connecticut Inc
Wallingford, CT — Page 89
Community Health Plan
Alhambra, CA — Page 42
Community Health Plan
St Joseph, MO — Page 245
Community Health Plan of Washington
Seattle, WA — Page 450
Community Medical Alliance
Boston, MA — Page 210
CommunityCare Managed Healthcare Plans of Oklahoma Inc
Tulsa, OK — Page 340

Index II: Health Maintenance Organizations

A

ABRI Health Plan Inc
West Allis, WI — Page 461
ACN Group
Golden Valley, MN — Page 233
ACN Group of California - Western Region
San Diego, CA — Page 31
Advantage Health Solutions Inc
Indianapolis, IN — Page 157
Aetna Health Inc
Houston, TX — Page 403
Aetna Health Inc - Colorado
Greenwood Village, CO — Page 77
Aetna Health Plans of Mid-Atlantic
Falls Church, VA — Page 441
Aetna Health of California Inc
Walnut Creek, CA — Page 31
Aetna Health of Illinois Inc
Chicago, IL — Page 143
Aetna Inc
Norwalk, CT — Page 87
Aetna Inc - Arizona
Phoenix, AZ — Page 11
Aetna Inc - Corporate Headquarters
Hartford, CT — Page 87
Aetna Inc - Corporate Headquarters
Blue Bell, PA — Page 355
Aetna Inc - Florida
Tampa, FL — Page 100
Aetna Inc - Georgia
Alpheretta, GA — Page 127
Aetna Inc - Jacksonville
Jacksonville, FL — Page 100
Aetna Inc - Louisiana
Metairie, LA — Page 189
Aetna Inc - Maine
Portland, ME — Page 195
Aetna Inc - Maryland
Linthicum, MD — Page 199
Aetna Inc - Massachusetts
Waltham, MA — Page 209
Aetna Inc - Michigan
Southfield, MI — Page 217
Aetna Inc - Missouri
Chesterfield, MO — Page 243
Aetna Inc - Nevada
Las Vegas, NV — Page 259
Aetna Inc - New Jersey
Mt Laurel, NJ — Page 267
Aetna Inc - New Jersey
Fairfield, NJ — Page 267
Aetna Inc - New York
New York, NY — Page 283
Aetna Inc - New York
Uniondale, NY — Page 283
Aetna Inc - Ohio
Richfield, OH — Page 319
Aetna Inc - Oklahoma
Oklahoma City, OK — Page 339
Aetna Inc - Pennsylvania
Pittsburgh, PA — Page 355
Aetna Inc - Pennsylvania
King of Prussia, PA — Page 355
Aetna Inc - Pennsylvania Region
Blue Bell, PA — Page 356
Aetna Inc - Plantation
Plantation, FL — Page 100
Aetna Inc - Tennessee
Memphis, TN — Page 391
Aetna Inc - Tulsa
Tulsa, OK — Page 339
Aetna Inc - Virginia
Richmond, VA — Page 441
Aetna Inc - Washington
Seattle, WA — Page 449
Aetna Inc of New England
Middletown, CT — Page 87
Aetna Inc of the Carolinas
Charlotte, NC — Page 309
Affinity Health Plan Inc
Bronx, NY — Page 283
Alameda Alliance for Health
Alameda, CA — Page 33
AlohaCare
Honolulu, HI — Page 137
Altius Health Plans
South Jordan, UT — Page 433
AmeriChoice of New York
New York, NY — Page 284
AmeriGroup - Arlington Health Plan
Arlington, TX — Page 404
AmeriGroup Community Care Ohio Inc
Cincinnati, OH — Page 319
AmeriGroup Community Careplan
New York, NY — Page 284
AmeriGroup Corporation
Virginia Beach, VA — Page 442
AmeriGroup District of Columbia
Washington, DC — Page 97
AmeriGroup Florida Inc
Tampa, FL — Page 101
AmeriGroup Maryland Inc
Linthicum, MD — Page 199
AmeriGroup New Jersey Inc
Edison, NJ — Page 268
AmeriGroup Tennessee Inc
Nashville, TN — Page 391
AmeriHealth Insurance Company
Wilmington, DE — Page 95
American Pioneer Health Plans Inc
Lake Mary, FL — Page 101
Americhoice of New Jersey
Newark, NJ — Page 268
Americhoice of Pennsylvania Inc
Philadelphia, PA — Page 356
Amerihealth Insurance Company - NJ North
Iselin, NJ — Page 269
Amerihealth Insurance Company - NJ South
Mt Laurel, NJ — Page 269
Anthem Blue Cross
Woodland Hills, CA — Page 34
Anthem Blue Cross Blue Shield of Colorado
Denver, CO — Page 77
Anthem Blue Cross Blue Shield of Maine
South Portland, ME — Page 195
Anthem Blue Cross Blue Shield of Missouri
St Louis, MO — Page 243
Anthem Blue Cross Blue Shield of Nevada
Reno, NV — Page 259
Anthem Blue Cross Blue Shield of Ohio
Mason, OH — Page 320
Anthem Blue Cross Blue Shield of Virginia Inc
Richmond, VA — Page 442
Anthem Blue Cross and Blue Shield of Kentucky (HMO Kentucky)
Louisville, KY — Page 183
Anthem Blue Cross and Blue Shield of Ohio
Cincinnati, OH — Page 320
Anthem Blue Cross/Blue Shield of Indiana
Indianapolis, IN — Page 157
Anthem Blue Cross/Blue Shield of New Hampshire
Manchester, NH — Page 265
Anthem Health Plan Inc dba: Anthem Blue Cross Blue Shield CT
North Haven, CT — Page 88
Arise Health Plan
Green Bay, WI — Page 461
Arkansas Community Care Inc
Little Rock, AR — Page 26
Arnett Health Plans
Lafayette, IN — Page 157
Arta Medicare Health Plan Inc
Irvine, CA — Page 34
Athens Area Health Plan Select Inc
Athens, GA — Page 127
Atlantis Health Plan
New York, NY — Page 285
Atrio Health Plans Inc
Roseburg, OR — Page 345
Aultcare
Canton, OH — Page 320
Av-Med Health Plan - Gainesville
Gainesville, FL — Page 102
Av-Med Health Plan - Jacksonville
Jacksonville, FL — Page 102
Av-Med Health Plan - Miami
Miami, FL — Page 103
Av-Med Health Plan - Orlando
Maitland, FL — Page 103
Av-Med Health Plan - Tampa
Tampa, FL — Page 103
Avera Health Plans Inc
Sioux Falls, SD — Page 387
Aveta Health Illinois Inc
Hillside, IL — Page 143
Aveta Inc
Fort Lee, NJ — Page 270

B

Baptist Health Services Group
Memphis, TN — Page 392
Blue Care Network of Michigan
Southfield, MI — Page 217
Blue Cross Blue Shield of Arizona
Phoenix, AZ — Page 12
Blue Cross Blue Shield of Delaware
Wilmington, DE — Page 95
Blue Cross Blue Shield of Florida & Health Options Inc
Miami, FL — Page 104
Blue Cross Blue Shield of Florida/ Health Options Inc
Jacksonville, FL — Page 104
Blue Cross Blue Shield of Illinois
Chicago, IL — Page 144
Blue Cross Blue Shield of Kansas
Topeka, KS — Page 177
Blue Cross Blue Shield of Kansas City
Kansas City, MO — Page 244
Blue Cross Blue Shield of Massachusetts
Boston, MA — Page 209
Blue Cross Blue Shield of Minnesota
St Paul, MN — Page 234
Blue Cross Blue Shield of Mississippi
Jackson, MS — Page 241
Blue Cross Blue Shield of Montana
Helena, MT — Page 253

Copyright MCIC -- The National Directory of Managed Care Organizations, Seventh Edition

Index II

Health Maintenance Organizations

Index I: Managed Care Organizations Alphabetically

University Health Care Inc - Passport Health Plan
Louisville, KY — Page 187
University Health Plans Inc
Newark, NJ — Page 277
UPMC Health Plan Univ of Pittsburgh Medical Center
Pittsburgh, PA — Page 374
Upper Peninsula Health Plan
Marquette, MI — Page 232
USA Managed Care Organization
Phoenix, AZ — Page 22
Utah Public Employees Health Program
Salt Lake City, UT — Page 438
UTMB Health Plans Inc
Galveston, TX — Page 431

V

Valley Baptist Insurance Company
Harlingen, TX — Page 431
Valley Health Plan Santa Clara County
San Jose, CA — Page 72
Valley Preferred
Allentown, PA — Page 375
Value Health Care
Wall, NJ — Page 277
ValueOptions - Corporate Headquarters
Norfolk, VA — Page 447
ValueOptions of California Inc
Cypress, CA — Page 72
ValueOptions of Texas Inc
Coppell, TX — Page 431
Vantage Health Plan Inc
Monroe, LA — Page 193
Vantage PPO
Meadville, PA — Page 375
Ventura County Foundation for Medical Care
Camarillo, CA — Page 73
Ventura County Health Care Plan
Ventura, CA — Page 73
Vermont Health Plans (Blue Care)
Montpelier, VT — Page 439
Virginia Health Network
Richmond, VA — Page 447
Virginia Premier Health Plans Inc
Richmond, VA — Page 447
Vision Care Network
Racine, WI — Page 471
Vision First Eye Care Inc
San Jose, CA — Page 73
Vision Health Management Systems
Chicago, IL — Page 155
Vision Insurance Plan of America Inc - Corp Headquarters
Milwaukee, WI — Page 471
Vision Plan of America
Los Angeles, CA — Page 75
Vision Service Plan
Rancho Cordova, CA — Page 75
Vision Service Plan
Denver, CO — Page 86
Vision Service Plan of Arizona
Phoenix, AZ — Page 22
Visioncare of California
San Diego, CA — Page 75
Vista Health Plan Inc
Hollywood, FL — Page 123
Vista Healthplan of South Florida Inc
Sunrise, FL — Page 123
Viva Health Inc
Birmingham, AL — Page 7
Volusia Health Network
Holly Hill, FL — Page 124

W

Washington Dental Service
Seattle, WA — Page 457
WelBorn Health Plans
Evansville, IN — Page 167
WellCare HMO Inc
Tampa, FL — Page 124
WellCare Health Plans Inc - Corporate Headquarters
Tampa, FL — Page 124
WellCare of New York
Poughkeepsie, NY — Page 307
WellPoint Inc - Corporate Headquarters
Indianapolis, IN — Page 167
Wellmark Blue Cross & Blue Shield of South Dakota
Sioux Falls, SD — Page 389
Wellmark Blue Cross Blue Shield of Iowa
Des Moines, IA — Page 174
Wellmark Health Plan of Iowa Inc
Des Moines, IA — Page 175
Wellmark Inc — Corporate Headquarters
Des Moines, IA — Page 175
Wellpath Select Inc
Morrisville, NC — Page 315
West Virginia Medical Institute
Charleston, WV — Page 460
Western Dental Services
Orange, CA — Page 75
Western Health
Rapid City, SD — Page 389
Western Health Advantage
Sacramento, CA — Page 75
Williamette Dental Group PC
Hillsboro, OR — Page 352
Williamette Dental of Washington Inc
Hillsboro, OR — Page 457
WINHealth Partners
Cheyenne, WY — Page 473
Windsor Health Plan of Tennessee Inc
Brentwood, TN — Page 401
Wisconsin Physician Services Insurance Company
Madison, WI — Page 471

X

XL Health
Baltimore, MD — Page 207

Y

Yale University Health Plan
New Haven, CT — Page 93

Z

Zurich Services Corporation
Schaumburg, IL — Page 155

Index I: Managed Care Organizations Alphabetically

Touchstone Health HMO Inc
New York, NY — Page 305
Triple-S Inc
San Juan, PR — Page 378
True Blue
Meridian, ID — Page 142
Trustmark Insurance Company
Lake Forest, IL — Page 153
Tufts Health Plan
Watertown, MA — Page 216

U

UAHC Health Plan of Tennessee
Memphis, TN — Page 399
Ucare Minnesota
Minneapolis, MN — Page 238
UDC Dental California Inc
San Diego, CA — Page 71
UDC Ohio Inc
Cincinnati, OH — Page 335
UHP Healthcare
Los Angeles, CA — Page 71
UlliCare
Washington, DC — Page 98
UniCare Health Plans of TX Inc
Houston, TX — Page 428
Unicare Health Plans of the Midwest Inc
Chicago, IL — Page 153
Unicare Life and Health Insurance Co Inc
Houston, TX — Page 428
Union Health Service Inc
Chicago, IL — Page 154
Union Labor Life Insurance Co
Mount Laurel, NJ — Page 276
Unipsych Systems
Hollywood, FL — Page 120
Unison Health Plan - Corporate Headquarters
Pittsburgh, PA — Page 372
Unison Health Plan of Ohio Inc
Cleveland, OH — Page 336
Unison Health Plan of Pennsylvania
Pittsburgh, PA — Page 373
Unison Health Plan of South Carolina Inc
Columbia, SC — Page 386
Unison Health Plan of Tennessee
Memphis, TN — Page 399
United Behavioral Health
Philadelphia, PA — Page 373
United Behavioral Health (UBH)
San Francisco, CA — Page 71
United Concordia Company Inc - Alabama
Birmingham, AL — Page 6
United Concordia Company Inc - Arizona
Phoenix, AZ — Page 21
United Concordia Company Inc - California
Woodland Hills, CA — Page 72
United Concordia Company Inc - Corporate Headquarters
Harrisburg, PA — Page 373
United Concordia Company Inc - Florida
Tampa, FL — Page 121
United Concordia Company Inc - Illinois
Chicago, IL — Page 154
United Concordia Company Inc - Maryland
Hunt Valley, MD — Page 206
United Concordia Company Inc - Michigan
Troy, MI — Page 231
United Concordia Company Inc - Missouri
Chesterfield, MO — Page 251
United Concordia Company Inc - New Mexico
Albuquerque, NM — Page 282
United Concordia Company Inc - New York
Plainview, NY — Page 306
United Concordia Company Inc - Pennsylvania
Pittsburgh, PA — Page 374
United Concordia Company Inc - Pennsylvania - Central
Harrisburg, PA — Page 374
United Concordia Company Inc - Texas
Dallas, TX — Page 429
United Concordia Company Inc - Virginia
Glen Allen, VA — Page 446
United Concordia Company Inc - Washington
Seattle, WA — Page 457
United Dental Care of Texas Inc - Assurant Employee Benefits
Addison, TX — Page 429
UnitedHealth Group—Corporate Headquarters
Minnetonka, MN — Page 238
UnitedHealthcare & Mid Atlantic Medical Services Inc
Rockville, MD — Page 206
UnitedHealthcare of Alabama
Birmingham, AL — Page 7
UnitedHealthcare of Arizona Inc
Phoenix, AZ — Page 21
UnitedHealthcare of Arkansas
Little Rock, AR — Page 28
UnitedHealthcare of Colorado
Centennial, CO — Page 85
UnitedHealthcare of Florida Inc
Jacksonville, FL — Page 121
UnitedHealthcare of Florida Inc
Maitland, FL — Page 121
UnitedHealthcare of Florida Inc
Tampa, FL — Page 122
UnitedHealthcare of Georgia
Norcross, GA — Page 134
UnitedHealthcare of Illinois Inc
Chicago, IL — Page 154
UnitedHealthcare of Kentucky
Lexington, KY — Page 186
UnitedHealthcare of Louisiana
Metairie, LA — Page 193
UnitedHealthcare of Massachusetts
Waltham, MA — Page 216
UnitedHealthcare of Mississippi Inc
Ridgeland, MS — Page 242
UnitedHealthcare of New England Inc
Warwick, RI — Page 381
UnitedHealthcare of New York Inc
East Syracuse, NY — Page 306
UnitedHealthcare of New York Metropolitan
New York, NY — Page 306
UnitedHealthcare of North Carolina Inc
Greensboro, NC — Page 315
UnitedHealthcare of Ohio Inc
Westerville, OH — Page 336
UnitedHealthcare of Ohio Inc-Cleveland
Cleveland, OH — Page 336
UnitedHealthcare of Oregon
Long Beach, CA — Page 352
UnitedHealthcare of SW Ohio Inc-Dayton/Cincinnati
Westchester, OH — Page 337
UnitedHealthcare of South Florida
Sunrise, FL — Page 122
UnitedHealthcare of Tennessee Inc
Brentwood, TN — Page 401
UnitedHealthcare of Texas Inc - Houston
Houston, TX — Page 429
UnitedHealthcare of Texas Inc - San Antonio
San Antonio, TX — Page 430
UnitedHealthcare of Texas Inc — Dallas
Plano, TX — Page 430
UnitedHealthcare of Utah
Salt Lake City, UT — Page 437
UnitedHealthcare of Virginia
Richmond, VA — Page 446
UnitedHealthcare of Washington
Mercer Island, WA — Page 457
UnitedHealthcare of Wisconsin Inc
Milwaukee, WI — Page 470
UnitedHealthcare of the Heartland States
Overland Park, KS — Page 182
UnitedHealthcare of the Midlands Inc
Omaha, NE — Page 257
UnitedHealthcare of the Midwest Inc
Maryland Heights, MO — Page 251
UnitedHealthcare Services Company of the River Valley Inc
Peoria, IL — Page 154
UnitedHealthcare Services Company of the River Valley Inc
Moline, IL — Page 154
UnitedHealthcare Services Company of the River Valley Inc
Bettendorf, IA — Page 172
UnitedHealthcare Services Company of the River Valley Inc
Dubuque, IA — Page 173
UnitedHealthcare Services Company of the River Valley Inc
Urbandale, IA — Page 173
UnitedHealthcare Services Company of the River Valley Inc
Waterloo, IA — Page 174
UnitedHealthcare Services Company of the River Valley Inc
Marion, IA — Page 173
UnitedHealthcare Services Company of the River Valley Inc
Kingsport, TN — Page 400
UnitedHealthcare Services Company of the River Valley Inc
Knoxville, TN — Page 400
UnitedHealthcare Services Company of the River Valley Inc
Chattanooga, TN — Page 400
Unity Dental Health Services
Lyndhurst, NJ — Page 277
Unity Health Insurance
Sauk City, WI — Page 470
Univera Community Health
Buffalo, NY — Page 307
Univera Healthcare of Western New York
Buffalo, NY — Page 307
Universal Health Care Inc
St Petersburg, FL — Page 122
Universal Health Network - Corporate Headquarters
Reno, NV — Page 264
University Family Care Health Plan
Tucson, AZ — Page 22
University Health Alliance
Honolulu, HI — Page 138

Index I: Managed Care Organizations Alphabetically

Quincy Health Care Management Inc
Quincy, IL — Page 153

R

Racine Dental Group SC
Racine, WI — Page 469
Rayant Insurance Company of New York
New York, NY — Page 304
Raytel Imaging Network
Collegeville, PA — Page 371
Regence Blue Cross Blue Shield of Oregon
Portland, OR — Page 351
Regence Blue Cross Blue Shield of Utah
Salt Lake City, UT — Page 436
Regence Blue Shield
Burlington, WA — Page 456
Regence Blue Shield
Seattle, WA — Page 456
Regence Blue Shield of Idaho
Lewiston, ID — Page 142
Regence Group, The — Corporate Headquarters
Portland, OR — Page 351
Regence Healthwise
Salt Lake City, UT — Page 436
Regence Valucare
Salt Lake City, UT — Page 436
Regencecare
Seattle, WA — Page 456
Renaissance Health Systems Inc
Wellington, FL — Page 119
Review Works
Farmington Hills, MI — Page 230
Robert T Dorris Associates
Westlake Village, CA — Page 66
Rocky Mountain Health Plans
Grand Junction, CO — Page 84
Rocky Mountain HealthCare Options Inc dba Healthcare Options
Grand Junction, CO — Page 84
Rocky Mountain Hosital & Medical Services Inc
Denver, CO — Page 85

S

S V S Visions Inc
Mt Clemens, MI — Page 231
Safeguard Health Enterprises Inc
Aliso Viejo, CA — Page 66
Safeguard Health Plans Inc
Ft Lauderdale, FL — Page 119
Safeguard Health Plans Inc
Dallas, TX — Page 424
Sagamore Health Network Inc
Carmel, IN — Page 164
Saint Mary's HealthFirst
Reno, NV — Page 263
Samaritan Health Plans Inc
Corvallis, OR — Page 352
San Francisco Health Plan
San Francisco, CA — Page 66
San Joaquin Foundation PPO
Murphys, CA — Page 67
Sanford Health Plan
Sioux Falls, SD — Page 388
Sanford Health Plan of Minnesota
Sioux Falls, SD — Page 238

Santa Barbara Regional Health Authority
Goleta, CA — Page 67
Santa Clara Family Health Plan
Campbell, CA — Page 67
Sante Community Physicians
Fresno, CA — Page 67
Scan Health Plan
Long Beach, CA — Page 68
Schc Total Care Inc
Syracuse, NY — Page 305
Scott & White Health Plan
Temple, TX — Page 424
Scripps Clinic Health Plan Services Inc
San Diego, CA — Page 68
Script Care Inc
Beaumont, TX — Page 425
Secure Health Plans of Georgia LLC
Macon, GA — Page 133
SecureCare Dental
Phoenix, AZ — Page 20
Security Health Plan of Wisconsin Inc
Marshfield, WI — Page 469
Select Circle Health Plan
Muncie, IN — Page 165
Select Health of South Carolina
North Charleston, SC — Page 385
SelectHealth
Salt Lake City, UT — Page 437
SelectHealth Network
Evansville, IN — Page 165
Selectcare Access Corporation
Pittsburgh, PA — Page 371
Sentinel Management Services - Corporate Headquarters
Lancaster, PA — Page 372
Seton Health Plan
Austin, TX — Page 425
Sharp Health Plan
San Diego, CA — Page 68
SHPS Healthcare Services
Scottsdale, AZ — Page 20
SHPS Inc
Louisville, KY — Page 186
Sierra Health Services Inc- Corporate Headquarters
Las Vegas, NV — Page 264
Signature Health Alliance
Nashville, TN — Page 398
Sloan's Lake Preferred Health Networks
Greenwood Village, CO — Page 85
SmileCare/Community Dental Services
Santa Ana, CA — Page 69
South Bay Independent Physicians Medical Group Inc
Torrance, CA — Page 69
South Central Preferred
York, PA — Page 372
Southcare/Healthcare Preferred
Atlanta, GA — Page 134
Southeastern Indiana Health Organization
Columbus, IN — Page 166
Southern Health Services Inc
Charlottesville, VA — Page 445
Southern Health Services Inc
Richmond, VA — Page 445
Southwest Health Alliance (SHALLC)
Austin, TX — Page 425
Spectera Vision Inc - Corporate Headquarters
Baltimore, MD — Page 206
Spectera Vision Inc - Indiana
Indianapolis, IN — Page 166
Spectera Vision Services of California Inc
Culver City, CA — Page 69

Spectrum Review Services Inc
Houston, TX — Page 426
Spectrum Vision Systems Inc
Overland Park, KS — Page 181
St Francis Optimum Health Network
Greenville, SC — Page 385
Standard Optical
Salt Lake City, UT — Page 437
Stanislaus Medical Society
Modesto, CA — Page 70
Staywell Insurance Guam Inc
Hagatna, GU — Page 135
Strategic Health Development Corporation
Miami Shores, FL — Page 119
Suburban Health Organization
Indianapolis, IN — Page 166
Suffolk Health Plan
Hauppauge, NY — Page 305
Summacare Inc
Akron, OH — Page 334
Summerlin Life & Health Insurance Company
Las Vegas, NV — Page 264
Summerline Life & Health Insurance Company
Honolulu, HI — Page 138
Summit Health Plan Inc
Hollywood, FL — Page 120
Sun Health Medisun
Sun City, AZ — Page 20
SuperMed Network
Cleveland, OH — Page 334
Superien Health Network Inc
Stow, OH — Page 335
Superior Dental Care Alliance
Dayton, OH — Page 335
Superior HealthPlan Inc
Austin, TX — Page 426
Superior Vision Services Inc
Laguna Hills, CA — Page 70
Susquehanna Health Care
Berwick, PA — Page 372

T

Talbert Health Plan
Costa Mesa, CA — Page 70
Tenet Choices Inc
Metaire, LA — Page 192
Tennessee Behavioral Health Inc
Nashville, TN — Page 399
Tennessee Healthcare LLC
Brentwood, TN — Page 399
Texas Childrens Health Plan
Houston, TX — Page 426
Texas Community Care
El Paso, TX — Page 427
Texas Dental Plan
San Antonio, TX — Page 427
Texas HealthSpring I LLC
Houston, TX — Page 427
Texas Medical Foundation Health Quality Institute
Austin, TX — Page 427
Texas True Choice
Plano, TX — Page 428
Total Dental Administrators Health Plan
Phoenix, AZ — Page 21
Total Health Care Inc
Detroit, MI — Page 231
Total Health Choice Inc
Miami, FL — Page 120

Index I: Managed Care Organizations Alphabetically

PacifiCare Dental & Vision
Santa Ana, CA — Page 61

PacifiCare Health Systems-Corporate Headquarters
Santa Ana, CA — Page 62

PacifiCare of Arizona
Phoenix, AZ — Page 19

PacifiCare of California
Cypress, CA — Page 62

PacifiCare of Colorado/United Healthcare
Greenwood Village, CO — Page 84

PacifiCare of Nevada
Las Vegas, NV — Page 263

PacifiCare of Oklahoma Inc/Secure Horizons
Tulsa, OK — Page 342

PacifiCare of Oregon
Lake Oswego, OR — Page 350

PacifiCare of Texas - Houston
Houston, TX — Page 422

PacifiCare of Texas Inc
Dallas, TX — Page 422

Pacific Health Alliance
Burlingame, CA — Page 62

Pacific IPA
El Monte, CA — Page 63

Pacific Union Dental Inc
Concord, CA — Page 63

Pacific Visioncare Washington Inc
Chehalis, WA — Page 453

PacificSource Health Plans
Springfield, OR — Page 350

Pacificare Life & Health Insurance Company
Cypress, CA — Page 63

ParadigmHealth
Upper Saddle River, NJ — Page 276

Paramount Advantage
Maumee, OH — Page 333

Paramount Care of Michigan
Dundee, MI — Page 228

Paramount Health Care Plan
Maumee, OH — Page 333

Parkland Community Health Plan Inc
Dallas, TX — Page 422

Parkview Signature Care
Ft Wayne, IN — Page 164

Partnercare Health Plan Inc
Tampa, FL — Page 117

Partners National Health Plans of North Carolina Inc
Winston-Salem, NC — Page 314

Partnership HealthPlan of California
Fairfield City, CA — Page 64

Peach State Health Plan
Smyrna, GA — Page 133

Pearle Vision Managed Care - HMO of Texas Inc
Dallas, TX — Page 423

Penn Highlands Health Plan
Johnstown, PA — Page 370

PerfectHealth Insurance Company
Staten Island, NY — Page 304

PersonalCare Insurance of Illinois Inc
Champaign, IL — Page 151

Phoebe Health Partners
Albany, GA — Page 133

Phoenix Health Plan - Community Connection
Phoenix, AZ — Page 19

PHP Companies Inc
Knoxville, TN — Page 397

Physical Therapy Provider Network
Delray Beach, FL — Page 117

Physicians Foundation for Medical Care
San Jose, CA — Page 64

Physicians Health Plan of Mid-Michigan
Lansing, MI — Page 228

Physicians Health Plan of Northern Indiana
Ft Wayne, IN — Page 164

Physicians Health Plan of South Michigan
Jackson, MI — Page 229

Physicians Plus Insurance Corporation
Madison, WI — Page 469

Physicians United Plan Inc
Orlando, FL — Page 118

PhysiciansPlus Baptist St Dominic Inc
Jackson, MS — Page 242

Pima Health Plan
Tucson, AZ — Page 19

Pioneer Health - The PPO
West Springfield, MA — Page 215

PPNM's Mastercare Network
Sparks, NV — Page 263

PPO USA Inc
Lee's Summit, MO — Page 250

ppoNEXT
Dallas, TX — Page 423

PPOPlus LLC
New Orleans, LA — Page 192

Prairie States Enterprises Inc
Chicago, IL — Page 152

Preferred Care
Rochester, NY — Page 304

Preferred Care Incorporated
Ft Washington, PA — Page 370

Preferred Care Partners Inc
Miami, FL — Page 118

Preferred Chiropractic Care Inc
Wichita, KS — Page 179

Preferred Dental Network (PDN)
Quincy, MA — Page 215

Preferred Health Alliance
Birmingham, AL — Page 6

Preferred Health Care
Lancaster, PA — Page 370

Preferred Health Plan Inc
Klamath Falls, OR — Page 350

Preferred Health Professionals
Overland Park, KS — Page 180

Preferred Health Systems
Wichita, KS — Page 180

Preferred Healthcare System Inc
Altoona, PA — Page 371

Preferred Medical Plan Inc
Coral Gables, FL — Page 118

Preferred Mental Health Management
Wichita, KS — Page 180

Preferred One
North Haven, CT — Page 93

Preferred One
Golden Valley, MN — Page 237

Preferred Plus of Kansas Inc
Wichita, KS — Page 181

Preferred Podiatrists of Oklahoma
Bethany, OK — Page 342

Preferred Podiatry Group
Northbrook, IL — Page 152

Preferred Provider Organization of Michigan (PPOM)
Southfield, MI — Page 229

Preferred Therapy Providers of America - Corp Headquarters
Phoenix, AZ — Page 19

Premera - Corporate Headquarters
Mountlake Terrace, WA — Page 454

Premera Blue Cross - Eastern
Spokane, WA — Page 454

Premera Blue Cross - Western
Mountlake Terrace, WA — Page 454

Premera Blue Cross Blue Shield of Alaska
Anchorage, AK — Page 9

Premier Behavioral Systems of Tennessee LLC
Nashville, TN — Page 398

Premier Health Networks of Alabama LLC
Huntsville, AL — Page 6

Presbyterian Health Plan
Alburquerque, NM — Page 281

Prevea Health Network
Green Bay, WI — Page 469

Primaris
Columbia, MO — Page 250

Primary Health Plan
Boise, ID — Page 142

Primary Provider Management Company Inc
San Diego, CA — Page 64

Prime Health Services Inc
Brentwood, TN — Page 398

Primecare Medical Network Inc
Ontario, CA — Page 65

Primetime Medical Health Plan
Canton, OH — Page 333

Principal Life Insurance Company
West Des Moines, IA — Page 172

Priority Health
Grand Rapids, MI — Page 230

Private Healthcare Systems - California
Irvine, CA — Page 65

Private Healthcare Systems - Corporate Headquarters
Waltham, MA — Page 215

Private Healthcare Systems - Georgia
Atlanta, GA — Page 133

Private Healthcare Systems - Illinois
Rosemont, IL — Page 153

Private Healthcare Systems - Missouri
Kansas City, MO — Page 251

Private Healthcare Systems - Texas
Dallas, TX — Page 423

Private Healthcare Systems - Washington
Bothell, WA — Page 455

PRO-Care Health Plan
Detroit, MI — Page 230

PRONJ, The Healthcare Quality Improvement Organization of NJ
East Brunswick, NJ — Page 276

ProviDRs Care Network
Wichita, KS — Page 181

Providence Health Plans
Beaverton, OR — Page 351

Provider Networks of America Inc
Arlington, TX — Page 424

PTPN - Corporate Headquarters
Calabasas, CA — Page 65

Pueblo Health Care
Pueblo, CO — Page 84

Puget Sound Health Partners
Lakewood, WA — Page 455

Q

QCA Health Plan Inc
Little Rock, AR — Page 28

QualCare Inc
Piscataway, NJ — Page 276

Qualis Health
Seattle, WA — Page 455

Quality Health Plan Inc
Holiday, FL — Page 119

Index I: Managed Care Organizations Alphabetically

Medwatch LLC
Lake Mary, FL — Page 116
Mega Life & Health Insurance Company
North Richland Hills, TX — Page 420
Memorial Hermann Health Network Providers
Houston, TX — Page 420
Memphis Managed Care Corp
Memphis, TN — Page 397
Mendocino and Lake Counties Foundation for Medical Care
Ukiah, CA — Page 59
Mental Health Consultants Inc
Jamison, PA — Page 369
Mercer First Choice
Sharon, PA — Page 369
Mercy Care Plan
Phoenix, AZ — Page 18
Mercy CarePlus
St Louis, MO — Page 249
Mercy Health Plans of Missouri Inc
Chesterfield, MO — Page 249
Mercy of Iowa City Regional PHO - Priority Health Network
Iowa City, IA — Page 172
Mercycare Health Plan Inc
Janesville, WI — Page 468
Meritain Health
Cleveland, OH — Page 330
Meritain Health Inc
Amherst, NY — Page 299
Metcare Health Plans Inc
West Palm Beach, FL — Page 116
MetroPlus Health Plan
New York, NY — Page 300
Metropolitan Health Plan
Minneapolis, MN — Page 237
Mid Atlantic Medical Services Inc (MAMSI)- Corp Headquarters
Rockville, MD — Page 204
Mid-Atlantic Managed Care Organization of Pennsylvania Inc
Gettysburg, PA — Page 369
Midlands Choice Inc
Omaha, NE — Page 256
Midwest Health Plan
Dearborn, MI — Page 226
Midwestern Dental Plans Inc
Dearborn, MI — Page 226
Mississippi Select Health Care
Gulfport, MS — Page 241
Missouri Care
Columbia, MO — Page 250
MIT Health Plan
Cambridge, MA — Page 214
MMM Healthcare Inc
San Juan, PR — Page 378
Molina Healthcare Inc - Corporate Headquarters
Long Beach, CA — Page 59
Molina Healthcare Inc of California
Long Beach, CA — Page 59
Molina Healthcare of Michigan Inc
Troy, MI — Page 227
Molina Healthcare of New Mexico
Albuquerque, NM — Page 281
Molina Healthcare of Ohio Inc
Columbus, OH — Page 330
Molina Healthcare of Texas Inc
Houston, TX — Page 421
Molina Healthcare of Utah Inc
Midvale, UT — Page 435
Molina Healthcare of Washington Inc
Bothell, WA — Page 453
Monroe Plan for Medical Care, The
Rochester, NY — Page 300

Mount Carmel Health Plan
Columbus, OH — Page 331
Mountain Medical Affiliates
Greenwood Village, CO — Page 83
Mountain Pacific Quality Health Foundation
Helena, MT — Page 254
Mountain State Blue Cross Blue Shield
Parkersburg, WV — Page 460
MPRO
Farmington Hills, MI — Page 227
MultiPlan Inc - Corporate Headquarters
New York, NY — Page 300
Mutual Assurance Administrators Inc
Oklahoma City, OK — Page 342
MVP Health Plan Inc
Schenectady, NY — Page 301
MVP Health Plan of New Hampshire
Bedford, NH — Page 266

N

NAMCI
Huntsville, AL — Page 6
National Capital PPO
Springfield, VA — Page 444
National Dental Consultants Inc
Islip, NY — Page 301
National Foot Care Program Inc
Lathrup Village, MI — Page 227
National Health Plan
New York, NY — Page 302
National Pacific Dental
Houston, TX — Page 421
Nationwide Better Health
Hunt Valley, MD — Page 204
Nationwide Health Plans
Columbus, OH — Page 331
NDC-West Inc dba NADENT
Fort Collins, CO — Page 83
Neighborhood Health Partnership
Miami, FL — Page 116
Neighborhood Health Plan
Boston, MA — Page 214
Neighborhood Health Plan of Rhode Island
Providence, RI — Page 380
Neighborhood Health Providers
New York, NY — Page 302
Network Health Plan Wisconsin
Menasha, WI — Page 468
Nevada Pacific Dental
Las Vegas, NV — Page 262
Nevada Preferred Professionals
Las Vegas, NV — Page 262
NevadaCare Inc
Las Vegas, NV — Page 262
New England Financial - Corporate Headquarters
Boston, MA — Page 214
New Mexico Medical Review Association
Albuquerque, NM — Page 281
New West Health Services
Helena, MT — Page 254
New York Compensation Managers Inc
Syracuse, NY — Page 302
New York Presbyterian Community Health Plan
New York, NY — Page 302
New York State Catholic Health Plan Inc
Rego Park, NY — Page 303

Newport Dental Plan
Santa Ana, CA — Page 60
North Dakota Health Care Review
Minot, ND — Page 318
Northeast Health Direct LLC
Marlborough, CT — Page 92
Northwest Rehab Alliance
Portland, OR — Page 349
Novasys Health Network
Little Rock, AR — Page 28
NYCHSRO/MedReview Inc
New York, NY — Page 303

O

ODS Health Plan
Portland, OR — Page 349
Ohio Health Choice
Akron, OH — Page 332
Ohio Kepro Inc
Seven Hills, OH — Page 332
Ohio State University Managed Health Care Systems Inc
Columbus, OH — Page 332
OhioHealth Group
Columbus, OH — Page 332
Oklahoma Foundation for Medical Quality
Oklahoma City, OK — Page 342
Olympus Managed Health Care Inc
Miami, FL — Page 117
OmniCare, A Coventry Health Plan
Detroit, MI — Page 228
On Lok Senior Health Services
San Francisco, CA — Page 60
One Call Medical Inc
Parsippany, NJ — Page 275
OneNet PPO
Rockville, MD — Page 205
Opticare Managed Vision
Rocky Mount, NC — Page 314
Optima Health Plan Inc
Virginia Beach, VA — Page 445
Optimum Choice Inc
Rockville, MD — Page 205
Optimum Choice of the Carolina Inc
Rockville, MD — Page 205
Optimum HealthCare Inc
Spring Hill, FL — Page 117
OraQuest Dental Plans
Sugarland, TX — Page 421
Orange County Health Authority
Orange, CA — Page 60
Orange County PPO
Orange, CA — Page 61
OSF Health Plans
Peoria, IL — Page 151
Outlook Vision Services
Mesa, AZ — Page 18
Oxford Health Plans Inc — Corporate Headquarters
Trumbell, CT — Page 92
Oxford Health Plans of New Jersey Inc
Iselin, NJ — Page 275
Oxford Health Plans of New York, Inc
New York, NY — Page 303
Oxford Health Plans-Connecticut
Trumbell, CT — Page 91

P

PacifiCare Behavioral Health
Santa Ana, CA — Page 61

Index I: Managed Care Organizations Alphabetically

Inland Empire Health Plan
San Bernardino, CA — Page 52
Innovative Care Management
Clackamas, OR — Page 347
Integra Group
Cincinnati, OH — Page 329
Integrated Health Plan Inc
St Petersburg, FL — Page 115
Inter Valley Health Plan Inc
Pomona, CA — Page 53
Interactive Medical Systems
Raleigh, NC — Page 313
Intercommunity Health Network
Corvallis, OR — Page 347
Intergroup Services Corporation
Malvern, PA — Page 367
Interplan Health Group
Stockton, CA — Page 53
Interplan Health Group
Arlington, TX — Page 419
Interplan Health Group - Corporate Headquarters
Farmington, CT — Page 91
Intracorp
Philadelphia, PA — Page 367
Iowa Foundation for Medical Care/ Encompass
West Des Moines, IA — Page 170
Iowa Health Solutions
Rock Island, IL — Page 171
IPRO
Lake Success, NY — Page 298

J

Jackson Memorial Health Plan
Miami, FL — Page 115
Jaimini Health Inc
Rancho Cucamonga, CA — Page 53
JP Farley Corporation
Westlake, OH — Page 329
JPS Benefits
Fort Worth, TX — Page 419

K

Kaiser Foundation Health Plan - Mid Atlantic States
Rockville, MD — Page 203
Kaiser Foundation Health Plan Northwest
Portland, OR — Page 347
Kaiser Foundation Health Plan of Colorado
Denver, CO — Page 83
Kaiser Foundation Health Plan of Georgia
Atlanta, GA — Page 132
Kaiser Foundation Health Plan of Northern California
Oakland, CA — Page 54
Kaiser Foundation Health Plan of Ohio
Cleveland, OH — Page 329
Kaiser Foundation Health Plan of Southern California
Pasadena, CA — Page 54
Kaiser Permanente - Kaiser Foundation Health Plan, Inc
Oakland, CA — Page 54
Kaiser Permanente Health Plan
Honolulu, HI — Page 137

Kansas Foundation Medical Care
Topeka, KS — Page 179
Keokuk Area Hospital Organized Delivery System Inc
Keokuk, IA — Page 171
Kepro
Harrisburg, PA — Page 367
Kern Family Health Care
Bakersfield, CA — Page 55
Kern Foundation/Preferred Provider Organization
Bakersfield, CA — Page 55
Keystone Health Plan Central
Harrisburg, PA — Page 367
Keystone Health Plan East Inc
Philadelphia, PA — Page 368
Keystone Health Plan West Inc
Pittsburgh, PA — Page 368
Keystone Mercy Health Plan
Philadelphia, PA — Page 368
KHS a KMG America Company
Lancaster, SC — Page 385
KPS Health Plans
Bremerton, WA — Page 452

L

LA Care Health Plan
Los Angeles, CA — Page 55
Lakewood Health Plan Inc
Lakewood, CA — Page 56
Landmark Healthcare Inc
Sacramento, CA — Page 56
Lane Oregon Health Plans
Eugene, OR — Page 347
Legacy Health Plan Inc
San Angelo, TX — Page 420
Leon Medical Centers Health Plan Inc
Miami, FL — Page 115
Liberty Dental Plan of California
Irvine, CA — Page 56
LifeWise Health Plan of Arizona
Scottsdale, AZ — Page 17
LifeWise Health Plan of Oregon
Portland, OR — Page 348
LifeWise Health Plan of Washington
Mountlake Terrace, WA — Page 453
Lifetime Healthcare Companies, The - Corporate Headquarters
Rochester, NY — Page 298
Lovelace Health Plan
Albuquerque, NM — Page 280
Lutheran Preferred/Three Rivers Preferred
Ft Wayne, IN — Page 162

M

M Plan Inc
Indianapolis, IN — Page 163
M-Care Inc
Ann Arbor, MI — Page 225
Magellan Behavioral Care of Iowa Inc
West Des Moines, IA — Page 171
Magellan Behavioral Health
Parsippany, NJ — Page 274
Magellan Health Services
Macon, GA — Page 132
Magellan Health Services Inc
Avon, CT — Page 91

MagnaCare
Garden City, NY — Page 298
Managed Care Consultants
Henderson, NV — Page 261
Managed Care of North America Inc
Ft Lauderdale, FL — Page 115
Managed Dental Care
Woodland Hills, CA — Page 57
Managed Health Network
Point Richmond, CA — Page 57
Managed Health Services Indiana Inc
Indianapolis, IN — Page 163
Managed Health Services Insurance Corporation
West Allis, WI — Page 467
Managed HealthCare Northwest Inc
Portland, OR — Page 348
March Vision Care Inc
Los Angeles, CA — Page 58
Maricopa Health Plan
Phoenix, AZ — Page 18
Marion Polk Community Health Plan Advantage
Salem, OR — Page 349
Martins Point Health Care
Portland, ME — Page 196
Masspro Inc
Waltham, MA — Page 213
McLaren Health Plan
Flint, MI — Page 226
MD-Individual Practice Association Inc (MD IPA)
Rockville, MD — Page 204
MDNY Healthcare Inc
Melville, NY — Page 299
MDWise
Indianapolis, IN — Page 163
MDX Hawaii
Honolulu, HI — Page 138
Med-Comp USA
Metairie, LA — Page 192
Med-Valu Inc
Hilliard, OH — Page 329
MedAvant National Preferred Provider Network
Middletown, NY — Page 299
MedSolutions
Franklin, TN — Page 396
Medco Health Solutions Inc
Franklin Lakes, NJ — Page 275
Medcore Health Plan
Stockton, CA — Page 58
Medcost LLC
Winston-Salem, NC — Page 313
Medfocus Radiology Network
Santa Monica, CA — Page 58
Medica Health Plans
Minnetonka, MN — Page 236
Medica Healthcare Plans Inc
Coral Gables, FL — Page 116
Medical Associates Clinic Health Plan of WI
Dubuque, IA — Page 467
Medical Associates Health Plans
Dubuque, IA — Page 172
Medical Card System
Hato Rey, PR — Page 377
Medical Care Referral Group
El Paso, TX — Page 420
Medical Eye Services Inc
Santa Ana, CA — Page 58
Medical Mutual of Ohio
Cleveland, OH — Page 330
Medical Network Inc
Portland, ME — Page 197
Medical Review Institute - Corporate Headquarters
Salt Lake City, UT — Page 435

Index I: Managed Care Organizations Alphabetically

**HealthAmerica Pennsylvania Inc -
Eastern Region**
Plymouth Meeting, PA — Page 365

**HealthAmerica Pennsylvania Inc -
Nortwestern**
Erie, PA — Page 365

**HealthAmerica Pennsylvania Inc -
Western Region**
Pittsburgh, PA — Page 365

HealthCare USA of Missouri LLC
St Louis, MO — Page 248

HealthCare Value Management Inc
Norwood, MA — Page 213

HealthChoice of Alabama
Birmingham, AL — Page 4

HealthEOS by MultiPlan
Brookfield, WI — Page 466

HealthEase of Florida Inc
Tampa, FL — Page 111

HealthFirst Inc
New York, NY — Page 295

HealthLink Inc
St Louis, MO — Page 248

**HealthLink Inc -
Corporate Headquarters**
St Louis, MO — Page 249

HealthLink of Arkansas Inc
North Little Rock, AR — Page 27

HealthNow New York Inc
Buffalo, NY — Page 295

HealthPartners Inc
Bloomington, MN — Page 236

HealthPlus of Michigan
Flint, MI — Page 224

HealthSmart Preferred Care
Lubbock, TX — Page 416

HealthSpring Inc - Corporate Headquarters
Franklin, TN — Page 395

HealthSpring Inc - Tennessee
Nashville, TN — Page 395

Healthcare Partners of East Texas Inc
Longview, TX — Page 416

Healthinsight
Salt Lake City, UT — Page 435

Healthnow
Memphis, TN — Page 395

Healthplex Inc
Uniondale, NY — Page 296

Healthplus Inc
Brooklyn, NY — Page 296

Healthspring of Alabama Inc
Birmingham, AL — Page 5

Healthsun Health Plans Inc
Miami, FL — Page 112

Healthy Palm Beaches Inc
West Palm Beach, FL — Page 112

Heart of America Health Plan
Rugby, ND — Page 317

Henry Ford OptimEyes
Madison Heights, MI — Page 224

Heritage Health Systems Inc
Houston, TX — Page 416

Heritage Provider Network Inc
Northridge, CA — Page 50

HFN Inc
Oak Brook, IL — Page 150

Highmark Inc
Pittsburgh, PA — Page 366

Hines & Associates Inc
Elgin, IL — Page 150

HIP Health Plan of New York
New York, NY — Page 296

HMO California
Signal Hill, CA — Page 51

HMO Health Ohio (Cleveland)
Cleveland, OH — Page 328

HMO Illinois
Chicago, IL — Page 150

HMO Louisiana Inc
Baton Rouge, LA — Page 191

HMO Nevada
Las Vegas, NV — Page 260

HMO New Mexico Inc
Albuquerque, NM — Page 280

HMS Colorado Inc
Greenwood Village, CO — Page 82

Holman Group, The
Northridge, CA — Page 51

Hometown Health Plan
Reno, NV — Page 260

Honored Citizen's Choice Health Plan
Beverly Hills, CA — Page 51

Horizon Behavioral Services
Lake Mary, FL — Page 112

Horizon Behavioral Services
Lewisville, TX — Page 417

Horizon Blue Cross/Blue Shield of NJ
Newark, NJ — Page 273

Horizon Health PPO
Henderson, NV — Page 261

Horizon Healthcare Dental Inc
Newark, NJ — Page 273

Horizon Healthcare Services Inc
Newark, NJ — Page 274

Horizon NJ Health
Trenton, NJ — Page 274

Hudson Health Plan
Tarrytown, NY — Page 297

Human Affairs International of California
El Segundo, CA — Page 52

Humana Health Benefit Plan of Louisiana
Metairie, LA — Page 191

Humana Health Care Plans of Arizona
Phoenix, AZ — Page 17

Humana Health Care Plans of Corpus Christi
Corpus Christi, TX — Page 417

Humana Health Care Plans of Dallas
Dallas, TX — Page 417

Humana Health Care Plans of Houston
Houston, TX — Page 418

Humana Health Care Plans of Illinois
Chicago, IL — Page 151

Humana Health Care Plans of Kansas & Missouri
Overland Park, KS — Page 179

Humana Health Care Plans of Lexington
Lexington, KY — Page 185

Humana Health Care Plans of San Antonio/Austin
San Antonio, TX — Page 418

Humana Health Plan - Jacksonville
Jacksonville, FL — Page 113

Humana Health Plan - Kentucky
Louisville, KY — Page 185

Humana Health Plan of Austin
Austin, TX — Page 419

Humana Health Plan of Ohio Inc
Cincinnati, OH — Page 328

Humana Health Plans of Georgia
Atlanta, GA — Page 132

Humana Inc - Arkansas
Louisville, KY — Page 27

Humana Inc - Colorado
Englewood, CO — Page 82

Humana Inc - Corporate Headquarters
Louisville, KY — Page 185

Humana Inc - District of Columbia
Louisville, KY — Page 98

Humana Inc - Grand Rapids Michigan
Grand Rapids, MI — Page 225

Humana Inc - Indiana
Indianapolis, IN — Page 161

Humana Inc - Iowa
Louisville, KY — Page 170

Humana Inc - Maryland
Louisville, KY — Page 203

Humana Inc - Mississippi
Louisville, KY — Page 241

Humana Inc - Nebraska
Louisville, KY — Page 256

Humana Inc - New Mexico
Louisville, KY — Page 280

Humana Inc - North Carolina
Charlotte, NC — Page 313

Humana Inc - North Dakota
Louisville, KY — Page 317

Humana Inc - Oklahoma
Louisville, KY — Page 341

Humana Inc - South Carolina
Louisville, KY — Page 384

Humana Inc - South Dakota
Louisville, KY — Page 388

Humana Inc - Tennessee
Memphis, TN — Page 396

Humana Inc - Utah
Louisville, KY — Page 435

Humana Inc - Wyoming
Laramie, WY — Page 473

Humana Inc/PCA - Puerto Rico
San Juan, PR — Page 377

Humana Insurance Co - Alabama
DePere, AL — Page 5

Humana Medical Plan - Central Florida
Tampa, FL — Page 113

Humana Medical Plan - Daytona
Daytona Beach, FL — Page 113

Humana Medical Plan Inc
Miramar, FL — Page 114

Humana Military Service Inc
Louisville, KY — Page 186

Humana Wisconsin Health Organization Inc
Waukesha, WI — Page 466

Hygeia Corporation
Miami Lakes, FL — Page 114

I

IBA Health Plans
Kalamazoo, MI — Page 225

Independence Blue Cross
Philadelphia, PA — Page 366

Independent Care Health Plan
Milwaukee, WI — Page 467

Independent Health Association Inc
Buffalo, NY — Page 297

Indiana Health Network
Indianapolis, IN — Page 161

Indiana Pro Health Network
Indianapolis, IN — Page 162

Individualized Care Management Inc
Lafayette, IN — Page 162

Initial Group Inc, The
Nashville, TN — Page 396

Inland Empire Foundation for Medical Care
Riverside, CA — Page 52

Index I: Managed Care Organizations Alphabetically

For Eyes Vision Plan Inc
Berkeley, CA — Page 47
Forte Managed Care
Austin, TX — Page 414
Fortified Provider Network Inc
Scottsdale, AZ — Page 15
Freedom Health Inc
St Petersburg, FL — Page 110

G

Galaxy Health Network
Arlington, TX — Page 414
Gateway Health Plan Inc
Pittsburgh, PA — Page 362
Geisinger Health Plan
Danville, PA — Page 363
GenWorth Life & Health Insurance Co
Windsor, CT — Page 90
GENEX Services
Wayne, PA — Page 363
GHI HMO Select Inc
New York, NY — Page 293
Global Health Inc
Oklahoma City, OK — Page 341
Global Medical Management
Davie, FL — Page 110
Golden Dental Plans Inc
Warren, MI — Page 221
Golden West Dental & Vision
Camarillo, CA — Page 47
Good Health HMO Inc
Kansas City, MO — Page 247
Grand Valley Health Plan
Grand Rapids, MI — Page 221
Great Expressions Dental Centers
Bloomfield Hills, MI — Page 222
Great Lakes Health Plan
Southfield, MI — Page 222
Great Lakes Medical Review
Sylvania, OH — Page 326
Great West Life Annuity Insurance Co
Greenwood Village, CO — Page 81
Great-West Healthcare - Corporate
Greenwood Village, CO — Page 81
Great-West Healthcare - New Jersey
Piscataway, NJ — Page 272
Great-West Healthcare of Arizona
Scottsdale, AZ — Page 16
Great-West Healthcare of California
Glendale, CA — Page 48
Great-West Healthcare of California - North
Pleasant Hill, CA — Page 48
Great-West Healthcare of Colorado
Greenwood Village, CO — Page 81
Great-West Healthcare of Florida
Tampa, FL — Page 111
Great-West Healthcare of Georgia
Atlanta, GA — Page 131
Great-West Healthcare of Illinois
Rosemont, IL — Page 148
Great-West Healthcare of Kansas/ Missouri
Overland Park, KS — Page 179
Great-West Healthcare of Maine
S Portland, ME — Page 196
Great-West Healthcare of Massachusetts
Waltham, MA — Page 212
Great-West Healthcare of Michigan
Southfield, MI — Page 223
Great-West Healthcare of Minnesota
Eden Prairie, MN — Page 236

Great-West Healthcare of New York
White Plains, NY — Page 294
Great-West Healthcare of New York
New York, NY — Page 294
Great-West Healthcare of North Carolina
Charlotte, NC — Page 313
Great-West Healthcare of Ohio
Columbus, OH — Page 326
Great-West Healthcare of Ohio
North Olmstead, OH — Page 326
Great-West Healthcare of Oregon
Portland, OR — Page 346
Great-West Healthcare of Pennsylvania
Media, PA — Page 363
Great-West Healthcare of Texas - Austin
Austin, TX — Page 414
Great-West Healthcare of Texas - Dallas
Dallas, TX — Page 415
Great-West Healthcare of Texas - Houston
Houston, TX — Page 415
Great-West Healthcare of Virginia Inc
Falls Church, VA — Page 444
Great-West Healthcare of Washington Inc
Bellevue, WA — Page 451
Group Health Cooperative
Coeur D'Alene, ID — Page 141
Group Health Cooperative
Spokane, WA — Page 451
Group Health Cooperative South Central Wisconsin
Madison, WI — Page 464
Group Health Cooperative of Eau Claire
Altoona, WI — Page 465
Group Health Cooperative of Puget Sound
Seattle, WA — Page 452
Group Health Options Inc
Seattle, WA — Page 452
Group Health Plan Inc
Earth City, MO — Page 248
GroupLink Inc
Indianapolis, IN — Page 160
Guardian Life Insurance Co of America
New York, NY — Page 294
Gulf Health Plans PPO Inc
Mobile, AL — Page 4
Gundersen Lutheran Health Plan Inc
La Crosse, WI — Page 465

H

Harmony Health Plan
Chicago, IL — Page 148
Harvard Pilgrim Health Care - Corporate Headquarters
Wellesley, MA — Page 212
Has Premier Providers Inc
Houston, TX — Page 415
Hawaii Management Alliance Association
Honolulu, HI — Page 137
Hawaii Medical Services Association - BC/BS of Hawaii
Honolulu, HI — Page 137
HCH Administration
Peoria, IL — Page 148
HDN PPO
Wilmette, IL — Page 149

Health Advantage
Little Rock, AR — Page 27
Health Alliance Medical Plans - Corporate Headquarters
Urbana, IL — Page 149
Health Alliance Plan of Michigan
Detroit, MI — Page 223
Health Care Evaluation
Stockton, CA — Page 48
Health Care Excel Incorporated
Indianapolis, IN — Page 160
Health Care Exchange Limited Company
Southfield, MI — Page 223
Health Care Resources Management
Manasquan, NJ — Page 272
Health Care Service Corporation - Corporate Headquarters
Chicago, IL — Page 149
Health Choice Arizona
Tempe, AZ — Page 16
Health Design Plus
Hudson, OH — Page 327
Health First Health Plans Inc
Rockledge, FL — Page 111
Health Management Network Inc
Tempe, AZ — Page 16
Health Net - Connecticut
Shelton, CT — Page 90
Health Net - New Jersey
Neptune, NJ — Page 272
Health Net - New York
White Plains, NY — Page 295
Health Net Health Plan of Oregon Inc
Tigard, OR — Page 346
Health Net Inc - Corporate Headquarters
Woodland Hills, CA — Page 49
Health Net Inc - Northeast Corporate Headquarters
Shelton, CT — Page 91
Health Net of Arizona
Tucson, AZ — Page 17
Health Net of California
Woodland Hills, CA — Page 49
Health New England
Springfield, MA — Page 212
Health Partners
Philadelphia, PA — Page 364
Health Plan of CareOregon Inc
Portland, OR — Page 346
Health Plan of Michigan
Southfield, MI — Page 224
Health Plan of Nevada Inc
Las Vegas, NV — Page 260
Health Plan of San Joaquin, The
French Camp, CA — Page 50
Health Plan of San Mateo
San Francisco, CA — Page 50
Health Plan of the Upper Ohio Valley
St Clairsville, OH — Page 327
Health Plan, The/Hometown Region
Massillon, OH — Page 327
Health Plans Inc
Westborough, MA — Page 213
Health Plus
Peoria, IL — Page 150
Health Plus of Louisiana Inc
Shreveport, LA — Page 191
Health Resources Inc
Evansville, IN — Page 161
Health Tradition Health Plans
Onalaska, WI — Page 466
HealthAmerica Pennsylvania Inc - Central Region
Harrisburg, PA — Page 364

Index I: Managed Care Organizations Alphabetically

Delta Dental Plan of Kentucky Inc
Louisville, KY — Page 184
Delta Dental Plan of Michigan Inc
Okemos, MI — Page 220
Delta Dental Plan of Minnesota
Eagan, MN — Page 235
Delta Dental Plan of Missouri
St Louis, MO — Page 246
Delta Dental Plan of New Hampshire
Concord, NH — Page 265
Delta Dental Plan of New Jersey
Parsippany, NJ — Page 271
Delta Dental Plan of New Mexico
Albuquerque, NM — Page 279
Delta Dental Plan of North Carolina
Raleigh, NC — Page 312
Delta Dental Plan of Ohio Inc
Westerville, OH — Page 324
Delta Dental Plan of Puerto Rico
Santruce, PR — Page 377
Delta Dental Plan of South Carolina
Columbia, SC — Page 384
Delta Dental Plan of South Dakota
Pierre, SD — Page 387
Delta Dental Plan of Tennessee
Nashville, TN — Page 394
Delta Dental Plan of Wisconsin
Racine, WI — Page 463
Delta Dental Plan of Wyoming
Cheyenne, WY — Page 473
Delta Dental Plans Association
Oak Brook Village, IL — Page 146
Delta Dental of Florida
Maitland, FL — Page 108
Delta Dental of Iowa
Ankeny, IA — Page 169
Delta Dental of Nebraska
Omaha, NE — Page 256
Delta Dental of Oklahoma
Oklahoma City, OK — Page 340
Delta Dental of Pennsylvania
Mechanicsburg, PA — Page 361
Delta Dental of Rhode Island
Providence, RI — Page 380
Delta Dental of Virginia
Roanoke, VA — Page 443
DeltaCare USA
Cerritos, CA — Page 44
Dencap Dental Plans
Detroit, MI — Page 220
DentCare Delivery Systems Inc
Uniondale, NY — Page 289
Denta Quest Mid-Atlantic Inc
Calverton, MD — Page 202
Denta Quest Ventures Inc
Boston, MA — Page 211
Dental Alliance Discount Plan
Torrance, CA — Page 45
Dental Benefit Providers Inc
Rockville, MD — Page 202
Dental Benefit Providers of CA Inc
San Francisco, CA — Page 45
Dental Care Plus Inc
Cincinnati, OH — Page 324
Dental Care of America Ltd
Buffalo Grove, IL — Page 146
Dental Group of New Jersey
Linden, NJ — Page 271
Dental Health Services
Long Beach, CA — Page 45
Dental Health Services Inc
Seattle, WA — Page 450
Dental Network of America
Oakbrook Terrace, IL — Page 146
Dentistat (Insurance Dentists of America)
Saratoga, CA — Page 45

Denver Health Medical Plan Inc
Denver, CO — Page 80
Deseret Healthcare
Salt Lake City, UT — Page 434
Devon Health Services Inc
King of Prussia, PA — Page 361
Dimension Health (PPO)
Miami Lakes, FL — Page 109
DMC Care
Detroit, MI — Page 221
DMS Dental Plan
Warwick, RI — Page 380
Dominion Dental Services - Corporate Headquarters
Alexandria, VA — Page 444
Doral Dental USA
Mequon, WI — Page 464
Driscoll Children's Health Plan
Corpus Christi, TX — Page 412

E

Easy Choice Health Plan Inc
Newport Beach, CA — Page 46
ECCA - Managed Vision Care Inc - Corporate Headquarters
San Antonio, TX — Page 413
Educators Health Care
Murray, UT — Page 434
EHP Inc
Lancaster, PA — Page 362
El Paso First Health Plans Inc
El Paso, TX — Page 413
Elderplan Inc
Brooklyn, NY — Page 289
Elderplan Inc - SHMO
Brooklyn, NY — Page 289
EM Risk Management, A POMCO Company
Endicott, NY — Page 290
EmblemHealth Inc
New York, NY — Page 290
Emerald Health Network Inc, The
Cleveland, OH — Page 325
Empire Blue Cross Blue Shield
New York, NY — Page 290
Employee Benefit Management Services Inc
Billings, MT — Page 253
Employee Benefits Corporation
Middletown, WI — Page 464
Employees Benefit Systems
Burlington, IA — Page 170
Employers Dental Services Inc
Tucson, AZ — Page 15
Encore Health Network
Indianapolis, IN — Page 160
Epoch Group LC, The
Leawood, KS — Page 178
Essence Inc
St Louis, MO — Page 246
Evercare Select
Phoenix, AZ — Page 15
Evercare of Texas LLC
Houston, TX — Page 413
Evergreen Medical Group LLC
Columbus, GA — Page 131
Evolutions Healthcare Systems Inc
New Port Richey, FL — Page 109
Excellus BlueCross BlueShield
Rochester, NY — Page 290
Excellus BlueCross BlueShield, Central NY Southern Tier
Syracuse, NY — Page 291

Excellus BlueCross BlueShield, Central New York Region
Syracuse, NY — Page 291
Excellus BlueCross BlueShield, Rochester Region
Rochester, NY — Page 292
Excellus BlueCross BlueShield, Utica Region
Utica, NY — Page 292
Exempla Healthcare LLC
Denver, CO — Page 81
Eye Care of Wisconsin Inc
Milwaukee, WI — Page 464
EyeMed Vision Care LLC
Mason, OH — Page 325
Eyexam of California Inc
Mission Viejo, CA — Page 46

F

Fallon Community Health Plan Inc
Worcester, MA — Page 211
Family Choice Health Alliance
Hackensack, NJ — Page 272
Family Health Partners
Kansas City, MO — Page 247
Fara Healthcare Management
Mandeville, LA — Page 190
Fidelio Insurance Company
Glenside, PA — Page 362
Fidelis Care New York
Rego Park, NY — Page 293
Fidelis SecureCare of Michigan Inc
Livonia, MI — Page 221
Fidelis SecureCare of North Carolina
Charlotte, NC — Page 312
Fidelis SecureCare of Texas
Houston, TX — Page 413
Fidelis SeniorCare Inc
Schaumburg, IL — Page 147
Finger Lakes Community Care Network
Canandaigua, NY — Page 293
First Choice Health Network
Seattle, WA — Page 451
First Choice of the Midwest Inc
Sioux Falls, SD — Page 388
First Commonwealth
Chicago, IL — Page 147
First Health — California
W Sacramento, CA — Page 46
First Health Group Corp
Downers Grove, IL — Page 147
First Health Network
San Diego, CA — Page 46
First Health Network (PPO Oklahoma Inc)
Oklahoma City, OK — Page 341
First Medical Health Plan of Florida
Miami, FL — Page 109
First Plan of Minnesota
Duluth, MN — Page 235
FirstCarolinaCare
Pinehurst, NC — Page 312
FirstSight Vision Services Inc
Upland, CA — Page 47
Fiserv Inc
Brookfield, WI — Page 464
Flora Health Network
Cleveland, OH — Page 325
Florida Health Care Plan Inc
Holly Hill, FL — Page 109
Florida Health Partners Inc
Tampa, FL — Page 110

Index I: Managed Care Organizations Alphabetically

CIGNA Healthcare of Louisiana
Houston, TX — Page 190
CIGNA Healthcare of Maine Inc
Falmouth, ME — Page 195
CIGNA Healthcare of Massachusetts
Newton, MA — Page 210
CIGNA Healthcare of Mid-Atlantic Inc
Columbia, MD — Page 201
CIGNA Healthcare of New Hampshire
Hooksett, NH — Page 265
CIGNA Healthcare of New York and New Jersey
Jersey City, NJ — Page 270
CIGNA Healthcare of North Carolina
Raleigh, NC — Page 311
CIGNA Healthcare of North Carolina Inc
Charlotte, NC — Page 311
CIGNA Healthcare of North Texas
Irving, TX — Page 409
CIGNA Healthcare of Ohio Inc
Cleveland, OH — Page 323
CIGNA Healthcare of Ohio Inc
Columbus, OH — Page 323
CIGNA Healthcare of PA
Blue Bell, PA — Page 360
CIGNA Healthcare of South Carolina
Greenville, SC — Page 384
CIGNA Healthcare of St Louis
St Louis, MO — Page 245
CIGNA Healthcare of Tennessee
Memphis, TN — Page 393
CIGNA Healthcare of Tennessee Inc
Franklin, TN — Page 394
CIGNA Healthcare of Texas Inc
Houston, TX — Page 409
CIGNA Healthcare of Virginia Inc - Richmond
Richmond, VA — Page 443
Cimro Quality Healthcare Solutions
Champaign, IL — Page 144
Citrus Health Care Inc
Tampa, FL — Page 108
Clear Choice Health Plans
Bend, OR — Page 345
Co/op Optical Services Inc
Detroit, MI — Page 219
Coalition America Inc
Atlanta, GA — Page 129
Coastal Healthcare Administrators
Salinas, CA — Page 41
Colorado Access
Denver, CO — Page 79
Colorado Choice Health Plana/San Luis Valley HMO Inc
Alamosa, CO — Page 79
Colorado Dental Service Inc, dba: Delta Dental Plan of CO
Denver, CO — Page 80
Colorado Health Networks LLC
Colorado Springs, CO — Page 80
Columbia United Providers
Vancouver, WA — Page 449
Combined Insurance Company of America
Glenview, IL — Page 145
Community Behavioral Healthcare Cooperative of Pennsylvania
Harrisburg, PA — Page 361
Community Choice Health Plan of Westchester Inc
Yonkers, NY — Page 287
Community Choice Michigan
Okemos, MI — Page 219
Community Clinical Services
Lewiston, ME — Page 196

Community First Health Plans Inc
San Antonio, TX — Page 410
Community Health Alliance
South Bend, IN — Page 159
Community Health Choice Inc
Houston, TX — Page 410
Community Health Group
Chula Vista, CA — Page 41
Community Health Network of Connecticut Inc
Wallingford, CT — Page 89
Community Health Plan
Alhambra, CA — Page 42
Community Health Plan
St Joseph, MO — Page 245
Community Health Plan of Washington
Seattle, WA — Page 450
Community Medical Alliance
Boston, MA — Page 210
CommunityCare Managed Healthcare Plans of Oklahoma Inc
Tulsa, OK — Page 340
CompBenefits - Denticare Inc
Houston, TX — Page 410
CompBenefits Corporation - Corporate Headquarters
Roswell, GA — Page 129
Complementary Healthcare Plans
Beaverton, OR — Page 345
Comprehensive Behavioral Care Inc
Tampa, FL — Page 108
Comprehensive Health Group
Duluth, GA — Page 129
Compsych Behavioral Health
Chicago, IL — Page 145
Concentra Operating Corporation
Addison, TX — Page 411
Concern: Employee Assistance Program
Mountain View, CA — Page 42
ConnectCare
Midland, MI — Page 219
Connecticare Inc
Farmington, CT — Page 89
Connecticare of Massachusetts Inc
Farmington, CT — Page 210
Connecticare of NY
Tarrytown, NY — Page 288
Contra Costa Health Plan
Martinez, CA — Page 43
Cooks Childrens Health Plan
Fort Worth, TX — Page 411
Coordinated Health Plan
Providence, RI — Page 379
Coordinated Health Systems
Bethlehem, PA — Page 361
Coreview
Minneapolis, MN — Page 235
CorpHealth Inc
Fort Worth, TX — Page 412
Corporate Care Management Inc
Binghamton, NY — Page 288
Corvel Corporation
Irvine, CA — Page 43
Corvel Corporation
Indianapolis, IN — Page 159
Corvel Corporation
West Des Moines, IA — Page 169
Corvel Corporation
Toledo, OH — Page 324
Coventry Health Care Inc — Carolinas
Charlotte, NC — Page 311
Coventry Health Care Inc — Corporate Headquarters
Bethesda, MD — Page 201

Coventry Health Care Inc — Delaware Inc
Wilmington, DE — Page 96
Coventry Health Care Inc — Georgia Inc
Atlanta, GA — Page 130
Coventry Health Care Inc — Iowa
Urbandale, IA — Page 169
Coventry Health Care Inc — Louisiana
Metairie, LA — Page 190
Coventry Health Care of Kansas - Wichita
Wichita, KS — Page 178
Coventry Health Care of Kansas Inc
Kansas City, MO — Page 245
Coventry Health Care of Nebraska Inc
Omaha, NE — Page 255
Coventry Health Care
Franklin, TN — Page 394
Cox Health Plans
Springfield, MO — Page 246
Crawford and Co - Corporate Headquarters
Atlanta, GA — Page 130

D

D C Chartered Health Plan Inc
Washington, DC — Page 97
DaVita VillageHealth of Michigan Inc
Brighton, MI — Page 220
DakotaCare
Sioux Falls, SD — Page 387
Davis Vision
Plainview, NY — Page 288
Deaconess Health Plans
Evansville, IN — Page 159
Dean Health Plan
Madison, WI — Page 463
Dedicated Dental Systems
Bakersfield, CA — Page 43
Delmarva Health Care Plan Inc
Easton, MD — Page 202
Delphi Card R
Fox River Grove, IL — Page 145
Delta Dental Insurance Company - Alabama
Birmingham, AL — Page 4
Delta Dental Insurance Company - Georgia
Alpharetta, GA — Page 131
Delta Dental Insurance Company - Nevada
Las Vegas, NV — Page 259
Delta Dental Insurance Company - Texas
Irving, TX — Page 412
Delta Dental Plan Inc - Utah
Salt Lake City, UT — Page 434
Delta Dental Plan of Arizona Inc
Phoenix, AZ — Page 14
Delta Dental Plan of Arkansas
Sherwood, AR — Page 26
Delta Dental Plan of California
San Francisco, CA — Page 44
Delta Dental Plan of Idaho
Boise, ID — Page 141
Delta Dental Plan of Illinois
Lisle, IL — Page 145
Delta Dental Plan of Indiana Inc
Indianapolis, IN — Page 159
Delta Dental Plan of Kansas
Wichita, KS — Page 178

Index I: Managed Care Organizations Alphabetically

**Blue Cross Blue Shield of Texas —
HMO Blue - Southeast**
Houston, TX   Page 407
**Blue Cross Blue Shield of Texas —
HMO Blue - West**
El Paso, TX   Page 407
Blue Cross Blue Shield of Vermont
Berlin, VT   Page 439
**Blue Cross Blue Shield of Western
New York**
Buffalo, NY   Page 285
Blue Cross Blue Shield of Wyoming
Cheyenne, WY   Page 473
Blue Cross of Idaho
Meridian, ID   Page 141
**Blue Cross of Puerto Rico/La Cruz
Azul de Puerto Rico**
San Juan, PR   Page 377
**Blue Preferred Plan-Blue Cross/
Blue Shield Michigan**
Detroit, MI   Page 218
Blue Ridge Health Network
Pottsville, PA   Page 357
Blue Shield of California
San Francisco, CA   Page 36
**BlueChoice Health Plan of South
Carolina Inc**
Columbia, SC   Page 383
**BlueCross of Northeastern
Pennsylvania**
Wilkes-Barre, PA   Page 358
BlueShield of Northeastern New York
Latham, NY   Page 286
Bluegrass Family Health Inc
Lexington, KY   Page 183
Bluelincs HMO
Tulsa, OK   Page 340
BMC HealthNet Plan
Boston, MA   Page 209
Bravo Health Inc
Baltimore, MD   Page 200
Bravo Health Mid-Atlantic Inc
Baltimore, MD   Page 200
Bravo Health Pennsylvania Inc
Philadelphia, PA   Page 358
Bravo Health Texas Inc
San Antonio, TX   Page 407
Brazos Valley Health Network
Waco, TX   Page 408
Broadspire Inc
Plantation, FL   Page 105
Buckeye Community Health Plan Inc
Columbus, OH   Page 321
**Bucks County
Physician Hospital Alliance**
Doylestown, PA   Page 358

C

California Benefits Dental Plan
Santa Ana, CA   Page 37
California Dental Network Inc
Santa Ana, CA   Page 37
Cambridge Managed Care Services
Rancho Cordova, CA   Page 38
Capital Blue Cross
Harrisburg, PA   Page 359
Capital District Physicians Health Plan
Albany, NY   Page 286
Capital Health Plan
Tallahassee, FL   Page 105
Capitol Administrators
Rancho Cordova, CA   Page 38

Care 1st Health Plan
Alhambra, CA   Page 38
Care 1st Health Plan Arizona Inc
Phoenix, AZ   Page 13
Care Choices
Farmington Hills, MI   Page 218
Care Network
Pittsburgh, PA   Page 359
Care-Plus Dental Plans Inc
Wauwatosa, WI   Page 462
CareFirst Blue Cross Blue Shield
Owings Mills, MD   Page 200
CareFirst BlueChoice Inc
Washington, DC   Page 97
CareGuide
Coral Springs, FL   Page 105
CareIQ
Miramar, FL   Page 106
CareMore Health Plan
Cerritos, CA   Page 38
CarePlus Health Plans Inc
Coral Gables, FL   Page 106
CareSource
Dayton, OH   Page 321
**Careington International -
The Dental Network**
Frisco, TX   Page 408
Carelink Health Plans
Wheeling, WV   Page 459
Carelink Health Plans
Charleston, WV   Page 459
Cariten Healthcare
Knoxville, TN   Page 393
Carolina Care Plan Inc
Columbia, SC   Page 383
**Carolinas Center for Medical
Excellence, The**
Cary, NC   Page 310
**Catalina Behavioral
Health Services Inc**
Mesa, AZ   Page 13
CBCA Care Management Inc
Dallas, TX   Page 408
Centene Corporation
St Louis, MO   Page 244
Center Care
Bowling Green, KY   Page 184
Centercare Inc
Rego Park, NY   Page 287
**Central Benefits Mutual
Insurance Company**
Columbus, OH   Page 321
Central Coast Alliance for Health
Scotts Valley, CA   Page 39
Central Health Plan of California Inc
Covina, CA   Page 39
**Central New York East HealthNow
New York Inc**
East Syracuse, NY   Page 287
**Central New York West HealthNow
New York Inc**
Rochester, NY   Page 287
**Central Susquehanna Healthcare
Providers**
Lewisburg, PA   Page 359
CHA Health - Humana
Lexington, KY   Page 184
Children's Community Health Plan Inc
Madison, WI   Page 462
Chinese Community Health Plan
San Francisco, CA   Page 39
ChiroSource - Corporate Headquarters
Concord, CA   Page 40
Chirocare of Minnesota INC
Shoreview, MN   Page 234
Chiropractic Arizona Network Inc
Phoenix, AZ   Page 13

CHN MCO
Independence, OH   Page 322
CHN Solutions
Hamilton, NJ   Page 270
ChoiceCare/Humana
Cincinnati, OH   Page 322
CIGNA Behavioral Health Inc
Glendale, CA   Page 40
CIGNA Behavioral Health Inc
Hartford, CT   Page 88
CIGNA Behavioral Health Inc
Irving, TX   Page 408
**CIGNA Behavioral Health Inc -
Corporate Headquarters**
Eden Prairie, MN   Page 234
**CIGNA Dental Health Inc -
Corporation Headquarters**
Sunrise, FL   Page 106
**CIGNA Dental Health Plan of
Arizona Inc**
Sunrise, FL   Page 14
CIGNA Dental Health of California Inc
Glendale, CA   Page 40
CIGNA Dental Health of Colorado
Sunrise, FL   Page 78
CIGNA Dental Health of Delaware Inc
Sunrise, FL   Page 95
CIGNA Dental Health of Florida
Sunrise, FL   Page 107
CIGNA Dental Health of Kansas Inc
Sunrise, FL   Page 177
CIGNA Dental Health of Maryland Inc
Sunrise, FL   Page 201
CIGNA Dental Health of New Jersey Inc
Sunrise, FL   Page 270
**CIGNA Dental Health of
North Carolina Inc**
Sunrise, FL   Page 310
CIGNA Dental Health of Ohio Inc
Sunrise, FL   Page 322
**CIGNA Dental Health of
Pennsylvania Inc**
Sunrise, FL   Page 360
CIGNA Dental Health of Texas Inc
Irving, TX   Page 409
CIGNA Dental Health of Virginia Inc
Sunrise, FL   Page 443
CIGNA Health Plan of Utah Inc
Salt Lake City, UT   Page 433
**CIGNA HealthCare —
Corporate Headquarters**
Philadelphia, PA   Page 360
CIGNA Healthcare
Burlington, VT   Page 439
CIGNA Healthcare - Cincinnati
Cincinnati, OH   Page 323
CIGNA Healthcare of Arizona
Phoenix, AZ   Page 14
CIGNA Healthcare of California
Glendale, CA   Page 41
CIGNA Healthcare of Colorado
Denver, CO   Page 79
CIGNA Healthcare of Connecticut
Hartford, CT   Page 89
CIGNA Healthcare of Florida
Tampa, FL   Page 107
CIGNA Healthcare of Florida
Sunrise, FL   Page 107
CIGNA Healthcare of Georgia
Atlanta, GA   Page 128
CIGNA Healthcare of Illinois Inc
Chicago, IL   Page 144
CIGNA Healthcare of Indiana
Indianapolis, IN   Page 158
CIGNA Healthcare of Kansas/Missouri
Overland Park, KS   Page 177

Index I: Managed Care Organizations Alphabetically

Anthem Blue Cross Blue Shield of Colorado
Denver, CO — Page 77

Anthem Blue Cross Blue Shield of Maine
South Portland, ME — Page 195

Anthem Blue Cross Blue Shield of Missouri
St Louis, MO — Page 243

Anthem Blue Cross Blue Shield of Nevada
Reno, NV — Page 259

Anthem Blue Cross Blue Shield of Ohio
Mason, OH — Page 320

Anthem Blue Cross Blue Shield of Virginia Inc
Richmond, VA — Page 442

Anthem Blue Cross Blue Shield of Wisconsin
Milwaukee, WI — Page 461

Anthem Blue Cross and Blue Shield of Kentucky (HMO Kentucky)
Louisville, KY — Page 183

Anthem Blue Cross and Blue Shield of Ohio
Cincinnati, OH — Page 320

Anthem Blue Cross/Blue Shield of Indiana
Indianapolis, IN — Page 157

Anthem Blue Cross/Blue Shield of New Hampshire
Manchester, NH — Page 265

Anthem Health Plan Inc dba: Anthem Blue Cross Blue Shield CT
North Haven, CT — Page 88

APS Healthcare Inc
Silver Springs, MD — Page 199

APS Healthcare Midwest Inc
Brookfield, WI — Page 461

APS Healthcare Northwest Inc
Missoula, MT — Page 253

Arise Health Plan
Green Bay, WI — Page 461

Arizona Foundation for Medical Care
Phoenix, AZ — Page 11

Arkansas Blue Cross/Blue Shield a Mutual Insurance Company
Little Rock, AR — Page 25

Arkansas Community Care Inc
Little Rock, AR — Page 26

Arkansas Foundation for Medical Care
Ft Smith, AR — Page 26

Arkansas Managed Care Organization
Little Rock, AR — Page 26

Arnett Health Plans
Lafayette, IN — Page 157

Arta Medicare Health Plan Inc
Irvine, CA — Page 34

Assurant Employee Benefits - Alabama
Birmingham, AL — Page 3

Assurant Employee Benefits - Arizona
Phoenix, AZ — Page 12

Assurant Employee Benefits - California
San Diego, CA — Page 35

Assurant Employee Benefits - Colorado
Greenwood Village, CO — Page 78

Assurant Employee Benefits - Corporate Office
Kansas City, MO — Page 244

Assurant Employee Benefits - Florida
Tampa, FL — Page 102

Assurant Employee Benefits - Georgia
Atlanta, GA — Page 127

Assurant Employee Benefits - Illinois
Oakbrook Terrace, IL — Page 143

Assurant Employee Benefits - Indiana
Mooresville, IN — Page 158

Assurant Employee Benefits - Michigan
Troy, MI — Page 217

Assurant Employee Benefits - New Mexico
Albuquerque, NM — Page 279

Assurant Employee Benefits - New York
New York, NY — Page 285

Assurant Employee Benefits - North Carolina
Raleigh, NC — Page 309

Assurant Employee Benefits - Pennsylvania
Radnor, PA — Page 357

Assurant Employee Benefits - Tennessee
Nashville, TN — Page 392

Assurant Employee Benefits - Washington
Seattle, WA — Page 449

Assurant Health - Corporate Headquarters
Milwaukee, WI — Page 462

Asuris Northwest Health
Spokane, WA — Page 449

Athens Area Health Plan Select Inc
Athens, GA — Page 127

AtlantiCare Health Plans Inc
Hammonton, NJ — Page 269

Atlantic Dental Inc
Coral Gables, FL — Page 102

Atlantic Integrated Health Inc
New Bern, NC — Page 309

Atlantis Health Plan
New York, NY — Page 285

Atrio Health Plans Inc
Roseburg, OR — Page 345

Aultcare
Canton, OH — Page 320

Av-Med Health Plan - Gainesville
Gainesville, FL — Page 102

Av-Med Health Plan - Jacksonville
Jacksonville, FL — Page 102

Av-Med Health Plan - Miami
Miami, FL — Page 103

Av-Med Health Plan - Orlando
Maitland, FL — Page 103

Av-Med Health Plan - Tampa
Tampa, FL — Page 103

Avante Behavioral Health Plan
Fresno, CA — Page 35

Avera Health Plans Inc
Sioux Falls, SD — Page 387

Avesis Inc
Phoenix, AZ — Page 12

Aveta Health Illinois Inc
Hillside, IL — Page 143

Aveta Inc
Fort Lee, NJ — Page 270

B

Baptist Health Services Group
Memphis, TN — Page 392

Basic Chiropractic Health Plan Inc
Stockton, CA — Page 35

Beech Street Corporation — Corporate Headquarters
Lake Forest, CA — Page 36

Behavioral Health Systems Inc
Birmingham, AL — Page 3

Behavioral Healthcare Inc
Centennial, CO — Page 78

Behavioral Healthcare Options Inc
Las Vegas, NV — Page 259

Berkley Administrators of Connecticut Inc
Farmington, CT — Page 88

Berkshire Health Partners/ Medicus Resource Management
Wyomissing, PA — Page 357

Best Health Plans
Irvine, CA — Page 36

Block Vision of Texas Inc
Dallas, TX — Page 405

Blue Care Network of Michigan
Southfield, MI — Page 217

Blue Cross Blue Shield of Alabama
Birmingham, AL — Page 3

Blue Cross Blue Shield of Arizona
Phoenix, AZ — Page 12

Blue Cross Blue Shield of Delaware
Wilmington, DE — Page 95

Blue Cross Blue Shield of Florida & Health Options Inc
Miami, FL — Page 104

Blue Cross Blue Shield of Florida/ Health Options Inc
Jacksonville, FL — Page 104

Blue Cross Blue Shield of Georgia
Atlanta, GA — Page 128

Blue Cross Blue Shield of Illinois
Chicago, IL — Page 144

Blue Cross Blue Shield of Kansas
Topeka, KS — Page 177

Blue Cross Blue Shield of Kansas City
Kansas City, MO — Page 244

Blue Cross Blue Shield of Louisiana Inc
Baton Rouge, LA — Page 189

Blue Cross Blue Shield of Massachusetts
Boston, MA — Page 209

Blue Cross Blue Shield of Minnesota
St Paul, MN — Page 234

Blue Cross Blue Shield of Mississippi
Jackson, MS — Page 241

Blue Cross Blue Shield of Montana
Helena, MT — Page 253

Blue Cross Blue Shield of Nebraska
Omaha, NE — Page 255

Blue Cross Blue Shield of New Mexico
Albuquerque, NM — Page 279

Blue Cross Blue Shield of North Carolina
Durham, NC — Page 310

Blue Cross Blue Shield of North Dakota
Fargo, ND — Page 317

Blue Cross Blue Shield of Oklahoma
Tulsa, OK — Page 339

Blue Cross Blue Shield of Rhode Island
Providence, RI — Page 379

Blue Cross Blue Shield of South Carolina - Corporate Hqtrs
Columbia, SC — Page 383

Blue Cross Blue Shield of Tennessee
Chattanooga, TN — Page 392

Blue Cross Blue Shield of Tennessee - Memphis
Memphis, TN — Page 393

Blue Cross Blue Shield of Texas — Corporate Headquarters
Richardson, TX — Page 406

Blue Cross Blue Shield of Texas — HMO Blue - Midwest TX
Austin, TX — Page 406

Index I: Managed Care Organizations Alphabetically

1st Medical Network
Atlanta, GA — Page 127
20/20 Eyecare Plan Inc
Ft Lauderdale, FL — Page 99
4MOST Health Network
Charleston, WV — Page 459

A

Abri Health Plan Inc
West Allis, WI — Page 461
Access Dental Services
Sacramento, CA — Page 31
ACN Group
Golden Valley, MN — Page 233
ACN Group of California - Western Region
San Diego, CA — Page 31
Action Health Care Management Services
Phoenix, AZ — Page 11
Active Health Management
Chantilly, VA — Page 441
Acumentra Health
Portland, OR — Page 345
Advantage Health Solutions Inc
Indianapolis, IN — Page 157
Advantica Eyecare Inc
Clearwater, FL — Page 99
AECC Total Vision Health Plan of Texas Inc
Dallas, TX — Page 403
Aetna Behavioral Health - Utah Care Management Center
Sandy, UT — Page 433
Aetna Dental Inc - New Jersey
Fairfield, NJ — Page 267
Aetna Health Inc
Houston, TX — Page 403
Aetna Health Inc - Colorado
Greenwood Village, CO — Page 77
Aetna Health Plans of Mid-Atlantic
Falls Church, VA — Page 441
Aetna Health of California Inc
Walnut Creek, CA — Page 31
Aetna Health of Illinois Inc
Chicago, IL — Page 143
Aetna Inc
Norwalk, CT — Page 87
Aetna Inc - Altamonte Springs
Altamonte Springs, FL — Page 99
Aetna Inc - Arizona
Phoenix, AZ — Page 11
Aetna Inc - Arkansas
Metairie, LA — Page 25
Aetna Inc - Arkansas
Little Rock, AR — Page 25
Aetna Inc - Corporate Headquarters
Hartford, CT — Page 87
Aetna Inc - Corporate Headquarters
Blue Bell, PA — Page 355
Aetna Inc - Dental Care of California
Thousand Oaks, CA — Page 32
Aetna Inc - Dental Plan of Texas
Dallas, TX — Page 403
Aetna Inc - Florida
Tampa, FL — Page 100
Aetna Inc - Georgia
Alpheretta, GA — Page 127
Aetna Inc - Jacksonville
Jacksonville, FL — Page 100
Aetna Inc - Louisiana
Metairie, LA — Page 189

Aetna Inc - Maine
Portland, ME — Page 195
Aetna Inc - Maryland
Linthicum, MD — Page 199
Aetna Inc - Massachusetts
Waltham, MA — Page 209
Aetna Inc - Michigan
Southfield, MI — Page 217
Aetna Inc - Missouri
Chesterfield, MO — Page 243
Aetna Inc - Nevada
Las Vegas, NV — Page 259
Aetna Inc - New Jersey
Mt Laurel, NJ — Page 267
Aetna Inc - New Jersey
Fairfield, NJ — Page 267
Aetna Inc - New York
New York, NY — Page 283
Aetna Inc - New York
Uniondale, NY — Page 283
Aetna Inc - Ohio
Richfield, OH — Page 319
Aetna Inc - Oklahoma
Oklahoma City, OK — Page 339
Aetna Inc - Pennsylvania
Pittsburgh, PA — Page 355
Aetna Inc - Pennsylvania
King of Prussia, PA — Page 355
Aetna Inc - Pennsylvania Region
Blue Bell, PA — Page 356
Aetna Inc - Plantation
Plantation, FL — Page 100
Aetna Inc - Tennessee
Memphis, TN — Page 391
Aetna Inc - Tennessee
Nashville, TN — Page 391
Aetna Inc - Tulsa
Tulsa, OK — Page 339
Aetna Inc - Virginia
Richmond, VA — Page 441
Aetna Inc - Washington
Seattle, WA — Page 449
Aetna Inc of New England
Middletown, CT — Page 87
Aetna Inc of the Carolinas
Charlotte, NC — Page 309
Affinity Dental Health Plans
Culver City, CA — Page 32
Affinity Health Plan Inc
Bronx, NY — Page 283
Aids Healthcare Foundation
Los Angeles, CA — Page 32
Alabama Quality Assurance Foundation
Birmingham, AL — Page 3
Alameda Alliance for Health
Alameda, CA — Page 33
Alignis Inc
Paramus, NJ — Page 268
All Florida PPO Inc
Pompano Beach, FL — Page 101
Alliance Regional Health Network
Amarillo, TX — Page 404
Allianz Life Insurance Company of North America
Minneapolis, MN — Page 233
AlohaCare
Honolulu, HI — Page 137
Alpha Dental Plan of Colorado
Denver, CO — Page 77
Alpha Dental Programs Inc
Flower Mound, TX — Page 404
Alternative Care Management Systems
Dublin, OH — Page 319
Altius Health Plans
South Jordan, UT — Page 433

Altus Dental Insurance Company Inc
Providence, RI — Page 379
AmeriChoice of New York
New York, NY — Page 284
AmeriGroup - Arlington Health Plan
Arlington, TX — Page 404
AmeriGroup Community Care Ohio Inc
Cincinnati, OH — Page 319
AmeriGroup Community Careplan
New York, NY — Page 284
AmeriGroup Corporation
Virginia Beach, VA — Page 442
AmeriGroup District of Columbia
Washington, DC — Page 97
AmeriGroup Florida Inc
Tampa, FL — Page 101
AmeriGroup Maryland Inc
Linthicum, MD — Page 199
AmeriGroup New Jersey Inc
Edison, NJ — Page 268
AmeriGroup Tennessee Inc
Nashville, TN — Page 391
AmeriHealth Insurance Company
Wilmington, DE — Page 95
American College of Medical Quality
Bethesda, MD — Page 199
American Dental Examiners
New Rochelle, NY — Page 284
American Healthcare Alliance
Kansas City, MO — Page 243
American Healthcare Group INC
Pittsburgh, PA — Page 356
American Healthguard Corporation
Arcadia, CA — Page 33
American LIFECARE - Louisiana
New Orleans, LA — Page 189
American LIFECARE - Mississippi
Jackson, MS — Page 241
American National Insurance Company
Galveston, TX — Page 405
American Pharmacy Services Corporation
Frankfort, KY — Page 183
American Pioneer Health Plans Inc
Lake Mary, FL — Page 101
American Preferred Provider Organization LLC
Irving, TX — Page 405
American Republic Insurance Company
Des Moines, IA — Page 169
American Specialty Health Plans Inc
San Diego, CA — Page 33
American WholeHealth Networks Inc
Sterling, VA — Page 442
Americas PPO
Bloomington, MN — Page 233
Americhoice of New Jersey
Newark, NJ — Page 268
Americhoice of Pennsylvania Inc
Philadelphia, PA — Page 356
Amerihealth Insurance Company - NJ North
Iselin, NJ — Page 269
Amerihealth Insurance Company - NJ South
Mt Laurel, NJ — Page 269
Ameritas Group Dental
Lincoln, NE — Page 255
Ameritas Managed Dental Plan Inc
Costa Mesa, CA — Page 34
Antares Management Solutions
Westlake, OH — Page 319
Anthem Blue Cross
Woodland Hills, CA — Page 34

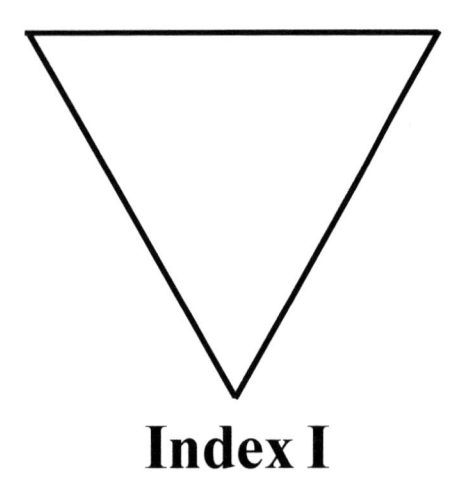

Index I

Managed Care Organizations (Alphabetically)

Directory of Healthcare Resources

The National Directory of Managed Care Organizations, Online. An online directory at your fingertips. More than 1,700 managed care plans. Call for more information and pricing, or visit our website (http://www.themcic.com) for a trial database. Call for Pricing. Address: The Managed Care Information Center, Dept. 14D7RS, 1913 Atlantic Ave., Suite F5, Manasquan, NJ 08736-1096; toll-free 888-THE-MCIC (888-843-6242), fax 888-FAX-MCIC (888-329-6242) www.healthresourcesonline.com.

The National Directory of Medical Directors, Database on CD-ROM is the Windows-based software program that includes more than 1,400 medical directors from managed care organizations and physician organizations. Program can export to other software programs. CD-ROM only. Cost: Call for Pricing. Address: The Managed Care Information Center, Dept. 14D7RS, 1913 Atlantic Ave., Suite F5, Manasquan, NJ 08736-1096; toll-free 888-THE-MCIC (888-843-6242), fax 888-FAX-MCIC (888-329-6242); www.healthresourcesonline.com.

The National Directory of Physician Organizations, Database on CD-ROM. You'll get detailed profiles on over 1,800 physician organizations. Listings include physician hospital organizations (PHOs), independent practice associations (IPAs), management services organizations (MSOs), and physician practice management companies (PPMCs). Key elements of the data profiled include: executive officers, year founded, profit status, state of incorporation, number of associated physicians, market area, market analysis, affiliated/participating hospitals, and management service organizations used. CD-ROM Database: Call for Pricing. Address: The Managed Care Information Center, Dept. 14D7RS, 1913 Atlantic Ave., Suite F5, Manasquan, NJ 08736-1096; toll-free 888-THE-MCIC (888-843-6242), fax 888-FAX-MCIC (888-329-6242); www.healthresourcesonline.com.

The National Directory of Physician Organizations, print on CD-ROM in PDF format in a searchable program. You'll get detailed profiles on over 1,800 physician organizations. Listings include physician hospital organizations (PHOs), independent practice associations (IPAs), management services organizations (MSOs), and physician practice management companies (PPMCs). Key elements of the data profiled include: executive officers, year founded, profit status, state of incorporation, number of associated physicians, market area, market analysis, affiliated/participating hospitals, and management service organizations used. Call for Pricing. Address: The Managed Care Information Center, Dept. 14D7RS, 1913 Atlantic Ave., Suite F5, Manasquan, NJ 08736-1096; toll-free 888-THE-MCIC (888-843-6242), fax 888-FAX-MCIC (888-329-6242); www.healthresourcesonline.com.

Pay for Performance Reporter will provide you with answers to questions you may have, with facts, news, insight and emerging P4P developments. Discover how early adopters achieve physician "buy in," the importance of leverage, how to choose your measures wisely and choose measures that are defensible, and why provider feedback is so important. Cost: $247 — 12 issues -- Save $150! Introductory Price - New Subscribers Only. Address: Managed Care Information Center, Dept. 14D7RS, 1913 Atlantic Ave., Suite F5, Manasquan, NJ 08736-1096; toll-free (888) 843-6242, fax (888) 329-6242; www.healthresourcesonline.com.

Wellness Program Management Advisor is a monthly newsletter that contains all the hard-to-find facts and figures you need to make those tough decisions on where your wellness program should be heading and to measure its effectiveness. You'll get the statistics you need to show that wellness programs are working at organizations throughout the country to control healthcare costs and improve participants' daily lives. Cost: $197 — 12 issues - Introductory Price - New Subscribers Only. Address: American Business Publishing, Dept. 14D7RS, 1913 Atlantic Ave., Suite F5, Manasquan, NJ 08736-1096; toll-free (888) 843-6242, fax (888) 329-6242, e-mail info@wellnessjunction.com, www.healthresourcesonline.com.

healthcare; managed healthcare plan trends; managed care partnerships; network developments; and how employers are making managed care work. Cost: $397 — 24 issues - Introductory Price - New Subscribers Only. Address: The Managed Care Information Center, Dept. 14D7RS, 1913 Atlantic Ave., Suite F5, Manasquan, NJ 08736-1096; toll-free 888-THE-MCIC (888-843-6242), fax 888-FAX-MCIC (888-329-6242); www.healthresourceonline.com.

The Executive Report on Physician Organizations. In one fast-reading, concise news briefing, you will get up-to-date information on physician hospital organizations, IPAs, physician practice management companies, and management services organizations, along with hard-to-come-by facts, statistics and comparative information. By spending a few minutes with The Executive Report on Physician Organizations, you can easily track who the "major players" are and even spot new organizations that have the potential to become major players. Cost: $197 - 12 issues - Introductory Price - New Subscribers Only. Address: The Managed Care Information Center, Dept. 14D7RS, 1913 Atlantic Ave., Suite F5, Manasquan, NJ 08736-1096; toll-free 888-THE-MCIC (888-843-6242), fax 888-FAX-MCIC (888-329-6242); or www.healthresourcesonline.com.

The National Directory of Health Systems, Hospitals, and Their Affiliates, Database on CD-ROM You'll get detailed profiles on more than 760 Integrated Healthcare Delivery Systems. Listings include: company name and address, telephone number, fax number, toll-free number, key contacts, revenues, enrollments, physicians (primary and specialists), outpatient and inpatient admissions, system affiliations and other pertinent information. CD-ROM Database: Call for Pricing. Address: The Managed Care Information Center, Dept. 14D7RS, 1913 Atlantic Ave., Suite F5, Manasquan, NJ 08736-1096; toll-free 888-THE-MCIC (888-843-6242), fax 888-FAX-MCIC (888-329-6242), www.healthresourcesonline.com.

The National Directory of Health Systems, Hospitals, and Their Affiliates print on CD-ROM in PDF format in a searchable program. You'll get detailed profiles on more than 760 Integrated Healthcare Delivery Systems. Listings include: company name and address, telephone number, fax number, toll-free number, key contacts, revenues, enrollments, physicians (primary and specialists), outpatient and inpatient admissions, system affiliations and other pertinent information. Call for Pricing. Address: The Managed Care Information Center, Dept. 14D7RS, 1913 Atlantic Ave., Suite F5, Manasquan, NJ 08736-1096; toll-free 888-THE-MCIC (888-843-6242), fax 888-FAX-MCIC (888-329-6242), www.healthresourcesonline.com.

The National Directory of Managed Care Organizations, Seventh Edition, print version, is a directory of more than 1,400 managed care plans. Profiles include: company name and address; parent company; "doing business as" name; telephone number, fax number, toll-free number; key contacts; model type (HMO, PPO, etc.); service area and other pertinent information. The organization model types include HMOs, PPOs, Specialty HMOs, Specialty PPOs, POS plans and utilization review organizations. Call for Pricing. Address: The Managed Care Information Center, Dept. 14D7RS, 1913 Atlantic Ave., Suite F5, Manasquan, NJ 08736-1096; toll-free 888-THE-MCIC (888-843-6242), fax 888-FAX-MCIC (888-329-6242); www.healthresourcesonline.com.

The National Directory of Managed Care Organizations, Seventh Edition, print on CD-ROM in PDF format in a searchable program is a directory of more than 1,500 managed care plans. Profiles include: company name and address; parent company; "doing business as" name; telephone number, fax number, toll-free number; key contacts; model type (HMO, PPO, etc.); service area and other pertinent information. The organization model types include HMOs, PPOs, Specialty HMOs, Specialty PPOs, POS plans and utilization review organizations. Call for Pricing. Address: The Managed Care Information Center, Dept. 14D7RS, 1913 Atlantic Ave., Suite F5, Manasquan, NJ 08736-1096; toll-free 888-THE-MCIC (888-843-6242), fax 888-FAX-MCIC (888-329-6242); www.healthresourcesonline.com.

The National Directory of Managed Care Organizations, Database on CD-ROM. A directory at your fingertips. More than 1,700 managed care plans. CD-ROM Standard Database: Cost: Call for Pricing. Includes 1 Free six-month update — Enrollment module (must be purchased with the standard module) includes statistical break downs by plan type, geographic, coverage, etc. Cost: Call for Pricing. Address: The Managed Care Information Center, Dept. 14D7RS, 1913 Atlantic Ave., Suite F5, Manasquan, NJ 08736-1096; toll-free 888-THE-MCIC (888-843-6242), fax 888-FAX-MCIC (888-329-6242); www.healthresourcesonline.com.

Pay for Performance: "How Millions of Dollars in Physician Bonus Incentives Linked to Improving Quality of Care May Be The Answer for Managed Care": During this 90-minute audio conference, we will cover how this new trend will affect MCOs, employers and health plan members, and how you could benefit from P4P programs. Hard Copy Report: Here's an insider look at the emerging $100 million provider pay for performance bonus incentive trend. The transcript of the recent audio conference on pay for performance programs is now available in a convenient, readable format including the complete text of speaker presentations and conference "handout" material.

Planning For Compliance With The Key Time Lines And Deadlines Of The Federal Mandates To Implement e-Healthcare Technology: A combination of federal health regulatory mandates are poised to force healthcare providers and payors to adopt e-health technological applications.

Proven Steps To A Cost Effective And Innovative Workplace Wellness Program: If you feel that your organization fights for a wellness program budget and has to justify its costs, you are not alone. According to the Wellness Program Management Advisor's ROI Survey, although wellness managers improve morale, reduce absenteeism and enhance performance, but worksite wellness programs must continue to justify their program's existence.

The Successful Privacy Officer: The Steps Every Privacy Officer Should be Taking To Lead Their HCO Toward Compliance: Learn how the privacy officers at two leading edge organizations are helping their organizations achieve HIPAA compliance during our audio-conference on CD-Rom

What's Fueling the Growth and Adoption of e-Healthcare Solutions In 2003: This conference, recorded on CD-ROM, will help your organization learn more about e-health trends in 2003 and how to deal with the changes.

What's Ahead for EAP: Employee assistance programs are becoming increasingly more common in today's worksites, and as the field grows, the responsibilities of employee assistance professionals are expanding as well. But many EAP experts have expressed deep concern over the numerous ethical and quality issues existing in the field today. Join Employee Assistence Program Management Letter for a review of the multiple forces shaping the EA industry in the 90-minute audio conference.

Wellness That Works! Strategies To Improve Your Wellness Program's ROI: This special audio conference on tape focused on the experiences of several organizations that have found wellness programs DO provide a great return on investment.

Winning Ideas in Health Plan Wellness and Health Improvement Programs: What's Working Today to Achieve Member Commitment and Participation on CD-ROM: Free personalized online lifestyle-improvement programs, rewards for health plan members who use health management and disease management programs, online health risk assessment and reimbursement for health club membership dues, are among the wellness initiatives that health plans are offering their employees and members. The growth and market adoption of consumer-driven health plans will continue to drive health plans to develop more widespread member health improvement initiatives. In fact, some plans are developing innovative approaches. Discover what's working in health plan wellness and health promotion programs, award winning and unique programs, best practices, ROI, and lessons learned in this special audio conference.

Workplace Wellness Program: 'What's in it for me?' How to Motivate Your Employees and Boost Participation: During this 90-minute audio conference, we will cover how companies have successfully used incentive programs to boost participation in employee wellness programs.

Employee Assistance Program Management Letter is a monthly briefing on the range of influences surrounding your EAP, including policy issues; coverages and limitations; dealing with and monitoring costs; case histories of successful programs; and how your program can mesh with your overall human resource goals. Cost: $137 — 12 issues - Introductory Price - New Subscribers Only. Address: American Business Publishing, Dept. 14D7RS, 1913 Atlantic Ave., Suite F4, Manasquan, NJ 08736-1096; toll-free (888) 843-6242, fax (888) 329-6242; www.healthresourcesonline.com.

The Executive Report on Managed Care is a twice-monthly newsletter covering the managed healthcare field, including: comparisons of premium increases; plan features and coverages; legislation affecting managed for a program that could mean hundreds of thousands of dollars for your organization. Find out how to submit approvable claims and how to successfully appeal denial of a claim.

How To Prove Disease Management's Value to Managed Care. Disease management professionals know DM is working. However, measuring disease management's ROI is no easy task. DM has a way to go before it is accepted as a means to pare down healthcare costs in managed care, according to an exclusive MCIC survey. How do you prove the ROI value? A new executive briefing audio conference aims to find the answers. Listen in to "How to Prove Disease Management's Value to Managed Care," now on CD-ROM.

Indicators of Excellence In Hospice: Secrets To The Key Best Practices In Today's Competitive Health and Palliative Care Environment: There are reasons why the best of breed hospices are the best, and why it's critical for hospice executives, your boards and management team to focus on your hospice's indicators of excellence. Join our special audio conference on the most important aspects of managing and measuring your hospice program.

The Managed Care Internet: How MCOs Are Shifting to Web-Enabled Applications: This special audio conference on tape is designed to serve the information needs of MCO senior management, strategists and executives charged with the responsibility of building out their plan's array of Web-based services.

The Managed Care Internet in 2003: The goal of this educational seminar on CD-ROM is to provide real-world, practical solutions and answers to professionals taking advantage of the Internet by increasing the number of members, to retain members, and to see a return on investment.

Management Briefing: Hospital Inpatient Prospective Payment System 2007 Final Rule Changes: The Centers for Medicare & Medicaid Services (CMS) has changed the method for reimbursing hospitals for inpatient stays for fiscal year (FY) 2007. It is the first significant change in the reimbursement system since it was first implemented in 1983. The revised payments will be effective for discharges on or after October 1st. Join the reimbursement experts of BESLER Consulting to get a better understanding of the new Medicare methodology and how it will affect your organization.

Management Briefing: New Medicare 2007 Outpatient and Reimbursement Final Rule Change: The Centers for Medicare & Medicaid Services (CMS) has announced its final rule for billing and coding outpatient and ASC services for Medicare payments effective on January 1, 2007. "Attend this 90-minute audio conference to get a better understanding of the new medicare coding and reimbursement changes for OPPS and how it will impact your organization.

Mergers and Acquisitions in the Managed Care Industry: The Trends, Issues and Impact on CD-ROM: During the first three quarters of 2005, $11.8 billion was committed to healthcare mergers and acquisitions. In the third quarter, $57.5 billion was committed to finance healthcare deals. And the managed care sector alone posted three billion dollar deals in the third quarter totaling $16.9 billion. Join speakers from three leading investment banking companies that focus on merger & acquisition services in the healthcare industry for both providers and payors to learn the current trends in M&A's, what are the issues, waht are state officials' issues, what acquirers are seeking in a suitable fit, the strategic buyer's interests, and finally, the impact on providers in a consolidated market. Hard Copy Report: The transcript of the recent teleconference on the mergers and acquisitions in the managed care industry is now available in a convenient, readable format including the complete text of speakers' presentations and conference "handout: material.

Online Disease Management: The Promise, The Potential and The Practical: 90-minute Audio Conference on Tape - Great for planning, training and orientation. You'll get insight and analysis from four of the leading experts in the rapidly growing field of online disease management. Featured presentations focus on disease management from the perspectives of payors, healthcare providers and vendors of online disease manage ment tools.

Nondiscrimination and Wellness Programs: What You Need to Know About the Final HIPAA Regulation: The final HIPAA nondiscrimination and wellness program regulations were jointly issued by The Departments of Treasury, Labor and Health and Human Services in December 2006. Join Wellness Program Management Advisor and experts from Jackson Lewis and Holtyn and Associates for a review of the final HIPAA nondiscrimination and wellness program regulations in this special 90-minute audio conference.

Healthcare Provider Portals: The Internet Strategy for Improving Provider Communications: This conference on CD-ROM will provide an opportunity to discover how healthcare organizations are implementing and developing provider portals to improve communication between the organization and providers.

HIPAA Auditing and Monitoring: Creating, Building and Testing a Strategy To Ensure Your Organization's Compliance, CD-Rom: All covered entities under the HIPAA regulations must monitor and audit their organizations compliance with the TCS and privacy regulations. To help your organization meet these requirements.

HIPAA Compliance: Working Through the Priorities. HIPAA is the single most pressing challenge facing healthcare providers, payors, and their vendors this year. In order for you company to fully understand the HIPAA demands you need to listen to this 90 minute audio conference on cassette. Discover what our panel of HIPAA experts are finding and get their latest thinking.

HIPAA For Healthcare Vendors: Suppliers, your staff, and your products and services need to be HIPAA ready. Only covered entities must be HIPAA compliant by the federal deadlines. But, your service or solution must be able to help your healthcare client covered entity become HIPAA compliant.

HIPAA For New Managers, Department Heads, Supervisors and Members of HIPAA Committees: The new management level staff you've hired maybe may not understand HIPAA and what it means to them, and your organization. To help your "newbies" and those who may not have grasped HIPAA yet, HIPAA Bulletin for Management has sponsored this audio conference on CD ROM to help organizations under stand the basic information HIPAA compliance.

HIPAA PROGRESS 2002. Your Work Plan Priorities for Compliance. This highly rated Audio Conference on CD-ROM can help your staff focus quickly on what must be done now. You can use the program for management awareness training and for planning implementation procedures. The 90-minute audio conference on CD-ROM comes with conference materials including definitions, slides, charts, checklists, and frequently asked questions. This conference is great for planning, training and orientation.

HIPAA Progress 2003: This is an audio conference, just recorded, to help your organization implement the various aspects of the law.

How To Identify Grant Funding Opportunities In a Changing Healthcare Environment: To help your organization learn more about grant funding opportunities and where to find them.

How to Implement Electronic Healthcare Technology to Improve Patient Care and Improve Your Bottom Line. Electronic healthcare technology developments and particularly e-prescribing, are at the forefront of solutions being embraced by health and managed care organizations. Stimulating the growth and keen interest in e-Healthcare technology is the Medicare Prescription Act that mandates e-Prescribing by 2008 with the first deadline due date of 2005.

How to Manage Your Physician Organization's Payor Relationships Under the Shadow of the FTC: A growing number of IPAs and PHOs have been stunned to learn they are the subjects of Federal Trade Commission antitrust violation investigations and charges. IPAs and PHOs in several states have been slapped with Federal Trade Commission complaints charging alleged price fixing violations. In fact, one New Mexico physicians' organization formally disbanded, following charges by the FTC that it fixed prices and restrained competition among area payors.

How To Maximize Your Organization's Grant Funding Readiness In Today's Healthcare Environment: Successful healthcare grant-seeking begins with quality research. Knowing what programs are available, what the grant-makers funding interests are, and the kinds of organizations being funded is the foundation of success. If you are involved in the management or development of your organization's grant seeking efforts, sign up now for what promises to be a valuable 90-minutes.

How to Optimize Your Organization's Cash Flow by Effective Denials Management An average of 18 percent of health claims are routinely denied by managed care plans, according to providers participating in a survey by The Managed Care Information Center (MCIC). 54.8 percent of respondents replied that denials are a problem for both physicians and hospitals. If you have ever had a claim denied, sign up now

AUDIO CONFERENCES: On CD-ROM. Call for Pricing. Speaker handouts and 30 minute question & answer session included with each audio conference. Address: Health Resources Publishing, Dept. 14D6RS, P.O. Box 559, Allenwood, NJ 08720; (888) 843-6242, fax (888) 329-6242, www.healthresourcesonline.com.

Beyond Mugs and T-Shirts: Wellness Incentives that Boost Participation and Health Improvement: Do incentives really improve participation and outcomes? And if they do, what kind of incentives gets the best results? Join Wellness Program Management Advisor to explore the types of incentives that work to boost participation and, most importantly, health improvement in this 90-minute audio conference.

Consumer Driven Plans Meet Managed Care: What the Future Holds: As out-of-pocket healthcare costs rise, more employers are starting to consider offering their employees consumer-driven options on their health plan menu. The trend is expected to continue, as employers require their workers to pay substantially more in premiums, deductibles, co-insurance and co-payments over the next several years.

Developing HIPAA Awareness an Training Programs For Your Staff, For organizations to achieve compliance, anyone who comes into contact with protected health information (PHI) needs to be educated about HIPAA compliance procedures, HIPAA experts say. Learn how to make the necessary changes within your workforce to create a HIPAA-compliant environment in which employees are made aware of the behavioral changes needed to adequately protect health information according to the legislation with this live 90-minute audio conference on CD-ROM.

Developing Your Organization's HIPAA Policies and Procedures Under the Final HIPAA Rules: To help you insure that your organization is on track to meet the policy and procedure requirements by next April, this audio conference has been recorded on CD-ROM.

e-Healthcare Trends- An Executive Briefing: The conference proceedings on tape include what providers, payors, tech companies and "dot.coms" are doing, a look at what types of business models may succeed and results of exclusive surveys. This briefing session is ideal for marketers, strategists, business development, planners, and other executives from healthcare technology companies, managed care organizations, health insurers, pharmaceutical manufacturers, and consulting firms.

eRx: How Healthcare is Adopting the Technology to Reduce Prescribing Errors, Enhance Safety, and Save $$$: During this 90-minute audio conference, we cover what's driving the adoption of ePrescribing; the impact of eRx on the managed care and pharmaceutical industries; and how organizations can use ePrescribing to better reduce prescribing errors and enhance patient care. Hard Copy Report: This convenient hard copy report takes the transcript of the above ePrescribing audio conference and provides it to you in a readable format, including the complete text of speakers' presentations and conference "handout" material.

Forecast: What's Ahead For Managed Care In 2007: The managed care industry faces a series of challenges in 2007 that may change how business is conducted for both health providers and payors. Pressures to lower healthcare costs and increase the quality of care, along with the growing army of uinsured, will all have an effect on plans. Join The Managed Care Information Center for a review of the challenges ahead in this special 90-minute audio conference.

The Future of Women's Healthcare - 2005. Today's health, wellness, managed care, and women's health professionals are increasingly aware of the gaps and challenges in providing comprehensive healthcare services to women. That's why "The Future of Women's Healthcare - 2005" was organized. This special teleconference, featured three highly respected leaders in the field, focused on new clinical and health research activities, then looks at what's working now and what's ahead for women's health programs.

Health Savings Accounts: The New Future For Managed Care And Consumer Driven Health Plans During this 90-minute audio conference, we will cover how the new HSA legislation, included in the Medicare Prescription Drug, Improvement and Modernization Act, will impact the managed care industry.

Healthcare Intranets 2002 How HCOs are Maximizing Efficiencies, Reducing Costs, Improving the Bottom Line: The 90-minute program on CD-ROM provides a cost-effective way to gather your key staff in a conference room to listen to this important information. Get a practical, real-world overview of how healthcare organizations (HCOs) are using their Intranets to maximize efficiencies, reduce costs and improve the bottom line.

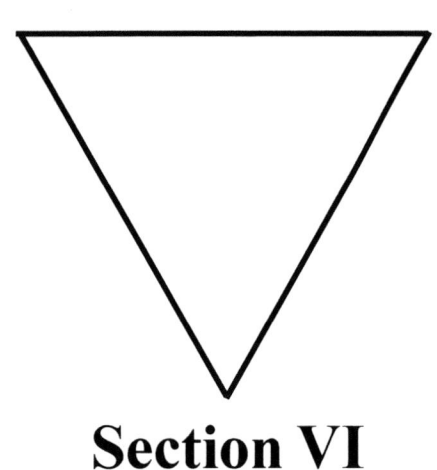

Section VI

Directory of Healthcare Resources

Healthcare Information and Management Systems Society, 230 East Ohio Street, #500, Chicago, Illinois 60611-3269; (312) 664-4467; fax: (312) 664-6143; http://www.himss.org

Hospice Association of America, 228 Seventh St SE, Washington, DC 20003; (202)546-4759; fax: (202) 547-9559; http://www.nahc.org

Joint Commission on Accreditation of Healthcare Organizations, 601 13th St NW, Suite 1150, Washington, DC, 20005; (202) 783-6655; fax: (202) 783-6888; http://www.jointcommission.org

Managed Care Information Center, 1913 Atlantic Avenue, Suite F5, Manasquan, New Jersey 08736; toll-free 888-THE-MCIC (888-843-6242), fax 888-FAX-MCIC (888-329-6242); http://www.themcic.com

Mental Health America (Formerly: National Mental Health Association), 2000 N Beauregard St, 6 Fl, Alexandria, Virginia 22311; (703) 684-7722; fax: (703) 684-5968; http://www.nmha.org

National Association of Health Data Organizations, 448 East 400 South, Suite 301, Salt Lake City, Utah, 84111; (801) 532-2299; fax: (801) 532-2228; http://www.nahdo.org

National Association for Home Care and Hospice, 228 Seventh St., SE, Washington, DC 20003; (202) 547-7424; fax: (202)547-3540; http://www.nahc.org

National Association of Psychiatric Health Systems, 701 13th Street NW, Ste 950, Washington, DC 20005; (202) 393-6700; fax: (202) 783-6041; http://www.naphs.org

National Committee for Quality Assurance (NCQA), 1100 13th Street NW, Ste 1000, Washington, DC 20036; (202) 955-3500, fax: (202) 955-3599; http:// www.ncqa.org

National Health Council, 1730 M Street NW, Suite 500, Washington, DC 20036; (202) 785-3910; fax: (202) 785-5923; http://www.nationalhealthcouncil.org

National Health Information Center, PO Box 1133, Washington, DC 20013-1133; (800) 336-4797; fax: (301) 984-4256; http://www.health.gov/nhic/

Pharmaceutical Care Management Association, 601 Pennsylvania Ave, NW Suite 740, Washington, DC 20004; (202) 207-3610, fax: (202) 207-3623; http://www.pcmanet.org

Utilization Review Accreditation Commission, 1220 L Street, Suite 400, Washington, DC 20005; (202) 216-9010; fax: (202) 216-9006; http://www.urac.org

Directory of Healthcare Associations

Accreditation Association for Ambulatory Health Care, Inc. 5250 Old Orchard Rd., Suite 200, Stokie, Illinois; 60077; (847) 853-6060; fax (847) 853-9028: http://www.aaahc.org

American Association of Preferred Provider Organizations, 222 S First St., Ste 303, Louisville, KY, 40202; (502) 403-1122, fax: (502) 403-1129; http://www.aappo.org

American College of Healthcare Executives, 1 North Franklin, Suite 1700, Chicago, Illinois 60606-3529; (312) 424-2800; fax: (312) 424-0023; http://www.ache.org

American College of Nurse Practitioners, 1501 Wilson Blvd., Suite 509, Arlington, VA 22209 (703) 740-2529, fax: (703) 740-2533, http://acnpweb.org

American Health Care Association, 1201 L Street NW, Washington, DC 20005; (202) 842-4444, fax: (202) 842-3860; http://www.ahcancal.org

American Health Insurance Plans, (Formerly AAHP & HIAA), 601 Pennsylvania Ave. NW, South Building, Ste 500; Washington, DC 20004; (202) 778-3200; fax: (202) 331-7487; http://www.ahip.org

American Health Planning Association, 7245 Arlington Blvd., Suite 300, Falls Church, Virginia 22042; (703) 573-3103, fax: (703) 573-3103; http://www.ahpanet.org

American Hospital Association, 1 North Franklin, Chicago, Illinois 60606-3421; (312) 422-3000, fax (312-422-4796); http://www.aha.org

American Medical Association, 515 North State Street, Chicago, Illinois 60610; (312) 464-5000; Toll-free: (800) 621-8335; http://www.ama-assn.org

American Nurses Association, 8515 Georgia Ave, Ste 400, Silver Springs, Maryland 20910; (301) 628-5000; fax: (301) 628-5001; Toll-free: (800) 274-4262; http://www.ana.org

American Osteopathic Association, 142 East Ontario St., Chicago, Illinois 60611; (800) 621-1773; (312) 202-8000; fax: (312) 202-8200; http://www.osteopathic.org

American Pharmacists Association, 1105 15th St, Ste 400, Washington, DC 20005-1707; (202)-628-4410; fax: (202) 783-2351; www.pharmacist.com

American Public Health Association, 800 I St NW, Washington, DC 20001-3710; (202-777-2742; fax: (202) 777-2534; http://www.apha.org

Association for Ambulatory Behavioral Healthcare, 247 Douglas Avenue, Portsmouth, Virginia, 23707; (757) 673-3741; fax: (757) 966-7734; http://www.aabh.org

Blue Cross and Blue Shield Association, 1310 G Street NW, Washington, DC 20005; (202) 626-4780; http://www.bcbs.com

Centers for Medicare & Medicaid Services (formerly HCFA), 7500 Security Blvd., Baltimore, Maryland 21244-1850; (877) 267-2323; (410) 786-3000; http://www.cms.gov

Healthcare Financial Management Association, 2 Westbrook Corporate Center, Suite 700, Westchester, Illinois 60154-5700; (800) 252-4362; (708) 531-9600; fax: (708) 531-0032; http://www.hfma.org

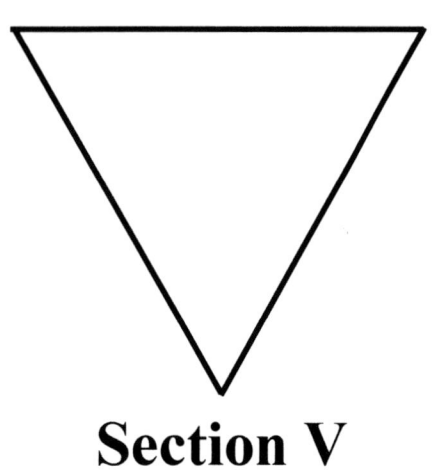

Section V

Directory of Healthcare Associations

Miscellaneous Organizations

Total Enrollment:
2000:		2003:	332	2006:	234
2001:	226	2004:	337	2007:	1,066
2002:	236	2005:	380		

SERVICE AREA:
WI;

Product Name: Wisconsin Partnership Program

PLAN TYPE: WI PARTNERSHIP PROGRAM

ELDER CARE HEALTH PLAN INC
2802 International Lane
Madison, WI 53704
Phone: 608-245-3016 Fax: 608-245-3077 Toll-Free:
Web site: www.eldercarehealthplan.org

Mailing Address:
ELDER CARE HEALTH PLAN INC
2802 International Lane
Madison, WI 53704

Key Executives:
Chief Executive Officer .... Karen Musser

Company Profile:
Parent Company Name: Elder Care of Wisconsin Inc
Contract Effective Date: 01/01/99
Nonprofit: [Y]   Forprofit: [ ]
Total Enrollment:
2000:		2003:	422	2006:	526
2001:	351	2004:	442	2007:	603
2002:	376	2005:	470		

SERVICE AREA:
WI;

Product Name: Wisconsin Partnership Program

PLAN TYPE: WI PARTNERSHIP PROGRAM

HEALTH PLAN FOR COMMUNITY LIVING INC
1414 MacArthur Rd
Madison, WI 53708-8028
Phone: 608-242-8335 Fax: 605-240-7060 Toll-Free:
Web site: www.cla-madison.org

Mailing Address:
HEALTH PLAN FOR COMM LIVING INC
1414 MacArthur Rd
Madison, WI 53708-8028

Key Executives:
Chief Executive Officer .... Owen McCusker

Company Profile:
Parent Company Name: Community Living Alliance
Contract Effective Date: 01/01/99
Nonprofit: [Y]   Forprofit: [ ]
Total Enrollment:
2000:		2003:	174	2006:	234
2001:	106	2004:	187	2007:	236
2002:	131	2005:	210		

SERVICE AREA:
WI;

Product Name: Wisconsin Partnership Program

PLAN TYPE: WI PARTNERSHIP PROGRAM

PARTNERSHIP HEALTH PLAN INC
2240 EastRidge Center
Eau Claire, WI 54701
Phone: 715-838-2900 Fax: 715-838-2910 Toll-Free: 800-842-1814
Web site: www.communityhealthpartnership.com

Managed Care Organization Profiles

Mailing Address:
PARTNERSHIP HEALTH PLAN INC
2240 EastRidge Ctr
Eau Claire, WI 54701

Key Executives:
Chief Executive Officer .... Karen Bulloch
Health Plan Director .... Brent Bauman
Director of Operations .... Steve Landkamer

Company Profile:
Parent Company Name: Community Health Partnership Inc
Contract Effective Date: 01/01/99
Nonprofit: [Y]   Forprofit: [ ]
Total Enrollment:
2000:		2003:	453	2006:	766
2001:	245	2004:	485	2007:	978
2002:	281	2005:	647		

SERVICE AREA:
WI;

Managed Care Organization Profiles — Miscellaneous Organizations

Total Enrollment:
- 2000:
- 2001:
- 2002:
- 2003:
- 2004:
- 2005:
- 2006:
- 2007: 138,384

SERVICE AREA:
TX;

Product Name: Unicare

PLAN TYPE: PRIVATE FEE-FOR-SERVICE PLAN

UNICARE HEALTH PLANS OF THE MIDWEST INC
233 S Wacker Dr Ste 3900
Chicago, IL 60606
Phone: 312-234-7000 Fax: 312-234-8001 Toll-Free: 877-864-2273
Web site: www.unicare.com

Mailing Address:
UNICARE HEALTH PLANS OF THE MIDWEST Inc
233 S Wacker Dr Ste 3900
Chicago, IL 60606

Key Executives:
Chief Executive Officer .... Sandra Van Trease
President .... David W Fields
Chief Financial Officer .... Tim Schryver

Company Profile:
Parent Company Name: Rush Presbyterian St Luke's Medical Ctr.
Contract Effective Date: 04/01/03
Nonprofit: [ ]   Forprofit: [Y]
Total Enrollment:
- 2000:
- 2001:
- 2002:
- 2003:
- 2004:
- 2005: 46,888
- 2006:
- 2007: 142,258

SERVICE AREA:
NW;

Product Name: Delaware Physicians Care Advantage

PLAN TYPE: PSO

DELAWARE PHYSICIANS CARE INC
252 Chapman Rd Ste 250
Newark, DE 19702
Phone: 866-543-2167 Fax: Toll-Free:
Web site: www.delawarephysicianscare.com

Mailing Address:
DELAWARE PHYSICIANS CARE INC
252 Chapman Rd Ste 250
Newark, DE 19702

Key Executives:
Compliance Manager .... Patricia Simpson

Company Profile:
Parent Company Name:
Contract Effective Date: 01/01/07
Nonprofit: [ ]   Forprofit: [Y]
Total Enrollment:
- 2000:
- 2001:
- 2002:
- 2003:
- 2004:
- 2005:
- 2006:
- 2007:

SERVICE AREA:
DE,

Product Name: Golden Advantage Plus

PLAN TYPE: PSO

MARYLAND CARE INC
509 Progress Dr
Linthicum, MD 21090
Phone: 866-651-7843 Fax: Toll-Free:
Web site: www.marylandphysicianscare.com

Mailing Address:
MARYLAND CARE INC
509 Progress Dr
Linthicum, MD 21090

Key Executives:
Member Services Representative .... Linda Dietsch

Company Profile:
Parent Company Name:
Contract Effective Date: 01/01/07
Nonprofit: [ ]   Forprofit: [ ]
Total Enrollment:
- 2000:
- 2001:
- 2002:
- 2003:
- 2004:
- 2005:
- 2006:
- 2007: 60

SERVICE AREA:
MD;

Product Name: SelectCare of Texas

PLAN TYPE: PSO

SELECTCARE OF TEXAS LLC
4888 Loop Central Dr Ste 300
Houston, TX 77081
Phone: 713-965-9444 Fax: 713-965-0433 Toll-Free: 800-544-5428
Web site: www.sctexas.com

Mailing Address:
SELECTCARE OF TEXAS LLC
4888 Loop Central Dr Ste 300
Houston, TX 77081

Key Executives:
Chief Executive Officer/President .... Theodore M Carpenter Jr
Chief Financial Officer .... Steven C Holman

Company Profile:
Parent Company Name: Universal American Corporation
Contract Effective Date: 03/01/01
Nonprofit: [ ]   Forprofit: [Y]
Total Enrollment:
- 2000:
- 2001: 1,222
- 2002: 8,968
- 2003: 15,497
- 2004: 15,982
- 2005: 24,090
- 2006: 63,161
- 2007: 38,415

SERVICE AREA:
TX (Beaumont, Houston);

Product Name: Wisconsin Partnership Program

PLAN TYPE: WI PARTNERSHIP PROGRAM

COMMUNITY CARE HEALTH PLAN INC
5228 W Fond du Lac Ave
Milwaukee, WI 53202
Phone: 414-536-2100 Fax: 414-536-2111 Toll-Free:
Web site: www.communitycareinc.org

Mailing Address:
COMMUNITY CARE HEALTH PLAN INC
5228 W Fond du Lac Ave
Milwaukee, WI 53202

Key Executives:
Chief Executive Officer .... Kirby Shoaf
Chief Financial Officer .... Lawrence J Paplham
Govrnm Rltns/Legislative Issue .... Paul F Soczynski
Associate Operating Officer .... Stephanie W Griggs

Company Profile:
Parent Company Name: Community Care Organization Inc
Contract Effective Date: 01/01/99
Nonprofit: [Y]   Forprofit: [ ]

Miscellaneous Organizations

Total Enrollment:
- 2000:
- 2001:
- 2002:
- 2003:
- 2004:
- 2005:
- 2006:
- 2007: 10

SERVICE AREA:
NY;

Product Name: Select Advantage

PLAN TYPE: PRIVATE FEE-FOR-SERVICE PLAN

QCC INSURANCE COMPANY
1901 Market St
Philadelphia, PA 19103
Phone: 800-331-0017   Fax: Toll-Free: 800-331-0017
Web site:
Mailing Address:
QCC INSURANCE COMPANY
1901 Market St
Philadelphia, PA 19103

Company Profile:
Parent Company Name: AmeriHealth Mercy Health Plan
Contract Effective Date: 01/01/08
Nonprofit: [ ]   Forprofit: [ ]
Total Enrollment:
- 2000:
- 2001:
- 2002:
- 2003:
- 2004:
- 2005:
- 2006:
- 2007: 83

SERVICE AREA:
PA;

Product Name: Sterling Option I

PLAN TYPE: PRIVATE FEE-FOR-SERVICE PLAN

STERLING LIFE INSURANCE COMPANY
PO Box 1917
Bellingham, WA 98227
Phone: 888-858-8572   Fax: 888-858-8552   Toll-Free: 888-858-8572
Web site: www.sterlingplans.com
Mailing Address:
STERLING LIFE INSURANCE CO
PO Box 1917
Bellingham, WA 98227

Key Executives:
President .... Steven E Lippai, FSA

Company Profile:
Parent Company Name:
Contract Effective Date: 07/01/00
Nonprofit: [ ]   Forprofit: [Y]
Total Enrollment:
- 2000:
- 2001: 19,835
- 2002: 22,728
- 2003: 18,677
- 2004: 30,195
- 2005: 33,259
- 2006:
- 2007: 98,891

SERVICE AREA:
AK; AR; AZ; DE; IA; ID; IL; KY; LA; MN; NE; NM; NV; OH; OK; OR; PA; SC; SD; TN; TX; UT; WA; WV;

Product Name: Today's Option

PLAN TYPE: PRIVATE FEE-FOR-SERVICE PLAN

AMERICAN PROGRESSIVE LIFE & INSURANCE COMPANY
6 International Dr
Rye Brook, NY 10573-1068
Phone: 800-332-3377   Fax: 914-934-1988   Toll-Free:
Web site: www.amerprog.com

Mailing Address:
AMERICAN PROGRESS LIFE & INS CO
6 International Dr
Rye Brook, NY 10573-1068

Key Executives:
Chief Executive Officer/President .... Richard A Barasch
Executive VP, Chief Financial Officer .... Robert A Waegelein
VP, Administration .... Judy M Borrell

Company Profile:
Parent Company Name: Universal American Financial Corporation
Contract Effective Date: 05/01/04
Nonprofit: [ ]   Forprofit: [Y]
Total Enrollment:
- 2000:
- 2001:
- 2002:
- 2003:
- 2004:
- 2005: 4,065
- 2006: 10,580
- 2007: 50,923

SERVICE AREA:
NY;

Product Name: Today's Option

PLAN TYPE: PRIVATE-FEE-FOR-SERVICE PLAN

MARQUETTE NATIONAL LIFE INSURANCE COMPANY
1001 Heathrow Park Lane
Lake Mary, FL 32746
Phone: 407-628-1776   Fax: Toll-Free:
Web site: www.todaysoption.com
Mailing Address:
MARQUETTE NATL LIFE INS CO
PO Box 958465
Lake Mary, FL 32746

Key Executives:
Chief Executive Officer/President .... Richard A Barasch

Company Profile:
Parent Company Name: Universal American Corporation
Contract Effective Date: 01/01/08
Nonprofit: [ ]   Forprofit: [Y]
Total Enrollment:
- 2000:
- 2001:
- 2002:
- 2003:
- 2004:
- 2005:
- 2006:
- 2007: 5,176

SERVICE AREA:
TX;

Product Name: Today's Option

PLAN TYPE: PRIVATE-FEE-FOR-SERVICE PLAN

PYRAMID LIFE INSURANCE COMPANY
1001 Heathrow Park Lane
Lake Mary, FL 32746
Phone: 407-628-1776   Fax: Toll-Free:
Web site: www.todaysoption.com
Mailing Address:
PYRAMID LIFE INSURANCE CO
PO Box 958465
Lake Mary, FL 32746

Key Executives:
Chief Executive Officer/President .... Richard A Barasch

Company Profile:
Parent Company Name: Universal American Corporation
Contract Effective Date: 08/01/05
Nonprofit: [ ]   Forprofit: [Y]

Managed Care Organization Profiles — Miscellaneous Organizations

Product Name: Medicare Plus Blue Option I

PLAN TYPE: PRIVATE FEE-FOR-SERVICE PLAN

BLUE PREFERRED PLAN-BLUE CROSS/BLUE SHIELD MICHIGAN
600 E Lafayette Blvd
Detroit, MI 48226-2927
Phone: 313-225-9000 Fax: 313-225-5629 Toll-Free:
Web site: www.bcbsmi.com

Mailing Address:
BLUE PREFERRED PLAN-BC/BS MI
600 E Lafayette Blvd
Detroit, MI 48226-2927

Key Executives:
Chief Executive Officer/President .... Richard E Whitmer
Chief Financial Officer .... Mark R Bartlett
Executive VP, Chief Operating Officer .... Robert Naffaly

Company Profile:
Parent Company Name: Blue Cross Blue Shield of Michigan
Contract Effective Date: 07/01/05
Nonprofit: [Y]   Forprofit: [ ]
Total Enrollment:
  2000:   2003:   2006: 23,110
  2001:   2004:   2007: 218,574
  2002:   2005: 3,193

SERVICE AREA:
MI;

Product Name: Mennonite Mutual Aid Association

PLAN TYPE: PRIVATE-FEE-FOR-SERVICE PLAN

MENNONITE MUTUAL AID ASSOCIATION
1110 N Main St
Goshen, IN 46527
Phone: 574-533-9511 Fax: 574-533-5264 Toll-Free: 800-348-7468
Web site: www.mma-online.org

Mailing Address:
MENNONITE MUTUAL AID ASSOC
PO Box 483
Goshen, IN 46527

Key Executives:
Chief Executive Officer/President .... Larry D Miller
Chief Financial Officer .... Mel Claassen
Senior VP, Administrative Services/Health .... Steve Garboden

Company Profile:
Parent Company Name: Mennonite Mutual Aid Association
Contract Effective Date: 01/01/08
Nonprofit: [Y]   Forprofit: [ ]
Total Enrollment:
  2000:   2003:   2006:
  2001:   2004:   2007: 26
  2002:   2005:

SERVICE AREA:
IN;

Product Name: SecureHorizons MedicareDirect

PLAN TYPE: PRIVATE FEE-FOR-SERVICE PLAN

PACIFICARE LIFE & HEALTH INSURANCE COMPANY
5995 Plaza Dr
Cypress, CA 90630
Phone: 714-952-1121 Fax: 714-226-3581 Toll-Free:
Web site: www.pacificare.com

Mailing Address:
PACIFICARE LIFE & HEALTH INS CO
5995 Plaza Dr MailStopCY20-462
Cypress, CA 90630

Key Executives:
Chief Executive Officer/President .... Howard G Phanstiel
Chief Financial Officer .... Gregory Scott

Company Profile:
Parent Company Name: UnitedHealth Group
Contract Effective Date: 09/01/05
Nonprofit: [ ]   Forprofit: [Y]
Total Enrollment:
  2000:   2003:   2006:
  2001:   2004:   2007: 76,100
  2002:   2005: 6,662

SERVICE AREA:
CA;

Product Name: SecureHorizons MedicareDirect

PLAN TYPE: PRIVATE FEE-FOR-SERVICE PLAN

UNITED HEALTHCARE INSURANCE COMPANY
9900 Bren Rd East
Minnetonka, MN 55343
Phone: 952-936-1300 Fax: 952-936-0044 Toll-Free:
Web site: www.uhc.com

Mailing Address:
UNITED HEALTHCARE INSURANCE CO
9900 Bren Rd East
Minnetonka, MN 55343

Key Executives:
Chief Executive Officer/President .... Stephen J Hemsley
Chief Financial Officer .... Patrick Erlandson

Company Profile:
Parent Company Name: UnitedHealth Group
Contract Effective Date: 09/01/04
Nonprofit: [ ]   Forprofit: [Y]
Total Enrollment:
  2000:   2003:   2006: 14,592
  2001:   2004:   2007: 16,286
  2002:   2005: 7,434

SERVICE AREA:
NW;

Product Name: SecureHorizons MedicareDirect

PLAN TYPE: PRIVATE FEE-FOR-SERVICE PLAN

UNITEDHEALTHCARE INSURANCE COMPANY OF NEW YORK
9900 Bren Rd East
Minnetonka, MN 55343
Phone: 888-867-5517 Fax: Toll-Free: 888-867-5517
Web site: www.uhc.com

Mailing Address:
UNITEDHEALTHCARE INS CO OF NY
9900 Bren Rd East
Minnetonka, MN 55343

Key Executives:
.... Erica Cimino

Company Profile:
Parent Company Name: UnitedHealth Group
Contract Effective Date: 01/01/07
Nonprofit: [ ]   Forprofit: [Y]

Miscellaneous Organizations   Managed Care Organization Profiles

Product Name: Humana Gold Choice

PLAN TYPE: PRIVATE FEE-FOR-SERVICE PLAN

HUMANA INC/PCA - PUERTO RICO
383 FD Roosevelt 3rd Fl
San Juan, PR 00918-2131
Phone: 787-282-7900 Fax: 787-282-6277 Toll-Free: 800-314-3121
Web site: www.pr.humana.com
Mailing Address:
   HUMANA INC PCA PUERTO RICO
   383 FD Roosevelt 3rd Fl
   San Juan, PR 00918-2131

Key Executives:
Chief Executive Officer/President .... Victor Gutierrez, MD
Executive VP, Chief Operating Officer .... David Krebs

Company Profile:
Parent Company Name: Humana Inc
Contract Effective Date: 06/01/05
Nonprofit: [ ]   Forprofit: [Y]
Total Enrollment:
   2000:   2003:   2006: 433
   2001:   2004:   2007: 337
   2002:   2005: 91

SERVICE AREA:
PR;

Product Name: Humana Gold Choice

PLAN TYPE: PRIVATE FEE-FOR-SERVICE PLAN

HUMANA INSURANCE COMPANY OF NEW YORK
500 W Main St
Louisville, KY 40202
Phone: 877-511-5000 Fax: Toll-Free: 800-852-9556
Web site: www.humana.com
Mailing Address:
   HUMANA INS CO OF NY
   101 E Main St
   Louisville, KY 40202

Key Executives:
Chief Executive Officer .... Michael B McCallister

Company Profile:
Parent Company Name: Humana Inc
Contract Effective Date: 01/01/07
Nonprofit: [ ]   Forprofit: [Y]
Total Enrollment:
   2000:   2003:   2006:
   2001:   2004:   2007: 1,672
   2002:   2005:

SERVICE AREA:
NY;

Product Name: Instil Incare

PLAN TYPE: PRIVATE FEE-FOR-SERVICE PLAN

INSTIL HEALTH
PO Box 100298
Columbia, SC 29202-3298
Phone: 877-446-7845 Fax: 800-503-3115 Toll-Free:
Web site: www.myinstil.com
Mailing Address:
   INSTIL HEALTH
   PO Box 100298
   Columbia, SC 29202-3298

Key Executives:
Chief Executive Officer/President .... Robert Johnson

Company Profile:
Parent Company Name:
Contract Effective Date: 04/01/05
Nonprofit: [ ]   Forprofit: [Y]
Total Enrollment:
   2000:   2003:   2006: 518
   2001:   2004:   2007: 5,562
   2002:   2005: 226

SERVICE AREA:
SC;

Product Name: Medica Advantage Solution

PLAN TYPE: PRIVATE FEE-FOR-SERVICE PLAN

MEDICA HEALTH PLANS
401 Carlson Pkwy
Minnetonka, MN 55305
Phone: 952-992-8013 Fax: 952-992-3554 Toll-Free:
Web site: www.medica.com
Mailing Address:
   MEDICA HEALTH PLANS
   401 Carlson Pkwy
   Minnetonka, MN 55305

Key Executives:
Chief Executive Officer/President .... David Tilford
Exectuive VP, CAO, Chief Financial Officer .... Aaron Reynolds
Chief Operating Officer .... Jana Johnson

Company Profile:
Parent Company Name: Medica Health Plans
Contract Effective Date: 08/01/05
Nonprofit: [Y]   Forprofit: [ ]
Total Enrollment:
   2000:   2003:   2006: 1,267
   2001:   2004:   2007: 2,374
   2002:   2005: 875

SERVICE AREA:
MN;

Product Name: Medica Advantage Solutions

PLAN TYPE: PRIVATE FEE-FOR-SERVICE PLAN

MEDICA HEALTH PLANS OF WISCONSIN
401 Carlson Pkwy
Minnetonka, MN 55305
Phone: 952-992-8013 Fax: 952-992-3554 Toll-Free:
Web site: www.medica.com
Mailing Address:
   MEDICA HEALTH PLANS OF WI
   401 Carlson Pkwy
   Minnetonka, MN 55305

Key Executives:
Chief Executive Officer/President .... David Tilford

Company Profile:
Parent Company Name: Medica Health Plans
Contract Effective Date: 07/01/05
Nonprofit: [Y]   Forprofit: [ ]
Total Enrollment:
   2000:   2003:   2006:
   2001:   2004:   2007: 294
   2002:   2005:

SERVICE AREA:
MN;

Managed Care Organization Profiles — Miscellaneous Organizations

Product Name: Blue Cross of California

PLAN TYPE: PRIVATE FEE-FOR-SERVICE PLAN

BLUE CROSS OF CALIFORNIA
21555 Oxnard St
Woodland Hills, CA 91367
Phone: 818-234-2345 Fax: 818-234-2848 Toll-Free:
Web site: www.bluecrossca.com
Mailing Address:
   BLUE CROSS OF CALIFORNIA
   21555 Oxnard St
   Woodland Hills, CA 91367

Key Executives:
Chief Executive Officer/President .... Brian A Sassi

Company Profile:
Parent Company Name: WellPoint Inc
Contract Effective Date: 02/01/05
Nonprofit: [ ]   Forprofit: [Y]
Total Enrollment:
   2000:   2003:   2006: 2,743
   2001:   2004:   2007: 6,226
   2002:   2005: 2,181

SERVICE AREA:
CA;

Product Name: Bravo Liberty Plan - Medicare Advantage

PLAN TYPE: PRIVATE FEE-FOR-SERVICE PLAN

BRAVO HEALTH MID-ATLANTIC INC
3601 O'Donnell St
Baltimore, MD 21224
Phone: 410-864-4557 Fax: Toll-Free: 800-235-9188
Web site: www.elderhealth.com
Mailing Address:
   BRAVO HEALTH MID-ATLANTIC
   3601 O'Donnell St
   Baltimore, MD 21224

Key Executives:
Chief Executive Officer .... Jeff Folick
VP, Executive Director .... Mary Ann Eull
Medical Director .... Ace M Hodgin, MD

Company Profile:
Parent Company Name:
Contract Effective Date: 01/01/07
Nonprofit: [ ]   Forprofit: [ ]
Total Enrollment:
   2000:   2003:   2006:
   2001:   2004:   2007: 220
   2002:   2005:

SERVICE AREA:
MD;

Product Name: HealthMarkets Care Assured

PLAN TYPE: PRIVATE-FEE-FOR-SERVICE PLAN

CHESAPEAKE LIFE INSURANCE COMPANY
9151 Blvd 26
North Richland Hills, TX 76180
Phone: 817-255-3100 Fax: 817-255-8130 Toll-Free: 877-219-5458
Web site: www.healthmarkets.com
Mailing Address:
   CHESAPEAKE LIFE INSURANCE CO
   9151 Blvd 26
   North Richland Hills, TX 76180

Key Executives:
Chief Executive Officer/President .... William J Gedwed

Company Profile:
Parent Company Name: HealthMarkets
Contract Effective Date: 01/01/08
Nonprofit: [ ]   Forprofit: [ ]
Total Enrollment:
   2000:   2003:   2006:
   2001:   2004:   2007: 6,590
   2002:   2005:

SERVICE AREA:
TX;

Product Name: Humana Gold Choice

PLAN TYPE: PRIVATE FEE-FOR-SERVICE PLAN

HUMANA HEALTH BENEFIT PLAN OF LOUISIANA
One Galleria Blvd Ste 850
Metairie, LA 70001
Phone: 504-836-6600 Fax: 504-219-5520 Toll-Free: 877-511-5000
Web site: www.ohpnow.com
Mailing Address:
   HUMANA HEALTH BENEFIT PLAN OF LA
   One Galleria Blvd Ste 850
   Metairie, LA 70001

Key Executives:
Chief Executive Officer .... Terry S Shilling
President .... James E Schlottman
Chief Financial Officer .... Lisa Blume
Senior VP of Operations .... Lynn Comeaux

Company Profile:
Parent Company Name: Humana Inc
Contract Effective Date: 05/01/05
Nonprofit: [ ]   Forprofit: [Y]
Total Enrollment:
   2000:   2003:   2006: 3,048
   2001:   2004:   2007: 4,985
   2002:   2005: 137

SERVICE AREA:
LA;

Product Name: Humana Gold Choice

PLAN TYPE: PRIVATE FEE-FOR-SERVICE PLAN

HUMANA HEALTH PLAN - KENTUCKY
1100 Employers Blvd
DePere, WI 54115
Phone: 502-580-5001 Fax: 502-580-5044 Toll-Free: 877-511-5000
Web site: www.humana.com
Mailing Address:
   HUMANA HEALTH PLAN - KY
   101 E Main St
   Louisville, KY 54115

Key Executives:
Market President .... Michael B McCallister

Company Profile:
Parent Company Name: Humana Inc
Contract Effective Date: 01/01/03
Nonprofit: [ ]   Forprofit: [Y]
Total Enrollment:
   2000:   2003:   2006: 654,392
   2001:   2004:   2007: 653,696
   2002:   2005: 101,785

SERVICE AREA:
KY;

Miscellaneous Organizations

Product Name: VIA Christi OutReach Program Elders Inc

PLAN TYPE: PACE

VIA CHRISTI HOPE INC
3720 East Bayley St
Wichita, KS 67218
Phone: 316-858-1111   Fax: 316-858-1166   Toll-Free:
Web site:

Mailing Address:
   VIA CHRISTI HOPE INC
   3720 E Bayley St
   Wichita, KS 67218

Key Executives:
Chief Executive Officer .... Mark Bailey

Company Profile:
Parent Company Name:
Contract Effective Date: 09/01/02
Nonprofit: [Y]   Forprofit: [ ]
Total Enrollment:
   2000:   2003:   80   2006: 174
   2001:   2004: 104   2007: 175
   2002:   2005: 157

SERVICE AREA:
KS;

Product Name: Advantra Freedom

PLAN TYPE: PRIVATE FEE-FOR-SERVICE PLAN

CAMBRIDGE LIFE INSURANCE COMPANY
3200 Highland Ave
Downers Grove, IL 60515
Phone: 866-386-2330   Fax: 866-386-2329   Toll-Free: 866-386-2330
Web site: www.cvty.com

Mailing Address:
   CAMBRIDGE LIFE INSURANCE CO
   PO Box 7154
   London, KY 60515

Key Executives:
Chief Executive Officer .... Dale B Wolf

Company Profile:
Parent Company Name: Coventry Health Care Inc
Contract Effective Date: 01/01/07
Nonprofit: [ ]   Forprofit: [Y]
Total Enrollment:
   2000:   2003:   2006:
   2001:   2004:   2007: 517
   2002:   2005:

SERVICE AREA:
IL;

Product Name: Aetna Medicare

PLAN TYPE: PRIVATE FEE-FOR-SERVICE PLAN

AETNA LIFE INSURANCE COMPANY
151 Farmington Ave
Hartford, CT 06156
Phone: 860-273-4888   Fax: 860-273-6675   Toll-Free: 800-445-1796
Web site: www.aetna.com

Mailing Address:
   AETNA LIFE INSURANCE COMPANY
   151 Farmington Ave
   Hartford, CT 06156

Managed Care Organization Profiles

Key Executives:
Chief Executive Officer .... Ronald A Williams

Company Profile:
Parent Company Name: Aetna Inc
Contract Effective Date: 01/01/06
Nonprofit: [ ]   Forprofit: [Y]
Total Enrollment:
   2000:   2003:   2006:
   2001:   2004:   2007: 163,538
   2002:   2005:

SERVICE AREA:
NW;

Product Name: Anthem SmartValue

PLAN TYPE: PRIVATE FEE-FOR-SERVICE PLAN

ANTHEM INSURANCE COMPANIES INC
1351 William Howard Taft Rd
Cincinnati, OH 45206-9974
Phone: 866-803-5169   Fax: Toll-Free:
Web site: www.anthem.com

Mailing Address:
   ANTHEM INSURANCE COMPANIES INC
   PO Box 9154
   Oxnard, CA 45206-9974

Key Executives:
President/Operations/Technology/Government Services ... Mark L Boxer

Company Profile:
Parent Company Name: WellPoint Inc
Contract Effective Date: 04/01/07
Nonprofit: [ ]   Forprofit: [Y]
Total Enrollment:
   2000:   2003:   2006:
   2001:   2004:   2007: 19,684
   2002:   2005:

SERVICE AREA:
IN; OH; KY;

Product Name: Avalon

PLAN TYPE: PRIVATE FEE-FOR-SERVICE PLAN

AVALON INSURANCE COMPANY
2500 Elmerton Ave
Harrisburg, PA 17177
Phone: Fax: Toll-Free:
Web site: www.avaloninsurance.com

Mailing Address:
   AVALON INSURANCE COMPANY
   PO Box 772610
   Harrisburg, PA 17177

Key Executives:
President/Chief Executive Officer .... Anita M Smith

Company Profile:
Parent Company Name: Capital Blue Cross
Contract Effective Date: 01/01/08
Nonprofit: [ ]   Forprofit: [Y]
Total Enrollment:
   2000:   2003:   2006:
   2001:   2004:   2007:
   2002:   2005:

SERVICE AREA:
PA,

Managed Care Organization Profiles — Miscellaneous Organizations

Product Name: Sutter Health Sacramento Sierra Region

PLAN TYPE: PACE

SUTTER SENIOR CARE
1234 U Street
Sacramento, CA 95818
Phone: 916-446-3100   Fax: Toll-Free:
Web site: www.suttermedicalcenter.org

Mailing Address:
   SUTTER HEALTH SACRAMENTO SIERRA
   1234 U St
   Sacramento, CA 95818

Key Executives:
Chief Executive Officer .... Sara Krebens

Company Profile:
Parent Company Name:
Contract Effective Date: 11/01/03
Nonprofit: [Y]   Forprofit: [ ]
Total Enrollment:
   2000:   2003:   207   2006: 192
   2001:   2004:   200   2007: 172
   2002:   2005:   208

SERVICE AREA:
CA;

Product Name: Total Community Care

PLAN TYPE: PACE

TOTAL COMMUNITY CARE
904-A Las Lomas Rd NE
Albuquerque, NM 87102-2633
Phone: 505-294-2650   Fax: Toll-Free:
Web site: www.totallongtermcare.org

Mailing Address:
   TOTAL COMMUNITY CARE
   904-A Las Lomas Rd NE
   Albuquerque, NM 87102-2633

Key Executives:
Revenue & Data integrity Analyst .... Matthew Zimmerman

Company Profile:
Parent Company Name:
Contract Effective Date: 06/01/04
Nonprofit: [Y]   Forprofit: [ ]
Total Enrollment:
   2000:   2003:   2006: 252
   2001:   2004:   2007: 297
   2002:   2005:   227

SERVICE AREA:
NM (Bernaliello, Sandoval);

Product Name: Total Long Term Care

PLAN TYPE: PACE

TOTAL LONG TERM CARE
200 E 9th Ave
Denver, CO 80202
Phone: 869-4664   Fax: Toll-Free:
Web site: www.totallongtermcare.org

Mailing Address:
   TOTAL LONG TERM CARE
   200 E 9th Ave
   Denver, CO 80202

Key Executives:
Executive Director .... David Reyes

Company Profile:
Parent Company Name:
Contract Effective Date: 04/01/03
Nonprofit: [Y]   Forprofit: [ ]
Total Enrollment:
   2000:   2003:   754   2006: 1,008
   2001:   2004:   842   2007: 1,118
   2002:   2005: 1,028

SERVICE AREA:
CO;

Product Name: TriHealth Senior Link

PLAN TYPE: PACE

TRIHEALTH SENIOR LINK
4750 Wesley Ave Ste J
Cincinnati, OH 45212
Phone: 513-531-5110   Fax: Toll-Free:
Web site:

Mailing Address:
   TRIHEALTH SENIOR LINK
   4750 Wesley Ave Ste J
   Cincinnati, OH 45212

Key Executives:
Director of Senior Health Business Development .... Brian Tilow

Company Profile:
Parent Company Name:
Contract Effective Date: 11/01/02
Nonprofit: [Y]   Forprofit: [ ]
Total Enrollment:
   2000:   2003:   226   2006: 333
   2001:   2004:   236   2007: 365
   2002:   365   2005:   327

SERVICE AREA:
OH (Clermont, Hamilton);

Product Name: Uphams Elder Service Plan

PLAN TYPE: PACE

UPHAMS CORNER HEALTH COMMITTEE INC
1140 Dorchester Ave
Boston, MA 02125-3305
Phone: 617-288-0970   Fax: 617-282-8625   Toll-Free:
Web site:

Mailing Address:
   UPHAMS CORNER HLTH COMM INC
   1140 Dorchester Ave
   Boston, MA 02125-3305

Key Executives:
Operations Manager .... Jagdeep Trivedi

Company Profile:
Parent Company Name:
Contract Effective Date: 11/01/02
Nonprofit: [Y]   Forprofit: [ ]
Total Enrollment:
   2000:   2003:   94   2006: 121
   2001:   2004:   106   2007: 133
   2002:   2005:   111

SERVICE AREA:
MA;

Miscellaneous Organizations / Managed Care Organization Profiles

Product Name: Providence ElderPlace - Seattle

PLAN TYPE: PACE

PROVIDENCE HEALTH SYSTEM
4515 Martin Lthr King Jr Way S
Seattle, WA 98118
Phone: 206-320-5325 Fax: Toll-Free:
Web site: www.providence.org

Mailing Address:
PROVIDENCE HEALTH SYSTEM
PO Box 18737
Seattle, WA 98118

Key Executives:
Director .... Michael Whitley

Company Profile:
Parent Company Name:
Contract Effective Date: 11/01/02
Nonprofit: [Y]   Forprofit: [ ]
Total Enrollment:
  2000:   2003: 158   2006: 208
  2001:   2004: 187   2007: 220
  2002:   2005: 211

SERVICE AREA:
WA (King); OR (Clark);

Product Name: Senior LIFE Johnstown

PLAN TYPE: PACE

PENNSYLVANIA PACE INC
401 Broad St
Johnstown, PA 15905
Phone: 814-535-6000 Fax: Toll-Free:
Web site: www.seniorlifejohnstown.com

Mailing Address:
PA PACE INC
401 Broad St
Johnstown, PA 15905

Key Executives:
Chief Operating Officer .... Mark Irwin

Company Profile:
Parent Company Name:
Contract Effective Date: 11/02/07
Nonprofit: [ ]   Forprofit: [Y]
Total Enrollment:
  2000:   2003:   2006:
  2001:   2004:   2007: 105
  2002:   2005:

SERVICE AREA:
PA;

Product Name: Sentara Senior Community Care

PLAN TYPE: PACE

SENTARA LIFE CARE CORPORATION INC
665 Newtown Rd #121
Virginia Beach, VA 23562
Phone: 757-892-5400 Fax: Toll-Free:
Web site: www.sentara.com

Mailing Address:
SENTARA LIFE CARE CORP INC
665 Newtown Rd #121
Virginia Beach, VA 23562

Key Executives:
Site Manager .... Laura R Gadsby

Company Profile:
Parent Company Name:
Contract Effective Date: 11/02/07
Nonprofit: [Y]   Forprofit: [ ]
Total Enrollment:
  2000:   2003:   2006:
  2001:   2004:   2007: 108
  2002:   2005:

SERVICE AREA:
VA;

Product Name: St Paul's PACE

PLAN TYPE: PACE

COMMUNITY ELDERCARE OF SAN DIEGO
328 Maple St
San Diego, CA 92103
Phone: 619-239-6900 Fax: 619-239-1256 Toll-Free:
Web site: www.stpaulspace.org

Mailing Address:
COMMUNITY ELDERCARE OF SAN DIEGO
328 Maple St
San Diego, CA 92103

Key Executives:
Executive Director .... John A Allgood

Company Profile:
Parent Company Name:
Contract Effective Date: 01/01/08
Nonprofit: [Y]   Forprofit: [ ]
Total Enrollment:
  2000:   2003:   2006:
  2001:   2004:   2007:
  2002:   2005:

SERVICE AREA:
CA;

Product Name: Summit ElderCare

PLAN TYPE: PACE

FALLON COMMUNITY HEALTH PLAN
10 Chestnut St
Worchester, MA 01608
Phone: 508-852-2026 Fax: Toll-Free:
Web site: www.summiteldercare.org

Mailing Address:
FALLON COMMUNITY HEALTH PLAN
10 Chestnut St
Worchester, MA 01608

Key Executives:
Chief Executive Officer .... Eric H Schultz

Company Profile:
Parent Company Name:
Contract Effective Date: 11/01/02
Nonprofit: [Y]   Forprofit: [ ]
Total Enrollment:
  2000:   2003: 174   2006: 283
  2001:   2004: 171   2007: 425
  2002: 153   2005: 228

SERVICE AREA:
MA;

Managed Care Organization Profiles

Miscellaneous Organizations

Product Name: PACE Greater New Orleans

PLAN TYPE: PACE

PACE GREATER NEW ORLEANS
4201 N Rampart St
New Orleans, LA 70113
Phone: 504-596-3099 Fax: Toll-Free:
Web site: www.archdiocese-no.org

Mailing Address:
> PACE GREATER NEW ORLEANS
> 4201 N Rampart St
> New Orleans, LA 70113

Key Executives:
Chief Executive Officer/President .... Mark Drennen
Administration .... Christopher Meguess

Company Profile:
Parent Company Name:
Contract Effective Date: 09/01/07
Nonprofit: [Y]   Forprofit: [ ]
Total Enrollment:
  2000:   2003:   2006:
  2001:   2004:   2007: 26
  2002:   2005:

SERVICE AREA:
LA;

Product Name: PACE Organization of Rhode Island

PLAN TYPE: PACE

PACE ORGANIZATION OF RHODE ISLAND
225 Chapman St
Providence, RI 02905
Phone: 401-490-6566 Fax: Toll-Free:
Web site:

Mailing Address:
> PACE ORG OF RHODE ISLAND
> 225 Chapman St
> Providence, RI 02905

Key Executives:
Marketing Director .... Jennifer Jaswell

Company Profile:
Parent Company Name:
Contract Effective Date: 12/01/05
Nonprofit: [Y]   Forprofit: [ ]
Total Enrollment:
  2000:   2003:   2006: 23
  2001:   2004:   2007: 76
  2002:   2005:

SERVICE AREA:
RI;

Product Name: PACE Vermont Inc

PLAN TYPE: PACE

PACE VERMONT INC
786 College Pkwy
Colchester, VT 05446
Phone: 802-655-6700 Fax: 802-655-6760 Toll-Free: 888-655-6706
Web site: www.pacevermont.org

Mailing Address:
> PACE VERMONT INC
> 786 College Pkwy
> Colchester, VT 05446

Key Executives:
President .... Janice Clements
Administration, Fiscal Services Manager .... Patricia Gratton

Company Profile:
Parent Company Name:
Contract Effective Date: 03/01/07
Nonprofit: [Y]   Forprofit: [ ]
Total Enrollment:
  2000:   2003:   2006:
  2001:   2004:   2007: 23
  2002:   2005:

SERVICE AREA:
VT;

Product Name: Palmetto SeniorCare

PLAN TYPE: PACE

PALMETTO SENIORCARE
15 Richland Medical Park #203
Columbia, SC 29203-6843
Phone: 803-434-3770 Fax: Toll-Free:
Web site: www.palmettohealth.org/richland/

Mailing Address:
> PALMETTO SENIORCARE
> 15 Richland Medical Park #203
> Columbia, SC 29203-6843

Key Executives:
Vice President .... Judy Baskins

Company Profile:
Parent Company Name:
Contract Effective Date: 11/01/03
Nonprofit: [ ]   Forprofit: [Y]
Total Enrollment:
  2000:   2003: 325   2006: 356
  2001:   2004: 311   2007: 336
  2002:   2005: 327

SERVICE AREA:
SC (Lexington, Richland);

Product Name: Providence Elder Place

PLAN TYPE: PACE

PROVIDENCE HEALTH SYSTEM - OREGON
13007 N E Glisan St
Portland, OR 97230
Phone: 503-215-6556 Fax: Toll-Free:
Web site: www.providence.org/elderplace

Mailing Address:
> PROVIDENCE HEALTH SYSTEM - OR
> 13007 N E Glisan St
> Portland, OR 97230

Key Executives:
Executive Director .... Don Keester

Company Profile:
Parent Company Name: Providence Health System
Contract Effective Date: 11/01/03
Nonprofit: [Y]   Forprofit: [ ]
Total Enrollment:
  2000:   2003: 536   2006: 672
  2001:   2004: 551   2007: 625
  2002: 133   2005: 666

SERVICE AREA:
OR (Clackamas, Multnomah, Washington);

Miscellaneous Organizations

Product Name: Life at Home LLC

PLAN TYPE: PACE

LIFE AT HOME LLC
101 E State St
Kennett Square, PA 19348
Phone: 610-925-4270 Fax: 610-925-4000 Toll-Free:
Web site: www.genesishcc.com

Mailing Address:
LIFE AT HOME LLC
101 E State St
Kennett Square, PA 19348

Key Executives:
Administration .... Christine Allen

Company Profile:
Parent Company Name:
Contract Effective Date: 07/01/07
Nonprofit: [ ]   Forprofit: [Y]
Total Enrollment:
2000:   2003:   2006:
2001:   2004:   2007: 24
2002:   2005:

SERVICE AREA:
PA;

Product Name: Living Independently for Elders

PLAN TYPE: PACE

UNIVERSITY OF PENNSYLVANIA, TRUSTEES
4101 Woodland Ave
Philadelphia, PA 19104-4510
Phone: 215-573-7200 Fax: 215-573-4442 Toll-Free:
Web site:

Mailing Address:
UNIVERSITY OF PENNSYLVANIA
4101 Woodland Ave
Philadelphia, PA 19104-4510

Key Executives:
Executive Director .... Carola Somers

Company Profile:
Parent Company Name:
Contract Effective Date: 01/01/02
Nonprofit: [Y]   Forprofit: [ ]
Total Enrollment:
2000:   2003: 142   2006: 268
2001:   2004: 162   2007: 213
2002:   2005: 246

SERVICE AREA:
PA (Philadelphia);

Product Name: Loretto Independent Living Srvs Inc

PLAN TYPE: PACE

INDEPENDENT LIVING SERVICES OF CENTRAL NEW YORK
100 Malta Lane
N Syracuse, NY 13212
Phone: 315-452-5800 Fax: Toll-Free:
Web site: www.lorettosystem.org

Mailing Address:
INDEPENDENT LVNG SRVS CNTRL NY
100 Malta Lane
N Syracuse, NY 13212

Managed Care Organization Profiles

Key Executives:
Executive Director .... Penny Abulencra

Company Profile:
Parent Company Name:
Contract Effective Date: 11/01/02
Nonprofit: [Y]   Forprofit: [ ]
Total Enrollment:
2000:   2003: 272   2006: 307
2001:   2004: 284   2007: 338
2002:   2005: 332

SERVICE AREA:
NY;

Product Name: Midland PACE

PLAN TYPE: PACE

MIDLAND CARE CONNECTION
200 SW Frazier Circle
Topeka, KS 66606
Phone: 785-232-2044 Fax: Toll-Free:
Web site: www.midlandcc.org

Mailing Address:
MIDLAND HOSPICE INC
200 SW Frazier Circle
Topeka, KS 66606

Key Executives:
IT Coordinator .... Dreux Doty

Company Profile:
Parent Company Name:
Contract Effective Date: 01/01/07
Nonprofit: [Y]   Forprofit: [ ]
Total Enrollment:
2000:   2003:   2006:
2001:   2004:   2007: 10
2002:   2005:

SERVICE AREA:
KS;

Product Name: ON Lok Senior Health Services

PLAN TYPE: PACE

ON LOK SENIOR HEALTH SERVICES
1333 Bush St
San Francisco, CA 94109-5611
Phone: 415-292-8883 Fax: 415-292-8745 Toll-Free: 888-866-6565
Web site: www.onlok.org

Mailing Address:
ON LOK SENIOR HEALTH SERVICES
1333 Bush St
San Francisco, CA 94109-5611

Key Executives:
Executive Director .... Jennie Chin Hansen, RN, MS
Director of Adminstration & Finance .... Sue Wong
Director, Policy & Government Relations .... Eileen Kunz, MPH

Company Profile:
Parent Company Name:
Contract Effective Date: 11/01/03
Nonprofit: [Y]   Forprofit: [ ]
Total Enrollment:
2000:   2003: 912   2006: 967
2001:   2004: 906   2007: 997
2002:   2005: 930

SERVICE AREA:
CA (Alameda, Marin, San Francisco);

Managed Care Organization Profiles

Miscellaneous Organizations

Product Name: Florida Pace Centers Inc

PLAN TYPE: PACE

FLORIDA PACE CENTERS INC
5200 Northeast Second Ave
Miami, FL 33137
Phone: 305-751-7223 Fax: 305-532-5848 Toll-Free:
Web site:

Mailing Address:
FLORIDA PACE CENTERS INC
5200 Northeast Second Ave
Miami, FL 33137

Key Executives:
Executive Director .... Jack Rutelberg
Chief Operating Officer .... Dr Dan Brady

Company Profile:
Parent Company Name:
Contract Effective Date: 01/01/03
Nonprofit: [Y]   Forprofit: [ ]
Total Enrollment:
  2000:   2003:   14   2006: 110
  2001:   2004:   45   2007: 143
  2002:   2005:   106

SERVICE AREA:
FL;

Product Name: Hopkins Elderplus

PLAN TYPE: PACE

JOHNS HOPKINS HEALTH SYSTEM INC
4940 Eastern Ave
Baltimore, MD 21224
Phone: 410-550-7044 Fax: Toll-Free:
Web site: www.jhbmc.jhu.edu

Mailing Address:
JOHNS HOPKINS HEALTH SYSTEM IN
4940 Eastern Ave
Baltimore, MD 21224

Key Executives:
Director .... Karen Armacost, RNC

Company Profile:
Parent Company Name: John Hopkins Bayview Medical Center
Contract Effective Date: 11/01/02
Nonprofit: [Y]   Forprofit: [ ]
Total Enrollment:
  2000:   2003:   143   2006: 133
  2001:   2004:   141   2007: 112
  2002:   121   2005:   140

SERVICE AREA:
MD;

Product Name: Independent Living for Seniors

PLAN TYPE: PACE

INDEPENDENT LIVING FOR SENIORS
2066 Hudson Ave
Rochester, NY 14617
Phone: 585-922-2800 Fax: Toll-Free:
Web site: www.viahealth.org

Mailing Address:
INDEPENDENT LVNG SRS
2066 Hudson Ave
Rochester, NY 14617

Key Executives:
Administrator .... Kathy McGuire

Company Profile:
Parent Company Name:
Contract Effective Date: 11/01/03
Nonprofit: [Y]   Forprofit: [ ]
Total Enrollment:
  2000:   2003:   326   2006: 336
  2001:   2004:   326   2007: 282
  2002:   2005:   317

SERVICE AREA:
NY;

Product Name: LIFE - Pittsburgh Inc

PLAN TYPE: PACE

LIFE - PITTSBURGH INC
875 Greentree Rd Ste 200
Pittsburgh, PA 15220
Phone: 412-388-8042 Fax: Toll-Free:
Web site:

Mailing Address:
LIFE PITTSBURGH INC
875 Greentree Rd Ste 200
Pittsburgh, PA 15220

Key Executives:
Director of Finance .... Laura Schmitt

Company Profile:
Parent Company Name:
Contract Effective Date: 05/01/05
Nonprofit: [Y]   Forprofit: [ ]
Total Enrollment:
  2000:   2003:   2006: 223
  2001:   2004:   2007: 245
  2002:   2005:   209

SERVICE AREA:
PA;

Product Name: LIFE - St Agnes

PLAN TYPE: PACE

ST AGNES MEDICAL CENTER
1500 S Columbus Blvd
Philadelphia, PA 19147
Phone: 215-339-4747 Fax: Toll-Free:
Web site:

Mailing Address:
LIFE ST AGNES MEDICAL CENTER
1500 S Columbus Blvd
Philadelphia, PA 19147

Key Executives:
Director, Quality Assurance/Compliance .... Susan Wilson

Company Profile:
Parent Company Name:
Contract Effective Date: 10/01/05
Nonprofit: [Y]   Forprofit: [ ]
Total Enrollment:
  2000:   2003:   2006: 102
  2001:   2004:   2007: 176
  2002:   2005:

SERVICE AREA:
PA;

Miscellaneous Organizations

Product Name: Elder Service Plan - Cambridge

PLAN TYPE: PACE

**ELDER SERVICE PLAN
OF THE CAMBRIDGE HEALTH ALLIANCE**
270 Green St
Cambridge, MA 02139
Phone: 617-381-7100   Fax: Toll-Free:
Web site:
Mailing Address:
  ELDER SRV PLN OF CAMBRIDGE HLT
  270 Green St
  Cambridge, MA 02139

Key Executives:
Chief Executive Officer .... Paul Vitale

Company Profile:
Parent Company Name:
Contract Effective Date: 11/01/02
Nonprofit: [Y]   Forprofit: [ ]
Total Enrollment:
  2000:   2003:   107   2006:   108
  2001:   2004:   102   2007:   137
  2002:   2005:   113

SERVICE AREA:
  MA;

Product Name: Elder Service Plan of E Boston

PLAN TYPE: PACE

**ELDER SERVICE PLAN
OF EAST BOSTON HEALTH CENTER**
10 Gove St
East Boston, MA 02128
Phone: 617-568-4602   Fax: Toll-Free:
Web site:
Mailing Address:
  ELDER SRV PN/E BOSTON HLTH CTR
  10 Gove St
  East Boston, MA 02128

Key Executives:
Chief Operating Officer .... Ginny Felice

Company Profile:
Parent Company Name:
Contract Effective Date: 11/01/03
Nonprofit: [Y]   Forprofit: [ ]
Total Enrollment:
  2000:   2003:   334   2006:   301
  2001:   2004:   299   2007:   294
  2002:   2005:   300

SERVICE AREA:
  MA;

Product Name: Elder Service Plan of Harbor Health Srvs Inc

PLAN TYPE: PACE

**ELDER SERVICE PLAN
OF HARBOR HEALTH SERVICES INC**
2216 Dorchester Ave
Dorchester, MA 02124-5607
Phone: 617-296-5100   Fax: Toll-Free:
Web site:
Mailing Address:
  ELDER SRV PLN OF HARBOR HLTH S
  2216 Dorchester Ave
  Dorchester, MA 02124-5607

Key Executives:
Administrator, Coordinator .... Jadeep Drivedi
Vice President .... Sheila R Morrison

Company Profile:
Parent Company Name:
Contract Effective Date: 11/01/02
Nonprofit: [Y]   Forprofit: [ ]
Total Enrollment:
  2000:   2003:   158   2006:   204
  2001:   2004:   176   2007:   206
  2002:   92   2005:   209

SERVICE AREA:
  MA;

Product Name: Elder Service Plan of the North Shore

PLAN TYPE: PACE

ELDER SERVICE PLAN OF THE NORTH SHORE
20 School St
Lynn, MA 01901
Phone: 781-581-7565   Fax: 781-581-2976   Toll-Free:
Web site:
Mailing Address:
  ELDER SRV PLN OF NORTH SHORE
  20 School St
  Lynn, MA 01901

Key Executives:
Executive Director .... Carol Suleski
Chief Financial Officer .... Robert Durante

Company Profile:
Parent Company Name:
Contract Effective Date: 11/01/03
Nonprofit: [Y]   Forprofit: [ ]
Total Enrollment:
  2000:   2003:   301   2006:   368
  2001:   2004:   307   2007:   424
  2002:   2005:   341

SERVICE AREA:
  MA;

Product Name: Elderhaus PACE

PLAN TYPE: PACE

ELDERHAUS INC
1950 Amphitheater Dr
Wilmington, NC 28401
Phone: 910-343-8209   Fax: 910-343-8836   Toll-Free: 888-343-8209
Web site: www.elderhaus.com
Mailing Address:
  ELDERHAUS INC
  1950 Amphitheater Dr
  Wilmington, NC 28401

Key Executives:
PACE Program Director/Chief Financial Officer .... Larry Reinhart
Social Worker .... Stacy Bullard

Company Profile:
Parent Company Name:
Contract Effective Date: 02/01/08
Nonprofit: [Y]   Forprofit: [ ]

SERVICE AREA:
  NC (New Hanover, Northern Brunswick);

Managed Care Organization Profiles — Miscellaneous Organizations

Product Name: Community Care's PACE Program

PLAN TYPE: PACE

COMMUNITY CARE ORGANIZATION INC
1555 South Layton Blvd
Milwaukee, WI 53215
Phone: 414-902-2401 Fax: Toll-Free:
Web site: www.cco-cce.org

Mailing Address:
COMMUNITY CARE ORG INC
1555 South Layton Blvd
Milwaukee, WI 53215

Key Executives:
Executive Director .... Kirby Shoaf

Company Profile:
Parent Company Name:
Contract Effective Date: 11/01/03
Nonprofit: [Y]   Forprofit: [ ]
Total Enrollment:
2000:	2003: 397	2006: 666
2001:	2004: 406	2007: 700
2002:	2005: 499	

SERVICE AREA:
WI;

Product Name: Community LIFE

PLAN TYPE: PACE

PITTSBURGH CARE PARTNERSHIP INC
2400 Ardmore Blvd Ste 700
Pittsburgh, PA 15221-5238
Phone: 412-436-1320 Fax: Toll-Free:
Web site:

Mailing Address:
PITTSBURGH CARE PARTNERSHIP IN
2400 Ardmore Blvd Ste 700
Pittsburgh, PA 15221-5238

Key Executives:
Outreach Coordinator .... Staci Kaczkowski

Company Profile:
Parent Company Name:
Contract Effective Date: 03/01/04
Nonprofit: [Y]   Forprofit: [ ]
Total Enrollment:
2000:	2003:	2006: 220
2001:	2004:	2007: 240
2002:	2005:	

SERVICE AREA:
PA;

Product Name: Comprehensive Care Management Corp

PLAN TYPE: PACE

COMPREHENSIVE CARE MANAGEMENT CORP
612 Allerton Ave
Bronx, NY 10467
Phone: 718-519-5925 Fax: Toll-Free:
Web site: www.bethabe.org/ccm.html

Mailing Address:
COMPREHENSIVE CARE MANAGEMENT
2401 White Plains Rd
Bronx, NY 10467

Key Executives:
Senior Vice President .... Susan Aldrich

Company Profile:
Parent Company Name:
Contract Effective Date: 11/01/03
Nonprofit: [Y]   Forprofit: [ ]
Total Enrollment:
2000:	2003: 1,063	2006: 1,645
2001:	2004: 1,120	2007: 1,860
2002:	2005: 1,487	

SERVICE AREA:
NY;

Product Name: Concordia Care

PLAN TYPE: PACE

CONCORDIA CARE
2373 Euclid Heights Blvd
Cleveland Heights, OH 44106
Phone: 216-791-3580 Fax: Toll-Free:
Web site: www.concordiacareohio.org

Mailing Address:
CONCORDIA CARE
2373 Euclid Heights Blvd
Cleveland Heights, OH 44106

Key Executives:
Marketing Manager .... Joseph Bandiera

Company Profile:
Parent Company Name:
Contract Effective Date: 11/01/02
Nonprofit: [Y]   Forprofit: [ ]
Total Enrollment:
2000:	2003: 215	2006: 261
2001:	2004: 220	2007: 230
2002: 169	2005: 258	

SERVICE AREA:
OH;

Product Name: EDDY Senior Care

PLAN TYPE: PACE

SENIOR CARE CONNECTION INC
504 State St
Schenectady, NY 12305
Phone: 518-382-3290 Fax: Toll-Free:
Web site: www.northeasthealth.com

Mailing Address:
SENIOR CARE CONNECTION INC
504 State St
Schenectady, NY 12305

Key Executives:
Executive Director .... Bernadette Hallam

Company Profile:
Parent Company Name: Senior Care Connection Inc
Contract Effective Date: 11/01/02
Nonprofit: [Y]   Forprofit: [ ]
Total Enrollment:
2000:	2003: 82	2006: 68
2001:	2004: 77	2007: 86
2002: 91	2005: 76	

SERVICE AREA:
NY;

Miscellaneous Organizations

Managed Care Organization Profiles

Product Name: Basics at Jan Werner, The

PLAN TYPE: PACE

AMARILLO MULTI SERVICE CENTER FOR THE AGING INC
3108 S Fillmore St
Amarillo, TX 79110
Phone: 806-374-5516 Fax: 806-373-9446 Toll-Free:
Web site: www.amaonline.com
Mailing Address:
  AMARILLO MULTI-SRV CTR AGING
  3108 S Fillmore St
  Amarillo, TX 79110

Key Executives:
Executive Director .... Alana Chilcote

Company Profile:
Parent Company Name:
Contract Effective Date: 03/01/04
Nonprofit: [Y]   Forprofit: [ ]
Total Enrollment:
  2000:   2003:   2006: 140
  2001:   2004: 46   2007: 138
  2002:   2005: 134

SERVICE AREA:
TX;

Product Name: Bienvivir Senior Health Services

PLAN TYPE: PACE

BIENVIVIR SENIOR HEALTH SERVICES
6000 Welch Ste A2
El Paso, TX 77905-1753
Phone: 915-599-8812 Fax: Toll-Free:
Web site:
Mailing Address:
  BIENVIVIR SENIOR HLTH SRVS
  6000 Welch Ste A2
  El Paso, TX 77905-1753

Key Executives:
Executive Director .... Rosemary Castillo

Company Profile:
Parent Company Name:
Contract Effective Date: 11/01/03
Nonprofit: [Y]   Forprofit: [ ]
Total Enrollment:
  2000:   2003: 648   2006: 731
  2001:   2004: 646   2007: 724
  2002:   2005: 763

SERVICE AREA:
TX (El Paso);

Product Name: Care Resources

PLAN TYPE: PACE

CARE RESOURCES INC
5363 44th St SE
Grand Rapids, MI 49512
Phone: 616-913-2014 Fax: Toll-Free:
Web site: www.care-resources.org
Mailing Address:
  CARE RESOURCES INC
  5363 44th St SE
  Grand Rapids, MI 49512

Key Executives:
Executive Director .... Thomas Muszynski

Company Profile:
Parent Company Name:
Contract Effective Date: 09/01/06
Nonprofit: [Y]   Forprofit: [ ]
Total Enrollment:
  2000:   2003:   2006:
  2001:   2004:   2007: 32
  2002:   2005:

SERVICE AREA:
MI;

Product Name: Center for Elders Independence

PLAN TYPE: PACE

CENTER FOR ELDERS INDEPENDENCE
510 17t St Ste 400
Oakland, CA 94612-1367
Phone: 510-433-1150 Fax: Toll-Free:
Web site: www.cei.elders.org
Mailing Address:
  CENTER FOR ELDERS INDEPENDENCE
  510 17th St Ste 400
  Oakland, CA 94612-1367

Key Executives:
Chief Executive Officer .... Peter Szuto

Company Profile:
Parent Company Name:
Contract Effective Date: 11/01/03
Nonprofit: [Y]   Forprofit: [ ]
Total Enrollment:
  2000:   2003: 319   2006: 267
  2001:   2004: 305   2007: 356
  2002:   2005: 272

SERVICE AREA:
CA;

Product Name: Center for Senior Independence

PLAN TYPE: PACE

HENRY FORD HEALTH SYSTEM
7800 W Outer Dr Ste 240
Detroit, MI 48235
Phone: 313-653-2020 Fax: Toll-Free:
Web site:
Mailing Address:
  HENRY FORD HEALTH SYSTEM
  7800 W Outer Dr Ste 240
  Detroit, MI 48235

Key Executives:
Executive Director .... Glenn Black

Company Profile:
Parent Company Name:
Contract Effective Date: 11/01/03
Nonprofit: [Y]   Forprofit: [ ]
Total Enrollment:
  2000:   2003: 164   2006: 170
  2001:   2004: 164   2007: 161
  2002:   2005: 184

SERVICE AREA:
MI;

Managed Care Organization Profiles — Miscellaneous Organizations

Product Name: Minnesota Senior Health Options

PLAN TYPE: MN SENIOR CARE OPTIONS

SOUTH COUNTRY HEALTH ALLIANCE
110 Fremont St W
Owatonna, MN 55060
Phone: 507-444-7770   Fax: Toll-Free:
Web site: www.mnscha.org
Mailing Address:
   SOUTH COUNTRY HEALTH ALLIANCE
   110 Fremont St W
   Owatonna, MN 55060

Key Executives:
Chief Executive Officer .... Brian A. Nasi
Chief Financial Officer .... John Gregoire

Company Profile:
Parent Company Name:
Contract Effective Date: 08/01/05
Nonprofit: [ ]   Forprofit: [ ]
Total Enrollment:
   2000:   2003:   2006: 1,924
   2001:   2004:   2007: 1,997
   2002:   2005:

SERVICE AREA:
MN;

Product Name: Minnesota Senior Health Options

PLAN TYPE: MN SENIOR HEALTH OPTIONS

UCARE OF MINNESOTA
2000 Summer St NE
Minneapolis, MN 55413
Phone: 612-676-6500   Fax: 612-676-6501   Toll-Free: 800-203-7225
Web site: www.ucare.org
Mailing Address:
   UCARE OF MINNESOTA
   PO Box 52
   St Paul, MN 55413

Key Executives:
Chief Executive Officer/President .... Nancy Feldman
Chief Financial Officer .... Mark Hudson
Chief Operating Officer .... Sharon A Carlin

Company Profile:
Parent Company Name:
Contract Effective Date: 01/01/97
Nonprofit: [Y]   Forprofit: [ ]
Total Enrollment:
   2000:   2003: 2,256   2006: 6,969
   2001:   2004: 2,345   2007: 7,563
   2002:   2005: 3,429

SERVICE AREA:
MN;

Product Name: Alexian Brothers Community Services

PLAN TYPE: PACE

ALEXIAN BROTHERS COMMUNITY SERVICES
3900 S Grand Blvd
St Louis, MO 63103
Phone: 314-771-7800   Fax: Toll-Free:
Web site: www.alexianbrothers.net
Mailing Address:
   ALEXIAN BROTHERS COMM SERVICES
   3900 S Grand Blvd
   St Louis, MO 63103

Key Executives:
Chief Executive Officer .... Victoria Steward-Alexander

Company Profile:
Parent Company Name:
Contract Effective Date: 11/01/01
Nonprofit: [Y]   Forprofit: [ ]
Total Enrollment:
   2000:   2003: 163   2006: 141
   2001:   2004: 164   2007: 143
   2002: 154   2005: 152

SERVICE AREA:
MO;

Product Name: Alexian Brothers Community Services

PLAN TYPE: PACE

ALEXIAN BROTHERS HEALTH SYSTEMS INC
425 Cumberland St Ste 110
Chattanooga, TN 37404-1905
Phone: 423-698-0802   Fax: Toll-Free:
Web site: www.alexianbrothers.net
Mailing Address:
   ALEXIAN BROTHERS HLT SYS INC
   425 Cumberland St Ste 110
   Chattanooga, TN 37404-1905

Key Executives:
Chief Executive Officer .... Viston Taylor

Company Profile:
Parent Company Name:
Contract Effective Date: 11/01/02
Nonprofit: [Y]   Forprofit: [ ]
Total Enrollment:
   2000:   2003: 240   2006: 279
   2001:   2004: 164   2007: 284
   2002:   2005: 287

SERVICE AREA:
TN (Hamilton);

Product Name: AltaMed Senior Buena Care

PLAN TYPE: PACE

ALTAMED HEALTH SERVICES CORPORATION
5425 E Pomona Blvd
Los Angeles, CA 90022-1716
Phone: 323-728-0411   Fax: 373-899-7399   Toll-Free:
Web site: www.altamed.org
Mailing Address:
   ALTAMED HEALTH SERVICES CORP
   5425 E Pomona Blvd
   Los Angeles, CA 90022-1716

Key Executives:
Chief Executive Officer/President .... Castulo de la Rocha

Company Profile:
Parent Company Name:
Contract Effective Date: 11/01/02
Nonprofit: [Y]   Forprofit: [ ]
Total Enrollment:
   2000:   2003: 202   2006: 264
   2001:   2004: 207   2007: 325
   2002: 148   2005: 258

SERVICE AREA:
CA;

Miscellaneous Organizations

Product Name: Minnesota Senior Health Options

PLAN TYPE: MN SENIOR CARE OPTIONS

HEALTHPARTNERS INC
8100 34th Ave South
Bloomington, MN 55425
Phone: 952-883-6000   Fax: 952-883-5380   Toll-Free: 888-470-4470
Web site: www.healthpartners.com

Mailing Address:
    HEALTHPARTNERS INC
    PO Box 1309
    Minneapolis, MN 55425

Key Executives:
Chief Executive Officer/President .... Mary Brainerd
Senior VP, Chief Financial Officer .... Kathy Cooney

Company Profile:
Parent Company Name:
Contract Effective Date: 05/01/05
Nonprofit: [Y]   Forprofit: [ ]
Total Enrollment:
    2000:   2003:   2006: 1,995
    2001:   2004:   2007: 2,535
    2002:   2005: 308

SERVICE AREA:
MN;

Product Name: Minnesota Senior Health Options

PLAN TYPE: MN SENIOR CARE OPTIONS

ITASCA MEDICAL CARE
1209 SE 2nd Ave
Grand Rapids, MN 55744
Phone: 218-327-6193   Fax: Toll-Free: 800-843-9536
Web site: www.co.itasca.mn.us

Mailing Address:
    ITASCA MEDICAL CARE
    1209 SE 2nd Ave
    Grand Rapids, MN 55744

Key Executives:
IMCare Director .... Karen Campbell

Company Profile:
Parent Company Name:
Contract Effective Date: 06/01/05
Nonprofit: [ ]   Forprofit: [ ]
Total Enrollment:
    2000:   2003:   2006: 422
    2001:   2004:   2007: 451
    2002:   2005:

SERVICE AREA:
MN;

Product Name: Minnesota Senior Health Options

PLAN TYPE: MN SENIOR HEALTH OPTIONS

MEDICA HEALTH PLANS
5601 Smetana Dr
Minnetonka, MN 55343
Phone: 952-992-2900   Fax: 952-992-3554   Toll-Free:
Web site: www.medica.com

Mailing Address:
    MEDICA HEALTH PLANS
    PO Box 9310
    Minneapolis, MN 55343

Managed Care Organization Profiles

Key Executives:
Chief Executive Officer .... David Tilford
President .... David R Strand
VP of Finance .... Patti Andreini-Arnold
Chief Operations Officer .... Karen Vigil

Company Profile:
Parent Company Name:
Contract Effective Date: 07/01/97
Nonprofit: [Y]   Forprofit: [ ]
Total Enrollment:
    2000:   2003: 2,214   2006: 8,867
    2001: 2,270   2004: 2,409   2007: 8,453
    2002: 2,322   2005: 2,558

SERVICE AREA:
MN;

Product Name: Minnesota Senior Health Options

PLAN TYPE: MN SENIOR HEALTH OPTIONS

METROPOLITAN HEALTH PLAN
400 S 4th St Ste 201
Minneapolis, MN 55415-1289
Phone: 612-347-8557   Fax: 612-904-4493   Toll-Free:
Web site: wwwa.co.hennepin.mn.us

Mailing Address:
    METROPOLITAN HEALTH PLAN
    400 S 4th St Ste 201
    Minneapolis, MN 55415-1289

Key Executives:
Chief Executive Officer .... David R Johnson
Chief Financial Officer .... Dave Edwards

Company Profile:
Parent Company Name:
Contract Effective Date: 01/01/97
Nonprofit: [ ]   Forprofit: [ ]
Total Enrollment:
    2000:   2003: 377   2006: 908
    2001: 352   2004: 374   2007: 844
    2002: 409   2005: 348

SERVICE AREA:
MN;

Product Name: Minnesota Senior Health Options

PLAN TYPE: MN SENIOR CARE OPTIONS

PRIMEWEST HEALTH SYSTEM
822 S 3rd St Ste 150
Minneapolis, MN 55415
Phone: 320-763-4135   Fax: Toll-Free:
Web site: www.primewest.org

Mailing Address:
    PRIMEWEST HEALTH SYSTEM
    822 S 3rd St Ste 150
    Minneapolis, MN 55415

Key Executives:
Chief Executive Officer .... Jim Przybilla
Director of Administrative Services .... Kathy Hungness

Company Profile:
Parent Company Name: Metropolitan Health Plan
Contract Effective Date: 07/01/05
Nonprofit: [ ]   Forprofit: [ ]
Total Enrollment:
    2000:   2003:   2006: 1,918
    2001:   2004:   2007: 2,035
    2002:   2005: 1,022

SERVICE AREA:
MN;

Managed Care Organization Profiles
Miscellaneous Organizations

Product Name: Massachusetts Senior Care Options

PLAN TYPE: MA SENIOR CARE OPTIONS
COMMONWEALTH CARE ALLIANCE INC
30 Winter St
Boston, MA 02108
Phone: 617-426-0600 Fax: 617-426-3097 Toll-Free:
Web site: www.commonwealthcare.org
Mailing Address:
　　COMMONWEALTH CARE ALLIANCE LLC
　　30 Winter St
　　Boston, MA 02108

Key Executives:
Chief Executive Officer/President .... Robert J Master, MD
Chief Financial Officer .... Robert Fallon
Chief Operating Officer .... Lois Simon

Company Profile:
Parent Company Name:
Contract Effective Date: 06/01/04
Nonprofit: [Y]　　　　Forprofit: [ ]
Total Enrollment:
　　2000:　　　　2003:　　　　　　2006: 700
　　2001:　　　　2004: 134　　　　2007: 991
　　2002:　　　　2005: 437

SERVICE AREA:
MA;

Product Name: Massachusetts Senior Care Options

PLAN TYPE: MA SENIOR CARE OPTIONS
SENIOR WHOLE HEALTH LLC
58 Charles St 2nd Fl
Cambridge, MA 02141
Phone: 617-494-5353 Fax: 617-494-5599 Toll-Free:
Web site: www.seniorwholehealth.com
Mailing Address:
　　SENIOR WHOLE HEALTH LLC
　　58 Charles St 2nd Fl
　　Cambridge, MA 02141

Key Executives:
Chief Executive Officer .... John Baackes

Company Profile:
Parent Company Name:
Contract Effective Date: 08/01/04
Nonprofit: [Y]　　　　Forprofit: [ ]
Total Enrollment:
　　2000:　　　　2003:　　　　　　2006: 1,848
　　2001:　　　　2004: 66　　　　 2007: 2,923
　　2002:　　　　2005: 875

SERVICE AREA:
MA;

Product Name: Minnesota Disability Health Options

PLAN TYPE: MN DISABILITY HEALTH OPTIONS
UCARE OF MINNESOTA
2000 Summer St NE
Minneapolis, MN 55413
Phone: 612-676-6500 Fax: 612-676-6501 Toll-Free: 800-203-7225
Web site: www.ucare.org
Mailing Address:
　　UCARE OF MINNESOTA
　　PO Box 52
　　St Paul, MN 55413

Key Executives:
Chief Executive Officer .... Nancy Feldman
Chief Financial Officer .... Mark Hudson
Chief Operating Officer .... Sharon A Carlin

Company Profile:
Parent Company Name:
Contract Effective Date: 11/01/01
Nonprofit: [Y]　　　　Forprofit: [ ]
Total Enrollment:
　　2000:　　　　2003: 145　　　　2006: 331
　　2001:　　　　2004: 167　　　　2007: 493
　　2002:　　　　2005: 277

SERVICE AREA:
MN;

Product Name: Minnesota Senior Health Options

PLAN TYPE: MN SENIOR CARE OPTIONS
BLUE CROSS BLUE SHIELD OF MINNESOTA
3535 Blue Cross Rd
St Paul, MN 55122
Phone: 651-662-1502 Fax: 651-662-1657 Toll-Free:
Web site: www.bluecrossmn.com
Mailing Address:
　　BLUE CROSS BLUE SHIELD MN
　　PO Box 64560
　　St Paul, MN 55122

Key Executives:
Chief Executive Officer/President .... Mark W Banks, MD
VP of Finance .... Timothy Peterson
Executive VP of Operations .... Colleen Reitan

Company Profile:
Parent Company Name: Blue Cross/Blue Shield
Contract Effective Date: 09/01/05
Nonprofit: [Y]　　　　Forprofit: [ ]
Total Enrollment:
　　2000:　　　　2003:　　　　　　2006: 9,070
　　2001:　　　　2004:　　　　　　2007: 9,836
　　2002:　　　　2005: 836

SERVICE AREA:
MN;

Product Name: Minnesota Senior Health Options

PLAN TYPE: MN SENIOR CARE OPTIONS
FIRST PLAN OF MINNESOTA
525 S Lake Ave Ste 222
Two Harbors, MN 55802
Phone: 218-834-7207 Fax: 218-834-6215 Toll-Free: 800-635-4159
Web site: www.firstplan.org
Mailing Address:
　　FIRST PLAN OF MINNESOTA
　　525 S Lake Ave Ste 222
　　Duluth, MN 55802

Key Executives:
Chief Executive Officer/President .... John S Bjorum
Chief Financial Officer .... Timothy Miller
Chief Operating Officer .... Julie Stone

Company Profile:
Parent Company Name: Blue Cross & Blue Shield
Contract Effective Date: 05/01/05
Nonprofit: [Y]　　　　Forprofit: [ ]
Total Enrollment:
　　2000:　　　　2003:　　　　　　2006:
　　2001:　　　　2004:　　　　　　2007: 918
　　2002:　　　　2005: 98

SERVICE AREA:
MN;

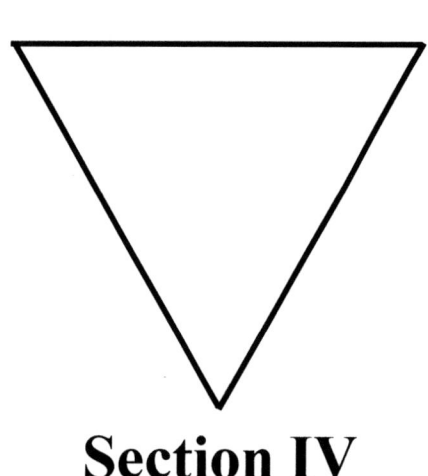

Section IV

Miscellaneous Organizations

Medicare Advantage Demonstration Projects

Product Name: ESRD II - HMOPOS

PLAN NAME: VILLAGEHEALTH

SCAN HEALTH PLAN
3800 Kilroy Airport Way #100
Long Beach, CA 90806
Phone: 562-989-5100 Fax: 562-989-5200 Toll-Free: 800-247-5091
Web site: www.scanhealthplan.com

Mailing Address:
   SCAN HEALTH PLAN
   3800 Kilroy Airport Way #100
   Long Beach, CA 90806

Key Executives:
Chief Executive Officer .... Dave Schmidt
Chief Financial Officer .... Dennis Eder

Company Profile:
Parent Company Name:
Contract Effective Date: 01/01/06
Nonprofit: [ ]   Forprofit: [Y]
Total Enrollment:
   2000:   2003:   2006:   195
   2001:   2004:   2007:   367
   2002:   2005:

SERVICE AREA:
   CA (Riverside, San Bernardino);

Product Name: ESRD II - PFFS

PLAN NAME: EVERCARE PLAN RD

EVERCARE HEALTH PLANS
3720 Davinci Court Ste 400
Norcross, GA 30092
Phone: 800-414-2015 Fax: Toll-Free: 800-414-2015
Web site: www.evercarehealthplans.com

Mailing Address:
   EVERCARE HEALTH PLANS
   9900 Bren Rd East
   Minnetonka, MN 30092

Key Executives:
Executive Director .... Rick McNatt

Company Profile:
Parent Company Name: UnitedHealth Group
Contract Effective Date: 09/01/05
Nonprofit: [ ]   Forprofit: [Y]
Total Enrollment:
   2000:   2003:   2006:   66
   2001:   2004:   2007:   97
   2002:   2005:

SERVICE AREA:
   GA (DeKalb, Fulton);

Managed Care Organization Profiles — Medicare Advantage Demonstration Projects

Product Name: Continuing Care Retirement Community

PLAN NAME: ERICKSON ADVANTAGE

UNITED HEALTHCARE INSURANCE COMPANY
9900 Bren Rd East
Minnetonka, MN 55343
Phone: 888-861-5518 Fax: Toll-Free: 888-861-5518
Web site: www.uhc.com

Mailing Address:
UNITED HEALTHCARE INS CO
9900 Bren Rd E - MN-008 W140
Minnetonka, MN 55343

Key Executives:
Contact .... Erica Cimino

Company Profile:
Parent Company Name: United Health Group
Contract Effective Date: 02/12/08
Nonprofit: [ ]   Forprofit: [Y]
Total Enrollment:
 2000:   2003:   2006:
 2001:   2004:   2007: 3,281
 2002:   2005:

SERVICE AREA:
CO; IL; KS; MA; MD; MI; NJ; PA; TX; VA;

Product Name: ESRD I - PFFS

PLAN NAME: FRESENIUS MEDICAL CARE HEALTH PLAN INC - NEW YORK

AMERICAN PROGRESSIVE LIFE & HEALTH OF NEW YORK
6 International Dr
Rye Brook, NY 10573-1068
Phone: 800-332-3377 Fax: 914-934-1988 Toll-Free:
Web site: www.amerprog.com

Mailing Address:
AMERICAN PROGRESS L & H OF NY
6 International Dr
Rye Brook, NY 10573-1068

Key Executives:
Chief Executive Officer .... Richard A Barasch
Executive VP, Chief Financial Officer .... Robert A Waegelein
VP, Administration .... Judy M Borrell

Company Profile:
Parent Company Name: Universal American Corporation
Contract Effective Date: 01/01/06
Nonprofit: [ ]   Forprofit: [Y]
Total Enrollment:
 2000:   2003:   2006: 83
 2001:   2004:   2007: 241
 2002:   2005:

SERVICE AREA:
NY;

Product Name: ESRD I - PFFS

PLAN NAME: FRESENIUS MEDICAL HEALTH PLAN INC - PENNSYLVANIA

STERLING LIFE INSURANCE COMPANY
2219 Rimland Dr
Bellingham, WA 98227-5348
Phone: 360-647-9080 Fax: 360-392-9074 Toll-Free:
Web site: www.sterlingplans.com

Mailing Address:
STERLING LIFE INSURANCE CO
PO Box 5348
Bellingham, WA 98227-5348

Key Executives:
Contact .... Mark Gilster

Company Profile:
Parent Company Name: AON Corporation
Contract Effective Date: 01/17/08
Nonprofit: [ ]   Forprofit: [Y]
Total Enrollment:
 2000:   2003:   2006:
 2001:   2004:   2007: 127
 2002:   2005:

SERVICE AREA:
PA;

Product Name: ESRD I - PFFS

PLAN NAME: FRESENIUS MEDICAL CARE HEALTH PLAN

PENNSYLVANIA LIFE INSURANCE COMPANY
4888 Loop Central Dr Ste 800
Houston, TX 77081
Phone: 866-660-4728 Fax: Toll-Free:
Web site: www.hhsi.com

Mailing Address:
PA LIFE INSURANCE CO
4888 Loop Central Dr Ste 800
Houston, TX 77081

Key Executives:
Contact .... P Matzelle

Company Profile:
Parent Company Name: Universal American Corporation
Contract Effective Date: 08/18/06
Nonprofit: [ ]   Forprofit: [Y]
Total Enrollment:
 2000:   2003:   2006:
 2001:   2004:   2007: 163
 2002:   2005:

SERVICE AREA:
TX;

Product Name: ESRD I - PFFS

PLAN NAME: FRESENIUS MEDICAL HEALTH PLAN INC - TEXAS

STERLING LIFE INSURANCE COMPANY
2219 Rimland Dr
Bellingham, WA 98227-5348
Phone: 360-647-9080 Fax: 360-392-9074 Toll-Free:
Web site: www.sterlingplans.com

Mailing Address:
STERLING LIFE INSURANCE CO
PO Box 5348
Bellingham, WA 98227-5348

Key Executives:
Contact .... Mark Gilster

Company Profile:
Parent Company Name: AON Corporation
Contract Effective Date: 01/01/06
Nonprofit: [Y]   Forprofit: [ ]
Total Enrollment:
 2000:   2003:   2006:
 2001:   2004:   2007: 200
 2002:   2005:

SERVICE AREA:
TX;

Introducing **Pay-for-Performance Reporter**

Your Authoritative Briefing on Pay-for-Performance

Pay for Performance Reporter is a monthly management briefing covering the news and key developments in P4P.

This newsletter will provide you with answers to questions you may have, with facts, news, insight and emerging P4P developments. Discover how early adopters achieved physician "buy in," the importance of leverage, how to choose your performance incentive measures wisely and choose measures that are defensible, and why provider feedback is so important. Every month you'll receive an objective, balanced report with current news and findings surrounding P4P.

When you subscribe today, save $50 and receive FREE our special bonus report "New Initiatives, Trends, and Results in Provider Pay-for-Performance," valued at $99.

For more information, visit: www.healthresourcesonline.com/managed_care/p4p.htm

---

PAY-FOR-PERFORMANCE REPORTER
Dept. 27NLD7AD, PO Box 559, Allenwood, NJ 08720
Call TOLL-FREE 888-THE-MCIC (888)-843-6242 or fax: 888- FAX-MCIC (888-329-6242)

Section III

Medicare Advantage Demonstration Project Participants

Mailing Address:
    WALGREENS HEALTH INITIATIVES
    1417 Lake Cook Rd MS L457
    Deerfield, IL 60015

Key Executives:
President .... Stanley B Blaylock

Statistics:
Parent Company Name: Walgreen Co
Doing Business As:
Year Founded: 1995
Nonprofit: [ ]   Forprofit: [Y]
Federally Qualified? [ ]

SERVICE AREA:
    IL;

WELLDYNE RX

7472 S Tucson Way Ste 100
Centennial, CO 80112
Phone: 720-895-3109 Fax: 303-645-2610 Toll-Free: 800-479-2000
Web site: www.welldynerx.com

Mailing Address:
    WELLDYNE RX
    PO Box 4517
    Englewood, CO 80112

Key Executives:
Chief Executive Officer/President .... Damien Lamendola
Chief Information Officer .... David King
Senior VP, Sales & Marketing .... Douglas A Taylor
Chief Operation Officer .... Susan Cain
VP, National Pharmacy Operations .... Michael Woodley, RPh

Statistics:
Parent Company Name: WellDyne Inc
Doing Business As:
Year Founded: 1990
Nonprofit: [ ]   Forprofit: [Y]
Federally Qualified? [ ]

SERVICE AREA:
    NW;

WELLPOINT NEXTRX

8407 Fallbrook Ave
West Hills, CA 91304
Phone: 818-313-5131 Fax: 818-313-5140 Toll-Free: 800-451-0433
Web site: www.wellpoint.com

Mailing Address:
    WELLPOINT NEXTRX
    8407 Fallbrook Ave
    West Hills, CA 91304

Key Executives:
Chairman .... Larry C Glasscock
Chief Executive Officer .... Angela F Braly
President - PBM .... Renwcyk Elder

Statistics:
Parent Company Name: WellPoint Health Networks
Doing Business As: Wellpoint NextRx
Year Founded: 1993
Nonprofit: [ ]   Forprofit: [Y]
Federally Qualified? [ ]

SERVICE AREA:
    CA;

WELLPOINT NEXTRX

8990 Duke Blvd
Mason, OH 45040-8943
Phone: 866-755-2776 Fax: 513-336-5142 Toll-Free: 800-221-6915
Web site: www.anthemprescription.com

Mailing Address:
    WELLPOINT NEXTRX
    8990 Duke Blvd - Mail# Pharmacy
    Mason, OH 45040-8943

Key Executives:
Chairman .... Larry C Glasscock
Chief Executive Officer .... Angela F Braly
President - PBM .... Renwcyk Elder

Statistics:
Parent Company Name: Anthem Inc/WellPoint
Doing Business As: WellPointNextRx
Year Founded: 1995
Nonprofit: [Y]   Forprofit: [ ]
Federally Qualified? [N]

SERVICE AREA:
    NW;

Pharmacy Benefit Management Companies | Managed Care Organization Profiles

Statistics:
Parent Company Name:
Doing Business As:
Year Founded:
Nonprofit: [ ]   Forprofit: [ ]
Federally Qualified? [ ]

SERVICE AREA:
TN;

TMESYS

5483 W Waters Ave Ste 1200
Tampa, FL 33634
Phone: 800-229-5000   Fax: Toll-Free: 800-229-5000
Web site: www.tmesys.com
Mailing Address:
    TMESYS
    5483 W Waters Ave Ste 1200
    Tampa, FL 33634

Key Executives:
President .... Mark Hollifield

Statistics:
Parent Company Name: PMSI-TMESYS
Doing Business As:
Year Founded: 1992
Nonprofit: [ ]   Forprofit: [ ]
Federally Qualified? [ ]

SERVICE AREA:
FL;

TOTAL SCRIPT

10901 W 120th Ave Ste 175
Broomfield, CO 80021
Phone: 800-752-2211   Fax: 303-438-9922 Toll-Free: 800-752-2211
Web site: www.totalscript.com
Mailing Address:
    TOTAL SCRIPT
    10901 W 120th Ave Ste 175
    Broomfield, CO 80021

Key Executives:
Vice President .... Janine Roeding

Statistics:
Parent Company Name:
Doing Business As:
Year Founded: 1997
Nonprofit: [ ]   Forprofit: [ ]
Federally Qualified? [ ]

SERVICE AREA:
NW;

UNITED DRUGS

7227 N 16th St Ste 160
Phoenix, AZ 85020
Phone: 602-678-1179   Fax: 602-678-0772 Toll-Free: 800-800-2988
Web site: www.uniteddrugs.com
Mailing Address:
    UNITED DRUGS
    7227 N 16th St Ste 160
    Phoenix, AZ 85020

Key Executives:
Chief Executive Officer .... Bruce A Semingson, RPh

Statistics:
Parent Company Name: American Associated Druggists Inc
Doing Business As: United Drugs
Year Founded: 1975
Nonprofit: [ ]   Forprofit: [Y]
Federally Qualified? [ ]

SERVICE AREA:
AZ;

US SCRIPT INC

2425 W Shaw Ave
Fresno, CA 93711
Phone: 559-244-3700   Fax: 559-244-3710 Toll-Free: 800-413-7721
Web site: www.usscript.com
Mailing Address:
    US SCRIPT INC
    2425 W Shaw Ave
    Fresno, CA 93711

Key Executives:
Sales & Marketing Manager .... Allison Gerrard

Statistics:
Parent Company Name: Centene Corp
Doing Business As: CenCorp Health Solutions
Year Founded: 1999
Nonprofit: [ ]   Forprofit: [ ]
Federally Qualified? [ ]

SERVICE AREA:
NW;

US-RX CARE

20 River Ct Ste 2908
Jersey City, NJ 07310
Phone: 201-386-9338   Fax: Toll-Free:
Web site: www.us-rxcare.com
Mailing Address:
    US-RX CARE
    20 River Ct Ste 2908
    Jersey City, NJ 07310

Key Executives:
President .... Renzo Luzzatti

Statistics:
Parent Company Name:
Doing Business As:
Year Founded:
Nonprofit: [ ]   Forprofit: [ ]
Federally Qualified? [ ]

SERVICE AREA:
NW;

WAL-MART STORES PHARMACY DIV

702 Southwest 8th St
Bentonville, AR 72716-9113
Phone: 479-273-4000   Fax: 479-277-4332 Toll-Free:
Web site: www.walmartstores.com
Mailing Address:
    WAL-MART STORES PHARMACY DIV
    702 Southwest 8th St
    Bentonville, AR 72716-9113

Key Executives:
VP Pharmacy Operations .... Ron Chomiuk

Statistics:
Parent Company Name:
Doing Business As:
Year Founded:
Nonprofit: [ ]   Forprofit: [ ]
Federally Qualified? [ ]

SERVICE AREA:
AR;

WALGREENS HEALTH INITIATIVES

1417 Lake Cook Rd MS L457
Deerfield, IL 60015
Phone: 847-940-2483   Fax: 847-940-9061 Toll-Free: 800-926-6779
Web site: www.walgreenshealth.com

Managed Care Organization Profiles / Pharmacy Benefit Management Companies

Statistics:
Parent Company Name:
Doing Business As:
Year Founded: 1989
Nonprofit: [ ]   Forprofit: [ ]
Federally Qualified? [ ]

SERVICE AREA:
    TX;

SCRIPTRAX

255 Charlois Blvd
Winston-Salem, NC 27103
Phone: 336-718-1043   Fax: 336-718-1465 Toll-Free: 877-774-8729
Web site: www.scriptrax.com
Mailing Address:
        SCRIPTRAX
        255 Charlois Blvd
        Winston-Salem, NC 27103

Key Executives:
Director, New Business Development .... Gerry Smith

Statistics:
Parent Company Name: Novant Health
Doing Business As:
Year Founded:
Nonprofit: [Y]   Forprofit: [ ]
Federally Qualified? [ ]

SERVICE AREA:
    NC;

SERVE YOU CUSTOM PRESCRIPTION MANAGEMENT

9051 West Heather Ave
Milwaukee, WI 53224
Phone: 414-410-8100   Fax: 414-410-8181 Toll-Free: 800-759-3203
Web site: www.serve-you-rx.com
Mailing Address:
        SERVE YOU CUSTOM PRESCRIPTION
        PO Box 240034
        Milwaukee, WI 53224

Key Executives:
President .... Sharon Murillo
Marketing Manager .... Cheryl DeShambo
VP of Operatiosn .... Michael Wade
Director Client Services & Cntrct .... Dennis W Crowley

Statistics:
Parent Company Name:
Doing Business As:
Year Founded: 1987
Nonprofit: [ ]   Forprofit: [Y]
Federally Qualified? [ ]

SERVICE AREA:
    Nationwide;

SOUTH DAKOTA PHARMACIST ASSOCIATION

320 E Capitol Ave
Pierre, SD 57501
Phone: 605-224-2338   Fax: 605-224-1280 Toll-Free:
Web site: www.sdpha.org
Mailing Address:
        SOUTH DAKOTA PHARMACIST ASSOC
        PO Box 518
        Pierre, SD 57501

Key Executives:
Executive Director .... Sue Schaefer
President .... Robert Reiswig, RPh

Statistics:
Parent Company Name:
Doing Business As:
Year Founded: 1987
Nonprofit: [Y]   Forprofit: [ ]
Federally Qualified? [ ]

SERVICE AREA:
    SD;

SUNRX INC

815 East Gate Dr #102
Mount Laurel, NJ 08054
Phone: 800-786-1791   Fax: 800-786-7550 Toll-Free: 800-786-1791
Web site: www.sunrx.com
Mailing Address:
        SUNRX INC
        815 East Gate Dr #102
        Mount Laurel, NJ 08054

Key Executives:
Chairman/Chief Executive Officer .... Gerard J Ferro
President .... Christine Serenelli
Chief Operating Officer .... Edward R Miersch

Statistics:
Parent Company Name:
Doing Business As:
Year Founded: 2002
Nonprofit: [ ]   Forprofit: [ ]
Federally Qualified? [ ]

SERVICE AREA:
    NW;

SXC HEALTH SOLUTIONS INC

2441 Warrenville Rd Ste 610
Lisle, IL 60532-3642
Phone: 630-577-3100   Fax: 630-577-3101 Toll-Free: 800-282-3232
Web site: www.sxc.com
Mailing Address:
        SXC HEALTH SOLUTIONS INC
        2441 Warrenville Rd Ste 610
        Lisle, IL 60532-3642

Key Executives:
Chairman/Chief Executive Officer .... Gordon S Glenn
President .... Mark A Thierer
Senior VP,Chief Financial Officer .... Jeffrey Park
Senior VP, Sales & Marketing .... Mike Meyer
Chief Operating Officer .... Mark A Thierer

Statistics:
Parent Company Name: SXC Health Solutions Inc, Canada
Doing Business As:
Year Founded: 1993
Nonprofit: [ ]   Forprofit: [ ]
Federally Qualified? [ ]

SERVICE AREA:
    NW;

TENNESSEE PHARMACIST ASSOCIATION

500 Church St Ste 650
Nashville, TN 37219
Phone: 615-255-9487   Fax: 615-255-9492 Toll-Free:
Web site: www.tnpharm.org
Mailing Address:
        TENNESSEE PHARMACIST ASSOC
        500 Church St Ste 650
        Nashville, TN 37219

Key Executives:
Executive Director .... Baeteena Black, RPh

Pharmacy Benefit Management Companies

Statistics:
Parent Company Name: Regence Group Inc
Doing Business As:
Year Founded:
Nonprofit: [Y]   Forprofit: [ ]
Federally Qualified? [ ]

SERVICE AREA:
ID; OR; Ut; WA;

RESTAT

724 Elm St
West Bend, WI 53095
Phone: 262-338-5760 Fax: 262-338-5767 Toll-Free: 800-926-5858
Web site: www.restat.com
Mailing Address:
RESTAT
PO Box 758
West Bend, WI 53095

Key Executives:
President .... Michael W Clark

Statistics:
Parent Company Name: The F Dohmen Co
Doing Business As:
Year Founded:
Nonprofit: [ ]   Forprofit: [ ]
Federally Qualified? [ ]

SERVICE AREA:
WI;

RITE AID HEALTH SOLUTIONS

30 Hunter Lane
Camp Hill, PA 17011
Phone: 866-828-5966 Fax: 717-214-2526 Toll-Free:
Web site: www.riteaidhealthsolutions.com
Mailing Address:
RITE AID HEALTH SOLUTIONS
30 Hunter Lane
Camp Hill, PA 17011

Key Executives:
VP, General Manager .... Greg Drew, RPh
VP, Sales .... Lance Aizen

Statistics:
Parent Company Name: Rite Aid Corporation
Doing Business As:
Year Founded:
Nonprofit: [ ]   Forprofit: [ ]
Federally Qualified? [ ]

SERVICE AREA:
NW;

RXAMERICA LLC

221 N Charles Lindbergh Dr
Salt Lake City, UT 84116
Phone: 801-961-6000 Fax: 801-961-6341 Toll-Free: 800-770-8014
Web site: www.rxamerica.com
Mailing Address:
RXAMERICA LLC
221 N Charles Lindbergh Dr
Salt Lake City, UT 84116

Key Executives:
Chief Executive Officer/President .... John Gardynik, PharmD, MBA
Chief Financial Officer .... Denis Muskat
Chief Medical Officer .... Ken McGrory
Chief Information Officer .... Jean Rolando
Chief Marketing Officer .... Mark SantaCroce
Chief Operating Officer .... Gary Purk

Managed Care Organization Profiles

Statistics:
Parent Company Name: Long Drug Stores
Doing Business As:
Year Founded: 1994
Nonprofit: [ ]   Forprofit: [ ]
Federally Qualified? [ ]

SERVICE AREA:
NW;

RXPLUS PHARMACIES INC

3660 Wadsworth Blvd
Wheat Ridge, CO 80033
Phone: 303-463-4875 Fax: 303-463-4880 Toll-Free:
Web site: www.rxplus.com
Mailing Address:
RXPLUS PHARMACIES INC
3660 Wadsworth Blvd
Wheat Ridge, CO 80033

Key Executives:
Executive Director .... Grant Kinn
Director Business Development .... Mike Mitchell

Statistics:
Parent Company Name:
Doing Business As:
Year Founded: 1982
Nonprofit: [ ]   Forprofit: [ ]
Federally Qualified? [ ]

SERVICE AREA:
CO; AK; NE; NM; WA; WY;

SCRIPNET

10050 Banburry Cross Dr #290
Las Vegas, NV 89144
Phone: 702-851-3816 Fax: 888-245-1745 Toll-Free: 888-880-8562
Web site: www.scripnet.com
Mailing Address:
SCRIPNET
PO Box 379037
Las Vegas, NV 89144

Key Executives:
Chief Executive Officer/President .... Dennis M Sponer
Chief Financial Officer .... Joachim Waechter
Director of Operations .... Jennifer Sponer
Director Human Resources .... Sharon Planchunas

Statistics:
Parent Company Name:
Doing Business As:
Year Founded: 1997
Nonprofit: [ ]   Forprofit: [Y]
Federally Qualified? [N]

SERVICE AREA:
NW;

SCRIPT CARE INC - TEXAS

6380 Folsom Dr
Beaumont, TX 77706
Phone: 409-832-3041 Fax: 409-832-3109 Toll-Free: 800-880-9988
Web site: www.scriptcare.com
Mailing Address:
SCRIPT CARE INC - TEXAS
6380 Folsom Dr
Beaumont, TX 77706

Key Executives:
Chief Executive Officer .... Jim Brown, RPh

Managed Care Organization Profiles
Pharmacy Benefit Management Companies

Key Executives:
Chief Executive Officer .... Kenneth Sack

Statistics:
Parent Company Name: Catalyst Rx
Doing Business As: Catalyst Rx
Year Founded: 1983
Nonprofit: [ ]   Forprofit: [Y]
Federally Qualified? [ ]

SERVICE AREA:
FL;

PREMIER PHARMACY PLAN

101 W Saint John St Ste 303
Spartanburg, SC 29306
Phone: 864-591-0025 Fax: 864-582-0819 Toll-Free: 800-247-4526
Web site: www.smithpremier.com
Mailing Address:
PREMIER PHARMACY PLAN
PO Box 5824
Spartanburg, SC 29306

Key Executives:
Chief Executive Officer .... Michael Webb

Statistics:
Parent Company Name: JM Smith Corp
Doing Business As: Premier Pharmacy Plan
Year Founded: 1985
Nonprofit: [ ]   Forprofit: [Y]
Federally Qualified? [ ]

SERVICE AREA:
SC;

PRESCRIPTION MANAGEMENT SERVICES INC

175 Kelsey Lane
Tampa, FL 33619
Phone: 800-237-7676 Fax: 813-664-0774 Toll-Free: 800-237-7676
Web site: www.tmesys.com
Mailing Address:
PRESCRIPTION MNGT SERVICES INC
PO Box 30054
Tampa, FL 33619

Key Executives:
President .... Mark Hollifield

Statistics:
Parent Company Name: Amerisource Bergen Corp
Doing Business As: PMSI-TMESYS
Year Founded: 1976
Nonprofit: [ ]   Forprofit: [Y]
Federally Qualified? [N]

SERVICE AREA:
FL;

PRESCRIPTION SOLUTIONS

2300 Main Street
Irvine, CA 92614
Phone: 714-825-3600 Fax: 714-825-3898 Toll-Free: 800-788-4863
Web site: www.rxsolutions.com
Mailing Address:
PRESCRIPTION SOLUTIONS
2300 Main Street
Irvine, CA 92614

Key Executives:
Chief Executive Officer/President .... Edward M Feaver, PharmD
Chief Financial Officer .... Paul R Miller, CPA
Chief Medical Officer .... Joseph Addiego, MD
VP, Operations .... William Mickle
VP Government Affairs, Pharmacy Policy .... John D Jones, RPh, JD

Statistics:
Parent Company Name: United Health Group Co
Doing Business As:
Year Founded: 1993
Nonprofit: [ ]   Forprofit: [Y]
Federally Qualified? [ ]

SERVICE AREA:
CA;

PRIME THERAPEUTICS

1305 Corporate Center Dr
Eagan, MN 55121
Phone: 651-414-4000 Fax: 651-286-4403 Toll-Free: 800-858-0723
Web site: www.primetherapeutics.com
Mailing Address:
PRIME THERAPEUTICS
PO Box 64812
St Paul, MN 55121

Key Executives:
Chief Executive Officer/President .... Timothy F Dickman
Chief Financial Officer .... Charles Roehrick
Senior VP,Chief Medical Officer .... James E Hartert, MD, MS, FACP
Chief Information Officer .... John Mielke
Senior VP, Business Development .... Matt S Yordy
Senior VP, Chief Operating Officer .... Kim Mageau
VP, Human Resources .... Erin Ascher
Senior VP, Client Services .... Cameron Olig
Senior VP, General Counsel .... Valerie Ruttenberg

Statistics:
Parent Company Name: Owned by 10 Blue Cross Blue Shield Plans
Doing Business As:
Year Founded: 1998
Nonprofit: [ ]   Forprofit: [Y]
Federally Qualified? [ ]

SERVICE AREA:
FL; IL; KS; MN; ND; NE; NM; OK; TX; WY;

RAMSELL HOLDING CORPORATION

200 Webster St Ste 200
Oakland, CA 94607
Phone: 510-587-2600 Fax: 510-663-6005 Toll-Free: 888-311-7632
Web site: www.rhsb.com
Mailing Address:
RAMSELL HOLDING CORPORATION
200 Webster St Ste 200
Oakland, CA 94607

Key Executives:
Chief Executive Officer/President .... Eric A Flowers, MBA

Statistics:
Parent Company Name:
Doing Business As:
Year Founded: 1967
Nonprofit: [ ]   Forprofit: [ ]
Federally Qualified? [ ]

SERVICE AREA:
CA; WA;

REGENCERX

100 Southwest Market St
Portland, OR 97207
Phone: 800-621-2155 Fax: 503-225-5274 Toll-Free: 800-621-2155
Web site: www.regencerx.com
Mailing Address:
REGENCERX
PO Box 1271 MSE12A
Portland, OR 97207

Key Executives:
Chief Executive Officer/President .... Mark B Ganz

Pharmacy Benefit Management Companies

PERFORMRX

200 Stevens Dr
Philadelphia, PA 19113
Phone: 866-456-1692   Fax: 800-684-5504   Toll-Free: 866-456-1692
Web site: www.performrx.com
Mailing Address:
   PERFORMRX
   PO Box 41535
   Philadelphia, PA 19113

Key Executives:
President .... Mesfin Tegenu, MS, RPh
VP, Corporate Communications .... Rick Buck

Statistics:
Parent Company Name: AmeriHealth Mercy
Doing Business As:
Year Founded:
Nonprofit: [ ]   Forprofit: [ ]
Federally Qualified? [ ]

SERVICE AREA:
   PA;

PHARMAVAIL BENEFIT MANAGEMENT COMPANY

3380 Trickum Rd Bld 500 Unit100
Woodstock, GA 31088
Phone: 678-236-0403   Fax: 678-236-0415   Toll-Free: 800-933-3734
Web site: www.pharmavailbenefits.com
Mailing Address:
   PHARMAVAIL BENEFIT MNGMNT CO
   3380 Trickum Rd Bld 500 Unit 100
   Woodstock, GA 31088

Key Executives:
Chief Executive Officer .... Charles Callahan, RPh, CDM
VP, Clinical Services .... Robyn Lon Dr

Statistics:
Parent Company Name:
Doing Business As:
Year Founded: 2001
Nonprofit: [ ]   Forprofit: [ ]
Federally Qualified? [ ]

SERVICE AREA:
   NW;

PHARMACY ASSOCIATION, THE

211 E Capitol Ave
Jefferson City, MO 65101
Phone: 573-636-7522   Fax: 573-636-7485   Toll-Free: 800-468-4672
Web site: www.morx.com
Mailing Address:
   PHARMACY ASSOCIATION, THE
   211 E Capitol Ave
   Jefferson City, MO 65101

Key Executives:
Chief Executive Officer .... Ron Fitzwater
Director of Marketing .... Travis Fitzwater

Statistics:
Parent Company Name: Missouri Pharmacy Association
Doing Business As:
Year Founded: 1879
Nonprofit: [ ]   Forprofit: [ ]
Federally Qualified? [ ]

SERVICE AREA:
   MO;

PHARMACY DATA MANAGEMENT INC

940 Windham Court Ste 1
Boardman, OH 44512
Phone: 800-767-4226   Fax: 330-629-7339   Toll-Free: 800-800-7364
Web site: www.pdmi.com

Managed Care Organization Profiles

Mailing Address:
   PHARMACY DATA MANAGEMENT INC
   940 Windham Court Ste 1
   Boardman, OH 44512

Key Executives:
Chief Executive Officer/President .... Douglas Wittenauer

Statistics:
Parent Company Name:
Doing Business As:
Year Founded: 1983
Nonprofit: [ ]   Forprofit: [Y]
Federally Qualified? [ ]

SERVICE AREA:
   NW;

PHARMACY PROVIDERS SERVICES CORP

3375 I Capital Circle NE
Tallahassee, FL 32308
Phone: 850-656-0100   Fax: 866-765-8415   Toll-Free: 888-778-9909
Web site: www.ppsconline.com
Mailing Address:
   PHARMACY PROVIDERS SERVICES CO
   3375 I Capital Circle NE
   Tallahassee, FL 32308

Key Executives:
President .... Cyndi Mincy
Comptroller .... Angela Guardia
Director of Sales & Marketing .... Carol Mitchell-Yon
Director Business Development/Clinical Pharmacy ..... Bill Mincy RPh
Director, Information Systems .... Ron Burnette

Statistics:
Parent Company Name: Pharmacy Provider Services Corporation
Doing Business As: PPSC
Year Founded: 1983
Nonprofit: [ ]   Forprofit: [Y]
Federally Qualified? [ ]

SERVICE AREA:
   FL;

PHARMACY PROVIDERS OF OKLAHOMA

PO Box 18204
Oklahoma City, OK 73154
Phone: 405-557-5700   Fax: 405-525-7523   Toll-Free: 877-557-5707
Web site: www.ppok.com
Mailing Address:
   PHARMACY PROVIDERS OF OKLAHOMA
   PO Box 18204
   Oklahoma City, OK 73154

Key Executives:
Executive Director .... Lonny Wilson

Statistics:
Parent Company Name: Mirixa
Doing Business As:
Year Founded: 1985
Nonprofit: [ ]   Forprofit: [ ]
Federally Qualified? [ ]

SERVICE AREA:
   OK;

PHARMACY SERVICES GROUP

6301 NW 5th Way Ste 5010
Fort Lauderdale, FL 33309
Phone: 954-938-9980   Fax: 954-938-7984   Toll-Free: 800-774-2002
Web site: www.psgpbm.com
Mailing Address:
   PHARMACY SERVICES GROUP
   6301 NW 5th Way Ste 5010
   Fort Lauderdale, FL 33309

Mailing Address:
   OVATIONS PHARMACY SOLUTIONS
   9900 Bren Rd East Opus Ctr
   Minnetonka, MN 55343

Key Executives:
Chief Executive Officer/President .... Stephen J Hemsley
Chief Financial Officer .... G Mike Mikan

Statistics:
Parent Company Name: UnitedHealth Group
Doing Business As:
Year Founded: 1974
Nonprofit: [ ]   Forprofit: [Y]
Federally Qualified? [ ]

SERVICE AREA:
   NW;

PARAGON BIOMEDICAL INC

9685 Research Dr
Irvine, CA 92618
Phone: 949-224-2800 Fax: 949-224-2811 Toll-Free: 800-6paragon
Web site: www.parabio.com
Mailing Address:
   PARAGON BIOMEDICAL INC
   9685 Research Dr
   Irvine, CA 92618

Key Executives:
Founder/Chief Executive Officer .... Gena H Reed
President .... Mark Havill
Chief Financial Officer .... Carol A O'Brien
Medical Director .... Liza DeAnnuntis, MD
Chief Information Officer .... Subash Sadanandan
VP Global Sales & Marketing .... William Blank
Chief Operating Officer .... Mark Harvill
Medical Lead - India .... Sachidananda Moorthy, MD
Medical Lead - CEE/Poland .... Marcin Koziej, MD

Statistics:
Parent Company Name: Paragon Biomedical Inc
Doing Business As:
Year Founded: 1989
Nonprofit: [ ]   Forprofit: [ ]
Federally Qualified? [ ]

SERVICE AREA:
   CA;

PARTNERS RX MANAGEMENT LLC

15950 N 76th St Ste 200
Scottsdale, AZ 85260
Phone: 480-624-9400 Fax: 480-624-9401 Toll-Free: 800-659-4112
Web site: www.partnersrx.com
Mailing Address:
   PARTNERS RX MANAGEMENT LLC
   15950 N 76th Ste 200
   Scottsdale, AZ 85260

Key Executives:
Chairman of the Board .... Mark V Mertel
Chief Executive Officer/President .... Robert W Field
Chief Financial Officer .... Edward T Printy CPA
Senior VP, Sales & Marketing .... Matthew P Ward
VP of Operations .... Lori Bymark, MSIA
Chief Pharmacy Officer .... Richard Bullard, RPh
VP, Managed Care .... Steven G Avey

Statistics:
Parent Company Name: Diversified Health Care Services Inc
Doing Business As:
Year Founded:
Nonprofit: [ ]   Forprofit: [ ]
Federally Qualified? [ ]

SERVICE AREA:
   NW;

PBA HEALTH

1575 N Universal Ave Ste 100
Kansas City, MO 64120
Phone: 816-245-5700 Fax: 816-245-5702 Toll-Free: 800-333-8097
Web site: www.pbahealth.com
Mailing Address:
   PBA HEALTH
   1575 N Universal Ave Ste 100
   Kansas City, MO 64120

Key Executives:
Chief Executive Officer .... Nick Smock
Chief Information Officer .... Clark Balcom

Statistics:
Parent Company Name: TrueCare Community Pharmacy
Doing Business As:
Year Founded:
Nonprofit: [ ]   Forprofit: [Y]
Federally Qualified? [N]

SERVICE AREA:
   KS;

PBM PLUS INC

300 TechneCenter Dr Ste B
Milford, OH 45150
Phone: 513-248-3071 Fax: 513-248-3079 Toll-Free: 888-863-1726
Web site: www.pbmplus.com
Mailing Address:
   PBM PLUS INC
   300 TechneCenter Dr Ste B
   Milford, OH 45150

Key Executives:
Chief Executive Officer/President .... Klaus A Hieber, RPh
Chief Operating Officer .... Nick Page, PharmD

Statistics:
Parent Company Name: Omnicare Inc
Doing Business As:
Year Founded:
Nonprofit: [ ]   Forprofit: [ ]
Federally Qualified? [ ]

SERVICE AREA:
   OH;

PEQUOT PHARMACEUTICAL NETWORK

1 Annie George Dr Bldg 3
Mashantucket, CT 06338
Phone: 860-396-6455 Fax: 860-396-6339 Toll-Free: 800-342-5779
Web site: www.prxn.com
Mailing Address:
   PEQUOT PHARMACEUTICAL NETWORK
   PO Box 3559
   Mashantucket, CT 06338

Key Executives:
President .... Karen Hatcher-Sneed
Executive Director, Finance & Operations .... Donna Dooley
Director Sales & Marketing .... Dawn Coley
MIS Director .... Barry Levine

Statistics:
Parent Company Name: Mashantucket Pequot Tribal Nation
Doing Business As: PRxn/Pequot Plus Health Benefits
Year Founded: 1991
Nonprofit: [ ]   Forprofit: [Y]
Federally Qualified? [ ]

SERVICE AREA:
   NW;

Pharmacy Benefit Management Companies

NAVITUS HEALTH SOLUTIONS

999 Fourier Dr Ste 301
Madison, WI 53717
Phone: 866-333-2757 Fax: 608-827-7527 Toll-Free: 877-571-7500
Web site: www.navitus.com
Mailing Address:
    NAVITUS HEALTH SOLUTIONS
    999 Fourier Dr Ste 301
    Madison, WI 53717

Key Executives:
Chief Executive Officer .... Robert Palmer
President .... Terry Seligman
VP, Chief Financial Officer .... Pete Beste
VP, Chief Information Officer .... Loran Lentz
Senior VP, Sales, Marketing, Client Services .... Byron Mickle
VP, Pharmacy Network Development .... Alan Van Amber
VP, Chief Compliance Officer .... Debbie Ludka

Statistics:
Parent Company Name:
Doing Business As:
Year Founded: 2003
Nonprofit: [ ]   Forprofit: [ ]
Federally Qualified? [ ]

SERVICE AREA:
    WI;

ND PHARMACY SERVICE CORP

1661 Capitol Way 102
Bismarck, ND 58501-2195
Phone: 701-258-4968 Fax: 701-258-9312 Toll-Free:
Web site: www.nodakpharmacy.net
Mailing Address:
    ND PHARMACY SERVICE CORP
    1661 Capitol Way 102
    Bismarck, ND 58501-2195

Key Executives:
Executive Vice President .... Michael Schwab

Statistics:
Parent Company Name:
Doing Business As:
Year Founded:
Nonprofit: [ ]   Forprofit: [ ]
Federally Qualified? [ ]

SERVICE AREA:
    ND;

NORTHEAST PHARMACY SERVICE CORP

1661 Worcester Rd Ste 405
Framingham, MA 01701
Phone: 508-875-1866 Fax: 508-875-6108 Toll-Free: 800-532-3742
Web site: www.northeastpharmacy.com
Mailing Address:
    NORTHEAST PHARMACY SERVICE COR
    1661 Worcester Rd Ste 405
    Framingham, MA 01701

Key Executives:
Chief Executive Officer/President .... Patricia Monaco
Director, Finance .... Mary Oram
Director, MIS .... Anna Yamaykina

Statistics:
Parent Company Name:
Doing Business As:
Year Founded: 1991
Nonprofit: [X]   Forprofit: [ ]
Federally Qualified? [ ]

SERVICE AREA:
    MA;

NORTHWEST PHARMACY SERVICES

929 E Main Ave Ste 310
Puyallup, WA 98372-3124
Phone: 253-840-5604 Fax: 253-840-5013 Toll-Free: 800-998-2611
Web site: www.nwpsrx.com
Mailing Address:
    NORTHWEST PHARMACY SERVICES
    929 E Main Ave Ste 310
    Puyallup, WA 98372-3124

Key Executives:
Marketing Director/Quality Assurance Director .... Floyd Monen

Statistics:
Parent Company Name: Northwest Pharmacy Services
Doing Business As:
Year Founded: 1985
Nonprofit: [Y]   Forprofit: [N]
Federally Qualified? [N]

SERVICE AREA:
    NW;

NPAX INC

1200 Rt 46 W
Clifton, NJ 07013
Phone: 973-574-2400 Fax: 973-574-2495 Toll-Free:
Web site: www.e-nva.com
Mailing Address:
    NPAX INC
    1200 Rte 46 W
    Clifton, NJ 07013

Key Executives:
Chief Executive Officer .... Richard O Ullman

Statistics:
Parent Company Name: National Vision Administrator Llc
Doing Business As: NPAX INC
Year Founded:
Nonprofit: [ ]   Forprofit: [ ]
Federally Qualified? [ ]

SERVICE AREA:
    NJ;

OMNICARE OF SOUTH FLORIDA

2955 W Corporate Lakes Blvd
Weston, FL 33331
Phone: 877-446-7828 Fax: 954-660-5560 Toll-Free: 877-446-7828
Web site: www.omnicare.com
Mailing Address:
    OMNICARE OF SOUTH FLORIDA
    2955 W Corp Lakes Blvd
    Weston, FL 33331

Key Executives:
General Manager .... Rubin Navarro

Statistics:
Parent Company Name: Omnicare Inc
Doing Business As:
Year Founded:
Nonprofit: [ ]   Forprofit: [ ]
Federally Qualified? [ ]

SERVICE AREA:
    AL; FL; LA; MS; OH;

OVATIONS PHARMACY SOLUTIONS

9900 Bren Rd East Opus Ctr
Minnetonka, MN 55343
Phone: 952-936-1300 Fax: 952-936-0044 Toll-Free:
Web site: www.uhc.com

Mailing Address:
    MEDCO HEALTH SOLUTIONS INC
    100 Parsons Pond Drive
    Franklin Lakes, NJ 07417

Key Executives:
Chairman of the Board/Chief Executive Officer .... David B Snow, Jr
President .... Kenneth O Klepper
Chief Financial Officer .... Richard J Rubino CPA
Senior VP Chief Medical Officer .... Robert S Epstein, MD, MS
Senior VP, Chief Marketing Officer .... Jack A Smith
Chief Operating Officer .... Kenneth O Klepper
Group President, Health Plans .... Brian T Griffin
Senior VP, Human Resources .... Karin Princivalle
Group President, Employee Account .... Bryan D Birch

Statistics:
Parent Company Name: Merck & Co Inc
Doing Business As:
Year Founded: 1985
Nonprofit: [ ]   Forprofit: [ ]
Federally Qualified? [ ]

SERVICE AREA:
    NW;

MEDICAP PHARMACIES INC

4350 Westown Pkwy Ste 400
West Des Moines, IA 50266-1061
Phone: 515-224-8400 Fax: 515-224-8415 Toll-Free: 800-445-2244
Web site: www.medshoppe.com
Mailing Address:
    MEDICAP PHARMACIES INC
    4350 Westown Pkwy Ste 400
    West Des Moines, IA 50266-1061

Key Executives:
President .... Terry Burnside

Statistics:
Parent Company Name: Cardinal Health Inc
Doing Business As: Medicine Shoppe International Inc
Year Founded: 1971
Nonprofit: [ ]   Forprofit: [ ]
Federally Qualified? [ ]

SERVICE AREA:
    NW;

MEMBERHEALTH INC

29100 Aurora Rd Ste 301
Solon, OH 44139
Phone: 440-248-8448 Fax: Toll-Free: 888-868-5854
Web site: www.mhrx.com
Mailing Address:
    MEMBERHEALTH INC
    PO Box 391180
    Cleveland, OH 44139

Key Executives:
Chief Executive Officer/President .... Charles E Hallberg, JD
Chief Financial Officer .... David S Azzolina
Chief Information Officer .... Len Ploskonka
General Counsel, Human Resources Dir .... Jane Koehl-Colling, Esq
VP, Clncial Operations .... Samuel Rajan, RPh
Senior VP, Corporate Developmnt .... D Alan Scantland
Deputy Director/Community Care Rx .... John G Kloss

Statistics:
Parent Company Name:
Doing Business As:
Year Founded: 1998
Nonprofit: [ ]   Forprofit: [ ]
Federally Qualified? [ ]

SERVICE AREA:
    NW;

MOLINA HEALTHCARE INC

200 Oceangate-Ste 100
Long Beach, CA 90802
Phone: 562-435-3666 Fax: 562-437-1335 Toll-Free: 888-562-5442
Web site: www.molinahealthcare.com
Mailing Address:
    MOLINA HEALTHCARE INC
    200 Oceangate-Ste 100
    Long Beach, CA 90802

Key Executives:
Chief Executive Officer/President .... J Mario Molina, MD
Executive VP, Chief Financial Officer .... John C Molina, JD
Chief Medical Officer .... James Howatt, MD
Chief Operating Officer .... Terry P Bayer MPH JD

Statistics:
Parent Company Name:
Doing Business As:
Year Founded: 1993
Nonprofit: [ ]   Forprofit: [Y]
Federally Qualified? [ ]

SERVICE AREA:
    CA; IN; MI; NM; OH; TX; UT; WA;

MYMATRIXX

PO Box 274070
Tampa, FL 33688
Phone: 813-247-2341 Fax: 813-247-3391 Toll-Free: 800-785-0884
Web site: www.mymatrixx.com
Mailing Address:
    MYMATRIXX
    PO Box 274070
    Tampa, FL 33688

Key Executives:
Chief Executive Officer .... Steven MacDonald
Business Manager .... Vikki Fritch
Medical Director .... Steven P Stanos, Jr, DO
Director of Information Technology .... Stuart Kime
VP of Sales .... Mike Bunkley
Senior VP, Pharmacy Operations .... Phil Walls, RPh
VP of Business Development .... Keith Marquez

Statistics:
Parent Company Name: Matrix Healthcare Services
Doing Business As: myMatrixx
Year Founded: 2001
Nonprofit: [ ]   Forprofit: [Y]
Federally Qualified? [N]

SERVICE AREA:
    NW;

NATIONAL MEDICAL HEALTH CARD SYSTEMS - CORPORATE HEADQUARTER

26 Harbor Park Dr
Port Washington, NY 11050
Phone: 516-626-0007 Fax: 516-621-4793 Toll-Free: 800-251-3883
Web site: www.nmhc.com
Mailing Address:
    NMHC- CORPORATE HEADQUARTERS
    26 Harbor Park Dr
    Port Washington, NY 11050

Key Executives:
Chief Financial Officer .... Stuart Diamond
Chief Marketing Officer .... Martin A Magill
Chief Specialty Pharmacy Officer .... Mark A Adkison

Statistics:
Parent Company Name:
Doing Business As: NMHCRx
Year Founded: 1981
Nonprofit: [ ]   Forprofit: [Y]
Federally Qualified? [Y]

SERVICE AREA:
    NW;

Pharmacy Benefit Management Companies

MANAGED PHARMACY CARE

28200 Hwy 189, Ste R-110
Lake Arrowhead, CA 92392
Phone: 909-336-9392 Fax: 909-336-9364 Toll-Free: 800-582-5889
Web site: www.mpcas.com
Mailing Address:
    MANAGED PHARMACY CARE
    PO Box 969
    Lake Arrowhead, CA 92392

Key Executives:
Chairman of the Board/President .... Charles Beeman, PharmD
Chief Operating Officer .... Gary Ellis

Statistics:
Parent Company Name:
Doing Business As:
Year Founded: 1991
Nonprofit: [ ]   Forprofit: [ ]
Federally Qualified? [ ]

SERVICE AREA:
    CA;

MANAGEMENT SCIENCES FOR HEALTH

4301 N Fairfax Dr Ste 400
Arlington, VA 22203
Phone: 703-524-6575 Fax: 703-524-7898 Toll-Free:
Web site: www.msh.org
Mailing Address:
    MANAGEMENT SCIENCES FOR HEALTH
    4301 N Fairfax Dr Ste 400
    Arlington, VA 22203

Key Executives:
Vice President .... Jim Rankin

Statistics:
Parent Company Name:
Doing Business As:
Year Founded:
Nonprofit: [ ]   Forprofit: [ ]
Federally Qualified? [ ]

SERVICE AREA:
    VA;

MAXOR PLUS

320 S Polk St Ste 100
Amarillo, TX 79101
Phone: 806-324-5400 Fax: 806-324-5495 Toll-Free: 800-658-6146
Web site: www.maxor.com
Mailing Address:
    MAXOR PLUS
    320 S Polk St Ste 100
    Amarillo, TX 79101

Key Executives:
Chairman .... Jerry Hodge, RPh
Chief Executive Officer .... John Ward
President .... Carl Birdsong, RPh
Chief Financial Officer .... Jerry Havard
VP Marketing & Sales .... John Fabrizio
VP, Operations .... Angelo Serio
Executive Vice President .... Steve Smith, RPh

Statistics:
Parent Company Name: Maxor National Pharmacy Services Corp
Doing Business As:
Year Founded: 1926
Nonprofit: [ ]   Forprofit: [ ]
Federally Qualified? [ ]

SERVICE AREA:
    TX;

Managed Care Organization Profiles

MCKESSON PHARMACY PROVIDER NETWORK

One Post St
San Francisco, CA 94104
Phone: 415-983-8300 Fax: 415-983-9400 Toll-Free:
Web site: www.mckesson.com
Mailing Address:
    MCKESSON PHARMACY PROVIDER NET
    One Post St
    San Francisco, CA 94104

Key Executives:
Chairman/Chief Executive Officer .... John Hammergren

Statistics:
Parent Company Name:
Doing Business As:
Year Founded: 1970
Nonprofit: [ ]   Forprofit: [ ]
Federally Qualified? [ ]

SERVICE AREA:
    NW;

MEDIMPACT HEALTHCARE SYSTEMS INC

10680 Treena St FL 5
San Diego, CA 92131
Phone: 858-566-2727 Fax: 858-621-5147 Toll-Free:
Web site: www.medimpact.com
Mailing Address:
    MEDIMPACT HLTHCARE SYSTEMS INC
    10680 Treena St FL 5
    San Diego, CA 92131

Key Executives:
Senior Vice President .... Jerry Parker
Senior VP, Chief Medical Officer .... Louis Brunetti Dr
Senior VP Business Development .... Dale Brown

Statistics:
Parent Company Name:
Doing Business As:
Year Founded:
Nonprofit: [ ]   Forprofit: [ ]
Federally Qualified? [ ]

SERVICE AREA:
    CA;

MEDSCRIPT

13185 Lakefront Dr
Earth City, MO 63045
Phone: 314-506-6066 Fax: 314-506-6067 Toll-Free: 800-274-8723
Web site: www.medscript.net
Mailing Address:
    MEDSCRIPT
    13185 Lakefront Dr
    Earth City, MO 63045

Key Executives:
Marketing Director .... Steve Sommer

Statistics:
Parent Company Name: Unity Health
Doing Business As:
Year Founded: 2003
Nonprofit: [ ]   Forprofit: [ ]
Federally Qualified? [ ]

SERVICE AREA:
    NW;

MEDCO HEALTH SOLUTIONS INC

100 Parsons Pond Dr
Franklin Lakes, NJ 07417
Phone: 201-269-3400 Fax: 201-269-1109 Toll-Free:
Web site: www.medco.com

Managed Care Organization Profiles | **Pharmacy Benefit Management Companies**

INNOVIANT INC

11 Scott St Ste 150
Wausau, WI 54403-4808
Phone: 952-922-0777 Fax: 952-920-6812 Toll-Free: 866-800-4321
Web site: www.innoviant.com

Mailing Address:
　　INNOVIANT INC
　　11 Scott St Ste 150
　　Wausau, WI 54403-4808

Key Executives:
Chief Executive Officer/President .... Mark Campbell, Pharm D
Chief Financial Officer .... Cullen Sloan, CPA
Chief Information Officer/Pharmacy Division .... Howard Drake
VP, Sales .... Rich Wipperfurth
VP, Operations .... Jamie Friedrich M S
VP, Clinical Services .... Mary Jenkins, Pharm D, MS
VP, Strategic Planning .... Rhonda Grabow
VP, Account Management .... Mike McGinnity

Statistics:
Parent Company Name: United Health Group
Doing Business As:
Year Founded:
Nonprofit: [　]   Forprofit: [　]
Federally Qualified? [　]

SERVICE AREA:
　　NW;

IOWA PHARMACISTS ASSOCIATION

8515 Douglas Ave Ste 16
Des Moines, IA 50322
Phone: 515-270-0713 Fax: 515-270-2979 Toll-Free:
Web site: www.iarx.org

Mailing Address:
　　IOWA PHARMACISTS ASSOCIATION
　　8515 Douglas Ave Ste 16
　　Des Moines, IA 50322

Key Executives:
Executive VP, Chief Executive Officer .... Thomas R Temple, RPh, MS
President .... Jay Currie

Statistics:
Parent Company Name:
Doing Business As:
Year Founded:
Nonprofit: [　]   Forprofit: [　]
Federally Qualified? [　]

SERVICE AREA:
　　IA;

KANSAS PHARMACY SERVICE CORPORATION

1020 SW Fairlawn Rd
Topeka, KS 66604-2019
Phone: 785-228-1695 Fax: 785-228-9147 Toll-Free: 800-279-3022
Web site: www.kspharmserv.com

Mailing Address:
　　KANSAS PHARMACY SERVICE CORP
　　1020 SW Fairlawn Td
　　Topeka, KS 66604-2019

Key Executives:
Executive Director .... Peter Stern

Statistics:
Parent Company Name:
Doing Business As:
Year Founded:
Nonprofit: [　]   Forprofit: [　]
Federally Qualified? [　]

SERVICE AREA:
　　KS;

KROGER PRESCRIPTION PLANS

1014 Vine St 3rd Fl
Cincinnati, OH 45202
Phone: 513-762-4000 Fax: 513-762-1547 Toll-Free: 800-221-4141
Web site: www.kroger.com

Mailing Address:
　　KROGER PRESCRIPTION PLANS
　　1014 Vine St 3rd Fl
　　Cincinnati, OH 45202

Key Executives:
VP of Pharmacy .... Lincoln Lutz

Statistics:
Parent Company Name:
Doing Business As: Kroger Inc
Year Founded: 1992
Nonprofit: [　]   Forprofit: [Y]
Federally Qualified? [　]

SERVICE AREA:
　　OH;

LDI PHARMACY BENEFIT MANAGEMENT

680 Craig Rd Ste 200
St Louis, MO 63103
Phone: 314-652-3121 Fax: 314-652-3126 Toll-Free: 800-652-9550
Web site: www.ldipbm.com

Mailing Address:
　　LDI PHARMACY BENEFIT MANAGEMEN
　　680 Craig Rd Ste 200
　　St Louis, MO 63103

Key Executives:
Executive Director .... Leonard S Dino, Jr, Pharm D
Chief Operating Officer .... Joseph M McHugh

Statistics:
Parent Company Name: Leehar Distributors Inc
Doing Business As: LDI Pharmacy
Year Founded:
Nonprofit: [　]   Forprofit: [　]
Federally Qualified? [　]

SERVICE AREA:
　　MO;

LEADERNET/LEADER DRUG STORES — CARDINAL HEALTH INC

7000 Cardinal Place
Dublin, OH 43017
Phone: 614-757-5000 Fax: 614-757-8702 Toll-Free:
Web site: www.cardinal-health.com

Mailing Address:
　　LEADERNET/LEADER DRUG STORES -
　　7000 Cardinal Place
　　Dublin, OH 43017

Key Executives:
Chairman of the Board/Chief Executive Officer .... Kerry Clark
Chief Financial Officer .... Jeff Henderson

Statistics:
Parent Company Name: Cardinal Health
Doing Business As:
Year Founded: 1971
Nonprofit: [　]   Forprofit: [　]
Federally Qualified? [　]

SERVICE AREA:
　　NW;

Pharmacy Benefit Management Companies

Statistics:
Parent Company Name:
Doing Business As: CatalystRx
Year Founded:
Nonprofit: [ ]   Forprofit: [ ]
Federally Qualified? [ ]

SERVICE AREA:
GA; NV; NM; OK; TX; NC; SC;

HEALTHPARTNERS

8170 34th Ave South
Bloomington, MN 55440
Phone: 952-883-5200   Fax: 952-883-5260 Toll-Free: 888-883-2177
Web site: www.healthpartners.com
Mailing Address:
HEALTHPARTNERS
PO Box 1309
Minneapolis, MN 55440

Key Executives:
Chief Executive Officer/President .... Mary Brainerd
Senior VP, Chief Financial Officer .... Kathy Cooney
Med Director, Chief Health Officer .... George Isham
Executive VP, Chief Marketing Officer .... Andrea Walsh
Senior VP, General Counsel .... Barb Tretheway
Medical Director Health Partners Medical Group .... Brian Rank MD

Statistics:
Parent Company Name:
Doing Business As:
Year Founded: 1957
Nonprofit: [Y]   Forprofit: [ ]
Federally Qualified? [Y]

SERVICE AREA:
MN (Anoka, Becker, Beltrami, Benton, Big Stone, Blue Earth, Brown, Carver, Cass, Chippewa, Chisago, Clay, Clearwater, Cottonwood, Crow Wing, Dakota, Dodge, Douglas, Faribault, Fillmore, Freeborn, Goodhue, Hennepin, Hubbard, Isanti, Jackson, Kandiyohi, Lac Qui Parle, Le Sueur, Lincoln, Lyon, Mahnomen, Martin, McLeod, Meeker, Mille Lacs, Morrison, Mower, Murray, Nicollet, Nobles, Norman, Olmsted, Otter Tail, Pipestone, Pope, Ramsey, Redwood, Renville, Rice, Scott, Sherburne, Sibley, Stearns, Steele, Stevens, Swift, Todd, Traverse, Wabasha, Waseca, Washington, Watonwan, Wilkin, Winona, Wright, Yellow Medicine); ND (Barnes, Cass, Grand Forks, LaMoure, Logan, McHenry, Nelson, Pembia, Ransom, Richland, Sargent, Steele, Stutsman, Traill, Walsh); WI (Ashland, Bayfield,Buffalo, Burnett, Douglas, Dunn, Iron, Pepin, Pierce, Polk, Saint Croix, Sawyer, Wasburn); IA (Lyon, Plymouth, Sioux); SD (Clay, Lincoln. Minnehaha, Moody, Turner, Union, Yankton);

HEALTHTRANS LLC

8300 E Maplewood Ave Ste 100
Greenwood Village, CO 80111
Phone: 800-950-9120   Fax: 303-221-7775 Toll-Free: 800-950-9120
Web site: www.healthtrans.com
Mailing Address:
HEALTHTRANS LLC
8300 E Maplewood Ave Ste 100
Greenwood Village, CO 80111

Key Executives:
Chief Executive Officer ....Jack McClurg
President .... Louis Hutchison Jr
Chief Financial Officer ....Christopher B Hanks
Senior VP, Sales .... Charles Donovan
Chief Operating Officer .... Steve Groover
VP, Business Services .... Kevin Donahue
Senior VP, Business Relations .... Linda Groover

Statistics:
Parent Company Name:
Doing Business As:
Year Founded: 2000
Nonprofit: [ ]   Forprofit: [ ]
Federally Qualified? [ ]

SERVICE AREA:
NW;

Managed Care Organization Profiles

HEALTHESYSTEMS

5109 W Lemon St Ste A
Tampa, FL 33609
Phone: 813-769-1880   Fax: 813-769-1881 Toll-Free: 800-921-1880
Web site: www.healthesystems.com
Mailing Address:
HEALTHESYSTEMS
5109 W Lemon St Ste A
Tampa, FL 33609

Key Executives:
Chief Executive Officer/President .... Daryl Corr
Pharmacy Director .... Ralph Kendall, PharmD

Statistics:
Parent Company Name:
Doing Business As:
Year Founded:
Nonprofit: [ ]   Forprofit: [ ]
Federally Qualified? [ ]

SERVICE AREA:
NW;

HUMANA INC

500 W Main St
Louisville, KY 40202
Phone: 502-580-1543   Fax: 502-508-4303 Toll-Free:
Web site: www.humana.com
Mailing Address:
HUMANA INC
500 W Main St
Louisville, KY 40202

Key Executives:
Chairman .... David A Jones Jr
Chief Executive Officer/President .... Michael B McCallister
Senior VP, Chief Finanacial Officer .... James H Bloem
Senior VP, Chief Service & Information Officer .... Bruce Goodman
Senior VP, Chief Marketing Officer .... Steve Moya
Chief Operating Officer .... Jim Murray
Senior VP, Chief Human Resource Officer .... Bonnie Hathcock

Statistics:
Parent Company Name:
Doing Business As:
Year Founded:
Nonprofit: [ ]   Forprofit: [ ]
Federally Qualified? [ ]

SERVICE AREA:
NW;

IMMEDIATE PHARMACEUTICAL SERVICES INC

33381 Walker Rd
Avon Lake, OH 44012
Phone: 800-233-3872   Fax: 440-930-5540 Toll-Free: 800-233-3872
Web site: www.ipsrx.com
Mailing Address:
IMMEDIATE PHARMACEUTICAL SRV
PO Box 166
Avon Lake, OH 44012

Key Executives:
President .... Thomas E Garvey
Regional VP of Sales .... Eric Singer
Director of Pharmacy .... William Davis, RPh
Regional VP of Sales .... Joseph McCormack

Statistics:
Parent Company Name: Discount Drug Mart Inc
Doing Business As:
Year Founded:
Nonprofit: [ ]   Forprofit: [ ]
Federally Qualified? [ ]

SERVICE AREA:
OH;

Key Executives:
Chairman/Chief Executive Officer .... George Paz
President .... George Paz
Executive VP, Chief Financial Officer .... Jeffrey Hall

Statistics:
Parent Company Name: Express Scripts Inc
Doing Business As:
Year Founded:
Nonprofit: [ ]   Forprofit: [ ]
Federally Qualified? [ ]

SERVICE AREA:
PA;

FIRST HEALTH RX

3200 Highland Ave
Downers Grove, IL 60515
Phone: 630-737-7900   Fax: 630-719-0076 Toll-Free: 800-455-1425
Web site: www.firsthealth.com
Mailing Address:
   FIRST HEALTH RX
   3200 Highland Ave
   Downers Grove, IL 60515

Key Executives:
Chief Executive Officer - Coventry .... Dale B Wolf

Statistics:
Parent Company Name: Coventry Healthcare Inc
Doing Business As:
Year Founded: 1982
Nonprofit: [ ]   Forprofit: [Y]
Federally Qualified? [ ]

SERVICE AREA:
NW;

FIRST HEALTH SERVICES CORP

4300 Cox Rd
Glen Allen, VA 23060
Phone: 804-965-7400   Fax: 804-527-6849 Toll-Free: 800-884-2822
Web site: www.fhsc.com
Mailing Address:
   FIRST HEALTH SERVICES CORP
   4300 Cox Rd
   Glen Allen, VA 23060

Key Executives:
Chief Operating Officer .... Peter Quinn

Statistics:
Parent Company Name: Coventry Health Care
Doing Business As: First Health Grp - Downers Grove Il
Year Founded: 1982
Nonprofit: [ ]   Forprofit: [Y]
Federally Qualified? [ ]

SERVICE AREA:
NW;

FIRST SCRIPT NETWORK SERVICES

155 N Rosemont Blvd Ste 201
Tucson, AZ 85711
Phone: 520-202-1290   Fax: 520-514-9348 Toll-Free: 800-766-2041
Web site: www.firstscript.com
Mailing Address:
   FIRST SCRIPT NETWORK SERVICES
   155 N Rosemont Blvd Ste 201
   Tucson, AR 85711

Key Executives:
Chief Executive Officer/President .... Charles Bavier

Statistics:
Parent Company Name: Coventry Health Care Workers Comp Inc
Doing Business As:
Year Founded:
Nonprofit: [ ]   Forprofit: [ ]
Federally Qualified? [ ]

SERVICE AREA:
NW;

GARDEN STATE PHARMACY OWNERS PROVIDER SERVICES

44 West Taylor Ave
Hamilton, NJ 08610
Phone: 800-778-8089   Fax: 609-439-0865 Toll-Free: 800-778-8089
Web site: www.gspops.com
Mailing Address:
   GARDEN STATE PHARMACY OWNERS P
   44 West Taylor Ave
   Hamilton, NJ 08610

Key Executives:
Executive Vice President .... Desmond Fitzgerald

Statistics:
Parent Company Name: GSPO
Doing Business As: GSPOPS
Year Founded: 1986
Nonprofit: [ ]   Forprofit: [Y]
Federally Qualified? [ ]

SERVICE AREA:
NJ;

HEALTH DELIVERY MANAGEMENT LLC

1725 West Harrison Ste 418
Chicago, IL 60612
Phone: 312-563-2244   Fax: 312-563-2247 Toll-Free:
Web site: www.rush.edu/patients/pharmacy
Mailing Address:
   HEALTH DELIVERY MANAGEMENT LLC
   1725 West Harrison Ste 418
   Chicago, IL 60612

Key Executives:
Pharmacy Manager .... Marilou Daza

Statistics:
Parent Company Name: Rush University
Doing Business As:
Year Founded:
Nonprofit: [ ]   Forprofit: [ ]
Federally Qualified? [ ]

SERVICE AREA:
IL;

HEALTHEXTRAS INC

800 King Farm Blvd
Rockville, MD 20850
Phone: 800-323-6640   Fax: 301-548-2991 Toll-Free: 800-323-6640
Web site: www.healthextras.com
Mailing Address:
   HEALTHEXTRAS INC
   800 King Farm Blvd
   Rockville, MD 20850

Key Executives:
Chairman of the Board .... Edward S Civera
Chief Executive Officer .... David T Blair
Executive VP, Chief Financial Officer .... MIchael P Donovan
Executive VP, Chief Operating Officer .... Nick J Grujich
General Counsel/Corp Secretary .... Thomas M Farah

Pharmacy Benefit Management Companies / Managed Care Organization Profiles

Mailing Address:
    EMPLOYEE HEALTH INSURANCE MNGT
    26711 Northwestern Hwy Ste 400
    Southfield, MI 48033

Key Executives:
Director of Marketing .... Marcy Hilton

Statistics:
Parent Company Name:
Doing Business As:
Year Founded:
Nonprofit: [ ]   Forprofit: [ ]
Federally Qualified? [ ]

SERVICE AREA:
   NW;

ENVISION PHARMACEUTICAL SERVICES INC

2181 E Aurora Rd Ste 201
Twinsburg, OH 44087
Phone: 330-405-8080 Fax: 330-405-8081 Toll-Free: 800-361-4542
Web site: www.envisionrx.com
Mailing Address:
    ENVISION PHARMACEUTICAL SRVS I
    2181 E Aurora Rd Ste 201
    Twinsburg, OH 44087

Key Executives:
Chief Executive Officer/President .... Kevin M Nagle
Chief Operating Officer .... Barry I Katz RPh
Pharmacy Director .... Amanda Peterson RPh

Statistics:
Parent Company Name:
Doing Business As: Envision Rx Options
Year Founded: 2000
Nonprofit: [ ]   Forprofit: [ ]
Federally Qualified? [ ]

SERVICE AREA:
   NW;

EPIC PHARMACY NETWORK INC

6501 Mechanicsville Trnpk #103
Mechanicsville, VA 23111-3698
Phone: 804-559-4597 Fax: 804-559-2038 Toll-Free: 800-876-3742
Web site: www.epicrx.com
Mailing Address:
    EPIC PHARMACY NETWORK INC
    6501 Mechanicsville Trnpk #103
    Mechanicsville, VA 23111-3698

Key Executives:
Executive Vice President .... Patrick M Berryman
President/Chief Executive Officer .... Angelo C Voxakis, PD

Statistics:
Parent Company Name: Maryland Professional Pharmacies, Inc.
Doing Business As: Epic Pharmacies Inc
Year Founded: 1992
Nonprofit: [ ]   Forprofit: [ ]
Federally Qualified? [ ]

SERVICE AREA:
   VA;

EXPRESS SCRIPTS INC - CORPORATE HEADQUARTERS

1 Express Way
St Louis, MO 63121
Phone: 314-996-0900 Fax: Toll-Free: 800-332-5455
Web site: www.express-scripts.com
Mailing Address:
    EXPRESS SCRIPTS INC - CORP
    1 Express Way
    St Louis, MO 63121

Key Executives:
Chairman/Chief Executive Officer .... George Paz
President .... George Paz
Executive VP, Chief Financial Officer .... Jeffrey Hall

Statistics:
Parent Company Name:
Doing Business As:
Year Founded:
Nonprofit: [ ]   Forprofit: [ ]
Federally Qualified? [ ]

SERVICE AREA:
   NW;

EXPRESS SCRIPTS INC - MINNESOTA

6625 W 78th St
Bloomington, MN 55439
Phone: 952-820-7000 Fax: 612-896-6944 Toll-Free: 800-233-8065
Web site: www.express-scripts.com
Mailing Address:
    EXPRESS SCRIPTS INC - MN
    6625 W 78th St
    Bloomington, MN 55439

Key Executives:
Chairman/Chief Executive Officer .... George Paz
President .... George Paz
Executive VP, Chief Financial Officer .... Jeffrey Hall

Statistics:
Parent Company Name:
Doing Business As:
Year Founded: 1992
Nonprofit: [ ]   Forprofit: [ ]
Federally Qualified? [ ]

SERVICE AREA:
   MN;

EXPRESS SCRIPTS INC - NEW JERSEY

711 Ridgedale Ave
East Hanover, NJ 07936
Phone: 800-451-6245 Fax: 973-503-1096 Toll-Free: 800-451-6245
Web site: www.express-scripts.com
Mailing Address:
    EXPRESS SCRIPTS INC - NJ
    711 Ridgedale Ave
    East Hanover, NJ 07936

Key Executives:
Chairman/Chief Executive Officer .... George Paz
President .... George Paz
Executive VP, Chief Financial Officer .... Jeffrey Hall

Statistics:
Parent Company Name: Express Scripts Inc
Doing Business As:
Year Founded:
Nonprofit: [ ]   Forprofit: [ ]
Federally Qualified? [ ]

SERVICE AREA:
   NJ;

EXPRESS SCRIPTS INC - PENNSYLVANIA

206 Welsh Rd
Horsham, PA 19044
Phone: 215-658-4000 Fax: 215-658-4030 Toll-Free: 800-233-8065
Web site: www.express-scripts.com
Mailing Address:
    EXPRESS SCRIPTS INC - PA
    206 Welsh Rd
    Horsham, PA 19044

Mailing Address:
CATALYST RX A HEALTHEXTRAS CO
800 King Farm Blvd Ste 400
Rockville, MD 20850

Key Executives:
Chief Executive Officer .... David T Blair
Executive VP, Chief Operating Officer .... Nick J Grujich

Statistics:
Parent Company Name: Health Extras Inc
Doing Business As:
Year Founded: 1994
Nonprofit: [ ]   Forprofit: [N]
Federally Qualified? [N]

SERVICE AREA:
NC;

CBCA

675 Foxon Rd Ste 204
East Haven, CT 06513
Phone: 877-903-6888 Fax: 203-468-8930 Toll-Free: 877-903-6888
Web site: www.cbcainc.com

Mailing Address:
CBCA
675 Foxon Rd Ste 204
East Haven, CT 06513

Key Executives:
Chief Executive Officer/Chief Operating Officer .... Kenneth Di Bella

Statistics:
Parent Company Name:
Doing Business As:
Year Founded:
Nonprofit: [ ]   Forprofit: [Y]
Federally Qualified? [ ]

SERVICE AREA:
NW;

CIGNA PHARMACY MANAGEMENT

900 Cottage Grove Rd S-128
Hartford, CT 06152-1118
Phone: 860-226-6000 Fax: 860-226-3535 Toll-Free: 800-345-9458
Web site: www.cigna.com

Mailing Address:
CIGNA PHARMACY MANAGEMENT
900 Cottage Grove Rd S-128
Hartford, CT 06152-1118

Key Executives:
President .... Eric A Elliott

Statistics:
Parent Company Name: CIGNA Corporation
Doing Business As:
Year Founded: 1985
Nonprofit: [ ]   Forprofit: [Y]
Federally Qualified? [Y]

SERVICE AREA:
NW;

COMMUNITYCARE MANAGED HEALTHCARE PLANS OF OKLAHOMA INC

218 W 6th St
Tulsa, OK 74119
Phone: 918-594-5200 Fax: 918-594-5367 Toll-Free: 800-278-7563
Web site: www.ccok.com

Mailing Address:
COMMUNITYCARE INC
218 W 6th St
Tulsa, OK 74119

Key Executives:
Chief Executive Officer/President .... Richard W Todd
Chief Financial Officer .... Earle Rice
Medical Director .... Jack Sommers, MD
Chief Information Officer .... Lorenzo Marquez
Executive Vice President .... Nancy Horstmann
Pharmacy Director .... Melanie Maxwell
MIS Director .... Lorenzo Marquez

Statistics:
Parent Company Name: St Francis Hlth Systems, St Johns Hlth Systems
Doing Business As:
Year Founded: 1994
Nonprofit: [ ]   Forprofit: [Y]
Federally Qualified? [Y]

SERVICE AREA:
OK (Ardmore, Bartlesville, Broken Arrow, Muckogee, Oklahoma City, Stillwater, Tulsa, Vinita);

CVS/CAREMARK - CORPORATE HEADQUARTERS

695 George Washington Hwy
Lincoln, RI 02865
Phone: 401-334-0069 Fax: 401-334-4995 Toll-Free: 800-237-6184
Web site: www.pharmacare.com

Mailing Address:
CVS/CAREMARK - CORP HDQRTRS
695 George Washington Hwy
Lincoln, RI 02865

Key Executives:
Chairman/Chief Executive Officer .... Thomas M Ryan
President .... Thomas M Ryan

Statistics:
Parent Company Name:
Doing Business As:
Year Founded: 1994
Nonprofit: [ ]   Forprofit: [Y]
Federally Qualified? [ ]

SERVICE AREA:
NW;

CYPRESS CARE

2736 Meadow Church RD Ste 300
Duluth, GA 30097
Phone: 678-730-1002 Fax: 678-730-1008 Toll-Free: 800-419-7191
Web site: www.cypresscare.com

Mailing Address:
CYPRESS CARE
PO Box 2829
Suwanee, GA 30097

Key Executives:
Chief Executive Officer .... David A George
President .... Tim Vroman
Chief Finanicial Officer .... George Dunaway
Chief Marketing Officer .... Robert Kulbick

Statistics:
Parent Company Name:
Doing Business As:
Year Founded:
Nonprofit: [ ]   Forprofit: [ ]
Federally Qualified? [ ]

SERVICE AREA:
GA;

EMPLOYEE HEALTH INSURANCE MANAGEMENT INC

26711 Northwestern Hwy Ste 400
Southfield, MI 48033
Phone: 248-948-9900 Fax: 248-948-9904 Toll-Free: 800-311-3446
Web site: www.ehimrx.com

Year Founded: 1937
Nonprofit: [Y]   Forprofit: [ ]
Federally Qualified? [ ]

SERVICE AREA:
   DC; MD; VA; DE;

CAREMARK/CVS - ARIZONA

9501 E Shea Blvd
Scottsdale, AZ 85260-6719
Phone: 480-391-4600   Fax: 480-451-7430 Toll-Free:
Web site: www.caremark.com
Mailing Address:
   CAREMARK/CVS - ARIZONA
   9501 E Shea Blvd
   Scottsdale, AZ 85260-6719

Key Executives:
Chairman/Chief Executive Officer .... Thomas M Ryan
President .... Thomas M Ryan

Statistics:
Parent Company Name: CVS/Caremark
Doing Business As:
Year Founded:
Nonprofit: [ ]   Forprofit: [ ]
Federally Qualified? [ ]

SERVICE AREA:
   AZ;

CAREMARK/CVS

2211 Sanders Rd
Northbrook, IL 60062
Phone: 847-559-4700   Fax: 847-559-3694 Toll-Free:
Web site: www.caremark.com
Mailing Address:
   CAREMARK/CVS
   2211 Sanders Rd
   Northbrook, IL 60062

Key Executives:
Chairman/Chief Executive Officer .... Thomas M Ryan
President .... Thomas M Ryan

Statistics:
Parent Company Name: CVS/Caremark Rx Inc
Doing Business As: Pharmacy Benefit Manager
Year Founded: 1977
Nonprofit: [ ]   Forprofit: [Y]
Federally Qualified? [ ]

SERVICE AREA:
   NW;

CAREMARK/CVS - TENNESSEE

211 Commerce St Ste 800
Nashville, TN 37201
Phone: 615-743-6600   Fax: 205-743-9780 Toll-Free: 800-633-9509
Web site: www.caremark.com
Mailing Address:
   CAREMARK/CVS - TENNESSEE
   211 Commerce St Ste 800
   Nashville, TN 37201

Key Executives:
Chairman/Chief Executive Officer .... Thomas M Ryan
President .... Thomas M Ryan

Statistics:
Parent Company Name: CVS/Caremark
Doing Business As:
Year Founded: 1993
Nonprofit: [ ]   Forprofit: [Y]
Federally Qualified? [ ]

SERVICE AREA:
   NW;

CAREMARK/CVS - TEXAS

750 E John Carpenter Frwy 1200
Irving, TX 75062
Phone: 469-524-4700   Fax: 469-524-4702 Toll-Free: 800-749-6199
Web site: www.caremark.com
Mailing Address:
   CAREMARK/CVS - TEXAS
   750 E John Carpenter Frwy 1200
   Irving, TX 75062

Key Executives:
Chairman/Chief Executive Officer .... Thomas M Ryan
President .... Thomas M Ryan

Statistics:
Parent Company Name: CVS/Caremark
Doing Business As:
Year Founded: 1986
Nonprofit: [ ]   Forprofit: [ ]
Federally Qualified? [ ]

SERVICE AREA:
   TX;

CAROLINA PHARMACY NETWORK

1350 Browning Rd
Columbia, SC 29201
Phone: 803-354-9977   Fax: 803-354-9207 Toll-Free: 800-532-4033
Web site: www.scrx.org
Mailing Address:
   CAROLINA PHARMACY NETWORK
   1350 Browning Rd
   Columbia, SC 29201

Key Executives:
Executive Vice President .... Carmelo Clinqueonce, MBA

Statistics:
Parent Company Name: South Carolina Pharmacy Association
Doing Business As:
Year Founded: 1876
Nonprofit: [ ]   Forprofit: [ ]
Federally Qualified? [ ]

SERVICE AREA:
   SC;

CATALYST RX, A HEALTHEXTRAS COMPANY

9225 Hillwood Dr Ste 100
Las Vegas, NV 89134
Phone: 702-869-4600   Fax: 240-268-3112 Toll-Free: 800-331-7108
Web site: www.catalystrx.com
Mailing Address:
   CATALYST RX A HEALTHEXTRAS CO
   9525 Hillwood Dr Ste 100
   Las Vegas, NV 89134

Key Executives:
Chief Executive Officer .... David T Blair

Statistics:
Parent Company Name: HealthExtras Inc
Doing Business As:
Year Founded:
Nonprofit: [ ]   Forprofit: [ ]
Federally Qualified? [ ]

SERVICE AREA:
   NV;

CATALYST RX, A HEALTHEXTRAS COMPANY

800 King Farm Blvd Ste400
Rockville, MD 20850
Phone: 919-876-4642   Fax: 919-876-1593 Toll-Free: 800-331-7108
Web site: www.catalystrx.com

Managed Care Organization Profiles — Pharmacy Benefit Management Companies

BAYER CORPORATION PHARMACEUTICAL DIVISION

400 Morgan Lane
West Haven, CT 06516
Phone: 800-468-0894   Fax: 203-812-5300   Toll-Free: 888-842-2937
Web site: www.bayerpharma-na.com

Mailing Address:
BAYER CORPORATION PHARMACEUTIC
400 Morgan Lane
West Haven, CT 06516

Key Executives:
Chief Executive Officer .... Helge Wehier
President/General Manager .... Gunner Riemann, MD

Statistics:
Parent Company Name: Bayer Corp
Doing Business As:
Year Founded:
Nonprofit: [ ]   Forprofit: [ ]
Federally Qualified? [ ]

SERVICE AREA:
NW;

BENESCRIPT SERVICES INC

3720 DaVinci Ct Ste 200
Norcross, GA 30092-3238
Phone: 770-448-4344   Fax: 770-810-2406   Toll-Free: 888-345-3189
Web site: www.benescript.com

Mailing Address:
BENESCRIPT SERVICES INC
PO Box 921229
Norcross, GA 30092-3238

Key Executives:
Chairman/Chief Executive Officer .... Paul Berube
President .... Larry Ethridge
Chief Financial Officer .... Mark Wells
VP, Marketing & Sales .... Viviana Brantley

Statistics:
Parent Company Name: BeneScript Services Inc
Doing Business As:
Year Founded: 1989
Nonprofit: [ ]   Forprofit: [ ]
Federally Qualified? [ ]

SERVICE AREA:
NW;

BIOSCRIP INC

100 Clearbrook Rd
Elmsford, NY 10523
Phone: 914-460-1600   Fax: 877-347-1448   Toll-Free: 800-899-4323
Web site: www.bioscrip.com

Mailing Address:
BIOSCRIP INC
100 Clearbrook Rd
Elmsford, NY 10523

Key Executives:
Chairman of the Board/Chief Executive Officer .. Richard H Friedman
Executive VP General Counsel .... Barry A Posner
Executive VP, Chief Financial Officer .... Stanley Rosenbaum
VP, Chief Information Officer .... Douglas A Lee
Executive VP, Marketing & Sales .... Scott W Friedman

Statistics:
Parent Company Name:
Doing Business As:
Year Founded:
Nonprofit: [ ]   Forprofit: [ ]
Federally Qualified? [ ]

SERVICE AREA:
NW;

BLUE CROSS & BLUE SHIELD OF NORTH CAROLINA

5901 Chapel Hill Rd
Durham, NC 27707
Phone: 919-489-7431   Fax: 919-765-3943   Toll-Free: 800-250-3630
Web site: www.bcbsnc.com

Mailing Address:
BLUE CROSS & BLUE SHIELD OF NC
P O Box 2291
Durham, NC 27707

Key Executives:
Chief Executive Officer/President .... Robert J Greczyn, Jr
Chief Financial Officer .... Daniel E Glaser
Senior VP, Chief Medical Officer .... Don Bradley, MD
Chief Sales & Marketing .... John T Roos
Chief Operating Officer - NC .... J Bradley Wilson
VP, Employee Health & Pharmacy .... Ron Smith, MD

Statistics:
Parent Company Name: BC/BS of North Carolina
Doing Business As:
Year Founded: 1985
Nonprofit: [Y]   Forprofit: [ ]
Federally Qualified? [Y]

SERVICE AREA:
NC;

BLUE CROSS AND BLUE SHIELD OF IL PHARMACY PROGRAMS

300 E Randolph St
Chicago, IL 60601
Phone: 312-653-6000   Fax: 312-946-1430   Toll-Free:
Web site: www.bcbsil.com

Mailing Address:
BC/BS OF IL PHARMACY PROGRAMS
300 E Randolph St
Chicago, IL 60601

Key Executives:
Chief Executive Officer -HCSC .... Raymond F McCaskey
President- BCBSIL .... Paul S Boulis

Statistics:
Parent Company Name: Health Care Service Corp
Doing Business As:
Year Founded:
Nonprofit: [ ]   Forprofit: [ ]
Federally Qualified? [ ]

SERVICE AREA:
IL;

CAREFIRST BLUE CROSS BLUE SHIELD

10455 Mill Run Circle
Owings Mills, MD 21117
Phone: 410-581-3000   Fax: 410-998-5732   Toll-Free:
Web site: www.carefirst.com

Mailing Address:
CAREFIRST BLUE CROSS BLUE SHIELD
10455 Mill Run Circle
Owings Mills, MD 21117

Key Executives:
Chairman .... Michael R Merson
Chief Executive Officer/President .... Chester Burrell
Executive VP, Chief Financial Officer .... G Mark Chaney
Senior VP, Chief Medical Officer .... Jon Shematek, MD
Senior VP, Chief Information Officer .... Ted Della Vecchia
Executive VP, Chief Marketing Officer .... Gregory A Devou

Statistics:
Parent Company Name: Care First Inc
Doing Business As:

Pharmacy Benefit Management Companies

AMERICAN HEALTH CARE

2217 Plaza Dr Ste 100
Rocklin, CA 95765
Phone: 916-773-7227 Fax: 916-773-7210 Toll-Free: 800-872-8276
Web site: www.americanhealthcare.com
Mailing Address:
　　AMERICAN HEALTH CARE
　　2217 Plaza Dr Ste 100
　　Rocklin, CA 95765

Key Executives:
President .... Grover C Lee, PharmD, BCMCM
Senior VP, Sales & Marketing .... David A Valerio, Esq
Executive VP, Pharmacy Director .... Christine V Lee, PharmD, CLS

Statistics:
Parent Company Name:
Doing Business As:
Year Founded: 1982
Nonprofit: [ ]　　Forprofit: [Y]
Federally Qualified? [N]

SERVICE AREA:
　　NW; PR;

AMERICAN PHARMACY SERVICES CORP

102 Enterprise Dr
Frankfort, KY 40601
Phone: 502-695-8899 Fax: 502-695-9912 Toll-Free:
Web site: www.apscnet.com
Mailing Address:
　　AMERICAN PHARMACY SERVICES COR
　　1228 US 127 S
　　Frankfort, KY 40601

Key Executives:
Chief Executive Officer/President ..... Ralph E Bouvette, RPh, PhD, JD
VP, Marketing/Group Purchasing .... Cathi Clark

Statistics:
Parent Company Name:
Doing Business As:
Year Founded: 1985
Nonprofit: [ ]　　Forprofit: [Y]
Federally Qualified? [N]

SERVICE AREA:
　　IL;IN;KY;MO;OH;TN;VA;WV;

AMERISOURCE BERGEN
PERFORMANCE PLUS NETWORK - CORPORATE

1300 Morris Dr Ste 100
Chesterbrook, PA 19482
Phone: 610-727-7000 Fax: 610-727-3600 Toll-Free: 800-829-3132
Web site: www.amerisourcebergen.com
Mailing Address:
　　AMERISOURCE BERGEN PERFORMANCE
　　1300 Morris Dr Ste 100
　　Chesterbrook, PA 19482

Key Executives:
Chairman .... Richard C Gozon
Chief Executive Officer/President .... R David Yost
Chief Operating Officer .... Kurt J Hilzinger

Statistics:
Parent Company Name:
Doing Business As:
Year Founded:
Nonprofit: [ ]　　Forprofit: [ ]
Federally Qualified? [ ]

SERVICE AREA:
　　NW;

Managed Care Organization Profiles

AMERISOURCE BERGEN
PERFORMANCE PLUS NETWORK - WEST

4000 Metropolitan Dr
Orange, CA 92868
Phone: 800-442-3040 Fax: 714-385-6920 Toll-Free: 800-442-3040
Web site: www.amerisourcebergen.com
Mailing Address:
　　AMERISOURCE BERGEN PERFRM WEST
　　4000 Metropolitan Dr
　　Orange, CA 92868

Key Executives:
Chief Executive Officer/President .... R David Yost
Senior VP, Chief Financial Officer .... Michael D DiCandilo
VP, Chief Information Officer .... Terrance P Haas
Chief Operating Officer .... Kurt J Hilzinger

Statistics:
Parent Company Name:
Doing Business As:
Year Founded:
Nonprofit: [ ]　　Forprofit: [ ]
Federally Qualified? [ ]

SERVICE AREA:
　　NW;

ARGUS HEALTH SYSTEM INC

1300 Washington Street
Kansas City, MO 64105-1433
Phone: 816-435-5400 Fax: 816-435-5499 Toll-Free: 800-792-7487
Web site: www.argushealth.com
Mailing Address:
　　ARGUS HEALTH SYSTEM INC
　　1300 Washington Street
　　Kansas City, MO 64105-1433

Key Executives:
Chief Executive Officer .... Charles W Schellhorn
President .... Jonathan Boehm
Senior VP, Sales & Marketing .... Michael Huffer
Senior VP, Operations .... Wayne Armstrong
Senior VP, Managed Care .... John Tobin

Statistics:
Parent Company Name: DST Systems INC & Financial Holding Corp
Doing Business As: Argus Health System
Year Founded:
Nonprofit: [ ]　　Forprofit: [Y]
Federally Qualified? [ ]

SERVICE AREA:
　　MO;

ARXCEL INC

6400 Sheridan Dr Ste 206
Williamsville, NY 14221
Phone: 716-204-3393 Fax: 716-204-3394 Toll-Free:
Web site: www.arxcel.com
Mailing Address:
　　ARXCEL INC
　　6400 Sheridan Dr Ste 206
　　Williamsville, NY 14221

Key Executives:
Chief Executive Officer .... Chris Robbins

Statistics:
Parent Company Name:
Doing Business As:
Year Founded:
Nonprofit: [ ]　　Forprofit: [ ]
Federally Qualified? [ ]

SERVICE AREA:
　　NY;

Managed Care Organization Profiles — Pharmacy Benefit Management Companies

4D PHARMACY MANAGEMENT SYSTEMS INC

2520 Industrial Row Dr
Troy, MI 48084
Phone: 249-540-8066 Fax: 248-540-0112 Toll-Free: 800-241-5103
Web site: www.4dpharmacy.com
Mailing Address:
  4D PHARMACY MANAGEMENT SYS INC
  2520 Industrial Row Dr
  Troy, MI 48084

Key Executives:
Chief Executive Officer/President .... Gerald C Borsand, RPh
Director, Information Systems & Technology .... Steve Goode
VP, Managed Care .... Sue Ann Syoen, RPh
VP, Account Management/Business Development .... Jeff Polter
Compliance Officer .... Jonathan D Borsand

Statistics:
Parent Company Name:
Doing Business As:
Year Founded:
Nonprofit: [ ]   Forprofit: [ ]
Federally Qualified? [ ]

SERVICE AREA:
  NW;

ACS GOVERNMENT HEALTHCARE SOLUTIONS

9040 Roswell Rd Ste 700
Atlanta, GA 30350
Phone: 770-594-7799 Fax: 770-552-6919 Toll-Free: 800-358-2381
Web site: www.acsstatehealthcare.com
Mailing Address:
  ACS GOVERNMENT HEALTHCARE SOLS
  9040 Roswell Rd Ste 700
  Atlanta, GA 30350

Key Executives:
Senior VP, Managing Director - DC .... Christopher Deelsnyder

Statistics:
Parent Company Name:
Doing Business As:
Year Founded: 1970
Nonprofit: [ ]   Forprofit: [Y]
Federally Qualified? [ ]

SERVICE AREA:
  GA;

AETNA PHARMACY MANAGEMENT - CORPORATE HEADQUARTERS

151 Farmington Ave MS MA61
Hartford, CT 06156-7317
Phone: 860-273-0123 Fax: 866-329-2779 Toll-Free: 800-872-3862
Web site: www.aetnapharmacy.com
Mailing Address:
  AETNA PHARMACY MANAGEMENT-CORP
  151 Farmington Ave MS MA61
  Hartford, CT 06156-7317

Key Executives:
Head of Pharmacy .... Steven C Meholic

Statistics:
Parent Company Name:
Doing Business As:
Year Founded:
Nonprofit: [ ]   Forprofit: [ ]
Federally Qualified? [ ]

SERVICE AREA:
  NW;

AETNA SPECIALTY PHARMACY

11675 Great Oaks Way
Alpharetta, GA 30022
Phone: 770-346-4300 Fax: 678-256-2045 Toll-Free: 866-782-2779
Web site: www.aetnapharmacy.com
Mailing Address:
  AETNA SPECIALTY PHARMACY
  11675 Great Oaks Way
  Alpharetta, GA 30022

Key Executives:
Clinical Pharmacy Manager .... Michael Brodeur

Statistics:
Parent Company Name: Aetna Inc & Priority Healthcare Corp
Doing Business As:
Year Founded: 2004
Nonprofit: [ ]   Forprofit: [ ]
Federally Qualified? [ ]

SERVICE AREA:
  NW;

ALLSCRIPTS PHARMACEUTICALS INC

222 Merchandise Mart Plz #2024
Chicago, IL 60654
Phone: 312-506-1200 Fax: 800-524-7572 Toll-Free: 800-548-5160
Web site: www.allscripts.com
Mailing Address:
  ALLSCRIPTS PHARMACEUTICALS INC
  222 Merchandise Mart Plz #2024
  Chicago, IL 60654

Key Executives:
Chairman of the Board/Chief Executive Officer .... Glen E Tullman
President .... Lee Shapiro
Chief Financial Officer .... William J Davis
Chief Medical Officer .... Douglas A Gentile, MD MBA
Chief Marketing Officer .... Dan Michelson
Chief Operating Officer .... Benjamin Bulkley
President, Medication Services Group .... John G Cull
Senior VP, Business Development .... Steven P Schwartz

Statistics:
Parent Company Name: Allscripts Healthcare Solutions
Doing Business As:
Year Founded:
Nonprofit: [ ]   Forprofit: [ ]
Federally Qualified? [ ]

SERVICE AREA:
  IL;

AMERISCRIPT INC

Stratford Pl 4301 Darrow Rd
Stow, OH 44224
Phone: 330-686-7010 Fax: 330-524-7572 Toll-Free: 800-681-6912
Web site: www.ameriscript.com
Mailing Address:
  AMERISCRIPT INC
  PO Box 2410
  Stow, OH 44224

Key Executives:
Chairman/Chief Executive Officer .... Paul W Glover
Chief Financial Officer .... Steven L Ditman
VP, Sales & Product Development .... Jim Wallace RPh
VP, PBM Operations .... John Baker
VP Clinical Resources - IHG .... Mary Romanchok

Statistics:
Parent Company Name: Interplan Health Group
Doing Business As: AmeriScript Inc
Year Founded: 1986
Nonprofit: [ ]   Forprofit: [Y]
Federally Qualified? [ ]

SERVICE AREA:
  NW;

Targeting Providers?
Point your sales force in the right direction with

The National Directory of Health Systems, Hospitals and Their Affiliates

"The ONLY nationwide compilation of key statistical data on more than 734 Integrated Healthcare Delivery Networks available today"

Your Sales Reference Tool for Greater Profits this Year

- Target over 5,300 Key Decision Makes
- Learn Revenue Figures
- Top 50 Rankings
- 11,000+ System Affiliates
- More than 734 Comprehensive System Profiles
- Includes over 3,600 hospitals

• You'll get carefully compiled in depth profiles by IHDN within each state

• Verified names of the system's key executives who can authorize technology purchasing decisions

• Important IHDN system statistics - critical for your background information on your prospects

• Thousands of IHDN system affiliates are identified including community hospital, home healthcare agencies and long term care facilities

**Call Toll-Free Today!
(888) THE-MCIC
or fax
(888) FAX-MCIC**

■ ■ Sample Profile ■ ■

OCEAN REGIONAL HEALTH SYSTEMS

1000 Garden Street
Healthtown, NJ
Phone: 908-555-1212   Fax: 908-555-1313   Toll-Free: 800-555-1212
Web Site:www.themcic.com

KEY EXECUTIVE PERSONNEL
Chief Executive Officer .... Larry Sanders
Chief Financial Officer .... Michael Simmons
Marketing Officer .... Cheyenne Hains
Pharmaceutical Purchasing Officer .... Donald Kilmore
Capital Equipment Purchasing Officer .... David Roberts
Network Development/Contracts Officer .... Michael Johnson

SYSTEM STATISTICS
Year Founded: 1999
Parent: Wellington Health Services
Tax Status: For-Profit?   Not-For-Profit? Y
Type of Integration: Horizontal: Vertical: X
Enrollment (Covered Lives): 68,000
Primary Physicians: 86
Physician Specialists: 221
Admissions (Visits):   Outpatient: 195,000   Inpatient: 12,000
Gross Revenue: $193,600,000
Number of Facilities Curently in Operation: 15
Number of Facilities Planned: 36

SYSTEM AFFILIATIONS
Ocean Regional Medical Center   H
100 Garden St
Healthtown, NJ 00000
Chief Executive Officer/President: Mary Floers
Telephone: 908-555-1212   Fax: 908-555-1313
Web: www.themcic.com
Hospitla Beds: 325
Amber Family Medicine Associations   PC
000 Safe St
Healthtown, NJ 00000
Chief Executive Officer/President: Mary Floers
Telephone: 908-555-1212   Fax: 908-555-1313

Available in PDF and Database formats

How we gather this information for your use . . .

All the data on the CD ROM has been collected directly from the organizations themselves, state agencies, other public sources of information, proprietary data files created and maintained by the Managed Care Information Center and extensive telephone interview research by our own staff.

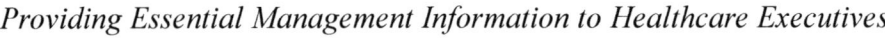
Managed Care Information Center
Providing Essential Management Information to Healthcare Executives

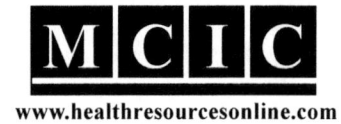
www.healthresourcesonline.com

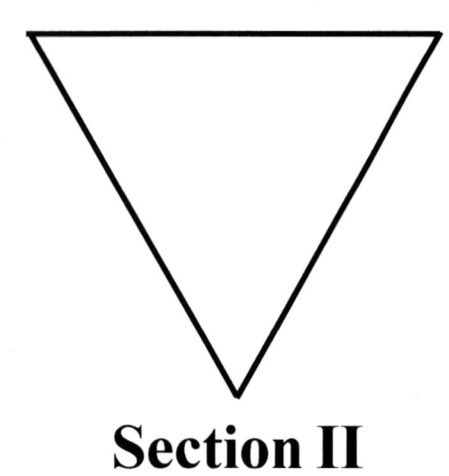

Section II

Pharmacy Benefit Management Companies
(Alphabetically)

WYOMING

COMPANY PROFILE:
Parent Company Name:
Doing Business As:
Year Founded: 1996   Federally Qualified: [N]
Forprofit: [ ]   Not-For-Profit: [Y]
Model Type: NETWORK
Accreditation: [ ] AAPPO [ ] JACHO [ ] NCQA [ ] URAC
Plan Type: HMO, PPO, POS, TPA, ASO, PBM
Total Revenue: 2005:   2006: 39,319,634
Net Income   2005:   2006:
Total Enrollment:
   2001: 10,100   2004: 9,660   2007: 0
   2002: 10,689   2005:
   2003: 10,474   2006:
Medical Loss Ratio: 2005:   2006: 81.50
Administrative Expense Ratio: 2005:   2006:

SERVICE AREA:
Nationwide: N
   WY;

TYPE OF COVERAGE:
Commercial: [Y] Individual: [ ] FEHBP: [ ] Indemnity: [ ]
Medicare: [ ] Medicaid: [ ] Supplemental Medicare: [ ]
Tricare   [ ]

Managed Care Organization Profiles

WYOMING

BLUE CROSS BLUE SHIELD OF WYOMING

4000 House Ave
Cheyenne, WY 82001
Phone: 307-634-1393 Fax: 307-634-5742 Toll-Free:
Web site: www.bcbswy.com

MAILING ADDRESS:
BC BS OF WYOMING
PO Box 2266
Cheyenne, WY 82001

KEY EXECUTIVES:
Chairman of the Board .... Cliff Kirk
Chief Executive Officer/President .... Tim J Crilly
Medical Director .... Darryl D Bindschadler, MD
Chief Operating Officer .... Karen Dobson
VP of Marketing .... Rick Schum
Director of Public & Provider Affairs .... Jane Stephen

COMPANY PROFILE:
Parent Company Name: Blue Cross/Blue Shield Association
Doing Business As:
Year Founded: 1976   Federally Qualified: [ ]
Forprofit: [ ]   Not-For-Profit: [Y]
Model Type:
Accreditation: [ ] AAPPO [ ] JACHO [ ] NCQA [ ] URAC
Plan Type: HMO, PPO, HDHP, HSA
Total Enrollment:
 2001: 67,282   2004: 65,737   2007: 100,000
 2002: 62,583   2005:
 2003: 65,909   2006:

SERVICE AREA:
Nationwide: N
 WY;

TYPE OF COVERAGE:
Commercial: [Y] Individual: [Y] FEHBP: [ ] Indemnity: [ ]
Medicare: [Y] Medicaid: [Y] Supplemental Medicare: [Y]
Tricare [ ]

CONSUMER-DRIVEN PRODUCTS
                          HSA Company
                          HSA Product
                          HSA Administrator
                          Consumer-Driven Health Plan
Blue Choice Personal   High Deductible Health Plan

DELTA DENTAL PLAN OF WYOMING

320 W 25th St Ste 100
Cheyenne, WY 82001-3069
Phone: 307-632-3313 Fax: 307-632-7309 Toll-Free: 800-735-3379
Web site: www.deltadentalwy.org

MAILING ADDRESS:
DELTA DENTAL PLAN OF WY
PO Box 29
Cheyenne, WY 82001-3069

KEY EXECUTIVES:
Chief Executive Officer .... Kerry Hall
Chief Financial Officer .... Stacy Zaftoupil
Dental Director .... Earl Kincheloe, DDS

COMPANY PROFILE:
Parent Company Name: Delta Dental Plan Association
Doing Business As:
Year Founded: Federally Qualified: [ ]
Forprofit: [ ]   Not-For-Profit: [ ]
Model Type:
Accreditation: [ ] AAPPO [ ] JACHO [ ] NCQA [ ] URAC
Plan Type: Specialty HMO

SERVICE AREA:
Nationwide: N
 WY;

TYPE OF COVERAGE:
Commercial: [Y] Individual: [ ] FEHBP: [ ] Indemnity: [ ]
Medicare: [ ] Medicaid: [ ] Supplemental Medicare: [ ]
Tricare [ ]

PLAN BENEFITS:
Alternative Medicine: [ ]   Behavioral Health: [ ]
Chiropractic: [ ]   Dental: [X]
Home Care: [ ]   Inpatient SNF: [ ]
Long-Term Care: [ ]   Pharm. Mail Order: [ ]
Physical Therapy: [ ]   Podiatry: [ ]
Psychiatric: [ ]   Transplant: [ ]
Vision: [ ]   Wellness: [ ]
Workers' Comp: [ ]
Other Benefits:

HUMANA INC - WYOMING

1465 N 4th St Ste 110
Laramie, WY 82072-2066
Phone: 307-745-3616 Fax: 307-745-3211 Toll-Free:
Web site: www.humana.com

MAILING ADDRESS:
HUMANA INC - WYOMING
500 W Main St
Louisville, KY 40201

KEY EXECUTIVES:
Chairman of the Board .... David A Jones Jr
Chief Executive Officer/President .... Michael B McCallister
Chief Financial Officer .... James H Bloem
VP, Medical Director .... Jonathan T Lord, MD
Senior VP, Chief Information Officer .... Bruce J Goodman
Senior VP, Human Resources .... Bonnie C Hathcock

COMPANY PROFILE:
Parent Company Name: Humana Inc
Doing Business As:
Year Founded: 1961   Federally Qualified: [Y]
Forprofit: [Y]   Not-For-Profit: [ ]
Model Type:
Accreditation: [ ] AAPPO [ ] JACHO [ ] NCQA [ ] URAC
Plan Type: PPO, CDHP, HDHP, HSA

SERVICE AREA:
Nationwide: N
 WY;

TYPE OF COVERAGE:
Commercial: [Y] Individual: [ ] FEHBP: [ ] Indemnity: [ ]
Medicare: [Y] Medicaid: [ ] Supplemental Medicare: [Y]
Tricare [ ]

CONSUMER-DRIVEN PRODUCTS
JP Morgan Chase   HSA Company
HumanaOne HSA   HSA ProductJP Morgan Chase
HSA Administrator
Personal Care Account   Consumer-Driven Health Plan
HumanaOne   High Deductible Health Plan

PLAN BENEFITS:
Alternative Medicine: [ ]   Behavioral Health: [ ]
Chiropractic: [X]   Dental: [X]
Home Care: [ ]   Inpatient SNF: [ ]
Long-Term Care: [ ]   Pharm. Mail Order: [X]
Physical Therapy: [ ]   Podiatry: [ ]
Psychiatric: [X]   Transplant: [X]
Vision: [ ]   Wellness: [X]
Workers' Comp: [X]
Other Benefits:

WIN HEALTH PARTNERS

1200 East 20th St Ste A
Cheyenne, WY 82001
Phone: 307-773-1300 Fax: 307-638-7701 Toll-Free: 800-868-7670
Web site: www.winhealthpartners.org

MAILING ADDRESS:
WIN HEALTH PARTNERS
1200 East 20th St Ste A
Cheyenne, WY 82001

KEY EXECUTIVES:
Chairman of the Board/President .... Richard E Torkelson, MD
Chief Executive Officer .... Beth A Wasson
Chief Financial Officer .... Lonny D Warren
Medical Director .... Vincent Miles, MD
Director of Information Technology .... David Unruh
Case Management Director .... Barbara Wild

WISCONSIN

SERVICE AREA:
Nationwide: N
　　WI;

TYPE OF COVERAGE:
Commercial: [Y] Individual: [Y] FEHBP: [ ] Indemnity: [ ]
Medicare: [ ] Medicaid: [ ] Supplemental Medicare: [ ]
Tricare [ ]

PLAN BENEFITS:
Alternative Medicine: [ ]　　　Behavioral Health: [ ]
Chiropractic: [X]　　　　　　　Dental: [X]
Home Care: [X]　　　　　　　　Inpatient SNF: [X]
Long-Term Care: [X]　　　　　　Pharm. Mail Order: [X]
Physical Therapy: [X]　　　　　Podiatry: [X]
Psychiatric: [X]　　　　　　　　Transplant: [X]
Vision: [X]　　　　　　　　　　Wellness: [X]
Workers' Comp: [ ]
Other Benefits:

Managed Care Organization Profiles **WISCONSIN**

SERVICE AREA:
Nationwide: N
  WI (Adams, Columbia, Crawford, Dane, Dodge, Fond du Lac, Grant, Green, Green Lake, Iowa, Jefferson, Juneau, Lafayette, Marquette, Richland, Rock, Sauk, Vernon, Walworth and Waushara);
TYPE OF COVERAGE:
Commercial: [Y] Individual: [Y] FEHBP: [ ] Indemnity: [ ]
Medicare: [ ] Medicaid: [Y] Supplemental Medicare: [ ]
Tricare   [ ]
PRODUCTS OFFERED:
Product Name:	Type:
	Medicare Elect
	U-Care Plus
Unity Medicaid	Medicaid HMO
Unity Health Plans	HMO
BadgerCare SCHIP	Medicaid

CONSUMER-DRIVEN PRODUCTS
HSA Bank	HSA Company
	HSA Product
HSA Bank	HSA Administrator
HMO Deductible	Consumer-Driven Health Plan
Choice POS	High Deductible Health Plan

PLAN BENEFITS:
Alternative Medicine: [ ]   Behavioral Health: [X]
Chiropractic: [X]   Dental: [X]
Home Care: [X]   Inpatient SNF: [X]
Long-Term Care: [ ]   Pharm. Mail Order: [ ]
Physical Therapy: [X]   Podiatry: [X]
Psychiatric: [X]   Transplant: [X]
Vision: [X]   Wellness: [X]
Workers' Comp: [ ]
Other Benefits:
Comments:
Unity is owned by University Health Care, Inc. (UHC) is affiliated with the University of Wisconsin Hopsital and Clinics and University of Wisconsin Medical Foundation, and does business as UW Health. Formerly Unity Health Plans.

VISION CARE NETWORK

1421 Washington Ave
Racine, WI 53403
Phone: 800-767-8801 Fax: 262-637-7958 Toll-Free: 800-767-8801
Web site:
MAILING ADDRESS:
  VISION CARE NETWORK
  1421 Washington Ave
  Racine, WI 53403

KEY EXECUTIVES:
Chief Executive Officer .... *Bruce A Savin, OD*
Medical Director .... *Rick D Anderson, OD*
Marketing Director .... *Dale Savin*

COMPANY PROFILE:
Parent Company Name:
Doing Business As:
Year Founded: 1989   Federally Qualified: [ ]
Forprofit: [Y]   Not-For-Profit: [ ]
Model Type: NETWORK
Accreditation: [ ] AAPPO [ ] JACHO [ ] NCQA [ ] URAC
Plan Type: Specialty HMO
SERVICE AREA:
Nationwide: N
  WI (Southeastern);
TYPE OF COVERAGE:
Commercial: [Y] Individual: [Y] FEHBP: [ ] Indemnity: [ ]
Medicare: [ ] Medicaid: [ ]   Supplemental Medicare: [ ]
Tricare   [ ]
PLAN BENEFITS:
Alternative Medicine: [ ]   Behavioral Health: [ ]
Chiropractic: [ ]   Dental: [ ]
Home Care: [ ]   Inpatient SNF: [ ]
Long-Term Care: [ ]   Pharm. Mail Order: [ ]
Physical Therapy: [ ]   Podiatry: [ ]
Psychiatric: [ ]   Transplant: [ ]
Vision: [X]   Wellness: [ ]
Workers' Comp: [ ]
Other Benefits:

VISION INSURANCE PLAN OF AMERICA INC - CORPORATE HEADQUARTERS

6737 W Washington St Ste 2202
Milwaukee, WI 53214-7077
Phone: 414-475-1875 Fax: 414-475-1599 Toll-Free: 800-883-5747
Web site: www.visionplans.com
MAILING ADDRESS:
  VISION INSURANCE PLAN OF AMERICA INC
  PO Box 44077
  Milwaukee, WI 53214-7077

KEY EXECUTIVES:
President .... *Dana Witter*
Director of Operations .... *Jenna Sabir*
Manager of Sales .... *Mark P Wallner*
Compliance Officer .... *Dana Bagnall*

COMPANY PROFILE:
Parent Company Name: Block Vision Inc
Doing Business As:
Year Founded: 1992   Federally Qualified: [N]
Forprofit: [Y]   Not-For-Profit: [ ]
Model Type: NETWORK
Accreditation: [ ] AAPPO [ ] JACHO [ ] NCQA [ ] URAC
Plan Type: Specialty HMO,
Total Enrollment:
  2001: 0   2004: 66,106   2007: 0
  2002: 50,774   2005:
  2003: 54,240   2006:
SERVICE AREA:
Nationwide: Y
  NW;
TYPE OF COVERAGE:
Commercial: [Y] Individual: [ ] FEHBP: [ ] Indemnity: [ ]
Medicare: [ ] Medicaid: [ ]   Supplemental Medicare: [ ]
Tricare   [ ]
PRODUCTS OFFERED:
Product Name:	Type:
Vision Insurance Plan	Specialty HMO

PLAN BENEFITS:
Alternative Medicine: [ ]   Behavioral Health: [ ]
Chiropractic: [ ]   Dental: [ ]
Home Care: [ ]   Inpatient SNF: [ ]
Long-Term Care: [ ]   Pharm. Mail Order: [ ]
Physical Therapy: [ ]   Podiatry: [ ]
Psychiatric: [ ]   Transplant: [ ]
Vision: [X]   Wellness: [ ]
Workers' Comp: [ ]
Other Benefits:

WISCONSIN PHYSICIAN SERVICES INSURANCE COMPANY

1717 W Broadway
Madison, WI 53713
Phone: 608-221-4711 Fax: 608-223-3603 Toll-Free:
Web site: www.wpsic.com
MAILING ADDRESS:
  WISCONSIN PHYSICIAN SERVICES INS CO
  PO Box 8190
  Madison, WI 53713

KEY EXECUTIVES:
Chief Executive Officer/President .... *James R Riordan*
Senior VP, Finance .... *William C Beisenstein*
Medical Director .... *David B Luce, MD*
Chief Operating Officer .... *William T Bathke*
Marketing Director .... *Bob Andrew*
Director, Information Systems .... *Jean M Kolowrat*
Compliance Officer/Provider Relations Director .. *Josephine W Musser*

COMPANY PROFILE:
Parent Company Name: WPS Wisconsin Physician Services
Doing Business As:
Year Founded: 1983   Federally Qualified: [N]
Forprofit: [ ]   Not-For-Profit: [Y]
Model Type: GROUP
Accreditation: [ ] AAPPO [ ] JACHO [ ] NCQA [ ] URAC
Plan Type: HMO, PPO, POS, EPO, HDHP, HSA

WISCONSIN

Plan Type: HMO,
Primary Physicians: 1,695 Physician Specialists:
Hospitals: 30
Total Revenue: 2005: 385,590,000 2006: 458,179,000
Net Income 2005: 13,823,000 2006: 9,837,000
Total Enrollment:
  2001: 117,786 2004: 112,821 2007: 0
  2002: 115,775 2005: 109,102
  2003: 117,926 2006: 122,480
Medical Loss Ratio: 2005: 89.60 2006: 90.70
Administrative Expense Ratio: 2005: 7.40 2006: 7.70

SERVICE AREA:
Nationwide: N
WI (Adams, Ashland, Barron, Chippewa, Clark, Dunn, Eau Claire, Clark, Forest, Iron, Jackson, Juneau, Langlade, Lincoln, Marathon, Milwaukee, Monroe, Oneida, Portage, Price, Rusk, Sawyer, Shawano, Taylor, Trempealeau, Vilas, Washburn, Waupaca, Vilas, Waupaca, Wood);

TYPE OF COVERAGE:
Commercial: [Y] Individual: [Y] FEHBP: [ ] Indemnity: [ ]
Medicare: [ ] Medicaid: [ ] Supplemental Medicare: [Y]
Tricare [ ]

PRODUCTS OFFERED:
Product Name:	Type:
Security Health	Medicaid HMO
BadgerCare SCHIP	Medicaid
Advocare By Security Health Plan	Medicare

PLAN BENEFITS:
Alternative Medicine: [ ] Behavioral Health: [X]
Chiropractic: [X] Dental: [ ]
Home Care: [X] Inpatient SNF: [X]
Long-Term Care: [ ] Pharm. Mail Order: [ ]
Physical Therapy: [X] Podiatry: [X]
Psychiatric: [X] Transplant: [X]
Vision: [X] Wellness: [X]
Workers' Comp: [ ]
Other Benefits:

UNITEDHEALTHCARE OF WISCONSIN INC

10701 W Research Dr
Milwaukee, WI 53226
Phone: 414-443-4000 Fax: 414-443-4750 Toll-Free: 800-879-0071
Web site: www.uhc.com

MAILING ADDRESS:
UNITEDHEALTHCARE OF WI INC
10701 W Research Dr
Milwaukee, WI 53226

KEY EXECUTIVES:
Non-Executive Chairman .... Richard T Burke
Chief Executive Officer/President .... Wendy Arnone
Chief Financial Officer/Chief Operating Officer .... Glenn Reinhardt
Medical Director .... James Hare, MD
Pharmacy Director .... Janet Edwards
Director Corporate Communications .... Susan Wesley
Director, Provider Services .... John Foley
Office Network Development .... Gary Hovila
Director Human Resources .... Randall Sannes
Directory Quality Management .... Wendy Potochnik
VP Marketing Middle Market .... Mike Derdzinski

COMPANY PROFILE:
Parent Company Name: UnitedHealth Group
Doing Business As: PrimeCare Health Inc
Year Founded: 1986 Federally Qualified: [N]
Forprofit: [Y] Not-For-Profit: [ ]
Model Type: MIXED
Accreditation: [ ] AAPPO [ ] JACHO [X] NCQA [ ] URAC
Plan Type: HMO, PPO, POS, ASO, CDHP, HDHP, HSA, HRA
Primary Physicians: 11,312 Physician Specialists:
Hospitals: 24
Total Revenue: 2005: 652,064,000 2006: 645,935,000
Net Income 2005: 42,130,000 2006: 23,057,000

Total Enrollment:
  2001: 285,055 2004: 311,510 2007: 0
  2002: 0 2005: 191,254
  2003: 71,602 2006: 177,459
Medical Loss Ratio: 2005: 79.30 2006: 83.90
Administrative Expense Ratio: 2005: 12.40 2006: 11.90

SERVICE AREA:
Nationwide: N
WI (Dodge Cty, Jefferson Cty, Kenosha Cty, Milwaukee Cty, Ozaukee Cty, Racine Cty, Rock, Walworth Cty, Washington, Waukesha Cty);

TYPE OF COVERAGE:
Commercial: [Y] Individual: [ ] FEHBP: [ ] Indemnity: [ ]
Medicare: [Y] Medicaid: [Y] Supplemental Medicare: [ ]
Tricare [ ]

PRODUCTS OFFERED:
Product Name:	Type:
Select HMO	Gatekeeper HMO
Select Plus	Gatekeeper POS
Choice HMO	Open Access HMO
Choice Plus	Open Access Point of
BadgerCare SCHIP	Medicaid
Primecare Gold	Medicare
Primecare	Medicaid

CONSUMER-DRIVEN PRODUCTS
Exante Bank/Golden Rule Ins Co	HSA Company
iPlan HSA	HSA Product
	HSA Administrator
	Consumer-Driven Health Plan
	High Deductible Health Plan

PLAN BENEFITS:
Alternative Medicine: [ ] Behavioral Health: [X]
Chiropractic: [X] Dental: [ ]
Home Care: [X] Inpatient SNF: [X]
Long-Term Care: [ ] Pharm. Mail Order: [X]
Physical Therapy: [X] Podiatry: [ ]
Psychiatric: [X] Transplant: [X]
Vision: [X] Wellness: [X]
Workers' Comp: [ ]
Other Benefits:

UNITY HEALTH INSURANCE

840 Carolina St
Sauk City, WI 53583-1374
Phone: 608-643-2491 Fax: 608-643-2564 Toll-Free: 800-362-3308
Web site: www.unityhealth.com

MAILING ADDRESS:
UNITY HEALTH INSURANCE
840 Carolina St
Sauk City, WI 53583-1374

KEY EXECUTIVES:
Chairman of the Board/Chief Executive Officer .... Terry Bolz
VP, Finance .... Radovan Bursac
Medical Director .... Dr Mary Pak
Pharmacy Director .... Patrick Cory, PharmD
VP, Operations .... Gail Midlikowski
VP, Sales .... Kurt Popp
Director Health Services & Quality Improvement .... Elaine Rosenblatt
Director, Medical Management .... Pat Senter
Compliance Officer .... Nancy Sielaff
Human Resources Director .... Karen Bender
Director, Underwriting .... Kathe DeVay
Director, Internet Application Support .... Dave Roughen
Director, Customer Relations/Quality .... Debbie Schiffman

COMPANY PROFILE:
Parent Company Name: University Health Care Inc
Doing Business As:
Year Founded: 1994 Federally Qualified: [N]
Forprofit: [Y] Not-For-Profit: [ ]
Model Type: MIXED
Accreditation: [ ] AAPPO [ ] JACHO [X] NCQA [ ] URAC
Plan Type: HMO, PPO, POS, TPA, CDHP, HDHP, HSA
Primary Physicians: 1,000 Physician Specialists: 2,500
Hospitals: 45
Total Revenue: 2005: 220,024,858 2006: 241,029,000
Net Income 2005: -5,007,410 2006: 2,173,000
Total Enrollment:
  2001: 73,725 2004: 74,744 2007: 0
  2002: 76,919 2005: 75,238
  2003: 80,178 2006: 76,338
Medical Loss Ratio: 2005: 92.90 2006: 89.90
Administrative Expense Ratio: 2005: 9.80 2006: 9.70

Managed Care Organization Profiles — WISCONSIN

PHYSICIANS PLUS INSURANCE CORPORATION

22 E Mifflin St #200
Madison, WI 53703-4220
Phone: 608-282-8900 Fax: 608-282-8365 Toll-Free: 800-545-5015
Web site: www.pplusic.com

MAILING ADDRESS:
    PHYSICIANS PLUS INS CORP
    PO Box 2078
    Madison, WI 53703-4220

KEY EXECUTIVES:
Chief Executive Officer/President .... Marty Preizler
Chief Financial Officer .... Mike Mohoney
Medical Director .... Ron Parton, MD
Pharmacy Director .... Bill Reay
Chief Operating Officer .... Bill Jollie
Marketing Director .... Katherine McGowan
Quality Assurance Director .... Dr John Martin

COMPANY PROFILE:
Parent Company Name: Meriter Health Services
Doing Business As:
Year Founded: 1986   Federally Qualified: [N]
Forprofit: [Y]   Not-For-Profit: [ ]
Model Type: NETWORK
Accreditation: [ ] AAPPO [ ] JACHO [X] NCQA [ ] URAC
Plan Type: HMO, HDHP, HSA
Primary Physicians: 1,616   Physician Specialists:
Hospitals: 22
Total Revenue: 2005: 268,083,000   2006: 295,820,000
Net Income   2005: 6,744,000   2006: 4,084,000
Total Enrollment:
  2001: 102,326   2004: 93,637   2007: 0
  2002: 97,519   2005: 91,912
  2003: 89,369   2006: 96,029
Medical Loss Ratio: 2005: 87.10   2006: 89.40
Administrative Expense Ratio: 2005: 9.90   2006: 9.30

SERVICE AREA:
Nationwide: N
    WI (Adams, Columbia, Dane, Dodge, Grant, Green, Iowa, Jackson, Jefferson, Juneau, Lafayette, Marquette, Milwaukee, Ozaukee, Richland, Rock, Sauk, Vernon, Walworth, Washington, Waukesha);

TYPE OF COVERAGE:
Commercial: [Y] Individual: [Y] FEHBP: [ ] Indemnity: [ ]
Medicare: [ ] Medicaid: [Y] Supplemental Medicare: [Y]
Tricare [ ]

PRODUCTS OFFERED:
Product Name:	Type:
	Medicaid
Physicians Plus HMO	HMO

PLAN BENEFITS:
Alternative Medicine: [ ]   Behavioral Health: [X]
Chiropractic: [X]   Dental: [X]
Home Care: [X]   Inpatient SNF: [X]
Long-Term Care: [ ]   Pharm. Mail Order: [ ]
Physical Therapy: [X]   Podiatry: [X]
Psychiatric: [X]   Transplant: [X]
Vision: [X]   Wellness: [X]
Workers' Comp: [ ]
Other Benefits:

PREVEA HEALTH NETWORK

2710 Executive Dr
Green Bay, WI 54304
Phone: 920-272-1100 Fax: 920-272-1120 Toll-Free:
Web site: www.preveappo.com

MAILING ADDRESS:
    PREVEA HEALTH NETWORK
    PO Box 11625
    Green Bay, WI 54304

KEY EXECUTIVES:
Chief Executive Officer/President .... Richard Rolston, MD, FAAP
Chief Financial Officer .... Mike Gilbert
Senior VP,Chief Medical Officer .... Ashok Rai, MD
Exec VP,Chief Operating Officer .... Dan Ramsey
VP, Human Resources .... Deb Mauthe
Director of Business Development .... Jim La Haye
Director of Clinic Operations .... Brian Charlier

COMPANY PROFILE:
Parent Company Name:
Doing Business As:
Year Founded: Federally Qualified: [ ]
Forprofit: [ ]   Not-For-Profit: [ ]
Model Type:
Accreditation: [ ] AAPPO [ ] JACHO [ ] NCQA [ ] URAC
Plan Type: PPO
Primary Physicians: 10,000   Physician Specialists:
Hospitals: 55

SERVICE AREA:
Nationwide:
    WI;

RACINE DENTAL GROUP SC

1320 S Green Bay Rd
Racine, WI 53406
Phone: 262-637-9371 Fax: 262-637-3071 Toll-Free:
Web site: www.racinedentalgroup.com

MAILING ADDRESS:
    RACINE DENTAL GROUP SC
    1320 S Green Bay Rd
    Racine, WI 53406

KEY EXECUTIVES:
Chief Executive Officer .... Earl W Newton

COMPANY PROFILE:
Parent Company Name:
Doing Business As:
Year Founded: 1969   Federally Qualified: [ ]
Forprofit: [Y]   Not-For-Profit: [ ]
Model Type:
Accreditation: [ ] AAPPO [ ] JACHO [ ] NCQA [ ] URAC
Plan Type: Specialty HMO, Specialty PPO

SERVICE AREA:
Nationwide: N
    WI (Kenosha, Racine);

TYPE OF COVERAGE:
Commercial: [Y] Individual: [Y] FEHBP: [ ] Indemnity: [ ]
Medicare: [ ] Medicaid: [ ] Supplemental Medicare: [ ]
Tricare [ ]

PLAN BENEFITS:
Alternative Medicine: [ ]   Behavioral Health: [ ]
Chiropractic: [ ]   Dental: [X]
Home Care: [ ]   Inpatient SNF: [ ]
Long-Term Care: [ ]   Pharm. Mail Order: [ ]
Physical Therapy: [ ]   Podiatry: [ ]
Psychiatric: [ ]   Transplant: [ ]
Vision: [ ]   Wellness: [ ]
Workers' Comp: [ ]
Other Benefits:

SECURITY HEALTH PLAN OF WISCONSIN INC

1515 Saint Joseph Ave
Marshfield, WI 54449-8000
Phone: 715-387-5621 Fax: 715-389-5799 Toll-Free: 800-472-2363
Web site: www.securityhealth.org

MAILING ADDRESS:
    SECURITY HEALTH PLAN OF WI INC
    PO Box 8000
    Marshfield, WI 54449-8000

KEY EXECUTIVES:
Chief Administrative Officer .... Steven Youso
Chief Financial Officer .... Barbara Johnson
Chief Medical Officer .... Lawrence G McFarlane, MD
Director of Pharmacy Services .... Twild R Johnson
Director of Operations .... Jeff Zriny
Marketing & Sales Director .... Charles Paine

COMPANY PROFILE:
Parent Company Name: Marshfield Clinic
Doing Business As:
Year Founded: 1986   Federally Qualified: [N]
Forprofit: [ ]   Not-For-Profit: [Y]
Model Type: GROUP
Accreditation: [ ] AAPPO [ ] JACHO [ ] NCQA [ ] URAC

WISCONSIN

Plan Type: HMO, FSA
Primary Physicians: 169   Physician Specialists:
Hospitals: 12
Total Revenue: 2005:   22,406,000   2006:   22,993,000
Net Income   2005:   54,000   2006:   20,642,000
Total Enrollment:
  2001: 6,158   2004: 6,854   2007: 0
  2002: 6,717   2005: 6,753
  2003: 7,346   2006: 6,662
Medical Loss Ratio: 2005: 90.80   2006: 89.70
Administrative Expense Ratio: 2005:   9.30   2006:   9.80

SERVICE AREA:
Nationwide: N
  WI;

TYPE OF COVERAGE:
Commercial: [Y] Individual: [ ] FEHBP: [ ] Indemnity: [ ]
Medicare: [Y] Medicaid: [ ] Supplemental Medicare: [ ]
Tricare   [ ]

PRODUCTS OFFERED:
Product Name:	Type:
HMO	HMO
Medicare Advantage	Medicare

PLAN BENEFITS:
Alternative Medicine: [ ]   Behavioral Health: [X]
Chiropractic: [X]   Dental: [ ]
Home Care: [X]   Inpatient SNF: [X]
Long-Term Care: [ ]   Pharm. Mail Order: [ ]
Physical Therapy: [X]   Podiatry: [X]
Psychiatric: [X]   Transplant: [X]
Vision: [X]   Wellness: [X]
Workers' Comp: [ ]
Other Benefits:

MERCYCARE HEALTH PLAN INC

3430 Palmer Dr
Janesville, WI 53547
Phone: 608-755-5362 Fax: 608-752-3751 Toll-Free: 800-752-3431
Web site: www.mercyhealthsystem.org

MAILING ADDRESS:
  MERCYCARE HEALTH PLAN INC
  PO Box 2770
  Janesville, WI 53547

KEY EXECUTIVES:
Chief Executive Officer .... Javon Bea
Chief Financial Officer .... Matt Hicks
Medical Director .... Phillip Bedrossian, MD
VP, Chief Operating Officer .... Joseph Nemeth
Sales, Marketing & Network Development .... DuWayne Severson
MIS Director .... Fred Terry
Medical Management Director .... Dr Phillip Bedrossian
Director of Compliance & Audit .... Barbara Johnson

COMPANY PROFILE:
Parent Company Name: Mercy Health Systems Inc
Doing Business As: MercyCare Insurance Company
Year Founded: 1994   Federally Qualified: [Y]
Forprofit: [Y]   Not-For-Profit: [ ]
Model Type: MIXED
Accreditation: [ ] AAPPO [ ] JACHO [X] NCQA [ ] URAC
Plan Type: HMO, POS, EPO
Primary Physicians: 296   Physician Specialists:
Hospitals: 5
Total Revenue: 2005: 81,496,000   2006: 84,454,000
Net Income   2005:   -38,000   2006: -4,955,000
Total Enrollment:
  2001: 29,072   2004: 31,478   2007: 0
  2002: 29,921   2005: 31,300
  2003:   8,091   2006: 30,970
Medical Loss Ratio: 2005: 95.20   2006: 99.50
Administrative Expense Ratio: 2005:   6.50   2006:   6.80

SERVICE AREA:
Nationwide: N
  WI (Dane, Green, Jefferson, Rock, Walworth);

TYPE OF COVERAGE:
Commercial: [Y] Individual: [ ] FEHBP: [ ] Indemnity: [ ]
Medicare: [ ] Medicaid: [Y] Supplemental Medicare: [Y]
Tricare   [ ]

PRODUCTS OFFERED:
Product Name:	Type:
Medigap	Medicaid
Mercycare HMO Inc	HMO
Mercycare	POS
BadgerCare SCHIP	Medicaid

PLAN BENEFITS:
Alternative Medicine: [ ]   Behavioral Health: [ ]
Chiropractic: [X]   Dental: [ ]
Home Care: [X]   Inpatient SNF: [X]
Long-Term Care: [ ]   Pharm. Mail Order: [ ]
Physical Therapy: [X]   Podiatry: [X]
Psychiatric: [X]   Transplant: [X]
Vision: [X]   Wellness: [X]
Workers' Comp: [ ]
Other Benefits:

NETWORK HEALTH PLAN WISCONSIN

1570 Midway Place
Menasha, WI 54952
Phone: 920-727-1900 Fax: 920-720-1756 Toll-Free: 800-826-0940
Web site: www.networkhealth.com

MAILING ADDRESS:
  NETWORK HEALTH PLAN WISCONSIN
  1570 Midway Place
  Menasha, WI 54952

KEY EXECUTIVES:
President .... Sheila Jenkins
Medical Director .... Edward Scanlon, MD
Chief Operating Officer .... Tim Temperly
MIS Director .... David Bloedorn
Public Relations Director .... Sandra Peterson

COMPANY PROFILE:
Parent Company Name: Affinity Health System
Doing Business As:
Year Founded: 1982   Federally Qualified: [N]
Forprofit: [Y]   Not-For-Profit: [ ]
Model Type: GROUP
Accreditation: [ ] AAPPO [ ] JACHO [X] NCQA [ ] URAC
Plan Type: HMO, PPO, UR, POS, HDHP, HSA
Primary Physicians: 1,158   Physician Specialists:
Hospitals: 14
Total Revenue: 2005:   2006:
Net Income   2005:   2006:
Total Enrollment:
  2001: 104,223   2004: 119,125   2007: 0
  2002: 111,847   2005: 120,661
  2003: 119,873   2006: 124,316
Medical Loss Ratio: 2005: 86.20   2006: 88.40
Administrative Expense Ratio: 2005: 10.90   2006: 10.00

SERVICE AREA:
Nationwide: N
  WI (Brown, Calumen, Dane, Dodge, Fond du Lac, Green Lake,
  Kewaunee, Manitowoc, Marathon, Marinette, Marquette,
  Menominee, Milwaukee, Oconto, Oneida, Outagamie, Ozaukee,
  Portage, Racine, Sawyer, Sheboygan, Washington, Waukesha,
  Waupaca, Waushara, Winnebago);

TYPE OF COVERAGE:
Commercial: [Y] Individual: [ ] FEHBP: [ ] Indemnity: [ ]
Medicare: [Y] Medicaid: [Y] Supplemental Medicare: [Y]
Tricare   [ ]

PRODUCTS OFFERED:
Product Name:	Type:
Network Health Plan	Medicaid HMO
BadgerCare SCHIP	Medicaid
Network Health Plan HMO	HMO
Network Senior Plus	Medicare

PLAN BENEFITS:
Alternative Medicine: [ ]   Behavioral Health: [ ]
Chiropractic: [X]   Dental: [X]
Home Care: [X]   Inpatient SNF: [X]
Long-Term Care: [X]   Pharm. Mail Order: [X]
Physical Therapy: [X]   Podiatry: [X]
Psychiatric: [X]   Transplant: [X]
Vision: [X]   Wellness: [X]
Workers' Comp: [ ]
Other Benefits:

Managed Care Organization Profiles — WISCONSIN

SERVICE AREA:
Nationwide: N
WI (Dodge, Douglas, Dunn, Eau Claire, Fond du Lac, Green, Jefferson, Kenosha, Manitowoc, Milwaukee, Ozaukee, Pierce, Polk, Racine, Rock, St Croix, Sheboygan, Walworth, Washington, Waukesha);

TYPE OF COVERAGE:
Commercial: [Y] Individual: [ ] FEHBP: [ ] Indemnity: [ ]
Medicare: [ ] Medicaid: [ ] Supplemental Medicare: [ ]
Tricare [ ]

PRODUCTS OFFERED:
Product Name: Type:
Humana Wisconsin Ins Co   HMO

CONSUMER-DRIVEN PRODUCTS
JP Morgan Chase   HSA Company
HumanaOne HSA   HSA Product
JP Morgan Chase   HSA Administrator
Personal Care Account   Consumer-Driven Health Plan
High Deductible Health Plan

PLAN BENEFITS:
Alternative Medicine: [ ]   Behavioral Health: [ ]
Chiropractic: [X]   Dental: [X]
Home Care: [ ]   Inpatient SNF: [ ]
Long-Term Care: [ ]   Pharm. Mail Order: [X]
Physical Therapy: [ ]   Podiatry: [ ]
Psychiatric: [X]   Transplant: [X]
Vision: [ ]   Wellness: [ ]
Workers' Comp: [X]
Other Benefits:

Comments:
Formerly Humana Employers Health Insurance.

INDEPENDENT CARE HEALTH PLAN

1555 N RiverCenter Dr Ste 202A
Milwaukee, WI 53212
Phone: 414-223-4847 Fax: 414-231-1092 Toll-Free: 800-777-4376
Web site: www.icare-wi.org

MAILING ADDRESS:
INDEPENDENT CARE HEALTH PLAN
1555 N RiverCenter Dr Ste 202A
Milwaukee, WI 53212

KEY EXECUTIVES:
Chief Executive Officer/President .... Patricia M Jerominski
Chief Financial Officer .... Donald J Slowik
Director, Marketing & Compliance .... William F Jensen
Executive Assistant .... Sandy Rozga

COMPANY PROFILE:
Parent Company Name:
Doing Business As:
Year Founded: 2003   Federally Qualified: [N]
Forprofit: [ ]   Not-For-Profit: [ ]
Model Type: MIXED
Accreditation: [ ] AAPPO [ ] JACHO [ ] NCQA [ ] URAC
Plan Type: HMO
Primary Physicians: 2,016   Physician Specialists:
Hospitals: 21
Total Revenue: 2005: 65,623,000   2006: 75,884,000
Net Income   2005: 1,590,000   2006: 806,000
Total Enrollment:
  2001: 0   2004: 6,046   2007: 0
  2002: 0   2005: 8,343
  2003: 6,007   2006: 8,565
Medical Loss Ratio: 2005: 87.80   2006: 87.90
Administrative Expense Ratio: 2005: 8.90   2006: 11.40

SERVICE AREA:
Nationwide:
WI;

TYPE OF COVERAGE:
Commercial: [ ] Individual: [ ] FEHBP: [ ] Indemnity: [ ]
Medicare: [ ]   Medicaid: [Y]   Supplemental Medicare: [ ]
Tricare [ ]

MANAGED HEALTH SERVICES INSURANCE CORPORATION

1205 S 70th St Ste 500
West Allis, WI 53214
Phone: 414-345-4600 Fax: 414-345-4670 Toll-Free: 800-547-1647
Web site: www.mhswi.com

MAILING ADDRESS:
MANAGED HEALTH SERVICES
1205 S 70th St Ste 500
West Allis, WI 53214

KEY EXECUTIVES:
Chief Executive Officer/President .... Kathleen R Crampton
Chief Financial Officer .... Karey L Witty, CPA
Medical Director .... Wayne Keiserman, MD
Provider Relations Director .... Kyla Kack
VP, Medical Management .... Jan Larson, RN
Director, Quality Improvement .... Janice Vele, MD

COMPANY PROFILE:
Parent Company Name: Centene Corporation Inc
Doing Business As:
Year Founded: 1990   Federally Qualified: [ ]
Forprofit: [Y]   Not-For-Profit: [ ]
Model Type: NETWORK
Accreditation: [ ] AAPPO [ ] JACHO [ ] NCQA [ ] URAC
Plan Type: HMO,
Primary Physicians: 1,958   Physician Specialists: 3,605
Hospitals: 56
Total Revenue: 2005: 230,618,000   2006: 242,088,000
Net Income   2005: 15,007,000   2006: 2,1478,000
Total Enrollment:
  2001: 89,281   2004: 165,800   2007: 0
  2002: 95,412   2005: 172,100
  2003: 157,800   2006: 110,708
Medical Loss Ratio: 2005: 83.90   2006: 86.70
Administrative Expense Ratio: 2005: 13.10   2006: 13.00

SERVICE AREA:
Nationwide: N
WI (Dane, Dodge, Eau Claire, Fond du Lac, Jefferson, Kenosha, Milwaukee, Ozaukee, Racine, Sheboygan, Walworth, Washington, Waukesha);

TYPE OF COVERAGE:
Commercial: [Y] Individual: [ ] FEHBP: [ ] Indemnity: [ ]
Medicare: [ ]   Medicaid: [Y]   Supplemental Medicare: [ ]
Tricare [ ]

PRODUCTS OFFERED:
Product Name: Type:
Medicaid HMO   Medicaid
BadgerCare SCHIP   Medicaid

PLAN BENEFITS:
Alternative Medicine: [ ]   Behavioral Health: [ ]
Chiropractic: [X]   Dental: [X]
Home Care: [X]   Inpatient SNF: [X]
Long-Term Care: [ ]   Pharm. Mail Order: [X]
Physical Therapy: [X]   Podiatry: [ ]
Psychiatric: [X]   Transplant: [X]
Vision: [X]   Wellness: [X]
Workers' Comp: [ ]
Other Benefits:

Comments:
Formerly Maxicare Health Company.

MEDICAL ASSOCIATES CLINIC HEALTH PLAN OF WISCONSIN

1605 Associates Dr Ste 101
Dubuque, IA 52002-2270
Phone: 563-556-8070 Fax: 563-556-5134 Toll-Free: 800-747-8900
Web site: www.mahealthcare.com

MAILING ADDRESS:
MEDICAL ASSOCIATES CLINIC HEALTH PLAN - WI
1605 Associates Dr Ste 101
Dubuque, IA 52002-2270

KEY EXECUTIVES:
Chief Executive Officer/President .... Alan Avery
Chief Financial Officer .... Ronald Fahey, CPA
Chief Medical Officer .... Edward Alt, MD
Marketing Director .... Julie Hoffmann

COMPANY PROFILE:
Parent Company Name: Medical Associates Health Plan Inc
Doing Business As:
Year Founded: 1985   Federally Qualified: [N]
Forprofit: [Y]   Not-For-Profit: [ ]
Model Type: GROUP
Accreditation: [ ] AAPPO [ ] JACHO [ ] NCQA [ ] URAC

WISCONSIN

PRODUCTS OFFERED:
Product Name: Type:
Senior Preferred   Medicare
Gunderson HMO   HMO

PLAN BENEFITS:
Alternative Medicine: [ ]   Behavioral Health: [ ]
Chiropractic: [X]   Dental: [ ]
Home Care: [X]   Inpatient SNF: [X]
Long-Term Care: [ ]   Pharm. Mail Order: [ ]
Physical Therapy: [X]   Podiatry: [X]
Psychiatric: [X]   Transplant: [X]
Vision: [X]   Wellness: [X]
Workers' Comp: [ ]
Other Benefits:

HEALTH TRADITION HEALTH PLANS

1808 E Main St
Onalaska, WI 54650
Phone: 608-781-9692 Fax: 608-781-9653 Toll-Free: 888-459-3020
Web site: www.healthtradition.com

MAILING ADDRESS:
HEALTH TRADITION HEALTH PLANS
PO Box 188
La Crosse, WI 54650

KEY EXECUTIVES:
Executive Director .... Steven M Kunes
Chief Financial Officer .... John Nemec
Director, Operations/Clinical Services .... Beverly Larson, RN
Director, Sales & Marketing .... Michael Eckstein
Medical Director .... Alan Krumholz, MD
Associate Medical Director .... Martha Binn, MD
Pharmacy Director .... John Johnson

COMPANY PROFILE:
Parent Company Name: Mayo Health System
Doing Business As:
Year Founded: 1986   Federally Qualified: [N]
Forprofit: [Y]   Not-For-Profit: [ ]
Model Type: GROUP
Accreditation: [ ] AAPPO [ ] JACHO [ ] NCQA [ ] URAC
Plan Type: HMO, POS
Primary Physicians: 894   Physician Specialists:
Hospitals: 19
Total Revenue: 2005: 86,866,000   2006: 101,096,000
Net Income   2005:   158,000   2006:   535,000
Total Enrollment:
  2001: 28,423   2004: 29,669   2007: 0
  2002: 28,173   2005: 29,071
  2003: 28,552   2006: 31,677
Medical Loss Ratio: 2005: 90.40   2006: 90.80
Administrative Expense Ratio: 2005: 9.60   2006: 8.80

SERVICE AREA:
Nationwide: N
  IA (Northeast); MN (Southeast); WI (Western); Buffalo, Crawford, Jackson, LaCrosse, Milwaukee, Trempealeau, Vernon

TYPE OF COVERAGE:
Commercial: [Y] Individual: [ ] FEHBP: [ ] Indemnity: [ ]
Medicare: [ ] Medicaid: [Y] Supplemental Medicare: [Y]
Tricare   [ ]

PRODUCTS OFFERED:
Product Name: Type:
Medicaid HMO   Medicaid
                                  HMO
Badgercare SCHIP   Medicaid

Comments:
Formerly called Greater La Crosse Health Plans.

HEALTHEOS BY MULTIPLAN

18650 West Corporate Dr #310
Brookfield, WI 53045-6344
Phone: 262-879-0100 Fax: 262-879-0876 Toll-Free: 800-952-8661
Web site: www.healtheos.com

MAILING ADDRESS:
HEALTHEOS BY MULTIPLAN
PO Box 981
Brookfield, WI 53045-6344

KEY EXECUTIVES:
Chief Executive Officer/President .... Bruce Lefko
Chief Financial Officer .... Curt Zoeller
VP Operations .... Trish Nienow
Marketing Director .... Bill Kersch
Provider Relations Director .... Jim Meyers

COMPANY PROFILE:
Parent Company Name: Multiplan Inc
Doing Business As:
Year Founded: Federally Qualified: [ ]
Forprofit: [Y]   Not-For-Profit: [ ]
Model Type: NETWORK
Accreditation: [ ] AAPPO [ ] JACHO [ ] NCQA [ ] URAC
Plan Type: PPO, PBM, UR
Primary Physicians: 17,000   Physician Specialists:
Hospitals: 159
Total Enrollment:
  2001: 0   2004: 0   2007: 0
  2002: 0   2005:
  2003: 0   2006: 1,200,000

SERVICE AREA:
Nationwide: N
  WI;

TYPE OF COVERAGE:
Commercial: [Y] Individual: [ ] FEHBP: [ ] Indemnity: [ ]
Medicare: [ ] Medicaid: [ ] Supplemental Medicare: [ ]
Tricare   [ ]

PLAN BENEFITS:
Alternative Medicine: [ ]   Behavioral Health: [ ]
Chiropractic: [X]   Dental: [X]
Home Care: [X]   Inpatient SNF: [ ]
Long-Term Care: [X]   Pharm. Mail Order: [ ]
Physical Therapy: [ ]   Podiatry: [X]
Psychiatric: [X]   Transplant: [X]
Vision: [X]   Wellness: [X]
Workers' Comp: [X]
Other Benefits:

Comments:
Combined Wisconsin Preferred Provider Network, Health Care Network of Wisconsin, Associates for Health Care to form HealthEOS/MultiPlan in 2006.

HUMANA WISCONSIN HEALTH ORGANIZATION INC

N19W24133 Riverwood Dr Ste 300
Waukesha, WI 53188
Phone: 262-951-2560 Fax: 262-951-2561 Toll-Free: 800-289-0260
Web site: www.humana.com

MAILING ADDRESS:
HUMANA WISCONSIN HEALTH ORG
N19W24133 Riverwood Dr Ste 300
Waukesha, WI 53188

KEY EXECUTIVES:
Chairman of the Board .... David A Jones Jr
Chief Executive Officer .... Larry Rambo
VP, WI Service Center .... Sandy Ganoni
Chief Medical Officer .... Lisa Weaver, MD
Sales Director .... Jim Nelson
Director Claims/Medical Mgntmnt .... Cathy Thompson

COMPANY PROFILE:
Parent Company Name: Humana Inc
Doing Business As:
Year Founded: 1985   Federally Qualified: [ ]
Forprofit: [Y]   Not-For-Profit: [ ]
Model Type: IPA
Accreditation: [ ] AAPPO [ ] JACHO [ ] NCQA [ ] URAC
Plan Type: HMO, CDHP, HDHP, HSA
Primary Physicians: 6,804   Physician Specialists:
Hospitals: 15
Total Revenue: 2005: 240,695,000   2006: 173,760,000
Net Income   2005:   9,980,000   2006:   6,611,000
Total Enrollment:
  2001: 68,523   2004: 85,120   2007: 0
  2002: 86,142   2005: 54,053
  2003: 83,667   2006: 53,302
Medical Loss Ratio: 2005: 86.00   2006: 88.80
Administrative Expense Ratio: 2005: 8.40   2006: 7.30

Managed Care Organization Profiles   **WISCONSIN**

KEY EXECUTIVES:
Chief Executive Officer/General Manager ....Peter Farrow
President ....Linda Wendt
Finance Director ....Steven Hofkes
Medical Director ....Lon Blaser, DO
Pharmacy Director ....Bob Wildenberg
Senior Account Representitive ....Mary J Glassbrenner
MIS Director ....John Brunstad
Credentialing Manager ....Kelly Grabara
Compliance Manager ....Wendy Bergh
Provider Relations/Education Coordinator ....Wendy Ross
Human Resources Manager ....Sue Kern
Quality Assurance Manager..Rhonda Thorson
Credentialing Manager ....Kelly Grabara
Director of Marketing ....Mike Konzen
Compliance Manager ....Wendy Bergh
MA Programs General Manager ....Carroll Carlson

COMPANY PROFILE:
Parent Company Name:
Doing Business As:
Year Founded: 1976   Federally Qualified: [N]
Forprofit: [ ]   Not-For-Profit: [Y]
Model Type: STAFF
Accreditation: [ ] AAPPO [ ] JACHO [ ] NCQA [ ] URAC
Plan Type: HMO
Primary Physicians: 4,117   Physician Specialists:
Hospitals: 34
Total Revenue: 2005: 60,026,000   2006: 92,435,000
Net Income   2005:   5,152,000   2006:   4,214,000
Total Enrollment:
   2001: 25,292   2004: 21,932   2007: 0
   2002: 24,934   2005: 20,697
   2003: 24,448   2006: 30,217
Medical Loss Ratio: 2005: 83.50   2006: 91.60
Administrative Expense Ratio: 2005: 12.10   2006: 11.60

SERVICE AREA:
Nationwide: N
    WI (Ashland, Barron, Bayfield, Buffalo, Burnett, Chippewa, Clark, Crawford, Douglas, Dunn, Eau Claire, Grant, Jackson, Juneau, La Crosse, Monroe, Pepin, Pierce, Polk, Richland, Rusk, Sawyer, St Croix, Taylor, Trempealeau, Vernon, Washburn);

TYPE OF COVERAGE:
Commercial: [Y] Individual: [Y] FEHBP: [ ] Indemnity: [ ]
Medicare: [ ] Medicaid: [Y] Supplemental Medicare: [ ]
Tricare   [ ]

PRODUCTS OFFERED:
Product Name: Type:
Medicaid HMO   Medicaid
Group Health Cooperative HMO   HMO
BadgerCare SCHIP   Medicaid

PLAN BENEFITS:
Alternative Medicine: [ ]   Behavioral Health: [ ]
Chiropractic: [X]   Dental: [X]
Home Care: [X]   Inpatient SNF: [X]
Long-Term Care: [ ]   Pharm. Mail Order: [X]
Physical Therapy: [X]   Podiatry: [X]
Psychiatric: [X]   Transplant: [X]
Vision: [X]   Wellness: [X]
Workers' Comp: [ ]
Other Benefits:

GROUP HEALTH COOPERATIVE SOUTH CENTRAL WISCONSIN

1265 John Q Hammins Dr
Madison, WI 53744-4971
Phone: 608-251-4156 Fax: 608-441-3291 Toll-Free: 800-605-4327
Web site: www.ghc-hmo.com
MAILING ADDRESS:
    GROUP HEALTH COOPERATEVE S CENTRAL WI
    PO Box 44971
    Madison, WI 53744-4971

KEY EXECUTIVES:
Chief Executive Officer..Lawrence J Zanoni
President ....Kenneth Machtan
Chief Financial Officer ....Edward Pautz
Medical Director ....Michael Ostrov
Pharmacy Director ....Paul Baum
Marketing Director ....Allen Wearing
MIS Director ....Gaylon Metz

COMPANY PROFILE:
Parent Company Name:
Doing Business As:
Year Founded: 1976   Federally Qualified: [Y]
Forprofit: [ ]   Not-For-Profit: [Y]
Model Type: STAFF
Accreditation: [ ] AAPPO [ ] JACHO [X] NCQA [ ] URAC
Plan Type: HMO
Primary Physicians: 4,117   Physician Specialists:
Hospitals: 7
Total Revenue: 2005: 159,123,000   2006: 177,467,000
Net Income   2005:   3,143,000   2006:   1,962,000
Total Enrollment:
   2001: 52,139   2004: 51,718   2007: 0
   2002: 52,790   2005: 54,918
   2003: 51,982   2006: 57,046
Medical Loss Ratio: 2005: 87.60   2006: 91.00
Administrative Expense Ratio: 2005: 10.80   2006: 9.10

SERVICE AREA:
Nationwide: N
    WI (Columbia, Dane, Dodge, Green, Iowa, Jefferson, Rock, Sauk);

TYPE OF COVERAGE:
Commercial: [Y] Individual: [Y] FEHBP: [ ] Indemnity: [ ]
Medicare: [ ] Medicaid: [Y] Supplemental Medicare: [Y]
Tricare   [ ]

PRODUCTS OFFERED:
Product Name: Type:
Medicaid HMO   Medicaid
                                       Medicare Select
BadgerCare SCHIP   Medicaid

PLAN BENEFITS:
Alternative Medicine: [ ]   Behavioral Health: [ ]
Chiropractic: [X]   Dental: [X]
Home Care: [X]   Inpatient SNF: [ ]
Long-Term Care: [ ]   Pharm. Mail Order: [X]
Physical Therapy: [ ]   Podiatry: [X]
Psychiatric: [ ]   Transplant: [X]
Vision: [X]   Wellness: [X]
Workers' Comp: [ ]
Other Benefits:

GUNDERSEN LUTHERAN HEALTH PLAN INC

1836 South Ave
La Crosse, WI 54601
Phone: 608-775-8000 Fax: 608-775-8042 Toll-Free: 800-370-9718
Web site: www.glhealthplan.org
MAILING ADDRESS:
    GUNDERSEN LUTHERAN HEALTH PLAN
    1836 South Ave
    La Crosse, WI 54601

KEY EXECUTIVES:
Executive Director ....Patrick Killeen
Finance Manager ....Tim Ferrier
Manager, Medical Management ....Jayne Spindler
Compliance Officer ....Kari Adank

COMPANY PROFILE:
Parent Company Name: Gundersen Clinic/Lutheran Hospital
Doing Business As: Gundersen Lutheran Health Plan
Year Founded: 1995   Federally Qualified: [N]
Forprofit: [ ]   Not-For-Profit: [Y]
Model Type: MIXED
Accreditation: [ ] AAPPO [ ] JACHO [ ] NCQA [ ] URAC
Plan Type: HMO, POS, TPA
Primary Physicians: 743   Physician Specialists:
Hospitals: 13
Total Revenue: 2005: 136,014,000   2006: 158,158,000
Net Income   2005:   109,000   2006:   1,571,000
Total Enrollment:
   2001: 31,750   2004: 27,114   2007: 0
   2002: 32,050   2005: 28,504
   2003: 32,878   2006: 28,531
Medical Loss Ratio: 2005: 93.10   2006: 93.10
Administrative Expense Ratio: 2005: 7.10   2006: 6.40

SERVICE AREA:
Nationwide: N
    WI;

TYPE OF COVERAGE:
Commercial: [Y] Individual: [ ] FEHBP: [ ] Indemnity: [ ]
Medicare: [Y] Medicaid: [ ] Supplemental Medicare: [ ]
Tricare   [ ]

WISCONSIN

Managed Care Organization Profiles

DORAL DENTAL USA

10201 N Port Washington Rd, #13W
Mequon, WI 53092
Phone: 262-241-7140 Fax: 262-241-7366 Toll-Free: 800-417-7140
Web site: www.doralusa.com
MAILING ADDRESS:
    DORAL DENTAL USA
    10201 N Port Washington Rd, #13W
    Mequon, WI 53092

KEY EXECUTIVES:
Chief Executive Officer .... Bob Hunter
President .... Steven Pollock
Chief Dental Officer .... Doyle Williams, DDS
Marketing Director .... Beth Richards
VP, Information Services .... Jeffrey E Warner
VP, Human Resources .... Angela S Kish
VP, Business Development .... Robert E Lynn
Media Contact .... Michael Pflughoeft

COMPANY PROFILE:
Parent Company Name: DentaQuest
Doing Business As:
Year Founded: 1993   Federally Qualified: [ ]
Forprofit: [Y]   Not-For-Profit: [ ]
Model Type:
Accreditation: [ ] AAPPO [ ] JACHO [ ] NCQA [ ] URAC
Plan Type: Specialty HMO, TPA
SERVICE AREA:
Nationwide: Y
  NW;
TYPE OF COVERAGE:
Commercial: [ ] Individual: [ ] FEHBP: [ ] Indemnity: [ ]
Medicare: [Y] Medicaid: [Y] Supplemental Medicare: [ ]
Tricare [ ]

EMPLOYEE BENEFITS CORPORATION

1350 Deming Way, Ste 200
Middleton, WI 53562-3536
Phone: 414-365-4600 Fax: 414-365-4610 Toll-Free:
Web site: www.ebcflex.com
MAILING ADDRESS:
    EMPLOYEE BENEFITS CORPORATION
    1350 Deming Way, Ste 200
    Middleton, WI 53562-3536

KEY EXECUTIVES:
Chief Executive Officer .... Bruce Flunker
Chief Financial Officer .... Susan Stablefeld
Marketing Director .... Tim Hussey

COMPANY PROFILE:
Parent Company Name: Safeco Life
Doing Business As: EBC
Year Founded: 1977   Federally Qualified: [ ]
Forprofit: [Y]   Not-For-Profit: [ ]
Model Type:
Accreditation: [ ] AAPPO [ ] JACHO [ ] NCQA [ ] URAC
Plan Type: PPO, POS, ASO, TPA, UR, FSA, HRA
SERVICE AREA:
Nationwide: Y
  NW;
CONSUMER-DRIVEN PRODUCTS
                        HSA Company
                        HSA Product
                        HSA Administrator
Bestflex Plan   Consumer-Driven Health Plan
                        High Deductible Health Plan

EYE CARE OF WISCONSIN INC

8633 North Port Washington Rd
Milwaukee, WI 53217-2213
Phone: 414-351-3030 Fax: 414-351-3603 Toll-Free: 800-373-6370
Web site:
MAILING ADDRESS:
    EYE CARE OF WISCONSIN INC
    8633 North Port Washington Rd
    Milwaukee, WI 53217-2213

KEY EXECUTIVES:
Chairman of the Board/Chief Executive Officer .... Patrick Cashin
President/Marketing Director .... Patrick Flanagan
Chief Financial Officer .... Patrick Cashin

COMPANY PROFILE:
Parent Company Name:
Doing Business As:
Year Founded: 1986   Federally Qualified: [Y]
Forprofit: [ ]   Not-For-Profit: [Y]
Model Type: IPA
Accreditation: [ ] AAPPO [ ] JACHO [ ] NCQA [ ] URAC
Plan Type: Specialty HMO, Specialty PPO
SERVICE AREA:
Nationwide: Y
  NW;
TYPE OF COVERAGE:
Commercial: [ ] Individual: [ ] FEHBP: [ ] Indemnity: [ ]
Medicare: [Y] Medicaid: [Y] Supplemental Medicare: [ ]
Tricare [ ]
PLAN BENEFITS:
Alternative Medicine: [ ]   Behavioral Health: [ ]
Chiropractic: [ ]   Dental: [ ]
Home Care: [ ]   Inpatient SNF: [ ]
Long-Term Care: [ ]   Pharm. Mail Order: [ ]
Physical Therapy: [ ]   Podiatry: [ ]
Psychiatric: [ ]   Transplant: [ ]
Vision: [X]   Wellness: [ ]
Workers' Comp: [ ]
Other Benefits: Laser Refractory

FISERV INC

255 Fiserv Dr
Brookfield, WI 53008
Phone: 262-879-5000 Fax: 262-879-5013 Toll-Free: 800-872-5013
Web site: www.fiserv.com
MAILING ADDRESS:
    FISERV INC
    PO Box 979
    Brookfield, WI 53008

KEY EXECUTIVES:
Chairman of the Board .... Donald F Dillon
Chief Executive Officer/President .... Leslie M Muma
Chief Financial Officer .... Kenneth R Jensen
Chief Operating Officer .... Norman J Balthasar
Group President, Marketing & Sales .... Dean C Schmelzer
Human Resources Director .... Gordon L Schroeder
VP for External Affairs .... Kim M Robak
General Counsel/Chief Administrative Officer .... Charles W Sprague

COMPANY PROFILE:
Parent Company Name:
Doing Business As:
Year Founded: 1984   Federally Qualified: [ ]
Forprofit: [Y]   Not-For-Profit: [ ]
Model Type:
Accreditation: [ ] AAPPO [ ] JACHO [ ] NCQA [X] URAC
Plan Type: UR
SERVICE AREA:
Nationwide: Y
  NW;
Comments:
Formerly Willis Administratives.

GROUP HEALTH COOPERATIVE OF EAU CLAIRE

2503 N Hillcrest Pkwy
Altoona, WI 54720-2602
Phone: 715-552-4300 Fax: 715-836-7683 Toll-Free: 888-203-7770
Web site: www.group-health.com
MAILING ADDRESS:
    GROUP HEALTH COOPERATIVE OF EAU CLAIRE
    2503 N Hillcrest Pkwy
    Altoona, WI 54720-2602

Managed Care Organization Profiles — WISCONSIN

MAILING ADDRESS:
   CHILDREN'S COMMUNITY HEALTH PLAN INC
   PO Box 56099
   Milwaukee, WI 53705

KEY EXECUTIVES:
Chief Executive Officer/President .... Craig Smith

COMPANY PROFILE:
Parent Company Name: Children's Hospital and Health System
Doing Business As:
Year Founded: 2006   Federally Qualified: [ ]
Forprofit: [ ]   Not-For-Profit: [ ]
Model Type: MIXED
Accreditation: [ ] AAPPO [ ] JACHO [ ] NCQA [ ] URAC
Plan Type: HMO
Primary Physicians: 2,817   Physician Specialists:
Hospitals: 25
Total Revenue: 2005:   2006: 4,993,000
Net Income   2005:   2006: -1,383,000
Total Enrollment:
   2001:   2004:   2007:
   2002:   2005:
   2003:   2006: 4,714
Medical Loss Ratio: 2005:   2006:   98.00
Administrative Expense Ratio: 2005:   2006:   22.60

SERVICE AREA:
Nationwide: N
   WI (Kenosha, Milwaukee, Ozaukee, Racine, Walworth, Washington, Waukesha);

TYPE OF COVERAGE:
Commercial: [ ]   Individual: [ ]   FEHBP: [ ]   Indemnity: [ ]
Medicare: [ ]   Medicaid: [Y]   Supplemental Medicare: [ ]
Tricare   [ ]

PRODUCTS OFFERED:
Product Name: Type:
BadgerCare Plus   Medicaid

Comments:
Affiliated with Dean Health Plan Southeast

DEAN HEALTH PLAN

1277 Deming Way
Madison, WI 53717
Phone: 608-836-1400 Fax: 608-836-9620 Toll-Free: 800-356-7344
Web site: www.deancare.com

MAILING ADDRESS:
   DEAN HEALTH PLAN
   PO Box 56099
   Madison, WI 53705-9399

KEY EXECUTIVES:
Chief Executive Officer/President .... Robert Palmer
Chief Medical Officer .... Tom Hirsch, MD
VP, Technology .... Karl Richards
Chief Operating Officer .... Lon Sprecher
VP, Sales .... Edward Pattarozzi
VP, Customer Operations .... Dan Edge
VP, Medical Affairs .... Thomas J Hirsch, MD
Senior VP, Planning & Development .... Robert Myers

COMPANY PROFILE:
Parent Company Name: Dean Health Systems/SSM Health Care Inc
Doing Business As: Dean Care HMO
Year Founded: 1984   Federally Qualified: [Y]
Forprofit: [Y]   Not-For-Profit: [ ]
Model Type: GROUP
Accreditation: [ ] AAPPO [ ] JACHO [X] NCQA [ ] URAC
Plan Type: HMO, PPO, POS,
Primary Physicians: 2,102   Physician Specialists:
Hospitals: 28
Total Revenue: 2005: 653,572,000   2006: 690,171,000
Net Income   2005:   2,767,000   2006:   2,057,000
Total Enrollment:
   2001: 200,029   2004: 214,373   2007: 0
   2002: 211,871   2005: 217,112
   2003: 215,912   2006: 215,340
Medical Loss Ratio: 2005: 93.00   2006: 93.80
Administrative Expense Ratio: 2005:   7.30   2006: 6.20

SERVICE AREA:
Nationwide: N
   WI (Adams, Columbia, Crawford, Dane, Dodge, Fond du Lac, Grant, Green, Green Lake, Iowa, Jefferson, Juneau, Kenosha, Lafayette, Marquette, Racine, Richland, Rock, Sauk, Walworth, Washington, Waukesha);

TYPE OF COVERAGE:
Commercial: [Y]   Individual: [Y]   FEHBP: [ ]   Indemnity: [ ]
Medicare: [Y]   Medicaid: [Y]   Supplemental Medicare: [Y]
Tricare   [ ]

PRODUCTS OFFERED:
Product Name: Type:
Deancare Gold   Medicare Select
                           Triple Option Plan
                           POS
Dean Care HMO   HMO
BadgerCare SCHIP   Medicaid

PLAN BENEFITS:
Alternative Medicine: [ ]   Behavioral Health: [X]
Chiropractic: [X]   Dental: [ ]
Home Care: [X]   Inpatient SNF: [X]
Long-Term Care: [ ]   Pharm. Mail Order: [X]
Physical Therapy: [X]   Podiatry: [X]
Psychiatric: [X]   Transplant: [X]
Vision: [X]   Wellness: [X]
Workers' Comp: [ ]
Other Benefits:

DELTA DENTAL PLAN OF WISCONSIN

1320 S Green Bay Rd
Racine, WI 53406
Phone: 262-637-9371 Fax: 715-344-2446 Toll-Free: 800-236-3713
Web site: www.deltadentalwi.com

MAILING ADDRESS:
   DELTA DENTAL PLAN OF WI
   PO Box 828
   Stevens Point, WI 54481

KEY EXECUTIVES:
Chief Executive Officer/President .... Dennis Brown
VP, Finance .... Patty Glennon
VP, Information Systems .... Lindie Landin
VP, Operations .... Karen Johnson
VP, Marketing .... Gary Rogers
Professional Relations Representative .... Lois Joswick
Corporate Communications Manager .... Bob Walker

COMPANY PROFILE:
Parent Company Name: Delta Dental Plan Association
Doing Business As:
Year Founded: 1962   Federally Qualified: [ ]
Forprofit: [ ]   Not-For-Profit: [Y]
Model Type:
Accreditation: [ ] AAPPO [ ] JACHO [ ] NCQA [ ] URAC
Plan Type: Specialty HMO, Specialty PPO, TPA, POS, ASO
Total Enrollment:
   2001: 114,855   2004: 147,224   2007: 0
   2002: 1,621,885   2005:
   2003: 1,676,984   2006:

SERVICE AREA:
Nationwide: N
   WI;

TYPE OF COVERAGE:
Commercial: [Y]   Individual: [ ]   FEHBP: [ ]   Indemnity: [ ]
Medicare: [ ]   Medicaid: [ ]   Supplemental Medicare: [ ]
Tricare   [ ]

PRODUCTS OFFERED:
Product Name: Type:
Delta Premier   Fee for Service
Delta Preferred Option   Dental PPO
DeltaCare   Dental HMO

PLAN BENEFITS:
Alternative Medicine: [ ]   Behavioral Health: [ ]
Chiropractic: [ ]   Dental: [X]
Home Care: [ ]   Inpatient SNF: [ ]
Long-Term Care: [ ]   Pharm. Mail Order: [ ]
Physical Therapy: [ ]   Podiatry: [ ]
Psychiatric: [ ]   Transplant: [ ]
Vision: [ ]   Wellness: [ ]
Workers' Comp: [ ]
Other Benefits:

WISCONSIN

Managed Care Organization Profiles

MAILING ADDRESS:
  ARISE HEALTH PLAN
  PO Box 11625
  Green Bay, WI 54304

KEY EXECUTIVES:
Chief Executive Officer/President/Chief Operating .... Mark Minsloff
Chief Financial Officer .... Vicki Lorge
Chief Medical Officer .... Jeffrey Young, MD
Pharmacy Director .... Mike Chester
Marketing Manager .... Tom Duffy
Compliance Officer .... Lori Turek
Manager of Network Development .... Karen Christel
Manager of Medical Management .... Connie Polasik
Member Services Manager .... Tina Rybak
Inderwriting Manager .... Bill Baeten
Director of PPO Development .... Tom Reimer

COMPANY PROFILE:
Parent Company Name: Wisconsin Physician Services Ins Co
Doing Business As:
Year Founded: 1996   Federally Qualified: [Y]
Forprofit: [Y]   Not-For-Profit: [ ]
Model Type: NETWORK
Accreditation: [ ] AAPPO [ ] JACHO [ ] NCQA [ ] URAC
Plan Type: HMO, PPO, POS, HDHP, HSA,
Primary Physicians: 1,795   Physician Specialists:
Hospitals:
Total Revenue: 2005: 55,598,000   2006: 85,532,000
Net Income   2005: -2,842,000   2006: 962,000
Total Enrollment:
  2001: 28,011   2004: 33,723   2007: 0
  2002: 25,837   2005: 30,169
  2003: 31,070   2006: 29,062
Medical Loss Ratio: 2005: 94.00   2006: 87.60
Administrative Expense Ratio: 2005: 11.60 2006: 11.70

SERVICE AREA:
Nationwide: N
  WI (Brown, Door, Kewaunee, Manitowoc, Marinette, Oconto, Shawano);

TYPE OF COVERAGE:
Commercial: [Y] Individual: [ ] FEHBP: [ ] Indemnity: [ ]
Medicare: [ ] Medicaid: [ ] Supplemental Medicare: [Y]
Tricare   [ ]

PRODUCTS OFFERED:
Product Name: Type:
Prevea HMO   HMO
Prevea POS   POS
State of WI Contract   HMO
Prevea 65 Plus   PPO

Comments:
Formerly Prevea Health Plan. Formerly WPS Health Plan Inc.

ASSURANT HEALTH - CORPORATE HEADQUARTERS

501 W Michigan Street
Milwaukee, WI 53201-0624
Phone: 414-299-8502 Fax: 414-299-8188 Toll-Free: 800-800-1212
Web site: www.assuranthealthbenefits.com

MAILING ADDRESS:
  ASSURANT HEALTH - CORP HDQTRS
  PO Box 3050
  Milwaukee, WI 53201-0624

KEY EXECUTIVES:
Chief Executive Officer/President .... Don Hamm
Chief Financial Officer .... Howard Miller
Chief Information Officer .... Lance Wilson
Executive VP, Chief Operating Officer .... Rajeev Bal
Senior VP, Marketing .... Debbie Kramer
Chief Sales Officer .... Laura Hohing

COMPANY PROFILE:
Parent Company Name: Assurant Health
Doing Business As:
Year Founded: 1892   Federally Qualified: [ ]
Forprofit: [Y]   Not-For-Profit: [ ]
Model Type:
Accreditation: [ ] AAPPO [ ] JACHO [ ] NCQA [ ] URAC
Plan Type: PPO, CDHP, HDHP, HSA,
Total Revenue: 2005: 7,497,675   2006:
Net Income   2005: 479,355   2006: 167,900,000
Total Enrollment:
  2001: 0   2004: 1,000,000   2007: 0
  2002: 0   2005: 1,000,000
  2003: 0   2006: 1,000,000

SERVICE AREA:
Nationwide: Y
  NW;

TYPE OF COVERAGE:
Commercial: [Y] Individual: [Y] FEHBP: [ ] Indemnity: [ ]
Medicare: [ ] Medicaid: [ ] Supplemental Medicare: [ ]
Tricare   [ ]

Comments:
Formerly Time Insurance Company.

CARE-PLUS DENTAL PLANS INC

11711 W Burleigh Street
Wauwatosa, WI 53222
Phone: 414-771-1711 Fax: 414-456-9911 Toll-Free:
Web site: www.dentalassociates.com

MAILING ADDRESS:
  CARE-PLUS DENTAL PLANS INC
  11711 W Burleigh Street
  Wauwatosa, WI 53222-3108

KEY EXECUTIVES:
Chairman .... John G Gonis
Chief Executive Officer .... Anthony G Vastardis
Chief Financial Officer .... Kurt W Schmidt
Chief Information Officer .... Don Whamond
Marketing Director .... John Krause
Human Resources Director .... Dan Egan
Fraud Prevention Director .... Bruce Spiewak

COMPANY PROFILE:
Parent Company Name: Dental Associates LTD
Doing Business As:
Year Founded: 1983   Federally Qualified: [ ]
Forprofit: [ ]   Not-For-Profit: [Y]
Model Type: STAFF
Accreditation: [ ] AAPPO [ ] JACHO [ ] NCQA [ ] URAC
Plan Type: Specialty HMO
Total Enrollment:
  2001: 61,961   2004: 60,032   2007: 0
  2002: 61,293   2005:
  2003: 60,967   2006:
Medical Loss Ratio: 2005: 99.00   2006:
Administrative Expense Ratio: 2005:   2006:

SERVICE AREA:
Nationwide: N
  WI (Brown, Calumet, Door, Fond du Lac, Kenosha, Kawaunee, Milwaukee, Oconto, Outagamie, Racine, Walworth, Washington, Waukesha, Winnebago);

PRODUCTS OFFERED:
Product Name: Type:
Care-Plus Prepaid
Care-Plus Premier
Care-Plus Gold
Care-Plus Supplement
Care-Plus VIP
Care Credit

PLAN BENEFITS:
Alternative Medicine: [ ]   Behavioral Health: [ ]
Chiropractic: [ ]   Dental: [X]
Home Care: [ ]   Inpatient SNF: [ ]
Long-Term Care: [ ]   Pharm. Mail Order: [ ]
Physical Therapy: [ ]   Podiatry: [ ]
Psychiatric: [ ]   Transplant: [ ]
Vision: [ ]   Wellness: [ ]
Workers' Comp: [ ]
Other Benefits:

CHILDREN'S COMMUNITY HEALTH PLAN INC

1277 Deming Way
Milwaukee, WI 53717
Phone: 414-266-6328 Fax: 608-827-4212 Toll-Free: 800-482-8010
Web site: www.childrenschp.com

Managed Care Organization Profiles — WISCONSIN

ABRI HEALTH PLAN INC

2400 S 102nd St Ste 103
West Allis, WI 53227
Phone: 414-347-1777 Fax: 262-946-1201 Toll-Free: 888-995-2404
Web site: www.abrihealthplan.com

MAILING ADDRESS:
ABRI HEALTH PLAN INC
2400 S 102nd St Ste 103
West Allis, WI 53227

KEY EXECUTIVES:
President .... Ron Scasny
Finance Manager .... Julie Tindall
Provider Relations Director .... Randy Westley
Quality Assurance Director .... Paula Lucier

COMPANY PROFILE:
Parent Company Name:
Doing Business As:
Year Founded: 2004   Federally Qualified: [ ]
Forprofit: [ ]   Not-For-Profit: [ ]
Model Type: Mixed
Accreditation: [ ] AAPPO [ ] JACHO [ ] NCQA [ ] URAC
Plan Type: HMO
Primary Physicians: 500   Physician Specialists: 1,100
Hospitals: 16
Total Revenue: 2005: 10,908,000   2006: 25,446,000
Net Income   2005: 178,000   2006: 1,093,000
Total Enrollment:
  2001: 0   2004: 55,153   2007: 0
  2002: 0   2005: 5,140
  2003: 0   2006: 17,779
Medical Loss Ratio: 2005: 71.10   2006: 78.60
Administrative Expense Ratio: 2005: 22.50   2006: 17.50

SERVICE AREA:
Nationwide:
WI (Kenesha, Milwaukee, Ozaukee, Racine, Waukesha);

TYPE OF COVERAGE:
Commercial: [ ] Individual: [ ] FEHBP: [ ] Indemnity: []
Medicare: [ ] Medicaid: [Y] Supplemental Medicare: [Y]
Tricare   [ ]

ANTHEM BLUE CROSS BLUE SHIELD OF WISCONSIN

N 17 W24340 Riverwood Dr
Waukesha, WI 53188
Phone: 262-523-4020 Fax: 262-523-4772 Toll-Free: 888-239-9514
Web site: www.bcbswi.com

MAILING ADDRESS:
ANTHEM BC BS OF WISCONSIN
N 17 W24340 Riverwood Dr
Waukesha, WI 53188

KEY EXECUTIVES:
General Manager, WI Group .... Steve Martenet
VP, Finance .... Craig Steffes
Medical Director .... Michael Jaeger, MD
Director, Public Relations .... Jill A Becher
VP, Health Services .... John J Foley

COMPANY PROFILE:
Parent Company Name: WellPoint Inc
Doing Business As: BC BS of WI, Compcare Health Services Ins Co
Year Founded: 1984   Federally Qualified: [Y]
Forprofit: [Y]   Not-For-Profit: [ ]
Model Type: NETWORK
Accreditation: [ ] AAPPO [ ] JACHO [ ] NCQA [ ] URAC
Plan Type: HMO, POS, HDHP, HSA,
Primary Physicians: 3,280   Physician Specialists:
Hospitals: 75
Total Revenue: 2005: 397,507,000   2006: 425,968,000
Net Income   2005: 43,418,000   2006: 12,137,000
Total Enrollment:
  2001: 357,831   2004: 200,294   2007: 0
  2002: 250,375   2005:
  2003: 227,779   2006: 89,624
Medical Loss Ratio: 2005: 87.50   2006: 86.30
Administrative Expense Ratio: 2005: 11.00   2006: 13.10

SERVICE AREA:
Nationwide: N
WI;

TYPE OF COVERAGE:
Commercial: [Y] Individual: [ ] FEHBP: [ ] Indemnity: [ ]
Medicare: [Y] Medicaid: [ ] Supplemental Medicare: [ ]
Tricare   [ ]

PRODUCTS OFFERED:
Product Name: **Type:**
CompcareBlue   HMO
CompcareBlue   POS

CONSUMER-DRIVEN PRODUCTS

Compcareblue HSA   HSA Company
                        HSA Product
                        HSA Administrator
                        Consumer-Driven Health Plan
                        High Deductible Health Plan

PLAN BENEFITS:
Alternative Medicine: [ ]   Behavioral Health: [ ]
Chiropractic: [X]   Dental: [ ]
Home Care: [X]   Inpatient SNF: [X]
Long-Term Care: [ ]   Pharm. Mail Order: [X]
Physical Therapy: [X]   Podiatry: [X]
Psychiatric: [X]   Transplant: [X]
Vision: [X]   Wellness: [X]
Workers' Comp: [ ]
Other Benefits:
Comments:
Formerly CompCare Health Services Insurance Corporation.

APS HEALTHCARE MIDWEST INC

300 North Executive Dr
Brookfield, WI 53005
Phone: 262-787-2200 Fax: 262-787-2501 Toll-Free: 800-499-0267
Web site: www.apshealthcare.com

MAILING ADDRESS:
APS HEALTHCARE MIDWEST INC
300 North Executive Dr
Brookfield, WI 53005

KEY EXECUTIVES:
Chief Executive Officer/President .... Eileen Auen, MD
Chief Financial Officer .... Brett McIntyre
Medical Director .... Kenneth Redlin, MD
Chief Information Officer .... Arthur Held
VP of National Medical Sales .... Tom McCormick
Human Resource Director .... Rosemary Finora
VP of Clinical Services .... Jack Melton, MD

COMPANY PROFILE:
Parent Company Name: APS Healthcare Inc
Doing Business As:
Year Founded: 1992   Federally Qualified: [ ]
Forprofit: [Y]   Not-For-Profit: [ ]
Model Type:
Accreditation: [ ] AAPPO [ ] JACHO [X] NCQA [X] URAC
Plan Type: Specialty HMO, Specialty PPO

SERVICE AREA:
Nationwide:
NW;

TYPE OF COVERAGE:
Commercial: [Y] Individual: [ ] FEHBP: [ ] Indemnity: [ ]
Medicare: [Y] Medicaid: [Y] Supplemental Medicare: [ ]
Tricare   [ ]

PLAN BENEFITS:
Alternative Medicine: [ ]   Behavioral Health: [X]
Chiropractic: [ ]   Dental: [ ]
Home Care: [ ]   Inpatient SNF: [ ]
Long-Term Care: [ ]   Pharm. Mail Order: [ ]
Physical Therapy: [ ]   Podiatry: [ ]
Psychiatric: [ ]   Transplant: [ ]
Vision: [ ]   Wellness: [ ]
Workers' Comp: [ ]
Other Benefits:

ARISE HEALTH PLAN

2710 Executive Dr
Green Bay, WI 54304
Phone: 920-490-6938 Fax: 920-490-6942 Toll-Free: 888-833-4988
Web site: www.pspreveahealthplan.com

WEST VIRGINIA

Managed Care Organization Profiles

PLAN BENEFITS:
Alternative Medicine:	[ ]	Behavioral Health:	[X]
Chiropractic:	[X]	Dental:	[ ]
Home Care:	[X]	Inpatient SNF:	[X]
Long-Term Care:	[X]	Pharm. Mail Order:	[X]
Physical Therapy:	[X]	Podiatry:	[ ]
Psychiatric:	[X]	Transplant:	[X]
Vision:	[X]	Wellness:	[X]
Workers' Comp:	[ ]		
Other Benefits:			

Comments:
Formerly Charleston Area Health Plan.

MOUNTAIN STATE BLUE CROSS BLUE SHIELD

700 Market Square
Parkersburg, WV 26102
Phone: 304-424-7700 Fax: 304-424-9878 Toll-Free:
Web site: www.msbcbs.com

MAILING ADDRESS:
MOUNTAIN STATE BC/BS
700 Market Square
Parkersburg, WV 26102

KEY EXECUTIVES:
Chairman of the Board .... Gregory K Smith
Chief Executive Officer/President .... Gregory K Smith
Chief Financial Officer .... J Mark Sengewalt
Senior VP, Operations .... JoAnn Morrison
Marketing Director .... J Fred Earley II
VP, Sales .... Scott N Swartz

COMPANY PROFILE:
Parent Company Name: Blue Cross Blue Shield Association
Doing Business As:
Year Founded: 1993   Federally Qualified: [ ]
Forprofit: [ ]   Not-For-Profit: [Y]
Model Type:
Accreditation: [ ] AAPPO [ ] JACHO [ ] NCQA [ ] URAC
Plan Type: PPO, POS, TPA
Total Revenue: 2005: 603,439   2006: 710,808
Net Income 2005: 22,574   2006: 17,503
Total Enrollment:
  2001: 153,734   2004: 173,110   2007: 0
  2002: 158,210   2005: 245,000
  2003: 164,725   2006:

SERVICE AREA:
Nationwide: N
  OH; WV;

TYPE OF COVERAGE:
Commercial: [Y] Individual: [Y] FEHBP: [ ] Indemnity: [ ]
Medicare: [ ] Medicaid: [ ] Supplemental Medicare: [Y]
Tricare [ ]

PRODUCTS OFFERED:
Product Name:	Type:
Super Blue Plus	PPO
Super Blue Select	POS
New Blue	Indemnity

PLAN BENEFITS:
Alternative Medicine:	[ ]	Behavioral Health:	[X]
Chiropractic:	[X]	Dental:	[X]
Home Care:	[X]	Inpatient SNF:	[X]
Long-Term Care:	[ ]	Pharm. Mail Order:	[ ]
Physical Therapy:	[X]	Podiatry:	[X]
Psychiatric:	[X]	Transplant:	[X]
Vision:	[X]	Wellness:	[X]
Workers' Comp:	[ ]		
Other Benefits:			

WEST VIRGINIA MEDICAL INSTITUTE

3001 Chesterfield Pl
Charleston, WV 25304
Phone: 304-346-9864 Fax: 304-346-9863 Toll-Free: 800-642-8686
Web site: www.wvmi.org

MAILING ADDRESS:
WEST VIRGINIA MED INSTITUTE
3001 Chesterfield Pl
Charleston, WV 25304

KEY EXECUTIVES:
Chief Executive Officer .... John C Wiesendanger
Chief Financial Officer .... Kathleen Merrill
Chief Medical Officer .... John G Brehm, MD, FACP
Chief Information Officer .... Gary Hamrick
Communications Director .... Marc McCombs
Director of Human Resources .... Laura Nauman

COMPANY PROFILE:
Parent Company Name:
Doing Business As:
Year Founded: 1973   Federally Qualified: [ ]
Forprofit: [ ]   Not-For-Profit: [Y]
Model Type:
Accreditation: [ ] AAPPO [ ] JACHO [ ] NCQA [ ] URAC
Plan Type: UR, PRO, EPO

SERVICE AREA:
Nationwide: Y
  NW;

Managed Care Organization Profiles — WEST VIRGINIA

4MOST HEALTH NETWORK

323 Call Rd
Charleston, WV 25312
Phone: 304-720-6801 Fax: 304-720-6810 Toll-Free: 888-258-6477
Web site: www.4most.com

MAILING ADDRESS:
4MOST HEALTH NETWORK
PO Box 13429
Charleston, WV 25312

KEY EXECUTIVES:
President .... John A Fischer
VP, Network & Financial Affairs .... Vince Sowards
Medical Director .... John P Lilly, MD
Senior Credentialing Manager .... Tammy Brown
HIPPA Compliance Officer .... Dianna R Hardin
Director of Network Affairs .... Brenda K Alexander
Director, Human Resources/Quality Assurance .... Lisa A Painter
VP, Business Development .... Gary C Shorter
Account Service Manager .... Dianna R Hardin

COMPANY PROFILE:
Parent Company Name: Physician Services LC
Doing Business As:
Year Founded: 1999   Federally Qualified: [ ]
Forprofit: [Y]   Not-For-Profit: [ ]
Model Type: MIXED
Accreditation: [ ] AAPPO [ ] JACHO [ ] NCQA [ ] URAC
Plan Type: PPO
Primary Physicians: 2,795   Physician Specialists: 7,932
Hospitals: 119
Total Enrollment:
  2001: 0   2004: 0   2007: 204,000
  2002: 0   2005:
  2003: 0   2006:

SERVICE AREA:
Nationwide:
  KY; MD; OH; PA; VA; WV;

TYPE OF COVERAGE:
Commercial: [Y] Individual: [Y] FEHBP: [ ] Indemnity: [ ]
Medicare: [ ] Medicaid: [ ] Supplemental Medicare: [ ]
Tricare [ ]

PRODUCTS OFFERED:
Product Name: Type:
4MOST Health PPO   PPO

PLAN BENEFITS:
Alternative Medicine: [ ]   Behavioral Health: [ ]
Chiropractic: [ ]   Dental: [X]
Home Care: [ ]   Inpatient SNF: [ ]
Long-Term Care: [ ]   Pharm. Mail Order: [ ]
Physical Therapy: [ ]   Podiatry: [ ]
Psychiatric: [ ]   Transplant: [ ]
Vision: [ ]   Wellness: [ ]
Workers' Comp: [X]
Other Benefits:

CARELINK HEALTH ASSURANCE

2001 Main St Ste 202
Wheeling, WV 26003
Phone: 304-234-5100 Fax: 304-234-5119 Toll-Free: 800-896-9612
Web site: www.chccarelink.com

MAILING ADDRESS:
CARELINK HEALTH ASSURANCE
2001 Main St Ste 202
Wheeling, WV 26003

KEY EXECUTIVES:
Chief Executive Officer .... Cosby M Davis, III
Executive Director/Plan Chief Operating Offr ...... Harold E Preston, Jr
Marketing Director .... Gene Kanter
Public Relations Director .... Mary Sandridge
Network Development Director .... Bruce Cash

COMPANY PROFILE:
Parent Company Name: Coventry Health Care Inc
Doing Business As: American Service Life Insurance Company
Year Founded: 1995   Federally Qualified: [N]
Forprofit: [Y]   Not-For-Profit: [ ]
Model Type: NETWORK
Accreditation: [ ] AAPPO [ ] JACHO [ ] NCQA [ ] URAC
Plan Type: HMO, PPO, POS
Hospitals: 60

SERVICE AREA:
Nationwide: N
  WV (Barbour, Brooke, Doddridge, Hancock, Harrison, Marshall, Monongalia, Ohio, Preston, Taylor);

TYPE OF COVERAGE:
Commercial: [Y] Individual: [ ] FEHBP: [ ] Indemnity: [ ]
Medicare: [Y] Medicaid: [ ] Supplemental Medicare: [ ]
Tricare [ ]

PRODUCTS OFFERED:
Product Name: Type:
HealthAssurance HMO   HMO

CONSUMER-DRIVEN PRODUCTS
Wells Fargo   HSA Company
                                    HSA Product
Corporate Benefits Services of America   HSA Administrator
                                    Consumer-Driven Health Plan
Open Access Plus Plan   High Deductible Health Plan

PLAN BENEFITS:
Alternative Medicine: [ ]   Behavioral Health: [ ]
Chiropractic: [X]   Dental: [X]
Home Care: [X]   Inpatient SNF: [X]
Long-Term Care: [X]   Pharm. Mail Order: [X]
Physical Therapy: [X]   Podiatry: [X]
Psychiatric: [X]   Transplant: [X]
Vision: [X]   Wellness: [X]
Workers' Comp: [ ]
Other Benefits:

CARELINK HEALTH PLANS

500 Virginia St Ste 400
Charleston, WV 25301
Phone: 304-348-2900 Fax: 304-348-2948 Toll-Free: 888-388-1744
Web site: www.chccarelink.com

MAILING ADDRESS:
CARELINK HEALTH PLANS
500 Virginia St Ste 400
Charleston, WV 25301

KEY EXECUTIVES:
Chief Executive Officer .... Cosby M Davis, III
Executive Director/Plan Chief Operating Offr ...... Harold E Preston, Jr
Marketing Director .... Gene Kanter
Network Development Director .... Bruce Cash
Quality Assurance Manager .... Patty Coffield

COMPANY PROFILE:
Parent Company Name: Coventry Health Care Inc
Doing Business As: Carelink Health Plans
Year Founded: 1994   Federally Qualified: [N]
Forprofit: [Y]   Not-For-Profit: [ ]
Model Type: MIXED
Accreditation: [ ] AAPPO [ ] JACHO [X] NCQA [X] URAC
Plan Type: HMO, PPO, POS, ASO, TPA
Primary Physicians: 3,165   Physician Specialists:
Hospitals: 67
Total Enrollment:
  2001: 88,990   2004: 49,293   2007: 0
  2002: 65,290   2005:
  2003: 59,501   2006:

SERVICE AREA:
Nationwide: N
  WV (Boone, Braxton, Calhoun, Clay, Fayette, Jackson, Kanawha, Lincoln, Logan, Marion, McDowell, Mingo, Monongalia, Monroe, Pocohontas, Preston, Putnam, Raleigh, Roane, Summers, Webster, Wood, Wyoming, Logan, Marion, Wirt.

TYPE OF COVERAGE:
Commercial: [Y] Individual: [ ] FEHBP: [ ] Indemnity: [ ]
Medicare: [Y] Medicaid: [Y] Supplemental Medicare: [Y]
Tricare [ ]

PRODUCTS OFFERED:
Product Name: Type:
PrimeOne HMO   HMO
Carelink's Gold Health Plan Medicare
Medicaid   MedicaidMedicare Wrap
Medicare
ASO
HealthAssurance PPO   PPO

WASHINGTON

KEY EXECUTIVES:
Chairman of the Board .... *Eugene Skourtes, DMD*
Chief Executive Officer/President .... *Stephen J Petruzelli*
Chief Financial Officer .... *Yuen Chin*
Medical Director .... *Gary Allen, DMD*
Sales & Marketing Consultant .... *Steve Malvick*
Director of Information Systems .... *John Shields*
Human Resources Director .... *Kris Holgerson*

COMPANY PROFILE:
Parent Company Name:
Doing Business As:
Year Founded: Federally Qualified: [ ]
Forprofit: [Y]   Not-For-Profit: [ ]
Model Type:
Accreditation: [ ] AAPPO [ ] JACHO [ ] NCQA [ ] URAC
Plan Type: Specialty HMO
Total Revenue: 2005: 10,503,300   2006: 11,281,946
Net Income   2005:   253,625   2006:   303,558
Total Enrollment:
   2001:   0   2004:   0   2007: 70,043
   2002:   0   2005: 68,525
   2003: 58,143   2006: 68,948

SERVICE AREA:
Nationwide: N
   WA;

TYPE OF COVERAGE:
Commercial: [Y] Individual: [ ]   FEHBP: [ ]   Indemnity: [ ]
Medicare: [ ] Medicaid: [ ]   Supplemental Medicare: [ ]
Tricare   [ ]

PLAN BENEFITS:
Alternative Medicine: [ ]   Behavioral Health: [ ]
Chiropractic: [ ]   Dental: [X]
Home Care: [ ]   Inpatient SNF: [ ]
Long-Term Care: [ ]   Pharm. Mail Order: [ ]
Physical Therapy: [ ]   Podiatry: [ ]
Psychiatric: [ ]   Transplant: [ ]
Vision: [ ]   Wellness: [ ]
Workers' Comp: [ ]
Other Benefits:

Comments:
Formerly Columbia Dental of Washington Inc.

UNITED CONCORDIA COMPANY INC - WASHINGTON

2200 Sixth Ave Ste 804
Seattle, WA 98121
Phone: 888-245-8224 Fax: 206-728-2740 Toll-Free: 888-245-8224
Web site: www.ucci.com
MAILING ADDRESS:
UNITED CONCORDIA CO INC - WA
2200 Sixth Ave Ste 804
Seattle, WA 98121

KEY EXECUTIVES:
Chief Executive Officer/President .... Thomas A Dzuryachko
Chief Financial Officer .... Daniel Wright
VP, National Dental Director .... Richard Klich, DMD
Director of Sales .... Troy Mundy

COMPANY PROFILE:
Parent Company Name: Highmark Inc
Doing Business As:
Year Founded: 1991   Federally Qualified: [ ]
Forprofit: [Y]   Not-For-Profit: [ ]
Model Type:
Accreditation: [ ] AAPPO [ ] JACHO [ ] NCQA [ ] URAC
Plan Type: Specialty HMO, Specialty PPO, POS, TPA
SERVICE AREA:
Nationwide: N
AK; ID; MT; OR; WA; WY;
TYPE OF COVERAGE:
Commercial: [Y] Individual: [ ] FEHBP: [ ] Indemnity: [ ]
Medicare: [ ] Medicaid: [ ] Supplemental Medicare: [ ]
Tricare   [ ]
PLAN BENEFITS:
Alternative Medicine: [ ]   Behavioral Health: [ ]
Chiropractic: [ ]   Dental: [X]
Home Care: [ ]   Inpatient SNF: [ ]
Long-Term Care: [ ]   Pharm. Mail Order: [ ]
Physical Therapy: [ ]   Podiatry: [ ]
Psychiatric: [ ]   Transplant: [ ]
Vision: [ ]   Wellness: [ ]
Workers' Comp: [ ]
Other Benefits:

UNITEDHEALTHCARE OF WASHINGTON

7525 SE 24th St
Mercer Island, WA 98040
Phone: 206-236-2500 Fax: 206-230-7496 Toll-Free: 800-829-2925
Web site: www.pacificare.com
MAILING ADDRESS:
UNITEDHEALTHCARE OF WASHINGTON
7525 SE 24th St
Mercer Island, WA 98040

KEY EXECUTIVES:
Chief Executive Officer/President .... Murphy J Hensley
Medical Director .... Roger Muller, MD
Chief Financial Officer .... Susan L Berkel

COMPANY PROFILE:
Parent Company Name: UnitedHealth Group
Doing Business As:
Year Founded: 1981   Federally Qualified: [Y]
Forprofit: [Y]   Not-For-Profit: [ ]
Model Type: IPA/GROUP
Accreditation: [ ] AAPPO [ ] JACHO [ ] NCQA   [ ]
URACPlan Type: HMO, POS, HSA
Total Revenue: 2005: 246,478,080   2006: 258,750,895
Net Income   2005: 15,146,757   2006: 19,715,798
Total Enrollment:
    2001: 135,901   2004: 94,207   2007: 52,399
    2002: 118,182   2005: 68,815
    2003: 117,964   2006: 62,159
SERVICE AREA:
Nationwide: N
WA (Chelan (parts), Clark, Cowlitz, Douglas (parts), Ferry, Grays Harbor, Island, King, Kitsap, Lewis, Mason, Okanogan, Pend Oreille, Pierce, San Juan, Skagit, Snohomish, Spokane, Stevens, Thurston, Walla Walla, Whitman);
TYPE OF COVERAGE:
Commercial: [Y] Individual: [ ] FEHBP: [ ] Indemnity: [ ]
Medicare: [Y] Medicaid: [ ] Supplemental Medicare: [ ]
Tricare   [ ]

PRODUCTS OFFERED:
Product Name: Type:
Secure Horizons   Medicare Advantage
Pacificare of WA HMO   HMO
PLAN BENEFITS:
Alternative Medicine: [ ]   Behavioral Health: [X]
Chiropractic: [X]   Dental: [X]
Home Care: [X]   Inpatient SNF: [X]
Long-Term Care: [ ]   Pharm. Mail Order: [X]
Physical Therapy: [X]   Podiatry: [X]
Psychiatric: [X]   Transplant: [X]
Vision: [X]   Wellness: [X]
Workers' Comp: [X]
Other Benefits:

WASHINGTON DENTAL SERVICE

9706 Fourth Ave NE
Seattle, WA 98115
Phone: 206-522-1300 Fax: 206-525-2330 Toll-Free: 800-367-4104
Web site: www.deltadentalwa.com
MAILING ADDRESS:
WASHINGTON DENTAL SERVICE
PO BOX 75983
Seattle, WA 98115

KEY EXECUTIVES:
Chief Executive Officer/President .... James D Dwyer
Chief Financial Officer .... Tracy Warner
Dental Director .... Ron Inge, DDS
Chief Information Officer .... Craig Gowdey
Marketing Director .... Kristin Merlo
Human Resources Director .... Larry Leopold

COMPANY PROFILE:
Parent Company Name: Delta Dental Plans Association
Doing Business As:
Year Founded: 1954   Federally Qualified: [ ]
Forprofit: [ ]   Not-For-Profit: [Y]
Model Type:
Accreditation: [ ] AAPPO [ ] JACHO [ ] NCQA [ ] URAC
Plan Type: Specialty PPO
Total Revenue: 2005: 165,381,224   2006: 173,862,015
Net Income   2005:   7,339,353   2006: 12,916,206
Total Enrollment:
    2001: 838,614   2004: 819,280   2007: 907,902
    2002: 822,156   2005: 544,183
    2003: 813,906   2006: 884,468
SERVICE AREA:
Nationwide: N
WA;
TYPE OF COVERAGE:
Commercial: [Y] Individual: [ ] FEHBP: [ ] Indemnity: [ ]
Medicare: [ ] Medicaid: [ ] Supplemental Medicare: [Y]
Tricare   [ ]
PLAN BENEFITS:
Alternative Medicine: [ ]   Behavioral Health: [ ]
Chiropractic: [ ]   Dental: [X]
Home Care: [ ]   Inpatient SNF: [ ]
Long-Term Care: [ ]   Pharm. Mail Order: [ ]
Physical Therapy: [ ]   Podiatry: [ ]
Psychiatric: [ ]   Transplant: [ ]
Vision: [ ]   Wellness: [ ]
Workers' Comp: [ ]
Other Benefits:

WILLIAMETTE DENTAL OF WASHINGTON INC

6950 NE Campus Way
Hillsboro, OR 97124-5611
Phone: 503-952-2000 Fax: 503-952-2200 Toll-Free: 800-460-7644
Web site: www.denkor.com
MAILING ADDRESS:
WILLIAMETTE DENTAL OF WA INC
6950 NE Campus Way
Hillsboro, OR 97124-5611

WASHINGTON

PLAN BENEFITS:
Alternative Medicine:	[ ]	Behavioral Health:	[X]
Chiropractic:	[X]	Dental:	[ ]
Home Care:	[X]	Inpatient SNF:	[X]
Long-Term Care:	[X]	Pharm. Mail Order:	[ ]
Physical Therapy:	[X]	Podiatry:	[X]
Psychiatric:	[X]	Transplant:	[X]
Vision:	[ ]	Wellness:	[ ]
Workers' Comp:	[X]		
Other Benefits:			

REGENCE BLUE SHIELD

1800 Ninth Ave
Seattle, WA 98101-1322
Phone: 206-464-3600 Fax: 206-292-9935 Toll-Free: 800-544-4246
Web site: www.wa.regence.com

MAILING ADDRESS:
REGENCE BLUE SHIELD
PO Box 21267
Seattle, WA 98101-1322

KEY EXECUTIVES:
Chairman of the Board .... Terry W Torgenrud, MD
President .... Mary O McWilliams
Senior VP, Chief Medical Officer/Healthcre ... Jeffrey A Robertson, MD
Assistant VP, Information Services .... Steve Swanson
VP, Provider Network Management .... John Wagner
VP, Human Resources .... Charles Pricknell
Senior Vice President .... Margaret Stanley
Senior Vice President .... John Pierre
VP, General Counsel .... JoAnne Long

COMPANY PROFILE:
Parent Company Name: The Regence Group
Doing Business As:
Year Founded: 1917   Federally Qualified: [N]
Forprofit: [ ]   Not-For-Profit: [Y]
Model Type: GROUP
Accreditation: [ ] AAPPO [ ] JACHO [ ] NCQA [X] URAC
Plan Type: HMO, PPO, POS, TPA, ASO, HDHP, HSA,
Total Enrollment:
 2001: 1,005,677   2004: 853,245   2007: 885,521
 2002: 1,017,729   2005:
 2003: 937,144   2006: 945,954

SERVICE AREA:
Nationwide: N
 WA (17 Counties);

TYPE OF COVERAGE:
Commercial: [Y] Individual: [Y] FEHBP: [ ] Indemnity: [ ]
Medicare: [ ] Medicaid: [Y] Supplemental Medicare: [Y]
Tricare [ ]

PRODUCTS OFFERED:
Product Name:	Type:
Regence BS	Medicaid

CONSUMER-DRIVEN PRODUCTS
	HSA Company
HSA 101	HSA Product
Wells Fargo	HSA Administrator
	Consumer-Driven Health Plan
	High Deductible Health Plan

PLAN BENEFITS:
Alternative Medicine:	[X]	Behavioral Health:	[X]
Chiropractic:	[X]	Dental:	[X]
Home Care:	[X]	Inpatient SNF:	[X]
Long-Term Care:	[X]	Pharm. Mail Order:	[X]
Physical Therapy:	[X]	Podiatry:	[X]
Psychiatric:	[X]	Transplant:	[X]
Vision:	[X]	Wellness:	[X]
Workers' Comp:	[ ]		
Other Benefits:			

Comments:
Formerly Grays Harbor Medical Bureau.

REGENCE BLUE SHIELD

333 Gilkey Rd
Burlington, WA 98233-2823
Phone: 360-527-4000 Fax: 206-389-5669 Toll-Free: 800-659-7229
Web site: www.wa.regence.com

MAILING ADDRESS:
REGENCE BLUE SHIELD
333 Gilkey Rd
Burlington, WA 98233-2823

KEY EXECUTIVES:
Chairman of the Board .... Terry W Torgenrud, MD
President .... Mary O McWilliams
Chief Medical Officer .... R Scott French, MD

COMPANY PROFILE:
Parent Company Name: The Regence Group
Doing Business As:
Year Founded: 1933   Federally Qualified: [ ]
Forprofit: [ ]   Not-For-Profit: [ ]
Model Type:
Accreditation: [ ] AAPPO [ ] JACHO [ ] NCQA [ ] URAC
Plan Type: PPO, UR, POS, HDHP, HSA,

SERVICE AREA:
Nationwide: N
 WA (Island, Skagit, San Juan);

TYPE OF COVERAGE:
Commercial: [Y] Individual: [Y] FEHBP: [ ] Indemnity: [ ]
Medicare: [ ] Medicaid: [Y] Supplemental Medicare: [Y]
Tricare [ ]

PLAN BENEFITS:
Alternative Medicine:	[ ]	Behavioral Health:	[X]
Chiropractic:	[X]	Dental:	[X]
Home Care:	[X]	Inpatient SNF:	[ ]
Long-Term Care:	[ ]	Pharm. Mail Order:	[ ]
Physical Therapy:	[ ]	Podiatry:	[X]
Psychiatric:	[X]	Transplant:	[X]
Vision:	[X]	Wellness:	[X]
Workers' Comp:	[ ]		
Other Benefits:			

Comments:
Formerly called Northwest Washington Medical Bureau.

REGENCECARE

1800 Ninth Ave
Seattle, WA 98101-1621
Phone: 206-464-3663 Fax: 206-389-5669 Toll-Free:
Web site: www.regence.com

MAILING ADDRESS:
REGENCECARE
1800 Ninth Ave
Seattle, WA 98101-1621

KEY EXECUTIVES:
Chief Executive Officer/President .... Mary O McWilliams
Chief Financial Officer .... Eric M Tanaka
Chief Medical Officer .... Jeffrey A Robertson, MD

COMPANY PROFILE:
Parent Company Name: Regence Blue Shield
Doing Business As:
Year Founded: 1986   Federally Qualified: [Y]
Forprofit: [Y]   Not-For-Profit: [ ]
Model Type:
Accreditation: [ ] AAPPO [ ] JACHO [ ] NCQA [ ] URAC
Plan Type: HMO, HDHP, HSA,
Total Enrollment:
 2001: 42,256   2004: 21,221   2007: 0
 2002: 37,560   2005:
 2003: 22,970   2006:

SERVICE AREA:
Nationwide: N
 WA (King, Pierce, Snohomish, Spokane);

TYPE OF COVERAGE:
Commercial: [Y] Individual: [Y] FEHBP: [ ] Indemnity: [ ]
Medicare: [Y] Medicaid: [ ] Supplemental Medicare: [ ]
Tricare [ ]

CONSUMER-DRIVEN PRODUCTS
	HSA Company
HSA 101	HSA Product
Wells Fargo	HSA Administrator
	Consumer-Driven Health Plan
	High Deductible Health Plan

Managed Care Organization Profiles — WASHINGTON

Model Type: MIXED
Accreditation: [ ] AAPPO [ ] JACHO [ ] NCQA [ ] URAC
Plan Type: HMO, PPO, POS, CDHP, HSA
Primary Physicians: 35,000   Physician Specialists:
Hospitals: 193
Total Enrollment:
   2001: 974,795   2004: 793,289   2007: 726,319
   2002: 912,444   2005:
   2003: 904,190   2006: 714,406

SERVICE AREA:
Nationwide: N
   WA;

TYPE OF COVERAGE:
Commercial: [Y] Individual: [Y] FEHBP: [ ] Indemnity: [ ]
Medicare: [Y] Medicaid: [ ] Supplemental Medicare: [Y]
Tricare [ ]

PRODUCTS OFFERED:
Product Name:	Type:
MSC Classic Care	Medicare
Premera Blue Cross	Medicaid

CONSUMER-DRIVEN PRODUCTS
	HSA Company
Personal Dimensions HSA	HSA Product
	HSA Administrator
Dimensions	Consumer-Driven Health Plan
Personal Dimensions	High Deductible Health Plan

PLAN BENEFITS:
Alternative Medicine: [ ]   Behavioral Health: [X]
Chiropractic: [X]   Dental: [X]
Home Care: [X]   Inpatient SNF: [ ]
Long-Term Care: [X]   Pharm. Mail Order: [X]
Physical Therapy: [ ]   Podiatry: [X]
Psychiatric: [X]   Transplant: [X]
Vision: [X]   Wellness: [X]
Workers' Comp: [ ]
Other Benefits:

PRIVATE HEALTHCARE SYSTEMS - WASHINGTON

19515 North Creek Pkwy #308
Bothell, WA 98011
Phone: 425-806-2626 Fax: 425-488-5610 Toll-Free: 800-253-4417
Web site: www.phcs.com

MAILING ADDRESS:
   PRIVATE HEALTHCARE SYSTEMS-WA
   1100 Winter St
   Waltham, MA 98011

KEY EXECUTIVES:
Chief Executive Officer/President .... Mark Tabak
Executive VP, Chief Financial Officer .... Richard Gerstein
Medical Director .... Dr Goldstein
Executive VP, Chief of Operations .... Michael Ferrante
Executive VP, Marketing .... Warren Handelman

COMPANY PROFILE:
Parent Company Name: MultiPlan Inc
Doing Business As:
Year Founded: 1991   Federally Qualified: [N]
Forprofit: [Y]   Not-For-Profit: [ ]
Model Type:
Accreditation: [ ] AAPPO [ ] JACHO [X] NCQA [X] URAC
Plan Type: PPO, POS, UR

SERVICE AREA:
Nationwide: N
   WA;

TYPE OF COVERAGE:
Commercial: [Y] Individual: [ ] FEHBP: [ ] Indemnity: [ ]
Medicare: [ ] Medicaid: [ ] Supplemental Medicare: [ ]
Tricare [ ]

PLAN BENEFITS:
Alternative Medicine: [X]   Behavioral Health: [X]
Chiropractic: [X]   Dental: [ ]
Home Care: [X]   Inpatient SNF: [X]
Long-Term Care: [X]   Pharm. Mail Order: [X]
Physical Therapy: [X]   Podiatry: [X]
Psychiatric: [X]   Transplant: [X]
Vision: [X]   Wellness: [ ]
Workers' Comp: [X]
Other Benefits:

Comments:
Acquired by MultiPlan, Inc. on October 18, 2006.

PUGET SOUND HEALTH PARTNERS

7502 Lakewood Dr W Ste A
Lakewood, WA 98499-8410
Phone: 253-779-8830 Fax: 253-658-2969 Toll-Free:
Web site: www.ourPSHP.com

MAILING ADDRESS:
   PUGET SOUND HEALTH PARTNERS
   7502 Lakewood Dr W Ste A
   Lakewood, WA 98499-8410

KEY EXECUTIVES:
Chief Executive Officer .... Lawrence W Sing Loo
Chief Financial Officer .... Sharon D Waymire
Chief Medical Officer .... Corinne E Jedynak-Bell, DO
Director, Operations .... Nancy Rickenbach
Director, Network Development/Sales & Marketing ..... Christine Turner

COMPANY PROFILE:
Parent Company Name:
Doing Business As:
Year Founded: 2007   Federally Qualified: [N]
Forprofit: [Y]   Not-For-Profit: [ ]
Model Type:
Accreditation: [ ] AAPPO [ ] JACHO [ ] NCQA [ ] URAC
Plan Type: HMO

SERVICE AREA:
Nationwide: N
   WA;

TYPE OF COVERAGE:
Commercial: [ ] Individual: [ ] FEHBP: [ ] Indemnity: [ ]
Medicare: [Y] Medicaid: [ ] Supplemental Medicare: [ ]
Tricare [ ]

QUALIS HEALTH

10700 Meridian Ave N Ste 100
Seattle, WA 98133-9075
Phone: 206-364-9700 Fax: 206-368-2419 Toll-Free: 800-949-7536
Web site: www.qualishealth.org

MAILING ADDRESS:
   QUALIS HEALTH
   PO Box 3340
   Seattle, WA 98133-9075

KEY EXECUTIVES:
Chief Executive Officer/President .... Jonathan Sugarman, MD, MPH
VP, Finance/Administration .... Robin Shuler, CPA, MBA
Senior Medical Director .... Lydia Bartholomew, MD, MHA, CPE
Chief Information Officer/MIS Director .... Mary Sellers
VP, Business Development .... Michael Garrett, MS, CCM
Privacy Officer .... Denise Perkins
Public Relations Director .... Evan Stults
Human Resources Director .... Joni Chenoweth
Chief Operating Officer .... Marci Weis, RN, MPH, CCM
Quality Assurance Director .... Loy Maslen, RNC, MSN, NNP
Risk & Financial Management Director .... Donna Christiansen
Compliance Officer .... Denise Perkins

COMPANY PROFILE:
Parent Company Name: Qualis Health
Doing Business As: Qualis Health
Year Founded: 1974   Federally Qualified: [N]
Forprofit: [ ]   Not-For-Profit: [Y]
Model Type:
Accreditation: [ ] AAPPO [ ] JACHO [ ] NCQA [X] URAC
Plan Type: UR

SERVICE AREA:
Nationwide: Y
   NW;

TYPE OF COVERAGE:
Commercial: [Y] Individual: [ ] FEHBP: [ ] Indemnity: [ ]
Medicare: [Y] Medicaid: [Y] Supplemental Medicare: [ ]
Tricare [ ]

PRODUCTS OFFERED:
Product Name:	Type:
Case Management	
Quality Improvement	
Utilization Management	
Systems Auditing	

WASHINGTON

Managed Care Organization Profiles

Total Enrollment:
2001: 0	2004: 5,053	2007: 2,850
2002: 1,997	2005: 4,744	
2003: 3,037	2006: 3,428	

SERVICE AREA:
Nationwide:
    WA:

TYPE OF COVERAGE:
Commercial: [ ] Individual: [ ] FEHBP: [ ] Indemnity: [ ]
Medicare: [ ] Medicaid: [ ] Supplemental Medicare: [ ]
Tricare [ ]

PRODUCTS OFFERED:
Product Name:	Type:
Pacificare VisionCare	Specialty PPO

PREMERA - CORPORATE HEADQUARTERS

7001 220th St SW
Mountlake Terrace, WA 98043-2124
Phone: 425-670-4000 Fax: 425-918-5575 Toll-Free: 800-840-8216
Web site: www.premera.com

MAILING ADDRESS:
    PREMERA - CORPORATE
    7001 220th St SW
    Mountlake Terrace, WA 98043-2124

KEY EXECUTIVES:
Chief Executive Officer/President .... HR Brereton Barlow
Executive VP, Finance/Chief Financial Officer .... Kent Marquardt
Senior VP, Chief Medical Officer .... John L Castiglia, MD
Director of Pharmacy .... Edward Wong, PharmD
Senior VP, Chief Information Officer .... Kirsten Simonitsch
Executive VP, Operations .... Karen Bartlett
Executive VP, Chief Marketing Executive .... Heyward Donigan
Senior VP, Human Resources .... Barbara Magusin
Chief Legal/Public Policy Officer .... Yori Milo
Executive VP, Strategic Development/Health Care Serv ... Brian Ancell
Senior VP, Health Care Delivery System .... Richard Maturi

COMPANY PROFILE:
Parent Company Name:
Doing Business As: Premera Blue Cross
Year Founded: 1933   Federally Qualified: [ ]
Forprofit: [ ]   Not-For-Profit: [Y]
Model Type:
Accreditation: [ ] AAPPO [ ] JACHO [ ] NCQA [ ] URAC
Plan Type: HMO, PPO, POS, CDHP, HDHP, HSA,
Primary Physicians: 35,000   Physician Specialists:
Hospitals: 193
Total Revenue 2005: 3,061,269,000 2006: 3,093,741,000
Net Income 2005: 90,928,000 2006: 121,360,000
Total Enrollment:
2001: 0	2004: 1,477,000	2007: 1,514,000
2002: 2,147,810	2005: 1,200,000	
2003: 1,550,000	2006: 1,570,000	

SERVICE AREA:
Nationwide:
    AK; AZ; OR; WA;

TYPE OF COVERAGE:
Commercial: [Y] Individual: [Y] FEHBP: [ ] Indemnity: [ ]
Medicare: [Y] Medicaid: [ ] Supplemental Medicare: [Y]
Tricare [ ]

PRODUCTS OFFERED:
Product Name:	Type:
LifeWise Health Plan of AZ	
LifeWise Health Plan of OR	
Premera Blue Cross of AK	
Premera BC of WA - Eastern	
Premera BC of WA - Western	

CONSUMER-DRIVEN PRODUCTS
HSA Bank	HSA Company
Personal Dimensions HSA	HSA Product
FlexBen and HSA Bank	HSA Administrator
Dimensions	Consumer-Driven Health Plan
Personal Dimensions	High Deductible Health Plan

PLAN BENEFITS:
Alternative Medicine:	[ ]	Behavioral Health:	[X]
Chiropractic:	[X]	Dental:	[X]
Home Care:	[X]	Inpatient SNF:	[ ]
Long-Term Care:	[X]	Pharm. Mail Order:	[X]
Physical Therapy:	[ ]	Podiatry:	[X]
Psychiatric:	[X]	Transplant:	[X]
Vision:	[X]	Wellness:	[X]
Workers' Comp:	[ ]		
Other Benefits:			

PREMERA BLUE CROSS - EASTERN

3900 E Sprague Ave
Spokane, WA 99202
Phone: 509-252-7460 Fax: 425-918-5575 Toll-Free: 800-572-0778
Web site: www.premera.com

MAILING ADDRESS:
    PREMERA BLUE CROSS - EASTERN
    3900 E Sprague Ave
    Spokane, WA 99202

KEY EXECUTIVES:
Chief Executive Officer/President .... HR Brereton Barlow
Executive VP, Finance/Chief Financial Officer .... Kent Marquardt
Senior VP, Chief Medical Officer .... John L Castiglia, MD
Director of Pharmacy .... Edward Wong, PharmD
Senior VP, Chief Information Officer .... Kirsten Simonitsch
Executive VP, Operations .... Karen Bartlett
Executive VP, Chief Marketing Executive .... Heyward Donigan
Senior VP, Human Resources .... Barbara Magusin
Chief Legal/Public Policy Officer .... Yori Milo
Executive VP, Strategic Development/Health Care Srv ..... Brian Ancell
Senior VP, Health Care Delivery System .... Richard Maturi
Senior VP, Chief Information Officer .... Alan Smit
Network Development .... Brent Stanyer

COMPANY PROFILE:
Parent Company Name: Premera Blue Cross
Doing Business As:
Year Founded: 1933   Federally Qualified: [ ]
Forprofit: [ ]   Not-For-Profit: [Y]
Model Type:
Accreditation: [ ] AAPPO [ ] JACHO [X] NCQA [ ] URAC
Plan Type: HMO, PPO, POS, CDHP, HDHP, HSA,:

SERVICE AREA:
Nationwide: N
    WA (Central and Eastern);

TYPE OF COVERAGE:
Commercial: [Y] Individual: [Y] FEHBP: [ ] Indemnity: [ ]
Medicare: [Y] Medicaid: [Y] Supplemental Medicare: [Y]
Tricare [ ]

PRODUCTS OFFERED:
Product Name:	Type:
Dimensions	

CONSUMER-DRIVEN PRODUCTS
Personal Dimensions HSA	HSA Company
	HSA Product
	HSA Administrator
Dimensions	Consumer-Driven Health Plan
Personal Dimensions	High Deductible Health Plan

Comments:
Formerly Medical Services Corporation (MSC).

PREMERA BLUE CROSS - WESTERN

7001 220th St SW
Mountlake Terrace, WA 98043-2124
Phone: 425-918-4000 Fax: 425-918-5575 Toll-Free: 800-840-8216
Web site: www.premera.com

MAILING ADDRESS:
    PREMERA BLUE CROSS - WESTERN
    7001 220th St SW
    Mountlake Terrace, WA 98043-2124

KEY EXECUTIVES:
Chief Executive Officer/President .... HR Brereton Barlow
Executive VP, Finance/Chief Financial Officer .... Kent Marquardt
Senior VP, Chief Medical Officer .... John L Castiglia, MD
Director of Pharmacy .... Edward Wong, PharmD
Senior VP, Chief Information Officer .... Kirsten Simonitsch
Executive VP, Operations .... Karen Bartlett
Executive VP, Chief Marketing Executive .... Heyward Donigan
Senior VP, Human Resources .... Barbara Magusin
Chief Legal/Public Policy Officer .... Yori Milo
Executive VP, Strategic Development/Health Care Serv ... Brian Ancell
Senior VP, Health Care Delivery System .... Richard Maturi

COMPANY PROFILE:
Parent Company Name: Premera Blue Cross
Doing Business As:
Year Founded: 1948   Federally Qualified: [ ]
Forprofit: [ ]   Not-For-Profit: [Y]

Managed Care Organization Profiles — WASHINGTON

TYPE OF COVERAGE:
Commercial: [Y] Individual: [Y] FEHBP: [Y] Indemnity: [ ]
Medicare: [ ] Medicaid: [ ] Supplemental Medicare: [Y]
Tricare [ ]

PRODUCTS OFFERED:

Product Name:	Type:
Group Comprehensive	Traditional PPO
Sound Harbor Basic	Traditional PPO
Shond Harbor Group	Traditional PPO
ASO Plans for Large Groups	ASO
Fed Employee Health Benefit Plans	HMO, PPO
Group Preferred Choice	Traditional PPO

CONSUMER-DRIVEN PRODUCTS

	HSA Company
The Healthy Investor	HSA Product
	HSA Administrator
	Consumer-Driven Health Plan
KPS Federal Employees HDHP	High Deductible Health Plan

PLAN BENEFITS:
Alternative Medicine: [X] Behavioral Health: [ ]
Chiropractic: [X] Dental: [X]
Home Care: [X] Inpatient SNF: [X]
Long-Term Care: [ ] Pharm. Mail Order: [ ]
Physical Therapy: [X] Podiatry: [X]
Psychiatric: [X] Transplant: [X]
Vision: [X] Wellness: [X]
Workers' Comp: [ ]
Other Benefits:
Comments:
Formerly Kitsap Physicians Service.

LIFEWISE HEALTH PLAN OF WASHINGTON

7001 220th St SW Bldg 3
Mountlake Terrace, WA 98043
Phone: 425-672-4777 Fax: 425-918-5628 Toll-Free: 800-592-6804
Web site: www.lifewisewa.com

MAILING ADDRESS:
LIFEWISE HEALTH PLAN OF WA
PO Box 91059
Seattle, WA 98043

KEY EXECUTIVES:
Chief Executive Officer/President .... Jeff Roe
Executive VP, Finance/Chief Financial Officer .... Kent Marquardt
Senior VP, Chief Medical Officer .... John L Castiglia, MD
Director of Pharmacy .... Edward Wong
Senior VP, Chief Information Officer .... Alan Smit
Senior VP, Operations .... Karen Bartlett
Executive VP, Chief Marketing Executive .... Heyward Donigan
Chief Legal/Public Policy Officer .... Yori Milo

COMPANY PROFILE:
Parent Company Name: Premera Blue Cross
Doing Business As:
Year Founded: 1933 Federally Qualified: [ ]
Forprofit: [ ] Not-For-Profit: [Y]
Model Type:
Accreditation: [ ] AAPPO [ ] JACHO [ ] NCQA [ ] URAC
Plan Type: PPO, CDHP, HDHP, HSA,
Total Revenue: 2005: 73,135,168 2006: 89,576,756
Net Income: 2005: 1,048,345 2006: 3,071,407
Total Enrollment:
 2001: 11,935 2004: 63,803 2007: 89,102
 2002: 33,193 2005: 83,829
 2003: 48,157 2006: 85,729

SERVICE AREA:
Nationwide:
 WA;

TYPE OF COVERAGE:
Commercial: [Y] Individual: [Y] FEHBP: [ ] Indemnity: [ ]
Medicare: [ ] Medicaid: [ ] Supplemental Medicare: [ ]
Tricare [ ]

CONSUMER-DRIVEN PRODUCTS

HSA Bank	HSA Company
	HSA Product
HSA Bank	HSA Administrator
	Consumer-Driven Health Plan
LifeWise Fund Plans	High Deductible Health Plan

MOLINA HEALTHCARE OF WASHINGTON INC

21540 30th Dr SE Ste 400
Bothell, WA 98041
Phone: 425-424-1100 Fax: 425-424-1132 Toll-Free: 800-869-7175
Web site: www.molinahealthcare.com

MAILING ADDRESS:
MOLINA HEALTHCARE OF WA INC
PO Box 1469
Bothell, WA 98041

KEY EXECUTIVES:
Chairman of the Board/Chief Executive Offr ..... Joseph M Molina, MD
President .... Dale C Ahlskog
Chief Financial Officer .... Jennifer Freeman, CPA
Chief Operating Officer .... Laurel A Lee, MSPH
Chief Medical Officer .... Ward B Hurlburt, MD MPH
Director of Contracts/Compliance .... Peggy Wanta, M Ed

COMPANY PROFILE:
Parent Company Name: Molina Healthcare Inc
Doing Business As:
Year Founded: Federally Qualified: [Y]
Forprofit: [Y] Not-For-Profit: [ ]
Model Type: IPA
Accreditation: [ ] AAPPO [ ] JACHO [ ] NCQA [ ] URAC
Plan Type: HMO, POS
Primary Physicians: 2,534 Physician Specialists: 5,693
Hospitals: 83
Total Enrollment:
 2001: 134,059 2004: 262,736 2007: 288,931
 2002: 160,839 2005: 285,000
 2003: 182,854 2006: 281,000

SERVICE AREA:
Nationwide: N
 WA;

TYPE OF COVERAGE:
Commercial: [Y] Individual: [ ] FEHBP: [ ] Indemnity: [ ]
Medicare: [Y] Medicaid: [Y] Supplemental Medicare: [Y]
Tricare [ ]

PRODUCTS OFFERED:

Product Name:	Type:
Molina	Medicaid

PLAN BENEFITS:
Alternative Medicine: [ ] Behavioral Health: [ ]
Chiropractic: [X] Dental: [ ]
Home Care: [X] Inpatient SNF: [ ]
Long-Term Care: [ ] Pharm. Mail Order: [ ]
Physical Therapy: [ ] Podiatry: [ ]
Psychiatric: [X] Transplant: [X]
Vision: [X] Wellness: [X]
Workers' Comp: [ ]
Other Benefits:

PACIFIC VISIONCARE WASHINGTON INC

2517 NE Kresky Ave
Chehalis, WA 98532
Phone: 360-748-8632 Fax: 360-748-3869 Toll-Free: 800-888-1146
Web site: www.pvcare.com

MAILING ADDRESS:
PACIFIC VISIONCARE WA INC
PO Box 1506
Chehalis, WA 98532

KEY EXECUTIVES:
Chief Executive Officer/President .... Debbie Eldredge
Finance Director .... Kathy L McWilliams
Vice President .... Marlin W Gimbel

COMPANY PROFILE:
Parent Company Name:
Doing Business As:
Year Founded: 1999 Federally Qualified: [ ]
Forprofit: [Y] Not-For-Profit: [ ]
Model Type: Network
Accreditation: [ ] AAPPO [ ] JACHO [ ] NCQA [ ] URAC
Plan Type: Specialty PPO
Primary Physicians: Physician Specialists: 272
Hospitals:
Total Revenue: 2005: 159,758 2006: 141,179
Net Income: 2005: -14,220 2006: -13,400

WASHINGTON

GROUP HEALTH COOPERATIVE OF PUGET SOUND

PO Box 34590
Seattle, WA 98124
Phone: 206-448-5528 Fax: 206-448-5105 Toll-Free: 800-442-4062
Web site: www.ghc.org

MAILING ADDRESS:
  GROUP HEALTH COOP PUGET SOUND
  PO Box 34590
  Seattle, WA 98124

KEY EXECUTIVES:
Chair .... Jerry Campbell
Chief Executive Officer/President .... Scott Armstrong
Chief Financial Officer .... Richard Magnuson
Medical Director .... Hugh Straley, MD
Executive VP/Chief Marketing Officer .... Maureen McLaughlin
VP of Public Affairs & Governance .... Pam MacEwan
VP & General Counsel .... Rick Woods
Executive Vice President .... Peter Morgan
Executive Medical Director .... Michael Soman, MD

COMPANY PROFILE:
Parent Company Name: Group Health Cooperative of Puget Sound
Doing Business As:
Year Founded: 1947   Federally Qualified: [N]
Forprofit: [ ]   Not-For-Profit: [Y]
Model Type: MIXED
Accreditation: [ ] AAPPO [ ] JACHO [X] NCQA [ ] URAC
Plan Type: HMO, POS,
Total Enrollment:
  2001: 442,312   2004: 420,668   2007: 0
  2002: 444,375   2005:
  2003: 435,482   2006:

SERVICE AREA:
Nationwide: N
  ID (Northern); WA;

TYPE OF COVERAGE:
Commercial: [Y] Individual: [Y] FEHBP: [Y] Indemnity: [ ]
Medicare: [Y] Medicaid: [Y] Supplemental Medicare: [ ]
Tricare   [ ]

PRODUCTS OFFERED:
Product Name: Type:
Group Health   HMO
Options   POS
Alliant Select   HMO
Alliant Plus   POS
GHC Medicare High Option Plan   Medicare Advantage

PLAN BENEFITS:
Alternative Medicine: [X]   Behavioral Health: [X]
Chiropractic: [X]   Dental: [X]
Home Care: [X]   Inpatient SNF: [X]
Long-Term Care: [X]   Pharm. Mail Order: [X]
Physical Therapy: [X]   Podiatry: [X]
Psychiatric: [X]   Transplant: [X]
Vision: [X]   Wellness: [X]
Workers' Comp: [X]
Other Benefits:

GROUP HEALTH OPTIONS INC

PO Box 34585
Seattle, WA 98124
Phone: 206-901-4636 Fax: 206-901-4612 Toll-Free: 888-901-4636
Web site: www.ghc.org

MAILING ADDRESS:
  GROUP HEALTH OPTIONS INC
  PO Box 34585
  Seattle, WA 98124

KEY EXECUTIVES:
Chair .... Scott E Armstrong
President .... April D Golenor
Chief Financial Officer .... Richard Magnuson
Medical Director .... Hugh Straley, MD
Chief Marketing Officer .... Maureen McLaughlin
Director, Provider Services .... Chuck Levine
VP & General Counsel .... Rick Woods

COMPANY PROFILE:
Parent Company Name: Group Health Cooperative of Puget Sound
Doing Business As:
Year Founded: 1990   Federally Qualified: [N]
Forprofit: [Y]   Not-For-Profit: [ ]
Model Type: GROUP
Accreditation: [ ] AAPPO [X] JACHO [X] NCQA [ ] URAC
Plan Type: POS, HDHP, HSA,
Total Revenue: 2005: 200,547,419   2006: 204,611,946
Net Income   2005: -1,112,892   2006:   1,381,945
Total Enrollment:
  2001: 144,201   2004: 114,145   2007: 103,491
  2002: 138,615   2005: 119,657
  2003: 114,819   2006: 107,413

SERVICE AREA:
Nationwide: N
  ID; WA;

TYPE OF COVERAGE:
Commercial: [Y] Individual: [ ] FEHBP: [ ] Indemnity: [ ]
Medicare: [Y] Medicaid: [ ] Supplemental Medicare: [ ]
Tricare   [ ]

PRODUCTS OFFERED:
Product Name: Type:
Options Health Care   Medicare

PLAN BENEFITS:
Alternative Medicine: [ ]   Behavioral Health: [X]
Chiropractic: [X]   Dental: [ ]
Home Care: [X]   Inpatient SNF: [X]
Long-Term Care: [X]   Pharm. Mail Order: [X]
Physical Therapy: [X]   Podiatry: [X]
Psychiatric: [X]   Transplant: [X]
Vision: [X]   Wellness: [X]
Workers' Comp: [ ]
Other Benefits:
Comments:
Formerly Options Health Care Inc.

KPS HEALTH PLANS

400 Warren Ave PO BOX 339
Bremerton, WA 98337-0039
Phone: 360-377-5576 Fax: 360-698-0982 Toll-Free: 800-552-7114
Web site: www.kpshealthplans.com

MAILING ADDRESS:
  KPS HEALTH PLANS
  PO Box 339 400 Warren Ave
  Bremerton, WA 98337-0039

KEY EXECUTIVES:
Chairman, Board of Directors .... Rick Woods
Chief Executive Officer/President .... Richard Marks
Chief Financial Officer .... Jim Page
Medical Director/Pharmacy Director .... David Hennes, MD
Chief Operating Officer .... John Woodall
Director of Marketing .... Ty Tabor
Director of Business Systems .... Pam Tirao
Credentialing Manager .... Gisela Mejia
VP, Contracts & Compliance .... Cris Krisologo-Elliott
Director, Provider Relations .... Stephen Braun
Director, Human Resources .... Debbie Laudenslager
Director Medical Management .... Lori Hudson
Credentialing Manager .... Gisela Mejia
Director Contracts & Compliance .... Debbie Stewart
Director, Member Services .... Carrie Debriae
Director Underwriting .... Bruce Brazier

COMPANY PROFILE:
Parent Company Name: Group Health Cooperative
Doing Business As: KPS Health Plan (wholly owned sub of GHC
Year Founded: 1946   Federally Qualified: [N]
Forprofit: [ ]   Not-For-Profit: [Y]
Model Type: IPA
Accreditation: [ ] AAPPO [ ] JACHO [ ] NCQA [ ] URAC
Plan Type: HMO, PPO, TPA, ASO, CDHP, HDHP, HSA,
Primary Physicians: 5,850   Physician Specialists: 8,332
Hospitals: 89
Total Revenue: 2005: 143,272,000   2006: 71,498,087
Net Income   2005:   6,625,000   2006: 3,444,282
Total Enrollment:
  2001: 42,656   2004: 52,552   2007: 45,740
  2002: 44,837   2005: 45,753
  2003: 51,788   2006: 43,106
Medical Loss Ratio: 2005: 81.71   2006: 81.79
Administrative Expense Ratio: 2005: 10.14   2006: 11.24

SERVICE AREA:
Nationwide: N
  WA;

Managed Care Organization Profiles — WASHINGTON

FIRST CHOICE HEALTH NETWORK

One Union Sq 600 Univ St #1400
Seattle, WA 98101-1838
Phone: 206-292-8255 Fax: 206-667-8062 Toll-Free: 800-467-5281
Web site: www.1stchoiceofwa.com

MAILING ADDRESS:
FIRST CHOICE HEALTH NETWORK
One Union Sq 600 Univ St #1400
Seattle, WA 98101-1838

KEY EXECUTIVES:
Chief Executive Officer/President .... Gary R Gannaway
Chief Financial Officer .... Kenneth Hamm
Chief Information Officer .... Stacy Kessel
Chief Marketing Officer .... Ross D Heyl

COMPANY PROFILE:
Parent Company Name:
Doing Business As:
Year Founded: 1984   Federally Qualified: [ ]
Forprofit: [Y]   Not-For-Profit: [ ]
Model Type:
Accreditation: [ ] AAPPO [ ] JACHO [ ] NCQA [ ] URAC
Plan Type: PPO, Specialty PPO, UR, PBM
Primary Physicians: 21,000   Physician Specialists:
Hospitals: 110
Total Revenue: 2005: 18,759,920   2006:
Net Income   2005: 2,591,649   2006:
Total Enrollment:
  2001: 0   2004: 0   2007: 0
  2002: 28,715   2005: 1,000,000
  2003: 1,100,000   2006:

SERVICE AREA:
Nationwide: N
AK; ID; MT; WA;

TYPE OF COVERAGE:
Commercial: [Y] Individual: [Y] FEHBP: [ ] Indemnity: [ ]
Medicare: [ ] Medicaid: [ ] Supplemental Medicare: [ ]
Tricare   [ ]

PRODUCTS OFFERED:
Product Name: Type:
First Choice Health Network's   PPO

PLAN BENEFITS:
Alternative Medicine: [ ]   Behavioral Health: [ ]
Chiropractic: [ ]   Dental: [X]
Home Care: [ ]   Inpatient SNF: [X]
Long-Term Care: [ ]   Pharm. Mail Order: [ ]
Physical Therapy: [X]   Podiatry: [X]
Psychiatric: [ ]   Transplant: [ ]
Vision: [ ]   Wellness: [ ]
Workers' Comp: [ ]
Other Benefits:

GREAT-WEST HEALTHCARE OF WASHINGTON INC

155 108th Ave NE #800
Bellevue, WA 98004
Phone: 425-827-2282 Fax: 425-827-2466 Toll-Free: 866-860-2225
Web site: www.greatwesthealthcare.com

MAILING ADDRESS:
GREAT-WEST HEALTHCARE OF WA IN
155 108th Ave NE #800
Bellevue, WA 98004

KEY EXECUTIVES:
Provider Relations Director .... Dennis Orvosh
VP of Network Management .... Teresa Davis
Medical Management Director .... Robert Allen, MD

COMPANY PROFILE:
Parent Company Name: Great West Life & Annuity Insurance Co
Doing Business As:
Year Founded: 1997   Federally Qualified: [ ]
Forprofit: [Y]   Not-For-Profit: [ ]
Model Type: NETWORK
Accreditation: [ ] AAPPO [ ] JACHO [ ] NCQA [X] URAC
Plan Type: PPO, POS, CDHP, HDHP, HSA,
Total Revenue: 2005: 520,483   2006: -2,959
Net Income   2005: 31,163   2006: 66,793
Total Enrollment:
  2001: 12,873   2004: 2,358   2007: 0
  2002: 5,781   2005:   222
  2003: 2,825   2006:

SERVICE AREA:
Nationwide: N
WA;

TYPE OF COVERAGE:
Commercial: [Y] Individual: [ ] FEHBP: [ ] Indemnity: [ ]
Medicare: [ ] Medicaid: [ ] Supplemental Medicare: [ ]
Tricare   [ ]

CONSUMER-DRIVEN PRODUCTS
Mellon HR Solutions LLC   HSA Company
                                HSA Product
                                HSA Administrator
                                Consumer-Driven Health Plan
                                High Deductible Health Plan

PLAN BENEFITS:
Alternative Medicine: [X]   Behavioral Health: [ ]
Chiropractic: [X]   Dental: [X]
Home Care: [X]   Inpatient SNF: [X]
Long-Term Care: [ ]   Pharm. Mail Order: [X]
Physical Therapy: [X]   Podiatry: [X]
Psychiatric: [X]   Transplant: [X]
Vision: [X]   Wellness: [X]
Workers' Comp: [ ]
Other Benefits:

GROUP HEALTH COOPERATIVE

5615 W Sunset Hwy
Spokane, WA 99210-0204
Phone: 509-838-9100 Fax: 509-458-0368 Toll-Free: 800-497-2210
Web site: www.ghc.org

MAILING ADDRESS:
GROUP HLTH COOPERATIVE
PO Box 204
Spokane, WA 99210-0204

KEY EXECUTIVES:
Chief Executive Officer/President .... Scott Armstrong
Chief Financial Officer .... Richard Magnuson
Medical Director .... Hugh Straley, MD
Pharmacy Director .... Kim Orchard, RPh
Chief Marketing Officer .... Maureen McLaughlin
Public Relations Director .... Pam MacEwan
District Administrator .... William Akers
VP & General Counsel .... Rick Woods

COMPANY PROFILE:
Parent Company Name: Kaiser Foundation
Doing Business As:
Year Founded: 1947   Federally Qualified: [Y]
Forprofit: [ ]   Not-For-Profit: [Y]
Model Type:
Accreditation: [ ] AAPPO [ ] JACHO [X] NCQA [ ] URAC
Plan Type: HMO, POS, HDHP, HSA,
Primary Physicians: 853   Physician Specialists: 45
Hospitals: 2
Total Revenue: 2005:   2006: 1,725,385,476
Net Income   2005:   2006:   188,406,430
Total Enrollment:
  2001: 0   2004: 547,691   2007: 401,888
  2002: 444,375   2005:
  2003: 435,482   2006: 400,867

SERVICE AREA:
Nationwide: N
ID; WA;

TYPE OF COVERAGE:
Commercial: [Y] Individual: [Y] FEHBP: [ ] Indemnity: [ ]
Medicare: [Y] Medicaid: [Y] Supplemental Medicare: [ ]
Tricare   [ ]

PRODUCTS OFFERED:
Product Name: Type:
Group Health Cooperative   Medicaid

PLAN BENEFITS:
Alternative Medicine: [ ]   Behavioral Health: [X]
Chiropractic: [X]   Dental: [ ]
Home Care: [X]   Inpatient SNF: [ ]
Long-Term Care: [ ]   Pharm. Mail Order: [ ]
Physical Therapy: [ ]   Podiatry: [X]
Psychiatric: [X]   Transplant: [X]
Vision: [X]   Wellness: [X]
Workers' Comp: [X]
Other Benefits:

WASHINGTON

MAILING ADDRESS:
   COLUMBIA UNITED PROVIDERS
   19120 SE 34th St Ste 201
   Vancouver, WA 98683

KEY EXECUTIVES:
Chief Executive Officer/President .... Ann Wheelock
Medical Director .... Thomas Culhane, MD
Director Information Services .... Janet Hamilton
Director, Provider Services .... Cindy Orth
Quality Assurance Director .... Diane Mowreader
Claims & Member Services Director .... Sharon Bryant

COMPANY PROFILE:
Parent Company Name:
Doing Business As: Southwest Washington Medical Directorect
Year Founded: 1994   Federally Qualified: [Y]
Forprofit: [Y]   Not-For-Profit: [ ]
Model Type: MIXED
Accreditation: [ ] AAPPO [ ] JACHO [ ] NCQA [ ] URAC
Plan Type: HMO,
Total Revenue: 2005: 34,476,195   2006: 35,774,459
Net Income   2005:   174,111   2006:   -606,545
Total Enrollment:
   2001: 40,254   2004: 34,898   2007: 35,681
   2002: 42,278   2005: 35,764
   2003: 40,433   2006: 35,251

SERVICE AREA:
Nationwide: N
   WA (Clark);

TYPE OF COVERAGE:
Commercial: [ ] Individual: [ ] FEHBP: [ ] Indemnity: [ ]
Medicare: [ ] Medicaid: [Y] Supplemental Medicare: [ ]
Tricare   [ ]

PRODUCTS OFFERED:
Product Name: Type:
Columbia United Providers   Medicaid
Columbia United Providers HMO   HMO

Comments:
Plan benefits are per State mandate.

COMMUNITY HEALTH PLAN OF WASHINGTON

720 Olive Way Ste 300
Seattle, WA 98101-1866
Phone: 206-521-8833 Fax: 206-521-8834 Toll-Free: 800-440-1561
Web site: www.chpw.org

MAILING ADDRESS:
   COMMUNITY HEALTH PLAN OF WA
   720 Olive Way Ste 300
   Seattle, WA 98101-1866

KEY EXECUTIVES:
Chief Executive Officer .... Darnell Dent
Acting,Chief Financial Officer .... Stacy Kessel
Senior VP,Chief Medical Officer .... Christopher Mathews, MD
Pharmacy Director .... Rachel Koh
Chief Information Officer .... Russell Sarbora
Director Marketing/Corporate Communications .... Kris Thompson
VP, Network Mngmnt/Clncl Support .... Abie Castillo
VP, Human Resources/Organization Effective .... Laura Boyd
Corporate Medical Director .... Keith Hurst
Assistant VP, Quality Management .... Helen Harte
VP, Corporate Compliance/Risk .... Maryan Schwab
Executive VP, Customer Care/External Affairs .... Marilee McGuire

COMPANY PROFILE:
Parent Company Name: Community Health Network of Washington
Doing Business As:
Year Founded: 1992   Federally Qualified: [ ]
Forprofit: [ ]   Not-For-Profit: [Y]
Model Type: NETWORK
Accreditation: [ ] AAPPO [ ] JACHO [ ] NCQA [ ] URAC
Plan Type: HMO,
Primary Physicians: 1,000   Physician Specialists: 8,000
Hospitals: 80
Total Revenue: 2005: 221,165,429   2006: 231,595,674
Net Income   2005:   8,112,916   2006:   1,374,526
Total Enrollment:
   2001: 193,492   2004: 205,819   2007: 232,579
   2002: 208,378   2005: 220,241
   2003: 191,244   2006: 222,608

SERVICE AREA:
Nationwide: N
   WA;

TYPE OF COVERAGE:
Commercial: [Y] Individual: [ ] FEHBP: [ ] Indemnity: [ ]
Medicare: [ ] Medicaid: [Y] Supplemental Medicare: [ ]
Tricare   [ ]

PRODUCTS OFFERED:
Product Name: Type:
Basic Health Plan   HMO
Healthy Option   Medicaid
Children's Health Ins Program   Medicaid
Public Employees Benefit   HMO

PLAN BENEFITS:
Alternative Medicine: [X]   Behavioral Health: [ ]
Chiropractic: [X]   Dental: [ ]
Home Care: [ ]   Inpatient SNF: [ ]
Long-Term Care: [ ]   Pharm. Mail Order: [X]
Physical Therapy: [ ]   Podiatry: [ ]
Psychiatric: [ ]   Transplant: [ ]
Vision: [ ]   Wellness: [X]
Workers' Comp: [ ]
Other Benefits:

DENTAL HEALTH SERVICES INC

936 North 34th St Ste 208
Seattle, WA 98133
Phone: 206-633-2300 Fax: 206-624-8755 Toll-Free: 800-248-8108
Web site: www.dentalhealthservices.com

MAILING ADDRESS:
   DENTAL HEALTH SERVICES INC
   936 North 34th St Ste 208
   Seattle, WA 98133

KEY EXECUTIVES:
Chief Executive Officer .... Gary Pernell
President .... Godfrey Pernell, DDS
Chief Financial Officer .... Mehdi Moussavi
VP, Health Services .... Robert Tillery, DDS
Director of Operations .... Joe Cannizzaro
Director of Communications .... Jeff Arnim
Professional Services Manager .... Edith Bravo
Dental Director/ QA Director .... John Hom, DDS
Vice President Sales & Service .... Josh Nace

COMPANY PROFILE:
Parent Company Name: Dental Health Services of America
Doing Business As:
Year Founded: 1984   Federally Qualified: [ ]
Forprofit: [Y]   Not-For-Profit: [ ]
Model Type: MIXED
Accreditation: [ ] AAPPO [ ] JACHO [ ] NCQA [ ] URAC
Plan Type: Specialty HMO, Specialty PPO, ASO, EPA, TPA
Total Revenue: 2005: 1,800,086   2006: 2,227,988
Net Income   2005:   89,471   2006:   -90,867
Total Enrollment:
   2001: 20,501   2004: 19,435   2007: 25,664
   2002: 20,151   2005: 19,755
   2003: 19,948   2006: 21,414

SERVICE AREA:
Nationwide: N
   WA;

TYPE OF COVERAGE:
Commercial: [Y] Individual: [Y] FEHBP: [ ] Indemnity: [ ]
Medicare: [Y] Medicaid: [ ] Supplemental Medicare: [ ]
Tricare   [ ]

PRODUCTS OFFERED:
Product Name: Type:
Dental Health Services PPO   Specialty PPO
Dental Health Services HMO   Specialty HMO

PLAN BENEFITS:
Alternative Medicine: [ ]   Behavioral Health: [ ]
Chiropractic: [ ]   Dental: [X]
Home Care: [ ]   Inpatient SNF: [ ]
Long-Term Care: [ ]   Pharm. Mail Order: [ ]
Physical Therapy: [ ]   Podiatry: [ ]
Psychiatric: [ ]   Transplant: [ ]
Vision: [ ]   Wellness: [ ]
Workers' Comp: [ ]
Other Benefits:

AETNA INC - WASHINGTON

601 Union St Ste 800
Seattle, WA 98101
Phone: 206-701-8000 Fax: 206-701-8177 Toll-Free: 800-654-3250
Web site: www.aetna.com

MAILING ADDRESS:
AETNA INC - WA
601 Union St Ste 800
Seattle, WA 98101

KEY EXECUTIVES:
Chairman of the Board/Chief Executive Officer .... Ronald A Williams
President .... Jeffrey Haas
Regional Financial Officer .... Lee Durham Aurich
Medical Director .... Donald Storey, MD
Marketing Director .... Norm Seabrooks
Controller .... James D Weiss

COMPANY PROFILE:
Parent Company Name: Aetna Inc
Doing Business As:
Year Founded: 1995   Federally Qualified: [N]
Forprofit: [Y]   Not-For-Profit: [ ]
Model Type:
Accreditation: [ ] AAPPO [ ] JACHO [ ] NCQA [X] URAC
Plan Type: HMO, PPO, UR, CDHP, HDHP, HSA,
Total Revenue: 2005: 18,429,154   2006: 18,342,048
Net Income   2005: -1,238,323   2006: 206,505
Total Enrollment:
   2001: 84,396   2004: 14,161   2007: 6,708
   2002: 43,490   2005: 11,796
   2003: 19,710   2006: 9,693

SERVICE AREA:
Nationwide: N
   AK; OR; WA;

TYPE OF COVERAGE:
Commercial: [Y] Individual: [ ] FEHBP: [ ] Indemnity: [ ]
Medicare: [ ] Medicaid: [ ] Supplemental Medicare: [ ]
Tricare   [ ]

CONSUMER-DRIVEN PRODUCTS
Aetna Life Insurance Co   HSA Company
Aetna HealthFund HSA   HSA Product
Aetna   HSA Administrator
Aetna HealthFund   Consumer-Driven Health Plan
PPO I; PPO II   High Deductible Health Plan

PLAN BENEFITS:
Alternative Medicine: [ ]   Behavioral Health: [X]
Chiropractic: [X]   Dental: [ ]
Home Care: [ ]   Inpatient SNF: [ ]
Long-Term Care: [X]   Pharm. Mail Order: [ ]
Physical Therapy: [ ]   Podiatry: [X]
Psychiatric: [ ]   Transplant: [X]
Vision: [X]   Wellness: [ ]
Workers' Comp: [ ]
Other Benefits:

Comments:
Aetna US Healthcare took over NYL Care and its subsidiaries August 98.

ASSURANT EMPLOYEE BENEFITS - WASHINGTON

1512 Plaza 600 Bldg
Seattle, WA 98121
Phone: 206-441-3133 Fax: 206-728-2509 Toll-Free: 800-331-6020
Web site: www.assurantemployeebenefits.com

MAILING ADDRESS:
ASSURANT EMPLOYEE BENEFITS - WA
1512 Plaza 600 Bldg
Seattle, WA 98121

KEY EXECUTIVES:
InterimChief Executive Officer/President .... John S Roberts
Chief Financial Officer .... Floyd F Chadee
VP, Medical Director .... Polly M Galbraith, MD
Chief Information Officer .... Karla J Schacht
Senior VP, Marketing .... Joseph A Sevcik
Privacy Officer .... John L Fortini
VP of Provider Services .... James A Barrett, DMD
Senior VP, Human Resources & Development .... Sylvia R Wagner
General Manager .... Todd Boyd
National Dental Director .... James A Barrett, DMD

COMPANY PROFILE:
Parent Company Name: Assurant Health
Doing Business As:
Year Founded: Federally Qualified: [ ]
Forprofit: [Y]   Not-For-Profit: [ ]
Model Type:
Accreditation: [ ] AAPPO [ ] JACHO [ ] NCQA [ ] URAC
Plan Type: Specialty HMO,

SERVICE AREA:
Nationwide:
   WA;

TYPE OF COVERAGE:
Commercial: [Y] Individual: [Y] FEHBP: [ ] Indemnity: [ ]
Medicare: [ ] Medicaid: [ ] Supplemental Medicare: [ ]
Tricare   [ ]

PLAN BENEFITS:
Alternative Medicine: [ ]   Behavioral Health: [ ]
Chiropractic: [ ]   Dental: [Y]
Home Care: [ ]   Inpatient SNF: [ ]
Long-Term Care: [ ]   Pharm. Mail Order: [ ]
Physical Therapy: [ ]   Podiatry: [ ]
Psychiatric: [ ]   Transplant: [ ]
Vision: [ ]   Wellness: [ ]
Workers' Comp: [ ]
Other Benefits:

Comments:
Formerly Fortis Benefits Dental.

ASURIS NORTHWEST HEALTH

528 E Spokane Falls Blvd #301
Spokane, WA 99202
Phone: 509-922-8072 Fax: 509-922-8264 Toll-Free: 888-344-5587
Web site: www.asurisnorthwesthealth.com

MAILING ADDRESS:
ASURIS NORTHWEST HEALTH
PO Box 91130
Seattle, WA 99202

KEY EXECUTIVES:
President - Washington .... Mary O McWilliams
President and CEO .... Mark B. Ganz
Chief Medical Officer .... Joe Gifford, MD

COMPANY PROFILE:
Parent Company Name: Regence Blue Shield
Doing Business As: ANH
Year Founded: 1984   Federally Qualified: [ ]
Forprofit: [N]   Not-For-Profit: [Y]
Model Type:
Accreditation: [ ] AAPPO [ ] JACHO [ ] NCQA [ ] URAC
Plan Type: PPO
Total Revenue: 2005: 39,454,762   2006: 70,470,201
Net Income   2005: 1,654,465   2006: -1,382,985
Total Enrollment:
   2001: 0   2004: 28,901   2007: 90,828
   2002: 33,134   2005: 31,677
   2003: 35,979   2006: 62,877

SERVICE AREA:
Nationwide: N
   WA;

TYPE OF COVERAGE:
Commercial: [Y] Individual: [Y] FEHBP: [ ] Indemnity: [ ]
Medicare: [ ] Medicaid: [ ] Supplemental Medicare: [Y]
Tricare   [ ]

PLAN BENEFITS:
Alternative Medicine: [ ]   Behavioral Health: [ ]
Chiropractic: [X]   Dental: [ ]
Home Care: [X]   Inpatient SNF: [X]
Long-Term Care: [ ]   Pharm. Mail Order: [ ]
Physical Therapy: [X]   Podiatry: [X]
Psychiatric: [X]   Transplant: [X]
Vision: [ ]   Wellness: [ ]
Workers' Comp: [ ]
Other Benefits:

COLUMBIA UNITED PROVIDERS

19120 SE 34th St Ste 201
Vancouver, WA 98683
Phone: 360-891-1520 Fax: 360-449-8881 Toll-Free: 800-315-7862
Web site: www.cuphealth.com

VIRGINIA

PRODUCTS OFFERED:

Product Name:	Type:
HMO	Medicare Risk
Medicaid	Medicaid
SCHIP	

PLAN BENEFITS:

Alternative Medicine:	[ ]	Behavioral Health:	[X]
Chiropractic:	[ ]	Dental:	[X]
Home Care:	[ ]	Inpatient SNF:	[ ]
Long-Term Care:	[ ]	Pharm. Mail Order:	[X]
Physical Therapy:	[ ]	Podiatry:	[ ]
Psychiatric:	[X]	Transplant:	[ ]
Vision:	[X]	Wellness:	[ ]
Workers' Comp:	[ ]		

Other Benefits:

Comments:
Changed name January 1st, 2001. Formerly called Virginia Chartered Health Plan Inc.

Managed Care Organization Profiles — VIRGINIA

PLAN BENEFITS:
Alternative Medicine:	[ ]	Behavioral Health:	[ ]
Chiropractic:	[X]	Dental:	[X]
Home Care:	[X]	Inpatient SNF:	[X]
Long-Term Care:	[X]	Pharm. Mail Order:	[ ]
Physical Therapy:	[X]	Podiatry:	[X]
Psychiatric:	[ ]	Transplant:	[X]
Vision:	[ ]	Wellness:	[X]
Workers' Comp:	[X]		

Other Benefits:
Comments:
Formerly Metrahealth.

VALUEOPTIONS - CORPORATE HEADQUARTERS

240 Corporate Blvd
Norfolk, VA 23502
Phone: 757-459-5200 Fax: 757-461-6481 Toll-Free: 800-236-4648
Web site: www.valueoptions.com

MAILING ADDRESS:
VALUEOPTIONS - CORP HDQTRS
240 Corporate Blvd
Norfolk, VA 23502

KEY EXECUTIVES:
Chairman of the Board .... Ronald I Dozoretz, MD
Chief Executive Officer .... Barbara B Hill
Chief Financial Officer .... E Paul Dunn, Jr
Chief Medical Officer .... Hal Levine, DO
Chief Information Officer .... Bob Esposito
Chief Operating Officer .... Michele D Alfano
VP of Commercial Sales .... Tom Shjerven
Senior VP, Human Resources .... Larry Anderson
Chief Administrative Officer .... Tom Brown
Chief Strategy Officer .... Kerry Mooney, ACSW
Senior VP, National & Health Plan Accounts .... Chris P Wilson
Executive VP, Public Sector .... Jeff D Emerson
Executive VP, National Network Operations .... Deb Adler

COMPANY PROFILE:
Parent Company Name: FHC Health Systems
Doing Business As: ValueOptions Inc
Year Founded: 1983   Federally Qualified: [Y]
Forprofit: [Y]   Not-For-Profit: [ ]
Model Type: NETWORK
Accreditation: [ ] AAPPO [ ] JACHO [X] NCQA [X] URAC
Plan Type: Specialty PPO, POS, PBN, ASO, UR
Total Enrollment:
  2001: 25,000,000   2004: 23,000,000   2007: 23,000,000
  2002: 0   2005: 24,000,000
  2003: 0   2006:

SERVICE AREA:
Nationwide: Y
  NW;

TYPE OF COVERAGE:
Commercial: [Y] Individual: [ ] FEHBP: [ ] Indemnity: [ ]
Medicare: [Y] Medicaid: [Y] Supplemental Medicare: [ ]
Tricare [ ]

PLAN BENEFITS:
Alternative Medicine:	[ ]	Behavioral Health:	[X]
Chiropractic:	[ ]	Dental:	[ ]
Home Care:	[ ]	Inpatient SNF:	[ ]
Long-Term Care:	[ ]	Pharm. Mail Order:	[ ]
Physical Therapy:	[ ]	Podiatry:	[ ]
Psychiatric:	[X]	Transplant:	[ ]
Vision:	[ ]	Wellness:	[X]
Workers' Comp:	[ ]		

Other Benefits: WPS, Employee Assist
Comments:
Formerly Value Behavioral Health Inc.

VIRGINIA HEALTH NETWORK

7400 Beaufont Springs Dr #505
Richmond, VA 23225
Phone: 804-320-3837 Fax: 804-320-5984 Toll-Free: 800-989-3837
Web site: www.vhn.com

MAILING ADDRESS:
VIRGINIA HEALTH NETWORK
7400 Beaufont Springs Dr #505
Richmond, VA 23225

KEY EXECUTIVES:
President .... James W Brittain
Medical Director .... Barry L Gross, MD
Marketing Vice President .... James L Gore
MIS Director .... Devonna Flora
VP of Provider Relations & Operations .... Judith K Southworth

COMPANY PROFILE:
Parent Company Name:
Doing Business As:
Year Founded: 1988   Federally Qualified: [N]
Forprofit: [Y]   Not-For-Profit: [ ]
Model Type: NETWORK
Accreditation: [ ] AAPPO [ ] JACHO [ ] NCQA [ ] URAC
Plan Type: PPO, POS
Primary Physicians: 4,097   Physician Specialists: 6,874
Hospitals: 83
Total Enrollment:
  2001: 150,000   2004: 133,000   2007: 0
  2002: 140,000   2005:
  2003: 146,000   2006: 126,000

SERVICE AREA:
Nationwide: N
  VA;

TYPE OF COVERAGE:
Commercial: [Y] Individual: [Y] FEHBP: [ ] Indemnity: [ ]
Medicare: [Y] Medicaid: [ ] Supplemental Medicare: [ ]
Tricare [ ]

PRODUCTS OFFERED:
Product Name:	Type:
Virginia Health PPO	PPO

VIRGINIA PREMIER HEALTH PLANS INC

600 E Broad St Ste 400
Richmond, VA 23219-5708
Phone: 804-819-5151 Fax: 804-819-5187 Toll-Free:
Web site: www.virginiapremier.com

MAILING ADDRESS:
VIRGINIA PREMIER HLTH PLAN INC
PO Box 5307
Richmond, VA 23219-5708

KEY EXECUTIVES:
Chief Executive Officer/President .... James S Parrott
Director Finance .... Tim Carpenter, CPA
Senior Medical Director .... Melvin T Pinn Jr, MD
Director of Systems Developmnt/MIS Director .... David Summers
Director, Quality Improvement/Credentialing .... Jamie McPherson
Privacy/Compliance Officer .... Gloria Reynolds
Director, Provider Relations .... Patrick McMahon
Human Resources Director .... Tonya Woodson
VP Medical Management .... Linda Hines

COMPANY PROFILE:
Parent Company Name: Doing Business As:
Year Founded: 1995   Federally Qualified: [N]
Forprofit: [Y]   Not-For-Profit: [ ]
Model Type: IPA
Accreditation: [ ] AAPPO [X] JACHO [ ] NCQA [ ] URAC
Plan Type: HMO, POS
Primary Physicians: 1,525   Physician Specialists: 4,233
Hospitals: 54
Total Revenue: 2005: 294,639,923   2006: 335,171,662
Net Income 2005: 11,922,991   2006: 13,818,300
Total Enrollment:
  2001: 0   2004: 89,515   2007: 109,494
  2002: 70,000   2005: 86,253
  2003: 64,673   2006: 109,353
Medical Loss Ratio: 2005: 85.50   2006:
Administrative Expense Ratio: 2005: 7.40   2006:

SERVICE AREA:
Nationwide: N
  VA (Accomack, Amelia, Brunswick, Charles City, Chesterfield, Dinwiddie, Essex, Goochland, Greensville, Hanover, Henrico, King & Queen, King William, Lancaster, Mathews, Middlesex, New Kent, Northampton, Northumberland, Nottoway, Powhatan, Prince Edward, Prince George, Richmond County, Southampton, Surry, Sussex);

TYPE OF COVERAGE:
Commercial: [ ] Individual: [Y] FEHBP: [ ] Indemnity: [ ]
Medicare: [ ] Medicaid: [Y] Supplemental Medicare: [ ]
Tricare [ ]

VIRGINIA

Managed Care Organization Profiles

Year Founded: 1984 Federally Qualified: [Y]
Forprofit: [Y] Not-For-Profit: [ ]
Model Type: IPA
Accreditation: [ ] AAPPO [ ] JACHO [X] NCQA [ ] URAC
Plan Type: HMO, POS, CDHP, HDHP, HSA,
Primary Physicians: 4,442 Physician Specialists: 7,202
Hospitals: 131
Total Revenue: 2005: 338,032,322 2006: 362,886,208
Net Income 2005: 2006: 31,420,036
Total Enrollment:
  2001: 165,146 2004: 163,145 2007: 179,501
  2002: 140,235 2005:
  2003: 160,000 2006:
Medical Loss Ratio: 2005: 2006: 80.40
Administrative Expense Ratio: 2005: 2006:
SERVICE AREA:
Nationwide: N
  VA (Albemarle, City of Alexandria, Alleghany, Amelia, Arlington, August, Bath, Bedford, City of Bedford, Bland, Botetourt, Buckingham, City of Buena Vista, Caroline, Charles City, Charlotte, City of Charlottesville, Chesterfield, Clarke, City of Clifton Forge, City of Colonial Heights, City of Covington, Craig, Culpeper, Cumberland, City of Danville, Dinwiddie, Essex, Fairfax, City of Fairfax, City of Falls Church, Fauquier, Floyd, Fluvanna, Franklin, Frederick, City of Fredericksburg, City of Galax, Giles, Goochland, Greene, Halifax, Hanover, City of Harrisonburg, Henrico, City of Hopewell, James City, King & Queen, King George, King William, Lancaster, City of Lexington, Loudoun, Louisa, Lunenburg, Madison, City of Manassas Park, City of Manassas, Mathews, Mecklenburg, Middlesex, Montgomery, Nelson, New Kent, Northumberland, Nottoway, Orange, Page, City of Petersburg, Pittsylvania, Powhatan, Prince Edward, Prince George, Prince William, Pulaski, City of Radford, Rappahannock, Richmond, City of Richmond, Roanoke, City of Roanoke, Rockbridge, Rockingham, City of Salem, Shenandoah, South Boston, Spotsylvania, Stafford, City of Staunton, Surry, Sussex, Tazewell, Warren, City of Waynesboro, Westmoreland, City of Williamsburg, Winchester, Wythe);
TYPE OF COVERAGE:
Commercial: [Y] Individual: [ ] FEHBP: [ ] Indemnity: [ ]
Medicare: [ ] Medicaid: [Y] Supplemental Medicare: [ ]
Tricare [ ]
PRODUCTS OFFERED:
Product Name: Type:
HMO
POS
Southern Health Services Medicaid
ASO ASO
PPO PPO
CONSUMER-DRIVEN PRODUCTS
Wells Fargo HSA Company
  HSA Product
Corporate Benefits Services of America HSA Administrator
  Consumer-Driven Health Plan
Open Access Plus Plan High Deductible Health Plan
PLAN BENEFITS:
Alternative Medicine: [ ] Behavioral Health: [ ]
Chiropractic: [X] Dental: [ ]
Home Care: [X] Inpatient SNF: [X]
Long-Term Care: [ ] Pharm. Mail Order: [X]
Physical Therapy: [X] Podiatry: [X]
Psychiatric: [X] Transplant: [X]
Vision: [X] Wellness: [X]
Workers' Comp: [ ]
Other Benefits:

UNITED CONCORDIA COMPANY INC - VIRGINIA

4860 Cox Rd Ste 200
Glen Allen, VA 23060
Phone: 800-454-3224 Fax: 804-217-8368 Toll-Free: 800-454-3224
Web site: www.ucci.com
MAILING ADDRESS:
  UNITED CONCORDIA CO INC - VA
  4860 Cox Rd Ste 200
  Glen Allen, VA 23060

KEY EXECUTIVES:
Regional Vice President .... Thomas A Dzuryachko
Sr VP, Finance .... Daniel Wright
VP, National Dental Director .... Richard Klich, DMD
VP, Sales & Marketing .... Ron Onda
MIS Director .... Jim Robins
Director, Provider Services .... Ted Pesano

COMPANY PROFILE:
Parent Company Name: Highmark Inc
Doing Business As:
Year Founded: 1991 Federally Qualified: [ ]
Forprofit: [Y] Not-For-Profit: [ ]
Model Type:
Accreditation: [ ] AAPPO [ ] JACHO [ ] NCQA [ ] URAC
Plan Type: Specialty HMO, Specialty PPO, POS, TPA
Total Revenue: 2005: 91,327,688 2006: 119,184,331
Net Income 2005: 4,541,662 2006: 5,110,854
SERVICE AREA:
Nationwide: N
  DC; DE; MD; VA;
TYPE OF COVERAGE:
Commercial: [Y] Individual: [ ] FEHBP: [ ] Indemnity: [ ]
Medicare: [ ] Medicaid: [ ] Supplemental Medicare: [ ]
Tricare [ ]
PLAN BENEFITS:
Alternative Medicine: [ ] Behavioral Health: [ ]
Chiropractic: [ ] Dental: [X]
Home Care: [ ] Inpatient SNF: [ ]
Long-Term Care: [ ] Pharm. Mail Order: [ ]
Physical Therapy: [ ] Podiatry: [ ]
Psychiatric: [ ] Transplant: [ ]
Vision: [ ] Wellness: [ ]
Workers' Comp: [ ]
Other Benefits:
Comments:
Formerly MIDA Dental Plans - UCCI Inc.

UNITEDHEALTHCARE OF MID ATLANTIC REGION

9020 Stony Point Pkwy Ste 400
Richmond, VA 23235
Phone: 804-267-5200 Fax: 804-267-5281 Toll-Free: 888-286-4908
Web site: www.uhc.com
MAILING ADDRESS:
  UNITEDHEALTHCARE OF MID ATLANTIC REGION
  9020 Stony Point Pkwy Ste 400
  Richmond, VA 23235

KEY EXECUTIVES:
Non-Executive Chairman .... Richard T Burke

COMPANY PROFILE:
Parent Company Name: UnitedHealth Group
Doing Business As: UnitedHealthcare of VA Inc
Year Founded: 1997 Federally Qualified: [ ]
Forprofit: [Y] Not-For-Profit: [ ]
Model Type: IPA
Accreditation: [ ] AAPPO [ ] JACHO [ ] NCQA [ ] URAC
Plan Type: HMO, PPO, POS, CDHP, HDHP, HSA, HRA,
Primary Physicians: Physician Specialists:
Hospitals:
Total Revenue: 2005: 109,791,524 2006: 469,541,210
Net Income 2005: 14,135,019 2006: 15,101,117
Medical Loss Ratio: 2005: 2006: 82.40
Administrative Expense Ratio: 2005: 2006:
SERVICE AREA:
Nationwide: N
  VA (Bedford, Botetourt, Charles City, Chesapeake, Chesterfield, Colonial Heights City, Craig, Dinwiddie, Floyd, Franklin, Gloucester, Goochland, Hampton, Hanover, Henrico, Hopewell, King William, Louisa, Montgomery, New Kent, Newport News, Norfolk, Petersburg, Portsmouth, Powhatan, Prince George, Pulaski, Richmond, Roanoke, Salem, Suffolk, Sussex, Virginia Beach, Williamsburg, York);
TYPE OF COVERAGE:
Commercial: [Y] Individual: [ ] FEHBP: [ ] Indemnity: [ ]
Medicare: [ ] Medicaid: [ ] Supplemental Medicare: [ ]
Tricare [ ]
PRODUCTS OFFERED:
Product Name: Type:
Choice HMO
Choice Plus
Fully Insured & Self Funded
CONSUMER-DRIVEN PRODUCTS
Exante Bank/Golden Rule Ins Co HSA Company
iPlan HSA HSA Product
  HSA Administrator
  Consumer-Driven Health Plan
  High Deductible Health Plan

Managed Care Organization Profiles

VIRGINIA

Year Founded: 1988
Forprofit: [Y]
Model Type: NETWORK
Accreditation: [ ] AAPPO [ ] JACHO [ ] NCQA [ ] URAC
Plan Type: PPO
Primary Physicians: 23,000   Physician Specialists: 11,000
Hospitals: 100
Total Enrollment:
  2001: 0   2004: 124,000   2007: 0
  2002: 0   2005: 123,000
  2003: 0   2006:
Federally Qualified: [N]
Not-For-Profit: [ ]

SERVICE AREA:
Nationwide: N
  DC; DE; MD; NJ; PA; VA;

OPTIMA HEALTH PLAN INC

4417 Corporation Lane
Virginia Beach, VA 23462-3162
Phone: 757-552-7401 Fax: 757-687-6031 Toll-Free: 877-552-7401
Web site: www.optimahealth.com

MAILING ADDRESS:
OPTIMA HEALTH PLAN INC
4417 Corporation Lane
Virginia Beach, VA 23462-3162

KEY EXECUTIVES:
President .... Michael Dudley
Senior Medical Director .... George K Heuser, MD
Pharmacy Director .... Tim Jennings
Chief Operating Officer .... Darleen Anderson
Director of Sales .... Rachel T Thomas
Manager, Provider Relations .... Ydsia Slagle
Director, Network Development .... Rachel Schneider
Director, Community Health & Prevention .... Terrina Thomas
Director, Medical Care Management .... Patricia Curtis
Director, Product Development .... Sharon Poulos

COMPANY PROFILE:
Parent Company Name: Sentara Health Care
Doing Business As: Optima Health
Year Founded: 1984   Federally Qualified: [Y]
Forprofit: [ ]   Not-For-Profit: [Y]
Model Type: NETWORK
Accreditation: [ ] AAPPO [ ] JACHO [X] NCQA [X] URAC
Plan Type: HMO, PPO, POS, ASO, CDHP, HDHP,
Primary Physicians: 1,531   Physician Specialists: 3,761
Hospitals: 21
Total Revenue: 2005: 703,735,940   2006: 781,674,346
Net Income   2005: 83,636,290   2006: 79,793,271
Total Enrollment:
  2001: 0   2004: 330,000   2007: 0
  2002: 299,390   2005: 226,961
  2003: 311,132   2006: 250,620
Medical Loss Ratio: 2005: 52.00   2006: 83.40
Administrative Expense Ratio: 2005: 6.90   2006: 8.40

SERVICE AREA:
Nationwide: N
  VA (Hampton Roads, Richmond);

TYPE OF COVERAGE:
Commercial: [Y] Individual: [ ] FEHBP: [ ] Indemnity: [ ]
Medicare: [Y] Medicaid: [Y] Supplemental Medicare: [ ]
Tricare   [ ]

PRODUCTS OFFERED:
Product Name:	Type:
Optima HMO	HMO
Sentara Family Plan	Medicaid
Optima POS	POS
Optima	PPO

PLAN BENEFITS:
Alternative Medicine:	[ ]	Behavioral Health:	[X]
Chiropractic:	[ ]	Dental:	[ ]
Home Care:	[X]	Inpatient SNF:	[X]
Long-Term Care:	[ ]	Pharm. Mail Order:	[X]
Physical Therapy:	[X]	Podiatry:	[ ]
Psychiatric:	[ ]	Transplant:	[ ]
Vision:	[X]	Wellness:	[X]
Workers' Comp:	[X]		
Other Benefits:

SOUTHERN HEALTH SERVICES INC

1000 Research Park Blvd
Charlottesville, VA 22911
Phone: 434-975-1212 Fax: 434-951-2551 Toll-Free: 800-975-1213
Web site: www.southernhealth.com

MAILING ADDRESS:
SOUTHERN HEALTH SERVICES INC
1000 Research Park Blvd
Charlottesville, VA 22911

KEY EXECUTIVES:
Chief Executive Officer .... Cosby M Davis III
Chief Financial Officer .... Drew A Joyce
Sr Medical Director .... Ian Bushnell, MD
VP Sales & Marketing Director .... Chris Fanning
VP, Network Management .... Matthew Meleski
Director of Human Resources .... Karol H Norman, PHR
VP of Health Services .... Karin Ferguson, RN

COMPANY PROFILE:
Parent Company Name: Coventry Health Care Inc
Doing Business As:
Year Founded: 1994   Federally Qualified: [N]
Forprofit: [Y]   Not-For-Profit: [ ]
Model Type: IPA
Accreditation: [ ] AAPPO [ ] JACHO [ ] NCQA [ ] URAC
Plan Type: HMO, PPO, POS, ASO, CDHP, HDHP, HSA
Total Enrollment:
  2001: 0   2004: 160,000   2007: 0
  2002: 97,836   2005:
  2003: 103,386   2006:

SERVICE AREA:
Nationwide: N
  VA;

TYPE OF COVERAGE:
Commercial: [Y] Individual: [ ] FEHBP: [ ] Indemnity: [ ]
Medicare: [Y] Medicaid: [ ] Supplemental Medicare: [ ]
Tricare   [ ]

CONSUMER-DRIVEN PRODUCTS
Wells Fargo   HSA Company
                                         HSA Product
Corporate Benefits Services of America   HSA Administrator
                                         Consumer-Driven Health Plan
Open Access Plus Plan   High Deductible Health Plan

PLAN BENEFITS:
Alternative Medicine:	[ ]	Behavioral Health:	[X]
Chiropractic:	[X]	Dental:	[X]
Home Care:	[X]	Inpatient SNF:	[X]
Long-Term Care:	[ ]	Pharm. Mail Order:	[X]
Physical Therapy:	[X]	Podiatry:	[X]
Psychiatric:	[X]	Transplant:	[X]
Vision:	[X]	Wellness:	[X]
Workers' Comp:	[ ]		
Other Benefits:

Comments:
Formerly Qualchoice of Virginia Health Plan.

SOUTHERN HEALTH SERVICES INC

9881 Mayland Dr
Richmond, VA 23233
Phone: 804-747-3700 Fax: 804-762-9349 Toll-Free: 800-424-0077
Web site: www.southernhealth.com

MAILING ADDRESS:
SOUTHERN HEALTH SERVICES INC
9881 Mayland Dr
Richmond, VA 23233

KEY EXECUTIVES:
Chief Executive Officer .... Cosby M Davis III
Chief Executive Officer .... Drew A Joyce
Senior Medical Director .... Ian W Bushnell, MD
VP of Marketing & Sales .... Chris Fanning
VP, Network Management .... Matthew Meleski
Human Resources Manager .... Karol H Morman, PHR
Medical Management Director .... Jill Mercier
Manager Quality Improvement .... Joyce Dayvault
VP, Health Services .... Karin Ferguson, RN

COMPANY PROFILE:
Parent Company Name: Coventry Health Care Inc
Doing Business As:

VIRGINIA

Managed Care Organization Profiles

COMPANY PROFILE:
Parent Company Name: Delta Dental Plan Association
Doing Business As:
Year Founded: 1964   Federally Qualified: [ ]
Forprofit: [ ]   Not-For-Profit: [Y]
Model Type:
Accreditation: [ ] AAPPO [ ] JACHO [ ] NCQA [ ] URAC
Plan Type: Specialty PPO, POS
Total Revenue: 2005: 90,039,364   2006: 111,481,090
Net Income   2005: 8,990,986   2006: 10,202,989
Total Enrollment:
    2001: 261,129   2004: 347,802   2007: 0
    2002: 260,691   2005:
    2003: 339,907   2006:

SERVICE AREA:
Nationwide: N
    VA;

TYPE OF COVERAGE:
Commercial: [Y] Individual: [ ] FEHBP: [ ] Indemnity: [ ]
Medicare: [ ] Medicaid: [ ] Supplemental Medicare: [ ]
Tricare   [ ]

PLAN BENEFITS:
Alternative Medicine: [ ]   Behavioral Health: [ ]
Chiropractic: [ ]   Dental: [X]
Home Care: [ ]   Inpatient SNF: [ ]
Long-Term Care: [ ]   Pharm. Mail Order: [ ]
Physical Therapy: [ ]   Podiatry: [ ]
Psychiatric: [ ]   Transplant: [ ]
Vision: [ ]   Wellness: [ ]
Workers' Comp: [ ]
Other Benefits:

DOMINION DENTAL SERVICES - CORPORATE HEADQUARTERS

115 S Union St Ste 300
Alexandria, VA 22314
Phone: 703-518-5000 Fax: 703-518-8849 Toll-Free: 888-681-5100
Web site: www.dominiondental.com
MAILING ADDRESS:
    DOMINION DENTAL SERVICES
    115 S Union St Ste 300
    Alexandria, VA 22314

KEY EXECUTIVES:
Chairman of the Board .... Mitchell E McGlynn
Chief Executive Officer/President .... Mitchell E McGlynn
Chief Financial Officer .... Patricia L Doyle
Dental Director .... Kenneth Stoner, DDS
Director of Finance & Information Systems .... Tracey McDaniel
Senior VP of Operations .... Michael Davis
Marketing Manager .... Michael Swinney
Director Accounting & Compliance .... Kara Greenhouse
Director of Professional Services .... Lori Hayes
Human Resources & Office Manager .... Sharene Cook
Director of New Product Development .... Michael Davis
VP of Business Development .... Jay Rausch

COMPANY PROFILE:
Parent Company Name: Dominion Dental USA, Inc
Doing Business As:
Year Founded: 1996   Federally Qualified: [N]
Forprofit: [Y]   Not-For-Profit: [ ]
Model Type: IPA
Accreditation: [ ] AAPPO [ ] JACHO [ ] NCQA [ ] URAC
Plan Type: Specialty HMO, ASO, TPA
Primary Physicians: 1,600   Physician Specialists:
Hospitals:
Total Revenue: 2005: 11,059,557   2006: 11,500,165
Net Income   2005:   2006: 297,976
Total Enrollment:
    2001: 0   2004: 121,623   2007: 60.20
    2002: 148,999   2005:
    2003: 128,323   2006:

SERVICE AREA:
Nationwide: N
    DC; MD; PA; VA;

TYPE OF COVERAGE:
Commercial: [Y] Individual: [Y] FEHBP: [ ] Indemnity: [Y]
Medicare: [Y] Medicaid: [Y] Supplemental Medicare: [ ]
Tricare   [ ]

GREAT-WEST HEALTHCARE OF VIRGINIA INC

7600 Leesburg Pike Ste 120 E
Falls Church, VA 22043
Phone: 703-356-1004 Fax: 703-356-1226 Toll-Free: 888-241-8614
Web site: www.greatwesthealthcare.com
MAILING ADDRESS:
    GREAT-WEST HEALTHCARE OF VA IN
    7600 Leesburg Pike Ste 120 E
    Falls Church, VA 22043

KEY EXECUTIVES:
Vice President .... William O'Donnell
Senior Executive .... Richard F Rivers

COMPANY PROFILE:
Parent Company Name: Great West Life & Annuity Insurance Co
Doing Business As:
Year Founded: Federally Qualified: [ ]
Forprofit: [Y]   Not-For-Profit: [ ]
Model Type:
Accreditation: [ ] AAPPO [ ] JACHO [ ] NCQA [ ] URAC
Plan Type: HMO, CDHP, HDHP, HSA,

SERVICE AREA:
Nationwide: N
    VA;

TYPE OF COVERAGE:
Commercial: [Y] Individual: [ ] FEHBP: [ ] Indemnity: [ ]
Medicare: [ ] Medicaid: [ ] Supplemental Medicare: [ ]
Tricare   [ ]

CONSUMER-DRIVEN PRODUCTS
Mellon HR Solutions LLC   HSA Company
                                 HSA Product
                                 HSA Administrator
                                 Consumer-Driven Health Plan
                                 High Deductible Health Plan

PLAN BENEFITS:
Alternative Medicine: [X]   Behavioral Health: [ ]
Chiropractic: [X]   Dental: [X]
Home Care: [X]   Inpatient SNF: [X]
Long-Term Care: [ ]   Pharm. Mail Order: [X]
Physical Therapy: [X]   Podiatry: [X]
Psychiatric: [X]   Transplant: [X]
Vision: [X]   Wellness: [X]
Workers' Comp: [ ]
Other Benefits:

NATIONAL CAPITAL PPO

6850 Versar Center Ste 420
Springfield, VA 22151
Phone: 703-914-5650 Fax: 703-914-5686 Toll-Free: 800-871-7888
Web site: www.ncppo.com
MAILING ADDRESS:
    NATIONAL CAPITAL PPO
    6850 Versar Center Ste 420
    Springfield, VA 22151

KEY EXECUTIVES:
Regional Vice President .... Gerald Young
Financial Services Manager .... Kathleen Chandra
Medical Director .... Fredric Garner, MD
Chief Operating Officer .... Gerald Young
Director of Marketing .... Mark Sucoloski
Manager of Network Services .... Brenda Faust-Thomas
Regional VP .... Jeanell Austin

COMPANY PROFILE:
Parent Company Name: WellPoint Inc
Doing Business As:

Managed Care Organization Profiles — VIRGINIA

TYPE OF COVERAGE:
Commercial: [Y] Individual: [Y] FEHBP: [ ] Indemnity: [ ]
Medicare: [ ] Medicaid: [ ] Supplemental Medicare: [Y]
Tricare [ ]

PRODUCTS OFFERED:

Product Name:	Type:
Healthkeepers Plus Inc	Medicaid
Blue Advantage	HMO/PPO
Healthkeepers Plus - Peninsula	Medicaid
Healthkeepers Plus - Priority	Medicaid
Trigon Healthkeepers Gold	Medicare

CONSUMER-DRIVEN PRODUCTS

JP Morgan Chase	HSA Company
Anthem ByDesign HSA	HSA Product
JP Morgan Chase	HSA Administrator
Blue Access Saver	Consumer-Driven Health Plan
Blue Access Economy Plans PPO	High Deductible Health Plan

PLAN BENEFITS:
Alternative Medicine: [ ]   Behavioral Health: [ ]
Chiropractic: [X]   Dental: [X]
Home Care: [X]   Inpatient SNF: [X]
Long-Term Care: [X]   Pharm. Mail Order: [X]
Physical Therapy: [X]   Podiatry: [X]
Psychiatric: [X]   Transplant: [X]
Vision: [X]   Wellness: [X]
Workers' Comp: [X]
Other Benefits:

CIGNA DENTAL HEALTH OF VIRGINIA

1571 Sawgrass Corporate Pksy
Sunrise, FL 33323
Phone: 954-514-6600 Fax: 954-514-6905 Toll-Free: 800-367-1037
Web site: www.cigna.com/dental

MAILING ADDRESS:
CIGNA DENTAL HEALTH OF VIRGINIA
1571 Sawgrass Corporate Pkwy
Sunrise, FL 33323

KEY EXECUTIVES:
President .... Karen S Rohan

COMPANY PROFILE:
Parent Company Name: CIGNA Corporation
Doing Business As:
Year Founded: 1995   Federally Qualified: [N]
Forprofit: [Y]   Not-For-Profit: [ ]
Model Type:
Accreditation: [ ] AAPPO [ ] JACHO [ ] NCQA [ ] URAC
Plan Type: Specialty HMO
Total Revenue: 2005:   2006: 7,466,045
Net Income: 2005:   2006: 1,337,870
Medical Loss Ratio: 2005:   2006: 59.30
Administrative Expense Ratio: 2005: 2006:

SERVICE AREA:
Nationwide: N
VA;

TYPE OF COVERAGE:
Commercial: [ ] Individual: [ ] FEHBP: [ ] Indemnity: [ ]
Medicare: [ ] Medicaid: [ ] Supplemental Medicare: [ ]
Tricare [ ]

PRODUCTS OFFERED:

Product Name:	Type:
CIGNA Dental Health of VA	Specialty HMO

PLAN BENEFITS:
Alternative Medicine: [ ]   Behavioral Health: [ ]
Chiropractic: [ ]   Dental: [X]
Home Care: [ ]   Inpatient SNF: [ ]
Long-Term Care: [ ]   Pharm. Mail Order: [ ]
Physical Therapy: [ ]   Podiatry: [ ]
Psychiatric: [ ]   Transplant: [ ]
Vision: [ ]   Wellness: [ ]
Workers' Comp: [ ]
Other Benefits:

CIGNA HEALTHCARE OF VIRGINIA INC - RICHMOND

7501 Boulders View Dr Ste 500
Richmond, VA 23225
Phone: 804-560-3959 Fax: 804-560-3907 Toll-Free: 800-533-1708
Web site: www.cigna.com

MAILING ADDRESS:
CIGNA HEALTHCARE OF VA INC-RCHMND
PO Box 31353
Richmond, VA 23225

KEY EXECUTIVES:
General Manager .... Thomas Martel
VP & Senior Medical Executive .... Z Colette Edwards, MD
Director, Provider Relations .... John Crowley
Director, Provider Relations .... Rob Smart
Medical Management Director .... Latricia Norris
Quality Improvement .... Alice Counts
Quality Improvement .... Judy French
Government Relations .... Jeffery Tindall
Pharmacy Benefits .... Nadia Assadi
General Company Information .... Lamonte Thomas

COMPANY PROFILE:
Parent Company Name: CIGNA Corporation
Doing Business As: CIGNA Health Plans Inc
Year Founded: 1984   Federally Qualified: [N]
Forprofit: [Y]   Not-For-Profit: [ ]
Model Type: IPA
Accreditation: [ ] AAPPO [ ] JACHO [X] NCQA [ ] URAC
Plan Type: HMO, PPO, POS, ASO, EPO, CDHP, HDHP, HSA, FSA, HRA,
Primary Physicians: 4,540   Physician Specialists: 8,197
Hospitals: 104
Total Revenue: 2005: 27,597,901   2006: 169,261,434
Net Income   2005: -304,089   2006: 4,201,215
Total Enrollment:
  2001: 69,609   2004: 28,696   2007: 338,694
  2002: 38,449   2005:
  2003: 334,006 2006:

SERVICE AREA:
Nationwide: N
VA (Albemarle, Amelia, Augusta, Botetourt, Caroline, Chesterfield, Cumberland, Dinwiddie, Franklin, Gloucester, Goochland, Hanover, Henrico, Isle of Wight, James City, King and Queen, King William, Louisa, Mathews, Middlesex, New Kent, Nottoway, Page, Patrick, Pittsylvania, Powhatan, Prince George, Richmond, Roanoke, Rockingham, Surry, Sussex, York, Hampton Roads,

TYPE OF COVERAGE:
Commercial: [Y] Individual: [ ] FEHBP: [ ] Indemnity: [ ]
Medicare: [Y] Medicaid: [ ] Supplemental Medicare: [ ]
Tricare [ ]

PRODUCTS OFFERED:

Product Name:	Type:
Cigna Healthcare HMO	HMO
Cigna Healthcare for Seniors	Medicare

CONSUMER-DRIVEN PRODUCTS

JP Morgan Chase	HSA Company
CIGNA Choice Fund	HSA Product
	HSA Administrator
Open Access Plus	Consumer-Driven Health Plan
PPO	High Deductible Health Plan

PLAN BENEFITS:
Alternative Medicine: [ ]   Behavioral Health:
[X]Chiropractic: [X]   Dental: [X]
Home Care: [X]   Inpatient SNF: [X]
Long-Term Care: [X]   Pharm. Mail Order: [X]
Physical Therapy: [X]   Podiatry: [X]
Psychiatric: [X]   Transplant: [X]
Vision: [X]   Wellness: [X]
Workers' Comp: [X]
Other Benefits:

DELTA DENTAL OF VIRGINIA

4818 Starkey Rd
Roanoke, VA 24018
Phone: 540-989-8000 Fax: 540-774-7574 Toll-Free: 800-237-6060
Web site: www.deltadentalva.com

MAILING ADDRESS:
DELTA DENTAL OF VIRGINIA
4818 Starkey Rd
Roanoke, VA 24018

KEY EXECUTIVES:
Chief Executive Officer .... George A Levicki, DDS
VP, Finance/CFO .... Mike Wise
VP, Marketing .... Dyke Davies
VP, Information Systems .... Oscar Bryant
VP, Operations .... Vicki Welsh

VIRGINIA Managed Care Organization Profiles

AMERIGROUP CORPORATION

4425 Corporation Lane
Virginia Beach, VA 23462
Phone: 757-490-6900 Fax: 757-518-3600 Toll-Free: 800-600-4441
Web site: www.amerigroupcorp.com

MAILING ADDRESS:
AMERIGROUP CORPORATION
4425 Corporation Lane
Virginia Beach, VA 23462

KEY EXECUTIVES:
Chairman of the Board .... Jeffrey L McWaters
Chief Executive Officer/President .... James G Carlson
Executive VP, Chief Financial Officer .... James W Truess
Senior VP, Chief Technology Officer .... Leon A Root, Jr
Executive VP, Chief Operating Officer .... Richard C Zoretic
Executive VP, Chief Marketing Officer .... Nancy L Grden
HIPAA Training Manager .... Theresa Collazo
VP, Corporate Development .... Timothy J Spillane
General Counsel & Secretary .... Stanley F Baldwin
Senior VP, Financial Controls .... Sherri E Lee, CPA

COMPANY PROFILE:
Parent Company Name:
Doing Business As: Amerigroup Community Care
Year Founded: 1994   Federally Qualified: [ ]
Forprofit: [Y]   Not-For-Profit: [ ]
Model Type:
Accreditation: [ ] AAPPO [ ] JACHO [ ] NCQA [ ] URAC
Plan Type: HMO
Primary Physicians: 10,122   Physician Specialists: 38,333
Hospitals: 432
Total Revenue: 2005: 2,329,909,000   2006: 2,835,089,000
Net Income   2005: 53,651,000   2006: 107,106,000
Total Enrollment:
  2001: 472,000   2004: 936,000   2007: 1,711,000
  2002: 510,000   2005: 1,129,000
  2003: 867,000   2006: 1,316,000
Medical Loss Ratio: 2005: 84.70   2006: 81.10
Administrative Expense Ratio: 2005: 11.10   2006: 13.00

TYPE OF COVERAGE:
Commercial: [ ] Individual: [ ] FEHBP: [ ] Indemnity: [ ]
Medicare: [ ] Medicaid: [Y] Supplemental Medicare: [ ]
Tricare [ ]

SERVICE AREA:
Nationwide: N
  DC; FL; MD; NJ; TX; VA;

PRODUCTS OFFERED:
Product Name: Type:
Americaid   Medicaid
Amerikids   SCHIP
Ameriplus
Amerifam

AMERICAN WHOLEHEALTH NETWORKS INC

46040 Center Oak Plaza Ste 130
Sterling, VA 20166
Phone: 703-430-2511 Fax: 703-430-9638 Toll-Free: 800-274-7526
Web site: www.americanwholehealth.com

MAILING ADDRESS:
AMERICAN WHOLEHEALTH NETWORKS
46040 Center Oak Plaza Ste 130
Sterling, VA 20166

KEY EXECUTIVES:
Chief Executive Officer .... William J Luben
Chief Financial Officer .... Dave Waldron
VP, Medical Affairs .... John Reed, MD
Director of Information Technology .... Billie York
Director of Operations .... Marty Stabelfeldt
VP of Sales .... Mary Anne Mason
Director, Quality Assurance/Medical Management .... Kathy Moore

COMPANY PROFILE:
Parent Company Name: Axia Health Management
Doing Business As:
Year Founded: 1988   Federally Qualified: [N]
Forprofit: [Y]   Not-For-Profit: [ ]
Model Type: NETWORK
Accreditation: [ ] AAPPO [ ] JACHO [ ] NCQA [ ] URAC
Plan Type: Specialty HMO, Specialty PPO, ASO, UR, PBM,
Primary Physicians: 30,000   Physician Specialists:
Total Enrollment:
  2001: 0   2004: 0   2007: 0
  2002: 0   2005: 47,000,000
  2003: 0   2006:

SERVICE AREA:
Nationwide: Y
  NW;

TYPE OF COVERAGE:
Commercial: [Y] Individual: [ ] FEHBP: [ ] Indemnity: [ ]
Medicare: [Y] Medicaid: [Y] Supplemental Medicare: [ ]
Tricare   [ ]

PRODUCTS OFFERED:
Product Name: Type:
AWHN Select   Capitated
AWHN Preferred   Fee for service
Wholehealth Living   Discount Card
Wholehealth Choices   Affinity products

PLAN BENEFITS:
Alternative Medicine: [X]   Behavioral Health: [ ]
Chiropractic: [X]   Dental: [ ]
Home Care: [ ]   Inpatient SNF: [ ]
Long-Term Care: [ ]   Pharm. Mail Order: [X]
Physical Therapy: [ ]   Podiatry: [ ]
Psychiatric: [ ]   Transplant: [ ]
Vision: [ ]   Wellness: [X]
Workers' Comp: [X]
Other Benefits:

Comments:
Formerly Chirohealth America Inc, National Employee Benefit Inc, Chiropractic Health Partners of America.

ANTHEM BLUE CROSS BLUE SHIELD OF VIRGINIA INC

2015 Staples Mill Road Ste 1
Richmond, VA 23230
Phone: 804-354-7000 Fax: 804-354-2029 Toll-Free:
Web site: www.anthem.com

MAILING ADDRESS:
ANTHEM BC/BS OF VIRGINIA INC
PO Box 27401
Richmond, VA 23230

KEY EXECUTIVES:
Chairman of the Board/Chief Executive Officer ... Thomas G Snead, Jr
President/Chief Operating Officer .... Thomas G Snead, Jr
Senior VP, President VA/Chief Financial Officer .... Thomas R Byrd
Medical Director .... Jay Schukman, MD
Pharmacy Director .... Pat Russo
Chief Information Officer .... Ralph T Bullock
Marketing Director .... Carl J Slone
MIS Director .... Phil Crowder
Director Security Compliance .... Jeff Walko
Director, Provider Services .... Sam Rhye

COMPANY PROFILE:
Parent Company Name: WellPoint Inc
Doing Business As:
Year Founded: 1983   Federally Qualified: [ ]
Forprofit: [Y]   Not-For-Profit: [ ]
Model Type:
Accreditation: [ ] AAPPO [ ] JACHO [ ] NCQA [X] URAC
Plan Type: HMO, PPO, POS, HDHP, HSA
Primary Physicians: 5,955   Physician Specialists: 9,440
Hospitals: 98
Total Revenue: 2005: 3,267,093,966   2006: 3,480,050,275
Net Income   2005: 307,085,077   2006: 349,705,539
Total Enrollment:
  2001: 2,410,330   2004: 0   2007: 2,494,184
  2002: 0   2005:
  2003: 1,905,615   2006:
Medical Loss Ratio: 2005:   2006: 79.30
Administrative Expense Ratio: 2005:   2006:

SERVICE AREA:
Nationwide: N
  VA;

Managed Care Organization Profiles — VIRGINIA

ACTIVE HEALTH MANAGEMENT

14155 Newbrook Dr Ste 400
Chantilly, VA 20151
Phone: 703-995-6300 Fax: 703-488-9663 Toll-Free: 800-422-7711
Web site: www.health-cost.com

MAILING ADDRESS:
ACTIVE HEALTH MANAGEMENT
14155 Newbrook Dr Ste 400
Chantilly, VA 20151

KEY EXECUTIVES:
Chief Executive Officer .... Lonny Reisman, MD
President/Chief Operating Officer .... Felicia F Norwood
Chief Financial Officer .... John Budnick
Chief Medical Officer .... Gregory Steinberg, MD
Chief Information Officer .... Frank C Norman Jr
Senior VP, Marketing .... Len Greer
Senior VP, Sales .... Rich Beland
Executive VP, Clinical Programs .... Ann Meyer, RN, MBA
Executive VP, Corporate Development .... Michael G Lenahan
Executive VP, Operations .... Anne Polese

COMPANY PROFILE:
Parent Company Name: Active Health Management
Doing Business As:
Year Founded: 1983   Federally Qualified: [ ]
Forprofit: [Y]   Not-For-Profit: [ ]
Model Type:
Accreditation: [ ] AAPPO [ ] JACHO [ ] NCQA [X] URAC
Plan Type: UR

SERVICE AREA:
Nationwide: Y
  NW;

TYPE OF COVERAGE:
Commercial: [Y] Individual: [ ] FEHBP: [ ] Indemnity: [ ]
Medicare: [Y] Medicaid: [Y] Supplemental Medicare: [ ]
Tricare   [ ]

Comments:
Formerly Health Cost Consultants and E-MEDX. Acquired by Aetna Inc May 2005.

AETNA HEALTH PLANS OF MID-ATLANTIC

7600A Leesburg Pike
Falls Church, VA 22043
Phone: 703-903-7100 Fax: 703-903-7026 Toll-Free:
Web site: www.aetna.com

MAILING ADDRESS:
AETNA HEALTH PLANS-MID-ATLANTIC
7600A Leesburg Pike
Falls Church, VA 22043

KEY EXECUTIVES:
Chairman of the Board/Chief Executive Officer .... Ronald A Williams
President .... Mark T Bertolini
Executive VP, Finance .... Joseph M Zubretsky
Medical Director .... William Fried, MD
Sales Manager .... James Mackrell
Provider Services .... Amy Turner
General Manager .... Jeffrey Lucht
Government Relations .... Linda Cooper

COMPANY PROFILE:
Parent Company Name: Aetna Inc
Doing Business As:
Year Founded: 1984   Federally Qualified: [N]
Forprofit: [Y]   Not-For-Profit: [ ]
Model Type: IPA
Accreditation: [ ] AAPPO [ ] JACHO [X] NCQA [ ] URAC
Plan Type: HMO, PPO, POS, UR, CDHP, HDHP, HSA,
Primary Physicians: 4,455   Physician Specialists: 8,228
Hospitals: 81
Total Enrollment:
  2001: 0   2004: 376,442   2007: 0
  2002: 0   2005:
  2003: 0   2006:

SERVICE AREA:
Nationwide: N
DC; MD (Anne Arundel, Baltimore, Carroll, Cecil, Charles, Frederick, Harford, Howard, Montgomery, Prince Georges, St Mary's, Wicomico, Washington, Worcester); VA (Alexandria, Arlington, Caroline, Fairfax, Falls Churck, Fredricksburg, King George, Loudoun, Manassas, Manassas Park, Prince William, Spotsilvania, Stafford, Westmoreland);

TYPE OF COVERAGE:
Commercial: [Y] Individual: [ ] FEHBP: [ ] Indemnity: [ ]
Medicare: [ ] Medicaid: [ ] Supplemental Medicare: [ ]
Tricare   [ ]

CONSUMER-DRIVEN PRODUCTS
Aetna Life Insurance Co   HSA Company
Aetna HealthFund HSA   HSA Product
Aetna   HSA Administrator
Aetna HealthFund   Consumer-Driven Health Plan
PPO I; PPO II   High Deductible Health Plan

PLAN BENEFITS:
Alternative Medicine: [ ]   Behavioral Health: [ ]
Chiropractic: [X]   Dental: [X]
Home Care: [X]   Inpatient SNF: [X]
Long-Term Care: [ ]   Pharm. Mail Order: [X]
Physical Therapy: [X]   Podiatry: [X]
Psychiatric: [X]   Transplant: [X]
Vision: [X]   Wellness: [X]
Workers' Comp: [X]
Other Benefits:

AETNA INC - VIRGINIA

1100 Boulders Pkwy Ste 750
Richmond, VA 23225
Phone: 804-323-0900 Fax: 804-330-8676 Toll-Free:
Web site: www.aetna.com

MAILING ADDRESS:
AETNA INC - VA
1100 Boulders Pkwy Ste 750
Richmond, VA 23225

KEY EXECUTIVES:
Chairman of the Board/Chief Executive Officer .... Ronald A Williams
President .... Mark T Bertolini
Executive VP, Finance .... Joseph M Zubretsky
Sales Manager .... James Mackrell

COMPANY PROFILE:
Parent Company Name: Aetna Inc
Doing Business As:
Year Founded: Federally Qualified: [ ]
Forprofit: [Y]   Not-For-Profit: [ ]
Model Type:
Accreditation: [ ] AAPPO [ ] JACHO [ ] NCQA [ ] URAC
Plan Type: HMO, PPO, CDHP, HSA
Primary Physicians: 2660   Physician Specialists: 7,738
Hospitals: 71
Total Revenue: 2005: 710,048,946   2006: 715,122,403
Net Income   2005: 51,752,638   2006: 37,707,704
Total Enrollment:
  2001: 2,410,330   2004: 0   2007:
  2002: 0   2005:
  2003: 1,905,615   2006: 162,719

SERVICE AREA:
Nationwide: N
  VA;

TYPE OF COVERAGE:
Commercial: [Y] Individual: [ ] FEHBP: [ ] Indemnity: [ ]
Medicare: [ ] Medicaid: [ ] Supplemental Medicare: [ ]
Tricare   [ ]

CONSUMER-DRIVEN PRODUCTS
Aetna Life Insurance Co   HSA Company
Aetna HealthFund HSA   HSA Product
Aetna   HSA Administrator
Aetna HealthFund   Consumer-Driven Health Plan
PPO I; PPO II   High Deductible Health Plan

VERMONT

Managed Care Organization Profiles

BLUE CROSS BLUE SHIELD OF VERMONT

445 Industrial Lane
Berlin, VT 05601-0186
Phone: 802-223-6131 Fax: 802-229-0511 Toll-Free:
Web site: www.bcbsvt.com

MAILING ADDRESS:
BLUE CROSS BLUE SHIELD OF VT
PO Box 186
Montpelier, VT 05602

KEY EXECUTIVES:
Chairman of the Board .... Guy Boyer
Chief Executive Officer/President .... William R Milnes, Jr
Financial Officer .... James W Du Charmes, CMA
Chief Operating Officer .... Walter Merrow
VP, Marketing & Sales .... David Krupa
VP, Human Resources .... Karen Saudek
General Counsel & Secretary .... Jeffrey Johnson
VP Managed Health Systems .... Don George
VP, External Affairs .... Kevin Goddard

COMPANY PROFILE:
Parent Company Name: Blue Cross/Blue Shield of Vermont
Doing Business As:
Year Founded: 1944   Federally Qualified: [14]
Forprofit: [ ]   Not-For-Profit: [Y]
Model Type:
Accreditation: [ ] AAPPO [ ] JACHO [ ] NCQA [ ] URAC
Plan Type: HMO, PPO, POS, HDHP, HSA,
Total Enrollment:
  2001: 126,821   2004: 143,667   2007: 0
  2002: 137,110   2005: 189,980
  2003: 138,902   2006:

SERVICE AREA:
Nationwide: N
  VT;

TYPE OF COVERAGE:
Commercial: [Y] Individual: [ ] FEHBP: [ ] Indemnity: [ ]
Medicare: [ ] Medicaid: [ ] Supplemental Medicare: [ ]
Tricare   [ ]

PRODUCTS OFFERED:
Product Name: Type:
Blue First   Medicaid

PLAN BENEFITS:
Alternative Medicine: [ ]   Behavioral Health: [ ]
Chiropractic: [X]   Dental: [ ]
Home Care: [ ]   Inpatient SNF: [ ]
Long-Term Care: [ ]   Pharm. Mail Order: [ ]
Physical Therapy: [ ]   Podiatry: [ ]
Psychiatric: [ ]   Transplant: [ ]
Vision: [X]   Wellness: [X]
Workers' Comp: [ ]
Other Benefits:

CIGNA HEALTHCARE - VERMONT

30 Main St Ste 130
Burlington, VT 05401
Phone: 800-531-4584 Fax: 802-603-7981 Toll-Free: 800-531-4584
Web site: www.cigna.com

MAILING ADDRESS:
CIGNA HEALTHCARE - VERMONT
30 Main St Ste 130
Burlington, VT 05401

KEY EXECUTIVES:
Chief Executive Officer .... Donald M Curry
Client Manager .... Mark Gagne
Account Manager, Sales .... Sandra McAllister
Media Contact .... Lindsay Shearer

COMPANY PROFILE:
Parent Company Name: CIGNA Corporation
Doing Business As:
Year Founded: 1995   Federally Qualified: [Y]
Forprofit: [Y]   Not-For-Profit: [ ]
Model Type: IPA
Accreditation: [ ] AAPPO [X] JACHO [X] NCQA [ ] URAC
Plan Type: HMO, PPO, Specialty PPO, POS, ASO, EPO, PBM, CDHP, HSA, FSA, HRA
Hospitals: 14

Total Enrollment:
  2001: 0   2004: 0   2007: 0
  2002: 80,000   2005:
  2003: 85,000   2006:

SERVICE AREA:
Nationwide: N
  NH; VT;

TYPE OF COVERAGE:
Commercial: [Y] Individual: [ ] FEHBP: [ ] Indemnity: [ ]
Medicare: [ ] Medicaid: [ ] Supplemental Medicare: [ ]
Tricare   [ ]

CONSUMER-DRIVEN PRODUCTS
JP Morgan Chase   HSA Company
CIGNA Choice Fund   HSA Product
                             HSA Administrator
Open Access Plus   Consumer-Driven Health Plan
PPO   High Deductible Health Plan

PLAN BENEFITS:
Alternative Medicine: [ ]   Behavioral Health: [ ]
Chiropractic: [X]   Dental: [X]
Home Care: [X]   Inpatient SNF: [X]
Long-Term Care: [X]   Pharm. Mail Order: [X]
Physical Therapy: [X]   Podiatry: [X]
Psychiatric: [X]   Transplant: [X]
Vision: [X]   Wellness: [X]
Workers' Comp: [ ]
Other Benefits:

VERMONT HEALTH PLANS (BLUE CARE)

PO Box 186
Montpelier, VT 05601-0186
Phone: 800-905-8427 Fax: 802-229-0511 Toll-Free: 800-905-8427
Web site: www.bcbsvt.com

MAILING ADDRESS:
VERMONT HEALTH PLANS
PO Box 186
Montpelier, VT 05601-0186

KEY EXECUTIVES:
Chief Executive Officer/President .... William R Milnes, Jr
Chief Financial Officer .... John Trifone
Corporate Medical Director .... Stephen Perkins, MD
Chief Operating Officer .... Walter Merrow
VP, Marketing .... David Krupa
VP, Human Resources .... Karen Saudek
General Counsel & Secretary .... Jeffrey Johnson

COMPANY PROFILE:
Parent Company Name: Blue Cross Blue Shield
Doing Business As:
Year Founded: Federally Qualified: [ ]
Forprofit: [ ]   Not-For-Profit: [ ]
Model Type:
Accreditation: [ ] AAPPO [ ] JACHO [ ] NCQA [ ] URAC
Plan Type: HMO, POS
Total Revenue: 2005:   2006:
Net Income   2005: 9,736,222   2006:
Total Enrollment:
  2001: 28,570   2004: 22,333   2007: 0
  2002: 27,651   2005: 171,000
  2003: 26,266   2006:

SERVICE AREA:
Nationwide: N
  VT;

TYPE OF COVERAGE:
Commercial: [Y] Individual: [ ] FEHBP: [ ] Indemnity: [ ]
Medicare: [ ] Medicaid: [ ] Supplemental Medicare: [ ]
Tricare   [ ]

PRODUCTS OFFERED:
Product Name: Type:
Blue Care   HMO
                           POS

UTAH   Managed Care Organization Profiles

KEY EXECUTIVES:
Executive Director .... Curt Howell
Medical Director .... Robert Beauchamp, MD

COMPANY PROFILE:
Parent Company Name: UnitedHealth Group
Doing Business As:
Year Founded: 1984   Federally Qualified: [N]
Forprofit: [Y]   Not-For-Profit: [ ]Model Type: IPA
Accreditation: [ ] AAPPO [ ] JACHO [ ] NCQA [ ] URAC
Plan Type: HMO, PPO, POS, CDHP, HSA, HRA
Primary Physicians: 1,254   Physician Specialists: 1,786
Hospitals:
Total Enrollment:
   2001: 120,469   2004: 16,498   2007: 57,583
   2002:   55,137   2005:
   2003:   31,353   2006: 56,990

SERVICE AREA:
Nationwide: N
   UT (Box Elder, David, Salt Lake City, Summit, Tooele, Utah, Wasatch, Weber);

TYPE OF COVERAGE:
Commercial: [Y] Individual: [ ] FEHBP: [ ] Indemnity: [ ]
Medicare: [ ] Medicaid: [Y] Supplemental Medicare: [ ]
Tricare   [ ]

PRODUCTS OFFERED:
Product Name: Type:
MedChoice   Medicaid

CONSUMER-DRIVEN PRODUCTS
Exante Bank/Golden Rule Ins Co   HSA Company
iPlan HSA   HSA Product
                                 HSA Administrator
                                 Consumer-Driven Health Plan
                                 High Deductible Health Plan

PLAN BENEFITS:
Alternative Medicine: Behavioral Health: [X]
Chiropractic: [X]   Dental: [ ]
Home Care: [X]   Inpatient SNF: [X]
Long-Term Care: [ ]   Pharm. Mail Order: [X]
Physical Therapy: [X]   Podiatry: [X]
Psychiatric: [X]   Transplant: [X]
Vision: [X]   Wellness: [X]
Workers' Comp: [ ]
Other Benefits:

TYPE OF COVERAGE:
Commercial: [Y] Individual: [ ] FEHBP: [ ] Indemnity: [ ]
Medicare: [ ] Medicaid: [ ] Supplemental Medicare: [Y]
Tricare   [ ]

PLAN BENEFITS:
Alternative Medicine: [ ]   Behavioral Health:
[X]Chiropractic: [X]   Dental: [X]
Home Care: [X]   Inpatient SNF: [X]
Long-Term Care: [X]   Pharm. Mail Order: [X]
Physical Therapy: [X]   Podiatry: [X]
Psychiatric: [X]   Transplant: [X]
Vision: [X]   Wellness: [X]
Workers' Comp: [ ]
Other Benefits:
Comments:
Open to Public Employees only.

UTAH PUBLIC EMPLOYEES HEALTH PROGRAM

560 E 200 South
Salt Lake City, UT 84102
Phone: 801-366-7555 Fax: 801-366-7596 Toll-Free:
Web site: www.pehp.org
MAILING ADDRESS:
   UTAH PUBLIC EMPLOYEES HEALTH PROGRAM
   560 E 200 South
   Salt Lake City, UT 84102

KEY EXECUTIVES:
Chief Executive Officer .... Linn Baker
Deputy Director .... Jeff Jensen
Financial Director .... Steve Broadhead
Medical Director .... Howard G McQuarrie, MD
Pharmacy Manager .... Deborah Webb
Operations Director .... Scott Hansen
Marketing Manager .... Carla Vandever
MIS Manager .... Rick Hanks
Provider Relations Manager .... Alicia Sylvies
Quality Assurance Manager .... Shelly Williams
Production Director .... Christy Simpson
Quality/Benefits Director .... Linda Parrish
Controller .... Randy Booth
Enrollment Manager .... Larry Herndon
LTD Manager .... Jalyn Outsen

COMPANY PROFILE:
Parent Company Name: State of Utah Retirement-PEHP
Doing Business As: Public Employees Health Plan
Year Founded: 1977   Federally Qualified: [ ]
Forprofit: [ ]   Not-For-Profit: [Y]
Model Type:
Accreditation: [ ] AAPPO [ ] JACHO [ ] NCQA [ ] URAC
Plan Type: PPO, TPA, HDHP, HSA,

SERVICE AREA:
Nationwide: N
   UT;

438   Copyright MCIC -- The National Directory of Managed Care Organizations, Seventh Edition

Managed Care Organization Profiles — UTAH

KEY EXECUTIVES:
Chief Executive Officer .... Mark B Ganz
Chief Financial Officer .... R Paul Warburton
Chief Medical Officer .... Paul Molchan, MD
Assistant VP, Pharmacy .... Terry Killilea
Assistant VP, Marketing & Sales .... Barbara Neilson

COMPANY PROFILE:
Parent Company Name: Regence Blue Cross Blueshield of UT
Doing Business As: Regence Blue Cross Blueshield of UT
Year Founded: 1984   Federally Qualified: [ ]
Forprofit: [ ]   Not-For-Profit: [Y]
Model Type: IPA
Accreditation: [ ] AAPPO [ ] JACHO [ ] NCQA [ ] URAC
Plan Type: HMO, PPO, PBM, TPA, HDHP, HSA,
Primary Physicians: 1,442   Physician Specialists: 2,797
Hospitals:

SERVICE AREA:
Nationwide: N
  UT;

TYPE OF COVERAGE:
Commercial: [Y] Individual: [Y] FEHBP: [ ] Indemnity: [ ]
Medicare: [ ]   Medicaid: [ ]   Supplemental Medicare: [ ]
Tricare [ ]

CONSUMER-DRIVEN PRODUCTS
HSA 101   HSA Company
Wells Fargo   HSA Product
                            HSA Administrator
                            Consumer-Driven Health Plan
                            High Deductible Health Plan

PLAN BENEFITS:
Alternative Medicine: [ ]   Behavioral Health: [X]
Chiropractic: [X]   Dental: [X]
Home Care: [X]   Inpatient SNF: [X]
Long-Term Care: [ ]   Pharm. Mail Order: [X]
Physical Therapy: [X]   Podiatry: [X]
Psychiatric: [X]   Transplant: [X]
Vision: [X]   Wellness: [X]
Workers' Comp: [ ]
Other Benefits:

SELECTHEALTH

4646 W Lake Park Blvd
Salt Lake City, UT 84120
Phone: 801-442-5000 Fax: 801-442-5183 Toll-Free: 800-538-5038
Web site: www.selecthealth.org

MAILING ADDRESS:
SELECTHEALTH
PO Box 30192
Salt Lake City, UT 84130-0912

KEY EXECUTIVES:
Chairman of the Board .... Thomas B Morgan
Chief Executive Officer/President .... Sidney C Paulson
Chief Financial Officer .... Bert R Zimmerli
Medical Director .... Stephen L Barlow, MD

COMPANY PROFILE:
Parent Company Name: Intermountain Health Care
Doing Business As: IHC Care, SelectMed, Hlth Chce, IHC Med
Year Founded: 1985   Federally Qualified: [N]
Forprofit: [ ]   Not-For-Profit: [Y]
Model Type: MIXED
Accreditation: [ ] AAPPO [ ] JACHO [X] NCQA [ ] URAC
Plan Type: HMO, PPO, POS, ASO, HDHP, HSA
Primary Physicians: 1,260   Physician Specialists: 2,025
Hospitals: 26
Total Enrollment:
  2001: 451,502   2004: 459,000   2007: 502,618
  2002: 323,006   2005:
  2003: 507,909   2006: 475,099

SERVICE AREA:
Nationwide: N
  ID (Southeastern); UT;

TYPE OF COVERAGE:
Commercial: [Y] Individual: [Y] FEHBP: [ ] Indemnity: [ ]
Medicare: [ ]   Medicaid: [ ]   Supplemental Medicare: [ ]
Tricare [ ]

PRODUCTS OFFERED:
Product Name: Type:
Health Choice   PPO
IHC Care   HMO/POS
Select Med   HMO
Self Funded   ASO
IHC Direct   HMO, POS
IHC Access   Medicaid
IHC MED   HMO

PLAN BENEFITS:
Alternative Medicine: [ ]   Behavioral Health: [ ]
Chiropractic: [X]   Dental: [X]
Home Care: [X]   Inpatient SNF: [X]
Long-Term Care: [X]   Pharm. Mail Order: [X]
Physical Therapy: [X]   Podiatry: [X]
Psychiatric: [X]   Transplant: [X]
Vision: [X]   Wellness: [X]
Workers' Comp: [X]
Other Benefits:

Comments:
DBA names: IHC Care, SelectMed, Health Choice, IHC Direct Care, IHC Med.

STANDARD OPTICAL

1901 W Parkway Blvd
Salt Lake City, UT 84119
Phone: 801-886-2020 Fax: 801-954-0054 Toll-Free: 800-363-0950
Web site: www.opticareofutah.com

MAILING ADDRESS:
STANDARD OPTICAL
1901 W Parkway Blvd
Salt Lake City, UT 84119

KEY EXECUTIVES:
Chief Executive Officer/President .... Stephen Schubach
Chief Financial Officer .... Kenneth Acker
Chief Operating Officer .... Aaron Schuback

COMPANY PROFILE:
Parent Company Name: Standard Optical
Doing Business As:
Year Founded: 1911   Federally Qualified: [N]
Forprofit: [Y]   Not-For-Profit: [ ]
Model Type: NETWORK
Accreditation: [ ] AAPPO [ ] JACHO [ ] NCQA [ ] URAC
Plan Type: Specialty HMO

SERVICE AREA:
Nationwide: N
  UT;

TYPE OF COVERAGE:
Commercial: [Y] Individual: [Y] FEHBP: [ ] Indemnity: [ ]
Medicare: [Y]   Medicaid: [Y]   Supplemental Medicare: [Y]
Tricare [ ]

PLAN BENEFITS:
Alternative Medicine: [ ]   Behavioral Health: [ ]
Chiropractic: [ ]   Dental: [ ]
Home Care: [ ]   Inpatient SNF: [ ]
Long-Term Care: [ ]   Pharm. Mail Order: [ ]
Physical Therapy: [ ]   Podiatry: [ ]
Psychiatric: [ ]   Transplant: [ ]
Vision: [X]   Wellness: [ ]
Workers' Comp: [ ]
Other Benefits: Optical Care

UNITEDHEALTHCARE OF UTAH

2525 Lake Park Blvd
Salt Lake City, UT 84120
Phone: 800-624-2942 Fax: 801-982-4550 Toll-Free: 800-624-2942
Web site: www.uhc.com

MAILING ADDRESS:
UNITEDHEALTHCARE OF UTAH
PO Box 71409
Salt Lake City, UT 84121

UTAH

Forprofit: [Y] Not-For-Profit: [ ]
Model Type: NETWORK
Accreditation: [ ] AAPPO [ ] JACHO [ ] NCQA [ ] URAC
Plan Type: HMO, TPA
Primary Physicians: 971 Physician Specialists: 804
Hospitals: 32
Total Revenue: 2005: 115,296,758 2006: 87,438,485
Net Income 2005: 673,447 2006: 513,000
Total Enrollment:
  2001: 16,187 2004: 49,463 2007: 0
  2002: 42,469 2005: 58,815
  2003: 45,340 2006: 52,000

SERVICE AREA:
Nationwide: N
  UT;

TYPE OF COVERAGE:
Commercial: [Y] Individual: [Y] FEHBP: [ ] Indemnity: [ ]
Medicare: [Y] Medicaid: [Y] Supplemental Medicare: [ ]
Tricare [ ]

PRODUCTS OFFERED:
Product Name:	Type:
Senior Security	Medicaid

PLAN BENEFITS:
Alternative Medicine:	[ ]	Behavioral Health:	[X]
Chiropractic:	[X]	Dental:	[ ]
Home Care:	[X]	Inpatient SNF:	[X]
Long-Term Care:	[ ]	Pharm. Mail Order:	[X]
Physical Therapy:	[X]	Podiatry:	[X]
Psychiatric:	[X]	Transplant:	[X]
Vision:	[X]	Wellness:	[X]
Workers' Comp:	[ ]		

Other Benefits:

Comments:
Formerly American Family Care of UT Inc.

REGENCE BLUE CROSS BLUE SHIELD OF UTAH

2890 E Cottonwood Pkwy
Salt Lake City, UT 84121
Phone: 801-333-2100 Fax: 801-333-6523 Toll-Free: 800-662-0876
Web site: www.ut.regence.com

MAILING ADDRESS:
REGENCE BC BS OF UT
PO Box 30270
Salt Lake City, UT 84121

KEY EXECUTIVES:
President .... D Scott Ideson
Chief Financial Officer .... R Paul Warburton
Chief Medical Officer .... Paul Molchan, MD
Pharmacy Director .... Jack Schiess
Chief Info Off/PR Director .... Kevin Bischoff
Senior VP, Sales & Marketing .... Donald E Smith
MIS Director .... Robert Johnston
Director, Provider Services .... Byron Clawson

COMPANY PROFILE:
Parent Company Name: The Regence Group
Doing Business As:
Year Founded: 1942 Federally Qualified: [Y]
Forprofit: [Y] Not-For-Profit: [ ]
Model Type: MIXED
Accreditation: [ ] AAPPO [ ] JACHO [ ] NCQA [ ] URAC
Plan Type: HMO, PPO, UR, CDHP, HDHP, HSA
Primary Physicians: 1,533 Physician Specialists: 2,901
Hospitals:
Total Enrollment:
  2001: 251,452 2004: 321,457 2007: 0
  2002: 332,281 2005:
  2003: 314,693 2006:

SERVICE AREA:
Nationwide: N
  UT;

TYPE OF COVERAGE:
Commercial: [Y] Individual: [Y] FEHBP: [ ] Indemnity: [ ]
Medicare: [ ] Medicaid: [Y] Supplemental Medicare: [Y]
Tricare [ ]

PRODUCTS OFFERED:
Product Name:	Type:
Healthpoint	HMO
Healthwise	HMO
Bluecare	HMO
ValueCare	PPO
Med-Utah	Medicaid

CONSUMER-DRIVEN PRODUCTS
Wells Fargo	HSA Company
Regence HSA	HSA Product
	HSA Administrator
	Consumer-Driven Health Plan
	High Deductible Health Plan

PLAN BENEFITS:
Alternative Medicine:	[ ]	Behavioral Health:	[X]
Chiropractic:	[X]	Dental:	[X]
Home Care:	[X]	Inpatient SNF:	[X]
Long-Term Care:	[ ]	Pharm. Mail Order:	[X]
Physical Therapy:	[X]	Podiatry:	[X]
Psychiatric:	[X]	Transplant:	[X]
Vision:	[X]	Wellness:	[ ]
Workers' Comp:	[X]		

Other Benefits:

REGENCE HEALTHWISE

PO Box 30804
Salt Lake City, UT 84130-0804
Phone: 801-333-2100 Fax: 801-333-6523 Toll-Free: 800-662-3398
Web site: www.ut.regence.com

MAILING ADDRESS:
REGENCE HEALTHWISE
PO Box 30804
Salt Lake City, UT 84130-0804

KEY EXECUTIVES:
President .... D Scott Ideson
Chief Financial Officer .... R Paul Warburton
Medical Director .... Paul Molchan, MD
Senior Vice President, Marketing .... Donald E Smith
Director, Provider Relations .... Byron Clawson

COMPANY PROFILE:
Parent Company Name: Blue Cross/Blue Shield
Doing Business As:
Year Founded: 1982 Federally Qualified: [Y]
Forprofit: [Y] Not-For-Profit: [ ]
Model Type: NETWORK
Accreditation: [ ] AAPPO [ ] JACHO [ ] NCQA [ ] URAC
Plan Type: HMO, HDHP, HSA,
Primary Physicians: 1,225 Physician Specialists: 2,407
Hospitals:
Total Enrollment:
  2001: 2,103 2004: 30,839 2007: 0
  2002: 17,312 2005:
  2003: 21,972 2006:

SERVICE AREA:
Nationwide: N
  UT (Davis, Salt Lake, Summit, Utah, Wasatch, Weber);

TYPE OF COVERAGE:
Commercial: [Y] Individual: [ ] FEHBP: [ ] Indemnity: [ ]
Medicare: [ ] Medicaid: [Y] Supplemental Medicare: [ ]
Tricare [ ]

PLAN BENEFITS:
Alternative Medicine:	[ ]	Behavioral Health:	[X]
Chiropractic:	[X]	Dental:	[ ]
Home Care:	[X]	Inpatient SNF:	[X]
Long-Term Care:	[ ]	Pharm. Mail Order:	[X]
Physical Therapy:	[X]	Podiatry:	[X]
Psychiatric:	[X]	Transplant:	[ ]
Vision:	[X]	Wellness:	[X]
Workers' Comp:	[ ]		

Other Benefits:

Comments:
Formerly Healthwise.

REGENCE VALUCARE

2890 E Cottonwood Pkwy
Salt Lake City, UT 84130
Phone: 801-333-2310 Fax: 801-333-6523 Toll-Free: 800-245-0026
Web site: www.ut.regence.com

MAILING ADDRESS:
REGENCE VALUCARE
PO Box 30270
Salt Lake City, UT 84130

Managed Care Organization Profiles — UTAH

HEALTHINSIGHT

348 E 4500 S Ste 300
Salt Lake City, UT 84170
Phone: 801-892-0155 Fax: 801-892-0160 Toll-Free:
Web site: www.healthinsight.org
MAILING ADDRESS:
　　HEALTHINSIGHT
　　348 E 4500 S Ste 300
　　Salt Lake City, UT 84170

KEY EXECUTIVES:
Chief Executive Officer/President .... Marc H Bennett
VP, Fiance/Administration/Chief Financial Officer ... Daniel Memmott
VP, Medical Affairs - Utah .... Kim Bateman, MD
VP, Medical Affairs - Nevada .... Robert W Shreck, MD, FAAFP
VP, Quality Assurance Director .... Lance N Coss, MS, MEd, CGC
VP, Strategy & Development .... Michael P Silver, MPH
VP, Quality Improvement .... Michelle Geis

COMPANY PROFILE:
Parent Company Name:
Doing Business As:
Year Founded: 1971　　　Federally Qualified: [N]
Forprofit: [ ]　　　　　　Not-For-Profit: [Y]
Model Type:
Accreditation: [ ] AAPPO [ ] JACHO [ ] NCQA [ ] URAC
Plan Type: PRO
SERVICE AREA:
Nationwide: N
　NV; UT;

HUMANA INC - UTAH

500 W Main St
Louisville, KY 40201
Phone: 502-580-5804 Fax: 502-980-8528 Toll-Free:
Web site: www.humana.com
MAILING ADDRESS:
　　HUMANA INC - UTAH
　　500 W Main St
　　Louisville, KY 40201

KEY EXECUTIVES:
Chairman of the Board .... David A Jones Jr
Chief Executive Officer/President .... Michael B McCallister
Chief Financial Officer .... James H Bloem
VP Medical Director .... Jonathan T Lord, MD
Senior VP, Chief Information Officer .... Bruce J Goodman
Senior VP, Human Resources .... Bonnie C Hathcock

COMPANY PROFILE:
Parent Company Name: Humana Inc
Doing Business As:
Year Founded: 1961　　　Federally Qualified: [Y]
Forprofit: [Y]　　　　　　Not-For-Profit: [ ]
Model Type:
Accreditation: [ ] AAPPO [ ] JACHO [ ] NCQA [ ] URAC
Plan Type: PPO, ASO, CDHP, HDHP, HSA,
SERVICE AREA:
Nationwide: N
　UT;
TYPE OF COVERAGE:
Commercial: [Y] Individual: [ ] FEHBP: [ ] Indemnity: [ ]
Medicare: [Y] Medicaid: [ ] Supplemental Medicare: [Y]
Tricare [ ]
CONSUMER-DRIVEN PRODUCTS
JP Morgan Chase　　　　　　HSA Company
HumanaOne HSA　　　　　　HSA Product
JP Morgan Chase　　　　　　HSA Administrator
Personal Care Account　　　Consumer-Driven Health Plan
HumanaOne　　　　　　　　High Deductible Health Plan
PLAN BENEFITS:
Alternative Medicine: [ ]　　Behavioral Health: [ ]
Chiropractic: [X]　　　　　　Dental: [X]
Home Care: [ ]　　　　　　　Inpatient SNF: [ ]
Long-Term Care: [ ]　　　　Pharm. Mail Order: [X]
Physicial Therapy: [ ]　　　Podiatry: [ ]
Psychiatric: [X]　　　　　　Transplant: [X]
Vision: [ ]　　　　　　　　　Wellness: [X]
Workers' Comp: [X]
Other Benefits:

MEDICAL REVIEW INSTITUTE - CORPORATE HEADQUARTERS

2875 S Decker Lake Dr Ste 550
Salt Lake City, UT 84119
Phone: 801-261-3003 Fax: 801-261-3189 Toll-Free: 800-654-2422
Web site: www.medicalopinions.com
MAILING ADDRESS:
　　MEDICAL REVIEW INSTITUTE
　　2875 S Decker Lake Dr Ste 550
　　Salt Lake City, UT 84119

KEY EXECUTIVES:
Chief Executive Officer/President .... William W Low
Chief Financial Officer .... William W Low
Corporate Medical Director .... Dick Creager, MD
Director of IT .... Don Murphy
Operations Manager .... Clara Tobin
Marketing Director .... Darren Rollins
Provider Relations Director .... Jeff Rollins
Quality Assurance Director .... Laura Daley

COMPANY PROFILE:
Parent Company Name: Medical Opinions Inc
Doing Business As: Medical Review Institute
Year Founded: 1982　　　Federally Qualified: [ ]
Forprofit: [Y]　　　　　　Not-For-Profit: [ ]
Model Type:
Accreditation: [ ] AAPPO [ ] JACHO [X] NCQA [X] URAC
Plan Type: UR, PRO
Primary Physicians:　　　　Physician Specialists: 750
Hospitals:
SERVICE AREA:
Nationwide: Y
　NW;
TYPE OF COVERAGE:
Commercial: [Y] Individual: [Y] FEHBP: [ ] Indemnity: [ ]
Medicare: [ ] Medicaid: [ ] Supplemental Medicare: [ ]
Tricare [ ]
PRODUCTS OFFERED:
Product Name:　　　　　　　Type:
Peer Review Nationwide　　Prospective, Concurr
PLAN BENEFITS:
Alternative Medicine: [ ]　　Behavioral Health: [X]
Chiropractic: [X]　　　　　　Dental: [X]
Home Care: [X]　　　　　　　Inpatient SNF: [X]
Long-Term Care: [X]　　　　Pharm. Mail Order: [ ]
Physical Therapy: [X]　　　Podiatry: [X]
Psychiatric: [X]　　　　　　Transplant: [X]
Vision: [X]　　　　　　　　　Wellness: [ ]
Workers' Comp: [X]
Other Benefits:

MOLINA HEALTHCARE OF UTAH INC

7050 Union Park Center Ste 200
Midvale, UT 84047
Phone: 801-858-0400 Fax: 801-858-0409 Toll-Free:
Web site: www.molinahealthcare.com
MAILING ADDRESS:
　　MOLINA HEALTHCARE OF UTAH
　　7050 Union Park Center Ste 200
　　Midvale, UT 84047

KEY EXECUTIVES:
Chairman of the Board .... Joseph M Molina, MD
Chief Executive Officer .... G Kirk Olsen
President .... Paul Muench
Director of Finance .... Farley Sowards
Medical Director .... Gary Call, MD
Director of Marketing .... Jason Worthen
Director of Provider Relations .... Michael Egbert
Humand Resources Director .... Francesca Sarvello
QI Director .... Karen Warren
Compliance Officer .... Brian Monsen
Vice Chairman .... George S Goldstein, PhD

COMPANY PROFILE:
Parent Company Name: Molina Healthcare Inc
Doing Business As:
Year Founded: 1998　　　Federally Qualified: [ ]

UTAH — Managed Care Organization Profiles

TYPE OF COVERAGE:
Commercial: [Y] Individual: [ ] FEHBP: [ ] Indemnity: [ ]
Medicare: [ ] Medicaid: [ ] Supplemental Medicare: [ ]
Tricare [ ]

CONSUMER-DRIVEN PRODUCTS
JP Morgan Chase   HSA Company
CIGNA Choice Fund   HSA Product
                               HSA Administrator
Open Access Plus   Consumer-Driven Health Plan
PPO   High Deductible Health Plan

PLAN BENEFITS:
Alternative Medicine: [ ]   Behavioral Health: [ ]
Chiropractic: [X]   Dental: [X]
Home Care: [X]   Inpatient SNF: [X]
Long-Term Care: [X]   Pharm. Mail Order: [X]
Physical Therapy: [X]   Podiatry: [X]
Psychiatric: [X]   Transplant: [X]
Vision: [X]   Wellness: [X]
Workers' Comp: [ ]
Other Benefits:

DELTA DENTAL INSURANCE COMPANY - UTAH

257 East 200 South Ste 375
Salt Lake City, UT 84111
Phone: 801-575-5168 Fax: 801-575-5171 Toll-Free: 800-453-5577
Web site: www.deltadental.com

MAILING ADDRESS:
DELTA DENTAL INSURANCE COMPANY - UTAH
257 East 200 South Ste 375
Salt Lake City, UT 84111

KEY EXECUTIVES:
Chief Executive Officer .... Gary D Radine
Chief Financial Officer .... Michael J Castro
Chief Information Officer .... Patrick S Steele
Marketing Director .... Sheila Ransdell

COMPANY PROFILE:
Parent Company Name: Delta Dental Plan of California
Doing Business As:
Year Founded: 1991   Federally Qualified: [ ]
Forprofit: [ ]   Not-For-Profit: [Y]
Model Type: NETWORK
Accreditation: [ ] AAPPO [ ] JACHO [ ] NCQA [ ] URAC
Plan Type: Specialty HMO
Total Enrollment:
  2001: 1,056   2004: 705   2007: 0
  2002: 1,067   2005:
  2003:   869   2006:

SERVICE AREA:
Nationwide: N
  UT (Salt Lake City);

TYPE OF COVERAGE:
Commercial: [Y] Individual: [Y] FEHBP: [ ] Indemnity: [ ]
Medicare: [ ] Medicaid: [ ] Supplemental Medicare: [ ]
Tricare [ ]

PLAN BENEFITS:
Alternative Medicine: [ ]   Behavioral Health: [ ]
Chiropractic: [ ]   Dental: [X]
Home Care: [ ]   Inpatient SNF: [ ]
Long-Term Care: [ ]   Pharm. Mail Order: [ ]
Physical Therapy: [ ]   Podiatry: [ ]
Psychiatric: [ ]   Transplant: [ ]
Vision: [ ]   Wellness: [ ]
Workers' Comp: [ ]
Other Benefits:

DESERET HEALTHCARE

60 East South Temple
Salt Lake City, UT 84111
Phone: 801-578-5600 Fax: 801-578-5905 Toll-Free: 800-777-3622
Web site: www.dmba.com

MAILING ADDRESS:
DESERET HEALTHCARE
PO Box 45530
Salt Lake City, UT 84111

KEY EXECUTIVES:
Chief Executive Officer/President .... Michael J Stapley
Chief Financial Officer .... Steve Felsted
Medical Director .... Larry Staker, MD
Pharmacy Director .... Jake Murdock
Chief Information Officer .... David Lewis
Director Health Care Systems .... Kent Whiting
Medical Management Director .... Marilyn Stewart, RN
Vice President Medical Plans .... David D Call
Director of Operations .... Ron Reed

COMPANY PROFILE:
Parent Company Name: Deseret Mutual
Doing Business As:
Year Founded: 1970   Federally Qualified: [N]
Forprofit: [ ]   Not-For-Profit: [Y]
Model Type: GROUP
Accreditation: [ ] AAPPO [ ] JACHO [ ] NCQA [ ] URAC
Plan Type: HMO, PPO, FSA
Primary Physicians: 707   Physician Specialists: 2,930
Hospitals:

SERVICE AREA:
Nationwide: Y
  NW;

TYPE OF COVERAGE:
Commercial: [Y] Individual: [ ] FEHBP: [ ] Indemnity: [ ]
Medicare: [Y] Medicaid: [ ] Supplemental Medicare: [Y]
Tricare [ ]

PLAN BENEFITS:
Alternative Medicine: [ ]   Behavioral Health: [ ]
Chiropractic: [X]   Dental: [X]
Home Care: [X]   Inpatient SNF: [X]
Long-Term Care: [ ]   Pharm. Mail Order: [X]
Physical Therapy: [X]   Podiatry: [X]
Psychiatric: [X]   Transplant: [X]
Vision: [X]   Wellness: [X]
Workers' Comp: [X]
Other Benefits:

EDUCATORS HEALTH CARE

852 E Arrowhead Ln
Murray, UT 84107-6399
Phone: 801-262-7476 Fax: 801-269-9734 Toll-Free: 800-662-5850
Web site: www.educatorsmutual.com

MAILING ADDRESS:
EDUCATORS HEALTH CARE
852 E Arrowhead Ln
Murray, UT 84107-6399

KEY EXECUTIVES:
Chief Executive Officer .... Rolando Galano
Chief Financial Officer .... David Glauser
Marketing Director .... Tom Busby

COMPANY PROFILE:
Parent Company Name:
Doing Business As:
Year Founded: 1979   Federally Qualified: [Y]
Forprofit: [ ]   Not-For-Profit: [Y]
Model Type: IPA
Accreditation: [ ] AAPPO [ ] JACHO [ ] NCQA [ ] URAC
Plan Type: HMO, FSA
Primary Physicians: 1,473   Physician Specialists: 3,001
Hospitals:
Total Enrollment:
  2001: 14,394   2004: 16,659   2007: 0
  2002: 10,684   2005:
  2003: 13,668   2006:

SERVICE AREA:
Nationwide: N
  UT;

TYPE OF COVERAGE:
Commercial: [Y] Individual: [ ] FEHBP: [ ] Indemnity: [ ]
Medicare: [ ] Medicaid: [ ] Supplemental Medicare: [ ]
Tricare [ ]

PRODUCTS OFFERED:
Product Name: Type:
Educators Care Plus   HMO
Educators Health Choice   PPO
Educators Select Care

Managed Care Organization Profiles UTAH

AETNA BEHAVIORAL HEALTH - UTAH CARE MANAGEMENT CENTER

10150 S Centennial Pkwy
Sandy, UT 84070
Phone: 801-256-7525 Fax: 801-256-7088 Toll-Free: 800-424-4047
Web site: www.aetna.com

MAILING ADDRESS:
AETNA BEHAVIORAL HEALTH- UTAH CMC
10150 S Centennial Pkwy
Sandy, UT 84070

KEY EXECUTIVES:
Chairman of the Board/Chief Executive Officer .... Ronald A Williams
Head - Aetna Behavioral Health .... Louise Murphy

COMPANY PROFILE:
Parent Company Name: Aetna Inc
Doing Business As:
Year Founded: Federally Qualified: [ ]
Forprofit: [Y]   Not-For-Profit: [ ]
Model Type:
Accreditation: [ ] AAPPO [ ] JACHO [ ] NCQA [ ] URAC
Plan Type: Specialty PPO
Primary Physicians: 65,000   Physician Specialists:
Hospitals:
Total Enrollment:
  2001: 0   2004: 0   2007: 0
  2002: 0   2005:
  2003: 0   2006: 12,000,000

SERVICE AREA:
Nationwide: N
  UT;

TYPE OF COVERAGE:
Commercial: [Y] Individual: [ ] FEHBP: [ ] Indemnity: [ ]
Medicare: [ ] Medicaid: [ ] Supplemental Medicare: [ ]
Tricare   [ ]

PRODUCTS OFFERED:
Product Name: Type:
Behavioral Health   Specialty PPO
Employee Assistance Program   EAP

PLAN BENEFITS:
Alternative Medicine: [ ]   Behavioral Health: [X]
Chiropractic: [ ]   Dental: [ ]
Home Care: [ ]   Inpatient SNF: [ ]
Long-Term Care: [ ]   Pharm. Mail Order: [ ]
Physical Therapy: [ ]   Podiatry: [ ]
Psychiatric: [ ]   Transplant: [ ]
Vision: [ ]   Wellness: [ ]
Workers' Comp: [ ]
Other Benefits:

Comments:
Purchased the assets of Magellan Health Services previously used to provide behavior health care services to Aetna's members.

ALTIUS HEALTH PLANS

10421 S Jordan Gateway Ste 400
South Jordan, UT 84095
Phone: 801-933-3412 Fax: 801-323-6100 Toll-Free: 800-365-1334
Web site: www.altiushealthplans.com

MAILING ADDRESS:
ALTIUS HEALTH PLANS
10421 S Jordan Gateway Ste 400
South Jordan, UT 84095

KEY EXECUTIVES:
Chief Executive Officer/President .... Michael Bahr
Chief Financial Officer .... Brett Clay
VP, Med Affrs,Chief Med Offr .... Dennis T Harston, MD, MBA
Pharmacy Director .... Robert Jaramillo
Director, Information Systems/MIS .... Russell Nelson
Operations Director .... Deborah Webster
Director, Marketing/Public Relations .... Debbie Rosenhan
Sales Director .... Bonnie Hansen
Credentialing Manager .... Collette Heaps
Privacy Officer .... Frank Kyle
Director, Provider Relations/Network Development .... Collette Heaps
Health Promotion Director .... Tanna Terrin
Human Resources Director .... Lani Anderson
Medical Management Director .... Tanna Ferrin
Quality Assurance Director .... Marsha Greenberg
Compliance Officer .... Frank Kyle

COMPANY PROFILE:
Parent Company Name: Coventry Health Care Inc
Doing Business As:
Year Founded: 1998   Federally Qualified: [Y]
Forprofit: [Y]   Not-For-Profit: [ ]
Model Type: MIXED
Accreditation: [ ] AAPPO [ ] JACHO [ ] NCQA [ ] URAC
Plan Type: HMO, PPO, POS, TPA, CDHP, HDHP, HSA, FSA
Primary Physicians: 1,568   Physician Specialists: 2,085
Hospitals: 46
Total Revenue: 2005:   2006:
Net Income   2005: 11,382,220   2006:
Total Enrollment:
  2001: 103,478   2004: 121,060   2007: 222,000
  2002: 160,282   2005: 207,722
  2003: 168,391   2006: 2,100,000

SERVICE AREA:
Nationwide: N
  ID; UT (Box Elder, Cache, Davis, Juab, Morgan, Salt Lake, Summit, Tooele, Utah, Wasatch, Washington, Weber); WY;

TYPE OF COVERAGE:
Commercial: [Y] Individual: [Y] FEHBP: [Y] Indemnity: [ ]
Medicare: [ ] Medicaid: [ ] Supplemental Medicare: [ ]
Tricare   [ ]

PRODUCTS OFFERED:
Product Name: Type:
Altius   HMO
Total Choice   POS
Altius   Medicaid
Peak Advantage

CONSUMER-DRIVEN PRODUCTS
Wells Fargo   HSA Company
                                     HSA Product
Corporate Benefits Servs of Am   HSA Administrator
                                     Consumer-Driven Health Plan
Open Access Plus Plan   High Deductible Health Plan

PLAN BENEFITS:
Alternative Medicine: [ ]   Behavioral Health: [X]
Chiropractic: [X]   Dental: [X]
Home Care: [X]   Inpatient SNF: [X]
Long-Term Care: [ ]   Pharm. Mail Order: [X]
Physical Therapy: [X]   Podiatry: [X]
Psychiatric: [X]   Transplant: [X]
Vision: [X]   Wellness: [X]
Workers' Comp: [ ]
Other Benefits:

Comments:
Formerly Pacificare of Utah. Purchased Integroup of Utah Inc.

CIGNA HEALTH PLAN OF UTAH INC

5295 S 320 West Ste 280
Salt Lake City, UT 84107
Phone: 801-265-2777 Fax: 801-261-7537 Toll-Free: 800-261-5731
Web site: www.cigna.com

MAILING ADDRESS:
CIGNA HEALTH PLAN OF UTAH INC
5295 S 320 West Ste 280
Salt Lake City, UT 84107

KEY EXECUTIVES:
General Manager .... Daryl W Edmonds
Medical Director .... Dennis Chong, MD
Regional Marketing Director .... Sallie A Vanasdale
Public Relations Director .... Gwyn Dilday

COMPANY PROFILE:
Parent Company Name: CIGNA Corporation
Doing Business As:
Year Founded: 1985   Federally Qualified: [Y]
Forprofit: [Y]   Not-For-Profit: [ ]
Model Type: IPA
Accreditation: [ ] AAPPO [ ] JACHO [ ] NCQA [ ] URAC
Plan Type: HMO, PPO, ASO, POS, CDHP, HDHP, HSA, FSA, HRA
Total Revenue: 2005:   2006:
Net Income   2005: 401,667   2006:
Total Enrollment:
  2001: 9,698   2004: 4,216   2007: 2,377
  2002: 6,716   2005:
  2003: 5,381   2006: 2,100

SERVICE AREA:
Nationwide: N
  UT (Box Elder, Cache, Davis, Morgan, Salt Lake, Summit, Tooele, Utah, Wasatch, Weber);

TEXAS — Managed Care Organization Profiles

SERVICE AREA:
Nationwide: N
  TX (Anderson, Angelina, Aransas, Archer, Atascosa, Bastrop, Bell, Bexar, Bowie, Brazoria, Brazos, Brown, Calhoun, Cameron, Chambers, Cherokee, Collin, Dallas, Denton, Ector, El Paso, Ellis, Fort Bend, Galveston, Gillespie, Gray, Grayson, Guadalupe, Harris, Hays, Henderson, Hidalgo, Hopkins, Houston, Howard, Hunt, Jefferson, Johnson, Jones, Kaufman, Kerr, Kleberg, Lamar, Liberty, Limestone, Lubbock, McLennan, Midland, Montgomery, Nacogdoches, Navarro, Nueces, Orange, Parker, Potter, Randall, Rockwall, Rusk, Smith, Tarrant, Taylor, Titus, Tom Green, Travis, Victoria, Walker, Washington, Wharton, Wichita, Williamson, Wise);

TYPE OF COVERAGE:
Commercial: [ ]   Individual: [ ]   FEHBP: [ ]   Indemnity: [ ]
Medicare: [ ]   Medicaid: [Y]   Supplemental Medicare: [ ]
Tricare: [ ]

PRODUCTS OFFERED:
Product Name: Type:
ValueOptions Medicaid   Medicaid

PLAN BENEFITS:
Alternative Medicine: [ ]   Behavioral Health: [X]
Chiropractic: [ ]   Dental: [ ]
Home Care: [ ]   Inpatient SNF: [ ]
Long-Term Care: [ ]   Pharm. Mail Order: [ ]
Physical Therapy: [ ]   Podiatry: [ ]
Psychiatric: [X]   Transplant: [ ]
Vision: [ ]   Wellness: [X]
Workers' Comp: [ ]
Other Benefits:

Managed Care Organization Profiles — TEXAS

SERVICE AREA:
Nationwide: N
  TX (Collin, Cooke, Dallas, Denton, Ellis, Erath, Fannin, Grayson, Hood, Hunt, Johnson, Kaufman, Palo Pinto, Parker, Rockwall, Somervell, Tarrant, Wise);
TYPE OF COVERAGE:
Commercial: [Y] Individual: [ ] FEHBP: [ ] Indemnity: [ ]
Medicare: [ ] Medicaid: [ ] Supplemental Medicare: [ ]
Tricare   [ ]
PRODUCTS OFFERED:

Product Name:	Type:
United HealthCare Choice	HMO
United HealthCare	HMO
United HealthCare	POS
United HealthCare	PPO
United HealthCare	Indemnity
Medicare Complete	Medicare

CONSUMER-DRIVEN PRODUCTS

Exante Bank/Golden Rule Ins Co	HSA Company
iPlan HSA	HSA Product
	HSA Administrator
	Consumer-Driven Health Plan
	High Deductible Health Plan

PLAN BENEFITS:

Alternative Medicine:	[ ]	Behavioral Health:	[ ]
Chiropractic:	[X]	Dental:	[X]
Home Care:	[X]	Inpatient SNF:	[X]
Long-Term Care:	[ ]	Pharm. Mail Order:	[X]
Physical Therapy:	[X]	Podiatry:	[X]
Psychiatric:	[X]	Transplant:	[X]
Vision:	[X]	Wellness:	[X]
Workers' Comp:	[ ]		

Other Benefits:
Comments:
Formerly Metrahealth Care Plan Inc.

UTMB HEALTH PLANS INC

301 University Blvd Rt 0985
Galveston, TX 77555-0985
Phone: 409-797-8010 Fax: 409-772-6216 Toll-Free:
Web site: www.utmb.edu
MAILING ADDRESS:
  UTMB HEALTHCARE SYSTEMS
  301 University Blvd Rt 0985
  Galveston, TX 77555-0985

KEY EXECUTIVES:
Chief Executive Officer/President .... Aurora B Mitchell
Chief Financial Officer .... Lawrence Revill
Medical Director .... Reuben Matalon, MD
MIS Director .... Gina Hightower
Compliance Officer .... Melba Stiefel
Provider Relations Director .... Jennifer Gabbard
Director of Human Resources .... Rhea Hernandez
Compliance Specialist .... Sandy Benigar

COMPANY PROFILE:
Parent Company Name:
Doing Business As: UTMB HealthCare Systems
Year Founded: 1998   Federally Qualified: [ ]
Forprofit: [ ]   Not-For-Profit: [Y]
Model Type:
Accreditation: [ ] AAPPO [ ] JACHO [ ] NCQA [ ] URAC
Plan Type: HMO
Total Revenue: 2005: 27,362,110   2006: 25,429,778
Net Income   2005:   1,070,810   2006:   2,118,416
Total Enrollment:
   2001: 40,515   2004: 28,689   2007: 789
   2002: 48,171   2005: 25,310
   2003: 52,000   2006: 22,303
SERVICE AREA:
Nationwide: N
  TX (Angelina, Austin, Brazoria, Brazos, Burleson, Chambers, Colorado, Fort Bend, Galveston, Grimes, Hardin, Harris, Houston, Jasper, Jefferson, Leon, Liberty, Madison, Matagorda, Montgomery, Nacogdoches, Newton, Orange, Polk, Robertson, Sabine, San Augustine, San Jacinto, Shelby, Trinity, Tyler, Walker, Waller, Washington, Wharton);
TYPE OF COVERAGE:
Commercial: [Y] Individual: [ ] FEHBP: [ ] Indemnity: [ ]
Medicare: [ ] Medicaid: [ ] Supplemental Medicare: [ ]
Tricare   [ ]
PRODUCTS OFFERED:

Product Name:	Type:
Utmb Healthcare Systems	HMO

VALLEY BAPTIST INSURANCE COMPANY

2005 Ed Carey Dr
Harlingen, TX 78550
Phone: 956-389-2273 Fax: 956-389-2281 Toll-Free: 877-422-4400
Web site: www.vbmc.org
MAILING ADDRESS:
  VALLEY BAPTIST INSURANCE CO
  2005 Ed Carey Dr
  Harlingen, TX 78550

KEY EXECUTIVES:
Chief Executive Officer/President .... Karen Pederson
Chief Financial Officer .... Danny Coyle
Chief Medical Officer .... Garner Klein, MD
Marketing Director .... Nick Espinola
Information Systems Director .... Mohammed Abbas
Privacy Officer .... Carol Hrobowchec

COMPANY PROFILE:
Parent Company Name: Valley Baptist Health Plan Inc
Doing Business As:
Year Founded: Federally Qualified: [N]
Forprofit: [ ]   Not-For-Profit: [ ]
Model Type: IPA
Accreditation: [ ] AAPPO [ ] JACHO [ ] NCQA [ ] URAC
Plan Type: HMO, POS, TPA, UR,
Total Revenue: 2005: 36,916,709   2006: 16,669,779
Net Income   2005:   248,310   2006:
Total Enrollment:
   2001: 11,421   2004: 12,059   2007: 0
   2002: 11,183   2005: 11,280
   2003:   9,658   2006: 14,267
SERVICE AREA:
Nationwide: N
  TX (Cameron, Hadalgo, Willacy);
TYPE OF COVERAGE:
Commercial: [Y] Individual: [ ] FEHBP: [ ] Indemnity: [ ]
Medicare: [ ] Medicaid: [ ] Supplemental Medicare: [ ]
Tricare   [ ]
PRODUCTS OFFERED:

Product Name:	Type:
Valley Health Plans	HMO

VALUEOPTIONS OF TEXAS INC

1199 S Beltline Ste 100
Coppell, TX 75019
Phone: 972-906-2500 Fax: 972-906-0846 Toll-Free: 800-535-0108
Web site: www.valueoptions.com
MAILING ADDRESS:
  VALUEOPTIONS OF TEXAS INC
  1199 S Beltline Ste 100
  Coppell, TX 75019

KEY EXECUTIVES:
Chairman of the Board/President .... Ronald I Dozoretz
Chief Executive Officer .... Barbara Hill
Chief Financial Officer .... Paul Dunn
Chief Clinical Officer .... Donald E Christensen, MD
Chief Information Officer .... Bob Esposito
Chief Operating Officer .... Michele D Alfano

COMPANY PROFILE:
Parent Company Name: FHC Health Systems
Doing Business As:
Year Founded: 1998   Federally Qualified: [ ]
Forprofit: [Y]   Not-For-Profit: [ ]
Model Type:
Accreditation: [ ] AAPPO [ ] JACHO [X] NCQA [X] URAC
Plan Type: Specialty HMO,
Total Revenue: 2005: 121,418,648   2006: 120,430,987
Net Income   2005:   -5,648   2006:   -13,877
Total Enrollment:
   2001: 144,841   2004: 262,697   2007: 266,206
   2002: 229,484   2005: 266,530
   2003: 244,034   2006: 261,833

TEXAS
Managed Care Organization Profiles

MAILING ADDRESS:
UNITEDHEALTHCARE OF TEXAS-HOUSTON
1333 West Loop South Ste 1100
Houston, TX 77027

KEY EXECUTIVES:
Non-Executive Chairman .... Richard T Burke
Chief Executive Officer .... Randy Giles
Medical Director .... Charles J Morris, MD
Chief Operating Officer .... Michael J Koehler
MIS Director .... Son Nguyen
Provider Portal Deployment Leader .... Audrey Mohr
Network Management Director .... Marcia Shea
Human Resource Director .... Lori Burggraff
Medical Expense Manager .... Prowess White
Quality Assurance Manager .... Lynn Schwaazenburg
Ancillary Benefits Director .... Marcia Shea
VP Small Business Sales .... Frederick Bricker

COMPANY PROFILE:
Parent Company Name: UnitedHealth Group
Doing Business As:
Year Founded: 1985   Federally Qualified: [ ]
Forprofit: [Y]   Not-For-Profit: [ ]
Model Type: NETWORK
Accreditation: [ ] AAPPO [ ] JACHO [X] NCQA [ ] URAC
Plan Type: HMO, PPO, UR, POS, CDHP, HDHP, HSA, HRA,
Primary Physicians: 2,514   Physician Specialists: 6,739
Hospitals: 96
Total Revenue: 2005: 61,679,413   2006: 10,173,039
Net Income   2005: 2,396,816   2006: -410,499
Total Enrollment:
  2001: 78,627   2004: 17,929   2007: 1,576
  2002: 382,916   2005: 16,439
  2003: 0   2006: 2,269
Medical Loss Ratio: 2005:   2006:
Administrative Expense Ratio: 2005:   2006:

SERVICE AREA:
Nationwide: N
  TX (Austin, Brazoria, Braxos, Burleson, Calhoun, Chambers, Fort Bend, Galveston, Grimes, Harris, Jackson, Liberty, Matagorda, Montgomery, Victoria, Waller, Walker, Wharton);

TYPE OF COVERAGE:
Commercial: [Y]   Individual: [ ]   FEHBP: [ ]   Indemnity: [ ]
Medicare: [ ]   Medicaid: [ ]   Supplemental Medicare: [ ]
Tricare   [ ]

PRODUCTS OFFERED:
Product Name: Type:
United HealthCare Choice   HMO
United HealthCare   HMO
United HealthCare   POS
United HealthCare   PPO
United HealthCare   Indemnity
Medicare Complete   Medicare

CONSUMER-DRIVEN PRODUCTS
Exante Bank/Golden Rule Ins Co   HSA Company
iPlan HSA   HSA Product
                                       HSA Administrator
                                       Consumer-Driven Health Plan
                                       High Deductible Health Plan

PLAN BENEFITS:
Alternative Medicine: [ ]   Behavioral Health: [ ]
Chiropractic: [X]   Dental: [X]
Home Care: [X]   Inpatient SNF: [X]
Long-Term Care: [ ]   Pharm. Mail Order: [X]
Physical Therapy: [X]   Podiatry: [X]
Psychiatric: [X]   Transplant: [X]
Vision: [X]   Wellness: [X]
Workers' Comp: [ ]
Other Benefits:

Comments:
Formerly Metrahealth Care Plan of Texas Inc.

UNITEDHEALTHCARE OF TEXAS INC - SAN ANTONIO

5959 Northwest Pkwy Ste 107
San Antonio, TX 78249-3340
Phone: 210-694-6850 Fax: 210-694-6868 Toll-Free: 800-842-0174
Web site: www.uhc.com

MAILING ADDRESS:
UNITEDHEALTHCARE OF TX
5959 Northwest Pkwy Ste 107
San Antonio, TX 78249-3340

KEY EXECUTIVES:
Non-Executive Chairman .... Richard T Burke
Chief Executive Officer .... Robert Herndon
Medical Director .... Michael Hawkins, MD
Director, Network Operations .... Jeffrey Cook

COMPANY PROFILE:
Parent Company Name: UnitedHealth Group
Doing Business As:
Year Founded: 1987   Federally Qualified: [Y]
Forprofit: [Y]   Not-For-Profit: [ ]
Model Type: IPA
Accreditation: [ ] AAPPO [ ] JACHO [ ] NCQA [ ] URAC
Plan Type: HMO, PPO, UR, POS, CDHP, HDHP, HSA,
Total Revenue: 2005: 26,911,932   2006: 261,744,002
Net Income   2005:   864,405   2006: -3,311,431
Total Enrollment:
  2001: 55,537   2004: 6,300   2007: 6,099
  2002: 38,137   2005: 10,712
  2003: 17,692   2006: 6,440

SERVICE AREA:
Nationwide: N
  TX (Atascosa, Bandera, Bastrop, Bell, Bexar, Blanco, Burnet, Caldwell, Comal, Fayette, Gillespie, Guadalupe, Hays, Kendall, Kerr, Lee, McLennan, Medina, Milam, Travis, Williamson, Wilson);

TYPE OF COVERAGE:
Commercial: [Y]   Individual: [ ]   FEHBP: [ ]   Indemnity: [ ]
Medicare: [ ]   Medicaid: [ ]   Supplemental Medicare: [ ]
Tricare   [ ]

PRODUCTS OFFERED:
Product Name: Type:
United HealthCare Choice   HMO
United HealthCare   HMO
United HealthCare   POS
United HealthCare   PPO
United HealthCare   Indemnity

CONSUMER-DRIVEN PRODUCTS
Exante Bank/Golden Rule Ins Co   HSA Company
iPlan HSA   HSA Product
                                       HSA Administrator
                                       Consumer-Driven Health Plan
                                       High Deductible Health Plan

PLAN BENEFITS:
Alternative Medicine: [ ]   Behavioral Health: [X]
Chiropractic: [X]   Dental: [X]
Home Care: [X]   Inpatient SNF: [X]
Long-Term Care: [ ]   Pharm. Mail Order: [X]
Physical Therapy: [X]   Podiatry: [X]
Psychiatric: [X]   Transplant: [X]
Vision: [X]   Wellness: [X]
Workers' Comp: [ ]
Other Benefits:

UNITEDHEALTHCARE OF TEXAS INC — DALLAS

5800 Granite Pkwy #900
Plano, TX 75024
Phone: 469-633-8500 Fax: 469-633-8815 Toll-Free: 800-458-5653
Web site: www.uhc.com

MAILING ADDRESS:
UNITEDHEALTHCARE OF TEXAS INC
5800 Granite Pkwy #900
Plano, TX 75024

KEY EXECUTIVES:
Non-Executive Chairman .... Richard T Burke
Chief Executive Officer .... Thomas Quirk
Medical Director .... Paul Solomon, MD
Vice President of Sales .... Martin Foster

COMPANY PROFILE:
Parent Company Name: UnitedHealth Group
Doing Business As: United HealthCare of Texas - Dallas
Year Founded: 1987   Federally Qualified: [N]
Forprofit: [Y]   Not-For-Profit: [ ]
Model Type: IPA
Accreditation: [ ] AAPPO [ ] JACHO [X] NCQA [ ] URAC
Plan Type: HMO, PPO, POS, ASO, EPO, CDHP, HDHP, HSA, HRA,
Total Revenue: 2005: 481,239,427   2006: 17,727,703
Net Income   2005: -110,570   2006:
Total Enrollment:
  2001: 120,776   2004: 40,028   2007: 4,813
  2002: 237,455   2005: 10,361
  2003: 1,100,000 2006: 3,137

Managed Care Organization Profiles — TEXAS

SERVICE AREA:
Nationwide: N
   TX;
TYPE OF COVERAGE:
Commercial: [Y]   Individual: [Y]   FEHBP: [ ]   Indemnity: [ ]
Medicare: [ ]   Medicaid: [ ]   Supplemental Medicare: [ ]
Tricare   [ ]
PRODUCTS OFFERED:
Product Name: Type:
Unicare PPO   PPO
CONSUMER-DRIVEN PRODUCTS
JP Morgan Chase   HSA Company
Complete Choice HealthFund   HSA Product
Arcus Enterprises Inc   HSA Administrator
                                       Consumer-Driven Health Plan
UniCare PPO HRA   High Deductible Health Plan
PLAN BENEFITS:
Alternative Medicine: [ ]   Behavioral Health: [X]
Chiropractic: [X]   Dental: [ ]
Home Care: [X]   Inpatient SNF: [X]
Long-Term Care: [ ]   Pharm. Mail Order: [X]
Physical Therapy: [X]   Podiatry: [X]
Psychiatric: [X]   Transplant: [X]
Vision: [ ]   Wellness: [X]
Workers' Comp: [ ]
Other Benefits:
Comments:
Pharmacy benefits are handled by WellPoint Pharmacy.

UNITED CONCORDIA COMPANY INC - TEXAS

8214 Westchester Dr Ste 600
Dallas, TX 75225
Phone: 214-378-6410 Fax: 214-378-6306 Toll-Free:
Web site: www.ucci.com
MAILING ADDRESS:
   UNITED CONCORDIA CO INC - TX
   8214 Westchester Dr Ste 600
   Dallas, TX 75225

KEY EXECUTIVES:
Chief Executive Officer/President .... Thomas A Dzuryachko
Senior VP, Finance .... Daniel Wright
VP, National Dental Director .... Richard Klich, DMD
Marketing Director .... Gretchen Stevenson
Regional Sales Manager .... Craig Martin
MIS Director .... Jim Robins
Dental Director .... Gary Delz, DDS

COMPANY PROFILE:
Parent Company Name: Highmark Inc
Doing Business As:
Year Founded: 1988   Federally Qualified: [ ]
Forprofit: [Y]   Not-For-Profit: [ ]
Model Type:
Accreditation: [ ] AAPPO [ ] JACHO [X] NCQA [ ] URAC
Plan Type: Specialty HMO, Specialty PPO, POS, TPA
Total Revenue: 2005:   2006:   737,928
Net Income   2005:   -76,749   2006:
Total Enrollment:
   2001: 3,235   2004: 3,799   2007: 4,280
   2002: 0   2005: 4,219
   2003: 3,463   2006: 4,513
SERVICE AREA:
Nationwide: N
   LA; OK; TX (Bastrop, Bell, Bexar, Brazoria, Brazos, Chambers,
   Collin, Comal, Dallas, Denton, El Paso, Ellis, Falls, Fort Bend,
   Galveston, Grayson, Grimes, Guadalupe, Harris, Hays, Hill,
   Jefferson, Johnson, Kaufman, Liberty, McLennan, Midland, Milam,
   Montgomery, Orange, Robertson, Rockwall, Smith, Tarrant, Tom
   Green, Travis, Upshur, Van Zandt, Walker, Waller, Webb,
   Williamson);
TYPE OF COVERAGE:
Commercial: [Y]   Individual: [ ]   FEHBP: [ ]   Indemnity: [ ]
Medicare: [ ]   Medicaid: [ ]   Supplemental Medicare: [ ]
Tricare   [ ]
PRODUCTS OFFERED:
Product Name: Type:
United Concordia Dental Plans   Specialty HMO

PLAN BENEFITS:
Alternative Medicine: [ ]   Behavioral Health: [ ]
Chiropractic: [ ]   Dental: [X]
Home Care: [ ]   Inpatient SNF: [ ]
Long-Term Care: [ ]   Pharm. Mail Order: [ ]
Physical Therapy: [ ]   Podiatry: [ ]
Psychiatric: [ ]   Transplant: [ ]
Vision: [ ]   Wellness: [ ]
Workers' Comp: [ ]
Other Benefits:
Comments:
Formerly Alternative Dental Care of Texas. For enrollment and
revenues see Corporate listing, Camp Hill, PA.

UNITED DENTAL CARE OF TEXAS INC - ASSURANT EMPLOYEE BENEFITS

16775 Addison Rd Ste 500
Addison, TX 75001
Phone: 214-258-1020 Fax: 214-258-1100 Toll-Free: 800-442-0911
Web site: www.assurantemployeebenefits.com
MAILING ADDRESS:
   UDC OF TEXAS INC - ASSURANT
   16775 Addison Rd Ste 500
   Addison, TX 75001

KEY EXECUTIVES:
Interim Chief Executive Officer/President .... John S Roberts
Chief Financial Officer .... Floyd F Chadee
VP, Medical Director .... Polly M Galbraith, MD
Chief Information Officer .... Karla J Schacht
Senior VP, Marketing .... Joseph A Sevcik
Privacy Officer .... John L Fortini
VP, Provider Services .... James A Barrett, DMD
Senior VP, Human Resources & Development .... Sylvia R Wagner
General Manager .... Todd Boyd
National Dental Director .... James A Barrett, DMD

COMPANY PROFILE:
Parent Company Name: Assurant Health
Doing Business As: United Dental Care of Texas Inc
Year Founded: 1975   Federally Qualified: [ ]
Forprofit: [Y]   Not-For-Profit: [ ]
Model Type:
Accreditation: [ ] AAPPO [ ] JACHO [ ] NCQA [ ] URAC
Plan Type: Specialty HMO
Total Revenue: 2005:   2006:   13,956,363
Net Income   2005:   2006:
Total Enrollment:
   2001: 0   2004: 0   2007: 101,988
   2002: 0   2005:
   2003: 0   2006: 133,299
SERVICE AREA:
Nationwide: N
   TX;
TYPE OF COVERAGE:
Commercial: [Y]   Individual: [Y]   FEHBP: [ ]   Indemnity: [ ]
Medicare: [ ]   Medicaid: [ ]   Supplemental Medicare: [ ]
Tricare   [ ]
PLAN BENEFITS:
Alternative Medicine: [ ]   Behavioral Health: [ ]
Chiropractic: [ ]   Dental: [X]
Home Care: [ ]   Inpatient SNF: [ ]
Long-Term Care: [ ]   Pharm. Mail Order: [ ]
Physical Therapy: [ ]   Podiatry: [ ]
Psychiatric: [ ]   Transplant: [ ]
Vision: [X]   Wellness: [ ]
Workers' Comp: [ ]
Other Benefits:
Comments:
Formerly Fortis Benefits Dental.

UNITEDHEALTHCARE OF TEXAS INC - HOUSTON

1333 West Loop South Ste 1100
Houston, TX 77027
Phone: 713-961-4300 Fax: 713-961-4431 Toll-Free:
Web site: www.uhc.com

TEXAS
Managed Care Organization Profiles

Year Founded: 1971
Forprofit: [ ]
Model Type:
Accreditation: [ ] AAPPO [ ] JACHO [ ] NCQA [ ] URAC
Plan Type: UR
Federally Qualified: [ ]
Not-For-Profit: [Y]
SERVICE AREA:
Nationwide: N
   TX;

TEXAS TRUE CHOICE

5000 Legacy Dr Ste 190
Plano, TX 75024
Phone: 469-443-3400 Fax: 469-443-3401 Toll-Free: 800-683-4856
Web site: www.texastruechoice.com
MAILING ADDRESS:
   TEXAS TRUE CHOICE
   5000 Legacy Dr Ste 190
   Plano, TX 75024

KEY EXECUTIVES:
Chief Executive Officer/President .... Michael Wilson
Chief Financial Officer .... Alan Scoggins
Director of Marketing .... Mark Jones
MIS Director .... Tim Powell
Senior VP, Provider Relations .... Devin Zakrzewski

COMPANY PROFILE:
Parent Company Name: Viant Inc
Doing Business As:
Year Founded: 1996
Forprofit: [Y]
Model Type: MIXED
Accreditation: [ ] AAPPO [ ] JACHO [ ] NCQA [ ] URAC
Plan Type: PPO, EPO
Primary Physicians: 36,000   Physician Specialists: 35,044
Hospitals: 350
Total Enrollment:
   2001: 420,000   2004: 0   2007: 820,000
   2002: 500,000   2005:
   2003: 0   2006:
Federally Qualified: [ ]
Not-For-Profit: [ ]
SERVICE AREA:
Nationwide: N
   TX;
TYPE OF COVERAGE:
Commercial: [Y] Individual: [ ] FEHBP: [ ] Indemnity: [ ]
Medicare: [ ] Medicaid: [ ] Supplemental Medicare: [ ]
Tricare [ ]
PRODUCTS OFFERED:
Product Name: Type:
Preferred Health Arrangement   PPO
PLAN BENEFITS:
Alternative Medicine: [X]   Behavioral Health: [X]
Chiropractic: [X]   Dental: [X]
Home Care: [X]   Inpatient SNF: [X]
Long-Term Care: [X]   Pharm. Mail Order: [X]
Physical Therapy: [X]   Podiatry: [X]
Psychiatric: [X]   Transplant: [X]
Vision: [X]   Wellness: [X]
Workers' Comp: [X]
Other Benefits:
Comments:
Purchased by Viant Inc 2007.

UNICARE HEALTH PLANS OF TX INC

2 Greenway Plaza Ste 500
Houston, TX 77046
Phone: 713-479-4100 Fax: 713-479-4473 Toll-Free:
Web site: www.unicare.com/texas
MAILING ADDRESS:
   UNICARE HEALTH PLANS OF TX INC
   2 Greenway Plaza Ste 500
   Houston, TX 77046

KEY EXECUTIVES:
Chief Executive Officer/President .... David W Fields
Chief Financial Officer .... Wayne S DeVeydt
Medical Director .... Stephen Nesbitt, DO
Chief Operating Officer .... Thomas McGeehan
Product Development & Sales .... Becky Korenek

COMPANY PROFILE:
Parent Company Name: WellPoint Inc
Doing Business As:
Year Founded: 1996
Forprofit: [Y]
Model Type: MIXED
Accreditation: [ ] AAPPO [ ] JACHO [ ] NCQA [ ] URAC
Plan Type: HMO, UR, PPO, CDHP, HDHP, HSA,
Total Revenue: 2005: 66,110,305 2006: 69,872,246
Net Income 2005: 3,300,228 2006: 6,622,074
Total Enrollment:
   2001: 81,984   2004: 21,328   2007: 35,936
   2002: 47,508   2005: 18,802
   2003: 26,788   2006: 31,923
Federally Qualified: [N]
Not-For-Profit: [ ]
SERVICE AREA:
Nationwide: N
   TX (Angelina, Aransas, Austin, Bee, Brazoria, Calhoun, Chambers, Cherokee, Colorado, DeWitt, Fayette, Fort Bend, Galveston, Goliad, Gonzales, Grimes, Hardin, Harris, Houston, Jackson, Jasper, Jefferson, Kames, Lavaca, Liberty, Madison, Matagorda, Montgomery, Nacogdoches, Newton, Orange, Polk, Refugio, Sabine, San Augustine, San Joacinto, Shelby, Trinity, Tyler, Victoria, Walker, Waller, Washington, Wharton);
TYPE OF COVERAGE:
Commercial: [Y] Individual: [Y] FEHBP: [ ] Indemnity: [ ]
Medicare: [Y] Medicaid: [Y] Supplemental Medicare: [ ]
Tricare [ ]
PRODUCTS OFFERED:
Product Name: Type:
Methodistcare 65 Plus   Medicare
Methodistcare   Medicaid
CONSUMER-DRIVEN PRODUCTS
JP Morgan Chase   HSA Company
Complete Choice HealthFund   HSA Product
Arcus Enterprises Inc   HSA Administrator
    Consumer-Driven Health
PlanUniCare PPO HRA   High Deductible Health Plan
PLAN BENEFITS:
Alternative Medicine: [ ]   Behavioral Health: [ ]
Chiropractic: [ ]   Dental: [ ]
Home Care: [X]   Inpatient SNF: [X]
Long-Term Care: [ ]   Pharm. Mail Order: [X]
Physical Therapy: [X]   Podiatry: [ ]
Psychiatric: [X]   Transplant: [X]
Vision: [ ]   Wellness: [X]
Workers' Comp: [ ]
Other Benefits:
Comments:
Formerly MethodistCare.

UNICARE LIFE AND HEALTH INSURANCE CO INC

2 Greenway Plaza Ste 500
Houston, TX 77046
Phone: 713-479-4100 Fax: 713-781-6308 Toll-Free: 800-451-0608
Web site: www.unicare.com
MAILING ADDRESS:
   UNICARE LIFE AND HEALTH INS CO
   2 Greenway Plaza Ste 500
   Houston, TX 77046

KEY EXECUTIVES:
President .... Jim Hickey
Chief Financial Officer .... Wayne S DeVeydt
Chief Operating Officer .... Thomas McGeehan
VP Network Services .... Janice Fagen

COMPANY PROFILE:
Parent Company Name: WellPoint Inc
Doing Business As:
Year Founded: 2001
Forprofit: [Y]
Model Type:
Accreditation: [ ] AAPPO [ ] JACHO [ ] NCQA [X] URAC
Plan Type: PPO, CDHP, HDHP, HSA,
Total Revenue: 2005: 2006:
Net Income 2005: 2006:
Total Enrollment:
   2001: 450,000   2004: 0   2007: 0
   2002: 0   2005:
   2003: 0   2006:
Federally Qualified: [ ]
Not-For-Profit: [ ]

Managed Care Organization Profiles   TEXAS

TEXAS COMMUNITY CARE

6070 Gateway East #105
El Paso, TX 79905
Phone: 915-843-4043 Fax: 915-843-2978 Toll-Free: 866-688-0644
Web site: www.texascommunitycare.com

MAILING ADDRESS:
  TEXAS COMMUNITY CARE
  6070 Gateway East #105
  El Paso, TX 79905

KEY EXECUTIVES:
Director, Sales .... Miquel Rossy

COMPANY PROFILE:
Parent Company Name: Arcadian Health Plan Inc
Doing Business As:
Year Founded: 2005   Federally Qualified: [ ]
Forprofit: [ ]   Not-For-Profit: [ ]
Model Type:
Accreditation: [ ] AAPPO [ ] JACHO [ ] NCQA [ ] URAC
Plan Type: HMO
Total Revenue: 2005:   2006:   80,025,887
Net Income   2005:   2006:   16,398,646
Total Enrollment:
  2001: 0   2004: 0   2007: 18,901
  2002: 0   2005:
  2003: 0   2006: 12,304

SERVICE AREA:
Nationwide: N
  TX (Anderson, Bowie, Camp, Cass, Cherokee, El Paso, Franklin, Freestone, Gregg, Harrison, Henderson, Hopkins, Houston, Kaufman, Lamar, Marion, Morris, Navarro, Panola, Red River, Rusk, Shelby, Smith, Titus, Travis, Trinity, Upshur, Van Zandt, Williamson);

TYPE OF COVERAGE:
Commercial: [ ] Individual: [ ] FEHBP: [ ] Indemnity: [ ]
Medicare: [Y] Medicaid: [ ]   Supplemental Medicare: [ ]
Tricare   [ ]

PRODUCTS OFFERED:
Product Name: Type:
Texas Community Care   Medicare Advantage

TEXAS DENTAL PLAN

85 Northeast Loop 410 Ste 603
San Antonio, TX 78216
Phone: 210-979-3940 Fax: 210-979-3982 Toll-Free: 800-721-0455
Web site: www.compbenefits.com

MAILING ADDRESS:
  TEXAS DENTAL PLAN
  85 Northeast Loop 410 Ste 603
  San Antonio, TX 78216

KEY EXECUTIVES:
Chief Executive Officer/President .... Kirk Rothrock
Chief Financial Officer .... George Dunaway
National Medical Director .... Kenneth J Hammer, DDS
Senior VP of Operations .... Mary Kay Gilbert
Senior VP, Marketing .... Judith Herron
Executive VP, General Counsel .... Bruce Mitchell

COMPANY PROFILE:
Parent Company Name: CompDent Corporation
Doing Business As: Summa HE
Year Founded: 1978   Federally Qualified: [N]
Forprofit: [Y]   Not-For-Profit: [ ]
Model Type: IPA
Accreditation: [ ] AAPPO [ ] JACHO [ ] NCQA [ ] URAC
Plan Type: Specialty PPO
Total Revenue: 2005:   2006:   12,392,355
Net Income   2005:   2006:
Total Enrollment:
  2001: 0   2004: 0   2007: 118,241
  2002: 0   2005:
  2003: 0   2006: 120,224

SERVICE AREA:
Nationwide: N
  TX;

TYPE OF COVERAGE:
Commercial: [Y] Individual: [Y] FEHBP: [ ] Indemnity: []
Medicare: [ ] Medicaid: [ ]   Supplemental Medicare: [Y]
Tricare   [ ]

PRODUCTS OFFERED:
Product Name: Type:
Dental Preferred Plan

PLAN BENEFITS:
Alternative Medicine: [ ]   Behavioral Health: [ ]
Chiropractic: [ ]   Dental: [X]
Home Care: [ ]   Inpatient SNF: [ ]
Long-Term Care: [ ]   Pharm. Mail Order: [ ]
Physical Therapy: [ ]   Podiatry: [ ]
Psychiatric: [ ]   Transplant: [ ]
Vision: [ ]   Wellness: [ ]
Workers' Comp: [ ]
Other Benefits:

TEXAS HEALTHSPRING I LLC

2900 North Loop West Ste 1300
Houston, TX 77092
Phone: 832-553-3300 Fax: 832-553-3400 Toll-Free: 877-213-6732
Web site: www.myhealthspring.com

MAILING ADDRESS:
  TEXAS HEALTHSPRING I LLC
  POBox 922002
  Houston, TX 77092

KEY EXECUTIVES:
Chief Executive Officer .... Greg Allen
President .... Murray Blackshear
VP, Sales & Marketing .... Peter Gardner

COMPANY PROFILE:
Parent Company Name:
Doing Business As:
Year Founded: 2002   Federally Qualified: [ ]
Forprofit: [Y]   Not-For-Profit: [ ]
Model Type: GROUP
Accreditation: [ ] AAPPO [ ] JACHO [ ] NCQA [ ] URAC
Plan Type: HMO
Total Revenue: 2005: 245,428,565   2006:   363,154,414
Net Income   2005: 15,607,671   2006:   46,934,196
Total Enrollment:
  2001: 0   2004: 21,079   2007: 36,503
  2002: 7,790   2005: 29,593
  2003: 15,785   2006: 57,386

SERVICE AREA:
Nationwide:
  TX;

TYPE OF COVERAGE:
Commercial: [ ] Individual: [ ] FEHBP: [ ] Indemnity: [ ]
Medicare: [Y] Medicaid: [ ]   Supplemental Medicare: [ ]
Tricare   [ ]

TEXAS MEDICAL FOUNDATION HEALTH QUALITY INSTITUTE

5918 W Courtyard Dr Ste 300
Austin, TX 78730-5036
Phone: 512-329-6610 Fax: 512-327-7159 Toll-Free: 800-725-9216
Web site: www.tmf.org

MAILING ADDRESS:
  TMF HEALTH QUALITY INSTITUTE
  5918 W Courtyard Dr Ste 300
  Austin, TX 78730-5036

KEY EXECUTIVES:
Chief Executive Officer .... Tom Manley
President Board .... Patrick Hanford MD
Senior VP, Chief Financial Officer .... Pamela Hoernis, CPA
Medical Director .... Abraham Delgado, MD, FACP
Senior VP, Business Development .... Thom Sloan
VP, Information Technology .... Judy Dooley
VP, Human Resources .... Leslie Froeschle, PHR
Senior VP, Quality Improvement .... Kevin Warren
VP Communications .... Emile Fennell
VP Business Development .... Debbie Lovata RN

COMPANY PROFILE:
Parent Company Name:
Doing Business As:

TEXAS

Managed Care Organization Profiles

SERVICE AREA:
Nationwide: N
TX (Andrews, Armstrong, Bailey, Bell, Borden, Bosque, Brazos, Brewster, Briscoe, Burleson, Burnet, Callahan, Carson, Castro, Childress, Cochran, Coke, Coleman, Collingsworth, Comanche, Concho, Coryell, Cottle, Crane, Crockett, Crosby, Dallam, Dawson, Deaf Smith, Dickens, Donley, Eastland, Ector, Falls, Fisher, Floyd, Freestone, Gaines, Garza, Glasscock, Gray, Grimes, Hale, Hall, Hamilton, Hansford, Hartley, Haskell, Hemphill, Hill, Hockley, Houston, Howard, Hutchinson, Irion, Jones, Kent, King, Knox, Lamb, Lampasas, Lee, Leon, Limestone, Lipscomb, Llano, Loving, Lubbock, Lynn, Madison, Martin, McCulloch, McLennan, Midland, Milam, Mills, Mitchell, Moore, Motley, Navarro, Nolan, Ochiltree, Oldham, Parmer, Pecos, Potter, Randall, Reagan, Reeves, Roberts, Robertson, Runnels, San Saba, Schleicher, Scurry, Shackelford, Sherman, Somervell, Stephens, Sterling, Stonewall, Sutton, Swisher, Taylor, Terry, Throckmorton, Tom Green, Upton, Walker, Ward, Washington, Wheeler, Winkler, Yoakum);

TYPE OF COVERAGE:
Commercial: [Y] Individual: [Y] FEHBP: [ ] Indemnity: [ ]
Medicare: [ ] Medicaid: [Y] Supplemental Medicare: [ ]
Tricare   [ ]

PRODUCTS OFFERED:
Product Name: Type:
HMO   Commercial
HMO   Individual
HMO   Medicaid
HMO   Self Funded
PPO
Firstcare   Medicare

PLAN BENEFITS:
Alternative Medicine: [ ]   Behavioral Health: [ ]
Chiropractic: [X]   Dental: [X]
Home Care: [X]   Inpatient SNF: [X]
Long-Term Care: [ ]   Pharm. Mail Order: [X]
Physical Therapy: [X]   Podiatry: [X]
Psychiatric: [X]   Transplant: [X]
Vision: [X]   Wellness: [X]
Workers' Comp: [ ]
Other Benefits:

SPECTRUM REVIEW SERVICES INC

14405 Walters Rd Ste 900
Houston, TX 77014
Phone: 281-444-2194 Fax: 281-444-2482 Toll-Free: 800-258-5055
Web site: www.spectrumreview.com

MAILING ADDRESS:
SPECTRUM REVIEW SERVICES INC
14405 Walters Rd Ste 900
Houston, TX 77014

KEY EXECUTIVES:
Chairman of the Board .... Frank J Berrier Jr, PhD
Chief Executive Officer/President .... Frank J Berrier Jr, PhD
Chief Financial Officer/Chief Operating Officer ... Ernest C Munshower
Medical Director .... John R Gerdas, MD, FACOG
VP, Marketing/Administration .... Brenda Dusenbury
Privacy Officer .... Frank J Berrier Jr, PhD
Director, Case Management/Utilization Review Rene Nettles RN, CCM

COMPANY PROFILE:
Parent Company Name:
Doing Business As:
Year Founded: 1991   Federally Qualified: [N]
Forprofit: [Y]   Not-For-Profit: [ ]
Model Type:
Accreditation: [ ] AAPPO [ ] JACHO [ ] NCQA [ ] URAC
Plan Type: UR

SERVICE AREA:
Nationwide: N
TX;

SUPERIOR HEALTHPLAN INC

2100 South IH 35 Ste 202
Austin, TX 78704
Phone: 512-692-1465 Fax: 512-692-1435 Toll-Free: 800-783-5386
Web site: www.superiorhealthplan.com

MAILING ADDRESS:
SUPERIOR HEALTHPLAN INC
2100 South IH 35 Ste 202
Austin, TX 78704

KEY EXECUTIVES:
Chief Executive Officer/President .... Christopher D Bowers
Chief Operating Officer .... William Baker
VP, Marketing & Business Development .... Holly Williams
Public Relations Director .... Sonia Villa
VP, Medical Management .... Terry Johnson, MD
Director, Quality Improvement .... Suzanne Feay, RN

COMPANY PROFILE:
Parent Company Name: Centene Corporation Inc
Doing Business As:
Year Founded: 1999   Federally Qualified: [ ]
Forprofit: [Y]   Not-For-Profit: [ ]
Model Type: NETWORK
Accreditation: [ ] AAPPO [ ] JACHO [ ] NCQA [ ] URAC
Plan Type: HMO
Primary Physicians: 4,715   Physician Specialists: 10,038
Hospitals: 324
Total Revenue: 2005: 228,114,644   2006: 269,960,786
Net Income   2005:   6,278,098   2006:   7,159
Total Enrollment:
    2001: 54,901   2004: 244,300   2007: 255,519
    2002: 117,989   2005: 242,000
    2003: 158,369   2006: 217,198

SERVICE AREA:
Nationwide: N
TX, (Harris, Culberson, El Paso, Hudspeth),

TYPE OF COVERAGE:
Commercial: [ ] Individual: [ ] FEHBP: [ ] Indemnity: [ ]
Medicare: [ ] Medicaid: [Y] Supplemental Medicare: [ ]
Tricare   [ ]

PRODUCTS OFFERED:
Product Name: Type:
Superior Healthplan HMO   Medicaid

TEXAS CHILDRENS HEALTH PLAN

2450 Holcombe Blvd Ste 34-L
Houston, TX 77021
Phone: 832-824-2600 Fax: 832-825-2836 Toll-Free: 800-990-8247
Web site: www.texaschildrenshospital.org

MAILING ADDRESS:
TEXAS CHILDRENS HEALTH PLAN
PO Box 301011 NB 8360
Houston, TX 77021

KEY EXECUTIVES:
Chief Executive Officer .... Chris Born
Chief Financial Officer .... Anna Mateja
Medical Director .... Angelo Giardino, MD
Chief Operating Officer .... Jan Scott
Director, Marketing/Network Development .... Sonja Beaty

COMPANY PROFILE:
Parent Company Name: Texas Childrens Hospital
Doing Business As:
Year Founded: 1996   Federally Qualified: [Y]
Forprofit: [ ]   Not-For-Profit: [Y]
Model Type: STAFF
Accreditation: [ ] AAPPO [ ] JACHO [ ] NCQA [ ] URAC
Plan Type: HMO,
Total Revenue: 2005: 166,161,621   2006: 204,648,139
Net Income   2005:   540,982   2006: 10,092,186
Total Enrollment:
    2001: 68,026   2004: 127,223   2007: 171,115
    2002: 92,494   2005: 135,389
    2003: 118,644   2006: 159,154
Medical Loss Ratio: 2005:   2006:
Administrative Expense Ratio: 2005:   2006:

SERVICE AREA:
Nationwide: N
TX (Austin, Bee, Brazoria, Chambers, Fort Bend, Galveston, Harris, Liberty, Matagorda, Montgomery, Waller);

TYPE OF COVERAGE:
Commercial: [Y] Individual: [ ] FEHBP: [ ] Indemnity: [ ]
Medicare: [ ] Medicaid: [Y] Supplemental Medicare: [ ]
Tricare   [ ]

Comments:
Formerly Kaiser Health Plan of Texas.

Managed Care Organization Profiles — TEXAS

Medical Loss Ratio: 2005: 94.00 2006:
Administrative Expense Ratio: 2005: 0.02 2006:
SERVICE AREA:
Nationwide: N
   TX (Bastrop, Bell, Blanco, Bosque, Brazos, Burleson, Burnet, Coryell, Falls, Fayette, Grimes, Hamilton, Lampasas, Lee, Leon, Llano, Madison, McLennan, Milam, Mills, Robertson, San Saba, Travis, Washington, Williamson);
TYPE OF COVERAGE:
Commercial: [Y] Individual: [Y] FEHBP: [ ] Indemnity: [ ]
Medicare: [Y] Medicaid: [ ] Supplemental Medicare: [ ]
Tricare [ ]
PRODUCTS OFFERED:
Product Name: Type:
Scott & White HMO   HMO
Health Plus   HMO
Sr Care Senior Preferred Plus   Medicare Advantage
Self-Insured   Individual
CONSUMER-DRIVEN PRODUCTS
HealthEquity   HSA Company
                                        HSA Product
HealthEquity   HSA Administrator
Consumer Choice   Consumer-Driven Health Plan
                                        High Deductible Health Plan
PLAN BENEFITS:
Alternative Medicine: [ ]   Behavioral Health: [ ]
Chiropractic: [ ]   Dental: [X]
Home Care: [X]   Inpatient SNF: [X]
Long-Term Care: [X]   Pharm. Mail Order: [X]
Physical Therapy: [X]   Podiatry: [X]
Psychiatric: [X]   Transplant: [X]
Vision: [X]   Wellness: [X]
Workers' Comp: [ ]
Other Benefits:

SCRIPT CARE INC

6380 Folsom Dr
Beaumont, TX 77706
Phone: 409-832-3041 Fax: 409-832-3109 Toll-Free: 800-880-9988
Web site: www.scriptcare.com
MAILING ADDRESS:
   SCRIPT CARE INC
   6380 Folsom Dr
   Beaumont, TX 77706

KEY EXECUTIVES:
Chief Executive Officer/Chief Financial Officer .... Jim Brown, RPh
Pharmacy Director .... Jim Brown, RPh
MIS Director .... Mike Sabochek

COMPANY PROFILE:
Parent Company Name:
Doing Business As:
Year Founded: 1988   Federally Qualified: [ ]
Forprofit: [Y]   Not-For-Profit: [ ]
Model Type:
Accreditation: [ ] AAPPO [ ] JACHO [ ] NCQA [ ] URAC
Plan Type: Specialty PPO
SERVICE AREA:
Nationwide: Y
   NW;
PLAN BENEFITS:
Alternative Medicine: [ ]   Behavioral Health: [ ]
Chiropractic: [ ]   Dental: [ ]
Home Care: [ ]   Inpatient SNF: [ ]
Long-Term Care: [ ]   Pharm. Mail Order: [X]
Physical Therapy: [ ]   Podiatry: [ ]
Psychiatric: [ ]   Transplant: [ ]
Vision: [ ]   Wellness: [ ]
Workers' Comp: [ ]
Other Benefits: Pharmacy Benefits

SETON HEALTH PLAN

7715 Chevy Chase Ste 225
Austin, TX 78752-1242
Phone: 512-324-3125 Fax: 512-324-3359 Toll-Free:
Web site: www.seton.net

MAILING ADDRESS:
   SETON HEALTH PLAN
   7715 Chevy Chase Ste 225
   Austin, TX 78752-1242

KEY EXECUTIVES:
Chief Executive Officer/President .... Charles J Barnett
Chief Financial Officer .... Douglas D Waite
Medical Director .... Gary Piefer, MD

COMPANY PROFILE:
Parent Company Name: Seton Health System
Doing Business As:
Year Founded: 1995   Federally Qualified: [ ]
Forprofit: [Y]   Not-For-Profit: [ ]
Model Type: MIXED
Accreditation: [ ] AAPPO [X] JACHO [ ] NCQA [ ] URAC
Plan Type: HMO, TPA
Total Revenue: 2005: 18,276,507   2006: 18,512,613
Net Income   2005:   857,934   2006:   2,206,995
Total Enrollment:
   2001: 0   2004: 17,121   2007: 11,044
   2002: 32,791   2005: 16,577
   2003: 21,373   2006: 14,466
SERVICE AREA:
Nationwide: N
   TX (Bastrop, Bell, Blanco, Bosque, Brazos, Burleson, Burnet, Caldwell, Colorado, Comal, Coryell, Falls, Fayette, Gonzales, Grimes, Guadalupe, Hays, Hill, Lampasas, Lee, Leon, Limestone, Llano, Madison, McLennan, Milam, Robertson, Travis, Washington, Williamson);
PRODUCTS OFFERED:
Product Name: Type:
Seton Health Plan   Medicaid
Seton Health Plan   Medicare
PLAN BENEFITS:
Alternative Medicine: [ ]   Behavioral Health: [X]
Chiropractic: [X]   Dental: [ ]
Home Care: [X]   Inpatient SNF: [X]
Long-Term Care: [ ]   Pharm. Mail Order: [X]
Physical Therapy: [X]   Podiatry: [ ]
Psychiatric: [X]   Transplant: [X]
Vision: [ ]   Wellness: [X]
Workers' Comp: [X]
Other Benefits:

SOUTHWEST HEALTH ALLIANCE (SHALLC)

12940 North Hwy 183
Austin, TX 78750
Phone: 512-257-6000 Fax: 512-257-6037 Toll-Free: 800-431-7737
Web site: www.firstcare.com
MAILING ADDRESS:
   SW HEALTH ALLIANCE (SHALLC)
   12940 North Hwy 183
   Austin, TX 78750

KEY EXECUTIVES:
Chief Executive Officer .... Keith Lundien
Chief Finanical Officer .... Keenan B Freeman
Chief Information Officer .... Martin Mikula
Chief Operating Officer .... Bill Thames
Provider Relations Director .... Pat Lorda

COMPANY PROFILE:
Parent Company Name: SHA LLC
Doing Business As: Firstcare
Year Founded: 1986   Federally Qualified: [Y]
Forprofit: [Y]   Not-For-Profit: [ ]
Model Type: IPA
Accreditation: [ ] AAPPO [ ] JACHO [ ] NCQA [ ] URAC
Plan Type: HMO, PPO, HDHP, HSA,
Total Revenue: 2005: 217,014,481   2006: 241,877,143
Net Income   2005: -1,463,376   2006: -2,224,677
Total Enrollment:
   2001: 78,014   2004: 90,864   2007: 99,631
   2002: 90,580   2005: 86,971
   2003: 88,834   2006: 98,633

TEXAS
Managed Care Organization Profiles

PLAN BENEFITS:
Alternative Medicine:	[X]	Behavioral Health:	[X]
Chiropractic:	[X]	Dental:	[ ]
Home Care:	[X]	Inpatient SNF:	[X]
Long-Term Care:	[X]	Pharm. Mail Order:	[X]
Physicial Therapy:	[X]	Podiatry:	[X]
Psychiatric:	[X]	Transplant:	[X]
Vision:	[X]	Wellness:	[ ]
Workers' Comp:	[X]		

Other Benefits:
Comments:
Acquired by MultiPlan, Inc. on October 18, 2006.

PROVIDER NETWORKS OF AMERICA INC

4300 Centreway
Arlington, TX 76018
Phone: 817-417-2830 Fax: 817-417-2839 Toll-Free:
Web site: www.providernetworks.com

MAILING ADDRESS:
PROVIDER NETWORKS OF AMERICA
4300 Centreway
Arlington, TX 76018

KEY EXECUTIVES:
Human Resources Director .... *Nicole Lammons*
New Product Development Officer .... *Patty White*
Managing Director .... *Karen Kinney*
Managing Director II .... *Kim Kindred*

COMPANY PROFILE:
Parent Company Name: Aetna Inc
Doing Business As:
Year Founded: 1989 Federally Qualified: [ ]
Forprofit: [Y] Not-For-Profit: [ ]
Model Type:
Accreditation: [ ] AAPPO [ ] JACHO [ ] NCQA [X] URAC
Plan Type: PPO

SERVICE AREA:
Nationwide: Y
  NW;

TYPE OF COVERAGE:
Commercial: [Y] Individual: [Y] FEHBP: [ ] Indemnity: [ ]
Medicare: [ ] Medicaid: [ ] Supplemental Medicare: [ ]
Tricare [ ]

PRODUCTS OFFERED:
Product Name: Type:
Utilization Management

SAFEGUARD HEALTH PLANS INC

5495 Beltline Rd #155
Dallas, TX 75254
Phone: 972-364-5000 Fax: 972-364-5015 Toll-Free: 800-880-1800
Web site: www.safeguard.net

MAILING ADDRESS:
SAFEGUARD HEALTH PLANS INC
5495 Beltline Rd #155
Dallas, TX 75254

KEY EXECUTIVES:
Chief Executive Officer .... *James E Buncher*
Chief Financial Officer .... *Dennis Sates*
Chief Information Officer .... *Mike Laufenburger*
Chief Operating Officer .... *Steve Baker*
Marketing Director .... *Andy Laderman*
Provider Relations Director .... *Rene Carales*
Executive President/Texas .... *Trei Wild*

COMPANY PROFILE:
Parent Company Name: Safeguard Health Enterprises
Doing Business As:
Year Founded: 1986 Federally Qualified: [ ]
Forprofit: [Y] Not-For-Profit: [ ]
Model Type:
Accreditation: [ ] AAPPO [ ] JACHO [ ] NCQA [ ] URAC
Plan Type: Specialty HMO,
Total Revenue: 2005: 9,782,000 2006: 11,200,932
Net Income 2005: 172,457 2006:

Total Enrollment:
  2001: 213,007 2004: 107,251 2007: 120,119
  2002: 205,000 2005: 114,948
  2003: 99,663   2006: 118,837

SERVICE AREA:
Nationwide: N
  TX (Anderson, Andrews, Angelina, Aransas, Archer, Armstrong, Atascosa, Austin, Bailey, Bandera, Bastrop, Baylor, Bee, Bell, Bexar, Blanco, Borden, Bosque, Bowie, Brazoria, Brazos, Brewster, Briscoe, Brooks, Brown, Burleston, Burnet, Caldwell, Calhoun, Callahan, Cameron, Camp, Carson, Cass, Castro, Chambers, Cherokee, Childress, Clay, Cochran, Coke, Coleman, Collin, Collingsworth, Colorado, Comal, Comanche, Concho, Cooke, Coryell, Cottle, Crane, Crockett, Crosby, Culberson, Dallam, Dallas, Dawson, DeWitt, Deaf Smith, Delta, Denton, Dickens, Dimmit, Donley, Duval, Eastland, Ector, Edwards, El Paso, Ellis, Erath, Falls, Fannin, Fayette, Fisher, Floyd, Foard, Fort Bend, Franklin, Freestone, Frio, Gaines, Galveston, Garza, Gillispie, Glasscock, Goliad, Gonzales, Gray, Grayson, Gregg, Grimes, Guadalupe, Hale, Hall, Hamilton, Hansford, Hardeman, Hardin, Harris, Harrisaon, Hartley, Haskell, Hays, Hemphill, Henderson, Hidalgo, Hill, Hockley, Hood, Hopkins, Houston, Howard, Hudspeth, Hunt, Hutchinson, Irion, Jack, Jackson, Jasper, Jeff, Davis, Jefferson, Jim, Hogg, Jim, Wells, Johnson, Jones, Karnes, Kufman, Kendall, Kenedy, Kent, Kerr, Kimble, King, Kinney, Kleberg, Knox, LaSalle, Lamar, Lamb, Lampases, Lavaca, Lee, Leon, Liberty, Limestone, Lipscomb, Live Oak, Llano, Loving, Lubbock, Lynn, Madison, Marion, Martin);

PRODUCTS OFFERED:
Product Name: Type:
Safeguard Health Plans Specialty HMO

PLAN BENEFITS:
Alternative Medicine:	[ ]	Behavioral Health:	[ ]
Chiropractic:	[ ]	Dental:	[X]
Home Care:	[ ]	Inpatient SNF:	[ ]
Long-Term Care:	[ ]	Pharm. Mail Order:	[ ]
Physical Therapy:	[ ]	Podiatry:	[ ]
Psychiatric:	[ ]	Transplant:	[ ]
Vision:	[X]	Wellness:	[ ]
Workers' Comp:	[ ]		

Other Benefits:

SCOTT & WHITE HEALTH PLAN

2401 S 31st St
Temple, TX 76508-0001
Phone: 254-298-3000 Fax: 254-298-3011 Toll-Free: 800-321-7947
Web site: www.sw.org

MAILING ADDRESS:
SCOTT & WHITE HEALTH PLAN
2401 S 31st St
Temple, TX 76508-0001

KEY EXECUTIVES:
Executive Director .... *Allan Einboden*
President .... *Alfred Knight, MD*
Chief Financial Officer .... *Dennis L Laraway*
Medical Director .... *Craig Clanton, MD*
Pharmacy Director .... *John Chaddick*
Director, MIS .... *Troy Stillwagon*
Associate Executive Director Operations .... *Marinan Williams*
Assistant Executive Director/Sales & Marketing .... *Lee Green*
Director, MIS .... *Troy Stillwagon*
Provider Relations Director .... *Kathy Lee*
Human Resources Director .... *Bambi Hester*
Health Services Director .... *Debbie Garrett*
Quality Improvement Director .... *Candus Ater*

COMPANY PROFILE:
Parent Company Name: Scott & White Health Plan
Doing Business As: Scott & White Health Plan
Year Founded: 1981 Federally Qualified: [Y]
Forprofit: [ ] Not-For-Profit: [Y]
Model Type: GROUP
Accreditation: [ ] AAPPO [ ] JACHO [X] NCQA [ ] URAC
Plan Type: HMO, PBM, POS, ASO, TPA, CDHP, HDHP,
Primary Physicians: 296 Physician Specialists: 394
Hospitals: 22
Total Revenue: 2005: 455,475,952 2006: 500,924,507
Net Income 2005: 3,942,933 2006: 5,064,388
Total Enrollment:
  2001: 182,451 2004: 166,410 2007: 190,324
  2002: 168,422 2005: 166,801
  2003: 169,656 2006: 174,171

Managed Care Organization Profiles — TEXAS

SERVICE AREA:
Nationwide: N
   TX (Collin, Dallas, Ellis, Hunt, Kaufman, Navarro, Rockwall);
TYPE OF COVERAGE:
Commercial: [ ]   Individual: [ ]   FEHBP: [ ]   Indemnity: [ ]
Medicare: [ ]   Medicaid: [Y]   Supplemental Medicare: [ ]
Tricare   [ ]
PRODUCTS OFFERED:
Product Name: Type:
Healthfirst   Medicaid
Kids First   CHIP
PLAN BENEFITS:
Alternative Medicine: [ ]   Behavioral Health: [X]
Chiropractic: [ ]   Dental: [ ]
Home Care: [X]   Inpatient SNF: [X]
Long-Term Care: [ ]   Pharm. Mail Order: [ ]
Physical Therapy: [X]   Podiatry: [X]
Psychiatric: [X]   Transplant: [X]
Vision: [X]   Wellness: [ ]
Workers' Comp: [ ]
Other Benefits:

PEARLE VISION MANAGED CARE - HMO OF TEXAS INC

2465 Joe Field Rd
Dallas, TX 75229-3479
Phone: 972-277-6000 Fax: 972-277-6422 Toll-Free: 800-267-9894
Web site:
MAILING ADDRESS:
   PEARLE VISION MANAGEDCARE-HMO
   2465 Joe Field Rd
   Dallas, TX 75229-3479

KEY EXECUTIVES:
President .... Stephen Holden
Treasurer .... Joseph Gaglioti
VP, Medical Director .... Ken Clanton, MD
Director of Operations .... Kevin Hilst
Director, Provider Network Management .... Bob Loerch
Director, Legal & Regulatory Affairs .... Colleen Shannon

COMPANY PROFILE:
Parent Company Name: Cole Managed Vision Corp
Doing Business As:
Year Founded: 1996   Federally Qualified: [ ]
Forprofit: [ ]   Not-For-Profit: [ ]
Model Type: NETWORK
Accreditation: [ ] AAPPO [ ] JACHO [ ] NCQA [ ] URAC
Plan Type: Specialty HMO
Total Revenue: 2005: 2,826,537   2006: 2,580,917
Net Income   2005:   540,723   2006:
Total Enrollment:
   2001: 954,551   2004: 308,954   2007: 66,524
   2002:   0   2005: 309,421
   2003: 234,809   2006: 191,198
SERVICE AREA:
Nationwide: N
   TX;
PRODUCTS OFFERED:
Product Name: Type:
HMO of Texas Inc   Specialty HMO
PLAN BENEFITS:
Alternative Medicine: [ ]   Behavioral Health: [ ]
Chiropractic: [ ]   Dental: [ ]
Home Care: [ ]   Inpatient SNF: [ ]
Long-Term Care: [ ]   Pharm. Mail Order: [ ]
Physical Therapy: [ ]   Podiatry: [ ]
Psychiatric: [ ]   Transplant: [ ]
Vision: [X]   Wellness: [ ]
Workers' Comp: [ ]
Other Benefits:

PPONEXT

8625 King George Dr Ste 300
Dallas, TX 75235
Phone: 214-267-3300 Fax: 214-267-3336 Toll-Free: 800-388-6799
Web site: www.pponext.com
MAILING ADDRESS:
   PPONEXT
   8625 King George Dr Ste 300
   Dallas, TX 75235

KEY EXECUTIVES:
Chief Executive Officer/President .... James M Pennington
Acting Chief Financial Officer .... Jim Iwanaga
Chief Marketing & Sales Officer .... Charles E Busch
Senior VP, Provider Services/Network Development .... Lynn Littleton
VP, Human Resources Director .... Joan Stokey
VP, Customer Care & Account Management .... Aaron A. Means III
Director - Claims .... Gary Evans

COMPANY PROFILE:
Parent Company Name: Viant Inc
Doing Business As:
Year Founded: 1984   Federally Qualified: [N]
Forprofit: [Y]   Not-For-Profit: [ ]
Model Type:
Accreditation: [ ] AAPPO [ ] JACHO [ ] NCQA [X] URAC
Plan Type: PPO, TPA, UR
Primary Physicians: 167,394   Physician Specialists: 382,306
Hospitals: 3,720
Total Enrollment:
   2001: 0   2004: 2,600,000   2007: 0
   2002: 0   2005: 2,800,000
   2003: 0   2006: 3,000,000
SERVICE AREA:
Nationwide: Y
   NW;
TYPE OF COVERAGE:
Commercial: [Y]   Individual: [ ]   FEHBP: [ ]   Indemnity: [ ]
Medicare: [ ]   Medicaid: [ ]   Supplemental Medicare: [ ]
Tricare   [ ]
PLAN BENEFITS:
Alternative Medicine: [ ]   Behavioral Health: [X]
Chiropractic: [X]   Dental: [X]
Home Care: [X]   Inpatient SNF: [X]
Long-Term Care: [ ]   Pharm. Mail Order: [ ]
Physical Therapy: [X]   Podiatry: [X]
Psychiatric: [ ]   Transplant: [X]
Vision: [ ]   Wellness: [X]
Workers' Comp: [X]
Other Benefits:
Comments:
Acquired Houston Healthcare Purchasing Organization September 1998.
Purchased by Beech Street Corporation.

PRIVATE HEALTHCARE SYSTEMS - TEXAS

1501 LBJ Parkway #650
Dallas, TX 75234-6800
Phone: 972-241-3330 Fax: 972-620-9650 Toll-Free:
Web site: www.phcs.com
MAILING ADDRESS:
   PRIVATE HEALTHCARE SYSTEMS-TX
   1100 Winter St
   Waltham, MA 75234-6800

KEY EXECUTIVES:
Chief Executive Officer .... Mark Tabak

COMPANY PROFILE:
Parent Company Name: MultiPlan Inc
Doing Business As:
Year Founded: 1986   Federally Qualified: [N]
Forprofit: [Y]   Not-For-Profit: [ ]
Model Type:
Accreditation: [ ] AAPPO [ ] JACHO [ ] NCQA [X] URAC
Plan Type: PPO, UR, POS
SERVICE AREA:
Nationwide: N
   TX;
TYPE OF COVERAGE:
Commercial: [Y]   Individual: [ ]   FEHBP: [ ]   Indemnity: [ ]
Medicare: [ ]   Medicaid: [ ]   Supplemental Medicare: [ ]
Tricare   [ ]

TEXAS
Managed Care Organization Profiles

PLAN BENEFITS:
Alternative Medicine: [ ]　　Behavioral Health: [ ]
Chiropractic: [ ]　　Dental: [X]
Home Care: [ ]　　Inpatient SNF: [ ]
Long-Term Care: [ ]　　Pharm. Mail Order: [ ]
Physical Therapy: [ ]　　Podiatry: [ ]
Psychiatric: [ ]　　Transplant: [ ]
Vision: [ ]　　Wellness: [ ]
Workers' Comp: [ ]
Other Benefits:
Comments:
Formerly Affordable Dental Plans.

PACIFICARE OF TEXAS - HOUSTON

1800 W Loop South Ste 350
Houston, TX 77027
Phone: 713-993-3012　Fax: 713-993-3295　Toll-Free: 800-825-9355
Web site: www.pacificare.com
MAILING ADDRESS:
PACIFICARE OF TEXAS - HOUSTON
1800 W Loop South Ste 350
Houston, TX 77027

KEY EXECUTIVES:
Chief Executive Officer/President .... George H Becker
Chief Financial Officer .... Daniel J Comrie
Medical Director .... Dan Stuckey, MD
Marketing Director .... Victor J Pluto

COMPANY PROFILE:
Parent Company Name: UnitedHealth Group
Doing Business As:
Year Founded: 1994　　Federally Qualified: [Y]
Forprofit: [Y]　　Not-For-Profit: [ ]
Model Type: IPA
Accreditation: [ ] AAPPO [ ] JACHO [ ] NCQA [ ] URAC
Plan Type: HMO, POS, HSA
Total Revenue: 2005:　　2006: 3,710,401
Net Income 2005: 105,784　2006: 212,217
Total Enrollment:
　2001: 56,657　　2004: 434　　2007: 0
　2002: 23,239　　2005: 385
　2003: 1,504　　2006: 891
SERVICE AREA:
Nationwide: N
TX (Austin, Brazoria, Chambers, Colorado, Fort Bend, Galveston, Grimes, Hardin, Harris, Jasper, Jefferson, Liberty, Matagorda, Montgomery, Newton, Orange, Polk, San Jacinto, Tyler, Walker, Waller, Washington, Wharton);
TYPE OF COVERAGE:
Commercial: [Y]　Individual: [ ]　FEHBP: [ ]　Indemnity: [ ]
Medicare: [Y]　Medicaid: [ ]　Supplemental Medicare: [ ]
Tricare [ ]
PLAN BENEFITS:
Alternative Medicine: [ ]　　Behavioral Health: [ ]
Chiropractic: [X]　　Dental: [X]
Home Care: [X]　　Inpatient SNF: [X]
Long-Term Care: [ ]　　Pharm. Mail Order: [X]
Physical Therapy: [X]　　Podiatry: [X]
Psychiatric: [X]　　Transplant: [X]
Vision: [X]　　Wellness: [X]
Workers' Comp: [X]
Other Benefits:
Comments:
Formerly Pacificare Secure Horizons.

PACIFICARE OF TEXAS INC

5001 LBJ Freeway Ste 600
Dallas, TX 75244
Phone: 800-908-9185　Fax: 972-866-1658　Toll-Free: 800-908-9185
Web site: www.pacificare.com
MAILING ADDRESS:
PACIFICARE OF TEXAS INC
5001 LBJ Freeway Ste 600
Dallas, TX 75244

KEY EXECUTIVES:
Regional Vice President .... George Becker
Chief Financial Officer .... Daniel J Comrie
VP of Sales & Marketing .... Victor J Pluto
VP, Public Affairs .... Joe Guinn
VP, Network Development .... Austin Pittman

COMPANY PROFILE:
Parent Company Name: UnitedHealth Group
Doing Business As:
Year Founded: 1986　　Federally Qualified: [Y]
Forprofit: [Y]　　Not-For-Profit: [ ]
Model Type: IPA
Accreditation: [ ] AAPPO [ ] JACHO [X] NCQA [ ] URAC
Plan Type: HMO, PPO, POS, UR, HSA
Total Revenue: 2005: 943,955,938　2006: 1,277,909,348
Net Income 2005: 16,003,445　2006: 92,456,516
Total Enrollment:
　2001: 330,000　　2004: 118,536　　2007: 0
　2002: 201,497　　2005: 132,117
　2003: 211,388　　2006: 138,252
SERVICE AREA:
Nationwide: N
TX (Atascosa, Bandera, Bexar, Comal, Guadalupe, Gonzales, Medina, Wilson);
TYPE OF COVERAGE:
Commercial: [Y]　Individual: [ ]　FEHBP: [ ]　Indemnity: [ ]
Medicare: [Y]　Medicaid: [ ]　Supplemental Medicare: [ ]
Tricare [ ]
PRODUCTS OFFERED:
Product Name:　　　　　　　　　Type:
Secure Horizons　　　　　　　　Medicare Advantage
Pacificare HMO　　　　　　　　　HMO
PLAN BENEFITS:
Alternative Medicine: [ ]　　Behavioral Health: [ ]
Chiropractic: [ ]　　Dental: [X]
Home Care: [X]　　Inpatient SNF: [X]
Long-Term Care: [X]　　Pharm. Mail Order: [X]
Physical Therapy: [X]　　Podiatry: [X]
Psychiatric: [X]　　Transplant: [X]
Vision: [X]　　Wellness: [X]
Workers' Comp: [X]
Other Benefits:

PARKLAND COMMUNITY HEALTH PLAN INC

2777 N Stemmons Fwy Ste 1750
Dallas, TX 75207
Phone: 214-266-2100　Fax: 214-266-2150　Toll-Free: 888-814-2352
Web site: www.parklandhmo.com
MAILING ADDRESS:
PARKLAND COMMUNITY HEALTH PLAN
2777 N Stemmons Fwy Ste 1750
Dallas, TX 75207

KEY EXECUTIVES:
Chief Executive Officer .... Ron J Anderson, MD
Executive Director .... Tim Bahe
Director of Finance .... Barbara Holmes
Medical Director .... Barry Lachman, MD
Health Data Director .... Robert Kowalski
Member Service Manager .... Joanne Tenery
Provider Relations Manager .... Patricia Carney
Associate Director of Quality .... Paula Bassett

COMPANY PROFILE:
Parent Company Name: Dallas County Hospital District
Doing Business As: Parkland Health and Hospital System
Year Founded: 1996　　Federally Qualified: [N]
Forprofit: [ ]　　Not-For-Profit: [Y]
Model Type: MIXED
Accreditation: [ ] AAPPO [ ] JACHO [ ] NCQA [ ] URAC
Plan Type: HMO,
Total Revenue: 2005: 192,595,746　2006: 234,626,966
Net Income 2005: 4,749,858　2006: 6,872,893
Total Enrollment:
　2001: 69,960　　2004: 109,820　　2007: 134,632
　2002: 98,514　　2005: 109,857
　2003: 110,448　　2006: 122,159
Medical Loss Ratio:　　　　2005: 82.00　　2006: 83.71
Administrative Expense Ratio:　2005: 14.50　　2006: 12.15

Managed Care Organization Profiles — TEXAS

KEY EXECUTIVES:
Chief Executive Officer .... Scott Fenn
Chief Financial Officer .... Stacey Bevil
Physician in Chief .... Richard Blakely, MD
Sales Director .... Brent Schultz
Provider Relations .... David Foley
Medical Director, Outpatient Services .... Robert Wallis, MD

COMPANY PROFILE:
Parent Company Name: Memorial Healthcare System
Doing Business As:
Year Founded: Federally Qualified: [ ]
Forprofit: [ ]   Not-For-Profit: [ ]
Model Type: IPA
Accreditation: [ ] AAPPO [ ] JACHO [ ] NCQA [ ] URAC
Plan Type: TPA,

SERVICE AREA:
Nationwide: N
   TX;

MOLINA HEALTHCARE OF TEXAS INC

3104 Edloe St Ste 350
Houston, TX 75027-6098
Phone: 972-343-3600 Fax: 972-352-6564 Toll-Free:
Web site: www.molinahealthcare.com

MAILING ADDRESS:
MOLINA HEALTHCARE OF TX INC
2505 N Hwy 360 Ste 300
Grand Prairie, TX 75027-6098

KEY EXECUTIVES:
Chairman/Chief Executive Officer .... Joseph M Molina, MD
Chief Executive Officer .... Joseph M Molina, MD
President .... Chuck Carroll
Finance Director .... Michael Young CPA
Medical Director .... Michael Basco, MD
Director Special Programs .... Margaret Young RN BSN MBA

COMPANY PROFILE:
Parent Company Name: Molina Healthcare Inc
Doing Business As:
Year Founded: 2005   Federally Qualified: [N]
Forprofit: [Y]   Not-For-Profit: [ ]
Model Type:
Accreditation: [ ] AAPPO [ ] JACHO [ ] NCQA [ ] URAC
Plan Type: HMO,
Primary Physicians: 668   Physician Specialists: 1,821
Hospitals: 24
Total Revenue: 2005:   2006:   4,839,376
Net Income   2005:   2006:   -3,115,617
Total Enrollment:
   2001: 0   2004: 0   2007: 31,146
   2002: 0   2005:
   2003: 0   2006: 18,944

SERVICE AREA:
Nationwide: N
   TX;

TYPE OF COVERAGE:
Commercial: [Y] Individual: [Y] FEHBP: [ ] Indemnity: [ ]
Medicare: [ ] Medicaid: [Y] Supplemental Medicare: [ ]
Tricare   [ ]

PLAN BENEFITS:
Alternative Medicine: [ ]   Behavioral Health: [ ]
Chiropractic: [X]   Dental: [ ]
Home Care: [X]   Inpatient SNF: [X]
Long-Term Care: [ ]   Pharm. Mail Order: [X]
Physical Therapy: [X]   Podiatry: [X]
Psychiatric: [X]   Transplant: [ ]
Vision: [X]   Wellness: [X]
Workers' Comp: [ ]
Other Benefits:

NATIONAL PACIFIC DENTAL

1445 North Loop West Ste 500
Houston, TX 77008
Phone: 713-862-8404 Fax: 713-861-0008 Toll-Free: 800-232-0990
Web site: www.natlpacificdental.com

MAILING ADDRESS:
NATIONAL PACIFIC DENTAL
1445 North Loop West Ste 500
Houston, TX 77008

KEY EXECUTIVES:
President .... Kenneth M Sheldon
Chief Financial Officer .... Randy A Brecher
Dental Director .... Robert Gohlke, DDS
Marketing Director .... Kenneth M Sheldon

COMPANY PROFILE:
Parent Company Name:
Doing Business As:
Year Founded: 1989   Federally Qualified: [ ]
Forprofit: [Y]   Not-For-Profit: [ ]
Model Type:
Accreditation: [ ] AAPPO [ ] JACHO [ ] NCQA   [ ]
URACPlan Type: Specialty HMO, TPA
Total Revenue: 2005: 16,630,615   2006: 16,179,590
Net Income   2005:   2006:
Total Enrollment:
   2001: 139,253   2004: 167,111   2007: 178,856
   2002: 158,844   2005: 174,645
   2003: 160,188   2006: 167,899

SERVICE AREA:
Nationwide: N
   TX; (Anderson, Bowie, Brazoria, Brazos, Brown, Carson,
   Chambers, Collin, Dallas, Deaf Smith, Delta, Denton, Ellis, Fannin,
   Fort Bend, Galveston, Gray, Grayson, Grimes, Harris, Harrison,
   Hood, Hopkins, Hunt, Hutchinson, Jefferson, Johnson, Kaufman,
   Lamar, Liberty, Montgomery, Moore, Nacogdoches, Orange,
   Parker, Potter, Randall, Rockwall, Tarrant, Walker, Waller);

PLAN BENEFITS:
Alternative Medicine: [ ]   Behavioral Health: [ ]
Chiropractic: [ ]   Dental: [X]
Home Care: [ ]   Inpatient SNF: [ ]
Long-Term Care: [ ]   Pharm. Mail Order: [ ]
Physical Therapy: [ ]   Podiatry: [ ]
Psychiatric: [ ]   Transplant: [ ]
Vision: [ ]   Wellness: [ ]
Workers' Comp: [ ]
Other Benefits:
Comments:
Formerly Spectra Dental.

ORAQUEST DENTAL PLANS

12946 Dairy Ashford Ste 360
Sugarland, TX 77478
Phone: 281-313-7170 Fax: 281-313-7155 Toll-Free: 800-660-6064
Web site: www.oraquest.com

MAILING ADDRESS:
ORAQUEST DENTAL PLANS
12946 Dairy Ashford Ste 360
Sugarland, TX 77478

KEY EXECUTIVES:
Chief Executive Officer/President .... James Taylor
Chief Financial Officer .... Patrick Stoner
Dental Director .... James Sanders

COMPANY PROFILE:
Parent Company Name: Dental Economics LLC
Doing Business As:
Year Founded: 1995   Federally Qualified: [N]
Forprofit: [Y]   Not-For-Profit: [ ]
Model Type:
Accreditation: [ ] AAPPO [ ] JACHO [ ] NCQA [ ] URAC
Plan Type: Specialty HMO
Total Revenue: 2005: 1,561,708   2006: 1,775,979
Net Income   2005:   20,889   2006:   14,782
Total Enrollment:
   2001: 3,150   2004: 35,238   2007: 116,935
   2002: 0   2005: 42,017
   2003: 5,222   2006: 46,051

SERVICE AREA:
Nationwide: N
   TX (Austin, Dallas, Houston, Ft Worth, San Antonio, Waco);

TYPE OF COVERAGE:
Commercial: [Y] Individual: [Y] FEHBP: [ ] Indemnity: [ ]
Medicare: [Y] Medicaid: [ ] Supplemental Medicare: [Y]
Tricare   [ ]

TEXAS
Managed Care Organization Profiles

PRODUCTS OFFERED:
Product Name: Type:
MetroWest Medicaid   Medicaid
Comments:
Formerly Metrowest Health Plan Inc.

LEGACY HEALTH PLAN INC

2018 Pulliam St
San Angelo, TX 76905
Phone: 325-658-7104   Fax: 325-659-7275 Toll-Free: 800-839-7198
Web site: www.legacyhealthplan.com
MAILING ADDRESS:
    LEGACY HEALTH PLAN INC
    2018 Pulliam St
    San Angelo, TX 76905

KEY EXECUTIVES:
President .... Marinan Williams
Chief Financial Officer .... Tom Martin
Director of Sales .... Julia Stout
Health Plan Consultant .... Jimmy Rodriguez
Health Plan Consultant .... Cynthia Sutton

COMPANY PROFILE:
Parent Company Name:
Doing Business As: Legacy Health Plan
Year Founded: 1999   Federally Qualified: [ ]
Forprofit: [ ]   Not-For-Profit: [ ]
Model Type:
Accreditation: [ ] AAPPO [ ] JACHO [ ] NCQA [ ] URAC
Plan Type: HMO, PPO, CDHP, HDHP, HSA
Total Revenue: 2005:   937,935   2006:   2,223,436
Net Income   2005:   -442,646   2006:   7,259
Total Enrollment:
    2001: 0   2004: 0   2007: 731
    2002: 0   2005: 602
    2003: 0   2006: 681
Medical Loss Ratio: 2005:   2006:
Administrative Expense Ratio: 2005:   2006:
SERVICE AREA:
Nationwide: N
    TX;
TYPE OF COVERAGE:
Commercial: [Y] Individual: [ ]   FEHBP: [ ]   Indemnity: [ ]
Medicare: [ ] Medicaid: [ ]   Supplemental Medicare: [ ]
Tricare   [ ]
PLAN BENEFITS:
Alternative Medicine: [ ]   Behavioral Health: [X]
Chiropractic: [X]   Dental: [ ]
Home Care: [X]   Inpatient SNF: [X]
Long-Term Care: [X]   Pharm. Mail Order: [X]
Physical Therapy: [X]   Podiatry: [ ]
Psychiatric: [X]   Transplant: [X]
Vision: [ ]   Wellness: [X]
Workers' Comp: [ ]
Other Benefits:

MEDICAL CARE REFERRAL GROUP

4100 Rio Bravo Ste 211
El Paso, TX 79902-1010
Phone: 915-532-2408   Fax: 915-532-1772 Toll-Free: 800-424-9919
Web site: www.mcrg.net
MAILING ADDRESS:
    MEDICAL CARE REFERRAL GROUP
    4100 Rio Bravo Ste 211
    El Paso, TX 79902-1010

KEY EXECUTIVES:
Chief Executive Officer/Chief Financial Officer .... Lorri Halow
Chief Operating Officer .... Angie Carrasco
VP, Marketing .... Joseph Halow
Credentialing .... Cindy Torres

COMPANY PROFILE:
Parent Company Name: Assured Benefits Administrators Inc
Doing Business As:
Year Founded: 1985   Federally Qualified: [ ]

Forprofit: [Y]   Not-For-Profit: [ ]
Model Type:
Accreditation: [ ] AAPPO [ ] JACHO [X] NCQA [ ] URAC
Plan Type: PPO, POS, EPO
Total Enrollment:
    2001: 70,000   2004: 0   2007: 0
    2002: 0   2005:
    2003: 0   2006:
SERVICE AREA:
Nationwide: N
    NM; TX;
TYPE OF COVERAGE:
Commercial: [Y] Individual: [ ]   FEHBP: [ ]   Indemnity: [ ]
Medicare: [ ] Medicaid: [ ]   Supplemental Medicare: [ ]
Tricare   [ ]
PLAN BENEFITS:
Alternative Medicine: [ ]   Behavioral Health: [X]
Chiropractic: [X]   Dental: [X]
Home Care: [X]   Inpatient SNF: [X]
Long-Term Care: [ ]   Pharm. Mail Order: [X]
Physical Therapy: [X]   Podiatry: [X]
Psychiatric: [X]   Transplant: [X]
Vision: [X]   Wellness: [X]
Workers' Comp: [X]
Other Benefits:

MEGA LIFE & HEALTH INSURANCE COMPANY

9151 Boulevard 26
North Richland Hills, TX 761802
Phone: 800-527-5504   Fax: 800-343-3702 Toll-Free: 800-527-5504
Web site: www.megainsurance.com
MAILING ADDRESS:
    MEGA LIFE & HEALTH INS CO
    PO Box 982010
    North Richland Hills, TX 761802

KEY EXECUTIVES:
Chief Executive Officer/President .... William J Gedwed
Chief Financial Officer .... Mark D Hauptman
Chief Investment Officer .... Derrick A. Duke
Marketing Director .... John Hearell
Controller .... Connie Palacios
General Counsel .... Michael A. Colliflower
VP of Administration .... Elaine Gress

COMPANY PROFILE:
Parent Company Name: UICI Insurance
Doing Business As:
Year Founded: Federally Qualified: [ ]
Forprofit: [ ]   Not-For-Profit: [ ]
Model Type:
Accreditation: [ ] AAPPO [ ] JACHO [ ] NCQA [ ] URAC
Plan Type: PPO
Total Enrollment:
    2001: 3,826   2004: 0   2007: 0
    2002: 0   2005:
    2003: 0   2006:
SERVICE AREA:
Nationwide: N
    NW (Excluding NY);
Comments:
Purchased PFL Life Insurance Company, Cedar Rapids, Iowa, Oregon
business as of August 2000.

MEMORIAL HERMANN
HEALTH NETWORK PROVIDERS

9301 Southwest Freeway #5000
Houston, TX 77074
Phone: 713-448-6464   Fax: 713-448-6489 Toll-Free: 888-642-5040
Web site: www.mhhnp.org
MAILING ADDRESS:
    MEMORIAL HERMANN HLTH NTWK PRV
    9301 Southwest Freeway #5000
    Houston, TX 77074

Managed Care Organization Profiles — TEXAS

HUMANA HEALTH PLAN OF AUSTIN

1221 S Mopac Blvd Ste 200
Austin, TX 78746
Phone: 512-338-6154 Fax: 512-338-2588 Toll-Free: 800-234-7912
Web site: www.humana.com/austin/austin.html

MAILING ADDRESS:
  HUMANA HEALTH PLAN OF AUSTIN
  1221 S Mopac Blvd Ste 200
  Austin, TX 78746

KEY EXECUTIVES:
Chairman of the Board .... David A Jones Jr
Chief Executive Officer .... Gary Goldstein, MD
President .... Michael B McCallister
Chief Financial Officer .... Jennifer King
Medical Director .... Scott Simpson, MD
Director Marketing Administration .... Dubie Cantu
VP of Sales .... Richard Willis
Director of Provider Contracting .... Alan Lahti
VP, Network Management .... Donnie Hromadka
Director of Medical Management .... Kathie Becque, RN
Mgr of Quality Management .... Torje Scott, RN
Director Marketing Administration .... Jodie Richardson
Director of Provider Contracting .... Donnie Hromadka

COMPANY PROFILE:
Parent Company Name: Humana Inc
Doing Business As:
Year Founded: 1961   Federally Qualified: [Y]
Forprofit: [Y]   Not-For-Profit: [ ]
Model Type: IPA
Accreditation: [ ] AAPPO [ ] JACHO [ ] NCQA [ ] URAC
Plan Type: HMO, PPO, ASO, CDHP, HDHP, HSA,
Total Revenue: 2005: 36,591,564   2006: 28,721,664
Net Income   2005:   161,562 2006:   189,749
Total Enrollment:
  2001: 78,056   2004: 16,840   2007: 17,874
  2002: 40,435   2005: 9,312
  2003: 35,856   2006: 10,264

SERVICE AREA:
Nationwide: N
  TX

TYPE OF COVERAGE:
Commercial: [Y] Individual: [ ] FEHBP: [ ] Indemnity: [ ]
Medicare: [Y] Medicaid: [Y] Supplemental Medicare: [Y]
Tricare   [ ]

PRODUCTS OFFERED:
Product Name: Type:
Humana HMO   HMO
Humana PPO   PPO
Humana   Medicare

CONSUMER-DRIVEN PRODUCTS
JP Morgan Chase   HSA Company
HumanaOne HSA   HSA Product
JP Morgan Chase   HSA Administrator
Personal Care Account   Consumer-Driven Health Plan
HumanaOne   High Deductible Health Plan

PLAN BENEFITS:
Alternative Medicine: [ ]   Behavioral Health: [ ]
Chiropractic: [X]   Dental: [X]
Home Care: [ ]   Inpatient SNF: [ ]
Long-Term Care: [ ]   Pharm. Mail Order: [X]
Physical Therapy: [ ]   Podiatry: [ ]
Psychiatric: [X]   Transplant: [X]
Vision: [ ]   Wellness: [X]
Workers' Comp: [X]
Other Benefits: Long Term Disability Care

INTERPLAN HEALTH GROUP

600 Six Flags Dr Ste 200
Arlington, TX 76011
Phone: 817-633-8335 Fax: 817-640-1009 Toll-Free: 800-613-1124
Web site: www.ahpppo.com

MAILING ADDRESS:
  INTERPLAN HEALTH GROUP
  600 Six Flags Dr Ste 200
  Arlington, TX 76011

KEY EXECUTIVES:
Chairman/Chief Exeuctive Officer .... Paul W Glover
Chief Financial Officer .... Steven L Ditman
Medical Director .... Roland Anderson, MD
Chief Information Officer .... Hamilton Chaffee
National Director of Operations/Managed Care ...... Eileen Romansky
Marketing Director .... Michael Schotz
MIS Director .... Michele Jennings
National Director of Network Development .... Patricia Kohn
Director of Operations .... Michele Jennings

COMPANY PROFILE:
Parent Company Name: Interplan Health
Doing Business As:
Year Founded: 1994   Federally Qualified: [ ] Forprofit: [Y]
Not-For-Profit: [ ]
Model Type: NETWORK
Accreditation: [ ] AAPPO [ ] JACHO [ ] NCQA [X] URAC
Plan Type: PPO, UR
Primary Physicians: 43,011   Physician Specialists: 95,805
Hospitals: 909
Total Enrollment:
  2001: 68,000   2004:   0   2007: 3,000,000
  2002: 268,000   2005:
  2003:   0   2006:

SERVICE AREA:
Nationwide: N
  AZ; OK; TX; AR;

TYPE OF COVERAGE:
Commercial: [Y] Individual: [Y] FEHBP: [ ] Indemnity: [ ]
Medicare: [ ] Medicaid: [ ] Supplemental Medicare: [ ]
Tricare   [ ]

PRODUCTS OFFERED:
Product Name: Type:
Accountable Health Plant PPO   PPO

PLAN BENEFITS:
Alternative Medicine: [ ]   Behavioral Health: [X]
Chiropractic: [X]   Dental: [ ]
Home Care: [X]   Inpatient SNF: [X]
Long-Term Care: [ ]   Pharm. Mail Order: [X]
Physical Therapy: [X]   Podiatry: [ ]
Psychiatric: [X]   Transplant: [X]
Vision: [X]   Wellness: [X]
Workers' Comp: [ ]
Other Benefits:
Comments:
Formerly Accountable Health Plans of America - Corporate.

JPS BENEFITS

1500 S Main St
Fort Worth, TX 76110
Phone: 817-921-3431 Fax: 817-924-1207 Toll-Free: 888-924-8852
Web site: www.jpshealthnet.org

MAILING ADDRESS:
  JPS BENEFITS
  1500 S Main St
  Fort Worth, TX 76110

KEY EXECUTIVES:
Chairman of the Board .... Harold Samuels
Chief Executive Officer/President .... David M Cecero
Chief Financial Officer .... Gale S Pileggi, MBA
Chief Medical Officer .... Jay Haynes, MD
Chief Operating Officer .... Ronald Stutes
VP, Human Resources .... Judith B Redd, MD

COMPANY PROFILE:
Parent Company Name: JPS Health Network
Doing Business As:
Year Founded: 1997   Federally Qualified: [ ]
Forprofit: [ ]   Not-For-Profit: [ ]
Model Type:
Accreditation: [ ] AAPPO [ ] JACHO [ ] NCQA [ ] URAC
Plan Type: Specialty HMO
Total Enrollment:
  2001: 4,336   2004: 12,136   2007: 0
  2002: 5,539   2005:
  2003: 12,661   2006:

SERVICE AREA:
Nationwide: N
  TX (Denton, Hood, Johnson, Parker, Tarrant, Wise);

TEXAS

Managed Care Organization Profiles

CONSUMER-DRIVEN PRODUCTS
JP Morgan Chase   HSA Company
HumanaOne HSA   HSA Product
JP Morgan Chase   HSA Administrator
Personal Care Account   Consumer-Driven Health Plan
HumanaOne   High Deductible Health Plan

PLAN BENEFITS:
Alternative Medicine: [ ]   Behavioral Health: [ ]
Chiropractic: [X]   Dental: [X]
Home Care: [ ]   Inpatient SNF: [ ]
Long-Term Care: [ ]   Pharm. Mail Order: [X]
Physical Therapy: [ ]   Podiatry: [ ]
Psychiatric: [X]   Transplant: [X]
Vision: [ ]   Wellness: [X]
Workers' Comp: [X]
Other Benefits: Long Term Disability Care

HUMANA HEALTH CARE PLANS OF HOUSTON

1980 Post Oak Blvd Ste 1900
Houston, TX 77056
Phone: 713-662-6639 Fax: 713-513-3949 Toll-Free: 877-603-5516
Web site: www.humana.com/houston/home.html

MAILING ADDRESS:
    HUMANA HEALTH CARE PLANS OF HOUSTON
    1980 Post Oak Blvd Ste 1900
    Houston, TX 77056

KEY EXECUTIVES:
Chairman of the Board .... David A Jones Jr
Chief Executive Officer-TX .... Gary Goldstein, MD
Market President .... Pattie D Tye
Chief Financial Officer .... Scott Herman
Medical Director .... Harvey Balthaser, MD
Vice President of Sales .... Lisa Rowland
Director Provider Relations .... Jim Hickey
VP of Network Operations .... Jack Smith
Human Resources Director .... Denice Pittman
Quality Management Director .... Nancy Royal
Quality Management Director .... Yvonne Trinchitella, RN
Marketing Administrative Director .... Tina Yost
Director of Contract .... Jack Smith
Director of Contract .... Bonnie Drake

COMPANY PROFILE:
Parent Company Name: Humana Inc
Doing Business As:
Year Founded: 1961   Federally Qualified: [Y]
Forprofit: [Y]   Not-For-Profit: [ ]
Model Type: IPA
Accreditation: [ ] AAPPO [ ] JACHO [ ] NCQA [ ] URAC
Plan Type: HMO, PPO, ASO, CDHP, HDHP, HSA,
Primary Physicians: 1,500   Physician Specialists: 5,000
Hospitals: 67
Total Revenue: 2005: 106,478,676   2006: 66,701,099
Net Income   2005: -1,333,708   2006: 8,350,855
Total Enrollment:
    2001: 161,973   2004: 49,438   2007: 22,672
    2002: 176,044   2005: 20,509
    2003: 95,429   2006: 17,981

SERVICE AREA:
Nationwide: N
    TX;

TYPE OF COVERAGE:
Commercial: [Y] Individual: [ ] FEHBP: [ ] Indemnity: [ ]
Medicare: [Y] Medicaid: [Y] Supplemental Medicare: [Y]
Tricare   [ ]

PRODUCTS OFFERED:
Product Name: Type:
Humana HMO   HMO
Humana PPO   PPO
Humana ASO   ASO

CONSUMER-DRIVEN PRODUCTS
JP Morgan Chase   HSA Company
HumanaOne HSA   HSA Product
JP Morgan Chase   HSA Administrator
Personal Care Account   Consumer-Driven Health Plan
HumanaOne   High Deductible Health Plan

PLAN BENEFITS:
Alternative Medicine: [ ]   Behavioral Health: [ ]
Chiropractic: [X]   Dental: [X]
Home Care: [ ]   Inpatient SNF: [ ]
Long-Term Care: [ ]   Pharm. Mail Order: [ ]
Physical Therapy: [ ]   Podiatry: [ ]
Psychiatric: [X]   Transplant: [X]
Vision: [ ]   Wellness: [X]
Workers' Comp: [X]
Other Benefits: Long Term Disability Care

HUMANA HEALTH CARE PLANS OF SAN ANTONIO

8431 Fredericksburg Rd Ste 570
San Antonio, TX 78229
Phone: 210-617-1001 Fax: 210-615-0090 Toll-Free: 800-486-2620
Web site: www.humana.com/louisville/home.html

MAILING ADDRESS:
    HUMANA HEALTH CARE PLANS OF TX
    8431 Fredericksburg Rd Ste 570
    San Antonio, TX 78229

KEY EXECUTIVES:
Chairman of the Board .... David A Jones Jr
Chief Executive Officer/Marketing .... Linda T Hummel
President .... Michael B McCallister
Chief Financial Officer .... Linda T Hummell
Medical Director .... George Smith, MD
Large Group Sales Manager .... Andrew Grove
Director of Provider Contracting .... Cathy Trlica
Manager of Quality Management .... Mary Weiss
Director Marketing Administration .... Linda Eigel
Director of Provider Contracting .... Matt Stedman

COMPANY PROFILE:
Parent Company Name: Humana Inc
Doing Business As:
Year Founded: 1982   Federally Qualified: [Y]
Forprofit: [Y]   Not-For-Profit: [ ]
Model Type: IPA
Accreditation: [ ] AAPPO [ ] JACHO [ ] NCQA [ ] URAC
Plan Type: HMO, PPO, POS, ASO, CDHP, HSA
Primary Physicians: 1,000   Physician Specialists: 2,200
Hospitals:
Total Revenue: 2005: 263,748,896   2006: 284,858,261
Net Income   2005:   9,949,332   2006: 36,138,516
Total Enrollment:
    2001: 224,947   2004: 58,031   2007: 63,376
    2002: 239,034   2005: 50,162
    2003: 81,815   2006: 48,691

SERVICE AREA:
Nationwide: N
    TX;

TYPE OF COVERAGE:
Commercial: [Y] Individual: [ ] FEHBP: [ ] Indemnity: [ ]
Medicare: [Y] Medicaid: [Y] Supplemental Medicare: [Y]
Tricare   [ ]

PRODUCTS OFFERED:
Product Name: Type:
Humana Gold Plus Plan   Medicare Advantage

CONSUMER-DRIVEN PRODUCTS
JP Morgan Chase   HSA Company
HumanaOne HSA   HSA Product
JP Morgan Chase   HSA Administrator
Personal Care Account   Consumer-Driven Health Plan
HumanaOne   High Deductible Health Plan

PLAN BENEFITS:
Alternative Medicine: [ ]   Behavioral Health: [ ]
Chiropractic: [X]   Dental: [X]
Home Care: [ ]   Inpatient SNF: [ ]
Long-Term Care: [ ]   Pharm. Mail Order: [X]
Physical Therapy: [ ]   Podiatry: [ ]
Psychiatric: [X]   Transplant: [X]
Vision: [ ]   Wellness: [X]
Workers' Comp: [X]
Other Benefits: Long Term Disability Care

Managed Care Organization Profiles — TEXAS

HORIZON BEHAVIORAL SERVICES

2941 South Lake Vista Dr
Lewisville, TX 75056
Phone: 800-931-4646 Fax: 972-420-8252 Toll-Free: 800-727-2407
Web site: www.horizoncare.net

MAILING ADDRESS:
   HORIZON BEHAVIORAL SERVICES
   2941 South Lake Vista Dr
   Lewisville, TX 75056

KEY EXECUTIVES:
Chief Executive Officer .... Ken Newman
President .... Jackie L James
Medical Director .... William Eckbert, MD
Chief Information Officer .... Zeke Zoccoli
VP of Operations .... Dorothy Harrison PhD

COMPANY PROFILE:
Parent Company Name: Horizon Health Corporation
Doing Business As: Horizon Behavioral Services Inc
Year Founded: 1989   Federally Qualified: [ ]
Forprofit: [Y]   Not-For-Profit: [ ]
Model Type: NETWORK/STAFF
Accreditation: [ ] AAPPO [ ] JACHO [X] NCQA [X] URAC
Plan Type: Specialty HMO, Specialty PPO, ASO, UR
Primary Physicians: Physician Specialists: 17,000
Total Enrollment:
   2001: 2,300,582   2004: 0   2007: 0
   2002: 0   2005:
   2003: 0   2006:

SERVICE AREA:
Nationwide: Y
   NW:

TYPE OF COVERAGE:
Commercial: [Y] Individual: [ ] FEHBP: [Y] Indemnity: [ ]
Medicare: [Y] Medicaid: [Y] Supplemental Medicare: [ ]
Tricare [ ]

PRODUCTS OFFERED:
Product Name: Type:
Employee Assistant Program
Managed Behavioral Health Prog
Administrative Services
Utilization Review   ASO
On Line Work Life Services   EAP

PLAN BENEFITS:
Alternative Medicine: [ ]   Behavioral Health: [X]
Chiropractic: [ ]   Dental: [ ]
Home Care: [ ]   Inpatient SNF: [ ]
Long-Term Care: [ ]   Pharm. Mail Order: [ ]
Physical Therapy: [ ]   Podiatry: [ ]
Psychiatric: [X]   Transplant: [ ]
Vision: [ ]   Wellness: [X]
Workers' Comp: [ ]
Other Benefits: On Line Work Life

HUMANA HEALTH CARE PLANS OF CORPUS CHRISTI

802 N Carancahua Ste 1700
Corpus Christi, TX 78470
Phone: 361-866-2200 Fax: 361-866-2299 Toll-Free: 800-269-1645
Web site: www.humana.com/corpuschristi/home.html

MAILING ADDRESS:
   HUMANA HC PLNS-CORPUS CHRISTI
   802 N Carancahua Ste 1700
   Corpus Christi, TX 78470

KEY EXECUTIVES:
Chairman of the Board .... David A Jones Jr
Market Chief Executive Officer .... Linda T Hummel
President .... Michael B McCallister
Chief Financial Officer .... James H Bloem
Medical Director .... Weston P Scott
Chief Service & Information Officer .... Bruce Goodman
Chief Operating Officer .... Jim Murray
Chief Marketing Officer .... Steve Moya
Director of Sales .... Andrew Grove
VP of Network Development .... Steven Bishop
Chief Human Resources Director .... Bonnie C Hathcock
Quality Management .... Mary Weiss
Utilization Management .... Jacqueline Shadron
Large Group Sales Director .... Andrew Grove
Small Group Sales Director .... Bart Ming

COMPANY PROFILE:
Parent Company Name: Humana Inc
Doing Business As:
Year Founded: 1961   Federally Qualified: [Y]
Forprofit: [Y]   Not-For-Profit: [ ]
Model Type: IPA
Accreditation: [ ] AAPPO [ ] JACHO [ ] NCQA [ ] URAC
Plan Type: HMO, PPO, ASO, CDHP, HSA
Total Revenue: 2005: 89,556,379   2006: 109,718,664
Net Income   2005: 12,059,669   2006: 21,829,785
Total Enrollment:
   2001: 54,000   2004: 10,836   2007: 13,135
   2002: 17,586   2005: 10,839
   2003: 13,914   2006: 11,112

SERVICE AREA:
Nationwide: N
   TX:

TYPE OF COVERAGE:
Commercial: [Y] Individual: [Y] FEHBP: [ ] Indemnity: [ ]
Medicare: [Y] Medicaid: [Y] Supplemental Medicare: [Y]
Tricare   [Y]

PRODUCTS OFFERED:
Product Name: Type:
Humana Gold Plus Plan   Medicare Advantage
HMO   HMO

CONSUMER-DRIVEN PRODUCTS
UMB Bank   HSA Company
HSA   HSA Product
UMB Bank   HSA Administrator
CoverageFirst   Consumer-Driven Health Plan
CoverageFirst HDHP   High Deductible Health Plan

PLAN BENEFITS:
Alternative Medicine: [ ]   Behavioral Health: [X]
Chiropractic: [X]   Dental: [X]
Home Care: [X]   Inpatient SNF: [ ]
Long-Term Care: [ ]   Pharm. Mail Order: [X]
Physical Therapy: [ ]   Podiatry: [ ]
Psychiatric: [X]   Transplant: [X]
Vision: [X]   Wellness: [X]
Workers' Comp: [X]
Other Benefits: Long Term Disability

HUMANA HEALTH CARE PLANS OF DALLAS

8111 LBJ Freeway Ste 1400
Dallas, TX 75251
Phone: 972-643-1600 Fax: 972-437-9245 Toll-Free: 800-651-9079
Web site: www.humana.com/dallas/home.html

MAILING ADDRESS:
   HUMANA HEALTH CARE PLANS OF TX
   8111 LBJ Freeway Ste 1400
   Dallas, TX 75251

KEY EXECUTIVES:
Chairman of the Board .... David A Jones Jr
Market President .... Gary Goldstein, MD
Chief Financial Officer .... Jennifer King
Medical Director .... Mark Netoskie, MD
Vice President Sales .... Gary M Cole
Network Development Director .... Sam Waugh
Human Resources Director .... Eric Talb
Director of Account Management .... Bill Comerford
Director of Small Group Sales .... Frank McCaffrey

COMPANY PROFILE:
Parent Company Name: Humana Inc
Doing Business As:
Year Founded: 1961   Federally Qualified: [Y]
Forprofit: [Y]   Not-For-Profit: [ ]
Model Type:
Accreditation: [ ] AAPPO [ ] JACHO [ ] NCQA [ ] URAC
Plan Type: PPO, ASO, CDHP, HSA
Total Enrollment:
   2001: 8,243   2004: 0   2007: 0
   2002: 50,000   2005:
   2003: 0   2006:

SERVICE AREA:
Nationwide: N
   TX;

TYPE OF COVERAGE:
Commercial: [Y] Individual: [Y] FEHBP: [Y] Indemnity: [ ]
Medicare: [Y] Medicaid: [ ] Supplemental Medicare: [Y]
Tricare   [ ]

TEXAS
Managed Care Organization Profiles

KEY EXECUTIVES:
Vice President .... Richard Hillyer
Chief Executive Officer .... Steve Gaven
Chief Financial Officer/Marketing Officer .... Mike Nicknish
Chief Medical Officer .... Steve Duvall
Chief Information Officer/MIS Director .... Mike Nicknish
Director, Provider Services .... David Loper

COMPANY PROFILE:
Parent Company Name: Cibiz Century Business Services
Doing Business As: H.A.S. Premier Providers Inc
Year Founded: 1984   Federally Qualified: [ ]
Forprofit: [ ]   Not-For-Profit: [ ]
Model Type:
Accreditation: [ ] AAPPO [ ] JACHO [ ] NCQA [ ] URAC
Plan Type: UR,
Hospitals: 49
Total Enrollment:
  2001: 0   2004: 140,000   2007: 0
  2002: 0   2005:
  2003: 0   2006:

SERVICE AREA:
Nationwide: N
  TX;

HEALTHSMART PREFERRED CARE

2002 W Loop 289 Ste 121
Lubbock, TX 79407
Phone: 806-687-0500 Fax: 806-473-2525 Toll-Free: 800-687-0500
Web site: www.healthsmart.net

MAILING ADDRESS:
HEALTHSMART PREFERRED CARE
2002 W Loop 289 Ste 121
Lubbock, TX 79407

KEY EXECUTIVES:
Chief Executive Officer .... David Adams
Medical Director .... Randall Treadwell, MD
Chief Information Officer .... John Farnsley
SR VP Operations .... Jane Williamson, RN
VP Sales & Marketing .... Bobby Clark

COMPANY PROFILE:
Parent Company Name: Healthsmart Preferred Care
Doing Business As:
Year Founded: 1986   Federally Qualified: [ ]
Forprofit: [ ]   Not-For-Profit: [Y]
Model Type: MIXED
Accreditation: [ ] AAPPO [ ] JACHO [ ] NCQA [ ] URAC
Plan Type: PPO, POS, EPO
Primary Physicians: 4,245   Physician Specialists: 4,762
Hospitals: 69
Total Enrollment:
  2001: 181,249   2004: 0   2007: 0
  2002: 138,401   2005:
  2003: 700,000   2006:

SERVICE AREA:
Nationwide: N
  TX (18 North central counties, including Dallas-Ft Worth area);

TYPE OF COVERAGE:
Commercial: [Y] Individual: [ ] FEHBP: [ ] Indemnity: [ ]
Medicare: [ ] Medicaid: [ ] Supplemental Medicare: [ ]
Tricare   [ ]

PRODUCTS OFFERED:
Product Name: Type:
N TX Healthcare Network PPO   PPO
N TX Healthcare Network GEPO   EPO
N TX Healthcare Network POS   POS

Comments:
Parent companies: Baylor Health Care System, Texas Health Resources, Methodist Hospitals of Dallas.

HEALTHCARE PARTNERS OF EAST TEXAS INC

426 N Center St
Longview, TX 75601
Phone: 903-238-8845 Fax: 903-757-6204 Toll-Free: 800-362-3041
Web site: www.hpet.org

MAILING ADDRESS:
HEALTHCARE PARTNERS OF EAST TX
PO Box 2749
Longview, TX 75601

KEY EXECUTIVES:
Chairman of the Board .... Bryant H. Krenek, JR
Chief Executive Officer/President .... Carolyn Hess
Chief Financial Officer .... Carolyn Hess
Operations Director .... Kathy Hale
Executive Director of Marketing .... Mark Hobgood
Credentialing Supervisor .... Joyce Bumbard
Director Contracting & Legal .... Steve Johnston

COMPANY PROFILE:
Parent Company Name: Health Care Partners of East Texas Inc
Doing Business As:
Year Founded: 1993   Federally Qualified: [ ]
Forprofit: [ ]   Not-For-Profit: [Y]
Model Type: NETWORK
Accreditation: [ ] AAPPO [ ] JACHO [ ] NCQA [ ] URAC
Plan Type: PPO
Primary Physicians: Physician Specialists:
Hospitals: 62
Total Enrollment:
  2001: 350,000   2004: 0   2007: 0
  2002: 0   2005:
  2003: 0   2006:

SERVICE AREA:
Nationwide: N
  TX (44 eastern counties);

TYPE OF COVERAGE:
Commercial: [Y] Individual: [Y] FEHBP: [Y] Indemnity: [ ]
Medicare: [ ] Medicaid: [ ] Supplemental Medicare: [ ]
Tricare   [Y]

PRODUCTS OFFERED:
Product Name: Type:
Network Access   PPO

PLAN BENEFITS:
Alternative Medicine: [ ]   Behavioral Health: [X]
Chiropractic: [X]   Dental: [ ]
Home Care: [X]   Inpatient SNF: [X]
Long-Term Care: [ ]   Pharm. Mail Order: [ ]
Physical Therapy: [X]   Podiatry: [X]
Psychiatric: [X]   Transplant: [X]
Vision: [ ]   Wellness: [X]
Workers' Comp: [X]
Other Benefits:

HERITAGE HEALTH SYSTEMS INC

4888 Loop Central Dr Ste 700
Houston, TX 77081
Phone: 800-544-5428 Fax: 713-965-0433 Toll-Free: 800-544-5428
Web site: www.hhsi.com

MAILING ADDRESS:
HERITAGE HEALTH SYSTEMS INC
4888 Loop Central Dr Ste 700
Houston, TX 77081

KEY EXECUTIVES:
Chief Executive Officer/President .... Theodore M. Carpenter, Jr

COMPANY PROFILE:
Parent Company Name: Universal American Financial Corporation
Doing Business As:
Year Founded: Federally Qualified: [ ]
Forprofit: [ ]   Not-For-Profit: [ ]
Model Type:
Accreditation: [ ] AAPPO [ ] JACHO [ ] NCQA [ ] URAC
Plan Type: HMO

SERVICE AREA:
Nationwide:
  FL; OK; TX; WI;

TYPE OF COVERAGE:
Commercial: [ ] Individual: [ ] FEHBP: [ ] Indemnity: [ ]
Medicare: [Y] Medicaid: [ ] Supplemental Medicare: [ ]
Tricare   [ ]

Managed Care Organization Profiles — TEXAS

SERVICE AREA:
Nationwide: N
   AR; NM; OK; TX (Western Panhandle, Austin, San Antonio, Central);
TYPE OF COVERAGE:
Commercial: [Y] Individual: [ ] FEHBP: [ ] Indemnity: [ ]
Medicare: [ ] Medicaid: [ ] Supplemental Medicare: [ ]
Tricare [ ]
CONSUMER-DRIVEN PRODUCTS
Mellon HR Solutions LLC   HSA Company   HSA Product
                           HSA Administrator
                           Consumer-Driven Health Plan
                           High Deductible Health Plan

PLAN BENEFITS:
Alternative Medicine: [X]   Behavioral Health: [ ]
Chiropractic: [X]   Dental: [X]
Home Care: [X]   Inpatient SNF: [X]
Long-Term Care: [ ]   Pharm. Mail Order: [X]
Physical Therapy: [X]   Podiatry: [X]
Psychiatric: [X]   Transplant: [X]
Vision: [X]   Wellness: [X]
Workers' Comp: [ ]
Other Benefits:

GREAT-WEST HEALTHCARE OF TEXAS - DALLAS

8350 N Central Expwy Ste M1000
Dallas, TX 75206
Phone: 972-813-7000 Fax: 214-363-9785 Toll-Free: 800-866-3136
Web site: www.greatwesthealthcare.com
MAILING ADDRESS:
   GREAT-WEST HEALTHCARE TX-DALLAS
   8350 N Central Expwy Ste M1000
   Dallas, TX 75206

KEY EXECUTIVES:
President .... Janice Faulk
Finance Director .... Julie MaGill
Chief Medical Officer .... Allan Kogan, MD
MIS Manager .... David Revels
Credentialing Manager .... Tracey Scott
Director, Provider Services .... Jennifer Reeves
VP, Network Development .... John McGuinness
Human Resources Director .... Andrea Nelson
Medical Management/Quality Assurance Director .... Mary Reichardt

COMPANY PROFILE:
Parent Company Name: Great West Life & Annuity Insurance Co
Doing Business As: Great-West Healthcare
Year Founded: 1995   Federally Qualified: [N]
Forprofit: [Y]   Not-For-Profit: [ ]
Model Type: MIXED
Accreditation: [ ] AAPPO [ ] JACHO [ ] NCQA [ ] URAC
Plan Type: HMO, PPO, POS, ASO, TPA, CDHP, HSA
Primary Physicians: 12,371   Physician Specialists: 28,221
Hospitals: 560
Total Revenue: 2005: 4,425,051   2006: 4,083,562
Net Income   2005: 323,264   2006: 575,052
Total Enrollment:
   2001: 259,018   2004: 12,106   2007: 3,247
   2002: 448,235   2005: 4,769
   2003: 15,806   2006: 3,532

SERVICE AREA:
Nationwide: N
   TX (Atascosa, Bastrop, Bexar, Blanco, Brazoria, Burnet, Caldwell, Chambers, Collin, Comal, Dallas, Denton, Ellis, Fort Bend, Frio, Galveston, Guadalupe, Harris, Hays, Hunt, Johnson, Kaufman, Liberty, Medina, Montgomery, Parker, Rockwall, San Jacinto, Tarrant, Travis, Williamson, Wilson);
TYPE OF COVERAGE:
Commercial: [Y] Individual: [ ] FEHBP: [ ] Indemnity: [Y]
Medicare: [ ] Medicaid: [ ] Supplemental Medicare: [ ]
Tricare [ ]
PRODUCTS OFFERED:
Product Name: Type:
Great-West Life HMO   HMO
Great-West Life PPO   PPO
Great-West Life POS   POS

CONSUMER-DRIVEN PRODUCTS
Mellon HR Solutions LLC   HSA Company
                           HSA Product
                           HSA Administrator
                           Consumer-Driven Health Plan
                           High Deductible Health Plan

PLAN BENEFITS:
Alternative Medicine: [X]   Behavioral Health: [X]
Chiropractic: [X]   Dental: [X]
Home Care: [X]   Inpatient SNF: [X]
Long-Term Care: [ ]   Pharm. Mail Order: [X]
Physical Therapy: [X]   Podiatry: [X]
Psychiatric: [X]   Transplant: [X]
Vision: [X]   Wellness: [X]
Workers' Comp: [ ]
Other Benefits:

GREAT-WEST HEALTHCARE OF TEXAS - HOUSTON

10111 Richmond Ave Ste 400
Houston, TX 77042
Phone: 832-252-7000 Fax: Toll-Free:
Web site: www.greatwesthealthcare.com
MAILING ADDRESS:
   GREAT-WEST HEALTHCARE TX-HOUSTON
   10111 Richmond Ave Ste 400
   Houston, TX 77042

KEY EXECUTIVES:
Chief Executive Officer/President .... Raymond L McFeetors
Medical Director .... Allan Kogan, MD
General Manager .... Dennis McDowell

COMPANY PROFILE:
Parent Company Name: Great West Life & Annuity Insurance Co
Doing Business As:
Year Founded: Federally Qualified: [ ]
Forprofit: [Y]   Not-For-Profit: [ ]
Model Type:
Accreditation: [ ] AAPPO [ ] JACHO [ ] NCQA [ ] URAC
Plan Type: HMO, CDHP, HDHP, HSA,
Total Revenue: 2005: 2,360,879   2006: 1,828,306
Net Income   2005: -6,144   2006: 132,226
Total Enrollment:
   2001: 17,391   2004: 4,338   2007: 1,501
   2002: 0   2005: 2,474
   2003: 6,933   2006: 1,665

SERVICE AREA:
Nationwide: N
   TX;
TYPE OF COVERAGE:
Commercial: [Y] Individual: [ ] FEHBP: [ ] Indemnity: [ ]
Medicare: [ ] Medicaid: [ ] Supplemental Medicare: [ ]
Tricare [ ]
CONSUMER-DRIVEN PRODUCTS
Mellon HR Solutions LLC   HSA Company
                           HSA Product
                           HSA Administrator
                           Consumer-Driven Health Plan
                           High Deductible Health Plan

PLAN BENEFITS:
Alternative Medicine: [X]   Behavioral Health: [ ]
Chiropractic: [X]   Dental: [X]
Home Care: [X]   Inpatient SNF: [X]
Long-Term Care: [ ]   Pharm. Mail Order: [X]
Physical Therapy: [X]   Podiatry: [X]
Psychiatric: [X]   Transplant: [X]
Vision: [X]   Wellness: [X]
Workers' Comp: [ ]
Other Benefits:

HAS PREMIER PROVIDERS INC

100 Glenborough Dr Ste 450
Houston, TX 77067-3610
Phone: 281-873-8682 Fax: 281-872-5351 Toll-Free: 800-749-2714
Web site: www.hasonline.com
MAILING ADDRESS:
   HAS PREMIER PROVIDERS INC
   100 Glenborough Dr Ste 450
   Houston, TX 77067-3610

TEXAS   Managed Care Organization Profiles

KEY EXECUTIVES:
Chief Executive Officer .... Samuel R Willcoxon
President - Texas .... Eddie Parades
Director of Clinical Services .... Maryell VanAssendelft, RN
Director of Operations .... Deborah Manning

COMPANY PROFILE:
Parent Company Name: Fidelis SeniorCare Inc
Doing Business As:
Year Founded: 2006   Federally Qualified: [Y]
Forprofit: [ ]   Not-For-Profit: [ ]
Model Type:
Accreditation: [ ] AAPPO [ ] JACHO [ ] NCQA [ ] URAC
Plan Type:
Total Enrollment:
    2001: 0   2004: 0   2007: 346
    2002: 0   2005:
    2003: 0   2006: 342

SERVICE AREA:
Nationwide:
    TX (Bexar, Brazoria, Chambers, Collin, Dallas, Denton, Fort Bend, Galveston, Grimes, Harris, Johnson, Liberty, Montgomery, Rockwall, San Jacinto, Tarrant, Travis, Walker, Waller);

TYPE OF COVERAGE:
Commercial: [ ] Individual: [ ] FEHBP: [ ] Indemnity: [ ]
Medicare: [Y] Medicaid: [ ] Supplemental Medicare: [ ]
Tricare   [ ]

FORTE MANAGED CARE

7600 Chevy Chase Dr Ste 200
Austin, TX 78752
Phone: 512-371-8100 Fax: 800-580-3123 Toll-Free: 800-580-4567
Web site: www.fortereview.com

MAILING ADDRESS:
    FORTE MANAGED CARE
    7600 Chevy Chase Dr Ste 200
    Austin, TX 78752

KEY EXECUTIVES:
President .... Frank Vidrick
Medical Director .... Joel Wilk, MD
Chief Operating Officer .... Dan Moore
VP Sales & Marketing Forte .... Mundy Hebert
VP of Operations .... Claire Onks

COMPANY PROFILE:
Parent Company Name: Ron Luke Associates
Doing Business As: Forte Managed Care
Year Founded: 1986   Federally Qualified: [ ]
Forprofit: [Y]   Not-For-Profit: [ ]
Model Type:
Accreditation: [ ] AAPPO [ ] JACHO [ ] NCQA [X] URAC
Plan Type: PPO, EPO, UR

SERVICE AREA:
Nationwide: Y
    FL; TX;

TYPE OF COVERAGE:
Commercial: [Y] Individual: [ ] FEHBP: [ ] Indemnity: [ ]
Medicare: [ ] Medicaid: [ ] Supplemental Medicare: [ ]
Tricare   [ ]

PLAN BENEFITS:
Alternative Medicine: [ ]   Behavioral Health: [ ]
Chiropractic: [ ]   Dental: [ ]
Home Care: [ ]   Inpatient SNF: [ ]
Long-Term Care: [ ]   Pharm. Mail Order: [ ]
Physical Therapy: [ ]   Podiatry: [ ]
Psychiatric: [ ]   Transplant: [ ]
Vision: [ ]   Wellness: [ ]
Workers' Comp: [X]
Other Benefits:

Comments:
Formerly Forte-Compkey.

GALAXY HEALTH NETWORK

631 106th Street
Arlington, TX 76011
Phone: 817-633-5822 Fax: 817-633-5729 Toll-Free: 800-975-3322
Web site: www.galaxyhealth.net

MAILING ADDRESS:
    GALAXY HEALTH NETWORK
    PO Box 201425
    Arlington, TX 76011

KEY EXECUTIVES:
President .... Paul J Shane, Jr
Chief Financial Officer .... Dan Shadle
Marketing Director .... Stacy Hollinger
MIS Director .... Stephen Ferraro
Credentialing Manager .... Chris Guerue
Network/Contracts Officer .... Susdey Sud
Human Resource Manager .... Ann Smith
Credentialing Manager .... Chris Guerue
National Acct. Rep. .... Lisa Maddox

COMPANY PROFILE:
Parent Company Name: American Health Network
Doing Business As:
Year Founded: 1993   Federally Qualified: [ ]
Forprofit: [Y]   Not-For-Profit: [ ]
Model Type:
Accreditation: [X] AAPPO [ ] JACHO [ ] NCQA [X] URAC
Plan Type: PPO
Primary Physicians: 400,000   Physician Specialists: 215,959
Hospitals: 2,700
Total Enrollment:
    2001: 3,200,000   2004: 0   2007: 0
    2002: 4,000,000   2005:
    2003: 3,500,000   2006: 3,500,000

SERVICE AREA:
Nationwide: N
    AL; AR; AZ; CA; CO; FL; GA; IL; IN; KS; KY; LA; MA; MI; MO; NC; NJ; NM; NY; NV; OH; OK; OR; PA; SC; TN; TX; WA;

TYPE OF COVERAGE:
Commercial: [Y] Individual: [Y] FEHBP: [ ] Indemnity: [ ]
Medicare: [Y] Medicaid: [ ] Supplemental Medicare: [Y]
Tricare   [ ]

PRODUCTS OFFERED:
Product Name: Type:
Community Programs   PPO

PLAN BENEFITS:
Alternative Medicine: [ ]   Behavioral Health: [ ]
Chiropractic: [X]   Dental: [X]
Home Care: [X]   Inpatient SNF: [X]
Long-Term Care: [X]   Pharm. Mail Order: [X]
Physical Therapy: [X]   Podiatry: [X]
Psychiatric: [X]   Transplant: [X]
Vision: [X]   Wellness: [X]
Workers' Comp: [X]
Other Benefits:

GREAT-WEST HEALTHCARE OF TEXAS - AUSTIN

4807 Spicewood Sprngs B4 #200B
Austin, TX 78759-8591
Phone: 512-345-9565 Fax: 512-795-2105 Toll-Free:
Web site: www.greatwesthealthcare.com

MAILING ADDRESS:
    GREAT-WEST HEALTHCARE TX-AUSTIN
    4807 Spicewood Sprngs B4 #200B
    Austin, TX 78759-8591

KEY EXECUTIVES:
President .... Janice Fagan
Finance Director .... Julie Magill
Chief Medical Officer .... Allan Kogan, MD
Public Relations Director .... Mary Dean

COMPANY PROFILE:
Parent Company Name: Great West Life & Annuity Insurance Co
Doing Business As:
Year Founded: Federally Qualified: [ ]
Forprofit: [Y]   Not-For-Profit: [ ]
Model Type:
Accreditation: [ ] AAPPO [ ] JACHO [ ] NCQA [ ] URAC
Plan Type: HMO, PPO, POS, CDHP, HDHP, HSA,
Total Revenue: 2005: 1,444,623   2006: 1,613,318
Net Income   2005:   87,745   2006:   160,400
Total Enrollment:
    2001: 15,576   2004: 2,087   2007: 1,254
    2002: 0   2005: 1,760
    2003: 2,404   2006: 1,525

Managed Care Organization Profiles — TEXAS

ECCA - MANAGED VISION CARE INC - CORPORATE HEADQUARTERS

11103 West Ave
San Antonio, TX 78213
Phone: 210-340-3531 Fax: 210-524-6587 Toll-Free: 800-669-1183
Web site: www.ecca.com

MAILING ADDRESS:
ECCA - MANAGED VISION CARE INC
11103 West Ave
San Antonio, TX 78213

KEY EXECUTIVES:
Chief Executive Officer/President .... David Holmberg
VP Chief Financial Officer .... Jennifer Kelly
Medical Director .... Charles Cummins, MD
VP, Information Services .... Epsy Miller
Chief Operating Officer .... James J. Denny
Senior VP, ECCA Managed Vision Care Sales .... Mark Jolly
Provider Relations Manager .... Jamie Acosta
VP, Managed Care Operations .... Emily Rogers

COMPANY PROFILE:
Parent Company Name: Highmark Inc
Doing Business As: ECCA - Managed Vision Care Inc
Year Founded: 1995   Federally Qualified: [ ]
Forprofit: [ ]   Not-For-Profit: [ ]
Model Type: IPA
Accreditation: [ ] AAPPO [ ] JACHO [ ] NCQA [ ] URAC
Plan Type: Specialty PPO,

SERVICE AREA:
Nationwide: N
AL; AZ; FL; GA; IA; ID; IN; KY; KS; LA; MD; MN; MO; MS; NC; ND; NE; NH; NJ; MV; OH; OK; OR; SC; SD; TN; TX; UT; VA; WA; WI

TYPE OF COVERAGE:
Commercial: [Y] Individual: [ ] FEHBP: [ ] Indemnity: [ ]
Medicare: [Y] Medicaid: [Y] Supplemental Medicare: [ ]
Tricare   [ ]

PLAN BENEFITS:
Alternative Medicine: [ ]   Behavioral Health: [ ]
Chiropractic: [ ]   Dental: [ ]
Home Care: [ ]   Inpatient SNF: [ ]
Long-Term Care: [ ]   Pharm. Mail Order: [ ]
Physical Therapy: [ ]   Podiatry: [ ]
Psychiatric: [ ]   Transplant: [ ]
Vision: [X]   Wellness: [ ]
Workers' Comp: [ ]
Other Benefits:

EL PASO FIRST HEALTH PLANS INC

2501 N Mesa St
El Paso, TX 79902
Phone: 915-532-3778 Fax: 915-532-2877 Toll-Free: 877-532-3778
Web site: www.epfirst.com

MAILING ADDRESS:
EL PASO FIRST HEALTH PLANS INC
2501 N Mesa St
El Paso, TX 79902

KEY EXECUTIVES:
Board Chairman .... James S DeGroat
Interim Chief Executive Officer .... Norberto Correa
Chief Financial Officer .... Brian Kieser
Medical Director .... John F Tures, MD
Chief Operating Officer .... Norberto Correa
Director of Marketing & Sales .... Soledad Basoco
IT Manager .... Sharon Perkins
Credentialing Coordinator .... Kathy Brown
Privacy & Security Officer .... Delores Smith-Clem
Public Relations Director .... Soledad Basoco
Provider Relations Director .... Jeff Sterling
Health Promotion Director .... Sandra Amaya
Human Resources Director .... Gilbert Blancas
Quality Improvement Manager .... Veronique Carrillo
Credentialing Coordinator .... Kathy Brown
Director of Compliance .... Delores Smith-Clem
Member Services Manager .... Sandra Amaya
Finance Manager .... Angela Truett
Claims Manager .... Mary Dominguez
Director of Government Programs & Reports ...... Mitchel Newberry

COMPANY PROFILE:
Parent Company Name:
Doing Business As:
Year Founded: 2000   Federally Qualified: [ ]
Forprofit: [ ]   Not-For-Profit: [Y]
Model Type: MIXED
Accreditation: [ ] AAPPO [ ] JACHO [ ] NCQA [ ] URAC
Plan Type: HMO
Total Revenue: 2005: 71,670,720   2006: 80,743,440
Net Income   2005:   64,707   2006: -1,558,534
Total Enrollment:
    2001: 26,981   2004: 41,554   2007: 51,101
    2002: 32,696   2005: 45,508
    2003: 38,479   2006: 51,072

SERVICE AREA:
Nationwide: N
TX;

TYPE OF COVERAGE:
Commercial: [Y] Individual: [ ] FEHBP: [ ] Indemnity: [ ]
Medicare: [ ] Medicaid: [Y] Supplemental Medicare: [ ]
Tricare   [ ]

EVERCARE OF TEXAS LLC

9700 Bissonnet Ste 2225
Houston, TX 77036
Phone: 713-778-8684 Fax: 713-778-8798 Toll-Free: 800-393-0993
Web site: www.evercareonline.com

MAILING ADDRESS:
EVERCARE OF TEXAS LLC
PO Box 4377
Houston, TX 77036

KEY EXECUTIVES:
Chief Executive Officer/President .... John R Mach Jr, MD
Medical Director .... Frederick Buckwold, MD
Chief Operating Officer .... Sheila E McMillan
VP Public Relations .... Peter Ashkenaz
Executive Director Evercare of Texas ...... Diane Schimmelbusch

COMPANY PROFILE:
Parent Company Name:
Doing Business As:
Year Founded: 2001   Federally Qualified: [N]
Forprofit: [ ]   Not-For-Profit: [ ]
Model Type:
Accreditation: [ ] AAPPO [ ] JACHO [X] NCQA [ ] URAC
Plan Type: HMO,
Primary Physicians: Physician Specialists:
Hospitals:
Total Revenue: 2005: 239,042,763   2006: 383,447,576
Net Income   2005: 15,208,343   2006: 32,598,333
Total Enrollment:
    2001:   0   2004: 33,782   2007: 93,357
    2002: 87,058   2005: 36,304
    2003: 31,701   2006: 62,864

SERVICE AREA:
Nationwide:
TX (Harris);

TYPE OF COVERAGE:
Commercial: [ ] Individual: [ ] FEHBP: [ ] Indemnity: [ ]
Medicare: [Y] Medicaid: [Y] Supplemental Medicare: [ ]
Tricare   [ ]

PRODUCTS OFFERED:
Product Name: Type:
Evercare of Texas   Medicare
Evercare of Texas   Medicaid

FIDELIS SECURECARE OF TEXAS

17625 El Camino Real Ste 210
Houston, TX 77058
Phone: 877-372-8901 Fax: 866-511-5906 Toll-Free:
Web site: www.fidelissc.com

MAILING ADDRESS:
FIDELIS SECURECARE OF TX
17625 El Camino Real Ste 210
Houston, TX 77058

TEXAS

CORPHEALTH INC

1300 Summit Ste 600
Fort Worth, TX 76102
Phone: 817-332-2519 Fax: 817-335-9100 Toll-Free: 800-383-2327
Web site: www.corphealth.com

MAILING ADDRESS:
    CORPHEALTH INC
    1300 Summit Ste 600
    Fort Worth, TX 76102

KEY EXECUTIVES:
Chief Executive Officer/President .... Patrick D Gotcher
Chief Financial Officer .... Michael G Baker
Chief Medical Officer .... Ken Hopper, MD
Chief Information Officer .... Jodie Creamer
Chief Operating Officer .... Brae D Jacobson, MA, LPC
Chief Business Development Officer .... Paul J Floyd
Credentialing Manager .... Rhesa Gray
Director of Compliance .... Hayley Ellington
VP, Human Resources .... C Shane Wilbanks
VP, Quality Improvement .... Melissa Hamilton
Credentialing Manager .... Rhesa Gray
VP, Account Srv/Implementation .... Anita L Poole
Director of Operations .... Janae Taliafenno
Chief Strategic Development Officer .... David L Redfield
VP, Arkansas Operation .... Sharon Marcum

COMPANY PROFILE:
Parent Company Name:
Doing Business As:
Year Founded: 1987   Federally Qualified: [N]
Forprofit: [Y]   Not-For-Profit: [ ]
Model Type: NETWORK
Accreditation: [ ] AAPPO [ ] JACHO [ ] NCQA [X] URAC
Plan Type: Specialty HMO, Specialty PPO, TPA, UR
Total Enrollment:
  2001: 1,300,000   2004: 0   2007: 0
  2002: 0   2005:
  2003: 0   2006:

SERVICE AREA:
Nationwide: Y
  NW;

TYPE OF COVERAGE:
Commercial: [Y] Individual: [ ] FEHBP: [ ] Indemnity: [ ]
Medicare: [Y] Medicaid: [Y] Supplemental Medicare: [ ]
Tricare [ ]

PRODUCTS OFFERED:
Product Name:	Type:
PsychCap	PPO
PsychCap	Indemnity
PsychCap	HMO
Corphealth	ASO

PLAN BENEFITS:
Alternative Medicine:	[ ]	Behavioral Health:	[X]
Chiropractic:	[ ]	Dental:	[ ]
Home Care:	[ ]	Inpatient SNF:	[ ]
Long-Term Care:	[ ]	Pharm. Mail Order:	[ ]
Physical Therapy:	[ ]	Podiatry:	[ ]
Psychiatric:	[ ]	Transplant:	[ ]
Vision:	[ ]	Wellness:	[ ]
Workers' Comp:	[ ]		
Other Benefits:			

DELTA DENTAL INSURANCE COMPANY - TEXAS

1431 Greenway Dr Ste 520
Irving, TX 75038
Phone: 972-580-1616 Fax: 972-580-1333 Toll-Free: 800-775-0523
Web site: www.deltadental.com

MAILING ADDRESS:
    DELTA DENTAL INSURANCE CO - TX
    1431 Greenway Dr Ste 520
    Irving, TX 75038

KEY EXECUTIVES:
Chief Executive Officer .... Robert B Elliott

COMPANY PROFILE:
Parent Company Name: Delta Dental Plan Association
Doing Business As:
Year Founded: Federally Qualified: [ ]
Forprofit: [ ]   Not-For-Profit: [ ] Model Type:
Accreditation: [ ] AAPPO [ ] JACHO [ ] NCQA [ ] URAC
Plan Type: Specialty HMO, Specialty PPO
Total Enrollment:
  2001: 0   2004: 119,208   2007: 0
  2002: 0   2005:
  2003: 119,993   2006:

SERVICE AREA:
Nationwide: N
  TX;

TYPE OF COVERAGE:
Commercial: [Y] Individual: [ ] FEHBP: [ ] Indemnity: [ ]
Medicare: [ ] Medicaid: [ ] Supplemental Medicare: [ ]
Tricare [ ]

PLAN BENEFITS:
Alternative Medicine:	[ ]	Behavioral Health:	[ ]
Chiropractic:	[ ]	Dental:	[X]
Home Care:	[ ]	Inpatient SNF:	[ ]
Long-Term Care:	[ ]	Pharm. Mail Order:	[ ]
Physical Therapy:	[ ]	Podiatry:	[ ]
Psychiatric:	[ ]	Transplant:	[ ]
Vision:	[ ]	Wellness:	[ ]
Workers' Comp:	[ ]		
Other Benefits:			

DRISCOLL CHILDREN'S HEALTH PLAN

615 N Upper Broadway, Ste 1621
Corpus Christi, TX 78477
Phone: 361-694-6781 Fax: 361-881-1349 Toll-Free:
Web site: www.dchpkids.com

MAILING ADDRESS:
    DRISCOLL CHILDREN'S HEALTH
    PO BOX 6609
    Corpus Christi, TX 78477

KEY EXECUTIVES:
Chief Executive Officer/President .... Mary Dale Peterson, MD
Medical Director .... Ernest Buck, MD
Chief Operating Officer .... Charles Carroll
Executive Director, Quality Assurance .... Judy Kraft RN, MSN

COMPANY PROFILE:
Parent Company Name: Driscoll Children's Hospital
Doing Business As: Driscoll Children's Health Plan
Year Founded: 1997   Federally Qualified: [ ]
Forprofit: [ ]   Not-For-Profit: [Y]
Model Type: MIXED
Accreditation: [ ] AAPPO [ ] JACHO [ ] NCQA [ ] URAC
Plan Type: HMO
Primary Physicians: 500   Physician Specialists: 230
Hospitals: 18
Total Revenue: 2005: 10,215,652   2006: 33,816,992
Net Income 2005: -464,931   2006: -6,780,245
Total Enrollment:
  2001: 18,876   2004: 11,470   2007: 43,877
  2002: 19,245   2005: 10,660
  2003: 16,092   2006: 43,878

SERVICE AREA:
Nationwide: N
  TX (Aransas, Bee, Brooks, Calhoun, Duval, Goliad, Jim Wells, Karnes, Kenedy, Kleberg, Live Oak, Nueces, Refugio, San Patricio, Victoria);

TYPE OF COVERAGE:
Commercial: [ ] Individual: [ ] FEHBP: [ ] Indemnity: [ ]
Medicare: [ ] Medicaid: [Y] Supplemental Medicare: [ ]
Tricare [ ]

PRODUCTS OFFERED:
Product Name:	Type:
CHIP	HMO

PLAN BENEFITS:
Alternative Medicine:	[ ]	Behavioral Health:	[ ]
Chiropractic:	[X]	Dental:	[ ]
Home Care:	[X]	Inpatient SNF:	[ ]
Long-Term Care:	[ ]	Pharm. Mail Order:	[ ]
Physical Therapy:	[ ]	Podiatry:	[ ]
Psychiatric:	[X]	Transplant:	[X]
Vision:	[X]	Wellness:	[ ]
Workers' Comp:	[ ]		
Other Benefits:			

Managed Care Organization Profiles — TEXAS

MAILING ADDRESS:
 COMPBENEFITS - DENTICARE INC
 2929 Briar Park Ste 314
 Houston, TX 77042

KEY EXECUTIVES:
Chief Executive Officer/President .... *Kirk E Rothrock*
Chief Financial Officer .... *George Dunaway*
National Dental Director .... *Kenneth J Hammer, DDS, MBA*
Senior VP, Operations .... *Mary Kay Gilbert*
Senior VP, Marketing .... *John E. Lumkins*
Executive VP, Sales .... *Steven K Isaacs, LLIF*
Executive VP, General Counsel .... *Bruce Mitchell*
President-Vision Division .... *Howard J Braverman, OD*
Executive VP, Chief Actuary .... *Alan Stewart*

COMPANY PROFILE:
Parent Company Name: CompDent, GA, CompBenefits Corporation
Doing Business As: Denticare Inc
Year Founded: 1988   Federally Qualified: [ ]
Forprofit: [Y]   Not-For-Profit: [ ]
Model Type:
Accreditation: [ ] AAPPO [ ] JACHO [ ] NCQA [ ] URAC
Plan Type: Specialty HMO
Total Revenue: 2005: 12,109,146   2006:
Net Income   2005:   946,720   2006:
Total Enrollment:
 2001: 144,534   2004: 123,520   2007: 113,491
 2002: 129,867   2005: 120,351
 2003: 119,993   2006:   2,088

SERVICE AREA:
Nationwide: N
 TX; (Anderson, Andrews, Angelina, Aransas, Archer, Armstrong, Atascosa, Austin, Bailey, Bandera, Bastrop, Baylor, Bee, Bell, Bexar, Blanco, Borden, Bosque, Bowie, Brazoria, Brazos, Brewster, Briscoe, Brooks, Brown, Burleson, Burnet, Caldwell, Calhoun, Callahan, Cameron, Camp, Carson, Cass, Castro, Chambers, Cherokee, Childress, Clay, Cochran, Coke, Coleman, Collin, Collingsworth, Colorado, Comal, Comanche, Concho, Cooke, Coryell, Cottle, Crane, Crockett, Crosby, Culberson, Dallam, Dallas, Dawson, DeWitt, Deaf, Smith, Delta, Denton, Dickens, Dimmit, Donley, Duval, Eastland, Ector, Edwards, El Paso, Ellis, Erath, Falls, Fannin, Fayette, Fisher, Floyd, Foard, Fort Bend, Franklin, Freestone, Frio, Gaines, Galveston, Garza, Gillespie, Glasscock, Goliad, Gonzales, Gray, Grayson, Gregg, Grimes, Guadalupe, Hale, Hall, Hamilton, Hansford, Hardeman, Hardin, Harris, Harrison, Hartley, Haskell, Hays, Hemphill, Henderson, Hidalgo, Hill, Hockley, Hood, Hopkins, Houston, Howard, Hudspeth, Hunt, Hutchinson, Irion, Jack, Jackson, Jasper, Jeff, Davis, Jefferson, Jim, Hogg, Jim, Wells, Johnson, Jones, Karnes, Kaufman Lee, Kendall, Kenedy, Kent, Kerr, Kimble, King, Kinney, Kleberg, Knox, LaSalle, Lamar, Lamb, Lampasas, Lavaca, Lee, Leon, Liberty, Limestone, Lipscomb, Live Oak, Llano, Loving, Lubbock, Lynn, Madison, Marion, Martin);

TYPE OF COVERAGE:
Commercial: [Y] Individual: [Y] FEHBP: [ ] Indemnity: [ ]
Medicare: [ ] Medicaid: [ ] Supplemental Medicare: [ ]
Tricare   [ ]

PRODUCTS OFFERED:
Product Name: Type:
Dental HMO   Specialty HMO

PLAN BENEFITS:
Alternative Medicine: [ ]   Behavioral Health: [ ]
Chiropractic: [ ]   Dental: [X]
Home Care: [ ]   Inpatient SNF: [ ]
Long-Term Care: [ ]   Pharm. Mail Order: [ ]
Physical Therapy: [ ]   Podiatry: [ ]
Psychiatric: [ ]   Transplant: [ ]
Vision: [ ]   Wellness: [ ]
Workers' Comp: [ ]
Other Benefits:

Comments:
Formerly called Denticare Inc.

CONCENTRA OPERATING CORPORATION

5080 Spectrum Dr Ste 1200 W
Addison, TX 75001
Phone: 972-364-8000 Fax: 972-387-0941 Toll-Free: 800-232-3550
Web site: www.concentra.com

MAILING ADDRESS:
 CONCENTRA OPERATING CORP
 5080 Spectrum Dr Ste 1200 W
 Addison, TX 75001

KEY EXECUTIVES:
Chief Executive Officer .... *Jim Greenwood*
President/Chief Operating Officer .... *W Keith Newton*
Chief Financial Officer .... *Thomas E Kiraly*
Chief Medical Officer .... *W Thomas Fogerty, MD*
Chief Information Officer .... *Suzanne C Sienik*
Chief Marketing Officer .... *Andrew R Daniels*
Director of Marketing/Communication .... *Vicki Bryant*

COMPANY PROFILE:
Parent Company Name: Concentra Inc
Doing Business As: Beech Street
Year Founded: 1987   Federally Qualified: [ ]
Forprofit: [Y]   Not-For-Profit: [ ]
Model Type:
Accreditation: [ ] AAPPO [ ] JACHO [ ] NCQA [ ] URAC
Plan Type: PPO, UR
Total Revenue: 2005:1,155,069,000   2006:
Net Income   2005:   53,801,000   2006:

SERVICE AREA:
Nationwide: N
 TX;

Comments:
MHB was acquired in October 1997 by Prompt Associates of Salt Lake City, Utah.

COOKS CHILDRENS HEALTH PLAN

801 Seventh Ave
Fort Worth, TX 76104-2796
Phone: 682-885-2247 Fax: 682-885-2148 Toll-Free: 800-964-2247
Web site: www.cookchp.org

MAILING ADDRESS:
 COOKS CHILDRENS HEALTH PLAN
 801 Seventh Ave
 Fort Worth, TX 76104-2796

KEY EXECUTIVES:
Board Chairman .... *Robert Mann, MD*
President .... *John Grigson*
VP, Finance .... *Doris Hunt*
Medical Director .... *Gregory Preston, MD*
Manager Network Development .... *Rob Robidon*
Director Care Management .... *Sandra Flinn, RN*
Director, Credentialing .... *Karen Baker*

COMPANY PROFILE:
Parent Company Name: Cooks Children's Health Care System
Doing Business As: Cooks Children's Health Plan
Year Founded: 1999   Federally Qualified: [N]
Forprofit: [ ]   Not-For-Profit: [Y]
Model Type: IPA/NETWRK
Accreditation: [ ] AAPPO [ ] JACHO [ ] NCQA [ ] URAC
Plan Type: HMO,
Total Revenue: 2005: 28,196,603   2006: 34,507,898
Net Income   2005:   -634,023   2006:   -289,282
Total Enrollment:
 2001: 40,266   2004: 28,464   2007: 41,019
 2002: 38,312   2005: 28,231
 2003: 35,790   2006: 39,508

SERVICE AREA:
Nationwide: N
 TX (Denton, Hood, Johnson, Parker, Tarrant, Wise)

TYPE OF COVERAGE:
Commercial: [ ] Individual: [ ] FEHBP: [ ] Indemnity: [ ]
Medicare: [ ] Medicaid: [Y] Supplemental Medicare: [ ]
Tricare   [ ]

PRODUCTS OFFERED:
Product Name: Type:
CHIP   HMO

PLAN BENEFITS:
Alternative Medicine: [X]   Behavioral Health: [ ]
Chiropractic: [X]   Dental: [ ]
Home Care: [X]   Inpatient SNF: [ ]
Long-Term Care: [X]   Pharm. Mail Order: [ ]
Physical Therapy: [ ]   Podiatry: [X]
Psychiatric: [X]   Transplant: [X]
Vision: [X]   Wellness: [X]
Workers' Comp: [ ]
Other Benefits:

TEXAS

Accreditation: [ ] AAPPO [ ] JACHO [ ] NCQA [ ] URAC
Plan Type: HMO, PPO, CDHP, HDHP, HSA, FSA, HRA,
Total Revenue: 2005: 98,001,958 2006: 221,056,716
Net Income 2005: 10,327,318 2006: 3,753,890
Total Enrollment:
   2001: 323,530   2004: 73,030   2007: 58,290
   2002: 202,537   2005: 66,554
   2003: 141,037   2006: 62,698

SERVICE AREA:
Nationwide: N
   TX (East Texas, Houston);

TYPE OF COVERAGE:
Commercial: [Y] Individual: [ ] FEHBP: [ ] Indemnity: [ ]
Medicare: [ ] Medicaid: [ ] Supplemental Medicare: [ ]
Tricare [ ]

PRODUCTS OFFERED:
Product Name:	Type:
Cigna Healthcare for Seniors	Medicare

CONSUMER-DRIVEN PRODUCTS
JP Morgan Chase	HSA Company
CIGNA Choice Fund	HSA Product
	HSA Administrator
Open Access Plus	Consumer-Driven Health Plan
PPO	High Deductible Health Plan

PLAN BENEFITS:
Alternative Medicine:	[X]	Behavioral Health:	[X]
Chiropractic:	[X]	Dental:	[X]
Home Care:	[X]	Inpatient SNF:	[X]
Long-Term Care:	[X]	Pharm. Mail Order:	[X]
Physical Therapy:	[X]	Podiatry:	[X]
Psychiatric:	[X]	Transplant:	[X]
Vision:	[X]	Wellness:	[X]
Workers' Comp:	[X]		
Other Benefits:			

COMMUNITY FIRST HEALTH PLANS INC

4801 NW Loop 410 Ste 1000
San Antonio, TX 78229
Phone: 210-227-2347 Fax: 210-358-6039 Toll-Free: 800-434-2347
Web site: www.cfhp.com

MAILING ADDRESS:
   COMMUNITY FIRST HEALTH PLANS
   4801 NW Loop 410 Ste 1000
   San Antonio, TX 78229

KEY EXECUTIVES:
Chief Executive Officer/President .... Charles L Kight
VP, Chief Financial Officer .... Tony LoBasso
Medical Director .... Mary Watson, MD
Pharmacist .... Maria Gonzalez
Information Systems Director .... Stephen T Bishop
VP, Operations .... Eileen Weigum
VP, Sales & Marketing .... Russell P Gantos Jr
Information Systems Director .... Stephen T Bishop
Public Relations Director .... Karen Glenney
Network Operations .... Martin Jimenez
Health Promotion/Prevention .... Susan Lomba
VP, Health Services Management .... Susan Dickerson
Quality Management Director .... Lisa Crow
Compliance Regultry Affairs Director .... Charles Cliett
Case Management Director .... Joan Trimble
Quality Assurance Nurse .... Karen Wiatrek
Member Services Director .... Mary Helen Gonzalez
Claims Director .... Eileen Weigum

COMPANY PROFILE:
Parent Company Name: Bexar County Hospital District
Doing Business As:
Year Founded: 1995   Federally Qualified: [N]
Forprofit: [ ]   Not-For-Profit: [Y] Model Type: MIXED
Accreditation: [ ] AAPPO [ ] JACHO [ ] NCQA [ ] URAC
Plan Type: HMO, EPO
Total Revenue: 2005: 127,953,231 2006: 153,578,584
Net Income 2005: 5,633,860 2006: -1,692,876
Total Enrollment:
   2001: 81,123   2004: 82,248   2007: 94,296
   2002: 97,606   2005: 77,265
   2003: 85,549   2006: 96,146

SERVICE AREA:
Nationwide: N
   TX (Atascosa, Bandera, Bexar, Comal, Guadalupe, Kendall, Kerr, Medina, Wilson);

TYPE OF COVERAGE:
Commercial: [Y] Individual: [ ] FEHBP: [ ] Indemnity: [ ]
Medicare: [ ] Medicaid: [Y] Supplemental Medicare: [ ]
Tricare [ ]

PRODUCTS OFFERED:
Product Name:	Type:
Community First HMO	HMO
Community First Medicaid	Medicaid

PLAN BENEFITS:
Alternative Medicine:	[ ]	Behavioral Health:	[ ]
Chiropractic:	[ ]	Dental:	[X]
Home Care:	[X]	Inpatient SNF:	[X]
Long-Term Care:	[ ]	Pharm. Mail Order:	[X]
Physical Therapy:	[X]	Podiatry:	[X]
Psychiatric:	[X]	Transplant:	[X]
Vision:	[X]	Wellness:	[X]
Workers' Comp:	[ ]		
Other Benefits:			

COMMUNITY HEALTH CHOICE INC

2636 S Loop West Ste 700
Houston, TX 77054
Phone: 713-746-6994 Fax: 713-566-4365 Toll-Free:
Web site: www.communityhealthchoice.org

MAILING ADDRESS:
   COMMUNITY HEALTH CHOICE INC
   2636 S Loop West Ste 700
   Houston, TX 77054

KEY EXECUTIVES:
Chairman of the Board .... Charles A Moore
Chief Executive Officer/President .... Glen R Johnson
VP, Finance .... Paul Tannos, CPA
Medical Director .... Dr Alcorn
VP, Operations .... Kim Nettleton

COMPANY PROFILE:
Parent Company Name: Harris County Hospital District
Doing Business As:
Year Founded: 1996   Federally Qualified: [N]
Forprofit: [ ]   Not-For-Profit: [Y]
Model Type: NETWORK
Accreditation: [ ] AAPPO [ ] JACHO [ ] NCQA [ ] URAC
Plan Type: HMO,
Total Revenue: 2005: 113,466,046 2006: 180,555,320
Net Income 2005: 7,601,249 2006: 7,203,697
Total Enrollment:
   2001: 11,003   2004: 46,694   2007: 109,655
   2002: 33,364   2005: 53,452
   2003: 46,810   2006: 83,768

SERVICE AREA:
Nationwide: N
   TX (Brazoria, Chambers, Fort Bend, Galveston, Harris, Liberty, Montgomery, Waller);

TYPE OF COVERAGE:
Commercial: [Y] Individual: [ ] FEHBP: [ ] Indemnity: [ ]
Medicare: [ ] Medicaid: [ ] Supplemental Medicare: [ ]
Tricare [ ]

PRODUCTS OFFERED:
Product Name:	Type:
Community Health Choice	Medicaid

PLAN BENEFITS:
Alternative Medicine:	[ ]	Behavioral Health:	[X]
Chiropractic:	[X]	Dental:	[X]
Home Care:	[X]	Inpatient SNF:	[X]
Long-Term Care:	[X]	Pharm. Mail Order:	[X]
Physical Therapy:	[X]	Podiatry:	[X]
Psychiatric:	[X]	Transplant:	[X]
Vision:	[X]	Wellness:	[X]
Workers' Comp:	[ ]		
Other Benefits:			

Comments:
Formerly Total Community Healthplan Inc.

COMPBENEFITS - DENTICARE INC

2929 Briar Park Ste 314
Houston, TX 77042
Phone: 713-784-7011 Fax: 713-784-9440 Toll-Free: 800-679-7883
Web site: www.compdent.com

Managed Care Organization Profiles TEXAS

TYPE OF COVERAGE:
Commercial: [Y] Individual: [ ] FEHBP: [ ] Indemnity: [ ]
Medicare: [Y] Medicaid: [ ] Supplemental Medicare: [Y]
Tricare [ ]
PRODUCTS OFFERED:
Product Name: Type:
Employee Assistance Programs
Managed Mental Health
PLAN BENEFITS:
Alternative Medicine: [ ]   Behavioral Health: [X]
Chiropractic: [ ]   Dental: [ ]
Home Care: [ ]   Inpatient SNF: [ ]
Long-Term Care: [ ]   Pharm. Mail Order: [ ]
Physical Therapy: [ ]   Podiatry: [ ]
Psychiatric: [X]   Transplant: [ ]
Vision: [ ]   Wellness: [X]
Workers' Comp: [ ]
Other Benefits:
Comments:
Formerly MCC Managed Behavioral Care Inc.

CIGNA DENTAL HEALTH OF TEXAS INC

6600 E Campus Circle Dr #400
Irving, TX 75063
Phone: 972-582-7201 Fax: 972-582-7201 Toll-Free: 800-367-1037
Web site: www.cigna.com/dental
MAILING ADDRESS:
   CIGNA DENTAL HEALTH OF TX INC
   6600 E Campus Circle Dr #400
   Irving, TX 75063

KEY EXECUTIVES:
President .... Karen S Rohan
Chief Financial Officer .... Michelle I Haas
Vice President .... John P Frey

COMPANY PROFILE:
Parent Company Name: CIGNA Dental Health Inc
Doing Business As: CIGNA Dental Health
Year Founded: 1987   Federally Qualified: [N]
Forprofit: [Y]   Not-For-Profit: [ ]
Model Type:
Accreditation: [ ] AAPPO [ ] JACHO [X] NCQA [ ] URAC
Plan Type: Specialty HMO
Total Revenue: 2005: 40,373,075   2006: 38,817,128
Net Income   2005:   6,955,404   2006:
Total Enrollment:
   2001: 344,824   2004: 274,695   2007: 236,163
   2002: 328,963   2005: 258,910
   2003: 306,537   2006: 232,779
SERVICE AREA:
Nationwide: N
   TX;
TYPE OF COVERAGE:
Commercial: [Y] Individual: [ ] FEHBP: [ ] Indemnity: [ ]
Medicare: [ ] Medicaid: [ ] Supplemental Medicare: [ ]
Tricare [ ]
PRODUCTS OFFERED:
Product Name: Type:
CIGNA Dental HMO   Specialty HMO
PLAN BENEFITS:
Alternative Medicine: [ ]   Behavioral Health: [ ]
Chiropractic: [ ]   Dental: [X]
Home Care: [ ]   Inpatient SNF: [ ]
Long-Term Care: [ ]   Pharm. Mail Order: [ ]
Physical Therapy: [ ]   Podiatry: [ ]
Psychiatric: [ ]   Transplant: [ ]
Vision: [ ]   Wellness: [ ]
Workers' Comp: [ ]
Other Benefits:

CIGNA HEALTHCARE OF NORTH TEXAS

6600 E Campus Circle Dr #400
Irving, TX 75063
Phone: 972-582-7200 Fax: 972-582-7618 Toll-Free: 800-772-4462
Web site: www.cigna.com

MAILING ADDRESS:
   CIGNA HEALTHCARE OF NORTH TX
   6600 E Campus Circle Dr #400
   Irving, TX 75063

KEY EXECUTIVES:
President-Texas .... David Toomey
Medical Director .... Kenneth J Phenow, MD, MPH
Director of Marketing .... Kelly Metzdorf
VP Sales, N Texas & OK .... Jason Motter

COMPANY PROFILE:
Parent Company Name: CIGNA Corporation
Doing Business As:
Year Founded: 1980   Federally Qualified: [ ]
Forprofit: [Y]   Not-For-Profit: [ ]
Model Type:
Accreditation: [ ] AAPPO [ ] JACHO [ ] NCQA [ ] URAC
Plan Type: HMO, PPO, CDHP, HSA, FSA, HRA
Total Revenue: 2005: 226,377,608   2006:
Net Income   2005:   6,253,409   2006:   5,090,834
Total Enrollment:
   2001: 0   2004: 74,350   2007: 0
   2002: 0   2005: 35,664
   2003: 0   2006: 63,160
SERVICE AREA:
Nationwide: N
   TX (Austin, Brazoria, Chambers, Collin, Dallas, Denton, Ellis,
   Fannin, Fort Bend, Galveston, Grayson, Grimes, Hardin, Harris,
   Hood, Hunt, Jasper, Jefferson, Johnson, Kaufman, Liberty,
   Matagorda, Montgomery, Orange, Parker, Rockwall, San Jacinto,
   Tarrant, Walker, Waller, Wharton, Wise);
TYPE OF COVERAGE:
Commercial: [Y] Individual: [ ] FEHBP: [ ] Indemnity: [ ]
Medicare: [ ] Medicaid: [ ] Supplemental Medicare: [ ]
Tricare [ ]
PRODUCTS OFFERED:
Product Name: Type:
Cigna Hlthcare for Seniors   Medicare
CONSUMER-DRIVEN PRODUCTS
JP Morgan Chase   HSA Company
CIGNA Choice Fund   HSA Product
                                 HSA Administrator
Open Access Plus   Consumer-Driven Health Plan
PPO   High Deductible Health Plan
PLAN BENEFITS:
Alternative Medicine: [ ]   Behavioral Health: [X]
Chiropractic: [X]   Dental: [X]
Home Care: [X]   Inpatient SNF: [X]
Long-Term Care: [X]   Pharm. Mail Order: [X]
Physical Therapy: [X]   Podiatry: [X]
Psychiatric: [X]   Transplant: [X]
Vision: [X]   Wellness: [X]
Workers' Comp: [X]
Other Benefits:

CIGNA HEALTHCARE OF TEXAS INC

2 River Way Ste 1200
Houston, TX 77056
Phone: 713-552-7600 Fax: 866-530-3585 Toll-Free: 800-772-4462
Web site: www.cigna.com
MAILING ADDRESS:
   CIGNA HEALTHCARE OF TX INC
   2 River Way Ste 1200
   Houston, TX 77056

KEY EXECUTIVES:
Chief Executive Officer .... H Edward Hanway
President -Cigna Healthcare .... David M. Cordani
Chief Financial Officer .... Michael Bell
Chief Information Officer .... Andrea Anania
Senior VP, Marketing .... James Lyski
Executive VP, Human Resources .... John Murabito
Chief Clinical Officer .... W Allen Schaffer, MD

COMPANY PROFILE:
Parent Company Name: CIGNA Corporation
Doing Business As:
Year Founded: 1980   Federally Qualified: [ ]
Forprofit: [Y]   Not-For-Profit: [ ]
Model Type: MIXED

TEXAS

BRAZOS VALLEY HEALTH NETWORK

7524 Bosque Blvd Ste L
Waco, TX 76712
Phone: 254-202-5320 Fax: 254-202-5310 Toll-Free:
Web site: www.hillcrest.net
MAILING ADDRESS:
    BRAZOS VALLEY HEALTH NETWORK
    7524 Bosque Blvd Ste L
    Waco, TX 76712

KEY EXECUTIVES:
Chief Medical Officer .... James Gray, MD
Chief Operating Officer/Director Provider Services . Christopher Green

COMPANY PROFILE:
Parent Company Name: Hillcrest Baptist Medical Center
Doing Business As: Brazos Valley Health Network
Year Founded: 1992   Federally Qualified: [ ]
Forprofit: [ ]   Not-For-Profit: [Y]
Model Type:
Accreditation: [ ] AAPPO [ ] JACHO [ ] NCQA [ ] URAC
Plan Type: PPO
Primary Physicians: 305   Physician Specialists: 209
Hospitals: 10
Total Enrollment:
   2001: 0   2004: 65,500   2007: 0
   2002: 0   2005: 65,300
   2003: 0   2006:
SERVICE AREA:
Nationwide: N
   TX (Central);
TYPE OF COVERAGE:
Commercial: [Y] Individual: [Y] FEHBP: [ ] Indemnity: [ ]
Medicare: [ ] Medicaid: [ ] Supplemental Medicare: [Y]
Tricare [ ]
PRODUCTS OFFERED:
Product Name: Type:
Brazos Valley Health Network   PPO
PLAN BENEFITS:
Alternative Medicine: [ ]   Behavioral Health: [ ]
Chiropractic: [ ]   Dental: [ ]
Home Care: [X]   Inpatient SNF: [ ]
Long-Term Care: [ ]   Pharm. Mail Order: [X]
Physicial Therapy: [ ]   Podiatry: [X]
Psychiatric: [X]   Transplant: [ ]
Vision: [X]   Wellness: [X]
Workers' Comp: [X]
Other Benefits:

CAREINGTON INTERNATIONAL - THE DENTAL NETWORK

7400 Gaylord Pkwy
Frisco, TX 75034
Phone: 972-335-6970 Fax: 800-247-4450 Toll-Free: 800-441-0380
Web site: www.careington.com
MAILING ADDRESS:
    CAREINGTON INTL THE DENTAL NTW
    PO Box 2568
    Frisco, TX 75034

KEY EXECUTIVES:
Chief Executive Officer/President .... Barbara Williams
Chief Financial Officer .... Melissa Burke
Dental Director .... Edie Kendall, DDS
Director, Call Center .... Jeremy Hendrick
Chief Operating Officer .... Tracy Berwick
VP, Sales, Marketing Manager .... Stewart Sweda

COMPANY PROFILE:
Parent Company Name:
Doing Business As:
Year Founded: 1979   Federally Qualified: [ ]
Forprofit: [ ]   Not-For-Profit: [ ]
Model Type:
Accreditation: [ ] AAPPO [ ] JACHO [ ] NCQA [ ] URAC
Plan Type: Specialty PPO
SERVICE AREA:
Nationwide: N
   TX;

PLAN BENEFITS:
Alternative Medicine: [ ]   Behavioral Health: [ ]
Chiropractic: [ ]   Dental: [X]
Home Care: [ ]   Inpatient SNF: [ ]
Long-Term Care: [ ]   Pharm. Mail Order: [ ]
Physical Therapy: [ ]   Podiatry: [ ]
Psychiatric: [ ]   Transplant: [ ]
Vision: [ ]   Wellness: [ ]
Workers' Comp: [ ]
Other Benefits:
Comments:
CAREington is a privately held discount healthcare company. They offer innovative programs to compliment traditional health insurance and provide substantial savings for under and uninsured individuals.

CBCA CARE MANAGEMENT INC

5001 LBJ Freeway Ste 175
Dallas, TX 75244
Phone: 972-385-9300 Fax: 972-385-8028 Toll-Free: 800-824-3882
Web site: www.cbca.com
MAILING ADDRESS:
    CBCA CARE MANAGEMENT INC
    5001 LBJ Freeway Ste 175
    Dallas, TX 75244

KEY EXECUTIVES:
Chairman of the Board .... George D Pillari
Chief Executive Officer .... Kenneth DiBella
President .... Steve Carpenter
Chief Financial Officer .... Doug Koo
Chief Operating Officer .... Steve Carpenter
Director of Quality Assurance .... Glenn Dixon
Vice President .... Annette Sparkman
Senior VP, General Counsel .... Barbra Rabinowitz

COMPANY PROFILE:
Parent Company Name: CBCA Administrators Inc
Doing Business As:
Year Founded: Federally Qualified: [ ]
Forprofit: [ ]   Not-For-Profit: [ ]
Model Type:
Accreditation: [ ] AAPPO [ ] JACHO [ ] NCQA [ ] URAC
Plan Type: UR
SERVICE AREA:
Nationwide: N
   NW;

CIGNA BEHAVIORAL HEALTH INC

6600 E Campus Circle Dr #110
Irving, TX 75063
Phone: 972-465-7000 Fax: 972-582-7618 Toll-Free: 800-433-5768
Web site: www.cignabehavioral.com
MAILING ADDRESS:
    CIGNA BEHAVIORAL HEALTH INC
    6600 E Campus Circle Dr #110
    Irving, TX 75063

KEY EXECUTIVES:
Chief Executive Officer/President .... Keith Dixon, PhD
Chief Financial Officer .... Randall Odzer, CPA, MBA
Chief Medical Officer .... Rhonda Robinson-Beale, MD
Chief Information Officer .... Michael Jones, MBA
Senior Counsel/Legal/Public Affairs .... Elizabeth George, JD
Senior VP, Operations .... Jodi Aronson Prohofsky
Senior Director, Network Perf Management .... Larry Gleit

COMPANY PROFILE:
Parent Company Name: CIGNA Behavioral Health Inc, MN
Doing Business As:
Year Founded: 1974   Federally Qualified: [Y]
Forprofit: [Y]   Not-For-Profit: [ ]
Model Type:
Accreditation: [ ] AAPPO [ ] JACHO [ ] NCQA [X] URAC
Plan Type: Specialty HMO
SERVICE AREA:
Nationwide: N
   TX;

Managed Care Organization Profiles   **TEXAS**

BLUE CROSS BLUE SHIELD OF TEXAS — HMO BLUE - SOUTHEAST

2425 W Loop S Ste 1000
Houston, TX 77027
Phone: 713-663-1157 Fax: 713-354-7003 Toll-Free: 800-637-0171
Web site: www.bcbstx.com
MAILING ADDRESS:
    BC/BS OF TX - HMO BLUE - SE
    2425 W Loop S Ste 1000
    Houston, TX 77027

KEY EXECUTIVES:
President .... Martin G Foster
Chief Financial Officer .... Edward Mount
Chief Medical Director .... Terry Sutton, MD
VP, Marketing & Sales .... Elliott Jones
VP, Physicians Relations .... Dee Whittlesey, MD

COMPANY PROFILE:
Parent Company Name: Health Care Service Corporation
Doing Business As: HMO Blue Texas
Year Founded: 1987   Federally Qualified: [ ]
Forprofit: [ ]   Not-For-Profit: [Y]
Model Type: IPA
Accreditation: [ ] AAPPO [ ] JACHO [ ] NCQA [ ] URAC
Plan Type: HMO, PPO, POS, CDHP, HDHP, HSA,
Total Revenue: 2005: 397,603,608   2006: 366,076,511
Net Income   2005: -7,757,822   2006: 286,469,910
Total Enrollment:
    2001: 0   2004: 77,250   2007: 94,176
    2002: 0   2005: 118,112
    2003: 22,927   2006: 99,481
SERVICE AREA:
Nationwide: N
    TX (Brazoria, Chambers, Fort Bend, Galveston, Hardin, Harris, Jefferson, Liberty, Montgomery, Orange, Waller, Wharton);
TYPE OF COVERAGE:
Commercial: [Y] Individual: [ ] FEHBP: [ ] Indemnity: [ ]
Medicare: [ ] Medicaid: [Y] Supplemental Medicare: [ ]
Tricare [ ]
PRODUCTS OFFERED:
Product Name: Type:
HMO Blue Texas   HMO
BlueChoice Plus   POS
BlueChoice   PPO
BlueEdge PPO   PPO
BestChoice   PPO
PPO SelectChoice   PPO
Select Blue Advantage   PPO
PLAN BENEFITS:
Alternative Medicine: [ ]   Behavioral Health: [ ]
Chiropractic: [ ]   Dental: [ ]
Home Care: [X]   Inpatient SNF: [X]
Long-Term Care: [ ]   Pharm. Mail Order: [ ]
Physical Therapy: [X]   Podiatry: [X]
Psychiatric: [X]   Transplant: [X]
Vision: [X]   Wellness: [X]
Workers' Comp: [ ]
Other Benefits:
Comments:
Additional products offered: Select 2000; Individual Indemnity; Blue Advantage; Long-term care; SelectTEMP;

BLUE CROSS BLUE SHIELD OF TEXAS — HMO BLUE - WEST

118 Mesa Park Dr
El Paso, TX 79902-1035
Phone: 915-496-6756 Fax: 915-496-6772 Toll-Free: 800-831-0576
Web site: www.bcbstx.com
MAILING ADDRESS:
    BC/BS OF TEXAS - HMO BLUE WEST
    118 Mesa Park Dr
    El Paso, TX 79902-1035

KEY EXECUTIVES:
President .... Martin G Foster
Chief Medical Director .... Paul Handel, MD
Chief Operating Officer .... Robert L English
Marketing Director .... Marty Foster
Provider Relations Director .... Dee Whittlesey, MD

COMPANY PROFILE:
Parent Company Name: Blue Cross Blue Shield of Texas
Doing Business As: HMO Blue, Rio Grande HMO Inc
Year Founded: 1987   Federally Qualified: [Y]
Forprofit: [ ]   Not-For-Profit: [Y]
Model Type: IPA
Accreditation: [ ] AAPPO [ ] JACHO [ ] NCQA [ ] URAC
Plan Type: HMO, PPO, POS, HDHP, HSA
Total Revenue: 2005: 6,539,517   2006: 5,680,991
Net Income   2005: 903,075   2006: 1,079,608
Total Enrollment:
    2001: 0   2004: 2,229   2007: 1,608
    2002: 0   2005: 2,179
    2003: 0   2006: 1.498
SERVICE AREA:
Nationwide: N
    TX (El Paso);
TYPE OF COVERAGE:
Commercial: [Y] Individual: [ ] FEHBP: [ ] Indemnity: [ ]
Medicare: [ ] Medicaid: [ ] Supplemental Medicare: [ ]
Tricare [ ]
PRODUCTS OFFERED:
Product Name: Type:
HMO Blue Texas   HMO
BlueChoice Plus   POS
BlueChoice   PPO
BlueEdge PPO   PPO
BestChoice   PPO
PPO SelectChoice   PPO
Select Blue Advantage   PPO
PLAN BENEFITS:
Alternative Medicine: [ ]   Behavioral Health: [ ]
Chiropractic: [X]   Dental: [ ]
Home Care: [X]   Inpatient SNF: [ ]
Long-Term Care: [ ]   Pharm. Mail Order: [X]
Physical Therapy: [X]   Podiatry: [X]
Psychiatric: [X]   Transplant: [X]
Vision: [ ]   Wellness: [X]
Workers' Comp: [ ]
Other Benefits:
Comments:
Additional products offered: Select 2000, Individual Indemnity; Blue Advantage, Long-term care; SelectTEMP;

BRAVO HEALTH TEXAS INC

7551 Callaghan Rd Ste 310
San Antonio, TX 78229
Phone: 210-321-7700 Fax: Toll-Free: 800-ELDERTX
Web site: www.elderhealth.com
MAILING ADDRESS:
    BRAVO HEALTH TEXAS INC
    7551 Callaghan Rd Ste 310
    San Antonio, TX 78229

KEY EXECUTIVES:
Chief Executive Officer .... Jeff Folick
VP, Executive Director .... Patrick Feyen
Chief Financial Officer .... Scott Tabakin
Executive VP, Chief Medcial Officer .... Ace M Hodgin, MD

COMPANY PROFILE:
Parent Company Name: Bravo Health Inc
Doing Business As:
Year Founded: 2005   Federally Qualified: [ ]
Forprofit: [Y]   Not-For-Profit: [ ]
Model Type:
Accreditation: [ ] AAPPO [ ] JACHO [ ] NCQA [ ] URAC
Plan Type: HMO
Total Revenue: 2005:   2006: 37,084,886
Net Income   2005:   2006: 588,340
Total Enrollment:
    2001: 0   2004: 0   2007: 22,630
    2002: 0   2005:
    2003: 0   2006: 21,739
SERVICE AREA:
Nationwide:
    TX;
TYPE OF COVERAGE:
Commercial: [ ] Individual: [ ] FEHBP: [ ] Indemnity: [ ]
Medicare: [Y] Medicaid: [ ] Supplemental Medicare: [ ]
Tricare [ ]
Comments:
Formerly Elder Health Inc.

Copyright MCIC -- The National Directory of Managed Care Organizations, Seventh Edition

TEXAS — Managed Care Organization Profiles

Primary Physicians:　　　　　Physician Specialists: 1,112
Hospitals:
Total Revenue:　2005:　7,978,080　　2006:　11,770,710
Net Income　　2005:　　　97,285　　2006:
Total Enrollment:
　2001:　409,946　　　2004:　485,932　　2007:　919,199
　2002:　　　　　0　　　2005:　717,245
　2003:　452,541　　　2006:　828,483
SERVICE AREA:
Nationwide:　N
　TX;
TYPE OF COVERAGE:
Commercial:　[Y]　Individual:　[ ]　FEHBP:　[ ]　Indemnity:　[ ]
Medicare:　　[Y]　Medicaid:　[Y]　Supplemental Medicare:　[ ]
Tricare　　　[ ]
PRODUCTS OFFERED:
Product Name:　　　　　　　　Type:
Block Vision　　　　　　　　　Specialty HMO
PLAN BENEFITS:
Alternative Medicine:　[ ]　　Behavioral Health:　[ ]
Chiropractic:　　　　　[ ]　　Dental:　　　　　　[ ]
Home Care:　　　　　　 [ ]　　Inpatient SNF:　　　[ ]
Long-Term Care:　　　　[ ]　　Pharm. Mail Order:　[ ]
Physical Therapy:　　　[ ]　　Podiatry:　　　　　 [ ]
Psychiatric:　　　　　 [ ]　　Transplant:　　　　 [ ]
Vision:　　　　　　　　[X]　　Wellness:　　　　　 [ ]
Workers' Comp:　　　　 [ ]
Other Benefits:

BLUE CROSS BLUE SHIELD OF TEXAS — CORPORATE HEADQUARTERS

901 S Central Expressway
Richardson, TX 75080
Phone:　877-299-2377　Fax:　972-766-6609 Toll-Free:　877-299-2377
Web site: www.bcbstx.com
MAILING ADDRESS:
　BC/BS OF TEXAS - CORP HDQTRS
　PO Box 833840
　Richardson, TX 75080

KEY EXECUTIVES:
President .... Martin G Foster
Chief Financial Officer .... Denise A Bujak
Chief Medical Officer .... Paul Handel, MD
Pharmacy Director .... Tom Tran
VP, Physician Relations .... Dee Whittlesey, MD
VP, Network Management .... Ted Haynes
VP, Human Resources .... Sue Hunt

COMPANY PROFILE:
Parent Company Name:　Health Care Service Corporation
Doing Business As:　HMO Blue Texas
Year Founded:　1987　　　Federally Qualified:　[N]
Forprofit:　[ ]　　　　　Not-For-Profit:　[Y]
Model Type:　IPA
Accreditation:　[ ] AAPPO　[ ] JACHO　[ ] NCQA　[ ] URAC
Plan Type:　HMO, PPO, POS, ASO, CDHP, HDHP, HSA,
Primary Physicians:　14,778　　Physician Specialists:　53,321
Hospitals:　664
Total Revenue:　2005:　2,897,973,562　　2006:　2,996,553,647
Net Income　　2005:　　184,733,512　　2006:　　308,093,846
Total Enrollment:
　2001:　　　　　　0　　2004:　4,009,656　　2007:
　2002:　3,646,334　　　2005:　1,033,825
　2003:　3,645,891　　　2006:　4,000,000
SERVICE AREA:
Nationwide:　N
　TX (Collin, Dallas, Denton, Ellis, Johnson, Kaufman, Rockwall, Tarrant);
TYPE OF COVERAGE:
Commercial:　[Y]　Individual:　[Y]　FEHBP:　[ ]　Indemnity:　[ ]
Medicare:　　[Y]　Medicaid:　[Y]　Supplemental Medicare:　[ ]
Tricare　　　[ ]
PRODUCTS OFFERED:
Product Name:　Type:
HMO Blue Texas　　　　　　HMO
BlueChoice Plus　　　　　　POS
BlueChoice　　　　　　　　 PPO
BlueEdge PPO　　　　　　　PPO
BestChoice　　　　　　　　 PPO
PPO SelectChoice　　　　　PPO
Select Blue Advantage　　PPO

CONSUMER-DRIVEN PRODUCTS
Blue Edge HSA　　　　　　　　HSA Company
　　　　　　　　　　　　　　　HSA Product
　　　　　　　　　　　　　　　HSA Administrator
Blue Edge PPO　　　　　　　　Consumer-Driven Health Plan
　　　　　　　　　　　　　　　High Deductible Health Plan
PLAN BENEFITS:
Alternative Medicine:　[ ]　　Behavioral Health:　[ ]
Chiropractic:　　　　　[X]　　Dental:　　　　　　[ ]
Home Care:　　　　　　 [X]　　Inpatient SNF:　　　[X]
Long-Term Care:　　　　[ ]　　Pharm. Mail Order:　[X]
Physical Therapy:　　　[X]　　Podiatry:　　　　　 [X]
Psychiatric:　　　　　 [X]　　Transplant:　　　　 [X]
Vision:　　　　　　　　[X]　　Wellness:　　　　　 [X]
Workers' Comp:　　　　 [ ]
Other Benefits:
Comments:
Additional products offered: Select 2000, Individual Indemnity; Blue Advantage, Long-term Care; SelectTEMP;

BLUE CROSS BLUE SHIELD OF TEXAS — HMO BLUE - MIDWEST TX

9020-II Capital TX Hwy N #400
Austin, TX 78759
Phone:　512-349-4800 Fax:　512-349-4884 Toll-Free:　800-336-5696
Web site: www.bcbstx.com
MAILING ADDRESS:
　BC/BS OF TX - HMO BLUE - CNTR
　9020-II Capital TX Hwy N #400
　Austin, TX 78759

KEY EXECUTIVES:
President .... Martin G Foster
VP &Chief Medical Officer .... Paul Handel, MD
Chief Operating Officer .... Sherman M Wolff
Marketing Director .... Jeff Jacobi

COMPANY PROFILE:
Parent Company Name:　Health Care Service Corporation
Doing Business As:　HMO Blue Texas
Year Founded:　1987　　　Federally Qualified:　[ ]
Forprofit:　[ ]　　　　　Not-For-Profit:　[Y]
Model Type:　IPA
Accreditation:　[ ] AAPPO　[ ] JACHO　[ ] NCQA　[ ] URAC
Plan Type:　HMO, PPO, CDHP, HDHP, HSA,
Total Revenue:　2005: 135,111,211　　2006:　164,632,221
Net Income　　2005:　　5,371,667　　2006:　　　-70,966
Total Enrollment:
　2001:　　0　　　　2004:　16,603　　2007:　35,439
　2002:　　0　　　　2005:　47,230
　2003:　　0　　　　2006:　41,965
SERVICE AREA:
Nationwide:　N
　TX (9 Southeastern Counties);
TYPE OF COVERAGE:
Commercial:　[Y]　Individual:　[Y]　FEHBP:　[ ]　Indemnity:　[ ]
Medicare:　　[ ]　Medicaid:　[ ]　Supplemental Medicare:　[ ]
Tricare　　　[ ]
PRODUCTS OFFERED:
Product Name:　　　　　　　　Type:
HMO Blue Texas　　　　　　　HMO
BlueChoice Plus　　　　　　POS
BlueChoice　　　　　　　　 PPO
BlueEdge PPO　　　　　　　 PPO
BestChoice　　　　　　　　 PPO
PPO SelectChoice　　　　　PPO
Select Blue Advantage　　PPO
PLAN BENEFITS:
Alternative Medicine:　[ ]　　Behavioral Health:　[ ]
Chiropractic:　　　　　[X]　　Dental:　　　　　　[ ]
Home Care:　　　　　　 [X]　　Inpatient SNF:　　　[X]
Long-Term Care:　　　　[ ]　　Pharm. Mail Order:　[ ]
Physical Therapy:　　　[X]　　Podiatry:　　　　　 [X]
Psychiatric:　　　　　 [X]　　Transplant:　　　　 [X]
Vision:　　　　　　　　[X]　　Wellness:　　　　　 [X]
Workers' Comp:　　　　 [ ]
Other Benefits:
Comments:
Additional products offered: Select 2000; Individual Indemnity; SelectTEMP; Blue Advantage, Long-Term Care.

Managed Care Organization Profiles — TEXAS

Model Type:
Accreditation: [ ] AAPPO [ ] JACHO [ ] NCQA [ ] URAC
Plan Type: HMO,
Total Revenue: 2005: 850,460,544   2006: 945,059,732
Net Income   2005: 20,743,851   2006: 66,283,353
Total Enrollment:
  2001: 205,737   2004: 393,916   2007: 449,941
  2002: 295,078   2005: 398,974
  2003: 343,327   2006: 405,850

SERVICE AREA:
Nationwide: N
  TX (Brazoria, Collin, Dallas, Denton, Ellis, Fort Bend, Galveston, Harris, Hood, Hunt, Johnson, Kaufman, Montgomery, Navarro, Parker, Rockwall, Tarrant, Waller, Wise);

TYPE OF COVERAGE:
Commercial: [ ]   Individual: [ ]   FEHBP: [ ]   Indemnity: [ ]
Medicare: [ ]   Medicaid: [Y]   Supplemental Medicare: [ ]
Tricare   [ ]

PRODUCTS OFFERED:
Product Name:	Type:
Americaid	Medicaid
Americaid - Star	Medicaid

PLAN BENEFITS:
Alternative Medicine: [ ]   Behavioral Health: [X]
Chiropractic: [X]   Dental: [ ]
Home Care: [X]   Inpatient SNF: [X]
Long-Term Care: [ ]   Pharm. Mail Order: [ ]
Physical Therapy: [X]   Podiatry: [ ]
Psychiatric: [X]   Transplant: [X]
Vision: [X]   Wellness: [X]
Workers' Comp: [ ]
Other Benefits:

AMERICAN NATIONAL INSURANCE COMPANY

One Moody Plaza
Galveston, TX 77550-7999
Phone: 409-763-4661 Fax: 409-766-6663 Toll-Free: 800-899-6503
Web site: www.anico.com

MAILING ADDRESS:
  AMERICAN NATIONAL INSURANCE CO
  One Moody Plaza
  Galveston, TX 77550-7999

KEY EXECUTIVES:
Chairman of the Board/Chief Executive Officer .... Robert L Moody
President/Chief Operating Officer .... G Richard Ferdinandtsen
Senior VP & Controller .... Stephen E Pavlicek
Medical Director .... Harry Kelso, Jr, MD
Director, Information Systems .... J D Johnson
Group/Health Compliance .... Morris Soler
Director of Managed Care .... Gary White
Senior VP, Health Insurance Operations .... Steven H Schouweiler

COMPANY PROFILE:
Parent Company Name:
Doing Business As:
Year Founded: 1905   Federally Qualified: [ ]
Forprofit: [Y]   Not-For-Profit: [ ]
Model Type:
Accreditation: [ ] AAPPO [ ] JACHO [ ] NCQA [ ] URAC
Plan Type: PPO, TPA

SERVICE AREA:
Nationwide: N
  NW (Excluding NY);

TYPE OF COVERAGE:
Commercial: [Y]   Individual: [Y]   FEHBP: [ ]   Indemnity: [Y]
Medicare: [Y]   Medicaid: [N]   Supplemental Medicare: [Y]
Tricare   [ ]

PLAN BENEFITS:
Alternative Medicine: [ ]   Behavioral Health: [ ]
Chiropractic: [X]   Dental: [X]
Home Care: [X]   Inpatient SNF: [X]
Long-Term Care: [X]   Pharm. Mail Order: [X]
Physical Therapy: [X]   Podiatry: [X]
Psychiatric: [X]   Transplant: [X]
Vision: [X]   Wellness: [X]
Workers' Comp: [ ]
Other Benefits:

AMERICAN PREFERRED PROVIDER ORGANIZATION LLC

600 E J.Carpenter Fwy Ste 170
Irving, TX 75062
Phone: 972-717-5200 Fax: 972-717-5209 Toll-Free: 877-223-3372
Web site: www.americanppo.com

MAILING ADDRESS:
  AMERICAN PPO INC
  600 E J.Carpenter Fwy Ste 170
  Irving, TX 75062

KEY EXECUTIVES:
Chief Executive Officer/President .... Michael Caolo
Marketing Director .... Shelly Caolo

COMPANY PROFILE:
Parent Company Name: American Preferred Provider Org INC
Doing Business As: American PPO
Year Founded: 2000   Federally Qualified: [ ]
Forprofit: [Y]   Not-For-Profit: [ ]
Model Type: MIXED
Accreditation: [ ] AAPPO [ ] JACHO [ ] NCQA [ ] URAC
Plan Type: PPO, UR, HDHP, HSA,
Primary Physicians: 8,500   Physician Specialists:
Hospitals: 225

SERVICE AREA:
Nationwide: N
  AR (Arkansas, Ashley, Baxter, Benton, Boone, Bradley, Calhoun, Carroll, Chicot, Clark, Clay, Cleburne, Cleveland, Conway, Craighead, Crawford, Crittenden, Cross, Dallas, Desha, Drew, Faulkner, Franklin, Fulton, Garland, Grant, Greene, Homestead, Hot Springs, Independence, Izard, Jackson, Jefferson, Lafayette, Lawrence, Lincoln, Logon, Lonoke, Madison, Marion, Miller, Mississippi, Monroe, Montgomery, Nevada, Ouachita, Perry, Pike, Poinsett, Polk, Prairie, Pulaski, Randolph, Saint Francis, Saline, Scott, Sebastian, Sevier, Sharp, Stone, Van Buren, Washington, White, Woodruff, Yell); LA; MO; MS; OK; TN; TX;

TYPE OF COVERAGE:
Commercial: [Y]   Individual: [Y]   FEHBP: [ ]   Indemnity: [ ]
Medicare: [ ]   Medicaid: [ ]   Supplemental Medicare: [ ]
Tricare   [ ]

PLAN BENEFITS:
Alternative Medicine: [ ]   Behavioral Health: [ ]
Chiropractic: [X]   Dental: [ ]
Home Care: [X]   Inpatient SNF: [ ]
Long-Term Care: [ ]   Pharm. Mail Order: [ ]
Physical Therapy: [ ]   Podiatry: [X]
Psychiatric: [X]   Transplant: [X]
Vision: [ ]   Wellness: [X]
Workers' Comp: [ ]
Other Benefits:
Comments:
Formerly called American Health Care Providers.

BLOCK VISION OF TEXAS INC

400 Alpha RD Ste 910
Dallas, TX 75244
Phone: 972-991-8816 Fax: 972-991-4704 Toll-Free: 800-914-9795
Web site: www.blockvision.com

MAILING ADDRESS:
  BLOCK VISION OF TEXAS INC
  400 Alpha Rd Ste 910
  Dallas, TX 75244

KEY EXECUTIVES:
Chief Executive Officer/President .... Andrew Alcorn
Medical Director .... Barry Davis, OD
Chief Information Officer .... James Burton
VP Chief Operating Officer .... Joy K Schreiber
Senior VP, Sales .... Stefanie J Crammond
VP of Legal Counsel .... Audrey Weinstein
Senior VP, Clinical Director .... Howard Levin, OD

COMPANY PROFILE:
Parent Company Name: Block Vision, Inc
Doing Business As:
Year Founded: 1996   Federally Qualified: [Y]
Forprofit: [Y]   Not-For-Profit: [ ]
Model Type: NETWORK
Accreditation: [ ] AAPPO [ ] JACHO [X] NCQA [ ] URAC
Plan Type: Specialty HMO, TPA

TEXAS

Guadalupe, Hale, Hall, Hami,lton, Hansfors, Hardeman, Hardin, Harris, Harrison Hartley, Haskell, Hays, Hemphil, Henderson, Hidalgo, Hill, Hockley, Hood, Hopkins, Houston, Howard, Hudspeth, Hunt, Hutchinson, Irion, Jack, Jackson, Jasper, Jeff Davis, Jefferson, Jim Hogg, Wells Johnson, Jones, Karnes, Kaufman Lee, Kendall, Kenedy, Kent, Kerr, Kimble, King, Kinney, Kleberg, Knox, LaSalle, Lamar, Lamb, Lampass, Lavaca, Lee, Leon, Liberty, Limestone, Lipscomb, Live Oak, Llano, Loving, Lubbock, Lynn, Madison, Marion, Martin, Mason, Matagorda, Maverick, McCulloch, McLennan, McMullen, Medina);

PRODUCTS OFFERED:
Product Name: Type:
Aetna Dental Plan HMO   Specialty HMO

CONSUMER-DRIVEN PRODUCTS
Aetna Life Insurance Co   HSA Company
Aetna HealthFund HSA   HSA Product
Aetna   HSA Administrator
Aetna HealthFund   Consumer-Driven Health Plan
PPO I; PPO II   High Deductible Health Plan

PLAN BENEFITS:
Alternative Medicine: [ ]   Behavioral Health: [ ]
Chiropractic: [ ]   Dental: [X]
Home Care: [ ]   Inpatient SNF: [ ]
Long-Term Care: [ ]   Pharm. Mail Order: [ ]
Physical Therapy: [ ]   Podiatry: [ ]
Psychiatric: [ ]   Transplant: [ ]
Vision: [ ]   Wellness: [ ]
Workers' Comp: [ ]
Other Benefits:

ALLIANCE REGIONAL HEALTH NETWORK

1501 S Coulter
Amarillo, TX 79106
Phone: 806-351-5151 Fax: 806-351-5159 Toll-Free: 800-687-8007
Web site: www.nwtexashealthcare.com

MAILING ADDRESS:
ALLIANCE REG HEALTH NETWORK
PO Box 51980
Amarillo, TX 79106

KEY EXECUTIVES:
Director of Operations .... Clay Weiss
Sales & Marketing Manager .... Scott Carlisle
Credentialing Coordinator .... Patsy Smith
Provider Relations Coordinator .... Diane Murrillo

COMPANY PROFILE:
Parent Company Name: Universal Healthcare Services
Doing Business As: Alliance Regional Health Network
Year Founded: 1986   Federally Qualified: [ ]
Forprofit: [Y]   Not-For-Profit: [ ]
Model Type: Network
Accreditation: [ ] AAPPO [ ] JACHO [ ] NCQA [ ] URAC
Plan Type: PPO, EPO
Primary Physicians: 640   Physician Specialists: 435
Hospitals: 25
Total Enrollment:
   2001: 60,000   2004: 0   2007: 0
   2002: 72,000   2005:
   2003: 78,000   2006:

SERVICE AREA:
Nationwide: N
   NM; OK; TX;

TYPE OF COVERAGE:
Commercial: [Y] Individual: [Y] FEHBP: [ ] Indemnity: [ ]
Medicare: [ ] Medicaid: [ ] Supplemental Medicare: [ ]
Tricare [ ]

PRODUCTS OFFERED:
Product Name: Type:
Alliance PPO   PPO

PLAN BENEFITS:
Alternative Medicine: [ ]   Behavioral Health: [ ]
Chiropractic: [X]   Dental: [X]
Home Care: [ ]   Inpatient SNF: [X]
Long-Term Care: [X]   Pharm. Mail Order: [ ]
Physical Therapy: [X]   Podiatry: [X]
Psychiatric: [X]   Transplant: [ ]
Vision: [ ]   Wellness: [X]
Workers' Comp: [X]
Other Benefits:

ALPHA DENTAL PROGRAMS INC

700 Parker Square Ste 150
Flower Mound, TX 75028
Phone: 972-410-3700 Fax: 972-410-3701 Toll-Free: 800-775-0523
Web site: www.deltadentalins.com

MAILING ADDRESS:
ALPHA DENTAL PROGRAMS INC
700 Parker Square Ste 150
Flower Mound, TX 75028

KEY EXECUTIVES:
President .... Robert B Elliott
Chief Operating Officer .... Robert Budd

COMPANY PROFILE:
Parent Company Name: Delta Dental of California
Doing Business As: Delta Care
Year Founded: 1989   Federally Qualified: [ ]
Forprofit: [Y]   Not-For-Profit: [ ]
Model Type: NETWORK
Accreditation: [ ] AAPPO [ ] JACHO [ ] NCQA [ ] URAC
Plan Type: Specialty HMO
Total Revenue: 2005: 4,477,508   2006: 5,270,880
Net Income 2005: 45,700   2006:
Total Enrollment:
   2001: 51,172   2004: 41,214   2007: 50,789
   2002: 46,562   2005: 38,138
   2003: 37,912   2006: 49,074

SERVICE AREA:
Nationwide: N
   TX (Armstrong, Bailey, Bowie, Brewster, Briscoe, Brown, Carson, Castro, Cochran, Coke, Coleman, Collingsworth, Concho, Crosby, Culberson, Dallam, Deaf Smith, Donley, Edwards, Floyd, Garza, Gray, Hale, Hansford, Hartley, Hemphill, Hockley, Hutchinson, Jasper, Jeff Davis, Kinney, Lamb, Lipscomb, Loving, Lubbock, McCulloch, Menard, Moore, Motley, Newton, Newton, Ochiltree, Oldham, Parmer, Pecos, Poeeter, Presidio, Randall, Reeves, Roberts, Runnels, Sabine, San Augustine, Schleicher, Shelby, Sherman, Sutton, Swisher, Terrell, Tom Green, Val Verde, Wheeler, Willacy);

TYPE OF COVERAGE:
Commercial: [Y] Individual: [Y] FEHBP: [ ] Indemnity: [ ]
Medicare: [ ] Medicaid: [ ] Supplemental Medicare: [ ]
Tricare [ ]

PRODUCTS OFFERED:
Product Name: Type:
Delta Care   Specialty HMO

PLAN BENEFITS:
Alternative Medicine: [ ]   Behavioral Health: [ ]
Chiropractic: [ ]   Dental: [X]
Home Care: [ ]   Inpatient SNF: [ ]
Long-Term Care: [ ]   Pharm. Mail Order: [ ]
Physical Therapy: [ ]   Podiatry: [ ]
Psychiatric: [ ]   Transplant: [ ]
Vision: [ ]   Wellness: [ ]
Workers' Comp: [ ]
Other Benefits:

AMERIGROUP - ARLINGTON HEALTH PLAN

1200 E Copeland Rd Ste 200
Arlington, TX 76011
Phone: 817-861-7700 Fax: 817-548-7125 Toll-Free: 800-839-6275
Web site: www.amerigroupcorp.com

MAILING ADDRESS:
AMERIGROUP TEXAS INC
1200 E Copeland Rd Ste 200
Arlington, TX 76011

KEY EXECUTIVES:
Chief Executive Officer/President .... Eric Yoder, MD, MBA
Medical Director .... David Layland, MD
Chief Operating Officer .... Patricia L Behrens
Marketing Director .... B Randy Johnson
Director, Provider Services .... Celia Manlove

COMPANY PROFILE:
Parent Company Name: Amerigroup Corporation
Doing Business As: Americaid Community Care
Year Founded: 1995   Federally Qualified: [Y]
Forprofit: [Y]   Not-For-Profit: [ ]

Managed Care Organization Profiles — TEXAS

AECC TOTAL VISION HEALTH PLAN OF TEXAS INC

3010 LBJ Freeway Ste 1410
Dallas, TX 75234
Phone: 972-620-8909 Fax: 972-620-9484 Toll-Free: 800-268-8847
Web site: www.opticare.com

MAILING ADDRESS:
AECC TOTAL VISION HEALTH PLAN
3010 LBJ Freeway Ste 1410
Dallas, TX 75234

KEY EXECUTIVES:
President of Managed Care .... Jason Harrold
VP, Finance .... David Lavely
National Medical Director .... Mark Ruchman, MD
VP, Information Systems ....Juan Marrero

COMPANY PROFILE:
Parent Company Name: Opticare
Doing Business As: Total Vision Health Plan
Year Founded: 1996   Federally Qualified: [N]
Forprofit: [Y]   Not-For-Profit: [ ]
Model Type:
Accreditation: [ ] AAPPO [ ] JACHO [X] NCQA [ ] URAC
Plan Type: Specialty HMO
Primary Physicians: Physician Specialists:
Hospitals:
Total Revenue: 2005: 8,536,239   2006: 7,825,837
Net Income   2005:   35,756   2006:   766,058
Total Enrollment:
  2001: 530,479   2004: 624,085   2007: 636,327
  2002: 767,025   2005: 629,630
  2003: 656,655   2006: 590,322

SERVICE AREA:
Nationwide: N
  TX;

TYPE OF COVERAGE:
Commercial: [ ] Individual: [Y] FEHBP: [ ] Indemnity: [ ]
Medicare: [ ] Medicaid: [ ] Supplemental Medicare: [ ]
Tricare   [ ]

PRODUCTS OFFERED:
Product Name: Type:
Total Vision Health Plan   Specialty HMO

PLAN BENEFITS:
Alternative Medicine: [ ]   Behavioral Health: [ ]
Chiropractic: [ ]   Dental: [ ]
Home Care: [ ]   Inpatient SNF: [ ]
Long-Term Care: [ ]   Pharm. Mail Order: [ ]
Physical Therapy: [ ]   Podiatry: [ ]
Psychiatric: [ ]   Transplant: [ ]
Vision: [X]   Wellness: [ ]
Workers' Comp: [ ]
Other Benefits:

AETNA HEALTH INC

3800 Buffalo Speedway Ste 150
Houston, TX 77098
Phone: 713-350-2000 Fax: 215-775-6790 Toll-Free: 800-876-7778
Web site: www.aetna.com

MAILING ADDRESS:
AETNA HEALTH INC
3800 Buffalo Speedway Ste 150
Houston, TX 77098

KEY EXECUTIVES:
Chairman of the Board/Chief Executive Officer .... Ronald A Williams
Regional Manager .... Carl King
Executive VP, Finance .... Joseph M Zubretsky
Medical Director .... Susan Mueller, MD
General Manager-Key Accounts .... Kate Begley
VP, Sales & Services .... Lisa Rowland
Senior Network Manager .... Joann Beck
Regional Manager of Product Development .... Michael Ciarocchi
General Manager-Select Account .... Laurie Brubaker
General Manager-Small Business .... Regina Hunter

COMPANY PROFILE:
Parent Company Name: Aetna Inc
Doing Business As:
Year Founded: 1975   Federally Qualified: [Y]
Forprofit: [Y]   Not-For-Profit: [ ]
Model Type: MIXED
Accreditation: [ ] AAPPO [ ] JACHO [X] NCQA [ ] URAC
Plan Type: HMO, PPO, POS, ASO, CDHP, HDHP, HSA,
Total Revenue: 2005: 968,361,051   2006: 976,665,368
Net Income   2005:   39,743,992   2006:   51,578,932
Total Enrollment:
  2001: 482,156   2004: 330,511   2007: 256,332
  2002: 469,982   2005: 293,557
  2003: 326,915   2006: 291,786

SERVICE AREA:
Nationwide: N
  TX (Brazoria, Fort Bend, Galveston, Harris, Montgomery, Waller);

TYPE OF COVERAGE:
Commercial: [Y] Individual: [ ] FEHBP: [ ] Indemnity: [ ]
Medicare: [Y] Medicaid: [ ] Supplemental Medicare: [ ]
Tricare   [ ]

PRODUCTS OFFERED:
Product Name: Type:
Aetna HMO   HMO

CONSUMER-DRIVEN PRODUCTS
Aetna Life Insurance Co   HSA Company
Aetna HealthFund HSA   HSA Product
Aetna   HSA Administrator
Aetna HealthFund   Consumer-Driven Health Plan
PPO I; PPO II   High Deductible Health Plan

PLAN BENEFITS:
Alternative Medicine: [ ]   Behavioral Health: [ ]
Chiropractic: [X]   Dental: [X]
Home Care: [X]   Inpatient SNF: [X]
Long-Term Care: [ ]   Pharm. Mail Order: [X]
Physical Therapy: [X]   Podiatry: [X]
Psychiatric: [X]   Transplant: [X]
Vision: [X]   Wellness: [X]
Workers' Comp: [ ]
Other Benefits:
Comments:
Formerly Prudential Healthcare of Houston.

AETNA INC - DENTAL PLAN OF TEXAS

2777 Stemmons Frwy
Dallas, TX 75207
Phone: 214-200-8000 Fax: 214-200-8916 Toll-Free: 800-825-7935
Web site: www.aetna.com

MAILING ADDRESS:
AETNA INC - DENTAL PLN OF TX
2777 Stemmons Frwy
Dallas, TX 75207

KEY EXECUTIVES:
Chairman of the Board/Chief Executive Officer .... Ronald A Williams
Regional Manager-West Central .... Charles T Brown
Executive VP, Finance .... Joseph M Zubretsky
Marketing Director .... Mike Ziogas

COMPANY PROFILE:
Parent Company Name: Aetna Inc
Doing Business As: Aetna Inc
Year Founded: 1985   Federally Qualified: [N]
Forprofit: [Y]   Not-For-Profit: [ ]
Model Type:
Accreditation: [ ] AAPPO [ ] JACHO [ ] NCQA [ ] URAC
Plan Type: Specialty HMO, Specialty PPO, CDHP, HSA,
Total Revenue: 2005: 73,367,395   2006: 713,767,315
Net Income   2005: 12,053,785   2006:
Total Enrollment:
  2001:   77,448   2004: 585,451   2007: 538,745
  2002: 607,080   2005: 576,929
  2003: 597,436   2006: 561,912

SERVICE AREA:
Nationwide: N
  TX (Anderson, Andrews, Angelina, Aransas, Archer, Armstrong,
  Atascosa, Austin, Bailey, Bandera, Bastrop, Baylor, Bee, Bell,
  Bexar, Blanco, Borden, Bosque, Bowie, Brazoria, Brazos, Brewster,
  Briscoe, Brooks, Brown, Burleson, Burnet, Caldwell, Calhoun
  Callahan, Cameron, Camp, Carson, Cass, Castro, Chambers,
  Cherokee, Childress, Clay, Cochran, Coke, Coleman, Collin,
  Collingworth, Colorado, Comal, Comanche, Concho, Cookie,
  Coryell, Cottle, Crane, Crockett, Crosby, Culberson, Dallam,
  Dallas, Dawson, DeWitt Deaf Smith, Delta, Denton, Dickens,
  Dimmit Donley, Duval, Eastland, Ector, Edwards, El Paso, Ellis,
  Erath, Falls, Fammin, Fayette, Fisher, Floyd, Foard, Fort Bend,
  Franklin, Freestone, Frio, Gaines, Galveston, Garza, Gillespie,
  Glasscock, Goliad, Gonzales, Gray, Grayson, Gregg, Grimes,

Managed Care Organization Profiles — TENNESSEE

KEY EXECUTIVES:
Non-Executive Chairman .... Richard T Burke
Chief Executive Officer .... Robert J Sheehy
President .... Richard L Bartsh, MD

COMPANY PROFILE:
Parent Company Name: UnitedHealth Group
Doing Business As: UHC Health Plan of the River Valley
Year Founded: 1985   Federally Qualified: [N]
Forprofit: [Y]   Not-For-Profit: [ ]
Model Type: IPA
Accreditation: [ ] AAPPO [ ] JACHO [X] NCQA [ ] URAC
Plan Type: HMO, POS, CDHP, HDHP, HSA,
Total Revenue: 2005: 664,290,228   2006: 555,973,955
Net Income   2005: 22,430,613   2006:   29,479,262
Total Enrollment:
   2001: 275,792   2004: 220,903   2007: 328,980
   2002: 206,584   2005: 185,971
   2003: 225,405   2006: 181,589
Medical Loss Ratio: 2005: 83.40   2006:
Administrative Expense Ratio: 2005:   2006:

SERVICE AREA:
Nationwide: N
   TN (Anderson, Bledsoe, Blount, Bradley, Campbell, Carter, Caliborne, Cocke, Franklin, Grundy, Grainger, Greene, Hamblen, Hamilton, Hancock, Hawkins, Jefferson, Johnson, Knox, Loudon, Marion, McMinn, Meigs, Monroe, Morgan, Polk, Rhea, Roane, Scott, Sequatchie, Sevier, Sullivan, Unicoi, Union, Washington);

TYPE OF COVERAGE:
Commercial: [Y] Individual: [ ] FEHBP: [ ] Indemnity: [ ]
Medicare: [Y] Medicaid: [Y] Supplemental Medicare: [ ]
Tricare   [ ]

PRODUCTS OFFERED:
Product Name: Type:
Secure Plus   Medicare
HMO   HMO

CONSUMER-DRIVEN PRODUCTS
Wells Fargo   HSA Company
Heritage Options HSA   HSA Product
Wells Fargo   HSA Administrator
                           Consumer-Driven Health Plan
                           High Deductible Health Plan

PLAN BENEFITS:
Alternative Medicine: [ ]   Behavioral Health: [X]
Chiropractic: [X]   Dental: [X]
Home Care: [ ]   Inpatient SNF: [X]
Long-Term Care: [ ]   Pharm. Mail Order: [X]
Physical Therapy: [X]   Podiatry: [X]
Psychiatric: [X]   Transplant: [X]
Vision: [X]   Wellness: [X]
Workers' Comp: [X]
Other Benefits:

Comments:
Formerly John Deere Health Plan, acquired by UnitedHealth on February 24, 2006.

UNITEDHEALTHCARE OF TENNESSEE INC

10 Cadillac Dr
Brentwood, TN 37027
Phone: 615-372-3622 Fax: 615-372-3640 Toll-Free: 800-695-1273
Web site: www.uhc.com

MAILING ADDRESS:
   UNITEDHEALTHCARE OF TN
   10 Cadillac Dr
   Brentwood, TN 37027

KEY EXECUTIVES:
Non-Executive Chairman .... Richard T Burke
Chief Executive Officer/President .... Garland G Scott, III
Vice President of Finance .... Wes Waters
VP of Network Management .... Larry Nall
Quality Assurance Director .... Kathy Cartwright

COMPANY PROFILE:
Parent Company Name: UnitedHealth Group
Doing Business As:
Year Founded: 1991   Federally Qualified: [N]
Forprofit: [Y]   Not-For-Profit: [ ]
Model Type: IPA
Accreditation: [ ] AAPPO [X] JACHO [ ] NCQA [ ] URAC
Plan Type: HMO, PPO, POS, CDHP, HDHP, HSA,
Total Enrollment:
   2001: 89,658   2004: 19,966   2007: 0
   2002: 59,804   2005:
   2003: 44,413   2006:

SERVICE AREA:
Nationwide: N
   TN (Anderson, Bedford, Benton, Bledsoe, Blount, Bradley, Cannon, Carroll, Cheatham, Chester, Cocke, Coffee, Crockett, Cumberland, Davidson, Decatur, DeKalb, Dickson, Dyer, Fayette, Franklin, Gibson, Giles, Grundy, Hamilton, Hardeman, Hardin, Haywood, Henderson, Hickman, Houston, Jackson, Knox, Lake, Lauderdale, Lawrence, Lewis, Lincoln, Loudin, Macon, Madison, Marion, Marshall, Maury, McMinn, McNairy, Meiges, Monroe, Moore, Overton, Perry, Polk, Putnam, Rhea, Roane, Robertson, Rutherford, Sequatchie, Sevier, Shelby, Smith, Steward, Sumner, Tipton, Trousdale, Van Buren, Warren, Wayne, White, Williamson, Wilson);

TYPE OF COVERAGE:
Commercial: [Y] Individual: [ ] FEHBP: [ ] Indemnity: [ ]
Medicare: [ ] Medicaid: [ ] Supplemental Medicare: [ ]
Tricare   [ ]

CONSUMER-DRIVEN PRODUCTS
Exante Bank/Golden Rule Ins Co   HSA Company
iPlan HSA   HSA Product
                                   HSA Administrator
                                   Consumer-Driven Health Plan
                                   High Deductible Health Plan

PLAN BENEFITS:
Alternative Medicine: [ ]   Behavioral Health: [X]
Chiropractic: [X]   Dental: [X]
Home Care: [X]   Inpatient SNF: [X]
Long-Term Care: [X]   Pharm. Mail Order: [X]
Physical Therapy: [X]   Podiatry: [X]
Psychiatric: [X]   Transplant: [X]
Vision: [X]   Wellness: [X]
Workers' Comp: [ ]
Other Benefits:

WINDSOR HEALTH PLAN OF TENNESSEE INC

7100 Commerce Way Ste 285
Brentwood, TN 37027
Phone: 615-782-7910 Fax: 615-782-7812 Toll-Free:
Web site: www.vhptn.com

MAILING ADDRESS:
   WINDSOR HEALTH PLAN OF TN INC
   7100 Commerce Way Ste 285
   Brentwood, TN 37027

KEY EXECUTIVES:
President .... Michael Bailey
Executive VP, Chief Financial Officer .... Willis E Jones, III
Director, Health Services .... Robin Conard, BSN, MBA
Manager, Provider Relations .... Susan Davis
Manager, Public Relations .... Amanda Woodhead

COMPANY PROFILE:
Parent Company Name: Windsor Health Group
Doing Business As: VHP CommunityCare
Year Founded: 1993   Federally Qualified: [ ]
Forprofit: [ ]   Not-For-Profit: [ ]
Model Type:
Accreditation: [ ] AAPPO [ ] JACHO [ ] NCQA [ ] URAC
Plan Type: HMO
Total Revenue: 2005:   2006: 50,702,115
Net Income   2005: 377,817   2006: 1,181,448
Total Enrollment:
   2001: 35,711   2004: 38,361   2007: 10,365
   2002: 26,632   2005: 40,951
   2003: 28,910   2006: 53,537

SERVICE AREA:
Nationwide:
   TN;

TYPE OF COVERAGE:
Commercial: [ ] Individual: [ ] FEHBP: [ ] Indemnity: [ ]
Medicare: [ ] Medicaid: [Y] Supplemental Medicare: [ ]
Tricare   [ ]

PRODUCTS OFFERED:
Product Name: Type:
VHP CommunityCare   Medicaid

TENNESSEE

MAILING ADDRESS:
UNISON HEALTH PLAN OF TN
1000 Ridgeway Loop Rd Ste 203
Memphis, TN 38120

KEY EXECUTIVES:
Chief Executive Officer/President .... John P Blank, MD
VP, Finance .... Leslie A Gelpi
Senior VP, Medical Operations .... Shirley J Blevins
VP, Pharmacy .... Jim Hancovsky
Chief Information Officer .... Steve Bugajski
Senior VP, Operations .... Fred O Madill
VP Network Development .... Heather Cianfrocco
Director, Human Resources .... Beverly Ludlum
VP, General Counsel .... David W Thomas
Compliance Officer .... John G Beck

COMPANY PROFILE:
Parent Company Name: Three River Holdings Inc
Doing Business As: Unison Health Plan of Tennessee
Year Founded: 2001   Federally Qualified: [N]
Forprofit: [Y]   Not-For-Profit: [ ]
Model Type: Mixed
Accreditation: [ ] AAPPO [ ] JACHO [ ] NCQA [ ] URAC
Plan Type: HMO
Total Revenue: 2005:   2006:
Net Income   2005: 402,250   2006:   480,361
Total Enrollment:
    2001: 40,910   2004: 0   2007: 941
    2002: 44,696   2005:
    2003: 0   2006:

SERVICE AREA:
Nationwide:
    TN;

TYPE OF COVERAGE:
Commercial: [ ] Individual: [ ] FEHBP: [ ] Indemnity: [ ]
Medicare: [ ] Medicaid: [Y] Supplemental Medicare: [ ]
Tricare   [ ]

UNITEDHEALTHCARE SERVICES COMPANY OF THE RIVER VALLEY INC

7213 Noah Reid Rd Ste 102
Chattanooga, TN 37421
Phone: 423-499-0673 Fax: 423-954-9907 Toll-Free: 800-747-1446
Web site: www.uhcrivervalley.com

MAILING ADDRESS:
UHC OF THE RIVER VALLEY INC
1300 River Dr Ste 200
Moline, IL 37421

KEY EXECUTIVES:
Non-Executive Chairman .... Richard T Burke
Chief Executive Officer .... Robert J Sheehy
President .... Richard L Bartsh, MD

COMPANY PROFILE:
Parent Company Name: UnitedHealth Group
Doing Business As: UHC Health Plan of the River Valley
Year Founded: 1985   Federally Qualified: [N]
Forprofit: [Y]   Not-For-Profit: [ ]
Model Type: IPA
Accreditation: [ ] AAPPO [ ] JACHO [X] NCQA [ ] URAC
Plan Type: HMO, POS, CDHP, HDHP, HSA,

SERVICE AREA:
Nationwide: N
    TN;

TYPE OF COVERAGE:
Commercial: [Y] Individual: [ ] FEHBP: [ ] Indemnity: [ ]
Medicare: [Y] Medicaid: [Y] Supplemental Medicare: [ ]
Tricare   [ ]

CONSUMER-DRIVEN PRODUCTS
Wells Fargo   HSA Company
Heritage Options HSA   HSA Product
Wells Fargo   HSA Administrator
                               Consumer-Driven Health Plan
                               High Deductible Health Plan

PLAN BENEFITS:
Alternative Medicine: [ ]   Behavioral Health: [X]
Chiropractic: [X]   Dental: [X]
Home Care: [ ]   Inpatient SNF: [X]
Long-Term Care: [ ]   Pharm. Mail Order: [X]
Physical Therapy: [X]   Podiatry: [X]
Psychiatric: [X]   Transplant: [X]
Vision: [X]   Wellness: [X]
Workers' Comp: [X]
Other Benefits:

Comments:
Formerly John Deere Health Plan, acquired by UnitedHealth on February 24, 2006. See Knoxville, TN for enrollment information.

UNITEDHEALTHCARE SERVICES COMPANY OF THE RIVER VALLEY INC

2033 Meadowview Lane Ste 300
Kingsport, TN 37660
Phone: 423-378-5122 Fax: 423-378-4752 Toll-Free: 800-747-1446
Web site: www.uhcrivervalley.com

MAILING ADDRESS:
UHC OF THE RIVER VALLEY INC
1300 River Dr Ste 200
Moline, IL 37660

KEY EXECUTIVES:
Non-Executive Chairman .... Richard T Burke
Chief Executive Officer .... Robert J Sheehy
President .... Richard L Bartsh, MD

COMPANY PROFILE:
Parent Company Name: UnitedHealth Group
Doing Business As: UHC Health Plan of the River Valley
Year Founded: 1985   Federally Qualified: [N]
Forprofit: [Y]   Not-For-Profit: [ ]
Model Type: IPA
Accreditation: [ ] AAPPO [ ] JACHO [X] NCQA [ ] URAC
Plan Type: HMO, POS, CDHP, HDHP, HSA,

SERVICE AREA:
Nationwide: N
    TN;

TYPE OF COVERAGE:
Commercial: [Y] Individual: [ ] FEHBP: [ ] Indemnity: [ ]
Medicare: [Y] Medicaid: [Y] Supplemental Medicare: [ ]
Tricare   [ ]

PRODUCTS OFFERED:
Product Name: Type:
John Deere Health Care   Medicaid
John Deere Health Care   HMO

CONSUMER-DRIVEN PRODUCTS
Wells Fargo   HSA Company
Heritage Options HSA   HSA Product
Wells Fargo   HSA Administrator
                               Consumer-Driven Health Plan
                               High Deductible Health Plan

PLAN BENEFITS:
Alternative Medicine: [ ]   Behavioral Health: [X]
Chiropractic: [X]   Dental: [X]
Home Care: [ ]   Inpatient SNF: [X]
Long-Term Care: [ ]   Pharm. Mail Order: [X]
Physical Therapy: [X]   Podiatry: [X]
Psychiatric: [X]   Transplant: [X]
Vision: [X]   Wellness: [X]
Workers' Comp: [X]
Other Benefits:

Comments:
Formerly John Deere Health Plan, acquired by UnitedHealth on February 24, 2006. See Knoxville, TN for enrollment information.

UNITEDHEALTHCARE SERVICES COMPANY OF THE RIVER VALLEY INC

408 N Cedar Bluff Rd Ste 400
Knoxville, TN 37923
Phone: 865-690-5572 Fax: 865-690-2741 Toll-Free: 800-747-1446
Web site: www.uhcrivervalley.com

MAILING ADDRESS:
UHC OF THE RIVER VALLEY INC
1300 River Dr Ste 200
Moline, IL 37923

Managed Care Organization Profiles   **TENNESSEE**

Accreditation: [X] AAPPO [ ] JACHO [ ] NCQA [ ] URAC
Plan Type: PPO, ASO, TPA
Primary Physicians: 5,131   Physician Specialists: 13,537
Hospitals: 196
Total Enrollment:
   2001: 200,000   2004: 200,000   2007: 54,641
   2002: 0   2005: 87,000
   2003: 0   2006: 62,000

SERVICE AREA:
Nationwide: N
    TN; and bordering counties;

TYPE OF COVERAGE:
Commercial: [Y] Individual: [Y] FEHBP: [Y] Indemnity: [ ]
Medicare: [ ] Medicaid: [ ] Supplemental Medicare: [ ]
Tricare [ ]

PLAN BENEFITS:
Alternative Medicine: [ ]   Behavioral Health: [Y]
Chiropractic: [Y]   Dental: [ ]
Home Care: [Y]   Inpatient SNF: [Y]
Long-Term Care: [ ]   Pharm. Mail Order: [ ]
Physical Therapy: [Y]   Podiatry: [Y]
Psychiatric: [Y]   Transplant: [Y]
Vision: [ ]   Wellness: [Y]
Workers' Comp: [ ]
Other Benefits:

TENNESSEE BEHAVIORAL HEALTH INC

222 Second Ave N Ste 220
Nashville, TN 37201
Phone: 410-953-1643   Fax: 410-953-5205   Toll-Free:
Web site: www.magellanhealth.com

MAILING ADDRESS:
    TN BEHAVIORAL HEALTH INC
    222 Second Ave N Ste 220
    Nashville, TN 37201

KEY EXECUTIVES:
President .... *Russell C Petrella, PhD*
Secretary .... *Andrew M Cummings*

COMPANY PROFILE:
Parent Company Name: Magellan Health Services
Doing Business As:
Year Founded: 1996   Federally Qualified: [ ]
Forprofit: [ ]   Not-For-Profit: [ ]
Model Type:
Accreditation: [ ] AAPPO [ ] JACHO [ ] NCQA [ ] URAC
Plan Type: Specialty HMO
Total Revenue: 2005:   2006: 141,839,443
Net Income 2005:   2006: 9,103,010
Total Enrollment:
   2001: 0   2004: 0   2007: 595,458
   2002: 0   2005: 0
   2003: 0   2006: 592,465

SERVICE AREA:
Nationwide: N
    TN;

TYPE OF COVERAGE:
Commercial: [ ] Individual: [ ] FEHBP: [ ] Indemnity: [ ]
Medicare: [ ] Medicaid: [Y] Supplemental Medicare: [ ]
Tricare [ ]

PLAN BENEFITS:
Alternative Medicine: [ ]   Behavioral Health: [X]
Chiropractic: [ ]   Dental: [ ]
Home Care: [ ]   Inpatient SNF: [ ]
Long-Term Care: [ ]   Pharm. Mail Order: [ ]
Physical Therapy: [ ]   Podiatry: [ ]
Psychiatric: [ ]   Transplant: [ ]
Vision: [ ]   Wellness: [ ]
Workers' Comp: [ ]
Other Benefits:

TENNESSEE HEALTHCARE LLC

1620 Westgate Circle Ste 225
Brentwood, TN 37027
Phone: 615-301-4500   Fax: 615-301-4501   Toll-Free:
Web site: www.tennesseehealthcare.com

MAILING ADDRESS:
    TENNESSEE HEALTHCARE LLC
    1620 Westgate Circle Ste 225
    Brentwood, TN 37027

KEY EXECUTIVES:
President .... *Tom McElroy*
Marketing Director .... *Greg McNair*

COMPANY PROFILE:
Parent Company Name:
Doing Business As: Group Health PPO
Year Founded: 1994   Federally Qualified: [ ]
Forprofit: [ ]   Not-For-Profit: [ ]
Model Type:
Accreditation: [ ] AAPPO [ ] JACHO [ ] NCQA [ ] URAC
Plan Type: PPO
Primary Physicians: 9,000   Physician Specialists:
Hospitals: 145

SERVICE AREA:
Nationwide: N
    AL; AR; GA; MO MS; NC; TN; VA;

UAHC HEALTH PLAN OF TENNESSEE

1769 Paragon Dr Ste 100
Memphis, TN 38132
Phone: 901-346-0064   Fax: 901-346-1032   Toll-Free: 800-346-0034
Web site: www.ochptn.com

MAILING ADDRESS:
    UAHC HEALTH PLAN OF TENNESSEE
    1769 Paragon Dr Ste 100
    Memphis, TN 38132

KEY EXECUTIVES:
Chief Executive Officer .... *Stephanie Dowell*
Chief Financial Officer .... *Stephen Harris*
Medical Director .... *Melrose Blackett, MD*
VP, Information Services .... *Stacey Hill*

COMPANY PROFILE:
Parent Company Name: United American Healthcare Corp
Doing Business As:
Year Founded: 1994   Federally Qualified: [Y]
Forprofit: [Y]   Not-For-Profit: [ ]
Model Type:
Accreditation: [ ] AAPPO [ ] JACHO [ ] NCQA [ ] URAC
Plan Type: HMO,
Primary Physicians: 1,372   Physician Specialists:
Hospitals: 68
Total Revenue: 2005: 538,850   2006: 360,956
Net Income 2005: 1,683,187   2006: 965,071
Total Enrollment:
   2001: 79,739   2004: 114,000   2007: 315,611
   2002: 0   2005: 122,260
   2003: 130,492   2006: 1,418,559
Medical Loss Ratio: 2005: 215.00   2006:
Administrative Expense Ratio: 2005:   2006:

SERVICE AREA:
Nationwide: N
    TN (Benton, Carroll, Chester, Crockett, Decatur, Dyer, Fayette, Gibson, Hardin, Hardeman, Haywood, Henderson, Henry, Lake, Lauderdale, Madison, McNairy, Shelby, Tipton, Weakley);

TYPE OF COVERAGE:
Commercial: [Y] Individual: [ ] FEHBP: [ ] Indemnity: [ ]
Medicare: [Y] Medicaid: [Y] Supplemental Medicare: [ ]
Tricare [ ]

PRODUCTS OFFERED:
Product Name: Type:
TennCare   Medicaid

Comments:
Formerly OmniCare Health Plan Inc.

UNISON HEALTH PLAN OF TENNESSEE

1000 Ridgeway Loop Rd Ste 203
Memphis, TN 38120
Phone: 412-858-4000   Fax: 412-457-1414   Toll-Free: 800-400-4003
Web site: www.unisonhealthplan.com

TENNESSEE
Managed Care Organization Profiles

PLAN BENEFITS:
Alternative Medicine:	[ ]	Behavioral Health:	[X]
Chiropractic:	[X]	Dental:	[X]
Home Care:	[X]	Inpatient SNF:	[X]
Long-Term Care:	[X]	Pharm. Mail Order:	[X]
Physical Therapy:	[X]	Podiatry:	[X]
Psychiatric:	[X]	Transplant:	[X]
Vision:	[X]	Wellness:	[X]
Workers' Comp:	[X]		

Other Benefits:

PREMIER BEHAVIORAL SYSTEMS OF TENNESSEE LLC

222 Second Ave N Ste 220
Nashville, TN 37201
Phone: 410-953-1643 Fax: 410-953-5205 Toll-Free:
Web site: www.magellanhealth.com

MAILING ADDRESS:
PREMIER BEHAVIORAL SYSTEMS OF TN LLC
222 Second Ave N Ste 220
Nashville, TN 37201

KEY EXECUTIVES:
President .... Russell C Petrella, PhD
Director .... William R Grimm

COMPANY PROFILE:
Parent Company Name: Magellan Health Services
Doing Business As:
Year Founded: 1996   Federally Qualified: [ ]
Forprofit: [ ]   Not-For-Profit: [ ]
Model Type:
Accreditation: [ ] AAPPO [ ] JACHO [ ] NCQA [ ] URAC
Plan Type: Specialty HMO
Total Revenue: 2005:   2006: 162,268,312
Net Income   2005:   2006: 12,792,111
Total Enrollment:
   2001: 0   2004: 0   2007: 245,749
   2002: 0   2005: 0
   2003: 0   2006: 606,786

SERVICE AREA:
Nationwide: N
   TN;

PRODUCTS OFFERED:
Product Name: Type:
TENNCare   Medicaid

TYPE OF COVERAGE:
Commercial: [ ] Individual: [ ] FEHBP: [ ] Indemnity: [ ]
Medicare: [ ] Medicaid: [Y]   Supplemental Medicare: [ ]
Tricare   [ ]

PLAN BENEFITS:
Alternative Medicine:	[ ]	Behavioral Health:	[X]
Chiropractic:	[ ]	Dental:	[ ]
Home Care:	[ ]	Inpatient SNF:	[ ]
Long-Term Care:	[ ]	Pharm. Mail Order:	[ ]
Physical Therapy:	[ ]	Podiatry:	[ ]
Psychiatric:	[ ]	Transplant:	[ ]
Vision:	[ ]	Wellness:	[ ]
Workers' Comp:	[ ]		

Other Benefits:

PRIME HEALTH SERVICES INC

7110 Crossroads Blvd Ste 100
Brentwood, TN 37027
Phone: 615-329-4098 Fax: 615-329-4751 Toll-Free: 866-348-3887
Web site: www.prime-health.net

MAILING ADDRESS:
PRIME HEALTH SERVICES INC
7110 Crossroads Blvd Ste 100
Brentwood, TN 37027

KEY EXECUTIVES:
Chief Executive Officer/President ... Brian A Sharp, MEd, CCM, CDMS
Medical Director .... Gilbert Woodall, Jr, MD
Chief Information Technology .... Brandon Sharp
VP of Business Development .... Bryan Hunziker, BS, MS
Senior Director Network Development .... Dorrence B Stovall
Director of Network Development .... Nicki Jolly
Credentialing Representative .... Tanya Ziebarth
Director of Business Development .... Bethany Cook
Account Manager .... Jennifer Pitoscia

COMPANY PROFILE:
Parent Company Name: Prime Health Services Inc
Doing Business As:
Year Founded: 1995   Federally Qualified: [N]
Forprofit: [Y]   Not-For-Profit: [ ]
Model Type: NETWORK
Accreditation: [ ] AAPPO [ ] JACHO [ ] NCQA [ ] URAC
Plan Type: PPO, EPO, CDHP, HSA
Primary Physicians: 125,000   Physician Specialists:
Hospitals: 2,500
Total Enrollment:
   2001: 0   2004: 1,500,000   2007: 0
   2002: 600,000   2005: 5,000,000
   2003: 0   2006:

SERVICE AREA:
Nationwide:
   NW;

TYPE OF COVERAGE:
Commercial: [Y] Individual: [ ] FEHBP: [ ] Indemnity: [ ]
Medicare: [ ] Medicaid: [ ]   Supplemental Medicare: [ ]
Tricare   [ ]

PRODUCTS OFFERED:
Product Name: Type:
Prime Health Services   PPO

CONSUMER-DRIVEN PRODUCTS
                                 HSA Company
                                 HSA Product
                                 HSA Administrator
Prime Discount Care Program   Consumer-Driven Health Plan
Prime Discount Care Program   High Deductible Health Plan

PLAN BENEFITS:
Alternative Medicine:	[ ]	Behavioral Health:	[X]
Chiropractic:	[X]	Dental:	[ ]
Home Care:	[X]	Inpatient SNF:	[X]
Long-Term Care:	[X]	Pharm. Mail Order:	[X]
Physical Therapy:	[X]	Podiatry:	[X]
Psychiatric:	[X]	Transplant:	[X]
Vision:	[X]	Wellness:	[X]
Workers' Comp:	[X]		

Other Benefits: Workers' Comp Pharmacy

SIGNATURE HEALTH ALLIANCE

44 Vantage Way Ste 410
Nashville, TN 37228
Phone: 615-401-4674 Fax: 615-401-4530 Toll-Free: 800-264-3060
Web site: www.signaturehealth.com

MAILING ADDRESS:
SIGNATURE HEALTH ALLIANCE
44 Vantage Way Ste 410
Nashville, TN 37228

KEY EXECUTIVES:
Chief Executive Officer .... Herbert A Fritch
President .... M Shawn Morris
Chief Financial Officer .... Kevin McNamara
Chief Medical Director .... Hardy Sorkin, MD
Chief Information Officer .... Andy Flatt
Chief Operating Officer .... Greg Allen
VP, Sales & Marketing .... Scott Clark
Credentialing Manager .... Lori Pegler
Manager, PPO Operations .... Victoria Prendergast
VP, Human Resources .... Sonny Terrill
Credentialing Manager .... Lori Pegler

COMPANY PROFILE:
Parent Company Name: HealthSpring of Tennessee
Doing Business As: Signature Health Alliance
Year Founded: 1985   Federally Qualified: [ ]
Forprofit: [Y]   Not-For-Profit: [ ]
Model Type: NETWORK

Managed Care Organization Profiles

TENNESSEE

COMPANY PROFILE:
Parent Company Name:
Doing Business As:
Year Founded: 1992   Federally Qualified: [ ]
Forprofit: [Y]   Not-For-Profit: [ ]
Model Type:
Accreditation: [X] AAPPO [ ] JACHO [X] NCQA [X] URAC
Plan Type: Specialty PPO, UM
Total Enrollment:
    2001: 5,000,000   2004: 0   2007: 0
    2002: 0   2005:
    2003: 0   2006:
SERVICE AREA:
Nationwide: Y
    NW;
PLAN BENEFITS:
Alternative Medicine:	[ ]	Behavioral Health:	[ ]
Chiropractic:	[ ]	Dental:	[ ]
Home Care:	[ ]	Inpatient SNF:	[ ]
Long-Term Care:	[ ]	Pharm. Mail Order:	[ ]
Physical Therapy:	[ ]	Podiatry:	[ ]
Psychiatric:	[ ]	Transplant:	[ ]
Vision:	[ ]	Wellness:	[ ]
Workers' Comp:	[ ]		

Other Benefits: Radiology

MEMPHIS MANAGED CARE CORP

1407 Union Ave Ste 210
Memphis, TN 38104
Phone: 901-725-7100 Fax: 901-725-2846 Toll-Free: 800-473-6523
Web site: www.mmcc-tlc.com
MAILING ADDRESS:
    MEMPHIS MANAGED CARE CORP
    1407 Union Ave Ste 210
    Memphis, TN 38104

KEY EXECUTIVES:
Chief Executive Officer/President .... Al King
Chief Financial Officer .... Jim Proctor
Medical Director .... Clarence Davis, Jr, MD
Director Disease Management .... Mark Stephens, PharmD
VP Administration/IS .... Michael Scarbrough
VP Operations .... Michael Jones
Director Information Systems .... Jarrel Thomas
Director Provider Relations .... Latasha Jones
Human Resources Director .... Kathy London
Director of Medical Management .... Edna Willingham
Quality Assurance Director .... Linda Bedrin
Fraud Prevention .... Art Ansert
Director Claims & Customer Service .... Michael Jones
VP of Medical Management .... Jamie Patterson
Director of Project & Process Improvement .... Steven Jenkins

COMPANY PROFILE:
Parent Company Name:
Doing Business As: TLC Family Care Health Plan
Year Founded: 1993   Federally Qualified: [ ]
Forprofit: [ ]   Not-For-Profit: [Y]
Model Type: NETWORK
Accreditation: [ ] AAPPO [ ] JACHO [ ] NCQA [ ] URAC
Plan Type: HMO
Primary Physicians: 3,500   Physician Specialists:
Hospitals:
Total Revenue: 2005:   2006:
Net Income   2005: 7,972,686   2006: 3,629,387
Total Enrollment:
    2001: 172,182   2004: 0   2007: 169,542
    2002: 0   2005: 2,246,795
    2003: 190,282   2006: 2,054,603
SERVICE AREA:
Nationwide: N
    21 counties in West Tennessee.
TYPE OF COVERAGE:
Commercial: [ ] Individual: [ ] FEHBP: [ ] Indemnity: [ ]
Medicare: [ ] Medicaid: [Y] Supplemental Medicare: [ ]
Tricare [ ]
PRODUCTS OFFERED:
Product Name: Type:
TLC Family Care Healthplan   HMO-Medicaid

PLAN BENEFITS:
Alternative Medicine:	[ ]	Behavioral Health:	[ ]
Chiropractic:	[ ]	Dental:	[X]
Home Care:	[X]	Inpatient SNF:	[ ]
Long-Term Care:	[ ]	Pharm. Mail Order:	[ ]
Physical Therapy:	[ ]	Podiatry:	[ ]
Psychiatric:	[ ]	Transplant:	[ ]
Vision:	[X]	Wellness:	[X]
Workers' Comp:	[ ]		

Other Benefits:
Comments:
TLC Family Care Healthplan is a Medicaid HMO.

PHP COMPANIES INC

1420 Centerpoint Blvd
Knoxville, TN 37932
Phone: 865-470-7460 Fax: 865-670-7255 Toll-Free: 800-793-1495
Web site: www.phpcompanies.com
MAILING ADDRESS:
    PHP COMPANIES INC
    1420 Centerpoint Blvd
    Knoxville, TN 37932

KEY EXECUTIVES:
Chief Executive Officer/President .... Lance Hunsinger
Chief Financial Officer .... Jeff Collake
Chief Medical Officer .... George Andrews, MD
Chief Operating Officer .... Doug Haaland
Director, Marketing .... Christy Newman
VP, MIS/Chief Information Officer Health Plan .... Barry Robbins
Manager Credentialing .... Vicki Weaver
Risk Analyst, Privacy Officer .... Mary Cogar
Director, Provider Services .... Pat Gillespie
Manager, Network Development .... Jonathan Wright
Director Medical Management .... Suzy Hanson
Director Quality Improvement .... Mary Woolley
Manager Credentialing .... Vicki Weaver
Investigations Specialist Coordinator .... Beverly Brown
Executive Director/Compliance Officer .... Peggy McCurry

COMPANY PROFILE:
Parent Company Name: Covenant Health Systems;
                     Mountain States Health Alliance
Doing Business As: Preferred Health Partnership, Cariten H
Year Founded: 1985   Federally Qualified: [Y]
Forprofit: [Y]   Not-For-Profit: [ ]
Model Type: NETWORK
Accreditation: [ ] AAPPO [ ] JACHO [X] NCQA [ ] URAC
Plan Type: HMO, PPO, POS, HDHP, TPA
Primary Physicians: 2,685   Physician Specialists: 10,227
Hospitals: 69
Total Revenue: 2005: 380,778,093   2006: 567,676,696
Net Income   2005: 27,257,079   2006: 23,562,373
Total Enrollment:
    2001: 117,787   2004: 645,600   2007: 596,464
    2002: 0   2005: 621,500
    2003: 129,238   2006: 614,286
Medical Loss Ratio: 2005: 86.60   2006: 90.50
Administrative Expense Ratio: 2005: 15.90   2006: 11.40
SERVICE AREA:
Nationwide: N
    TN (Anderson, Bedford, Benton, Bledsoe, Blount, Bradley,
    Campbell, Carroll, Carter, Cheatham, Claiborne, Cocke, Coffee,
    Crockett, Dickson, Dyer, Franklin, Gibson, Giles, Grainger, Greene,
    Grundy, Hamblen, Hamilton, Hancock, Hawkins, Henry, Hickman,
    Houston, Humphreys, Jefferson, Johnson, Knox, Lake, Lawrence,
    Lincoln, Loudon, Marion, Marshall, Maury, McMinn, Meigs,
    Monroe, Montgomery, Moore, Morgan, Obion, Perry, Polk,
    Rhea, Roane, Robertson, Rutherford, Scott, Sequatchie, Sevier,
    Shelby, Stewart, Sullivan, Sumner, Trousdale, Unicoi, Union,
    Washington, Wayne, Weakley, Williamson, Wilson); GA; VA;
TYPE OF COVERAGE:
Commercial: [Y] Individual: [Y] FEHBP: [ ] Indemnity: [ ]
Medicare: [Y] Medicaid: [Y] Supplemental Medicare: [ ]
Tricare [ ]
PRODUCTS OFFERED:
Product Name: Type:
Preferred Health Partnership   Medicaid

TENNESSEE

Year Founded: 2000
Forprofit: [Y]
Model Type:
Accreditation: [ ] AAPPO [ ] JACHO [ ] NCQA [ ] URAC
Plan Type: HMO, PPO, UR, POS, TPA, EPO
Primary Physicians: 1,439   Physician Specialists: 4,368
Hospitals: 57
Total Enrollment:
  2001: 350,909   2004: 0   2007: 61,556
  2002: 0   2005: 143,050
  2003: 0   2006: 75,602

Federally Qualified: [N]
Not-For-Profit: [ ]

SERVICE AREA:
Nationwide: N
  AL; FL; IL; MS; TN; TX;

TYPE OF COVERAGE:
Commercial: [Y] Individual: [ ] FEHBP: [ ] Indemnity: [ ]
Medicare: [Y] Medicaid: [ ] Supplemental Medicare: [ ]
Tricare [ ]

PLAN BENEFITS:
Alternative Medicine: [ ]   Behavioral Health: [ ]
Chiropractic: [X]   Dental: [ ]
Home Care: [ ]   Inpatient SNF: [ ]
Long-Term Care: [ ]   Pharm. Mail Order: [ ]
Physical Therapy: [ ]   Podiatry: [X]
Psychiatric: [ ]   Transplant: [ ]
Vision: [ ]   Wellness: [ ]
Workers' Comp: [X]
Other Benefits:

HUMANA INC - TENNESSEE

6075 Poplar Ave Ste 221
Memphis, TN 38119
Phone: 901-685-8351 Fax: 901-685-0194 Toll-Free:
Web site: www.humana.com

MAILING ADDRESS:
  HUMANA INC - TENNESSEE
  PO Box 740036
  Louisville, KY 38119

KEY EXECUTIVES:
Chairman of the Board .... David A Jones Jr
Chief Executive Officer/President .... Michael B McCallister
Market President .... C Evans Looney
Chief Financial Officer .... James H Bloem
VP, Medical Director .... Jonathan T Lord, MD
Senior VP, Chief Information Officer .... Bruce J Goodman
Manager of Sales .... Bryan Wenger
Senior VP, Human Resources .... Bonnie C Hathrock
ChoiceCare Area Director .... Jane Raymond
Manager of Sales Administration .... Jo Ellen Seyerle

COMPANY PROFILE:
Parent Company Name: Humana Inc
Doing Business As:
Year Founded: 1961   Federally Qualified: [Y]
Forprofit: [Y]   Not-For-Profit: [ ]
Model Type: IPA
Accreditation: [ ] AAPPO [ ] JACHO [ ] NCQA [X] URAC
Plan Type: PPO, ASO, CDHP, HDHP, HSA,
Total Enrollment:
  2001: 0   2004: 0   2007: 0
  2002: 35,000   2005:
  2003: 131,000   2006:

SERVICE AREA:
Nationwide: N
  TN (Bradley, Cocke, Davidson, DeKalb, Grainger, Hamblen, Hamilton, Hancock, Hawkins, Jefferson, Macon, Smith, Shelby, Tipton, Trousdale, Wilson)

TYPE OF COVERAGE:
Commercial: [Y] Individual: [ ] FEHBP: [ ] Indemnity: [ ]
Medicare: [ ] Medicaid: [ ] Supplemental Medicare: [Y]
Tricare [Y]

CONSUMER-DRIVEN PRODUCTS
JP Morgan Chase   HSA Company
HumanaOne HSA   HSA Product
JP Morgan Chase   HSA Administrator
Personal Care Account   Consumer-Driven Health Plan
HumanaOne   High Deductible Health Plan

PLAN BENEFITS:
Alternative Medicine: [ ]   Behavioral Health: [X]
Chiropractic: [X]   Dental: [X]
Home Care: [ ]   Inpatient SNF: [ ]
Long-Term Care: [ ]   Pharm. Mail Order: [X]
Physical Therapy: [ ]   Podiatry: [ ]
Psychiatric: [X]   Transplant: [X]
Vision: [ ]   Wellness: [ ]
Workers' Comp: [X]
Other Benefits: Long Term Disability Care

INITIAL GROUP INC, THE

95 Whitebridge Rd Ste 317
Nashville, TN 37205
Phone: 615-352-8721 Fax: 615-352-8782 Toll-Free: 866-571-0933
Web site: www.initialgroup.com

MAILING ADDRESS:
  INITIAL GROUP INC, THE
  95 Whitebridge Rd Ste 317
  Nashville, TN 37205

KEY EXECUTIVES:
Chief Executive Officer .... Carl Papp
President, Chief Operating Officer .... Mike Miller
Medical Director .... Robert C Ripley, MD

COMPANY PROFILE:
Parent Company Name:
Doing Business As:
Year Founded: 1991   Federally Qualified: [N]
Forprofit: [Y]   Not-For-Profit: [ ]
Model Type: NETWORK
Accreditation: [ ] AAPPO [ ] JACHO [ ] NCQA [ ] URAC
Plan Type: PPO, POS
Primary Physicians: 1,721   Physician Specialists: 4,257
Hospitals: 68
Total Enrollment:
  2001: 94,702   2004: 110,000   2007: 0
  2002: 117,636   2005:
  2003: 130,000   2006:

SERVICE AREA:
Nationwide: N
  TN (Eastern & national access);

TYPE OF COVERAGE:
Commercial: [Y] Individual: [Y] FEHBP: [ ] Indemnity: [ ]
Medicare: [ ] Medicaid: [ ] Supplemental Medicare: [ ]
Tricare [ ]

PRODUCTS OFFERED:
Product Name: Type:
Initial Group   PPO

PLAN BENEFITS:
Alternative Medicine: [ ]   Behavioral Health: [X]
Chiropractic: [X]   Dental: [X]
Home Care: [X]   Inpatient SNF: [X]
Long-Term Care: [X]   Pharm. Mail Order: [ ]
Physical Therapy: [X]   Podiatry: [X]
Psychiatric: [X]   Transplant: [X]
Vision: [X]   Wellness: [X]
Workers' Comp: [X]
Other Benefits:

MEDSOLUTIONS

730 Cool Springs Blvd Ste 800
Franklin, TN 37067
Phone: 615-468-4000 Fax: 615-468-4001 Toll-Free: 800-467-6424
Web site: www.medsolutions.com

MAILING ADDRESS:
  MEDSOLUTIONS
  730 Cool Springs Blvd Ste 800
  Franklin, TN 37067

KEY EXECUTIVES:
Chief Executive Officer/President .... Curt Thorne
Chief Financial Officer .... Steve Mengert
Medical Director .... Gregg Allen, MD
Chief Information Officer .... Steve Wise
Executive VP, Sales & Marketing .... Steve Janicak
VP, Account Management .... David Smith
VP, Sales .... Suzanne M Kane

Managed Care Organization Profiles — TENNESSEE

Forprofit: [ ] Not-For-Profit: [Y]
Model Type: GROUP
Accreditation: [ ] AAPPO [ ] JACHO [ ] NCQA [ ] URAC
Plan Type: PPO, Specialty PPO, POS, ASO,
Total Revenue: 2005: 161,628,783 2006: 189,129,661
Net Income 2005: 2006:
Total Enrollment:
  2001: 0   2004: 693,000   2007: 0
  2002: 0   2005: 697,000
  2003: 0   2006: 788,000

SERVICE AREA:
Nationwide: N
  TN;
TYPE OF COVERAGE:
Commercial: [Y] Individual: [ ] FEHBP: [ ] Indemnity: [ ]
Medicare: [ ] Medicaid: [ ] Supplemental Medicare: [ ]
Tricare [ ]
CONSUMER-DRIVEN PRODUCTS
                      HSA Company
                      HSA Product
First Tennessee   HSA Administrator
                      Consumer-Driven Health Plan
                      High Deductible Health Plan

PLAN BENEFITS:
Alternative Medicine: [ ]   Behavioral Health: [ ]
Chiropractic: [ ]   Dental: [X]
Home Care: [ ]   Inpatient SNF: [ ]
Long-Term Care: [ ]   Pharm. Mail Order: [ ]
Physical Therapy: [ ]   Podiatry: [ ]
Psychiatric: [ ]   Transplant: [ ]
Vision: [ ]   Wellness: [ ]
Workers' Comp: [ ]
Other Benefits:

HEALTHNOW

5959 Park Ave
Memphis, TN 38119
Phone: 901-765-3190 Fax: 901-765-3179 Toll-Free:
Web site: www.saintfrancishosp.com
MAILING ADDRESS:
  HEALTHNOW
  5959 Park Ave
  Memphis, TN 38119

KEY EXECUTIVES:
Chief Executive Officer .... David Archer
Chief Financial Officer .... Edwin Bode
Chief Information Officer/MIS Director .... Michael Hadley
Marketing Director .... Marilyn Robinson
Human Resources Director .... Laura Adler
Director, Quality Assurance/Case Management .... Brenda Ray
VP, Managed Care/Compliance Officer .... Delores Voigt

COMPANY PROFILE:
Parent Company Name: Tenet Health Care
Doing Business As: St Francis Hospital
Year Founded: 1974   Federally Qualified: [ ]
Forprofit: [Y]   Not-For-Profit: [ ]
Model Type:
Accreditation: [ ] AAPPO [X] JACHO [X] NCQA [ ] URAC
Plan Type: HMO, PPO
SERVICE AREA:
Nationwide: N
  TN;
TYPE OF COVERAGE:
Commercial: [Y] Individual: [Y] FEHBP: [ ] Indemnity: [ ]
Medicare: [Y] Medicaid: [Y] Supplemental Medicare: [Y]
Tricare [ ]
PLAN BENEFITS:
Alternative Medicine: [ ]   Behavioral Health: [X]
Chiropractic: [ ]   Dental: [ ]
Home Care: [X]   Inpatient SNF: [ ]
Long-Term Care: [ ]   Pharm. Mail Order: [ ]
Physical Therapy: [ ]   Podiatry: [ ]
Psychiatric: [X]   Transplant: [ ]
Vision: [ ]   Wellness: [ ]
Workers' Comp: [ ]
Other Benefits: Full Service Hospital

HEALTHSPRING INC- CORPORATE HEADQUARTERS

9009 Carothers Pkwy Ste 501
Franklin, TN 37067
Phone: 615-236-6100 Fax: Toll-Free: 800-243-2336
Web site: www.healthspring.com
MAILING ADDRESS:
  HEALTHSPRING INC - CORP HDQTRS
  9009 Carothers Pkwy Ste 501
  Franklin, TN 37067

KEY EXECUTIVES:
Chairman/Chief Executive Officer .... Herbert A Fritch
President .... Herbert A Fritch
Executive VP, Chief Operating Officer .... Gerald V Coil
Executive VP, Chief Financial Officer .... Kevin M McNamara
Senior VP, Chief Marketing Officer .... Craig S Schub
Senior VP, Corporate General Counsel .... J Gentry Barden
Senior VP, Chief Actuary .... David L Terry, Jr
Senior VP, Managed Care Operations .... Mark A Tulloch
Senior VP, Chief Medical Officer .... Dirk O Wales, MD

COMPANY PROFILE:
Parent Company Name:
Doing Business As:
Year Founded: 2000   Federally Qualified: [N]
Forprofit: [Y]   Not-For-Profit: [ ]
Model Type:
Accreditation: [ ] AAPPO [ ] JACHO [ ] NCQA [ ] URAC
Plan Type: HMO, PPO, UR, POS, TPA, EPO
Primary Physicians: 3,800   Physician Specialists: 10,828
Hospitals: 202
Total Revenue: 2005: 857,000,000 2006: 1,308,956,000
Net Income   2005:   2006: 80,836,000
Total Enrollment:
  2001: 350,909   2004: 0   2007: 164,998
  2002: 0   2005: 143,050
  2003: 0   2006: 147,102
Medical Loss Ratio: 2005: 78.40 2006: 78.80
Administrative Expense Ratio: 2005:   2006:
SERVICE AREA:
Nationwide: N
  AL; FL; IL; MS; TN; TX;
TYPE OF COVERAGE:
Commercial: [Y] Individual: [ ] FEHBP: [ ] Indemnity: [ ]
Medicare: [Y] Medicaid: [ ] Supplemental Medicare: [ ]
Tricare [ ]
PLAN BENEFITS:
Alternative Medicine: [ ]   Behavioral Health: [ ]
Chiropractic: [X]   Dental: [ ]
Home Care: [ ]   Inpatient SNF: [ ]
Long-Term Care: [ ]   Pharm. Mail Order: [ ]
Physical Therapy: [ ]   Podiatry: [X]
Psychiatric: [ ]   Transplant: [ ]
Vision: [ ]   Wellness: [ ]
Workers' Comp: [X]
Other Benefits: Auto

HEALTHSPRING INC - TENNESSEE

44 Vantage Way Ste 300
Nashville, TN 37228
Phone: 615-291-7000 Fax: 615-291-2664 Toll-Free: 866-206-5565
Web site: www.myhealthspring.com
MAILING ADDRESS:
  HEALTHSPRING INC - TENNESSEE
  44 Vantage Way Ste 300
  Nashville, TN 37228

KEY EXECUTIVES:
Chairman/Chief Executive Officer .... Herbert A Fritch
President .... Shawn Morris
Executive VP, Chief Operating Officer .... Gerald V Coil
Executive VP, Chief Financial Officer .... Kevin M McNamara
Senior VP, Chief Marketing Officer .... Craig S Schub
Senior VP, Corporate General Counsel .... J Gentry Barden
Senior VP, Chief Actuary .... David L Terry, Jr
Senior VP, Managed Care Operations .... Mark A Tulloch
Senior VP, Chief Medical Officer .... Dirk O Wales, MD

COMPANY PROFILE:
Parent Company Name: HealthSpring Inc
Doing Business As:

TENNESSEE

KEY EXECUTIVES:
Regional Director .... Melissa Bode

COMPANY PROFILE:
Parent Company Name: CIGNA Corporation
Doing Business As:
Year Founded: 1987   Federally Qualified: [Y]
Forprofit: [Y]   Not-For-Profit: [ ]
Model Type: IPA
Accreditation: [ ] AAPPO [ ] JACHO [X] NCQA [ ] URAC
Plan Type: HMO, PPO, POS, CDHP, HDHP, HSA,
Total Enrollment:
   2001: 0   2004: 0   2007: 0
   2002: 72,831   2005:
   2003: 85,399   2006:

SERVICE AREA:
Nationwide: N
   AR; MS (DeSoto); TN (Fayette, Shelby, Tipton);

TYPE OF COVERAGE:
Commercial: [Y] Individual: [ ] FEHBP: [ ] Indemnity: [ ]
Medicare: [ ] Medicaid: [ ] Supplemental Medicare: [ ]
Tricare   [ ]

PRODUCTS OFFERED:
Product Name: Type:
Cigna Healthcare HMO   HMO
Cigna Healthcare for Seniors
CONSUMER-DRIVEN PRODUCTS
JP Morgan Chase   HSA Company
CIGNA Choice Fund   HSA Product
                                 HSA Administrator
Open Access Plus   Consumer-Driven Health Plan
PPO   High Deductible Health Plan

PLAN BENEFITS:
Alternative Medicine: [ ]   Behavioral Health: [X]
Chiropractic: [X]   Dental: [X]
Home Care: [X]   Inpatient SNF: [X]
Long-Term Care: [X]   Pharm. Mail Order: [X]
Physical Therapy: [X]   Podiatry: [X]
Psychiatric: [X]   Transplant: [X]
Vision: [X]   Wellness: [X]
Workers' Comp: [ ]
Other Benefits:

CIGNA HEALTHCARE OF TENNESSEE INC

1000 Corporate Ctr Dr Ste 500
Franklin, TN 37067
Phone: 615-595-3000 Fax: 615-595-3287 Toll-Free: 800-492-2224
Web site: www.cigna.com
MAILING ADDRESS:
   CIGNA HEALTHCARE OF TN INC
   1000 Corporate Ctr Dr Ste 500
   Franklin, TN 37067

KEY EXECUTIVES:
Chief Executive Officer .... H Edward Hanway
President .... John W Sorrow

COMPANY PROFILE:
Parent Company Name: CIGNA Corporation
Doing Business As:
Year Founded: 1985   Federally Qualified: [ ]
Forprofit: [Y]   Not-For-Profit: [ ]
Model Type:
Accreditation: [ ] AAPPO [ ] JACHO [X] NCQA [ ] URAC
Plan Type: HMO, POS, CDHP, HDHP, HSA, FSA, HRA
Total Enrollment:
   2001: 83,406   2004: 81,582   2007: 0
   2002: 72,831   2005:
   2003: 85,399   2006:

SERVICE AREA:
Nationwide: N
   TN; (Anderson, Bledsoe, Blount, Bradley, Cannon, Campbell,
   Carter, Cheatham, Coffee, Claiborne, Cocke, Davidson, DeKalb,
   Dickson, Fayette, Franklin, Grainger, Greene, Hamblen, Hamilton,
   Hancock, Hawkins, Hickman, Jefferson, Johnson, Knox, Loudon,
   Macon, Marion, Maury, McKinn, Meigs, Monroe, Montgomery,
   Morgan, Overton, Polk, Rhea, Roane, Robertson, Rutherford,
   Scott, Sequatchie, Sevier, Shelby, Smith, Sullivan, Sumner, Tipton,
   Unicoi, Union, Warren, Washington Williamson, Wilson).

TYPE OF COVERAGE:
Commercial: [Y] Individual: [ ] FEHBP: [ ] Indemnity: [ ]
Medicare: [ ] Medicaid: [ ] Supplemental Medicare: [ ]
Tricare   [ ]

PRODUCTS OFFERED:
Product Name: Type:
Cigna Healthcare HMO   HMO
FlexCare   Exclusive Provider
Cigna Health Access
FlexCare   Designated Provider
Cigna Healthcare for Seniors   Medicare
CONSUMER-DRIVEN PRODUCTS
JP Morgan Chase   HSA Company
CIGNA Choice Fund   HSA Product
                                 HSA Administrator
Open Access Plus   Consumer-Driven Health Plan
PPO   High Deductible Health Plan

PLAN BENEFITS:
Alternative Medicine: [ ]   Behavioral Health: [X]
Chiropractic: [X]   Dental: [X]
Home Care: [X]   Inpatient SNF: [ ]
Long-Term Care: [X]   Pharm. Mail Order: [X]
Physical Therapy: [ ]   Podiatry: [ ]
Psychiatric: [X]   Transplant: [X]
Vision: [X]   Wellness: [X]
Workers' Comp: [ ]
Other Benefits:

COVENTRY HEALTHCARE

720 Cool Springs Blvd Ste 300
Franklin, TN 37067
Phone: 615-778-4000 Fax: 615-778-0915 Toll-Free: 800-243-2336
Web site: www.cvty.com
MAILING ADDRESS:
   COVENTRY HEALTHCARE
   720 Cool Springs Blvd Ste 300
   Franklin, TN 37067

KEY EXECUTIVES:
Chief Executive Officer/President .... Dale B Wolf
Chief Medical Officer .... Dwight Robertson, MD

COMPANY PROFILE:
Parent Company Name:
Doing Business As:
Year Founded: 1986   Federally Qualified: [N]
Forprofit: [Y]   Not-For-Profit: [ ]
Model Type:
Accreditation: [ ] AAPPO [ ] JACHO [ ] NCQA [ ] URAC
Plan Type: PPO

SERVICE AREA:
Nationwide: N
   TN;

TYPE OF COVERAGE:
Commercial: [Y] Individual: [ ] FEHBP: [ ] Indemnity: [ ]
Medicare: [ ] Medicaid: [ ] Supplemental Medicare: [ ]
Tricare   [ ]

DELTA DENTAL PLAN OF TENNESSEE

240 Venture Circle
Nashville, TN 37228
Phone: 615-255-3175 Fax: 615-244-8108 Toll-Free: 800-223-3104
Web site: www.deltadentaltn.com
MAILING ADDRESS:
   DELTA DENTAL PLAN OF TN
   240 Venture Circle
   Nashville, TN 37228

KEY EXECUTIVES:
Chairman of the Board .... John Collier
Chief Executive Officer/President .... Philip Wenk, DDS
Senior VP, Chief Financial Officer .... J Thomas Perry
Senior VP, Operations .... Liz Cheek
Senior VP Marketing .... Charles N Young
VP Underwriting .... Jay Reavis
VP Professional Relations .... Dr Henry Ramer
Senior VP, Human Resources .... Pam Dishman

COMPANY PROFILE:
Parent Company Name: Delta Dental Plan Association
Doing Business As:
Year Founded: 1965   Federally Qualified: [N]

Managed Care Organization Profiles — TENNESSEE

CONSUMER-DRIVEN PRODUCTS
HSA Company
HSA Product
HSA Administrator
BluePartner   Consumer-Driven Health Plan
                      High Deductible Health Plan

PLAN BENEFITS:
Alternative Medicine:	[ ]	Behavioral Health:	[ ]
Chiropractic:	[X]	Dental:	[X]
Home Care:	[X]	Inpatient SNF:	[X]
Long-Term Care:	[ ]	Pharm. Mail Order:	[X]
Physical Therapy:	[X]	Podiatry:	[ ]
Psychiatric:	[X]	Transplant:	[X]
Vision:	[X]	Wellness:	[X]
Workers' Comp:	[ ]		

Other Benefits:
Comments:
Formerly Southern Health Plan Inc.

BLUE CROSS BLUE SHIELD OF TENNESSEE - MEMPHIS

85 N Danny Thomas Blvd
Memphis, TN 38103-2398
Phone: 901-544-2226 Fax: 901-544-2220 Toll-Free:
Web site: www.bcbst.com

MAILING ADDRESS:
BC/BS OF TENNESSEE - MEMPHIS
85 N Danny Thomas Blvd
Memphis, TN 38103-2398

KEY EXECUTIVES:
Chairman of the Board .... Herbert H Hilliard
Chief Executive Officer/President .... Vicky Gregg
Chief Financial Officer .... David Deal
Chief Medical Officer .... Steven Coulter, MD
Chief Public Relations Director .... Calvin Anderson
Chief Marketing Officer .... Joan Harp
Director, Provider Services .... Whit Deacon
Network Development Director .... Mark Austin
Chief Human Resources Officer .... Dan Blomberg
Senior VP, General Counsel .... Bill Young

COMPANY PROFILE:
Parent Company Name: BC & BS of Tennessee
Doing Business As:
Year Founded: 1981   Federally Qualified: [Y] Forprofit: [ ]
Not-For-Profit: [Y]
Model Type: IPA
Accreditation: [ ] AAPPO [ ] JACHO [ ] NCQA [ ] URAC
Plan Type: HMO, PPO, POS, HDHP, HSA,
Total Enrollment:
   2001: 775,332   2004: 955,890   2007: 0
   2002: 824,451   2005:
   2003: 847,594   2006:

SERVICE AREA:
Nationwide: N
TN;

TYPE OF COVERAGE:
Commercial: [Y] Individual: [Y] FEHBP: [ ] Indemnity: [ ]
Medicare: [Y] Medicaid: [ ] Supplemental Medicare: [Y]
Tricare: [ ]

Comments:
Formerly Memphis Hospital Services Surgical Association.

CARITEN HEALTHCARE

1420 Centerpoint Blvd
Knoxville, TN 37932
Phone: 865-470-7470 Fax: 865-670-7255 Toll-Free: 800-793-1495
Web site: www.cariten.com

MAILING ADDRESS:
CARITEN HEALTHCARE
1420 Centerpoint Blvd
Knoxville, TN 37932

KEY EXECUTIVES:
Chief Executive Officer/President .... Lance Hunsinger
Chief Financial Officer .... Jeff Collake
Medical Director .... George Andrews, MD
VP, MIS/Chief Information Officer .... Barry Robbins
Chief Operating Officer .... Doug Haaland
Marketing Director .... Christy Newman
Manager, Supervisor .... Vicki Weaver
Risk Analyst, Privacy Officer .... Mary Cogar
Marketing Director .... Christy Newman
Director of Provider Relations .... Pat Gillespie
Director of Medical Management .... Suzy Hanson
Quality Improvement Director .... Mary Woolley
Investigations Specialist Coordinator .... Beverly Brown
Executive Director/Compliance Officer .... Peggy McCurry

COMPANY PROFILE:
Parent Company Name: Covenant Health
Doing Business As: Cariten Healthcare
Year Founded: 1985   Federally Qualified: [N]
Forprofit: [Y]   Not-For-Profit: [ ]
Model Type: NETWORK
Accreditation: [ ] AAPPO [ ] JACHO [X] NCQA [ ] URAC
Plan Type: HMO, PPO, POS, HDHP, TPA
Primary Physicians: 2,685   Physician Specialists: 10,227
Hospitals: 69
Total Revenue: 2005: 380,778,093   2006: 567,676,696
Net Income   2005: 27,257,079   2006: 23,562,373
Total Enrollment:
   2001: 447,017   2004: 645,600   2007: 596,464
   2002: 0   2005: 621,500
   2003: 550,000   2006: 614,286
Medical Loss Ratio: 2005: 86.60   2006: 90.50
Administrative Expense Ratio: 2005: 15.90   2006: 11.40

SERVICE AREA:
Nationwide: N
TN (Anderson, Bedford, Benton, Bledsoe, Blount, Bradley, Campbell, Carroll, Carter, Cheatham, Claiborne, Cocke, Coffee, Crockett, Dickson, Dyer, Franklin, Gibson, Giles, Grainger, Greene, Grundy, Hamblen, Hamilton, Hancock, Hawkins, Henry, Hickman, Houston, Humphreys, Jefferson, Johnson, Knox, Lake, Lawrence, Lincoln, Loudon, Marion, Marshall, Maury, McMinn, Meigs, Monroe, Montgomery, Moore, Morgan, Obion, Perry, Polk, Rhea, Roane, Robertson, Rutherford, Scott, Sequatchie, Sevier, Shelby, Stewart, Sullivan, Sumner, Trousdale, Unicoi, Union, Washington, Wayne, Weakley, Williamson, Wilson); GA; VA;

TYPE OF COVERAGE:
Commercial: [Y] Individual: [Y] FEHBP: [ ] Indemnity: [ ]
Medicare: [Y] Medicaid: [Y] Supplemental Medicare: [ ]
Tricare: [ ]

PRODUCTS OFFERED:
Product Name:	Type:
Cariten Health Plan	HMO Cariten Senior Health
Medicare	HMO
Cariten TPA Services	ASO
Cariten Preferred	PPO
Cariten Select	POS
Cariten Workers' Comp	Workers' Comp

PLAN BENEFITS:
Alternative Medicine:	[ ]	Behavioral Health:	[X]
Chiropractic:	[X]	Dental:	[X]
Home Care:	[X]	Inpatient SNF:	[X]
Long-Term Care:	[X]	Pharm. Mail Order:	[X]
Physical Therapy:	[X]	Podiatry:	[ ]
Psychiatric:	[X]	Transplant:	[X]
Vision:	[X]	Wellness:	[X]
Workers' Comp:	[X]		

Other Benefits:
Comments:
Individual coverage is for medicare only.

CIGNA HEALTHCARE OF TENNESSEE

660 Primacy Pkwy Ste 420
Memphis, TN 38119
Phone: 901-818-1260 Fax: 901-818-1265 Toll-Free: 800-832-3211
Web site: www.cigna.com

MAILING ADDRESS:
CIGNA HEALTHCARE OF TN
660 Primacy Pkwy Ste 420
Memphis, TN 38119

TENNESSEE

Managed Care Organization Profiles

ASSURANT EMPLOYEE BENEFITS - TENNESSEE

3322 West End Ave Ste 210
Nashville, TN 30205
Phone: 615-279-3500 Fax: 615-279-5599 Toll-Free: 800-285-6812
Web site: www.assurantemployeebenefits.com

MAILING ADDRESS:
ASSURANT EMPLOYEE BNFTS - TN
3322 West End Ave Ste 210
Nashville, TN 30205

KEY EXECUTIVES:
Interim Chief Executive Officer/President .... John S Roberts
Chief Financial Officer .... Floyd F Chadee
VP, Medical Director .... Polly M Galbraith, MD
Chief Information Officer .... Karla J Schacht
Senior VP, Marketing .... Joseph A Sevcik
Privacy Officer .... John L Fortini
VP of Provider Services .... James A Barrett, DMD
Senior VP, Human Resources & Development .... Sylvia R Wagner
General Manager .... Todd Boyd
National Dental Director .... James A Barrett, DMD

COMPANY PROFILE:
Parent Company Name: Assurant Health
Doing Business As: DentiCare Inc
Year Founded: 1986   Federally Qualified: [ ]
Forprofit: [Y]   Not-For-Profit: [ ]
Model Type:
Accreditation: [ ] AAPPO [ ] JACHO [ ] NCQA [ ] URAC
Plan Type: Specialty HMO
Total Enrollment:
2001: 1,430   2004: 0   2007: 0
2002: 0   2005:
2003: 0   2006:

SERVICE AREA:
Nationwide: N
AR (Conway, Crittenden, Faulkner, Garland, Jefferson, Logan, Lonoke, Pulaski, Saline, Sebastian, Washington, White); TN;

TYPE OF COVERAGE:
Commercial: [Y] Individual: [Y] FEHBP: [ ] Indemnity: [ ]
Medicare: [ ] Medicaid: [ ] Supplemental Medicare: [ ]
Tricare   [ ]

PRODUCTS OFFERED:
Product Name: Type:
Protective Dental   HMO

PLAN BENEFITS:
Alternative Medicine: [ ]   Behavioral Health: [ ]
Chiropractic: [ ]   Dental: [X]
Home Care: [ ]   Inpatient SNF: [ ]
Long-Term Care: [ ]   Pharm. Mail Order: [ ]
Physical Therapy: [ ]   Podiatry: [ ]
Psychiatric: [ ]   Transplant: [ ]
Vision: [ ]   Wellness: [ ]
Workers' Comp: [ ]
Other Benefits:
Comments:
Formerly Fortis Benefits Dental.

BAPTIST HEALTH SERVICES GROUP

350 N Humphreys Blvd 4th Fl
Memphis, TN 38120
Phone: 901-227-2474 Fax: 901-759-9700 Toll-Free: 800-522-2474
Web site: www.bmhcc.org

MAILING ADDRESS:
BAPTIST HEALTH SERVICES GROUP
350 N Humphreys Blvd 4th Fl
Memphis, TN 38120

KEY EXECUTIVES:
Chief Executive Officer .... David Elliot
Chief Financial Officer .... William Griffin
Marketing Director .... Kim Manning

COMPANY PROFILE:
Parent Company Name: Baptist Memorial Health Care Corporation
Doing Business As: B & PIDS and BHSG
Year Founded: 1995   Federally Qualified: [N]
Forprofit: [ ]   Not-For-Profit: [Y]
Model Type:
Accreditation: [ ] AAPPO [ ] JACHO [ ] NCQA [ ] URAC
Plan Type: HMO, PPO, POS, TPA, EPO,
Primary Physicians: 2,700   Physician Specialists:
Hospitals: 40

SERVICE AREA:
Nationwide: N
AR; TN; MS;

TYPE OF COVERAGE:
Commercial: [Y] Individual: [ ] FEHBP: [ ] Indemnity: [ ]
Medicare: [Y] Medicaid: [ ] Supplemental Medicare: [ ]
Tricare   [ ]

PRODUCTS OFFERED:
Product Name: Type:
Baptist & Physicians PPO   PPO
Baptist & Physicians TPA   TPA
Baptist & Physicians HMO   HMO
Baptist & Physicians POS   POS

PLAN BENEFITS:
Alternative Medicine: [ ]   Behavioral Health: [ ]
Chiropractic: [ ]   Dental: [X]
Home Care: [X]   Inpatient SNF: [X]
Long-Term Care: [ ]   Pharm. Mail Order: [X]
Physical Therapy: [X]   Podiatry: [ ]
Psychiatric: [X]   Transplant: [X]
Vision: [ ]   Wellness: [X]
Workers' Comp: [ ]
Other Benefits:

BLUE CROSS BLUE SHIELD OF TENNESSEE

801 Pine St
Chattanooga, TN 37402
Phone: 423-755-5600 Fax: 423-755-6355 Toll-Free:
Web site: www.bcbst.com

MAILING ADDRESS:
BLUE CROSS BLUE SHIELD OF TN
801 Pine St
Chattanooga, TN 37402

KEY EXECUTIVES:
Chairman of the Board .... DeWitt Ezell, Jr
Chief Executive Officer/President .... Vicky Gregg
Executive VP, Chief Financial Officer .... John Giblien
Chief Medical Officer .... Kenneth Patric, MD
Executive VP, President, Commecial Business/Markets .... Joan Harp
Regional Sales Director .... G Henry Smith
Network Development Director .... Mark Austin
Chief Human Resources Officer .... Dan Blomberg
Senior VP, Chief Compliance Officer .... Bill Young

COMPANY PROFILE:
Parent Company Name:
Doing Business As:
Year Founded: 1945   Federally Qualified: [Y]
Forprofit: [ ]   Not-For-Profit: [Y]
Model Type: IPA
Accreditation: [ ] AAPPO [ ] JACHO [X] NCQA [X] URAC
Plan Type: HMO, PPO, Specialty PPO, POS, ASO, TPA, HDHP, HSA
Primary Physicians: 17,500   Physician Specialists:
Hospitals: 150
Total Enrollment:
2001: 4,300,000   2004: 4,600,000   2007: 5,000,000
2002: 4,200,000   2005: 5,000,000
2003: 4,600,000   2006: 5,000,000

SERVICE AREA:
Nationwide: N
TN (Fayette, Haywood, Lauderdale, Madison, Shelby, Tipton);

TYPE OF COVERAGE:
Commercial: [Y] Individual: [ ] FEHBP: [ ] Indemnity: [ ]
Medicare: [ ] Medicaid: [ ] Supplemental Medicare: [ ]
Tricare   [ ]

PRODUCTS OFFERED:
Product Name: Type:
BasicBlue
TennCare
BlueCross65
Multi-Plan Approach
Multi-Pak Health Plans
ValuePak Health Plans

Managed Care Organization Profiles — TENNESSEE

AETNA INC - TENNESSEE

3150 Lenox Park Blvd Ste 110
Memphis, TN 38115
Phone: 901-541-9400 Fax: 901-541-9343 Toll-Free:
Web site: www.aetna.com

MAILING ADDRESS:
  AETNA INC - TN
  3150 Lenox Park Blvd Ste 110
  Memphis, TN 38115

KEY EXECUTIVES:
Chairman of the Board/Chief Executive Officer .... Ronald A Williams
Regional Manager-South East .... Charles A Peck, MD
Executive VP, Finance .... Joseph M Zubretsky
Medical Director .... Troyen A Brennan, MD
Chief Information Officer .... Wei-Tih Cheng, PhD
Senior VP, Human Resources .... Elease E Wright

COMPANY PROFILE:
Parent Company Name: Aetna Inc
Doing Business As:
Year Founded: 1982   Federally Qualified: [Y]
Forprofit: [Y]   Not-For-Profit: [ ]
Model Type:
Accreditation: [ ] AAPPO [ ] JACHO [ ] NCQA [ ] URAC
Plan Type: HMO, POS, ASO, CDHP, HDHP, HSA,

SERVICE AREA:
Nationwide: N
  AR; MS; TN (Cheatham, Coffee, Crockett, Davidson, Dickson, Dyer, Fayette, Hardeman, Haywood, Lauderdale, Madison, Marshall, Maury, Montgomery, Robertson, Rutherford, Shelby, Smith, Sumner, Tipton, Trousdale, Williamson, Wilson);

TYPE OF COVERAGE:
Commercial: [Y] Individual: [ ] FEHBP: [ ] Indemnity: [ ]
Medicare: [ ] Medicaid: [ ] Supplemental Medicare: [ ]
Tricare   [ ]

PRODUCTS OFFERED:
Product Name: Type:
Aetna Inc   Medicaid

CONSUMER-DRIVEN PRODUCTS
Aetna Life Insurance Co   HSA Company
Aetna HealthFund HSA   HSA Product
Aetna   HSA Administrator
Aetna HealthFund   Consumer-Driven Health Plan
PPO I; PPO II   High Deductible Health Plan

PLAN BENEFITS:
Alternative Medicine: [ ]   Behavioral Health: [ ]
Chiropractic: [ ]   Dental: [ ]
Home Care: [X]   Inpatient SNF: [X]
Long-Term Care: [ ]   Pharm. Mail Order: [X]
Physical Therapy: [X]   Podiatry: [X]
Psychiatric: [X]   Transplant: [X]
Vision: [X]   Wellness: [X]
Workers' Comp: [ ]
Other Benefits:
Comments:
Formerly Prudential Healthcare.

AETNA INC - TENNESSEE

1801 West End Ave Ste 500
Nashville, TN 37203
Phone: 615-322-1600 Fax: 615-322-1649 Toll-Free:
Web site: www.aetna.com

MAILING ADDRESS:
  AETNA INC - TN
  1801 West End Ave Ste 500
  Nashville, TN 37203

KEY EXECUTIVES:
Chairman of the Board/Chief Executive Officer .... Ronald A Williams
President .... Mark T Bertolini
Executive VP, Finance .... Joseph M Zubretsky
Medical Director .... Gregg Cannella, MD
Chief Information Officer .... Wei-Tih Cheng, PhD
Marketing Director .... Scott Bowlenbaugh
VP, Human Resources .... Elease E Wright

COMPANY PROFILE:
Parent Company Name: Aetna Inc
Doing Business As:
Year Founded: 1988   Federally Qualified: [ ]
Forprofit: [Y]   Not-For-Profit: [ ]
Model Type: NETWORK
Accreditation: [ ] AAPPO [ ] JACHO [ ] NCQA [ ] URAC
Plan Type: PPO, POS, CDHP, HDHP, HSA,
Total Enrollment:
  2001: 22,520   2004: 27,685   2007: 0
  2002: 33,568   2005:
  2003: 30,152   2006:

SERVICE AREA:
Nationwide: N
  TN (Bedford, Cannon, Cheatham, Coffee, Davidson, DeKalb, Dickson, Franklin, Giles, Hickman, Humphreys, Lawrence, Lewis, Lincoln, Macon, Marshall, Maury, Montgomery, Moore, Perry, Robertson, Rutherford, Smith, Sumner, Trousdale, Wayne, Williamson, Wilson) ; AR (Eastern); GA (Northwest); MI (Northern); VA (Southwest);

TYPE OF COVERAGE:
Commercial: [Y] Individual: [ ] FEHBP: [ ] Indemnity: [ ]
Medicare: [ ] Medicaid: [ ] Supplemental Medicare: [ ]
Tricare   [ ]

CONSUMER-DRIVEN PRODUCTS
Aetna Life Insurance Co   HSA Company
Aetna HealthFund HSA   HSA Product
Aetna   HSA Administrator
Aetna HealthFund   Consumer-Driven Health Plan
PPO I; PPO II   High Deductible Health Plan

PLAN BENEFITS:
Alternative Medicine: [ ]   Behavioral Health: [ ]
Chiropractic: [X]   Dental: [X]
Home Care: [X]   Inpatient SNF: [X]
Long-Term Care: [X]   Pharm. Mail Order: [X]
Physical Therapy: [X]   Podiatry: [X]
Psychiatric: [X]   Transplant: [X]
Vision: [X]   Wellness: [X]
Workers' Comp: [ ]
Other Benefits:

AMERIGROUP TENNESSEE INC

22 Century Blvd Ste 310
Nashville, TN 37214
Phone: 615-231-6065 Fax: 615-883-5218 Toll-Free:
Web site: www.amerigroup.com

MAILING ADDRESS:
  AMERIGROUP TENNESSEE INC
  22 Century Blvd Ste 310
  Nashville, TN 37214

KEY EXECUTIVES:
Chief Executive Officer/President .... Charles Brian Shipp
VP, Chief Operating Officer .... Lorena Jean Stanley
VP, Treasurer .... James W Truess
VP, Medical Director .... Carol A Churchill, MD

COMPANY PROFILE:
Parent Company Name: Amerigroup Inc
Doing Business As: Amerigroup Community Care
Year Founded: Federally Qualified: [ ]
Forprofit: [ ]   Not-For-Profit: [ ]
Model Type:
Accreditation: [ ] AAPPO [ ] JACHO [ ] NCQA [ ] URAC
Plan Type: HMO
Total Enrollment:
  2001:   2004:   2007: 185,365
  2002:   2005:
  2003:   2006:

SERVICE AREA:
Nationwide: N
  TN;

TYPE OF COVERAGE:
Commercial: [ ] Individual: [ ] FEHBP: [ ] Indemnity: [ ]
Medicare: [ ] Medicaid: [Y] Supplemental Medicare: [ ]
Tricare   [ ]

PRODUCTS OFFERED:
Product Name: Type:
TENNCare   Medicaid

Medical Loss Ratio: 2005: 86.20 2006:
Administrative Expense Ratio: 2005: 2006:
SERVICE AREA:
Nationwide: N
IA; MN; SD;
TYPE OF COVERAGE:
Commercial: [Y] Individual: [ ] FEHBP: [Y] Indemnity: [ ]
Medicare: [ ] Medicaid: [ ] Supplemental Medicare: [Y]
Tricare [ ]
PRODUCTS OFFERED:
Product Name:	Type:
Sioux Valley Health Plan of IA	HMO
Sioux Valley Health Plan of SD	HMO
Valley Choice Basic Plan	Medicare Advantage
Valley Choice Plus Plan	Medicare Advantage

Comments:
Formerly Sioux Valley Health Plan. Changed name February 2007.

WELLMARK BLUE CROSS & BLUE SHIELD OF SOUTH DAKOTA

1601 W Madison St
Sioux Falls, SD 57104
Phone: 605-373-7200 Fax: 605-373-7497 Toll-Free: 800-952-1976
Web site: www.wellmark.com
MAILING ADDRESS:
WELLMARK BC & BS OF SD
1601 W Madison St
Sioux Falls, SD 57104

KEY EXECUTIVES:
Chairman of the Board/Chief Executive Officer .... John D Forsyth
President/Chief Operating Officer .... Philip M Davis
SVP, Finance .... Richard C Anderson
Chief Medical Officer .... Dale J Andringa, MD
Chief Information Officer .... Denis J Roy
VP, Marketing .... Danielle Slifka
VP, Information Systems .... Sandy J Nelson
VP, Sales .... Lyndon T Peterson
Senior VP, Human Resources .... Laura Jackson

COMPANY PROFILE:
Parent Company Name: Wellmark Inc
Doing Business As: Wellmark BC & BS of South Dakota
Year Founded: 1948 Federally Qualified: [ ]
Forprofit: [Y] Not-For-Profit: [ ]
Model Type:
Accreditation: [ ] AAPPO [ ] JACHO [X] NCQA [ ] URAC
Plan Type: PPO, CDHP, HDHP, HSA,
Total Enrollment:
  2001: 250,212   2004: 0   2007: 301,000
  2002: 0   2005:
  2003: 263,092   2006: 293,750
SERVICE AREA:
Nationwide: N
SD;
TYPE OF COVERAGE:
Commercial: [Y] Individual: [Y] FEHBP: [Y] Indemnity: [Y]
Medicare: [ ] Medicaid: [ ] Supplemental Medicare: [Y]
Tricare [Y]
PRODUCTS OFFERED:
Product Name:	Type:
Blue Select	PPO
Blue Street Options	PPO
Senior Blue	Medicare Supplement
Senior Blue Options	Medicare
Classic Blue	Indemnity
Blue Rx	

CONSUMER-DRIVEN PRODUCTS
MSAver Resources, LLC	HSA Company
Blue Priority HSA	HSA Product
MSAver Resouces, LLC	HSA Administrator
	Consumer-Driven Health Plan
Alliance Select	High Deductible Health Plan

PLAN BENEFITS:
Alternative Medicine: [ ]   Behavioral Health: [ ]
Chiropractic: [X]   Dental: [X]
Home Care: [X]   Inpatient SNF: [X]
Long-Term Care: [ ]   Pharm. Mail Order: [X]
Physical Therapy: [X]   Podiatry: [X]
Psychiatric: [X]   Transplant: [X]
Vision: [X]   Wellness: [ ]
Workers' Comp: [ ]
Other Benefits:

WESTERN HEALTH

529 Kansas City Ste 200
Rapid City, SD 57701
Phone: 605-716-4600 Fax: 605-716-8401 Toll-Free: 888-341-1766
Web site: www.mywellnessadvantage.com
MAILING ADDRESS:
WESTERN HEALTH
529 Kansas City Ste 200
Rapid City, SD 57701

KEY EXECUTIVES:
Executive Director .... Joseph Sluka
Medical Director .... Michael P Elston, MD

COMPANY PROFILE:
Parent Company Name:
Doing Business As:
Year Founded: Federally Qualified: [ ]
Forprofit: [ ]   Not-For-Profit: [ ]
Model Type:
Accreditation: [ ] AAPPO [ ] JACHO [ ] NCQA [ ] URAC
Plan Type: ASO
SERVICE AREA:
Nationwide: N
SD;

SOUTH DAKOTA

Managed Care Organization Profiles

Forprofit: [ ] Not-For-Profit: [Y]
Model Type:
Accreditation: [ ] AAPPO [ ] JACHO [ ] NCQA [ ] URAC
Plan Type: Specialty PPO,
Dentists: 40
Total Enrollment:
   2001: 0   2004: 149,625   2007: 255,000
   2002: 129,285 2005:
   2003: 135,861 2006:

SERVICE AREA:
Nationwide: N
SD;

TYPE OF COVERAGE:
Commercial: [Y] Individual: [ ] FEHBP: [ ] Indemnity: [ ]
Medicare: [ ] Medicaid: [ ] Supplemental Medicare: [ ]
Tricare   [ ]
Alternative Medicine: [ ]   Behavioral Health: [ ]
Chiropractic: [ ]   Dental: [X]
Home Care: [ ]   Inpatient SNF: [ ]
Long-Term Care: [ ]   Pharm. Mail Order: [ ]
Physical Therapy: [ ]   Podiatry: [ ]
Psychiatric: [ ]   Transplant: [ ]
Vision: [ ]   Wellness: [ ]
Workers' Comp: [ ]
Other Benefits:

FIRST CHOICE OF THE MIDWEST INC

100 S Spring Ave Ste 220
Sioux Falls, SD 57104
Phone: 605-332-5955 Fax: 605-332-5953 Toll-Free: 888-246-9949
Web site: www.1choicem.com

MAILING ADDRESS:
   FIRST CHOICE OF THE MIDWEST
   PO Box 5078
   Sioux Falls, SD 57104

KEY EXECUTIVES:
Chief Executive Officer .... Michael Hagert
Sales & Marketing Director .... Susie Eiesland
Credentialing Manager/Provider Relations .... Kristina Pyle
Office Manager .... Suzy Welch
Credentialing Manager .... Kristina Pyle
Claims Manager .... Tricia Parker

COMPANY PROFILE:
Parent Company Name:
Doing Business As:
Year Founded: 1997   Federally Qualified: [ ]
Forprofit: [Y]   Not-For-Profit: [ ]
Model Type: NETWORK
Accreditation: [ ] AAPPO [ ] JACHO [ ] NCQA [ ] URAC
Plan Type: PPO,
Total Enrollment:
   2001: 35,000   2004: 0   2007: 0
   2002: 0   2005:
   2003: 42,000   2006:

SERVICE AREA:
Nationwide: N
   SD; IA; MN; WY; ND; CO; MT; NE; UT; ID;

TYPE OF COVERAGE:
Commercial: [Y] Individual: [ ] FEHBP: [ ] Indemnity: [ ]
Medicare: [ ] Medicaid: [ ] Supplemental Medicare: [ ]
Tricare   [ ]

PRODUCTS OFFERED:
Product Name: Type:
First Choice of the Midwest   PPO

HUMANA INC - SOUTH DAKOTA

500 W Main St
Louisville, KY 40201
Phone: 502-580-5804 Fax: 502-580-5044 Toll-Free:
Web site: www.humana.com

MAILING ADDRESS:
   HUMANA INC - SOUTH DAKOTA
   500 W Main St
   Louisville, KY 40201

KEY EXECUTIVES:
Chairman of the Board .... David A Jones Jr
Chief Executive Officer/President .... Michael B McCallister
Chief Financial Officer .... James H Bloem
Medicare Director .... Darrell Russell

COMPANY PROFILE:
Parent Company Name: Humana Inc
Doing Business As:
Year Founded: 1961   Federally Qualified: [Y]
Forprofit: [Y]   Not-For-Profit: [ ]
Model Type:
Accreditation: [ ] AAPPO [ ] JACHO [ ] NCQA [ ] URAC
Plan Type: PPO, CDHP, HDHP, HSA,
Total Enrollment:
   2001: 0   2004: 0   2007: 38,000
   2002: 0   2005:
   2003: 0   2006:

SERVICE AREA:
Nationwide: N
SD;

TYPE OF COVERAGE:
Commercial: [Y] Individual: [ ] FEHBP: [ ] Indemnity: [ ]
Medicare: [Y] Medicaid: [ ] Supplemental Medicare: [Y]
Tricare   [ ]

PRODUCTS OFFERED:
Product Name: Type:

CONSUMER-DRIVEN PRODUCTS
JP Morgan Chase   HSA Company
HumanaOne HSA   HSA Product
JP Morgan Chase   HSA Administrator
Personal Care Account   Consumer-Driven Health Plan
HumanaOne   High Deductible Health Plan

PLAN BENEFITS:
Alternative Medicine: [ ]   Behavioral Health: [ ]
Chiropractic: [X]   Dental: [X]
Home Care: [ ]   Inpatient SNF: [ ]
Long-Term Care: [ ]   Pharm. Mail Order: [X]
Physical Therapy: [ ]   Podiatry: [ ]
Psychiatric: [X]   Transplant: [X]
Vision: [ ]   Wellness: [X]
Workers' Comp: [X]
Other Benefits:

SANFORD HEALTH PLAN

300 Cherapa Pl Ste 201
Sioux Falls, SD 57103
Phone: 605-328-6868 Fax: 605-328-6811 Toll-Free: 800-752-5863
Web site: www.sanfordhealth.org

MAILING ADDRESS:
   SANFORD HEALTH PLAN
   300 Cherapa Pl Ste 201
   Sioux Falls, SD 57103

KEY EXECUTIVES:
Chief Executive Officer/President .... Ruth Krystopolski
Chief Financial Officer .... Cecily Tucker
Chief Medical Officer .... Michael Crandel, MD
Chief Operating Officer .... Trixy Burgess
Client Services Director .... Toni McEntee
Provider Relations Director .... Ryan Bahy
Quality Assurance Director .... Lynn Thomas
Compliance Officer .... Lisa Carlson

COMPANY PROFILE:
Parent Company Name: Sanford Health
Doing Business As:
Year Founded: 1998   Federally Qualified: [Y]
Forprofit: [ ]   Not-For-Profit: [Y]
Model Type: IPA
Accreditation: [ ] AAPPO [ ] JACHO [X] NCQA [ ] URAC
Plan Type: HMO, FSA
Primary Physicians: Physician Specialists:
Hospitals:
Total Revenue: 2005: 65,912,462   2006:
Net Income   2005: 3,393,546   2006:
Total Enrollment:
   2001: 31,701   2004: 24,254   2007: 0
   2002: 47,139   2005: 25,140
   2003: 59,493   2006:

Managed Care Organization Profiles — SOUTH DAKOTA

AVERA HEALTH PLANS INC

3816 S Elmwood Ave Ste 100
Sioux Falls, SD 57105-6538
Phone: 605-322-4545 Fax: 605-322-4535 Toll-Free:
Web site: www.averahealthplans.com

MAILING ADDRESS:
AVERA HEALTH PLANS INC
3816 S Elmwood Ave Ste 100
Sioux Falls, SD 57105-6538

KEY EXECUTIVES:
Chief Executive Officer/President .... Robin O Bates
Chief Financial Officer/Chief Operating Officer .... Ted Weinberg
Medical Director .... Rick Miller, DO
Sales Manager .... Nathan van Roekel
Credentialing Specialist .... Patricia Olson
Director Network Services .... Debra Muller
Director Health Services .... Nancy Beaumont
Credentialing Specialist .... Patricia Olson
Finance Manager .... Tanna Gries
Claims Manager .... Margaret Solma
Client Services Manager .... Kevin Fahy

COMPANY PROFILE:
Parent Company Name: Avera Health
Doing Business As: Avera Health Plans
Year Founded: 1999   Federally Qualified: [N]
Forprofit: [Y]   Not-For-Profit: [ ]
Model Type: Mixed
Accreditation: [ ] AAPPO [ ] JACHO [ ] NCQA [ ] URAC
Plan Type: HMO, POS, HDHP, HSA, FSA
Primary Physicians: 569   Physician Specialists: 915
Hospitals: 37
Total Revenue: 2005: 41,894,880   2006:
Net Income   2005:   971,411   2006:
Total Enrollment:
  2001: 11,288   2004: 19,541   2007: 17,337
  2002: 25,088   2005: 19,767
  2003: 30,173   2006: 18,694
Medical Loss Ratio: 2005: 83.00 2006:
Administrative Expense Ratio: 2005:   2006:

SERVICE AREA:
Nationwide: N
  IA; MN; NE; SD;

TYPE OF COVERAGE:
Commercial: [Y] Individual: [ ] FEHBP: [Y] Indemnity: [ ]
Medicare: [ ] Medicaid: [ ] Supplemental Medicare:
[Y]Tricare [ ]

PRODUCTS OFFERED:
Product Name: Type:
Avera Preferred   HMO
Avera Advantage   POS
Avera Choice   POS

CONSUMER-DRIVEN PRODUCTS
Wells Fargo Bank   HSA Company
Avera HSA   HSA Product
                             HSA Administrator
Avera Choice High Deductible Consumer-Driven Health Plan
                             High Deductible Health Plan

PLAN BENEFITS:
Alternative Medicine: [ ]   Behavioral Health: [X]
Chiropractic: [X]   Dental: [ ]
Home Care: [ ]   Inpatient SNF: [X]
Long-Term Care: [ ]   Pharm. Mail Order: [X]
Physical Therapy: [X]   Podiatry: [ ]
Psychiatric: [ ]   Transplant: [X]
Vision: [X]   Wellness: [X]
Workers' Comp: [X]
Other Benefits:

DAKOTACARE

2600 W 49th St
Sioux Falls, SD 57117-7406
Phone: 605-334-4000 Fax: 605-336-0270 Toll-Free: 800-325-5598
Web site: www.dakotacare.com

MAILING ADDRESS:
DAKOTACARE
PO Box 7406
Sioux Falls, SD 57117-7406

KEY EXECUTIVES:
Board Chairman/President .... Thomas Krafka, MD
Chief Executive Officer .... Kirk I Zimmer
Chief Financial Officer .... Mike North
Medical Director .... Paul Amundson, MD
Pharmacy Director .... Christine Lounsbery, PharmD
Chief Information Officer .... Brian Meyer
VP of Sales & Marketing .... Thomas Nicholson
VP Provider Relations .... Scott Jamison
Human Resources Director .... Teresa Gevens
VP, Medical Management .... Rich Jones, RN
Quality Assurance Director/Compliance Officer .... Jacque Cole, RN
Voluntary Benefits Specialist .... Dan Aberson
HMO Sales Manager .... Wade Ericson

COMPANY PROFILE:
Parent Company Name: South Dakota State Med Holding Co Inc
Doing Business As: DakotaCare
Year Founded: 1986   Federally Qualified: [N]
Forprofit: [Y]   Not-For-Profit: [ ]
Model Type: IPA
Accreditation: [ ] AAPPO [ ] JACHO [ ] NCQA [ ] URAC
Plan Type: HMO, POS, ASO, TPA, UR, CDHP, HDHP, HSA, FSA
Primary Physicians: 780   Physician Specialists: 1,100
Hospitals: 72
Total Revenue: 2005: 86,000,000   2006: 43,700,000
Net Income   2005: 3,300,000   2006: 2,100,000
Total Enrollment:
  2001: 91,834   2004: 109,071   2007: 0
  2002: 103,000   2005: 108,170
  2003: 105,000   2006: 109,390

SERVICE AREA:
Nationwide: N
  SD;

TYPE OF COVERAGE:
Commercial: [Y] Individual: [Y] FEHBP: [ ] Indemnity: [ ]
Medicare: [Y] Medicaid: [ ] Supplemental Medicare: [ ]
Tricare [ ]

PRODUCTS OFFERED:
Product Name: Type:
Dakotacare   HMO
Dakotacare Self-Funded   ASO
Dakotacare Dental   Dental

CONSUMER-DRIVEN PRODUCTS
First Horizon   HSA Company
Dakotacare Reserve   HSA Product
MSAver   HSA Administrator
Dakotacare Flex   Consumer-Driven Health Plan
Dakotacare Reserve   High Deductible Health Plan

PLAN BENEFITS:
Alternative Medicine: [ ]   Behavioral Health: [X]
Chiropractic: [X]   Dental: [ ]
Home Care: [X]   Inpatient SNF: [X]
Long-Term Care: [ ]   Pharm. Mail Order: [X]
Physical Therapy: [X]   Podiatry: [X]
Psychiatric: [X]   Transplant: [X]
Vision: [X]   Wellness: [X]
Workers' Comp: [ ]
Other Benefits:

DELTA DENTAL PLAN OF SOUTH DAKOTA

720 N Euclid Ave
Pierre, SD 57501
Phone: 605-224-7345 Fax: 605-224-0909 Toll-Free: 800-627-3961
Web site: www.deltadentalsd.com

MAILING ADDRESS:
DELTA DENTAL PLAN OF SD
PO Box 1157
Pierre, SD 57501

KEY EXECUTIVES:
Chairman of the Board .... Dale Gibson, DDS
Chief Executive Officer/President .... Scott Jones
Chief Financial Officer .... Kirby Scott
VP, Operations .... Mick Heckenlaible
Marketing Director .... Sid Gran
VP, Professional Relations .... Nance Orsbon

COMPANY PROFILE:
Parent Company Name: Delta Dental Plan Association
Doing Business As:
Year Founded: 1963   Federally Qualified: [ ]

SOUTH CAROLINA

PLAN BENEFITS:
Alternative Medicine:	[ ]	Behavioral Health:	[ ]
Chiropractic:	[ ]	Dental:	[ ]
Home Care:	[X]	Inpatient SNF:	[X]
Long-Term Care:	[ ]	Pharm. Mail Order:	[ ]
Physical Therapy:	[X]	Podiatry:	[X]
Psychiatric:	[X]	Transplant:	[X]
Vision:	[ ]	Wellness:	[X]
Workers' Comp:	[X]		

Other Benefits:

UNISON HEALTH PLAN OF SOUTH CAROLINA INC

100 Executive Center Dr #A-1
Columbia, SC 29210
Phone: 803-798-6210 Fax: 866-546-0889 Toll-Free: 800-414-9025
Web site: www.unisonhealthplan.com

MAILING ADDRESS:
  UNISON HEALTH PLAN OF SC INC
  100 Executive Center Dr #A-1
  Columbia, SC 29210

KEY EXECUTIVES:
President .... Daniel Gallagher
Medical Director .... Brenna DeLaine, MD

COMPANY PROFILE:
Parent Company Name: Three Rivers Health Plan
Doing Business As:
Year Founded: 2004   Federally Qualified: [N]
Forprofit: [Y]   Not-For-Profit: [ ]
Model Type: IPA
Accreditation: [ ] AAPPO [ ] JACHO [ ] NCQA [ ] URAC
Plan Type: HMO
Total Enrollment:
  2001: 0   2004: 271   2007: 0
  2002: 0   2005: 4,048
  2003: 0   2006:

SERVICE AREA:
Nationwide:
  SC,

TYPE OF COVERAGE:
Commercial: [ ] Individual: [ ] FEHBP: [ ] Indemnity: [ ]
Medicare: [ ] Medicaid: [ ] Supplemental Medicare: [ ]
Tricare   [ ]

PRODUCTS OFFERED:
Product Name:	Type:
HMO	HMO

Managed Care Organization Profiles — SOUTH CAROLINA

CONSUMER-DRIVEN PRODUCTS
JP Morgan Chase	HSA Company
HumanaOne HSA	HSA Product
JP Morgan Chase	HSA Administrator
Personal Care Account	Consumer-Driven Health Plan
HumanaOne	High Deductible Health Plan

PLAN BENEFITS:
Alternative Medicine:	[ ]	Behavioral Health:	[X]
Chiropractic:	[X]	Dental:	[X]
Home Care:	[ ]	Inpatient SNF:	[ ]
Long-Term Care:	[ ]	Pharm. Mail Order:	[X]
Physical Therapy:	[ ]	Podiatry:	[ ]
Psychiatric:	[X]	Transplant:	[X]
Vision:	[ ]	Wellness:	[ ]
Workers' Comp:	[X]		

Other Benefits: Long Term Disability Care

KHS A KMG AMERICA COMPANY

210 S Lancaster St
Lancaster, SC 29720
Phone: 803-822-1274 Fax: 803-283-5488 Toll-Free: 800-822-1274
Web site: www.khsonline.com

MAILING ADDRESS:
KHS A KMG AMERICA COMPANY
PO Box 610
Lancaster, SC 29720

KEY EXECUTIVES:
Chief Executive Officer/Senior VP, Marketing/Sales ...... Scott MacEwen
Chief Financial Officer .... Robert Matthews
Medical Director .... Joseph Whalen, MD
MIS Director .... Ron Groover
2nd VP Managed Care .... Patricia England
Human Resource Director .... Debbie Jaillette

COMPANY PROFILE:
Parent Company Name: Kanawha Insurance Company
Doing Business As:
Year Founded: 1996   Federally Qualified: [N]
Forprofit: [Y]   Not-For-Profit: [ ]
Model Type:
Accreditation: [ ] AAPPO [ ] JACHO [ ] NCQA [X] URAC
Plan Type: PPO, ASO, TPA, UR, CDHP, HSA

SERVICE AREA:
Nationwide: N
SC; NC;

TYPE OF COVERAGE:
Commercial: [Y] Individual: [Y] FEHBP: [ ] Indemnity: [ ]
Medicare: [ ] Medicaid: [ ] Supplemental Medicare: [Y]
Tricare [ ]

PLAN BENEFITS:
Alternative Medicine:	[ ]	Behavioral Health:	[X]
Chiropractic:	[ ]	Dental:	[X]
Home Care:	[X]	Inpatient SNF:	[X]
Long-Term Care:	[X]	Pharm. Mail Order:	[X]
Physical Therapy:	[X]	Podiatry:	[ ]
Psychiatric:	[X]	Transplant:	[X]
Vision:	[X]	Wellness:	[X]
Workers' Comp:	[ ]		

Other Benefits:
Comments:
Formerly Coordinated Health Care Management Inc.

SELECT HEALTH OF SOUTH CAROLINA

4390 Bella Oaks Dr
North Charleston, SC 29405
Phone: 843-569-1759 Fax: 843-569-7222 Toll-Free: 800-741-6605
Web site: www.selecthealthofsc.com

MAILING ADDRESS:
SELECT HEALTH OF SOUTH CAROLINA
4390 Bella Oaks Dr
North Charleston, SC 29405

KEY EXECUTIVES:
Chief Executive Officer/President .... J Michael Jernigan
Chief Financial Officer .... Clark Phillip
Associate Medical Director .... Stuart A Hamilton, MD
VP, Chief Operating Officer .... Cindy Hellings
Associate VP, Marketing .... Ismael Hernandez
Director of Provider Relations .... Philip Fairchild
Director of Network Management .... Peggy Vickery
Director of Human Resources .... Michelle Powell
Senior Director of Quality Improvement .... Rebecca Engelman
Community Liaison Director .... Terry Jones Davenport
Associate Medical Director .... James G Baldwin, Jr, MD
Director Member Services .... Kevin Vaugh
Director of Operations Support .... John McFadden

COMPANY PROFILE:
Parent Company Name: AmeriHealth Mercy Health Plan
Doing Business As:
Year Founded: 1996   Federally Qualified: [N]
Forprofit: [Y]   Not-For-Profit: [ ]
Model Type: IPA
Accreditation: [ ] AAPPO [ ] JACHO [X] NCQA [ ] URAC
Plan Type: HMO
Total Enrollment:
2001: 36,625	2004: 54,335	2007: 0
2002: 54,739	2005: 62,060	
2003: 51,478	2006:	

SERVICE AREA:
Nationwide: N
SC;

TYPE OF COVERAGE:
Commercial: [ ] Individual: [ ] FEHBP: [ ] Indemnity: [ ]
Medicare: [ ] Medicaid: [Y] Supplemental Medicare: [ ]
Tricare [ ]

PRODUCTS OFFERED:
Product Name:	Type:
Select Health Medicaid	Medicaid

ST FRANCIS OPTIMUM HEALTH NETWORK

One St Francis Dr
Greenville, SC 29601
Phone: 864-213-4989 Fax: 864-213-4928 Toll-Free:
Web site: www.stfrancishealth.org

MAILING ADDRESS:
ST FRANCIS OPTIMUM HEALTH NETWORK
One St Francis Dr
Greenville, SC 29601

KEY EXECUTIVES:
Chief Executive Officer .... Valinda Rutledge
Chief Financial Officer .... Ronnie Hyatt
Medical Director .... Mary Jo Cagle, MD
Marketing Director/Managed Care Director .... Steve Poole

COMPANY PROFILE:
Parent Company Name: St Francis Health System
Doing Business As:
Year Founded: 1993   Federally Qualified: [ ]
Forprofit: [Y]   Not-For-Profit: [ ]
Model Type:
Accreditation: [ ] AAPPO [ ] JACHO [ ] NCQA [X] URAC
Plan Type: PPO
Primary Physicians: 181   Physician Specialists: 353
Hospitals:
Total Enrollment:
2001: 40,000	2004: 0	2007: 25,000
2002: 0	2005:	
2003: 0	2006:	

SERVICE AREA:
Nationwide: N
SC;

TYPE OF COVERAGE:
Commercial: [Y] Individual: [Y] FEHBP: [ ] Indemnity: [ ]
Medicare: [ ] Medicaid: [ ] Supplemental Medicare: [ ]
Tricare [ ]

SOUTH CAROLINA

Total Enrollment:
  2001: 104,348   2004: 67,571   2007: 0
  2002: 89,698   2005: 70,352
  2003: 70,108   2006:
SERVICE AREA:
Nationwide: N
  SC;
TYPE OF COVERAGE:
Commercial: [Y] Individual: [ ] FEHBP: [ ] Indemnity: [ ]
Medicare: [ ] Medicaid: [ ] Supplemental Medicare: [ ]
Tricare   [ ]
PRODUCTS OFFERED:
Product Name: Type:
Carolina Care Plan Inc   HMO
CONSUMER-DRIVEN PRODUCTS
                                       HSA Company
                                       HSA Product
American Benefit Services LLC   HSA Administrator
Carolina HSA 80/3500   Consumer-Driven Health Plan
Carolina HSA 50/200   High Deductible Health Plan
Comments:
Formerly Physicians Health Plan Inc.

CIGNA HEALTHCARE OF SOUTH CAROLINA

250 Commonwealth Dr Ste 110
Greenville, SC 29615-4847
Phone: 864-234-7768 Fax: 864-987-1389 Toll-Free: 800-949-0325
Web site: www.cigna.com
MAILING ADDRESS:
  CIGNA HEALTHCARE OF SC
  250 Commonwealth Dr Ste 110
  Greenville, SC 29615-4847

KEY EXECUTIVES:
President, General Manager .... Charles C Pitts
VP, Sales .... Steve Parham

COMPANY PROFILE:
Parent Company Name: CIGNA Corporation
Doing Business As:
Year Founded: 1994   Federally Qualified: [ ]
Forprofit: [Y]   Not-For-Profit: [ ]
Model Type: IPA
Accreditation: [ ] AAPPO [ ] JACHO [ ] NCQA   [ ]
URACPlan Type: HMO, CDHP, FSA, HRA, HSA
Total Enrollment:
  2001: 88,479   2004: 28,128   2007: 0
  2002: 55,442   2005: 28,743
  2003: 39,809   2006:
SERVICE AREA:
Nationwide: N
  SC;
TYPE OF COVERAGE:
Commercial: [Y] Individual: [ ] FEHBP: [ ] Indemnity: [ ]
Medicare: [ ] Medicaid: [ ] Supplemental Medicare: [ ]
Tricare   [ ]
PRODUCTS OFFERED:
Product Name: Type:
CIGNA HMO   HMO
CIGNA POS   POS
CONSUMER-DRIVEN PRODUCTS
JP Morgan Chase   HSA Company
CIGNA Choice Fund   HSA Product
                                       HSA Administrator
Open Access Plus   Consumer-Driven Health Plan
PPO   High Deductible Health Plan
PLAN BENEFITS:
Alternative Medicine: [ ]   Behavioral Health: [ ]
Chiropractic: [X]   Dental: [X]
Home Care: [X]   Inpatient SNF: [X]
Long-Term Care: [X]   Pharm. Mail Order: [X]
Physical Therapy: [X]   Podiatry: [X]
Psychiatric: [X]   Transplant: [X]
Vision: [X]   Wellness: [X]
Workers' Comp: [ ]
Other Benefits:

DELTA DENTAL PLAN OF SOUTH CAROLINA

200 Center Point Circle Ste 150
Columbia, SC 29210
Phone: 803-731-2495 Fax: 803-731-0273 Toll-Free: 800-529-3268
Web site: www.deltadentalsc.com
MAILING ADDRESS:
  DELTA DENTAL PLAN OF SC
  200 Center Point Circle Ste 150
  Columbia, SC 29210

KEY EXECUTIVES:
Chairman of the Board .... Richard J Haffner, DDS
Chief Executive Officer/President .... Steve P Gaal, III
Regional VP .... Nancy Spencer

COMPANY PROFILE:
Parent Company Name: Delta Dental Plan Association
Doing Business As:
Year Founded: Federally Qualified: [ ]
Forprofit: [ ]   Not-For-Profit: [ ]
Model Type:
Accreditation: [ ] AAPPO [ ] JACHO [ ] NCQA [ ] URAC
Plan Type: Specialty HMO
SERVICE AREA:
Nationwide: N
  SC;
TYPE OF COVERAGE:
Commercial: [Y] Individual: [ ] FEHBP: [ ] Indemnity: [ ]
Medicare: [ ] Medicaid: [ ] Supplemental Medicare: [ ]
Tricare   [ ]
PLAN BENEFITS:
Alternative Medicine: [ ]   Behavioral Health: [ ]
Chiropractic: [ ]   Dental: [X]
Home Care: [ ]   Inpatient SNF: [ ]
Long-Term Care: [ ]   Pharm. Mail Order: [ ]
Physical Therapy: [ ]   Podiatry: [ ]
Psychiatric: [ ]   Transplant: [ ]
Vision: [ ]   Wellness: [ ]
Workers' Comp: [ ]
Other Benefits:

HUMANA INC - SOUTH CAROLINA

500 W Main St
Louisville, KY 40201-7436
Phone: 502-580-1000 Fax: 859-232-8557 Toll-Free: 800-281-6918
Web site: www.humana.com
MAILING ADDRESS:
  HUMANA INC - SOUTH CAROLINA
  PO Box 740036
  Louisville, KY 40201-7436

KEY EXECUTIVES:
Chairman of the Board .... David A Jones Jr
Chief Executive Officer/President .... Michael B McCallister
Chief Financial Officer .... James H Bloem
Chief Medical Officer .... Jonathan T Lord, MD
Marketing Director .... John Dammon
Media Relations .... Mitch Lubitz

COMPANY PROFILE:
Parent Company Name: Humana Inc
Doing Business As:
Year Founded: 1961   Federally Qualified: [Y]
Forprofit: [Y]   Not-For-Profit: [ ]
Model Type: IPA
Accreditation: [ ] AAPPO [ ] JACHO [ ] NCQA [ ] URAC
Plan Type: PPO, ASO, Champus, CDHP, HDHP, HSA,
Total Enrollment:
  2001: 0   2004: 0   2007: 0
  2002: 0   2005:
  2003: 138,100   2006:
SERVICE AREA:
Nationwide: N
  SC;
TYPE OF COVERAGE:
Commercial: [Y] Individual: [ ] FEHBP: [ ] Indemnity: [ ]
Medicare: [ ] Medicaid: [ ] Supplemental Medicare: [ ]
Tricare   [Y]

Managed Care Organization Profiles — SOUTH CAROLINA

BLUE CROSS BLUE SHIELD OF SOUTH CAROLINA - CORPORATE HEADQUATERS

I-20 E at Alpine Rd
Columbia, SC 29219
Phone: 803-788-0222 Fax: 803-736-9289 Toll-Free: 800-288-2227
Web site: www.southcarolinablues.com

MAILING ADDRESS:
BLUE CROSS BLUE SHIELD OF SC
I-20 E at Alpine Rd
Columbia, SC 29219

KEY EXECUTIVES:
Chairman of the Board/Chief Executive Officer .... M Edward Sellers
President/Chief Operating Officer .... David S Pankau
Chief Financial Officer .... Robert A Leichtle
VP, Chief Medical Officer .... John M Little, MD
Chief Information Officer .... Steven K Wiggins
Senior VP, Major Group Division .... James Deyling
Executive VP, Chief Legal Officer .... Judith M Davis
VP, Chief Actuary .... Will Shrader
Senior VP, Group & Individual Divsion .... Jim Hart
Senior VP, Federal Affairs/Brand Compliance .... George Johnson

COMPANY PROFILE:
Parent Company Name: Blue Cross/Blue Shield of South Carolina
Doing Business As: BlueCross BlueShield of South Carolina
Year Founded: 1984   Federally Qualified: [N]
Forprofit: [ ]   Not-For-Profit: [ ]
Model Type: NETWORK
Accreditation: [ ] AAPPO [ ] JACHO [ ] NCQA [ ] URAC
Plan Type: HMO, PPO, POS, ASO, TPA, HSA
Total Enrollment:
  2001: 0   2004: 0   2007: 1,000,000
  2002: 0   2005:
  2003: 0   2006:

SERVICE AREA:
Nationwide: N
SC;

TYPE OF COVERAGE:
Commercial: [Y] Individual: [Y] FEHBP: [Y] Indemnity: [ ]
Medicare: [Y] Medicaid: [Y] Supplemental Medicare: [Y]
Tricare [Y]

PRODUCTS OFFERED:
Product Name: Type:
Preferred Blue   PPO
HMO Blue   HMO
BlueChoice Health Plan   HMO
Medicare Advantage   PFFS

CONSUMER-DRIVEN PRODUCTS
HSA Bank   HSA Company
Blue Health Fund HSA   HSA Product
HSA Bank   HSA Administrator
                              Consumer-Driven Health Plan
Blue Health Fund   High Deductible Health Plan

PLAN BENEFITS:
Alternative Medicine: [X]   Behavioral Health: [X]
Chiropractic: [X]   Dental: [X]
Home Care: [X]   Inpatient SNF: [X]
Long-Term Care: [X]   Pharm. Mail Order: [X]
Physical Therapy: [X]   Podiatry: [X]
Psychiatric: [X]   Transplant: [X]
Vision: [X]   Wellness: [X]
Workers' Comp: [X]
Other Benefits:

Comments:
A Mutual Insurance Company.

BLUECHOICE HEALTH PLAN OF SOUTH CAROLINA INC

4101 Percical Rd
Columbia, SC 29223
Phone: 803-786-8466 Fax: 803-714-6461 Toll-Free: 800-327-3183
Web site: www.bluechoicesc.com

MAILING ADDRESS:
BLUECHOICE HEALTH PLAN OF SC INC
4101 Percical Rd
Columbia, SC 29223

KEY EXECUTIVES:
Chief Executive Officer .... M Edward Sellers
President .... Mary Mazzola Spivey
Chief Medical Officer .... Laura Long, MD
Chief Operating Officer .... Mary Mazzola Spivey
VP of Marketing .... Bill Ferguson
VP of Provider Ntwk Services .... Ann Burnett

COMPANY PROFILE:
Parent Company Name: Blue Cross Blue Shield of SC
Doing Business As: BlueChoice Health Plan
Year Founded: 1984   Federally Qualified: [Y]
Forprofit: [Y]   Not-For-Profit: [ ]
Model Type: IPA
Accreditation: [ ] AAPPO [ ] JACHO [X] NCQA [ ] URAC
Plan Type: HMO, PPO, POS, HDHP, HSA,
Primary Physicians: 7,000   Physician Specialists:
Hospitals:
Total Enrollment:
  2001: 88,441   2004: 78,998   2007: 212,000
  2002: 88,710   2005: 85,875
  2003: 72,244   2006:

SERVICE AREA:
Nationwide: N
SC;

TYPE OF COVERAGE:
Commercial: [Y] Individual: [Y] FEHBP: [ ] Indemnity: [ ]
Medicare: [ ] Medicaid: [ ] Supplemental Medicare: [ ]
Tricare [ ]

PRODUCTS OFFERED:
Product Name: Type:
BlueChoice HMO   HMO
Choices   POS
Blueadvantage   Open access POS
Prime Companion   Medicare

PLAN BENEFITS:
Alternative Medicine: [X]   Behavioral Health: [ ]
Chiropractic: [X]   Dental: [X]
Home Care: [X]   Inpatient SNF: [X]
Long-Term Care: [X]   Pharm. Mail Order: [X]
Physical Therapy: [X]   Podiatry: [X]
Psychiatric: [X]   Transplant: [X]
Vision: [X]   Wellness: [X]
Workers' Comp: [ ]
Other Benefits:

Comments:
Formerly Companion Healthcare Corporation. Changed name July 1, 2005.

CAROLINA CARE PLAN INC

201 Executive Ctr Dr Ste 300
Columbia, SC 29210-8406
Phone: 803-750-7400 Fax: 803-750-7476 Toll-Free: 800-868-6734
Web site: www.carolinacareplan.com

MAILING ADDRESS:
CAROLINA CARE PLAN INC
201 Executive Ctr Dr Ste 300
Columbia, SC 29210-8406

KEY EXECUTIVES:
President .... Carson Meehan
Chief Financial Officer .... Mark T Corcoran
Medical Director .... Edward D Hutt, MD, MBA
Director, Pharmacy Operations .... Malissa Binley
Chief Information Officer .... Buster Elrod
VP of Operations & Medical Affairs .... Belinda Cox, RN, CPHQ
VP, Sales & Marketing .... Dave Olaka
VP, Network Management .... Donald Pifer

COMPANY PROFILE:
Parent Company Name: Managed by United Healthcare
Doing Business As:
Year Founded: 1985   Federally Qualified: [N]
Forprofit: [Y]   Not-For-Profit: [ ]
Model Type: IPA
Accreditation: [ ] AAPPO [ ] JACHO [ ] NCQA [ ] URAC
Plan Type: HMO, POS, HDHP, HSA,
Primary Physicians: Physician Specialists:
Hospitals: 61
Total Revenue: 2005: 102,416,407   2006:
Net Income   2005:   2006:

PLAN BENEFITS:
Alternative Medicine:	[X]	Behavioral Health:	[X]
Chiropractic:	[X]	Dental:	[ ]
Home Care:	[X]	Inpatient SNF:	[X]
Long-Term Care:	[ ]	Pharm. Mail Order:	[X]
Physical Therapy:	[X]	Podiatry:	[X]
Psychiatric:	[X]	Transplant:	[X]
Vision:	[X]	Wellness:	[X]
Workers' Comp:	[ ]		

Other Benefits:
Comments:
Acquiring Harvard Pilgrim's Rhode Island members.

UNITEDHEALTHCARE OF NEW ENGLAND INC

475 Kilvert St Ste 310
Warwick, RI 02886-1392
Phone: 401-737-6900 Fax: 401-732-7536 Toll-Free: 800-447-1245
Web site: www.uhc.com

MAILING ADDRESS:
UNITEDHEALTHCARE OF NE INC
475 Kilvert St Ste 310
Warwick, RI 02886-1392

KEY EXECUTIVES:
Non-Executive Chairman .... Richard T Burke
Chief Executive Officer/Chief Financial Officer .... Stephen J Farrell
Medical Director .... Neal Galinko, MD
Director of Pharmacy Services .... Scott Enos
Marketing Vice President .... Eric Swain
VP Finance & Assistant Treasurer .... Robert N Dellacorte

COMPANY PROFILE:
Parent Company Name: UnitedHealth Group
Doing Business As:
Year Founded: 1978   Federally Qualified: [N]
Forprofit: [Y]   Not-For-Profit: [ ]
Model Type: IPA
Accreditation: [ ] AAPPO [ ] JACHO [ ] NCQA [ ] URAC
Plan Type: HMO, PPO, POS, EPO, ASO, CDHP, HDHP, HSA,
Total Revenue: 2005: 345,030,172   2006: 362,528,833
Net Income   2005: 5,469,858   2006: 16,809,229
Total Enrollment:
   2001: 168,317   2004: 145,757   2007: 108,881
   2002: 155,153   2005: 131,112
   2003: 157,136   2006: 113,746
Medical Loss Ratio: 2005:   2006: 81.03

SERVICE AREA:
Nationwide: N
   MA (Barnstable, Bristol, Norfolk, Plymouth, Suffolk, Worcester);
   RI;

TYPE OF COVERAGE:
Commercial: [Y] Individual: [ ] FEHBP: [ ] Indemnity: [ ]
Medicare: [Y] Medicaid: [Y] Supplemental Medicare: [ ]
Tricare [ ]

PRODUCTS OFFERED:
Product Name:	Type:
Medicare Complete	Medicare Advantage
United Hlth Medicaid	Medicaid

CONSUMER-DRIVEN PRODUCTS
Exante Bank/Golden Rule Ins Co	HSA Company
iPlan HSA	HSA Product
	HSA Administrator
	Consumer-Driven Health Plan
	High Deductible Health Plan

PLAN BENEFITS:
Alternative Medicine:	[ ]	Behavioral Health:	[X]
Chiropractic:	[X]	Dental:	[ ]
Home Care:	[X]	Inpatient SNF:	[X]
Long-Term Care:	[ ]	Pharm. Mail Order:	[X]
Physical Therapy:	[X]	Podiatry:	[X]
Psychiatric:	[X]	Transplant:	[X]
Vision:	[X]	Wellness:	[X]
Workers' Comp:	[ ]		

Other Benefits:

RHODE ISLAND

DELTA DENTAL OF RHODE ISLAND

10 Charles St 3rd Fl
Providence, RI 02904-2208
Phone: 401-752-6000 Fax: 401-752-6060 Toll-Free: 800-598-6684
Web site: www.deltadentalri.com

MAILING ADDRESS:
DELTA DENTAL OF RI
PO Box 1517
Providence, RI 02904-2208

KEY EXECUTIVES:
Chairman of the Board .... Colin A MacGillivray
Chief Executive Officer/President .... Joseph A Nagle
VP, Finance .... Richard A Fritz
Dental Director .... Diane Monti-Markowski, DMD
VP Operations/Administration .... Stephen J Sperandio
VP of Marketing & Sales .... Angelo Pezzullo
Public Relations Coordinator .... Ann Corrado

COMPANY PROFILE:
Parent Company Name: Delta Dental Plan Association
Doing Business As:
Year Founded: 1959   Federally Qualified: [ ]
Forprofit: [ ]   Not-For-Profit: [ ]
Model Type:
Accreditation: [ ] AAPPO [ ] JACHO [ ] NCQA [ ] URAC
Plan Type: Specialty HMO
Total Revenue: 2005: 96,630,306   2006: 112,016,568
Net Income 2005: 5,002,585   2006: 4,689,338
Total Enrollment:
  2001: 490,782   2004: 541,446   2007: 330,481
  2002: 539,526   2005: 322,989
  2003: 548,822   2006: 363,678
Medical Loss Ratio: 2005: 83.10   2006: 85.70
Administrative Expense Ratio: 2005:   2006:

SERVICE AREA:
Nationwide: N
  RI;

TYPE OF COVERAGE:
Commercial: [Y] Individual: [ ] FEHBP: [ ] Indemnity: [ ]
Medicare: [ ] Medicaid: [ ] Supplemental Medicare: [ ]
Tricare

PLAN BENEFITS:
Alternative Medicine: [ ]   Behavioral Health: [ ]
Chiropractic: [ ]   Dental: [X]
Home Care: [ ]   Inpatient SNF: [ ]
Long-Term Care: [ ]   Pharm. Mail Order: [ ]
Physical Therapy: [ ]   Podiatry: [ ]
Psychiatric: [ ]   Transplant: [ ]
Vision: [ ]   Wellness: [ ]
Workers' Comp: [ ]
Other Benefits:

DMS DENTAL PLAN

1429 Warwick Ave
Warwick, RI 02888
Phone: 401-463-5116 Fax: 401-463-6059 Toll-Free: 800-456-8715
Web site:
MAILING ADDRESS:
DMS DENTAL PLAN
1429 Warwick Ave
Warwick, RI 02888

KEY EXECUTIVES:
Chief Executive Officer/Chief Financial Officer .... Linda S Kinney
Medical Director .... Christopher Walinski, MD
Chief Information Officer/Marketing Director .... James T Kinney

COMPANY PROFILE:
Parent Company Name: Dental Maintenance Service Inc
Doing Business As:
Year Founded: 1986   Federally Qualified: [ ]
Forprofit: [Y]   Not-For-Profit: [ ]
Model Type: NETWORK
Accreditation: [ ] AAPPO [ ] JACHO [ ] NCQA [ ] URAC
Plan Type: Specialty HMO

SERVICE AREA:
Nationwide: N
  MA; RI;

TYPE OF COVERAGE:
Commercial: [Y] Individual: [ ] FEHBP: [ ] Indemnity: [ ]
Medicare: [ ] Medicaid: [ ] Supplemental Medicare: [ ]
Tricare   [ ]

PLAN BENEFITS:
Alternative Medicine: [ ]   Behavioral Health: [ ]
Chiropractic: [ ]   Dental: [X]
Home Care: [ ]   Inpatient SNF: [ ]
Long-Term Care: [ ]   Pharm. Mail Order: [ ]
Physical Therapy: [ ]   Podiatry: [ ]
Psychiatric: [ ]   Transplant: [ ]
Vision: [X]   Wellness: [ ]
Workers' Comp: [ ]
Other Benefits:

NEIGHBORHOOD HEALTH PLAN OF RHODE ISLAND

299 Promenade St
Providence, RI 02908
Phone: 401-459-6000 Fax: 401-459-6175 Toll-Free: 800-963-1001
Web site: www.nhpri.org
MAILING ADDRESS:
NEIGHBORHOOD HLTH PLN OF RI
299 Promenade St
Providence, RI 02908

KEY EXECUTIVES:
Chairman of the Board .... Raymond Lavoie
Chief Executive Officer .... Mark Reynolds
Chief Financial Officer .... Scott O'Gorman
Medical Director .... L McTyeire Johnston, MD
Pharmacy Director .... Peter Vargas
Chief Operating Officer .... Nancy Coburn
MIS Director .... Sin Mei Ko
Credentialing Manager .... Patricia Huschie
Public Relations Director .... Brenda Whittle
Provider Relations/Network Development Director ..... Nancy Hermniz
Human Resources Director .... Frank Tabela
Quality Assurance Director .... Beth Marootian
Fraud Prevention Director .... Tracy McCaughey

COMPANY PROFILE:
Parent Company Name:
Doing Business As:
Year Founded: 1994   Federally Qualified: [N]
Forprofit: [ ]   Not-For-Profit: [Y]
Model Type: NETWORK
Accreditation: [ ] AAPPO [ ] JACHO [X] NCQA [ ] URAC
Plan Type: HMO
Total Revenue: 2005: 170,305,090   2006: 183,200,683
Net Income 2005: 9,104,628   2006: 7,880,820
Total Enrollment:
  2001: 74,603   2004: 68,206   2007: 66,056
  2002: 70,857   2005: 68,413
  2003: 66,505   2006: 68,294
Medical Loss Ratio: 2005:   2006: 89.50
Administrative Expense Ratio: 2005:   2006:

SERVICE AREA:
Nationwide: N
  RI;

TYPE OF COVERAGE:
Commercial: [Y] Individual: [ ] FEHBP: [ ] Indemnity: [ ]
Medicare: [ ] Medicaid: [Y] Supplemental Medicare: [ ]
Tricare   [ ]

PRODUCTS OFFERED:
Product Name: Type:
Neighborhood Health Plan   Medicaid

Managed Care Organization Profiles **RHODE ISLAND**

ALTUS DENTAL INSURANCE COMPANY INC

10 Charles St 3rd Fl
Providence, RI 02904-2208
Phone: 877-223-0577 Fax: 401-752-6060 Toll-Free: 800-598-6684
Web site: www.altusdental.com
MAILING ADDRESS:
 ALTUS DENTAL INSURANCE CO INC
 10 Charles St 3rd Fl
 Providence, RI 02904-2208

KEY EXECUTIVES:
Chairman of the Board .... Colin A MacGillivray
Chief Executive Officer/President .... Joseph A Nagle
VP, Finance .... Richard A Fritz
VP, Operations/Administration .... Stephen J Sperandio
VP, Sales .... Joseph Perroni

COMPANY PROFILE:
Parent Company Name: Delta Dental Plan Association
Doing Business As:
Year Founded: 2000   Federally Qualified: [ ]
Forprofit: [ ]   Not-For-Profit: [ ]
Model Type:
Accreditation: [ ] AAPPO [ ] JACHO [ ] NCQA [ ] URAC
Plan Type: Specialty HMO,
Total Revenue: 2005: 12,387,280   2006: 16,094,054
Net Income   2005: 406,872   2006: 108,398
Total Enrollment:
  2001: 0   2004: 30,097   2007: 60,338
  2002: 11,558   2005: 39,173
  2003: 19,671   2006: 57,156
Medical Loss Ratio: 2005:   2006: 81.20
Administrative Expense Ratio: 2005:   2006:
SERVICE AREA:
Nationwide: N
 RI;
TYPE OF COVERAGE:
Commercial: [Y] Individual: [ ] FEHBP: [ ] Indemnity: [ ]
Medicare: [ ] Medicaid: [ ] Supplemental Medicare: [ ]
Tricare   [ ]
PLAN BENEFITS:
Alternative Medicine: [ ]   Behavioral Health: [ ]
Chiropractic: [ ]   Dental: [X]
Home Care: [ ]   Inpatient SNF: [ ]
Long-Term Care: [ ]   Pharm. Mail Order: [ ]
Physical Therapy: [ ]   Podiatry: [ ]
Psychiatric: [ ]   Transplant: [ ]
Vision: [ ]   Wellness: [ ]
Workers' Comp: [ ]
Other Benefits:

BLUE CROSS BLUE SHIELD OF RHODE ISLAND

444 Westminster St
Providence, RI 02903
Phone: 401-459-1000 Fax: 401-455-6990 Toll-Free: 800-637-3718
Web site: www.bcbsri.com
MAILING ADDRESS:
 BLUE CROSS BLUE SHIELD OF RI
 444 Westminster St
 Providence, RI 02903

KEY EXECUTIVES:
Chief Executive Officer/President .... James E Purcell, Esq
Chief Financial Officer .... James J Joy
Chief of Communications .... Christopher J Medici
VP, Sales & Marketing .... Matthew T Brannigan
VP, Information Technology .... Everett J Sutherladn
VP, Human Resources .... Eric Gasbarro
VP, Community Relations .... Linda H Newton
VP, Strategic Planning/Communications .... Dale D Huff
VP, Government Relations .... Scott A Frazer
VP, Health & Wellness Services .... Michael H Samuelson
VP, Underwriting .... Thomas A Boyd
VP, General Counsel .... Michele B Lederberg
VP, Operations .... John H Gorman

COMPANY PROFILE:
Parent Company Name:
Doing Business As: BlueCHiP
Year Founded: 1939   Federally Qualified: [ ]
Forprofit: [ ]   Not-For-Profit: [Y]
Model Type:
Accreditation: [ ] AAPPO [ ] JACHO [X] NCQA [X] URAC
Plan Type: HMO, PPO
Total Revenue: 2005:1,586,311,420   2006: 1,696,753,816
Net Income   2005: 31,054,531   2006: 49,979,879
Total Enrollment:
  2001: 0   2004: 680,000   2007: 510,609
  2002: 364,553   2005: 443,447
  2003: 670,000   2006: 465,262
Medical Loss Ratio: 2005: 87.60   2006: 85.50
Administrative Expense Ratio: 2005:   2006:
SERVICE AREA:
Nationwide: N
 RI;
TYPE OF COVERAGE:
Commercial: [Y] Individual: [Y] FEHBP: [ ] Indemnity: [ ]
Medicare: [ ] Medicaid: [ ] Supplemental Medicare: [ ]
Tricare   [ ]
PRODUCTS OFFERED:
Product Name: Type:
HealthMate Coast-to-Coast   PPO
BlueChip   HMO
Classic Blue   Trad
Blue Cross Dental   Dental
Pharmacy   PBM
PLAN BENEFITS:
Alternative Medicine: [ ]   Behavioral Health: [X]
Chiropractic: [X]   Dental: [X]
Home Care: [X]   Inpatient SNF: [X]
Long-Term Care: [ ]   Pharm. Mail Order: [ ]
Physical Therapy: [X]   Podiatry: [X]
Psychiatric: [X]   Transplant: [X]
Vision: [X]   Wellness: [X]
Workers' Comp: [X]
Other Benefits: X

COORDINATED HEALTH PLAN

444 Westminster St
Providence, RI 02903-3279
Phone: 401-459-5601 Fax: 401-459-5586 Toll-Free: 800-564-0888
Web site: www.bcbsri.com
MAILING ADDRESS:
 COORDINATED HEALTH PLAN
 444 Westminster St
 Providence, RI 02903-3279

KEY EXECUTIVES:
Chief Executive Officer/President .... James E Purcell
Chief Financial Officer .... James J Joy
Chief Information Officer .... E J Southerland
Communications Director .... Dale D Huff
Chief of Communications .... Christopher Medici
VP, Sales & Marketing .... Matthew T Brannigan
Assistant VP, Public Relations .... Kim Keough
AVP, Medical Management .... Mary Hickey

COMPANY PROFILE:
Parent Company Name: Blue Cross Blue Shield of Rhode Island
Doing Business As: BlueChip, Coordinated Health Partners
Year Founded: 1987   Federally Qualified: [Y]
Forprofit: [Y]   Not-For-Profit: [ ]
Model Type: IPA
Accreditation: [ ] AAPPO [ ] JACHO [X] NCQA [X] URAC
Plan Type: HMO, PPO, POS:
Total Enrollment:
  2001: 116,496   2004: 106,969   2007: 0
  2002: 123,715   2005:
  2003: 112,723   2006:
SERVICE AREA:
Nationwide: N
 RI;
TYPE OF COVERAGE:
Commercial: [Y] Individual: [ ] FEHBP: [ ] Indemnity: [ ]
Medicare: [Y] Medicaid: [Y] Supplemental Medicare: [ ]
Tricare   [ ]
PRODUCTS OFFERED:
Product Name: Type:
BlueCHiP Commercial   HMO
BlueCHiP for Medicare   Medicare Advantage
BlueCHiP for Rite Care   Medicaid

PUERTO RICO

COMPANY PROFILE:
Parent Company Name: Medical Card System Inc
Doing Business As: Medical Card System
Year Founded: 1982 Federally Qualified: [N]
Forprofit: [Y] Not-For-Profit: [ ]
Model Type: IPA
Accreditation: [ ] AAPPO [ ] JACHO [ ] NCQA [ ] URAC
Plan Type: HMO, PPO, Specialty PPO, UR, POS, TPA, ASO, EPO
Primary Physicians: 729 Physician Specialists: 2,088
Hospitals: 44
Total Enrollment:
2001: 0   2004: 750,000   2007: 750,000
2002: 549,380   2005: 278,334
2003: 0   2006:

SERVICE AREA:
Nationwide: N
PR;

TYPE OF COVERAGE:
Commercial: [Y] Individual: [Y] FEHBP: [ ] Indemnity: [ ]
Medicare: [ ] Medicaid: [Y] Supplemental Medicare: [ ]
Tricare [ ]

PLAN BENEFITS:
Alternative Medicine: [ ] Behavioral Health: [X]
Chiropractic: [X] Dental: [X]
Home Care: [X] Inpatient SNF: [ ]
Long-Term Care: [X] Pharm. Mail Order: [X]
Physical Therapy: [ ] Podiatry: [X]
Psychiatric: [X] Transplant: [X]
Vision: [X] Wellness: [ ]
Workers' Comp: [ ]
Other Benefits:

MMM HEALTHCARE INC

350 Chardon Ave Ste 500
San Juan, PR 00918
Phone: 787-622-3000 Fax: 787-620-2399 Toll-Free:
Web site: www.aveta.com

MAILING ADDRESS:
MMM HEALTHCARE INC
350 Chardon Ave Ste 500
San Juan, PR 00936-3628

KEY EXECUTIVES:
Chief Executive Officer .... Val Dean, MD
President .... Julio F Julia
VP, Chief Medical Officer .... David Scanavino

COMPANY PROFILE:
Parent Company Name:
Doing Business As:
Year Founded: Federally Qualified: [ ]
Forprofit: [Y] Not-For-Profit: [ ]
Model Type: GROUP
Accreditation: [ ] AAPPO [ ] JACHO [ ] NCQA [ ] URAC
Plan Type: HMO
Total Enrollment:
2001: 2,389   2004: 73,123   2007: 0
2002: 17,534   2005:
2003: 38,754   2006:

SERVICE AREA:
Nationwide:
PR;

TYPE OF COVERAGE:
Commercial: [ ] Individual: [ ] FEHBP: [ ] Indemnity: [ ]
Medicare: [Y] Medicaid: [ ] Supplemental Medicare: [ ]
Tricare [ ]

PRODUCTS OFFERED:
Product Name: Type:
Medicare & Mucho Mas (MMM) Medicare

TRIPLE-S INC

1441 FD Roosevelt Ave
San Juan, PR 00920
Phone: 787-749-4949 Fax: 787-706-4006 Toll-Free: 787-749-4193
Web site: www.ssspr.com

MAILING ADDRESS:
TRIPLE-S INC
PO Box 363628
San Juan, PR 00920

KEY EXECUTIVES:
President .... Socotto Rivas
Treasurer .... Vincente J Leon Irizarry, CPA
Compliance Director .... Julia Lopez
VP of Human Resources .... Arturo Delahongra

COMPANY PROFILE:
Parent Company Name: Blue Cross Blue Shield
Doing Business As:
Year Founded: 1959 Federally Qualified: [N]
Forprofit: [Y] Not-For-Profit: [ ]
Model Type:
Accreditation: [ ] AAPPO [ ] JACHO [ ] NCQA [ ] URAC
Plan Type: HMO, PPO,
Total Enrollment:
2001: 1,319,012   2004: 1,237,012   2007: 1,200,000
2002: 1,273,256   2005: 337,626
2003: 1,236,799   2006:

SERVICE AREA:
Nationwide: N
PR;

TYPE OF COVERAGE:
Commercial: [Y] Individual: [ ] FEHBP: [ ] Indemnity: [ ]
Medicare: [Y] Medicaid: [Y] Supplemental Medicare: [ ]
Tricare [ ]

PRODUCTS OFFERED:
Product Name: Type:
Triple-S Medicaid Medicaid

Managed Care Organization Profiles — **PUERTO RICO**

BLUE CROSS OF PUERTO RICO/ LA CRUZ AZUL DE PUERTO RICO

Carr Estatal #1 Km.17.3
San Juan, PR 00927
Phone: 787-272-9898 Fax: 787-272-7867 Toll-Free: 888-272-9078
Web site: www.cruzazul.com
MAILING ADDRESS:
   BLUE CROSS OF PUERTO RICO
   PO Box 366038
   San Juan, PR 00927

KEY EXECUTIVES:
Chief Executive Officer .... Oscar Garcia Romain
President .... Zoraida Marchany
VP Medical Director .... Arcilio Alvarado
VP Operations .... Zloria Zibes

COMPANY PROFILE:
Parent Company Name:
Doing Business As:
Year Founded: 1940   Federally Qualified: [ ]
Forprofit: [ ]   Not-For-Profit: [ ]
Model Type:
Accreditation: [ ] AAPPO [ ] JACHO [ ] NCQA [ ] URAC
Plan Type: HMO
Primary Physicians: 7,314   Physician Specialists:
Hospitals: 59

SERVICE AREA:
Nationwide: N
   PR;

TYPE OF COVERAGE:
Commercial: [Y] Individual: [ ] FEHBP: [ ] Indemnity: [ ]
Medicare: [ ] Medicaid: [ ] Supplemental Medicare: [ ]
Tricare   [ ]
PRODUCTS OFFERED:
Product Name: Type:
La Cruz Azul de Puerto Rico   Medicaid

DELTA DENTAL PLAN OF PUERTO RICO

75 DeDiego Ave, Cornr Loiza St
Santruce, PR 00902
Phone: 877-728-6120 Fax: 787-728-9618 Toll-Free:
Web site: www.deltapr.com
MAILING ADDRESS:
   DELTA DENTAL PLAN OF PR
   PO Box 9020992
   San Juan, PR 00902

COMPANY PROFILE:
Parent Company Name: Delta Dental Plan Association
Doing Business As:
Year Founded: 1984   Federally Qualified: [ ]
Forprofit: [ ]   Not-For-Profit: [ ]
Model Type:
Accreditation: [ ] AAPPO [ ] JACHO [ ] NCQA [ ] URAC
Plan Type: Specialty HMO,
Total Enrollment:
   2001: 0   2004: 309,997   2007: 0
   2002: 226,461   2005:
   2003: 225,399   2006:

SERVICE AREA:
Nationwide: N
   PR;

TYPE OF COVERAGE:
Commercial: [Y] Individual: [ ] FEHBP: [ ] Indemnity: [ ]
Medicare: [ ] Medicaid: [ ] Supplemental Medicare: [ ]
Tricare   [ ]
PLAN BENEFITS:
Alternative Medicine: [ ]   Behavioral Health: [ ]
Chiropractic: [ ]   Dental: [X]
Home Care: [ ]   Inpatient SNF: [ ]
Long-Term Care: [ ]   Pharm. Mail Order: [ ]
Physical Therapy: [ ]   Podiatry: [ ]
Psychiatric: [ ]   Transplant: [ ]
Vision: [ ]   Wellness: [ ]
Workers' Comp: [ ]
Other Benefits:

HUMANA INC/PCA - PUERTO RICO

383 FD Roosevelt 3rd Fl
San Juan, PR 00918-2131
Phone: 787-622-5555 Fax: 787-282-6277 Toll-Free: 800-314-3121
Web site: www.humana.prcom
MAILING ADDRESS:
   HUMANA INC PCA PUERTO RICO
   383 FD Roosevelt 3rd Fl
   San Juan, PR 00918-2131

KEY EXECUTIVES:
Chairman/Chief Executive Officer .... Victor Gutierrez, MD
President/Chief Operating Officer .... David M Krebs
VP, Provider Network Operations .... Angel L Cordero
Human Resources Director .... Arlene Marrero
Marketing/Public Relations Director .... Sandra Estada
Government Relations Director .... Hector Mujica

COMPANY PROFILE:
Parent Company Name: Humana Inc
Doing Business As:
Year Founded: 1961   Federally Qualified: [Y]
Forprofit: [Y]   Not-For-Profit: [ ]
Model Type: IPA
Accreditation: [ ] AAPPO [ ] JACHO [ ] NCQA [ ] URAC
Plan Type: HMO, PPO, CDHP, HDHP, HSA,
Total Enrollment:
   2001: 198,248   2004: 417,284   2007: 0
   2002: 430,000   2005: 216,056
   2003: 490,400   2006:

SERVICE AREA:
Nationwide: N
   PR:

TYPE OF COVERAGE:
Commercial: [Y] Individual: [ ] FEHBP: [ ] Indemnity: [ ]
Medicare: [ ] Medicaid: [Y] Supplemental Medicare: [ ]
Tricare   [ ]
PRODUCTS OFFERED:
Product Name: Type:
Humana Medicaid   Medicaid
CONSUMER-DRIVEN PRODUCTS
JP Morgan Chase   HSA Company
HumanaOne HSA   HSA Product
JP Morgan Chase   HSA Administrator
Personal Care Account   Consumer-Driven Health Plan
HumanaOne   High Deductible Health Plan
PLAN BENEFITS:
Alternative Medicine: [ ]   Behavioral Health: [X]
Chiropractic: [X]   Dental: [X]
Home Care: [ ]   Inpatient SNF: [ ]
Long-Term Care: [ ]   Pharm. Mail Order: [X]
Physical Therapy: [ ]   Podiatry: [ ]
Psychiatric: [X]   Transplant: [X]
Vision: [ ]   Wellness: [ ]
Workers' Comp: [X]
Other Benefits: Long Term Disability Care

MEDICAL CARD SYSTEM

255 Ponce De Leon Ave Ste 1600
Hato Rey, PR 00917
Phone: 787-758-2500 Fax: 787-250-0380 Toll-Free:
Web site: www.mcs.com.pr
MAILING ADDRESS:
   MEDICAL CARD SYSTEM
   255 Ponce De Leon Ave Ste 1600
   Hato Rey, PR 00917

KEY EXECUTIVES:
Executive Chairman .... Carlos A Munoz-Bravo, PhD
Chief Executive Officer .... Gregory H Wolf
Chief Operating Officer .... Madeline Hernandez-Urquiza, CPA
Chief Financial Officer .... Mark Rishell
Chie Medical Officer .... Mary Davis, MD
VP, Information Systems/Technology .... Gerald Lopez De Choudens
Chief Sales & Marketing .... Jose Abreu
VP, Finance .... David Schaffer
VP, Business Development & Marketing .... Roberto Pando
Group Sales .... Jaime Pericas
VP, Individual Sales .... Richard Luna
VP, Network Administration .... Edmuno Caban
Medical Management .... Eddie Ortiz, MD
UM, Health Management .... Ines Hernandez, MD
VP, Claims & Quality Assurance Operations .... Ing Pedro Aponte

PENNSYLVANIA

TYPE OF COVERAGE:
Commercial: [Y] Individual: [ ] FEHBP: [ ] Indemnity: [ ]
Medicare: [ ] Medicaid: [ ] Supplemental Medicare: [ ]
Tricare [ ]

PRODUCTS OFFERED:
Product Name:	Type:
Vantage PPO	PPO

Comments:
Formerly Crawford Health Plan.

Managed Care Organization Profiles PENNSYLVANIA

KEY EXECUTIVES:
Chairman of the Board .... G Nicholas Beckwith, III
Chief Executive Officer/President .... Diane P Holder
Acting Chief Financial Officer .... Scott Lammie
Chief Medical Officer .... Ann Boland Docimo, MD
Director, Clinical Pharmacy .... Rae Ann Maxwell
VP of Information Systems .... Joyce Metnick
Director Operations & System Support .... Mary Beth Jenkins
Exec Director, Sales/Marketing/Communications .. Anthony Benevento
Chief Information Officer .... Ed McCallister
Director, Legal Services/Chief Compliance Offr .... Daniel Vukmer, Esq
Communications Director .... Bill Sawchak
Director, Network Management .... Rita Orr
Seniorr Program Manager .... Susan Dachille
Manager, Human Resources .... Sharon Cayzewski
Senior Director of Medical Management .... Colleen Walsh
Director, Quality Management & Improvement .... Debra Rose Horn
Director Quality Audit, Fraud, Abuse .... Bill Gedman
Manager, Product Development .... Connie Koch
Acting VP, Clinical & Network Service .... Debra Rose Horn
VP, Medicaid Programs, Children's Health .... John Lovelace
VP, Medical Affairs .... Michael Culyba, MD
VP, EAP Solutions .... Richard S Citrin, PhD, MBA

COMPANY PROFILE:
Parent Company Name: University of Pittsburgh Medical Center
Doing Business As: UPMC Health Plan
Year Founded: 1996   Federally Qualified: [ ]
Forprofit: [Y]   Not-For-Profit: [ ]
Model Type: Network
Accreditation: [ ] AAPPO [ ] JACHO [X] NCQA [ ] URAC
Plan Type: HMO, POS
Primary Physicians: 2,568   Physician Specialists: 3,947
Hospitals: 76
Total Revenue: 2005:   1,600,000,000   2006:
Net Income   2005:   41,000,000   2006:
Total Enrollment:
    2001: 72,764   2004: 307,403   2007: 297,988
    2002: 346,268   2005: 288,101
    2003: 321,628   2006: 281,640

SERVICE AREA:
Nationwide: N
    PA (Armstrong, Allegheny, Beaver, Bedford, Blair, Butler, Cambria, Fayette, Greene, Indiana, Lawrence, McKean, Mercer, Washington, Westmoreland);

TYPE OF COVERAGE:
Commercial: [Y] Individual: [ ] FEHBP: [ ] Indemnity: [ ]
Medicare: [ ] Medicaid: [Y] Supplemental Medicare: [Y]
Tricare   [ ]

PRODUCTS OFFERED:
Product Name: Type:
Enhanced Access HMO   HMO
Traditional   HMO
Enhanced Access POS   POS
UPMC For You   Medicaid
UPMC For Life   Medicare
UPMC Health Plan   Medicare Advantage
Self-Funded Traditional   HMO

PLAN BENEFITS:
Alternative Medicine: [ ]   Behavioral Health: [X]
Chiropractic: [X]   Dental: [ ]
Home Care: [X]   Inpatient SNF: [X]
Long-Term Care: [ ]   Pharm. Mail Order: [X]
Physical Therapy: [X]   Podiatry: [X]
Psychiatric: [X]   Transplant: [X]
Vision: [X]   Wellness: [X]
Workers' Comp: [ ]
Other Benefits:

VALLEY PREFERRED

1605 N Cedar Crest Blvd Ste 411
Allentown, PA 18104-2351
Phone: 610-969-0480 Fax: 610-969-0439 Toll-Free: 800-955-6620
Web site: www.valleypreferred.com
MAILING ADDRESS:
    VALLEY PREFERRED
    1605 N Cedar Crest Blvd Ste 411
    Allentown, PA 18104-2351

KEY EXECUTIVES:
Executive Director .... Gregory Kile
Executive Medical Director .... John Jaffe, MD
Chief Information Officer .... Louis Bottitta
Director of Operations .... Joseph Felix
General Manager .... Laura Mertz
Director Provider Relations .... Patricia Sarik
Medical Director .... Jack Lenhart, MD

COMPANY PROFILE:
Parent Company Name: Lehigh Valley Physician Hospital Org Inc
Doing Business As: Valley Preferred
Year Founded: 1993   Federally Qualified: [N]
Forprofit: [ ]   Not-For-Profit: [Y]
Model Type: NETWORK
Accreditation: [X] AAPPO [ ] JACHO [ ] NCQA [ ] URAC
Plan Type: PPO, Specialty PPO
Primary Physicians: 768   Physician Specialists: 2,654
Hospitals: 18
Total Enrollment:
    2001: 83,482   2004: 0   2007: 186,201
    2002: 83,658   2005:
    2003: 0   2006: 186,000

SERVICE AREA:
Nationwide: N
    PA (Bucks, Carbon, Columbia, Lehigh, Luzerne, Montgomery, Northampton);

TYPE OF COVERAGE:
Commercial: [Y] Individual: [Y] FEHBP: [ ] Indemnity: [ ]
Medicare: [ ] Medicaid: [ ]   Supplemental Medicare: [ ]
Tricare   [ ]

PRODUCTS OFFERED:
Product Name: Type:
Valley Preferred   PPO

PLAN BENEFITS:
Alternative Medicine: [ ]   Behavioral Health: [X]
Chiropractic: [ ]   Dental: [X]
Home Care: [X]   Inpatient SNF: [X]
Long-Term Care: [X]   Pharm. Mail Order: [X]
Physical Therapy: [X]   Podiatry: [X]
Psychiatric: [X]   Transplant: [X]
Vision: [X]   Wellness: [X]
Workers' Comp: [ ]
Other Benefits: MRI, Trauma Unit

VANTAGE PPO

11031 Perry Hwy Ste 105
Meadville, PA 16335
Phone: 814-333-8533 Fax: 814-337-8777 Toll-Free:
Web site: www.vhcn.com
MAILING ADDRESS:
    VANTAGE PPO
    11031 Perry Hwy Ste 105
    Meadville, PA 16335

KEY EXECUTIVES:
Chief Executive Officer .... Gerald Alonge
Chief Financial Officer .... Michael Mosbacher
Medical Director .... Ken Challener, MD
Chief Operating Officer .... Cheryl Sedlak
Marketing/Communications Director .... Tom Surman

COMPANY PROFILE:
Parent Company Name: Vantage Healthcare Network
Doing Business As:
Year Founded: 1992   Federally Qualified: [ ]
Forprofit: [Y]   Not-For-Profit: [ ]
Model Type:
Accreditation: [X] AAPPO [ ] JACHO [ ] NCQA [ ] URAC
Plan Type: PPO
Total Enrollment:
    2001: 0   2004: 30,000   2007: 0
    2002: 0   2005:
    2003: 0   2006:

SERVICE AREA:
Nationwide: N
    PA (Crawford and its contiguous counties);

PENNSYLVANIA

KEY EXECUTIVES:
Chairperson of the Board .... Thomas A Dzuryachko
Chief Executive Officer/President .... Thomas A Dzuryachko
Senior VP, Finance .... Daniel Wright
VP, National Dental Director .... Richard Klich, DMD
Senior VP, Operations .... Jon Seltenheim
Senior VP, Chief Marketing Officer .... Chip Merkel
Senior VP, Sales .... Jan Jewett
Corp VP, Professional Relations .... Karen Whitesel
VP, Human Resources .... Harlon Robinson
Corp VP, TRICARE Dental Program .... Dr Lawrence McKinley

COMPANY PROFILE:
Parent Company Name: Highmark Inc
Doing Business As:
Year Founded: 1992   Federally Qualified: [ ]
Forprofit: [Y]   Not-For-Profit: [ ]
Model Type:
Accreditation: [ ] AAPPO [ ] JACHO [ ] NCQA [ ] URAC
Plan Type: Specialty HMO, Specialty PPO, POS, ASO, TPA
Primary Physicians: 362   Physician Specialists:
Hospitals:
Total Revenue: 2005:   2006: 1,188,991,000
Net Income   2005:   2006: 56,904,000
Total Enrollment:
  2001: 6,500,000   2004: 0   2007: 7,300,000
  2002: 0   2005: 7,000,000
  2003: 6,000,000   2006: 7,200,000

SERVICE AREA:
Nationwide: Y
  AZ; CO; HI; NV; NM; UT; AK; ID; MT; OR; WA; WY;
  LA; OK; TX; PA; NY; MD; ME; MA; NH; VT; KY; VA;
  WV; VA; IL; IN; MI; WI; AL; FL' GA; MS; NC; PR;
  SC; IL; IA; MN; NE; ND; SD; CA;

TYPE OF COVERAGE:
Commercial: [Y] Individual: [ ] FEHBP: [ ] Indemnity: [ ]
Medicare: [ ] Medicaid: [ ] Supplemental Medicare: [ ]
Tricare   [Y]

PLAN BENEFITS:
Alternative Medicine: [ ]   Behavioral Health: [ ]
Chiropractic: [ ]   Dental: [X]
Home Care: [ ]   Inpatient SNF: [ ]
Long-Term Care: [ ]   Pharm. Mail Order: [ ]
Physical Therapy: [ ]   Podiatry: [ ]
Psychiatric: [ ]   Transplant: [ ]
Vision: [ ]   Wellness: [ ]
Workers' Comp: [ ]
Other Benefits:

Comments:
Formerly MIDA Dental Plans - UCCI Inc. Listing reflects corporate office and nationwide enrollment and revenue information.

UNITED CONCORDIA COMPANY INC - PENNSYLVANIA

120 5th Ave Ste P2503
Pittsburgh, PA 15222
Phone: 412-544-3650 Fax: 412-544-2380 Toll-Free:
Web site: www.ucci.com
MAILING ADDRESS:
  UNITED CONCORDIA CO INC - PA
  120 5th Ave Ste P2503
  Pittsburgh, PA 15222

KEY EXECUTIVES:
Chief Executive Officer/President .... Thomas A Dzuryachko
Senior VP, Finance .... Daniel Wright
VP, National Dental Director .... Richard Klich, DMD
Regional Sales Director .... Vince Pinzotto

COMPANY PROFILE:
Parent Company Name: Highmark Inc
Doing Business As:
Year Founded: 1991   Federally Qualified: [ ]
Forprofit: [Y]   Not-For-Profit: [ ]
Model Type:
Accreditation: [ ] AAPPO [ ] JACHO [ ] NCQA [ ] URAC
Plan Type: Specialty HMO, Specialty PPO, POS, TPA

SERVICE AREA:
Nationwide: N
  KY; MI; OH; PA (Western); WV;

TYPE OF COVERAGE:
Commercial: [Y] Individual: [ ] FEHBP: [ ] Indemnity: [ ]
Medicare: [ ] Medicaid: [ ] Supplemental Medicare: [ ]
Tricare   [ ]

PLAN BENEFITS:
Alternative Medicine: [ ]   Behavioral Health: [ ]
Chiropractic: [ ]   Dental: [X]
Home Care: [ ]   Inpatient SNF: [ ]
Long-Term Care: [ ]   Pharm. Mail Order: [ ]
Physical Therapy: [ ]   Podiatry: [ ]
Psychiatric: [ ]   Transplant: [ ]
Vision: [ ]   Wellness: [ ]
Workers' Comp: [ ]
Other Benefits:

UNITED CONCORDIA COMPANY INC - PENNSYLVANIA - CENTRAL

4401 Deer Path Rd - Northwoods
Harrisburg, PA 17011
Phone: 717-260-6800 Fax: 717-260-7485 Toll-Free: 800-972-4191
Web site: www.ucci.com
MAILING ADDRESS:
  UNITED CONCORDIA CO INC - PA
  4401 Deer Path Rd
  Harrisburg, PA 17011

KEY EXECUTIVES:
Chief Executive Officer/President .... Thomas A Dzuryachko
Senior VP, Finance .... Daniel Wright
VP, National Dental Director .... Richard Klich, DMD
Regional Sales Director .... Vince Pinzotto

COMPANY PROFILE:
Parent Company Name: Highmark Inc
Doing Business As:
Year Founded: 1991   Federally Qualified: [ ]
Forprofit: [Y]   Not-For-Profit: [ ]
Model Type:
Accreditation: [ ] AAPPO [ ] JACHO [ ] NCQA [ ] URAC
Plan Type: Specialty HMO, Specialty PPO, POS, TPA
Total Enrollment:
  2001: 1,505,396   2004: 1,613,137 2007: 0
  2002: 1,548,171   2005:
  2003: 1,581,025   2006:

SERVICE AREA:
Nationwide:
  PA (Central);

TYPE OF COVERAGE:
Commercial: [Y] Individual: [ ] FEHBP: [ ] Indemnity: [ ]
Medicare: [ ] Medicaid: [ ] Supplemental Medicare: [ ]
Tricare   [ ]

PLAN BENEFITS:
Alternative Medicine: [ ]   Behavioral Health: [ ]
Chiropractic: [ ]   Dental: [X]
Home Care: [ ]   Inpatient SNF: [ ]
Long-Term Care: [ ]   Pharm. Mail Order: [ ]
Physical Therapy: [ ]   Podiatry: [ ]
Psychiatric: [ ]   Transplant: [ ]
Vision: [ ]   Wellness: [ ]
Workers' Comp: [ ]
Other Benefits:

UPMC HEALTH PLAN
UNIVERSITY OF PITTSBURGH MEDICAL CENTER

1 Chatham Ctr 112 Washington P
Pittsburgh, PA 15219
Phone: 412-454-7500 Fax: 412-454-7711 Toll-Free:
Web site: www.upmchealthplan.com
MAILING ADDRESS:
  UPMC HEALTH PLAN
  1 Chatham Ctr 112 Washington P
  Pittsburgh, PA 15219

MAILING ADDRESS:
    UNISON HEALTH PLAN- CORP HQTRS
    1001 Brinton Rd
    Pittsburgh, PA 15221

KEY EXECUTIVES:
Chief Executive Officer .... John P Blank, MD
Chief Financial Officer .... Leslie A Gelpi
VP, Senior Medical Director .... Mark Mahler, MD
Pharmacy Director .... Jim Hancovsky
Chief Information Officer .... Steve Bugajski
Senior VP, Operations .... Fred O Madill
Senior VP, Medical Operations .... Shirley Blevins
Compliance Officer/Senior Counsel .... John G Beck
VP, Network Administration .... Heather Cianfrocco
Director, Marketing .... Brandon Moser
VP/General Counsel .... David Thomas, Esq
VP, Medicare Products .... Keith Vollberg

COMPANY PROFILE:
Parent Company Name: Three Rivers Holdings Inc
Doing Business As: Unison Advantage
Year Founded: 1995   Federally Qualified: [N]
Forprofit: [Y]   Not-For-Profit: [ ]
Model Type: MIXED
Accreditation: [ ] AAPPO [ ] JACHO [X] NCQA [ ] URAC
Plan Type: HMO
SERVICE AREA:
Nationwide: N
    AR; DE; MS; OH; PA; SC; TN;
TYPE OF COVERAGE:
Commercial: [ ] Individual: [ ] FEHBP: [ ] Indemnity: [ ]
Medicare: [Y] Medicaid: [Y] Supplemental Medicare: [ ]
Tricare [ ]
Comments:
Formerly known as: Three Rivers Health Plan

UNISON HEALTH PLAN OF PENNSYLVANIA

1388 Beulah Rd Bldg 801 4th Fl
Pittsburgh, PA 15235
Phone: 412-858-4000 Fax: 412-457-1414 Toll-Free: 800-414-9025
Web site: www.trhp.com
MAILING ADDRESS:
    UNISON HEALTH PLAN OF PA
    c/o TRAS 300 Oxford Dr
    Monroeville, PA 15235

KEY EXECUTIVES:
President - Pennsylvania .... Jennifer Kessler
Medical Director .... Joseph Sheridan, DO

COMPANY PROFILE:
Parent Company Name: Three Rivers Holdings Inc
Doing Business As: Unison Advantage
Year Founded: 1995   Federally Qualified: [N]
Forprofit: [Y]   Not-For-Profit: [ ]
Model Type: MIXED
Accreditation: [ ] AAPPO [ ] JACHO [X] NCQA [ ] URAC
Plan Type: HMO
Primary Physicians: 2,676   Physician Specialists: 7,541
Hospitals: 118
Total Enrollment:
    2001: 0   2004: 217,813   2007: 180,575
    2002: 190,703   2005: 223,823
    2003: 205,899   2006: 198,401
SERVICE AREA:
Nationwide: N
    PA (Allegheny, Armstrong, Beaver, Blair, Butler, Erie, Fayette, Green, Indian, Lockawanna, Lawrence, Mercer, Schuylkill, Washington, Westmoreland);
TYPE OF COVERAGE:
Commercial: [ ] Individual: [ ] FEHBP: [ ] Indemnity: [ ]
Medicare: [Y] Medicaid: [Y] Supplemental Medicare: [ ]
Tricare [ ]
PRODUCTS OFFERED:

Product Name:	Type:
Unison Family Health Plan PA	HMO
Unison Health Plan of PA	Medicare
Unison Health Plan of PA	Medicaid

PLAN BENEFITS:
Alternative Medicine: [ ]   Behavioral Health: [ ]
Chiropractic: [X]   Dental: [X]
Home Care: [X]   Inpatient SNF: [X]
Long-Term Care: [X]   Pharm. Mail Order: [ ]
Physicial Therapy: [X]   Podiatry: [X]
Psychiatric: [X]   Transplant: [X]
Vision: [X]   Wellness: [X]
Workers' Comp: [ ]
Other Benefits: Med Plus Miracles
Comments:
Formerly known as: Three Rivers Health Plan and Three Rivers Children's Health Plan.

UNITED BEHAVIORAL HEALTH

100 E Penn Sq Ste 400
Philadelphia, PA 19107
Phone: 215-557-6126 Fax: 215-557-5761 Toll-Free: 800-842-1311
Web site: www.unitedbehavioralhealth.com
MAILING ADDRESS:
    UNITED BEHAVIORAL HEALTH
    100 E Penn Sq Ste 400
    Phildelphia, PA 19107

KEY EXECUTIVES:
Chairman of the Board/Chief Executive Officer ..... Saul Feldman, MD
President .... Jim Hudak
Chief Financial Officer .... Karen Schievelbein
Chief Clinical Officer .... Robert Fusco, MD
Chief Operating Officer .... Jim Hudak
Director, Provider Services .... Chris Paules
VP Employee Division .... Michael Golinkoff, MD
Facilities Coordinator .... Colleen Canacan

COMPANY PROFILE:
Parent Company Name: UnitedHealth Group
Doing Business As: United Behavioral Health
Year Founded: 1988   Federally Qualified: [Y]
Forprofit: [Y]   Not-For-Profit: [ ]
Model Type:
Accreditation: [ ] AAPPO [ ] JACHO [ ] NCQA [ ] URAC
Plan Type: Specialty PPO, PPO, POS
SERVICE AREA:
Nationwide: N
    DE; NJ (South Jersey); PA (Philadelphia);
TYPE OF COVERAGE:
Commercial: [Y] Individual: [ ] FEHBP: [ ] Indemnity: [ ]
Medicare: [ ] Medicaid: [ ] Supplemental Medicare: [ ]
Tricare [ ]
PLAN BENEFITS:
Alternative Medicine: [ ]   Behavioral Health: [ ]
Chiropractic: [X]   Dental: [ ]
Home Care: [ ]   Inpatient SNF: [ ]
Long-Term Care: [ ]   Pharm. Mail Order: [ ]
Physicial Therapy: [ ]   Podiatry: [ ]
Psychiatric: [ ]   Transplant: [ ]
Vision: [ ]   Wellness: [ ]
Workers' Comp: [ ]
Other Benefits:
Comments:
Formerly MetraHealth.

UNITED CONCORDIA COMPANY INC - CORPORATE HEADQUARTERS

4401 Deer Path Rd - Northwoods
Harrisburg, PA 17110
Phone: 717-260-6800 Fax: 717-260-7485 Toll-Free: 800-972-4191
Web site: www.ucci.com
MAILING ADDRESS:
    UNITED CONCORDIA CO INC - CORP
    4401 Deer Path Rd
    Harrisburg, PA 17110

PENNSYLVANIA — Managed Care Organization Profiles

SENTINEL MANAGEMENT SERVICES - CORPORATE HEADQUARTERS

1871 Santa Barbara Drive
Lancaster, PA 17601
Phone: 717-581-1245 Fax: 717-581-8841 Toll-Free: 800-432-8877
Web site:

MAILING ADDRESS:
SENTINEL MANAGEMENT SERVICES
PO Box 8377
Lancaster, PA 17601

KEY EXECUTIVES:
President .... Robert Hettrick
Medical Director .... Robert Scott, MD
MIS Director .... Kathy Shaffer
Case Manager .... Karen Hermann

COMPANY PROFILE:
Parent Company Name:
Doing Business As:
Year Founded: 1988   Federally Qualified: [N]
Forprofit: [Y]   Not-For-Profit: [ ]
Model Type:
Accreditation: [ ] AAPPO [ ] JACHO [ ] NCQA [X] URAC
Plan Type: UR

SERVICE AREA:
Nationwide: Y
  NW;

TYPE OF COVERAGE:
Commercial: [Y] Individual: [Y] FEHBP: [ ] Indemnity: [ ]
Medicare: [ ] Medicaid: [ ] Supplemental Medicare: [ ]
Tricare   [ ]

PLAN BENEFITS:
Alternative Medicine: [ ]   Behavioral Health: [ ]
Chiropractic: [X]   Dental: [ ]
Home Care: [X]   Inpatient SNF: [X]
Long-Term Care: [X]   Pharm. Mail Order: [X]
Physical Therapy: [X]   Podiatry: [X]
Psychiatric: [X]   Transplant: [X]
Vision: [ ]   Wellness: [ ]
Workers' Comp: [X]
Other Benefits:

SOUTH CENTRAL PREFERRED

1803 Mount Rose Ave Ste B5
York, PA 17403
Phone: 717-851-6800 Fax: 717-851-6775 Toll-Free: 800-842-1768
Web site: www.scp-ppo.com

MAILING ADDRESS:
SOUTH CENTRAL PREFERRED
1803 Mount Rose Ave Ste B5
York, PA 17403

KEY EXECUTIVES:
Executive Director .... Charles Chodroff, MD
Manager Finance .... William Smith
Medical Director .... Neal Friedman
Chief Operating Officer .... James Cochran
Marketing Director .... Andrew Seebolt
Manager, Information Systems .... Christina Eckert
Manager, Provider Relations .... Jane Grove
Manager, Medical Management .... Vicki Armstrong
Director, TPA Operations .... Lynn Boyd
Manager, Claims .... Deborah Kehres
Manager, Customer Service .... Rebecca Timmermans

COMPANY PROFILE:
Parent Company Name: Wellspan Health System
Doing Business As: York Health Plan (So Central Preferred)
Year Founded: 1991   Federally Qualified: [ ]
Forprofit: [ ]   Not-For-Profit: [Y]
Model Type:
Accreditation: [ ] AAPPO [ ] JACHO [ ] NCQA [ ] URAC
Plan Type: PPO, TPA
Primary Physicians: 514   Physician Specialists: 1,005
Hospitals: 13

Total Enrollment:
  2001: 0   2004: 55,211   2007: 0
  2002: 0   2005: 50,080
  2003: 0   2006: 46,326

SERVICE AREA:
Nationwide: N
  PA (Adams, Franklin, York);

TYPE OF COVERAGE:
Commercial: [Y] Individual: [ ] FEHBP: [ ] Indemnity: [ ]
Medicare: [ ] Medicaid: [ ] Supplemental Medicare: [ ]
Tricare   [ ]

PLAN BENEFITS:
Alternative Medicine: [ ]   Behavioral Health: [X]
Chiropractic: [X]   Dental: [X]
Home Care: [X]   Inpatient SNF: [X]
Long-Term Care: [ ]   Pharm. Mail Order: [ ]
Physical Therapy: [X]   Podiatry: [X]
Psychiatric: [X]   Transplant: [X]
Vision: [X]   Wellness: [X]
Workers' Comp: [ ]
Other Benefits:
Comments:
Formerly York Health Plan.

SUSQUEHANNA HEALTH CARE

109 N Mulberry St
Berwick, PA 18603-4706
Phone: 570-759-1702 Fax: 570-759-2559 Toll-Free:
Web site:

MAILING ADDRESS:
SUSQUEHANNA HEALTH CARE
109 N Mulberry St
Berwick, PA 18603-4706

KEY EXECUTIVES:
Chief Executive Officer/President .... William Cusatis
Marketing Director .... James Cusatis
Provider Relations/Human Resources Director ... Ginger Bartholomew

COMPANY PROFILE:
Parent Company Name: Susquehanna Healthcare
Doing Business As: Susquehanna Healthcare
Year Founded: 1986   Federally Qualified: [N]
Forprofit: [Y]   Not-For-Profit: [ ]
Model Type: MIXED
Accreditation: [ ] AAPPO [ ] JACHO [ ] NCQA [ ] URAC
Plan Type: PPO, Specialty PPO
Primary Physicians: 225   Physician Specialists: 1,025
Hospitals: 32
Total Enrollment:
  2001: 32,000   2004: 0   2007: 0
  2002: 34,000   2005:
  2003: 42,000   2006:

SERVICE AREA:
Nationwide: N
  PA (Clinton, Columbia, Lycoming, Luzerne, Montour,
  Norrhumberland, Schuylkill, Snyder, Union); Carbon, Pike,
  Sullivan, Susgushanna, Wayne, Wyoming, Lackawanna,

TYPE OF COVERAGE:
Commercial: [Y] Individual: [Y] FEHBP: [ ] Indemnity: [ ]
Medicare: [ ] Medicaid: [ ] Supplemental Medicare: [Y]
Tricare   [ ]

PLAN BENEFITS:
Alternative Medicine: [ ]   Behavioral Health: [X]
Chiropractic: [X]   Dental: [X]
Home Care: [X]   Inpatient SNF: [X]
Long-Term Care: [ ]   Pharm. Mail Order: [X]
Physical Therapy: [X]   Podiatry: [X]
Psychiatric: [X]   Transplant: [X]
Vision: [ ]   Wellness: [X]
Workers' Comp: [ ]
Other Benefits: MRI, Transport, Hospital

UNISON HEALTH PLAN - CORPORATE HEADQUARTER

1001 Brinton Rd
Pittsburgh, PA 15221
Phone: 412-858-4000 Fax: 412-457-1414 Toll-Free: 800-414-9025
Web site: www.unisonhealthplan.com

Managed Care Organization Profiles — PENNSYLVANIA

COMPANY PROFILE:
Parent Company Name: PHC
Doing Business As:
Year Founded: 1984   Federally Qualified: [N]
Forprofit: [ ]   Not-For-Profit: [Y]
Model Type: NETWORK
Accreditation: [ ] AAPPO [ ] JACHO [ ] NCQA [ ] URAC
Plan Type: PPO
Total Enrollment:
  2001: 0   2004: 0   2007: 0
  2002: 0   2005:
  2003: 0   2006: 71,200

SERVICE AREA:
Nationwide: N
  PA (Lancaster, Chester);

TYPE OF COVERAGE:
Commercial: [Y] Individual: [Y] FEHBP: [ ] Indemnity: [ ]
Medicare: [ ] Medicaid: [ ] Supplemental Medicare: [ ]
Tricare [ ]

PRODUCTS OFFERED:
Product Name: Type:
Preferred Health Care   PPO

PLAN BENEFITS:
Alternative Medicine: [ ]   Behavioral Health: [X]
Chiropractic: [ ]   Dental: [ ]
Home Care: [X]   Inpatient SNF: [X]
Long-Term Care: [ ]   Pharm. Mail Order: [ ]
Physical Therapy: [X]   Podiatry: [X]
Psychiatric: [X]   Transplant: [X]
Vision: [ ]   Wellness: [ ]
Workers' Comp: [X]
Other Benefits:

PREFERRED HEALTHCARE SYSTEM INC

620 Howard Ave
Altoona, PA 16601
Phone: 814-889-3166 Fax: 814-889-3009 Toll-Free: 800-238-9900
Web site: www.phsppo.com

MAILING ADDRESS:
  PREFERRED HEALTHCARE SYSTEM
  620 Howard Ave
  Altoona, PA 16601

KEY EXECUTIVES:
Chief Executive Director/Chief Financial Offr .... Joseph R Fromknecht
Medical Director .... David Cowyer, MD
Marketing Representative .... Brian Brumbaugh
Provider Services Director .... Jeff Coltabaugh
Marketing Representative .... Maureen Frucella

COMPANY PROFILE:
Parent Company Name: Preferred Healthcare System Inc
Doing Business As:
Year Founded: 1985   Federally Qualified: [N]
Forprofit: [Y]   Not-For-Profit: [ ]
Model Type: NETWORK
Accreditation: [ ] AAPPO [ ] JACHO [ ] NCQA [ ] URAC
Plan Type: PPO, UR
Primary Physicians: 350   Physician Specialists: 560
Hospitals: 12
Total Enrollment:
  2001: 25,000   2004: 0   2007: 0
  2002: 25,000   2005:
  2003: 0   2006: 21,000

SERVICE AREA:
Nationwide: N
  PA (Bedford, Blair, Cambria, Centra, Clearfield, Fulton, Huntingdon, Juniata, Mifflin, Somerset);

TYPE OF COVERAGE:
Commercial: [Y] Individual: [Y] FEHBP: [ ] Indemnity: [ ]
Medicare: [ ] Medicaid: [ ] Supplemental Medicare: [ ]
Tricare [ ]

PLAN BENEFITS:
Alternative Medicine: [ ]   Behavioral Health: [ ]
Chiropractic: [X]   Dental: [X]
Home Care: [X]   Inpatient SNF: [X]
Long-Term Care: [ ]   Pharm. Mail Order: [ ]
Physical Therapy: [X]   Podiatry: [X]
Psychiatric: [X]   Transplant: [X]
Vision: [X]   Wellness: [X]
Workers' Comp: [ ]
Other Benefits:

RAYTEL IMAGING NETWORK

430 Park Ave Ste 102
Collegeville, PA 19406
Phone: 610-831-1112 Fax: 610-831-1122 Toll-Free: 800-453-0574
Web site: www.raytel.com

MAILING ADDRESS:
  RAYTEL IMAGING NETWORK
  430 Park Ave Ste 102
  Collegeville, PA 19406

KEY EXECUTIVES:
Chief Executive Officer/Marketing Director .... Jeff Flanegin
Director of Sales .... Cindy Pirozzi

COMPANY PROFILE:
Parent Company Name: SHL Telemedicine
Doing Business As:
Year Founded: 1992   Federally Qualified: [ ]
Forprofit: [Y]   Not-For-Profit: [ ]
Model Type:
Accreditation: [ ] AAPPO [ ] JACHO [ ] NCQA [ ] URAC
Plan Type: Specialty PPO

SERVICE AREA:
Nationwide: N
  Mid-Atlantic Region;

TYPE OF COVERAGE:
Commercial: [Y] Individual: [ ] FEHBP: [ ] Indemnity: [ ]
Medicare: [ ] Medicaid: [ ] Supplemental Medicare: [ ]
Tricare [ ]

PLAN BENEFITS:
Alternative Medicine: [ ]   Behavioral Health: [ ]
Chiropractic: [ ]   Dental: [ ]
Home Care: [ ]   Inpatient SNF: [ ]
Long-Term Care: [ ]   Pharm. Mail Order: [ ]
Physical Therapy: [ ]   Podiatry: [ ]
Psychiatric: [ ]   Transplant: [ ]
Vision: [ ]   Wellness: [ ]
Workers' Comp: [ ]
Other Benefits: Diagnostic Imaging

SELECTCARE ACCESS CORPORATION

820 Parish St
Pittsburgh, PA 15220
Phone: 412-922-0780 Fax: 412-922-3071 Toll-Free: 800-922-4966
Web site: www.mcoa.com

MAILING ADDRESS:
  SELECTCARE ACCESS CORPORATION
  820 Parish St
  Pittsburgh, PA 15220

KEY EXECUTIVES:
Chief Executive Officer .... Phyllis Shehab
President .... Jay R Ver Hulst
Chief Financial Officer .... Patrick Forrest

COMPANY PROFILE:
Parent Company Name: Managed Care of America
Doing Business As:
Year Founded: 1991   Federally Qualified: [ ]
Forprofit: [Y]   Not-For-Profit: [ ]
Model Type:
Accreditation: [ ] AAPPO [ ] JACHO [ ] NCQA [ ] URAC
Plan Type: PPO, UR, TPA, HSA

SERVICE AREA:
Nationwide: N
  PA;

TYPE OF COVERAGE:
Commercial: [Y] Individual: [ ] FEHBP: [ ] Indemnity: [ ]
Medicare: [ ] Medicaid: [ ] Supplemental Medicare: [ ]
Tricare [ ]

Comments:
Select Access Corp is a PPO for self funded employer groups and TPA's of group health benefits. Because of this, benefit plans vary for each employer.

PENNSYLVANIA

COMPANY PROFILE:
Parent Company Name:
Doing Business As:
Year Founded: 1993 Federally Qualified: [N]
Forprofit: [Y] Not-For-Profit: [ ]
Model Type: NETWORK
Accreditation: [ ] AAPPO [ ] JACHO [ ] NCQA [ ] URAC
Plan Type: PPO, ASO
SERVICE AREA:
Nationwide: N
  PA (Allegheny, Armstrong, Beaver, Bedford, Berks, Blair, Bucks, Butler, Cambria, Cameron, Carbon, Centre, Chester, Clarion, Clearfield, Clinton, Columbia, Crawford, Cumberland, Dauphin, Delaware, Elk, Erie, Fayette, Forest, Huntingdon, Jefferson, Juniata, Lackswanna, Lancaster, Lawrence, LeHigh, Luzerne, Lycoming, McLean, Mercer, Mifflin, Montgomery, Montour, Northampton, Northumberland, Perry, Philadelphia, Schuylkill, Snyder, Union, Venango, Warren, Washington, Westmoreland, Wyoming);
TYPE OF COVERAGE:
Commercial: [Y] Individual: [ ] FEHBP: [ ] Indemnity: [ ]
Medicare: [ ] Medicaid: [ ] Supplemental Medicare: [ ]
Tricare   [ ]

PENN HIGHLANDS HEALTH PLAN

1086 Franklin St
Johnstown, PA 15905
Phone: 814-536-7525 Fax: 814-533-1544 Toll-Free: 888-722-0805
Web site: www.conemaugh.org
MAILING ADDRESS:
  PENN HIGHLANDS HEALTH PLAN
  1086 Franklin St
  Johnstown, PA 15905

KEY EXECUTIVES:
President .... Jack D Lipomi
Chief Financial Officer .... Ed DePasquale
Medical Director .... Richard Wozniak, MD
Marketing Director .... Jack D Lipomi

COMPANY PROFILE:
Parent Company Name:
Doing Business As:
Year Founded: 1986 Federally Qualified: [N]
Forprofit: [Y] Not-For-Profit: [ ]
Model Type: NETWORK
Accreditation: [X] AAPPO [ ] JACHO [ ] NCQA [ ] URAC
Plan Type: PPO, POS, HDHP, HSA
Primary Physicians: 180   Physician Specialists: 245
Hospitals: 7
Total Enrollment:
  2001: 18,500   2004: 0   2007: 0
  2002: 17,500   2005:
  2003: 18,400   2006:
SERVICE AREA:
Nationwide: N
  PA (Bedford, Blair, Cambria, Somerset);
TYPE OF COVERAGE:
Commercial: [Y] Individual: [ ] FEHBP: [ ] Indemnity: [ ]
Medicare: [ ] Medicaid: [Y] Supplemental Medicare: [ ]
Tricare   [ ]
PRODUCTS OFFERED:
Product Name: Type:
Penn Highlands Choice   Fully Insured
Directorect   Self Funded
Commercial Insurance   HMO, PPO, POS
CONSUMER-DRIVEN PRODUCTS
                                 HSA Company
Penn Highslands Choice   HSA Product
Managed Care of America   HSA Administrator
                                 Consumer-Driven Health Plan
                                 High Deductible Health Plan
PLAN BENEFITS:
Alternative Medicine: [ ]   Behavioral Health: [X]
Chiropractic: [ ]   Dental: [ ]
Home Care: [X]   Inpatient SNF: [X]
Long-Term Care: [X]   Pharm. Mail Order: [X]
Physical Therapy: [X]   Podiatry: [X]
Psychiatric: [X]   Transplant: [X]
Vision: [ ]   Wellness: [X]
Workers' Comp: [ ]
Other Benefits:

PREFERRED CARE INCORPORATED

1300 Virginia Dr Ste 315
Ft Washington, PA 19034
Phone: 215-639-6208 Fax: 215-639-2672 Toll-Free: 800-222-3085
Web site: www.preferredcareinc.net
MAILING ADDRESS:
  PREFERRED CARE INCORPORATED
  1300 Virginia Dr Ste 315
  Ft Washington, PA 19034

KEY EXECUTIVES:
President .... Richard Wehr, CLU
President PPO .... Richard L Matthew
Treasurer .... Robert Koch
VP Operations .... Denise Rosetti
Marketing Director .... Patrick McGovern
Provider Administrator/Human Resources .... Carole Chapman
Claims Manager .... Maureen Renson

COMPANY PROFILE:
Parent Company Name:
Doing Business As:
Year Founded: 1985 Federally Qualified: [ ]
Forprofit: [Y] Not-For-Profit: [ ]
Model Type:
Accreditation: [ ] AAPPO [X] JACHO [X] NCQA [ ] URAC
Plan Type: PPO, TPA, HSA
SERVICE AREA:
Nationwide: N
  PA (Bucks, Chester, Delaware, LeHigh, Montgomery, Philadelphia, North Hampton);
TYPE OF COVERAGE:
Commercial: [Y] Individual: [Y] FEHBP: [ ] Indemnity: [ ]
Medicare: [ ] Medicaid: [ ] Supplemental Medicare: [ ]
Tricare   [ ]
PRODUCTS OFFERED:
Product Name: Type:
The Preferred Care PPO Plan
The Crew Health Crew Plan
Network Access for other plus
CONSUMER-DRIVEN PRODUCTS
Leesport Bank   HSA Company
CHAMP Plan   HSA Product
Preferred Care Inc   HSA Administrator
                                 Consumer-Driven Health Plan
CHAMP Plan   High Deductible Health Plan
PLAN BENEFITS:
Alternative Medicine: [ ]   Behavioral Health: [X]
Chiropractic: [X]   Dental: [X]
Home Care: [X]   Inpatient SNF: [X]
Long-Term Care: [X]   Pharm. Mail Order: [X]
Physical Therapy: [X]   Podiatry: [X]
Psychiatric: [X]   Transplant: [X]
Vision: [X]   Wellness: [X]
Workers' Comp: [ ]
Other Benefits:

PREFERRED HEALTH CARE

20 D East Roseville Rd
Lancaster, PA 17601
Phone: 717-560-9290 Fax: 717-560-2312 Toll-Free:
Web site: www.phcunity.com
MAILING ADDRESS:
  PREFERRED HEALTH CARE
  PO Box 4824
  Lancaster, PA 17601

KEY EXECUTIVES:
Chief Executive Officer/President .... Eric E Buck
Financial/Employee Services Administration .... Bruce White
Medical Director .... David Bowers, MD
VP of Operations .... Sherry Wolgemuth
Network Affairs Representative .... Roger Milner
Director, Client & Provider Relations .... Eric E Buck
Financial/Employee Services Administration .... Karen Haines

Managed Care Organization Profiles

PENNSYLVANIA

KEY EXECUTIVES:
Chief Executive Officer/President .... Daniel J Hilferty
Senior VP, Finance/Chief Financial Officer .... Alan Krigstein
Senior VP, Medical Affairs/Chief Medical Officer .... Jay Feldstein DO
Senior VP, Pharmacy Director .... Mesfin Tegenu, MS RPh
VP, Strategic Planning & Execution .... Betsy Scarcelli
Exec VP, Chief Operating Officer .... Michael A Rashid
Senior VP, Public Affairs/Marketing .... Maria Pajil Battle
Senior VP, Network Management .... Bruce Herdman, MBA, PhD
Senior VP Human Resources .... Regina Heffernan
VP, Chief Compliance Officer .... Barbara G Jones
Communications .... Rick Buck

COMPANY PROFILE:
Parent Company Name: Independence Blue Cross
Doing Business As:
Year Founded: 1983   Federally Qualified: [ ]
Forprofit: [ ]   Not-For-Profit: [Y]
Model Type:
Accreditation: [ ] AAPPO [ ] JACHO [X] NCQA [ ] URAC
Plan Type: HMO
Primary Physicians: 2,105   Physician Specialists: 6,798
Hospitals: 60
Total Revenue: 2005:   1,633,253,907   2006:   1,475,135,691
Net Income   2005:   2,304,297   2006:   3,637,347
Total Enrollment:
  2001: 0   2004: 300,000   2007: 378,143
  2002: 243,980   2005: 390,847
  2003: 268,000   2006: 356,285
Medical Loss Ratio: 2005:   2006:
Administrative Expense Ratio: 2005:   2006:

SERVICE AREA:
Nationwide: N
  PA (Bucks, Chester, Delaware, Montgomery, Philadelphia);

TYPE OF COVERAGE:
Commercial: [ ] Individual: [ ] FEHBP: [ ] Indemnity: [ ]
Medicare: [ ] Medicaid: [X] Supplemental Medicare: [ ]
Tricare   [ ]

PRODUCTS OFFERED:
Product Name: Type:
Vista Health Plan Inc   Medicaid

PLAN BENEFITS:
Alternative Medicine: [ ]   Behavioral Health: [ ]
Chiropractic: [X]   Dental: [X]
Home Care: [X]   Inpatient SNF: [X]
Long-Term Care: [X]   Pharm. Mail Order: [X]
Physical Therapy: [X]   Podiatry: [X]
Psychiatric: [X]   Transplant: [X]
Vision: [X]   Wellness: [X]
Workers' Comp: [X]
Other Benefits:

MENTAL HEALTH CONSULTANTS INC

2500 York Rd Ste 110
Jamison, PA 18929
Phone: 215-343-8987 Fax: 215-343-8983 Toll-Free:
Web site: www.mhconsultants.com

MAILING ADDRESS:
M H CONSULTANTS INC
2500 York Rd Ste 110
Jamison, PA 18929

KEY EXECUTIVES:
Chief Executive Officer/President .... Edward J Haaz
Chief Financial Officer .... Edward J Haaz
Director of Operations .... Lynn Zeitenberg
Marketing Director .... Edward Haaz
Director of Provider Relations .... Gary Nightingale
Director of Case Management .... Debby Dichter

COMPANY PROFILE:
Parent Company Name:
Doing Business As:
Year Founded: 1980   Federally Qualified: [ ]
Forprofit: [Y]   Not-For-Profit: [ ]
Model Type: NETWORK
Accreditation: [ ] AAPPO [ ] JACHO [ ] NCQA [ ] URAC
Plan Type: Specialty PPO
Primary Physicians: 926   Physician Specialists: 154
Hospitals: 123
Total Enrollment:
  2001: 0   2004: 0   2007: 2,300,000
  2002: 0   2005:
  2003: 0   2006: 2,200,000

SERVICE AREA:
Nationwide: N
  NJ; PA(eastern)

TYPE OF COVERAGE:
Commercial: [Y] Individual: [ ] FEHBP: [ ] Indemnity: [ ]
Medicare: [ ] Medicaid: [ ] Supplemental Medicare: [ ]
Tricare   [ ]

PLAN BENEFITS:
Alternative Medicine: [ ]   Behavioral Health: [X]
Chiropractic: [ ]   Dental: [ ]
Home Care: [ ]   Inpatient SNF: [ ]
Long-Term Care: [ ]   Pharm. Mail Order: [ ]
Physical Therapy: [ ]   Podiatry: [ ]
Psychiatric: [X]   Transplant: [ ]
Vision: [ ]   Wellness: [ ]
Workers' Comp: [ ]
Other Benefits:

MERCER FIRST CHOICE

740 E State St
Sharon, PA 16146
Phone: 724-983-5654 Fax: 724-983-3824 Toll-Free:
Web site:

MAILING ADDRESS:
MERCER FIRST CHOICE
740 E State St
Sharon, PA 16146

KEY EXECUTIVES:
President .... Matthew Liburdi
Chief Financial Officer .... Raymond Schauer
Medical Director .... Shani Vaturi, MD
Marketing Director .... Ed Newmeyer

COMPANY PROFILE:
Parent Company Name:
Doing Business As:
Year Founded: 1994   Federally Qualified: [ ]
Forprofit: [Y]   Not-For-Profit: [ ]
Model Type:
Accreditation: [ ] AAPPO [ ] JACHO [ ] NCQA [ ] URAC
Plan Type: PPO

SERVICE AREA:
Nationwide: N
  PA (Lawrence, Mercer);

TYPE OF COVERAGE:
Commercial: [Y] Individual: [ ] FEHBP: [ ] Indemnity: [ ]
Medicare: [ ] Medicaid: [ ] Supplemental Medicare: [ ]
Tricare   [ ]

MID-ATLANTIC MANAGED CARE ORGANIZATION OF PENNSYLVANIA INC

404 Baltimore St
Gettysburg, PA 17325
Phone: 717-334-9247 Fax: 717-334-9167 Toll-Free: 800-497-4474
Web site: www.mamcoppo.net

MAILING ADDRESS:
MID-ATLANTIC MANAGED CARE ORG
PO Box 1060
Gettysburg, PA 17325

KEY EXECUTIVES:
Chief Executive Officer/President .... Ronald E Pack, CLU
Chief Financial Officer .... Curtis L Winger
VP, Chief Operating Officer, Information Technology .... Dan Kelly
Marketing Director .... Ronald E Pack, CLU
Chief Counsel .... Babette L Madison
New Product Development .... Matthew Crowner

PENNSYLVANIA

MAILING ADDRESS:
KEYSTONE HEALTH PLAN CENTRAL
2500 Elmerton Ave
Harrisburg, PA 17177

KEY EXECUTIVES:
Chairman of the Board .... William Lehr
Chief Executive Officer/President .... Anita M Smith
VP, Finance & CFO .... Gary St Hilare
Chief Medical Officer .... Morton Orman, MD
Communications, Media Speclts .... Joseph Butora
Chief Operating Officer .... Anita M Smith
Privacy Officer .... Kathy Kelly

COMPANY PROFILE:
Parent Company Name: Capital Blue Cross
Doing Business As:
Year Founded: 1988   Federally Qualified: [N]
Forprofit: [ ]   Not-For-Profit: [Y]
Model Type:
Accreditation: [ ] AAPPO [ ] JACHO [X] NCQA [ ] URAC
Plan Type: HMO,
Total Enrollment:
   2001: 158,479   2004: 204,665   2007: 157,050
   2002: 222,800   2005: 174,112
   2003: 211,692   2006: 159,365

SERVICE AREA:
Nationwide: N
   PA (Adams, Berks, Centre, Columbia, Cumberland, Dauphin, Juniata, Lebanon, LeHigh, Mifflin, Montour, Northampton, Northumberland, Perry, Schuylkill, Snyder, Union, York);

TYPE OF COVERAGE:
Commercial: [ ]   Individual: [ ]   FEHBP: [ ]   Indemnity: [ ]
Medicare: [ ]   Medicaid: [Y]   Supplemental Medicare: [ ]
Tricare   [ ]

PRODUCTS OFFERED:
Product Name:	Type:
Senior Blue Option1	Medicare
Senior Blue Option2	Medicare
Senior Blue Option3	Medicare
Senior Blue Option4	Medicare
Senior Blue ER w RX	Medicare
Senior Blue ER without RX	Medicare

PLAN BENEFITS:
Alternative Medicine: [ ]   Behavioral Health: [ ]
Chiropractic: [X]   Dental: [X]
Home Care: [X]   Inpatient SNF: [X]
Long-Term Care: [X]   Pharm. Mail Order: [X]
Physical Therapy: [X]   Podiatry: [X]
Psychiatric: [X]   Transplant: [X]
Vision: [X]   Wellness: [X]
Workers' Comp: [X]
Other Benefits:

KEYSTONE HEALTH PLAN EAST INC

1901 Market St
Philadelphia, PA 19103
Phone: 215-636-9559 Fax: 215-241-2017 Toll-Free: 800-555-1514
Web site: www.khpe.com

MAILING ADDRESS:
KEYSTONE HEALTH PLAN EAST INC
1901 Market St
Philadelphia, PA 19103

KEY EXECUTIVES:
Chief Executive Officer/President .... Joseph A Frick
Chief Financial Officer .... John G Foos
Chief Medical Officer .... Steven Udvaryhelyi, MD
Pharmacy Director .... Mark Strollo
Director of Operations .... Neil T Canavan
Chief Marketing Executive .... Christopher D Butler
VP, Corporate/Public Affairs .... Butch Ward
Sr Director of Medicare Operations .... Michelle Barry

COMPANY PROFILE:
Parent Company Name: Independence Blue Cross
Doing Business As:
Year Founded: 1988   Federally Qualified: [Y]

Managed Care Organization Profiles

Forprofit: [Y]   Not-For-Profit: [ ]
Model Type: IPA
Accreditation: [ ] AAPPO [ ] JACHO [X] NCQA [ ] URAC
Plan Type: HMO, PPO, Specialty HMO, POS
Total Enrollment:
   2001: 2,873,882   2004: 869,996   2007: 869,382
   2002: 1,227,000   2005: 854,181
   2003: 1,180,652   2006: 882,848

SERVICE AREA:
Nationwide: N
   PA (Bucks, Chester, Delaware, Montgomery, Philadelphia);

TYPE OF COVERAGE:
Commercial: [ ]   Individual: [ ]   FEHBP: [ ]   Indemnity: [ ]
Medicare: [Y]   Medicaid: [Y]   Supplemental Medicare: [ ]
Tricare   [ ]

PRODUCTS OFFERED:
Product Name:	Type:
Personal Choice	PPO
Keystone Health Plan East	POS
Personal Choice 65	PPO Medicare
Keystone HMO	HMO
Keystone Specialty HMO	Specialty HMO
Keystone HMO	Medicaid
Keystone 65	Medicare Advantage

PLAN BENEFITS:
Alternative Medicine: [ ]   Behavioral Health: [ ]
Chiropractic: [X]   Dental: [X]
Home Care: [X]   Inpatient SNF: [X]
Long-Term Care: [X]   Pharm. Mail Order: [X]
Physical Therapy: [X]   Podiatry: [X]
Psychiatric: [X]   Transplant: [X]
Vision: [X]   Wellness: [X]
Workers' Comp: [X]
Other Benefits:

KEYSTONE HEALTH PLAN WEST INC

120 Fifth Ave Ste 938
Pittsburgh, PA 15222
Phone: 412-544-7000 Fax: 412-544-6911 Toll-Free: 800-547-9378
Web site: www.highmarkbcbs.com

MAILING ADDRESS:
KEYSTONE HEALTH PLAN WEST INC
PO Box 226
Pittsburgh, PA 15222

KEY EXECUTIVES:
Chief Executive Officer/President .... Kenneth R Melani, MD
VP, Contractor, Medical Director .... Andrew Bloschichak, MD

COMPANY PROFILE:
Parent Company Name: Highmark Inc
Doing Business As:
Year Founded: Federally Qualified: [ ]
Forprofit: [Y]   Not-For-Profit: [ ]
Model Type: IPA
Accreditation: [ ] AAPPO [ ] JACHO [ ] NCQA [ ] URAC
Plan Type: HMO, POS,
Total Enrollment:
   2001: 372,969   2004: 907,726   2007: 373,811
   2002: 1,324,419 2005: 783,652
   2003: 1,159,108 2006: 570,383

SERVICE AREA:
Nationwide:
   PA;

TYPE OF COVERAGE:
Commercial: [ ]   Individual: [ ]   FEHBP: [ ]   Indemnity: [ ]
Medicare: [Y]   Medicaid: [ ]   Supplemental Medicare: [ ]
Tricare   [ ]

KEYSTONE MERCY HEALTH PLAN

200 Stevens Dr
Philadelphia, PA 19113
Phone: 215-937-8000 Fax: 215-863-5673 Toll-Free:
Web site: www.keystonemercy.com

MAILING ADDRESS:
KEYSTONE MERCY HEALTH PLAN
200 Stevens Dr
Philadelphia, PA 19113

Managed Care Organization Profiles — PENNSYLVANIA

PLAN BENEFITS:
Alternative Medicine:	[X]	Behavioral Health:	[X]
Chiropractic:	[X]	Dental:	[X]
Home Care:	[X]	Inpatient SNF:	[X]
Long-Term Care:	[X]	Pharm. Mail Order:	[X]
Physical Therapy:	[X]	Podiatry:	[X]
Psychiatric:	[X]	Transplant:	[X]
Vision:	[X]	Wellness:	[X]
Workers' Comp:	[X]		
Other Benefits:			

INTERGROUP SERVICES CORPORATION

101 Lindenwood Dr Ste 150
Malvern, PA 19355
Phone: 610-640-0646 Fax: 610-647-5383 Toll-Free: 800-537-9389
Web site: www.igs-ppo.com

MAILING ADDRESS:
INTERGROUP SERVICES CORP
101 Lindenwood Dr Ste 150
Malvern, PA 19355

KEY EXECUTIVES:
Chairman of the Board/Chief Executive Officer .... G Martin Dudley
President .... John A George
Chief Financial Officer .... G Martin Dudley
Manager of Information System/MIS Director .... Gregory Dudley
Marketing Director .... Joseph McLaughlin
VP Provider Relations/Network/Contracts .... Gregory Dudley
Office Manager .... Julie Odabashian

COMPANY PROFILE:
Parent Company Name:
Doing Business As: Intergroup Services Corporation
Year Founded: 1984   Federally Qualified: [N]
Forprofit: [Y]   Not-For-Profit: [ ]
Model Type: NETWORK
Accreditation: [ ] AAPPO [ ] JACHO [ ] NCQA [ ] URAC
Plan Type: PPO, PBM
Primary Physicians: 16,212   Physician Specialists: 38,016
Hospitals: 380
Total Enrollment:
  2001: 1,483,847   2004: 1,000,000   2007: 700,000
  2002: 0   2005: 540,000
  2003: 1,000,000   2006: 650,000

SERVICE AREA:
Nationwide: N
NJ; WV; PA; DE;

TYPE OF COVERAGE:
Commercial: [Y] Individual: [ ] FEHBP: [ ] Indemnity: [ ]
Medicare: [ ] Medicaid: [ ] Supplemental Medicare: [ ]
Tricare [ ]

PRODUCTS OFFERED:
Product Name:	Type:
Intergroup Services	PPO

PLAN BENEFITS:
Alternative Medicine:	[ ]	Behavioral Health:	[ ]
Chiropractic:	[X]	Dental:	[ ]
Home Care:	[X]	Inpatient SNF:	[X]
Long-Term Care:	[ ]	Pharm. Mail Order:	[ ]
Physical Therapy:	[X]	Podiatry:	[X]
Psychiatric:	[X]	Transplant:	[X]
Vision:	[X]	Wellness:	[ ]
Workers' Comp:	[X]		
Other Benefits:			

INTRACORP

1601 Chestnut St 2 Liberty Pl
Philadelphia, PA 19192-2116
Phone: 215-761-7100 Fax: 215-761-7458 Toll-Free: 800-345-1075
Web site: www.intracorp.com

MAILING ADDRESS:
INTRACORP
1601 Chestnut St 2 Liberty Pl
Philadelphia, PA 19192-2116

KEY EXECUTIVES:
President .... T Mark Farrerll
Senior VP, Chief Financial Officer .... Jonathan Winderman
National Medical Director .... Allen Woolf, MD
VP, Products & Marketing .... Betsy Robinson
VP, Human Resources ....Stacy Conti
General Counsel .... Tracy Kilcullin, Esq
Chief Technology Officer .... Tony Cuva
VP, Case Management .... Margaret Aslakson

COMPANY PROFILE:
Parent Company Name: CIGNA Corporation
Doing Business As:
Year Founded: 1970   Federally Qualified: [ ]
Forprofit: [Y]   Not-For-Profit: [ ]
Model Type:
Accreditation: [ ] AAPPO [ ] JACHO [ ] NCQA [X] URAC
Plan Type: UR,

SERVICE AREA:
Nationwide: N

TYPE OF COVERAGE:
Commercial: [ ] Individual: [ ] FEHBP: [ ] Indemnity: [ ]
Medicare: [ ] Medicaid: [ ] Supplemental Medicare: [ ]
Tricare

PLAN BENEFITS:
Alternative Medicine:	[ ]	Behavioral Health:	[ ]
Chiropractic:	[ ]	Dental:	[ ]
Home Care:	[ ]	Inpatient SNF:	[ ]
Long-Term Care:	[ ]	Pharm. Mail Order:	[ ]
Physical Therapy:	[ ]	Podiatry:	[ ]
Psychiatric:	[ ]	Transplant:	[ ]
Vision:	[ ]	Wellness:	[ ]
Workers' Comp:	[X]		
Other Benefits:			

KEPRO

777 E Park Dr
Harrisburg, PA 17105
Phone: 717-564-8288 Fax: 717-564-3862 Toll-Free:
Web site: www.kepro.org

MAILING ADDRESS:
KEPRO
PO Box 8310
Harrisburg, PA 17105

KEY EXECUTIVES:
Chairman, Board of Directors .... Frederick G Brown, MD
Chief Executive Officer .... Joseph Dougher
President .... Donald E Harrop, MD
Chief Financial Officer .... Scott Bohner
Chief Medical Officer .... Alice Stollenwerk Petrulis
Chief Information Officer .... Chris Bouvier
Chief Operating Officer .... Mary Kay Kohut
Chief Development Officer .... Andrew Wientraub
Public Relations Director .... Joanne Benteler
VP, Corporate Human Resources .... Rose Ungaro Ciullo
VP, Public Programs - State .... Nancy Kohler

COMPANY PROFILE:
Parent Company Name: Keystone Peer Review Org Inc
Doing Business As:
Year Founded: Federally Qualified: [ ]
Forprofit: [Y]   Not-For-Profit: [ ]
Model Type:
Accreditation: [ ] AAPPO [ ] JACHO [ ] NCQA [ ] URAC
Plan Type: UR

SERVICE AREA:
Nationwide: Y
NW;

TYPE OF COVERAGE:
Commercial: [ ] Individual: [ ] FEHBP: [ ] Indemnity: [ ]
Medicare: [ ] Medicaid: [ ] Supplemental Medicare: [ ]
Tricare [ ]

KEYSTONE HEALTH PLAN CENTRAL

2500 Elmerton Ave
Harrisburg, PA 17177
Phone: 717-541-7000 Fax: 717-541-6072 Toll-Free: 800-547-2583
Web site: www.khpc.com

PENNSYLVANIA — Managed Care Organization Profiles

PRODUCTS OFFERED:
Product Name: Advantra
Type: Medicare Advantage

CONSUMER-DRIVEN PRODUCTS
Wells Fargo — HSA Company, HSA Product
Corporate Benefits Services of America — HSA Administrator, Consumer-Driven Health Plan
Open Access Plus Plan — High Deductible Health Plan

PLAN BENEFITS:
Alternative Medicine: [ ]   Behavioral Health: [ ]
Chiropractic: [X]   Dental: [X]
Home Care: [X]   Inpatient SNF: [X]
Long-Term Care: [X]   Pharm. Mail Order: [X]
Physical Therapy: [X]   Podiatry: [ ]
Psychiatric: [X]   Transplant: [X]
Vision: [ ]   Wellness: [X]
Workers' Comp: [ ]
Other Benefits:

Comments:
See HealthAmerica of Central Pennsylvania for enrollment figures.

HIGHMARK INC

120 Fifth Ave Pl
Pittsburgh, PA 15222-3099
Phone: 412-544-7000 Fax: 412-544-5318 Toll-Free: 800-235-4999
Web site: www.highmark.com

MAILING ADDRESS:
HIGHMARK INC
120 Fifth Ave Pl
Pittsburgh, PA 15222-3099

KEY EXECUTIVES:
Board Chairman .... J Robert Baum, PhD
Chief Executive Officer/President .... Kenneth R Melani, MD
Executive VP, Chief Financial Officer .... Nanette P DeTurk
Chief Medical Officer .... Donald Fischer, MD
VP, Pharmacy Affairs .... Robert Wanovich
Senior VP, Chief Information Officer .... Thomas R Tabor
Senior VP, Marketing & Product Management ...... Thomas W Kerr
Chief Privacy Officer .... Kimberly S Gray, Esq, CIPP
Director, Corp Communications .... John McDermott
Senior VP, Provider Services .... Sandra Tomlinson
VP & Executive Director, Health Ed Center .... W Bradley Pifalo, MD
Executive VP, HR/Administrative Service .... S Tyrone Alexander
Executive VP, Health Services .... James M Klingensmith, ScD
Executive VP, Government Services .... David O'Brien
Senior VP, Corporate Affairs .... Aaron A Walton
Senior VP, Gen Counsel & Corp Secretary .... Gary R Truitt, ESQ

COMPANY PROFILE:
Parent Company Name: Highmark Inc
Doing Business As:
Year Founded: 1992   Federally Qualified: [ ]
Forprofit: [ ]   Not-For-Profit: [Y]
Model Type:
Accreditation: [ ] AAPPO [ ] JACHO [X] NCQA [ ] URAC
Plan Type: HMO, PPO, POS, CDHP, HDHP, HSA
Total Revenue: 2005: 9,847,298,000 2006: 11,083,803,000
Net Income 2005: 341,597,000 2006: 398,290,000
Total Enrollment:
2001: 5,712,723   2004: 4,100,000   2007: 4,600,000
2002: 3,678,090   2005: 4,600,000
2003: 3,404,644   2006: 4,100,000

SERVICE AREA:
Nationwide: N
PA (Allegheny, Armstrong, Beaver, Bedford, Blair, Butter, Cambria, Cameron, Centre, Clarion, Clearfield, Crawford, Elk, Erie, Fayette, Forest, Greene, Huntingdon, Indiana, Jefferson, Lawrence, McKean, Mercer, Potter, Somerset, Venango, Warren, Washington, Westmoreland);

TYPE OF COVERAGE:
Commercial: [Y] Individual: [Y] FEHBP: [ ] Indemnity: [ ]
Medicare: [Y] Medicaid: [Y] Supplemental Medicare: [Y]
Tricare: [ ]

PRODUCTS OFFERED:
Product Name: Type:
Keystone Health Plan West Inc HMO
FreedomBlue Medicare

CONSUMER-DRIVEN PRODUCTS
PFPC Trust Company — HSA Company
BlueAccount HSA — HSA Product, HSA Administrator
BlueAccount FSA — Consumer-Driven Health Plan, High Deductible Health Plan

PLAN BENEFITS:
Alternative Medicine: [ ]   Behavioral Health: [X]
Chiropractic: [X]   Dental: [ ]
Home Care: [X]   Inpatient SNF: [X]
Long-Term Care: [ ]   Pharm. Mail Order: [X]
Physical Therapy: [X]   Podiatry: [X]
Psychiatric: [X]   Transplant: [X]
Vision: [ ]   Wellness: [X]
Workers' Comp: [ ]
Other Benefits: Carve out Dental & Vision

INDEPENDENCE BLUE CROSS

1901 Market St
Philadelphia, PA 19103-1480
Phone: 215-241-2400 Fax: 215-241-4746 Toll-Free: 800-555-1514
Web site: www.ibx.com

MAILING ADDRESS:
INDEPENDENCE BLUE CROSS
1901 Market St
Philadelphia, PA 19103-1480

KEY EXECUTIVES:
Chief Executive Officer/President .... Joseph A Frick
Chief Financial Officer .... John G Foos
Senior VP, Chief Medical Officer .... Steven Udvaryhalyi, MD
Pharmacy Director .... Paul Urick
Chief Marketing Officer .... Christopher D Butler
HIPAA Project Executive .... Kenneth W Fody
VP, Public Affairs .... Butch Ward
Senior VP, Contracting & Provider Network ...... Donna O Moore
VP Health Services .... Daniel Lyons, MD
Senior VP, General Counsel .... Paul A Tufano
Senior VP, Corp & Public Affairs .... Christopher Cashman

COMPANY PROFILE:
Parent Company Name: Independence Blue Cross
Doing Business As:
Year Founded: 1938   Federally Qualified: [ ]
Forprofit: [ ]   Not-For-Profit: [Y]
Model Type:
Accreditation: [ ] AAPPO [X] JACHO [X] NCQA [X] URAC
Plan Type: HMO, PPO, POS, CDHP, HDHP, HSA
Primary Physicians: 34,553   Physician Specialists:
Hospitals: 171
Total Revenue: 2005:   2006: 10,700,000,000
Net Income 2005: 167,485,000 2006: 210,860,000
Total Enrollment:
2001: 2,481,352   2004: 24,178   2007: 0
2002: 2,481,352   2005: 3,500,000
2003: 2,800,000   2006: 3,400,000

SERVICE AREA:
Nationwide: N
PA;

TYPE OF COVERAGE:
Commercial: [Y] Individual: [Y] FEHBP: [ ] Indemnity: [ ]
Medicare: [Y] Medicaid: [Y] Supplemental Medicare: [Y]
Tricare: [ ]

PRODUCTS OFFERED:
Product Name: Type:
Keystone Health Plan East HMO
Keystone Point-Of-Service POS
Personal Choice PPO
Keystone 65 Medicare Advantage
Personal Choice 65 Medicare Advantage

CONSUMER-DRIVEN PRODUCTS
Bankcore — HSA Company
Personal Choice HSA — HSA Product, HSA Administrator, Consumer-Driven Health Plan, High Deductible Health Plan

Managed Care Organization Profiles — PENNSYLVANIA

HEALTHAMERICA PENNSYLVANIA INC - EASTERN REGION

401 Plymouth Rd, Ste 350
Plymouth Meeting, PA 19462
Phone: 610-729-7500 Fax: Toll-Free: 866-522-3886
Web site: www.healthamericacvty.com

MAILING ADDRESS:
HEALTHAMERICA PA INC - EASTERN REGION
401 Plymouth Rd, Ste 350
Plymouth Meeting, PA 19462

KEY EXECUTIVES:
Chief Executive Officer/President .... Kirk E Rothrock
Chief Financial Officer .... Stephen R Dengler
VP, Medical Affairs .... John C Wallendjack, MD
VP, Business Development .... N Timothy Guarneschelli
Director, Sales .... Douglas Callenberger
Network Management Leader .... Kathy Kleese

COMPANY PROFILE:
Parent Company Name: Coventry Health Care Inc
Doing Business As: HealthAssurance; Advantra
Year Founded: 1984   Federally Qualified: [Y]
Forprofit: [Y]   Not-For-Profit: [ ]
Model Type: MIXED
Accreditation: [ ] AAPPO [ ] JACHO [X] NCQA [ ] URAC
Plan Type: HMO, PPO, POS, CDHP, HDHP, HSA, MSA

SERVICE AREA:
Nationwide: N
  PA;

TYPE OF COVERAGE:
Commercial: [Y] Individual: [ ] FEHBP: [ ] Indemnity: [ ]
Medicare: [Y] Medicaid: [ ] Supplemental Medicare: [ ]
Tricare   [ ]

PRODUCTS OFFERED:
Product Name: Type:
Advantra   Medicare Advantage

CONSUMER-DRIVEN PRODUCTS
Wells Fargo   HSA Company
                                  HSA Product
Corporate Benefits Services of America HSA Administrator
                                  Consumer-Driven Health Plan
Open Access Plus Plan   High Deductible Health Plan

PLAN BENEFITS:
Alternative Medicine: [ ]   Behavioral Health: [ ]
Chiropractic: [X]   Dental: [ ]
Home Care: [X]   Inpatient SNF: [X]
Long-Term Care: [X]   Pharm. Mail Order: [X]
Physical Therapy: [X]   Podiatry: [ ]
Psychiatric: [X]   Transplant: [X]
Vision: [ ]   Wellness: [X]
Workers' Comp: [ ]
Other Benefits:

HEALTHAMERICA PENNSYLVANIA INC - NORTHWESTERN

5473 Village Common Dr #204
Erie, PA 16506-4961
Phone: 814-878-1700 Fax: 717-541-5739 Toll-Free: 800-255-4281
Web site: www.newalliancehealth.com

MAILING ADDRESS:
HEALTHAMERICA PENNSYLVANIA INC - NORTHWESTERN
5473 Village Common Dr #204
Erie, PA 16506-4961

KEY EXECUTIVES:
Chief Executive Officer/President .... Kirk E Rothrock
Regional President .... Mary Lou Osborne
Chief Financial Officer .... Stephen R Dengler
VP, Medical Affairs .... Eugene Sun, MD
VP, Marketing .... Darrin Hayes
VP, Business Development .... N Timothy Guarneschelli

COMPANY PROFILE:
Parent Company Name: Coventry Health Care Inc
Doing Business As: New Alliance Health Plan
Year Founded: 1994   Federally Qualified: [N]
Forprofit: [Y]   Not-For-Profit: [ ]
Model Type: NETWORK
Accreditation: [ ] AAPPO [ ] JACHO [X] NCQA [ ] URAC
Plan Type: HMO, PPO, POS, CDHP, HDHP, HSA, MSA
Total Enrollment:
  2001: 50,297   2004: 0   2007: 0
  2002: 0   2005:
  2003: 700,000   2006:

SERVICE AREA:
Nationwide: N
  PA (Northwestern);

TYPE OF COVERAGE:
Commercial: [Y] Individual: [ ] FEHBP: [ ] Indemnity: [ ]
Medicare: [ ] Medicaid: [ ] Supplemental Medicare: [Y]
Tricare   [ ]

PRODUCTS OFFERED:
Product Name: Type:
New Alliance HMO   HMO
New Alliance ASO   ASO
New Alliance POS   POS

CONSUMER-DRIVEN PRODUCTS
Wells Fargo   HSA Company
                                  HSA Product
Corporate Benefits Servs of Am   HSA Administrator
                                  Consumer-Driven Health Plan
Open Access Plus Plan   High Deductible Health Plan

PLAN BENEFITS:
Alternative Medicine: [ ]   Behavioral Health: [X]
Chiropractic: [X]   Dental: [X]
Home Care: [X]   Inpatient SNF: [X]
Long-Term Care: [ ]   Pharm. Mail Order: [ ]
Physical Therapy: [X]   Podiatry: [X]
Psychiatric: [X]   Transplant: [X]
Vision: [X]   Wellness: [X]
Workers' Comp: [ ]
Other Benefits:

Comments:
Acquired by Coventry Health Care Inc May 1, 2002. Formerly called Alliance Health Network Inc.

HEALTHAMERICA PENNSYLVANIA INC - WESTERN REGION

11 Stanwix St Ste 2300
Pittsburgh, PA 15222
Phone: 412-553-7522 Fax: 412-553-7523 Toll-Free: 800-735-4404
Web site: www.healthamerica.cvty.com

MAILING ADDRESS:
HEALTHAMERICA PA INC - WESTERN
11 Stanwix St Ste 2300
Pittsburgh, PA 15222

KEY EXECUTIVES:
Chief Executive Officer/President .... Kirk E Rothrock
Chief Financial Officer .... Steven R Dengler
VP, Medical Affairs .... Eugene Sun, MD
Pharmacy Director .... Bob Gilkin
VP, Sales .... Darin Hayes
VP, Health Services .... Angel Oddo

COMPANY PROFILE:
Parent Company Name: Coventry Health Care Inc
Doing Business As: HealthAssurance; Advantra
Year Founded: 1975   Federally Qualified: [Y]
Forprofit: [Y]   Not-For-Profit: [ ]
Model Type: MIXED
Accreditation: [ ] AAPPO [ ] JACHO [X] NCQA [ ] URAC
Plan Type: HMO, PPO, POS, CDHP, HDHP, HSA, MSA
Total Enrollment:
  2001: 485,798   2004: 728,219   2007: 437,614
  2002: 646,252   2005: 723,000
  2003: 0   2006:

SERVICE AREA:
Nationwide: N
  OH; PA (Armstrong, Beaver, Butler, Cambria, Fayette, Greene, Indiana, Lawrence, Mercer, Somerset, Washington, Westmoreland);

TYPE OF COVERAGE:
Commercial: [Y] Individual: [ ] FEHBP: [ ] Indemnity: [Y]
Medicare: [Y] Medicaid: [Y] Supplemental Medicare: [ ]
Tricare   [ ]

PENNSYLVANIA

MAILING ADDRESS:
GREAT-WEST HEALTHCARE OF PA
1023 E Baltimore Pike, Ste 200
Media, PA 19063-5126

KEY EXECUTIVES:
Executive Director .... William O'Donnell
President .... Joan Russo
Director of Provider Relations .... Vicki Williamson

COMPANY PROFILE:
Parent Company Name: Great West Life & Annuity Insurance Co
Doing Business As:
Year Founded: 1998   Federally Qualified: [ ]
Forprofit: [Y]   Not-For-Profit: [ ]
Model Type: MIXED
Accreditation: [ ] AAPPO [ ] JACHO [ ] NCQA [X] URAC
Plan Type: HMO, PPO, POS, CDHP, HDHP, HSA,
Primary Physicians: 8,910   Physician Specialists: 13,175
Hospitals: 165
Total Enrollment:
    2001: 52,000   2004: 0   2007: 0
    2002: 67,000   2005:
    2003: 0   2006:

SERVICE AREA:
Nationwide: N
    PA (Philadelphia; central PA)

TYPE OF COVERAGE:
Commercial: [Y]   Individual: [ ]   FEHBP: [ ]   Indemnity: [ ]
Medicare: [ ]   Medicaid: [ ]   Supplemental Medicare: [ ]
Tricare   [ ]

PRODUCTS OFFERED:
Product Name: Type:
                                                              PPO

CONSUMER-DRIVEN PRODUCTS
Mellon HR Solutions LLC   HSA Company
                                                   HSA Product
                                                   HSA Administrator
                                                   Consumer-Driven Health Plan
                                                   High Deductible Health Plan

PLAN BENEFITS:
Alternative Medicine: [X]   Behavioral Health: [X]
Chiropractic: [X]   Dental: [X]
Home Care: [X]   Inpatient SNF: [X]
Long-Term Care: [X]   Pharm. Mail Order: [X]
Physical Therapy: [X]   Podiatry: [X]
Psychiatric: [X]   Transplant: [X]
Vision: [X]   Wellness: [X]
Workers' Comp: [ ]
Other Benefits:
Comments:
Formerly One Health Plan of Pennsylvania.

HEALTH PARTNERS

901 Market St Ste 500
Philadelphia, PA 19107
Phone: 215-849-9606 Fax: 215-849-9636 Toll-Free: 800-553-0784
Web site: www.healthpart.com

MAILING ADDRESS:
HEALTH PARTNERS
901 Market St Ste 500
Philadelphia, PA 19107

KEY EXECUTIVES:
Chief Executive Officer/President .... William S George
Senior VP & Chief Medical Officer .... Mary K Stom, MD
Senior VP, Pharmacy .... Donald Daddario
Senior VP, Operations/Chief Operating Officer .... Debra A Kircher
VP, Sales & Marketing .... John Roehm
VP, Corp Communications/Public Affairs .... Teresa L Heavens
Provider Relations Director .... William Hunt
Senior VP, Resources Management\Compliance .... Vickie L Sessoms
Senior VP, Business Development .... Judy B Harrington

COMPANY PROFILE:
Parent Company Name:
Doing Business As:
Year Founded: 1985   Federally Qualified: [Y]
Forprofit: [ ]   Not-For-Profit: [Y]
Model Type: NETWORK
Accreditation: [ ] AAPPO [ ] JACHO [ ] NCQA [ ] URAC
Plan Type: HMO, HDHP, HSA,
Total Enrollment:
    2001: 136,129   2004: 155,360   2007: 138,322
    2002: 147,942   2005: 166,656
    2003: 147,028   2006: 157,013

SERVICE AREA:
Nationwide: N
    PA (Bucks, Delaware, Montgomery, Philadelphia);

TYPE OF COVERAGE:
Commercial: [ ]   Individual: [ ]   FEHBP: [ ]   Indemnity: [ ]
Medicare: [Y]   Medicaid: [Y]   Supplemental Medicare: [ ]
Tricare   [ ]

PRODUCTS OFFERED:
Product Name: Type:
Health Partners Medicaid   Medicaid
Health Partners Medicare   Medicare

HEALTHAMERICA PENNSYLVANIA INC - CENTRAL REGION

3721 TecPort Dr
Harrisburg, PA 17106-7103
Phone: 717-540-4260 Fax: 717-541-5739 Toll-Free: 800-788-6445
Web site: www.healthamericacvty.com

MAILING ADDRESS:
HEALTHAMERICA PA INC - CENTRAL REGION
PO Box 67103
Harrisburg, PA 17106-7103

KEY EXECUTIVES:
Chief Executive Officer/President .... Kirk E Rothrock
Chief Financial Officer .... Stephen R Dengler
VP, Medical Affairs .... John C Wallendjack, MD
VP, Business Development .... N Timothy Guarneschelli
VP, Sales .... Connie Erney

COMPANY PROFILE:
Parent Company Name: Coventry Health Care Inc
Doing Business As: HealthAssurance; Advantra
Year Founded: 1984   Federally Qualified: [Y]
Forprofit: [Y]   Not-For-Profit: [ ]
Model Type: MIXED
Accreditation: [ ] AAPPO [ ] JACHO [X] NCQA [ ] URAC
Plan Type: HMO, PPO, POS, CDHP, HDHP, HSA, MSA
Total Enrollment:
    2001: 196,513   2004: 251,325   2007: 0
    2002: 489,642   2005: 501,796
    2003: 265,894   2006: 496,166

SERVICE AREA:
Nationwide: N
    PA (Adams, Berks, Blair, Centre, Clinton, Columbia, Cumberland,
    Dauphin, Huntingdon, Juniata, Lancaster, Lebanon, Luzerne,
    Lycoming, Mifflin, Northumberland, Perry, Schuylkill,
    Snyder, Union, York);

TYPE OF COVERAGE:
Commercial: [Y]   Individual: [ ]   FEHBP: [ ]   Indemnity: [ ]
Medicare: [Y]   Medicaid: [ ]   Supplemental Medicare: [ ]
Tricare   [ ]

PRODUCTS OFFERED:
Product Name: Type:
Advantra   Medicare Advantage

CONSUMER-DRIVEN PRODUCTS
Wells Fargo   HSA Company
                                                                HSA Product
Corporate Benefits Services of America   HSA Administrator
                                                                Consumer-Driven Health Plan
Open Access Plus Plan   High Deductible Health Plan

PLAN BENEFITS:
Alternative Medicine: [ ]   Behavioral Health: [ ]
Chiropractic: [X]   Dental: [ ]
Home Care: [X]   Inpatient SNF: [X]
Long-Term Care: [X]   Pharm. Mail Order: [X]
Physical Therapy: [X]   Podiatry: [ ]
Psychiatric: [X]   Transplant: [X]
Vision: [ ]   Wellness: [X]
Workers' Comp: [ ]
Other Benefits:

Managed Care Organization Profiles PENNSYLVANIA

KEY EXECUTIVES:
Chief Executive Officer/President .... Michael Blackwood
VP, Chief Financial Officer .... C Eric Huss
Chief Medical Officer .... Bob Mirsky, MD
Pharmacy Director...Dennis Sebastian
Marketing Director .... Marcia Martin
MIS Director ....George Galbraith
Compliance Officer .... Mary Craig
VP Operations .... Margaret Worek
Human Resource Director .... Monica Porter
VP, Medical Management .... Vicki Huffman
VP, General Counsel .... Karen Barringer

COMPANY PROFILE:
Parent Company Name: Mercy Health Plan/Highmark Inc/Gateway
Doing Business As: Gateway Health Plan Inc
Year Founded: 1992   Federally Qualified: [N]
Forprofit: [Y]   Not-For-Profit: [ ]
Model Type: NETWORK
Accreditation: [ ] AAPPO [ ] JACHO [X] NCQA [ ] URAC
Plan Type: HMO
Total Enrollment:
 2001: 0   2004: 260,796   2007: 269,443
 2002: 225,659   2005: 266,415
 2003: 241,912   2006: 243,689

SERVICE AREA:
Nationwide: N
  PA; OH;

TYPE OF COVERAGE:
Commercial: [ ] Individual: [ ] FEHBP: [ ] Indemnity: [ ]
Medicare: [ ] Medicaid: [Y] Supplemental Medicare:
[Y]Tricare [ ]

PRODUCTS OFFERED:
Product Name: Type:
Gateway Health Plan   Medicaid

GEISINGER HEALTH PLAN

100 North Academy Ave
Danville, PA 17822-3020
Phone: 717-271-8760 Fax: 570-826-7882 Toll-Free: 800-631-1656
Web site: www.thehealthplan.com
MAILING ADDRESS:
   GEISINGER HEALTH PLAN
   100 North Academy Ave
   Danville, PA 17822-3020

KEY EXECUTIVES:
Chief Executive Officer/President .... Richard Gilfillan, MD
VP, Finance .... Sharon Duncan
VP, Chief Medical Officer .... Duane E Davis, MD
VP, Medical Operations .... Janet F Tomcavage, RN, MSN
Executive VP, Interim .... Frank Trembulak
VP Sales & Marketing .... Thomas Qualley
Public Relations Coordinator .... Amy Bowen
VP, Provider Network Management .... Teresa Willard
Director Care Coordination .... Sabrina Girolami RN, BSN
VP Medical Management .... Lila Sobel, RN
Quality Assurance Director .... David Evans
Product Development Director .... David Jani
VP Medicare/Indemnity Insurance .... Richard Slaughter
VP External Operations .... Anne McDow
VP Internal Operations .... George Kutz
Director of Utilization Management .... Faye Jeffries, RN

COMPANY PROFILE:
Parent Company Name: Geisinger Health System
Doing Business As:
Year Founded: 1985   Federally Qualified: [N]
Forprofit: [ ]   Not-For-Profit: [Y]
Model Type: Network
Accreditation: [ ] AAPPO [ ] JACHO [X] NCQA [ ] URAC
Plan Type: HMO, PPO, TPA, POS
Primary Physicians: 1,832   Physician Specialists: 9,095
Hospitals: 62
Total Revenue: 2005:   2006:
Net Income   2005:   2006: 156,297,011

Total Enrollment:
 2001: 282,337   2004: 233,241   2007: 181,866
 2002: 258,787   2005: 180,252
 2003: 238,653   2006: 190,419
Medical Loss Ratio: 2005:   2006: 79.40
Administrative Expense Ratio: 2005:   2006:

SERVICE AREA:
Nationwide: N
  PA (Bedford, Berks, Blair, Bradford, Cambria,Cameron, Carbon, Centre, Clearfield, Clinton, Columbia, Cumberland, Dauphin, Elk, Huntingdon,Jefferson, Juniata, Lackawanna,Lancaster, Lebanon, Luzerne, Lycoming, Mifflin, Monroe, Montour, Northumberland, Perry, Pike, Potter, Schuylkill, Snyder, Sullivan, Susquehanna, Tioga, Union, Wayne, Wyoming, York);

TYPE OF COVERAGE:
Commercial: [Y] Individual: [Y] FEHBP: [ ] Indemnity: [ ]
Medicare: [Y] Medicaid: [Y] Supplemental Medicare: [ ]
Tricare [ ]

PRODUCTS OFFERED:
Product Name: Type:
Geisinger Health Plan HMO   HMO
Geisinger Health Options   TPA
Geisinger Health Plan POS   POS
Geiginger Select Care PPO   PPO
Geisinger Gold   Medicare Advantage

PLAN BENEFITS:
Alternative Medicine: [ ]   Behavioral Health: [X]
Chiropractic: [X]   Dental: [X]
Home Care: [X]   Inpatient SNF: [X]
Long-Term Care: [ ]   Pharm. Mail Order: [X]
Physical Therapy: [X]   Podiatry: [X]
Psychiatric: [X]   Transplant: [X]
Vision: [X]   Wellness: [X]
Workers' Comp: [ ]
Other Benefits: Transportation
Comments:
Formerly Geisinger Health Plan.

GENEX SERVICES

440 E Swedesford Rd Ste 1000
Wayne, PA 19087
Phone: 610-964-5100 Fax: 610-964-1919 Toll-Free: 800-GO-ENEX
Web site: www.genexservices.com
MAILING ADDRESS:
   GENEX SERVICES
   440 E Swedesford Rd Ste 1000
   Wayne, PA 19087

KEY EXECUTIVES:
Chief Executive Officer/President .... Peter C Madeja
Chief Financial Officer .... John Keohane
VP, Information Systems & Services .... Christopher D Darrell
Exec VP, Operations .... Delphia G Frisch
Senior VP, Sales & Marketing .... Stanley S Jakubowski
VP, Human Resources .... Debbi Bromley
VP, Product Management & Development .... Ronald Skrocki
VP, National Sales .... Paul E Neff
President, OCI .... Dan Blaney

COMPANY PROFILE:
Parent Company Name: Stone Point Capital LLC
Doing Business As: GENEX
Year Founded: 1978   Federally Qualified: [ ]
Forprofit: [Y]   Not-For-Profit: [ ]
Model Type:
Accreditation: [ ] AAPPO [ ] JACHO [ ] NCQA [X] URAC
Plan Type: Specialty PPO, UR,

SERVICE AREA:
Nationwide: N
   Nationwide, Canada, Puerto Rico;

GREAT-WEST HEALTHCARE OF PENNSYLVANIA

1023 E Baltimore Pike, Ste 200
Media, PA 19063-5126
Phone: 610-744-1010 Fax: 610-466-1327 Toll-Free:
Web site: www.greatwesthealthcare.com

PENNSYLVANIA

MAILING ADDRESS:
DEVON HEALTH SERVICES INC
1100 1st Ave Ste 100
King of Prussia, PA 19406

KEY EXECUTIVES:
President .... Charles Falcone
Chief Financial Officer .... George Clark
Chief Operating Officer .... Brian Atkinson
Director, Marketing & Communicatins .... Darren M Behuniak
VP, Network Development .... Bill Bruce
Human Resources Manager .... Felicia Moffa-Sipio
Senior VP, Operations .... Andrea Fisher

COMPANY PROFILE:
Parent Company Name: Devon Health Services Inc
Doing Business As: Health Care Cost Mgmt Company & a PPO
Year Founded: 1991   Federally Qualified: [ ]
Forprofit: [Y]   Not-For-Profit: [ ]
Model Type:
Accreditation: [ ] AAPPO [ ] JACHO [ ] NCQA [ ] URAC
Plan Type: PPO
Primary Physicians: 140,225   Physician Specialists: 30,608
Hospitals: 476
Total Enrollment:
  2001: 0   2004: 0   2007: 3,000,000
  2002: 3,000,000   2005:
  2003: 3,000,000   2006:

SERVICE AREA:
Nationwide:
  DE; NJ; NY; OH; PA;
TYPE OF COVERAGE:
Commercial: [Y] Individual: [ ] FEHBP: [ ] Indemnity: [ ]
Medicare: [Y] Medicaid: [ ] Supplemental Medicare: [ ]
Tricare   [ ]
PRODUCTS OFFERED:
Product Name: Type:
Devon Health Services Inc   PPO
PLAN BENEFITS:
Alternative Medicine: [ ]   Behavioral Health: [X]
Chiropractic: [X]   Dental: [X]
Home Care: [X]   Inpatient SNF: [ ]
Long-Term Care: [ ]   Pharm. Mail Order: [X]
Physical Therapy: [ ]   Podiatry: [X]
Psychiatric: [X]   Transplant: [X]
Vision: [X]   Wellness: [ ]
Workers' Comp: [X]
Other Benefits:

EHP INC

1871 Santa Barbara Dr
Lancaster, PA 17603
Phone: 717-735-7760 Fax: 717-399-1693 Toll-Free:
Web site: www.ehpservices.com
MAILING ADDRESS:
EHP INC
PO Box 8737
Lancaster, PA 17603

KEY EXECUTIVES:
Chief Executive Officer .... David R Smith
Medical Director .... Jon Schrock, MD
Data & Technical Services Manager .... Andy Osika
Credentialing Manager .... Kris Danz
Director, Provider Relations .... Renee Connor
Credentialing Manager .... Kris Danz

COMPANY PROFILE:
Parent Company Name:
Doing Business As:
Year Founded: 1996   Federally Qualified: [N]
Forprofit: [Y]   Not-For-Profit: [ ]
Model Type: IPA
Accreditation: [ ] AAPPO [ ] JACHO [ ] NCQA [ ] URAC
Plan Type: PPO, HSA
Primary Physicians: 8,000   Physician Specialists: 28,000
Hospitals: 276

SERVICE AREA:
Nationwide: N
  PA (Berks, Lancaster, York);
TYPE OF COVERAGE:
Commercial: [Y] Individual: [ ] FEHBP: [ ] Indemnity: [ ]
Medicare: [ ] Medicaid: [ ] Supplemental Medicare: [ ]
Tricare   [ ]
PRODUCTS OFFERED:
Product Name: Type:
Alliance Health Plan   PPO
PLAN BENEFITS:
Alternative Medicine: [ ]   Behavioral Health: [X]
Chiropractic: [X]   Dental: [ ]
Home Care: [X]   Inpatient SNF: [X]
Long-Term Care: [X]   Pharm. Mail Order: [ ]
Physical Therapy: [X]   Podiatry: [X]
Psychiatric: [X]   Transplant: [X]
Vision: [X]   Wellness: [ ]
Workers' Comp: [ ]
Other Benefits:
Comments:
Formerly Alliance Health Plan.

FIDELIO INSURANCE COMPANY

2826 Mt Carmel Ave
Glenside, PA 19038
Phone: 215-885-2443 Fax: 215-576-5849 Toll-Free:
Web site: www.fideliodental.com
MAILING ADDRESS:
FIDELIO INSURANCE COMPANY
2826 Mt Carmel Ave
Glenside, PA 19038

KEY EXECUTIVES:
Chief Executive Officer\Marketing Director .... Mario Mele
Chief Medical Officer .... Mike Wilson
Director/Network Operations/Dev .... Michael Mele

COMPANY PROFILE:
Parent Company Name:
Doing Business As:
Year Founded: 1988   Federally Qualified: [ ]
Forprofit: [ ]   Not-For-Profit: [ ]
Model Type:
Accreditation: [ ] AAPPO [ ] JACHO [ ] NCQA [ ] URAC
Plan Type: Specialty PPO
SERVICE AREA:
Nationwide: N
  PA (Montgomery, Philadelphia);
TYPE OF COVERAGE:
Commercial: [ ] Individual: [ ] FEHBP: [ ] Indemnity: [ ]
Medicare: [ ] Medicaid: [ ] Supplemental Medicare: [ ]
Tricare   [ ]
PLAN BENEFITS:
Alternative Medicine: [ ]   Behavioral Health: [ ]
Chiropractic: [ ]   Dental: [X]
Home Care: [ ]   Inpatient SNF: [ ]
Long-Term Care: [ ]   Pharm. Mail Order: [ ]
Physical Therapy: [ ]   Podiatry: [ ]
Psychiatric: [ ]   Transplant: [ ]
Vision: [ ]   Wellness: [ ]
Workers' Comp: [ ]
Other Benefits:

GATEWAY HEALTH PLAN INC

600 Grant Street
Pittsburgh, PA 15219-2704
Phone: 412-255-4640 Fax: 412-255-4334 Toll-Free: 800-392-1147
Web site: www.gatewayhealthplan.com
MAILING ADDRESS:
GATEWAY HEALTH PLAN INC
600 Grant Street
Pittsburgh, PA 15219-2704

Managed Care Organization Profiles — PENNSYLVANIA

PLAN BENEFITS:
Alternative Medicine:	[ ]	Behavioral Health:	[X]
Chiropractic:	[X]	Dental:	[X]
Home Care:	[ ]	Inpatient SNF:	[ ]
Long-Term Care:	[ ]	Pharm. Mail Order:	[X]
Physical Therapy:	[ ]	Podiatry:	[ ]
Psychiatric:	[ ]	Transplant:	[ ]
Vision:	[X]	Wellness:	[ ]
Workers' Comp:	[ ]		
Other Benefits:			

COMMUNITY BEHAVIORAL HEALTHCARE COOPERATIVE OF PENNSYLVANIA

8040 Carlson Rd
Harrisburg, PA 17112
Phone: 717-671-6500 Fax: 717-671-6521 Toll-Free:
Web site: www.cbhnp.org

MAILING ADDRESS:
COMMUNITY BEHAVIORAL HEALTHCARE
PO Box 6600
Harrisburg, PA 17112

KEY EXECUTIVES:
Chief Executive Officer/President .... Richard S Edley, PhD
Chief Financial Officer .... Robert Bickford
Chief Medical Officer .... Rajnikant Lad, MD
Chief Operating Officer .... Scott Daubert, PhD
VP Strategic Initatives .... Sarah Eyster, LSW
VP Administration/Privacy Officer .... Malcolm R West, MA
Clinial Manager, Commercial & Medicare .... Burt Reilly, MA
Director, Provider/Network Operations .... Sheryl Swanson, MBA
Director, Human Resources .... Jason LaFrance, MA
Director, Quality Improvement .... Laurie Cross
Director of Clinical Development .... Alan Petroski, PhD
Mgr/Consumer & Family Affairs .... Anthony House
Communications Manager .... Gema Nelson

COMPANY PROFILE:
Parent Company Name: AmeriHealth Mercy Company
Doing Business As: Community Behavioral HlthCr Ntwk of PA
Year Founded: 1995   Federally Qualified: [ ]
Forprofit: [ ]   Not-For-Profit: [Y]
Model Type: NETWORK
Accreditation: [ ] AAPPO [ ] JACHO [ ] NCQA [ ] URAC
Plan Type: Specialty PPO
Total Enrollment:
   2001: 0   2004: 0   2007: 3,400,000
   2002: 586,000   2005:
   2003: 662,000   2006:

SERVICE AREA:
Nationwide: N
   PA;

TYPE OF COVERAGE:
Commercial: [Y] Individual: [ ] FEHBP: [ ] Indemnity: [ ]
Medicare: [Y] Medicaid: [Y] Supplemental Medicare: [ ]
Tricare [ ]

PLAN BENEFITS:
Alternative Medicine:	[ ]	Behavioral Health:	[X]
Chiropractic:	[ ]	Dental:	[ ]
Home Care:	[ ]	Inpatient SNF:	[ ]
Long-Term Care:	[ ]	Pharm. Mail Order:	[ ]
Physical Therapy:	[ ]	Podiatry:	[ ]
Psychiatric:	[ ]	Transplant:	[ ]
Vision:	[ ]	Wellness:	[ ]
Workers' Comp:	[ ]		
Other Benefits:			

Comments:
Acquired by AmeriHealth Mercy.

COORDINATED HEALTH SYSTEMS

2775 Schoenersville Rd
Bethlehem, PA 18017
Phone: 610-861-88080 Fax: 610-807-0366 Toll-Free: 877-247-8080
Web site: www.chs4health.com

MAILING ADDRESS:
COORDINATED HEALTH SYSTEMS
2775 Schoenersville Rd
Bethlehem, PA 18017

KEY EXECUTIVES:
Chief Executive Officer .... Emil DiLorio, MD
Chief Financial Officer .... David Weikel
Medical Director .... Carl Weiss, Jr, MD
Senior VP of Operations .... Robert Savers
MIS Director .... Jeff Cascino

COMPANY PROFILE:
Parent Company Name: Coordinated Health Systems
Doing Business As: American Health Plan Mgmt Inc
Year Founded: 1993   Federally Qualified: [ ]
Forprofit: [Y]   Not-For-Profit: [ ]
Model Type:
Accreditation: [ ] AAPPO [ ] JACHO [ ] NCQA [ ] URAC
Plan Type: HMO, PPO

SERVICE AREA:
Nationwide: N
   PA (Bucks, Carbon, LeHigh, Monroe, Northampton);

TYPE OF COVERAGE:
Commercial: [Y] Individual: [ ] FEHBP: [ ] Indemnity: [ ]
Medicare: [ ] Medicaid: [ ] Supplemental Medicare: [ ]
Tricare [ ]

Comments:
Formerly American Healthplan Management Inc.

DELTA DENTAL OF PENNSYLVANIA

One Delta Dr
Mechanicsburg, PA 17055-6999
Phone: 717-766-8500 Fax: 717-766-8719 Toll-Free:
Web site: www.deltadentalpa.org

MAILING ADDRESS:
DELTA DENTAL OF PA
One Delta Dr
Mechanicsburg, PA 17055-6999

KEY EXECUTIVES:
Chief Executive Officer/President .... Gary D Radine
Chief Financial Officer .... Michael J Castro
Chief Information Officer .... Patrick S Steele

COMPANY PROFILE:
Parent Company Name: Delta Dental Plan Association
Doing Business As:
Year Founded: Federally Qualified: [ ]
Forprofit: [ ]   Not-For-Profit: [ ]
Model Type:
Accreditation: [ ] AAPPO [ ] JACHO [ ] NCQA [ ] URAC
Plan Type: Specialty HMO
Total Enrollment:
   2001: 334,635   2004: 437,861   2007: 0
   2002: 375,494   2005:
   2003: 390,982   2006:

SERVICE AREA:
Nationwide: N
   DC; DE; MD; NY; PA; WV;

TYPE OF COVERAGE:
Commercial: [Y] Individual: [ ] FEHBP: [ ] Indemnity: [ ]
Medicare: [ ] Medicaid: [ ] Supplemental Medicare: [ ]
Tricare [ ]

PLAN BENEFITS:
Alternative Medicine:	[ ]	Behavioral Health:	[ ]
Chiropractic:	[ ]	Dental:	[X]
Home Care:	[ ]	Inpatient SNF:	[ ]
Long-Term Care:	[ ]	Pharm. Mail Order:	[ ]
Physical Therapy:	[ ]	Podiatry:	[ ]
Psychiatric:	[ ]	Transplant:	[ ]
Vision:	[ ]	Wellness:	[ ]
Workers' Comp:	[ ]		
Other Benefits:			

DEVON HEALTH SERVICES INC

1100 1st Ave Ste 100
King of Prussia, PA 19406
Phone: 800-431-2273 Fax: 800-221-0002 Toll-Free: 800-431-2273
Web site: www.devonhealth.com

PENNSYLVANIA — Managed Care Organization Profiles

CIGNA DENTAL HEALTH OF PENNSYLVANIA INC

1571 Sawgrass Corporate Pkwy
Sunrise, FL 33323
Phone: 954-514-6600 Fax: 954-514-6905 Toll-Free: 800-367-1037
Web site: www.cigna.com/dental

MAILING ADDRESS:
CIGNA DENTAL HEALTH OF PA INC
1571 Sawgrass Corporate Pkwy
Sunrise, FL 33323

KEY EXECUTIVES:
Chairman/Chief Executive Officer .... H Edward Hanway
President .... Karen S Rohan

COMPANY PROFILE:
Parent Company Name: CIGNA Dental Health Inc
Doing Business As: CIGNA Dental
Year Founded: 1985   Federally Qualified: [N]
Forprofit: [Y]   Not-For-Profit: [ ]
Model Type:
Accreditation: [ ] AAPPO [ ] JACHO [ ] NCQA [ ] URAC
Plan Type: Specialty HMO
Total Enrollment:
  2001: 52,534   2004: 38,625   2007: 0
  2002: 58,568   2005:
  2003: 56,812   2006:

SERVICE AREA:
Nationwide: N
  PA;

TYPE OF COVERAGE:
Commercial: [Y] Individual: [ ] FEHBP: [ ] Indemnity: [ ]
Medicare: [ ] Medicaid: [ ] Supplemental Medicare: [ ]
Tricare   [ ]

PLAN BENEFITS:
Alternative Medicine: [ ]   Behavioral Health: [ ]
Chiropractic: [ ]   Dental: [X]
Home Care: [ ]   Inpatient SNF: [ ]
Long-Term Care: [ ]   Pharm. Mail Order: [ ]
Physical Therapy: [ ]   Podiatry: [ ]
Psychiatric: [ ]   Transplant: [ ]
Vision: [ ]   Wellness: [ ]
Workers' Comp: [ ]
Other Benefits:

CIGNA HEALTHCARE — CORPORATE HEADQUARTERS

One Liberty Place
1650 Market St
Philadelphia, PA 19192
Phone: 215-761-1000 Fax: 215-761-5517 Toll-Free:
Web site: www.cigna.com

MAILING ADDRESS:
CIGNA HEALTHCARE — CORP HDQTR
One Liberty Place
1650 Market St
Philadelphia, PA 19192

KEY EXECUTIVES:
Chairman/Chief Executive Officer .... H Edward Hanway
President .... David M Cordani
Chief Financial Officer .... Michael W Bell
Chief Medical Officer, Group .... Allen Woolf, MD
Chief Information Officer .... Juan Conde
Senior VP, Marketing .... James Lyski
Executive VP, Human Resources .... John Murabito
Senior VP, Medical Management .... Matt Manders
Chief Counsel .... John Perlstein

COMPANY PROFILE:
Parent Company Name: CIGNA Corporation
Doing Business As: CIGNA Healthcare
Year Founded: 1982   Federally Qualified: [Y]
Forprofit: [Y]   Not-For-Profit: [ ]
Model Type: IPA
Accreditation: [ ] AAPPO [ ] JACHO [ ] NCQA [ ] URAC
Plan Type: HMO, PPO, POS, UR, CDHP, HDHP, HSA, FSA, HRA

Total Revenue: 2005: 16,684,000   2006:
Net Income   2005: 1,625,000   2006:
Total Enrollment:
  2001: 14,318,000   2004: 9,701,000   2007: 0
  2002: 13,300,000   2005: 9,006,000
  2003: 12,300,000   2006: 9,389,000
Medical Loss Ratio: 2005:   2006:
Administrative Expense Ratio: 2005:   2006:

SERVICE AREA:
Nationwide: Y
  NW;

TYPE OF COVERAGE:
Commercial: [Y] Individual: [Y] FEHBP: [ ] Indemnity: [ ]
Medicare: [Y] Medicaid: [Y] Supplemental Medicare: [Y]
Tricare   [ ]

PRODUCTS OFFERED:
Product Name: Type:

CONSUMER-DRIVEN PRODUCTS
JP Morgan Chase   HSA CompanyCIGNA Choice
Fund   HSA Product
                           HSA Administrator
Open Access Plus   Consumer-Driven Health Plan
PPO   High Deductible Health Plan

PLAN BENEFITS:
Alternative Medicine: [ ]   Behavioral Health: [ ]
Chiropractic: [X]   Dental: [X]
Home Care: [X]   Inpatient SNF: [X]
Long-Term Care: [ ]   Pharm. Mail Order: [X]
Physical Therapy: [X]   Podiatry: [X]
Psychiatric: [X]   Transplant: [X]
Vision: [X]   Wellness: [X]
Workers' Comp: [X]
Other Benefits:

CIGNA HEALTHCARE OF PA

1777 Sentry Pkwy W Ste 100
Blue Bell, PA 19422
Phone: 215-283-3300 Fax: 215-283-3920 Toll-Free:
Web site: www.cigna.com

MAILING ADDRESS:
CIGNA HEALTHCARE OF PA
1777 Sentry Pkwy Ste 100
Blue Bell, PA 19422

KEY EXECUTIVES:
Business Manager .... Vince Sobocinski

COMPANY PROFILE:
Parent Company Name: CIGNA Corporation
Doing Business As: CIGNA Healthcare
Year Founded: 1989   Federally Qualified: [ ]
Forprofit: [Y]   Not-For-Profit: [ ]
Model Type: IPA
Accreditation: [ ] AAPPO [ ] JACHO [ ] NCQA [X] URAC
Plan Type: HMO, PPO, POS, CDHP, HSA, FSA, HRA, HDHP
Total Enrollment:
  2001: 0   2004: 43,308   2007: 18,914
  2002: 0   2005: 13,408
  2003: 54,699   2006: 14,148

SERVICE AREA:
Nationwide: N
  PA; DE;

TYPE OF COVERAGE:
Commercial: [Y] Individual: [ ] FEHBP: [ ] Indemnity: [ ]
Medicare: [ ] Medicaid: [ ] Supplemental Medicare: [ ]
Tricare   [ ]

PRODUCTS OFFERED:
Product Name: Type:
Cigna Hlthcare for Seniors   Medicare

CONSUMER-DRIVEN PRODUCTS
JP Morgan Chase   HSA Company
CIGNA Choice Fund   HSA Product
                           HSA Administrator
Open Access Plus   Consumer-Driven Health Plan
PPO   High Deductible Health Plan

Managed Care Organization Profiles **PENNSYLVANIA**

PLAN BENEFITS:
Alternative Medicine:	[ ]	Behavioral Health:	[X]
Chiropractic:	[X]	Dental:	[ ]
Home Care:	[X]	Inpatient SNF:	[X]
Long-Term Care:	[ ]	Pharm. Mail Order:	[ ]
Physical Therapy:	[X]	Podiatry:	[X]
Psychiatric:	[X]	Transplant:	[X]
Vision:	[ ]	Wellness:	[X]
Workers' Comp:	[X]		
Other Benefits:			

CAPITAL BLUE CROSS

2500 Elmerton Ave
Harrisburg, PA 17110
Phone: 717-541-7000 Fax: 717-541-6915 Toll-Free: 800-958-5558
Web site: www.capbluecross.com
MAILING ADDRESS:
　　CAPITAL BLUE CROSS
　　2500 Elmerton Ave
　　Harrisburg, PA 17110

KEY EXECUTIVES:
Chairman of the Board .... William Lehr, Jr
Chief Executive Officer/President .... Anita M Smith
Senior VP, Chief Financial Officer .... Gary D St Hilarie
Senior VP, Operations & Human Resource .... Debra B Cohen

COMPANY PROFILE:
Parent Company Name:
Doing Business As:
Year Founded: 1938　　　Federally Qualified: [ ]
Forprofit: [ ]　　　Not-For-Profit: [Y]
Model Type: IPA
Accreditation: [ ] AAPPO [ ] JACHO [ ] NCQA [ ] URAC
Plan Type: HMO, PPO, POS, ASO, HDHP, HSA
Primary Physicians: 8,300　　Physician Specialists: 37
Hospitals:
Total Revenue: 2005:　　2006: 291,124,411
Net Income 2005:　　2006:
Total Enrollment:
　2001: 927,907　　2004: 152,547　　2007: 0
　2002: 1,100,000　　2005:
　2003: 1,000,000　　2006: 1,000,000
Medical Loss Ratio: 2005:　　2006: 93.10
Administrative Expense Ratio: 2005:　　2006:
SERVICE AREA:
Nationwide: N
　PA (Adams, Berks, Centre, Columbia, Cumberland, Dauphin, Franklin, Fulton, Juniata, Lancaster, Lebanon, LeHigh, Mifflin, Montour, Northampton, Northumberland, Perry, Schuylkill, Snyder, Union, York);
TYPE OF COVERAGE:
Commercial: [Y] Individual: [Y] FEHBP: [ ] Indemnity: [ ]
Medicare:　[Y] Medicaid: [Y] Supplemental Medicare: [Y]
Tricare　　[ ]
PRODUCTS OFFERED:
Product Name:	Type:
Capital Advantage Insurance Company	GPPO
Keystone Health Plan Central	Medicare Advantage

CONSUMER-DRIVEN PRODUCTS
	HSA Company
	HSA Product
	HSA Administrator
	Consumer-Driven Health Plan
Simply Select	High Deductible Health Plan

CARE NETWORK

820 Parish St
Pittsburgh, PA 15220
Phone: 412-922-4616 Fax: 412-922-9461 Toll-Free: 800-233-5216
Web site: www.pennhighlands.com
MAILING ADDRESS:
　　CARE NETWORK
　　820 Parish St
　　Pittsburgh, PA 15220

KEY EXECUTIVES:
Chief Executive Officer .... Phyllis Shehab
President .... Jay R Ver Hulst
Chief Financial Officer .... Patrick Forrest
Medical Director .... Roland Griggs, MD
VP, Utilization Management .... Deborah Immel, RN
MIS Director .... Jeff Stanley
Director of Utilization Management .... Jan MacDonald, RN
VP, Legal .... John Beck

COMPANY PROFILE:
Parent Company Name: Managed Care of America
Doing Business As:
Year Founded: 1986　　　Federally Qualified: [ ]
Forprofit: [Y]　　　Not-For-Profit: [ ]
Model Type:
Accreditation: [ ] AAPPO [ ] JACHO [ ] NCQA [X] URAC
Plan Type: UR
SERVICE AREA:
Nationwide: Y
　NW;
TYPE OF COVERAGE:
Commercial: [Y] Individual: [ ] FEHBP: [ ] Indemnity: [ ]
Medicare:　[ ] Medicaid: [ ] Supplemental Medicare: [ ]
Tricare　　[ ]

CENTRAL SUSQUEHANNA HEALTHCARE PROVIDERS

1 Hospital Dr
Lewisburg, PA 17837
Phone: 570-522-2748 Fax: 570-522-4072 Toll-Free: 866-890-2747
Web site: www.cshpnetwork.com
MAILING ADDRESS:
　　CENTRAL SUSQUEHANNA HEALTHCARE
　　1 Hospital Dr
　　Lewisburg, PA 17837

KEY EXECUTIVES:
Chairman/Medical Director .... J Lawrence Ginsberg, MD
Director of Managed Care .... Matt Romania, RN
President/Controller .... Michael O'Keefe
Treasurer .... James Stopper
Managed Care Coordinator .... Jason S Beach

COMPANY PROFILE:
Parent Company Name: Evangelical Hospital, Sunbury Hospital
Doing Business As:
Year Founded: 1987　　　Federally Qualified: [ ]
Forprofit: [ ]　　　Not-For-Profit: [Y]
Model Type: NETWORK
Accreditation: [ ] AAPPO [ ] JACHO [ ] NCQA [ ] URAC
Plan Type: PPO
Primary Physicians: 272　　Physician Specialists: 873
Hospitals: 8
Total Enrollment:
　2001: 12,908　　2004: 11,308　　2007: 0
　2002: 0　　2005:
　2003: 10,618　　2006: 10,000
SERVICE AREA:
Nationwide: N
　PA (Lycoming, Northumberland, Snyder, Union);
TYPE OF COVERAGE:
Commercial: [Y] Individual: [ ] FEHBP: [ ] Indemnity: [ ]
Medicare:　[ ] Medicaid: [ ] Supplemental Medicare: [ ]
]Tricare　　[ ]
PRODUCTS OFFERED:
Product Name:	Type:
Central Susquehanna PPO	PPO

PLAN BENEFITS:
Alternative Medicine:	[ ]	Behavioral Health:	[ ]
Chiropractic:	[ ]	Dental:	[ ]
Home Care:	[X]	Inpatient SNF:	[ ]
Long-Term Care:	[ ]	Pharm. Mail Order:	[ ]
Physical Therapy:	[ ]	Podiatry:	[X]
Psychiatric:	[X]	Transplant:	[X]
Vision:	[ ]	Wellness:	[ ]
Workers' Comp:	[ ]		
Other Benefits:			

PENNSYLVANIA

Accreditation: [ ] AAPPO [ ] JACHO [ ] NCQA [ ] URAC
Plan Type: PPO
Primary Physicians: Physician Specialists:
Hospitals: 14
SERVICE AREA:
Nationwide: N
   PA (Carbon, Schuylkill, and Lebanon);
TYPE OF COVERAGE:
Commercial: [Y] Individual: [Y] FEHBP: [ ] Indemnity: [ ]
Medicare: [ ] Medicaid: [ ] Supplemental Medicare: [ ]
Tricare   [ ]
PLAN BENEFITS:
Alternative Medicine: [ ]   Behavioral Health: [X]
Chiropractic: [ ]   Dental: [ ]
Home Care: [X]   Inpatient SNF: [X]
Long-Term Care: [X]   Pharm. Mail Order: [ ]
Physical Therapy: [X]   Podiatry: [X]
Psychiatric: [X]   Transplant: [X]
Vision: [ ]   Wellness: [X]
Workers' Comp: [ ]
Other Benefits:

BLUECROSS OF NORTHEASTERN PENNSYLVANIA

19 N Main St
Wilkes-Barre, PA 18711
Phone: 570-200-4300 Fax: 570-200-6710 Toll-Free:
Web site: www.bcnepa.com
MAILING ADDRESS:
   BLUECROSS OF NORTHEASTERN PA
   19 N Main St
   Wilkes-Barre, PA 18711

KEY EXECUTIVES:
Chairman .... John P Moses
Chief Executive Officer/President .... Denise S Cesare
Chief Financial Officer .... Ken Suchoski
Chief Medical Officer .... Leo Hartz
Chief Information Officer .... Thomas Druby

COMPANY PROFILE:
Parent Company Name: Blue Cross/Blue Shield Association
Doing Business As:
Year Founded: 1938   Federally Qualified: [ ]
Forprofit: [ ]   Not-For-Profit: [Y]
Model Type:
Accreditation: [ ] AAPPO [ ] JACHO [ ] NCQA [ ] URAC
Plan Type: HMO, PPO, POS
Total Revenue: 2005:   721,867,000   2006:
Net Income   2005:   3,408,000   2006:
Total Enrollment:
   2001: 0   2004: 600,000   2007: 114,649
   2002: 550,000   2005: 180,252
   2003: 600,000   2006: 600,000
SERVICE AREA:
Nationwide:
   PA (Bradford, Carbon, Clinton, Lackawanna, Luzerne, Lycoming, Monroe, Pike, Sullivan, Susquehanna, Tioga, Wayne, Wyoming):
TYPE OF COVERAGE:
Commercial: [Y] Individual: [ ] FEHBP: [ ] Indemnity: [ ]
Medicare: [ ] Medicaid: [ ] Supplemental Medicare: [Y]
Tricare   [ ]
PRODUCTS OFFERED:
Product Name: Type:
First Priority Health   HMO
First Priority Health Plus   POS
Access Care II   PPO
Traditional Plans
65-Spec   Medicare Supplement

BRAVO HEALTH PENNSYLVANIA INC

1500 Spring Garden St Ste 800
Philadelphia, PA 19130
Phone: 215-606-6355 Fax: 215-606-6402 Toll-Free: 888-776-8851
Web site: www.elderhealth.com/pa

MAILING ADDRESS:
   BRAVO HEALTH PA INC
   1500 Spring Garden St Ste 800
   Philadelphia, PA 19130

KEY EXECUTIVES:
Chief Executive Officer .... Jeff Folick
VP, Executive Director .... Don Fox
Chief Financial Officer .... Scott Tabakin
Medical Director .... David Yalowitz, MD
Pharmacy Director .... David Yoder, MD
Chief Information Officer .... Greg Pontius

COMPANY PROFILE:
Parent Company Name: Bravo Health Inc
Doing Business As:
Year Founded: 2002   Federally Qualified: [ ]
Forprofit: [Y]   Not-For-Profit: [ ]
Model Type: GROUP
Accreditation: [ ] AAPPO [ ] JACHO [ ] NCQA [ ] URAC
Plan Type: HMO, CDHP, HDHP, HSA,
Total Enrollment:
   2001: 0   2004: 5,305   2007: 36,684
   2002: 3,232   2005: 13,836
   2003: 3,635   2006: 14,148
SERVICE AREA:
Nationwide:
   PA;
TYPE OF COVERAGE:
Commercial: [ ] Individual: [ ] FEHBP: [ ] Indemnity: [ ]
Medicare: [Y] Medicaid: [ ] Supplemental Medicare: [ ]
Tricare   [ ]
PRODUCTS OFFERED:
Product Name: Type:
Bravo Eldercare   Medicare
Comments:
Formerly Elder Health Pennsylvania HMO Inc.

BUCKS COUNTY PHYSICIAN HOSPITAL ALLIANCE

252 W Swamp Rd Ste 5
Doylestown, PA 18901
Phone: 267-880-1235 Fax: 267-489-5271 Toll-Free:
Web site: www.bcpha.com
MAILING ADDRESS:
   BUCKS COUNTY PHYICIAN HOSPITAL ALLIANCE
   252 W Swamp Rd Ste 5
   Doylestown, PA 18901

KEY EXECUTIVES:
Chief Executive Officer/President .... Sheri M Putnam
Chief Financial Officer .... William Smith
Medical Director .... Jon Walheim, MD
Chief Information Officer .... Ron Watson
Director of Provider Services .... Nancy L Pericone

COMPANY PROFILE:
Parent Company Name: Doylestown Hosp/Doylestown Independent
Doing Business As:
Year Founded: 1989   Federally Qualified: [ ]
Forprofit: [Y]   Not-For-Profit: [ ]
Model Type: GROUP
Accreditation: [ ] AAPPO [ ] JACHO [ ] NCQA [ ] URAC
Plan Type: PPO
Total Enrollment:
   2001: 0   2004: 0   2007: 0
   2002: 0   2005:
   2003: 125,000   2006:
SERVICE AREA:
Nationwide: N
   PA (Bucks, Carbon, LeHigh, Luzerne, Monroe, Montgomery, Schuylkill);
TYPE OF COVERAGE:
Commercial: [Y] Individual: [ ] FEHBP: [ ] Indemnity: [ ]
Medicare: [ ] Medicaid: [ ] Supplemental Medicare: [ ]
Tricare   [ ]

Managed Care Organization Profiles — PENNSYLVANIA

KEY EXECUTIVES:
Chief Executive Officer .... Mary McSorley
Finance .... Dan O'Brien
Medical Director .... Sandra Nichols

COMPANY PROFILE:
Parent Company Name: UnitedHealth Group
Doing Business As:
Year Founded: 1989   Federally Qualified: [ ]
Forprofit: [Y]   Not-For-Profit: [ ]
Model Type: GROUP
Accreditation: [ ] AAPPO [ ] JACHO [ ] NCQA [ ] URAC
Plan Type: HMO,
Total Enrollment:
   2001: 112,079   2004: 115,096   2007: 79,458
   2002: 115,507   2005: 103,439
   2003: 115,507   2006: 92,722

SERVICE AREA:
Nationwide:
  PA (Philadelphia, Bucks, Chester, Delaware, Montgomery);

TYPE OF COVERAGE:
Commercial: [ ] Individual: [ ] FEHBP: [ ] Indemnity: [ ]
Medicare: [Y] Medicaid: [ ] Supplemental Medicare: [ ]
Tricare

PRODUCTS OFFERED:
Product Name: Type:
Americhoice Personal Care Plus   Medicaid
Children's Health Insurance Plan   CHIP

ASSURANT EMPLOYEE BENEFITS - PENNSYLVANIA

150 N Radnor Chester Rd
Radnor, PA 19087
Phone: 610-660-8070 Fax: 484-582-1218 Toll-Free: 800-220-1957
Web site: www.assurantemployeebenefits.com

MAILING ADDRESS:
   ASSURANT EMPLOYEE BNFTS - PA
   150 N Radnor Chester Rd
   Radnor, PA 19087

KEY EXECUTIVES:
Interim Chief Executive Officer/President .... John S Roberts
Chief Financial Officer .... Floyd F Chadee
VP, Medical Director .... Polly M Galbraith, MD
Chief Information Officer .... Karla J Schacht
Senior VP, Marketing .... Joseph A Sevcik
Privacy Officer .... John L Fortini
VP of Provider Services .... James A Barrett, DMD
Senior VP, Human Resources & Development .... Sylvia R Wagner
General Manager .... Todd Boyd
National Dental Director .... James A Barrett, DMD

COMPANY PROFILE:
Parent Company Name: Assurant Health
Doing Business As:
Year Founded: 1986   Federally Qualified: [ ]
Forprofit: [Y]   Not-For-Profit: [ ]
Model Type:
Accreditation: [ ] AAPPO [ ] JACHO [ ] NCQA [ ] URAC
Plan Type: Specialty HMO

SERVICE AREA:
Nationwide: N
  CT; DE; MD; ME; MS; NH; NJ; RI; PA; VT; WV;

TYPE OF COVERAGE:
Commercial: [Y] Individual: [Y] FEHBP: [ ] Indemnity: [ ]
Medicare: [ ] Medicaid: [ ] Supplemental Medicare: [ ]
Tricare

PLAN BENEFITS:
Alternative Medicine: [ ]   Behavioral Health: [ ]
Chiropractic: [ ]   Dental: [X]
Home Care: [ ]   Inpatient SNF: [ ]
Long-Term Care: [ ]   Pharm. Mail Order: [ ]
Physical Therapy: [ ]   Podiatry: [ ]
Psychiatric: [ ]   Transplant: [ ]
Vision: [ ]   Wellness: [ ]
Workers' Comp: [ ]
Other Benefits:

Comments:
Formerly Fortis Benefits Dental.

BERKSHIRE HEALTH PARTNERS/ MEDICUS RESOURCE MANAGEMENT

50 Commerce Drive
Wyomissing, PA 19610
Phone: 610-372-8044 Fax: 610-372-3036 Toll-Free:
Web site: www.bhp.org

MAILING ADDRESS:
   BERKSHIRE HLTH PTN/MEDICUS RES
   50 Commerce Drive
   Wyomissing, PA 19610

KEY EXECUTIVES:
President .... Charles Wills
Controller .... Dennis Wolfe
Medical Director .... Eugene J Fellin, DO
Manager of Information Systems .... Dan Scott
Director of Operations .... Tanya Glouner
Director, Business Development/Marketing .... Natalie Zimmerman
MIS Director .... Dan Scott
Credentialing Manager .... Travonya Quarles
Manager, Utilization Management/HIPAA .... Robin J Riegner, RN
Director of Medical Management .... Dawn Dreibelbis, RN
Credentialing Manager .... Travonya Quarles

COMPANY PROFILE:
Parent Company Name:
Doing Business As:
Year Founded: 1986   Federally Qualified: [N]
Forprofit: [ ]   Not-For-Profit: [Y]
Model Type: NETWORK
Accreditation: [ ] AAPPO [ ] JACHO [ ] NCQA [ ] URAC
Plan Type: PPO, UR
Primary Physicians: 789   Physician Specialists: 1,546
Hospitals: 14
Total Enrollment:
   2001: 68,146   2004: 95,818   2007: 91,852
   2002: 68,779   2005: 102,584
   2003: 84,186   2006: 105,753

SERVICE AREA:
Nationwide: N
  PA (Berks, Buck, Carbon, Lancaster, Lehigh, Montgomery, Northampton, Schuylkill);

TYPE OF COVERAGE:
Commercial: [Y] Individual: [Y] FEHBP: [ ] Indemnity: [ ]
Medicare: [ ] Medicaid: [ ] Supplemental Medicare: [ ]
Tricare

PLAN BENEFITS:
Alternative Medicine: [ ]   Behavioral Health: [X]
Chiropractic: [X]   Dental: [ ]
Home Care: [X]   Inpatient SNF: [X]
Long-Term Care: [X]   Pharm. Mail Order: [ ]
Physical Therapy: [X]   Podiatry: [X]
Psychiatric: [X]   Transplant: [X]
Vision: [ ]   Wellness: [ ]
Workers' Comp: [X]
Other Benefits:

BLUE RIDGE HEALTH NETWORK

1900 West End Ave
Pottsville, PA 17901
Phone: 570-628-2236 Fax: 570-628-1880 Toll-Free: 800-730-0134
Web site: www.blueridgehealthnetwork.com

MAILING ADDRESS:
   BLUE RIDGE HEALTH NETWORK
   1900 West End Ave
   Pottsville, PA 17901

KEY EXECUTIVES:
President .... Robert E Jones
Chief Financial Officer/Principal .... Lisa Laudeman
Medical Director .... Samuel Burlock
Marketing Director .... Robert E Jones
MIS Director .... Lisa A Laudeman

COMPANY PROFILE:
Parent Company Name:
Doing Business As:
Year Founded: 1995   Federally Qualified: [ ]
Forprofit: [Y]   Not-For-Profit: [ ]
Model Type:

PENNSYLVANIA   Managed Care Organization Profiles

COMPANY PROFILE:
Parent Company Name: Aetna Inc
Doing Business As: Aetna Inc
Year Founded: 1974   Federally Qualified: [Y]
Forprofit: [Y]   Not-For-Profit: [ ]
Model Type: IPA
Accreditation: [ ] AAPPO [ ] JACHO [X] NCQA [X] URAC
Plan Type: HMO, PPO, POS, CDHP, HDHP, HSA,
SERVICE AREA:
Nationwide: N
    PA;
TYPE OF COVERAGE:
Commercial: [Y] Individual: [ ] FEHBP: [ ] Indemnity: [ ]
Medicare: [Y] Medicaid: [Y] Supplemental Medicare: [ ]
Tricare   [ ]
PRODUCTS OFFERED:
Product Name: Type:
Golden Medicare   Medicare
CONSUMER-DRIVEN PRODUCTS
Aetna Life Insurance Co   HSA Company
Aetna HealthFund HSA   HSA Product
Aetna   HSA Administrator
Aetna HealthFund   Consumer-Driven Health Plan
PPO I; PPO II   High Deductible Health Plan
PLAN BENEFITS:
Alternative Medicine: [ ]   Behavioral Health: [X]
Chiropractic: [X]   Dental: [X]
Home Care: [ ]   Inpatient SNF: [ ]
Long-Term Care: [ ]   Pharm. Mail Order: [ ]
Physical Therapy: [ ]   Podiatry: [X]
Psychiatric: [X]   Transplant: [X]
Vision: [X]   Wellness: [X]
Workers' Comp: [X]
Other Benefits: AD&D, Life, LTD, STD
Comments:
Formerly Aetna Life Insurance Company.

AETNA INC - PENNSYLVANIA REGION

980 Jolly Rd
Blue Bell, PA 19422-1962
Phone: 215-775-4800 Fax: 860-952-2017 Toll-Free:
Web site: www.aetna.com
MAILING ADDRESS:
    AETNA INC - PA REGION
    PO Box 1109
    Blue Bell, PA 19422-1962

KEY EXECUTIVES:
Chairman of the Board/Chief Executive Officer .... Ronald A Williams
Regional Manager-Mid Atlantic .... Felicia Norwood
Executive VP, Finance .... Joseph M Zubretsky
Medical Director .... Troyen A Brennan, MD

COMPANY PROFILE:
Parent Company Name: Aetna Inc
Doing Business As:
Year Founded: 1976   Federally Qualified: [Y]
Forprofit: [Y]   Not-For-Profit: [ ]
Model Type: IPA
Accreditation: [ ] AAPPO [ ] JACHO [ ] NCQA [ ] URAC
Plan Type: HMO, PPO, POS, CDHP, HDHP, HSA,
Total Enrollment:
    2001: 873,056   2004: 651,242   2007: 564,740
    2002: 583,408   2005: 651,321
    2003: 602,061   2006: 606,425
SERVICE AREA:
Nationwide: N
    PA;
TYPE OF COVERAGE:
Commercial: [ ] Individual: [ ] FEHBP: [ ] Indemnity: [ ]
Medicare: [Y] Medicaid: [ ] Supplemental Medicare: [ ]
Tricare   [ ]
PRODUCTS OFFERED:
Product Name: Type:
Golden Medicare   Medicare
CONSUMER-DRIVEN PRODUCTS
Aetna Life Insurance Co   HSA Company
Aetna HealthFund HSA   HSA Product
Aetna   HSA Administrator
Aetna HealthFund   Consumer-Driven Health Plan
PPO I; PPO II   High Deductible Health Plan

PLAN BENEFITS:
Alternative Medicine: [ ]   Behavioral Health: [ ]
Chiropractic: [X]   Dental: [X]
Home Care: [X]   Inpatient SNF: [X]
Long-Term Care: [X]   Pharm. Mail Order: [X]
Physical Therapy: [X]   Podiatry: [X]
Psychiatric: [X]   Transplant: [X]
Vision: [X]   Wellness: [X]
Workers' Comp: [ ]
Other Benefits:

AMERICAN HEALTHCARE GROUP INC

1910 Cochran Rd 1 Manor Oak #600
Pittsburgh, PA 15220
Phone: 412-563-8800 Fax: 412-563-8319 Toll-Free:
Web site: www.american-healthcare.net
MAILING ADDRESS:
    AMERICAN HEALTHCARE GROUP INC
    1910 Cochran Rd 1 Manor Oak #600
    Pittsburgh, PA 15220

KEY EXECUTIVES:
Chief Executive Officer .... Robert E Hagan, Jr, CPA
Fininical Operations, Human Resources Mngr .... Lynn Datsko Hagan
Chief Medical Officer .... Joseph C Maroon, MD
Health Benefits Services Manager .... Erin E Hart Hagan
Marketing Manager .... Mary Hagan Double
Medical Management Director .... Sarah D Steranka
Wellness Program Manager .... Liz Hagan Kanche

COMPANY PROFILE:
Parent Company Name:
Doing Business As:
Year Founded: 1994   Federally Qualified: [ ]
Forprofit: [Y]   Not-For-Profit: [ ]
Model Type:
Accreditation: [ ] AAPPO [ ] JACHO [ ] NCQA [ ] URAC
Plan Type: PPO, PBM
Primary Physicians: 900   Physician Specialists: 2,000
Hospitals: 15
Total Enrollment:
    2001: 0   2004: 0   2007: 0
    2002: 120,000   2005:
    2003: 65,000   2006:
SERVICE AREA:
Nationwide: N
    PA (Southwestern);
TYPE OF COVERAGE:
Commercial: [Y] Individual: [ ] FEHBP: [ ] Indemnity: [ ]
Medicare: [ ] Medicaid: [ ] Supplemental Medicare: [ ]
Tricare   [ ]
PLAN BENEFITS:
Alternative Medicine: [ ]   Behavioral Health: [ ]
Chiropractic: [X]   Dental: [X]
Home Care: [ ]   Inpatient SNF: [ ]
Long-Term Care: [ ]   Pharm. Mail Order: [ ]
Physical Therapy: [ ]   Podiatry: [X]
Psychiatric: [ ]   Transplant: [ ]
Vision: [X]   Wellness: [ ]
Workers' Comp: [ ]
Other Benefits:
Comments:
Formerly Metro Health Plan.

AMERICHOICE OF PENNSYLVANIA INC

100 Penn Square East Ste 900
Philadelphia, PA 19107
Phone: 215-832-4500 Fax: 215-832-4644 Toll-Free: 800-514-9410
Web site: www.americhoice.com
MAILING ADDRESS:
    AMERICHOICE OF PA INC
    PO Box 41566
    Philadelphia, PA 19101-1566

356   Copyright MCIC -- The National Directorectory of Managed Care Organizations, Seventh Edition

Managed Care Organization Profiles PENNSYLVANIA

AETNA INC - CORPORATE HEADQUARTERS

980 Jolly Road
Blue Bell, PA 19422-1962
Phone: 215-775-4800 Fax: 860-952-2017 Toll-Free: 800-872-3862
Web site: www.aetna.com

MAILING ADDRESS:
   AETNA INC - CORP HEADQUARTERS
   PO Box 1109
   Blue Bell, PA 19422-1962

KEY EXECUTIVES:
Chairman of the Board/Chief Executive Officer .... Ronald A Williams
President .... Mark T Bertolini
Executive VP, Finance .... Joseph M Zubretsky
Medical Director .... Troyen A Brennan, MD
Head of Pharmacy .... Robyn S Walsh

COMPANY PROFILE:
Parent Company Name: Aetna Inc
Doing Business As:
Year Founded: 1976   Federally Qualified: [ ]
Forprofit: [Y]   Not-For-Profit: [ ]
Model Type: IPA
Accreditation: [ ] AAPPO [ ] JACHO [ ] NCQA [ ] URAC
Plan Type: HMO, PPO, POS, CDHP, HDHP, HSA,
Primary Physicians: 458,000   Physician Specialists: 212,198
Hospitals: 4,681
Total Revenue   2005: 19,616,100,000   2006: 22,240,500,000
Net Income   2005: 1,493,900,000   2006: 1,525,500,000
Total Enrollment:
   2001: 14,318,000   2004: 13,570,000   2007: 17,593,000
   2002: 13,300,000   2005: 15,433,000
   2003: 12,300,000   2006: 16,109,000

SERVICE AREA:
Nationwide: Y
   NW;

TYPE OF COVERAGE:
Commercial: [Y] Individual: [ ] FEHBP: [ ] Indemnity: [ ]
Medicare: [Y] Medicaid: [ ] Supplemental Medicare: [ ]
Tricare   [ ]

PRODUCTS OFFERED:
Product Name: Type:
Aetna Medicare Plan   Medicare
Aetna Medicaid   Medicaid
Aetna HMO   HMO
Aetna Preferred Provider   PPO
Aetna Dental   Dental
Aetna Indemnity   Indemnity
Aetna POS   POS

CONSUMER-DRIVEN PRODUCTS
Aetna Life Insurance Co   HSA Company
Aetna HealthFund HSA   HSA Product
Aetna   HSA Administrator
Aetna HealthFund   Consumer-Driven Health Plan
PPO I; PPO II   High Deductible Health Plan

PLAN BENEFITS:
Alternative Medicine: [ ]   Behavioral Health: [ ]
Chiropractic: [X]   Dental: [X]
Home Care: [X]   Inpatient SNF: [X]
Long-Term Care: [X]   Pharm. Mail Order: [X]
Physical Therapy: [X]   Podiatry: [X]
Psychiatric: [X]   Transplant: [X]
Vision: [X]   Wellness: [X]
Workers' Comp: [X]
Other Benefits:

AETNA INC - PENNSYLVANIA

2201 Renaissance Blvd
King of Prussia, PA 19406
Phone: 484-322-2000 Fax: 866-223-2041 Toll-Free: 800-872-3862
Web site: www.aetna.com

MAILING ADDRESS:
   AETNA INC - PA
   2201 Renaissance Blvd
   King of Prussia, PA 19406

KEY EXECUTIVES:
Chairman of the Board/Chief Executive Officer .... Ronald A Williams
Regional Manager-Mid Atlantic .... Felicia Norwood
Executive VP, Finance .... Joseph M Zubretsky
Medical Director .... Richard Rosen, MD
Pharmacy Director .... George Fleszar
Public Relations Director .... Kevin Heine
Sales Director .... Neal Brown
Director, Provider Services .... Karen Piacentini

COMPANY PROFILE:
Parent Company Name: Aetna Inc
Doing Business As:
Year Founded: 1988   Federally Qualified: [Y]
Forprofit: [Y]   Not-For-Profit: [ ]
Model Type: MIXED
Accreditation: [ ] AAPPO [ ] JACHO [X] NCQA [ ] URAC
Plan Type: HMO, PPO, POS, CDHP, HDHP, HSA,
Total Enrollment:
   2001: 0   2004: 620,232   2007: 0
   2002: 0   2005: 636,155
   2003: 0   2006:

SERVICE AREA:
Nationwide: N
   DE (New Castle); NJ (Atlantic, Burlington, Camden, Cape May,
     Cumberland, Gloucester, Mercer, Salem); PA (Bucks, Chester,
     Delaware, Lehigh, Montgomery, Northampton, Philadelphia);

TYPE OF COVERAGE:
Commercial: [Y] Individual: [ ] FEHBP: [ ] Indemnity: [ ]
Medicare: [ ] Medicaid: [ ] Supplemental Medicare: [ ]
Tricare   [ ]

CONSUMER-DRIVEN PRODUCTS
Aetna Life Insurance Co   HSA Company
Aetna HealthFund HSA   HSA Product
Aetna   HSA Administrator
Aetna HealthFund   Consumer-Driven Health Plan
PPO I; PPO II   High Deductible Health Plan

PLAN BENEFITS:
Alternative Medicine: [ ]   Behavioral Health: [X]
Chiropractic: [X]   Dental: [ ]
Home Care: [X]   Inpatient SNF: [X]
Long-Term Care: [ ]   Pharm. Mail Order: [X]
Physical Therapy: [X]   Podiatry: [ ]
Psychiatric: [X]   Transplant: [X]
Vision: [X]   Wellness: [X]
Workers' Comp: [ ]
Other Benefits:
Comments:
Formerly PruCare of Philadelphia.

AETNA INC - PENNSYLVANIA

730 Holiday Dr Bldg 8
Pittsburgh, PA 15220
Phone: 412-875-7000 Fax: 412-875-7861 Toll-Free: 800-422-8742
Web site: www.aetna.com

MAILING ADDRESS:
   AETNA INC - PENNSYLVANIA
   730 Holiday Dr Bldg 8
   Pittsburgh, PA 15220

KEY EXECUTIVES:
Chairman of the Board/Chief Executive Officer .... Ronald A Williams
President .... Mark T Bertolini
Executive VP, Finance .... Joseph M Zubretsky
Chief Medical Officer .... Troyen A Brennan, MD
Aetna Pharmacy Management .... Mark Rubino, RPh, MHA
Senior VP, Chief Infomation Officer .... Margaret McCarthy
Executive VP Strategy & Finance .... David Kelso
Middle Market Accounts & Health Delivery .... Mary Claire Bonner
Director Sales & Service-Pittsburgh .... William Jesserer
National Quality Management .... Mary Beth Krovisky
Chief Privacy Officer .... Thomas Young
Product Development .... Robin Downey
Medical Cost Management/Promotion/Education .... Sue Peters
Senior Vice President .... Elease E Wright
USQA Aetna Health .... Tina Brown-Stevenson
National Quality Management .... Mary Beth Krovisky
VP Counsel & Chief Compliance .... Thomas Strohmenger
New Product Development Director .... Robyn Walsh
Medical Director-Pittsburgh .... Michael Mesoras
Network Market Lead-Pittsburgh .... Donna Bell

Managed Care Organization Profiles **OREGON**

Forprofit: [Y]　　　　　　Not-For-Profit: [ ]
Model Type: STAFF
Accreditation: [ ] AAPPO　[ ] JACHO　[ ] NCQA　[ ] URAC
Plan Type: Specialty HMO
Total Enrollment:
　2001: 0　　　　　2004: 0　　　　2007: 0
　2002: 0　　　　　2005: 59,103
　2003: 41,836　　 2006:

SERVICE AREA:
Nationwide: N
　OR; WA;

TYPE OF COVERAGE:
Commercial: [Y]　Individual: [Y]　FEHBP: [ ]　Indemnity: [ ]
Medicare: [ ]　Medicaid: [ ]　Supplemental Medicare: [ ]
Tricare [ ]

PRODUCTS OFFERED:
Product Name:	Type:
Dental Plus	Individual
Williamette Health Service, In	Group

PLAN BENEFITS:
Alternative Medicine:	[ ]	Behavioral Health:	[ ]
Chiropractic:	[ ]	Dental:	[X]
Home Care:	[ ]	Inpatient SNF:	[ ]
Long-Term Care:	[ ]	Pharm. Mail Order:	[ ]
Physical Therapy:	[ ]	Podiatry:	[ ]
Psychiatric:	[ ]	Transplant:	[ ]
Vision:	[ ]	Wellness:	[ ]
Workers' Comp:	[ ]		

Other Benefits:

Forprofit: [Y]　　　　　　Not-For-Profit: [ ]

OREGON

Managed Care Organization Profiles

SERVICE AREA:
Nationwide: N
   WA; ID; OR; UT;
TYPE OF COVERAGE:
Commercial: [Y] Individual: [Y] FEHBP: [ ] Indemnity: [ ]
Medicare: [Y] Medicaid: [ ] Supplemental Medicare: [Y]
Tricare [ ]
PRODUCTS OFFERED:
Product Name: Type:
Regence Blue Shield of Idaho
Regence BC BS of Oregon
Regence Blue Shield
Regence BC BS of Utah
CONSUMER-DRIVEN PRODUCTS
                        HSA Company
HSA 101   HSA Product
Wells Fargo   HSA Administrator
                        Consumer-Driven Health Plan
                        High Deductible Health Plan

PLAN BENEFITS:
Alternative Medicine: [ ]   Behavioral Health: [X]
Chiropractic: [ ]   Dental: [ ]
Home Care: [X]   Inpatient SNF: [X]
Long-Term Care: [X]   Pharm. Mail Order: [X]
Physical Therapy: [X]   Podiatry: [X]
Psychiatric: [X]   Transplant: [X]
Vision: [X]   Wellness: [X]
Workers' Comp: [ ]
Other Benefits:

SAMARITAN HEALTH PLANS INC

3600 NW Samaritan Dr
Corvallis, OR 97330
Phone: 541-757-5377 Fax: 541-768-5011 Toll-Free: 800-757-5114
Web site: www.samhealth.org
MAILING ADDRESS:
    SAMARITAN HEALTH PLANS INC
    3600 NW Samaritan Dr
    Corvallis, OR 97330

KEY EXECUTIVES:
Chairman of the Board .... Larry A Mullins, DHA
Chief Executive Officer.. Kelley C Kaiser, MPH
Chief Financial Officer .... Ronald S Stevens, MBA
Chief Operations Officer .... Kim R Whitley, MPA

COMPANY PROFILE:
Parent Company Name: Samaritan Health Services
Doing Business As:
Year Founded: 1993   Federally Qualified: [ ]
Forprofit: [ ]   Not-For-Profit: [Y]
Model Type:
Accreditation: [ ] AAPPO [ ] JACHO [ ] NCQA [ ] URAC
Plan Type: HMO
Primary Physicians: 1,2000   Physician Specialists:
Hospitals: 12
Total Revenue: 2005:   2006: 29,172,458
Net Income 2005:   2006:
Total Enrollment:
   2001: 0   2004: 0   2007: 0
   2002: 0   2005: 16,000
   2003: 0   2006:
Medical Loss Ratio: 2005:   2006: 96.20
Administrative Expense Ratio: 2005:   2006:
SERVICE AREA:
Nationwide:
   OR (Benton, Linn, Lincoln, Marion, Polk);
TYPE OF COVERAGE:
Commercial: [ ] Individual: [ ] FEHBP: [ ] Indemnity: [ ]
Medicare: [ ] Medicaid: [Y] Supplemental Medicare: [ ]
Tricare [ ]
PRODUCTS OFFERED:
Product Name: Type:
InterCommunity Health Network   Medicaid
Samaritan Choice Plans   Self-funded
Samaritan Advantage Health Plan   Medicare Advantage
Samaritan Select

UNITEDHEALTHCARE OF OREGON

180 E Ocean Blvd Ste 500
Long Beach, CA 90802
Phone: 562-951-6400 Fax: 562-951-6885 Toll-Free: 800-325-6651
Web site: www.uhc.com
MAILING ADDRESS:
    UNITEDHEALTHCARE OF OR
    180 E Ocean Blvd Ste 500
    Long Beach, CA 90802

KEY EXECUTIVES:
Non-Executive Chairman .... Richard T Burke
Chief Executive Officer .... Emery Dameron
Chief Operating Officer .... Kathleen Lynaugh

COMPANY PROFILE:
Parent Company Name: UnitedHealth Group
Doing Business As:
Year Founded: Federally Qualified: [ ]
Forprofit: [Y]   Not-For-Profit: [ ]
Model Type:
Accreditation: [ ] AAPPO [ ] JACHO [ ] NCQA [ ] URAC
Plan Type: HMO, PPO, POS, EPO, CDHP, HSA, HRA
Total Enrollment:
   2001: 0   2004: 0   2007: 0
   2002: 0   2005: 903
   2003: 0   2006:
SERVICE AREA:
Nationwide: N
   OR;
TYPE OF COVERAGE:
Commercial: [Y] Individual: [ ] FEHBP: [ ] Indemnity: [ ]
Medicare: [ ] Medicaid: [ ] Supplemental Medicare: [ ]
Tricare [ ]
PRODUCTS OFFERED:
Product Name: Type:
HMO Choice   HMO
CONSUMER-DRIVEN PRODUCTS
Exante Bank/Golden Rule Ins Co   HSA Company
iPlan HSA   HSA Product
                       HSA Administrator
                       Consumer-Driven Health Plan
                       High Deductible Health Plan

PLAN BENEFITS:
Alternative Medicine: [ ]   Behavioral Health: [ ]
Chiropractic: [X]   Dental: [X]
Home Care: [X]   Inpatient SNF: [X]
Long-Term Care: [ ]   Pharm. Mail Order: [X]
Physical Therapy: [X]   Podiatry: [X]
Psychiatric: [X]   Transplant: [X]
Vision: [X]   Wellness: [X]
Workers' Comp: [ ]
Other Benefits:

WILLIAMETTE DENTAL GROUP PC

6950 NE Campus Way
Hillsboro, OR 97124-5611
Phone: 503-925-2000 Fax: 503-952-2200 Toll-Free: 800-460-7644
Web site: www.denkor.com
MAILING ADDRESS:
    WILLIAMETTE DENTAL GROUP PC
    6950 NE Campus Way
    Hillsboro, OR 97124-5611

KEY EXECUTIVES:
Chairman of the Board .... Eugene C Skourtes
Chief Executive Officer/President .... Steve Petruzelli
Chief Medical Officer .... Gary Allen, DMD
Chief Information Officer .... John Shields
Chief Operating Officer .... Yuen Chin
Marketing Director .... Doug Wohlman
Human Resources Director .... Kris Holgerson
VP of Administration.. April Kniess

COMPANY PROFILE:
Parent Company Name: Williamette Dental Management Co
Doing Business As: Managed Care Dental Group
Year Founded: 1970   Federally Qualified: [ ]

Managed Care Organization Profiles **OREGON**

PROVIDENCE HEALTH PLANS

3601 SW Murry Blvd Ste 10
Beaverton, OR 97005
Phone: 503-574-7426 Fax: 503-574-8600 Toll-Free: 800-826-7218
Web site: www.providencehealthplans.org
MAILING ADDRESS:
    PROVIDENCE HEALTH PLANS
    3601 SW Murry Blvd Ste 10
    Beaverton, OR 97005

KEY EXECUTIVES:
Chief Executive Officer .... Russ Danielson
Chief Financial Officer .... Shelly Handkins
Chief Medical Director .... Kevin Keck, MD
Pharmacy Director .... Helen Noonan Harnsberger
Chief Information Officer .... Bruce Wilkinson
Marketing Director .... Barb Christensen
Director, Provider Services .... Phil Jackson

COMPANY PROFILE:
Parent Company Name: Providence Health System
Doing Business As: Providence Health Plans
Year Founded: 1984   Federally Qualified: [Y]
Forprofit: [ ]   Not-For-Profit: [Y]
Model Type: MIXED
Accreditation: [ ] AAPPO [ ] JACHO [X] NCQA [ ] URAC
Plan Type: HMO, PPO, POS, EPO, HDHP, HSA,
Total Revenue: 2005:   2006: 753,623,427
Net Income 2005:   2006:
Total Enrollment:
    2001: 208,994   2004: 146,208   2007: 222,715
    2002: 148,986   2005:
    2003: 148,019   2006: 217,035
Medical Loss Ratio: 2005:   2006: 82.30
Administrative Expense Ratio: 2005:   2006:
SERVICE AREA:
Nationwide: N
    OR; WA (Southwest);
TYPE OF COVERAGE:
Commercial: [Y] Individual: [ ] FEHBP: [ ] Indemnity: [ ]
Medicare: [Y] Medicaid: [Y] Supplemental Medicare: [ ]
Tricare [ ]
PRODUCTS OFFERED:
Product Name:	Type:
Providence Medicare Extra	Medicare Advantage
Providence Medicaid	Medicaid

PLAN BENEFITS:
Alternative Medicine:	[ ]	Behavioral Health:	[X]
Chiropractic:	[X]	Dental:	[ ]
Home Care:	[X]	Inpatient SNF:	[X]
Long-Term Care:	[X]	Pharm. Mail Order:	[X]
Physical Therapy:	[X]	Podiatry:	[X]
Psychiatric:	[X]	Transplant:	[X]
Vision:	[X]	Wellness:	[X]
Workers' Comp:	[ ]		
Other Benefits:			

REGENCE BLUE CROSS BLUE SHIELD OF OREGON

100 Southwest Market St
Portland, OR 97201
Phone: 503-225-5221 Fax: 503-225-4848 Toll-Free: 800-452-7390
Web site: www.or.regence.com
MAILING ADDRESS:
    REGENCE BC BS OF OREGON
    PO Box 1271
    Portland, OR 97201

KEY EXECUTIVES:
Chief Executive Officer .... Mark B Ganz
President .... Bart McMullan, MD
Chief Financial Officer .... Steven Hooker
VP, Chief Medical Officer .... Ralph Prows, MD
Pharmacy Director .... Patty Church
Chief Information Officer .... Cheron Vail
Marketing Communications Director .... MaryAnne Harmer
Director, Provider Services .... John Hutchison
Human Resources Director .... Thomas F Kennedy

COMPANY PROFILE:
Parent Company Name: The Regence Group
Doing Business As:
Year Founded: 1976   Federally Qualified: [Y]
Forprofit: [ ]   Not-For-Profit: [Y]
Model Type: IPA
Accreditation: [ ] AAPPO [ ] JACHO [ ] NCQA [ ] URAC
Plan Type: HMO, PPO, POS, CDHP, HDHP, HSA,
Total Revenue: 2005:   2006: 2,092,665,946
Net Income 2005:   2006:
Total Enrollment:
    2001: 620,053   2004: 985,889   2007: 712,081
    2002: 1,017,720   2005:
    2003: 951,367   2006: 660,082
Medical Loss Ratio: 2005:   2006: 87.10
Administrative Expense Ratio: 2005:   2006:
SERVICE AREA:
Nationwide: N
    OR; WA (Southwestern);
TYPE OF COVERAGE:
Commercial: [Y] Individual: [Y] FEHBP: [ ] Indemnity: [ ]
Medicare: [Y] Medicaid: [ ] Supplemental Medicare: [ ]
Tricare [ ]
PRODUCTS OFFERED:
Product Name:	Type:
Preferred Choice Sixty- Five	HMO
First Choice 65	Medicare
PPO	PPO
Traditional	

PLAN BENEFITS:
Alternative Medicine:	[ ]	Behavioral Health:	[X]
Chiropractic:	[ ]	Dental:	[ ]
Home Care:	[X]	Inpatient SNF:	[X]
Long-Term Care:	[X]	Pharm. Mail Order:	[X]
Physical Therapy:	[X]	Podiatry:	[X]
Psychiatric:	[X]	Transplant:	[X]
Vision:	[X]	Wellness:	[X]
Workers' Comp:	[ ]		
Other Benefits:			

REGENCE GROUP, THE — CORPORATE HEADQUARTERS

200 Southwest Market St
Portland, OR 97207
Phone: 503-225-5221 Fax: 503-225-5274 Toll-Free: 800-452-7278
Web site: www.regence.com
MAILING ADDRESS:
    REGENCE GROUP, THE — CORP HQTRS
    PO Box 1071
    Portland, OR 97207

KEY EXECUTIVES:
Chairman of the Board .... Jack G Struther
Chief Executive Officer/President .... Mark B Ganz
Senior VP, Chief Financial Officer .... Steven L Hooker
Executive VP & Chief Marketing Executive .... Mohandas Nair
Chief Medical Officer .... Jeffrey A Robertson, MD
Senior VP, Chief Information Officer .... Cheron R Vail
Health Care Operations .... William C Barr
Health Care Services .... Thomas F Kennedy

COMPANY PROFILE:
Parent Company Name:
Doing Business As:
Year Founded: 1946   Federally Qualified: [Y]
Forprofit: [ ]   Not-For-Profit: [Y]
Model Type: IPA
Accreditation: [ ] AAPPO [ ] JACHO [X] NCQA [ ] URAC
Plan Type: HMO, PPO, TPA, UR, HDHP, HSA, PBM
Primary Physicians: 38,532   Physician Specialists:
Hospitals:
Total Revenue: 2005: 6,728,611,000   2006: 7,551,298,000
Net Income 2005: 327,800,000   2006: 240,600,000
Total Enrollment:
    2001: 0   2004: 2,808,349   2007: 0
    2002: 0   2005: 2,567,066
    2003: 3,000,000   2006: 2,767,833
Medical Loss Ratio: 2005:   2006:
Administrative Expense Ratio: 2005: 9.60   2006: 9.30

OREGON — Managed Care Organization Profiles

PACIFICARE OF OREGON

Five Centerpointe Dr #600
Lake Oswego, OR 97035-8650
Phone: 503-603-7355 Fax: 503-603-7377 Toll-Free: 800-922-1444
Web site: www.pacificare.com

MAILING ADDRESS:
PACIFICARE OF OREGON
Five Centerpointe Dr #600
Lake Oswego, OR 97035-8650

KEY EXECUTIVES:
VP, General Manager .... David Hansen
Chief Financial Officer .... Susan L Berkel
Director of Sales & Services .... Carol Kotonias-Ray
Director of Sales .... Kendall Thiemann

COMPANY PROFILE:
Parent Company Name: UnitedHealth Group
Doing Business As:
Year Founded: 1985   Federally Qualified: [Y]
Forprofit: [Y]   Not-For-Profit: [ ]
Model Type: MIXED
Accreditation: [ ] AAPPO [ ] JACHO [X] NCQA [ ] URAC
Plan Type: HMO, PPO, POS, HDHP, HSA,
Total Revenue: 2005:   2006: 319,210,553
Net Income   2005:   2006:
Total Enrollment:
   2001: 120,001   2004: 63,942   2007: 39,221
   2002: 93,333   2005:
   2003: 82,172   2006: 46,265
Medical Loss Ratio: 2005:   2006: 80.00
Administrative Expense Ratio: 2005:   2006:

SERVICE AREA:
Nationwide: N
OR (Benton, Clackamas, Clare, Columbia, Jackson, Josephine, Lane, Linn, Marion, Multonmah, Polk, Washington, Yamhill);

TYPE OF COVERAGE:
Commercial: [Y] Individual: [Y] FEHBP: [ ] Indemnity: [ ]
Medicare: [Y] Medicaid: [ ] Supplemental Medicare: [ ]
Tricare [ ]

PRODUCTS OFFERED:
Product Name: Type:
Secure Horizons   Medicare Advantage
Pacificare HMO   HMO

PLAN BENEFITS:
Alternative Medicine: [ ]   Behavioral Health: [X]
Chiropractic: [X]   Dental: [X]
Home Care: [X]   Inpatient SNF: [X]
Long-Term Care: [ ]   Pharm. Mail Order: [X]
Physical Therapy: [X]   Podiatry: [X]
Psychiatric: [X]   Transplant: [X]
Vision: [X]0   Wellness: [X]
Workers' Comp: [X]
Other Benefits:

PACIFICSOURCE HEALTH PLANS

110 International Pkwy
Springfield, OR 97477
Phone: 541-686-1242 Fax: 541-485-0915 Toll-Free: 800-624-6052
Web site: www.pacificsource.com

MAILING ADDRESS:
PACIFICSOURCE HEALTH PLANS
110 International Pkwy
Springfield, OR 97477

KEY EXECUTIVES:
Chief Executive Officer/President .... Kenneth Provencher
Chief Financial Officer .... Steven Ord
Medical Director .... Steven Marks, MD
Pharmacy Director .... Dennis Rogers
Chief Operating Officer .... Sujata Sanghui
Marketing Director .... Troy Kirk
VP of Information Systems .... Erick Doolen
Community Development Director .... Laura Brennan
Community Development Director .... Sandie Longtin
Human Resources Director .... Paul Wynkoop
Health Management Services Manager .... Kathy Blain
Compliance Manager .... Jim Gravette

COMPANY PROFILE:
Parent Company Name: Pacific Hospital Association
Doing Business As:
Year Founded: 1933   Federally Qualified: [N]
Forprofit: [ ]   Not-For-Profit: [Y]
Model Type:
Accreditation: [ ] AAPPO [ ] JACHO [ ] NCQA [ ] URAC
Plan Type: HMO, PPO, CDHP, HSA
Primary Physicians: 9,000   Physician Specialists:
Hospitals:
Total Revenue: 2005:   2006: 123,513,415
Net Income   2005:   2006:
Total Enrollment:
   2001: 110,521   2004: 148,113   2007: 151,000
   2002: 115,500   2005:
   2003: 146,063   2006: 135,396
Medical Loss Ratio: 2005:   2006: 85.60
Administrative Expense Ratio: 2005:   2006:

SERVICE AREA:
Nationwide: N
OR;

TYPE OF COVERAGE:
Commercial: [Y] Individual: [Y] FEHBP: [ ] Indemnity: [ ]
Medicare: [Y] Medicaid: [ ] Supplemental Medicare: [ ]
Tricare [ ]

PRODUCTS OFFERED:
Product Name: Type:
FlexPerks   CDHP
Preferred   PPO
Prime
Choice

CONSUMER-DRIVEN PRODUCTS
HSA Bank   HSA Company
                        HSA Product
HSA Bank   HSA Administrator
                        Consumer-Driven Health Plan
FlexPerks   High Deductible Health Plan

PLAN BENEFITS:
Alternative Medicine: [ ]   Behavioral Health: [X]
Chiropractic: [X]   Dental: [ ]
Home Care: [X]   Inpatient SNF: [X]
Long-Term Care: [ ]   Pharm. Mail Order: [X]
Physical Therapy: [X]   Podiatry: [X]
Psychiatric: [X]   Transplant: [X]
Vision: [X]   Wellness: [X]
Workers' Comp: [ ]
Other Benefits:

PREFERRED HEALTH PLAN INC

2909 Daggett Ave Ste 275
Klamath Falls, OR 97601-0383
Phone: 541-882-1466 Fax: 541-882-1447 Toll-Free: 800-303-8680
Web site:

MAILING ADDRESS:
PREFERRED HEALTH PLAN INC
PO Box 9
Klamath Falls, OR 97601-0383

KEY EXECUTIVES:
Chief Executive Officer/President .... Greg Clark
Chief Medical Officer .... Ken Webb-Bowen

COMPANY PROFILE:
Parent Company Name:
Doing Business As:
Year Founded: Federally Qualified: [ ]
Forprofit: [ ]   Not-For-Profit: [ ]
Model Type:
Accreditation: [ ] AAPPO [ ] JACHO [ ] NCQA [ ] URAC
Plan Type: PPO
Total Revenue: 2005:   2006: 21,368,498
Net Income   2005:   2006:
Total Enrollment:
   2001:   2004:   2007: 4,153
   2002:   2005: 7,000
   2003:   2006: 4,191
Medical Loss Ratio: 2005:   2006: 96.20
Administrative Expense Ratio: 2005:   2006:

SERVICE AREA:
Nationwide: N
OR (Klamath, Lane);

Managed Care Organization Profiles — OREGON

MARION POLK COMMUNITY HEALTH PLAN

245 Commerical St SE Ste 200
Salem, OR 97301
Phone: 503-371-7701 Fax: 503-371-8046 Toll-Free:
Web site: www.mvipa.org
MAILING ADDRESS:
   MARION POLK COMMUNITY HEALTH PLAN
   245 Commerical St SE Ste 200
   Salem, OR 97301

KEY EXECUTIVES:
Plan Administrator/Chief Executive Officer .... Jan L Buffa, PhD, MBA
Chief Financial Officer .... Chad Niegel
Operations Manager .... Dean Andretta

COMPANY PROFILE:
Parent Company Name: Mid Valley Independent Physicians Association
Doing Business As:
Year Founded: 2001   Federally Qualified: [ ]
Forprofit: [ ]   Not-For-Profit: [ ]
Model Type:
Accreditation: [ ] AAPPO [ ] JACHO [ ] NCQA [ ] URAC
Plan Type: HMO
otal Revenue: 2005:   2006:   42,395,991
Net Income   2005:   2006:
Total Enrollment:
   2001:   2004:   2007: 3,311
   2002:   2005:
   2003:   2006:
Medical Loss Ratio: 2005:   2006: 87.60
Administrative Expense Ratio: 2005:   2006:
SERVICE AREA:
Nationwide: N
   OR (Clackamas, Linn, Marion, Polk, Yamhill);
TYPE OF COVERAGE:
Commercial: [ ] Individual: [ ] FEHBP: [ ] Indemnity: [ ]
Medicare: [Y] Medicaid: [ ] Supplemental Medicare: [ ]
Tricare   [ ]

NORTHWEST REHAB ALLIANCE

11481 SW Hall Blvd Ste 201
Portland, OR 97223
Phone: 503-626-7724 Fax: 888-224-9578 Toll-Free:
Web site: www.nwrehab.com
MAILING ADDRESS:
   NORTHWEST REHAB ALLIANCE
   11481 SW Hall Blvd Ste 201
   Portland, OR 97223

KEY EXECUTIVES:
Chief Executive Officer .... Richard Katz, PT
President ....John Mckinnon
Secretary .... J'Anna Post

COMPANY PROFILE:
Parent Company Name: Therapeutic Associates—Mgmt Service Org
Doing Business As: Rehab Alliance
Year Founded: 1953   Federally Qualified: [ ]
Forprofit: [ ]   Not-For-Profit: [Y]
Model Type: NETWORK
Accreditation: [ ] AAPPO [ ] JACHO [ ] NCQA [ ] URAC
Plan Type: Specialty PPO
SERVICE AREA:
Nationwide: N
   WA, OR,
TYPE OF COVERAGE:
Commercial: [Y] Individual: [Y] FEHBP: [ ] Indemnity: [ ]
Medicare: [Y] Medicaid: [Y] Supplemental Medicare: [Y]
Tricare   [ ]
PRODUCTS OFFERED:
Product Name: Type:
Outpatient Physical Therapy
Occupational Therapy
Speech Language Pathology

PLAN BENEFITS:
Alternative Medicine: [ ]   Behavioral Health: [ ]
Chiropractic: [ ]   Dental: [ ]
Home Care: [ ]   Inpatient SNF: [ ]
Long-Term Care: [ ]   Pharm. Mail Order: [ ]
Physical Therapy: [ ]   Podiatry: [ ]
Psychiatric: [ ]   Transplant: [ ]
Vision: [ ]   Wellness: [ ]
Workers' Comp: [ ]
Other Benefits: Specialty Pathology,
Comments:
A horizontally based specialty PPO network of outpatient providers delivering physical therapy, occupational therapy and speech therapy services.

ODS HEALTH PLAN

601 S W Second Ave
Portland, OR 97204-3154
Phone: 503-228-6554 Fax: 503-948-5558 Toll-Free: 800-852-5195
Web site: www.odshp.com
MAILING ADDRESS:
   ODS HEALTH PLAN
   PO Box 40384
   Portland, OR 97204-3154

KEY EXECUTIVES:
Chief Executive Officer/President .... Robert Gootee
Chief Financial Officer ....Jon Jurevic
Chief Medical Officer ....Csaba Mera
Pharmacy Director .... Karen Beauchamp
Vice President of Operations .... Andrew Franklin
Chief Marketing Executive .... CJ McLeod
VP, Information Systems .... Bill Hockett
Senior VP, Dental Services .... Bill Ten Pas
Director of Corporate Communication .... Charlie LaTourette

COMPANY PROFILE:
Parent Company Name: Oregon Dental Services
Doing Business As: Oregon Health Plan
Year Founded: 1955   Federally Qualified: [ ]
Forprofit: [ ]   Not-For-Profit: [ ]
Model Type:
Accreditation: [ ] AAPPO [ ] JACHO [ ] NCQA [ ] URAC
Plan Type: PPO, POS, CDHP, HDHP, HSA
Total Revenue: 2005:   2006:   144,355,823
Net Income   2005:   2006:
Total Enrollment:
   2001: 77,626   2004: 35,313   2007: 0
   2002: 42,282   2005:
   2003: 29,653   2006: 171,180
Medical Loss Ratio: 2005:   2006: 83.80
Administrative Expense Ratio: 2005:   2006:
SERVICE AREA:
Nationwide: N
   OR; WA (southwest region)
TYPE OF COVERAGE:
Commercial: [Y] Individual: [ ] FEHBP: [ ] Indemnity: [ ]
Medicare: [ ] Medicaid: [ ] Supplemental Medicare: [ ]
Tricare   [ ]
PRODUCTS OFFERED:
Product Name: Type:
Senior Select
CONSUMER-DRIVEN PRODUCTS
Wells Fargo   HSA Company
ODS HSA   HSA Product
                            HSA Administrator
                            Consumer-Driven Health Plan
                            High Deductible Health Plan

PLAN BENEFITS:
Alternative Medicine: [ ]   Behavioral Health: [ ]
Chiropractic: [ ]   Dental: [X]
Home Care: [ ]   Inpatient SNF: [ ]
Long-Term Care: [ ]   Pharm. Mail Order: [ ]
Physical Therapy: [ ]   Podiatry: [ ]
Psychiatric: [ ]   Transplant: [ ]
Vision: [ ]   Wellness: [ ]
Workers' Comp: [ ]
Other Benefits:

| OREGON | Managed Care Organization Profiles |

MAILING ADDRESS:
    LANE OREGON HEALTH PLANS
    PO Box 11740
    Eugene, OR 97440

KEY EXECUTIVES:
Chief Executive Officer .... Terry W Coplin
Chief Financial Officer .... David L Cole
Senior Medical Director .... John Sattenspiel, MD
Chief Operations Officer .... Rhonda Busek

COMPANY PROFILE:
Parent Company Name:
Doing Business As:
Year Founded: 1977   Federally Qualified: [ ]
Forprofit: [Y]   Not-For-Profit: [ ]
Model Type: IPA
Accreditation: [ ] AAPPO [ ] JACHO [ ] NCQA [ ] URAC
Plan Type: HMO
Total Enrollment:
    2001: 0   2004: 0   2007: 0
    2002: 0   2005: 28,447
    2003: 55,294   2006:

SERVICE AREA:
Nationwide: N
    OR (Lane);

TYPE OF COVERAGE:
Commercial: [Y] Individual: [Y] FEHBP: [ ] Indemnity: [ ]
Medicare: [Y] Medicaid: [Y] Supplemental Medicare: [Y]
Tricare [ ]

PRODUCTS OFFERED:
Product Name: Type:
Lane IPA MHO   Medicaid

Comments:
Formerly Lane IPA.

LIFEWISE HEALTH PLAN OF OREGON

2020 SW 4th Ave Ste 1000
Portland, OR 97201-0000
Phone: 503-295-6707 Fax: 503-279-5295 Toll-Free: 800-926-6707
Web site: www.lifewisehealth.com

MAILING ADDRESS:
    LIFEWISE HEALTH PLAN OF OR
    2020 SW 4th Ave Ste 1000
    Portland, OR 97201-0000

KEY EXECUTIVES:
Chief Executive Officer/President .... Majd El-Azma
Chief Financial Officer .... Kent Marquardt
Chief Medical Officer .... Eric M Wall, MD, MPH
VP, Operations .... Tom Hebner
VP, Sales & Marketing .... David Lechner
Communications Director .... Deana Strunk
Director Health Care Delivery Services .... Allison Bechtol
Compliance Officer .... Nancy Nevins
Director of Underwriting .... Sharon Howe

COMPANY PROFILE:
Parent Company Name: Premera Blue Cross
Doing Business As:
Year Founded: 1986   Federally Qualified: [ ]
Forprofit: [Y]   Not-For-Profit: [ ]
Model Type: NETWORK
Accreditation: [ ] AAPPO [ ] JACHO [ ] NCQA [ ] URAC
Plan Type: PPO, ASO, TPA, CDHP, HDHP, HSA,
Primary Physicians: 1,856   Physician Specialists: 5,491
Hospitals: 59
Total Revenue: 2005: 371,288,053   2006: 324,831,435
Net Income 2005: 11,869,831   2006: 7,551,090
Total Enrollment:
    2001: 136,654   2004: 163,709   2007: 116,993
    2002: 159,413   2005: 132,408
    2003: 146,360   2006: 121,119
Medical Loss Ratio: 2005:   2006: 78.20
Administrative Expense Ratio: 2005:   2006:

SERVICE AREA:
Nationwide: N
    OR;

TYPE OF COVERAGE:
Commercial: [Y] Individual: [Y] FEHBP: [ ] Indemnity: [Y]
Medicare: [ ] Medicaid: [ ] Supplemental Medicare: [Y]
Tricare [ ]

PRODUCTS OFFERED:
Product Name: Type:
LifeWise Health Plan of OR   PPO

CONSUMER-DRIVEN PRODUCTS
HSA Bank   HSA Company
     HSA Product
HSA Bank   HSA Administrator
     Consumer-Driven Health Plan
LifeWise Fund Plans   High Deductible Health Plan

PLAN BENEFITS:
Alternative Medicine: [X]   Behavioral Health: [X]
Chiropractic: [X]   Dental: [X]
Home Care: [X]   Inpatient SNF: [X]
Long-Term Care: [ ]   Pharm. Mail Order: [X]
Physical Therapy: [X]   Podiatry: [ ]
Psychiatric: [X]   Transplant: [X]
Vision: [X]   Wellness: [X]
Workers' Comp: [ ]
Other Benefits:

Comments:
Formerly Pacific Health & Life.

MANAGED HEALTHCARE NORTHWEST INC

1120 NW 20th Ave #200
Portland, OR 97209
Phone: 503-413-5800 Fax: 503-413-5801 Toll-Free: 800-648-6356
Web site: www.mhninc.com

MAILING ADDRESS:
    MANAGED HEALTHCARE NORTHWEST
    1120 NW 20th Ave #200
    Portland, OR 97209

KEY EXECUTIVES:
Chief Executive Officer/President .... Dolores Russell
Finance Director .... David Pyle
Medical Director .... Frank Wong, MD
Information Services Director .... David Pyle
Marketing Manager .... Jody Ordway
Provider Relations/Human Resources Director .... Jennifer Kirk

COMPANY PROFILE:
Parent Company Name: Legacy Hlth System/Adventist Med Center
Doing Business As: Managed HealthCare Northwest Inc
Year Founded: 1988   Federally Qualified: [ ]
Forprofit: [Y]   Not-For-Profit: [ ]
Model Type: NETWORK
Accreditation: [ ] AAPPO [ ] JACHO [ ] NCQA [ ] URAC
Plan Type: PPO, Specialty PPO, UR, EPO
Primary Physicians: 1,131   Physician Specialists: 2,589
Hospitals: 19
Total Enrollment:
    2001: 49,300   2004: 527,822   2007: 0
    2002: 450,000   2005:
    2003: 445,000   2006:

SERVICE AREA:
Nationwide: N
    OR (Clackamas, Columbia, Coos, Hood River, Lane, Multnomah, Wasco, Washington, Yamhill); WA (Clark, Cowlitz, Klickitat, Skamania).

TYPE OF COVERAGE:
Commercial: [Y] Individual: [ ] FEHBP: [ ] Indemnity: [ ]
Medicare: [ ] Medicaid: [ ] Supplemental Medicare: [ ]
Tricare [ ]

PLAN BENEFITS:
Alternative Medicine: [ ]   Behavioral Health: [ ]
Chiropractic: [ ]   Dental: [ ]
Home Care: [ ]   Inpatient SNF: [ ]
Long-Term Care: [ ]   Pharm. Mail Order: [ ]
Physical Therapy: [ ]   Podiatry: [ ]
Psychiatric: [ ]   Transplant: [ ]
Vision: [ ]   Wellness: [ ]
Workers' Comp: [X]
Other Benefits:

Managed Care Organization Profiles   OREGON

Forprofit: [ ]   Not-For-Profit: [Y]
Model Type:
Accreditation: [ ] AAPPO [ ] JACHO [ ] NCQA [ ] URAC
Plan Type: HMO
Primary Physicians: 950   Physician Specialists: 3,000
Hospitals: 33
Total Revenue: 2005:   2006:   66,408,329
Net Income   2005:   2006:
Total Enrollment:
   2001: 0   2004: 0   2007: 5,390
   2002: 0   2005:
   2003: 0   2006: 5,641
Medical Loss Ratio: 2005:   2006: 85.40
Administrative Expense Ratio: 2005:   2006:
SERVICE AREA:
Nationwide:
   OR;
TYPE OF COVERAGE:
Commercial: [ ] Individual: [ ] FEHBP: [ ] Indemnity: [ ]
Medicare: [ ] Medicaid: [Y] Supplemental Medicare: [ ]
Tricare   [ ]

INNOVATIVE CARE MANAGEMENT

10121 SE Sunnyside Rd Ste 208
Clackamas, OR 97015
Phone: 503-654-9447 Fax: 503-654-8570 Toll-Free: 800-862-3338
Web site: www.innovativecare.com
MAILING ADDRESS:
   INNOVATIVE CARE MANAGEMENT
   10121 SE Sunnyside Rd Ste 208
   Clackamas, OR 97015

KEY EXECUTIVES:
Chief Executive Officer .... Ed O'Mara
President .... Kristine M Hallock
Chief Financial Officer .... James Shepperd
Medical Director .... Linda Lewis, MD
Chief Operating Officer .... Marion Shipley
VP Sales & Marketing .... Jay Dee Banasky
Director, Provider Services .... Kristine M Hallock
Director Case Management .... Wendy Howell
Executive Vice President .... Sherry Chenell

COMPANY PROFILE:
Parent Company Name:
Doing Business As:
Year Founded: 1990   Federally Qualified: [N]
Forprofit: [Y]   Not-For-Profit: [ ]
Model Type:
Accreditation: [ ] AAPPO [ ] JACHO [ ] NCQA [X] URAC
Plan Type: UR
SERVICE AREA:
Nationwide: N
   NW;

INTERCOMMUNITY HEALTH NETWORK

3600 NW Samaritan Dr
Corvallis, OR 97330
Phone: 541-757-5377 Fax: 541-768-5011 Toll-Free: 800-757-5114
Web site: www.samhealth.org
MAILING ADDRESS:
   INTERCOMMUNITY HEALTH NETWORK
   3600 NW Samaritan Dr
   Corvallis, OR 97330

KEY EXECUTIVES:
Chief Executive Officer/President .... Larry A Mullins, DHA

COMPANY PROFILE:
Parent Company Name: Samaritan Health Services
Doing Business As:
Year Founded: 1993   Federally Qualified: [ ]
Forprofit: [ ]   Not-For-Profit: [Y]
Model Type:

Accreditation: [ ] AAPPO [ ] JACHO [ ] NCQA [ ] URAC
Plan Type: HMO
Total Enrollment:
   2001: 0   2004: 0   2007: 0
   2002: 0   2005:
   2003: 0   2006: 16,000
SERVICE AREA:
Nationwide:
   OR (Linn, Benton)'
TYPE OF COVERAGE:
Commercial: [ ] Individual: [ ] FEHBP: [ ] Indemnity: [ ]
Medicare: [ ] Medicaid: [Y] Supplemental Medicare: [ ]
Tricare   [ ]

KAISER FOUNDATION HEALTH PLAN NORTHWEST

500 NE Multnomah Ste 100
Portland, OR 97232-1191
Phone: 503-813-2800 Fax: 503-813-4967 Toll-Free:
Web site: www.kp.org
MAILING ADDRESS:
   KAISER FOUNDATION HLTH PLAN NW
   500 NE Multnomah Ste 100
   Portland, OR 97232-1191

KEY EXECUTIVES:
Regional President - Northwest .... Andrew R McCullough
Chief Financial Officer .... Frank Hemeon
Medical Director .... Andrew Lum, MD
Pharmacy Director .... Michael Kanard
Chief Operating Officer .... Cynthia Finter
Marketing Director .... Gary Morgan

COMPANY PROFILE:
Parent Company Name: Kaiser Permanente
Doing Business As:
Year Founded: 1946   Federally Qualified: [Y]
Forprofit: [ ]   Not-For-Profit: [Y]
Model Type: GROUP
Accreditation: [ ] AAPPO [ ] JACHO [ ] NCQA [ ] URAC
Plan Type: HMO, HDHP, HSA,
Total Revenue: 2005:   2006:   1,994,707,714
Net Income   2005:   2006:
Total Enrollment:
   2001: 477,056   2004: 453,288   2007: 483,552
   2002: 446,407   2005: 477,929
   2003: 434,468   2006: 485,000
Medical Loss Ratio: 2005:   2006: 94.10
Administrative Expense Ratio: 2005:   2006:
SERVICE AREA:
Nationwide: N
   OR; WA;
TYPE OF COVERAGE:
Commercial: [Y] Individual: [Y] FEHBP: [ ] Indemnity: [ ]
Medicare: [Y] Medicaid: [Y] Supplemental Medicare: [Y]
Tricare   [ ]
PRODUCTS OFFERED:
Product Name: Type:
KP Senior Advantage   Medicare Advantage
KP Medicaid   Medicaid
Kaiser HMO   HMO
Senior Advantage II   Medicare Advantage
PLAN BENEFITS:
Alternative Medicine: [ ]   Behavioral Health: [ ]
Chiropractic: [X]   Dental: [X]
Home Care: [ ]   Inpatient SNF: [X]
Long-Term Care: [ ]   Pharm. Mail Order: [ ]
Physical Therapy: [X]   Podiatry: [X]
Psychiatric: [ ]   Transplant: [ ]
Vision: [X]   Wellness: [ ]
Workers' Comp: [ ]
Other Benefits:

LANE OREGON HEALTH PLANS

PO Box 11740
Eugene, OR 97440
Phone: 541-485-2155 Fax: 541-434-1109 Toll-Free:
Web site: www.lipa.net

OREGON | **Managed Care Organization Profiles**

SERVICE AREA:
Nationwide: N
    OR; WA;
TYPE OF COVERAGE:
Commercial: [Y] Individual: [ ] FEHBP: [ ] Indemnity: [ ]
Medicare: [ ] Medicaid: [ ] Supplemental Medicare: [ ]
Tricare   [ ]
PRODUCTS OFFERED:
Product Name: Type:
ChiroNet   Chiropractic
AcuMed Net   Acupuncture
Naturnet   Naturopathy
Complementary Healthcare Plans   Specialty PPO
PLAN BENEFITS:
Alternative Medicine: [X]   Behavioral Health: [ ]
Chiropractic: [X]   Dental: [ ]
Home Care: [ ]   Inpatient SNF: [ ]
Long-Term Care: [ ]   Pharm. Mail Order: [ ]
Physical Therapy: [ ]   Podiatry: [ ]
Psychiatric: [ ]   Transplant: [ ]
Vision: [ ]   Wellness: [ ]
Workers' Comp: [ ]
Other Benefits:

GREAT-WEST HEALTHCARE OF OREGON

121 SW Morrison St Ste 400
Portland, OR 97204-3190
Phone: 503-224-0143 Fax: 503-222-3253 Toll-Free:
Web site: www.greatwesthealthcare.com
MAILING ADDRESS:
    GREAT-WEST HEALTHCARE OF OR
    121 SW Morrison St Ste 400
    Portland, OR 97204-3190

KEY EXECUTIVES:
General Manager .... Nam Lewis

COMPANY PROFILE:
Parent Company Name: Great West Life & Annuity Insurance Co
Doing Business As:
Year Founded: Federally Qualified: [ ]
Forprofit: [Y]   Not-For-Profit: [ ]
Model Type:
Accreditation: [ ] AAPPO [ ] JACHO [ ] NCQA [ ] URAC
Plan Type: PPO, POS, CDHP, HDHP, HSA,
Total Enrollment:
    2001: 14,962   2004: 3,521   2007: 0
    2002: 9,820   2005:
    2003: 4,972   2006:
SERVICE AREA:
Nationwide: N
    OR;
TYPE OF COVERAGE:
Commercial: [Y] Individual: [ ] FEHBP: [ ] Indemnity: [ ]
Medicare: [ ] Medicaid: [ ] Supplemental Medicare: [ ]
Tricare   [ ]
CONSUMER-DRIVEN PRODUCTS
Mellon HR Solutions LLC   HSA Company
                               HSA Product
                               HSA Administrator
                               Consumer-Driven Health Plan
                               High Deductible Health Plan
PLAN BENEFITS:
Alternative Medicine: [X]   Behavioral Health: [ ]
Chiropractic: [X]   Dental: [X]
Home Care: [X]   Inpatient SNF: [X]
Long-Term Care: [ ]   Pharm. Mail Order: [X]
Physical Therapy: [X]   Podiatry: [X]
Psychiatric: [X]   Transplant: [X]
Vision: [X]   Wellness: [X]
Workers' Comp: [ ]
Other Benefits:

HEALTH NET HEALTH PLAN OF OREGON INC

13221 SW 68th Pkwy Ste 200
Tigard, OR 97223
Phone: 888-802-7001 Fax: 503-213-2800 Toll-Free: 888-802-7001
Web site: www.health.net

MAILING ADDRESS:
    HEALTH NET HEALTH PLAN OF OR
    13221 SW 68th Pkwy Ste 200
    Tigard, OR 97223

KEY EXECUTIVES:
Regional President .... Stephen Lynch
President .... Chris Ellertson
Chief Financial Officer .... Scott Weiner
Medical Director .... Andrew Glass, MD
Pharmacy Director .... Lynn Petit
Marketing Director .... Matt Gougler
Credentialing Manager .... Linda Baker
Public Relations Director .... Lezli Goheen
Medical Management Director .... Renee Hayburn
Underwriting Director .... Linda Harrison
Regional Chief Medical Officer .... William P Bracciodieta, MD

COMPANY PROFILE:
Parent Company Name: Health Net Inc
Doing Business As:
Year Founded: 1985   Federally Qualified: [Y]
Forprofit: [Y]   Not-For-Profit: [ ]
Model Type: MIXED
Accreditation: [ ] AAPPO [ ] JACHO [ ] NCQA [ ] URAC
Plan Type: HMO, PPO, POS, HDHP, HSA
Total Revenue: 2005: 359,003,838   2006: 368,720,158
Net Income: 2005:   10,707,851   2006:
Total Enrollment:
    2001: 75,447   2004: 127,979   2007: 156,000
    2002: 79,368   2005: 155,000
    2003: 120,347   2006: 153,000
Medical Loss Ratio: 2005:   2006: 82.40
Administrative Expense Ratio: 2005:   2006:
SERVICE AREA:
Nationwide: N
    OR; WA (Southwest);
TYPE OF COVERAGE:
Commercial: [Y] Individual: [Y] FEHBP: [ ] Indemnity: [ ]
Medicare: [ ] Medicaid: [ ] Supplemental Medicare: [Y]
Tricare   [ ]
PRODUCTS OFFERED:
Product Name: Type:
Health Net OR - HMO   HMO
Health Net OR - PPO   PPO
Health Net OR - POS   POS
Health Net OR - SpMdc   Supplementl Medicare
PLAN BENEFITS:
Alternative Medicine: [ ]   Behavioral Health: [X]
Chiropractic: [X]   Dental: [X]
Home Care: [X]   Inpatient SNF: [X]
Long-Term Care: [X]   Pharm. Mail Order: [X]
Physical Therapy: [X]   Podiatry: [X]
Psychiatric: [X]   Transplant: [X]
Vision: [X]   Wellness: [X]
Workers' Comp: [X]
Other Benefits:
Comments:
Formerly called Qual-Med Oregon Health Plan.

HEALTH PLAN OF CAREOREGON INC

315 SW Fifth Ave Ste 900
Portland, OR 97204
Phone: 503-416-4100 Fax: 504-416-3668 Toll-Free: 800-224-4840
Web site: www.careoregon.org
MAILING ADDRESS:
    HEALTH PLAN OF CAREOREGON INC
    315 SW Fifth Ave Ste 900
    Portland, OR 97204

KEY EXECUTIVES:
Chief Executive Officer .... David Ford
Medical Director .... David Labnby, MD
Director of Provider Services .... Peter McGarry
Director of Claims & Member Service .... Tom DeVaney

COMPANY PROFILE:
Parent Company Name:
Doing Business As:
Year Founded: Federally Qualified: [ ]

Managed Care Organization Profiles

OREGON

ACUMENTRA HEALTH

2020 SW 4th Ave Ste 520
Portland, OR 97201-4960
Phone: 503-279-0100 Fax: 503-279-0190 Toll-Free:
Web site: www.acumentra.org

MAILING ADDRESS:
  ACUMENTRA HEALTH
  2020 SW 4th Ave Ste 520
  Portland, OR 97201-4960

KEY EXECUTIVES:
Chief Executive Officer/President .... Jon Mitchell, FACHE
Director of Finance .... Tim Dragila, CPA
Medical Director .... Ruth Medack, MD
Marketing Director .... Leslie Peltz
Communications Director .... Leslie Peltz
Network & System Administrator .... Laurie Christopher
Human Resources Manager .... Judith Wilson
Director Medicare Quality Services .... Stacy Aguas, RN, MBA
Compliance Officer .... Laurie Christopher
Director State & Private Services .... Michael Cooper, RN, MN

COMPANY PROFILE:
Parent Company Name:
Doing Business As:
Year Founded: 1984   Federally Qualified: [Y]
Forprofit: [ ]   Not-For-Profit: [Y]
Model Type:
Accreditation: [ ] AAPPO [ ] JACHO [ ] NCQA [ ] URAC
Plan Type: PRO, UR

SERVICE AREA:
Nationwide: N

Comments:
  Formerly known as Oregon Medical Professional Review Association, April 2006.

ATRIO HEALTH PLANS INC

500 SE Cass Ave 230
Roseburg, OR 97470
Phone: 541-672-8620 Fax: 541-672-8670 Toll-Free:
Web site: www.atriohp.com

MAILING ADDRESS:
  ATRIO HEALTH PLANS INC
  500 SE Cass Ave 230
  Roseburg, OR 97470

KEY EXECUTIVES:
Chief Executive Officer .... Eam Johnson
Chief Financial Officer .... Susan Wingaurd

COMPANY PROFILE:
Parent Company Name:
Doing Business As:
Year Founded: 2004   Federally Qualified: [ ]
Forprofit: [ ]   Not-For-Profit: [ ]
Model Type:
Accreditation: [ ] AAPPO [ ] JACHO [ ] NCQA [ ] URAC
Plan Type: HMO
Total Revenue: 2005:   2006: 38,653,992
Net Income   2005:   2006:
Total Enrollment:
  2001: 0   2004: 0   2007: 3,267
  2002: 0   2005:
  2003: 0   2006: 3,199
Medical Loss Ratio: 2005:   2006: 88.90
Administrative Expense Ratio: 2005:   2006:

SERVICE AREA:
Nationwide:
  OR (Coos, Douglas, Klamath);

TYPE OF COVERAGE:
Commercial: [ ] Individual: [ ] FEHBP: [ ] Indemnity: [ ]
Medicare: [Y] Medicaid: [ ] Supplemental Medicare: [ ]
Tricare   [ ]

PRODUCTS OFFERED:
Product Name: Type:
Atrio Health Plans   Medicare Advantage

Comments:
Atrio was formed by three provider-sponsored organizations.

CLEAR CHOICE HEALTH PLANS

2650 NE Courtney Dr
Bend, OR 97701
Phone: 541-385-5315 Fax: 541-382-3407 Toll-Free: 888-575-0334
Web site: www.clearchoicehp.com

MAILING ADDRESS:
  CLEAR CHOICE HEALTH PLANS
  2650 NE Courtney Dr
  Bend, OR 97701

KEY EXECUTIVES:
Executive Director/President .... Pat Gibford
Chief Financial Officer .... Gunnar Hansen
VP, Information Technology .... Sandra Loder

COMPANY PROFILE:
Parent Company Name: Central OR Independent Health Services
Doing Business As:
Year Founded: Federally Qualified: [ ]
Forprofit: [Y]   Not-For-Profit: [ ]
Model Type: GROUP
Accreditation: [ ] AAPPO [ ] JACHO [ ] NCQA [ ] URAC
Plan Type: HMO,
Total Revenue: 2005:   2006: 118,946,098
Net Income   2005:   2006:
Total Enrollment:
  2001: 31,575   2004: 11,767   2007: 44,811
  2002: 33,621   2005:
  2003: 28,468   2006: 43,892
Medical Loss Ratio: 2005:   2006: 86.90
Administrative Expense Ratio: 2005:   2006:

SERVICE AREA:
Nationwide:
  OR;

TYPE OF COVERAGE:
Commercial: [ ] Individual: [ ] FEHBP: [ ] Indemnity: [ ]
Medicare: [Y] Medicaid: [ ] Supplemental Medicare: [ ]
Tricare   [ ]

COMPLEMENTARY HEALTHCARE PLANS

6600 SW 105th Ave #115
Beaverton, OR 97008
Phone: 503-203-8333 Fax: 503-644-0442 Toll-Free: 800-449-9479
Web site: www.chpplans.us

MAILING ADDRESS:
  COMPLEMENTARY HEALTHCARE PLANS
  6600 SW 105th Ave #115
  Beaverton, OR 97008

KEY EXECUTIVES:
Chairman .... Arthur Walker, DC
Chief Executive Officer .... Pamella J Marchand
Director of Finance .... Chuck Adams
Chief Medical Officer .... Charles A Simpson, DC
Provider Services Manager .... Amy King
Director of Provider Services .... Juanita Neibert
VP, Sales & Marketing .... Jeff Akers
Chief Operating Officer .... Linda Voelsch
Operations Director .... David Hein

COMPANY PROFILE:
Parent Company Name: Complementary Healthcare Plans Inc
Doing Business As:
Year Founded: 1989   Federally Qualified: [N]
Forprofit: [Y]   Not-For-Profit: [ ]
Model Type: NETWORK
Accreditation: [ ] AAPPO [ ] JACHO [ ] NCQA [ ] URAC
Plan Type: PPO, Specialty PPO, ASO
Primary Physicians: Physician Specialists: 1,700
Hospitals:
Total Enrollment:
  2001: 1,550,000   2004: 0   2007: 0
  2002: 1,600,000   2005:
  2003: 480,000   2006:

Managed Care Organization Profiles   **OKLAHOMA**

TYPE OF COVERAGE:
Commercial: [Y] Individual: [Y] FEHBP: [ ] Indemnity: [ ]
Medicare: [Y] Medicaid: [ ] Supplemental Medicare: [Y]
Tricare [ ]

PLAN BENEFITS:

Alternative Medicine:	[ ]	Behavioral Health:	[ ]
Chiropractic:	[ ]	Dental:	[ ]
Home Care:	[ ]	Inpatient SNF:	[ ]
Long-Term Care:	[ ]	Pharm. Mail Order:	[ ]
Physical Therapy:	[ ]	Podiatry:	[X]
Psychiatric:	[ ]	Transplant:	[ ]
Vision:	[ ]	Wellness:	[ ]
Workers' Comp:	[ ]		

Other Benefits: Podiatry

OKLAHOMA

PLAN BENEFITS:

Alternative Medicine:	[ ]	Behavioral Health:	[ ]
Chiropractic:	[X]	Dental:	[X]
Home Care:	[ ]	Inpatient SNF:	[ ]
Long-Term Care:	[ ]	Pharm. Mail Order:	[X]
Physical Therapy:	[ ]	Podiatry:	[ ]
Psychiatric:	[X]	Transplant:	[X]
Vision:	[ ]	Wellness:	[X]
Workers' Comp:	[X]		

Other Benefits:

MUTUAL ASSURANCE ADMINISTRATORS INC

3121 Quail Springs Pkwy
Oklahoma City, OK 73134
Phone: 405-840-0882 Fax: 405-607-2694 Toll-Free:
Web site: www.maa-tpa.com

MAILING ADDRESS:
MUTUAL ASSURANCE ADMINISTRATOR
3121 Quail Springs Pkwy
Oklahoma City, OK 73134

KEY EXECUTIVES:
Chairman of the Board .... Richard E Carllson
Chief Executive Officer/President .... Todd Archer
Chief Financial Officer .... Carl Denning
Executive Director of IT .... Jason Shiflett
Chief Operating Officer .... Clint Wilson
Marketing Director .... Eric Wright
Executive Director of IS .... Jeff Knox
Executive Director of Client Solutions .... Kelly Haynes
Human Resources Direcctor .... Denise Sivigliano
Executive Director of Quality & Automation .... Linda Wilson
Vice President Operations .... Carol Montgomery
Human Resources Director .... Shelli Smart
Executive Director of Client Solutions .... Jan White
Executive Director of Disability Management .... Cyndi Norris
Executive Director of Client Services .... Sandy Locke

COMPANY PROFILE:
Parent Company Name: Mutual Assurance Administrators
Doing Business As: Mutual Assurance Advantage
Year Founded: 1975   Federally Qualified: [ ]
Forprofit: [Y]   Not-For-Profit: [ ]
Model Type:
Accreditation: [ ] AAPPO [ ] JACHO [ ] NCQA [ ] URAC
Plan Type: UR, TPA

SERVICE AREA:
Nationwide: N
   OK;

OKLAHOMA FOUNDATION FOR MEDICAL QUALITY

14000 Quail Springs Pkwy #400
Oklahoma City, OK 73134-2627
Phone: 405-840-2891 Fax: 405-840-1343 Toll-Free: 800-522-3414
Web site: www.ofmq.com

MAILING ADDRESS:
OK FOUNDATION FOR MEDICAL QUALITY
14000 Quail Springs Pkwy #400
Oklahoma City, OK 73134-2627

KEY EXECUTIVES:
Chief Executive Officer .... Jim L Williams
Chief Financial Officer .... Gregg Koehn
Chief Operating Officer .... Claudette Greenway, RN
Health Care Quality Project Manager .... Cheryl Hays
Communications Manager .... Tracie LaGere-Litsch

COMPANY PROFILE:
Parent Company Name:
Doing Business As:
Year Founded: 1972   Federally Qualified: [ ]
Forprofit: [ ]   Not-For-Profit: [Y]
Model Type:
Accreditation: [ ] AAPPO [ ] JACHO [ ] NCQA [ ] URAC
Plan Type: UR

SERVICE AREA:
Nationwide: N
   OK;

PACIFICARE OF OKLAHOMA INC/SECURE HORIZONS

7666 E 61st St Ste 500
Tulsa, OK 74133
Phone: 918-459-1100 Fax: 918-459-1452 Toll-Free: 800-297-9355
Web site: www.pacificare.com

MAILING ADDRESS:
PACIFICARE OF OK/SECURE HRZNS
7666 E 61st St Ste 500
Tulsa, OK 74133

KEY EXECUTIVES:
Chief Executive Officer/President .... George H Becker
Chief Financial Officer .... Daniel J Comrie
VP, Sales & Marketing .... Victor J Pluto
General Manager & VP, Network Management .... Austin Pittman

COMPANY PROFILE:
Parent Company Name: UnitedHealth Group
Doing Business As: PacifiCare of Oklahoma
Year Founded: 1986   Federally Qualified: [Y]
Forprofit: [Y]   Not-For-Profit: [ ]
Model Type: GROUP
Accreditation: [ ] AAPPO [ ] JACHO [X] NCQA [ ] URAC
Plan Type: HMO, HDHP, HSA,
Total Enrollment:
   2001: 121,564   2004: 82,379   2007: 0
   2002: 120,891   2005:
   2003: 123,027   2006:

SERVICE AREA:
Nationwide: N
   OK (Lawton, Oklahoma City, Tulsa);

TYPE OF COVERAGE:
Commercial: [Y] Individual: [ ] FEHBP: [ ] Indemnity: [ ]
Medicare: [Y] Medicaid: [ ] Supplemental Medicare: [ ]
Tricare   [ ]

PRODUCTS OFFERED:

Product Name:	Type:
Pacificare OK HMO	HMO
Secure Horizons	Medicare Advantage

PLAN BENEFITS:

Alternative Medicine:	[ ]	Behavioral Health:	[X]
Chiropractic:	[X]	Dental:	[ ]
Home Care:	[X]	Inpatient SNF:	[X]
Long-Term Care:	[ ]	Pharm. Mail Order:	[X]
Physical Therapy:	[X]	Podiatry:	[X]
Psychiatric:	[X]	Transplant:	[X]
Vision:	[X]	Wellness:	[X]
Workers' Comp:	[X]		

Other Benefits:

PREFERRED PODIATRISTS OF OKLAHOMA

3818 N Rockwell St
Bethany, OK 73008-3350
Phone: 405-787-8820 Fax: 405-495-6523 Toll-Free:
Web site:

MAILING ADDRESS:
PREFERRED PODIATRISTS OF OK
3818 N Rockwell St
Bethany, OK 73008-3350

KEY EXECUTIVES:
Chief Executive Officer .... Richard J Traczyk, DPM
Chief Financial Officer/Medical Director .... Richard J Traczyk, DPM

COMPANY PROFILE:
Parent Company Name: Richard J Traczyk, DPM
Doing Business As: Bethany Foot Clinic, Ltd
Year Founded: 1995   Federally Qualified: [N]
Forprofit: [Y]   Not-For-Profit: [ ]
Model Type: IPA
Accreditation: [ ] AAPPO [ ] JACHO [ ] NCQA [ ] URAC
Plan Type: Specialty HMO

SERVICE AREA:
Nationwide: N
   OK;

Managed Care Organization Profiles   **OKLAHOMA**

KEY EXECUTIVES:
Chief Executive Officer .... *John Gladden*
VP of Operations .... *Barbara Fennell*
VP of Marketing .... *Kenneth McGuire*

COMPANY PROFILE:
Parent Company Name: Delta Dental Plan Association
Doing Business As:
Year Founded: Federally Qualified: [ ]
Forprofit: [ ]   Not-For-Profit: [ ]
Model Type:
Accreditation: [ ] AAPPO [ ] JACHO [ ] NCQA [ ] URAC
Plan Type: Specialty HMO
Total Enrollment:
  2001: 0   2004: 458,133   2007: 0
  2002: 145,259   2005:
  2003: 148,210   2006:

SERVICE AREA:
Nationwide: N
  OK;

TYPE OF COVERAGE:
Commercial: [Y] Individual: [ ] FEHBP: [ ] Indemnity: [ ]
Medicare: [ ] Medicaid: [ ] Supplemental Medicare: [ ]
Tricare   [ ]

PLAN BENEFITS:
Alternative Medicine: [ ]   Behavioral Health: [ ]
Chiropractic: [ ]   Dental: [X]
Home Care: [ ]   Inpatient SNF: [ ]
Long-Term Care: [ ]   Pharm. Mail Order: [ ]
Physical Therapy: [ ]   Podiatry: [ ]
Psychiatric: [ ]   Transplant: [ ]
Vision: [ ]   Wellness: [ ]
Workers' Comp: [ ]
Other Benefits:

FIRST HEALTH NETWORK (PPO OKLAHOMA INC)

3503 NW 63rd St Ste 304
Oklahoma City, OK 73116
Phone: 405-843-9551 Fax: 405-843-0956 Toll-Free:
Web site: www.ppooklahoma.com
MAILING ADDRESS:
       FIRST HEALTH NETWORK
       PO Box 20040
       Oklahoma City, OK 73116

KEY EXECUTIVES:
Vice President/Chief Medical Director .... *Kim Sizemore*
Provider Services/Network/Contracts Director .... *Kim Sizemore*
Office Manager .... *Judy Lesnewski*

COMPANY PROFILE:
Parent Company Name: Coventry Health Care Inc
Doing Business As:
Year Founded: Federally Qualified: [ ]
Forprofit: [ ]   Not-For-Profit: [ ]
Model Type:
Accreditation: [ ] AAPPO [ ] JACHO [ ] NCQA [ ] URAC
Plan Type: PPO
SERVICE AREA:
Nationwide: N
  OK;

TYPE OF COVERAGE:
Commercial: [Y] Individual: [Y] FEHBP: [ ] Indemnity: [ ]
Medicare: [Y] Medicaid: [ ] Supplemental Medicare: [ ]
Tricare   [ ]

PLAN BENEFITS:
Alternative Medicine: [ ]   Behavioral Health: [X]
Chiropractic: [X]   Dental: [ ]
Home Care: [X]   Inpatient SNF: [X]
Long-Term Care: [ ]   Pharm. Mail Order: [ ]
Physical Therapy: [X]   Podiatry: [X]
Psychiatric: [X]   Transplant: [X]
Vision: [X]   Wellness: [X]
Workers' Comp: [X]
Other Benefits:
Comments:
Formerly PPO Oklahoma Inc.

GLOBAL HEALTH INC

701 NE 10th St Ste 300
Oklahoma City, OK 73104
Phone: 405-280-5656 Fax: 405-280-5894 Toll-Free: 877-280-5600
Web site: www.globalhealth.cc/
MAILING ADDRESS:
       GLOBAL HEALTH INC
       PO Box 1747
       Oklahoma City, OK 73104

KEY EXECUTIVES:
Chairman .... *John Bell, MD*
Chief Executive Officer .... *Denise Semands Suttles*
Medical Director .... *Don Wilber, MD*

COMPANY PROFILE:
Parent Company Name:
Doing Business As:
Year Founded: 2002   Federally Qualified: [ ]
Forprofit: [Y]   Not-For-Profit: [ ]
Model Type: GROUP
Accreditation: [ ] AAPPO [ ] JACHO [ ] NCQA [ ] URAC
Plan Type: HMO
Total Enrollment:
  2001: 0   2004: 2,507   2007: 0
  2002: 0   2005:
  2003: 406   2006:

SERVICE AREA:
Nationwide: N
  FL;

TYPE OF COVERAGE:
Commercial: [ ] Individual: [ ] FEHBP: [ ] Indemnity: [ ]
Medicare: [Y] Medicaid: [ ] Supplemental Medicare: [ ]
Tricare   [ ]

HUMANA INC - OKLAHOMA

500 W Main St
Louisville, KY 40201
Phone: 502-580-5804 Fax: 502-980-8528 Toll-Free:
Web site: www.humana.com
MAILING ADDRESS:
       HUMANA INC - OKLAHOMA
       500 W Main St
       Louisville, KY 40201

KEY EXECUTIVES:
Chairman of the Board .... *David A Jones Jr*
Chief Executive Officer/President .... *Michael B McCallister*
Chief Financial Officer .... *James H Bloem*
VP Medical Director .... *Jonathan T Lord, MD*
Senior VP, Chief Information Officer .... *Bruce J Goodman*
Senior VP, Human Resources .... *Bonnie C Hathcock*

COMPANY PROFILE:
Parent Company Name: Humana Inc
Doing Business As:
Year Founded: 1961   Federally Qualified: [Y]
Forprofit: [Y]   Not-For-Profit: [ ]
Model Type:
Accreditation: [ ] AAPPO [ ] JACHO [ ] NCQA [ ] URAC
Plan Type: HMO, PPO, ASO, CDHP, HDHP, HSA,
SERVICE AREA:
Nationwide: N
  OK;

TYPE OF COVERAGE:
Commercial: [Y] Individual: [ ] FEHBP: [ ] Indemnity: [ ]
Medicare: [Y] Medicaid: [ ] Supplemental Medicare: [Y]
Tricare   [ ]
CONSUMER-DRIVEN PRODUCTS
JP Morgan Chase   HSA Company
HumanaOne HSA   HSA Product
JP Morgan Chase   HSA Administrator
Personal Care Account   Consumer-Driven Health Plan
HumanaOne   High Deductible Health Plan

OKLAHOMA

SERVICE AREA:
Nationwide: N
OK;

TYPE OF COVERAGE:
Commercial: [ ]   Individual: [Y]   FEHBP: [Y]   Indemnity: [Y]
Medicare: [ ]   Medicaid: [ ]   Supplemental Medicare: [Y]
Tricare

PRODUCTS OFFERED:

Product Name:	Type:
Bluelincs HMO	HMO
BlueChoice PPO	PPO
BluePreferred PPO	PPO
BlueTraditional	Individual
Health Check Select Care	Individual
Plan65	Supplemental Medicar
Blue Plan65 Select	Supplementl Medicare

PLAN BENEFITS:
Alternative Medicine: [ ]   Behavioral Health: [X]
Chiropractic: [X]   Dental: [X]
Home Care: [X]   Inpatient SNF: [X]
Long-Term Care: [X]   Pharm. Mail Order: [X]
Physical Therapy: [X]   Podiatry: [X]
Psychiatric: [X]   Transplant: [X]
Vision: [X]   Wellness: [X]
Workers' Comp: [ ]
Other Benefits:

BLUELINCS HMO

1400 South Boston
Tulsa, OK 74119-3618
Phone: 918-561-9900 Fax: 918-560-3380 Toll-Free: 800-250-9020
Web site: www.bcbsok.com

MAILING ADDRESS:
BLUELINCS HMO
1400 South Boston
Tulsa, OK 74119-3618

KEY EXECUTIVES:
Chairman of the Board .... Ronald F King
Chief Executive Officer .... Rodney I Huey MD
VP, Bluelincs .... Lyndle Ellis
Corporate Medical Director .... Joe Nicholson, MD
Pharmacy Director .... Tom Kaye RPh
Chief Infomation Officer .... Jerry D Scherer
VP of Marketing .... Lisa Putt
MIS Director .... Dennis Timms
Director of Provider Services .... Wayne Wallace
General Counsel .... Jacqueline Haglund
Group VP, Blue Lincs HMO .... Lyndle Ellis

COMPANY PROFILE:
Parent Company Name: Blue Cross Blue Shield of Oklahoma
Doing Business As:
Year Founded: 1983   Federally Qualified: [Y]
Forprofit: [Y]   Not-For-Profit: [ ]
Model Type: IPA
Accreditation: [ ] AAPPO [ ] JACHO [X] NCQA [ ] URAC
Plan Type: HMO
Total Enrollment:
2001: 32,566   2004: 0   2007: 0
2002: 30,400   2005:
2003: 0   2006:

SERVICE AREA:
Nationwide: N
OK (Metro Areas, Oklahoma City, Tulsa);

TYPE OF COVERAGE:
Commercial: [Y]   Individual: [ ]   FEHBP: [ ]   Indemnity: [ ]
Medicare: [Y]   Medicaid: [ ]   Supplemental Medicare: [ ]
Tricare [ ]

PRODUCTS OFFERED:

Product Name:	Type:
Bluelincs HMO	HMO
Bluelincs Senior	Medicare

PLAN BENEFITS:
Alternative Medicine: [ ]   Behavioral Health: [X]
Chiropractic: [X]   Dental: [ ]
Home Care: [X]   Inpatient SNF: [ ]
Long-Term Care: [ ]   Pharm. Mail Order: [X]
Physical Therapy: [ ]   Podiatry: [X]
Psychiatric: [X]   Transplant: [X]
Vision: [X]   Wellness: [X]
Workers' Comp: [ ]
Other Benefits:

COMMUNITYCARE MANAGED HEALTHCARE PLANS OF OKLAHOMA INC

218 W Sixth St
Tulsa, OK 74119-1004
Phone: 918-594-5200 Fax: 918-594-5260 Toll-Free: 800-278-7563
Web site: www.cchp.com

MAILING ADDRESS:
COMMUNITYCARE
PO Box 3249
Tulsa, OK 74119-1004

KEY EXECUTIVES:
Chief Executive Officer/President .... Richard W Todd
Chief Financial Officer .... Earle Rice
Medical Director .... Jack Sommers, MD
Pharmacy Director .... Melanie Maxwell
Chief Information Officer .... Lorenzo Marquez
Chief Operating Officer .... Nancy Horstmann
Marketing Director .... Cindy Giddings
MIS Director .... Lorenzo Marquez
Corporate Communications Director .... Hollace Fugate
Director, Provider Services .... Kelly Ross
Human Resource Director .... Candia Fields
Fraud Prevention/Investigation .... Rem Beitel

COMPANY PROFILE:
Parent Company Name: St Francis Hlth System, St John Hlth Sys
Doing Business As: Commty Care HMO, Preferred Commty Choice
Year Founded: 1994   Federally Qualified: [Y]
Forprofit: [Y]   Not-For-Profit: [ ]
Model Type: IPA
Accreditation: [ ] AAPPO [X] JACHO [ ] NCQA [ ] URAC
Plan Type: HMO, PPO, POS, EPO, UR, PBM, HDHP, HSA,
Total Enrollment:
2001: 118,639   2004: 103,114   2007: 0
2002: 111,441   2005:
2003: 95,825   2006:

SERVICE AREA:
Nationwide: N
OK (Ardmore, Bartlesville, Broken Arrow, Muckogee, Oklahoma City, Stillwater, Tulsa, Vinita);

TYPE OF COVERAGE:
Commercial: [Y]   Individual: [ ]   FEHBP: [ ]   Indemnity: [ ]
Medicare: [Y]   Medicaid: [Y]   Supplemental Medicare: [Y]
Tricare [ ]

PRODUCTS OFFERED:

Product Name:	Type:
CommunityCare HMO	HMO
Preferred CommunityChoice	PPO
Work Net	CWMP
Senior Health Plan	Medicare
ExcelCare	UR
SoonerCare	Medicaid

PLAN BENEFITS:
Alternative Medicine: [ ]   Behavioral Health: [X]
Chiropractic: [X]   Dental: [X]
Home Care: [X]   Inpatient SNF: [X]
Long-Term Care: [X]   Pharm. Mail Order: [X]
Physical Therapy: [X]   Podiatry: [X]
Psychiatric: [X]   Transplant: [X]
Vision: [X]   Wellness: [X]
Workers' Comp: [X]
Other Benefits:

Comments:
Formerly Community Care HMO. Owned and operated by four hospitals: Mercy Health Systems, St Anthony Hospital, St Francis Hospital and St Johns Hospital.

DELTA DENTAL OF OKLAHOMA

16 NW 63rd St Ste 301
Oklahoma City, OK 73116
Phone: 800-522-0188 Fax: 405-607-2190 Toll-Free:
Web site: www.deltadentalok.com

MAILING ADDRESS:
DELTA DENTAL OF OK
PO Box 54709
Oklahoma City, OK 73116

Managed Care Organization Profiles   **OKLAHOMA**

AETNA INC - OKLAHOMA

4013 NW Expressway Ste 300
Oklahoma City, OK 73116
Phone: 405-475-6500 Fax: 405-879-7180 Toll-Free:
Web site: www.aetna.com

MAILING ADDRESS:
    AETNA INC - OK
    4013 NW Expressway Ste 300
    Oklahoma City, OK 73116

KEY EXECUTIVES:
Chairman of the Board .... Ronald A Williams
Chief Executive Officer .... Jim McNaughton
Regional Manager-West Central .... Charles T Brown
Executive VP, Finance .... Joseph M Zubretsky
Pharmacy Director .... Doug McCann
Marketing Director .... Tim McFall
Director, Provider Services .... Robert Warren

COMPANY PROFILE:
Parent Company Name: Aetna Inc
Doing Business As:
Year Founded: 1981   Federally Qualified: [Y]
Forprofit: [Y]   Not-For-Profit: [ ]
Model Type: GROUP
Accreditation: [ ] AAPPO [ ] JACHO [X] NCQA [ ] URAC
Plan Type: HMO, POS, CDHP, HSA
Total Enrollment:
   2001: 37,187   2004: 0   2007: 0
   2002: 6,294   2005:
   2003: 0   2006:

SERVICE AREA:
Nationwide: N
OK;

TYPE OF COVERAGE:
Commercial: [Y] Individual: [ ] FEHBP: [ ] Indemnity: [ ]
Medicare: [ ] Medicaid: [ ] Supplemental Medicare: [ ]
Tricare [ ]

PRODUCTS OFFERED:
Product Name: Type:
Aetna Prudential HMO   HMO

CONSUMER-DRIVEN PRODUCTS
Aetna Life Insurance Co   HSA Company
Aetna HealthFund HSA   HSA Product
Aetna   HSA Administrator
Aetna HealthFund   Consumer-Driven Health Plan
PPO I; PPO II   High Deductible Health Plan

PLAN BENEFITS:
Alternative Medicine: [ ]   Behavioral Health: [ ]
Chiropractic: [X]   Dental: [ ]
Home Care: [X]   Inpatient SNF: [X]
Long-Term Care: [ ]   Pharm. Mail Order: [X]
Physical Therapy: [X]   Podiatry: [X]
Psychiatric: [X]   Transplant: [X]
Vision: [X]   Wellness: [X]
Workers' Comp: [ ]
Other Benefits:
Comments:
Formerly Prudential Health Care of Oklahoma.

AETNA INC - TULSA

6120 S Yale Ste 350
Tulsa, OK 74136
Phone: 918-624-4700 Fax: 860-273-9806 Toll-Free: 800-435-8310
Web site: www.aetna.com

MAILING ADDRESS:
    AETNA INC - TULSA
    6120 S Yale Ste 350
    Tulsa, OK 74136

KEY EXECUTIVES:
Chairman of the Board .... Ronald A Williams
Chief Executive Officer .... Melissa Lawrence
Regional Manager-West Central .... Charles T Brown
Executive VP, Finance .... Joseph M Zubretsky
Pharmacy Director .... John Spoon, RPh
Marketing Director .... Brian Forbes
Director, Provider Services .... Michelle Crawford

COMPANY PROFILE:
Parent Company Name: Aetna Inc
Doing Business As:
Year Founded: 1983   Federally Qualified: [Y]
Forprofit: [Y]   Not-For-Profit: [ ]
Model Type: GROUP
Accreditation: [ ] AAPPO [ ] JACHO [X] NCQA [ ] URAC
Plan Type: HMO, PPO, POS, CDHP, HDHP, HSA,
Total Enrollment:
   2001: 50,576   2004: 41,966   2007: 0
   2002: 72,327   2005:
   2003: 50,345   2006:

SERVICE AREA:
Nationwide: N
   OK (Creek, Okmulgee, Osage, Rogers, Wagoner, Washington);

TYPE OF COVERAGE:
Commercial: [Y] Individual: [ ] FEHBP: [ ] Indemnity: [ ]
Medicare: [ ] Medicaid: [ ] Supplemental Medicare: [ ]
Tricare [ ]

PRODUCTS OFFERED:
Product Name: Type:
Aetna US Healthcare HMO   HMO
Aetna US Healthcare   POS

CONSUMER-DRIVEN PRODUCTS
Aetna Life Insurance Co   HSA Company
Aetna HealthFund HSA   HSA Product
Aetna   HSA Administrator
Aetna HealthFund   Consumer-Driven Health Plan
PPO I; PPO II   High Deductible Health Plan

PLAN BENEFITS:
Alternative Medicine: [ ]   Behavioral Health: [X]
Chiropractic: [X]   Dental: [ ]
Home Care: [X]   Inpatient SNF: [X]
Long-Term Care: [ ]   Pharm. Mail Order: [X]
Physical Therapy: [X]   Podiatry: [X]
Psychiatric: [X]   Transplant: [X]
Vision: [X]   Wellness: [X]
Workers' Comp: [ ]
Other Benefits:
Comments:
Formerly Prudential Healthcare of Tulsa.

BLUE CROSS BLUE SHIELD OF OKLAHOMA

1215 S Boulder
Tulsa, OK 74102
Phone: 918-560-3500 Fax: 918-560-2095 Toll-Free: 800-942-5837
Web site: www.bcbsok.com

MAILING ADDRESS:
    BLUE CROSS BLUE SHIELD OF OK
    PO Box 3283
    Tulsa, OK 74102

KEY EXECUTIVES:
Chairperson .... Ronald F King
President .... Rodney I Huey, MD
Medical Director .... R Joseph Cunningham, MD
Chief Information Officer .... Jerry D Scherer
Marketing Director .... Lisa Putt
MIS Director .... Chuck Rygiel
General Counsel .... Jacqueline Haglund
Public Relations Director .... Linda Sponsler
Provider Relations Director .... C Wayne Wallace
Group Vice President .... Lyndle Ellis
Executive VP .... Mike Rhoads
Division VP, Marketing & Sales .... Greg Burn

COMPANY PROFILE:
Parent Company Name: Group Health Services
Doing Business As: Blue Lincs
Year Founded: 1940   Federally Qualified: [Y]
Forprofit: [ ]   Not-For-Profit: [Y]
Model Type: NETWORK
Accreditation: [ ] AAPPO [ ] JACHO [X] NCQA [X] URAC
Plan Type: HMO, PPO, TPA, CDHP, HDHP, HSA,
Total Enrollment:
   2001: 445,000   2004: 0   2007: 0
   2002: 846,856   2005:
   2003: 0   2006:

Managed Care Organization Profiles — OHIO

COMPANY PROFILE:
Parent Company Name: UnitedHealth Group
Doing Business As:
Year Founded: 1979 Federally Qualified: [N]
Forprofit: [Y] Not-For-Profit: [ ]
Model Type: IPA
Accreditation: [ ] AAPPO [ ] JACHO [ ] NCQA [ ] URAC
Plan Type: HMO, PPO, POS, CDHP, HDHP, HSA, HRA,

SERVICE AREA:
Nationwide: N

OH; (Adams, Allen, Ashland, Ashtabula, Athens, Auglaize, Belmont, Brown, Butler, Carroll, Champaign, Clark, Clemont, Clinton, Columbiana, Coshocton, Crawford, Cuyahoga, Darke, Delaware, Erie, Fairfield, Fayette, Franklin, Gallia, Geauga, Greene, Guernsey, Hamilton, Hardin, Harrison, Highland, Hocking, Holmes, Huron, Jackson, Jefferson, Knox, Lake, Lawrence, Licking, Logan, Lorain, Lucas, Madison, Mahoning, Marion, Medina, Meigs, Mercer, Miami, Monroe, Montgomery, Morgan, Morrow, Muskingum, Noble, Ottawa, Perry, Pickaway, Pike, Portage, Preble, Richland, Ross, Sandusky, Scioto, Seneca, Shelby, Stark, Summit, Trumbull, Tuscarawas, Union, Vinton, Warren, Washington, wayne, Wood, Wyandot),

TYPE OF COVERAGE:
Commercial: [Y] Individual: [ ] FEHBP: [ ] Indemnity: [ ]
Medicare: [Y] Medicaid: [ ] Supplemental Medicare: [ ]
Tricare [ ]

PRODUCTS OFFERED:
Product Name: Type:
Choice HMO

CONSUMER-DRIVEN PRODUCTS
Exante Bank/Golden Rule Ins Co HSA Company
iPlan HSA HSA Product
  HSA Administrator
  Consumer-Driven Health Plan
  High Deductible Health Plan

PLAN BENEFITS:
Alternative Medicine: [ ] Behavioral Health: [ ]
Chiropractic: [ ] Dental: [ ]
Home Care: [X] Inpatient SNF: [X]
Long-Term Care: [ ] Pharm. Mail Order: [X]
Physical Therapy: [X] Podiatry: [X]
Psychiatric: [X] Transplant: [X]
Vision: [X] Wellness: [X]
Workers' Comp: [ ]
Other Benefits:

Comments:
See United Healthcare of Ohio Inc, Westerville, OH for enrollment figures.

UNITEDHEALTHCARE OF SW OHIO INC-DAYTON/CINCINNATI

9050 Centre Pointe Dr Ste 400
Westchester, OH 45069
Phone: 513-603-6200 Fax: 513-603-6271 Toll-Free:
Web site: www.unitedhealthgroup.com

MAILING ADDRESS:
UNITEDHEALTHCARE OF SW OH INC
9050 Centre Pointe Dr Ste 400
Westchester, OH 45069

KEY EXECUTIVES:
Chairman/Chief Executive Officer/President........ Robert C Falkenberg
Executive Director .... Paul Brophy
Chief Financial Officer National Public Sector........ Dorothy Coleman
Medical Director .... Richard Shonk
Senior Director, ASO Sales .... L Aaron Adkins
Information Systems Director .... Matt Rye

COMPANY PROFILE:
Parent Company Name: UnitedHealth Group
Doing Business As:
Year Founded: 1979 Federally Qualified: [N]
Forprofit: [Y] Not-For-Profit: [ ]
Model Type: IPA
Accreditation: [ ] AAPPO [ ] JACHO [X] NCQA [ ] URAC
Plan Type: HMO, PPO, POS, TPA, EPO, CDHP, HSA, HRA

SERVICE AREA:
Nationwide: N
OH;

TYPE OF COVERAGE:
Commercial: [Y] Individual: [Y] FEHBP: [ ] Indemnity: [ ]
Medicare: [Y] Medicaid: [Y] Supplemental Medicare: [ ]
Tricare [ ]

PRODUCTS OFFERED:
Product Name: Type:
Choice HMO

CONSUMER-DRIVEN PRODUCTS
Exante Bank/Golden Rule Ins Co HSA Company
iPlan HSA HSA Product
  HSA Administrator
  Consumer-Driven Health Plan
  High Deductible Health Plan

PLAN BENEFITS:
Alternative Medicine: [ ] Behavioral Health: [X]
Chiropractic: [ ] Dental: [X]
Home Care: [X] Inpatient SNF: [X]
Long-Term Care: [ ] Pharm. Mail Order: [X]
Physical Therapy: [X] Podiatry: [X]
Psychiatric: [X] Transplant: [X]
Vision: [ ] Wellness: [X]
Workers' Comp: [ ]
Other Benefits:

Comments:
See United Healthcare of Ohio Inc, Westerville, OH for enrollment figures.

OHIO

Managed Care Organization Profiles

Total Enrollment:
  2001: 0   2004: 0   2007: 12,587
  2002: 0   2005: 17,640
  2003: 0   2006: 13,470
Medical Loss Ratio: 2005: 58.10   2006: 55.60
Administrative Expense Ratio: 2005:   2006:

SERVICE AREA:
Nationwide: N
  OH;

TYPE OF COVERAGE:
Commercial: [Y] Individual: [Y] FEHBP: [ ] Indemnity: [ ]
Medicare: [ ] Medicaid: [ ] Supplemental Medicare: [ ]
Tricare   [ ]

PLAN BENEFITS:
Alternative Medicine: [ ]   Behavioral Health: [ ]
Chiropractic: [ ]   Dental: [X]
Home Care: [ ]   Inpatient SNF: [ ]
Long-Term Care: [ ]   Pharm. Mail Order: [ ]
Physical Therapy: [ ]   Podiatry: [ ]
Psychiatric: [ ]   Transplant: [ ]
Vision: [ ]   Wellness: [ ]
Workers' Comp: [ ]
Other Benefits:
Comments:
Formerly Fortis Benefits Dental.

UNISON HEALTH PLAN OF OHIO INC

1300 E Ninth St
Cleveland, OH 44114
Phone: 412-898-400 Fax: Toll-Free:
Web site: www.unisonhealthplan.com

MAILING ADDRESS:
    UNISON HEALTH PLAN OF OHIO INC
    Unison Plaza 1001 Brinton Rd
    Pittsburgh, PA 44114

KEY EXECUTIVES:
Chief Executive Officer .... *John P Blank, MD*
President .... *Scott A Bowers*
Treasurer .... *Leslie A Gelpi*
Medical Director .... *Linda L Post, MD*

COMPANY PROFILE:
Parent Company Name: Unison Health Holdings of Ohio Inc
Doing Business As:
Year Founded: 2004   Federally Qualified: [N]
Forprofit: [Y]   Not-For-Profit: [ ]
Model Type:
Accreditation: [ ] AAPPO [ ] JACHO [ ] NCQA [ ] URAC
Plan Type: HMO
Total Revenue: 2005:   3,999,266   2006:   50,694,342
Net Income   2005:   38,284   2006:   195,181
Total Enrollment:
  2001: 0   2004: 0   2007: 77,965
  2002: 0   2005: 11,459
  2003: 0   2006: 60,143
Medical Loss Ratio: 2005: 85.74   2006: 81.45
Administrative Expense Ratio: 2005: 14.00   2006: 17.88

SERVICE AREA:
Nationwide: N
  OH;

TYPE OF COVERAGE:
Commercial: [ ] Individual: [ ] FEHBP: [ ] Indemnity: [ ]
Medicare: [ ] Medicaid: [Y] Supplemental Medicare: [ ]
Tricare   [ ]

PRODUCTS OFFERED:
Product Name: Type:
Unison   Medicaid

PLAN BENEFITS:
Alternative Medicine: [ ]   Behavioral Health: [X]
Chiropractic: [ ]   Dental: [X]
Home Care: [ ]   Inpatient SNF: [ ]
Long-Term Care: [ ]   Pharm. Mail Order: [ ]
Physical Therapy: [ ]   Podiatry: [ ]
Psychiatric: [ ]   Transplant: [ ]
Vision: [X]   Wellness: [ ]
Workers' Comp: [ ]
Other Benefits:

UNITEDHEALTHCARE OF OHIO INC

9200 Worthington Rd
Westerville, OH 43082
Phone: 614-410-7000 Fax: 614-410-7119 Toll-Free: 888-328-8835
Web site: www.uhc.com

MAILING ADDRESS:
    UNITEDHEALTHCARE OF OHIO INC
    9200 Worthington Rd
    Westerville, OH 43082

KEY EXECUTIVES:
Chairman/Chief Executive Officer/President .... *Robert C Falkenberg*
Chief Financial Officer .... *Richard G Dunlop*
Medical Director .... *Owen Johnson, MD*
Chief Operating Officer .... *Stevan Garcia*

COMPANY PROFILE:
Parent Company Name: UnitedHealth Group
Doing Business As:
Year Founded: 1980   Federally Qualified: [Y]
Forprofit: [Y]   Not-For-Profit: [ ]
Model Type: IPA
Accreditation: [ ] AAPPO [ ] JACHO [X] NCQA [ ] URAC
Plan Type: HMO, PPO, CDHP, HSA, HRA
Total Revenue: 2005:   1,017,842,297   2006:   908,790,307
Net Income   2005:   5,246,119   2006:   22,047,810
Total Enrollment:
  2001: 678,562   2004: 330,971   2007: 98,111
  2002: 513,132   2005: 232,935
  2003: 407,338   2006: 141,659
Medical Loss Ratio: 2005: 84.30   2006: 83.60
Administrative Expense Ratio: 2005:   2006:

SERVICE AREA:
Nationwide: N
  KY; OH;

TYPE OF COVERAGE:
Commercial: [Y] Individual: [Y] FEHBP: [ ] Indemnity: [ ]
Medicare: [Y] Medicaid: [ ] Supplemental Medicare: [ ]
Tricare   [ ]

PRODUCTS OFFERED:
Product Name: Type:
United Healthcare Select   HMO
Select Plus   HMO
Choice/Choice Plus
Medicare Complete   Medicare
Evercare   Medicare
CONSUMER-DRIVEN PRODUCTS
Exante Bank/Golden Rule Ins Co   HSA Company
iPlan HSA   HSA Product
                                    HSA Administrator
                                    Consumer-Driven Health Plan
                                    High Deductible Health Plan

PLAN BENEFITS:
Alternative Medicine: [ ]   Behavioral Health: [ ]
Chiropractic: [ ]   Dental: [ ]
Home Care: [X]   Inpatient SNF: [ ]
Long-Term Care: [ ]   Pharm. Mail Order: [ ]
Physical Therapy: [ ]   Podiatry: [X]
Psychiatric: [X]   Transplant: [X]
Vision: [ ]   Wellness: [X]
Workers' Comp: [ ]
Other Benefits:

UNITEDHEALTHCARE OF OHIO INC-CLEVELAND

1001 Lakeside Ave Ste 1000
Cleveland, OH 44114-1158
Phone: 800-468-5001 Fax: 216-771-1737 Toll-Free: 800-468-5001
Web site: www.uhc.com

MAILING ADDRESS:
    UNITEDHEALTHCARE OF OHIO INC
    1001 Lakeside Ave Ste 1000
    Cleveland, OH 44114-1158

KEY EXECUTIVES:
Chairman/Chief Executive Officer/President .... *Robert C Falkenberg*
Chief Financial Officer .... *Joy Pascoe*
Medical Director .... *Charles Stemple, MD*
Marketing Director .... *Roger Griswold*
Medical Officer .... *Odell Owens, MD*

Managed Care Organization Profiles — OHIO

PRODUCTS OFFERED:

Product Name:	Type:
Super Med HMO	HMO
Super Med PPO	PPO
Super Med Select	POS
Supermed HMO	Medicaid

PLAN BENEFITS:

Alternative Medicine:	[ ]	Behavioral Health:	[ ]
Chiropractic:	[X]	Dental:	[X]
Home Care:	[X]	Inpatient SNF:	[X]
Long-Term Care:	[ ]	Pharm. Mail Order:	[ ]
Physical Therapy:	[X]	Podiatry:	[X]
Psychiatric:	[X]	Transplant:	[X]
Vision:	[X]	Wellness:	[X]
Workers' Comp:	[ ]		

Other Benefits:

SUPERIEN HEALTH NETWORK INC

4301 Darrow Rd Stratford Pl
Stow, OH 44224
Phone: 330-689-7025 Fax: 330-686-7087 Toll-Free: 888-315-6045
Web site: www.superienhealthnetwork.com

MAILING ADDRESS:
SUPERIEN HEALTH NETWORK INC
4301 Darrow Rd Stratford Pl
Stow, OH 44224

KEY EXECUTIVES:
Chief Executive Officer .... Paul Glover
President .... Joseph Manheim
Chief Financial Officer .... Steven L Ditman
Chief Medical Officer .... Michael Cohen, MD
VP, Pharmacy Services .... Michael Dlugos
Chief Operating Officer .... Eileen Romansky
Chief Sales & Marketing Director .... Michael D Schotz
Manager, Network Operations .... Verdis Norwood
Senior VP, Provider Networks .... Cornelia Outten
Controller .... Kelli Swanson-Pico
Senior VP, Med & Case Mgnt/Product Development ...... Maureen Star
VP, Direct Medical Management .... Mary Romanchok
VP, Client Services .... Kathy Polenske
National Director, Superien Health Network .... Jen Dietch

COMPANY PROFILE:
Parent Company Name: Interplan Health Group (formerly IPACQ)
Doing Business As:
Year Founded: 1997   Federally Qualified: [ ]
Forprofit: [Y]   Not-For-Profit: [ ]
Model Type: Network
Accreditation: [ ] AAPPO [ ] JACHO [ ] NCQA [ ] URAC
Plan Type: PPO, EPO, PBM, UR
Primary Physicians: 191,084   Physician Specialists: 412,064
Hospitals: 4,903
Total Enrollment:
  2001: 0   2004: 0   2007: 0
  2002: 0   2005:
  2003: 485,886   2006:

SERVICE AREA:
Nationwide: Y
  NW;

TYPE OF COVERAGE:
Commercial: [Y] Individual: [ ] FEHBP: [ ] Indemnity: [ ]
Medicare: [ ] Medicaid: [ ] Supplemental Medicare: [ ]
Tricare   [ ]

SUPERIOR DENTAL CARE INC

6683 Centerville Business Pkwy
Dayton, OH 45459
Phone: 937-438-0283 Fax: 937-438-0288 Toll-Free: 800-762-3159
Web site: www.superiordental.com

MAILING ADDRESS:
SUPERIOR DENTAL CARE INC
6683 Centerville Business Pkwy
Dayton, OH 45459

KEY EXECUTIVES:
Chairman .... Richard W Portune, DDS
Executive VP, Chief Executive Officer .... Rebecca York
Controller .... Wendy Glover
Director of Sales & Service .... Traci Harrell
MIS Manager .... Neda Bahrani
Privacy Officer .... Bettina Imes
Manager/Dentist Relations/Member Services .... Bettina Imes
Director of Administration .... Jane Fullmer

COMPANY PROFILE:
Parent Company Name:
Doing Business As:
Year Founded: 1985   Federally Qualified: [N]
Forprofit: [Y]   Not-For-Profit: [ ]
Model Type: IPA
Accreditation: [ ] AAPPO [ ] JACHO [ ] NCQA [ ] URAC
Plan Type: Specialty HMO
Total Revenue: 2005:   23,012,938   2006:   26,229,980
Net Income   2005:   465,356   2006:   599,029
Total Enrollment:
  2001: 0   2004: 109,566   2007: 132,560
  2002: 0   2005: 1,198,930
  2003: 104,586   2006: 129,365
Medical Loss Ratio: 2005: 80.30   2006: 80.40
Administrative Expense Ratio: 2005:   2006:

SERVICE AREA:
Nationwide: N
  KY; OH;

TYPE OF COVERAGE:
Commercial: [Y] Individual: [ ] FEHBP: [ ] Indemnity: [ ]
Medicare: [ ] Medicaid: [ ] Supplemental Medicare: [ ]
Tricare   [ ]

PLAN BENEFITS:

Alternative Medicine:	[ ]	Behavioral Health:	[ ]
Chiropractic:	[ ]	Dental:	[X]
Home Care:	[ ]	Inpatient SNF:	[ ]
Long-Term Care:	[ ]	Pharm. Mail Order:	[ ]
Physical Therapy:	[ ]	Podiatry:	[ ]
Psychiatric:	[ ]	Transplant:	[ ]
Vision:	[ ]	Wellness:	[ ]
Workers' Comp:	[ ]		

Other Benefits:
Comments:
  Changed company name in 2006 from Superior Dental Health Inc. to Superior Dental Health Alliance.

UDC OHIO INC

312 Elm St Ste 1500
Cincinnati, OH 45202
Phone: 513-621-1924 Fax: 513-621-4553 Toll-Free: 800-543-7266
Web site: www.assurantemployeebenefits.com

MAILING ADDRESS:
UDC OHIO INC
312 Elm St Ste 1500
Cincinnati, OH 45202

KEY EXECUTIVES:
President .... James R Gimarelli, Jr
VP, Treasurer .... Stacia N Almquist

COMPANY PROFILE:
Parent Company Name: Assurant Employee Benefits
Doing Business As:
Year Founded: 1986   Federally Qualified: [ ]
Forprofit: [Y]   Not-For-Profit: [ ]
Model Type:
Accreditation: [ ] AAPPO [ ] JACHO [ ] NCQA [ ] URAC
Plan Type: Specialty HMO
Total Revenue: 2005:   2,094,208   2006:   1,595,041
Net Income   2005:   125,984   2006:   47,781

OHIO

MAILING ADDRESS:
PRIMETIME HEALTH PLAN
PO Box 6905
Canton, OH 44706

KEY EXECUTIVES:
Chief Executive Officer .... Rick L Haines
Chief Financial Officer .... George Film
Medical Director .... Gregory Haban, MD

COMPANY PROFILE:
Parent Company Name: Aultman
Doing Business As: Primetime Health Plan
Year Founded: Federally Qualified: [ ]
Forprofit: [ ]   Not-For-Profit: [ ]
Model Type:
Accreditation: [ ] AAPPO [ ] JACHO [ ] NCQA [ ] URAC
Plan Type: HMO
Total Enrollment:
   2001: 0   2004: 45,377   2007: 0
   2002: 30,031   2005:
   2003: 36,561   2006:

SERVICE AREA:
Nationwide:
   OH;

PRODUCTS OFFERED:
Product Name: Type:
Primetime Health Plan Medicare   Medicare Advantage

SUMMACARE INC

10 N Main St
Akron, OH 44308
Phone: 330-996-8410 Fax: 330-996-8454 Toll-Free: 800-996-8411
Web site: www.summacare.com

MAILING ADDRESS:
SUMMACARE INC
PO Box 3620
Akron, OH 44308

KEY EXECUTIVES:
Chief Executive Officer/President .... Martin Hauser
Chief Medical Officer .... Teresa Koening, MD
Director, Pharmacy .... Tim Colligan
Chief Information Officer .... Mark Robinson
Sr VP Chief Operating Officer .... Claude Vincenti
VP of Sales & Marketing .... Tracy Kimaitas
Director, Technical Services .... Norman Tipton
VP, Sales & Marketing .... Kevin Cavalier
VP, Operations & Network Development .... Anne Armao
VP, Health Services .... Nancy Markle
Human Resources Manager .... Andrea Verroca
VP, Corporate Services .... Judith Marco
VP, Sales & Marketing .... Kevin Cavalier

COMPANY PROFILE:
Parent Company Name: Summa Health System
Doing Business As: SummaCare, Inc
Year Founded: 1993   Federally Qualified: [N]
Forprofit: [Y]   Not-For-Profit: [ ]
Model Type: IPA
Accreditation: [ ] AAPPO [ ] JACHO [ ] NCQA [ ] URAC
Plan Type: HMO, PPO, POS, ASO, EPO, TPA, UR, HDHP, HSA
Primary Physicians: 1,400   Physician Specialists: 3,348
Hospitals: 46
Total Revenue: 2005:   262,900,000   2006:   118,500,000
Net Income   2005:   32,800,000   2006:   7,300,000
Total Enrollment:
   2001: 86,296   2004: 134,413   2007: 115,000
   2002: 102,023   2005: 133,430
   2003: 95,364   2006: 94,500
Medical Loss Ratio: 2005: 87.00   2006: 85.00
Administrative Expense Ratio: 2005:   2006:

SERVICE AREA:
Nationwide: N
   OH (Ashtabula, Carroll, Cuyahoga, Erie, Geauga, Huron, Lorain, Mahoning, Medina, Ottawa, Portage, Sandnsky, Stark, Summit, Trumbell, Tuscawaras, Wayne);

TYPE OF COVERAGE:
Commercial: [Y] Individual: [ ] FEHBP: [ ] Indemnity: [ ]
Medicare: [Y] Medicaid: [Y] Supplemental Medicare: [Y]
Tricare   [ ]

PRODUCTS OFFERED:
Product Name: Type:
Summacare Secure   Medicare
Summacare   Medicaid
SummaCare Secure   Medicare Advantage

CONSUMER-DRIVEN PRODUCTS
MSAver Resources, LLC   HSA Company
MSAver HSA   HSA Product
MSAver Resources, LLC   HSA Administrator
                                Consumer-Driven Health Plan
PPO HDHP   High Deductible Health Plan

PLAN BENEFITS:
Alternative Medicine: [ ]   Behavioral Health: [ ]
Chiropractic: [X]   Dental: [ ]
Home Care: [X]   Inpatient SNF: [X]
Long-Term Care: [X]   Pharm. Mail Order: [X]
Physical Therapy: [X]   Podiatry: [X]
Psychiatric: [X]   Transplant: [X]
Vision: [X]   Wellness: [X]
Workers' Comp: [ ]
Other Benefits:

SUPERMED NETWORK

2060 East Ninth Street
Cleveland, OH 44115-1355
Phone: 216-687-7000 Fax: 216-687-7274 Toll-Free: 800-700-2583
Web site: www.supermednetwork.com

MAILING ADDRESS:
SUPERMED NETWORK
2060 East Ninth Street
Cleveland, OH 44115-1355

KEY EXECUTIVES:
Chairman of the Board .... Kent W Clapp
Chief Executive Officer/President .... Kent W Clapp
Chief Financial Officer .... Susan Tyler
Medical Director .... Robert Rzewnicki, MD
Chief Marketing Officer .... Errol D Brick
VP, Corporate Communications .... Jared P Chaney
Director, Provider Services/Network/Contracts .... Michael Taddeo
Fraud Prevention/Investigation .... John Dorrell

COMPANY PROFILE:
Parent Company Name: Medical Mutual of Ohio
Doing Business As: Super Med
Year Founded: 1994   Federally Qualified: [N]
Forprofit: [ ]   Not-For-Profit: [Y]
Model Type: MIXED
Accreditation: [ ] AAPPO [ ] JACHO [X] NCQA [X] URAC
Plan Type: PPO
Primary Physicians: 19,250   Physician Specialists: 13,926
Hospitals: 208
Total Revenue: 2005: 1,754,802,929   2006: 1,916,061,473
Net Income   2005:   58,071,532   2006:   91,077,056
Total Enrollment:
   2001: 0   2004: 1,1723,124   2007: 1,122,787
   2002: 0   2005: 1,183,946
   2003: 1,222,173   2006: 1,158,266
Medical Loss Ratio: 2005: 82.60   2006: 80.80
Administrative Expense Ratio: 2005:   2006:

SERVICE AREA:
Nationwide: N
   OH (Northeast; Cleveland, Akron, Youngstown areas);

TYPE OF COVERAGE:
Commercial: [Y] Individual: [Y] FEHBP: [ ] Indemnity: [ ]
Medicare: [ ] Medicaid: [Y] Supplemental Medicare: [ ]
Tricare   [ ]

Managed Care Organization Profiles — OHIO

SERVICE AREA:
Nationwide: N
OH; (Adams, Allen, Ashland, Athens, Belmont, Carroll, Champaign, Clark, Coshocton, Crawford, Delaware, Fairfield, Fayette, Franklin, Gallia, Guemsey, Hancock, Hardin, Harrison, Highland, Hocking, Huron, Jackson, Knox, Lawrence, Licking, Logan, Madison, Marion, Meigs, Monroe, Morgan, Muskingum, Noble, Perry, Pickaway, Pike, Richland, Ross, Scioto, Tuscarawas, Union, Vinton, Washington, Wyandot),

TYPE OF COVERAGE:
Commercial: [Y] Individual: [ ] FEHBP: [ ] Indemnity: [ ]
Medicare: [Y] Medicaid: [ ] Supplemental Medicare: [ ]
Tricare   [ ]

PRODUCTS OFFERED:
Product Name:	Type:
Healthpledge	HMO
Healthpledge Plus	POS
Healthreach	PPO
Healthreach RX	PBN
Health Pact	PPO

PLAN BENEFITS:
Alternative Medicine: [ ]   Behavioral Health: [X]
Chiropractic: [X]   Dental: [X]
Home Care: [X]   Inpatient SNF: [ ]
Long-Term Care: [ ]   Pharm. Mail Order: [X]
Physical Therapy: [ ]   Podiatry: [X]
Psychiatric: [X]   Transplant: [X]
Vision: [ ]   Wellness: [X]
Workers' Comp: [ ]
Other Benefits:

Comments:
Formerly US Health Plan.

PARAMOUNT ADVANTAGE

1901 Indian Wood Circle
Maumee, OH 43537-4068
Phone: 419-887-2500 Fax: 419-887-2530 Toll-Free: 800-462-3589
Web site: www.paramounthealthcare.com

MAILING ADDRESS:
PARAMOUNT ADVANTAGE
1901 Indian Wood Circle
Maumee, OH 43537-4068

KEY EXECUTIVES:
Chief Executive Officer .... John C Randolph
Chief Financial Officer .... Gary Akenberger
Chief Medical Officer .... Neeraj Kanwal, MD
Chief Information Officer/Marketing Director .... Mark H Moser

COMPANY PROFILE:
Parent Company Name: ProMedica Health System
Doing Business As:
Year Founded: 2005   Federally Qualified: [N]
Forprofit: [ ]   Not-For-Profit: [ ]
Model Type:
Accreditation: [ ] AAPPO [ ] JACHO [X] NCQA [ ] URAC
Plan Type: HMO,
Total Revenue: 2005:   7,545,794   2006:   103,601,016
Net Income   2005:   -397,829   2006:   45,874
Total Enrollment:
  2001:   2004:   2007: 54,645
  2002:   2005: 39,890
  2003:   2006: 60,513
Medical Loss Ratio: 2005: 94.00   2006: 86.00
Administrative Expense Ratio: 2005:   2006:

SERVICE AREA:
Nationwide: N
OH (Allen, Ashland, Crawford, Defiance, Delaware, Erie, Fulton, Hancock, Hardin, Henry, Huron, Knox, Lorain, Lucas, Marion, Morrow, Ottawa, Paulding, Putnam, Richland, Sandusky, Seneca, Williams, Wood, Wyandot);

TYPE OF COVERAGE:
Commercial: [ ] Individual: [ ] FEHBP: [ ] Indemnity: [ ]
Medicare: [Y] Medicaid: [ ] Supplemental Medicare: [ ]
Tricare   [ ]

PRODUCTS OFFERED:
Product Name:	Type:
Paramount Advantage	Medicare Advantage

PLAN BENEFITS:
Alternative Medicine: [ ]   Behavioral Health: [X]
Chiropractic: [X]   Dental: [X]
Home Care: [ ]   Inpatient SNF: [ ]
Long-Term Care: [ ]   Pharm. Mail Order: [X]
Physical Therapy: [X]   Podiatry: [X]
Psychiatric: [X]   Transplant: [X]
Vision: [X]   Wellness: [X]
Workers' Comp: [X]
Other Benefits:

PARAMOUNT HEALTH CARE PLAN

1901 Indian Wood Circle
Maumee, OH 43537-4068
Phone: 419-887-2500 Fax: 419-887-2530 Toll-Free: 800-462-3589
Web site: www.paramounthealthcare.com

MAILING ADDRESS:
PARAMOUNT HEALTH CARE PLAN
1901 Indian Wood Circle
Maumee, OH 43537-4068

KEY EXECUTIVES:
Chief Executive Officer .... John C Randolph
Chief Financial Officer .... Gary Akenberger
Chief Medical Officer .... Neeraj Kanwal, MD
Chief Information Officer/Marketing Director .... Mark H Moser

COMPANY PROFILE:
Parent Company Name: ProMedica Health System
Doing Business As:
Year Founded: 1988   Federally Qualified: [N]
Forprofit: [Y]   Not-For-Profit: [ ]
Model Type: IPA
Accreditation: [ ] AAPPO [ ] JACHO [X] NCQA [ ] URAC
Plan Type: HMO, PPO, UR, POS, TPA
Total Revenue: 2005:   475,376,918   2006:   420,072,730
Net Income   2005:   8,177,095   2006:   14,963,1814
Total Enrollment:
  2001: 161,224   2004: 154,336   2007: 81,845
  2002: 170,991   2005: 100,821
  2003: 146,617   2006: 92,240
Medical Loss Ratio: 2005: 91.00   2006: 88.00
Administrative Expense Ratio: 2005:   2006:

SERVICE AREA:
Nationwide: N
OH (Allen, Ashland, Crawford, Defiance, Delaware, Erie, Fulton, Hancock, Hardin, Henry, Huron, Knox, Lorain, Lucas, Marion, Morrow, Ottawa, Paulding, Putnam, Richland, Sandusky, Seneca, Williams, Wood, Wyandot);

TYPE OF COVERAGE:
Commercial: [Y] Individual: [Y] FEHBP: [ ] Indemnity: [ ]
Medicare: [Y] Medicaid: [Y]   Supplemental Medicare: [ ]
Tricare   [ ]

PRODUCTS OFFERED:
Product Name:	Type:
Paramount Elite	Medicare
Paramount Health Care	Medicaid
Paramount Standard Plan	Medicare Advantage

PLAN BENEFITS:
Alternative Medicine: [ ]   Behavioral Health: [X]
Chiropractic: [X]   Dental: [X]
Home Care: [ ]   Inpatient SNF: [X]
Long-Term Care: [ ]   Pharm. Mail Order: [X]
Physical Therapy: [X]   Podiatry: [X]
Psychiatric: [X]   Transplant: [X]
Vision: [X]   Wellness: [X]
Workers' Comp: [X]
Other Benefits:

PRIMETIME HEALTH PLAN

2600 6th St SW
Canton, OH 44710
Phone: 330-438-6360 Fax: 330-438-2911 Toll-Free:
Web site: www.aultman.com

OHIO

OHIO HEALTH CHOICE

168 E Main St
Akron, OH 44309
Phone: 330-996-8200 Fax: 330-996-8201 Toll-Free: 800-554-0027
Web site: www.ohiohealthchoice.com

MAILING ADDRESS:
OHIO HEALTH CHOICE
PO Box 2090
Akron, OH 44309-2090

KEY EXECUTIVES:
President .... Bryan Kennedy

COMPANY PROFILE:
Parent Company Name: Summa Health Systems, Mercy Medical Ctr
Doing Business As: Ohio Health Choice
Year Founded: 1982   Federally Qualified: [ ]
Forprofit: [Y]   Not-For-Profit: [ ]
Model Type:
Accreditation: [ ] AAPPO [ ] JACHO [ ] NCQA [X] URAC
Plan Type: PPO, POS, EPO, UR
Primary Physicians: 28,000   Physician Specialists:
Hospitals: 199
Total Enrollment:
  2001: 0   2004: 0   2007: 370,000
  2002: 0   2005:
  2003: 370,000   2006:

SERVICE AREA:
Nationwide: N
  OH;

TYPE OF COVERAGE:
Commercial: [ ] Individual: [Y] FEHBP: [ ] Indemnity: [ ]
Medicare: [ ] Medicaid: [ ] Supplemental Medicare: [ ]
Tricare   [ ]

PRODUCTS OFFERED:
Product Name: Type:
Ohio Health Choice PPO Network   PPO
Accessible Health Alliance   Indemnity
Ohio Health Choice Workers Com   Workers' Comp
Ohio Health Choice EPO   EPO

OHIO KEPRO INC

5700 Lombardo Center Dr
Seven Hills, OH 44131
Phone: 216-447-9604 Fax: 216-447-7925 Toll-Free:
Web site: www.ohiokeproinc.com

MAILING ADDRESS:
OHIO KEPRO INC
5700 Lombardo Center Dr
Seven Hills, OH 44131

KEY EXECUTIVES:
Director, Ohio Operations .... Gayle Smith
Medical Director .... Alice Stollenwerk Petrulis, MD
Project Director, Ohio Operations .... Meghan Harris, MS
Director, Community Based Services . Betty Pilous, RN, MHSA, CPHQ
Medical Director, Quality Improvement .... Ronald A Savrin, MD
Director, Acute Care/HPMP .... Rita Bowling, RN, MSN, MBA, CPHQ

COMPANY PROFILE:
Parent Company Name: Keyston Peer Review, Harrisburg, PA
Doing Business As:
Year Founded: 1999   Federally Qualified: [ ]
Forprofit: [Y]   Not-For-Profit: [ ]
Model Type:
Accreditation: [ ] AAPPO [ ] JACHO [ ] NCQA [ ] URAC
Plan Type: PRO

SERVICE AREA:
Nationwide: N
  OH;

OHIO STATE UNIVERSITY MANAGED HEALTH CARE SYSTEMS INC

700 Ackerman Rd Ste 580
Columbus, OH 43202
Phone: 614-292-4700 Fax: 614-292-1166 Toll-Free: 800-678-6269
Web site: www.osumhcs.com

MAILING ADDRESS:
OH STATE UNIV MANAGED HEALTH CARE SYSTEMS
700 Ackerman Rd Ste 580
Columbus, OH 43202

KEY EXECUTIVES:
Chief Executive Officer/Executive Director .... Scott Streator
President .... Fred Sanfilippo, MD, PhD
Director, Information Technology & Finance .... Tom VonderBrink
Interim Medical Director .... Glen Aukerman, MD
Pharmacy Benefit Manager .... Brian Lehman
Associate Executive Director .... Judy Kadja
Communication Manager .... Joni Bentz Seal
Credentialing Coordinator .... Tamara Tuttle
Director Provider Relations .... Maureen Cahill
Medical Director Wellness Program .... Stephanie Cook, DO
Director Medical Management .... Lorena Owings, RN
Quality Improvement Manager/Compliance Officer .... Kim Kivimaki
Credentialing Coordinator .... Tamara Tuttle

COMPANY PROFILE:
Parent Company Name: The Ohio State University
Doing Business As: OSU Managed Health Care Systems Inc
Year Founded: 1991   Federally Qualified: [N]
Forprofit: [ ]   Not-For-Profit: [Y]
Model Type:
Accreditation: [ ] AAPPO [ ] JACHO [ ] NCQA [ ] URAC
Plan Type: PPO, EPO

SERVICE AREA:
Nationwide: N
  OH;

TYPE OF COVERAGE:
Commercial: [Y] Individual: [ ] FEHBP: [ ] Indemnity: [ ]
Medicare: [ ] Medicaid: [ ] Supplemental Medicare: [ ]
Tricare   [ ]

PRODUCTS OFFERED:
Product Name: Type:
University Prime Care   EPO
OSU Health Plan   PPO

PLAN BENEFITS:
Alternative Medicine: [X]   Behavioral Health: [X]
Chiropractic: [X]   Dental: [ ]
Home Care: [X]   Inpatient SNF: [X]
Long-Term Care: [ ]   Pharm. Mail Order: [X]
Physical Therapy: [X]   Podiatry: [X]
Psychiatric: [X]   Transplant: [X]
Vision: [ ]   Wellness: [X]
Workers' Comp: [ ]
Other Benefits:

OHIOHEALTH GROUP

445 Hutchinson Ave Ste 300
Columbus, OH 43235
Phone: 614-566-0123 Fax: 614-566-0400 Toll-Free: 800-635-7207
Web site: www.ohiohealthgroup.com

MAILING ADDRESS:
OHIOHEALTH GROUP
445 Hutchinson Ave Ste 300
Columbus, OH 43235

KEY EXECUTIVES:
Chief Executive Officer .... Thomas Thompson
Medical Director .... Bruce Wall, MD
Pharmacy Director .... Eileen Murphy
Chief Operating Officer .... Kathy Savenko
MIS Director .... Morgan Jackson

COMPANY PROFILE:
Parent Company Name: OhioHealth Corp & Medical Group of OH
Doing Business As:
Year Founded: 1981   Federally Qualified: [N]
Forprofit: [Y]   Not-For-Profit: [ ]
Model Type: IPA
Accreditation: [ ] AAPPO [ ] JACHO [ ] NCQA [ ] URAC
Plan Type: PPO, UR, PBM
Total Enrollment:
  2001: 0   2004: 0   2007: 0
  2002: 0   2005:
  2003: 42,159   2006:

Managed Care Organization Profiles — OHIO

Primary Physicians: 1,481   Physician Specialists: 4,861
Hospitals: 83
Total Revenue: 2005:   38,396   2006:   94,148,037
Net Income   2005:   -994,814   2006:   -3,845,229
Total Enrollment:
   2001: 0   2004: 0   2007: 137,726
   2002: 0   2005: 215
   2003: 0   2006: 76,390
Medical Loss Ratio: 2005: 94.00   2006: 89.20
Administrative Expense Ratio: 2005:   2006:

SERVICE AREA:
Nationwide: N
   OH;

TYPE OF COVERAGE:
Commercial: [ ]   Individual: [ ]   FEHBP: [ ]   Indemnity: [ ]
Medicare: [ ]   Medicaid: [Y]   Supplemental Medicare: [ ]
Tricare [ ]

PLAN BENEFITS:
Alternative Medicine: [ ]   Behavioral Health: [ ]
Chiropractic: [X]   Dental: [ ]
Home Care: [X]   Inpatient SNF: [X]
Long-Term Care: [ ]   Pharm. Mail Order: [X]
Physical Therapy: [X]   Podiatry: [X]
Psychiatric: [X]   Transplant: [ ]
Vision: [ ]   Wellness: [ ]
Workers' Comp: [ ]
Other Benefits:

MOUNT CARMEL HEALTH PLAN

6150 E Broad St Ste EE 320
Columbus, OH 43213
Phone: 614-546-3152   Fax: 614-546-3131   Toll-Free: 800-255-0726
Web site: www.medigold.com

MAILING ADDRESS:
    MOUNT CARMEL HEALTH PLAN
    6150 E Broad St Ste EE 320
    Columbus, OH 43213

KEY EXECUTIVES:
Chief Executive Officer .... Mark Richardson
Chief Financial Officer .... Veronica Szydlowski
Medical Director .... Greg Wise, MD
Chief Operating Officer .... Veronica Szydlowski
Marketing Director .... Doug Alfred
Director of Managed Care Information Systems .... Jim Armstrong
Director, Provider Services .... Marisa Dennis
Senior Director Medical Management .... Karen Allenbach
Compliance Officer .... Jen Calder

COMPANY PROFILE:
Parent Company Name: Mount Carmel Health System
Doing Business As:
Year Founded: 1996   Federally Qualified: [N]
Forprofit: [N]   Not-For-Profit: [Y]
Model Type: IPA
Accreditation: [ ] AAPPO [ ] JACHO [ ] NCQA [ ] URAC
Plan Type: HMO
Primary Physicians: 500   Physician Specialists: 1,000
Hospitals: 10
Total Revenue: 2005:   165,793,343   2006:   223,150,070
Net Income   2005:   11,375,680   2006:   28,399,728
Total Enrollment:
   2001: 18,008   2004: 17,023   2007: 21,776
   2002: 15,384   2005: 19,055
   2003: 15,393   2006: 20,473
Medical Loss Ratio: 2005: 84.90   2006: 78.95
Administrative Expense Ratio: 2005:   2006:

SERVICE AREA:
Nationwide: N
   OH (Clark, Delaware, Franklin, Fairfield, Fayette, Greene, Knox, Licking, Madison, Montgomery, Pickaway, Ross, Union);

TYPE OF COVERAGE:
Commercial: [ ]   Individual: [ ]   FEHBP: [ ]   Indemnity: [ ]
Medicare: [Y]   Medicaid: [ ]   Supplemental Medicare: [ ]
Tricare [ ]

PRODUCTS OFFERED:
Product Name: Type:
MediGold   Medicare

PLAN BENEFITS:
Alternative Medicine: [ ]   Behavioral Health: [X]
Chiropractic: [ ]   Dental: [X]
Home Care: [X]   Inpatient SNF: [X]
Long-Term Care: [ ]   Pharm. Mail Order: [X]
Physical Therapy: [X]   Podiatry: [ ]
Psychiatric: [X]   Transplant: [X]
Vision: [X]   Wellness: [X]
Workers' Comp: [ ]
Other Benefits:

NATIONWIDE HEALTH PLANS

5525 Park Center Circle
Columbus, OH 43017-3685
Phone: 614-854-3001   Fax: 614-854-3648   Toll-Free: 800-826-9017
Web site: www.nationwidehealthplans.com

MAILING ADDRESS:
    NATIONWIDE HEALTH PLANS
    5525 Park Center Circle
    Columbus, OH 43017-3685

KEY EXECUTIVES:
Chief Executive Officer .... Joe SanFilippo
Chief Financial Officer .... Jeff McDaniel
Medical Director .... Glen Ackermen, MD
Chief Operating Officer .... Susan Hatfield
Marketing Director .... Mike Medwid
MIS Director .... Karen Cairo
Network/Contracts Officer .... Barbara Hyre

COMPANY PROFILE:
Parent Company Name: Nationwide Life Insurance
Doing Business As:
Year Founded: 1985   Federally Qualified: [N]
Forprofit: [Y]   Not-For-Profit: [ ]
Model Type: IPA
Accreditation: [ ] AAPPO [ ] JACHO [X] NCQA [X] URAC
Plan Type: HMO, PPO, POS, UR, ASO, HSA
Total Enrollment:
   2001: 15,886   2004: 0   2007: 0
   2002: 0   2005:
   2003: 80,000   2006:

SERVICE AREA:
Nationwide: N
   OH; (Adams, Allen, Ashland, Ashtabula, Auglaize, Butler, Brown, Carroll, Champaign, Clermont, Clinton, Clark, Columbiana, Coshocton, Crawford, Cuyahoga, Delaware, Darke, Erie, Fairfield, Fayette, Franklin, Fulton, Gallia, Geauga, Greene, Guernsey, Hamilton, Hancock, Hardin, Henry, Highland, Hocking, Holmes, Huron, Jackson, Knox, Lake, Lawrence, Licking, Logan, Lorain, Lucas, Madison, Mahoning, Marion, Medina, Meigs, Miami, Montgomery, Morgan, Morrow, Muskingum, Noble, Ottawa, Perry, Pickaway, Pike, Portage, Preble, Putnam, Richland, Ross, Sandusky, Scioto, Seneca, Shelby, Stark, Summit, Union, Trunbell, Tuscarawas, Vinton, Warren, Wayne, Wood, Wyandot); CA;

TYPE OF COVERAGE:
Commercial: [Y]   Individual: [Y]   FEHBP: [ ]   Indemnity: [ ]
Medicare: [Y]   Medicaid: [ ]   Supplemental Medicare: [ ]
Tricare [ ]

CONSUMER-DRIVEN PRODUCTS
My Health 2 HSA   HSA Company
    HSA Product
    HSA Administrator
    Consumer-Driven Health Plan
My Health 2   High Deductible Health Plan

PLAN BENEFITS:
Alternative Medicine: [ ]   Behavioral Health: [X]
Chiropractic: [X]   Dental: [X]
Home Care: [X]   Inpatient SNF: [ ]
Long-Term Care: [ ]   Pharm. Mail Order: [X]
Physical Therapy: [ ]   Podiatry: [X]
Psychiatric: [X]   Transplant: [X]
Vision: [X]   Wellness: [X]
Workers' Comp: [X]
Other Benefits:

OHIO
Managed Care Organization Profiles

COMPANY PROFILE:
Parent Company Name:
Doing Business As:
Year Founded: 1987   Federally Qualified: [ ]
Forprofit: [Y]   Not-For-Profit: [ ]
Model Type: NETWORK
Accreditation: [ ] AAPPO [ ] JACHO [ ] NCQA [X] URAC
Plan Type: UR, TPA, PRO
SERVICE AREA:
Nationwide: Y
 NW;

MEDICAL MUTUAL OF OHIO

2060 East 9th St
Cleveland, OH 44115
Phone: 216-687-7000 Fax: 216-687-6164 Toll-Free: 800-700-2583
Web site: www.mmoh.com
MAILING ADDRESS:
 MEDICAL MUTUAL OF OHIO
 2060 East 9th St
 Cleveland, OH 44115

KEY EXECUTIVES:
Chairman of the Board .... Kent W Clapp
Chief Executive Officer/President .... Kent W Clapp
Executive VP, Chief Financial Officer .... Susan M Tyler
Medical Director .... Robert Rzewnicki, MD
Executive VP IS, President AMS .... Kenneth Sidon
Chief Marketing Officer .... Errol D Brick
VP, ET Development & Management Innovation .... Paul B Apostle
VP, National Network Development .... Michael Taddeo
Corp Counsel & VP Legal Affair .... John Dorrell
Chief Communications Officer .... Jared P Chaney
VP, Human Resources .... Thomas E Greene
VP, Care Management .... Paula M Sauer
Executive VP, Statewide Operations .... Linda Johnson
Executive VP & Executive Assistant to President .... Joseph C Krysh

COMPANY PROFILE:
Parent Company Name:
Doing Business As:
Year Founded: 1934   Federally Qualified: [Y]
Forprofit: [ ]   Not-For-Profit: [Y]
Model Type: MIXED
Accreditation: [ ] AAPPO [ ] JACHO [X] NCQA [X] URAC
Plan Type: HMO, PPO, POS, CDHP, HDHP, HSA,
Total Revenue: 2005: 1,754,802,929   2006: 2,000,000,000
Net Income   2005: 58,071,532   2006:
Total Enrollment:
 2001: 0   2004: 1,173,124   2007: 3,900,000
 2002: 66,635   2005: 1,183,946
 2003: 1,222,173 2006:
Medical Loss Ratio: 2005: 82.60   2006:
Administrative Expense Ratio: 2005:   2006:
SERVICE AREA:
Nationwide: N
 OH;
TYPE OF COVERAGE:
Commercial: [Y] Individual: [Y] FEHBP: [ ] Indemnity: [ ]
Medicare: [Y] Medicaid: [ ] Supplemental Medicare: [Y]
Tricare   [ ]
PRODUCTS OFFERED:
Product Name:	Type:
Traditional	Traditional Indemnit
Supermed Classic	Hospital Network
Supermed Plus	PPO
Supermed Select	POS
Supermed HMO	HMOHMO Health Ohio
HMO	
Supermed Works	Workers' Comp

CONSUMER-DRIVEN PRODUCTS
National City Corporation	HSA Company
SuperMed HSA	HSA Product
MSAver	HSA Administrator
	Consumer-Driven Health Plan
	High Deductible Health Plan

PLAN BENEFITS:
Alternative Medicine:	[ ]	Behavioral Health:	[ ]
Chiropractic:	[ ]	Dental:	[X]
Home Care:	[X]	Inpatient SNF:	[X]
Long-Term Care:	[ ]	Pharm. Mail Order:	[X]
Physical Therapy:	[X]	Podiatry:	[ ]
Psychiatric:	[X]	Transplant:	[ ]
Vision:	[X]	Wellness:	[X]
Workers' Comp:	[X]		

Other Benefits:

MERITAIN HEALTH

19800 Detroit Rd
Cleveland, OH 44116
Phone: 440-356-8212 Fax: 440-356-0140 Toll-Free: 800-356-6226
Web site: www.meritain.com
MAILING ADDRESS:
 MERITAIN HEALTH
 19800 Detroit Rd
 Cleveland, OH 44116

KEY EXECUTIVES:
Chairman .... Jacob L Canova
Chief Executive Officer/President .... Jacob L Canova
Sr VP, Finance/Controller .... Vincent DiMura, CPA
Chief Medical Officer .... Larry J Luter, MD, FAAFP
President, National Sales .... Richard Bukovinsky

COMPANY PROFILE:
Parent Company Name: North American Benefits Network Inc
Doing Business As: Gateway Health Management Services
Year Founded: 1962   Federally Qualified: [ ]
Forprofit: [Y]   Not-For-Profit: [ ]
Model Type: MIXED
Accreditation: [ ] AAPPO [ ] JACHO [ ] NCQA [X] URAC
Plan Type: Specialty HMO, TPA, UR, HSA
SERVICE AREA:
Nationwide: N
 OH;
PLAN BENEFITS:
Alternative Medicine:	[ ]	Behavioral Health:	[X]
Chiropractic:	[X]	Dental:	[X]
Home Care:	[ ]	Inpatient SNF:	[ ]
Long-Term Care:	[ ]	Pharm. Mail Order:	[X]
Physical Therapy:	[ ]	Podiatry:	[X]
Psychiatric:	[X]	Transplant:	[X]
Vision:	[X]	Wellness:	[X]
Workers' Comp:	[ ]		

Other Benefits:

MOLINA HEALTHCARE OF OHIO INC

8101 N High St Ste 210
Columbus, OH 43235
Phone: 614-781-4300 Fax: 614-781-1410 Toll-Free:
Web site: www.molinahealthcare.com
MAILING ADDRESS:
 MOLINA HEALTHCARE OF OHIO INC
 8101 N High St Ste 210
 Columbus, OH 43235

KEY EXECUTIVES:
President .... Kathy Mancini
Chief Operating Officer .... Amy Schultz Clubbs
Chief Financial Officer .... Ernest E Humbert
Chief Medical Officer .... Kevin Smith, MD, MBA

COMPANY PROFILE:
Parent Company Name: Molina Healthcare Inc
Doing Business As:
Year Founded: 2005   Federally Qualified: [N]
Forprofit: [Y]   Not-For-Profit: [ ]
Model Type:
Accreditation: [ ] AAPPO [ ] JACHO [ ] NCQA [ ] URAC
Plan Type: HMO,

Managed Care Organization Profiles — OHIO

INTEGRA GROUP

16 Triangle Park Dr Ste 1600
Cincinnati, OH 45246
Phone: 513-326-5600 Fax: 513-326-5614 Toll-Free: 800-424-8384
Web site: www.integragrp.com

MAILING ADDRESS:
   INTEGRA GROUP
   16 Triangle Park Dr Ste 1600
   Cincinnati, OH 45246

KEY EXECUTIVES:
President .... Kathleen J Lutz
Director Information Systems .... Mark Warner
Manager Administrative Support .... Janet Theado
Manager Customer Service .... Melissa Fookes

COMPANY PROFILE:
Parent Company Name: Integra Group
Doing Business As:
Year Founded: 1988   Federally Qualified: [ ]
Forprofit: [Y]   Not-For-Profit: [ ]
Model Type: NETWORK
Accreditation: [ ] AAPPO [ ] JACHO [ ] NCQA [ ] URAC
Plan Type: PPO, UR
Total Enrollment:
   2001: 1,077,067   2004: 0   2007: 0
   2002: 0   2005:
   2003: 0   2006:

SERVICE AREA:
Nationwide: Y
   NW;

TYPE OF COVERAGE:
Commercial: [Y] Individual: [ ] FEHBP: [ ] Indemnity: [ ]
Medicare: [ ] Medicaid: [ ] Supplemental Medicare: [ ]
Tricare [ ]

PRODUCTS OFFERED:
Product Name: Type:
Integra Home   PPO

PLAN BENEFITS:
Alternative Medicine: [ ]   Behavioral Health: [ ]
Chiropractic: [ ]   Dental: [ ]
Home Care: [ ]   Inpatient SNF: [ ]
Long-Term Care: [ ]   Pharm. Mail Order: [ ]
Physical Therapy: [ ]   Podiatry: [ ]
Psychiatric: [ ]   Transplant: [ ]
Vision: [ ]   Wellness: [ ]
Workers' Comp: [ ]
Other Benefits: Ancillary Home Health

JP FARLEY CORP

29055 Clemens Rd
Westlake, OH 44145
Phone: 440-250-4300 Fax: 440-250-4301 Toll-Free: 800-634-0173
Web site: www.jpfarley.com

MAILING ADDRESS:
   JP FARLEY CORP
   29055 Clemens Rd
   Westlake, OH 44145

KEY EXECUTIVES:
Chief Executive Officer/President .... James P Farley
Chief Financial Officer .... Robert Bernath, CPA
VP, Director of Account Mngmnt/Sales .... Patricia Hannigan-Farley
Client Services .... Beth Whelan
Director of Information Systems .... Rob Moeller
Director of Operations .... Tim Catron
Utilization Management .... Pam Queen

COMPANY PROFILE:
Parent Company Name:
Doing Business As:
Year Founded: 1979   Federally Qualified: [ ]
Forprofit: [Y]   Not-For-Profit: [ ]
Model Type:
Accreditation: [ ] AAPPO [ ] JACHO [ ] NCQA [ ] URAC
Plan Type: UR, TPA, PBM

KAISER FOUNDATION HEALTH PLAN OF OHIO

1001 Lakeside Ave Ste 1200
Cleveland, OH 44114
Phone: 216-621-5600 Fax: 216-623-8776 Toll-Free: 800-524-7371
Web site: www.kaiserpermanente.com

MAILING ADDRESS:
   KAISER FOUNDATION HLTH PLN-OH
   1001 Lakeside Ave Ste 1200
   Cleveland, OH 44114

KEY EXECUTIVES:
Regional Chief Executive Officer .... Patricia Kennedy-Scott
Executive VP, Chief Financial Officer .... Kathy Lancaster
Executive VP, Health Plan Operations .... Arthur M Southarn, MD

COMPANY PROFILE:
Parent Company Name: Kaiser Permanente
Doing Business As:
Year Founded: 1964   Federally Qualified: [Y]
Forprofit: [ ]   Not-For-Profit: [Y]
Model Type: GROUP
Accreditation: [ ] AAPPO [ ] JACHO [X] NCQA [ ] URAC
Plan Type: HMO, POS, HDHP, HSA
Total Revenue: 2005: 500,304,331   2006: 545,582,445
Net Income   2005: -31,046,035   2006: -18,488,585
Total Enrollment:
   2001: 170,830   2004: 143,645   2007: 147,393
   2002: 158,322   2005: 145,962
   2003: 145,767   2006: 149,745
Medical Loss Ratio: 2005: 97.90   2006: 96.50
Administrative Expense Ratio: 2005:   2006:

SERVICE AREA:
Nationwide: N
   OH (Northeastern);

TYPE OF COVERAGE:
Commercial: [Y] Individual: [Y] FEHBP: [ ] Indemnity: [ ]
Medicare: [Y] Medicaid: [ ] Supplemental Medicare: [ ]
Tricare [ ]

PRODUCTS OFFERED:
Product Name: Type:
Kaiser Medicare Plus   Medicare
Kaiser HMO   HMO
Medicare Plus II   Medicare Advantage

PLAN BENEFITS:
Alternative Medicine: [ ]   Behavioral Health: [X]
Chiropractic: [ ]   Dental: [ ]
Home Care: [X]   Inpatient SNF: [X]
Long-Term Care: [X]   Pharm. Mail Order: [X]
Physical Therapy: [X]   Podiatry: [X]
Psychiatric: [X]   Transplant: [X]
Vision: [X]   Wellness: [X]
Workers' Comp: [X]
Other Benefits:

MED-VALU INC

3962-C Brown Park Dr
Hilliard, OH 43026
Phone: 614-684-2364 Fax: 614-684-2361 Toll-Free: 800-447-3459
Web site: www.medvalu.com

MAILING ADDRESS:
   MED-VALU INC
   3962-C Brown Park Dr
   Hilliard, OH 43026

KEY EXECUTIVES:
Chief Executive Officer/President .... Michael Linde
Chief Financial Officer .... David O'Brien
Chief Medical Officer .... Albert Scheff, MD
VP, Sales & Marketing .... Lynda Davis
Information Systems .... Laurie Peck
Human Resources Director .... Joan Estep
Quality Assurance Administrator .... Anita O'Donnell, RN
Director of Nursing .... Jeannette Hopkins

OHIO

Total Revenue: 2005: 93,647,088 2006: 26,743,549
Net Income 2005: 11,046,406 2006: 6,742,409
Total Enrollment:
 2001: 50,550 2004: 22,057 2007: 20,113
 2002: 84,000 2005: 20,475
 2003: 25,845 2006: 380,000
SERVICE AREA:
Nationwide: N
 OH (Ashland, Carroll, Columbiana, Coshocton, Cuyahoga, Geauga, Guernsey, Harrison, Holmes, Knox, Lorain, Mahoning, Medina, Muskingum, Portage, Richland, Stark, Summit, Trumbull, Tuscarawas, Wayne);
TYPE OF COVERAGE:
Commercial: [Y] Individual: [Y] FEHBP: [ ] Indemnity: [ ]
Medicare: [ ] Medicaid: [ ] Supplemental Medicare: [Y]
Tricare [ ]
PRODUCTS OFFERED:
Product Name: Type:
Hometown Securecare Medicare
Hometown HMO HMO
Hometown ASO ASO
PLAN BENEFITS:
Alternative Medicine: [X] Behavioral Health: [X]
Chiropractic: [X] Dental: [X]
Home Care: [X] Inpatient SNF: [X]
Long-Term Care: [X] Pharm. Mail Order: [X]
Physical Therapy: [X] Podiatry: [X]
Psychiatric: [X] Transplant: [X]
Vision: [X] Wellness: [X]
Workers' Comp: [X]
Other Benefits:

HMO HEALTH OHIO (CLEVELAND)

2060 East Ninth Street
Cleveland, OH 44115-1355
Phone: 216-687-7000 Fax: 216-687-7274 Toll-Free: 800-700-2583
Web site: www.medmutual.com
MAILING ADDRESS:
 HMO HEALTH OHIO (CLEVELAND)
 2060 East Ninth Street
 Cleveland, OH 44115-1355
KEY EXECUTIVES:
Chairman of the Board .... Kent W Clapp
Chief Executive Officer/President .... Kent W Clapp
Chief Financial Officer .... Susan Tyler
Medical Director .... Robert Rzewnicki, MD
Chief Communication Officer .... Jared P Chaney
Chief Marketing Officer .... Errol D Brick
VP, Corporate Communications .... Jared Chaney
Director, Provider Services/Network/Contracts .... Michael Taddeo
Fraud Prevention Director .... John Dorrell
COMPANY PROFILE:
Parent Company Name: Medical Mutual of Ohio
Doing Business As: HMO Health Ohio
Year Founded: 1978 Federally Qualified: [N]
Forprofit: [ ] Not-For-Profit: [Y]
Model Type: MIXED
Accreditation: [ ] AAPPO [ ] JACHO [ ] NCQA [X] URAC
Plan Type: HMO, HDHP, HSA,
Hospitals: 173
Total Revenue: 2005: 91,938,045 2006: 92,809,670
Net Income 2005: 6,114,362 2006: 8,850,693
Total Enrollment:
 2001: 100,860 2004: 29,846 2007: 26,161
 2002: 59,579 2005: 22,328
 2003: 33,084 2006: 19,773
Medical Loss Ratio: 2005: 87.80 2006: 80.60
Administrative Expense Ratio: 2005: 2006:
SERVICE AREA:
Nationwide: N
 OH (Butler, Clark, Franklin, Greene, Hamilton, Montgomery, Pickaway);
TYPE OF COVERAGE:
Commercial: [Y] Individual: [Y] FEHBP: [ ] Indemnity: [ ]
Medicare: [ ] Medicaid: [Y] Supplemental Medicare: [Y]
Tricare [ ]

PRODUCTS OFFERED:
Product Name: Type:
HMO Health Medicaid
CONSUMER-DRIVEN PRODUCTS
  HSA Company
  HSA Product
National City Corporation HSA Administrator
  Consumer-Driven Health Plan
  High Deductible Health Plan
PLAN BENEFITS:
Alternative Medicine: [ ] Behavioral Health: [ ]
Chiropractic: [X] Dental: [X]
Home Care: [X] Inpatient SNF: [X]
Long-Term Care: [ ] Pharm. Mail Order: [X]
Physical Therapy: [X] Podiatry: [X]
Psychiatric: [X] Transplant: [X]
Vision: [X] Wellness: [X]
Workers' Comp: [ ]
Other Benefits:

HUMANA HEALTH PLAN OF OHIO INC

655 Eden Park Dr
Cincinnati, OH 45202
Phone: 513-784-5200 Fax: 502-580-5044 Toll-Free: 800-543-7158
Web site: www.humana.com
MAILING ADDRESS:
 HUMANA HEALTH PLAN OF OHIO INC
 655 Eden Park Dr
 Cincinnati, OH 45202
KEY EXECUTIVES:
Chairman of the Board .... David A Jones Jr
Chief Executive Officer .... Michael B McCallister
President .... Larry Savage
Chief Financial Director .... James H Bloem
Chief Medical Officer .... Derek Van Amerongen, MD, MS
Marketing Director .... John Timothy Cappel
Small Group Sales Manager .... Mike Brooks
COMPANY PROFILE:
Parent Company Name: Humana Inc
Doing Business As:
Year Founded: 1961 Federally Qualified: [Y]
Forprofit: [Y] Not-For-Profit: [ ]
Model Type: IPA
Accreditation: [ ] AAPPO [ ] JACHO [Y] NCQA [Y] URAC
Plan Type: HMO, PPO, POS, EPO, ASO, CDHP, HSA
Primary Physicians: 2,116 Physician Specialists:
Hospitals:
Total Revenue: 2005: 309,502,866 2006: 186,171,984
Net Income 2005: -26,872,897 2006: 14,031,274
Total Enrollment:
 2001: 0 2004: 133,494 2007: 53,191
 2002: 166,022 2005: 102,626
 2003: 586,372 2006: 63,532
Medical Loss Ratio: 2005: 90.80 2006: 84.80
Administrative Expense Ratio: 2005: 2006:
SERVICE AREA:
Nationwide: N
 OH; IN;
TYPE OF COVERAGE:
Commercial: [Y] Individual: [Y] FEHBP: [ ] Indemnity: [ ]
Medicare: [Y] Medicaid: [ ] Supplemental Medicare: [Y]
Tricare [ ]
PRODUCTS OFFERED:
Product Name: Type:
Humana Gold Plus Plan Medicare Advantage
CONSUMER-DRIVEN PRODUCTS
JP Morgan Chase HSA Company
HumanaOne HSA HSA Product
JP Morgan Chase HSA AdministratorPersonal
Care Account Consumer-Driven Health Plan
HumanaOne High Deductible Health Plan
PLAN BENEFITS:
Alternative Medicine: [ ] Behavioral Health: [X]
Chiropractic: [X] Dental: [X]
Home Care: [ ] Inpatient SNF: [ ]
Long-Term Care: [ ] Pharm. Mail Order: [X]
Physical Therapy: [ ] Podiatry: [ ]
Psychiatric: [X] Transplant: [X]
Vision: [ ] Wellness: [ ]
Workers' Comp: [X]
Other Benefits: Long Term Disability Care

Managed Care Organization Profiles — OHIO

CONSUMER-DRIVEN PRODUCTS
Mellon HR Solutions LLC
HSA Company
HSA Product
HSA Administrator
Consumer-Driven Health Plan
High Deductible Health Plan

PLAN BENEFITS:
Alternative Medicine: [X] Behavioral Health: [ ]
Chiropractic: [X] Dental: [X]
Home Care: [X] Inpatient SNF: [X]
Long-Term Care: [ ] Pharm. Mail Order: [X]
Physical Therapy: [X] Podiatry: [X]
Psychiatric: [X] Transplant: [X]
Vision: [X] Wellness: [X]
Workers' Comp: [ ]
Other Benefits:

HEALTH DESIGN PLUS

1755 Georgetown Rd
Hudson, OH 44236
Phone: 330-656-1072 Fax: 330-656-9387 Toll-Free: 800-877-5843
Web site: www.hdplus.com

MAILING ADDRESS:
HEALTH DESIGN PLUS
1755 Georgetown Rd
Hudson, OH 44236

KEY EXECUTIVES:
Chief Executive Officer/President .... M Ruth Coleman, RN, MA
Chief Financial Officer .... Louis Castellano, CPA
Medical Director .... Alan Hirsh, MD
Chief Information Officer .... John Strickland, BS, MCSE
Chief Operating Officer .... John Perkins, PhD
VP, Sales & Marketing .... Melissa Kozmon, BA
Director, Plan Operations .... Charles W Leach, MBA
Director, Network Analytics .... Jennifer Deitch
Director, Compliance & Recovery .... Francis Fikes, BA
VP, Client Services .... Roberta Kordish, RN, MSN

COMPANY PROFILE:
Parent Company Name: Health Design Plus
Doing Business As:
Year Founded: 1989 Federally Qualified: [N]
Forprofit: [Y] Not-For-Profit: [ ]
Model Type:
Accreditation: [ ] AAPPO [ ] JACHO [ ] NCQA [ ] URAC
Plan Type: PPO, FSA,

SERVICE AREA:
Nationwide: Y
NW;

TYPE OF COVERAGE:
Commercial: [Y] Individual: [ ] FEHBP: [ ] Indemnity: [ ]
Medicare: [ ] Medicaid: [ ] Supplemental Medicare: [ ]
Tricare [ ]

HEALTH PLAN OF THE UPPER OHIO VALLEY

52160 National Road East
St Clairsville, OH 43950
Phone: 740-695-3585 Fax: 740-695-5297 Toll-Free: 800-624-6961
Web site: www.healthplan.org

MAILING ADDRESS:
HEALTH PLAN OF THE UPPER OHIO
52160 National Road East
Saint Clairsville, OH 43950

KEY EXECUTIVES:
Chief Executive Officer/President .... Phil Wright
Chief Financial Officer .... John Yeager
Medical Director .... Kenneth Allen, MD
Pharmacy Director .... Steve Neal
Marketing Director .... Dave Mathieu
Chief Information Officer .... Bob Roset
Director, Provider Services .... Bonnie Cook

COMPANY PROFILE:
Parent Company Name:
Doing Business As: The Health Plan
Year Founded: 1979 Federally Qualified: [Y]
Forprofit: [ ] Not-For-Profit: [Y]
Model Type: IPA
Accreditation: [ ] AAPPO [ ] JACHO [X] NCQA [ ] URAC
Plan Type: HMO
Total Enrollment:
2001: 102,538   2004: 92,025   2007: 0
2002: 95,146   2005:
2003: 92,812   2006:
Medical Loss Ratio: 2005:   2006:
Administrative Expense Ratio: 2005:   2006:

SERVICE AREA:
Nationwide: N
OH; WV;

TYPE OF COVERAGE:
Commercial: [Y] Individual: [Y] FEHBP: [ ] Indemnity: [ ]
Medicare: [Y] Medicaid: [Y] Supplemental Medicare: [Y]
Tricare [ ]

PRODUCTS OFFERED:
Product Name: Type:
The Health Plan   Commercial HMO
Mountain Health Trust   WV Medicaid
Medicare Plus   Medicare (Cost)
Employer Funded Plan   ASO
Health Partnership Program   Workers' Comp
Medicare Plus - High Option   Medicare Advantage
Health Plan Medicare Choice   Medicare

PLAN BENEFITS:
Alternative Medicine: [ ] Behavioral Health: [ ]
Chiropractic: [X] Dental: [ ]
Home Care: [X] Inpatient SNF: [X]
Long-Term Care: [ ] Pharm. Mail Order: [X]
Physical Therapy: [X] Podiatry: [X]
Psychiatric: [X] Transplant: [X]
Vision: [X] Wellness: [ ]
Workers' Comp: [X]
Other Benefits:

HEALTH PLAN, THE/HOMETOWN REGION

100 Lillian Gish Blvd
Massillon, OH 44648
Phone: 330-834-2200 Fax: 330-837-6869 Toll-Free: 877-236-2289
Web site: www.healthplan.org

MAILING ADDRESS:
HEALTH PLAN, THE/HOMETOWN REGN
PO Box 4816
Massillon, OH 44648

KEY EXECUTIVES:
Chief Executive Officer/President .... Phil Wright
Chief Financial Officer .... Jeff Knight
Director of Finance .... John Strah
Medical Director .... Carl J Kite, MD
Pharmacy Director .... Steve Neal
Chief Information Officer .... Bob Roset
Chief Operating Officer .... Patti Fast
VP of Sales/Marketing .... Dave Mathieu
Credentialing Manager .... Jane Webb
Marketing & Communications Manager .... Janie Pavlek
Provider Relations Director .... Bonnie Cook
Assistant Director, Network Development .... Tim Oprzadek
Human Resources Director .... Mary Ann Saunders
Medical Management Director .... Jennifer Ault
Quality Assurance Director .... Judy Karpinski
Credentialing Manager .... Jane Webb
Compliance Officer .... Jennifer Johnston
VP, Legal .... Bob Kota
Medical Director .... Kenneth Allan, MD
Medical Director .... Linda Stark, MD

COMPANY PROFILE:
Parent Company Name: The Health Plan of the Upper Ohio Valley
Doing Business As: The Health Plan (Hometown Region)
Year Founded: 1987 Federally Qualified: [N]
Forprofit: [ ] Not-For-Profit: [Y]
Model Type: NETWORK
Accreditation: [ ] AAPPO [ ] JACHO [Y] NCQA [ ] URAC
Plan Type: HMO, PPO, POS, ASO, TPA, EPO, UR, CDHP
Primary Physicians: 2,500 Physician Specialists: 1,500
Hospitals: 63

OHIO   Managed Care Organization Profiles

KEY EXECUTIVES:
Chairman/Chief Executive Officer .... Jeff Connolly
President .... Christopher Crowley
Chief Financial Officer .... Jeff Connolly
Chief Information Officer .... Lisa Stevens
Chief Operating Officer .... Tracey Jaycox
Human Resources Director .... Juliet Hafford
VP Business Development .... Bill Shuman

COMPANY PROFILE:
Parent Company Name: PPOM
Doing Business As: Flora Midwest
Year Founded: 1993   Federally Qualified: [ ]
Forprofit: [Y]   Not-For-Profit: [ ]
Model Type: NETWORK
Accreditation: [ ] AAPPO [ ] JACHO [ ] NCQA [ ] URAC
Plan Type: PPO, EPO, POS
Primary Physicians: 13,476   Physician Specialists: 22,755
Hospitals: 186
Total Enrollment:
   2001: 270,000   2004: 0   2007: 0
   2002: 266,000   2005:
   2003: 256,000   2006:

SERVICE AREA:
Nationwide: N
   KY; OH; PA; WV;

TYPE OF COVERAGE:
Commercial: [Y] Individual: [ ] FEHBP: [ ] Indemnity: [ ]
Medicare: [ ] Medicaid: [ ] Supplemental Medicare: [ ]
Tricare   [ ]

PRODUCTS OFFERED:
Product Name:	Type:
PPOM	PPO
Flora Midwest	EPO

PLAN BENEFITS:
Alternative Medicine:	[ ]	Behavioral Health:	[ ]
Chiropractic:	[X]	Dental:	[X]
Home Care:	[X]	Inpatient SNF:	[X]
Long-Term Care:	[X]	Pharm. Mail Order:	[ ]
Physical Therapy:	[X]	Podiatry:	[X]
Psychiatric:	[X]	Transplant:	[X]
Vision:	[ ]	Wellness:	[ ]
Workers' Comp:	[X]		

Other Benefits: Varies by Client

GREAT LAKES MEDICAL REVIEW

5600 Monroe St
Sylvania, OH 43560
Phone: 419-882-0546 Fax: 419-885-3581 Toll-Free:
Web site:

MAILING ADDRESS:
   GREAT LAKES MEDICAL REVIEW
   5600 Monroe St
   Sylvania, OH 43560

KEY EXECUTIVES:
Chief Executive Officer/Marketing Director .... Ann Hansen

COMPANY PROFILE:
Parent Company Name:
Doing Business As:
Year Founded: 1974   Federally Qualified: [N]
Forprofit: [Y]   Not-For-Profit: [ ]
Model Type:
Accreditation: [ ] AAPPO [ ] JACHO [ ] NCQA [ ] URAC
Plan Type: UR

SERVICE AREA:
Nationwide: N
   OH;

GREAT-WEST HEALTHCARE OF OHIO

25000 Country Club Blvd #255B
North Olmstead, OH 44070
Phone: 440-716-1777 Fax: 440-716-1221 Toll-Free: 800-644-9335
Web site: www.greatwesthealthcare.com

MAILING ADDRESS:
   GREAT-WEST HEALTHCARE OF OH
   25000 Country Club Blvd #255B
   North Olmstead, OH 44070

KEY EXECUTIVES:
Chief Executive Officer/President .... Raymond L McFeetors
Chief Medical Officer .... Terry L Fouts, MD
Chief Information Officer .... John R Gabbert
Chief Operating Officer .... Donna Goldin

COMPANY PROFILE:
Parent Company Name: Great West Life & Annuity Insurance Co
Doing Business As:
Year Founded: Federally Qualified: [ ]
Forprofit: [Y]   Not-For-Profit: [ ]
Model Type:
Accreditation: [ ] AAPPO [ ] JACHO [ ] NCQA [ ] URAC
Plan Type: HMO, PPO, POS, CDHP, HDHP, HSA,
Total Revenue: 2005:   641   2006:
Net Income   2005:   158,401   2006:
Total Enrollment:
   2001: 9,973   2004: 1,394   2007: 0
   2002: 4,047   2005:
   2003: 2,748   2006:

SERVICE AREA:
Nationwide: N
   OH;

TYPE OF COVERAGE:
Commercial: [Y] Individual: [ ] FEHBP: [ ] Indemnity: [ ]
Medicare: [ ] Medicaid: [ ] Supplemental Medicare: [ ]
Tricare   [ ]

CONSUMER-DRIVEN PRODUCTS
Mellon HR Solutions LLC   HSA Company
                                    HSA Product
                                    HSA Administrator
                                    Consumer-Driven Health Plan
                                    High Deductible Health Plan

PLAN BENEFITS:
Alternative Medicine:	[X]	Behavioral Health:	[ ]
Chiropractic:	[X]	Dental:	[X]
Home Care:	[X]	Inpatient SNF:	[X]
Long-Term Care:	[ ]	Pharm. Mail Order:	[X]
Physical Therapy:	[X]	Podiatry:	[X]
Psychiatric:	[X]	Transplant:	[X]
Vision:	[X]	Wellness:	[X]
Workers' Comp:	[ ]		

Other Benefits:

GREAT-WEST HEALTHCARE OF OHIO

100 E Campus View Blvd Ste 200
Columbus, OH 43235
Phone: 614-848-5369 Fax: 614-848-3593 Toll-Free:
Web site: www.greatwesthealthcare.com

MAILING ADDRESS:
   GREAT-WEST HEALTHCARE OF OH
   100 E Campus View Blvd Ste 200
   Columbus, OH 43235

KEY EXECUTIVES:
Chief Executive Officer/President .... Raymond L McFeetors
Medical Director .... Terry L Fouts, MD
Chief Information Officer .... John R Gabbert
Senior VP, Operations .... Donna Goldin

COMPANY PROFILE:
Parent Company Name: Great West Life & Annuity Insurance Co
Doing Business As:
Year Founded: Federally Qualified: [ ]
Forprofit: [Y]   Not-For-Profit: [ ]
Model Type:
Accreditation: [ ] AAPPO [ ] JACHO [ ] NCQA [ ] URAC
Plan Type: HMO, PPO, CDHP, HDHP, HSA,

SERVICE AREA:
Nationwide: N
   OH;

TYPE OF COVERAGE:
Commercial: [Y] Individual: [ ] FEHBP: [ ] Indemnity: [ ]
Medicare: [ ] Medicaid: [ ] Supplemental Medicare: [ ]
Tricare   [ ]

Managed Care Organization Profiles — OHIO

KEY EXECUTIVES:
Chairman .... Stephen T Schuler, DMD
Chief Executive Officer/President .... Anthony A Cook, MBA, MS
VP, Chief Financial Officer .... Robert C Hodgkins, Jr
Dental Consultant .... Dennis Nabors, DDS
Director, Operations .... Cindy Law
Chief Information & Technology Officer .... Laura Hemmer
Chief Sales & Marketing Officer .... Ann Young
Director, Provider Relations .... Libby Allen
Assistant Controller .... Laura Taylor
Credentialing .... Deborah Williams
Director of Claims/Customer Service .... Jodi Fronczek
Accounts Receivable Manager .... Sarah McCoy
Corporate Communications .... Allison Dubbs

COMPANY PROFILE:
Parent Company Name:
Doing Business As: Dental Care Plus
Year Founded: 1986 Federally Qualified: [ ]
Forprofit: [Y] Not-For-Profit: [ ]
Model Type: IPA
Accreditation: [ ] AAPPO [ ] JACHO [ ] NCQA [ ] URAC
Plan Type: HMO
Primary Physicians: 724 Physician Specialists: 216
Hospitals:
Total Revenue: 2005: 34,838,803 2006: 38,586,760
Net Income 2005: 310,620 2006: 175,402
Total Enrollment:
 2001: 143,774 2004: 163,702 2007: 223,633
 2002: 138,322 2005: 180,191
 2003: 154,959 2006: 200,616
Medical Loss Ratio: 2005: 79.90 2006: 80.80
Administrative Expense Ratio: 2005: 2006:

SERVICE AREA:
Nationwide:
 KY; OH; IN;

EMERALD HEALTH NETWORK INC, THE

1301 E Ninth St 24th Fl
Cleveland, OH 44114-1888
Phone: 216-479-2030 Fax: 216-479-2039 Toll-Free: 800-683-6830
Web site: www.emeraldhealth.com

MAILING ADDRESS:
EMERALD HEALTH NETWORK INC, THE
1301 E Ninth St 24th Fl
Cleveland, OH 44114-1888

KEY EXECUTIVES:
Chief Executive Officer .... Peter R Osenar
President .... Paul W Glover, III
Secretary & Treasurer .... Steven L Ditman
Assistant Secretary .... Paul A Hughes, ESQ

COMPANY PROFILE:
Parent Company Name: Interplan Health Group
Doing Business As: Emerald Health Network Inc, The
Year Founded: 1983 Federally Qualified: [N]
Forprofit: [Y] Not-For-Profit: [ ]
Model Type: NETWORK
Accreditation: [X] AAPPO [ ] JACHO [ ] NCQA [ ] URAC
Plan Type: PPO, PBM, EPO, UR, HSA,
Primary Physicians: 25,000 Physician Specialists:
Hospitals: 205
Total Enrollment:
 2001: 325,000 2004: 0 2007: 0
 2002: 0 2005:
 2003: 0 2006:

SERVICE AREA:
Nationwide: N
 OH; PA; KY; IN;

TYPE OF COVERAGE:
Commercial: [Y] Individual: [ ] FEHBP: [ ] Indemnity: [ ]
Medicare: [Y] Medicaid: [Y] Supplemental Medicare: [ ]
Tricare [ ]

PLAN BENEFITS:
Alternative Medicine: [X] Behavioral Health: [X]
Chiropractic: [X] Dental: [ ]
Home Care: [X] Inpatient SNF: [X]
Long-Term Care: [ ] Pharm. Mail Order: [ ]
Physicial Therapy: [X] Podiatry: [X]
Psychiatric: [X] Transplant: [X]
Vision: [X] Wellness: [X]
Workers' Comp: [X]
Other Benefits:

Comments:
Formerly Emerald PPO Inc.

EYEMED VISION CARE LLC

4000 Luxottica Place
Mason, OH 45040
Phone: 513-765-6000 Fax: 513-765-6388 Toll-Free: a88-439-3633
Web site: www.eyemedvisioncare.com

MAILING ADDRESS:
EYEMED VISION CARE LLC
4000 Luxottica Place
Mason, OH 45040

KEY EXECUTIVES:
Chief Executive Officer .... Kerry Bradley
Vice President .... Liz DiGiandomenico
Senior Director of Finance .... Steve Rogier
Medical Director .... John Lahr, MD
Chief Operating Officer .... Kerry Bradley
Senior Marketing Director .... Wendy Hauteman
Associate VP of Sales .... Greg T Rudisill
Vice President IT .... Mitch Spring
Provider Relations Director .... Linda Denham

COMPANY PROFILE:
Parent Company Name: Luxottica
Doing Business As: Eyemed Vision Care
Year Founded: 1983 Federally Qualified: [ ]
Forprofit: [Y] Not-For-Profit: [ ]
Model Type:
Accreditation: [ ] AAPPO [ ] JACHO [ ] NCQA [ ] URAC
Plan Type: Specialty PPO
Total Enrollment:
 2001: 0 2004: 120,000,000 2007: 0
 2002: 35,000,000 2005:
 2003: 40,000,000 2006:

SERVICE AREA:
Nationwide: Y
 NW;

TYPE OF COVERAGE:
Commercial: [Y] Individual: [ ] FEHBP: [ ] Indemnity: [ ]
Medicare: [ ] Medicaid: [ ] Supplemental Medicare: [ ]
Tricare [ ]

PLAN BENEFITS:
Alternative Medicine: [ ] Behavioral Health: [ ]
Chiropractic: [ ] Dental: [ ]
Home Care: [ ] Inpatient SNF: [ ]
Long-Term Care: [ ] Pharm. Mail Order: [ ]
Physicial Therapy: [ ] Podiatry: [ ]
Psychiatric: [ ] Transplant: [ ]
Vision: [X] Wellness: [ ]
Workers' Comp: [ ]
Other Benefits:

FLORA HEALTH NETWORK

4511 Rockside Rd Ste 320
Cleveland, OH 44131
Phone: 216-642-8575 Fax: 616-956-9862 Toll-Free: 800-966-0200
Web site: www.floramidwest.com

MAILING ADDRESS:
FLORA HEALTH NETWORK
4511 Rockside Rd Ste 320
Cleveland, OH 44131

OHIO

Managed Care Organization Profiles

SERVICE AREA:
Nationwide: N
KS (Douglas, Franklin, Jackson, Jefferson, Johnson, Leavenworth, Miami, Osage, Shawnee, Wyandotte); OH (NE OHIO), Ashtabula, Cuyahoga, Geauga, Lake, Lorain, Mahoning, Medina, Portage, Stark, Summit, Trumbull, Wayne, (NC OHIO), Ashland, Crawford, Huron, Richland, (Columbus), Delaware, Fairfield, Franklin, Licking, Madison, Muskingum, Pickaway, Ross, (Cincinnati), Allen, Auglaize, Butler, Clermont, Hamilton, Warren; MO (Andrew, Barry, Buchanan, Cass, Christian, Clay, Clinton, DeKalb, Greene, Jackson, Jasper, Lafayette, Lawrence, Newton, Platte, Polk, Ray, Webster);

TYPE OF COVERAGE:
Commercial: [Y] Individual: [Y] FEHBP: [ ] Indemnity: [ ]
Medicare: [ ] Medicaid: [ ] Supplemental Medicare: [ ]
Tricare [ ]

PRODUCTS OFFERED:
Product Name:	Type:
Cigna HMO	HMO
Cigna PPO	PPO
Cigna Healthcare for Seniors	Medicare

CONSUMER-DRIVEN PRODUCTS
JP Morgan Chase	HSA Company
CIGNA Choice Fund	HSA Product
	HSA Administrator
Open Access Plus	Consumer-Driven Health Plan
PPO	High Deductible Health Plan

PLAN BENEFITS:
Alternative Medicine: [ ]   Behavioral Health: [ ]
Chiropractic: [X]   Dental: [X]
Home Care: [X]   Inpatient SNF: [X]
Long-Term Care: [X]   Pharm. Mail Order: [X]
Physical Therapy: [X]   Podiatry: [X]
Psychiatric: [X]   Transplant: [X]
Vision: [X]   Wellness: [X]
Workers' Comp: [ ]
Other Benefits:

CORVEL CORPORATION

5555 Airport Hwy Suite 145
Toledo, OH 43615
Phone: 419-865-6444 Fax: 419-865-6841 Toll-Free: 800-275-6463
Web site: www.corvel.com
MAILING ADDRESS:
CORVEL CORPORATION
5555 Airport Hwy Ste 145
Toledo, OH 43615

KEY EXECUTIVES:
Chairman of the Board/Chief Executive Officer .... Gordon Clemons
President/Chief Operating Officer .... Daniel J Starck
Chief Financial Officer .... Scott McCloud
VP, Chief Information Officer .... Don McFarlane
VP, Information Systems .... Tom Benson
Director, Legal Services .... Sharon O'Connor

COMPANY PROFILE:
Parent Company Name:
Doing Business As:
Year Founded: Federally Qualified: [ ]
Forprofit: [Y]   Not-For-Profit: [ ] Model Type: IPA
Accreditation: [ ] AAPPO [ ] JACHO [ ] NCQA [ ] URAC
Plan Type: Specialty PPO, UR

SERVICE AREA:
Nationwide: N
OH (Nothwestern);

TYPE OF COVERAGE:
Commercial: [Y] Individual: [ ] FEHBP: [ ] Indemnity: [ ]
Medicare: [ ] Medicaid: [ ] Supplemental Medicare: [ ]
Tricare [ ]

PLAN BENEFITS:
Alternative Medicine: [ ]   Behavioral Health: [ ]
Chiropractic: [X]   Dental: [X]
Home Care: [X]   Inpatient SNF: [X]
Long-Term Care: [ ]   Pharm. Mail Order: [X]
Physical Therapy: [X]   Podiatry: [X]
Psychiatric: [X]   Transplant: [X]
Vision: [X]   Wellness: [X]
Workers' Comp: [ ]
Other Benefits: MRI, Transportation

DELTA DENTAL PLAN OF OHIO INC

550 Polaris Pkwy Ste 550
Westerville, OH 43082
Phone: 614-890-1117 Fax: 614-890-1274 Toll-Free: 800-537-5527
Web site: www.deltadentaloh.com
MAILING ADDRESS:
DELTA DENTAL PLAN OF OH INC
550 Polaris Pkwy Ste 550
Westerville, OH 43082

KEY EXECUTIVES:
Chairperson of the Board............................ Laura O Stearns
Chief Executive Officer/President .... Thomas J Fleszar, DDS, MS
Chief Financial Officer .... Laura L Czelada, CPA
Dental Director .... Jed J Jacobson, DDS, MPH
VP, Corp & Public Affairs Director .... Nancy E Hostetler
VP, Information Systems .... Timothy DeWeese
VP, Operations .... Sherry L Crisp
VP, Marketing .... E Craig Lesley
VP, Sales .... Charles D Floyd
Professional Relation Director .... Cathy Kiernan
Quality Assurance Director .... Amos Ford
Labor/Market Relations Director .... Richard Karas
VP, Administration .... Patrick D Cahill
VP, New Business Development .... Lonell D Rice
VP, Chief Actuary .... William T Billard

COMPANY PROFILE:
Parent Company Name: Delta Dental Plan of Michigan Inc
Doing Business As:
Year Founded: 1964   Federally Qualified: [ ]
Forprofit: [ ]   Not-For-Profit: [Y]
Model Type: NETWORK
Accreditation: [ ] AAPPO [ ] JACHO [ ] NCQA [ ] URAC
Plan Type: Specialty HMO, Specialty PPO, POS
Total Revenue: 2005:   122,733,114   2006:   133,797,319
Net Income   2005:   1,170,680   2006:   11,865,742
Total Enrollment:
  2001: 0   2004: 520,847   2007: 473,017
  2002: 0   2005: 539,935
  2003: 520,786   2006: 499,682
Medical Loss Ratio: 2005: 86.00   2006: 85.00
Administrative Expense Ratio: 2005:   2006:

SERVICE AREA:
Nationwide: N
OH;

TYPE OF COVERAGE:
Commercial: [Y] Individual: [ ] FEHBP: [ ] Indemnity: [ ]
Medicare: [ ] Medicaid: [ ] Supplemental Medicare: [ ]
Tricare [ ]

PRODUCTS OFFERED:
Product Name:	Type:
Delta Premier	Managed Fee for Serv
Delta Preferred Option Standar	PPO
Delta Preferred Option Point o	PPO
DeltaCare	HMO

PLAN BENEFITS:
Alternative Medicine: [ ]   Behavioral Health: [ ]
Chiropractic: [ ]   Dental: [X]
Home Care: [ ]   Inpatient SNF: [ ]
Long-Term Care: [ ]   Pharm. Mail Order: [ ]
Physical Therapy: [ ]   Podiatry: [ ]
Psychiatric: [ ]   Transplant: [ ]
Vision: [ ]   Wellness: [ ]
Workers' Comp: [ ]
Other Benefits:

DENTAL CARE PLUS INC

100 Crown Pointe Place
Cincinnati, OH 45241
Phone: 513-554-1100 Fax: 513-554-3187 Toll-Free: 800-367-9466
Web site: www.dentalcareplus.com
MAILING ADDRESS:
DENTAL CARE PLUS INC
100 Crown Pointe Place
Cincinnati, OH 45241

Managed Care Organization Profiles — OHIO

CIGNA HEALTHCARE - CINCINNATI

7 West 7th St Ste 1402
Cincinnati, OH 45202-2417
Phone: 800-832-3211 Fax: 513-629-2675 Toll-Free:
Web site: www.cigna.com

MAILING ADDRESS:
   CIGNA HEALTHCARE - CINCINNATI
   7 West 7th St Ste 1402
   Cincinnati, OH 45202-2417

KEY EXECUTIVES:
Chief Executive Officer .... H Edward Hanway
President/General Manager .... Jeanne McCarthy
Medical Director .... Jennifer Harper, MD
Pharmacy Director .... David Marsola, RPH
Sales Manager .... Steve Biats
Medical Management Director .... Cathy Eck
Regional Controller .... Cheryl Colles
Regional VP of Operations .... Ron Dziedzicki

COMPANY PROFILE:
Parent Company Name: CIGNA Corporation
Doing Business As:
Year Founded: 1987   Federally Qualified: [N]
Forprofit: [Y]   Not-For-Profit: [ ]
Model Type: MIXED
Accreditation: [ ] AAPPO [ ] JACHO [X] NCQA [ ] URAC
Plan Type: HMO, PPO, POS, ASO, CDHP, HDHP, HSA, FSA, HRA

SERVICE AREA:
Nationwide: N
   OH; (Ashtubula, Cuyahoga, Geagua, Lake, Lorain, Mahoning, Medina, Portage, Stark, Summit, Trumbell, Wayne, Ashland, Crawford, Huron, Richland, Delaware, Fairfield, Franklin, Licking, Madison, Muskingum, Pickaway, Ross, Allen, Auglaize, Bitler, Clermont, Hamilton, Warren.)

TYPE OF COVERAGE:
Commercial: [Y] Individual: [Y] FEHBP: [ ] Indemnity: [ ]
Medicare: [ ] Medicaid: [ ] Supplemental Medicare: [ ]
Tricare [ ]

CONSUMER-DRIVEN PRODUCTS
                                 HSA Company
CIGNA Choice Fund   HSA Product
                                 HSA Administrator
Open Access Plus   Consumer-Driven Health
PlanPPO   High Deductible Health Plan

PLAN BENEFITS:
Alternative Medicine: [ ]   Behavioral Health: [ ]
Chiropractic: [X]   Dental: [X]
Home Care: [X]   Inpatient SNF: [X]
Long-Term Care: [X]   Pharm. Mail Order: [X]
Physical Therapy: [X]   Podiatry: [X]
Psychiatric: [X]   Transplant: [X]
Vision: [X]   Wellness: [X]
Workers' Comp: [ ]
Other Benefits:

CIGNA HEALTHCARE OF OHIO INC

1000 Polaris Parkway
Columbus, OH 43240-2005
Phone: 614-785-1310 Fax: 614-985-4233 Toll-Free: 800-542-7526
Web site: www.cigna.com

MAILING ADDRESS:
   CIGNA HEALTHCARE OF OH INC
   1000 Polaris Parkway
   Columbus, OH 43240-2005

KEY EXECUTIVES:
President/General Manager .... Joseph C Gregor
Medical Director .... Z Colette Edwards, MD
Pharmacy Director .... Matt Houser, RPh
Sales Manager .... Steve Biats
VP, Provider Services .... Noreen Nageotte
VP, Provider Contracting .... Karen Shullick
Medical Management Director .... Cathy Eck
Regional Controller .... Cheryl Colles

COMPANY PROFILE:
Parent Company Name: CIGNA Corporation
Doing Business As:
Year Founded: 1985   Federally Qualified: [ ]
Forprofit: [Y]   Not-For-Profit: [ ]
Model Type: MIXED
Accreditation: [ ] AAPPO [ ] JACHO [X] NCQA [ ] URAC
Plan Type: PPO, POS, ASO, EPO, CDHP, HDHP, HSA, FSA, HRA
Total Revenue: 2005: 12,667,537 2006: 16,071,036
Net Income   2005: 2,018,949   2006: 86,242
Total Enrollment:
   2001: 0   2004: 5,359   2007: 2,610
   2002: 0   2005: 4,145
   2003: 7,125   2006: 5,915
Medical Loss Ratio: 2005: 67.40   2006: 88.00
Administrative Expense Ratio: 2005:   2006:

SERVICE AREA:
Nationwide: N
   OH (Ashtabula, Cuyahoga, Geauga, Lake, Lorain, Mahoning, Medina, Portage, Stark, Summit, Trumbull, Wayne, Ashland, Crawford, Huron, Richland, Delaware, Fairfield, Franklin, Kicking, Madison, Muskinggum, Pickaway, Ross, Allen, Auglaize, Butler, Clermont, Hamilton, Warren).

TYPE OF COVERAGE:
Commercial: [Y] Individual: [Y] FEHBP: [ ] Indemnity: [ ]
Medicare: [ ] Medicaid: [ ] Supplemental Medicare: [ ]
Tricare [ ]

PRODUCTS OFFERED:
Product Name: Type:
CHMO
DPP
EPP
PPA
PPO

CONSUMER-DRIVEN PRODUCTS
JP Morgan Chase   HSA Company
CIGNA Choice Fund   HSA Product
                                 HSA Administrator
Open Access Plus   Consumer-Driven Health Plan
PPO   High Deductible Health Plan

PLAN BENEFITS:
Alternative Medicine: [ ]   Behavioral Health: [ ]
Chiropractic: [X]   Dental: [X]
Home Care: [X]   Inpatient SNF: [X]
Long-Term Care: [X]   Pharm. Mail Order: [X]
Physical Therapy: [X]   Podiatry: [X]
Psychiatric: [X]   Transplant: [X]
Vision: [X]   Wellness: [X]
Workers' Comp: [ ]
Other Benefits:

CIGNA HEALTHCARE OF OHIO INC

5005 Rockside Rd Ste 700
Cleveland, OH 44131
Phone: 216-642-2920 Fax: 216-642-2990 Toll-Free: 800-647-7748
Web site: www.cigna.com

MAILING ADDRESS:
   CIGNA HEALTHCARE OF OH INC
   5005 Rockside Rd Ste 700
   Cleveland, OH 44131

KEY EXECUTIVES:
President/General Manager .... Joseph C Gregor
Medical Director .... Z Colette Edwards, MD
Pharmacy Director .... Matt Houser, RPh
Sales Manager .... Steve Biats
VP, Provider Services .... Karen Shullick
VP, Network Development .... Noreen Nageotte
Human Resources Director .... Lisa Kilcher
Compliance Officer .... Lynn Gruber

COMPANY PROFILE:
Parent Company Name: CIGNA Corporation
Doing Business As:
Year Founded: 1987   Federally Qualified: [N]
Forprofit: [Y]   Not-For-Profit: [ ]
Model Type: MIXED
Accreditation: [ ] AAPPO [ ] JACHO [X] NCQA [ ] URAC
Plan Type: HMO, PPO, POS, ASO, EPO, CDHP, HDHP, HSA
Total Enrollment:
   2001: 18,894   2004: 5,359   2007: 0
   2002: 10,736   2005:
   2003: 7,125   2006:

OHIO

Forprofit: [ ]   Not-For-Profit: [ ]
Model Type:
Accreditation: [ ] AAPPO [ ] JACHO [ ] NCQA [ ] URAC
Plan Type: PPO, TPA
SERVICE AREA:
Nationwide: N
  OH;
PLAN BENEFITS:
Alternative Medicine: [ ]   Behavioral Health: [X]
Chiropractic: [ ]   Dental: [ ]
Home Care: [X]   Inpatient SNF: [X]
Long-Term Care: [X]   Pharm. Mail Order: [ ]
Physical Therapy: [X]   Podiatry: [X]
Psychiatric: [X]   Transplant: [ ]
Vision: [ ]   Wellness: [ ]
Workers' Comp: [ ]
Other Benefits:

CHN MCO

6000 W Creek Rd Ste 20
Independence, OH 44131
Phone: 216-986-1200 Fax: 216-328-7551 Toll-Free:
Web site: www.chnetwork.com
MAILING ADDRESS:
    CHN MCO
    6000 W Creek Rd Ste 20
    Independence, OH 44131

KEY EXECUTIVES:
Chief Executive Officer/President .... Martin Hauser
Chief Financial Officer/Chief Operating Officer .... Dennis Pijor
Medical Director .... Alan London, MD
Director, Provider Services/Network Operations .... Rita Drvenkar
Human Resources Director .... Deb Jewell
Medical Management Director .... Kathy Miller
Plan/Communications Director .... Mary Schnitzer

COMPANY PROFILE:
Parent Company Name: Cleveland Health Network
Doing Business As:
Year Founded: 2003   Federally Qualified: [ ]
Forprofit: [ ]   Not-For-Profit: [ ]
Model Type:
Accreditation: [ ] AAPPO [ ] JACHO [ ] NCQA [ ] URAC
Plan Type: HMO, PPO, POS, HSA,
SERVICE AREA:
Nationwide: N
  OH (Cuyahoga, Summit, Lorain, Mohoning, Lake City, Trumbell,
  Erie, Wayne, Medina, Stark, Ashtabula, Portage, Huron Counties);
TYPE OF COVERAGE:
Commercial: [Y] Individual: [ ] FEHBP: [ ] Indemnity: [ ]
Medicare: [Y] Medicaid: [Y] Supplemental Medicare: [ ]
Tricare   [ ]

CHOICECARE/HUMANA

655 Eden Park Dr Ste 400
Cincinnati, OH 45202-6056
Phone: 513-784-5200 Fax: 513-357-6906 Toll-Free: 800-521-3508
Web site: www.choicecare.com
MAILING ADDRESS:
    CHOICECARE/HUMANA
    655 Eden Park Dr Ste 400
    Cincinnati, OH 45202-6056

KEY EXECUTIVES:
Executive Director/President .... Larry Savage
Chief Financial Officer .... James Eldred
Chief Medical Officer .... Derek Van Amerongen, MD, MS
Pharmacy Director .... Peter Reeme, PharmD
Quality Management Manager .... Patti Bliss, RN
Utilization Management/Medical Director .... Mike Vossmeyer, MD
Medical Director/OB/GYN .... Randy Slinger, MD

COMPANY PROFILE:
Parent Company Name:
Doing Business As:
Year Founded: 1978   Federally Qualified: [Y]
Forprofit: [Y]   Not-For-Profit: [ ]
Model Type: MIXED

Accreditation: [ ] AAPPO [ ] JACHO [X] NCQA [ ] URAC
Plan Type: HMO, PPO, POS, ASO, HSA
Primary Physicians: 1,700   Physician Specialists: 2,800
Hospitals:
Total Enrollment:
    2001: 172,815   2004: 0   2007: 0
    2002: 177,769   2005:
    2003: 157,572   2006:
SERVICE AREA:
Nationwide: N
  IN (Adams, Ashland, Brown, Butler, Champaign, Clark, Clermont,
  Clinton, Darke, Delaware, Fairfield, Fayette, Franklin, Greene,
  Hamilton, Highland, Hocking, Jackson, Knox, Lawrence, Licking,
  Madison, Marion, Miami, Montgomery, Morrow, Muskingum,
  Pickaway, Pike, Preble, Richland, Ross, Scioto, Union, Vinton,
  Warren);
TYPE OF COVERAGE:
Commercial: [Y] Individual: [Y] FEHBP: [ ] Indemnity: [ ]
Medicare: [Y] Medicaid: [ ] Supplemental Medicare: [ ]
Tricare   [ ]
PRODUCTS OFFERED:
Product Name: Type:
Senior Health by Choicecare   Medicare
PLAN BENEFITS:
Alternative Medicine: [ ]   Behavioral Health: [ ]
Chiropractic: [X]   Dental: [ ]
Home Care: [X]   Inpatient SNF: [X]
Long-Term Care: [X]   Pharm. Mail Order: [X]
Physical Therapy: [X]   Podiatry: [X]
Psychiatric: [X]   Transplant: [X]
Vision: [X]   Wellness: [X]
Workers' Comp: [X]
Other Benefits:

CIGNA DENTAL HEALTH OF OHIO INC

1300 East 9th St
Cleveland, OH 44114
Phone: 954-514-6600 Fax: 954-514-6905 Toll-Free: 800-367-1037
Web site: www.cigna.com/dental
MAILING ADDRESS:
    CIGNA DENTAL HEALTH OF OHIO INC
    1571 Sawgrass Corporate Pkwy
    Sunrise, FL 33323

KEY EXECUTIVES:
President .... Karen S Rohan
Chief Financial Officer .... Michelle I Haas
Marketing Director .... Judith Herron
MIS Director .... Laurel A Flebotte

COMPANY PROFILE:
Parent Company Name: CIGNA Dental Health Inc
Doing Business As: CIGNA Dental
Year Founded: 1974   Federally Qualified: [N]
Forprofit: [Y]   Not-For-Profit: [ ]
Model Type:
Accreditation: [ ] AAPPO [ ] JACHO [ ] NCQA [ ] URAC
Plan Type: Specialty HMO
Total Revenue: 2005:   11,228,461   2006: 10,722,814
Net Income   2005:   1,563,460   2006: 1,562,539
Total Enrollment:
    2001: 0   2004: 74,698   2007: 52,741
    2002: 88,372   2005: 69,214
    2003: 78,940   2006: 64,550
Medical Loss Ratio: 2005: 64.60   2006: 64.90
Administrative Expense Ratio: 2005:   2006:
SERVICE AREA:
Nationwide: N
  FL;
TYPE OF COVERAGE:
Commercial: [Y] Individual: [ ] FEHBP: [ ] Indemnity: [ ]
Medicare: [ ] Medicaid: [ ] Supplemental Medicare: [ ]
Tricare   [ ]
PLAN BENEFITS:
Alternative Medicine: [ ]   Behavioral Health: [ ]
Chiropractic: [ ]   Dental: [X]
Home Care: [ ]   Inpatient SNF: [ ]
Long-Term Care: [ ]   Pharm. Mail Order: [ ]
Physical Therapy: [ ]   Podiatry: [ ]
Psychiatric: [ ]   Transplant: [ ]
Vision: [ ]   Wellness: [ ]
Workers' Comp: [ ]
Other Benefits:

Managed Care Organization Profiles — OHIO

Model Type: GROUP
Accreditation: [ ] AAPPO [ ] JACHO [ ] NCQA [ ] URAC
Plan Type: HMO, PPO, CDHP, HDHP, HSA,
Total Enrollment:
    2001: 4,711   2004: 500,000   2007: 0
    2002: 5,525   2005:
    2003: 4,946   2006:

SERVICE AREA:
Nationwide: N
    OH (Carroll, Columbiana, Holmes, Mahoning, Portage, Stark, Summit, Tuscarawas, Wayne);

TYPE OF COVERAGE:
Commercial: [Y] Individual: [ ] FEHBP: [ ] Indemnity: [ ]
Medicare: [ ] Medicaid: [ ] Supplemental Medicare: [ ]
Tricare [ ]

PRODUCTS OFFERED:
Product Name:	Type:
Aultcare HMO	HMO
Aultcare PPO	PPO

BUCKEYE COMMUNITY HEALTH PLAN INC

175 S 3rd St Ste 1200
Columbus, OH 43215
Phone: 614-220-4900 Fax: 614-221-7726 Toll-Free: 866-246-4356
Web site: www.bchpohio.com

MAILING ADDRESS:
BUCKEYE COMMUNITY HEALTH PLAN
175 S 3rd St Ste 1200
Columbus, OH 43215

KEY EXECUTIVES:
Chairman .... Kathleen R Crampton
Chief Executive Officer/President .... Richard L Fredrickson
Senior VP, Chief Financial Officer .... William Scheffel
VP, Medical Affairs .... Christopher G Sivak, MD
VP, Contracting & Network Development .... Debra Collins
VP, Medical Management .... Lori Mulichak
VP, Regulatory Affairs .... David Amerine

COMPANY PROFILE:
Parent Company Name: Centene Corporation Inc
Doing Business As:
Year Founded: 2004   Federally Qualified: [ ]
Forprofit: [ ]   Not-For-Profit: [ ]
Model Type:
Accreditation: [ ] AAPPO [ ] JACHO [ ] NCQA [ ] URAC
Plan Type: HMO,
Primary Physicians: 508   Physician Specialists: 1,980
Hospitals: 9
Total Revenue: 2005: 97,399,296 2006: 33,196,798
Net Income: 2005: -4,034,270 2006: 386,984
Total Enrollment:
    2001: 0   2004: 23,767   2007: 126,770
    2002: 0   2005: 58,707
    2003: 0   2006: 108,428

SERVICE AREA:
Nationwide:
    OH;

TYPE OF COVERAGE:
Commercial: [ ] Individual: [ ] FEHBP: [ ] Indemnity: [ ]
Medicare: [ ] Medicaid: [Y] Supplemental Medicare: [ ]
Tricare [ ]

PRODUCTS OFFERED:
Product Name:	Type:
Buckeye Community Health Plan	Medicaid

Comments:
Acquired the Medicaid-related assets from Family Health Plan, owned by Mercy Health Partners, Toledo, OH, January, 2004.

CARESOURCE

1 South Main St Ste 900
Dayton, OH 45402-2016
Phone: 937-224-3300 Fax: 937-224-3383 Toll-Free: 800-488-0134
Web site: www.caresource-ohio.com

MAILING ADDRESS:
CARESOURCE
1 South Main St Ste 900
Dayton, OH 45402-2016

KEY EXECUTIVES:
Chief Executive Officer/President .... Pamela B Morris
Chief Financial Officer .... Pamela Sedmark
Chief Medical Officer .... Terence P Torbeck, MD
Chief Information Officer .... Mike Knellinger
Chief Operating Officer .... Daniel Paquin
VP, Marketing .... Kevin Wells
Human Resources Director .... Adele Perry
Quality Improvement Director .... Salli Duncan, RN
New Product Development .... Janet Grant
Regulatory Compliance Officer .... Cathy Potisuk

COMPANY PROFILE:
Parent Company Name: CareSource Management Group
Doing Business As:
Year Founded: 1989   Federally Qualified: [N]
Forprofit: [ ]   Not-For-Profit: [Y]
Model Type: MIXED
Accreditation: [ ] AAPPO [ ] JACHO [ ] NCQA [Y] URAC
Plan Type: HMO
Primary Physicians: 1,855   Physician Specialists: 4,400
Hospitals: 89
Total Revenue: 2005: 762,920,262 2006: 230,657,853
Net Income: 2005: 15,786,060 2006: 16,879,957
Total Enrollment:
    2001: 139,513   2004: 345,935   2007: 544,000
    2002: 245,731   2005: 391,318
    2003: 320,233   2006: 428,698
Medical Loss Ratio: 2005: 92.80   2006:
Administrative Expense Ratio: 2005:   2006:

SERVICE AREA:
Nationwide: N
    OH (Butler, Clark, Cuyahoga, Franklin, Greene, Hamilton, Marion, Mahoning, Miami, Montgomery, Pickaway, Summit); MI;

TYPE OF COVERAGE:
Commercial: [Y] Individual: [ ] FEHBP: [ ] Indemnity: [ ]
Medicare: [ ] Medicaid: [Y] Supplemental Medicare: [ ]
Tricare [ ]

PRODUCTS OFFERED:
Product Name:	Type:
Caresource	Medicaid

PLAN BENEFITS:
Alternative Medicine:	[ ]	Behavioral Health:	[X]
Chiropractic:	[X]	Dental:	[X]
Home Care:	[X]	Inpatient SNF:	[ ]
Long-Term Care:	[ ]	Pharm. Mail Order:	[ ]
Physical Therapy:	[ ]	Podiatry:	[X]
Psychiatric:	[X]	Transplant:	[ ]
Vision:	[X]	Wellness:	[X]
Workers' Comp:	[ ]		

Other Benefits:
Comments:
Company formerly known as Dayton Area Health Plan.

CENTRAL BENEFITS MUTUAL INSURANCE COMPANY

716 Mt Airyshire Blvd
Columbus, OH 43235
Phone: 614-797-5200 Fax: 614-797-5268 Toll-Free: 800-333-5711
Web site: www.centralbenefits.com

MAILING ADDRESS:
CENTRAL BENEFITS MUT INS CO
PO Box 16526
Columbus, OH 43235

KEY EXECUTIVES:
Chief Executive Officer .... William C Mechling
Chief Financial Officer .... Joseph H Hoffman
Director, Provider Services .... Patricia Cabrera

COMPANY PROFILE:
Parent Company Name:
Doing Business As: Central Benefits Mutual Ins Co
Year Founded: 1938   Federally Qualified: [ ]

OHIO

COMPANY PROFILE:
Parent Company Name: Medical Mutual of Ohio
Doing Business As:
Year Founded: 1997
Forprofit: [Y]
Federally Qualified: [ ]
Not-For-Profit: [ ]
Model Type:
Accreditation: [ ] AAPPO [ ] JACHO [ ] NCQA [ ] URAC
Plan Type: UR, TPA

SERVICE AREA:
Nationwide: N
OH;

TYPE OF COVERAGE:
Commercial: [Y] Individual: [ ] FEHBP: [ ] Indemnity: [ ]
Medicare: [ ] Medicaid: [ ] Supplemental Medicare: [ ]
Tricare [ ]

Comments:
Formerly called Medical Mutual Services LLC.

ANTHEM BLUE CROSS BLUE SHIELD OF OHIO

4361 Irwin Simpson Rd
Mason, OH 45040
Phone: 513-872-8100 Fax: 513-336-5599 Toll-Free: 800-442-1832
Web site: www.80.anthem.com

MAILING ADDRESS:
ANTHEM BC/BS OF OHIO
4361 Irwin Simpson Rd
Mason, OH 45040

KEY EXECUTIVES:
Chief Executive Officer .... Angela F Braly
President - Ohio .... Chuck Slater
Chief Financial Officer .... Mike Smith
Medical Director .... Samuel Nussbaum, MD
Pharmacy Director-President APM .... Marjorie W Dorr
Marketing Director .... Eric Neuville
MIS Vice President .... Cecilia Claudio

COMPANY PROFILE:
Parent Company Name: WellPoint Inc
Doing Business As:
Year Founded: 1995
Forprofit: [ ]
Federally Qualified: [N]
Not-For-Profit: [Y]
Model Type: MIXED
Accreditation: [ ] AAPPO [ ] JACHO [X] NCQA [ ] URAC
Plan Type: HMO, PPO, HDHP, HSA
Total Revenue: 2005: 2006: 53,626,186
Net Income 2005: 2006: -4,200,233
Total Enrollment:
  2001: 320,647   2004: 304,109   2007: 142,962
  2002: 334,208   2005:
  2003: 278,955   2006: 85,081
Medical Loss Ratio: 2005: 2006: 89.3
Administrative Expense Ratio: 2005: 2006:

SERVICE AREA:
Nationwide: N
OH; (Adams, Allen, Bartholomew, Benton, Blackford, Boone, Brown, Carroll, Cass, Clark, Clay, Clinton, Crawford, Daviess, Decatur, Dekalb, Delaware, Dubois, Elkhart, Fayette, Floyd, Fountain, Fulton, Gibson, Grant, Greene, Hamilton, Hancock, Harrison, Hendricks, Henry, Howard, Huntington, Jackson, Jasper, Jay, Jefferson, Jennings, Johnson, Knox, Kosciusko, Lagrange, Lake, Laporte, Lawrence, Madison, Marion, Marshall, Martin, Miami, Monroe, Montgomery, Morgan, Newton, Noble, Orange, Owen, Parke, Perry, Pike, Porter, Posey, Pulaski, Putnam, Randolph, Ripley, Rush, St Joseph, Scott, Shelby, Spencer, Starke, Steuben, Sullivan, Tippecanoe, Tipton, Vanderburgh, Vermillion, Vigo, Wabash, Warren, Warrick, Washington, Wayne, Wells, White, Whitley);

TYPE OF COVERAGE:
Commercial: [Y] Individual: [Y] FEHBP: [ ] Indemnity:[]Medicare: [Y] Medicaid: [ ] Supplemental Medicare: [Y]
Tricare [ ]

PRODUCTS OFFERED:
Product Name:	Type:
Anthem Senior Advantage	Medicare Advantage

CONSUMER-DRIVEN PRODUCTS
JP Morgan Chase	HSA Company
Anthem ByDesign HSA	HSA Product
JP Morgan Chase	HSA Administrator
Blue Access Saver	Consumer-Driven Health Plan
Blue Access Economy Plans PPO	High Deductible Health Plan

Comments:
Enrollment reflects HMP and Anthem Premier 100.

ANTHEM BLUE CROSS AND BLUE SHIELD OF OHIO

1351 William H Taft Rd
Cincinnati, OH 45206
Phone: 513-475-2973 Fax: 513-336-6021 Toll-Free:
Web site: www.anthem.com

MAILING ADDRESS:
ANTHEM BLUE CROSS/BLUE SHIELD
1351 William H Taft Rd
Cincinnati, OH 45206

KEY EXECUTIVES:
Chief Executive Officer .... Angela F Braly
President - Ohio .... Chuck Slater
Chief Financial Officer .... Mike Smith
Medical Director .... Samuel Nussbaum, MD

COMPANY PROFILE:
Parent Company Name: WellPoint Inc
Doing Business As:
Year Founded: 1975
Forprofit: [ ]
Federally Qualified: [ ]
Not-For-Profit: [Y]
Model Type: MIXED
Accreditation: [ ] AAPPO [ ] JACHO [ ] NCQA [ ] URAC
Plan Type: HMO, PPO, POS, EPO, HDHP, HSA
Total Enrollment:
  2001: 0   2004: 81,717   2007: 0
  2002: 0   2005:
  2003: 0   2006:

SERVICE AREA:
Nationwide: N
IN; KY; OH (Allen, Ashland, Ashtabula, Athens, Brown, Butler, Carroll, Champaign, Clark, Clermont, Clinton, Columbiana, Coshocton, Cuyahoga, Darke, Defiance, Delaware, Erie, Fairfield, Fayette, Franklin, Fulton, Geauga, Greene, Hamilton, Hancock, Harrison, Henry, Highland, Holmes, Huron, Jefferson, Lake, Licking, Logan, Lorain, Lucas, Madison, Mahoning, Medina, Miami, Montgomery, Ottawa, Paulding, Pickaway, Portage, Preble, Putnam, Sandusky, Seneca, Shelby, Stark, Summit, Trumbull, Tuscarawas, Union, Van Wert, Warren, Washington, Wayne, Williams, Wood);

TYPE OF COVERAGE:
Commercial: [Y] Individual: [Y] FEHBP: [ ] Indemnity: [ ]
Medicare: [Y] Medicaid: [ ] Supplemental Medicare: [Y]
Tricare [ ]

PRODUCTS OFFERED:
Product Name:	Type:
Anthem Senior Advantage	Medicare

CONSUMER-DRIVEN PRODUCTS
JP Morgan Chase	HSA Company
Anthem ByDesign HSA	HSA Product
JP Morgan Chase	HSA Administrator
Blue Access Saver	Consumer-Driven Health Plan
Blue Access Economy Plans PPO	High Deductible Health Plan

AULTCARE

2600 6th St SW
Canton, OH 44710-1799
Phone: 330-438-6390 Fax: 330-454-7845 Toll-Free: 800-344-8858
Web site: www.aultcare.com

MAILING ADDRESS:
AULTCARE
2600 6th St SW
Canton, OH 44710-1799

KEY EXECUTIVES:
Chief Executive Officer .... Rick L Haines
Chief Medical Officer .... Gregory Haban, MD
Pharmacy Director .... Kevin Pete
Chief Information Officer .... Brian Burley
Marketing Director .... Robin Clark

COMPANY PROFILE:
Parent Company Name: Aultman Health Services Association
Doing Business As:
Year Founded: 1985
Forprofit: [ ]
Federally Qualified: [ ]
Not-For-Profit: [Y]

Managed Care Organization Profiles

OHIO

AETNA INC - OHIO

4059 Kinross Lakes Pkwy
Richfield, OH 42286
Phone: 330-659-8000 Fax: 330-659-8034 Toll-Free: 800-458-3940
Web site: www.aetna.com

MAILING ADDRESS:
AETNA INC - OH
4059 Kinross Lakes Pkwy
Richfield, OH 42286

KEY EXECUTIVES:
Chairman of the Board/Chief Executive Officer .... Ronald A Williams
Regional Manager-Midwest .... Edward Dulik
Executive VP, Finance .... Joseph M Zubretsky
Medical Director .... Mark Studebaker, MD

COMPANY PROFILE:
Parent Company Name: Aetna Inc
Doing Business As: Prudential Health Care Plan Inc
Year Founded: 1985   Federally Qualified: [ ]
Forprofit: [Y]   Not-For-Profit: [ ]
Model Type: GROUP
Accreditation: [ ] AAPPO [ ] JACHO [X] NCQA [ ] URAC
Plan Type: HMO, POS, CDHP, HDHP, HSA,
Primary Physicians: 443,660   Physician Specialists:
Hospitals:
Total Revenue: 2005:   286,439,647   2006:   310,445,230
Net Income   2005:   5,976,550   2006:   2,413,415
Total Enrollment:
   2001: 16,464   2004: 105,373   2007: 88,801
   2002: 0   2005: 91,146
   2003: 108,301   2006: 85,498
Medical Loss Ratio: 2005: 82.50   2006: 83.50
Administrative Expense Ratio: 2005:   2006:

SERVICE AREA:
Nationwide: N
OH (Ashland, Ashtabula, Brown, Clark, Clermont, Clinton, Columbiana, Coshocton, Crawford, Cuyahoga, Delaware, Fairfield, Franklin, Geauga, Greene, Hamilton, Hardin, Knox, Lake, Licking, Logan, Lorain, Madison, Mahoning, Marion, Medina, Miami, Montgomery, Morrow, Muskingum, Pickaway, Portage, Stark, Summit, Trumbull, Union, Warren, Wayne, Wyandot);

TYPE OF COVERAGE:
Commercial: [Y] Individual: [ ] FEHBP: [ ] Indemnity: [ ]
Medicare: [Y] Medicaid: [ ] Supplemental Medicare: [ ]
Tricare   [ ]

PRODUCTS OFFERED:
Product Name: Type:
Aetna US Healthcare Golden Medic   Medicare
Prudential Healthcare Senircare   Medicare

CONSUMER-DRIVEN PRODUCTS
Aetna Life Insurance Co   HSA Company
Aetna HealthFund HSA   HSA Product
Aetna   HSA Administrator
Aetna HealthFund   Consumer-Driven Health Plan
PPO I; PPO II   High Deductible Health Plan

PLAN BENEFITS:
Alternative Medicine: [ ]   Behavioral Health: [X]
Chiropractic: [X]   Dental: [X]
Home Care: [X]   Inpatient SNF: [X]
Long-Term Care: [X]   Pharm. Mail Order: [X]
Physical Therapy: [X]   Podiatry: [X]
Psychiatric: [X]   Transplant: [X]
Vision: [X]   Wellness: [X]
Workers' Comp: [ ]
Other Benefits:

Comments:
Formerly Prudential Healthcare Plan.

ALTERNATIVE CARE MANAGEMENT SYSTEMS

4789 Rings Rd Ste 100
Dublin, OH 43017-0956
Phone: 614-761-0035 Fax: 614-761-0452 Toll-Free: 800-831-6677
Web site: www.ebmconline.com

MAILING ADDRESS:
ALTERNATIVE CARE MANAGEMENT SYSTEMS
P O Box 9056
Dublin, OH 43017-0956

KEY EXECUTIVES:
VP, Sales & Marketing .... Greg Hubbell

COMPANY PROFILE:
Parent Company Name: Employee Benefits Managment Corporation
Doing Business As:
Year Founded: Federally Qualified: [ ]
Forprofit: [ ]   Not-For-Profit: [ ]
Model Type:
Accreditation: [ ] AAPPO [ ] JACHO [ ] NCQA [ ] URAC
Plan Type: UR,

SERVICE AREA:
Nationwide: Y
   NW;

PRODUCTS OFFERED:
Product Name: Type:
Utilization Review   Self Funded
Case Management
Disability Management

AMERIGROUP COMMUNITY CARE OHIO INC

10123 Alliance Rd Ste 104
Cincinnati, OH 45242
Phone: 513-733-2300 Fax: 513-733-0516 Toll-Free:
Web site: www.amerigroupcorp.com

MAILING ADDRESS:
AMERIGROUP COMMUNITY CARE OHIO
10123 Alliance Rd Ste 104
Cincinnati, OH 45242

KEY EXECUTIVES:
Chairman of the Board .... Jeffrey L McWaters
Chief Executive Officer/President .... Gary Hall Fletcher
Executive VP, Chief Financial Officer .... James Ware Truess

COMPANY PROFILE:
Parent Company Name: Amerigroup Corporation
Doing Business As:
Year Founded: 2005   Federally Qualified: [ ]
Forprofit: [Y]   Not-For-Profit: [ ]
Model Type:
Accreditation: [ ] AAPPO [ ] JACHO [ ] NCQA [ ] URAC
Plan Type: HMO
Total Revenue: 2005:   10,381,617   2006:   81,834,743
Net Income   2005:   -1,580,532   2006:   -4,594,233
Total Enrollment:
   2001: 0   2004: 0   2007: 50,635
   2002: 0   2005: 22,269
   2003: 0   2006: 46,099
Medical Loss Ratio: 2005:   2006: 88.00
Administrative Expense Ratio: 2005:   2006:

SERVICE AREA:
Nationwide:
   OH;

TYPE OF COVERAGE:
Commercial: [ ] Individual: [ ] FEHBP: [ ] Indemnity: [ ]
Medicare: [ ] Medicaid: [Y] Supplemental Medicare: [ ]
Tricare   [ ]

ANTARES MANAGEMENT SOLUTIONS

24650 Center Ridge Rd B 2 #400
Westlake, OH 44145-5620
Phone: 440-414-2100 Fax: 440-414-2101 Toll-Free: 866-268-2737
Web site: www.antaressolutions.com

MAILING ADDRESS:
ANTARES MANAGEMENT SOLUTIONS
24650 Center Ridge Rd B 2 #400
Westlake, OH 44145-5620

KEY EXECUTIVES:
Chief Executive Officer .... Ed Hartzell
President, US Operations .... Ken Sidon
VP, Finance .... Tom Stepec
VP, Marketing .... Jeff Perry
VP, Enterprise Tech Development, Innovations .... Paul B Apostle
VP, US Operations .... Jim Harless

NORTH DAKOTA HEALTH CARE REVIEW

800 31st Ave SW
Minot, ND 58701
Phone: 701-852-4231 Fax: 701-838-6009 Toll-Free:
Web site: www.ndhcri.org

MAILING ADDRESS:
    NORTH DAKOTA HEALTH CARE REVIEW
    800 31st Ave SW
    Minot, ND 58701

KEY EXECUTIVES:
Chairman of the Board .... David J Glatt, MD
Chief Executive Officer .... Dave Remillard
Director of Finance .... Rich Haugen, CPA
Medical Director .... Michael Goldstone, MD
Director, HCQIP & Communications .... Barbara Groutt, MSA
Director, Information Systems & Analysis .... Richard Bubach, MSA
Director of Review .... Julie Thrailkill, RHIT

COMPANY PROFILE:
Parent Company Name:
Doing Business As:
Year Founded: Federally Qualified: [ ]
Forprofit: [ ]   Not-For-Profit: [ ]
Model Type:
Accreditation: [ ] AAPPO [ ] JACHO [ ] NCQA [ ] URAC
Plan Type: UR

SERVICE AREA:
Nationwide: N
    ND;

Managed Care Organization Profiles — NORTH DAKOTA

BLUE CROSS BLUE SHIELD OF NORTH DAKOTA

4510 13th Ave S
Fargo, ND 58121-0001
Phone: 701-282-1100 Fax: 701-277-2132 Toll-Free: 800-342-4718
Web site: www.bcbsnd.com

MAILING ADDRESS:
BC BS OF NORTH DAKOTA
4510 13th Ave S
Fargo, ND 58121-0001

KEY EXECUTIVES:
Chairperson of the Board .... Robert Grossman, MD
Chief Executive Officer/President .... Michael B Unhjem
Senior VP,Chief Financial Officer .... David Breuer
Senior VP,Chief Medical Officer .... Jon Rice, MD
Senior VP, IS,Chief Information Officer .... Darrell Vanyo
Senior VP, Chief Marketing Officer .... Chad Niles
Senior VP, IS,Chief Information Officer .... Darryl Vanyo
VP, Provider Relations/Reimbursemt .... Charley Hundley
VP, Human Resources .... Randy Johnson
Executive VP, Health Operations .... Tim Huckle
VP, Corporate Communications .... Larry Gauper

COMPANY PROFILE:
Parent Company Name: Noridian Mutual Insurance Company
Doing Business As: CareChoice
Year Founded: 1985   Federally Qualified: [N]
Forprofit: [ ]   Not-For-Profit: [Y]
Model Type:
Accreditation: [ ] AAPPO [ ] JACHO [ ] NCQA [ ] URAC
Plan Type: HMO
Total Revenue: 2005:   2006: 1,050,269,000
Net Income   2005:   2006: 3,927,000
Total Enrollment:
  2001: 0   2004: 0   2007: 450,000
  2002: 400,000   2005:
  2003: 0   2006:

SERVICE AREA:
Nationwide: N
  MN (Central); ND (Central and Northeast);

TYPE OF COVERAGE:
Commercial: [Y] Individual: [Y] FEHBP: [ ] Indemnity: [ ]
Medicare: [ ] Medicaid: [ ] Supplemental Medicare: [ ]Tricare
[ ]

PRODUCTS OFFERED:
Product Name: Type:
Blue Care   Medicare

PLAN BENEFITS:
Alternative Medicine: [ ]   Behavioral Health: [X]
Chiropractic: [X]   Dental: [ ]
Home Care: [X]   Inpatient SNF: [X]
Long-Term Care: [ ]   Pharm. Mail Order: [X]
Physical Therapy: [X]   Podiatry: [X]
Psychiatric: [X]   Transplant: [X]
Vision: [ ]   Wellness: [X]
Workers' Comp: [ ]
Other Benefits:

HEART OF AMERICA HEALTH PLAN

810 S Main Ave
Rugby, ND 58368
Phone: 701-776-5848 Fax: 701-776-5425 Toll-Free: 800-525-5661
Web site: www.hoahp.com

MAILING ADDRESS:
HEART OF AMERICA HEALTH PLAN
810 S Main Ave
Rugby, ND 58368

KEY EXECUTIVES:
Chief Executive Officer/President .... Jerry Jurena
Chief Financial Officer .... Mary Ann Jaeger
Medical Director .... Ron Skipper, MD
Marketing Director .... Chad Hager

COMPANY PROFILE:
Parent Company Name:
Doing Business As: Heart of America HMO
Year Founded: 1983   Federally Qualified: [ ]
Forprofit: [ ]   Not-For-Profit: [Y]
Model Type:
Accreditation: [ ] AAPPO [ ] JACHO [ ] NCQA [ ] URAC
Plan Type: HMO
Total Revenue: 2005:   2006: 4,793,911
Net Income   2005:   2006:
Total Enrollment:
  2001: 2,300   2004: 2,060   2007: 0
  2002: 2,233   2005:
  2003: 2,101   2006:
Medical Loss Ratio: 2005:   2006: 88.90
Administrative Expense Ratio: 2005:   2006:

SERVICE AREA:
Nationwide: N
  ND (Rugby, Minot);

TYPE OF COVERAGE:
Commercial: [ ] Individual: [Y] FEHBP: [ ] Indemnity: [ ]
Medicare: [Y] Medicaid: [ ] Supplemental Medicare: [ ]
Tricare   [ ]

PRODUCTS OFFERED:
Product Name: Type:
Medicare Coordinated Care Plan   Medicare Advantage

HUMANA INC - NORTH DAKOTA

500 W Main St
Louisville, KY 40201
Phone: 502-580-5804 Fax: 502-580-5044 Toll-Free:
Web site: www.humana.com

MAILING ADDRESS:
HUMANA INC - NORTH DAKOTA
500 W Main St
Louisville, KY 40201

KEY EXECUTIVES:
Chairman of the Board .... David A Jones Jr
Chief Executive Officer/President .... Michael B McCallister
Chief Financial Officer .... James H Bloem
Chief Clinical Strategy .... Jonathan T Lord, MD
Senior VP Chief Information Officer .... Bruce J Goodman
Chief Operating Officer .... Jim Murray
Chief Marketing Officer .... Steve Moya
Senior VP Human Resources .... Bonnie C Hathcock
New Product Development Director .... Tom Liston
Senior VP, General Counsel .... Art Hipwell
Senior VP, Corporate Communications .... Tom Noland

COMPANY PROFILE:
Parent Company Name: Humana Inc
Doing Business As:
Year Founded: 1961   Federally Qualified: [Y]
Forprofit: [Y]   Not-For-Profit: [ ]
Model Type:
Accreditation: [ ] AAPPO [ ] JACHO [ ] NCQA [ ] URAC
Plan Type: PPO, ASO, CDHP, HDHP, HSA,

SERVICE AREA:
Nationwide: N
  ND;

TYPE OF COVERAGE:
Commercial: [Y] Individual: [ ] FEHBP: [ ] Indemnity: [ ]
Medicare: [Y] Medicaid: [ ] Supplemental Medicare: [Y]
Tricare   [ ]

CONSUMER-DRIVEN PRODUCTS
JP Morgan Chase   HSA Company
HumanaOne HSA   HSA Product
JP Morgan Chase   HSA Administrator
Personal Care Account   Consumer-Driven Health Plan
HumanaOne   High Deductible Health Plan

PLAN BENEFITS:
Alternative Medicine: [ ]   Behavioral Health: [ ]
Chiropractic: [X]   Dental: [X]
Home Care: [ ]   Inpatient SNF: [ ]
Long-Term Care: [ ]   Pharm. Mail Order: [X]
Physical Therapy: [ ]   Podiatry: [ ]
Psychiatric: [X]   Transplant: [X]
Vision: [ ]   Wellness: [X]
Workers' Comp: [X]
Other Benefits:

Managed Care Organization Profiles — NORTH CAROLINA

PRODUCTS OFFERED:
Product Name:	Type:
Partners HMO	HMO
Partners POS	POS
Partners ASO	ASO
Partners Medicare Choice	Medicare

PLAN BENEFITS:
Alternative Medicine:	[X]	Behavioral Health:	[ ]
Chiropractic:	[X]	Dental:	[X]
Home Care:	[X]	Inpatient SNF:	[X]
Long-Term Care:	[X]	Pharm. Mail Order:	[ ]
Physical Therapy:	[X]	Podiatry:	[X]
Psychiatric:	[X]	Transplant:	[X]
Vision:	[X]	Wellness:	[X]
Workers' Comp:	[ ]		
Other Benefits:			

UNITEDHEALTHCARE OF NORTH CAROLINA INC

3803 N Elm St
Greensboro, NC 27455
Phone: 336-282-0900 Fax: 336-288-5206 Toll-Free: 800-521-2603
Web site: www.uhc.com

MAILING ADDRESS:
UNITEDHEALTHCARE OF NC INC
3803 N Elm St
Greensboro, NC 27455

KEY EXECUTIVES:
Non-Executive Chairman .... Richard T Burke
Chief Executive Officer .... Jane Rollinson
Chief Financial Officer .... Jack Shields
Medical Director .... Leonard A Wilkerson, DO
Public Relations Director .... Roger Rollman
VP, Network Management .... Anita Bachmann
Quality Assurance Director .... Mary Snider

COMPANY PROFILE:
Parent Company Name: UnitedHealth Group
Doing Business As:
Year Founded: 1985   Federally Qualified: [N]
Forprofit: [Y]   Not-For-Profit: [ ]
Model Type: IPA
Accreditation: [ ] AAPPO [ ] JACHO [X] NCQA [ ] URAC
Plan Type: HMO, CDHP, HDHP, HSA, HRA,
Primary Physicians: 6,377   Physician Specialists:
Hospitals:
Total Revenue: 2005: 887,573,563 2006: 882,781,245
Net Income   2005: 36,373,563 2006: 27,090,634
Total Enrollment:
  2001: 319,923   2004: 257,287   2007: 0
  2002: 272,746   2005: 188,724
  2003: 264,115   2006: 129,081
Medical Loss Ratio: 2005:   2006: 81.10
Administrative Expense Ratio: 2005:   2006:

SERVICE AREA:
Nationwide: N
NC;

TYPE OF COVERAGE:
Commercial: [Y] Individual: [ ] FEHBP: [ ] Indemnity: [ ]
Medicare: [Y] Medicaid: [ ] Supplemental Medicare: [ ]
Tricare: [ ]

PRODUCTS OFFERED:
Product Name:	Type:
Medicare Complete	Medicare Advantage
United Healthcare Medicaid	Medicaid
United Healthcare HMO	HMO
United Healthcare PPO	PPO

CONSUMER-DRIVEN PRODUCTS
Exante Bank/Golden Rule Ins Co	HSA Company
iPlan HSA	HSA Product
	HSA Administrator
	Consumer-Driven Health Plan
	High Deductible Health Plan

PLAN BENEFITS:
Alternative Medicine:	[ ]	Behavioral Health:	[X]
Chiropractic:	[X]	Dental:	[X]
Home Care:	[X]	Inpatient SNF:	[X]
Long-Term Care:	[ ]	Pharm. Mail Order:	[X]
Physical Therapy:	[X]	Podiatry:	[X]
Psychiatric:	[X]	Transplant:	[X]
Vision:	[X]	Wellness:	[X]
Workers' Comp:	[ ]		
Other Benefits:			

Comments:
Formerly PHP Inc of North Carolina.

WELLPATH SELECT INC

2801 Slater Rd #200
Morrisville, NC 27560
Phone: 866-935-7284 Fax: 877-204-8727 Toll-Free:
Web site: www.wellpathonline.com

MAILING ADDRESS:
WELLPATH SELECT INC
2801 Slater Rd #200
Morrisville, NC 27560

KEY EXECUTIVES:
Chief Executive Officer/President .... Tracy H Baker
Chief Financial Officer .... Dewey Brown
VP, Medical Affairs .... Daniel Barco, MD
Pharmacy Director .... Tim Kurek
Chief Operating Officer .... Peter Chauncey
VP, Sales & Marketing .... John Eutledge
VP, Sales & Marketing II .... Dave McClain
VP, Network Management .... Matt Ungs
VP, Quality Management .... Esther Watson RN
Director Product Development & Regulatory Affairs ...... Cheryl Harris

COMPANY PROFILE:
Parent Company Name: Coventry Health Care Inc
Doing Business As:
Year Founded: 1995   Federally Qualified: [ ]
Forprofit: [Y]   Not-For-Profit: [ ]
Model Type: IPA
Accreditation: [ ] AAPPO [ ] JACHO [ ] NCQA [X] URAC
Plan Type: HMO, PPO, POS, ASO, CDHP, HSA, HDHP
Total Revenue: 2005: 204,129,677 2006: 201,143,980
Net Income   2005: 13,111,986 2006: 18,971,691
Total Enrollment:
  2001: 35,924   2004: 121,628   2007: 0
  2002: 109,146   2005: 132,845
  2003: 76,482   2006: 100,000
Medical Loss Ratio: 2005:   2006: 74.50
Administrative Expense Ratio: 2005:   2006:

SERVICE AREA:
Nationwide: N
NC; SC;

TYPE OF COVERAGE:
Commercial: [Y] Individual: [ ] FEHBP: [ ] Indemnity: [Y]
Medicare: [ ] Medicaid: [ ] Supplemental Medicare: [Y]
Tricare: [ ]

PRODUCTS OFFERED:
Product Name:	Type:
WellPath Select Inc	HMO
WellPath Select Plus	POS
WellPath Preferred	PPO
WellPath 65 Health Plan	Medicare

CONSUMER-DRIVEN PRODUCTS
Wells Fargo	HSA Company
	HSA Product
Corporate Benefits Services of America	HSA Administrator
	Consumer-Driven Health Plan
Open Access Plus Plan	High Deductible Health Plan

PLAN BENEFITS:
Alternative Medicine:	[ ]	Behavioral Health:	[ ]
Chiropractic:	[ ]	Dental:	[X]
Home Care:	[X]	Inpatient SNF:	[ ]
Long-Term Care:	[X]	Pharm. Mail Order:	[X]
Physical Therapy:	[ ]	Podiatry:	[X]
Psychiatric:	[X]	Transplant:	[X]
Vision:	[X]	Wellness:	[X]
Workers' Comp:	[ ]		
Other Benefits:			

NORTH CAROLINA

MAILING ADDRESS:
  MEDCOST LLC
  PO Box 25347
  Winston-Salem, NC 27103

KEY EXECUTIVES:
Chief Executive Officer .... William D Ketner
VP, Finance .... Joel Groce
Chief Medical Officer .... William B Lorentz, Jr, MD
Director Information Services .... Kevin Barnette
Director of Marketing Services .... Laura Patterson
Director of Information Services .... Kevin Barnette
Provider Relations Director .... Paul Stetson
Medical Management Director .... Ann Culp
VP of Business Development & Quality .... Kathryn Showalter
Director of Network Claims/Customer Services .... Wanda Owen

COMPANY PROFILE:
Parent Company Name: Carolinas Med Ctr-Charlotte/NC Baptist H
Doing Business As:
Year Founded: 1983   Federally Qualified: [ ]
Forprofit: [Y]   Not-For-Profit: [ ]
Model Type: NETWORK
Accreditation: [ ] AAPPO [ ] JACHO [ ] NCQA [X] URAC
Plan Type: PPO, UR
Primary Physicians: 10,557   Physician Specialists: 20,068
Hospitals: 1,012
Total Enrollment:
  2001: 860,969   2004: 778,027   2007: 0
  2002: 881,012   2005:
  2003: 0   2006: 819,000

SERVICE AREA:
Nationwide: N
  NC; SC;

TYPE OF COVERAGE:
Commercial: [Y] Individual: [Y] FEHBP: [ ] Indemnity: [ ]
Medicare: [ ] Medicaid: [ ] Supplemental Medicare: [ ]
Tricare   [ ]

PRODUCTS OFFERED:
Product Name: Type:
MedCost PPO   PPO

Comments:
Acquired Health Care Savings, Inc. July 18, 2006.

OPTICARE MANAGED VISION

112 Zebulon Ct
Rocky Mount, NC 27804
Phone: 252-937-6650 Fax: 252-451-2171 Toll-Free: 800-334-3937
Web site: www.opticare.com

MAILING ADDRESS:
  OPTICARE MANAGED VISION
  PO Box 7548
  Rocky Mount, NC 27804

KEY EXECUTIVES:
President, Managed Vision .... Jason Harrold
Medical Director I .... Mark Ruchman, MD
Senior VP, Operations .... Larry Keeley
Senior VP of Information Systems .... Juan Marrero
VP of Provider Affairs .... Jeremy Myers
VP of Medical Management .... Connie Cook
Managed Care Development Dir .... Marigene McHale
Medical Director II .... David R Haas, MD
Medical Director III .... Shawn Putnam, MD
Senior VP, Opticare Vision Plan .... David Lavely

COMPANY PROFILE:
Parent Company Name: OptiCare Health Systems Inc
Doing Business As: Opticare Eye Health Network, Total Visio
Year Founded: Federally Qualified: [N]
Forprofit: [Y]   Not-For-Profit: [ ]
Model Type: NETWORK
Accreditation: [ ] AAPPO [ ] JACHO [X] NCQA [ ] URAC
Plan Type: Specialty HMO, ASO, TPA, UR

SERVICE AREA:
Nationwide: N
  All States except NY for OptiCare Vision Plans, OptiCare Managed Vision in multiple states;

TYPE OF COVERAGE:
Commercial: [Y] Individual: [ ] FEHBP: [ ] Indemnity: [ ]
Medicare: [Y] Medicaid: [Y] Supplemental Medicare: [ ]
Tricare   [ ]

PLAN BENEFITS:
Alternative Medicine: [ ]   Behavioral Health: [ ]
Chiropractic: [ ]   Dental: [ ]
Home Care: [ ]   Inpatient SNF: [ ]
Long-Term Care: [ ]   Pharm. Mail Order: [ ]
Physical Therapy: [ ]   Podiatry: [ ]
Psychiatric: [ ]   Transplant: [ ]
Vision: [X]   Wellness: [ ]
Workers' Comp: [ ]
Other Benefits:

Comments:
Name changed from Opticare Eye Health Network. Formerly Association for Eyecare Centers & Opticare Health Systems.

PARTNERS NATIONAL HEALTH PLANS OF NORTH CAROLINA INC

5660 University Parkway
Winston-Salem, NC 27105
Phone: 336-760-4822 Fax: 336-760-3198 Toll-Free: 800-942-5695
Web site: www.partnershealth.com

MAILING ADDRESS:
  PARTNERS NATL HLTH PLANS OF NC
  PO Box 17509
  Winston-Salem, NC 27116-7509

KEY EXECUTIVES:
Chief Executive Officer/President .... Robert Grezcyn
Medical Director .... Tom Lanava, MD
VP, Operations .... Marianella Perdomo

COMPANY PROFILE:
Parent Company Name: Blue Cross Blue Shield of NC
Doing Business As: Partners National Health Plans of NC
Year Founded: 1986   Federally Qualified: [N]
Forprofit: [Y]   Not-For-Profit: [ ]
Model Type: MIXED
Accreditation: [ ] AAPPO [ ] JACHO [X] NCQA [ ] URAC
Plan Type: HMO, PPO, POS,
Total Revenue: 2005:   326,311,686   2006:   374,674,563
Net Income   2005:   21,692,145   2006:   20,372,773
Total Enrollment:
  2001: 295,992   2004: 37,035   2007: 0
  2002: 36,303   2005: 39,000
  2003: 75,521   2006:
Medical Loss Ratio: 2005:   2006: 84.10
Administrative Expense Ratio: 2005:   2006:

SERVICE AREA:
Nationwide: N
  NC (Alamance, Alexander, Alleghany, Anson, Ashe, Avery, Beaufort,Bertie, Bladen, Brunswick, Buncombe, Burke, Cabarrus, Caldwell, Camden, Carteret, Caswell, Catawba, Chatham, Cherokee, Chowan, Clay, Cleveland, Craven, Columbus, Cumberland, Currituck, Dare, Davidson, Davie, Duplin, Durham, Edgecombe, Forsyth, Franklin, Gaston, Gates, Graham, Granville, Greene, Guilford, Halifax, Harnett, Haywood, Henderson, Hertford, Hoke, Hyde, Iredell, Jackson, Johnston, Jones, Lee, Lenoir, Lincoln, Macon, Madison, Martin, McDowell, Mecklenburg, Mitchell, Montgomery, Moore, Nash,New Hanover, Northampton, Onslow, Orange, Pamlico, Pasquotank, Pender, Perquimans, Person, Pitt, Polk, Randolph, Richmond, Robeson, Rockingham, Rowan, Rutherford, Sampson, Scotland, Stanly, Stokes, Surry, Swain, Transylvania, Tyrrell, Union, Vance, Wake, Warren, Washington, Watauga, Wayne, Wilkes, Wilson, Yadkin, Yancey); SC (Anderson, Cherokee, Chester, Darlington, Dillon, Fairfield, Florence, Greenville, Lancaster, Lee, Lexington, Pickens,Richland, Spartanburg, Union, Williamsburg, York); VA (Bedford, Botetourt, Campbell, Carroll, Craig, Floyd, Franklin, Giles, Grayson, Henry, Montgomery, Patrick, Pittsylvania, Pulaski, Roanoke, Rockbridge, Wythe).

TYPE OF COVERAGE:
Commercial: [Y] Individual: [ ] FEHBP: [ ] Indemnity: [ ]
Medicare: [Y] Medicaid: [ ] Supplemental Medicare: [ ]
Tricare   [ ]

Managed Care Organization Profiles — NORTH CAROLINA

GREAT-WEST HEALTHCARE OF NORTH CAROLINA

5970 Fairview Rd Ste 650
Charlotte, NC 28210
Phone: 704-556-9033 Fax: 704-552-7042 Toll-Free: 800-663-8081
Web site: www.greatwesthealthcare.com

MAILING ADDRESS:
GREAT-WEST HEALTHCARE OF NC
5970 Fairview Rd Ste 650
Charlotte, NC 28210

KEY EXECUTIVES:
Chief Executive Officer/President .... Raymond L McFeetors
President, SE Region .... Steve A White
Director, Network Development .... Daniel Tubaugh

COMPANY PROFILE:
Parent Company Name: Great West Life & Annuity Insurance Co
Doing Business As:
Year Founded: Federally Qualified: [N]
Forprofit: [Y]   Not-For-Profit: [ ]
Model Type:
Accreditation: [ ] AAPPO [ ] JACHO [ ] NCQA [X] URAC
Plan Type: PPO, POS, UR, CDHP, HSA
Total Enrollment:
  2001: 4,719   2004: 162   2007: 0
  2002: 1,438   2005:
  2003: 667   2006:

SERVICE AREA:
Nationwide: N
NC;

TYPE OF COVERAGE:
Commercial: [Y] Individual: [ ] FEHBP: [ ] Indemnity: [ ]
Medicare: [ ] Medicaid: [ ] Supplemental Medicare: [ ]
Tricare   [ ]

PRODUCTS OFFERED:
Product Name: Type:
Great West Life PPO   PPO

CONSUMER-DRIVEN PRODUCTS
Mellon HR Solutions LLC   HSA Company
                                    HSA Product
                                    HSA Administrator
                                    Consumer-Driven Health Plan
                                    High Deductible Health Plan

PLAN BENEFITS:
Alternative Medicine: [X]   Behavioral Health: [ ]
Chiropractic: [X]   Dental: [X]
Home Care: [X]   Inpatient SNF: [X]
Long-Term Care: [ ]   Pharm. Mail Order: [X]
Physical Therapy: [X]   Podiatry: [X]
Psychiatric: [X]   Transplant: [X]
Vision: [X]   Wellness: [X]
Workers' Comp: [ ]
Other Benefits:

HUMANA INC - NORTH CAROLINA

6100 Fairview Rd Ste 750
Charlotte, NC 28210
Phone: 704-643-0400 Fax: 704-643-0306 Toll-Free: 800-234-9761
Web site: www.humana.com

MAILING ADDRESS:
HUMANA INC - NORTH CAROLINA
500 W Main St
Louisville, KY 28210

KEY EXECUTIVES:
Chairman of the Board .... David A Jones Jr
Chief Executive Officer/President .... Michael B McCallister
Chief Financial Officer .... James H Bloem
Senior VP, Chief Information Officer .... Bruce J Goodman
Sales Director .... Gary Greenwald
Senior VP, Human Resources .... Bonnie C Hathcock
Media Relations Manager .... Mitch Lubitz

COMPANY PROFILE:
Parent Company Name: Humana Inc
Doing Business As:
Year Founded: 1961   Federally Qualified: [Y]
Forprofit: [Y]   Not-For-Profit: [ ]
Model Type:
Accreditation: [ ] AAPPO [ ] JACHO [ ] NCQA [ ] URAC
Plan Type: HMO, PPO, ASO, CDHP, HSA
Total Enrollment:
  2001: 23,843   2004: 10,100   2007: 0
  2002: 30,700   2005: 3,962
  2003: 167,100   2006:

SERVICE AREA:
Nationwide: N
NC;

TYPE OF COVERAGE:
Commercial: [Y] Individual: [ ] FEHBP: [ ] Indemnity:[ ]Medicare: [Y] Medicaid: [ ] Supplemental Medicare: [Y]
Tricare   [Y]

CONSUMER-DRIVEN PRODUCTS
JP Morgan Chase   HSA Company
HumanaOne HSA   HSA Product
JP Morgan Chase   HSA Administrator
Personal Care Account   Consumer-Driven Health Plan
HumanaOne   High Deductible Health Plan

PLAN BENEFITS:
Alternative Medicine: [ ]   Behavioral Health: [ ]
Chiropractic: [X]   Dental: [X]
Home Care: [ ]   Inpatient SNF: [ ]
Long-Term Care: [ ]   Pharm. Mail Order: [X]
Physical Therapy: [ ]   Podiatry: [ ]
Psychiatric: [X]   Transplant: [X]
Vision: [ ]   Wellness: [X]
Workers' Comp: [X]
Other Benefits:

INTERACTIVE MEDICAL SYSTEMS

5621 Departure Dr Ste 117
Raleigh, NC 27616
Phone: 919-877-9933 Fax: 919-877-0615 Toll-Free: 800-426-8739
Web site: www.ims-tpa.com

MAILING ADDRESS:
INTERACTIVE MEDICAL SYSTEMS
PO Box 19108
Raleigh, NC 27616

KEY EXECUTIVES:
Vice President .... Brent Monroe
President .... Eric Ludwig
Chief Financial Officer .... Judy Paulakuhn
Chief Operating Officer .... Brent Monroe
Marketing Director/Account Manager .... Suzanne Bishoff
Senior Account Manager .... Wyndin Sheen
Claims Manager .... Judith A Hall

COMPANY PROFILE:
Parent Company Name:
Doing Business As:
Year Founded: Federally Qualified: [ ]
Forprofit: [Y]   Not-For-Profit: [ ]
Model Type:
Accreditation: [ ] AAPPO [ ] JACHO [ ] NCQA [ ] URAC
Plan Type: TPA

SERVICE AREA:
Nationwide: N
NC;

TYPE OF COVERAGE:
Commercial: [Y] Individual: [ ] FEHBP: [ ] Indemnity: [ ]
Medicare: [ ] Medicaid: [ ] Supplemental Medicare: [ ]
Tricare   [ ]

MEDCOST LLC

165 Kimel Park Drive
Winston-Salem, NC 27103
Phone: 336-760-3090 Fax: 336-760-2352 Toll-Free:
Web site: www.medcost.com

NORTH CAROLINA

Total Enrollment:
2001: 33,807   2004: 0   2007: 0
2002: 0   2005: 118,000
2003: 40,210   2006:
Medical Loss Ratio: 2005:   2006: 82.30
Administrative Expense Ratio: 2005:   2006:

SERVICE AREA:
Nationwide: N
NC (Cabarrus, Gaston, Mecklenburg, Union); SC (York);

TYPE OF COVERAGE:
Commercial: [Y] Individual: [ ] FEHBP: [ ] Indemnity: [ ]
Medicare: [ ] Medicaid: [ ] Supplemental Medicare: [ ]
Tricare   [ ]

PRODUCTS OFFERED:
Product Name: Type:
Coventry Healthcare HMO   HMO

CONSUMER-DRIVEN PRODUCTS
Wells Fargo   HSA Company
                                       HSA Product
Corporate Benefits Services of America HSA Administrator
                                       Consumer-Driven Health Plan
Open Access Plus Plan   High Deductible Health Plan

PLAN BENEFITS:
Alternative Medicine: [ ]   Behavioral Health: [X]
Chiropractic: [X]   Dental: [X]
Home Care: [X]   Inpatient SNF: [X]
Long-Term Care: [ ]   Pharm. Mail Order: [X]
Physical Therapy: [X]   Podiatry: [X]
Psychiatric: [X]   Transplant: [X]
Vision: [X]   Wellness: [X]
Workers' Comp: [ ]
Other Benefits:

Comments:
Formerly Principal Health Care of the Carolinas Inc.

DELTA DENTAL PLAN OF NORTH CAROLINA

343 Six Forks Rd Ste 180
Raleigh, NC 27609
Phone: 919-832-6015 Fax: 919-832-6061 Toll-Free: 800-662-8856
Web site: www.deltadentalnc.org

MAILING ADDRESS:
DELTA DENTAL PLAN OF NC
343 Six Forks Rd Ste 180
Raleigh, NC 27609

KEY EXECUTIVES:
Chief Executive Officer/President .... Robert Rosenthal, DDS
Controller .... Steve Dudash
VP, Marketing .... Kevin Simpson

COMPANY PROFILE:
Parent Company Name: Delta Dental Plan Association
Doing Business As:
Year Founded: 1954   Federally Qualified: [ ]
Forprofit: [ ]   Not-For-Profit: [ ]
Model Type:
Accreditation: [ ] AAPPO [ ] JACHO [ ] NCQA [ ] URAC
Plan Type: Specialty HMO
Total Revenue: 2005:   2006:
Net Income   2005:   2006: -1,452,393
Total Enrollment:
2001: 0   2004: 58,928   2007: 0
2002: 48,372   2005:
2003: 59,366   2006:
Medical Loss Ratio: 2005:   2006: 80.3
Administrative Expense Ratio: 2005:   2006:

SERVICE AREA:
Nationwide: N
NC;

TYPE OF COVERAGE:
Commercial: [Y] Individual: [ ] FEHBP: [ ] Indemnity: [ ]
Medicare: [ ] Medicaid: [ ] Supplemental Medicare: [ ]
Tricare   [ ]

PLAN BENEFITS:
Alternative Medicine: [ ]   Behavioral Health: [ ]
Chiropractic: [ ]   Dental: [X]
Home Care: [ ]   Inpatient SNF: [ ]
Long-Term Care: [ ]   Pharm. Mail Order: [ ]
Physical Therapy: [ ]   Podiatry: [ ]
Psychiatric: [ ]   Transplant: [ ]
Vision: [ ]   Wellness: [ ]
Workers' Comp: [ ]
Other Benefits:

FIDELIS SECURECARE OF NORTH CAROLINA

9300 Harris Corners Pkwy #100
Charlotte, NC 28269
Phone: 877-372-8080 Fax: 877-372-8081 Toll-Free:
Web site: www.fidelissc.com

MAILING ADDRESS:
FIDELIS SECURECARE OF NC
9300 Harris Corners Pkwy #100
Charlotte, NC 28269

KEY EXECUTIVES:
Chief Executive Officer .... Samuel R Willcoxon
President - North Carolina .... Robert Dunlap
Director of Operations .... C L Nelson
Director of Sales .... Neal Lail
Director of Provider Relations .... David Kaplan
Director of Clinical Services .... Karen Walker, RN

COMPANY PROFILE:
Parent Company Name: Fidelis SeniorCare Inc
Doing Business As:
Year Founded: 2006   Federally Qualified: [Y]
Forprofit: [ ]   Not-For-Profit: [ ]
Model Type:
Accreditation: [ ] AAPPO [ ] JACHO [ ] NCQA [ ] URAC
Plan Type: HMO
Primary Physicians: Physician Specialists:
Hospitals:
Total Revenue: 2005:   2006: 2,249,672
Net Income   2005:   2006: -1,914,672
Medical Loss Ratio: 2005: 2006: 88.50
Administrative Expense Ratio: 2005: 2006:

SERVICE AREA:
Nationwide:
NC (Alamance, Cabarrus, Davidson, Davie, Durham, Forsyth,
Guilford, Iredell, Mecklenburg, Rowan, Stanly, Union, Wake);

TYPE OF COVERAGE:
Commercial: [ ] Individual: [ ] FEHBP: [ ] Indemnity: [ ]
Medicare: [Y] Medicaid: [ ] Supplemental Medicare: [ ]
Tricare   [ ]

FIRSTCAROLINACARE

42 Memorial Dr Ste 1
Pinehurst, NC 28370
Phone: 910-715-8100 Fax: 910-715-8101 Toll-Free: 800-574-8556
Web site: www.firstcarolinacare.com

MAILING ADDRESS:
FIRSTCAROLINACARE
PO Box 909
Pinehurst, NC 28370

KEY EXECUTIVES:
Executive Director .... Kenneth J Lewis
Corporate Medical Director .... Sandra Morris, MD

COMPANY PROFILE:
Parent Company Name: FirstHealth of the Carolinas
Doing Business As:
Year Founded: 2000   Federally Qualified: [ ]
Forprofit: [Y]   Not-For-Profit: [ ]
Model Type:
Accreditation: [ ] AAPPO [ ] JACHO [ ] NCQA [ ] URAC
Plan Type: HMO,
Total Revenue: 2005:   2006: 40,989,870
Net Income   2005: 978,081   2006: 950,780
Total Enrollment:
2001: 6,186   2004: 10,536   2007: 0
2002: 7,043   2005: 11,227
2003: 8,091   2006: 11,227
Medical Loss Ratio: 2005:   2006: 83.20
Administrative Expense Ratio: 2005:   2006:

SERVICE AREA:
Nationwide:
NC;

TYPE OF COVERAGE:
Commercial: [Y] Individual: [ ] FEHBP: [ ] Indemnity: [ ]
Medicare: [ ] Medicaid: [ ] Supplemental Medicare: [ ]
Tricare   [ ]

Managed Care Organization Profiles — NORTH CAROLINA

PRODUCTS OFFERED:
Product Name: Type:
CIGNA Dental HMO   Specialty HMO

PLAN BENEFITS:
Alternative Medicine: [ ]   Behavioral Health: [ ]
Chiropractic: [ ]   Dental: [X]
Home Care: [ ]   Inpatient SNF: [ ]
Long-Term Care: [ ]   Pharm. Mail Order: [ ]
Physical Therapy: [ ]   Podiatry: [ ]
Psychiatric: [ ]   Transplant: [ ]
Vision: [ ]   Wellness: [ ]
Workers' Comp: [ ]
Other Benefits:

CIGNA HEALTHCARE OF NORTH CAROLINA

701 Corporate Center Dr
Raleigh, NC 27607
Phone: 919-854-7000   Fax: 919-854-7100   Toll-Free: 800-849-9300
Web site: www.cigna.com

MAILING ADDRESS:
    CIGNA HEALTHCARE OF NC
    701 Corporate Center Dr
    Raleigh, NC 27607

KEY EXECUTIVES:
President .... Charles Pitts
Medical Director .... Scott T Josephs, MD
Director of Provider Services .... Chutamar Altizer

COMPANY PROFILE:
Parent Company Name: CIGNA Corporation
Doing Business As: HealthSource NC Inc
Year Founded: 1986   Federally Qualified: [N]
Forprofit: [Y]   Not-For-Profit: [ ]
Model Type: IPA
Accreditation: [ ] AAPPO [ ] JACHO [X] NCQA [ ] URAC
Plan Type: HMO, POS, TPA, CDHP, HDHP, HSA, FSA, HRA
Total Revenue: 2005:   2006: 230,247,996
Net Income: 2005:   2006: 7,384,438
Total Enrollment:
   2001: 0   2004: 88,971   2007: 0
   2002: 195,357   2005:
   2003: 122,253   2006:
Medical Loss Ratio: 2005:   2006: 82.60
Administrative Expense Ratio: 2005:   2006:

SERVICE AREA:
Nationwide: N
   NC;

TYPE OF COVERAGE:
Commercial: [Y]   Individual: [ ]   FEHBP: [ ]   Indemnity: [ ]
Medicare: [ ]   Medicaid: [ ]   Supplemental Medicare: [ ]
Tricare [ ]

PRODUCTS OFFERED:
Product Name: Type:
Cigna HMO   HMO

CONSUMER-DRIVEN PRODUCTS
JP Morgan Chase   HSA Company
CIGNA Choice Fund   HSA Product
    HSA Administrator
Open Access Plus   Consumer-Driven Health Plan
PPO   High Deductible Health Plan

PLAN BENEFITS:
Alternative Medicine: [ ]   Behavioral Health: [X]
Chiropractic: [X]   Dental: [ ]
Home Care: [X]   Inpatient SNF: [X]
Long-Term Care: [X]   Pharm. Mail Order: [ ]
Physical Therapy: [X]   Podiatry: [X]
Psychiatric: [X]   Transplant: [X]
Vision: [X]   Wellness: [X]
Workers' Comp: [ ]
Other Benefits:

CIGNA HEALTHCARE OF NORTH CAROLINA INC

207 Regency Executive Dr
Charlotte, NC 28217
Phone: 704-586-0708   Fax: 919-854-8135   Toll-Free: 800-235-5707
Web site: www.cigna.com

MAILING ADDRESS:
    CIGNA HEALTHCARE OF NC
    207 Regency Executive Dr
    Charlotte, NC 28217

KEY EXECUTIVES:
Chief Executive Officer .... Edward Hanway
President .... Charles Pitts
Medical Director .... Scott Josephs, MD

COMPANY PROFILE:
Parent Company Name: CIGNA Corporation
Doing Business As:
Year Founded: 1986   Federally Qualified: [N]
Forprofit: [Y]   Not-For-Profit: [ ]
Model Type: IPA
Accreditation: [ ] AAPPO [ ] JACHO [X] NCQA [ ] URAC
Plan Type: HMO, PPO, POS, CDHP, HSA, FSA, HRA
Total Revenue: 2005: 241,234,556   2006:
Net Income: 2005: 11,938,135   2006:
Total Enrollment:
   2001: 231,046   2004: 88,971   2007: 0
   2002: 195,357   2005: 76,803
   2003: 122,253   2006:

SERVICE AREA:
Nationwide: N
   NC (Greater Metropolitan areas and surrounding counties); SC (Greater Metropolitan areas and surrounding counties);

TYPE OF COVERAGE:
Commercial: [Y]   Individual: [ ]   FEHBP: [ ]   Indemnity: [ ]
Medicare: [ ]   Medicaid: [ ]   Supplemental Medicare: [ ]
Tricare [ ]

PRODUCTS OFFERED:
Product Name: Type:
Healthsource   HMO

CONSUMER-DRIVEN PRODUCTS
JP Morgan Chase   HSA Company
CIGNA Choice Fund   HSA Product
    HSA Administrator
Open Access Plus   Consumer-Driven Health Plan
PPO   High Deductible Health Plan

PLAN BENEFITS:
Alternative Medicine: [ ]   Behavioral Health: [X]
Chiropractic: [X]   Dental: [X]
Home Care: [X]   Inpatient SNF: [X]
Long-Term Care: [X]   Pharm. Mail Order: [X]
Physical Therapy: [X]   Podiatry: [X]
Psychiatric: [X]   Transplant: [X]
Vision: [X]   Wellness: [X]
Workers' Comp: [ ]
Other Benefits:

COVENTRY HEALTH CARE INC — CAROLINAS

2815 Coliseum Ctr Dr Ste 550
Charlotte, NC 28217
Phone: 704-357-1421   Fax: 704-357-3164   Toll-Free: 800-470-4523
Web site: www.cvty.com

MAILING ADDRESS:
    COVENTRY HEALTHCARE — CAROLINAS
    2815 Coliseum Ctr Dr Ste 550
    Charlotte, NC 28217

KEY EXECUTIVES:
Chief Executive Officer .... Tracy H Baker
Chief Financial Officer .... Dewey Brown
Chief Medical Officer .... Daniel Barco, MD
VP, Sales & Marketing .... Cory Scott

COMPANY PROFILE:
Parent Company Name: Coventry Health Care Inc
Doing Business As:
Year Founded: 1995   Federally Qualified: [Y]
Forprofit: [Y]   Not-For-Profit: [ ]
Model Type: IPA
Accreditation: [ ] AAPPO [ ] JACHO [ ] NCQA [ ] URAC
Plan Type: HMO, PPO, POS, CDHP, HDHP, HSA
Total Revenue: 2005:   2006: 26,962,968
Net Income: 2005:   2006:

NORTH CAROLINA

Managed Care Organization Profiles

Accreditation: [ ] AAPPO [ ] JACHO [ ] NCQA [ ] URAC
Plan Type: PPO,
Primary Physicians: 1,600 Physician Specialists: 2,400
Hospitals: 35
Total Enrollment:
  2001: 0   2004: 0   2007: 0
  2002: 40,000   2005:
  2003: 0   2006:
SERVICE AREA:
Nationwide: N
  NC;

BLUE CROSS BLUE SHIELD OF NORTH CAROLINA

5901 Chapel Hill Rd
Durham, NC 27702-2291
Phone: 919-489-7431 Fax: 919-765-3943 Toll-Free: 800-250-3630
Web site: www.bcbsnc.com
MAILING ADDRESS:
  BLUE CROSS BLUE SHIELD OF NC
  PO Box 2291
  Durham, NC 27702-2291

KEY EXECUTIVES:
Chairman .... E Rhone Sasser
Chief Executive Officer/President .... Robert J Greczyn, Jr
Senior VP, Chief Financial Officer .... Daniel E Glaser
Senior VP, Chief Medical Officer .... Don Bradley
Chief Information Officer .... John Sternbergh
Chief Operating Officer .... J Bradley Wilson
Senior VP Sales & Marketing .... John T Roos
VP Corp Communications .... Lynne Garrison
Senior VP, Human Resources .... Robert T Vavrina
Senior VP, Government Operations .... Ken Lerner

COMPANY PROFILE:
Parent Company Name: BC & BS of North Carolina
Doing Business As:
Year Founded: 1985   Federally Qualified: [Y]
Forprofit: [ ]   Not-For-Profit: [Y]
Model Type: IPA
Accreditation: [ ] AAPPO [ ] JACHO [X] NCQA [ ] URAC
Plan Type: PPO, POS, ASO, HMO, TPA, PBM, HDHP, HSA
Primary Physicians: 4,790 Physician Specialists: 14,932
Hospitals: 114
Total Revenue: 2005: 3,822,808,000 2006: 3,666,949,935
Net Income   2005: 119,271,981   2006: 125,393,669
Total Enrollment:
  2001: 2,500,000   2004: 3,100,000 2007: 0
  2002: 2,733,330   2005: 3,300,000
  2003: 2,900,000   2006: 3,435,785
Medical Loss Ratio: 2005: 80.10   2006: 80.70
Administrative Expense Ratio: 2005: 20.50 2006:
SERVICE AREA:
Nationwide: N
  NC;
TYPE OF COVERAGE:
Commercial: [Y] Individual: [Y] FEHBP: [ ] Indemnity: [ ]
Medicare: [ ] Medicaid: [ ] Supplemental Medicare: [Y]
Tricare   [ ]
PRODUCTS OFFERED:
Product Name: Type:
BC/BS Personal Plan   HMO
BC/BS PPO   PPO
CONSUMER-DRIVEN PRODUCTS
                           HSA Company
Blue HSA   HSA Product
Mellon Financial Corporation HSA Administrator
                           Consumer-Driven Health Plan
Blue Options PPO   High Deductible Health Plan
PLAN BENEFITS:
Alternative Medicine: [X] Behavioral Health: [X]
Chiropractic: [X] Dental: [X]
Home Care: [X] Inpatient SNF: [X]
Long-Term Care: [ ] Pharm. Mail Order: [X]
Physical Therapy: [X] Podiatry: [X]
Psychiatric: [X] Transplant: [X]
Vision: [X] Wellness: [X]
Workers' Comp: [ ]
Other Benefits:

CAROLINAS CENTER FOR MEDICAL EXCELLENCE, THE

100 Regency Forest Dr Ste 200
Cary, NC 27511-8598
Phone: 919-380-9860 Fax: 919-380-7637 Toll-Free: 800-682-2650
Web site: www.thecarolinascenter.org
MAILING ADDRESS:
  CAROLINAS CTR FOR MEDICAL EXCL
  100 Regency Forest Dr Ste 200
  Cary, NC 27511-8598

KEY EXECUTIVES:
Chief Executive Officer .... Charles Riddick
Chief Financial Officer .... Kathy Tapp
Principal Clinical Coordinator .... Ross J Simpson Jr, MD
Chief Operating Officer .... Robert Weiser
Chief Communications Officer .... Peg O'Connell

COMPANY PROFILE:
Parent Company Name: Medical Review of North Carolina Inc
Doing Business As: Carolinas Ctr for Medical Excellence,The
Year Founded: 1983   Federally Qualified: [ ]
Forprofit: [ ]   Not-For-Profit: [Y]
Model Type:
Accreditation: [ ] AAPPO [ ] JACHO [ ] NCQA [ ] URAC
Plan Type: UR, PRO
SERVICE AREA:
Nationwide: N
  NC; SC;

CIGNA DENTAL HEALTH OF NORTH CAROLINA INC

1571 Sawgrass Corporate Pkwy
Sunrise, FL 33323
Phone: 954-514-6600 Fax: 954-514-6905 Toll-Free: 800-367-1037
Web site: www.cigna.com/dental
MAILING ADDRESS:
  CIGNA DENTAL HEALTH OF NC INC
  1571 Sawgrass Corporate Pkwy
  Sunrise, FL 33323

KEY EXECUTIVES:
Chief Executive Officer .... Randee Lehrer
President .... Karen S Rohan
Chief Financial Officer .... Michelle I Haas
Dental Director .... Miles Hall, DDS
Marketing Director .... Judith Herron
MIS Director .... Laurel A Flebotte

COMPANY PROFILE:
Parent Company Name: CIGNA Dental Health Inc
Doing Business As: CIGNA Dental
Year Founded: 1992   Federally Qualified: [N]
Forprofit: [Y]   Not-For-Profit: [ ]
Model Type:
Accreditation: [ ] AAPPO [ ] JACHO [ ] NCQA [ ] URAC
Plan Type: Specialty HMO
Dentists: 81   Dental Specialists: 25
Hospitals:
Total Revenue: 2005: 2,851,260   2006: 2,993,775
Net Income   2005: -25,263   2006: -151,822
Total Enrollment:
  2001: 25,892   2004: 17,614   2007: 0
  2002: 25,801   2005: 18,860
  2003: 20,235   2006: 18,265
Medical Loss Ratio: 2005:   2006: 95.30
Administrative Expense Ratio: 2005:   2006:
SERVICE AREA:
Nationwide: N
  NC (Alamance, Buncombe, Cabarrus, Catawba, Chatham,
  Cumberland, Davidson, Davie, Durham, Edgecombe, Forsyth,
  Gaston, Granville, Guilford, Harnett, Iredell, Johnston, Lee,
  Mecklenburg, Nash, New Hanover, Orange, Pitt, Randolph, Rowan,
  Union, Wake);
TYPE OF COVERAGE:
Commercial: [Y] Individual: [ ] FEHBP: [ ] Indemnity: [ ]
Medicare: [ ] Medicaid: [ ] Supplemental Medicare: [ ]
Tricare   [ ]

Managed Care Organization Profiles — NORTH CAROLINA

AETNA INC OF THE CAROLINAS

13860 Ballantyne Corp Pl #250
Charlotte, NC 28277
Phone: 704-544-5716 Fax: 704-544-5756 Toll-Free:
Web site: www.aetna.com

MAILING ADDRESS:
    AETNA INC OF THE CAROLINAS
    13860 Ballantyne Corp Pl #250
    Charlotte, NC 28277

KEY EXECUTIVES:
Chairman of the Board/Chief Executive Officer .... Ronald A Williams
President .... Mark T Bertolini
Executive VP, Finance .... Joseph M Zubretsky
Medical Director .... Troyen A Brennan, MD
Chief Information Officer .... Margaret McCarthy
Marketing Director .... Brian Shields
Senior VP, Communications .... Roger Bolton
Senior VP, Human Resources .... Elease E Wright

COMPANY PROFILE:
Parent Company Name: Aetna Inc
Doing Business As:
Year Founded: 1995   Federally Qualified: [ ]
Forprofit: [Y]   Not-For-Profit: [ ]
Model Type: IPA
Accreditation: [ ] AAPPO [ ] JACHO [ ] NCQA [ ] URAC
Plan Type: HMO, PPO, POS, CDHP, HDHP, HSA,
Primary Physicians: 2,926   Physician Specialists: 6,491
Hospitals: 53
Total Revenue: 2005: 40,334,089   2006: 43,105,001
Net Income   2005:   1,736,079   2006:   1,451,553
Total Enrollment:
    2001: 61,441   2004: 14,755   2007: 0
    2002: 23,792   2005: 25,582
    2003: 14,824   2006: 12,076
Medical Loss Ratio: 2005:   2006: 83.70
Administrative Expense Ratio: 2005:   2006:

SERVICE AREA:
Nationwide: N
    NC; SC;

TYPE OF COVERAGE:
Commercial: [Y] Individual: [ ] FEHBP: [ ] Indemnity: [ ]
Medicare: [ ] Medicaid: [ ] Supplemental Medicare: [ ]
Tricare   [ ]

PRODUCTS OFFERED:
Product Name: Type:
HMO NC   HMO
HMO SC   HMO

CONSUMER-DRIVEN PRODUCTS
Aetna Life Insurance Co   HSA Company
Aetna HealthFund HSA   HSA Product
Aetna   HSA Administrator
Aetna HealthFund   Consumer-Driven Health Plan
PPO I; PPO II   High Deductible Health Plan

PLAN BENEFITS:
Alternative Medicine: [ ]   Behavioral Health: [ ]
Chiropractic: [X]   Dental: [X]
Home Care: [X]   Inpatient SNF: [X]
Long-Term Care: [X]   Pharm. Mail Order: [X]
Physical Therapy: [X]   Podiatry: [X]
Psychiatric: [X]   Transplant: [X]
Vision: [X]   Wellness: [ ]
Workers' Comp: [ ]
Other Benefits:

ASSURANT EMPLOYEE BENEFITS - NORTH CAROLINA

3700 National Dr
Raleigh, NC 27612
Phone: 704-553-7609 Fax: 704-553-7821 Toll-Free: 800-772-6809
Web site: www.assurantemployeebenefits.com

MAILING ADDRESS:
    ASSURANT EMPLOYEE BENEFITS - NC
    3700 National Dr
    Raleigh, NC 27612

KEY EXECUTIVES:
Interim Chief Executive Officer/President .... John S Roberts
Chief Financial Officer .... Floyd F Chadee
VP, Medical Director .... Polly M Galbraith, MD
Chief Information Officer .... Karla J Schacht
Senior VP, Marketing .... Joseph A Sevcik
Privacy Officer .... John L Fortini
VP, Provider Services .... James A Barrett, DMD
Senior VP, Human Resources & Development .... Sylvia R Wagner
General Manager .... Todd Boyd
National Dental Director .... James A Barrett, DMD
VP Sales (NC) .... Peter Cook
Local Senior Account Executive (NC) .... Pete Stam

COMPANY PROFILE:
Parent Company Name: Assurant Health
Doing Business As: DentiCare Inc
Year Founded: 1975   Federally Qualified: [ ]
Forprofit: [Y]   Not-For-Profit: [ ]
Model Type:
Accreditation: [ ] AAPPO [ ] JACHO [ ] NCQA [ ] URAC
Plan Type: Specialty PPO
Total Enrollment:
    2001: 0   2004: 0   2007: 0
    2002: 0   2005:
    2003: 3,473   2006:

SERVICE AREA:
Nationwide: N
    NC; VA;

TYPE OF COVERAGE:
Commercial: [Y] Individual: [Y] FEHBP: [ ] Indemnity: [ ]
Medicare: [ ] Medicaid: [ ] Supplemental Medicare: [ ]
Tricare   [ ]

PRODUCTS OFFERED:
Product Name: Type:
                             DHMO
                             Vision

PLAN BENEFITS:
Alternative Medicine: [ ]   Behavioral Health: [ ]
Chiropractic: [ ]   Dental: [X]
Home Care: [ ]   Inpatient SNF: [ ]
Long-Term Care: [ ]   Pharm. Mail Order: [ ]
Physical Therapy: [ ]   Podiatry: [ ]
Psychiatric: [ ]   Transplant: [ ]
Vision: [ ]   Wellness: [ ]
Workers' Comp: [ ]
Other Benefits:
Comments:
Formerly Fortis Benefits Dental.

ATLANTIC INTEGRATED HEALTH INC

The Beacon Co 1308 Commerce Dr
New Bern, NC 28562
Phone: 252-514-0057 Fax: 252-514-0750 Toll-Free: 877-514-0057
Web site: www.aihinc.com

MAILING ADDRESS:
    ATLANTIC INTEGRATED HEALTH INC
    The Beacon Co 1308 Commerce Dr
    New Bern, NC 28562

KEY EXECUTIVES:
Chairman of the Board .... James Stackhouse, MD
Chief Executive Officer .... Kerry A Willis, MD
President .... Phil Mahaney, MD
Chief Financial Officer .... Steve Nuckols
Medical Director/Medical Management Director .. Robert Meyers, MD
Chief Operating Officer .... Wayne Williams, COO
Director of Marketing .... Michael Rice
Credentialing Manager .... Mimi Maassen
Public Relations Director .... Margaret Jarmon
Provider Relations Director .... George Sterns
Financial Manager .... Alice Fielder
Office Manager .... Renessa Denney

COMPANY PROFILE:
Parent Company Name:
Doing Business As: The Beacon Company
Year Founded: 1996   Federally Qualified: [ ]
Forprofit: [Y]   Not-For-Profit: [ ]
Model Type: NETWORK

NEW YORK — Managed Care Organization Profiles

Total Enrollment:
- 2001: 19,582
- 2002: 42,943
- 2003: 55,666
- 2004: 68,978
- 2005: 95,001
- 2006:
- 2007: 85,000

Medical Loss Ratio: 2005:   2006: 73.70
Administrative Expense Ratio: 2005:   2006:

SERVICE AREA:
Nationwide: N
CT; NY;

TYPE OF COVERAGE:
Commercial: [Y] Individual: [ ] FEHBP: [ ] Indemnity: [ ]
Medicare: [Y] Medicaid: [Y] Supplemental Medicare: [ ]
Tricare: [ ]

PRODUCTS OFFERED:

Product Name:	Type:
HealthChoice	Medicaid HMO
Child Health Plus	Medicaid
Senior Health Plan	Medicare
Family Health Plus	Medicaid

Managed Care Organization Profiles — **NEW YORK**

PLAN BENEFITS:
Alternative Medicine:	[ ]	Behavioral Health:	[ ]
Chiropractic:	[X]	Dental:	[ ]
Home Care:	[ ]	Inpatient SNF:	[ ]
Long-Term Care:	[ ]	Pharm. Mail Order:	[X]
Physical Therapy:	[ ]	Podiatry:	[X]
Psychiatric:	[X]	Transplant:	[X]
Vision:	[X]	Wellness:	[X]
Workers' Comp:	[X]		
Other Benefits:			

UNIVERA COMMUNITY HEALTH

205 Park Club Ln
Buffalo, NY 14221-5239
Phone: 716-857-4410 Fax: 716-857-6224 Toll-Free:
Web site: www.univeracommunityhealth.org
MAILING ADDRESS:
   UNIVERA COMMUNITY HEALTH
   205 Park Club Ln
   Buffalo, NY 14221-5239

KEY EXECUTIVES:
Executive Director .... Michael C Holvey, Jr
Medical Director .... Richard P Vienne, Jr, DO
Manager of Operations .... Linda Tempeny
Marketing & Sales Manager .... Oliver C Miller
Project Analyst .... Gary Whiteford
Director .... Laura P Mongeon
Communications Manager .... Kandis R Fuller, APR

COMPANY PROFILE:
Parent Company Name: The Lifetime Healthcare Companies Inc
Doing Business As: Buffalo Community Health
Year Founded: 1996   Federally Qualified: [ ]
Forprofit: [ ]   Not-For-Profit: [Y]
Model Type: NETWORK
Accreditation: [ ] AAPPO [ ] JACHO [ ] NCQA [ ] URAC
Plan Type: HMO, HSA
Total Enrollment:
   2001: 0   2004: 22,937   2007: 0
   2002: 13,109   2005: 28,147
   2003: 13,260   2006:

SERVICE AREA:
Nationwide: N
   NY;

PRODUCTS OFFERED:
Product Name:	Type:
Plus Med	Medicaid
Child Health Plus	Medicaid
Family Health Plus	Medicaid

Comments:
Formerly Buffalo Community Health.

UNIVERA HEALTHCARE OF WESTERN NEW YORK

205 Park Club Lane
Buffalo, NY 14221-5239
Phone: 716-847-0881 Fax: 716-847-1257 Toll-Free: 800-628-8451
Web site: www.univerahealthcare.com
MAILING ADDRESS:
   UNIVERA HEALTHCARE WESTERN NY
   205 Park Club Lane
   Buffalo, NY 14221-5239

KEY EXECUTIVES:
Chairman .... John G Doyle, Jr
Chief Executive Officer .... David H Klein
Regional President .... Mary Lee Campbell-Wisley
Chief Financial Officer .... Emil D Duda
Chief Medical Officer .... Robert J Holzhauer, MD, MBA
Chief Information Officer .... David C McDowell
VP, Communications .... Peter B Kates
VP, Provider Contracting/Relations .... Jeffrey K Lowry
VP, Human Resources .... Timothy M McNamara
Government Relations .... Valerie J Rosenhoch
Senior VP, Healthcare Affairs ... Martin Hickey, MD, MS, CPE, FACPE

COMPANY PROFILE:
Parent Company Name: The Lifetime Healthcare Companies Inc
Doing Business As:
Year Founded: 1976   Federally Qualified: [Y]
Forprofit: [ ]   Not-For-Profit: [Y]
Model Type: NETWORK
Accreditation: [ ] AAPPO [ ] JACHO [X] NCQA [ ] URAC
Plan Type: HMO, PPO, POS, ASO, CDHP, HSA
Primary Physicians: 3,020   Physician Specialists:
Hospitals:
Total Enrollment:
   2001: 0   2004: 200,000   2007: 0
   2002: 185,000   2005: 135,177
   2003: 165,000   2006:

SERVICE AREA:
Nationwide: N
   NY (Allegany, Cattaraugus, Chautauqua, Erie, Genesee. Niagara, Orleans, Wyoming);

TYPE OF COVERAGE:
Commercial: [Y] Individual: [Y] FEHBP: [ ] Indemnity: [ ]
Medicare: [Y] Medicaid: [Y] Supplemental Medicare: [ ]
Tricare [ ]

PRODUCTS OFFERED:
Product Name:	Type:
SeniorChoice	Medicare
Choicecare	

CONSUMER-DRIVEN PRODUCTS
	HSA Company
	HSA Product
	HSA Administrator
Univera 4Front	Consumer-Driven Health Plan
	High Deductible Health Plan

PLAN BENEFITS:
Alternative Medicine:	[ ]	Behavioral Health:	[ ]
Chiropractic:	[X]	Dental:	[X]
Home Care:	[X]	Inpatient SNF:	[X]
Long-Term Care:	[ ]	Pharm. Mail Order:	[X]
Physical Therapy:	[X]	Podiatry:	[ ]
Psychiatric:	[X]	Transplant:	[X]
Vision:	[X]	Wellness:	[X]
Workers' Comp:	[ ]		
Other Benefits:			

Comments:
Formerly Healthcare Plan (HCP).

WELLCARE OF NEW YORK

One Civic Center
Poughkeepsie, NY 12601
Phone: 845-566-6069 Fax: 845-566-6056 Toll-Free:
Web site: www.wellcare.com
MAILING ADDRESS:
   WELLCARE OF NEW YORK
   One Civic Center
   Poughkeepsie, NY 12601

KEY EXECUTIVES:
Executive Chairman .... Charles G Berg
Chief Executive Officer/President .... Heath Schiesser
President - New York .... Dan Parietti
Chief Medical Officer .... William Kerr, MD
Chief Information Officer .... Anil Kottoor
VP, Operations .... Darcy Shepard
Marketing Manager .... Thomas Mercklein
VP, Provider Relations .... Diane Wilkosz
VP, Human Resources .... Gretchen Demartini

COMPANY PROFILE:
Parent Company Name: WellCare Health Plans Inc
Doing Business As:
Year Founded: 1987   Federally Qualified: [ ]
Forprofit: [Y]   Not-For-Profit: [ ]
Model Type: IPA
Accreditation: [ ] AAPPO [ ] JACHO [ ] NCQA [ ] URAC
Plan Type: HMO
Total Revenue: 2005:   2006: 296,370,887
Net Income: 2005:   2006:

NEW YORK

UNITED CONCORDIA COMPANY INC - NEW YORK

159 Express St
Plainview, NY 11803
Phone: 516-827-6720 Fax: 516-827-6618 Toll-Free:
Web site: www.ucci.com

MAILING ADDRESS:
UNITED CONCORDIA CO INC - NY
159 Express St
Plainview, NY 11803

KEY EXECUTIVES:
Chief Executive Officer/President .... Thomas A Dzuryachko
Senior VP, Finance .... Daniel Wright
VP, National Dental Director .... Richard Klich, DMD
Director, Provider Services .... Ted Pesano

COMPANY PROFILE:
Parent Company Name: Highmark Inc
Doing Business As:
Year Founded: 1991   Federally Qualified: [ ]
Forprofit: [Y]   Not-For-Profit: [ ]
Model Type:
Accreditation: [ ] AAPPO [ ] JACHO [ ] NCQA [ ] URAC
Plan Type: Specialty HMO, Specialty PPO, POS, TPA
Total Revenue: 2005:   2006: 9,580,872
Net Income   2005:   2006:
Medical Loss Ratio: 2005:   2006: 76.20
Administrative Expense Ratio: 2005:   2006:

SERVICE AREA:
Nationwide: N
CT; MA; ME; NH; NJ; NY; PA; RI; VT;

TYPE OF COVERAGE:
Commercial: [Y] Individual: [ ] FEHBP: [ ] Indemnity: [ ]
Medicare: [ ] Medicaid: [ ] Supplemental Medicare: [ ]
Tricare   [ ]

PLAN BENEFITS:
Alternative Medicine: [ ]   Behavioral Health: [ ]
Chiropractic: [ ]   Dental: [X]
Home Care: [ ]   Inpatient SNF: [ ]
Long-Term Care: [ ]   Pharm. Mail Order: [ ]
Physical Therapy: [ ]   Podiatry: [ ]
Psychiatric: [ ]   Transplant: [ ]
Vision: [ ]   Wellness: [ ]
Workers' Comp: [ ]
Other Benefits:

UNITEDHEALTHCARE OF NEW YORK INC

5015 Campuswood Dr Ste 107
East Syracuse, NY 13057
Phone: 800-339-5380 Fax: 315-433-5779 Toll-Free: 800-339-5380
Web site: www.uhc.com

MAILING ADDRESS:
UNITEDHEALTHCARE OF NY INC
5015 Campuswood Dr Ste 107
East Syracuse, NY 13057

KEY EXECUTIVES:
Non-Executive Chairman .... Richard T Burke
Director of Provider Services/Network Operations .... Paul Marchetti
Quality Assurance Director .... Anne Marie O'Brien
Case Management Director .... Helen Noonan

COMPANY PROFILE:
Parent Company Name: UnitedHealth Group
Doing Business As: United HealthCare
Year Founded: 1986   Federally Qualified: [Y]
Forprofit: [Y]   Not-For-Profit: [ ]
Model Type: IPA
Accreditation: [ ] AAPPO [ ] JACHO [X] NCQA [ ] URAC
Plan Type: HMO, POS, CDHP, HDHP, HSA, HRA,
Total Revenue: 2005:   2006: 412,845,420
Net Income   2005:   2006:
Total Enrollment:
  2001:   0   2004: 124,633   2007: 0
  2002:   33,940   2005:
  2003:   124,013   2006:
Medical Loss Ratio: 2005:   2006: 86.70
Administrative Expense Ratio: 2005:   2006:

SERVICE AREA:
Nationwide: N
NY;

TYPE OF COVERAGE:
Commercial: [Y] Individual: [Y] FEHBP: [ ] Indemnity: [ ]
Medicare: [ ] Medicaid: [Y] Supplemental Medicare: [Y]
Tricare   [ ]

PRODUCTS OFFERED:
Product Name: Type:
United Hlthcare Medicaid   Medicaid
Medicare Complete   Medicare

CONSUMER-DRIVEN PRODUCTS
Exante Bank/Golden Rule Ins Co   HSA Company
iPlan HSA   HSA Product
                                       HSA Administrator
                                       Consumer-Driven Health Plan
                                       High Deductible Health Plan

PLAN BENEFITS:
Alternative Medicine: [ ]   Behavioral Health: [X]
Chiropractic: [X]   Dental: [ ]
Home Care: [X]   Inpatient SNF: [X]
Long-Term Care: [X]   Pharm. Mail Order: [X]
Physical Therapy: [X]   Podiatry: [X]
Psychiatric: [X]   Transplant: [X]
Vision: [X]   Wellness: [X]
Workers' Comp: [ ]
Other Benefits:
Comments:
Formerly UnitedHealthcare Upstate New York.

UNITEDHEALTHCARE OF NEW YORK METROPOLITAN

One Penn Plaza 8th Floor
New York, NY 10119
Phone: 212-216-6400 Fax: 212-216-6604 Toll-Free:
Web site: www.uhc.com

MAILING ADDRESS:
UNITEDHEALTHCARE — METRO NY
One Penn Plaza 8th Floor
New York, NY 10119

KEY EXECUTIVES:
Non-Executive Chairman .... Richard T Burke
Chief Executive Officer/President .... Michael A Turpin
Senior VP, Sales .... William Golden

COMPANY PROFILE:
Parent Company Name: UnitedHealth Group
Doing Business As:
Year Founded: 1986   Federally Qualified: [N]
Forprofit: [Y]   Not-For-Profit: [ ]
Model Type: IPA
Accreditation: [ ] AAPPO [ ] JACHO [ ] NCQA [ ] URAC
Plan Type: HMO, PPO, POS, EPO, CDHP, HDHP, HSA, HRA,
Total Enrollment:
  2001:   83,085   2004: 138,198   2007: 0
  2002:   162,012   2005: 127,189
  2003:   138,700   2006:

SERVICE AREA:
Nationwide: N
CT (Fairfield); NJ (Atlantic, Bergen Burlington, Camden, Cape May, Cumberland, Essex, Gloucester, Hudson, Hunterdon, Mercer, Middlesex, Monmouth, Morris, Ocean, Passaic, Salem, Somerset, Sussex, Union, Warren); NY (Bronx, Brooklyn, Dutchess, Kings, Manhattan, Nassau, Orange, Queens, Putnam, Richmond, Rockland, Suffolk, Ulster, Westchester);

TYPE OF COVERAGE:
Commercial: [Y] Individual: [Y] FEHBP: [ ] Indemnity: [ ]
Medicare: [Y] Medicaid: [Y] Supplemental Medicare: [ ]
Tricare   [ ]

PRODUCTS OFFERED:
Product Name: Type:
Medicare Complete   Medicare Advantage
United Behavioral Health   Mental health & chem
Optum Care24   24 hour access to co
United Resource Networks   Transplant Benefit M

CONSUMER-DRIVEN PRODUCTS
Exante Bank/Golden Rule Ins Co   HSA Company
iPlan HSA   HSA Product
                                       HSA Administrator
                                       Consumer-Driven Health Plan
                                       High Deductible Health Plan

Managed Care Organization Profiles — NEW YORK

Model Type:
Accreditation: [ ] AAPPO [ ] JACHO [ ] NCQA [ ] URAC
Plan Type: HMO
Total Revenue: 2005:   2006: 168,20,195
Net Income   2005:   2006:
Total Enrollment:
  2001: 0   2004: 474   2007: 0
  2002: 470   2005:
  2003: 316   2006:
Medical Loss Ratio: 2005:   2006: 99.4
Administrative Expense Ratio: 2005:   2006:

SERVICE AREA:
Nationwide:
  NY (Bronx, Kings, Nassau, New York, Orange, Queens, Richmond, Rockland, Suffolk, Westchester); PA;

TYPE OF COVERAGE:
Commercial: [Y] Individual: [ ] FEHBP: [ ] Indemnity: [ ]
Medicare: [ ] Medicaid: [ ] Supplemental Medicare: [ ]
Tricare   [ ]

PRODUCTS OFFERED:
Product Name: Type:
Horizon HealthCare of NY Inc   HMO

Comments:
Formerly known as Horizon Healthcare Ins Company of New York.

SCHC TOTAL CARE INC

819 S Salina St
Syracuse, NY 13202-3527
Phone: 315-634-5555 Fax: 315-475-1448 Toll-Free: 800-223-7242
Web site:

MAILING ADDRESS:
SCHC TOTAL CARE INC
PO Box 11507
Syracuse, NY 13202-3527

KEY EXECUTIVES:
Chief Executive Officer .... Ruben P Cowart, DDS
Director of Finance .... John DiPaula
Medical Director/Pharmacy Director .... Diane Green-El, MD
Director Customer Operation .... Michael Broader
Chief Operating Officer .... Angela Zeppetello
Marketing Director .... Eleanor Fitzgerald
Provider Relations/Contracting Coordinator .... Maria Stala
Corporate Counsel .... Jennifer Bolster
Chief Operating Officer .... Angela Zeppetello
Corporate Human Resource Director .... Craig Williams
Assistant Medical Director .... Felipe Diaz, MD
Quality Assurance/UR Nurse Manager .... Cathy Brigden

COMPANY PROFILE:
Parent Company Name: SCHC Companies Inc
Doing Business As: Total Care
Year Founded: 1987   Federally Qualified: [N]
Forprofit: [ ]   Not-For-Profit: [Y]
Model Type: MIXED
Accreditation: [ ] AAPPO [ ] JACHO [ ] NCQA [ ] URAC
Plan Type: Specialty HMO
Total Enrollment:
  2001: 0   2004: 20,890   2007: 0
  2002: 16,664   2005: 22,769
  2003: 21,262   2006: 24,171

SERVICE AREA:
Nationwide: N
  NY (Onondaga, Oswego, Tompkins);

TYPE OF COVERAGE:
Commercial: [ ] Individual: [ ] FEHBP: [ ] Indemnity: [ ]
Medicare: [ ] Medicaid: [Y] Supplemental Medicare: [ ]
Tricare   [ ]

PRODUCTS OFFERED:
Product Name: Type:
Syracuse PHSP   Medicaid
Child Health Plus   Medicaid
Family Health Plus   Medicaid

PLAN BENEFITS:
Alternative Medicine: [ ]   Behavioral Health: [X]
Chiropractic: [ ]   Dental: [X]
Home Care: [X]   Inpatient SNF: [ ]
Long-Term Care: [ ]   Pharm. Mail Order: [ ]
Physical Therapy: [ ]   Podiatry: [X]
Psychiatric: [X]   Transplant: [X]
Vision: [X]   Wellness: [X]
Workers' Comp: [ ]
Other Benefits:

SUFFOLK HEALTH PLAN

H Lee Dennison Blgd 3rd Fl
100 Veterans Memorial Hwy PO 6100
Hauppauge, NY 11788
Phone: 631-853-2982 Fax: 631-853-2927 Toll-Free: 800-763-9132
Web site: www.suffolkhealthplan.com

MAILING ADDRESS:
SUFFOLK HEALTH PLAN
PO Box 6100
Hauppauge, NY 11788

KEY EXECUTIVES:
Chief Executive Officer .... Matthew Miner
Chief Financial Officer .... Margaret Bermel
Chief Operating Officer .... Fred Weimann
Medical Director .... Maureen Crowley, MD, MPH

COMPANY PROFILE:
Parent Company Name: Suffolk County Dept of Health Services
Doing Business As:
Year Founded: 1995   Federally Qualified: [ ]
Forprofit: [ ]   Not-For-Profit: [Y]
Model Type:
Accreditation: [ ] AAPPO [ ] JACHO [ ] NCQA [ ] URAC
Plan Type: HMO
Total Enrollment:
  2001: 0   2004: 13,922   2007: 0
  2002: 14,994   2005: 16,317
  2003: 13,330   2006:

SERVICE AREA:
Nationwide:
  NY (Suffolk);

TYPE OF COVERAGE:
Commercial: [ ] Individual: [ ] FEHBP: [ ] Indemnity: [ ]
Medicare: [ ] Medicaid: [Y] Supplemental Medicare: [ ]
Tricare   [ ]

PRODUCTS OFFERED:
Product Name: Type:
Prepaid Health Services Plan   Medicaid
Child Health Plus   Medicaid

TOUCHSTONE HEALTH HMO INC

14 Wall St 9th Fl
New York, NY 10005
Phone: 212-294-6996 Fax: 212-294-8210 Toll-Free:
Web site: www.touchstone-health.com

MAILING ADDRESS:
TOUCHSTONE HEALTH HMO INC
14 Wall St 9th Fl
New York, NY 10005

KEY EXECUTIVES:
Chief Executive Officer/President .... Michael A Muchnicki
VP, Marketing .... Jill Tobin

COMPANY PROFILE:
Parent Company Name: Touchstone Health Partnership Inc
Doing Business As:
Year Founded: 2007   Federally Qualified: [ ]
Forprofit: [ ]   Not-For-Profit: [Y]
Model Type:
Accreditation: [ ] AAPPO [ ] JACHO [ ] NCQA [ ] URAC
Plan Type: HMO, PSO
Total Enrollment:
  2001:   2004:   2007: 9,898
  2002:   2005:
  2003:   2006:

SERVICE AREA:
Nationwide:
  NY (Bronx, Broome, Chenango, Delaware, Kings, Onondaga, Orange, Queens, Richmond, Westchester);

TYPE OF COVERAGE:
Commercial: [ ] Individual: [ ] FEHBP: [ ] Indemnity: [ ]
Medicare: [Y] Medicaid: [ ] Supplemental Medicare: [ ]
Tricare   [ ]

PRODUCTS OFFERED:
Product Name: Type:
Touchstone Health   HMO
Touchstone Health   PSO

NEW YORK

Total Revenue: 2005: 2006: 2,705,938,353
Net Income 2005: 2006:
Total Enrollment:
  2001: 73,574 2004: 729,579 2007: 0
  2002: 969,501 2005: 601,664
  2003: 900,173 2006:
Medical Loss Ratio: 2005: 2006: 77.70
Administrative Expense Ratio: 2005: 2006:

SERVICE AREA:
Nationwide: N
NY;

TYPE OF COVERAGE:
Commercial: [Y] Individual: [Y] FEHBP: [ ] Indemnity: [ ]
Medicare: [Y] Medicaid: [Y] Supplemental Medicare: [ ]
Tricare [ ]

PRODUCTS OFFERED:
Product Name:	Type:
Oxford Medicare Advantage	Medicare Advantage
Oxford HMO	HMO
Liberty Plan	POS
Freedom Plan	POS
Oxford Indemnity	Indemnity

PLAN BENEFITS:
Alternative Medicine: [X] Behavioral Health: [X]
Chiropractic: [X] Dental: [X]
Home Care: [X] Inpatient SNF: [X]
Long-Term Care: [X] Pharm. Mail Order: [X]
Physical Therapy: [X] Podiatry: [ ]
Psychiatric: [X] Transplant: [X]
Vision: [X] Wellness: [X]
Workers' Comp: [X]
Other Benefits:

PERFECTHEALTH INSURANCE COMPANY

1200 South Ave Ste 301
Staten Island, NY 10314
Phone: 718-370-5380 Fax: 718-370-5386 Toll-Free: 877-455-0294
Web site: www.perfectny.com

MAILING ADDRESS:
PERFECTHEALTH INSURANCE CO
PO Box 140724
Staten Island, NY 10314

KEY EXECUTIVES:
President .... Carmine Morano
VP, Chief Administration Officer .... Linda A Farren
VP, Finance & Underwriting .... Joseph D'Apolito
Medical Director .... Stephen Ford, MD
VP, Sales & Marketing .... Robert McCord
Manager of Provider Services .... Doug Murray
Executive Vice President .... William Thomas
Director, HSA Claims & Services .... Antoinette Lapetina

COMPANY PROFILE:
Parent Company Name: MultiPlan Inc
Doing Business As:
Year Founded: 1997 Federally Qualified: [ ]
Forprofit: [ ] Not-For-Profit: [ ]
Model Type:
Accreditation: [ ] AAPPO [X] JACHO [ ] NCQA [ ] URAC
Plan Type: PPO, HDHP, HSA,

SERVICE AREA:
Nationwide: N
NY (Nassau, New York City (all five boroughs), Orange, Putnam, Rockland, Suffolk, Westchester);

Comments:
Formerly Anthem Health Network.

PREFERRED CARE

259 Monroe Ave
Rochester, NY 14607-3699
Phone: 585-325-3920 Fax: 585-327-2298 Toll-Free: 800-933-3920
Web site: www.preferredcare.org

MAILING ADDRESS:
PREFERRED CARE
259 Monroe Ave
Rochester, NY 14607-3699

KEY EXECUTIVES:
Chief Executive Officer/President .... David W Oliker
Chief Financial Officer .... Thomas J Combs
Medical Director .... Steven Cohen, MD
Pharmacy Director .... Wendy Colin, MD
Chief Operations Officer .... Lisa Brubaker
VP, Marketing & Sales .... Patrick Glavey
VP, Information Technology .... Kevin Husted
Manager, Credentialing .... Jan Richardson
Director, Professional Relations .... Rosemary Bond
VP, Network Operations .... Matthew MacKinnon
Director, Health Resource Management .... Brian Shapley
VP, Medical Qualtiy Management .... Dominic Galanate, MD
VP, Underwriting .... Carl Maleri
Director, Operations/Service .... Jane Gentile

COMPANY PROFILE:
Parent Company Name:
Doing Business As:
Year Founded: 1979 Federally Qualified: [Y]
Forprofit: [ ] Not-For-Profit: [Y]
Model Type:
Accreditation: [ ] AAPPO [ ] JACHO [X] NCQA [ ] URAC
Plan Type: HMO, PPO, POS, ASO
Primary Physicians: 4,500 Physician Specialists:
Hospitals:
Total Enrollment:
  2001: 32,223 2004: 251,789 2007: 0
  2002: 147,020 2005: 184,543
  2003: 219,883 2006:

SERVICE AREA:
Nationwide: N
NY (Livingston, Monroe, Ontario, Orleans, Seneca, Wyoming, Yates);

TYPE OF COVERAGE:
Commercial: [Y] Individual: [Y] FEHBP: [ ] Indemnity: [ ]
Medicare: [Y] Medicaid: [Y] Supplemental Medicare: [ ]
Tricare [ ]

PRODUCTS OFFERED:
Product Name:	Type:
Rochester HMO	HMO
Preferred Care Gold	Medicare Advantage

PLAN BENEFITS:
Alternative Medicine: [ ] Behavioral Health: [X]
Chiropractic: [X] Dental: [ ]
Home Care: [X] Inpatient SNF: [X]
Long-Term Care: [ ] Pharm. Mail Order: [X]
Physical Therapy: [X] Podiatry: [X]
Psychiatric: [X] Transplant: [X]
Vision: [X] Wellness: [X]
Workers' Comp: [ ]
Other Benefits:

Comments:
Preferred Care and MVP Health Plans merged January 2006.

RAYANT INSURANCE COMPANY OF NEW YORK

1180 Ave of the Americas 8th F
New York, NY 10036
Phone: 212-626-2900 Fax: 212-626-2910 Toll-Free:
Web site: www.horizon-healthcare.com

MAILING ADDRESS:
RAYANT INSURANCE CO OF NY
1180 Ave of the Americas 8th F
New York, NY 10036

KEY EXECUTIVES:
Chief Medical Officer .... Naim Munir, MD
Chief Operating Officer .... Minal Patel
VP of Sales/Account Management .... Raymond M Boscio

COMPANY PROFILE:
Parent Company Name:
Doing Business As: Horizon Healthcare Services Inc, NJ
Year Founded: 1999 Federally Qualified: [ ]
Forprofit: [Y] Not-For-Profit: [ ]

Managed Care Organization Profiles — NEW YORK

COMPANY PROFILE:
Parent Company Name: New York-Presbyterian System
Doing Business As:
Year Founded: 1995   Federally Qualified: [N]
Forprofit: [ ]   Not-For-Profit: [Y]
Model Type: MIXED
Accreditation: [ ] AAPPO [ ] JACHO [ ] NCQA [ ] URAC
Plan Type: HMO
Total Enrollment:
   2001: 0   2004: 0   2007: 105,000
   2002: 33,000 2005: 64,901
   2003: 50,000 2006: 61,000

SERVICE AREA:
Nationwide: N
   NY (Kings, New York, Queens);

TYPE OF COVERAGE:
Commercial: [ ]   Individual: [ ]   FEHBP: [ ]   Indemnity: [ ]
Medicare: [ ]   Medicaid: [Y]   Supplemental Medicare: [ ]
Tricare [ ]

PRODUCTS OFFERED:
Product Name: Type:
NY-Presbyterian Community H P   Medicaid
Child Health Plus   Medicaid
Family Health Plus   Medicaid

PLAN BENEFITS:
Alternative Medicine:	[ ]	Behavioral Health:	[X]
Chiropractic:	[ ]	Dental:	[ ]
Home Care:	[X]	Inpatient SNF:	[X]
Long-Term Care:	[ ]	Pharm. Mail Order:	[ ]
Physical Therapy:	[X]	Podiatry:	[X]
Psychiatric:	[X]	Transplant:	[X]
Vision:	[X]	Wellness:	[X]
Workers' Comp:	[X]		

Other Benefits:

NEW YORK STATE CATHOLIC HEALTH PLAN INC

95-25 Queens Blvd
Rego Park, NY 11374
Phone: 718-896-6500 Fax: 718-896-1920 Toll-Free: 888-343-3547
Web site: www.fideliscareny.org

MAILING ADDRESS:
   NY STATE CATHOLIC HEALTH PLAN INC
   95-25 Queens Blvd
   Rego Park, NY 11374

KEY EXECUTIVES:
Chairman of the Board .... Rev Joseph M Sullivan
Chief Executive Officer/President .... Mark L Lane
Chief Financial Officer .... Dana Sorka
Chief Medical Officer .... Marco Michaelson, MD
Chief Operating Officer .... Patrick J Frawley
Marketing Manager .... Pamela Hassen
Public Relations Coordinator .... Jayson R White
Provider Relations Director .... Gloria Wong
Vice President .... Mary Ellen Connington
Vice President .... Laura Scoones
Strategic Planning/Development .... David Thomas
Director of Legal Affairs .... Pamela McNair

COMPANY PROFILE:
Parent Company Name:
Doing Business As: Fidelis Care New York
Year Founded: 1994   Federally Qualified: [Y]
Forprofit: [ ]   Not-For-Profit: [Y]
Model Type:
Accreditation: [ ] AAPPO [ ] JACHO [ ] NCQA [ ] URAC
Plan Type: Specialty HMO, Specialty PPO
Total Enrollment:
   2001: 0   2004: 213,599   2007: 298,000
   2002: 177,293 2005:
   2003: 194,032 2006: 290,000
Medical Loss Ratio: 2005:   2006:
Administrative Expense Ratio: 2005:   2006:

SERVICE AREA:
Nationwide: N
   NY (Albany, Chautaugua, Erie, Nassau, Niagara, Onondaga, Rensselaer, Rockland, Schenectady, Suffolk, Westchester);

TYPE OF COVERAGE:
Commercial: [ ]   Individual: [ ]   FEHBP: [ ]   Indemnity: [ ]
Medicare: [ ]   Medicaid: [Y]   Supplemental Medicare: [Y]
Tricare [ ]

PRODUCTS OFFERED:
Product Name: Type:
New York State Catholic Health Plan   Medicaid
Child Health Plus   Medicaid
Family Health Plus   Medicaid

PLAN BENEFITS:
Alternative Medicine:	[ ]	Behavioral Health:	[X]
Chiropractic:	[ ]	Dental:	[X]
Home Care:	[X]	Inpatient SNF:	[ ]
Long-Term Care:	[ ]	Pharm. Mail Order:	[ ]
Physical Therapy:	[ ]	Podiatry:	[X]
Psychiatric:	[X]	Transplant:	[X]
Vision:	[X]	Wellness:	[X]
Workers' Comp:	[ ]		

Other Benefits:

NYCHSRO/MEDREVIEW INC

199 Water St 27th Fl
New York, NY 10038
Phone: 212-897-6000 Fax: 212-897-6062 Toll-Free:
Web site: www.nychsro-medreview.com

MAILING ADDRESS:
   NYCHSRO/MEDREVIEW INC
   199 Water St 27th Fl
   New York, NY 10038

KEY EXECUTIVES:
Chairman .... Albert F Keegan, MD
Chief Executive Officer/President .... Joseph B Stamm
Chief Financial Officer .... Helen Mutchler
Medical Director .... Juanita Everetez, MD
Chief Operating Officer .... Terry Patterson
VP, Plan & Development .... George Bopp
VP, Government Contracts .... Harriet Starr, MD
VP, Legal Affairs .... Robert Rosenbloom, Esq

COMPANY PROFILE:
Parent Company Name: NY County Health Services Review Org
Doing Business As:
Year Founded: 1974   Federally Qualified: [ ]
Forprofit: [ ]   Not-For-Profit: [Y]
Model Type:
Accreditation: [ ] AAPPO [ ] JACHO [X] NCQA [ ] URAC
Plan Type: UR

SERVICE AREA:
Nationwide: N
   NY;

OXFORD HEALTH PLANS OF NEW YORK, INC

One Penn Plaza 8th Fl
New York, NY 10119
Phone: 203-459-9100 Fax: 203-601-8001 Toll-Free: 800-444-6222
Web site: www.oxhp.com

MAILING ADDRESS:
   OXFORD HEALTH PLANS OF NY
   One Penn Plaza 8th Fl
   New York, NY 10119

KEY EXECUTIVES:
Chief Executive Officer/President .... Michael A Turpin
Medical Director .... Alan M Muney, MD, MHA

COMPANY PROFILE:
Parent Company Name: Oxford Health Plans, CT
Doing Business As:
Year Founded: 1984   Federally Qualified: [Y]
Forprofit: [Y]   Not-For-Profit: [ ]
Model Type: IPA
Accreditation: [ ] AAPPO [ ] JACHO [X] NCQA [ ] URAC
Plan Type: HMO, PPO, POS, TPA, CDHP

NEW YORK

NATIONAL HEALTH PLAN

11 Penn Plaza Ste 330
New York, NY 10001
Phone: 212-279-3232 Fax: 212-629-0749 Toll-Free: 800-647-2677
Web site: www.nationalhealthplan.com
MAILING ADDRESS:
NATIONAL HEALTH PLAN
PO Box 2319
New York, NY 10001-2006

KEY EXECUTIVES:
Chairman/Chief Executive Officer .... Alvin Konigsberg
President .... David Konigsberg
Pharmacy Director .... Teresita Visaya
Chief Operating, Privacy, Compliance Officer .... David Zaback

COMPANY PROFILE:
Parent Company Name:
Doing Business As:
Year Founded: 1975   Federally Qualified: [ ]
Forprofit: [Y]   Not-For-Profit: [ ]
Model Type: NETWORK
Accreditation: [ ] AAPPO [ ] JACHO [ ] NCQA [ ] URAC
Plan Type: PPO, UR, POS, CDHP, HDHP, HSA,
Primary Physicians: 3,000   Physician Specialists: 12,000
Hospitals: 150
SERVICE AREA:
Nationwide: N
    NJ; NY;
TYPE OF COVERAGE:
Commercial: [Y] Individual: [ ] FEHBP: [ ] Indemnity: [ ]
Medicare: [ ] Medicaid: [ ] Supplemental Medicare: [ ]
Tricare   [ ]
PRODUCTS OFFERED:
Product Name: Type:
National Health Plan   PPO
CONSUMER-DRIVEN PRODUCTS
                                         HSA Company
                                         HSA Product
MSAver Resources LLC   HSA Administrator
                                         Consumer-Driven Health Plan
PPO Choice Saver Plus Plan   High Deductible Health Plan
PLAN BENEFITS:
Alternative Medicine: [ ]   Behavioral Health: [ ]
Chiropractic: [X]   Dental: [X]
Home Care: [X]   Inpatient SNF: [X]
Long-Term Care: [ ]   Pharm. Mail Order: [X]
Physical Therapy: [X]   Podiatry: [X]
Psychiatric: [X]   Transplant: [X]
Vision: [X]   Wellness: [ ]
Workers' Comp: [ ]
Other Benefits:

NEIGHBORHOOD HEALTH PROVIDERS

521 5th Ave, 3rd Fl
New York, NY 10175
Phone: 212-883-0883 Fax: 212-808-4772 Toll-Free:
Web site: www.getnhp.com
MAILING ADDRESS:
NEIGHBORHOOD HEALTH PROVIDERS
521 5th Ave, 3rd Fl
New York, NY 10175

KEY EXECUTIVES:
Chief Executive Officer/President .... Steven Boryy
Chief Financial Officer .... Ronald Arfin
Medical Director .... Raul Coronado, MD
Chief Operating Officer .... Catherine Weigle
VP, Marketing .... Regina Morris
VP, MIS .... Robert Lowry
Network Development Director .... James Kramer
General Counsel .... Traci Kosak

COMPANY PROFILE:
Parent Company Name:
Doing Business As: Neighborhood Health Providers
Year Founded: 1995   Federally Qualified: [ ]
Forprofit: [Y]   Not-For-Profit: [ ]
Model Type: MIXED
Accreditation: [ ] AAPPO [ ] JACHO [ ] NCQA [ ] URAC
Plan Type: Specialty HMO
Primary Physicians: 1,911   Physician Specialists: 4,509
Hospitals: 37
Total Enrollment:
    2001: 53,222   2004: 96,791   2007: 0
    2002: 75,713   2005: 105,449
    2003: 81,104   2006:
SERVICE AREA:
Nationwide: N
    NY (Kings, Queens);
TYPE OF COVERAGE:
Commercial: [ ] Individual: [ ] FEHBP: [ ] Indemnity: [ ]
Medicare: [Y] Medicaid: [Y] Supplemental Medicare: [ ]
Tricare   [ ]
PRODUCTS OFFERED:
Product Name: Type:
Neighborhood Health Providers   Medicaid
Child Health Plus   Medicaid
Family Health Plus   Medicaid
PLAN BENEFITS:
Alternative Medicine: [ ]   Behavioral Health: [X]
Chiropractic: [ ]   Dental: [ ]
Home Care: [X]   Inpatient SNF: [ ]
Long-Term Care: [ ]   Pharm. Mail Order: [ ]
Physical Therapy: [ ]   Podiatry: [X]
Psychiatric: [X]   Transplant: [X]
Vision: [X]   Wellness: [X]
Workers' Comp: [ ]
Other Benefits:

NEW YORK COMPENSATION MANAGERS INC

6250 South Bay Rd
Syracuse, NY 13220
Phone: 315-699-8475 Fax: 315-699-1438 Toll-Free: 888-352-4456
Web site: www.workerscomp.com
MAILING ADDRESS:
NY COMPENSATION MANAGERS INC
PO Box 3580
Syracuse, NY 13220

KEY EXECUTIVES:
Chief Executive Officer .... David Francey
Chief Financial Officer .... Ed Coombs, CPA
Director of IT .... David Laribee
General Counsel/Director of Operations .... Christopher R Mason
Director, Claims Management .... Cathy Marsden
Director, Underwriting .... Peg McChesney

COMPANY PROFILE:
Parent Company Name:
Doing Business As:
Year Founded: Federally Qualified: [ ]
Forprofit: [ ]   Not-For-Profit: [ ]
SERVICE AREA:
Nationwide: N
    NY;

NEW YORK-PRESBYTERIAN COMMUNITY HEALTH PLAN

525 East 68th St Box 182
New York, NY 10016
Phone: 212-297-5514 Fax: 212-297-5923 Toll-Free:
Web site: www.nyp.org/healthplan
MAILING ADDRESS:
NY-PRESBYTERIAN COMMUNITY HEALTH PLAN
525 E 68th St Box 182
New York, NY 10016

KEY EXECUTIVES:
Chief Executive Officer .... J Emilio Carrillo, MD, MPH
Chief Financial Officer .... Phyllis Lantos
Chief Medical Officer .... J Emilio Carrillo, MD, MPH
Chief Information Officer .... Chuck Merlino
Chief Operating Officer .... Jane Murnane
Marketing Director .... Michael Simone
Network Development Director .... Angela Scott
Medical Management Director .... Judith Wimmer, RN
Quality Assurance Director .... Terri Welch, RN

Managed Care Organization Profiles — NEW YORK

MAILING ADDRESS:
   MULTIPLAN INC - CORP HDQTRS
   115 Fifth Ave 7th Fl
   New York, NY 10003-1004

KEY EXECUTIVES:
Chief Executive Officer .... Mark Tabak
Executive VP, Chief Financial Officer .... Richard Gerstein
Executive VP, Chief of Operations .... Michael Ferrante
Executive VP, Marketing .... Warren Handelman
Executive VP, Sales & Account Management .... Dale White
VP General Counsel .... Marcy Feller

COMPANY PROFILE:
Parent Company Name: The Caryle Group
Doing Business As:
Year Founded: 1970   Federally Qualified: [N]
Forprofit: [Y]   Not-For-Profit: [ ]
Model Type: NON-RISK
Accreditation: [ ] AAPPO [ ] JACHO [ ] NCQA [ ] URAC
Plan Type: PPO, UR
Primary Physicians: 450,000   Physician Specialists:
Hospitals: 4,300
Total Enrollment:
  2001: 0   2004: 25,000,000   2007: 0
  2002: 0   2005: 70,000,000
  2003: 0   2006: 27,000,000

SERVICE AREA:
Nationwide: Y
  NW;

TYPE OF COVERAGE:
Commercial: [Y] Individual: [ ] FEHBP: [ ] Indemnity:[ ] Medicare: [ ] Medicaid: [ ] Supplemental Medicare: [ ]
Tricare [ ]

PRODUCTS OFFERED:
Product Name: Type:
National PPO Network   Commercial
Utilization Review   Commercial

PLAN BENEFITS:
Alternative Medicine: [ ]   Behavioral Health: [X]
Chiropractic: [X]   Dental: [X]
Home Care: [X]   Inpatient SNF: [X]
Long-Term Care: [X]   Pharm. Mail Order: [ ]
Physical Therapy: [X]   Podiatry: [X]
Psychiatric: [X]   Transplant: [X]
Vision: [X]   Wellness: [X]
Workers' Comp: [ ]
Other Benefits: Podiatric

MVP HEALTH PLAN INC

625 State St
Schenectady, NY 12305
Phone: 518-370-4793 Fax: 518-386-7869 Toll-Free: 800-777-4793
Web site: www.mvphealthcare.com

MAILING ADDRESS:
   MVP HEALTH PLAN INC
   PO Box 2207
   Schenectady, NY 12305

KEY EXECUTIVES:
Chief Executive Officer/President .... David W Oliker
Chief Financial Officer .... Thomas Combs
Executive VP, Chie Operations Officer .... David Field
Chief Medical Officer .... Dennis Allen, MD
VP, Pharmacy Programs .... James Hopsicker
Chief Marketing Officer .... Scott W Averill
VP, Clinical Qlty Imprvmnt .... Jerry Salkowe, MD
Executive VP, Chief Legal Officer .... Denise Gonick, Esq

COMPANY PROFILE:
Parent Company Name:
Doing Business As: MVP Health Plan Inc, MVP Health Ins Co
Year Founded: 1983   Federally Qualified: [Y]
Forprofit: [Y]   Not-For-Profit: [Y]
Model Type: IPA
Accreditation: [ ] AAPPO [ ] JACHO [X] NCQA [ ] URAC
Plan Type: HMO, PPO, ASO, EPO, POS, TPA, HDHP, HSA
Total Revenue: 2005: 1,120,000,000   2006:
Net Income: 2005: 39,700,000   2006:
Total Enrollment:
  2001: 449,000   2004: 550,000   2007: 650,000
  2002: 477,000   2005: 710,000
  2003: 340,940   2006: 660,000

SERVICE AREA:
Nationwide: N
  NH; NY (Albany, Broome, Chenango, Columbia, Delaware, Dutchess, Fulton, Greene, Hamilton, Herkimer, Lewis, Madison, Montgomery, Oneida, Onandaga, Orange, Otsego, Putnam, Renssaeler, Saratoga, Schenectady, Schohaire, Tioga, Ulster, Warren, Washington); VT;

TYPE OF COVERAGE:
Commercial: [Y] Individual: [Y] FEHBP: [ ] Indemnity: [ ]
Medicare: [ ] Medicaid: [Y] Supplemental Medicare: [ ]
Tricare [ ]

PRODUCTS OFFERED:
Product Name: Type:
MVP Health Plan Inc   HMO
MVP Health Insurance Co   PPO, EPO,
MVP Select Care Inc   ASO, TPA,

CONSUMER-DRIVEN PRODUCTS
    HSA Company
    HSA Product
Mellon Financial   HSA Administrator
    Consumer-Driven Health Plan
Personal Rx   High Deductible Health Plan

PLAN BENEFITS:
Alternative Medicine: [ ]   Behavioral Health: [ ]
Chiropractic: [X]   Dental: [X]
Home Care: [X]   Inpatient SNF: [X]
Long-Term Care: [ ]   Pharm. Mail Order: [ ]
Physical Therapy: [X]   Podiatry: [ ]
Psychiatric: [X]   Transplant: [X]
Vision: [X]   Wellness: [X]
Workers' Comp: [ ]
Other Benefits:

Comments:
Preferred Care & MVP Health Plans merged January 2006.

NATIONAL DENTAL CONSULTANTS INC

355 Main Street
Islip, NY 11751
Phone: 800-632-3444 Fax: 631-581-2772 Toll-Free: 800-632-3444
Web site: www.nadent.com

MAILING ADDRESS:
   NATIONAL DENTAL CONSULTANTS
   PO Box 10
   Islip, NY 11751

KEY EXECUTIVES:
Chief Executive Officer .... Charles Silberstein
IT Specialist .... Gerry Depace
Chief Operating Officer .... Milagros Robles
Marketing Director .... David Silberstein
Corporate Communications .... Nina Silberstein
Human Resources Director .... Jody Vega

COMPANY PROFILE:
Parent Company Name:
Doing Business As:
Year Founded: Federally Qualified: [ ]
Forprofit: [ ]   Not-For-Profit: [ ]
Model Type:
Accreditation: [ ] AAPPO [ ] JACHO [ ] NCQA [ ] URAC
Plan Type: Specialty PPO

SERVICE AREA:
Nationwide: N
  NY;

PLAN BENEFITS:
Alternative Medicine: [ ]   Behavioral Health: [ ]
Chiropractic: [ ]   Dental: [X]
Home Care: [ ]   Inpatient SNF: [ ]
Long-Term Care: [ ]   Pharm. Mail Order: [ ]
Physicial Therapy: [ ]   Podiatry: [ ]
Psychiatric: [ ]   Transplant: [ ]
Vision: [ ]   Wellness: [ ]
Workers' Comp: [ ]
Other Benefits:

NEW YORK

Managed Care Organization Profiles

KEY EXECUTIVES:
Chairman/Chief Executive Officer .... Jacob L Canova
Senior VP, Finance/Controller .... Vincent DiMura, CPA
Chief Medical Officer .... Larry J Luter, MD, FAAFP
Chief Information Officer/Sr VP, Strategic Initiatives .... Peter Fianu
President, National Sales .... Richard Bukovinsky
Senior VP, Operations .... Christine Calarco
Senior VP, Cost Management Strategies .... Tracie A Canby
Senior VP, Sales .... David C Parker
Senior VP, Client Relations .... Margie DeGrace
President, Business Development/Client Relations .... Brent Hiller
VP, Associate General Counsel .... Timothy J Quinlivan, Esq
Senior VP, Product and Service Innovation .... Janice L Rahm
Senior VP, Corporate Development .... Todd Squilanti
Senior VP, Underwriting .... John T Sullivan

COMPANY PROFILE:
Parent Company Name: Prodigy Health Group Inc
Doing Business As: Meritain Health
Year Founded: 1988   Federally Qualified: [ ]
Forprofit: [Y]   Not-For-Profit: [ ]
Model Type: NETWORK
Accreditation: [ ] AAPPO [ ] JACHO [ ] NCQA [ ] URAC
Plan Type: PPO, POS, TPA, CDHP, HDHP, HSA,
SERVICE AREA:
Nationwide: N
   NY; GA; MA; TX; TN; NJ; MO;
TYPE OF COVERAGE:
Commercial: [Y] Individual: [ ] FEHBP: [ ] Indemnity: [ ]
Medicare: [ ] Medicaid: [ ] Supplemental Medicare: [ ]
Tricare   [ ]
PLAN BENEFITS:
Alternative Medicine: [ ]   Behavioral Health: [X]
Chiropractic: [X]   Dental: [X]
Home Care: [X]   Inpatient SNF: [X]
Long-Term Care: [X]   Pharm. Mail Order: [X]
Physical Therapy: [X]   Podiatry: [X]
Psychiatric: [X]   Transplant: [X]
Vision: [X]   Wellness: [X]
Workers' Comp: [ ]
Other Benefits:
Comments:
Network is North American Preferred.

METROPLUS HEALTH PLAN

160 Water Street
New York, NY 10038
Phone: 212-908-8600 Fax: 212-908-8601 Toll-Free: 800-475-6387
Web site: www.metroplus.org
MAILING ADDRESS:
   METROPLUS HEALTH PLAN
   160 Water Street
   New York, NY 10038

KEY EXECUTIVES:
President .... Arnold Saperstein, MD
Chief Financial Officer .... John Cuda
Medical Director .... Van Dunn, MD
Director of Communications .... Mari S Gold
Chief Operating Officer .... Philip Passantino
Marketing Director .... Roger Milliner
Chief Information Officer .... Michael Mattola
Privacy Officer .... Angela Adetola
Provider Relations/Contracting .... Robert Ethinger
Health Promotion/Prevention .... Virgilina Gonzalez
Human Resources Director .... Ryan Harris
Quality Assurance Director .... Debra Corbett
Compliance Officer .... Angela Adetola
Associate Medical Director .... Sanjiv Shah
Compliance Department .... Toni Cassetta
Deputy Director, Customer Service,
   Human Resources, Organizational Development,
   Intergovernmental Relations .... Gail Smith

COMPANY PROFILE:
Parent Company Name: NYC Health & Hospital Corp
Doing Business As:
Year Founded: 1985   Federally Qualified: [ ]
Forprofit: [ ]   Not-For-Profit: [Y]
Model Type: NETWORK
Accreditation: [ ] AAPPO [ ] JACHO [ ] NCQA [ ] URAC
Plan Type: HMO
Total Enrollment:
   2001:   0   2004: 224,777   2007: 260,532
   2002: 135,599   2005: 244,316
   2003: 179,965   2006: 247,125
SERVICE AREA:
Nationwide: N
   NY (NYC - Brooklyn, Bronx, Manhattan, Queens boroughs)
TYPE OF COVERAGE:
Commercial: [Y] Individual: [ ] FEHBP: [ ] Indemnity: [ ]
Medicare: [ ] Medicaid: [Y] Supplemental Medicare: [ ]
Tricare   [ ]
PRODUCTS OFFERED:
Product Name: Type:
MDNY Medicaid   Medicaid
Child Health Plus   Medicaid
Citycaid   HMO
Metroplus Gold (Commercial)   HMO
PLAN BENEFITS:
Alternative Medicine: [ ]   Behavioral Health: [ ]
Chiropractic: [ ]   Dental: [ ]
Home Care: [X]   Inpatient SNF: [ ]
Long-Term Care: [ ]   Pharm. Mail Order: [ ]
Physical Therapy: [ ]   Podiatry: [X]
Psychiatric: [ ]   Transplant: [ ]
Vision: [X]   Wellness: [X]
Workers' Comp: [ ]
Other Benefits:

MONROE PLAN FOR MEDICAL CARE, THE

2700 Elmwood Ave
Rochester, NY 14618
Phone: 585-244-5550 Fax: 585-244-9647 Toll-Free:
Web site: www.monroeplan.com
MAILING ADDRESS:
   MONROE PLN FOR MEDICAL CARE, THE
   2700 Elmwood Ave
   Rochester, NY 14618

KEY EXECUTIVES:
Chairman .... Peter Szilagyi, MD, MPH
Chief Executive Officer/President .... Robert H Thompson

COMPANY PROFILE:
Parent Company Name:
Doing Business As:
Year Founded: 1974   Federally Qualified: [ ]
Forprofit: [ ]   Not-For-Profit: [Y]
Model Type:
Accreditation: [ ] AAPPO [ ] JACHO [ ] NCQA [ ] URAC
Plan Type: HMO,
Primary Physicians: 4,500   Physician Specialists:
Hospitals:
Total Enrollment:
   2001: 0   2004: 0   2007: 0
   2002: 0   2005:
   2003: 0   2006: 90,000
SERVICE AREA:
Nationwide:
   NY;
TYPE OF COVERAGE:
Commercial: [ ] Individual: [ ] FEHBP: [ ] Indemnity: [ ]
Medicare: [ ] Medicaid: [Y] Supplemental Medicare: [ ]
Tricare   [ ]
PRODUCTS OFFERED:
Product Name: Type:
Monroe Plan for Medical Care   Medicaid

MULTIPLAN INC - CORPORATE HEADQUARTERS

115 Fifth Ave 7th Floor
New York, NY 10003-1004
Phone: 212-539-8086 Fax: 212-529-6381 Toll-Free: 800-677-1098
Web site: www.multiplan.com

Managed Care Organization Profiles — NEW YORK

KEY EXECUTIVES:
Chief Executive Officer/President .... Joseph Berardo, Jr
Chief Medical Officer .... Catherine Marino, MD
VP, Operations .... Naren Lulla
VP, Sales & Marketing .... Heather Suris
VP, Information Systems .... Arun Bhatia
Compliance Officer/General Counsel .... Craig B Greenfield

COMPANY PROFILE:
Parent Company Name: Preferred Choice Management Systems
Doing Business As: Magnacare
Year Founded: 1990   Federally Qualified: [N]
Forprofit: [Y]   Not-For-Profit: [ ]
Model Type: NETWORK
Accreditation: [ ] AAPPO [ ] JACHO [ ] NCQA [ ] URAC
Plan Type: HMO, PPO, UR, POS, TPA
Primary Physicians: Physician Specialists:
Hospitals: 260
Total Enrollment:
  2001: 0   2004: 153   2007: 0
  2002: 0   2005:
  2003: 170   2006:

SERVICE AREA:
Nationwide: N
  NJ; NY;

TYPE OF COVERAGE:
Commercial: [Y] Individual: [ ] FEHBP: [ ] Indemnity: [ ]
Medicare: [ ] Medicaid: [ ] Supplemental Medicare: [ ]
Tricare   [ ]

PLAN BENEFITS:
Alternative Medicine: [ ]   Behavioral Health: [X]
Chiropractic: [X]   Dental: [X]
Home Care: [X]   Inpatient SNF: [X]
Long-Term Care: [ ]   Pharm. Mail Order: [X]
Physical Therapy: [X]   Podiatry: [X]
Psychiatric: [X]   Transplant: [ ]
Vision: [ ]   Wellness: [ ]
Workers' Comp: [X]
Other Benefits:

MDNY HEALTHCARE INC

One Huntington Quad Ste 4C01
Melville, NY 11747
Phone: 631-454-1900 Fax: 631-454-1914 Toll-Free: 800-707-6369
Web site: www.mdnyhealthcare.org
MAILING ADDRESS:
  MDNY HEALTHCARE INC
  One Huntington Quad Ste 4C01
  Melville, NY 11747

KEY EXECUTIVES:
Chief Executive Officer .... Paul T Accardi
Chief Financial Officer .... Concetta A Pryor
Chief Medical Officer .... Ronald Perrone, MD, MBA
VP, Claims/Information Technology .... Lucy Oliva
VP, Health Services/Operations .... Cheryl McAndrew
Customer Service/Compliance Officer .... Denise L Munson

COMPANY PROFILE:
Parent Company Name: LIPH Inc
Doing Business As: MDNY Healthcare, Inc
Year Founded: 1995   Federally Qualified: [N]
Forprofit: [Y]   Not-For-Profit: [ ]
Model Type: IPA
Accreditation: [ ] AAPPO [ ] JACHO [ ] NCQA [X] URAC
Plan Type: HMO, POS
Primary Physicians: 7,100   Physician Specialists:
Hospitals:
Total Revenue: 2005:   2006: 93,830,233
Net Income   2005:   2006:
Total Enrollment:
  2001: 0   2004: 39,670   2007: 0
  2002: 61,178   2005: 32,455
  2003: 46,533   2006:
Medical Loss Ratio: 2005:   2006: 92.60
Administrative Expense Ratio: 2005:   2006:

SERVICE AREA:
Nationwide: N
  NY;

TYPE OF COVERAGE:
Commercial: [Y] Individual: [Y] FEHBP: [ ] Indemnity: [ ]
Medicare: [Y] Medicaid: [ ] Supplemental Medicare: [ ]
Tricare   [ ]

PRODUCTS OFFERED:
Product Name: Type:
MDNY HMO   HMO
MDNY POS   POS

PLAN BENEFITS:
Alternative Medicine: [ ]   Behavioral Health: [X]
Chiropractic: [X]   Dental: [X]
Home Care: [X]   Inpatient SNF: [X]
Long-Term Care: [ ]   Pharm. Mail Order: [X]
Physical Therapy: [X]   Podiatry: [X]
Psychiatric: [X]   Transplant: [X]
Vision: [X]   Wellness: [ ]
Workers' Comp: [ ]
Other Benefits:

MEDAVANT NATIONAL PREFERRED PROVIDER NETWORK

419 East Main Street
Middletown, NY 10940
Phone: 845-343-1600 Fax: 845-343-6113 Toll-Free: 800-863-3320
Web site: www.planvista.com
MAILING ADDRESS:
  MEDAVANT NATIONAL
  PREFERRED PROVIDER NETWORK
  419 East Main Street
  Middletown, NY 10940

KEY EXECUTIVES:
Chief Executive Officer .... John G Lettko
Chief Financial Officer .... Gerard M Hayden, Jr
Executive VP, Information Technology .... Adnane Khalil
Executive VP, Marketing/Corp Communications .... Teresa D Stubbs
Executive VP, Human Resources .... Allison W Myers
Executive VP, Business Operations .... Lonnie W Hardin
Executive VP, Product Management .... Eric D Arnson
General Counsel, Secretary .... Peter E Flemming, III
Executive VP, Sales/Account Management .... Emily J Pietrzak

COMPANY PROFILE:
Parent Company Name: MedAvant Healthcare Solutions
Doing Business As:
Year Founded: 1993   Federally Qualified: [ ]
Forprofit: [Y]   Not-For-Profit: [ ]
Model Type: NETWORK
Accreditation: [X] AAPPO [ ] JACHO [ ] NCQA [ ] URAC
Plan Type: PPO
Total Enrollment:
  2001: 5,000,000   2004: 0   2007: 0
  2002: 0   2005:
  2003: 0   2006:

SERVICE AREA:
Nationwide: Y
  NW;

TYPE OF COVERAGE:
Commercial: [Y] Individual: [ ] FEHBP: [ ] Indemnity: [ ]
Medicare: [ ] Medicaid: [ ] Supplemental Medicare: [ ]
Tricare   [ ]

PRODUCTS OFFERED:
Product Name: Type:
Plan Vista Solutions PPO   PPO

MERITAIN HEALTH INC

300 Corporate Pkwy
Amherst, NY 14226
Phone: 716-446-5500 Fax: 716-319-5732 Toll-Free: 800-828-6922
Web site: www.meritain.com
MAILING ADDRESS:
  MERITAIN HEALTH INC
  PO Box 9501
  Amherst, NY 14226

NEW YORK

Managed Care Organization Profiles

SERVICE AREA:
Nationwide: N
  NY (Allegany, Charaugus, Chautauqua, Erie, Genesee, Niagara, Orleans, Wyoming);

TYPE OF COVERAGE:
Commercial: [Y] Individual: [Y] FEHBP: [ ] Indemnity: [ ]
Medicare: [Y] Medicaid: [Y] Supplemental Medicare: [ ]
Tricare [ ]

PRODUCTS OFFERED:

Product Name:	Type:
Encompass	Commercial & Point
MediSource	Medicaid Program
Encompass 65	Medicare Plus Choice

PLAN BENEFITS:
Alternative Medicine:	[ ]	Behavioral Health:	[ ]
Chiropractic:	[X]	Dental:	[X]
Home Care:	[X]	Inpatient SNF:	[X]
Long-Term Care:	[ ]	Pharm. Mail Order:	[ ]
Physical Therapy:	[X]	Podiatry:	[X]
Psychiatric:	[X]	Transplant:	[X]
Vision:	[X]	Wellness:	[X]
Workers' Comp:	[ ]		

Other Benefits:

IPRO

1979 Marcus Ave Ste 105
Lake Success, NY 11042-1002
Phone: 516-326-7767 Fax: 516-328-2310 Toll-Free:
Web site: www.ipro.org

MAILING ADDRESS:
  IPRO
  1979 Marcus Ave Ste 105
  Lake Success, NY 11042-1002

KEY EXECUTIVES:
Chief Executive Officer .... Theodore O Will
President .... Thomas J Sheehy, Jr
Chief Financial Officer .... Alan King
Senior VP/Chief Medical Officer .... Clare B Bradley, MD, MPH
Chief Information Officer .... Richard A Alfieri
VP, Communications/Corp Development .... Spencer Vibbert
Healthcae Quality Improvement .... Thomas Hartman
VP, Managed Care .... Virginia Hill

COMPANY PROFILE:
Parent Company Name:
Doing Business As:
Year Founded: 1982   Federally Qualified: [ ]
Forprofit: [ ]   Not-For-Profit: [Y]
Model Type:
Accreditation: [ ] AAPPO [ ] JACHO [X] NCQA [ ] URAC
Plan Type: UR

SERVICE AREA:
Nationwide: N
  NY;

LIFETIME HEALTHCARE COMPANIES, THE - CORPORATE HEADQUARTERS

165 Court St
Rochester, NY 14647
Phone: 585-454-1700 Fax: 585-238-3659 Toll-Free: 800-347-1200
Web site: www.lifethc.com

MAILING ADDRESS:
  LIFETIME HEALTHCARE CO, THE
  165 Court St
  Rochester, NY 14647

KEY EXECUTIVES:
Chairman .... John G Doyle, Jr
Chief Executive Officer/President .... David H Klein
SEVP/Chief Financial Officer .... Emil D Duda
Executive VP, Med Affairs/Chief Med Officer .... Martin Lustick, MD
Chief Pharmacy Officer .... Joel Owerbach, PharmD
Senior VP, Chief Information Officer .... David C McDowell
Chief Operating Officer .... Paul von Ebers
Senior VP, Marketing, Excellus .... Paul von Ebers
Sales Director .... Kevin O'Keefe
Credentialing Manager .... Barbara McClain
Senior VP, Corporate Relations .... David J Mack
Director, Provider Relations .... Mary Maar
VP, Network Development & Strategy .... Kathleen Faulk
Health Promotion Director .... Jill Wilbert
Senior VP, Human Resources .... Ginger E Parysek
VP, UM & Medical Management .... Karen Eckert
Director Special Investigations Unit .... Flora Allen
VP, Business & Product Development .... Gary Ward
Senior VP, Corp Administration/Compliance .... Keith A Volkmar
Senior VP, Corporate Communication .... Geoffrey E Taylor
CAO Executive VP, Corp General Counsel... Christopher C Booth, Esq
Chief Actuary .... Robert A Toczynski

COMPANY PROFILE:
Parent Company Name:
Doing Business As: Excellus BC BS; Univera Healthcare;
Year Founded: Federally Qualified: [ ]
Forprofit: [ ]   Not-For-Profit: [Y]
Model Type: MIXED
Accreditation: [ ] AAPPO [ ] JACHO [Y] NCQA [ ] URAC
Plan Type: HMO, PPO, POS, ASO, CDHP, HDHP, HSA, EPO, TPA, PBM
Primary Physicians: 4,500   Physician Specialists: 8,500
Hospitals: 110
Total Revenue: 2005: 4,445,825,000   2006: 4,814,000,000
Net Income   2005: 197,876,000   2006: 152,000,000
Total Enrollment:
  2001: 0   2004: 0   2007: 2,000,000
  2002: 0   2005: 1,838,514
  2003: 2,000,000   2006: 1,881,000
Medical Loss Ratio: 2005: 85.50   2006:
Administrative Expense Ratio: 2005:   2006:

SERVICE AREA:
Nationwide: N
  NY;

TYPE OF COVERAGE:
Commercial: [Y] Individual: [Y] FEHBP: [ ] Indemnity: [Y]
Medicare: [Y] Medicaid: [Y] Supplemental Medicare: [Y]
Tricare [ ]

PRODUCTS OFFERED:

Product Name:	Type:
Univera Community Health Inc	Medicaid HMO
Excellus BC BS of Rochester A	HMO, POS
Excellus BC BS of Central NY	HMO
Excellus BC BS of Central NY So Tier	HMO, POS
Excellus BC BS of Utica/Watertown	HMO, POS, PPO
Univera Healthcare	
SeniorChoice	

CONSUMER-DRIVEN PRODUCTS

HSA Bank	HSA Company
Blue PPO HSA, Univera PPO HSA	HSA Product
HSA Bank	HSA Administrator
FourFront, 4Front	Consumer-Driven Health Plan
Blue PPO HSA, Univera PPO HSA	High Deductible Health Plan

PLAN BENEFITS:
Alternative Medicine:	[ ]	Behavioral Health:	[X]
Chiropractic:	[X]	Dental:	[X]
Home Care:	[X]	Inpatient SNF:	[X]
Long-Term Care:	[X]	Pharm. Mail Order:	[X]
Physical Therapy:	[X]	Podiatry:	[X]
Psychiatric:	[X]	Transplant:	[X]
Vision:	[X]	Wellness:	[X]
Workers' Comp:	[ ]		

Other Benefits:

MAGNACARE

825 East Gate Blvd Suite 200
Garden City, NY 11530
Phone: 516-282-8000 Fax: 516-227-6967 Toll-Free:
Web site: www.magnacare.com

MAILING ADDRESS:
  MAGNACARE
  825 East Gate Blvd Suite 200
  Garden City, NY 11530

Managed Care Organization Profiles — NEW YORK

COMPANY PROFILE:
Parent Company Name: Health Insurance Plan of Greater NY
Doing Business As: HIP Health Plan of New York
Year Founded: 1947 Federally Qualified: [N]
Forprofit: [ ] Not-For-Profit: [Y]
Model Type: GROUP
Accreditation: [ ] AAPPO [ ] JACHO [X] NCQA [ ] URAC
Plan Type: HMO, PPO, ASO, POS, TPA, CDHP, HRA
Primary Physicians: 19,000   Physician Specialists:
Hospitals: 160
Total Revenue: 2005: 4,599,802 2006: 5,039,667
Net Income 2005: 115,333 2006: 205,106
Total Enrollment:
   2001: 740,391   2004: 868,745   2007: 1,300,000
   2002: 814,409   2005: 905,399
   2003: 861,277   2006:

SERVICE AREA:
Nationwide: N
   NY; (Manhattan, Brooklyn, Bronx, Westchester, Staten Island, Queens, Rockland, Nassau, Suffolk, Orange).

TYPE OF COVERAGE:
Commercial: [Y] Individual: [Y] FEHBP: [ ] Indemnity: [ ]
Medicare: [Y] Medicaid: [Y] Supplemental Medicare: [Y]
Tricare [ ]

PRODUCTS OFFERED:
Product Name:	Type:
HIP	HMO
HIP	POS
HIP VIP Medicare Plan	Medicare
HIP Prime	EPO/PPO
HIP Access I & II	Medicaid
HIP Prime	Dental

CONSUMER-DRIVEN PRODUCTS
	HSA Company
	HSA Product
	HSA Administrator
	Consumer-Driven Health Plan
MyFund	High Deductible Health Plan

PLAN BENEFITS:
Alternative Medicine: [ ]   Behavioral Health: [X]
Chiropractic: [X]   Dental: [X]
Home Care: [X]   Inpatient SNF: [X]
Long-Term Care: [ ]   Pharm. Mail Order: [X]
Physical Therapy: [X]   Podiatry: [X]
Psychiatric: [X]   Transplant: [X]
Vision: [X]   Wellness: [X]
Workers' Comp: [X]
Other Benefits:
Comments:
Sold HIP Healthplan of Florida in 2000. Acquired Vytra Health Plans, NY, November 2001. Closed Vytra Health Plans, 2006.

HUDSON HEALTH PLAN

303 South Broadway Ste 321
Tarrytown, NY 10591
Phone: 914-631-1611 Fax: 914-631-1615 Toll-Free: 800-339-4557
Web site: www.hudsonhealthplan.org

MAILING ADDRESS:
   HUDSON HEALTH PLAN
   303 South Broadway Ste 321
   Tarrytown, NY 10591

KEY EXECUTIVES:
Chief Executive Officer/President .... Georganne Chapin
Chief Financial Officer .... Howard Birnbawn
Chief Medical Officer .... Janet Sullivan, MD
VP for Information Systems .... Toni Bonde
Chief Operating Officer .... Kevin Nelson
Senior VP of Marketing .... Mark Santiago
Director of Regulatory Affairs .... Frank DiGiovanni
VP, PR & Communication .... Ted Herman
Provider Relations Director .... Doris Carril
VP, Human Resources .... Julie Levin
Medical Director .... Carolyn Leihbacher
Chief Compliance Officer .... Kevin Nelson
Senior VP, Corp Development/Strategy .... Cathy Clancey

COMPANY PROFILE:
Parent Company Name:
Doing Business As: Hudson Health Plan
Year Founded: 1987 Federally Qualified: [Y]
Forprofit: [ ] Not-For-Profit: [Y]
Model Type: MIXED
Accreditation: [ ] AAPPO [ ] JACHO [ ] NCQA [ ] URAC
Plan Type: HMO
Total Enrollment:
   2001: 32,572   2004: 40,152   2007: 62,157
   2002: 42,057   2005: 56,270
   2003: 48,285   2006: 60,214

SERVICE AREA:
Nationwide: N
   NY (Dutchess, Orange, Rockland, Sullivan, Ulster, Westchester);

TYPE OF COVERAGE:
Commercial: [ ] Individual: [ ] FEHBP: [ ] Indemnity: [ ]
Medicare: [ ] Medicaid: [Y] Supplemental Medicare: [ ]
Tricare [ ]

PRODUCTS OFFERED:
Product Name:	Type:
Hudson Health Plan	Medicaid
Child Health Plus	Medicaid
Family Health Plus	Medicaid

PLAN BENEFITS:
Alternative Medicine: [ ]   Behavioral Health: [X]
Chiropractic: [ ]   Dental: [X]
Home Care: [X]   Inpatient SNF: [X]
Long-Term Care: [ ]   Pharm. Mail Order: [X]
Physical Therapy: [X]   Podiatry: [X]
Psychiatric: [X]   Transplant: [X]
Vision: [X]   Wellness: [X]
Workers' Comp: [ ]
Other Benefits: Transportation
Comments:
Formerly Westchester Prepaid Health Services Plan Inc.

INDEPENDENT HEALTH

511 Farber Lakes Dr
Buffalo, NY 14221
Phone: 716-631-3001 Fax: 716-631-0430 Toll-Free: 800-247-1466
Web site: www.independenthealth.com

MAILING ADDRESS:
   INDEPENDENT HEALTH
   511 Farber Lakes Dr
   Buffalo, NY 14221

KEY EXECUTIVES:
Chief Executive Officer/President .... Michael Cropp, MD
Chief Financial Officer .... Mark Johnson
Chief Medical Officer .... John Gillespie, MD
Pharmacy Director .... John Rodgers
Chief Information Officer .... Robert Hoover
Chief Marketing Officer .... Scott Averill
Health Promotion/Care Management .... Pamela Meynard
VP, Sales, Strategic Planning .... William McHugh
Director of Provider Services .... Carm Caruana
Director of Wellness/Prevention .... Cathy Basacci
VP, Human Resources .... Judy Boyle
Technical Services Director .... David Rogers
VP, Internal Operations .... Jill Syracuse
Senior VP, General Counsel .... Fred Cohen
Executive Director of Independent Foundation .... Carrie Meyer

COMPANY PROFILE:
Parent Company Name:
Doing Business As:
Year Founded: 1980 Federally Qualified: [Y]
Forprofit: [ ] Not-For-Profit: [Y]
Model Type: IPA
Accreditation: [ ] AAPPO [ ] JACHO [X] NCQA [ ] URAC
Plan Type: HMO, PPO, POS, ASO, TPA, CDHP, HDHP, FSA, HSA,
Total Enrollment:
   2001: 349,525   2004: 291,227   2007: 360,000
   2002: 343,378   2005: 267,555
   2003: 321,128   2006:

NEW YORK — Managed Care Organization Profiles

Medical Loss Ratio: 2005:   2006: 86.70
Administrative Expense Ratio: 2005:   2006:

SERVICE AREA:
Nationwide:
   NY;

TYPE OF COVERAGE:
Commercial: [Y] Individual: [Y] FEHBP: [ ] Indemnity: [ ]
Medicare: [Y] Medicaid: [Y]   Supplemental Medicare: [Y]
Tricare

PLAN BENEFITS:
Alternative Medicine:	[ ]	Behavioral Health:	[ ]
Chiropractic:	[X]	Dental:	[X]
Home Care:	[X]	Inpatient SNF:	[X]
Long-Term Care:	[X]	Pharm. Mail Order:	[ ]
Physical Therapy:	[X]	Podiatry:	[X]
Psychiatric:	[X]	Transplant:	[X]
Vision:	[X]	Wellness:	[X]
Workers' Comp:	[ ]		

Other Benefits:

HEALTHPLEX INC

333 Earle Ovington Blvd #300
Uniondale, NY 11553
Phone: 516-542-2200 Fax: 516-794-3186 Toll-Free: 800-468-0608
Web site: www.healthplex.com

MAILING ADDRESS:
   HEALTHPLEX INC
   333 Earle Ovington Blvd #300
   Uniondale, NY 11553

KEY EXECUTIVES:
Chairman of the Board .... Stephen Cuchel, MD
President .... Martin Kane, MD
Chief Information Officer .... Christopher Schmidt
Chief Operating Officer .... Bruce H Safran
Marketing Director .... Bob Richardson
MIS Director .... Phillip Rizzuto
Credentialing Manager .... Kelly Andron
Privacy Officer .... Bruce H Safran
Director of Provider Services .... Sharon Zelkind
Human Reosources Director .... Lisa Yaeger

COMPANY PROFILE:
Parent Company Name:
Doing Business As:
Year Founded: 1984   Federally Qualified: [ ]
Forprofit: [ ]   Not-For-Profit: [Y]
Model Type: MIXED
Accreditation: [ ] AAPPO [ ] JACHO [X] NCQA [ ] URAC
Plan Type: Specialty HMO, Specialty PPO, POS, ASO, TPA, UR
Primary Physicians: 3,000   Physician Specialists: 1,500
Hospitals:
Total Enrollment:
   2001: 0   2004: 0   2007: 0
   2002: 1,400,000   2005:
   2003: 1,300,000   2006:

SERVICE AREA:
Nationwide: N
   NJ; NY;

TYPE OF COVERAGE:
Commercial: [Y] Individual: [Y] FEHBP: [ ] Indemnity: [ ]
Medicare: [Y] Medicaid: [Y]   Supplemental Medicare: [ ]
Tricare [ ]

PLAN BENEFITS:
Alternative Medicine:	[ ]	Behavioral Health:	[ ]
Chiropractic:	[ ]	Dental:	[X]
Home Care:	[ ]	Inpatient SNF:	[ ]
Long-Term Care:	[ ]	Pharm. Mail Order:	[ ]
Physical Therapy:	[ ]	Podiatry:	[ ]
Psychiatric:	[ ]	Transplant:	[ ]
Vision:	[ ]	Wellness:	[ ]
Workers' Comp:	[ ]		

Other Benefits:

HEALTHPLUS INC

241 37th St Ste 412
Brooklyn, NY 11232
Phone: 718-745-0030 Fax: 718-745-1180 Toll-Free:
Web site: www.healthplus-ny.org

MAILING ADDRESS:
   HEALTHPLUS INC
   241 37th St Ste 412
   Brooklyn, NY 11232

KEY EXECUTIVES:
Chairman of the Board .... Howard Smith
Chief Executive Officer .... Thomas Early
Chief Financial Officer .... Rolondo Portocarrero
Chief Medical Officer .... Cliff Marbut, MD
Chief Operating Officer .... Michael Brown
Chief Marketing Officer .... Ada Rodriguez
Director, Provider Services .... Sylvia D'Allesandro
Quality Assurance Director .... Rick Weinberg

COMPANY PROFILE:
Parent Company Name:
Doing Business As:
Year Founded: 1984   Federally Qualified: [Y]
Forprofit: [ ]   Not-For-Profit: [Y]
Model Type:
Accreditation: [ ] AAPPO [ ] JACHO [ ] NCQA [ ] URAC
Plan Type: HMO
Primary Physicians: 2,000   Physician Specialists: 5,000
Hospitals: 50
Total Enrollment:
   2001: 120,000   2004: 219,785   2007: 0
   2002: 175,042   2005: 271,556
   2003: 195,717   2006:

SERVICE AREA:
Nationwide: N
   NY (all of NYC);

TYPE OF COVERAGE:
Commercial: [ ] Individual: [ ] FEHBP: [ ] Indemnity: [ ]
Medicare: [ ] Medicaid: [Y]   Supplemental Medicare: [ ]
Tricare [ ]

PRODUCTS OFFERED:
Product Name:	Type:
Health Plus Inc	Medicaid
Child Health Plus	Medicaid
Family Health Plus	Medicaid

PLAN BENEFITS:
Alternative Medicine:	[ ]	Behavioral Health:	[X]
Chiropractic:	[ ]	Dental:	[X]
Home Care:	[X]	Inpatient SNF:	[ ]
Long-Term Care:	[ ]	Pharm. Mail Order:	[ ]
Physical Therapy:	[ ]	Podiatry:	[ ]
Psychiatric:	[X]	Transplant:	[X]
Vision:	[X]	Wellness:	[ ]
Workers' Comp:	[ ]		

Other Benefits: Child Health Plus

HIP HEALTH PLAN OF NEW YORK

55 Water St
New York, NY 10041-8190
Phone: 646-447-5900 Fax: 646-447-3011 Toll-Free: 800-447-8255
Web site: www.hipusa.com

MAILING ADDRESS:
   HIP HEALTH PLAN OF NEW YORK
   55 Water St
   New York, NY 10041-8190

KEY EXECUTIVES:
Chairman of the Board/Chief Executive Officer .... Anthony L Watson
President/Chief Operating Officer .... Daniel T McGowan
Executive VP, Chief Financial Officer .... Michael D Fullwood, Esq
Executive VP, Corp Chief Medical Officer .... Dan J Dragalin, MD
VP, Chief Pharmacy Officer .... Araksi H Sarafian
Executive VP, Operations/Chief Info Officer .... John H Steber
Senior VP, Sales & Marketing .... Dewitt M Smith
Senior VP, IT .... Pedro Villabba
VP, Provider Relations .... Judy A Kohn
Senior VP, Human Resources .... Fred Blickman
Senior VP, Underwriting/Actuarial Srv .... Leslie Strassberg, FSA
Senior VP, Strategic Planning .... Edward A Lucy
Senior VP, Public Policy/Regulatory .... David Abernethy
Senior VP, External Affairs .... Arthur Barnes
Senior VP, General Counsel .... Michael D Fullwood, ESQ
Senior VP, Finance/Corporate Controller .... Dominic F D'Adamo

Managed Care Organization Profiles — NEW YORK

PLAN BENEFITS:

Alternative Medicine:	[ ]	Behavioral Health:	[ ]
Chiropractic:	[X]	Dental:	[X]
Home Care:	[X]	Inpatient SNF:	[X]
Long-Term Care:	[X]	Pharm. Mail Order:	[X]
Physical Therapy:	[X]	Podiatry:	[X]
Psychiatric:	[X]	Transplant:	[X]
Vision:	[X]	Wellness:	[X]
Workers' Comp:	[ ]		

Other Benefits:
Comments:
Guardian Lifes CDHP is limited to IL, MD, VA, and DC.

HEALTH NET - NEW YORK

399 Knollwood Rd #212
White Plains, NY 10603-1914
Phone: 203-225-8559 Fax: 212-856-4648 Toll-Free: 800-748-2559
Web site: www.healthnet.com

MAILING ADDRESS:
HEALTH NET - NEW YORK
399 Knollwood Rd #212
White Plains, NY 10603-1914

KEY EXECUTIVES:
Chief Executive Officer .... Jay M Gellert
President .... Anju Sikka, MD
Chief Financial Officer .... William Lamoreaux
Medical Director .... Anju Sikka, MD
Pharmacy Director .... Julee Oh
Director of IS .... David Anderson
Senior VP of Sales & Marketing .... Steven Calabrese

COMPANY PROFILE:
Parent Company Name: Health Net Inc, NE Corp Hdqrts
Doing Business As: Health Net
Year Founded: 1987   Federally Qualified: [Y]
Forprofit: [Y]   Not-For-Profit: [ ]
Model Type: IPA
Accreditation: [ ] AAPPO [ ] JACHO [ ] NCQA [X] URAC
Plan Type: HMO, POS, HDHP, HSA
Total Revenue: 2005:   2006: 519,108,931
Net Income: 2005:   2006:
Total Enrollment:
   2001: 268,059   2004: 265,000   2007: 250,000
   2002: 240,117   2005: 244,000
   2003: 217,991   2006: 247,000
Medical Loss Ratio: 2005:   2006: 81.20
Administrative Expense Ratio: 2005:   2006:

SERVICE AREA:
Nationwide: N
NJ;

TYPE OF COVERAGE:
Commercial: [Y] Individual: [ ] FEHBP: [ ] Indemnity: [ ]
Medicare: [ ]   Medicaid: [Y]   Supplemental Medicare: [ ]
Tricare: [ ]

PRODUCTS OFFERED:
Product Name: Type:
Health Net SmartChoice   Medicare

PLAN BENEFITS:

Alternative Medicine:	[ ]	Behavioral Health:	[X]
Chiropractic:	[ ]	Dental:	[ ]
Home Care:	[X]	Inpatient SNF:	[X]
Long-Term Care:	[ ]	Pharm. Mail Order:	[X]
Physical Therapy:	[X]	Podiatry:	[X]
Psychiatric:	[X]	Transplant:	[X]
Vision:	[X]	Wellness:	[X]
Workers' Comp:	[ ]		

Other Benefits:

HEALTHFIRST INC

25 Broadway 9th Fl
New York, NY 10004
Phone: 212-801-6000 Fax: 212-801-3245 Toll-Free: 800-225-5477
Web site: www.healthfirstny.com

MAILING ADDRESS:
HEALTHFIRST INC
25 Broadway 9th Fl
New York, NY 10004

KEY EXECUTIVES:
Chief Executive Officer/President .... Paul Dickstein
Senior VP, Chief Medical Officer .... Jay Schechtman, MD
Senior VP, Chief Information Officer .... Steve Sakovits
Acting Chief Operating Officer .... Thomas Bergdall
VP, Human Resources .... Andrea Forino
VP, Medical Management Director .... Maria Oliveri
Quality Assurance Director .... Lani Alison
General Counsel .... Thomas W Bergdall, Esq

COMPANY PROFILE:
Parent Company Name:
Doing Business As: Managed Health Inc
Year Founded: 1994   Federally Qualified: [Y]
Forprofit: [ ]   Not-For-Profit: [Y]
Model Type:
Accreditation: [ ] AAPPO [ ] JACHO [ ] NCQA [ ] URAC
Plan Type: HMO, PPO, TPA
Total Enrollment:
   2001: 0   2004: 258,250   2007: 0
   2002: 156,236   2005: 335,284
   2003: 223,467   2006:

SERVICE AREA:
Nationwide: N
NY (Bronx, Kings, Nassau, New York, Queens, Suffolk);

TYPE OF COVERAGE:
Commercial: [ ] Individual: [ ] FEHBP: [ ] Indemnity: [ ]
Medicare: [ ]   Medicaid: [Y]   Supplemental Medicare: [ ]
Tricare: [ ]

PRODUCTS OFFERED:
Product Name: Type:
Managed Health Inc   HMO
Managed Health 65 Plus   Medicare
Health First   Medicaid

Comments:
Formerly Managed Health Inc.

HEALTHNOW NEW YORK INC

257 W Genesee St
Buffalo, NY 14202
Phone: 716-887-6900 Fax: 716-887-8981 Toll-Free: 800-856-0480
Web site: www.healthnowny.com

MAILING ADDRESS:
HEALTHNOW NEW YORK INC
PO Box 15013
Buffalo, NY 12212-5013

KEY EXECUTIVES:
Chairman of the Board .... Joseph J Castiglio
Chief Executive Officer/President .... Alphonso O'Neil-White
VP, Finance .... James Dickerson
Senior VP, Chief Medical Officer .. Jay I Pomerantz, MD, MMM, FACP
Self Insurance/Brokerage Accounts .... Nora K McGuire
General Manager .... Steve Manzelli
VP, Chief Information Officer .... Pau Stoddard
VP, Government Affairs .... Donald R Ingalls

COMPANY PROFILE:
Parent Company Name: HealthNow New York Inc
Doing Business As:
Year Founded: 1985   Federally Qualified: [N]
Forprofit: [ ]   Not-For-Profit: [Y]
Model Type:
Accreditation: [ ] AAPPO [ ] JACHO [ ] NCQA [ ] URAC
Plan Type: HMO, PPO, POS, ASO,
Primary Physicians: 6,000   Physician Specialists:
Hospitals: 3,400
Total Revenue: 2005:   2006: 2,110,474,431
Net Income: 2005:   2006:
Total Enrollment:
   2001: 0   2004: 0   2007: 0
   2002: 0   2005: 900,000
   2003: 0   2006: 1,000,000

NEW YORK

TYPE OF COVERAGE:
Commercial: [Y] Individual: [Y] FEHBP: [ ] Indemnity: [ ]
Medicare: [ ] Medicaid: [ ] Supplemental Medicare: [Y]
Tricare [ ]

PRODUCTS OFFERED:
Product Name:	Type:
GHI HMO Select	HMO
GHI HMO POS	POS
GHI Medicaid	Medicaid

PLAN BENEFITS:
Alternative Medicine: [X]   Behavioral Health: [X]
Chiropractic: [X]   Dental: [ ]
Home Care: [X]   Inpatient SNF: [X]
Long-Term Care: [X]   Pharm. Mail Order: [X]
Physical Therapy: [X]   Podiatry: [X]
Psychiatric: [X]   Transplant: [X]
Vision: [X]   Wellness: [X]
Workers' Comp: [ ]
Other Benefits:

Comments:
In June 1999, Wellcare of New York sold its commercial HMO New York State business to GHI (Group Health Incorporated).

GREAT-WEST HEALTHCARE OF NEW YORK

475 Park Ave S 23rd Fl
New York, NY 10016
Phone: 212-685-5999 Fax: 212-685-6446 Toll-Free:
Web site: www.greatwesthealthcare.com

MAILING ADDRESS:
GREAT-WEST HEALTHCARE OF NY
475 Park Ave S 23rd Fl
New York, NY 10016

KEY EXECUTIVES:
Executive Director .... Joan Russo

COMPANY PROFILE:
Parent Company Name: Great West Life & Annuity Insurance Co
Doing Business As:
Year Founded: Federally Qualified: [ ]
Forprofit: [Y]   Not-For-Profit: [ ]
Model Type:
Accreditation: [ ] AAPPO [ ] JACHO [ ] NCQA [ ] URAC
Plan Type: HMO, CDHP, HSA

SERVICE AREA:
Nationwide: N
NY;

TYPE OF COVERAGE:
Commercial: [Y] Individual: [ ] FEHBP: [ ] Indemnity: [ ]
Medicare: [ ] Medicaid: [ ] Supplemental Medicare: [ ]
Tricare [ ]

CONSUMER-DRIVEN PRODUCTS
Mellon HR Solutions LLC   HSA Company
    HSA Product
    HSA Administrator
    Consumer-Driven Health Plan
    High Deductible Health Plan

PLAN BENEFITS:
Alternative Medicine: [X]   Behavioral Health: [ ]
Chiropractic: [X]   Dental: [X]
Home Care: [X]   Inpatient SNF: [X]
Long-Term Care: [ ]   Pharm. Mail Order: [X]
Physical Therapy: [X]   Podiatry: [X]
Psychiatric: [X]   Transplant: [X]
Vision: [X]   Wellness: [X]
Workers' Comp: [ ]
Other Benefits:

GREAT-WEST HEALTHCARE OF NEW YORK

50 Main St 9th Fl
White Plains, NY 10606
Phone: 914-682-0159 Fax: 914-682-0409 Toll-Free: 800-736-0700
Web site: www.greatwesthealthcare.com

MAILING ADDRESS:
GREAT-WEST HEALTHCARE OF NY
50 Main St 9th Fl
White Plains, NY 10606

KEY EXECUTIVES:
Regional Group Manager .... Garrison Hudkins

COMPANY PROFILE:
Parent Company Name: Great West Life & Annuity Insurance Co
Doing Business As:
Year Founded: Federally Qualified: [ ]
Forprofit: [Y]   Not-For-Profit: [ ]
Model Type:
Accreditation: [ ] AAPPO [ ] JACHO [ ] NCQA [ ] URAC
Plan Type: PPO, HDHP, HSA,

SERVICE AREA:
Nationwide: N
NY;

TYPE OF COVERAGE:
Commercial: [Y] Individual: [ ] FEHBP: [ ] Indemnity: [ ]
Medicare: [ ] Medicaid: [ ] Supplemental Medicare: [ ]
Tricare [ ]

PLAN BENEFITS:
Alternative Medicine: [X]   Behavioral Health: [ ]
Chiropractic: [X]   Dental: [X]
Home Care: [X]   Inpatient SNF: [X]
Long-Term Care: [ ]   Pharm. Mail Order: [X]
Physical Therapy: [X]   Podiatry: [X]
Psychiatric: [X]   Transplant: [X]
Vision: [X]   Wellness: [X]
Workers' Comp: [ ]
Other Benefits:

GUARDIAN LIFE INSURANCE CO OF AMERICA

7 Hanover Sq
New York, NY 10004
Phone: 212-598-8000 Fax: 212-919-2423 Toll-Free: 888-600-4667
Web site: www.guardianlife.com

MAILING ADDRESS:
GUARDIAN LIFE INSURANCE CO
7 Hanover Sq
New York, NY 10004

KEY EXECUTIVES:
Chief Executive Officer/President .... Dennis J Manning, CLU, CHFC
Chief Financial Officer .... Robert E Broatch
Chief Information Officer .... Frank Wander
Senior VP, Corporate Marketing .... Nancy Rogers
VP Healthcare Quality .... Edward Kane
Chief Investment Officer .... Thomas G Sorell, CFA
Senior VP, Human Resources .... James D Ranton
VP, General Counsel .... John Peluso, CLU, JD
Senior VP, Individual Markets .... David W Allen, FSA

COMPANY PROFILE:
Parent Company Name:
Doing Business As:
Year Founded: 1860   Federally Qualified: [Y]
Forprofit: [Y]   Not-For-Profit: [ ]
Model Type:
Accreditation: [ ] AAPPO [ ] JACHO [ ] NCQA [ ] URAC
Plan Type: HMO, PPO, POS, HDHP, HSA
Total Revenue: 2005:   2006: 7,491,000
Net Income 2005:   2006: 376,000
Total Enrollment:
    2001: 50,117   2004: 0   2007: 0
    2002: 0   2005:
    2003: 0   2006: 5,000,000

SERVICE AREA:
Nationwide: Y
NW;

TYPE OF COVERAGE:
Commercial: [Y] Individual: [ ] FEHBP: [ ] Indemnity: [ ]
Medicare: [ ] Medicaid: [ ] Supplemental Medicare: [ ]
Tricare [ ]

CONSUMER-DRIVEN PRODUCTS
    HSA Company
    HSA Product
    HSA Administrator
    Consumer-Driven Health Plan
Destiny Health Plan   High Deductible Health Plan

FIDELIS CARE NEW YORK

95-25 Queens Blvd
Rego Park, NY 11374
Phone: 718-896-6500 Fax: 718-896-1920 Toll-Free: 888-343-3547
Web site: www.fideliscare.com
MAILING ADDRESS:
    FIDELIS CARE NEW YORK
    95-25 Queens Blvd
    Rego Park, NY 11374

KEY EXECUTIVES:
Chief Executive Officer/President .... Mark L Lane
Chief Financial Officer .... Dina Soroka
Medical Director .... Marco Michaelson, MD
Pharmacy Director .... Liya Davydov
Chief Operating Officer .... Patrick J Frawley
Marketing Manager .... Rupert Brady

COMPANY PROFILE:
Parent Company Name: New York State Catholic Hlth Pln, The
Doing Business As: Fidelis Care New York
Year Founded: 1993   Federally Qualified: [ ]
Forprofit: [ ]   Not-For-Profit: [Y]
Model Type:
Accreditation: [ ] AAPPO [ ] JACHO [ ] NCQA [ ] URAC
Plan Type: HMO
Total Enrollment:
    2001: 75,592   2004: 227,000   2007: 298,000
    2002: 0   2005:
    2003: 0   2006: 290,000
SERVICE AREA:
Nationwide: N
    NY (Albany, Chautauqua, Erie, Nassau, New York City, Niagara, Onondaga, Rensselaer, Rockland, Schenectady, Suffolk, Westchester);
TYPE OF COVERAGE:
Commercial: [ ] Individual: [ ] FEHBP: [ ] Indemnity: [ ]
Medicare: [ ] Medicaid: [Y] Supplemental Medicare: [Y]
Tricare [ ]
PRODUCTS OFFERED:
Product Name: Type:
Catholic Services Health Plan   Medicaid
Fidelis Medicare Advantage   Medicare
PLAN BENEFITS:
Alternative Medicine: [ ]   Behavioral Health: [X]
Chiropractic: [ ]   Dental: [X]
Home Care: [X]   Inpatient SNF: [ ]
Long-Term Care: [ ]   Pharm. Mail Order: [ ]
Physical Therapy: [ ]   Podiatry: [ ]
Psychiatric: [X]   Transplant: [X]
Vision: [X]   Wellness: [X]
Workers' Comp: [ ]
Other Benefits: X
Comments:
Formerly Better Health Plan Inc, Amherst, NY.

FINGER LAKES COMMUNITY CARE NETWORK

3170 West Street Ste 150
Canandaigua, NY 14424
Phone: 585-396-6463 Fax: 585-396-6674 Toll-Free: 888-758-7658
Web site: www.thompsonhealth.com
MAILING ADDRESS:
    FINGER LAKES COMMUNITY CARE
    3170 West Street Ste 150
    Canandaigua, NY 14424

KEY EXECUTIVES:
Chief Executive Officer .... Linda Janczak
Senior VP, FLCCN .... Bonnie Ross
Medical Director .... Robert Ostrander, MD
Dir, Business Development Thompson Health .... Sheila Rossi
Contracts Manager .... Sally Bagley

COMPANY PROFILE:
Parent Company Name: Thompson Health Systems
Doing Business As:
Year Founded: 1992   Federally Qualified: [N]
Forprofit: [Y]   Not-For-Profit: [ ]
Model Type: NETWORK
Accreditation: [ ] AAPPO [ ] JACHO [ ] NCQA [ ] URAC
Plan Type: PPO
Total Enrollment:
    2001: 5,400   2004: 0   2007: 0
    2002: 0   2005:
    2003: 0   2006:
SERVICE AREA:
Nationwide: N
    NY (Ontario, Seneca, Wayne, Yates);
TYPE OF COVERAGE:
Commercial: [Y] Individual: [Y] FEHBP: [ ] Indemnity: [ ]
Medicare: [ ] Medicaid: [ ] Supplemental Medicare: [ ]
Tricare [ ]
PRODUCTS OFFERED:
Product Name: Type:
Finger Lakes Health Plan   PPO
PLAN BENEFITS:
Alternative Medicine: [ ]   Behavioral Health: [ ]
Chiropractic: [X]   Dental: [ ]
Home Care: [X]   Inpatient SNF: [ ]
Long-Term Care: [ ]   Pharm. Mail Order: [X]
Physical Therapy: [ ]   Podiatry: [X]
Psychiatric: [X]   Transplant: [X]
Vision: [X]   Wellness: [X]
Workers' Comp: [X]
Other Benefits:

GHI HMO SELECT INC

441 Ninth Ave
New York, NY 10001-1686
Phone: 212-615-0000 Fax: 212-563-8567 Toll-Free: 877-244-4466
Web site: www.ghi.com
MAILING ADDRESS:
    GHI HMO SELECT INC
    441 Ninth Ave
    New York, NY 10001-1686

KEY EXECUTIVES:
Chairman of the Board .... James F Gill, Esq
Chief Executive Officer .... Frank J Branchini
Corporate Treasurer .... Michael Palmateer
President/Chief Operating Officer .... Aran Ron, MD
Medical Director .... Maria Martins-Lopes, MD
Chief Marketing Officer .... David Henderson
VP, Sales .... Justin Fieldler
Corporate Communications .... John Demers
Provider Services Manager .... Denise Becker
VP, Human Resources .... Mariann Drohan
Medical Management Director .... Cathy Kania
Quality Assurance Director .... Cathy Kania

COMPANY PROFILE:
Parent Company Name: Group Health Incorporated
Doing Business As:
Year Founded: 1999   Federally Qualified: [N]
Forprofit: [Y]   Not-For-Profit: [ ]
Model Type: IPA
Accreditation: [ ] AAPPO [ ] JACHO [X] NCQA [ ] URAC
Plan Type: HMO, POS
Primary Physicians: 79,000   Physician Specialists:
Hospitals:
Total Revenue: 2005:   2006: 2,741.540,000
Net Income: 2005:   2006: 33,754,000
Total Enrollment:
    2001: 0   2004: 47,566   2007: 2,600,000
    2002: 32,150   2005: 67,910
    2003: 35,646   2006:
Medical Loss Ratio: 2005:   2006: 90.00
Administrative Expense Ratio: 2005:   2006:
SERVICE AREA:
Nationwide: N
    NY (Albany, Bronx, Broome, Columbia, Delaware, Dutchess, Fulton, Greene, Kings, Montgomery, New York, Orange, Otsego, Putnam, Queens, Rensselaer, Rockland, Saratoga, Schenectady, Schoharie, Sullivan, Ulster, Warren, Washington, Westchester);

NEW YORK — Managed Care Organization Profiles

CONSUMER-DRIVEN PRODUCTS
HSA Bank
BluePPOHSA
HSA Bank
HSA Company
HSA Product
HSA Administrator
Consumer-Driven Health Plan
High Deductible Health Plan

PLAN BENEFITS:
Alternative Medicine:	[ ]	Behavioral Health:	[ ]
Chiropractic:	[X]	Dental:	[ ]
Home Care:	[X]	Inpatient SNF:	[X]
Long-Term Care:	[ ]	Pharm. Mail Order:	[X]
Physical Therapy:	[X]	Podiatry:	[ ]
Psychiatric:	[X]	Transplant:	[ ]
Vision:	[X]	Wellness:	[X]
Workers' Comp:	[X]		
Other Benefits:			

EXCELLUS BLUECROSS BLUESHIELD, ROCHESTER REGION

165 Court St
Rochester, NY 14647
Phone: 585-454-1700 Fax: 585-238-4233 Toll-Free: 800-347-1200
Web site: www.excellus.com
MAILING ADDRESS:
EXCELLUS BC BS, ROCHESTER REGION
165 Court St
Rochester, NY 14647

KEY EXECUTIVES:
Chairman .... John G Doyle, Jr
Chief Executive Officer .... David H Klein
Regional President .... Scott G Ellsworth
Chief Financial Officer .... Emil D Duda
VP, Chief Medical Director .... Martin Lustick, MD
VP, Chief Pharmacy Officer .... Joel Owerbach, PharmD
VP Communications .... James Redmond
Senior VP, Operations .... Paul von Ebers
VP, Human Resources .... Richard Nangreave
Regional VP, Sales .... Todd Muscatello
General Counsel .... Ralph W Cox, Esq

COMPANY PROFILE:
Parent Company Name: The Lifetime Healthcare Companies Inc
Doing Business As:
Year Founded: 1985   Federally Qualified: [N]
Forprofit: [ ]   Not-For-Profit: [Y]
Model Type: MIXED
Accreditation: [ ] AAPPO [ ] JACHO [X] NCQA [X] URAC
Plan Type: HMO, PPO, EPO, CDHP, HDHP, HSA,
Total Enrollment:
 2001: 800,000   2004: 18,418   2007: 0
 2002: 525,782   2005: 419,339
 2003: 161,855   2006:

SERVICE AREA:
Nationwide: N
NY (Livingston, Monroe, Ontario, Seneca, Wayne, Yates);

TYPE OF COVERAGE:
Commercial: [Y] Individual: [Y] FEHBP: [Y] Indemnity: [Y]
Medicare: [Y] Medicaid: [Y] Supplemental Medicare: [Y]
Tricare [ ]

PRODUCTS OFFERED:
Product Name:	Type:
Blue Choice	HMO
ViaHealth Plan	HMO
StrongCare	HMO
Blue Choice Option	Medicaid HMO
Blue Choice Senior/Seniorcare	Medicare

CONSUMER-DRIVEN PRODUCTS
HSA Bank
BluePPOHSA
HSA Bank
HSA Company
HSA Product
HSA Administrator
Consumer-Driven Health Plan
High Deductible Health Plan

PLAN BENEFITS:
Alternative Medicine:	[ ]	Behavioral Health:	[ ]
Chiropractic:	[X]	Dental:	[ ]
Home Care:	[X]	Inpatient SNF:	[X]
Long-Term Care:	[ ]	Pharm. Mail Order:	[X]
Physical Therapy:	[X]	Podiatry:	[ ]
Psychiatric:	[X]	Transplant:	[ ]
Vision:	[X]	Wellness:	[X]
Workers' Comp:	[X]		
Other Benefits:			

Comments:
FEHBP-enrollment 5,860.

EXCELLUS BLUECROSS BLUESHIELD, UTICA REGION

12 Rhoads Dr
Utica, NY 13502-6398
Phone: 315-798-4200 Fax: 315-797-4298 Toll-Free: 800-722-7884
Web site: www.bcbsuw.com
MAILING ADDRESS:
EXCELLUS BC BS, UTICA REGION
12 Rhoads Dr
Utica, NY 13502-6398

KEY EXECUTIVES:
Chairman .... David T Griffith
Chief Executive Officer .... David H Klein
Regional President .... Cynthia C Hummel
Chief Financial Officer .... Emil D Duda
VP, Chief Medical Officer .... Frank Dubeck, MD
VP, Communications .... Stephanie K Davis
VP, Marketing .... Mark Ruszczyk
VP, Network Management .... Kathy Horn
General Counsel .... Margaret M Cassady, Esq
VP, Chief Medical Officer .... Arthur Verullo, MD
VP, Administration .... Eve Van de Wal

COMPANY PROFILE:
Parent Company Name: The Lifetime Healthcare Companies Inc
Doing Business As: HMO Blue
Year Founded: 1986   Federally Qualified: [N]
Forprofit: [ ]   Not-For-Profit: [Y]
Model Type: IPA
Accreditation: [ ] AAPPO [ ] JACHO [ ] NCQA [ ] URAC
Plan Type: HMO, POS, ASO, CDHP, HDHP, HSA,
Total Enrollment:
 2001: 300,000   2004: 0   2007: 0
 2002: 37,518   2005:
 2003: 0   2006:

SERVICE AREA:
Nationwide: N
NY (Clinton, Delaware, Essex, Franklin, Fulton, Hamilton, Herkimer, Madison, Montgomery, Oneida, Otsego);

TYPE OF COVERAGE:
Commercial: [Y] Individual: [Y] FEHBP: [ ] Indemnity: [ ]
Medicare: [ ] Medicaid: [ ] Supplemental Medicare: [ ]
Tricare [ ]

PRODUCTS OFFERED:
Product Name:	Type:
HMO Blue	HMO

CONSUMER-DRIVEN PRODUCTS
HSA Bank
BluePPOHSA
HSA Bank
HSA Company
HSA Product
HSA Administrator
Consumer-Driven Health Plan
High Deductible Health Plan

PLAN BENEFITS:
Alternative Medicine:	[ ]	Behavioral Health:	[X]
Chiropractic:	[X]	Dental:	[ ]
Home Care:	[X]	Inpatient SNF:	[X]
Long-Term Care:	[ ]	Pharm. Mail Order:	[X]
Physical Therapy:	[X]	Podiatry:	[ ]
Psychiatric:	[X]	Transplant:	[X]
Vision:	[X]	Wellness:	[X]
Workers' Comp:	[X]		
Other Benefits:			

Managed Care Organization Profiles — **NEW YORK**

Plan Type: HMO, PPO, EPO, POS, CDHP, HDHP, HSA
Total Revenue: 2005:   2006: 4,811,946,510
Net Income   2005:   2006:   151,722,000

Total Enrollment:
  2001: 1,750,000   2004: 1,867,481   2007: 1,400,000
  2002: 2,001,806   2005:
  2003: 1,890,430   2006:
Medical Loss Ratio: 2005:   2006: 87.00
Administrative Expense Ratio: 2005:   2006:

SERVICE AREA:
Nationwide: N
  NY (Broome, Cayuga, Chemug, Chenango, Clinton, Cortland, Delaware, Essex, Franklin, Fulton, Hamilton, Herkimer, Jefferson, Livingston, Lewis, Madison, Monroe, Montgomery, Oneida, Onondaga, Ontario, Oswego, Otsego, Schuyler, Seneca, St Lawrence, Steuben, Tioga, Tompkins, Wayne, Yates);

TYPE OF COVERAGE:
Commercial: [Y] Individual: [Y] FEHBP: [ ] Indemnity: [Y]
Medicare: [Y] Medicaid: [Y] Supplemental Medicare: [Y]
Tricare   [ ]

PRODUCTS OFFERED:
Product Name:	Type:
Excellus BC BS, Rochester Area	HMO
Excellus BC BS, Central NY	HMO
Excellus BC BS, Utica	HMO
Excellus BC BS, Central NY Southern	HMO
SeniorChoice	Medicare
BlueChoice Senior/Seniorcare	Medicare Advantge
Excellus	Medicaid

CONSUMER-DRIVEN PRODUCTS
HSA Bank   HSA Company
BluePPOHSA   HSA Product
HSA Bank   HSA Administrator
                    Consumer-Driven Health Plan
                    High Deductible Health Plan

PLAN BENEFITS:
Alternative Medicine: [ ]   Behavioral Health: [ ]
Chiropractic: [X]   Dental: [ ]
Home Care: [X]   Inpatient SNF: [X]
Long-Term Care: [ ]   Pharm. Mail Order: [X]
Physical Therapy: [X]   Podiatry: [ ]
Psychiatric: [X]   Transplant: [ ]
Vision: [X]   Wellness: [X]
Workers' Comp: [X]
Other Benefits:

Comments:
Parent of: Excellus Blue Cross Blue Shield of Rochester Area; Excellus Blue Cross Blue Shield of Utica-Watertown; Excellus Blue Cross Blue Shield, Central New York Southern Region; Excellus Blue Cross Blue Shield of Central New York;

EXCELLUS BLUECROSS BLUESHIELD, CENTRAL NEW YORK REGION

344 S Warren St
Syracuse, NY 13221
Phone: 315-671-6400 Fax: 315-671-6799 Toll-Free: 800-252-2209
Web site: www.excellusbcbs.com

MAILING ADDRESS:
EXCELLUS BC BS, CENTRAL NEW YORK REGION
PO Box 4809
Syracuse, NY 13221

KEY EXECUTIVES:
Chairman of the Board .... Casper F Sedgwick
Chief Executive Officer .... David H Klein
Regional Vice President .... James R Smith
Chief Financial Officer .... Emil D Duda
VP, Chief Medical Officer .... Arthur Vercillo, MD
VP, Communications .... Elizabeth Martin
VP, Sales East .... James Reed
VP, Network Management .... Wendy D Kotcamp
VP, Human Resources .... Ellen G Wilson
General Counsel .... Margaret M Cassady, Esq
VP, Chief Medical Officer, Quality .... Norman Lindenmuth, MD

COMPANY PROFILE:
Parent Company Name: The Lifetime Healthcare Companies Inc
Doing Business As: Excellus Health Plan Inc DBA Upstate HMO
Year Founded: 1984   Federally Qualified: [N]
Forprofit: [Y]   Not-For-Profit: [Y]
Model Type: IPA
Accreditation: [ ] AAPPO [ ] JACHO [X] NCQA [ ] URAC
Plan Type: HMO, CDHP, HDHP, HSA,
Total Enrollment:
  2001: 650,000   2004: 0   2007: 0
  2002: 0   2005:
  2003: 0   2006:

SERVICE AREA:
Nationwide: N
  NY (Cayuga, Cortland, Jefferson, Lewis, Onondaga, Oswego, St Lawrence, Tompkins);

TYPE OF COVERAGE:
Commercial: [Y] Individual: [Y] FEHBP: [ ] Indemnity: [ ]
Medicare: [ ] Medicaid: [ ] Supplemental Medicare: [ ]
Tricare   [ ]

PRODUCTS OFFERED:
Product Name:	Type:
HMO-CNY	HMO

CONSUMER-DRIVEN PRODUCTS
HSA Bank   HSA Company
BluePPOHSA   HSA Product
HSA Bank   HSA Administrator
                    Consumer-Driven Health Plan
                    High Deductible Health Plan

PLAN BENEFITS:
Alternative Medicine: [ ]   Behavioral Health: [ ]
Chiropractic: [ ]   Dental: [ ]
Home Care: [X]   Inpatient SNF: [X]
Long-Term Care: [ ]   Pharm. Mail Order: [ ]
Physical Therapy: [X]   Podiatry: [ ]
Psychiatric: [X]   Transplant: [X]
Vision: [ ]   Wellness: [X]
Workers' Comp: [ ]
Other Benefits:

EXCELLUS BLUECROSS BLUESHIELD, CENTRAL NEW YORK SOUTHERN TIER

150 North Main St Ste 1
Elmira, NY 13901
Phone: 607-734-1551 Fax: 607-732-7624 Toll-Free:
Web site: www.excellus.com

MAILING ADDRESS:
EXCELLUS BC BS, CENTRAL NEW YORK SOUTHERN
150 North Main St Ste 1
Elmira, NY 13901

KEY EXECUTIVES:
Chairman .... Thomas S Coughlin
Chief Executive Officer .... David H Klein
Regional President .... Kevin J McGurgan
Chief Financial Officer .... Emil D Duda
Medical Director .... Steven Goldberg, MD
VP of Sales & Marketing .... James Reed
General Counsel .... Lisa Santelli, Esq
Director of Communications .... Stephanie K Davis
Director, Physician/Ancillary Contracting .... Nancy Dorfman

COMPANY PROFILE:
Parent Company Name: The Lifetime Healthcare Companies Inc
Doing Business As:
Year Founded: Federally Qualified: [N]
Forprofit: [ ]   Not-For-Profit: [Y]
Model Type:
Accreditation: [ ] AAPPO [ ] JACHO [X] NCQA [ ] URAC
Plan Type: HMO, CDHP, HSA
Total Enrollment:
  2001: 0   2004: 0   2007: 0
  2002: 35,993   2005:
  2003: 0   2006:

SERVICE AREA:
Nationwide: N
  NY (Broome, Chemug, Chenango, Schuyler, Steuben, Tioga);

TYPE OF COVERAGE:
Commercial: [Y] Individual: [Y] FEHBP: [ ] Indemnity: [ ]
Medicare: [Y] Medicaid: [Y] Supplemental Medicare: [Y]
Tricare   [ ]

NEW YORK — Managed Care Organization Profiles

EM RISK MANAGEMENT, A POMCO COMPANY

111 Grant Ave Ste 206
Endicott, NY 13760
Phone: 607-786-9700 Fax: 607-786-3470 Toll-Free: 800-934-2459
Web site: www.emmgt.com
MAILING ADDRESS:
    EM RISK MANAGEMENT, A POMCO COMPANY
    111 Grant Ave Ste 206
    Endicott, NY 13760

KEY EXECUTIVES:
President/Chief Executive Officer .... Robert W Pomfry
Vice President .... David Price
Senior VP, Chief Financial Officer .... Terrence C Dowd, Jr
Medical Director .... Dennis Daly, MD
Senior VP, Chief Operating Officer .... Donald P Napier
VP of Marketing .... Marc Flood
VP, Information Systems .... Bruce Peterson
Medical Management Director .... Sharon Miller
Quality Assurance/Case Management Director .... Sharon Miller
Workers Compensation Director .... Bryan Thompson

COMPANY PROFILE:
Parent Company Name: Maurice Pomfry & Associates, LTD
Doing Business As:
Year Founded: 1987   Federally Qualified: [ ]
Forprofit: [Y]   Not-For-Profit: [ ]
Model Type:
Accreditation: [ ] AAPPO [ ] JACHO [ ] NCQA [ ] URAC
Plan Type: PPO, Specialty PPO, ASO, TPA, UR
SERVICE AREA:
Nationwide: N
    NY;
PRODUCTS OFFERED:
Product Name: Type:
Health Management Services
Utilization review
Utilization Management
TPA Services
Medical Billing Auditing
Case Management
PLAN BENEFITS:
Alternative Medicine: [ ]   Behavioral Health: [ ]
Chiropractic: [X]   Dental: [ ]
Home Care: [X]   Inpatient SNF: [X]
Long-Term Care: [X]   Pharm. Mail Order: [ ]
Physical Therapy: [X]   Podiatry: [ ]
Psychiatric: [X]   Transplant: [X]
Vision: [ ]   Wellness: [ ]
Workers' Comp: [X]
Other Benefits:
Comments:
Coverage type is Self-insured.

EMPIRE BLUE CROSS BLUE SHIELD

One Liberty Plaza 165 Broadway
New York, NY 10006
Phone: 212-476-1000 Fax: 212-476-1430 Toll-Free:
Web site: www.empireblue.com
MAILING ADDRESS:
    EMPIRE BLUE CROSS BLUE SHIELD
    One Liberty Plaza 165 Broadway
    New York, NY 10006

KEY EXECUTIVES:
President .... Mark Wagnar

COMPANY PROFILE:
Parent Company Name: WellPoint Inc
Doing Business As: Empire Healthchoice HMO Inc
Year Founded: 1936   Federally Qualified: [Y]
Forprofit: [Y]   Not-For-Profit: [ ]
Model Type: NETWORK
Accreditation: [ ] AAPPO [ ] JACHO [X] NCQA [ ] URAC
Plan Type: HMO, PPO, ASO, TPA, EPO, POS, CDHP, HSA
Primary Physicians: 25,338   Physician Specialists: 60,000
Hospitals: 228
Total Revenue: 2005:   2006: 2,541,672,073
Net Income: 2005:   2006:
Total Enrollment:
    2001: 4,383,354   2004: 4,950,000   2007: 5,000,000
    2002: 4,644,000   2005: 5,000,000
    2003: 4,800,000   2006:
Medical Loss Ratio: 2005:   2006: 83.60
Administrative Expense Ratio: 2005:   2006:
SERVICE AREA:
Nationwide: N
    CT (Fairfield, Litchfield); NJ (Bergen, Essex, Hudson, Monmouth, Middlesex, Passaic, Sussex, Union); NY (Albany, Bronx, Clinton, Columbia, Delaware, Dutchess, Essex, Fulton, Greene, Kings, Manhattan, Montgomery, Nassau, Orange, Putnam, Queens, Rennsselear, Richmond, Rockland, Saratoga, Schenectady, Schoharie, Suffolk, Sullivan, Ulster, Warren, Washington, Westchester);
TYPE OF COVERAGE:
Commercial: [Y] Individual: [Y] FEHBP: [Y] Indemnity: [ ]
Medicare: [Y] Medicaid: [ ] Supplemental Medicare: [Y]
Tricare   [ ]
PRODUCTS OFFERED:
Product Name: Type:
BlueChoice HMO   HMO
Direct Connection HMO   HMO
Empire Deluxe PPO   PPO
Direct Connection EPO   EPO
BlueChoice Senior Plan   Medicare
Empire HealthChoice HMO   HMO
CONSUMER-DRIVEN PRODUCTS
Mellon Financial   HSA Company
Total Blue   HSA Product
                                       HSA Administrator
Total Blue   Consumer-Driven Health Plan
                                       High Deductible Health Plan
PLAN BENEFITS:
Alternative Medicine: [ ]   Behavioral Health: [ ]
Chiropractic: [X]   Dental: [X]
Home Care: [X]   Inpatient SNF: [X]
Long-Term Care: [ ]   Pharm. Mail Order: [X]
Physical Therapy: [X]   Podiatry: [X]
Psychiatric: [X]   Transplant: [X]
Vision: [X]   Wellness: [X]
Workers' Comp: [ ]
Other Benefits:
Comments:
Formerly HealthNet.

EXCELLUS BLUECROSS BLUESHIELD

165 Court St
Rochester, NY 14647
Phone: 585-454-1700 Fax: 585-238-3659 Toll-Free: 800-847-1200
Web site: www.bcbsroch.com
MAILING ADDRESS:
    EXCELLUS BC BS
    165 Court St
    Rochester, NY 14647

KEY EXECUTIVES:
Chairman of the Board .... John G Doyle, Jr
Chief Executive Officer .... David H Klein
Regional President .... Kevin N Hill
Chief Financial Officer .... Emil D Duda
Chief Medical Officer .... Jonathan S Kaplan, MD
Chief Information Officer .... David C McDowell
Chief Operating Officer .... Kevin N Hill
Senior VP, Marketing .... Paul M von Ebers
VP, Provider Operations .... Daniel Aaronson
Senior VP, Network Management Support .... Jack Sieber
VP, Human Resources .... Richard Nangreave
VP, Quality Management Admin .... Kathleen Curtin
VP, Business & Product Development .... Leon D Lamoreaux
VP, Health Plan Adminstration .... Carolyn Schofield
VP, Medicare Division .... Donna C McDonald
VP, Excellus Rx .... Anne Ruflin
General Counsel .... Ralph W Cox, ESQ

COMPANY PROFILE:
Parent Company Name: The Lifetime Healthcare Companies Inc
Doing Business As: Excellus BC BS Companies
Year Founded: 1998   Federally Qualified: [N]
Forprofit: [ ]   Not-For-Profit: [Y]
Model Type:
Accreditation: [ ] AAPPO [ ] JACHO [X] NCQA [ ] URAC

Managed Care Organization Profiles — NEW YORK

TYPE OF COVERAGE:
Commercial: [Y] Individual: [ ] FEHBP: [Y] Indemnity: [ ]
Medicare: [Y] Medicaid: [Y] Supplemental Medicare: [ ]
Tricare   [ ]

PRODUCTS OFFERED:
Product Name:	Type:
The Eyecare Advantage	PPO
Affinity Discount	PPO

PLAN BENEFITS:
Alternative Medicine:	[ ]	Behavioral Health:	[ ]
Chiropractic:	[ ]	Dental:	[ ]
Home Care:	[ ]	Inpatient SNF:	[ ]
Long-Term Care:	[ ]	Pharm. Mail Order:	[ ]
Physical Therapy:	[ ]	Podiatry:	[ ]
Psychiatric:	[ ]	Transplant:	[ ]
Vision:	[X]	Wellness:	[ ]
Workers' Comp:	[ ]		
Other Benefits:			

DENTCARE DELIVERY SYSTEMS INC

333 Earle Ovington Blvd #300
Uniondale, NY 11553
Phone: 516-542-2200 Fax: 516-794-3186 Toll-Free: 800-468-0608
Web site: www.dentcaredeliverysystems.org

MAILING ADDRESS:
DENTCARE DELIVERY SYSTEMS INC
333 Earle Ovington Blvd #300
Uniondale, NY 11553

KEY EXECUTIVES:
Chief Executive Officer/President .... Stephen Cuchel, MD
Chief Information Officer .... Christopher Schmidt
Chief Operating Officer .... Bruce H Safran
Marketing Director .... Mario Masciandaro
MIS Director .... Phillip Rizzuto

COMPANY PROFILE:
Parent Company Name:
Doing Business As:
Year Founded: 1978   Federally Qualified: [ ]
Forprofit: [ ]   Not-For-Profit: [Y]
Model Type: IPA
Accreditation: [ ] AAPPO [ ] JACHO [ ] NCQA [ ] URAC
Plan Type: Specialty HMO, Specialty PPO, POS, ASO, TPA:
Total Enrollment:
  2001: 0   2004: 368,361   2007: 0
  2002: 415,604   2005:
  2003: 373,725   2006:

SERVICE AREA:
Nationwide: N
 NJ; NY;

TYPE OF COVERAGE:
Commercial: [Y] Individual: [Y] FEHBP: [ ] Indemnity: [ ]
Medicare: [Y] Medicaid: [Y] Supplemental Medicare: [ ]
Tricare   [ ]

PLAN BENEFITS:
Alternative Medicine:	[ ]	Behavioral Health:	[ ]
Chiropractic:	[ ]	Dental:	[X]
Home Care:	[ ]	Inpatient SNF:	[ ]
Long-Term Care:	[ ]	Pharm. Mail Order:	[ ]
Physical Therapy:	[ ]	Podiatry:	[ ]
Psychiatric:	[ ]	Transplant:	[ ]
Vision:	[ ]	Wellness:	[ ]
Workers' Comp:	[ ]		
Other Benefits:			

ELDERPLAN INC

6323 Seventh Ave
Brooklyn, NY 11220
Phone: 718-921-7898 Fax: 718-630-2565 Toll-Free: 800-353-3765
Web site: www.elderplan.org

MAILING ADDRESS:
ELDERPLAN INC
6323 Seventh Ave
Brooklyn, NY 11220

KEY EXECUTIVES:
Chief Executive Officer/President .... Eli S Feldman
Chief Financial Officer .... Alex Balko
Executive VP, Chief Operating Officer .... Barry Volin
Marketing Director/Publics Relations .... Janet Rothman

COMPANY PROFILE:
Parent Company Name:
Doing Business As:
Year Founded: 1985   Federally Qualified: [Y]
Forprofit: [ ]   Not-For-Profit: [Y]
Model Type: NETWORK
Accreditation: [ ] AAPPO [ ] JACHO [ ] NCQA [ ] URAC
Plan Type: Specialty HMO
Total Enrollment:
  2001: 9,391   2004: 13,733   2007: 0
  2002: 10,127   2005: 16,180
  2003: 12,620   2006:

SERVICE AREA:
Nationwide: N
 NY (Kings);

TYPE OF COVERAGE:
Commercial: [ ] Individual: [Y] FEHBP: [ ] Indemnity: [ ]
Medicare: [Y] Medicaid: [Y] Supplemental Medicare: [ ]
Tricare   [ ]

PRODUCTS OFFERED:
Product Name:	Type:
Elderplan Medicaid	Medicaid
Elderplan Medicare	Medicare

PLAN BENEFITS:
Alternative Medicine:	[ ]	Behavioral Health:	[X]
Chiropractic:	[X]	Dental:	[X]
Home Care:	[X]	Inpatient SNF:	[X]
Long-Term Care:	[X]	Pharm. Mail Order:	[X]
Physical Therapy:	[X]	Podiatry:	[X]
Psychiatric:	[X]	Transplant:	[X]
Vision:	[X]	Wellness:	[X]
Workers' Comp:	[ ]		
Other Benefits:			

ELDERPLAN INC - SHMO

6323 7th Ave
Brooklyn, NY 11220-4711
Phone: 718-921-7898 Fax: 718-630-2565 Toll-Free:
Web site: www.elderplan.org

MAILING ADDRESS:
ELDERPLAN INC - SHMO
6323 7th Ave
Brooklyn, NY 11220-4711

KEY EXECUTIVES:
Chief Executive Officer .... Eli S Feldman
Chief Financial Officer .... Alex Balko
Executive VP, Chief Operating Officer .... Dam Kasle

COMPANY PROFILE:
Parent Company Name: Metropolitan Jewish Health System
Doing Business As:
Year Founded: Federally Qualified: [ ]
Forprofit: [ ]   Not-For-Profit: [Y]
Model Type:
Accreditation: [ ] AAPPO [ ] JACHO [ ] NCQA [ ] URAC
Plan Type: HMO
Total Enrollment:
  2001: 9,301   2004: 13,660   2007: 16,693
  2002: 10,699   2005: 15,712
  2003: 12,376   2006: 3,008

SERVICE AREA:
Nationwide:
 NY (Kings, New York, Queens, Richmond, Suffolk);

TYPE OF COVERAGE:
Commercial: [ ] Individual: [ ] FEHBP: [ ] Indemnity: [ ]
Medicare: [ ] Medicaid: [ ] Supplemental Medicare: [ ]
Tricare   [ ]

NEW YORK

SERVICE AREA:
Nationwide: N
  NY (Westchester);
TYPE OF COVERAGE:
Commercial: [ ] Individual: [ ] FEHBP: [ ] Indemnity: [ ]
Medicare: [ ] Medicaid: [Y] Supplemental Medicare: [ ]
Tricare   [ ]
PRODUCTS OFFERED:
Product Name: Type:
Community Choice Health Plan   Medicaid
Child Health Plus   Medicaid
Family Health Plus   Medicaid
PLAN BENEFITS:
Alternative Medicine: [ ]   Behavioral Health: [X]
Chiropractic: [ ]   Dental: [X]
Home Care: [X]   Inpatient SNF: [ ]
Long-Term Care: [ ]   Pharm. Mail Order: [ ]
Physical Therapy: [ ]   Podiatry: [ ]
Psychiatric: [ ]   Transplant: [ ]
Vision: [ ]   Wellness: [ ]
Workers' Comp: [ ]
Other Benefits:

CONNECTICARE OF NY

560 White Plains Rd Ste 410
Tarrytown, NY 10591
Phone: 860-674-2075 Fax: 860-674-5728 Toll-Free: 800-846-8578
Web site: www.connecticare.com
MAILING ADDRESS:
  CONNECTICARE OF NY
  560 White Plains Rd Ste 410
  Tarrytown, NY 10591

KEY EXECUTIVES:
Chairman .... Anthony L Watson
Chief Executive Officer/President .... Michael E Herbert
Senior VP, Chief Medical Officer .... Paul A Bluestein, MD
Executive VP, Chief Information Officer .... Michael Wise
Director, Pharmacy .... Jeffrey Casberg
VP, Chief Information Officer .... Mark G Dixon
Chief Marketing Officer .... Paul M Philpott
Senior VP, Chief Sales Officer .... Jim Buccheri
VP, Large Group Sales .... Carol Dosdall
Public Relations Director .... Stephen Jewett
Senior VP, Human Resources .... Richard Rogers
Director, Quality Improvement .... Pam Spinazola

COMPANY PROFILE:
Parent Company Name: Health Insurance Plan of New York
Doing Business As:
Year Founded: 1995   Federally Qualified: [N]
Forprofit: [Y]   Not-For-Profit: [ ]
Model Type:
Accreditation: [ ] AAPPO [ ] JACHO [ ] NCQA [ ] URAC
Plan Type: HMO, PPO, POS, ASO, HDHP, HSA
Total Enrollment:
  2001: 3   2004: 3   2007: 0
  2002: 4   2005: 17
  2003: 4   2006:
SERVICE AREA:
Nationwide: N
  NY;
TYPE OF COVERAGE:
Commercial: [Y] Individual: [ ] FEHBP: [ ] Indemnity: [ ]
Medicare: [ ] Medicaid: [ ] Supplemental Medicare: [ ]
Tricare   [ ]
Comments:
Formerly Amerihealth Health Plan Inc.

CORPORATE CARE MANAGEMENT INC

1 Kattelville Rd Ste 7
Binghamton, NY 13901
Phone: 607-648-3400 Fax: 607-648-3444 Toll-Free: 800-541-7403
Web site: www.corporatecaremgmt.com
MAILING ADDRESS:
  CORPORATE CARE MANAGEMENT INC
  1 Kattelville Rd Ste 7
  Binghamton, NY 13901

KEY EXECUTIVES:
Chief Executive Officer/President .... Barbara Kane, MSN, BSN, CCM
Medical Director .... John Harding, MD
Chief Information Officer .... Alesia Hurban
Marketing Director .... Barbara Kane
Senior VP, Director of Provider Services ...... Dawn M Bigney
Senior VP, ... Deborah Clough-Gitchell

COMPANY PROFILE:
Parent Company Name:
Doing Business As:
Year Founded: 1976   Federally Qualified: [ ]
Forprofit: [Y]   Not-For-Profit: [ ]
Model Type:
Accreditation: [ ] AAPPO [ ] JACHO [ ] NCQA [X] URAC
Plan Type: PPO, UR
SERVICE AREA:
Nationwide: Y
  NW;
TYPE OF COVERAGE:
Commercial: [Y] Individual: [ ] FEHBP: [ ] Indemnity: [ ]
Medicare: [ ] Medicaid: [Y] Supplemental Medicare: [ ]
Tricare   [ ]
PLAN BENEFITS:
Alternative Medicine: [ ]   Behavioral Health: [X]
Chiropractic: [X]   Dental: [X]
Home Care: [X]   Inpatient SNF: [X]
Long-Term Care: [X]   Pharm. Mail Order: [ ]
Physical Therapy: [X]   Podiatry: [X]
Psychiatric: [X]   Transplant: [X]
Vision: [X]   Wellness: [ ]
Workers' Comp: [X]
Other Benefits:

DAVIS VISION

159 Express Street
Plainview, NY 11803
Phone: 516-932-9500 Fax: 516-932-9770 Toll-Free: 800-328-4728
Web site: www.davisvision.com
MAILING ADDRESS:
  DAVIS VISION
  159 Express Street
  Plainview, NY 11803

KEY EXECUTIVES:
Chief Executive Officer/President ... Joseph Carlomusto, ABOC, FNAO
Chief Financial Officer .... Larry Gabel, CPA
Senior VP, Professional Affairs/Quality Mngmnt .... Joseph Wende, MD
Senior VP, Chief Information Officer .... Michael Thibdeau, CPA
Chief Operating Officer .... Larry Gabel, CPA
Senior VP, Corp Marketing & Client Relations .... Dale Paustian
Director, Credentialing .... Jodi Wolf
VP Business Development & Provider Relations ... Robert Elsas
Network Development Director .... Ray Thomas
Human Resources Director .... David Negron
Director, Quality Assurance .... Nicole Carroll
Senior VP Manufacturing .... Michael O'Connor
Senior VP & GM, PVC Retail Operation .... Thomas J Rosa, ABOC

COMPANY PROFILE:
Parent Company Name: Highmark Inc
Doing Business As: Davis Vision
Year Founded: 1964   Federally Qualified: [ ]
Forprofit: [Y]   Not-For-Profit: [ ]
Model Type: NETWORK
Accreditation: [ ] AAPPO [X] JACHO [X] NCQA [X] URAC
Plan Type: Specialty PPO
Total Enrollment:
  2001: 0   2004: 0   2007: 50,000,000
  2002: 0   2005:
  2003: 0   2006: 40,000,000
SERVICE AREA:
Nationwide: Y
  Nationwide (all 50 states, Washington, DC., Puerto Rico, Guam, Saipan, The Dominican Republic);

Managed Care Organization Profiles NEW YORK

CENTERCARE INC

95-25 Queens Blvd
Rego Park, NY 11374
Phone: 212-293-9200 Fax: 212-293-9256 Toll-Free: 800-454-0571
Web site: www.centercare.org
MAILING ADDRESS:
    CENTERCARE INC
    95-25 Queens Blvd
    Rego Park, NY 11374

KEY EXECUTIVES:
Chief Executive Officer/President .... *Mark Lane*
Chief Financial Officer .... *Dina Soroka*
Chief Information Officer .... *Patrick Garland*
Chief Operating Officer .... *Rev. Patrick J Frawley*
Vice President of Marketing .... *Pamela Hassen*

COMPANY PROFILE:
Parent Company Name: Ryan Community Health Network
Doing Business As:
Year Founded: 1988   Federally Qualified: [Y]
Forprofit: [ ]   Not-For-Profit: [Y]
Model Type: MIXED
Accreditation: [ ] AAPPO [ ] JACHO [ ] NCQA [ ] URAC
Plan Type: HMO
Primary Physicians: Physician Specialists:
Hospitals: 45
Total Enrollment:
    2001: 0   2004: 79,813   2007: 0
    2002: 60,850   2005: 80,796
    2003: 80,208   2006:

SERVICE AREA:
Nationwide: N
    NY (New York City - Bronx, Brooklyn, Manhattan, Queens, Richmond);

PRODUCTS OFFERED:
Product Name: Type:
Manhattan PHSP   Medicaid

CENTRAL NEW YORK EAST HEALTHNOW NEW YORK INC

4983 Brittonfield Pkwy Ste 203
East Syracuse, NY 13057
Phone: 315-431-3620 Fax: 315-463-2454 Toll-Free:
Web site: www.healthnowny.com
MAILING ADDRESS:
    CENTRAL NY EAST HEALTHNOW NY
    4983 Brittonfield Pkwy Ste 203
    East Syracuse, NY 13057

KEY EXECUTIVES:
Senior VP, Chief Medical Officer ...*Jay I Pomerantz, MD, MMM, FACP*

COMPANY PROFILE:
Parent Company Name: HealthNow New York Inc
Doing Business As:
Year Founded: 1985   Federally Qualified: [N]
Forprofit: [ ]   Not-For-Profit: [Y]
Model Type:
Accreditation: [ ] AAPPO [ ] JACHO [ ] NCQA [ ] URAC
Plan Type: HMO, PPO, POS, ASO,
SERVICE AREA:
Nationwide:
    NY;
TYPE OF COVERAGE:
Commercial: [Y] Individual: [Y] FEHBP: [ ] Indemnity: [ ]
Medicare: [Y] Medicaid: [Y] Supplemental Medicare: [Y]
Tricare   [ ]
PLAN BENEFITS:
Alternative Medicine: [ ]   Behavioral Health: [ ]
Chiropractic: [X]   Dental: [X]
Home Care: [X]   Inpatient SNF: [X]
Long-Term Care: [X]   Pharm. Mail Order: [ ]
Physical Therapy: [X]   Podiatry: [X]
Psychiatric: [X]   Transplant: [X]
Vision: [X]   Wellness: [X]
Workers' Comp: [ ]
Other Benefits:

CENTRAL NEW YORK WEST HEALTHNOW NEW YORK INC

46 Prince St 2nd Fl
Rochester, NY 14607
Phone: 585-241-0900 Fax: 315-463-2454 Toll-Free:
Web site: www.healthnowny.com
MAILING ADDRESS:
    CENTRAL NY WEST HEALTHNOW NY
    46 Prince St 2nd Fl
    Rochester, NY 14607

KEY EXECUTIVES:
Senior VP,Chief Medical Officer ...*Jay I Pomerantz, MD, MMM, FACP*

COMPANY PROFILE:
Parent Company Name: HealthNow New York Inc
Doing Business As:
Year Founded: 1985   Federally Qualified: [N]
Forprofit: [ ]   Not-For-Profit: [Y]
Model Type:
Accreditation: [ ] AAPPO [ ] JACHO [ ] NCQA [ ] URAC
Plan Type: HMO, PPO, POS, ASO,
SERVICE AREA:
Nationwide:
    NY;
TYPE OF COVERAGE:
Commercial: [Y] Individual: [Y] FEHBP: [ ] Indemnity: [ ]
Medicare: [Y] Medicaid: [Y] Supplemental Medicare: [Y]
Tricare   [ ]
PLAN BENEFITS:
Alternative Medicine: [ ]   Behavioral Health: [ ]
Chiropractic: [X]   Dental: [X]
Home Care: [X]   Inpatient SNF: [X]
Long-Term Care: [X]   Pharm. Mail Order: [ ]
Physical Therapy: [X]   Podiatry: [X]
Psychiatric: [X]   Transplant: [X]
Vision: [X]   Wellness: [X]
Workers' Comp: [ ]
Other Benefits:

COMMUNITY CHOICE HEALTH PLAN OF WESTCHESTER INC

30 S Broadway #4
Yonkers, NY 10701-3712
Phone: 914-377-0710 Fax: 914-709-8590 Toll-Free:
Web site: www.cchphealth.com
MAILING ADDRESS:
    COMMUNITY CHOICE HEALTH PLAN WESTCHESTER
    30 S Broadway #4
    Yonkers, NY 10701-3712

KEY EXECUTIVES:
Chief Executive Officer .... *Le Dice W Murphy*
Board President .... *Carole Morris*
Chief Financial Officer .... *Abraham Benitez*
Medical Director .... *Carl Richie, MD*
Marketing Director .... *Harold Morris*
MIS Director .... *Egal Sanchez*
Chief Compliance Officer .... *Lynette Powell-Wick*
Provider Education/Support Manager .... *Thomas Martinez*
Human Resources Director .... *Rayman Ritchie*
Director of Medical Management .... *Cathy Moon*
Director of Quality Managmenet .... *Roween Woodley*

COMPANY PROFILE:
Parent Company Name:
Doing Business As:
Year Founded: 1995   Federally Qualified: [ ]
Forprofit: [ ]   Not-For-Profit: [Y]
Model Type: NETWORK
Accreditation: [ ] AAPPO [ ] JACHO [ ] NCQA [ ] URAC
Plan Type: HMO, Specialty HMO
Total Enrollment:
    2001: 11,000   2004: 14,526   2007: 0
    2002: 17,000   2005: 18,443
    2003: 13,528   2006:

NEW YORK

SERVICE AREA:
Nationwide: N
  NY (Allegany, Cattaraugus, Chautauqua, Erie, Genesee, Niagara, Orleans, Wyoming);

TYPE OF COVERAGE:
Commercial: [Y] Individual: [Y] FEHBP: [ ] Indemnity: [ ]
Medicare: [ ] Medicaid: [Y] Supplemental Medicare: [Y]
Tricare [ ]

PRODUCTS OFFERED:
Product Name:	Type:
HealthNow New York Inc	HMO
Community Blue	Medicaid
Senior Blue	Medicare Advantage

CONSUMER-DRIVEN PRODUCTS
Wells Fargo	HSA Company
eElect HSA	HSA Product
Wells Fargo	HSA Administrator
	Consumer-Driven Health Plan
Traditional Blue PPO	High Deductible Health Plan

PLAN BENEFITS:
Alternative Medicine:	[ ]	Behavioral Health:	[ ]
Chiropractic:	[X]	Dental:	[X]
Home Care:	[X]	Inpatient SNF:	[X]
Long-Term Care:	[X]	Pharm. Mail Order:	[ ]
Physical Therapy:	[X]	Podiatry:	[X]
Psychiatric:	[X]	Transplant:	[X]
Vision:	[X]	Wellness:	[X]
Workers' Comp:	[ ]		

Other Benefits:

BLUESHIELD OF NORTHEASTERN NEW YORK

30 Century Hill Dr
Latham, NY 12110
Phone: 518-220-5700 Fax: 716-887-8981 Toll-Free:
Web site: www.bsneny.com

MAILING ADDRESS:
BLUESHIELD OF NORTHEASTERN NY
PO Box 15013
Albany, NY 12110

KEY EXECUTIVES:
Chief Marketing Officer .... Brian G O'Grady

COMPANY PROFILE:
Parent Company Name: HealthNow New York Inc
Doing Business As:
Year Founded: 1985   Federally Qualified: [N]
Forprofit: [ ]   Not-For-Profit: [Y]
Model Type:
Accreditation: [ ] AAPPO [ ] JACHO [ ] NCQA [ ] URAC
Plan Type: HMO, PPO, POS, ASO,
Total Enrollment:
  2001: 0   2004: 0   2007: 0
  2002: 0   2005: 170,000
  2003: 0   2006:

SERVICE AREA:
Nationwide:
  NY;

TYPE OF COVERAGE:
Commercial: [Y] Individual: [Y] FEHBP: [ ] Indemnity: [ ]
Medicare: [Y] Medicaid: [Y] Supplemental Medicare: [Y]
Tricare [ ]

PLAN BENEFITS:
Alternative Medicine:	[ ]	Behavioral Health:	[ ]
Chiropractic:	[X]	Dental:	[X]
Home Care:	[X]	Inpatient SNF:	[X]
Long-Term Care:	[X]	Pharm. Mail Order:	[ ]
Physical Therapy:	[X]	Podiatry:	[X]
Psychiatric:	[X]	Transplant:	[X]
Vision:	[X]	Wellness:	[X]
Workers' Comp:	[ ]		

Other Benefits:

CAPITAL DISTRICT PHYSICIANS HEALTH PLAN

1223 Washington Ave
Albany, NY 12206
Phone: 518-641-3000 Fax: 518-641-3507 Toll-Free: 800-993-7299
Web site: www.cdphp.com

MAILING ADDRESS:
CAPITAL DISTRICT PHYSICIAN HEALTH PLAN
1223 Washington Ave
Albany, NY 12206

KEY EXECUTIVES:
Chairman of the Board .... John D Bennett, MD
Chief Executive Officer/President .... William J Cromie, MD, MBA
Senior VP, Chief Financial Officer .... James DuCharme
Senior VP, Med Affairs/Chief Med Officer . Bruce D Nash, MD, FACHE
Senior Medical Director .... Clifford R Waldman, MD
Medical Director .... Hugh Kelley Riley, MD, MBA
Medical Director .... Martin R Symansky, MD
Medical Director .... James Figge, MD
Chief Information Officer .... Linda Navarro
Senior VP, Corp Operations, Chief of Staff .... Barbara Downs, RN
Senior Vice President, Sales .... Carole Montepare
Manager, Credentialing/Provider File Maintenance .... Lisa Baum
Manager, Security Information .... Christine Kittrell
VP, Government/External Relations .... Robert Hinckley
Director, Provider Services .... Judy Fitzgerald
VP, Network & Contracting Development .... Cynthia Wicks
Manager, Disease Management/Wellness .... Sheila Hoorwitz
VP, Human Resources .... Scott Klenk
Director, Quality/Regulatory Cmplnc .... Patricia Weafer
Manager/Special Investigative Unit .... Richard Moscheo
Manager, Strategy & Business Development .... Jennifer Quinn
Director, Corporate Compliance .... Randy Rothstein
Legal Affairs, General Counsel .... Frederick B Galt

COMPANY PROFILE:
Parent Company Name: Capital District Physicians Health Plan
Doing Business As: Capital District Physicians Health Plan
Year Founded: 1984   Federally Qualified: [N]
Forprofit: [ ]   Not-For-Profit: [Y]
Model Type: IPA
Accreditation: [ ] AAPPO [ ] JACHO [X] NCQA [ ] URAC
Plan Type: HMO, PPO, PBM, POS, ASO, EPO, TPA, HDHP, HSA,
Total Revenue: 2005:   2006: 844,040,951
Net Income   2005:   2006:
Total Enrollment:
  2001: 286,985   2004: 297,186   2007: 0
  2002: 317,794   2005: 254,761
  2003: 302,835   2006:
Medical Loss Ratio: 2005:   2006: 86.30
Administrative Expense Ratio: 2005: 2006:

SERVICE AREA:
Nationwide: N
  NY (Albany, Broome, Chenango, Clinton, Columbia, Delaware, Dutchess, Essex, Franklin, Fulton, Greene, Hamilton, Herkimer, Jefferson, Lewis, Madison, Montgomery, Oneida, Orange, Otsego, Rensselaer, Saratoga, Schenectady, Schoharie, St Lawrence, Tioga, Ulster, Warren, Washington); VT (Addison, Chittenden, Franklin, Lamoille, Rutland, Washington, Windham);

TYPE OF COVERAGE:
Commercial: [Y] Individual: [Y] FEHBP: [ ] Indemnity: [ ]
Medicare: [Y] Medicaid: [Y] Supplemental Medicare: [ ]
Tricare [ ]

PRODUCTS OFFERED:
Product Name:	Type:
Medicare Choice	Medicare Advantage
Capital District Physician Health	Medicaid

CONSUMER-DRIVEN PRODUCTS
Mellon Financial Corporation	HSA Company
	HSA Product
HSA Bank	HSA Administrator
	Consumer-Driven Health Plan
AchievaCare High Deductble PPO	High Deductible Health Plan

PLAN BENEFITS:
Alternative Medicine:	[ ]	Behavioral Health:	[ ]
Chiropractic:	[X]	Dental:	[X]
Home Care:	[X]	Inpatient SNF:	[X]
Long-Term Care:	[ ]	Pharm. Mail Order:	[X]
Physical Therapy:	[X]	Podiatry:	[X]
Psychiatric:	[X]	Transplant:	[X]
Vision:	[X]	Wellness:	[X]
Workers' Comp:	[ ]		

Other Benefits:

Comments:
Kaiser Permanente New York commercial members have been aquisitioned by Capital District.

Managed Care Organization Profiles — NEW YORK

ASSURANT EMPLOYEE BENEFITS - NEW YORK

1633 Broadway Ste 2020
New York, NY 10019
Phone: 212-471-2075 Fax: 212-471-2076 Toll-Free: 888-424-0030
Web site: www.assurantemployeebenefits.com

MAILING ADDRESS:
ASSURANT EMPLOYEE BNFTS - NY
1633 Broadway Ste 2020
New York, NY 10019

KEY EXECUTIVES:
Interim Chief Executive Officer/President .... John S Roberts
Chief Financial Officer .... Floyd F Chadee
VP, Medical Director .... Polly M Galbraith, MD
Chief Information Officer .... Karla J Schacht
Senior VP, Marketing .... Joseph A Sevcik
Privacy Officer .... John L Fortini
VP of Provider Services .... James A Barrett, DMD
Senior VP, Human Resources & Development .... Sylvia R Wagner
General Manager .... Todd Boyd
National Dental Director .... James A Barrett, DMD

COMPANY PROFILE:
Parent Company Name: Assurant Health
Doing Business As:
Year Founded: Federally Qualified: [ ]
Forprofit: [Y]   Not-For-Profit: [ ]
Model Type:
Accreditation: [ ] AAPPO [ ] JACHO [ ] NCQA [ ] URAC
Plan Type: Specialty HMO

SERVICE AREA:
Nationwide: N
NY,

TYPE OF COVERAGE:
Commercial: [Y] Individual: [Y] FEHBP: [ ] Indemnity: [ ]
Medicare: [Y] Medicaid: [Y] Supplemental Medicare: [ ]
Tricare   [ ]

PRODUCTS OFFERED:
Product Name: Type:
                                     DHMO
                                     Vision

PLAN BENEFITS:
Alternative Medicine: [ ]   Behavioral Health: [ ]
Chiropractic: [ ]   Dental: [X]
Home Care: [ ]   Inpatient SNF: [ ]
Long-Term Care: [ ]   Pharm. Mail Order: [ ]
Physical Therapy: [ ]   Podiatry: [ ]
Psychiatric: [ ]   Transplant: [ ]
Vision: [X]   Wellness: [ ]
Workers' Comp: [ ]
Other Benefits:

Comments:
Formerly Fortis Benefits Dental.

ATLANTIS HEALTH PLAN

39 Broadway Ste 1240
New York, NY 10006
Phone: 212-747-0877 Fax: 212-747-0843 Toll-Free: 888-258-1498
Web site: www.atlantishp.com

MAILING ADDRESS:
ATLANTIS HEALTH PLAN
PO Box 873 Bowling Green Stn
New York, NY 10006

KEY EXECUTIVES:
Chairman .... Sury Anand, MD
Chief Executive Officer/President .... Sury Anand, MD
Executive VP, Chief Financial Officer .... Thomas Dwyer
Medical Director .... Delia Baquiran, MD
Medical Director II .... Jean Claude Lemoine, MD
VP of Information Technology .... Abraham Wachsman
Executive VP, Chief Operating Officer .... Thomas Dwyer
Senior VP, Chief Marketing Officer .... Steven Denes
VP Provider Relations .... Frank Bove
Human Resources Manager .... Janneth Torres
Senior Vice President .... John Muney
Senior VP Operations .... Patrick Dodge

COMPANY PROFILE:
Parent Company Name:
Doing Business As:
Year Founded: 1995   Federally Qualified: [ ]
Forprofit: [Y]   Not-For-Profit: [ ]
Model Type: NETWORK
Accreditation: [ ] AAPPO [ ] JACHO [ ] NCQA [ ] URAC
Plan Type: HMO, POS,
Total Revenue: 2005:   2006: 26,789,125
Net Income   2005:   2006:
Total Enrollment:
   2001: 18,353   2004: 6,327   2007: 0
   2002: 10,723   2005:
   2003: 7,502   2006:
Medical Loss Ratio: 2005:   2006: 68.90
Administrative Expense Ratio: 2005:   2006:

SERVICE AREA:
Nationwide: N
NY;

TYPE OF COVERAGE:
Commercial: [Y] Individual: [ ] FEHBP: [ ] Indemnity: [ ]
Medicare: [ ] Medicaid: [ ] Supplemental Medicare: [ ]
Tricare   [ ]

PRODUCTS OFFERED:
Product Name: Type:
Atlantis Health Plan   HMO
Atlantis POS   POS

PLAN BENEFITS:
Alternative Medicine: [ ]   Behavioral Health: [ ]
Chiropractic: [X]   Dental: [X]
Home Care: [ ]   Inpatient SNF: [ ]
Long-Term Care: [ ]   Pharm. Mail Order: [X]
Physical Therapy: [ ]   Podiatry: [X]
Psychiatric: [X]   Transplant: [X]
Vision: [X]   Wellness: [X]
Workers' Comp: [ ]
Other Benefits:

BLUE CROSS BLUE SHIELD OF WESTERN NEW YORK

257 West Genesee St
Buffalo, NY 14202
Phone: 716-887-6900 Fax: 716-887-8981 Toll-Free: 800-544-2583
Web site: www.bcbswny.com

MAILING ADDRESS:
BC BS OF WESTERN NEW YORK
PO Box 80
Buffalo, NY 14240-0080

KEY EXECUTIVES:
Chairman of the Board .... Joseph J Castiglia
Chief Executive Officer .... Alphonso O'Neil-White
Chief Financial Officer .... James Dickerson
Medical Director .... Jay I Pomerantz, MD, MMM, FACP
Chief Information Officer .... Paul Stoddard
Manager of Credentialing .... Barbara McCroskey
Privacy Officer .... Nancy Schoellkopf
Sr Dir, Public Relations, Communications ..... Karen Merkel-liberatore
Director of Network Management .... Lisa Meyers-Alessi
VP of Human Resources .... Ralph Volpe
VP of Quality Assurance .... Phil Smeltzer
Manager of Credentialing .... Barbara McCroskey
Fraud/Special Investigation .... Scott Kovel
New Product Development .... Kerri Garrison

COMPANY PROFILE:
Parent Company Name: HealthNow New York Inc
Doing Business As: Community Blue, HMO of BCBSWNY
Year Founded: 1985   Federally Qualified: [N]
Forprofit: [ ]   Not-For-Profit: [Y]
Model Type: IPA
Accreditation: [ ] AAPPO [ ] JACHO [X] NCQA [ ] URAC
Plan Type: HMO, PPO, POS, ASO, HDHP, HSA,
Primary Physicians: 1,262   Physician Specialists: 3,228
Hospitals: 32
Total Enrollment:
   2001: 403,653   2004: 413,061   2007: 0
   2002: 380,809   2005: 571,000
   2003: 414,393   2006:

NEW YORK
Managed Care Organization Profiles

PLAN BENEFITS:
Alternative Medicine:	[ ]	Behavioral Health:	[X]
Chiropractic:	[ ]	Dental:	[ ]
Home Care:	[X]	Inpatient SNF:	[ ]
Long-Term Care:	[ ]	Pharm. Mail Order:	[ ]
Physical Therapy:	[ ]	Podiatry:	[X]
Psychiatric:	[X]	Transplant:	[X]
Vision:	[ ]	Wellness:	[X]
Workers' Comp:	[ ]		

Other Benefits:
Comments:
Formerly The Bronx Health Plan.

AMERICHOICE OF NEW YORK

7 Hanover Square 5th Fl
New York, NY 10004
Phone: 212-509-5999 Fax: 212-898-7967 Toll-Free:
Web site: www.americhoice.com

MAILING ADDRESS:
AMERICHOICE OF NY
7 Hanover Square 5th Fl
New York, NY 10004

KEY EXECUTIVES:
Chairman of the Board .... Anthony Welters
Chief Executive Officer .... Ernest Monfifetto
President .... Thelma Duggin
Chief Financial Officer .... Pat Celli
Medical Director .... Robert Scelletar, MD
Pharmacy Director .... Marion Pardes
Chief Operating Officer .... Donald Langer
VP, Marketing .... Craig Hueben
Marketing Director .... Linda Goldsworthy

COMPANY PROFILE:
Parent Company Name: UnitedHealth Group
Doing Business As: Managed Healthcare Systems of New York
Year Founded: 1993   Federally Qualified: [N]
Forprofit: [Y]   Not-For-Profit: [ ]
Model Type:
Accreditation: [ ] AAPPO [ ] JACHO [ ] NCQA [ ] URAC
Plan Type: HMO
Primary Physicians: Physician Specialists:
Hospitals:
Total Revenue: 2005:   2006: 254,298,717
Net Income 2005:   2006:
Total Enrollment:
 2001: 59,182   2004: 111,351   2007: 0
 2002: 62,990   2005: 115,692
 2003: 99,916   2006:
Medical Loss Ratio: 2005:   2006: 82.30
Administrative Expense Ratio: 2005:   2006:

SERVICE AREA:
Nationwide: N
NY (Brooklyn, Bronx);

TYPE OF COVERAGE:
Commercial: [ ] Individual: [ ] FEHBP: [ ] Indemnity: [ ]
Medicare: [ ] Medicaid: [Y] Supplemental Medicare: [ ]
Tricare: [ ]

PRODUCTS OFFERED:
Product Name:	Type:
AmeriChoice Personal Care Plus	Medicare
Managed Healthcare System of NY	Medicaid
AmeriChoice Individual	HMO

AMERICAN DENTAL EXAMINERS

277 North Ave 2nd Fl
New Rochelle, NY 10801
Phone: 914-712-0100 Fax: 914-576-3077 Toll-Free:
Web site: www.ade1.com

MAILING ADDRESS:
AMERICAN DENTAL EXAMINERS
277 North Ave 2nd Fl
New Rochelle, NY 10801

KEY EXECUTIVES:
Chief Executive Officer .... Robert Leaf
Chief Financial/Operating Officer .... Brenda Prunty
Executive Secretary .... Elaine Riggs

COMPANY PROFILE:
Parent Company Name:
Doing Business As:
Year Founded: 1976   Federally Qualified: [ ]
Forprofit: [Y]   Not-For-Profit: [ ]
Model Type:
Accreditation: [ ] AAPPO [ ] JACHO [ ] NCQA [ ] URAC
Plan Type: UR

SERVICE AREA:
Nationwide: Y
NW;

PLAN BENEFITS:
Alternative Medicine:	[ ]	Behavioral Health:	[ ]
Chiropractic:	[ ]	Dental:	[X]
Home Care:	[ ]	Inpatient SNF:	[ ]
Long-Term Care:	[ ]	Pharm. Mail Order:	[ ]
Physical Therapy:	[ ]	Podiatry:	[ ]
Psychiatric:	[ ]	Transplant:	[ ]
Vision:	[ ]	Wellness:	[ ]
Workers' Comp:	[ ]		

Other Benefits:

AMERIGROUP COMMUNITY CARE

360 W 31st St 5th Fl
New York, NY 10001-2727
Phone: 212-563-5570 Fax: 212-563-5975 Toll-Free:
Web site: www.careplus.net

MAILING ADDRESS:
AMERIGROUP COMMUNITY CARE
360 W 31st St 5th Fl
New York, NY 10001-2727

KEY EXECUTIVES:
Chief Executive Officer/President .... Nasry Michelen
Chief Financial Officer .... Vince Achillare
Medical Director .... Marie Casalino, MD
Chief Operating Officer .... Nasry Michelen
Marketing Director .... Jill Tobin
Director of MIS .... Chris Bouvier
Public Relations Director .... Jill Tobin
Director of Ntwrk Development & Management .... Mariella Fermin

COMPANY PROFILE:
Parent Company Name: Doing Business As:
Year Founded: Federally Qualified: [ ]
Forprofit: [Y]   Not-For-Profit: [ ]
Model Type: IPA
Accreditation: [ ] AAPPO [ ] JACHO [ ] NCQA [ ] URAC
Plan Type: HMO
Total Enrollment:
 2001: 0   2004: 89,599   2007: 0
 2002: 74,049   2005: 135,484
 2003: 77,105   2006:

SERVICE AREA:
Nationwide: N
NY;

TYPE OF COVERAGE:
Commercial: [ ] Individual: [ ] FEHBP: [ ] Indemnity: [ ]
Medicare: [ ] Medicaid: [Y] Supplemental Medicare: [ ]
Tricare: [ ]

PRODUCTS OFFERED:
Product Name:	Type:
Amerigroup Community Care	Medicaid
Child Health Plus	Medicaid
Family Health Plus	Medicaid

PLAN BENEFITS:
Alternative Medicine:	[ ]	Behavioral Health:	[X]
Chiropractic:	[ ]	Dental:	[X]
Home Care:	[X]	Inpatient SNF:	[ ]
Long-Term Care:	[ ]	Pharm. Mail Order:	[ ]
Physical Therapy:	[ ]	Podiatry:	[X]
Psychiatric:	[X]	Transplant:	[X]
Vision:	[X]	Wellness:	[X]
Workers' Comp:	[ ]		

Other Benefits:
Comments:
Formerly called Careplus Health Plan.

Managed Care Organization Profiles — NEW YORK

AETNA INC - NEW YORK

333 Earle Ovington Blvd Ste104
Uniondale, NY 11553
Phone: 516-794-6565 Fax: 516-794-2389 Toll-Free: 800-322-8742
Web site: www.aetna.com

MAILING ADDRESS:
AETNA INC - NY
333 Earle Ovington Blvd Ste104
Uniondale, NY 11553

KEY EXECUTIVES:
Chairman of the Board .... Ronald A Williams
Chief Executive Officer/President .... Robert J Nolan
Executive VP, Finance .... Joseph M Zubretsky
Medical Director .... Gordon W Grundy, MD
Human Resources Director .... Elease E Wright
Senior Network Manager/Provider Relations .... John Catalan
General Manager .... James Reid

COMPANY PROFILE:
Parent Company Name: Aetna Inc
Doing Business As:
Year Founded: 1987 Federally Qualified: [Y]
Forprofit: [Y] Not-For-Profit: [ ]
Model Type: MIXED
Accreditation: [ ] AAPPO [ ] JACHO [X] NCQA [ ] URAC
Plan Type: HMO, PPO, CDHP, HDHP, HSA,
Total Revenue: 2005:   2006:
Net Income 2005:   2006:
Total Enrollment:
Total Enrollment:
  2001: 747,146   2004: 0   2007: 0
  2002: 586,811   2005: 231,281
  2003: 375,492   2006:
Medical Loss Ratio: 2005:   2006:
Administrative Expense Ratio: 2005:   2006:

SERVICE AREA:
Nationwide: N
NY (Armed Forces, Bronx, Dutchess, Kings, Nassau, New York, Orange, Putnam, Queens, Richmond, Rockland, Suffolk, Sullivan, Ulster, Westchester).

TYPE OF COVERAGE:
Commercial: [Y] Individual: [ ] FEHBP: [ ] Indemnity: [ ]
Medicare: [Y] Medicaid: [ ] Supplemental Medicare: [ ]
Tricare [ ]

PRODUCTS OFFERED:
Product Name:	Type:
Aetna US Healthcare Golden Med	Medicare

CONSUMER-DRIVEN PRODUCTS
Aetna Life Insurance Co	HSA Company
Aetna HealthFund HSA	HSA Product
Aetna	HSA Administrator
Aetna HealthFund	Consumer-Driven Health Plan
PPO I; PPO II	High Deductible Health Plan

PLAN BENEFITS:
Alternative Medicine: [ ]   Behavioral Health: [ ]
Chiropractic: [X]   Dental: [X]
Home Care: [X]   Inpatient SNF: [ ]
Long-Term Care: [X]   Pharm. Mail Order: [X]
Physical Therapy: [ ]   Podiatry: [X]
Psychiatric: [X]   Transplant: [ ]
Vision: [X]   Wellness: [ ]
Workers' Comp: [ ]
Other Benefits:
Comments:
Formerly US Healthcare (New York).

AETNA INC - NEW YORK

99 Park Avenue
New York, NY 10016
Phone: 212-457-0700 Fax: 212-457-0306 Toll-Free:
Web site: www.aetna.com

MAILING ADDRESS:
AETNA INC - NEW YORK
99 Park Avenue
New York, NY 10016

KEY EXECUTIVES:
Chairman of the Board/Chief Executive Officer .... Ronald A Williams
President .... Mark T Bertolini
Executive VP, Finance .... Joseph M Zubretsky

COMPANY PROFILE:
Parent Company Name: Aetna Inc
Doing Business As: Aetna US Healthcare Inc
Year Founded: 1986 Federally Qualified: [ ]
Forprofit: [Y] Not-For-Profit: [ ]
Model Type:
Accreditation: [ ] AAPPO [ ] JACHO [ ] NCQA [ ] URAC
Plan Type: HMO, CDHP, HDHP, HSA,
Total Enrollment:
  2001: 0   2004: 0   2007: 0
  2002: 0   2005:
  2003: 774,960   2006:

SERVICE AREA:
Nationwide:
NY;

CONSUMER-DRIVEN PRODUCTS
Aetna Life Insurance Co	HSA Company
Aetna HealthFund HSA	HSA Product
Aetna	HSA Administrator
Aetna HealthFund	Consumer-Driven Health Plan
PPO I; PPO II	High Deductible Health Plan

AFFINITY HEALTH PLAN INC

2500 Halsey St
Bronx, NY 10461
Phone: 718-794-7700 Fax: 718-794-7800 Toll-Free:
Web site: www.affinityplan.org

MAILING ADDRESS:
AFFINITY HEALTH PLAN INC
2500 Halsey St
Bronx, NY 10461

KEY EXECUTIVES:
Chief Executive Officer/President .... Maura Bluestone
Chief Financial Officer .... Jean Lobban
Senior VP, Chief Medical Officer .... Susan J Beane, MD
Senior VP, Chief Operating Officer .... Barbara Kelman
VP, Marketing .... Kel Ritter
VP, Information Services .... James Carmona
Director Provider Relations .... Alice King
Director Network Development/Contracting .... Eleanor Chin-Wardwell
Director Human Resources .... Ann Van Etten
Director Utilization Management .... Carol Feeney, RN
Director Quality Management .... Barbara Hurley, RN
VP Public Affairs .... Abenaa Abboa-Offei
VP Care Delivery .... Denise Marchese, RN
Director, Compliance & Finance Control .... Caron Cullen

COMPANY PROFILE:
Parent Company Name:
Doing Business As:
Year Founded: 1987 Federally Qualified: [N]
Forprofit: [ ] Not-For-Profit: [Y]
Model Type: MIXED
Accreditation: [ ] AAPPO [ ] JACHO [ ] NCQA [ ] URAC
Plan Type: HMO
Total Enrollment:
  2001: 0   2004: 181,376   2007: 0
  2002: 143,661   2005: 210,870
  2003: 176,093   2006: 105,201

SERVICE AREA:
Nationwide: N
NY (Bronx, Manhattan);

TYPE OF COVERAGE:
Commercial: [ ] Individual: [ ] FEHBP: [ ] Indemnity: [ ]
Medicare: [ ] Medicaid: [Y] Supplemental Medicare: [ ]
Tricare [ ]

PRODUCTS OFFERED:
Product Name:	Type:
Affinity Health Plan	Medicaid
Child Health Plus	Medicaid
Family Health Plus	Medicaid

PLAN BENEFITS:
Alternative Medicine:	[X]	Behavioral Health:	[ ]
Chiropractic:	[X]	Dental:	[X]
Home Care:	[X]	Inpatient SNF:	[X]
Long-Term Care:	[ ]	Pharm. Mail Order:	[X]
Physical Therapy:	[X]	Podiatry:	[X]
Psychiatric:	[X]	Transplant:	[X]
Vision:	[X]	Wellness:	[X]
Workers' Comp:	[ ]		
Other Benefits:			

UNITED CONCORDIA COMPANY INC - NEW MEXICO

6301 Indian School Rd NE #200
Albuquerque, NM 87110
Phone: 505-883-0007 Fax: 505-883-1668 Toll-Free: 877-654-2124
Web site: www.ucci.com

MAILING ADDRESS:
UNITED CONCORDIA CO INC - NM
6301 Indian School Rd NE #200
Albuquerque, NM 87110

KEY EXECUTIVES:
Chief Executive Officer/President .... Thomas A Dzuryachko
Senior VP, Finance .... Daniel Wright
VP, National Dental Director .... Richard Klich, DMD
Marketing Director .... Larry Adams
Vice President, Sales & Marketing .... Ron Onda
MIS Director .... Jim Robins
Director, Provider Services .... Ted Pesano

COMPANY PROFILE:
Parent Company Name: Highmark Inc
Doing Business As:
Year Founded: 1991   Federally Qualified: [ ]
Forprofit: [Y]   Not-For-Profit: [ ]
Model Type:
Accreditation: [ ] AAPPO [ ] JACHO [ ] NCQA [ ] URAC
Plan Type: Specialty HMO, Specialty PPO, POS, TPA

SERVICE AREA:
Nationwide: N
KY;

TYPE OF COVERAGE:
Commercial: [Y] Individual: [ ] FEHBP: [ ] Indemnity: [ ]
Medicare: [ ] Medicaid: [ ] Supplemental Medicare: [ ]
Tricare [ ]

PLAN BENEFITS:
Alternative Medicine:	[ ]	Behavioral Health:	[ ]
Chiropractic:	[ ]	Dental:	[X]
Home Care:	[ ]	Inpatient SNF:	[ ]
Long-Term Care:	[ ]	Pharm. Mail Order:	[ ]
Physical Therapy:	[ ]	Podiatry:	[ ]
Psychiatric:	[ ]	Transplant:	[ ]
Vision:	[ ]	Wellness:	[ ]
Workers' Comp:	[ ]		
Other Benefits:			

Comments:
For enrollment and revenue information see corporate listing, Camp Hill, Pennsylvania.

Managed Care Organization Profiles — NEW MEXICO

PRODUCTS OFFERED:
Product Name:	Type:
Lovelace Senior Plan	Medicare
Lovelace Community Health Plan	
Salud	Medicaid

PLAN BENEFITS:
Alternative Medicine:	[ ]	Behavioral Health:	[ ]
Chiropractic:	[X]	Dental:	[ ]
Home Care:	[X]	Inpatient SNF:	[X]
Long-Term Care:	[X]	Pharm. Mail Order:	[X]
Physical Therapy:	[X]	Podiatry:	[X]
Psychiatric:	[X]	Transplant:	[X]
Vision:	[X]	Wellness:	[X]
Workers' Comp:	[X]		
Other Benefits:			

MOLINA HEALTHCARE OF NEW MEXICO

8801 Horizon Blvd NE
Albuquerque, NM 87113
Phone: 505-342-4681 Fax: 505-798-7380 Toll-Free: 800-580-2811
Web site: www.molinahealthcare.com

MAILING ADDRESS:
MOLINA HEALTHCARE OF NM
8801 Horizon Blvd NE
Albuquerque, NM 87113

KEY EXECUTIVES:
Chairman of the Board .... Joseph M Molina, MD
Chief Executive Officer/President .... Ann Wehr, MD
Chief Financial Officer .... Anita Mullins
Corporate Medical Officer .... Catharine Kincaid
Pharmacy Director .... Gary Gijsbers
VP MIS .... Bruce Lorenz
Credentialing Manager .... Diane Madrid
Provider Services Contracts .... Lynn Allen
Medical Mgmt Director .... Sharon Huerta
Fraud Prevention/Invest Coord .... Mary Alice Garcia

COMPANY PROFILE:
Parent Company Name: Molina Healthcare Inc
Doing Business As:
Year Founded: 1993   Federally Qualified: [ ]
Forprofit: [Y]   Not-For-Profit: [ ]
Model Type: NETWORK
Accreditation: [ ] AAPPO [ ] JACHO [X] NCQA [ ] URAC
Plan Type: HMO, POS
Primary Physicians: 1,490   Physician Specialists: 6,849
Hospitals: 54
Total Enrollment:
  2001: 123,000   2004: 65,000   2007: 0
  2002: 0   2005: 60,000
  2003: 0   2006: 65,000

SERVICE AREA:
Nationwide: N
NM;

PRODUCTS OFFERED:
Product Name:	Type:
Salud Managed Care	Medicaid
SCHIP	

PLAN BENEFITS:
Alternative Medicine:	[ ]	Behavioral Health:	[ ]
Chiropractic:	[X]	Dental:	[ ]
Home Care:	[X]	Inpatient SNF:	[X]
Long-Term Care:	[ ]	Pharm. Mail Order:	[X]
Physical Therapy:	[X]	Podiatry:	[X]
Psychiatric:	[X]	Transplant:	[X]
Vision:	[X]	Wellness:	[X]
Workers' Comp:	[ ]		
Other Benefits:			

Comments:
Molina Healthcare purchased Health Care Horizons, the parent company of Cimarron Health Plans. Molina sold the commercial members to Lovelace Health Plan, August 1st, 2004.

NEW MEXICO MEDICAL REVIEW ASSOCIATION

5801 Osuna NE Ste 200
Albuquerque, NM 87109
Phone: 505-998-9898 Fax: 505-998-9899 Toll-Free:
Web site: www.nmmra.org

MAILING ADDRESS:
NEW MEXICO MEDICAL REVIEW ASSN
5801 Osuna NE Ste 200
Albuquerque, NM 87109

KEY EXECUTIVES:
Chief Executive Officer .... Dan Jaco, MA, MSPH
Director of Finance .... David Bagby
Medical Director .... John Seibel, MD
Chief Operating Officer .... Boyd Kleefisch
Human Resources & Facilities Director .... Dawn Miller
EQRO Program Director .... Patty Kehoe

COMPANY PROFILE:
Parent Company Name:
Doing Business As:
Year Founded: 1971   Federally Qualified: [ ]
Forprofit: [ ]   Not-For-Profit: [Y]
Model Type:
Accreditation: [ ] AAPPO [ ] JACHO [ ] NCQA [ ] URAC
Plan Type: PRO, UR

SERVICE AREA:
Nationwide: N
NM;

PRESBYTERIAN HEALTH PLAN

2501 Buena Vista SE
Alburquerque, NM 87106
Phone: 505-923-5700 Fax: 505-923-5277 Toll-Free: 800-356-2884
Web site: www.phs.org

MAILING ADDRESS:
PRESBYTERIAN HEALTH PLAN
PO Box 27489
Alburquerque, NM 87106

KEY EXECUTIVES:
Chairman/Chief Executive Officer .... James H Hinton
President .... David R Scrase, MD
Chief Financial Officer .... Dale Maxwell
Senior VP, Chief Medical Officer .... Dale Anderson, MD
Pharmacy Director .... Larry Georgopoulous
Chief Information Officer .... Robert Skinner
Chief Operating Officer .... Jim Brown
Executive Director, Commercial Products/Sales ... Sue Nelson
Executive Director Provider Services .... Rebecca Kohl
Admin Director Health Management .... Revathi A Davidson
VP Human Resources .... Renee Reimer
Health Services Director .... Diane Hice
Quality Assurance Director .... Rhonda Ryba
VP Executive Director Secure Horizons .... Karen Smith
Corporate Counsel .... Gabriel Parra

COMPANY PROFILE:
Parent Company Name: Presbyterian Healthcare Services
Doing Business As: Presbyterian Health Plan
Year Founded: 1986   Federally Qualified: [Y]
Forprofit: [Y]   Not-For-Profit: [ ]
Model Type: MIXED
Accreditation: [ ] AAPPO [ ] JACHO [ ] NCQA [ ] URAC
Plan Type: HMO, PPO, POS, ASO, TPA
Primary Physicians: 300   Physician Specialists:
Hospitals:
Total Enrollment:
  2001: 222,046   2004: 244,490   2007: 0
  2002: 225,736   2005:
  2003: 241,683   2006:

SERVICE AREA:
Nationwide:
NM;

TYPE OF COVERAGE:
Commercial: [Y] Individual: [Y] FEHBP: [ ] Indemnity: [ ]
Medicare: [ ] Medicaid: [Y] Supplemental Medicare: [Y]
Tricare: [ ]

PRODUCTS OFFERED:
Product Name:	Type:
Presbterian Salud	Medicaid
Secure Horizons Pacificare	Medicare
Presbyterian Senior Care	Medicare Advantage

NEW MEXICO

HMO NEW MEXICO INC

12800 Indian School Road NE
Albuquerque, NM 87112
Phone: 505-291-3500 Fax: 505-816-5324 Toll-Free: 800-423-1630
Web site: www.bcbsnm.com

MAILING ADDRESS:
HMO NEW MEXICO INC
PO Box 27630
Albuquerque, NM 87112

KEY EXECUTIVES:
Chief Executive Officer .... Raymond McCaskey
President .... Elizabeth A Watrin
Chief Financial Officer .... Kurt Shipley
Medical Director .... Lawrence Wilson, MD
Pharmacy Director .... Doug Lohkamp
Director Marketing & Community Relations .... Alfonso Trujillo
Director, Quality Management & Improvement ... Peggy Mohoric, RN
Network/Contracts Director .... Karen Smoot
Manager, Human Resources/Dir Health Promotion ..... Thomas Frock
Director, Health Care Management .... Kathy Boyle, RN
Medical Management Director .... Kathy Stanley

COMPANY PROFILE:
Parent Company Name: New Mexico Blue Cross/Blue Shield
Doing Business As: HMO New Mexico
Year Founded: 1986   Federally Qualified: [Y]
Forprofit: [ ]   Not-For-Profit: [Y]
Model Type: IPA
Accreditation: [ ] AAPPO [ ] JACHO [X] NCQA [ ] URAC
Plan Type: HMO, POS
Total Revenue: 2005:   101,293,014   2006:   6,989,590
Net Income   2005:   2,239,144   2006:   1,632,024
Total Enrollment:
  2001: 0   2004: 33,594   2007: 0
  2002: 31,627   2005: 31,271
  2003: 34,548   2006: 25,747
Medical Loss Ratio: 2005: 84.30   2006: 81.70
Administrative Expense Ratio: 2005:   2006:

SERVICE AREA:
Nationwide: N
  NM;

TYPE OF COVERAGE:
Commercial: [Y] Individual: [ ] FEHBP: [ ] Indemnity: [ ]
Medicare: [Y] Medicaid: [ ] Supplemental Medicare: [ ]
Tricare   [ ]

PLAN BENEFITS:
Alternative Medicine:	[ ]	Behavioral Health:	[X]
Chiropractic:	[X]	Dental:	[X]
Home Care:	[X]	Inpatient SNF:	[X]
Long-Term Care:	[ ]	Pharm. Mail Order:	[X]
Physical Therapy:	[X]	Podiatry:	[X]
Psychiatric:	[X]	Transplant:	[X]
Vision:	[X]	Wellness:	[X]
Workers' Comp:	[ ]		
Other Benefits:			

HUMANA INC - NEW MEXICO

500 W Main St
Louisville, KY 40201
Phone: 502-580-5804 Fax: 502-580-5044 Toll-Free:
Web site: www.humana.com

MAILING ADDRESS:
HUMANA INC - NEW MEXICO
500 W Main St
Louisville, KY 40201

KEY EXECUTIVES:
Chairman of the Board .... David A Jones Jr
Chief Executive Officer/President .... Michael B McCallister
Chief Financial Officer .... James H Bloem
VP Medical Director .... Jonathan T Lord, MD
Senior VP Chief Information Officer .... Bruce J Goodman
Senior VP Human Resources .... Bonnie C Hathcock

COMPANY PROFILE:
Parent Company Name: Humana Inc
Doing Business As:
Year Founded: 1961   Federally Qualified: [Y]
Forprofit: [Y]   Not-For-Profit: [ ]
Model Type:
Accreditation: [ ] AAPPO [ ] JACHO [ ] NCQA [ ] URAC
Plan Type: PPO, ASO, CDHP, HSA

SERVICE AREA:
Nationwide: N
  NM;

TYPE OF COVERAGE:
Commercial: [ ] Individual: [ ] FEHBP: [ ] Indemnity: [ ]
Medicare: [Y] Medicaid: [ ] Supplemental Medicare: [Y]
Tricare   [ ]

CONSUMER-DRIVEN PRODUCTS
JP Morgan Chase	HSA Company
HumanaOne HSA	HSA Product
JP Morgan Chase	HSA Administrator
Personal Care Account	Consumer-Driven Health Plan
HumanaOne	High Deductible Health Plan

PLAN BENEFITS:
Alternative Medicine:	[ ]	Behavioral Health:	[ ]
Chiropractic:	[X]	Dental:	[X]
Home Care:	[ ]	Inpatient SNF:	[ ]
Long-Term Care:	[ ]	Pharm. Mail Order:	[X]
Physical Therapy:	[ ]	Podiatry:	[ ]
Psychiatric:	[X]	Transplant:	[X]
Vision:	[ ]	Wellness:	[X]
Workers' Comp:	[X]		
Other Benefits:			

LOVELACE HEALTH PLAN

4101 Indian School Rd NE #110
Albuquerque, NM 87110
Phone: 505-262-7363 Fax: 505-262-7545 Toll-Free: 800-808-7363
Web site: www.lovelacehealthplan.com

MAILING ADDRESS:
LOVELACE HEALTH PLAN
4101 Indian School Rd NE #110
Albuquerque, NM 87110

KEY EXECUTIVES:
Chief Executive Officer .... Gayle Adams
Chief Financial Officer .... Sharon Charlton
Acting Medical Director .... Jeanette Velarde
Pharmacy Director .... Larry Pesko
Chief Operating Officer .... Robert Simmons
Marketing Director .... Ann McKinney
Credentialing Manager .... Sean Pettis
Director, Provider Services .... Kevin Kandalaft
Human Resources Director .... Carol Shelton
Medical Management Director .... Cheryl Lopez
Quality Assurance Director .... Linda Hubbard
Credentialing Manager .... Sean Pettis
Compliance Officer .... Ann Greenberg

COMPANY PROFILE:
Parent Company Name: Ardent Health Services
Doing Business As: Lovelace Health Plan
Year Founded: 1973   Federally Qualified: [Y]
Forprofit: [Y]   Not-For-Profit: [ ]
Model Type: MIXED
Accreditation: [ ] AAPPO [X] JACHO [X] NCQA [ ] URAC
Plan Type: HMO, PPO, POS, ASO,
Total Enrollment:
  2001: 0   2004: 250,000   2007: 0
  2002: 167,700   2005: 190,000
  2003: 60,000   2006:

SERVICE AREA:
Nationwide: N
  NM;

TYPE OF COVERAGE:
Commercial: [Y] Individual: [ ] FEHBP: [Y] Indemnity: [ ]
Medicare: [Y] Medicaid: [Y] Supplemental Medicare: [Y]
Tricare   [ ]

Managed Care Organization Profiles NEW MEXICO

ASSURANT EMPLOYEE BENEFITS - NEW MEXICO

1128 Pennsylvania St NE Ste210
Albuquerque, NM 87110
Phone: 505-266-7709 Fax: 505-265-3576 Toll-Free: 800-269-5415
Web site: www.assurantemployeebenefits.com
MAILING ADDRESS:
    ASSURANT EMPLOYEE BNFTS - NM
    1128 Pennsylvania St NE Ste210
    Albuquerque, NM 87110

KEY EXECUTIVES:
Interim Chief Executive Officer/President .... John S Roberts
Chief Financial Officer .... Floyd F Chadee
VP, Medical Director .... Polly M Galbraith, MD
Chief Information Officer .... Karla J Schacht
Senior VP, Marketing .... Mark J Bohen
Privacy Officer .... John L Fortini
VP of Provider Services .... James A Barrett, DMD
Senior VP, Human Resources & Development .... Sylvia R Wagner
General Manager .... Todd Boyd
National Dental Director .... James A Barrett, DMD

COMPANY PROFILE:
Parent Company Name: Assurant Health
Doing Business As:
Year Founded: 1986   Federally Qualified: [ ]
Forprofit: [Y]   Not-For-Profit: [ ]
Model Type:
Accreditation: [ ] AAPPO [ ] JACHO [ ] NCQA [ ] URAC
Plan Type: Specialty HMO, Specialty PPO, POS
SERVICE AREA:
Nationwide: N
    NM;
TYPE OF COVERAGE:
Commercial: [Y] Individual: [Y] FEHBP: [ ] Indemnity: [ ]
Medicare: [Y] Medicaid: [Y] Supplemental Medicare: [ ]
Tricare   [ ]
PLAN BENEFITS:
Alternative Medicine: [ ]   Behavioral Health: [ ]
Chiropractic: [ ]   Dental: [X]
Home Care: [ ]   Inpatient SNF: [ ]
Long-Term Care: [ ]   Pharm. Mail Order: [ ]
Physical Therapy: [ ]   Podiatry: [ ]
Psychiatric: [ ]   Transplant: [ ]
Vision: [X]   Wellness: [ ]
Workers' Comp: [ ]
Other Benefits:
Comments:
Formerly Fortis Benefits Dental.

BLUE CROSS BLUE SHIELD OF NEW MEXICO

12800 Indian School Road
Albuquerque, NM 87112
Phone: 505-291-3500 Fax: 505-816-5324 Toll-Free: 800-835-8699
Web site: www.bcbsnm.com
MAILING ADDRESS:
    BC/BS OF NEW MEXICO
    12800 Indian School Rd
    Albuquerque, NM 87112

KEY EXECUTIVES:
Chief Executive Officer-HCSC .... Raymond McCaskey
President - New Mexico .... Elizabeth A Watrin
VP New Mexico Business .... Kurt Shipley
Medical Director .... Lawrence Wilson, MD
Pharmacy Manager .... Doug Lohcamp
Director Sales & Marketing .... Dorane Wintermeyer
Public Relations Coordinator .... Lydia Ashanin
Director Network Services .... Karen Smott
VP Health Care Management .... Tom MacLean
Manager Human Resources .... Tom Frock
Director Quality & Improvement .... Peggy Mohoric, RN
New Product Development .... Margie Crow
Subscriber Services Division .... Linda Amburn
VP & General Counsel .... Deborah Dorman-Rodriguez

COMPANY PROFILE:
Parent Company Name: Health Care Service Corporation
Doing Business As:
Year Founded: 1940   Federally Qualified: [Y]
Forprofit: [ ]   Not-For-Profit: [Y]
Model Type: IPA
Accreditation: [ ] AAPPO [ ] JACHO [X] NCQA [ ] URAC
Plan Type: HMO, PPO, UR, POS, CDHP, HSA
Primary Physicians: 8,600   Physician Specialists:
Hospitals:
Total Enrollment:
    2001: 0   2004: 237,000   2007: 0
    2002: 0   2005:
    2003: 220,000   2006:
SERVICE AREA:
Nationwide: N
    NM;
TYPE OF COVERAGE:
Commercial: [Y] Individual: [ ] FEHBP: [ ] Indemnity: [ ]
Medicare: [ ] Medicaid: [Y] Supplemental Medicare: [ ]
Tricare   [ ]
PRODUCTS OFFERED:
Product Name: Type:
HMO New Mexico   HMO
Blue Cross POS Plan   POS
PLAN BENEFITS:
Alternative Medicine: [ ]   Behavioral Health: [ ]
Chiropractic: [X]   Dental: [X]
Home Care: [X]   Inpatient SNF: [X]
Long-Term Care: [X]   Pharm. Mail Order: [ ]
Physical Therapy: [X]   Podiatry: [X]
Psychiatric: [X]   Transplant: [X]
Vision: [ ]   Wellness: [ ]
Workers' Comp: [X]
Other Benefits:

DELTA DENTAL PLAN OF NEW MEXICO

2500 Louisiana Blvd NE Ste 600
Albuquerque, NM 87110
Phone: 505-883-4777 Fax: 505-883-7444 Toll-Free: 800-999-0963
Web site: www.deltadentalnm.com
MAILING ADDRESS:
    DELTA DENTAL PLAN OF NM
    2500 Louisiana Blvd NE Ste 600
    Albuquerque, NM 87110

KEY EXECUTIVES:
Chief Executive Officer/President .... Walter Bolic
Chief Financial Officer .... Edwin J Harris
Marketing Director .... Maggie Nevins
IT Manager .... Michael Maynard

COMPANY PROFILE:
Parent Company Name: Delta Dental Plan Association
Doing Business As:
Year Founded: Federally Qualified: [ ]
Forprofit: [ ]   Not-For-Profit: [ ]
Model Type:
Accreditation: [ ] AAPPO [ ] JACHO [ ] NCQA [ ] URAC
Plan Type: Specialty HMO
Total Enrollment:
    2001: 115,715   2004: 113,022   2007: 0
    2002: 121,682   2005:
    2003: 103,583   2006:
SERVICE AREA:
Nationwide: N
    NM;
TYPE OF COVERAGE:
Commercial: [Y] Individual: [ ] FEHBP: [ ] Indemnity: [ ]
Medicare: [ ] Medicaid: [ ] Supplemental Medicare: [ ]
Tricare   [ ]
PLAN BENEFITS:
Alternative Medicine: [ ]   Behavioral Health: [ ]
Chiropractic: [ ]   Dental: [X]
Home Care: [ ]   Inpatient SNF: [ ]
Long-Term Care: [ ]   Pharm. Mail Order: [ ]
Physical Therapy: [ ]   Podiatry: [ ]
Psychiatric: [ ]   Transplant: [ ]
Vision: [ ]   Wellness: [ ]
Workers' Comp: [ ]
Other Benefits:

NEW JERSEY

MAILING ADDRESS:
VALUE HEALTH CARE
PO Box 1442
Wall, NJ 07719

KEY EXECUTIVES:
Chief Executive Officer .... Phyllis Millrowe
Chief Financial Officer .... Lisa Nawhert
Marketing Director .... Dawn Mustel

COMPANY PROFILE:
Parent Company Name:
Doing Business As:
Year Founded: 1977　　Federally Qualified: [ ]
Forprofit: [ ]　　Not-For-Profit: [ ]
Model Type:
Accreditation: [ ] AAPPO　[ ] JACHO　[ ] NCQA　[ ] URAC
Plan Type: Specialty HMO

SERVICE AREA:
Nationwide:
　NJ;

TYPE OF COVERAGE:
Commercial: [Y]　Individual: [ ]　FEHBP: [ ]　Indemnity: [ ]
Medicare: [ ]　Medicaid: [ ]　Supplemental Medicare: [ ]
Tricare [ ]

PLAN BENEFITS:
Alternative Medicine: [ ]　　Behavioral Health: [ ]
Chiropractic: [ ]　　　　　　 Dental: [ ]
Home Care: [ ]　　　　　　　Inpatient SNF: [ ]
Long-Term Care: [X]　　　　 Pharm. Mail Order: [X]
Physical Therapy: [ ]　　　　Podiatry: [ ]
Psychiatric: [ ]　　　　　　　Transplant: [ ]
Vision: [ ]　　　　　　　　　Wellness: [X]
Workers' Comp: [ ]
Other Benefits:

Managed Care Organization Profiles — NEW JERSEY

MAILING ADDRESS:
UNION LABOR LIFE INSURANCE CO
700 E Gate Dr Ste 115
Mount Laurel, NJ 08054

KEY EXECUTIVES:
Chairman of the Board .... Joseph J Hunt
President/Chief Executive Officer .... Mark E Singleton
Acting Chief Financial Officer .... Damon Gasque
Senior VP, Marketing Development .... James J Kennedy Jr
Chief Information Officer .... James Tierney
Senior VP, Chief of Corporate Operations .... James M Paul
Senior VP, General Counsel/Chief Compliance .... Teresa E Valentine

COMPANY PROFILE:
Parent Company Name: ULLICO
Doing Business As:
Year Founded: 1929   Federally Qualified: [Y]
Forprofit: [Y]   Not-For-Profit: [ ]
Model Type: NETWORK
Accreditation: [ ] AAPPO [ ] JACHO [ ] NCQA [ ] URAC
Plan Type: Specialty PPO

SERVICE AREA:
Nationwide: N
CT; MA; ME; NH; NJ; NY; PA; RI; VT;

TYPE OF COVERAGE:
Commercial: [Y] Individual: [ ] FEHBP: [ ] Indemnity: [ ]
Medicare: [ ] Medicaid: [ ] Supplemental Medicare: [ ]
Tricare [ ]

PRODUCTS OFFERED:
Product Name: Type:
Union Life Health   SPECPPO
Union Life Dental   Specialty PPO

PLAN BENEFITS:
Alternative Medicine: [X]   Behavioral Health: [X]
Chiropractic: [X]   Dental: [X]
Home Care: [X]   Inpatient SNF: [X]
Long-Term Care: [X]   Pharm. Mail Order: [X]
Physical Therapy: [X]   Podiatry: [X]
Psychiatric: [X]   Transplant: [X]
Vision: [X]   Wellness: [X]
Workers' Comp: [X]
Other Benefits:
Comments:
Provides Union insurance.

UNITY DENTAL HEALTH SERVICES

1099 Wall St West Ste 317
Lyndhurst, NJ 07071
Phone: 201-635-3033 Fax: 201-635-3035 Toll-Free: 877-558-6489
Web site: www.unitydentalcompanies.com

MAILING ADDRESS:
UNITY DENTAL HEALTH SERVICES
1099 Wall St West Ste 317
Lyndhurst, NJ 07071

KEY EXECUTIVES:
Chief Executive Officer .... Robert Dubman, MD
Treasurer .... Richard E Fox

COMPANY PROFILE:
Parent Company Name:
Doing Business As:
Year Founded: 1985   Federally Qualified: [N]
Forprofit: [ ]   Not-For-Profit: [ ]
Model Type:
Accreditation: [ ] AAPPO [ ] JACHO [ ] NCQA [ ] URAC
Plan Type: Specialty HMO, Specialty PPO, TPA, UR
Total Enrollment:
  2001: 0   2004: 494   2007: 0
  2002: 12,985   2005: 1,417
  2003: 652   2006:

SERVICE AREA:
Nationwide: N
NJ;

TYPE OF COVERAGE:
Commercial: [Y] Individual: [ ] FEHBP: [ ] Indemnity: [ ]
Medicare: [ ] Medicaid: [ ] Supplemental Medicare: [ ]
Tricare [ ]

PRODUCTS OFFERED:
Product Name: Type:
Choice   HMO

PLAN BENEFITS:
Alternative Medicine: [ ]   Behavioral Health: [ ]
Chiropractic: [ ]   Dental: [X]
Home Care: [ ]   Inpatient SNF: [ ]
Long-Term Care: [ ]   Pharm. Mail Order: [ ]
Physical Therapy: [ ]   Podiatry: [ ]
Psychiatric: [ ]   Transplant: [ ]
Vision: [ ]   Wellness: [ ]
Workers' Comp: [ ]
Other Benefits:

UNIVERSITY HEALTH PLANS INC

550 Broad St 17th Fl
Newark, NJ 07102-4599
Phone: 973-623-8700 Fax: 973-623-7306 Toll-Free: 800-TRI-UHP1
Web site: www.uhpnet.com

MAILING ADDRESS:
UNIVERSITY HEALTH PLANS INC
550 Broad St 17th Fl
Newark, NJ 07102-4599

KEY EXECUTIVES:
Chief Executive Officer/President .... Alexander H McLean
Chief Financial Officer .... James P Dalessio
Medical Director .... Sebastian F Dovi, MD
Plan Pharmacist .... Michael Pica
Marketing Director .... Frank Alkin
Director of Provider Relations .... William Van Gieson
Medical Management Director .... Eileen Hooven
VP of Marketing .... Jack Rohfritch

COMPANY PROFILE:
Parent Company Name: Centene Corporation Inc
Doing Business As:
Year Founded: 1993   Federally Qualified: [N]
Forprofit: [Y]   Not-For-Profit: [ ]
Model Type: NETWORK
Accreditation: [ ] AAPPO [ ] JACHO [ ] NCQA [ ] URAC
Plan Type: HMO, PPO, POS, PBM
Primary Physicians: 1,848   Physician Specialists: 4,213
Hospitals: 78
Total Revenue: 2005:   2006: 137,057,972
Net Income   2005:   2006:
Total Enrollment:
  2001: 57,285   2004: 52,847   2007: 58,098
  2002: 52,969   2005: 55,339
  2003: 53,960   2006: 57,865
Medical Loss Ratio: 2005:   2006: 86.80
Administrative Expense Ratio: 2005:   2006:

SERVICE AREA:
Nationwide: N
NJ;

TYPE OF COVERAGE:
Commercial: [Y] Individual: [ ] FEHBP: [ ] Indemnity: [ ]
Medicare: [ ] Medicaid: [Y] Supplemental Medicare: [ ]
Tricare [ ]

PRODUCTS OFFERED:
Product Name: Type:
Groupcare   Commercial HMO & POS
Family Care   Medicaid HMO
Kid Care   CHIP

PLAN BENEFITS:
Alternative Medicine: [ ]   Behavioral Health: [ ]
Chiropractic: [X]   Dental: [X]
Home Care: [X]   Inpatient SNF: [X]
Long-Term Care: [ ]   Pharm. Mail Order: [X]
Physical Therapy: [X]   Podiatry: [X]
Psychiatric: [X]   Transplant: [X]
Vision: [X]   Wellness: [X]
Workers' Comp: [ ]
Other Benefits:

VALUE HEALTH CARE

PO Box 1442
Wall, NJ 07719
Phone: Fax: 908-292-1111 Toll-Free: 800-516-4343
Web site:

NEW JERSEY — Managed Care Organization Profiles

Total Revenue: 2005:   2006: 550,086,108
Net Income 2005:   2006:
Total Enrollment:
   2001: 170,641   2004: 159,576   2007: 136,336
   2002: 157,902   2005: 173,811
   2003: 129,198   2006: 144,509
Medical Loss Ratio: 2005:   2006: 74.20
Administrative Expense Ratio: 2005:   2006:

SERVICE AREA:
Nationwide: N
   NJ;

TYPE OF COVERAGE:
Commercial: [Y] Individual: [Y] FEHBP: [ ] Indemnity: [ ]
Medicare: [Y] Medicaid: [ ] Supplemental Medicare: [ ]
Tricare [ ]

PRODUCTS OFFERED:
Product Name:	Type:
Oxford Medicare Advantage	Medicare Advantage
Freedom Plan	POS
Oxford HMO	HMO
Oxford PPO	PPO

PLAN BENEFITS:
Alternative Medicine:	[X]	Behavioral Health:	[X]
Chiropractic:	[X]	Dental:	[X]
Home Care:	[X]	Inpatient SNF:	[X]
Long-Term Care:	[X]	Pharm. Mail Order:	[X]
Physical Therapy:	[X]	Podiatry:	[ ]
Psychiatric:	[X]	Transplant:	[X]
Vision:	[X]	Wellness:	[X]
Workers' Comp:	[X]		

Other Benefits:
Comments:
UnitedHealth Group merged with Oxford in 2004.

PARADIGMHEALTH

10 Mountainview Rd
Upper Saddle River, NJ 07458-1933
Phone: 201-934-0017 Fax: 201-934-4953 Toll-Free:
Web site: www.paradigmhealth.com

MAILING ADDRESS:
   PARADIGMHEALTH
   10 Mountainview Rd
   Upper Saddle River, NJ 07458-1933

KEY EXECUTIVES:
Chairman of the Board/Chief Executive Officer .... John Penrose
President .... Michael Burcham
Chief Financial Officer .... Ferdie Schmitz
Medical Director .... Albert Holt
Chief Operating Officer .... Thomas Hagan
Marketing Director .... Mark Patton
Senior VP, Care Management Services .... Jeanne Clement, RN, MPH

COMPANY PROFILE:
Parent Company Name:
Doing Business As:
Year Founded: Federally Qualified: [ ]
Forprofit: [ ]   Not-For-Profit: [ ]
Model Type:
Accreditation: [ ] AAPPO [ ] JACHO [ ] NCQA [ ] URAC
Plan Type: UR
Administrative Expense Ratio: 2005: 2006:

SERVICE AREA:
Nationwide: Y
   NW;

Comments:
Formerly Franklin Health Inc.

PRONJ, THE HEALTHCARE QUALITY IMPROVEMENT ORGANIZATION OF NJ

557 Cranbury Rd Ste 21
East Brunswick, NJ 08816
Phone: 732-238-5570 Fax: 732-238-9157 Toll-Free:
Web site: www.pronj.org

MAILING ADDRESS:
   PRONJ, THE HEALTHCARE QUALITY IMPR NJ
   557 Cranbury Rd Ste 21
   East Brunswick, NJ 08816

KEY EXECUTIVES:
Chief Executive Officer .... Martin P Margolies
Chief Financial Officer .... James Anderson
Chief Operating Officer .... Mary Jane Brubaker
Communications Director .... Cari Miller

COMPANY PROFILE:
Parent Company Name:
Doing Business As:
Year Founded: Federally Qualified: [ ]
Forprofit: [ ]   Not-For-Profit: [ ]
Model Type:
Accreditation: [ ] AAPPO [ ] JACHO [ ] NCQA [ ] URAC
Plan Type: UR, PRO

SERVICE AREA:
Nationwide: N
   NJ;

QUALCARE INC

30 Knightsbridge Rd
Piscataway, NJ 08854-3754
Phone: 732-562-0833 Fax: 732-562-2833 Toll-Free: 800-992-6613
Web site: www.qualcareinc.com

MAILING ADDRESS:
   QUALCARE INC
   30 Knightsbridge Rd
   Piscataway, NJ 08854-3754

KEY EXECUTIVES:
Chief Executive Officer/President .... Annette Catino
Chief Financial Officer/Chief Information Officer .... John McSorley
Medical Director .... Bruce Fisher, MD
Medical Director .... Mark Cukierman, MD
Chief Operating Officer .... Sharon Seitzman
VP, Client Services .... Allison Hofmann
Assistant VP, Sales .... Jerry Eisenberg
VP, Provider Services .... Kevin Joyce
VP Finance & Controller .... Janet Buggle
VP, Workers' Comp .... Ann Noble
Assistant VP, Claims .... Charlene Renollet

COMPANY PROFILE:
Parent Company Name: QualCare Inc
Doing Business As: QualCare Inc
Year Founded: 1993   Federally Qualified: [N]
Forprofit: [Y]   Not-For-Profit: [ ]
Model Type: NETWORK
Accreditation: [ ] AAPPO [ ] JACHO [ ] NCQA [ ] URAC
Plan Type: HMO, PPO, POS, EPO, TPA, UR
Primary Physicians: 8,400   Physician Specialists: 22,000
Hospitals: 87
Total Enrollment:
   2001: 0   2004: 441,000   2007: 0
   2002: 480,000   2005:
   2003: 0   2006:

SERVICE AREA:
Nationwide: N
   NJ;

TYPE OF COVERAGE:
Commercial: [Y] Individual: [ ] FEHBP: [ ] Indemnity: [ ]
Medicare: [ ] Medicaid: [ ] Supplemental Medicare: [ ]
Tricare [ ]

PLAN BENEFITS:
Alternative Medicine:	[ ]	Behavioral Health:	[X]
Chiropractic:	[X]	Dental:	[ ]
Home Care:	[X]	Inpatient SNF:	[X]
Long-Term Care:	[ ]	Pharm. Mail Order:	[X]
Physical Therapy:	[X]	Podiatry:	[X]
Psychiatric:	[X]	Transplant:	[X]
Vision:	[X]	Wellness:	[X]
Workers' Comp:	[X]		

Other Benefits:

UNION LABOR LIFE INSURANCE CO

700 E Gate Dr Ste 115
Mount Laurel, NJ 08054
Phone: 856-727-9200 Fax: 856-727-3763 Toll-Free: 800-526-6648
Web site: www.ullico.com

Managed Care Organization Profiles — NEW JERSEY

KEY EXECUTIVES:
Chairman of the Board/Chief Executive Officer .... Steven J Shulman
President/Chief Operating Officer .... Rene Lerer, MD
Executive VP/Chief Financial Officer .... Mark S Demilio
Chief Clinical Officer/Marketing Officer .... Anthony M Kotin, MD
Chief Information Officer .... Jeff D Emerson
Chief Communications Officer .... Christopher W Cooney
Chief Human Resources Officer .... Caskie Lewis-Clapper

COMPANY PROFILE:
Parent Company Name: Magellan Health Services Inc
Doing Business As:
Year Founded: Federally Qualified: [ ]
Forprofit: [Y]   Not-For-Profit: [ ]
Model Type:
Accreditation: [ ] AAPPO [ ] JACHO [X] NCQA [ ] URAC
Plan Type: Specialty PPO
SERVICE AREA:
Nationwide: N
  NJ;
TYPE OF COVERAGE:
Commercial: [Y] Individual: [ ] FEHBP: [ ] Indemnity: [ ]
Medicare: [ ] Medicaid: [ ] Supplemental Medicare: [ ]
Tricare   [ ]
PLAN BENEFITS:
Alternative Medicine: [ ]   Behavioral Health: [X]
Chiropractic: [ ]   Dental: [ ]
Home Care: [ ]   Inpatient SNF: [ ]
Long-Term Care: [ ]   Pharm. Mail Order: [ ]
Physical Therapy: [ ]   Podiatry: [ ]
Psychiatric: [X]   Transplant: [ ]
Vision: [ ]   Wellness: [X]
Workers' Comp: [ ]
Other Benefits:

MEDCO HEALTH SOLUTIONS INC

100 Parsons Pond Dr
Franklin Lakes, NJ 07417
Phone: 201-269-3400 Fax: 201-269-2874 Toll-Free: 800-248-2268
Web site: www.medcohealth.com
MAILING ADDRESS:
  MEDCO HEALTH SOLUTIONS INC
  100 Parsons Pond Dr
  Franklin Lakes, NJ 07417

KEY EXECUTIVES:
Chairman/Chief Executive Officer .... David B Snow
President/Chief Operating Officer .... Kenneth Klepper
Chief Financial Officer .... JoAnn Reed
Medical Director .... Robert S Epstein, MD, MS

COMPANY PROFILE:
Parent Company Name:
Doing Business As:
Year Founded: 1967   Federally Qualified: [ ]
Forprofit: [Y]   Not-For-Profit: [ ]
Model Type:
Accreditation: [ ] AAPPO [ ] JACHO [ ] NCQA [ ] URAC
Plan Type: Specialty PPO
Total Revenue: 2005:   2006:   42,543,700,000
Net Income   2005:   2006:   630,200,000
SERVICE AREA:
Nationwide: Y
  NW;
TYPE OF COVERAGE:
Commercial: [Y] Individual: [ ] FEHBP: [ ] Indemnity: [ ]
Medicare: [ ] Medicaid: [ ] Supplemental Medicare: [ ]
Tricare   [ ]
PLAN BENEFITS:
Alternative Medicine: [ ]   Behavioral Health: [ ]
Chiropractic: [ ]   Dental: [ ]
Home Care: [ ]   Inpatient SNF: [ ]
Long-Term Care: [ ]   Pharm. Mail Order: [X]
Physical Therapy: [ ]   Podiatry: [ ]
Psychiatric: [ ]   Transplant: [ ]
Vision: [ ]   Wellness: [ ]
Workers' Comp: [ ]
Other Benefits:
Comments:
Formerly Paid Prescriptions Inc.

ONE CALL MEDICAL INC

20 Waterview Blvd
Parsippany, NJ 07054-0614
Phone: 973-257-1000 Fax: 973-257-0044 Toll-Free: 800-872-2875
Web site: www.onecallmedical.com
MAILING ADDRESS:
  ONE CALL MEDICAL INC
  20 Waterview Blvd
  Parsippany, NJ 07054-0614

KEY EXECUTIVES:
Chief Executive Officer/President .... Kent Spafford
Chief Financial Officer .... Warren Green
Chief Operating Officer .... Don Duford
Executive VP, Marketing .... Ray Tamkorini
Senior VP, Human Resources .... Jerry Masin
Director, Client Relations .... Thomas Toohey
VP, Provider Development .... Steve Ellerman
Regional VP .... Mathew Dougherty

COMPANY PROFILE:
Parent Company Name:
Doing Business As:
Year Founded: 1992   Federally Qualified: [ ]
Forprofit: [Y]   Not-For-Profit: [ ]
Model Type:
Accreditation: [ ] AAPPO [ ] JACHO [ ] NCQA [ ] URAC
Plan Type: Specialty PPO
SERVICE AREA:
Nationwide: Y
  NW;
TYPE OF COVERAGE:
Commercial: [Y] Individual: [ ] FEHBP: [ ] Indemnity: [ ]
Medicare: [ ] Medicaid: [ ] Supplemental Medicare: [ ]
Tricare   [ ]
PRODUCTS OFFERED:
Product Name: Type:
EMG Referrals
MRI & CT Referrals
PLAN BENEFITS:
Alternative Medicine: [ ]   Behavioral Health: [ ]
Chiropractic: [ ]   Dental: [ ]
Home Care: [ ]   Inpatient SNF: [ ]
Long-Term Care: [ ]   Pharm. Mail Order: [ ]
Physical Therapy: [ ]   Podiatry: [ ]
Psychiatric: [ ]   Transplant: [ ]
Vision: [ ]   Wellness: [ ]
Workers' Comp: [X]
Other Benefits: MRI & CT Imaging
Comments:
Nationwide steerage program for Workers Comp.

OXFORD HEALTH PLANS OF NEW JERSEY INC

111 Wood Ave S Ste 2
Iselin, NJ 08830
Phone: 203-459-6000 Fax: 203-459-6464 Toll-Free: 800-889-4694
Web site: www.oxhp.com
MAILING ADDRESS:
  OXFORD HEALTH PLANS OF NJ
  111 Wood Ave S Ste 2
  Iselin, NJ 08830

KEY EXECUTIVES:
Chief Executive Officer/President .... Michael Turpin
Medical Director .... Alan M Muney, MD, MHA
Regional VP, Sales .... Darrell Farkus

COMPANY PROFILE:
Parent Company Name: UnitedHealth GroupDoing Business As:
Year Founded: 1984   Federally Qualified: [Y]
Forprofit: [Y]   Not-For-Profit: [ ]
Model Type: IPA
Accreditation: [ ] AAPPO [ ] JACHO [ ] NCQA [ ] URAC
Plan Type: HMO, PPO, POS, TPA, CDHP
Primary Physicians: 16,185   Physician Specialists:
Hospitals: 84

NEW JERSEY

MAILING ADDRESS:
   HORIZON HEALTHCARE DENTAL INC
   3 Penn Plaza East PP-15D
   Newark, NJ 07105

KEY EXECUTIVES:
Chief Executive Officer .... William J Marino

COMPANY PROFILE:
Parent Company Name: Horizon Healthcare Services Inc
Doing Business As:
Year Founded: 1986   Federally Qualified: [ ]
Forprofit: [N]   Not-For-Profit: [Y]
Model Type:
Accreditation: [ ] AAPPO [ ] JACHO [ ] NCQA [ ] URAC
Plan Type: Specialty HMO,
Total Revenue: 2005:   2006:   18,586,798
Net Income   2005:   2006:
Total Enrollment:
   2001: 69,107   2004: 95,991   2007: 0
   2002: 81,471   2005:
   2003: 91,978   2006: 99,327
Medical Loss Ratio: 2005:   2006: 80.00
Administrative Expense Ratio: 2005:   2006:

SERVICE AREA:
Nationwide: N
   NJ, NY,

TYPE OF COVERAGE:
Commercial: [ ] Individual: [ ] FEHBP: [ ] Indemnity: [ ]
Medicare: [ ] Medicaid: [ ] Supplemental Medicare: [ ]
Tricare   [ ]

PRODUCTS OFFERED:
Product Name: Type:
Horizon Healthcare Dental   Specialty HMO

PLAN BENEFITS:
Alternative Medicine: [ ]   Behavioral Health: [ ]
Chiropractic: [ ]   Dental: [X]
Home Care: [ ]   Inpatient SNF: [ ]
Long-Term Care: [ ]   Pharm. Mail Order: [ ]
Physical Therapy: [ ]   Podiatry: [ ]
Psychiatric: [ ]   Transplant: [ ]
Vision: [ ]   Wellness: [ ]
Workers' Comp: [ ]
Other Benefits:

HORIZON HEALTHCARE SERVICES INC

3 Penn Plaza East PP-15D
Newark, NJ 07105
Phone: 973-466-6669 Fax: 973-466-6645 Toll-Free: 888-667-4547
Web site: www.horizonblue.com

MAILING ADDRESS:
   HORIZON HEALTHCARE SRVS INC
   3 Penn Plaza East PP-15D
   Newark, NJ 07105

KEY EXECUTIVES:
Chief Executive Officer/President .... William J Marino
VP, Chief Medical Officer .... Richard G Popiel, MD
Senior VP Chief Information Officer .... Charles C Emery Jr

COMPANY PROFILE:
Parent Company Name:
Doing Business As: Horizon BC/BS; Horizon NJ Health;
Year Founded: 1986   Federally Qualified: [ ]
Forprofit: [N]   Not-For-Profit: [Y]
Model Type:
Accreditation: [ ] AAPPO [ ] JACHO [X] NCQA [X] URAC
Plan Type: HMO, PPO, POS, CDHP, HDHP, HSA
Total Revenue: 2005: 6,025,277,000 2006: 6,887,845,000
Net Income   2005:   213,751,000 2006:   180,066,000
Total Enrollment:
   2001: 0   2004: 3,100,000   2007: 3,300,000
   2002: 0   2005: 3,200,000
   2003: 0   2006: 3,200,000
Medical Loss Ratio: 2005:   2006: 86.40
Administrative Expense Ratio: 2005:   2006:

SERVICE AREA:
Nationwide: N
   NJ, NY, PA,

TYPE OF COVERAGE:
Commercial: [Y] Individual: [Y] FEHBP: [ ] Indemnity: [ ]
Medicare: [Y] Medicaid: [Y] Supplemental Medicare: [ ]
Tricare   [ ]

PLAN BENEFITS:
Alternative Medicine: [ ]   Behavioral Health: [ ]
Chiropractic: [X]   Dental: [X]
Home Care: [X]   Inpatient SNF: [X]
Long-Term Care: [ ]   Pharm. Mail Order: [X]
Physical Therapy: [X]   Podiatry: [X]
Psychiatric: [ ]   Transplant: [X]
Vision: [X]   Wellness: [X]
Workers' Comp: [ ]
Other Benefits:

HORIZON NJ HEALTH

210 Silvia St
Trenton, NJ 08628-3242
Phone: 609-538-0700 Fax: 609-538-0833 Toll-Free: 800-682-9092
Web site: www.horizon-mercy.com

MAILING ADDRESS:
   HORIZON NJ HEALTH
   210 Silvia St
   Trenton, NJ 08628-3242

KEY EXECUTIVES:
President/Chief Operating Officer .... Karen L Clark
Chief Financial Officer .... James P Dalessio
Chief Medical Officer .... Philip M Bonaparte, MD
Marketing Director .... Leonard Kudgis
Dental Director .... Brian J Bastecki, DMD

COMPANY PROFILE:
Parent Company Name: Horizon Healthcare Services Inc
Doing Business As:
Year Founded: 1994   Federally Qualified: [ ]
Forprofit: [ ]   Not-For-Profit: [ ]
Model Type:
Accreditation: [ ] AAPPO [ ] JACHO [ ] NCQA [ ] URAC
Plan Type: HMO
Total Enrollment:
   2001: 0   2004: 276,000   2007: 0
   2002: 0   2005:
   2003: 278,000   2006: 314,000

SERVICE AREA:
Nationwide: N
   NJ;

TYPE OF COVERAGE:
Commercial: [ ] Individual: [ ] FEHBP: [ ] Indemnity: [ ]
Medicare: [ ] Medicaid: [Y] Supplemental Medicare: [ ]
Tricare   [ ]

PLAN BENEFITS:
Alternative Medicine: [ ]   Behavioral Health: [ ]
Chiropractic: [X]   Dental: [X]
Home Care: [X]   Inpatient SNF: [X]
Long-Term Care: [ ]   Pharm. Mail Order: [X]
Physical Therapy: [X]   Podiatry: [X]
Psychiatric: [ ]   Transplant: [X]
Vision: [X]   Wellness: [X]
Workers' Comp: [ ]
Other Benefits:
Comments:
Formerly Horizon Mercy.

MAGELLAN BEHAVIORAL HEALTH

199 Pomerly
Parsippany, NJ 07054
Phone: 973-515-5010 Fax: 973-515-2012 Toll-Free:
Web site: www.magellanhealth.com

MAILING ADDRESS:
   MAGELLAN BEHAVIORAL HEALTH
   199 Pomerly
   Parsippany, NJ 07054

Managed Care Organization Profiles — NEW JERSEY

Doing Business As: Health Net
Year Founded: 1993   Federally Qualified: [Y]
Forprofit: [Y]   Not-For-Profit: [ ]
Model Type: NETWORK
Accreditation: [ ] AAPPO [ ] JACHO [ ] NCQA [ ] URAC
Plan Type: HMO, POS, CDHP, HDHP, HSA
Primary Physicians: 13,529   Physician Specialists:
Hospitals:
Total Revenue: 2005: 454,924,000   2006: 385,503,697
Net Income   2005:   1,846,000   2006:
Total Enrollment:
  2001: 316,417   2004: 251,550   2007: 130,297
  2002: 348,005   2005: 166,249
  2003: 339,405   2006: 149,032
Medical Loss Ratio: 2005: 84.30   2006: 80.00
Administrative Expense Ratio: 2005: 11.70   2006:

SERVICE AREA:
Nationwide: N
  NJ;

TYPE OF COVERAGE:
Commercial: [Y] Individual: [Y] FEHBP: [ ] Indemnity: [ ]
Medicare: [ ] Medicaid: [Y] Supplemental Medicare: [Y]
Tricare   [ ]

PRODUCTS OFFERED:
Product Name: Type:
HealthNet NJ HMO   HMO
HealthNet NJ   Medicaid

PLAN BENEFITS:
Alternative Medicine: [ ]   Behavioral Health: [ ]
Chiropractic: [X]   Dental: [X]
Home Care: [X]   Inpatient SNF: [X]
Long-Term Care: [X]   Pharm. Mail Order: [X]
Physical Therapy: [X]   Podiatry: [X]
Psychiatric: [X]   Transplant: [X]
Vision: [X]   Wellness: [X]
Workers' Comp: [X]
Other Benefits:

Comments:
Formerly First Option Health Plan of New Jersey.

HOPE RESOURCES PROVIDERS (HRP)

PO Box 456
Allenwood, NJ 08720
Phone: Fax: 732-292-0620   Toll-Free: 800-516-4343
Web site:
MAILING ADDRESS:
  HOPE RESOURCES PROVIDERS (HRP)
  PO Box 456
  Allenwood, NJ 08720

KEY EXECUTIVES:
Chairperson of the Board .... Barbara Mille
Chief Executive Officer .... Robert Tulkes
Medical Director .... Amy Camise

COMPANY PROFILE:
Parent Company Name: Our Lady of Hope Health Alliance
Doing Business As:
Year Founded: 1998   Federally Qualified: [ ]
Forprofit: [Y]   Not-For-Profit: [ ]
Model Type:
Accreditation: [ ] AAPPO [ ] JACHO [ ] NCQA [ ] URAC
Plan Type: Specialty PPO, TPA

SERVICE AREA:
Nationwide: N
  NJ;

TYPE OF COVERAGE:
Commercial: [Y] Individual: [ ] FEHBP: [ ] Indemnity: [ ]
Medicare: [ ] Medicaid: [ ] Supplemental Medicare: [ ]
Tricare   [ ]

PLAN BENEFITS:
Alternative Medicine: [ ]   Behavioral Health: [X]
Chiropractic: [X]   Dental: [X]
Home Care: [X]   Inpatient SNF: [X]
Long-Term Care: [X]   Pharm. Mail Order: [X]
Physical Therapy: [X]   Podiatry: [X]
Psychiatric: [X]   Transplant: [X]
Vision: [X]   Wellness: [X]
Workers' Comp: [X]
Other Benefits:

HORIZON BLUE CROSS/BLUE SHIELD OF NJ

3 Penn Plaza East PP13K
Newark, NJ 07015-2200
Phone: 973-466-6669 Fax: 973-466-6645 Toll-Free: 888-667-4547
Web site: www.horizonblue.com
MAILING ADDRESS:
  HORIZON BC/BS OF NJ HMO BLUE
  3 Penn Plaza East PP13K
  Newark, NJ 07015-2200

KEY EXECUTIVES:
Chief Executive Officer/President .... William J Marino
Chief Financial Officer .... Robert J Pures
VP, Chief Medical Officer .... Richard G Popiel, MD
Senior VP, IT, Chief Information Officer .... Mark Barnard
Director of Corp Marketing .... Lawrence B Altman
HIPAA Education & Awareness Coordinator .... Micki Jackson
Director, Provider Services .... Ann Sylvestro
Senior VP, Market Business Units .... Robert A Marino
VP Human Resources .... Margaret Coors
Senior VP, Healthcare Management .... Christy Bell W
Senior VP, General Counsel .... John W Campbell
Med Dir, Clinical Network Management .... Paul Krentzlin, MD MBA
Senior VP, Service .... Patrick J Geraghty
Senior VP, Market Business Units .... Robert A Marino

COMPANY PROFILE:
Parent Company Name: Horizon Healthcare Services Inc
Doing Business As: HMO Blue
Year Founded: 1986   Federally Qualified: [ ]
Forprofit: [ ]   Not-For-Profit: [Y]
Model Type: IPA
Accreditation: [ ] AAPPO [ ] JACHO [X] NCQA [X] URAC
Plan Type: HMO, PPO, POS, CDHP, HDHP, HSA
Primary Physicians: 23,080   Physician Specialists:
Hospitals:
Total Revenue: 2005: 1,666,979,000   2006: 1,919,077,423
Net Income   2005:   65,680,000   2006:
Total Enrollment:
  2001: 478,644   2004: 473,492   2007: 567,002
  2002: 505,568   2005: 483,492
  2003: 455,219   2006: 562,362
Medical Loss Ratio: 2005: 84.40   2006: 82.90
Administrative Expense Ratio: 2005: 11.70   2006:

SERVICE AREA:
Nationwide: N
  NJ;

TYPE OF COVERAGE:
Commercial: [Y] Individual: [Y] FEHBP: [ ] Indemnity: [ ]
Medicare: [Y] Medicaid: [Y] Supplemental Medicare: [ ]
Tricare   [ ]

PRODUCTS OFFERED:
Product Name: Type:
Horizon HMO Blue   HMO
Horizon POS   POS
Horizon PPO   PPO
Horizon Direct Access   Open Access
Medicare Blue   Medicare Advantage
Traditional Indemnity Plans
                           Medicaid

PLAN BENEFITS:
Alternative Medicine: [ ]   Behavioral Health: [ ]
Chiropractic: [ ]   Dental: [X]
Home Care: [ ]   Inpatient SNF: [ ]
Long-Term Care: [ ]   Pharm. Mail Order: [ ]
Physical Therapy: [ ]   Podiatry: [ ]
Psychiatric: [ ]   Transplant: [ ]
Vision: [ ]   Wellness: [ ]
Workers' Comp: [ ]
Other Benefits:

HORIZON HEALTHCARE DENTAL INC

3 Penn Plaza East PP-15D
Newark, NJ 07105
Phone: 973-466-6669 Fax: 973-466-6645 Toll-Free: 800-433-6825
Web site: www.horizonblue.com

NEW JERSEY | Managed Care Organization Profiles

FAMILY CHOICE HEALTH ALLIANCE

401 Hackensack Ave 9th Fl
Hackensack, NJ 07601-6411
Phone: 201-487-6002 Fax: 201-487-1116 Toll-Free: 800-732-7892
Web site: www.familychoicehealth.com

MAILING ADDRESS:
FAMILY CHOICE HEALTH ALLIANCE
401 Hackensack Ave 9th Fl
Hackensack, NJ 07601-6411

KEY EXECUTIVES:
Chief Executive Officer .... Andrew Baker
President ....Karen Piotti
Medical Director .... Rodney C Armstead, MD
Chief Information Officer .... Frank Xie
Director of Provider Services .... Eileen Feldman
Director Network Development .... Karen Spector-Piotti
Claims Manager .... Zule Ka Felix

COMPANY PROFILE:
Parent Company Name: Medical Diagnostic Management Inc
Doing Business As: PCHA
Year Founded: 1989   Federally Qualified: [ ]
Forprofit: [Y]   Not-For-Profit: [ ]
Model Type: NETWORK
Accreditation: [ ] AAPPO [ ] JACHO [ ] NCQA [ ] URAC
Plan Type: PPO

SERVICE AREA:
Nationwide: N
NJ;

TYPE OF COVERAGE:
Commercial: [Y] Individual: [ ] FEHBP: [ ] Indemnity: [ ]
Medicare: [ ] Medicaid: [ ] Supplemental Medicare: [ ]
Tricare   [ ]

PLAN BENEFITS:
Alternative Medicine: [ ]   Behavioral Health: [ ]
Chiropractic: [X]   Dental: [ ]
Home Care: [ ]   Inpatient SNF: [ ]
Long-Term Care: [ ]   Pharm. Mail Order: [ ]
Physical Therapy: [ ]   Podiatry: [X]
Psychiatric: [X]   Transplant: [ ]
Vision: [ ]   Wellness: [ ]
Workers' Comp: [ ]
Other Benefits:
Comments:
Formerly Preferred Health Strategies.

GREAT-WEST HEALTHCARE - NEW JERSEY

One Centennial Ave 1st Fl
Piscataway, NJ 08855
Phone: 732-357-2783 Fax: 732-357-2509 Toll-Free: 800-644-9175
Web site: www.greatwesthealthcare.com

MAILING ADDRESS:
GREAT-WEST HEALTHCARE - NJ
One Centennial Ave 1st Fl
Piscataway, NJ 08855

KEY EXECUTIVES:
Regional President ....Joan Russo
Provider Relations .... Helen Greenberg

COMPANY PROFILE:
Parent Company Name: Great West Life & Annuity Insurance Co
Doing Business As: Great West Life
Year Founded: Federally Qualified: [ ]
Forprofit: [Y]   Not-For-Profit: [ ]
Model Type:
Accreditation: [ ] AAPPO [ ] JACHO [ ] NCQA [ ] URAC
Plan Type: PPO, POS, CDHP, HDHP, HSA,
Primary Physicians: 14,854   Physician Specialists:
Hospitals:
Total Enrollment:
  2001: 5,784   2004: 13   2007: 0
  2002: 2,288   2005:
  2003: 375   2006:

SERVICE AREA:
Nationwide: N
NJ;

TYPE OF COVERAGE:
Commercial: [Y] Individual: [ ] FEHBP: [ ] Indemnity: [Y]
Medicare: [ ] Medicaid: [ ] Supplemental Medicare: [ ]
Tricare   [ ]

PRODUCTS OFFERED:
Product Name: Type:
Great-West Healthcare   HMO

CONSUMER-DRIVEN PRODUCTS
Mellon HR Solutions LLC   HSA Company
                                      HSA Product
                                      HSA Administrator
                                      Consumer-Driven Health Plan
High Deductible Health Plan

PLAN BENEFITS:
Alternative Medicine: [X]   Behavioral Health: [ ]
Chiropractic: [X]   Dental: [X]
Home Care: [X]   Inpatient SNF: [X]
Long-Term Care: [ ]   Pharm. Mail Order: [X]
Physical Therapy: [X]   Podiatry: [X]
Psychiatric: [X]   Transplant: [X]
Vision: [X]   Wellness: [X]
Workers' Comp: [ ]
Other Benefits:
Comments: In the process of being bought out by CIGNA Healthcare.

HEALTH CARE RESOURCES MANAGEMENT

1913 Atlantic Ave Ste F4
Manasquan, NJ 08736
Phone: 800-516-4343 Fax: Toll-Free:
Web site:

MAILING ADDRESS:
HEALTH CARE RESOURCES MNMNGT
1913 Atlantic Ave Ste F4
Manasquan, NJ 08736

KEY EXECUTIVES:
Chief Executive Officer.. Ellen Seirely

COMPANY PROFILE:
Parent Company Name:
Doing Business As:
Year Founded: Federally Qualified: [ ]
Forprofit: [ ]   Not-For-Profit: [ ]
Model Type:
Accreditation: [ ] AAPPO [ ] JACHO [ ] NCQA [ ] URAC
Plan Type: UR

SERVICE AREA:
Nationwide: N
NJ;

HEALTH NET - NEW JERSEY

90 Matawan Rd
Old Bridge, NJ 07747
Phone: 732-353-7400 Fax: 732-353-7511 Toll-Free: 800-848-4747
Web site: www.health.net

MAILING ADDRESS:
HEALTH NET - NEW JERSEY
90 Matawan Rd
Old Bridge, NJ 07747

KEY EXECUTIVES:
President .... Anju Sikka, MD
Chief Financial Officer .... Carol Richey
Chief Medical Officer .... Robert Grossman, MD
Pharmacy Director .... Julee Oh
Director of IS .... David Anderson
Chief Operating Officer .... William Limoreaux
Marketing Director .... Steven Calabrese

COMPANY PROFILE:
Parent Company Name: Health Net Inc, NE Corp Hdqrts

Managed Care Organization Profiles — NEW JERSEY

COMPANY PROFILE:
Parent Company Name: CIGNA Corporation
Doing Business As:
Year Founded: 1988   Federally Qualified: [Y]
Forprofit: [Y]   Not-For-Profit: [ ]
Model Type: MIXED
Accreditation: [ ] AAPPO [ ] JACHO [X] NCQA [ ] URAC
Plan Type: HMO, PPO, POS, CDHP, HDHP, HSA, FSA, HRA
Primary Physicians: 17,398   Physician Specialists:
Hospitals:
Total Revenue: 2005:   2006: 148,799,904
Net Income: 2005:   2006:
Total Enrollment:
  2001: 81,602   2004: 57,101   2007: 16,522
  2002: 149,356   2005: 53,240
  2003: 153,022   2006: 34,335
Medical Loss Ratio: 2005:   2006: 84.80
Administrative Expense Ratio: 2005:   2006:

SERVICE AREA:
Nationwide: N
  NJ; NY;

TYPE OF COVERAGE:
Commercial: [Y] Individual: [Y] FEHBP: [ ] Indemnity: [ ]
Medicare: [Y] Medicaid: [ ] Supplemental Medicare: [ ]
Tricare   [ ]

PRODUCTS OFFERED:
Product Name: Type:
Cigna HMO   HMO

CONSUMER-DRIVEN PRODUCTS
JP Morgan Chase   HSA Company
CIGNA Choice Fund   HSA Product
                                HSA Administrator
Open Access Plus   Consumer-Driven Health Plan
PPO   High Deductible Health Plan

PLAN BENEFITS:
Alternative Medicine: [ ]   Behavioral Health: [X]
Chiropractic: [X]   Dental: [X]
Home Care: [X]   Inpatient SNF: [X]
Long-Term Care: [ ]   Pharm. Mail Order: [X]
Physical Therapy: [X]   Podiatry: [X]
Psychiatric: [X]   Transplant: [X]
Vision: [X]   Wellness: [X]
Workers' Comp: [ ]
Other Benefits:
Comments:
Formerly CIGNA Healthcare of Northern New Jersey.

DELTA DENTAL PLAN OF NEW JERSEY

1639 Rte 10
Parsippany, NJ 07054-0222
Phone: 973-285-4000 Fax: 973-285-4162 Toll-Free: 800-848-3524
Web site: www.deltadentalnj.com
MAILING ADDRESS:
  DELTA DENTAL PLAN OF NJ
  PO Box 222
  Parsippany, NJ 07054-0222

KEY EXECUTIVES:
Chairman of the Board .... Gerald A Sydell, DDS
Chief Executive Officer/President .... Walter Van Brunt
Senior VP, Chief Financial Officer .... Jim Suleski
Dental Director .... D Scott Navarro, DDS
VP, Marketing .... Mark Nadeau
MIS Director .... Steve Stoll
VP, Corporate Communications/Chief Information Offr .... Diane Belle
VP, Provider Services/Network Development .... D Scott Navarro, DDS
VP, Human Resources .... Kathleen Fennell
Senior VP, General Counsel .... Douglas Sanborn Esq
Senior VP Claims/Customer Service .... Bruce Silverman

COMPANY PROFILE:
Parent Company Name:
Doing Business As:
Year Founded: 1968   Federally Qualified: [ ]
Forprofit: [ ]   Not-For-Profit: [Y]
Model Type: MIXED
Accreditation: [ ] AAPPO [ ] JACHO [ ] NCQA [ ] URAC
Plan Type: Specialty HMO, Specialty PPO, POS, UR
Primary Dentists: 338   Dental Specialists: 295
Hospitals:
Total Enrollment:
  2001: 645,000   2004: 656,599   2007: 0
  2002: 667,407   2005:
  2003: 673,761   2006: 605,369

SERVICE AREA:
Nationwide: N
  CT; NJ;

TYPE OF COVERAGE:
Commercial: [Y] Individual: [ ] FEHBP: [ ] Indemnity: [ ]
Medicare: [ ] Medicaid: [ ] Supplemental Medicare: [ ]
Tricare   [ ]

PRODUCTS OFFERED:
Product Name: Type:
Delta Dental PPO   Specialty PPO

PLAN BENEFITS:
Alternative Medicine: [ ]   Behavioral Health: [ ]
Chiropractic: [ ]   Dental: [X]
Home Care: [ ]   Inpatient SNF: [ ]
Long-Term Care: [ ]   Pharm. Mail Order: [ ]
Physical Therapy: [ ]   Podiatry: [ ]
Psychiatric: [ ]   Transplant: [ ]
Vision: [ ]   Wellness: [ ]
Workers' Comp: [ ]
Other Benefits:

DENTAL GROUP OF NEW JERSEY

924 N Wood Ave
Linden, NJ 07036
Phone: 908-925-6022 Fax: 908-925-4416 Toll-Free:
Web site: www.dgnj.com
MAILING ADDRESS:
  DENTAL GROUP OF NEW JERSEY
  924 N Wood Ave
  Linden, NJ 07036

KEY EXECUTIVES:
Chief Executive Officer .... Richard J Lukenda, DMD
Chief Financial Officer .... James Sosinski
Administrator .... Susan Lukenda

COMPANY PROFILE:
Parent Company Name: Dental Group of New Jersey
Doing Business As:
Year Founded: 1990   Federally Qualified: [ ]
Forprofit: [ ]   Not-For-Profit: [ ]
Model Type:
Accreditation: [ ] AAPPO [ ] JACHO [ ] NCQA [ ] URAC
Plan Type: Specialty PPO
Total Enrollment:
  2001: 0   2004: 821   2007: 0
  2002: 595   2005:
  2003: 703   2006: 718

SERVICE AREA:
Nationwide: N
  NJ;

TYPE OF COVERAGE:
Commercial: [Y] Individual: [Y] FEHBP: [ ] Indemnity: [ ]
Medicare: [ ] Medicaid: [ ] Supplemental Medicare: [ ]
Tricare   [ ]

PRODUCTS OFFERED:
Product Name: Type:
Low Cost Dental Insurance   DPO/PPO

PLAN BENEFITS:
Alternative Medicine: [ ]   Behavioral Health: [ ]
Chiropractic: [ ]   Dental: [X]
Home Care: [ ]   Inpatient SNF: [ ]
Long-Term Care: [ ]   Pharm. Mail Order: [ ]
Physical Therapy: [ ]   Podiatry: [ ]
Psychiatric: [ ]   Transplant: [ ]
Vision: [ ]   Wellness: [ ]
Workers' Comp: [ ]
Other Benefits:

NEW JERSEY   Managed Care Organization Profiles

AVETA INC

173 Bridge Plaza North
Fort Lee, NJ 07024
Phone: 201-346-8400 Fax: 201-969-2339 Toll-Free:
Web site: www.aveta.com
MAILING ADDRESS:
    AVETA INC
    173 Bridge Plaza North
    Fort Lee, NJ 07024

KEY EXECUTIVES:
Chairman of the Board/Chief Executive Officer .... Daniel E Straus
President .... Richard Shinto
Executive VP, Chief Operating Officer .... Robert G. Torricelli
Vice President & Corporate Controller .... Lawrence M. Dunn
Senior Vice President and General Counsel .... Jonathan P. Rich

COMPANY PROFILE:
Parent Company Name:
Doing Business As:
Year Founded: Federally Qualified: [ ]
Forprofit: [Y]   Not-For-Profit: [ ]
Model Type:
Accreditation: [ ] AAPPO [ ] JACHO [ ] NCQA [ ] URAC
Plan Type: HMO
Total Revenue   2005:   938,200,000   2006:
Net Income   2005:   12,137,000   2006:
Total Enrollment:
    2001: 0   2004: 99,100   2007: 0
    2002: 0   2005: 130,500
    2003: 0   2006:
Medical Loss Ratio: 2005: 80.10   2006:
Administrative Expense Ratio: 2005: 11.00   2006:
SERVICE AREA:
Nationwide: N
    CA; IL; NJ; PR;
TYPE OF COVERAGE:
Commercial: [ ] Individual: [ ] FEHBP: [ ] Indemnity: [ ]
Medicare: [Y] Medicaid: [ ] Supplemental Medicare: [ ]
Tricare   [ ]

CHN SOLUTIONS

3525 Quakerbridge Rd
Hamilton, NJ 08619
Phone: 609-631-0474 Fax: 609-584-8052 Toll-Free: 800-225-4246
Web site: www.chn.com
MAILING ADDRESS:
    CHN SOLUTIONS
    3525 Quakerbridge Rd
    Hamilton, NJ 08619

KEY EXECUTIVES:
Chief Executive Officer/President .... Leonard V Weinman
Chief Financial Officer .... Mary Ann Nagy
Chief Medical Officer .... M Leonide Sipski
VP of Sales .... G Roger Eiler
Credentialing Manager .... Nancy Provenzano
Public Relations Director .... Missy Pudimott
Director, Network Operations .... Cara Ianniello
Senior VP, Network Operations .... Dick Heyman
Human Resources Director .... Randy Defazio
Credentialing Manager .... Nancy Provenzano

COMPANY PROFILE:
Parent Company Name: Selective Insurance Company
Doing Business As: Consumer Health Network
Year Founded: 1988   Federally Qualified: [ ]
Forprofit: [Y]   Not-For-Profit: [ ]
Model Type: NETWORK
Accreditation: [ ] AAPPO [ ] JACHO [ ] NCQA [X] URAC
Plan Type: PPO
SERVICE AREA:
Nationwide: N
    CT; NJ; NY;
TYPE OF COVERAGE:
Commercial: [Y] Individual: [Y] FEHBP: [ ] Indemnity: [ ]
Medicare: [ ] Medicaid: [ ] Supplemental Medicare: [ ]
Tricare   [ ]

PLAN BENEFITS:
Alternative Medicine: [ ]   Behavioral Health: [X]
Chiropractic: [X]   Dental: [ ]
Home Care: [X]   Inpatient SNF: [X]
Long-Term Care: [ ]   Pharm. Mail Order: [ ]
Physical Therapy: [X]   Podiatry: [X]
Psychiatric: [X]   Transplant: [X]
Vision: [ ]   Wellness: [X]
Workers' Comp: [X]
Other Benefits: Student Accident, MRI

CIGNA DENTAL HEALTH OF NEW JERSEY INC

1571 Sawgrass Corporate Pkwy
Sunrise, FL 33323
Phone: 954-514-6600 Fax: 954-514-6905 Toll-Free: 800-367-1037
Web site: www.cigna.com/dental
MAILING ADDRESS:
    CIGNA DENTAL HEALTH OF NJ INC
    1571 Sawgrass Corporate Pkwy
    Sunrise, FL 33323

KEY EXECUTIVES:
President .... Karen S Rohan

COMPANY PROFILE:
Parent Company Name: CIGNA Dental Health Inc
Doing Business As: CIGNA Dental
Year Founded: 1983   Federally Qualified: [N]
Forprofit: [Y]   Not-For-Profit: [ ]
Model Type:
Accreditation: [ ] AAPPO [ ] JACHO [ ] NCQA [ ] URAC
Plan Type: Specialty PPO
Total Revenue   2005:   2006: 12,528,372
Net Income   2005:   2006:
Total Enrollment:
    2001: 0   2004: 0   2007: 0
    2002: 0   2005:
    2003: 0   2006: 80,308
SERVICE AREA:
Nationwide: N
    NJ;
TYPE OF COVERAGE:
Commercial: [Y] Individual: [ ] FEHBP: [ ] Indemnity: [ ]
Medicare: [ ] Medicaid: [ ] Supplemental Medicare: [ ]
Tricare   [ ]
PRODUCTS OFFERED:
Product Name: Type:
Cigna Dental Health of NJ   Specialty HMO
PLAN BENEFITS:
Alternative Medicine: [ ]   Behavioral Health: [ ]
Chiropractic: [ ]   Dental: [X]
Home Care: [ ]   Inpatient SNF: [ ]
Long-Term Care: [ ]   Pharm. Mail Order: [ ]
Physical Therapy: [ ]   Podiatry: [ ]
Psychiatric: [ ]   Transplant: [ ]
Vision: [ ]   Wellness: [ ]
Workers' Comp: [ ]
Other Benefits:

CIGNA HEALTHCARE OF NEW YORK AND NEW JERSEY

499 Washington Blvd
Jersey City, NJ 07310
Phone: 201-533-7000 Fax: 201-533-7164 Toll-Free:
Web site: www.cigna.com
MAILING ADDRESS:
    CIGNA HEALTHCARE OF NY AND NJ
    499 Washington Blvd
    Jersey City, NJ 07310

KEY EXECUTIVES:
President/General Manager .... Charles Catalano
Executive VP, Chief Financial Officer .... Michael W Bell
Medical Director .... Dan Nichol, MD
MIS Director .... Charlene Renollet
Director, Provider Services .... Tom Garvey

Managed Care Organization Profiles — NEW JERSEY

PRODUCTS OFFERED:
Product Name:	Type:
AmeriChoice Personal Care Plus	Medicare
AmeriChoice Medicaid	Medicaid

Comments:
Purchased Liberty Health Plan Inc.

AMERIHEALTH INSURANCE COMPANY - NJ NORTH

485 C US Hwy 1 S Ste 300
Iselin, NJ 08830
Phone: 732-726-6700 Fax: 732-726-6753 Toll-Free:
Web site: www.amerihealth.com

MAILING ADDRESS:
 AMERIHEALTH INS CO - NJ NORTH
 485 C US Hwy 1 S Ste 300
 Iselin, NJ 08830

KEY EXECUTIVES:
Chief Executive Officer .... *William F Haggett*
Chief Financial Officer .... *Marty Brill*
Regional Medical Director .... *Allan Goldstein, MD*
VP of Sales & Marketing .... *Susan Sendlewski*

COMPANY PROFILE:
Parent Company Name: Independence Blue Cross
Doing Business As: AmeriHealth HMO Inc
Year Founded: Federally Qualified: [ ]
Forprofit: [Y]   Not-For-Profit: [ ]
Model Type:
Accreditation: [ ] AAPPO [ ] JACHO [X] NCQA [ ] URAC
Plan Type: HMO, PPO, POS

SERVICE AREA:
Nationwide: N
 NJ;

TYPE OF COVERAGE:
Commercial: [Y] Individual: [ ] FEHBP: [ ] Indemnity: [ ]
Medicare: [Y] Medicaid: [Y] Supplemental Medicare: [ ]
Tricare   [ ]

PRODUCTS OFFERED:
Product Name:	Type:
Amerihealth HMO	HMO
Personal Choice	PPO
Amerihealth 65	Medicare
Amerihealth POS	POS
Amerihealth CMM	Traditional

Comments:
For enrollment figures, see AmeriHealth HMO Inc-NJ South.

AMERIHEALTH INSURANCE COMPANY - NJ SOUTH

8000 Midlantic Dr Ste 333
Mt Laurel, NJ 08054-1560
Phone: 856-778-6500 Fax: 856-778-6550 Toll-Free: 800-454-7651
Web site: www.amerihealth.com

MAILING ADDRESS:
 AMERIHEALTH INS CO - NJ SOUTH
 8000 Midlantic Dr Ste 333
 Mt Laurel, NJ 08054-1560

KEY EXECUTIVES:
Chief Executive Officer/President .... *William F Haggett*
Chief Financial Officer .... *Marty Brill*
Regional Medical Director .... *Allan Goldstein, MD*
VP of Sales & Marketing .... *Susan Sendlewski*

COMPANY PROFILE:
Parent Company Name: Independence Blue Cross
Doing Business As: AmeriHealth HMO Inc
Year Founded: 1976   Federally Qualified: [N]
Forprofit: [Y]   Not-For-Profit: [ ]
Model Type: IPA
Accreditation: [ ] AAPPO [X] JACHO [X] NCQA [X] URAC
Plan Type: HMO, PPO, POS
Primary Physicians: 20,161   Physician Specialists:
Hospitals:

Total Revenue: 2005: 424,555,000 2006: 229,670,505
Net Income   2005: -9,800   2006:
Total Enrollment:
 2001: 156,666   2004: 234,038   2007: 96,024
 2002: 172,758   2005: 126,098
 2003: 138,193   2006: 114,719
Medical Loss Ratio: 2005: 89.70   2006: 78.80
Administrative Expense Ratio: 2005: 14.30   2006:

SERVICE AREA:
Nationwide: N
 DE; NJ; PA; (Philadelphia- metro area);

TYPE OF COVERAGE:
Commercial: [Y] Individual: [Y] FEHBP: [ ] Indemnity: [ ]
Medicare: [Y] Medicaid: [Y] Supplemental Medicare: [ ]
Tricare   [ ]

PRODUCTS OFFERED:
Product Name:	Type:
Amerihealth HMO	HMO
Personal Choice	PPO
Amerihealth 65	Medicare
Amerihealth POS	POS
Amerihealth CMM	Traditional

PLAN BENEFITS:
Alternative Medicine:	[ ]	Behavioral Health:	[ ]
Chiropractic:	[X]	Dental:	[X]
Home Care:	[X]	Inpatient SNF:	[X]
Long-Term Care:	[ ]	Pharm. Mail Order:	[X]
Physical Therapy:	[X]	Podiatry:	[X]
Psychiatric:	[X]	Transplant:	[X]
Vision:	[X]	Wellness:	[X]
Workers' Comp:	[ ]		

Other Benefits:

ATLANTICARE HEALTH PLANS INC

1001 S Grand St
Hammonton, NJ 08037-0941
Phone: 800-272-5995 Fax: 609-567-5079 Toll-Free: 800-272-5995
Web site: www.atlanticare.org

MAILING ADDRESS:
 ATLANTICARE HEALTH PLANS INC
 1001 S Grand St
 Hammonton, NJ 08037-0941

KEY EXECUTIVES:
Chief Executive Officer/President .... *Pat Koeling*
Chief Financial Officer .... *Pat Koeling*
Medical Director .... *Henry Wu, MD*

COMPANY PROFILE:
Parent Company Name: Horizon BC/BS NJ&AtlantiCare Hlth System
Doing Business As:
Year Founded: 1994   Federally Qualified: [N]
Forprofit: [ ]   Not-For-Profit: [Y]
Model Type: IPA
Accreditation: [ ] AAPPO [ ] JACHO [ ] NCQA [ ] URAC
Plan Type: PPO, TPA
Primary Physicians: 4,000   Physician Specialists:
Hospitals: 36
Total Enrollment:
 2001: 3,968   2004: 0   2007: 0
 2002: 198   2005:
 2003: 60,000 2006:

SERVICE AREA:
Nationwide: N
 NJ (Atlantic, Cape May, Cumberland);

TYPE OF COVERAGE:
Commercial: [Y] Individual: [ ] FEHBP: [ ] Indemnity: [ ]
Medicare: [ ] Medicaid: [ ] Supplemental Medicare: [ ]
Tricare   [ ]

PRODUCTS OFFERED:
Product Name:	Type:
AtlantiCare PPO	PPO

PLAN BENEFITS:
Alternative Medicine:	[ ]	Behavioral Health:	[X]
Chiropractic:	[X]	Dental:	[X]
Home Care:	[X]	Inpatient SNF:	[X]
Long-Term Care:	[X]	Pharm. Mail Order:	[X]
Physical Therapy:	[X]	Podiatry:	[X]
Psychiatric:	[X]	Transplant:	[X]
Vision:	[X]	Wellness:	[X]
Workers' Comp:	[ ]		

Other Benefits: X

NEW JERSEY — Managed Care Organization Profiles

ALIGNIS INC - HEALTHWAYS

1 Kalisa Way Ste 210
Paramus, NJ 07652
Phone: 201-322-0413 Fax: 201-322-0425 Toll-Free: 800-863-2932
Web site: www.alignis.com

MAILING ADDRESS:
ALIGNIS INC - HEALTHWAYS
1 Kalisa Way Ste 210
Paramus, NJ 07652

KEY EXECUTIVES:
Chief Executive Officer/President .... William P Dorney, DC
Controller .... Lori Piccioni
Medical Director .... William P Dorney, DC
VP of Operations .... Vincent J Love
Chief Marketing Officer .... Peter A Day
Chief Technology Officer .... Amrish Macedo

COMPANY PROFILE:
Parent Company Name: American Wholehealth Networks
Doing Business As:
Year Founded: 1994   Federally Qualified: [ ]
Forprofit: [Y]   Not-For-Profit: [ ]
Model Type: MIXED
Accreditation: [ ] AAPPO [ ] JACHO [ ] NCQA [X] URAC
Plan Type: Specialty HMO, Specialty PPO, POS, TPA, U

SERVICE AREA:
Nationwide: N
AZ; CA; FL; MN; NJ; NY; NV; PA;

TYPE OF COVERAGE:
Commercial: [Y] Individual: [Y] FEHBP: [ ] Indemnity: [ ]
Medicare: [Y] Medicaid: [Y] Supplemental Medicare: [ ]
Tricare   [ ]

PLAN BENEFITS:
Alternative Medicine: [X]   Behavioral Health: [ ]
Chiropractic: [X]   Dental: [ ]
Home Care: [ ]   Inpatient SNF: [ ]
Long-Term Care: [ ]   Pharm. Mail Order: [ ]
Physical Therapy: [ ]   Podiatry: [X]
Psychiatric: [ ]   Transplant: [ ]
Vision: [ ]   Wellness: [ ]
Workers' Comp: [X]
Other Benefits:

Comments:
Alignis Inc is a privately held specialty managed care company focused on organizing and managing musculoskeletal providers.

AMERIGROUP NEW JERSEY INC

399 Thornall St 9th Fl
Edison, NJ 08818
Phone: 732-452-6000 Fax: 732-452-0407 Toll-Free:
Web site: www.amerigroupcorp.com

MAILING ADDRESS:
AMERIGROUP NEW JERSEY INC
399 Thornall St 9th Fl
Edison, NJ 08818

KEY EXECUTIVES:
Chief Executive Officer/President .... Peter D Haytaian, Esq
Chief Financial Officer .... E Paul Dunn Jr
Medical Director .... Eric Berman, MD
Senior VP, Medical Management .... Janet Pizzelanti
Chief Information Officer .... Leon A Root, Jr
Marketing Director .... Adam Mintz
Director, Provider Services .... Patricia Warren

COMPANY PROFILE:
Parent Company Name: Amerigroup Corporation
Doing Business As: Americaid Community Care
Year Founded: 1995   Federally Qualified: [N]
Forprofit: [Y]   Not-For-Profit: [ ]
Model Type: MIXED
Accreditation: [ ] AAPPO [ ] JACHO [ ] NCQA [ ] URAC
Plan Type: HMO
Primary Physicians: 8,804   Physician Specialists:
Hospitals:
Total Revenue: 2005:   2006: 234,485,258
Net Income   2005:   2006:
Total Enrollment:
  2001: 87,789   2004: 105,575   2007: 98,763
  2002: 99,024   2005: 108,922
  2003: 99,478   2006: 101,924
Medical Loss Ratio: 2005:   2006: 73.60
Administrative Expense Ratio: 2005:   2006:

SERVICE AREA:
Nationwide: N
NJ;

TYPE OF COVERAGE:
Commercial: [ ] Individual: [ ] FEHBP: [ ] Indemnity: [ ]
Medicare: [ ] Medicaid: [Y] Supplemental Medicare: [ ]
Tricare   [ ]

PRODUCTS OFFERED:
Product Name: Type:
Amerigroup   Medicaid

PLAN BENEFITS:
Alternative Medicine: [ ]   Behavioral Health: [ ]
Chiropractic: [X]   Dental: [X]
Home Care: [X]   Inpatient SNF: [X]
Long-Term Care: [ ]   Pharm. Mail Order: [ ]
Physical Therapy: [X]   Podiatry: [X]
Psychiatric: [ ]   Transplant: [X]
Vision: [X]   Wellness: [X]
Workers' Comp: [ ]
Other Benefits:

Comments:
49 States including Washington DC (Not NY). Formerly Americaid New Jersey.

AMERICHOICE OF NEW JERSEY

4 Gateway Center 13th Fl
Newark, NJ 07102
Phone: 973-297-5500 Fax: 973-297-5580 Toll-Free: 800-941-4647
Web site: www.americhoice.com

MAILING ADDRESS:
AMERICHOICE OF NJ
PO Box 200098
Newark, NJ 07102

KEY EXECUTIVES:
Chief Executive Officer/President .... Pat Celli
Medical Director .... Donald Wernsing, MD
Pharmacy Director .... Marion Pardes
Marketing Director .... Allison Manning
MIS Manager .... Rash Patel

COMPANY PROFILE:
Parent Company Name: UnitedHealth Group
Doing Business As: Managed Healthcare Systems of NJ
Year Founded: 1995   Federally Qualified: [N]
Forprofit: [Y]   Not-For-Profit: [ ]
Model Type: IPA
Accreditation: [ ] AAPPO [ ] JACHO [ ] NCQA [ ] URAC
Plan Type: HMO
Primary Physicians: 10,375   Physician Specialists:
Hospitals:
Total Revenue: 2005:   2006: 477,742,825
Net Income   2005:   2006:
Total Enrollment:
  2001: 195,348   2004: 167,332   2007: 208,871
  2002: 179,341   2005: 177,039
  2003: 175,405   2006: 204,210
Medical Loss Ratio: 2005:   2006: 83.00
Administrative Expense Ratio: 2005:   2006:

SERVICE AREA:
Nationwide: N
NJ (Atlantic, Bergen, Burlington, Camden, Cape May, Cumberland, Essex, Gloucester; Hudson, Hunterdon, Mercer, Middlesex, Monmouth, Morris, Ocean, Passaic, Salem, Somerset, Sussex, Union, Warren);

TYPE OF COVERAGE:
Commercial: [Y] Individual: [ ] FEHBP: [ ] Indemnity: [ ]
Medicare: [ ] Medicaid: [Y] Supplemental Medicare: [ ]
Tricare   [ ]

Managed Care Organization Profiles **NEW JERSEY**

AETNA DENTAL INC - NEW JERSEY

55 Lane Rd
Fairfield, NJ 07004
Phone: 973-244-3900 Fax: 973-244-3990 Toll-Free: 800-852-0629
Web site: www.aetna.com
MAILING ADDRESS:
    AETNA DENTAL INC - NJ
    55 Lane Rd
    Fairfield, NJ 07004

KEY EXECUTIVES:
Chairman of the Board .... Ronald A Williams

COMPANY PROFILE:
Parent Company Name: Aetna Inc
Doing Business As:
Year Founded: 1974   Federally Qualified: [Y]
Forprofit: [Y]   Not-For-Profit: [ ]
Model Type: IPA
Accreditation: [ ] AAPPO [ ] JACHO [ ] NCQA [ ] URAC
Plan Type: Specialty HMO, Specialty PPO, CDHP, HDHP, HSA
Total Revenue: 2005:   12,212,000   2006:   13,265,730
Net Income   2005:   2006:
Total Enrollment:
    2001: 726,969   2004: 680,141   2007:
    2002: 530,549   2005: 204,030
    2003: 548,721   2006: 203,970
Medical Loss Ratio: 2005: 91.80   2006: 86.80
Administrative Expense Ratio: 2005:   2006:

SERVICE AREA:
Nationwide:
    NJ;

TYPE OF COVERAGE:
Commercial: [Y] Individual: [ ] FEHBP: [ ] Indemnity: [ ]
Medicare: [Y] Medicaid: [Y] Supplemental Medicare: [ ]
Tricare   [ ]

PLAN BENEFITS:
Alternative Medicine: [ ]   Behavioral Health: [ ]
Chiropractic: [ ]   Dental: [Y]
Home Care: [ ]   Inpatient SNF: [ ]
Long-Term Care: [ ]   Pharm. Mail Order: [ ]
Physical Therapy: [ ]   Podiatry: [ ]
Psychiatric: [ ]   Transplant: [ ]
Vision: [ ]   Wellness: [ ]
Workers' Comp: [ ]
Other Benefits:

AETNA INC - NEW JERSEY

55 Lane Rd
Fairfield, NJ 07004
Phone: 973-575-5600 Fax: 973-244-3990 Toll-Free: 800-852-0629
Web site: www.aetna.com
MAILING ADDRESS:
    AETNA INC - NJ
    55 Lane Rd
    Fairfield, NJ 07004

KEY EXECUTIVES:
Chairman of the Board/Chief Executive Officer .... Ronald A Williams
President .... Mark T Bertolini
Executive VP, Finance .... Joseph M Zubretsky

COMPANY PROFILE:
Parent Company Name: Aetna Inc
Doing Business As: Aetna Inc
Year Founded: 1975   Federally Qualified: [Y]
Forprofit: [Y]   Not-For-Profit: [ ]
Model Type: IPA
Accreditation: [ ] AAPPO [X] JACHO [X] NCQA [X] URAC
Plan Type: HMO, PPO, POS, CDHP
Total Enrollment:
    2001: 0   2004: 680,141   2007: 478,014
    2002: 0   2005: 716,682
    2003: 548,721   2006: 543,887

SERVICE AREA:
Nationwide: N
    NJ;

TYPE OF COVERAGE:
Commercial: [Y] Individual: [ ] FEHBP: [ ] Indemnity: [ ]
Medicare: [ ] Medicaid: [ ] Supplemental Medicare: [ ]
Tricare   [ ]

PLAN BENEFITS:
Alternative Medicine: [ ]   Behavioral Health: [X]
Chiropractic: [X]   Dental: [X]
Home Care: [ ]   Inpatient SNF: [ ]
Long-Term Care: [ ]   Pharm. Mail Order: [ ]
Physical Therapy: [ ]   Podiatry: [ ]
Psychiatric: [X]   Transplant: [X]
Vision: [X]   Wellness: [X]
Workers' Comp: [X]
Other Benefits: AD&D, Life, LTD, Emp
Comments:
See Aetna Healthcare NJ Mt Laurel for enrollment figures.

AETNA INC - NEW JERSEY

8000 Mid Atlantic Dr Ste 100N
Mt Laurel, NJ 08054
Phone: 856-222-5560 Fax: 856-727-8490 Toll-Free:
Web site: www.aetna.com
MAILING ADDRESS:
    AETNA INC - NJ
    8000 Mid Atlantic Dr Ste 100N
    Mt Laurel, NJ 08054

KEY EXECUTIVES:
Chairman of the Board/Chief Executive Officer .... Ronald A Williams
Executive VP, Finance .... Joseph M Zubretsky
Mid-Atlantic Regional Medical Director .... William Fried, MD
Chief Information Officer .... Margaret McCarthy
Marketing Director .... Robert M Mead
General Manager .... Russell Dickhart
Director, Provider Services .... Laurie Kleman

COMPANY PROFILE:
Parent Company Name: Aetna Inc
Doing Business As: Aetna Inc
Year Founded: 1974   Federally Qualified: [Y]
Forprofit: [Y]   Not-For-Profit: [ ]
Model Type: IPA
Accreditation: [ ] AAPPO [ ] JACHO [X] NCQA [X] URAC
Plan Type: HMO, PPO, POS, CDHP, HDHP, HSA,
Primary Physicians: 16,443   Physician Specialists:
Hospitals:
Total Revenue: 2005:   2006: 2,341,619,279
Net Income   2005:   2006:   75,912,000
Total Enrollment:
    2001: 725,969   2004: 680,141   2007: 521,320
    2002: 530,549   2005: 716,682
    2003: 548,721   2006: 543,887
Medical Loss Ratio: 2005:   2006: 80.90
Administrative Expense Ratio: 2005:   2006:

SERVICE AREA:
Nationwide: N
    NJ;

TYPE OF COVERAGE:
Commercial: [Y] Individual: [ ] FEHBP: [ ] Indemnity: [ ]
Medicare: [Y] Medicaid: [Y] Supplemental Medicare: [ ]
Tricare   [ ]

PRODUCTS OFFERED:
Product Name: Type:
Golden Medicare Plan   Medicare
Aetna US Healthcare   HMO
CONSUMER-DRIVEN PRODUCTS
Aetna Life Insurance Co   HSA Company
Aetna HealthFund HSA   HSA Product
Aetna   HSA Administrator
Aetna HealthFund   Consumer-Driven Health Plan
PPO I; PPO II   High Deductible Health Plan

PLAN BENEFITS:
Alternative Medicine: [ ]   Behavioral Health: [X]
Chiropractic: [X]   Dental: [X]
Home Care: [ ]   Inpatient SNF: [ ]
Long-Term Care: [ ]   Pharm. Mail Order: [ ]
Physical Therapy: [ ]   Podiatry: [X]
Psychiatric: [X]   Transplant: [X]
Vision: [X]   Wellness: [X]
Workers' Comp: [X]
Other Benefits: AD&D, Life, LTD, STD
Comments:
Formerly Aetna Health Plans - New Jersey.

NEW HAMPSHIRE

PLAN BENEFITS:
Alternative Medicine:	[ ]	Behavioral Health:	[ ]
Chiropractic:	[ ]	Dental:	[X]
Home Care:	[ ]	Inpatient SNF:	[ ]
Long-Term Care:	[ ]	Pharm. Mail Order:	[ ]
Physical Therapy:	[ ]	Podiatry:	[ ]
Psychiatric:	[ ]	Transplant:	[ ]
Vision:	[ ]	Wellness:	[ ]
Workers' Comp:	[ ]		

Other Benefits:

HARVARD PILGRAM HEALTH CARE OF NEW ENGLAND

Go to the State of Massachusetts.

MVP HEALTH PLAN OF NEW HAMPSHIRE

One Club Acre Lane
Bedford, NH 03110
Phone: 603-6477181   Fax: 603-647-9607   Toll-Free: 866-687-6364
Web site: www.mvphealthcare.com

MAILING ADDRESS:
MVP HEALTH PLAN OF NEW HAMPSHIRE
One Club Acre Lane
Bedford, NH 03110

KEY EXECUTIVES:
Chief Executive Officer/President .... David W Oliker
Vice President - New Hampshire .... Chris Henchey

COMPANY PROFILE:
Parent Company Name: MVP Health Plan
Doing Business As:
Year Founded: 2004   Federally Qualified: [Y]
Forprofit: [Y]   Not-For-Profit: [Y]
Model Type:
Accreditation: [ ] AAPPO [ ] JACHO [X] NCQA [ ] URAC
Plan Type: HMO, PPO, ASO, EPO, POS, TPA, HDHP, HSA
Total Revenue: 2005:   2006:   1,701,394
Net Income   2005:   2006:
Total Enrollment:
    2001:   2004:   2006:
    2002:   2005:
    2003:   2006:
Medical Loss Ratio: 2005:   2006: 79.80
Administrative Expense Ratio: 2005:   2006:

SERVICE AREA:
Nationwide: N
NH;

TYPE OF COVERAGE:
Commercial: [Y] Individual: [Y] FEHBP: [ ] Indemnity: [ ]
Medicare: [ ] Medicaid: [Y]   Supplemental Medicare: [ ]
Tricare   [ ]

PRODUCTS OFFERED:
Product Name:	Type:
HMO Basix	HMO
HMO Options	HMO
TriVantage	Preferred EPO
	Preferred PPO
MVP Gold	Medicare

PLAN BENEFITS:
Alternative Medicine:	[ ]	Behavioral Health:	[ ]
Chiropractic:	[X]	Dental:	[X]
Home Care:	[X]	Inpatient SNF:	[X]
Long-Term Care:	[ ]	Pharm. Mail Order:	[ ]
Physical Therapy:	[X]	Podiatry:	[ ]
Psychiatric:	[X]	Transplant:	[X]
Vision:	[X]	Wellness:	[X]
Workers' Comp:	[ ]		

Other Benefits:

Managed Care Organization Profiles — NEW HAMPSHIRE

ANTHEM BLUE CROSS/BLUE SHIELD OF NEW HAMPSHIRE

3000 Goffs Falls Rd
Manchester, NH 03111-0001
Phone: 603-695-7000 Fax: 603-695-7304 Toll-Free:
Web site: www.anthembcbsnh.com

MAILING ADDRESS:
ANTHEM BLUE CROSS/BLUE SHIELD
3000 Goffs Falls Rd
Manchester, NH 03111-0001

KEY EXECUTIVES:
President .... Lisa M Guertin
Chief Medical Officer .... Elizabeth Malko, MD
Pharmacy Director .... Robert Lenza
Chief Information Officer .... Chris Dugan
Director of Network Management .... Robert J Noonan
VP Health Care Management - Northeast .... Richard D Lynch

COMPANY PROFILE:
Parent Company Name: WellPoint Inc
Doing Business As: Matthew Thornton Health Plans Inc
Year Founded: 1942   Federally Qualified: [N]
Forprofit: [ ]   Not-For-Profit: [Y]
Model Type: MIXED
Accreditation: [ ] AAPPO [ ] JACHO [X] NCQA [X] URAC
Plan Type: HMO, PPO, POS, ASO, TPA, HDHP, HSA,
Total Revenue: 2005:   2006:   430,811,229
Net Income   2005:   2006:
Total Enrollment:
  2001: 47,587   2004: 117,286   2007: 0
  2002: 88,632   2005:
  2003: 101,801   2006:
Medical Loss Ratio: 2005:   2006: 84.40
Administrative Expense Ratio: 2005:   2006:

SERVICE AREA:
Nationwide: N
  NH;

TYPE OF COVERAGE:
Commercial: [Y] Individual: [Y] FEHBP: [ ] Indemnity: [ ]
Medicare: [ ] Medicaid: [Y] Supplemental Medicare: [Y]
Tricare   [ ]

CONSUMER-DRIVEN PRODUCTS
JP Morgan Chase   HSA Company
Anthem ByDesign HSA   HSA Product
JP Morgan Chase   HSA Administrator
Blue Access Saver   Consumer-Driven Health Plan
Blue Access Economy Plans PPO High Deductible Health Plan

PLAN BENEFITS:
Alternative Medicine: [ ]   Behavioral Health: [ ]
Chiropractic: [X]   Dental: [ ]
Home Care: [X]   Inpatient SNF: [X]
Long-Term Care: [ ]   Pharm. Mail Order: [X]
Physical Therapy: [X]   Podiatry: [X]
Psychiatric: [X]   Transplant: [X]
Vision: [X]   Wellness: [X]
Workers' Comp: [X]
Other Benefits:

CIGNA HEALTHCARE OF NEW HAMPSHIRE

Two College Park Dr
Hooksett, NH 03106
Phone: 603-268-7000 Fax: 603-268-7981 Toll-Free: 800-531-4584
Web site: www.cigna.com

MAILING ADDRESS:
CIGNA HEALTHCARE OF NH
Two College Park Dr
Hooksett, NH 03106

KEY EXECUTIVES:
Chief Executive Officer/President .... Donald M Curry
Medical Director .... Jeffrey Kang, MD

COMPANY PROFILE:
Parent Company Name: CIGNA Corporation
Doing Business As:
Year Founded: 1985   Federally Qualified: [Y]
Forprofit: [Y]   Not-For-Profit: [ ]
Model Type: IPA
Accreditation: [ ] AAPPO [ ] JACHO [X] NCQA [X] URAC
Plan Type: HMO, PPO, POS, CDHP, HDHP, HSA, FSA, HRA
Total Revenue: 2005:   2006:   138,596,101
Net Income   2005:   2006:
Total Enrollment:
  2001: 0   2004: 49,209   2007: 0
  2002: 94,222   2005:
  2003: 69,585   2006:
Medical Loss Ratio: 2005:   2006: 91.20
Administrative Expense Ratio: 2005:   2006:

SERVICE AREA:
Nationwide: N
  MA (Essex, Franklin, Middlesex, Norfolk, Worcester); NH;

TYPE OF COVERAGE:
Commercial: [Y] Individual: [ ] FEHBP: [ ] Indemnity: [ ]
Medicare: [Y] Medicaid: [Y] Supplemental Medicare: [ ]
Tricare   [ ]

PRODUCTS OFFERED:
Product Name: Type:
Healthsource for Seniors   Medicare

CONSUMER-DRIVEN PRODUCTS
JP Morgan Chase   HSA Company
CIGNA Choice Fund   HSA Product
                               HSA Administrator
Open Access Plus   Consumer-Driven Health Plan
PPO   High Deductible Health Plan

PLAN BENEFITS:
Alternative Medicine: [ ]   Behavioral Health: [X]
Chiropractic: [X]   Dental: [X]
Home Care: [X]   Inpatient SNF: [X]
Long-Term Care: [X]   Pharm. Mail Order: [X]
Physical Therapy: [X]   Podiatry: [X]
Psychiatric: [X]   Transplant: [X]
Vision: [X]   Wellness: [X]
Workers' Comp: [X]
Other Benefits:

DELTA DENTAL PLAN OF NEW HAMPSHIRE

One Delta Drive
Concord, NH 03302
Phone: 603-223-1000 Fax: 603-223-1199 Toll-Free: 800-537-1715
Web site: www.nedelta.com

MAILING ADDRESS:
DELTA DENTAL PLAN OF NH
PO Box 2002
Concord, NH 03302

KEY EXECUTIVES:
Chairman of the Board .... David Hedstrom, DDS
Chief Executive Officer/President .... Thomas Raffio, FLMI
Chief Financial Officer .... Helen T Biglin
Senior VP, Operations .... William H Lambrukos
VP, Marketing .... Gene Emery
MIS Director .... Michael D Bourbeau
VP, Human Resources .... Connie M Roy-Czyzowski
General Counsel .... Kenneth L Robinson Jr, Esq

COMPANY PROFILE:
Parent Company Name: Delta Dental Plan Association
Doing Business As:
Year Founded: Federally Qualified: [ ]
Forprofit: [Y]   Not-For-Profit: [ ]
Model Type:
Accreditation: [ ] AAPPO [ ] JACHO [ ] NCQA [ ] URAC
Plan Type: Specialty HMO, Specialty PPO

SERVICE AREA:
Nationwide: N
  ME; NH; VT;

TYPE OF COVERAGE:
Commercial: [Y] Individual: [ ] FEHBP: [ ] Indemnity: [ ]
Medicare: [ ] Medicaid: [ ] Supplemental Medicare: [ ]
Tricare   [ ]

NEVADA

SIERRA HEALTH SERVICES INC-CORPORATE HEADQUARTERS

2724 N Teneya Way
Las Vegas, NV 89128
Phone: 702-242-7000 Fax: 702-242-7915 Toll-Free:
Web site: www.sierrahealth.com

MAILING ADDRESS:
SIERRA HEALTH SERVICES INC.
PO Box 15645
Las Vegas, NV 89128

KEY EXECUTIVES:
Chairman of the Board/Chief Executive Officer . Anthony Marlon, MD
President/Chief Operating Officer .... Jonathan W Bunker
Senior VP, Chief Financial Officer .... Marc R Briggs
VP, Medical Affairs/CMO ....Joseph A Kaufman, MD
VP, Chief Information Officer .... Robert L Schaich
Senior VP, Sales & Marketing.............................. Donald J Giancursio
VP, Provider Relations .... Scott G Cassano
VP, Human Resources ....Daniel A Kruger
VP, Public & Investor Relations ....Peter O'Neill
Senior VP, Operations.. Darren G D Sivertsen

COMPANY PROFILE:
Parent Company Name: Sierra Health Services Inc
Doing Business As:
Year Founded: 1972   Federally Qualified: [N]
Forprofit: [Y]   Not-For-Profit: [ ]
Model Type: GROUP
Accreditation: [ ] AAPPO [X] JACHO [ ] NCQA [ ] URAC
Plan Type: HMO, PPO, POS, ASO, UR
Total Revenue: 2005:   1,385,040,000   2006:   1,718,892,000
Net Income   2005:   120,020,000   2006:   140,471,000
Total Enrollment:
   2001: 1,282,100   2004: 580,000   2007: 876,800
   2002: 0   2005: 637,900
   2003: 550,000   2006: 838,700

SERVICE AREA:
Nationwide: N
   NV (Las Vegas, Reno); TX (Houston, Dallas, Ft. Worth); AZ (Northern);

TYPE OF COVERAGE:
Commercial: [Y] Individual: [ ]   FEHBP: [Y]   Indemnity: [ ]
Medicare: [Y] Medicaid: [ ]   Supplemental Medicare: [Y]
Tricare   [ ]

PRODUCTS OFFERED:
Product Name:	Type:
Sierra Health & Life	PPO
Senior Dimensions	Medicare
Sierra Choice	POS
Health Plan of Nevada	HMO
Sierra Healthcare Options	UR/ASO
Texas Health Choice LC	HMO
Sierra Military Health Choices	Tricare

PLAN BENEFITS:
Alternative Medicine: [ ]   Behavioral Health: [X]
Chiropractic: [X]   Dental: [X]
Home Care: [X]   Inpatient SNF: [X]
Long-Term Care: [X]   Pharm. Mail Order: [X]
Physical Therapy: [X]   Podiatry: [X]
Psychiatric: [X]   Transplant: [X]
Vision: [X]   Wellness: [X]
Workers' Comp: [ ]
Other Benefits:

Comments:
Acquired Kaiser - Texas.

SUMMERLIN LIFE & HEALTH INSURANCE COMPANY

10600 West Charleston Blvd
Las Vegas, NV 89135
Phone: 702-304-5500 Fax: 702-474-7592 Toll-Free:
Web site: www.summerlinlifeandhealth.com

MAILING ADDRESS:
SUMMERLIN LIFE & HEALTH INS CO
10600 West Charleston Blvd
Las Vegas, NV 89135

KEY EXECUTIVES:
Chief Executive Officer/President .... James D Dyer

COMPANY PROFILE:
Parent Company Name: The i/mX Company
Doing Business As:
Year Founded: 2003   Federally Qualified: [ ]
Forprofit: [Y]   Not-For-Profit: [ ]
Model Type:
Accreditation: [ ] AAPPO [ ] JACHO [ ] NCQA [ ] URAC
Plan Type: PPO, PBM, POS, ASO
Total Enrollment:
   2001: 0   2004: 6,552   2007: 0
   2002: 0   2005:
   2003: 0   2006:

SERVICE AREA:
Nationwide: N
   NV;

TYPE OF COVERAGE:
Commercial: [ ] Individual: [ ]   FEHBP: [ ]   Indemnity: [ ]
Medicare: [ ] Medicaid: [ ]   Supplemental Medicare: [ ]
Tricare   [ ]

UNIVERSAL HEALTH NETWORK - CORPORATE HEADQUARTERS

639 Isbell Rd Ste 400
Reno, NV 89509
Phone: 775-356-1159 Fax: 775-352-8207 Toll-Free: 800-776-6959
Web site: www.uhnppo.com

MAILING ADDRESS:
UNIVERSAL HEALTH NETWORK-CORP
PO Box 30007
Reno, NV 89509

KEY EXECUTIVES:
Vice President .... Mary Hoover
Controller .... Linda Barnes
Medical Director .... Daniel Spogan, MD
Director of Marketing & Business Development .... Jim Kroft
Director of Contracting/Client Relations............... Charmaane Buehrle
Network Management/Human Resources Department ... Cheryl Lyman
Director, Utilization Management .... Gaye Nichols

COMPANY PROFILE:
Parent Company Name: UHS
Doing Business As:
Year Founded: 1991   Federally Qualified: [N]
Forprofit: [Y]   Not-For-Profit: [ ]
Model Type: NETWORK
Accreditation: [ ] AAPPO [ ] JACHO [ ] NCQA [ ] URAC
Plan Type: PPO, EPO, CDHP, HDHP, HSA
Primary Physicians: 1,115   Physician Specialists: 1,617
Hospitals: 31
Total Enrollment:
   2001: 160,000   2004: 0   2007: 0
   2002: 187,000   2005:
   2003: 185,000   2006:

SERVICE AREA:
Nationwide: N
   NV;

TYPE OF COVERAGE:
Commercial: [Y] Individual: [Y]   FEHBP: [ ]   Indemnity: [ ]
Medicare: [ ] Medicaid: [ ]   Supplemental Medicare: [ ]
Tricare   [ ]

PLAN BENEFITS:
Alternative Medicine: [ ]   Behavioral Health: [X]
Chiropractic: [X]   Dental: [ ]
Home Care: [X]   Inpatient SNF: [X]
Long-Term Care: [X]   Pharm. Mail Order: [ ]
Physical Therapy: [X]   Podiatry: [X]
Psychiatric: [X]   Transplant: [X]
Vision: [ ]   Wellness: [ ]
Workers' Comp: [X]
Other Benefits:

Managed Care Organization Profiles **NEVADA**

PACIFICARE OF NEVADA

700 E Warm Springs Rd
Las Vegas, NV 89119-4323
Phone: 702-269-7500 Fax: 702-269-2649 Toll-Free: 800-826-4347
Web site: www.pacificare.com

MAILING ADDRESS:
 PACIFICARE OF NEVADA
 700 E Warm Springs Rd
 Las Vegas, NV 89119-4323

KEY EXECUTIVES:
Chief Executive Officer/Medical Director .... *Bard H Coats, MD*
VP, Commercial Sales .... *Michael E Clark*
VP, Network Management .... *Thomas P Smith*
Director, Commercial Sales .... *Bruce Huyghue*
Business Manager .... *Todd Mays*

COMPANY PROFILE:
Parent Company Name: UnitedHealth Group
Doing Business As:
Year Founded: 1978   Federally Qualified: [Y]
Forprofit: [Y]   Not-For-Profit: [ ]
Model Type: MIXED
Accreditation: [ ] AAPPO [ ] JACHO [X] NCQA [ ] URAC
Plan Type: HMO, PPO, POS, HDHP, HSA,
Primary Physicians: 267   Physician Specialists: 805
Hospitals: 7
Total Revenue: 2005:   2006: 374,461,835
Net Income 2005:   2006:
Total Enrollment:
 2001: 67,000   2004: 72,314   2007: 66,738
 2002: 51,693   2005: 75,679
 2003: 51,031   2006: 79,665
Medical Loss Ratio: 2005:   2006: 84.40
Administrative Expense Ratio: 2005:   2006:

SERVICE AREA:
Nationwide: N
 AZ; NV;

TYPE OF COVERAGE:
Commercial: [Y] Individual: [Y] FEHBP: [ ] Indemnity: [ ]
Medicare: [Y] Medicaid: [ ] Supplemental Medicare: [ ]
Tricare [ ]

PRODUCTS OFFERED:
Product Name:	Type:
Pacificare of Nevada	HMO
Secure Horizons	Medicare
Pacificare of Nevada	PPO

PLAN BENEFITS:
Alternative Medicine: [ ]   Behavioral Health: [X]
Chiropractic: [X]   Dental: [X]
Home Care: [X]   Inpatient SNF: [X]
Long-Term Care: [X]   Pharm. Mail Order: [X]
Physical Therapy: [X]   Podiatry: [X]
Psychiatric: [X]   Transplant: [X]
Vision: [X]   Wellness: [X]
Workers' Comp: [X]
Other Benefits:
Comments:
Formerly FHP Inc.

PPNM'S MASTERCARE NETWORK

1605 Freeport Blvd
Sparks, NV 89431
Phone: 775-359-3732 Fax: 775-359-0162 Toll-Free: 888-283-3687
Web site: www.dentsppo.com

MAILING ADDRESS:
 PPNM'S MASTERCARE NETWORK
 1605 Freeport Blvd
 Sparks, NV 89431

KEY EXECUTIVES:
Chief Executive Officer/Medical Director .... *Joseph Evans, MD*
Chief Financial Officer .... *Nancy Evans*
Marketing Director .... *Diane Neuweiler*

COMPANY PROFILE:
Parent Company Name:
Doing Business As:
Year Founded: 1985   Federally Qualified: [ ]
Forprofit: [Y]   Not-For-Profit: [ ]
Model Type:
Accreditation: [ ] AAPPO [ ] JACHO [ ] NCQA [ ] URAC
Plan Type: Specialty PPO
Primary Physicians: Physician Specialists: 100
Hospitals:

SERVICE AREA:
Nationwide: N
 NV (Northern);

TYPE OF COVERAGE:
Commercial: [Y] Individual: [ ] FEHBP: [ ] Indemnity: [ ]
Medicare: [ ] Medicaid: [ ] Supplemental Medicare: [ ]
Tricare   [ ]

PLAN BENEFITS:
Alternative Medicine: [ ]   Behavioral Health: [ ]
Chiropractic: [ ]   Dental: [X]
Home Care: [ ]   Inpatient SNF: [ ]
Long-Term Care: [ ]   Pharm. Mail Order: [ ]
Physical Therapy: [ ]   Podiatry: [ ]
Psychiatric: [ ]   Transplant: [ ]
Vision: [ ]   Wellness: [ ]
Workers' Comp: [ ]
Other Benefits:

SAINT MARY'S HEALTHFIRST

1510 Meadow Wood Lane
Reno, NV 89502
Phone: 775-770-6230 Fax: 775-770-6253 Toll-Free:
Web site: www.saintmaryshealthplans.com

MAILING ADDRESS:
 SAINT MARY'S HEALTHFIRST
 1510 Meadow Wood Lane
 Reno, NV 89502

KEY EXECUTIVES:
President .... *Lawrence O'Brien*
VP, Chief Financial Officer/Chief Operating .... *M Donald Kowitz*
Medical Director .... *Dennis Schuman, MD*
Manager, Provider Services .... *Kevin Brizendine*
Manager, Health Management .... *Victoria Simmon, RN*
Vice President .... *Jennifer Schultz*
Medical Management .... *Denise Epperson, RN*
Manager, Quality Assurance .... *Barbara Slick, RN*
Director HMO PPO Administration .... *Lois Paynter*
Compliance Specialties/Product Development .... *Scott Heinz*

COMPANY PROFILE:
Parent Company Name: Saint Mary's Health Network
Doing Business As: Saint Mary's Health Plans
Year Founded: 1993   Federally Qualified: [N]
Forprofit: [Y]   Not-For-Profit: [ ]
Model Type: MIXED
Accreditation: [ ] AAPPO [ ] JACHO [X] NCQA [ ] URAC
Plan Type: HMO, PPO, POS, TPA
Primary Physicians: 112   Physician Specialists: 725
Hospitals: 12
Total Revenue: 2005:   2006: 99,777,220
Net Income 2005:   2006:
Total Enrollment:
 2001: 26,661   2004: 30,252   2007: 27,523
 2002: 30,225   2005: 28,185
 2003: 30,217   2006: 43,141
Medical Loss Ratio: 2005:   2006: 79.30
Administrative Expense Ratio: 2005:   2006:

SERVICE AREA:
Nationwide: N
 NV (Carson City, Churchill, Douglas, Elko, Eureka, Humboldt, Lander, Lyon, Mineral, Pershing, Storey, White Pine, Washoe);

TYPE OF COVERAGE:
Commercial: [Y] Individual: [ ] FEHBP: [ ] Indemnity: [ ]
Medicare: [ ] Medicaid: [ ] Supplemental Medicare: [ ]
Tricare   [ ]

NEVADA

NEVADA PACIFIC DENTAL

1432 South Jones Blvd
Las Vegas, NV 89102-1231
Phone: 702-737-8900 Fax: 702-259-0904 Toll-Free: 800-926-0925
Web site: www.nevadapacificdental.com

MAILING ADDRESS:
NEVADA PACIFIC DENTAL
1432 South Jones Blvd
Las Vegas, NV 89102-1231

KEY EXECUTIVES:
Chairman of the Board .... John Gaebel, DDS
Chief Executive Officer .... Randy Brecher
Regional President .... R Dennis Spain, DDS
Dental Director/Quality Assurance Director ... O Guy Humphries, DDS
VP, Marketing .... Jim Fuhrman
Credentialing Manager .... Susy Storms
Privacy Officer/Human Resources Director .... Ellen Willingham
Director, Provider Relations/Network Development ... Tammy Ishibashi
VP, Health Services .... Dan Maher
Regional Vice President .... Ted DeCorte
Client & Member Services Director .... Cathie Davenport

COMPANY PROFILE:
Parent Company Name: PacificDental Benefits Inc (PDBI)
Doing Business As:
Year Founded: 1987   Federally Qualified: [N]
Forprofit: [Y]   Not-For-Profit: [ ]
Model Type:
Accreditation: [ ] AAPPO [ ] JACHO [ ] NCQA [ ] URAC
Plan Type: Specialty HMO, Specialty PPO, POS, ASO, TPA
Total Enrollment:
  2001: 0   2004: 156,625   2007: 0
  2002: 114,880   2005:
  2003: 119,228   2006:

SERVICE AREA:
Nationwide: N
NV;

TYPE OF COVERAGE:
Commercial: [Y] Individual: [ ] FEHBP: [ ] Indemnity: [ ]
Medicare: [ ] Medicaid: [ ] Supplemental Medicare: [ ]
Tricare [ ]

PLAN BENEFITS:
Alternative Medicine: [ ]   Behavioral Health: [ ]
Chiropractic: [ ]   Dental: [X]
Home Care: [ ]   Inpatient SNF: [ ]
Long-Term Care: [ ]   Pharm. Mail Order: [ ]
Physical Therapy: [ ]   Podiatry: [ ]
Psychiatric: [ ]   Transplant: [ ]
Vision: [ ]   Wellness: [ ]
Workers' Comp: [ ]
Other Benefits:

NEVADA PREFERRED PROFESSIONALS

4170 South Decator Blvd A-8
Las Vegas, NV 89103
Phone: 702-384-3366 Fax: 702-384-9781 Toll-Free:
Web site: www.nvpp.com

MAILING ADDRESS:
NEVADA PREFERRED PROFESSIONALS
4170 South Dacator Blvd A-8
Las Vegas, NV 89103

KEY EXECUTIVES:
Vice President .... Mary Hoover
Controller .... Linda Barnes
Director of Marketing & Business Development .... Jim Kroft
Director of Contracting/Client Relations .... Charmaane Buehrle
Network Management/Human Resources Department ... Cheryl Lyman
Director, Utilization Management .... Gaye Nichols

COMPANY PROFILE:
Parent Company Name: UHN/UHS
Doing Business As:
Year Founded: 1982   Federally Qualified: [ ]
Forprofit: [Y]   Not-For-Profit: [ ]
Model Type: NETWORK
Accreditation: [ ] AAPPO [ ] JACHO [ ] NCQA [ ] URAC
Plan Type: PPO, Specialty PPO, EPO
Primary Physicians: 1,168   Physician Specialists: 1,691
Hospitals: 44
Total Enrollment:
  2001: 24,000   2004: 0   2007: 0
  2002: 33,000   2005:
  2003: 33,000   2006:

SERVICE AREA:
Nationwide: N
NV;

TYPE OF COVERAGE:
Commercial: [Y] Individual: [ ] FEHBP: [ ] Indemnity: [ ]
Medicare: [ ] Medicaid: [ ] Supplemental Medicare: [ ]
Tricare [ ]

PLAN BENEFITS:
Alternative Medicine: [X]   Behavioral Health: [ ]
Chiropractic: [X]   Dental: [ ]
Home Care: [X]   Inpatient SNF: [X]
Long-Term Care: [ ]   Pharm. Mail Order: [ ]
Physical Therapy: [X]   Podiatry: [X]
Psychiatric: [X]   Transplant: [X]
Vision: [ ]   Wellness: [ ]
Workers' Comp: [ ]
Other Benefits:

NEVADACARE INC

10600 W Charleston Blvd
Las Vegas, NV 89102-2320
Phone: 702-474-7241 Fax: 702-474-7592 Toll-Free:
Web site: www.nevadacare.com

MAILING ADDRESS:
NEVADACARE INC
10600 W Charleston Blvd
Las Vegas, NV 89102-2320

KEY EXECUTIVES:
Chief Executive Officer/President .... Todd Meek
Chief Financial Officer .... Paul C Carter
Medical Director .... Kenneth Osgood, MD
Marketing Director .... Eddie Burkhart

COMPANY PROFILE:
Parent Company Name: The i/mX Companies
Doing Business As:
Year Founded: 1991   Federally Qualified: [N]
Forprofit: [Y]   Not-For-Profit: [ ]
Model Type: IPA
Accreditation: [ ] AAPPO [ ] JACHO [ ] NCQA [ ] URAC
Plan Type: HMO
Total Revenue: 2005:   128,623,004   2006:   94,908,174
Net Income   2005:   130,587   2006:   -407,774
Total Enrollment:
  2001: 101,048   2004: 168,826   2007: 7,808
  2002: 107,210   2005: 62,679
  2003: 118,229   2006: 20,871
Medical Loss Ratio: 2005: 82.40   2006: 82.30
Administrative Expense Ratio: 2005:   2006:

SERVICE AREA:
Nationwide: N
AZ; CO; IA; IL; NV (Clark, Washoe);

TYPE OF COVERAGE:
Commercial: [Y] Individual: [ ] FEHBP: [ ] Indemnity: [ ]
Medicare: [ ] Medicaid: [Y] Supplemental Medicare: [ ]
Tricare [ ]

PRODUCTS OFFERED:
Product Name: Type:
Nevada Health Solutions   Medicaid
Iowa Health Solutiions   HMO

PLAN BENEFITS:
Alternative Medicine: [ ]   Behavioral Health: [X]
Chiropractic: [X]   Dental: [X]
Home Care: [X]   Inpatient SNF: [X]
Long-Term Care: [X]   Pharm. Mail Order: [X]
Physical Therapy: [X]   Podiatry: [X]
Psychiatric: [X]   Transplant: [X]
Vision: [X]   Wellness: [X]
Workers' Comp: [X]
Other Benefits:

Managed Care Organization Profiles — NEVADA

MAILING ADDRESS:
    HOMETOWN HEALTH PLAN
    830 Harvard Way
    Reno, NV 89502

KEY EXECUTIVES:
Chairman of the Board .... Nazir Ansari
Chief Executive Officer .... Jim Miller
Vice President .... Troy Smith
Finance Director .... Jeff Butcher
Medical Director .... Linda Ash-Jackson, MD
Pharmacy Director .... Judy Britt
Information Resource Director .... Bob Farrar
Chief Operating Officer .... Jeff Snyder
Marketing Director .... Ty Windfeldt
Provider Services Director .... Denise Lipinski
Human Resources .... Suzanne Oetgen
Quality Assurance Director/Credentialing Manager .... Yvonne Riggan

COMPANY PROFILE:
Parent Company Name: Washoe Health Systems
Doing Business As: Hometown Health
Year Founded: 1988   Federally Qualified: [Y]
Forprofit: [ ]   Not-For-Profit: [Y]
Model Type: MIXED
Accreditation: [ ] AAPPO [ ] JACHO [ ] NCQA [ ] URAC
Plan Type: HMO, PPO, CDHP
Total Revenue: 2005:   2006: 127,793,640
Net Income 2005:   2006:
Total Enrollment:
  2001: 45,576   2004: 90,187   2007: 101,385
  2002: 35,145   2005: 97,188
  2003: 33,166   2006: 103,939
Medical Loss Ratio: 2005:   2006: 88.30
Administrative Expense Ratio: 2005:   2006:

SERVICE AREA:
Nationwide: N
  NV (Carson City, Churchill, Douglas, Elko, Eureka, Humboldt, Lander, Lyon, Mineral, Pershing, Storey, Washoe);

TYPE OF COVERAGE:
Commercial: [Y] Individual: [ ] FEHBP: [ ] Indemnity: [ ]
Medicare: [Y] Medicaid: [ ] Supplemental Medicare: [ ]
Tricare [ ]

PRODUCTS OFFERED:
Product Name:	Type:
Senior Care Plus Health Plan	Medicare
Hometown Health Plan	Medicaid
Seniorr Care Plus - Senior Plan 2002	Medicare Advantage

PLAN BENEFITS:
Alternative Medicine: [ ]   Behavioral Health: [X]
Chiropractic: [X]   Dental: [X]
Home Care: [X]   Inpatient SNF: [X]
Long-Term Care: [ ]   Pharm. Mail Order: [X]
Physical Therapy: [X]   Podiatry: [X]
Psychiatric: [X]   Transplant: [X]
Vision: [X]   Wellness: [X]
Workers' Comp: [ ]
Other Benefits:

HORIZON HEALTH PPO

321 North Pecos Rd Ste 500
Henderson, NV 89074
Phone: 702-367-2222 Fax: 702-247-4758 Toll-Free: 800-884-6875
Web site: www.horizonhealthppo.com

MAILING ADDRESS:
    HORIZON HEALTH PPO
    321 North Pecos Rd Ste 500
    Henderson, NV 89074

KEY EXECUTIVES:
Executive Director .... Joseph Lawreno
Executive Vice President .... Gerald W Kring
Chief Financial Officer .... Paul Rheinberger
Medical Director .... Joel Davidson, MD
MIS Director .... Greg McFarland

COMPANY PROFILE:
Parent Company Name: CIGNA Inc
Doing Business As:
Year Founded: 1978   Federally Qualified: [N]
Forprofit: [Y]   Not-For-Profit: [ ]
Model Type: NETWORK
Accreditation: [ ] AAPPO [ ] JACHO [ ] NCQA [ ] URAC
Plan Type: PPO, EPO,
Primary Physicians: 2,400   Physician Specialists:
Hospitals:

SERVICE AREA:
Nationwide: N
  NV;

TYPE OF COVERAGE:
Commercial: [Y] Individual: [ ] FEHBP: [ ] Indemnity: [ ]
Medicare: [ ] Medicaid: [ ] Supplemental Medicare: [ ]
Tricare [ ]

PLAN BENEFITS:
Alternative Medicine: [ ]   Behavioral Health: [X]
Chiropractic: [X]   Dental: [ ]
Home Care: [X]   Inpatient SNF: [X]
Long-Term Care: [ ]   Pharm. Mail Order: [ ]
Physical Therapy: [X]   Podiatry: [ ]
Psychiatric: [X]   Transplant: [X]
Vision: [X]   Wellness: [ ]
Workers' Comp: [X]
Other Benefits: MRI, Special Transportation

MANAGED CARE CONSULTANTS

311 N Pecos Rd Ste 100
Henderson, NV 89074
Phone: 702-792-2994 Fax: 702-933-6672 Toll-Free: 800-748-6842
Web site: www.mccnevada.com

MAILING ADDRESS:
    MANAGED CARE CONSULTANTS
    311 N Pecos Rd Ste 100
    Henderson, NV 89074

KEY EXECUTIVES:
Chief Executive Officer .... Joseph Lawrence
Executive Vice President .... Gerald W Kring
Chief Financial Officer .... Paul Rheinberger
Medical Director .... Joel Davidson, MD
MIS Director .... Greg McFarland
Privacy Officer .... Kenneth Land
Corporate Communications Manger .... Stefanie Van Aken
Director of Contracting/Provider Relations .... Marcy Platt
Executive Director Horizon Health .... Marcy Platt

COMPANY PROFILE:
Parent Company Name: Managed Care Consultants Inc
Doing Business As:
Year Founded: 1988   Federally Qualified: [Y]
Forprofit: [Y]   Not-For-Profit: [ ]
Model Type: NETWORK
Accreditation: [X] AAPPO [ ] JACHO [ ] NCQA [ ] URAC
Plan Type: PPO, POS, TPA, ASO
Primary Physicians: 1,444   Physician Specialists: 4,145
Hospitals: 42
Total Enrollment:
  2001: 0   2004: 0   2007: 0
  2002: 145,000   2005:
  2003: 0   2006:

SERVICE AREA:
Nationwide: N
  NV;

TYPE OF COVERAGE:
Commercial: [Y] Individual: [Y] FEHBP: [ ] Indemnity: [ ]
Medicare: [ ] Medicaid: [ ] Supplemental Medicare: [ ]
Tricare [ ]

PLAN BENEFITS:
Alternative Medicine: [ ]   Behavioral Health: [X]
Chiropractic: [X]   Dental: [X]
Home Care: [X]   Inpatient SNF: [X]
Long-Term Care: [X]   Pharm. Mail Order: [X]
Physical Therapy: [X]   Podiatry: [X]
Psychiatric: [X]   Transplant: [X]
Vision: [X]   Wellness: [X]
Workers' Comp: [X]
Other Benefits:

NEVADA — **Managed Care Organization Profiles**

MAILING ADDRESS:
DELTA DENTAL INSURANCE CO - NV
3012 W Charleston Blvd Ste 120
Las Vegas, NV 89102

KEY EXECUTIVES:
Chief Executive Officer/President .... Robert B Elliott
Chief Medical Officer .... Marilyn Belleck
Chief Information Officer .... Patrick S Steele
Director of Public Affairs .... Jeff Album

COMPANY PROFILE:
Parent Company Name: Delta Dental Plan Association
Doing Business As:
Year Founded: Federally Qualified: [ ]
Forprofit: [Y]   Not-For-Profit: [ ]
Model Type:
Accreditation: [ ] AAPPO [ ] JACHO [ ] NCQA [ ] URAC
Plan Type: Specialty HMO, Specialty PPO
Total Enrollment:
  2001: 0   2004: 0   2007: 0
  2002: 0   2005:
  2003: 76,000   2006:

SERVICE AREA:
Nationwide: N
  NV;

TYPE OF COVERAGE:
Commercial: [Y] Individual: [ ] FEHBP: [ ] Indemnity: [ ]
Medicare: [ ] Medicaid: [ ] Supplemental Medicare: [ ]
Tricare [ ]

PLAN BENEFITS:
Alternative Medicine: [ ]   Behavioral Health: [ ]
Chiropractic: [ ]   Dental: [X]
Home Care: [ ]   Inpatient SNF: [ ]
Long-Term Care: [ ]   Pharm. Mail Order: [ ]
Physical Therapy: [ ]   Podiatry: [ ]
Psychiatric: [ ]   Transplant: [ ]
Vision: [ ]   Wellness: [ ]
Workers' Comp: [ ]
Other Benefits:

HEALTH PLAN OF NEVADA INC

2720 N Tenaya Way
Las Vegas, NV 89128
Phone: 702-242-7242 Fax: 702-240-4824 Toll-Free: 800-777-1840
Web site: www.healthplanofnevada.com

MAILING ADDRESS:
HEALTH PLAN OF NEVADA INC
PO Box 15645
Las Vegas, NV 89128

KEY EXECUTIVES:
President Managed Healthcare Division .... Jonathon W Bunker
VP, Chief Financial Officer .... Paul H Palmer
VP, Chief Medical Officer .... Christine A Petersen, MD
VP/COO Managed Healthcare Division .... Rudy Cardenas
VP Sales .... Donald J Giancursio
VP Chief Information Officer .... Robert L Schaich
VP Network Development/Contracts .... Scott Cassano
VP Health Care Quality & Education .... Allan Ebbib, MD

COMPANY PROFILE:
Parent Company Name: Sierra Health Services Inc
Doing Business As:
Year Founded: 1982   Federally Qualified: [Y]
Forprofit: [Y]   Not-For-Profit: [ ]
Model Type: MIXED
Accreditation: [ ] AAPPO [X] JACHO [X] NCQA [X] URAC
Plan Type: HMO, POS
Primary Physicians: 528   Physician Specialists: 1,191
Hospitals:
Total Revenue: 2005:   2006: 1,313,262,805
Net Income   2005:   2006:
Total Enrollment:
  2001: 234,218   2004: 355,882   2007: 396,625
  2002: 271,137   2005: 393,176
  2003: 283,099   2006: 429,897
Medical Loss Ratio: 2005:   2006: 77.70
Administrative Expense Ratio: 2005:   2006:

SERVICE AREA:
Nationwide: N
  AZ; NV (Clark, Washoe, Nye, Esmeralda, Lyon)

TYPE OF COVERAGE:
Commercial: [Y] Individual: [Y] FEHBP: [ ] Indemnity: [ ]
Medicare: [Y] Medicaid: [Y] Supplemental Medicare: [ ]
Tricare [ ]

PRODUCTS OFFERED:
Product Name: Type:
Senior Dimensions Medicare   Medicare
Health Plan Medicaid   Medicaid
Health Plan HMO   HMO
Health Plan PPO   PPO

PLAN BENEFITS:
Alternative Medicine: [ ]   Behavioral Health: [X]
Chiropractic: [X]   Dental: [X]
Home Care: [X]   Inpatient SNF: [X]
Long-Term Care: [ ]   Pharm. Mail Order: [X]
Physical Therapy: [X]   Podiatry: [X]
Psychiatric: [X]   Transplant: [X]
Vision: [X]   Wellness: [X]
Workers' Comp: [ ]
Other Benefits:

HMO NEVADA

6900 Westcliff Dr Ste 600
Las Vegas, NV 89145
Phone: 702-228-2583 Fax: 702-228-1259 Toll-Free: 800-438-5270
Web site: www.anthem-inc.com

MAILING ADDRESS:
HMO NEVADA
6900 Westcliff Dr Ste 600
Las Vegas, NV 89145

KEY EXECUTIVES:
Medical Director .... William Bannen, MD

COMPANY PROFILE:
Parent Company Name: HMO Colorado
Doing Business As: HMO Nevada
Year Founded: 1992   Federally Qualified: [Y]
Forprofit: [ ]   Not-For-Profit: [Y]
Model Type: GROUP
Accreditation: [ ] AAPPO [X] JACHO [ ] NCQA [ ] URAC
Plan Type: HMO
Total Enrollment:
  2001: 146,174   2004: 224,943   2007: 58,710
  2002: 0   2005: 11,035
  2003: 0   2006: 231,971

SERVICE AREA:
Nationwide: N
  NV (Carson City, Clark, Douglas, Esmeralda, Eureka, Humboldt, Lincoln, Lyon, Nye, Storey, Washoe);

TYPE OF COVERAGE:
Commercial: [Y] Individual: [ ] FEHBP: [ ] Indemnity: [ ]
Medicare: [ ] Medicaid: [ ] Supplemental Medicare: [ ]
Tricare [ ]

PRODUCTS OFFERED:
Product Name: Type:
HMO   HMO
PPO   PPO

PLAN BENEFITS:
Alternative Medicine: [ ]   Behavioral Health: [ ]
Chiropractic: [X]   Dental: [ ]
Home Care: [X]   Inpatient SNF: [X]
Long-Term Care: [ ]   Pharm. Mail Order: [X]
Physical Therapy: [X]   Podiatry: [X]
Psychiatric: [X]   Transplant: [X]
Vision: [ ]   Wellness: [X]
Workers' Comp: [ ]
Other Benefits:

HOMETOWN HEALTH PLAN

830 Harvard Way
Reno, NV 89502
Phone: 775-982-3000 Fax: 775-982-3746 Toll-Free:
Web site: www.hometownhealth.com

Managed Care Organization Profiles — NEVADA

AETNA INC - NEVADA

4040 S Eastern Ave Ste 240
Las Vegas, NV 89119
Phone: 702-650-8200 Fax: 702-650-8256 Toll-Free:
Web site: www.aetna.com

MAILING ADDRESS:
AETNA INC - NV
4040 S Eastern Ave Ste 240
Las Vegas, NV 89119

KEY EXECUTIVES:
Chairman of the Board/Chief Executive Officer .... Ronald A Williams
Regional Manager-Western .... Thomas R Williams
Executive VP, Finance .... Joseph M Zubretsky
Chief Medical Officer .... Richard Jones

COMPANY PROFILE:
Parent Company Name: Aetna Inc
Doing Business As:
Year Founded: 1997   Federally Qualified: [ ]
Forprofit: [Y]   Not-For-Profit: [ ]
Model Type:
Accreditation: [ ] AAPPO [ ] JACHO [ ] NCQA [ ] URAC
Plan Type: HMO, CDHP, HDHP, HSA,
Net Income 2005:   2006:
Total Enrollment:
  2001: 50,432   2004: 11,733   2007: 14,598
  2002: 0   2005: 10,363
  2003: 0   2006: 9,108

SERVICE AREA:
Nationwide: N
NV;

TYPE OF COVERAGE:
Commercial: [Y] Individual: [ ] FEHBP: [ ] Indemnity: [ ]
Medicare: [ ] Medicaid: [ ] Supplemental Medicare: [ ]
Tricare   [ ]

CONSUMER-DRIVEN PRODUCTS
Aetna Life Insurance Co   HSA Company
Aetna HealthFund HSA   HSA Product
Aetna   HSA Administrator
Aetna HealthFund   Consumer-Driven Health Plan
PPO I; PPO II   High Deductible Health Plan

ANTHEM BLUE CROSS BLUE SHIELD OF NEVADA

5250 S Virginia St
Reno, NV 89502
Phone: 775-448-4000 Fax: 775-448-4040 Toll-Free: 800-992-6907
Web site: www.anthem.com

MAILING ADDRESS:
ANTHEM BC BS OF NV
5250 S Virginia St
Reno, NV 89502

KEY EXECUTIVES:
Chairman of the Board .... Larry C Glasscock
Chief Executive Officer .... Angela F Braly
President, Anthem West .... Caroline S Matthews
Medical Director .... William Bannen, MD
Sales Director .... Gabrielle Sansome

COMPANY PROFILE:
Parent Company Name: WellPoint Inc
Doing Business As:
Year Founded: Federally Qualified: [ ]
Forprofit: [ ]   Not-For-Profit: [Y]
Model Type:
Accreditation: [ ] AAPPO [ ] JACHO [ ] NCQA [ ] URAC
Plan Type: HMO, PPO, CDHP, HDHP, HSA,
Total Enrollment:
  2001: 0   2004: 214,942   2007: 267,923
  2002: 0   2005: 239,363
  2003: 0   2006:

SERVICE AREA:
Nationwide: N
NV;

TYPE OF COVERAGE:
Commercial: [Y] Individual: [Y] FEHBP: [ ] Indemnity: [ ]
Medicare: [ ] Medicaid: [ ] Supplemental Medicare: [Y]
Tricare   [ ]

PRODUCTS OFFERED:
Product Name: Type:
PPO   PPO

CONSUMER-DRIVEN PRODUCTS
JP Morgan Chase   HSA Company
Anthem ByDesign HSA   HSA Product
JP Morgan Chase   HSA Administrator
Blue Access Saver   Consumer-Driven Health Plan
Blue Access Economy Plans PPO   High Deductible Health Plan

PLAN BENEFITS:
Alternative Medicine: [ ]   Behavioral Health: [ ]
Chiropractic: [X]   Dental: [X]
Home Care: [X]   Inpatient SNF: [X]
Long-Term Care: [ ]   Pharm. Mail Order: [X]
Physical Therapy: [X]   Podiatry: [X]
Psychiatric: [X]   Transplant: [X]
Vision: [ ]   Wellness: [ ]
Workers' Comp: [ ]
Other Benefits:

BEHAVIORAL HEALTHCARE OPTIONS INC

2716 N Tenaya Way
Las Vegas, NV 89128
Phone: 877-393-6094 Fax: 702-242-5864 Toll-Free: 800-873-2246
Web site: www.behavioralhealthcareoptions.com

MAILING ADDRESS:
BEHAVIORAL HEALTHCARE OPTIONS
PO Box 15645
Las Vegas, NV 89128

KEY EXECUTIVES:
Chief Executive Officer/President .... Michael R Adams, ACSW
Director of Finance .... Brad Ellerman
Medical Director ....George Westerman, MD
Provider Relations Specialist .... Annetta Crider
Director Quality Assurance & Provider Relations .... Susan Hockenson
Director of Utilization Management .... Kathy Boehning
Director of Clinical Services .... Alec McCosh, PhD
Compliance Officer .... Stephen E Shoop

COMPANY PROFILE:
Parent Company Name: Sierra Health Services Inc
Doing Business As:
Year Founded: 1991   Federally Qualified: [Y]
Forprofit: [Y]   Not-For-Profit: [ ]
Model Type: MIXED
Accreditation: [ ] AAPPO [ ] JACHO [X] NCQA [X] URAC
Plan Type: Specialty HMO, Specialty PPO, UR, POS

SERVICE AREA:
Nationwide: N
NV;

TYPE OF COVERAGE:
Commercial: [Y] Individual: [Y] FEHBP: [ ] Indemnity: [ ]
Medicare: [Y] Medicaid: [Y] Supplemental Medicare: [Y]
Tricare   [ ]

PLAN BENEFITS:
Alternative Medicine: [ ]   Behavioral Health: [X]
Chiropractic: [ ]   Dental: [ ]
Home Care: [ ]   Inpatient SNF: [ ]
Long-Term Care: [ ]   Pharm. Mail Order: [ ]
Physical Therapy: [ ]   Podiatry: [ ]
Psychiatric: [X]   Transplant: [ ]
Vision: [ ]   Wellness: [ ]
Workers' Comp: [ ]
Other Benefits: Employee Assistance

DELTA DENTAL INSURANCE COMPANY - NEVADA

3012 W Charleston Blvd Ste 120
Las Vegas, NV 89102
Phone: 702-870-6860 Fax: 702-870-0644 Toll-Free:
Web site: www.deltadentalins.com

Managed Care Organization Profiles — NEBRASKA

PLAN BENEFITS:
Alternative Medicine:	[ ]	Behavioral Health:	[X]
Chiropractic:	[X]	Dental:	[ ]
Home Care:	[X]	Inpatient SNF:	[X]
Long-Term Care:	[ ]	Pharm. Mail Order:	[ ]
Physical Therapy:	[X]	Podiatry:	[X]
Psychiatric:	[X]	Transplant:	[X]
Vision:	[ ]	Wellness:	[X]
Workers' Comp:	[ ]		

Other Benefits:

UNITEDHEALTHCARE OF THE MIDLANDS INC

2717 N 118th Circle
Omaha, NE 68164-9672
Phone: 402-445-5000 Fax: 402-445-5575 Toll-Free: 800-284-0626
Web site: www.uhc.com

MAILING ADDRESS:
UNITEDHEALTHCARE OF MIDLANDS
2717 N 118th Circle
Omaha, NE 68164-9672

KEY EXECUTIVES:
Non-Executive Chairman .... Richard T Burke
Chief Executive Officer/President .... William C Tracy
Medical Director .... Deb Esser, MD
Midwest Communications Contact .... Greg Thompson

COMPANY PROFILE:
Parent Company Name: UnitedHealth Group
Doing Business As:
Year Founded: 1984   Federally Qualified: [ ]
Forprofit: [Y]   Not-For-Profit: [ ]
Model Type: IPA
Accreditation: [ ] AAPPO [ ] JACHO [ ] NCQA [ ] URAC
Plan Type: HMO, PPO, Specialty HMO, POS, ASO, TPA, CDHP, HSA, HRA, HDHP
Total Revenue: 2005:   165,844,939   2006:   167,004,678
Net Income   2005:   7,135,096   2006:   3,256,111
Total Enrollment:
  2001: 66,714   2004: 49,511   2007: 45,638
  2002: 60,916   2005: 46,877
  2003: 56,718   2006: 46,171
Medical Loss Ratio: 2005: 81.30   2006: 85.20
Administrative Expense Ratio: 2005:   2006:

SERVICE AREA:
Nationwide: N
  IA (Harrison, Mills, Pottawattamie); NE;

TYPE OF COVERAGE:
Commercial: [Y] Individual: [ ] FEHBP: [ ] Indemnity: [ ]
Medicare: [Y] Medicaid: [Y] Supplemental Medicare: [ ]
Tricare [ ]

PRODUCTS OFFERED:
Product Name:	Type:
Choice Plus	PPO
United Medicare PPO	Medicare
Medicare Complete	Medicare
United Healthcare Choice -IA	HMO
United Healthcare Choice - NE	HMO
United Healthcare Select Plus	POS
Share Advantage	Medicaid

CONSUMER-DRIVEN PRODUCTS
Exante Bank/Golden Rule Ins Co	HSA Company
iPlan HSA	HSA Product
	HSA Administrator
	Consumer-Driven Health Plan
	High Deductible Health Plan

PLAN BENEFITS:
Alternative Medicine:	[ ]	Behavioral Health:	[X]
Chiropractic:	[X]	Dental:	[ ]
Home Care:	[X]	Inpatient SNF:	[X]
Long-Term Care:	[ ]	Pharm. Mail Order:	[X]
Physical Therapy:	[X]	Podiatry:	[X]
Psychiatric:	[X]	Transplant:	[X]
Vision:	[X]	Wellness:	[X]
Workers' Comp:	[ ]		

Other Benefits:

NEBRASKA
Managed Care Organization Profiles

PLAN BENEFITS:
Alternative Medicine:	[ ]	Behavioral Health:	[X]
Chiropractic:	[X]	Dental:	[X]
Home Care:	[X]	Inpatient SNF:	[X]
Long-Term Care:	[ ]	Pharm. Mail Order:	[X]
Physical Therapy:	[X]	Podiatry:	[ ]
Psychiatric:	[X]	Transplant:	[X]
Vision:	[X]	Wellness:	[X]
Workers' Comp:	[ ]		

Other Benefits:
Comments:
Formerly Principal Health Care of Nebraska Inc.

DELTA DENTAL OF NEBRASKA

11235 Davenport St Ste 105
Omaha, NE 68154
Phone: 402-397-4878 Fax: 402-397-6401 Toll-Free: 800-736-0710
Web site: www.deltadentalne.org

MAILING ADDRESS:
DELTA DENTAL OF NE
11235 Davenport St STe 105
Omaha, NE 68154

KEY EXECUTIVES:
Chief Executive Officer .... Michael F Walsh
Chief Marketing Officer .... Chris Earl
Dental Director of Nebraska .... Richard Hastreiter, DDS

COMPANY PROFILE:
Parent Company Name: Delta Dental Plan Association
Doing Business As:
Year Founded: 1985   Federally Qualified: [ ]
Forprofit: [Y]   Not-For-Profit: [ ]
Model Type:
Accreditation: [ ] AAPPO [ ] JACHO [ ] NCQA [ ] URAC
Plan Type: Specialty HMO, Specialty PPO
Total Revenue: 2005:   2006: 6,123,081
Net Income 2005:   2006: 4,343,804
Total Enrollment:
  2001: 0   2004: 28,661   2007: 0
  2002: 20,438   2005:
  2003: 24,524   2006:
Medical Loss Ratio: 2005:   2006: 72.30
Administrative Expense Ratio: 2005:   2006:

SERVICE AREA:
Nationwide: N
  NE;

TYPE OF COVERAGE:
Commercial: [Y] Individual: [ ] FEHBP: [ ] Indemnity: [ ]
Medicare: [ ] Medicaid: [ ] Supplemental Medicare: [ ]
Tricare [ ]

PLAN BENEFITS:
Alternative Medicine:	[ ]	Behavioral Health:	[ ]
Chiropractic:	[ ]	Dental:	[X]
Home Care:	[ ]	Inpatient SNF:	[ ]
Long-Term Care:	[ ]	Pharm. Mail Order:	[ ]
Physical Therapy:	[ ]	Podiatry:	[ ]
Psychiatric:	[ ]	Transplant:	[ ]
Vision:	[ ]	Wellness:	[ ]
Workers' Comp:	[ ]		

Other Benefits:

HUMANA INC - NEBRASKA

500 W Main St
Louisville, KY 40202
Phone: 502-580-5005 Fax: 502-580-5044 Toll-Free:
Web site: www.humana.com

MAILING ADDRESS:
HUMANA INC - NEBRASKA
PO Box 740036
Louisville, KY 40202

KEY EXECUTIVES:
Chairman of the Board .... David A Jones Jr
Chief Executive Officer/President .... Michael B McCallister
Chief Financial Officer .... James H Bloem
VP Medical Director .... Jonathan T Lord, MD
Senior VP, Chief Information Officer .... Bruce J Goodman
Senior VP, Human Resources .... Bonnie C Hathcock

COMPANY PROFILE:
Parent Company Name: Humana Inc
Doing Business As:
Year Founded: 1961   Federally Qualified: [Y]
Forprofit: [Y]   Not-For-Profit: [ ]
Model Type: IPA
Accreditation: [ ] AAPPO [ ] JACHO [ ] NCQA [ ] URAC
Plan Type: PPO, ASO, CDHP, HSA
Total Revenue: 2005:   2006:
Net Income 2005:   2006: 205,420,689

SERVICE AREA:
Nationwide: N
  NE;

TYPE OF COVERAGE:
Commercial: [Y] Individual: [Y] FEHBP: [ ] Indemnity: [ ]
Medicare: [Y] Medicaid: [ ] Supplemental Medicare: [Y]
Tricare [ ]

CONSUMER-DRIVEN PRODUCTS
JP Morgan Chase	HSA Company
HumanaOne HSA	HSA Product
JP Morgan Chase	HSA Administrator
Personal Care Account	Consumer-Driven Health Plan
HumanaOne	High Deductible Health Plan

PLAN BENEFITS:
Alternative Medicine:	[ ]	Behavioral Health:	
[X]Chiropractic:	[X]	Dental:	[X]
Home Care:	[ ]	Inpatient SNF:	[ ]
Long-Term Care:	[ ]	Pharm. Mail Order:	[X]
Physical Therapy:	[ ]	Podiatry:	[ ]
Psychiatric:	[X]	Transplant:	[X]
Vision:	[ ]	Wellness:	[ ]
Workers' Comp:	[X]		

Other Benefits: Long Term Disability Care

MIDLANDS CHOICE INC

8420 W Dodge Rd Ste 210
Omaha, NE 68114
Phone: 402-390-8233 Fax: 402-390-8239 Toll-Free: 800-605-8259
Web site: www.midlandschoice.com

MAILING ADDRESS:
MIDLANDS CHOICE INC
8420 W Dodge Rd Ste 210
Omaha, NE 68114

KEY EXECUTIVES:
Chief Executive Officer/President .... Thomas E Press
Chief Financial Officer .... Jackie Joaquin
Medical Director .... Michael Romano, MD
MIS Director .... Bob Hood
VP Operations .... Carmen Backman
Director, Business Development & Communications ...... Kelly Nieman
Director, Legal Services & Credentialing .... Timothy A Waggoner, JD
Director, Medical Economics .... Daniel McCulley
Director, Administration .... Sharon Rasmussen
Communications Specialist .... Rita Shelley

COMPANY PROFILE:
Parent Company Name: Midlands Health Partners
Doing Business As:
Year Founded: 1997   Federally Qualified: [ ]
Forprofit: [Y]   Not-For-Profit: [ ]
Model Type:
Accreditation: [ ] AAPPO [ ] JACHO [ ] NCQA [X] URAC
Plan Type: PPO
Primary Physicians: 20,000   Physician Specialists:
Hospitals: 301
Total Enrollment:
  2001: 0   2004: 0   2007: 635,000
  2002: 0   2005:
  2003: 0   2006:

SERVICE AREA:
Nationwide: N
  IA; NE; SD;

TYPE OF COVERAGE:
Commercial: [Y] Individual: [ ] FEHBP: [ ] Indemnity: [ ]
Medicare: [ ] Medicaid: [ ] Supplemental Medicare: [ ]
Tricare [ ]

Managed Care Organization Profiles   **NEBRASKA**

AMERITAS GROUP DENTAL

5900 O St
Lincoln, NE 68501-1889
Phone: 402-467-1122 Fax: 402-467-7338 Toll-Free: 800-659-2223
Web site: www.ameritasgroup.com

MAILING ADDRESS:
   AMERITAS GROUP DENTAL
   PO Box 81889
   Lincoln, NE 68501-1889

KEY EXECUTIVES:
Chairman of the Board/Chief Executive Officer .... Lawrence J Arth
President/Chief Financial Officer .... JoAnn Martin
Chief Operating Officer .... JoAnn Martin
VP Group Marketing & Managed Care .... Karen Gustin

COMPANY PROFILE:
Parent Company Name: Ameritas Acacia Mutual Holding Company
Doing Business As: Ameritas Life Insurance Corp
Year Founded: 1887   Federally Qualified: [ ]
Forprofit: [Y]   Not-For-Profit: [ ]
Model Type: IPA
Accreditation: [ ] AAPPO [ ] JACHO [ ] NCQA [ ] URAC
Plan Type: Specialty PPO, ASO
Primary Physicians: 34,319   Physician Specialists: 11,183
Hospitals:
Total Enrollment:
   2001: 0   2004: 2,000,000   2007: 0
   2002: 0   2005: 2,000,000
   2003: 0   2006: 3,000,000

SERVICE AREA:
Nationwide: Y
   NW;

TYPE OF COVERAGE:
Commercial: [Y] Individual: [ ]   FEHBP: [ ]   Indemnity: [ ]
Medicare: [ ] Medicaid: [ ]   Supplemental Medicare: [ ]
Tricare   [ ]

PRODUCTS OFFERED:
Product Name: Type:
Ameritas Group Dental   Specialty PPO

PLAN BENEFITS:
Alternative Medicine: [ ]   Behavioral Health: [ ]
Chiropractic: [ ]   Dental: [X]
Home Care: [ ]   Inpatient SNF: [ ]
Long-Term Care: [ ]   Pharm. Mail Order: [ ]
Physical Therapy: [ ]   Podiatry: [ ]
Psychiatric: [ ]   Transplant: [ ]
Vision: [X]   Wellness: [ ]
Workers' Comp: [ ]
Other Benefits:

BLUE CROSS BLUE SHIELD OF NEBRASKA

7261 Mercy Rd
Omaha, NE 68180-0001
Phone: 402-390-1800 Fax: 402-398-3737 Toll-Free: 800-642-8980
Web site: www.bcbsne.com

MAILING ADDRESS:
   BLUE CROSS BLUE SHIELD OF NE
   PO Box 3248
   Omaha, NE 68180-0001

KEY EXECUTIVES:
Chief Executive Officer/President .... Steven S Martin
Chief Financial Officer .... Duane Wilson
Medical Director .... William Minier, MD
Pharmacy Director .... Clint Williams, MD
Senior VP, Marketing .... Steven Harm
Senior VP, Information Services .... Steven Grandfield
VP, Public Relations & Corp Communications .... Celann LaGreca
Senior VP, Manage Care Networks .... Steve Lorenzen
Executive VP of Organizational Relations .... Micki Baldino
Senior VP, Benefits .... Karen Hollingsworth
Chief Underwriting Officer .... Jim Pusateri
Compliance Officer .... Sarah Waldman

COMPANY PROFILE:
Parent Company Name: Blue Cross Blue Shield of Nebraska
Doing Business As:
Year Founded: 1987   Federally Qualified: [ ]
Forprofit: [ ]   Not-For-Profit: [N]
Model Type:
Accreditation: [ ] AAPPO [ ] JACHO [ ] NCQA [ ] URAC
Plan Type: HMO, PPO, POS, ASO, HDHP, HSA
Total Revenue: 2005:   2006:
Net Income   2005:   2006: 439,352,782
Total Enrollment:
   2001: 640,000   2004: 285,935   2007: 0
   2002: 0   2005: 550,000
   2003: 700,000   2006: 717,000

SERVICE AREA:
Nationwide: N
   NE;

TYPE OF COVERAGE:
Commercial: [Y] Individual: [ ]   FEHBP: [ ]   Indemnity: [Y]
Medicare: [ ] Medicaid: [ ]   Supplemental Medicare: [Y]
Tricare   [ ]

Comments:
A Mutual Insurance Company.

COVENTRY HEALTH CARE OF NEBRASKA INC

13305 Birch Dr Ste 100
Omaha, NE 68164
Phone: 402-498-9030 Fax: 402-498-9706 Toll-Free: 800-471-0240
Web site: www.chcnebraska.com

MAILING ADDRESS:
   COVENTRY HEALTH CARE OF NE INC
   PO Box 541210
   Omaha, NE 68164

KEY EXECUTIVES:
Chief Executive Officer .... Kathy A Mallatt
Chief Medical Officer .... Robert Masterson, DO, MBA
Chief Financial Officer .... Deanna H Gray
Chief Operating Officer .... Barbara A Witte
Market Vice President .... Michael Nelson, DO
Director of Network Development .... Donna Jennings
VP Business Development .... Brian Wise

COMPANY PROFILE:
Parent Company Name: Coventry Health Care Inc
Doing Business As:
Year Founded: 1987   Federally Qualified: [ ]
Forprofit: [Y]   Not-For-Profit: [ ]
Model Type:
Accreditation: [ ] AAPPO [ ] JACHO [ ] NCQA [ ] URAC
Plan Type: HMO, PPO, POS, CDHP, HDHP, HSA
Total Revenue: 2005:   2006: 131,605,708
Net Income   2005:   2006: 7,252,308
Total Enrollment:
   2001: 44,507   2004: 44,293   2007: 52,672
   2002: 32,451   2005: 47,000
   2003: 41,679   2006: 54,782
Medical Loss Ratio: 2005:   2006: 82.50
Administrative Expense Ratio: 2005:   2006:

SERVICE AREA:
Nationwide: N
   IA (Cherokee, Crawford, Harrison, Ida, Lyon, Mills, Monona, O'Brien, Osceola, Plymouth, Page, Pottawattamie, Sioux and Woodbury); NE (Antelope, Burt, Cass, Cedar, Cuming, Dakota, Dixon, Dodge, Douglas, Lancaster, Madison, Otoe, Pierce, Sarpy, Sounders, Stanton, Thurston, Washington and Wayne);

TYPE OF COVERAGE:
Commercial: [Y] Individual: [ ]   FEHBP: [ ]   Indemnity: [ ]
Medicare: [ ] Medicaid: [ ]   Supplemental Medicare: [ ]
Tricare   [ ]

CONSUMER-DRIVEN PRODUCTS
Wells Fargo   HSA Company
                                                          HSA Product
Corporate Benefits Services of America   HSA Administrator
                                                          Consumer-Driven Health Plan
Open Access Plus Plan   High Deductible Health Plan

MONTANA

PLAN BENEFITS:
Alternative Medicine: [ ]   Behavioral Health: [ ]
Chiropractic: [X]   Dental: [X]
Home Care: [X]   Inpatient SNF: [X]
Long-Term Care: [X]   Pharm. Mail Order: [X]
Physical Therapy: [X]   Podiatry: [X]
Psychiatric: [X]   Transplant: [X]
Vision: [X]   Wellness: [X]
Workers' Comp: [ ]
Other Benefits:

MOUNTAIN PACIFIC QUALITY HEALTH FOUNDATION

3404 Cooney Dr
Helena, MT 59602
Phone: 406-443-4020 Fax: 406-443-4585 Toll-Free: 800-497-8235
Web site: www.mpqhf.org
MAILING ADDRESS:
   MOUNTAIN PACIFIC QUALITY HEALTH
   3404 Cooney Dr
   Helena, MT 59602

KEY EXECUTIVES:
Chief Executive Officer .... Janice Connors
Corporate Medical Director .... John W McMahon Sr, MD
Chief Operating Officer .... Sara Medley

COMPANY PROFILE:
Parent Company Name:
Doing Business As:
Year Founded: 1973   Federally Qualified: [ ]
Forprofit: [ ]   Not-For-Profit: [ ]
Model Type:
Accreditation: [ ] AAPPO [ ] JACHO [ ] NCQA [ ] URAC
Plan Type: PRO, TPA, UR
SERVICE AREA:
Nationwide: N
   MT;
TYPE OF COVERAGE:
Commercial: [ ] Individual: [ ] FEHBP: [ ] Indemnity: [ ]
Medicare: [Y] Medicaid: [Y] Supplemental Medicare: [ ]
Tricare   [ ]

NEW WEST HEALTH SERVICES

130 Neill Ave
Helena, MT 59602
Phone: 406-457-2200 Fax: 406-457-2299 Toll-Free: 800-500-3355
Web site: www.newwesthealth.com
MAILING ADDRESS:
   NEW WEST HEALTH SERVICES
   130 Neill Ave
   Helena, MT 59602

KEY EXECUTIVES:
Chief Executive Officer .... David Kibbe
Chief Financial Officer .... Angela Huschka
Medical Director .... Robert M Shepard
Marketing Director .... Jeff Ireland
Compliance Officer .... Denise Pizzini
Director of Operations .... Paul Marchant
Director of Information Technology .... Marc Best
Director/Healthcare Access Programs .... Colleen Senterfitt
Director of Care Management .... Casey Clark

COMPANY PROFILE:
Parent Company Name:
Doing Business As: New West Health Plan,
Year Founded: 1997   Federally Qualified: [ ]
Forprofit: [ ]   Not-For-Profit: [Y]
Model Type:
Accreditation: [ ] AAPPO [ ] JACHO [ ] NCQA [ ] URAC
Plan Type: HMO, PPO, POS, ASO,
Primary Physicians: 1,400   Physician Specialists:
Total Revenue: 2005:   2006: 68,674,955
Net Income: 2005:   2006:

Total Enrollment:
   2001: 0   2004: 24,784   2007: 0
   2002: 14,240   2005:
   2003: 16,296   2006: 33,000
Medical Loss Ratio: 2005:   2006: 74.80
Administrative Expense Ratio: 2005:   2006:
SERVICE AREA:
Nationwide: N
   MT (Beaverhead, Bis Horn, Blaine, Broadwater, Carbon, Choteau,
   Custer, Garfield, Golden Valley, Granite, Hill, Jefferson, Lake, Lewis
   & Clark, Meagher, Mineral, Missoula, Musselshell, Park, Phillips,
   Powell, Ravalli, Rosebud, Sanders, Stillwater, Sweet Grass, Treasure,
   Wheatland, Yellowstone);
TYPE OF COVERAGE:
Commercial: [Y] Individual: [ ] FEHBP: [ ] Indemnity: [ ]
Medicare: [ ] Medicaid: [ ] Supplemental Medicare: [ ]
Tricare   [ ]
PRODUCTS OFFERED:
Product Name: Type:
ValCare   HMO
WestCare   HMO
ValCare Plus   HMO
WestCare Plus   HMO
Innovations   PPO
Health Connections
CareMarkRx

CONSUMER-DRIVEN PRODUCTS
                                 HSA Company
New West Select   HSA Product
Wells Fargo   HSA Administrator
                                 Consumer-Driven Health Plan
New West Select   High Deductible Health Plan

Managed Care Organization Profiles — MONTANA

APS HEALTHCARE NORTHWEST INC

3010 Santa Fe Court
Missoula, MT 59801
Phone: 406-327-7000 Fax: 406-327-7386 Toll-Free: 800-330-8565
Web site: www.apshealthcare.com

MAILING ADDRESS:
APS HEALTHCARE NORTHWEST INC
PO Box 16090
Missoula, MT 59808-6090

KEY EXECUTIVES:
Chairman of the Board .... Ken Kessler, MD
Chief Executive Officer .... Eileen O'Shea Auen, MBA
Chief Financial Officer .... Brett McIntyre
Senior VP, Chief Information Officer .... Arthur Held
Executive VP, Sales & Marketing .... Richard Kodora, MBA
Senior VP of Medical Management .... Cheryl Stacy
President APS Public Division .... David Hunsaker
President, Product Development .... Kristin Blasko
President/Behavioral Health Division .... Roderick J Hafer, PhD

COMPANY PROFILE:
Parent Company Name: APS Healthcare Inc
Doing Business As:
Year Founded: 1992   Federally Qualified: [ ]
Forprofit: [Y]   Not-For-Profit: [ ]
Model Type:
Accreditation: [ ] AAPPO [ ] JACHO [X] NCQA [X] URAC
Plan Type: Specialty HMO, Specialty PPO, UR, POS, EPO

SERVICE AREA:
Nationwide: Y
 NW;

TYPE OF COVERAGE:
Commercial: [Y] Individual: [ ] FEHBP: [ ] Indemnity: [Y]
Medicare: [Y] Medicaid: [Y] Supplemental Medicare: [ ]
Tricare [ ]

PLAN BENEFITS:
Alternative Medicine: [ ]   Behavioral Health: [X]
Chiropractic: [ ]   Dental: [ ]
Home Care: [ ]   Inpatient SNF: [ ]
Long-Term Care: [ ]   Pharm. Mail Order: [ ]
Physical Therapy: [ ]   Podiatry: [ ]
Psychiatric: [X]   Transplant: [ ]
Vision: [ ]   Wellness: [ ]
Workers' Comp: [ ]
Other Benefits: Employee Assistance

BLUE CROSS BLUE SHIELD OF MONTANA

560 North Park Ave
Helena, MT 59601-5006
Phone: 406-444-8200 Fax: 406-444-8961 Toll-Free: 800-447-7828
Web site: www.bcbsmt.com

MAILING ADDRESS:
BC/BS OF MONTANA
PO Box 4309
Helena, MT 59601-5006

KEY EXECUTIVES:
Chairman of the Board .... Jerry Lusk
Chief Executive Officer/President .... Sherry L Cladouhos
Chief Financial Officer .... Eric Schinaler
Corporate Medical Director .... Fred Olson, MD
Chief Operating Officer .... Sheila Shapiro
Executive VP, General Counsel .... Terry Cosgrove
VP, Marketing & Sales .... Jared Short
Chief Administrative Officer .... Michael Frank
Director of Provider Services .... Mark Burzynski
Director, Corporate Communications .... Linda McGillen

COMPANY PROFILE:
Parent Company Name: Blue Cross and Blue Shield of Montana
Doing Business As: HMO Montana
Year Founded: 1987   Federally Qualified: [N]
Forprofit: [ ]   Not-For-Profit: [Y]
Model Type: NETWORK
Accreditation: [ ] AAPPO [ ] JACHO [ ] NCQA [ ] URAC
Plan Type: HMO, PPO, POS,
Primary Physicians: 1,700   Physician Specialists:
Hospitals: 59
Total Revenue: 2005: 536,425,534 2006: 480,178,059
Net Income 2005: 2006:
Total Enrollment:
 2001: 170,033   2004: 228,344   2007: 235,000
 2002: 204,217   2005: 230,000
 2003: 233,038   2006: 240,000
Medical Loss Ratio: 2005: 2006: 85.60
Administrative Expense Ratio: 2005: 2006:

SERVICE AREA:
Nationwide: N
 MT;

TYPE OF COVERAGE:
Commercial: [Y] Individual: [ ] FEHBP: [ ] Indemnity: [ ]
Medicare: [Y] Medicaid: [ ] Supplemental Medicare: [ ]
Tricare [ ]

PRODUCTS OFFERED:
Product Name: Type:
HMO Montana   HMO
Montana Care
Montana Health
Blue Choice
Blue Select
Health First Direct
Medicare Bluesm Rx

PLAN BENEFITS:
Alternative Medicine: [ ]   Behavioral Health: [ ]
Chiropractic: [X]   Dental: [ ]
Home Care: [X]   Inpatient SNF: [X]
Long-Term Care: [ ]   Pharm. Mail Order: [X]
Physical Therapy: [X]   Podiatry: [ ]
Psychiatric: [X]   Transplant: [X]
Vision: [ ]   Wellness: [ ]
Workers' Comp: [ ]
Other Benefits:
Comments:
Nationwide coverage available through HMO Blue USA.

EMPLOYEE BENEFIT MANAGEMENT SERVICES INC

2075 Overland Ave
Billings, MT 59102
Phone: 406-245-3575 Fax: 406-652-5380 Toll-Free: 800-777-3575
Web site: www.ebms.com

MAILING ADDRESS:
EMPLOYEE BENEFIT MGMT SERVICES
P O Box 21367
Billings, MT 59102

KEY EXECUTIVES:
Chief Executive Officer .... Rick Larson
President .... Nicki Larson
Controller .... Al Galt
Medical Director .... Luanne Ricks
Chief Information Officer .... Rod Kaselitz
MIS Director .... Andrew Lindley
Provider Relations Director .... Kirsten Mailloux
Human Resources Director .... Bob Burnaugh
Quality Assurance Director .... Vikki Fosjord
Managed Care Director .... Luanne Ricks

COMPANY PROFILE:
Parent Company Name: Computer Claims Administrators
Doing Business As: Employee Benefit Management Services Inc
Year Founded: 1980   Federally Qualified: [N]
Forprofit: [Y]   Not-For-Profit: [ ]
Model Type: IPA
Accreditation: [ ] AAPPO [ ] JACHO [ ] NCQA [ ] URAC
Plan Type: Specialty PPO, UR, POS, TPA, ASO

SERVICE AREA:
Nationwide: N
 AK; CA; CO; ID; MT; NC; NE; NV; OR; UT; WA; WY;

TYPE OF COVERAGE:
Commercial: [Y] Individual: [ ] FEHBP: [ ] Indemnity: [Y]
Medicare: [ ] Medicaid: [ ] Supplemental Medicare: [Y]
Tricare [ ]

MISSOURI

SERVICE AREA:
Nationwide: N
IL (Bond, Calhoun, Clinton, Gteene, Jersey, Macoupin, Madison, Monroe, Montgomery, Randolph, St Clair, Williamson); KS (Anderson, Atchison, Douglas, Franklin, Jackson, Jefferson, Johnson, Leavenworth, Linn, Miami, Osage, Sedgewick, Shawnee, Wyandotte); MO (Adair, Audrain, Barry, Bollinger, Boone, Butler, Callaway, Camden, Cape Girardeau, Carter, Cass, Chariton, Christian, Clay, Cooper, Crawford, Dade, Dallas, Dent, Dunklin, Franklin, Gasconade, Greene, Howell, Howard, Iron, Jackson, Jasper, Jefferson, Johnson, Knox, Laclede, Lafayette, Lawrence, Lewis, Linn, Lincoln, Macon, Madison, Maries, McDonald, Miller, Mississippi, Moniteau, Monroe, Montgomery, Morgan, New Madrid, Newton, Oregon, Osage, Pemiscot, Perry, Pettis, Phelps, Pike, Platte, Pulaske, Randolph, Raymond, Reynolds, Ripley, Saline, St Charles, St Francois, Ste Genevieve, St Louis City, St Louis, Schuyler, Scott, Scotland, Shannon, Shelby, Stoddard, Stone, Sullivan, Taney, Texas, Warren, Washington, Wayne, Webster, Wright);

TYPE OF COVERAGE:
Commercial: [Y] Individual: [Y] FEHBP: [ ] Indemnity: [ ]
Medicare: [Y] Medicaid: [ ] Supplemental Medicare: [ ]
Tricare   [ ]

PRODUCTS OFFERED:
Product Name: Type:
Medicare Complete   Medicare Advantage
Select/Select Plus
Choice/Choice Plus

CONSUMER-DRIVEN PRODUCTS
Exante Bank/Golden Rule Ins Co   HSA Company
iPlan HSA   HSA Product
                                   HSA Administrator
                                   Consumer-Driven Health Plan
                                   High Deductible Health Plan

PLAN BENEFITS:
Alternative Medicine: [ ]   Behavioral Health: [X]
Chiropractic: [ ]   Dental: [X]
Home Care: [X]   Inpatient SNF: [ ]
Long-Term Care: [ ]   Pharm. Mail Order: [X]
Physical Therapy: [ ]   Podiatry: [ ]
Psychiatric: [X]   Transplant: [X]
Vision: [X]   Wellness: [X]
Workers' Comp: [ ]
Other Benefits:

Comments:
Formerly Goddard Medical Association.

Managed Care Organization Profiles **MISSOURI**

COMPANY PROFILE:
Parent Company Name:
Doing Business As:
Year Founded: 1983   Federally Qualified: [Y]
Forprofit: [ ]   Not-For-Profit: [Y]
Model Type:
Accreditation: [ ] AAPPO [ ] JACHO [X] NCQA [X] URAC
Plan Type: PRO, UR
SERVICE AREA:
Nationwide: N
    MO;
TYPE OF COVERAGE:
Commercial: [ ] Individual: [ ] FEHBP: [ ] Indemnity: [ ]
Medicare: [Y] Medicaid: [ ] Supplemental Medicare: [ ]
Tricare   [ ]
Comments:
Formerly Missouri Patient Care Review.

PRIVATE HEALTHCARE SYSTEMS - MISSOURI

2405 Grand Blvd Ste 1030
Kansas City, MO 64108
Phone: 816-221-4455 Fax: 816-221-4466 Toll-Free: 800-253-4417
Web site: www.phcs.com
MAILING ADDRESS:
    PRIVATE HEALTHCARE SYSTEMS-MO
    1100 Winter St
    Waltham, MA 64108

KEY EXECUTIVES:
Chief Executive Officer/President .... Mark Tabak
Executive VP, Chief Financial Officer .... Richard Gerstein
Medical Director .... Dr Goldstein
Executive VP, Chief of Operations .... Michael Ferrante
Executive VP, Marketing .... Warren Handelman

COMPANY PROFILE:
Parent Company Name: MultiPlan Inc
Doing Business As:
Year Founded: 1987   Federally Qualified: [N]
Forprofit: [Y]   Not-For-Profit: [ ]
Model Type:
Accreditation: [ ] AAPPO [ ] JACHO [ ] NCQA [X] URAC
Plan Type: PPO, UR, POS
SERVICE AREA:
Nationwide: N
    MO;
TYPE OF COVERAGE:
Commercial: [Y] Individual: [ ] FEHBP: [ ] Indemnity: [ ]
Medicare: [ ] Medicaid: [ ] Supplemental Medicare: [ ]
Tricare   [ ]
PLAN BENEFITS:
Alternative Medicine: [X]   Behavioral Health: [X]
Chiropractic: [X]   Dental: [ ]
Home Care: [X]   Inpatient SNF: [X]
Long-Term Care: [X]   Pharm. Mail Order: [X]
Physical Therapy: [X]   Podiatry: [X]
Psychiatric: [X]   Transplant: [X]
Vision: [X]   Wellness: [ ]
Workers' Comp: [X]
Other Benefits: X
Comments:
Acquired by MultiPlan, Inc. on October 18, 2006.

UNITED CONCORDIA COMPANY INC - MISSOURI

390 South Woods Mill Rd Ste175
Chesterfield, MO 63017
Phone: 314-205-9605 Fax: 314-205-9601 Toll-Free: 888-245-8224
Web site: www.ucci.com
MAILING ADDRESS:
    UNITED CONCORDIA CO INC - MO
    390 South Woods Mill Rd Ste 175
    Chesterfield, MO 63017

KEY EXECUTIVES:
Chief Executive Officer/President .... Thomas A Dzuryachko
Senior VP, Finance .... Daniel Wright
VP, National Dental Director .... Richard Klich, DMD
Marketing Director .... Philip McCullum
MIS Director .... Jim Robins
Director, Provider Services .... Ted Pesano

COMPANY PROFILE:
Parent Company Name: Highmark Inc
Doing Business As:
Year Founded: 1991   Federally Qualified: [ ]
Forprofit: [Y]   Not-For-Profit: [ ]
Model Type:
Accreditation: [ ] AAPPO [ ] JACHO [ ] NCQA [ ] URAC
Plan Type: Specialty HMO, Specialty PPO, POS, TPA
SERVICE AREA:
Nationwide: N
    IA; KS; MO; ND; NE; SD;
TYPE OF COVERAGE:
Commercial: [Y] Individual: [ ] FEHBP: [ ] Indemnity: [ ]
Medicare: [ ] Medicaid: [ ] Supplemental Medicare: [ ]
Tricare   [ ]
PLAN BENEFITS:
Alternative Medicine: [ ]   Behavioral Health: [ ]
Chiropractic: [ ]   Dental: [X]
Home Care: [ ]   Inpatient SNF: [ ]
Long-Term Care: [ ]   Pharm. Mail Order: [ ]
Physical Therapy: [ ]   Podiatry: [ ]
Psychiatric: [ ]   Transplant: [ ]
Vision: [ ]   Wellness: [ ]
Workers' Comp: [ ]
Other Benefits:

UNITEDHEALTHCARE OF THE MIDWEST INC

13655 Riverport Dr
Maryland Heights, MO 63043-8560
Phone: 314-592-7000 Fax: 314-592-7157 Toll-Free: 800-535-9291
Web site: www.uhc.com
MAILING ADDRESS:
    UNITEDHEALTHCARE MIDWEST INC
    PO Box 2560
    Maryland Heights, MO 63043-8560

KEY EXECUTIVES:
Non-Executive Chairman .... Richard T Burke
Chief Executive Officer/President .... Steve C Walli
Director, Finance .... Barbara C Bentrup
Medical Director .... Jordan Ginsburg, MD
Executive Director .... Edward Graves
VP, Key Account & Sales Administration .... David Milich
Director, Network Management .... Michelle Grimm
Director, Quality Management .... Kathy Zilligen

COMPANY PROFILE:
Parent Company Name: UnitedHealth Group
Doing Business As:
Year Founded: 1986   Federally Qualified: [N]
Forprofit: [Y]   Not-For-Profit: [ ]
Model Type: IPA
Accreditation: [ ] AAPPO [X] JACHO [ ] NCQA [X] URAC
Plan Type: HMO, POS, CDHP, HSA, HRA
Primary Physicians: 3,082   Physician Specialists: 8,304
Hospitals: 100
Total Revenue: 2005:   521,080,309   2006:   545,409,340
Net Income   2005:   32,550,335   2006:   31,134,447
Total Enrollment:
    2001: 532,746   2004: 141,278   2007: 0
    2002: 436,259   2005: 107,255
    2003: 251,239   2006:   92,737
Medical Loss Ratio: 2005: 79.00   2006: 80.70
Administrative Expense Ratio: 2005: 12.00   2006: 11.50

MISSOURI

Plan Type: HMO, PPO, POS, ASO, TPA, HDHP
Total Revenue: 2005: 592,349,000 2006: 418,111,021
Net Income 2005: 21,200,000 2006: 563,710
Total Enrollment:
   2001: 207,199   2004: 230,830   2007: 0
   2002: 202,880   2005: 249,169
   2003: 211,388   2006: 57,973
Medical Loss Ratio: 2005: 85.80   2006: 90.30
Administrative Expense Ratio: 2005: 5.90   2006: 6.10

SERVICE AREA:
Nationwide: N
   AR; IL; KS; MO (Audrain, Barry, Barton, Benton, Boone, Callaway, Camden, Cedar, Chariton, Christian, Clinton, Cole, Cooper, Crawford, Dave, Dallas, Dent, Douglas, Franklin, Gasconade, Greene, Hickory, Howard, Howell, Iron, Jasper, Jefferson, Jersey, Laclede, Lawrence, Lincoln, Linn, Macon, Madison, Maries, McDonald, Miller, Maniteau, Monroe, Montgomery, Morgan, Newton, Osage, Ozark, Pettis, Phelps, Pike, Polk, Pulaski, Ralls, Randolph, Reynolds, Saline, Shannon, StCharles, St Clair, St Francois, St Louis, Stone, Taney, Texas, Warren, Washington, Webster, Wright); TX (Jim Hogg, Webb, Zapata);

TYPE OF COVERAGE:
Commercial: [Y] Individual: [ ] FEHBP: [Y] Indemnity: [ ]
Medicare: [Y] Medicaid: [ ] Supplemental Medicare: [Y]
Tricare   [ ]

PRODUCTS OFFERED:
Product Name:	Type:
Mercy Care Plus	Medicare
Mercy Premier Plus	Medicare
Mercy Health Plan	Medicaid
St Johns PremierPlus	Medicare Advantage

CONSUMER-DRIVEN PRODUCTS
	HSA Company
	HSA Product
	HSA Administrator
	Consumer-Driven Health Plan
MyChoice	High Deductible Health Plan

PLAN BENEFITS:
Alternative Medicine: [ ]   Behavioral Health: [X]
Chiropractic: [X]   Dental: [ ]
Home Care: [X]   Inpatient SNF: [X]
Long-Term Care: [ ]   Pharm. Mail Order: [X]
Physical Therapy: [X]   Podiatry: [X]
Psychiatric: [X]   Transplant: [X]
Vision: [X]   Wellness: [X]
Workers' Comp: [ ]
Other Benefits:

MISSOURI CARE

2404 Forum Blvd
Columbia, MO 65203
Phone: 573-441-2100 Fax: 573-441-2199 Toll-Free: 800-322-6027
Web site: www.missouricare.com

MAILING ADDRESS:
   MISSOURI CARE
   2404 Forum Blvd
   Columbia, MO 65203

KEY EXECUTIVES:
Chief Executive Officer .... Donna Checkett
Chief Financial Officer .... Susan Christy
Chief Medical Officer .... Andrew Matera, MD
Secretary .... Hank Wells

COMPANY PROFILE:
Parent Company Name:
Doing Business As:
Year Founded: 1997   Federally Qualified: [ ]
Forprofit: [ ]   Not-For-Profit: [Y]
Model Type:
Accreditation: [ ] AAPPO [ ] JACHO [ ] NCQA [ ] URAC
Plan Type: HMO, PRO, UR,
Primary Physicians: 1,000   Physician Specialists:
Hospitals: 18
Total Revenue: 2005: 79,616,609 2006: 76,089,021
Net Income   2005: 2,280,608   2006: -2,318,172
Total Enrollment:
   2001: 0   2004: 35,607   2007: 0
   2002: 30,393   2005: 32,492
   2003: 33,246   2006: 29,808

Medical Loss Ratio: 2005: 83.00   2006: 86.60
Administrative Expense Ratio: 2005: 12.30   2006: 13.50

SERVICE AREA:
Nationwide:
   MO, (Audrain, Boone, Callaway, Camden, Chariton, Cole, Cooper, Gasconade, Howard, Miller, Moniteau, Monroe, Montgomery, Morgan, Osage, Pettis, Randolph, Saline);

PPO USA INC

310 N E Mulberry
Lee's Summit, MO 64086
Phone: 816-434-4408 Fax: 816-434-4422 Toll-Free: 877-477-6872
Web site: www.ppousa.com

MAILING ADDRESS:
   PPO USA INC
   310 N E Mulberry
   Lee's Summit, MO 64086

KEY EXECUTIVES:
Chief Executive Officer .... Joseph Witkowski
Marketing Director .... Joseph Witkowski

COMPANY PROFILE:
Parent Company Name: Government Employees Hospital Assoc Inc
Doing Business As:
Year Founded: 1997   Federally Qualified: [ ]
Forprofit: [Y]   Not-For-Profit: [ ]
Model Type: Network
Accreditation: [ ] AAPPO [ ] JACHO [ ] NCQA [ ] URAC
Plan Type: PPO
Total Enrollment:
   2001: 500,000   2004: 435,000   2007: 0
   2002: 0   2005: 531,605
   2003: 0   2006:

SERVICE AREA:
Nationwide: Y
   Dental, Vision, Hearing, Nationwide; Medical: AK, AL, CO, IA, ID, LA, MN, MS, MT, ND, NE, NM, NV, OK, SD, TN, UT, WI, WV, WY;

TYPE OF COVERAGE:
Commercial: [Y] Individual: [ ] FEHBP: [ ] Indemnity: [ ]
Medicare: [ ] Medicaid: [ ] Supplemental Medicare: [ ]
Tricare   [ ]

PRODUCTS OFFERED:
Product Name:	Type:
PPO	PPO
Connection Dental	
Connection Hearing	
Connection Vision	

PLAN BENEFITS:
Alternative Medicine: [ ]   Behavioral Health: [ ]
Chiropractic: [ ]   Dental: [X]
Home Care: [ ]   Inpatient SNF: [ ]
Long-Term Care: [ ]   Pharm. Mail Order: [ ]
Physical Therapy: [ ]   Podiatry: [ ]
Psychiatric: [ ]   Transplant: [ ]
Vision: [X]   Wellness: [ ]
Workers' Comp: [ ]
Other Benefits:

PRIMARIS

200 N Keene St
Columbia, MO 65201
Phone: 573-817-8300 Fax: 573-817-8330 Toll-Free: 800-735-6776
Web site: www.primaris.com

MAILING ADDRESS:
   PRIMARIS
   200 N Keene St
   Columbia, MO 65201

KEY EXECUTIVES:
Chairman of the Board .... James T Rogers
Chief Executive Officer .... Richard A Royer
Chief Financial Officer .... Timothy J Schultz, MBA, CPA, MBS, MS
Medical Director .... Gregg R Laiben, MD
Director, Physician Services .... Deborah K Finley, MPA
Human Resources Director .... Carlene Johnson
Manager, Information Technology .... Jason Isaacs, BS

Managed Care Organization Profiles — MISSOURI

Total Enrollment:
  2001: 9,089   2004: 15,076   2007: 0
  2002: 1,188,183   2005:
  2003: 960,956   2006: 95
Medical Loss Ratio: 2005: 84.40   2006: 87.80
Administrative Expense Ratio: 2005: 58.00   2006: 39.40
SERVICE AREA:
Nationwide: N
  MO;
TYPE OF COVERAGE:
Commercial: [Y] Individual: [Y] FEHBP: [ ] Indemnity: [ ]
Medicare: [ ] Medicaid: [ ] Supplemental Medicare: [ ]
Tricare   [ ]
PRODUCTS OFFERED:
Product Name: Type:
HealthLink HMO   HMO
HealthLink PPO   PPO
PLAN BENEFITS:
Alternative Medicine: [ ]   Behavioral Health: [X]
Chiropractic: [ ]   Dental: [X]
Home Care: [ ]   Inpatient SNF: [X]
Long-Term Care: [ ]   Pharm. Mail Order: [X]
Physical Therapy: [X]   Podiatry: [X]
Psychiatric: [X]   Transplant: [ ]
Vision: [X]   Wellness: [X]
Workers' Comp: [ ]
Other Benefits:

HEALTHLINK INC - CORPORATE HEADQUARTERS

12443 Olive Blvd
St Louis, MO 63141
Phone: 314-989-6000 Fax: 314-989-6620 Toll-Free: 877-284-0101
Web site: www.healthlink.com
MAILING ADDRESS:
  HEALTHLINK INC - CORP HDQTRS
  12443 Olive Blvd
  St Louis, MO 63141

KEY EXECUTIVES:
Chief Executive Officer/President .... Dennis Casey
Staff VP, Finance .... Tim Neyer
VP, Medical Director .... John J Seidenfeld, MD
Staff VP, Information Tchnlgy .... Gary Siemen
VP Operations/IT .... Lynn Yearwood
VP, Marketing .... Courtney B Walter

COMPANY PROFILE:
Parent Company Name: WellPoint Inc
Doing Business As: HealthLink Inc
Year Founded: 1985   Federally Qualified: [N]
Forprofit: [Y]   Not-For-Profit: [ ]
Model Type: NETWORK
Accreditation: [ ] AAPPO [ ] JACHO [ ] NCQA [X] URAC
Plan Type: HMO, PPO, Specialty PPO, ASO, POS, TPA, PBM
Primary Physicians: 25,000   Physician Specialists: 14,000
Hospitals: 300
Total Enrollment:
  2001: 2,000,000   2004: 1,000,000   2007: 0
  2002: 0   2005:
  2003: 1,200,000   2006: 1,000,000
SERVICE AREA:
Nationwide: N
  AR; IA; IL; IN; KY; MO; WV;
TYPE OF COVERAGE:
Commercial: [Y] Individual: [ ] FEHBP: [ ] Indemnity: [ ]
Medicare: [ ] Medicaid: [ ] Supplemental Medicare: [ ]
Tricare   [ ]
PRODUCTS OFFERED:
Product Name: Type:
HealthLink HMO   HMO
HealthLink PPO   PPO
HealthLink CompManagement   Workers' Comp
HealthLink Open Access   Open Access
PLAN BENEFITS:
Alternative Medicine: [ ]   Behavioral Health: [X]
Chiropractic: [ ]   Dental: [X]
Home Care: [ ]   Inpatient SNF: [X]
Long-Term Care: [ ]   Pharm. Mail Order: [X]
Physical Therapy: [X]   Podiatry: [X]
Psychiatric: [X]   Transplant: [ ]
Vision: [X]   Wellness: [X]
Workers' Comp: [X]
Other Benefits:

MERCY CAREPLUS

14528 S Outer 40 Ste 300
St Louis, MO 63132
Phone: 314-214-8100 Fax: 314-214-8101 Toll-Free:
Web site:
MAILING ADDRESS:
  MERCY CAREPLUS
  14528 S Outer 40 Ste 300
  St Louis, MO 63132

KEY EXECUTIVES:
Chief Executive Officer/President .... Jerry Linder
Director of Finance .... Ed Oswald
Chief Medical Officer .... Rajendra Parikh, MD
Pharmacy Director .... Beverly Thompson, MD
Chief Operating Officer .... Cris Cristea
Marketing Director .... Marcia Aldridge
MIS Manager .... Jim Lamkin
Provider Relations Director .... Cris Cristea
Human Resources Director .... Ron Port

COMPANY PROFILE:
Parent Company Name: Molina Healthcare Inc
Doing Business As: Alliance For Community Health, LLC
Year Founded: 1995   Federally Qualified: [Y]
Forprofit: [ ]   Not-For-Profit: [Y]
Model Type:
Accreditation: [ ] AAPPO [ ] JACHO [ ] NCQA [ ] URAC
Plan Type: HMO
Total Revenue: 2005:   85,487,331   2006: 124,237,316
Net Income   2005:   460,995   2006:   9,400,623
Total Enrollment:
  2001: 34,239   2004: 47,298   2007: 67,800
  2002: 0   2005: 45,017
  2003: 46,674   2006: 69,874
Medical Loss Ratio: 2005: 90.60   2006: 81.00
Administrative Expense Ratio: 2005: 4.60   2006: 5.10
SERVICE AREA:
Nationwide: N
  MO;
TYPE OF COVERAGE:
Commercial: [Y] Individual: [ ] FEHBP: [ ] Indemnity: [ ]
Medicare: [ ] Medicaid: [ ] Supplemental Medicare: [ ]
Tricare   [ ]
PRODUCTS OFFERED:
Product Name: Type:
Community Care Plus   Medicaid
Comments:
Community Care Plus and Alliance for Community Care and Mercy
Health Plan merged July 1, 2006 to create Mercy Care Plus. Acquired by
Molina Healthcare Inc, November 1, 2007.

MERCY HEALTH PLANS OF MISSOURI INC

14528 Outer 40 Dr
Chesterfield, MO 63017-5705
Phone: 314-214-8100 Fax: 314-214-8101 Toll-Free: 800-830-1918
Web site: www.mercyhealthplans.com
MAILING ADDRESS:
  MERCY HEALTH PLANS OF MO INC
  14528 Outer 40 Dr
  Chesterfield, MO 63017-5705

KEY EXECUTIVES:
Chief Executive Officer/President .... Michael G Murphy
Chief Financial Officer .... George Schneider, CPA, CMCP
Chief Medical Officer .... Deborah Zimmerman, MD
Clinical Pharmacy Manager .... Catherine Linsin, PhD
Vice President .... Gary Levine
VP, Human Resources .... Donna McDaniel
VP, General Counsel .... Charles Gilham
Executive Director, St Louis Region .... Carl Schultz
Executive Director, Controller .... Steve Jansen
Executive Director, Arkansas Region .... Brett Kirkman
Executive Director, Texas Region .... Ernesto Sequra

COMPANY PROFILE:
Parent Company Name: Mercy Health Plans, Inc
Doing Business As: Premier Health Plans, Mercy MC + Inc
Year Founded: 1994   Federally Qualified: [N]
Forprofit: [Y]   Not-For-Profit: [ ]
Model Type: NETWORK
Accreditation: [ ] AAPPO [ ] JACHO [ ] NCQA [ ] URAC

MISSOURI — Managed Care Organization Profiles

GROUP HEALTH PLAN INC

111 Corporate Office Dr #400
Earth City, MO 63045
Phone: 314-506-1700 Fax: 314-506-1767 Toll-Free: 800-755-3901
Web site: www.ghp.com

MAILING ADDRESS:
GROUP HEALTH PLAN INC
111 Corporate Office Dr #400
Earth City, MO 63045

KEY EXECUTIVES:
Chief Executive Officer/President .... Charles R Stark
Chief Financial Officer .... Barbara Witte
Medical Director .... Richard Sanchez, MD
Chief Operating Officer .... Claudia Bjerre
VP, Sales & Marketing .... Frank D'Antonio
Provider Services VP .... Bonnie Kitson
VP, Network Operations .... Ryan Voisey
Human Resource VP .... Lisa Williams
Health Services VP .... Rebecca Sanborn
Quality Assurance VP .... Laura Ruzas

COMPANY PROFILE:
Parent Company Name: Coventry Health Care Inc
Doing Business As:
Year Founded: 1982   Federally Qualified: [Y]
Forprofit: [Y]   Not-For-Profit: [ ]
Model Type: IPA
Accreditation: [ ] AAPPO [ ] JACHO [ ] NCQA [ ] URAC
Plan Type: HMO, PPO, POS, CDHP, HDHP, HSA
Total Revenue: 2005:   524,739,385   2006:   517,275,130
Net Income   2005:   40,283,277   2006:   38,497,372
Total Enrollment:
   2001: 249,798   2004: 200,048   2007: 0
   2002: 221,046   2005: 110,797
   2003: 195,161   2006: 297,000
Medical Loss Ratio: 2005: 81.60   2006: 83.70
Administrative Expense Ratio: 2005:   5.90   2006:   5.20

SERVICE AREA:
Nationwide: N
MO (St Louis, Mid-MO); IL (Southern & Central);

TYPE OF COVERAGE:
Commercial: [Y] Individual: [Y] FEHBP: [ ] Indemnity: [ ]
Medicare: [Y] Medicaid: [ ] Supplemental Medicare: [ ]
Tricare   [ ]

PRODUCTS OFFERED:
Product Name: Type:
Access, Exclusive & Sensicare   HMO
Access Plus, Exclusive Plus   POS
Advantra   Medicare Advantage
CMR   TPA
CONSUMER-DRIVEN PRODUCTS
Wells Fargo   HSA Company
                                     HSA Product
Corporate Benefits Services of America   HSA Administrator
                                     Consumer-Driven Health Plan
Open Access Plus Plan   High Deductible Health Plan

PLAN BENEFITS:
Alternative Medicine: [X]   Behavioral Health: [X]
Chiropractic: [X]   Dental: [X]
Home Care: [X]   Inpatient SNF: [X]
Long-Term Care: [ ]   Pharm. Mail Order: [X]
Physical Therapy: [X]   Podiatry: [X]
Psychiatric: [X]   Transplant: [X]
Vision: [X]   Wellness: [X]
Workers' Comp: [ ]
Other Benefits:
Comments:
Formerly called Partners HMO.

HEALTHCARE USA OF MISSOURI LLC

10 S Broadway #1200
St Louis, MO 63102
Phone: 314-241-5300 Fax: 314-241-8010 Toll-Free: 800-213-7792
Web site: www.cvty.com

MAILING ADDRESS:
HEALTHCARE USA OF MISSOURI
10 S Broadway #1200
St Louis, MO 63102

KEY EXECUTIVES:
Chief Executive Officer/President .... Claudia Bjerre
Medical Director .... Carl G Bynum, MD
VP, Health Services .... Linda Whaley

COMPANY PROFILE:
Parent Company Name: Coventry Health Care Inc
Doing Business As:
Year Founded: 1995   Federally Qualified: [N]
Forprofit: [Y]   Not-For-Profit: [ ]Model Type:
Accreditation: [ ] AAPPO [ ] JACHO [ ] NCQA [ ] URAC
Plan Type: HMO
Total Revenue: 2005:   34,285,244   2006:   324,586,616
Net Income   2005:   17,360,349   2006:   12,328,754
Total Enrollment:
   2001: 137,719   2004: 185,375   2007: 0
   2002: 154,902   2005: 162,470
   2003: 188,815   2006: 150,748
Medical Loss Ratio: 2005: 83.20   2006: 87.50
Administrative Expense Ratio: 2005:   7.50   2006:   6.80

SERVICE AREA:
Nationwide: N
MO (Audrain, Boone, Callaway, Camden, Cass, Chariton, Clay, Cole, Cooper, Franklin, Gasconade, Henry, Howard, Jackson, Jefferson, Johnson, Lafayette, Lincoln, Miller, Moniteau, Monroe, Montgomery, Morgan, Osage, Pettis, Platte, Randolph, Ray, Saline, St Charles, St Clair, St Francois, St Louis City, St Louis County, Ste Genevieve, Warren, Washington);

TYPE OF COVERAGE:
Commercial: [ ] Individual: [ ] FEHBP: [ ] Indemnity: [ ]
Medicare: [ ] Medicaid: [Y] Supplemental Medicare: [ ]
Tricare   [ ]

PRODUCTS OFFERED:
Product Name: Type:
Healthcare USA   Medicaid

PLAN BENEFITS:
Alternative Medicine: [ ]   Behavioral Health: [X]
Chiropractic: [ ]   Dental: [X]
Home Care: [X]   Inpatient SNF: [ ]
Long-Term Care: [ ]   Pharm. Mail Order: [ ]
Physical Therapy: [ ]   Podiatry: [ ]
Psychiatric: [X]   Transplant: [ ]
Vision: [X]   Wellness: [X]
Workers' Comp: [ ]
Other Benefits:
Comments:
Purchased FirstGuard Health Plans, December 2006.

HEALTHLINK INC

12443 Olive Blvd
St Louis, MO 63141
Phone: 314-989-6000 Fax: 314-989-6620 Toll-Free: 800-624-2356
Web site: www.healthlink.com

MAILING ADDRESS:
HEALTHLINK INC
12443 Olive Blvd
St Louis, MO 63141

KEY EXECUTIVES:
Chief Executive Officer/President .... David W Fields
VP & Chief Financial Officer .... Larry Glasscock
VP & Medical Director .... John J Seidenfeld, MD
General Manager, WPM .... Michael A Nameth, RPh, MBA
Staff Vice President .... Gary Sieman
VP Marketing .... Courtney B Walter

COMPANY PROFILE:
Parent Company Name: HealthLink Inc
Doing Business As: Healthlink HMO, HealthLink PPO
Year Founded: 1993   Federally Qualified: [N]
Forprofit: [Y]   Not-For-Profit: [ ]
Model Type: IPA
Accreditation: [ ] AAPPO [ ] JACHO [ ] NCQA [ ] URAC
Plan Type: HMO, PPO, PBM, POS, UR
Primary Physicians: 6,121   Physician Specialists: 12,204
Hospitals: 251
Total Revenue: 2005:   66,074   2006:   52,201
Net Income   2005:   -7,211   2006:   -1,519

Managed Care Organization Profiles   **MISSOURI**

KEY EXECUTIVES:
President .... Charles J Willey, MD
Chief Financial Officer .... Paul Meuttenmuller
Chief Medical Officer .... Thomas Hastings, MD

COMPANY PROFILE:
Parent Company Name: American Multispecialty Group Inc
Doing Business As:
Year Founded: 2003   Federally Qualified: [ ]
Forprofit: [Y]   Not-For-Profit: [ ]
Model Type:
Accreditation: [ ] AAPPO [ ] JACHO [ ] NCQA [ ] URAC
Plan Type: HMO,
Total Revenue: 2005: 12,981,628   2006: 31,997,110
Net Income   2005: -1,281,287   2006: 824,493
Total Enrollment:
   2001: 0   2004: 256   2007: 0
   2002: 0   2005: 3,003
   2003: 0   2006: 4,862
Medical Loss Ratio: 2005: 74.50   2006: 76.40
Administrative Expense Ratio: 2005: 24.40   2006: 15.90

SERVICE AREA:
Nationwide:
   MO (Jefferson, St Charles, St Louis City, St Louis County):

TYPE OF COVERAGE:
Commercial: [ ] Individual: [ ] FEHBP: [ ] Indemnity: [ ]
Medicare: [Y] Medicaid: [ ] Supplemental Medicare: [ ]
Tricare   [ ]

FAMILY HEALTH PARTNERS

215 W Pershing Rd 6th Fl
Kansas City, MO 64108
Phone: 816-855-1888 Fax: 816-855-1890 Toll-Free: 800-347-9363
Web site: www.fhp.org
MAILING ADDRESS:
   FAMILY HEALTH PARTNERS
   215 W Pershing Rd 6th Fl
   Kansas City, MO 64108

KEY EXECUTIVES:
Chief Executive Officer .... Bob Finuf
President .... Jo Stueve
Director of Finance .... Suzie Dunaway
Medical Director .... Ben Rubin, MD
Director Community & Government Relations .... Taira Green
Director of Information Technology .... Bob Clark
Director Community & Government Relations .... Tara Miller
Director of Operations .... Linda Steinke
Quality Improvement Manager .... Jenny Hainey RN
Compliance Officer .... Mikki Massey
Health Services Director .... Ma'ata Touslee

COMPANY PROFILE:
Parent Company Name: Children's Mercy Hospital
Doing Business As:
Year Founded: 1996   Federally Qualified: [ ]
Forprofit: [ ]   Not-For-Profit: [Y]
Model Type: IPA
Accreditation: [ ] AAPPO [ ] JACHO [X] NCQA [ ] URAC
Plan Type: HMO, PPO, PBM, POS, ASO, PRO, EPO, TPA, UR, CDHP, HDHP, HSA, FSA, HRA
Primary Physicians: 310   Physician Specialists: 1,200
Hospitals: 31
Total Revenue: 2005: 109,420,014   2006: 96,763,173
Net Income   2005: 3,698,481   2006: 1,135,977
Total Enrollment:
   2001:   2004:   2007:
   2002:   2005: 31,343
   2003:   2006: 27,865
Medical Loss Ratio: 2005: 87.10   2006: 84.80
Administrative Expense Ratio: 2005: 6.70   2006: 11.50

SERVICE AREA:
Nationwide: N
   MO (Cass, Clay, Henry, Jackson, Johnson, Lafayette, Platte, Ray, St Clair);

TYPE OF COVERAGE:
Commercial: [ ] Individual: [ ] FEHBP: [ ] Indemnity: [ ]
Medicare: [ ] Medicaid: [Y] Supplemental Medicare: [ ]
Tricare   [ ]

PRODUCTS OFFERED:
Product Name: Type:
MCT Program   HMO
Healthwave Program   HMO
Family Health Partners   Medicaid

PLAN BENEFITS:
Alternative Medicine: [ ]   Behavioral Health: [X]
Chiropractic: [ ]   Dental: [X]
Home Care: [X]   Inpatient SNF: [X]
Long-Term Care: [ ]   Pharm. Mail Order: [ ]
Physical Therapy: [X]   Podiatry: [X]
Psychiatric: [X]   Transplant: [ ]
Vision: [X]   Wellness: [X]
Workers' Comp: [ ]
Other Benefits: X

GOOD HEALTH HMO INC

2301 Main St
Kansas City, MO 64108-2428
Phone: 816-395-2222 Fax: 816-395-2726 Toll-Free:
Web site: www.bcbskc.com
MAILING ADDRESS:
   GOOD HEALTH HMO INC
   PO Box 419163
   Kansas City, MO 64108-2428

KEY EXECUTIVES:
Chairman of the Board .... Ben D McCallister, MD
Chief Executive Officer/President .... Tom Bowser
Chief Operations Officer .... John W Kennedy
Chief Financial Officer .... Marilyn T Tromans
Chief Medical Officer .... Blake Williamson, MD
Chief Information Officer .... Kevin P Sparks
Chief Marketing Officer .... Roger L Foreman
VP, Information Access .... Darren C Taylor

COMPANY PROFILE:
Parent Company Name: Blue Cross Blue Shield of Kansas City
Doing Business As: Blue Care Inc
Year Founded: 1988   Federally Qualified: [N]
Forprofit: [Y]   Not-For-Profit: [ ]
Model Type: IPA
Accreditation: [ ] AAPPO [ ] JACHO [X] NCQA [X] URAC
Plan Type: HMO, PPO, HDHP, HSA,
Primary Physicians: 3,250   Physician Specialists:
Hospitals: 32
Total Revenue: 2005: 224,569,406   2006: 269,995.833
Net Income   2005: 986,446   2006: 341,211
Total Enrollment:
   2001: 0   2004: 64,416   2007: 58,600
   2002: 0   2005: 45,990
   2003: 0   2006: 53,541
Medical Loss Ratio: 2005: 88.40   2006: 89.80
Administrative Expense Ratio: 2005: 8.80   2006: 8.20

SERVICE AREA:
Nationwide: N
   MO (Andrew, Buchanan, Cass, Clay, Jackson, Johnson, Lafayette, Platte, Ray); KS (Johnson, Wyandotte);

TYPE OF COVERAGE:
Commercial: [Y] Individual: [ ] FEHBP: [ ] Indemnity: [ ]
Medicare: [Y] Medicaid: [ ] Supplemental Medicare: [ ]
Tricare   [ ]

PRODUCTS OFFERED:
Product Name: Type:
Total Healthcare 65   Medicare

CONSUMER-DRIVEN PRODUCTS
                              HSA Company
                              HSA Product
Wells Fargo   HSA Administrator
                              Consumer-Driven Health Plan
Blue Saver   High Deductible Health Plan

Comments:
Formerly Total Healthcare.

MISSOURI

KEY EXECUTIVES:
Chief Executive Officer/President .... George B Wheeler
Chief Financial Officer .... James M Maxwell
Chief Medical Officer .... William R Rooney, MD

COMPANY PROFILE:
Parent Company Name: Coventry Health Care Inc
Doing Business As:
Year Founded: 1981   Federally Qualified: [N]
Forprofit: [Y]   Not-For-Profit: [ ]
Model Type: MIXED
Accreditation: [ ] AAPPO [ ] JACHO [ ] NCQA [X] URAC
Plan Type: HMO, PPO, POS,
Total Revenue: 2005:   459,270,660   2006:   480,019,717
Net Income   2005:   48,361,977   2006:   43,079,757
Total Enrollment:
   2001: 144,210   2004: 155,374   2007: 0
   2002: 258,591   2005: 209,000
   2003: 168,555   2006: 76,113
Medical Loss Ratio: 2005: 74.50   2006: 76.40
Administrative Expense Ratio: 2005:   9.80   2006: 10.00

SERVICE AREA:
Nationwide: N
   KS (Allen, Anderson, Atchison, Bourbon, Brown, Butler, Chase, Chautauqua); IL (Cook, DuPage, Lake, Madison, McHenry, Peoria, Sangamon, Whiteside); MO (Andrew, Barton, Benton, Buchanan, Caldwell, Carroll, Cass, Christian, Clay, Clinton, Dade, Dallas, Daviess, DeKalb, Gentry, Green, Grundy, Henry, Jackson, Jasper, Johnson, Lafayette, Livingston, Newton, Pettis, Platte, Polk, Ray, Vernon, Webster);

TYPE OF COVERAGE:
Commercial: [Y] Individual: [ ]   FEHBP: [ ]   Indemnity: [ ]
Medicare: [Y] Medicaid: [ ]   Supplemental Medicare: [ ]
Tricare   [ ]

PRODUCTS OFFERED:
Product Name: Type:
Advantra 65   Medicare Advantage
CONSUMER-DRIVEN PRODUCTS
Wells Fargo   HSA Company
                                       HSA Product
Corporate Benefits Servs of Am   HSA Administrator
                                       Consumer-Driven Health Plan
Open Access Plus Plan   High Deductible Health Plan

Comments:
Formerly Principal Health Care of Kansas Inc - Kansas City.

COX HEALTH PLANS

3200 S National Ste B
Springfield, MO 65807
Phone: 417-269-4679 Fax: 417-269-4667 Toll-Free: 800-205-7665
Web site: www.coxhealthplans.com
MAILING ADDRESS:
   COX HEALTH PLANS
   3200 S National Ste B
   Springfield, MO 65807

KEY EXECUTIVES:
Chief Executive Officer/President .... Jeffrey C Bond
Chief Financial Officer .... Matthew Aug
Chief Medical Officer .... Kerry Randolph, MD
Chief Operating Officer .... Kurt Scherer
VP, Marketing .... Jacob Salinas

COMPANY PROFILE:
Parent Company Name: Cox Health Systems
Doing Business As: Cox Health Plans
Year Founded: 1996   Federally Qualified: [N]
Forprofit: [Y]   Not-For-Profit: [ ]
Model Type: NETWORK
Accreditation: [ ] AAPPO [ ] JACHO [ ] NCQA [ ] URAC
Plan Type: HMO, PPO, POS,
Primary Physicians: 385   Physician Specialists: 784
Hospitals: 14
Total Revenue: 2005:   12,268,587   2006:   21,003,766
Net Income   2005:   -1,993,089   2006:   -2,453,632
Total Enrollment:
   2001: 18,395   2004: 3,349   2007: 0
   2002: 18,137   2005: 5,498
   2003: 14,653   2006: 7,999
Medical Loss Ratio: 2005: 103.60   2006: 99.80
Administrative Expense Ratio: 2005: 11.70   2006: 10.90

SERVICE AREA:
Nationwide: N
   MO (Barry, Barton, Cedar, Christian, Dade, Dallas, Douglas, Greene, Hickory, Howell, Jasper, Laclede, Lawrence, McDonald, Newton, Oregon, Ozark, Polk, Shannon, Stone, Taney, Texas, Vernon, Webster, Wright);

TYPE OF COVERAGE:
Commercial: [Y] Individual: [ ]   FEHBP: [ ]   Indemnity: [ ]
Medicare: [ ] Medicaid: [ ]   Supplemental Medicare: [ ]
Tricare   [ ]

PRODUCTS OFFERED:
Product Name: Type:
Cox Health HMO   HMO
Cox Health POS   POS

DELTA DENTAL PLAN OF MISSOURI

12399 Gravois Rd
St Louis, MO 63126-0690
Phone: 314-656-3000 Fax: 314-656-2900 Toll-Free: 800-392-1167
Web site: www.deltadentalmo.com
MAILING ADDRESS:
   DELTA DENTAL PLAN OF MO
   PO Box 8690
   St Louis, MO 63126-0690

KEY EXECUTIVES:
Chairman of the Board .... Richard J Haffner, DDS
Chief Executive Officer/President .... Steve P Gaal, III
Chief Financial Officer .... David Haynes
Chief Information Officer .... Karl Mudra
Senior VP, Chief Operating Officer .... Pam Martin
Marketing Director .... Richard Klassen

COMPANY PROFILE:
Parent Company Name: Delta Dental Plan Association
Doing Business As:
Year Founded: 1958   Federally Qualified: [N]
Forprofit: [ ]   Not-For-Profit: [Y]
Model Type:
Accreditation: [ ] AAPPO [ ] JACHO [ ] NCQA [ ] URAC
Plan Type: Specialty PPO, POS
Total Enrollment:
   2001:   0   2004: 386,094   2007: 0
   2002: 351,317   2005:
   2003: 351,265   2006:

SERVICE AREA:
Nationwide: N
   MO;

TYPE OF COVERAGE:
Commercial: [Y] Individual: [ ]   FEHBP: [ ]   Indemnity: [ ]
Medicare: [ ] Medicaid: [ ]   Supplemental Medicare: [ ]
Tricare   [ ]

PRODUCTS OFFERED:
Product Name: Type:
Delta Dental Plan of MO   Specialty PPO
Delta Dental Plan of MO   Indemnity

PLAN BENEFITS:
Alternative Medicine: [ ]   Behavioral Health: [ ]
Chiropractic: [ ]   Dental: [X]
Home Care: [ ]   Inpatient SNF: [ ]
Long-Term Care: [ ]   Pharm. Mail Order: [ ]
Physicial Therapy: [ ]   Podiatry: [ ]
Psychiatric: [ ]   Transplant: [ ]
Vision: [ ]   Wellness: [ ]
Workers' Comp: [ ]
Other Benefits:

ESSENCE INC

12655 Olive Blvd 4th Fl
St Louis, MO 63141
Phone: 314-851-1000 Fax: 314-851-4445 Toll-Free:
Web site:
MAILING ADDRESS:
   ESSENCE INC
   12655 Olive Blvd 4th Fl
   St Louis, MO 63141

Managed Care Organization Profiles — MISSOURI

SERVICE AREA:
Nationwide: N
  IN; KS; MO; NJ; OH; TX; WI;
TYPE OF COVERAGE:
Commercial: [ ] Individual: [ ] FEHBP: [ ] Indemnity: [ ]
Medicare: [ ] Medicaid: [Y] Supplemental Medicare: [ ]
Tricare [ ]
PRODUCTS OFFERED:

Product Name:	Type:
Coordinated Care Corp	Medicaid
University Health Plan Inc	Medicaid
Buckeye Community Health Plan	Medicaid
Superior Health Plan	Medicaid
Managed Health Services WI Inc	Medicaid
Peach State Health Plan	Medicaid
Total Carolina Care Inc	Medicaid

CIGNA HEALTHCARE OF ST LOUIS

One North Brentwood Blvd
St Louis, MO 63105
Phone: 314-726-7850 Fax: 314-726-7820 Toll-Free: 800-832-3211
Web site: www.cigna.com
MAILING ADDRESS:
  CIGNA HEALTHCARE OF ST LOUIS
  One North Brentwood Blvd
  St Louis, MO 63105

KEY EXECUTIVES:
President .... Frank A Monahan
Chief Financial Officer .... Vincent L Shreckengast
Chief Medical Officer .... Aslam Mohammad Khan, MD, MM
COMPANY PROFILE:
Parent Company Name: CIGNA Corporation
Doing Business As:
Year Founded: 1986   Federally Qualified: [Y]
Forprofit: [Y]   Not-For-Profit: [ ]
Model Type: IPA
Accreditation: [ ] AAPPO [ ] JACHO [X] NCQA [ ] URAC
Plan Type: HMO, PPO, PBM, POS, ASO, PRO, EPO, TPA, UR, CDHP, HDHP, HSA, FSA, HRA
Total Revenue: 2005:   16,129,326   2006:   16,077,079
Net Income   2005:   1,535,999   2006:   993,042
Total Enrollment:
  2001: 1,924   2004: 4,106   2007: 0
  2002: 10,781   2005: 4,335
  2003: 7,558   2006: 4,292
Medical Loss Ratio: 2005: 82.40   2006: 81.80
Administrative Expense Ratio: 2005:   3.70   2006:   8.40
SERVICE AREA:
Nationwide: N
  MO (Crawford, Franklin, Gasconade, Jefferson, Lincoln, Montgomery, Pike, St Charles, St Francois, St Louis City, St Louis County, Ste Genevieve, Warren, Washington); IL (Bond, Calhoun, Clinton, Greene, Jersey, Macoupin, Madison, Monroe, Montgomery, Randolph, St Clair, Washington);
TYPE OF COVERAGE:
Commercial: [Y] Individual: [ ] FEHBP: [ ] Indemnity: [ ]
Medicare: [ ] Medicaid: [ ] Supplemental Medicare: [ ]
Tricare [ ]
CONSUMER-DRIVEN PRODUCTS

JP Morgan Chase	HSA Company
CIGNA Choice Fund	HSA Product
	HSA Administrator
Open Access Plus	Consumer-Driven Health Plan
PPO	High Deductible Health Plan

PLAN BENEFITS:

Alternative Medicine:	[ ]	Behavioral Health:	[ ]
Chiropractic:	[X]	Dental:	[X]
Home Care:	[X]	Inpatient SNF:	[X]
Long-Term Care:	[X]	Pharm. Mail Order:	[X]
Physical Therapy:	[X]	Podiatry:	[X]
Psychiatric:	[X]	Transplant:	[X]
Vision:	[X]	Wellness:	[X]
Workers' Comp:	[ ]		
Other Benefits:			

COMMUNITY HEALTH PLAN

137 N Belt Hwy
St Joseph, MO 64506
Phone: 816-271-1247 Fax: 816-271-1248 Toll-Free: 800-990-9247
Web site: www.mychp.com
MAILING ADDRESS:
  COMMUNITY HEALTH PLAN
  137 N Belt Hwy
  St Joseph, MO 64506

KEY EXECUTIVES:
Chief Executive Officer .... Lowell Kruse
Team Leader: Finance .... Stan Vaughan
Medical Director .... Jay McMillen, MD
Pharmacy Director .... Casey Nelson
Plan Administrator .... Linda Bahrke
Team Leader: Sales .... Dick Pugh
MIS Director .... Milisa Suckow
Public Relations Director .... Amy Owens
Network Development Director .... Audrey Shandley
Health Promotion Director .... Kim McManus
Team Leader Care Management/Call Center .... Cheryl Daniels
Quality Improvement Manager .... Stacey Counts
Credentialing Manager/Claims Team Leader .... Audrey Shandley
COMPANY PROFILE:
Parent Company Name: Heartland Health
Doing Business As:
Year Founded: 1994   Federally Qualified: [N]
Forprofit: [ ]   Not-For-Profit: [Y]
Model Type: NETWORK
Accreditation: [ ] AAPPO [ ] JACHO [ ] NCQA [ ] URAC
Plan Type: HMO, PPO, POS, ASO, CDHP, HDHP, HSA, TPA, EPO
Primary Physicians: 600   Physician Specialists: 1,900
Hospitals: 36
Total Revenue: 2005:   62,076,378   2006:   45,527,917
Net Income   2005:   196,000   2006:   -2,745,576
Total Enrollment:
  2001: 28,068   2004: 18,578   2007: 26,529
  2002: 29,846   2005: 213,492
  2003: 19,527   2006: 144,036
Medical Loss Ratio: 2005: 88.50   2006: 93.40
Administrative Expense Ratio: 2005: 11.80   2006: 13.70
SERVICE AREA:
Nationwide: N
  MO (Andrew, Atchison, Buchanan, Caldwell, Carroll, Cass, Clay, Clinton, Daviess, DeKalb, Gentry, Grundy, Harrison, Henry, Holt, Jackson, Johnson, Lafayette, Livingston, Mercer, Nodaway, Platte, Putnam, Ray, Saline, Sullivan, Worth); KS (Atchison, Brown, Doniphan, Johnson, Leavenworth, Wyandotte);
TYPE OF COVERAGE:
Commercial: [Y] Individual: [Y] FEHBP: [ ] Indemnity: [ ]
Medicare: [ ] Medicaid: [ ] Supplemental Medicare: [ ]
Tricare [ ]
PRODUCTS OFFERED:

Product Name:	Type:
Community Health Plan	HMO
Community Health Plan	POS

PLAN BENEFITS:

Alternative Medicine:	[ ]	Behavioral Health:	[X]
Chiropractic:	[X]	Dental:	[X]
Home Care:	[X]	Inpatient SNF:	[X]
Long-Term Care:	[ ]	Pharm. Mail Order:	[ ]
Physical Therapy:	[X]	Podiatry:	[X]
Psychiatric:	[X]	Transplant:	[X]
Vision:	[X]	Wellness:	[X]
Workers' Comp:	[ ]		
Other Benefits:			

COVENTRY HEALTH CARE OF KANSAS INC

8320 Ward Parkway
Kansas City, MO 64114
Phone: 816-941-3030 Fax: 816-941-4597 Toll-Free: 800-969-3343
Web site: www.chckansas.com
MAILING ADDRESS:
  COVENTRY HEALTH CARE OF KS INC
  8320 Ward Parkway
  Kansas City, MO 64114

MISSOURI — Managed Care Organization Profiles

ASSURANT EMPLOYEE BENEFITS - CORPORATE OFFICE

2323 Grand Blvd
Kansas City, MO 64108
Phone: 816-474-2345 Fax: 816-881-8996 Toll-Free: 800-456-9194
Web site: www.assurantemployeebenefits.com

MAILING ADDRESS:
ASSURANT EMPLOYEE BENEFITS - CORP
2323 Grand Blvd
Kansas City, MO 64108

KEY EXECUTIVES:
Interim Chief Executive Officer/President ...... John S Roberts
Chief Financial Officer ...... Floyd F Chadee
VP, Medical Director ...... Polly M Galbraith, MD
Chief Information Officer ...... Karla J Schacht
Senior VP, Marketing ...... Joseph A Sevcik
VP of Provider Services ...... James A Barrett, DMD
Senior VP, Human Resources & Development ...... Sylvia R Wagner
National Dental Director ...... James A Barrett, DMD

COMPANY PROFILE:
Parent Company Name: Assurant Health
Doing Business As:
Year Founded: Federally Qualified: [ ] Forprofit: [Y]
Not-For-Profit: [ ]
Model Type:
Accreditation: [ ] AAPPO [ ] JACHO [ ] NCQA [ ] URAC
Plan Type: Specialty HMO
SERVICE AREA:
Nationwide: N
  AL; AZ; CA; CO; FL; GA; IL; IN; MI; ND; NM; NY;
  OH; OK; PA; TN; TX; WA;
TYPE OF COVERAGE:
Commercial: [Y] Individual: [Y] FEHBP: [ ] Indemnity: [ ]
Medicare: [ ] Medicaid: [ ] Supplemental Medicare: [ ]
Tricare [ ]
PLAN BENEFITS:
Alternative Medicine: [ ]   Behavioral Health: [ ]
Chiropractic: [ ]   Dental: [X]
Home Care: [ ]   Inpatient SNF: [ ]
Long-Term Care: [ ]   Pharm. Mail Order: [ ]
Physical Therapy: [ ]   Podiatry: [ ]
Psychiatric: [ ]   Transplant: [ ]
Vision: [ ]   Wellness: [ ]
Workers' Comp: [ ]
Other Benefits:
Comments:
Formerly Fortis Benefits Dental.

BLUE CROSS BLUE SHIELD OF KANSAS CITY

2301 Main St
Kansas City, MO 64108-2428
Phone: 816-395-2222 Fax: 816-395-2035 Toll-Free:
Web site: www.bcbskc.com

MAILING ADDRESS:
BC/BS OF KANSAS CITY
2301 Main St
Kansas City, MO 64108-2428

KEY EXECUTIVES:
Chairman of the Board ...... Ben D McCallister, MD
Chief Executive Officer/President ...... Tom Bowser
Chief Financial Officer ...... Marilyn T Tromans
Senior VP, Chief Medical Officer ...... Frank DiTirro, PhD, MD, FCCP
VP Information Systems ...... Kevin P Sparks
Executive VP, Chief Operating Officer ...... John W Kennedy
Executive VP, Chief Marketing Officer ...... Roger L Foreman
VP Information Systems ...... Kevin Sparks
VP of Human Resources ...... Sherri Enright
Executive VP/Chief Administration ...... Peter K Yelorda
VP & General Counsel ...... Richard J Kastner
Executive VP, Chief Member Services ...... David R Gentile

COMPANY PROFILE:
Parent Company Name:
Doing Business As:
Year Founded: 1938   Federally Qualified: [N]
Forprofit: [ ]   Not-For-Profit: [Y]
Model Type: IPA
Accreditation: [ ] AAPPO [ ] JACHO [ ] NCQA [ ] URAC
Plan Type: HMO, PPO, HSA
Total Revenue: 2005: 170,770,479   2006: 113,519,629
Net Income   2005:   1,758,525   2006:   -2,962,217
Total Enrollment:
  2001: 805,000   2004: 67,614   2007: 0
  2002: 830,000   2005: 75,901
  2003:   71,678   2006: 880,000
Medical Loss Ratio: 2005: 85.90   2006: 90.50
Administrative Expense Ratio: 2005:   8.80   2006:   8.20
SERVICE AREA:
Nationwide: N
  KS (Johnson, Wyandotte); MO;
TYPE OF COVERAGE:
Commercial: [Y] Individual: [Y] FEHBP: [ ] Indemnity: [ ]
Medicare: [Y] Medicaid: [Y] Supplemental Medicare: [Y]
Tricare   [ ]
PRODUCTS OFFERED:
Product Name: Type:
Blue-Advantage 65   Medicare
Blue-Advantage+Plus   Medicare Risk
Preferred Health Professionals   Workers' Comp
Blue Advantage Plus of Kansas City   HMO
Blue Care Open Access
Preferred Care Blue
New Directorections Behavioral Health
PLAN BENEFITS:
Alternative Medicine: [ ]   Behavioral Health: [ ]
Chiropractic: [X]   Dental: [X]
Home Care: [X]   Inpatient SNF: [X]
Long-Term Care: [X]   Pharm. Mail Order: [X]
Physical Therapy: [X]   Podiatry: [X]
Psychiatric: [X]   Transplant: [X]
Vision: [X]   Wellness: [X]
Workers' Comp: [X]
Other Benefits:
Comments:
The Company has three HMO's and two PPO's. BC/BS of Kansas City is providing coverage to HMO and POS members of the Mutual of Omaha Company.

CENTENE CORPORATION

7711 Carondelet Ave Ste 800
St Louis, MO 63105
Phone: 314-725-4477 Fax: 314-558-2428 Toll-Free: 800-225-2573
Web site: www.centene.com

MAILING ADDRESS:
CENTENE CORPORATION
7711 Carondelet Ave Ste 800
St Louis, MO 63105

KEY EXECUTIVES:
Chairman of the Board/Chief Executive Officer ...... Michael F Neidorff
Executive VP, Chief Financial Officer ...... Eric R Slusser
Senior VP, Chief Medical Officer ...... Mary V Mason, MD
Senior VP, Operations ...... Patricia J Darnley
Senior VP, Health Plan Business Unit ...... Christopher D Bowers
Executive VP, Chief Administrative Officer ...... Carol E Goldman
Executive VP, Health Plans ...... Mark W Eggert
Senior VP, Medical Affairs ...... Robert C Packman, MD
Senior VP, Business Management & Integration ...... Cary D Hobbs
Senior VP, Corporate Development ...... Jesse N Hunter

COMPANY PROFILE:
Parent Company Name:
Doing Business As:
Year Founded: 1984   Federally Qualified: [ ]
Forprofit: [ ]   Not-For-Profit: [Y]
Model Type:
Accreditation: [ ] AAPPO [ ] JACHO [ ] NCQA [ ] URAC
Plan Type: HMO
Primary Physicians: 11,486   Physician Specialists: 27,364
Hospitals: 713
Total Revenue: 2005:   1,505,864   2006: 2,279,020,000
Net Income   2005:   55,632   2006:   -43,629,000
Total Enrollment:
  2001:   0   2004: 772,700   2007: 1,103,300
  2002: 409,600   2005: 871,900
  2003: 489,600   2006: 1,232,000

Managed Care Organization Profiles — **MISSOURI**

AETNA INC - MISSOURI

1350 Elbridge Payne Rd Ste 201
Chesterfield, MO 63017
Phone: 636-534-2100 Fax: 859-455-8650 Toll-Free: 800-624-0756
Web site: www.aetna.com
MAILING ADDRESS:
  AETNA INC - MO
  1350 Elbridge Payne Rd Ste 201
  Chesterfield, MO 63017

KEY EXECUTIVES:
Chairman of the Board/Chief Executive Officer .... *Ronald A Williams*
President .... *Allan I Greenberg*
Executive VP, Finance .... *Joseph M Zubretsky*
Chief Medical Officer .... *Burton Vanderlaan, MD*

COMPANY PROFILE:
Parent Company Name: Aetna Inc
Doing Business As:
Year Founded: 1998   Federally Qualified: [N]
Forprofit: [Y]   Not-For-Profit: [ ]
Model Type: MIXED
Accreditation: [ ] AAPPO [ ] JACHO [ ] NCQA [ ] URAC
Plan Type: HMO, PPO, POS, CDHP, HDHP, HSA
Total Revenue: 2005:   86,220,764   2006:   69,736,263
Net Income   2005:   -940,860   2006:   -774,727
Total Enrollment:
  2001: 79,158   2004: 32,352   2007: 0
  2002: 31,095   2005: 26,816
  2003: 26,537   2006: 13,791
Medical Loss Ratio: 2005: 83.30   2006: 85.20
Administrative Expense Ratio: 2005: 12.00   2006: 14.00
SERVICE AREA:
Nationwide: N
  MO (Buchanan, Cass, Clay, Jackson, Jefferson, Lafayette, Platte, Ray, St Charles, St Louis, St Louis City); KS(Atchison, Douglas, Franklin, Johnson, Leavenworth, Miami, Shawnee, Wyandotte);
TYPE OF COVERAGE:
Commercial: [Y] Individual: [ ] FEHBP: [ ] Indemnity: [ ]
Medicare: [ ] Medicaid: [ ] Supplemental Medicare: [ ]
Tricare   [ ]
PRODUCTS OFFERED:
Product Name: Type:
Prudential Health Care Plan   HMO
Aetna US Healthcare   HMO
CONSUMER-DRIVEN PRODUCTS
Aetna Life Insurance Co   HSA Company
Aetna HealthFund HSA   HSA Product
Aetna   HSA Administrator
Aetna HealthFund   Consumer-Driven Health Plan
PPO I; PPO II   High Deductible Health Plan
PLAN BENEFITS:
Alternative Medicine: [ ]   Behavioral Health: [ ]
Chiropractic: [X]   Dental: [X]
Home Care: [X]   Inpatient SNF: [X]
Long-Term Care: [X]   Pharm. Mail Order: [X]
Physical Therapy: [X]   Podiatry: [X]
Psychiatric: [X]   Transplant: [X]
Vision: [X]   Wellness: [X]
Workers' Comp: [ ]
Other Benefits:

AMERICAN HEALTHCARE ALLIANCE

9229 Ward Pkwy Ste 300
Kansas City, MO 64114
Phone: 816-523-7799 Fax: 816-523-1098 Toll-Free:
Web site: www.aha.ppo.net
MAILING ADDRESS:
  AMERICAN HEALTHCARE ALLIANCE
  9229 Ward Pkwy Ste 300
  Kansas City, MO 64114

KEY EXECUTIVES:
Chief Executive Officer .... *Ed Cosler*
Chief Financial Officer .... *John Termini*
Marketing Director/MIS Director .... *Mark Winner*

COMPANY PROFILE:
Parent Company Name:
Doing Business As:
Year Founded: 1986   Federally Qualified: [ ]
Forprofit: [Y]   Not-For-Profit: [ ]
Model Type:
Accreditation: [ ] AAPPO [ ] JACHO [ ] NCQA [ ] URAC
Plan Type: PPO
Total Enrollment:
  2001: 0   2004: 0   2007: 0
  2002: 0   2005:
  2003: 16,500,000   2006:
SERVICE AREA:
Nationwide: Y
  NW;
TYPE OF COVERAGE:
Commercial: [Y] Individual: [ ] FEHBP: [ ] Indemnity: [ ]
Medicare: [ ] Medicaid: [ ] Supplemental Medicare: [ ]
Tricare   [ ]

ANTHEM BLUE CROSS BLUE SHIELD OF MISSOURI

1831 Chestnut Street
St Louis, MO 63103-2275
Phone: 314-923-4444 Fax: 314-923-8907 Toll-Free: 800-366-2583
Web site: www.bcbsmo.com
MAILING ADDRESS:
  ANTHEM BC/BS OF MISSOURI
  1831 Chestnut Street
  St Louis, MO 63103-2275

KEY EXECUTIVES:
President .... *Stuart Campbell*
Chief Financial Officer .... *Wayne S DeVeydt*
Medical Director .... *John J Seidenfeld, MD*
Pharmacy Director .... *Michael Donze*
Marketing Director .... *Dennis Matheis*

COMPANY PROFILE:
Parent Company Name: Wellpoint Inc
Doing Business As: HMO Missouri Inc
Year Founded: 1988   Federally Qualified: [Y]
Forprofit: [ ]   Not-For-Profit: [Y]
Model Type: IPA
Accreditation: [ ] AAPPO [ ] JACHO [ ] NCQA [ ] URAC
Plan Type: HMO, PPO, POS, HDHP, HSA
Total Revenue: 2005:   332,873,176   2006:   388,008,409
Net Income   2005:   18,009,319   2006:   18,887,849
Total Enrollment:
  2001: 0   2004: 387,161   2007: 0
  2002: 0   2005:
  2003: 375,663   2006: 1,100,000
Medical Loss Ratio: 2005: 82.70   2006: 82.90
Administrative Expense Ratio: 2005: 9.80   2006: 9.20
SERVICE AREA:
Nationwide: N
  MO;
TYPE OF COVERAGE:
Commercial: [Y] Individual: [Y] FEHBP: [ ] Indemnity: [ ]
Medicare: [Y] Medicaid: [Y] Supplemental Medicare: [Y]
Tricare   [ ]
PRODUCTS OFFERED:
Product Name: Type:
HMO Missouri Inc, Blue Choice   HMO
RightCHOICE Managed Care   PPO
Bluechoice Senior   Medicare
BlueChoice POS   POS
Blue Horizons   Medicare
Blue Horizons   Supplemental Medicare
PLAN BENEFITS:
Alternative Medicine: [ ]   Behavioral Health: [ ]
Chiropractic: [X]   Dental: [X]
Home Care: [X]   Inpatient SNF: [X]
Long-Term Care: [ ]   Pharm. Mail Order: [X]
Physical Therapy: [X]   Podiatry: [ ]
Psychiatric: [X]   Transplant: [X]
Vision: [X]   Wellness: [X]
Workers' Comp: [ ]
Other Benefits:

MISSISSIPPI

SERVICE AREA:
Nationwide: N
  MS (Adams, Amite, Franklin, George, Hancock, Harrison, Jackson, Lawrence, Lincoln, Pearl River, Pike, Stone, Walthall, Wilkinson);

TYPE OF COVERAGE:
Commercial: [Y] Individual: [ ] FEHBP: [ ] Indemnity: [ ]
Medicare: [ ] Medicaid: [ ] Supplemental Medicare: [ ]
Tricare [ ]

PRODUCTS OFFERED:
Product Name:	Type:
Mississippi Select HMO	HMO
POS	
PPO	

PLAN BENEFITS:
Alternative Medicine:	[ ]	Behavioral Health:	[X]
Chiropractic:	[ ]	Dental:	[X]
Home Care:	[X]	Inpatient SNF:	[X]
Long-Term Care:	[ ]	Pharm. Mail Order:	[X]
Physical Therapy:	[X]	Podiatry:	[X]
Psychiatric:	[X]	Transplant:	[X]
Vision:	[X]	Wellness:	[X]
Workers' Comp:	[ ]		
Other Benefits:			

PHYSICIANSPLUS BAPTIST & ST DOMINIC INC

969 Lakeland Dr
Jackson, MS 39216
Phone: 601-200-6840 Fax: 601-200-6854 Toll-Free:
Web site:

MAILING ADDRESS:
  PHYSICIANSPLUS BAPTIST & ST DOMINIC INC
  969 Lakeland Dr
  Jackson, MS 39216

KEY EXECUTIVES:
Chief Executive Officer .... Senior Mary Dorothea Sondgeroth
Treasurer .... Frank Quiriconi
Chief Medical Officer .... Tom Herrin, MD
SVP, Human Resources .... Lamar Nesbit

COMPANY PROFILE:
Parent Company Name:
Doing Business As:
Year Founded: Federally Qualified: [ ]
Forprofit: [ ]   Not-For-Profit: [ ]
Model Type:
Accreditation: [ ] AAPPO [ ] JACHO [ ] NCQA [ ] URAC
Plan Type: HMO

SERVICE AREA:
Nationwide: N
  MS (Copiah, Hinds, Madison, Rankin);

TYPE OF COVERAGE:
Commercial: [Y] Individual: [ ] FEHBP: [ ] Indemnity: [ ]
Medicare: [ ] Medicaid: [ ] Supplemental Medicare: [ ]
Tricare [ ]

UNITEDHEALTHCARE OF MISSISSIPPI INC

800 Woodlands Pkwy Ste 102
Ridgeland, MS 39157
Phone: 504-549-1603 Fax: 601-957-1306 Toll-Free: 800-264-3639
Web site: www.uhc.com

MAILING ADDRESS:
  UNITEDHEALTHCARE OF MS INC
  800 Woodlands Pkwy Ste 102
  Ridgeland, MS 39157

KEY EXECUTIVES:
Non-Executive Chairman .... Richard T Burke
Chief Executive Officer/President-Gulf State Region ...... T David Lewis
Chief Financial Officer .... Tom Lindquist
Senior Medical Director .... Larry B Amacker, MD
Director of Marketing .... Stan Neese

COMPANY PROFILE:
Parent Company Name: UnitedHealth Group
Doing Business As:
Year Founded: 1993   Federally Qualified: [N]
Forprofit: [Y]   Not-For-Profit: [ ]
Model Type:
Accreditation: [ ] AAPPO [ ] JACHO [ ] NCQA [ ] URAC
Plan Type: HMO, PPO, POS, EPO, ASO, CDHP, HDHP, HSA, HRA
Total Enrollment:
  2001: 30,290   2004: 175   2007: 0
  2002: 23,248   2005:
  2003: 14,344   2006:

SERVICE AREA:
Nationwide: N
  MS;

TYPE OF COVERAGE:
Commercial: [Y] Individual: [ ] FEHBP: [ ] Indemnity: [ ]
Medicare: [Y] Medicaid: [ ] Supplemental Medicare: [ ]
Tricare [ ]

PRODUCTS OFFERED:
Product Name:	Type:
United Healthcare of MS	HMO

CONSUMER-DRIVEN PRODUCTS
Exante Bank/Golden Rule Ins Co	HSA Company
iPlan HSA	HSA Product
	HSA Administrator
	Consumer-Driven Health Plan
	High Deductible Health Plan

PLAN BENEFITS:
Alternative Medicine:	[ ]	Behavioral Health:	[ ]
Chiropractic:	[X]	Dental:	[X]
Home Care:	[X]	Inpatient SNF:	[X]
Long-Term Care:	[X]	Pharm. Mail Order:	[X]
Physical Therapy:	[X]	Podiatry:	[X]
Psychiatric:	[X]	Transplant:	[X]
Vision:	[X]	Wellness:	[X]
Workers' Comp:	[ ]		
Other Benefits:			

Managed Care Organization Profiles — **MISSISSIPPI**

AMERICAN LIFECARE - MISSISSIPPI

1675 Lakeland Dr Ste 550
Jackson, MS 39216
Phone: 601-713-1930 Fax: 601-713-1931 Toll-Free: 877-460-0352
Web site: www.americanlifecare.com

MAILING ADDRESS:
AMERICAN LIFECARE - MS
1675 Lakeland Dr Ste 550
Jackson, MS 39216

KEY EXECUTIVES:
Chief Executive Officer/President .... Joseph Driscoll
Sales Consultant .... Don Foote
Provider Relations .... Glen Gregory
Claims Representative .... Cornelius D Evans

COMPANY PROFILE:
Parent Company Name: Private Healthcare Systems
Doing Business As:
Year Founded: 1983   Federally Qualified: [N]
Forprofit: [Y]   Not-For-Profit: [ ]
Model Type: NETWORK
Accreditation: [ ] AAPPO [ ] JACHO [ ] NCQA [ ] URAC
Plan Type: PPO

SERVICE AREA:
Nationwide: N
  MS;

TYPE OF COVERAGE:
Commercial: [Y] Individual: [ ] FEHBP: [ ] Indemnity: [ ]
Medicare: [ ] Medicaid: [ ] Supplemental Medicare: [ ]
Tricare   [ ]

PLAN BENEFITS:
Alternative Medicine: [ ]   Behavioral Health: [X]
Chiropractic: [X]   Dental: [X]
Home Care: [X]   Inpatient SNF: [X]
Long-Term Care: [X]   Pharm. Mail Order: [X]
Physical Therapy: [X]   Podiatry: [X]
Psychiatric: [X]   Transplant: [X]
Vision: [X]   Wellness: [X]
Workers' Comp: [X]
Other Benefits:

BLUE CROSS BLUE SHIELD OF MISSISSIPPI

3545 Lakeland Dr
Jackson, MS 39232
Phone: 601-932-3704 Fax: 601-939-7035 Toll-Free: 800-222-8046
Web site: www.bcbsms.com

MAILING ADDRESS:
BLUE CROSS BLUE SHIELD OF MS
PO Box 1043
Jackson, MS 39232

KEY EXECUTIVES:
Chief Executive Officer .... Richard Hale
Chief Financial Officer .... Jeff Leber
Medical Director .... Fred May, MD
Pharmacy Director .... Jennifer Wilson
Chief Information Officer .... John Sewall
Marketing Director .... Steve Gregory

COMPANY PROFILE:
Parent Company Name:
Doing Business As: HMO of Mississippi Inc
Year Founded: 1947   Federally Qualified: [Y]
Forprofit: [ ]   Not-For-Profit: [Y]
Model Type:
Accreditation: [ ] AAPPO [ ] JACHO [ ] NCQA [ ] URAC
Plan Type: HMO, PPO, POS, HDHP, HSA,

SERVICE AREA:
Nationwide: N
  MS;

TYPE OF COVERAGE:
Commercial: [Y] Individual: [Y] FEHBP: [ ] Indemnity: [ ]
Medicare: [ ] Medicaid: [ ] Supplemental Medicare: [Y]
Tricare   [ ]

PRODUCTS OFFERED:
Product Name: Type:
HMO of Mississippi Inc   HMO

HUMANA INC - MISSISSIPPI

500 W Main St
Louisville, KY 40201
Phone: 502-580-5804 Fax: 502-580-5044 Toll-Free:
Web site: www.humana.com

MAILING ADDRESS:
HUMANA INC - MISSISSIPPI
500 W Main St
Louisville, KY 40201

KEY EXECUTIVES:
Chairman of the Board .... David A Jones Jr
Chief Executive Officer/President .... Michael B McCallister
Chief Financial Officer .... James H Bloem
Senior VP, Chief Innovation Officer .... Jonathan T Lord, MD
Senior VP Chief Information Officer .... Bruce J Goodman
Senior VP Human Resources .... Bonnie C Hathcock

COMPANY PROFILE:
Parent Company Name: Humana Inc
Doing Business As:
Year Founded: 1961   Federally Qualified: [Y]
Forprofit: [Y]   Not-For-Profit: [ ]
Model Type:
Accreditation: [ ] AAPPO [ ] JACHO [ ] NCQA [ ] URAC
Plan Type: PPO, ASO, CDHP, HDHP, HSA,
Total Enrollment:
  2001: 0   2004: 0   2007: 0
  2002: 0   2005:
  2003: 78,600   2006:

SERVICE AREA:
Nationwide: N
  MS;

TYPE OF COVERAGE:
Commercial: [Y] Individual: [ ] FEHBP: [ ] Indemnity: [ ]
Medicare: [Y] Medicaid: [ ] Supplemental Medicare: [Y]
Tricare   [Y]

CONSUMER-DRIVEN PRODUCTS
JP Morgan Chase   HSA Company
HumanaOne HSA   HSA ProductJP Morgan Chase
HSA Administrator
Personal Care Account   Consumer-Driven Health Plan
HumanaOne   High Deductible Health Plan

PLAN BENEFITS:
Alternative Medicine: [ ]   Behavioral Health: [ ]
Chiropractic: [X]   Dental: [X]
Home Care: [ ]   Inpatient SNF: [ ]
Long-Term Care: [ ]   Pharm. Mail Order: [X]
Physical Therapy: [ ]   Podiatry: [ ]
Psychiatric: [X]   Transplant: [X]
Vision: [ ]   Wellness: [X]
Workers' Comp: [X]
Other Benefits:

MISSISSIPPI SELECT HEALTH CARE

14110 Airport Rd Ste 100
Gulfport, MS 39503
Phone: 228-865-0514 Fax: 228-865-0550 Toll-Free: 800-847-6621
Web site: www.hmhs.com

MAILING ADDRESS:
MISSISSIPPI SELECT HEALTH CARE
14110 Airport Rd Ste 100
Gulfport, MS 39503

KEY EXECUTIVES:
Chief Executive Officer/Chief Financial Officer .... George Rea Montjoy
Medical Director .... Joseph Mitchell

COMPANY PROFILE:
Parent Company Name: Select Administrative Services
Doing Business As:
Year Founded: 1997   Federally Qualified: [ ]
Forprofit: [Y]   Not-For-Profit: [ ]
Model Type: NETWORK
Accreditation: [ ] AAPPO [ ] JACHO [ ] NCQA [ ] URAC
Plan Type: POS

Managed Care Organization Profiles **MINNESOTA**

TYPE OF COVERAGE:
Commercial: [Y] Individual: [Y] FEHBP: [ ] Indemnity: [ ]
Medicare: [Y] Medicaid: [Y] Supplemental Medicare: [Y]
Tricare   [ ]

PRODUCTS OFFERED:
Product Name:	Type:
Select/Select Plus	HMO
Option PPO	PPO
Point of Service Options	POS
Managed Indemnity	Indemnity

CONSUMER-DRIVEN PRODUCTS
Exante Bank/Golden Rule Ins Co	HSA Company
iPlan HSA	HSA Product
	HSA Administrator
	Consumer-Driven Health Plan
	High Deductible Health Plan

PLAN BENEFITS:
Alternative Medicine:	[ ]	Behavioral Health:	[X]
Chiropractic:	[X]	Dental:	[X]
Home Care:	[X]	Inpatient SNF:	[X]
Long-Term Care:	[X]	Pharm. Mail Order:	[X]
Physical Therapy:	[X]	Podiatry:	[X]
Psychiatric:	[X]	Transplant:	[X]
Vision:	[X]	Wellness:	[X]
Workers' Comp:	[X]		

Other Benefits:

Comments:
Formerly UHC MGMT CO Inc. Acquired PacifiCareHealth Systems, Inc. in December 2005. Oxford Health Plans, Inc. in July 2004. Mid Atlantic Medical Services, Inc, in February 2004. Also acquried John Deere Health Plans.

MINNESOTA

Managed Care Organization Profiles

PRODUCTS OFFERED:
Product Name:	Type:
Preferred One Community Health	HMO

PLAN BENEFITS:
Alternative Medicine:	[X]	Behavioral Health:	[X]
Chiropractic:	[X]	Dental:	[X]
Home Care:	[X]	Inpatient SNF:	[X]
Long-Term Care:	[X]	Pharm. Mail Order:	[X]
Physical Therapy:	[X]	Podiatry:	[X]
Psychiatric:	[X]	Transplant:	[X]
Vision:	[X]	Wellness:	[X]
Workers' Comp:	[ ]		

Other Benefits:

SANFORD HEALTH PLAN OF MINNESOTA

300 Cherapa Pl Ste 201
Sioux Falls, SD 57103
Phone: 605-328-6800 Fax: 605-328-6811 Toll-Free: 800-752-5863
Web site: www.sanfordhealth.org

MAILING ADDRESS:
SANFORD HEALTH PLAN OF MN
PO Box 91110
Sioux Falls, SD 57103

KEY EXECUTIVES:
Chief Executive Officer/President .... Ruth Krystopolski

COMPANY PROFILE:
Parent Company Name: Sanford Health
Doing Business As:
Year Founded: 1998   Federally Qualified: [ ]
Forprofit: [ ]   Not-For-Profit: [Y]
Model Type:
Accreditation: [ ] AAPPO [ ] JACHO [ ] NCQA [ ] URAC
Plan Type: HMO,
Primary Physicians: Physician Specialists:
Hospitals:
Total Revenue: 2005:   2006: 1,601,019
Net Income   2005:   2006:
Total Enrollment:
    2001:   0   2004: 0   2007: 0
    2002:   0   2005:
    2003:   0   2006: 3,249
Medical Loss Ratio: 2005:   2006: 92.80
Administrative Expense Ratio: 2005:   2006:

SERVICE AREA:
Nationwide:
    MN (Cottonwood, Jackson, Lac Qui Parle, Lincoln, Lyon, Martin, Murray, Nobles, Pipestone, Redwood, Rock, Watonwan, Yellow Medicine);

Comments:
Formerly Sioux Valley Health Plan.

UCARE MINNESOTA

2000 Summer St NE
Minneapolis, MN 55413
Phone: 612-676-6500 Fax: 612-603-6501 Toll-Free: 800-203-7225
Web site: www.ucare.org

MAILING ADDRESS:
UCARE MINNESOTA
PO Box 52
Minneapolis, MN 55413

KEY EXECUTIVES:
Chief Executive Officer/President .... Nancy Feldman
Chief Financial Officer .... Mark Hudson
Medical Director .... Barry Baines, MD
Chief Operating Officer .... Sharon A Carlin
VP, Public Affairs & Development .... Ghita Worcester
Provider Relations Director .... Marilyn Halseth
Health Promotion Manager .... Marie Maslowski
VP, Human Resources .... Terry Chism
Quality Management Director .... Carolyn Calomeni
General Counsel .... Mark Traynor
New Product Development .... Michele Fedderly
Compliance Manager .... Mary deRanitz

COMPANY PROFILE:
Parent Company Name:
Doing Business As:
Year Founded: 1998   Federally Qualified: [N]
Forprofit: [ ]   Not-For-Profit: [Y]
Model Type: NETWORK
Accreditation: [ ] AAPPO [ ] JACHO [ ] NCQA [ ] URAC
Plan Type: HMO
Total Enrollment:
    2001: 89,959   2004: 131,397   2007: 0
    2002: 129,970   2005: 118,341
    2003: 123,084   2006: 127,601

SERVICE AREA:
Nationwide: N
    MN;

TYPE OF COVERAGE:
Commercial: [ ] Individual: [ ] FEHBP: [ ] Indemnity: [ ]
Medicare: [Y] Medicaid: [Y] Supplemental Medicare: [ ]
Tricare   [ ]

PRODUCTS OFFERED:
Product Name:	Type:
UCARE for Seniors	Medicare
UCARE Medicaid	Medicaid

PLAN BENEFITS:
Alternative Medicine:	[ ]	Behavioral Health:	[X]
Chiropractic:	[X]	Dental:	[X]
Home Care:	[X]	Inpatient SNF:	[X]
Long-Term Care:	[X]	Pharm. Mail Order:	[ ]
Physical Therapy:	[X]	Podiatry:	[X]
Psychiatric:	[X]	Transplant:	[X]
Vision:	[X]	Wellness:	[X]
Workers' Comp:	[ ]		

Other Benefits:

UNITEDHEALTH GROUP — CORPORATE HEADQUARTERS

9900 Bren Rd East
Minnetonka, MN 55343
Phone: 952-936-1300 Fax: 952-936-0044 Toll-Free:
Web site: www.unitedhealthgroup.com

MAILING ADDRESS:
UNITEDHEALTH GROUP - CORP HQR
9900 Bren Rd East
Minnetonka, MN 55343

KEY EXECUTIVES:
Non-Executive Chairman .... Richard T Burke
Chief Executive Officer/President .... Stephen J Hemsley
Chief Financial Officer .... Patrick Erlandson
Pharmacy Director .... Eric L Bergen
Chief Operating Officer .... Stephen J Hemsley
Marketing Director .... Jay Silverstein
Public Relations Director .... Philip Soucheray
VP of Human Resources .... Peggy Bernhardt
General Counsel .... David J Lubben

COMPANY PROFILE:
Parent Company Name:
Doing Business As:
Year Founded: 1974   Federally Qualified: [ ]
Forprofit: [Y]   Not-For-Profit: [ ]
Model Type: NETWORK
Accreditation: [X] AAPPO [X] JACHO [X] NCQA [X] URAC
Plan Type: HMO, PPO, UR, POS, PBM, CDHP, HSA, HRA
Primary Physicians: 400,000   Physician Specialists: 520,000
Hospitals: 4,700
Total Revenue: 2005: 45,365,000,000   2006: 71,542,000,000
Net Income   2005:   3,300,000   2006:   4,159,000,000
Total Enrollment:
    2001: 8,540,000   2004: 55,000,000 2007: 0
    2002: 9,040,000   2005: 65,000,000
    2003: 9,630,000   2006: 70,000,000
Medical Loss Ratio: 2005:   2006: 81.20
Administrative Expense Ratio: 2005:   2006:

SERVICE AREA:
Nationwide: Y
    NW;

Managed Care Organization Profiles MINNESOTA

KEY EXECUTIVES:
Chairman of the Board .... John Buck
Chief Executive Officer/President .... David Tilford
Executive VP, CAO, CFO .... Aaron Reynolds
Senior VP, Chief Medical Officer .... Charles Fazio, MD
VP of Pharmacy .... Kerry Bendel
Senior VP, Chief Information Officer .... Scott Booher
Chief Operating Officer .... Jana Johnson
Senior VP, Marketing .... Robert Longendyke
Marketing & Communications Director .... Larry Bussey
SVP of Human Resources .... Deb Knutson
Quality Assurance Director .... Leslie Frank
Fraud Prevention/Investigation .... Rick Munson
Case Management Director .... Ann Earl
VP, Health Management .... Patricia Dennis

COMPANY PROFILE:
Parent Company Name: Allina Health System
Doing Business As: Medica Health Plans
Year Founded: 1974   Federally Qualified: [N]
Forprofit: [ ]   Not-For-Profit: [Y]
Model Type: IPA
Accreditation: [ ] AAPPO [ ] JACHO [X] NCQA [ ] URAC
Plan Type: HMO, PPO, ASO, POS, HDHP, HSA
Total Revenue: 2005:   2006:   1,026,507,296
Net Income   2005:   2006:
Total Enrollment:
  2001:   97,937   2004: 378,639   2007: 0
  2002: 494,332   2005: 262,770
  2003: 484,931   2006: 186,832
Medical Loss Ratio: 2005:   2006: 97.00
Administrative Expense Ratio: 2005:   2006:

SERVICE AREA:
Nationwide: N
  MN; ND (Eastern); SD (Eastern); WI (Western);

TYPE OF COVERAGE:
Commercial: [Y] Individual: [Y] FEHBP: [ ] Indemnity: [ ]
Medicare: [Y] Medicaid: [Y] Supplemental Medicare: [ ]
Tricare   [ ]

PRODUCTS OFFERED:
Product Name:	Type:
Select Care	PPO
Medica Premier	HMO
Medica Choice/MAC	Medicaid
Medica Self Insurer	ASO
Medica Primary	HMO
Medica Elect	
Medica Seniors	Medicare

PLAN BENEFITS:
Alternative Medicine:	[ ]	Behavioral Health:	[X]
Chiropractic:	[X]	Dental:	[X]
Home Care:	[X]	Inpatient SNF:	[X]
Long-Term Care:	[ ]	Pharm. Mail Order:	[X]
Physical Therapy:	[X]	Podiatry:	[X]
Psychiatric:	[X]	Transplant:	[X]
Vision:	[X]	Wellness:	[X]
Workers' Comp:	[X]		
Other Benefits:			

METROPOLITAN HEALTH PLAN

400 S 4th St Ste 201
Minneapolis, MN 55415-1289
Phone: 612-347-8557 Fax: 612-904-3198 Toll-Free: 800-647-0550
Web site: www.co.hennepin.mn.us

MAILING ADDRESS:
  METROPOLITAN HEALTH PLAN
  400 S 4th St Ste 201
  Minneapolis, MN 55415-1289

KEY EXECUTIVES:
Executive Director .... David R Johnson
Director of Fiscal Services .... Dave Edwards
Medical Director .... Joseph C Horozaniecki, MD
Director of Information Services .... Kay Hendrikson
Director, Marketing/Public Relations .... Bonnie Hays
Compliance Officer .... Angela Kaiser
Public Relations Director .... Bonnie Hays
Provider Relations/Network Development Director .... Hannah LaMere
Human Resource Liason .... Angela Kaiser
Quality Assurance Director .... Ned Moore
Director Fraud Prevention/Investigation .... Doris Safo

COMPANY PROFILE:
Parent Company Name: Hennepin County Government
Doing Business As:
Year Founded: 1983   Federally Qualified: [ ]
Forprofit: [ ]   Not-For-Profit: [Y]
Model Type: NETWORK
Accreditation: [ ] AAPPO [ ] JACHO [ ] NCQA [ ] URAC
Plan Type: HMO
Total Enrollment:
  2001:   0   2004: 18,261   2007: 0
  2002: 20,900   2005: 17,733
  2003: 32,125   2006: 16,941

SERVICE AREA:
Nationwide: N
  MN (Anoka, Carver, Hennepin, Scott);

TYPE OF COVERAGE:
Commercial: [ ] Individual: [ ] FEHBP: [ ] Indemnity: [ ]
Medicare: [Y] Medicaid: [Y] Supplemental Medicare: [ ]
Tricare   [ ]

PRODUCTS OFFERED:
Product Name:	Type:
MIP Health Plan	HMO
Metropolitan Health Plan	Medicaid

PLAN BENEFITS:
Alternative Medicine:	[ ]	Behavioral Health:	[X]
Chiropractic:	[X]	Dental:	[X]
Home Care:	[X]	Inpatient SNF:	[X]
Long-Term Care:	[X]	Pharm. Mail Order:	[X]
Physical Therapy:	[X]	Podiatry:	[X]
Psychiatric:	[X]	Transplant:	[X]
Vision:	[X]	Wellness:	[ ]
Workers' Comp:	[ ]		
Other Benefits:			

PREFERRED ONE

6105 Golden Hills Dr
Golden Valley, MN 55416
Phone: 763-847-3201 Fax: 763-847-4010 Toll-Free:
Web site: www.preferredone.com

MAILING ADDRESS:
  PREFERRED ONE
  6105 Golden Hills Dr
  Golden Valley, MN 55416

KEY EXECUTIVES:
Chief Executive Officer .... Marcus Merz
Chief Financial Officer .... Mike Umland
Medical Director .... John Fredrick, MD
Marketing Director .... Dennis Fenster
MIS Director .... John Hofflander
VP Provider Services .... Darcee Weber
General Counsel .... Mike McKim
Chief Marketing Officer .... Paul Geiwitz
VP, Insurance Services .... Bob Gadola
VP, Account Management .... Renee Ambrosia

COMPANY PROFILE:
Parent Company Name: Preferred One Administrative Services
Doing Business As: Preferred One Community Health Plan
Year Founded: 1984   Federally Qualified: [N]
Forprofit: [ ]   Not-For-Profit: [Y]
Model Type: MIXED
Accreditation: [X] AAPPO [ ] JACHO [X] NCQA [X] URAC
Plan Type: HMO, PPO, TPA, HSA, POS, ASO, CDHP, HDHP, FSA
Primary Physicians: 6,300   Physician Specialists: 6,400
Hospitals: 240
Total Enrollment:
  2001: 650,000   2004: 48,277   2007: 0
  2002:   33,278   2005: 48,380
  2003: 536,000   2006: 50,540

SERVICE AREA:
Nationwide: N
  MN (Upper Midwest);

TYPE OF COVERAGE:
Commercial: [Y] Individual: [Y] FEHBP: [ ] Indemnity: [ ]
Medicare: [ ] Medicaid: [ ] Supplemental Medicare: [ ]
Tricare   [ ]

MINNESOTA

PLAN BENEFITS:

Alternative Medicine:	[ ]	Behavioral Health:	[X]
Chiropractic:	[X]	Dental:	[ ]
Home Care:	[X]	Inpatient SNF:	[ ]
Long-Term Care:	[ ]	Pharm. Mail Order:	[ ]
Physical Therapy:	[ ]	Podiatry:	[ ]
Psychiatric:	[X]	Transplant:	[X]
Vision:	[X]	Wellness:	[X]
Workers' Comp:	[ ]		
Other Benefits:			

GREAT-WEST HEALTHCARE OF MINNESOTA

11095 Viking Dr Ste 300
Eden Prairie, MN 55344
Phone: 952-942-7565 Fax: 952-944-3974 Toll-Free: 877-809-8211
Web site: www.greatwesthealthcare.com

MAILING ADDRESS:
GREAT-WEST HEALTHCARE OF MN
11095 Viking Dr Ste 300
Minneapolis, MN 55344

KEY EXECUTIVES:
Chief Executive Officer/President .... Raymond L McFeetors

COMPANY PROFILE:
Parent Company Name: Great West Life & Annuity Insurance Co
Doing Business As:
Year Founded: Federally Qualified: [ ]
Forprofit: [Y] Not-For-Profit: [ ]
Model Type:
Accreditation: [ ] AAPPO [ ] JACHO [ ] NCQA [ ] URAC
Plan Type: HMO, CDHP, HSA

SERVICE AREA:
Nationwide: N
MN;

TYPE OF COVERAGE:
Commercial: [Y] Individual: [ ] FEHBP: [ ] Indemnity: [ ]
Medicare: [ ] Medicaid: [ ] Supplemental Medicare: [ ]
Tricare [ ]

PLAN BENEFITS:

Alternative Medicine:	[X]	Behavioral Health:	[ ]
Chiropractic:	[X]	Dental:	[X]
Home Care:	[X]	Inpatient SNF:	[X]
Long-Term Care:	[ ]	Pharm. Mail Order:	[X]
Physical Therapy:	[X]	Podiatry:	[X]
Psychiatric:	[X]	Transplant:	[X]
Vision:	[X]	Wellness:	[X]
Workers' Comp:	[ ]		
Other Benefits:			

HEALTHPARTNERS INC

8100 34th Ave South
Bloomington, MN 55425
Phone: 952-883-6000 Fax: 952-883-5380 Toll-Free: 888-470-4470
Web site: www.healthpartners.com

MAILING ADDRESS:
HEALTHPARTNERS INC
PO Box 1309
Minneapolis, MN 55425

KEY EXECUTIVES:
Chairperson .... Alan Fletcher
Chief Executive Officer/President .... Mary Brainerd
Senior VP & Chief Financial Officer .... Kathy Cooney
Med Director/Chief Health Officer .... George Isham, MD
Director Pharmacy Operations .... Rick Bruzek
Senior VP & Chief Information Officer .... Alan Abramson
Executive VP, Chief Marketing Director .... Andrea Walsh
VP Primary Care Clinics Operations .... Beth Waterman
Credentialing Manager .... Marilee Forsberg
VP Corporate Compliance .... Tobi Tanzer
Senior Director Corp Communications .... Shannon Beaodin Klein
Senior VP, Health & Care Management .... Babette Apland
VP Center for Health Promotion .... Nico Pronk PhD
VP & Chief Human Resources Officer .... Calvin Allen
Senior Director, Health Plan Quality .... Kathy Ohmann
Credentialing Manager .... Marilee Forsberg
Senior VP, Customer Service/Product Innovation .... Scott Aebischer
Case Management Director .... Karen Kraemer
Senior VP General Counsel .... Barb Tretheway
Med Director Health Partners Medical Group .... Brian Rank MD
Senior VP Health Partners Medical Group .... Nancy McClure

COMPANY PROFILE:
Parent Company Name:
Doing Business As: HealthPartners Inc, Group Health Inc
Year Founded: 1957 Federally Qualified: [Y]
Forprofit: [ ] Not-For-Profit: [Y]
Model Type: MIXED
Accreditation: [ ] AAPPO [ ] JACHO [X] NCQA [ ] URAC
Plan Type: HMO, PPO, PBM, HSA, HDHP
Total Revenue: 2005: 2006:
Net Income 2005: 2006:
Total Enrollment:
    2001: 657,675   2004: 575,421   2007: 0
    2002: 655,956   2005: 340,612
    2003: 349,070   2006: 579,688

SERVICE AREA:
Nationwide: N
MN (Anoka, Becker, Beltrami, Benton, Big Stone, Blue Earth, Brown, Carver, Cass, Chippewa, Chisago, Clay, Clearwater, Cottonwood, Crow Wing, Dakota, Dodge, Douglas, Faribault, Fillmore, Freeborn, Goodhue, Hennepin, Hubbard, Isanti, Jackson, Kandiyohi, Lac Qui Parle, Le Sueur, Lincoln, Lyon, Mahnomen, Martin, McLeod, Meeker, Mille Lacs, Morrison, Mower, Murray, Nicollet, Nobles, Norman, Olmsted, Otter Tail, Pipestone, Pope, Ramsey, Redwood, Renville, Rice, Scott, Sherburne, Sibley, Stearns, Steele, Stevens, Swift, Todd, Traverse, Wabasha, Waseca, Washington, Watonwan, Wilkin, Winona, Wright, Yellow Medicine); ND (Barnes, Cass, Grand Forks, LaMoure, Logan, McHenry, Nelson, Pembia, Ransom, Richland, Sargent, Steele, Stutsman, Traill, Walsh); WI (Ashland, Bayfield, Buffalo, Burnett, Douglas, Dunn, Iron, Pepin, Pierce, Polk, Saint Croix, Sawyer, Wasburn); IA (Lyon, Plymoouth, Sioux); SD (Clay, Lincoln. Minnehaha, Moody, Turner, Union, Yankton);

TYPE OF COVERAGE:
Commercial: [Y] Individual: [Y] FEHBP: [Y] Indemnity: [Y]
Medicare: [Y] Medicaid: [Y] Supplemental Medicare: [Y]
Tricare [ ]

PRODUCTS OFFERED:

Product Name:	Type:
Total Medicare	Medicare
Total at Risk	Medicare
Total HMO/POS	POS
Total PPO	PPO-Self-insured
Group Health Seniors	Medicaid
Group Health Seniors	Medicare
HealthPartners	Other

PLAN BENEFITS:

Alternative Medicine:	[X]	Behavioral Health:	[X]
Chiropractic:	[X]	Dental:	[X]
Home Care:	[X]	Inpatient SNF:	[ ]
Long-Term Care:	[ ]	Pharm. Mail Order:	[X]
Physical Therapy:	[ ]	Podiatry:	[ ]
Psychiatric:	[X]	Transplant:	[X]
Vision:	[X]	Wellness:	[X]
Workers' Comp:	[X]		
Other Benefits:			

MEDICA HEALTH PLANS

401 Carlson Pkwy
Minnetonka, MN 55305
Phone: 952-992-8013 Fax: 952-992-3554 Toll-Free:
Web site: www.medica.com

MAILING ADDRESS:
MEDICA HEALTH PLANS
PO Box 9310 RTE 0501
Minneapolis, MN 55440-9310

Managed Care Organization Profiles — MINNESOTA

PRODUCTS OFFERED:
Product Name: Type:
Employee Assistance Programs   EAP
Managed Mental Health

PLAN BENEFITS:
Alternative Medicine: [ ]   Behavioral Health: [X]
Chiropractic: [ ]   Dental: [ ]
Home Care: [ ]   Inpatient SNF: [ ]
Long-Term Care: [ ]   Pharm. Mail Order: [ ]
Physical Therapy: [ ]   Podiatry: [ ]
Psychiatric: [X]   Transplant: [ ]
Vision: [ ]   Wellness: [X]
Workers' Comp: [ ]
Other Benefits:

Comments:
Formerly called MCC Managed Behavioral Care Inc.

COREVIEW

3300 County Road 10 Ste 500
Minneapolis, MN 55429
Phone: 763-560-8818 Fax: 763-560-5103 Toll-Free:
Web site:

MAILING ADDRESS:
 COREVIEW
 3300 County Road 10 Ste 500
 Minneapolis, MN 55429

KEY EXECUTIVES:
Chief Executive Officer .... Jennifer Sherman
Chief Medical Officer .... Rashid Khan

COMPANY PROFILE:
Parent Company Name:
Doing Business As:
Year Founded: Federally Qualified: [ ]
Forprofit: [Y]   Not-For-Profit: [ ]
Model Type:
Accreditation: [ ] AAPPO [ ] JACHO [ ] NCQA [ ] URAC
Plan Type: UR

SERVICE AREA:
Nationwide: N
 MN;

DELTA DENTAL PLAN OF MINNESOTA

3560 Delta Dental Dr
Eagan, MN 55122-3166
Phone: 651-406-5900 Fax: 651-406-5936 Toll-Free: 800-328-1188
Web site: www.deltadentalmn.org

MAILING ADDRESS:
 DELTA DENTAL PLAN OF MN
 PO Box 9304
 Minneapolis, MN 55122-3166

KEY EXECUTIVES:
Chief Executive Officer/President .... Michael F Walsh
Executive VP Finance & Business Development .... Dani Fjelstad
Dental Director .... Richard Hastreiter, DDS
Executive VP Operations .... Norman Storbakken
Executive VP Sales & Marketing .... Mark Moksnes
Senior VP Professional Services .... Nancy McMorran
Senior VP Human Resources .... Mary Stacke
Fraud Prevention Director .... Karen Haarala
New Product Development Director .... Patti Bruntgen
Senior VP, Operations .... Gary Ballman
General Counsel .... David B Morse
Compliance Officer .... Joseph Lally

COMPANY PROFILE:
Parent Company Name: Delta Dental Plan of Minnesota
Doing Business As:
Year Founded: 1969   Federally Qualified: [ ]
Forprofit: [ ]   Not-For-Profit: [Y]
Model Type: MIXED
Accreditation: [ ] AAPPO [ ] JACHO [ ] NCQA [ ] URAC
Plan Type: Specialty HMO, Specialty PPO, PPO, POS, ASO, TPA,
Total Revenue: 2005:   158,669,290   2006:   157,335,747
Net Income   2005:   2006:
Total Enrollment:
 2001: 664,827   2004: 548,846   2007: 0
 2002: 632,513   2005:
 2003: 546,061   2006:
Medical Loss Ratio: 2005: 80.80   2006:
Administrative Expense Ratio: 2005:   2006:

SERVICE AREA:
Nationwide: N
 MN; NE; WY;

TYPE OF COVERAGE:
Commercial: [Y] Individual: [ ] FEHBP: [ ] Indemnity: [ ]
Medicare: [Y] Medicaid: [Y] Supplemental Medicare: [Y]
Tricare   [ ]

PLAN BENEFITS:
Alternative Medicine: [ ]   Behavioral Health: [ ]
Chiropractic: [ ]   Dental: [X]
Home Care: [ ]   Inpatient SNF: [ ]
Long-Term Care: [ ]   Pharm. Mail Order: [ ]
Physical Therapy: [ ]   Podiatry: [ ]
Psychiatric: [ ]   Transplant: [ ]
Vision: [ ]   Wellness: [ ]
Workers' Comp: [ ]
Other Benefits:

FIRST PLAN OF MINNESOTA

525 S Lake Ave Ste 222
Duluth, MN 55802
Phone: 218-724-3083 Fax: 218-834-6215 Toll-Free: 800-635-4159
Web site: www.firstplan.org

MAILING ADDRESS:
 FIRST PLAN OF MINNESOTA
 525 S Lake Ave Ste 222
 Duluth, MN 55802

KEY EXECUTIVES:
Chairman of the Board .... Milt Larson
Chief Executive Officer/President .... John S Bjorum
Chief Financial Officer .... Timothy Miller
Medical Director .... Douglas Hiza, MD
Pharmacy Director .... Roger McDannold
Director of Communications .... Cathy Nevanen
Chief Operating Officer .... Julie Stone
Director of Marketing .... Cheryl Macheledt
Director Human Resources .... Annette Forsell
Director Strategic Planning .... Nancy Ojard
Director Clinical Operations .... Kathy McNamara

COMPANY PROFILE:
Parent Company Name: Blue Cross & Blue Shield
Doing Business As:
Year Founded: 1944   Federally Qualified: [N]
Forprofit: [ ]   Not-For-Profit: [Y]
Model Type: MIXED
Accreditation: [ ] AAPPO [ ] JACHO [ ] NCQA [ ] URAC
Plan Type: HMO, POS, TPA
Primary Physicians: 200   Physician Specialists:
Hospitals:
Total Enrollment:
 2001: 0   2004: 1,495   2007: 0
 2002: 13,430   2005: 6,500
 2003: 15,400   2006:

SERVICE AREA:
Nationwide: N
 MN (Northeastern);

TYPE OF COVERAGE:
Commercial: [Y] Individual: [Y] FEHBP: [ ] Indemnity: [ ]
Medicare: [Y] Medicaid: [Y] Supplemental Medicare: [Y]
Tricare   [ ]

PRODUCTS OFFERED:
Product Name: Type:
First Plan   HMO
First Plan Plus   POS
Seniors First   Medicare
Government Health Plans
Third Party Administration
First Plan   Medicaid

MINNESOTA

BLUE CROSS BLUE SHIELD OF MINNESOTA

3535 Blue Cross Rd
St Paul, MN 55122
Phone: 651-662-1502 Fax: 651-662-2138 Toll-Free:
Web site: www.bluecrossmn.com
MAILING ADDRESS:
  BLUE CROSS BLUE SHIELD MN
  PO Box 64560
  St Paul, MN 55122

KEY EXECUTIVES:
Chief Executive Officer/President .... Mark W Banks, MD
VP of Finance .... Timothy Peterson
Senior VP, Chief Medical Officer .... David Plocher, MD
Chief Operations Officer .... Colleen Reitan
Senior VP, Chief Marketing Officer .... Richard P Neuner
Senior VP, Human Resources/Facilities Service .... Roger W Kleppe
Senior VP, Operations .... Denise McKenna
VP, Public Affairs .... Kathleen Mock

COMPANY PROFILE:
Parent Company Name: Blue Cross/Blue Shield
Doing Business As:
Year Founded: 1933   Federally Qualified: [Y] Forprofit: [ ]
Not-For-Profit: [Y]
Model Type: NETWORK
Accreditation: [ ] AAPPO [ ] JACHO [X] NCQA [ ] URAC
Plan Type: HMO, PPO, POS, CDHP, HSA
Total Revenue: 2005: 7,115,307,000 2006: 7,865,816,000
Net Income 2005: 55,577,000 2006: 4,921,000
Total Enrollment:
  2001: 2,015,382   2004: 2,632,799   2007: 2,700,000
  2002: 2,419,176   2005: 2,698,286
  2003: 2,584,468   2006: 2,707,023
SERVICE AREA:
Nationwide: N
  MN;
TYPE OF COVERAGE:
Commercial: [Y] Individual: [Y] FEHBP: [ ] Indemnity: [ ]
Medicare: [Y] Medicaid: [Y] Supplemental Medicare: [Y]
Tricare   [ ]
PRODUCTS OFFERED:
Product Name: Type:
Blue Plus, Inc   HMO
Preferred Seniors   Medicare
Blue Plus   Medicaid
PLAN BENEFITS:
Alternative Medicine: [ ]   Behavioral Health: [ ]
Chiropractic: [X]   Dental: [ ]
Home Care: [X]   Inpatient SNF: [X]
Long-Term Care: [X]   Pharm. Mail Order: [X]
Physical Therapy: [X]   Podiatry: [X]
Psychiatric: [X]   Transplant: [X]
Vision: [X]   Wellness: [X]
Workers' Comp: [X]
Other Benefits:
Comments:
Enrollment figures include Indemnity coverage.

CHIROCARE OF MINNESOTA

1000 County Rd E Ste 230
Shoreview, MN 55156
Phone: 763-595-3200 Fax: 763-595-3333 Toll-Free: 800-873-4575
Web site: www.chirocaremn.org
MAILING ADDRESS:
  CHIROCARE OF MINNESOTA
  1000 County Rd E Ste 230
  Shoreview, MN 55156

KEY EXECUTIVES:
Chief Executive Officer .... William A Barrett, DC

COMPANY PROFILE:
Parent Company Name: Landmark Healthcare
Doing Business As: ChiroCare
Year Founded: 1984   Federally Qualified: [ ]
Forprofit: [Y]   Not-For-Profit: [ ]
Model Type:
Accreditation: [ ] AAPPO [ ] JACHO [ ] NCQA [ ] URAC
Plan Type: Specialty PPO
Primary Physicians: Physician Specialists: 700
Hospitals:
Total Enrollment:
  2001: 0   2004: 0   2007: 1,500,000
  2002: 0   2005:
  2003: 0   2006:
SERVICE AREA:
Nationwide: N
  MN;
TYPE OF COVERAGE:
Commercial: [Y] Individual: [ ] FEHBP: [ ] Indemnity: [ ]
Medicare: [Y] Medicaid: [Y] Supplemental Medicare: [Y]
Tricare   [ ]
PLAN BENEFITS:
Alternative Medicine: [ ]   Behavioral Health: [ ]
Chiropractic: [X]   Dental: [ ]
Home Care: [ ]   Inpatient SNF: [ ]
Long-Term Care: [ ]   Pharm. Mail Order: [ ]
Physical Therapy: [ ]   Podiatry: [ ]
Psychiatric: [ ]   Transplant: [ ]
Vision: [ ]   Wellness: [ ]
Workers' Comp: [ ]
Other Benefits:
Comments:
Also reflects American Complementary CareNetwork.

CIGNA BEHAVIORAL HEALTH INC - CORPORATE HEADQUARTERS

11905 Viking Dr Ste 350
Eden Prairie, MN 55344-7234
Phone: 952-996-2000 Fax: 952-996-2579 Toll-Free: 800-433-5768
Web site: www.cignabehavioral.com
MAILING ADDRESS:
  CIGNA BEHAVRL HLTH INC - CORP
  11905 Viking Dr Ste 350
  Eden Prairie, MN 55344-7234

KEY EXECUTIVES:
Chief Executive Officer/President .... Keith Dixon, PhD
Chief Financial Officer .... David Bourdon, MBA
Chief Medical Director .... Doug Nemecek, MD
Chief Information Officer .... David Peterson, BS
Senior VP, Operations .... Jodi Aronson Prohofsky, PhD
Marketing Director .... Nelia Infante
VP, Network Services, Provider Relations Director .... Julie Vayer
Health Promotion Director .... Nance Moeller-Roy
Medical Management Director .... Nancy Hedstrom
Quality Assurance Director .... Susan Sheridan
Medical Director .... Craig Coenson, MD
Customer Advocacy .... Karen Cierzan

COMPANY PROFILE:
Parent Company Name:
Doing Business As:
Year Founded: 1974   Federally Qualified: [Y]
Forprofit: [Y]   Not-For-Profit: [ ]
Model Type: NETWORK
Accreditation: [ ] AAPPO [ ] JACHO [X] NCQA [X] URAC
Plan Type: Specialty PPO, Specialty HMO
Total Enrollment:
  2001: 13,500,000   2004: 0   2007: 18,000,000
  2002: 14,100,000   2005:
  2003: 17,300,000   2006:
SERVICE AREA:
Nationwide: Y
  AI; AK; AR; AZ; CA; CO; CT; DC; DE; FI; GA; HI; IA; ID; IL; IN;
  KS; KY; LA; MA; MD; ME; MI; MN; MO; MS; MT; NC; ND; NE;
  NH; NJ; NM; NV; NY; OH; OK; OR; PA; PR; RI; SC; SD; TN; TX;
  UT; VA; VT; WA; WI; WV; WY;
TYPE OF COVERAGE:
Commercial: [Y] Individual: [ ] FEHBP: [Y] Indemnity: [ ]
Medicare: [Y] Medicaid: [ ] Supplemental Medicare: [ ]
Tricare   [ ]

Managed Care Organization Profiles — **MINNESOTA**

ACN GROUP

6300 Olson Memorial Hwy
Golden Valley, MN 55427
Phone: 763-595-3496 Fax: 763-595-3333 Toll-Free: 800-873-4575
Web site: www.theacngroup.com

MAILING ADDRESS:
   ACN GROUP
   6300 Olson Memorial Hwy
   Golden Valley, MN 55427

KEY EXECUTIVES:
Chief Executive Officer .... Thomas J Allenburg, DC
Chief Financial Officer .... Scott Dreyling
Senior VP of Clinical Products .... David Elton, DC
VP of Information Technology .... David Carufel
Chief Operating Officer .... John DeSmet
National CRM Chair .... Gary LeDuc
Professional Relations .... RT Donahue
Director Network Strategy & Policy .... Victor Feldman
Human Capital Partner .... Dana Nueheisel
National CRM Chair .... Gary LeDuc
Senior Director, Compliance .... Laurie Berry
Director of Product Development .... Betty Lake
National Chief Clinical Officer .... Bruce Hoffmann, DC
Regional Chief Clinical Officer - MN .... Kecia Erickson
Regional Chief Clinical Officer - NY .... Tom Kosloff
Regional Chief Clinical Officer - CA .... Brett Sullivan

COMPANY PROFILE:
Parent Company Name: UnitedHealth Group
Doing Business As: American Chiropractic Network
Year Founded: 1987   Federally Qualified: [ ]
Forprofit: [Y]   Not-For-Profit: [ ]
Model Type: MIXED
Accreditation: [ ] AAPPO [ ] JACHO [X] NCQA [X] URAC
Plan Type: HMO, PPO, Specialty HMO, Specialty PPO, ASO, UR

SERVICE AREA:
Nationwide: Y
   NW;

TYPE OF COVERAGE:
Commercial: [Y] Individual: [ ] FEHBP: [ ] Indemnity: [ ]
Medicare: [Y] Medicaid: [Y] Supplemental Medicare: [ ]
Tricare   [ ]

PLAN BENEFITS:
Alternative Medicine: [X]   Behavioral Health: [ ]
Chiropractic: [X]   Dental: [ ]
Home Care: [ ]   Inpatient SNF: [ ]
Long-Term Care: [ ]   Pharm. Mail Order: [ ]
Physical Therapy: [ ]   Podiatry: [ ]
Psychiatric: [ ]   Transplant: [ ]
Vision: [ ]   Wellness: [X]
Workers' Comp: [X]
Other Benefits:

ALLIANZ LIFE INSURANCE COMPANY OF NORTH AMERICA

5701 Golden Hills Dr
Minneapolis, MN 55416-1297
Phone: 763-765-6500 Fax: 763-765-6657 Toll-Free: 800-950-5872
Web site: www.allianzlife.com

MAILING ADDRESS:
   ALLIANZ LIFE INS CO OF NORTH AMERICA
   PO Box 1344
   Minneapolis, MN 55416-1297

KEY EXECUTIVES:
Chairman of the Board .... Jan Carendi
Chief Executive Officer/President .... Gary C Bhojwani
Executive VP, Chief Financial Officer .... Jill Paterson
Medical Director .... Robert W Watson
Chief Information Officer/Chief Operating Officer .. Douglas Reynolds
Chief Marketing Officer .... Patrick M Foley
Human Resources .... Cary Brinkley
Chief Actuary .... Neil McKay
Senior VP, Corporate Communications .... Juli Wall

COMPANY PROFILE:
Parent Company Name: Allianz AG Holding
Doing Business As:
Year Founded: 1896   Federally Qualified: [ ]
Forprofit: [Y]   Not-For-Profit: [ ]
Model Type:
Accreditation: [ ] AAPPO [ ] JACHO [ ] NCQA [ ] URAC
Plan Type: PPO
Total Enrollment:
   2001: 3,684   2004: 0   2007: 0
   2002: 0   2005:
   2003: 1,388   2006:

SERVICE AREA:
Nationwide: Y
   AL; AK; AR; AZ; CA; CO; CT; DC; DE; FL; GA; HI; IA; ID; IL; IN;
   KS; KY; LA; MA; MD; ME; MI; MN; MO; MS; MT; NC; ND; NE;
   NH; NJ; NM; NV; NY; OH; OK; OR; PA; RI; SC; SD; TN; TX; UT;
   VA; VT; WA; WI; WV; WY;

TYPE OF COVERAGE:
Commercial: [Y] Individual: [ ] FEHBP: [ ] Indemnity: [ ]
Medicare: [ ] Medicaid: [ ] Supplemental Medicare: [ ]
Tricare   [ ]

AMERICAS PPO

7201 West 78 St Ste 100
Bloomington, MN 55437-3800
Phone: 952-896-1200 Fax: 952-896-4888 Toll-Free: 800-444-3005
Web site: www.americasppo.com

MAILING ADDRESS:
   AMERICAS PPO
   7201 West 78 St Ste 100
   Bloomington, MN 55437-3800

KEY EXECUTIVES:
Chief Executive Officer .... Nazie Eftekhari
President .... Amir Eftekhari
Chief Financial Officer .... Lee Marwede
Medical Director .... Brian Ebeling, MD
Chief Information Officer .... Chaker Khatib
Marketing Director .... Tim Bode
Director of Provider Services .... Rich Henriksen
Human Resource Director .... Tricia Belfield
Medical Management Director .... Jean Grangaard
Provider Services Manager .... Tammy Smithson

COMPANY PROFILE:
Parent Company Name: The Araz Group
Doing Business As:
Year Founded: 1982   Federally Qualified: [N]
Forprofit: [Y]   Not-For-Profit: [ ]
Model Type: MIXED
Accreditation: [ ] AAPPO [ ] JACHO [ ] NCQA [X] URAC
Plan Type: Specialty PPO, UR, POS
Primary Physicians: 7,386   Physician Specialists: 8,671
Hospitals: 290
Total Enrollment:
   2001: 250,000   2004: 0   2007: 0
   2002: 0   2005:
   2003: 0   2006:

SERVICE AREA:
Nationwide: N
   IA; MN; ND; SD; WI; ND;

TYPE OF COVERAGE:
Commercial: [Y] Individual: [Y] FEHBP: [ ] Indemnity: [ ]
Medicare: [ ] Medicaid: [ ] Supplemental Medicare: [Y]
Tricare   [ ]

PRODUCTS OFFERED:
Product Name: Type:
Utilization Management
Large Corp Management
Maternity Management
Disability Management
Large Claims Management

PLAN BENEFITS:
Alternative Medicine: [X]   Behavioral Health: [X]
Chiropractic: [X]   Dental: [ ]
Home Care: [X]   Inpatient SNF: [ ]
Long-Term Care: [ ]   Pharm. Mail Order: [X]
Physical Therapy: [ ]   Podiatry: [X]
Psychiatric: [X]   Transplant: [X]
Vision: [ ]   Wellness: [X]
Workers' Comp: [X]
Other Benefits:

MICHIGAN

UPPER PENINSULA HEALTH PLAN

228 W Washington St
Marquette, MI 49855
Phone: 906-225-7500 Fax: 906-225-7690 Toll-Free: 800-835-2556
Web site: www.uphp.com

MAILING ADDRESS:
UPPER PENINSULA HEALTH PLAN
228 W Washington St
Marquette, MI 49855

KEY EXECUTIVES:
Chief Executive Officer .... Dennis H Smith
Chief Financial Officer .... Greg A Gustafson
Medical Director .... Michael Mlsna, MD
Director of Operations .... Beth Casady
MIS Director .... Paula Johnson
Human Resources Manager .... Tanya Jennings
Clinical Services Director .... Marcie Jones, RN

COMPANY PROFILE:
Parent Company Name: UP Managed Care LLC
Doing Business As: Upper Peninsula Health Plan
Year Founded: 1997   Federally Qualified: [N]
Forprofit: [Y]   Not-For-Profit: [ ]
Model Type: NETWORK
Accreditation: [ ] AAPPO [ ] JACHO [X] NCQA [ ] URAC
Plan Type: HMO
Total Revenue: 2005:   48,623,941   2006:   48,498,038
Net Income   2005:   67,862   2006:   2,858,337
Total Enrollment:
   2001: 18,245   2004: 26,025   2007: 24,834
   2002: 19,052   2005: 25,942
   2003: 26,195   2006: 25,447
Medical Loss Ratio: 2005: 86.20   2006: 81.80
Administrative Expense Ratio: 2005:   2006:

SERVICE AREA:
Nationwide: N
   MI;

TYPE OF COVERAGE:
Commercial: [ ] Individual: [Y] FEHBP: [ ] Indemnity: [ ]
Medicare: [ ] Medicaid: [Y] Supplemental Medicare: [ ]
Tricare   [ ]

PRODUCTS OFFERED:
Product Name:	Type:
Upper Peninsula Health Plan HMO	Medicaid

Managed Care Organization Profiles — MICHIGAN

Accreditation: [ ] AAPPO [ ] JACHO [ ] NCQA [ ] URAC
Plan Type: UR
SERVICE AREA:
Nationwide: N
  MI;

S V S VISIONS INC

140 Macomb St
Mt Clemens, MI 48043-5651
Phone: 586-468-7612 Fax: 586-468-7682 Toll-Free: 800-225-3095
Web site: www.svsvision.com
MAILING ADDRESS:
  S V S VISIONS INC
  140 Macomb St
  Mt Clemens, MI 48043-5651

KEY EXECUTIVES:
Chief Executive Officer/President .... Robert G Farrell Jr
Chief Financial Officer .... Kenneth J Starn
Chief Operating Officer .... William F Miller
Business Development Director .... James Madaus, OD
Director of Otometry .... Robert G Farrell, Jr

COMPANY PROFILE:
Parent Company Name:
Doing Business As:
Year Founded: 1974   Federally Qualified: [N]
Forprofit: [Y]   Not-For-Profit: [ ]
Model Type:
Accreditation: [ ] AAPPO [ ] JACHO [ ] NCQA [ ] URAC
Plan Type: Specialty HMO
Total Enrollment:
  2001: 0   2004: 462,458   2007: 0
  2002: 473,690   2005:
  2003: 469,228   2006:
SERVICE AREA:
Nationwide: N
  IL; IN; KY; MI;
TYPE OF COVERAGE:
Commercial: [Y] Individual: [Y] FEHBP: [ ] Indemnity: [ ]
Medicare: [ ] Medicaid: [Y] Supplemental Medicare: [ ]
Tricare   [ ]
PLAN BENEFITS:
Alternative Medicine: [ ]   Behavioral Health: [ ]
Chiropractic: [ ]   Dental: [ ]
Home Care: [ ]   Inpatient SNF: [ ]
Long-Term Care: [ ]   Pharm. Mail Order: [ ]
Physical Therapy: [ ]   Podiatry: [ ]
Psychiatric: [ ]   Transplant: [ ]
Vision: [X]   Wellness: [ ]
Workers' Comp: [ ]
Other Benefits:

TOTAL HEALTH CARE INC

3011 W Grand Blvd Ste 1600
Detroit, MI 48202
Phone: 313-871-2000 Fax: 313-871-0196 Toll-Free:
Web site: www.totalhealthcareonline.com
MAILING ADDRESS:
  TOTAL HEALTH CARE INC
  3011 W Grand Blvd Ste 1600
  Detroit, MI 48202

KEY EXECUTIVES:
Executive Director .... Lyle E Algate
Controller .... Brian Efrusy
Medical Director .... Robyn J Arrington, Jr, MD
Chief Operating Officer .... Randy A Narowitz
Marketing & Sales Manager .... Mitchell Mcmurren
Compliance Officer .... Karen W Connolly, RN

COMPANY PROFILE:
Parent Company Name:
Doing Business As: THC
Year Founded: 1973   Federally Qualified: [Y]
Forprofit: [ ]   Not-For-Profit: [Y]
Model Type: IPA
Accreditation: [ ] AAPPO [X] JACHO [ ] NCQA [ ] URAC
Plan Type: HMO
Total Revenue: 2005:   131,223,881   2006:
Net Income   2005:   -1,422,398   2006:
Total Enrollment:
  2001: 54,639   2004: 63,584   2007: 55,503
  2002: 53,327   2005: 51,654
  2003: 55,867   2006: 54,270
Medical Loss Ratio: 2005: 81.00   2006: 78.00
Administrative Expense Ratio: 2005:   2006:
SERVICE AREA:
Nationwide: N
  MI (Genesee, Macomb, Oakland, Wayne);
TYPE OF COVERAGE:
Commercial: [Y] Individual: [ ] FEHBP: [ ] Indemnity: [ ]
Medicare: [ ] Medicaid: [Y] Supplemental Medicare: [ ]
Tricare   [ ]
PRODUCTS OFFERED:
Product Name: Type:
Total Health Care   HMO
Total Health Care   Medicaid
MIChild   HMO
PLAN BENEFITS:
Alternative Medicine: [ ]   Behavioral Health: [X]
Chiropractic: [X]   Dental: [ ]
Home Care: [X]   Inpatient SNF: [X]
Long-Term Care: [ ]   Pharm. Mail Order: [ ]
Physical Therapy: [X]   Podiatry: [X]
Psychiatric: [X]   Transplant: [ ]
Vision: [X]   Wellness: [X]
Workers' Comp: [ ]
Other Benefits: Disease Management

UNITED CONCORDIA COMPANY INC - MICHIGAN

3250 W Big Beaver Ste 327
Troy, MI 48084
Phone: 248-458-1580 Fax: 248-458-1136 Toll-Free: 800-944-6432
Web site: www.ucci.com
MAILING ADDRESS:
  UNITED CONCORDIA CO INC - MI
  3250 W Big Beaver Ste 327
  Troy, MI 48084

KEY EXECUTIVES:
Chief Executive Officer/President .... Thomas A Dzuryachko
Sr VP, Finance .... Daniel Wright
VP, National Dental Director .... Richard Klich, DMD
MIS Director .... Tom Rice
Director, Provider Services .... Ted Pesano

COMPANY PROFILE:
Parent Company Name: Highmark Inc
Doing Business As:
Year Founded: 1991   Federally Qualified: [ ]
Forprofit: [Y]   Not-For-Profit: [ ]
Model Type:
Accreditation: [ ] AAPPO [ ] JACHO [ ] NCQA [ ] URAC
Plan Type: Specialty HMO, Specialty PPO, POS, TPA
SERVICE AREA:
Nationwide: N
  KY; MI; OH; PA (Western); WV;
TYPE OF COVERAGE:
Commercial: [Y] Individual: [ ] FEHBP: [ ] Indemnity: [ ]
Medicare: [ ] Medicaid: [Y] Supplemental Medicare: [ ]
Tricare   [ ]
PLAN BENEFITS:
Alternative Medicine: [ ]   Behavioral Health: [ ]
Chiropractic: [ ]   Dental: [X]
Home Care: [ ]   Inpatient SNF: [ ]
Long-Term Care: [ ]   Pharm. Mail Order: [ ]
Physical Therapy: [ ]   Podiatry: [ ]
Psychiatric: [ ]   Transplant: [ ]
Vision: [ ]   Wellness: [ ]
Workers' Comp: [ ]
Other Benefits:
Comments:
Formerly Mida Dental Plans - UCCI Inc. For enrollment and revenue information see corporate listing, Camp Hill, Pennsylvania.

MICHIGAN | Managed Care Organization Profiles

PRIORITY HEALTH

1231 East Beltline NE
Grand Rapids, MI 49525
Phone: 616-942-0954 Fax: 616-942-5651 Toll-Free: 800-942-0954
Web site: www.priority-health.com

MAILING ADDRESS:
PRIORITY HEALTH
1231 East Beltline NE
Grand Rapids, MI 49525

KEY EXECUTIVES:
Chief Executive Officer/President .... Kimberly K Horn
Chief Financial Officer .... Gregory Hawkins
Chief Medical Officer .... James J Byrne, MD
Director, Pharmacy .... Rhonda Wassom
Chief Information Officer .... James S Slubowski
VP Operations .... Guy S Gauthier
VP Marketing .... George Conte
Senior Manager, Credentialing .... Karen Dugan
Senior Manager, Legal .... Terry Somerville
Associate VP Market & Commncations .... Rob Pocock
Assoc VP, Provider Network Management .... Kim Suarez
Chief Administrative Officer .... Thea Reigler
Director, Health Management .... Marnie Byers
Director, Corp Quality Improvement .... Bob VanEck
Senior Manager, Credentialing .... Karen Dugan
Manager, Cost Recovery .... Brenda Gross

COMPANY PROFILE:
Parent Company Name: Spectrum Health/Holland Community Hospital/Munson
Doing Business As: Priority Health
Year Founded: 1986 Federally Qualified: [N]
Forprofit: [ ] Not-For-Profit: [Y]
Model Type: IPA
Accreditation: [ ] AAPPO [ ] JACHO [X] NCQA [ ] URAC
Plan Type: HMO, PPO, POS, ASO, EPO, TPA, CDHP, HDHP, HSA, FSA
Primary Physicians: 1,068   Physician Specialists: 1,848
Hospitals: 35
Total Revenue: 2005: 1,048,491,582 2006: 1,084,042,080
Net Income 2005: 37,187,853 2006: 41,263,399
Total Enrollment:
  2001: 268,585 2004: 363,563 2007: 399,474
  2002: 288,535 2005: 372,107
  2003: 335,480 2006: 344,469
Medical Loss Ratio: 2005: 2006:
Administrative Expense Ratio: 2005: 2006:

SERVICE AREA:
Nationwide: N
MI (Alcona, Allegan, Alpena, Barry, Bay, Benzie, Berrien, Calhoun, Charlevoix, Cheboygan, Clinton, Crawford, Eaton, Emmet, Genesee, Grand Traverse, Gratiot, Ionia, Isabella, Kalamazoo, Kalkaska, Kent, Lake, Leelanau, Mackinac, Manistee, Mason, Mecosta, Missaukee, Montcalm, Montmorency, Muskegon, Newaygo, Oceana, Osceola, Oscoda, Otsego, Ottawa, Presque Isle, Roscommon, Saginaw, Tuscola, Van Buren, Wexford);

TYPE OF COVERAGE:
Commercial: [Y] Individual: [Y] FEHBP: [Y] Indemnity: [ ]
Medicare: [Y] Medicaid: [Y] Supplemental Medicare: [Y]
Tricare [ ]

PRODUCTS OFFERED:
Product Name:	Type:
Priority Health	HMO
Priority Health	POS
Priority Health	PPO
Priority Health	Medicaid
MIChild	HMO

CONSUMER-DRIVEN PRODUCTS
Mellon Trust of New England	HSA Company
PriorityHSA	HSA Product
	HSA Administrator
	Consumer-Driven Health Plan
PriorityHRA	High Deductible Health Plan

PLAN BENEFITS:
Alternative Medicine: [ ] Behavioral Health: [X]
Chiropractic: [X] Dental: [ ]
Home Care: [X] Inpatient SNF: [ ]
Long-Term Care: [ ] Pharm. Mail Order: [X]
Physical Therapy: [ ] Podiatry: [X]
Psychiatric: [X] Transplant: [X]
Vision: [X] Wellness: [X]
Workers' Comp: [ ]
Other Benefits:

Comments:
DBA names: Spectrum Health, Holland Community Hospital, Munson Healthcare and Healthshare Inc.

PRO-CARE HEALTH PLAN

3956 Mt Elliot St
Detroit, MI 48207
Phone: 313-925-4607 Fax: 313-925-0472 Toll-Free:
Web site:

MAILING ADDRESS:
PRO-CARE HEALTH PLAN
3956 Mt Elliot St
Detroit, MI 48207

KEY EXECUTIVES:
Chief Executive Officer .... Augustine Kole-James, MD, FACP
Chief Financial Officer .... Harold Montgomery, CPA
Medical Director .... Augustine Kole-James, MD, FACP
Chief Operating Officer .... Deborah Hall-Turner, RN, BSN

COMPANY PROFILE:
Parent Company Name:
Doing Business As:
Year Founded: 1995 Federally Qualified: [N]
Forprofit: [ ] Not-For-Profit: [ ]
Model Type:
Accreditation: [ ] AAPPO [ ] JACHO [ ] NCQA [ ] URAC
Plan Type: HMO
Total Revenue: 2005: 476,296 2006: 604 004
Net Income 2005: -368,307 2006: -367,356
Total Enrollment:
  2001: 0 2004: 63,584 2007: 0
  2002: 0 2005:
  2003: 55,867 2006:

SERVICE AREA:
Nationwide: N
MI;

TYPE OF COVERAGE:
Commercial: [ ] Individual: [ ] FEHBP: [ ] Indemnity: [ ]
Medicare: [ ] Medicaid: [Y] Supplemental Medicare: [ ]
Tricare [ ]

PRODUCTS OFFERED:
Product Name:	Type:
ProCare Health Plan	Medicaid

REVIEW WORKS

33533 W 12 Mile Rd Ste 200
Farminton Hills, MI 48331
Phone: 248-848-5100 Fax: 248-848-9505 Toll-Free: 800-443-1320
Web site: www.reviewworks.com

MAILING ADDRESS:
REVIEW WORKS
33533 W 12 Mile Rd Ste 200
Farmington Hills, MI 48331

KEY EXECUTIVES:
Chief Executive Officer/President .... Carolyn LaHousse
Medical Director .... Kastytis Buitkus, MD
Marketing Director/MIS Director .... Robert Bartlett

COMPANY PROFILE:
Parent Company Name: LaHousse-Bartlett Disability Management
Doing Business As: Reviewworks
Year Founded: 1989 Federally Qualified: [ ]
Forprofit: [Y] Not-For-Profit: [ ]
Model Type:

Managed Care Organization Profiles **MICHIGAN**

KEY EXECUTIVES:
Chief Executive Officer/President .... Scott Wilkerson
Chief Financial Officer .... Daid L Vis
Medical Director .... Howard Burgess, II, MD
VP of Sales & Marketing .... David Olako
Provider Services Director .... Greg England
Care Coordination Director .... Terrie Boggus, RN
Quality Assurance Director .... Julie Griffith

COMPANY PROFILE:
Parent Company Name:
Doing Business As: PHPMM
Year Founded: 1981   Federally Qualified: [Y]
Forprofit: [ ]   Not-For-Profit: [Y]
Model Type: IPA
Accreditation: [ ] AAPPO [ ] JACHO [X] NCQA [ ] URAC
Plan Type: HMO, POS, HSA
Primary Physicians: 416   Physician Specialists: 768
Hospitals: 11
Total Revenue: 2005:   214,379,719   2006:   230,417,691
Net Income   2005:   9,835,374   2006:   7,562,435
Total Enrollment:
   2001: 126,218   2004: 67,286   2007: 49,231
   2002: 100,126   2005: 72,755
   2003: 69,426   2006: 65,692
Medical Loss Ratio: 2005: 89.10   2006: 88.70
Administrative Expense Ratio: 2005:   2006:

SERVICE AREA:
Nationwide: N
   MI;

TYPE OF COVERAGE:
Commercial: [Y] Individual: [ ] FEHBP: [ ] Indemnity: [ ]
Medicare: [ ] Medicaid: [Y] Supplemental Medicare: [ ]
Tricare   [ ]

PRODUCTS OFFERED:
Product Name:	Type:
Physicians Health Plan of South	HMO
Physicians Health Plan of Mid	HMO
Physicians Health Plan of South	HMO
Physicians Health Plan of West	HMO
Physicians Health Plan	Medicaid

PHYSICIANS HEALTH PLAN OF SOUTH MICHIGAN

One Jackson Square
Jackson, MI 49201
Phone: 517-782-7154 Fax: 517-782-4512 Toll-Free:
Web site: www.phpcares.com

MAILING ADDRESS:
   PHYSICIANS HEALTH PLAN OF S MI
   One Jackson Square
   Jackson, MI 49201

KEY EXECUTIVES:
Interim President/Chief Financial Officer .... Wynn Hazen

COMPANY PROFILE:
Parent Company Name: Physicians Health Plan of So Mich, Inc
Doing Business As:
Year Founded: 2000   Federally Qualified: [N]
Forprofit: [ ]   Not-For-Profit: [Y]
Model Type: IPA
Accreditation: [ ] AAPPO [ ] JACHO [ ] NCQA [ ] URAC
Plan Type: HMO, PPO, POS, HSA
Total Revenue: 2005:   86,008,943   2006:   80,387,080
Net Income   2005:   2,615,917   2006:   351,004
Total Enrollment:
   2001: 126,218   2004: 67,286   2007: 17,582
   2002: 100,126   2005: 28,156
   2003: 69,426   2006: 21,857
Medical Loss Ratio: 2005: 89.10   2006: 88.70
Administrative Expense Ratio: 2005:   2006:

SERVICE AREA:
Nationwide: N
   MI (Hillsdale, Jackson, Washtenaw);

TYPE OF COVERAGE:
Commercial: [Y] Individual: [ ] FEHBP: [ ] Indemnity: [ ]
Medicare: [Y] Medicaid: [Y] Supplemental Medicare: [ ]
Tricare   [ ]

PRODUCTS OFFERED:
Product Name:	Type:
Physicians Health Plan of S MI	HMO

CONSUMER-DRIVEN PRODUCTS

	HSA Company
	HSA Product
Wells Fargo Health Benefit Service	HSA Administrator
	Consumer-Driven Health Plan
Plans 4 Health	High Deductible Health Plan

PLAN BENEFITS:
Alternative Medicine: [ ]   Behavioral Health: [X]
Chiropractic: [X]   Dental: [X]
Home Care: [X]   Inpatient SNF: [X]
Long-Term Care: [ ]   Pharm. Mail Order: [X]
Physical Therapy: [X]   Podiatry: [X]
Psychiatric: [X]   Transplant: [X]
Vision: [X]   Wellness: [X]
Workers' Comp: [ ]
Other Benefits:

PREFERRED PROVIDER ORGANIZATION OF MICHIGAN (PPOM)

28588 Northwestern Hwy
Southfield, MI 48034-8318
Phone: 248-357-7766 Fax: 248-357-2418 Toll-Free: 800-878-7766
Web site: www.ppom.com

MAILING ADDRESS:
   PREFERRED PROVIDER ORG MI(PPOM
   28588 Northwestern Hwy
   Southfield, MI 48034-8318

KEY EXECUTIVES:
Chief Executive Officer/President .... Christopher Crowley
VP of Finance .... Mark O'Neill
Senior VP & Chief Operating Officer .... Kelly Wright
Mktg/Communications Director .... Deborah Wilson
VP of Corporate Sales .... Tiffany Otis
VP of Provider Services .... Mike Andreshak
Director of Corporate Development .... Faith Lavine

COMPANY PROFILE:
Parent Company Name: Aetna Inc
Doing Business As: PPOM LP
Year Founded: 1984   Federally Qualified: [N]
Forprofit: [Y]   Not-For-Profit: [ ]
Model Type:
Accreditation: [X] AAPPO [ ] JACHO [ ] NCQA [X] URAC
Plan Type: PPO

SERVICE AREA:
Nationwide: N
   IN; KY; MI; OH; WI;

TYPE OF COVERAGE:
Commercial: [Y] Individual: [ ] FEHBP: [ ] Indemnity: [ ]
Medicare: [ ] Medicaid: [ ] Supplemental Medicare: [ ]
Tricare   [ ]

PRODUCTS OFFERED:
Product Name:	Type:
PPO	
SelectCare PPO	PPO
SelectCare POS	POS

PLAN BENEFITS:
Alternative Medicine: [ ]   Behavioral Health: [ ]
Chiropractic: [X]   Dental: [X]
Home Care: [X]   Inpatient SNF: [ ]
Long-Term Care: [X]   Pharm. Mail Order: [ ]
Physical Therapy: [ ]   Podiatry: [X]
Psychiatric: [X]   Transplant: [ ]
Vision: [X]   Wellness: [ ]
Workers' Comp: [X]
Other Benefits:

Comments:
Purchased SelectCare's PPO & certain POS product lines, March 12th, 2001.

MICHIGAN

COMPANY PROFILE:
Parent Company Name:
Doing Business As:
Year Founded: 1984 Federally Qualified: [N]
Forprofit: [Y] Not-For-Profit: [ ]
Model Type: NETWORK
Accreditation: [ ] AAPPO [ ] JACHO [ ] NCQA [ ] URAC
Plan Type: Specialty PPO
Primary Physicians: 215 Physician Specialists:
Hospitals:
Total Enrollment:
  2001: 0   2004: 450,000   2007: 0
  2002: 0   2005:
  2003: 389,303   2006:

SERVICE AREA:
Nationwide: Y
  NW;

TYPE OF COVERAGE:
Commercial: [Y] Individual: [ ] FEHBP: [ ] Indemnity: [ ]
Medicare: [ ] Medicaid: [ ] Supplemental Medicare: [ ]
Tricare   [ ]

PRODUCTS OFFERED:
Product Name: Type:
All PPO

PLAN BENEFITS:
Alternative Medicine: [ ]   Behavioral Health: [ ]
Chiropractic: [ ]   Dental: [ ]
Home Care: [ ]   Inpatient SNF: [ ]
Long-Term Care: [ ]   Pharm. Mail Order: [ ]
Physical Therapy: [ ]   Podiatry: [X]
Psychiatric: [ ]   Transplant: [ ]
Vision: [ ]   Wellness: [ ]
Workers' Comp: [ ]
Other Benefits:

OMNICARE, A COVENTRY HEALTH PLAN

1333 Gratiot Ave Ste 400
Detroit, MI 48207
Phone: 313-465-1564 Fax: 313-465-1605 Toll-Free: 866-316-3784
Web site: www.cvty.com

MAILING ADDRESS:
  OMNICARE, A COVENTRY HEALTH PL
  1333 Gratiot Ave Ste 400
  Detroit, MI 48207

KEY EXECUTIVES:
Chief Executive Officer .... Beverly A Allen
Chief Financial Officer .... Kenyata J Rogers
Medical Director .... Joseph L Blount, MD
Pharmacy Director .... Le Thal Dillard
Chief Information Officer .... Michele Vasconcellos
Chief Operating Officer .... Gloria Larkins
VP of Marketing .... James Lee
MIS Director .... Norman Smith
Provider Relations Director .... Sandra Hooks
Human Resources Director .... LaZandra Reid
VP of Medical Affairs .... Vernal Blankley

COMPANY PROFILE:
Parent Company Name: Coventry Health Care Inc
Doing Business As: Omnicare
Year Founded: 1973 Federally Qualified: [Y]
Forprofit: [ ] Not-For-Profit: [Y]
Model Type: IPA
Accreditation: [ ] AAPPO [ ] JACHO [X] NCQA [ ] URAC
Plan Type: HMO, POS
Primary Physicians: 480 Physician Specialists: 2,000
Hospitals: 41
Total Revenue: 2005:   146,324,958   2006:   137,961,012
Net Income   2005:   8,122,054   2006:   13,476,025
Total Enrollment:
  2001: 94,218   2004: 62,455   2007: 56,943
  2002: 78,665   2005: 60,965
  2003: 77,255   2006: 57,945
Medical Loss Ratio: 2005: 78.00   2006: 73.20
Administrative Expense Ratio: 2005:   2006:

SERVICE AREA:
Nationwide: N
  MI (Macomb, Monroe, Oakland, Wayne, Washtanaw Counties);

TYPE OF COVERAGE:
Commercial: [Y] Individual: [ ] FEHBP: [ ] Indemnity: [ ]
Medicare: [ ] Medicaid: [Y] Supplemental Medicare: [ ]
Tricare   [ ]

PRODUCTS OFFERED:
Product Name: Type:
OmniCare Plus   POS
OmniCare Health Plan   HMO
OmniCare   Medicaid

PLAN BENEFITS:
Alternative Medicine: [ ]   Behavioral Health: [ ]
Chiropractic: [X]   Dental: [ ]
Home Care: [X]   Inpatient SNF: [X]
Long-Term Care: [ ]   Pharm. Mail Order: [ ]
Physical Therapy: [X]   Podiatry: [X]
Psychiatric: [X]   Transplant: [X]
Vision: [X]   Wellness: [X]
Workers' Comp: [ ]
Other Benefits:

PARAMOUNT CARE OF MICHIGAN

106 Park Place
Dundee, MI 48131
Phone: 888-241-5604 Fax: 734-529-8896 Toll-Free: 888-241-5604
Web site: www.paramountcareofmichigan.com

MAILING ADDRESS:
  PARAMOUNT CARE OF MICHIGAN
  106 Park Place
  Dundee, MI 48131

KEY EXECUTIVES:
Chief Executive Officer/President .... John C Randolph
Senior VP, Finance & Operations .... Gary Akenberger
Chief Medical Officer .... Neeraj Kanwal, MD
Pharmacy Director .... Craig Bogner
VP of Marketing .... Mark Henry Moser
Secretary .... Jeffrey Craig Kuhn

COMPANY PROFILE:
Parent Company Name: Promedica
Doing Business As:
Year Founded: 1996 Federally Qualified: [N]
Forprofit: [ ] Not-For-Profit: [ ]
Model Type:
Accreditation: [ ] AAPPO [ ] JACHO [ ] NCQA [ ] URAC
Plan Type: HMO
Total Revenue: 2005: 30,743,039   2006: 34,469,375
Net Income   2005:   -97,988   2006:   1,021,332
Total Enrollment:
  2001: 3,241   2004: 8,171   2007: 8,175
  2002: 4,504   2005: 8,101
  2003: 7,623   2006: 8,403
Medical Loss Ratio: 2005: 91.00   2006: 88.00
Administrative Expense Ratio: 2005:   2006:

SERVICE AREA:
Nationwide: N
  MI (Monroe);

TYPE OF COVERAGE:
Commercial: [Y] Individual: [ ] FEHBP: [ ] Indemnity: [ ]
Medicare: [Y] Medicaid: [ ] Supplemental Medicare: [ ]
Tricare   [ ]

PRODUCTS OFFERED:
Product Name: Type:
Elite   Medicare
Paramount   HMO

PHYSICIANS HEALTH PLAN OF MID-MICHIGAN

1400 E Michigan Ave
Lansing, MI 48912
Phone: 517-364-8400 Fax: 517-364-8280 Toll-Free: 800-661-8299
Web site: www.phpmm.org

MAILING ADDRESS:
  PHYSICIANS HEALTH PLAN OF MID-MI
  PO Box 30377
  Lansing, MI 48912

Managed Care Organization Profiles — MICHIGAN

COMPANY PROFILE:
Parent Company Name:
Doing Business As:
Year Founded: 1989   Federally Qualified: [N]
Forprofit: [Y]   Not-For-Profit: [ ]
Model Type:
Accreditation: [ ] AAPPO [ ] JACHO [ ] NCQA [ ] URAC
Plan Type: Specialty HMO
Total Enrollment:
   2001: 0   2004: 59,612   2007: 0
   2002: 65,006   2005:
   2003: 60,763   2006:

SERVICE AREA:
Nationwide: N
   MI (Southeastern & Greater Lansing Area);

TYPE OF COVERAGE:
Commercial: [Y] Individual: [Y] FEHBP: [ ] Indemnity: [ ]
Medicare: [ ] Medicaid: [ ] Supplemental Medicare: [ ]
Tricare [ ]

PRODUCTS OFFERED:
Product Name: Type:
Midwestern Dental Plans Inc   Dental

PLAN BENEFITS:
Alternative Medicine:	[ ]	Behavioral Health:	[ ]
Chiropractic:	[ ]	Dental:	[X]
Home Care:	[ ]	Inpatient SNF:	[ ]
Long-Term Care:	[ ]	Pharm. Mail Order:	[ ]
Physical Therapy:	[ ]	Podiatry:	[ ]
Psychiatric:	[ ]	Transplant:	[ ]
Vision:	[ ]	Wellness:	[ ]
Workers' Comp:	[ ]		

Other Benefits:

MOLINA HEALTHCARE OF MICHIGAN INC

100 W Big Beaver Rd Ste 600
Troy, MI 48084-5209
Phone: 248-925-1700 Fax: 248-925-1709 Toll-Free: 888-898-7969
Web site: www.molinahealthcare.com

MAILING ADDRESS:
   MOLINA HEALTHCARE OF MI INC
   100 W Big Beaver Rd Ste 600
   Troy, MI 48084-5209

KEY EXECUTIVES:
Chairman of the Board .... Joseph M Molina, MD
Chief Executive Officer .... Roman T Kulich
President .... Jesse Thomas
Chief Financial Officer .... Thomas Murar
Chief Medical Director .... James Forshee, MD
Director of Pharmacy .... James N Clarke, RPh, MS
Chief Operations Officer .... Nancy Wanchik
Chief Information Officer/MIS Director .... Amer Sanjak
Director, Provider Services/Community Affairs .... Dennis Rogissart
Director of Network Services .... Ron Szumski
Regional Director, Human Resources .... Amy O'Donnell
Director, Quality Improvement .... Marianne Thomas-Brown, RN
Vice Chairman .... George S Goldstein, PhD

COMPANY PROFILE:
Parent Company Name: Molina Healthcare Inc
Doing Business As:
Year Founded: 1998   Federally Qualified: [N]
Forprofit: [Y]   Not-For-Profit: [ ]
Model Type: NETWORK
Accreditation: [ ] AAPPO [ ] JACHO [X] NCQA [ ] URAC
Plan Type: HMO
Primary Physicians: 1,942   Physician Specialists: 4,349
Hospitals: 49
Total Revenue: 2005: 472,713,213   2006: 468,568,961
Net Income: 2005: 10,768,567   2006: 23,187,316
Total Enrollment:
   2001: 25,732   2004: 157,998   2007: 211,279
   2002: 34,581   2005: 232,425
   2003: 81,661   2006: 227,797
Medical Loss Ratio: 2005: 82.40   2006: 77.40
Administrative Expense Ratio: 2005:   2006:

SERVICE AREA:
Nationwide: N
   MI;

TYPE OF COVERAGE:
Commercial: [ ] Individual: [ ] FEHBP: [ ] Indemnity: [ ] Medicare: [ ] Medicaid: [Y] Supplemental Medicare: [ ]
Tricare [ ]

PRODUCTS OFFERED:
Product Name: Type:
Molina Healthcare of MI   Medicaid

PLAN BENEFITS:
Alternative Medicine:	[ ]	Behavioral Health:	[X]
Chiropractic:	[X]	Dental:	[ ]
Home Care:	[X]	Inpatient SNF:	[X]
Long-Term Care:	[ ]	Pharm. Mail Order:	[ ]
Physical Therapy:	[X]	Podiatry:	[X]
Psychiatric:	[X]	Transplant:	[X]
Vision:	[X]	Wellness:	[X]
Workers' Comp:	[ ]		

Other Benefits:

Comments:
Merged with Good Health Plan.

MPRO

22670 Haggerty Rd Ste 100
Farmington Hills, MI 48335-2611
Phone: 248-465-7300 Fax: 248-465-7428 Toll-Free:
Web site: www.mpro.org

MAILING ADDRESS:
   MPRO
   22670 Haggerty Rd Ste 100
   Farmington Hills, MI 48335-2611

KEY EXECUTIVES:
Board Chairman .... Charles Barone II, MD
Chief Executive Officer/President .... Debra L Moss, MD MBA
Medical Director .... Jeffrey Deitch, DO
Director, Marketing & Public Relations .... Susan Burns, BA
Director, IT/Corp Compliance Manager .... Ken Oishi, BA
Human Resource Director .... Patricia Headley
Senior VP, Quality/Review Operations .... Colleen Cieszkowski, RN, MA
VP, Marketing/Communications/Business Dev ...... Thomas Leyden, BA

COMPANY PROFILE:
Parent Company Name:
Doing Business As: Quality Improvement Organization
Year Founded: 1984   Federally Qualified: [Y]
Forprofit: [ ]   Not-For-Profit: [Y]
Model Type:
Accreditation: [ ] AAPPO [ ] JACHO [ ] NCQA [X] URAC
Plan Type: UR, PRO

SERVICE AREA:
Nationwide: N
   MI;

TYPE OF COVERAGE:
Commercial: [ ] Individual: [ ] FEHBP: [ ] Indemnity: [ ]
Medicare: [Y] Medicaid: [Y] Supplemental Medicare: [ ]
Tricare [ ]

Comments:
Michigan Peer Review Organization is the federally-designated quality improvement organization of Michigan.

NATIONAL FOOT CARE PROGRAM INC

PO Box 760547
Lathrup Village, MI 48076
Phone: 248-559-2579 Fax: 248-423-1077 Toll-Free: 800-922-1695
Web site: www.nationalfootcare.com

MAILING ADDRESS:
   NATIONAL FOOT CARE PROGRAM INC
   PO Box 760547
   Lathrup Village, MI 48076

KEY EXECUTIVES:
Chief Executive Officer/President .... Claude Oster, DO
Chief Financial Officer .... John Homeister
VP Medical Affairs .... Scott Oster, Do
Chief Operating Officer .... Terri Mulligan
MIS Director .... Andrew Nelson
Executive Vice President .... Jim Chatfield

MICHIGAN

COMPANY PROFILE:
Parent Company Name: Blue Care Network/BC BS of Michigan
Doing Business As: M-CARE
Year Founded: 1986 Federally Qualified: [Y]
Forprofit: [ ] Not-For-Profit: [Y] Model Type: MIXED
Accreditation: [ ] AAPPO [ ] JACHO [X] NCQA [ ] URAC
Plan Type: HMO, PPO, POS, HSA, HDHP
Primary Physicians: Physician Specialists:
Hospitals: 40
Total Revenue: 2005: 462,248,418 2006: 467,340,828
Net Income 2005: 14,973,159 2006: 52,652,970
Total Enrollment:
    2001: 197,721   2004: 183,355   2007: 121,307
    2002: 205,170   2005: 180,882
    2003: 191,548   2006: 163,701
Medical Loss Ratio: 2005: 90.40 2006: 86.90
Administrative Expense Ratio: 2005: 2006:

SERVICE AREA:
Nationwide: N
MI (Clinton, Eaton, Genesee, Hillsdale, Ingham, Jackson, Lapeer, Livingston, Macomb, Monroe, Oakland, Saginaw, Shiawassee, St Clair, Washtenaw, Wayne, Tuscola, Barry, Calhoun, Kalamazoo);

TYPE OF COVERAGE:
Commercial: [Y] Individual: [Y] FEHBP: [ ] Indemnity: [ ]
Medicare: [ ] Medicaid: [Y] Supplemental Medicare: [ ]
Tricare: [ ]

PRODUCTS OFFERED:
Product Name:	Type:
M-Care Senior Plan	Medicare
M-Care Medicaid	Medicaid
M-Care	HMO
M-Care	POS
MIChild	HMO

CONSUMER-DRIVEN PRODUCTS
	HSA Company
	HSA Product
Mellon Financial	HSA Administrator
	Consumer-Driven Health Plan
	High Deductible Health Plan

PLAN BENEFITS:
Alternative Medicine:	[X]	Behavioral Health:	[X]
Chiropractic:	[ ]	Dental:	[ ]
Home Care:	[X]	Inpatient SNF:	[X]
Long-Term Care:	[ ]	Pharm. Mail Order:	[ ]
Physical Therapy:	[X]	Podiatry:	[X]
Psychiatric:	[X]	Transplant:	[X]
Vision:	[X]	Wellness:	[X]
Workers' Comp:	[ ]		
Other Benefits:			

MCLAREN HEALTH PLAN

G-3245 Beecher Rd Ste 200
Flint, MI 48532
Phone: 810-733-9722 Fax: 810-733-9645 Toll-Free: 888-327-0671
Web site: www.mclarenhealthplan.org

MAILING ADDRESS:
MCLAREN HEALTH PLAN
PO Box 1511
Flint, MI 48532

KEY EXECUTIVES:
Chief Executive Officer/President .... Kathy Kendall
VP, Chief Financial Officer .... Michael G Grodus
Chief Medical Officer .... Thomas Petroff, DO
VP, Chief Information Officer .... Carol Soloman
VP, Medical Management .... Beth Caughlin
VP, Provider Services .... Sue Bayer
Dir of Human Resources .... Carissa Haring
VP, Marketing .... Ed Harden

COMPANY PROFILE:
Parent Company Name: McLaren Health Care Corporation
Doing Business As:
Year Founded: 1998 Federally Qualified: [N]
Forprofit: [ ] Not-For-Profit: [ ]
Model Type:
Accreditation: [ ] AAPPO [ ] JACHO [X] NCQA [ ] URAC
Plan Type: HMO
Total Revenue: 2005: 102,070,328 2006: 115,094,861
Net Income 2005: 5,157,371 2006: 7,695,234
Total Enrollment:
    2001: 15,881   2004: 46,495   2007: 61,197
    2002: 20,830   2005: 52,530
    2003: 29,464   2006: 56,307
Medical Loss Ratio: 2005: 84.00 2006: 83.00
Administrative Expense Ratio: 2005: 2006:

SERVICE AREA:
Nationwide: N
MI;

TYPE OF COVERAGE:
Commercial: [ ] Individual: [ ] FEHBP: [ ] Indemnity: [ ]
Medicare: [ ] Medicaid: [Y] Supplemental Medicare: [ ]
Tricare: [ ]

PRODUCTS OFFERED:
Product Name:	Type:
McLaren Health Plan	Medicaid

MIDWEST HEALTH PLAN

5050 Schaefer Rd
Dearborn, MI 48126
Phone: 313-581-3700 Fax: 313-581-2780 Toll-Free: 888-654-2200
Web site: www.midwesthealthplan.com

MAILING ADDRESS:
MIDWEST HEALTH PLAN
5050 Schaefer Rd
Dearborn, MI 48126

KEY EXECUTIVES:
President .... Mark B Saffer, DPM
VP, Chief Financial Officer .... Allen A Kessler, CPA
Medical Director .... Mark H Tucker, MD
Pharmacy Director .... Ellen Anderson, RN
Chief Information Officer .... Refaat Shulaiba

COMPANY PROFILE:
Parent Company Name:
Doing Business As:
Year Founded: 1994 Federally Qualified: [N]
Forprofit: [ ] Not-For-Profit: [ ]
Model Type:
Accreditation: [ ] AAPPO [ ] JACHO [X] NCQA [ ] URAC
Plan Type: HMO, TPA
Total Revenue: 2005: 117,777,219 2006: 121,367,001
Net Income 2005: 5,704,094 2006: 6,009,219
Total Enrollment:
    2001: 35,477   2004: 55,065   2007: 63,855
    2002: 40,316   2005: 55,700
    2003: 48,729   2006: 59,381
Medical Loss Ratio: 2005: 81.00 2006: 80.00
Administrative Expense Ratio: 2005: 2006:

SERVICE AREA:
Nationwide: N
MI (Macomb, Oakland, Washtenew, Wayne);

TYPE OF COVERAGE:
Commercial: [ ] Individual: [ ] FEHBP: [ ] Indemnity: [ ]
Medicare: [ ] Medicaid: [Y] Supplemental Medicare: [ ]
Tricare: [ ]

PRODUCTS OFFERED:
Product Name:	Type:
Midwest Health Plan	Medicaid

MIDWESTERN DENTAL PLANS INC

5050 Schaefer Road
Dearborn, MI 48126-3221
Phone: 313-582-8150 Fax: 313-582-6015 Toll-Free: 800-544-6374
Web site: www.midwesterndentalplans.com

MAILING ADDRESS:
MIDWESTERN DENTAL PLANS INC
5050 Schaefer Road
Dearborn, MI 48126-3221

KEY EXECUTIVES:
VP, Administration/President .... John Morgan, Jr
Treasurer .... Joel Sharenow

Managed Care Organization Profiles — MICHIGAN

SERVICE AREA:
Nationwide: N
 MI;
TYPE OF COVERAGE:
Commercial: [Y] Individual: [ ] FEHBP: [ ] Indemnity: [ ]
Medicare: [Y] Medicaid: [Y] Supplemental Medicare: [ ]
Tricare [ ]
PLAN BENEFITS:
Alternative Medicine: [ ]   Behavioral Health: [ ]
Chiropractic: [ ]   Dental: [ ]
Home Care: [ ]   Inpatient SNF: [ ]
Long-Term Care: [ ]   Pharm. Mail Order: [ ]
Physical Therapy: [ ]   Podiatry: [ ]
Psychiatric: [ ]   Transplant: [ ]
Vision: [X]   Wellness: [ ]
Workers' Comp: [ ]
Other Benefits:
Comments:
Formerly First Optometry Vision Plans Inc. First Optometry and Henry Ford Health System joined together under the name OptimEyes.

HUMANA INC - GRAND RAPIDS MICHIGAN

5555 Glenwood Hills Pkwy Ste 150
Grand Rapids, MI 49503
Phone: 616-336-0011 Fax: 616-336-5161 Toll-Free: 800-991-1953
Web site: www.humana.com
MAILING ADDRESS:
 HUMANA INC - GRAND RAPIDS MI
 5555 Glenwood Hills Pkwy Ste 150
 Grand Rapids, MI 49503

KEY EXECUTIVES:
Chairman of the Board .... David A Jones Jr
Chief Executive Officer .... Michael B McCallister
Market President .... Denise Christy
Sr VP, Chief Innovation Officer .... Jonathan T Lord, MD
VP of Sales .... John Crusse
Manager of Sales Administratn .... LaShaundia Abner
Sales Coordinator .... Arin Blankenship
Sales Coordinator .... Jill Tafel

COMPANY PROFILE:
Parent Company Name: Humana Inc
Doing Business As:
Year Founded: 1961   Federally Qualified: [Y]
Forprofit: [Y]   Not-For-Profit: [ ]
Model Type:
Accreditation: [ ] AAPPO [ ] JACHO [ ] NCQA [ ] URAC
Plan Type: PPO, CDHP, HSA
Total Enrollment:
 2001: 0   2004: 52,000   2007: 172,000
 2002: 0   2005:
 2003: 0   2006:
SERVICE AREA:
Nationwide:
 WI;
TYPE OF COVERAGE:
Commercial: [Y] Individual: [ ] FEHBP: [ ] Indemnity: [ ]
Medicare: [ ] Medicaid: [ ] Supplemental Medicare: [ ]
Tricare [Y]
CONSUMER-DRIVEN PRODUCTS
JP Morgan Chase   HSA Company
HumanaOne HSA   HSA Product
JP Morgan Chase   HSA Administrator
Personal Care Account   Consumer-Driven Health Plan
HumanaOne   High Deductible Health Plan
PLAN BENEFITS:
Alternative Medicine: [ ]   Behavioral Health: [ ]
Chiropractic: [X]   Dental: [X]
Home Care: [ ]   Inpatient SNF: [ ]
Long-Term Care: [ ]   Pharm. Mail Order: [X]
Physical Therapy: [ ]   Podiatry: [ ]
Psychiatric: [X]   Transplant: [X]
Vision: [ ]   Wellness: [ ]
Workers' Comp: [X]
Other Benefits:

IBA HEALTH PLANS

106 Farmers Alley Ste 300
Kalamazoo, MI 49005-1100
Phone: 269-216-2168 Fax: 269-341-6832 Toll-Free:
Web site: www.ibahealthplans.com
MAILING ADDRESS:
 IBA HEALTH PLANS
 PO Box 51100
 Kalamazoo, MI 49005-1100

KEY EXECUTIVES:
Chief Executive Officer .... David Kibbe
Chief Financial Officer .... David Vis
Pharmacy Director .... Scott Musial
Marketing Director .... Cindy Crandel
VP Sales & Service .... Tamara Schumacher
Director Network Services .... Judy Klein
Compliance Officer .... Sue Morgan
VP Operations .... Scott Musial

COMPANY PROFILE:
Parent Company Name: UnitedHealth Group
Doing Business As: IBA Health and Life Assurance Company
Year Founded: 1967   Federally Qualified: [Y]
Forprofit: [ ]   Not-For-Profit: [Y]
Model Type:
Accreditation: [ ] AAPPO [Y] JACHO [ ] NCQA [ ] URAC
Plan Type: HMO, PPO, ASO, TPA
Total Enrollment:
 2001: 0   2004: 85,000   2007: 0
 2002: 0   2005:
 2003: 83,000   2006: 80,000
SERVICE AREA:
Nationwide: N
 MI (Allegan, Barry, Berrien, Branch, Cass, Calhoun, Kalamazoo, St Joseph, Van Buren);
TYPE OF COVERAGE:
Commercial: [Y] Individual: [ ] FEHBP: [ ] Indemnity: [Y]
Medicare: [ ] Medicaid: [Y] Supplemental Medicare: [ ]
Tricare [ ]
PRODUCTS OFFERED:
Product Name: Type:
IBA PPO   PPO
IBA Managed Indemnity
PLAN BENEFITS:
Alternative Medicine: [ ]   Behavioral Health: [ ]
Chiropractic: [X]   Dental: [ ]
Home Care: [X]   Inpatient SNF: [X]
Long-Term Care: [ ]   Pharm. Mail Order: [X]
Physical Therapy: [X]   Podiatry: [X]
Psychiatric: [X]   Transplant: [X]
Vision: [ ]   Wellness: [ ]
Workers' Comp: [ ]
Other Benefits:
Comments:
Purchased by UnitedHealthcare in 2006.

M-CARE INC

2301 Commonwealth Blvd
Ann Arbor, MI 48105-2945
Phone: 734-747-8700 Fax: 734-332-2195 Toll-Free: 888-269-7755
Web site: www.mcare.org
MAILING ADDRESS:
 M-CARE INC
 2301 Commonwealth Blvd
 Ann Arbor, MI 48105-2945

KEY EXECUTIVES:
Chief Executive Officer/President .... Zelda Geyer-Sylvia
Chief Financial Officer .... Gregory A Hawkins
Medical Director .... Robert P Kelch, MD
Chief Information Officer/MIS Director .... Dolph Courchaine
Marketing Director .... Tim George
Senior Director .... Joseph Katulic
Manager, Medical Managt .... Martha Richard
Director, Quality Improvement .... Linda Ziesmer

MICHIGAN — Managed Care Organization Profiles

PLAN BENEFITS:
Alternative Medicine: [ ] Behavioral Health: [ ]
Chiropractic: [ ] Dental: [X]
Home Care: [ ] Inpatient SNF: [ ]
Long-Term Care: [ ] Pharm. Mail Order: [ ]
Physical Therapy: [ ] Podiatry: [ ]
Psychiatric: [ ] Transplant: [ ]
Vision: [ ] Wellness: [ ]
Workers' Comp: [ ]
Other Benefits:

HEALTH PLAN OF MICHIGAN

17515 W Nine Mile Rd Ste 650
Southfield, MI 48075
Phone: 248-557-3700 Fax: 248-569-4702 Toll-Free: 888-773-2647
Web site: www.hpmich.com

MAILING ADDRESS:
HEALTH PLAN OF MI
17515 W Nine Mile Rd Ste 650
Southfield, MI 48075

KEY EXECUTIVES:
Chief Executive Officer/President .... David B Cotton, MD
Chief Financial Officer .... Janice Torosian
Medical Director .... Gregory Berger, MD
Chief Information Officer .... Thomas Lauzon
Chief Operating Officer .... Sheryl L Cotton
Director, Provider Services .... Raymond D Pitera
Quality Assurance Director .... Geriann Finnegan, RN, MSA

COMPANY PROFILE:
Parent Company Name:
Doing Business As:
Year Founded: 1995 Federally Qualified: [N]
Forprofit: [Y] Not-For-Profit: [ ]
Model Type:
Accreditation: [ ] AAPPO [ ] JACHO [X] NCQA [ ] URAC
Plan Type: HMO,
Total Revenue: 2005: 180,127,438 2006: 204,725,815
Net Income 2005: 12,953,446 2006: 11,997,772
Total Enrollment:
  2001: 33,434 2004: 87,325 2007: 130,550
  2002: 46,845 2005: 100,349
  2003: 68,568 2006: 119,149
Medical Loss Ratio: 2005: 77.00 2006: 78.00
Administrative Expense Ratio: 2005: 2006:
SERVICE AREA:
Nationwide: N
  MI;
TYPE OF COVERAGE:
Commercial: [ ] Individual: [ ] FEHBP: [ ] Indemnity: [ ]
Medicare: [ ] Medicaid: [Y] Supplemental Medicare: [ ]
Tricare [ ]
PRODUCTS OFFERED:
Product Name: Type:
Health Plan Medicaid

HEALTHPLUS OF MICHIGAN

2050 S Linden Rd
Flint, MI 48532
Phone: 810-230-2000 Fax: 810-230-2208 Toll-Free: 800-332-9161
Web site: www.healthplus.com

MAILING ADDRESS:
HEALTHPLUS OF MICHIGAN
PO Box 1700
Flint, MI 48532

KEY EXECUTIVES:
Chairman of the Board .... Jack Berry, MD
Chief Executive Officer/President .... David Crosby
VP of Finance & Operations .... Matthew A Mendrygal, CPA
VP/Chief Medical Officer .... John Saalwaechter, MD
Director of Pharmacy Services .... Carrie Germain RPh
Senior Director of Information Systems .... Julie Boyer
VP of Sales & Product Development .... Nancy Jenkins
VP of Sales & Product Development .... Nancy Jenkins
Director of Quality Management .... Gloria Snidersich
Compliance & Privacy Official .... Theresa Schurmann
Director Public Relations .... Rich Swenson
Director, Provider Network Management .... Elyse Berry, Greater Flint
VP of Regional Operations & Business Development .... Bruce Hill
Director of Human Resources .... Kathy Verros
Director of Medical Systems .... Margaret Kokoszka
Sr Director of Utilization Mngmnt .... Meg Pointon
Director of Quality Management .... Gloria Snidersich
Director of Marketing & Corp Accounts .... Nancy Starks-Jenkins
Director of Utilization Management .... Carla Parkes
Director, Provider Network Management Jeanne Visuri, Tri-City Region
Director of Customer Service .... Jeannine Lemonds

COMPANY PROFILE:
Parent Company Name:
Doing Business As:
Year Founded: 1979 Federally Qualified: [Y]
Forprofit: [ ] Not-For-Profit: [Y]
Model Type: NETWORK
Accreditation: [ ] AAPPO [ ] JACHO [X] NCQA [ ] URAC
Plan Type: HMO, TPA, POS
Primary Physicians: 440 Physician Specialists: 857
Hospitals: 10
Total Revenue: 2005: 389,252,995 2006: 402,271,797
Net Income 2005: 10,857,347 2006: 10,017,851
Total Enrollment:
  2001: 159,145 2004: 103,266 2007: 152,252
  2002: 163,673 2005: 99,269
  2003: 107,616 2006: 156,723
Medical Loss Ratio: 2005: 90.00 2006: 89.00
Administrative Expense Ratio: 2005: 2006:
SERVICE AREA:
Nationwide: N
  Mid MI;
TYPE OF COVERAGE:
Commercial: [Y] Individual: [Y] FEHBP: [ ] Indemnity: [ ]
Medicare: [Y] Medicaid: [Y] Supplemental Medicare: [Y]
Tricare [ ]
PRODUCTS OFFERED:
Product Name: Type:
Health Plus Options HMO/POS
MIChild HMO
Health Plus Senior Medicare Risk
Health Plus Senior Program Medicare Supplementa
HealthPlus Partners Inc Medicaid
PLAN BENEFITS:
Alternative Medicine: [ ] Behavioral Health: [X]
Chiropractic: [X] Dental: [ ]
Home Care: [X] Inpatient SNF: [X]
Long-Term Care: [X] Pharm. Mail Order: [ ]
Physical Therapy: [X] Podiatry: [X]
Psychiatric: [X] Transplant: [X]
Vision: [ ] Wellness: [X]
Workers' Comp: [ ]
Other Benefits:

HENRY FORD OPTIMEYES

655 West 13 Mile Rd
Madison Heights, MI 48071
Phone: 248-588-9300 Fax: 248-588-3355 Toll-Free: 800-792-3262
Web site: www.optimeyes.com

MAILING ADDRESS:
HENRY FORD OPTIMEYES
655 West 13 Mile Rd
Madison Heights, MI 48071

KEY EXECUTIVES:
Medical Director .... Ranald Mackenzie, MD
Marketing Director .... Katie Darr

COMPANY PROFILE:
Parent Company Name: Henry Ford Health System
Doing Business As:
Year Founded: 1980 Federally Qualified: [ ]
Forprofit: [Y] Not-For-Profit: [ ]
Model Type:
Accreditation: [ ] AAPPO [ ] JACHO [ ] NCQA [ ] URAC
Plan Type: Specialty PPO

Managed Care Organization Profiles — MICHIGAN

GREAT-WEST HEALTHCARE OF MICHIGAN

1 Town Sq Oakland Ste 1500
Southfield, MI 48076
Phone: 248-355-3919 Fax: 248-355-5488 Toll-Free:
Web site: www.greatwesthealthcare.com

MAILING ADDRESS:
GREAT-WEST HEALTHCARE OF MI
1 Town Sq Oakland Ste 1500
Southfield, MI 48076

KEY EXECUTIVES:
Chief Executive Officer/President .... Raymond L McFeetors
Provider Relations Coordinator .... Shannon Dishneau
VP Network Development .... Gretchen Kline

COMPANY PROFILE:
Parent Company Name: CIGNA Inc
Doing Business As:
Year Founded: Federally Qualified: [ ]
Forprofit: [Y]   Not-For-Profit: [ ]
Model Type:
Accreditation: [ ] AAPPO [ ] JACHO [ ] NCQA [ ] URAC
Plan Type: HMO, PPO, POS, CDHP, HSA

SERVICE AREA:
Nationwide: N
 MI;

TYPE OF COVERAGE:
Commercial: [Y] Individual: [ ] FEHBP: [ ] Indemnity: [ ]
Medicare: [ ] Medicaid: [ ] Supplemental Medicare: [ ]
Tricare   [ ]

CONSUMER-DRIVEN PRODUCTS
Mellon HR Solutions LLC   HSA Company
                                 HSA Product
                                 HSA Administrator
                                 Consumer-Driven Health Plan
                                 High Deductible Health Plan

PLAN BENEFITS:
Alternative Medicine: [X]   Behavioral Health: [ ]
Chiropractic: [X]   Dental: [X]
Home Care: [X]   Inpatient SNF: [X]
Long-Term Care: [ ]   Pharm. Mail Order: [X]
Physical Therapy: [X]   Podiatry: [X]
Psychiatric: [X]   Transplant: [X]
Vision: [X]   Wellness: [X]
Workers' Comp: [ ]
Other Benefits:
Comments: Acquired by CIGNA Inc April 1, 2008.

HEALTH ALLIANCE PLAN OF MICHIGAN

2850 West Grand Blvd
Detroit, MI 48202
Phone: 313-872-8100 Fax: 313-664-8433 Toll-Free: 800-422-4641
Web site: www.hap.org

MAILING ADDRESS:
HEALTH ALLIANCE PLAN OF MI
2850 West Grand Blvd
Detroit, MI 48202

KEY EXECUTIVES:
Chief Executive Officer/President .... Francine Parker
Senior VP, Chief Financial Officer .... Ronald Berry
Chief Medical Officer .... Mary Beth Bolton, MD
VP Sales & Marketing .... Scott W Averill
VP Human Resources & Support Service .... Donald Davis, Jr
VP, General Counsel .... Maurice E McMurray

COMPANY PROFILE:
Parent Company Name:
Doing Business As: HAP
Year Founded: 1979   Federally Qualified: [Y]
Forprofit: [ ]   Not-For-Profit: [Y]
Model Type: MIXED
Accreditation: [ ] AAPPO [ ] JACHO [X] NCQA [ ] URAC
Plan Type: HMO, PPO, POS, EPO, CDHP, HSA
Primary Physicians: 2,100   Physician Specialists: 3,800
Hospitals: 44
Total Revenue: 2005:   1,507,239,774   2006:   1,587,239,857
Net Income   2005:   34,213,133   2006:   48,891,712
Total Enrollment:
 2001: 462,085   2004: 460,919   2007: 403,432
 2002: 485,154   2005: 449,656
 2003: 471,150   2006: 430,864
Medical Loss Ratio: 2005: 91.10   2006: 91.00
Administrative Expense Ratio: 2005:   2006:

SERVICE AREA:
Nationwide: N
 MI;

TYPE OF COVERAGE:
Commercial: [Y] Individual: [ ] FEHBP: [ ] Indemnity: [ ]
Medicare: [Y] Medicaid: [ ] Supplemental Medicare: [Y]
Tricare   [ ]

PRODUCTS OFFERED:
Product Name: Type:
Health Alliance Plan HMO   HMO
HAP Senior Plus   Medicare
Health Alliance Plan   MedicaidSelectCare HMO
HMO
SelectCare HMO   HMO Plus
SelectCare Medicare Gold   Medicare

CONSUMER-DRIVEN PRODUCTS
                                 HSA Company
                                 HSA Product
Mellon Bank   HSA Administrator
                                 Consumer-Driven Health Plan
                                 High Deductible Health Plan

PLAN BENEFITS:
Alternative Medicine: [ ]   Behavioral Health: [ ]
Chiropractic: [ ]   Dental: [ ]
Home Care: [X]   Inpatient SNF: [X]
Long-Term Care: [ ]   Pharm. Mail Order: [X]
Physical Therapy: [X]   Podiatry: [X]
Psychiatric: [X]   Transplant: [X]
Vision: [X]   Wellness: [X]
Workers' Comp: [ ]
Other Benefits:
Comments:
Purchased SelectCare's HMO, HMO Plus and Medicare Gold product lines.

HEALTH CARE EXCHANGE LIMITED COMPANY

28588 Northwestern Hwy Ste 450
Southfield, MI 48034
Phone: 248-327-9200 Fax: 248-327-9201 Toll-Free: 800-752-1547
Web site: www.dentemax.com

MAILING ADDRESS:
HEALTH CARE EXCHANGE LTD CO
28588 Northwestern Hwy Ste 450
Southfield, MI 48034

KEY EXECUTIVES:
Chief Executive Officer/President .... Rick Morrone
Chief Financial Officer .... Amy Sherman
Marketing Director .... Kim Sharbatz

COMPANY PROFILE:
Parent Company Name: Doing Business As: Dentemax Inc
Year Founded: 1985   Federally Qualified: [N]
Forprofit: [Y]   Not-For-Profit: [ ]
Model Type: MIXED
Accreditation: [ ] AAPPO [ ] JACHO [ ] NCQA [ ] URAC
Plan Type: PPO, Specialty PPO, POS, PPO
Total Enrollment:
 2001: 0   2004: 0   2007: 4,500,000
 2002: 0   2005:
 2003: 0   2006:

SERVICE AREA:
Nationwide: N
 NW (48 states);

TYPE OF COVERAGE:
Commercial: [Y] Individual: [Y] FEHBP: [ ] Indemnity: [ ]
Medicare: [Y] Medicaid: [ ] Supplemental Medicare: [ ]
Tricare   [ ]

MICHIGAN — Managed Care Organization Profiles

KEY EXECUTIVES:
Chief Executive Officer/President .... Roland Palmer
Medical Director .... James Kerby, MD
Pharmacy Director .... Ann Kozal
Director of Operations/Marketing Director .... Pam Silva
IS Manager .... William Jones
Public Relations Manager .... Kristen Cichon
Contract & Vendor Relations Manager .... Steve Hekman
Human Resources Manager .... Jan Jones
Quality Assurance Manager .... Barbara Luskin
Managed Care Director/Compliance Officer .... Janet Lederman

COMPANY PROFILE:
Parent Company Name:
Doing Business As:
Year Founded: 1982   Federally Qualified: [N]
Forprofit: [Y]   Not-For-Profit: [ ]
Model Type: STAFF
Accreditation: [ ] AAPPO [ ] JACHO [X] NCQA [ ] URAC
Plan Type: HMO
Total Revenue: 2005:   45,531,744   2006:   39,390,085
Net Income   2005:   -439,045   2006:   407,302
Total Enrollment:
  2001: 20,503   2004: 17,946   2007: 9,689
  2002: 19,561   2005: 15,546
  2003: 18,874   2006: 11,566
Medical Loss Ratio: 2005: 93.70   2006: 88.70
Administrative Expense Ratio: 2005:   2006:

SERVICE AREA:
Nationwide: N
  MI; (Allegan, Kent, Ottawa);

TYPE OF COVERAGE:
Commercial: [Y] Individual: [Y] FEHBP: [ ] Indemnity: [ ]
Medicare: [ ] Medicaid: [ ] Supplemental Medicare: [Y]
Tricare   [ ]

PRODUCTS OFFERED:
Product Name:	Type:
Grand Valley Health Plan	HMO
Grand Valley Health Plan	POS

PLAN BENEFITS:
Alternative Medicine:	[X]	Behavioral Health:	[X]
Chiropractic:	[X]	Dental:	[X]
Home Care:	[X]	Inpatient SNF:	[X]
Long-Term Care:	[ ]	Pharm. Mail Order:	[X]
Physical Therapy:	[X]	Podiatry:	[X]
Psychiatric:	[X]	Transplant:	[X]
Vision:	[X]	Wellness:	[X]
Workers' Comp:	[ ]		

Other Benefits:

GREAT EXPRESSIONS DENTAL CENTERS

300 E Long Lake Rd Ste 311
Bloomfield Hills, MI 48304
Phone: 248-203-1100 Fax: 248-594-6587 Toll-Free: 888-764-5380
Web site: www.greatexpressions.com

MAILING ADDRESS:
  GREAT EXPRESSIONS DENTAL CENTERS
  300 E Long Lake Rd Ste 311
  Bloomfield Hills, MI 48304

KEY EXECUTIVES:
Chairman of the Board .... Walter Kynsz, Jr, MD
Chief Executive Officer .... Richard Beckman
Chief Financial Officer .... Guy Flannery, CPA
Chief Dental Director .... James Sarcheck, DDS
MIS Director .... Don Kulka
Provider Relations Director .... Megan Bildstein
Human Resource Director .... Vicki Gorlitz
Executive Vice President .... Janet Kynsz, MD

COMPANY PROFILE:
Parent Company Name:
Doing Business As:
Year Founded: 1981   Federally Qualified: [ ]
Forprofit: [ ]   Not-For-Profit: [ ]
Model Type: GROUP
Accreditation: [ ] AAPPO [ ] JACHO [ ] NCQA [ ] URAC
Plan Type: Specialty HMO, Specialty PPO

SERVICE AREA:
Nationwide: N
  MI;

PLAN BENEFITS:
Alternative Medicine:	[ ]	Behavioral Health:	[ ]
Chiropractic:	[ ]	Dental:	[X]
Home Care:	[ ]	Inpatient SNF:	[ ]
Long-Term Care:	[ ]	Pharm. Mail Order:	[ ]
Physical Therapy:	[ ]	Podiatry:	[ ]
Psychiatric:	[ ]	Transplant:	[ ]
Vision:	[ ]	Wellness:	[ ]
Workers' Comp:	[ ]		

Other Benefits:

GREAT LAKES HEALTH PLAN

17117 W Nine Mile Rd Ste 1600
Southfield, MI 48075-2127
Phone: 248-559-5656 Fax: 248-559-4640 Toll-Free: 800-903-5253
Web site: www.glhp.com

MAILING ADDRESS:
  GREAT LAKES HEALTH PLAN
  17117 W Nine Mile Rd Ste 1600
  Southfield, MI 48075-2127

KEY EXECUTIVES:
President .... Chris A Scherer
Director, Financial Operations .... Scott Schumann
VP, Medical Director .... Steven Stein, MD
Chief Information Officer .... Steve Washburn
General Counsel .... Eric Wexler
VP, Government & Public Relations .... Dawn Koehler
VP, Customer Operations .... Lisa Gray
Manager Contracting .... Shelley Turcu
VP Health Services .... Rachel Godwin
Manager Quality Improvement .... Mary Ellen Gies

COMPANY PROFILE:
Parent Company Name: AmeriChoice
Doing Business As: Great Lakes Health Plan
Year Founded: 1994   Federally Qualified: [N]
Forprofit: [Y]   Not-For-Profit: [ ]
Model Type: IPA
Accreditation: [ ] AAPPO [X] JACHO [ ] NCQA [ ] URAC
Plan Type: HMO
Primary Physicians: 726   Physician Specialists: 3,000
Hospitals: 52
Total Revenue: 2005:   235,741,232   2006:   261,943,980
Net Income   2005:   5,777,080   2006:   1,391,290
Total Enrollment:
  2001: 82,404   2004: 107,564   2007: 157,987
  2002: 92,553   2005: 108,034
  2003: 96,299   2006: 142,619
Medical Loss Ratio: 2005: 79.10   2006: 82.30
Administrative Expense Ratio: 2005:   2006:

SERVICE AREA:
Nationwide: N
  MI (Branch, Berrien, Calhoun, Cass, Hillsdale, Huron, Jackson, Kalamazoo, Lenawee, Livingston, Macomb, Oakland, Saginaw, Sanilac, St Clair, St Joseph, Tuscola, Van Buren, Wayne);

TYPE OF COVERAGE:
Commercial: [ ] Individual: [ ] FEHBP: [ ] Indemnity: [ ]
Medicare: [ ] Medicaid: [Y] Supplemental Medicare: [ ]
Tricare   [ ]

PRODUCTS OFFERED:
Product Name:	Type:
Great Lakes Health Plan	Medicaid
MIChild	HMO

PLAN BENEFITS:
Alternative Medicine:	[ ]	Behavioral Health:	[ ]
Chiropractic:	[X]	Dental:	[ ]
Home Care:	[X]	Inpatient SNF:	[X]
Long-Term Care:	[ ]	Pharm. Mail Order:	[ ]
Physical Therapy:	[X]	Podiatry:	[ ]
Psychiatric:	[ ]	Transplant:	[X]
Vision:	[X]	Wellness:	[X]
Workers' Comp:	[ ]		

Other Benefits:

Comments:
Acquired Thumb Area Health Plan in June 1999. Acquired Physicians Health Plan of Southwest Michigan September 1, 2006.

Managed Care Organization Profiles MICHIGAN

Total Enrollment:
2001: 0   2004: 10,313   2007: 0
2002: 17,052   2005:
2003: 14,501   2006:
SERVICE AREA:
Nationwide: N
  MI;
TYPE OF COVERAGE:
Commercial: [Y] Individual: [Y] FEHBP: [ ] Indemnity: [ ]
Medicare: [ ] Medicaid: [ ] Supplemental Medicare: [ ]
Tricare   [ ]
PRODUCTS OFFERED:
Product Name: Type:
Dencap Dental   HMO
PLAN BENEFITS:
Alternative Medicine: [ ]   Behavioral Health: [ ]
Chiropractic: [ ]   Dental: [X]
Home Care: [ ]   Inpatient SNF: [ ]
Long-Term Care: [ ]   Pharm. Mail Order: [ ]
Physical Therapy: [ ]   Podiatry: [ ]
Psychiatric: [ ]   Transplant: [ ]
Vision: [ ]   Wellness: [ ]
Workers' Comp: [ ]
Other Benefits:

DMC CARE

PO Box 44290
Detroit, MI 48244
Phone: 800-543-0161 Fax: Toll-Free:
Web site: www.dmc-care.org
MAILING ADDRESS:
  DMC CARE
  PO Box 44290
  Detroit, MI 48244

KEY EXECUTIVES:
Chief Executive Officer/President DMC .... Michael Duggan

COMPANY PROFILE:
Parent Company Name: Detroit Medical Center
Doing Business As:
Year Founded: Federally Qualified: [ ]
Forprofit: [ ]   Not-For-Profit: [ ]
Model Type:
Accreditation: [ ] AAPPO [ ] JACHO [ ] NCQA [ ] URAC
Plan Type: PPO
SERVICE AREA:
Nationwide:
  MI;
TYPE OF COVERAGE:
Commercial: [ ] Individual: [ ] FEHBP: [ ] Indemnity: [ ]
Medicare: [ ] Medicaid: [ ] Supplemental Medicare: [ ]
Tricare   [ ]

FIDELIS SECURECARE OF MICHIGAN INC

38777 W Six Mile Rd Ste 207
Livonia, MI 48152
Phone: 734-779-1680 Fax: 734-779-1681 Toll-Free: 800-931-7211
Web site: www.fidelissc.com
MAILING ADDRESS:
  FIDELIS SECURECARE OF MI INC
  38777 W Six Mile Rd Ste 207
  Livonia, MI 48152

KEY EXECUTIVES:
Chief Executive Officer .... Samuel R Willcoxon
President - Michigan .... Catherine Kiley, DO, CMD
Director of Operations .... Jodi Siegel, RN

COMPANY PROFILE:
Parent Company Name: Fidelis SeniorCare Inc
Doing Business As:
Year Founded: 2004   Federally Qualified: [Y]
Forprofit: [ ]   Not-For-Profit: [ ]
Model Type:
Accreditation: [ ] AAPPO [ ] JACHO [ ] NCQA [ ] URAC
Plan Type: HMO
Total Revenue: 2005:   814,647   2006:   8,756,847
Net Income   2005:   2006:   57,551
Total Enrollment:
2001: 0   2004: 0   2007: 891
2002: 0   2005: 192
2003: 0   2006: 672
Medical Loss Ratio: 2005: 91.70   2006: 97.30
Administrative Expense Ratio: 2005:   2006:
SERVICE AREA:
Nationwide:
  MI;
TYPE OF COVERAGE:
Commercial: [ ] Individual: [ ] FEHBP: [ ] Indemnity: [ ]
Medicare: [Y] Medicaid: [ ] Supplemental Medicare: [ ]
Tricare   [ ]

GOLDEN DENTAL PLANS INC

29377 Hoover Rd
Warren, MI 48093-3475
Phone: 800-451-5918 Fax: 586-573-8720 Toll-Free: 800-451-5918
Web site: www.goldendentalplans.com
MAILING ADDRESS:
  GOLDEN DENTAL PLANS INC
  29377 Hoover Rd
  Warren, MI 48093-3475

KEY EXECUTIVES:
Chairman of the Board .... Sam Lentine
Chief Executive Officer .... Joseph S Lentine
Vice President .... Anthony Lentine
Dental Director .... John Valenti, DDS
Marketing Director .... Gary Bingaman
Professional Relations Manager .... Suzanne Dinkel

COMPANY PROFILE:
Parent Company Name: Golden Dental Plans of America
Doing Business As:
Year Founded: 1983   Federally Qualified: [ ]
Forprofit: [Y]   Not-For-Profit: [ ]
Model Type:
Accreditation: [ ] AAPPO [ ] JACHO [ ] NCQA [ ] URAC
Plan Type: Specialty HMO
Total Enrollment:
2001: 0   2004: 0   2007: 0
2002: 49,173   2005:
2003: 47,785   2006:
SERVICE AREA:
Nationwide: N
  DC; IL; KY; MD; MI;
TYPE OF COVERAGE:
Commercial: [Y] Individual: [Y] FEHBP: [ ] Indemnity: [ ]
Medicare: [ ] Medicaid: [ ] Supplemental Medicare: [ ]
Tricare   [ ]
PLAN BENEFITS:
Alternative Medicine: [ ]   Behavioral Health: [ ]
Chiropractic: [ ]   Dental: [X]
Home Care: [ ]   Inpatient SNF: [ ]
Long-Term Care: [ ]   Pharm. Mail Order: [ ]
Physical Therapy: [ ]   Podiatry: [ ]
Psychiatric: [ ]   Transplant: [ ]
Vision: [ ]   Wellness: [ ]
Workers' Comp: [ ]
Other Benefits:

GRAND VALLEY HEALTH PLAN

829 Forest Hills Ave SE
Grand Rapids, MI 49546-3697
Phone: 616-949-2410 Fax: 616-949-4978 Toll-Free:
Web site: www.gvhpchoosewell.com
MAILING ADDRESS:
  GRAND VALLEY HEALTH PLAN
  829 Forest Hills Ave SE
  Grand Rapids, MI 49546-3697

MICHIGAN

Total Enrollment:
2001: 0	2004: 36,738	2007: 43,347
2002: 39,980	2005: 39,876	
2003: 36,158	2006: 44,588	

SERVICE AREA:
Nationwide: N
MI;

TYPE OF COVERAGE:
Commercial: [Y] Individual: [ ] FEHBP: [ ] Indemnity: [Y]
Medicare: [Y] Medicaid: [ ] Supplemental Medicare: [ ]
Tricare   [ ]

PRODUCTS OFFERED:
Product Name:	Type:
ConnectCare PPO	PPO
ConnectCare Traditional	Indemnity
ConnectiCare Medicare	Medicare
Connecticare Contracting	

PLAN BENEFITS:
Alternative Medicine:	[ ]	Behavioral Health:	[X]
Chiropractic:	[X]	Dental:	[ ]
Home Care:	[ ]	Inpatient SNF:	[X]
Long-Term Care:	[ ]	Pharm. Mail Order:	[ ]
Physical Therapy:	[X]	Podiatry:	[ ]
Psychiatric:	[X]	Transplant:	[X]
Vision:	[ ]	Wellness:	[X]
Workers' Comp:	[ ]		
Other Benefits:			

DAVITA VILLAGEHEALTH OF MICHIGAN INC

7960 W Grand River Rd Ste 200
Brighton, MI 48114
Phone: 810-225-2304 Fax: 866-660-9726 Toll-Free:
Web site: www.davita.com

MAILING ADDRESS:
DAVITA VILLAGEHEALTH OF MI INC
945 Lakeview Pkwy Ste 110
Vernon Hills, IL 48114

KEY EXECUTIVES:
President .... Andrew Hayek
Treasurer .... Jess Parks
Chief Medical Officer .... Allen Nissenson, MD, FACP

COMPANY PROFILE:
Parent Company Name: DaVita Corporation
Doing Business As:
Year Founded: 2007   Federally Qualified: [N]
Forprofit: [ ]   Not-For-Profit: [ ]
Model Type:
Accreditation: [ ] AAPPO [ ] JACHO [ ] NCQA [ ] URAC
Plan Type: HMO
Total Revenue   2005:   2006:
Net Income   2005:   2006: 33,987

SERVICE AREA:
Nationwide:
MI;

TYPE OF COVERAGE:
Commercial: [ ] Individual: [ ] FEHBP: [ ] Indemnity: [ ]
Medicare: [ ] Medicaid: [ ] Supplemental Medicare: [Y]
Tricare   [ ]

PLAN BENEFITS:
Alternative Medicine:	[ ]	Behavioral Health:	[ ]
Chiropractic:	[ ]	Dental:	[ ]
Home Care:	[ ]	Inpatient SNF:	[ ]
Long-Term Care:	[ ]	Pharm. Mail Order:	[ ]
Physical Therapy:	[ ]	Podiatry:	[ ]
Psychiatric:	[ ]	Transplant:	[ ]
Vision:	[ ]	Wellness:	[ ]
Workers' Comp:	[ ]		
Other Benefits:			

DELTA DENTAL PLAN OF MICHIGAN INC

4100 Okemos Rd
Okemos, MI 48864
Phone: 517-349-6000 Fax: 517-347-5237 Toll-Free: 800-524-0149
Web site: www.ddpmi.com

MAILING ADDRESS:
DELTA DENTAL PLAN OF MI
PO Box 30146
Lansing, MI 48864

KEY EXECUTIVES:
Chairperson .... Robert A Anthony, DDS
Chief Executive Officer/President .... Thomas J Fleszar, DDS, MS
Chief Financial Officer .... Laura L Czelada, CPA
VP Prof Srvcs & Dental Director .... Jed J Jacobson, DDS, MPH
Vice President Operations .... Sherry L Crisp
Director, Marketing/VP of Sales .... Charles E Floyd
Director of Information Systems .... Brend Laird
VP New Business Development .... Lonell D Rice
VP Labor Market Relations .... Rick Karas
Vice President Actuary .... William T Billard
Executive Vice President .... Judge Patrick T Cahill
VP Corporate & Public Affairs .... Nancy E Hostetler

COMPANY PROFILE:
Parent Company Name:
Doing Business As:
Year Founded: 1968   Federally Qualified: [N]
Forprofit: [ ]   Not-For-Profit: [Y]
Model Type: NETWORK
Accreditation: [ ] AAPPO [ ] JACHO [ ] NCQA [ ] URAC
Plan Type: Specialty HMO, Specialty PPO, POS
Total Enrollment:
2001: 4,600,000	2004: 1,107,297	2007: 0
2002: 993,111	2005:	
2003: 1,133,715	2006:	

SERVICE AREA:
Nationwide: N
IN; OH; MI;

TYPE OF COVERAGE:
Commercial: [Y] Individual: [ ] FEHBP: [ ] Indemnity: [ ]
Medicare: [ ] Medicaid: [ ] Supplemental Medicare: [ ]
Tricare   [ ]

PRODUCTS OFFERED:
Product Name:	Type:
Delta Premier	Managed Fee for Serv
Delta Preferred Option Standar	PPO
Delta Preferred Option Point of Service	PPO
DeltaCare	HMO

PLAN BENEFITS:
Alternative Medicine:	[ ]	Behavioral Health:	[ ]
Chiropractic:	[ ]	Dental:	[X]
Home Care:	[ ]	Inpatient SNF:	[ ]
Long-Term Care:	[ ]	Pharm. Mail Order:	[ ]
Physical Therapy:	[ ]	Podiatry:	[ ]
Psychiatric:	[ ]	Transplant:	[ ]
Vision:	[ ]	Wellness:	[ ]
Workers' Comp:	[ ]		
Other Benefits:			

DENCAP DENTAL PLANS

45 East Milwaukee Ave
Detroit, MI 48202
Phone: 313-972-1400 Fax: 313-972-4662 Toll-Free: 800-875-2400
Web site: www.dencap.com

MAILING ADDRESS:
DENCAP DENTAL PLANS
45 East Milwaukee Ave
Detroit, MI 48202

KEY EXECUTIVES:
Chief Executive Officer/President .... Joseph T Lentine
Dental Director .... James Feldman, DDS
Marketing Director .... Roger Roberts

COMPANY PROFILE:
Parent Company Name: Dencap Dental Plans
Doing Business As:
Year Founded: 1984   Federally Qualified: [N]
Forprofit: [Y]   Not-For-Profit: [ ]
Model Type: IPA
Accreditation: [ ] AAPPO [ ] JACHO [ ] NCQA [ ] URAC
Plan Type: Specialty HMO,

Managed Care Organization Profiles — MICHIGAN

PRODUCTS OFFERED:
Product Name:	Type:
Care Choices HMO	Commercial HMO
Care Choices Senior	Medicare Advantage
Preferred Choices PPO	PPO
Care Choices PPO	

CONSUMER-DRIVEN PRODUCTS
	HSA Company
	HSA Product
	HSA Administrator
	Consumer-Driven Health Plan
Care Choices HMO	High Deductible Health Plan

PLAN BENEFITS:
Alternative Medicine:	[X]	Behavioral Health:	[X]
Chiropractic:	[X]	Dental:	[ ]
Home Care:	[ ]	Inpatient SNF:	[X]
Long-Term Care:	[ ]	Pharm. Mail Order:	[X]
Physical Therapy:	[X]	Podiatry:	[X]
Psychiatric:	[X]	Transplant:	[ ]
Vision:	[X]	Wellness:	[X]
Workers' Comp:	[ ]		
Other Benefits:			

CO/OP OPTICAL SERVICES INC

2424 E 8 Mile Rd
Detroit, MI 48234-1010
Phone: 313-366-5100 Fax: 313-366-2246 Toll-Free:
Web site: www.coopoptical.com

MAILING ADDRESS:
CO/OP OPTICAL SERVICES INC
2424 E 8 Mile Rd
Detroit, MI 48234-1010

KEY EXECUTIVES:
Chairman of the Board .... Ken Morris
Chief Executive Officer/President .... Jackee Smith
Marketing Director .... Ethelle King
Sales Director .... Dan Reedy
Executive Vice President .... Cynthia Mearnic
Executive Director Retail Operation .... Benjamin Edwards
Executive Director Manufacturing .... Charles Benson
Facilities Director .... Tom Dick

COMPANY PROFILE:
Parent Company Name:
Doing Business As: Co/op Optical
Year Founded: 1961   Federally Qualified: [Y]
Forprofit: [ ]   Not-For-Profit: [Y]
Model Type: Mixed
Accreditation: [ ] AAPPO [ ] JACHO [ ] NCQA [ ] URAC
Plan Type: Specialty HMO, PBM
Total Enrollment:
  2001: 218,000   2004: 0   2007: 0
  2002: 176,131   2005:
  2003: 250,000   2006: 250,000

SERVICE AREA:
Nationwide: N
  MI; OH;

TYPE OF COVERAGE:
Commercial: [Y] Individual: [ ] FEHBP: [ ] Indemnity: [ ]
Medicare: [ ] Medicaid: [ ] Supplemental Medicare: [ ]
Tricare   [ ]

PRODUCTS OFFERED:
Product Name:	Type:
CO/OP Optical Services Inc	HMO

PLAN BENEFITS:
Alternative Medicine:	[ ]	Behavioral Health:	[ ]
Chiropractic:	[ ]	Dental:	[ ]
Home Care:	[ ]	Inpatient SNF:	[ ]
Long-Term Care:	[ ]	Pharm. Mail Order:	[ ]
Physical Therapy:	[ ]	Podiatry:	[ ]
Psychiatric:	[ ]	Transplant:	[ ]
Vision:	[X]	Wellness:	[ ]
Workers' Comp:	[ ]		
Other Benefits:			

COMMUNITY CHOICE MICHIGAN

2369 Woodlake Dr Ste 200
Okemos, MI 48864
Phone: 517-349-9922 Fax: 517-349-5343 Toll-Free: 800-390-7102
Web site: www.ccmhmo.org

MAILING ADDRESS:
COMMUNITY CHOICE MICHIGAN
2369 Woodlake Dr Ste 200
Okemos, MI 48864

KEY EXECUTIVES:
Chief Executive Officer .... Karl Kovacs
President .... Christine Baumgardner
Chief Financial Officer .... Roger Blackwell
Medical Director .... Paul M Daker, MD
Director of Operations .... Mary Anne Sesti
Network Administration .... Aaron Atkinson
Director of Medical Services .... Terrie Boggus

COMPANY PROFILE:
Parent Company Name: Caresource Management Group
Doing Business As:
Year Founded: 1996   Federally Qualified: [N]
Forprofit: [ ]   Not-For-Profit: [Y]
Model Type:
Accreditation: [ ] AAPPO [X] JACHO [ ] NCQA [ ] URAC
Plan Type: HMO
Primary Physicians: 428   Physician Specialists: 2,241
Hospitals: 49
Total Revenue: 2005:   95,697,827   2006:   97,391,392
Net Income   2005:   6,884,721   2006:   3,591,702
Total Enrollment:
  2001: 74,999   2004: 49,047   2007: 48,490
  2002: 67,926   2005: 46,995
  2003: 56,312   2006: 49,163
Medical Loss Ratio: 2005: 77.70   2006: 80.30
Administrative Expense Ratio: 2005:   2006:

SERVICE AREA:
Nationwide: N
  MI;

TYPE OF COVERAGE:
Commercial: [Y] Individual: [ ] FEHBP: [ ] Indemnity: [ ]
Medicare: [ ] Medicaid: [ ] Supplemental Medicare: [ ]
Tricare   [ ]

PRODUCTS OFFERED:
Product Name:	Type:
Community Choice	Medicaid
MIChild	HMO

CONNECTCARE

4009 Orchard Dr Ste 3021
Midland, MI 48640
Phone: 989-839-1600 Fax: 989-839-1626 Toll-Free: 888-646-2429
Web site: www.connectcare.com

MAILING ADDRESS:
CONNECTCARE
4009 Orchard Dr Ste 3021
Midland, MI 48640

KEY EXECUTIVES:
Chief Executive Officer/President .... Brian Rodgers
Chief Financial Officer .... Victor Morgan
Medical Director .... Dan Sorenson, MD
Director of Operations .... Janis Bond, RN, CMCN
Director of Marketing .... Gary LeForge
Privacy Officer .... Joyce Cook, RN, CHCM, CLNC
Dir, Provider Services/Medical Management .. Janis Bond, RN, CMCN

COMPANY PROFILE:
Parent Company Name: MidMichigan Health Network
Doing Business As: ConnectCare
Year Founded: 1993   Federally Qualified: [ ]
Forprofit: [ ]   Not-For-Profit: [Y]
Model Type: NETWORK
Accreditation: [ ] AAPPO [ ] JACHO [ ] NCQA [ ] URAC
Plan Type: PPO, POS, UR
Primary Physicians: 109   Physician Specialists: 269
Hospitals: 27

MICHIGAN

PRODUCTS OFFERED:
Product Name:	Type:
Blue Care Network	HMO
Medicare Blue	Medicare
	Medicare Supplement
	FEHBP

CONSUMER-DRIVEN PRODUCTS
Blue HSAsm	HSA Company
	HSA Product
	HSA Administrator
	Consumer-Driven Health Plan
Healthy Blue PPOs	High Deductible Health Plan

PLAN BENEFITS:
Alternative Medicine: [ ]   Behavioral Health: [ ]
Chiropractic: [ ]   Dental: [ ]
Home Care: [ ]   Inpatient SNF: [ ]
Long-Term Care: [ ]   Pharm. Mail Order: [X]
Physical Therapy: [ ]   Podiatry: [ ]
Psychiatric: [X]   Transplant: [ ]
Vision: [ ]   Wellness: [X]
Workers' Comp: [ ]
Other Benefits: Substance Abuse

Comments:
On February 1, 1998, the Michigan Insurance Bureau approved the merger of four separate BCN HMO's into a single HMO-Blue Care Network of Michigan.

BLUE PREFERRED PLAN-BLUE CROSS/BLUE SHIELD MICHIGAN

600 E Lafayette Blvd
Detroit, MI 48226-2927
Phone: 313-225-9000 Fax: 313-225-5629 Toll-Free:
Web site: www.bcbsmi.com

MAILING ADDRESS:
BLUE PREFERRED PLAN-BC/BS MI
600 E Lafayette Blvd
Detroit, MI 48226-2927

KEY EXECUTIVES:
Chairman of the Board .... Gregory Sudderth
Chief Executive Officer/President .... Daniel J Loepp
Chief Financial Officer .... Mark R Bartlett
Medical Director .... Thomas L Simmer, MD
Executive VP, Operations/Chief Information Officer ... William P Smith
Group Sales & Corporate Marketing .... Kenneth R Dallafior
Senior VP, Human Resources .... Darrell E Middleton

COMPANY PROFILE:
Parent Company Name: Blue Cross Blue Shield of Michigan
Doing Business As:
Year Founded: 1983   Federally Qualified: [ ]
Forprofit: [ ]   Not-For-Profit: [Y]
Model Type: IPA
Accreditation: [ ] AAPPO [ ] JACHO [ ] NCQA [ ]
URACPlan Type: PPO, HSA
Total Enrollment:
2001: 0   2004: 0   2007: 0
2002: 0   2005:
2003: 4,800,000   2006: 4,700,000

SERVICE AREA:
Nationwide: N
MI Ctys-(Alger, Allegan, Alpena, Antrim, Arenac, Baraga, BArry, Bay, Benzie, Berrien, Branch, Calhoun, Cass, Charlevoux, Cheboygan, Chippwea, Clare, Clinton, Crawford, Delta, Dickinson, Eaton, Emmet, Genesee, Gladwin, Gogebic, Grand Traverse, Gratiot, Hillsdale, Houghton, Huron, Ingham, Ionia, Iosco, Iron, Isabella, Jackson, Kalamazoo, Kalkaska, Kent, Lake, Lapeer, Leelanau, Lenawee, Livingston, Luce, Mackinac, Missaukee, Macomb, Manistee, Marquette, Mason, Mecosta, Midland, Menominee, Monroe, Montcalm, Montgomery, Muskegon, Newaygo, Oakland, Oceana, Ogemaw, Ontonagon, Osceola, Oscoda, Otsego, Ottawa, Presque, Isle, Roscommon, Saginaw, St Clair, Saint Joseph, Sanilac, Shiawassee, Tuscola, Van Buren, Washtenaw, Wayne, Wexford. Cities- (Detroit, Flint, Saginaw, Lansing, Grand Rapids, Battle Creek, Muskegon, Traverse City, Alpena, Hastings, Oscoda) Metro Area- SE MI. (Metro Detroit Area) Grand Rapids, Tri-cities, Flint, Saginaw area, Traverse City.

TYPE OF COVERAGE:
Commercial: [Y]   Individual: [Y]   FEHBP: [ ]   Indemnity: [ ]
Medicare: [ ]   Medicaid: [ ]   Supplemental Medicare: [ ]
Tricare [ ]

PRODUCTS OFFERED:
Product Name:	Type:
Blue Preferred	PPO
Community Blue	PPO

CONSUMER-DRIVEN PRODUCTS
Blue HSAsm	HSA Company
	HSA Product
	HSA Administrator
	Consumer-Driven Health Plan
HealthyBlue PPOs	High Deductible Health Plan

PLAN BENEFITS:
Alternative Medicine: [ ]   Behavioral Health: [X]
Chiropractic: [X]   Dental: [ ]
Home Care: [X]   Inpatient SNF: [X]
Long-Term Care: [ ]   Pharm. Mail Order: [ ]
Physical Therapy: [X]   Podiatry: [X]
Psychiatric: [X]   Transplant: [X]
Vision: [ ]   Wellness: [X]
Workers' Comp: [ ]
Other Benefits: Preventive Care

CARE CHOICES

34605 Twelve Mile Rd
Farmington Hills, MI 48331
Phone: 248-489-6203 Fax: 248-489-6280 Toll-Free: 800-852-9780
Web site: www.carechoices.com

MAILING ADDRESS:
CARE CHOICES
34605 Twelve Mile Road
Farmington Hills, MI 48331

KEY EXECUTIVES:
Chief Executive Officer/President .... William R Alvin
Chief Finacial Officer .... Michael R Koziara
Chief Medical Officer .... Gilbert Burgos, MD
Director, Pharmacy Programs .... Steven Marciniak
Director Managed Care Information Services .... Tammy Rupp
Chief Administrative Officer .... Laurie Westfall
Chief Marketing Officer .... Jelka Petrovic
Director, Communications, Public Affairs, Training .... Ellen Downey
Director of Provider Relations .... Deborah Spencer
Director, Provider Network Contract .... Carol Mroue
Director Health & Life Styles .... Alice Easterling
Human Resource Manager .... Jene Allen
Director of Care Management .... Rachel Godwin
Director Quality Development & Clinical Information .... Ed Tuller
Director of Product Development .... Graham Smith

COMPANY PROFILE:
Parent Company Name: Trinity Health Plans
Doing Business As: Care Choices HMO, PPO, Prfrd Choice PPO
Year Founded: 1986   Federally Qualified: [Y]
Forprofit: [ ]   Not-For-Profit: [Y]
Model Type: IPA
Accreditation: [ ] AAPPO [ ] JACHO [X] NCQA [ ] URAC
Plan Type: HMO, PPO, HDHP
Primary Physicians: 11,700   Physician Specialists:
Hospitals: 83
Total Revenue: 2005: 296,014,942   2006: 305,312,846
Net Income   2005: 6,297,436   2006: 1,862,657
Total Enrollment:
2001: 193,341   2004: 146,000   2007: 87,361
2002: 120,679   2005: 144,170
2003: 150,631   2006: 91,888
Medical Loss Ratio: 2005: 89.00   2006: 91.00
Administrative Expense Ratio: 2005:   2006:

SERVICE AREA:
Nationwide: N
MI (Allegan, Barry, Calhoun, Clinton, Crawford, Eaton, Genesee, Grand Traverse, Huron, Ionia, Ingham, Jackson, Kalamazoo, Kent, Livingston, Maconb, Monroe, Monroe, Montcalm, Muskegon, Newaygo, Oakland, Oceana, Ottawa, Sanilac, Shiawassee, St Clair, Washtenaw, Wayne, Wexford).

TYPE OF COVERAGE:
Commercial: [Y]   Individual: [ ]   FEHBP: [ ]   Indemnity: [ ]
Medicare: [ ]   Medicaid: [ ]   Supplemental Medicare: [ ]
Tricare [ ]

Managed Care Organization Profiles — **MICHIGAN**

AETNA INC - MICHIGAN

26933 Northwestern Hwy Ste 100
Southfield, MI 48034
Phone: 248-208-8600 Fax: 248-208-8633 Toll-Free:
Web site: www.aetna.com

MAILING ADDRESS:
AETNA INC - MI
26933 Northwestern Hwy Ste 100
Southfield, MI 48034

KEY EXECUTIVES:
Chairman of the Board/Chief Executive Officer .... Ronald A Williams
President .... Mark T Bertolini
Executive VP, Finance .... Joseph M Zubretsky

COMPANY PROFILE:
Parent Company Name: Aetna Inc
Doing Business As:
Year Founded: 1998   Federally Qualified: [N]
Forprofit: [Y]   Not-For-Profit: [ ]
Model Type:
Accreditation: [ ] AAPPO [ ] JACHO [ ] NCQA [ ] URAC
Plan Type: HMO, POS, EPO, PRO, CDHP, HSA
Total Revenue: 2005:   7,844,661   2006:   6,135,417
Net Income   2005:   320,070   2006:   340,325
Total Enrollment:
    2001: 21,964   2004: 2,941   2007: 939
    2002: 8,166   2005: 2,313
    2003: 4,062   2006: 1,710
Medical Loss Ratio: 2005: 86.50   2006: 77.00
Administrative Expense Ratio: 2005:   2006:

SERVICE AREA:
Nationwide: N
    MI (Lower two-thirds of the lower peninsula);

TYPE OF COVERAGE:
Commercial: [Y] Individual: [ ] FEHBP: [ ] Indemnity: [ ]
Medicare: [ ] Medicaid: [ ] Supplemental Medicare: [ ]
Tricare   [ ]

PRODUCTS OFFERED:
Product Name: Type:
Aetna HMO   HMO
Aetna POS   POS

CONSUMER-DRIVEN PRODUCTS
Aetna Life Insurance Co   HSA Company
Aetna HealthFund HSA   HSA Product
Aetna   HSA Administrator
Aetna HealthFund   Consumer-Driven Health Plan
PPO I; PPO II   High Deductible Health Plan

PLAN BENEFITS:
Alternative Medicine: [ ]   Behavioral Health: [ ]
Chiropractic: [X]   Dental: [X]
Home Care: [X]   Inpatient SNF: [X]
Long-Term Care: [X]   Pharm. Mail Order: [X]
Physical Therapy: [X]   Podiatry: [X]
Psychiatric: [X]   Transplant: [X]
Vision: [X]   Wellness: [X]
Workers' Comp: [X]
Other Benefits:

ASSURANT EMPLOYEE BENEFITS - MICHIGAN

3001 W Big Beaver Rd Ste 330
Troy, MI 48084
Phone: 248-649-4410 Fax: 248-649-1210 Toll-Free: 800-488-0410
Web site: www.assurantemployeebenefits.com

MAILING ADDRESS:
ASSURANT EMPLOYEE BNFTS - MI
3001 W Big Beaver Rd Ste 330
Troy, MI 48084

KEY EXECUTIVES:
Interim Chief Executive Officer/Interim President .... John S Roberts
Chief Financial Officer .... Floyd F Chadee
VP, Medical Director .... Polly M Galbraith, MD
Chief Information Officer .... Karla J Schacht
Senior VP, Marketing .... Mark J Bohen
Privacy Officer .... Carol Deadrick
VP of Provider Services .... James A Barrett, DMD
Senior VP, Human Resources & Development .... Sylvia R Wagner
2nd VP, Voluntary Segment Market .... Joseph A Sevcik
National Dental Director .... James A Barrett, DMD

COMPANY PROFILE:
Parent Company Name: Assurant Health
Doing Business As:
Year Founded: 1957   Federally Qualified: [ ]
Forprofit: [Y]   Not-For-Profit: [ ]
Model Type:
Accreditation: [ ] AAPPO [ ] JACHO [ ] NCQA [ ] URAC
Plan Type: PPO, ASO, Specialty HMO,

SERVICE AREA:
Nationwide: N
    MI;

TYPE OF COVERAGE:
Commercial: [Y] Individual: [Y] FEHBP: [ ] Indemnity: [ ]
Medicare: [ ] Medicaid: [ ] Supplemental Medicare: [ ]
Tricare   [ ]

PLAN BENEFITS:
Alternative Medicine: [ ]   Behavioral Health: [ ]
Chiropractic: [ ]   Dental: [X]
Home Care: [ ]   Inpatient SNF: [ ]
Long-Term Care: [ ]   Pharm. Mail Order: [ ]
Physical Therapy: [ ]   Podiatry: [ ]
Psychiatric: [ ]   Transplant: [ ]
Vision: [X]   Wellness: [ ]
Workers' Comp: [ ]
Other Benefits:
Comments:
Formerly Fortis Benefits Dental.

BLUE CARE NETWORK OF MICHIGAN

20500 Civic Center Dr
Southfield, MI 48086
Phone: 800-662-6667 Fax: 248-799-6979 Toll-Free: 800-662-2667
Web site: www.bcbsmi.com/bcn

MAILING ADDRESS:
BLUE CARE NTWRK OF MICHIGAN
20500 Civic Center Dr
Southfield, MI 48086

KEY EXECUTIVES:
Chairman of the Board .... Frank Garrison
Chief Executive Officer/President .... Jeanne H Carlson
Chief Financial Officer .... Susan A Kluge
Chief Medical Officer .... Douglas R Woll, MD
Pharmacy Director .... James Lang, PharmD
VP, Chief Information Officer .... Janet Maquiren
Chief Operating Officer .... Laurie Westfall
Provider Services Director .... Steve Goldberg
VP of Human Resources .... Sandra Boozer
Quality Management Director .... Pam Reinert RN
VP Customer Service/Business .... Gail Ross
VP of Quality Improvement .... Jamie Fleming RN
VP Health & Medical Affairs .... Carla Chambers

COMPANY PROFILE:
Parent Company Name: Blue Cross/Blue Shield of Michigan
Doing Business As:
Year Founded: 1998   Federally Qualified: [Y]
Forprofit: [ ]   Not-For-Profit: [Y]
Model Type: MIXED
Accreditation: [ ] AAPPO [ ] JACHO [X] NCQA [ ] URAC
Plan Type: HMO, HDHP, HSA
Primary Physicians: 3,100   Physician Specialists: 7,600
Hospitals: 110
Total Revenue: 2005:   1,439,429,414   2006:   1,567,047,772
Net Income   2005:   78,396,434   2006:   28,289,203
Total Enrollment:
    2001: 572,422   2004: 460,516   2007: 0
    2002: 518,946   2005: 452,163
    2003: 478,043   2006: 482,998
Medical Loss Ratio: 2005: 80.10   2006: 85.80
Administrative Expense Ratio: 2005:   2006:

SERVICE AREA:
Nationwide: N
    MI (East, West, Southeast and Mid Michigan);

TYPE OF COVERAGE:
Commercial: [Y] Individual: [ ] FEHBP: [ ] Indemnity: [ ]
Medicare: [Y] Medicaid: [Y] Supplemental Medicare: [ ]
Tricare   [ ]

MASSACHUSETTS

TUFTS HEALTH PLAN

705 Mt Auburn St
Watertown, MA 02471
Phone: 781-466-9400 Fax: 781-466-8504 Toll-Free:
Web site: www.tufts-health.com

MAILING ADDRESS:
TUFTS HEALTH PLAN
705 Mt Auburn St
Watertown, MA 02471

KEY EXECUTIVES:
Chairman .... Davey Scoon
Chief Executive Officer/President .... James Roosevelt, Jr
Chief Financial Officer .... J Andy Hilbert
Senior VP, Chief Medical Officer .... Allen J Hinkle, MD
Senior VP, Operations/Chief Information Officer .... Patricia Trebino
Chief Operating Officer .... Thomas A Croswell
Senior VP, Marketing & Product Development............. Robert D Egan
Senior VP, Sales & Client Services .... Brian P Pagliaro
Senior VP, Human Resources/Compliance Officer .. Lois Dehis Cornell
Senior VP, Planning & Development .... Jon M Kingsdale, PhD
Senior VP, General Counsel .... Lois Dehls Cornell

COMPANY PROFILE:
Parent Company Name: Tufts Associated Health Plans, Inc.
Doing Business As:
Year Founded: 1981   Federally Qualified: [Y]
Forprofit: [ ]   Not-For-Profit: [Y]
Model Type: IPA
Accreditation: [X] AAPPO [X] JACHO [X] NCQA [X] URAC
Plan Type: HMO, PPO, POS, EPO, HSA
Primary Physicians: 22,000   Physician Specialists:
Hospitals: 85
Total Revenue: 2005:   2006: 1,900,000,000
Net Income   2005:   2006:   78,000,000
Total Enrollment:
   2001: 624,406   2004: 698,000   2007: 654,116
   2002: 729,012   2005: 620,000
   2003: 585,436   2006: 606,000
Medical Loss Ratio: 2005: 86.60   2006:
Administrative Expense Ratio: 2005:   2006:

SERVICE AREA:
Nationwide: N
   MA; ME; NH;

TYPE OF COVERAGE:
Commercial: [Y] Individual: [Y] FEHBP: [ ] Indemnity: [ ]
Medicare: [Y] Medicaid: [Y] Supplemental Medicare: [Y]
Tricare   [ ]

PRODUCTS OFFERED:
Product Name: Type:
Secure Horizons Tufts Health Services Medicare Advantage
Tufts Seniors Product   Medicare
Tufts Associated Health Plans   Medicaid

PLAN BENEFITS:
Alternative Medicine: [ ]   Behavioral Health: [ ]
Chiropractic: [X]   Dental: [X]
Home Care: [X]   Inpatient SNF: [X]
Long-Term Care: [ ]   Pharm. Mail Order: [X]
Physical Therapy: [X]   Podiatry: [X]
Psychiatric: [X]   Transplant: [X]
Vision: [X]   Wellness: [X]
Workers' Comp: [ ]
Other Benefits:

UNITEDHEALTHCARE OF MASSACHUSETTS

281 Winter St Ste 301
Waltham, MA 02154
Phone: 781-768-2200 Fax: 781-768-2288 Toll-Free:
Web site: www.evercareonline.com

MAILING ADDRESS:
UNITEDHEALTHCARE OF MA
281 Winter St Ste 301
Waltham, MA 02154

KEY EXECUTIVES:
Executive Director .... John Mach

COMPANY PROFILE:
Parent Company Name: United Health Group
Doing Business As:
Year Founded: Federally Qualified: [ ]
Forprofit: [Y]   Not-For-Profit: [ ]
Model Type:
Accreditation: [ ] AAPPO [ ] JACHO [ ] NCQA [ ] URAC
Plan Type: HMO
Total Enrollment:
   2001: 4,464   2004: 5,831   2007: 2,312
   2002: 5,077   2005:   924
   2003: 5,759   2006: 1,411

SERVICE AREA:
Nationwide:
   MA (Barnstable, Bristol, Essex, Middlesex, Norfolk, Plymouth,
   Suffolk, Worcester); NH (Hillsborough, Rockingham);

TYPE OF COVERAGE:
Commercial: [ ] Individual: [ ] FEHBP: [ ] Indemnity: [ ]
Medicare: [Y] Medicaid: [ ] Supplemental Medicare: [ ]
Tricare   [ ]

Managed Care Organization Profiles — MASSACHUSETTS

Forprofit: [ ]   Not-For-Profit: [ ]
Model Type:
Accreditation: [ ] AAPPO [ ] JACHO [ ] NCQA [ ] URAC
Plan Type: PPO,
SERVICE AREA:
Nationwide: Y
  NW;
TYPE OF COVERAGE:
Commercial: [Y] Individual: [ ] FEHBP: [ ] Indemnity: [ ]
Medicare: [ ] Medicaid: [ ] Supplemental Medicare: [ ]
Tricare   [ ]
Comments:
Formerly New England, The.

PIONEER HEALTH - THE PPO

123 Interstate Dr
West Springfield, MA 01090
Phone: 413-539-9900 Fax: 413-265-2780 Toll-Free: 800-423-4586
Web site: www.pioneerhealth.com
MAILING ADDRESS:
  PIONEER HEALTH - THE PPO
  PO Box 9040
  West Springfield, MA 01090

KEY EXECUTIVES:
Chief Executive Officer/Finance Director .... Bruce E Suchy
Information Services Director .... Jed Provjansky
Marketing Director .... Bruce E Suchy
VP of Provider Relations .... Roland Malboeuf
Human Resources .... Marilyn Greenwood
VP Quality/Utilization Management .... Kay Monnihan
Chief Legal Counsel .... Lisa Crouser

COMPANY PROFILE:
Parent Company Name: Pioneer Management Systems Inc
Doing Business As:
Year Founded: 1983   Federally Qualified: [ ]
Forprofit: [Y]   Not-For-Profit: [ ]
Model Type: NETWORK
Accreditation: [ ] AAPPO [ ] JACHO [ ] NCQA [ ] URAC
Plan Type: PPO, EPO, PBM, FSA
SERVICE AREA:
Nationwide: N
  MA; CT; NC;
TYPE OF COVERAGE:
Commercial: [Y] Individual: [Y] FEHBP: [ ] Indemnity: [ ]
Medicare: [ ] Medicaid: [ ] Supplemental Medicare: [ ]
Tricare   [ ]
PLAN BENEFITS:
Alternative Medicine: [ ]   Behavioral Health: [ ]
Chiropractic: [X]   Dental: [X]
Home Care: [X]   Inpatient SNF: [X]
Long-Term Care: [X]   Pharm. Mail Order: [X]
Physical Therapy: [X]   Podiatry: [X]
Psychiatric: [X]   Transplant: [X]
Vision: [X]   Wellness: [X]
Workers' Comp: [X]
Other Benefits:

PREFERRED DENTAL NETWORK (PDN)

300 Congress St
Quincy, MA 02169
Phone: 888-225-0522 Fax: 617-471-6323 Toll-Free: 888-225-0522
Web site: www.medicalclaimsservice.com
MAILING ADDRESS:
  PREFERRED DENTAL NETWORK (PDN)
  300 Congress St
  Quincy, MA 02169

KEY EXECUTIVES:
Chief Executive Officer/Chief Financial Officer ..... William G McKelvey
Marketing Director .... Judith Reed

COMPANY PROFILE:
Parent Company Name: Medical Claims Service Inc
Doing Business As:
Year Founded: 1993   Federally Qualified: [N]
Forprofit: [Y]   Not-For-Profit: [ ]

Model Type:
Accreditation: [ ] AAPPO [ ] JACHO [ ] NCQA [ ] URAC
Plan Type: Specialty PPO, TPA
Total Enrollment:
  2001: 0   2004: 45,000   2007: 0
  2002: 0   2005:
  2003: 40,000   2006:
SERVICE AREA:
Nationwide: N
  MA;
TYPE OF COVERAGE:
Commercial: [Y] Individual: [ ] FEHBP: [ ] Indemnity: [ ]
Medicare: [ ] Medicaid: [ ] Supplemental Medicare: [ ]
Tricare   [ ]
PLAN BENEFITS:
Alternative Medicine: [ ]   Behavioral Health: [ ]
Chiropractic: [ ]   Dental: [X]
Home Care: [ ]   Inpatient SNF: [ ]
Long-Term Care: [ ]   Pharm. Mail Order: [ ]
Physical Therapy: [ ]   Podiatry: [ ]
Psychiatric: [ ]   Transplant: [ ]
Vision: [ ]   Wellness: [ ]
Workers' Comp: [ ]
Other Benefits:

PRIVATE HEALTHCARE SYSTEMS - CORPORATE HEADQUARTERS

1100 Winter St
Waltham, MA 02451
Phone: 781-895-7500 Fax: 781-895-3458 Toll-Free: 800-253-4417
Web site: www.phcs.com
MAILING ADDRESS:
  PRIVATE HEALTHCARE SYSTEMS
  1100 Winter St
  Waltham, MA 02451

KEY EXECUTIVES:
Chief Executive Officer .... Mark Tabak
Executive VP, Chief Financial Officer .... Richard Gerstein
Executive VP, Chief of Operations .... Michael Ferrante
Executive VP, Marketing .... Warren Handelman
Executive VP, Sales & Account Management .... Dale White
VP General Counsel .... Marcy Feller

COMPANY PROFILE:
Parent Company Name: MultiPlan Inc
Doing Business As:
Year Founded: 1985   Federally Qualified: [N]
Forprofit: [Y]   Not-For-Profit: [ ]
Model Type: MIXED
Accreditation: [ ] AAPPO [ ] JACHO [X] NCQA [X] URAC
Plan Type: PPO, POS, UR
Primary Physicians: 450,000   Physician Specialists: 270,288
Hospitals: 4,000
Total Enrollment:
  2001: 0   2004: 16,000,000   2007: 0
  2002: 6,500,000   2005:
  2003: 15,000,000   2006: 16,000,000
SERVICE AREA:
Nationwide: Y
  NW;
TYPE OF COVERAGE:
Commercial: [Y] Individual: [ ] FEHBP: [ ] Indemnity: [ ]
Medicare: [ ] Medicaid: [ ] Supplemental Medicare: [ ]
Tricare   [ ]
PRODUCTS OFFERED:
Product Name: Type:
Healthy Directions
National Advantage
Access Advantage
Open Access
PLAN BENEFITS:
Alternative Medicine: [X]   Behavioral Health: [X]
Chiropractic: [X]   Dental: [X]
Home Care: [X]   Inpatient SNF: [X]
Long-Term Care: [X]   Pharm. Mail Order: [X]
Physical Therapy: [X]   Podiatry: [X]
Psychiatric: [X]   Transplant: [X]
Vision: [X]   Wellness: [ ]
Workers' Comp: [X]
Other Benefits: X
Comments:
Acquired by MultiPlan, Inc. on October 18, 2006.

MASSACHUSETTS — Managed Care Organization Profiles

KEY EXECUTIVES:
Chairman .... Gregg S Meyer, MD, MSC
Chief Executive Officer/President .... Jeffrey East
VP/Chief Operating Officer .... Robert B Palardy, CPA
Senior VP, Chief Medical Officer .... Kenneth A LaBresh, MD, FAHA
VP, Strategy & Operations .... Laura N Moore, MPA
Director of Marketing .... Heidi R Sporel
Director of IS .... Brian M McCarthy
Director of Human Resources .... James P Fitzgerald
General Counsel, Chief Compliance .... Joseph E Mullaney III, Esq
Med Director Medicare + Priv Review .... William S Kaden, MD
Medical Director for Medicaid .... Barbara Chase MD
Corporate Communications Specialist .... Monique Cassidy, MA
Chief Technology Officer .... Charles Parker

COMPANY PROFILE:
Parent Company Name: Massachussetts Medical Society
Doing Business As:
Year Founded: 1986 Federally Qualified: [Y]
Forprofit: [ ] Not-For-Profit: [Y]
Model Type:
Accreditation: [ ] AAPPO [ ] JACHO [ ] NCQA [ ] URAC
Plan Type: PRO

SERVICE AREA:
Nationwide: N
  MA;

MIT HEALTH PLAN

77 Massachusetts Ave Bldg E23
Cambridge, MA 02139
Phone: 617-253-1322 Fax: 617-253-6558 Toll-Free:
Web site: web.mit.edu/medical

MAILING ADDRESS:
MIT HEALTH PLAN
77 Massachusetts Ave Bldg E23
Cambridge, MA 02139

KEY EXECUTIVES:
Chief Executive Officer .... Annette Jacobs
Chief Financial Officer .... Eileen O'Keefe
Medical Director .... William Kettyle, MD
Pharmacy Director .... Deborah Friscino

COMPANY PROFILE:
Parent Company Name: Massachussetts Institute of Technology
Doing Business As:
Year Founded: 1972 Federally Qualified: [N]
Forprofit: [ ] Not-For-Profit: [Y]
Model Type: STAFF
Accreditation: [ ] AAPPO [X] JACHO [ ] NCQA [ ] URAC
Plan Type: HMO

SERVICE AREA:
Nationwide: N
  MA;

TYPE OF COVERAGE:
Commercial: [ ] Individual: [Y] FEHBP: [ ] Indemnity: [ ]
Medicare: [Y] Medicaid: [ ] Supplemental Medicare: [ ]
Tricare [ ]

PLAN BENEFITS:
Alternative Medicine:	[ ]	Behavioral Health:	[ ]
Chiropractic:	[ ]	Dental:	[X]
Home Care:	[X]	Inpatient SNF:	[X]
Long-Term Care:	[ ]	Pharm. Mail Order:	[X]
Physical Therapy:	[X]	Podiatry:	[X]
Psychiatric:	[X]	Transplant:	[X]
Vision:	[X]	Wellness:	[X]
Workers' Comp:	[X]		

Other Benefits:

NEIGHBORHOOD HEALTH PLAN

253 Summer St
Boston, MA 02210
Phone: 617-772-5500 Fax: 617-478-7153 Toll-Free: 800-433-5556
Web site: www.nhp.org

MAILING ADDRESS:
NEIGHBORHOOD HEALTH PLAN
253 Summer St
Boston, MA 02210

KEY EXECUTIVES:
Chairman .... Robert J Ingala
Chief Executive Officer/President .... Deborah Enos
Chief Financial Officer .... Harold Putnam
Chief Medical Officer .... Paul Mendis, MD
Chief Information Officer .... Marilyn Daly
VP, Operations .... Joanne Landry
Marketing/Communications Director .... Sonia Javier-Obinger
VP of Provider Network Management .... Thankam Rangala
Human Resources Director .... Roberta Goldman-Wilkinson
VP, Quality & Compliance .... Pamela Siren

COMPANY PROFILE:
Parent Company Name:
Doing Business As: Neighborhood Health Plan
Year Founded: 1986 Federally Qualified: [Y]
Forprofit: [ ] Not-For-Profit: [Y]
Model Type: IPA
Accreditation: [ ] AAPPO [ ] JACHO [X] NCQA [ ] URAC
Plan Type: HMO
Primary Physicians: 10,436 Physician Specialists: 2,000
Hospitals: 50
Total Revenue: 2005: 2006: 526,669,731
Net Income 2005: 2006:
Total Enrollment:
  2001: 126,836 2004: 124,021 2007: 147,946
  2002: 112,718 2005: 130,102
  2003: 116,436 2006: 141,785
Medical Loss Ratio: 2005: 89.40 2006: 88.00
Administrative Expense Ratio: 2005: 2006:

SERVICE AREA:
Nationwide: N
  MA (Barnstable, Bristol, Essex, Franklin, Hampden, Hampshire, Middlesex, Norfolk, Plymouth Suffolk, Worcester);

TYPE OF COVERAGE:
Commercial: [Y] Individual: [ ] FEHBP: [ ] Indemnity: [ ]
Medicare: [ ] Medicaid: [Y] Supplemental Medicare: [ ]
Tricare [ ]

PRODUCTS OFFERED:
Product Name: Type:
Neighborhood Health Plan Medicaid

PLAN BENEFITS:
Alternative Medicine:	[ ]	Behavioral Health:	[X]
Chiropractic:	[ ]	Dental:	[X]
Home Care:	[X]	Inpatient SNF:	[X]
Long-Term Care:	[X]	Pharm. Mail Order:	[X]
Physical Therapy:	[X]	Podiatry:	[X]
Psychiatric:	[X]	Transplant:	[X]
Vision:	[X]	Wellness:	[X]
Workers' Comp:	[ ]		

Other Benefits:

NEW ENGLAND FINANCIAL - CORPORATE HEADQUARTERS

One Financial Center
Boston, MA 02111
Phone: 617-578-2000 Fax: 617-578-6852 Toll-Free: 800-388-4000
Web site: www.nefn.com

MAILING ADDRESS:
NEW ENGLAND FINANCIAL
One Financial Center
Boston, MA 02111

KEY EXECUTIVES:
President .... Brian Breneman
Chief Financial Officer .... Eric Steingerwalt
Chief Operating Officer .... Robert Henrickson
AVP, Marketing .... Dan Sheehan

COMPANY PROFILE:
Parent Company Name: MetLife
Doing Business As:
Year Founded: 1990 Federally Qualified: [N]

Managed Care Organization Profiles — MASSACHUSETTS

MAILING ADDRESS:
  HEALTH NEW ENGLAND
  One Monarch Place
  Springfield, MA 01144-1006

KEY EXECUTIVES:
Chief Executive Officer/President .... Peter F Straley
Chief Financial Officer .... Robert A Kosior
Chief Medical Officer .... Thomas H Ebert, MD
VP of Marketing & Busnss Development .... Maura McCaffrey
VP of Sales .... Juan Campbell
VP of Information Technology .... Philip M LaCombe
Compliance & Privacy Officer .... Renee Wroth
Public Relations Manager .... Mark Morris
Network Operation/Development Management .... Pam Zagorski
Health Promotion Manager .... Lynn Ostrowski
VP of Human Resources .... Amy Trombley
VP & General Counsel .... James S Kessler

COMPANY PROFILE:
Parent Company Name: Baystate Health Systems & Harvard
Doing Business As:
Year Founded: 1986   Federally Qualified: [Y]
Forprofit: [Y]   Not-For-Profit: [ ]
Model Type: IPA
Accreditation: [ ] AAPPO [ ] JACHO [X] NCQA [ ] URAC
Plan Type: HMO, PPO, POS
Total Revenue: 2005:   2006: 247,690,116
Net Income   2005:   2006:
Total Enrollment:
  2001: 67,262   2004: 68,929   2007: 66,850
  2002: 74,401   2005: 62,088
  2003: 71,358   2006: 62,690
Medical Loss Ratio: 2005: 83.50   2006: 85.20
Administrative Expense Ratio: 2005:   2006:

SERVICE AREA:
Nationwide: N
  CT (Hartford, Litchfield, Tolland); MA (Berkshire, Franklin, Hampden, Hampshire, Worcester);

TYPE OF COVERAGE:
Commercial: [Y] Individual: [ ]   FEHBP: [ ]   Indemnity: [ ]
Medicare: [ ] Medicaid: [ ]   Supplemental Medicare: [ ]
Tricare   [ ]

PRODUCTS OFFERED:
Product Name: Type:
Health New England   HMO
Health New England   POS

PLAN BENEFITS:
Alternative Medicine: [ ]   Behavioral Health: [X]
Chiropractic: [X]   Dental: [ ]
Home Care: [X]   Inpatient SNF: [X]
Long-Term Care: [X]   Pharm. Mail Order: [X]
Physical Therapy: [X]   Podiatry: [X]
Psychiatric: [X]   Transplant: [X]
Vision: [X]   Wellness: [X]
Workers' Comp: [ ]
Other Benefits:
Comments:
Kaiser Permanente Massachusetts commercial members have been acquisitioned by Health New England.

HEALTH PLANS INC

1500 W Park Dr Ste 330
Westborough, MA 01581
Phone: 508-752-2480 Fax: 508-754-9664 Toll-Free: 800-343-7674
Web site: www.healthplansinc.com

MAILING ADDRESS:
  HEALTH PLANS INC
  PO Box 5199
  Westborough, MA 01581

KEY EXECUTIVES:
Chief Executive Officer/President .... William Briedenbach
Medical Director .... Linda McInerny, MD
Chief Operating Officer .... Deb Hovagimian
VP Marketing .... Debbie Hodges

COMPANY PROFILE:
Parent Company Name: Harvard Health Plans Inc
Doing Business As:
Year Founded: 1981   Federally Qualified: [N]
Forprofit: [Y]   Not-For-Profit: [ ]
Model Type:
Accreditation: [ ] AAPPO [ ] JACHO [ ] NCQA [ ] URAC
Plan Type: PPO

SERVICE AREA:
Nationwide: N
  MA;

TYPE OF COVERAGE:
Commercial: [Y] Individual: [ ]   FEHBP: [ ]   Indemnity: [ ]
Medicare: [ ] Medicaid: [ ]   Supplemental Medicare: [ ]
Tricare   [ ]

PLAN BENEFITS:
Alternative Medicine: [ ]   Behavioral Health: [ ]
Chiropractic: [ ]   Dental: [X]
Home Care: [X]   Inpatient SNF: [ ]
Long-Term Care: [ ]   Pharm. Mail Order: [X]
Physical Therapy: [X]   Podiatry: [X]
Psychiatric: [X]   Transplant: [X]
Vision: [X]   Wellness: [ ]
Workers' Comp: [ ]
Other Benefits:

HEALTHCARE VALUE MANAGEMENT INC

100 River Ridge Drive
Norwood, MA 02062
Phone: 781-762-5511 Fax: 781-762-5518 Toll-Free:
Web site: www.hcvm.com

MAILING ADDRESS:
  HEALTHCARE VALUE MANAGEMENT INC
  100 River Ridge Drive
  Norwood, MA 02062

KEY EXECUTIVES:
Chief Executive Officer .... Dale B Wolf

COMPANY PROFILE:
Parent Company Name: First Health Group Corp
Doing Business As:
Year Founded: 1990   Federally Qualified: [ ]
Forprofit: [Y]   Not-For-Profit: [ ]
Model Type: NETWORK
Accreditation: [X] AAPPO [ ] JACHO [ ] NCQA [ ] URAC
Plan Type: PPO
Primary Physicians: 12,954   Physician Specialists: 16,992
Hospitals: 242
Total Enrollment:
  2001: 600,000   2004: 0   2007: 0
  2002: 625,000   2005:
  2003: 0   2006:

SERVICE AREA:
Nationwide: N
  MA; NH; RI; CT; ME; VT

TYPE OF COVERAGE:
Commercial: [Y] Individual: [ ]   FEHBP: [ ]   Indemnity: [ ]
Medicare: [ ] Medicaid: [ ]   Supplemental Medicare: [ ]
Tricare   [ ]

PRODUCTS OFFERED:
Product Name: Type:
Healthcare Value Management PPO   PPO

Comments:
Healthcare Value Management Inc was bought out by First Health Group Corp, so the officers are the same as First Health Group Corp.

MASSPRO INC

245 Winter St
Waltham, MA 02154-1231
Phone: 781-890-0011 Fax: 781-487-0083 Toll-Free:
Web site: www.masspro.org

MAILING ADDRESS:
  MASSPRO INC
  235 Wyman St
  Waltham, MA 02154-1231

MASSACHUSETTS

PRODUCTS OFFERED:

Product Name:	Type:
Fallon HMO	HMO
Fallon Senior Plan	Medicare Advantage
The Independent Plan	Guarantee IssueFallon Flex
POS	
Fallon Major Medical	Indemnity
Fallon Medicaid	Medicaid

CONSUMER-DRIVEN PRODUCTS

Sovereign Bank	HSA Company
FCHP Direct Care Choice	HSA Product
Fallon Community Health Plan	HSA Administrator
FCHP Select Care Choice	Consumer-Driven Health Plan
Fallon Preferred Care Choice	High Deductible Health Plan

PLAN BENEFITS:

Alternative Medicine:	[ ]	Behavioral Health:	[X]
Chiropractic:	[X]	Dental:	[X]
Home Care:	[X]	Inpatient SNF:	[X]
Long-Term Care:	[ ]	Pharm. Mail Order:	[X]
Physical Therapy:	[X]	Podiatry:	[X]
Psychiatric:	[X]	Transplant:	[X]
Vision:	[X]	Wellness:	[X]
Workers' Comp:	[ ]		

Other Benefits:

GREAT-WEST HEALTHCARE OF MASSACHUSETTS

130 Turner St Bldg 3 Ste 610
Waltham, MA 02453
Phone: 781-893-0370 Fax: 781-647-0132 Toll-Free: 800-234-2040
Web site: www.greatwesthealthcare.com

MAILING ADDRESS:
GREAT-WEST HEALTHCARE OF MA
130 Turner St Bldg 3 Ste 610
Waltham, MA 02453

KEY EXECUTIVES:
Regional Group Manager .... Michael Brian
President .... Deborah L Origer

COMPANY PROFILE:
Parent Company Name: CIGNA Inc
Doing Business As:
Year Founded: Federally Qualified: [ ]
Forprofit: [Y]   Not-For-Profit: [ ]
Model Type:
Accreditation: [ ] AAPPO [ ] JACHO [ ] NCQA [ ] URAC
Plan Type: PPO, CDHP, HDHP, HSA,
Total Enrollment:
  2001: 0   2004: 3   2007: 0
  2002: 1,725   2005:
  2003: 348   2006:

SERVICE AREA:
Nationwide: N
  MA;

TYPE OF COVERAGE:
Commercial: [Y] Individual: [ ] FEHBP: [ ] Indemnity: [ ]
Medicare: [ ] Medicaid: [ ] Supplemental Medicare: [ ]
Tricare [ ]

CONSUMER-DRIVEN PRODUCTS

Mellon HR Solutions LLC	HSA Company
	HSA Product
	HSA Administrator
	Consumer-Driven Health Plan
	High Deductible Health Plan

PLAN BENEFITS:

Alternative Medicine:	[X]	Behavioral Health:	[ ]
Chiropractic:	[X]	Dental:	[X]
Home Care:	[X]	Inpatient SNF:	[X]
Long-Term Care:	[ ]	Pharm. Mail Order:	[X]
Physical Therapy:	[X]	Podiatry:	[X]
Psychiatric:	[X]	Transplant:	[X]
Vision:	[X]	Wellness:	[X]
Workers' Comp:	[ ]		

Other Benefits:
Comments: Acquired by CIGNA Inc April 1, 2008

HARVARD PILGRIM HEALTH CARE - CORPORATE HEADQUARTERS

93 Worcester St
Wellesley, MA 02481
Phone: 781-263-6000 Fax: 617-509-2515 Toll-Free: 800-742-8326
Web site: www.hphc.org

MAILING ADDRESS:
HARVARD PILGRIM HEALTH CARE
93 Worcester St
Wellesley, MA 02481

KEY EXECUTIVES:
Chief Executive Officer/President .... Charles D Baker
Senior VP, Health Services, Chief Med Officer .... Roberta Herman, MD
Senior VP/Chief Information Officer .... Deborah A Norton
Chief Operating Officer .... Bruce M Bullen
Senior VP Sales & Marketing .... Vincent Capozzi
Senior VP, Network Services/Operations .... Leanne Berge
VP, Human Resources .... Deborah Hicks
Senior VP Medical Management & Quality .... Roberta Herman, MD
Pharmacy Director .... Nancy P Davis

COMPANY PROFILE:
Parent Company Name: Harvard Pilgrim Health Care Inc
Doing Business As:
Year Founded: 1969   Federally Qualified: [Y]
Forprofit: [ ]   Not-For-Profit: [Y]
Model Type: IPA
Accreditation: [ ] AAPPO [ ] JACHO [X] NCQA [ ] URAC
Plan Type: HMO, PPO, POS, CDHP, HDHP, HSA,
Total Revenue: 2005: 2,035,646,003 2006: 2,198,190,404
Net Income   2005:   64,983,595 2006:   68,354,069
Total Enrollment:
  2001: 729,168   2004: 785,000   2007: 1,012,000
  2002: 560,745   2005: 892,598
  2003: 803,959   2006: 975,000
Medical Loss Ratio: 2005: 84.35   2006:
Administrative Expense Ratio: 2005: 8.05   2006:

SERVICE AREA:
Nationwide: N
  CT; MA; ME; NH; NY; VT;

TYPE OF COVERAGE:
Commercial: [Y] Individual: [Y] FEHBP: [ ] Indemnity: [ ]
Medicare: [Y] Medicaid: [Y] Supplemental Medicare: [Y]
Tricare [ ]

PRODUCTS OFFERED:

Product Name:	Type:
First Seniority	Medicare Advantage
Seniorcare	Medicare
Harvard Pilgrim HMO	HMO
Harvard Pilgrim POS	
Harvard Pilgrim PPO	

CONSUMER-DRIVEN PRODUCTS

	HSA Company
Best Buy HSA	HSA Product
Mellon Bank	HSA Administrator
	Consumer-Driven Health Plan
Best Buy HSA PPO	High Deductible Health Plan

PLAN BENEFITS:

Alternative Medicine:	[ ]	Behavioral Health:	[ ]
Chiropractic:	[X]	Dental:	[X]
Home Care:	[X]	Inpatient SNF:	[X]
Long-Term Care:	[X]	Pharm. Mail Order:	[X]
Physical Therapy:	[X]	Podiatry:	[X]
Psychiatric:	[X]	Transplant:	[X]
Vision:	[X]	Wellness:	[X]
Workers' Comp:	[X]		

Other Benefits:
Comments:
HCHP 1969, PHC 1981, HPHC 1995.

HEALTH NEW ENGLAND

One Monarch Place Ste 1500
Springfield, MA 01144-1006
Phone: 413-787-4000 Fax: 413-731-5275 Toll-Free: 800-842-4464
Web site: www.hne.com

Managed Care Organization Profiles — MASSACHUSETTS

COMPANY PROFILE:
Parent Company Name: Health Insurance Plan of New York
Doing Business As:
Year Founded: 1982   Federally Qualified: [ ]
Forprofit: [N]   Not-For-Profit: [ ]
Model Type:
Accreditation: [ ] AAPPO [ ] JACHO [ ] NCQA [ ] URAC
Plan Type: HMO, PPO, POS, ASO, HDHP, HSA
Total Revenue: 2005:   2006: 26,115,335
Net Income   2005:   2006:
Total Enrollment:
  2001: 0   2004: 0   2007: 6,131
  2002: 0   2005: 4,710
  2003: 0   2006: 5,318
Medical Loss Ratio: 2005:   2006: 78.10
Administrative Expense Ratio: 2005:   2006:
SERVICE AREA:
Nationwide: N
  MA (Berkshire, Franklin, Hampden, Hampshire);
TYPE OF COVERAGE:
Commercial: [Y] Individual: [ ] FEHBP: [ ] Indemnity: [ ]
Medicare: [ ] Medicaid: [ ] Supplemental Medicare: [ ]
Tricare   [ ]
PLAN BENEFITS:
Alternative Medicine: [ ]   Behavioral Health: [X]
Chiropractic: [X]   Dental: [ ]
Home Care: [X]   Inpatient SNF: [X]
Long-Term Care: [ ]   Pharm. Mail Order: [X]
Physical Therapy: [X]   Podiatry: [X]
Psychiatric: [X]   Transplant: [X]
Vision: [X]   Wellness: [X]
Workers' Comp: [ ]
Other Benefits:

DENTA QUEST VENTURES INC

465 Medford St
Boston, MA 02129
Phone: 617-886-1000 Fax: 617-886-1500 Toll-Free: 888-788-8600
Web site: www.dentaquest.com
MAILING ADDRESS:
  DENTA QUEST VENTURES INC
  465 Medford St
  Boston, MA 02129

KEY EXECUTIVES:
Chairman .... Hassell McClellan
Chief Executive Officer/President .... Fay Donohue
Chief Financial Officer .... Scott O'Gorman
Chief Dental Officer .... Doyle Williams, DDS
Executive VP .... William Bradford
Chief Operating Officer .... Fay Donohue
Marketing Director .... Dennis Leonard
VP, Sales - Mid Atlantic Region .... Mark Haraway
VP, Human Resources .... Frances Gallitano
VP & General Counsel .... Patricia Ma

COMPANY PROFILE:
Parent Company Name: Dental Service of Massachusetts
Doing Business As: Delta Dental Plan of Massachusetts
Year Founded: 2001   Federally Qualified: [N]
Forprofit: [Y]   Not-For-Profit: [ ]
Model Type: MIXED
Accreditation: [ ] AAPPO [ ] JACHO [ ] NCQA [ ] URAC
Plan Type: Specialty HMO, Specialty PPO
Total Enrollment:
  2001: 1,889,122   2004: 1,960,185   2007: 0
  2002: 1,846,428   2005:
  2003: 1,888,229   2006:
SERVICE AREA:
Nationwide: N
  MA;
TYPE OF COVERAGE:
Commercial: [Y] Individual: [ ] FEHBP: [ ] Indemnity: [ ]
Medicare: [ ] Medicaid: [Y] Supplemental Medicare: [ ]
Tricare   [ ]
PRODUCTS OFFERED:
Product Name: Type:
Dental Plans

PLAN BENEFITS:
Alternative Medicine: [ ]   Behavioral Health: [ ]
Chiropractic: [ ]   Dental: [X]
Home Care: [ ]   Inpatient SNF: [ ]
Long-Term Care: [ ]   Pharm. Mail Order: [ ]
Physical Therapy: [ ]   Podiatry: [ ]
Psychiatric: [ ]   Transplant: [ ]
Vision: [ ]   Wellness: [ ]
Workers' Comp: [ ]
Other Benefits:
Comments:
Formerly Delta Dental Plan of Massachusetts.

FALLON COMMUNITY HEALTH PLAN INC

10 Chestnut St
Worcester, MA 01608-2810
Phone: 508-799-2100 Fax: 508-368-9164 Toll-Free: 800-333-2535
Web site: www.fchp.org
MAILING ADDRESS:
  FALLON COMMUNITY HEALTH PLAN
  10 Chestnut St
  Worcester, MA 01608-2810

KEY EXECUTIVES:
Chairman of the Board .... Richard P Houlihan, Esq
Chief Executive Officer/President .... Eric H Schultz
Senior VP, Chief Financial Officer .... Charles Goheen
Senior VP, Chief Medical Officer .... Dennis Batay, MD
Pharmacy Director .... Leslie Fish, PharmD
Chief Information Officer .... Jean Politakis
VP & Chief Operating Officer .... Mark Fisher
VP, Chief Marketing Officer .... Jennifer Eardley
Information Technology Director .... Michael Benita
Director Credentialing/Provider Information ...... Margo Ferro
Privacy Officer .... Jeannette Frey
VP Public Affairs & Business Planning .... Richard P Burke
Provider Relations Director .... Lisa Mancini-Peare
AVP Network Development & Management .... Daniel Concaugh
Health Promotion Manager .... Emily Eaton
Senior VP, Chief Human Resource Officer .... Teena Osgood
AVP, Care Management Operations .... Kelly Cummings
AVP, Quality & Health Management ...... AnnMarie Sciammacco
Director Credentialing/Provider Information ...... Margo Ferro
Manager, Internal Audit .... Wendy Vitkauskas
Director of Product Development .... Beth Helenius
Senior VP, Compliance Officer .... Anne Doyle
AVP Administrative Operations .... John Monte
AVP Underwriting/Actuarial Service .... Charles Bouton
AVP Finance .... Kevin McGovern

COMPANY PROFILE:
Parent Company Name:
Doing Business As: Fallon Community Health Plan
Year Founded: 1977   Federally Qualified: [Y]
Forprofit: [ ]   Not-For-Profit: [Y]
Model Type: MIXED
Accreditation: [ ] AAPPO [ ] JACHO [X] NCQA [ ] URAC
Plan Type: HMO, PPO, POS, ASO, HDHP, HSA
Primary Physicians: 1,618   Physician Specialists: 3,638
Hospitals: 40
Total Revenue: 2005: 781,433,328   2006: 414,173,977
Net Income   2005: 15,645,809   2006:   7,914,789
Total Enrollment:
  2001: 193,000   2004: 175,393   2007: 154,283
  2002: 185,960   2005: 171,500
  2003: 178,545   2006: 155,669
Medical Loss Ratio: 2005:   2006: 90.40
Administrative Expense Ratio: 2005:   2006:
SERVICE AREA:
Nationwide: N
  MA; (Boston/Greater Boston Region, Central/Western Region,
  Northeast/Southeast Region);
TYPE OF COVERAGE:
Commercial: [Y] Individual: [Y] FEHBP: [Y] Indemnity: [Y]
Medicare: [Y] Medicaid: [Y] Supplemental Medicare: [ ]
Tricare   [ ]

MASSACHUSETTS

Forprofit: [ ]   Not-For-Profit: [ ]
Model Type:
Accreditation: [ ] AAPPO [ ] JACHO [ ] NCQA [ ] URAC
Plan Type: HMO
Primary Physicians: Physician Specialists:
Hospitals: 30
Total Enrollment:
  2001: 0   2004: 0   2007: 180,000
  2002: 0   2005: 160,000
  2003: 0   2006: 200,000

SERVICE AREA:
Nationwide:
  MA;

TYPE OF COVERAGE:
Commercial: [ ] Individual: [ ] FEHBP: [ ] Indemnity: [ ]
Medicare: [Y] Medicaid: [Y] Supplemental Medicare: [ ]
Tricare   [ ]

PRODUCTS OFFERED:
Product Name: Type:
MassHealth   Medicaid
Commonwealth Care

CIGNA HEALTHCARE OF MASSACHUSETTS

2223 Washington St Ste 200
Newton, MA 02462
Phone: 617-630-4300 Fax: 617-630-4383 Toll-Free:
Web site: www.cigna.com

MAILING ADDRESS:
  CIGNA HEALTHCARE OF MA
  2223 Washington St Ste 200
  Newton, MA 02462

KEY EXECUTIVES:
President .... Donald M Curry
Medical Director .... Imre Toth, MD
Marketing Director .... Linda Griffiths

COMPANY PROFILE:
Parent Company Name: CIGNA Corporation
Doing Business As:
Year Founded: 1986   Federally Qualified: [Y]
Forprofit: [Y]   Not-For-Profit: [ ]
Model Type: IPA
Accreditation: [ ] AAPPO [ ] JACHO [ ] NCQA [ ] URAC
Plan Type: HMO, PPO, POS, CDHP, HSA
Total Revenue: 2005:   2006: 32,235,636
Net Income   2005:   2006:
Total Enrollment:
  2001: 0   2004: 34,520   2007: 2,966
  2002: 61,251   2005: 7,306
  2003: 11,496   2006: 5,661
Medical Loss Ratio: 2005: 72.20   2006: 84.80
Administrative Expense Ratio: 2005:   2006:

SERVICE AREA:
Nationwide: N
  MA;

TYPE OF COVERAGE:
Commercial: [Y] Individual: [ ] FEHBP: [ ] Indemnity: [ ]
Medicare: [ ] Medicaid: [ ] Supplemental Medicare: [ ]
Tricare   [ ]

CONSUMER-DRIVEN PRODUCTS
JP Morgan Chase   HSA Company
CIGNA Choice Fund   HSA Product
                          HSA Administrator
Open Access Plus   Consumer-Driven Health Plan
PPO   High Deductible Health Plan

PLAN BENEFITS:
Alternative Medicine: [ ]   Behavioral Health: [ ]
Chiropractic: [X]   Dental: [ ]
Home Care: [X]   Inpatient SNF: [X]
Long-Term Care: [X]   Pharm. Mail Order: [X]
Physical Therapy: [X]   Podiatry: [X]
Psychiatric: [X]   Transplant: [X]
Vision: [X]   Wellness: [X]
Workers' Comp: [ ]
Other Benefits:

COMMUNITY MEDICAL ALLIANCE

253 Summer St
Boston, MA 02210
Phone: 617-423-0040 Fax: 617-772-5519 Toll-Free: 800-462-5449
Web site: www.nhp.org

MAILING ADDRESS:
  COMMUNITY MEDICAL ALLIANCE
  253 Summer St
  Boston, MA 02210

KEY EXECUTIVES:
Chief Executive Officer .... Jim Hooley
President .... Deborah Enos
Chief Financial Officer .... Harold Putnam
Chief Medical Officer .... Paul Mendis, MD
Chief Information Officer .... Ned Spadani
Member Services Manager .... Joann Landry
Provider Relations Director .... Ramona Bourgvignon
VP, Provider Network Management .... Thankam Rangala
Director of Human Resources .... Roberta Goldman-Wilkinson
Quality Assurance Director .... Richard Dropski
Fraud Prevention Director .... Willie Mae
Compliance Officer .... Pamela Siren

COMPANY PROFILE:
Parent Company Name: Neighborhood Health Plan
Doing Business As:
Year Founded: 1986   Federally Qualified: [ ]
Forprofit: [ ]   Not-For-Profit: [Y]
Model Type:
Accreditation: [ ] AAPPO [ ] JACHO [ ] NCQA [ ] URAC
Plan Type: HMO, Specialty HMO, PBM, HDHP
Primary Physicians: 1,900   Physician Specialists: 9,000
Hospitals: 41
Total Enrollment:
  2001: 0   2004: 124,000   2007: 0
  2002: 0   2005:
  2003: 120,000   2006:

SERVICE AREA:
Nationwide: N
  MA;

TYPE OF COVERAGE:
Commercial: [Y] Individual: [Y] FEHBP: [ ] Indemnity: [ ]
Medicare: [ ] Medicaid: [ ] Supplemental Medicare: [ ]
Tricare   [ ]

CONSUMER-DRIVEN PRODUCTS
                          HSA Company
                          HSA Product
                          HSA Administrator
                          Consumer-Driven Health Plan
NHP Care 1000   High Deductible Health Plan

PLAN BENEFITS:
Alternative Medicine: [ ]   Behavioral Health: [ ]
Chiropractic: [ ]   Dental: [ ]
Home Care: [ ]   Inpatient SNF: [ ]
Long-Term Care: [ ]   Pharm. Mail Order: [ ]
Physical Therapy: [ ]   Podiatry: [ ]
Psychiatric: [ ]   Transplant: [ ]
Vision: [ ]   Wellness: [ ]
Workers' Comp: [ ]
Other Benefits:

CONNECTICARE OF MASSACHUSETTS INC

175 Scott Swamp Rd
Farmington, CT 06032
Phone: 860-674-5700 Fax: 860-674-2030 Toll-Free: 800-923-2822
Web site: www.connecticare.com

MAILING ADDRESS:
  CONNECTICARE OF MA INC
  175 Scott Swamp Rd
  Farmington, CT 06032

KEY EXECUTIVES:
Chairman .... Anthony L Watson
Chief Executive Officer/President .... Michael E Herbert
Senior VP, Chief Medical Officer .... Paul A Bluestein, MD
Director, Pharmacy .... Jeffrey Casberg
VP & Chief Information Officer .... Mark G Dixon
Senior VP, Human Resources .... Richard Rogers
Director, Quality Improvement .... Pam Spinazola

Managed Care Organization Profiles **MASSACHUSETTS**

AETNA INC - MASSACHUSETTS

400-1 Totten Pond Rd
Waltham, MA 02451
Phone: 781-902-3800 Fax: 781-530-2001 Toll-Free: 800-435-8742
Web site: www.aetna.com
MAILING ADDRESS:
   AETNA INC - MA
   400-1 Totten Pond Rd
   Waltham, MA 02451

KEY EXECUTIVES:
Chairman of the Board/Chief Executive Officer .... Ronald A Williams
President .... Charles A Peck, MD
Principal Financial Officer .... Emanuel F Germano
Senior Medical Officer .... Gordon W Grundy, MD

COMPANY PROFILE:
Parent Company Name: Aetna Inc
Doing Business As:
Year Founded: 1987   Federally Qualified: [N]
Forprofit: [Y]   Not-For-Profit: [ ]
Model Type: IPA
Accreditation: [ ] AAPPO [ ] JACHO [ ] NCQA [ ] URAC
Plan Type: HMO, CDHP, HDHP, HSA,
Total Revenue: 2005:   2006:   35,421,153
Net Income   2005:   2006:
Total Enrollment:
   2001: 75,139   2004: 12,705   2007: 4,122
   2002: 28,910   2005:   7,015
   2003: 15,831   2006:   4,926
Medical Loss Ratio: 2005: 74.50   2006: 75.40
Administrative Expense Ratio: 2005:   2006:
SERVICE AREA:
Nationwide: N
   MA;
TYPE OF COVERAGE:
Commercial: [Y] Individual: [ ] FEHBP: [ ] Indemnity: [ ]
Medicare: [Y] Medicaid: [ ] Supplemental Medicare: [ ]
Tricare   [ ]
PRODUCTS OFFERED:
Product Name: Type:
US Hlthcare Medicare Hlth Plan   Medicare
Aetna Health   HMO
Aetna Health   POS
CONSUMER-DRIVEN PRODUCTS
Aetna Life Insurance Co   HSA Company
Aetna HealthFund HSA   HSA Product
Aetna   HSA Administrator
Aetna HealthFund   Consumer-Driven Health Plan
PPO I; PPO II   High Deductible Health Plan
PLAN BENEFITS:
Alternative Medicine: [ ]   Behavioral Health: [ ]
Chiropractic: [X]   Dental: [X]
Home Care: [X]   Inpatient SNF: [X]
Long-Term Care: [X]   Pharm. Mail Order: [X]
Physical Therapy: [X]   Podiatry: [X]
Psychiatric: [X]   Transplant: [X]
Vision: [X]   Wellness: [X]
Workers' Comp: [ ]
Other Benefits:

BLUE CROSS BLUE SHIELD OF MASSACHUSETTS

401 Park Drive
Boston, MA 02115-3326
Phone: 617-246-5000 Fax: 617-246-3353 Toll-Free:
Web site: www.bluecrossma.com
MAILING ADDRESS:
   BLUE CROSS BLUE SHIELD OF MA
   401 Park Drive
   Boston, MA 02115-3326

KEY EXECUTIVES:
Chairman .... William C Van Faasen
Chief Executive Officer/President .... Cleve L Killingsworth
Chief Financial Officer .... Allen Maltz
Senior VP, Chief Physician Exective .John A Fallon, MD, MBA, FACP
Chief Information Officer .... Carl Ascenzo
Executive VP, Sales, Marketing/Services .... Stephen J Booma
Senior VP, Corporate Relations .... Fredi Shonkoff
Senior VP, Chief Information Officer .... Joseph Patrnchak
Executive VP, Health Care Services .... Andrew Dreyfus
Executive VP, Chief Legal Officer .... Sandra L Jesse
Executive VP, Corporate Affairs................................... Peter Meade
Senior VP, Chief Strategy Officer .... Vinod K Sahney, PhD
Chief of Staff, Executive Officer .... John Schoenbaum

COMPANY PROFILE:
Parent Company Name:
Doing Business As:
Year Founded: 1992   Federally Qualified: [N]
Forprofit: [ ]   Not-For-Profit: [Y]
Model Type: NETWORK
Accreditation: [ ] AAPPO [ ] JACHO [X] NCQA [ ] URAC
Plan Type: HMO, PPO, POS, HDHP, HSA
Primary Physicians: 18,114   Physician Specialists:
Hospitals: 69
Total Revenue: 2005: 1,976,829,000   2006:
Net Income   2005:   127,723,000   2006:
Total Enrollment:
   2001: 2,392,283   2004: 2,661,417   2007: 3,000,000
   2002: 2,411,154   2005: 2,820,000
   2003: 2,492,276   2006: 2,900,000
SERVICE AREA:
Nationwide: N
   MA;
TYPE OF COVERAGE:
Commercial: [Y] Individual: [Y] FEHBP: [ ] Indemnity: [ ]
Medicare: [ ] Medicaid: [ ] Supplemental Medicare: [ ]
Tricare   [ ]
PRODUCTS OFFERED:
Product Name: Type:
Blue Choice   POS
HMO Blue   HMO
Blue Care Elect   PPO
Blue Care 65   Medicare
Medex   Medicare Supplement
Medicare Advantage   PFFS
CONSUMER-DRIVEN PRODUCTS
Wells Fargo   HSA Company
Blue Saver   HSA Product
Wells Fargo Health Bnft Services   HSA Administrator
                                       Consumer-Driven Health Plan
PPO Basic Blue Direct   High Deductible Health Plan
PLAN BENEFITS:
Alternative Medicine: [ ]   Behavioral Health: [X]
Chiropractic: [X]   Dental: [ ]
Home Care: [X]   Inpatient SNF: [X]
Long-Term Care: [ ]   Pharm. Mail Order: [X]
Physical Therapy: [X]   Podiatry: [X]
Psychiatric: [X]   Transplant: [X]
Vision: [X]   Wellness: [X]
Workers' Comp: [ ]
Other Benefits:

BMC HEALTHNET PLAN

Two Copley Pl Ste 600
Boston, MA 02116
Phone: 617-748-6000 Fax: 617-748-6132 Toll-Free: 800-792-4355
Web site: www.bmchp.org
MAILING ADDRESS:
   BMC HEALTHNET PLAN
   Two Copley Pl Ste 600
   Boston, MA 02116

KEY EXECUTIVES:
Chief Executive Officer.. Elaine Ullian
Executive Director/Interium Chief Financial Officer .... Jean Haynes
Chief Medical Officer/S E Region.............................Andrea Gelzer, MD
Chief Information Officer .... Marie Maloney
Chief Operating Officer .... Michele Lepore
Chief Compliance Officer .... Katherine McGrath
General Counsel .... Susan Coakley
Vice President .... Thomas Traylor

COMPANY PROFILE:
Parent Company Name: Boston Medical Center
Doing Business As:
Year Founded: 1997   Federally Qualified: [ ]

Managed Care Organization Profiles — **MARYLAND**

PRODUCTS OFFERED:
Product Name:	Type:
Medicare Complete	Medicare Advantage
United Hlth Care Medicaid	Medicaid
United Health Care HMO	HMO

CONSUMER-DRIVEN PRODUCTS
Exante Bank/Golden Rule Ins Co	HSA Company
iPlan HSA	HSA Product
	HSA Administrator
	Consumer-Driven Health Plan
	High Deductible Health Plan

PLAN BENEFITS:
Alternative Medicine:	[ ]	Behavioral Health:	[ ]
Chiropractic:	[X]	Dental:	[X]
Home Care:	[X]	Inpatient SNF:	[X]
Long-Term Care:	[ ]	Pharm. Mail Order:	[X]
Physical Therapy:	[X]	Podiatry:	[X]
Psychiatric:	[X]	Transplant:	[X]
Vision:	[X]	Wellness:	[X]
Workers' Comp:	[ ]		

Other Benefits: X

Comments:
Formerly Cheaspeake Health Plan.

XL HEALTH

351 W Camden St Ste 100
Baltimore, MD 21201
Phone: 410-625-2200 Fax: 410-625-2244 Toll-Free:
Web site: www.xlhealth.com

MAILING ADDRESS:
XL HEALTH
351 W Camden St Ste 100
Baltimore, MD 21201

KEY EXECUTIVES:
Chairman/President .... Patrick Hervy, MBA
Chief Financial Officer .... Robert L Cinquegrana, CPA
Chief Medical Officer .... Harry L Leider, MD, MBA
Chief Information Officer .... Suresh Ramakrishnan
VP, Operations .... Leslie Young
Senior Human Resources Manager .... Lyda E Prack
Executive VP .... Paul A Serini, Esq.
VP, Government Affairs .... Robb A Cohen, MBA
Senior Director of Administration & Associate Counsel .... Sue Dent

COMPANY PROFILE:
Parent Company Name:
Doing Business As:
Year Founded: Federally Qualified: [ ]
Forprofit: [Y]   Not-For-Profit: [ ]
Model Type: GROUP
Accreditation: [ ] AAPPO [ ] JACHO [ ] NCQA [ ] URAC
Plan Type: HMO

SERVICE AREA:
Nationwide:
    MD;

TYPE OF COVERAGE:
Commercial: [ ] Individual: [ ] FEHBP: [ ] Indemnity: [ ]
Medicare: [Y] Medicaid: [ ] Supplemental Medicare: [ ]
Tricare [ ]

PLAN BENEFITS:
Alternative Medicine:	[ ]	Behavioral Health:	[ ]
Chiropractic:	[ ]	Dental:	[ ]
Home Care:	[ ]	Inpatient SNF:	[ ]
Long-Term Care:	[ ]	Pharm. Mail Order:	[ ]
Physical Therapy:	[ ]	Podiatry:	[ ]
Psychiatric:	[ ]	Transplant:	[ ]
Vision:	[ ]	Wellness:	[ ]
Workers' Comp:	[ ]		

Other Benefits: Disease Management

MARYLAND

SERVICE AREA:
Nationwide:
  NC; SC;
TYPE OF COVERAGE:
Commercial: [Y] Individual: [ ] FEHBP: [ ] Indemnity: [ ]
Medicare: [ ] Medicaid: [ ] Supplemental Medicare: [ ]
Tricare [ ]

SPECTERA VISION INC - CORPORATE HEADQUARTERS

2811 Lord Baltimore Dr
Baltimore, MD 21244
Phone: 443-896-0427 Fax: 410-265-5872 Toll-Free: 800-638-3895
Web site: www.spectera.com
MAILING ADDRESS:
  SPECTERA VISION INC-CORPORATE
  2811 Lord Baltimore Dr
  Baltimore, MD 21244

KEY EXECUTIVES:
Executive VP, Chief Executive Officer .... Paul Grosand
Senior VP, Marketing .... Susan E Cox
VP of Care Programs/MIS Director .... Michael Pham
VP, Corporate Communications .... Jeannette Duerr

COMPANY PROFILE:
Parent Company Name: UnitedHealth Group-Specialized Care Service
Doing Business As: Spectera Inc/Care Programs
Year Founded: 1964   Federally Qualified: [ ]
Forprofit: [Y]   Not-For-Profit: [ ]
Model Type:
Accreditation: [ ] AAPPO [ ] JACHO [ ] NCQA [X] URAC
Plan Type: Specialty HMO, UR
Total Enrollment:
  2001: 0   2004: 0   2007: 17,000,000
  2002: 0   2005:
  2003: 0   2006:
SERVICE AREA:
Nationwide: Y
  NW;
TYPE OF COVERAGE:
Commercial: [Y] Individual: [ ] FEHBP: [ ] Indemnity: [ ]
Medicare: [Y] Medicaid: [Y] Supplemental Medicare: [Y]
Tricare [ ]
PLAN BENEFITS:
Alternative Medicine: [ ]   Behavioral Health: [X]
Chiropractic: [X]   Dental: [X]
Home Care: [X]   Inpatient SNF: [X]
Long-Term Care: [X]   Pharm. Mail Order: [ ]
Physical Therapy: [X]   Podiatry: [X]
Psychiatric: [X]   Transplant: [X]
Vision: [X]   Wellness: [ ]
Workers' Comp: [X]
Other Benefits: X
Comments:
Formerly Care Programs.

UNITED CONCORDIA COMPANY INC - MARYLAND

309 International Circle #130
Hunt Valley, MD 21030
Phone: 800-272-8865 Fax: 443-886-9525 Toll-Free: 800-272-8865
Web site: www.ucci.com
MAILING ADDRESS:
  UNITED CONCORDIA CO INC - MD
  309 International Circle #130
  Hunt Valley, MD 21030

KEY EXECUTIVES:
Chief Executive Officer/President .... Thomas A Dzuryachko
Senior VP, Finance .... Daniel Wright
VP, National Dental Director .... Richard Klich, DMD
Vice President, Sales & Marketing .... Martha Hamnick
Vice President, Sales & Marketing .... Wayne Paul

COMPANY PROFILE:
Parent Company Name: Highmark Inc
Doing Business As:
Year Founded: 1987   Federally Qualified: [ ]
Forprofit: [Y]   Not-For-Profit: [ ]
Model Type:
Accreditation: [ ] AAPPO [ ] JACHO [ ] NCQA [ ] URAC
Plan Type: Specialty HMO, Specialty PPO, POS, TPA
Total Revenue: 2005:   2006: 19,523,919
Net Income   2005:   2006:
Total Enrollment:
  2001: 0   2004: 227,243   2007: 0
  2002: 0   2005:
  2003: 229,090 2006:
Medical Loss Ratio: 2005:   2006: 70.80
Administrative Expense Ratio: 2005:   2006:
SERVICE AREA:
Nationwide: N
  DC, DE, MD, VA;
TYPE OF COVERAGE:
Commercial: [Y] Individual: [ ] FEHBP: [ ] Indemnity: [ ]
Medicare: [ ] Medicaid: [ ] Supplemental Medicare: [ ]
Tricare [ ]
PLAN BENEFITS:
Alternative Medicine: [ ]   Behavioral Health: [ ]
Chiropractic: [ ]   Dental: [X]
Home Care: [ ]   Inpatient SNF: [ ]
Long-Term Care: [ ]   Pharm. Mail Order: [ ]
Physical Therapy: [ ]   Podiatry: [ ]
Psychiatric: [ ]   Transplant: [ ]
Vision: [ ]   Wellness: [ ]
Workers' Comp: [ ]
Other Benefits:
Comments:
For enrollment and revenue information see corporate listing, Camp Hill, Pennsylvania.

UNITEDHEALTHCARE & MID ATLANTIC MEDICAL SERVICES INC

10 Taft Court
Rockville, MD 20850
Phone: 301-545-5575 Fax: 301-545-5394 Toll-Free: 800-321-3192
Web site: www.uhc.com
MAILING ADDRESS:
  UNITEDHEALTHCARE & MAMSI
  10 Taft Court
  Rockville, MD 20850

KEY EXECUTIVES:
Non-Executive Chairman .... Richard T Burke
Chief Executive Officer/President .... Thomas P Barbera
Chief Financial Officer .... George L Mikan
Chief Medical Director .... Vera C Dvorak, MD
VP of Sales .... Sue Schenk

COMPANY PROFILE:
Parent Company Name: UnitedHealth Group
Doing Business As:
Year Founded: 1977   Federally Qualified: [Y]
Forprofit: [Y]   Not-For-Profit: [ ]
Model Type: IPA
Accreditation: [ ] AAPPO [ ] JACHO [X] NCQA [ ] URAC
Plan Type: HMO, PPO, POS, EPO, CDHP, HSA, HRA
Total Revenue: 2005:   2006: 469,541,210
Net Income   2005:   2006:
Total Enrollment:
  2001: 0   2004: 177,602   2007: 0
  2002: 187,224 2005:
  2003: 185,902 2006:
Medical Loss Ratio: 2005:   2006: 82.40
Administrative Expense Ratio: 2005:   2006:
SERVICE AREA:
Nationwide: N
  DC; DE; MD; VA;
TYPE OF COVERAGE:
Commercial: [Y] Individual: [Y] FEHBP: [ ] Indemnity: [ ]
Medicare: [Y] Medicaid: [Y] Supplemental Medicare: [Y]
Tricare [ ]

Managed Care Organization Profiles — MARYLAND

SERVICE AREA:
Nationwide: Y
NW:
TYPE OF COVERAGE:
Commercial: [Y] Individual: [ ] FEHBP: [ ] Indemnity: [ ]
Medicare: [ ] Medicaid: [ ] Supplemental Medicare: [ ]
Tricare [ ]
PRODUCTS OFFERED:
Product Name: Type:
Patient Centered Risk Manageme
Utilizaton Management
Disease Management
Individual Large Case Manageme
Telephone Triage & Physician R
Comments:
Former FutureHealth Corporation.

ONENET PPO

4 Taft Court
Rockville, MD 20850
Phone: 301-360-8063 Fax: 301-545-5380 Toll-Free: 800-342-2102
Web site: www.mamsi.com
MAILING ADDRESS:
   ONENET PPO
   4 Taft Court
   Rockville, MD 20850

KEY EXECUTIVES:
Chairman of the Board .... Mark D Groban, MD
Chief Executive Officer .... Thomas P Barbera
President .... John DeRosa
VP Marketing .... Robert Tallent
VP Corporate Communications .... Elizabeth Sammis
VP, Physician Liaison .... Gloria Pilgrim
VP Network Operations/Development .... Robert White
VP of Human Resources .... Judy Graham
VP Quality Improvement .... Sally Duran
VP Claims .... Cathy Fridell
Medical Director Quality Improvemt .... Michael Rosnick MD

COMPANY PROFILE:
Parent Company Name: UnitedHealth Group
Doing Business As: Alliance PPO LLC
Year Founded: 1989   Federally Qualified: [N]
Forprofit: [Y]   Not-For-Profit: [ ]
Model Type: NETWORK
Accreditation: [ ] AAPPO [ ] JACHO [ ] NCQA [ ] URAC
Plan Type: PPO, TPA
Total Enrollment:
   2001: 1,800,000   2004: 0   2007: 0
   2002: 0   2005:
   2003: 0   2006:
SERVICE AREA:
Nationwide: N
   DC; DE; MD; NC; PA; VA; WV;
TYPE OF COVERAGE:
Commercial: [Y] Individual: [ ] FEHBP: [ ] Indemnity: [ ]
Medicare: [ ] Medicaid: [ ] Supplemental Medicare: [ ]
Tricare [ ]
PRODUCTS OFFERED:
Product Name: Type:
Alliance PPO LLC   PPO
PLAN BENEFITS:
Alternative Medicine: [ ]   Behavioral Health: [X]
Chiropractic: [X]   Dental: [X]
Home Care: [X]   Inpatient SNF: [ ]
Long-Term Care: [ ]   Pharm. Mail Order: [X]
Physical Therapy: [ ]   Podiatry: [X]
Psychiatric: [X]   Transplant: [X]
Vision: [X]   Wellness: [X]
Workers' Comp: [X]
Other Benefits: Outpatient SNF

OPTIMUM CHOICE INC

4 Taft Court
Rockville, MD 20850
Phone: 301-360-8040 Fax: 301-545-5394 Toll-Free: 800-544-2853
Web site: www.mamsi.com
MAILING ADDRESS:
   OPTIMUM CHOICE INC
   4 Taft Court
   Rockville, MD 20850

KEY EXECUTIVES:
Chairman of the Board .... Mark D Groban, MD
Chief Executive Officer/President .... Thomas P Barbera
Chief Financial Officer .... Robert Foss
Pharmacy Director .... Wendy Toler
Chief Information Officer .... L Gray Johnson, Jr
Marketing Director .... Susan A Goff
VP of Corporate Comm .... Elizabeth Sammis
Provider Services Director .... Anita Bitter
Network Development/Contracts .... J Stevens DuFresne
VP of Human Resources .... Judy Graham
VP of Quality Assurance .... Sally Duran
VP of Marketing .... Debbie Hulen

COMPANY PROFILE:
Parent Company Name: UnitedHealth Group
Doing Business As:
Year Founded: 1987   Federally Qualified: [N]
Forprofit: [Y]   Not-For-Profit: [ ]
Model Type: IPA
Accreditation: [ ] AAPPO [ ] JACHO [X] NCQA [ ] URAC
Plan Type: HMO
Total Enrollment:
   2001: 0   2004: 0   2007: 0
   2002: 444,238   2005:
   2003: 427,818   2006:
SERVICE AREA:
Nationwide: N
   DC; DE; MD; NC; PA; VA; WV;
TYPE OF COVERAGE:
Commercial: [Y] Individual: [Y] FEHBP: [ ] Indemnity: [ ]
Medicare: [Y] Medicaid: [Y] Supplemental Medicare: [ ]
Tricare [ ]
PRODUCTS OFFERED:
Product Name: Type:
Optimum Choice Advantage   Medicare
Optimum Choice Inc   Medicaid
PLAN BENEFITS:
Alternative Medicine: [ ]   Behavioral Health: [X]
Chiropractic: [X]   Dental: [X]
Home Care: [X]   Inpatient SNF: [ ]
Long-Term Care: [ ]   Pharm. Mail Order: [X]
Physical Therapy: [ ]   Podiatry: [X]
Psychiatric: [X]   Transplant: [X]
Vision: [X]   Wellness: [X]
Workers' Comp: [ ]
Other Benefits: Outpatient SNF

OPTIMUM CHOICE OF THE CAROLINA INC

4 Taft Court
Rockville, MD 20850
Phone: 301-545-5914 Fax: 301-545-5385 Toll-Free: 800-347-1965
Web site: www.uhc.com
MAILING ADDRESS:
   OPTIMUM CHOICE OF CAROLINAS
   4 Taft Court
   Rockville, MD 20850

KEY EXECUTIVES:
Chief Executive Officer .... Thomas P Barbera
President .... Thomas P Barbera
Medical Director .... C Franklin Church, MD

COMPANY PROFILE:
Parent Company Name: UnitedHealth Group
Doing Business As:
Year Founded: 1995   Federally Qualified: [ ]
Forprofit: [Y]   Not-For-Profit: [ ]
Model Type:
Accreditation: [ ] AAPPO [ ] JACHO [ ] NCQA [ ] URAC
Plan Type: HMO,
Total Enrollment:
   2001: 0   2004: 8,379   2007: 0
   2002: 0   2005:
   2003: 12,988   2006:

MARYLAND

MD-INDIVIDUAL PRACTICE ASSOCIATION INC (MD IPA)

4 Taft Court
Rockville, MD 20850
Phone: 301-762-8205 Fax: 301-545-5388 Toll-Free: 800-544-2853
Web site: www.mamsi.com

MAILING ADDRESS:
MD-INDIVIDUAL PRACTICE ASSOCIATION INC
4 Taft Court
Rockville, MD 20850

KEY EXECUTIVES:
Chairman of the Board .... Mark D Groban, MD
Chief Executive Officer .... Thomas P Barbera
President .... Susan A Goff
Chief Financial Officer .... Christopher E Mackail
Chief Information Officer .... Larry Mauzy
Chief Operating Officer .... Catherine Ramey
Senior VP of Corp Communications .... Elizabeth Sammis
Provider Services Director .... Anita Gray
Senior VP of Network Operations/Development .... Robert White
VP of Human Resources .... Judy Graham
Senior VP of Quality Improvement .... Sally Duran
Senior VP of Marketing .... Debbie Hulen
Medical Director Quality Improvement .... Michael Rosnick MD

COMPANY PROFILE:
Parent Company Name: UnitedHealth Group
Doing Business As:
Year Founded: 1979   Federally Qualified: [Y]
Forprofit: [Y]   Not-For-Profit: [ ]
Model Type: IPA
Accreditation: [ ] AAPPO [ ] JACHO [X] NCQA [ ] URAC
Plan Type: HMO, PPO
Total Revenue: 2005:   2006:   11,184,836
Net Income   2005:   2006:   44,381,870
Total Enrollment:
  2001: 832,300   2004: 208,643   2007: 0
  2002: 176,319   2005: 3,039
  2003: 204,262   2006: 3,167

SERVICE AREA:
Nationwide: N
  DC; MD; VA;

TYPE OF COVERAGE:
Commercial: [Y] Individual: [ ] FEHBP: [ ] Indemnity: [ ]
Medicare: [ ] Medicaid: [ ] Supplemental Medicare: [ ]
Tricare   [ ]

PRODUCTS OFFERED:
Product Name: Type:
Alliance PPO LLC   PPO
Optimum Choice Inc   HMO

PLAN BENEFITS:
Alternative Medicine: [ ]   Behavioral Health: [X]
Chiropractic: [X]   Dental: [X]
Home Care: [X]   Inpatient SNF: [ ]
Long-Term Care: [ ]   Pharm. Mail Order: [X]
Physical Therapy: [ ]   Podiatry: [X]
Psychiatric: [X]   Transplant: [X]
Vision: [X]   Wellness: [X]
Workers' Comp: [X]
Other Benefits: Outpatient SNF

MID ATLANTIC MEDICAL SERVICES INC (MAMSI)-CORPORATE HEADQUARTERS

10 Taft Court
Rockville, MD 20850
Phone: 301-762-8205 Fax: 301-738-1230 Toll-Free:
Web site: www.mamsi.com

MAILING ADDRESS:
MID ATLANTIC MED SERVICES INC
10 Taft Court
Rockville, MD 20850

KEY EXECUTIVES:
Chairman of the Board .... Mark D Groban, MD
Chief Executive Officer/President .... Thomas P Barbera
Chief Financial Officer .... Robert Foss
Chief Information Officer .... Larry Mauzy
Executive VP, Marketing .... Susan A Goff
Senior VP, Corp Communicatons .... Elizabeth Sammis
Senior VP, Provider Networks .... Robert White
VP of Human Resources .... Judy Graham
Senior VP, Quality Improvement .... Sally Duran
Senior VP, Marketing .... Debra Hulen
Med Dir of Quality Improvement .... Michael Rosnick, MD

COMPANY PROFILE:
Parent Company Name: UnitedHealth Group
Doing Business As: Alliance PPO, LLC
Year Founded: 1987   Federally Qualified: [Y]
Forprofit: [Y]   Not-For-Profit: [ ]
Model Type: IPA
Accreditation: [ ] AAPPO [ ] JACHO [X] NCQA [ ] URAC
Plan Type: HMO, PPO, POS
Total Enrollment:
  2001: 1,800,000   2004: 1,900,000 2007: 0
  2002: 0   2005:
  2003: 0   2006:

SERVICE AREA:
Nationwide: N
  DC; DE; MD; NC; PA; VA; WV;

TYPE OF COVERAGE:
Commercial: [Y] Individual: [Y] FEHBP: [ ] Indemnity: [ ]
Medicare: [Y] Medicaid: [Y] Supplemental Medicare: [Y]
Tricare   [ ]

PRODUCTS OFFERED:
Product Name: Type:
Alliance PPO, LLC
Optimum Choice Inc
MD IPA
MAMSI Life and Health Insuranc

NATIONWIDE BETTER HEALTH

300 Clubhouse Rd Ste 100
Hunt Valley, MD 21031
Phone: 410-891-3300 Fax: 410-329-1940 Toll-Free:
Web site: www.nwbetterhealth.com

MAILING ADDRESS:
NATIONWIDE BETTER HEALTH
300 Clubhouse Rd Ste 100
Hunt Valley, MD 21031

KEY EXECUTIVES:
Chairman .... Claire B Rosse
Chief Executive Officer/President .... Claire B Rosse
Controller .... Donna Stewart
Corporate Medical Director .... Neil Gordan, MD
Chief Operating Officer .... Vishu Jhaveri, MD
Chief Marketing Officer .... Steve Hart
VP Sales .... Pat Curran
Director of Communications .... Kristen Barber
VP, Human Resources .... Jim Waller
VP, Quality Assurance .... Jodi Dunn
VP of Client Services .... John Kunkle
Vice Chairman Board .... Carl Sardegna
VP of Client Services .... Kim Tawney
VP of Client Services .... Paula M Hrr

COMPANY PROFILE:
Parent Company Name:
Doing Business As:
Year Founded: 1992   Federally Qualified: [ ]
Forprofit: [Y]   Not-For-Profit: [ ]
Model Type:
Accreditation: [ ] AAPPO [ ] JACHO [ ] NCQA [X] URAC
Plan Type: UR
Total Enrollment:
  2001: 450,000   2004: 0   2007: 0
  2002: 0   2005:
  2003: 0   2006:

Managed Care Organization Profiles — MARYLAND

KEY EXECUTIVES:
Chief Executive Officer .... Paul Gustrand
President .... Karen Schievelbein
Chief Financial Officer .... Mete Sahin
Chief Operating Officer .... Karen Schievelbein
Senior VP Marketing .... Susan E Cox
Director of Provider Services .... Jill Schultze-Evans

COMPANY PROFILE:
Parent Company Name: UnitedHealth Group
Doing Business As: Dental Benefit Providers
Year Founded: 1984   Federally Qualified: [N]
Forprofit: [Y]   Not-For-Profit: [ ]
Model Type: NETWORK
Accreditation: [ ] AAPPO [ ] JACHO [ ] NCQA [ ] URAC
Plan Type: Specialty HMO, Specialty PPO, ASO, POS, EPO,
Total Revenue: 2005:   2006: 4,667,284
Net Income   2005:   2006:
Total Enrollment:
   2001: 2,000,000   2004: 7,070   2007: 6,600,000
   2002: 0   2005:
   2003: 7,600   2006: 5,000,000
Medical Loss Ratio: 2005:   2006: 87.30
Administrative Expense Ratio: 2005:   2006:

SERVICE AREA:
Nationwide: N
   CA; CO; CT; DC; FL; GA; IA; ID; IL; IN; KS; KY; MA; MD; MI; MO; NH; NJ; NY; OH; PA; RI; TX; VA; WA;

TYPE OF COVERAGE:
Commercial: [Y] Individual: [ ] FEHBP: [ ] Indemnity: [Y]
Medicare: [Y] Medicaid: [Y] Supplemental Medicare: [ ]
Tricare   [ ]

PLAN BENEFITS:
Alternative Medicine: [ ]   Behavioral Health: [ ]
Chiropractic: [ ]   Dental: [X]
Home Care: [ ]   Inpatient SNF: [ ]
Long-Term Care: [ ]   Pharm. Mail Order: [ ]
Physical Therapy: [ ]   Podiatry: [ ]
Psychiatric: [ ]   Transplant: [ ]
Vision: [ ]   Wellness: [ ]
Workers' Comp: [ ]
Other Benefits:

HUMANA INC - MARYLAND

201 W Main St 6th Fl
Louisville, KY 40202
Phone: 502-580-5005 Fax: 502-580-5044 Toll-Free:
Web site: www.humana.com

MAILING ADDRESS:
   HUMANA INC - MARYLAND
   PO Box 740023
   Louisville, KY 40202

KEY EXECUTIVES:
Chairman of the Board .... David A Jones Jr
Chief Executive Officer/President .... Michael B McCallister
Chief Financial Officer .... James H Bloem
Senior VP, Chief Innovation Officer .... Jonathan T Lord, MD
Senior VP Chief Information Officer .... Bruce J Goodman
Chief Operating Officer .... Jim Murray
Chief Marketing Officer .... Steve Moya
Senior VP Human Resources .... Bonnie C Hathcock

COMPANY PROFILE:
Parent Company Name: Humana Inc
Doing Business As:
Year Founded: 1961   Federally Qualified: [Y]
Forprofit: [Y]   Not-For-Profit: [ ]
Model Type: IPA
Accreditation: [ ] AAPPO [ ] JACHO [ ] NCQA [ ] URAC
Plan Type: PPO, ASO, CDHP, HSA

SERVICE AREA:
Nationwide: N
   MD;

TYPE OF COVERAGE:
Commercial: [Y] Individual: [ ] FEHBP: [ ] Indemnity: [ ]
Medicare: [ ] Medicaid: [ ] Supplemental Medicare: [ ]
Tricare   [ ]

CONSUMER-DRIVEN PRODUCTS
JP Morgan Chase   HSA Company
HumanaOne HSA   HSA Product
JP Morgan Chase   HSA Administrator
Personal Care Account   Consumer-Driven Health Plan
HumanaOne   High Deductible Health Plan

PLAN BENEFITS:
Alternative Medicine: [ ]   Behavioral Health: [ ]
Chiropractic: [X]   Dental: [X]
Home Care: [ ]   Inpatient SNF: [ ]
Long-Term Care: [ ]   Pharm. Mail Order: [X]
Physical Therapy: [ ]   Podiatry: [ ]
Psychiatric: [X]   Transplant: [X]
Vision: [ ]   Wellness: [X]
Workers' Comp: [X]
Other Benefits: Long Term Disability Care

KAISER FOUNDATION HEALTH PLAN - MID ATLANTIC STATES

2101 E Jefferson St
Rockville, MD 20853
Phone: 301-816-2424 Fax: 301-816-7470 Toll-Free: 800-368-5784
Web site: www.kp.org

MAILING ADDRESS:
   KAISER FNDTN HLTH PLN-MID ATL
   2101 E Jefferson St
   Rockville, MD 20853

KEY EXECUTIVES:
Chief Executive Officer/President .... Marilyn Kowamura
Chief Financial Officer .... Andee Petersen
Medical Director of Mid-Atlantic .... Philip S Carney, MD
Director, Provider Services .... Cynthia Marquardt

COMPANY PROFILE:
Parent Company Name: Kaiser Permanente
Doing Business As:
Year Founded: 1972   Federally Qualified: [Y]
Forprofit: [ ]   Not-For-Profit: [Y]
Model Type: GROUP
Accreditation: [ ] AAPPO [ ] JACHO [X] NCQA [ ] URAC
Plan Type: HMO, POS, HSA
Total Revenue: 2005:   2006: 1,721,645,373
Net Income   2005:   2006:
Total Enrollment:
   2001: 545,064   2004: 485,045   2007: 507,630
   2002: 507,543   2005: 500,194
   2003: 493,436   2006:
Medical Loss Ratio: 2005:   2006: 90.60
Administrative Expense Ratio: 2005:   2006:

SERVICE AREA:
Nationwide: N
   DC; MD; VA;

TYPE OF COVERAGE:
Commercial: [Y] Individual: [Y] FEHBP: [ ] Indemnity: [ ]
Medicare: [Y] Medicaid: [ ] Supplemental Medicare: [ ]
Tricare   [ ]

PRODUCTS OFFERED:
Product Name: Type:
Kaiser Permanente
Kaiser HMO
Senior Advantage   Medicare Advantage
Medicare Plus   Medicare

PLAN BENEFITS:
Alternative Medicine: [ ]   Behavioral Health: [X]
Chiropractic: [X]   Dental: [X]
Home Care: [X]   Inpatient SNF: [X]
Long-Term Care: [ ]   Pharm. Mail Order: [X]
Physical Therapy: [X]   Podiatry: [X]
Psychiatric: [X]   Transplant: [X]
Vision: [X]   Wellness: [X]
Workers' Comp: [ ]
Other Benefits:

MARYLAND

Managed Care Organization Profiles

COMPANY PROFILE:
Parent Company Name:
Doing Business As:
Year Founded: 1998 Federally Qualified: [ ]
Forprofit: [Y] Not-For-Profit: [ ]
Model Type:
Accreditation: [ ] AAPPO [ ] JACHO [ ] NCQA [ ] URAC
Plan Type: HMO, PPO, POS, CDHP, HDHP, HSA
Total Revenue: 2005: 6,611,246,000 2006: 7,733,756,000
Net Income 2005: 501,639,000 2006: 560,045,000
Total Enrollment:
    2001: 1,840,726 2004: 2,509,000 2007: 4,090,000
    2002: 2,035,000 2005: 2,546,000
    2003: 2,383,000 2006: 4,077,000
Medical Loss Ratio: 2005: 79.40 2006: 78.40
Administrative Expense Ratio: 2005: 12.00 2006: 17.30

SERVICE AREA:
Nationwide: N
    DE; GA; IA; IL; IN; LA; KS; MO; NC; NE; OH; PA; VA; WV;

TYPE OF COVERAGE:
Commercial: [Y] Individual: [ ] FEHBP: [ ] Indemnity: [Y]
Medicare: [Y] Medicaid: [Y] Supplemental Medicare: [ ]
Tricare [ ]

CONSUMER-DRIVEN PRODUCTS
Wells Fargo HSA Company
      HSA Product
Corporate Benefits Srvs of Am HSA Administrator Consumer-Driven Health Plan
Open Access Plus Plan High Deductible Health Plan

PLAN BENEFITS:
Alternative Medicine: [ ] Behavioral Health: [X]
Chiropractic: [X] Dental: [X]
Home Care: [X] Inpatient SNF: [X]
Long-Term Care: [X] Pharm. Mail Order: [X]
Physical Therapy: [X] Podiatry: [X]
Psychiatric: [X] Transplant: [X]
Vision: [X] Wellness: [ ]
Workers' Comp: [ ]
Other Benefits:

Comments:
Acquisitions: American Service Company, 1987; HealthAmerica Pennsylvania Inc, 1988; Group Health Plan Inc, St Louis, MO 1990;

DELMARVA HEALTH CARE PLAN INC

301 Bay St Ste 401
Easton, MD 21401
Phone: 410-822-7223 Fax: 410-822-8152 Toll-Free: 800-334-3427
Web site: www.delmarvahealthplan.com
MAILING ADDRESS:
    DELMARVA HEALTH CARE PLAN INC
    10455 Mill Run Circle
    Owings Mills, MD 21401

KEY EXECUTIVES:
Chairman .... Michael R Merson
Chief Executive Officer/President .... Chester Burrell
Chief Financial Officer .... G Mark Chaney
Senior VP Chief Medical Officer .... Jon Shematek, MD
Pharmacy Director .... Winston Wong, PharmD
Senior VP, Chief Information Officer .... Ted Dellavecchia
Executive VP, Operations .... Leon Kaplan
Executive VP & Chief Marketing Officer .... Gregory A Devou
Executive VP, Med Systems Corp Development .... David D Wolf
VP, Corporate Communications .... Maria Harris Tildon

COMPANY PROFILE:
Parent Company Name: CareFirst Inc
Doing Business As: CareFirst BlueCross BlueShield
Year Founded: 1982 Federally Qualified: [N]
Forprofit: [Y] Not-For-Profit: [ ]
Model Type: IPA
Accreditation: [ ] AAPPO [ ] JACHO [ ] NCQA [ ] URAC
Plan Type: HMO, POS
Total Enrollment:
    2001: 12,510 2004: 42 2007: 0
    2002: 1,273 2005:
    2003: 45 2006:

SERVICE AREA:
Nationwide: N
    DE (Kent, New Castle, Sussex); MD (Caroline, Cecil, Dorchester, Harford, Kent, Queen Annes, Somerset, Talbot, Wicomico, Worcester);

TYPE OF COVERAGE:
Commercial: [Y] Individual: [Y] FEHBP: [ ] Indemnity: [ ]
Medicare: [ ] Medicaid: [ ] Supplemental Medicare: [Y]
Tricare [ ]

PRODUCTS OFFERED:
Product Name: Type:
Delmarva Health Plan HMO

PLAN BENEFITS:
Alternative Medicine: [ ] Behavioral Health: [X]
Chiropractic: [ ] Dental: [X]
Home Care: [X] Inpatient SNF: [X]
Long-Term Care: [X] Pharm. Mail Order: [X]
Physical Therapy: [X] Podiatry: [X]
Psychiatric: [X] Transplant: [X]
Vision: [X] Wellness: [X]
Workers' Comp: [ ]
Other Benefits:

DENTA QUEST MID-ATLANTIC INC

4061 Powder Mill Rd #325
Calverton, MD 20705
Phone: 301-937-4447 Fax: 301-937-0245 Toll-Free: 800-879-0288
Web site: www.dentaquest.com
MAILING ADDRESS:
    DENTA QUEST MID-ATLANTIC INC
    4061 Powder Mill Rd #325
    Calverton, MD 20705

KEY EXECUTIVES:
President .... Christopher J Niceley
Treasurer .... Scott F O'Gorman
Chief Dental Officer .... Doyle Williams, DDS
Marketing Director .... Dennis Leonard
Director, Provider Services/Quality Assurance .... Trina Gotkin
Administration Director .... Lynn Redmond

COMPANY PROFILE:
Parent Company Name: Denta Quest Ventures Inc
Doing Business As:
Year Founded: 1980 Federally Qualified: [N]
Forprofit: [Y] Not-For-Profit: [ ]
Model Type:
Accreditation: [ ] AAPPO [ ] JACHO [ ] NCQA [ ] URAC
Plan Type: Specialty HMO, Specialty PPO, ASO
Total Revenue: 2005: 2006: 15,853,897
Net Income 2005: 2006:
Total Enrollment:
    2001: 102,435 2004: 130,471 2007: 0
    2002: 120,096 2005:
    2003: 110,344 2006:
Medical Loss Ratio: 2005: 2006: 56.90
Administrative Expense Ratio: 2005: 2006:

SERVICE AREA:
Nationwide: N
    MD; VA;

PLAN BENEFITS:
Alternative Medicine: [ ] Behavioral Health: [ ]
Chiropractic: [ ] Dental: [X]
Home Care: [ ] Inpatient SNF: [ ]
Long-Term Care: [ ] Pharm. Mail Order: [ ]
Physical Therapy: [ ] Podiatry: [ ]
Psychiatric: [ ] Transplant: [ ]
Vision: [ ] Wellness: [ ]
Workers' Comp: [ ]
Other Benefits:

Comments:
Formerly Consumer Dental Care Company.

DENTAL BENEFIT PROVIDERS INC

800 King Farm Blvd Ste 600
Rockville, MD 20850
Phone: 240-632-8000 Fax: 240-632-8100 Toll-Free: 800-445-9090
Web site: www.dbp-inc.com
MAILING ADDRESS:
    DENTAL BENEFIT PROVIDERS INC
    800 King Farm Blvd Ste 600
    Rockville, MD 20850

Managed Care Organization Profiles   MARYLAND

Total Revenue: 2005: 5,168,942,000 2006: 5,510,184,000
Net Income   2005:   118,503,000 2006:   164,256,000
Total Enrollment:
   2001: 3,101,535   2004: 3,300,000   2007: 3,100,000
   2002: 6,100,000   2005: 3,400,000
   2003: 3,200,000   2006: 3,000,000
Medical Loss Ratio: 2005:   2006:
Administrative Expense Ratio: 2005:   2006:

SERVICE AREA:
Nationwide: N
   DC; MD; VA; DE;

TYPE OF COVERAGE:
Commercial: [Y] Individual: [Y] FEHBP: [Y] Indemnity: [Y]
Medicare: [Y] Medicaid: [ ] Supplemental Medicare: [Y]
Tricare   [ ]

PRODUCTS OFFERED:
Product Name:	Type:
CareFirst PPO	PPO
CareFirst Blue Choice	HMO
Preferred Health Network	HMO
Delmarva	HMO
FreeState	HMO

CONSUMER-DRIVEN PRODUCTS
	HSA Company
CareFirst HSA	HSA Product
	HSA Administrator
	Consumer-Driven Health Plan
	High Deductible Health Plan

PLAN BENEFITS:
Alternative Medicine: [X]   Behavioral Health: [ ]
Chiropractic: [X]   Dental: [X]
Home Care: [X]   Inpatient SNF: [ ]
Long-Term Care: [ ]   Pharm. Mail Order: [X]
Physical Therapy: [ ]   Podiatry: [X]
Psychiatric: [X]   Transplant: [X]
Vision: [X]   Wellness: [X]
Workers' Comp: [ ]
Other Benefits:

Comments:
CareFirst Inc completed acquisition of Blue Cross Blue Shield of Delaware in March, 2000.

CIGNA DENTAL HEALTH OF MARYLAND INC

1571 Sawgrass Corporate Pkwy
Sunrise, FL 33323
Phone: 954-514-6600 Fax: 954-423-5491 Toll-Free: 800-367-1037
Web site: www.cigna.com/dental

MAILING ADDRESS:
   CIGNA DENTAL HEALTH OF MD INC
   1571 Sawgrass Corporate Pkwy
   Sunrise, FL 33323

KEY EXECUTIVES:
Chief Executive Officer .... H Edward Hanway
President .... Karen S Rohan
Dental Director .... Ed Schooley, DDS
Marketing Director .... Samantha Snyder
MIS Director .... Laurel A Flebotte

COMPANY PROFILE:
Parent Company Name: CIGNA Dental Health Inc
Doing Business As: CIGNA Dental
Year Founded: 1986   Federally Qualified: [N]
Forprofit: [Y]   Not-For-Profit: [ ]
Model Type:
Accreditation: [ ] AAPPO [ ] JACHO [ ] NCQA [ ] URAC
Plan Type: Specialty HMO
Total Revenue: 2005:   2006: 14,152,212
Net Income   2005:   2006:
Total Enrollment:
   2001: 0   2004: 0   2007: 0
   2002: 94,991   2005:
   2003: 0   2006:
Medical Loss Ratio: 2005:   2006: 52.30
Administrative Expense Ratio: 2005:   2006:

SERVICE AREA:
Nationwide: N
   MD;

TYPE OF COVERAGE:
Commercial: [Y] Individual: [ ] FEHBP: [ ] Indemnity: [ ]
Medicare: [ ] Medicaid: [ ] Supplemental Medicare: [ ]
Tricare   [ ]

PRODUCTS OFFERED:
Product Name:	Type:
Cigna Dental Health	HMO

PLAN BENEFITS:
Alternative Medicine: [ ]   Behavioral Health: [ ]
Chiropractic: [ ]   Dental: [X]
Home Care: [ ]   Inpatient SNF: [ ]
Long-Term Care: [ ]   Pharm. Mail Order: [ ]
Physical Therapy: [ ]   Podiatry: [ ]
Psychiatric: [ ]   Transplant: [ ]
Vision: [ ]   Wellness: [ ]
Workers' Comp: [ ]
Other Benefits:

CIGNA HEALTHCARE OF MID-ATLANTIC INC

10490 Little Patuxent Pkwy 400
Columbia, MD 21044
Phone: 410-884-2500 Fax: 410-720-5860 Toll-Free:
Web site: www.cigna.com

MAILING ADDRESS:
   CIGNA HLTHCR OF MID-ATL INC
   10490 Little Patuxent Pkwy 400
   Columbia, MD 21044

KEY EXECUTIVES:
President .... Thomas Martel
Medical Director .... Richard M Fornadel, MD
Market Medical Executive .... Collette Edwards, MD

COMPANY PROFILE:
Parent Company Name: CIGNA Corporation
Doing Business As:
Year Founded: Federally Qualified: [ ]
Forprofit: [ ]   Not-For-Profit: [ ]
Model Type:
Accreditation: [ ] AAPPO [ ] JACHO [ ] NCQA [ ] URAC
Plan Type: HMO
Total Revenue: 2005:   2006: 469,261,434
Net Income   2005:   2006:
Total Enrollment:
   2001: 0   2004: 16,687   2007: 0
   2002: 0   2005:
   2003: 0   2006:
Medical Loss Ratio: 2005:   2006: 84.70
Administrative Expense Ratio: 2005:   2006:

SERVICE AREA:
Nationwide:
   DC; MD; VA;

TYPE OF COVERAGE:
Commercial: [ ] Individual: [ ] FEHBP: [ ] Indemnity: [ ]
Medicare: [ ] Medicaid: [ ] Supplemental Medicare: [ ]
Tricare   [ ]

COVENTRY HEALTH CARE INC — CORPORATE HEADQUARTERS

6705 Rockledge Dr Ste 900
Bethesda, MD 20817
Phone: 301-581-0600 Fax: 301-493-0700 Toll-Free:
Web site: www.cvty.com

MAILING ADDRESS:
   COVENTRY HEALTH CARE INC
   6705 Rockledge Dr Ste 900
   Bethesda, MD 20817

KEY EXECUTIVES:
Chairman of the Board .... John H Austin, MD
Chief Executive Officer .... Dale B Wolf
President .... Thomas P McDonough
Executive VP, Chief Financial Officer .... Shawn M Guertin
Senior VP, Chief Medical Officer .... Bernard J Mansheim, MD
Executive VP, Chief Information Officer .... Harvey C DeMovick, Jr
Executive VP Chief Operating Officer .... Thomas P McDonough
Senior VP, Chief Marketing & Sales .... J Stewart Lavelle
VP, Chief Human Resources Officer .... Patrisha L Davis
Executive VP, Health Plan Operations .... Francis S Soistman Jr
VP Investors Relations .... Drew Asher
VP of Business Development .... John J Stelben
VP Decision Support/Product Development .... Peter Clay
VP, Pharmaceutical Services .... James R Hailey

MARYLAND

COMPANY PROFILE:
Parent Company Name:
Doing Business As:
Year Founded: 1992   Federally Qualified: [ ]
Forprofit: [Y]   Not-For-Profit: [ ]
Model Type:
Accreditation: [ ] AAPPO [ ] JACHO [X] NCQA [X] URAC
Plan Type: Specialty HMO, Specialty PPO, ASO
Total Enrollment:
    2001: 0   2004: 12,000,000   2007: 20,000,000
    2002: 0   2005: 20,000,000
    2003: 9,300,000   2006: 20,000,000
SERVICE AREA:
Nationwide:
    NW;
TYPE OF COVERAGE:
Commercial: [Y] Individual: [ ] FEHBP: [ ] Indemnity: [ ]
Medicare: [Y] Medicaid: [Y] Supplemental Medicare: [ ]
Tricare   [ ]
PLAN BENEFITS:
Alternative Medicine:	[ ]	Behavioral Health:	[X]
Chiropractic:	[ ]	Dental:	[ ]
Home Care:	[ ]	Inpatient SNF:	[ ]
Long-Term Care:	[ ]	Pharm. Mail Order:	[ ]
Physical Therapy:	[ ]	Podiatry:	[ ]
Psychiatric:	[ ]	Transplant:	[ ]
Vision:	[ ]	Wellness:	[ ]
Workers' Comp:	[ ]		

Other Benefits:

BRAVO HEALTH INC

3601 O'Donnell St
Baltimore, MD 21224
Phone: 410-864-4460 Fax: 410-864-4467 Toll-Free: 888-863-3637
Web site: www.elderhealth.com
MAILING ADDRESS:
    BRAVO HEALTH INC
    3601 O'Donnell St
    Baltimore, MD 21224

KEY EXECUTIVES:
Chief Executive Officer .... Jeff Folick
Chief Financial Officer .... Scott Tabakin
Executive VP, Chief Medical Officer .... Ace M Hodgin, MD
Chief Information Officer .... Greg Pontius
Executive VP, Sales & Marketing .... Scott Ptacek
VP, Network Development .... Paul Staudenmeier
VP, Human Resources .... Susan Coe
Executive VP, Health Care Delivery .... Jason Feuerman
VP, Part D Program .... Tom Rim
VP, Senior Medical Director .... David Yalowitz, MD

COMPANY PROFILE:
Parent Company Name:
Doing Business As:
Year Founded: 1996   Federally Qualified: [ ]
Forprofit: [Y]   Not-For-Profit: [ ]
Model Type:
Accreditation: [ ] AAPPO [ ] JACHO [ ] NCQA [ ] URAC
Plan Type: HMO
Total Enrollment:
    2001: 0   2004: 0   2007: 71,000
    2002: 0   2005:
    2003: 0   2006:
SERVICE AREA:
Nationwide:
    CA; DC; DE; FL; IL; MD; MI; NJ; NY; OH; PA; TX; WV;
TYPE OF COVERAGE:
Commercial: [ ] Individual: [ ] FEHBP: [ ] Indemnity: [ ]
Medicare: [Y] Medicaid: [ ] Supplemental Medicare: [ ]
Tricare   [ ]
Comments:
Formerly Elder Health Inc.

BRAVO HEALTH MID-ATLANTIC INC

3601 O'Donnell St
Baltimore, MD 21224
Phone: 410-864-4460 Fax: 410-864-4467 Toll-Free: 888-863-3637
Web site: www.elderhealth.com
MAILING ADDRESS:
    BRAVO HEALTH MID-ATLANTIC INC
    3601 O'Donnell St
    Baltimore, MD 21224

KEY EXECUTIVES:
Chief Executive Officer .... Jeff Folick
VP, Executive Director .... Mary Ann Eull
Chief Financial Officer .... Scott Tabakin
Executive VP, Chief Medical Officer .... Ace M Hodgin, MD
VP, Sales & Marketing .... Scott Ptacek

COMPANY PROFILE:
Parent Company Name: Bravo Health Inc
Doing Business As:
Year Founded: 1996   Federally Qualified: [ ]
Forprofit: [Y]   Not-For-Profit: [ ]
Model Type:
Accreditation: [ ] AAPPO [ ] JACHO [ ] NCQA [ ] URAC
Plan Type: HMO
Total Enrollment:
    2001: 0   2004: 4,410   2007: 0
    2002: 2,443   2005: 6,975
    2003: 3,113   2006: 7,971
SERVICE AREA:
Nationwide:
    DC; DE; MD;
TYPE OF COVERAGE:
Commercial: [ ] Individual: [ ] FEHBP: [ ] Indemnity: [ ]
Medicare: [Y] Medicaid: [ ] Supplemental Medicare: [ ]
Tricare   [ ]
PRODUCTS OFFERED:
Product Name:	Type:
Medichoice of Baltimore	Medicare
Medichoice of Maryland	Medicare

Comments:
Formerly Elder Health Inc.

CAREFIRST BLUE CROSS BLUE SHIELD

10455 Mill Run Circle
Owings Mills, MD 21117
Phone: 410-581-3000 Fax: 410-998-5351 Toll-Free:
Web site: www.carefirst.com
MAILING ADDRESS:
    CAREFIRST BLUE CROSS/BLUE SHIELD
    10455 Mill Run Circle
    Owings Mills, MD 21117

KEY EXECUTIVES:
Chairman .... Michael R Merson
Chief Executive Officer/President .... Chester Burrell
Chief Financial Officer .... G Mark Chaney
Senior VP Chief Medical Officer .... Jon Shematek, MD
Pharmacy Director .... Winston Wong, PharmD
Senior VP, Chief Information Officer .... Ted Dellavecchia
Executive VP, Operations .... Leon Kaplan
ExecutiveVP & Chief Marketing Officer .... Gregory A Devou
ExecutiveVP, Med Systems Corp Development .... David D Wolf
VP, Corporate Communications .... Maria Tildon
Director Provider Network Management .... Stacy Breidenstein
VP Network Management .... Bruce Edwards
Director Health Communications/Commun Relations .. Karen Pointon
Senior VP Human Resources .... Sharon Vecchioni
Director of Quality Assurance .... Wanda Lessner
Director New Business Development .... Sandy Beard
Senior VP & General Auditor .... Gwendoyln Skillern
Senior VP Strategic Marketing & Analysis .... Rita Costello
VP, Senior Med Director, Med Affairs .... Daniel Winn, MD

COMPANY PROFILE:
Parent Company Name: CareFirst Inc
Doing Business As: CareFirst BC/BS
Year Founded: 1937   Federally Qualified: [ ]
Forprofit: [ ]   Not-For-Profit: [Y]
Model Type: MIXED
Accreditation: [ ] AAPPO [ ] JACHO [X] NCQA [ ] URAC
Plan Type: HMO, POS, ASO, TPA, PBM, CDHP, HSA
Primary Physicians: 4,500   Physician Specialists:
Hospitals: 165

Managed Care Organization Profiles **MARYLAND**

AETNA INC - MARYLAND

1302 Concourse Dr Ste 402
Linthicum, MD 21090
Phone: 410-691-1080 Fax: 410-691-1198 Toll-Free: 800-328-8742
Web site: www.aetna.com
MAILING ADDRESS:
   AETNA INC - MARYLAND
   1302 Concourse Dr Ste 402
   Linthicum, MD 21090

KEY EXECUTIVES:
Chairman of the Board/Chief Executive Officer .... Ronald A Williams
President .... Mark T Bertolini
Executive VP, Finance .... Joseph M Zubretsky
Senior Medical Director .... Rick Fornadel, MD

COMPANY PROFILE:
Parent Company Name: Aetna Inc
Doing Business As:
Year Founded: 1987   Federally Qualified: [Y]
Forprofit: [Y]   Not-For-Profit: [ ]
Model Type: IPA
Accreditation: [ ] AAPPO [ ] JACHO [ ] NCQA [ ] URAC
Plan Type: HMO, PPO, POS, CDHP, HSA
Total Revenue: 2005:   2006: 715,122,403
Net Income 2005:   2006:
Total Enrollment:
   2001: 0   2004: 233,251   2007: 0
   2002: 289,198   2005:
   2003: 233,681   2006:
Medical Loss Ratio: 2005:   2006: 80.00
Administrative Expense Ratio: 2005:   2006:
SERVICE AREA:
Nationwide: N
   MD;
TYPE OF COVERAGE:
Commercial: [Y] Individual: [ ] FEHBP: [ ] Indemnity: [ ]
Medicare: [ ] Medicaid: [ ] Supplemental Medicare: [ ]
Tricare   [ ]
CONSUMER-DRIVEN PRODUCTS
Aetna Life Insurance Co   HSA Company
Aetna HealthFund HSA   HSA Product
Aetna   HSA Administrator
Aetna HealthFund   Consumer-Driven Health Plan
PPO I; PPO II   High Deductible Health Plan
PLAN BENEFITS:
Alternative Medicine: [ ]   Behavioral Health: [ ]
Chiropractic: [X]   Dental: [X]
Home Care: [X]   Inpatient SNF: [X]
Long-Term Care: [X]   Pharm. Mail Order: [X]
Physical Therapy: [X]   Podiatry: [X]
Psychiatric: [X]   Transplant: [X]
Vision: [X]   Wellness: [X]
Workers' Comp: [X]
Other Benefits:
Comments:
See other Aetna US HealthCare listings for additional markets.

AMERIGROUP MARYLAND INC

857 Elkridge Landing Rd
Linthicum, MD 21090
Phone: 410-859-5800 Fax: 410-981-4070 Toll-Free:
Web site: www.amerigroupcorp.com
MAILING ADDRESS:
   AMERIGROUP - MD
   857 Elkridge Landing Rd
   Linthicum, MD 21090

KEY EXECUTIVES:
Chief Executive Officer .... Julie Locke
President .... Steven B Larson
Medical Director .... Sandra D Bruce-Nichols, MD
Chief Operating Officer .... Kenneth M Puente
Marketing Director .... Kenneth Brown
Physician Advisor .... Ginny Moore, MD

COMPANY PROFILE:
Parent Company Name: Amerigroup Corporation
Doing Business As:
Year Founded: Federally Qualified: [ ]
Forprofit: [Y]   Not-For-Profit: [ ]
Model Type:
Accreditation: [ ] AAPPO [ ] JACHO [ ] NCQA [ ] URAC
Plan Type: HMO
Total Revenue: 2005:   2006: 575,407,755
Net Income   2005:   2006:
Total Enrollment:
   2001: 118,000   2004: 170,859   2007: 0
   2002: 162,770   2005: 141,000
   2003: 161,659   2006:
Medical Loss Ratio: 2005:   2006: 81.30
Administrative Expense Ratio: 2005:   2006:
SERVICE AREA:
Nationwide:
   MD;
TYPE OF COVERAGE:
Commercial: [ ] Individual: [ ] FEHBP: [ ] Indemnity: [ ]
Medicare: [ ] Medicaid: [Y] Supplemental Medicare: [ ]
Tricare   [ ]
PRODUCTS OFFERED:
Product Name: Type:
Amerigroup HMO   Medicaid

AMERICAN COLLEGE OF MEDICAL QUALITY

4334 Montgomery Ave Ste B
Bethesda, MD 20814
Phone: 301-913-9149 Fax: 301-913-9142 Toll-Free: 800-924-2149
Web site: www.acmq.org
MAILING ADDRESS:
   AMERICAN COLLEGE MEDICAL QUAL
   4334 Montgomery Ave Ste B
   Bethesda, MD 20814

KEY EXECUTIVES:
Chief Executive Officer .... Robert F Pendrak, MD
President .... Donald E Fetterolf, MD
Marketing Director .... Kim Goodman
Public Relations Director .... Stacy Anderson
Executive Vice President .... Bridget Brodie

COMPANY PROFILE:
Parent Company Name:
Doing Business As:
Year Founded: 1972   Federally Qualified: [ ]
Forprofit: [ ]   Not-For-Profit: [Y]
Model Type:
Accreditation: [ ] AAPPO [ ] JACHO [ ] NCQA [ ] URAC
Plan Type: UR
SERVICE AREA:
Nationwide: N
   MD;

APS HEALTHCARE INC

8403 Colesville Rd Ste 1600
Silver Springs, MD 20910
Phone: 301-563-5633 Fax: 301-563-7338 Toll-Free: 800-305-3720
Web site: www.apshealthcare.com
MAILING ADDRESS:
   APS HEALTHCARE INC
   8403 Colesville Rd Ste 1600
   Silver Spring, MD 20910

KEY EXECUTIVES:
Chairman of the Board/Chief Executive Officer .... Gregory W Scott
President .... Jerome V Vaccaro, MD
Chief Financial Officer .... Brett McIntyre
Chief Medical Officer/Pres APS .... Christopher Gorton, MD, MHSA
Chief Information Officer .... Roger Jaffe
Chief Operating Officer .... Jerome V Vaccaro, MD
Executive VP, Sales & Marketing .... Richard Kodora, MBA
Senior VP, Human Resources .... Lynne Frazier
President, Behavioral Health .... Roderick J Hafer, PhD
President, APS Public Div .... David Hunsaker
Executive VP, General Counsel .... Laura F Tarantino, CPA
President/CEO Puerto Rico Division .... Alexis Cardona

Managed Care Organization Profiles MAINE

TYPE OF COVERAGE:
Commercial: [Y] Individual: [Y] FEHBP: [ ] Indemnity: [ ]
Medicare: [Y] Medicaid: [ ] Supplemental Medicare: [ ]
Tricare   [ ]

PLAN BENEFITS:
Alternative Medicine:	[ ]	Behavioral Health:	[ ]
Chiropractic:	[X]	Dental:	[ ]
Home Care:	[X]	Inpatient SNF:	[X]
Long-Term Care:	[ ]	Pharm. Mail Order:	[X]
Physical Therapy:	[X]	Podiatry:	[X]
Psychiatric:	[X]	Transplant:	[X]
Vision:	[X]	Wellness:	[X]
Workers' Comp:	[ ]		
Other Benefits:			

Comments:
Licensed a HMO in April, 2006.

MEDICAL NETWORK INC

59 Middle St 3rd FL
Portland, ME 04101
Phone: 207-773-5116 Fax: 207-773-1739 Toll-Free: 800-556-1144
Web site: www.mainemednet.com

MAILING ADDRESS:
   MEDICAL NETWORK INC
   PO Box 15253
   Portland, ME 04101

KEY EXECUTIVES:
Chief Executive Officer .... Robert Hillman
President .... Vincent Furey, Jr
Controller .... Lisa Liponis
Director of Operations & Network Development .... Robert Hillman
Credentialing Coordinator .... Carole Belliveau
Provider Relations Director .... Steven Maxcy
Credentialing Coordinator .... Carole Belliveau
Claims Status .... Jeff Morin

COMPANY PROFILE:
Parent Company Name:
Doing Business As:
Year Founded: 1986   Federally Qualified: [ ]
Forprofit: [Y]   Not-For-Profit: [ ]
Model Type: IPA
Accreditation: [ ] AAPPO [ ] JACHO [ ] NCQA [ ] URAC
Plan Type: PPO, POS
Total Enrollment:
   2001: 75,000   2004: 75,000   2007: 0
   2002: 0   2005:
   2003: 103,645   2006:

SERVICE AREA:
Nationwide: N
   ME;

TYPE OF COVERAGE:
Commercial: [Y] Individual: [Y] FEHBP: [ ] Indemnity: [ ]
Medicare: [ ] Medicaid: [ ] Supplemental Medicare: [ ]
Tricare   [ ]

PRODUCTS OFFERED:
Product Name:	Type:
Medical Network Inc PPO	PPO
Medical Network Inc HMO	HMO

PLAN BENEFITS:
Alternative Medicine:	[ ]	Behavioral Health:	[X]
Chiropractic:	[X]	Dental:	[ ]
Home Care:	[X]	Inpatient SNF:	[X]
Long-Term Care:	[ ]	Pharm. Mail Order:	[ ]
Physical Therapy:	[X]	Podiatry:	[X]
Psychiatric:	[X]	Transplant:	[X]
Vision:	[X]	Wellness:	[ ]
Workers' Comp:	[ ]		
Other Benefits:			

MAINE

Managed Care Organization Profiles

Total Enrollment:
- 2001: 65,104
- 2002: 46,250
- 2003: 32,392
- 2004: 21,797
- 2005: 17,925
- 2006: 13,427
- 2007: 6,635

Medical Loss Ratio: 2005: 81.34 2006: 89.65
Administrative Expense Ratio: 2005: 5.25 2006: 7.84

SERVICE AREA:
Nationwide: N
ME;

TYPE OF COVERAGE:
Commercial: [Y] Individual: [Y] FEHBP: [ ] Indemnity: [ ]
Medicare: [ ] Medicaid: [ ] Supplemental Medicare: [ ]
Tricare [ ]

PRODUCTS OFFERED:
Product Name:	Type:
CIGNA HMO	HMO

CONSUMER-DRIVEN PRODUCTS
JP Morgan Chase	HSA Company
CIGNA Choice Fund	HSA Product
	HSA Administrator
Open Access Plus	Consumer-Driven Health Plan
PPO	High Deductible Health Plan

PLAN BENEFITS:
Alternative Medicine:	[ ]	Behavioral Health:	[ ]
Chiropractic:	[X]	Dental:	[ ]
Home Care:	[X]	Inpatient SNF:	[ ]
Long-Term Care:	[ ]	Pharm. Mail Order:	[ ]
Physical Therapy:	[ ]	Podiatry:	[ ]
Psychiatric:	[X]	Transplant:	[X]
Vision:	[X]	Wellness:	[X]
Workers' Comp:	[ ]		
Other Benefits:			

COMMUNITY CLINICAL SERVICES

95 Campus Ave Ste 27
Lewiston, ME 04240
Phone: 207-777-8841 Fax: 207-777-8847 Toll-Free:
Web site: www.communityclinicalservices.com

MAILING ADDRESS:
COMMUNITY CLINICAL SERVICES
95 Campus Ave Ste 27
Lewiston, ME 04240

KEY EXECUTIVES:
Chief Executive Officer .... James E Cassidy
Chief Financial Officer .... Carolyn Kasabian
Medical Director .... Ralph Harder, MD
Director of Operations .... Eric Small
Marketing Director .... Russ Donahue
Vice President .... Susan Keiler

COMPANY PROFILE:
Parent Company Name: Sisters of Charity Health Systems
Doing Business As:
Year Founded: 1988   Federally Qualified: [Y]
Forprofit: [Y]   Not-For-Profit: [ ]
Model Type: NETWORK
Accreditation: [ ] AAPPO [ ] JACHO [ ] NCQA [ ] URAC
Plan Type: HMO

SERVICE AREA:
Nationwide: N
ME (Androscoggin);

TYPE OF COVERAGE:
Commercial: [Y] Individual: [ ] FEHBP: [ ] Indemnity: [ ]
Medicare: [ ] Medicaid: [ ] Supplemental Medicare: [ ]
Tricare [ ]

GREAT-WEST HEALTHCARE OF MAINE

100 Foden Rd E Ste 202
S Portland, ME 04106
Phone: 207-828-5084 Fax: 207-828-4672 Toll-Free:
Web site: www.greatwesthealthcare.com

MAILING ADDRESS:
GREAT-WEST HEALTHCARE OF ME
100 Foden Rd E Ste 202
S Portland, ME 04106

KEY EXECUTIVES:
Office & Sales Manager .... Thomas Griffin
Provider Relations Manager .... Amy Johnson
Manager of Network Development .... Mark Simpson

COMPANY PROFILE:
Parent Company Name: Great West Life & Annuity Insurance Co
Doing Business As: Great-West Healthcare
Year Founded: Federally Qualified: [ ]
Forprofit: [Y]   Not-For-Profit: [ ]
Model Type:
Accreditation: [ ] AAPPO [ ] JACHO [ ] NCQA [ ] URAC
Plan Type: PPO, CDHP, HSA

SERVICE AREA:
Nationwide: N
ME; NH; VT;

TYPE OF COVERAGE:
Commercial: [Y] Individual: [ ] FEHBP: [ ] Indemnity: [ ]
Medicare: [ ] Medicaid: [ ] Supplemental Medicare: [ ]
Tricare [ ]

CONSUMER-DRIVEN PRODUCTS
Mellon HR Solutions LLC	HSA Company
	HSA Product
	HSA Administrator
	Consumer-Driven Health Plan
	High Deductible Health Plan

PLAN BENEFITS:
Alternative Medicine:	[X]	Behavioral Health:	[ ]
Chiropractic:	[X]	Dental:	[X]
Home Care:	[X]	Inpatient SNF:	[X]
Long-Term Care:	[ ]	Pharm. Mail Order:	[X]
Physical Therapy:	[X]	Podiatry:	[X]
Psychiatric:	[X]	Transplant:	[X]
Vision:	[X]	Wellness:	[X]
Workers' Comp:	[ ]		
Other Benefits:			

MARTINS POINT HEALTH CARE

891 Washington Ave
Portland, ME 04103
Phone: 207-828-2436 Fax: 207-828-2446 Toll-Free:
Web site: www.martinspoint.com

MAILING ADDRESS:
MARTINS POINT HEALTH CARE
891 Washington Ave
Portland, ME 04103

KEY EXECUTIVES:
Chief Executive Officer/President .... David H Howes, MD
Chief Financial Officer .... Mark McAulifee
Chief Medical Officer .... David H Howes, MD
Chief Information Officer/Chief Operating Officer ...... Doug Smith
Human Resources Director .... Suanne William-Lindgren
Director of Strategic Planning .... Angela Wheaton

COMPANY PROFILE:
Parent Company Name: PBMA
Doing Business As:
Year Founded: 1981   Federally Qualified: [N]
Forprofit: [ ]   Not-For-Profit: [Y]
Model Type:
Accreditation: [ ] AAPPO [X] JACHO [ ] NCQA [ ] URAC
Plan Type: HMO, PPO,
Total Revenue: 2005:   2006: 2,758,900
Net Income: 2005:   2006: -630,711
Total Enrollment:
- 2001: 0
- 2002: 0
- 2003: 0
- 2004: 0
- 2005:
- 2006:
- 2007: 303

SERVICE AREA:
Nationwide: N
ME; NH;

Managed Care Organization Profiles

MAINE

AETNA INC - MAINE

174 Running Hill Rd Ste 301
Portland, ME 04106-3220
Phone: 207-879-1995 Fax: 207-879-0191 Toll-Free:
Web site: www.aetna.com

MAILING ADDRESS:
AETNA INC - ME
174 Running Hill Rd Ste 301
Portland, ME 04106-3220

KEY EXECUTIVES:
Chairman of the Board/Chief Executive Officer .... Ronald A Williams
President .... Michael E Morris
Principal Financial Officer .... Deborah M Wightman
Senior Medical Director .... Mary T McCluskey, MD
Marketing Manager .... Christine Haslam
Provider Services Director .... Mark Granzier
General Manager .... Daniel Fishbein MD

COMPANY PROFILE:
Parent Company Name: Aetna Inc
Doing Business As:
Year Founded: 1996 Federally Qualified: [N]
Forprofit: [Y] Not-For-Profit: [ ]
Model Type: NETWORK
Accreditation: [ ] AAPPO [ ] JACHO [ ] NCQA [ ] URAC
Plan Type: HMO, PPO, POS, CDHP, HSA
Total Revenue: 2005: 174,775,154 2006: 175,272,207
Net Income 2005: 14,518,280 2006: 62,825,001
Total Enrollment:
  2001: 72,813 2004: 45,591 2007: 0
  2002: 40,799 2005:
  2003: 43,095 2006: 43,128
Medical Loss Ratio: 2005: 75.14 2006: 80.87
Administrative Expense Ratio: 2005: 11.81 2006: 13.59

SERVICE AREA:
Nationwide: N
  ME;

TYPE OF COVERAGE:
Commercial: [Y] Individual: [Y] FEHBP: [ ] Indemnity: [ ]
Medicare: [ ] Medicaid: [Y] Supplemental Medicare: [ ]Tricare [ ]

PRODUCTS OFFERED:
Product Name:	Type:
Nylcare 65	Medicare
Aetna	HMO

CONSUMER-DRIVEN PRODUCTS
Aetna Life Insurance Co	HSA Company
Aetna HealthFund HSA	HSA Product
Aetna	HSA Administrator
Aetna HealthFund	Consumer-Driven Health Plan
PPO I; PPO II	High Deductible Health Plan

PLAN BENEFITS:
Alternative Medicine:	[ ]	Behavioral Health:	[ ]
Chiropractic:	[X]	Dental:	[ ]
Home Care:	[X]	Inpatient SNF:	[ ]
Long-Term Care:	[ ]	Pharm. Mail Order:	[X]
Physical Therapy:	[ ]	Podiatry:	[ ]
Psychiatric:	[X]	Transplant:	[ ]
Vision:	[X]	Wellness:	[X]
Workers' Comp:	[ ]		

Other Benefits:

ANTHEM BLUE CROSS BLUE SHIELD OF MAINE

2 Gannett Drive
South Portland, ME 04106-6911
Phone: 207-822-7000 Fax: 207-822-7375 Toll-Free:
Web site: www.anthem.com

MAILING ADDRESS:
ANTHEM BC/BS OF MAINE
2 Gannett Drive
South Portland, ME 04106-6911

KEY EXECUTIVES:
Chairman of the Board .... Larry C Glasscock
President .... Angela F Braly
President, Maine .... Erin Hoeflinger
Medical Director .... Jeff Holmstrom, MD
Public Relations Director .... Carol Morris
Manager of Provider Relations .... Robin Allen
Health Promotion/Prevention .... Meredith Tipton
Human Resources Manager .... Jack Quirk
Fraud Prevention/Investigation .... Don Sirois
VP, General Manager, Health Care Management ...... Douglas Wenners
VP of Case Management .... Terry Garrett
VP Health Care Management/NE .... Richard D Lynch

COMPANY PROFILE:
Parent Company Name: WellPoint Inc
Doing Business As:
Year Founded: 2000 Federally Qualified: [Y]
Forprofit: [ ] Not-For-Profit: [Y]
Model Type: GROUP
Accreditation: [ ] AAPPO [ ] JACHO [X] NCQA [ ] URAC
Plan Type: HMO, PPO, POS, HSA
Total Revenue: 2005: 402,418,046 2006: 428,171,165
Net Income 2005: 17,521,306 2006: 25,753,492
Total Enrollment:
  2001: 113,473 2004: 282,994 2007: 313,165
  2002: 290,688 2005: 474,423
  2003: 266,135 2006: 320,618
Medical Loss Ratio: 2005: 84.86 2006: 85.27
Administrative Expense Ratio: 2005: 5.66 2006: 4.11

SERVICE AREA:
Nationwide: N
  ME;

TYPE OF COVERAGE:
Commercial: [Y] Individual: [Y] FEHBP: [ ] Indemnity: [ ]
Medicare: [ ] Medicaid: [ ] Supplemental Medicare: [ ]
Tricare [ ]

PRODUCTS OFFERED:
Product Name:	Type:
HMO Maine	HMO

CONSUMER-DRIVEN PRODUCTS
JP Morgan Chase	HSA Company
Anthem ByDesign HSA	HSA Product
JP Morgan Chase	HSA Administrator
Blue Access Saver	Consumer-Driven Health Plan
Blue Access Economy Plans PPO	High Deductible Health Plan

Comments:
Anthem Blue Cross/Blue Shield co-owns Maine Partners Health Plan Inc and Central Maine Partners Health Plan.

CIGNA HEALTHCARE OF MAINE INC

6 Fundy Rd Ste 300
Falmouth, ME 04105
Phone: 207-781-6800 Fax: 207-781-6836 Toll-Free: 800-642-5551
Web site: www.cigna.com

MAILING ADDRESS:
CIGNA HEALTHCARE OF MAINE INC
6 Fundy Rd Ste 300
Falmouth, ME 04105

KEY EXECUTIVES:
President .... Donald M Curry
Medical Director .... Robert Hockmuth, MD
Pharmacy Director .... James Demosthenes

COMPANY PROFILE:
Parent Company Name: CIGNA Corporation
Doing Business As:
Year Founded: 1987 Federally Qualified: [Y]
Forprofit: [Y] Not-For-Profit: [ ]
Model Type: IPA
Accreditation: [ ] AAPPO [ ] JACHO [X] NCQA [ ] URAC
Plan Type: HMO, PPO, POS, CDHP, HSA, FSA, HRA
Total Revenue: 2005: 64,283,954 2006: 56,330,789
Net Income 2005: 6,266,606 2006: -232,555

Managed Care Organization Profiles — LOUISIANA

COMPANY PROFILE:
Parent Company Name:
Doing Business As: Peoples Health
Year Founded: 1997   Federally Qualified: [N]
Forprofit: [Y]   Not-For-Profit: [ ]
Model Type:
Accreditation: [ ] AAPPO [ ] JACHO [ ] NCQA [ ] URAC
Plan Type: HMO, PPO, POS,
Total Revenue: 2005:   2006:   397,767,399
Net Income   2005:   2006:
Total Enrollment:
  2001: 26,784   2004: 38,725   2007: 0
  2002: 32,721   2005:
  2003: 34,910   2006: 36,000
Medical Loss Ratio: 2005:   2006: 85.00
Administrative Expense Ratio: 2005:   2006:

SERVICE AREA:
Nationwide: N
   LA

TYPE OF COVERAGE:
Commercial: [Y] Individual: [ ] FEHBP: [ ] Indemnity: [ ]
Medicare: [Y] Medicaid: [ ] Supplemental Medicare: [ ]
Tricare   [ ]

PRODUCTS OFFERED:
Product Name: Type:
Tenet Choice 65   Medicare
New Orleans Choice Plan   Commercial
Tenet Choices   Commercial
Tenet Choices 65   Medicare Advantage

UNITEDHEALTHCARE OF LOUISIANA

3838 N Causeway Blvd Ste 2600
Metairie, LA 70002
Phone: 504-849-1609 Fax: 504-849-3551 Toll-Free: 800-349-1999
Web site: www.uhc.com

MAILING ADDRESS:
   UNITEDHEALTHCARE — LA
   3838 N Causeway Blvd Ste 2600
   Metairie, LA 70002

KEY EXECUTIVES:
Non-Executive Chairman .... Richard T Burke
Chief Executive Officer/President .... Glen J Golemi
Chief Financial Officer .... Frank Ulibarri
Medical Director .... Larry B Amacker, MD
VP, Large Group Sales .... Kim Lewis
Compliance Officer .... Harry Beaudoin
Public Relations Director .... Roger Rollman
Network Management Director .... Bob Humphrey
Human Resources Director .... Cheryl Lippert
VP, Network Management .... Jeff Wedin
VP, Key Accounts .... Kim Lewis
VP, Small Business .... Aaron Brace

COMPANY PROFILE:
Parent Company Name: UnitedHealth Group
Doing Business As:
Year Founded: 1986   Federally Qualified: [N]
Forprofit: [Y]   Not-For-Profit: [ ]
Model Type: IPA
Accreditation: [ ] AAPPO [ ] JACHO [ ] NCQA [ ] URAC
Plan Type: HMO, PPO, POS, CDHP, HSA, HRA
Total Revenue: 2005:   2006: 21,682,302
Net Income   2005:   2006:
Total Enrollment:
  2001: 87,231   2004: 17,396   2007: 0
  2002: 92,347   2005:
  2003: 60,280   2006:
Medical Loss Ratio: 2005:   2006: 64.30
Administrative Expense Ratio: 2005:   2006:

SERVICE AREA:
Nationwide: N
   LA (Acadia, Allen, Ascension, Assumption, Avoyelles, Bienville, Bossier, Caddo, Cathoula, Concordia, DeSoto, East Baton Rouge, East Feliciana, Evangeline, Grant, Iberia, Iberville, Jefferson, Lafayette, Lafourche, LaSalle, Livingston, Natchitoches, Orleans, Plaquemines, Pointe Coupee, Rapides, Red River, Savine, St Bernard, St Charles, St Helena, St Landry, St Martin, St Mary, St James, St John the Baptist, St Tammany, Tangipahoa, Terrebonne, Vermillion, Vernon, Washington, West Baton Rouge, West Feliciana);

TYPE OF COVERAGE:
Commercial: [Y] Individual: [ ] FEHBP: [ ] Indemnity: [ ]
Medicare: [Y] Medicaid: [ ] Supplemental Medicare: [ ]
Tricare   [ ]

PRODUCTS OFFERED:
Product Name: Type:
Medicare Complete   Medicare Advantage

CONSUMER-DRIVEN PRODUCTS
Exante Bank/Golden Rule Ins Co   HSA Company
iPlan HSA   HSA Product
                                      HSA Administrator
                                      Consumer-Driven Health Plan
                                      High Deductible Health Plan

PLAN BENEFITS:
Alternative Medicine: [ ]   Behavioral Health: [ ]
Chiropractic: [X]   Dental: [X]
Home Care: [X]   Inpatient SNF: [X]
Long-Term Care: [X]   Pharm. Mail Order: [X]
Physical Therapy: [X]   Podiatry: [ ]
Psychiatric: [X]   Transplant: [X]
Vision: [X]   Wellness: [X]
Workers' Comp: [ ]
Other Benefits:

VANTAGE HEALTH PLAN INC

130 DiSiard St Ste 300
Monroe, LA 71201
Phone: 318-361-0900 Fax: 318-361-2159 Toll-Free: 888-823-1910
Web site: www.vhpla.com

MAILING ADDRESS:
   VANTAGE HEALTH PLAN INC
   130 DiSiard St Ste 300
   Monroe, LA 71201

KEY EXECUTIVES:
Chief Executive Officer/President .... Patrick G Jones, MD
Chief Financial Officer .... Rhonda Haygood
Medical Director .... Patrick G Jones, MD
VP, Finance & Operations .... Mike W Breard
Marketing Director .... William Justice
MIS Director .... Sam Rainer
Compliance Officer .... Keith McRee
Director of Provider Services .... Annette Napier
Human Resources Director .... Jody Maynard
Medical Management Director .... Melissa Halley

COMPANY PROFILE:
Parent Company Name:
Doing Business As:
Year Founded: 1994   Federally Qualified: [N]
Forprofit: [Y]   Not-For-Profit: [ ]
Model Type: GROUP
Accreditation: [ ] AAPPO [ ] JACHO [ ] NCQA [ ] URAC
Plan Type: HMO, PPO, UR, PRO, HDHP, HSA
Total Revenue: 2005: 45,340,065   2006: 56,959,948
Net Income   2005:   1,911,452   2006:   4,505,245
Total Enrollment:
  2001: 0   2004: 12,761   2007: 17,306
  2002: 13,507   2005: 14,654
  2003: 15,079   2006: 16,380
Medical Loss Ratio: 2005: 84.20   2006: 78.60
Administrative Expense Ratio: 2005: 11.59   2006: 11.85

SERVICE AREA:
Nationwide: N
   LA (Northeast);

TYPE OF COVERAGE:
Commercial: [Y] Individual: [Y] FEHBP: [ ] Indemnity: [ ]
Medicare: [ ] Medicaid: [ ] Supplemental Medicare: [ ]
Tricare   [ ]

PRODUCTS OFFERED:
Product Name: Type:
Vantage Health Plan   HMO

PLAN BENEFITS:
Alternative Medicine: [ ]   Behavioral Health: [ ]
Chiropractic: [X]   Dental: [ ]
Home Care: [X]   Inpatient SNF: [X]
Long-Term Care: [X]   Pharm. Mail Order: [ ]
Physical Therapy: [X]   Podiatry: [ ]
Psychiatric: [X]   Transplant: [X]
Vision: [X]   Wellness: [X]
Workers' Comp: [ ]
Other Benefits:

LOUISIANA

Managed Care Organization Profiles

KEY EXECUTIVES:
Chairman of the Board .... David A Jones Jr
Chief Executive Officer .... Terry S Shilling
President .... James E Schlottman
Chief Financial Officer .... Lisa Blume
Medical Director .... Larry Cortez, MD
Pharmacy Director .... Gionne McLean
Chief Information Officer (Interium) .... Robert Stallings
Senior VP of Operations .... Lynn Comeaux
Senior VP Administration .... George Renaudin II
Provider Relations Director .... Mary Armstrong
VP of Network Contracting .... John Blake
Health Services Director .... Cheryl DeBold
Quality Management Director .... Ann E Corrigan
VP, Large Group .... Jay Fielder
VP, Provider Contracting .... Jeffrey Fernandez
Director of Account Management .... Jerri Alexander
Commerical Finance .... Rhonda Bagby

COMPANY PROFILE:
Parent Company Name: Humana Inc
Doing Business As:
Year Founded: 1985   Federally Qualified: [Y]
Forprofit: [Y]   Not-For-Profit: [ ]
Model Type: MIXED
Accreditation: [ ] AAPPO [X] JACHO [X] NCQA [ ] URAC
Plan Type: HMO, POS, TPA, CDHP, HSA
Primary Physicians: 4,400   Physician Specialists:
Hospitals: 69
Total Revenue: 2005:   2006: 910,111,931
Net Income   2005:   2006:
Total Enrollment:
  2001: 186,644   2004: 185,528   2007: 0
  2002: 204,076   2005: 195,000
  2003: 191,138   2006:
Medical Loss Ratio: 2005:   2006: 80.50
Administrative Expense Ratio: 2005:   2006:

SERVICE AREA:
Nationwide: N
  LA (Acadia, Allen, Ascension, Assumption, Avoyelles, Beauregard, Bienville, Bossier, Caddo, Calcasieu, Cameron, Catahoula, Claiborne, Concordia, DeSoto, East Baton Rouge, East Feliciana, Evangeline, Grant, Iberia, Iberville, Jackson, Jefferson, Jefferson Davis, LaSalle, Lafayette, LaFourche, Lincoln, Livingston, Natchitoches, Orleans, Plaquamines, Pointe Coupee, Rapides, Red River, Sabine, St Bernard, St Charles, St Helena, St James, St John the Baptist, St Landry, St Martin, St Mary, Tangipahoa, Terrebonne, Vermilion, Vernon, Washington, Webster, West Baton Rouge, West Feliciana, Winn);

TYPE OF COVERAGE:
Commercial: [Y] Individual: [Y] FEHBP: [ ] Indemnity: [ ]
Medicare: [Y] Medicaid: [ ] Supplemental Medicare: [ ]
Tricare   [ ]

PRODUCTS OFFERED:
Product Name: Type:
Total Health Choice & Total He   HMO
Total Health One   HMO
Total Health Plus & Total Heal   POS
Kids First   HMO
Total Health 65   Medicare Advantage

CONSUMER-DRIVEN PRODUCTS
JP Morgan Chase   HSA Company
HumanaOne HSA   HSA Product
JP Morgan Chase   HSA Administrator Personal
Care Account   Consumer-Driven Health Plan
HumanaOne   High Deductible Health Plan

PLAN BENEFITS:
Alternative Medicine: [ ]   Behavioral Health: [X]
Chiropractic: [X]   Dental: [X]
Home Care: [ ]   Inpatient SNF: [X]
Long-Term Care: [ ]   Pharm. Mail Order: [X]
Physical Therapy: [X]   Podiatry: [X]
Psychiatric: [X]   Transplant: [X]
Vision: [X]   Wellness: [X]
Workers' Comp: [ ]
Other Benefits:

MED-COMP USA

2901 N Causeway Blvd Ste 202
Metairie, LA 70002
Phone: 504-832-4106 Fax: 504-835-1079 Toll-Free: 800-869-1098
Web site: www.medcompusa.com

MAILING ADDRESS:
MED-COMP USA
2901 N Causeway Blvd Ste 202
Metairie, LA 70002

KEY EXECUTIVES:
Chief Executive/Chief Operating Officer .... Michael P McCrossen
Chief Financial Officer .... W H Jones
Marketing Director .... B J Parrish
Director of Provider Services .... Erin Maura
Director of Quality Assurance .... Carol Fife
Director of Self Funded Plans .... Adam Christopher

COMPANY PROFILE:
Parent Company Name: Med Comp USA
Doing Business As:
Year Founded: 1987   Federally Qualified: [N]
Forprofit: [Y]   Not-For-Profit: [ ]
Model Type: MIXED
Accreditation: [ ] AAPPO [ ] JACHO [ ] NCQA [ ] URAC
Plan Type: Specialty PPO

SERVICE AREA:
Nationwide: Y
  NW;

PLAN BENEFITS:
Alternative Medicine: [ ]   Behavioral Health: [X]
Chiropractic: [X]   Dental: [ ]
Home Care: [ ]   Inpatient SNF: [ ]
Long-Term Care: [ ]   Pharm. Mail Order: [ ]
Physical Therapy: [ ]   Podiatry: [ ]
Psychiatric: [X]   Transplant: [ ]
Vision: [ ]   Wellness: [ ]
Workers' Comp: [X]
Other Benefits:

PPOPLUS LLC

400 Poydras St Ste 2040
New Orleans, LA 70130
Phone: 504-566-9501 Fax: 504-566-9509 Toll-Free:
Web site: www.ppoplus.com

MAILING ADDRESS:
PPOPLUS LLC
400 Poydras St Ste 2040
New Orleans, LA 70130

KEY EXECUTIVES:
President .... Catherine Hill

COMPANY PROFILE:
Parent Company Name:
Doing Business As:
Year Founded: 2001   Federally Qualified: [ ]
Forprofit: [ ]   Not-For-Profit: [ ]
Model Type: NETWORK
Accreditation: [ ] AAPPO [ ] JACHO [ ] NCQA [ ] URAC
Plan Type: PPO

SERVICE AREA:
Nationwide:
  AR; LA; MS;

TENET CHOICES INC

3838 N Causeway Blvd Ste 2200
Metairie, LA 70002
Phone: 504-849-4500 Fax: 504-849-6983 Toll-Free: 800-984-6565
Web site: www.tenetchoices.com

MAILING ADDRESS:
TENET CHOICES INC
3838 N Causeway Blvd Ste 2200
Metairie, LA 70002

KEY EXECUTIVES:
Chief Executive Officer/President .... Carol A Solomon
Chief Financial Officer .... Kim Eller
Medical Director .... Eric Joel Pesetski, MD
Chief Operating Officer .... Gerald Parton
Marketing & Sales Director .... Mike Putiak
MIS Director .... Colin Hulin
Secretary/Director .... Stephen L Newman MD
Director .... Robert Shackleton, MD
Director .... Frank N Deus, MD

Managed Care Organization Profiles — LOUISIANA

Alternative Medicine: [ ]
Chiropractic: [X]
Home Care: [X]
Long-Term Care: [X]
Physical Therapy: [X]
Psychiatric: [X]
Vision: [ ]
Workers' Comp: [X]
Other Benefits:

Behavioral Health: [ ]
Dental: [X]
Inpatient SNF: [X]
Pharm. Mail Order: [X]
Podiatry: [ ]
Transplant: [X]
Wellness: [X]

HEALTH PLUS OF LOUISIANA INC

2219 Line Ave
Shreveport, LA 71104
Phone: 318-212-8800 Fax: 318-212-8520 Toll-Free: 800-331-5055
Web site: www.wkhealthplus.com

MAILING ADDRESS:
HEALTH PLUS OF LOUISIANA INC
PO Box 32625
Shreveport, LA 71104

KEY EXECUTIVES:
Chairman .... James K Elrod
President .... Patrick F Bicknell
VP/Chief Financial Officer .... Larry D Knighton
VP/Chief Medical Officer .... Carey C Allison, MD
Pharmacy Director .... James M Frantz
Information Technology Manager .... Lewis Wooten
Director of Operations .... James M Frantz
Director of Marketing .... Tony J Papa
Provider Relations Director/Network Development Mgr . Sandy Brown
Director of Care Management .... Stephanie Roberts
Director of Compliance .... James M Frantz

COMPANY PROFILE:
Parent Company Name: Willis Knighton Health System
Doing Business As: Health Plus
Year Founded: 1995   Federally Qualified: [N]
Forprofit: [Y]   Not-For-Profit: [ ]
Model Type: IPA
Accreditation: [ ] AAPPO [ ] JACHO [ ] NCQA [ ] URAC
Plan Type: HMO, POS, ASO, TPA, CDHP, HDHP, HSA, FSA
Primary Physicians: 288   Physician Specialists: 580
Hospitals: 14
Total Enrollment:
  2001: 32,554   2004: 18,607   2007: 29,974
  2002: 27,606   2005: 29,968
  2003: 19,807   2006: 28,968

SERVICE AREA:
Nationwide: N
  LA; (Northwest Louisiana including the follwing Parishes - Bienville, Caddo, Claiborne, Bossier, DeSoto, Jackson, Lincoln, Natchitoches, Ouchita, Red River, Sabine, Union, Webster, Winn);

TYPE OF COVERAGE:
Commercial: [Y] Individual: [ ] FEHBP: [ ] Indemnity: [ ]
Medicare: [ ] Medicaid: [ ] Supplemental Medicare: [ ]
Tricare [ ]

PRODUCTS OFFERED:
Product Name: Type:
Health Plus   HMO
POS
Open Access

CONSUMER-DRIVEN PRODUCTS
Bank of America   HSA Company
Health Plus HSA   HSA Product
DST Health Solutions   HSA Administrator
                             Consumer-Driven Health
PlanHealth Plus HDHP   High Deductible Health Plan

PLAN BENEFITS:
Alternative Medicine: [ ]
Chiropractic: [X]
Home Care: [X]
Long-Term Care: [ ]
Physical Therapy: [X]
Psychiatric: [X]
Vision: [X]
Workers' Comp: [ ]
Other Benefits:

Behavioral Health: [X]
Dental: [ ]
Inpatient SNF: [X]
Pharm. Mail Order: [X]
Podiatry: [X]
Transplant: [X]
Wellness: [X]

HMO LOUISIANA INC

5525 Reitz Ave
Baton Rouge, LA 70809
Phone: 225-295-3307 Fax: 225-295-2054 Toll-Free: 800-376-7741
Web site: www.bcbsla.com

MAILING ADDRESS:
HMO LOUISIANA INC
PO Box 98029
Baton Rouge, LA 70809

KEY EXECUTIVES:
Chairman of the Board .... Virgil Robinson
Chief Executive Officer/President .... Gery J Berry
Chief Financial Officer .... Mark A Rishell
Chief Medical Officer .... James J Carney, MD
Manager of Pharmacy Services .... Milam Ford
Chief Information Officer .... Worachote 'Ob' Soonthornsima
Director, Marketing Support .... Eric Harrington
Privacy Officer .... Darrel Langlois
VP Corporate Communications .... John Maginnis
VP Provider Contracting .... Dawn Cantrell
Director of Network Operations .... Gina Laird
VP of Human Resources .... Sandra Smith
Associate Medical Director .... Dwight Brower
Manager Health & Quality Management .... Patty Daniel
Care Management Director .... Cynthia Hallam
Associate Medical Director II .... Julie Samuels

COMPANY PROFILE:
Parent Company Name: Louisiana Health Service & Indemnity Co
Doing Business As: HMO Louisiana Inc
Year Founded: 1986   Federally Qualified: [N]
Forprofit: [Y]   Not-For-Profit: [ ]
Model Type: NETWORK
Accreditation: [ ] AAPPO [ ] JACHO [ ] NCQA [X] URAC
Plan Type: HMO, PPO, POS, ASO, HDHP
Total Revenue: 2005:   2006: 289,704,889
Net Income 2005:   2006:
Total Enrollment:
  2001: 78,011   2004: 103,390   2007: 0
  2002: 105,601   2005:
  2003: 103,391   2006:
Medical Loss Ratio: 2005:   2006: 82.20
Administrative Expense Ratio: 2005:   2006:

SERVICE AREA:
Nationwide: N
  LA;

TYPE OF COVERAGE:
Commercial: [Y] Individual: [Y] FEHBP: [Y] Indemnity: [ ]
Medicare: [Y] Medicaid: [ ] Supplemental Medicare: [Y]
Tricare [ ]

PRODUCTS OFFERED:
Product Name: Type:
Louisiana Blue Health Plan   HMO
Louisiana Blue Health Plan ASO   ASO

PLAN BENEFITS:
Alternative Medicine: [ ]
Chiropractic: [X]
Home Care: [X]
Long-Term Care: [X]
Physical Therapy: [X]
Psychiatric: [X]
Vision: [X]
Workers' Comp: [ ]
Other Benefits:

Behavioral Health: [X]
Dental: [ ]
Inpatient SNF: [X]
Pharm. Mail Order: [X]
Podiatry: [ ]
Transplant: [X]
Wellness: [X]

HUMANA HEALTH BENEFIT PLAN OF LOUISIANA

One Galleria Blvd Ste 850
Metairie, LA 70001
Phone: 504-219-6600 Fax: 504-219-6530 Toll-Free: 888-882-9806
Web site: www.ohpnow.com

MAILING ADDRESS:
HUMANA HEALTH BENEFIT PLAN OF LA
One Galleria Blvd Ste 850
Metairie, LA 70001

LOUISIANA

Managed Care Organization Profiles

CIGNA HEALTHCARE OF LOUISIANA

2 Riverway Ste 1200
Houston, TX 77036-2036
Phone: 866-244-8081 Fax: 866-530-3585 Toll-Free: 800-244-8081
Web site: www.cigna.com

MAILING ADDRESS:
CIGNA HEALTHCARE OF LA
2 Riverway Ste 1200
Houston, TX 77036-2036

KEY EXECUTIVES:
General Manager, Irving Office .... David Toomey

COMPANY PROFILE:
Parent Company Name: CIGNA Corporation
Doing Business As:
Year Founded: 1986   Federally Qualified: [N]
Forprofit: [Y]   Not-For-Profit: [ ]
Model Type:
Accreditation: [ ] AAPPO [X] JACHO [ ] NCQA [ ] URAC
Plan Type: PPO, CDHP, FSA, HRA

SERVICE AREA:
Nationwide: N
LA (Acadia, Allen, Ascension, Assumption, Baton Rouge, Beaugard, Calcasieu, Cameron, East Feliciana, Iberia, Jefferson, Jefferson Davis, Lafayette, Lafouche, Livington, Orleans, Plaguemines, Pointe Coupee, St Bernard, St Charles, St Helena, St James, St John the Baptist, St Landry, St Mary, St Tammany, Tangipahoa, Terrebonne, Vermilion, West Feliciana);

TYPE OF COVERAGE:
Commercial: [Y] Individual: [ ] FEHBP: [ ] Indemnity: [ ]
Medicare: [ ] Medicaid: [ ] Supplemental Medicare: [ ]
Tricare   [ ]

CONSUMER-DRIVEN PRODUCTS
JP Morgan Chase   HSA Company
CIGNA Choice Fund   HSA Product
                               HSA Administrator
Open Access Plus   Consumer-Driven Health Plan
PPO   High Deductible Health Plan

PLAN BENEFITS:
Alternative Medicine: [ ]   Behavioral Health: [X]
Chiropractic: [X]   Dental: [ ]
Home Care: [X]   Inpatient SNF: [X]
Long-Term Care: [ ]   Pharm. Mail Order: [X]
Physical Therapy: [X]   Podiatry: [X]
Psychiatric: [X]   Transplant: [X]
Vision: [X]   Wellness: [X]
Workers' Comp: [ ]
Other Benefits:

COVENTRY HEALTH CARE INC — LOUISIANA

3838 N Causeway Blvd Ste 3350
Metairie, LA 70002
Phone: 504-834-0840 Fax: 504-834-2694 Toll-Free: 800-341-6613
Web site: www.cvty.com

MAILING ADDRESS:
COVENTRY HEALTH CARE — LA INC
3838 N Causeway Blvd Ste 3350
Metairie, LA 70002

KEY EXECUTIVES:
Chief Executive Officer .... George Bucher
Chief Financial Officer/Chief Operating Officer .... Angie Meoli
Director of Sales .... Al Tredway
Director of Network Operations .... Tom Graves
Director of Health Services .... Lee Reilley

COMPANY PROFILE:
Parent Company Name: Coventry Health Care Inc
Doing Business As:
Year Founded: 1985   Federally Qualified: [N]
Forprofit: [Y]   Not-For-Profit: [ ]
Model Type: IPA
Accreditation: [ ] AAPPO [ ] JACHO [ ] NCQA [ ] URAC
Plan Type: HMO, PPO, POS, CDHP, HDHP, HSA, ASO, FSA, MSA,

Total Revenue: 2005:   2006: 150,641,644
Net Income   2005:   2006:
Total Enrollment:
    2001: 60,298   2004: 71,919   2007: 0
    2002: 71,089   2005: 76,000
    2003: 71,456   2006:
Medical Loss Ratio: 2005:   2006: 64.40
Administrative Expense Ratio: 2005:   2006:

SERVICE AREA:
Nationwide: N
LA (Ascension, Assumption, East Baton Rouge, East Feliciana, Iberville, Jefferson, Livingston, Orleans, Plaquemines, Pointe Coupee, St. Bernard, St. Charles, St. Helena, St. James, St. John the Baptist, St. Tammany, TAngipahoa, Vermillion, Washington, West Baton Rouge, West Feliciana);

TYPE OF COVERAGE:
Commercial: [Y] Individual: [ ] FEHBP: [Y] Indemnity: [ ]
Medicare: [Y] Medicaid: [ ] Supplemental Medicare: [ ]
Tricare   [ ]

PRODUCTS OFFERED:
Product Name: Type:
Coventry Health Care of LA   HMO

CONSUMER-DRIVEN PRODUCTS
Wells Fargo   HSA Company
                                      HSA Product
Corporate Benefits Servs of Am   HSA Administrator
Open Access Plus Plan   Consumer-Driven Health Plan
Health Assurance   High Deductible Health Plan

PLAN BENEFITS:
Alternative Medicine: [ ]   Behavioral Health: [X]
Chiropractic: [X]   Dental: [ ]
Home Care: [X]   Inpatient SNF: [X]
Long-Term Care: [ ]   Pharm. Mail Order: [X]
Physical Therapy: [X]   Podiatry: [X]
Psychiatric: [X]   Transplant: [X]
Vision: [X]   Wellness: [X]
Workers' Comp: [ ]
Other Benefits:

Comments:
Formerly Principal Health Care of Louisiana Inc. Purchased Maxicare Louisiana Inc in August 2000.

FARA HEALTHCARE MANAGEMENT

1625 W Causeway Approach
Mandeville, LA 70471
Phone: 985-624-8383 Fax: 985-624-8489 Toll-Free: 800-259-8388
Web site: www.fara.com

MAILING ADDRESS:
FARA HEALTHCARE MANAGEMENT
1625 W Causeway Approach
Mandeville, LA 70471

KEY EXECUTIVES:
Chief Executive Officer/President .... M Todd Richard
Chief Financial Officer .... Louis R Dubuc
VP, Information Technology .... David M Richard
Chief Operating Officer .... Reed A Bell
VP of Sales & Marketing .... Eric Knudsen
Provider Relations Director .... Bridgette Hammant
Human Resources Director .... Michelle Boullion
VP, Healthcare Management .... Kay Martin
VP of Administration .... Camilla Q Davis

COMPANY PROFILE:
Parent Company Name: F A Richard & Assoc Inc
Doing Business As:
Year Founded: 1992   Federally Qualified: [ ]Forprofit: [Y]
Not-For-Profit: [ ]
Model Type:
Accreditation: [ ] AAPPO [ ] JACHO [ ] NCQA [ ] URAC
Plan Type: PPO, UR, POS, TPA

SERVICE AREA:
Nationwide: N
    NW;

TYPE OF COVERAGE:
Commercial: [Y] Individual: [ ] FEHBP: [ ] Indemnity: [ ]
Medicare: [ ] Medicaid: [ ] Supplemental Medicare: [ ]
Tricare   [ ]

PLAN BENEFITS:

Managed Care Organization Profiles — LOUISIANA

AETNA INC - LOUISIANA

3900 N Causeway Blvd Ste 1460
Metairie, LA 70002
Phone: 504-830-5600 Fax: 504-837-6571 Toll-Free: 800-685-4857
Web site: www.aetna.com
MAILING ADDRESS:
   AETNA INC - LA
   3900 N Causeway Blvd Ste 1460
   Metairie, LA 70002

KEY EXECUTIVES:
Chairman of the Board/Chief Executive Officer .... Ronald A Williams
Regional Manager-Southeast .... Joseph Blanford
Executive VP, Finance .... Joseph M Zubretsky
Public Relations Director .... Danla Geraci
Quality Manager .... Shirley Divinty

COMPANY PROFILE:
Parent Company Name: Aetna Inc
Doing Business As:
Year Founded: 1987   Federally Qualified: [N]
Forprofit: [Y]   Not-For-Profit: [ ]
Model Type: MIXED
Accreditation: [ ] AAPPO [ ] JACHO [ ] NCQA [ ] URAC
Plan Type: HMO, POS, CDHP, HSA
Total Enrollment:
   2001: 0   2004: 0   2007: 0
   2002: 168   2005:
   2003: 0   2006:

SERVICE AREA:
Nationwide: N
   LA;

TYPE OF COVERAGE:
Commercial: [Y] Individual: [Y] FEHBP: [ ] Indemnity: [ ]
Medicare: [ ] Medicaid: [ ] Supplemental Medicare: [ ]
Tricare   [ ]

CONSUMER-DRIVEN PRODUCTS
Aetna Life Insurance Co   HSA Company
Aetna HealthFund HSA   HSA Product
Aetna   HSA Administrator
Aetna HealthFund   Consumer-Driven Health Plan
PPO I; PPO II   High Deductible Health Plan

PLAN BENEFITS:
Alternative Medicine: [ ]   Behavioral Health: [ ]
Chiropractic: [X]   Dental: [X]
Home Care: [ ]   Inpatient SNF: [ ]
Long-Term Care: [ ]   Pharm. Mail Order: [X]
Physical Therapy: [ ]   Podiatry: [ ]
Psychiatric: [ ]   Transplant: [ ]
Vision: [X]   Wellness: [ ]
Workers' Comp: [ ]
Other Benefits:

AMERICAN LIFECARE - LOUISIANA

1100 Poydras St Ste 2600
New Orleans, LA 70163-2602
Phone: 504-681-3600 Fax: 504-681-3611 Toll-Free:
Web site: www.phcs.com
MAILING ADDRESS:
   AMERICAN LIFECARE - LA
   1100 Poydras St Ste 2600
   New Orleans, LA 70163-2602

KEY EXECUTIVES:
Chief Executive Officer/President .... Mark Tabak
Executive VP, Chief Financial Officer .... Richard Gerstein
Medical Director .... Dr Goldstein
Executive VP, Chief of Operations .... Michael Ferrante
Executive VP, Marketing .... Warren Handelman

COMPANY PROFILE:
Parent Company Name: MultiPlan Inc
Doing Business As:
Year Founded: 1985   Federally Qualified: [N]
Forprofit: [Y]   Not-For-Profit: [ ]
Model Type: MIXED
Accreditation: [ ] AAPPO [ ] JACHO [X] NCQA [X] URAC
Plan Type: PPO, POS, UR
Primary Physicians: 3,082   Physician Specialists: 5,889
Hospitals: 142
Total Enrollment:
   2001: 0   2004: 68,000   2007: 0
   2002: 694,000   2005: 72,000
   2003: 0   2006:

SERVICE AREA:
Nationwide: N
   LA;

TYPE OF COVERAGE:
Commercial: [Y] Individual: [ ] FEHBP: [ ] Indemnity: [ ]
Medicare: [ ] Medicaid: [ ] Supplemental Medicare: [ ]
Tricare

PLAN BENEFITS:
Alternative Medicine: [ ]   Behavioral Health: [X]
Chiropractic: [X]   Dental: [X]
Home Care: [X]   Inpatient SNF: [X]
Long-Term Care: [X]   Pharm. Mail Order: [X]
Physical Therapy: [X]   Podiatry: [X]
Psychiatric: [X]   Transplant: [X]
Vision: [X]   Wellness: [X]
Workers' Comp: [X]
Other Benefits:
Comments:
Acquired by MultiPlan, Inc. on October 18, 2006.

BLUE CROSS BLUE SHIELD OF LOUISIANA INC

5525 Reitz Ave
Baton Rouge, LA 70898-9024
Phone: 225-295-3307 Fax: 225-295-2054 Toll-Free: 800-599-2583
Web site: www.bcbsla.com
MAILING ADDRESS:
   BC/BS OF LOUISIANA INC
   PO Box 98024
   Baton Rouge, LA 70898-9024

KEY EXECUTIVES:
Chairman Board of Directors .... C Richard Atkins, DDS
Chief Executive Officer/President .... Gery J Barry
Executive VP, Chief Financial Officer .... Peggy Scott
Chief Medical Officer .... James J Carney, MD
Senior VP Chief Information Officer ... Worachote 'Ob' Soonthornsima
Chief Marketing Officer .... Mike Reitz
VP Corp Communications .... John Maginnis
VP Provider Contracting/Network Administrator .... Dawn Cantrell
Senior VP, Human Resources .... Todd Schexnayder
Director of Case Management .... Dwight Brower
Manager Health & Quality Management .... Danis Daigle
Fraud Prevention/Investigation .... Darrel Langlois
Director New Product Development .... Eric Harrington
Manager Retro Review & Managed Care .... Dawn Clayton

COMPANY PROFILE:
Parent Company Name: Louisiana Health Service & Indemnity Co
Doing Business As: Blue Cross/Blue Shield of Louisiana
Year Founded: 1934   Federally Qualified: [ ]
Forprofit: [ ]   Not-For-Profit: [Y]
Model Type: NETWORK
Accreditation: [ ] AAPPO [ ] JACHO [ ] NCQA [ ] URAC
Plan Type: PPO, ASO, POS, HDHP, HSA
Total Revenue: 2005:   2006: 1,764,000,000
Net Income   2005:   2006: 78,000,000
Total Enrollment:
   2001: 0   2004: 986,947   2007: 0
   2002: 899,755   2005: 1,018,150
   2003: 910,530   2006: 1,070,453

SERVICE AREA:
Nationwide: N
   LA;

TYPE OF COVERAGE:
Commercial: [Y] Individual: [Y] FEHBP: [Y] Indemnity: [Y]
Medicare: [ ] Medicaid: [ ] Supplemental Medicare: [Y]
Tricare   [ ]

PRODUCTS OFFERED:
Product Name: Type:
Preferred Care PPO   PPO

Managed Care Organization Profiles — KENTUCKY

Year Founded: 1986 Federally Qualified: [N]
Forprofit: [Y] Not-For-Profit: [ ]
Model Type: IPA
Accreditation: [ ] AAPPO [ ] JACHO [ ] NCQA [ ] URAC
Plan Type: HMO, PPO, POS, CDHP, HDHP, HSA, HRA,
Total Revenue: 2005: 2006: 67,546,250
Net Income 2005: 2006:
Total Enrollment:
   2001: 0 2004: 29,907 2007: 0
   2002: 83,041 2005:
   2003: 50,446 2006:
Medical Loss Ratio: 2005: 2006: 83.40
Administrative Expense Ratio: 2005: 2006:

SERVICE AREA:
Nationwide: N
   KY (Clark, Crawford, Floyd, Harrison);

TYPE OF COVERAGE:
Commercial: [Y] Individual: [ ] FEHBP: [ ] Indemnity: [ ]
Medicare: [ ] Medicaid: [ ] Supplemental Medicare: [ ]
Tricare [ ]

PRODUCTS OFFERED:
Product Name: Type:
United Healthcare of KY HMO

CONSUMER-DRIVEN PRODUCTS
Exante Bank/Golden Rule Ins Co HSA Company
iPlan HSA HSA Product
   HSA Administrator
   Consumer-Driven Health Plan
   High Deductible Health Plan

PLAN BENEFITS:
Alternative Medicine: [ ] Behavioral Health: [ ]
Chiropractic: [X] Dental: [X]
Home Care: [X] Inpatient SNF: [X]
Long-Term Care: [ ] Pharm. Mail Order: [ ]
Physical Therapy: [X] Podiatry: [X]
Psychiatric: [X] Transplant: [X]
Vision: [X] Wellness: [X]
Workers' Comp: [ ]
Other Benefits:
Comments:
Formerly Healthwise of Kentucky.

UNIVERSITY HEALTH CARE INC - PASSPORT HEALTH PLAN

305 W Broadway 3rd Fl
Louisville, KY 40202
Phone: 502-585-7900 Fax: 502-585-7985 Toll-Free: 800-578-0603
Web site: www.passporthealthplan.com

MAILING ADDRESS:
   UNIVERSITY HEALTH CARE INC/PP
   305 W Broadway 3rd Fl
   Louisville, KY 40202

KEY EXECUTIVES:
Chairman of the Board/Chief Executive Officer .... Larry N Cook, MD
President .... Joyce S Hagen
Chief Financial Officer .... David A Stanley
Chief Medical Officer .... Jacqueline Roberts Simmons, MD
Chief Operating Officer .... Ruth Atkins
Vice President Public Affairs .... Jill Joseph Bell
Director Provider Services .... Lois Dailey

COMPANY PROFILE:
Parent Company Name: University Health Care Inc
Doing Business As: Passport Health Plan
Year Founded: 2000 Federally Qualified: [N]
Forprofit: [ ] Not-For-Profit: [Y]
Model Type:
Accreditation: [ ] AAPPO [ ] JACHO [ ] NCQA [ ] URAC
Plan Type: HMO
Primary Physicians: 718 Physician Specialists: 2,219
Hospitals: 33
Total Revenue: 2005: 2006: 716,434,659
Net Income 2005: 2006:
Total Enrollment:
   2001: 0 2004: 135,912 2007: 0
   2002: 129,262 2005:
   2003: 132,579 2006: 140,625
Medical Loss Ratio: 2005: 2006: 86.60
Administrative Expense Ratio: 2005: 2006:

SERVICE AREA:
Nationwide: N
   KY;

TYPE OF COVERAGE:
Commercial: [ ] Individual: [ ] FEHBP: [ ] Indemnity: [ ]
Medicare: [ ] Medicaid: [Y] Supplemental Medicare: [ ]
Tricare [ ]

PRODUCTS OFFERED:
Product Name: Type:
Passport Health Plan Medicaid HMO

KENTUCKY

COMPANY PROFILE:
Parent Company Name: Humana Inc
Doing Business As:
Year Founded: 1961   Federally Qualified: [Y]
Forprofit: [Y]   Not-For-Profit: [ ]
Model Type: MIXED
Accreditation: [Y] AAPPO [ ] JACHO [Y] NCQA [Y] URAC
Plan Type: HMO, PPO, Specialty HMO, Specialty PPO, PBM, POS, EPO, ASO, CDHP, HSA, TPA
Primary Physicians: Physician Specialists:
Hospitals: 4,015
Total Revenue: 2005: 14,418,127,000   2006: 21,416,537,000
Net Income   2005:   296,730,000   2006:   487,423,000
Total Enrollment:
  2001: 6,435,800   2004: 8,740,900   2007: 11,282,400
  2002: 6,647,100   2005: 7,075,600
  2003: 6,769,600   2006: 11,272,100
Medical Loss Ratio: 2005: 83.20   2006: 84.00
Administrative Expense Ratio: 2005: 15.40   2006: 17.30

SERVICE AREA:
Nationwide: N
  AK; AL; AR; AZ; CA; CO; DC; DE; FL; GA; HI; IA; ID; IL; IN; KS; KY; MA; MD; ME; MI; MN; MO; NC; NE; NH; NJ; NM; NY; NV; OH; PR; TN; TX; VA; WI;

TYPE OF COVERAGE:
Commercial: [Y] Individual: [Y] FEHBP: [Y] Indemnity: [Y]
Medicare: [Y] Medicaid: [Y] Supplemental Medicare: [Y]
Tricare   [Y]

PRODUCTS OFFERED:
Product Name:	Type:
Humana HMO	HMO
Humana PPO	PPO
Humana Medicare Advantage	Medicare
Humana Tricare	Tricare
Humana ASO	ASO
Humana Tricare ASO	ASO
Humana	Medicaid

CONSUMER-DRIVEN PRODUCTS
UMB Bank	HSA Company
HDHP with HSA	HSA Product
UMB Bank	HSA Administrator
Personal Care Account	Consumer-Driven Health Plan
SmartSuite HDHP and PCA	High Deductible Health Plan

PLAN BENEFITS:
Alternative Medicine: [ ]   Behavioral Health: [X]
Chiropractic: [X]   Dental: [X]
Home Care: [X]   Inpatient SNF: [X]
Long-Term Care: [X]   Pharm. Mail Order: [X]
Physical Therapy: [X]   Podiatry: [X]
Psychiatric: [X]   Transplant: [X]
Vision: [ ]   Wellness: [X]
Workers' Comp: [X]
Other Benefits: Long Term Disability

Comments:
To meet the needs of its members, Humana offers discounts on complementary and alternative medicine (CAM) services that include chiropractic care, acupuncture, and massage. Please note that CAM services are not insurance products.

HUMANA MILITARY SERVICE INC

500 W Main St Humana Bldg
Louisville, KY 40201
Phone: 502-580-5804 Fax: 502-580-5044 Toll-Free:
Web site: www.humana-military.com

MAILING ADDRESS:
  HUMANA MILITARY SERVICE INC
  500 W Main St Humana Bldg
  Louisville, KY 40201

KEY EXECUTIVES:
Chairman of the Board .... David A Jones Jr
Chief Executive Officer/President .... David Baker
Chief Financial Officer .... Ray Pryor
Chief Medical Officer .... John Crum, MD
Chief Operating Officer .... Orie Mullen

COMPANY PROFILE:
Parent Company Name: Humana Inc
Doing Business As:
Year Founded: 1993   Federally Qualified: [Y]
Forprofit: [Y]   Not-For-Profit: [ ]
Model Type:
Accreditation: [ ] AAPPO [ ] JACHO [ ] NCQA [ ] URAC
Plan Type: HMO, PPO, POS, ASO, CDHP, HSA
Total Enrollment:
  2001: 0   2004: 2,871,800   2007: 0
  2002: 0   2005:
  2003: 2,906,900   2006:

SERVICE AREA:
Nationwide: N
  AL; FL; GA; LA; MS; SC; TN;

CONSUMER-DRIVEN PRODUCTS
JP Morgan Chase	HSA Company
HumanaOne HSA	HSA Product
JP Morgan Chase	HSA Administrator
Personal Care Account	Consumer-Driven Health Plan
HumanaOne	High Deductible Health Plan

SHPS INC

9200 Shelbyville Rd
Louisville, KY 40222
Phone: 502-267-4900 Fax: 502-263-5610 Toll-Free: 888-421-7477
Web site: www.shps.net

MAILING ADDRESS:
  SHPS INC
  9200 Shelbyville Rd
  Louisville, KY 40222

KEY EXECUTIVES:
Chief Executive Officer/President .... Rishabh Mehrotra
Chief Financial Officer .... John McCarty
Chief Medical Officer .... Gerald E Osband, MD
Chief Technology Officer/MIS Director .... Amin Kassem
Chief Operating Officer .... Keith Stoneback
Chief Strategy & Marketing Officer .... Chris Ryan
Privacy Officer .... David Lee
Director, Corporate Communications .... Sarah Bovine
Senior Vice President, Healthcare Operations .... Jim Beck
Director of Human Resources .... Irene Wong
Chief Quality Officer .... Susan Lemons
Vice President, Product Management, Healthcare .... Janis Moebus
President/Health Management Solutions .... Reed Keller

COMPANY PROFILE:
Parent Company Name:
Doing Business As:
Year Founded: 1997   Federally Qualified: [ ]
Forprofit: [Y]   Not-For-Profit: [ ]
Model Type:
Accreditation: [ ] AAPPO [ ] JACHO [ ] NCQA [ ] URAC
Plan Type: UR

SERVICE AREA:
Nationwide:
  NW;

Comments:
Acquired National Health Services and Landacorp Inc in 2004.

UNITEDHEALTHCARE OF KENTUCKY

2424 Harrodsburg Rd Ste 300
Lexington, KY 40504-3329
Phone: 859-296-6000 Fax: 859-224-3732 Toll-Free: 800-495-5283
Web site: www.uhc.com

MAILING ADDRESS:
  UNITEDHEALTHCARE OF KENTUCKY
  2424 Harrodsburg Rd Ste 300
  Lexington, KY 40504-3329

KEY EXECUTIVES:
Non-Executive Chairman .... Richard T Burke
Chief Executive Officer/President .... Larry J Kissner
President .... Larry J Kissner
Chief Financial Officer .... Steven McCowan
Medical Director .... Alan Grimes, MD

COMPANY PROFILE:
Parent Company Name: UnitedHealth Group
Doing Business As:

Managed Care Organization Profiles   **KENTUCKY**

Medical Loss Ratio: 2005:   2006: 82.60
Administrative Expense Ratio: 2005:   2006:
SERVICE AREA:
Nationwide: N
   KY;
TYPE OF COVERAGE:
Commercial: [Y] Individual: [Y] FEHBP: [ ] Indemnity: [ ]
Medicare: [ ] Medicaid: [ ] Supplemental Medicare: [ ]
Tricare   [ ]
PRODUCTS OFFERED:
Product Name: Type:
Delta Premier   Indemnity
Delta Preferred Option   PPO
Delta Care   DHMO
PLAN BENEFITS:
Alternative Medicine: [ ]   Behavioral Health: [ ]
Chiropractic: [ ]   Dental: [X]
Home Care: [ ]   Inpatient SNF: [ ]
Long-Term Care: [ ]   Pharm. Mail Order: [ ]
Physical Therapy: [ ]   Podiatry: [ ]
Psychiatric: [ ]   Transplant: [ ]
Vision: [X]   Wellness: [ ]
Workers' Comp: [ ]
Other Benefits:

HUMANA HEALTH CARE PLANS OF LEXINGTON

300 W Vine St
Lexington, KY 40507
Phone: 859-263-1400 Fax: 859-263-1488 Toll-Free: 800-221-8390
Web site: www.humana.com
MAILING ADDRESS:
   HUMANA HEALTH CARE PLANS LEXINGTON
   300 W Vine St
   Lexington, KY 40507

KEY EXECUTIVES:
Chairman of the Board .... David A Jones Jr
Chief Executive Officer .... Michael B McCallister
President .... Jeff Bringardner
Vice President of Sales .... Charles Ritz

COMPANY PROFILE:
Parent Company Name: Humana Inc
Doing Business As:
Year Founded: 1961   Federally Qualified: [Y]
Forprofit: [Y]   Not-For-Profit: [ ]
Model Type: MIXED
Accreditation: [ ] AAPPO [ ] JACHO [ ] NCQA [X] URAC
Plan Type: HMO, PPO, POS, EPO, ASO, CDHP, HSA
Total Enrollment:
   2001: 0   2004: 0   2007: 0
   2002: 300,000   2005:
   2003: 421,500   2006:
SERVICE AREA:
Nationwide: N
   KY;
TYPE OF COVERAGE:
Commercial: [Y] Individual: [ ] FEHBP: [ ] Indemnity: [ ]
Medicare: [ ] Medicaid: [ ] Supplemental Medicare: [ ]
Tricare   [ ]
CONSUMER-DRIVEN PRODUCTS
JP Morgan Chase   HSA Company
HumanaOne HSA   HSA Product
JP Morgan Chase   HSA Administrator
Personal Care Account   Consumer-Driven Health Plan
HumanaOne   High Deductible Health Plan
PLAN BENEFITS:
Alternative Medicine: [ ]   Behavioral Health: [X]
Chiropractic: [X]   Dental: [X]
Home Care: [ ]   Inpatient SNF: [ ]
Long-Term Care: [ ]   Pharm. Mail Order: [X]
Physical Therapy: [ ]   Podiatry: [ ]
Psychiatric: [X]   Transplant: [X]
Vision: [ ]   Wellness: [ ]
Workers' Comp: [X]
Other Benefits: Long Term Disability
Comments:
See Humana Health Plan-Kentucky for enrollment figures.

HUMANA HEALTH PLAN - KENTUCKY

321 W Main St
Louisville, KY 40202
Phone: 502-476-5001 Fax: 502-580-5044 Toll-Free: 800-448-0222
Web site: www.humana.com
MAILING ADDRESS:
   HUMANA HEALTH PLAN - KY
   321 W Main St
   Louisville, KY 40202

KEY EXECUTIVES:
Chairman of the Board .... David A Jones Jr
Market President .... Jeff Bringardner
Vice President of Clinical Innovations .... Bryan Loy, MD
Regional Marketing Leader .... Shelley Richter
Vice President of Sales .... Carla Whaley
Network Development Director .... Bill Niehaus
Human Capital Consultant .... A J Hubbard
Compliance Officer .... Nancy Walsh
Communications/Media Relations .... Jim Turner

COMPANY PROFILE:
Parent Company Name: Humana Inc
Doing Business As:
Year Founded: 1961   Federally Qualified: [Y]
Forprofit: [Y]   Not-For-Profit: [ ]
Model Type: GROUP
Accreditation: [ ] AAPPO [ ] JACHO [X] NCQA [X] URAC
Plan Type: HMO, PPO, POS, EPO, ASO, CDHP, HDHP, HSA
Total Enrollment:
   2001: 0   2004: 580,582   2007: 0
   2002: 782,573   2005:
   2003: 686,877   2006:
SERVICE AREA:
Nationwide: N
   KY; Southern IN;
TYPE OF COVERAGE:
Commercial: [Y] Individual: [Y] FEHBP: [ ] Indemnity: [ ]
Medicare: [Y] Medicaid: [ ] Supplemental Medicare: [Y]
Tricare   [ ]
PRODUCTS OFFERED:
Product Name: Type:
Humana Gold Plus Plan   Medicare Advantage
CONSUMER-DRIVEN PRODUCTS
JP Morgan Chase   HSA Company
HumanaOne HSA   HSA Product
JP Morgan Chase   HSA Administrator
Personal Care Account   Consumer-Driven Health Plan
HumanaOne   High Deductible Health Plan
PLAN BENEFITS:
Alternative Medicine: [ ]   Behavioral Health: [X]
Chiropractic: [X]   Dental: [X]
Home Care: [ ]   Inpatient SNF: [ ]
Long-Term Care: [ ]   Pharm. Mail Order: [X]
Physical Therapy: [ ]   Podiatry: [ ]
Psychiatric: [X]   Transplant: [X]
Vision: [ ]   Wellness: [ ]
Workers' Comp: [X]
Other Benefits: Long Term Disability

HUMANA INC - CORPORATE HEADQUARTERS

500 W Main St
Louisville, KY 40202
Phone: 502-580-1000 Fax: 502-580-3677 Toll-Free:
Web site: www.humana.com
MAILING ADDRESS:
   HUMANA INC - CORPORATE HDQTRS
   500 W Main St
   Louisville, KY 40202

KEY EXECUTIVES:
Chairman of the Board .... David A Jones Jr
Chief Executive Officer/President .... Michael B McCallister
Chief Financial Officer .... James H Bloem
Senior VP, Chief Innovation Officer .... Jonathan T Lord, MD
Senior VP, Chief Service Information Officer .... Bruce J Goodman
Chief Operating Officer .... James E Murray
Senior Vice President Chief Marketing Officer .... Steven O Moya
SR Vice President of Human Resources .... Bonnie C Hathcock
Senior Vice President, Government Relations .... Heidi S Margulis

KENTUCKY
Managed Care Organization Profiles

PLAN BENEFITS:

Alternative Medicine:	[ ]	Behavioral Health:	[X]
Chiropractic:	[X]	Dental:	[ ]
Home Care:	[ ]	Inpatient SNF:	[X]
Long-Term Care:	[X]	Pharm. Mail Order:	[X]
Physical Therapy:	[X]	Podiatry:	[X]
Psychiatric:	[X]	Transplant:	[X]
Vision:	[X]	Wellness:	[ ]
Workers' Comp:	[X]		

Other Benefits:

CENTER CARE

1225 Fairway St
Bowling Green, KY 42103
Phone: 270-745-1517 Fax: 270-796-2106 Toll-Free: 800-972-7038
Web site: www.centercare.com

MAILING ADDRESS:
CENTER CARE
PO Box 148
Bowling Green, KY 42103

KEY EXECUTIVES:
Chief Executive Officer .... Ron Fowell
Senior Vice President .... John Mark Fones
Medical Director .... John Blackburn
Senior Applications Analyst .... Larecia Denning-Bell
Vice President of Operations .... Teresa Wilson
Vice President of Market Development .... Sean McGuinness
Director of Member Services .... Kim Mitchell

COMPANY PROFILE:
Parent Company Name: Commonwealth Health Corporation
Doing Business As: Center Care Health Benefit Programs
Year Founded: 1990   Federally Qualified: [ ]
Forprofit: [ ]   Not-For-Profit: [Y]
Model Type: NETWORK
Accreditation: [ ] AAPPO [ ] JACHO [ ] NCQA [ ] URAC
Plan Type: PPO, POS, TPA, EPO, UR

SERVICE AREA:
Nationwide: N
KY;

TYPE OF COVERAGE:
Commercial: [Y] Individual: [ ] FEHBP: [ ] Indemnity: [ ]
Medicare: [ ] Medicaid: [ ] Supplemental Medicare: [ ]
Tricare [ ]

PRODUCTS OFFERED:

Product Name:	Type:
Center Care	PPO
Center Care Plus	POS
Community Health Plans	EPO
Complink	Workers' Comp

PLAN BENEFITS:

Alternative Medicine:	[ ]	Behavioral Health:	[ ]
Chiropractic:	[ ]	Dental:	[X]
Home Care:	[ ]	Inpatient SNF:	[ ]
Long-Term Care:	[ ]	Pharm. Mail Order:	[ ]
Physical Therapy:	[ ]	Podiatry:	[ ]
Psychiatric:	[ ]	Transplant:	[ ]
Vision:	[X]	Wellness:	[X]
Workers' Comp:	[X]		

Other Benefits:

Comments:
Network only at this time. TPA services in development as well as Network expansion.

CHA HEALTH - HUMANA

300 W Vine St 16th Fl
Lexington, KY 40503
Phone: 859-232-8686 Fax: 859-232-8557 Toll-Free: 800-277-1088
Web site: www.cha-health.com

MAILING ADDRESS:
CHA HEALTH - HUMANA
300 W Vine St 16th Fl
Lexington, KY 40503

KEY EXECUTIVES:
Chairman .... David A Jones, Jr
Chief Executive Officer/President .... Michael B McCallister

COMPANY PROFILE:
Parent Company Name: Humana Inc
Doing Business As: CHA Health
Year Founded: 1995   Federally Qualified: [ ]
Forprofit: [Y]   Not-For-Profit: [ ]
Model Type: MIXED
Accreditation: [ ] AAPPO [ ] JACHO [ ] NCQA [ ] URAC
Plan Type: HMO, POS, TPA
Total Revenue: 2005:   2006: 181,417,076
Net Income   2005:   2006:
Total Enrollment:
   2001: 0   2004: 122,012   2007: 0
   2002: 78,712   2005:
   2003: 114,947   2006: 600,000
Medical Loss Ratio: 2005:   2006: 90.90
Administrative Expense Ratio: 2005:   2006:

SERVICE AREA:
Nationwide: N
KY (Adair, Allen, Anderson, Ballard, Barren, Bath, Bell, Boone, Bourbon, Boyd, Boyle, Bracken, Breathitt, Butler, Caldwell, Calloway, Campbell, Carlisle, Carter, Casey, Clark, Clay, Clinton, Crittenden, Cumberland, Edmonson, Elliott, Estill, Fayette, Fleming, Floyd, Franklin, Fulton, Gallatin, Garrard, Grant, Graves, Greenup, Harlan, Harrison, Hart, Hickman, Jackson, Jessamine, Johnson, Kenton, Knott, Knox, Laurel, Lawrence, Lee, Leslie, Letcher, Lewis, Lincoln, Livingston, Logan, Lyon, Madison, Magoffin, Marshall, Martin, Mason, Mc Cracken, Menifee, Mercer, Metcalfe, Monroe, Montgomery, Morgan, Nicholas, Owen, Owsley, Pendleton, Perry, Pike, Powell, Robertson, Rockcastle, Rowan, Russell, Scott, Simpson, Trigg, Washington, Warren, Whitley, Wolfe, Woodford);

TYPE OF COVERAGE:
Commercial: [Y] Individual: [ ] FEHBP: [ ] Indemnity: [ ]
Medicare: [ ] Medicaid: [ ] Supplemental Medicare: [ ]
Tricare [ ]

PLAN BENEFITS:

Alternative Medicine:	[ ]	Behavioral Health:	[ ]
Chiropractic:	[X]	Dental:	[X]
Home Care:	[X]	Inpatient SNF:	[X]
Long-Term Care:	[X]	Pharm. Mail Order:	[ ]
Physical Therapy:	[X]	Podiatry:	[X]
Psychiatric:	[X]	Transplant:	[X]
Vision:	[X]	Wellness:	[X]
Workers' Comp:	[ ]		

Other Benefits:

DELTA DENTAL PLAN OF KENTUCKY INC

9901 Linn Station Rd
Louisville, KY 40223
Phone: 502-736-4621 Fax: 502-736-4826 Toll-Free: 800-955-2030
Web site: www.deltadentalky.com

MAILING ADDRESS:
DELTA DENTAL PLAN OF KY
PO Box 242810
Louisville, KY 40223

KEY EXECUTIVES:
Chief Executive Officer/President .... Clifford T Maesaka, Jr, DDS
Chief Financial Officer .... Curtis R Ladig
Chief Marketing Officer .... Stephen C Day
Director of Provider Services .... Angie Nenni

COMPANY PROFILE:
Parent Company Name: Delta Dental Plan of Kentucky Inc
Doing Business As: Delta Dental Plan of Kentucky Inc
Year Founded: 1966   Federally Qualified: [N]
Forprofit: [ ]   Not-For-Profit: [Y] Model Type:
Accreditation: [ ] AAPPO [ ] JACHO [ ] NCQA [ ] URAC
Plan Type: Specialty PPO, TPA
Total Revenue: 2005:   2006: 61,469,514
Net Income   2005:   2006:
Total Enrollment:
   2001: 0   2004: 135,396   2007: 0
   2002: 101,789   2005:
   2003: 82,265   2006:

Managed Care Organization Profiles — KENTUCKY

AMERICAN PHARMACY SERVICES CORPORATION

102 Enterprise Dr
Frankfort, KY 40601-6514
Phone: 502-695-8899 Fax: 502-695-9912 Toll-Free: 800-928-2228
Web site: www.apscnet.com

MAILING ADDRESS:
AMERICAN PHARMACY SRVCS CORP
102 Enterprise Dr
Frankfort, KY 40601-6514

KEY EXECUTIVES:
Chairman ....Dominic Bartone
Executive Vice President .... Ralph E Bouvette, RPA, PhD, JD
Business Administrator .... Teresa Doris
Vice President, Marketing/Group Purchasing .... Cathi Clark
Vice President, Professional Affairs .... J D Hammond, PharmD
Vice President, Professional Affairs .... Cathy Hanna
Administrative Assistant .... Amanda Jefferson

COMPANY PROFILE:
Parent Company Name: APSC (American Pharmacy Service Corp)
Doing Business As:
Year Founded: 1985   Federally Qualified: [N]
Forprofit: [Y]   Not-For-Profit: [ ]
Model Type:
Accreditation: [ ] AAPPO [ ] JACHO [ ] NCQA [ ] URAC
Plan Type: Specialty PPO, PBM

SERVICE AREA:
Nationwide: N
    IL; IN; KY; MO; OH; TN; VA; WV;

TYPE OF COVERAGE:
Commercial: [ ] Individual: [Y] FEHBP: [ ] Indemnity: [ ]
Medicare: [ ] Medicaid: [ ] Supplemental Medicare: [ ]
Tricare   [ ]

PLAN BENEFITS:
Alternative Medicine: [ ]   Behavioral Health: [ ]
Chiropractic: [ ]   Dental: [ ]
Home Care: [ ]   Inpatient SNF: [ ]
Long-Term Care: [ ]   Pharm. Mail Order: [ ]
Physical Therapy: [ ]   Podiatry: [ ]
Psychiatric: [ ]   Transplant: [ ]
Vision: [ ]   Wellness: [ ]
Workers' Comp: [ ]
Other Benefits: Pharmacy Cooperative

ANTHEM BLUE CROSS AND BLUE SHIELD OF KENTUCKY (HMO KENTUCKY)

13550 Triton Park Blvd
Louisville, KY 40223
Phone: 502-889-2111 Fax: 502-329-8559 Toll-Free: 800-880-2583
Web site: www.anthem.com

MAILING ADDRESS:
ANTHEM BLUE CROSS BLUE SHIELD
13550 Triton Park Blvd
Louisville, KY 40223

KEY EXECUTIVES:
Chief Executive Officer/President .... Deborah W Moessner
Provider Services Director .... Kathy Lower

COMPANY PROFILE:
Parent Company Name: WellPoint Inc
Doing Business As:
Year Founded: Federally Qualified: [ ]
Forprofit: [Y]   Not-For-Profit: [ ]
Model Type:
Accreditation: [ ] AAPPO [ ] JACHO [ ] NCQA [ ] URAC
Plan Type: HMO, PPO, POS, HSA
Total Revenue: 2005:   2006:   1,528,805,051
Net Income   2005:   2006:
Total Enrollment:
    2001: 0   2004: 625,351   2007: 0
    2002: 568,000   2005:
    2003: 590,410   2006: 1,200,000

SERVICE AREA:
Nationwide: N
    KY;

TYPE OF COVERAGE:
Commercial: [Y] Individual: [ ] FEHBP: [ ] Indemnity: [ ]
Medicare: [ ] Medicaid: [ ] Supplemental Medicare: [ ]
Tricare   [ ]

PRODUCTS OFFERED:
Product Name: Type:
Anthem Senior Advantage   Medicare

CONSUMER-DRIVEN PRODUCTS
JP Morgan Chase   HSA Company
Anthem ByDesign HSA   HSA Product
JP Morgan Chase   HSA Administrator
Blue Access Saver   Consumer-Driven Health Plan
Blue Access Economy Plans PPO   High Deductible Health Plan

BLUEGRASS FAMILY HEALTH INC

651 Perimeter Dr Ste 300
Lexington, KY 40517
Phone: 859-269-4475 Fax: 859-335-3750 Toll-Free:
Web site: www.bgfh.com

MAILING ADDRESS:
BLUEGRASS FAMILY HEALTH INC
651 Perimeter Dr Ste 300
Lexington, KY 40517

KEY EXECUTIVES:
Chief Executive Officer/President .... James S Fritz
Chief Financial Officer .... Art Lowe
Chief Medical Officer .... Jaudon Behrman, MD
Director of Pharmacy .... Joe Vennari
Information Technology Director .... Preston Gorman
Chief Marketing Officer .... Garry Ramsey
Director of Sales & Marketing .... Nancy Atkins
Director of Information Technology .... Preston Gorman
Credentialing Coordinator .... Barbara Farrell
Director of Compliance .... Jessica Kearney
Director Network Development/Provider Relations .... Spencer Boyer
Human Resources Director .... Carole Owen
Vice President Healthcare Management .... Peter Gurk, MD
Credentialing Coordinator .... Barbara Farrell
Director of Customer Service .... Jetta Jones
Healthcare Operations Director .... Angela Parker
Marketing/Sales Administrator .... Faith Powers

COMPANY PROFILE:
Parent Company Name: Baptist Healthcare System
Doing Business As:
Year Founded: 1993   Federally Qualified: [N]
Forprofit: [ ]   Not-For-Profit: [Y]
Model Type: IPA
Accreditation: [ ] AAPPO [ ] JACHO [ ] NCQA [ ] URAC
Plan Type: HMO, PPO, POS, HDHP, HSA
Primary Physicians: 7,915   Physician Specialists: 10,514
Hospitals: 289
Total Revenue: 2005: 492,588,115   2006: 80,560,414
Net Income   2005:   13,594,781   2006:   4,427,205
Total Enrollment:
    2001: 0   2004: 136,506   2007: 50,214
    2002: 123,039   2005: 136,223
    2003: 136,455   2006: 51,003
Medical Loss Ratio: 2005:   2006: 84.00
Administrative Expense Ratio: 2005:   2006: 10.00

SERVICE AREA:
Nationwide: N
    KY (Central & Eastern);

TYPE OF COVERAGE:
Commercial: [Y] Individual: [ ] FEHBP: [ ] Indemnity: [ ]
Medicare: [ ] Medicaid: [ ] Supplemental Medicare: [ ]
Tricare   [ ]

CONSUMER-DRIVEN PRODUCTS
Fifth Third Bank   HSA Company
                                       HSA Product
1 Point Solution   HSA Administrator
                                       Consumer-Driven Health Plan
                                       High Deductible Health Plan

KANSAS

Managed Care Organization Profiles

SERVICE AREA:
Nationwide: Y
  NW;
TYPE OF COVERAGE:
Commercial: [Y] Individual: [Y] FEHBP: [ ] Indemnity: [ ]
Medicare: [ ] Medicaid: [ ] Supplemental Medicare: [ ]
Tricare   [ ]
PLAN BENEFITS:
Alternative Medicine: [ ]   Behavioral Health: [ ]
Chiropractic: [ ]   Dental: [X]
Home Care: [ ]   Inpatient SNF: [ ]
Long-Term Care: [ ]   Pharm. Mail Order: [ ]
Physical Therapy: [ ]   Podiatry: [ ]
Psychiatric: [ ]   Transplant: [ ]
Vision: [X]   Wellness: [X]
Workers' Comp: [ ]
Other Benefits:

UNITEDHEALTHCARE OF THE HEARTLAND STATES

9900 W 109th St Ste 200
Overland Park, KS 66210-2002
Phone: 913-663-6500 Fax: 314-592-7600 Toll-Free: 888-340-9716
Web site: www.uhc.com
MAILING ADDRESS:
  UNITEDHEALTHCARE OF HEARTLND STATES
  9900 W 109th St Ste 200
  Overland Park, KS 66210-2002

KEY EXECUTIVES:
Non-Executive Chairman .... Richard T Burke
Chief Executive Officer .... William C Tracy
Chief Financial Officer .... Keith Wisdom
Marketing Director .... Greg Thompson

COMPANY PROFILE:
Parent Company Name: UnitedHealth Group
Doing Business As:
Year Founded: 1987   Federally Qualified: [N]
Forprofit: [Y]   Not-For-Profit: [ ]
Model Type: IPA
Accreditation: [X] AAPPO [ ] JACHO [ ] NCQA [X] URAC
Plan Type: HMO, PPO, POS, CDHP, HDHP, HRA, HSA,
Total Enrollment:
  2001: 0   2004: 0   2007: 0
  2002: 436,259   2005:
  2003: 251,239   2006:
SERVICE AREA:
Nationwide: N
  KS (Anderson, Atchison, Douglas, Franklin, Jackson, Jefferson,
  Johnson, Leavenworth, Linn, Miami, Osage, Segwick, Shawnee,
  Wyandotte); MO (Cass, Clay, Jackson, Lafayette, Platt, Ray);
TYPE OF COVERAGE:
Commercial: [Y] Individual: [Y] FEHBP: [ ] Indemnity: [ ]
Medicare: [ ] Medicaid: [ ] Supplemental Medicare: [ ]
Tricare   [ ]
PRODUCTS OFFERED:

Product Name:	Type:
United HealthCare Choice Select Plus	HMO
United HealthCare Medicare Complete	HMO MedicareUnited
HealthCare Preferred Provider	PPO

CONSUMER-DRIVEN PRODUCTS

Exante Bank/Golden Rule Ins Co	HSA Company
iPlan HSA	HSA Product
	HSA Administrator
	Consumer-Driven Health Plan
	High Deductible Health Plan

PLAN BENEFITS:
Alternative Medicine: [ ]   Behavioral Health: [X]
Chiropractic: [X]   Dental: [ ]
Home Care: [X]   Inpatient SNF: [X]
Long-Term Care: [ ]   Pharm. Mail Order: [X]
Physical Therapy: [X]   Podiatry: [X]
Psychiatric: [X]   Transplant: [X]
Vision: [X]   Wellness: [X]
Workers' Comp: [ ]
Other Benefits:
Comments:
Formerly Metrahealth Care Plan Kansas City.

Managed Care Organization Profiles — KANSAS

MAILING ADDRESS:
PREFERRED MENTAL HEALTH MGNMT
401 E Douglas Ste 300
Wichita, KS 67202-3411

KEY EXECUTIVES:
Chief Executive Officer/President .... Les Ruthven, PhD
Executive Vice President .... Courtney Ruthven, PhD
Chief Psychologist .... R Lance Parker, PhD
Director of Operations .... Melissa Smith
Marketing Director .... Teri Bjostad
Director of Provider Services .... Patrick McMurphy

COMPANY PROFILE:
Parent Company Name:
Doing Business As:
Year Founded: 1987   Federally Qualified: [ ]
Forprofit: [Y]   Not-For-Profit: [ ]
Model Type:
Accreditation: [ ] AAPPO [X] JACHO [ ] NCQA [ ] URAC
Plan Type: Specialty PPO, UR

SERVICE AREA:
Nationwide: Y
NW;

TYPE OF COVERAGE:
Commercial: [Y] Individual: [ ] FEHBP: [ ] Indemnity: [ ]
Medicare: [ ] Medicaid: [ ] Supplemental Medicare: [ ]
Tricare [ ]

PLAN BENEFITS:
Alternative Medicine: [ ]   Behavioral Health: [X]
Chiropractic: [ ]   Dental: [ ]
Home Care: [ ]   Inpatient SNF: [ ]
Long-Term Care: [ ]   Pharm. Mail Order: [ ]
Physical Therapy: [ ]   Podiatry: [ ]
Psychiatric: [ ]   Transplant: [ ]
Vision: [ ]   Wellness: [ ]
Workers' Comp: [ ]
Other Benefits:

PREFERRED PLUS OF KANSAS INC

8535 E 21st St N
Wichita, KS 67206
Phone: 316-609-2345 Fax: 316-609-2346 Toll-Free: 800-990-0345
Web site: www.phsystems.com

MAILING ADDRESS:
PREFERRED PLUS OF KS INC
8535 E 21st Street N
Wichtia, KS 67206

KEY EXECUTIVES:
President/Chief Executive Officer .... Marion Dauner

COMPANY PROFILE:
Parent Company Name: Preferred Health Systems
Doing Business As: Preferred Plus of Kansas
Year Founded: 1992   Federally Qualified: [N]
Forprofit: [Y]   Not-For-Profit: [ ]
Model Type:
Accreditation: [ ] AAPPO [ ] JACHO [ ] NCQA [ ] URAC
Plan Type: HMO
Total Revenue: 2005:   2006: 230,084,255
Net Income   2005:   2006:
Total Enrollment:
  2001: 0   2004: 0   2007: 0
  2002: 0   2005:
  2003: 0   2006:
Medical Loss Ratio: 2005:   2006: 88.40
Administrative Expense Ratio: 2005:   2006:

SERVICE AREA:
Nationwide: N
KS (Brown, Pottawatomie, Shawnee, Jefferson, Segwick, Butler, Cowley, Chautauqua, Sumner, Kingman, Harvey, McPherson, Marion, Jackson, Nemaha);

TYPE OF COVERAGE:
Commercial: [ ] Individual: [ ] FEHBP: [ ] Indemnity: [ ]
Medicare: [ ] Medicaid: [ ] Supplemental Medicare: [ ]
Tricare [ ]

PROVIDRS CARE NETWORK

1102 S Hillside
Wichita, KS 67211-4004
Phone: 316-683-4111 Fax: 316-683-6255 Toll-Free: 800-801-9772
Web site: www.proviDRsCare.net

MAILING ADDRESS:
PROVIDERS CARE NETWORK
1102 S Hillside
Wichita, KS 67211-4004

KEY EXECUTIVES:
Chief Executive Officer .... Jan Rosell
Marketing Representative .... Serena Lubbers
Credentialing Manager .... Mary Ann Morand
Director of Provider Services .... Marsha Fisher
Network Development Coordinator .... Erika McGuire
Program Administrator .... Jodi Smith

COMPANY PROFILE:
Parent Company Name: Medical Society Medical Review Fndtn
Doing Business As:
Year Founded: 1985   Federally Qualified: [ ]
Forprofit: [Y]   Not-For-Profit: [ ]
Model Type:
Accreditation: [ ] AAPPO [ ] JACHO [ ] NCQA [X] URAC
Plan Type: PPO, POS, UR, CDHP, HDHP, HSA
Primary Physicians: 1,615   Physician Specialists: 2,527
Hospitals: 139
Total Enrollment:
  2001: 142,000   2004: 141,778   2007: 0
  2002: 133,399   2005:
  2003: 134,432   2006:

SERVICE AREA:
Nationwide: N
KS;

TYPE OF COVERAGE:
Commercial: [Y] Individual: [Y] FEHBP: [ ] Indemnity: [ ]
Medicare: [ ] Medicaid: [ ] Supplemental Medicare: [ ]
Tricare [ ]

PRODUCTS OFFERED:
Product Name: Type:
WPPA PPO   PPO

PLAN BENEFITS:
Alternative Medicine: [ ]   Behavioral Health: [X]
Chiropractic: [X]   Dental: [ ]
Home Care: [X]   Inpatient SNF: [X]
Long-Term Care: [ ]   Pharm. Mail Order: [ ]
Physical Therapy: [X]   Podiatry: [X]
Psychiatric: [X]   Transplant: [X]
Vision: [ ]   Wellness: [ ]
Workers' Comp: [X]
Other Benefits:
Comments:
Formerly known as WPPA, Inc.

SPECTRUM VISION SYSTEMS INC

7101 College Blvd Ste 520
Overland Park, KS 66210
Phone: 913-451-1672 Fax: 913-451-1704 Toll-Free: 800-635-7874
Web site: www.preferredvisioncare.com

MAILING ADDRESS:
SPECTRUM VISION SYSTEMS INC
PO Box 26025
Overland Park, KS 66210

KEY EXECUTIVES:
Chief Executive Officer .... Paul Disser
Chief Financial Officer .... Thomas Mulland, CPA
Marketing Director .... Evan J Disser
Quality Assurance Director .... Hollace M Disser

COMPANY PROFILE:
Parent Company Name:
Doing Business As: Preferred Vision Care
Year Founded: 1983   Federally Qualified: [ ]
Forprofit: [Y]   Not-For-Profit: [ ]
Model Type:
Accreditation: [X] AAPPO [ ] JACHO [X] NCQA [ ] URAC
Plan Type: Specialty PPO, POS, TPA

KANSAS

Managed Care Organization Profiles

MAILING ADDRESS:
PREFERRED CHIROPRACTIC CARE
555 N McLean Blvd Ste 200
Wichita, KS 67203

KEY EXECUTIVES:
Chief Executive Officer/Chief Financial Officer .... Mark Dopps
President/Medical Director .... Brad Dopps
Vice President of Marketing .... Brad Dopps
Director, Provider Services .... Kay Lukens
Director of Marketing .... Beth Dauner

COMPANY PROFILE:
Parent Company Name: Preferred Chiropractic Care Inc
Doing Business As:
Year Founded: 1984   Federally Qualified: [ ]
Forprofit: [Y]   Not-For-Profit: [ ]
Model Type:
Accreditation: [ ] AAPPO [ ] JACHO [ ] NCQA [ ] URAC
Plan Type: PPO, Specialty PPO, UR
Total Enrollment:
  2001: 26,000,000   2004: 0   2007: 0
  2002: 300,000   2005:
  2003: 0   2006: 5,000,000

SERVICE AREA:
Nationwide: Y
  NW;

TYPE OF COVERAGE:
Commercial: [Y] Individual: [ ] FEHBP: [ ] Indemnity: [ ]
Medicare: [ ] Medicaid: [ ] Supplemental Medicare: [ ]
Tricare   [ ]

PLAN BENEFITS:
Alternative Medicine: [ ]   Behavioral Health: [ ]
Chiropractic: [X]   Dental: [ ]
Home Care: [ ]   Inpatient SNF: [ ]
Long-Term Care: [ ]   Pharm. Mail Order: [ ]
Physical Therapy: [ ]   Podiatry: [ ]
Psychiatric: [ ]   Transplant: [ ]
Vision: [ ]   Wellness: [ ]
Workers' Comp: [X]
Other Benefits:

PREFERRED HEALTH PROFESSIONALS

9393 W 110th St Ste 200
Overland Park, KS 66210-1422
Phone: 913-685-6300 Fax: 913-685-6355 Toll-Free: 800-544-3014
Web site: www.phpkc.com

MAILING ADDRESS:
PREFERRED HEALTH PROFESSIONALS
9393 W 110th St Ste 200
Overland Park, KS 66210-1422

KEY EXECUTIVES:
Chief Financial Officer .... Joseph Intfen
Chief Operating Officer .... Roberta Suenram
Vice President, Marketing & Sales .... Robert Herduin
Director of IS .... Ray Panfil
Director of Health Services .... Nadine Yacos
Director, Claims & Customer Service .... Tim Randol
Supervisor of Claims Department .... Sherry Patton

COMPANY PROFILE:
Parent Company Name: BC & BS Kansas City
Doing Business As: PHP
Year Founded: 1983   Federally Qualified: [N]
Forprofit: [ ]   Not-For-Profit: [Y]
Model Type: NETWORK
Accreditation: [ ] AAPPO [ ] JACHO [ ] NCQA [X] URAC
Plan Type: PPO, UR
Primary Physicians: 7,814   Physician Specialists:
Hospitals: 70

SERVICE AREA:
Nationwide: N
  KS; MO;

TYPE OF COVERAGE:
Commercial: [Y] Individual: [ ] FEHBP: [ ] Indemnity: [ ]
Medicare: [ ] Medicaid: [ ] Supplemental Medicare: [ ]
Tricare   [ ]

PRODUCTS OFFERED:
Product Name: Type:
Preferred Health Professionals   PPO

PREFERRED HEALTH SYSTEMS

8535 E 21st St N
Wichita, KS 67206
Phone: 316-609-2345 Fax: 316-609-2346 Toll-Free: 800-990-0345
Web site: www.phsystems.com

MAILING ADDRESS:
PREFERRED HEALTH SYSTEMS
8535 E 21st Street N
Wichtia, KS 67206

KEY EXECUTIVES:
Chief Executive Officer/President .... Marlon R Dauner
Chief Financial Officer .... Todd Kasitz
Chief Medical Officer .... Jill Sumfest, MD
Pharmacy Director .... Warren Burge
SVP Operations .... Brad Clothier
Director, Sales & Marketing .... Brian Rose
Director Systems Development .... Cheryl Seibert
Director Provider Services .... Christine Jones
Human Resources Officer .... Raedina Hupman
Director Quality Resource Management .... Cynthia Houser
Quality Assurance Associate Director .... Mary Scott
Compliance Officer .... Bruce Witt

COMPANY PROFILE:
Parent Company Name: Preferred Health Systems
Doing Business As: Preferred Plus, PHS Ins Co, Preferred Be
Year Founded: 1992   Federally Qualified: [N]
Forprofit: [Y]   Not-For-Profit: [ ]
Model Type: IPA
Accreditation: [ ] AAPPO [X] JACHO [ ] NCQA [ ] URAC
Plan Type: HMO, PPO, POS, CDHP, HDHP, HSA,
Total Revenue: 2005:   2006: 128,607,143
Net Income   2005:   2006:
Total Enrollment:
  2001: 82,944   2004: 98,224   2007: 0
  2002: 95,756   2005:
  2003: 96,886   2006:
Medical Loss Ratio: 2005:   2006: 90.80
Administrative Expense Ratio: 2005:   2006:

SERVICE AREA:
Nationwide: N
  KS (Brown, Pottawatomie, Shawnee, Jefferson, Segwick, Butler,
  Cowley, Chautauqua, Sumner, Kingman, Harvey, McPherson,
  Marion, Jackson, Nemaha);

TYPE OF COVERAGE:
Commercial: [Y] Individual: [Y] FEHBP: [Y] Indemnity: [ ]
Medicare: [Y] Medicaid: [ ] Supplemental Medicare: [Y]
Tricare   [ ]

PRODUCTS OFFERED:
Product Name: Type:
Preferred Plus of Kansas   HMO
Preferred Senior Care   Medicare HMO
Preferred Health Systems PPO   PPO
Preferred Health Systems POS   POS
Preferred Healthcare PPO TBN   TBN

CONSUMER-DRIVEN PRODUCTS

Preferred Health Systems HDHP   HSA Company
                                    HSA Product
                                    HSA Administrator
                                    Consumer-Driven Health Plan
Preferred Health Systems HSA   High Deductible Health Plan

PLAN BENEFITS:
Alternative Medicine: [X]   Behavioral Health: [X]
Chiropractic: [X]   Dental: [X]
Home Care: [X]   Inpatient SNF: [X]
Long-Term Care: [ ]   Pharm. Mail Order: [X]
Physical Therapy: [X]   Podiatry: [X]
Psychiatric: [X]   Transplant: [X]
Vision: [X]   Wellness: [X]
Workers' Comp: [ ]
Other Benefits:

PREFERRED MENTAL HEALTH MANAGEMENT

401 E Douglas Ste 300
Wichita, KS 67202-3411
Phone: 316-262-0444 Fax: 316-262-5723 Toll-Free: 800-264-7496
Web site: www.pmhm.com

Managed Care Organization Profiles   **KANSAS**

GREAT-WEST HEALTHCARE OF KANSAS/MISSOURI

10851 Mastin Blvd Bldg 82 #200
Overland Park, KS 66210
Phone: 913-491-9436 Fax: 913-491-9417 Toll-Free: 800-678-8287
Web site: www.greatwesthealthcare.com

MAILING ADDRESS:
  GREAT-WEST HEALTHCARE OF KS/MO
  10851 Mastin Blvd Bldg 82 #200
  Overland Park, KS 66210

KEY EXECUTIVES:
Chief Executive Officer/President .... Raymond L McFeetors
Chief Financial Officer .... Mitchell Graye
Senior Vice President, Chief Medical Officer .... Terry L Fouts, MD
Senior Vice President, Chief Information Officer .... John R Gabbert
Senior Vice President, Operations .... Donna Goldin
Vice President, Human Resources .... George C Bogdewiecz

COMPANY PROFILE:
Parent Company Name: CIGNA Inc
Doing Business As:
Year Founded: 2001   Federally Qualified: [N]
Forprofit: [Y]   Not-For-Profit: [ ]
Model Type:
Accreditation: [ ] AAPPO [ ] JACHO [ ] NCQA [ ] URAC
Plan Type: HMO, PPO, CDHP, HDHP, HSA,
Total Enrollment:
  2001: 1,210   2004: 1,107   2007: 0
  2002: 1,259   2005:
  2003: 3,888   2006:

SERVICE AREA:
Nationwide: N
  KS;

TYPE OF COVERAGE:
Commercial: [Y] Individual: [ ] FEHBP: [ ] Indemnity: [ ]
Medicare: [ ] Medicaid: [ ] Supplemental Medicare: [ ]
Tricare   [ ]

CONSUMER-DRIVEN PRODUCTS
Mellon HR Solutions LLC   HSA Company
                               HSA Product
                               HSA Administrator
                               Consumer-Driven Health Plan
                               High Deductible Health Plan

PLAN BENEFITS:
Alternative Medicine: [X]   Behavioral Health: [ ]
Chiropractic: [X]   Dental: [X]
Home Care: [X]   Inpatient SNF: [X]
Long-Term Care: [ ]   Pharm. Mail Order: [X]
Physical Therapy: [X]   Podiatry: [X]
Psychiatric: [X]   Transplant: [X]
Vision: [X]   Wellness: [X]
Workers' Comp: [ ]
Other Benefits:
Comments: Acquired by CIGNA Inc April 1, 2008

HUMANA HEALTH CARE PLANS OF KANSAS & MISSOURI

7311 W 132nd St Ste 200
Overland Park, KS 66213-1134
Phone: 913-217-3300 Fax: 913-217-3241 Toll-Free: 800-842-6188
Web site: www.humana.com/kansascity/home.html

MAILING ADDRESS:
  HUMANA HEALTH CARE PLAN KANSAS CITY
  500 W Main St
  Louisville, KY 66213-1134

KEY EXECUTIVES:
Chairman of the Board .... David A Jones Jr
Chief Executive Officer .... Michael B McCallister
President .... David Miller
Chief Financial Director .... Kevin Edwards
Medical Director .... Roger Diemert, MD
Director of Large Group Sales .... Jeremy Gaskill
Compliance Director .... Carlene Marra
Vice President of Provider Contracts .... Randa Anderson-Stice
Manager Director Quality/Utilization .... Brenda Sinclair
Director of Small Group Sales .... John Prue

COMPANY PROFILE:
Parent Company Name: Humana Inc
Doing Business As: Humana Inc
Year Founded: 1961   Federally Qualified: [Y]
Forprofit: [Y]   Not-For-Profit: [ ]
Model Type: MIXED
Accreditation: [ ] AAPPO [ ] JACHO [X] NCQA [X] URAC
Plan Type: HMO, PPO, POS, EPO, ASO, CDHP, HSA
Total Enrollment:
  2001: 42,256   2004: 580,582   2007: 0
  2002: 0   2005:
  2003: 130,985   2006: 68,000
Medical Loss Ratio: 2005:   2006:
Administrative Expense Ratio: 2005:   2006:

SERVICE AREA:
Nationwide: N
  KS (Atchison, Jefferson, Johnson, Leavenworth, Linn, Miami,
  Wyandotte,); MO (Cass, Clay, Henry, Jackson, Johnson,
  Layfayette, Platte, Ray);

TYPE OF COVERAGE:
Commercial: [Y] Individual: [Y] FEHBP: [Y] Indemnity: [ ]
Medicare: [Y] Medicaid: [ ] Supplemental Medicare: [Y]
Tricare   [ ]

PRODUCTS OFFERED:
Product Name: Type:
Humana Gold Plus Plan   Medicare Advantage

CONSUMER-DRIVEN PRODUCTS
JP Morgan Chase   HSA Company
HumanaOne HSA   HSA Product
JP Morgan Chase   HSA Administrator
Personal Care Account   Consumer-Driven Health Plan
HumanaOne   High Deductible Health Plan

PLAN BENEFITS:
Alternative Medicine: [ ]   Behavioral Health: [X]
Chiropractic: [X]   Dental: [X]
Home Care: [ ]   Inpatient SNF: [ ]
Long-Term Care: [ ]   Pharm. Mail Order: [X]
Physical Therapy: [ ]   Podiatry: [ ]
Psychiatric: [X]   Transplant: [X]
Vision: [ ]   Wellness: [ ]
Workers' Comp: [X]
Other Benefits: Long Term Disability

KANSAS FOUNDATION MEDICAL CARE

2947 SW Wanamaker Dr
Topeka, KS 66614
Phone: 785-273-2552 Fax: 785-273-5130 Toll-Free: 800-432-0770
Web site: www.kfmc.org

MAILING ADDRESS:
  KANSAS FOUNDATION MEDICAL CARE
  2947 SW Wanamaker Dr
  Topeka, KS 66614

KEY EXECUTIVES:
Chief Executive Officer/President .... Larry W Pitman
Senior Vice President Administration .... Patricia Evans, CPA
Medical Director .... Jeffrey Wheeler, MD, JD
Senior Vice President Community Relations .... Connie Hubbell
IS, HIT, HIE, Director .... Steve Rosebrook
Director Communications .... Lisa Williams
Information Systems Director .... Kevin Cronister
Human Resources Director .... Evelyn Stevener
Senior Vice President Quality Improvement .... Sam Markello, PhD

COMPANY PROFILE:
Parent Company Name: KFMC
Doing Business As:
Year Founded: 1972   Federally Qualified: [ ]
Forprofit: [ ]   Not-For-Profit: [Y]
Model Type:
Accreditation: [ ] AAPPO [ ] JACHO [ ] NCQA [ ] URAC
Plan Type: UR, PRO

SERVICE AREA:
Nationwide: N
  KS;

PREFERRED CHIROPRACTIC CARE INC

555 N McLean Blvd Ste 200
Wichita, KS 67203
Phone: 316-263-7800 Fax: 316-263-7814 Toll-Free:
Web site: www.pccnetwork.com

KANSAS

PLAN BENEFITS:
Alternative Medicine:	[ ]	Behavioral Health:	[ ]
Chiropractic:	[X]	Dental:	[X]
Home Care:	[X]	Inpatient SNF:	[X]
Long-Term Care:	[X]	Pharm. Mail Order:	[X]
Physical Therapy:	[X]	Podiatry:	[X]
Psychiatric:	[X]	Transplant:	[X]
Vision:	[X]	Wellness:	[X]
Workers' Comp:	[ ]		

Other Benefits:

COVENTRY HEALTH CARE OF KANSAS - WICHITA

8301 E 21st St N #300
Wichita, KS 67206
Phone: 316-634-1222 Fax: 316-634-1266 Toll-Free: 800-664-9251
Web site: www.cvty.com

MAILING ADDRESS:
COVENTRY HLTH CARE OF KANSAS
8301 E 21st St N #300
Wichita, KS 67206

KEY EXECUTIVES:
Chief Executive Officer/President .... George Wheeler
Director, Provider Services .... Bruce Cash

COMPANY PROFILE:
Parent Company Name: Coventry Health Care Inc
Doing Business As:
Year Founded: 1981   Federally Qualified: [ ]
Forprofit: [Y]   Not-For-Profit: [ ]
Model Type:
Accreditation: [ ] AAPPO [ ] JACHO [X] NCQA [ ] URAC
Plan Type: HMO, PPO, POS, TPA, CDHP, HDHP, HSA
Total Enrollment:
  2001: 43,238   2004: 155,374   2007: 0
  2002: 188,450   2005:
  2003: 168,555   2006:

SERVICE AREA:
Nationwide: N
KS (Butler, Cowley, Dickson, Elsworth, Greenwood, Harper, Harvey, Kingman, Lincoln, Marion, McPherson, Ottowa, Reno, Saline, Sedgwick, Sumner);

TYPE OF COVERAGE:
Commercial: [Y] Individual: [ ] FEHBP: [ ] Indemnity: [ ]
Medicare: [ ] Medicaid: [ ] Supplemental Medicare: [ ]
Tricare [ ]

PRODUCTS OFFERED:
Product Name:	Type:
Advantra 65	Medicare Advantage

CONSUMER-DRIVEN PRODUCTS
Wells Fargo	HSA Company
	HSA Product
Corporate Benefits Servs of Am	HSA Administrator
	Consumer-Driven Health Plan
Open Access Plus Plan	High Deductible Health Plan

PLAN BENEFITS:
Alternative Medicine:	[ ]	Behavioral Health:	[X]
Chiropractic:	[X]	Dental:	[X]
Home Care:	[X]	Inpatient SNF:	[ ]
Long-Term Care:	[ ]	Pharm. Mail Order:	[X]
Physical Therapy:	[ ]	Podiatry:	[ ]
Psychiatric:	[ ]	Transplant:	[X]
Vision:	[X]	Wellness:	[X]
Workers' Comp:	[ ]		

Other Benefits:

Comments:
Formerly Principal Healthcare of Kansas Inc, Wichita.

DELTA DENTAL PLAN OF KANSAS

1619 N Waterfront Pkwy
Wichita, KS 67278-9769
Phone: 316-264-1099 Fax: 316-462-3393 Toll-Free: 877-511-5113
Web site: www.deltadentalks.com

MAILING ADDRESS:
DELTA DENTAL PLAN OF KS
PO Box 789769
Wichita, KS 67278-9769

KEY EXECUTIVES:
Chief Executive Officer/President .... Michael Clark
Chief Financial Officer .... Michael Herbert
Dental Director .... Christina Gore, DDS
Chief Operating Officer .... Linda Brantner
Vice President, Marketing/Sales .... Dean Newton
Privacy Officer .... Lisa Ward
Human Resources Director .... Amy Ellison
Consultant .... Dr Ronald Whitcomb
Consultant .... Dr A Edward Hall
Vice President of Professional Relations .... Junetta Everett

COMPANY PROFILE:
Parent Company Name: Delta Dental Plan Association
Doing Business As:
Year Founded: 1973   Federally Qualified: [N]
Forprofit: [ ]   Not-For-Profit: [Y]
Model Type:
Accreditation: [ ] AAPPO [ ] JACHO [ ] NCQA [ ] URAC
Plan Type: Specialty HMO, Specialty PPO, FSA,
Total Revenue: 2005:   2006: 56,824,715
Net Income   2005:   2006:
Total Enrollment:
  2001: 0   2004: 190,827   2007: 0
  2002: 339,427   2005:
  2003: 189,346   2006:
Medical Loss Ratio: 2005:   2006: 80.50
Administrative Expense Ratio: 2005:   2006:

SERVICE AREA:
Nationwide: N
KS;

TYPE OF COVERAGE:
Commercial: [Y] Individual: [ ] FEHBP: [ ] Indemnity: [ ]
Medicare: [ ] Medicaid: [ ] Supplemental Medicare: [ ]
Tricare [ ]

PRODUCTS OFFERED:
Product Name:	Type:
Delta Dental Plan of KS	Dental

PLAN BENEFITS:
Alternative Medicine:	[ ]	Behavioral Health:	[ ]
Chiropractic:	[ ]	Dental:	[X]
Home Care:	[ ]	Inpatient SNF:	[ ]
Long-Term Care:	[ ]	Pharm. Mail Order:	[ ]
Physical Therapy:	[ ]	Podiatry:	[ ]
Psychiatric:	[ ]	Transplant:	[ ]
Vision:	[X]	Wellness:	[ ]
Workers' Comp:	[ ]		

Other Benefits:

EPOCH GROUP LC, THE

2020 W 89th St
Leawood, KS 66206
Phone: 913-362-0040 Fax: 913-362-0041 Toll-Free: 800-255-6065
Web site: www.epochgroup.com

MAILING ADDRESS:
EPOCH GROUP LC, THE
2020 W 89th St
Leawood, KS 66206

KEY EXECUTIVES:
Chief Executive Officer/President .... Paul Stucky
Chief Financial Officer .... Jeff Rudell
Executive Vice President .... Mark Williams

COMPANY PROFILE:
Parent Company Name:
Doing Business As:
Year Founded: 1974   Federally Qualified: [N]
Forprofit: [Y]   Not-For-Profit: [ ]
Model Type:
Accreditation: [ ] AAPPO [ ] JACHO [ ] NCQA [ ] URAC
Plan Type: TPA
Total Enrollment:
  2001: 0   2004: 0   2007: 0
  2002:   2005:
  2003: 0   2006: 90,000

SERVICE AREA:
Nationwide: N
KS; MO;

Managed Care Organization Profiles KANSAS

BLUE CROSS BLUE SHIELD OF KANSAS

1133 SW Topeka Blvd
Topeka, KS 66629-0001
Phone: 785-291-4180 Fax: 785-291-8295 Toll-Free: 800-432-3990
Web site: www.bcbsks.com
MAILING ADDRESS:
    BLUE CROSS BLUE SHIELD OF KANSAS
    1133 SW Topeka Blvd
    Topeka, KS 66629-0001

KEY EXECUTIVES:
Chief Executive Officer/President .... Andrew C Corbin
Vice President of Finance .... Bebo Lowery-Born
Vice President of Medical Affairs .... Ralph Weber, MD
Vice President Information Services & Claims .... William J Wallace
Vice President, Group Sales & Marketing .... Mark G Dulsky
Vice President Information Services & Claims .... William J Wallace
Vice President, Public Relations .... S Graham Bailey
Vice President, Provider Affairs/Medical Affairs ... Fredrick D Palenske
Vice President, Human Rsrc, Government Relations ...... Matthew D All
Senior Vice President.. William Pitsenberger
Vice President, Internal Sales/Member Relations .... Shelley Pittman

COMPANY PROFILE:
Parent Company Name: Blue Cross Blue Shield Association
Doing Business As:
Year Founded: Federally Qualified: [ ]
Forprofit: [ ]   Not-For-Profit: [ ]
Model Type:
Accreditation: [ ] AAPPO [ ] JACHO [ ] NCQA [ ] URAC
Plan Type: HMO, PPO, CDHP, HDHP, HSA
Total Enrollment:
   2001: 715,000   2004: 625,000   2007: 1,658,230
   2002: 0   2005:
   2003: 0   2006:
SERVICE AREA:
Nationwide: N
   KS,(all counties except Johnson and Wyandotte);
TYPE OF COVERAGE:
Commercial: [Y] Individual: [Y] FEHBP: [ ] Indemnity: [ ]
Medicare: [ ] Medicaid: [ ] Supplemental Medicare: [Y]
Tricare [ ]
PRODUCTS OFFERED:
Product Name: Type:
Premier Health Inc/Premier Blu   HMO
Blue Select   POS
CONSUMER-DRIVEN PRODUCTS
                                   HSA Company
BluebyDesign HSA   HSA Product
MII Life   HSA Administrator
                                   Consumer-Driven Health Plan
BluebyDesign   High Deductible Health Plan
PLAN BENEFITS:
Alternative Medicine: [ ]   Behavioral Health: [ ]
Chiropractic: [ ]   Dental: [X]
Home Care: [ ]   Inpatient SNF: [ ]
Long-Term Care: [ ]   Pharm. Mail Order: [ ]
Physical Therapy: [ ]   Podiatry: [ ]
Psychiatric: [ ]   Transplant: [ ]
Vision: [ ]   Wellness: [ ]
Workers' Comp: [ ]
Other Benefits:
Comments:
A Mutual Insurance Company.

CIGNA DENTAL HEALTH OF KANSAS INC

1571 Sawgrass Corporate Pkwy
Sunrise, FL 33323
Phone: 954-514-6600 Fax: 954-514-6905 Toll-Free: 800-367-1037
Web site: www.cigna.com/dental
MAILING ADDRESS:
    CIGNA DENTAL HEALTH OF KS INC
    1571 Sawgrass Corporate Pkwy
    Sunrise, FL 33323

KEY EXECUTIVES:
Chief Executive Officer... Barbara Demaio
President .... Karen S Rohan
Dental Director .... Ed Schooley, DDS
Marketing Director .... Samantha Snyder
MIS Director .... Laurel A Flebotte

COMPANY PROFILE:
Parent Company Name: CIGNA Dental Health Inc
Doing Business As: CIGNA Dental
Year Founded: 1985   Federally Qualified: [N]
Forprofit: [Y]   Not-For-Profit: [ ]
Model Type:
Accreditation: [ ] AAPPO [ ] JACHO [ ] NCQA [ ] URAC
Plan Type: Specialty HMO
Total Revenue: 2005:   2006: 1,974,232
Net Income   2005:   2006:
Total Enrollment:
   2001: 0   2004: 0   2007: 0
   2002: 20,249   2005:
   2003: 21,834   2006:
Medical Loss Ratio: 2005:   2006: 72.70
Administrative Expense Ratio: 2005:   2006:
SERVICE AREA:
Nationwide: N
   KS; NE;
TYPE OF COVERAGE:
Commercial: [Y] Individual: [ ] FEHBP: [ ] Indemnity: [ ]
Medicare: [ ] Medicaid: [ ] Supplemental Medicare: [ ]
Tricare [ ]
PLAN BENEFITS:
Alternative Medicine: [ ]   Behavioral Health: [ ]
Chiropractic: [ ]   Dental: [X]
Home Care: [ ]   Inpatient SNF: [ ]
Long-Term Care: [ ]   Pharm. Mail Order: [ ]
Physical Therapy: [ ]   Podiatry: [ ]
Psychiatric: [ ]   Transplant: [ ]
Vision: [ ]   Wellness: [ ]
Workers' Comp: [ ]
Other Benefits:

CIGNA HEALTHCARE OF KANSAS/MISSOURI

7400 W 110th Street Ste 400
Overland Park, KS 66210
Phone: 913-339-4700 Fax: 913-339-4705 Toll-Free:
Web site: www.cigna.com
MAILING ADDRESS:
    CIGNA HEALTHCARE OF KS/MO
    7400 W 110th Street Ste 400
    Overland Park, KS 66210

KEY EXECUTIVES:
President & General Manager .... Frank A Monahan
Director, Client Strategy .... Cynthia Davis
Network Development .... Evan Peters
Director, Client Management...................................... Gary Godin
Compliance Officer .... Cheryl Chamorro

COMPANY PROFILE:
Parent Company Name: CIGNA Corporation
Doing Business As:
Year Founded: 1981   Federally Qualified: [Y]
Forprofit: [Y]   Not-For-Profit: [ ]
Model Type: IPA
Accreditation: [ ] AAPPO [ ] JACHO [X] NCQA [ ] URAC
Plan Type: HMO, PPO, POS, ASO, EPO, CDHP, HDHP, HSA, FSA,
   HRA
Total Enrollment:
   2001: 178,696   2004: 0   2007: 0
   2002: 0   2005:
   2003: 0   2006:
SERVICE AREA:
Nationwide: N
   KS; MO; NE;
TYPE OF COVERAGE:
Commercial: [Y] Individual: [ ] FEHBP: [ ] Indemnity: [Y]
Medicare: [ ] Medicaid: [ ] Supplemental Medicare: [ ]
Tricare [ ]
PRODUCTS OFFERED:
Product Name: Type:
Cigna Healthcare for Seniors   Medicare
CONSUMER-DRIVEN PRODUCTS
JP Morgan Chase   HSA Company
CIGNA Choice Fund   HSA Product
                                   HSA Administrator
Open Access Plus   Consumer-Driven Health Plan
PPO   High Deductible Health Plan

Managed Care Organization Profiles — IOWA

WELLMARK HEALTH PLAN OF IOWA INC

636 Grand Ave
Des Moines, IA 50309-2565
Phone: 515-245-4500 Fax: 515-248-5617 Toll-Free:
Web site: www.wellmark.com

MAILING ADDRESS:
WELLMARK HEALTH PLAN OF IOWA INC
636 Grand Ave
Des Moines, IA 50309-2565

KEY EXECUTIVES:
Chairman of the Board/Chief Executive Officer .... John D Forsyth
Chief Financial Officer .... David N Southwell
Chief Medical Officer .... Dale J Andringa, MD
Chief Information Officer .... Denis J Roy
Vice President, Marketing .... Tim Weber
Vice President, Information Systems .... Sandy J Nelson
Vice President, Provider Relations .... Mike Fay
Senior Vice President, Human Resources .... Laura Jackson

COMPANY PROFILE:
Parent Company Name: Wellmark Inc
Doing Business As:
Year Founded: 1997   Federally Qualified: [N]
Forprofit: [ ]   Not-For-Profit: [ ]
Model Type:
Accreditation: [ ] AAPPO [ ] JACHO [ ] NCQA [X] URAC
Plan Type: HMO, POS,
Total Revenue: 2005:   2006: 267,842,615
Net Income   2005:   2006: 10,001,306
Total Enrollment:
   2001: 0   2004: 97,804   2007: 119,281
   2002: 67,361   2005: 106,942
   2003: 79,884   2006: 95,976
Medical Loss Ratio: 2005:   2006: 86.50
Administrative Expense Ratio: 2005:   2006:

SERVICE AREA:
Nationwide: N
   IA;

TYPE OF COVERAGE:
Commercial: [Y] Individual: [Y] FEHBP: [ ] Indemnity: [ ]
Medicare: [ ] Medicaid: [ ] Supplemental Medicare: [ ]
Tricare   [ ]

PRODUCTS OFFERED:
Product Name: Type:
Classic Blue

CONSUMER-DRIVEN PRODUCTS
MSAver Resources, LLC   HSA Company
Blue Priority HSA   HSA Product
MSAver Resouces, LLC   HSA Administrator
                              Consumer-Driven Health Plan
Alliance Select   High Deductible Health Plan

PLAN BENEFITS:
Alternative Medicine:	[ ]	Behavioral Health:	[ ]
Chiropractic:	[X]	Dental:	[X]
Home Care:	[X]	Inpatient SNF:	[X]
Long-Term Care:	[ ]	Pharm. Mail Order:	[X]
Physical Therapy:	[X]	Podiatry:	[X]
Psychiatric:	[X]	Transplant:	[X]
Vision:	[X]	Wellness:	[X]
Workers' Comp:	[ ]		

Other Benefits:

WELLMARK INC — CORPORATE HEADQUARTERS

636 Grand Ave
Des Moines, IA 50309-2565
Phone: 515-245-4500 Fax: 515-248-5617 Toll-Free:
Web site: www.wellmark.com

MAILING ADDRESS:
WELLMARK INC
636 Grand Ave
Des Moines, IA 50309-2565

KEY EXECUTIVES:
Chairman of the Board .... John D Forsyth
Chief Executive Officer/President .... John D Forsyth
Group VP Finance Officer & Treasurer .... David N Southwell
Vice President, Medical Director .... Dale J Andringa, MD
Senior Vice President, Chief Information Officer .... Denis J Roy
Group VP Operations Quality/Customer Satisfaction .... Ellen Gaucher
Vice President, Marketing .... Tim Weber
Senior Vice President, Sales .... Matthew M Shaffer
Vice President, IS Applications .... Sandy J Nelson
Vice President Corp & Marketing Communications .... Dana McNeill
Group Vice President, PR & Health Management ...... Peter W Roberts
Vice President, Health Networks .... Mike Fay
Senior Vice President, Human Resources .... Laura Jackson
President Wellmark Health Plan of Iowa .... Clifford D Gold
Vice President, Health Networks .... Mike Fay
Senior Vice President, General Counsel .... George B Hanna

COMPANY PROFILE:
Parent Company Name: Wellmark Inc
Doing Business As: BC BS of Iowa, BC BS of South Dakota
Year Founded: 1939   Federally Qualified: [N]
Forprofit: [Y]   Not-For-Profit: [ ]
Model Type: NETWORK
Accreditation: [ ] AAPPO [ ] JACHO [ ] NCQA [X] URAC
Plan Type: HMO, PPO, UR, POS, TPA, HSA
Total Revenue: 2005: 1,821,540,302   2006: 1,478,740,715
Net Income   2005:   102,938,176   2006:   84,997,636
Total Enrollment:
   2001: 1,676,151   2004: 1,912,961   2007: 2,148,706
   2002: 0   2005: 1,182,102
   2003: 1,799,449   2006: 1,979,915

SERVICE AREA:
Nationwide: N
   IA; SD;

TYPE OF COVERAGE:
Commercial: [Y] Individual: [Y] FEHBP: [ ] Indemnity: [ ]
Medicare: [ ] Medicaid: [ ] Supplemental Medicare: [Y]
Tricare   [ ]

PRODUCTS OFFERED:
Product Name:	Type:
Classic Blue	Indemnity
Alliance Select	PPO
Blue Select	PPO
Blue Advantage	HMO Gatekeeper
Blue Access	HMO Open Access
Blue Choice	HMO-POS

CONSUMER-DRIVEN PRODUCTS
MSAver Resources, LLC	HSA Company
Blue Priority HSA	HSA Product
MSAver Resouces, LLC	HSA Administrator
	Consumer-Driven Health Plan
Alliance Select	High Deductible Health Plan

PLAN BENEFITS:
Alternative Medicine:	[ ]	Behavioral Health:	[ ]
Chiropractic:	[X]	Dental:	[X]
Home Care:	[X]	Inpatient SNF:	[X]
Long-Term Care:	[ ]	Pharm. Mail Order:	[X]
Physical Therapy:	[X]	Podiatry:	[X]
Psychiatric:	[X]	Transplant:	[X]
Vision:	[X]	Wellness:	[X]Workers'
Comp:	[ ]		

Other Benefits:

IOWA

KEY EXECUTIVES:
Non-Executive Chairman .... Richard T Burke
Chief Executive Officer .... Robert J Sheehy

COMPANY PROFILE:
Parent Company Name: UnitedHealth Group
Doing Business As: UHC Health Plan of the River Valley
Year Founded: 1985   Federally Qualified: [N]
Forprofit: [Y]   Not-For-Profit: [ ]
Model Type: IPA
Accreditation: [ ] AAPPO [ ] JACHO [X] NCQA [ ] URAC
Plan Type: HMO, POS, CDHP, HDHP, HSA,
Total Revenue: 2005: 163,561,683 2006: 184,893,494
Net Income 2005: -1,446,443 2006: 11,425,970
Total Enrollment:
  2001: 0   2004: 0   2007: 0
  2002: 0   2005: 185,971
  2003: 35,327   2006: 183,761

SERVICE AREA:
Nationwide: N
  IA;

TYPE OF COVERAGE:
Commercial: [Y] Individual: [ ] FEHBP: [ ] Indemnity: [ ]
Medicare: [Y] Medicaid: [Y] Supplemental Medicare: [ ]
Tricare   [ ]

CONSUMER-DRIVEN PRODUCTS
Wells Fargo   HSA Company
Heritage Options HSA   HSA Product
Wells Fargo   HSA Administrator
                               Consumer-Driven Health Plan
                               High Deductible Health Plan

PLAN BENEFITS:
Alternative Medicine: [ ]   Behavioral Health: [X]
Chiropractic: [X]   Dental: [X]
Home Care: [ ]   Inpatient SNF: [X]
Long-Term Care: [ ]   Pharm. Mail Order: [X]
Physical Therapy: [X]   Podiatry: [X]
Psychiatric: [X]   Transplant: [X]
Vision: [X]   Wellness: [X]
Workers' Comp: [X]
Other Benefits:
Comments:
Formerly John Deere Health Plan, acquired by UnitedHealth on February 24, 2006.

UNITEDHEALTHCARE SERVICES COMPANY OF THE RIVER VALLEY INC

3022 Airport Blvd
Waterloo, IA 50704
Phone: 319-291-3291 Fax: 319-291-7838 Toll-Free: 800-747-1446
Web site: www.uhcrivervalley.com
MAILING ADDRESS:
  UHC OF THE RIVER VALLEY INC
  PO Box 9000
  Waterloo, IA 50704

KEY EXECUTIVES:
Non-Executive Chairman .... Richard T Burke
Chief Executive Officer .... Robert J Sheehy

COMPANY PROFILE:
Parent Company Name: UnitedHealth Group
Doing Business As: UHC Health Plan of the River Valley
Year Founded: 1985   Federally Qualified: [N]
Forprofit: [Y]   Not-For-Profit: [ ]
Model Type: IPA
Accreditation: [ ] AAPPO [ ] JACHO [X] NCQA [ ] URAC
Plan Type: HMO, POS, CDHP, HDHP, HSA,

SERVICE AREA:
Nationwide: N
  IA;

TYPE OF COVERAGE:
Commercial: [Y] Individual: [ ] FEHBP: [ ] Indemnity: [ ]
Medicare: [Y] Medicaid: [Y] Supplemental Medicare: [ ]
Tricare   [ ]

CONSUMER-DRIVEN PRODUCTS
Wells Fargo   HSA Company
Heritage Options HSA   HSA Product
Wells Fargo   HSA Administrator
                               Consumer-Driven Health Plan
                               High Deductible Health Plan

PLAN BENEFITS:
Alternative Medicine: [ ]   Behavioral Health: [X]
Chiropractic: [X]   Dental: [X]
Home Care: [ ]   Inpatient SNF: [X]
Long-Term Care: [ ]   Pharm. Mail Order: [X]
Physical Therapy: [X]   Podiatry: [X]
Psychiatric: [X]   Transplant: [X]
Vision: [X]   Wellness: [X]
Workers' Comp: [X]
Other Benefits:
Comments:
Formerly John Deere Health Plan, acquired by UnitedHealth on February 24, 2006.

WELLMARK BLUE CROSS BLUE SHIELD OF IOWA

636 Grand Ave
Des Moines, IA 50309-2565
Phone: 515-245-4500 Fax: 515-248-5617 Toll-Free:
Web site: www.wellmark.com
MAILING ADDRESS:
  WELLMARK BC BS OF IA
  636 Grand Ave
  Des Moines, IA 50309-2565

KEY EXECUTIVES:
Chairman of the Board/Chief Executive Officer .... John D Forsyth
President .... Clifford D Gold
Chief Financial Officer .... David N Southwell
Chief Medical Officer .... Dale J Andringa, MD
Chief Information Officer .... Denis J Roy
Vice President, Marketing .... Tim Weber
Vice President, Information Systems .... Sandy J Nelson
Vice President, Provider Relations .... Mike Fay
Senior Vice President, Human Resources .... Laura Jackson

COMPANY PROFILE:
Parent Company Name: Wellmark Inc
Doing Business As: Blue Cross & Blue Shield of Iowa
Year Founded: 1939   Federally Qualified: [N]
Forprofit: [Y]   Not-For-Profit: [ ]
Model Type:
Accreditation: [ ] AAPPO [ ] JACHO [ ] NCQA [X] URAC
Plan Type: HMO, PPO, UR, POS, TPA, EPO, PBM, HDHP, HSA
Total Revenue: 2005: 273,731,101 2006: 190,905,614
Net Income 2005: 6,924,100 2006: 136,583,301
Total Enrollment:
  2001: 1,392,873   2004: 1,643,314   2007: 1,246,246
  2002: 67,361   2005: 1,182,102
  2003: 1,536,357   2006: 1,240,767

SERVICE AREA:
Nationwide: N
  IA;

TYPE OF COVERAGE:
Commercial: [Y] Individual: [Y] FEHBP: [ ] Indemnity: [ ]
Medicare: [ ] Medicaid: [ ] Supplemental Medicare: [Y]
Tricare   [ ]

PRODUCTS OFFERED:
Product Name: Type:
Blue Advantage   HMO
Blue Choice   POS
Blue Access   Blue RX, Blue Vision
Unity Choice   HMO
Blue Advantage   HMO
Unity Choice 2   POS
Alliance Select   PPO

CONSUMER-DRIVEN PRODUCTS
MSAver Resources, LLC   HSA Company
Blue Priority HSA   HSA ProductMSAver Resouces,
LLC   HSA Administrator
                               Consumer-Driven Health Plan
Alliance Select   High Deductible Health Plan

PLAN BENEFITS:
Alternative Medicine: [ ]   Behavioral Health: [ ]
Chiropractic: [X]   Dental: [X]
Home Care: [X]   Inpatient SNF: [X]
Long-Term Care: [ ]   Pharm. Mail Order: [X]
Physical Therapy: [X]   Podiatry: [X]
Psychiatric: [X]   Transplant: [X]
Vision: [X]   Wellness: [X]
Workers' Comp: [ ]
Other Benefits:

Managed Care Organization Profiles — IOWA

KEY EXECUTIVES:
Non-Executive Chairman .... Richard T Burke
Chief Executive Officer .... Robert J Sheehy

COMPANY PROFILE:
Parent Company Name: UnitedHealth Group
Doing Business As: UHC Health Plan of the River Valley
Year Founded: 1985   Federally Qualified: [N]
Forprofit: [Y]   Not-For-Profit: [ ]
Model Type: IPA
Accreditation: [ ] AAPPO [ ] JACHO [X] NCQA [ ] URAC
Plan Type: HMO, POS, CDHP, HDHP, HSA,

SERVICE AREA:
Nationwide: N
   IA;

TYPE OF COVERAGE:
Commercial: [Y] Individual: [ ] FEHBP: [ ] Indemnity: [ ]
Medicare: [Y] Medicaid: [Y] Supplemental Medicare: [ ]
Tricare   [ ]

CONSUMER-DRIVEN PRODUCTS
Wells Fargo   HSA Company
Heritage Options HSA   HSA Product
Wells Fargo   HSA Administrator
                                                Consumer-Driven Health Plan
                                                High Deductible Health Plan

PLAN BENEFITS:
Alternative Medicine:	[ ]	Behavioral Health:	[ ]
Chiropractic:	[X]	Dental:	[X]
Home Care:	[ ]	Inpatient SNF:	[X]
Long-Term Care:	[ ]	Pharm. Mail Order:	[X]
Physicial Therapy:	[X]	Podiatry:	[X]
Psychiatric:	[X]	Transplant:	[X]
Vision:	[X]	Wellness:	[X]
Workers' Comp:	[X]		

Other Benefits:
Comments:
Formerly John Deere Health Plan, acquired by UnitedHealth on February 24, 2006.

UNITEDHEALTHCARE SERVICES COMPANY OF THE RIVER VALLEY INC

1660 Embassy W Dr Ste 150
Dubuque, IA 52002
Phone: 563-588-2831 Fax: 319-291-7838 Toll-Free: 800-747-1446
Web site: www.uhcrivervalley.com
MAILING ADDRESS:
   UHC OF THE RIVER VALLEY INC
   1300 River Dr Ste 200
   Moline, IL 52002

KEY EXECUTIVES:
Non-Executive Chairman .... Richard T Burke
Chief Executive Officer .... Robert J Sheehy

COMPANY PROFILE:
Parent Company Name: UnitedHealth Group
Doing Business As: UHC Health Plan of the River Valley
Year Founded: 1985   Federally Qualified: [N]
Forprofit: [Y]   Not-For-Profit: [ ]
Model Type: IPA
Accreditation: [ ] AAPPO [ ] JACHO [X] NCQA [ ] URAC
Plan Type: HMO, POS, CDHP, HDHP, HSA,

SERVICE AREA:
Nationwide: N
   IA;

TYPE OF COVERAGE:
Commercial: [Y] Individual: [ ] FEHBP: [ ] Indemnity: [ ]
Medicare: [Y] Medicaid: [Y] Supplemental Medicare: [ ]
Tricare   [ ]

CONSUMER-DRIVEN PRODUCTS
Wells Fargo   HSA Company
Heritage Options HSA   HSA Product
Wells Fargo   HSA Administrator
                                                Consumer-Driven Health Plan
                                                High Deductible Health Plan

UNITEDHEALTHCARE SERVICES COMPANY OF THE RIVER VALLEY INC

1195 E Post Rd, Ste 1
Marion, IA 52302
Phone: 800-747-1446 Fax: 319-291-7838 Toll-Free: 800-747-1446
Web site: www.uhcrivervalley.com
MAILING ADDRESS:
   UHC OF THE RIVER VALLEY INC
   1300 River Dr Ste 200
   Moline, IL 52302

KEY EXECUTIVES:
Non-Executive Chairman .... Richard T Burke
Chief Executive Officer .... Robert J Sheehy

COMPANY PROFILE:
Parent Company Name: UnitedHealth Group
Doing Business As: UHC Health Plan of the River Valley
Year Founded: 1985   Federally Qualified: [N]
Forprofit: [Y]   Not-For-Profit: [ ]
Model Type: IPA
Accreditation: [ ] AAPPO [ ] JACHO [X] NCQA [ ] URAC
Plan Type: HMO, POS, CDHP, HDHP, HSA,

SERVICE AREA:
Nationwide: N
   IA;

TYPE OF COVERAGE:
Commercial: [Y] Individual: [ ] FEHBP: [ ] Indemnity: [ ]
Medicare: [Y] Medicaid: [Y] Supplemental Medicare: [ ]
Tricare   [ ]

CONSUMER-DRIVEN PRODUCTS
Wells Fargo   HSA Company
Heritage Options HSA   HSA Product
                                                HSA Administrator
                                                Consumer-Driven Health Plan
                                                High Deductible Health Plan

PLAN BENEFITS:
Alternative Medicine:	[ ]	Behavioral Health:	[X]
Chiropractic:	[X]	Dental:	[X]
Home Care:	[ ]	Inpatient SNF:	[X]
Long-Term Care:	[ ]	Pharm. Mail Order:	[X]
Physicial Therapy:	[X]	Podiatry:	[X]
Psychiatric:	[X]	Transplant:	[X]
Vision:	[X]	Wellness:	[X]
Workers' Comp:	[X]		

Other Benefits:
Comments:
Formerly John Deere Health Plan, acquired by UnitedHealth on February 24, 2006.

UNITEDHEALTHCARE SERVICES COMPANY OF THE RIVER VALLEY INC

11141 Aurora Ave
Urbandale, IA 50322
Phone: 515-327-2000 Fax: 515-327-1128 Toll-Free: 800-747-1446
Web site: www.uhcrivervalley.com
MAILING ADDRESS:
   UHC OF THE RIVER VALLEY INC
   1300 River Dr Ste 200
   Moline, IL 50322

IOWA — Managed Care Organization Profiles

PRODUCTS OFFERED:
Product Name: Type:
Amerigroup Community Care   Medicaid
PLAN BENEFITS:
Alternative Medicine: [ ]   Behavioral Health: [X]
Chiropractic: [ ]   Dental: [ ]
Home Care: [ ]   Inpatient SNF: [ ]
Long-Term Care: [ ]   Pharm. Mail Order: [ ]
Physical Therapy: [ ]   Podiatry: [ ]
Psychiatric: [ ]   Transplant: [ ]
Vision: [ ]   Wellness: [ ]
Workers' Comp: [ ]
Other Benefits:

MEDICAL ASSOCIATES HEALTH PLANS

1605 Associates Dr Ste 101
Dubuque, IA 52002-2270
Phone: 563-556-8070 Fax: 563-556-5134 Toll-Free: 800-747-8900
Web site: www.mahealthcare.com
MAILING ADDRESS:
  MEDICAL ASSOCIATES HEALTH PLAN
  1605 Associates Dr Ste 101
  Dubuque, IA 52002-2270

KEY EXECUTIVES:
Chairman/President .... Andrea Ries, MD
Chief Executive Officer .... John Tallent
Chief Financial Officer .... Ronald Fahey, CPA
Chief Medical Officer .... Edward Alt, MD
Pharmacy Director .... Mary Leary
Chief Information Officer .... Gary Sewell
Chief Operating Officer .... Brian Schatz
Executive Director & Marketing Director .... Alan Avery

COMPANY PROFILE:
Parent Company Name:
Doing Business As: Medical Associates Health Plans
Year Founded: 1987   Federally Qualified: [N]
Forprofit: [Y]   Not-For-Profit: [ ]
Model Type: NETWORK
Accreditation: [ ] AAPPO [ ] JACHO [X] NCQA [ ] URAC
Plan Type: HMO, POS
Total Revenue   2005:   47,784,804   2006:   71,724,243
Net Income   2005:   2,289,188   2006:   1,184,826
Total Enrollment:
  2001: 25,257   2004: 26,774   2007: 23,454
  2002: 25,846   2005: 22,136
  2003: 27,002   2006: 22,949
SERVICE AREA:
Nationwide: N
  IA (Clayton, Delaware, Dubuque, Jackson, Jones); IL (JoDaviess);
  WI (Crawford, Grant, Iowa, Lafayette);
TYPE OF COVERAGE:
Commercial: [Y] Individual: [ ] FEHBP: [ ] Indemnity: [ ]
Medicare: [Y] Medicaid: [ ] Supplemental Medicare: [Y]
Tricare   [ ]
PRODUCTS OFFERED:
Product Name: Type:
Medicare Advantage Plan   Medicare Advantage
HMO   HMO
PLAN BENEFITS:
Alternative Medicine: [ ]   Behavioral Health: [X]
Chiropractic: [X]   Dental: [ ]
Home Care: [X]   Inpatient SNF: [X]
Long-Term Care: [ ]   Pharm. Mail Order: [ ]
Physical Therapy: [X]   Podiatry: [X]
Psychiatric: [X]   Transplant: [X]
Vision: [X]   Wellness: [X]
Workers' Comp: [ ]
Other Benefits:

MERCY OF IOWA CITY REGIONAL PHO - PRIORITY HEALTH NETWORK

625 S Gilbert St Ste 2
Iowa City, IA 52245
Phone: 319-339-3992 Fax: 319-358-2628 Toll-Free: 800-358-2767
Web site: www.mercyicpho.org
MAILING ADDRESS:
  MERCY OF IOWA CITY REGL PHO
  625 S Gilbert St Ste 2
  Iowa City, IA 52245

KEY EXECUTIVES:
Executive Director .... Hodge Carter, CHE

COMPANY PROFILE:
Parent Company Name: Mercy of Iowa City Regional PHO
Doing Business As: Priority Health Network
Year Founded: 1994   Federally Qualified: [ ]
Forprofit: [ ]   Not-For-Profit: [ ]
Model Type:
Accreditation: [ ] AAPPO [ ] JACHO [ ] NCQA [ ] URAC
Plan Type: PPO,
Primary Physicians: 145   Physician Specialists:
Hospitals: 1
SERVICE AREA:
Nationwide: N
  IA;

PRINCIPAL LIFE INSURANCE COMPANY

7780 Office Plz Dr S, Mon #112
West Des Moines, IA 50266
Phone: 515-223-4961 Fax: 515-223-4931 Toll-Free: 877-340-7755
Web site: www.principal.com
MAILING ADDRESS:
  PRINCIPAL LIFE INS CO
  7780 Office Plz Dr S, Mon #112
  Des Moines, IA 50266

KEY EXECUTIVES:
Chairman of the Board .... J Barry Griswell
Chief Executive Officer/President .... J Barry Griswell
Chief Financial Officer .... Michael H Gersie
Chief Medical Officer .... Greg Haessler, MD
Chief Information Officer .... Gary P Scholten
Chief Marketing Officer .... Mary A O'Keefe
EVP, General Counsel .... Karen E Shaff

COMPANY PROFILE:
Parent Company Name: Principal Life Insurance Co
Doing Business As:
Year Founded: Federally Qualified: [ ]
Forprofit: [Y]   Not-For-Profit: [ ]
Model Type:
Accreditation: [ ] AAPPO [ ] JACHO [ ] NCQA [ ] URAC
Plan Type: PPO, HDHP, HSA
SERVICE AREA:
Nationwide: N
  NW;
TYPE OF COVERAGE:
Commercial: [Y] Individual: [Y] FEHBP: [ ] Indemnity: [ ]
Medicare: [ ] Medicaid: [ ] Supplemental Medicare: [ ]
Tricare   [ ]
PRODUCTS OFFERED:
Product Name: Type:
Classic PPO   PPO
Classic Value PPO   PPO
Classic Plus PPO   PPO

UNITEDHEALTHCARE SERVICES COMPANY OF THE RIVER VALLEY INC

3740 Utica Ridge Rd Ste A
Bettendorf, IA 52722
Phone: 563-344-4500 Fax: 319-291-7838 Toll-Free: 800-747-1446
Web site: www.uhcrivervalley.com
MAILING ADDRESS:
  UHC OF THE RIVER VALLEY INC
  1300 River Dr Ste 200
  Moline, IL 52722

Managed Care Organization Profiles — IOWA

KEY EXECUTIVES:
Chief Executive Officer .... Keith Vander Kolk
Medical Director for Encompass ....Jeffrey Stahl, MD
Chief Information Officer .... Sue Nesbit-Fisher
National Sales Director ....Michael Larson
MIS Director .... Greg Gesaman
Director, Provider Services ....Elodie Opstad
Compliance Officer .... Terry Miller
Group President, Quality Management .... Peg Mason

COMPANY PROFILE:
Parent Company Name: Iowa Foundation For Medical Care
Doing Business As:
Year Founded: 1985   Federally Qualified: [N]
Forprofit: [Y]   Not-For-Profit: [ ]
Model Type:
Accreditation: [ ] AAPPO [ ] JACHO [ ] NCQA [X] URAC
Plan Type: PPO, Specialty PPO, UR, POS
Total Enrollment:
    2001: 0   2004: 0   2007: 0
    2002: 0   2005:
    2003: 0   2006: 2,000,000

SERVICE AREA:
Nationwide: N
    IA;

TYPE OF COVERAGE:
Commercial: [Y] Individual: [Y] FEHBP: [ ] Indemnity: [ ]
Medicare: [ ] Medicaid: [ ] Supplemental Medicare: [ ]
Tricare   [ ]

PLAN BENEFITS:
Alternative Medicine: [ ]   Behavioral Health: [ ]
Chiropractic: [X]   Dental: [ ]
Home Care: [X]   Inpatient SNF: [X]
Long-Term Care: [X]   Pharm. Mail Order: [X]
Physical Therapy: [X]   Podiatry: [ ]
Psychiatric: [X]   Transplant: [X]
Vision: [ ]   Wellness: [X]
Workers' Comp: [X]
Other Benefits:

IOWA HEALTH SOLUTIONS

1830 Second Ave Ste 100
Rock Island, IA 61201
Phone: 309-283-0930 Fax: 309-283-0937 Toll-Free: 800-928-8004
Web site: www.imxinc.lcom/wps/portal/IAHS

MAILING ADDRESS:
    IOWA HEALTH SOLUTIONS
    1830 Second Ave Ste 100
    Rock Island, IA 61201

KEY EXECUTIVES:
Chairman of the Board .... James D Dyer
Chief Executive Officer/President .... Todd Meek
Chief Financial Officer .... Paul Carter
Medical Director .... Richard O'Connor
Chief Operating Officer .... Bob Wilcox

COMPANY PROFILE:
Parent Company Name: Nevada Healthcare
Doing Business As:
Year Founded: Federally Qualified: [ ]
Forprofit: [Y]   Not-For-Profit: [ ]
Model Type: IPA/NETWORK
Accreditation: [ ] AAPPO [X] JACHO [ ] NCQA [ ] URAC
Plan Type: HMO, Specialty HMO, ASO
Total Enrollment:
    2001: 28,124   2004: 29,454   2007: 0
    2002: 29,819   2005:
    2003: 43,411   2006:

SERVICE AREA:
Nationwide: N
    IA;

TYPE OF COVERAGE:
Commercial: [Y] Individual: [ ] FEHBP: [ ] Indemnity: [ ]
Medicare: [ ] Medicaid: [ ] Supplemental Medicare: [ ]
Tricare   [ ]

PRODUCTS OFFERED:
Product Name: Type:
Hawkeye   HMO
Hawki   Kids
Iowa Medicaid   Medicaid

KEOKUK AREA HOSPITAL ORGANIZED DELIVERY SYSTEM INC

1600 Morgan St
Keokuk, IA 56232
Phone: 319-524-7150 Fax: 319-524-5317 Toll-Free:
Web site: www.keokukhealthsystem.org

MAILING ADDRESS:
    KEOKUK AREA HOSPITAL ORGANIZED DELIVERY
    1600 Morgan St
    Keokuk, IA 56232

KEY EXECUTIVES:
Chief Executive Officer/President .... Allan W Zastrow
Chief Financial Officer .... Walter H Winkler
Chief Information Officer .... Linda Schaffner
Marketing Director .... Ronda Schreck

COMPANY PROFILE:
Parent Company Name: Keokuk Health System
Doing Business As:
Year Founded: 1998   Federally Qualified: [N]
Forprofit: [ ]   Not-For-Profit: [ ]
Model Type:
Accreditation: [ ] AAPPO [X] JACHO [ ] NCQA [ ] URAC
Plan Type: HMO
Total Revenue: 2005:   2006: 1,779,910
Net Income   2005:   2006:   440,988
Total Enrollment:
    2001: 0   2004: 0   2007: 705
    2002: 0   2005: 891
    2003: 1,094   2006: 718

SERVICE AREA:
Nationwide:
    IA;

MAGELLAN BEHAVIORAL CARE OF IOWA INC

2600 Westown Pkwy Ste 200
West Des Moines, IA 50266
Phone: 515-223-0306 Fax: 314-387-5407 Toll-Free:
Web site: www.magellanhealth.com

MAILING ADDRESS:
    MAGELLAN BEHAVIORAL CARE OF IOWA
    2600 Westown Pkwy Ste 200
    West Des Moines, IA 50266

KEY EXECUTIVES:
President .... Russell Petrella
Chief Financial Officer .... William Grimm
Medical Director .... Charles Wadle, DO
Chief Operating Officer .... Joan Discher

COMPANY PROFILE:
Parent Company Name: Magellan Behavioral Health
Doing Business As:
Year Founded: Federally Qualified: [ ]
Forprofit: [ ]   Not-For-Profit: [ ]
Model Type:
Accreditation: [ ] AAPPO [ ] JACHO [ ] NCQA [ ] URAC
Plan Type: Specialty HMO
Total Revenue: 2005: 89,129,765   2006: 29,912,776
Net Income   2005: 1,353,512   2006:   528,575
Total Enrollment:
    2001: 0   2004: 0   2007: 282,047
    2002: 0   2005:
    2003: 0   2006: 280,281

SERVICE AREA:
Nationwide:
    IA;

IOWA Managed Care Organization Profiles

MAILING ADDRESS:
DELTA DENTAL OF IA
2401 SE Tones Dr Ste 13
Ankeny, IA 50021

KEY EXECUTIVES:
Chairman of the Board .... Jeff Plagge
Chief Executive Officer/President .... Donn Hutchinson
Chief Financial Officer .... Tamera K Robinson, CPA
Dental Director .... Edwin Schooley, DDS, MHS

COMPANY PROFILE:
Parent Company Name: Delta Dental Plan Association
Doing Business As:
Year Founded: Federally Qualified: [ ]
Forprofit: [Y]   Not-For-Profit: [ ]
Model Type:
Accreditation: [ ] AAPPO [ ] JACHO [ ] NCQA [ ] URAC
Plan Type: Specialty PPO,
Total Revenue: 2005:   31,494,574   2006:   11,087,735
Net Income   2005:   2,591,313   2006:   696,752
Total Enrollment:
  2001: 0   2004: 171,657   2007: 190,703
  2002: 156,930   2005: 169,389
  2003: 154,105   2006: 191,198

SERVICE AREA:
Nationwide: N
  IA;

TYPE OF COVERAGE:
Commercial: [Y] Individual: [ ] FEHBP: [ ] Indemnity: [ ]
Medicare: [ ] Medicaid: [ ] Supplemental Medicare: [ ]
Tricare   [ ]

PLAN BENEFITS:
Alternative Medicine: [ ]   Behavioral Health: [ ]
Chiropractic: [ ]   Dental: [X]
Home Care: [ ]   Inpatient SNF: [ ]
Long-Term Care: [ ]   Pharm. Mail Order: [ ]
Physical Therapy: [ ]   Podiatry: [ ]
Psychiatric: [ ]   Transplant: [ ]
Vision: [ ]   Wellness: [ ]
Workers' Comp: [ ]
Other Benefits:

EMPLOYEES BENEFIT SYSTEMS

214 N Main St
Burlington, IA 52601
Phone: 319-752-3200 Fax: 319-753-6114 Toll-Free: 800-373-1327
Web site: www.ebs-tpa.com

MAILING ADDRESS:
EMPLOYEES BENEFIT SYSTEMS
214 N Main St
Burlington, IA 52601

KEY EXECUTIVES:
Chief Executive Officer/Chief Financial Officer .... Richard Archer
Marketing Director .... William Kelly

COMPANY PROFILE:
Parent Company Name:
Doing Business As:
Year Founded: 1991   Federally Qualified: [ ]
Forprofit: [ ]   Not-For-Profit: [Y]
Model Type:
Accreditation: [ ] AAPPO [ ] JACHO [ ] NCQA [ ] URAC
Plan Type: TPA
Total Enrollment:
  2001: 18,000   2004: 0   2007: 0
  2002: 0   2005:
  2003: 0   2006:

SERVICE AREA:
Nationwide: N
  IA (Southeast); IL (Western);

TYPE OF COVERAGE:
Commercial: [Y] Individual: [ ] FEHBP: [ ] Indemnity: [ ]
Medicare: [ ] Medicaid: [ ] Supplemental Medicare: [Y]
Tricare   [ ]

PLAN BENEFITS:
Alternative Medicine: [ ]   Behavioral Health: [ ]
Chiropractic: [X]   Dental: [X]
Home Care: [X]   Inpatient SNF: [X]
Long-Term Care: [ ]   Pharm. Mail Order: [X]
Physical Therapy: [X]   Podiatry: [X]
Psychiatric: [X]   Transplant: [X]
Vision: [X]   Wellness: [X]
Workers' Comp: [ ]
Other Benefits:

HUMANA INC - IOWA

500 W Main St
Louisville, KY 40202
Phone: 502-580-5005 Fax: 859-232-8557 Toll-Free:
Web site: www.humana.com

MAILING ADDRESS:
HUMANA INC - IOWA
PO Box 740036
Louisville, KY 40202

KEY EXECUTIVES:
Chairman of the Board .... David A Jones Jr
Chief Executive Officer/President .... Michael B McCallister
Senior VP Chief Financial Officer .... James H Bloem
Vice President Medical Director .... Lisa Weaver, MD
Senior VP Chief Information Officer .... Bruce J Goodman
Senior VP Human Resources .... Bonnie C Hathcock

COMPANY PROFILE:
Parent Company Name: Humana Inc
Doing Business As:
Year Founded: 1961   Federally Qualified: [Y]
Forprofit: [Y]   Not-For-Profit: [ ]
Model Type: IPA
Accreditation: [ ] AAPPO [ ] JACHO [ ] NCQA [ ] URAC
Plan Type: PPO, ASO, CDHP, HDHP, HSA,
Total Enrollment:
  2001: 0   2004: 0   2007: 600,000
  2002: 0   2005:
  2003: 0   2006:

SERVICE AREA:
Nationwide: N
  IA;

TYPE OF COVERAGE:
Commercial: [Y] Individual: [Y] FEHBP: [ ] Indemnity: [ ]
Medicare: [ ] Medicaid: [ ] Supplemental Medicare: [Y]
Tricare   [ ]

CONSUMER-DRIVEN PRODUCTS
JP Morgan Chase   HSA Company
HumanaOne HSA   HSA Product
JP Morgan Chase   HSA Administrator
Personal Care Account   Consumer-Driven Health Plan
HumanaOne   High Deductible Health Plan

PLAN BENEFITS:
Alternative Medicine: [ ]   Behavioral Health: [X]
Chiropractic: [X]   Dental: [X]
Home Care: [ ]   Inpatient SNF: [ ]
Long-Term Care: [ ]   Pharm. Mail Order: [X]
Physical Therapy: [ ]   Podiatry: [ ]
Psychiatric: [X]   Transplant: [X]
Vision: [ ]   Wellness: [ ]
Workers' Comp: [X]
Other Benefits: Long Term Disability

IOWA FOUNDATION FOR MEDICAL CARE/ ENCOMPASS

6000 Westown Pkwy
West Des Moines, IA 50266-7771
Phone: 515-223-2900 Fax: 515-222-2407 Toll-Free: 800-383-2856
Web site: www.ifmc.org

MAILING ADDRESS:
IOWA FOUNDATION FOR MEDICAL/ENCOMPASS
6000 Westown Pkwy
West Des Moines, IA 50266-7771

Managed Care Organization Profiles — IOWA

AMERICAN REPUBLIC INSURANCE COMPANY

601 6th Ave
Des Moines, IA 50309
Phone: 515-245-2000 Fax: 515-245-2305 Toll-Free: 800-247-2190
Web site: www.aric.com

MAILING ADDRESS:
   AMERICAN REPUBLIC INS CO
   PO Box 1
   Des Moines, IA 50309

KEY EXECUTIVES:
Chief Executive Officer/President .... Michael E Abbott
Chief Medical Officer .... Andy McGuire, MD
Chief Information Officer .... John Klinkner
Chief Operations Officer .... Tom Peterson
Vice President, Marketing .... Kevin Pendergast
Chief Human Resources Officer .... Kevin Spitzig
COO, American Republic Sales .... Doug Baraket
COO, Direct Marketing .... Lorenzo Battani
Chief Actuary .... Dick Garner

COMPANY PROFILE:
Parent Company Name:
Doing Business As:
Year Founded: 1929   Federally Qualified: [ ]
Forprofit: [Y]   Not-For-Profit: [ ]
Model Type:
Accreditation: [ ] AAPPO [ ] JACHO [ ] NCQA [ ] URAC
Plan Type: PPO, HDHP
Total Enrollment:
   2001: 12,963   2004: 0   2007: 0
   2002: 0   2005:
   2003: 5,013   2006: 230,000

SERVICE AREA:
Nationwide: Y
AL; AK; AR; AZ; CA; CO; CT; DE; DC; FL; GA; HI; IA; ID; IL; IN; KS; KY; LA; ME; MD; MA; MI; MN; MS; MO; MT; NE; NV; NH; NJ; NM; NY; NC; ND; OH; OK; OR; PA; RI; SC; SD; TN; TX; UT; VA; VT; WA; WV; WI; WY;

TYPE OF COVERAGE:
Commercial: [ ] Individual: [Y] FEHBP: [ ] Indemnity: [ ]
Medicare: [ ]   Medicaid: [ ]   Supplemental Medicare: [Y]
Tricare   [ ]

CORVEL CORPORATION

1701 48th St Ste 275
West Des Moines, IA 50266
Phone: 515-333-4700 Fax: 515-333-4701 Toll-Free: 800-929-1160
Web site: www.corvel.com

MAILING ADDRESS:
   CORVEL CORPORATION
   1701 48th St Ste 275
   West Des Moines, IA 50266

KEY EXECUTIVES:
Chairman of the Board .... Gordon Clemons
Chief Executive Officer/President .... Gordon Clemons
Marketing Director .... Laura Schumacher
Human Resources Director .... Sharon O'Connor
District Manager .... Mary Ann Cullen

COMPANY PROFILE:
Parent Company Name:
Doing Business As:
Year Founded: 1992   Federally Qualified: [ ]
Forprofit: [Y]   Not-For-Profit: [ ]
Model Type:
Accreditation: [ ] AAPPO [ ] JACHO [ ] NCQA [ ] URAC
Plan Type: PPO

SERVICE AREA:
Nationwide: N
   IA;

TYPE OF COVERAGE:
Commercial: [Y] Individual: [ ] FEHBP: [ ] Indemnity: [ ]
Medicare: [ ]   Medicaid: [ ]   Supplemental Medicare: [ ]
Tricare   [ ]

COVENTRY HEALTH CARE INC — IOWA

4320 114th St
Urbandale, IA 50322-5408
Phone: 515-225-1234 Fax: 515-223-0097 Toll-Free: 800-470-6352
Web site: www.chciowa.com

MAILING ADDRESS:
   COVENTRY HEALTH CARE — IA
   4320 114th St
   Urbandale, IA 50322-5408

KEY EXECUTIVES:
Chief Executive Officer/President .... Michael W Teachout
Chief Financial Officer .... Deanna H Gray
Medical Director .... Jerry LeMar, DO
Vice President, Network Management .... Gary Busack
Human Resources Manager .... Tami Rubino
Quality Improvement Manager .... Nancy Mundy

COMPANY PROFILE:
Parent Company Name: Coventry Health Care Inc
Doing Business As:
Year Founded: 1985   Federally Qualified: [N]
Forprofit: [Y]   Not-For-Profit: [ ]
Model Type: IPA
Accreditation: [ ] AAPPO [ ] JACHO [X] NCQA [ ] URAC
Plan Type: HMO, PPO, Specialty HMO, Specialty PPO, PBM, POS, ASO, EPO, CDHP, HDHP, HSA
Total Revenue: 2005: 142,166,471   2006: 115,501,700
Net Income   2005:   5,328,934   2006:   9,555,207
Total Enrollment:
   2001: 85,239   2004: 72,568   2007: 48,505
   2002: 66,393   2005: 53,594
   2003: 70,328   2006: 52,379
Medical Loss Ratio: 2005:   2006:
Administrative Expense Ratio: 2005:   2006:

SERVICE AREA:
Nationwide: N
IA; (Adair, Benton, Black Hawk, Boone, Bremer, Butler, Calhoun, Carroll, Cerro Gordo, Cherokee, Clarke, Clay, Clinton, Crawford, Dallas, Davis, Decatur, Delaware, Fayette, Floyd, Franklin, Greene, Grundy, Guthrie, Hamilton, Hancock, Hardin, Ida, Jasper, Jefferson, Kossuth, Lyon, Lucas, Madison, Marion, Mitchell, Monona, Monroe, Montgomery, O'Brien, Osceola, Palo Alto, Plymouth, Pocahontas, Polk, Poewshiek, Ringgold, Sac, Scott, Sioux, Story, Tama, Wapello, Warren, Wayne, Webster, Winnebago, Woodbury and Worth); SD;

TYPE OF COVERAGE:
Commercial: [Y] Individual: [ ] FEHBP: [Y] Indemnity: [ ]
Medicare: [Y]   Medicaid: [Y]   Supplemental Medicare: [ ]
Tricare   [ ]

PRODUCTS OFFERED:
Product Name:	Type:
HMO Open Access Network	HMO
HMO Primary Care Network	HMO
HMO Point of Service	HMO
Healthcare Preferred	PPO

CONSUMER-DRIVEN PRODUCTS
Wells Fargo	HSA Company
	HSA Product
Corporate Benefits Services of America	HSA Administrator
PPO QHDHP	Consumer-Driven Health Plan
Choice QHDHP	High Deductible Health Plan

PLAN BENEFITS:
Alternative Medicine:	[ ]	Behavioral Health:	[X]
Chiropractic:	[X]	Dental:	[X]
Home Care:	[X]	Inpatient SNF:	[X]
Long-Term Care:	[X]	Pharm. Mail Order:	[X]
Physical Therapy:	[X]	Podiatry:	[X]
Psychiatric:	[X]	Transplant:	[X]
Vision:	[X]	Wellness:	[X]
Workers' Comp:	[ ]		

Other Benefits:
Comments:
Formerly Principal Health Care of Iowa Inc.

DELTA DENTAL OF IOWA

2401 SE Tones Dr Ste 13
Ankeny, IA 50021
Phone: 515-261-5500 Fax: 515-261-5609 Toll-Free:
Web site: www.deltadentalia.com

Managed Care Organization Profiles — **INDIANA**

SERVICE AREA:
Nationwide: N
  Central Indiana,

WELBORN HEALTH PLANS

101 S E Third St
Evansville, IN 47708
Phone: 812-426-6600 Fax: 812-434-7928 Toll-Free: 800-521-0265
Web site: www.welbornhealthplans.com

MAILING ADDRESS:
  WELBORN HEALTH PLANS
  101 S E Third St
  Evansville, IN 47708

KEY EXECUTIVES:
Chairman of the Board/Chief Executive Officer .... William Macko
President .... Christopher Reef
Medical Director .... Roy Arnold, MD
Pharmacy Manager .... Jama Wallace PharmD
Chief Operating Officer .... Claudia Winslett
Sales & Marketing Manager .... Janet Burnett
IS Manager .... Jeremy Mathews
Hlth Promotion& Wellness Manager .... Candy Harper
Health Services Director .... Julie Girten, RN
Chief Administrator Officer .... Ali Kalor

COMPANY PROFILE:
Parent Company Name: Welborn Clinic
Doing Business As: Welborn Hlth Plns, Welborn Hlth Opts Slt
Year Founded: 1986   Federally Qualified: [Y]
Forprofit: [Y]   Not-For-Profit: [ ]
Model Type: MIXED
Accreditation: [ ] AAPPO [ ] JACHO [ ] NCQA [ ] URAC
Plan Type: HMO, POS, ASO, TPA
Primary Physicians: 725   Physician Specialists:
Hospitals: 11
Total Enrollment:
  2001: 39,157   2004: 28,749   2007: 0
  2002: 38,651   2005:
  2003: 33,594   2006: 25,000

SERVICE AREA:
Nationwide: N
  IN (Davies, Dubois, Gibson, Knox, Perry, Pike, Posey, Spencer, Vanderburgh, Warrick);

TYPE OF COVERAGE:
Commercial: [Y] Individual: [ ] FEHBP: [Y] Indemnity: [ ]
Medicare: [Y] Medicaid: [ ] Supplemental Medicare: [ ]
Tricare   [ ]

PRODUCTS OFFERED:
Product Name:	Type:
Welborn HMO	HMO
Welborn POS	POS
Welborn Medicare	Medicare
Welborn Health Plus Plan	Medicare Advantage

PLAN BENEFITS:
Alternative Medicine: [ ]   Behavioral Health: [ ]
Chiropractic: [X]   Dental: [ ]
Home Care: [X]   Inpatient SNF: [X]
Long-Term Care: [ ]   Pharm. Mail Order: [X]
Physicial Therapy: [X]   Podiatry: [X]
Psychiatric: [X]   Transplant: [X]
Vision: [X]   Wellness: [X]
Workers' Comp: [ ]
Other Benefits: Oral Surgery

Comments:
DBA Names: Welborn Health Plans, Welborn Health Options, Welborn Health Options-Select.

WELLPOINT INC - CORPORATE HEADQUARTERS

120 Monument Circle
Indianapolis, IN 46204
Phone: 317-532-6000 Fax: 317-488-6028 Toll-Free:
Web site: www.wellpoint.com

MAILING ADDRESS:
  WELLPOINT INC - CORP HDQTRS
  120 Monument Circle
  Indianpolis, IN 46204

KEY EXECUTIVES:
Chairperson of the Board .... Larry C Glasscock
Chief Executive Officer/President .... Angela F Braly
Executive Vice President, Chief Financial Officer ...... Wayne S DeVeydt
Chief Medical Officer .... Samuel R Nussbaum, MD
President/CEO Operation Tech, Government Services .... Mark L Boxer
Wellpoint Foundation .... Caroline S Matthews
Senior VP Human Resources .... Randy L Brown
President, Specialty Business .... Joan E Herman
President, Anthem Virginia .... Thomas Byrd

COMPANY PROFILE:
Parent Company Name:
Doing Business As: Blue Cross Blue Shield
Year Founded: Federally Qualified: [ ]
Forprofit: [Y]   Not-For-Profit: [ ]   Model Type:
Accreditation: [ ] AAPPO [ ] JACHO [ ] NCQA [ ] URAC
Plan Type: HMO, PPO, POS, HDHP, HSA
Total Revenue: 2005: 44,541,300,000   2006: 57,038,800,000
Net Income   2005: 2,463,800,000   2006: 3,094,900,000
Total Enrollment:
  2001: 7,883,000   2004: 27,728,000   2007: 34,809,000
  2002: 11,053,000   2005: 33,856,000
  2003: 11,927,000   2006: 34,101,000

SERVICE AREA:
Nationwide: N
  CO; CT; IN; KY; ME; NH; NV; OH;

TYPE OF COVERAGE:
Commercial: [Y] Individual: [ ] FEHBP: [ ] Indemnity: [ ]
Medicare: [ ] Medicaid: [ ] Supplemental Medicare: [ ]
Tricare   [ ]

PLAN BENEFITS:
Alternative Medicine: [ ]   Behavioral Health: [ ]
Chiropractic: [X]   Dental: [ ]
Home Care: [X]   Inpatient SNF: [X]
Long-Term Care: [ ]   Pharm. Mail Order: [X]
Physical Therapy: [X]   Podiatry: [ ]
Psychiatric: [X]   Transplant: [X]
Vision: [ ]   Wellness: [X]
Workers' Comp: [ ]
Other Benefits:

INDIANA

PRODUCTS OFFERED:
Product Name: Type:
St. Marys Managed Care Service   PPO
PLAN BENEFITS:
Alternative Medicine: [ ]   Behavioral Health: [X]
Chiropractic: [X]   Dental: [ ]
Home Care: [X]   Inpatient SNF: [X]
Long-Term Care: [ ]   Pharm. Mail Order: [ ]
Physical Therapy: [X]   Podiatry: [X]
Psychiatric: [X]   Transplant: [ ]
Vision: [ ]   Wellness: [ ]
Workers' Comp: [ ]
Other Benefits:

SOUTHEASTERN INDIANA HEALTH ORGANIZATION

417 Washington St
Columbus, IN 47201
Phone: 812-378-7000 Fax: 812-348-4592 Toll-Free:
Web site: www.siho.org
MAILING ADDRESS:
   SOUTHEASTERN INDIANA HEALTH ORGANIZATION
   PO Box 1787
   Columbus, IN 47201

KEY EXECUTIVES:
Chief Executive Officer/President .... David Barker
Senior VP/Chief Financial Officer .... Marc E Rothbart
Medical Director ....Joseph Sheehy, MD
Pharmacy Manager .... Nancy Burns
Manager, Provider Relations, Marketing ....Chris Asher
Vice President IS/IT/Compliance .... Mike Clancy
Network Services .... Randy Mills
Senior Vice President, Provider Relations .... Marc E Rothbart
Senior Vice President, Human Resources ....Bill Whisman
Manager, Medical Management .... Angela Hilycord
Vice President Client Services .... Jennifer Cutsinger

COMPANY PROFILE:
Parent Company Name:
Doing Business As: SIHO Insurance Services
Year Founded: 1987   Federally Qualified: [N]
Forprofit: [ ]   Not-For-Profit: [Y]
Model Type: IPA
Accreditation: [ ] AAPPO [ ] JACHO [ ] NCQA [ ] URAC
Plan Type: HMO, PPO, POS, TPA, PBM, EPO, HDHP, HSA
Primary Physicians: 8,100   Physician Specialists:
Hospitals:
Total Revenue: 2005:   44,400,000   2006:   47,200,000
Net Income   2005:   2006:
Total Enrollment:
   2001: 85,000   2004: 0   2007: 59,571
   2002: 45,000   2005: 64,346
   2003: 65,000   2006: 60,725
Medical Loss Ratio: 2005: 84.00   2006: 86.00
Administrative Expense Ratio: 2005: 16.00   2006: 15.00
SERVICE AREA:
Nationwide: N
   IN; (Bartholomew, Brown, Clark, Dearborn, Decatur, Floyd,
   Franklin, Harrison, Jackson, Jasper, Jefferson, Jennings, Johnson,
   Lawrence, Monroe, Ohio, Orange, Ripley, Rush, Scott, Shelby,
   Switzerland, Washington).
TYPE OF COVERAGE:
Commercial: [Y] Individual: [ ] FEHBP: [ ] Indemnity: [ ]
Medicare: [Y] Medicaid: [ ] Supplemental Medicare: [ ]
Tricare   [ ]
PRODUCTS OFFERED:
Product Name: Type:
Prime Care   POS
Southeastern Self Funded Mana   PPO
HMO   HMO
CONSUMER-DRIVEN PRODUCTS
Irwin Union Bank   HSA Company
SIHO HSA   HSA Product
                                    HSA Administrator
                                    Consumer-Driven Health Plan
SIHO Select Savings HDHP   High Deductible Health Plan

PLAN BENEFITS:
Alternative Medicine: [ ]   Behavioral Health: [ ]
Chiropractic: [X]   Dental: [X]
Home Care: [X]   Inpatient SNF: [X]
Long-Term Care: [ ]   Pharm. Mail Order: [X]
Physical Therapy: [X]   Podiatry: [X]
Psychiatric: [X]   Transplant: [X]
Vision: [X]   Wellness: [X]
Workers' Comp: [ ]
Other Benefits:

SPECTERA VISION INC - INDIANA

5975 Castle Creek Pkwy Ste 150
Indianapolis, IN 46250
Phone: 317-577-5155 Fax: 317-577-5160 Toll-Free: 800-668-6143
Web site: www.spectera.com
MAILING ADDRESS:
   SPECTERA VISION INC - IN
   5975 Castle Creek Pkwy Ste 150
   Indianapolis, IN 46250

KEY EXECUTIVES:
Chief Executive Officer/President .... Paul Gaulstrand
Chief Financial Officer .... Kyle Stern
Vice President, Corporate Communications .... Jeannette Duerr
Chief Operating Officer .... Tom Rekart
Chief Marketing Officer .... Jim Fuhrman
Sales Executive .... Laurinda Mackenzie
MIS Director .... Michael Pham
Director of Account Management- NY .... Kim Thompson

COMPANY PROFILE:
Parent Company Name: UnitedHealth Group
Doing Business As:
Year Founded: Federally Qualified: [ ]
Forprofit: [Y]   Not-For-Profit: [ ]
Model Type:
Accreditation: [ ] AAPPO [ ] JACHO [ ] NCQA [ ] URAC
Plan Type: Specialty HMO
Primary Physicians: 302   Physician Specialists:
Hospitals:
Total Enrollment:
   2001: 0   2004: 0   2007: 0
   2002: 0   2005:
   2003: 55,832   2006:
SERVICE AREA:
Nationwide: N
   IN;

SUBURBAN HEALTH ORGANIZATION

2780 Waterfront Pkwy E Dr #300
Indianapolis, IN 46214
Phone: 317-692-5222 Fax: 317-692-5233 Toll-Free: 800-570-7816
Web site: www.suburbanhealth.com
MAILING ADDRESS:
   SUBURBAN HEALTH ORGANIZATION
   2780 Waterfront Pkwy E Dr #300
   Indianapolis, IN 46214

KEY EXECUTIVES:
Chief Executive Officer.. Julie Carmichael
Director of Finance .... Keith Barnhart
Director Information Systems .... Dan Davis
President of Surb. Phys. Org .... Lynn Bowers MD

COMPANY PROFILE:
Parent Company Name:
Doing Business As:
Year Founded: Federally Qualified: [ ]
Forprofit: [ ]   Not-For-Profit: [ ]
Model Type:
Accreditation: [ ] AAPPO [ ] JACHO [ ] NCQA [ ] URAC
Plan Type: HMO
Primary Physicians: 1,600   Physician Specialists:
Hospitals: 8

Managed Care Organization Profiles — INDIANA

KEY EXECUTIVES:
Chief Executive Officer/President .... *Greg Yust*
Medical Director .... *Michael Shirley, MD*
Vice President of Operations .... *Kris Weber*
Director of Sales .... *Patti Thielking*
VP of MIS .... *Doug Pearson*
Director of Network Developmnt .... *Jackie Lee-McCord*
Director of Human Resources .... *Janet Hedlund*
Director of Medical Management .... *Becky Richey*
VP of Network Development & Contracting .... *Jon Anderson*
VP, General Counsel .... *Sharon Paulus*

COMPANY PROFILE:
Parent Company Name: CIGNA Healthcare
Doing Business As:
Year Founded: 1985   Federally Qualified: [N]
Forprofit: [Y]   Not-For-Profit: [ ]
Model Type: MIXED
Accreditation: [ ] AAPPO [ ] JACHO [ ] NCQA [X] URAC
Plan Type: PPO, POS, UR
Primary Physicians: 9,400   Physician Specialists: 26,600
Hospitals: 222
Total Enrollment:
  2001: 0   2004: 0   2007: 0
  2002: 0   2005:
  2003: 725,000   2006:

SERVICE AREA:
Nationwide: N
IL (Clark, Cook, Crawford, Cumberland, Douglas, Edgar, Edwards, Gallatin, Jasper, Lawrence, Richland, Saline, Will);IN (Adams, Allen, Bartholomew, Benton, Blackford, Boone, Brown, Carroll, Cass, Clark, Clay, Clinton, Crawford, Davies, Dearborn, Decatur, DeKalb, Delaware, Dubois, Elkhart, Fayette, Floyd, Fountain, Franklin, Fulton, Gibson, Grant, Greene, Hamilton, Hancock, Harrison, Hendricks, Henry, Howard, Huntington, Jackson, Jasper, Jay, Jefferson, Jennings, Johnson, Knox, Kosciusko, LaGrange, Lake, LaPorte, Lawrence, Madison, Marion, Marshall, Martin, Miami, Monroe, Montgomery, Morgan, Newton, Noble, Ohio, Orange, Owen, Parke, Perry, Pike, Porter, Posey, Pulaski, Putnam, Randolph, Ripley, Rush, St Joseph, Scott, Shelby, Spencer, Starke, Steuben, Sullivan, Switzerland, Tippecanoe, Tipton, Union, Vanderburgh, Vermillion, Vigo, Wabash, Warren, Warrick, Washington, Wayne, Wells, White, Whitley);

TYPE OF COVERAGE:
Commercial: [Y] Individual: [Y] FEHBP: [ ] Indemnity: [ ]
Medicare: [ ] Medicaid: [ ] Supplemental Medicare: [ ]
Tricare   [ ]

PRODUCTS OFFERED:
Product Name: Type:
Sagamore Senior Care   Medicare

PLAN BENEFITS:
Alternative Medicine: [ ]   Behavioral Health: [ ]
Chiropractic: [ ]   Dental: [ ]
Home Care: [ ]   Inpatient SNF: [ ]
Long-Term Care: [ ]   Pharm. Mail Order: [ ]
Physical Therapy: [ ]   Podiatry: [X]
Psychiatric: [ ]   Transplant: [ ]
Vision: [X]   Wellness: [X]
Workers' Comp: [ ]
Other Benefits:

Comments:
Purchased Family Health Plans of Indiana Inc.

SELECT CIRCLE HEALTH PLAN

300 N Pauline Ave
Muncie, IN 47303
Phone: 765-286-2150 Fax: 765-751-3061 Toll-Free:
Web site: www.cardinalcare.com

MAILING ADDRESS:
SELECT CIRCLE HEALTH PLAN
300 N Pauline Ave
Muncie, IN 47303

KEY EXECUTIVES:
President .... *Karen Popovich*
Chief Financial Officer .... *Kathy Edwards*
Medical Director .... *Charles Routh MD*
Pharmacy Director .... *Terry Pence, RPh*
Credentialing Manager .... *Tiffany Ridge*
Case Management Director .... *Pam Miller, RN*

COMPANY PROFILE:
Parent Company Name: Cardinal Health Alliance, LLC
Doing Business As:
Year Founded: 1995   Federally Qualified: [N]
Forprofit: [Y]   Not-For-Profit: [ ]
Model Type:
Accreditation: [ ] AAPPO [ ] JACHO [ ] NCQA [ ] URAC
Plan Type: PPO
Total Enrollment:
  2001: 67,000   2004: 60,000   2007: 0
  2002: 0   2005:
  2003: 65,000   2006:

SERVICE AREA:
Nationwide: N
IN;

TYPE OF COVERAGE:
Commercial: [Y] Individual: [ ] FEHBP: [ ] Indemnity: [ ]
Medicare: [ ] Medicaid: [ ] Supplemental Medicare: [ ]
Tricare   [ ]

PRODUCTS OFFERED:
Product Name: Type:
Select Circle Health Plan   PPO

PLAN BENEFITS:
Alternative Medicine: [ ]   Behavioral Health:
[X]Chiropractic: [ ]   Dental: [ ]
Home Care: [X]   Inpatient SNF: [X]
Long-Term Care: [ ]   Pharm. Mail Order: [ ]
Physical Therapy: [X]   Podiatry: [ ]
Psychiatric: [X]   Transplant: [ ]
Vision: [ ]   Wellness: [X]
Workers' Comp: [X]
Other Benefits:

SELECTHEALTH NETWORK

1400 Professional Blvd Ste 100
Evansville, IN 47714
Phone: 812-485-6992 Fax: 812-485-7995 Toll-Free: 800-200-6862
Web site:

MAILING ADDRESS:
SELECTHEALTH NETWORK
1400 Professional Blvd Ste 100
Evansville, IN 47714

KEY EXECUTIVES:
Director .... *Candace Adye*
Chief Financial Officer .... *Mike Browning, MBA, CPA*
Medical Director .... *Ken Spear, MD*
Marketing Director .... *Cathy Fulkerson*
Medical Manager .... *Barbara Rutkowski, EdD, MN*
Director, Managed Care Services .... *Mike Hassel*

COMPANY PROFILE:
Parent Company Name: St Marys Health System
Doing Business As: SelectHealth Network
Year Founded: 1992   Federally Qualified: [ ]
Forprofit: [ ]   Not-For-Profit: [Y]
Model Type: NETWORK
Accreditation: [ ] AAPPO [ ] JACHO [ ] NCQA [X] URAC
Plan Type: PPO, UR
Primary Physicians: 100   Physician Specialists: 800
Hospitals: 27
Total Enrollment:
  2001: 0   2004: 0   2007: 0
  2002: 140,000   2005:
  2003: 0   2006: 100,000

SERVICE AREA:
Nationwide: N
IL; IN; KY;

TYPE OF COVERAGE:
Commercial: [Y] Individual: [ ] FEHBP: [ ] Indemnity: [ ]
Medicare: [ ] Medicaid: [ ] Supplemental Medicare: [ ]
Tricare   [ ]

INDIANA   Managed Care Organization Profiles

Total Enrollment:
  2001: 0   2004: 0   2007: 280,000
  2002: 0   2005: 120,071
  2003: 106,207   2006: 122,000
Medical Loss Ratio: 2005:   2006: 92.00
Administrative Expense Ratio: 2005:   2006:
SERVICE AREA:
Nationwide: N
  IN;
TYPE OF COVERAGE:
Commercial: [ ]   Individual: [ ]   FEHBP: [ ]   Indemnity: [ ]
Medicare: [ ]   Medicaid: [Y]   Supplemental Medicare: [ ]
Tricare   [ ]
PRODUCTS OFFERED:
Product Name: Type:
Hoosier Healthwise Health Plan   Medicaid :
Comments:
Formerly Central Indiana Managed Care Organization. Purchased IU Health Plan December 28, 2006.

PARKVIEW SIGNATURE CARE

10501 Corporate Drive
Ft Wayne, IN 46845
Phone: 260-373-9100 Fax: 260-373-9004 Toll-Free: 800-666-4449
Web site: www.signaturecareppo.com
MAILING ADDRESS:
  PARKVIEW SIGNATURE CARE
  PO Box 5548
  Ft Wayne, IN 46845

KEY EXECUTIVES:
Executive Director .... Lisa Schambacher
Director of Finance .... Karen Dailey
Medical Director .... Dave Johnson, MD
Director of Sales .... Ned Hart
MIS Manager .... Dan Schneider
Provider Services Manager .... Wendy McConnell
Director of Medical Management .... Phil Henneman

COMPANY PROFILE:
Parent Company Name: Parkview Health System
Doing Business As: Signature Care PPO
Year Founded: 1996   Federally Qualified: [ ]
Forprofit: [Y]   Not-For-Profit: [ ]
Model Type: NETWORK
Accreditation: [ ] AAPPO [ ] JACHO [ ] NCQA [ ] URAC
Plan Type: PPO, UR, TPA
Total Enrollment:
  2001: 89,000   2004: 0   2007: 0
  2002: 0   2005:
  2003: 0   2006:
SERVICE AREA:
Nationwide: N
  IN; OH (DeFiance, Paulding, Van Wert, Williams);
TYPE OF COVERAGE:
Commercial: [Y]   Individual: [ ]   FEHBP: [ ]   Indemnity: [ ]
Medicare: [ ]   Medicaid: [ ]   Supplemental Medicare: [ ]
Tricare   [ ]
PRODUCTS OFFERED:
Product Name: Type:
Signature Care PPO   PPO
PLAN BENEFITS:
Alternative Medicine: [ ]   Behavioral Health: [X]
Chiropractic: [X]   Dental: [ ]
Home Care: [X]   Inpatient SNF: [X]
Long-Term Care: [X]   Pharm. Mail Order: [ ]
Physical Therapy: [X]   Podiatry: [X]
Psychiatric: [X]   Transplant: [X]
Vision: [X]   Wellness: [X]
Workers' Comp: [X]
Other Benefits:
Comments:
Formerly Parkview Health Plan Services.

PHYSICIANS HEALTH PLAN OF NORTHERN INDIANA

8101 W Jefferson Blvd
Ft Wayne, IN 46804-4163
Phone: 260-432-6690 Fax: 260-432-0493 Toll-Free: 800-982-6257
Web site: www.phpni.com

MAILING ADDRESS:
  PHYSICIANS HEALTH PLAN OF NORTHERN INDIANA
  8101 W Jefferson Blvd
  Ft Wayne, IN 46804-4163

KEY EXECUTIVES:
Chairman of the Board .... Michael McArdle, MD
Chief Executive Officer/President .... Jay M Gilbert
Chief Financial Officer .... Randy Kummer
Medical Director .... Philip Wright, MD
Assistant VP Pharmacy/Ancillary Svcs .... Dale Bultemeier
Chief Information Officer .... Karen Lihott
Assistant VP of Operations .... Gail Doran
Director of Marketing .... Vicki Lee Johnson
Assistant VP Sales/Service .... Angela Pippin
Privacy Officer .... Laura Carrico
Health Services Director .... Phyllis Borders
Human Resources Director .... Denise SzelisDirector
Medical Management .... Phyllis Borders
Assistant VP Chief Actuary .... Bruce Palmer

COMPANY PROFILE:
Parent Company Name: Physicians Health Plan of Northern IN
Doing Business As:
Year Founded: 1983   Federally Qualified: [Y]
Forprofit: [ ]   Not-For-Profit: [Y]
Model Type: IPA
Accreditation: [ ] AAPPO [ ] JACHO [ ] NCQA [ ] URAC
Plan Type: HMO, POS, HDHP, FSA
Total Revenue: 2005:   2006: 117,378,196
Net Income   2005:   2006:
Total Enrollment:
  2001: 0   2004: 52,327   2007: 0
  2002: 63,966   2005:
  2003: 60,088   2006:
Medical Loss Ratio: 2005:   2006: 83.20
Administrative Expense Ratio: 2005:   2006:
SERVICE AREA:
Nationwide: N
  IN (Adams, Allen, Blackford, DeKalb, Elkhart, Grant, Huntington, Jay, Kosciusko, LaGrange, Marshall, Noble, Saint Joseph, Steuben, Wabash, Wells, Whitley);
TYPE OF COVERAGE:
Commercial: [Y]   Individual: [ ]   FEHBP: [Y]   Indemnity: [ ]
Medicare: [ ]   Medicaid: [ ]   Supplemental Medicare: [ ]
Tricare   [ ]
PRODUCTS OFFERED:
Product Name: Type:
Physicians HMO   HMO
Health Choice   POS
Physician Point of Service
CONSUMER-DRIVEN PRODUCTS
Wells Fargo Bank   HSA Company
Wells Fargo HSA   HSA Product
Wells Fargo Health Benefits Services HSA Administrator
                                      Consumer-Driven Health Plan
Plans4Health   High Deductible Health Plan
PLAN BENEFITS:
Alternative Medicine: [ ]   Behavioral Health: [ ]
Chiropractic: [ ]   Dental: [X]
Home Care: [X]   Inpatient SNF: [X]
Long-Term Care: [ ]   Pharm. Mail Order: [X]
Physical Therapy: [X]   Podiatry: [X]
Psychiatric: [X]   Transplant: [X]
Vision: [X]   Wellness: [X]
Workers' Comp: [ ]
Other Benefits:

SAGAMORE HEALTH NETWORK INC

11555 N Meridian St Ste 400
Carmel, IN 46032
Phone: 317-573-2900 Fax: 317-580-8488 Toll-Free: 800-632-0353
Web site: www.sagamorehn.com
MAILING ADDRESS:
  SAGAMORE HEALTH NETWORK INC
  11555 N Meridian St Ste 400
  Carmel, IN 46032

Managed Care Organization Profiles — INDIANA

M PLAN INC

8802 North Meridian St Ste 100
Indianapolis, IN 46260-5371
Phone: 317-571-5300 Fax: 317-571-5306 Toll-Free: 800-878-8802
Web site: www.mplan.com

MAILING ADDRESS:
M PLAN INC
8802 North Meridian St Ste 100
Indianapolis, IN 46260-5371

KEY EXECUTIVES:
Chairman of the Board .... Alex Slabosky
Chief Executive Officer/President/Director .... Alex Slabosky
VP of Finance .... Constance Brown
Medical Director .... John Ellis, MD
Pharmacy Director .... Chuck Mihalik
Vice President Marketing .... Rick Altstadt
Public Relations Director .... Andrew Stoner
VP of Network Planning/Development .... LeAnn Donovan
Human Resources Director .... Troy Taylor
VP of Quality & Risk Management .... Rosemarie Byrd
VP Operations/Provider Relations .... Kathy O'Farrell

COMPANY PROFILE:
Parent Company Name: The Healthcare Group LLC
Doing Business As:
Year Founded: 1989   Federally Qualified: [N]
Forprofit: [Y]   Not-For-Profit: [ ]
Model Type: NETWORK
Accreditation: [ ] AAPPO [ ] JACHO [X] NCQA [ ] URAC
Plan Type: HMO, PPO, POS, HDHP
Total Revenue: 2005:   617,168,904   2006:   605,342,305
Net Income   2005:   7,556,236   2006:   3,415,833
Total Enrollment:
 2001: 172,769   2004: 182,308   2007: 0
 2002: 180,733   2005: 163,571
 2003: 188,409   2006: 156,554
Medical Loss Ratio: 2005:   2006: 90.40
Administrative Expense Ratio: 2005:   2006:

SERVICE AREA:
Nationwide: N
IN; (Adams, Allen, Bartholomew, Boone, Brown, Carroll, Cass, Clark, Clay, Clinton, Crawford, Daviess, Decatur, DeKalb, Delaware, Dubois, Elkhart, Floyd, Fulton, Gibson, Grant, Greene, Hamilton, Hanock, Harrison, Hendricks, Henry, Howard, Huntington, Jackson, Jennings, Johnson, Knox, Kosciusko, Lagrnage, Lawrence, Madison, Marion, Marshall, Martin, Miami, Monroe, Montgomery, Morgan, Noble, Orange, Owen, Parke, Perry, Pike, Posey, Putnam, Rush, St Joseph, Shelby, Spencer, Steuben, Sullivan, Tippecanoe, Tipton, Vanderburgh, Vermillion, Vigo, Wabash, Warrick, Washington, Wells, White, Whitley);

TYPE OF COVERAGE:
Commercial: [Y] Individual: [ ] FEHBP: [Y] Indemnity: [ ]
Medicare: [Y] Medicaid: [Y] Supplemental Medicare: [ ]
Tricare   [ ]

PRODUCTS OFFERED:
Product Name:	Type:
M-Plan	HMO
Senior Smart Choice	Medicare Advantage
Senior Securecare	Medicare

PLAN BENEFITS:
Alternative Medicine: [ ]   Behavioral Health: [X]
Chiropractic: [X]   Dental: [ ]
Home Care: [X]   Inpatient SNF: [X]
Long-Term Care: [ ]   Pharm. Mail Order: [X]
Physical Therapy: [X]   Podiatry: [X]
Psychiatric: [X]   Transplant: [X]
Vision: [X]   Wellness: [X]
Workers' Comp: [ ]
Other Benefits:

MANAGED HEALTH SERVICES INDIANA INC

1099 N Meridian St Ste 400
Indianapolis, IN 46204
Phone: 317-684-9478 Fax: 317-684-0297 Toll-Free: 877-647-4848
Web site: www.managedhealthservices.com

MAILING ADDRESS:
MANAGED HEALTH SERVICES IN INC
7711 Carondelet Ave Ste 800
St Louis, MO 46204

KEY EXECUTIVES:
Chairman of the Board .... Shelly Stewart
Chief Executive Officer/President .... Rita Johnson-Mills
Associate Medical Director .... John T Young
Pharmacy Director .... Larry Harrison
Chief Operating Officer .... Amy Williams
Manager, Provider & Member Services .... Jacquelyn Shearer
Director, Quality Improvement .... Linda Baker

COMPANY PROFILE:
Parent Company Name: Centene Corporation Inc
Doing Business As:
Year Founded: 1996   Federally Qualified: [ ]
Forprofit: [Y]   Not-For-Profit: [ ]
Model Type: NETWORK
Accreditation: [ ] AAPPO [ ] JACHO [ ] NCQA [ ] URAC
Plan Type: HMO, Specialty HMO
Primary Physicians: 793   Physician Specialists: 1,243
Hospitals: 40
Total Enrollment:
 2001: 55,220   2004: 150,600   2007: 0
 2002:   0   2005: 193,300
 2003: 119,400   2006: 161,700

SERVICE AREA:
Nationwide: N
IN (Adams, Allen, Bartholomew, Benton, Blackford, Boone, Brown, Carroll, Cass, Clark, Clay, Clinton, Crawford, Daviess, Dearborn, Decatur, Dekalb, Delaware, Dubois, Elkhart, Fayette, Floyd, Fountain, Franklin, Fulton, Gibson, Grant, Greene, Hamilton, Hancock, Harrison, Hendricks, Henry, Howard, Huntington, Jackson, Jasper, Jay, Jefferson, Jennings, Johnson, Knox, Kosciusko, Lagrange, Lake, Laporte, Lawrence, Madison, Marion, Marshall, Martin, Miami, Monroe, Montgomery, Morgan, Newton, Noble, Ohio, Orange, Owen, Parke, Perry, Pike, Porter, Posey, Pulaski, Putnam, Randolph, Ripley, Rush, Saint Joseph, Scott, Shelby, Spencer, Starke, Steuben, Sullivan, Switzerland, Tippecanoe, Tipton, Union, Vanderburgh, Vermillion, Vigo, Wabash, Warren, Warrick, Washington, Wayne, Wells, White, Whitley);

TYPE OF COVERAGE:
Commercial: [ ] Individual: [ ] FEHBP: [ ] Indemnity: [ ]
Medicare: [ ] Medicaid: [Y] Supplemental Medicare: [ ]
Tricare   [ ]

Comments:
Also known as Coordinated Care Corporation Indiana Inc.

MDWISE

1099 N Meridian St Ste 320
Indianapolis, IN 46204
Phone: 317-630-2828 Fax: 317-630-2835 Toll-Free: 800-356-1204
Web site: www.mdwise.org

MAILING ADDRESS:
MDWISE
PO Box 441423
Indianapolis, IN 46204

KEY EXECUTIVES:
Chief Executive Officer/President .... Charlotte Macbeth, JD
Chief Financial Officer .... Terry Cole, CPA
Medical Director .... Tony Pelezo, MD
VP of Information Services .... Jean Caster
VP of Legal Affairs .... Katherine Wentworth, JD
VP of Quality Improvement .... Barbara Wilder, MBA

COMPANY PROFILE:
Parent Company Name: Clarian Health Partners Inc
Doing Business As:
Year Founded: 1994   Federally Qualified: [ ]
Forprofit: [ ]   Not-For-Profit: [Y]
Model Type:
Accreditation: [ ] AAPPO [ ] JACHO [ ] NCQA [ ] URAC
Plan Type: HMO
Primary Physicians: 1,400   Physician Specialists: 2,800
Hospitals: 7
Total Revenue: 2005:   2006: 227,946,074
Net Income   2005:   2006:

INDIANA — Managed Care Organization Profiles

KEY EXECUTIVES:
Chief Executive Officer .... Jim Shelton
President .... Bruce Smiley
Medical Director .... David Cook, MD

COMPANY PROFILE:
Parent Company Name:
Doing Business As:
Year Founded: Federally Qualified: [ ]
Forprofit: [ ]   Not-For-Profit: [ ]
Model Type:
Accreditation: [ ] AAPPO [ ] JACHO [ ] NCQA [ ] URAC
Plan Type: PPO
Primary Physicians: 20,000   Physician Specialists:
Hospitals: 142

SERVICE AREA:
Nationwide: N
    IN,

INDIANA PRO HEALTH NETWORK

8180 Clearvista Pkwy Ste 230
Indianapolis, IN 46256
Phone: 800-344-8672 Fax: 317-621-7470 Toll-Free: 800-344-8672
Web site: www.ecommunity.com
MAILING ADDRESS:
    INDIANA PRO HEALTH NETWORK
    8180 Clearvista Pkwy Ste 230
    Indianapolis, IN 46256

KEY EXECUTIVES:
Chief Executive Officer/President .... William E Corley
Chief Financial Officer .... David Delaney
Medical Director .... Thomas Petrin, MD
MIS Director .... Chad Bailey
Director, Provider Relations .... Judy Bourquin
Medical Management Director .... Vivian Rice, RN
Executive Director .... Julie Pheqley

COMPANY PROFILE:
Parent Company Name: Community Hospitals of Indianapolis
Doing Business As: Indiana Pro Health Network
Year Founded: 1986   Federally Qualified: [N]
Forprofit: [ ]   Not-For-Profit: [Y]
Model Type: PHO
Accreditation: [ ] AAPPO [ ] JACHO [X] NCQA [ ] URAC
Plan Type: HMO, PPO, UR

SERVICE AREA:
Nationwide: N
    IN (Central);

TYPE OF COVERAGE:
Commercial: [Y] Individual: [ ] FEHBP: [ ] Indemnity: [ ]
Medicare: [Y] Medicaid: [Y] Supplemental Medicare: [ ]
Tricare   [ ]

INDIVIDUALIZED CARE MANAGEMENT INC

60 Professional Ct
Lafayette, IN 47905-6298
Phone: 765-448-1864 Fax: 765-447-8335 Toll-Free: 800-728-0327
Web site: www.indcaremgmt.com
MAILING ADDRESS:
    INDIVIDUALIZED CARE MGMT INC
    PO Box 6298
    Lafayette, IN 47905-6298

KEY EXECUTIVES:
Chief Executive Officer/Principal .... Ann H Roberts, BSN
Medical Director .... Martin J Maassen, MD
Director of Operations .... Anne Brown
Director of Clinical Affairs .... Trina Boston
Corporate Counsel .... Rebekah N Plowman
Marketing Director South .... Joyce Wittman

COMPANY PROFILE:
Parent Company Name: Individualized Care Management, Inc
Doing Business As: Net Pro
Year Founded: 1992   Federally Qualified: [ ]
Forprofit: [Y]   Not-For-Profit: [ ]
Model Type:
Accreditation: [ ] AAPPO [ ] JACHO [ ] NCQA [X] URAC
Plan Type: PPO, UR
Total Enrollment:
    2001: 0   2004: 0   2007: 0
    2002: 0   2005:
    2003: 0   2006: 300,000

SERVICE AREA:
Nationwide: N
    IN;

TYPE OF COVERAGE:
Commercial: [Y] Individual: [ ] FEHBP: [ ] Indemnity: [ ]
Medicare: [ ] Medicaid: [ ] Supplemental Medicare: [Y]
Tricare   [ ]

PLAN BENEFITS:
Alternative Medicine: [ ]   Behavioral Health: [X]
Chiropractic: [X]   Dental: [ ]
Home Care: [X]   Inpatient SNF: [X]
Long-Term Care: [ ]   Pharm. Mail Order: [ ]
Physical Therapy: [X]   Podiatry: [X]
Psychiatric: [X]   Transplant: [X]
Vision: [X]   Wellness: [ ]
Workers' Comp: [X]
Other Benefits:

LUTHERAN PREFERRED/THREE RIVERS PREFERRED

7950 West Jefferson Blvd
Ft Wayne, IN 46804
Phone: 260-435-7768 Fax: 260-435-6940 Toll-Free: 800-258-0974
Web site: www.lutheranpreferred.com
MAILING ADDRESS:
    LUTHERAN PREFERRED/THREE RIVER PREFERRED
    7950 West Jefferson Blvd
    Ft Wayne, IN 46804

KEY EXECUTIVES:
Chief Executive Officer .... Paul Moss
Marketing Director .... Beth Fremion
Medical Management Director .... Linda Pickerman
Director of Lutheran Preferred .... Karla Barnhart

COMPANY PROFILE:
Parent Company Name: Lutheran Hospital of Indiana
Doing Business As:
Year Founded: 1995   Federally Qualified: [ ]
Forprofit: [Y]   Not-For-Profit: [ ]
Model Type: NETWORK
Accreditation: [ ] AAPPO [ ] JACHO [ ] NCQA [ ] URAC
Plan Type: PPO, POS, EPO, UR
Primary Physicians: 3,000   Physician Specialists: 6,500
Hospitals: 38
Total Enrollment:
    2001: 57,000   2004: 0   2007: 0
    2002: 0   2005:
    2003: 60,000   2006:

SERVICE AREA:
Nationwide: N
    IL (Adams, Allen, Blackford, DeKalb, Grant, Huntington, Jay,
    Kosciusko, LaGrange, Miami, Noble, Steuben, Wabash, Wells,
    Whitley); IN; NE; OH(Defiance, Mercer, Paulding, Van Wert,
    Williams);

TYPE OF COVERAGE:
Commercial: [Y] Individual: [Y] FEHBP: [ ] Indemnity: [ ]
Medicare: [ ] Medicaid: [ ] Supplemental Medicare: [ ]
Tricare   [ ]

PLAN BENEFITS:
Alternative Medicine: [ ]   Behavioral Health: [ ]
Chiropractic: [ ]   Dental: [ ]
Home Care: [X]   Inpatient SNF: [ ]
Long-Term Care: [ ]   Pharm. Mail Order: [ ]
Physical Therapy: [ ]   Podiatry: [ ]
Psychiatric: [X]   Transplant: [X]
Vision: [ ]   Wellness: [X]
Workers' Comp: [X]
Other Benefits:

Managed Care Organization Profiles — INDIANA

MAILING ADDRESS:
HEALTH CARE EXCEL INCORPORATED
2629 Waterfront Pkwy East Dr
Indianapolis, IN 46214

KEY EXECUTIVES:
Chief Executive Officer .... Sharon Smith
Human Resources Director .... Sherrie Nicholson
Executive Director Medicare Q10 .... Mitzi Daffron
Director, Project Manager .... Carl Osborn

COMPANY PROFILE:
Parent Company Name:
Doing Business As:
Year Founded: 1974   Federally Qualified: [ ]
Forprofit: [ ]   Not-For-Profit: [Y]
Model Type:
Accreditation: [ ] AAPPO [ ] JACHO [ ] NCQA [ ] URAC
Plan Type: PRO, UR

SERVICE AREA:
Nationwide: N
   IN;

HEALTH RESOURCES INC

5010 Carriage Dr
Evansville, IN 47716-0660
Phone: 812-424-1444 Fax: 812-424-2096 Toll-Free: 800-727-1444
Web site: www.hri-dho.com

MAILING ADDRESS:
HEALTH RESOURCES INC
PO Box 15660
Evansville, IN 47716-0660

KEY EXECUTIVES:
Chairman of the Board .... Edward L Fritz, DDS
Chief Executive Officer/President .... Allan L Reid, DMD
Chief Operating Officer .... Cynthia A Kuester
Director, Marketing & Sales .... Chad Decker
Director of Provider Development/Relations .... Terry Bawel

COMPANY PROFILE:
Parent Company Name:
Doing Business As:
Year Founded: 1986   Federally Qualified: [N]
Forprofit: [Y]   Not-For-Profit: [ ]
Model Type: GROUP
Accreditation: [ ] AAPPO [ ] JACHO [ ] NCQA [ ] URAC
Plan Type: Specialty HMO, PPO
Primary Physicians: 900   Physician Specialists:
Hospitals:
Total Revenue   2005:   2006: 35,156,261
Net Income   2005:   2006:
Total Enrollment:
   2001: 100,000   2004: 121,000   2007: 0
   2002: 0   2005:
   2003: 69,525   2006: 160,000

SERVICE AREA:
Nationwide: N
   IN (Clay, Crawford, Davies, Dubois, Elkhart, Gibson, Greene, Knox, LaPorte, Lawrence, Marion, Marshall, Martin, Monroe, Orange, Owen, Parke, Perry, Pike, Posey, Putnam, Spencer, St Joseph, Sullivan, Vanderburgh, Vermillion, Vigo, Warrick, Washington); KY (Allen, Barren, Breckinridge, Butler, Caldwell, Calloway, Christian, Crittenden, Daviess, Edmonson, Graves, Grayson, Hancock, Hardin, Hart, Henderson, Hopkins, Larue, Logan, Lyon, Marshall, McCracken, McLean, Monroe, Muhlenburg, Nelson, Ohio, Simpson, Trigg, Union, Warren, Webster);

TYPE OF COVERAGE:
Commercial: [Y] Individual: [ ] FEHBP: [ ] Indemnity: [ ]
Medicare: [ ] Medicaid: [ ] Supplemental Medicare: [ ]
Tricare   [ ]

PRODUCTS OFFERED:
Product Name: Type:
Dental Health Options   Specialty HMO

PLAN BENEFITS:
Alternative Medicine: [ ]   Behavioral Health: [ ]
Chiropractic: [ ]   Dental: [X]
Home Care: [ ]   Inpatient SNF: [ ]
Long-Term Care: [ ]   Pharm. Mail Order: [ ]
Physical Therapy: [ ]   Podiatry: [ ]
Psychiatric: [ ]   Transplant: [ ]
Vision: [ ]   Wellness: [ ]
Workers' Comp: [ ]
Other Benefits:

HUMANA INC - INDIANA

8888 Keystone Crossing Ste 700
Indianapolis, IN 46240
Phone: 317-573-1020 Fax: 317-573-1030 Toll-Free: 800-444-9137
Web site: www.humana.com

MAILING ADDRESS:
HUMANA INC - INDIANA
8888 Keystone Crossing Ste 700
Indianapolis, IN 46240

KEY EXECUTIVES:
Chairman of the Board .... David A Jones Jr
Chief Executive Officer .... Michael B McCallister
Market President .... Veronica Martin
Director of Account Management .... Laura Waldo
Market Medical Officer .... Tricia Nguyen, MD
Senior VP Chief Information Officer .... Bruce J Goodman
Large Group, Director of Sales .... John Sadtler
Small Group, Director of Sales .... James Bryant
Senior VP of Human Resources .... Bonnie C Hathcock
VP, Provider Contracting .... John Johnson

COMPANY PROFILE:
Parent Company Name: Humana Inc
Doing Business As:
Year Founded: 1961   Federally Qualified: [Y]
Forprofit: [Y]   Not-For-Profit: [ ]
Model Type: IPA
Accreditation: [ ] AAPPO [ ] JACHO [ ] NCQA [ ] URAC
Plan Type: HMO, PPO, ASO, CDHP, HDHP, HSA,
Total Enrollment:
   2001: 617,022   2004: 0   2007: 0
   2002: 52,000   2005:
   2003: 102,500   2006: 260,000

SERVICE AREA:
Nationwide: N
   IN; (Boone, Carroll, Clark, Dubois, Fayette, Floyd, Franklin, Gibson, Grant, Harrison, Henry, Jefferson, Knox, Madison, Marion, Owen, Pike, Posey, Scott, Shelby, Spencer, Vanderburgh, Warrick, Washington),

TYPE OF COVERAGE:
Commercial: [Y] Individual: [Y] FEHBP: [ ] Indemnity: [ ]
Medicare: [Y] Medicaid: [ ] Supplemental Medicare: [Y]
Tricare   [Y]

PRODUCTS OFFERED:
Product Name: Type:
Humana Gold Plus   Medicare
Humana HMO   HMO
Humana PPO   PPO

CONSUMER-DRIVEN PRODUCTS
JP Morgan Chase   HSA Company
HumanaOne HSA   HSA Product
JP Morgan Chase   HSA Administrator
Personal Care Account   Consumer-Driven Health Plan
HumanaOne   High Deductible Health Plan

PLAN BENEFITS:
Alternative Medicine: [ ]   Behavioral Health: [X]
Chiropractic: [X]   Dental: [X]
Home Care: [ ]   Inpatient SNF: [ ]
Long-Term Care: [ ]   Pharm. Mail Order: [X]
Physical Therapy: [ ]   Podiatry: [ ]
Psychiatric: [X]   Transplant: [X]
Vision: [ ]   Wellness: [ ]
Workers' Comp: [X]
Other Benefits: Long Term Disability

INDIANA HEALTH NETWORK

8330 Allison Pointe Trail
Indianapolis, IN 46250
Phone: 317-284-7171 Fax: 317-284-7278 Toll-Free: 888-446-6670
Web site: www.ihnppo.com

MAILING ADDRESS:
INDIANA HEALTH NETWORK
8330 Allison Pointe Trail
Indianapolis, IN 46250

INDIANA   Managed Care Organization Profiles

COMPANY PROFILE:
Parent Company Name:
Doing Business As:
Year Founded: 1984   Federally Qualified: [Y]
Forprofit: [ ]   Not-For-Profit: [Y]
Model Type: MIXED
Accreditation: [ ] AAPPO [ ] JACHO [ ] NCQA [ ] URAC
Plan Type: Specialty HMO, Specialty PPO, POS
Primary Physicians: 742   Physician Specialists: 158
Hospitals:
Total Revenue: 2005:   2006: 1,567,029
Net Income   2005:   2006:
Total Enrollment:
  2001: 0   2004: 0   2007: 0
  2002: 302,261   2005:
  2003: 306,000   2006:

SERVICE AREA:
Nationwide: N
  IN;
TYPE OF COVERAGE:
Commercial: [Y] Individual: [ ] FEHBP: [ ] Indemnity: [ ]
Medicare: [ ] Medicaid: [Y] Supplemental Medicare: [ ]
Tricare   [ ]
PRODUCTS OFFERED:
Product Name: Type:
Delta Premier   Managed Fee for Serv
Delta Preferred Option Standard   PPO
Delta Preferred Option Point of Service PPO
DeltaCare   HMO
PLAN BENEFITS:
Alternative Medicine: [ ]   Behavioral Health: [ ]
Chiropractic: [ ]   Dental: [X]
Home Care: [ ]   Inpatient SNF: [ ]
Long-Term Care: [ ]   Pharm. Mail Order: [ ]
Physical Therapy: [ ]   Podiatry: [ ]
Psychiatric: [ ]   Transplant: [ ]
Vision: [ ]   Wellness: [ ]
Workers' Comp: [ ]
Other Benefits:

ENCORE HEALTH NETWORK

8802 N Meridian Ste 100
Indianapolis, IN 46260
Phone: 317-705-3280 Fax: 317-705-3281 Toll-Free: 888-446-5584
Web site: www.encoreconnect.com
MAILING ADDRESS:
  ENCORE HEALTH NETWORK
  8802 N Meridian Ste 100
  Indianapolis, IN 46260

KEY EXECUTIVES:
Chairman of the Board .... Mark A Hochstetler, MD
President .... Alex Slabosky
VP of Finance .... Constance Brown
VP & Chief Operating Officer .... Michelle Lobe
AVP/Marketing & Product Development .... Kathy O'Farrell
Credentialing Coordinator .... Allen Boswell
Compliance Officer .... Susan Mann
Provider Relations Director .... Lori Tomey
Human Resources Director .... Steve Jones
Credentialing Coordinator .... Allen Boswell
AVP, Marketing & Product Development .... Kathy O'Farrell
VP, PPO Networks .... Michelle Lobe

COMPANY PROFILE:
Parent Company Name: Healthcare Group LLC
Doing Business As: Encore Health Network
Year Founded: 1987   Federally Qualified: [ ]Forprofit: [ ]
Not-For-Profit: [Y]
Model Type: NETWORK
Accreditation: [ ] AAPPO [ ] JACHO [ ] NCQA [ ] URAC
Plan Type: Specialty PPO, PPO
Primary Physicians: 6,536   Physician Specialists: 19,549
Hospitals: 170
Total Enrollment:
  2001: 268,000   2004: 609,938   2007: 0
  2002: 0   2005:
  2003: 405,753   2006:

SERVICE AREA:
Nationwide: N
  IN; KY; IL; OH; MI;
TYPE OF COVERAGE:
Commercial: [Y] Individual: [Y] FEHBP: [ ] Indemnity: [ ]
Medicare: [ ] Medicaid: [ ] Supplemental Medicare: [ ]
Tricare   [ ]
PRODUCTS OFFERED:
Product Name: Type:
Encore Health Network PPO   PPO
PLAN BENEFITS:
Alternative Medicine: [X]   Behavioral Health: [X]
Chiropractic: [X]   Dental: [ ]
Home Care: [X]   Inpatient SNF: [X]
Long-Term Care: [ ]   Pharm. Mail Order: [X]
Physical Therapy: [X]   Podiatry: [X]
Psychiatric: [X]   Transplant: [X]
Vision: [X]   Wellness: [X]
Workers' Comp: [ ]
Other Benefits:

GROUPLINK INC

6612 E 75th St Ste 200
Indianapolis, IN 46250
Phone: 317-578-7128 Fax: 317-578-7306 Toll-Free: 800-935-2009
Web site: www.grouplinktpa.com
MAILING ADDRESS:
  GROUPLINK INC
  6612 E 75th St Ste 200
  Indianapolis, IN 46250

KEY EXECUTIVES:
President .... Roger W Skinner
VP of Operations .... Roger Brackett
VP, Sales & Marketing .... David Skinner
IS Director .... Keith Lollar
HIPAA Compliance Officer .... Roger Brackett
Director of Claims .... Ketrina Lollar
Director of Client Services .... Trisha Parker

COMPANY PROFILE:
Parent Company Name: GroupLink Inc
Doing Business As:
Year Founded: 1983   Federally Qualified: [N]
Forprofit: [Y]   Not-For-Profit: [ ]
Model Type:
Accreditation: [ ] AAPPO [ ] JACHO [ ] NCQA [ ] URAC
Plan Type: PPO, Specialty PPO, POS, ASO, TPA, EPO
Total Enrollment:
  2001: 0   2004: 0   2007: 0
  2002: 55,000   2005:
  2003: 80,000   2006:
SERVICE AREA:
Nationwide: N
  IN;
TYPE OF COVERAGE:
Commercial: [Y] Individual: [Y] FEHBP: [ ] Indemnity: [ ]
Medicare: [ ] Medicaid: [ ] Supplemental Medicare: [ ]
Tricare   [ ]
PRODUCTS OFFERED:
Product Name: Type:
DentaVest   Discount Fee for den
PLAN BENEFITS:
Alternative Medicine: [ ]   Behavioral Health: [ ]
Chiropractic: [ ]   Dental: [X]
Home Care: [ ]   Inpatient SNF: [ ]
Long-Term Care: [ ]   Pharm. Mail Order: [ ]
Physical Therapy: [ ]   Podiatry: [ ]
Psychiatric: [ ]   Transplant: [ ]
Vision: [ ]   Wellness: [ ]
Workers' Comp: [ ]
Other Benefits:

HEALTH CARE EXCEL INCORPORATED

2629 Waterfront Pkwy East Dr
Indianapolis, IN 46214
Phone: 317-347-4500 Fax: 317-347-4545 Toll-Free:
Web site: www.hce.org

Managed Care Organization Profiles   INDIANA

COMMUNITY HEALTH ALLIANCE

3355 Douglas Rd
South Bend, IN 46635
Phone: 574-647-1820 Fax: 574-647-1825 Toll-Free:
Web site: www.chanetwork.com
MAILING ADDRESS:
    COMMUNITY HEALTH ALLIANCE
    3355 Douglas Rd
    South Bend, IN 46635

KEY EXECUTIVES:
Chief Executive Officer .... Diane Maas
Chief Financial Officer .... Jeff Costello
Medical Director .... Sandra Brown, MD
Customer Sales .... Angela Latkowski
Credentialing Specialist .... Barb Garrett
Medical Management/Quality Assurance Director .... Kelly Foster
Contract/Credentialing Specialist .... Barb Garrett

COMPANY PROFILE:
Parent Company Name:
Doing Business As:
Year Founded: 1994   Federally Qualified: [N]
Forprofit: [ ]   Not-For-Profit: [Y]
Model Type: IPA
Accreditation: [ ] AAPPO [ ] JACHO [ ] NCQA [ ] URAC
Plan Type: PPO, UR
Primary Physicians: 8,584   Physician Specialists:
Hospitals: 70
Total Revenue: 2005:   2006:
Net Income   2005:   2006:
Total Enrollment:
    2001: 0   2004: 125,285   2007: 0
    2002: 110,000   2005:
    2003: 126,000   2006: 122,000
SERVICE AREA:
Nationwide: N
IN;
TYPE OF COVERAGE:
Commercial: [Y] Individual: [ ] FEHBP: [ ] Indemnity: [ ]
Medicare: [ ] Medicaid: [ ] Supplemental Medicare: [ ]
Tricare   [ ]

CORVEL CORPORATION

800 E 96th St Ste 450
Indianapolis, IN 46240
Phone: 317-816-6996 Fax: 317-816-6990 Toll-Free: 800-959-7958
Web site: www.corvel.com
MAILING ADDRESS:
    CORVEL CORPORATION
    800 E 96th St Ste 450
    Indianapolis, IN 46240

KEY EXECUTIVES:
Chief Executive Officer/President .... Gordon Clemons
Chief Financial Officer .... Scott McCloud
Chief Information Officer .... Don McFarlane
VP of Regional Sales .... Jayna Dunning
Director of Provider Services .... Sally Ferguson
Director, Legal Services .... Sharon O'Connor
District Manager .... Rhonda Moran
VP Information Systems .... Tom Benson

COMPANY PROFILE:
Parent Company Name: Corvel Corporation
Doing Business As:
Year Founded: 1981   Federally Qualified: [ ]
Forprofit: [Y]   Not-For-Profit: [ ]
Model Type:
Accreditation: [ ] AAPPO [ ] JACHO [ ] NCQA [ ] URAC
Plan Type: PPO, UR
Total Revenue: 2005:   2006: 26,650,400
Net Income   2005:   2006: 9,753,000
SERVICE AREA:
Nationwide: Y
    NW;
TYPE OF COVERAGE:
Commercial: [Y] Individual: [ ] FEHBP: [ ] Indemnity: [ ]
Medicare: [ ] Medicaid: [ ] Supplemental Medicare: [ ]
Tricare   [ ]

DEACONESS HEALTH PLANS

350 W Columbia St Ste 400
Evansville, IN 47710
Phone: 812-450-7265 Fax: 812-450-2030 Toll-Free: 800-374-8993
Web site: www.deaconesshealthplans.com
MAILING ADDRESS:
    DEACONESS HEALTH PLANS
    350 W Columbia St Ste 400
    Evansville, IN 47710

KEY EXECUTIVES:
Chief Executive Officer .... Joyce Hudson
Sales & Marketing .... Tina Hazelip
Sales & Marketing .... Beth Deters
Credentialing Coordinator .... Kimberly Catt, RN
Provider Relations Representative .... Sandra Ambrose
Account Executive .... Tina Hazelip

COMPANY PROFILE:
Parent Company Name: Deaconess Health System
Doing Business As: Deaconess Health Plans
Year Founded: 1985   Federally Qualified: [N]
Forprofit: [Y]   Not-For-Profit: [ ]
Model Type: NETWORK
Accreditation: [ ] AAPPO [ ] JACHO [ ] NCQA [ ] URAC
Plan Type: PPO
Primary Physicians: 900   Physician Specialists: 612
Hospitals: 16
Total Enrollment:
    2001: 133,000   2004: 227,092   2007: 0
    2002: 140,000   2005:
    2003: 146,940   2006:
SERVICE AREA:
Nationwide: N
IL; IN; KY;
TYPE OF COVERAGE:
Commercial: [Y] Individual: [ ] FEHBP: [ ] Indemnity: [ ]
Medicare: [ ] Medicaid: [ ] Supplemental Medicare: [ ]
Tricare   [ ]
PRODUCTS OFFERED:
Product Name: Type:
Deaconess PPO   PPO
PLAN BENEFITS:
Alternative Medicine: [ ]   Behavioral Health: [X]
Chiropractic: [X]   Dental: [ ]
Home Care: [X]   Inpatient SNF: [X]
Long-Term Care: [ ]   Pharm. Mail Order: [X]
Physical Therapy: [X]   Podiatry: [X]
Psychiatric: [X]   Transplant: [X]
Vision: [ ]   Wellness: [X]
Workers' Comp: [X]
Other Benefits:

DELTA DENTAL PLAN OF INDIANA INC

5875 Castle Creek Pkwy N # 191
Indianapolis, IN 46250-4327
Phone: 517-349-6000 Fax: 517-381-5572 Toll-Free: 800-382-5404
Web site: www.deltadentalin.com
MAILING ADDRESS:
    DELTA DENTAL PLAN OF IN
    5875 Castle Creek Pkwy N # 191
    Indianapolis, IN 46250-4327

KEY EXECUTIVES:
Chairperson .... Robert A Anthony, DDS
Chief Executive Officer/President .... Thomas J Fleszar, DDS, MS
Executive VP, Chief Financial Officer .... Laura L Czelada, CPA
VP Professional Services & Dental Dir ..... Jed J Jacobson, DDS, MPH
Executive VP, Chief Information Officer .... Laura L Czelada, CPA
Vice President Operations .... Sherry L Crisp
Marketing & New Business Development .... Lonell D Rice
Executive VP, Acturial, Underwriting, Sales .... Charles E Floyd, CEBS
VP, Quality Assurance & Informatics .... Karen M Green
VP, New Business Development .... Lonell D Rice
Vice President Actuary .... Mr William T Billard
Executive Vice President .... Judge Patrick T Cahill
VP Corporate & Public Affairs .... Nancy E Hostetler
VP Labor Market Relations .... Mr Rick Karas

INDIANA

Managed Care Organization Profiles

COMPANY PROFILE:
Parent Company Name:
Doing Business As:
Year Founded: 1985   Federally Qualified: [Y]
Forprofit: [Y]   Not-For-Profit: [ ]
Model Type: GROUP
Accreditation: [ ] AAPPO [ ] JACHO [X] NCQA [ ] URAC
Plan Type: HMO, TPA, POS,
Total Revenue: 2005:   2006: 158,831,939
Net Income   2005:   2006:
Total Enrollment:
    2001: 0   2004: 56,491   2007: 0
    2002: 56,695   2005:
    2003: 58,538   2006:
Medical Loss Ratio: 2005:   2006: 92.10
Administrative Expense Ratio: 2005:   2006:

SERVICE AREA:
Nationwide: N
    IN (Benton, Boone, Carroll, Cass, Clinton, Fountain, Fulton, Howard, Jasper, Miami, Montgomery, Newton, Pulaski, Putnam, Tippecanoe, Tipton, Warren, White);

TYPE OF COVERAGE:
Commercial: [Y] Individual: [ ] FEHBP: [ ] Indemnity: [ ]
Medicare: [Y] Medicaid: [ ] Supplemental Medicare: [ ]
Tricare   [ ]

PRODUCTS OFFERED:
Product Name: Type:
Arnett Gold   Medicare
Arnett   HMO
Arnett HMO   Medicare Advantage

Comments:
Formerly Arnett Managed Health Plans.

ASSURANT EMPLOYEE BENEFITS - INDIANA

1394 Sugarberry Ct
Mooresville, IN 46158-7637
Phone: 317-834-4665 Fax: 317-291-5188 Toll-Free: 800-996-4900
Web site: www.assurantemployeebenefits.com

MAILING ADDRESS:
    ASSURANT EMPLOYEE BNFTS - IN
    1394 Sugarberry Ct
    Mooresville, IN 46158-7637

KEY EXECUTIVES:
Interim Chief Executive Officer/President .... John S Roberts
Chief Financial Officer .... Floyd F Chadee
VP, Medical Director .... Polly M Galbraith, MD
Chief Information Officer .... Karla J Schacht
Senior VP, Marketing .... Jospeh A Sevcik
Privacy Officer .... John L Fortini
VP of Provider Services .... James V Barrett, DMD
Senior VP, Human Resources & Development .... Sylvia R Wagner
National Dental Director ....James V Barrett, DMD

COMPANY PROFILE:
Parent Company Name: Assurant Health
Doing Business As:
Year Founded: 1986   Federally Qualified: [N]
Forprofit: [Y]   Not-For-Profit: [ ]
Model Type: IPA
Accreditation: [ ] AAPPO [ ] JACHO [ ] NCQA [ ] URAC
Plan Type: Specialty HMO

SERVICE AREA:
Nationwide: N
    IN;

TYPE OF COVERAGE:
Commercial: [Y] Individual: [Y] FEHBP: [ ] Indemnity: [ ]
Medicare: [ ] Medicaid: [ ] Supplemental Medicare: [ ]
Tricare   [ ]

PRODUCTS OFFERED:
Product Name: Type:
                           DHMO
                           Vision

PLAN BENEFITS:
Alternative Medicine: [ ]   Behavioral Health: [ ]
Chiropractic: [ ]   Dental: [X]
Home Care: [ ]   Inpatient SNF: [ ]
Long-Term Care: [ ]   Pharm. Mail Order: [ ]
Physical Therapy: [ ]   Podiatry: [ ]
Psychiatric: [ ]   Transplant: [ ]
Vision: [ ]   Wellness: [ ]
Workers' Comp: [ ]
Other Benefits:
Comments:
Formerly Fortis Benefits Dental.

CIGNA HEALTHCARE OF INDIANA

429 N Pennsylvania St Ste 301
Indianapolis, IN 46204
Phone: 317-615-1200 Fax: 317-615-1301 Toll-Free: 800-276-0363
Web site: www.cigna.com

MAILING ADDRESS:
    CIGNA HEALTHCARE OF INDIANA
    429 N Pennsylvania St Ste 301
    Indianapolis, IN 46204

COMPANY PROFILE:
Parent Company Name: CIGNA Corporation
Doing Business As:
Year Founded: 1986   Federally Qualified: [N]
Forprofit: [Y]   Not-For-Profit: [ ]
Model Type:
Accreditation: [ ] AAPPO [ ] JACHO [ ] NCQA [ ] URAC
Plan Type: HMO, PPO, POS, TPA, CDHP, HDHP, HSA,
Primary Physicians: 5,030   Physician Specialists:
Hospitals:
Total Revenue: 2005:   2006: 45,183,276
Net Income   2005:   2006:
Total Enrollment:
    2001: 0   2004: 18,101   2007: 0
    2002: 34,120   2005:
    2003: 29,174   2006:
Medical Loss Ratio: 2005:   2006: 96.00
Administrative Expense Ratio: 2005:   2006:

SERVICE AREA:
Nationwide: N
    IN (Adams, Allen, Bartholonew, Benton, Blackford, Boone, Brown, Carroll, Cass, Clark, Clay, Clinton, Crawford, Davies, Dearborn, Decatur, DeKalb, Delaware, Dubois, Elkhart, Fayette, Floyd, Fountain, Franklin, Fulton, Gibson, Grant, Greene, Hamilton, Hancock, Harrison, Hendricks, Henry, Howard, Huntington, Jackson, Jasper, Jay, Jefferson, Jennings, Johnson, Knox, Kosciusko, LaGrange, Lake, LaPorte, Lawrence, Madison, Marion, Marshall, Martin, Miami, Monroe, Montgomery, Morgan, Newton, Noble, Ohio, Orange, Owen, Parke, Perry, Pike, Porter, Posey, Pulaski, Putnam, Randolph, Ripley, Rush, St Joseph, Scott, Shelby, Spencer, Starke, Steuben, Sullivan, Switzerland, Tippecanoe, Tipton, Union, Vanderburgh, Vermillion, Vigo, Wabash, Warren, Warrick, Washington, Wayne, Wells, White, Whitley);

TYPE OF COVERAGE:
Commercial: [Y] Individual: [Y] FEHBP: [ ] Indemnity: [ ]
Medicare: [ ] Medicaid: [ ] Supplemental Medicare: [ ]
Tricare   [ ]

PRODUCTS OFFERED:
Product Name: Type:
CIGNA Healthcare of IN   HMO
CIGNA Healthcare of IN   POS

CONSUMER-DRIVEN PRODUCTS
JP Morgan Chase   HSA Company
CIGNA Choice Fund   HSA Product
                           HSA Administrator
Open Access Plus   Consumer-Driven Health Plan
PPO   High Deductible Health Plan

PLAN BENEFITS:
Alternative Medicine: [X]   Behavioral Health: [ ]
Chiropractic: [X]   Dental: [X]
Home Care: [X]   Inpatient SNF: [X]
Long-Term Care: [X]   Pharm. Mail Order: [X]
Physical Therapy: [X]   Podiatry: [X]
Psychiatric: [X]   Transplant: [X]
Vision: [X]   Wellness: [X]
Workers' Comp: [ ]
Other Benefits:

Managed Care Organization Profiles — **INDIANA**

ADVANTAGE HEALTH SOLUTIONS INC

9490 Priority Way West Dr
Indianapolis, IN 46240
Phone: 317-573-2700 Fax: 317-580-8009 Toll-Free: 877-903-2237
Web site: www.advantageplan.com

MAILING ADDRESS:
　　ADVANTAGE HEALTH SOLUTIONS INC
　　9490 Priority Way West Dr
　　Indianapolis, IN 46240

KEY EXECUTIVES:
Chairman of the Board .... Vincent Caponi
Chief Executive Officer/President .... Vicki F Perry
Chief Financial Officer .... Jennifer Ponski
Director, Medical Affairs/Medical Management .... Anthony Akosa, MD
Pharmacy Director .... Brian Musial
Chief Operating Officer/Vice President of Compliance .... Jan Teal
Director of Sales .... Lenny Cavender
Quality Assurance Director .... Kay Zimmerman
Dir of Business Development .... Gary Hinkle
Vice President External Reporting .... Jan Teal
Dir of Government Programs .... Amy Brown

COMPANY PROFILE:
Parent Company Name:
Doing Business As:
Year Founded: 2000　　Federally Qualified: [Y]
Forprofit: [Y]　　Not-For-Profit: [ ]
Model Type: MIXED
Accreditation: [ ] AAPPO　[ ] JACHO　[X] NCQA　[ ] URAC
Plan Type: HMO, POS, HDHP, HSA, TPA,
Primary Physicians: 1,272　　Physician Specialists: 3,832
Hospitals: 22
Total Revenue:　2005:　201,764,098　2006:　232,881,202
Net Income　2005:　3,940,125　2006:　473,792
Total Enrollment:
　2001: 50,313　　2004: 65,784　　2007: 0
　2002: 53,297　　2005:
　2003: 62,697　　2006:
Medical Loss Ratio:　2005:　　2006: 92.00
Administrative Expense Ratio:　2005:　　2006:

SERVICE AREA:
Nationwide: N
IN (Adams, Allen, Bartholomew, Benton, Blackford, Boone, Brown, Carroll, Cass, Clark, Clay, Clinton, Crawford, Daviess, Dearborn, Decatur, Dekalb, Delaware, Dubois, Elkhart, Fayette, Floyd, Fountain, Franklin, Fulton, Gibson, Grant, Greene, Hamilton, Hancock, Harrison, Hendricks, Henry, Howard, Huntington, Jackson, Jasper, Jay, Jefferson, Jennings, Johnson, Knox, Kosciusko, Lagrange, Lake, Laporte, Lawrence, Madison, Marshall, Martin, Miami, Monroe, Montgomerty, Morgan, Newton, Noble, Ohio, Orange, Owen, Parke, Perry, Pike, Porter, Posey, Pulaski, Putnam, Randoplh, Ripley, Rush, Saint Joseph, Scott, Shelby, Spencer, Starke, Steuben, Sullivan, Switzerland, Tippecanoe, Tipton, Union, Vanderbaugh, Vermillion, Vigo, Wabash, Warren, Warrick, Washington, Wayne, Wells, White, Whitley);

TYPE OF COVERAGE:
Commercial: [Y]　Individual: [ ]　FEHBP: [ ]　Indemnity: [ ]
Medicare:　[Y]　Medicaid: [ ]　Supplemental Medicare: [ ]
Tricare　[ ]

PRODUCTS OFFERED:
Product Name:　　　　　　　　　Type:
Advantage Health Plan HMO　　　HMO
Advantage Medicare+Choice　　　Medicare
Advantage POS　　　　　　　　　POS

CONSUMER-DRIVEN PRODUCTS
Fifth Third Bank　　　　　　　　HSA Company
Advantage HDHP Option　　　　HSA Product
Canopy Financial　　　　　　　　HSA Administrator
Advantage HDHP Option　　　　Consumer-Driven Health Plan
Advantage HDHP Option　　　　High Deductible Health Plan

PLAN BENEFITS:
Alternative Medicine: [ ]　　Behavioral Health: [X]
Chiropractic: [X]　　　　　　Dental: [X]
Home Care: [X]　　　　　　　Inpatient SNF: [X]
Long-Term Care: [ ]　　　　　Pharm. Mail Order: [X]
Physical Therapy: [X]　　　　Podiatry: [X]
Psychiatric: [X]　　　　　　　Transplant: [X]
Vision: [X]　　　　　　　　　Wellness: [X]
Workers' Comp: [ ]
Other Benefits:

Comments:
Formerly Sagamore Advantege HMO Inc. Also formerly Advantage Health Plans Inc.

ANTHEM BLUE CROSS/BLUE SHIELD OF INDIANA

220 Virginia Ave
Indianapolis, IN 46204
Phone: 317-488-6000 Fax: 317-488-6891 Toll-Free: 800-367-4207
Web site: www.80.anthem.com

MAILING ADDRESS:
　　ANTHEM BLUE CROSS/BLUE SHIELD
　　220 Virginia Ave
　　Indianapolis, IN 46204

KEY EXECUTIVES:
President .... Robert W Hillman
Chief Financial Officer .... Wayne DeVyet
Medical Director - Indiana .... Randy Howard, MD
Chief Operating Officer .... Jane Niederberger
Marketing Director .... Jerry Mallicoat

COMPANY PROFILE:
Parent Company Name: WellPoint Inc
Doing Business As: Key Health Plan, Anthem Hlth Plan of IN
Year Founded: 1991　　Federally Qualified: [ ]
Forprofit: [Y]　　Not-For-Profit: [ ]
Model Type: IPA
Accreditation: [ ] AAPPO　[ ] JACHO　[ ] NCQA　[ ] URAC
Plan Type: HMO, PPO, POS, HDHP, HSA,
Total Revenue:　2005:　　2006:　165,179,608
Net Income　2005:　　2006:

SERVICE AREA:
Nationwide: N
IN;

TYPE OF COVERAGE:
Commercial: [Y]　Individual: [ ]　FEHBP: [ ]　Indemnity: [ ]
Medicare:　[Y]　Medicaid: [ ]　Supplemental Medicare: [ ]
Tricare　[ ]

PRODUCTS OFFERED:
Product Name:　　　　　　　　　Type:
Anthem Sr Advantage (Community　Medicare
Anthem Advantage of IN　　　　　Medicare

CONSUMER-DRIVEN PRODUCTS
JP Morgan Chase　　　　　　　　HSA Company
Anthem ByDesign HSA　　　　　　HSA Product
JP Morgan Chase　　　　　　　　HSA Administrator
Blue Access Saver　　　　　　　　Consumer-Driven Health Plan
Blue Access Economy Plans PPO　High Deductible Health Plan

PLAN BENEFITS:
Alternative Medicine: [ ]　　Behavioral Health: [ ]
Chiropractic: [X]　　　　　　Dental: [ ]
Home Care: [X]　　　　　　　Inpatient SNF: [X]
Long-Term Care: [ ]　　　　　Pharm. Mail Order: [X]
Physical Therapy: [X]　　　　Podiatry: [ ]
Psychiatric: [X]　　　　　　　Transplant: [X]
Vision: [ ]　　　　　　　　　Wellness: [X]
Workers' Comp: [ ]
Other Benefits:

ARNETT HEALTH PLANS

415 N 26th St Ste 101
Lafayette, IN 47903
Phone: 765-448-7400 Fax: 765-448-7700 Toll-Free:
Web site: www.arnettplans.com

MAILING ADDRESS:
　　ARNETT HEALTH PLANS
　　PO Box 6108
　　Lafayette, IN 47903

KEY EXECUTIVES:
Chief Executive Officer .... Robert Paskowski
Chief Financial Officer .... Debra English
Medical Director .... Jeffrey Beardmore, MD
Chief Operating Officer .... Robert Paskowski
Marketing Director .... Marshall Powell
MIS Director .... Suzanne Fisk
Director of Provider Services .... Marcy Hart
Director of Health Services .... Mary Anne Sloan

ILLINOIS

VISION HEALTH MANAGEMENT SYSTEMS

5401 S Wentworth Ave Ste 14C
Chicago, IL 60609
Phone: 773-924-5292 Fax: 773-924-5241 Toll-Free:
Web site: www.planovision.org

MAILING ADDRESS:
VISION HEALTH MANAGEMENT SYSTM
5401 S Wentworth Ave Ste 14C
Chicago, IL 60609

KEY EXECUTIVES:
Chief Executive Officer/President .... Robert L Johnson, OD, MS
Finance Manager .... Mary Taylor
Medical Director .... Joseph W McCray Jr, OD
Office Manager .... Addie Davis

COMPANY PROFILE:
Parent Company Name: Plano Vision
Doing Business As:
Year Founded: 1978   Federally Qualified: [ ]
Forprofit: [Y]   Not-For-Profit: [ ]
Model Type:
Accreditation: [ ] AAPPO [ ] JACHO [ ] NCQA [ ] URAC
Plan Type: Specialty PPO

SERVICE AREA:
Nationwide: N
  IL;

TYPE OF COVERAGE:
Commercial: [ ]   Individual: [Y]   FEHBP: [ ]   Indemnity: [ ]
Medicare: [Y]   Medicaid: [Y]   Supplemental Medicare: [Y]
Tricare   [ ]

PLAN BENEFITS:
Alternative Medicine: [ ]   Behavioral Health: [ ]
Chiropractic: [ ]   Dental: [ ]
Home Care: [ ]   Inpatient SNF: [ ]
Long-Term Care: [ ]   Pharm. Mail Order: [ ]
Physical Therapy: [ ]   Podiatry: [ ]
Psychiatric: [ ]   Transplant: [ ]
Vision: [X]   Wellness: [ ]
Workers' Comp: [ ]
Other Benefits:

ZURICH SERVICES CORPORATION

1400 American Lane
Schaumburg, IL 60196-1056
Phone: 847-605-6000 Fax: 847-706-2608 Toll-Free: 800-382-2150
Web site: www.zurichna.com

MAILING ADDRESS:
ZURICH SERVICES CORPORATION
1400 American Lane
Schaumburg, IL 60196-1056

KEY EXECUTIVES:
Vice President .... Duane Perkins
President .... Frank Patalano
Medical Director .... Avrum Simon, MD
VP Marketing .... Christina Preisig
MIS Director .... Larry Kening
VP Medical Management .... Mark Johnson
Quality Assurance Director .... Cyndy Howry
Fraud Prevention Director .... Brian Wilson
VP Product & Business Development .... Christina Preisig
VP of Managed Care .... Duane Perkins

COMPANY PROFILE:
Parent Company Name: Zurich Holding Co of America
Doing Business As: Zurich Services Corp
Year Founded: Federally Qualified: [ ]
Forprofit: [ ]   Not-For-Profit: [ ]
Model Type:
Accreditation: [ ] AAPPO [ ] JACHO [ ] NCQA [ ] URAC
Plan Type: TPA, UR

SERVICE AREA:
Nationwide: Y
  NW,

TYPE OF COVERAGE:
Commercial: [Y]   Individual: [ ]   FEHBP: [ ]   Indemnity: [ ]
Medicare: [ ]   Medicaid: [ ]   Supplemental Medicare: [ ]
Tricare   [ ]

PLAN BENEFITS:
Alternative Medicine: [ ]   Behavioral Health: [ ]
Chiropractic: [ ]   Dental: [ ]
Home Care: [ ]   Inpatient SNF: [ ]
Long-Term Care: [ ]   Pharm. Mail Order: [ ]
Physical Therapy: [ ]   Podiatry: [ ]
Psychiatric: [ ]   Transplant: [ ]
Vision: [ ]   Wellness: [ ]
Workers' Comp: [X]
Other Benefits:

Managed Care Organization Profiles — ILLINOIS

Model Type: IPA
Accreditation: [ ] AAPPO [ ] JACHO [X] NCQA [ ] URAC
Plan Type: HMO, PPO, POS, CDHP, HDHP, HSA
Total Enrollment:
  2001: 38,345   2004: 0   2007: 0
  2002: 0   2005:
  2003: 0   2006:

SERVICE AREA:
Nationwide: N
  IL;

TYPE OF COVERAGE:
Commercial: [Y] Individual: [ ] FEHBP: [ ] Indemnity: [ ]
Medicare: [Y]   Medicaid: [Y]   Supplemental Medicare: [ ]
Tricare [ ]

PRODUCTS OFFERED:
Product Name:	Type:
Senior Care Basic	Medicare Advantage

CONSUMER-DRIVEN PRODUCTS
Wells Fargo	HSA Company
Heritage Options HSA	HSA Product
Wells Fargo	HSA Administrator
	Consumer-Driven Health Plan
	High Deductible Health Plan

PLAN BENEFITS:
Alternative Medicine:	[ ]	Behavioral Health:	[X]
Chiropractic:	[X]	Dental:	[X]
Home Care:	[ ]	Inpatient SNF:	[X]
Long-Term Care:	[ ]	Pharm. Mail Order:	[X]
Physical Therapy:	[X]	Podiatry:	[X]
Psychiatric:	[X]	Transplant:	[X]
Vision:	[X]	Wellness:	[X]
Workers' Comp:	[X]		

Other Benefits:

Comments:
Formerly John Deere Health Plan, acquired by UnitedHealth on February 24, 2006.

UNITEDHEALTHCARE SERVICES COMPANY OF THE RIVER VALLEY INC

1300 River Dr Ste 200
Moline, IL 61265
Phone: 309-765-1200 Fax: 309-609-3165 Toll-Free: 800-747-1446
Web site: www.uhcrivervalley.com

MAILING ADDRESS:
UHC OF THE RIVER VALLEY INC
1300 River Dr Ste 200
Moline, IL 61265

KEY EXECUTIVES:
Non-Executive Chairman .... Richard T Burke
Chief Executive Officer .... Robert J Sheehy

COMPANY PROFILE:
Parent Company Name: UnitedHealth Group
Doing Business As: UHC Health Plan of River Valley, UHC Ins Co of RV
Year Founded: 1985   Federally Qualified: [N]
Forprofit: [Y]   Not-For-Profit: [ ]
Model Type: IPA
Accreditation: [ ] AAPPO [ ] JACHO [X] NCQA [ ] URAC
Plan Type: HMO, PPO, POS, CDHP, HDHP, HSA
Total Revenue: 2005: 664,290,228   2006:
Net Income: 2005: 22,430,613   2006:
Total Enrollment:
  2001: 251,834   2004: 239,213   2007: 0
  2002: 206,584   2005: 220,903
  2003: 225,405   2006: 178,582

SERVICE AREA:
Nationwide: N
  IA; IL; TN; VA;

TYPE OF COVERAGE:
Commercial: [Y] Individual: [ ] FEHBP: [ ] Indemnity: [ ]
Medicare: [Y]   Medicaid: [Y]   Supplemental Medicare: [ ]
Tricare [ ]

PRODUCTS OFFERED:
Product Name:	Type:
Senior Care Basic	Medicare Advantage

CONSUMER-DRIVEN PRODUCTS
Wells Fargo	HSA Company
Heritage Options HSA	HSA Product
Wells Fargo	HSA Administrator
	Consumer-Driven Health Plan
	High Deductible Health Plan

PLAN BENEFITS:
Alternative Medicine:	[ ]	Behavioral Health:	[X]
Chiropractic:	[X]	Dental:	[X]
Home Care:	[ ]	Inpatient SNF:	[X]
Long-Term Care:	[ ]	Pharm. Mail Order:	[X]
Physical Therapy:	[X]	Podiatry:	[X]
Psychiatric:	[X]	Transplant:	[X]
Vision:	[X]	Wellness:	[X]
Workers' Comp:	[X]		

Other Benefits:

Comments:
Formerly John Deere Health Plan, acquired by UnitedHealth on February 24, 2006.

UNITEDHEALTHCARE OF ILLINOIS INC

233 N Michigan Ave
Chicago, IL 60601
Phone: 312-424-4460 Fax: 312-424-4448 Toll-Free:
Web site: www.uhc.com

MAILING ADDRESS:
UNITEDHEALTHCARE OF ILLINOIS
233 N Michigan Ave
Chicago, IL 60601

KEY EXECUTIVES:
Non-Executive Chairman .... Richard T Burke
Chief Executive Officer/President .... Thomas P Wiffler
Chief Financial Officer .... Mark Napier
Medical Director .... David O Wiechers, MD, MS, MBA

COMPANY PROFILE:
Parent Company Name: UnitedHealth Group
Doing Business As:
Year Founded: 1976   Federally Qualified: [Y]
Forprofit: [Y]   Not-For-Profit: [ ]
Model Type: NETWORK
Accreditation: [ ] AAPPO [ ] JACHO [ ] NCQA [ ] URAC
Plan Type: HMO, PPO, POS, CDHP, HSA, HRA
Total Revenue: 2005:   2006: 101,063,030
Net Income: 2005:   2006:
Total Enrollment:
  2001: 137,233   2004: 68,787   2007: 0
  2002: 69,445   2005: 38,764
  2003: 874,935   2006: 26,537
Medical Loss Ratio: 2005:   2006: 81.60
Administrative Expense Ratio: 2005:   2006:

SERVICE AREA:
Nationwide: N
  IL(Lake, Laporte, Porter);

TYPE OF COVERAGE:
Commercial: [Y] Individual: [Y] FEHBP: [ ] Indemnity: [ ]
Medicare: [Y]   Medicaid: [Y]   Supplemental Medicare: [ ]
Tricare [ ]

PRODUCTS OFFERED:
Product Name:	Type:
United Healthcare Select HMO	HMO
United Healthcare HMO	HMO
United Healthcare Premier HMO	HMO
United Hlthcare Medicare Compl	Medicare
United Healthcare Options	PPO
United Healthcare Plus	POS
United Healthcare Open Access	

CONSUMER-DRIVEN PRODUCTS
Exante Bank/Golden Rule Ins Co	HSA Company
iPlan HSA	HSA Product
	HSA Administrator
	Consumer-Driven Health Plan
	High Deductible Health Plan

PLAN BENEFITS:
Alternative Medicine:	[ ]	Behavioral Health:	[X]
Chiropractic:	[X]	Dental:	[X]
Home Care:	[X]	Inpatient SNF:	[X]
Long-Term Care:	[X]	Pharm. Mail Order:	[X]
Physical Therapy:	[X]	Podiatry:	[X]
Psychiatric:	[X]	Transplant:	[X]
Vision:	[X]	Wellness:	[X]
Workers' Comp:	[X]		

Other Benefits:

ILLINOIS   **Managed Care Organization Profiles**

SERVICE AREA:
Nationwide: N
   IL (Cook, DuPage, Kankakee, Kane, Kendall, Lake, McHenry, Will); IN (Lake, LaPorte, Porter);
TYPE OF COVERAGE:
Commercial: [Y]   Individual: [ ]   FEHBP: [ ]   Indemnity: [ ]
Medicare: [Y]   Medicaid: [ ]   Supplemental Medicare: [ ]
Tricare   [ ]
PRODUCTS OFFERED:

Product Name:	Type:
Rush Prudential HMO	HMO
Rush Prudential POS	POS
Rush Prudential Open Network	PPO
First Choice	Medicare

CONSUMER-DRIVEN PRODUCTS

JP Morgan Chase	HSA Company
Complete Choice HealthFund	HSA Product
Arcus Enterprises Inc	HSA Administrator
	Consumer-Driven Health Plan
UniCare PPO HRA	High Deductible Health Plan

PLAN BENEFITS:
Alternative Medicine: [X]   Behavioral Health: [ ]
Chiropractic: [X]   Dental: [ ]
Home Care: [X]   Inpatient SNF: [X]
Long-Term Care: [ ]   Pharm. Mail Order: [X]
Physical Therapy: [X]   Podiatry: [X]
Psychiatric: [X]   Transplant: [X]
Vision: [X]   Wellness: [X]
Workers' Comp: [ ]
Other Benefits:

UNION HEALTH SERVICE INC

1634 W Polk St
Chicago, IL 60612
Phone: 312-829-4224 Fax: 312-423-4326 Toll-Free:
Web site: www.unionhealth.org
MAILING ADDRESS:
   UNION HEALTH SERVICE INC
   1634 W Polk St
   Chicago, IL 60612

KEY EXECUTIVES:
Administrator .... W Joe Garrett
President .... Leon Wolin
Medical Director .... Angelo P Creticos, MD
Director of Information Systems .... Elizabeth Garnes
Director of Operations .... Ramesh Joshi
Director of Medical Management .... Joyce Valentine
Director of Health Services .... Nancy Swenson
Director of Member Services .... Derrick Branch
Dental Director .... Norman Dabiri, DDS

COMPANY PROFILE:
Parent Company Name:
Doing Business As:
Year Founded: 1955   Federally Qualified: [N]
Forprofit: [ ]   Not-For-Profit: [Y]
Model Type: STAFF
Accreditation: [ ] AAPPO [ ] JACHO [ ] NCQA [ ] URAC
Plan Type: HMO
Total Revenue: 2005:   2006: 36,963,775
Net Income 2005:   2006:
Total Enrollment:
   2001: 25,356   2004: 34,928   2007: 0
   2002: 30,109   2005: 35,625
   2003: 35,521   2006: 37,925
Medical Loss Ratio: 2005:   2006: 85.50
Administrative Expense Ratio: 2005:   2006:
SERVICE AREA:
Nationwide: N
   IL (Cook, DuPage);
TYPE OF COVERAGE:
Commercial: [Y]   Individual: [ ]   FEHBP: [ ]   Indemnity: [ ]
Medicare: [Y]   Medicaid: [ ]   Supplemental Medicare: [ ]
Tricare   [ ]
PRODUCTS OFFERED:

Product Name:	Type:
HMO	HMO
Voluntary Health Service Plan	Physician Only
Medicare Cost Plan	

PLAN BENEFITS:
Alternative Medicine: [ ]   Behavioral Health: [ ]
Chiropractic: [ ]   Dental: [X]
Home Care: [ ]   Inpatient SNF: [ ]
Long-Term Care: [ ]   Pharm. Mail Order: [ ]
Physical Therapy: [ ]   Podiatry: [ ]
Psychiatric: [ ]   Transplant: [ ]
Vision: [X]   Wellness: [ ]
Workers' Comp: [ ]
Other Benefits:

UNITED CONCORDIA COMPANY INC - ILLINOIS

10 S Riverside Plz Ste 1800
Chicago, IL 60606
Phone: 312-474-7852 Fax: 312-474-7851 Toll-Free: 800-332-0366
Web site: www.ucci.com
MAILING ADDRESS:
   UNITED CONCORDIA CO INC - IL
   10 S Riverside Plz Ste 1800
   Chicago, IL 60606

KEY EXECUTIVES:
Chief Executive Officer .... Thomas A Dzuryachko
Senior VP, Finance .... Daniel Wright
Corporate Dental Director .... Claude Padgett, DDS

COMPANY PROFILE:
Parent Company Name: Highmark Inc
Doing Business As:
Year Founded: 1991   Federally Qualified: [ ]
Forprofit: [Y]   Not-For-Profit: [ ]
Model Type:
Accreditation: [ ] AAPPO [ ] JACHO [ ] NCQA [ ] URAC
Plan Type: Specialty HMO, Specialty PPO, TPA
SERVICE AREA:
Nationwide: N
   IL; MN; WI;
TYPE OF COVERAGE:
Commercial: [Y]   Individual: [ ]   FEHBP: [ ]   Indemnity: [ ]
Medicare: [ ]   Medicaid: [ ]   Supplemental Medicare: [ ]
Tricare   [ ]
PLAN BENEFITS:
Alternative Medicine: [ ]   Behavioral Health: [ ]
Chiropractic: [ ]   Dental: [X]
Home Care: [ ]   Inpatient SNF: [ ]
Long-Term Care: [ ]   Pharm. Mail Order: [ ]
Physical Therapy: [ ]   Podiatry: [ ]
Psychiatric: [ ]   Transplant: [ ]
Vision: [ ]   Wellness: [ ]
Workers' Comp: [ ]
Other Benefits:
Comments:
For enrollment and revenue information see corporate listing, Camp Hill, Pennsylvania.

UNITEDHEALTHCARE SERVICES COMPANY OF THE RIVER VALLEY INC

7210 N Villa Lake Drive Ste A
Peoria, IL 61614
Phone: 309-692-2160 Fax: 309-692-3165 Toll-Free: 800-747-1446
Web site: www.uhcrivervalley.com
MAILING ADDRESS:
   UHC OF THE RIVER VALLEY INC
   1300 River Dr Ste 200
   Moline, IL 61614

KEY EXECUTIVES:
Non-Executive Chairman .... Richard T Burke
Chief Executive Officer .... Robert J Sheehy

COMPANY PROFILE:
Parent Company Name: UnitedHealth Group
Doing Business As: UHC Health Plan of River Valley, UHC Ins Co of RV
Year Founded: 1985   Federally Qualified: [N]
Forprofit: [Y]   Not-For-Profit: [ ]

Managed Care Organization Profiles — ILLINOIS

PRIVATE HEALTHCARE SYSTEMS - ILLINOIS

9701 W Higgins Rd Ste 700
Rosemont, IL 60018
Phone: 847-292-6700 Fax: 847-292-6736 Toll-Free: 800-253-4417
Web site: www.phcs.com
MAILING ADDRESS:
   PRIVATE HEALTHCARE SYSTEMS-IL
   1100 Winter St
   Waltham, MA 60018

KEY EXECUTIVES:
Chief Executive Officer/President .... Mark Tabak

COMPANY PROFILE:
Parent Company Name: MultiPlan Inc
Doing Business As:
Year Founded: 1986   Federally Qualified: [N]
Forprofit: [Y]   Not-For-Profit: [ ]
Model Type:
Accreditation: [ ] AAPPO [ ] JACHO [ ] NCQA [X] URAC
Plan Type: PPO, UR, POS

SERVICE AREA:
Nationwide: N
   IL;

TYPE OF COVERAGE:
Commercial: [Y] Individual: [ ] FEHBP: [ ] Indemnity:[ ] Medicare: [ ] Medicaid: [ ] Supplemental Medicare: [ ]
Tricare [ ]

PLAN BENEFITS:
Alternative Medicine:	[X]	Behavioral Health:	[X]
Chiropractic:	[X]	Dental:	[ ]
Home Care:	[X]	Inpatient SNF:	[X]
Long-Term Care:	[X]	Pharm. Mail Order:	[X]
Physical Therapy:	[X]	Podiatry:	[X]
Psychiatric:	[X]	Transplant:	[X]
Vision:	[X]	Wellness:	[ ]
Workers' Comp:	[X]		

Other Benefits:
Comments:
Acquired by MultiPlan, Inc. on October 18, 2006.

QUINCY HEALTH CARE MANAGEMENT INC

1246 Broadway
Quincy, IL 62301
Phone: 217-222-9157 Fax: 217-222-1732 Toll-Free: 800-637-7100
Web site: www.riverquestnetwork.com
MAILING ADDRESS:
   QUINCY HEALTH CARE MNGMNT INC
   PO Box 5126
   Quincy, IL 62301

KEY EXECUTIVES:
Executive Director .... Suzanne Ellerbrock

COMPANY PROFILE:
Parent Company Name:
Doing Business As: River Quest Network
Year Founded: 1992   Federally Qualified: [N]
Forprofit: [Y]   Not-For-Profit: [ ]
Model Type: NETWORK
Accreditation: [X] AAPPO [ ] JACHO [ ] NCQA [ ] URAC
Plan Type: PPO, POS,
Primary Physicians: 1,636   Physician Specialists:
Hospitals: 54
Total Enrollment:
   2001: 35,000   2004: 0   2007: 0
   2002: 0   2005:
   2003: 0   2006: 23,000

SERVICE AREA:
Nationwide: N
   IA; IL; MO;

TYPE OF COVERAGE:
Commercial: [Y] Individual: [ ] FEHBP: [ ] Indemnity: [ ]
Medicare: [ ] Medicaid: [ ] Supplemental Medicare: [ ]
Tricare [ ]

PRODUCTS OFFERED:
Product Name: Type:
PPO   PPO

TRUSTMARK INSURANCE COMPANY

400 Field Dr
Lake Forest, IL 60045
Phone: 847-615-1500 Fax: 847-615-3907 Toll-Free: 800-621-4784
Web site: www.trustmarkins.com
MAILING ADDRESS:
   TRUSTMARK INSURANCE CO
   400 Field Dr
   Lake Forest, IL 60045

KEY EXECUTIVES:
Chairman .... J Grover Thomas Jr
Chief Executive Officer/President .... Dave McDonough
Chief Financial Officer .... Brinke Marcuccilli
Medical Director .... Deborah Smart, MD
MIS Director .... Steven Penney
Privacy Officer .... Catherine Bresler
Human Resources Director .... Robert Worobow
Fraud Prevention Director .... Kelli Garvanian
Sales Executive .... Tim Hakanson
Sales Executive .... Dale Kumpula
Sales Executive .... Nancy Strangle
Sales Executive .... Mark Vana

COMPANY PROFILE:
Parent Company Name:
Doing Business As:
Year Founded: 1913   Federally Qualified: [N]
Forprofit: [Y]   Not-For-Profit: [ ]
Model Type: MIXED
Accreditation: [ ] AAPPO [ ] JACHO [ ] NCQA [ ] URAC
Plan Type: PPO, CDHP, HDHP, HSA,

SERVICE AREA:
Nationwide: Y
   NW;

TYPE OF COVERAGE:
Commercial: [ ] Individual: [ ] FEHBP: [ ] Indemnity: [Y]
Medicare: [ ] Medicaid: [ ] Supplemental Medicare: [ ]
Tricare [ ]

UNICARE HEALTH PLANS OF THE MIDWEST INC

233 S Wacker Dr Ste 3900
Chicago, IL 60606
Phone: 312-234-7000 Fax: 312-234-8001 Toll-Free: 877-864-2273
Web site: www.unicare.com
MAILING ADDRESS:
   UNICARE HEALTH PLANS OF THE MIDWEST INC
   233 S Wacker Dr Ste 3900
   Chicago, IL 60606

KEY EXECUTIVES:
Chief Executive Officer .... Sandra Van Trease
Chief Financial Officer .... Tim Schryver
Medical Director .... Alan Rosenberg
Vice President of Sales/Marketing .... Denny Lavia
Vice President of Sales/Marketing .... Lee B Green
Provider Services Director .... Christine Stoll
Network/Contracts Officer .... Lenore Holt-Darcy
Human Resources Director .... Mike Gyton

COMPANY PROFILE:
Parent Company Name: WellPoint Inc
Doing Business As:
Year Founded: 1993   Federally Qualified: [N]
Forprofit: [Y]   Not-For-Profit: [ ]
Model Type: MIXED
Accreditation: [ ] AAPPO [ ] JACHO [X] NCQA [ ] URAC
Plan Type: HMO, PPO, POS, CDHP, HDHP, HSA
Total Revenue: 2005:   2006: 377,786,628
Net Income: 2005:   2006:
Total Enrollment:
   2001: 173,099   2004: 152,739   2007: 0
   2002: 163,430   2005: 132,420
   2003: 155,015   2006: 125,779
Medical Loss Ratio: 2005:   2006: 87.40
Administrative Expense Ratio: 2005:   2006:

ILLINOIS **Managed Care Organization Profiles**

MAILING ADDRESS:
    PERSONALCARE INS OF IL INC
    2110 Fox Dr
    Champaign, IL 61820

KEY EXECUTIVES:
Chief Executive Officer/President .... Todd Petersen
Chief Financial Officer .... Jamey Maxwell
Corporate Medical Director .... Richard G Grassy, MD
VP Marketing & Sales Director .... Darcy Sementi
Corporate Communications Manager .... Tom Drabelle
Provider Relations Manager .... Sallie Miller
Human Resources Director .... Cindy Guthrie
Quality Improvement Director .... Dawn Smith

COMPANY PROFILE:
Parent Company Name: Coventry Health Care Inc
Doing Business As:
Year Founded: 1984   Federally Qualified: [Y]
Forprofit: [Y]   Not-For-Profit: [ ]
Model Type: NETWORK
Accreditation: [ ] AAPPO [ ] JACHO [X] NCQA [ ] URAC
Plan Type: HMO, PPO, POS, CDHP, HDHP, HSA
Total Revenue: 2005:   2006: 277,267,797
Net Income 2005:   2006:
Total Enrollment:
    2001: 72,524   2004: 85,884   2007: 0
    2002: 68,353   2005: 56,580
    2003: 61,140   2006: 54,523
Medical Loss Ratio: 2005:   2006: 80.80
Administrative Expense Ratio: 2005:   2006:
SERVICE AREA:
Nationwide: N
    IL (Central & Eastern);
TYPE OF COVERAGE:
Commercial: [Y] Individual: [Y] FEHBP: [ ] Indemnity: [ ]
Medicare: [ ] Medicaid: [ ] Supplemental Medicare: [Y]
Tricare [ ]
PRODUCTS OFFERED:
Product Name: Type:
PersonalCare HMO   HMO
CONSUMER-DRIVEN PRODUCTS
Wells Fargo   HSA Company
    HSA Product
Corporate Benefits Services of America HSA Administrator
    Consumer-Driven Health Plan
Open Access Plus Plan   High Deductible Health Plan
PLAN BENEFITS:
Alternative Medicine: [ ]   Behavioral Health: [ ]
Chiropractic: [X]   Dental: [ ]
Home Care: [X]   Inpatient SNF: [X]
Long-Term Care: [ ]   Pharm. Mail Order: [ ]
Physical Therapy: [X]   Podiatry: [X]
Psychiatric: [X]   Transplant: [X]
Vision: [X]   Wellness: [X]
Workers' Comp: [ ]
Other Benefits:
Comments:
Acquired by Coventry Health Care Inc, February 1, 2003.

PRAIRIE STATES ENTERPRISES INC

101 W Grand Ave Ste 404
Chicago, IL 60610
Phone: 312-464-1888 Fax: 312-464-0097 Toll-Free:
Web site: www.prairieontheweb.com
MAILING ADDRESS:
    PRAIRIE STATES ENTERPRISES INC
    101 W Grand Ave Ste 404
    Chicago, IL 60610

KEY EXECUTIVES:
Chief Executive Officer .... Felicia Wilhelm, RN
Chief Financial Officer .... Jay Borden
Medical Director .... Lorie Rath

COMPANY PROFILE:
Parent Company Name:
Doing Business As:
Year Founded: Federally Qualified: [ ]
Forprofit: [Y]   Not-For-Profit: [ ]
Model Type:
Accreditation: [ ] AAPPO [ ] JACHO [ ] NCQA [X] URAC
Plan Type: TPA
SERVICE AREA:
Nationwide: N
    IL;
PLAN BENEFITS:
Alternative Medicine: [ ]   Behavioral Health: [ ]
Chiropractic: [X]   Dental: [X]
Home Care: [X]   Inpatient SNF: [X]
Long-Term Care: [ ]   Pharm. Mail Order: [ ]
Physical Therapy: [X]   Podiatry: [ ]
Psychiatric: [X]   Transplant: [X]
Vision: [X]   Wellness: [X]
Workers' Comp: [ ]
Other Benefits:
Comments:
Self-funded.

PREFERRED PODIATRY GROUP

425 Huehl Rd
Northbrook, IL 60062
Phone: 847-504-5000 Fax: 847-504-5015 Toll-Free: 800-654-3772
Web site: www.preferredpodiatry.com
MAILING ADDRESS:
    PREFERRED PODIATRY GROUP
    425 Huehl Rd, Unit 13
    Northbrook, IL 60062

KEY EXECUTIVES:
President .... Sanford Mason, DPM
Chief Financial Officer .... Melanie Michaels
Co-Medical Director - Illinois .... Randy Pachnik, DPM
Medical Director - Indiana .... Todd Mann, DPM
Director of Operations .... Tony Torres
Marketing Director .... Jay Kracik
MIS Director .... Marvin Bero
Credentialing Manager/Privacy Officer .... Tony Torres
Human Resources Director/Compliance Officer .... Tony Torres
General Counsel .... Melanie Michaels

COMPANY PROFILE:
Parent Company Name: Preferred Podiatry Group PC
Doing Business As: PPG
Year Founded: 1972   Federally Qualified: [N]
Forprofit: [Y]   Not-For-Profit: [ ]
Model Type: STAFF
Accreditation: [ ] AAPPO [ ] JACHO [ ] NCQA [ ] URAC
Plan Type: Specialty PPO, HDHP, HSA
Hospitals: 2
Total Enrollment:
    2001: 0   2004: 0   2007: 83,800
    2002: 73,000   2005:
    2003: 75,000   2006:
SERVICE AREA:
Nationwide: N
    IL; IN; MO; WI;
TYPE OF COVERAGE:
Commercial: [Y] Individual: [Y] FEHBP: [ ] Indemnity: [ ]
Medicare: [Y] Medicaid: [Y] Supplemental Medicare: [Y]
Tricare [ ]
PRODUCTS OFFERED:
Product Name: Type:
Preferred Podiatry Group   Specialty PPO
CONSUMER-DRIVEN PRODUCTS
BCBS of Illinois   HSA Company
BC BS of IL   HSA Product
New Central Bank   HSA Administrator
    Consumer-Driven Health Plan
BC BS of IL   High Deductible Health Plan
PLAN BENEFITS:
Alternative Medicine: [ ]   Behavioral Health: [ ]
Chiropractic: [ ]   Dental: [ ]
Home Care: [ ]   Inpatient SNF: [ ]
Long-Term Care: [X]   Pharm. Mail Order: [ ]
Physical Therapy: [ ]   Podiatry: [X]
Psychiatric: [ ]   Transplant: [ ]
Vision: [ ]   Wellness: [ ]
Workers' Comp: [ ]
Other Benefits: Audiology

Managed Care Organization Profiles — ILLINOIS

SERVICE AREA:
Nationwide: N
IL (Bond, Boone, Brown, Bureau, Calhoun, Carroll, Cass, Champaign, Christian, Clark, Clay, Clinton, Coles, Cook, Crawford, Cumberland, DeKalb, DeWitt, Douglas, DuPage, Edwards, Edgar, Effingham, Fayette, Ford, Franklin, Fulton, Gallatin, Greene, Grundy, Hamilton, Hardin, Henry, Heyworth, Iroquois, Jackson, Jasper, Jefferson, Jersey, Jo Daviess, Johnson, Kane, Kankakee, Kendall, Lake, LaSalle, Lawrence, Lee, Livingston, Logan, Macon, Macoupin, Madison, Marion, Mason, McDonough, McHenry, McLean, Menard, Monroe, Montgomery, Morgan, Moultrie, Ogle, Peoria, Perry, Pike, Pope, Pulaski, Randolph, Richard, Saline, Sangamon, Schuyler, Scott, Shelby, St Clair, Stephenson, Tazewell, Union, Vermilion, Wabash, Washington, Wayne, Whiteside, Will, Williamson, Winnebago); IN (Benton, Daviess, Fountain, Gibson, Greene, Hammond, Jasper, Knox, Lake, LaPorte, Montgomery, Newton, Parke, Pike, Porter, Posey, Starke, Sullivan, Tippecanoe, Vermilion, Warren); KY (Livingston, Union); MO (Bollinger, Cape Girardeau, Franklin, Jefferson, Perry, St Charles, St Francois, St Louis, St Louis City, St Genevieve); WI (Kenosha, LaFayette, Milwaukee, Racine, Rock, Walworth, Waukesha);

TYPE OF COVERAGE:
Commercial: [Y] Individual: [ ] FEHBP: [ ] Indemnity: [ ]
Medicare: [ ] Medicaid: [ ] Supplemental Medicare: [Y]
Tricare

PLAN BENEFITS:
Alternative Medicine: [ ]   Behavioral Health: [ ]
Chiropractic: [X]   Dental: [ ]
Home Care: [ ]   Inpatient SNF: [X]
Long-Term Care: [ ]   Pharm. Mail Order: [X]
Physical Therapy: [X]   Podiatry: [X]
Psychiatric: [X]   Transplant: [X]
Vision: [X]   Wellness: [X]
Workers' Comp: [ ]
Other Benefits:

HUMANA HEALTH CARE PLANS OF ILLINOIS

550 West Adams 7th FL
Chicago, IL 60661
Phone: 312-627-8500 Fax: 312-441-5086 Toll-Free: 800-230-6825
Web site: www.humana.com/illinois/home.html
MAILING ADDRESS:
HUMANA HEALTHCARE PLANS - IL
550 West Adams 7th FL
Chicago, IL 60661

KEY EXECUTIVES:
Chairman of the Board .... David A Jones Jr
Chief Executive Officer .... Hassan Rifaat, MD
Market President - Illinois .... Mike Kasper
Chief Financial Officer .... Sanjoy Musunuri
Senior VP & Chief Clinical Strategy .... David Steele, MD
VP, Sales .... Dave Reynolds
VP, Network Development .... Paul Maxwell
Medical Director, Chicago .... Edward Leary, MD
Quality Management/Utilization Director .... Laura Hatfield, RN

COMPANY PROFILE:
Parent Company Name: Humana Inc
Doing Business As:
Year Founded: 1972   Federally Qualified: [Y]
Forprofit: [Y]   Not-For-Profit: [ ]
Model Type: MIXED
Accreditation: [ ] AAPPO [ ] JACHO [X] NCQA [ ] URAC
Plan Type: HMO, PPO, POS, ASO, CDHP, HSA
Total Enrollment:
  2001: 720,092   2004: 37,393   2007: 0
  2002: 377,376   2005: 406,256
  2003: 314,741   2006: 332,179

SERVICE AREA:
Nationwide: N
IL; (Cook, DuPage, Kane, Kankakee, Kendall, Lake, McHenry, Will),

TYPE OF COVERAGE:
Commercial: [Y] Individual: [ ] FEHBP: [ ] Indemnity: [ ]
Medicare: [Y] Medicaid: [Y] Supplemental Medicare: [Y]
Tricare [Y]

PRODUCTS OFFERED:
Product Name:	Type:
Humana Gold Plus Plan	Medicare Advantage
Humana Medicaid	Medicaid

CONSUMER-DRIVEN PRODUCTS
JP Morgan Chase	HSA Company
HumanaOne HSA	HSA Product
JP Morgan Chase	HSA Administrator
Personal Care Account	Consumer-Driven Health Plan
HumanaOne	High Deductible Health Plan

PLAN BENEFITS:
Alternative Medicine: [ ]   Behavioral Health: [X]
Chiropractic: [X]   Dental: [X]
Home Care: [ ]   Inpatient SNF: [ ]
Long-Term Care: [ ]   Pharm. Mail Order: [X]
Physical Therapy: [ ]   Podiatry: [ ]
Psychiatric: [X]   Transplant: [X]
Vision: [ ]   Wellness: [ ]
Workers' Comp: [X]
Other Benefits: Long Term Disability

OSF HEALTH PLANS

7915 N Hale Ave Ste D
Peoria, IL 61615-2047
Phone: 309-677-8200 Fax: 309-677-8338 Toll-Free: 800-673-4699
Web site: www.osfhealthplans.com
MAILING ADDRESS:
OSF HEALTH PLANS
7915 N Hale Ave Ste D
Peoria, IL 61615-2047

KEY EXECUTIVES:
Chairperson .... Sister Judith Ann Duvall, OSF
Chief Executive Officer .... Robert C Sehring
President .... Kevin D Schoeplein
Chief Financial Officer .... Jeff Dillon
Medical Director .... Ralph Velazquez, MD
VP Operations .... John Evancho
VP of Marketing/Communications .... Melody Berry
MIS Director .... Joe McIntire
Marketing Communications Manager .... Jeff Koch
Associate Medical Director .... William Marshall, MD
Human Resources Director .... Nancy Wright
Quality Management Director .... Nalini Ambrose
Compliance Manager .... Mary Anne Nieukirk

COMPANY PROFILE:
Parent Company Name: OSF Healthcare System
Doing Business As:
Year Founded: 1994   Federally Qualified: [N]
Forprofit: [Y]   Not-For-Profit: [ ]
Model Type: IPA
Accreditation: [ ] AAPPO [ ] JACHO [Y] NCQA [ ] URAC
Plan Type: HMO, PPO, POS, ASO, TPA, CDHP, HDHP, HSA
Hospitals: 28
Total Revenue: 2005:   2006: 3,273,084
Net Income   2005:   2006:
Total Enrollment:
  2001: 60,609   2004: 80,000   2007: 0
  2002: 66,700   2005: 66,959
  2003: 61,874   2006: 90,576

SERVICE AREA:
Nationwide: N
IL (Central and Northwest);

TYPE OF COVERAGE:
Commercial: [Y] Individual: [ ] FEHBP: [ ] Indemnity: [ ]
Medicare: [Y] Medicaid: [ ] Supplemental Medicare: [ ]
Tricare [ ]

PRODUCTS OFFERED:
Product Name:	Type:
OSF Healthplans HMO	HMO
OSF Healthplans POS	POS
OSF Care Advantage	Medicare Advantage

PERSONALCARE INSURANCE OF ILLINOIS INC

2110 Fox Dr
Champaign, IL 61820
Phone: 217-366-1226 Fax: 217-366-5410 Toll-Free: 888-366-6730
Web site: www.personalcare.org

ILLINOIS

Managed Care Organization Profiles

PLAN BENEFITS:
Alternative Medicine:	[ ]	Behavioral Health:	[ ]
Chiropractic:	[ ]	Dental:	[ ]
Home Care:	[X]	Inpatient SNF:	[X]
Long-Term Care:	[X]	Pharm. Mail Order:	[X]
Physical Therapy:	[X]	Podiatry:	[X]
Psychiatric:	[ ]	Transplant:	[ ]
Vision:	[ ]	Wellness:	[ ]
Workers' Comp:	[ ]		

Other Benefits:
Comments:
Purchased Blue Cross Blue Shield of Texas December 31, 1998.

HEALTH PLUS

5409 N Knoxville Ave
Peoria, IL 61614
Phone: 309-689-8600 Fax: 309-689-8601 Toll-Free:
Web site: www.healthpluspeoria.org
MAILING ADDRESS:
HEALTH PLUS
5409 N Knoxville Ave
Peoria, IL 61614

KEY EXECUTIVES:
Adminstrative Director .... Linda Beckman
Chief Financial Officer .... Dave Underwood
Medical Director .... Jack Domintz, MD
Marketing Director .... Mike Grover
Provider Relations Manager .... Cindy Bumeter

COMPANY PROFILE:
Parent Company Name:
Doing Business As:
Year Founded: 1991   Federally Qualified: [ ]
Forprofit: [Y]   Not-For-Profit: [ ]
Model Type: MIXED
Accreditation: [ ] AAPPO [ ] JACHO [ ] NCQA [ ] URAC
Plan Type: PPO, POS, TPA
SERVICE AREA:
Nationwide: N
IL;
TYPE OF COVERAGE:
Commercial: [Y] Individual: [ ] FEHBP: [ ] Indemnity: [ ]
Medicare: [ ] Medicaid: [ ] Supplemental Medicare: [Y]
Tricare [ ]
PRODUCTS OFFERED:
Product Name:	Type:
Health Plus PPO	PPO

PLAN BENEFITS:
Alternative Medicine:	[ ]	Behavioral Health:	[X]
Chiropractic:	[X]	Dental:	[ ]
Home Care:	[X]	Inpatient SNF:	[X]
Long-Term Care:	[ ]	Pharm. Mail Order:	[X]
Physical Therapy:	[X]	Podiatry:	[X]
Psychiatric:	[X]	Transplant:	[X]
Vision:	[X]	Wellness:	[X]
Workers' Comp:	[X]		

Other Benefits:

HFN INC

1315 W 22nd St Ste 300
Oak Brook, IL 60523
Phone: 630-954-1232 Fax: 630-954-1308 Toll-Free:
Web site: www.hfninc.com
MAILING ADDRESS:
HFN INC
1315 W 22nd St Ste 300
Oak Brook, IL 60523

KEY EXECUTIVES:
Chief Executive Officer .... David Kolb
Senior VP, Human Resources/Finance .... Sharon Williams
VP Operations, Information Services .... Robert Rykacezeski

COMPANY PROFILE:
Parent Company Name:
Doing Business As:
Year Founded: 1985   Federally Qualified: [ ]
Forprofit: [ ]   Not-For-Profit: [ ]
Model Type:
Accreditation: [ ] AAPPO [ ] JACHO [ ] NCQA [ ] URAC
Plan Type: PPO
SERVICE AREA:
Nationwide:
IL;

HINES & ASSOCIATES INC

115 E Highland Ave
Elgin, IL 60120
Phone: 847-741-1291 Fax: 847-742-2781 Toll-Free: 800-735-1200
Web site: www.hinesassoc.com
MAILING ADDRESS:
HINES & ASSOCIATES INC
115 E Highland Ave
Elgin, IL 60120

KEY EXECUTIVES:
Chief Executive Officer/President .... Judith Hines
Controller .... Mark Rundle
Medical Director .... William L Nelson, MD
Executive VP Operations .... Eileen Zurblis
VP, Marketing & Operations .... Lynn Breitbach
Director of IT .... Carl Valiulis
Human Resources .... Sylvia Potts

COMPANY PROFILE:
Parent Company Name:
Doing Business As:
Year Founded: 1987   Federally Qualified: [ ]
Forprofit: [Y]   Not-For-Profit: [ ]
Model Type:
Accreditation: [ ] AAPPO [ ] JACHO [ ] NCQA [X] URAC
Plan Type: UR
SERVICE AREA:
Nationwide: Y
NW;
PRODUCTS OFFERED:
Product Name:	Type:
Utilization Review	
Case Management	
Disability Management	
Diabetes Management	

HMO ILLINOIS

300 E Randolph St
Chicago, IL 60601
Phone: 312-653-6000 Fax: 312-819-1220 Toll-Free:
Web site: www.bcbsil.com
MAILING ADDRESS:
HMO ILLINOIS
300 E Randolph St
Chicago, IL 60601

KEY EXECUTIVES:
Chief Executive Officer .... Raymond McCaskey
President of IL .... Paul S Boulis
Chief Information Officer .... John Obon
Marketing Director .... Dennis Hooker
MIS Director .... Karen A Chesrown
Director, Provider Services .... Frank E Nicholson

COMPANY PROFILE:
Parent Company Name: Health Care Service Corporation
Doing Business As: Blue Cross & Blue Shield of Illinois
Year Founded: 1977   Federally Qualified: [N]
Forprofit: [ ]   Not-For-Profit: [Y]
Model Type: NETWORK
Accreditation: [ ] AAPPO [ ] JACHO [X] NCQA [ ] URAC
Plan Type: HMO, CDHP, HDHP, HSA,
Primary Physicians: Physician Specialists:
Hospitals: 101
Total Enrollment:
2001: 0	2004: 97	2007: 0
2002: 0	2005: 718,211	
2003: 0	2006: 716,861	

Managed Care Organization Profiles — **ILLINOIS**

PLAN BENEFITS:
Alternative Medicine: [ ] Behavioral Health: [ ]
Chiropractic: [X] Dental: [X]
Home Care: [X] Inpatient SNF: [X]
Long-Term Care: [ ] Pharm. Mail Order: [X]
Physical Therapy: [X] Podiatry: [X]
Psychiatric: [X] Transplant: [X]
Vision: [X] Wellness: [X]
Workers' Comp: [X]
Other Benefits:

HDN PPO

204 17th St
Wilmette, IL 60091
Phone: 847-920-9052 Fax: 847-920-9053 Toll-Free:
Web site: www.healthdynamics.com
MAILING ADDRESS:
 HDN PPO
 204 17th St
 Wilmette, IL 60091

KEY EXECUTIVES:
Chief Executive Officer .... Joseph N Mohr

COMPANY PROFILE:
Parent Company Name:
Doing Business As:
Year Founded: 1987 Federally Qualified: [N]
Forprofit: [Y] Not-For-Profit: [ ]
Model Type:
Accreditation: [ ] AAPPO [ ] JACHO [ ] NCQA [ ] URAC
Plan Type: PPO, UR, EPO, CDHP, HDHP, HSA,
Total Enrollment:
 2001: 0 2004: 0 2007: 260,000
 2002: 0 2005:
 2003: 0 2006:
SERVICE AREA:
Nationwide: N
 IA; IL; IN; KS; MO; NC; VA; NY; AR;
TYPE OF COVERAGE:
Commercial: [Y] Individual: [ ] FEHBP: [ ] Indemnity: [ ]
Medicare: [ ] Medicaid: [ ] Supplemental Medicare: [ ]
Tricare [ ]
PLAN BENEFITS:
Alternative Medicine: [ ] Behavioral Health: [X]
Chiropractic: [X] Dental: [ ]
Home Care: [X] Inpatient SNF: [X]
Long-Term Care: [ ] Pharm. Mail Order: [ ]
Physical Therapy: [X] Podiatry: [X]
Psychiatric: [X] Transplant: [X]
Vision: [ ] Wellness: [ ]
Workers' Comp: [X]
Other Benefits:

HEALTH ALLIANCE MEDICAL PLANS - CORPORATE HEADQUARTERS

301 S Vine St
Urbana, IL 61801
Phone: 217-337-8000 Fax: 217-337-8093 Toll-Free: 800-851-3379
Web site: www.healthalliance.org
MAILING ADDRESS:
 HEALTH ALLIANCE MEDICAL PLANS
 301 S Vine St
 Urbana, IL 61801

KEY EXECUTIVES:
Chief Executive Officer/President .... Jeffrey C Ingrum, MD
Chief Financial Officer .... Gordon W Salm
Medical Director .... Robert Scully, MD
Pharmacy Director .... Christina Barrington
Chief Operating Officer .... Robin Winskas
VP of Marketing .... MaryAnn Tournoux

COMPANY PROFILE:
Parent Company Name: Carle Clinic
Doing Business As:
Year Founded: 1980 Federally Qualified: [Y]
Forprofit: [Y] Not-For-Profit: [ ]
Model Type: MIXED
Accreditation: [ ] AAPPO [ ] JACHO [X] NCQA [ ] URAC
Plan Type: HMO, PPO, POS, EPO, CDHP, HDHP, HSA, FSA, TPA
Total Revenue: 2005: 2006: 1,497,811
Net Income 2005: 2006: 75,283
Total Enrollment:
 2001: 147,011 2004: 246,726 2007: 0
 2002: 234,110 2005: 143,079
 2003: 247,646 2006: 240,000
SERVICE AREA:
Nationwide: N
 IA; IL;
TYPE OF COVERAGE:
Commercial: [Y] Individual: [Y] FEHBP: [Y] Indemnity: [ ]
Medicare: [Y] Medicaid: [ ] Supplemental Medicare: [Y]
Tricare [ ]
PRODUCTS OFFERED:
Product Name: Type:
Secure Plus Medicare
Health Alliance Premier Choice Medicare Advantage
PLAN BENEFITS:
Alternative Medicine: [ ] Behavioral Health: [ ]
Chiropractic: [X] Dental: [ ]
Home Care: [X] Inpatient SNF: [X]
Long-Term Care: [ ] Pharm. Mail Order: [ ]
Physical Therapy: [X] Podiatry: [X]
Psychiatric: [X] Transplant: [X]
Vision: [X] Wellness: [X]
Workers' Comp: [ ]
Other Benefits:

HEALTH CARE SERVICE CORPORATION - CORPORATE HEADQUARTERS

300 E Randolph St
Chicago, IL 60601-5099
Phone: 312-653-6000 Fax: 312-819-1220 Toll-Free:
Web site: www.hcsc.net
MAILING ADDRESS:
 HEALTHCARE SERVICE CORPORATION -
 CORP HDQTRS
 300 E Randolph St
 Chicago, IL 60601-5099

KEY EXECUTIVES:
Chairman of the Board .... Milton Carroll
Chief Executive Officer .... Raymond McCaskey
President, Chief Operating Officer .... Patricia A Hemingway Hall
Senior VP, Chief Financial Officer .... Denise A Bujak
Chief Medical Officer .... Paul Handel, MD
Chief Information Officer .... John A Oborn
President/Life&Subsidiary Operations Officer .... Larry J Newsom
Director, Provider Services .... Frank E Nicholson
Chief Human Resources Officer .... Patrick F O'Connor

COMPANY PROFILE:
Parent Company Name:
Doing Business As: BC BS of Illinois, BC BS of Texas
Year Founded: Federally Qualified: [Y]
Forprofit: [ ] Not-For-Profit: [Y]
Model Type:
Accreditation: [ ] AAPPO [ ] JACHO [ ] NCQA [ ] URAC
Plan Type: HMO, PPO, POS
Total Revenue: 2005: 11,713,900 2006:
Net Income 2005: 1,145,600 2006:
Total Enrollment:
 2001: 826,156 2004: 10,400,000 2007: 0
 2002: 3,600,000 2005: 11,000,000
 2003: 9,500,000 2006: 11,500,000
SERVICE AREA:
Nationwide: N
 IL; TX;
TYPE OF COVERAGE:
Commercial: [Y] Individual: [Y] FEHBP: [ ] Indemnity: [ ]
Medicare: [ ] Medicaid: [ ] Supplemental Medicare: [Y]
Tricare [ ]
PRODUCTS OFFERED:
Product Name: Type:
HMO HMO

ILLINOIS

SERVICE AREA:
Nationwide: Y
  NW;
TYPE OF COVERAGE:
Commercial: [Y] Individual: [ ] FEHBP: [Y] Indemnity: [ ]
Medicare: [ ] Medicaid: [ ] Supplemental Medicare: [ ]
Tricare   [ ]
PRODUCTS OFFERED:
Product Name: Type:
The First Health Network   PPO
CCN Network   PPO
First Health Care Support   Disease Management
First Health Rx   PBM
PLAN BENEFITS:
Alternative Medicine: [ ]   Behavioral Health: [X]
Chiropractic: [X]   Dental: [X]
Home Care: [X]   Inpatient SNF: [ ]
Long-Term Care: [ ]   Pharm. Mail Order: [X]
Physical Therapy: [ ]   Podiatry: [X]
Psychiatric: [X]   Transplant: [X]
Vision: [X]   Wellness: [X]
Workers' Comp: [X]
Other Benefits:
Comments:
Acquired by Coventry Health Care Inc., January 2005.

GREAT-WEST HEALTHCARE OF ILLINOIS

6250 River Rd #3030
Rosemont, IL 60018
Phone: 847-292-0024 Fax: 847-292-0015 Toll-Free:
Web site: www.greatwesthealthcare.com
MAILING ADDRESS:
  GREAT-WEST HEALTHCARE OF IL
  6250 River Rd #3030
  Rosemont, IL 60018

KEY EXECUTIVES:
Chief Executive Officer/President .... Raymond L McFeetors
President, Georgia .... Donald A Franke
Chief Financial Officer .... Mitchell Graye
Medical Director .... Terry L Fouts, MD

COMPANY PROFILE:
Parent Company Name: CIGNA Inc
Doing Business As:
Year Founded: Federally Qualified: [ ]
Forprofit: [Y]   Not-For-Profit: [ ]
Model Type:
Accreditation: [ ] AAPPO [ ] JACHO [ ] NCQA [ ] URAC
Plan Type: HMO, PPO, CDHP, HDHP, HSA,
Total Revenue: 2005:   2006: 2,013,960
Net Income   2005:   2006:
Total Enrollment:
   2001: 0   2004: 9,207   2007: 0
   2002: 16,371   2005: 9,207
   2003: 11,577   2006: 4,254
SERVICE AREA:
Nationwide: N
  IL;
TYPE OF COVERAGE:
Commercial: [Y] Individual: [ ] FEHBP: [ ] Indemnity: [ ]
Medicare: [ ] Medicaid: [ ] Supplemental Medicare: [ ]
Tricare   [ ]
CONSUMER-DRIVEN PRODUCTS
Mellon HR Solutions LLC   HSA Company
                                 HSA Product
                                 HSA Administrator
                                 Consumer-Driven Health Plan
                                 High Deductible Health Plan
PLAN BENEFITS:
Alternative Medicine: [X]   Behavioral Health: [ ]
Chiropractic: [X]   Dental: [X]
Home Care: [X]   Inpatient SNF: [X]
Long-Term Care: [ ]   Pharm. Mail Order: [X]
Physical Therapy: [X]   Podiatry: [X]
Psychiatric: [X]   Transplant: [X]
Vision: [X]   Wellness: [X]
Workers' Comp: [ ]
Other Benefits:
Comments:
Acquired by CIGNA Inc April 1, 2008.

HARMONY HEALTH PLAN

200 W Adams St Ste 800
Chicago, IL 60606-4420
Phone: 312-516-4900 Fax: 312-630-2022 Toll-Free: 888-684-2026
Web site: www.harmonyhpi.com
MAILING ADDRESS:
  HARMONY HEALTH PLAN
  200 W Adams St Ste 800
  Chicago, IL 60606-4420

KEY EXECUTIVES:
Chief Executive Officer .... Heath Schiesser
President .... Keith Kudla
Medical Director .... Tammaji Kuckarni, MD

COMPANY PROFILE:
Parent Company Name: WellCare Health Plans Inc
Doing Business As:
Year Founded: 1996   Federally Qualified: [N]
Forprofit: [Y]   Not-For-Profit: [ ]
Model Type:
Accreditation: [ ] AAPPO [ ] JACHO [ ] NCQA [ ] URAC
Plan Type: HMO,
Total Revenue: 2005:   2006: 263,999,393
Net Income   2005:   2006: 8,824,190
Total Enrollment:
   2001: 43,733   2004: 112,275   2007: 0
   2002: 77,330   2005: 176,916
   2003: 82,604   2006: 171,814
Medical Loss Ratio: 2005:   2006: 84.30
Administrative Expense Ratio: 2005:   2006:
SERVICE AREA:
Nationwide: N
  IL; IN;
TYPE OF COVERAGE:
Commercial: [Y] Individual: [ ] FEHBP: [ ] Indemnity: [ ]
Medicare: [ ] Medicaid: [Y] Supplemental Medicare: [ ]
Tricare   [ ]
PRODUCTS OFFERED:
Product Name: Type:
Harmony Health Plan   Medicaid
Harmony Health Plan   Medicare

HCH ADMINISTRATION

209 W R B Garrett Ave
Peoria, IL 61605
Phone: 309-673-7330 Fax: 309-673-7369 Toll-Free: 800-322-1516
Web site: www.hchadministration.com
MAILING ADDRESS:
  HCH ADMINISTRATION
  PO Box 1986
  Peoria, IL 61605

KEY EXECUTIVES:
President .... James Stevenson
Director Utilization Mangement .... Linda Walker
VP Operations .... Paul Wann
VP Sales & Marketing .... R Scott Ried
MIS Director .... Chaker Khatib

COMPANY PROFILE:
Parent Company Name: Health-Care Horizons Inc
Doing Business As: HCH Administration
Year Founded: 1982   Federally Qualified: [ ]
Forprofit: [Y]   Not-For-Profit: [ ]
Model Type:
Accreditation: [ ] AAPPO [ ] JACHO [ ] NCQA [ ] URAC
Plan Type: UR, TPA
SERVICE AREA:
Nationwide: Y
  NW;
TYPE OF COVERAGE:
Commercial: [Y] Individual: [ ] FEHBP: [ ] Indemnity: [ ]
Medicare: [ ] Medicaid: [Y] Supplemental Medicare: [ ]
Tricare   [ ]

Managed Care Organization Profiles   **ILLINOIS**

KEY EXECUTIVES:
Chief Executive Officer/President .... *Steve Klister*
Chief Financial Officer .... *Craig Simunza*
Dental Director .... *Tim Custer, DDS*
Director of Marketing .... *Lynne Culberson*
Executive Director of IT Management .... *Tom Kimrey*
Manager, Network Administration .... *Ted Cerven*
Quality Assurance Director .... *Thomas McNally*
VP, Professional Services .... *Greg Stobbe*
VP, Sales .... *John Doyle*
Executive Director, Risk Management .... *Charley Renfro*

COMPANY PROFILE:
Parent Company Name: HCSC (Health Care Service Corporation)
Doing Business As: Dental Network of America
Year Founded: 1985   Federally Qualified: [ ]
Forprofit: [Y]   Not-For-Profit: [ ]
Model Type:
Accreditation: [ ] AAPPO [ ] JACHO [ ] NCQA [ ] URAC
Plan Type: Specialty HMO, Specialty PPO, TPA
Total Enrollment:
  2001: 3,100,000   2004: 0   2007: 0
  2002: 0   2005:
  2003: 0   2006: 2,600,000

SERVICE AREA:
Nationwide: Y
  NW;

TYPE OF COVERAGE:
Commercial: [Y] Individual: [ ] FEHBP: [ ] Indemnity: [Y]
Medicare: [ ] Medicaid: [Y] Supplemental Medicare: [ ]
Tricare   [ ]

PLAN BENEFITS:
Alternative Medicine: [ ]   Behavioral Health: [ ]
Chiropractic: [ ]   Dental: [X]
Home Care: [ ]   Inpatient SNF: [ ]
Long-Term Care: [ ]   Pharm. Mail Order: [ ]
Physical Therapy: [ ]   Podiatry: [ ]
Psychiatric: [ ]   Transplant: [ ]
Vision: [ ]   Wellness: [ ]
Workers' Comp: [ ]
Other Benefits:

FIDELIS SECURECARE INC

1700 East Golf Road
Schaumburg, IL 60173
Phone: 847-605-0501 Fax: Toll-Free:
Web site: www.www.fidelissc.com
MAILING ADDRESS:
    FIDELIS SECURECARE INC
    1700 East Golf Road
    Schaumburg, IL 60173

KEY EXECUTIVES:
Chief Executive Officer/President .... *Samuel R Willcoxon*
Chief Financial/Compliance Officer .... *David Goltz*
Senior VP, Sales & Marketing .... *Beattie DeLong*
Chief Medical Officer .... *Scott Sarran, MD*
Director of Pharmacy .... *Jay Gandhi, PharmD, CDM*
VP, Health Services .... *Jean Foltin, RN*
VP, Opertions .... *Kathy Cortez*

COMPANY PROFILE:
Parent Company Name:
Doing Business As:
Year Founded: 2006   Federally Qualified: [Y]
Forprofit: [ ]   Not-For-Profit: [ ]
Model Type:
Accreditation: [ ] AAPPO [ ] JACHO [ ] NCQA [ ] URAC
Plan Type: HMO
SERVICE AREA:
Nationwide:
  MI; NC; TX;
TYPE OF COVERAGE:
Commercial: [ ] Individual: [ ] FEHBP: [ ] Indemnity: [ ]
Medicare: [Y] Medicaid: [ ] Supplemental Medicare: [ ]
Tricare   [ ]

FIRST COMMONWEALTH

559 W Jackson Ste 800
Chicago, IL 60661
Phone: 312-279-5111 Fax: 312-279-5140 Toll-Free: 800-562-1366
Web site: www.firstcommonwealth.net
MAILING ADDRESS:
    FIRST COMMONWEALTH
    559 W Jackson Ste 800
    Chicago, IL 60661

KEY EXECUTIVES:
Acting President .... *Richard Goren, DDS*
Dental Director .... *Paul Chaitkin, DDS*
Director of Network Management .... *Ann Hunt*

COMPANY PROFILE:
Parent Company Name: Guardian
Doing Business As: First Commonwealth
Year Founded: 1990   Federally Qualified: [N]
Forprofit: [Y]   Not-For-Profit: [ ]
Model Type: IPA
Accreditation: [ ] AAPPO [ ] JACHO [ ] NCQA [ ] URAC
Plan Type: Specialty HMO, Specialty PPO
Total Enrollment:
  2001: 0   2004: 0   2007: 0
  2002: 4,751   2005:
  2003: 4,116   2006:
SERVICE AREA:
Nationwide: N
  IL; IN; MI; MO; WI;
TYPE OF COVERAGE:
Commercial: [Y] Individual: [ ] FEHBP: [ ] Indemnity: [ ]
Medicare: [ ] Medicaid: [ ] Supplemental Medicare: [ ]
Tricare   [ ]
PLAN BENEFITS:
Alternative Medicine: [ ]   Behavioral Health: [ ]
Chiropractic: [ ]   Dental: [X]
Home Care: [ ]   Inpatient SNF: [ ]
Long-Term Care: [ ]   Pharm. Mail Order: [ ]
Physical Therapy: [ ]   Podiatry: [ ]
Psychiatric: [ ]   Transplant: [ ]
Vision: [ ]   Wellness: [ ]
Workers' Comp: [ ]
Other Benefits:

FIRST HEALTH GROUP CORP

3200 Highland Ave
Downers Grove, IL 60515
Phone: 630-737-7900 Fax: 630-737-7856 Toll-Free: 800-455-1425
Web site: www.firsthealth.com
MAILING ADDRESS:
    FIRST HEALTH GROUP CORP
    3200 Highland Ave
    Downers Grove, IL 60515

KEY EXECUTIVES:
Chief Executive Officer .... *Dale B Wolf*
President .... *John Langenus*
Executive Vice President .... *Shawn M Guertin*

COMPANY PROFILE:
Parent Company Name: Coventry Health Care Inc
Doing Business As:
Year Founded: 1982   Federally Qualified: [N]
Forprofit: [Y]   Not-For-Profit: [ ]
Model Type: NETWORK
Accreditation: [ ] AAPPO [ ] JACHO [ ] NCQA [X] URAC
Plan Type: PPO, TPA, UR, PBM
Primary Physicians: 152,676   Physician Specialists:
Hospitals: 4,451
Total Enrollment:
  2001: 9,100,000   2004: 0   2007: 0
  2002: 7,900,000   2005:
  2003: 0   2006:

ILLINOIS   **Managed Care Organization Profiles**

MAILING ADDRESS:
   DELTA DENTAL PLAN OF IL
   801 Ogden Ave
   Lisle, IL 60532

KEY EXECUTIVES:
Chairman of the Board .... Frank A Maggio, DDS
Chief Executive Officer/President .... Robert E Dennison, DMD
Chief Financial Officer .... Tamera K Robinson, CPA
Chief Marketing Officer .... Thomas J Colgan
VP, Sales .... Jeanette Battista
VP, Information Technology .... Ross Gosnell
Privacy Officer .... Hazel Fisher-Gable
Provider Relations Manager .... Jan Ross
Director, Product Development .... Michael White

COMPANY PROFILE:
Parent Company Name: Delta Dental Plan of Illinois
Doing Business As:
Year Founded: 1967   Federally Qualified: [ ]
Forprofit: [ ]   Not-For-Profit: [Y]
Model Type:
Accreditation: [ ] AAPPO [ ] JACHO [ ] NCQA [ ] URAC
Plan Type: Specialty HMO, Specialty PPO, POS, ASO
Total Enrollment:
   2001: 313,307   2004: 257,289   2007: 0
   2002: 275,905   2005:
   2003: 239,746   2006:

SERVICE AREA:
Nationwide: N
   IL;

TYPE OF COVERAGE:
Commercial: [Y] Individual: [ ] FEHBP: [ ] Indemnity: [ ]
Medicare: [ ] Medicaid: [ ] Supplemental Medicare: [ ]
Tricare [ ]

PRODUCTS OFFERED:
Product Name: Type:
Delta Preferred Option   PPO
Delta Care   DHMO

PLAN BENEFITS:
Alternative Medicine: [ ]   Behavioral Health: [ ]
Chiropractic: [ ]   Dental: [X]
Home Care: [ ]   Inpatient SNF: [ ]
Long-Term Care: [ ]   Pharm. Mail Order: [ ]
Physical Therapy: [ ]   Podiatry: [ ]
Psychiatric: [ ]   Transplant: [ ]
Vision: [ ]   Wellness: [ ]
Workers' Comp: [ ]
Other Benefits:

DELTA DENTAL PLANS ASSOCIATION

1515 W 22nd St Ste 1200
Oak Brook Village, IL 60523
Phone: 630-574-6001 Fax: 630-574-6999 Toll-Free:
Web site: www.deltadental.com
MAILING ADDRESS:
   DELTA DENTAL PLANS ASSOCIATION
   1515 W 22nd St Ste 1200
   Oak Brook Village, IL 60523

KEY EXECUTIVES:
Chief Executive Officer/President .... Kim Volk
Chief Financial Officer .... Stephen White
National Oral Health Advisor .... Max Anderson, DDS
VP, Technology .... Karron Callaghan
VP, Marketing .... Tom Dolatowski
Director, Network & Product Development .... Janis Oshensky
VP, Communications & Public Policy .... Susan Morris
Corporate Administrator .... Stefany Soutor
Director, Education & Meeting Planning .... Lucia Clark

COMPANY PROFILE:
Parent Company Name:
Doing Business As:
Year Founded: 1954   Federally Qualified: [ ]
Forprofit: [ ]   Not-For-Profit: [ ]
Model Type:
Accreditation: [ ] AAPPO [ ] JACHO [ ] NCQA [ ] URAC
Plan Type: Specialty HMO, Specialty PPO, TPA, POS, ASO
Total Enrollment:
   2001: 0   2004: 0   2007: 0
   2002: 0   2005:
   2003: 0   2006: 47,000,000

SERVICE AREA:
Nationwide: Y
   Nationwide;

TYPE OF COVERAGE:
Commercial: [Y] Individual: [ ] FEHBP: [ ] Indemnity: [ ]
Medicare: [ ] Medicaid: [ ] Supplemental Medicare: [ ]
Tricare [ ]

PLAN BENEFITS:
Alternative Medicine: [ ]   Behavioral Health: [ ]
Chiropractic: [ ]   Dental: [X]
Home Care: [ ]   Inpatient SNF: [ ]
Long-Term Care: [ ]   Pharm. Mail Order: [ ]
Physical Therapy: [ ]   Podiatry: [ ]
Psychiatric: [ ]   Transplant: [ ]
Vision: [ ]   Wellness: [ ]
Workers' Comp: [ ]
Other Benefits:

DENTAL CARE OF AMERICA LTD

360 Red Bud Place
Buffalo Grove, IL 60089-1854
Phone: 847-520-3390 Fax: 847-520-8161 Toll-Free:
Web site:
MAILING ADDRESS:
   DENTAL CARE OF AMERICA LTD
   PO Box 4869
   Buffalo Grove, IL 60089-1854

KEY EXECUTIVES:
Chief Executive Officer/President .... Angelo Lendino
Chief Financial Officer .... Angelo Lendino
Dental Director .... Michael White, DDS

COMPANY PROFILE:
Parent Company Name:
Doing Business As:
Year Founded: 1983   Federally Qualified: [N]
Forprofit: [Y]   Not-For-Profit: [ ]
Model Type:
Accreditation: [ ] AAPPO [ ] JACHO [ ] NCQA [ ] URAC
Plan Type: Specialty PPO

SERVICE AREA:
Nationwide: N
   FL; IL; IN; MA; MI; NJ; NY; WI;

TYPE OF COVERAGE:
Commercial: [Y] Individual: [Y] FEHBP: [ ] Indemnity: [ ]
Medicare: [ ] Medicaid: [ ] Supplemental Medicare: [ ]
Tricare [ ]

PLAN BENEFITS:
Alternative Medicine: [ ]   Behavioral Health: [ ]
Chiropractic: [ ]   Dental: [X]
Home Care: [ ]   Inpatient SNF: [ ]
Long-Term Care: [ ]   Pharm. Mail Order: [ ]
Physical Therapy: [ ]   Podiatry: [ ]
Psychiatric: [ ]   Transplant: [ ]
Vision: [ ]   Wellness: [ ]
Workers' Comp: [ ]
Other Benefits:

DENTAL NETWORK OF AMERICA

2 TransAm Plz Dr Ste 500
Oakbrook Terrace, IL 60181
Phone: 630-691-1133 Fax: 630-495-0575 Toll-Free: 800-323-6840
Web site: www.dnoa.com
MAILING ADDRESS:
   DENTAL NETWORK OF AMERICA
   2 TransAm Plz Dr Ste 500
   Oakbrook Terrace, IL 60181

Managed Care Organization Profiles ILLINOIS

PRODUCTS OFFERED:
Product Name: Type:
Utilization & Quality Manageme
Quality Assurance Oversight/Ex
Comments:
Name has been changed. Formerly known as Central Illinois Medical Review Organization.

COMBINED INSURANCE COMPANY OF AMERICA

1000 N Milwaukee Ave
Glenview, IL 60025
Phone: 847-953-2025 Fax: 847-953-8030 Toll-Free: 800-225-4500
Web site: www.combined.com
MAILING ADDRESS:
   COMBINED INS CO OF AMERICA
   1000 N Milwaukee Ave
   Glenview, IL 60025

KEY EXECUTIVES:
Chairman of the Board .... Richard Ravin
Chief Executive Officer .... Douglas R Wendt
Chief Financial Officer .... Jim Hom
Chief Information Officer .... Koorosh Beigian
Executive Vice President .... Michael Conway
Owner/Founder .... W Clement Stone
Corporate Communications Manager .... Pamela Birch
Executive VP, Chief Actuary .... Steve Lippai

COMPANY PROFILE:
Parent Company Name: AON Corporation
Doing Business As:
Year Founded: 1919   Federally Qualified: [ ]
Forprofit: [Y]   Not-For-Profit: [ ]
Model Type:
Accreditation: [ ] AAPPO [ ] JACHO [ ] NCQA [ ] URAC
Plan Type: HMO
Total Revenue: 2005:   2006: 1,355,421,156
Net Income   2005:   2006:
Total Enrollment:
   2001: 0   2004: 400,000   2007: 0
   2002: 0   2005: 5,000,000
   2003: 0   2006:
SERVICE AREA:
Nationwide: Y
   NW;
TYPE OF COVERAGE:
Commercial: [ ] Individual: [ ] FEHBP: [ ] Indemnity: [ ]
Medicare: [ ] Medicaid: [ ] Supplemental Medicare: [Y]
Tricare   [ ]
PRODUCTS OFFERED:
Product Name: Type:
Golden Life Plus   Supplemental Medicare
Golden Advantage Plus   Supplemental Medicare

COMPSYCH BEHAVIORAL HEALTH

NBC T 13th Fl 455 N City Front
Chicago, IL 60611-5532
Phone: 312-595-4000 Fax: 312-595-3125 Toll-Free: 800-851-1714
Web site: www.compsych.com
MAILING ADDRESS:
   COMPSYCH CORPORATION
   NBC T 13th Fl 455 N City Front
   Chicago, IL 60611-5532

KEY EXECUTIVES:
Chairman/Chief Executive Officer .... Richard Chaifetz, PhD
Chief Financial Officer .... Robert Jacobson
VP, Marketing .... Mary Paskell

COMPANY PROFILE:
Parent Company Name:
Doing Business As:
Year Founded: 1984   Federally Qualified: [Y]
Forprofit: [Y]   Not-For-Profit: [ ]
Model Type:
Accreditation: [ ] AAPPO [ ] JACHO [ ] NCQA [ ] URAC
Plan Type: Specialty PPO, ASO, TPA, UR
Total Enrollment:
   2001: 6,800,000   2004: 0   2007: 0
   2002: 0   2005:
   2003: 0   2006:
SERVICE AREA:
Nationwide: Y
   NW;
TYPE OF COVERAGE:
Commercial: [Y] Individual: [ ] FEHBP: [ ] Indemnity: [ ]
Medicare: [Y] Medicaid: [ ] Supplemental Medicare: [ ]
Tricare   [ ]
PLAN BENEFITS:
Alternative Medicine: [ ]   Behavioral Health: [X]
Chiropractic: [ ]   Dental: [ ]
Home Care: [ ]   Inpatient SNF: [ ]
Long-Term Care: [ ]   Pharm. Mail Order: [ ]
Physical Therapy: [ ]   Podiatry: [ ]
Psychiatric: [X]   Transplant: [ ]
Vision: [ ]   Wellness: [X]
Workers' Comp: [ ]
Other Benefits:

DELPHI CARD R

960 Rt 22 Ste 215
Fox River Grove, IL 60021
Phone: 847-516-9592 Fax: 847-777-6630 Toll-Free:
Web site: www.delphicard.com
MAILING ADDRESS:
   DELPHI CARD R
   PO Box 677
   Cary, IL 60021

KEY EXECUTIVES:
Chief Executive Officer .... Randall Preston
Chief Financial Officer .... Carol Rogers
Medical Director .... Joel Shalowitz, MD
Marketing, Provider Services Director .... William Houy

COMPANY PROFILE:
Parent Company Name: The Preston Group Inc
Doing Business As:
Year Founded: 1990   Federally Qualified: [N]
Forprofit: [Y]   Not-For-Profit: [ ]
Model Type:
Accreditation: [ ] AAPPO [ ] JACHO [ ] NCQA [ ] URAC
Plan Type: Specialty PPO, UR, POS, PR0, TPA
Total Enrollment:
   2001: 0   2004: 0   2007: 0
   2002: 0   2005:
   2003: 30,000   2006:
SERVICE AREA:
Nationwide: Y
   NW;
TYPE OF COVERAGE:
Commercial: [Y] Individual: [Y] FEHBP: [ ] Indemnity: [ ]
Medicare: [ ] Medicaid: [ ] Supplemental Medicare: [ ]
Tricare   [ ]
PLAN BENEFITS:
Alternative Medicine: [ ]   Behavioral Health: [X]
Chiropractic: [X]   Dental: [X]
Home Care: [X]   Inpatient SNF: [X]
Long-Term Care: [X]   Pharm. Mail Order: [X]
Physical Therapy: [X]   Podiatry: [X]
Psychiatric: [X]   Transplant: [X]
Vision: [X]   Wellness: [X]
Workers' Comp: [X]
Other Benefits:

DELTA DENTAL PLAN OF ILLINOIS

801 Ogden Ave
Lisle, IL 60532
Phone: 630-964-2400 Fax: 630-964-2596 Toll-Free: 800-343-1743
Web site: www.deltadentalil.com

ILLINOIS

BLUE CROSS BLUE SHIELD OF ILLINOIS

300 E Randolph St
Chicago, IL 60601
Phone: 312-938-6000 Fax: 312-819-1628 Toll-Free:
Web site: www.bcbsil.com

MAILING ADDRESS:
BLUE CROSS BLUE SHIELD OF IL
300 E Randolph St
Chicago, IL 60601

KEY EXECUTIVES:
Chief Executive Officer .... Raymond McCaskey
President of IL .... Paul S Boulis
Senior VP, Chief Financial Officer .... Denise A Bujak
Chief Information Officer .... John A Oborn
Chief Operating Officer .... Sherman M Wolff
Marketing Director .... Dennis Hooker
MIS Director .... Karen A Chesrown
Director, Provider Services .... Frank E Nicholson

COMPANY PROFILE:
Parent Company Name: Health Care Service Corporation
Doing Business As: Blue Cross & Blue Shield of Illinois
Year Founded: 1985   Federally Qualified: [N]
Forprofit: [ ]   Not-For-Profit: [Y]
Model Type:
Accreditation: [ ] AAPPO [X] JACHO [ ] NCQA [ ] URAC
Plan Type: HMO, PPO, POS, CDHP, HDHP, HSA,
Total Enrollment:
   2001: 4,500,000   2004: 97   2007: 0
   2002: 127   2005:
   2003: 111   2006:

SERVICE AREA:
Nationwide: N
   IL;

TYPE OF COVERAGE:
Commercial: [Y] Individual: [Y] FEHBP: [ ] Indemnity: [ ]
Medicare: [Y] Medicaid: [ ] Supplemental Medicare: [Y]
Tricare   [ ]

PRODUCTS OFFERED:
Product Name: Type:
BCI HMO   HMO

PLAN BENEFITS:
Alternative Medicine: [ ]   Behavioral Health: [ ]
Chiropractic: [X]   Dental: [ ]
Home Care: [ ]   Inpatient SNF: [X]
Long-Term Care: [ ]   Pharm. Mail Order: [ ]
Physical Therapy: [X]   Podiatry: [X]
Psychiatric: [X]   Transplant: [ ]
Vision: [ ]   Wellness: [X]
Workers' Comp: [ ]
Other Benefits:

Comments:
Acquired Oxford Health Plan business during 1998. Oxford acquired Compare Health Care Plans during 1997.

CIGNA HEALTHCARE OF ILLINOIS INC

525 W Monroe St Ste 300
Chicago, IL 60661-3629
Phone: 312-648-2460 Fax: 312-648-3617 Toll-Free: 800-541-7526
Web site: www.cigna.com

MAILING ADDRESS:
CIGNA HEALTHCARE OF IL
525 W Monroe St Ste 300
Chicago, IL 60661-3629

KEY EXECUTIVES:
Chairman/Chief Executive Officer .... H Edward Hanway
Chief Executive Officer .... H Edward Hanway
Market Leader .... Robert S Fry, Jr
Medical Director .... Cynthia Alston, MD

COMPANY PROFILE:
Parent Company Name: CIGNA Corporation
Doing Business As:
Year Founded: 1986   Federally Qualified: [Y]
Forprofit: [Y]   Not-For-Profit: [ ]
Model Type: IPA
Accreditation: [ ] AAPPO [ ] JACHO [X] NCQA [ ] URAC
Plan Type: HMO, POS, CDHP, HDHP, HSA, FSA, HRA
Total Revenue: 2005:   2006: 14,856,934
Net Income   2005:   2006:
Total Enrollment:
   2001: 11,080   2004: 5,306   2007: 0
   2002: 7,586   2005: 4,591
   2003: 6,060   2006: 4,331
Medical Loss Ratio: 2005:   2006: 80.40
Administrative Expense Ratio: 2005:   2006:

SERVICE AREA:
Nationwide: N
   IL; (Lake, Laporte, Porter); IA;

TYPE OF COVERAGE:
Commercial: [Y] Individual: [ ] FEHBP: [ ] Indemnity: [ ]
Medicare: [ ] Medicaid: [ ] Supplemental Medicare: [Y]
Tricare   [ ]

PRODUCTS OFFERED:
Product Name: Type:

CONSUMER-DRIVEN PRODUCTS
JP Morgan Chase   HSA Company
CIGNA Choice Fund   HSA Product
                                 HSA Administrator
Open Access Plus   Consumer-Driven Health Plan
PPO   High Deductible Health Plan

PLAN BENEFITS:
Alternative Medicine: [ ]   Behavioral Health: [ ]
Chiropractic: [X]   Dental: [X]
Home Care: [X]   Inpatient SNF: [X]
Long-Term Care: [ ]   Pharm. Mail Order: [X]
Physical Therapy: [X]   Podiatry: [X]
Psychiatric: [X]   Transplant: [X]
Vision: [X]   Wellness: [X]
Workers' Comp: [ ]
Other Benefits:

CIMRO QUALITY HEALTHCARE SOLUTIONS

100 Trade Centre Dr Ste 401
Champaign, IL 61820-7237
Phone: 217-352-1060 Fax: 217-353-7583 Toll-Free: 800-635-9407
Web site: www.cimro.com

MAILING ADDRESS:
CIMRO QUALITY HEALTHCARE SOLUTIONS
100 Trade Centre Dr Ste 401
Champaign, IL 61820-7237

KEY EXECUTIVES:
Chairman of the Board .... Barry Slotky, MD
Chief Executive Officer .... Tina Georgy, RN, MS
Chief Financial Officer .... Julia Overstreet, CPA
Medical Director .... Jay A Yambert, MD, FACP, FACEP
Manager Information Technology . Jeremy Anderson BA, MBA, MCSE
Managed Care Director .... Judy Kinkelaar, RN, BSN
Senior VP Medicaid Services .... Jennifer Kirkland, RN,BS,CPHQ
Director, Review Services .... April Oglei, RN, MS

COMPANY PROFILE:
Parent Company Name: CIMRO
Doing Business As: Peer Review Organ & Quality Improvement
Year Founded: 1972   Federally Qualified: [ ]
Forprofit: [ ]   Not-For-Profit: [Y]
Model Type:
Accreditation: [ ] AAPPO [ ] JACHO [ ] NCQA [X] URAC
Plan Type: UR, PRO
Total Enrollment:
   2001: 0   2004: 0   2007: 0
   2002: 0   2005:
   2003: 0   2006: 2,000,000

SERVICE AREA:
Nationwide: N
   IL; MO; (Midwest Region);

TYPE OF COVERAGE:
Commercial: [Y] Individual: [ ] FEHBP: [ ] Indemnity: [ ]
Medicare: [Y] Medicaid: [Y] Supplemental Medicare: [ ]
Tricare   [ ]

Managed Care Organization Profiles **ILLINOIS**

AETNA HEALTH OF ILLINOIS INC

100 North Riverside Plaza 20Fl
Chicago, IL 60606-1518
Phone: 312-928-3108 Fax: 312-928-3232 Toll-Free: 800-627-5039
Web site: www.aetna.com
MAILING ADDRESS:
    AETNA HEALTH OF ILLINOIS INC
    100 North Riverside Plaza 20Fl
    Chicago, IL 60606-1518

KEY EXECUTIVES:
Chairman of the Board/Chief Executive Officer .... Ronald A Williams
Regional Manager-Midwest .... Edward Dulik
Executive VP, Finance .... Joseph M Zubretsky
VP, Chief Medical Officer .... Burton Vanderlaan, MD
Pharmacy Director .... Richard Wolson
Regional Chief Information Officer .... Stacey Jones
Regional Marketing Director .... Amy Scavo
MIS Director .... R Max Gould
Regional Director, Provider Services .... Jeff Murphy
Communications .... Wendy Morphew

COMPANY PROFILE:
Parent Company Name: Aetna Inc
Doing Business As: Aetna Inc
Year Founded: 1853   Federally Qualified: [Y]
Forprofit: [Y]   Not-For-Profit: [ ]
Model Type: IPA
Accreditation: [ ] AAPPO [ ] JACHO [X] NCQA [ ] URAC
Plan Type: HMO, PPO, UR, POS, EP0, CDHP, HSA
Total Revenue: 2005:   2006:   195,668,582
Net Income   2005:   2006:
Total Enrollment:
    2001: 118,811   2004: 57,861   2007: 0
    2002: 54,982   2005: 65,121
    2003: 149,364   2006: 64,056
Medical Loss Ratio: 2005:   2006: 81.60
Administrative Expense Ratio: 2005:   2006:
SERVICE AREA:
Nationwide: N
    IL (Adams, Bartholomew, Boone, Brown, Cass, Clinton Cook, DeKalb, DuPage, Grant, Greene, Hamilton, Hancock, Hendricks, Henry, Huntington, Johnson, Kane, Kosciusko, Lake, LaPorte, Lawrence, Madison, Marion, McHenry, Miami, Monroe, Morgan, Noble, Posey, Shelby, Steuben, Tipton, Vanderburgh, Vermilion, Vigo, Wabash, Warrick, Wells, Whitley, Will); IN (Lake, LaPorte);
TYPE OF COVERAGE:
Commercial: [Y] Individual: [ ] FEHBP: [ ] Indemnity: [ ]
Medicare: [Y] Medicaid: [ ] Supplemental Medicare: [ ]
Tricare   [ ]
PRODUCTS OFFERED:

Product Name:	Type:
Aetna HMO	HMO
Aetna US Healthcare Golden Medicare	Medicare
Quality Point of Service	POS
Elect Choice EPO	EPO
Managed Choice POS	POS
Open Choice PPO	PPO
Advantage/Advantage Plus	Dental

CONSUMER-DRIVEN PRODUCTS

Aetna Life Insurance Co	HSA Company
Aetna HealthFund HSA	HSA Product
Aetna	HSA Administrator
Aetna HealthFund	Consumer-Driven Health Plan
PPO I; PPO II	High Deductible Health Plan

PLAN BENEFITS:
Alternative Medicine: [ ]   Behavioral Health: [X]
Chiropractic: [X]   Dental: [X]
Home Care: [X]   Inpatient SNF: [X]
Long-Term Care: [X]   Pharm. Mail Order: [X]
Physical Therapy: [X]   Podiatry: [X]
Psychiatric: [X]   Transplant: [X]
Vision: [X]   Wellness: [X]
Workers' Comp: [ ]
Other Benefits: X

ASSURANT EMPLOYEE BENEFITS - ILLINOIS

140 Butterfield Rd Ste 1250
Oakbrook Terrace, IL 60181
Phone: 630-954-5700 Fax: 630-954-1365 Toll-Free: 888-773-4220
Web site: www.assurantemployeebenefits.com

MAILING ADDRESS:
    ASSURANT EMPLOYEE BENEFITS - IL
    140 Butterfield Rd Ste 1250
    Oakbrook Terrace, IL 60181

KEY EXECUTIVES:
Chief Executive Officer/President .... Michael J Peninger
Chief Financial Officer .... Floyd F Chadee
VP, Medical Director .... Polly M Galbraith, MD
Chief Information Officer .... Karla J Schacht
Senior VP, Marketing .... Joseph A Sevcik
Privacy Officer .... John L Fortini
VP of Provider Services .... James A Barrett, DMD
Senior VP, Human Resources & Development .... Sylvia R Wagner
General Manager .... Todd Boyd
National Dental Director .... James A Barrett, DMD

COMPANY PROFILE:
Parent Company Name: Assurant Health
Doing Business As:
Year Founded: 1986   Federally Qualified: [ ]
Forprofit: [Y]   Not-For-Profit: [ ]
Model Type:
Accreditation: [ ] AAPPO [ ] JACHO [ ] NCQA [ ] URAC
Plan Type: Specialty HMO
SERVICE AREA:
Nationwide: N
    ID; IL; MI; MN; MT; ND; SD; WY;
TYPE OF COVERAGE:
Commercial: [Y] Individual: [Y] FEHBP: [ ] Indemnity: [ ]
Medicare: [ ] Medicaid: [ ] Supplemental Medicare: [ ]
Tricare
PLAN BENEFITS:
Alternative Medicine: [ ]   Behavioral Health: [ ]
Chiropractic: [ ]   Dental: [X]
Home Care: [ ]   Inpatient SNF: [ ]
Long-Term Care: [ ]   Pharm. Mail Order: [ ]
Physical Therapy: [ ]   Podiatry: [ ]
Psychiatric: [ ]   Transplant: [ ]
Vision: [ ]   Wellness: [ ]
Workers' Comp: [ ]
Other Benefits:
Comments:
Formerly Fortis Benefits Dental.

AVETA HEALTH ILLINOIS INC

4415 W Harrison St Ste 300
Hillside, IL 60162
Phone: 708-432-1700 Fax: 708-432-0185 Toll-Free: 800-660-7421
Web site: www.avetacarepartners.com
MAILING ADDRESS:
    AVETA HEALTH ILLINOIS INC
    4415 W Harrison St Ste 300
    Hillside, IL 60162

KEY EXECUTIVES:
Chief Executive Officer/President .... Wayne Aardsma

COMPANY PROFILE:
Parent Company Name:
Doing Business As: Aveta CarePartners
Year Founded: 2006   Federally Qualified: [ ]
Forprofit: [Y]   Not-For-Profit: [ ]
Model Type:
Accreditation: [ ] AAPPO [ ] JACHO [ ] NCQA [ ] URAC
Plan Type: HMO
Total Revenue: 2005:   2006:   652,797
Net Income   2005:   2006:
Total Enrollment:
    2001: 0   2004: 0   2007: 0
    2002: 0   2005:
    2003: 0   2006: 179
Medical Loss Ratio: 2005:   2006: 95.00
Administrative Expense Ratio: 2005:   2006:
SERVICE AREA:
Nationwide: N
    IL (Cook);
TYPE OF COVERAGE:
Commercial: [ ] Individual: [ ] FEHBP: [ ] Indemnity: [ ]
Medicare: [Y] Medicaid: [ ] Supplemental Medicare: [ ]
Tricare   [ ]

IDAHO — Managed Care Organization Profiles

PRIMARY HEALTH PLAN

800 Park Blvd Ste 760
Boise, ID 83712
Phone: 208-344-1811 Fax: 208-344-4262 Toll-Free: 800-688-5008
Web site: www.primaryhealth.com

MAILING ADDRESS:
PRIMARY HEALTH PLAN
800 Park Blvd Ste 760
Boise, ID 83712

KEY EXECUTIVES:
Chairman of the Board .... Barbara Santry
Chief Executive Officer .... Elwood Kleaver
President .... David Self
Chief Financial Officer .... Dennis Bruns, CPA
Medical Director .... Robert Friedman, MD
Director, Information Technology .... Mike Hronek
Director of Operations, Health Plan .... David Self
Executive Director, Physicians Network .... Linda Duer
Human Resources Director .... Susan Miller
Director of Operations, Medical Group .... Tracy Morris
Director of Plan Operations .... Mark Ammons

COMPANY PROFILE:
Parent Company Name: Primary Health Inc
Doing Business As:
Year Founded: 1996   Federally Qualified: [N]
Forprofit: [Y]   Not-For-Profit: [ ]
Model Type: NETWORK
Accreditation: [ ] AAPPO [ ] JACHO [ ] NCQA [ ] URAC
Plan Type: HMO, PPO, POS, UR, HDHP, HSA
Total Revenue: 2005:   2006: 27,769,135
Net Income   2005:   2006:
Total Enrollment:
  2001: 0   2004: 137,486   2007: 0
  2002: 0   2005:
  2003: 149,402   2006:
Medical Loss Ratio: 2005:   2006: 80.00
Administrative Expense Ratio: 2005:   2006:

SERVICE AREA:
Nationwide: N
  ID;

TYPE OF COVERAGE:
Commercial: [Y] Individual: [ ] FEHBP: [ ] Indemnity: [ ]
Medicare: [ ] Medicaid: [ ] Supplemental Medicare: [ ]
Tricare   [ ]

REGENCE BLUE SHIELD OF IDAHO

1602 21st Ave
Lewiston, ID 83501
Phone: 208-746-2671 Fax: 208-798-2097 Toll-Free:
Web site: www.id.regence.com

MAILING ADDRESS:
REGENCE BLUE SHIELD OF IDAHO
PO Box 1106
Lewiston, ID 83501

KEY EXECUTIVES:
Chairman of the Board .... Greg Charlton
Chief Executive Officer .... Mark B Ganz
President .... John Stellmon
Chief Medical Officer .... Richard Rainey, MD
Assistant Director of Communications .... Georganne Benjamin
VP of Sales .... Chris Larsen
Managed Care Director .... Carol Steinbrecher-Loera

COMPANY PROFILE:
Parent Company Name:
Doing Business As: Healthsense
Year Founded: 1996   Federally Qualified: [ ]
Forprofit: [ ]   Not-For-Profit: [ ]
Model Type:
Accreditation: [ ] AAPPO [ ] JACHO [ ] NCQA [ ] URAC
Plan Type: POS, HDHP, HSA
Primary Physicians: 4,455   Physician Specialists:
Hospitals:
Total Enrollment:
  2001: 0   2004: 244,945   2007: 0
  2002: 0   2005:
  2003: 0   2006:

SERVICE AREA:
Nationwide: N
  ID;

TYPE OF COVERAGE:
Commercial: [ ] Individual: [ ] FEHBP: [ ] Indemnity: [ ]
Medicare: [Y] Medicaid: [ ] Supplemental Medicare: [ ]
Tricare   [ ]

PRODUCTS OFFERED:
Product Name:	Type:
Healthsense	POS
Healthsense 65	POS
HealthSense 65 Plus	Medicare Advantage
HealthSense 65 Plus Rx	Medicare Advantage

CONSUMER-DRIVEN PRODUCTS
Wells Fargo	HSA Company
Individual HSA	HSA Product
	HSA Administrator
	Consumer-Driven Health Plan
	High Deductible Health Plan

Comments:
No longer provide HMO-dropped at beginning of year. Only provide POS.

TRUE BLUE

3000 E Pine Ave
Meridian, ID 83642
Phone: 208-395-8200 Fax: 208-387-6811 Toll-Free:
Web site: www.bcidaho.com

MAILING ADDRESS:
TRUE BLUE
PO Box 7408
Meridian, ID 83642

KEY EXECUTIVES:
Chief Executive Officer/President .... Ray Flachbart
Chief Financial Officer .... Jack A Myers
Senior VP & Medical Director .... Douglas Dammrose, MD
Director, Pharmacy Management .... Steve Brocksome
Chief Operating Officer .... Gary M Dyer
Chief Marketing Officer .... Jerry Dworak
VP, Information Systems .... Mike D Cannon

COMPANY PROFILE:
Parent Company Name: Blue Cross of Idaho
Doing Business As:
Year Founded: Federally Qualified: [ ]
Forprofit: [ ]   Not-For-Profit: [Y]
Model Type: IPA
Accreditation: [ ] AAPPO [ ] JACHO [ ] NCQA [ ] URAC
Plan Type: HMO
Total Enrollment:
  2001: 0   2004: 10,889   2007: 0
  2002: 7,742   2005:
  2003: 9,849   2006:
Medical Loss Ratio: 2005:   2006:
Administrative Expense Ratio: 2005:   2006:

SERVICE AREA:
Nationwide:
  ID;

TYPE OF COVERAGE:
Commercial: [ ] Individual: [ ] FEHBP: [ ] Indemnity: [ ]
Medicare: [Y] Medicaid: [ ] Supplemental Medicare: [ ]
Tricare   [ ]

PRODUCTS OFFERED:
Product Name:	Type:
True Blue	Medicare
Workers' Comp: [ ]	

Managed Care Organization Profiles **IDAHO**

BLUE CROSS OF IDAHO

3000 E Pine Ave
Meridian, ID 83707
Phone: 208-345-4550 Fax: 208-331-7311 Toll-Free: 800-274-4018
Web site: www.bcidaho.com
MAILING ADDRESS:
   BLUE CROSS OF IDAHO
   PO Box 7408
   Boise, ID 83707

KEY EXECUTIVES:
Chairman of the Board .... Jack Gustavel
Chief Executive Officer/President .... Raymond Flachbart
Chief Financial Officer .... Jack A Myers
Senior VP & Medical Director .... Douglas Dammrose, MD
Director Pharmacy Management .... Steve Brocksome
Executive Vice President .... Gary M Dyer
Senior VP, Sales & Marketing .... Richard M Armstrong
VP Information Services .... Mike D Cannon
Information Privacy Officer .... Jane Lindsay
Director, Provider Services .... Jeff Crouch
VP, HR & Administration Services .... Debra M Henry
Director Medical/Quality Management .... Mary Jo Kleinfeldt
Director, Dental, Vision, Ancillary .... Carol Rosebrock
Director Internal Audit .... Rod Stiller

COMPANY PROFILE:
Parent Company Name:
Doing Business As:
Year Founded: 1990   Federally Qualified: [ ]
Forprofit: [ ]   Not-For-Profit: [Y]
Model Type: MIXED
Accreditation: [ ] AAPPO [ ] JACHO [ ] NCQA [ ] URAC
Plan Type: PPO, POS, ASO, CDHP, HDHP, HSA,
Primary Physicians: Physician Specialists:
Hospitals: 27
Total Enrollment:
   2001: 303,163   2004: 321,100   2007: 445,000
   2002: 306,109   2005:
   2003: 317,341   2006:

SERVICE AREA:
Nationwide: N
   ID;

TYPE OF COVERAGE:
Commercial: [Y] Individual: [ ] FEHBP: [Y] Indemnity: [ ]
Medicare: [ ] Medicaid: [ ] Supplemental Medicare:
[Y]Tricare   [ ]

PRODUCTS OFFERED:
Product Name: Type:
                                 HMO
Preferred Blue   PPO
Blue Works   Indemnity
True Blue   Medicare
CONSUMER-DRIVEN PRODUCTS
                                 HSA Company
HSA Blue PPO   HSA Product
American Health Value   HSA Administrator
                                 Consumer-Driven Health Plan
                                 High Deductible Health Plan

PLAN BENEFITS:
Alternative Medicine: [ ]   Behavioral Health: [X]
Chiropractic: [X]   Dental: [X]
Home Care: [X]   Inpatient SNF: [X]
Long-Term Care: [X]   Pharm. Mail Order: [X]
Physicial Therapy: [X]   Podiatry: [X]
Psychiatric: [X]   Transplant: [X]
Vision: [X]   Wellness: [X]
Workers' Comp: [ ]
Other Benefits:

DELTA DENTAL PLAN OF IDAHO

555 E Parkcenter Blvd
Boise, ID 83706
Phone: 208-344-4546 Fax: 208-489-3557 Toll-Free: 800-388-3490
Web site: www.deltadentalid.com
MAILING ADDRESS:
   DELTA DENTAL PLAN OF ID
   PO Box 2870
   Boise, ID 83706

KEY EXECUTIVES:
Chief Executive Officer .... Tamara Bramstenner

COMPANY PROFILE:
Parent Company Name: Delta Dental Plan Association
Doing Business As:
Year Founded: 1972   Federally Qualified: [ ]
Forprofit: [ ]   Not-For-Profit: [ ]
Model Type:
Accreditation: [ ] AAPPO [ ] JACHO [ ] NCQA [ ] URAC
Plan Type: Specialty HMO, Specialty PPO
SERVICE AREA:
Nationwide: N
   ID;
TYPE OF COVERAGE:
Commercial: [Y] Individual: [ ] FEHBP: [ ] Indemnity: [ ]
Medicare: [ ] Medicaid: [ ] Supplemental Medicare: [ ]
Tricare   [ ]
PLAN BENEFITS:
Alternative Medicine: [ ]   Behavioral Health: [ ]
Chiropractic: [ ]   Dental: [X]
Home Care: [ ]   Inpatient SNF: [ ]
Long-Term Care: [ ]   Pharm. Mail Order: [ ]
Physicial Therapy: [ ]   Podiatry: [ ]
Psychiatric: [ ]   Transplant: [ ]
Vision: [ ]   Wellness: [ ]
Workers' Comp: [ ]
Other Benefits:

GROUP HEALTH COOPERATIVE

2010 N Lakewood Dr
Coeur D'Alene, ID 83814-2635
Phone: 208-664-5174 Fax: 208-664-9315 Toll-Free: 800-497-2210
Web site: www.ghc.org
MAILING ADDRESS:
   GROUP HEALTH COOPERATIVE
   2010 N Lakewood Dr
   Coeur D'Alene, ID 83814-2635

KEY EXECUTIVES:
Chief Executive Officer/President .... Scott Armstrong
Chief Financial Officer .... Richard Magnuson
Medical Director .... Hugh Straley, MD
Pharmacy Director .... Kim Orchard RPh
Chief Marketing Officer .... Maureen McLaughlin
Public Relations Director .... Pam MacEwan
VP & General Counsel .... Rick Woods

COMPANY PROFILE:
Parent Company Name: Group Health Cooperative
Doing Business As:
Year Founded: 1977   Federally Qualified: [Y]
Forprofit: [ ]   Not-For-Profit: [Y]
Model Type: MIXED
Accreditation: [ ] AAPPO [ ] JACHO [X] NCQA [ ] URAC
Plan Type: HMO, POS
SERVICE AREA:
Nationwide: N
   ID; WA;
TYPE OF COVERAGE:
Commercial: [Y] Individual: [Y] FEHBP: [ ] Indemnity: [ ]
Medicare: [Y] Medicaid: [Y] Supplemental Medicare: [ ]
Tricare   [ ]
PLAN BENEFITS:
Alternative Medicine: [ ]   Behavioral Health: [X]
Chiropractic: [X]   Dental: [ ]
Home Care: [X]   Inpatient SNF: [X]
Long-Term Care: [ ]   Pharm. Mail Order: [ ]
Physicial Therapy: [X]   Podiatry: [X]
Psychiatric: [X]   Transplant: [X]
Vision: [X]   Wellness: [X]
Workers' Comp: [ ]
Other Benefits:
Comments:
Formerly Group Health Northwest.

Managed Care Organization Profiles HAWAII

COMPANY PROFILE:
Parent Company Name:
Doing Business As:
Year Founded: 1988 Federally Qualified: [N]
Forprofit: [ ] Not-For-Profit: [ ]
Model Type: NETWORK
Accreditation: [ ] AAPPO [ ] JACHO [ ] NCQA [X] URAC
Plan Type: PPO
Total Revenue: 2005: 83,691,555 2006: 47,331,954
Net Income 2005: 2006:
Total Enrollment:
   2001: 0 2004: 31,047 2007: 40,000
   2002: 0 2005: 35,972
   2003: 0 2006: 37,247

SERVICE AREA:
Nationwide:
   HI;

TYPE OF COVERAGE:
Commercial: [Y] Individual: [ ] FEHBP: [ ] Indemnity: [ ]
Medicare: [ ] Medicaid: [ ] Supplemental Medicare: [ ]
Tricare [ ]

PLAN BENEFITS:
Alternative Medicine: [X] Behavioral Health: [X]
Chiropractic: [X] Dental: [ ]
Home Care: [X] Inpatient SNF: [X]
Long-Term Care: [ ] Pharm. Mail Order: [ ]
Physical Therapy: [X] Podiatry: [X]
Psychiatric: [X] Transplant: [X]
Vision: [ ] Wellness: [X]
Workers' Comp: [ ]
Other Benefits:

Comments:
Mutual Benefit Society.

HAWAII

KEY EXECUTIVES:
Regional President .... Janice L Head
Chief Financial Officer .... Dave Delaney
VP, Marketing/Brands/Public Affairs .... Bill Corba
Human Resources .... Winona White

COMPANY PROFILE:
Parent Company Name: Kaiser Permanente
Doing Business As:
Year Founded: Federally Qualified: [Y]
Forprofit: [ ]   Not-For-Profit: [Y]
Model Type: MIXED
Accreditation: [ ] AAPPO [ ] JACHO [ ] NCQA [ ] URAC
Plan Type: HMO, HDHP, HSA
Total Revenue: 2005:   2006: 217,100,000
Net Income   2005:   2006: 1,500,000
Total Enrollment:
  2001: 220,261   2004: 231,179   2007: 219,000
  2002: 233,646   2005: 226,653
  2003: 235,192   2006: 225,000

SERVICE AREA:
Nationwide: N
HI;

TYPE OF COVERAGE:
Commercial: [ ] Individual: [ ] FEHBP: [ ] Indemnity: [ ]
Medicare: [Y] Medicaid: [ ] Supplemental Medicare: [ ]
Tricare   [ ]

PRODUCTS OFFERED:
Product Name:	Type:
Permanente Senior Adantage	Medicare Advantage
Kaiser Permanente	Medicaid
Kaiser HMO	HMO

MDX HAWAII

500 Ala Moana Blvd Ste 2-200
Honolulu, HI 96813
Phone: 808-522-7560 Fax: 808-522-7561 Toll-Free:
Web site: www.mdxhawaii.com
MAILING ADDRESS:
  MDX HAWAII
  500 Ala Moana Blvd Ste 2-200
  Honolulu, HI 96813

KEY EXECUTIVES:
Chief Executive Officer .... Rick Jackson
Account Manager .... Evelyn Misech
Medical Director .... Ron Morton, MD
Director, Operations .... Jeff Kakuno
MIS Manager .... Bruce Kan
Manager, Provider Services .... Jodi Lining
Medical Management Director .... Susan Ellis, RN

COMPANY PROFILE:
Parent Company Name: Medical Data Exchange
Doing Business As:
Year Founded: 1985   Federally Qualified: [N]
Forprofit: [Y]   Not-For-Profit: [ ]
Model Type: MIXED
Accreditation: [ ] AAPPO [ ] JACHO [ ] NCQA [ ] URAC
Plan Type: TPA
Primary Physicians: 840   Physician Specialists:
Hospitals: 24
Total Enrollment:
  2001: 16,000   2004: 0   2007: 0
  2002: 0   2005:
  2003: 25,000   2006:

SERVICE AREA:
Nationwide: N
HI;

TYPE OF COVERAGE:
Commercial: [Y] Individual: [ ] FEHBP: [ ] Indemnity: [ ]
Medicare: [ ] Medicaid: [ ] Supplemental Medicare: [ ]
Tricare   [ ]

PRODUCTS OFFERED:
Product Name:	Type:
Queen's Hawaii Care	Medicaid
Queen's Hawaii Care HMO	HMO

PLAN BENEFITS:
Alternative Medicine:	[ ]	Behavioral Health:	[X]
Chiropractic:	[ ]	Dental:	[ ]
Home Care:	[X]	Inpatient SNF:	[X]
Long-Term Care:	[ ]	Pharm. Mail Order:	[X]
Physical Therapy:	[X]	Podiatry:	[ ]
Psychiatric:	[X]	Transplant:	[X]
Vision:	[X]	Wellness:	[X]
Workers' Comp:	[ ]		
Other Benefits: X			

Comments:
Formerly Queens Island Care.

SUMMERLINE LIFE & HEALTH INSURANCE COMPANY

1440 Kapiolani Blvd Ste 1020
Honolulu, HI 96814
Phone: 808-951-4645 Fax: 866-206-5689 Toll-Free:
Web site: www.summerlinlifeandhealth.com
MAILING ADDRESS:
  SUMMERLINE LIFE & HEALTH INS C
  1440 Kapiolani Blvd Ste 1020
  Honolulu, HI 96814

KEY EXECUTIVES:
Chairman/Chief Executive Officer .... James D Dyer

COMPANY PROFILE:
Parent Company Name: i/mx Company, The
Doing Business As:
Year Founded: 2004   Federally Qualified: [N]
Forprofit: [ ]   Not-For-Profit: [ ]
Model Type:
Accreditation: [ ] AAPPO [ ] JACHO [ ] NCQA [ ] URAC
Plan Type: PPO
Total Enrollment:
  2001: 0   2004: 0   2007: 0
  2002: 0   2005: 3,733
  2003: 0   2006:

SERVICE AREA:
Nationwide:
HI;

TYPE OF COVERAGE:
Commercial: [Y] Individual: [ ] FEHBP: [ ] Indemnity: [ ]
Medicare: [ ] Medicaid: [Y] Supplemental Medicare: [ ]
Tricare   [ ]

PLAN BENEFITS:
Alternative Medicine:	[ ]	Behavioral Health:	[X]
Chiropractic:	[X]	Dental:	[X]
Home Care:	[X]	Inpatient SNF:	[X]
Long-Term Care:	[X]	Pharm. Mail Order:	[X]
Physical Therapy:	[X]	Podiatry:	[X]
Psychiatric:	[X]	Transplant:	[X]
Vision:	[X]	Wellness:	[X]
Workers' Comp:	[X]		
Other Benefits:			

UNIVERSITY HEALTH ALLIANCE

Topa Fin Ctr, 700 Bishop St
Honolulu, HI 96813-4100
Phone: 808-532-4000 Fax: 808-522-8894 Toll-Free:
Web site: www.uhahealth.com
MAILING ADDRESS:
  UNIVERSITY HEALTH ALLIANCE
  Topa Fin Ctr 700 Bishop St 300
  Honolulu, HI 96813-4100

KEY EXECUTIVES:
Chairman .... Max G Botticelli, MD
Chief Executive Officer/President .... Max G Botticelli, MD
Chief Financial Officer .... Charles Murray
Chief Medical Officer .... Richard Ridao, MD
Chief Information Officer .... Chad Lee
VP,Chief Operating Officer .... Howard KF Lee
Chief Marketing Officer/Administrative Secretary .... Linda Kalahiki

Managed Care Organization Profiles **HAWAII**

ALOHACARE

1357 Kapiolani Blvd Ste 1250
Honolulu, HI 96814
Phone: 808-973-6395 Fax: Toll-Free:
Web site: www.alohacarehawaii.org
MAILING ADDRESS:
  ALOHACARE
  1357 Kapiolani Blvd Ste 1250
  Honolulu, HI 96814

KEY EXECUTIVES:
Chief Executive Officer .... John E McComas
Medical Director .... Rio Banner, MD
Marketing/Public Relations Coordinator .... Noe Foster

COMPANY PROFILE:
Parent Company Name:
Doing Business As: AlohaCare, Quest Health Plan
Year Founded: Federally Qualified: [ ]
Forprofit: [ ]   Not-For-Profit: [Y]
Model Type:
Accreditation: [ ] AAPPO [ ] JACHO [ ] NCQA [ ] URAC
Plan Type: HMO
Total Enrollment:
  2001: 0   2004: 0   2007: 0
  2002: 0   2005: 31,937
  2003: 0   2006: 50,000

SERVICE AREA:
Nationwide:
  HI;

TYPE OF COVERAGE:
Commercial: [ ] Individual: [ ] FEHBP: [ ] Indemnity: [ ]
Medicare: [Y] Medicaid: [Y] Supplemental Medicare: [ ]
Tricare   [ ]

PRODUCTS OFFERED:
Product Name: Type:
AlohaCare   Medicare QUEST
AlohaCare Advantage   Medicare Advantage
AlohaCare Advantage Plus   Medicare Advantage

HAWAII MANAGEMENT ALLIANCE ASSOCIATION

737 Bishop St Ste 1200
Honolulu, HI 96813
Phone: 808-591-0088 Fax: 808-591-0463 Toll-Free:
Web site: www.hmaa.com
MAILING ADDRESS:
  HAWAII MANAGEMENT ALLIANCE ASSOCIATION
  737 Bishop St Ste 1200
  Honolulu, HI 96813

KEY EXECUTIVES:
President .... Arnie Baptiste

COMPANY PROFILE:
Parent Company Name:
Doing Business As:
Year Founded: 1989   Federally Qualified: [ ]
Forprofit: [ ]   Not-For-Profit: [ ]
Model Type:
Accreditation: [ ] AAPPO [ ] JACHO [ ] NCQA [ ] URAC
Plan Type: PPO,
Total Enrollment:
  2001: 0   2004: 0   2007: 0
  2002: 0   2005: 31,937
  2003: 0   2006:

SERVICE AREA:
Nationwide:
  HI;

PRODUCTS OFFERED:
Product Name: Type:
Option Plus One
Option Plus Two
Prescription Drug
Vision

HAWAII MEDICAL SERVICES ASSOCIATION - BC/BS OF HAWAII

818 Keeaumoku St
Honolulu, HI 96814
Phone: 808-948-6297 Fax: 808-948-5567 Toll-Free: 800-648-3190
Web site: www.hmsa.com
MAILING ADDRESS:
  HAWAII MEDICAL SERVICES ASSOCIATION
  PO Box 860
  Honolulu, HI 96814

KEY EXECUTIVES:
Chairman of the Board .... Allan R Lanoon
Chief Eecutive Officer/President .... Robert P Hiam
Exec VP, Chief Financial Officer .... Steve Van Ribbink
VP Medical Director .... John T Berthiaume, MD
SVP &Chief Information Officer .... Gordon R Hilton
Exec VP,Chief Operating Officer .... Michael A Gold
VP, Marketing .... John L Jacobs
VP, Provider Services .... James P Walsh
Health Services .... Myra L Williams
VP, Human Resources .... Michael WC Wong
VP, Medical Management .... William J Osheroff, MD
Compliance & Ethics Officer .... Norman S Matthews, Jr
VP, Corporate Communications .... Michael B Stoller

COMPANY PROFILE:
Parent Company Name: Hawaii Medical Service Association
Doing Business As:
Year Founded: 1938   Federally Qualified: [Y]
Forprofit: [ ]   Not-For-Profit: [Y]
Model Type:
Accreditation: [ ] AAPPO [ ] JACHO [X] NCQA [ ] URAC
Plan Type: HMO, PPO, POS, TPA
Total Revenue: 2005:   2006: 452,600,000
Net Income   2005:   2006: -7,200,000
Total Enrollment:
  2001: 629,329   2004: 692,786   2007: 0
  2002: 668,493   2005: 707,100
  2003: 677,140   2006: 557,900

SERVICE AREA:
Nationwide: N
  HI;

TYPE OF COVERAGE:
Commercial: [Y] Individual: [Y] FEHBP: [ ] Indemnity: [ ]
Medicare: [Y] Medicaid: [Y] Supplemental Medicare: [Y]
Tricare   [ ]

PRODUCTS OFFERED:
Product Name: Type:
Health Plan Hawaii   HMO
Preferred Provider   PPO
65C Plus Plan   Medicare Advantage
HMSA Medicaid   Medicaid

PLAN BENEFITS:
Alternative Medicine: [ ]   Behavioral Health: [ ]
Chiropractic: [X]   Dental: [X]
Home Care: [X]   Inpatient SNF: [X]
Long-Term Care: [X]   Pharm. Mail Order: [X]
Physical Therapy: [X]   Podiatry: [X]
Psychiatric: [X]   Transplant: [X]
Vision: [X]   Wellness: [X]
Workers' Comp: [ ]
Other Benefits:

KAISER PERMANENTE HEALTH PLAN

711 Kapiolani Blvd
Honolulu, HI 96813-5249
Phone: 808-432-5955 Fax: 808-983-4989 Toll-Free:
Web site: www.kaiserpermanente.org
MAILING ADDRESS:
  KAISER PERMANENTE HEALTH PLAN
  711 Kapiolani Blvd
  Honolulu, HI 96813-5249

STAYWELL INSURANCE GUAM INC

430 West Soledad Ave
Hagatna, GU 96910
Phone: 671-477-5091 Fax: 671-477-5096 Toll-Free:
Web site: www.staywellguam.com

MAILING ADDRESS:
STAYWELL INSURANCE GUAM INC
430 West Soledad Ave
Hagatna, GU 96910

KEY EXECUTIVES:
Acting Chief Executive Officer/President .... Maria D R Taitano
Chief Financial Officer/Administrator . Taling M Taitano, CPA, CGFM
Medical Director/Assoc Admin .... Lee G Saltzgaber, MD, MPH, CPE

COMPANY PROFILE:
Parent Company Name:
Doing Business As:
Year Founded: 1982   Federally Qualified: [ ]
Forprofit: [ ]   Not-For-Profit: []
Model Type:
Accreditation: [ ] AAPPO [ ] JACHO [ ] NCQA [ ] URAC
Plan Type: PPO
Total Enrollment:
  2001: 0   2004: 0   2007: 0
  2002: 0   2005:
  2003: 0   2006: 30,000

SERVICE AREA:
Nationwide:
  Guam; Commonwealth Northern Mariana Islands;

Comments:
Backed by Zurich Insurance Company.

GEORGIA

MAILING ADDRESS:
SECURE HEALTH PLANS OF GEORGIA
PO Box 4088
Macon, GA 31210

KEY EXECUTIVES:
Chief Executive Officer .... Rob Morton
Director of IS and Finance .... Cindy Tidwell
Medical Director .... Sharon Ash, MD
Director of Operations .... Karen Manning
Director of Sales & Marketing .... Sam Macfie
Human Resources .... Cherry Carr
Director of Health Services .... Laura Hart

COMPANY PROFILE:
Parent Company Name:
Doing Business As:
Year Founded: 1992   Federally Qualified: [N]
Forprofit: [Y]   Not-For-Profit: [ ]
Model Type:
Accreditation: [ ] AAPPO [ ] JACHO [ ] NCQA [ ] URAC
Plan Type: PPO, POS, EPO, TPA, UR
Primary Physicians: 320   Physician Specialists:
Hospitals: 21
Total Enrollment:
  2001: 0   2004: 0   2007: 0
  2002: 29,000   2005:
  2003: 0   2006:

SERVICE AREA:
Nationwide: N
  GA (Baldwin, Bibb, Bleckley, Crawford, Crisp, Dodge, Dooly, Hancock, Houston, Jasper, Jones, Lamar, Laurens, Macon, Monroe, Peach, Pike, Pulaski, Putnam, Taylor, Twiggs, Upson, Washington, Wilcox, Wilkinson, Worth);

TYPE OF COVERAGE:
Commercial: [Y] Individual: [ ] FEHBP: [ ] Indemnity: [ ]
Medicare: [ ] Medicaid: [Y] Supplemental Medicare: [ ]
Tricare   [ ]

PLAN BENEFITS:
Alternative Medicine: [ ]   Behavioral Health: [X]
Chiropractic: [X]   Dental: [ ]
Home Care: [ ]   Inpatient SNF: [ ]
Long-Term Care: [ ]   Pharm. Mail Order: [X]
Physical Therapy: [ ]   Podiatry: [ ]
Psychiatric: [X]   Transplant: [ ]
Vision: [ ]   Wellness: [X]
Workers' Comp: [X]
Other Benefits:

SOUTHCARE/HEALTHCARE PREFERRED

1100 Circle 75 Pkwy Ste 1400
Atlanta, GA 30339
Phone: 678-202-2100 Fax: 678-202-2193 Toll-Free: 800-470-2004
Web site: www.southcareppo.com

MAILING ADDRESS:
SOUTHCARE/HEALTHCARE PREFERRED
1100 Circle 75 Pkwy Ste 1400
Atlanta, GA 30339

KEY EXECUTIVES:
Chief Executive Officer .... Thomas A Davis
Chief Financial Officer .... Paul Farrell
Medical Director .... Bernie Cohen, MD
Chief Operating Officer .... Marc Malloy
Marketing Director .... Cory Scott

COMPANY PROFILE:
Parent Company Name: Coventry Health Care Inc
Doing Business As:
Year Founded: 1987   Federally Qualified: [ ]
Forprofit: [Y]   Not-For-Profit: [ ]
Model Type:
Accreditation: [ ] AAPPO [ ] JACHO [ ] NCQA [ ] URAC
Plan Type: PPO, UR

SERVICE AREA:
Nationwide: N
  AL; DE; FL; GA; IA; IL; KS; MD; MO; NC; NE; NJ; PA; SC; SD; TN;

TYPE OF COVERAGE:
Commercial: [Y] Individual: [ ] FEHBP: [ ] Indemnity:[ ]
Medicare: [ ] Medicaid: [ ] Supplemental Medicare: [ ]
Tricare [ ]

PLAN BENEFITS:
Alternative Medicine: [ ]   Behavioral Health: [ ]
Chiropractic: [X]   Dental: [ ]
Home Care: [ ]   Inpatient SNF: [ ]
Long-Term Care: [ ]   Pharm. Mail Order: [ ]
Physical Therapy: [ ]   Podiatry: [ ]
Psychiatric: [ ]   Transplant: [ ]
Vision: [ ]   Wellness: [X]
Workers' Comp: [X]
Other Benefits:

UNITEDHEALTHCARE OF GEORGIA

3720 DaVinci Ct Ste 300
Norcross, GA 30092
Phone: 770-300-3501 Fax: 770-300-4362 Toll-Free: 800-842-6219
Web site: www.uhc.com

MAILING ADDRESS:
UNITEDHEALTHCARE OF GEORGIA
3720 DaVinci Ct Ste 300
Norcross, GA 30092

KEY EXECUTIVES:
Non-Executive Chairman .... Richard T Burke
Chief Executive Officer/President .... Dan L Ohman
Chief Financial Officer .... Robert Friedrichs
Medical Director .... Catherine L Palmier, MD
Executive Director/Chief Operating Officer .... Cindy Follmer
Marketing Director .... Jamie Holt
Public Relations Director .... Roger Rollman
Network/Contracts Officer .... Victoria Wachowiak

COMPANY PROFILE:
Parent Company Name: UnitedHealth Group
Doing Business As:
Year Founded: 1985   Federally Qualified: [N]
Forprofit: [Y]   Not-For-Profit: [ ]
Model Type: IPA
Accreditation: [ ] AAPPO [ ] JACHO [X] NCQA [ ] URAC
Plan Type: HMO, PPO, POS, ASO, CDHP, HDHP, HSA, HRA
Total Enrollment:
  2001: 0   2004: 54,266   2007: 0
  2002: 79,171   2005:
  2003: 55,701   2006:
Medical Loss Ratio: 2005:   2006: 81.60
Administrative Expense Ratio: 2005:   2006:

SERVICE AREA:
Nationwide: N
  GA (Baker, Banks, Bartow, Bibb, Bleckley, Bryan, Bulloch, Butts, Calhoun, Carroll, Chatham, Chattahoochee, Chattooga, Cherokee, Clay, Clayton, Cobb, Columbia, Coweta, Crawford, Dawson, DeKalb, Dooly, Dougherty, Douglas, Effingham, Fayette, Floyd, Forsyth, Fulton, Gordon, Gwinnett, Hall, Haralson, Harris, Heard, Henry, Houston, Jones, Lamar, Lee, Liberty, Marion, Meriwether, Mitchell, Monroe, Muscogee, Newton, Paulding, Pickens, Pike, Polk, Pulaski, Quitman, Randolph, Richmond, Rockdale, Spalding, Stewart, Talbot, Terrell, Twiggs, Walton, Webster, Wilcox, Worth);

TYPE OF COVERAGE:
Commercial: [Y] Individual: [ ] FEHBP: [ ] Indemnity: [ ]
Medicare: [ ] Medicaid: [ ] Supplemental Medicare: [ ]
Tricare   [ ]

PRODUCTS OFFERED:
Product Name: Type:
PPO of Georgia   PPO
United for Seniors   Medicare
United Healthcare of GA   HMO

CONSUMER-DRIVEN PRODUCTS
Exante Bank/Golden Rule Ins Co   HSA Company
iPlan HSA   HSA Product
                                   HSA Administrator
                                   Consumer-Driven Health Plan
                                   High Deductible Health Plan

PLAN BENEFITS:
Alternative Medicine: [ ]   Behavioral Health: [X]
Chiropractic: [X]   Dental: [X]
Home Care: [X]   Inpatient SNF: [X]
Long-Term Care: [ ]   Pharm. Mail Order: [X]
Physical Therapy: [X]   Podiatry: [X]
Psychiatric: [X]   Transplant: [X]
Vision: [X]   Wellness: [X]
Workers' Comp: [ ]
Other Benefits:

Managed Care Organization Profiles **GEORGIA**

Doing Business As:
Year Founded: Federally Qualified: [ ]
Forprofit: [Y]   Not-For-Profit: [ ]
Model Type:
Accreditation: [ ] AAPPO [ ] JACHO [ ] NCQA [ ] URAC
Plan Type: Specialty HMO, Specialty PPO, POS
SERVICE AREA:
Nationwide: N
  GA;
TYPE OF COVERAGE:
Commercial: [Y] Individual: [ ] FEHBP: [ ] Indemnity: [ ]
Medicare: [ ] Medicaid: [ ] Supplemental Medicare: [ ]
Tricare   [ ]

PEACH STATE HEALTH PLAN

3200 Highlands Pkwy SE Ste 300
Smyrna, GA 30082
Phone: 678-556-2300 Fax: Toll-Free:
Web site: www.pshgeorgia.com
MAILING ADDRESS:
   PEACH STATE HEALTH PLAN
   3200 Highlands Pkwy SE Ste 300
   Smyrna, GA 30082

KEY EXECUTIVES:
Chief Executive Officer/President .... Michael Cadger
Chief Financial Officer .... Scott Foster
Interim VP, Medical Affairs .... Anthony Newell, MD
VP, Operations .... Jonna Kirkwood
VP, Member & Provider Services .... Debra Peterson-Smith
VP, Medical Management .... Jacqueline Jones
Director of Government Affairs .... Diane Hutchins

COMPANY PROFILE:
Parent Company Name:
Doing Business As:
Year Founded: 2006   Federally Qualified: [ ]
Forprofit: [ ]   Not-For-Profit: [ ]
Model Type:
Accreditation: [ ] AAPPO [ ] JACHO [ ] NCQA [ ] URAC
Plan Type: HMO
Medical Loss Ratio: 2005:   2006: 84.40
Administrative Expense Ratio: 2005:   2006:
SERVICE AREA:
Nationwide:
  GA (Atkinson, Baker, Baldwin, Barrow, Bartow, Ben Hill, Berrien,
  Bibb, Bleckley, Brooks, Butts, Calhoun, Carroll, Chattahoochee,
  Cherokee, Clay, Clayton, Clinch, Cobb, Coffee, Colquitt, Cook,
  Coweta, Crawford, Crisp, Decatur, DeKalb, Dodge, Dooly,
  Dougherty, Douglas, Early, Echols, Fayette, Forsyth, Fulton, Grady,
  Gwinnett, Haralson, Harris, Heard, Henry, Houston, Irwin, Jasper,
  Johnson, Jones, Lamar, Lanier, Lee, Lowndes, Macon, Marion,
  Meriwether, Miller, Mitchell, Monroe, Muscogee, Newton,
  Paulding, Peach, Pickens, Pike, Pulaski, Quitman, Randolph,
  Rockdale, Schley, Seminole, Spalding, Stewart, Sumter, Talbot,
  Telfair, Terrell, Thomas, Tift, Treutlen, Troup, Turner, Twiggs,
  Upson, Walton, Webster, Wheeler, Wilcox, Wilkinson, Worth);
TYPE OF COVERAGE:
Commercial: [ ] Individual: [ ] FEHBP: [ ] Indemnity: [ ]
Medicare: [ ] Medicaid: [Y] Supplemental Medicare: [ ]
Tricare   [ ]

PHOEBE HEALTH PARTNERS

306 Third Ave
Albany, GA 31701
Phone: 229-312-8061 Fax: 229-312-8068 Toll-Free: 800-474-6323
Web site: www.phoebehealthpartners.com
MAILING ADDRESS:
   PHOEBE HEALTH PARTNERS
   PO Box 1828
   Albany, GA 31701

KEY EXECUTIVES:
Executive Director .... Pat Sumner, RN
Chief Financial Officer .... Kerry Loudermilk
Medical Director .... Frank F Middleton, III, MD
Sales & Marketing Manager .... Gail Korpal
Sales & Marketing Manager .... Sharon Gross
Credentialing Specialist .... Charis Phelps, CPCS
Manager, Provider Relations .... Lisa Hamslay, RN

COMPANY PROFILE:
Parent Company Name: Phoebe Health Partners Inc
Doing Business As:
Year Founded: 1995   Federally Qualified: [ ]
Forprofit: [ ]   Not-For-Profit: [Y]
Model Type: PHO
Accreditation: [ ] AAPPO [ ] JACHO [ ] NCQA [X] URAC
Plan Type: PPO
Primary Physicians: 176   Physician Specialists:
Hospitals: 11
Total Enrollment:
   2001: 0   2004: 0   2007: 0
   2002: 0   2005: 67,300
   2003: 0   2006: 70,000
SERVICE AREA:
Nationwide: N
  GA (Albany);
TYPE OF COVERAGE:
Commercial: [Y] Individual: [ ] FEHBP: [ ] Indemnity: [ ]
Medicare: [ ] Medicaid: [ ] Supplemental Medicare: [ ]
Tricare   [ ]
PLAN BENEFITS:
Alternative Medicine: [ ]   Behavioral Health: [X]
Chiropractic: [ ]   Dental: [ ]
Home Care: [X]   Inpatient SNF: [X]
Long-Term Care: [ ]   Pharm. Mail Order: [ ]
Physical Therapy: [X]   Podiatry: [X]
Psychiatric: [X]   Transplant: [ ]
Vision: [X]   Wellness: [X]
Workers' Comp: [ ]
Other Benefits:
Comments:
Formerly Health Choice of Georgia.

PRIVATE HEALTHCARE SYSTEMS - GEORGIA

5660 New Northside Dr Ste 700
Atlanta, GA 30328
Phone: 770-818-9048 Fax: 770-818-9101 Toll-Free: 800-253-4417
Web site: www.phcs.com
MAILING ADDRESS:
   PRIVATE HEALTHCARE SYSTEMS-GA
   1100 Winter St
   Waltham, MA 30328

KEY EXECUTIVES:
Chief Executive Officer .... Mark Tabak

COMPANY PROFILE:
Parent Company Name: MultiPlan Inc
Doing Business As:
Year Founded: 1986   Federally Qualified: [N]
Forprofit: [Y]   Not-For-Profit: [ ]
Model Type:
Accreditation: [ ] AAPPO [ ] JACHO [X] NCQA [X] URAC
Plan Type: PPO, UR, POS
SERVICE AREA:
Nationwide: N
  NW;
TYPE OF COVERAGE:
Commercial: [Y] Individual: [ ] FEHBP: [ ] Indemnity: [ ]
Medicare: [ ] Medicaid: [ ] Supplemental Medicare: [ ]
Tricare
PLAN BENEFITS:
Alternative Medicine: [X]   Behavioral Health: [X]
Chiropractic: [X]   Dental: [ ]
Home Care: [X]   Inpatient SNF: [X]
Long-Term Care: [X]   Pharm. Mail Order: [X]
Physical Therapy: [X]   Podiatry: [X]
Psychiatric: [X]   Transplant: [X]
Vision: [X]   Wellness: [ ]
Workers' Comp: [X]
Other Benefits: X
Comments:
Acquired by MultiPlan, Inc. on October 18, 2006.

SECURE HEALTH PLANS OF GEORGIA LLC

3920 Arkwright Rd Ste 405
Macon, GA 31210
Phone: 478-314-2400 Fax: 478-314-2428 Toll-Free: 800-648-7563
Web site: www.shpg.com

GEORGIA

Managed Care Organization Profiles

PLAN BENEFITS:
Alternative Medicine:	[X]	Behavioral Health:	[X]
Chiropractic:	[X]	Dental:	[X]
Home Care:	[X]	Inpatient SNF:	[X]
Long-Term Care:	[X]	Pharm. Mail Order:	[X]
Physical Therapy:	[X]	Podiatry:	[X]
Psychiatric:	[X]	Transplant:	[X]
Vision:	[X]	Wellness:	[X]
Workers' Comp:	[ ]		

Other Benefits:
Comments:
Acquired by CIGNA Inc April 1, 2008.

HUMANA HEALTH PLANS OF GEORGIA

900 Ashwood Pkwy Ste 400
Atlanta, GA 30338
Phone: 770-393-9226 Fax: 770-393-2845 Toll-Free: 800-234-3486
Web site: www.humana.com/georgia/home.html

MAILING ADDRESS:
HUMANA HEALTH PLANS OF GA
900 Ashwood Pkwy Ste 400
Atlanta, GA 30338

KEY EXECUTIVES:
Chairman of the Board .... David A Jones Jr
Chief Executive Officer .... Michael B McCallister
Market President .... Dan Feruck
President .... Greg Powell
Dental Director .... Alan Wood
Marketing Director- Small Group .... John Dammon
Vice President of Sales .... Jillian M Frenkel
Commerical Market President .... Dan Feruck

COMPANY PROFILE:
Parent Company Name: Humana Inc
Doing Business As:
Year Founded: 1961   Federally Qualified: [Y]
Forprofit: [Y]   Not-For-Profit: [ ]
Model Type: IPA
Accreditation: [ ] AAPPO [ ] JACHO [ ] NCQA [ ] URAC
Plan Type: HMO, PPO, POS, ASO, CDHP, HSA
Total Enrollment:
    2001: 66,233   2004: 18,380   2007: 0
    2002: 0   2005:
    2003: 330,800   2006: 500,000
Medical Loss Ratio: 2005:   2006: 73.30
Administrative Expense Ratio: 2005:   2006:

SERVICE AREA:
Nationwide: N
GA (Barrow, Bartow, Cherokee, Clayton, Cobb, Coweta, DeKalb, Douglas, Fayette, Fulton, Gwinnett, Henry, Newton, Paulding, Rockdale);

TYPE OF COVERAGE:
Commercial: [Y] Individual: [Y] FEHBP: [ ] Indemnity: [ ]
Medicare: [Y] Medicaid: [ ] Supplemental Medicare: [Y]
Tricare [Y]

PRODUCTS OFFERED:
Product Name:	Type:
Humana HMO	HMO
Humana PPO	PPO

CONSUMER-DRIVEN PRODUCTS
JP Morgan Chase	HSA Company
HumanaOne HSA	HSA Product
JP Morgan Chase	HSA Administrator
Personal Care Account	Consumer-Driven Health Plan
HumanaOne	High Deductible Health Plan

PLAN BENEFITS:
Alternative Medicine:	[ ]	Behavioral Health:	
[X]Chiropractic:	[X]	Dental:	[X]
Home Care:	[ ]	Inpatient SNF:	[ ]
Long-Term Care:	[ ]	Pharm. Mail Order:	[X]
Physical Therapy:	[ ]	Podiatry:	[ ]
Psychiatric:	[X]	Transplant:	[X]
Vision:	[ ]	Wellness:	[ ]
Workers' Comp:	[X]		

Other Benefits: Long Term Disability

KAISER FOUNDATION HEALTH PLAN OF GEORGIA

3495 Piedmont Rd NE Bldg 9
Atlanta, GA 30305-1736
Phone: 404-364-7000 Fax: 404-364-4791 Toll-Free:
Web site: www.kaiserpermanente.org

MAILING ADDRESS:
KAISER FOUNDATION HEALTH PLAN OF GA
3495 Piedmont Rd NE Bldg 9
Atlanta, GA 30305-1736

KEY EXECUTIVES:
Chief Executive Officer/President .... Carolyn Kenny
VP of Finance .... Merrill Boone
Medical Director .... Bruce Perry MD, MPH
Pharmacy Director .... Adrienne Washington
Regional Chief Information Officer .... Larry Panatera
Public Affairs Director .... Beverly Thomas
Director, Provider Relations .... Lourdes Quinones
VP of Human Resources .... Tammy Jones

COMPANY PROFILE:
Parent Company Name: Kaiser Permanente
Doing Business As:
Year Founded: 1985   Federally Qualified: [Y]
Forprofit: [ ]   Not-For-Profit: [Y]
Model Type: GROUP
Accreditation: [ ] AAPPO [ ] JACHO [X] NCQA [ ] URAC
Plan Type: HMO, POS, HSA
Total Enrollment:
    2001: 0   2004: 275,458   2007: 283,001
    2002: 275,458   2005: 279,394
    2003: 275,458   2006: 268,000
Medical Loss Ratio: 2005:   2006: 93.30
Administrative Expense Ratio: 2005:   2006:

SERVICE AREA:
Nationwide: N
GA (Barrow, Bartow, Butts, Cherokee, Clayton, Cobb, Coweta, DeKalb, Douglas, Fayette, Forsyth, Fulton, Hall, Gwinnett, Henry, Newton, Paulding, Rockdale, Spalding, Walton);

TYPE OF COVERAGE:
Commercial: [Y] Individual: [Y] FEHBP: [ ] Indemnity: [ ]
Medicare: [Y] Medicaid: [ ] Supplemental Medicare: [ ]
Tricare [ ]

PRODUCTS OFFERED:
Product Name:	Type:
Kaiser Foundation Health Plan	HMO
Senior Advantage	Medicare

CONSUMER-DRIVEN PRODUCTS
Wells Fargo	HSA Company
Carepay HSA	HSA Product
	HSA Administrator
	Consumer-Driven Health Plan
	High Deductible Health Plan

PLAN BENEFITS:
Alternative Medicine:	[ ]	Behavioral Health:	[ ]
Chiropractic:	[ ]	Dental:	[ ]
Home Care:	[X]	Inpatient SNF:	[ ]
Long-Term Care:	[ ]	Pharm. Mail Order:	[ ]
Physical Therapy:	[ ]	Podiatry:	[X]
Psychiatric:	[X]	Transplant:	[X]
Vision:	[X]	Wellness:	[X]
Workers' Comp:	[ ]		

Other Benefits:

MAGELLAN HEALTH SERVICES

125 Plantation Center Dr
Macon, GA 31210
Phone: 478-405-7943 Fax: 478-474-9065 Toll-Free:
Web site: www.magellanhealth.com

MAILING ADDRESS:
MAGELLAN HEALTH SERVICES
125 Plantation Center Dr
Macon, GA 31210

KEY EXECUTIVES:
Chairman of the Board/Chief Executive Officer .... Steven J Shulman
President .... Rene Lerer, MD
Executive VP/Chief Financial Officer .... Mark S Demilio
Chief Medical Officer, Chief Marketing Officer .. Anthony M Kotin, MD
Chief Information Officer .... Jeff D Emerson
Chief Operating Officer .... Russell C Petrella, PhD
VP Corporate Communications .... Jody Buffington
Executive VP, Chief Clinical Officer .... Clarissa C Marques, PhD
Chief Human Resources Director .... Caskie Lewis-Clapper, MS
Senior VP Corporate Medical Director .... Alan M Elkins, MD
President/Health Plan Solutions .... Dennis Moody, MBA

COMPANY PROFILE:
Parent Company Name: Magellan Health Services Inc

Managed Care Organization Profiles **GEORGIA**

DELTA DENTAL INSURANCE COMPANY - GEORGIA

1000 Mansell Exchn W B100 #100
Alpharetta, GA 30022
Phone: 770-645-8700 Fax: 770-518-4757 Toll-Free: 800-521-2651
Web site: www.deltadentalga.com
MAILING ADDRESS:
  DELTA DENTAL INSURANCE CO - GA
  1000 Mansell Exchn W B100 #100
  Alpharetta, GA 30022

KEY EXECUTIVES:
Vice President, Operations .... Tom Toon
President/Chief Financial Officer .... Robert B Elliott
Medical Director .... Mindy Broda, DDS
Vice President of Marketing .... Debbie Reeves
Director of Marketing/Texas .... Jill Balboni
Public Relations Director .... Jeff Album
Director of Human Resources .... Ruth Miller
VP, Eastern Region .... Dick Aracich
Director of Marketing/Georgia .... Bill Zvelke
Director of Marketing/Florida .... Bob Luman
VP, Western Region .... Robert Budd

COMPANY PROFILE:
Parent Company Name: Delta Dental Plan of California
Doing Business As:
Year Founded: 1970   Federally Qualified: [ ]
Forprofit: [Y]   Not-For-Profit: [ ]
Model Type: NETWORK
Accreditation: [ ] AAPPO [ ] JACHO [ ] NCQA [ ] URAC
Plan Type: Specialty HMO, Specialty PPO
SERVICE AREA:
Nationwide: N
  GA;
TYPE OF COVERAGE:
Commercial: [Y] Individual: [Y]   FEHBP: [ ]   Indemnity: [ ]
Medicare: [ ] Medicaid: [ ]   Supplemental Medicare: [ ]
Tricare   [ ]
PRODUCTS OFFERED:
Product Name: Type:
Delta Premier/DPO   PPO/Fee for Service
DeltaCare   Dental HMO
PLAN BENEFITS:
Alternative Medicine: [ ]   Behavioral Health: [ ]
Chiropractic: [ ]   Dental: [X]
Home Care: [ ]   Inpatient SNF: [ ]
Long-Term Care: [ ]   Pharm. Mail Order: [ ]
Physical Therapy: [ ]   Podiatry: [ ]
Psychiatric: [ ]   Transplant: [ ]
Vision: [ ]   Wellness: [ ]
Workers' Comp: [ ]
Other Benefits:

EVERGREEN MEDICAL GROUP LLC

707 Center St Ste 110
Columbus, GA 31901
Phone: 706-660-6175 Fax: 706-660-6515 Toll-Free: 888-294-9451
Web site: www.evergreenhealthplan.com
MAILING ADDRESS:
  EVERGREEN MEDICAL GROUP LLC
  707 Center St Ste 110
  Columbus, GA 31901

KEY EXECUTIVES:
Chief Executive Officer .... Mike Hill
Chief Operating Officer .... Allen Holladay
Marketing Director .... Kristy Herrera
Provider Relations Supervisor .... Sharon Blaxton

COMPANY PROFILE:
Parent Company Name:
Doing Business As:
Year Founded: 1997   Federally Qualified: [N]
Forprofit: [Y]   Not-For-Profit: [ ]
Model Type:
Accreditation: [ ] AAPPO [ ] JACHO [ ] NCQA [ ] URAC
Plan Type: HMO, PPO, POS
Total Revenue: 2005:   28,548,380   2006:   14,846,281
Net Income   2005:   -140,378   2006:   300,745
Total Enrollment:
  2001: 10,744   2004: 12,254   2007: 0
  2002: 11,491   2005:
  2003: 11,741   2006:
Medical Loss Ratio: 2005:   2006: 91.00
Administrative Expense Ratio: 2005:   2006:
SERVICE AREA:
Nationwide: N
  AL; GA;
TYPE OF COVERAGE:
Commercial: [Y] Individual: [ ]   FEHBP: [ ]   Indemnity: [ ]
Medicare: [ ] Medicaid: [ ]   Supplemental Medicare: [ ]
Tricare   [ ]
PRODUCTS OFFERED:
Product Name: Type:
Evergreen Health Plan   HMO
Evergreen Health Plan   POS
CONSUMER-DRIVEN PRODUCTS
Columbus Bank & Trust Co   HSA Company
                                     HSA Product
                                     HSA Administrator
                                     Consumer-Driven Health Plan
Classic High Deductible Plan   High Deductible Health Plan
PLAN BENEFITS:
Alternative Medicine: [ ]   Behavioral Health: [X]
Chiropractic: [ ]   Dental: [ ]
Home Care: [X]   Inpatient SNF: [X]
Long-Term Care: [X]   Pharm. Mail Order: [X]
Physical Therapy: [X]   Podiatry: [X]
Psychiatric: [X]   Transplant: [X]
Vision: [X]   Wellness: [X]
Workers' Comp: [X]
Other Benefits:

GREAT-WEST HEALTHCARE OF GEORGIA

245 Perimeter Ctr Pkwy 10th Fl
Atlanta, GA 30346
Phone: 770-290-7000 Fax: 770-290-7022 Toll-Free: 800-511-3899
Web site: www.greatwesthealthcare.com
MAILING ADDRESS:
  GREAT-WEST HEALTHCARE OF GA
  245 Perimeter Ctr Pkwy 10th Fl
  Atlanta, GA 30346

KEY EXECUTIVES:
Chief Executive Officer/President .... Steven White
Chief Financial Officer .... Tim King
Chief Medical Director .... Dean Greeson, MD
Director Provider Network .... Chris Buka

COMPANY PROFILE:
Parent Company Name: CIGNA Inc
Doing Business As:
Year Founded: 1995   Federally Qualified: [N]
Forprofit: [Y]   Not-For-Profit: [ ]
Model Type:
Accreditation: [ ] AAPPO [ ] JACHO [ ] NCQA [X] URAC
Plan Type: HMO, PPO, UR, POS, CDHP, HSA
Total Enrollment:
  2001: 0   2004: 0   2007: 0
  2002: 7,564   2005:
  2003: 7,564   2006:
Medical Loss Ratio: 2005:   2006: 32.00
Administrative Expense Ratio: 2005:   2006:
SERVICE AREA:
Nationwide: N
  GA (Barrow, Bartow, Cherokee, Clark, Clayton, Cobb, Coweta,
  Dawson, Dekalb, Douglas, Fayette, Floyd, Forsyth, Fulton, Gilmer,
  Gwinnett, Hall, Henry, Jackson, Lumpkin, Newton, Oconee,
  Pickerns, Polk, Paulding, Rockdale, Walton);
TYPE OF COVERAGE:
Commercial: [Y] Individual: [ ]   FEHBP: [ ]   Indemnity: [ ]
Medicare: [ ] Medicaid: [ ]   Supplemental Medicare: [ ]
Tricare   [ ]
PRODUCTS OFFERED:
Product Name: Type:
One Health Plan of GA   HMO
CONSUMER-DRIVEN PRODUCTS
Dreyfus Corp, a Mellon Co   HSA Company
Mellon HSA   HSA Product
                                     HSA Administrator
                                     Consumer-Driven Health Plan
                                     High Deductible Health Plan

GEORGIA

KEY EXECUTIVES:
President .... George E Spalding Jr, CPA
VP of Provider Relations .... John Wood
VP of Employer Services .... Tim Stewert

COMPANY PROFILE:
Parent Company Name:
Doing Business As: CorpSavers HealthCare, Allied Hlth Bnfts
Year Founded: 1992   Federally Qualified: [ ]
Forprofit: [Y]   Not-For-Profit: [ ]
Model Type: MIXED
Accreditation: [ ] AAPPO [ ] JACHO [X] NCQA [ ] URAC
Plan Type: Specialty PPO,

SERVICE AREA:
Nationwide: Y
    NW;

TYPE OF COVERAGE:
Commercial: [Y] Individual: [Y] FEHBP: [ ] Indemnity: [ ]
Medicare: [ ] Medicaid: [ ] Supplemental Medicare: [ ]
Tricare   [ ]

PRODUCTS OFFERED:
Product Name:	Type:
Allied Good Health Card	Medical Benefits
CHG Chiropractic Network	Chiropractic
Employer Assistance Group	Collections

CONSUMER-DRIVEN PRODUCTS
	HSA Company
Allied Health Benefits HSA	HSA Product
Time Life Insurance Co	HSA Administrator
Allied Health Benefits CDHP	Consumer-Driven Health Plan
Allied Health Benefits HDHP	High Deductible Health Plan

PLAN BENEFITS:
Alternative Medicine: [X]   Behavioral Health: [ ]
Chiropractic: [X]   Dental: [X]
Home Care: [X]   Inpatient SNF: [ ]
Long-Term Care: [X]   Pharm. Mail Order: [X]
Physical Therapy: [ ]   Podiatry: [X]
Psychiatric: [X]   Transplant: [ ]
Vision: [X]   Wellness: [X]
Workers' Comp: [ ]
Other Benefits: All are a discount plan

COVENTRY HEALTH CARE INC — GEORGIA INC

1100 Circle 75 Pkwy Ste 1400
Atlanta, GA 30339
Phone: 678-202-210 Fax: 678-202-2196 Toll-Free: 800-470-2004
Web site: www.cvty.com

MAILING ADDRESS:
    COVENTRY HEALTH CARE — GA
    1100 Circle 75 Pkwy Ste 1400
    Atlanta, GA 30339

KEY EXECUTIVES:
Chief Executive Officer/President .... Thomas A Davis
Chief Financial Officer .... Paul Farrell
Medical Director .... Bernie Cohen, MD
Chief Operating Officer .... Marc Malloy
Marketing Director .... Cory Scott

COMPANY PROFILE:
Parent Company Name: Coventry Health Care Inc
Doing Business As:
Year Founded: 1994   Federally Qualified: [N]
Forprofit: [Y]   Not-For-Profit: [ ]
Model Type: IPA
Accreditation: [ ] AAPPO [ ] JACHO [ ] NCQA [ ] URAC
Plan Type: HMO, PPO, POS, CDHP, HDHP, HSA
Primary Physicians: Physician Specialists:
Hospitals: 65
Total Enrollment:
    2001: 54,218   2004: 79,906   2007: 0
    2002: 80,000   2005: 70,000
    2003: 80,000   2006: 100,000
Medical Loss Ratio: 2005: 00.00   2006: 69.90
Administrative Expense Ratio: 2005:   2006:

SERVICE AREA:
Nationwide: N
    FL; GA (Barrow, Bartow, Cherokee, Coweta, Clayton, Cobb, Dekalb, Douglas, Fayette, Forsyth, Fulton, Gwinnett, Hall, Henry, Jackson, Newton, Paulding, Rockdale, Spalding, Walton);

TYPE OF COVERAGE:
Commercial: [Y] Individual: [ ] FEHBP: [ ] Indemnity: [ ]
Medicare: [ ] Medicaid: [ ] Supplemental Medicare: [ ]
Tricare   [ ]

PRODUCTS OFFERED:
Product Name:	Type:
Coventry HMO	HMO

CONSUMER-DRIVEN PRODUCTS
Wells Fargo	HSA Company
	HSA Product
Corporate Benefits Servs of Am	HSA Administrator
	Consumer-Driven Health Plan
Open Access Plus Plan	High Deductible Health Plan

PLAN BENEFITS:
Alternative Medicine: [ ]   Behavioral Health: [X]
Chiropractic: [X]   Dental: [X]
Home Care: [X]   Inpatient SNF: [X]
Long-Term Care: [X]   Pharm. Mail Order: [X]
Physical Therapy: [X]   Podiatry: [X]
Psychiatric: [X]   Transplant: [X]
Vision: [X]   Wellness: [X]
Workers' Comp: [ ]
Other Benefits:
Comments:
Formerly Principal Health Care of Georgia Inc.

CRAWFORD AND CO - CORPORATE HEADQUARTERS

5620 Glenridge Drive NE
Atlanta, GA 30342
Phone: 404-256-0830 Fax: 404-937-8229 Toll-Free: 800-241-2541
Web site: www.crawfordandcompany.com

MAILING ADDRESS:
    CRAWFORD AND CO
    PO Box 5047
    Atlanta, GA 30342

KEY EXECUTIVES:
Chairman .... Grover Davis
Chief Executive Officer/President .... Thomas W Crawford
Chief Financial Officer .... Bruce Swaine
Branch Manager .... Sherri Palish
Chief Information Officer .... Nick Coussoule
Marketing Director .... Kara Grady
Human Resource Director .... Bill Beach
Quality Assurance Director .... John Fleming
Fraud Prevention/Investigation .... Bryan Mapnet
Executive VP, Healthcare Management .... Vicki Holland
Executive VP, Risk Management Services .... Annette Sanchez
Executive VP, Claims Services .... Marshall Long

COMPANY PROFILE:
Parent Company Name: Crawford & Co
Doing Business As: Crawford & Co
Year Founded: 1941   Federally Qualified: [Y]
Forprofit: [Y]   Not-For-Profit: [ ]
Model Type:
Accreditation: [ ] AAPPO [ ] JACHO [ ] NCQA [X] URAC
Plan Type: UR, TPA
Total Revenue: 2005:   2006: 900,380,000
Net Income   2005:   2006: 15,011,000

SERVICE AREA:
Nationwide: Y
    Nationwide;

PRODUCTS OFFERED:
Product Name:	Type:
Medical Case Management	
Long Term Care	
Workers Compensation Claims Ad	
Utilization Pension	
Provider Bill Audit	

PLAN BENEFITS:
Alternative Medicine: [ ]   Behavioral Health: [ ]
Chiropractic: [ ]   Dental: [ ]
Home Care: [ ]   Inpatient SNF: [ ]
Long-Term Care: [ ]   Pharm. Mail Order: [ ]
Physical Therapy: [ ]   Podiatry: [ ]
Psychiatric: [ ]   Transplant: [ ]
Vision: [ ]   Wellness: [ ]
Workers' Comp: [X]
Other Benefits:

Managed Care Organization Profiles **GEORGIA**

Medical Loss Ratio: 2005: 2006: 84.90
Administrative Expense Ratio: 2005: 2006:
SERVICE AREA:
Nationwide: N
AL: GA (Atlanta and Augusta Areas Barrow, Bartow, Bibb, Butts, Catoosa, Chattooga, Chattahoochee, Cherokee, Clarke, Clayton, Cobb, Columbia, Coweta, Dekalb, Douglas, Elbert, Fayette, Floyd, Forsyth, Franklin, Fulton, Gordon, Greene, Gwinnett, Hall, Henry, Houston, Jackson, Jones, Madison, Meriwether, Muscogee, Newton, Oconee, Oglethorpe, Paulding, Peach, Polk, Richmond, Rockdale, Spalding, Stewart, Talbot, Troup, Twiggs, Upson, Walker, Walton, Webster, White, Wilkes, Wilkerson, Savannah Area Appling, Bacon, Brantley, Bryan, Bulloch, Camden, Candler, Chatham, Charlton, Clinch, Coffee, Effingham, Emanuel, Evans, Glynn, Jeff Davis, Jenkins, Liberty, Long, McIntosh, Montgomery, Pierce, Screven, Tattinall, Toombs, Treutlen, Ware, Wayne, Wheeler);

TYPE OF COVERAGE:
Commercial: [Y] Individual: [ ] FEHBP: [ ] Indemnity: [ ]
Medicare: [Y] Medicaid: [ ] Supplemental Medicare: [ ]
Tricare [ ]

PRODUCTS OFFERED:
Product Name: Type:
Cigna Healthcare for Seniors Medicare

CONSUMER-DRIVEN PRODUCTS
JP Morgan Chase HSA Company
CIGNA Choice Fund HSA Product
 HSA Administrator
Open Access Plus Consumer-Driven Health Plan
PPO High Deductible Health Plan

PLAN BENEFITS:
Alternative Medicine: [ ] Behavioral Health: [ ]
Chiropractic: [X] Dental: [X]
Home Care: [X] Inpatient SNF: [X]
Long-Term Care: [X] Pharm. Mail Order: [X]
Physical Therapy: [X] Podiatry: [X]
Psychiatric: [X] Transplant: [X]
Vision: [X] Wellness: [X]
Workers' Comp: [ ]
Other Benefits:

COALITION AMERICA INC

Two Concourse Pkwy Ste 300
Atlanta, GA 30328
Phone: 404-459-7201 Fax: 404-459-6645 Toll-Free:
Web site: www.coalitionamerica.com
MAILING ADDRESS:
COALITION AMERICA INC
Two Concourse Pkwy Ste 300
Atlanta, GA 30328

KEY EXECUTIVES:
Chairman of the Board/Chief Executive Officer .... Sean Smith
Executive Vice President .... Scott Smith, Senior
Chief Financial Officer .... Anthony Levinson
Chief Operating Officer .... Tina Ellex
Director of Marketing .... Libby Roper
Chief Technology Officer .... Steve Alford
Director of Public Relations .... Libby Roper
Director, Strategic Business Development .... Corte Larossi
Human Resources Director .... Monica Hembrick

COMPANY PROFILE:
Parent Company Name:
Doing Business As:
Year Founded: 1995 Federally Qualified: [N]
Forprofit: [Y] Not-For-Profit: [ ]
Model Type:
Accreditation: [Y] AAPPO [ ] JACHO [ ] NCQA [ ] URAC
Plan Type: PPO, Specialty PPO, EPO, UR
Total Enrollment:
 2001: 0 2004: 0 2007: 0
 2002: 0 2005:
 2003: 0 2006:
SERVICE AREA:
Nationwide: Y
 NW;
TYPE OF COVERAGE:
Commercial: [Y] Individual: [ ] FEHBP: [ ] Indemnity: [ ]
Medicare: [ ] Medicaid: [ ] Supplemental Medicare: [ ]
Tricare [ ]

PLAN BENEFITS:
Alternative Medicine: [ ] Behavioral Health: [X]
Chiropractic: [X] Dental: [X]
Home Care: [X] Inpatient SNF: [X]
Long-Term Care: [X] Pharm. Mail Order: [X]
Physical Therapy: [X] Podiatry: [X]
Psychiatric: [X] Transplant: [X]
Vision: [X] Wellness: [X]
Workers' Comp: [X]
Other Benefits: X

COMPBENEFITS CORPORATION - CORPORATE HEADQUARTERS

100 Mansell Court East Ste 400
Roswell, GA 30076
Phone: 770-998-8936 Fax: 770-998-6871 Toll-Free: 800-633-1262
Web site: www.compbenefits.com
MAILING ADDRESS:
COMPBENEFITS CORP - CORP HQRT
100 Mansell Court East Ste 400
Roswell, GA 30076

KEY EXECUTIVES:
Chairman of the Board .... David R Klock, MD
Chief Financial Officer .... George Dunaway
Medical Director .... Kenneth J Hammer, DDS, MBA
Chief Information Officer .... Ron Wood
Senior VP, Operations .... Mary Kay Gilbert
Marketing, Strategy Director .... John Arnold
MIS Director .... Ron Wood
Human Resource Director .... Karen Mitchell
Compliance Officer .... Cindy Bolovrelchi

COMPANY PROFILE:
Parent Company Name: Humana Inc
Doing Business As:
Year Founded: 1978 Federally Qualified: [N]
Forprofit: [Y] Not-For-Profit: [ ]
Model Type: MIXED
Accreditation: [ ] AAPPO [ ] JACHO [ ] NCQA [ ] URAC
Plan Type: Specialty HMO, Specialty PPO, ASO
Total Enrollment:
 2001: 0 2004: 4,500,000 2007: 0
 2002: 4,500,000 2005: 5,000,000
 2003: 0 2006:
SERVICE AREA:
Nationwide: N
 AL; AR; CO; FL; GA; IL; IN; KS; KY; LA; MA; MD; MO; MS; NC; NJ; OH; OK; PA; SC; TN; TX; VA; WV;
TYPE OF COVERAGE:
Commercial: [Y] Individual: [Y] FEHBP: [ ] Indemnity: [ ]
Medicare: [ ] Medicaid: [ ] Supplemental Medicare: [ ]
Tricare [ ]
PLAN BENEFITS:
Alternative Medicine: [ ] Behavioral Health: [ ]
Chiropractic: [ ] Dental: [X]
Home Care: [ ] Inpatient SNF: [ ]
Long-Term Care: [ ] Pharm. Mail Order: [X]
Physical Therapy: [ ] Podiatry: [ ]
Psychiatric: [ ] Transplant: [ ]
Vision: [X] Wellness: [ ]
Workers' Comp: [ ]
Other Benefits:
Comments:
American Dental Plan, HealthStream, CompDent, American PrePaid Dental Plan, Texas Dental Plan, DentiCare (Texas), National Dental Plans. Acquired by Humana Inc October 1, 2007.

COMPREHENSIVE HEALTH GROUP

6479 E Johns Crossing Ste 170
Duluth, GA 30097
Phone: 770-448-4677 Fax: 770-448-4749 Toll-Free: 800-669-8682
Web site: www.chgallied.com
MAILING ADDRESS:
COMPREHENSIVE HEALTH GROUP
6479 E Johns Crossing Ste 170
Norcross, GA 30097

GEORGIA

KEY EXECUTIVES:
Executive Director .... Jeffrey A Kunkle
President .... Larry Webb
Chief Financial Officer .... Rob Aubrey
Medical Director .... Jeff Cole, MD
Chief Operating Officer .... Raymond Donovan
Director/Quality/Utilization Mgmnt .... Christie Baxter

COMPANY PROFILE:
Parent Company Name: Athens Regional Health Services Inc
Doing Business As: Health Plan Select
Year Founded: 1996   Federally Qualified: [N]
Forprofit: [ ]   Not-For-Profit: [Y]
Model Type: NETWORK
Accreditation: [ ] AAPPO [ ] JACHO [ ] NCQA [Y] URAC
Plan Type: HMO, POS, TPA, CDHP, HDHP, HSA
Primary Physicians: 329   Physician Specialists: 515
Hospitals: 15
Total Revenue: 2005:   44,071,230   2006:   47,024,721
Net Income   2005:   -5,752,852   2006:   -839,747
Total Enrollment:
   2001: 0   2004: 15,588   2007: 24,385
   2002: 16,572   2005: 21,964
   2003: 15,695   2006: 24,385
Medical Loss Ratio: 2005: 99.31   2006: 89.16
Administrative Expense Ratio: 2005: 14.69   2006: 13.98

SERVICE AREA:
Nationwide: N
GA (Banks, Barrow, Clarke, Elbert, Franklin, Greene, Habersham, Hart, Jackson, Madison, Morgan, Oconee, Ogelthorpe, Taliaferro, Walton, Wilkes);

TYPE OF COVERAGE:
Commercial: [Y]   Individual: [ ]   FEHBP: [ ]   Indemnity: [ ]
Medicare: [ ]   Medicaid: [ ]   Supplemental Medicare: [ ]
Tricare   [ ]

PRODUCTS OFFERED:
Product Name: Type:
Athens Health Plan   HMO
Athens Point of Service   POS

CONSUMER-DRIVEN PRODUCTS
                                    HSA Company
DHP1, DHP2, DHP5   HSA Product
Athens Area Health Plan Select I   HSA Administrator
                                    Consumer-Driven Health Plan
DHP1, DHP2, DHP5   High Deductible Health Plan

PLAN BENEFITS:
Alternative Medicine: [ ]   Behavioral Health: [X]
Chiropractic: [ ]   Dental: [X]
Home Care: [X]   Inpatient SNF: [X]
Long-Term Care: [ ]   Pharm. Mail Order: [ ]
Physical Therapy: [X]   Podiatry: [X]
Psychiatric: [X]   Transplant: [X]
Vision: [ ]   Wellness: [X]
Workers' Comp: [ ]
Other Benefits:

BLUE CROSS BLUE SHIELD OF GEORGIA

3350 Peachtree Rd NE
Atlanta, GA 30326
Phone: 404-842-8000 Fax: 404-842-8822 Toll-Free: 877-868-7950
Web site: www.bcbsga.com

MAILING ADDRESS:
   BLUE CROSS BLUE SHIELD OF GA
   PO Box 4445
   Atlanta, GA 30326

KEY EXECUTIVES:
Chief Executive Officer .... Monye Connolly
President/General Manager .... Monye Connolly
Staff VP, Finance .... Lynn Welborn
VP, Medical Director .... Sandra L White, MD
Staff VP, Operations .... Doris Anderson
VP, Information Systems .... Douglas Brown
VP, Public Affairs .... Charles E Harman
Provider Services Director .... Moyne Connolly
Regional VP, Network Development .... Ron Lawrence
VP of Human Resources .... Darlene Andrews
Medical Management Director .... Sandra L White, MD
Case Manager .... Joaquin Thompson
Director, Corporate Communications .... Cindy Sanders

COMPANY PROFILE:
Parent Company Name: Wellpoint Inc
Doing Business As:
Year Founded: 1984   Federally Qualified: [N]
Forprofit: [Y]   Not-For-Profit: [ ]
Model Type: IPA
Accreditation: [ ] AAPPO [ ] JACHO [ ] NCQA [X] URAC
Plan Type: PPO, CDHP, HDHP, HSA,
Total Enrollment:
   2001: 0   2004: 622,501   2007: 0
   2002: 0   2005:
   2003: 622,501   2006: 3,200,000

SERVICE AREA:
Nationwide: N
GA; (Bacon, Baker, Baldwin, Banks, Barrow, Bartow, Ben Hill, Bibb, Bleckley, Brantley, Brooks, Bryan, Burke, Butts, Camden, Candler, Carroll, Catoosa, Charlton, Chatham, Chattahoochee, Chattooga, Cherokee, Clarke, Clayton, Cobb, Colquitt, Columbia, Coweta, Crawford, Crisp, Dade, Dawson, Decatur, DeKalb, Dodge, Dooly, Dougherty, Douglas, Early, Effingham, Elbert, Evans, Fayette, Floyd, Forsyth, Franklin, Fulton, Glascock, Gordon, Grady, Greene, Gwinnett, Habersham, Hall, Hancock, Haralson, Harris, Hart, Heard, Henry, Houston, Jackson, Jefferson, Jenkins, Johnson, Jones, Lamar, Laurens, Lee, Liberty, Lincoln, Lumpkin, Macon, Madison, Marion, McDuffie, Meriwether, Mitchell, Monroe, Morgan, Murray, Muscogee, Newton, Oconee, Ogelthorpe, Paulding, Peach, Pierce, Pike, Polk, Pulaski, Putnam, Quitman, Randolph, Richmond, Rockdale, Schley, Seminole, Spalding, Sumter, Talbot, Taliaferro, Telfair, Terrell, Thomas, Tift, Treutlen, Troup, Twiggs, Union, Upson, Walker, Walton, Ware, Warren, Washington, White, Wilkes, Wilkinson, Worth);

TYPE OF COVERAGE:
Commercial: [Y]   Individual: [ ]   FEHBP: [ ]   Indemnity: [ ]
Medicare: [Y]   Medicaid: [ ]   Supplemental Medicare: [ ]
Tricare   [ ]

PRODUCTS OFFERED:
Product Name: Type:
BlueChoice PPO   PPO
BlueChoice Platinum   Medicare

CONSUMER-DRIVEN PRODUCTS
                                    HSA Company
                                    HSA Product
                                    HSA Administrator
                                    Consumer-Driven Health Plan
Blue Choice PPO   High Deductible Health Plan

PLAN BENEFITS:
Alternative Medicine: [ ]   Behavioral Health: [X]
Chiropractic: [ ]   Dental: [ ]
Home Care: [X]   Inpatient SNF: [X]
Long-Term Care: [X]   Pharm. Mail Order: [ ]
Physical Therapy: [X]   Podiatry: [ ]
Psychiatric: [X]   Transplant: [X]
Vision: [ ]   Wellness: [X]
Workers' Comp: [ ]
Other Benefits:

CIGNA HEALTHCARE OF GEORGIA

2 Sc Ctr 3500 Piedmont NE #200
Atlanta, GA 30305
Phone: 404-443-8800 Fax: 404-443-8932 Toll-Free:
Web site: www.cigna.com

MAILING ADDRESS:
   CIGNA HEALTHCARE OF GA
   2 Sc Ctr 3500 Piedmont NE #200
   Atlanta, GA 30305

KEY EXECUTIVES:
President/General Manager .... Scott Evelyn

COMPANY PROFILE:
Parent Company Name: CIGNA Corporation
Doing Business As: CIGNA Healthcare of Georgia
Year Founded: 1985   Federally Qualified: [Y]
Forprofit: [Y]   Not-For-Profit: [ ]
Model Type: IPA
Accreditation: [ ] AAPPO [ ] JACHO [X] NCQA [ ] URAC
Plan Type: HMO, PPO, POS, CDHP, HDHP, HSA
Total Enrollment:
   2001: 0   2004: 25,325   2007: 0
   2002: 0   2005:
   2003: 29,993   2006:

Managed Care Organization Profiles   GEORGIA

1ST MEDICAL NETWORK

1899 Powers Ferry Rd Ste 400
Atlanta, GA 30339
Phone: 678-742-9100 Fax: 678-742-9180 Toll-Free:
Web site: www.1stmn.com

MAILING ADDRESS:
    1ST MEDICAL NETWORK
    1899 Powers Ferry Rd Ste 400
    Atlanta, GA 30339

KEY EXECUTIVES:
Chairman of the Board .... Doug Patten, MD
Chief Executive Officer/President .... Gary Hutchins
Chief Financial Officer .... Stephen Braden
Medical Director .... Mark Lefler, MD
Chief Operating Officer .... Debra Peterson-Smith
Chief Marketing Officer .... John Wofford
Network Management Officer .... Jonna Kirkwood

COMPANY PROFILE:
Parent Company Name:
Doing Business As:
Year Founded: 2002   Federally Qualified: [ ]
Forprofit: [ ]   Not-For-Profit: [ ]
Model Type: NETWORK
Accreditation: [ ] AAPPO [ ] JACHO [ ] NCQA [X] URAC
Plan Type: PPO,
Hospitals: 150
Total Enrollment:
    2001: 0   2004: 0   2007: 0
    2002: 0   2005: 640,000
    2003: 0   2006: 200,000

SERVICE AREA:
Nationwide:
    GA;

AETNA INC - GEORGIA

11675 Great Oaks Way
Alpheretta, GA 30022
Phone: 770-346-4300 Fax: 678-256-2045 Toll-Free: 800-346-3778
Web site: www.aetna.com

MAILING ADDRESS:
    AETNA INC - GA
    11675 Great Oaks Way MS F350
    Alpheretta, GA 30022

KEY EXECUTIVES:
Chairman of the Board/Chief Executive Officer .... Ronald A Williams
President .... Clarence C King, II
Principal Financial Officer .... Deborah M Wightman
Senior Medical Director .... William E Hauser Jr, MD
Chief Information Officer .... Timothy A Holt
Public Relations Director .... Marlene Baltar

COMPANY PROFILE:
Parent Company Name: Aetna Inc
Doing Business As: Prudential
Year Founded: Federally Qualified: [Y]
Forprofit: [Y]   Not-For-Profit: [ ]
Model Type:
Accreditation: [ ] AAPPO [ ] JACHO [ ] NCQA [ ] URAC
Plan Type: HMO, PPO, POS, CDHP, HSA,
Total Enrollment:
    2001: 204,692   2004: 162,163   2007: 0
    2002: 196,685   2005:
    2003: 174,071   2006:
Medical Loss Ratio: 2005:   2006: 81.60
Administrative Expense Ratio: 2005:   2006:

SERVICE AREA:
Nationwide: N
    GA (Barrow, Bartow, Bibb, Butts, Cherokee, Clayton, Cobb, Coweta, Crawford, Dekalb, Douglas, Fayette, Floyd, Forsyth, Fulton, Gwinnett, Hall, Henry, Houston, Jones, Monroe, Newton, Paulding, Peach, Rockdale, Spalding, Twiggs, Walton, Wilkinson); MS;

TYPE OF COVERAGE:
Commercial: [Y] Individual: [ ] FEHBP: [ ] Indemnity: [ ]
Medicare: [ ] Medicaid: [ ] Supplemental Medicare: [ ]
Tricare   [ ]

PRODUCTS OFFERED:
Product Name: Type:
Prudential Healthcare Seniorcare   Medicare
CONSUMER-DRIVEN PRODUCTS
Aetna Life Insurance Co   HSA Company
Aetna HealthFund HSA   HSA Product
Aetna   HSA Administrator
Aetna HealthFund   Consumer-Driven Health Plan
PPO I; PPO II   High Deductible Health Plan

PLAN BENEFITS:
Alternative Medicine: [ ]   Behavioral Health: [X]
Chiropractic: [X]   Dental: [X]
Home Care: [X]   Inpatient SNF: [X]
Long-Term Care: [X]   Pharm. Mail Order: [X]
Physical Therapy: [X]   Podiatry: [X]
Psychiatric: [X]   Transplant: [ ]
Vision: [ ]   Wellness: [ ]
Workers' Comp: [ ]
Other Benefits: Preventive Dental
Comments:
Formerly Prudential Health Care Systems.

ASSURANT EMPLOYEE BENEFITS - GEORGIA

780 Johnson Ferry Rd Ste 450
Atlanta, GA 30342
Phone: 404-303-2160 Fax: 404-303-2175 Toll-Free: 800-553-3348
Web site: www.assurantemployeebenefits.com

MAILING ADDRESS:
    ASSURANT EMPLOYEE BNFTS - GA
    780 Johnson Ferry Rd Ste 450
    Atlanta, GA 30342

KEY EXECUTIVES:
Interim Chief Executive Officer/President .... John S Roberts
Chief Financial Officer .... Floyd F Chadee
VP, Medical Director .... Polly M Galbraith, MD
Chief Information Officer .... Karla J Schacht
Senior VP, Marketing .... Joseph A Sevcik
Privacy Officer .... John L Fortini
VP of Provider Services .... James A Barrett, DMD
Senior VP, Human Resources & Development .... Sylvia R Wagner
General Manager .... Todd Boyd
National Dental Director .... James A Barrett, DMD

COMPANY PROFILE:
Parent Company Name: Assurant Health
Doing Business As: DentiCare Inc
Year Founded: 1975   Federally Qualified: [ ]
Forprofit: [Y]   Not-For-Profit: [ ]
Model Type:
Accreditation: [ ] AAPPO [ ] JACHO [ ] NCQA [ ] URAC
Plan Type: Specialty HMO

SERVICE AREA:
Nationwide: N
    GA;

TYPE OF COVERAGE:
Commercial: [Y] Individual: [Y] FEHBP: [ ] Indemnity: [ ]
Medicare: [ ] Medicaid: [ ] Supplemental Medicare: [ ]
Tricare   [ ]

PLAN BENEFITS:
Alternative Medicine: [ ]   Behavioral Health: [ ]
Chiropractic: [ ]   Dental: [X]
Home Care: [ ]   Inpatient SNF: [ ]
Long-Term Care: [ ]   Pharm. Mail Order: [ ]
Physical Therapy: [ ]   Podiatry: [ ]
Psychiatric: [ ]   Transplant: [ ]
Vision: [X]   Wellness: [ ]
Workers' Comp: [ ]
Other Benefits:

ATHENS AREA HEALTH PLAN SELECT INC

295 W Clayton St
Athens, GA 30601
Phone: 706-549-0549 Fax: 706-549-8004 Toll-Free: 800-293-6260
Web site: www.aahps.com

MAILING ADDRESS:
    ATHENS AREA HEALTH PLAN SELECT
    295 W Clayton St
    Athens, GA 30601

Managed Care Organization Profiles   **FLORIDA**

Total Enrollment:
2001: 0	2004: 747,000	2007: 2,300,000
2002: 0	2005: 855,300	
2003: 555,000	2006: 2,011,000	

SERVICE AREA:
Nationwide:
   CT; FL; IL; IN; NY;

TYPE OF COVERAGE:
Commercial: [Y] Individual: [Y] FEHBP: [ ] Indemnity: [ ]
Medicare: [Y] Medicaid: [Y] Supplemental Medicare: [ ]
Tricare   [ ]

PRODUCTS OFFERED:

Product Name:	Type:
Healthease of Florida	Medicaid
Staywell Health Plan	Medicaid
Preferred Care - CT	Medicaid
Harmony Health Plan - IL	Medicaid
Harmony Health Management - IN	Medicaid
WellCare of NY	Medicaid
WellCare of Texas	Medicare

PLAN BENEFITS:
Alternative Medicine: [ ]   Behavioral Health: [X]
Chiropractic: [ ]   Dental: [X]
Home Care: [ ]   Inpatient SNF: [ ]
Long-Term Care: [ ]   Pharm. Mail Order: [ ]
Physical Therapy: [ ]   Podiatry: [ ]
Psychiatric: [ ]   Transplant: [ ]
Vision: [X] Wellness: [ ]
Workers' Comp: [ ]
Other Benefits:

FLORIDA — Managed Care Organization Profiles

PLAN BENEFITS:

Alternative Medicine:	[ ]	Behavioral Health:	[X]
Chiropractic:	[X]	Dental:	[X]
Home Care:	[X]	Inpatient SNF:	[X]
Long-Term Care:	[ ]	Pharm. Mail Order:	[X]
Physical Therapy:	[X]	Podiatry:	[X]
Psychiatric:	[X]	Transplant:	[X]
Vision:	[X]	Wellness:	[X]
Workers' Comp:	[ ]		
Other Benefits:			

Comments:
Formerly known as Foundation Health, A Florida Health Plan Inc. Formerly owned by Health Net, CA.

VOLUSIA HEALTH NETWORK

1340 Ridgewood Ave Ste 700
Holly Hill, FL 32117
Phone: 386-258-4896 Fax: 386-253-2756 Toll-Free:
Web site: www.vhnonline.com

MAILING ADDRESS:
VOLUSIA HEALTH NETWORK
1340 Ridgewood Ave Ste 700
Daytona Beach, FL 32117

KEY EXECUTIVES:
Chairman, Board of Directors .... Charles Burkett, MD
Medical Director .... Lane Jennings, MD
Provider Relations Coordinator .... Jean Carroll
Operation Manager .... Karen Aalbregtse

COMPANY PROFILE:
Parent Company Name: Halifax Community Health System
Doing Business As:
Year Founded: 1984   Federally Qualified: [ ]
Forprofit: [ ]   Not-For-Profit: [Y] Model Type:
Accreditation: [ ] AAPPO [ ] JACHO [ ] NCQA [ ] URAC
Plan Type: PPO, UR, TPA, EPO
Total Enrollment:
2001: 0   2004: 0   2007: 0
2002: 25,000   2005:
2003: 0   2006:

SERVICE AREA:
Nationwide: N
FL (Flagler, Seminole, Volusia);

TYPE OF COVERAGE:
Commercial: [Y] Individual: [ ] FEHBP: [ ] Indemnity: [ ]
Medicare: [ ]   Medicaid: [ ]   Supplemental Medicare: [ ]
Tricare [ ]

PLAN BENEFITS:

Alternative Medicine:	[ ]	Behavioral Health:	[X]
Chiropractic:	[X]	Dental:	[ ]
Home Care:	[X]	Inpatient SNF:	[X]
Long-Term Care:	[X]	Pharm. Mail Order:	[ ]
Physical Therapy:	[X]	Podiatry:	[X]
Psychiatric:	[X]	Transplant:	[X]
Vision:	[X]	Wellness:	[ ]
Workers' Comp:	[ ]		
Other Benefits:			

WELL CARE HMO INC

8735 Henderson Rd Renaissance1
Tampa, FL 33634
Phone: 813-290-6219 Fax: 813-262-2802 Toll-Free: 800-610-4466
Web site: www.wellcarehmo.com

MAILING ADDRESS:
WELL CARE HMO INC
8735 Henderson Rd Renaissance1
Tampa, FL 33634

KEY EXECUTIVES:
Executive Chairman .... Charles G Berg
President/Chief Executive Officer .... Heath Schiesser
Senior VP, Market Expansion .... Rupesh Shah
VP, Human Resources .... Gretchen DiMartini

COMPANY PROFILE:
Parent Company Name: WellCare Health Plans Inc
Doing Business As: WellCare, Staywell Health Plan of FL
Year Founded: 1985   Federally Qualified: [N]
Forprofit: [Y]   Not-For-Profit: [ ]
Model Type: IPA
Accreditation: [ ] AAPPO [ ] JACHO [ ] NCQA [ ] URAC
Plan Type: HMO
Total Revenue: 2005:   2006: 468,693,685
Net Income   2005:   2006: 5,023,613
Total Enrollment:
2001: 186,548   2004: 300,652   2007: 0
2002: 211,330   2005: 310,780
2003: 272,419   2006: 310,224

SERVICE AREA:
Nationwide: N
FL (Broward, Clay, Dade, Duval, Hernando, Hillsborough, Lee, Manatee, Nassau, Okeechobee, Orange, Osceola, Palm Beach, Pasco, Pinellas, Polk, Seminole, St Lucie, Volusia);

TYPE OF COVERAGE:
Commercial: [Y] Individual: [Y] FEHBP: [ ] Indemnity: [ ]
Medicare: [ ]   Medicaid: [Y]   Supplemental Medicare: [Y]
Tricare [ ]

PRODUCTS OFFERED:
Product Name:	Type:
Well Care Choice Plan	Medicare Advantage
Well Care & Staywell Health	Medicaid
HealthyKids	HMO

PLAN BENEFITS:

Alternative Medicine:	[ ]	Behavioral Health:	[ ]
Chiropractic:	[ ]	Dental:	[X]
Home Care:	[ ]	Inpatient SNF:	[ ]
Long-Term Care:	[ ]	Pharm. Mail Order:	[ ]
Physical Therapy:	[ ]	Podiatry:	[ ]
Psychiatric:	[ ]	Transplant:	[ ]
Vision:	[X]	Wellness:	[ ]
Workers' Comp:	[ ]		
Other Benefits:			

WELLCARE HEALTH PLANS INC - CORPORATE HEADQUARTERS

8735 Henderson Rd Renaissance1
Tampa, FL 33634
Phone: 813-290-6200 Fax: 813-262-2802 Toll-Free: 800-610-4466
Web site: www.wellcare.com

MAILING ADDRESS:
WELLCARE HLTH PLNS INC - CORP
8735 Henderson Rd Renaissance1
Tampa, FL 33634

KEY EXECUTIVES:
Executive Chairman .... Charles G Berg
President/Chief Executive Officer .... Heath Schiesser
President, Illinois .... Keith Kudla
Senior VP, Chief Medical Officer .... William Kerr, MD
VP Pharmacy .... John Sirera
Senior VP, Chief Information Officer .... Anil Kottoor
Senior VP, Market Expansion .... Rupesh Shah
Senior VP, Health Services .... Randall D Zomermaand
VP, Human Resources .... Gretchen Demartini
President, Texas .... Cesar D Martinez
VP, Connecticut .... Doug Hayward
VP, New York .... Dan Parietti
Chief Operating Officer, Georgia .... Michael Cotton

COMPANY PROFILE:
Parent Company Name:
Doing Business As:
Year Founded: 2004   Federally Qualified: [Y]
Forprofit: [Y]   Not-For-Profit: [ ]
Model Type:
Accreditation: [ ] AAPPO [ ] JACHO [ ] NCQA [ ] URAC
Plan Type: HMO
Primary Physicians: 20,000   Physician Specialists:
Hospitals:
Total Revenue: 2005: 205,539,332   2006: 3,762,926
Net Income   2005: 2,070,720   2006: 139,187

Managed Care Organization Profiles — **FLORIDA**

KEY EXECUTIVES:
Chief Executive Officer/President .... Akshay Desai, MD
Chief Operating Officer .... Phil Sheesley
Director of Provider Services .... Charlene Brash-Sorensen

COMPANY PROFILE:
Parent Company Name:
Doing Business As:
Year Founded: 2002   Federally Qualified: [Y]
Forprofit: [Y]   Not-For-Profit: [ ]
Model Type:
Accreditation: [ ] AAPPO [ ] JACHO [ ] NCQA [ ] URAC
Plan Type: HMO
Total Revenue: 2005:   2006:   136,125,290
Net Income   2005:   2006:   2,160,573
Total Enrollment:
  2001: 0   2004: 6,166   2007: 0
  2002: 0   2005: 14,790
  2003: 1,147   2006: 48,116

SERVICE AREA:
Nationwide:
  FL;

TYPE OF COVERAGE:
Commercial: [Y] Individual: [Y] FEHBP: [ ] Indemnity: [ ]
Medicare: [Y] Medicaid: [Y] Supplemental Medicare: [Y]
Tricare   [ ]

PRODUCTS OFFERED:
Product Name: Type:
Medicare Masterpiece Plan   Medicare
U-First   Medicaid
Universal Individual Hlth Plns
Healthy Kids   Medicaid

VISTA HEALTH PLAN INC

300 South Park Road
Hollywood, FL 33021
Phone: 954-962-3008 Fax: 954-839-1381 Toll-Free:
Web site: www.vistahealthplan.com
MAILING ADDRESS:
    VISTA HEALTH PLAN INC
    300 South Park Road
    Hollywood, FL 33021

KEY EXECUTIVES:
Chief Executive Officer .... Steven M Scott, MD
Chief Financial Officer .... Jack Greenman
Corporate Communications .... Michelle Johnson
VP of Operations .... Kim O'Connor
VP, Communications .... Kathy Aguirre
Executive Director of Medical Affairs .... Ronald Platt, MD
VP of Medical Operations .... Patricia Jamison
Compliance Officer .... Darcy Gartner

COMPANY PROFILE:
Parent Company Name: Coventry Health Care Inc
Doing Business As:
Year Founded: 1985   Federally Qualified: [X]
Forprofit: [ ]   Not-For-Profit: [Y]
Model Type: IPA
Accreditation: [ ] AAPPO [ ] JACHO [X] NCQA [ ] URAC
Plan Type: HMO, PPO, POS
Total Revenue: 2005:   2006:   336,087,305
Net Income   2005:   2006:   12,654,264
Total Enrollment:
  2001: 192,410   2004: 240,664   2007: 0
  2002: 166,902   2005: 222,135
  2003: 259,615   2006: 207,625

SERVICE AREA:
Nationwide: N
  FL (Broward, Dade, Hernando, Hillsborough, Pasco, Palm Beach, Pinellas);

TYPE OF COVERAGE:
Commercial: [Y] Individual: [ ] FEHBP: [ ] Indemnity: [ ]
Medicare: [Y] Medicaid: [Y] Supplemental Medicare: [ ]
Tricare   [ ]

PRODUCTS OFFERED:
Product Name: Type:
HIP VIP Medicare Plan   Medicare
HealthyKids   HMO
Vista HMO   HMO
Vista FEHBP   HMO
Medicare Advantage   Medicare Advantage
Vista   Medicaid

PLAN BENEFITS:
Alternative Medicine: [ ]   Behavioral Health: [X]
Chiropractic: [X]   Dental: [X]
Home Care: [ ]   Inpatient SNF: [X]
Long-Term Care: [ ]   Pharm. Mail Order: [X]
Physical Therapy: [X]   Podiatry: [X]
Psychiatric: [X]   Transplant: [X]
Vision: [X]   Wellness: [X]
Workers' Comp: [ ]
Other Benefits:
Comments:
Formerly HIP Health Plan of Florida, Inc.

VISTA HEALTHPLAN OF SOUTH FLORIDA INC

1340 Concord Terrace
Sunrise, FL 33323
Phone: 954-858-3000 Fax: 954-846-0331 Toll-Free: 800-422-7335
Web site: www.vistahealthplan.com
MAILING ADDRESS:
    VISTA HEALTHPLAN OF SO FL INC
    1340 Concord Terrace
    Sunrise, FL 33323

KEY EXECUTIVES:
Chief Executive Officer .... Steven M Scott, MD
Chief Financial Officer .... Jack Greenman
Corporate Communications Director .... Michelle Johnson
VP of Operations .... Kim O'Connor
Marketing Director .... Kathy Aguirre
Provider Services Director .... Linda Barbanell
Health Services Director .... Janice Valesey
Director of Human Resources .... Linda Prickman
Director of Quality Assurance .... Lucielle Soltesz
Senior Health Education Specialist .... Kathy LaMagna
Director of Product Development .... Stephanie Jones
National Director .... Kate Strautman
Compliance Officer .... Darcy Gartner
Manager of Application & Operation .... Myer Kwavnick
Provider Services Director .... Judi Ryder

COMPANY PROFILE:
Parent Company Name: Coventry Health Care Inc
Doing Business As:
Year Founded: 1984   Federally Qualified: [ ]
Forprofit: [Y]   Not-For-Profit: [ ]
Model Type: IPA
Accreditation: [ ] AAPPO [ ] JACHO [X] NCQA [ ] URAC
Plan Type: HMO, PPO, POS
Total Revenue: 2005:   2006:   193,453,203
Net Income   2005:   2006:   -1,918,903
Total Enrollment:
  2001: 155,974   2004: 70,857   2007: 0
  2002: 107,851   2005: 74,073
  2003: 77,356   2006: 77,232

SERVICE AREA:
Nationwide: N
  FL (Brevard, Broward, Charlotte, Clay, Dade, Dural, Hillsborough, Lee, Martin, Okeechobee, Orange, Osceola, Palm Beach, Pasco, Pinellas, Polk, Putnam, Seminole, St Lucie, Volusia);

TYPE OF COVERAGE:
Commercial: [Y] Individual: [Y] FEHBP: [Y] Indemnity: [Y]
Medicare: [Y] Medicaid: [Y] Supplemental Medicare: [ ]
Tricare   [ ]

PRODUCTS OFFERED:
Product Name: Type:
Foundation Senior Plan   Medicare Advantage
Foundation Hlth Medicaid   Medicaid
HMO   HMO
FEHBP   HMO

FLORIDA   **Managed Care Organization Profiles**

CONSUMER-DRIVEN PRODUCTS
Exante Bank/Golden Rule Ins Co   HSA Company
iPlan HSA   HSA Product
   HSA Administrator
   Consumer-Driven Health Plan
   High Deductible Health Plan

PLAN BENEFITS:
Alternative Medicine: [ ]   Behavioral Health: [X]
Chiropractic: [X]   Dental: [ ]
Home Care: [X]   Inpatient SNF: [X]
Long-Term Care: [ ]   Pharm. Mail Order: [X]
Physical Therapy: [X]   Podiatry: [X]
Psychiatric: [X]   Transplant: [X]
Vision: [X]   Wellness: [X]
Workers' Comp: [ ]
Other Benefits: Optum 24, UBH,
Comments:
See United Healthcare, Orlando, FL for enrollment figures.

UNITEDHEALTHCARE OF FLORIDA INC

495 N Keller Rd Ste 200
Maitland, FL 32751
Phone: 407-659-6900 Fax: 407-659-6930 Toll-Free: 800-899-6500
Web site: www.uhc.com
MAILING ADDRESS:
   UNITEDHEALTHCARE OF FLORIDA
   495 N Keller Rd Ste 200
   Maitland, FL 32751

KEY EXECUTIVES:
Non-Executive Chairman .... Richard T Burke
Chief Executive Officer/President .... Matthew M Davies
Chief Financial Officer .... Robyn Cerio
Medical Director .... Dennis Young, MD
Pharmacy Director .... Jeff Olson
MIS Director .... Ron Fava
VP Network Management .... Gregg MacDonald

COMPANY PROFILE:
Parent Company Name: UnitedHealth Group
Doing Business As:
Year Founded: 1984   Federally Qualified: [N]
Forprofit: [Y]   Not-For-Profit: [ ]
Model Type: MIXED
Accreditation: [ ] AAPPO [X] JACHO [ ] NCQA [ ] URAC
Plan Type: HMO, PPO, POS, ASO, EPO, CDHP, HSA, HRA
Total Revenue: 2005:   2006: 893,951,933
Net Income 2005:   2006: 27,479,087
Total Enrollment:
   2001: 872,327   2004: 527,923   2007: 0
   2002: 687,868   2005: 436,925
   2003: 659,980   2006: 4,138,555
SERVICE AREA:
Nationwide: N
   FL (Broward, Dade, Hernando, Hillsborough, Lake, Orange, Osceloa, Palm Beach, Pasco, Pinellas, Polk, Sarasota, Seminole, Volusia);
TYPE OF COVERAGE:
Commercial: [Y] Individual: [Y] FEHBP: [ ] Indemnity: [ ]
Medicare: [Y] Medicaid: [Y] Supplemental Medicare: [ ]
Tricare [ ]
PRODUCTS OFFERED:
Product Name: Type:
Medicare Complete   Medicare Advantage
United Hlthcare   Medicaid
HealthyKid   HMO
United Healthcare   HMO
Evercare Florida   HMO Demostration
CONSUMER-DRIVEN PRODUCTS
Exante Bank/Golden Rule Ins Co   HSA Company
iPlan HSA   HSA Product
   HSA Administrator
   Consumer-Driven Health Plan
   High Deductible Health Plan

PLAN BENEFITS:
Alternative Medicine: [ ]   Behavioral Health: [X]
Chiropractic: [X]   Dental: [X]
Home Care: [X]   Inpatient SNF: [X]
Long-Term Care: [ ]   Pharm. Mail Order: [X]
Physical Therapy: [X]   Podiatry: [X]
Psychiatric: [X]   Transplant: [X]
Vision: [X]   Wellness: [X]
Workers' Comp: [ ]
Other Benefits:

UNITEDHEALTHCARE OF SOUTH FLORIDA

13621 NW 12th St
Sunrise, FL 33323
Phone: 954-858-4000 Fax: 954-858-3815 Toll-Free:
Web site: www.uhc.com
MAILING ADDRESS:
   UNITEDHEALTHCARE OF SOUTH FL
   13621 NW 12th St
   Sunrise, FL 33323

KEY EXECUTIVES:
Non-Executive Chairman .... Richard T Burke
Chief Executive Officer .... Daniel Rosenthal
Medical Director .... Dr Manuel Selva
Human Resources Director .... Tom Kurpiel

COMPANY PROFILE:
Parent Company Name: UnitedHealth Group
Doing Business As:
Year Founded: 1970   Federally Qualified: [Y]
Forprofit: [Y]   Not-For-Profit: [ ]
Model Type: STAFF
Accreditation: [ ] AAPPO [ ] JACHO [ ] NCQA [ ] URAC
Plan Type: HMO, PPO, POS, CDHP, HSA, HRA
Total Enrollment:
   2001: 0   2004: 10,871   2007: 0
   2002: 0   2005:
   2003: 10,557   2006:
SERVICE AREA:
Nationwide: N
   FL (Broward, Dade, Palm Beach);
TYPE OF COVERAGE:
Commercial: [Y] Individual: [Y] FEHBP: [ ] Indemnity: [ ]
Medicare: [Y] Medicaid: [Y] Supplemental Medicare: [ ]
Tricare [ ]
PRODUCTS OFFERED:
Product Name: Type:
Medicare Complete   Medicare Advantage
CONSUMER-DRIVEN PRODUCTS
Exante Bank/Golden Rule Ins Co   HSA Company
iPlan HSA   HSA Product
   HSA Administrator
   Consumer-Driven Health Plan
   High Deductible Health Plan

PLAN BENEFITS:
Alternative Medicine: [ ]   Behavioral Health: [X]
Chiropractic: [X]   Dental: [X]
Home Care: [X]   Inpatient SNF: [X]
Long-Term Care: [ ]   Pharm. Mail Order: [X]
Physical Therapy: [X]   Podiatry: [X]
Psychiatric: [X]   Transplant: [X]
Vision: [X]   Wellness: [X]
Workers' Comp: [ ]
Other Benefits:

UNIVERSAL HEALTH CARE INC

150 2nd Ave N Ste 400
St Petersburg, FL 33701
Phone: 727-822-3446 Fax: 727-822-3556 Toll-Free: 866-690-4842
Web site: www.univhc.com
MAILING ADDRESS:
   UNIVERSAL HEALTH CARE INC
   150 2nd Ave N Ste 400
   St Petersburg, FL 33701

UNITED CONCORDIA COMPANY INC - FLORIDA

2202 N Westshore Blvd Ste 200
Tampa, FL 33607
Phone: 813-288-4633 Fax: 813-288-4638 Toll-Free:
Web site: www.ucci.com

MAILING ADDRESS:
    UNITED CONCORDIA CO INC - FL
    2202 N Westshore Blvd Ste 200
    Tampa, FL 33607

KEY EXECUTIVES:
Chief Executive Officer .... Thomas A Dzuryachko
Senior VP, Finance .... Daniel Wright
Dental Director .... Mark Schulman, DDS
Senior VP of Sales/Marketing .... John Tearcy
MIS Director .... Jim Robins
Regional Public Relations Director .... Cecelia Muller
Director, Provider Services .... Ted Pesano
Provider Analyst .... Diane Tyson

COMPANY PROFILE:
Parent Company Name: Highmark Inc
Doing Business As: Highmark
Year Founded: 1991   Federally Qualified: [ ]
Forprofit: [Y]   Not-For-Profit: [ ]
Model Type:
Accreditation: [ ] AAPPO [ ] JACHO [ ] NCQA [ ] URAC
Plan Type: Specialty HMO, Specialty PPO, POS, TPA
Total Enrollment:
    2001: 0   2004: 755   2007: 0
    2002: 0   2005:
    2003: 0   2006:
SERVICE AREA:
Nationwide: N
    FL;
TYPE OF COVERAGE:
Commercial: [Y] Individual: [ ] FEHBP: [ ] Indemnity: [ ]
Medicare: [ ] Medicaid: [ ] Supplemental Medicare: [ ]
Tricare [ ]
PLAN BENEFITS:
Alternative Medicine: [ ]   Behavioral Health: [ ]
Chiropractic: [ ]   Dental: [X]
Home Care: [ ]   Inpatient SNF: [ ]
Long-Term Care: [ ]   Pharm. Mail Order: [ ]
Physical Therapy: [ ]   Podiatry: [ ]
Psychiatric: [ ]   Transplant: [ ]
Vision: [ ]   Wellness: [ ]
Workers' Comp: [ ]
Other Benefits:
Comments:
For enrollment and revenue information see corporate listing, Camp Hill, Pennsylvania.

UNITEDHEALTHCARE OF FLORIDA INC

9009 Corporate Lake Dr
Tampa, FL 33624
Phone: 813-890-4500 Fax: 813-890-4510 Toll-Free: 800-595-0440
Web site: www.uhc.com

MAILING ADDRESS:
    UNITEDHEALTHCARE OF FLORIDA
    9009 Corporate Lake Dr
    Tampa, FL 33624

KEY EXECUTIVES:
Non-Executive Chairman .... Richard T Burke
Chief Executive Officer .... Ken L Hoverman
Chief Financial Officer .... Robyn Cerio
Medical Director .... Robert Shaw, MD
Marketing Director .... Katie McCarey
MIS Director .... Mike Hanson
Public Relations Director .... Roger Rollman
Director of Provider Services .... Patty Hesson
Network/Operations Development .... Jeffrey Antihik
Medical Management Director .... Kathy Marjar

COMPANY PROFILE:
Parent Company Name: UnitedHealth Group
Doing Business As: United Healthcare of Florida Inc
Year Founded: 1974   Federally Qualified: [N]
Forprofit: [Y]   Not-For-Profit: [ ]
Model Type: MIXED
Accreditation: [ ] AAPPO [ ] JACHO [ ] NCQA [ ] URAC
Plan Type: HMO, PPO, POS, EPO, CDHP, HSA
Total Enrollment:
    2001: 58,689   2004: 300,000   2007: 0
    2002: 0   2005:
    2003: 34,796   2006:
SERVICE AREA:
Nationwide: N
    FL (Brevard, Broward, Charlotte, Clay, Dade, DeSoto, Duval, Escambia, Flagler, Hernando, Highlands, Hillsborough, Lake, Lee, Manatee, Okaloosa, Okeechobee, Orange, Osceola, Palm Beach, Pasco, Pinellas, Polk, Santa Rosa, Sarasota, Seminole, St Johns, Volusia);
TYPE OF COVERAGE:
Commercial: [Y] Individual: [Y] FEHBP: [ ] Indemnity: [ ]
Medicare: [Y] Medicaid: [Y] Supplemental Medicare: [ ]
Tricare [ ]
PRODUCTS OFFERED:
Product Name: Type:
Choice HMO   HMO
Choice Plus POS   POS
Medicare Choice HMO   HMO
Medicare Complete   Medicare
CONSUMER-DRIVEN PRODUCTS
Exante Bank/Golden Rule Ins Co   HSA Company
iPlan HSA   HSA Product
    HSA Administrator
    Consumer-Driven Health Plan
    High Deductible Health Plan

PLAN BENEFITS:
Alternative Medicine: [ ]   Behavioral Health: [X]
Chiropractic: [X]   Dental: [X]
Home Care: [X]   Inpatient SNF: [ ]
Long-Term Care: [ ]   Pharm. Mail Order: [X]
Physical Therapy: [ ]   Podiatry: [X]
Psychiatric: [X]   Transplant: [X]
Vision: [X]   Wellness: [X]
Workers' Comp: [ ]
Other Benefits:

UNITEDHEALTHCARE OF FLORIDA INC

7077 Bonneval Rd Ste 130
Jacksonville, FL 32216
Phone: 904-296-1332 Fax: 904-296-2649 Toll-Free: 800-250-6178
Web site: www.uhc.com

MAILING ADDRESS:
    UNITEDHEALTHCARE OF FLORIDA
    7077 Bonneval Rd Ste 130
    Jacksonville, FL 32216

KEY EXECUTIVES:
Non-Executive Chairman .... Richard T Burke
Chief Executive Officer .... Matthew M Davies
Chief Financial Officer .... Jon Schwarz
Medical Director .... Dennis Young, MD
VP, Small Business Sales .... Eric Sauby
VP, Network Management .... Gregg MacDonald

COMPANY PROFILE:
Parent Company Name: UnitedHealth Group
Doing Business As:
Year Founded: Federally Qualified: [ ]
Forprofit: [Y]   Not-For-Profit: [ ]
Model Type:
Accreditation: [ ] AAPPO [X] JACHO [ ] NCQA [ ] URAC
Plan Type: HMO, PPO, CDHP, HSA, HRA
SERVICE AREA:
Nationwide: N
    FL (Clay, Duval, St Johns);
TYPE OF COVERAGE:
Commercial: [Y] Individual: [Y] FEHBP: [ ] Indemnity: [Y]
Medicare: [Y] Medicaid: [Y] Supplemental Medicare: [ ]
Tricare [ ]

FLORIDA — Managed Care Organization Profiles

COMPANY PROFILE:
Parent Company Name:
Doing Business As:
Year Founded: 1985   Federally Qualified: [ ]
Forprofit: [Y]   Not-For-Profit: [ ]
Model Type:
Accreditation: [ ] AAPPO [ ] JACHO [ ] NCQA [X] URAC
Plan Type: UR
SERVICE AREA:
Nationwide: N
   FL;

SUMMIT HEALTH PLAN INC

300 S Park Rd
Hollywood, FL 33021
Phone: 954-962-3008 Fax: Toll-Free: 800-356-7485
Web site: www.summithealthplan.com
MAILING ADDRESS:
   SUMMIT HEALTH PLAN INC
   M Stop 1290/1340 Concord Terr
   Sunrise, FL 33021

KEY EXECUTIVES:
Chief Executive Officer/President .... Stephen Scott, MD

COMPANY PROFILE:
Parent Company Name: Vista Health Plans
Doing Business As:
Year Founded: 2005   Federally Qualified: [ ]
Forprofit: [ ]   Not-For-Profit: [ ]
Model Type:
Accreditation: [ ] AAPPO [ ] JACHO [ ] NCQA [ ] URAC
Plan Type: HMO
Total Revenue: 2005:   2006: 3,619,422
Net Income 2005:   2006: 164,377
Total Enrollment:
   2001: 0   2004: 0   2007: 0
   2002: 0   2005:
   2003: 0   2006: 1,224
SERVICE AREA:
Nationwide:
   FL (Broward, Martin, Miami-Dade, Palm Beach, St Lucie);
TYPE OF COVERAGE:
Commercial: [ ]   Individual: [ ]   FEHBP: [ ]   Indemnity: [ ]
Medicare: [Y]   Medicaid: [ ]   Supplemental Medicare: [ ]
Tricare [ ]

TOTAL HEALTH CHOICE INC

N Kendall Dr & SW 137th Ave
Miami, FL 33283-0010
Phone: 305-408-5700 Fax: 305-408-5710 Toll-Free: 800-887-6888
Web site: www.totalhealthchoiceonline.com
MAILING ADDRESS:
   TOTAL HEALTH CHOICE INC
   PO Box 830010
   Miami, FL 33283-0010

KEY EXECUTIVES:
Chief Executive Officer .... Lyle E Algate
Chief Medical Officer .... Robyn J Arrington Jr, MD
Marketing Director .... Carlos A Martinez
Director of Network/Contracts .... Francine Orta
Director of Medical Management .... Michael Ross RN

COMPANY PROFILE:
Parent Company Name: Total HealthCare Inc
Doing Business As: Total Health
Year Founded: 1997   Federally Qualified: [N]
Forprofit: [ ]   Not-For-Profit: [Y]
Model Type: MIXED
Accreditation: [ ] AAPPO [ ] JACHO [ ] NCQA [ ] URAC
Plan Type: HMO
Total Revenue: 2005:   2006: 19,913,773
Net Income 2005:   2006: -190,769
Total Enrollment:
   2001: 17,717   2004: 14,980   2007: 0
   2002: 20,337   2005: 12,189
   2003: 16,830   2006: 10,205
SERVICE AREA:
Nationwide: N
   FL (Broward, Dade, Palm Beach);
TYPE OF COVERAGE:
Commercial: [Y]   Individual: [Y]   FEHBP: [ ]   Indemnity: [ ]
Medicare: [ ]   Medicaid: [ ]   Supplemental Medicare: [ ]
Tricare [ ]
PRODUCTS OFFERED:
Product Name: Type:
Total Individual   HMO
Total Plus 5,10,15   HMO
FEHBP   HMO
PLAN BENEFITS:
Alternative Medicine: [ ]   Behavioral Health: [X]
Chiropractic: [X]   Dental: [X]
Home Care: [X]   Inpatient SNF: [X]
Long-Term Care: [ ]   Pharm. Mail Order: [ ]
Physical Therapy: [X]   Podiatry: [X]
Psychiatric: [X]   Transplant: [X]
Vision: [X]   Wellness: [ ]
Workers' Comp: [ ]
Other Benefits:
Comments:
Formerly Pacificare of Florida Inc.

UNIPSYCH SYSTEMS

7777 Davie Rd Ext Ste 100
Hollywood, FL 33024-2515
Phone: 954-704-8686 Fax: 954-704-8677 Toll-Free: 800-272-3626
Web site: www.unipsych.com
MAILING ADDRESS:
   UNIPSYCH SYSTEMS
   7777 Davie Rd Ext Ste 100
   Hollywood, FL 33024-2515

KEY EXECUTIVES:
Chief Executive Officer .... Leo Bradman, PsyD
Chief Financial Officer .... Zena Beadle
Medical Director .... Rahul Mehra, MD
Director of Operations .... Celissa Kunder
Marketing Director .... Denise Scott

COMPANY PROFILE:
Parent Company Name: Bradman Network, The
Doing Business As:
Year Founded: 1986   Federally Qualified: [ ] Forprofit: [Y]
Not-For-Profit: [ ]
Model Type: NETWORK
Accreditation: [ ] AAPPO [ ] JACHO [ ] NCQA [ ] URAC
Plan Type: Specialty PPO, UR, EPO, EAP
Total Revenue: 2005:   2006:
Net Income 2005:   2006:
Total Enrollment:
   2001: 1,000,000   2004: 0   2007: 0
   2002: 0   2005:
   2003: 1,000,000   2006:
SERVICE AREA:
Nationwide: Y
   NW;
TYPE OF COVERAGE:
Commercial: [Y]   Individual: [ ]   FEHBP: [ ]   Indemnity: [ ]
Medicare: [ ]   Medicaid: [ ]   Supplemental Medicare: [ ]
Tricare [ ]
PLAN BENEFITS:
Alternative Medicine: [ ]   Behavioral Health: [X]
Chiropractic: [ ]   Dental: [ ]
Home Care: [ ]   Inpatient SNF: [ ]
Long-Term Care: [ ]   Pharm. Mail Order: [ ]
Physical Therapy: [ ]   Podiatry: [ ]
Psychiatric: [X]   Transplant: [ ]
Vision: [ ]   Wellness: [ ]
Workers' Comp: [ ]
Other Benefits:

Managed Care Organization Profiles FLORIDA

PRODUCTS OFFERED:
Product Name: Type:
Preferred Medical Plan   Medicaid
HMO   HMO

QUALITY HEALTH PLAN INC

2435 US Hwy 19, Ste 470
Holiday, FL 34691
Phone: 727-945-8400 Fax: 727-945-8434 Toll-Free: 866-747-2700
Web site: www.qualityhealthplan.com
MAILING ADDRESS:
    QUALITY HEALTH PLAN INC
    2435 US Hwy 19 Ste 470
    Holiday, FL 34691

KEY EXECUTIVES:
Chief Executive Officer .... Nazeer H Khan, MD
President .... Haider A Khan, MD
Director of Finance .... David A Sherwin, CPA
Medical Director .... Nazeer H Khan, MD
Pharmacy Director .... John McDowell, RPh, MBA
Chief Operating Officer .... Sabiha Khan
Medical Director .... Michael Yanuk, MD
Medical Director .... Trevor Rose, MD, MS, MMM
Director, Medical Affairs .... Lisa Cierpka, RN, BSN
Corporate Servics Manager .... Farrah Sanabria, PHR

COMPANY PROFILE:
Parent Company Name:
Doing Business As:
Year Founded: 2002   Federally Qualified: [Y]
Forprofit: [Y]   Not-For-Profit: [ ]
Model Type:
Accreditation: [ ] AAPPO [ ] JACHO [ ] NCQA [ ] URAC
Plan Type: HMO
Total Revenue: 2005:   2006:   25,939,460
Net Income   2005:   2006:   807,158
Total Enrollment:
    2001: 0   2004: 5,736   2007: 0
    2002: 0   2005: 5,046
    2003: 34,133   2006: 6,487
SERVICE AREA:
Nationwide:
    FL;
TYPE OF COVERAGE:
Commercial: [ ] Individual: [ ] FEHBP: [ ] Indemnity: [ ]
Medicare: [Y] Medicaid: [ ] Supplemental Medicare: [ ]
Tricare   [ ]
PRODUCTS OFFERED:
Product Name: Type:
Seniors Choice   Medicare
Seniors Select   Medicare

RENAISSANCE HEALTH SYSTEMS INC

3420 Fairlane Farms Rd Ste C
Wellington, FL 33414
Phone: 877-778-9300 Fax: 561-828-7786 Toll-Free: 877-778-9300
Web site: www.RHSFL.com
MAILING ADDRESS:
    RENAISSANCE HEALTH SYSTEMS INC
    3420 Fairlane Farms Rd Ste C
    Wellington, FL 33414

KEY EXECUTIVES:
Chairperson of the Board .... Noel J Guillama
Chief Executive Officer/President .... Noel J Guillama
Chief Financial Officer .... Donald C Cohen
VP, Strategic Development/Public Relations Dir .... Danielle Amodio
Director of Technology Solutions .... Lorenzo Wright
Credentialing Manager .... Marcia M Potere
Provider Resources Manager/Human Resources .... Susan D Guillama
Chief Administrative Officer .... Susan D Guillama
VP, Provider Operations .... Barbara Roqueta
Patient Care Manager .... Erlinda Longalong-Coz
Corporate Development .... Ron Smith

COMPANY PROFILE:
Parent Company Name: Quantum Group, Inc, The
Doing Business As: Renaissance Health Systems Inc
Year Founded: 2000   Federally Qualified: [Y]
Forprofit: [Y]   Not-For-Profit: [ ]
Model Type: MIXED
Accreditation: [ ] AAPPO [ ] JACHO [ ] NCQA [ ] URAC
Plan Type: Specialty PPO
SERVICE AREA:
Nationwide:
    FL (East Coast);

SAFEGUARD HEALTH PLANS INC

8100 N University Dr Ste 200
Ft Lauderdale, FL 33321
Phone: 954-718-6200 Fax: 954-358-5101 Toll-Free: 800-204-0463
Web site: www.safeguard.net
MAILING ADDRESS:
    SAFEGUARD HEALTH PLANS INC
    8100 N University Dr Ste 200
    Ft Lauderdale, FL 33321

KEY EXECUTIVES:
Chairman of the Board .... James E Buncher
Chief Executive Officer .... James E Buncher

COMPANY PROFILE:
Parent Company Name:
Doing Business As:
Year Founded: 1990   Federally Qualified: [ ]
Forprofit: [Y]   Not-For-Profit: [ ]
Model Type:
Accreditation: [ ] AAPPO [ ] JACHO [ ] NCQA [ ] URAC
Plan Type: Specialty HMO, Specialty PPO, ASO
Total Enrollment:
    2001: 41,622   2004: 290,949   2007: 0
    2002: 281,647   2005:
    2003: 262,389   2006:
SERVICE AREA:
Nationwide:
    FL;
PLAN BENEFITS:
Alternative Medicine: [ ]   Behavioral Health: [ ]
Chiropractic: [ ]   Dental: [X]
Home Care: [ ]   Inpatient SNF: [ ]
Long-Term Care: [ ]   Pharm. Mail Order: [ ]
Physical Therapy: [ ]   Podiatry: [ ]
Psychiatric: [ ]   Transplant: [ ]
Vision: [ ]   Wellness: [ ]
Workers' Comp: [ ]
Other Benefits:

STRATEGIC HEALTH DEVELOPMENT CORPORATION

9501 NE 2nd Ave
Miami Shores, FL 33138
Phone: 305-754-7933 Fax: 305-751-1029 Toll-Free: 800-874-2378
Web site: www.strategichealthcorp.com
MAILING ADDRESS:
    STRATEGIC HEALTH DVLPMT CORP
    9501 NE 2nd Ave
    Miami Shores, FL 33138

KEY EXECUTIVES:
Chief Executive Officer/President .... Nigel Wallbank
Medical Director .... Barbara Freeman, MD, FAAFP
VP Operations .... Merry Gann
Director of Contracts .... Glenda Ortiz
Human Resources Director .... Gretchen Grote
Utilization/Precertification .... Myrna Hert
Case Management/Transplant Network .... Inda Leftwich
Utilization Management .... Rosella Villanveva
Director of Audit .... Nicolle Dugan

FLORIDA   Managed Care Organization Profiles

MAILING ADDRESS:
    PHYSICAL THERAPY PROVIDER NTWK
    4800 Linton Blvd Ste F-116
    Delray Beach, FL 33445

KEY EXECUTIVES:
Chief Executive Officer/President .... Linda Zane
Chief Financial Officer/Chief Operating Officer .... Linda Zane
Marketing Director .... Ira Fiebert

COMPANY PROFILE:
Parent Company Name: Physical Therapy Provider Network of CA
Doing Business As: PTPN
Year Founded: 1992   Federally Qualified: [N]
Forprofit: [Y]   Not-For-Profit: [ ]
Model Type: NETWORK
Accreditation: [ ] AAPPO   [ ] JACHO [ ] NCQA [ ] URAC
Plan Type: Specialty PPO

SERVICE AREA:
Nationwide: Y
    NW;

TYPE OF COVERAGE:
Commercial: [Y] Individual: [Y]   FEHBP: [ ]   Indemnity: [ ]
Medicare: [Y] Medicaid: [Y]   Supplemental Medicare: [Y]
Tricare

PLAN BENEFITS:
Alternative Medicine: [ ]   Behavioral Health: [ ]
Chiropractic: [ ]   Dental: [ ]
Home Care: [ ]   Inpatient SNF: [ ]
Long-Term Care: [ ]   Pharm. Mail Order: [ ]
Physical Therapy: [ ]   Podiatry: [ ]
Psychiatric: [ ]   Transplant: [ ]
Vision: [ ]   Wellness: [ ]
Workers' Comp: [ ]
Other Benefits: Occupational Therapy

PHYSICIANS UNITED PLAN INC

6220 S Orange Blossom Trl #199
Orlando, FL 32809
Phone: 866-571-0693 Fax: Toll-Free:
Web site: www.pupcorp.com

MAILING ADDRESS:
    PHYSICIANS UNITED PLAN INC
    6220 S Orange Blossom Trl #199
    Orlando, FL 32809

KEY EXECUTIVES:
Chief Executive Officer .... Dan Kollefrath
Medical Director .... Jose A Torres, MD
Chief Operating Officer .... Steve Arkin
Compliance Officer .... Paul A Christy

COMPANY PROFILE:
Parent Company Name:
Doing Business As:
Year Founded: 2005   Federally Qualified: [ ]
Forprofit: [ ]   Not-For-Profit: [ ]
Model Type:
Accreditation: [ ] AAPPO [ ] JACHO [ ] NCQA [ ] URAC
Plan Type: HMO,
Total Revenue: 2005:   2006: 2,163,202
Net Income   2005:   2006: -1,053,826
Total Enrollment:
    2001: 0   2004: 0   2007: 0
    2002: 0   2005:
    2003: 0   2006: 789

SERVICE AREA:
Nationwide:
    FL (Lake, Marion, Orange, Osceola, Polk, Seminole, Sumter);

TYPE OF COVERAGE:
Commercial: [ ] Individual: [ ]   FEHBP: [ ]   Indemnity: [ ]
Medicare: [Y] Medicaid: [ ]   Supplemental Medicare: [ ]
Tricare   [ ]

PREFERRED CARE PARTNERS INC

9100 S Dadeland Blvd Ste 1250
Miami, FL 33156
Phone: 305-670-8440 Fax: 305-670-2312 Toll-Free: 800-872-9750
Web site: www.psohealth.com

MAILING ADDRESS:
    PREFERRED CARE PARTNERS INC
    9100 S Dadeland Blvd Ste 1250
    Miami, FL 33156

KEY EXECUTIVES:
Chairman, Chief Medical Officer .... Orlando Lopez-Fernandez, MD
Chief Executive Officer .... Joseph Caruncho
President .... Justo L Pozo
Chief Financial Officer .... Eladio Gil
Chief Information Officer .... Doug Cormany
Chief Operating Officer .... Roger Rodriguez
Marketing Manager .... Arlene Montesino
Senior VP, General Counsel .... Annette C Onorati

COMPANY PROFILE:
Parent Company Name:
Doing Business As:
Year Founded: 2002   Federally Qualified: [Y]
Forprofit: [Y]   Not-For-Profit: [ ]
Model Type:
Accreditation: [ ] AAPPO [ ] JACHO [ ] NCQA [X] URAC
Plan Type: HMO
Total Revenue: 2005:   2006: 131,154,638
Net Income   2005:   2006: 3,719,481
Total Enrollment:
    2001: 0   2004: 7,187   2007: 22,905
    2002: 1,563   2005: 25,170
    2003: 4,919   2006: 22,687

SERVICE AREA:
Nationwide:
    FL;

TYPE OF COVERAGE:
Commercial: [ ] Individual: [ ]   FEHBP: [ ]   Indemnity: [ ]
Medicare: [Y] Medicaid: [ ]   Supplemental Medicare: [ ]
Tricare   [ ]

PRODUCTS OFFERED:
Product Name: Type:
PSO Health Plan   Medicare

PREFERRED MEDICAL PLAN INC

4950 SW 8th St
Coral Gables, FL 33134
Phone: 305-648-4000 Fax: 305-447-4959 Toll-Free: 800-767-5551
Web site: www.preferredmedicalplan.com

MAILING ADDRESS:
    PREFERRED MEDICAL PLAN INC
    4950 SW 8th St
    Coral Gables, FL 33134

KEY EXECUTIVES:
Chief Executive Officer/President .... Tamara Meyerson
Chief Financial Officer .... Albert Arca
Medical Director .... Gabriel Novoa, MD
Director of Operations .... Nancy Garcia
Marketing Director .... Juan Munoz
Director of Information Systems .... Ernie Pritz

COMPANY PROFILE:
Parent Company Name:
Doing Business As:
Year Founded: 1975   Federally Qualified: [N]
Forprofit: [Y]   Not-For-Profit: [ ]
Model Type: STAFF
Accreditation: [ ] AAPPO [ ] JACHO [ ] NCQA [ ] URAC
Plan Type: HMO
Total Revenue: 2005:   2006: 54,900,788
Net Income   2005:   2006: 5,523,877
Total Enrollment:
    2001: 41,349   2004: 56,098   2007: 0
    2002: 46,386   2005: 57,579
    2003: 49,593   2006: 56,541

SERVICE AREA:
Nationwide: N
    FL (Broward, Dade);

TYPE OF COVERAGE:
Commercial: [Y] Individual: [Y]   FEHBP: [ ]   Indemnity: [ ]
Medicare: [ ] Medicaid: [Y]   Supplemental Medicare: [ ]
Tricare   [ ]

Managed Care Organization Profiles   **FLORIDA**

MAILING ADDRESS:
   NEIGHBORHOOD HEALTH PARTNERSHIP
   7600 Corporate Center Dr
   Miami, FL 33126

KEY EXECUTIVES:
Chief Executive Officer/President .... Joseph Papa
Senior VP & Chief Financial Officer .... David Pollack
Senior VP & Chief Medical Officer .... Mayda Antun, MD
Chief Information Officer .... John Hurt
Senior VP & Chief Operating Officer .... Charles Ricevuto
Marketing Director .... Lisa Kofsky
Executive Vice President .... John Fries

COMPANY PROFILE:
Parent Company Name:
Doing Business As:
Year Founded: 1992   Federally Qualified: [Y]
Forprofit: [Y]   Not-For-Profit: [ ]
Model Type: IPA
Accreditation: [ ] AAPPO [ ] JACHO [X] NCQA [ ] URAC
Plan Type: HMO, POS, HDHP, HSA
Primary Physicians: 1,398   Physician Specialists:
Hospitals: 41
Total Revenue: 2005:   2006: 212,009,701
Net Income   2005:   2006: -1,897,484
Total Enrollment:
   2001: 156,511   2004: 177,403   2007: 0
   2002: 177,884   2005: 131,318
   2003: 218,755   2006: 120,042

SERVICE AREA:
Nationwide: N
   FL (Broward, Dade, Palm Beach);

TYPE OF COVERAGE:
Commercial: [Y] Individual: [ ] FEHBP: [ ] Indemnity: [ ]
Medicare: [Y] Medicaid: [ ] Supplemental Medicare: [ ]
Tricare   [ ]

PRODUCTS OFFERED:
Product Name: Type:
The Senior Plan   Medicare
Senior Health Choice   Medicare Advantage
HMO   HMO

CONSUMER-DRIVEN PRODUCTS
    HSA Company
    HSA Product
    HSA Administrator
    Consumer-Driven Health Plan
NHP HSA   High Deductible Health Plan

OLYMPUS MANAGED HEALTH CARE INC

777 Brickell Ave Penthouse 70
Miami, FL 33131
Phone: 305-530-8600 Fax: 305-530-0766 Toll-Free:
Web site: www.omhc.com

MAILING ADDRESS:
   OLYMPUS MANAGED HEALTH CARE IN
   777 Brickell Ave Penthouse 70
   Miami, FL 33131

KEY EXECUTIVES:
Chairman/Chief Executive Officer .... Stephen W Jacobson
Chief Financial Officer .... Ronald A Davis
Chief Information Officer .... David M Lopilato
Director of Operations .... Caridad S Acevedo, RN, BSN,CCM
Director of Sales .... Jim Anderson
Case Management Director .... Alejandro Sanchez, RN,BSN,CCM
Director of Call Center .... Roberto Ruadez

COMPANY PROFILE:
Parent Company Name:
Doing Business As:
Year Founded: Federally Qualified: [ ]
Forprofit: [Y]   Not-For-Profit: [ ]
Model Type:
Accreditation: [ ] AAPPO [ ] JACHO [ ] NCQA [ ] URAC
Plan Type: PPO

SERVICE AREA:
Nationwide:
   NW;

OPTIMUM HEALTHCARE INC

5478 Spring Hill Dr
Spring Hill, FL 34606
Phone: 866-245-5360 Fax: 352-688-6375 Toll-Free: 866-662-1220
Web site: www.youroptimumhealthcare.com

MAILING ADDRESS:
   OPTIMUM HEALTHCARE INC
   5478 Spring Hill Dr
   Spring Hill, FL 34606

KEY EXECUTIVES:
Marketing Director .... Michael McDonald
Director, Provider Relations .... Lynne Huey
Director of Compliance .... Carole Frank, RN
Claims Manager .... Carolyn White

COMPANY PROFILE:
Parent Company Name:
Doing Business As:
Year Founded: 2005   Federally Qualified: [ ]
Forprofit: [ ]   Not-For-Profit: [N]
Model Type:
Accreditation: [ ] AAPPO [ ] JACHO [ ] NCQA [ ] URAC
Plan Type: HMO
Total Revenue: 2005:   2006:
Net Income   2005:   2006: -428,562

SERVICE AREA:
Nationwide:
   FL (Hernando, Sumter);

PARTNERCARE HEALTH PLAN INC

5501 W Waters Ave Ste 401
Tampa, FL 33634
Phone: 813-901-9208 Fax: 813-901-9209 Toll-Free:
Web site: www.partnercarehealthplan.com

MAILING ADDRESS:
   PARTNERCARE HEALTH PLAN INC
   5501 W Waters Ave Ste 401
   Tampa, FL 33634

KEY EXECUTIVES:
Head of Internal Control .... Adrian Ramicez
Executive Director .... Robin Thomashaver

COMPANY PROFILE:
Parent Company Name:
Doing Business As:
Year Founded: 2005   Federally Qualified: [ ]
Forprofit: [ ]   Not-For-Profit: [ ]
Model Type:
Accreditation: [ ] AAPPO [ ] JACHO [ ] NCQA [ ] URAC
Plan Type: HMO,
Total Revenue: 2005:   2006: 984,265
Net Income   2005:   2006: -1,406,013
Total Enrollment:
   2001: 0   2004: 0   2007: 0
   2002: 0   2005:
   2003: 0   2006: 147

SERVICE AREA:
Nationwide:
   FL;

TYPE OF COVERAGE:
Commercial: [ ] Individual: [ ] FEHBP: [ ] Indemnity: [ ]
Medicare: [X] Medicaid: [ ] Supplemental Medicare: [ ]
Tricare   [ ]

PHYSICAL THERAPY PROVIDER NETWORK

4800 Linton Blvd Ste F-116
Delray Beach, FL 33445
Phone: 561-498-1446 Fax: 561-499-9190 Toll-Free:
Web site: www.ptinstitute.com

FLORIDA

Total Enrollment:
2001: 0   2004: 5,104   2007: 0
2002: 0   2005:
2003: 5,740 2006:

SERVICE AREA:
Nationwide:
  FL;

PLAN BENEFITS:
Alternative Medicine: [ ]   Behavioral Health: [ ]
Chiropractic: [ ]   Dental: [X]
Home Care: [ ]   Inpatient SNF: [ ]
Long-Term Care: [ ]   Pharm. Mail Order: [ ]
Physical Therapy: [ ]   Podiatry: [ ]
Psychiatric: [ ]   Transplant: [ ]
Vision: [ ]   Wellness: [ ]
Workers' Comp: [ ]
Other Benefits:

MEDICA HEALTHCARE PLANS INC

4000 Ponce de Leon Blvd #650
Coral Gables, FL 33146
Phone: 305-460-0600 Fax: 305-460-0613 Toll-Free: 800-407-9069
Web site: www.medicaplans.com

MAILING ADDRESS:
  MEDICA HEALTHCARE PLANS INC
  4000 Ponce de Leon Blvd #650
  Coral Gables, FL 33146

KEY EXECUTIVES:
Chief Executive Officer .... Raphael Perez
Chief Financial Officer .... Martin Perez
Medical Director .... Enrique Acevedo
VP, Marketing .... Nilda Lopez

COMPANY PROFILE:
Parent Company Name:
Doing Business As:
Year Founded: 2005   Federally Qualified: [ ]
Forprofit: [ ]   Not-For-Profit: [ ]
Model Type:
Accreditation: [ ] AAPPO [ ] JACHO [ ] NCQA [ ] URAC
Plan Type: HMO, PSO
Total Revenue: 2005:   2006: 38,703,608
Net Income   2005:   2006: -354,284
Total Enrollment:
  2001: 0   2004: 0   2007: 11,178
  2002: 0   2005: 4,945
  2003: 0   2006: 7,561

SERVICE AREA:
Nationwide:
  FL;

TYPE OF COVERAGE:
Commercial: [ ] Individual: [ ] FEHBP: [ ] Indemnity: [ ]
Medicare: [Y] Medicaid: [ ] Supplemental Medicare: [ ]
Tricare   [ ]

PRODUCTS OFFERED:
Product Name: Type:
Medica Healthcare   Medicare

MEDWATCH LLC

120 International Pkwy
Lake Mary, FL 32746
Phone: 407-333-8166 Fax: 407-333-8928 Toll-Free: 800-432-8421
Web site: www.urmedwatch.com

MAILING ADDRESS:
  MEDWATCH LLC
  PO Box 952679
  Lake Mary, FL 32746

KEY EXECUTIVES:
Chief Executive Officer/President .... Judy Garber, RN
Chief Financial Director .... Vince Butler
Medical Director .... Brenda Salter, MD
Marketing Director .... Judy Garber, RN
Medical Management Director .... Denise Davis RN
Case Management Director .... Nancy Leone RN

COMPANY PROFILE:
Parent Company Name: Alliance Underwriters
Doing Business As:
Year Founded: 1987   Federally Qualified: [ ]
Forprofit: [Y]   Not-For-Profit: [ ]
Model Type:
Accreditation: [ ] AAPPO [ ] JACHO [ ] NCQA [X] URAC
Plan Type: UR

SERVICE AREA:
Nationwide: Y
  NW;

PLAN BENEFITS:
Alternative Medicine: [ ]   Behavioral Health: [ ]
Chiropractic: [X]   Dental: [ ]
Home Care: [X]   Inpatient SNF: [X]
Long-Term Care: [X]   Pharm. Mail Order: [ ]
Physical Therapy: [X]   Podiatry: [X]
Psychiatric: [X]   Transplant: [X]
Vision: [ ]   Wellness: [ ]
Workers' Comp: [X]
Other Benefits:

METCARE HEALTH PLANS INC

250 S Australian Ave Ste 400
West Palm Beach, FL 33401
Phone: 561-805-8500 Fax: 561-805-8501 Toll-Free: 888-663-8227
Web site: www.metcare.com

MAILING ADDRESS:
  METCARE HEALTH PLANS INC
  250 S Australian Ave Ste 400
  West Palm Beach, FL 33401

KEY EXECUTIVES:
Chairman/Chief Executive Officer .... Michael M Earley
President .... Debra A Finnel
Chief Financial Officer .... Robert J Sabo
Chief Medical Officer-AdvantageCare .... Jose A Guethon, MD, MBA
Senior VP, Chief Information Officer .... Roman G Fisher, MS, LLM
Chief Operating Officer .... Debra A Finnel
VP, Human Resources .... Sharon Munroe
VP, Quality Management .... Lucille Soltesz
Chief Medical Officer-Metcare of FL 1 .... Hymin Zucker, MD
VP, Network Operations .... Brenton Hood
VP, Utilization Management .... Gary Baine

COMPANY PROFILE:
Parent Company Name:
Doing Business As: Metcare of Florida Inc & AdvantageCare
Year Founded: 2005   Federally Qualified: [ ]
Forprofit: [ ]   Not-For-Profit: [ ]
Model Type:
Accreditation: [ ] AAPPO [ ] JACHO [ ] NCQA [ ] URAC
Plan Type: HMO,
Total Revenue: 2005:   2006: 11,233,591
Net Income   2005:   2006: -4,169,868
Total Enrollment:
  2001: 0   2004: 0   2007: 0
  2002: 0   2005: 22,269
  2003: 0   2006: 27,000

SERVICE AREA:
Nationwide:
  FL;

TYPE OF COVERAGE:
Commercial: [ ] Individual: [ ] FEHBP: [ ] Indemnity: [ ]
Medicare: [Y] Medicaid: [ ] Supplemental Medicare: [ ]
Tricare   [ ]

PRODUCTS OFFERED:
Product Name: Type:
Metcare Health Plans Inc   Medicare Advantage

NEIGHBORHOOD HEALTH PARTNERSHIP

7600 Corporate Center Dr
Miami, FL 33126
Phone: 305-715-2200 Fax: 305-715-4306 Toll-Free: 800-354-0222
Web site: www.neighborhood-health.com

Managed Care Organization Profiles   **FLORIDA**

INTEGRATED HEALTH PLAN INC

4020 Park St N
St Petersburg, FL 33709
Phone: 727-345-8614 Fax: 727-345-7680 Toll-Free: 888-640-8707
Web site: www.ihplan.com
MAILING ADDRESS:
    INTEGRATED HEALTH PLAN INC
    4020 Park St N
    St Petersburg, FL 33709

KEY EXECUTIVES:
Chief Executive Officer/President .... Linda J Plaster
Director of Information Technology .... Rich Wheat
Chief Operating Officer .... Tommy L Tharp
Director of Provider Relations .... Laurie Casler
Executive Director of Network Development .... JoAnn Sadler
Chief Administrator Officer .... Judy Cadoret
Executive Director of Business Development .... Christian Clark
Director of Professional Relations .... Adrienne Cromwell

COMPANY PROFILE:
Parent Company Name:
Doing Business As:
Year Founded: Federally Qualified: [ ]
Forprofit: [Y]   Not-For-Profit: [ ]
Model Type:
Accreditation: [ ] AAPPO [ ] JACHO [ ] NCQA [ ] URAC
Plan Type: PPO,
Total Enrollment:
    2001: 0   2004: 0   2007: 0
    2002: 0   2005: 12,500,000
    2003: 0   2006: 12,500,000
SERVICE AREA:
Nationwide:
    NW;

JACKSON MEMORIAL HEALTH PLAN

1801 NW 9th Ave Ste 700
Miami, FL 33129-2610
Phone: 305-575-3700 Fax: 305-545-5212 Toll-Free: 800-721-2993
Web site: www.um-jmh.org
MAILING ADDRESS:
    JACKSON MEMORIAL HEALTH PLAN
    1801 NW 9th Ave Ste 700
    Miami, FL 33129-2610

KEY EXECUTIVES:
Chief Executive Officer .... Joseph Rogers
Chief Financial Officer .... Asif Jamal
Medical Director .... Clarence Smith, MD
Commercial Account Representative .... Vanessa Reeves
MIS Director .... Todd Roberts
Credentialing Manager .... Betty Larkin
Provider Relations Director .... John Ferkan
Medical Management Director .... Grace SubLaban
Member Services Manager .... Serge Boisette

COMPANY PROFILE:
Parent Company Name: Public Health Trust of Dade County, FL
Doing Business As: JMH Health Plan
Year Founded: 1985   Federally Qualified: [N]
Forprofit: [ ]   Not-For-Profit: [Y]
Model Type: MIXED
Accreditation: [ ] AAPPO [ ] JACHO [ ] NCQA [ ] URAC
Plan Type: HMO
Primary Physicians: 450   Physician Specialists:
Hospitals: 22
Total Revenue: 2005:   2006: 39,442,696
Net Income: 2005:   2006: 3,624,400
Total Enrollment:
    2001: 43,200   2004: 28,277   2007: 0
    2002: 44,360   2005: 26,265
    2003: 43,623   2006: 24,899
SERVICE AREA:
Nationwide: N
    FL (Dade County);

TYPE OF COVERAGE:
Commercial: [Y] Individual: [Y] FEHBP: [ ] Indemnity: [ ]
Medicare: [ ] Medicaid: [Y] Supplemental Medicare: [ ]
Tricare [ ]
PRODUCTS OFFERED:
Product Name: Type:
JMH Health Plan - Medicaid   Medicaid
JMH Health Plan   HMO
PLAN BENEFITS:
Alternative Medicine: [X]   Behavioral Health: [ ]
Chiropractic: [X]   Dental: [X]
Home Care: [X]   Inpatient SNF: [ ]
Long-Term Care: [ ]   Pharm. Mail Order: [X]
Physicial Therapy: [ ]   Podiatry: [X]
Psychiatric: [X]   Transplant: [X]
Vision: [X]   Wellness: [ ]
Workers' Comp: [ ]
Other Benefits:

LEON MEDICAL CENTERS HEALTH PLAN INC

101 SW 27th Ave 3rd Fl
Miami, FL 33135-1428
Phone: 305-642-5366 Fax: 305-642-1658 Toll-Free:
Web site:
MAILING ADDRESS:
    HEALTHSPRING INC
    101 SW 27th Ave 3rd Fl
    Miami, FL 33135-1428

KEY EXECUTIVES:
President/Administrator .... Benjamin Leon, Jr
Chief Financial Officer .... Albert Maury
Chief Medical Officer .... Alena Campos

COMPANY PROFILE:
Parent Company Name: HealthSpring Inc, TN
Doing Business As:
Year Founded: 2002   Federally Qualified: [ ]
Forprofit: [Y]   Not-For-Profit: [ ]
Model Type:
Accreditation: [ ] AAPPO [ ] JACHO [ ] NCQA [ ] URAC
Plan Type: HMO
Total Revenue: 2005:   2006: 131,533,254
Net Income: 2005:   2006: 9,218,985
Total Enrollment:
    2001: 0   2004: 0   2007: 0
    2002: 0   2005: 16,505
    2003: 0   2006: 22,849
SERVICE AREA:
Nationwide:
    FL;
Comments:
Acquired by HealthSpring, TN, October 1, 2007;

MANAGED CARE OF NORTH AMERICA INC

3230 W Commercial Blvd Ste 190
Ft Lauderdale, FL 33309
Phone: 954-730-7131 Fax: 954-730-7875 Toll-Free:
Web site: www.mcna.net
MAILING ADDRESS:
    MANAGED CARE OF N AMERICA INC
    3230 W Commercial Blvd Ste 190
    Ft Lauderdale, FL 33309

KEY EXECUTIVES:
Chief Executive Officer .... Glenn Feingold

COMPANY PROFILE:
Parent Company Name:
Doing Business As:
Year Founded: 1992   Federally Qualified: [ ]
Forprofit: [Y]   Not-For-Profit: [ ]
Model Type:
Accreditation: [ ] AAPPO [ ] JACHO [ ] NCQA [ ] URAC
Plan Type: Specialty HMO

FLORIDA — Managed Care Organization Profiles

MAILING ADDRESS:
   HUMANA MEDICAL PLAN DAYTONA
   135 Executive Circle
   Daytona Beach, FL 32114

KEY EXECUTIVES:
Chairman of the Board	David A Jones Jr
Chief Executive Officer	Craig Drablos
President	Scott Latimer, MD
VP & Chief Financial Officer	John Barger
Chief Medical Officer	Steve Lee, MD
VP Commercial Sales	Carson Meehan
Provider Contracting Operation	Sharon Glass
Quality Management Director	Mary Jane Eranch RN
Associate Medical Director	Lee Campbell MD
Utilization Manager	Grace Hodge RN

COMPANY PROFILE:
Parent Company Name: Humana Inc   Doing Business As:
Year Founded: 1961   Federally Qualified: [Y]
Forprofit: [Y]   Not-For-Profit: [ ]
Model Type: IPA
Accreditation: [ ] AAPPO [ ] JACHO [X] NCQA [X] URAC
Plan Type: HMO, PPO, CDHP, HSA

SERVICE AREA:
Nationwide: N
   FL (Volusia, Flagler);

TYPE OF COVERAGE:
Commercial: [Y] Individual: [ ] FEHBP: [ ] Indemnity: [ ]
Medicare: [ ] Medicaid: [ ] Supplemental Medicare: [ ]
Tricare [

CONSUMER-DRIVEN PRODUCTS
JP Morgan Chase	HSA Company
HumanaOne HSA	HSA Product
JP Morgan Chase	HSA Administrator
Personal Care Account	Consumer-Driven Health Plan
HumanaOne	High Deductible Health Plan

PLAN BENEFITS:
Alternative Medicine:	[ ]	Behavioral Health:	[X]
Chiropractic:	[X]	Dental:	[X]
Home Care:	[ ]	Inpatient SNF:	[ ]
Long-Term Care:	[ ]	Pharm. Mail Order:	[X]
Physical Therapy:	[ ]	Podiatry:	[ ]
Psychiatric:	[X]	Transplant:	[X]
Vision:	[ ]	Wellness:	[ ]
Workers' Comp:	[X]		

Other Benefits: Long Term Disability

HUMANA MEDICAL PLAN INC

3501 SW 160th Ave
Miramar, FL 33027
Phone: 305-626-5499 Fax: 502-508-8543 Toll-Free: 800-442-5555
Web site: www.humana.com

MAILING ADDRESS:
   HUMANA MEDICAL PLAN INC
   3501 SW 160th Ave
   Miramar, FL 33027

KEY EXECUTIVES:
Chairman of the Board	David A Jones Jr
Chief Executive Officer/South East Region	Craig Drablos
President, South Florida	Colin P D'Arcy
Chief Financial Officer	Scott Richardson
Chief Medical Director	Jill M Sumfest, MD, MS, FACS, FAS
Pharmacy Directory	Daniel Sihkin, RPh
Director of Operations & Business Development	Neil E Berman
Director of Marketing	Madeleine Arritola
VP Sales	Bill Condon
Statewide Director Regulatory Affairs	Terry Martinez
VP Network Management	Peter Martin
Human Resources Consultant	Lesley Shelton
Quality Management Director	Susan Hoffman RN
Director Commercial Sales	Shawn Thanert
Utilization Management Director	Sheri Ivey

COMPANY PROFILE:
Parent Company Name: Humana Inc
Doing Business As:
Year Founded: 1987   Federally Qualified: [Y]
Forprofit: [Y]   Not-For-Profit: [ ]
Model Type: MIXED
Accreditation: [ ] AAPPO [ ] JACHO [ ] NCQA [X] URAC
Plan Type: HMO, HDHP, HSA
Primary Physicians: 1,500   Physician Specialists:
Hospitals: 51
Total Revenue: 2005:   2006: 168,461,118
Net Income   2005:   2006: 97,880,992
Total Enrollment:
   2001: 425,237   2004: 455,056   2007: 156,441
   2002: 302,146   2005: 457,761
   2003: 464,115   2006: 463,851

SERVICE AREA:
Nationwide: N
   FL (Dade, Broward, Palm Beach, Monroe, Martin, St Lucie, Indian River, Okeechobee, Brevard, Lee, Collier, Charlotte, Desoto, Glades, Hendry, Highlands, Hardee);

TYPE OF COVERAGE:
Commercial: [Y] Individual: [Y] FEHBP: [ ] Indemnity: [ ]
Medicare: [Y] Medicaid: [Y] Supplemental Medicare: [ ]
Tricare [ ]

PRODUCTS OFFERED:
Product Name:	Type:
Humana Gold Plus Plan	Medicare Advantage
Humana Medicaid	Medicaid
FEHBP	HMO
HMO	HMO
Humana Gold Classic	Medicare Advantage

CONSUMER-DRIVEN PRODUCTS
JP Morgan Chase	HSA Company HumanaOne
HSA	HSA Product
JP Morgan Chase	HSA Administrator
Personal Care Account	Consumer-Driven Health Plan
HumanaOne	High Deductible Health Plan

PLAN BENEFITS:
Alternative Medicine:	[ ]	Behavioral Health:	[X]
Chiropractic:	[X]	Dental:	[X]
Home Care:	[ ]	Inpatient SNF:	[ ]
Long-Term Care:	[ ]	Pharm. Mail Order:	[X]
Physical Therapy:	[ ]	Podiatry:	[ ]
Psychiatric:	[X]	Transplant:	[X]
Vision:	[ ]	Wellness:	[ ]
Workers' Comp:	[X]		

Other Benefits: Long Term Disability

HYGEIA CORPORATION

15500 New Barn Rd Ste 200
Miami Lakes, FL 33014
Phone: 305-594-9291 Fax: 305-594-9293 Toll-Free: 877-540-9788
Web site: www.hygeia.net

MAILING ADDRESS:
   HYGEIA CORPORATION
   15500 New Barn Rd Ste 200
   Miami Lakes, FL 33014

KEY EXECUTIVES:
Chief Executive Officer	Virgil Bretz
Chief Financial Ofcier	Frank J Gnisci
Chief Information Officer	Roderick Hamilton
Chief Operating Officer	Joseph P Radigan
Chief Marketing Officer	Larry Taylor
Director of Business Development	Victor Mehra
General Counsel	Gary C Matzner

COMPANY PROFILE:
Parent Company Name:
Doing Business As:
Year Founded: 1994   Federally Qualified: [ ]
Forprofit: [Y]   Not-For-Profit: [ ]
Model Type:
Accreditation: [ ] AAPPO [X] JACHO [ ] NCQA [ ] URAC
Plan Type: PPO
Medical Loss Ratio: 2005:   2006:
Administrative Expense Ratio: 2005:   2006:

SERVICE AREA:
Nationwide:
   NW;

Managed Care Organization Profiles — FLORIDA

TYPE OF COVERAGE:
Commercial: [Y] Individual: [ ] FEHBP: [ ] Indemnity: [ ]
Medicare: [Y] Medicaid: [Y] Supplemental Medicare: [ ]
Tricare [ ]

PRODUCTS OFFERED:
Product Name:	Type:
Employee Assistant Program	
Managed Behavioral Health Program	
Administrative Services Only	
Utilization review	ASO
On Line Work Life Services	EAP

PLAN BENEFITS:
Alternative Medicine: [ ]   Behavioral Health: [X]
Chiropractic: [ ]   Dental: [ ]
Home Care: [ ]   Inpatient SNF: [ ]
Long-Term Care: [ ]   Pharm. Mail Order: [ ]
Physical Therapy: [ ]   Podiatry: [ ]
Psychiatric: [X]   Transplant: [ ]
Vision: [ ]   Wellness: [X]
Workers' Comp: [ ]
Other Benefits: Employee Assistance

Comments:
See Horizon Health Corp, Lewisville, TX for enrollment statistics- Orlando.

HUMANA HEALTH PLAN - JACKSONVILLE

76 South Laura St 16th Fl
Jacksonville, FL 32202
Phone: 904-376-1100   Fax: 502-508-8543   Toll-Free: 800-945-7703
Web site: www.humana.com

MAILING ADDRESS:
HUMANA HEALTH PLAN JACKSONVILLE
76 South Laura St 16th Fl
Jacksonville, FL 32202

KEY EXECUTIVES:
Chairman of the Board .... David A Jones Jr
Chief Executive Officer .... Craig Drablos
President .... Bruno Littleton
VP, Chief Financial Officer .... Rhonda Bagby
Medical Director .... Miguel Fernandez
Provider Contracts Director .... Ron Dobson
VP, Network Operations .... Lee Bowers
Quality Management Manager .... Patti Deguio RN
Clinical RX .... Cynthia Griffin
Associate Medical Director .... Eric Stewart
Service Center Director .... Cindy Carlton

COMPANY PROFILE:
Parent Company Name: Humana Inc
Doing Business As:
Year Founded: 1961   Federally Qualified: [Y]
Forprofit: [Y]   Not-For-Profit: [ ]
Model Type: IPA
Accreditation: [ ] AAPPO [ ] JACHO [ ] NCQA [X] URAC
Plan Type: HMO, PPO, POS, ASO, EPO, CDHP, HSA
Primary Physicians: 1,000   Physician Specialists:
Hospitals:
Total Enrollment:
  2001: 0   2004: 59,500   2007: 0
  2002: 36,341   2005:
  2003: 0   2006: 59,500

SERVICE AREA:
Nationwide: N
  FL;

TYPE OF COVERAGE:
Commercial: [Y] Individual: [Y] FEHBP: [ ] Indemnity: [ ]
Medicare: [Y] Medicaid: [Y] Supplemental Medicare: [Y]
Tricare [Y]

CONSUMER-DRIVEN PRODUCTS
JP Morgan Chase	HSA Company
HumanaOne HSA	HSA Product
JP Morgan Chase	HSA Administrator
Personal Care Account	Consumer-Driven Health Plan
HumanaOne	High Deductible Health Plan

PLAN BENEFITS:
Alternative Medicine: [ ]   Behavioral Health: [X]
Chiropractic: [X]   Dental: [X]
Home Care: [ ]   Inpatient SNF: [ ]
Long-Term Care: [ ]   Pharm. Mail Order: [X]
Physical Therapy: [ ]   Podiatry: [ ]
Psychiatric: [X]   Transplant: [X]
Vision: [ ]   Wellness: [ ]
Workers' Comp: [X]
Other Benefits: Long Term Disability

HUMANA MEDICAL PLAN - CENTRAL FLORIDA

5401 W Kennedy Blvd Ste 161
Tampa, FL 33609
Phone: 813-286-8829   Fax: 813-207-0995   Toll-Free: 800-568-3333
Web site: www.humana.com

MAILING ADDRESS:
HUMANA MEDICAL PLAN-CENTRAL FL
5401 W Kennedy Blvd Ste 161
Tampa, FL 33609

KEY EXECUTIVES:
Chairman of the Board .... David A Jones Jr
Chief Executive Officer, South East .... Reg Craig Drablos
President/Chief Operating Officer .... Scott Latimer, MD
VP & Chief Financial Officer .... John Barger
Chief Medical Officer .... Steve Lee, MD
VP of Commercial Sales .... Carson Meehan
VP of Network Operations .... Elizabeth Strombom
Quality Management Director .... Vicki Neupauer RN
Utilization Management .... Abby Marenger RN
VP of Consumer Advocacy .... Judy Woodworth

COMPANY PROFILE:
Parent Company Name: Humana Inc
Doing Business As:
Year Founded: 1961   Federally Qualified: [Y]
Forprofit: [Y]   Not-For-Profit: [ ]
Model Type: IPA
Accreditation: [ ] AAPPO [ ] JACHO [X] NCQA [ ] URAC
Plan Type: HMO, HDHP, HSA,
Primary Physicians: 1,400   Physician Specialists:
Hospitals: 65
Total Enrollment:
  2001: 0   2004: 0   2007: 0
  2002: 0   2005:
  2003: 0   2006: 242,000

SERVICE AREA:
Nationwide: N
  FL (Hillsborough, Pinellas, Pasco, Hernando, Citrus, Pock, Manatee, Sarasota),

TYPE OF COVERAGE:
Commercial: [Y] Individual: [ ] FEHBP: [ ] Indemnity: [ ]
Medicare: [ ] Medicaid: [ ] Supplemental Medicare: [ ]
Tricare [ ]

CONSUMER-DRIVEN PRODUCTS
JP Morgan Chase	HSA Company
HumanaOne HSA	HSA Product
JP Morgan Chase	HSA Administrator
Personal Care Account	Consumer-Driven Health Plan
HumanaOne	High Deductible Health Plan

PLAN BENEFITS:
Alternative Medicine: [ ]   Behavioral Health: [X]
Chiropractic: [X]   Dental: [X]
Home Care: [ ]   Inpatient SNF: [ ]
Long-Term Care: [ ]   Pharm. Mail Order: [X]
Physical Therapy: [ ]   Podiatry: [ ]
Psychiatric: [X]   Transplant: [X]
Vision: [ ]   Wellness: [ ]
Workers' Comp: [X]
Other Benefits: Long Term Disability

HUMANA MEDICAL PLAN - DAYTONA

135 Executive Circle
Daytona Beach, FL 32114
Phone: 386-676-1800   Fax: 502-580-2099   Toll-Free: 800-320-9565
Web site: www.humana.com

FLORIDA — Managed Care Organization Profiles

COMPANY PROFILE:
Parent Company Name: WellCare Health Plans Inc
Doing Business As:
Year Founded: 2000   Federally Qualified: [N]
Forprofit: [Y]   Not-For-Profit: [ ]
Model Type:
Accreditation: [ ] AAPPO [ ] JACHO [ ] NCQA [ ] URAC
Plan Type: HMO
Total Revenue: 2005:   2006: 221,206,245
Net Income   2005:   2006: 10,072,464
Total Enrollment:
  2001: 128,374   2004: 229,055   2007: 0
  2002: 159,438   2005: 232,401
  2003: 200,868   2006: 219,085

SERVICE AREA:
Nationwide: N
  FL;

TYPE OF COVERAGE:
Commercial: [ ] Individual: [ ] FEHBP: [ ] Indemnity: [ ]
Medicare: [ ] Medicaid: [Y] Supplemental Medicare: [ ]
Tricare   [ ]

PRODUCTS OFFERED:
Product Name:	Type:
Healtheast of FL	Medicaid
HealthyKids	HMO

Comments:
Formerly known as Tampa General Healthplan Inc.

HEALTHSUN HEALTH PLANS INC

1205 SW 37th Ave
Miami, FL 33135
Phone: 305-234-9292 Fax: 305-444-9148 Toll-Free: 877-207-4900
Web site: www.health-sun.com

MAILING ADDRESS:
  HEALTHSUN HEALTH PLANS INC
  1205 SW 37th Ave
  Miami, FL 33135

COMPANY PROFILE:
Parent Company Name:
Doing Business As:
Year Founded: 2005   Federally Qualified: [ ]
Forprofit: [ ]   Not-For-Profit: [ ]
Model Type:
Accreditation: [ ] AAPPO [ ] JACHO [ ] NCQA [ ]
URACPlan Type: HMO,
Total Revenue: 2005:   2006: 10,703,802
Net Income   2005:   2006: 362,062
Total Enrollment:
  2001: 0   2004: 0   2007: 0
  2002: 0   2005: 1,666
  2003: 0   2006: 1,884

SERVICE AREA:
Nationwide:
  FL;

TYPE OF COVERAGE:
Commercial: [ ] Individual: [ ] FEHBP: [ ] Indemnity: [ ]
Medicare: [Y] Medicaid: [ ] Supplemental Medicare: [ ]
Tricare   [ ]

PRODUCTS OFFERED:
Product Name:	Type:
Healthsun	Medicare
SunPlus Advantage	Medicare Advantage

HEALTHY PALM BEACHES INC

324 Datura St Ste 401
West Palm Beach, FL 33401
Phone: 561-659-1270 Fax: 561-659-4620 Toll-Free: 866-930-0035
Web site: www.healthypalmbeaches.org

MAILING ADDRESS:
  HEALTHY PALM BEACHES INC
  324 Datura St Ste 401
  West Palm Beach, FL 33401

KEY EXECUTIVES:
Chief Executive Officer .... Dwight Chenette
Chief Financial Officer .... Craig Jenkins
Chief Medical Officer .... Ronald Wiewora, MD
Chief Operating Officer .... Debi Gavras
Director of Communications .... Sherry Weinschenk
Compliance Officer .... Steve Fowler

COMPANY PROFILE:
Parent Company Name: Health Care District of Palm Beach Cnty
Doing Business As: Healthy Palm Beaches Inc
Year Founded: 1996   Federally Qualified: [N]
Forprofit: [ ]   Not-For-Profit: [Y]
Model Type:
Accreditation: [ ] AAPPO [ ] JACHO [ ] NCQA [ ] URAC
Plan Type: HMO,
Total Revenue: 2005:   2006: 3,004,440
Net Income   2005:   2006: 56,473
Total Enrollment:
  2001: 7,116   2004: 5,148   2007: 0
  2002: 5,826   2005: 5,186
  2003: 9,146   2006: 4,790

SERVICE AREA:
Nationwide: N
  FL; (Palm Beach)

TYPE OF COVERAGE:
Commercial: [Y] Individual: [ ] FEHBP: [ ] Indemnity: [ ]
Medicare: [ ] Medicaid: [Y] Supplemental Medicare: [ ]
Tricare   [ ]

PRODUCTS OFFERED:
Product Name:	Type:
Healthy Palm Beaches	Medicaid

HORIZON BEHAVIORAL SERVICES

1035 Greenwood Ste 201
Lake Mary, FL 32746
Phone: 407-647-6153 Fax: 407-915-0052 Toll-Free: 800-400-2606
Web site: www.horizoncare.net

MAILING ADDRESS:
  HORIZON BEHAVIORAL SERVICES
  1035 Greenwood Ste 201
  Lake Mary, FL 32746

KEY EXECUTIVES:
Chairman of the Board .... James Ken Newman
Chief Executive Officer/President/Director .... Jackie L James
Senior VP, CFO, Treasurer & Assistant Secretary ...... Ronald C Drabik
Medical Director .... William Eckbert, MD
Director of Information Technology .... John Anzalmo
President .... Jackie L James
Senior VP, Sales .... Dave Tingue
Director of Information Technology .... John Anzalmo
Network Services Manager .... Julie Osmanski-Harmon
HIPAA Compliance Officer .... Carol Sparks
Director of Operations, HBS Orlando .... Lupe Rivero
VP, Human Resources .... Ric Shriver
Director, Quality Management .... Eileen Bascombe
Director, Business Affairs .... Susan Bellofatto
VP of Operations HBS Denver/San Diego .... Peggy Wagner
VP of Operations, HBS Nashville .... Cindy Sherrif
VP of Operations, HBS Philadelphia .... Dorothy Harrison, PhD

COMPANY PROFILE:
Parent Company Name: Horizon Health Corporation
Doing Business As: Horizon Behavioral Services, Inc.
Year Founded: 1989   Federally Qualified: [Y]
Forprofit: [Y]   Not-For-Profit: [ ]
Model Type: MIXED
Accreditation: [ ] AAPPO [ ] JACHO [X] NCQA [X] URAC
Plan Type: Specialty PPO
Primary Physicians: 2,924   Physician Specialists:
Hospitals: 564
Total Enrollment:
  2001: 0   2004: 0   2007: 0
  2002: 2,349,000   2005:
  2003: 2,940,000   2006:

SERVICE AREA:
Nationwide: N
  FL;

Managed Care Organization Profiles   **FLORIDA**

GREAT-WEST HEALTHCARE OF FLORIDA

1511 N Westshore Blvd Ste 700
Tampa, FL 33607
Phone: 813-207-0216 Fax: 813-207-0613 Toll-Free: 800-533-0919
Web site: www.greatwesthealthcare.com

MAILING ADDRESS:
   GREAT-WEST HEALTHCARE OF FL
   1511 N Westshore Blvd Ste 700
   Tampa, FL 33607

KEY EXECUTIVES:
Chief Executive Officer/President .... Raymond L McFeetors
Vice President .... Susan Griffin
President .... Steven White
Medical Director .... Thomas Morrow, MD
Provider Relations Director .... Kelly Bock

COMPANY PROFILE:
Parent Company Name: CIGNA Inc
Doing Business As:
Year Founded: 1996   Federally Qualified: [N]
Forprofit: [Y]   Not-For-Profit: [ ]
Model Type: IPA
Accreditation: [ ] AAPPO [ ] JACHO [X] NCQA [ ] URAC
Plan Type: HMO, PPO, POS, CDHP, HDHP, HSA
Total Revenue: 2005:   2006: 759,020
Net Income   2005:   2006: 223,169
Total Enrollment:
   2001: 9,297   2004: 1,802   2007: 0
   2002: 6,456   2005: 1,143
   2003: 2,330   2006: 391

SERVICE AREA:
Nationwide: N
   FL (Hillsborough, Orange, Osceola, Pasco, Pinellas, Polk, Seminole)

TYPE OF COVERAGE:
Commercial: [Y] Individual: [ ] FEHBP: [ ] Indemnity: [ ]
Medicare: [Y] Medicaid: [ ] Supplemental Medicare: [ ]
Tricare   [ ]

PRODUCTS OFFERED:
Product Name: Type:
One Health Plan of FL   HMO

CONSUMER-DRIVEN PRODUCTS
Mellon HR Solutions LLC   HSA Company
                                      HSA Product
                                      HSA Administrator
                                      Consumer-Driven Health Plan
                                      High Deductible Health Plan

PLAN BENEFITS:
Alternative Medicine: [X]   Behavioral Health: [ ]
Chiropractic: [X]   Dental: [X]
Home Care: [X]   Inpatient SNF: [X]
Long-Term Care: [ ]   Pharm. Mail Order: [X]
Physical Therapy: [X]   Podiatry: [X]
Psychiatric: [X]   Transplant: [X]
Vision: [X]   Wellness: [X]
Workers' Comp: [ ]
Other Benefits:

Comments: Acquired by CIGNA Inc, April 1, 2008

HEALTH FIRST HEALTH PLANS INC

6450 US Hwy 1
Rockledge, FL 32955-5747
Phone: 321-434-5600 Fax: 321-434-4270 Toll-Free: 800-716-7737
Web site: www.health-first.org

MAILING ADDRESS:
   HEALTH FIRST HEALTH PLANS INC
   6450 US Hwy 1
   Rockledge, FL 32955-5747

KEY EXECUTIVES:
Chief Executive Officer .... Jerry Senne
President .... Peter Weiss, MD
Financial Services Manager .... Steve Lewis
Medical Director .... Joseph Collins, MD
Pharmacy Director .... Bill Anderson
Director Information Services .... Christi Rushnell
Chief Operating Officer .... Peter Weiss, MD
Vice President .... Angela Handa
MIS Manager .... Bruce Tate
Credentialing Coordinator .... Tammy Muzzy
Privacy Officer .... Beth Fleming
Director Provider Relations .... Katie Fleming
VP of Clinical Services .... Joy Gilbert
Credentialing Coordinator .... Tammy Muzzy
VP, Operations .... Betty Kennard

COMPANY PROFILE:
Parent Company Name: Health First Inc
Doing Business As:
Year Founded: 1995   Federally Qualified: [N]
Forprofit: [Y]   Not-For-Profit: [ ]
Model Type: IPA
Accreditation: [ ] AAPPO [ ] JACHO [X] NCQA [ ] URAC
Plan Type: HMO, POS, TPA, CDHP, HDHP, HSA
Primary Physicians: 183   Physician Specialists:
Hospitals: 5
Total Revenue: 2005: 254,873,722   2006: 308,513,635
Net Income   2005:   8,118,410   2006:   8,778,023
Total Enrollment:
   2001: 46,613   2004: 54,781   2007: 0
   2002: 58,378   2005: 50,774
   2003: 58,271   2006: 54,698

SERVICE AREA:
Nationwide: N
   FL (Brevard, Indian River);

TYPE OF COVERAGE:
Commercial: [Y] Individual: [ ] FEHBP: [ ] Indemnity: [ ]
Medicare: [Y] Medicaid: [ ] Supplemental Medicare: [ ]
Tricare   [ ]

PRODUCTS OFFERED:
Product Name: Type:
Health First Medicare Plan   Medicare Advantage
Health First Health Plan   HMO
HealthyKids   HMO

CONSUMER-DRIVEN PRODUCTS
Sun Trust   HSA Company
HSA   HSA Product
Sun Trust   HSA Administrator
                                      Consumer-Driven Health Plan
Consumer Engagement Series   High Deductible Health Plan

PLAN BENEFITS:
Alternative Medicine: [X]   Behavioral Health: [ ]
Chiropractic: [X]   Dental: [ ]
Home Care: [X]   Inpatient SNF: [X]
Long-Term Care: [X]   Pharm. Mail Order: [X]
Physical Therapy: [X]   Podiatry: [X]
Psychiatric: [X]   Transplant: [X]
Vision: [X]   Wellness: [X]
Workers' Comp: [ ]
Other Benefits:

HEALTHEASE OF FLORIDA INC

8735 Henderson Rd Renaissance2
Tampa, FL 33634
Phone: 813-290-6236 Fax: 813-290-6332 Toll-Free: 800-278-0656
Web site: www.wellcare.com

MAILING ADDRESS:
   HEALTHEASE OF FLORIDA INC
   8735 Henderson Rd Renaissance2
   Tampa, FL 33634

KEY EXECUTIVES:
Executive Chairman .... Charles G Berg
Chief Executive Officer/President .... Heath Schiesser
VP of Operations .... Steven Ogilvie
Senior VP, Marketing .... Heith Schieffer
Senior VP, Sales in Florida .... Rupesh Shah
Vp, Provider Relations .... Diane Wilkosz
Human Resources Director .... Gretchen Demartini

FLORIDA
Managed Care Organization Profiles

Primary Physicians: 73 Physician Specialists:
Hospitals: 7
Total Revenue: 2005:   2006: 152,041,512
Net Income   2005:   2006:   7,272,355
Total Enrollment:
   2001: 55,903   2004: 65,561   2007: 0
   2002: 61,763   2005: 64,767
   2003: 65,579   2006: 61,800

SERVICE AREA:
Nationwide: N
   FL (Flagler, Seminole, Volusia);

TYPE OF COVERAGE:
Commercial: [Y] Individual: [ ] FEHBP: [ ] Indemnity: [ ]
Medicare: [Y] Medicaid: [ ] Supplemental Medicare: [ ]
Tricare   [ ]

PRODUCTS OFFERED:
Product Name:	Type:
Senior Care	Medicare
HealthyKids	HMO
HMO	HMO
FL Health Care Plan	Medicare Advantage

CONSUMER-DRIVEN PRODUCTS
Bank of America	HSA Company
	HSA Product
	HSA Administrator
	Consumer-Driven Health Plan
	High Deductible Health Plan

PLAN BENEFITS:
Alternative Medicine: [ ]   Behavioral Health: [X]
Chiropractic: [X]   Dental: [X]
Home Care: [X]   Inpatient SNF: [X]
Long-Term Care: [ ]   Pharm. Mail Order: [X]
Physical Therapy: [X]   Podiatry: [X]
Psychiatric: [X]   Transplant: [ ]
Vision: [X]   Wellness: [X]
Workers' Comp: [ ]
Other Benefits:

FLORIDA HEALTH PARTNERS INC

8906 Britiany Way
Tampa, FL 33619
Phone: 800-808-3236 Fax: 813-246-7222 Toll-Free: 800-808-8033
Web site: www.floridahealthpartners.com

MAILING ADDRESS:
   FLORIDA HEALTH PARTNERS INC
   8906 Britiany Way
   Tampa, FL 33619

KEY EXECUTIVES:
Office Manager .... Bernie Roy
Medical Director .... David Moore, MD

COMPANY PROFILE:
Parent Company Name: ValueOptions Inc, FL Behavioral Hlth Inc
Doing Business As:
Year Founded: 1998   Federally Qualified: [ ]
Forprofit: [Y]   Not-For-Profit: [ ]
Model Type:
Accreditation: [ ] AAPPO [ ] JACHO [ ] NCQA [ ] URAC
Plan Type: Specialty HMO
Total Enrollment:
   2001: 0   2004: 67,200   2007: 0
   2002: 0   2005: 66,783
   2003: 56,505   2006:

SERVICE AREA:
Nationwide:
   FL;

TYPE OF COVERAGE:
Commercial: [ ] Individual: [ ] FEHBP: [ ] Indemnity: [ ]
Medicare: [ ] Medicaid: [Y] Supplemental Medicare: [ ]
Tricare   [ ]

PLAN BENEFITS:
Alternative Medicine: [ ]   Behavioral Health: [ ]
Chiropractic: [ ]   Dental: [ ]
Home Care: [ ]   Inpatient SNF: [ ]
Long-Term Care: [ ]   Pharm. Mail Order: [ ]
Physical Therapy: [ ]   Podiatry: [ ]
Psychiatric: [X]   Transplant: [ ]
Vision: [ ]   Wellness: [ ]
Workers' Comp: [ ]
Other Benefits: Prepaid Mental Health Plan

FREEDOM HEALTH INC

5501 49th St N
St Petersburg, FL 33709
Phone: 727-471-2101 Fax: 671-646-6923 Toll-Free: 727-471-2108
Web site: www.freedomhealth.com

MAILING ADDRESS:
   FREEDOM HEALTH INC
   PO Box 1162
   Pinnellas Park, FL 33709

KEY EXECUTIVES:
Chief Executive Officer .... Daviah Pagidipati
Marketing Director .... Robin Flores

COMPANY PROFILE:
Parent Company Name:
Doing Business As:
Year Founded: 2005   Federally Qualified: [ ]
Forprofit: [ ]   Not-For-Profit: [ ]
Model Type:
Accreditation: [ ] AAPPO [ ] JACHO [ ] NCQA [ ] URAC
Plan Type: HMO,
Total Revenue: 2005:   2006: 11,528,612
Net Income   2005:   2006:   102,013
Total Enrollment:
   2001: 0   2004: 0   2007: 0
   2002: 0   2005: 388
   2003: 0   2006: 3,471

SERVICE AREA:
Nationwide:
   FL;

TYPE OF COVERAGE:
Commercial: [ ] Individual: [ ] FEHBP: [ ] Indemnity: [ ]
Medicare: [Y] Medicaid: [ ] Supplemental Medicare: [ ]
Tricare   [ ]

GLOBAL MEDICAL MANAGEMENT

7901 SW 36th St Ste 100
Davie, FL 33328-1914
Phone: 954-370-6404 Fax: 954-370-6301 Toll-Free: 800-682-6065
Web site: www.gmmusa.com

MAILING ADDRESS:
   GLOBAL MEDICAL MANAGEMENT
   7901 SW 36th St Ste 100
   Davie, FL 33328-1914

KEY EXECUTIVES:
Chief Executive Officer/President .... Martin Smith
Director of Finance & Administration .... Melody Sharet
Medical Director .... Wayne Lee, MD
Information Technology Manager .... Dave Tepper
Chief Operating Officer .... Raija Itzchaki
Assistant VP .... Manuela Pujals
New Business Development .... Brian Piper
Director Health Care Services .... Zaydee Capo
Assistant VP, Client Accounts .... Monica Rummelhoff

COMPANY PROFILE:
Parent Company Name: Heusinkveld Group
Doing Business As: Global Medical Management Inc
Year Founded: 1991   Federally Qualified: [ ]
Forprofit: [Y]   Not-For-Profit: [ ]
Model Type:
Accreditation: [ ] AAPPO [ ] JACHO [ ] NCQA [ ] URAC
Plan Type: Specialty PPO

SERVICE AREA:
Nationwide: N
   FL;

PLAN BENEFITS:
Alternative Medicine: [ ]   Behavioral Health: [ ]
Chiropractic: [ ]   Dental: [ ]
Home Care: [ ]   Inpatient SNF: [ ]
Long-Term Care: [ ]   Pharm. Mail Order: [ ]
Physical Therapy: [ ]   Podiatry: [ ]
Psychiatric: [ ]   Transplant: [ ]
Vision: [ ]   Wellness: [ ]
Workers' Comp: [ ]
Other Benefits: Travel Health

Managed Care Organization Profiles — FLORIDA

DIMENSION HEALTH (PPO)

5881 N W 151 St #201
Miami Lakes, FL 33014
Phone: 305-823-7664 Fax: 305-818-8814 Toll-Free: 800-483-4992
Web site: www.dimensionhealth.com

MAILING ADDRESS:
DIMENSION HEALTH (PPO)
5881 N W 151 St #201
Miami Lakes, FL 33014

KEY EXECUTIVES:
Chief Executive Officer/President ....Charles Lindgren
Medical Director .... Ray Mummery, MD
Credentialing Manager/Provider Relations Director .... Creta Diehs
Network Development/Managed Care Director .... Leslie Glazer

COMPANY PROFILE:
Parent Company Name: Dimension Health Inc
Doing Business As:
Year Founded: 1985   Federally Qualified: [N]
Forprofit: [ ]   Not-For-Profit: [Y]
Model Type: NETWORK
Accreditation: [ ] AAPPO [ ] JACHO [ ] NCQA [ ] URAC
Plan Type: PPO, EPO
Primary Physicians: 1,740   Physician Specialists:
Hospitals: 50
Total Enrollment:
  2001: 559,945   2004: 0   2007: 0
  2002: 440,000   2005:   2003: 435,000
2006: 460,000

SERVICE AREA:
Nationwide: N
  FL (South East, Fl)

TYPE OF COVERAGE:
Commercial: [Y] Individual: [Y] FEHBP: [ ] Indemnity: [ ]
Medicare: [Y] Medicaid: [Y] Supplemental Medicare: [Y]
Tricare   [ ]

PRODUCTS OFFERED:
Product Name: Type:
Dimension Health Plan   PPO

PLAN BENEFITS:
Alternative Medicine: [ ]   Behavioral Health: [X]
Chiropractic: [X]   Dental: [ ]
Home Care: [X]   Inpatient SNF: [X]
Long-Term Care: [ ]   Pharm. Mail Order: [ ]
Physical Therapy: [X]   Podiatry: [X]
Psychiatric: [X]   Transplant: [X]
Vision: [X]   Wellness: [X]
Workers' Comp: [X]
Other Benefits:

EVOLUTIONS HEALTHCARE SYSTEMS INC

7916 Evolutions Way
New Port Richey, FL 34655
Phone: 727-938-2222 Fax: 727-938-2880 Toll-Free: 800-881-4474
Web site: www.ehsppo.com

MAILING ADDRESS:
EVOLUTIONS HEALTHCARE SYS INC
7916 Evolutions Way
New Port Richey, FL 34655

KEY EXECUTIVES:
Chairman .... Allen K Cranford
Chief Executive Officer .... Ed Johnes
President .... Allen K Cranford
Chief Financial Officer .... Jere Gulau
Chief Medical Officer .... Ed Johnes
Chief Operating Officer .... Debra Suarez

COMPANY PROFILE:
Parent Company Name:
Doing Business As:
Year Founded: 1992   Federally Qualified: [ ]
Forprofit: [Y]   Not-For-Profit: [ ]
Model Type: NETWORK
Accreditation: [ ] AAPPO [ ] JACHO [ ] NCQA [ ] URAC
Plan Type: PPO
Primary Physicians: 143,205   Physician Specialists:
Hospitals: 4,000
Total Enrollment:
  2001: 0   2004: 0   2007: 0
  2002: 0   2005:
  2003: 1,200,000   2006:

SERVICE AREA:
Nationwide:
  FL;

FIRST MEDICAL HEALTH PLAN OF FLORIDA

5960 NW 7th St
Miami, FL 33126-3155
Phone: 305-269-7995 Fax: 305-269-9582 Toll-Free:
Web site:

MAILING ADDRESS:
FIRST MEDICAL HEALTH PLAN OF FL
5960 NW 7th St
Miami, FL 33126-3155

COMPANY PROFILE:
Parent Company Name:
Doing Business As:
Year Founded: 2007   Federally Qualified: [ ]
Forprofit: [ ]   Not-For-Profit: [ ]
Model Type:
Accreditation: [ ] AAPPO [ ] JACHO [ ] NCQA [ ] URAC
Plan Type: HMO,

SERVICE AREA:
Nationwide:
  FL; PR;

TYPE OF COVERAGE:
Commercial: [ ] Individual: [ ] FEHBP: [ ] Indemnity: [ ]
Medicare: [Y] Medicaid: [ ] Supplemental Medicare: [ ]
Tricare   [ ]

Comments:
Accreditation due 2009

FLORIDA HEALTH CARE PLAN INC

1340 Ridgewood Ave
Holly Hill, FL 32117
Phone: 386-676-7110 Fax: 386-676-7119 Toll-Free: 800-232-0578
Web site: www.floridahealthcares.com

MAILING ADDRESS:
FLORIDA HEALTH CARE PLAN INC
1340 Ridgewood Ave
Holly Hill, FL 32117

KEY EXECUTIVES:
Chief Executive Officer .... Edward Simpson Jr
President .... Wendy Myers, MD
Chief Financial Officer .... David Schandel
Chief Medical Officer .... Wendy Myers, MD
Pharmacy Director .... Gary Klein
Chief Operating Officer .... David Schandel
Marketing Director .... Pamela Mims
MIS Director .... James W Bare, Jr
Compliance Officer .... Rob Gilliland
Advertising & Public Relations Manager .... Bissy Holden
Administrator, Provider Services .... Sherrie Hutchinson
Human Resources Director .... Kathy Evans
Quality Management Director .... Sandra O'Neal
New Product Development Director .... Pamala McIntire
Deputy Compliance Officer .... Rob Gilliland

COMPANY PROFILE:
Parent Company Name: Halifax Health
Doing Business As: Florida Health Care Plans
Year Founded: 1974   Federally Qualified: [Y]
Forprofit: [ ]   Not-For-Profit: [Y]
Model Type: MIXED
Accreditation: [ ] AAPPO [ ] JACHO [ ] NCQA [X] URAC
Plan Type: HMO, POS, CDHP, HDHP,

FLORIDA
Managed Care Organization Profiles

CITRUS HEALTH CARE INC

5420 Bay Center Dr Ste 250
Tampa, FL 33609
Phone: 813-490-8900 Fax: 813-490-8909 Toll-Free:
Web site: www.citrushc.com

MAILING ADDRESS:
CITRUS HEALTH CARE INC
5420 Bay Center Dr Ste 250
Tampa, FL 33609

KEY EXECUTIVES:
President .... Don Hairston
Executive VP, Medical Director .... Jayant Patel, MD
Medicaid Marketing Director .... Ramon Rios
MIS Director .... Leonard Mallard
Network Development Director .... Jean McDade
Human Resources Director .... Charmaine Thames-Conley
Medical Management Director .... Maureen Parker
Compliance/Quality Management .... Patricia Thorbin
Customer Servcie Director .... Deborah Waddell
Claims Director .... Maureen Lach
Medicare Marketing Director .... Steve Snider
Executive Director, Long Term Care .... JoAnne Dutcher

COMPANY PROFILE:
Parent Company Name: CEF Holdings, LLC
Doing Business As:
Year Founded: 2003   Federally Qualified: [N]
Forprofit: [Y]   Not-For-Profit: [ ]
Model Type: IPA
Accreditation: [ ] AAPPO [ ] JACHO [ ] NCQA [ ] URAC
Plan Type: HMO, CDHP
Total Revenue: 2005: 29,081,272   2006: 45,233,228
Net Income   2005:   380,506   2006:   744,515
Total Enrollment:
   2001: 0   2004: 7,712   2007: 16,920
   2002: 0   2005: 11,864
   2003: 0   2006: 16,237

SERVICE AREA:
Nationwide: N
FL;

TYPE OF COVERAGE:
Commercial: [Y] Individual: [Y] FEHBP: [ ] Indemnity: [ ]
Medicare: [Y] Medicaid: [Y] Supplemental Medicare: [ ]
Tricare   [ ]

PLAN BENEFITS:
Alternative Medicine: [ ]   Behavioral Health: [X]
Chiropractic: [ ]   Dental: [ ]
Home Care: [ ]   Inpatient SNF: [ ]
Long-Term Care: [X]   Pharm. Mail Order: [ ]
Physical Therapy: [ ]   Podiatry: [ ]
Psychiatric: [ ]   Transplant: [ ]
Vision: [ ]   Wellness: [ ]
Workers' Comp: [ ]
Other Benefits:

COMPREHENSIVE BEHAVIORAL CARE INC

3405 W Dr Martin Luther King #101
Tampa, FL 33609
Phone: 813-288-4808 Fax: 813-288-4844 Toll-Free:
Web site: www.compcare.com

MAILING ADDRESS:
COMPREHENSIVE BEHAVIORAL CARE
3405 W Dr Martin Luther King #101
Tampa, FL 33609

KEY EXECUTIVES:
Chief Executive Officer/President .... Mary Jane Johnson, RN, MBA
Chief Financial Officer .... Robert Landis
Marketing Coordinator .... Angela White Crane
MIS Director .... Ed Gorczycd
Director of Provider Services .... Arda Curtis
Director of Human Resources .... Leslie Fairweather
Senior VP, Clinical Service .... Paul Patti, PhD

COMPANY PROFILE:
Parent Company Name: Comprehensive Care Inc
Doing Business As: Comprehensive Behavioral Care Inc
Year Founded: 1990   Federally Qualified: [ ] Forprofit: [Y]
Not-For-Profit: [ ]
Model Type:
Accreditation: [ ] AAPPO [ ] JACHO [ ] NCQA [ ] URAC
Plan Type: Specialty HMO
Total Revenue: 2005: 24,473,000   2006:
Net Income   2005:   -268,000   2006:
Total Enrollment:
   2001: 1,000,000   2004: 0   2007: 0
   2002: 0   2005:
   2003: 0   2006: 10,700,000
Medical Loss Ratio: 2005: 2006:
Administrative Expense Ratio: 2005: 2006:

SERVICE AREA:
Nationwide: Y
NW;

TYPE OF COVERAGE:
Commercial: [Y] Individual: [ ] FEHBP: [ ] Indemnity: [ ]
Medicare: [Y] Medicaid: [Y] Supplemental Medicare: [ ]
Tricare   [ ]

PRODUCTS OFFERED:
Product Name: Type:
Comprehensive Behavioral Care   Specialty HMO

PLAN BENEFITS:
Alternative Medicine: [ ]   Behavioral Health: [X]
Chiropractic: [ ]   Dental: [ ]
Home Care: [ ]   Inpatient SNF: [X]
Long-Term Care: [ ]   Pharm. Mail Order: [ ]
Physical Therapy: [X]   Podiatry: [ ]
Psychiatric: [X]   Transplant: [ ]
Vision: [ ]   Wellness: [ ]
Workers' Comp: [ ]
Other Benefits:

Comments:
Plan type also includes EAP.

DELTA DENTAL OF FLORIDA

258 Southhall Lane Ste 350
Maitland, FL 32751
Phone: 407-660-9034 Fax: 407-660-2899 Toll-Free: 800-662-9034
Web site: www.deltadentalins.com

MAILING ADDRESS:
DELTA DENTAL OF FLORIDA
258 Southhall Lane Ste 350
Maitland, FL 32751

KEY EXECUTIVES:
President .... Robert B Elliott

COMPANY PROFILE:
Parent Company Name: Delta Dental Plan of California
Doing Business As:
Year Founded: 1970   Federally Qualified: [ ]
Forprofit: [ ]   Not-For-Profit: [Y]
Model Type:
Accreditation: [ ] AAPPO [ ] JACHO [ ] NCQA [ ] URAC
Plan Type: Specialty HMO, Specialty PPO
Total Enrollment:
   2001: 0   2004: 0   2007: 0
   2002: 0   2005:
   2003: 242,187   2006:

SERVICE AREA:
Nationwide: N
FL;

TYPE OF COVERAGE:
Commercial: [Y] Individual: [ ] FEHBP: [ ] Indemnity: [ ]
Medicare: [ ] Medicaid: [ ] Supplemental Medicare: [ ]
Tricare   [ ]

PLAN BENEFITS:
Alternative Medicine: [ ]   Behavioral Health: [ ]
Chiropractic: [ ]   Dental: [X]
Home Care: [ ]   Inpatient SNF: [ ]
Long-Term Care: [ ]   Pharm. Mail Order: [ ]
Physical Therapy: [ ]   Podiatry: [ ]
Psychiatric: [ ]   Transplant: [ ]
Vision: [ ]   Wellness: [ ]
Workers' Comp: [ ]
Other Benefits:

Managed Care Organization Profiles — FLORIDA

CIGNA DENTAL HEALTH OF FLORIDA

1571 Sawgrass Corporate Pkwy
Sunrise, FL 33323
Phone: 954-514-6600 Fax: 954-514-6905 Toll-Free: 800-367-1037
Web site: www.cigna.com/dental

MAILING ADDRESS:
CIGNA DENTAL HEALTH OF FL INC
1571 Sawgrass Corporate Pkwy
Sunrise, FL 33323

KEY EXECUTIVES:
President .... Karen S Rohan
Chief Financial Officer .... Michelle I Haas
Marketing Director .... Aaron Groffman
MIS Director .... Laurel A Flebotte

COMPANY PROFILE:
Parent Company Name: CIGNA Dental Health Inc
Doing Business As: CIGNA Dental
Year Founded: 1974   Federally Qualified: [N]
Forprofit: [Y]   Not-For-Profit: [ ]
Model Type:
Accreditation: [ ] AAPPO [ ] JACHO [ ] NCQA [ ] URAC
Plan Type: Specialty HMO
Total Enrollment:
  2001: 0   2004: 288,448   2007: 0
  2002: 339,374   2005:
  2003: 325,704   2006:

SERVICE AREA:
Nationwide: N
FL;

TYPE OF COVERAGE:
Commercial: [Y] Individual: [ ] FEHBP: [ ] Indemnity: [ ]
Medicare: [ ] Medicaid: [ ]   Supplemental Medicare: [ ]
Tricare   [ ]

PLAN BENEFITS:
Alternative Medicine: [ ]   Behavioral Health: [ ]
Chiropractic: [ ]   Dental: [X]
Home Care: [ ]   Inpatient SNF: [ ]
Long-Term Care: [ ]   Pharm. Mail Order: [ ]
Physical Therapy: [ ]   Podiatry: [ ]
Psychiatric: [ ]   Transplant: [ ]
Vision: [ ]   Wellness: [ ]
Workers' Comp: [ ]
Other Benefits:

CIGNA HEALTHCARE OF FLORIDA

3101 W Martin Luther King Blvd #200
Tampa, FL 33607
Phone: 813-353-4400 Fax: 813-353-4411 Toll-Free: 800-942-2471
Web site: www.cigna.com

MAILING ADDRESS:
CIGNA HEALTHCARE OF FL
3101 W Martin Luther King Blvd #200
Tampa, FL 33607

KEY EXECUTIVES:
Chief Executive Officer/President .... Andrew D Crooks
Chief Financial Officer .... Andrew D Crooks
Chief Operating Officer .... Mary Atkinson
Director of Provider Services .... Phil Wasden
Human Resources Director .... Steven Haigler
Quality Assurance Director .... George Andrews, MD

COMPANY PROFILE:
Parent Company Name: CIGNA Corporation
Doing Business As:
Year Founded: 1974   Federally Qualified: [N]
Forprofit: [Y]   Not-For-Profit: [ ]
Model Type: MIXED
Accreditation: [ ] AAPPO [ ] JACHO [X] NCQA [ ] URAC
Plan Type: HMO, PPO, POS, ASO, EPO, CDHP, HSA, FSA, HRA
Total Revenue: 2005: 178,629,059   2006: 130,404,865
Net Income   2005:   3,490,771   2006:   -1,075,648

Total Enrollment:
  2001: 125,800   2004: 81,764   2007: 0
  2002: 121,720   2005: 78,147
  2003: 94,668   2006: 78,147

SERVICE AREA:
Nationwide: N
FL (Baker, Broward, Clay, Dade, Duval, Hillsborough, Lake, Manatee, Martin, Nassau, Orange, Osceola, Palm Beach, Pasco, Pinellas, Seminole, Volusia);

TYPE OF COVERAGE:
Commercial: [Y] Individual: [ ] FEHBP: [ ] Indemnity: [ ]
Medicare: [Y] Medicaid: [ ]   Supplemental Medicare: [ ]
Tricare   [ ]

PRODUCTS OFFERED:
Product Name: Type:
Fully Insured HMO/POS
Experience Rates HMO/POS

CONSUMER-DRIVEN PRODUCTS
JP Morgan Chase   HSA Company
CIGNA Choice Fund   HSA Product
                             HSA Administrator
Open Access Plus   Consumer-Driven Health Plan
PPO   High Deductible Health Plan

PLAN BENEFITS:
Alternative Medicine: [ ]   Behavioral Health: [ ]
Chiropractic: [X]   Dental: [ ]
Home Care: [X]   Inpatient SNF: [X]
Long-Term Care: [ ]   Pharm. Mail Order: [X]
Physical Therapy: [X]   Podiatry: [X]
Psychiatric: [X]   Transplant: [X]
Vision: [X]   Wellness: [X]
Workers' Comp: [X]
Other Benefits:

CIGNA HEALTHCARE OF FLORIDA

1580 Sawgrass Corp Pkwy Ste200
Sunrise, FL 33323
Phone: 954-693-7500 Fax: 954-693-7540 Toll-Free:
Web site: www.cigna.com

MAILING ADDRESS:
CIGNA HEALTHCARE OF FL
1580 Sawgrass Corp Pkwy Ste200
Sunrise, FL 33323

KEY EXECUTIVES:
Regional Vice President South East .... Andrew D Crooks
President/General Manager South FL .... Susan Knapp Pinnas
Chief Financial Officer .... Andrew D Crooks
Medical Director .... Robert Kropp, MD
Marketing Director .... William Antonello

COMPANY PROFILE:
Parent Company Name: CIGNA Corporation
Doing Business As:
Year Founded: 1984   Federally Qualified: [Y]
Forprofit: [Y]   Not-For-Profit: [ ]
Model Type: MIXED
Accreditation: [ ] AAPPO [ ] JACHO [ ] NCQA [ ] URAC
Plan Type: HMO, PPO, POS, CDHP, HSA, FSA, HRA

SERVICE AREA:
Nationwide: N
FL (Orange, Osceola, Seminole, Volusia);

TYPE OF COVERAGE:
Commercial: [Y] Individual: [ ] FEHBP: [ ] Indemnity: [ ]
Medicare: [ ] Medicaid: [ ]   Supplemental Medicare: [ ]
Tricare   [ ]

CONSUMER-DRIVEN PRODUCTS
JP Morgan Chase   HSA Company
CIGNA Choice Fund   HSA Product
                             HSA Administrator
Open Access Plus   Consumer-Driven Health Plan
PPO   High Deductible Health Plan

PLAN BENEFITS:
Alternative Medicine: [ ]   Behavioral Health: [ ]
Chiropractic: [ ]   Dental: [X]
Home Care: [X]   Inpatient SNF: [X]
Long-Term Care: [ ]   Pharm. Mail Order: [X]
Physical Therapy: [X]   Podiatry: [X]
Psychiatric: [X]   Transplant: [X]
Vision: [X]   Wellness: [X]
Workers' Comp: [ ]
Other Benefits:

FLORIDA

Managed Care Organization Profiles

CAREIQ

3450 Lakeside Dr Ste 610
Miramar, FL 33027
Phone: 954-441-7600 Fax: 954-441-0398 Toll-Free: 800-414-4674
Web site: www.careiq.com
MAILING ADDRESS:
    CAREIQ
    3450 Lakeside Dr Ste 610
    Miramar, FL 33027

KEY EXECUTIVES:
Chief Executive Officer/President .... Gordon Clemons
Branch Manager .... Arlene Chejanovski
System Manager .... Leigh Valdimer

COMPANY PROFILE:
Parent Company Name:
Doing Business As:
Year Founded: 1994   Federally Qualified: [ ]
Forprofit: [Y]   Not-For-Profit: [ ]
Model Type: NETWORK
Accreditation: [ ] AAPPO [ ] JACHO [ ] NCQA [ ] URAC
Plan Type: PPO, Specialty PPO
Total Enrollment:
    2001: 63,000   2004: 0   2007: 0
    2002: 0   2005:
    2003: 0   2006:
SERVICE AREA:
Nationwide: Y
    NW;
TYPE OF COVERAGE:
Commercial: [Y] Individual: [ ] FEHBP: [ ] Indemnity: [ ]
Medicare: [ ] Medicaid: [ ] Supplemental Medicare: [ ]
Tricare   [ ]
PRODUCTS OFFERED:
Product Name: Type:
AnciCare PPO   PPO
PLAN BENEFITS:
Alternative Medicine: [ ]   Behavioral Health: [ ]
Chiropractic: [ ]   Dental: [ ]
Home Care: [ ]   Inpatient SNF: [ ]
Long-Term Care: [ ]   Pharm. Mail Order: [ ]
Physical Therapy: [ ]   Podiatry: [ ]
Psychiatric: [ ]   Transplant: [ ]
Vision: [ ]   Wellness: [ ]
Workers' Comp: [X]
Other Benefits:
Comments:
Formerly AnciCare PPO.

CAREPLUS HEALTH PLANS INC

55 Alhambra Plaza 7th Fl
Coral Gables, FL 33134
Phone: 800-794-4105 Fax: 813-829-8308 Toll-Free:
Web site: www.careplus-hp.com
MAILING ADDRESS:
    CAREPLUS HEALTH PLANS INC
    55 Alhambra Plaza 7th Fl
    Coral Gables, FL 33134

KEY EXECUTIVES:
Chief Executive Officer/President .... David Jarboe
Chief Financial Officer .... Frederick Brown
Medical Director .... Maria LaBarga, MD
Chief Operating Officer .... Peter Jimenez
Marketing Director .... Tony Alverez

COMPANY PROFILE:
Parent Company Name: Humana Inc
Doing Business As: Florida 1st Health Plan Inc
Year Founded: 1985   Federally Qualified: [Y]
Forprofit: [Y]   Not-For-Profit: [ ]
Model Type:
Accreditation: [ ] AAPPO [ ] JACHO [ ] NCQA [ ] URAC
Plan Type: HMO
Total Revenue: 2005:   420,009,523   2006:   43,276,777
Net Income   2005:   11,760,875   2006:   9,784,988
Total Enrollment:
    2001: 0   2004: 49,881   2007: 0
    2002: 37,653   2005: 49,380
    2003: 43,750   2006: 52,747
SERVICE AREA:
Nationwide:
    FL;
TYPE OF COVERAGE:
Commercial: [ ] Individual: [ ] FEHBP: [ ] Indemnity: [ ]
Medicare: [Y]   Medicaid: [ ] Supplemental Medicare: [ ]
Tricare   [ ]
PRODUCTS OFFERED:
Product Name: Type:
Physicians Care Plus   Medicare
PLAN BENEFITS:
Alternative Medicine: [ ]   Behavioral Health: [ ]
Chiropractic: [ ]   Dental: [ ]
Home Care: [ ]   Inpatient SNF: [ ]
Long-Term Care: [ ]   Pharm. Mail Order: [ ]
Physical Therapy: [ ]   Podiatry: [ ]
Psychiatric: [ ]   Transplant: [ ]
Vision: [ ]   Wellness: [ ]
Workers' Comp: [ ]
Other Benefits:
Comments:
Acquired by Humana Inc. February 2005.

CIGNA DENTAL HEALTH INC - CORPORATION HEADQUARTERS

1571 Sawgrass Corporate Pksy
Sunrise, FL 33323
Phone: 954-514-6600 Fax: 954-514-6905 Toll-Free: 800-367-1037
Web site: www.cigna.com/dental
MAILING ADDRESS:
    CIGNA DENTAL HEALTH INC - CORP
    1571 Sawgrass Corporate Pkwy
    Sunrise, FL 33323

KEY EXECUTIVES:
President .... Karen S Rohan
Chief Financial Officer .... Michelle I Haas
Marketing Director .... Aaron Groffman
MIS Director .... Laurel A Flebotte

COMPANY PROFILE:
Parent Company Name:
Doing Business As: CIGNA Dental
Year Founded: 1982   Federally Qualified: [N]
Forprofit: [Y]   Not-For-Profit: [ ]
Model Type:
Accreditation: [ ] AAPPO [ ] JACHO [ ] NCQA [ ] URAC
Plan Type: Specialty HMO;
Total Enrollment:
    2001: 0   2004: 0   2007: 0
    2002: 0   2005:
    2003: 0   2006: 10,700,000
SERVICE AREA:
Nationwide: N
    AL; AR; CT; DC; FL; GA; IA; ID; IN; LA; MA; MI; MN; MO; MS; NY; OK; OR; SC; TN; UT; VA; WA; WI; WV;
TYPE OF COVERAGE:
Commercial: [Y] Individual: [ ] FEHBP: [ ] Indemnity: [ ]
Medicare: [ ] Medicaid: [ ] Supplemental Medicare: [ ]
Tricare   [ ]
PRODUCTS OFFERED:
Product Name: Type:
CIGNA Dental   HMO
CIGNA Dental   Indemnity
PLAN BENEFITS:
Alternative Medicine: [ ]   Behavioral Health: [ ]
Chiropractic: [ ]   Dental: [X]
Home Care: [ ]   Inpatient SNF: [ ]
Long-Term Care: [ ]   Pharm. Mail Order: [ ]
Physical Therapy: [ ]   Podiatry: [ ]
Psychiatric: [ ]   Transplant: [ ]
Vision: [ ]   Wellness: [ ]
Workers' Comp: [ ]
Other Benefits:

Managed Care Organization Profiles — FLORIDA

BROADSPIRE INC

1601 Southwest 80th Terrace
Plantation, FL 33324-4036
Phone: 954-452-4000 Fax: 954-382-4585 Toll-Free: 800-726-8898
Web site: www.choosebroadspire.com

MAILING ADDRESS:
BROADSPIRE INC
1601 Southwest 80th Terrace
Plantation, FL 33324-4036

KEY EXECUTIVES:
Chief Executive Officer/President .... Dennis Replogle
VP,Chief Medical Officer .... Jacob Iazarovic, MD
Chief Operating Officer .... Ed Mullen
VP, Marketing.. Stephanie Zercher
Senior VP of Casualty Claims Serv .... Donnie Gray

COMPANY PROFILE:
Parent Company Name: Crawford & Co
Doing Business As: Broadspire
Year Founded: Federally Qualified: [ ]
Forprofit: [Y]   Not-For-Profit: [ ]
Model Type:
Accreditation: [ ] AAPPO [ ] JACHO [ ] NCQA [X] URAC
Plan Type: PPO, UR, TPA
Total Revenue: 2005:   2006:   68,160,000
Net Income   2005:   2006:

SERVICE AREA:
Nationwide: Y
NW;

TYPE OF COVERAGE:
Commercial: [Y] Individual: [ ] FEHBP: [ ] Indemnity: [ ]
Medicare: [ ] Medicaid: [ ] Supplemental Medicare: [ ]
Tricare   [ ]

PLAN BENEFITS:
Alternative Medicine: [ ]   Behavioral Health: [ ]
Chiropractic: [ ]   Dental: [ ]
Home Care: [ ]   Inpatient SNF: [ ]
Long-Term Care: [ ]   Pharm. Mail Order: [ ]
Physical Therapy: [ ]   Podiatry: [ ]
Psychiatric: [ ]   Transplant: [ ]
Vision: [ ]   Wellness: [ ]
Workers' Comp: [X]
Other Benefits:

Comments:
Formerly Kemper National Services PPO.

CAPITAL HEALTH PLAN

2140 Centerville Rd
Tallahassee, FL 32308-4300
Phone: 850-383-3333 Fax: 850-383-3497 Toll-Free: 800-390-1434
Web site: www.capitalhealth.com

MAILING ADDRESS:
CAPITAL HEALTH PLAN
2140 Centerville Rd
Tallahassse, FL 32308-4300

KEY EXECUTIVES:
Chief Executive Officer .... John M Hogan
Chief Financial Officer .... Sabin Bass
Medical Director .... Nancy Van Vessem, MD
Marketing Director .... Susan Conte

COMPANY PROFILE:
Parent Company Name: Blue Cross/Blue Shield
Doing Business As: Capital Health Plan
Year Founded: 1982   Federally Qualified: [Y]
Forprofit: [ ]   Not-For-Profit: [Y]
Model Type: MIXED
Accreditation: [ ] AAPPO [ ] JACHO [ ] NCQA [ ] URAC
Plan Type: HMO
Total Revenue: 2005: 289,878,732   2006: 213,635,661
Net Income   2005:   29,782,615   2006:   16,657,766

Total Enrollment:
2001: 108,233   2004: 110,799   2007: 0
2002: 110,000   2005: 112,876
2003: 107,909   2006: 112,876

SERVICE AREA:
Nationwide: N
FL (Gadsden, Jefferson, Leon, Taylor, Wakulla);

TYPE OF COVERAGE:
Commercial: [Y] Individual: [ ] FEHBP: [ ] Indemnity: [ ]
Medicare: [Y] Medicaid: [ ] Supplemental Medicare: [ ]
Tricare   [ ]

PRODUCTS OFFERED:
Product Name: Type:
Capital Small Group   HMO
Capital FEHBP   FEHBP
HMO   Medicare
Capital Large Group   HMO

PLAN BENEFITS:
Alternative Medicine: [ ]   Behavioral Health: [ ]
Chiropractic: [X]   Dental: [ ]
Home Care: [X]   Inpatient SNF: [ ]
Long-Term Care: [ ]   Pharm. Mail Order: [ ]
Physical Therapy: [ ]   Podiatry: [X]
Psychiatric: [ ]   Transplant: [X]
Vision: [X]   Wellness: [X]
Workers' Comp: [ ]
Other Benefits:

CAREGUIDE

12301 NW 39th St
Coral Springs, FL 33065
Phone: 888-721-9797 Fax: 954-796-3703 Toll-Free: 888-721-9797
Web site: www.careguide.com

MAILING ADDRESS:
CAREGUIDE
12301 NW 39th St
Coral Springs, FL 33065

KEY EXECUTIVES:
Chairman of the Board .... Albert Waxman, PhD
Chief Executive Officer/President .... Chris Patterson
Chief Financial Officer .... Glen A Spence
Medical Director .... James Jones, MD
Chief Information Officer .... Dale Brown
Senior VP, General Counsel .... Don Parisi
VP, Business Development.. Steve Gutman

COMPANY PROFILE:
Parent Company Name: Coordinated Care Solutions, FL
Doing Business As:
Year Founded: 1998   Federally Qualified: [ ]
Forprofit: [ ]   Not-For-Profit: [ ]
Model Type:
Accreditation: [ ] AAPPO [ ] JACHO [ ] NCQA [ ] URAC
Plan Type: Specialty HMO
Total Enrollment:
2001: 15,562   2004: 0   2007: 0
2002: 4,433   2005:
2003:   0   2006:

SERVICE AREA:
Nationwide: N
CT; FL; NY;

TYPE OF COVERAGE:
Commercial: [ ] Individual: [ ] FEHBP: [ ] Indemnity: [ ]
Medicare: [ ] Medicaid: [ ] Supplemental Medicare: [ ]
Tricare   [ ]

PLAN BENEFITS:
Alternative Medicine: [ ]   Behavioral Health: [X]
Chiropractic: [ ]   Dental: [ ]
Home Care: [ ]   Inpatient SNF: [ ]
Long-Term Care: [ ]   Pharm. Mail Order: [ ]
Physical Therapy: [ ]   Podiatry: [ ]
Psychiatric: [ ]   Transplant: [ ]
Vision: [ ]   Wellness: [ ]
Workers' Comp: [ ]
Other Benefits:

Comments:
Formerly Coordinated Care Solutions.

FLORIDA

Managed Care Organization Profiles

KEY EXECUTIVES:
Chief Executive Officer .... Douglas G Cueny
Chief Financial Officer .... Michael Gallagher
Medical Officer .... Kirk Cianciolo, DO
Pharmacy Director .... Shawn Barger
Chief Information Officer .... John R Higbee
MIS Director .... Winston Lonsdale
Director, Provider Services .... Barry Wagner
Director, Client Services .... Bill Mazza

COMPANY PROFILE:
Parent Company Name:
Doing Business As:
Year Founded: 1969   Federally Qualified: [Y]
Forprofit: [ ]   Not-For-Profit: [Y]
Model Type: IPA
Accreditation: [ ] AAPPO [ ] JACHO [X] NCQA [ ] URAC
Plan Type: HMO, POS, CDHP, HSA,
Total Enrollment:
  2001: 0   2004: 0   2007: 220,000
  2002: 0   2005:
  2003: 0   2006:

SERVICE AREA:
Nationwide: N
  FL;

TYPE OF COVERAGE:
Commercial: [Y] Individual: [ ] FEHBP: [ ] Indemnity: [ ]
Medicare: [Y] Medicaid: [ ] Supplemental Medicare: [ ]
Tricare   [ ]

CONSUMER-DRIVEN PRODUCTS
Health Equity   HSA Company
AvMed Consumer HSA   HSA Product
                                      HSA Administrator Con-
sumer-Driven Health Plan
                                      High Deductible Health Plan

PLAN BENEFITS:
Alternative Medicine: [X]   Behavioral Health: [X]
Chiropractic: [X]   Dental: [X]
Home Care: [X]   Inpatient SNF: [X]
Long-Term Care: [ ]   Pharm. Mail Order: [X]
Physical Therapy: [X]   Podiatry: [X]
Psychiatric: [ ]   Transplant: [X]
Vision: [X]   Wellness: [X]
Workers' Comp: [ ]
Other Benefits:

BLUE CROSS BLUE SHIELD OF FLORIDA & HEALTH OPTIONS INC

8400 NW 33rd St Ste 100
Miami, FL 33122-1932
Phone: 305-591-9955 Fax: 203-239-7742 Toll-Free:
Web site: www.bcbsfl.com
MAILING ADDRESS:
  BC/BS-FLORIDA & HEALTH OPTIONS
  PO Box 02-5314
  Miami, FL 33122-1932

KEY EXECUTIVES:
Chief Executive Officer .... Robert I Lufrano, MD
Senior VP & General Manager .... Ken Sellers
Chief Financial Officer .... R Chris Doerr
Medical Director .... Steven Singer
Chief Information Officer .... Duke Livermore
Director of Market Development .... Kenneth Berkowitz
Vice President of Sales .... Armando Luna
VP of Care & Network Development .... Melvyn Fletcher
Human Resources Director .... Lynn Capaldo

COMPANY PROFILE:
Parent Company Name: BC & BS of Florida
Doing Business As: BC & BS of Florida & Health Options
Year Founded: 1944   Federally Qualified: [Y]
Forprofit: [Y]   Not-For-Profit: [Y]
Model Type: IPA
Accreditation: [ ] AAPPO [ ] JACHO [X] NCQA [ ] URAC
Plan Type: HMO, PPO, POS, ASO, TPA, HDHP, HSA

Total Enrollment:
  2001: 50,953   2004: 0   2007: 0
  2002: 796,662   2005: 433,032
  2003: 0   2006: 334,514

SERVICE AREA:
Nationwide: N
  FL;

TYPE OF COVERAGE:
Commercial: [Y] Individual: [Y] FEHBP: [ ] Indemnity: [ ]
Medicare: [Y] Medicaid: [ ] Supplemental Medicare: [Y]
Tricare   [ ]

PRODUCTS OFFERED:
Product Name: Type:
Health Options Medicare   Medicare Advantage
HealthyKids   HMO
Health Options HMO   HMO

CONSUMER-DRIVEN PRODUCTS
                                      HSA Company
                                      HSA Product
                                      HSA Administrator
                                      Consumer-Driven Health Plan
Blue Options   High Deductible Health Plan

BLUE CROSS BLUE SHIELD OF FLORIDA/ HEALTH OPTIONS INC

4800 Deerwood Campus Pkwy
Jacksonville, FL 32246-8273
Phone: 904-791-6111 Fax: 904-905-6638 Toll-Free: 800-477-3736
Web site: www.bcbsfl.com
MAILING ADDRESS:
  BC BS OF FLORIDA/HEALTH OPTION
  PO Box 1798
  Jacksonville, FL 32246-8273

KEY EXECUTIVES:
Chairman/Chief Executive Officer .... Robert I Lufrano, MD
Chief Financial Officer .... R Chris Doerr
Public Relations/Corporate Communications .... Rick Curran
Chief Human Resources Officer .... Robert E Wall
VP Corporate Communications .... Sharon Wamble-King
VP Medical Operations .... Jonathan B Gavras, MD

COMPANY PROFILE:
Parent Company Name: Blue Cross-Blue Shield of Florida Inc
Doing Business As:
Year Founded: 1944   Federally Qualified: [Y]
Forprofit: [ ]   Not-For-Profit: [Y]
Model Type: NETWORK
Accreditation: [ ] AAPPO [ ] JACHO [X] NCQA [ ] URAC
Plan Type: HMO, PPO, Specialty HMO, Specialty PPO, POS, ASO, UR, CDHP, HDHP, HSA,
Total Revenue: 2005:   2006: 7,475,000,000
Net Income   2005:   2006: 311,000,000
Total Enrollment:
  2001: 0   2004: 7,000,000   2007: 4,100,000
  2002: 773,466   2005:
  2003: 6,000,000   2006: 3,794,000

SERVICE AREA:
Nationwide: N
  FL;

TYPE OF COVERAGE:
Commercial: [Y] Individual: [Y] FEHBP: [Y] Indemnity: [ ]
Medicare: [Y] Medicaid: [ ] Supplemental Medicare: [ ]
Tricare   [ ]

PRODUCTS OFFERED:
Product Name: Type:
Health Options, Inc   HMO
HealthyKid   HMO
Medicare   Medicare

PLAN BENEFITS:
Alternative Medicine: [ ]   Behavioral Health: [ ]
Chiropractic: [ ]   Dental: [ ]
Home Care: [ ]   Inpatient SNF: [ ]
Long-Term Care: [ ]   Pharm. Mail Order: [ ]
Physical Therapy: [ ]   Podiatry: [ ]
Psychiatric: [ ]   Transplant: [ ]
Vision: [ ]   Wellness: [ ]
Workers' Comp: [ ]
Other Benefits:

Comments:
Acquired Principal Health Care of Florida.

Managed Care Organization Profiles   FLORIDA

MAILING ADDRESS:
    AV-MED HEALTH PLAN JACKSONVILLE
    1300 Riverplace Blvd #2001
    Jacksonville, FL 32207-9054

KEY EXECUTIVES:
Chief Executive Officer .... Douglas G Cueny
Chief Financial Officer .... Michael Gallagher
Pharmacy Director .... Shawn Barger
Chief Information Officer .... John R Higbee
MIS Director .... Winston Lonsdale

COMPANY PROFILE:
Parent Company Name: Av-Med
Doing Business As:
Year Founded: 1986   Federally Qualified: [Y]
Forprofit: [Y]   Not-For-Profit: [ ]
Model Type: IPA
Accreditation: [ ] AAPPO [ ] JACHO [X] NCQA [ ] URAC
Plan Type: HMO, PPO, POS, CDHP, HDHP, HSA,
Total Enrollment:
    2001: 0   2004: 0   2007: 0
    2002: 0   2005:
    2003: 30,418   2006:

SERVICE AREA:
Nationwide: N
    FL;

TYPE OF COVERAGE:
Commercial: [Y] Individual: [ ] FEHBP: [ ] Indemnity: [ ]
Medicare: [Y] Medicaid: [ ] Supplemental Medicare: [ ]
Tricare [ ]

PLAN BENEFITS:
Alternative Medicine: [ ]   Behavioral Health: [ ]
Chiropractic: [X]   Dental: [X]
Home Care: [ ]   Inpatient SNF: [ ]
Long-Term Care: [ ]   Pharm. Mail Order: [X]
Physical Therapy: [ ]   Podiatry: [X]
Psychiatric: [X]   Transplant: [X]
Vision: [X]   Wellness: [X]
Workers' Comp: [ ]
Other Benefits:
Comments:
See Av-Med Gainesville, FL for enrollment figures.

AV-MED HEALTH PLAN - MIAMI

9400 S Dadeland Blvd
Miami, FL 33156
Phone: 305-671-5437 Fax: 305-671-4764 Toll-Free: 800-432-6676
Web site: www.avmed.com
MAILING ADDRESS:
    AV-MED HEALTH PLAN - MIAMI
    9400 S Dadeland Blvd
    Miami, FL 33156

KEY EXECUTIVES:
Chief Executive Officer .... Douglas G Cueny
Chief Financial Officer .... Michael Gallagher
Pharmacy Director .... Shawn Barger
Chief Information Officer .... John R Higbee
MIS Director .... Winston Lonsdale
Public Relations Director .... Valerie Rubin

COMPANY PROFILE:
Parent Company Name: Av-Med Health Plan
Doing Business As:
Year Founded: 1969   Federally Qualified: [Y]
Forprofit: [ ]   Not-For-Profit: [Y]
Model Type: IPA
Accreditation: [ ] AAPPO [ ] JACHO [X] NCQA [ ] URAC
Plan Type: HMO, POS, CDHP, HSA,
Total Revenue: 2005: 568,214,113   2006: 435,049,142
Net Income 2005: 21,637,567   2006: 12,799,478
Total Enrollment:
    2001: 252,770   2004: 188,622   2007: 0
    2002: 278,644   2005: 196,903
    2003: 210,777   2006: 205,278

SERVICE AREA:
Nationwide: N
    FL;

TYPE OF COVERAGE:
Commercial: [Y] Individual: [ ] FEHBP: [ ] Indemnity: [ ]
Medicare: [Y] Medicaid: [ ] Supplemental Medicare: [ ]
Tricare [ ]

PLAN BENEFITS:
Alternative Medicine: [ ]   Behavioral Health: [ ]
Chiropractic: [X]   Dental: [X]
Home Care: [X]   Inpatient SNF: [X]
Long-Term Care: [X]   Pharm. Mail Order: [X]
Physical Therapy: [X]   Podiatry: [X]
Psychiatric: [X]   Transplant: [X]
Vision: [X]   Wellness: [X]
Workers' Comp: [ ]
Other Benefits:

AV-MED HEALTH PLAN - ORLANDO

541 S Orlando Ave Ste 205
Maitland, FL 32751
Phone: 407-539-0007 Fax: 407-975-1623 Toll-Free:
Web site: www.avmed.com
MAILING ADDRESS:
    AV-MED HEALTH PLAN - ORLANDO
    541 Orlando Ave Ste 205
    Maitland, FL 32751

KEY EXECUTIVES:
Chief Executive Officer .... Douglas G Cueny
Chief Financial Officer .... Michael Gallagher
Pharmacy Director .... Shawn Barger
Chief Information Officer .... John R Higbee
MIS Director .... Winston Lonsdale
Public Relations Director .... Valerie Rubin

COMPANY PROFILE:
Parent Company Name: Av-Med
Doing Business As: AvMed Health Plan
Year Founded: 1969   Federally Qualified: [Y]
Forprofit: [ ]   Not-For-Profit: [Y]
Model Type: IPA
Accreditation: [ ] AAPPO [ ] JACHO [X] NCQA [ ] URAC
Plan Type: HMO, PPO, POS

SERVICE AREA:
Nationwide: N
    FL;

TYPE OF COVERAGE:
Commercial: [Y] Individual: [ ] FEHBP: [ ] Indemnity: [ ]
Medicare: [Y] Medicaid: [ ] Supplemental Medicare: [ ]
Tricare [ ]

PLAN BENEFITS:
Alternative Medicine: [ ]   Behavioral Health: [X]
Chiropractic: [X]   Dental: [ ]
Home Care: [X]   Inpatient SNF: [X]
Long-Term Care: [ ]   Pharm. Mail Order: [ ]
Physical Therapy: [X]   Podiatry: [X]
Psychiatric: [X]   Transplant: [X]
Vision: [X]   Wellness: [X]
Workers' Comp: [ ]
Other Benefits:
Comments:
See Av-Med Gainesville, FL for enrollment figures.

AV-MED HEALTH PLAN - TAMPA

1511 N Westshore Blvd Ste 700
Tampa, FL 33607
Phone: 813-281-5650 Fax: 813-281-0659 Toll-Free: 800-257-2273
Web site: www.avmed.com
MAILING ADDRESS:
    AV-MED HEALTH PLAN - TAMPA
    1511 N Westshore Blvd Ste 700
    Tampa, FL 33607

FLORIDA

Managed Care Organization Profiles

MAILING ADDRESS:
ASSURANT EMPLOYEE BENEFITS - FL
5401 W Kennedy Blvd Ste 760
Tampa, FL 33609-2447

KEY EXECUTIVES:
Chief Executive Officer/President .... Michael J Peninger
Chief Financial Officer .... Floyd F Chadee
VP, Medical Director .... Polly M Galbraith, MD
Chief Information Officer .... Karla J Schacht
Senior VP, Marketing .... Joseph A Sevcik
Privacy Officer .... John L Fortini
VP of Provider Services .... James A Barrett, DMD
Senior VP, Human Resources & Development .... Sylvia R Wagner
General Manager .... Todd Boyd
National Dental Director .... James A Barrett, DMD

COMPANY PROFILE:
Parent Company Name: Assurant Health
Doing Business As:
Year Founded: 1982   Federally Qualified: [ ]
Forprofit: [Y]   Not-For-Profit: [ ]
Model Type: IPA
Accreditation: [ ] AAPPO [ ] JACHO [ ] NCQA [ ] URAC
Plan Type: Specialty HMO

SERVICE AREA:
Nationwide: N
FL;

TYPE OF COVERAGE:
Commercial: [Y] Individual: [Y] FEHBP: [ ] Indemnity: [ ]
Medicare: [ ] Medicaid: [ ] Supplemental Medicare: [ ]
Tricare   [ ]

PRODUCTS OFFERED:
Product Name: Type:
                                  DHMO
                                  Vision

PLAN BENEFITS:
Alternative Medicine: [ ]   Behavioral Health: [ ]
Chiropractic: [ ]   Dental: [X]
Home Care: [ ]   Inpatient SNF: [ ]
Long-Term Care: [ ]   Pharm. Mail Order: [ ]
Physical Therapy: [ ]   Podiatry: [ ]
Psychiatric: [ ]   Transplant: [ ]
Vision: [X]   Wellness: [ ]
Workers' Comp: [ ]
Other Benefits:
Comments:
Formerly Fortis Benefits Dental.

ATLANTIC DENTAL INC

2100 Ponce De Leon Blvd Ste950
Coral Gables, FL 33134
Phone: 305-443-3111 Fax: 305-443-1926 Toll-Free:
Web site:

MAILING ADDRESS:
ATLANTIC DENTAL INC
2100 Ponce De Leon Blvd Ste950
Coral Gables, FL 33134

KEY EXECUTIVES:
Chief Executive Officer/President .... Marcio Cabrera
Director of Dental Operations .... Frank Manteiga, DDS
Chief Operating Officer .... Lordes Rivas

COMPANY PROFILE:
Parent Company Name:
Doing Business As:
Year Founded: 1997   Federally Qualified: [ ]
Forprofit: [Y]   Not-For-Profit: [ ]
Model Type:
Accreditation: [ ] AAPPO [ ] JACHO [ ] NCQA [ ] URAC
Plan Type: Specialty HMO
Total Enrollment:
  2001: 0   2004: 399,856   2007: 0
  2002: 0   2005: 209,806
  2003: 0   2006:

SERVICE AREA:
Nationwide:
FL;

PLAN BENEFITS:
Alternative Medicine: [ ]   Behavioral Health: [ ]
Chiropractic: [ ]   Dental: [X]
Home Care: [ ]   Inpatient SNF: [ ]
Long-Term Care: [ ]   Pharm. Mail Order: [ ]
Physical Therapy: [ ]   Podiatry: [ ]
Psychiatric: [ ]   Transplant: [ ]
Vision: [ ]   Wellness: [ ]
Workers' Comp: [ ]
Other Benefits:

AV-MED HEALTH PLAN - GAINESVILLE

4300 NW 89th Blvd
Gainesville, FL 32606
Phone: 352-372-8400 Fax: 352-337-8726 Toll-Free: 800-346-0231
Web site: www.avmed.com

MAILING ADDRESS:
AV-MED HEALTH PLAN GAINESVILLE
PO Box 749
Gainesville, FL 32606

KEY EXECUTIVES:
Chief Executive Officer .... Douglas G Cueny
Chief Financial Officer .... Michael Gallagher
Pharmacy Director .... Shawn Barger
Chief Information Officer .... John R Higbee
MIS Director .... Winston Lonsdale
Public Relations Director .... Valerie Rubin

COMPANY PROFILE:
Parent Company Name:
Doing Business As:
Year Founded: 1969   Federally Qualified: [Y]
Forprofit: [ ]   Not-For-Profit: [Y]
Model Type: IPA
Accreditation: [ ] AAPPO [ ] JACHO [X] NCQA [ ] URAC
Plan Type: HMO, CDHP, HDHP, HSA

SERVICE AREA:
Nationwide: N
    FL (Alachua, Baker, Bradford, Brevard, Broward, Citrus, Clay,
    Columbia, Dade, Dixie, Duval, Gilchrist, Hamilton, Hernando,
    Hillsborough, Lee, Levy, Marion, Nassau, Orange, Osceloa, Palm
    Beach, Pasco, Pinellas, Polk, Sarasota, Seminole, St Johns,
    Suwannee, Union, Volusia);

TYPE OF COVERAGE:
Commercial: [Y] Individual: [ ] FEHBP: [ ] Indemnity: [ ]
Medicare: [Y] Medicaid: [ ] Supplemental Medicare: [ ]
Tricare   [ ]

PRODUCTS OFFERED:
Product Name: Type:
Av-Med Medicare Plan   Medicare
Av-Med HMO
Av-Med Federal Employees   FEHBP

CONSUMER-DRIVEN PRODUCTS
                                 HSA Company
                                 HSA Product
                                 HSA Administrator
ChoicePlan   Consumer-Driven Health Plan
                                 High Deductible Health Plan

PLAN BENEFITS:
Alternative Medicine: [ ]   Behavioral Health: [ ]
Chiropractic: [X]   Dental: [X]
Home Care: [X]   Inpatient SNF: [X]
Long-Term Care: [X]   Pharm. Mail Order: [X]
Physical Therapy: [X]   Podiatry: [X]
Psychiatric: [X]   Transplant: [X]
Vision: [X]   Wellness: [X]
Workers' Comp: [ ]
Other Benefits:

AV-MED HEALTH PLAN - JACKSONVILLE

1300 Riverplace Blvd #2001
Jacksonville, FL 32207-9054
Phone: 904-858-1300 Fax: 904-858-1355 Toll-Free:
Web site: www.avmed.com

Managed Care Organization Profiles — FLORIDA

CONSUMER-DRIVEN PRODUCTS
Aetna Life Insurance Co
Aetna HealthFund HSA
Aetna
Aetna HealthFund
PPO I; PPO II
HSA Company
HSA Product
HSA Administrator
Consumer-Driven Health Plan
High Deductible Health Plan

PLAN BENEFITS:
Alternative Medicine: [ ]   Behavioral Health: [X]
Chiropractic: [X]   Dental: [X]
Home Care: [X]   Inpatient SNF: [X]
Long-Term Care: [X]   Pharm. Mail Order: [X]
Physical Therapy: [X]   Podiatry: [X]
Psychiatric: [X]   Transplant: [X]
Vision: [X]   Wellness: [X]
Workers' Comp: [ ]
Other Benefits: X

Comments:
Formerly Prudential Healthcare of South Florida.

ALL FLORIDA PPO INC

500 S Cypress Rd Ste 8
Pompano Beach, FL 33060
Phone: 954-946-5183 Fax: 954-946-0978 Toll-Free: 800-831-9710
Web site:

MAILING ADDRESS:
ALL FLORIDA PPO INC
500 S Cypress Rd Ste 8
Pompano Beach, FL 33060

KEY EXECUTIVES:
Chief Executive Officer/President .... Reg Watkins
Marketing Director .... Reg Watkins

COMPANY PROFILE:
Parent Company Name:
Doing Business As:
Year Founded: 1992   Federally Qualified: [N]
Forprofit: [Y]   Not-For-Profit: [ ]
Model Type: NETWORK
Accreditation: [ ] AAPPO [ ] JACHO [ ] NCQA [ ] URAC
Plan Type: PPO
Total Enrollment:
  2001: 378,950   2004: 0   2007: 0
  2002: 0   2005:
  2003: 0   2006:

SERVICE AREA:
Nationwide: N
  FL;

TYPE OF COVERAGE:
Commercial: [Y] Individual: [ ] FEHBP: [ ] Indemnity: [ ]
Medicare: [ ] Medicaid: [ ] Supplemental Medicare: [ ]
Tricare   [ ]

PLAN BENEFITS:
Alternative Medicine: [ ]   Behavioral Health: [ ]
Chiropractic: [X]   Dental: [ ]
Home Care: [X]   Inpatient SNF: [X]
Long-Term Care: [X]   Pharm. Mail Order: [X]
Physical Therapy: [X]   Podiatry: [X]
Psychiatric: [X]   Transplant: [X]
Vision: [X]   Wellness: [X]
Workers' Comp: [X]
Other Benefits:

AMERIGROUP FLORIDA INC

4200 W Cypress St
Tampa, FL 33607
Phone: 813-830-6900 Fax: 813-314-2050 Toll-Free: 800-873-7474
Web site: www.amerigroupcorp.com

MAILING ADDRESS:
AMERIGROUP FLORIDA INC
4200 W Cypress St
Tampa, FL 33607

KEY EXECUTIVES:
Chief Executive Officer .... William McHugh
President .... James G Carlson
Treasurer .... Donald Van Gilmore
Vice President, Sales .... Jose Valosin

COMPANY PROFILE:
Parent Company Name: Amerigroup Corporation
Doing Business As:
Year Founded: 1993   Federally Qualified: [N]
Forprofit: [Y]   Not-For-Profit: [ ]
Model Type: IPA
Accreditation: [ ] AAPPO [ ] JACHO [X] NCQA [ ] URAC
Plan Type: HMO, POS
Total Revenue: 2005: 293,260,820   2006: 190,212,317
Net Income   2005: -1,407,298   2006: 4,107,314
Total Enrollment:
  2001: 167,006   2004: 228,467   2007: 0
  2002: 193,652   2005: 219,000
  2003: 221,651   2006: 204,270

SERVICE AREA:
Nationwide: N
  FL (Broward, Charlotte, Dade, Hillsborough, Lee, Manatie, Marion, Orange, Osceola, Palm Beach, Pasco, Pinellas, Polk, Sarasota, Seminole, Valusia);

TYPE OF COVERAGE:
Commercial: [Y] Individual: [Y] FEHBP: [ ] Indemnity: [ ]
Medicare: [ ] Medicaid: [Y] Supplemental Medicare: [ ]
Tricare   [ ]

PRODUCTS OFFERED:
Product Name: Type:
Physicians Care Plus   Medicare Advantage
Physicians Healthcare Plans   Medicaid
HealthyKids   HMO
HMO   HMO

PLAN BENEFITS:
Alternative Medicine: [ ]   Behavioral Health: [ ]
Chiropractic: [X]   Dental: [X]
Home Care: [X]   Inpatient SNF: [X]
Long-Term Care: [X]   Pharm. Mail Order: [X]
Physical Therapy: [X]   Podiatry: [X]
Psychiatric: [X]   Transplant: [X]
Vision: [X]   Wellness: [X]
Workers' Comp: [ ]
Other Benefits:

Comments:
Formerly known as Physicians Healthcare Plans Inc.

AMERICAN PIONEER HEALTH PLANS INC

1001 Heathrow Park Lane #5001
Lake Mary, FL 32746
Phone: 800-538-1053 Fax: 800-999-2224 Toll-Free: 800-538-1053
Web site: www.amphp.com

MAILING ADDRESS:
AMERICAN PIONEER HLTH PLANS IN
1001 Heathrow Park Lane #5001
Lake Mary, FL 32746

KEY EXECUTIVES:
Chairman of the Board .... Richard A Barasch
Chief Executive Officer/President .... Gary W Bryant, CPA
Executive VP, Chief Financial Officer .... Robert A Waegelein
VP, Marketing .... Harry Jenkins
Senior VP, Managed Care .... Gary M Jacobs

COMPANY PROFILE:
Parent Company Name: Universal American Financial Group
Doing Business As:
Year Founded: 2006   Federally Qualified: [ ]
Forprofit: [ ]   Not-For-Profit: [ ]
Model Type: HMO
Accreditation: [ ] AAPPO [ ] JACHO [ ] NCQA [ ] URAC
Plan Type: HMO

SERVICE AREA:
Nationwide:
  FL (Miami-Dade, Broward, Jacksonville);

ASSURANT EMPLOYEE BENEFITS - FLORIDA

5401 W Kennedy Blvd Ste 760
Tampa, FL 33609-2447
Phone: 813-286-7736 Fax: 813-289-8315 Toll-Free: 800-654-7808
Web site: www.assurantemployeebenefits.com

FLORIDA

AETNA INC - FLORIDA

4630 Woodlands Corp Blvd
Tampa, FL 33614
Phone: 813-775-0000 Fax: 813-775-0600 Toll-Free: 800-232-2385
Web site: www.aetna.com

MAILING ADDRESS:
AETNA INC - FL
4630 Woodlands Corp Blvd
Tampa, FL 33614

KEY EXECUTIVES:
Chairman of the Board/Chief Executive Officer .... Ronald A Williams
Regional Mgr - SE & SW Region .... Carl King
Executive VP, Finance .... Joseph M Zubretsky

COMPANY PROFILE:
Parent Company Name: Aetna Inc
Doing Business As:
Year Founded: 1985   Federally Qualified: [ ]
Forprofit: [Y]   Not-For-Profit: [ ] Model Type: IPA
Accreditation: [ ] AAPPO [ ] JACHO [ ] NCQA [ ] URAC
Plan Type: HMO, PPO, POS, CDHP, HDHP, HSA
Total Revenue: 2005:   1,397,451,784   2006:   1,018,545,300
Net Income   2005:   104,955,095   2006:   18,564,387
Total Enrollment:
  2001: 599,625   2004: 554,315   2007: 0
  2002: 537,211   2005: 575,751
  2003: 511,367   2006: 591,774

SERVICE AREA:
Nationwide: N
  FL;

TYPE OF COVERAGE:
Commercial: [Y] Individual: [ ] FEHBP: [ ] Indemnity: [ ]
Medicare: [Y] Medicaid: [ ] Supplemental Medicare: [ ]
Tricare   [ ]

PRODUCTS OFFERED:
Product Name:	Type:
HMO	HMO
US Access	
Quality Point of Service	POS
Elect Choice	EPO
Managed Choice	POS
Open Choice	PPO
Advantage Plus	Managed Dental

CONSUMER-DRIVEN PRODUCTS
Aetna Life Insurance Co	HSA Company
Aetna HealthFund HSA	HSA Product
Aetna	HSA Administrator
Aetna HealthFund	Consumer-Driven Health Plan
PPO I; PPO II	High Deductible Health Plan

PLAN BENEFITS:
Alternative Medicine: [ ]   Behavioral Health: [ ]
Chiropractic: [X]   Dental: [X]
Home Care: [X]   Inpatient SNF: [X]
Long-Term Care: [X]   Pharm. Mail Order: [X]
Physical Therapy: [X]   Podiatry: [X]
Psychiatric: [X]   Transplant: [X]
Vision: [X]   Wellness: [X]
Workers' Comp: [ ]
Other Benefits:

AETNA INC - JACKSONVILLE

841 Prudential Dr
Jacksonville, FL 32207
Phone: 904-351-3000 Fax: 904-351-3730 Toll-Free:
Web site: www.aetna.com

MAILING ADDRESS:
AETNA INC - JACKSONVILLE
841 Prudential Dr
Jacksonville, FL 32207

KEY EXECUTIVES:
Chairman of the Board/Chief Executive Officer .... Ronald A Williams
Regional Manager-SE & SW .... Carl King
Executive VP, Finance .... Joseph M Zubretsky

COMPANY PROFILE:
Parent Company Name: Aetna Inc
Doing Business As:
Year Founded: 1984   Federally Qualified: [Y]
Forprofit: [Y]   Not-For-Profit: [ ]
Model Type: MIXED
Accreditation: [ ] AAPPO [ ] JACHO [ ] NCQA [ ] URAC
Plan Type: HMO, PPO, POS, CDHP, HDHP, HSA

SERVICE AREA:
Nationwide: N
  FL;

TYPE OF COVERAGE:
Commercial: [Y] Individual: [ ] FEHBP: [ ] Indemnity: [ ]
Medicare: [Y] Medicaid: [ ] Supplemental Medicare: [Y]
Tricare   [ ]

PRODUCTS OFFERED:
Product Name:	Type:
HMO	
ASO	
POS/PPO	
Medicare Risk HMO	
Seniorcare	Medicare

CONSUMER-DRIVEN PRODUCTS
Aetna Life Insurance Co	HSA Company
Aetna HealthFund HSA	HSA Product
Aetna	HSA Administrator
Aetna HealthFund	Consumer-Driven Health Plan
PPO I; PPO II	High Deductible Health Plan

PLAN BENEFITS:
Alternative Medicine: [ ]   Behavioral Health: [ ]
Chiropractic: [X]   Dental: [X]
Home Care: [X]   Inpatient SNF: [X]
Long-Term Care: [ ]   Pharm. Mail Order: [X]
Physical Therapy: [X]   Podiatry: [X]
Psychiatric: [X]   Transplant: [X]
Vision: [X]   Wellness: [X]
Workers' Comp: [ ]
Other Benefits:
Comments:
Formerly Prudential Healthcare.

AETNA INC - PLANTATION

8201 Peters Road Ste 2001
Plantation, FL 33324
Phone: 954-382-8100 Fax: 954-424-4448 Toll-Free:
Web site: www.aetna.com

MAILING ADDRESS:
AETNA INC - PLANTATION
8201 Peters Road Ste 2001
Plantation, FL 33324

KEY EXECUTIVES:
Chairman of the Board/Chief Executive Officer .... Ronald A Williams
Regional Manager- SE & SW .... Carl King
Executive VP, Finance .... Joseph M Zubretsky
Medical Director .... Valerie Beckies, MD
Marketing Director .... Todd Slawter
Provider Relations Director .... Ron Timonere

COMPANY PROFILE:
Parent Company Name: Aetna Inc
Doing Business As:
Year Founded: 1986   Federally Qualified: [Y]
Forprofit: [Y]   Not-For-Profit: [ ]
Model Type: NETWORK
Accreditation: [ ] AAPPO [ ] JACHO [X] NCQA [ ] URAC
Plan Type: HMO, PPO, POS, UR, CDHP, HDHP, HSA

SERVICE AREA:
Nationwide: N
  FL (Broward, Dade, Palm Beach);

TYPE OF COVERAGE:
Commercial: [Y] Individual: [ ] FEHBP: [ ] Indemnity: [ ]
Medicare: [Y] Medicaid: [ ] Supplemental Medicare: [ ]
Tricare   [ ]

PRODUCTS OFFERED:
Product Name:	Type:
Prudential Healthcare Seniorcare	Medicare

Managed Care Organization Profiles   **FLORIDA**

20/20 EYECARE PLAN INC

2900 W Cypress Creek Rd Ste 4
Ft Lauderdale, FL 33309-1715
Phone: 954-563-4101 Fax: 954-772-0137 Toll-Free:
Web site: www.2020eyecareplan.com

MAILING ADDRESS:
    20/20 EYECARE PLAN INC
    2900 W Cypress Creek Rd Ste 4
    Ft Lauderdale, FL 33309-1715

KEY EXECUTIVES:
President .... Robert C Coppola
Chief Information Officer .... Mike Statner
Provider Relations/Network Development Director .. Wanda Schroeder
Human Resources .... Diane Anderson
Quality Assurance Director/Compliance Officer .... Deb Arasi

COMPANY PROFILE:
Parent Company Name:
Doing Business As:
Year Founded: 1999   Federally Qualified: [ ]
Forprofit: [Y]   Not-For-Profit: [ ]
Model Type: MIXED
Accreditation: [ ] AAPPO [ ] JACHO [ ] NCQA [ ] URAC
Plan Type: Specialty HMO, Specialty PPO, HDHP
Total Enrollment:
    2001: 0   2004: 50,000   2007: 0
    2002: 0   2005:
    2003: 0   2006:

SERVICE AREA:
Nationwide:
    FL;

TYPE OF COVERAGE:
Commercial: [Y] Individual: [Y] FEHBP: [ ] Indemnity: [ ]
Medicare: [ ] Medicaid: [ ] Supplemental Medicare: [ ]
Tricare [ ]

PLAN BENEFITS:
Alternative Medicine: [ ]   Behavioral Health: [ ]
Chiropractic: [ ]   Dental: [ ]
Home Care: [ ]   Inpatient SNF: [ ]
Long-Term Care: [ ]   Pharm. Mail Order: [ ]
Physical Therapy: [ ]   Podiatry: [ ]
Psychiatric: [ ]   Transplant: [ ]
Vision: [X]   Wellness: [ ]
Workers' Comp: [ ]
Other Benefits:

ADVANTICA EYECARE INC

19321-C US Hwy 19 N
Clearwater, FL 33764
Phone: 727-363-1460 Fax: 727-538-4255 Toll-Free: 866-354-2020
Web site: www.alliedeyecare.com

MAILING ADDRESS:
    ADVANTICA EYECARE INC
    19321-C US Hwy 19 N
    Clearwater, FL 33764

KEY EXECUTIVES:
Chief Executive Officer/President .... Richard L Sanchez
Chief Financial Officer .... Joseph V Price
Chief Operating Officer .... Linda S Sayer

COMPANY PROFILE:
Parent Company Name: Allied Eyecare LLC
Doing Business As:
Year Founded: 2003   Federally Qualified: [ ]
Forprofit: [Y]   Not-For-Profit: [ ]
Model Type:
Accreditation: [ ] AAPPO [ ] JACHO [ ] NCQA [ ] URAC
Plan Type: Specialty HMO, Specialty PPO
Total Enrollment:
    2001: 0   2004: 800,000   2007: 0
    2002: 0   2005:
    2003: 0   2006:

SERVICE AREA:
Nationwide:
    FL; MD;

TYPE OF COVERAGE:
Commercial: [Y] Individual: [ ] FEHBP: [ ] Indemnity: [ ]
Medicare: [Y] Medicaid: [Y] Supplemental Medicare: [ ]
Tricare [ ]

PLAN BENEFITS:
Alternative Medicine: [ ]   Behavioral Health: [ ]
Chiropractic: [ ]   Dental: [ ]
Home Care: [ ]   Inpatient SNF: [ ]
Long-Term Care: [ ]   Pharm. Mail Order: [ ]
Physical Therapy: [ ]   Podiatry: [ ]
Psychiatric: [ ]   Transplant: [ ]
Vision: [X]   Wellness: [ ]
Workers' Comp: [ ]
Other Benefits:

AETNA INC - ALTAMONTE SPRINGS

385 Douglas Ave Ste 3350
Altamonte Springs, FL 32714
Phone: 407-618-2500 Fax: 407-618-2514 Toll-Free: 888-422-2128
Web site: www.aetna.com

MAILING ADDRESS:
    AETNA INC - ALTAMONTE SPRINGS
    385 Douglas Ave Ste 3350
    Altamonte Springs, FL 32714

KEY EXECUTIVES:
Chairman of the Board/Chief Executive Officer .... Ronald A Williams
Regional Manager-SE & SW .... Carl King
Executive VP, Finance .... Joseph M Zubretsky
Director, Provider Services .... Paula Kendall

COMPANY PROFILE:
Parent Company Name: Aetna Inc
Doing Business As:
Year Founded: 1986   Federally Qualified: [ ]
Forprofit: [Y]   Not-For-Profit: [ ]
Model Type: GROUP
Accreditation: [ ] AAPPO [X] JACHO [X] NCQA [ ] URAC
Plan Type: POS, CDHP, HDHP, HSA
Total Enrollment:
    2001: 175,281   2004: 0   2007: 0
    2002: 0   2005:
    2003: 0   2006:

SERVICE AREA:
Nationwide: N
    FL (Baker, Brevard, Broward, Clay, Dade, Duval, Hillsborough,
    Lake, Nassau, Orange, Osceola, Palm Beach, Pasco, Pinellas, Polk,
    Seminole, St Johns, Volusia);

TYPE OF COVERAGE:
Commercial: [Y] Individual: [ ] FEHBP: [ ] Indemnity: [ ]
Medicare: [Y] Medicaid: [ ] Supplemental Medicare: [ ]
Tricare [ ]

PRODUCTS OFFERED:
Product Name: Type:
Seniorcare   Medicare
HMO   HMO

CONSUMER-DRIVEN PRODUCTS
Aetna Life Insurance Co   HSA Company
Aetna HealthFund HSA   HSA Product
Aetna   HSA Administrator
Aetna HealthFund   Consumer-Driven Health Plan
PPO I; PPO II   High Deductible Health Plan

PLAN BENEFITS:
Alternative Medicine: [ ]   Behavioral Health: [ ]
Chiropractic: [X]   Dental: [X]
Home Care: [X]   Inpatient SNF: [X]
Long-Term Care: [ ]   Pharm. Mail Order: [X]
Physical Therapy: [X]   Podiatry: [X]
Psychiatric: [X]   Transplant: [X]
Vision: [X]   Wellness: [X]
Workers' Comp: [ ]
Other Benefits:
Comments:
Formerly Prudential Healthcare Plan.

DISTRICT OF COLUMBIA

HUMANA INC - DISTRICT OF COLUMBIA

500 W Main St
Louisville, KY 40202
Phone: 502-580-5005 Fax: 502-580-8543 Toll-Free: 800-558-4444
Web site: www.humana.com

MAILING ADDRESS:
HUMANA INC - DC
PO Box 740036
Louisville, KY 40202

KEY EXECUTIVES:
Chairman of the Board .... David A Jones Jr
Chief Executive Officer/President .... Michael B McCallister
Chief Financial Officer .... James H Bloem
Chief Clinical Strategy .... Jonathan T Lord, MD
Senior VP, Chief Information Officer .... Bruce J Goodman
Chief Operating Officer .... Jim Murray
Chief Marketing Officer .... Steve Moya
Senior VP, Human Resources .... Bonnie C Hathcock
New Product Development Director .... Tom Liston
Senior VP, General Counsel .... Art Hipwell
Senior VP, Corporate Communications .... Tom Noland

COMPANY PROFILE:
Parent Company Name: Humana Inc
Doing Business As:
Year Founded: 1961   Federally Qualified: [Y]
Forprofit: [Y]   Not-For-Profit: [ ]
Model Type: IPA
Accreditation: [ ] AAPPO [ ] JACHO [ ] NCQA [ ] URAC
Plan Type: PPO, CDHP, HDHP, HSA

SERVICE AREA:
Nationwide: N
   DC,

TYPE OF COVERAGE:
Commercial: [Y] Individual: [Y] FEHBP: [ ]   Indemnity: [ ]
Medicare: [ ] Medicaid: [ ] Supplemental Medicare: [ ]
Tricare   [ ]

CONSUMER-DRIVEN PRODUCTS
JP Morgan Chase   HSA Company
HumanaOne HSA   HSA Product
JP Morgan Chase   HSA Administrator
Personal Care Account   Consumer-Driven Health Plan
HumanaOne   High Deductible Health Plan

PLAN BENEFITS:
Alternative Medicine: [ ]   Behavioral Health: [X]
Chiropractic: [X]   Dental: [X]
Home Care: [ ]   Inpatient SNF: [ ]
Long-Term Care: [ ]   Pharm. Mail Order: [X]
Physical Therapy: [ ]   Podiatry: [ ]
Psychiatric: [X]   Transplant: [X]
Vision: [ ]   Wellness: [ ]
Workers' Comp: [X]
Other Benefits: Long Term Disability

Model Type:
Accreditation: [ ] AAPPO [ ] JACHO [ ] NCQA [X] URAC
Plan Type: UR

SERVICE AREA:
Nationwide: Y
   NW;

TYPE OF COVERAGE:
Commercial: [Y] Individual: [ ] FEHBP: [ ]   Indemnity: [ ]
Medicare: [ ] Medicaid: [ ] Supplemental Medicare: [ ]
Tricare   [ ]

ULLICARE

1625 Eye Street NW
Washington, DC 20001
Phone: 202-682-7911 Fax: 202-962-8854 Toll-Free: 800-848-9200
Web site: www.ullico.com

MAILING ADDRESS:
ULLICARE
1625 Eye Street NW
Washington, DC 20001

KEY EXECUTIVES:
Chairman of the Board/Chief Executive Officer . Terence M O'Sullivan
President .... Edward Grebow
Controller .... Damon Gasque
Senior VP, Marketing & Operations .... James J Kennedy Jr
Compliance Officer .... Teresa E Valentine
Senior VP, Human Resources .... James M Paul
Senior VP, General Counsel .... Theodore T Green
VP, Corporate Communications .... Pamela Greenwalt

COMPANY PROFILE:
Parent Company Name: Union Labor Life Insurance
Doing Business As:
Year Founded: 1984   Federally Qualified: [ ]
Forprofit: [Y]   Not-For-Profit: [ ]

Managed Care Organization Profiles **DISTRICT OF COLUMBIA**

AMERIGROUP DISTRICT OF COLUMBIA

750 First St NE Ste 1120
Washington, DC 20002
Phone: 202-218-4900 Fax: 202-783-0786 Toll-Free:
Web site: www.amerigroupcorp.com
MAILING ADDRESS:
    AMERIGROUP - DC
    750 First St NE Ste 1120
    Washington, DC 20002

KEY EXECUTIVES:
Chief Executive Officer .... Carolyn W Colvin
Chief Financial Officer .... Nancy Djordjevic
Medical Director .... Barry Cohen, MD
Assistant VP, Marketing .... Ken Howze
VP, Provider Relations .... Ed Walburn
Network Development Director .... Deborah Wilson
AssistantVP, Health Promotion Director .... Lisa Truitt
Director of Associates Services .... Deidre Carroll
Assistant VP, Healthcare Management Service .... Rosalyn Stephens
Assistant VP, Quality Management .... Sheila Taylor
Director, Health Plan Operations .... Tim Spooner
Assistant VP, HCMS-Behavioral Health .... Anne Clements
VP, Government Relations .... Karen Squarrell Shablin

COMPANY PROFILE:
Parent Company Name: Amerigroup Corporation
Doing Business As: Amerigroup DC, Americaid Community Care
Year Founded: 1999   Federally Qualified: [N]
Forprofit: [Y]   Not-For-Profit: [ ]
Model Type: NETWORK
Accreditation: [ ] AAPPO [ ] JACHO [ ] NCQA [X] URAC
Plan Type: HMO
Primary Physicians: 283   Physician Specialists:
Hospitals: 7
Total Enrollment:
    2001: 13,000   2004: 41,000   2007: 0
    2002: 36,500   2005: 40,247
    2003: 32,670   2006: 40,000
SERVICE AREA:
Nationwide:
    DC;
TYPE OF COVERAGE:
Commercial: [ ] Individual: [ ] FEHBP: [ ] Indemnity: [ ]
Medicare: [ ] Medicaid: [Y] Supplemental Medicare: [ ]
Tricare   [ ]
PRODUCTS OFFERED:
Product Name: Type:
Amerigroup HMO   Medicaid

CAREFIRST BLUECHOICE INC

840 First St NE
Washington, DC 20065
Phone: 202-479-8000 Fax: 410-872-4107 Toll-Free: 888-579-8969
Web site: www.carefirst.com
MAILING ADDRESS:
    CAREFIRST BLUECHOICE INC
    10455 Mill Run Circle
    Owings Mills, MD 20065

KEY EXECUTIVES:
Chairman .... Michael R Merson
Chief Executive Officer/President .... Chester Burrell
Chief Financial Officer .... G Mark Chaney
Chief Medical Officer .... Jon Shematek, MD
Pharmacy Director .... Winston Wong, PharmD
Senior VP, Chief Information Officer .... Theodore BellaVecchia
Executive VP, Operations .... Leon Kaplan
Marketing Director .... Gregory A Devou
Executive VP, Med Systems Corporate Development .... David D Wolf
VP, Corporate Communications .... Maria Tildon
Medical Director, Medical Affairs .... Linton Wray, MD

COMPANY PROFILE:
Parent Company Name: CareFirst Inc
Doing Business As: CareFirst BlueCross BlueShield
Year Founded: 1985   Federally Qualified: [N]
Forprofit: [Y]   Not-For-Profit: [ ]
Model Type: IPA
Accreditation: [ ] AAPPO [ ] JACHO [ ] NCQA [ ] URAC
Plan Type: HMO, POS, CDHP, HDHP, HSA,
Total Enrollment:
    2001: 288,781   2004: 405,576   2007: 0
    2002: 309,664   2005:
    2003: 370,326   2006:
SERVICE AREA:
Nationwide: N
    DC; MD (Montgomery, Prince George's); Northern VA (Arlington, Fairfax, Prince William);
TYPE OF COVERAGE:
Commercial: [Y] Individual: [ ] FEHBP: [Y] Indemnity: [ ]
Medicare: [ ] Medicaid: [ ] Supplemental Medicare: [ ]
Tricare   [ ]
PRODUCTS OFFERED:
Product Name: Type:
Capital Care   HMO
CONSUMER-DRIVEN PRODUCTS
    HSA Company
    HSA Product
    HSA Administrator
Personal Care Account   Consumer-Driven Health Plan
    High Deductible Health Plan
PLAN BENEFITS:
Alternative Medicine: [ ]   Behavioral Health: [ ]
Chiropractic: [X]   Dental: [X]
Home Care: [X]   Inpatient SNF: [ ]
Long-Term Care: [ ]   Pharm. Mail Order: [X]
Physicial Therapy: [ ]   Podiatry: [X]
Psychiatric: [X]   Transplant: [X]
Vision: [X]   Wellness: [X]
Workers' Comp: [ ]
Other Benefits:
Comments:
Formerly BC BS the national capital area.

D C CHARTERED HEALTH PLAN INC

1025 15th St NW
Washington, DC 20005
Phone: 202-408-3966 Fax: 202-408-4710 Toll-Free: 800-799-4710
Web site: www.chartered-health.com
MAILING ADDRESS:
    D C CHARTERED HEALTH PLN INC
    1025 15th St NW
    Washington, DC 20005

KEY EXECUTIVES:
Chairman of the Board .... Charles Bowles Jr, MD
Chief Executive Officer/President .... Tamara A Smith
Chief Financial Officer .... Gabriel J Hanna
Chief Medical Officer .... Joshua Holloway, MD
Chief Information Officer .... Khalil Bouharoun
Chief Operating Officer .... Cesar Martinez
VP Marketing .... Ronald V Joiner
Medical Director for Alliance .... Nieves M Zaldivar, MD, FAAP

COMPANY PROFILE:
Parent Company Name:
Doing Business As:
Year Founded: 1986   Federally Qualified: [N]
Forprofit: [ ]   Not-For-Profit: [Y]
Model Type: MIXED
Accreditation: [ ] AAPPO [ ] JACHO [ ] NCQA [ ] URAC
Plan Type: HMO
Total Enrollment:
    2001: 26,130   2004: 38,412   2007: 0
    2002: 34,385   2005: 38,002
    2003: 36,203   2006:
SERVICE AREA:
Nationwide: N
    DC;
TYPE OF COVERAGE:
Commercial: [Y] Individual: [ ] FEHBP: [ ] Indemnity: [ ]
Medicare: [ ] Medicaid: [Y] Supplemental Medicare: [ ]
Tricare   [ ]
PRODUCTS OFFERED:
Product Name: Type:
DC Chartered Health Plan   Medicaid

COVENTRY HEALTH CARE INC — DELAWARE INC

2751 Centerville Rd Ste 400
Wilmington, DE 19808
Phone: 302-995-6100 Fax: 302-633-4145 Toll-Free: 800-727-9951
Web site: www.cvty.com

MAILING ADDRESS:
COVENTRY HEALTH CARE — DE
2751 Centerville Rd Ste 400
Wilmington, DE 19808

KEY EXECUTIVES:
Chief Executive Officer/President .... Timothy E Nolan
Chief Financial Officer ....James Hynek
Regional Pharmacy Director ....Bob Gilkin
Marketing and Sales VP .... P Scott Fad
Compliance Officer .... Michael Herman
Manager of Communications ....Celia Bloom
VP Network Management .... Kevin Davis
Human Resources Manager .... Karen Vargas
Quality Director ....Cyndie Ganc
VP, Health Services... Maureen Cunningham

COMPANY PROFILE:
Parent Company Name: Coventry Health Care Inc
Doing Business As:
Year Founded: 1986   Federally Qualified: [N]
Forprofit: [Y]   Not-For-Profit: [ ]
Model Type: IPA
Accreditation: [ ] AAPPO [ ] JACHO [ ] NCQA [X] URAC
Plan Type: HMO, PPO, POS, CDHP, HDHP, HSA
Total Enrollment:
   2001: 154,139   2004: 104,000   2007: 0
   2002: 50,925   2005: 101,000
   2003: 103,388   2006:

SERVICE AREA:
Nationwide: N
   DE (Kent, New Castle, Sussex); MD (All Counties);

TYPE OF COVERAGE:
Commercial: [Y] Individual: [ ] FEHBP: [ ] Indemnity: [ ]
Medicare: [Y] Medicaid: [Y] Supplemental Medicare: [ ]
Tricare   [ ]

PRODUCTS OFFERED:
Product Name:	Type:
Advantra	Medicare Advantage
Delaware Care	Medicaid

CONSUMER-DRIVEN PRODUCTS
Wells Fargo	HSA Company
	HSA Product
Corporate Benefits Servs of Am	HSA Administrator
Coventry Flex Choice	Consumer-Driven Health Plan
Open Access Plus Plan	High Deductible Health Plan

PLAN BENEFITS:
Alternative Medicine:	[X]	Behavioral Health:	[X]
Chiropractic:	[X]	Dental:	[X]
Home Care:	[X]	Inpatient SNF:	[X]
Long-Term Care:	[X]	Pharm. Mail Order:	[X]
Physical Therapy:	[X]	Podiatry:	[X]
Psychiatric:	[X]	Transplant:	[X]
Vision:	[X]	Wellness:	[X]
Workers' Comp:	[ ]		

Other Benefits:
Comments:
Formerly Principal Health Care of Delaware Inc.

Managed Care Organization Profiles — DELAWARE

AMERIHEALTH INSURANCE COMPANY

919 N Market-Mellon Ctr #1200
Wilmington, DE 19801-3021
Phone: 302-777-6400 Fax: 302-777-6444 Toll-Free: 800-275-2583
Web site: www.amerihealth.com

MAILING ADDRESS:
AMERIHEALTH INSURANCE COMPANY
919 N Market-Mellon Ctr #1200
Wilmington, DE 19801-3021

KEY EXECUTIVES:
Marketing Director .... Mark Sweetsler

COMPANY PROFILE:
Parent Company Name: Independence Blue Cross
Doing Business As: Amerihealth HMO Inc/AmeriHealth Ins Co
Year Founded: 1983   Federally Qualified: [Y]
Forprofit: [Y]   Not-For-Profit: [ ]
Model Type: IPA
Accreditation: [ ] AAPPO [ ] JACHO [X] NCQA [ ] URAC
Plan Type: HMO, PPO, POS, ASO, TPA
Total Enrollment:
  2001: 12,822   2004: 0   2007: 0
  2002: 0   2005:
  2003: 0   2006:

SERVICE AREA:
Nationwide: N
  DE; NJ; 9 Counties in PA; Selected Counties in MD; 4 Counties in NY;

TYPE OF COVERAGE:
Commercial: [Y] Individual: [ ] FEHBP: [ ] Indemnity: [ ]
Medicare: [ ] Medicaid: [ ] Supplemental Medicare: [Y]
Tricare   [ ]

PRODUCTS OFFERED:
Product Name: Type:
Amerihealth HMO Inc   HMO
Amerihealth Personal Choice   PPO
Amerihealth POS   POS

PLAN BENEFITS:
Alternative Medicine: [ ]   Behavioral Health: [ ]
Chiropractic: [X]   Dental: [X]
Home Care: [X]   Inpatient SNF: [X]
Long-Term Care: [ ]   Pharm. Mail Order: [X]
Physical Therapy: [X]   Podiatry: [X]
Psychiatric: [X]   Transplant: [X]
Vision: [X]   Wellness: [X]
Workers' Comp: [ ]
Other Benefits:

BLUE CROSS BLUE SHIELD OF DELAWARE

One Brandywine Gateway
Wilmington, DE 19899-1991
Phone: 302-421-3000 Fax: 302-421-3461 Toll-Free:
Web site: www.bcbsde.com

MAILING ADDRESS:
BC/BS OF DE
PO Box 1991
Wilmington, DE 19899-1991

KEY EXECUTIVES:
Chief Executive Officer/President .... Timothy J Constantine
Corporate Controller, Treasurer .... Philip Carter
Chief Medical Officer .... Paul Kaplan, MD
VP Operations .... George H English, Jr
VP Corporate Marketing .... Christine L Alrich
Public Relations Director .... Darelle Riabov
VP, Network & Medical Management .... Paul Kaplan, MD

COMPANY PROFILE:
Parent Company Name: Care First Blue Cross Blue Shield
Doing Business As:
Year Founded: 1935   Federally Qualified: [ ]
Forprofit: [Y]   Not-For-Profit: [ ]
Model Type: IPA
Accreditation: [ ] AAPPO [ ] JACHO [X] NCQA [ ] URAC
Plan Type: HMO, PPO, POS, CDHP, HSA, HDHP,
Total Enrollment:
  2001: 281,894   2004: 94,052   2007: 482,000
  2002: 325,628   2005:
  2003: 88,325   2006: 388,000

SERVICE AREA:
Nationwide: N
  DE;

TYPE OF COVERAGE:
Commercial: [Y] Individual: [Y] FEHBP: [ ] Indemnity: [ ]
Medicare: [ ] Medicaid: [ ] Supplemental Medicare: [Y]
Tricare   [ ]

PRODUCTS OFFERED:
Product Name: Type:
Independent Practice Associati   IPA
HMO Delaware   HMO
Blue Choice   PPO
Blue Select

PLAN BENEFITS:
Alternative Medicine: [ ]   Behavioral Health: [ ]
Chiropractic: [ ]   Dental: [X]
Home Care: [ ]   Inpatient SNF: [ ]
Long-Term Care: [ ]   Pharm. Mail Order: [ ]
Physical Therapy: [ ]   Podiatry: [ ]
Psychiatric: [ ]   Transplant: [ ]
Vision: [ ]   Wellness: [ ]
Workers' Comp: [ ]
Other Benefits:

CIGNA DENTAL HEALTH OF DELAWARE INC

1571 Sawgrass Corporate Pkwy
Sunrise, FL 33323
Phone: 954-514-6600 Fax: 954-514-6905 Toll-Free: 800-367-1037
Web site: www.cigna.com/dental

MAILING ADDRESS:
CIGNA DENTAL HEALTH OF DE INC
1571 Sawgrass Corporate Pkwy
Sunrise, FL 33323

KEY EXECUTIVES:
Chief Executive Officer .... Benjamin K Haynes
President .... Karen S Rohan
Chief Financial Director .... Frank Lucia
Dental Director .... Ed Schooley, DDS
Marketing Director .... Aaron Groffman
MIS Director .... Laurel A Flebotte

COMPANY PROFILE:
Parent Company Name: CIGNA Dental Health Inc
Doing Business As: CIGNA Dental
Year Founded: 1985   Federally Qualified: [N]
Forprofit: [Y]   Not-For-Profit: [ ]
Model Type:
Accreditation: [ ] AAPPO [ ] JACHO [ ] NCQA [ ] URAC
Plan Type: Specialty HMO
Total Enrollment:
  2001: 205   2004: 23   2007: 0
  2002: 65   2005:
  2003: 8,800   2006:

SERVICE AREA:
Nationwide: N
  DE;

TYPE OF COVERAGE:
Commercial: [Y] Individual: [ ] FEHBP: [ ] Indemnity: [ ]
Medicare: [ ] Medicaid: [ ] Supplemental Medicare: [ ]
Tricare   [ ]

PRODUCTS OFFERED:
Product Name: Type:
CIGNA Dental Health of DE   Specialty HMO

PLAN BENEFITS:
Alternative Medicine: [ ]   Behavioral Health: [ ]
Chiropractic: [ ]   Dental: [X]
Home Care: [ ]   Inpatient SNF: [ ]
Long-Term Care: [ ]   Pharm. Mail Order: [ ]
Physical Therapy: [ ]   Podiatry: [ ]
Psychiatric: [ ]   Transplant: [ ]
Vision: [ ]   Wellness: [ ]
Workers' Comp: [ ]
Other Benefits:

Managed Care Organization Profiles   **CONNECTICUT**

MAILING ADDRESS:
   OXFORD HEALTH PLANS-CT
   48 Monroe Turnpike
   Trumbell, CT 06611

KEY EXECUTIVES:
Chief Executive Officer/President .... Michael Turpin
Executive VP Chief Medical Officer .... Alan M Muney, MD, MHA
Chief Information Officer .... Steven H Black
Executive VP, Operations .... Steven H Black
Regional VP of Sales .... Brendan Kerrigan
Director of Gov't Relations .... Tim Myers
VP Legal .... Jeff Boyd
Health Care Services .... Paul Conlin

COMPANY PROFILE:
Parent Company Name: UnitedHealth Group
Doing Business As:
Year Founded: 1993   Federally Qualified: [ ]
Forprofit: [Y]   Not-For-Profit: [ ]
Model Type: IPA
Accreditation: [ ] AAPPO [ ] JACHO [X] NCQA [ ] URAC
Plan Type: HMO, POS, TPA, CDHP
Primary Physicians: 3,012   Physician Specialists: 9,128
Hospitals:
Total Revenue: 2005:   2006: 243,426,002
Net Income   2005:   2006:
Total Enrollment:
   2001: 59,755   2004: 71,223   2007: 0
   2002: 83,505   2005: 67,889
   2003: 84,137   2006: 51,895

SERVICE AREA:
Nationwide: N
   CT;

TYPE OF COVERAGE:
Commercial: [Y] Individual: [Y] FEHBP: [ ] Indemnity: [ ]
Medicare: [Y] Medicaid: [ ] Supplemental Medicare: [ ]
Tricare   [ ]

PRODUCTS OFFERED:
Product Name: Type:
Oxford Freedom Plan   POS
Liberty Plan   POS
Medicare Advantage   Medicare Advantage
Oxford HMO   HMO

PLAN BENEFITS:
Alternative Medicine: [ ]   Behavioral Health: [X]
Chiropractic: [X]   Dental: [ ]
Home Care: [X]   Inpatient SNF: [X]
Long-Term Care: [X]   Pharm. Mail Order: [X]
Physical Therapy: [X]   Podiatry: [X]
Psychiatric: [X]   Transplant: [X]
Vision: [X]   Wellness: [X]
Workers' Comp: [X]
Other Benefits:

PREFERRED ONE

116 Washington Ave 2nd Fl
North Haven, CT 06473
Phone: 203-239-7444 Fax: 203-239-5308 Toll-Free: 800-925-3606
Web site: www.wellcare.com

MAILING ADDRESS:
   PREFERRED ONE
   116 Washington Ave 2nd Fl
   North Haven, CT 06473

KEY EXECUTIVES:
Executive Chairman .... Charles G Berg
Chief Executive Officer/President .... Heath Schiesser
Medical Director .... David Wilcox, MD
VP, Pharmacy .... John Sirera
Senior Vp, Chief Information Officer .... Anil Kottoor
Senior VP, Marketing Expansion .... Rupesh Shah
Human Resources Director .... Gretchen DeMartini
Utilization Management .... Linda Schofield
Member Services Manager .... JoAnn Villano
Sub Contracting Affr Manager .... Denise Consiglio

COMPANY PROFILE:
Parent Company Name: WellCare Health Plans-Health Choice CT
Doing Business As: WellCare of Connecticut Inc
Year Founded: Federally Qualified: [ ]
Forprofit: [Y]   Not-For-Profit: [ ]
Model Type:
Accreditation: [ ] AAPPO [ ] JACHO [ ] NCQA [ ] URAC
Plan Type: HMO, UR
Total Enrollment:
   2001: 22,347   2004: 33,733   2007: 0
   2002: 17,401   2005:
   2003: 24,164   2006:

SERVICE AREA:
Nationwide: N
   CT;

TYPE OF COVERAGE:
Commercial: [ ] Individual: [ ] FEHBP: [ ] Indemnity: [ ]
Medicare: [ ] Medicaid: [Y] Supplemental Medicare: [ ]
Tricare   [ ]

PRODUCTS OFFERED:
Product Name: Type:
Preferred One   Medicaid

Comments:
July 2004, WellCare Group Inc. and WellCare Holdings, LLC. merged and became WellCare Health Plans Inc.

YALE UNIVERSITY HEALTH PLAN

17 Hillhouse Ave
New Haven, CT 06520
Phone: 203-432-0076 Fax: 203-432-7289 Toll-Free:
Web site: www.yale.edu/uhs

MAILING ADDRESS:
   YALE UNIVERSITY HEALTH PLAN
   PO Box 208237
   New Haven, CT 06520

KEY EXECUTIVES:
Chief Executive Director .... Paul Genecin MD
Chief Financial Officer .... Robert Henry
Medical Director .... Michael Rigsby, MD
Deputy Director .... Judy Madeaux

COMPANY PROFILE:
Parent Company Name: Yale University
Doing Business As: Yale University Health Services
Year Founded: 1971   Federally Qualified: [ ]
Forprofit: [ ]   Not-For-Profit: [Y]
Model Type: STAFF
Accreditation: [ ] AAPPO [ ] JACHO [ ] NCQA [ ] URAC
Plan Type: HMO

SERVICE AREA:
Nationwide: N
   CT (New Haven);

TYPE OF COVERAGE:
Commercial: [Y] Individual: [Y] FEHBP: [ ] Indemnity: [ ]
Medicare: [Y] Medicaid: [ ] Supplemental Medicare: [ ]
Tricare   [ ]

PRODUCTS OFFERED:
Product Name: Type:
Yale Preferred Health Plan
Yale Faculty Practice Plan

PLAN BENEFITS:
Alternative Medicine: [ ]   Behavioral Health: [ ]
Chiropractic: [ ]   Dental: [ ]
Home Care: [ ]   Inpatient SNF: [X]
Long-Term Care: [ ]   Pharm. Mail Order: [ ]
Physical Therapy: [X]   Podiatry: [X]
Psychiatric: [X]   Transplant: [X]
Vision: [ ]   Wellness: [ ]
Workers' Comp: [X]
Other Benefits:

CONNECTICUT — Managed Care Organization Profiles

MAILING ADDRESS:
MAGELLAN HEALTH SERVICES INC
55 Nod Rd
Avon, CT 06001

KEY EXECUTIVES:
Chairman of the Board/Chief Executive Officer .... Steven J Shulman
President .... Rene Lerer, MD
Executive VP/Chief Financial Officer .... Mark S Demilio
Chief Medical Officer .... Alex R Rodriguez, MD
Chief Information Officer .... Jeff D Emerson
COO, Public Sector Solutions .... Russell C Petrella, PhD
Chief Sales & Marketing Officer .... Michael Majerik
Executive VP/Chief Clinical Officer .... Deborah Trout, PhD
VP, Investor Relations .... Melissa Rose, MBA
Chief Human Resources Director .... Caskie Lewis-Clapper, MS
Chief Clinical Officer .... Anthony M Kotin, MD
Corporate Compliance Officer .... Craig Harriger, MBA, JD
Executive VP Business Operations .... Dennis Moody, MBA
Executive VP & General Counsel .... Megan M Arthur, JD
Executive VP, Workplace Division .... William C Barr, MA
COO, Public Sector Division .... Russell C Petrella, PhD

COMPANY PROFILE:
Parent Company Name: Magellan Health Services Inc
Doing Business As:
Year Founded: 1989   Federally Qualified: [ ]
Forprofit: [Y]   Not-For-Profit: [ ]
Model Type:
Accreditation: [ ] AAPPO [ ] JACHO [X] NCQA [ ] URAC
Plan Type: Specialty HMO, Specialty PPO, UR, POS
Primary Physicians: Physician Specialists:
Hospitals:
Total Revenue: 2005:   2006:   1,230,000,000
Net Income   2005:   2006:   63,800,000
Total Enrollment:
  2001: 69,300,000   2004: 60,000,000   2007: 0
  2002: 68,000,000   2005: 55,000,000
  2003: 60,000,000   2006: 60,300,000
Medical Loss Ratio: 2005:   2006:
Administrative Expense Ratio: 2005:   2006:

SERVICE AREA:
Nationwide: Y
  NW;

TYPE OF COVERAGE:
Commercial: [Y] Individual: [ ] FEHBP: [ ] Indemnity: [ ]
Medicare: [Y] Medicaid: [Y] Supplemental Medicare: [ ]
Tricare   [ ]

PLAN BENEFITS:
Alternative Medicine: [ ]   Behavioral Health: [X]
Chiropractic: [ ]   Dental: [ ]
Home Care: [ ]   Inpatient SNF: [ ]
Long-Term Care: [ ]   Pharm. Mail Order: [ ]
Physical Therapy: [ ]   Podiatry: [ ]
Psychiatric: [ ]   Transplant: [ ]
Vision: [ ]   Wellness: [ ]
Workers' Comp: [ ]
Other Benefits:

NORTHEAST HEALTH DIRECT LLC

359 North Main St
Marlborough, CT 06447
Phone: 860-295-8261 Fax: 860-295-8679 Toll-Free: 800-423-6619
Web site: www.nehealthdirect.com

MAILING ADDRESS:
NORTHEAST HEALTH DIRECT LLC
PO Box 435
Marlborough, CT 06447

KEY EXECUTIVES:
Public Relations Director .... Missy Pudeman
Provider Relations Manager .... Janice McDonald
Network Development Director .... Jamie Kirdzik
Public Relations .... Maureen Moran

COMPANY PROFILE:
Parent Company Name: Consumer Health Network, NJ
Doing Business As: Northeast Health Direct LLC
Year Founded: 1995   Federally Qualified: [ ]
Forprofit: [Y]   Not-For-Profit: [ ]
Model Type: NETWORK
Accreditation: [ ] AAPPO [ ] JACHO [ ] NCQA [X] URAC
Plan Type: PPO
Total Enrollment:
  2001: 45,000   2004: 0   2007: 0
  2002: 0   2005:
  2003: 0   2006:

SERVICE AREA:
Nationwide: N
  CT; MA; NH; VT; RI;

TYPE OF COVERAGE:
Commercial: [Y] Individual: [ ] FEHBP: [ ] Indemnity: [ ]
Medicare: [ ] Medicaid: [ ] Supplemental Medicare: [ ]
Tricare   [ ]

PRODUCTS OFFERED:
Product Name: Type:
Northeast Direct   PPO

OXFORD HEALTH PLANS INC — CORPORATE HEADQUARTERS

48 Monroe Turnpike
Trumbell, CT 06611
Phone: 800-889-7658 Fax: 203-459-6464 Toll-Free: 800-889-7658
Web site: www.oxhp.com

MAILING ADDRESS:
OXFORD HEALTH PLANS INC CORP
48 Monroe Turnpike
Trumbell, CT 06611

KEY EXECUTIVES:
Chief Executive Officer/President .... Michael Turpin
Executive VP Chief Medical Officer .... Alan M Muney, MD, MHA
Senior VP, Chief Information Officer .... Steven H Black
Executive VP, Operations .... Steven H Black
Compliance Officer .... Donna Marie Stanley
Executive VP, General Counsel .... Daniel N Gregoire

COMPANY PROFILE:
Parent Company Name: UnitedHealth Group Doing Business As:
Year Founded: 1984   Federally Qualified: [N]
Forprofit: [Y]   Not-For-Profit: [ ]
Model Type: IPA
Accreditation: [ ] AAPPO [ ] JACHO [ ] NCQA [ ] URAC
Plan Type: HMO, PPO, POS, TPA, CDHP, HDHP
Total Enrollment:
  2001: 1,510,100   2004: 2,075,543   2007: 0
  2002: 1,601,500   2005:
  2003: 1,539,200   2006:

SERVICE AREA:
Nationwide: N
  CT; NJ; NY;

TYPE OF COVERAGE:
Commercial: [Y] Individual: [Y] FEHBP: [ ] Indemnity: [ ]
Medicare: [Y] Medicaid: [Y] Supplemental Medicare: [ ]
Tricare   [ ]

PRODUCTS OFFERED:
Product Name: Type:
Oxford Freedom Plan   POS
Liberty Plan   POS
Medicaid Health Start
Oxford HMO   HMO
Medicare Advantage   Medicare

PLAN BENEFITS:
Alternative Medicine: [X]   Behavioral Health: [X]
Chiropractic: [X]   Dental: [X]
Home Care: [X]   Inpatient SNF: [X]
Long-Term Care: [X]   Pharm. Mail Order: [X]
Physical Therapy: [X]   Podiatry: [X]
Psychiatric: [X]   Transplant: [X]
Vision: [X]   Wellness: [X]
Workers' Comp: [X]
Other Benefits:

OXFORD HEALTH PLANS-CONNECTICUT

48 Monroe Trnpke
Trumbell, CT 06611
Phone: 203-459-6000 Fax: 203-459-6464 Toll-Free:
Web site: www.oxhp.com

Managed Care Organization Profiles

CONNECTICUT

TYPE OF COVERAGE:
Commercial: [Y] Individual: [ ] FEHBP: [ ] Indemnity: [ ]
Medicare: [ ] Medicaid: [ ] Supplemental Medicare: [ ]
Tricare [ ]
PRODUCTS OFFERED:
Product Name:	Type:
Health Net HMO	HMO
Kaiser Health Plan of CT	HMO
Health Options	Medicaid
SmartChoice	Medicare

CONSUMER-DRIVEN PRODUCTS
                              HSA Company
                              HSA Product
                              HSA Administrator
                              Consumer-Driven Health Plan
Health Net Smart Choice   High Deductible Health Plan

PLAN BENEFITS:
Alternative Medicine:	[ ]	Behavioral Health:	[X]
Chiropractic:	[X]	Dental:	[ ]
Home Care:	[X]	Inpatient SNF:	[X]
Long-Term Care:	[X]	Pharm. Mail Order:	[X]
Physical Therapy:	[X]	Podiatry:	[X]
Psychiatric:	[X]	Transplant:	[ ]
Vision:	[ ]	Wellness:	[X]
Workers' Comp:	[ ]		

Other Benefits:
Comments:
Merger between MD Health Plans & Physician Health Services of Connecticut Inc.

HEALTH NET INC - NORTHEAST CORPORATE HEADQUARTERS

One Far Mill Crossing
Shelton, CT 06484
Phone: 203-402-4200 Fax: 203-225-4000 Toll-Free: 800-848-4747
Web site: www.healthnet.com
MAILING ADDRESS:
    HEALTH NET INC - NE CORPORATE
    PO Box 904
    Shelton, CT 06484

KEY EXECUTIVES:
Chief Executive Officer .... Jay M Gillert
President - NE Region .... Paul S Lambdin
Regional Financial Officer .... Peter Gladitsch
Medicare Medical Officer .... Steve Calabrese
Senior VP, Chief Information Officer .... David Anderson
Chief Operating Officer .... William Lamoreaux
Chief Sales Officer .... Rick Kaplan
Medicare Medical Officer .... Krista Bowers
VP, Business Analysis/Integra .... Charles Nostrand
VP, Application Development .... Jay Woloszynski
VP, Technolony Management .... Al Milazzo
Reg VP/Bus Retention/Devlpmnt .... Susan Ross

COMPANY PROFILE:
Parent Company Name: Health Net Inc
Doing Business As: Health Net
Year Founded: 1975 Federally Qualified: [Y]
Forprofit: [Y] Not-For-Profit: [ ]
Model Type: IPA
Accreditation: [ ] AAPPO [ ] JACHO [X] NCQA [ ] URAC
Plan Type: HMO, PPO, POS, HDHP, HSA
Total Enrollment:
   2001: 1,006,370 2004: 862,674 2007: 729,000
   2002: 0 2005: 826,000
   2003: 897,436 2006: 783,000
SERVICE AREA:
Nationwide: N
   CT; NJ; NY;
TYPE OF COVERAGE:
Commercial: [Y] Individual: [ ] FEHBP: [ ] Indemnity: [ ]
Medicare: [ ] Medicaid: [ ] Supplemental Medicare: [ ]
Tricare [ ]
PRODUCTS OFFERED:
Product Name:	Type:
SmartChoice	Medicare
Commercial HMO, PPO	
Health Net Medicaid	Medicaid
Health Net	ASO

CONSUMER-DRIVEN PRODUCTS
                              HSA Company
                              HSA Product
                              HSA Administrator
Healthcare Solutions Outlook   Consumer-Driven Health Plan
Health Smart Health Choice   High Deductible Health Plan

PLAN BENEFITS:
Alternative Medicine:	[ ]	Behavioral Health:	[X]
Chiropractic:	[X]	Dental:	[ ]
Home Care:	[X]	Inpatient SNF:	[X]
Long-Term Care:	[X]	Pharm. Mail Order:	[X]
Physical Therapy:	[X]	Podiatry:	[X]
Psychiatric:	[X]	Transplant:	[ ]
Vision:	[ ]	Wellness:	[X]
Workers' Comp:	[ ]		

Other Benefits:
Comments:
Physicians Health Services was the Northeast Division for Foundation Health Services. Foundation Health became Health Net.

INTERPLAN HEALTH GROUP - CORPORATE HEADQUARTERS

20 Waterside Dr
Farmington, CT 06032
Phone: 860-678-7877 Fax: 860-678-7719 Toll-Free: 800-799-8933
Web site: www.interplanhealth.com
MAILING ADDRESS:
    INTERPLAN HEALTH GROUP - CORP
    20 Waterside Dr
    Farmington, CT 06032

KEY EXECUTIVES:
Chairman/Chief Executive Officer .... Paul W Glover
President, Midwest Region .... Peter R Osenar
Chief Financial Officer .... Steven L Ditman
Chief Information Officer .... Hamilton Chaffee
Chief Operating Officer .... Eileen Romansky
Chief Sales & Marketing Officer .... Michael D Schotz

COMPANY PROFILE:
Parent Company Name:
Doing Business As:
Year Founded: 2001 Federally Qualified: [ ]
Forprofit: [Y] Not-For-Profit: [ ]
Model Type:
Accreditation: [ ] AAPPO [ ] JACHO [ ] NCQA [ ] URAC
Plan Type: PPO, PBM, EPO, UR
Total Enrollment:
   2001: 460,000 2004: 3,000,000 2007: 0
   2002: 0 2005:
   2003: 0 2006: 3,000,000
SERVICE AREA:
Nationwide: N
   NW;
TYPE OF COVERAGE:
Commercial: [Y] Individual: [Y] FEHBP: [ ] Indemnity: [ ]
Medicare: [ ] Medicaid: [ ] Supplemental Medicare: [ ]
Tricare [ ]
PLAN BENEFITS:
Alternative Medicine:	[X]	Behavioral Health:	[X]
Chiropractic:	[X]	Dental:	[ ]
Home Care:	[X]	Inpatient SNF:	[X]
Long-Term Care:	[X]	Pharm. Mail Order:	[X]
Physical Therapy:	[X]	Podiatry:	[X]
Psychiatric:	[X]	Transplant:	[X]
Vision:	[X]	Wellness:	[X]
Workers' Comp:	[X]		

Other Benefits:
Comments:
Formerly Northwest One.

MAGELLAN HEALTH SERVICES INC

55 Nod Rd
Avon, CT 06001
Phone: 860-507-1900 Fax: 410-953-5209 Toll-Free: 800-458-2740
Web site: www.magellanhealth.com

CONNECTICUT — Managed Care Organization Profiles

Senior VP, Health Services .... Paul Bluestein, MD
Director, Pharmacy .... Jeff Casberg
VP & Chief Information Officer .... Mark G Dixon
VP Operations .... Ida Schnipper
Senior VP & Chief Marketing Officer .... Paul M Philpott
Senior VP, Chief Sales Officer .... Jim Buccheri
Manager, Credentialing .... Joyce Vagts
Director, Compliance .... Maria Stiefel
Director, Public Relations .... Stephen Jewett
Manager, Provider Services .... Kathleen Gauthier
VP, Network Operations .... Kathleen Madden
Human Resources Director .... Richard Rogers
Director, Medical Operations .... Lauren Williams
Director, Quality Improvement .... Pam Spinazola
Manager, Credentialing .... Joyce Vagts
Director, Compliance .... Maria Stiefel
Director, Marketing Operations .... Leah Katz
VP, General Counsel .... Gail Bogossian
VP, Marketing & Chief of Staff .... Patrick Yung

COMPANY PROFILE:
Parent Company Name: ConnectiCare Holding Co Inc
Doing Business As: ConnectiCare Inc & Affiliates
Year Founded: 1982   Federally Qualified: [Y]
Forprofit: [Y]   Not-For-Profit: [ ]
Model Type: IPA
Accreditation: [ ] AAPPO [ ] JACHO [X] NCQA [ ] URAC
Plan Type: HMO, PPO, POS, ASO, HDHP, HSA
Primary Physicians: 4,879   Physician Specialists: 10,755
Hospitals: 78
Total Revenue: 2005: 718,888,021   2006: 750,000,000
Net Income   2005: 26,905,429   2006: 10,722,481
Total Enrollment:
  2001: 243,890   2004: 216,945   2007: 0
  2002: 223,601   2005: 240,499
  2003: 218,690   2006: 234,144
Medical Loss Ratio: 2005: 80.30   2006: 81.10
Administrative Expense Ratio: 2005: 14.90   2006: 15.50

SERVICE AREA:
Nationwide: N
  CT; MA (Hampden, Hampshire, Franklin);

TYPE OF COVERAGE:
Commercial: [Y] Individual: [ ] FEHBP: [ ] Indemnity: [ ]
Medicare: [ ] Medicaid: [ ] Supplemental Medicare: [ ]
Tricare   [ ]

PRODUCTS OFFERED:
Product Name:	Type:
HMO Open Access	HMO
HMO Personal Care Plan	HMO
POS Personal Care Plan	POS
Connecticare 65	Medicare

CONSUMER-DRIVEN PRODUCTS
	HSA Company
HMO/POS Open Access HDHP	HSA Product
First HSA Inc	HSA Administrator
	Consumer-Driven Health Plan
HMO/POS Open Access HDHP	High Deductible Health Plan

PLAN BENEFITS:
Alternative Medicine:	[ ]	Behavioral Health:	[X]
Chiropractic:	[X]	Dental:	[ ]
Home Care:	[X]	Inpatient SNF:	[X]
Long-Term Care:	[ ]	Pharm. Mail Order:	[X]
Physical Therapy:	[X]	Podiatry:	[X]
Psychiatric:	[X]	Transplant:	[X]
Vision:	[X]	Wellness:	[X]
Workers' Comp:	[ ]		

Other Benefits:
Comments:
Kaiser Permanente Northeast division Connecticut commercial membership has been acquisitioned by ConnectiCare.

GENWORTH LIFE & HEALTH INSURANCE CO

175 Addison Rd
Windsor, CT 06095-0725
Phone: 860-737-2198 Fax: 860-737-6598 Toll-Free: 800-451-2513
Web site: www.genworth.com
MAILING ADDRESS:
  GENWORTH LIFE & HEALTH INS CO
  PO Box 725
  Windsor, CT 06095-0725

KEY EXECUTIVES:
President .... K Rone Baldwin
Chief Financial Officer .... Edward Pike
Chief Compliance Officer .... Paul Finnegan
VP Human Resources .... Shawn Von Hassel
VP, Quality Assurance .... Sharon Van Wyk
Fraud: Claims Compliance/SIU .... Alanda Gamache
Compliance Manager, EBG Records, ... Thea Cardamone

COMPANY PROFILE:
Parent Company Name: Genworth Financial
Doing Business As:
Year Founded: 1973   Federally Qualified: [ ]
Forprofit: [Y]   Not-For-Profit: [ ]
Model Type:
Accreditation: [ ] AAPPO [ ] JACHO [X] NCQA [X] URAC
Plan Type: PPO, UR, TPA, EPO,
Total Enrollment:
  2001: 0   2004: 996   2007: 0
  2002: 0   2005:
  2003: 0   2006:

SERVICE AREA:
Nationwide: Y
  NW;

TYPE OF COVERAGE:
Commercial: [Y] Individual: [ ] FEHBP: [ ] Indemnity: [ ]
Medicare: [ ] Medicaid: [ ] Supplemental Medicare: [ ]
Tricare   [ ]

PLAN BENEFITS:
Alternative Medicine:	[ ]	Behavioral Health:	[X]
Chiropractic:	[X]	Dental:	[X]
Home Care:	[X]	Inpatient SNF:	[X]
Long-Term Care:	[ ]	Pharm. Mail Order:	[X]
Physical Therapy:	[X]	Podiatry:	[X]
Psychiatric:	[X]	Transplant:	[X]
Vision:	[X]	Wellness:	[X]
Workers' Comp:	[ ]		

Other Benefits:
Comments:
Formerly GE Group Life Assurance Company.

HEALTH NET - CONNECTICUT

One Far Mill Crossing
Shelton, CT 06484-0914
Phone: 203-402-4200 Fax: 203-225-4000 Toll-Free: 800-848-4747
Web site: www.health.net
MAILING ADDRESS:
  HEALTH NET - CONNECTICUT
  PO Box 904
  Shelton, CT 06484-0914

KEY EXECUTIVES:
President .... Jay M Gellert
Chief Financial Officer .... Carol Richey
Medical Director .... Timothy J Moore, MD, MS
Pharmacy Director .... Julee Oh
Director of IS .... David Anderson
Chief Marketing Officer .... Krista Bowers

COMPANY PROFILE:
Parent Company Name: Health Net Inc, NE Corp Hdqrts
Doing Business As: Health Net
Year Founded: 1975   Federally Qualified: [N]
Forprofit: [Y]   Not-For-Profit: [ ]
Model Type:
Accreditation: [ ] AAPPO [ ] JACHO [ ] NCQA [ ] URAC
Plan Type: HMO, PPO, POS, HDHP, HSA,
Primary Physicians: 2,588   Physician Specialists: 6,379
Hospitals:
Total Revenue: 2005:   2006: 124
Net Income   2005:   2006:
Total Enrollment:
  2001: 457,144   2004: 352,489   2007: 328,000
  2002: 494,491   2005: 391,000
  2003: 280,859   2006: 362,891

SERVICE AREA:
Nationwide: N
  CT;

Managed Care Organization Profiles — CONNECTICUT

Year Founded: 1974   Federally Qualified: [Y]
Forprofit: [Y]   Not-For-Profit: [ ]
Model Type:
Accreditation: [ ] AAPPO [ ] JACHO [ ] NCQA [X] URAC
Plan Type: Specialty HMO
SERVICE AREA:
Nationwide: N
   CT; DE; MA; ME; NH; NJ; NY; PA; RI; VT;
TYPE OF COVERAGE:
Commercial: [Y] Individual: [ ] FEHBP: [ ] Indemnity: [ ]
Medicare: [Y] Medicaid: [ ] Supplemental Medicare: [Y]
Tricare   [ ]
PRODUCTS OFFERED:
Product Name: Type:
Employee Assistance Programs
Managed Mental Health
PLAN BENEFITS:
Alternative Medicine: [ ]   Behavioral Health: [X]
Chiropractic: [ ]   Dental: [ ]
Home Care: [ ]   Inpatient SNF: [ ]
Long-Term Care: [ ]   Pharm. Mail Order: [ ]
Physical Therapy: [ ]   Podiatry: [ ]
Psychiatric: [X]   Transplant: [ ]
Vision: [ ]   Wellness: [X]
Workers' Comp: [ ]
Other Benefits:
Comments:
Formerly MCC Managed Behavioral Care Inc.

CIGNA HEALTHCARE OF CONNECTICUT

900 Cottage Grove Rd S-314
Hartford, CT 06152-1118
Phone: 860-226-2300 Fax: 860-226-2333 Toll-Free: 800-345-9458
Web site: www.cigna.com
MAILING ADDRESS:
   CIGNA HEALTHCARE OF CT
   900 Cottage Grove Rd S-314
   Hartford, CT 06152-1118

KEY EXECUTIVES:
Chief Executive Officer .... H Edward Hanway
Financial Director .... Elizabeth Henry
Chief Medical Officer .... Jeffery Kang, MD
Pharmacy Director .... John Poniatowski
VP Sales .... Michael Showalter
VP Sales .... Brian Cuddaback
MIS Director .... Scott A Storrer
Director, Provider Services .... Tom Garvey

COMPANY PROFILE:
Parent Company Name: CIGNA Corporation
Doing Business As:
Year Founded: 1985   Federally Qualified: [Y]
Forprofit: [Y]   Not-For-Profit: [ ]
Model Type: IPA
Accreditation: [ ] AAPPO [ ] JACHO [X] NCQA [ ] URAC
Plan Type: HMO, PPO, UR, POS, CDHP, HDHP, HSA, FSA, HRA
Primary Physicians: 2,368   Physician Specialists: 6,211
Hospitals:
Total Enrollment:
   2001: 35,218   2004: 86,096   2007: 0
   2002: 18,926   2005: 21,432
   2003: 45,936   2006:
SERVICE AREA:
Nationwide: N
   CT;
TYPE OF COVERAGE:
Commercial: [Y] Individual: [Y] FEHBP: [ ] Indemnity: [ ]
Medicare: [Y] Medicaid: [ ] Supplemental Medicare: [ ]
Tricare   [ ]
PRODUCTS OFFERED:
Product Name: Type:
CIGNA Healthcare for Seniors   Medicare
CIGNA HMO   HMO
CIGNA POS   POS
CONSUMER-DRIVEN PRODUCTS
JP Morgan Chase   HSA Company
CIGNA Choice Fund   HSA Product
                                    HSA Administrator
Open Access Plus   Consumer-Driven Health Plan
PPO   High Deductible Health Plan

PLAN BENEFITS:
Alternative Medicine: [ ]   Behavioral Health: [X]
Chiropractic: [X]   Dental: [X]
Home Care: [X]   Inpatient SNF: [ ]
Long-Term Care: [ ]   Pharm. Mail Order: [X]
Physical Therapy: [ ]   Podiatry: [X]
Psychiatric: [X]   Transplant: [X]
Vision: [X]   Wellness: [X]
Workers' Comp: [ ]
Other Benefits:
Comments:
Enrollment statistics cover Tri-State area: Connecticut, New Jersey, New York.

COMMUNITY HEALTH NETWORK OF CONNECTICUT INC

11 Fairfield Blvd
Wallingford, CT 06492
Phone: 203-949-4000 Fax: 203-265-2970 Toll-Free: 800-859-9889
Web site: www.chnct.org
MAILING ADDRESS:
   COMMUNITY HEALTH NETWORK OF CT
   11 Fairfield Blvd
   Wallingford, CT 06492

KEY EXECUTIVES:
Chief Executive Officer/President .... Sylvia Kelly
Chief Financial, VP .... Anthony Bruno
Medical Director .... John Federico, MD
Chief Information Officer .... John Kaukas
Operations VP .... Mark Scapellati
MIS Director .... Stuart MacDonald
Compliance Officer .... Cory Ludington
Provider Relations Director .... Jack Huber
VP, Human Resources .... Jim Karl
VP, Health Services .... Lynn Childs
Quality Assurance Director .... Judith Greene
Director, Member Services .... Tressa Spears
Director, Finance .... Dina Blaney
Director, Claims .... LeAnn Olson
Director, Quality Improvement .... Roberta Geller, RN, Esq

COMPANY PROFILE:
Parent Company Name:
Doing Business As:
Year Founded: 1995   Federally Qualified: [Y]
Forprofit: [ ]   Not-For-Profit: [Y]
Model Type:
Accreditation: [ ] AAPPO [ ] JACHO [ ] NCQA [ ] URAC
Plan Type: HMO
Total Enrollment:
   2001: 0   2004: 55,749   2007: 0
   2002: 52,064   2005: 55,822
   2003: 53,000   2006:
SERVICE AREA:
Nationwide: N
   CT;
PRODUCTS OFFERED:
Product Name: Type:
Community Health Network of CT   Medicaid
Comments:
Gatekeeper.

CONNECTICARE INC

175 Scott Swamp Rd
Farmington, CT 06032
Phone: 860-674-5700 Fax: 860-674-2030 Toll-Free: 800-923-2822
Web site: www.connecticare.com
MAILING ADDRESS:
   CONNECTICARE INC
   175 Scott Swamp Rd
   Farmington, CT 06032

KEY EXECUTIVES:
Chairman .... Anthony L Watson
Chief Executive Officer/President .... Michael E Herbert
Senior VP & Chief Financial Officer .... Michael R Wise

CONNECTICUT — Managed Care Organization Profiles

SERVICE AREA:
Nationwide: N
   CT; NH; RI; MA; ME; VT;
TYPE OF COVERAGE:
Commercial: [Y] Individual: [Y] FEHBP: [ ] Indemnity: [ ]
Medicare: [Y] Medicaid: [ ] Supplemental Medicare: [ ]
Tricare   [ ]
PRODUCTS OFFERED:
Product Name:	Type:
Golden Medicare Plan	Medicare
Aetna HMO	HMO

CONSUMER-DRIVEN PRODUCTS
Aetna Life Insurance Co	HSA Company Aetna
HealthFund HSA	HSA Product
Aetna	HSA Administrator
Aetna HealthFund	Consumer-Driven Health Plan
PPO I; PPO II	High Deductible Health Plan

PLAN BENEFITS:
Alternative Medicine:	[ ]	Behavioral Health:	[X]
Chiropractic:	[X]	Dental:	[X]
Home Care:	[X]	Inpatient SNF:	[X]
Long-Term Care:	[X]	Pharm. Mail Order:	[X]
Physical Therapy:	[X]	Podiatry:	[X]
Psychiatric:	[X]	Transplant:	[X]
Vision:	[X]	Wellness:	[X]
Workers' Comp:	[X]		

Other Benefits:

ANTHEM HEALTH PLAN INC
DBA: ANTHEM BLUE CROSS BLUE SHIELD CT

370 Bassett Road
North Haven, CT 06473
Phone: 203-239-4911 Fax: 203-985-7918 Toll-Free:
Web site: www.80.anthem.com
MAILING ADDRESS:
   ANTHEM HEALTH PLAN INC
   370 Bassett Road
   North Haven, CT 06473

KEY EXECUTIVES:
Chief Executive Officer .... Marjorie W Dorr
Medical Director .... Russell J Munson, MD
Marketing Director .... Alex Ungerlieder
HIPAA Program Manager .... Katherine Grussi
Medical Director .... Russell J Munson, MD

COMPANY PROFILE:
Parent Company Name: WellPoint Inc
Doing Business As: Anthem Blue Cross Blue Shield of CT
Year Founded: 1936   Federally Qualified: [ ]
Forprofit: [ ]   Not-For-Profit: [Y]
Model Type: IPA
Accreditation: [ ] AAPPO [ ] JACHO [X] NCQA [ ] URAC
Plan Type: HMO, PPO, UR, POS, HSA, HDHP
Primary Physicians: 2,497   Physician Specialists: 4,864
Hospitals:
Total Enrollment:
   2001: 690,818   2004: 814,386   2007: 0
   2002: 763,342   2005: 543,739
   2003: 802,547   2006:
SERVICE AREA:
Nationwide: N
   CT;
TYPE OF COVERAGE:
Commercial: [Y] Individual: [Y] FEHBP: [ ] Indemnity: [ ]
Medicare: [ ] Medicaid: [Y] Supplemental Medicare: [Y]
Tricare   [ ]
PRODUCTS OFFERED:
Product Name:	Type:
Medicare Blue Connecticut	Medicare
Blue Care Direct	HMO
Blue Care	Medicaid
Century Preferred Direct	PPO

CONSUMER-DRIVEN PRODUCTS
JP Morgan Chase	HSA Company
Century Preferred Direct HSA	HSA Product
JP Morgan Chase	HSA Administrator
Blue Access Saver	Consumer-Driven Health Plan
Century Preferred Direct	High Deductible Health Plan

PLAN BENEFITS:
Alternative Medicine:	[ ]	Behavioral Health:	[ ]
Chiropractic:	[X]	Dental:	[X]
Home Care:	[X]	Inpatient SNF:	[X]
Long-Term Care:	[ ]	Pharm. Mail Order:	[X]
Physical Therapy:	[X]	Podiatry:	[X]
Psychiatric:	[X]	Transplant:	[X]
Vision:	[X]	Wellness:	[X]
Workers' Comp:	[X]		

Other Benefits: LIFE, AD&D

BERKLEY ADMINISTRATORS OF CONNECTICUT INC

195 Scott Swamp Rd
Farmington, CT 06032
Phone: 860-409-2300 Fax: 866-303-1398 Toll-Free: 800-611-8535
Web site: www.berkleyrisk.com
MAILING ADDRESS:
   BERKLEY ADMINISTRATORS CT INC
   PO Box 4012
   Farmington, CT 06032

KEY EXECUTIVES:
President .... Rick McKenna
Medical Director .... Peter Amato, MD
Credentialing Manager, Provider Services Director .... Gina Barresi
Network Development Director .... Gina Barresi

COMPANY PROFILE:
Parent Company Name: Berkley Care Network/W R Berkley Corp
Doing Business As:
Year Founded: 1993   Federally Qualified: [ ]
Forprofit: [Y]   Not-For-Profit: [ ]
Model Type:
Accreditation: [ ] AAPPO [ ] JACHO [ ] NCQA [ ] URAC
Plan Type: Specialty PPO, UR
SERVICE AREA:
Nationwide: N
   Northeast & Mid-Atlantic States;
TYPE OF COVERAGE:
Commercial: [Y] Individual: [ ] FEHBP: [ ] Indemnity: [ ]
Medicare: [ ] Medicaid: [ ] Supplemental Medicare: [ ]
Tricare   [ ]
PLAN BENEFITS:
Alternative Medicine:	[ ]	Behavioral Health:	[ ]
Chiropractic:	[ ]	Dental:	[ ]
Home Care:	[ ]	Inpatient SNF:	[ ]
Long-Term Care:	[ ]	Pharm. Mail Order:	[ ]
Physical Therapy:	[ ]	Podiatry:	[ ]
Psychiatric:	[ ]	Transplant:	[ ]
Vision:	[ ]	Wellness:	[ ]
Workers' Comp:	[X]		

Other Benefits:

CIGNA BEHAVIORAL HEALTH INC

900 Cottage Grove Rd
Hartford, CT 06152-2317
Phone: 800-873-7904 Fax: 952-996-2579 Toll-Free: 800-873-7904
Web site: www.cignabehavioral.com
MAILING ADDRESS:
   CIGNA BEHAVIORAL HEALTH INC
   900 Cottage Grove Rd
   Hartford, CT 06152-2317

KEY EXECUTIVES:
Chief Executive Officer/President .... Keith Dixon, PhD
Chief Financial Officer .... David Bourdon, MBA
Chief Medical Officer .... Doug Nemecek, MD
Chief Information Officer .... David Peterson, BS Finance
Senior VP, Operations .... Jodi Aronson Prohofsky, PhD
Marketing Director .... Nelia Infante
VP, Network Services .... Julie Vayer
Human Resoures Officer .... Heather Daniels
Medical Management Director .... Nancy Hedstrom

COMPANY PROFILE:
Parent Company Name: CIGNA Behavioral Health Inc, MN
Doing Business As:

Managed Care Organization Profiles   **CONNECTICUT**

AETNA INC - CONNECTICUT

20 Glover Ave 4th Fl
Norwalk, CT 06850
Phone: 800-722-7315 Fax: Toll-Free:
Web site: www.aetna.com

MAILING ADDRESS:
   AETNA INC - CONNECTICUT
   20 Glover Ave 4th Fl
   Norwalk, CT 06850

KEY EXECUTIVES:
Chairman of the Board/Chief Executive Officer .... Ronald A Williams
President .... Mark T Bertolini
Regional Manager-Northeast .... Mary Claire Bonner
Executive VP, Finance .... Joseph M Zubretsky
Human Resources Director ....Elease E Wright
Senior Network Manager/Provider Relations .... John Catalan

COMPANY PROFILE:
Parent Company Name: Aetna Inc
Doing Business As:
Year Founded: Federally Qualified: [ ]
Forprofit: [Y]   Not-For-Profit: [ ]
Model Type: MIXED
Accreditation: [ ] AAPPO [ ] JACHO [ ] NCQA [ ] URAC
Plan Type: HMO, PPO, POS, CDHP, HDHP, HSA,
Primary Physicians: 2,337   Physician Specialists: 5,423
Hospitals:
Total Enrollment:
   2001: 0   2004: 0   2007: 0
   2002: 0   2005: 43,389
   2003: 0   2006:

SERVICE AREA:
Nationwide: N
   NY (Westchester, Rockland, Orange, Putnam, Dutchess, Sullivan);

TYPE OF COVERAGE:
Commercial: [Y] Individual: [ ]   FEHBP: [ ]   Indemnity: [ ]
Medicare: [Y] Medicaid: [ ]   Supplemental Medicare: [ ]
Tricare   [ ]

CONSUMER-DRIVEN PRODUCTS
Aetna Life Insurance Co   HSA Company
Aetna HealthFund HSA   HSA Product
Aetna   HSA Administrator
Aetna HealthFund   Consumer-Driven Health Plan
PPO I; PPO II   High Deductible Health Plan

PLAN BENEFITS:
Alternative Medicine: [ ]   Behavioral Health: [ ]
Chiropractic: [X]   Dental: [X]
Home Care: [X]   Inpatient SNF: [ ]
Long-Term Care: [X]   Pharm. Mail Order: [ ]
Physical Therapy: [ ]   Podiatry: [X]
Psychiatric: [ ]   Transplant: [ ]
Vision: [X]   Wellness: [X]
Workers' Comp: [ ]
Other Benefits:

AETNA INC - CORPORATE HEADQUARTERS

151 Farmington Ave
Hartford, CT 06156-1000
Phone: 860-273-0123 Fax: 860-273-3971 Toll-Free: 800-225-2949
Web site: www.aetna.com

MAILING ADDRESS:
   AETNA INC - CORP HEADQUARTERS
   151 Farmington Ave
   Hartford, CT 06156-1000

KEY EXECUTIVES:
Chairman of the Board/Chief Executive Officer .... Ronald A Williams
President .... Mark T Bertolini
Executive VP, Finance .... Joseph M Zubretsky
Chief Medical Director .... Troyen A Brennan, MD
Head of Pharmacy .... Robyn S Walsh
Senior VP, Chief Information Officer .... Margaret McCarthy
Senior VP, Marketing Strategic/Communications .... Robert M Mead
VP of Public Relations .... Roy Clason Jr
Head of Human Resources .... Elease E Wright
Dental Director .... George Koumaras

COMPANY PROFILE:
Parent Company Name: Aetna Inc
Doing Business As:
Year Founded: Federally Qualified: [.]
Forprofit: [Y]   Not-For-Profit: [ ]
Model Type: IPA
Accreditation: [ ] AAPPO [ ] JACHO [ ] NCQA [ ] URAC
Plan Type: HMO, PPO, POS, CDHP, HSA, HDHP
Primary Physicians: 431,200   Physician Specialists:
Hospitals: 4,300
Total Revenue: 2005: 22,491,900,000   2006: 34,700,000,000
Net Income   2005: 1,573,300,000   2006: 1,701,700,000
Total Enrollment:
   2001: 42,639,000   2004: 47,500,000   2007: 41,526,000
   2002: 38,200,000   2005: 40,218,000
   2003: 44,600,000   2006: 39,900,000
Medical Loss Ratio: 2005:   2006: 80.20
Administrative Expense Ratio: 2005:   2006:

SERVICE AREA:
Nationwide: Y
   NW;

TYPE OF COVERAGE:
Commercial: [Y] Individual: [ ]   FEHBP: [ ]   Indemnity: [ ]
Medicare: [ ] Medicaid: [ ]   Supplemental Medicare: [ ]
Tricare   [ ]

PRODUCTS OFFERED:
Product Name: Type:
Aetna HMO   HMO
Aetna POS   POS
Aetna PPO   PPO
Aenta Indemnity   Indemnity
Medicare   HMO
Medicaid   HMO
Aetna Dental

CONSUMER-DRIVEN PRODUCTS
Aetna Life Insurance Co   HSA Company
Aetna HealthFund HSA   HSA Product
Aetna   HSA Administrator
Aetna HealthFund   Consumer-Driven Health Plan
PPO I; PPO II   High Deductible Health Plan

PLAN BENEFITS:
Alternative Medicine: [ ]   Behavioral Health: [ ]
Chiropractic: [X]   Dental: [X]
Home Care: [X]   Inpatient SNF: [X]
Long-Term Care: [X]   Pharm. Mail Order: [X]
Physical Therapy: [X]   Podiatry: [X]
Psychiatric: [X]   Transplant: [X]
Vision: [X]   Wellness: [X]
Workers' Comp: [X]
Other Benefits:

AETNA INC OF NEW ENGLAND

1000 Middle St
Middletown, CT 06457-3342
Phone: 860-273-0123 Fax: 860-273-6872 Toll-Free:
Web site: www.aetna.com

MAILING ADDRESS:
   AETNA INC OF NEW ENGLAND
   1000 Middle St
   Middletown, CT 06457-3342

KEY EXECUTIVES:
Chairman of the Board/Chief Executive Officer .... Ronald A Williams
Regional President .... Charles Peck, MD
Principal Financial Officer .... Emanuel F Germano
VP of Public Relations .... Roy Clason, Jr
Dental Director .... George Koumaras

COMPANY PROFILE:
Parent Company Name: Aetna Inc
Doing Business As:
Year Founded: 1987   Federally Qualified: [N]
Forprofit: [Y]   Not-For-Profit: [ ]
Model Type: IPA
Accreditation: [ ] AAPPO [ ] JACHO [ ] NCQA [ ] URAC
Plan Type: HMO, PPO, POS, CDHP, HSA, HDHP
Total Enrollment:
   2001: 144,791   2004: 0   2007: 0
   2002: 156,016   2005:
   2003: 0   2006:

COLORADO

Managed Care Organization Profiles

MAILING ADDRESS:
UNITEDHEALTHCARE OF COLORADO
6465 S Greenwood Plz Blvd #300
Centennial, CO 80111

KEY EXECUTIVES:
Non-Executive Chairman .... Richard T Burke
Chief Executive Officer/President .... Elizabeth K Soberg
VP, Finance .... Donald A Powers
Medical Director .... Jacqueline E Stiff, MD
Chief Operating Officer .... Jeri Jones
Senior VP, Sales .... Tom Elliot
VP, Small Group Sales .... Jim Berman

COMPANY PROFILE:
Parent Company Name: UnitedHealth Group
Doing Business As: UnitedHealthcare of CO
Year Founded: 1986 Federally Qualified: [N]
Forprofit: [Y] Not-For-Profit: [ ]
Model Type: MIXED
Accreditation: [ ] AAPPO [ ] JACHO [X] NCQA [X] URAC
Plan Type: HMO, PPO, ASO, EPO, POS, UR, CDHP, HSA, HDHP, HRA
Total Revenue: 2005:   2006:   19,896,796
Net Income   2005:   2006:   391,713
Total Enrollment:
  2001: 0   2004: 28,826   2007: 4,564
  2002: 93,543   2005: 16,851
  2003: 54,838   2006: 6,948

SERVICE AREA:
Nationwide: N
  CO;

TYPE OF COVERAGE:
Commercial: [Y] Individual: [ ] FEHBP: [ ] Indemnity: [ ]
Medicare: [ ] Medicaid: [ ] Supplemental Medicare: [ ]
Tricare   [ ]

PRODUCTS OFFERED:
Product Name:	Type:
Managed Indemnity	
HMO	Gatekeeper and Open
United Hlthcare	Medicaid
Point of Service	
CHP+	
Medicare Complete	Medicare

CONSUMER-DRIVEN PRODUCTS
Exante Bank/Golden Rule Ins Co	HSA Company
iPlan HSA	HSA Product
	HSA Administrator
	Consumer-Driven Health Plan
	High Deductible Health Plan

PLAN BENEFITS:
Alternative Medicine: [ ]   Behavioral Health: [X]
Chiropractic: [X]   Dental: [X]
Home Care: [X]   Inpatient SNF: [X]
Long-Term Care: [ ]   Pharm. Mail Order: [X]
Physical Therapy: [X]   Podiatry: [X]
Psychiatric: [X]   Transplant: [X]
Vision: [X]   Wellness: [X]
Workers' Comp: [X]
Other Benefits:

VISION SERVICE PLAN

1050 17th St Ste 1885
Denver, CO 80265
Phone: 303-892-7663 Fax: 303-892-7768 Toll-Free:
Web site: www.vsp.com

MAILING ADDRESS:
VISION SERVICE PLAN
1050 17th St Ste 1885
Denver, CO 80265

KEY EXECUTIVES:
Chairman .... Dan L Mannen, OD
Chief Executive Officer .... Robert Lynch
Regional Manager .... Tom Swartzbaugh
Chief Financial Officer .... Patricia Cochran
Senior VP of Operations .... Gary Brooks
VP of Marketing .... Kate Renwick-Espinosa
VP of Sales .... Richard W Steere
VP of Information Systems .... Steve Scott
VP of Provider Relations .... Don Price
VP of Human Resources .... Elaine Leuchars
Account Executive .... Jennifer Nobles

COMPANY PROFILE:
Parent Company Name: Vision Service Plan, CA
Doing Business As:
Year Founded: 1970 Federally Qualified: [ ]
Forprofit: [ ] Not-For-Profit: [Y]
Model Type:
Accreditation: [ ] AAPPO [ ] JACHO [ ] NCQA [ ] URAC
Plan Type: Specialty PPO

SERVICE AREA:
Nationwide: N
  CO;

TYPE OF COVERAGE:
Commercial: [Y] Individual: [ ] FEHBP: [ ] Indemnity: [ ]
Medicare: [ ] Medicaid: [ ] Supplemental Medicare: [ ]
Tricare   [ ]

PLAN BENEFITS:
Alternative Medicine: [ ]   Behavioral Health: [ ]
Chiropractic: [ ]   Dental: [ ]
Home Care: [ ]   Inpatient SNF: [ ]
Long-Term Care: [ ]   Pharm. Mail Order: [ ]
Physical Therapy: [ ]   Podiatry: [ ]
Psychiatric: [ ]   Transplant: [ ]
Vision: [X]   Wellness: [ ]
Workers' Comp: [ ]
Other Benefits:

Managed Care Organization Profiles — COLORADO

MAILING ADDRESS:
ROCKY MOUNTAIN HEALTHCARE OPTIONS
PO Box 10600
Grand Junction, CO 81506

KEY EXECUTIVES:
Chief Executive Officer/President .... John P Hopkins, RPh
Chief Financial Officer .... Patrick Duncan
Chief Medical Director .... David S Herr, MD, FAAP
Chief Operating Officer .... Laurel Walters
Human Resources Director .... Jan Rohr

COMPANY PROFILE:
Parent Company Name: Rocky Mountain Health Plans
Doing Business As: HealthCare Options Inc
Year Founded: 1974   Federally Qualified: [N]
Forprofit: [ ]   Not-For-Profit: [Y]
Model Type:
Accreditation: [ ] AAPPO [ ] JACHO [ ] NCQA [ ] URAC
Plan Type: PPO
Total Revenue: 2005: 99,083,897   2006: 57,955,462
Net Income   2005: 1,795,207   2006: 498,264
Total Enrollment:
  2001: 0   2004: 0   2007: 38,236
  2002: 0   2005: 536,909
  2003: 0   2006: 556,300

SERVICE AREA:
Nationwide: N
  CO;

ROCKY MOUNTAIN HOSITAL & MEDICAL SERVICES INC

700 Broadway 7th Fl
Denver, CO 80273
Phone: 303-831-2000 Fax: 303-764-7160 Toll-Free:
Web site: www.anthem.com

MAILING ADDRESS:
ROCKY MTN HOSP & MED SRVS INC
700 Broadway 7th Fl
Denver, CO 80273

KEY EXECUTIVES:
Chairman of the Board .... Larry C Glasscock
Chief Executive Officer .... Angela F Braly
President .... John Martie
Chief Medical Officer .... Lisa Latts, MD
Pharmacy Director .... Jim Thorne
Chief Information Officer .... Brent Brown
Chief Operating Officer .... Donna Boeing
HIPAA Program Manager .... Anthony Carlson
VP of Healthcare Management .... Robert London, MD

COMPANY PROFILE:
Parent Company Name: Anthem Inc
Doing Business As:
Year Founded: 1978   Federally Qualified: [Y]
Forprofit: [ ]   Not-For-Profit: [Y]
Model Type:
Accreditation: [ ] AAPPO [ ] JACHO [ ] NCQA [ ] URAC
Plan Type: HMO, PPO, POS, PRO, ASO, UR CDHP, HDHP, HSA
Total Revenue: 2005:   2006: 558,692,429
Net Income   2005:   2006: 50,423,667
Total Enrollment:
  2001: 0   2004: 0   2007: 604,484
  2002: 0   2005:
  2003: 0   2006: 603,353

SERVICE AREA:
Nationwide:
  CO;

TYPE OF COVERAGE:
Commercial: [Y] Individual: [Y] FEHBP: [ ] Indemnity: [ ]
Medicare: [Y] Medicaid: [Y] Supplemental Medicare: [Y]
Tricare   [ ]

CONSUMER-DRIVEN PRODUCTS
JP Morgan Chase   HSA Company
Anthem ByDesign HSA   HSA Product
Lumenos   HSA Administrator
Blue Access Saver   Consumer-Driven Health Plan
Blue Access Economy Plan PPO High Deductible Health Plan

PLAN BENEFITS:
Alternative Medicine: [ ]   Behavioral Health: [X]
Chiropractic: [X]   Dental: [X]
Home Care: [X]   Inpatient SNF: [X]
Long-Term Care: [ ]   Pharm. Mail Order: [X]
Physical Therapy: [X]   Podiatry: [X]
Psychiatric: [X]   Transplant: [X]
Vision: [X]   Wellness: [X]
Workers' Comp: [X]
Other Benefits:

SLOAN'S LAKE PREFERRED HEALTH NETWORKS

6501 S Fiddlers Green Cir #300
Greenwood Village, CO 80111
Phone: 303-691-2200 Fax: 303-504-5321 Toll-Free: 800-457-2345
Web site: www.sloanslake.com

MAILING ADDRESS:
SLOAN'S LAKE PREFERRED HLTH NT
PO Box 241323
Denver, CO 80111

KEY EXECUTIVES:
Chairman of the Board .... Blair Tikker
Chief Executive Officer .... Rick Hale
VP, Finance .... Shelly Justice
Chief Medical Officer .... Larry Wolk, MD
VP, Chief Information Officer .... Al Armijo
VP, Marketing .... Jackie Driscoll
Director of Provider Services .... Bonita Burris
Assistant VP of Human Resources .... Rich Hegstad
VP, Utilization Management .... Barbara Mulcahy
VP, Provider Contracts & Services .... Dean Grohskopf

COMPANY PROFILE:
Parent Company Name: HMS Colorado
Doing Business As: Sloans Lake Preferred Health Networks
Year Founded: 1978   Federally Qualified: [N]
Forprofit: [Y]   Not-For-Profit: [ ]
Model Type: GROUP
Accreditation: [ ] AAPPO [ ] JACHO [ ] NCQA [X] URAC
Plan Type: PPO, UR, CDHP
Total Enrollment:
  2001: 0   2004: 500,000   2007: 0
  2002: 0   2005:
  2003: 375,000 2006:

SERVICE AREA:
Nationwide: N
  CO;

TYPE OF COVERAGE:
Commercial: [Y] Individual: [ ] FEHBP: [ ] Indemnity: [ ]
Medicare: [ ] Medicaid: [ ] Supplemental Medicare: [ ]
Tricare   [ ]

PRODUCTS OFFERED:
Product Name: Type:
Freedom Series HMO   HMO
Schooner Plan   HMO
Yacht Plan   HMO
Centura Employee   HMO
POS Plan Option   POS
Sloans Preferred Provider

PLAN BENEFITS:
Alternative Medicine: [X]   Behavioral Health: [X]
Chiropractic: [X]   Dental: [ ]
Home Care: [X]   Inpatient SNF: [X]
Long-Term Care: [ ]   Pharm. Mail Order: [ ]
Physical Therapy: [X]   Podiatry: [X]
Psychiatric: [X]   Transplant: [X]
Vision: [X]   Wellness: [X]
Workers' Comp: [ ]
Other Benefits: Disease Management E

UNITEDHEALTHCARE OF COLORADO

6465 S Greenwood Plz Blvd #300
Centennial, CO 80111
Phone: 303-267-3300 Fax: 303-267-3599 Toll-Free: 800-518-3344
Web site: www.uhc.com

COLORADO
Managed Care Organization Profiles

SERVICE AREA:
Nationwide: N
  CO;

PACIFICARE OF COLORADO/UNITED HEALTHCARE

6455 S Yosemite St
Greenwood Village, CO 80111
Phone: 303-220-5800 Fax: 303-714-3998 Toll-Free: 800-877-6685
Web site: www.pacificare.com
MAILING ADDRESS:
  PACIFICARE OF COLORADO/UHC
  6455 S Yosemite St
  Greenwood Village, CO 80111

KEY EXECUTIVES:
Chief Executive Officer/President .... *Elizabeth K Soberg*
VP, Finance .... *Donald A Powers*
VP of Health Services .... *John Rush, MD*
Pharmacy Director .... *Cliff Hardesty*
VP, Network Development .... *Scott Keim*
Quality Assurance Director .... *Colleen Campbell*
Director of New Products Development .... *Paul Jackson*

COMPANY PROFILE:
Parent Company Name: UnitedHealth Group
Doing Business As:
Year Founded: 1974   Federally Qualified: [Y]
Forprofit: [Y]   Not-For-Profit: [ ]
Model Type: MIXED
Accreditation: [ ] AAPPO [ ] JACHO [X] NCQA [ ] URAC
Plan Type: HMO, PPO, Specialty HMO, Specialty PPO, POS, TPA, HDHP, HSA
Total Revenue: 2005:   2006:   510,957,617
Net Income   2005:   2006:   19,161,457
Total Enrollment:
  2001: 262,600   2004: 330,000   2007: 132,641
  2002: 229,948   2005: 190,690
  2003: 226,319   2006: 165,965
SERVICE AREA:
Nationwide: N
  CO; (Adams, Arapahoe, Bent, Boulder, Cheyenne, Clear, Creek, Crowley, Denver, Douglas, Elbert);
TYPE OF COVERAGE:
Commercial: [Y] Individual: [Y] FEHBP: [ ] Indemnity: [ ]
Medicare: [Y] Medicaid: [ ] Supplemental Medicare: [Y]
Tricare   [ ]
PRODUCTS OFFERED:
Product Name:	Type:
Secure Horizons	Medicare Advantage
Pacificare HMO	HMO
Pacificare Dental of CO	Specialty HMO Dental
Pacificare POS	POS
	High Deductible Health Plan

PLAN BENEFITS:
Alternative Medicine: [ ]   Behavioral Health: [X]
Chiropractic: [X]   Dental: [X]
Home Care: [X]   Inpatient SNF: [X]
Long-Term Care: [X]   Pharm. Mail Order: [X]
Physical Therapy: [X]   Podiatry: [X]
Psychiatric: [X]   Transplant: [X]
Vision: [X]   Wellness: [X]
Workers' Comp: [X]
Other Benefits:
Comments:
Formerly Comprecare. Antero Health Plans merged into PacifiCare of Colorado.

PUEBLO HEALTH CARE

400 W 16th St
Pueblo, CO 81003
Phone: 719-584-4806 Fax: 719-584-4038 Toll-Free:
Web site: www.pueblohealthcare.com
MAILING ADDRESS:
  PUEBLO HEALTH CARE
  400 W 16th St
  Pueblo, CO 81003

KEY EXECUTIVES:
Executive Director .... *Ryan Lown*
Provider Relations Manager .... *Ann Bellah*
Administrative Assistant .... *Rose Jubert*

COMPANY PROFILE:
Parent Company Name:
Doing Business As:
Year Founded: Federally Qualified: [ ]
Forprofit: [ ]   Not-For-Profit: [ ]
Model Type:
Accreditation: [ ] AAPPO [ ] JACHO [ ] NCQA [ ] URAC
Plan Type: PPO
SERVICE AREA:
Nationwide: N
  CO;

ROCKY MOUNTAIN HEALTH PLANS

2775 Crossroads Blvd
Grand Junction, CO 81506
Phone: 970-244-7760 Fax: 970-244-7880 Toll-Free: 800-843-0719
Web site: www.rmhp.org
MAILING ADDRESS:
  ROCKY MOUNTAIN HEALTH PLANS
  PO Box 10600
  Grand Junction, CO 81506

KEY EXECUTIVES:
Chief Executive Officer/President .... *John P Hopkins, RPh*
Chief Financial Officer .... *Patrick Duncan*
Chief Medical Director .... *David S Herr, MD, FAAP*
Chief Operating Officer .... *Laurel Walters*
Marketing Director .... *Jerry Hayes*
IT Director .... *Gwen Costello*
Communications Manager .... *Deborah Dawes*
Provider Relations Director .... *Dorien Rawlinson*
Human Resources Director .... *Jan Rohr*
Director of Medical Direction .... *David S Herr, MD, FAAP*
Director of Medical Quality .... *Lori Stephenson RN*

COMPANY PROFILE:
Parent Company Name:
Doing Business As: Rocky Mountain HMO Inc
Year Founded: 1974   Federally Qualified: [Y]
Forprofit: [ ]   Not-For-Profit: [Y]
Model Type: IPA
Accreditation: [ ] AAPPO [ ] JACHO [X] NCQA [ ] URAC
Plan Type: HMO, POS
Total Revenue: 2005: 206,838,867   2006: 107,887,448
Net Income   2005: 10,154,390   2006:   4,116,263
Total Enrollment:
  2001: 27,016   2004: 21,018   2007: 175,905
  2002: 122,956   2005: 87,316
  2003: 112,000   2006: 83,117
SERVICE AREA:
Nationwide: N
  CO;
TYPE OF COVERAGE:
Commercial: [Y] Individual: [Y] FEHBP: [ ] Indemnity: [ ]
Medicare: [Y] Medicaid: [Y] Supplemental Medicare: [ ]
Tricare   [ ]
PRODUCTS OFFERED:
Product Name:	Type:
Rocky Mountain Care	Medicaid
Rocky Mountain HMO	HMO
Rocky Mountain Medicare	Medicare
RMHMO Medicare	Medicare Advantage

Comments:
Formerly Rocky Mountain HMO.

ROCKY MOUNTAIN HEALTHCARE OPTIONS INC
DBA: HEALTHCARE OPTIONS

2775 Crossroads Blvd
Grand Junction, CO 81506
Phone: 970-244-7760 Fax: 970-244-7880 Toll-Free: 800-843-0719
Web site: www.rmhp.org

Managed Care Organization Profiles **COLORADO**

CONSUMER-DRIVEN PRODUCTS
JP Morgan Chase   HSA Company
HumanaOne HSA   HSA Product
JP Morgan Chase   HSA Administrator
Personal Care Account   Consumer-Driven Health Plan
HumanaOne   High Deductible Health Plan
PLAN BENEFITS:
Alternative Medicine: [ ]   Behavioral Health: [X]
Chiropractic: [X]   Dental: [X]
Home Care: [ ]   Inpatient SNF: [ ]
Long-Term Care: [ ]   Pharm. Mail Order: [X]
Physical Therapy: [ ]   Podiatry: [ ]
Psychiatric: [X]   Transplant: [X]
Vision: [ ]   Wellness: [ ]
Workers' Comp: [X]
Other Benefits: Long Term Disability

KAISER FOUNDATION HEALTH PLAN OF COLORADO

10350 E Dakota Ave
Denver, CO 80231
Phone: 303-338-3800 Fax: 303-344-7956 Toll-Free: 800-632-9700
Web site: www.kaiserpermanente.org
MAILING ADDRESS:
   KAISER FNDTN HLTH PLAN OF CO
   10350 E Dakota Ave
   Denver, CO 80231

KEY EXECUTIVES:
Chairman/Chief Executive Officer .... George C Halvorson
Regional President .... Donna Lynne
Executive VP,Chief Financial Officer .... Rick Newsome
Executive Medical Director .... John H Cochran, Jr, MD
VP, Marketing, Sales & Bus Development .... Leo Tokar
VP, Marketing, Sales & Bus Development .... Wade Overgaard
VP, Human Resources .... Robin Sadler
VP, Quality & Public Affairs .... Kristin Snyder

COMPANY PROFILE:
Parent Company Name: Kaiser Permanente
Doing Business As:
Year Founded: 1971   Federally Qualified: [Y]
Forprofit: [ ]   Not-For-Profit: [Y]
Model Type: GROUP
Accreditation: [ ] AAPPO [ ] JACHO [ ] NCQA [ ] URAC
Plan Type: HMO, HSA, HDHP
Total Revenue: 2005:   2006: 899,305,904
Net Income   2005:   2006: 24,388,606
Total Enrollment:
   2001: 371,752   2004: 420,774   2007: 480,734
   2002: 402,043   2005: 453,245
   2003: 409,141   2006: 475,913
SERVICE AREA:
Nationwide: N
   CO (Boulder,Colorado Springs area, Denver, Langmont);
TYPE OF COVERAGE:
Commercial: [ ] Individual: [Y] FEHBP: [ ] Indemnity: [ ]
Medicare: [Y] Medicaid: [Y] Supplemental Medicare: [Y]
Tricare   [ ]
PRODUCTS OFFERED:
Product Name: Type:
KP Senior Advantage   Medicare Advantage
Kaiser HMO   HMO
Senior Advantage Silver   Medicare Advantage
Kaiser POS   POS
PLAN BENEFITS:
Alternative Medicine: [ ]   Behavioral Health: [ ]
Chiropractic: [ ]   Dental: [ ]
Home Care: [ ]   Inpatient SNF: [ ]
Long-Term Care: [ ]   Pharm. Mail Order: [X]
Physical Therapy: [ ]   Podiatry: [ ]
Psychiatric: [ ]   Transplant: [ ]
Vision: [X]   Wellness: [ ]
Workers' Comp: [ ]
Other Benefits:

MOUNTAIN MEDICAL AFFILIATES

5889 S Greenwood Plz Blvd #200
Greenwood Village, CO 80111
Phone: 303-290-9696 Fax: Toll-Free: 800-647-1856
Web site: www.mma.bp.com
MAILING ADDRESS:
   MOUNTAIN MEDICAL AFFILIATES
   5889 S Greenwood Plz Blvd #200
   Greenwood Village, CO 80111

KEY EXECUTIVES:
President/Director .... Doug Wilson
VP of Finance .... Mark O'Neill
VP Operations & IT .... Chris Crowley
VP Sales & Marketing .... Leigh Hull
VP Provider Contracts & Services .... Dean Grohskopf
Senior Project Manager .... Allita Parlette

COMPANY PROFILE:
Parent Company Name: HMS Colorado Inc
Doing Business As:
Year Founded: 1980   Federally Qualified: [ ]
Forprofit: [Y]   Not-For-Profit: [ ]
Model Type:
Accreditation: [ ] AAPPO [ ] JACHO [ ] NCQA [ ] URAC
Plan Type: PPO
Primary Physicians: Physician Specialists:
Hospitals: 78
SERVICE AREA:
Nationwide: N
   CO;
TYPE OF COVERAGE:
Commercial: [Y] Individual: [ ] FEHBP: [ ] Indemnity: [ ]
Medicare: [ ] Medicaid: [ ] Supplemental Medicare: [ ]
Tricare   [ ]
PRODUCTS OFFERED:
Product Name: Type:
Value Added Delivery System
Community Based Health Plan
PLAN BENEFITS:
Alternative Medicine: [ ]   Behavioral Health: [ ]
Chiropractic: [X]   Dental: [ ]
Home Care: [X]   Inpatient SNF: [X]
Long-Term Care: [X]   Pharm. Mail Order: [ ]
Physical Therapy: [X]   Podiatry: [X]
Psychiatric: [X]   Transplant: [X]
Vision: [X]   Wellness: [X]
Workers' Comp: [X]
Other Benefits:

NDC-WEST INC DBA NADENT

333 W Drake Rd Ste 21
Fort Collins, CO 80526
Phone: 800-367-7390 Fax: 970-226-0249 Toll-Free:
Web site: www.nadent.com
MAILING ADDRESS:
   NDC-WEST INC DBA NADENT
   PO Box 270430
   Fort Collins, CO 80526

KEY EXECUTIVES:
Chief Executive Officer .... Joseph C Tomlinson, DMD
Director of Operations .... Aurora Delatorre
Marketing Director .... David Silberstein
Corporate Communications .... Nina Silberstein

COMPANY PROFILE:
Parent Company Name:
Doing Business As:
Year Founded: Federally Qualified: [ ]
Forprofit: [ ]   Not-For-Profit: [ ]
Model Type:
Accreditation: [ ] AAPPO [ ] JACHO [ ] NCQA [ ] URAC
Plan Type: UR
Primary Physicians: 600   Physician Specialists:
Hospitals:

COLORADO | Managed Care Organization Profiles

GREAT-WEST HEALTHCARE OF COLORADO

8515 East Orchard Rd
Greenwood Village, CO 80111
Phone: 303-737-3000   Fax: 303-737-3198 Toll-Free:
Web site: www.greatwesthealthcare.com
MAILING ADDRESS:
    GREAT-WEST HEALTHCARE OF CO
    8515 East Orchard Rd
    Greenwood Village, CO 80111

KEY EXECUTIVES:
Chief Executive Officer .... Raymond L McFeetors
Presidnet .... Mark J Carley
Chief Financial Officer .... Mitchell Graye
VP, West Region Medical Director .... Pierre M Malek, MD
Chief Information Officer .... Mark A Marusin

COMPANY PROFILE:
Parent Company Name: CIGNA Inc
Doing Business As: Great-West Healthcare
Year Founded: 1990   Federally Qualified: [ ]
Forprofit: [Y]   Not-For-Profit: [ ]
Model Type: NETWORK
Accreditation: [ ] AAPPO [ ] JACHO [ ] NCQA [X] URAC
Plan Type: HMO, PPO, POS, CDHP, HDHP, HSA
Total Revenue: 2005:   7,452,292   2006:   2,777,282
Net Income   2005:   855,465   2006:   186,529
Total Enrollment:
   2001:   47,336   2004:   0   2007: 5,191
   2002:   31,572   2005:   7,140
   2003:   16,063   2006:   5,504
Medical Loss Ratio: 2005:   79.10   2006:
Administrative Expense Ratio: 2005:   2006:
SERVICE AREA:
Nationwide: N
   CO;
TYPE OF COVERAGE:
Commercial: [Y] Individual: [ ]   FEHBP: [ ]   Indemnity: [ ]
Medicare: [ ] Medicaid: [ ]   Supplemental Medicare: [ ]
Tricare   [ ]
PRODUCTS OFFERED:
Product Name: Type:
One Health Plan HMO   HMO
Great West/New England PPO
Great West/New England POS
Great West Indemnity
CONSUMER-DRIVEN PRODUCTS
Mellon HR Solutions LLC   HSA Company
                                    HSA Product
                                    HSA Administrator
                                    Consumer-Driven Health Plan
                                    High Deductible Health Plan
PLAN BENEFITS:
Alternative Medicine: [X]   Behavioral Health: [X]
Chiropractic: [X]   Dental: [X]
Home Care: [X]   Inpatient SNF: [X]
Long-Term Care: [ ]   Pharm. Mail Order: [X]
Physical Therapy: [X]   Podiatry: [X]
Psychiatric: [X]   Transplant: [X]
Vision: [X]   Wellness: [X]
Workers' Comp: [ ]
Other Benefits:
Comments:
Great-West Healthcare purchased New England Financial, CO in 2003. Acquired by CIGNA Inc April 1, 2008.

HMS COLORADO INC

6501 S Fiddlers Green Cir #300
Greenwood Village, CO 80111
Phone: 303-504-5701 Fax: 303-504-5321 Toll-Free: 800-457-2345
Web site: www.sloanslake.com
MAILING ADDRESS:
    HMS COLORADO INC
    6501 S Fiddlers Green Cir #300
    Greenwood Hills, CO 80111

KEY EXECUTIVES:
Chairman of the Board .... Blair Tikker
Chief Executive Officer... Rick Hale
VP, Finance .... Shelly Justice
Chief Medical Officer .... Larry Wolk, MD
VP, Chief Operating Officer .... Al Armijo
VP, Marketing .... Jackie Driscoll
Director of Provider Services .... Bonita Burris
Asst VP of Human Resources .... Rich Hegstad
VP, Utilization Management .... Barbara Mulcahy
VP, Provider Contracts & Services .... Dean Grohskopf

COMPANY PROFILE:
Parent Company Name:
Doing Business As: Sloans Lake Preferred Health Network
Year Founded: 1978   Federally Qualified: [N]
Forprofit: [Y]   Not-For-Profit: [ ]
Model Type: NETWORK
Accreditation: [ ] AAPPO [ ] JACHO [ ] NCQA [ ] URAC
Plan Type: PPO, UR
Total Enrollment:
   2001:   0   2004:   0   2007: 0
   2002:   0   2005:   500,000
   2003:   0   2006:
SERVICE AREA:
Nationwide:
   CO;
TYPE OF COVERAGE:
Commercial: [Y] Individual: [ ]   FEHBP: [ ]   Indemnity: [ ]
Medicare: [ ] Medicaid: [ ]   Supplemental Medicare: [ ]
Tricare   [ ]

HUMANA INC - COLORADO

8400 E Prentice Ave Ste 1400
Englewood, CO 80111
Phone: 303-694-1044 Fax: 303-694-1105 Toll-Free: 800-825-7496
Web site: www.humana.com
MAILING ADDRESS:
    HUMANA INC - COLORADO
    PO Box 740036
    Louisville, KY 80111

KEY EXECUTIVES:
Chairman of the Board .... David A Jones Jr
Chief Executive Officer/President .... Michael B McCallister
VP, Colorado .... Leslie H Andrews
Chief Financial Officer .... James H Bloem
Chief Clinical Strategy .... Jonathan T Lord, MD
Senior VP Chief Information Officer .... Bruce J Goodman
Chief Operating Officer .... Jim Murray
Chief Marketing Officer .... Steve Moya
Manager of Sales Administration .... Ellen Tawson
Vice President of Provider Contracting .... Rich Powers
Senior VP Human Resources .... Bonnie C Hathcock
New Product Development Director .... Tom Liston
Senior VP & General Counsel .... Art Hipwell
Senior VP, Corporate Communications .... Tom Noland

COMPANY PROFILE:
Parent Company Name: Humana Inc
Doing Business As:
Year Founded: 1987   Federally Qualified: [Y]
Forprofit: [Y]   Not-For-Profit: [ ]
Model Type:
Accreditation: [ ] AAPPO [ ] JACHO [ ] NCQA [ ] URAC
Plan Type: PPO, Specialty HMO, CDHP, HDHP, HSA
Total Enrollment:
   2001:   0   2004:   40,960   2007: 40,960
   2002:   52,239   2005:
   2003:   41,500   2006:   1,359
SERVICE AREA:
Nationwide: N
   CO;
TYPE OF COVERAGE:
Commercial: [Y] Individual: [Y]   FEHBP: [ ]   Indemnity: [ ]
Medicare: [ ] Medicaid: [ ]   Supplemental Medicare: [ ]
Tricare   [ ]

Managed Care Organization Profiles   COLORADO

EXEMPLA HEALTHCARE LLC

2420 W 26th Ave Ste 100-D
Denver, CO 80211
Phone: 303-813-5000 Fax: 303-813-5001 Toll-Free:
Web site: www.exempla.org
MAILING ADDRESS:
   EXEMPLA HEALTHCARE LLC
   2420 W 26th Ave Ste 100-D
   Denver, CO 80211

KEY EXECUTIVES:
Chairman of the Board .... Thomas Grimshaw
Chief Executive Officer/President .... Jeffrey D Selberg
Chief Financial Officer .... Ned Borgstrom Jr
Chief Medical Info Officer .... Robert W Beardall, MD
Chief Information Officer .... David Pecoraro
VP Communications & Marketing .... Kay Taylor
Public Relations Manager .... Pat Barker
Network Development Director .... Debbie Welle-Powell, CMPE
VP Human Resources Director .... Edward Freysinger
Quality Assurance Director .... Kristen Burkett

COMPANY PROFILE:
Parent Company Name: Lutheran Medical Ctr/Sisters of Charity
Doing Business As:
Year Founded: 1997   Federally Qualified: [ ]
Forprofit: [ ]   Not-For-Profit: [Y]
Model Type:
Accreditation: [ ] AAPPO [ ] JACHO [ ] NCQA [ ] URAC
Plan Type: PPO
SERVICE AREA:
Nationwide: N
   CO (Adams, Arapahoe, Boulder, Denver, Douglas, Jefferson);
TYPE OF COVERAGE:
Commercial: [Y] Individual: [ ] FEHBP: [ ] Indemnity: [ ]
Medicare: [ ] Medicaid: [ ] Supplemental Medicare: [ ]
Tricare   [ ]

GREAT WEST LIFE ANNUITY INSURANCE CO

8515 East Orchard Rd Tower 1
Greenwood Village, CO 80111
Phone: 303-737-3000 Fax: 303-737-3198 Toll-Free:
Web site: www.greatwesthealthcare.com
MAILING ADDRESS:
   GREAT-WEST LIFE ANNUITY INS CO
   PO Box 1700
   Denver, CO 80111

KEY EXECUTIVES:
Chairman of the Board .... Robert Gratton
Chief Executive Officer/President .... Raymond L McFeetors
Executive VP,Chief Financial Officer .... Mitchell T G Graye
Senior VP,Chief Medical Officer .... Terry L Fouts, MD
Senior VP,Chief Information Officer .... John R Gabbert
VP, Human Resources .... George C Bogdewiecz
Senior VP, Controller .... Glen R Derback

COMPANY PROFILE:
Parent Company Name: CIGNA Inc
Doing Business As:
Year Founded: 1986   Federally Qualified: [ ]
Forprofit: [Y]   Not-For-Profit: [ ]
Model Type:
Accreditation: [ ] AAPPO [ ] JACHO [ ] NCQA [X] URAC
Plan Type: HMO, PPO, POS, ASO, PBM, CDHP, HDHP, HSA
Total Revenue: 2005:2,402,069,000   2006: 2,402,069,000
Net Income   2005: 132,313,000   2006:
Total Enrollment:
   2001: 2,600,000   2004: 1,948,000   2007: 0
   2002: 0   2005: 1,965,000
   2003: 0   2006: 2,000,000
SERVICE AREA:
Nationwide: Y
   NW;
TYPE OF COVERAGE:
Commercial: [Y] Individual: [ ] FEHBP: [ ] Indemnity: [ ]
Medicare: [ ] Medicaid: [ ] Supplemental Medicare: [ ]
Tricare   [ ]
PRODUCTS OFFERED:
Product Name: Type:
Great West PPO   PPO
One Health Plan   HMO

CONSUMER-DRIVEN PRODUCTS
Mellon HR Solutions LLC   HSA Company
                                       HSA Product
                                       HSA Administrator
                                       Consumer-Driven Health Plan
                                       High Deductible Health Plan
PLAN BENEFITS:
Alternative Medicine: [X]   Behavioral Health: [X]
Chiropractic: [X]   Dental: [X]
Home Care: [X]   Inpatient SNF: [X]
Long-Term Care: [ ]   Pharm. Mail Order: [X]
Physicial Therapy: [X]   Podiatry: [X]
Psychiatric: [X]   Transplant: [X]
Vision: [X]   Wellness: [X]
Workers' Comp: [ ]
Other Benefits:
Comments:
Acquired by CIGNA Inc April 1, 2008.

GREAT-WEST HEALTHCARE - CORPORATE

8515 E Orchard Rd
Greenwood Village, CO 80111
Phone: 303-737-3000 Fax: 303-737-3146 Toll-Free: 800-537-2033
Web site: www.greatwesthealthcare.com
MAILING ADDRESS:
   GREAT-WEST HEALTHCARE - CORP
   PO Box 1700
   Denver, CO 80111

KEY EXECUTIVES:
Chief Executive Officer/President .... Raymond L McFeetors
Senior VP, Finance .... Martin Rosenbaum
Chief Medical Officer .... Terry L Fouts, MD
Senior VP &Chief Information Officer .... John R Gabbert
Senior VP, Healthcare Operations .... Donna A Goldin
VP Sales, Select & Mid-Markets .... Marc Neely
Executive Vice President .... Richard F Rivers
Senior VP, Healthcare Management .... Chris Knackstedt

COMPANY PROFILE:
Parent Company Name: CIGNA Inc
Doing Business As:
Year Founded: 1986   Federally Qualified: [ ]
Forprofit: [Y]   Not-For-Profit: [ ]
Model Type: MIXED
Accreditation: [ ] AAPPO [ ] JACHO [X] NCQA [X] URAC
Plan Type: HMO, PPO, POS, ASO, TPA, UR, CDHP, HDHP, HSA
Primary Physicians: 578,000   Physician Specialists:
Hospitals: 4,275
Total Revenue: 2005:   2006: 3,634,200,000
Net Income   2005:   2006: 337,200,000
Total Enrollment:
   2001: 0   2004: 2,021,000   2007: 2,200,000
   2002: 0   2005: 1,965,000
   2003: 0   2006: 2,051,000
SERVICE AREA:
Nationwide: N
   CO;
TYPE OF COVERAGE:
Commercial: [Y] Individual: [ ] FEHBP: [ ] Indemnity: [ ]
Medicare: [ ] Medicaid: [ ] Supplemental Medicare: [ ]
Tricare   [ ]
CONSUMER-DRIVEN PRODUCTS
Mellon HR Solutions LLC   HSA Company
                                       HSA Product
                                       HSA Administrator
                                       Consumer-Driven Health Plan
                                       High Deductible Health Plan
PLAN BENEFITS:
Alternative Medicine: [X]   Behavioral Health: [X]
Chiropractic: [X]   Dental: [X]
Home Care: [X]   Inpatient SNF: [X]
Long-Term Care: [ ]   Pharm. Mail Order: [X]
Physicial Therapy: [X]   Podiatry: [X]
Psychiatric: [X]   Transplant: [X]
Vision: [X]   Wellness: [X]
Workers' Comp: [ ]
Other Benefits:
Comments:
Administrative Office for One Health Plans. Acquired by CIGNA Inc April 1, 2008.

COLORADO

COLORADO DENTAL SERVICE INC, DBA: DELTA DENTAL PLAN OF CO

4582 S Ulster Pkwy Ste 800
Denver, CO 80237-2621
Phone: 303-741-9300 Fax: 303-741-9350 Toll-Free:
Web site: www.deltadentalco.com

MAILING ADDRESS:
COLORADO DENTAL SERVICE INC
4582 S Ulster Pkwy Ste 800
Denver, CO 80237-2621

KEY EXECUTIVES:
Chief Executive Officer .... Kate Paul
Chief Financial Officer .... Russell Schreier
Dental Director .... Maxwell Anderson, DDS
Chief Operating Officer .... Linda Arneson
VP, Marketing .... Jean Lawhead

COMPANY PROFILE:
Parent Company Name: Delta Dental Plan Association
Doing Business As: Delta Dental Plan of Colorado
Year Founded: 1966   Federally Qualified: [N]
Forprofit: [ ]   Not-For-Profit: [Y]
Model Type: IPA
Accreditation: [ ] AAPPO [ ] JACHO [ ] NCQA [ ] URAC
Plan Type: Specialty HMO, Specialty PPO, POS, ASO, EPO,
Total Revenue: 2005: 96,207,518   2006: 95,025,017
Net Income   2005: 2,838,647   2006: 3,595,236
Total Enrollment:
  2001: 229,071   2004: 577,670   2007: 447,200
  2002: 638,309   2005: 465,918
  2003: 0   2006: 481,740
Medical Loss Ratio: 2005: 82.00   2006:
Administrative Expense Ratio: 2005:   2006:

SERVICE AREA:
Nationwide: N
  CO;

TYPE OF COVERAGE:
Commercial: [Y] Individual: [ ] FEHBP: [ ] Indemnity: [ ]
Medicare: [ ] Medicaid: [ ] Supplemental Medicare: [ ]
Tricare   [ ]

PLAN BENEFITS:
Alternative Medicine: [ ]   Behavioral Health: [ ]
Chiropractic: [ ]   Dental: [X]
Home Care: [ ]   Inpatient SNF: [ ]
Long-Term Care: [ ]   Pharm. Mail Order: [ ]
Physical Therapy: [ ]   Podiatry: [ ]
Psychiatric: [ ]   Transplant: [ ]
Vision: [Y]   Wellness: [ ]
Workers' Comp: [ ]
Other Benefits:

COLORADO HEALTH NETWORKS LLC

7150 Campus Dr Ste 300
Colorado Springs, CO 80920
Phone: 719-538-1430 Fax: 719-538-1433 Toll-Free: 800-804-5040
Web site: www.chnpartnerships.com

MAILING ADDRESS:
COLORADO HEALTH NETWORKS LLC
7150 Campus Dr Ste 300
Colorado Springs, CO 80920

KEY EXECUTIVES:
Executive Director .... Arnold Salazar
Director of Finance .... Tina McCrory
Medical Director .... Stephen Holsenbeck, MD
MIS Director .... Chet Phelps
Human Resources/Compliance Director .... Maggie Tilley
Director of Quality Assurance .... Erica Arnold-Miller, MBA
Director of Clinical Services .... Stephen Dixon, PhD

COMPANY PROFILE:
Parent Company Name: Value Options
Doing Business As: Colorado Health Network
Year Founded: 1995   Federally Qualified: [ ]
Forprofit: [ ]   Not-For-Profit: [Y]
Model Type:
Accreditation: [ ] AAPPO [ ] JACHO [ ] NCQA [ ] URAC
Plan Type: Specialty HMO

Total Revenue: 2005:   2006:
Net Income   2005:   2006:
Total Enrollment:
  2001: 85,634   2004: 59,275   2007: 0
  2002: 101,653   2005:
  2003: 74,058   2006:

SERVICE AREA:
Nationwide: N
  CO (43 counties);

TYPE OF COVERAGE:
Commercial: [Y] Individual: [ ] FEHBP: [ ] Indemnity: [ ]
Medicare: [ ] Medicaid: [Y] Supplemental Medicare: [ ]
Tricare   [ ]

PRODUCTS OFFERED:
Product Name: Type:
Pikes Peak - Options   SPECHMO
SyCare - Options   Specialty HMO
West Slope - Options   Specialty HMO

DENVER HEALTH MEDICAL PLAN INC

777 Bannock St
Denver, CO 80204
Phone: 303-436-7253 Fax: 303-436-5714 Toll-Free:
Web site: www.denverhealth.org

MAILING ADDRESS:
DENVER HEALTH MEDICAL PLAN INC
777 Bannock St, MC 6000
Denver, CO 80204

KEY EXECUTIVES:
DHMP Inc Board Chairman .... Dawn Bookhardt
Interim Chief Executive Officer/Executive Director .... Peg Burnette
Treasurer .... Stephanie Thomas
Chief Information Officer .... Gregg Veltri
Chief Operating Officer .... Stefanie Thomas
Marketing Director .... Laurie Goss
MIS Director .... Deborah Markson
Compliance Officer .... Daniel Schirmer
Provider Relations Director .... Ronald Aguilar
Medical Management Director .... David Brody, MD
Credentialing Manager/Director .... Mary Pinkney
Managed Care Director/Officer .... Douglas Clinkscales

COMPANY PROFILE:
Parent Company Name: Denver Health & Hospital Authority
Doing Business As:
Year Founded: 1997   Federally Qualified: [N]
Forprofit: [ ]   Not-For-Profit: [Y]
Model Type: MIXED
Accreditation: [ ] AAPPO [ ] JACHO [ ] NCQA [ ] URAC
Plan Type: HMO,
Total Revenue: 2005: 29,547,201   2006: 22,118,700
Net Income   2005: -851,085   2006: 1,669,396
Total Enrollment:
  2001: 9,477   2004: 10,968   2007: 14,504
  2002: 10,950   2005: 11,700
  2003: 11,221   2006: 13,579
Medical Loss Ratio: 2005: 94.18   2006: 88.70
Administrative Expense Ratio: 2005: 8.62   2006: 9.00

SERVICE AREA:
Nationwide: N
  CO; (Adams, Araphoe, Denver, Jefferson);

TYPE OF COVERAGE:
Commercial: [Y] Individual: [ ] FEHBP: [ ] Indemnity: [ ]
Medicare: [Y] Medicaid: [ ] Supplemental Medicare: [ ]
Tricare   [ ]

PRODUCTS OFFERED:
Product Name: Type:
Denver Health Medical Plan   HMO

PLAN BENEFITS:
Alternative Medicine: [ ]   Behavioral Health: [ ]
Chiropractic: [X]   Dental: [ ]
Home Care: [X]   Inpatient SNF: [X]
Long-Term Care: [ ]   Pharm. Mail Order: [ ]
Physical Therapy: [X]   Podiatry: [X]
Psychiatric: [X]   Transplant: [X]
Vision: [X]   Wellness: [X]
Workers' Comp: [ ]
Other Benefits:

Managed Care Organization Profiles — COLORADO

CIGNA HEALTHCARE OF COLORADO

3900 E Mexico Ave Ste 1100
Denver, CO 80210
Phone: 303-782-1500 Fax: 602-371-2374 Toll-Free: 800-832-3211
Web site: www.cigna.com
MAILING ADDRESS:
   CIGNA HEALTHCARE OF CO
   3900 E Mexico Ave Ste 1100
   Denver, CO 80210

KEY EXECUTIVES:
Chief Executive Officer/President .... Daryl W Edmonds
Medical Director .... Lawrence Wolk, MD

COMPANY PROFILE:
Parent Company Name: CIGNA Corporation
Doing Business As:
Year Founded: 1985   Federally Qualified: [N]
Forprofit: [Y]   Not-For-Profit: [ ]
Model Type: IPA
Accreditation: [ ] AAPPO [ ] JACHO [X] NCQA [ ] URAC
Plan Type: HMO, PPO, POS, CDHP, HDHP, HSA, FSA, HRA
Total Revenue: 2005: 128,992,637   2006:   62,018,149
Net Income   2005:   5,095,096   2006:   1,713,530
Total Enrollment:
   2001: 85,634   2004: 59,275   2007: 29,512
   2002: 101,653   2005: 36,602
   2003: 74,058   2006: 31,625
Medical Loss Ratio: 2005: 86.30   2006: 84.00
Administrative Expense Ratio: 2005:   2006:

SERVICE AREA:
Nationwide: N
   CO;

TYPE OF COVERAGE:
Commercial: [Y] Individual: [ ] FEHBP: [ ] Indemnity: [ ]
Medicare: [Y] Medicaid: [ ] Supplemental Medicare: [ ]
Tricare   [ ]

PRODUCTS OFFERED:
Product Name: Type:
Cigna Hlthcare for Seniors   Medicare
CIGNA HMO   HMO
CIGNA POS   POS
CONSUMER-DRIVEN PRODUCTS
JP Morgan Chase   HSA Company
CIGNA Choice Fund   HSA Product
                                       HSA Administrator
Open Access Plus   Consumer-Driven Health Plan
PPO   High Deductible Health Plan

PLAN BENEFITS:
Alternative Medicine: [ ]   Behavioral Health: [ ]
Chiropractic: [X]   Dental: [X]
Home Care: [ ]   Inpatient SNF: [ ]
Long-Term Care: [ ]   Pharm. Mail Order: [X]
Physical Therapy: [ ]   Podiatry: [ ]
Psychiatric: [ ]   Transplant: [ ]
Vision: [X]   Wellness: [X]
Workers' Comp: [ ]
Other Benefits:

COLORADO ACCESS

10065 E Harvard Ave Ste 600
Denver, CO 80231
Phone: 720-744-5100 Fax: 303-751-9048 Toll-Free: 800-511-5010
Web site: www.coaccess.com
MAILING ADDRESS:
   COLORADO ACCESS
   10065 E Harvard Ave Ste 600
   Denver, CO 80231

KEY EXECUTIVES:
Chief Executive Officer/President .... Marshall Thomas, MD
Chief Medical Officer .... Marshall Thomas, MD
Chief Operating Officer .... Marie Steckbeck
Marketing Director .... LeNore Ralston
Compliance Officer .... Molly McCoy

COMPANY PROFILE:
Parent Company Name:
Doing Business As:
Year Founded: 1995   Federally Qualified: [N]
Forprofit: [ ]   Not-For-Profit: [Y]
Model Type:
Accreditation: [ ] AAPPO [ ] JACHO [ ] NCQA [ ] URAC
Plan Type: HMO
Total Revenue: 2005: 157,869,312   2006:   94,713,049
Net Income   2005: -10,988,878   2006:   2,107,781
Total Enrollment:
   2001: 96,000   2004: 188,506   2007: 97,104
   2002: 206,869   2005: 131,695
   2003: 188,722   2006: 95,839
Medical Loss Ratio: 2005: 88.90   2006:
Administrative Expense Ratio: 2005:   2006:

SERVICE AREA:
Nationwide: N
   CO;

TYPE OF COVERAGE:
Commercial: [ ] Individual: [ ] FEHBP: [ ] Indemnity: [ ]
Medicare: [Y] Medicaid: [Y] Supplemental Medicare: [ ]
Tricare   [ ]

PRODUCTS OFFERED:
Product Name: Type:
Colorado Access   Medicaid
Colorado HMO   Medicare

PLAN BENEFITS:
Alternative Medicine: [ ]   Behavioral Health: [X]
Chiropractic: [ ]   Dental: [ ]
Home Care: [ ]   Inpatient SNF: [ ]
Long-Term Care: [ ]   Pharm. Mail Order: [ ]
Physical Therapy: [ ]   Podiatry: [ ]
Psychiatric: [ ]   Transplant: [ ]
Vision: [ ]   Wellness: [ ]
Workers' Comp: [ ]
Other Benefits:

COLORADO CHOICE HEALTH PLANS
SAN LUIS VALLEY HMO INC

700 Main St Ste 100
Alamosa, CO 81101-2540
Phone: 719-589-3696 Fax: 719-589-4901 Toll-Free: 800-475-8466
Web site: www.slvhmo.com
MAILING ADDRESS:
   COLORADO CHOICE HEALTH PLANS
   700 Main St Ste 100
   Alamosa, CO 81101-2540

KEY EXECUTIVES:
Chairman .... Michael E Stewart
Chief Executive Officer .... Cynthia Palmer
Chief Financial Officer .... Lisa Sandoval, CPA
Chief Medical Director .... Betsy Thompson, MD
Sr Director of Operations .... Joyce F Little
Director, Sales & Marketing .... David Buckley
Vice President Development .... Lynn Borup

COMPANY PROFILE:
Parent Company Name:
Doing Business As: San Luis Valley HMO Inc
Year Founded: 1975   Federally Qualified: [Y]
Forprofit: [ ]   Not-For-Profit: [Y] Model Type:
NETWORK
Accreditation: [ ] AAPPO [ ] JACHO [ ] NCQA [ ] URAC
Plan Type: HMO, ASO, TPA, HDHP, HSA
Total Revenue: 2005:   3,668,591   2006:   7,372,674
Net Income   2005:   195,809   2006:   566,398
Total Enrollment:
   2001:   0   2004:   5,504   2007:   5,352
   2002: 5,404   2005:   5,096
   2003: 5,256   2006:   5,377
Medical Loss Ratio: 2005:   2006:
Administrative Expense Ratio: 2005:   2006:

SERVICE AREA:
Nationwide: N
   CO;

TYPE OF COVERAGE:
Commercial: [Y] Individual: [Y] FEHBP: [ ] Indemnity: [ ]
Medicare: [Y] Medicaid: [ ] Supplemental Medicare: [ ]
Tricare   [ ]

PRODUCTS OFFERED:
Product Name: Type:
HMO Health Plans Inc   Medicare

COLORADO	Managed Care Organization Profiles

ASSURANT EMPLOYEE BENEFITS - COLORADO

5350 S Roslyn St Ste 450
Greenwood Village, CO 80111
Phone: 303-796-7990 Fax: 303-796-2769 Toll-Free: 800-445-0979
Web site: www.assurantemployeebenefits.com
MAILING ADDRESS:
    ASSURANT EMPLOYEE BNFTS - CO
    5350 S Roslyn St Ste 450
    Greenwood Village, CO 80111

KEY EXECUTIVES:
Interim Chief Executive Officer/President .... John S Roberts
Chief Financial Officer .... Floyd F Chadee
VP, Medical Director .... Polly M Galbraith, MD
Chief Information Officer .... Karla J Schacht
Senior VP, Marketing .... Joseph A Sevcik
Privacy Officer .... John L Fortini
VP of Provider Services .... James A Barrett, DMD
Senior VP, Human Resources & Development .... Sylvia R Wagner
General Manager .... Todd Boyd
National Dental Director .... James A Barrett, DMD

COMPANY PROFILE:
Parent Company Name: Assurant Health
Doing Business As:
Year Founded: 1989   Federally Qualified: [ ]
Forprofit: [Y]   Not-For-Profit: [ ]
Model Type:
Accreditation: [ ] AAPPO [ ] JACHO [ ] NCQA [ ] URAC
Plan Type: Specialty HMO
SERVICE AREA:
Nationwide: N
    CO;
TYPE OF COVERAGE:
Commercial: [Y] Individual: [Y] FEHBP: [ ] Indemnity: [ ]
Medicare: [ ] Medicaid: [ ] Supplemental Medicare: [ ]
Tricare   [ ]
PRODUCTS OFFERED:
Product Name: Type:
United Dental Care   SPEC HMO
PLAN BENEFITS:
Alternative Medicine: [ ]   Behavioral Health: [ ]
Chiropractic: [ ]   Dental: [X]
Home Care: [ ]   Inpatient SNF: [ ]
Long-Term Care: [ ]   Pharm. Mail Order: [ ]
Physical Therapy: [ ]   Podiatry: [ ]
Psychiatric: [ ]   Transplant: [ ]
Vision: [ ]   Wellness: [ ]
Workers' Comp: [ ]
Other Benefits:
Comments:
Formerly Fortis Benefits Dental.

BEHAVIORAL HEALTHCARE INC

6801 S Yosemite St Ste 201
Centennial, CO 80112
Phone: 303-889-4805 Fax: 303-889-4808 Toll-Free:
Web site: www.bhicares.org
MAILING ADDRESS:
    BEHAVIORAL HEALTHCARE INC
    6801 S Yosemite St Ste 201
    Centennial, CO 80112

KEY EXECUTIVES:
Chief Executive Officer .... Randy Stith
Chief Financial Officer .... Mary Dice
Medical Director .... Marv Robbins, MD
Chief Operating Officer .... Julie Holtz
MIS Director .... John Stevens
Quality Improvement Director .... Ann Torres

COMPANY PROFILE:
Parent Company Name:
Doing Business As:
Year Founded: 1997   Federally Qualified: [ ]
Forprofit: [ ]   Not-For-Profit: [Y]
Model Type:
Accreditation: [ ] AAPPO [ ] JACHO [ ] NCQA [ ] URAC
Plan Type: Specialty HMO

Total Enrollment:
    2001: 0   2004: 76,698   2007: 0
    2002: 0   2005: 86,033
    2003: 64,785   2006:
SERVICE AREA:
Nationwide: N
    CO;
TYPE OF COVERAGE:
Commercial: [Y] Individual: [ ] FEHBP: [ ] Indemnity: [ ]
Medicare: [ ] Medicaid: [Y] Supplemental Medicare: [ ]
Tricare   [ ]
PRODUCTS OFFERED:
Product Name: Type:
Behavioral Care Medicaid   Medicaid
PLAN BENEFITS:
Alternative Medicine: [ ]   Behavioral Health: [X]
Chiropractic: [ ]   Dental: [ ]
Home Care: [ ]   Inpatient SNF: [ ]
Long-Term Care: [ ]   Pharm. Mail Order: [ ]
Physical Therapy: [ ]   Podiatry: [ ]
Psychiatric: [ ]   Transplant: [ ]
Vision: [ ]   Wellness: [ ]
Workers' Comp: [ ]
Other Benefits:

CIGNA DENTAL HEALTH OF COLORADO

1571 Sawgrass Corporate Pkwy
Sunrise, FL 33323
Phone: 954-514-6600 Fax: 954-514-6905 Toll-Free: 800-367-1037
Web site: www.cigna.com/dental
MAILING ADDRESS:
    CIGNA DENTAL HEALTH OF CO INC
    1571 Sawgrass Corporate Pkwy
    Sunrise, FL 33323

KEY EXECUTIVES:
Chief Executive Officer .... Benjamin K Haynes
President .... Karen S Rohan
Chief Financial Officer .... Frank Lucia
Dental Director .... Kazu Takiki DDS
Marketing Director .... Aaron Groffman
MIS Director .... Laurel A Flebotte

COMPANY PROFILE:
Parent Company Name: CIGNA Dental Health Inc
Doing Business As: CIGNA Dental
Year Founded: 1988   Federally Qualified: [N]
Forprofit: [Y]   Not-For-Profit: [ ]
Model Type:
Accreditation: [ ] AAPPO [ ] JACHO [ ] NCQA [ ] URAC
Plan Type: Specialty HMO, Specialty PPO
Total Enrollment:
    2001: 69,143   2004: 53,983   2007: 0
    2002: 64,649   2005:
    2003: 62,712   2006:
SERVICE AREA:
Nationwide: N
    CO;
TYPE OF COVERAGE:
Commercial: [Y] Individual: [ ] FEHBP: [ ] Indemnity: [ ]
Medicare: [ ] Medicaid: [ ] Supplemental Medicare: [ ]
Tricare   [ ]
PRODUCTS OFFERED:
Product Name: Type:
CIGNA Dental Health of CO   Specialty HMO
PLAN BENEFITS:
Alternative Medicine: [ ]   Behavioral Health: [ ]
Chiropractic: [ ]   Dental: [X]
Home Care: [ ]   Inpatient SNF: [ ]
Long-Term Care: [ ]   Pharm. Mail Order: [ ]
Physical Therapy: [ ]   Podiatry: [ ]
Psychiatric: [ ]   Transplant: [ ]
Vision: [ ]   Wellness: [ ]
Workers' Comp: [ ]
Other Benefits:
Comments:
Corporate address. Enrollment figures reflect Colorado only.

Managed Care Organization Profiles

COLORADO

AETNA HEALTH INC - COLORADO

6430 S Fiddlers Green Circle #200
Greenwood Village, CO 80111
Phone: 303-793-2500 Fax: Toll-Free: 800-872-3862
Web site: www.aetna.com
MAILING ADDRESS:
    AETNA HEALTH INC - COLORADO
    6430 S Fiddlers Green Circle #200
    Greenwood Village, CO 80111

KEY EXECUTIVES:
Chairman of the Board/Chief Executive Officer .... Ronald A Williams
President .... Allan I Greenberg
Executive VP, Finance .... Joseph M Zubretsky

COMPANY PROFILE:
Parent Company Name: Aetna Inc
Doing Business As:
Year Founded: 1995   Federally Qualified: [N]
Forprofit: [Y]   Not-For-Profit: [ ]
Model Type:
Accreditation: [ ] AAPPO [ ] JACHO [ ] NCQA [ ] URAC
Plan Type: HMO, PPO, POS, EPO, CDHP, HSA
Total Revenue: 2005: 110,584,262   2006: 57,320,785
Net Income 2005: 8,202,084   2006: 105,078
Total Enrollment:
    2001: 181,370   2004: 35,899   2007: 44,704
    2002: 51,982   2005: 35,324
    2003: 34,932   2006: 34,799
Medical Loss Ratio: 2005: 79.50   2006: 79.50
Administrative Expense Ratio: 2005:   2006:
SERVICE AREA:
Nationwide:
    CO;
TYPE OF COVERAGE:
Commercial: [Y] Individual: [ ] FEHBP: [ ] Indemnity: [Y]
Medicare: [Y] Medicaid: [ ] Supplemental Medicare: [ ]
Tricare [ ]
CONSUMER-DRIVEN PRODUCTS
Aetna Life Insurance Co   HSA Company
Aetna HealthFund HSA   HSA Product
Aetna   HSA Administrator
Aetna HealthFund   Consumer-Driven Health Plan
PPO I; PPO II   High Deductible Health Plan

ALPHA DENTAL PLAN OF COLORADO

9725 E Hampden Ave Ste 400
Denver, CO 80231
Phone: 303-744-3007 Fax: 303-744-2890 Toll-Free: 800-807-0706
Web site: www.alphadentalplan.com
MAILING ADDRESS:
    ALPHA DENTAL PLAN OF CO
    9725 E Hampden Ave Ste 400
    Denver, CO 80231

KEY EXECUTIVES:
Owner .... Donald L Miloni
Chief Executive Officer .... Kay McFarland
President/VP of Marketing .... Rod Henningson

COMPANY PROFILE:
Parent Company Name: Beta Health Association Inc
Doing Business As:
Year Founded: 1990   Federally Qualified: [ ]
Forprofit: [Y]   Not-For-Profit: [ ]
Model Type: NETWORK
Accreditation: [ ] AAPPO [ ] JACHO [ ] NCQA [ ] URAC
Plan Type: Specialty PPO
Total Enrollment:
    2001: 0   2004: 0   2007: 0
    2002: 0   2005:
    2003: 84,000   2006: 92,000
SERVICE AREA:
Nationwide: N
    CO;
TYPE OF COVERAGE:
Commercial: [Y] Individual: [ ] FEHBP: [ ] Indemnity: [ ]
Medicare: [ ] Medicaid: [ ] Supplemental Medicare: [ ]
Tricare [ ]
PLAN BENEFITS:
Alternative Medicine: [ ]   Behavioral Health: [ ]
Chiropractic: [ ]   Dental: [X]
Home Care: [ ]   Inpatient SNF: [ ]
Long-Term Care: [ ]   Pharm. Mail Order: [ ]
Physicial Therapy: [ ]   Podiatry: [ ]
Psychiatric: [ ]   Transplant: [ ]
Vision: [X]   Wellness: [ ]
Workers' Comp: [ ]
Other Benefits:

ANTHEM BLUE CROSS BLUE SHIELD OF COLORADO

700 Broadway 7th Fl
Denver, CO 80273
Phone: 303-831-2000 Fax: 303-764-7160 Toll-Free:
Web site: www.anthem.com
MAILING ADDRESS:
    ANTHEM BC BS OF COLORADO
    700 Broadway 7th Fl
    Denver, CO 80273

KEY EXECUTIVES:
Chairman of the Board .... Larry C Glasscock
Chief Executive Officer .... Angela F Braly
President .... John Martie
Chief Medical Officer .... Lisa Latts, MD
Pharmacy Director .... Jim Thorne
Chief Information Officer .... Brent Brown
Chief Operating Officer .... Donna Boeing
HIPAA Program Manager .... Anthony Carlson
VP of Healthcare Management .... Robert London, MD
VP, Health Services .... Mike Ramseier

COMPANY PROFILE:
Parent Company Name: WellPoint Inc
Doing Business As: Rocky Mountain Hospital & Medical Srvs I
Year Founded: 1978   Federally Qualified: [Y]
Forprofit: [ ]   Not-For-Profit: [Y]
Model Type: NETWORK
Accreditation: [ ] AAPPO [ ] JACHO [ ] NCQA [ ] URAC
Plan Type: HMO, PPO, POS, PRO, ASO, UR, CDHP, HDHP, HSA
Total Revenue: 2005:   2006: 102,691,157
Net Income 2005:   2006: 8,417,708
Total Enrollment:
    2001: 0   2004: 74,263   2007: 111,318
    2002: 104,902   2005: 66,603
    2003: 85,282   2006: 104,288
SERVICE AREA:
Nationwide: N
    CO;
TYPE OF COVERAGE:
Commercial: [Y] Individual: [Y] FEHBP: [ ] Indemnity: [ ]
Medicare: [Y] Medicaid: [Y] Supplemental Medicare: [Y]
Tricare [ ]
PRODUCTS OFFERED:
Product Name: Type:
Blue Advantage
HMO Colorado   HMO
BlueAdvantage for Seniors   Medicare
CONSUMER-DRIVEN PRODUCTS
JP Morgan Chase   HSA CompanyAnthem
ByDesign HSA   HSA Product
JP Morgan Chase   HSA Administrator
Blue Access Saver   Consumer-Driven Health Plan
Blue Access Economy Plans PPO   High Deductible Health Plan
PLAN BENEFITS:
Alternative Medicine: [ ]   Behavioral Health: [X]
Chiropractic: [X]   Dental: [X]
Home Care: [X]   Inpatient SNF: [X]
Long-Term Care: [ ]   Pharm. Mail Order: [X]
Physical Therapy: [X]   Podiatry: [X]
Psychiatric: [X]   Transplant: [X]
Vision: [X]   Wellness: [X]
Workers' Comp: [ ]
Other Benefits:

Managed Care Organization Profiles — CALIFORNIA

Accreditation: [ ] AAPPO [ ] JACHO [ ] NCQA [ ] URAC
Plan Type: Specialty HMO
Total Revenue: 2005:   3,417,133   2006:   3,427,647
Net Income   2005:   75,173   2006:   34,462
Total Enrollment:
   2001: 66,509   2004: 66,317   2007: 58,167
   2002: 73,644   2005: 68,750
   2003: 70,932   2006: 58,778
Medical Loss Ratio: 2005: 82.03   2006: 86.79
Administrative Expense Ratio: 2005: 16.18   2006: 13.04

SERVICE AREA:
Nationwide: N
   CA;

TYPE OF COVERAGE:
Commercial: [Y] Individual: [ ] FEHBP: [ ] Indemnity: [ ]
Medicare: [ ] Medicaid: [ ] Supplemental Medicare: [ ]
Tricare   [ ]

PRODUCTS OFFERED:
Product Name: Type:
Comprehensive Eye Exam   Specialty HMO

PLAN BENEFITS:
Alternative Medicine: [ ]   Behavioral Health: [ ]
Chiropractic: [ ]   Dental: [ ]
Home Care: [ ]   Inpatient SNF: [ ]
Long-Term Care: [ ]   Pharm. Mail Order: [ ]
Physical Therapy: [ ]   Podiatry: [ ]
Psychiatric: [ ]   Transplant: [ ]
Vision: [X]   Wellness: [ ]
Workers' Comp: [ ]
Other Benefits: Optometry

WESTERN DENTAL SERVICES

530 S Main St
Orange, CA 92868
Phone: 714-480-3000 Fax: 714-480-3001 Toll-Free: 800-417-4444
Web site: www.westerndental.com

MAILING ADDRESS:
WESTERN DENTAL SERVICES
530 S Main St
Orange, CA 92868

KEY EXECUTIVES:
Chief Executive Officer/President .... Samuel Gruenbaum
Chief Financial Officer .... David Joe
Chief Dental Director .... Louis J Amendola
Chief Information Officer .... Joseph Minksy
Senior VP & Chief Sales Officer .... Wayne Butts
Director, Provider Services .... Zina Smart
Quality Assurance Director .... David L Forney
Executive Vice President .... Stanley J Andrakowicz
General Counsel .... Susan Rule Sandler

COMPANY PROFILE:
Parent Company Name: Western Dental Services
Doing Business As: Western Dental Plan
Year Founded: 1985   Federally Qualified: [Y]
Forprofit: [Y]   Not-For-Profit: [ ]
Model Type:
Accreditation: [ ] AAPPO [ ] JACHO [ ] NCQA [ ] URAC
Plan Type: Specialty HMO
Total Revenue: 2005: 294,608,555   2006: 339,849,603
Net Income   2005:   932,455   2006: -26,671,577
Total Enrollment:
   2001: 311,447   2004: 399,613   2007: 555,278
   2002: 315,181   2005: 493,910
   2003: 327,718   2006: 541,755
Medical Loss Ratio: 2005: 82.37   2006: 85.62
Administrative Expense Ratio: 2005: 15.81   2006: 19.93

SERVICE AREA:
Nationwide: N
   CA; AZ;

TYPE OF COVERAGE:
Commercial: [Y] Individual: [Y] FEHBP: [ ] Indemnity: [ ]
Medicare: [Y] Medicaid: [Y] Supplemental Medicare: [ ]
Tricare   [ ]

PRODUCTS OFFERED:
Product Name: Type:
Western Dental Plan   Dental

PLAN BENEFITS:
Alternative Medicine: [ ]   Behavioral Health: [ ]
Chiropractic: [ ]   Dental: [X]
Home Care: [ ]   Inpatient SNF: [ ]
Long-Term Care: [ ]   Pharm. Mail Order: [ ]
Physical Therapy: [ ]   Podiatry: [ ]
Psychiatric: [ ]   Transplant: [ ]
Vision: [ ]   Wellness: [ ]
Workers' Comp: [ ]
Other Benefits:

WESTERN HEALTH ADVANTAGE

1331 Garden Hwy Ste 100
Sacramento, CA 95833
Phone: 916-563-2200 Fax: 916-563-3182 Toll-Free: 888-563-2250
Web site: www.westernhealth.com

MAILING ADDRESS:
WESTERN HEALTH ADVANTAGE
1331 Garden Hwy Ste 100
Sacramento, CA 95833

KEY EXECUTIVES:
Chief Executive Officer/President .... Garry Maisel
Chief Financial Officer .... Rita Ruecker
Chief Medical Officer .... Don Hufford, MD
Chief Administrative Officer/Marketing Director .... Bill Figenshu
Director/Regulatory Compliance/Center .... Christine Williams

COMPANY PROFILE:
Parent Company Name:
Doing Business As:
Year Founded: 1997   Federally Qualified: [ ]
Forprofit: [ ]   Not-For-Profit: [Y]
Model Type: MIXED
Accreditation: [ ] AAPPO [ ] JACHO [X] NCQA [ ] URAC
Plan Type: HMO, HDHP, HSA,
Total Revenue: 2005: 56,997,556   2006: 61,061,978
Net Income   2005:   181,579   2006: -247,455
Total Enrollment:
   2001: 52,619   2004: 73,063   2007: 94,886
   2002: 61,029   2005: 82,767
   2003: 65,366   2006: 89,282
Medical Loss Ratio: 2005: 90.44   2006: 90.45
Administrative Expense Ratio: 2005: 9.42   2006: 9.15

SERVICE AREA:
Nationwide: N
   CA (Colusa, Sacramento, Solano, Yolo, Western El Dorado, Western Placer);

TYPE OF COVERAGE:
Commercial: [Y] Individual: [ ] FEHBP: [ ] Indemnity: [ ]
Medicare: [ ] Medicaid: [Y] Supplemental Medicare: [Y]
Tricare   [ ]

PRODUCTS OFFERED:
Product Name: Type:
Western Hlth Advantage   Medicaid
Western Health Advantage CarePlus   Medicare Advantage
Western Health   HMO

PLAN BENEFITS:
Alternative Medicine: [ ]   Behavioral Health: [X]
Chiropractic: [X]   Dental: [ ]
Home Care: [X]   Inpatient SNF: [X]
Long-Term Care: [ ]   Pharm. Mail Order: [X]
Physical Therapy: [X]   Podiatry: [X]
Psychiatric: [X]   Transplant: [X]
Vision: [X]   Wellness: [X]
Workers' Comp: [ ]
Other Benefits:

CALIFORNIA

PLAN BENEFITS:

Alternative Medicine:	[ ]	Behavioral Health:	[ ]
Chiropractic:	[ ]	Dental:	[ ]
Home Care:	[ ]	Inpatient SNF:	[ ]
Long-Term Care:	[ ]	Pharm. Mail Order:	[ ]
Physical Therapy:	[ ]	Podiatry:	[ ]
Psychiatric:	[ ]	Transplant:	[ ]
Vision:	[X]	Wellness:	[ ]
Workers' Comp:	[ ]		

Other Benefits:

VISION PLAN OF AMERICA

3255 Wilshire Blvd Ste 1610
Los Angeles, CA 90010
Phone: 213-384-2600 Fax: 213-384-0084 Toll-Free: 800-400-4872
Web site: www.visionplanofamerica.com

MAILING ADDRESS:
VISION PLAN OF AMERICA
3255 Wilshire Blvd Ste 1610
Los Angeles, CA 90010

KEY EXECUTIVES:
Chief Executive Officer .... Stuart Needleman, OD
Chief Financial Officer .... Maya Pushin
Clinical Director .... Gerald Nankin, OD
Marketing Director/Compliance Officer .... Phillip Needleman
MIS Director .... Paula Marroquin
Credentialing Manager .... Gerald Nankin, OD
Network Development/Qualtiy Assurance Director .... Mario Viteri

COMPANY PROFILE:
Parent Company Name:
Doing Business As:
Year Founded: 1985   Federally Qualified: [N]
Forprofit: [Y]   Not-For-Profit: [ ]
Model Type: IPA
Accreditation: [ ] AAPPO [ ] JACHO [ ] NCQA [ ] URAC
Plan Type: Specialty HMO, Specialty PPO
Total Revenue: 2005:   377,277   2006:   337,583
Net Income   2005:   3,345   2006:   -21,298
Total Enrollment:
  2001: 37,949   2004: 31,059   2007: 26,015
  2002: 40,099   2005: 27,115
  2003: 45,223   2006: 24,537
Medical Loss Ratio: 2005: 22.08   2006: 30.52
Administrative Expense Ratio: 2005: 77.78   2006: 64.53

SERVICE AREA:
Nationwide: N
  CA;

TYPE OF COVERAGE:
Commercial: [Y] Individual: [Y] FEHBP: [ ] Indemnity: [ ]
Medicare: [ ] Medicaid: [ ] Supplemental Medicare: [ ]
Tricare   [ ]

PRODUCTS OFFERED:
Product Name:	Type:
Vision	Specialty HMO

PLAN BENEFITS:

Alternative Medicine:	[X]	Behavioral Health:	[ ]
Chiropractic:	[ ]	Dental:	[X]
Home Care:	[ ]	Inpatient SNF:	[ ]
Long-Term Care:	[ ]	Pharm. Mail Order:	[ ]
Physical Therapy:	[ ]	Podiatry:	[ ]
Psychiatric:	[ ]	Transplant:	[ ]
Vision:	[X]	Wellness:	[ ]
Workers' Comp:	[ ]		

Other Benefits:

VISION SERVICE PLAN

3333 Quality Drive
Rancho Cordova, CA 95670
Phone: 916-851-5000 Fax: 916-858-5329 Toll-Free: 800-852-7600
Web site: www.vsp.com

MAILING ADDRESS:
VISION SERVICE PLAN
3333 Quality Drive
Rancho Cordova, CA 95670

KEY EXECUTIVES:
Chief Executive Officer/President .... Rob Lynch
Chief Financial Officer .... Patricia C Cochran
Medical Director .... Douglas Cooper, MD
VP of Information Systems .... Steve Scott
Senior VP of Operations .... Gary Brooks
VP, Marketing .... Kate Renwick-Espinosa
VP, Sales .... Ric Steere
HIPAA Project Manager .... Julie Ramos
VP of Customer Service .... Laura Costa
VP of Provider Relations .... Don Price
VP of Health Care Services .... Cheryl Johnson
VP of Human Resources .... Elaine Leuchars
VP of General Counsel .... Thomas Fessler
VP of Client Services .... Mary Ann Cavanagh
VP of Ophthalmic & Claim Services .... Bill Conner
VP of Eastern Operations Center .... Judy Klein

COMPANY PROFILE:
Parent Company Name:
Doing Business As:
Year Founded: 1955   Federally Qualified: [N]
Forprofit: [ ]   Not-For-Profit: [Y]
Model Type:
Accreditation: [ ] AAPPO [ ] JACHO [ ] NCQA [ ] URAC
Plan Type: Specialty HMO, Specialty PPO
Total Revenue: 2005: 176,866,075   2006: 754,866,843
Net Income   2005: -2,674,429   2006:   15,341,949
Total Enrollment:
  2001: 8,510,683   2004: 9,048,143   2007: 8,771,153
  2002: 8,632,670   2005: 8,580,940
  2003: 7,602,357   2006: 8,538,745
Medical Loss Ratio: 2005: 83.74   2006: 89.05
Administrative Expense Ratio: 2005: 22.46   2006: 12.96

SERVICE AREA:
Nationwide: Y
  NW;

TYPE OF COVERAGE:
Commercial: [Y] Individual: [ ] FEHBP: [ ] Indemnity: [ ]
Medicare: [Y] Medicaid: [Y] Supplemental Medicare: [ ]
Tricare   [ ]

PLAN BENEFITS:

Alternative Medicine:	[ ]	Behavioral Health:	[ ]
Chiropractic:	[ ]	Dental:	[ ]
Home Care:	[ ]	Inpatient SNF:	[ ]
Long-Term Care:	[ ]	Pharm. Mail Order:	[ ]
Physical Therapy:	[ ]	Podiatry:	[ ]
Psychiatric:	[ ]	Transplant:	[ ]
Vision:	[X]	Wellness:	[ ]
Workers' Comp:	[ ]		

Other Benefits: Medical Eyecare
Comments:
Formerly California Vision Service. Corporate Information.

VISIONCARE OF CALIFORNIA

9625 Black Mountain Rd Ste 311
San Diego, CA 92126
Phone: 858-831-9322 Fax: 858-831-0225 Toll-Free:
Web site: www.sterlingvisioncare.com

MAILING ADDRESS:
VISIONCARE OF CALIFORNIA
9625 Black Mountain Rd Ste 311
San Diego, CA 92126

KEY EXECUTIVES:
President/Chief Operating Officer .... Nick Shashati, OD
Chief Financial Officer .... Richard Vardaro
Medical Director .... Stephen Dentone, MD
Managed Care Director .... Nick Shashati, OD
Credentialing Manager .... Nick Shashati, OD
Compliance/Privacy Officer .... Nick Shashati, OD
Provider Relations Director .... Nick Shashati, OD
Quality Assurance Director .... Stephen Dentone, MD
Fraud Prevention Director .... Richard Vardaro

COMPANY PROFILE:
Parent Company Name: VisionCare of California
Doing Business As: Sterling Visioncare
Year Founded: 1986   Federally Qualified: [N]
Forprofit: [Y]   Not-For-Profit: [ ]
Model Type: STAFF

Managed Care Organization Profiles CALIFORNIA

Medical Loss Ratio: 2005: 146.50 2006: 80.81
Administrative Expense Ratio: 2005: 37.38 2006:
SERVICE AREA:
Nationwide: N
   CA;
PLAN BENEFITS:
Alternative Medicine: [ ]   Behavioral Health: [ ]
Chiropractic: [ ]   Dental: [ ]
Home Care: [ ]   Inpatient SNF: [ ]
Long-Term Care: [ ]   Pharm. Mail Order: [ ]
Physical Therapy: [ ]   Podiatry: [ ]
Psychiatric: [X]   Transplant: [ ]
Vision: [ ]   Wellness: [ ]
Workers' Comp: [ ]
Other Benefits:

VENTURA COUNTY FOUNDATION FOR MEDICAL CARE

365 Willis Ave
Camarillo, CA 93010
Phone: 805-383-9740 Fax: 805-482-5561 Toll-Free: 800-232-9043
Web site: www.cfmcnet.org
MAILING ADDRESS:
   VENTURA CNTY FDN FOR MED CARE
   365 Willis Ave
   Camarillo, CA 93010

KEY EXECUTIVES:
Chief Executive Officer .... Richard E Michel
Chief Financial Officer .... Kay Craig
Medical Director .... Richard S Loft, MD
VP Contracting & Network Development .... Sandra Grimes

COMPANY PROFILE:
Parent Company Name:
Doing Business As: Ventura Insurance Administrators
Year Founded: 1971   Federally Qualified: [N]
Forprofit: [Y]   Not-For-Profit: [ ]
Model Type:
Accreditation: [ ] AAPPO [X] JACHO [ ] NCQA [ ] URAC
Plan Type: PPO, Speciality PPO, EPO
Hospitals: 400
Total Enrollment:
   2001: 0   2004: 40,000   2007: 0
   2002: 0   2005:
   2003: 0   2006:
SERVICE AREA:
Nationwide: N
   CA;
TYPE OF COVERAGE:
Commercial: [Y] Individual: [Y] FEHBP: [ ] Indemnity: [ ]
Medicare: [Y] Medicaid: [ ] Supplemental Medicare: [Y]
Tricare [ ]
PLAN BENEFITS:
Alternative Medicine: [ ]   Behavioral Health: [ ]
Chiropractic: [X]   Dental: [X]
Home Care: [X]   Inpatient SNF: [X]
Long-Term Care: [X]   Pharm. Mail Order: [X]
Physical Therapy: [X]   Podiatry: [X]
Psychiatric: [X]   Transplant: [X]
Vision: [X]   Wellness: [X]
Workers' Comp: [X]
Other Benefits:

VENTURA COUNTY HEALTH CARE PLAN

2323 Knoll Dr Ste 417
Ventura, CA 93003
Phone: 805-677-8787 Fax: 805-677-5179 Toll-Free: 800-600-8247
Web site: www.vchca.org/hcp
MAILING ADDRESS:
   VENTURA COUNTY HEALTH CARE PLN
   2323 Knoll Dr Ste 417
   Ventura, CA 93003

KEY EXECUTIVES:
Administrator .... Larry Keller
President .... Pierre Durand, DPA
Chief Financial Officer .... Karen Davis
Medical Director .... Cynthian Wilhelmy, MD
Service Administrator & Marketing .... Pamela Linderman

COMPANY PROFILE:
Parent Company Name: County of Ventura
Doing Business As:
Year Founded: 1993   Federally Qualified: [N]
Forprofit: [ ]   Not-For-Profit: [Y]
Model Type: MIXED
Accreditation: [ ] AAPPO [ ] JACHO [ ] NCQA [ ] URAC
Plan Type: HMO
Total Revenue: 2005: 4,626,120   2006: 6,225,905
Net Income   2005:   4,342   2006:   258,766
Total Enrollment:
   2001: 10,182   2004: 10,120   2007: 11,685
   2002: 10,724   2005: 9,723
   2003: 11,032   2006: 11,722
Medical Loss Ratio: 2005: 86.29 2006:
Administrative Expense Ratio: 2005: 14.10 2006: 11.11
SERVICE AREA:
Nationwide: N
   CA (Ventura);
TYPE OF COVERAGE:
Commercial: [Y] Individual: [ ] FEHBP: [ ] Indemnity: [ ]
Medicare: [ ] Medicaid: [ ] Supplemental Medicare: [ ]
Tricare [ ]
PRODUCTS OFFERED:
Product Name: Type:
Ventura County Health Plan   HMO
PLAN BENEFITS:
Alternative Medicine: [ ]   Behavioral Health: [ ]
Chiropractic: [ ]   Dental: [ ]
Home Care: [X]   Inpatient SNF: [X]
Long-Term Care: [X]   Pharm. Mail Order: [X]
Physical Therapy: [X]   Podiatry: [X]
Psychiatric: [X]   Transplant: [X]
Vision: [ ]   Wellness: [ ]
Workers' Comp: [ ]
Other Benefits:

VISION FIRST EYE CARE INC

1937-A Tully Rd
San Jose, CA 95122
Phone: 408-923-0400 Fax: 408-923-3303 Toll-Free:
Web site: www.visionfirsteye.com
MAILING ADDRESS:
   VISION FIRST EYE CARE INC
   1937-A Tully Rd Ste 1610
   San Jose, CA 95122

KEY EXECUTIVES:
President/Chief Information Officer .... James K Eu, OD, PhD

COMPANY PROFILE:
Parent Company Name:
Doing Business As:
Year Founded: Federally Qualified: [ ]
Forprofit: [ ]   Not-For-Profit: [ ]
Model Type:
Accreditation: [ ] AAPPO [ ] JACHO [ ] NCQA [ ] URAC
Plan Type: Specialty HMO
Total Revenue: 2005:   996,907   2006: 3,589,292
Net Income   2005:   34,424   2006:   50,134
Total Enrollment: 2001: 2,126   2004: 1,387
2007: 17,547
   2002: 1,702   2005: 1,851
   2003: 1,311   2006: 1,662
Medical Loss Ratio: 2005: 62.04 2006: 58.69
Administrative Expense Ratio: 2005: 34.56 2006: 38.68
SERVICE AREA:
Nationwide: N
   CA;
PRODUCTS OFFERED:
Product Name: Type:
Vision First Eye Care, Inc   Specialty HMO

CALIFORNIA

SERVICE AREA:
Nationwide: Y
  NW;
TYPE OF COVERAGE:
Commercial: [Y] Individual: [ ] FEHBP: [ ] Indemnity: [ ]
Medicare: [Y] Medicaid: [ ] Supplemental Medicare: [ ]
Tricare [ ]
PLAN BENEFITS:
Alternative Medicine:	[ ]	Behavioral Health:	[X]
Chiropractic:	[ ]	Dental:	[ ]
Home Care:	[ ]	Inpatient SNF:	[ ]
Long-Term Care:	[ ]	Pharm. Mail Order:	[ ]
Physical Therapy:	[ ]	Podiatry:	[ ]
Psychiatric:	[X]	Transplant:	[ ]
Vision:	[ ]	Wellness:	[ ]
Workers' Comp:	[ ]		

Other Benefits:

UNITED CONCORDIA COMPANY INC - CALIFORNIA

21700 Oxnard Ste 500
Woodland Hills, CA 91367-3642
Phone: 818-731-2532 Fax: 818-704-5033 Toll-Free: 800-876-6432
Web site: www.ucci.com
MAILING ADDRESS:
  UNITED CONCORDIA CO INC - CA
  21700 Oxnard Ste 500
  Woodland Hills, CA 91367-3642

KEY EXECUTIVES:
Chairperson of the Board .... Thomas A Dzuryachko
Chief Executive Officer/President .... Thomas A Dzuryachko
Senior VP, Finance .... Daniel Wright
VP, National Dental Director .... Richard Klich, DMD
Senior VP, Operations .... Jon Seltenheim
Senior VP, Chief Marketing Officer .... Chip Merkel
Senior VP, Sales .... Jan Jewett
Corp VP, Professional Relatins .... Karen Whitesel
VP, Human Resources .... Harlon Robinson
Regional VP .... Laurie Laspina
Corp VP, TRICARE Dental Progrm .... Dr Lawrence McKinley

COMPANY PROFILE:
Parent Company Name: Highmark Inc
Doing Business As: United Concordia Company Inc
Year Founded: 1991   Federally Qualified: [ ]
Forprofit: [Y]   Not-For-Profit: [ ]
Model Type:
Accreditation: [ ] AAPPO [ ] JACHO [ ] NCQA [ ] URAC
Plan Type: Specialty HMO, Specialty PPO, POS, TPA
Total Revenue: 2005: 9,803,019   2006: 40,530,741
Net Income   2005: 354,613   2006: 727,932
Total Enrollment:
  2001: 291,106   2004: 262,003   2007: 246,092
  2002: 286,014   2005: 258,208
  2003: 279,080   2006: 248,852
Medical Loss Ratio: 2005: 70.54   2006: 71.88
Administrative Expense Ratio: 2005: 31.47   2006: 30.26
SERVICE AREA:
Nationwide: N
  CA;
TYPE OF COVERAGE:
Commercial: [Y] Individual: [ ] FEHBP: [ ] Indemnity: [ ]
Medicare: [ ] Medicaid: [ ] Supplemental Medicare: [ ]
Tricare [ ]
PRODUCTS OFFERED:
Product Name: Type:
United Concordia   Specialty HMO
PLAN BENEFITS:
Alternative Medicine:	[ ]	Behavioral Health:	[ ]
Chiropractic:	[ ]	Dental:	[X]
Home Care:	[ ]	Inpatient SNF:	[ ]
Long-Term Care:	[ ]	Pharm. Mail Order:	[ ]
Physical Therapy:	[ ]	Podiatry:	[ ]
Psychiatric:	[ ]	Transplant:	[ ]
Vision:	[ ]	Wellness:	[ ]
Workers' Comp:	[ ]		

Other Benefits:
Comments:
Formerly Oral Health Services Inc.

VALLEY HEALTH PLAN SANTA CLARA COUNTY

2325 Enborg Lane Ste 290
San Jose, CA 95128
Phone: 408-885-4760 Fax: 408-885-4425 Toll-Free:
Web site: www.valleyhealthplan.org
MAILING ADDRESS:
  VALLEY HLTH PLN SANTA CLARA CT
  2325 Enborg Lane Ste 290
  San Jose, CA 95128

KEY EXECUTIVES:
Chief Executive Officer .... Greg Price
Finanical Director .... Kim Roberts
Medical Director .... Kent Imai, MD

COMPANY PROFILE:
Parent Company Name: Santa Clara County
Doing Business As: Valley Health Plan
Year Founded: 1985   Federally Qualified: [N]
Forprofit: [ ]   Not-For-Profit: [Y]
Model Type: STAFF
Accreditation: [ ] AAPPO [ ] JACHO [ ] NCQA [ ] URAC
Plan Type: HMO
Total Revenue: 2005: 23,498,504   2006: 24,062,353
Net Income   2005: 99,966   2006: -339,810
Total Enrollment:
  2001: 51,138   2004: 57,383   2007: 61,737
  2002: 51,125   2005: 57,297
  2003: 57,755   2006: 59,936
Medical Loss Ratio: 2005: 91.66   2006:
Administrative Expense Ratio: 2005: 8.46   2006: 9.78
SERVICE AREA:
Nationwide: N
  CA (Santa Clara);
TYPE OF COVERAGE:
Commercial: [Y] Individual: [ ] FEHBP: [ ] Indemnity: [ ]
Medicare: [ ] Medicaid: [ ] Supplemental Medicare: [ ]
Tricare [ ]
PRODUCTS OFFERED:
Product Name: Type:
Valley Health Plan   HMO
PLAN BENEFITS:
Alternative Medicine:	[ ]	Behavioral Health:	[ ]
Chiropractic:	[ ]	Dental:	[ ]
Home Care:	[X]	Inpatient SNF:	[X]
Long-Term Care:	[ ]	Pharm. Mail Order:	[ ]
Physical Therapy:	[X]	Podiatry:	[X]
Psychiatric:	[X]	Transplant:	[X]
Vision:	[X]	Wellness:	[X]
Workers' Comp:	[ ]		

Other Benefits: Acute Detoxification

VALUEOPTIONS OF CALIFORNIA INC

10805 Holder St Ste 300
Cypress, CA 90630
Phone: 714-763-2427 Fax: 714-763-2504 Toll-Free: 800-228-1286
Web site: www.valueoptions.com
MAILING ADDRESS:
  VALUEOPTIONS OF CA INC
  10805 Holder St Ste 300
  Cypress, CA 90630

KEY EXECUTIVES:
Executive Director .... Steven Rockowitz, PsyD
Medical Director .... Joseph Hullett, MD

COMPANY PROFILE:
Parent Company Name:
Doing Business As:
Year Founded: 1996   Federally Qualified: [ ]
Forprofit: [Y]   Not-For-Profit: [ ]
Model Type:
Accreditation: [ ] AAPPO [ ] JACHO [ ] NCQA [ ] URAC
Plan Type: Specialty HMO, ASO
Total Revenue: 2005: 4,456,269   2006: 16,009,211
Net Income   2005: 182,356   2006: 213,338
Total Enrollment:
  2001: 249,659   2004: 379,088   2007: 416,605
  2002: 250,910   2005: 417,864
  2003: 300,560   2006: 428,555

Managed Care Organization Profiles — **CALIFORNIA**

SERVICE AREA:
Nationwide:
   CA;
TYPE OF COVERAGE:
Commercial: [ ] Individual: [ ] FEHBP: [ ] Indemnity: [ ]
Medicare: [ ] Medicaid: [ ] Supplemental Medicare: [ ]
Tricare [ ]

UDC DENTAL CALIFORNIA INC

450 B St Ste 880
San Diego, CA 92101
Phone: 619-236-9595 Fax: 619-233-8669 Toll-Free: 800-443-2995
Web site: www.udcdentalcalifornia.com
MAILING ADDRESS:
   UDC DENTAL CALIFORNIA INC
   450 B St Ste 880
   San Diego, CA 92101

KEY EXECUTIVES:
President .... Janet Clark Stanley
Chief Financial Officer .... Brenda Deann Alexander
Quality Improvement Specialist .... Christian Cortez

COMPANY PROFILE:
Parent Company Name: Assurant Employee Benefits
Doing Business As:
Year Founded: 1988   Federally Qualified: [ ]
Forprofit: [ ]   Not-For-Profit: [ ]
Model Type:
Accreditation: [ ] AAPPO [ ] JACHO [ ] NCQA [ ] URAC
Plan Type: Specialty HMO
Total Revenue: 2005:   825,824   2006:   3,241,309
Net Income   2005:   154,617   2006:   481,477
Total Enrollment:
   2001: 0   2004: 24,857   2007: 30,310
   2002: 18,646   2005: 26,427
   2003: 25,563   2006: 25,782
Medical Loss Ratio: 2005: 54.73   2006: 61.57
Administrative Expense Ratio: 2005: 19.64   2006: 18.78
SERVICE AREA:
Nationwide:
   CA;
PLAN BENEFITS:
Alternative Medicine: [ ]   Behavioral Health: [ ]
Chiropractic: [ ]   Dental: [X]
Home Care: [ ]   Inpatient SNF: [ ]
Long-Term Care: [ ]   Pharm. Mail Order: [ ]
Physical Therapy: [ ]   Podiatry: [ ]
Psychiatric: [ ]   Transplant: [ ]
Vision: [ ]   Wellness: [ ]
Workers' Comp: [ ]
Other Benefits:

UHP HEALTHCARE

5959 Century Blvd Ste 739-741
Los Angeles, CA 90045
Phone: 310-671-3361 Fax: 310-412-5796 Toll-Free: 800-847-1222
Web site: www.uhphealthcare.com
MAILING ADDRESS:
   UHP HEALTHCARE
   PO Box 5127
   Los Angeles, CA 90045

KEY EXECUTIVES:
Chairman of the Board .... Johnny D Griggs
Chief Executive Officer .... Curtis Owens
Chief Financial Officer .... Sharon Isaac
Medical Director .... Albert Young, MD
Pharmacy Director .... Chris Nee
EVP/Chief Operations Officer .... Alan Bloom
Senior VP/Chief Information Officer .... Michael Rowan
Privacy Officer .... Michael Rowan
Public Relations Director .... Harold Hambrick
Provider Relations Director .... Sylvia Grantham
Network Development Director .... Cassandra Sams
Human Resources Director .... Micah Mullins
VP of Managed Care Services .... Pat Johnson
Compliance Officer .... Sianam Khan

COMPANY PROFILE:
Parent Company Name: Watts Health Foundation Inc
Doing Business As: UHP Health Care
Year Founded: 1971   Federally Qualified: [Y]
Forprofit: [ ]   Not-For-Profit: [Y]
Model Type: MIXED
Accreditation: [ ] AAPPO [X] JACHO [ ] NCQA [ ] URAC
Plan Type: HMO
Total Revenue: 2005: 42,033,000   2006: 43,069,000
Net Income   2005: 637,000   2006: -1,298,000
Total Enrollment:
   2001: 101,585   2004: 93,842   2007: 1
   2002: 108,482   2005: 80,977
   2003: 108,711   2006: 78,896
Medical Loss Ratio: 2005: 81.34   2006: 78.00
Administrative Expense Ratio: 2005: 17.82   2006: 27.68
SERVICE AREA:
Nationwide: N
   CA;
TYPE OF COVERAGE:
Commercial: [Y] Individual: [Y] FEHBP: [ ] Indemnity: [ ]
Medicare: [Y] Medicaid: [Y] Supplemental Medicare: [ ]
Tricare [ ]
PRODUCTS OFFERED:
Product Name: Type:
United Health Plan for Seniors   Medicare Advantage
PLAN BENEFITS:
Alternative Medicine: [ ]   Behavioral Health: [ ]
Chiropractic: [X]   Dental: [X]
Home Care: [X]   Inpatient SNF: [ ]
Long-Term Care: [ ]   Pharm. Mail Order: [ ]
Physical Therapy: [ ]   Podiatry: [X]
Psychiatric: [ ]   Transplant: [ ]
Vision: [X]   Wellness: [X]
Workers' Comp: [ ]
Other Benefits:

UNITED BEHAVIORAL HEALTH (UBH)

425 Market Street 27th Fl
San Francisco, CA 94105
Phone: 415-547-5000 Fax: 415-547-6100 Toll-Free:
Web site: www.unitedbehavioralhealth.com
MAILING ADDRESS:
   UNITED BEHAVIORAL HEALTH (UBH)
   425 Market Street 27th Fl
   San Francisco, CA 94105

KEY EXECUTIVES:
Chairman of the Board .... Saul Feldman, MD
Chief Executive Officer .... Gregory A Bayer, PhD
President .... Jim Hudak
Executive VP/Chief Financial Officr .... Karen Schievelbein
Chief Clinical Officer .... Robert Fusco, MD
Pharmacy Director .... Bernice Friscan
Chief Information Officer .... Michael Swanson
Chief Operating Officer .... Jim Hudak
Senior VP, Sales & Marketing .... Julian Cohen
Public Relations Director .... Pamela Beach
Director of Provider Services .... Carol Shaw
Human Resource Director .... Pam Russo
VP, Product Development & Marketing .... Kara Dornig

COMPANY PROFILE:
Parent Company Name: UnitedHealth Group
Doing Business As: UBG
Year Founded: 1979   Federally Qualified: [ ]
Forprofit: [Y]   Not-For-Profit: [ ]
Model Type: NETWORK
Accreditation: [ ] AAPPO [X] JACHO [X] NCQA [X] URAC
Plan Type: Specialty HMO, Specialty PPO, POS, ASO, EPO
Total Revenue: 2005: 125,314,761   2006: 129,361,805
Net Income   2005: 21,582,021   2006: 15,170,855
Total Enrollment:
   2001: 0   2004: 2,319,016   2007: 0
   2002: 1,870,059   2005: 2,636,378
   2003: 0   2006: 2,565,857
Medical Loss Ratio: 2005: 64.42   2006:
Administrative Expense Ratio: 2005: 7.18   2006:

CALIFORNIA   Managed Care Organization Profiles

MAILING ADDRESS:
   SPECTERA VISION SERVICES OF CA
   100 Corporate Point Ste #380
   Culver City, CA 90230

KEY EXECUTIVES:
President .... Paige Sanders
Optometrist Director .... Frank Giardina
Member Service Manager .... Deanna Brown

COMPANY PROFILE:
Parent Company Name: Spectera Vision Services of CA Inc
Doing Business As:
Year Founded: 1983   Federally Qualified: [ ]
Forprofit: [Y]   Not-For-Profit: [ ]
Model Type:
Accreditation: [ ] AAPPO [ ] JACHO [ ] NCQA [ ] URAC
Plan Type: Specialty HMO
Total Revenue: 2005: 4,052,653   2006: 4,350,734
Net Income   2005: -316,752   2006: 783,393
Total Enrollment:
   2001: 67,360   2004: 111,362   2007: 199,318
   2002: 133,295   2005: 160,311
   2003: 114,577   2006: 257,733
Medical Loss Ratio: 2005: 97.05   2006: 52.89
Administrative Expense Ratio: 2005: 15.96   2006: 17.63
SERVICE AREA:
Nationwide: N
  CA (Southern);
TYPE OF COVERAGE:
Commercial: [Y] Individual: [Y] FEHBP: [ ] Indemnity: [ ]
Medicare: [ ] Medicaid: [ ] Supplemental Medicare: [ ]
Tricare   [ ]
PRODUCTS OFFERED:
Product Name: Type:
Eye Care Service Plan   Specialty HMO
PLAN BENEFITS:
Alternative Medicine: [ ]   Behavioral Health: [ ]
Chiropractic: [ ]   Dental: [ ]
Home Care: [ ]   Inpatient SNF: [ ]
Long-Term Care: [ ]   Pharm. Mail Order: [ ]
Physical Therapy: [ ]   Podiatry: [ ]
Psychiatric: [ ]   Transplant: [ ]
Vision: [X]   Wellness: [ ]
Workers' Comp: [ ]
Other Benefits:
Comments:
Formerly Eyecare Service Plan Inc.

STANISLAUS MEDICAL SOCIETY

2339 St Paul's Way
Modesto, CA 95355
Phone: 209-527-1704 Fax: 209-527-5861 Toll-Free:
Web site: www.stanislausmedicalsociety.com
MAILING ADDRESS:
   STANISLAUS MEDICAL SOCIETY
   PO Box 576007
   Modesto, CA 95355

KEY EXECUTIVES:
President .... David Shiba, MD
Treasurer .... Alan Yates, MD

COMPANY PROFILE:
Parent Company Name:
Doing Business As:
Year Founded: Federally Qualified: [ ]
Forprofit: [ ]   Not-For-Profit: [Y]
Model Type:
Accreditation: [ ] AAPPO [ ] JACHO [ ] NCQA [ ] URAC
Plan Type: PPO, TPA, EPO
SERVICE AREA:
Nationwide: N
  CA;
TYPE OF COVERAGE:
Commercial: [Y] Individual: [Y] FEHBP: [ ] Indemnity: [ ]
Medicare: [Y] Medicaid: [ ] Supplemental Medicare: [Y]
Tricare   [ ]

PLAN BENEFITS:
Alternative Medicine: [ ]   Behavioral Health: [X]
Chiropractic: [X]   Dental: [X]
Home Care: [X]   Inpatient SNF: [X]
Long-Term Care: [X]   Pharm. Mail Order: [X]
Physical Therapy: [X]   Podiatry: [X]
Psychiatric: [X]   Transplant: [X]
Vision: [X]   Wellness: [X]
Workers' Comp: [X]
Other Benefits:

SUPERIOR VISION SERVICES INC

24012 Calle de la Plata #470
Laguna Hills, CA 92653-7624
Phone: 949-461-3300 Fax: 949-461-3311 Toll-Free: 800-923-6766
Web site: www.superiorvision.com
MAILING ADDRESS:
   SUPERIOR VISION SERVICES INC
   24012 Calle de la Plata #470
   Laguna Hills, CA 92653-7624

KEY EXECUTIVES:
Chief Executive Officer/President .... Rick P Corbett
VP of Finance .... Joanna Freeman
Chief Operating Officer .... Kimberly Hess
VP, Account Management, Marketing .... Karen O'Brien
VP, Product Development Compliance .. Lori Hemmingsen-Souza, RN
Senior VP, Business Development .... Wayne F Muller
VP Human Resources/Strategic Planning .... Gina Dickey

COMPANY PROFILE:
Parent Company Name:
Doing Business As:
Year Founded: 1993   Federally Qualified: [ ]
Forprofit: [Y]   Not-For-Profit: [ ]
Model Type:
Accreditation: [ ] AAPPO [ ] JACHO [ ] NCQA [ ] URAC
Plan Type: Specialty PPO
SERVICE AREA:
Nationwide: Y
  NW;
TYPE OF COVERAGE:
Commercial: [Y] Individual: [ ] FEHBP: [ ] Indemnity: [ ]
Medicare: [Y] Medicaid: [ ] Supplemental Medicare: [Y]
Tricare   [ ]
PLAN BENEFITS:
Alternative Medicine: [ ]   Behavioral Health: [ ]
Chiropractic: [ ]   Dental: [ ]
Home Care: [ ]   Inpatient SNF: [ ]
Long-Term Care: [ ]   Pharm. Mail Order: [ ]
Physical Therapy: [ ]   Podiatry: [ ]
Psychiatric: [ ]   Transplant: [ ]
Vision: [X]   Wellness: [ ]
Workers' Comp: [ ]
Other Benefits:

TALBERT HEALTH PLAN

1665 Scenic Ave Ste 100
Costa Mesa, CA 92626
Phone: 714-436-4890 Fax: 714-436-4889 Toll-Free:
Web site: www.talbertmedical.com
MAILING ADDRESS:
   TALBERT HEALTH PLAN
   1665 Scenic Ave Ste 100
   Costa Mesa, CA 92626

KEY EXECUTIVES:
Chief Executive Officer/President .... Keith Wilson, MD

COMPANY PROFILE:
Parent Company Name:
Doing Business As:
Year Founded: 2007   Federally Qualified: [ ]
Forprofit: [ ]   Not-For-Profit: [ ]
Model Type:
Accreditation: [ ] AAPPO [ ] JACHO [ ] NCQA [ ] URAC
Plan Type: HMO

Managed Care Organization Profiles — CALIFORNIA

MAILING ADDRESS:
SHARP HEALTH PLAN
4305 University Ave Ste 200
San Diego, CA 92105-1601

KEY EXECUTIVES:
Chief Executive Officer/President .... Melissa Hayden-Cook
Chief Financial Officer .... Rita Oatko
VP, Chief Medical Officer. Pharmacy Director .... Nora Faine, MD
VP, Chief Operating Officer .... Leslie Pels-Beck
VP, Business Development Officer .... Janet Hoy
Regulatory Compliance Officer .... Paul Belton
Public Relations Director .... Stephen Chin
VPChief Medical Officer .... Nora Faine MD
Director Quality Improvement .... Sandra Parkington
Regulatory Compliance Officer .... Paul Belton
VP, Business Development Officer .... Janet Hoy

COMPANY PROFILE:
Parent Company Name: San Diego Hospital Association
Doing Business As: Sharp Healthcare
Year Founded: 1992   Federally Qualified: [ ]
Forprofit: [ ]   Not-For-Profit: [Y]
Model Type: MIXED
Accreditation: [ ] AAPPO [ ] JACHO [ ] NCQA [ ] URAC
Plan Type: HMO
Total Revenue: 2005: 133,103,000   2006: 146,030,000
Net Income   2005: 23,182,000   2006: 746,000
Total Enrollment:
 2001: 101,429   2004: 123,447   2007: 43,816
 2002: 124,200   2005: 51,346
 2003: 126,668   2006: 48,466
Medical Loss Ratio: 2005: 86.65   2006: 90.98
Administrative Expense Ratio: 2005: 7.85   2006: 9.20

SERVICE AREA:
Nationwide: N
 CA (San Diego);

TYPE OF COVERAGE:
Commercial: [Y] Individual: [ ] FEHBP: [ ] Indemnity: [ ]
Medicare: [ ] Medicaid: [Y] Supplemental Medicare: [ ]
Tricare   [ ]

PRODUCTS OFFERED:
Product Name: Type:
Multiple Plans   HMO
Medi-Cal   Medicaid
Healthy Families   HMO
Focus   HMO
Aim   HMO

PLAN BENEFITS:
Alternative Medicine: [X]   Behavioral Health: [X]
Chiropractic: [X]   Dental: [ ]
Home Care: [X]   Inpatient SNF: [X]
Long-Term Care: [ ]   Pharm. Mail Order: [X]
Physical Therapy: [X]   Podiatry: [X]
Psychiatric: [X]   Transplant: [X]
Vision: [X]   Wellness: [X]
Workers' Comp: [ ]
Other Benefits:

SMILECARE/COMMUNITY DENTAL SERVICES

2 MacArthur Pl Ste 700
Santa Ana, CA 92707
Phone: 714-708-5360 Fax: 714-708-5399 Toll-Free: 800-764-5393
Web site: www.smilecare.com

MAILING ADDRESS:
SMILECARE/COMMUNITY DENTAL SRV
PO Box 92009
Los Angeles, CA 92707

KEY EXECUTIVES:
Principal .... Daniel D Crowley
President .... Joseph Sivori
Chief Financial Officer .... Robert Mathuny
Medical Director .... Ivan Berger, DDS, MAGD
VP, Information Systems .... Preet Takkar
Executive VP,Chief Operating Officer .... Patricia Mahony
Senior VP, Bus Development, Marketing/Sales .... Susan Klarner
Plan Operations Director .... Amy Adamo
VP, Human Resources .... Hal Nutter

COMPANY PROFILE:
Parent Company Name:
Doing Business As: Smilecare
Year Founded: 1982   Federally Qualified: [N]
Forprofit: [Y]   Not-For-Profit: [ ]
Model Type:
Accreditation: [ ] AAPPO [ ] JACHO [ ] NCQA [ ] URAC
Plan Type: Specialty HMO, Specialty PPO
Total Revenue: 2005: 22,726,000   2006: 25,968,000
Net Income   2005: -3,147,000   2006: -1,375,000
Total Enrollment:
 2001: 34,487   2004: 326,974   2007: 215,078
 2002: 115,523   2005: 230,260
 2003: 136,450   2006: 211,817
Medical Loss Ratio: 2005: 100.25   2006:
Administrative Expense Ratio: 2005: 13.60   2006:

SERVICE AREA:
Nationwide: N
 CA; NV;

TYPE OF COVERAGE:
Commercial: [Y] Individual: [ ] FEHBP: [ ] Indemnity: [ ]
Medicare: [ ] Medicaid: [ ] Supplemental Medicare: [ ]
Tricare   [ ]

PRODUCTS OFFERED:
Product Name: Type:
Community Dental Services   Specialty HMO

PLAN BENEFITS:
Alternative Medicine: [ ]   Behavioral Health: [ ]
Chiropractic: [ ]   Dental: [X]
Home Care: [ ]   Inpatient SNF: [ ]
Long-Term Care: [ ]   Pharm. Mail Order: [ ]
Physical Therapy: [ ]   Podiatry: [ ]
Psychiatric: [ ]   Transplant: [ ]
Vision: [ ]   Wellness: [ ]
Workers' Comp: [ ]
Other Benefits:

SOUTH BAY INDEPENDENT PHYSICIANS MEDICAL GROUP INC

3480 Torrance Blvd #220
Torrance, CA 90503
Phone: 310-543-8805 Fax: 310-543-8811 Toll-Free:
Web site: www.sbipmedicalgroup.com

MAILING ADDRESS:
SOUTH BAY INDEPENDENT
PHYSICIANS MEDICAL GROUP
3480 Torrance Blvd #220
Torrance, CA 90503

KEY EXECUTIVES:
Executive Director .... William T Ross
President .... Thomas LaGralious
Director/Finance & Member Services ...... Samm M List, CPHQ, CPCS
Director of Operations .... Lisa M DiLeva
Human Resources Director .... Samm M List

COMPANY PROFILE:
Parent Company Name:
Doing Business As:
Year Founded: 1984   Federally Qualified: [ ]
Forprofit: [Y]   Not-For-Profit: [ ]
Model Type: NETWORK
Accreditation: [ ] AAPPO [ ] JACHO [ ] NCQA [ ] URAC
Plan Type: PPO, POS, EPO
Total Enrollment:
 2001: 979,000   2004: 0   2007: 0
 2002: 0   2005:
 2003: 0   2006:

SERVICE AREA:
Nationwide: N
 CA; (Los Angeles, Marina Del Ray, South Bay);

TYPE OF COVERAGE:
Commercial: [Y] Individual: [Y] FEHBP: [ ] Indemnity: [ ]
Medicare: [ ] Medicaid: [ ] Supplemental Medicare: [Y]
Tricare   [ ]

SPECTERA VISION SERVICES OF CALIFORNIA INC

100 Corporate Point Ste #380
Culver City, CA 90230
Phone: 310-242-6200 Fax: 310-242-6222 Toll-Free:
Web site: www.spectera.com

CALIFORNIA　　　　　　　　　　　　　　　　　　　　　　　　　　　　　　　　Managed Care Organization Profiles

KEY EXECUTIVES:
Chief Executive Officer .... Scott Wells
President .... Mateo De Soto, MD
Chief Financial Officer .... Chris Cheney
Medical Director .... Daniel Bluestone, MD
Chief Information Officer .... Alice Allman
Marketing Manager .... Christi Rolff
MIS Director .... JP Muro

COMPANY PROFILE:
Parent Company Name: Community Hospitals
Doing Business As:
Year Founded: 1994　　　　　Federally Qualified: [N]
Forprofit: [Y]　　　　　　　　Not-For-Profit: [ ]
Model Type: IPA
Accreditation: [ ] AAPPO [ ] JACHO [ ] NCQA [ ] URAC
Plan Type: HMO, POS, TPA
Total Enrollment:
　2001: 140,000　　2004: 0　　　2007: 0
　2002: 0　　　　　2005:
　2003: 0　　　　　2006:

SERVICE AREA:
Nationwide: N
　CA (Fresno, Madera, Kings);

TYPE OF COVERAGE:
Commercial: [Y] Individual: [ ]　FEHBP: [ ]　Indemnity: [ ]
Medicare:　[Y] Medicaid: [ ]　Supplemental Medicare: [ ]
Tricare　　[ ]

PLAN BENEFITS:
Alternative Medicine:　[ ]　　Behavioral Health:　[ ]
Chiropractic:　　　　　[ ]　　Dental:　　　　　　[ ]
Home Care:　　　　　　[ ]　　Inpatient SNF:　　　[ ]
Long-Term Care:　　　　[ ]　　Pharm. Mail Order:　[ ]
Physical Therapy:　　　 [ ]　　Podiatry:　　　　　[X]
Psychiatric:　　　　　　[ ]　　Transplant:　　　　[ ]
Vision:　　　　　　　　[ ]　　Wellness:　　　　　[ ]
Workers' Comp:　　　　[X]
Other Benefits:

SCAN HEALTH PLAN

3800 Kilroy Airport Way #100
Long Beach, CA 90806
Phone: 562-989-5100　Fax: 562-989-5200　Toll-Free: 800-247-5091
Web site: www.scanhealthplan.com

MAILING ADDRESS:
　SCAN HEALTH PLAN
　3800 Kilroy Airport Way #100
　Long Beach, CA 90806

KEY EXECUTIVES:
Chairman of the Board .... Mike Noel
Chief Executive Officer .... Dave Schmidt
Chief Financial Officer .... Dennis Eder
Chief Medical Officer .... Timothy Schwab, MD
Pharmacy Director .... Sharon Bakshi, PharmD
Chief Information Officer .... Roy Swackhamer
Marketing Senior VP .... Sherry Stanislaw
VP, MIS .... Allan Shiraishi
Senior VP, Compliance Officer .... Rebecca Learner
Senior VP, Network Management .... Elizabeth Russell
Senior VP, Human Resources .... Marc Radner
VP Internal Audit .... Christian Zorn
Senior VP, General Counsel .... Douglas Jaques
Senior VP, Sales/Membership .... Roger Lapp
Senior VP, Health Care Services .... Deborah Miller
Senior VP, Business Development .... Hank Osowski

COMPANY PROFILE:
Parent Company Name: SCAN Health Plan
Doing Business As:
Year Founded: 1985　　　　Federally Qualified: [ ]
Forprofit: [ ]　　　　　　　Not-For-Profit: [Y]
Model Type: IPA
Accreditation: [ ] AAPPO [ ] JACHO [ ] NCQA [ ] URAC
Plan Type: HMO
Total Revenue:　2005: 975,285,418　　2006: 1,326,135,424
Net Income　　 2005: 140,717,464　　2006: 184,807,973

Total Enrollment:
　2001: 52,863　　2004: 65,482　　2007: 101,464
　2002: 55,419　　2005: 78,493
　2003: 52,945　　2006: 90,213
Medical Loss Ratio:　　　　　　2005: 90.11　　2006: 82.48
Administrative Expense Ratio:　2005:　7.35　　2006:　6.98

SERVICE AREA:
Nationwide: N
　CA (Kern, Los Angeles, Orange, Riverside, San Bernardino, San Diego, Ventura); AZ (Maricopa);

TYPE OF COVERAGE:
Commercial: [ ] Individual: [ ]　FEHBP: [ ]　Indemnity: [ ]
Medicare:　[Y] Medicaid: [ ]　Supplemental Medicare: [ ]
Tricare　　[ ]

PRODUCTS OFFERED:
Product Name:　　　　　　　　　Type:
Smartcare Health　　　　　　　　Medicare Advantage
Medi-Cal　　　　　　　　　　　　Medicaid

PLAN BENEFITS:
Alternative Medicine:　[ ]　　Behavioral Health:　[ ]
Chiropractic:　　　　　[ ]　　Dental:　　　　　　[ ]
Home Care:　　　　　　[X]　　Inpatient SNF:　　　[ ]
Long-Term Care:　　　　[ ]　　Pharm. Mail Order:　[ ]
Physical Therapy:　　　 [ ]　　Podiatry:　　　　　[ ]
Psychiatric:　　　　　　[ ]　　Transplant:　　　　[ ]
Vision:　　　　　　　　[ ]　　Wellness:　　　　　[ ]
Workers' Comp:　　　　[ ]
Other Benefits:

SCRIPPS CLINIC HEALTH PLAN SERVICES INC

10170 Sorrento Valley Rd SV4
San Diego, CA 92121
Phone: 858-784-5961　Fax: 858-784-5837　Toll-Free:
Web site: www.scrippsclinic.com

MAILING ADDRESS:
　SCRIPPS CLINIC HLTH PLN SRVS
　10170 Sorrento Valley Rd SV4
　San Diego, CA 92121

KEY EXECUTIVES:
Chief Executive Officer .... Larry J Harrison, MBA
Director of Finance/Compliance .... Chris Fritz
Medical Director .... Dan Dworsky, MD
Compliance Officer .... Kirsten L Patalano

COMPANY PROFILE:
Parent Company Name:
Doing Business As:
Year Founded: 1999　　　　Federally Qualified: [ ]
Forprofit: [ ]　　　　　　　Not-For-Profit: [Y]
Model Type:
Accreditation: [ ] AAPPO [ ] JACHO [ ] NCQA [ ] URAC
Plan Type: HMO,
Total Revenue:　2005: 33,847,129　　2006: 35,616,272
Net Income　　 2005: -34,611　　　　2006: -7,092
Total Enrollment:
　2001: 174,013　　2004: 40,098　　2007: 47,610
　2002: 141,752　　2005: 38,523
　2003: 71,229　　 2006: 37,600
Medical Loss Ratio:　　　　　　2005: 100.08　　2006: 100.55
Administrative Expense Ratio:　2005:　5.32　　 2006:　5.20

SERVICE AREA:
Nationwide: N
　CA;

PRODUCTS OFFERED:
Product Name:　　　　　　　　　　　Type:
Scripps Clinic Health Plan Services　　HMO
Scripps Clinic Health Plan Services　　Medicare

SHARP HEALTH PLAN

4305 University Ave Ste 200
San Diego, CA 92105-1601
Phone: 619-228-2300　Fax: 619-228-2444　Toll-Free: 800-359-2002
Web site: www.sharp.com

Managed Care Organization Profiles — CALIFORNIA

SAN JOAQUIN FOUNDATION PPO

PO Box 779
Murphys, CA 95247
Phone: 209-952-5299 Fax: 209-952-5298 Toll-Free:
Web site:

MAILING ADDRESS:
SAN JOAQUIN FOUNDATION PPO
PO Box 779
Murphys, CA 95247

KEY EXECUTIVES:
Executive Director ....Dorothy Anderson
President .... Michael Williams, Esq
Chief Financial Officer ....Randit Singh
Medical Director ....Roland Hart, MD
Marketing Director .... Gary Anderson
Credentialing Manager/Provider Services Director . Dorothy Anderson
Associate Executive Director ....Dianne Maness

COMPANY PROFILE:
Parent Company Name:
Doing Business As:
Year Founded: 1953   Federally Qualified: [ ]
Forprofit: [ ]   Not-For-Profit: [Y]
Model Type: NETWORK
Accreditation: [ ] AAPPO [ ] JACHO [ ] NCQA [ ] URAC
Plan Type: PPO, UR, EPO

SERVICE AREA:
Nationwide: N
  CA;

TYPE OF COVERAGE:
Commercial: [Y] Individual: [Y] FEHBP: [ ] Indemnity: [ ]
Medicare: [Y] Medicaid: [Y] Supplemental Medicare: [Y]
Tricare   [ ]

PLAN BENEFITS:
Alternative Medicine:	[ ]	Behavioral Health:	[X]
Chiropractic:	[X]	Dental:	[ ]
Home Care:	[X]	Inpatient SNF:	[X]
Long-Term Care:	[X]	Pharm. Mail Order:	[X]
Physical Therapy:	[X]	Podiatry:	[X]
Psychiatric:	[X]	Transplant:	[X]
Vision:	[X]	Wellness:	[X]
Workers' Comp:	[X]		

Other Benefits:
:

SANTA BARBARA REGIONAL HEALTH AUTHORITY

110 Castilian Dr
Goleta, CA 93117-3028
Phone: 805-685-9525 Fax: 805-685-8292 Toll-Free:
Web site: www.sbrha.org

MAILING ADDRESS:
SANTA BARBARA REGIONAL HEALTH AUTHORITY
110 Castilian Dr
Goleta, CA 93117-3028

KEY EXECUTIVES:
Chief Financial Officer .... Elaine Bowling
Medical Director .... Karen Moyes, MD
Pharmacy Director .... Randy Seifert
Director of Information Technology .... Michael Schrader
Chief Operating Officer .... Robert Freeman
Director of Provider Services ....Jacqueline Wright
Director of Human Resources... Betsy Redfield

COMPANY PROFILE:
Parent Company Name:
Doing Business As:
Year Founded: 1983   Federally Qualified: [ ]
Forprofit: [ ]   Not-For-Profit: [ ]
Model Type:
Accreditation: [ ] AAPPO [ ] JACHO [ ] NCQA [ ] URAC
Plan Type: HMO
Total Revenue: 2005: 39,634,425   2006: 37,303,204
Net Income   2005: -2,763,860   2006:   3,054,152
Total Enrollment:
  2001: 0   2004: 56,157   2007: 57,983
  2002: 52,398   2005: 56,281
  2003: 54,726   2006: 56,824
Medical Loss Ratio: 2005: 100.81   2006: 94.95
Administrative Expense Ratio: 2005:   6.92   2006: 7.07

SERVICE AREA:
Nationwide: N
  CA;

TYPE OF COVERAGE:
Commercial: [ ] Individual: [ ] FEHBP: [ ] Indemnity: [ ]
Medicare: [ ] Medicaid: [Y] Supplemental Medicare: [ ]
Tricare   [ ]

PRODUCTS OFFERED:
Product Name: Type:
Medi-Cal   Medicaid

SANTA CLARA FAMILY HEALTH PLAN

210 E Hacienda Ave
Campbell, CA 95008
Phone: 408-376-2000 Fax: 408-874-1955 Toll-Free: 800-260-2055
Web site: www.scfhp.com

MAILING ADDRESS:
SANTA CLARA FAMILY HLTH PLN
210 E Hacienda Ave
Campbell, CA 95008

KEY EXECUTIVES:
Chief Executive Officer ....Leona M Butler
Chief Financial Officer ....Ronald Wojtaszek
Medical Director .... Dennis Collins, MD
Chief Information Officer .... John Pawlyshyn
Marketing Director .... Mary Ellen Sweeney
Director, Community Relations .... Marta Avelar
Director of Provider Services ....Pamela Bohlmann
Health Education Manager .... Susana Razo
Human Resources Director ....Barbara Elsea
Quality Assurance Director ....Christine Gerbo
VP of Health Affairs .... Lisa Kraymer
VP of Gvrnmnt Affairs/General Counsel......................Sheila Maloney
Member Service Director .... Pat Posey
Utilization Management Director ....Carrie Tice

COMPANY PROFILE:
Parent Company Name: Santa Clara County Health Authority
Doing Business As: Santa Clara Family Health Plan
Year Founded: 1995   Federally Qualified: [N]
Forprofit: [ ]   Not-For-Profit: [Y]
Model Type: STAFF
Accreditation: [ ] AAPPO [ ] JACHO [ ] NCQA [ ] URAC
Plan Type: HMO
Total Revenue: 2005: 35,194,917   2006: 36,119,587
Net Income   2005:   631,462   2006:   597,677
Total Enrollment:
  2001: 57,613   2004: 95,621   2007: 100,975
  2002: 83,973   2005: 95,332
  2003: 95,943   2006: 98,296
Medical Loss Ratio: 2005: 97.65   2006: 97.96
Administrative Expense Ratio: 2005: 11.32   2006: 12.12

SERVICE AREA:
Nationwide: N
  CA (Santa Clara);

TYPE OF COVERAGE:
Commercial: [Y] Individual: [ ] FEHBP: [ ] Indemnity: [ ]
Medicare: [ ] Medicaid: [Y] Supplemental Medicare: [ ]
Tricare   [ ]

PRODUCTS OFFERED:
Product Name: Type:
Medi-Cal   Medicaid
                                       HMO

SANTE COMMUNITY PHYSICIANS

1180 E Shaw Ave Ste 201
Fresno, CA 93710
Phone: 559-228-4206 Fax: 559-224-8461 Toll-Free: 800-652-2900
Web site:

MAILING ADDRESS:
SANTE COMMUNITY PHYSICIANS
1180 E Shaw Ave Ste 201
Fresno, CA 93710

CALIFORNIA   Managed Care Organization Profiles

ROBERT T DORRIS ASSOCIATES

31416 Agoura Rd Ste 180
Westlake Village, CA 91361
Phone: 818-707-0544 Fax: 818-707-0496 Toll-Free:
Web site: www.dorris.com
MAILING ADDRESS:
  ROBERT T DORRIS ASSOCIATES
  31416 Agoura Rd Ste 180
  Westlake Village, CA 91361

KEY EXECUTIVES:
Chief Executive Officer .... Robert T Dorris, Jr

COMPANY PROFILE:
Parent Company Name:
Doing Business As:
Year Founded: Federally Qualified: [ ]
Forprofit: [ ]   Not-For-Profit: [ ]
Model Type:
Accreditation: [ ] AAPPO [ ] JACHO [ ] NCQA [ ] URAC
Plan Type: Specialty HMO
Total Revenue: 2005:   400,564   2006:   1,959,818
Net Income   2005:   -54,014   2006:   97,112
Total Enrollment:
  2001: 0   2004: 138   2007: 14,750
  2002: 0   2005: 3,020
  2003: 0   2006: 4,428
Medical Loss Ratio: 2005: 67.84   2006: 66.88
Administrative Expense Ratio: 2005: 48.20   2006: 32.66
SERVICE AREA:
Nationwide:
  CA;
PRODUCTS OFFERED:
Product Name: Type:
                                    HMO
PLAN BENEFITS:
Alternative Medicine: [ ]   Behavioral Health: [ ]
Chiropractic: [ ]   Dental: [ ]
Home Care: [ ]   Inpatient SNF: [ ]
Long-Term Care: [ ]   Pharm. Mail Order: [ ]
Physical Therapy: [ ]   Podiatry: [ ]
Psychiatric: [X]   Transplant: [ ]
Vision: [ ]   Wellness: [ ]
Workers' Comp: [ ]
Other Benefits:

SAFEGUARD HEALTH ENTERPRISES INC

95 Enterprise Ste 100
Aliso Viejo, CA 92656-2601
Phone: 949-425-4300 Fax: 949-425-4587 Toll-Free: 800-204-0463
Web site: www.safeguard.net
MAILING ADDRESS:
  SAFEGUARD HEALTH ENTERPRISES
  95 Enterprise Ste 100
  Aliso Viejo, CA 92656-2601

KEY EXECUTIVES:
Chief Executive Officer/President .... Stephen Baker
Senior VPChief Financial Officer .... Dennis Gates
Dental Director .... Raymond Osbrink, MD
Chief Information Officer .... Mike Lauffenburger
Executive VP, Chief Operating Officer .... Steve Baker
VP, Marketing/Chief Marketing Officer .... Ken Keating
VP, Provider Relations .... Judy M Deal
Director Network Management .... Tyrette Hamilton
VP, Service Center Operations .... Barbara Lucci
Senior VP, General Counsel .... Ronald I Brendzel

COMPANY PROFILE:
Parent Company Name: Safeguard Health Enterprises, Inc
Doing Business As:
Year Founded: 1974   Federally Qualified: [N]
Forprofit: [Y]   Not-For-Profit: [ ]
Model Type: NETWORK
Accreditation: [ ] AAPPO [ ] JACHO [ ] NCQA [ ] URAC
Plan Type: Specialty HMO, Specialty PPO, ASO
Total Revenue: 2005: 26,005,000   2006: 106,224,000
Net Income   2005:   1,334,000   2006:   8,521,000
Total Enrollment:
  2001: 310,526   2004: 750,497   2007: 1,030,452
  2002: 275,234   2005: 1,040,900
  2003: 300,356   2006: 1,085,630
Medical Loss Ratio: 2005: 69.17   2006: 65.18
Administrative Expense Ratio: 2005: 22.56   2006: 21.50
SERVICE AREA:
Nationwide: N
  AZ; CA; CO; IL; KA; MO; NV; OK; TX;
TYPE OF COVERAGE:
Commercial: [Y] Individual: [Y] FEHBP: [ ] Indemnity: [ ]
Medicare: [ ] Medicaid: [ ] Supplemental Medicare: [ ]
Tricare   [ ]
PRODUCTS OFFERED:
Product Name: Type:
Medi-Cal   Medicaid
Safeguard   Medicare
Safeguard   HMO
PLAN BENEFITS:
Alternative Medicine: [ ]   Behavioral Health: [ ]
Chiropractic: [ ]   Dental: [X]
Home Care: [ ]   Inpatient SNF: [ ]
Long-Term Care: [ ]   Pharm. Mail Order: [ ]
Physical Therapy: [ ]   Podiatry: [ ]
Psychiatric: [ ]   Transplant: [ ]
Vision: [X]   Wellness: [ ]
Workers' Comp: [ ]
Other Benefits:
Comments:
Purchased GE Dental & Vision, 2005. Acquired Smile Saver Dental & Vision of California.

SAN FRANCISCO HEALTH PLAN

201 Third St 7th Fl
San Francisco, CA 94103
Phone: 415-547-7818 Fax: 415-547-7826 Toll-Free: 800-288-5555
Web site: www.sfhp.org
MAILING ADDRESS:
  SAN FRANCISCO HEALTH PLAN
  201 Third St 7th Fl
  San Francisco, CA 94103

KEY EXECUTIVES:
Governing Board Chair .... Mitchell Katz, MD
Chief Executive Officer .... Jean S Frasier
Chief Financial Officer .... Kelvin Quan
Medical Director .... Michael Van Duren, MD
Clinical Pharmacist .... Allison Lun
Provider Relations Manager .... Taylor Winston
Director of Human Resources .... Victoria Carovello
Medical Management Director .... Betsy Price, MD

COMPANY PROFILE:
Parent Company Name:
Doing Business As:
Year Founded: 1994   Federally Qualified: [ ]
Forprofit: [ ]   Not-For-Profit: [Y]
Model Type:
Accreditation: [ ] AAPPO [ ] JACHO [ ] NCQA [ ] URAC
Plan Type: HMO
Total Revenue: 2005: 23,166,990   2006: 23,135,760
Net Income   2005:   1,287,105   2006: -2,744,420
Total Enrollment:
  2001: 34,404   2004: 48,523   2007: 53,152
  2002: 40,151   2005: 51,262
  2003: 45,013   2006: 51,660
Medical Loss Ratio: 2005: 89.32   2006: 91.49
Administrative Expense Ratio: 2005:   8.45   2006:   9.00
SERVICE AREA:
Nationwide: N
  CA (San Francisco);
TYPE OF COVERAGE:
Commercial: [ ] Individual: [ ] FEHBP: [ ] Indemnity:[ ]Medi-
care: [Y] Medicaid: [Y] Supplemental Medicare: [ ]
Tricare   [ ]
PRODUCTS OFFERED:
Product Name: Type:
Medi-Cal   Medicaid
San Francisco Health Plan   HMO

Managed Care Organization Profiles — CALIFORNIA

TYPE OF COVERAGE:
Commercial: [ ] Individual: [ ] FEHBP: [ ] Indemnity: [ ]
Medicare: [Y] Medicaid: [ ] Supplemental Medicare: [ ]
Tricare [ ]
PRODUCTS OFFERED:
Product Name: Type:
Access Health Direct   PPO
PLAN BENEFITS:
Alternative Medicine: [ ]   Behavioral Health: [ ]
Chiropractic: [X]   Dental: [ ]
Home Care: [ ]   Inpatient SNF: [X]
Long-Term Care: [ ]   Pharm. Mail Order: [ ]
Physical Therapy: [X]   Podiatry: [X]
Psychiatric: [X]   Transplant: [ ]
Vision: [X]   Wellness: [X]
Workers' Comp: [X]
Other Benefits: X

PRIMECARE MEDICAL NETWORK INC

3281 E Guasti Rd 7th Fl
Ontario, CA 91761
Phone: 909-605-8000 Fax: 909-605-8031 Toll-Free: 800-864-7500
Web site: www.nammcal.com
MAILING ADDRESS:
  PRIMECARE MEDICAL NETWORK INC
  3281 E Guasti Rd 7th Fl
  Ontario, CA 91761

KEY EXECUTIVES:
Chief Executive Officer/President .... Richard Shinto
Chief Financial Officer .... Julian Santoyo
Medical Director .... Rod St Clair, MD
Chief Information Officer .... Scott Thompson
Senior VP, Chief Operating Officer .... Leigh Hutchins
Marketing Director .... David Mellentine
VP, Human Resources .... Patricia Gutierrez
VP, Chief Administrator .... Karen Gee
VP, Legal Affairs, Corporate Counsl .... Elizabeth Haughton, JD
VP, Transactional Services .... Judi McGee

COMPANY PROFILE:
Parent Company Name: Primecare Internation & N American Med M
Doing Business As: Primecare Medical Network Inc
Year Founded: 1998   Federally Qualified: [Y]
Forprofit: [Y]   Not-For-Profit: [ ]
Model Type: MIXED
Accreditation: [ ] AAPPO [ ] JACHO [ ] NCQA [ ] URAC
Plan Type: HMO, POS
Total Revenue: 2005: 71,511,270   2006: 312,171,099
Net Income   2005:   11,307   2006: -1,326,718
Total Enrollment:
  2001: 246,258   2004: 234,766   2007: 215,166
  2002: 262,401   2005: 230,814
  2003: 240,336   2006: 220,236
Medical Loss Ratio: 2005: 66.61   2006: 80.90
Administrative Expense Ratio: 2005: 33.20   2006: 15.59
SERVICE AREA:
Nationwide: N
  CA;
TYPE OF COVERAGE:
Commercial: [Y] Individual: [Y] FEHBP: [ ] Indemnity: [ ]
Medicare: [Y] Medicaid: [Y] Supplemental Medicare: [Y]
Tricare [ ]

PRIVATE HEALTHCARE SYSTEMS - CALIFORNIA

3345 Michelson Dr Ste 200
Irvine, CA 92612
Phone: 949-476-9816 Fax: 949-476-0650 Toll-Free: 800-253-4417
Web site: www.phcs.com
MAILING ADDRESS:
  PRIVATE HEALTHCARE SYSTEMS-CA
  1100 Winter St
  Waltham, MA 92612

KEY EXECUTIVES:
Chief Executive Officer/President .... Mark Tabak
Executive VP, Chief Financial Officer .... Richard Gerstein
Medical Director .... Dr Goldstein
Executive VP, Chief of Operations .... Michael Ferrante
Executive VP, Marketing .... Warren Handelman

COMPANY PROFILE:
Parent Company Name: MultiPlan Inc
Doing Business As:
Year Founded: 1985   Federally Qualified: [N]
Forprofit: [Y]   Not-For-Profit: [ ]
Model Type:
Accreditation: [X] AAPPO [ ] JACHO [X] NCQA [X] URAC
Plan Type: PPO, UR, POS
SERVICE AREA:
Nationwide: N
  NW;
TYPE OF COVERAGE:
Commercial: [Y] Individual: [ ] FEHBP: [ ] Indemnity: [ ]
Medicare: [ ] Medicaid: [ ] Supplemental Medicare: [ ]
Tricare [ ]
PLAN BENEFITS:
Alternative Medicine: [X]   Behavioral Health: [X]
Chiropractic: [X]   Dental: [ ]
Home Care: [X]   Inpatient SNF: [X]
Long-Term Care: [X]   Pharm. Mail Order: [X]
Physical Therapy: [X]   Podiatry: [X]
Psychiatric: [X]   Transplant: [X]
Vision: [X]   Wellness: [ ]
Workers' Comp: [X]
Other Benefits: X
Comments:
Acquired by MultiPlan, Inc. on October 18, 2006.

PTPN - CORPORATE HEADQUARTERS

26635 W Agoura Rd #250
Calabasas, CA 91302
Phone: 818-883-7876 Fax: 818-737-0260 Toll-Free: 800-766-7876
Web site: www.ptpn.com
MAILING ADDRESS:
  PTPN - CORPORATE HEADQUARTERS
  26635 W Agoura Rd #250
  Calabasas, CA 91302

KEY EXECUTIVES:
Chief Executive Officer/President .... Michael Weinper, MPH, PT
Information Systems Director .... Kevin Gentry
Vice President .... Nancy Rothenberg
Marketing Director .... Stephen Moore
Provider Services Manager .... Dena Frost
Quality Assurance Director .... Mitchel Kaye, PT

COMPANY PROFILE:
Parent Company Name:
Doing Business As: PTPN
Year Founded: 1985   Federally Qualified: [N]
Forprofit: [Y]   Not-For-Profit: [ ]
Model Type: NETWORK
Accreditation: [ ] AAPPO [ ] JACHO [X] NCQA [ ] URAC
Plan Type: Specialty PPO
Primary Physicians: Physician Specialists: 4,400
SERVICE AREA:
Nationwide: Y
  NW;
TYPE OF COVERAGE:
Commercial: [Y] Individual: [ ] FEHBP: [ ] Indemnity: [ ]
Medicare: [ ] Medicaid: [ ] Supplemental Medicare: [ ]
Tricare [ ]
PLAN BENEFITS:
Alternative Medicine: [ ]   Behavioral Health: [ ]
Chiropractic: [ ]   Dental: [ ]
Home Care: [ ]   Inpatient SNF: [ ]
Long-Term Care: [ ]   Pharm. Mail Order: [ ]
Physical Therapy: [ ]   Podiatry: [ ]
Psychiatric: [ ]   Transplant: [ ]
Vision: [ ]   Wellness: [ ]
Workers' Comp: [ ]
Other Benefits: Occupational Therapy, Speech Therapy

CALIFORNIA

COMPANY PROFILE:
Parent Company Name:
Doing Business As:
Year Founded: Federally Qualified: [ ]
Forprofit: [Y]   Not-For-Profit: [ ]
Model Type: GROUP
Accreditation: [ ] AAPPO [ ] JACHO [ ] NCQA [ ] URAC
Plan Type: HMO, HDHP, HSA,
SERVICE AREA:
Nationwide:
  CA;
TYPE OF COVERAGE:
Commercial: [ ] Individual: [ ] FEHBP: [ ] Indemnity: [ ]
Medicare: [Y] Medicaid: [ ] Supplemental Medicare: [ ]
Tricare   [ ]

PARTNERSHIP HEALTHPLAN OF CALIFORNIA

360 Campus Lane Ste 100
Fairfield City, CA 94534
Phone: 707-863-4100 Fax: 707-863-4117 Toll-Free: 800-863-4155
Web site: www.partnershiphp.org
MAILING ADDRESS:
  PARTNERSHIP HEALTHPLAN OF CA
  360 Campus Lane Ste 100
  Fairfield City, CA 94534

KEY EXECUTIVES:
Chief Executive Officer .... Jack Horn
Chief Financial Officer .... Gary Erickson
Medical Director .... Chris Cammisa, MD
Pharmacy Services Director .... John Krainert
Chief Information Officer .... Lyman Dennis
Privacy Officer/Health Services Director .... Terri Stanley, RN, MPA
Provider Relations Director .... Mary Kerlin
Director of Administration .... Sue Monez
Member Services Director .... Debbie Shafer
Government Relations Director .... Liz Gibboney
Claims Director .... Paula Frederickson

COMPANY PROFILE:
Parent Company Name:
Doing Business As: Solano-Napa-Yolo Commssn on Medical Care
Year Founded: 1994   Federally Qualified: [N]
Forprofit: [ ]   Not-For-Profit: [Y]
Model Type:
Accreditation: [ ] AAPPO [ ] JACHO [ ] NCQA [ ] URAC
Plan Type: HMO
Total Revenue: 2005:   2006:   66,168,047
Net Income   2005:   2006:   -4,979,905
Total Enrollment:
  2001: 74,000   2004: 0   2007: 9,028
  2002: 0   2005:
  2003: 0   2006: 88,424
Medical Loss Ratio: 2005:   2006: 103.97
Administrative Expense Ratio: 2005:   2006:   5.51
SERVICE AREA:
Nationwide: N
  CA (Napa, Solano, Yolo);
TYPE OF COVERAGE:
Commercial: [ ] Individual: [Y] FEHBP: [ ] Indemnity: [ ]
Medicare: [Y] Medicaid: [Y] Supplemental Medicare: [ ]
Tricare   [ ]
PRODUCTS OFFERED:
Product Name: Type:
Medi-Cal   Medicaid
PLAN BENEFITS:
Alternative Medicine: [ ]   Behavioral Health: [ ]
Chiropractic: [X]   Dental: [ ]
Home Care: [ ]   Inpatient SNF: [X]
Long-Term Care: [X]   Pharm. Mail Order: [ ]
Physical Therapy: [X]   Podiatry: [ ]
Psychiatric: [ ]   Transplant: [ ]
Vision: [X]   Wellness: [ ]
Workers' Comp: [ ]
Other Benefits:

PHYSICIANS FOUNDATION FOR MEDICAL CARE

1112 Bascom Ave
San Jose, CA 95128
Phone: 408-248-9400 Fax: 951-686-1692 Toll-Free:
Web site: www.cfmcnet.org
MAILING ADDRESS:
  PHYSICIANS FOUNADTION MEDICAL CARE
  PO Box 5760
  San Jose, CA 95128

KEY EXECUTIVES:
Chief Executive Officer .... Jim Reikes
Chief Financial Officer .... Michael Ulrich
Medical Director .... Don Allari, MD
Marketing Director .... Jacquelyn Sullivan

COMPANY PROFILE:
Parent Company Name:
Doing Business As:
Year Founded: 1960   Federally Qualified: [N]
Forprofit: [Y]   Not-For-Profit: [ ]
Model Type:
Accreditation: [ ] AAPPO [X] JACHO [X] NCQA [ ] URAC
Plan Type: PPO, EPO:
Total Enrollment:
  2001: 0   2004: 0   2007: 0
  2002: 59,000   2005:
  2003: 51,000   2006:
Medical Loss Ratio: 2005:   2006:
Administrative Expense Ratio: 2005:   2006:
SERVICE AREA:
Nationwide: N
  CA;
TYPE OF COVERAGE:
Commercial: [Y] Individual: [ ] FEHBP: [ ] Indemnity: [ ]
Medicare: [ ] Medicaid: [ ] Supplemental Medicare: [ ]
Tricare   [ ]
PRODUCTS OFFERED:
Product Name: Type:
Physicians Fndtn Medical Care   PPO
PLAN BENEFITS:
Alternative Medicine: [ ]   Behavioral Health: [X]
Chiropractic: [X]   Dental: [ ]
Home Care: [X]   Inpatient SNF: [X]
Long-Term Care: [ ]   Pharm. Mail Order: [ ]
Physical Therapy: [X]   Podiatry: [X]
Psychiatric: [X]   Transplant: [X]
Vision: [ ]   Wellness: [X]
Workers' Comp: [X]
Other Benefits:

PRIMARY PROVIDER MANAGEMENT COMPANY INC

9275 Sky Park Ct Ste 400
San Diego, CA 92123
Phone: 858-467-7600 Fax: 858-467-7649 Toll-Free:
Web site: www.ppmcinc.com
MAILING ADDRESS:
  PRIMARY PROVIDER MANAGEMENT CO INC
  9275 Sky Park Ct Ste 400
  San Diego, CA 92123

KEY EXECUTIVES:
Chief Executive Officer .... R W Dukes, MD
President .... Jay Zybelman
Chief Financial Officer .... Bennett O Voit
Medical Director .... Nick Marciano, MD
Chief Information Officer .... Michael Chipperfield
Director of Operations .... Linda Hernandez
Human Resources Director .... Sandy Fuerish

COMPANY PROFILE:
Parent Company Name:
Doing Business As:
Year Founded: 1983   Federally Qualified: [ ]
Forprofit: [Y]   Not-For-Profit: [ ]
Model Type: IPA
Accreditation: [ ] AAPPO [ ] JACHO [ ] NCQA [ ] URAC
Plan Type: PPO, TPA
SERVICE AREA:
Nationwide: N
  CA;

Managed Care Organization Profiles CALIFORNIA

MAILING ADDRESS:
   PACIFIC HEALTH ALLIANCE
   1350 Old Bayshore Hwy #560
   Burlingame, CA 94010

KEY EXECUTIVES:
Chief Executive Officer .... Lawrence W Cappel, PhD
Medical Director .... Steven Slack
Executive VP & Chief Operating Officer .... Robert Mackler
Marketing Director .... Brian Thornberry
Director of Provider Services .... Allison Sparks

COMPANY PROFILE:
Parent Company Name:
Doing Business As:
Year Founded: 1986   Federally Qualified: [N]
Forprofit: [Y]   Not-For-Profit: [ ]
Model Type:
Accreditation: [ ] AAPPO [ ] JACHO [ ] NCQA [ ] URAC
Plan Type: PPO, UR

SERVICE AREA:
Nationwide: N
   CA; NV;

TYPE OF COVERAGE:
Commercial: [Y] Individual: [ ] FEHBP: [ ] Indemnity: [ ]
Medicare: [ ] Medicaid: [ ] Supplemental Medicare: [ ]
Tricare [ ]

PLAN BENEFITS:
Alternative Medicine: [ ]   Behavioral Health: [X]
Chiropractic: [X]   Dental: [ ]
Home Care: [X]   Inpatient SNF: [X]
Long-Term Care: [ ]   Pharm. Mail Order: [ ]
Physical Therapy: [X]   Podiatry: [X]
Psychiatric: [X]   Transplant: [X]
Vision: [X]   Wellness: [ ]
Workers' Comp: [X]
Other Benefits:

PACIFIC IPA

9700 Flair Dr
El Monte, CA 91731
Phone: 626-652-3500 Fax: 626-401-1676 Toll-Free: 888-888-PIPA
Web site: www.pacificipa.com

MAILING ADDRESS:
   PACIFIC IPA
   9700 Flair Dr
   El Monte, CA 91731

KEY EXECUTIVES:
Chairman .... Ronald Akaski, MD
Executive Director .... Peter Lindbion
President .... Thomas Chiu, MD
Controller .... Lili Shen
Medical Director .... Musa Nasir, MD
Marketing Director .... Wer Ling Antoire
IS Manager .... Richard Pagan
Provider Services VP .... Jamie Situ
OI/Credentialing Manager .... Amy Hung

COMPANY PROFILE:
Parent Company Name:
Doing Business As:
Year Founded: 1986   Federally Qualified: [N]
Forprofit: [Y]   Not-For-Profit: [ ]
Model Type: IPA
Accreditation: [ ] AAPPO [ ] JACHO [ ] NCQA [ ] URAC
Plan Type: HMO,

SERVICE AREA:
Nationwide: N
   CA (San Gabriel Valley);

TYPE OF COVERAGE:
Commercial: [Y] Individual: [Y] FEHBP: [ ] Indemnity: [ ]
Medicare: [Y] Medicaid: [ ] Supplemental Medicare: [ ]
Tricare [ ]

PLAN BENEFITS:
Alternative Medicine: [ ]   Behavioral Health: [ ]
Chiropractic: [ ]   Dental: [ ]
Home Care: [X]   Inpatient SNF: [X]
Long-Term Care: [ ]   Pharm. Mail Order: [ ]
Physical Therapy: [X]   Podiatry: [X]
Psychiatric: [ ]   Transplant: [ ]
Vision: [X]   Wellness: [X]
Workers' Comp: [ ]
Other Benefits:

PACIFIC UNION DENTAL INC

1390 Willow Poss Rd #800
Concord, CA 94520
Phone: 925-363-6000 Fax: 925-363-6099 Toll-Free: 800-999-3367
Web site: www.pdbi.com

MAILING ADDRESS:
   PACIFIC UNION DENTAL INC
   1390 Willow Poss Rd #800
   Concord, CA 94520

KEY EXECUTIVES:
Chief Executive Officer/President .... John Gaebel, DDS
Chief Financial Officer .... Randy A Brecher
Dental Director .... Dr Dugan
Chief Information Officer .... Doug Elloway
Vice President Operations .... Nilesh Patel
VP Marketing & Sales .... James Fuhrman
Human Resources Director .... Ellen Willingham

COMPANY PROFILE:
Parent Company Name:
Doing Business As: California Pacific Dental Inc
Year Founded: 1996   Federally Qualified: [ ]
Forprofit: [Y]   Not-For-Profit: [ ]
Model Type: MIXED
Accreditation: [ ] AAPPO [ ] JACHO [ ] NCQA [ ] URAC
Plan Type: Specialty HMO, Specialty PPO, ASO
Total Revenue: 2005:   8,927,156   2006: 36,002,484
Net Income   2005:   522,423   2006:   344,415
Total Enrollment:
   2001: 630,000   2004: 223,522   2007: 261,396
   2002: 237,784   2005: 238,316
   2003: 244,547   2006: 212,245
Medical Loss Ratio: 2005: 72.14   2006: 72.46
Administrative Expense Ratio: 2005: 21.97   2006: 27.99

SERVICE AREA:
Nationwide: N
   CA; NV; TX; IL;

TYPE OF COVERAGE:
Commercial: [Y] Individual: [Y] FEHBP: [ ] Indemnity: [ ]
Medicare: [Y] Medicaid: [ ] Supplemental Medicare: [Y]
Tricare [ ]

PRODUCTS OFFERED:
Product Name: Type:
Specialty HMO
EPO
ASO
PPO
Network Leasing

PLAN BENEFITS:
Alternative Medicine: [ ]   Behavioral Health: [ ]
Chiropractic: [ ]   Dental: [X]
Home Care: [ ]   Inpatient SNF: [ ]
Long-Term Care: [ ]   Pharm. Mail Order: [ ]
Physical Therapy: [ ]   Podiatry: [ ]
Psychiatric: [ ]   Transplant: [ ]
Vision: [ ]   Wellness: [ ]
Workers' Comp: [ ]
Other Benefits:
Comments:
Formerly California Pacific Dental Inc.

PACIFICARE LIFE & HEALTH INSURANCE COMPANY

5995 Plaza Dr
Cypress, CA 90630
Phone: 714-952-1121 Fax: 714-226-3581 Toll-Free:
Web site: www.pacificare.com

MAILING ADDRESS:
   PACIFICARE LIFE & HLTH INS CO
   5995 Plaza Dr MailStopCY20-462
   Cypress, CA 90630

KEY EXECUTIVES:
Chief Executive Officer/President .... Howard G Phanstiel
Chief Financial Officer .... Gregory Scott
Medical Director .... Sam N Ho, MD
Pharmacy Director .... Ed Feaver
Chief Information Officer .... Sharon Garrett
Senior VP Marketing & Product Dev .... Rich Roge

Copyright MCIC -- The National Directory of Managed Care Organizations, Seventh Edition

CALIFORNIA

Total Enrollment:
- 2001: 560,871
- 2002: 687,300
- 2003: 716,566
- 2004: 835,201
- 2005:
- 2006: 297,908
- 2007: 276,277

Medical Loss Ratio: 2005: 2006: 49.98
Administrative Expense Ratio: 2005: 2006: 33.35

SERVICE AREA:
Nationwide: N
AZ; CA; CO; NV; OK; OR; TX; WA;

TYPE OF COVERAGE:
Commercial: [Y] Individual: [Y] FEHBP: [Y] Indemnity: [Y]
Medicare: [Y] Medicaid: [ ] Supplemental Medicare: [ ]
Tricare [ ]

PRODUCTS OFFERED:
Product Name:	Type:
390, 490, 590, Dental	HMO
Dental PPO	PPO
Full Service Vision	PPO
Eye Wear Only Vision	PPO

PLAN BENEFITS:
Alternative Medicine:	[ ]	Behavioral Health:	[ ]
Chiropractic:	[ ]	Dental:	[X]
Home Care:	[ ]	Inpatient SNF:	[ ]
Long-Term Care:	[ ]	Pharm. Mail Order:	[ ]
Physical Therapy:	[ ]	Podiatry:	[ ]
Psychiatric:	[ ]	Transplant:	[ ]
Vision:	[X]	Wellness:	[ ]
Workers' Comp:	[ ]		
Other Benefits:			

Comments:
Formerly PacifiCare Dental and Vision.

PACIFICARE HEALTH SYSTEMS- CORPORATE HEADQUARTERS

3120 Lake Center Dr
Santa Ana, CA 92704
Phone: 714-952-1121 Fax: 714-825-2201 Toll-Free: 800-624-8822
Web site: www.pacificare.com

MAILING ADDRESS:
PACIFICARE HEALTH SYS-CORP HQT
PO Box 25186
Santa Ana, CA 92704

KEY EXECUTIVES:
Chairman of the Board/Chief Executive Officer ... Howard G Phanstiel
Executive Vice President/Health Plan Division President . Brad Bowlus
Ex VPChief Financial Officer .... Gregory W Scott
Chief Medical Officer .... Sam N Ho, MD
EVP, Pharmaceutical Services .... Jacqueline Kosecoff, PhD
Marketing Director .... Judy Richards
VP Public Relations .... Ben Singer
VP Network Development .... Ferial Behremand
Senior VP Human Resources .... Judy Ehrenreich
Senior VP Medical Management .... Ferial Behremand
VP Audit .... Linda Dannels
Chief Strategic Officer .... Bary Bailey, EVP, CSO

COMPANY PROFILE:
Parent Company Name: UnitedHealth Group
Doing Business As:
Year Founded: 1978 Federally Qualified: [Y]
Forprofit: [Y] Not-For-Profit: [ ]
Model Type:
Accreditation: [ ] AAPPO [ ] JACHO [X] NCQA [ ] URAC
Plan Type: HMO, PPO, POS, HDHP, HSA,
Total Enrollment:
- 2001: 3,479,900
- 2002: 12,474,400
- 2003: 12,275,300
- 2004: 13,779,200
- 2005:
- 2006: 13,000,000
- 2007: 0

SERVICE AREA:
Nationwide: N
AZ; CA; CO; KY; NV; OH; OK; OR; TX; UT; WA;

TYPE OF COVERAGE:
Commercial: [Y] Individual: [ ] FEHBP: [ ] Indemnity: [ ]
Medicare: [Y] Medicaid: [ ] Supplemental Medicare: [ ]
Tricare [ ]

PRODUCTS OFFERED:
Product Name:	Type:
Pacificare HMO	HMO
Secure Horizons	Medicare Advantage

PLAN BENEFITS:
Alternative Medicine:	[ ]	Behavioral Health:	[X]
Chiropractic:	[X]	Dental:	[X]
Home Care:	[X]	Inpatient SNF:	[X]
Long-Term Care:	[X]	Pharm. Mail Order:	[X]
Physical Therapy:	[X]	Podiatry:	[X]
Psychiatric:	[X]	Transplant:	[X]
Vision:	[X]	Wellness:	[X]
Workers' Comp:	[X]		
Other Benefits:			

PACIFICARE OF CALIFORNIA

5701 Katella Ave
Cypress, CA 90630-5028
Phone: 714-952-1121 Fax: 714-226-3581 Toll-Free: 800-624-8822
Web site: www.pacificare.com

MAILING ADDRESS:
PACIFICARE OF CALIFORNIA
5701 Katella Ave
Cypress, CA 90630-5028

KEY EXECUTIVES:
Chief Executive Officer/President .... Howard G Phanstiel
Chief Financial Officer .... Gregory Scott
Medical Director .... Sam N Ho, MD
Pharmacy Director .... Ed Feaver
Senior VP, Comm Marketing & Product Development .... Rich Roge

COMPANY PROFILE:
Parent Company Name: UnitedHealth Group
Doing Business As: Secure Horizons Health Plan
Year Founded: 1978 Federally Qualified: [Y]
Forprofit: [Y] Not-For-Profit: [ ]
Model Type: MIXED
Accreditation: [ ] AAPPO [ ] JACHO [X] NCQA [ ] URAC
Plan Type: HMO, PPO, POS, HDHP, HSA,
Total Revenue: 2005: 1,677,883,000 2006: 1,814,048,000
Net Income 2005: 32,134,000 2006: 291,035,000
Total Enrollment:
- 2001: 2,066,000
- 2002: 1,929,076
- 2003: 1,681,389
- 2004: 1,728,838
- 2005: 1,644,098
- 2006: 1,663,085
- 2007: 1,607,574

Medical Loss Ratio: 2005: 88.76 2006: 86.17
Administrative Expense Ratio: 2005: 8.66 2006: 7.75

SERVICE AREA:
Nationwide: N
CA (Alameda, Amador, Butte, Colusa, Contra Costa, El Dorado, Fresno, Glenn, Humboldt, Imperial, Kern, Kings, Lake, Los Angeles, Madera, Marin, Mariposa, Mendocino, Merced, Monterey, Napa, Nevada, Orange, Placer, Riverside, Sacramento, San Bernardino, San Diego, San Francisco, San Joaquin, San Luis Obispo, San Mateo, Santa Barbara, Santa Clara, Santa Cruz, Shasta, Solano, Sonoma, Stanislaus, Sutter, Tehama, Trinity, Tulare, Ventura, Yolo, Yuba).

TYPE OF COVERAGE:
Commercial: [Y] Individual: [Y] FEHBP: [ ] Indemnity: [ ]
Medicare: [Y] Medicaid: [ ] Supplemental Medicare: [ ]
Tricare [ ]

PRODUCTS OFFERED:
Product Name:	Type:
Secure Horizons	Medicare Advantage
PacifiCare HMO	HMO

PLAN BENEFITS:
Alternative Medicine:	[ ]	Behavioral Health:	[X]
Chiropractic:	[X]	Dental:	[X]
Home Care:	[X]	Inpatient SNF:	[X]
Long-Term Care:	[ ]	Pharm. Mail Order:	[X]
Physical Therapy:	[X]	Podiatry:	[X]
Psychiatric:	[X]	Transplant:	[X]
Vision:	[X]	Wellness:	[X]
Workers' Comp:	[X]		
Other Benefits:			

Comments:
Formerly FHP Health Care.

PACIFIC HEALTH ALLIANCE

1350 Old Bayshore Hwy #560
Burlingame, CA 94010
Phone: 650-375-5800 Fax: 650-375-5820 Toll-Free: 800-533-4742
Web site: www.pacifichealthalliance.com

Managed Care Organization Profiles — **CALIFORNIA**

COMPANY PROFILE:
Parent Company Name: Orange County Foundation for Medical Care
Doing Business As:
Year Founded: 1984 Federally Qualified: [N]
Forprofit: [ ] Not-For-Profit: [Y]
Model Type:
Accreditation: [ ] AAPPO [ ] JACHO [ ] NCQA [ ] URAC
Plan Type: PPO, EPO
SERVICE AREA:
Nationwide: N
  CA (Orange);
TYPE OF COVERAGE:
Commercial: [Y] Individual: [ ] FEHBP: [ ] Indemnity: [ ]
Medicare: [ ] Medicaid: [ ] Supplemental Medicare: [ ]
Tricare [ ]
PLAN BENEFITS:
Alternative Medicine: [ ] Behavioral Health: [ ]
Chiropractic: [X] Dental: [ ]
Home Care: [X] Inpatient SNF: [X]
Long-Term Care: [ ] Pharm. Mail Order: [ ]
Physicial Therapy: [X] Podiatry: [X]
Psychiatric: [X] Transplant: [X]
Vision: [ ] Wellness: [X]
Workers' Comp: [ ]
Other Benefits:

ORANGE PREVENTION & TREATMENT INTEGRATED

1120 W La Veta Ave
Orange, CA 92868
Phone: 714-246-8400 Fax: 714-246-8492 Toll-Free:
Web site: www.caloptima.org
MAILING ADDRESS:
  ORANGE PREVENTION & TREATMENT INTEGRATED
  PO Box 11033
  Orange, CA 92868

KEY EXECUTIVES:
Chief Executive Officer .... Richard Chambers
Chief Financial Officer .... Keith Quinlivan
Chief Medical Officer .... Trudi Carter, MD
Director of Clinical Pharmacy Management .... Kris Gericke, PharmD
Chief Information Officer .... Bill Farry
Interim Chief Operating Officer .... Greg Buchert, MD
Provider Relations Director .... Estela Martinez
Quality Management & Improvement .... Linda Lee
Chief Administrative Officer .... Kim Cunningham
Executive Director of OneCare .... Kurt Hubler
Medical Director .... Martha Tasinga, MD
Medical Director .... Richard Sax, MD

COMPANY PROFILE:
Parent Company Name:
Doing Business As: CalOptima
Year Founded: Federally Qualified: [ ]
Forprofit: [ ] Not-For-Profit: [ ]
Model Type: NETWORK
Accreditation: [ ] AAPPO [ ] JACHO [ ] NCQA [ ] URAC
Plan Type: HMO
Primary Physicians: 3,700 Physician Specialists:
Hospitals:
Total Revenue: 2005: 816,332,420 2006: 922,894,632
Net Income 2005: -24,374,130 2006: -24,308,105
Total Enrollment:
  2001: 266,535 2004: 325,992 2007: 333,924
  2002: 307,940 2005: 323,917
  2003: 323,343 2006: 333,030
Medical Loss Ratio: 2005: 98.56 2006: 100.32
Administrative Expense Ratio: 2005: 4.21 2006: 2.84
SERVICE AREA:
Nationwide: N
  CA;
TYPE OF COVERAGE:
Commercial: [ ] Individual: [ ] FEHBP: [ ] Indemnity: [ ]
Medicare: [ ] Medicaid: [Y] Supplemental Medicare: [ ]
Tricare [ ]
PRODUCTS OFFERED:
Product Name: Type:
CalOptima Medicaid HMO

PACIFICARE BEHAVIORAL HEALTH

3120 Lake Center Dr
Santa Ana, CA 92704-6917
Phone: 818-623-9585 Fax: 818-782-1846 Toll-Free:
Web site: www.pbhi.com
MAILING ADDRESS:
  PACIFICARE BEHAVIORAL HEALTH
  PO Box 25186
  Santa Ana, CA 92704-6917

KEY EXECUTIVES:
Chief Executive Officer/President .... Jerome V Vaccaro, MD
Chief Financial Officer .... Kenneth L Watkins
VP Corp Medical Director .... Robert Burchuk, MD
VP of Operations .... Kerry Matsumoto
VP, Marketing & Sales .... Ann McClanathan

COMPANY PROFILE:
Parent Company Name: UnitedHealth Group
Doing Business As:
Year Founded: 1986 Federally Qualified: [Y]
Forprofit: [Y] Not-For-Profit: [ ]
Model Type:
Accreditation: [ ] AAPPO [ ] JACHO [ ] NCQA [ ] URAC
Plan Type: Specialty HMO, Specialty PPO, ASO, POS,
Total Revenue: 2005: 40,443,299 2006: 175,701,332
Net Income 2005: 1,568,432 2006: 29,656,781
Total Enrollment:
  2001: 1,818,915 2004: 1,571,024 2007: 1,725,125
  2002: 3,876,000 2005: 1,568,432
  2003: 3,660,100 2006: 1,542,283
Medical Loss Ratio: 2005: 59.79 2006: 53.92
Administrative Expense Ratio: 2005: 32.00 2006: 20.27
SERVICE AREA:
Nationwide: Y
  NW;
TYPE OF COVERAGE:
Commercial: [Y] Individual: [ ] FEHBP: [ ] Indemnity: [ ]
Medicare: [Y] Medicaid: [ ] Supplemental Medicare: [ ]
Tricare [ ]
PLAN BENEFITS:
Alternative Medicine: [ ] Behavioral Health: [X]
Chiropractic: [ ] Dental: [ ]
Home Care: [ ] Inpatient SNF: [ ]
Long-Term Care: [ ] Pharm. Mail Order: [ ]
Physicial Therapy: [ ] Podiatry: [ ]
Psychiatric: [X] Transplant: [ ]
Vision: [ ] Wellness: [ ]
Workers' Comp: [ ]
Other Benefits:
Comments:
Formerly Lifeline Inc Psychology Systems.

PACIFICARE DENTAL & VISION

3110 Lake Center Dr
Santa Ana, CA 92704
Phone: 714-513-6494 Fax: 714-513-6380 Toll-Free: 800-228-3384
Web site: www.pacificare-dental.com
MAILING ADDRESS:
  PACIFICARE DENTAL & VISION
  PO Box 25187
  Santa Ana, CA 92704

KEY EXECUTIVES:
Chief Executive Officer/President .... Kelly McCrann
VP/Chief Financial Officer .... Christopher D Boles
VP, Sales & Marketing .... John W Whalley
Director, Information Systems .... Shankar Rao

COMPANY PROFILE:
Parent Company Name: UnitedHealth Group
Doing Business As: PacifiCare Dental & Vision
Year Founded: 1972 Federally Qualified: [Y]
Forprofit: [Y] Not-For-Profit: [ ]
Model Type: MIXED
Accreditation: [ ] AAPPO [ ] JACHO [ ] NCQA [ ] URAC
Plan Type: Specialty HMO, Specialty PPO, ASO, TPA, EPO
Total Revenue: 2005: 2006: 41,943,288
Net Income 2005: 2006: 4,285,216

CALIFORNIA

Medical Loss Ratio: 2005: 2006: 167.26
Administrative Expense Ratio: 2005: 2006: 15.25
SERVICE AREA:
Nationwide: N
CA;
TYPE OF COVERAGE:
Commercial: [Y] Individual: [ ] FEHBP: [ ] Indemnity: [ ]
Medicare: [ ] Medicaid: [Y] Supplemental Medicare: [ ]
Tricare [ ]
PRODUCTS OFFERED:
Product Name: Type:
Molina Health Care Inc HMO
PLAN BENEFITS:
Alternative Medicine: [ ] Behavioral Health: [ ]
Chiropractic: [X] Dental: [ ]
Home Care: [X] Inpatient SNF: [X]
Long-Term Care: [ ] Pharm. Mail Order: [ ]
Physical Therapy: [X] Podiatry: [X]
Psychiatric: [ ] Transplant: [ ]
Vision: [X] Wellness: [ ]
Workers' Comp: [ ]
Other Benefits:

NEWPORT DENTAL PLAN

201 E Sandpointe Ste 800
Santa Ana, CA 92707
Phone: 714-668-1300 Fax: 714-428-1300 Toll-Free: 800-347-6453
Web site: www.brightnow.com
MAILING ADDRESS:
NEWPORT DENTAL PLAN
201 E Sandpointe Ste 800
Santa Ana, CA 92707

KEY EXECUTIVES:
Chief Executive Officer/President .... Steven C Bilt
Chief Financial Officer .... Bradley E Schmidt
Dental Director .... Charles E Stirewalt, DMD
Chief Operating Officer .... Roy D Smith, DDS
Senior VP Marketing & Sales .... Rick Brown
Senior VP Marketing & Sales .... Kevin J Callahan
Vice President Human Resources .... Catherine R Crow
Vice President Dental Affairs .... Charles Stirewalt, DMD
Dental Plan Administrator .... Kathleen Kuretich

COMPANY PROFILE:
Parent Company Name: Consumer Health Inc
Doing Business As: Newport Dental Plan, Newport Dental Ctrs
Year Founded: 1985 Federally Qualified: [ ]
Forprofit: [Y] Not-For-Profit: [ ]
Model Type: MIXED
Accreditation: [ ] AAPPO [ ] JACHO [ ] NCQA [ ] URAC
Plan Type: Specialty HMO, Specialty PPO
Total Revenue: 2005: 7,318,959 2006: 33,911,137
Net Income 2005: 17,419 2006: 2,915,235
Total Enrollment:
2001: 39,272 2004: 0 2007: 57,895
2002: 46,840 2005: 60,360
2003: 0 2006: 60,265
Medical Loss Ratio: 2005: 89.60 2006: 75.67
Administrative Expense Ratio: 2005: 10.33 2006: 10.33
SERVICE AREA:
Nationwide: N
CA (Southern);
TYPE OF COVERAGE:
Commercial: [Y] Individual: [Y] FEHBP: [ ] Indemnity: [ ]
Medicare: [Y] Medicaid: [ ] Supplemental Medicare: [Y]
Tricare [ ]
PRODUCTS OFFERED:
Product Name: Type:
Newport Dental Plan 2011 PPO
Misc Group Products HMO
PLAN BENEFITS:
Alternative Medicine: [ ] Behavioral Health: [ ]
Chiropractic: [ ] Dental: [X]
Home Care: [ ] Inpatient SNF: [ ]
Long-Term Care: [ ] Pharm. Mail Order: [ ]
Physical Therapy: [ ] Podiatry: [ ]
Psychiatric: [ ] Transplant: [ ]
Vision: [ ] Wellness: [ ]
Workers' Comp: [ ]
Other Benefits: Orthodontics

ON LOK SENIOR HEALTH SERVICES

1333 Bush St
San Francisco, CA 94109-5611
Phone: 415-292-8888 Fax: 415-292-8745 Toll-Free: 888-886-6565
Web site: www.onlok.org
MAILING ADDRESS:
ON LOK SENIOR HEALTH SERVICES
1333 Bush St
San Francisco, CA 94109-5611

KEY EXECUTIVES:
President of the Board .... Wellman Tsang, MD
Chief Executive Officer .... Robert Edmonson
Health Plan Director .... Amy Shin
Chief Financial Officer .... Sue Wong
Medical Director .... Catherine Eng, MD
Director of Operations .... Grace Li, MHA
Marketing Director .... Sharon Kawaguchi
Human Resources Officer .... Deborah Stuart-Middleton
Compliance Officer .... Cheryle Bernard-Shaw, JD

COMPANY PROFILE:
Parent Company Name: On Lok Senior Health Services
Doing Business As: On Lok Senior Health
Year Founded: 1972 Federally Qualified: [Y]
Forprofit: [ ] Not-For-Profit: [Y]
Model Type: STAFF
Accreditation: [ ] AAPPO [ ] JACHO [ ] NCQA [ ] URAC
Plan Type: Specialty HMO
Total Revenue: 2005: 15,958,628 2006: 19,448,266
Net Income 2005: 879,987 2006: 1,643,070
Total Enrollment:
2001: 883 2004: 940 2007: 1,049
2002: 891 2005: 960
2003: 939 2006: 1,045
Medical Loss Ratio: 2005: 90.98 2006: 84.77
Administrative Expense Ratio: 2005: 7.28 2006: 6.83
SERVICE AREA:
Nationwide: N
CA (San Francisco);
TYPE OF COVERAGE:
Commercial: [ ] Individual: [ ] FEHBP: [ ] Indemnity: [ ]
Medicare: [Y] Medicaid: [Y] Supplemental Medicare: [ ]
Tricare [ ]
PRODUCTS OFFERED:
Product Name: Type:
On Lok Medicaid Medicaid
Medicare
PLAN BENEFITS:
Alternative Medicine: [X] Behavioral Health: [ ]
Chiropractic: [ ] Dental: [X]
Home Care: [X] Inpatient SNF: [X]
Long-Term Care: [X] Pharm. Mail Order: [ ]
Physical Therapy: [X] Podiatry: [X]
Psychiatric: [ ] Transplant: [ ]
Vision: [X] Wellness: [ ]
Workers' Comp: [ ]
Other Benefits:

ORANGE COUNTY PPO

300 South Flower St
Orange, CA 92668
Phone: 714-978-5048 Fax: 714-634-9655 Toll-Free: 800-345-8643
Web site: www.cfmcnet.org
MAILING ADDRESS:
ORANGE COUNTY PPO
300 South Flower St
Orange, CA 92668

KEY EXECUTIVES:
Chairman of the Board .... Mark E Krugman
Executive Director .... Elizabeth Ciaccio, RN, MBA
Chief Financial Officer .... Kenneth Karjala
Medical Director .... James Strebig, MD
Provider Service Director .... Joanne Stewart
Director of Medical Management .... Karl Gilbody, RN
Quality Assurance Director .... Margaret House, LVP, CPHQ

Managed Care Organization Profiles — **CALIFORNIA**

Doing Business As:
Year Founded: 1976   Federally Qualified: [ ]
Forprofit: [ ]   Not-For-Profit: [ ]
Model Type:
Accreditation: [ ] AAPPO [ ] JACHO [ ] NCQA [ ] URAC
Plan Type: PPO, Specialty PPO, Specialty HMO, ASO, TPA
Total Revenue: 2005:   1,293,831   2006:   3,803,068
Net Income   2005:   207,868   2006:   267,956
Total Enrollment:
  2001: 74,641   2004: 81,860   2007: 55,004
  2002: 100,304   2005: 77,686
  2003: 81,061   2006: 57,497
Medical Loss Ratio: 2005: 53.75   2006: 56.16
Administrative Expense Ratio: 2005: 27.99   2006: 36.24

SERVICE AREA:
Nationwide: N
  CA;

TYPE OF COVERAGE:
Commercial: [Y]   Individual: [ ]   FEHBP: [ ]   Indemnity: [Y]
Medicare: [ ]   Medicaid: [ ]   Supplemental Medicare: [ ]
Tricare [ ]

PRODUCTS OFFERED:
Product Name: Type:
    Specialty HMO

PLAN BENEFITS:
Alternative Medicine: [ ]   Behavioral Health: [ ]
Chiropractic: [ ]   Dental: [ ]
Home Care: [ ]   Inpatient SNF: [ ]
Long-Term Care: [ ]   Pharm. Mail Order: [ ]
Physical Therapy: [ ]   Podiatry: [ ]
Psychiatric: [ ]   Transplant: [ ]
Vision: [X]   Wellness: [ ]
Workers' Comp: [ ]
Other Benefits:

MENDOCINO AND LAKE COUNTIES FOUNDATION FOR MEDICAL CARE

216 W Henry St
Ukiah, CA 95482-4355
Phone: 707-462-7607 Fax: 707-462-1206 Toll-Free:
Web site:
MAILING ADDRESS:
  MENDOCINO & LAKE CTY FNDTN MED
  PO Box 1030
  Ukiah, CA 95482-4355

KEY EXECUTIVES:
Chief Executive Officer/President .... Robert Faulk
Chief Financial Officer/Medical Director .... Robert Faulk

COMPANY PROFILE:
Parent Company Name: Blue Cross/Blue Shield of California
Doing Business As:
Year Founded: Federally Qualified: [ ]
Forprofit: [ ]   Not-For-Profit: [ ]Model Type:
Accreditation: [ ] AAPPO [ ] JACHO [ ] NCQA [ ] URAC
Plan Type: PPO

SERVICE AREA:
Nationwide: N
  CA;

MOLINA HEALTHCARE INC - CORPORATE HEADQUARTERS

1 Golden Shore
Long Beach, CA 90802
Phone: 562-435-3666 Fax: 562-495-7770 Toll-Free: 800-526-8196
Web site: www.molinahealthcare.com
MAILING ADDRESS:
  MOLINA HEALTHCARE INC - CORP
  1 Golden Shore
  Long Beach, CA 90802

KEY EXECUTIVES:
Chairman of the Board .... Joseph M Molina, MD
Chief Executive Officer/President .... Joseph M Molina, MD
VPChief Financial Officer .... John C Molina, JD
Chief Medical Officer .... James W Howatt, MD
Chief Operating Officer .... Terry Bayer, BS, MPH, JD
Human Resources & Marketing .... Sheila K Shapiro, BS, MBA
AVP Human Resources .... Terry Bayer, BS, MPH, JD
VP, Utilization Mgnt/Quality .... Michael Siegel, MD
Executive VP, Business Services .... John C Molina, JD
Executive VP, Legal Affairs .... Mark L Andrews, ESQ
Executive VP, Health Plan Operations .... Terry Bayer, BS, MPH, JD
Research & Development .... Martha Bernaditt, MD

COMPANY PROFILE:
Parent Company Name:
Doing Business As:
Year Founded: 1980   Federally Qualified: [ ]
Forprofit: [Y]   Not-For-Profit: [ ]
Model Type:
Accreditation: [ ] AAPPO [ ] JACHO [X] NCQA [ ] URAC
Plan Type: HMO
Primary Physicians: 11,757   Physician Specialists: 31,052
Hospitals: 406
Total Revenue: 2005: 1,650,058,000   2006: 2,004,995,000
Net Income   2005: 27,596,000   2006: 45,727,000
Total Enrollment:
  2001: 0   2004: 788,000   2007: 1,074,000
  2002: 286,180   2005: 893,000
  2003: 564,000   2006: 1,077,000
Medical Loss Ratio: 2005: 86.90   2006: 84.60
Administrative Expense Ratio: 2005: 9.90   2006: 11.40

SERVICE AREA:
Nationwide: N
  CA; MI; NM; OH; TX; UT; WA;

TYPE OF COVERAGE:
Commercial: [ ]   Individual: [ ]   FEHBP: [ ]   Indemnity: [ ]
Medicare: [ ]   Medicaid: [Y]   Supplemental Medicare: [ ]
Tricare

PLAN BENEFITS:
Alternative Medicine: [ ]   Behavioral Health: [ ]
Chiropractic: [X]   Dental: [ ]
Home Care: [X]   Inpatient SNF: [X]
Long-Term Care: [ ]   Pharm. Mail Order: [ ]
Physical Therapy: [X]   Podiatry: [X]
Psychiatric: [ ]   Transplant: [ ]
Vision: [X]   Wellness: [X]
Workers' Comp: [ ]
Other Benefits:

MOLINA HEALTHCARE INC OF CALIFORNIA

1 Golden Shore
Long Beach, CA 90802
Phone: 562-435-3666 Fax: 562-951-1514 Toll-Free: 800-562-5442
Web site: www.molinahealthcare.com
MAILING ADDRESS:
  MOLINA HEALTHCARE INC OF CA
  1 Golden Shore
  Long Beach, CA 90802

KEY EXECUTIVES:
Chairman of the Board .... Joseph M Molina, MD
Chief Executive Officer .... Joann Zarza-Garrido
President .... Stephen T O'Dell
Chief Finanical Officer .... Greg Hamblin, BS, CPA
VPChief Medical Officer .... Long Dang, MD
Chief Operating Officer .... Roberta Holtzman, MBA
VP, Human Resources .... Richard J Hondel
Executive VP, Business Services .... John C Molina, JD
Executive VP, Legal Affairs .... Mark L Andrews, ESQ
Executive VP, Health Plan Operations .... George S Goldstein, PhD

COMPANY PROFILE:
Parent Company Name: Molina Healthcare Inc
Doing Business As:
Year Founded: 1980   Federally Qualified: [ ]
Forprofit: [Y]   Not-For-Profit: [ ]
Model Type: MIXED
Accreditation: [ ] AAPPO [ ] JACHO [X] NCQA [ ] URAC
Plan Type: HMO
Primary Physicians: 2,671   Physician Specialists: 6,675
Hospitals: 81
Total Revenue: 2005:   2006: 374,082,481
Net Income   2005:   2006: -15,510,889
Total Enrollment:
  2001: 405,454   2004: 252,737   2007: 290,834
  2002: 286,180   2005: 321,000
  2003: 254,393   2006: 294,122

CALIFORNIA   Managed Care Organization Profiles

PLAN BENEFITS:
Alternative Medicine:	[ ]	Behavioral Health:	[X]
Chiropractic:	[ ]	Dental:	[ ]
Home Care:	[ ]	Inpatient SNF:	[ ]
Long-Term Care:	[ ]	Pharm. Mail Order:	[ ]
Physical Therapy:	[ ]	Podiatry:	[ ]
Psychiatric:	[X]	Transplant:	[ ]
Vision:	[ ]	Wellness:	[ ]
Workers' Comp:	[ ]		
Other Benefits:			

Comments:
Formerly California Wellness Plan.

MARCH VISION CARE INC

6701 Center Dr W Ste 790
Los Angeles, CA 90045
Phone: 310-216-2300 Fax: Toll-Free: 888-493-4070
Web site: www.marchvisioncare.com
MAILING ADDRESS:
    MARCH VISION CARE INC
    6701 Center Dr W Ste 790
    Los Angeles, CA 90045

KEY EXECUTIVES:
Chief Executive Officer/President .... Glenville A March Jr, MD
Executive Vice President .... Cabrini T March, MD

COMPANY PROFILE:
Parent Company Name:
Doing Business As:
Year Founded: 2006   Federally Qualified: [ ]
Forprofit: [ ]   Not-For-Profit: [ ]
Model Type:
Accreditation: [ ] AAPPO [ ] JACHO [ ] NCQA [ ] URAC
Plan Type: HMO,
SERVICE AREA:
Nationwide:
    NW;
TYPE OF COVERAGE:
Commercial: [Y] Individual: [ ] FEHBP: [ ] Indemnity: [ ]
Medicare: [Y] Medicaid: [Y] Supplemental Medicare: [ ]
Tricare   [ ]
PLAN BENEFITS:
Alternative Medicine:	[ ]	Behavioral Health:	[ ]
Chiropractic:	[ ]	Dental:	[ ]
Home Care:	[ ]	Inpatient SNF:	[ ]
Long-Term Care:	[ ]	Pharm. Mail Order:	[ ]
Physical Therapy:	[ ]	Podiatry:	[ ]
Psychiatric:	[ ]	Transplant:	[ ]
Vision:	[X]	Wellness:	[ ]
Workers' Comp:	[ ]		
Other Benefits:			

MEDCORE HEALTH PLAN

509 W Weber Ave Ste 200
Stockton, CA 95203
Phone: 209-320-2650 Fax: 209-320-2644 Toll-Free: 800-320-5688
Web site: www.medcoreipa.com
MAILING ADDRESS:
    MEDCORE HEALTH PLAN
    509 W Weber Ave Ste 200
    Stockton, CA 95203

KEY EXECUTIVES:
President .... Kirit Patel, MD
Chief Financial Officer .... Lora Lagorio
Medical Director .... Gerry Yucht, MD
Chief Information Officer .... Douglas Chard
Chief Operating Officer .... Sheila Stevens
Marketing Director .... Nicole McGrath
Secretary .... George Westin, MD
Treasurer .... George Herron, MD

COMPANY PROFILE:
Parent Company Name: OMNI IPA, Medcore Management Inc
Doing Business As: Medcare Health Plan
Year Founded: 1996   Federally Qualified: [ ]
Forprofit: [ ]   Not-For-Profit: [ ]
Model Type:
Accreditation: [ ] AAPPO [ ] JACHO [ ] NCQA [ ] URAC
Plan Type: HMO
Total Revenue: 2005:   2006: 6,439,358
Net Income   2005:   2006: -904,956
Total Enrollment:
    2001: 0   2004: 0   2007: 1,169
    2002: 0   2005:
    2003: 0   2006: 587
Medical Loss Ratio: 2005:   2006: 77.64
Administrative Expense Ratio: 2005:   2006: 56.04
SERVICE AREA:
Nationwide:
    CA;
Comments:
Formerly Medcore HP.

MEDFOCUS RADIOLOGY NETWORK

2811 Wilshire Blvd Ste 900
Santa Monica, CA 90403
Phone: 310-828-4472 Fax: 310-829-3366 Toll-Free: 800-950-4700
Web site: www.medfocus.net
MAILING ADDRESS:
    MEDFOCUS RADIOLOGY NETWORK
    2811 Wilshire Blvd Ste 900
    Santa Monica, CA 90403

KEY EXECUTIVES:
Chief Executive Officer/Chief Financial Officer .... Catherine Lewis
President/Medical Director .... Stephen B Meisel, MD
Chief Operating Officer .... Catherine Lewis
Marketing Director .... Pat McCutcheon
MIS Director .... Shawn Harris
Credentialing Manager .... Michelle Friedman
Director of Provider Services .... Steven Casper
Director of Operations .... Karen Byrd

COMPANY PROFILE:
Parent Company Name: Medfocus
Doing Business As:
Year Founded: 1986   Federally Qualified: [ ]
Forprofit: [Y]   Not-For-Profit: [ ]
Model Type: NETWORK
Accreditation: [ ] AAPPO [ ] JACHO [X] NCQA [ ] URAC
Plan Type: Specialty PPO
SERVICE AREA:
Nationwide: N
    CA;
TYPE OF COVERAGE:
Commercial: [Y] Individual: [ ] FEHBP: [ ] Indemnity: [ ]
Medicare: [ ] Medicaid: [ ] Supplemental Medicare: [ ]
Tricare   [ ]
PLAN BENEFITS:
Alternative Medicine:	[ ]	Behavioral Health:	[ ]
Chiropractic:	[ ]	Dental:	[ ]
Home Care:	[ ]	Inpatient SNF:	[ ]
Long-Term Care:	[ ]	Pharm. Mail Order:	[ ]
Physical Therapy:	[ ]	Podiatry:	[ ]
Psychiatric:	[ ]	Transplant:	[ ]
Vision:	[ ]	Wellness:	[ ]
Workers' Comp:	[X]		
Other Benefits: Radiology Network			

MEDICAL EYE SERVICES INC

PO Box 25209
Santa Ana, CA 92799-5209
Phone: 714-619-4660 Fax: 714-619-4662 Toll-Free: 800-877-6372
Web site: www.mesvision.com
MAILING ADDRESS:
    MEDICAL EYE SERVICES INC
    PO Box 25209
    Santa Ana, CA 92799-5209

KEY EXECUTIVES:
Chief Executive Officer/President .... Aspasia Shappet
Chief Financial Officer .... Charles Kupfer
VP of Sales .... Mike Schell

COMPANY PROFILE:
Parent Company Name:

Managed Care Organization Profiles   **CALIFORNIA**

MAILING ADDRESS:
   LIBERTY DENTAL PLAN OF CA
   PO Box 26110
   Irvine, CA 92799

KEY EXECUTIVES:
Chairman of the Board/Chief Executive Officer .... Amir Neshat, DDS
Chief Financial Officer .... Maja Kapic
Dental Director .... Richard Hague, DMD
Director of Operations .... Marsha Hazlewood
Director of Sales & Finance .... Jason Park
Director of Provider Relations .... Machelle Madden
VP, New Business Development .... Hugh Hazlewood

COMPANY PROFILE:
Parent Company Name:
Doing Business As: Personal Dental Services
Year Founded: 1978   Federally Qualified: [ ]
Forprofit: [ ]   Not-For-Profit: [ ]
Model Type:
Accreditation: [ ] AAPPO [ ] JACHO [ ] NCQA [ ] URAC
Plan Type: Specialty HMO, CDHP
Total Revenue: 2005:   1,162,830   2006:   1,809,334
Net Income   2005:   -3,958   2006:   16,961
Total Enrollment:
   2001:   10,828   2004:   16,676   2007:   76,475
   2002:   5,626   2005:   51,561
   2003:   13,026   2006:   70,598
Medical Loss Ratio: 2005:   48.95   2006:   52.60
Administrative Expense Ratio: 2005:   51.70   2006:   45.85
SERVICE AREA:
Nationwide: N
   CA;
TYPE OF COVERAGE:
Commercial: [Y] Individual: [Y] FEHBP: [ ] Indemnity: [ ]
Medicare: [ ] Medicaid: [Y] Supplemental Medicare: [ ]
Tricare   [ ]
PRODUCTS OFFERED:
Product Name: Type:
Liberty HMO   Specialty HMO
CONSUMER-DRIVEN PRODUCTS
                                           HSA Company
                                           HSA Product
                                           HSA Administrator
CA80   Consumer-Driven Health Plan
                                           High Deductible Health Plan
PLAN BENEFITS:
Alternative Medicine: [ ]   Behavioral Health: [ ]
Chiropractic: [ ]   Dental: [X]
Home Care: [ ]   Inpatient SNF: [ ]
Long-Term Care: [ ]   Pharm. Mail Order: [ ]
Physical Therapy: [ ]   Podiatry: [ ]
Psychiatric: [ ]   Transplant: [ ]
Vision: [ ]   Wellness: [ ]
Workers' Comp: [ ]
Other Benefits:

MANAGED DENTAL CARE

6200 Canoga Ave Ste 100
Woodland Hills, CA 91367
Phone: 818-598-6599 Fax: 818-598-8653 Toll-Free: 800-273-3330
Web site:
MAILING ADDRESS:
   MANAGED DENTAL CARE
   6200 Canoga Ave Ste 100
   Woodland Hills, CA 91367

KEY EXECUTIVES:
President .... Candee Bolyog
Chief Financial Officer .... Jennifer Althaus
National Dental Director .... Richard Goren, DDS
Dental Director .... William Slavin, DDS

COMPANY PROFILE:
Parent Company Name: Guardian Life Insurance Co of NY
Doing Business As: Managed Dental Care of California
Year Founded: 1991   Federally Qualified: [ ]
Forprofit: [Y]   Not-For-Profit: [ ]
Model Type: NETWORK
Accreditation: [ ] AAPPO [ ] JACHO [ ] NCQA [ ] URAC

Plan Type: Specialty HMO
Total Revenue: 2005:   3,846,365   2006:   16,429,013
Net Income   2005:   89,909   2006:   847,602
Total Enrollment:
   2001:   54,601   2004: 115,328   2007: 129,433
   2002:   70,464   2005: 125,464
   2003:   89,867   2006: 122,474
Medical Loss Ratio: 2005:   78.08   2006:   72.69
Administrative Expense Ratio: 2005:   19.20   2006:   19.17
SERVICE AREA:
Nationwide: N
   CA (Alameda, Contra Costa, Los Angeles, Orange, Riverside,
   Sacramento, San Bernardino, San Diego, Santa Clara, San Francisco,
   San Mateo);
TYPE OF COVERAGE:
Commercial: [Y] Individual: [ ] FEHBP: [ ] Indemnity: [ ]
Medicare: [ ] Medicaid: [ ] Supplemental Medicare: [ ]
Tricare   [ ]
PRODUCTS OFFERED:
Product Name: Type:
Dental HMO   Specialty HMO
PLAN BENEFITS:
Alternative Medicine: [ ]   Behavioral Health: [ ]
Chiropractic: [ ]   Dental: [X]
Home Care: [ ]   Inpatient SNF: [ ]
Long-Term Care: [ ]   Pharm. Mail Order: [ ]
Physical Therapy: [ ]   Podiatry: [ ]
Psychiatric: [ ]   Transplant: [ ]
Vision: [ ]   Wellness: [ ]
Workers' Comp: [ ]
Other Benefits:

MANAGED HEALTH NETWORK

503 Canal Drive
Point Richmond, CA 94804
Phone: 510-620-6400 Fax: 818-676-8591 Toll-Free: 800-327-7526
Web site: www.mhn.com
MAILING ADDRESS:
   MANAGED HEALTH NETWORK
   503 Canal Drive
   Point Richmond, CA 94804

KEY EXECUTIVES:
Chief Executive Officer/President .... Steven Sell
VP of Finance/Chief Financial .... Gregory S Pence
Chief Medical Officer .... Ian A Shaffer, MD
Senior VP of Information Systems .... Bob Glas
Chief Operating Officer .... Jaunell Hefner
VP of Health Plan Services/Clinical Operations .... Judy Y Kubel

COMPANY PROFILE:
Parent Company Name: Health Net Inc
Doing Business As: Managed Health Network
Year Founded: 1972   Federally Qualified: [Y]
Forprofit: [Y]   Not-For-Profit: [ ]
Model Type: NETWORK
Accreditation: [ ] AAPPO [ ] JACHO [ ] NCQA [X] URAC
Plan Type: Specialty HMO, Specialty PPO, POS
Total Revenue: 2005:   2006:   13,298,8225
Net Income   2005:   2006:   9,856,503
Total Enrollment:
   2001: 2,398,390   2004: 2,759,778   2007: 3,112,160
   2002:   0   2005:
   2003: 7,100,000   2006: 3,129,537
Medical Loss Ratio: 2005:   2006:   70.32
Administrative Expense Ratio: 2005:   2006:   18.09
SERVICE AREA:
Nationwide: Y
   NW;
TYPE OF COVERAGE:
Commercial: [Y] Individual: [ ] FEHBP: [ ] Indemnity: [ ]
Medicare: [Y] Medicaid: [ ] Supplemental Medicare: [ ]
Tricare   [ ]
PRODUCTS OFFERED:
Product Name: Type:
EAP
Managed Care

CALIFORNIA — Managed Care Organization Profiles

Manager Provider Communication .... Mark Martinez
Senior Director, Human Resources .... Barbara Cook
Senior Medical Director .... Richard Seidman, MD
Chief of Managed Care Operations .... Dorothy Seleski
Chief Legal Counsel .... Augustavia Haydel, JD
Legislative Strategies .... Cherie Fields

COMPANY PROFILE:
Parent Company Name: Local Initiative Health Auth for LA Co
Doing Business As: LA Care Health Plan
Year Founded: 1994   Federally Qualified: [N]
Forprofit: [ ]   Not-For-Profit: [Y]
Model Type: NETWORK
Accreditation: [ ] AAPPO [ ] JACHO [ ] NCQA [ ] URAC
Plan Type: HMO
Total Revenue: 2005: 255,967,143   2006: 251,309,037
Net Income   2005:   7,252,733   2006:   7,570,583
Total Enrollment:
   2001: 747,973   2004: 785,743   2007: 790,035
   2002: 830,049   2005: 794,972
   2003: 801,963   2006: 799,275
Medical Loss Ratio: 2005: 95.40   2006: 96.44
Administrative Expense Ratio: 2005: 4.08   2006: 3.77

SERVICE AREA:
Nationwide: N
   CA; (Los Angeles Cty);

TYPE OF COVERAGE:
Commercial: [ ] Individual: [ ] FEHBP: [ ] Indemnity: [ ]
Medicare: [ ] Medicaid: [Y] Supplemental Medicare: [ ]
Tricare   [ ]

PRODUCTS OFFERED:
Product Name: Type:
Medi-Cal   Medicaid
Healthy Families   CHIP
CaliforniaKids

PLAN BENEFITS:
Alternative Medicine: [ ]   Behavioral Health: [X]
Chiropractic: [ ]   Dental: [X]
Home Care: [X]   Inpatient SNF: [X]
Long-Term Care: [X]   Pharm. Mail Order: [ ]
Physical Therapy: [X]   Podiatry: [X]
Psychiatric: [X]   Transplant: [X]
Vision: [X]   Wellness: [X]
Workers' Comp: [ ]
Other Benefits:

LAKEWOOD HEALTH PLAN INC

4909 Lakewood Blvd Ste 200
Lakewood, CA 90712
Phone: 562-602-1563 Fax: 562-531-0937 Toll-Free: 877-602-1563
Web site: www.coasthealthcare.net
MAILING ADDRESS:
   LAKEWOOD HEALTH PLAN INC
   4909 Lakewood Blvd Ste 200
   Lakewood, CA 90712

KEY EXECUTIVES:
Chairman/Chief Executive Officer .... Mansoor Shah, MD
Chief Financial/Chief Operating Officer .... Cynthia Guzman, CPA
Medical Director .... David Neer, MD, JD
Marketing Manager .... John Lopez
Provider Relations Manager .... Ava Holmes
Director Contracting/Reimburs .... Lili Tran, MHA
Director of Clinical Operations .... Susie Foley, RN, MSN
Quality Manager .... Gloria Calhoun-Davis, LVN
Controller .... Ceaser Abutin
Claims Supervisor .... Pam Dean
Utilization Coordinator .... Diane Rodriguez
Administrative Supervisor .... Kathryn Hogan

COMPANY PROFILE:
Parent Company Name:
Doing Business As:
Year Founded: 1986   Federally Qualified: [ ]
Forprofit: [Y]   Not-For-Profit: [ ]
Model Type: IPA
Accreditation: [ ] AAPPO [ ] JACHO [ ] NCQA [ ] URAC
Plan Type: HMO, PPO, POS

SERVICE AREA:
Nationwide: N
   CA; Long Beach and vicinity.

TYPE OF COVERAGE:
Commercial: [Y] Individual: [Y] FEHBP: [ ] Indemnity: [ ]
Medicare: [ ] Medicaid: [ ] Supplemental Medicare: [ ]
Tricare   [ ]

PLAN BENEFITS:
Alternative Medicine: [ ]   Behavioral Health: [ ]
Chiropractic: [ ]   Dental: [ ]
Home Care: [X]   Inpatient SNF: [X]
Long-Term Care: [X]   Pharm. Mail Order: [ ]
Physical Therapy: [X]   Podiatry: [X]
Psychiatric: [X]   Transplant: [X]
Vision: [X]   Wellness: [X]
Workers' Comp: [ ]
Other Benefits:

LANDMARK HEALTHCARE INC

1750 Howe Ave Ste 300
Sacramento, CA 95825
Phone: 916-646-3477 Fax: 916-929-2293 Toll-Free: 800-638-4557
Web site: www.landmarkhealthcare.com
MAILING ADDRESS:
   LANDMARK HEALTHCARE INC
   1750 Howe Ave Ste 300
   Sacramento, CA 95825

KEY EXECUTIVES:
Chief Executive Officer/President .... George W Vieth, Jr
Chief Financial Officer .... Tom Klammer
Chief Medical Officer .... John Gore, MD
Chief Operating Officer .... Debra Tull
VP Sales & Marketing .... Guy Shields
VP Sales & Marketing .... Robert Dickes
Senior VP Strategic Development .... Marvin C Cobern
Chief Medical Officer .... Joel Stevans, DC
VP Clinical/Quality Administration .... Debbie Enigl

COMPANY PROFILE:
Parent Company Name: Landmark Healthcare Inc
Doing Business As:
Year Founded: 1985   Federally Qualified: [ ]
Forprofit: [ ]   Not-For-Profit: [ ]
Model Type: NETWORK
Accreditation: [ ] AAPPO [ ] JACHO [ ] NCQA [ ] URAC
Plan Type: Specialty HMO, Specialty PPO, POS, ASO, EPO, UR
Total Revenue: 2005:   2006: 3,415,940
Net Income   2005:   2006:   457,120
Total Enrollment:
   2001: 300,389   2004: 177,313   2007: 172,291
   2002: 272,858   2005:
   2003: 153,043   2006: 170,237
Medical Loss Ratio: 2005:   2006: 36.83
Administrative Expense Ratio: 2005:   2006: 50.75

SERVICE AREA:
Nationwide: N
   AZ; CA; CO; CT; DC; HI; MA; MD; MI; NV; NJ; NM;
   NY; PA; TX; VT; VA;

TYPE OF COVERAGE:
Commercial: [Y] Individual: [ ] FEHBP: [ ] Indemnity: [ ]
Medicare: [Y] Medicaid: [ ] Supplemental Medicare: [ ]
Tricare   [ ]

PRODUCTS OFFERED:
Product Name: Type:
Landmark Health   Specialty HMO

PLAN BENEFITS:
Alternative Medicine: [X]   Behavioral Health: [ ]
Chiropractic: [X]   Dental: [ ]
Home Care: [ ]   Inpatient SNF: [ ]
Long-Term Care: [ ]   Pharm. Mail Order: [ ]
Physical Therapy: [ ]   Podiatry: [ ]
Psychiatric: [ ]   Transplant: [ ]
Vision: [ ]   Wellness: [ ]
Workers' Comp: [ ]
Other Benefits:

LIBERTY DENTAL PLAN OF CALIFORNIA

3200 El Camino Rd Ste 290
Irvine, CA 92799
Phone: 949-223-0007 Fax: 949-223-0011 Toll-Free: 888-703-6999
Web site: www.libertydentalplan.com

Managed Care Organization Profiles — CALIFORNIA

Senior VP,Chief Information Officer .... Philip Fasano
Health Plan Operations .... Arthur M Southam, MD
Senior VP/Quality & Automated Medical Records .. Louise Liang, MD
Senior VP/Health Plan Operations .... Leslie A Margolin
Senior VP/Health Plan Manager .... Jerry C Fleming
Senior VP/Chief Compliance Officer .... Daniel P Garcia

COMPANY PROFILE:
Parent Company Name: Kaiser Permanente
Doing Business As: Kaiser Permanente
Year Founded: 1946   Federally Qualified: [ ]
Forprofit: [ ]   Not-For-Profit: [Y]
Model Type:
Accreditation: [ ] AAPPO [X] JACHO [X] NCQA [ ] URAC
Plan Type: HMO, HDHP, HSA
Primary Physicians: 13,729   Physician Specialists:
Hospitals: 32
Total Revenue: 2005:   2006: 34,400,000,000
Net Income: 2005:   2006: 1,400,000,000
Total Enrollment:
  2001: 8,148,817   2004: 8,200,000   2007: 8,658,288
  2002: 8,370,154   2005: 8,400,000
  2003: 8,200,000   2006: 8,700,000

SERVICE AREA:
Nationwide: N
  CA; CO; DC; GA; HI; MD; OH; OR; VA; WA;

TYPE OF COVERAGE:
Commercial: [Y] Individual: [Y] FEHBP: [ ] Indemnity: [ ]
Medicare: [Y] Medicaid: [Y] Supplemental Medicare: [ ]
Tricare [ ]

PRODUCTS OFFERED:
Product Name: Type:
KP Senior Advantage   Medicare Advantage

PLAN BENEFITS:
Alternative Medicine: [ ]   Behavioral Health: [ ]
Chiropractic: [X]   Dental: [X]
Home Care: [X]   Inpatient SNF: [X]
Long-Term Care: [X]   Pharm. Mail Order: [X]
Physicial Therapy: [X]   Podiatry: [X]
Psychiatric: [X]   Transplant: [X]
Vision: [X]   Wellness: [X]
Workers' Comp: [X]
Other Benefits:

KERN FAMILY HEALTH CARE

9700 Stockdale Hwy
Bakersfield, CA 93311
Phone: 661-664-5000 Fax: 661-664-5151 Toll-Free: 800-391-2000
Web site: www.kernfamilyhealthcare.com
MAILING ADDRESS:
  KERN FAMILY HEALTH CARE
  9700 Stockdale Hwy
  Bakersfield, CA 93311

KEY EXECUTIVES:
Chief Executive Officer .... Carol Sorrell, RN
Chief Financial Officer .... Dave Shaffer
Medical Director .... Lon Graves, MD
Pharmacy Director .... Hal Stewart
Chief Information Officer .... Bob Woodard
Director of Operations .... Becky Davenport
Marketing Director .... Janet Sanders
MIS Manager .... Frank Ripepi
Director of Provider Services .... Stacie Reeves
Director of Health Services .... Anne Watkins
Chief Compliance Officer .... Anita Perrine, RN

COMPANY PROFILE:
Parent Company Name: Kern Health Systems
Doing Business As: Kern Family Health Care
Year Founded: 1996   Federally Qualified: [N]
Forprofit: [ ]   Not-For-Profit: [Y]
Model Type: NETWORK
Accreditation: [ ] AAPPO [ ] JACHO [ ] NCQA [ ] URAC
Plan Type: HMO
Total Revenue: 2005: 31,233,768   2006: 126,476,374
Net Income: 2005: -1,577,980   2006: -439,807
Total Enrollment:
  2001: 67,847   2004: 92,689   2007: 90,902
  2002: 74,712   2005: 90,842
  2003: 79,791   2006: 92,102

Medical Loss Ratio: 2005: 97.91   2006: 95.96
Administrative Expense Ratio: 2005: 8.60   2006: 7.44

SERVICE AREA:
Nationwide: N
  CA;

TYPE OF COVERAGE:
Commercial: [ ] Individual: [Y] FEHBP: [ ] Indemnity: [ ]
Medicare: [Y] Medicaid: [Y] Supplemental Medicare: [ ]
Tricare [ ]

PRODUCTS OFFERED:
Product Name: Type:
Medi-Cal   Medicaid
Kern Family Health Care   HMO

KERN FOUNDATION/PREFERRED PROVIDER ORGANIZATION

333 Palmer Dr Ste 200
Bakersfield, CA 93309
Phone: 661-327-7581 Fax: 661-327-5129 Toll-Free:
Web site: www.kernfmc.com
MAILING ADDRESS:
  KERN FOUNDATION/PPO
  333 Palmer Dr Ste 200
  Bakersfield, CA 93309

KEY EXECUTIVES:
Chief Executive Officer .... Carolyn J Temple
Administration & Finance Services .... Elizabeth Maynard
Chief Operating Officer .... Janet Clary
Chief Marketing Officer .... George Stephenson II
Provider Relations Coordinator .... Jeanne Simpson

COMPANY PROFILE:
Parent Company Name:
Doing Business As: Foundation for Medical Care/Kern/Santa Barbara
Year Founded: 1959   Federally Qualified: [N]
Forprofit: [ ]   Not-For-Profit: [Y]
Model Type:
Accreditation: [ ] AAPPO [ ] JACHO [ ] NCQA [ ] URAC
Plan Type: PPO, UR, TPA, EPO

SERVICE AREA:
Nationwide: N
  CA (Kern, Santa Barbara);

TYPE OF COVERAGE:
Commercial: [ ] Individual: [ ] FEHBP: [ ] Indemnity: [ ]
Medicare: [ ] Medicaid: [Y] Supplemental Medicare: [ ]
Tricare [ ]

PLAN BENEFITS:
Alternative Medicine: [ ]   Behavioral Health: [ ]
Chiropractic: [X]   Dental: [X]
Home Care: [X]   Inpatient SNF: [X]
Long-Term Care: [X]   Pharm. Mail Order: [X]
Physicial Therapy: [X]   Podiatry: [X]
Psychiatric: [X]   Transplant: [X]
Vision: [X]   Wellness: [X]
Workers' Comp: [X]
Other Benefits:

LA CARE HEALTH PLAN

555 W 5th St 29th Fl
Los Angeles, CA 90013-3036
Phone: 213-694-1250 Fax: 213-694-1246 Toll-Free: 888-452-2273
Web site: www.lacare.org
MAILING ADDRESS:
  LA CARE HEALTH PLAN
  555 W 5th St 29th Fl
  Los Angeles, CA 90013-3036

KEY EXECUTIVES:
Chairman of the Board .... Jim Lott
Chief Executive Officer .... Howard A Kahn
Chief Financial Officer .... W Randy Stone, MBA
Chief Medical Officer .... Elaine Batchlor, MD
Chief Information Officer .... Dan Sun
Chief of Managed Care Operations .... Dorothy Seleski
Director of Information Systems .... Sunny Cooper
Manager of Credentialing .... Penny Tunney
Program Manager & Privacy Official .... Karen Louise Elliott

CALIFORNIA

Managed Care Organization Profiles

PRODUCTS OFFERED:
Product Name: Type:
Jaimini Health Inc   Specialty HMO
PLAN BENEFITS:
Alternative Medicine: [ ]   Behavioral Health: [ ]
Chiropractic: [ ]   Dental: [X]
Home Care: [ ]   Inpatient SNF: [ ]
Long-Term Care: [ ]   Pharm. Mail Order: [ ]
Physical Therapy: [ ]   Podiatry: [ ]
Psychiatric: [ ]   Transplant: [ ]
Vision: [ ]   Wellness: [ ]
Workers' Comp: [ ]
Other Benefits:
Comments:
Formerly HealthDent of California Inc.

KAISER FOUNDATION HEALTH PLAN OF NORTHERN CALIFORNIA

1950 Franklin St
Oakland, CA 94612
Phone: 510-987-1000 Fax: 510-625-3278 Toll-Free: 800-464-4000
Web site: www.kaiserpermanente.org
MAILING ADDRESS:
    KAISER FOUNDATION HEALTH PLAN NO CA
    1950 Franklin St
    Oakland, CA 94612

KEY EXECUTIVES:
Chief Executive Officer .... George C Halvorsen
President, North CA Region .... Mary Ann Thode
Chief Financial Officer .... George Di Salvo
Medical Director .... Robert M Pearl, MD

COMPANY PROFILE:
Parent Company Name: Kaiser Permanente
Doing Business As:
Year Founded: 1946   Federally Qualified: [Y]
Forprofit: [ ]   Not-For-Profit: [Y]
Model Type: GROUP
Accreditation: [ ] AAPPO [ ] JACHO [ ] NCQA [ ] URAC
Plan Type: HMO, HDHP, HSA
Total Revenue: 2005:   2006: 34,851,506,000
Net Income   2005:   2006:   1,351,829,000
Total Enrollment:
    2001: 6,132,515   2004: 6,425,749   2007: 3,286,230
    2002: 6,567,050   2005: 3,236,785
    2003: 6,453,906   2006: 6,758,447
Medical Loss Ratio: 2005:   2006: 94.79
Administrative Expense Ratio: 2005:   2006:   3.65
SERVICE AREA:
Nationwide: N
    CA (Northern);
TYPE OF COVERAGE:
Commercial: [Y] Individual: [ ] FEHBP: [ ] Indemnity: [ ]
Medicare: [Y] Medicaid: [Y] Supplemental Medicare: [ ]
Tricare   [ ]
PRODUCTS OFFERED:
Product Name: Type:
Kaiser Foundation   Medicaid
Kaiser HMO   HMO
Senior Advantage   Medicare Advantage
CONSUMER-DRIVEN PRODUCTS
Wells Fargo   HSA Company
CarePay HSA   HSA Product
                                       HSA Administrator
                                       Consumer-Driven Health Plan
                                       High Deductible Health Plan
PLAN BENEFITS:
Alternative Medicine: [ ]   Behavioral Health: [ ]
Chiropractic: [X]   Dental: [ ]
Home Care: [X]   Inpatient SNF: [X]
Long-Term Care: [ ]   Pharm. Mail Order: [X]
Physical Therapy: [X]   Podiatry: [X]
Psychiatric: [X]   Transplant: [X]
Vision: [X]   Wellness: [X]
Workers' Comp: [X]
Other Benefits:

KAISER FOUNDATION HEALTH PLAN OF SOUTHERN CALIFORNIA

393 E Walnut St
Pasadena, CA 91188
Phone: 626-405-5890 Fax: 626-405-3176 Toll-Free:
Web site: www.kaiserpermanente.org
MAILING ADDRESS:
    KAISER FOUNDATION HEALTH PLAN SO CA
    393 E Walnut St
    Pasadena, CA 91188

KEY EXECUTIVES:
Chairman of the Board .... Jeffrey A Weisz, MD
Chief Executive Officer .... George C Halvorson
President-South Region .... Benjamin Chu, MD
Chief Financial Officer .... Kathy Lancaster
Executive Medical Director .... Jeffrey A Weisz, MD
Chief Information Officer .... Philip Fasano
VP Market & Business Dev .... William B Caswell
Assoc Director, Corporate Communications . Cynthia M Harding, APR
Human Resources Director .... Laurence G O'Neil

COMPANY PROFILE:
Parent Company Name: Kaiser Permanente
Doing Business As:
Year Founded: 1946   Federally Qualified: [ ]
Forprofit: [ ]   Not-For-Profit: [Y]
Model Type:
Accreditation: [ ] AAPPO [ ] JACHO [ ] NCQA [ ] URAC
Plan Type: HMO, HDHP, HSA
Total Enrollment:
    2001: 0   2004: 3,566   2007: 3,248,933
    2002: 0   2005: 3,125,072
    2003: 0   2006:
SERVICE AREA:
Nationwide: N
    CA (Southern);
TYPE OF COVERAGE:
Commercial: [Y] Individual: [ ] FEHBP: [ ] Indemnity: [ ]
Medicare: [Y] Medicaid: [Y] Supplemental Medicare: [ ]
Tricare   [ ]
PRODUCTS OFFERED:
Product Name: Type:
Kaiser South Medicare   Medicare
                                       Medicaid
CONSUMER-DRIVEN PRODUCTS
Wells Fargo   HSA Company
CarePay HSA   HSA Product
                                       HSA Administrator
                                       Consumer-Driven Health Plan
                                       High Deductible Health Plan
PLAN BENEFITS:
Alternative Medicine: [ ]   Behavioral Health: [ ]
Chiropractic: [X]   Dental: [ ]
Home Care: [X]   Inpatient SNF: [X]
Long-Term Care: [ ]   Pharm. Mail Order: [X]
Physical Therapy: [X]   Podiatry: [X]
Psychiatric: [X]   Transplant: [X]
Vision: [X]   Wellness: [X]
Workers' Comp: [X]
Other Benefits:

KAISER PERMANENTE - KAISER FOUNDATION HEALTH PLAN, INC

One Kaiser Plaza
Oakland, CA 94612
Phone: 510-271-2377 Fax: 510-271-5820 Toll-Free:
Web site: www.kaiserpermanente.org
MAILING ADDRESS:
    KAISER PERMANENTE
    One Kaiser Plaza
    Oakland, CA 94612

KEY EXECUTIVES:
Chairman of the Board .... George C Halvorson
Chief Executive Officer/President .... George C Halvorson
Chief Financial Officer .... Kathy Lancaster
Medical Director .... Francis J Crosson, MD

Managed Care Organization Profiles — CALIFORNIA

INTER VALLEY HEALTH PLAN INC

300 S Park Ave Ste 300
Pomona, CA 91769-6002
Phone: 909-623-6333 Fax: 909-622-2907 Toll-Free: 800-255-6882
Web site: www.ivhp.com
MAILING ADDRESS:
  INTER VALLEY HEALTH PLAN INC
  PO Box 6002
  Pomona, CA 91769-6002

KEY EXECUTIVES:
Chairman of the Board .... Richard Kirkendall, PhD
Chief Executive Officer .... Ronald Bolding
Chief Financial Officer .... Donald McCain
MIS Director .... Bill Chen
VP of Human Resources .... Trish Jacobson
VP of Health Services, UM/CM Manager .... Susan Tenorio, RN
Director Corporate Communications .... Cyndle O'Brien

COMPANY PROFILE:
Parent Company Name:
Doing Business As: Pomona Valley Health Plan Inc
Year Founded: 1979   Federally Qualified: [Y]
Forprofit: [ ]   Not-For-Profit: [Y]
Model Type: IPA
Accreditation: [ ] AAPPO [ ] JACHO [ ] NCQA [ ] URAC
Plan Type: HMO
Total Revenue: 2005: 116,602,000   2006: 32,367,496
Net Income   2005: 4,432,000   2006: 1,243,641
Total Enrollment:
  2001: 69,159   2004: 13,111   2007: 12,705
  2002: 15,372   2005: 12,996
  2003: 14,337   2006: 12,269
Medical Loss Ratio: 2005: 97.30   2006: 89.03
Administrative Expense Ratio: 2005: 8.60   2006: 8.64
SERVICE AREA:
Nationwide: N
  CA (Los Angeles, Orange, Riverside, San Bernardino, Santa Barbara, Ventura);
TYPE OF COVERAGE:
Commercial: [ ] Individual: [ ] FEHBP: [ ] Indemnity: [ ]
Medicare: [Y] Medicaid: [ ] Supplemental Medicare: [ ]
Tricare   [ ]
PRODUCTS OFFERED:
Product Name: Type:
Service to Seniors   Medicare Advantage
Premier 100
Premier 80
Nova 100
Nova 80
Vista 100
Vista 80
PLAN BENEFITS:
Alternative Medicine: [ ]   Behavioral Health: [X]
Chiropractic: [ ]   Dental: [ ]
Home Care: [X]   Inpatient SNF: [X]
Long-Term Care: [ ]   Pharm. Mail Order: [X]
Physical Therapy: [X]   Podiatry: [X]
Psychiatric: [X]   Transplant: [X]
Vision: [X]   Wellness: [X]
Workers' Comp: [ ]
Other Benefits:
Comments:
Formerly Pomona Valley Health Plan Inc.

INTERPLAN HEALTH GROUP

2575 Grand Canal Blvd Ste 100
Stockton, CA 95207
Phone: 209-473-0811 Fax: 209-473-0863 Toll-Free: 800-444-4036
Web site: www.interplanhealth.com
MAILING ADDRESS:
  INTERPLAN HEALTH GROUP
  2575 Grand Canal Blvd Ste 100
  Stockton, CA 95207

KEY EXECUTIVES:
Chairman/Chief Executive Officer .... Paul W Glover
President .... Joseph Manheim
Chief Financial Officer .... Steven L Ditman
Chief Medical Officer .... Michael Cohen, MD
VP, Pharmacy Services .... Michael Dlugos
Information Systems Officer .... Hamilton Chaffee
Chief Operating Officer .... Eileen Romansky
Chief Sales & Marketing Officer .... Michael D Schotz
Manager, Network Operations .... Verdis Norwood
Sr, VP of Provider Networks .... Cornelia Outten
Controller .... Kelli Swanson-Pico
Senior VP, Medical & Case Management, Prod Dvlp ... Maureen Starr
Manager, Network Operations .... Verdis Norwood
VP, Direct Medical Management .... Mary Romanchok
VP of Client Services .... Kathy Polenske

COMPANY PROFILE:
Parent Company Name: Interplan Health Group (formerly IPACQ)
Doing Business As:
Year Founded: 1984   Federally Qualified: [ ]
Forprofit: [Y]   Not-For-Profit: [ ]
Model Type: Network
Accreditation: [ ] AAPPO [ ] JACHO [ ] NCQA [X] URAC
Plan Type: PPO, UR, EPO
Total Enrollment:
  2001: 2,100,000   2004: 1,788,000   2007: 0
  2002: 2,340,000   2005: 3,000,000
  2003: 0   2006:
SERVICE AREA:
Nationwide: N
  CA; NV; WA;
TYPE OF COVERAGE:
Commercial: [Y] Individual: [ ] FEHBP: [ ] Indemnity: [ ]
Medicare: [ ] Medicaid: [ ] Supplemental Medicare: [ ]
Tricare
PLAN BENEFITS:
Alternative Medicine: [ ]   Behavioral Health: [X]
Chiropractic: [X]   Dental: [X]
Home Care: [X]   Inpatient SNF: [ ]
Long-Term Care: [X]   Pharm. Mail Order: [ ]
Physicial Therapy: [ ]   Podiatry: [X]
Psychiatric: [X]   Transplant: [X]
Vision: [ ]   Wellness: [X]
Workers' Comp: [X]
Other Benefits:

JAIMINI HEALTH INC

9500 Haven Ave #125
Rancho Cucamonga, CA 91730
Phone: 909-483-8310 Fax: 909-483-5351 Toll-Free: 800-937-3400
Web site: www.jaminihealth.com
MAILING ADDRESS:
  JAIMINI HEALTH INC
  9500 Haven Ave #125
  Rancho Cucamonga, CA 91730

KEY EXECUTIVES:
President .... Mohander Narula, DDS
Chief Financial Officer .... Mahesh Manchandia
Dental Director .... Robert Anderson, DDS
Chief Operating Officer .... Sandra Martinez
VP, Sales & Marketing .... Dan Baker
VP, Sales & Marketing .... Sandra Martinez
Director of Provider Services .... Cindy Semkiw

COMPANY PROFILE:
Parent Company Name: Jaimini Health Inc
Doing Business As: Healthdent of California
Year Founded: 1983   Federally Qualified: [N]
Forprofit: [Y]   Not-For-Profit: [ ]
Model Type: GROUP
Accreditation: [ ] AAPPO [ ] JACHO [ ] NCQA [ ] URAC
Plan Type: Specialty HMO
Total Revenue: 2005: 131,217   2006: 478,134
Net Income   2005: -87,713   2006: -164,868
Total Enrollment:
  2001: 17,000   2004: 8,161   2007: 5,542
  2002: 11,802   2005: 7,261
  2003: 9,890   2006: 6,043
Medical Loss Ratio: 2005: 90.30   2006: 40.45
Administrative Expense Ratio: 2005: 8.19   2006: 93.99
SERVICE AREA:
Nationwide: N
  CA;
TYPE OF COVERAGE:
Commercial: [Y] Individual: [Y] FEHBP: [ ] Indemnity: [ ]
Medicare: [ ] Medicaid: [ ] Supplemental Medicare: [ ]
Tricare   [ ]

CALIFORNIA   **Managed Care Organization Profiles**

HUMAN AFFAIRS INTERNATIONAL OF CALIFORNIA

300 Continental Blvd Ste 240
El Segundo, CA 90245
Phone: 310-726-7000 Fax: 310-726-7055 Toll-Free:
Web site: www.magellanhealth.com
MAILING ADDRESS:
    HUMAN AFFAIRS INTL OF CA
    300 Continental Blvd Ste 240
    El Segundo, CA 90245

KEY EXECUTIVES:
Chief Executive Officer/President .... Flora Vivaldo
Chief Financial Officer .... John Vieira

COMPANY PROFILE:
Parent Company Name: Magellan Health Services Inc
Doing Business As: HAI, HAI-CA
Year Founded: Federally Qualified: [Y]
Forprofit: [Y]   Not-For-Profit: [ ]
Model Type:
Accreditation: [ ] AAPPO [ ] JACHO [X] NCQA [ ] URAC
Plan Type: Specialty HMO
Total Revenue: 2005:   5,442,211   2006:   2,625,084
Net Income   2005:   183,984   2006:   505,936
Total Enrollment:
    2001: 1,336,031   2004: 978,766   2007: 624,206
    2002: 1,038,577   2005: 1,025,232
    2003:   939,428   2006:   650,454
Medical Loss Ratio: 2005: 63.13   2006: 49.56
Administrative Expense Ratio: 2005: 32.84   2006: 31.59
SERVICE AREA:
Nationwide: Y
    NW:
TYPE OF COVERAGE:
Commercial: [Y] Individual: [ ] FEHBP: [ ] Indemnity: [ ]
Medicare: [ ] Medicaid: [ ] Supplemental Medicare: [ ]
Tricare   [ ]
PRODUCTS OFFERED:
Product Name: Type:
                                 HMO
PLAN BENEFITS:
Alternative Medicine: [ ]   Behavioral Health: [X]
Chiropractic: [ ]   Dental: [ ]
Home Care: [ ]   Inpatient SNF: [ ]
Long-Term Care: [ ]   Pharm. Mail Order: [ ]
Physical Therapy: [ ]   Podiatry: [ ]
Psychiatric: [X]   Transplant: [ ]
Vision: [ ]   Wellness: [X]
Workers' Comp: [ ]
Other Benefits:

INLAND EMPIRE FOUNDATION FOR MEDICAL CARE

3993 Jurupa Ave
Riverside, CA 92506
Phone: 951-686-9049 Fax: 951-686-1692 Toll-Free: 800-334-7341
Web site: www.cfmcnet.org
MAILING ADDRESS:
    INLAND EMPIRE FDN FOR MED CRE
    3993 Jurupa Ave
    Riverside, CA 92506

KEY EXECUTIVES:
Chief Executive Officer .... Dolores L Green
President .... Steven E Larson, MD
Chief Financial Officer .... James L Merson, MD
Chief Operating Officer .... Teresa Herrera
Director of Marketing .... Ester Sanchez
MIS Director .... Debbie Kellenberger
Credentialing Manager/Provider Relations Director .... Mary Barnes
Vice President .... Alonso R Ojeda, MD

COMPANY PROFILE:
Parent Company Name: Statewide Ntwk: CA Fdn for Medical Care
Doing Business As:
Year Founded: 1960   Federally Qualified: [N]
Forprofit: [ ]   Not-For-Profit: [Y]
Model Type: NETWORK
Accreditation: [ ] AAPPO [ ] JACHO [ ] NCQA [ ] URAC
Plan Type: PPO, TPA, EPO

Primary Physicians: 600   Physician Specialists: 1,200
Hospitals: 27
Total Enrollment:
    2001: 0   2004: 75,000   2007: 1,200,000
    2002: 0   2005:
    2003: 0   2006: 1,200,000
SERVICE AREA:
Nationwide: N
    CA;
TYPE OF COVERAGE:
Commercial: [Y] Individual: [ ] FEHBP: [ ] Indemnity: [ ]
Medicare: [ ] Medicaid: [ ] Supplemental Medicare: [ ]
Tricare   [ ]
PLAN BENEFITS:
Alternative Medicine: [ ]   Behavioral Health: [X]
Chiropractic: [X]   Dental: [X]
Home Care: [X]   Inpatient SNF: [X]
Long-Term Care: [X]   Pharm. Mail Order: [X]
Physical Therapy: [X]   Podiatry: [X]
Psychiatric: [X]   Transplant: [X]
Vision: [X]   Wellness: [ ]
Workers' Comp: [X]
Other Benefits: COBRA, Flex 125, HIP
Comments:
Formerly Riverside County Foundation for Medical Care.

INLAND EMPIRE HEALTH PLAN

303 E Vanderbilt Way Ste 400
San Bernardino, CA 92408
Phone: 909-890-2000 Fax: 909-890-2019 Toll-Free:
Web site: www.IEHP.org
MAILING ADDRESS:
    INLAND EMPIRE HEALTH PLAN
    303 E Vanderbilt Way Ste 400
    San Bernardino, CA 92408

KEY EXECUTIVES:
Chief Executive Officer .... Richard Bruno
Chief Financial Officer .... Chet Uma
Executive Officer, Chief Medical Officer .... Brad Gilbert, MD
Director of Operations .... Phil Branstetter
Chief Marketing Officer .... Carl Marier
Chief Network Officer .... Eric Haden

COMPANY PROFILE:
Parent Company Name:
Doing Business As:
Year Founded: 1994   Federally Qualified: [N] Forprofit: [ ]
Not-For-Profit: [Y]
Model Type: IPA/Direct
Accreditation: [ ] AAPPO [ ] JACHO [Y] NCQA [ ] URAC
Plan Type: HMO
Total Revenue: 2005: 77,533,130   2006: 77,406,080
Net Income   2005: -2,236,205   2006: -1,972,841
Total Enrollment:
    2001: 217,419   2004: 277,742   2007: 320,854
    2002: 253,212   2005: 248,184
    2003: 265,148   2006: 302,705
Medical Loss Ratio: 2005: 95.61   2006: 93.77
Administrative Expense Ratio: 2005:   7.29   2006:   7.81
SERVICE AREA:
Nationwide: N
    CA (San Bernardino, Riverside);
TYPE OF COVERAGE:
Commercial: [Y] Individual: [ ] FEHBP: [ ] Indemnity: [ ]
Medicare: [ ] Medicaid: [Y] Supplemental Medicare: [ ]
Tricare   [ ]
PRODUCTS OFFERED:
Product Name: Type:
Inland Empire Hlth Plan   Medicaid
PLAN BENEFITS:
Alternative Medicine: [ ]   Behavioral Health: [ ]
Chiropractic: [ ]   Dental: [ ]
Home Care: [ ]   Inpatient SNF: [X]
Long-Term Care: [ ]   Pharm. Mail Order: [X]
Physical Therapy: [X]   Podiatry: [ ]
Psychiatric: [ ]   Transplant: [X]
Vision: [X]   Wellness: [X]
Workers' Comp: [ ]
Other Benefits:

Managed Care Organization Profiles — CALIFORNIA

Total Revenue: 2005: 178,694,960   2006: 800,103,198
Net Income   2005:   455,276   2006:   488,895
Total Enrollment:
  2001: 171,018   2004: 261,130   2007: 272,241
  2002: 194,574   2005: 257,882
  2003: 257,189   2006: 262,449
Medical Loss Ratio: 2005: 94.24   2006: 93.71
Administrative Expense Ratio: 2005: 8.56   2006: 8.19

SERVICE AREA:
Nationwide: N
  CA;

TYPE OF COVERAGE:
Commercial: [ ]   Individual: [ ]   FEHBP: [ ]   Indemnity: [ ]
Medicare: [ ]   Medicaid: [ ]   Supplemental Medicare: [ ]
Tricare   [ ]

PRODUCTS OFFERED:
Product Name:	Type:
Heritage HMO	HMO

HMO CALIFORNIA

1600 E Hill St
Signal Hill, CA 90806
Phone: 562-424-6200 Fax: 562-981-5818 Toll-Free: 866-255-4795
Web site: www.universalcare.com

MAILING ADDRESS:
  HMO CALIFORNIA
  1600 E Hill St
  Signal Hill, CA 90806

KEY EXECUTIVES:
Chief Executive Officer .... Howard E Davis
Chief Financial Officer .... Richard Schreiber
Chief Medical Officer .... John Adams, MD
Chief Operating Officer .... Jeffrey V Davis
Marketing Director .... Jay D Davis
VP Provider Contracting .... Laura Carmona

COMPANY PROFILE:
Parent Company Name: Health Net Inc
Doing Business As: Universal Care
Year Founded: 1983   Federally Qualified: [N]
Forprofit: [Y]   Not-For-Profit: [ ]
Model Type: MIXED
Accreditation: [ ] AAPPO [ ] JACHO [X] NCQA [ ] URAC
Plan Type: HMO, POS
Total Revenue: 2005: 13,940,333   2006: 12,477,810
Net Income   2005:   -441,068   2006:   13,444
Total Enrollment:
  2001: 329,085   2004: 463,288   2007: 188,526
  2002: 339,939   2005: 437,549
  2003: 492,240   2006: 190,385
Medical Loss Ratio: 2005: 94.77   2006: 88.32
Administrative Expense Ratio: 2005: 3.88   2006: 10.87

SERVICE AREA:
Nationwide: N
  CA (Los Angeles, Orange, Riverside, San Bernardino, San Diego);

TYPE OF COVERAGE:
Commercial: [Y]   Individual: [Y]   FEHBP: [ ]   Indemnity: [ ]
Medicare: [ ]   Medicaid: [Y]   Supplemental Medicare: [ ]
Tricare   [ ]

PRODUCTS OFFERED:
Product Name:	Type:
Universal Care Medicaid HMO	Medicaid
Universal Care HMO	HMO
Universal Care Health Advantag	Medicare
Universal Care POS	POS

PLAN BENEFITS:
Alternative Medicine:	[ ]	Behavioral Health:	[ ]
Chiropractic:	[X]	Dental:	[X]
Home Care:	[X]	Inpatient SNF:	[X]
Long-Term Care:	[ ]	Pharm. Mail Order:	[X]
Physical Therapy:	[X]	Podiatry:	[X]
Psychiatric:	[X]	Transplant:	[ ]
Vision:	[X]	Wellness:	[X]
Workers' Comp:	[ ]		
Other Benefits:			

Comments:
Health Net Inc acquired March 31, 2006.

HOLMAN GROUP, THE

9451 Corbin Ave Ste 100
Northridge, CA 91324
Phone: 818-704-1444 Fax: 818-704-9339 Toll-Free:
Web site: www.holmangroup.com

MAILING ADDRESS:
  HOLMAN GROUP, THE
  9451 Corbin Ave Ste 100
  Northridge, CA 91324

KEY EXECUTIVES:
Chief Executive Officer .... Ron Holmon
Senior Vice President .... Marcus Sola
Chief Financial Officer .... Linda Holmon
Medical Director .... Steven Cleven, MD

COMPANY PROFILE:
Parent Company Name:
Doing Business As:
Year Founded: 1985   Federally Qualified: [ ]
Forprofit: [ ]   Not-For-Profit: [ ]
Model Type:
Accreditation: [ ] AAPPO [ ] JACHO [ ] NCQA [ ] URAC
Plan Type: Specialty HMO
Total Revenue: 2005: 1,583,004   2006: 3,791,570
Net Income   2005: -180,506   2006:   43,873
Total Enrollment:
  2001: 200,219   2004: 188,150   2007: 136,758
  2002: 196,378   2005: 173,607
  2003: 205,321   2006: 156,231
Medical Loss Ratio: 2005: 71.90   2006: 72.81
Administrative Expense Ratio: 2005: 39.90   2006: 26.88

SERVICE AREA:
Nationwide: N
  CA;

PLAN BENEFITS:
Alternative Medicine:	[ ]	Behavioral Health:	[ ]
Chiropractic:	[ ]	Dental:	[ ]
Home Care:	[ ]	Inpatient SNF:	[ ]
Long-Term Care:	[ ]	Pharm. Mail Order:	[ ]
Physical Therapy:	[ ]	Podiatry:	[ ]
Psychiatric:	[X]	Transplant:	[ ]
Vision:	[ ]	Wellness:	[ ]
Workers' Comp:	[ ]		
Other Benefits:			

HONORED CITIZEN'S CHOICE HEALTH PLAN

9025 Wilshire Blvd Ste 301
Beverly Hills, CA 90211
Phone: 323-273-8220 Fax: 323-725-6933 Toll-Free:
Web site: www.citizenschoicehealth.com

MAILING ADDRESS:
  HONORED CITIZENS CHOICE HLT PL
  9025 Wilshire Blvd Ste 301
  Beverly Hills, CA 90211

KEY EXECUTIVES:
President/Chief Operating Officer .... Parvis Kahen

COMPANY PROFILE:
Parent Company Name:
Doing Business As:
Year Founded: 2004   Federally Qualified: [ ]
Forprofit: [ ]   Not-For-Profit: [ ]
Model Type:
Accreditation: [ ] AAPPO [ ] JACHO [ ] NCQA [ ] URAC
Plan Type: HMO
Total Revenue: 2005: 283,563   2006: 16,598,333
Net Income   2005: -575,101   2006:   -711,047
Total Enrollment:
  2001: 0   2004: 0   2007: 3,138
  2002: 0   2005: 141
  2003: 0   2006: 1,906
Medical Loss Ratio: 2005: 99.30   2006: 79.88
Administrative Expense Ratio: 2005: 207.00   2006: 25.24

SERVICE AREA:
Nationwide:
  CA;

CALIFORNIA — Managed Care Organization Profiles

PRODUCTS OFFERED:
Product Name:	Type:
Health Net HMO	HMO
Health Net PPO	PPO
Health Net	PPO
Select	POS
Seniority Plus HMO	Medicare Advantage
Seniority Plus POS	Medicare Supplement
Flex Net	Indemnity

PLAN BENEFITS:
Alternative Medicine:	[ ]	Behavioral Health:	[X]
Chiropractic:	[X]	Dental:	[X]
Home Care:	[X]	Inpatient SNF:	[X]
Long-Term Care:	[ ]	Pharm. Mail Order:	[X]
Physical Therapy:	[X]	Podiatry:	[X]
Psychiatric:	[X]	Transplant:	[X]
Vision:	[X]	Wellness:	[X]
Workers' Comp:	[X]		

Other Benefits: Acupuncture (Rider)
Comments:
Merged with Foundation Health.

HEALTH PLAN OF SAN JOAQUIN, THE

7757 S Manthey Rd
French Camp, CA 95231
Phone: 209-939-3500 Fax: 209-942-6305 Toll-Free:
Web site: www.hpsj.com
MAILING ADDRESS:
 HEALTH PLAN OF SAN JOAQUIN
 PO Box 30490
 Stockton, CA 95231

KEY EXECUTIVES:
Chief Executive Officer .... John Hackworth
Chief Financial Officer .... Chet Uma
Medical Director .... Sylvia Carlisle, MD
Director of Marketing .... David Hurst
MIS Director .... Adi Kremer
Director Communications/Public Affairs .... Perfecto Munoz
Supervisor, Provider Services .... Linda Reynolds
Senior Health Educator .... Robin Morrow
Medical Management Director .... Mary Jordan RN
Quality Improvement Manager .... Sharon Steely
Director Fraud Prvntn/Investigation .... Steve Cox
Compliance Officer .... Nancy Raymond
Utilization Management Manager .... Janet Braun, RN
Executive Assistant .... Penny Schenken

COMPANY PROFILE:
Parent Company Name: San Joaquin County Health Commission
Doing Business As:
Year Founded: 1996 Federally Qualified: [ ]
Forprofit: [ ] Not-For-Profit: [Y]
Model Type: NETWORK
Accreditation: [ ] AAPPO [ ] JACHO [ ] NCQA [ ] URAC
Plan Type: HMO,
Total Revenue: 2005: 22,193,250 2006: 22,167,570
Net Income 2005: 646,924 2006: 16,751
Total Enrollment:
  2001: 57,739 2004: 76,218 2007: 78,288
  2002: 63,926 2005: 74,576
  2003: 66,999 2006: 75,545
Medical Loss Ratio: 2005: 90.23 2006:
Administrative Expense Ratio: 2005: 10.26 2006: 10.74
SERVICE AREA:
Nationwide: N
  CA (San Joaquin);
TYPE OF COVERAGE:
Commercial: [Y] Individual: [ ] FEHBP: [ ] Indemnity: [ ]
Medicare: [ ] Medicaid: [Y] Supplemental Medicare: [ ]
Tricare [ ]
PRODUCTS OFFERED:
Product Name:	Type:
Medi-Cal	Medicaid HMO

PLAN BENEFITS:
Alternative Medicine:	[ ]	Behavioral Health:	[ ]
Chiropractic:	[ ]	Dental:	[ ]
Home Care:	[ ]	Inpatient SNF:	[X]
Long-Term Care:	[ ]	Pharm. Mail Order:	[ ]
Physical Therapy:	[X]	Podiatry:	[X]
Psychiatric:	[ ]	Transplant:	[ ]
Vision:	[X]	Wellness:	[ ]
Workers' Comp:	[ ]		

Other Benefits:

HEALTH PLAN OF SAN MATEO

701 Gateway Blvd Ste 400
San Francisco, CA 94080
Phone: 650-616-0050 Fax: 650-616-0060 Toll-Free: 800-750-4776
Web site: www.hpsm.org
MAILING ADDRESS:
 HEALTH PLAN OF SAN MATEO
 701 Gateway Blvd Ste 400
 San Francisco, CA 94080

KEY EXECUTIVES:
Executive Director .... Maya Altman
Finance & Admnstrtve Services Director .... Ron Robinson
Medical Director .... Mary Giammona, MD
MIS Director .... Eben Yong
Health & Provider Services Director .... Mari Baca

COMPANY PROFILE:
Parent Company Name: San Mateo Health Commission
Doing Business As:
Year Founded: 1987 Federally Qualified: [N]
Forprofit: [ ] Not-For-Profit: [Y]
Model Type: IPA
Accreditation: [ ] AAPPO [ ] JACHO [X] NCQA [ ] URAC
Plan Type: HMO
Total Revenue: 2005: 32,770,872 2006: 251,744,181
Net Income 2005: -1,714,191 2006: 2,586,679
Total Enrollment:
  2001: 39,106 2004: 56,655 2007: 67,496
  2002: 46,784 2005: 57,527
  2003: 52,944 2006: 67,545
Medical Loss Ratio: 2005: 102.95 2006:
Administrative Expense Ratio: 2005: 9.77 2006: 6.49
SERVICE AREA:
Nationwide: N
  CA (San Mateo);
TYPE OF COVERAGE:
Commercial: [ ] Individual: [ ] FEHBP: [ ] Indemnity: [ ]
Medicare: [ ] Medicaid: [Y] Supplemental Medicare: [ ]
Tricare [ ]
PRODUCTS OFFERED:
Product Name:	Type:
Medi-Cal	Medicaid HMO

PLAN BENEFITS:
Alternative Medicine:	[ ]	Behavioral Health:	[ ]
Chiropractic:	[X]	Dental:	[ ]
Home Care:	[X]	Inpatient SNF:	[ ]
Long-Term Care:	[ ]	Pharm. Mail Order:	[ ]
Physical Therapy:	[ ]	Podiatry:	[X]
Psychiatric:	[ ]	Transplant:	[X]
Vision:	[X]	Wellness:	[X]
Workers' Comp:	[ ]		

Other Benefits:

HERITAGE PROVIDER NETWORK INC

8510 Balboa Blvd Ste 285
Northridge, CA 91325
Phone: 818-654-3461 Fax: 818-654-3460 Toll-Free:
Web site: www.heritageprovidernetwork.com
MAILING ADDRESS:
 HERITAGE PROVIDER NETWORK INC
 8510 Balboa Blvd Ste 285
 Northridge, CA 91325

KEY EXECUTIVES:
Chief Executive Officer/Founder .... Richard Merkin
Chief Financial Officer .... Jaya Kurian

COMPANY PROFILE:
Parent Company Name:
Doing Business As:
Year Founded: 1997 Federally Qualified: [ ]
Forprofit: [ ] Not-For-Profit: [ ]
Model Type:
Accreditation: [ ] AAPPO [ ] JACHO [ ] NCQA [ ] URAC
Plan Type: HMO

Managed Care Organization Profiles — **CALIFORNIA**

SERVICE AREA:
Nationwide: Y
NW;
TYPE OF COVERAGE:
Commercial: [Y] Individual: [ ] FEHBP: [ ] Indemnity: [ ]
Medicare: [ ] Medicaid: [ ] Supplemental Medicare: [ ]
Tricare [ ]
PLAN BENEFITS:
Alternative Medicine: [ ]   Behavioral Health: [ ]
Chiropractic: [X]   Dental: [X]
Home Care: [X]   Inpatient SNF: [X]
Long-Term Care: [X]   Pharm. Mail Order: [ ]
Physical Therapy: [X]   Podiatry: [X]
Psychiatric: [X]   Transplant: [X]
Vision: [X]   Wellness: [X]
Workers' Comp: [X]
Other Benefits:

HEALTH NET INC - CORPORATE HEADQUARTERS

21650 Oxnard Street
Woodland Hills, CA 91367
Phone: 818-676-6000 Fax: 818-676-8591 Toll-Free: 800-291-6911
Web site: www.healthnet.com
MAILING ADDRESS:
    HEALTH NET INC - CORP HDQRTS
    21650 Oxnard Street
    Woodland Hills, CA 91367

KEY EXECUTIVES:
Chairman of the Board .... Roger F Greaves
Chief Executive Officer/President .... Jay M Gellert
Chief Financial Officer .... Joseph C Capezza, CPA
Chief Medical Officer .... Jonathan Scheff, MD
Chief Information Officer .... Rick Simmons
Chief Operating Officer .... James Woys
Senior VP, Corporate Communications .... David W Olson
Privacy Officer .... Toni Schiavo
Senior VP, Corporate Communitications .... David W Olson
Senior VP/Organization Effectiveness .... Karin B Mayhew
Chief Compliance Officer .... Phillip G Davis
Chief Senior Products Officer .... Mark El-Tawil
President, HealthNet Northeast .... Steve Nelson
VP, Government Relations .... Adrienne Morrell
President, Health Plan Division .... Stephen D Lynch
Senior VP, General Counsel & Secretary .... Linda Tiano
President, Government/Specialty Division .... James Woys

COMPANY PROFILE:
Parent Company Name: Health Net Inc
Doing Business As: Health Net of AZ, CA, NE, OR & Fed Srvcs
Year Founded: 1979   Federally Qualified: [Y]
Forprofit: [Y]   Not-For-Profit: [ ]
Model Type: MIXED
Accreditation: [ ] AAPPO [ ] JACHO [X] NCQA [X] URAC
Plan Type: HMO, PPO, POS, ASO, HSA, HDHP
Primary Physicians: 50,924   Physician Specialists: 125,647
Hospitals:
Total Revenue: 2005: 11,940,533,000   2006: 12,908,350,000
Net Income   2005:   229,785,000   2006:   329,313,000
Total Enrollment:
   2001: 3,987,959   2004: 3,605,000   2007: 6,600,000
   2002: 5,400,000   2005: 5,300,000
   2003: 3,835,992   2006: 4,582,000
Medical Loss Ratio: 2005: 82.50   2006: 83.30
Administrative Expense Ratio: 2005: 11.40   2006: 11.40
SERVICE AREA:
Nationwide: N
   AZ; CA; CT; DE; DC; IL; IN; IA; KY; ME; MD; MA;
   MI; MO; NH; NJ; NY; NC; OH; OR; PA; RI; TN; VT;
   VA; WA; WV; WI;
TYPE OF COVERAGE:
Commercial: [Y] Individual: [Y] FEHBP: [ ] Indemnity: [ ]
Medicare: [Y] Medicaid: [Y] Supplemental Medicare: [Y]
Tricare   [Y]
PRODUCTS OFFERED:
Product Name: Type:
Seniority Plus   MedicaidHealthNet HMO
CONSUMER-DRIVEN PRODUCTS
Wells Fargo   HSA Company
HNOR Individual PPO HSA Plan   HSA Product
                                    HSA Administrator
                                    Consumer-Driven Health Plan
PPO Value Basic 2500   High Deductible Health Plan

PLAN BENEFITS:
Alternative Medicine: [ ]   Behavioral Health: [X]
Chiropractic: [X]   Dental: [X]
Home Care: [ ]   Inpatient SNF: [ ]
Long-Term Care: [ ]   Pharm. Mail Order: [X]
Physical Therapy: [ ]   Podiatry: [X]
Psychiatric: [ ]   Transplant: [ ]
Vision: [X]   Wellness: [X]
Workers' Comp: [X]
Other Benefits:
Comments:
Changed company name November 6, 2000 from Foundation Health Systems Inc. Other DBA names: MHN, Health Net Pharmaceutical Services (HNPS).

HEALTH NET OF CALIFORNIA

21281 Burbank Blvd
Woodland Hills, CA 91367
Phone: 818-676-6775 Fax: 818-676-6982 Toll-Free: 800-522-0088
Web site: www.healthnet.com
MAILING ADDRESS:
    HEALTH NET OF CALIFORNIA
    21281 Burbank Blvd
    Woodland Hills, CA 91367

KEY EXECUTIVES:
President .... Stephen D Lynch
Chief Financial Officer .... Robert Beltch
Senior VP, Chief Medical Officer .... Jennifer M Gutzmore, MD
Associate VP Pharmacy .... Neil Higashida PharmD
VP, Chief Information Officer .... Tom Fleishman
Chief Operating Officer .... Hugh A Jones
VP, Marketing .... Vicki McDonald
Senior VP, Chief Sales Officer .... David W Anderson
VP Information Systems .... Dave Golonski
Ancillary Benefits Director .... Monica Alvarenga
Associate VP, Public Relations .... Lisa Kalustian
Provider Services Manager .... Kay Merrill
VP, Network Management-South .... Lorie Ballerdine
Health Promotion/Prevention .... Cindy Keitel
VP, Human Resources .... Sharon Maguire
VP, Medical Management .... Anna DeGroote
Quality Assurance Director .... Vicky Cuevas
Fraud Prevention Manager .... Mike Brandt
Director of New Product Development .... Robin Brown
Case Management Director .... Toni Schiavo
VP, Product Development .... Beverly Bandini
VP, Network Management-North .... David Koury
Regional Chief Medical Officer .... William P Bracciodieta, MD

COMPANY PROFILE:
Parent Company Name: Health Net Inc
Doing Business As: Health Net of California
Year Founded: 1979   Federally Qualified: [Y]
Forprofit: [Y]   Not-For-Profit: [ ]
Model Type: MIXED
Accreditation: [ ] AAPPO [ ] JACHO [X] NCQA [ ] URAC
Plan Type: HMO, PPO, POS, HDHP, HSA
Total Revenue: 2005: 1,603,601,362   2006: 7,201,076,080
Net Income   2005:   52,367,156   2006:   216,851,068
Total Enrollment:
   2001: 2,600,745   2004: 2,355,000   2007: 2,105,626
   2002: 2,392,664   2005: 2,028,638
   2003: 3,031,569   2006: 2,303,000
Medical Loss Ratio: 2005: 85.04   2006: 85.70
Administrative Expense Ratio: 2005: 10.38   2006: 10.20
SERVICE AREA:
Nationwide: N
   CA (Alameda, Amador, Butte, Calaveras, Colusa, Contra Costa, El
   Dorado, Fresno, Glenn, Humboldt, Kern, Kings, Lake, Lassen, Los
   Angeles, Madera, Marin, Mariposa, Mendocino, Merced, Napa,
   Nevada, Orange, Placer, Plumas, Riverside, Sacramento, San
   Bernardino, San Diego,, San Francisco, San Joaquin, San Luis
   Obispo, San Mateo, Santa Barbara, Santa Clara, Santa Cruz, Shasta,
   Sierra, Solano, Sonoma, Stanislaus, Sutter, Tehama, Trinity, Tulare,
   Tuolumme, Ventura, Yolo, Yuba);
TYPE OF COVERAGE:
Commercial: [Y] Individual: [Y] FEHBP: [Y] Indemnity: [Y]
Medicare: [Y] Medicaid: [Y] Supplemental Medicare: [Y]
Tricare   [ ]

CALIFORNIA

Total Enrollment:
- 2001: 270,654
- 2002: 250,592
- 2003: 247,277
- 2004: 222,910
- 2005: 219,721
- 2006: 210,941
- 2007: 196,785

Medical Loss Ratio: 2005: 63.99 2006: 59.71
Administrative Expense Ratio: 2005: 31.11 2006: 2738.29

SERVICE AREA:
Nationwide: N
CA;

TYPE OF COVERAGE:
Commercial: [Y] Individual: [Y] FEHBP: [ ] Indemnity: [ ]
Medicare: [ ] Medicaid: [ ] Supplemental Medicare: [ ]
Tricare [ ]

PRODUCTS OFFERED:
Product Name:	Type:
Dental & Vision	Specialty HMO

PLAN BENEFITS:
Alternative Medicine: [ ]   Behavioral Health: [ ]
Chiropractic: [ ]   Dental: [X]
Home Care: [ ]   Inpatient SNF: [ ]
Long-Term Care: [ ]   Pharm. Mail Order: [ ]
Physical Therapy: [ ]   Podiatry: [ ]
Psychiatric: [ ]   Transplant: [ ]
Vision: [X]   Wellness: [ ]
Workers' Comp: [ ]
Other Benefits:

Comments:
WellPoint acquired Golden West Dental & Vision June 30, 2003.

GREAT-WEST HEALTHCARE OF CALIFORNIA

655 N Central Ave 19th Fl
Glendale, CA 91203-3905
Phone: 818-409-0880 Fax: 818-409-0881 Toll-Free: 800-877-9102
Web site: www.greatwesthealthcare.com

MAILING ADDRESS:
GREAT-WEST HEALTHCARE OF CA
655 N Central Ave 19th Fl
Glendale, CA 91203-3905

KEY EXECUTIVES:
Chief Executive Officer/President .... Raymond L McFeetors
Regional Manager .... Tim Closson
Financial Director .... Anand Raghavan
Manager, Public Relations .... Loren Finkelstein
Office Manager .... Lisa Pearl

COMPANY PROFILE:
Parent Company Name: CIGNA Inc
Doing Business As:
Year Founded: 1996   Federally Qualified: [ ]
Forprofit: [Y]   Not-For-Profit: [ ]
Model Type:
Accreditation: [ ] AAPPO [ ] JACHO [ ] NCQA [ ] URAC
Plan Type: HMO, PPO, CDHP, HDHP, HSA
Total Revenue: 2005: 44,139,772   2006: 188,871,675
Net Income   2005: 5,255,563   2006: 16,032,042
Total Enrollment:
- 2001: 0
- 2002: 59,015
- 2003: 53,815
- 2004: 58,800
- 2005: 60,131
- 2006: 53,380
- 2007: 47,589

Medical Loss Ratio: 2005: 84.31 2006: 76.75
Administrative Expense Ratio: 2005: 14.19 2006: 32.87

SERVICE AREA:
Nationwide: N
CA;

TYPE OF COVERAGE:
Commercial: [Y] Individual: [ ] FEHBP: [ ] Indemnity: [ ]
Medicare: [ ] Medicaid: [ ] Supplemental Medicare: [ ]
Tricare [ ]

PRODUCTS OFFERED:
Product Name:	Type:
One Health Plan of CA Inc	HMO

CONSUMER-DRIVEN PRODUCTS
Mellon HR Solutions LLC   HSA Company
                           HSA Product
                           HSA Administrator
                           Consumer-Driven Health Plan
                           High Deductible Health Plan

PLAN BENEFITS:
Alternative Medicine: [X]   Behavioral Health: [ ]
Chiropractic: [X]   Dental: [X]
Home Care: [X]   Inpatient SNF: [X]
Long-Term Care: [ ]   Pharm. Mail Order: [X]
Physical Therapy: [X]   Podiatry: [X]
Psychiatric: [X]   Transplant: [X]
Vision: [X]   Wellness: [X]
Workers' Comp: [ ]
Other Benefits:

Comments: Acquired by CIGNA Inc April 1, 2008.

GREAT-WEST HEALTHCARE OF CALIFORNIA - NORTH

3480 Buskirk Ave Ste 350
Pleasant Hill, CA 94523
Phone: 925-938-7788 Fax: 925-938-0381 Toll-Free:
Web site: www.greatwesthealthcare.com

MAILING ADDRESS:
GREAT-WEST HEALTHCARE OF CA-NO
3480 Buskirk Ave Ste 350
Pleasant Hill, CA 94523

KEY EXECUTIVES:
Regional Manager .... Marlene Matsuoka
Regional President .... Susan Hallet

COMPANY PROFILE:
Parent Company Name: CIGNA Inc
Doing Business As:
Year Founded: 1996   Federally Qualified: [ ]
Forprofit: [Y]   Not-For-Profit: [ ]
Model Type:
Accreditation: [ ] AAPPO [ ] JACHO [ ] NCQA [ ] URAC
Plan Type: HMO, PPO, POS, CDHP, HDHP, HSA

SERVICE AREA:
Nationwide: N
CA;

TYPE OF COVERAGE:
Commercial: [Y] Individual: [ ] FEHBP: [ ] Indemnity: [ ]
Medicare: [ ] Medicaid: [ ] Supplemental Medicare: [ ]
Tricare [ ]

CONSUMER-DRIVEN PRODUCTS
Mellon HR Solutions LLC   HSA Company
                           HSA Product
                           HSA Administrator
                           Consumer-Driven Health Plan
                           High Deductible Health Plan

PLAN BENEFITS:
Alternative Medicine: [X]   Behavioral Health: [ ]
Chiropractic: [X]   Dental: [X]
Home Care: [X]   Inpatient SNF: [X]
Long-Term Care: [ ]   Pharm. Mail Order: [X]
Physical Therapy: [X]   Podiatry: [X]
Psychiatric: [X]   Transplant: [X]
Vision: [X]   Wellness: [X]
Workers' Comp: [ ]
Other Benefits:

Comments: Acquired by CIGNA Inc April 1, 2008.

HEALTH CARE EVALUATION

6702 N Inglewood Ave Ste G
Stockton, CA 95207
Phone: 209-951-6711 Fax: 209-951-2731 Toll-Free:
Web site: www.pponext.com

MAILING ADDRESS:
HEALTH CARE EVALUATION
6702 N Inglewood Ave Ste G
Stockton, CA 95207

KEY EXECUTIVES:
Chief Executive Officer.. Jim Pennington

COMPANY PROFILE:
Parent Company Name: Concentra Inc
Doing Business As:
Year Founded: 1968   Federally Qualified: [N]
Forprofit: [Y]   Not-For-Profit: [ ]
Model Type:
Accreditation: [ ] AAPPO [ ] JACHO [ ] NCQA [X] URAC
Plan Type: UR;

Managed Care Organization Profiles — CALIFORNIA

COMPANY PROFILE:
Parent Company Name: Coventry Health Care Inc
Doing Business As: First Health Network
Year Founded: 1984 Federally Qualified: [N]
Forprofit: [Y] Not-For-Profit: [ ]
Model Type: NETWORK
Accreditation: [ ] AAPPO [ ] JACHO [ ] NCQA [X] URAC
Plan Type: PPO, UR, POS
Total Enrollment:
  2001: 10,340,882 2004: 0 2007: 0
  2002: 5,800,000 2005: 3,500,000
  2003: 3,500,000 2006:
Medical Loss Ratio: 2005: 2006:
Administrative Expense Ratio: 2005: 2006:
SERVICE AREA:
Nationwide: Y
AL; AK; AR; AZ; CA; CO; CT; DC; DE; FL; GA; HI; IA; ID; IL; IN; KS; KY; LA; MA; MD; ME; MI; MN; MO; MT; MS; NC; ND; NE; NH; NJ; NM; NV; NY; OH; OK; OR; PA; RI; SC; SD; TN; TX; UT; VA; VT; WA; WI; WV; WY;
TYPE OF COVERAGE:
Commercial: [Y] Individual: [ ] FEHBP: [ ] Indemnity: [ ]
Medicare: [ ] Medicaid: [ ] Supplemental Medicare: [ ]
Tricare [ ]
PLAN BENEFITS:
Alternative Medicine: [ ] Behavioral Health: [ ]
Chiropractic: [X] Dental: [X]
Home Care: [X] Inpatient SNF: [X]
Long-Term Care: [X] Pharm. Mail Order: [ ]
Physical Therapy: [X] Podiatry: [X]
Psychiatric: [X] Transplant: [X]
Vision: [ ] Wellness: [ ]
Workers' Comp: [X]
Other Benefits:
Comments:
Purchased by First Health Group Corporation on August 16, 2001. As of January 1, 2007, the CCN Network has integrated into the First Health Network.

FIRSTSIGHT VISION SERVICES INC

1202 Monte Vista Ave Ste 17
Upland, CA 91786
Phone: 800-841-2790 Fax: 909-932-0062 Toll-Free: 800-841-2470
Web site: www.nval-vcs.com
MAILING ADDRESS:
  FIRSTSIGHT VISION SERVICES INC
  1202 Monte Vista Ave Ste 17
  Upland, CA 91786

KEY EXECUTIVES:
Chief Executive Officer/President .... Robert K Patton
Chief Financial Officer .... Joseph T Heidelman
Director, Quality Assurance .... Anh Nguyen, OD

COMPANY PROFILE:
Parent Company Name:
Doing Business As:
Year Founded: 1995 Federally Qualified: [ ]
Forprofit: [ ] Not-For-Profit: [ ]
Model Type:
Accreditation: [ ] AAPPO [ ] JACHO [ ] NCQA [ ] URAC
Plan Type: Specialty HMO
Total Revenue: 2005: 2006: 3,868,543
Net Income 2005: 2006: 141,652
Total Enrollment:
  2001: 0 2004: 0 2007: 216,367
  2002: 48,677 2005:
  2003: 150,862 2006: 216,696
Medical Loss Ratio: 2005: 2006: 95.85
Administrative Expense Ratio: 2005: 2006: 24.08
SERVICE AREA:
Nationwide:
  CA;
PLAN BENEFITS:
Alternative Medicine: [ ] Behavioral Health: [ ]
Chiropractic: [ ] Dental: [ ]
Home Care: [ ] Inpatient SNF: [ ]
Long-Term Care: [ ] Pharm. Mail Order: [ ]
Physical Therapy: [ ] Podiatry: [ ]
Psychiatric: [ ] Transplant: [ ]
Vision: [X] Wellness: [ ]
Workers' Comp: [ ]
Other Benefits:
Comments:
Formerly called NVAL Visioncare Systems of California, Inc.

FOR EYES VISION PLAN INC

2112 Shattuck Ave
Berkeley, CA 94704
Phone: 510-843-3200 Fax: 510-843-2597 Toll-Free:
Web site:
MAILING ADDRESS:
  FOR EYES VISION PLAN INC
  2112 Shattuck Ave
  Berkeley, CA 94704

KEY EXECUTIVES:
Chief Executive Officer/President .... Fred Hjerpe, MD
Chief Financial Officer/Medical Director .... Fred Hjerpe, MD

COMPANY PROFILE:
Parent Company Name:
Doing Business As:
Year Founded: 1996 Federally Qualified: [ ]
Forprofit: [ ] Not-For-Profit: [ ]
Model Type:
Accreditation: [ ] AAPPO [ ] JACHO [ ] NCQA [ ] URAC
Plan Type: Specialty HMO
Total Revenue: 2005: 443,692 2006: 1,890,068
Net Income 2005: 14,623 2006: 121,562
Total Enrollment:
  2001: 21,413 2004: 21,720 2007: 18,843
  2002: 21,600 2005: 20,421
  2003: 21,904 2006: 19,273
Medical Loss Ratio: 2005: 13.48 2006: 100.34
Administrative Expense Ratio: 2005: 15.89 2006: 15.72
SERVICE AREA:
Nationwide: N
  CA;
PRODUCTS OFFERED:
Product Name: Type:
For Eyes Vision Plan, Inc Specialty HMO
PLAN BENEFITS:
Alternative Medicine: [ ] Behavioral Health: [ ]
Chiropractic: [ ] Dental: [ ]
Home Care: [ ] Inpatient SNF: [ ]
Long-Term Care: [ ] Pharm. Mail Order: [ ]
Physical Therapy: [ ] Podiatry: [ ]
Psychiatric: [ ] Transplant: [ ]
Vision: [X] Wellness: [ ]
Workers' Comp: [ ]
Other Benefits:

GOLDEN WEST DENTAL & VISION

5171 Verdugo Way
Camarillo, CA 93010
Phone: 805-384-3895 Fax: 805-987-2205 Toll-Free: 800-995-4124
Web site: www.goldenwestdental.com
MAILING ADDRESS:
  GOLDEN WEST DENTAL & VISION
  PO Box 5347
  Oxnard, CA 93010

KEY EXECUTIVES:
Chief Executive Officer .... Derek Bridges
Dental Director .... Karen Feldman, DDS
Marketing Director .... Chris McCarthy
Director of Provider Services .... Vince Williams
Quality Assurance Director/Credentialing Mgr .. Karen Feldman, DDS

COMPANY PROFILE:
Parent Company Name: WellPoint Inc
Doing Business As: Golden West Dental and Vision
Year Founded: 1978 Federally Qualified: [N]
Forprofit: [Y] Not-For-Profit: [ ]
Model Type: NETWORK
Accreditation: [ ] AAPPO [ ] JACHO [ ] NCQA [ ] URAC
Plan Type: Specialty HMO, Specialty PPO, ASO, TPA
Total Revenue: 2005: 5,635,279 2006: 22,249,122
Net Income 2005: 474,420 2006: 1,680,645

CALIFORNIA

COMPANY PROFILE:
Parent Company Name: Dentistat
Doing Business As:
Year Founded: 1983   Federally Qualified: [N]
Forprofit: [Y]   Not-For-Profit: [ ]
Model Type:
Accreditation: [ ] AAPPO [ ] JACHO [ ] NCQA [ ] URAC
Plan Type: Specialty PPO, UR
SERVICE AREA:
Nationwide: Y
  NW;
TYPE OF COVERAGE:
Commercial: [Y] Individual: [ ] FEHBP: [ ] Indemnity: [ ]
Medicare: [ ] Medicaid: [ ] Supplemental Medicare: [ ]
Tricare [ ]
PLAN BENEFITS:
Alternative Medicine: [ ]   Behavioral Health: [ ]
Chiropractic: [ ]   Dental: [X]
Home Care: [ ]   Inpatient SNF: [ ]
Long-Term Care: [ ]   Pharm. Mail Order: [ ]
Physical Therapy: [ ]   Podiatry: [ ]
Psychiatric: [ ]   Transplant: [ ]
Vision: [ ]   Wellness: [ ]
Workers' Comp: [ ]
Other Benefits:

EASY CHOICE HEALTH PLAN INC

20411 SW Birch St Ste 200
Newport Beach, CA 92660
Phone: 949-999-3748 Fax: 949-999-3848 Toll-Free:
Web site: www.easychoicehealthplan.com
MAILING ADDRESS:
  EASY CHOICE HEALTH PLAN INC
  20411 SW Birch St Ste 200
  Newport Beach, CA 92660

KEY EXECUTIVES:
President .... Eric Spencer

COMPANY PROFILE:
Parent Company Name:
Doing Business As: EZ Choice Health Plan Inc
Year Founded: 2007   Federally Qualified: [ ]
Forprofit: [ ]   Not-For-Profit: [ ]
Model Type:
Accreditation: [ ] AAPPO [ ] JACHO [ ] NCQA [ ] URAC
Plan Type: HMO,
SERVICE AREA:
Nationwide:
  CA;
TYPE OF COVERAGE:
Commercial: [ ] Individual: [ ] FEHBP: [ ] Indemnity: [ ]
Medicare: [Y] Medicaid: [Y] Supplemental Medicare: [ ]
Tricare [ ]

EYEXAM OF CALIFORNIA INC

27000 Crown Valley Pkwy
Mission Viejo, CA 92691-6513
Phone: 949-364-2515 Fax: 949-364-0265 Toll-Free:
Web site: www.eyemedvisioncare.com
MAILING ADDRESS:
  EYEXAM OF CALIFORNIA INC
  27000 Crown Valley Pkwy
  Mission Viejo, CA 92691-6513

KEY EXECUTIVES:
Chief Executive Officer .... Yvon Wagner
Controller .... Lisa Roberts
Chief Financial Officer .... Liz DiGiandomenico
Medical Director .... Kim Villegan, OD
Exec Optometric Director .... Elliot Grossman
Marketing Director .... Kathy Dury

COMPANY PROFILE:
Parent Company Name: Luxottica (affiliated with Lenscrafters)
Doing Business As: EYEMED, Inc

Year Founded: 1986   Federally Qualified: [ ]
Forprofit: [Y]   Not-For-Profit: [ ]
Model Type:
Accreditation: [ ] AAPPO [ ] JACHO [ ] NCQA [ ] URAC
Plan Type: Specialty HMO
Total Revenue: 2005: 11,190,061   2006: 12,737,848
Net Income   2005:   34,670   2006:   12,612
Total Enrollment:
  2001: 683,872   2004:   0   2007: 380,455
  2002: 344,578   2005: 368,925
  2003:   0   2006: 379,444
Medical Loss Ratio: 2005: 134.81   2006: 138.93
Administrative Expense Ratio: 2005:   5.46   2006:   6.94
SERVICE AREA:
Nationwide: N
  CA (35 counties from San Francisco Bay area to Mexico);
TYPE OF COVERAGE:
Commercial: [Y] Individual: [Y] FEHBP: [ ] Indemnity: [ ]
Medicare: [ ] Medicaid: [ ] Supplemental Medicare: [ ]
Tricare [ ]
PRODUCTS OFFERED:
Product Name: Type:
EyeExam2000 of CA Inc   Specialty PPO
PLAN BENEFITS:
Alternative Medicine: [ ]   Behavioral Health: [ ]
Chiropractic: [ ]   Dental: [ ]
Home Care: [ ]   Inpatient SNF: [ ]
Long-Term Care: [ ]   Pharm. Mail Order: [ ]
Physical Therapy: [ ]   Podiatry: [ ]
Psychiatric: [ ]   Transplant: [ ]
Vision: [X]   Wellness: [ ]
Workers' Comp: [ ]
Other Benefits:

FIRST HEALTH — CALIFORNIA

750 Riverpoint Dr
W Sacramento, CA 95605
Phone: 916-374-4600 Fax: 916-374-4634 Toll-Free: 800-374-6824
Web site: www.firsthealth.com
MAILING ADDRESS:
  FIRST HEALTH — CA
  750 Riverpoint Dr
  W Sacramento, CA 95605

KEY EXECUTIVES:
Chief Executive Officer .... Edward L Wristen
National Medical Director .... Scott Smith, MD
Communications Director .... Andrea Hird

COMPANY PROFILE:
Parent Company Name: First Health, IL
Doing Business As:
Year Founded: 1983   Federally Qualified: [ ]
Forprofit: [Y]   Not-For-Profit: [ ]
Model Type:
Accreditation: [ ] AAPPO [ ] JACHO [ ] NCQA [ ] URAC
Plan Type: PPO, TPA, CDHP
SERVICE AREA:
Nationwide: N
  CA;
TYPE OF COVERAGE:
Commercial: [Y] Individual: [ ] FEHBP: [ ] Indemnity: [ ]
Medicare: [ ] Medicaid: [ ] Supplemental Medicare: [ ]
Tricare [ ]

FIRST HEALTH NETWORK

10260 Meanley Dr
San Diego, CA 92131
Phone: 858-547-2500 Fax: 858-547-2750 Toll-Free: 800-226-5116
Web site: www.firsthealth.com
MAILING ADDRESS:
  FIRST HEALTH NETWORK
  3200 Highland Ave
  Downers Grove, IL 92131

KEY EXECUTIVES:
Marketing Director .... Lisa Chu

Managed Care Organization Profiles — CALIFORNIA

DENTAL ASSOCIATES OF TORRANCE

21229 Hawthorne Blvd
Torrance, CA 90503
Phone: 310-792-5600 Fax: 310-792-5628 Toll-Free:
Web site: www.dentalassociatesoftorrence.com
MAILING ADDRESS:
   DENTAL ASSOCIATES OF TORRANCE
   21229 Hawthorne Blvd
   Torrance, CA 90503

KEY EXECUTIVES:
Regional Manager .... Ramona Colbert

COMPANY PROFILE:
Parent Company Name:
Doing Business As:
Year Founded: Federally Qualified: [ ]
Forprofit: [ ]   Not-For-Profit: [ ]
Model Type:
Accreditation: [ ] AAPPO [ ] JACHO [ ] NCQA [ ] URAC
Plan Type: Membership Benefit Program
SERVICE AREA:
Nationwide: N
   CA;
PLAN BENEFITS:
Alternative Medicine: [ ]   Behavioral Health: [ ]
Chiropractic: [ ]   Dental: [X]
Home Care: [ ]   Inpatient SNF: [ ]
Long-Term Care: [ ]   Pharm. Mail Order: [ ]
Physical Therapy: [ ]   Podiatry: [ ]
Psychiatric: [ ]   Transplant: [ ]
Vision: [ ]   Wellness: [ ]
Workers' Comp: [ ]
Other Benefits:

DENTAL BENEFIT PROVIDERS OF CA INC

425 Market St 12th Fl
San Francisco, CA 94105
Phone: 415-778-3800 Fax: 415-778-3833 Toll-Free:
Web site: www.dbp-inc.com
MAILING ADDRESS:
   DENTAL BENEFIT PROVIDERS OF CA
   425 Market St 12th CA035-1200
   San Francisco, CA 94105

KEY EXECUTIVES:
Chief Executive Officer .... David T Hall
President .... Kevin J Ruth
Chief Financial Officer .... Heather C White
Medical Director .... David S Wichmann
Chief Operating Officer .... Kevin Schievelbein

COMPANY PROFILE:
Parent Company Name:
Doing Business As: Dental Choice of California Inc
Year Founded: 1984   Federally Qualified: [ ]
Forprofit: [ ]   Not-For-Profit: [ ]
Model Type:
Accreditation: [ ] AAPPO [ ] JACHO [ ] NCQA [ ] URAC
Plan Type: Specialty HMO, Specialty PPO, ASO, EPO
Total Revenue: 2005: 8,685,512   2006: 35,129,370
Net Income   2005:   638,875   2006: 3,115,682
Total Enrollment:
   2001: 0   2004: 185,821   2007: 257,188
   2002: 123,544   2005: 217,660
   2003: 146,576   2006: 194,849
Medical Loss Ratio: 2005: 53.11   2006: 56.49
Administrative Expense Ratio: 2005: 13.08   2006: 12.51
SERVICE AREA:
Nationwide:
   CA;
TYPE OF COVERAGE:
Commercial: [ ] Individual: [ ] FEHBP: [ ] Indemnity: [ ]
Medicare: [ ] Medicaid: [ ] Supplemental Medicare: [ ]
Tricare   [ ]
PRODUCTS OFFERED:
Product Name: Type:
Dental Choice of CA Inc   Specialty HMO

DENTAL HEALTH SERVICES

3833 Atlantic Ave
Long Beach, CA 90807-3505
Phone: 562-595-6000 Fax: 562-424-0150 Toll-Free:
Web site: www.dentalhealthservices.com
MAILING ADDRESS:
   DENTAL HEALTH SERVICES
   3833 Atlantic Ave
   Long Beach, CA 90807-3505

KEY EXECUTIVES:
Chairman of the Board .... Godfrey Pernell, DDS
Chief Executive Officer .... Gary Pernell, DDS
Chief Financial Officer .... Michael Fenton
VP of Sales & Services .... Josh Nace
VP, Dental Service/Compliance .... Skip Ayers, DDS

COMPANY PROFILE:
Parent Company Name: Dental Health Services of America, Inc
Doing Business As:
Year Founded: 1974   Federally Qualified: [ ]
Forprofit: [Y]   Not-For-Profit: [ ]
Model Type: GROUP
Accreditation: [ ] AAPPO [ ] JACHO [ ] NCQA [ ] URAC
Plan Type: Specialty HMO, Specialty PPO
Total Revenue: 2005: 13,376,794   2006: 2,985,079
Net Income   2005:   180,267   2006:   107,034
Total Enrollment:
   2001: 85,000   2004: 0   2007: 69,173
   2002: 81,839   2005: 73,779
   2003: 83,000   2006: 68,088
Medical Loss Ratio: 2005: 73.66   2006: 65.77
Administrative Expense Ratio: 2005: 24.97   2006: 27.50
SERVICE AREA:
Nationwide: N
   CA; OR; WA;
TYPE OF COVERAGE:
Commercial: [ ] Individual: [Y] FEHBP: [ ] Indemnity: [ ]
Medicare: [ ] Medicaid: [ ] Supplemental Medicare: [ ]
Tricare   [ ]
PLAN BENEFITS:
Alternative Medicine: [ ]   Behavioral Health: [ ]
Chiropractic: [ ]   Dental: [X]
Home Care: [ ]   Inpatient SNF: [ ]
Long-Term Care: [ ]   Pharm. Mail Order: [ ]
Physical Therapy: [ ]   Podiatry: [ ]
Psychiatric: [ ]   Transplant: [ ]
Vision: [ ]   Wellness: [ ]
Workers' Comp: [ ]
Other Benefits:

DENTISTAT (INSURANCE DENTISTS OF AMERICA)

18805 Cox Ave Ste 250
Saratoga, CA 95070
Phone: 408-376-3801 Fax: 408-376-3535 Toll-Free: 800-336-8250
Web site: www.dentistat.com
MAILING ADDRESS:
   DENTISTAT (IDOA)
   18805 Cox Ave Ste 250
   Saratoga, CA 95070

KEY EXECUTIVES:
President .... Bret W Guenther, CEBS
Dental Director .... John Luther, MD
Chief Information Officer .... Sondra Zambino
Director of Operations .... John Kotecki

CALIFORNIA

Total Enrollment:
- 2001: 42,201
- 2002: 39,183
- 2003: 31,524
- 2004: 28,742
- 2005: 26,544
- 2006: 24,100
- 2007: 21,402

Medical Loss Ratio: 2005: 87.59 2006: 86.29
Administrative Expense Ratio: 2005: 11.86 2006: 10.42

SERVICE AREA:
Nationwide: N
 CA (Southern San Joaquin Valley);

TYPE OF COVERAGE:
Commercial: [Y] Individual: [Y] FEHBP: [ ] Indemnity: [ ]
Medicare: [ ] Medicaid: [ ] Supplemental Medicare: [ ]
Tricare [ ]

PRODUCTS OFFERED:
Product Name:	Type:
Dedicated Dental Systems, Inc	Specialty HMO

PLAN BENEFITS:
Alternative Medicine: [ ] Behavioral Health: [ ]
Chiropractic: [ ] Dental: [X]
Home Care: [ ] Inpatient SNF: [ ]
Long-Term Care: [ ] Pharm. Mail Order: [ ]
Physical Therapy: [ ] Podiatry: [ ]
Psychiatric: [ ] Transplant: [ ]
Vision: [ ] Wellness: [ ]
Workers' Comp: [ ]
Other Benefits:

Comments:
Formerly K & R Dental Plan.

DELTA DENTAL PLAN OF CALIFORNIA

100 First St
San Francisco, CA 94105
Phone: 415-972-8300 Fax: 415-972-8466 Toll-Free: 888-335-8227
Web site: www.deltadentalca.org

MAILING ADDRESS:
DELTA DENTAL PLAN OF CA
PO Box 7736
San Francisco, CA 94105

KEY EXECUTIVES:
Chief Executive Officer/President .... Gary D Radine
Chief Financial Officer .... Michael J Castro
Chief Dental Officer .... Marilynn G Belek, DMD
Chief Information Officer .... Patrick F Steele
Chief Operating Officer .... Tony Barth
Public Relations Director .... Jeff Album
VP, Network Development Director .... Daniel Crowley
Human Resources Director .... Teri Forestieri
Fraud Prevention/Investigation .... Sara Marcoux
Director of New Product Development .... Lynette Crosby
Commercial Operations .... Rohan Reid
Senior Vice President .... Anthony Barth
Senior Vice President .... Jerry Holcombe
Senior Vice President .... Michael Kaufmann
Senior Vice President .... Lowell Daun

COMPANY PROFILE:
Parent Company Name: Delta Dental Plan of California
Doing Business As: California Dental Services
Year Founded: 1955 Federally Qualified: [N]
Forprofit: [ ] Not-For-Profit: [Y]
Model Type: NETWORK
Accreditation: [ ] AAPPO [ ] JACHO [ ] NCQA [ ] URAC
Plan Type: Specialty HMO, Specialty PPO, POS, TPA, UR
Total Revenue: 2005: 524,441,000 2006: 2,249,430,000
Net Income 2005: 1,570,000 2006: 14,562,000
Total Enrollment:
- 2001: 15,900,000
- 2002: 14,384,000
- 2003: 14,933,000
- 2004: 14,405,000
- 2005: 14,561,000
- 2006: 14,700,000
- 2007: 16,500,000

Medical Loss Ratio: 2005: 85.81 2006: 16.72
Administrative Expense Ratio: 2005: 17.79 2006: 16.72

SERVICE AREA:
Nationwide: N
 CA;

TYPE OF COVERAGE:
Commercial: [Y] Individual: [ ] FEHBP: [ ] Indemnity: [ ]
Medicare: [Y] Medicaid: [Y] Supplemental Medicare: [ ]
Tricare [ ]

PRODUCTS OFFERED:
Product Name:	Type:
Delta Premier	Standard FFS
Delta Preferred Option	Dental PPO
Delta Care	Dental HMO
DeltaCare Point of Service	Dental POS
Delta Premier Table Program	Table Program
Delta Vision	Vision HMO
Delta Dental Medicaid	Medicaid

PLAN BENEFITS:
Alternative Medicine: [ ] Behavioral Health: [ ]
Chiropractic: [ ] Dental: [X]
Home Care: [ ] Inpatient SNF: [ ]
Long-Term Care: [ ] Pharm. Mail Order: [ ]
Physical Therapy: [ ] Podiatry: [ ]
Psychiatric: [ ] Transplant: [ ]
Vision: [X] Wellness: [ ]
Workers' Comp: [ ]
Other Benefits:

Comments:
Formerly California Dental Services.

DELTACARE USA

12898 Towne Ctr Dr
Cerritos, CA 90703
Phone: 562-924-8311 Fax: 562-924-8039 Toll-Free: 800-422-4234
Web site: www.deltadentalca.org/pmi

MAILING ADDRESS:
DELTACARE USA
100 First St
San Francisco, CA 90703

KEY EXECUTIVES:
President .... Robert B Elliott
Chief Financial Officer/Chief Information Officer .... Philip Runnoe
Public Relations Director .... Jeff Album
Provider Services Director .... Kay Kabarsky

COMPANY PROFILE:
Parent Company Name: Delta Dental Plan of California
Doing Business As: Private Medical-Care Inc, PMI
Year Founded: 1968 Federally Qualified: [ ]
Forprofit: [ ] Not-For-Profit: [Y]
Model Type: NETWORK
Accreditation: [ ] AAPPO [ ] JACHO [X] NCQA [ ] URAC
Plan Type: Specialty HMO, POS
Total Revenue: 2005: 36,527,516 2006: 158,153,286
Net Income 2005: 727,613 2006: 7,856,651
Total Enrollment:
- 2001: 1,258,227
- 2002: 1,284,256
- 2003: 1,009,267
- 2004: 0
- 2005: 957,617
- 2006: 1,035,357
- 2007: 0

Medical Loss Ratio: 2005: 66.61 2006: 68.64
Administrative Expense Ratio: 2005: 33.20 2006:

SERVICE AREA:
Nationwide: N
 CA, FL, GA, NV, NY, TX, UT,

TYPE OF COVERAGE:
Commercial: [Y] Individual: [Y] FEHBP: [ ] Indemnity: [ ]
Medicare: [Y] Medicaid: [ ] Supplemental Medicare: [Y]
Tricare [ ]

PRODUCTS OFFERED:
Product Name:	Type:
Delta Care	Dental HMO
DeltaCare Point of Service	Dental POS
Delta Vision	Vision HMO
PMI Dental Health Plan	Specialty HMO

PLAN BENEFITS:
Alternative Medicine: [ ] Behavioral Health: [ ]
Chiropractic: [ ] Dental: [X]
Home Care: [ ] Inpatient SNF: [ ]
Long-Term Care: [ ] Pharm. Mail Order: [ ]
Physical Therapy: [ ] Podiatry: [ ]
Psychiatric: [ ] Transplant: [ ]
Vision: [X] Wellness: [ ]
Workers' Comp: [ ]
Other Benefits:

Comments:
Delta Dental combined with PMI Dental Health Plan, January 1, 2007.

Managed Care Organization Profiles — CALIFORNIA

PLAN BENEFITS:
Alternative Medicine:	[ ]	Behavioral Health:	[ ]
Chiropractic:	[ ]	Dental:	[ ]
Home Care:	[ ]	Inpatient SNF:	[ ]
Long-Term Care:	[ ]	Pharm. Mail Order:	[ ]
Physical Therapy:	[ ]	Podiatry:	[ ]
Psychiatric:	[X]	Transplant:	[ ]
Vision:	[ ]	Wellness:	[ ]
Workers' Comp:	[ ]		

Other Benefits:

CONTRA COSTA HEALTH PLAN

595 Center Ave Ste 100
Martinez, CA 94553
Phone: 925-313-6000 Fax: 925-313-6002 Toll-Free:
Web site: www.cchealth.org

MAILING ADDRESS:
CONTRA COSTA HEALTH PLAN
595 Center Ave Ste 100
Martinez, CA 94553

KEY EXECUTIVES:
Chief Executive Officer .... Patricia Tanquary
Chief Financial Officer .... Pat Godley
Medical Director .... Jim Tysell, MD
Pharmacy Director .... Adeebeh Fakurnejad
Chief Information Officer .... Jeff Wanger
Chief Operating Officer .... Richard Harrison
Director Marketng and Member Services .... Judith Louro
Privacy Officer/Public Relations Director .... Teresa Snook O'Riva
Director Provider Services/Credentlaling .... Richard Harrison
Provider Liaison .... Beverly Jacobs
Director of Health & Resources Management .... Ellen Lent
HSD Personnel Director .... Shelly Pighin
Medical Director .... Jim Tysell, MD
Director of Quality Assurance .... Ken Tilly
Fraud Prevention Director .... Frank Lee
New Product Development Director .... Judith Louro
Case Management Director .... Florance Chan
Director of Government Relations .... Frank Lee
Planning Director .... Teresa Snook O'Riva

COMPANY PROFILE:
Parent Company Name: Contra Costa County Medical Services
Doing Business As: Contra Costa Health Plan
Year Founded: 1973   Federally Qualified: [Y]
Forprofit: [ ]   Not-For-Profit: [Y]
Model Type: MIXED
Accreditation: [ ] AAPPO [ ] JACHO [ ] NCQA [X] URAC
Plan Type: HMO
Total Revenue: 2005: 38,379,316   2006: 38,038,486
Net Income   2005:   -533,937   2006:   -302,790
Total Enrollment:
  2001: 57,834   2004: 64,140   2007: 66,493
  2002: 59,397   2005: 62,614
  2003: 61,634   2006: 62,427
Medical Loss Ratio: 2005: 121.06   2006: 119.04
Administrative Expense Ratio: 2005:   7.88   2006:   7.25

SERVICE AREA:
Nationwide: N
CA (Contra Costa);

TYPE OF COVERAGE:
Commercial: [Y] Individual: [Y] FEHBP: [ ] Indemnity: [ ]
Medicare: [Y] Medicaid: [Y] Supplemental Medicare: [Y]
Tricare   [ ]

PRODUCTS OFFERED:
Product Name:	Type:
Contra Costa Health Plan	Medicaid
Senior Health	Medicare
Contra Costa Health Plan	HMO

PLAN BENEFITS:
Alternative Medicine:	[X]	Behavioral Health:	[ ]
Chiropractic:	[X]	Dental:	[X]
Home Care:	[ ]	Inpatient SNF:	[ ]
Long-Term Care:	[X]	Pharm. Mail Order:	[ ]
Physical Therapy:	[ ]	Podiatry:	[X]
Psychiatric:	[X]	Transplant:	[ ]
Vision:	[X]	Wellness:	[X]
Workers' Comp:	[ ]		

Other Benefits:

CORVEL CORPORATION

2010 Main St Ste 600
Irvine, CA 92614
Phone: 949-851-1473 Fax: 949-851-1469 Toll-Free: 888-726-7835
Web site: www.corvel.com

MAILING ADDRESS:
CORVEL CORPORATION
2010 Main St Ste 600
Irvine, CA 92614

KEY EXECUTIVES:
Chairman of the Board/Chief Executive Officer ...... V Gordon Clemons
President .... Daniel J Starck
Chief Financial Officer .... Scott McCloud
Chief Information Officer .... Don McFarlane
Chief Operating Officer .... Daniel J Starck
VP, Marketing .... Heather Burnham
VP, Information Technology .... Tom Benson
Director of Human Resources .... Sharon O'Connor
VP, Business Development .... Peter Flynn
Director of Finance .... Richard Schweppe

COMPANY PROFILE:
Parent Company Name:
Doing Business As:
Year Founded: 1987 Federally Qualified: [ ]
Forprofit: [Y]   Not-For-Profit: [ ]
Model Type:
Accreditation: [ ] AAPPO [ ] JACHO [ ] NCQA [X] URAC
Plan Type: PPO, UR
Total Revenue: 2005: 291,000,000   2006: 266,504,000
Net Income   2005: 10,157,000   2006:   9,753,000
Total Enrollment:

SERVICE AREA:
Nationwide: N
CA;

TYPE OF COVERAGE:
Commercial: [Y] Individual: [ ] FEHBP: [ ] Indemnity: [ ]
Medicare: [ ] Medicaid: [ ] Supplemental Medicare: [ ]
Tricare   [ ]

PLAN BENEFITS:
Alternative Medicine:	[ ]	Behavioral Health:	[ ]
Chiropractic:	[X]	Dental:	[ ]
Home Care:	[X]	Inpatient SNF:	[X]
Long-Term Care:	[X]	Pharm. Mail Order:	[ ]
Physical Therapy:	[X]	Podiatry:	[X]
Psychiatric:	[X]	Transplant:	[ ]
Vision:	[ ]	Wellness:	[ ]
Workers' Comp:	[X]		

Other Benefits:

DEDICATED DENTAL SYSTEMS

3990 Ming Ave
Bakersfield, CA 93309
Phone: 661-397-2895 Fax: 661-397-2888 Toll-Free: 800-277-1112
Web site: www.dedicated-dental.com

MAILING ADDRESS:
DEDICATED DENTAL SYSTEMS
3990 Ming Ave
Bakerfield, CA 93309

KEY EXECUTIVES:
Chief Executive Officer .... Robert Hill
Dental Director .... Alan Slutsky, DMD
Chief Operating Officer .... David Spence, MBA
Quality Assurance Director .... Heather Martinez

COMPANY PROFILE:
Parent Company Name:
Doing Business As: DDS Inc; DDSI
Year Founded: 1986   Federally Qualified: [ ]
Forprofit: [Y]   Not-For-Profit: [ ]
Model Type:
Accreditation: [ ] AAPPO [ ] JACHO [ ] NCQA [ ] URAC
Plan Type: Specialty HMO
Total Revenue: 2005: 2,925,547   2006: 10,848,750
Net Income   2005:   -24,375   2006:   252,049

CALIFORNIA — Managed Care Organization Profiles

Chief Information Officer .... Jonathan Tamayo
Chief of Operations .... Francisca Chavey
Public Relations Director .... Joseph A Garcia
Provider & Network Administrtor .... Ann Warren
Director of Operations .... Melissa Sterns
Health Promotions/Prevention Manager Martha Jazo-Bajet RN, MPH
Human Resources Director .... Patty Urbina
CQI Manager .... Carol Anderson RN

COMPANY PROFILE:
Parent Company Name:
Doing Business As:
Year Founded: 1982   Federally Qualified: [N]
Forprofit: [ ]   Not-For-Profit: [Y]
Model Type: MIXED
Accreditation: [ ] AAPPO [ ] JACHO [ ] NCQA [ ] URAC
Plan Type: HMO
Total Revenue: 2005: 33,840,616   2006: 29,643,235
Net Income   2005:   1,018,426   2006:   7,554,097
Total Enrollment:
  2001: 86,906   2004: 100,114   2007: 93,583
  2002: 95,817   2005: 99,660
  2003: 103,414   2006: 91,836
Medical Loss Ratio: 2005: 86.01   2006: 85.26
Administrative Expense Ratio: 2005: 11.82   2006:

SERVICE AREA:
Nationwide: N
  CA (San Diego);

TYPE OF COVERAGE:
Commercial: [Y] Individual: [ ] FEHBP: [ ] Indemnity: [ ]
Medicare: [ ] Medicaid: [Y] Supplemental Medicare: [ ]
Tricare   [ ]

PRODUCTS OFFERED:
Product Name: Type:
Premier 5   HMO
Premier 10   HMO
Preferred 10   HMO
Preferred 15   HMO
Advantage 15   HMO
Advantage 20   HMO
Community Hlth Grp   Medicaid

PLAN BENEFITS:
Alternative Medicine: [ ]   Behavioral Health: [X]
Chiropractic: [X]   Dental: [ ]
Home Care: [X]   Inpatient SNF: [X]
Long-Term Care: [ ]   Pharm. Mail Order: [X]
Physical Therapy: [X]   Podiatry: [X]
Psychiatric: [X]   Transplant: [ ]
Vision: [X]   Wellness: [X]
Workers' Comp: [ ]
Other Benefits:

COMMUNITY HEALTH PLAN

1000 S Fremont Ave Bldg A9 2nd
Alhambra, CA 91803-1323
Phone: 626-299-5300 Fax: 626-458-6761 Toll-Free:
Web site: www.ladhs.org/chp

MAILING ADDRESS:
  COMMUNITY HEALTH PLAN
  1000 S Fremont Ave Bldg A9 2nd
  Alhambra, CA 91803-1323

KEY EXECUTIVES:
Chief Executive Officer .... Teri Daly Lauenstein
Chief Financial Officer .... Dave Beck
Chief Medical Officer .... Mary Abbott, MD
Pharmacy Director .... Duane Asao Pharm D
Chief Information Officer .... Laura Williams
ActingChief Operating Officer .... Mario Reyes
Acting Marketng/Communcations Manager ... Laura Lathrop-Warriner
Credentialing Manager .... Conception Said, RN
Provider Relations Manager .... Elisa Estrella
Contract Administration Director .... Chris Kawate
Administrative Services Manager .... Rosemarie Lugo
Director of Medical Administration .... Sobha Naimpally, MD
Quality Management Manager .... Grace Ibanuz, RN
Interim Compliance Officer .... Raub Mathias
Utilization/Case Management Manager .... Pam Ricks-Hawkins
Member Services Manager .... Charlotte Piggee
AssistantChief Financial Officer .... Rogers Moody

COMPANY PROFILE:
Parent Company Name: County of Los Angeles Dept of Health Services
Doing Business As: Community Health Plan
Year Founded: 1985   Federally Qualified: [Y]
Forprofit: [ ]   Not-For-Profit: [Y]
Model Type: STAFF/NETWORK
Accreditation: [ ] AAPPO [ ] JACHO [ ] NCQA [ ] URAC
Plan Type: HMO
Total Revenue: 2005: 202,458,236   2006: 214,103,386
Net Income   2005: 12,290,146   2006: 21,555,400
Total Enrollment:
  2001: 145,386   2004: 160,981   2007: 165,656
  2002: 179,137   2005: 157,797
  2003: 173,471   2006: 156,572
Medical Loss Ratio: 2005: 82.80   2006: 78.79
Administrative Expense Ratio: 2005: 11.13   2006: 11.14

SERVICE AREA:
Nationwide: N
  CA (Los Angeles);

TYPE OF COVERAGE:
Commercial: [Y] Individual: [ ] FEHBP: [ ] Indemnity: [ ]
Medicare: [ ] Medicaid: [Y] Supplemental Medicare: [ ]
Tricare   [ ]

PRODUCTS OFFERED:
Product Name: Type:
Medi-Cal   Medicaid
Healthy Families   HMO
County Temporary Employers   HMO
PASC-SELH Homecare Workers   HMO

PLAN BENEFITS:
Alternative Medicine: [ ]   Behavioral Health: [X]
Chiropractic: [ ]   Dental: [ ]
Home Care: [X]   Inpatient SNF: [X]
Long-Term Care: [X]   Pharm. Mail Order: [ ]
Physical Therapy: [X]   Podiatry: [ ]
Psychiatric: [X]   Transplant: [X]
Vision: [X]   Wellness: [X]
Workers' Comp: [ ]
Other Benefits:

CONCERN: EMPLOYEE ASSISTANCE PROGRAM

1503 Grant Rd Ste 120
Mountain View, CA 94040
Phone: 650-940-7100 Fax: 650-965-2849 Toll-Free: 888-533-6015
Web site: www.concern-eap.com

MAILING ADDRESS:
  CONCERN: EMPLOYEE ASSISTANCE P
  1503 Grant Rd Ste 120
  Mountain View, CA 94040

KEY EXECUTIVES:
Chief Executive Director .... Cecile Currier
Chief Financial Officer .... Marla Gularte
Medical Director .... Thomas Havel, MD
Director of Business Development .... Paulette Hannah

COMPANY PROFILE:
Parent Company Name: El Camino Hospital
Doing Business As:
Year Founded: 1961   Federally Qualified: [ ]
Forprofit: [ ]   Not-For-Profit: [Y]
Model Type: NETWORK
Accreditation: [ ] AAPPO [ ] JACHO [ ] NCQA [ ] URAC
Plan Type: Specialty HMO
Total Revenue: 2005:   1,401,174   2006:   1,359,121
Net Income   2005:   203,350   2006:   332,528
Total Enrollment:
  2001:   0   2004: 84,562   2007: 119,677
  2002: 54,199   2005: 89,420
  2003: 59,453   2006: 94,534
Medical Loss Ratio: 2005: 48.65   2006: 59.31
Administrative Expense Ratio: 2005: 46.53   2006: 38.45

SERVICE AREA:
Nationwide:
  NW;

TYPE OF COVERAGE:
Commercial: [Y] Individual: [ ] FEHBP: [ ] Indemnity: [ ]
Medicare: [ ] Medicaid: [ ] Supplemental Medicare: [ ]
Tricare   [ ]

Managed Care Organization Profiles   **CALIFORNIA**

TYPE OF COVERAGE:
Commercial: [Y] Individual: [ ] FEHBP: [ ] Indemnity: [ ]
Medicare: [ ] Medicaid: [ ] Supplemental Medicare: [ ]
Tricare [ ]
PRODUCTS OFFERED:
Product Name: Type:
CIGNA Dental Health of CA, Inc   Specialty HMO
PLAN BENEFITS:
Alternative Medicine: [ ]   Behavioral Health: [ ]
Chiropractic: [ ]   Dental: [X]
Home Care: [ ]   Inpatient SNF: [ ]
Long-Term Care: [ ]   Pharm. Mail Order: [ ]
Physical Therapy: [ ]   Podiatry: [ ]
Psychiatric: [ ]   Transplant: [ ]
Vision: [ ]   Wellness: [ ]
Workers' Comp: [ ]
Other Benefits:

CIGNA HEALTHCARE OF CALIFORNIA

400 N Brand Blvd Ste 400
Glendale, CA 91203
Phone: 818-500-6262 Fax: 818-500-6365 Toll-Free: 800-344-7421
Web site: www.cigna.com/healthcare
MAILING ADDRESS:
    CIGNA HEALTHCARE OF CA
    PO Box 2125
    Glendale, CA 91203

KEY EXECUTIVES:
President .... Christopher DeRosa
Chief Medical Officer .... James Wang, MD
Marketing Manager .... Lincoln Acholonu
Public Relations Director .... Gwyn Dilday
VP of Network Operations .... Randy Mathews
Human Resources Director .... Juliette Argwin
Director of Health Services .... Jan Ogle, RN
Quality Mgmt Director .... Kathy Gies
Director of Credentialing .... Kelli Santana

COMPANY PROFILE:
Parent Company Name: CIGNA Corporation
Doing Business As:
Year Founded: 1979   Federally Qualified: [Y]
Forprofit: [Y]   Not-For-Profit: [ ]
Model Type: NETWORK
Accreditation: [ ] AAPPO [ ] JACHO [X] NCQA [ ] URAC
Plan Type: HMO, POS, CDHP, HDHP, HSA, FSA, HRA
Total Revenue: 2005: 221,562,493   2006: 121,995,649
Net Income   2005:   2,577,143   2006:   3,101,676
Total Enrollment:
    2001: 671,184   2004: 427,118   2007: 289,276
    2002: 634,568   2005: 342,463
    2003: 546,692   2006: 312,960
Medical Loss Ratio: 2005: 96.23   2006: 95.18
Administrative Expense Ratio: 2005: 3.70   2006: 6.33
SERVICE AREA:
Nationwide: N
    Southern CA; (Kern, Los Angeles, Orange, Riverside, San Bernardino, San Luis Obispo, Santa Barbara, Ventura), Northern CA; (Alameda, Butte, Contra Costa, El Dorado, Fresno, Glenn, Kings, Marin, Merced, Monterey, Placer, Sacramento, San Francisco, San Joaquin, San Mateo, Santa Clara, Santa Cruz, Solano, Stanislaus, Tulare, Yolo); (San Diego, Imperial-PPO only)
TYPE OF COVERAGE:
Commercial: [Y] Individual: [Y] FEHBP: [ ] Indemnity: [ ]
Medicare: [Y] Medicaid: [ ] Supplemental Medicare: [ ]
Tricare [ ]
PRODUCTS OFFERED:
Product Name: Type:
HMO
POS
CONSUMER-DRIVEN PRODUCTS
JP Morgan Chase   HSA Company
CIGNA Choice Fund   HSA Product
                         HSA AdministratorOpen
Access Plus   Consumer-Driven Health Plan
PPO   High Deductible Health Plan

PLAN BENEFITS:
Alternative Medicine: [X]   Behavioral Health: [X]
Chiropractic: [X]   Dental: [X]
Home Care: [X]   Inpatient SNF: [X]
Long-Term Care: [ ]   Pharm. Mail Order: [X]
Physical Therapy: [X]   Podiatry: [X]
Psychiatric: [X]   Transplant: [X]
Vision: [X]   Wellness: [X]
Workers' Comp: [ ]
Other Benefits:

COASTAL HEALTHCARE ADMINISTRATORS

928 East Blanco Rd Ste 235
Salinas, CA 93901
Phone: 831-754-3800 Fax: 831-754-3830 Toll-Free: 800-564-7475
Web site: www.coastalmgmt.com
MAILING ADDRESS:
    COASTAL HEALTHCARE ADMINISTRATORSS
    928 East Blanco Rd Ste 235
    Salinas, CA 93901

KEY EXECUTIVES:
Chief Executive Officer/President .... Debi Hardwick
Medical Director .... Thomas Kehl, MD
Marketing Director .... Debi Hardwick
Director of Client Services .... Sidney Tolleson
Director of Network Management .... Betty Yancey

COMPANY PROFILE:
Parent Company Name: Bay Services Inc
Doing Business As: Coastal Healthcare Administrators
Year Founded: 1961   Federally Qualified: [N]
Forprofit: [Y]   Not-For-Profit: [ ]
Model Type: NETWORK
Accreditation: [ ] AAPPO [ ] JACHO [ ] NCQA [ ] URAC
Plan Type: PPO
Primary Physicians: 545   Physician Specialists: 673
Hospitals: 11
Total Enrollment:
    2001: 25,525   2004: 0   2007: 0
    2002: 29,512   2005:
    2003: 90,000   2006:
SERVICE AREA:
Nationwide: N
    CA (Monterey, Santa Benito, San Luis Obispo, Santa Cruz);
TYPE OF COVERAGE:
Commercial: [Y] Individual: [ ] FEHBP: [ ] Indemnity: [Y]
Medicare: [ ] Medicaid: [ ] Supplemental Medicare: [ ]
Tricare [ ]
PRODUCTS OFFERED:
Product Name: Type:
Coastal Healthcare Admns   PPO
PLAN BENEFITS:
Alternative Medicine: [ ]   Behavioral Health: [X]
Chiropractic: [ ]   Dental: [X]
Home Care: [ ]   Inpatient SNF: [X]
Long-Term Care: [ ]   Pharm. Mail Order: [ ]
Physical Therapy: [X]   Podiatry: [ ]
Psychiatric: [ ]   Transplant: [ ]
Vision: [X]   Wellness: [ ]
Workers' Comp: [X]
Other Benefits:

COMMUNITY HEALTH GROUP

740 Bay Boulevard 2nd Floor
Chula Vista, CA 91910
Phone: 619-422-0422 Fax: 619-422-5930 Toll-Free: 800-640-4662
Web site: www.chgsd.com
MAILING ADDRESS:
    COMMUNITY HEALTH GROUP
    740 Bay Boulevard 2nd Fl
    Chula Vista, CA 91910

KEY EXECUTIVES:
Chief Executive Officer .... Norma A Diaz
Chief Financial Officer .... William Rice
Chief Medical Officer .... Rafael Amaro, MD
Pharmacy Director .... Noreen Koizumi

CALIFORNIA

Managed Care Organization Profiles

TYPE OF COVERAGE:
Commercial: [Y] Individual: [Y] FEHBP: [ ] Indemnity: [ ]
Medicare: [Y] Medicaid: [ ] Supplemental Medicare: [ ]
Tricare [ ]

PRODUCTS OFFERED:
Product Name: Type:
CCHP-Senior Program A/B Plan   Medicare Advantage
CCHP HMO   HMO

PLAN BENEFITS:
Alternative Medicine: [ ]   Behavioral Health: [ ]
Chiropractic: [ ]   Dental: [ ]
Home Care: [X]   Inpatient SNF: [X]
Long-Term Care: [ ]   Pharm. Mail Order: [ ]
Physical Therapy: [X]   Podiatry: [X]
Psychiatric: [X]   Transplant: [X]
Vision: [X]   Wellness: [X]
Workers' Comp: [ ]
Other Benefits:

CHIROSOURCE - CORPORATE HEADQUARTERS

5356 Clayton Rd Ste 201
Concord, CA 94521
Phone: 925-844-8101 Fax: 925-844-3124 Toll-Free: 800-680-9997
Web site: www.chirosource.com

MAILING ADDRESS:
CHIROSOURCE
PO Box 130
Clayton, CA 94521

KEY EXECUTIVES:
Chief Executive Officer/President .... Ronald S Cataldo, DC
Chief Financial Officer .... Jeanette M Cataldo
Medical Director .... Ronald S Cataldo, DC
Vice President .... Todd Cataldo

COMPANY PROFILE:
Parent Company Name: Chiropractic Health Plan of California
Doing Business As: ChiroSource Inc
Year Founded: 1997   Federally Qualified: [ ]
Forprofit: [Y]   Not-For-Profit: [ ]
Model Type: NETWORK
Accreditation: [ ] AAPPO [ ] JACHO [ ] NCQA [ ] URAC
Plan Type: PPO, Specialty HMO, Specialty PPO, POS, ASO, EPO, TPA, UR

SERVICE AREA:
Nationwide: Y
NW;

TYPE OF COVERAGE:
Commercial: [Y] Individual: [Y] FEHBP: [ ] Indemnity: [Y]
Medicare: [Y] Medicaid: [ ] Supplemental Medicare: [ ]
Tricare [ ]

PLAN BENEFITS:
Alternative Medicine: [ ]   Behavioral Health: [ ]
Chiropractic: [X]   Dental: [ ]
Home Care: [ ]   Inpatient SNF: [ ]
Long-Term Care: [ ]   Pharm. Mail Order: [ ]
Physical Therapy: [ ]   Podiatry: [ ]
Psychiatric: [ ]   Transplant: [ ]
Vision: [ ]   Wellness: [ ]
Workers' Comp: [X]
Other Benefits: Health Benefits & Pe

CIGNA BEHAVIORAL HEALTH INC

450 N Brand Blvd Ste 400
Glendale, CA 91203
Phone: 818-551-2200 Fax: 818-551-2786 Toll-Free: 800-234-3596
Web site: www.cignabehavioral.com

MAILING ADDRESS:
CIGNA BEHAVIORAL HEALTH INC
450 N Brand Blvd Ste 400
Glendale, CA 91203

KEY EXECUTIVES:
Chief Executive Officer .... Susan Urbanski
President .... Keith Dixon, PhD
Chief Financial Officer .... William Palmer
Medical Director .... Michael Glasser MD
Director of Provider Services .... Leticia Fenton
Quality Assurance Director .... Jim Scjeel

COMPANY PROFILE:
Parent Company Name: CIGNA Behavioral Health Inc, MN
Doing Business As:
Year Founded: 1989   Federally Qualified: [Y]
Forprofit: [Y]   Not-For-Profit: [ ]
Model Type:
Accreditation: [ ] AAPPO [ ] JACHO [ ] NCQA [X] URAC
Plan Type: Specialty HMO
Total Revenue: 2005: 4,108,336   2006: 86,255,935
Net Income   2005: 581,244   2006: 2,662,146
Total Enrollment:
    2001: 558,833   2004: 321,702   2007: 231,583
    2002: 542,271   2005: 261,292
    2003: 467,226   2006: 243,242
Medical Loss Ratio: 2005: 78.82   2006: 71.78
Administrative Expense Ratio: 2005: 6.22   2006: 6.38

SERVICE AREA:
Nationwide: N
CA;

TYPE OF COVERAGE:
Commercial: [Y] Individual: [ ] FEHBP: [ ] Indemnity: [ ]
Medicare: [Y] Medicaid: [ ] Supplemental Medicare: [Y]
Tricare [ ]

PRODUCTS OFFERED:
Product Name: Type:
Employee Assistance Programs
Managed Mental Health

PLAN BENEFITS:
Alternative Medicine: [ ]   Behavioral Health: [X]
Chiropractic: [ ]   Dental: [ ]
Home Care: [ ]   Inpatient SNF: [ ]
Long-Term Care: [ ]   Pharm. Mail Order: [ ]
Physical Therapy: [ ]   Podiatry: [ ]
Psychiatric: [X]   Transplant: [ ]
Vision: [ ]   Wellness: [X]
Workers' Comp: [ ]
Other Benefits:

Comments:
Formerly MCC Managed Behavioral Care Inc.

CIGNA DENTAL HEALTH OF CALIFORNIA INC

400 N Brand Blvd Ste 400
Glendale, CA 91203
Phone: 818-546-5100 Fax: 818-546-5102 Toll-Free: 800-342-5234
Web site: www.cigna.com/dental

MAILING ADDRESS:
CIGNA DENTAL HEALTH OF CA INC
PO Box 2125
Glendale, CA 91203

KEY EXECUTIVES:
President .... Karen S Rohan
Chief Financial Officer .... Ahmed Ukani
Dental Director .... Cary Sun, DDS
Marketing Director .... Aaron Groffman
MIS Director .... Laurel A Flebotte
VP, Network Operations .... Nancy Pe Quilino

COMPANY PROFILE:
Parent Company Name: CIGNA Dental Health Inc
Doing Business As: CIGNA Dental Health
Year Founded: 1985   Federally Qualified: [N]
Forprofit: [Y]   Not-For-Profit: [ ]
Model Type: IPA
Accreditation: [ ] AAPPO [ ] JACHO [ ] NCQA [ ] URAC
Plan Type: Specialty HMO
Total Revenue: 2005: 12,095,187   2006: 39,896,374
Net Income   2005: 3,640,478   2006: 11,840,541
Total Enrollment: 2001: 436,442   2004: 313,365
2007:   214,466
    2002: 414,257   2005: 276,832
    2003: 380,438   2006: 218,812
Medical Loss Ratio: 2005: 42.84   2006: 41.41
Administrative Expense Ratio: 2005: 13.04   2006: 13.24

SERVICE AREA:
Nationwide: N
CA (Alameda, Contra Costa, Fresno, Kern, Kings, Los Angeles, Madera, Orange, Placer, Riverside, Sacramento, San Bernardino, San Diego, San Luis Obispo, San Francisco, San Joaquin, San Mateo, Santa Barbara, Santa Clara, Santa Cruz, Stanislaus, Sonoma, Ventura);

Managed Care Organization Profiles — CALIFORNIA

KEY EXECUTIVES:
Chief Executive Officer .... Alan Hoops
President .... Leeba Lessin
Chief Financial Officer .... Sergio Zaldivar
Chief Medical Officer .... Donald S Furman, MD, MBA
Senior VP of Operations .... Chuck Weber
VP, Chief of Sales & Marketing .... Dawn C Maroney

COMPANY PROFILE:
Parent Company Name:
Doing Business As: California Health Plan
Year Founded: 2002   Federally Qualified: [ ]
Forprofit: [ ]   Not-For-Profit: [ ]
Model Type:
Accreditation: [ ] AAPPO [ ] JACHO [ ] NCQA [ ] URAC
Plan Type: HMO,
Total Revenue: 2005:   2006: 24,989,000
Net Income   2005:   2006: 25,369,000
Total Enrollment:
  2001: 0   2004: 0   2007: 24,670
  2002: 0   2005:
  2003: 0   2006: 22,630
Medical Loss Ratio: 2005:   2006: 68.93
Administrative Expense Ratio: 2005:   2006: 14.49

SERVICE AREA:
Nationwide:
  CA;

TYPE OF COVERAGE:
Commercial: [ ] Individual: [ ] FEHBP: [ ] Indemnity: [ ]
Medicare: [Y] Medicaid: [ ]   Supplemental Medicare: [ ]
Tricare   [ ]

CENTRAL COAST ALLIANCE FOR HEALTH

1600 Green Hills Rd
Scotts Valley, CA 95066-9998
Phone: 831-430-5500 Fax: 831-430-5852 Toll-Free: 800-700-3874
Web site: www.ccah-alliance.org

MAILING ADDRESS:
CENTRAL COAST ALLIANCE FOR HEALTH
1600 Green Hills Rd
Scotts Valley, CA 95066-9998

KEY EXECUTIVES:
Executive Director .... Alan McKay
Finance Director .... Patti McFarland
Medical Director .... Barbara Palla, MD
IT Director .... Bob Chernis
Human Resources Director .... Scott Fortner

COMPANY PROFILE:
Parent Company Name: Santa Cruz-Monteray Mngd Care Commision
Doing Business As: Central Coast Alliance for Health
Year Founded: 2000   Federally Qualified: [ ]
Forprofit: [ ]   Not-For-Profit: [Y]
Model Type:
Accreditation: [ ] AAPPO [ ] JACHO [ ] NCQA [ ] URAC
Plan Type: HMO,
Total Revenue: 2005: 63,263,607   2006: 245,851,261,
Net Income   2005: -2,978,256   2006: 4,709,962
Total Enrollment:
  2001: 72,707   2004: 83,877   2007: 88,341
  2002: 85,098   2005: 85,944
  2003: 81,901   2006: 88,296
Medical Loss Ratio: 2005: 101.40   2006: 93.37
Administrative Expense Ratio: 2005: 5.70   2006: 5.64

SERVICE AREA:
Nationwide: N
  CA (Santa Cruz and Monterey);

TYPE OF COVERAGE:
Commercial: [ ] Individual: [ ] FEHBP: [ ] Indemnity: [ ]
Medicare: [ ] Medicaid: [Y]   Supplemental Medicare: [ ]
Tricare   [ ]

PRODUCTS OFFERED:
Product Name: Type:
Medi-Cal   Medicaid

Comments:
Formerly Santa Cruz-Monteray Managed Medical Care Commission.

CENTRAL HEALTH PLAN OF CALIFORNIA INC

1051 Parkview Dr Ste 120
Covina, CA 91724
Phone: 626-388-2300 Fax: 626-388-2329 Toll-Free:
Web site: www.centralhealthplan.com

MAILING ADDRESS:
CENTRAL HEALTH PLAN OF CA INC
1051 Parkview Dr Ste 120
Covina, CA 91724

KEY EXECUTIVES:
Chairman .... Sam Kam
Chief Executive Officer/President .... Sam Kam
Chief Financial Officer .... Larry Keller
Medical Director .... Edwin Chuong

COMPANY PROFILE:
Parent Company Name:
Doing Business As:
Year Founded: 2004   Federally Qualified: [ ]
Forprofit: [ ]   Not-For-Profit: [ ]
Model Type: NETWORK
Accreditation: [ ] AAPPO [ ] JACHO [ ] NCQA [ ] URAC
Plan Type: HMO,
Total Enrollment:
  2001: 0   2004: 0   2007: 1,795
  2002: 0   2005:
  2003: 0   2006: 408
Medical Loss Ratio: 2005:   2006: 54.83
Administrative Expense Ratio: 2005:   2006: 149.32

SERVICE AREA:
Nationwide:
  CA (Los Angeles);

PLAN BENEFITS:
Alternative Medicine: [ ]   Behavioral Health: [X]
Chiropractic: [X]   Dental: [X]
Home Care: [X]   Inpatient SNF: [X]
Long-Term Care: [X]   Pharm. Mail Order: [X]
Physical Therapy: [X]   Podiatry: [X]
Psychiatric: [X]   Transplant: [X]
Vision: [X]   Wellness: [X]
Workers' Comp: [ ]
Other Benefits:

CHINESE COMMUNITY HEALTH PLAN

445 Grant Ave Ste 700
San Francisco, CA 94108
Phone: 415-955-8800 Fax: 415-955-8817 Toll-Free:
Web site: www.cchphmo.com

MAILING ADDRESS:
CHINESE COMMUNITY HEALTH PLAN
445 Grant Ave Ste 700
San Francisco, CA 94108

KEY EXECUTIVES:
Chief Executive Officer/Administrator .... Richard Loos
Chief Financial Officer .... Steve Tsang
Medical Director .... Edward Chow, MD
Pharmacy Director .... Adrian Wong
Marketing Director .... Yolanda Lee
MIS Director .... JC Tucker

COMPANY PROFILE:
Parent Company Name: Chinese Hospital Association
Doing Business As: CCHP
Year Founded: 1987   Federally Qualified: [N]
Forprofit: [Y]   Not-For-Profit: [ ]
Model Type: IPA
Accreditation: [ ] AAPPO [ ] JACHO [ ] NCQA [ ] URAC
Plan Type: HMO
Total Revenue: 2005: 17,071,527   2006: 86,255,935
Net Income   2005: 326,536   2006: 1,957,206
Total Enrollment:
  2001: 8,458   2004: 11,115   2007: 13,315
  2002: 10,734   2005: 12,540
  2003: 11,237   2006: 13,231
Medical Loss Ratio: 2005: 87.04   2006: 87.85
Administrative Expense Ratio: 2005: 12.38   2006: 10.51

SERVICE AREA:
Nationwide: N
  CA (Los Angeles, San Francisco);

CALIFORNIA — Managed Care Organization Profiles

CAMBRIDGE MANAGED CARE SERVICES

11120 White Rock Dr 1st Fl
Rancho Cordova, CA 95670-6072
Phone: 916-853-5932 Fax: 916-853-5911 Toll-Free:
Web site:

MAILING ADDRESS:
CAMBRIDGE MANAGED CARE SRVCS
11120 White Rock Dr 1st Fl
Rancho Cordova, CA 95670-6072

KEY EXECUTIVES:
Chief Executive Officer .... Christopher A Sinclair
Marketing Director .... Lisa DeRitis
Co-president Managed Care Services .... Fred Crim
Co-president Managed Care Services .... Joan Baetz

COMPANY PROFILE:
Parent Company Name: Presidium Inc
Doing Business As:
Year Founded: 1985   Federally Qualified: [ ]
Forprofit: [ ]   Not-For-Profit: [ ]
Model Type:
Accreditation: [ ] AAPPO [ ] JACHO [ ] NCQA [X] URAC
Plan Type: UR

SERVICE AREA:
Nationwide: N
CA;

PLAN BENEFITS:
Alternative Medicine: [ ]   Behavioral Health: [ ]
Chiropractic: [ ]   Dental: [ ]
Home Care: [ ]   Inpatient SNF: [ ]
Long-Term Care: [ ]   Pharm. Mail Order: [ ]
Physical Therapy: [ ]   Podiatry: [ ]
Psychiatric: [ ]   Transplant: [ ]
Vision: [ ]   Wellness: [ ]
Workers' Comp: [X]
Other Benefits:
Comments:
Formerly Business Health Services.

CAPITOL ADMINISTRATORS

2920 Prospect Park Dr Ste 210
Rancho Cordova, CA 95670
Phone: 916-669-2570 Fax: 916-669-0576 Toll-Free: 800-654-6701
Web site: www.capitoladm.com

MAILING ADDRESS:
CAPITOL ADMINISTRATORS
2920 Prospect Park Dr Ste 210
Rancho Cordova, CA 95670

KEY EXECUTIVES:
Chief Executive Officer/President .... David Reynolds
Chief Financial Officer .... David Yee
Operations Manager .... Ginger Regotti
Marketing Director .... David Reynolds
MIS Director .... Russ Sutherland
Medical Management Director .... Sue Meador
Claims Manager .... Mindi Bertonellit
Senior Account Manager .... Renee Stout

COMPANY PROFILE:
Parent Company Name: Privately Held
Doing Business As: Capitol Administrators Inc
Year Founded: 1999   Federally Qualified: [Y]
Forprofit: [Y]   Not-For-Profit: [ ]
Model Type:
Accreditation: [ ] AAPPO [ ] JACHO [ ] NCQA [ ] URAC
Plan Type: PPO, Specialty PPO, PBM, POS, EPO, ASO, TPA, HSA, HDHP, FSA
Total Enrollment:
  2001: 0   2004: 0   2007: 0
  2002: 17,000   2005:
  2003: 0   2006:

SERVICE AREA:
Nationwide: Y
NW;

TYPE OF COVERAGE:
Commercial: [Y] Individual: [ ] FEHBP: [ ] Indemnity: [ ]
Medicare: [Y] Medicaid: [Y] Supplemental Medicare: [Y]
Tricare   [ ]

PRODUCTS OFFERED:
Product Name: Type:
Capital Administrators   TPA
PLAN BENEFITS:
Alternative Medicine: [ ]   Behavioral Health: [X]
Chiropractic: [X]   Dental: [X]
Home Care: [X]   Inpatient SNF: [X]
Long-Term Care: [ ]   Pharm. Mail Order: [X]
Physical Therapy: [X]   Podiatry: [X]
Psychiatric: [X]   Transplant: [X]
Vision: [X]   Wellness: [X]
Workers' Comp: [ ]
Other Benefits:
Comments:
Self funded benefit and IPA/PHO administration services.

CARE 1ST HEALTH PLAN

1000 S Fremont Ave #A-11 U-22
Alhambra, CA 91803
Phone: 626-299-4299 Fax: 626-458-0651 Toll-Free: 800-468-9935
Web site: www.care1st.com

MAILING ADDRESS:
CARE 1ST HEALTH PLAN
1000 S Fremont Ave #A-11 U-22
Alhambra, CA 91803

KEY EXECUTIVES:
Chairman of the Board .... SR Wong
Chief Executive Officer .... Anna Tran
Chief Financial Officer .... Janet Jan
Medical Director .... Jorge Weingarten, MD
Director of Pharmacy .... Jamie Ueoka, PharmD
Chief Information Officer/MIS Director .... Herbert Woo
Director, Marketing .... Felicia DePuch
Director, Provider Network Operatns .... Dolores Olague
Human Resources Director .... Ellen Smart
VP Administration/Corporate Compliance Officer .... Brooks Jones
VP, Medical Services .... Josie Wong, RN
VP, Business Development .... Walter Gray

COMPANY PROFILE:
Parent Company Name:
Doing Business As:
Year Founded: 1995   Federally Qualified: [N]
Forprofit: [Y]   Not-For-Profit: [ ]
Model Type:
Accreditation: [ ] AAPPO [ ] JACHO [X] NCQA [ ] URAC
Plan Type: HMO
Total Revenue: 2005: 78,278,781   2006: 370,363,892
Net Income   2005: 1,659,565   2006:   7,106,709
Total Enrollment:
  2001: 85,581   2004: 161,150   2007: 281,287
  2002: 196,616   2005: 159,803
  2003: 177,825   2006: 266,187
Medical Loss Ratio: 2005: 97.13   2006: 87.48
Administrative Expense Ratio: 2005: 10.94   2006: 10.79

SERVICE AREA:
Nationwide: N
CA (Los Angeles);

TYPE OF COVERAGE:
Commercial: [ ] Individual: [ ] FEHBP: [ ] Indemnity: [ ]
Medicare: [ ] Medicaid: [Y] Supplemental Medicare: [ ]
Tricare   [ ]

PRODUCTS OFFERED:
Product Name: Type:
Care 1st Health Plan   HMO
Care 1st Health Plan Dental   Medicaid

CAREMORE HEALTH PLAN

12900 Park Plz Ste 150
Cerritos, CA 90703
Phone: 562-741-4340 Fax: 562-741-4394 Toll-Free:
Web site: www.caremorehealthplan.com

MAILING ADDRESS:
CAREMORE HEALTH PLAN
12900 Park Plz Ste 150
Cerritos, CA 90703

Managed Care Organization Profiles   **CALIFORNIA**

VP Public Affairs .... Tom Epstein
Director, Provider Services .... Lisa Farnan
Senior VP/Network Management .... David Joyner
Senior VP of Human Resources .... Marianne Jackson
Statewide Medical Director .... Andy Halpert, MD
Senior Medical Director/Quality Managmt . Gifford Boyce-Smith, MD
Manager, Special Investigation .... Lou Lovato
VP Strategic & Product Development .... Betsy Stone
VP General Counsel/Chief Compliance Officer .... Chuck Sweeris
Director Accreditation & Credntlng .... Sheila Muller

COMPANY PROFILE:
Parent Company Name: California Physicians' Services
Doing Business As: Blue Shield of California
Year Founded: 1939   Federally Qualified: [N]
Forprofit: [ ]   Not-For-Profit: [Y]
Model Type: MIXED
Accreditation: [ ] AAPPO [ ] JACHO [ ] NCQA [X] URAC
Plan Type: HMO, PPO, POS, ASO, CDHP, HDHP, HSA
Total Revenue: 2005: 1,913,689,000   2006: 7,854,106,000
Net Income   2005:   66,658,000   2006:   381,585,000
Total Enrollment:
   2001: 2,314,760   2004: 2,775,624   2007: 2,597,851
   2002: 2,298,399   2005: 2,721,481
   2003: 2,701,377   2006: 2,621,060
Medical Loss Ratio: 2005: 86.35   2006:   85.74
Administrative Expense Ratio: 2005: 12.72   2006:   11.01
SERVICE AREA:
Nationwide: N
   CA;
TYPE OF COVERAGE:
Commercial: [Y] Individual: [Y]   FEHBP: [Y]   Indemnity: [Y]
Medicare: [Y] Medicaid: [ ]   Supplemental Medicare: [Y]
Tricare   [ ]
PRODUCTS OFFERED:
Product Name: Type:
Blue Shield Preferred   PPO
Blue Shield POS   POS
Blue Shield 65+   Medicare Advantage
Blue Shield Access + HMO   HMO
Blue Shield IFP   Individual
CONSUMER-DRIVEN PRODUCTS
Wells Fargo HSA   HSA Company
                                                              HSA Product
                                                              HSA Administrator
                                                              Consumer-Driven Health Plan
Shield Spectrum PPO Savings Plan   High Deductible Health Plan
PLAN BENEFITS:
Alternative Medicine: [ ]   Behavioral Health: [ ]
Chiropractic: [X]   Dental: [X]
Home Care: [X]   Inpatient SNF: [X]
Long-Term Care: [X]   Pharm. Mail Order: [X]
Physical Therapy: [X]   Podiatry: [X]
Psychiatric: [X]   Transplant: [X]
Vision: [X]   Wellness: [X]
Workers' Comp: [X]
Other Benefits:
Comments:
CareAmerica Health Plans was aquired and consolidated into California Physicians, dba Blue Shield of California.

CALIFORNIA BENEFITS DENTAL PLAN

3611 S Harbor Blvd Ste 150
Santa Ana, CA 92704-6928
Phone: 714-540-4255 Fax: 714-540-4754 Toll-Free: 800-350-3999
Web site:
MAILING ADDRESS:
   CALIFORNIA BENEFITS DENTAL PLN
   3611 S Harbor Blvd Ste 150
   Santa Ana, CA 92704-6928

KEY EXECUTIVES:
Chief Executive Officer/President .... Valerie A Clark
Dental Director .... Edward J Olivarez, DDS

COMPANY PROFILE:
Parent Company Name: Genworth Financial
Doing Business As:
Year Founded: 1992   Federally Qualified: [ ]
Forprofit: [Y]   Not-For-Profit: [ ]
Model Type:

Accreditation: [ ] AAPPO [ ] JACHO [ ] NCQA [ ] URAC
Plan Type: Specialty HMO
Total Revenue: 2005:   513,373   2006:   2,314,763
Net Income   2005:   -50,442   2006:   49,553
Total Enrollment:
   2001: 31,651   2004: 22,930   2007: 23,486
   2002: 29,373   2005: 21,418
   2003: 23,819   2006: 24,279
Medical Loss Ratio: 2005: 35.74   2006:   38.95
Administrative Expense Ratio: 2005: 83.68   2006:   59.03
SERVICE AREA:
Nationwide: N
   CA (Southern);
TYPE OF COVERAGE:
Commercial: [Y] Individual: [Y]   FEHBP: [ ]   Indemnity: [ ]
Medicare: [ ] Medicaid: [ ]   Supplemental Medicare: [ ]
Tricare   [ ]
PRODUCTS OFFERED:
Product Name: Type:
CA Benefits Dental Plan   Specialty HMO
PLAN BENEFITS:
Alternative Medicine: [ ]   Behavioral Health: [ ]
Chiropractic: [ ]   Dental: [X]
Home Care: [ ]   Inpatient SNF: [ ]
Long-Term Care: [ ]   Pharm. Mail Order: [ ]
Physical Therapy: [ ]   Podiatry: [ ]
Psychiatric: [ ]   Transplant: [ ]
Vision: [ ]   Wellness: [ ]
Workers' Comp: [ ]
Other Benefits:

CALIFORNIA DENTAL NETWORK INC

1971 E 4th St Ste 184
Santa Ana, CA 92705
Phone: 714-479-0777 Fax: 714-479-0779 Toll-Free:
Web site: www.caldental.net
MAILING ADDRESS:
   CALIFORNIA DENTAL NETWORK INC
   1971 E 4th St Ste 184
   Santa Ana, CA 92705

KEY EXECUTIVES:
Board Chairman .... James R Lindsey
Chief Executive Officer/President .... Stephen R Casey
Medical Director Officer .... Elizabeth Henderson, DDS
Director of Operations .... Jacki Houghton

COMPANY PROFILE:
Parent Company Name: Pacific Dental Network Inc
Doing Business As:
Year Founded: 1988   Federally Qualified: [ ]
Forprofit: [ ]   Not-For-Profit: [ ]
Model Type: NETWORK
Accreditation: [ ] AAPPO [ ] JACHO [ ] NCQA [ ] URAC
Plan Type: Specialty HMO
Total Revenue: 2005: 1,119,736   2006:   7,864,151
Net Income   2005:   31,209   2006:   -21,947
Total Enrollment:
   2001: 23,314   2004: 35,444   2007: 36,928
   2002: 26,874   2005: 34,459
   2003: 31,521   2006: 38,819
Medical Loss Ratio: 2005: 48.03   2006:   52.56
Administrative Expense Ratio: 2005: 50.12   2006:   48.92
SERVICE AREA:
Nationwide: N
   CA;
TYPE OF COVERAGE:
Commercial: [Y] Individual: [Y]   FEHBP: [ ]   Indemnity: [ ]
Medicare: [ ] Medicaid: [ ]   Supplemental Medicare: [ ]
Tricare   [ ]
PRODUCTS OFFERED:
Product Name: Type:
CA Dental Network, Inc   Specialty HMO
PLAN BENEFITS:
Alternative Medicine: [ ]   Behavioral Health: [ ]
Chiropractic: [ ]   Dental: [X]
Home Care: [ ]   Inpatient SNF: [ ]
Long-Term Care: [ ]   Pharm. Mail Order: [ ]
Physical Therapy: [ ]   Podiatry: [ ]
Psychiatric: [ ]   Transplant: [ ]
Vision: [ ]   Wellness: [ ]
Workers' Comp: [ ]
Other Benefits:

CALIFORNIA   Managed Care Organization Profiles

COMPANY PROFILE:
Parent Company Name:
Doing Business As:
Year Founded: 1999   Federally Qualified: [ ]
Forprofit: [ ]   Not-For-Profit: [ ]
Model Type:
Accreditation: [ ] AAPPO [ ] JACHO [ ] NCQA [ ] URAC
Plan Type: Specialty HMO
Total Revenue: 2005:   8,951   2006:   7,340
Net Income   2005: -76,804   2006: -91,009
Total Enrollment:
   2001: 0   2004: 316   2007: 145
   2002: 239   2005: 221
   2003: 355   2006: 137
Medical Loss Ratio: 2005: -177.49   2006:   77.98
Administrative Expense Ratio: 2005: 666.00   2006: 1279.55
SERVICE AREA:
Nationwide:
   CA;
TYPE OF COVERAGE:
Commercial: [ ] Individual: [ ] FEHBP: [ ] Indemnity: [ ]
Medicare: [ ] Medicaid: [ ] Supplemental Medicare: [ ]
Tricare   [ ]
PRODUCTS OFFERED:
Product Name: Type:
Basic Chiropractic Health Plan   Specialty HMO
PLAN BENEFITS:
Alternative Medicine: [ ]   Behavioral Health: [ ]
Chiropractic: [Y]   Dental: [ ]
Home Care: [ ]   Inpatient SNF: [ ]
Long-Term Care: [ ]   Pharm. Mail Order: [ ]
Physical Therapy: [ ]   Podiatry: [ ]
Psychiatric: [ ]   Transplant: [ ]
Vision: [ ]   Wellness: [ ]
Workers' Comp: [ ]
Other Benefits:

BEECH STREET CORPORATION — CORPORATE HEADQUARTERS

25500 Commercentre Dr
Lake Forest, CA 92630
Phone: 949-672-1000 Fax: 949-672-1111 Toll-Free: 800-877-1666
Web site: www.beechstreet.com
MAILING ADDRESS:
   BEECH STREET CORP HEADQUARTERS
   25500 Commercentre Dr
   Lake Forest, CA 92630

KEY EXECUTIVES:
Chief Executive Officer .... Daniel Thomas
President .... Thomas Bartlett

COMPANY PROFILE:
Parent Company Name: Viant Inc
Doing Business As: Beech Street
Year Founded: 1951   Federally Qualified: [ ]
Forprofit: [Y]   Not-For-Profit: [ ]
Model Type:
Accreditation: [ ] AAPPO [ ] JACHO [ ] NCQA [X] URAC
Plan Type: PPO, UR
Total Enrollment:
   2001: 0   2004: 0   2007: 16,000,000
   2002: 16,000,000   2005:
   2003: 16,000,000   2006:
SERVICE AREA:
Nationwide: Y
   NW;
TYPE OF COVERAGE:
Commercial: [Y] Individual: [Y] FEHBP: [ ] Indemnity: [ ]
Medicare: [ ] Medicaid: [ ] Supplemental Medicare: [Y]
Tricare   [ ]
PRODUCTS OFFERED:
Product Name: Type:
Health Benefits PPO Network   PPO
Workers Compensation PPO Network   Workers' Comp
Auto Medical PPO Network   PPO
Beech Street Utilization Management   UM
Beech Street Case Management   Case Management
Beech Street Disease Managemen   Maternity Options

PLAN BENEFITS:
Alternative Medicine: [X]   Behavioral Health: [X]
Chiropractic: [X]   Dental: [ ]
Home Care: [X]   Inpatient SNF: [X]
Long-Term Care: [X]   Pharm. Mail Order: [ ]
Physical Therapy: [X]   Podiatry: [X]
Psychiatric: [X]   Transplant: [X]
Vision: [ ]   Wellness: [ ]
Workers' Comp: [X]
Other Benefits:
Comments:
In 1999 Beech Street merged with CAPP Care Corporation. Acquired by Concentra Operating Corporation on October 3, 2005. Concentra Operating Corporation changed name to Viant Inc.

BEST HEALTH PLANS

2505 McCabe Way
Irvine, CA 92614-6243
Phone: 949-253-4080 Fax: 949-553-0883 Toll-Free: 800-854-7417
Web site: www.besthealthplans.com
MAILING ADDRESS:
   BEST HEALTH PLANS
   2505 McCabe Way
   Irvine, CA 92614-6243

KEY EXECUTIVES:
Chief Executive Officer-Best Life .... Donald R Lawrenz
President-Best Life .... Steve Course
VP,Chief Financial Officer .... Alan Koransky
Pharmacy Director .... Carolyn Johnson
Marketing Communications Coord .... Kori Jones
Privacy/Compliance Officer .... Paul Peatross
Human Resources Director .... Carolyn Johnson
Fraud Prevention Officer .... Paul Peatross
Claims Director .... Vicki MIller
Chief Administrative Officer .... James Stumpfel

COMPANY PROFILE:
Parent Company Name: Best Life & Health Insurance Company
Doing Business As:
Year Founded: 1970   Federally Qualified: [ ]
Forprofit: [ ]   Not-For-Profit: [ ]
Model Type:
Accreditation: [ ] AAPPO [ ] JACHO [ ] NCQA [ ] URAC
Plan Type: PPO
SERVICE AREA:
Nationwide:
   CA;
TYPE OF COVERAGE:
Commercial: [ ] Individual: [ ] FEHBP: [ ] Indemnity: [Y]
Medicare: [ ] Medicaid: [ ] Supplemental Medicare: [ ]
Tricare   [ ]
CONSUMER-DRIVEN PRODUCTS
Bancorp   HSA Company
                                  HSA Product
Bancorp   HSA Administrator
                                  Consumer-Driven Health Plan
HealthSolutions HDHP   High Deductible Health Plan

BLUE SHIELD OF CALIFORNIA

50 Beale Street
San Francisco, CA 94105
Phone: 415-229-5000 Fax: 415-229-5056 Toll-Free:
Web site: www.mylifepath.com/bsc
MAILING ADDRESS:
   BLUE SHIELD OF CALIFORNIA
   PO Box 7168
   San Francisco, CA 94105

KEY EXECUTIVES:
Chairman of the Board .... Bruce G Bodaken
Chief Executive Officer/President .... Bruce G Bodaken
Chief Financial Officer .... Heidi Kunz
Senior VP, Medical Director .... Alan Sokolow, MD
VP, Pharmacy Services .... Nancy Stalker
Chief Information Officer .... Elinor MacKinnon
Corporate Marketing/Customer Service .... Bob Novelli
VP Coporate Marketing .... Doug Biehn
VP Sales and Marketing .... Peter G Duncan

Managed Care Organization Profiles — CALIFORNIA

COMPANY PROFILE:
Parent Company Name:
Doing Business As: Arta
Year Founded: 2006   Federally Qualified: [ ]
Forprofit: [ ]   Not-For-Profit: [ ]
Model Type:
Accreditation: [ ] AAPPO [ ] JACHO [ ] NCQA [ ] URAC
Plan Type: HMO
Primary Physicians: 800   Physician Specialists:
Hospitals:
Total Enrollment:
  2001: 0   2004: 0   2007: 272
  2002: 0   2005:
  2003: 0   2006:

SERVICE AREA:
Nationwide:
  CA;

TYPE OF COVERAGE:
Commercial: [ ] Individual: [ ] FEHBP: [ ] Indemnity: [ ]
Medicare: [Y] Medicaid: [ ] Supplemental Medicare: [ ]
Tricare   [ ]

PRODUCTS OFFERED:
Product Name: Type:
Medicare

ASSURANT EMPLOYEE BENEFITS - CALIFORNIA

450 B St Ste 880
San Diego, CA 92101
Phone: 619-236-9595 Fax: 619-236-8151 Toll-Free: 800-821-1294
Web site: www.assurantemployeebenefits.com

MAILING ADDRESS:
  ASSURANT EMPLOYEE BNFTS - CA
  450 B St Ste 880
  San Diego, CA 92101

KEY EXECUTIVES:
Interim Chief Executive Officer/President .... John S Roberts
Chief Financial Officer .... Floyd F Chadee
VP, Medical Director .... Polly M Galbraith, MD
Chief Information Officer .... Karla J Schacht
Senior VP, Marketing .... Joseph A Sevcik
Privacy Officer .... John L Fortini
VP of Provider Services .... James A Barrett, DMD
Senior VP, Human Resources & Development .... Sylvia R Wagner
General Manager .... Todd Boyd
National Dental Director .... James A Barrett, DMD

COMPANY PROFILE:
Parent Company Name: Assurant Health
Doing Business As:
Year Founded: 1989   Federally Qualified: [ ]
Forprofit: [Y]   Not-For-Profit: [ ]
Model Type:
Accreditation: [ ] AAPPO [ ] JACHO [ ] NCQA [ ] URAC
Plan Type: Specialty HMO
Total Enrollment:
  2001: 20,062   2004: 0   2007: 0
  2002: 0   2005:
  2003: 0   2006:

SERVICE AREA:
Nationwide: N
  CA; HI;

TYPE OF COVERAGE:
Commercial: [Y] Individual: [Y] FEHBP: [ ] Indemnity: [ ]
Medicare: [ ] Medicaid: [ ] Supplemental Medicare: [ ]
Tricare   [ ]

PLAN BENEFITS:
Alternative Medicine: [ ]   Behavioral Health: [ ]
Chiropractic: [ ]   Dental: [X]
Home Care: [ ]   Inpatient SNF: [ ]
Long-Term Care: [ ]   Pharm. Mail Order: [ ]
Physical Therapy: [ ]   Podiatry: [ ]
Psychiatric: [ ]   Transplant: [ ]
Vision: [ ]   Wellness: [ ]
Workers' Comp: [ ]
Other Benefits:

Comments:
Formerly Fortis Benefits Dental.

AVANTE BEHAVIORAL HEALTH PLAN

1111 E Herndon Ave #308
Fresno, CA 93720-3100
Phone: 559-261-9060 Fax: 559-261-9073 Toll-Free: 800-498-9055
Web site: www.avantehealth.com

MAILING ADDRESS:
  AVANTE BEHAVIORAL HEALTH PLAN
  1111 E Herndon Ave #308
  Fresno, CA 93720-3100

KEY EXECUTIVES:
Chairman .... Bradley Schuyler
Chief Executive Officer/President .... D Duane Oswald
Chief Financial Officer .... Brent Lindquist
Medical Director .... Alan Drucker, MD
Marketing & Account Representative .... Keely Coyle
Director Information Systems, Claims .... Tara Lindlahr
Compliance Officer .... Tara Lindlahr
Director of Business Development .... Jeremy Oswald

COMPANY PROFILE:
Parent Company Name: Avante Health
Doing Business As:
Year Founded: 1999   Federally Qualified: [N]
Forprofit: [Y]   Not-For-Profit: [ ]
Model Type: MIXED
Accreditation: [ ] AAPPO [ ] JACHO [ ] NCQA [ ] URAC
Plan Type: Specialty HMO, Specialty PPO
Total Revenue: 2005: 374,513   2006: 1,489,872
Net Income   2005:   33,863   2006:   30,868
Total Enrollment:
  2001: 0   2004: 15,042   2007: 17,114
  2002: 1,032   2005: 15,069
  2003: 11,836   2006: 16,601
Medical Loss Ratio: 2005: 56.32   2006: 65.10
Administrative Expense Ratio: 2005: 56.49   2006: 56.84

SERVICE AREA:
Nationwide:
  CA (Central);

TYPE OF COVERAGE:
Commercial: [Y] Individual: [ ] FEHBP: [ ] Indemnity: [ ]
Medicare: [ ] Medicaid: [ ] Supplemental Medicare: [ ]
Tricare   [ ]

PRODUCTS OFFERED:
Product Name: Type:
Avante Behavioral Health Plan   Specialty HMO

PLAN BENEFITS:
Alternative Medicine: [ ]   Behavioral Health: [X]
Chiropractic: [ ]   Dental: [ ]
Home Care: [ ]   Inpatient SNF: [ ]
Long-Term Care: [ ]   Pharm. Mail Order: [ ]
Physical Therapy: [ ]   Podiatry: [ ]
Psychiatric: [X]   Transplant: [ ]
Vision: [ ]   Wellness: [ ]
Workers' Comp: [ ]
Other Benefits:

BASIC CHIROPRACTIC HEALTH PLAN INC

2027 Grand Canal Blvd Ste 21
Stockton, CA 95207
Phone: 209-957-9601 Fax: 209-956-6808 Toll-Free:
Web site: www.bchpinc.com

MAILING ADDRESS:
  BASIC CHIROPRACTIC HEALTH PLAN
  2027 Grand Canal Blvd Ste 21
  Stockton, CA 95207

KEY EXECUTIVES:
Chief Executive Officer/President .... Don Smallie, DC
Chief Financial Officer .... David Moscovic
Medical Director .... Don Smallie, DC
Chief Operating Officer/Marketing Director .... Ron Cataldo, Jr
Credentialing Manager/Compliance Officer .... Todd Cataldo
Network Development Director .... Ron Cataldo, Jr
Credentialing Manager .... Todd Cataldo
Director of Utilization Management .... Ron Cataldo, DC
Financial Oversight Director .... Jeanette M Cataldo

CALIFORNIA — Managed Care Organization Profiles

Total Revenue: 2005: 17,004,493 2006: 71,903,986
Net Income 2005: 938,902 2006: 6,974,461
Total Enrollment:
    2001: 4,259,683   2004: 4,182,321   2007: 4,349,290
    2002: 4,053,315   2005: 4,267,781
    2003: 3,981,361   2006: 4,350,518
Medical Loss Ratio: 2005: 49.78   2006: 48.92
Administrative Expense Ratio: 2005: 40.91   2006: 34.95

SERVICE AREA:
Nationwide: N
CA;

TYPE OF COVERAGE:
Commercial: [Y]   Individual: [Y]   FEHBP: [ ]   Indemnity: [ ]
Medicare: [Y]   Medicaid: [ ]   Supplemental Medicare: [Y]
Tricare [ ]

PLAN BENEFITS:
Alternative Medicine: [X]   Behavioral Health: [ ]
Chiropractic: [X]   Dental: [ ]
Home Care: [ ]   Inpatient SNF: [ ]
Long-Term Care: [ ]   Pharm. Mail Order: [ ]
Physical Therapy: [ ]   Podiatry: [ ]
Psychiatric: [ ]   Transplant: [ ]
Vision: [ ]   Wellness: [ ]
Workers' Comp: [X]
Other Benefits: Acupuncture

Comments:
Health Plans contracted with: Aetna, Blue Shield HMO, Blue Cross/California Care; CIGNA; Healthnet; Health Plan of the Redwoods; Kaiser Permanente.

AMERITAS MANAGED DENTAL PLAN INC

151 Kalmus Dr Ste J4
Costa Mesa, CA 92626-5988
Phone: 714-641-1800 Fax: 714-641-4800 Toll-Free: 800-336-6661
Web site: www.ameritasgroup.com

MAILING ADDRESS:
    AMERITAS MANAGED DENTAL PLAN
    151 Kalmus Dr Ste J4
    Costa Mesa, CA 92626-5988

KEY EXECUTIVES:
President/Chief Operating Officer .... Sherry Hobbs
Marketing Director .... Nicole Wallstrom
VP, Group Field Sales .... Todd Reimers
Assistant VP, Corporate Communications .... Scott Stuckey
Senior VP, Group Division .... Ken VanCleave

COMPANY PROFILE:
Parent Company Name: Ameritas Life Insurance Corp
Doing Business As:
Year Founded: 1963   Federally Qualified: [ ]
Forprofit: [Y]   Not-For-Profit: [ ]
Model Type: NETWORK
Accreditation: [ ] AAPPO [ ] JACHO [ ] NCQA [ ] URAC
Plan Type: Specialty PPO
Total Enrollment:
    2001: 0   2004: 0   2007: 0
    2002: 32,039   2005:
    2003: 0   2006:

SERVICE AREA:
Nationwide: N
CA;

TYPE OF COVERAGE:
Commercial: [Y]   Individual: [Y]   FEHBP: [ ]   Indemnity: [ ]
Medicare: [ ]   Medicaid: [ ]   Supplemental Medicare: [ ]
Tricare [ ]

PRODUCTS OFFERED:
Product Name: Type:
Ameritas Managed Dental Plan   Specialty HMO

PLAN BENEFITS:
Alternative Medicine: [ ]   Behavioral Health: [ ]
Chiropractic: [ ]   Dental: [X]
Home Care: [ ]   Inpatient SNF: [ ]
Long-Term Care: [ ]   Pharm. Mail Order: [ ]
Physical Therapy: [ ]   Podiatry: [ ]
Psychiatric: [ ]   Transplant: [ ]
Vision: [ ]   Wellness: [ ]
Workers' Comp: [ ]
Other Benefits:

Comments:
Formerly Consolidated Health Services Inc.

ANTHEM BLUE CROSS

21555 Oxnard St
Woodland Hills, CA 91367
Phone: 818-234-2345 Fax: 818-234-2848 Toll-Free:
Web site: www.bluecrossca.com

MAILING ADDRESS:
    ANTHEM BLUE CROSS
    21555 Oxnard St
    Woodland Hills, CA 91367

KEY EXECUTIVES:
Chief Executive Officer/President .... Brian A Sassi
EVP, Financial Services .... Wayne S DeVeydt
Chief Medical Officer .... Ivan Jeffrey Kamil
Director, Corporate Communications .... Michael Chee
Director, Provider Services .... Andrew Allocco
Senior VP, Network Development .... Josh Valdez

COMPANY PROFILE:
Parent Company Name: WellPoint Inc
Doing Business As: Anthem Blue Cross
Year Founded: 1937   Federally Qualified: [N]
Forprofit: [Y]   Not-For-Profit: [ ]
Model Type: MIXED
Accreditation: [ ] AAPPO [X] JACHO [X] NCQA [ ] URAC
Plan Type: HMO, PPO, UR, POS, EPO, CDHP, HDHP, HSA
Total Revenue: 2005: 2,949,393,000 2006: 11,452,685,000
Net Income 2005: 219,069,000 2006: 635,347,000
Total Enrollment:
    2001: 4,312,176   2004: 4,595,259   2007: 4,244,001
    2002: 4,836,701   2005: 4,550,212
    2003: 6,727,650   2006: 4,397,820
Medical Loss Ratio: 2005: 81.54   2006: 81.53
Administrative Expense Ratio: 2005: 10.13   2006: 11.43

SERVICE AREA:
Nationwide: N
CA;

TYPE OF COVERAGE:
Commercial: [Y]   Individual: [Y]   FEHBP: [ ]   Indemnity: [ ]
Medicare: [Y]   Medicaid: [Y]   Supplemental Medicare: [Y]
Tricare [ ]

PRODUCTS OFFERED:
Product Name:	Type:
Blue Cross Senior Secure	Medicare Advantage
Prudent Buyer	PPO
CaliforniaCare	HMO
Blue Cross of CA	Medicaid

CONSUMER-DRIVEN PRODUCTS
JP Morgan Chase   HSA Company
    HSA Product
    HSA Administrator
    Consumer-Driven Health Plan
Power HealthFund PPO   High Deductible Health Plan

PLAN BENEFITS:
Alternative Medicine: [ ]   Behavioral Health: [X]
Chiropractic: [X]   Dental: [X]
Home Care: [X]   Inpatient SNF: [X]
Long-Term Care: [ ]   Pharm. Mail Order: [X]
Physical Therapy: [X]   Podiatry: [X]
Psychiatric: [X]   Transplant: [X]
Vision: [ ]   Wellness: [X]
Workers' Comp: [X]
Other Benefits:

Comments:
Formerly Blue Cross of California

ARTA MEDICARE HEALTH PLAN INC

3333 Michelson Dr Ste 750
Irvine, CA 92612
Phone: 949-260-6520 Fax: 949-567-0216 Toll-Free:
Web site: www.artamedicare.com

MAILING ADDRESS:
    ARTA MEDICARE HEALTH PLAN INC
    3333 Michelson Dr Ste 750
    Irvine, CA 92612

KEY EXECUTIVES:
Chief Executive Officer/President .... Baruch Fogel

Managed Care Organization Profiles — **CALIFORNIA**

PLAN BENEFITS:
Alternative Medicine:	[X]	Behavioral Health:	[X]
Chiropractic:	[ ]	Dental:	[X]
Home Care:	[X]	Inpatient SNF:	[X]
Long-Term Care:	[ ]	Pharm. Mail Order:	[X]
Physical Therapy:	[X]	Podiatry:	[ ]
Psychiatric:	[ ]	Transplant:	[ ]
Vision:	[ ]	Wellness:	[ ]
Workers' Comp:	[ ]		

Other Benefits:

ALAMEDA ALLIANCE FOR HEALTH

1240 South Loop Rd
Alameda, CA 94502
Phone: 510-747-4500 Fax: 510-747-4502 Toll-Free:
Web site: www.alamedaalliance.com

MAILING ADDRESS:
ALAMEDA ALLIANCE FOR HEALTH
1240 South Loop Rd
Alameda, CA 94502

KEY EXECUTIVES:
Chief Executive Officer .... Ingrid Lamirault
Chief Financial Officer .... John Volkober
Chief Medical Officer .... Arthur Chen, MD
Director, Pharmacy Services .... Anna Yang, PharmD
Chief Information Officer .... Craig Elsdon'Dew
Member Services & Marketing Director .... Troy Lam
Credentialing Supervisor .... Melinda Garcia
Manager, Provider Services .... Diane Rigoletto
Human Resource Diretor .... Mark Roche
Quality Improvement Director .... Claudia Mundy
Director, Communications .... Amanda Flores-Witte
Director, Membership Accounting .... Zina Glover

COMPANY PROFILE:
Parent Company Name: Alameda Alliance for Health
Doing Business As:
Year Founded: 1995   Federally Qualified: [ ]
Forprofit: [ ]   Not-For-Profit: [Y]
Model Type: MIXED
Accreditation: [ ] AAPPO [ ] JACHO [ ] NCQA [ ] URAC
Plan Type: HMO
Total Revenue: 2005: 36,514,547   2006: 36,009,426
Net Income   2005: 2,455,301   2006: 645,691
Total Enrollment:
  2001: 75,000   2004: 92,628   2007: 88,201
  2002: 87,926   2005: 89,066
  2003: 95,472   2006: 90,198
Medical Loss Ratio: 2005: 84.69   2006: 86.89
Administrative Expense Ratio: 2005: 9.47   2006: 9.16

SERVICE AREA:
Nationwide: N
  CA (Alameda);

TYPE OF COVERAGE:
Commercial: [ ] Individual: [ ] FEHBP: [ ] Indemnity: [ ]
Medicare: [ ] Medicaid: [Y] Supplemental Medicare: [ ]
Tricare [ ]

PRODUCTS OFFERED:
Product Name:	Type:
Alameda Alliance for Health	Medicaid

PLAN BENEFITS:
Alternative Medicine:	[ ]	Behavioral Health:	[ ]
Chiropractic:	[ ]	Dental:	[ ]
Home Care:	[X]	Inpatient SNF:	[ ]
Long-Term Care:	[ ]	Pharm. Mail Order:	[ ]
Physical Therapy:	[ ]	Podiatry:	[X]
Psychiatric:	[ ]	Transplant:	[ ]
Vision:	[X]	Wellness:	[X]
Workers' Comp:	[ ]		

Other Benefits: Multiple Specialties

AMERICAN HEALTHGUARD CORPORATION

30 E Santa Clara Ste D
Arcadia, CA 91006
Phone: 626-821-5500 Fax: 626-821-5514 Toll-Free: 800-727-6453
Web site:

MAILING ADDRESS:
AMERICAN HEALTHGUARD CORP
30 E Santa Clara Ste D
Arcadia, CA 91006

KEY EXECUTIVES:
Chief Executive Officer/President .... David Kutner
Chief Financial Officer .... Stacey Pearlman
VP Sales & Marketing .... Michael Hershberger
MIS Director .... David Kutner

COMPANY PROFILE:
Parent Company Name:
Doing Business As: Centaguard Dental Plan
Year Founded: 1985   Federally Qualified: [N]
Forprofit: [Y]   Not-For-Profit: [ ]
Model Type:
Accreditation: [ ] AAPPO [ ] JACHO [ ] NCQA [ ] URAC
Plan Type: Specialty HMO
Total Revenue: 2005:   2006: 675,324
Net Income   2005:   2006: -25,337
Total Enrollment:
  2001: 18,085   2004: 0   2007: 28,241
  2002: 26,492   2005:
  2003: 0   2006: 19,971
Medical Loss Ratio: 2005:   2006: 67.06
Administrative Expense Ratio: 2005:   2006: 34.09

SERVICE AREA:
Nationwide: N
  CA (Orange, Los Angeles, Riverside, San Bernardino, San Diego, Ventura);

TYPE OF COVERAGE:
Commercial: [Y] Individual: [Y] FEHBP: [ ] Indemnity: [ ]
Medicare: [ ] Medicaid: [ ] Supplemental Medicare: [ ]
Tricare [ ]

PRODUCTS OFFERED:
Product Name:	Type:
American Healthguard	Medicaid

PLAN BENEFITS:
Alternative Medicine:	[ ]	Behavioral Health:	[ ]
Chiropractic:	[ ]	Dental:	[X]
Home Care:	[ ]	Inpatient SNF:	[ ]
Long-Term Care:	[ ]	Pharm. Mail Order:	[ ]
Physical Therapy:	[ ]	Podiatry:	[ ]
Psychiatric:	[ ]	Transplant:	[ ]
Vision:	[ ]	Wellness:	[ ]
Workers' Comp:	[ ]		

Other Benefits:

AMERICAN SPECIALTY HEALTH PLANS INC

777 Front St
San Diego, CA 92101
Phone: 619-578-2000 Fax: 619-237-3859 Toll-Free: 800-848-3555
Web site: www.americanspecialtyhp.com

MAILING ADDRESS:
AMERICAN SPECIALTY HEALTH PLNS
777 Front St
San Diego, CA 92101

KEY EXECUTIVES:
Chief Executive Officer/President .... George T DeVries, III
Chief Financial Officer .... Dennis N Beal
Chief Medical Officer .... Robert Crocker, MD
Chief Operating Officer .... Robert P White
Marketing Director .... Michael Finnerty
Chief Information Officer .... Kevin Kujawa
Director, Provider Services .... Susan Smith
Network/Contracts Director .... Phyllis Maeyher
Human Resource Director .... Katherine Mayer
Quality Assurance Director .... Monica Vagas
Case Management Director .... Kurt Hegschweiler DC
Chief Health Services Officer .... R Douglas Metz, DC

COMPANY PROFILE:
Parent Company Name:
Doing Business As: ACN/American Chiropractic Ntwrk Inc/ASHP
Year Founded: 1987   Federally Qualified: [N]
Forprofit: [Y]   Not-For-Profit: [ ]
Model Type: NETWORK
Accreditation: [ ] AAPPO [ ] JACHO [ ] NCQA [ ] URAC
Plan Type: Specialty HMO, Specialty PPO, POS

CALIFORNIA — Managed Care Organization Profiles

PLAN BENEFITS:
Alternative Medicine:	[ ]	Behavioral Health:	[X]
Chiropractic:	[X]	Dental:	[X]
Home Care:	[X]	Inpatient SNF:	[X]
Long-Term Care:	[ ]	Pharm. Mail Order:	[X]
Physical Therapy:	[X]	Podiatry:	[X]
Psychiatric:	[X]	Transplant:	[X]
Vision:	[X]	Wellness:	[X]
Workers' Comp:	[ ]		

Other Benefits:

AETNA INC - DENTAL CARE OF CALIFORNIA

2545 W Hillcrest Dr BldgC #700
Thousand Oaks, CA 91320
Phone: 925-543-9000 Fax: Toll-Free:
Web site: www.aetna.com

MAILING ADDRESS:
AETNA INC - DENTAL CARE OF CA
2545 W Hillcrest Dr BldgC #700
Thousand Oaks, CA 91320

KEY EXECUTIVES:
Chairman of the Board/Chief Executive Officer .... Ronald A Williams
Regional Manager-Western .... Thomas R Williams
Executive VP, Finance .... Joseph M Zubretsky
Chief Medical Officer .... Milton Schwartz, MD
Regional Information Technology Manager .... Liana Myers
Regional Marketing Head .... Cindy Ryan
Provider Communications Director .... Karen Havlicek
Regional Human Resources Director .... Dorian Linkogle

COMPANY PROFILE:
Parent Company Name: Aetna Inc
Doing Business As: Aetna Inc - Dental Care of CA Inc
Year Founded: Federally Qualified: [ ]
Forprofit: [Y] Not-For-Profit: [ ]
Model Type:
Accreditation: [ ] AAPPO [ ] JACHO [ ] NCQA [ ] URAC
Plan Type: Specialty HMO, CDHP, HSA
Total Revenue: 2005: 16,725,128 2006: 59,935,810
Net Income 2005: 4,224,126 2006: 14,311,771
Total Enrollment:
  2001: 99,162 2004: 271,746 2007: 261,393
  2002: 274,691 2005: 286,935
  2003: 271,475 2006: 272,368
Medical Loss Ratio: 2005: 42.75 2006: 45.90
Administrative Expense Ratio: 2005: 13.99 2006: 13.46

SERVICE AREA:
Nationwide: N
CA;

TYPE OF COVERAGE:
Commercial: [Y] Individual: [ ] FEHBP: [ ] Indemnity: [Y]
Medicare: [ ] Medicaid: [ ] Supplemental Medicare: [ ]
Tricare [ ]

PRODUCTS OFFERED:
Product Name:	Type:
Aetna US Healthcare Dental CA	Specialty HMO

CONSUMER-DRIVEN PRODUCTS
Aetna Life Insurance Co	HSA Company
Aetna HealthFund HSA	HSA Product
Aetna	HSA Administrator
Aetna HealthFund	Consumer-Driven Health Plan
PPO I; PPO II	High Deductible Health Plan

PLAN BENEFITS:
Alternative Medicine:	[ ]	Behavioral Health:	[ ]
Chiropractic:	[ ]	Dental:	[X]
Home Care:	[ ]	Inpatient SNF:	[ ]
Long-Term Care:	[ ]	Pharm. Mail Order:	[ ]
Physical Therapy:	[ ]	Podiatry:	[ ]
Psychiatric:	[ ]	Transplant:	[ ]
Vision:	[ ]	Wellness:	[ ]
Workers' Comp:	[ ]		

Other Benefits:

AFFINITY DENTAL HEALTH PLANS

6035 Bristol Pkwy Ste 200
Culver City, CA 90230
Phone: 866-960-2347 Fax: 888-492-2900 Toll-Free:
Web site: www.affinitydentalplan.com

MAILING ADDRESS:
AFFINITY DENTAL HEALTH PLANS
6035 Bristol Pkwy Ste 200
Culver City, CA 90230

KEY EXECUTIVES:
Chief Executive Officer/President .... Alexander Gladkov, DDS

COMPANY PROFILE:
Parent Company Name:
Doing Business As:
Year Founded: 2007 Federally Qualified: [ ]
Forprofit: [ ] Not-For-Profit: [ ]
Model Type:
Accreditation: [ ] AAPPO [ ] JACHO [ ] NCQA [ ] URAC
Plan Type: Specialty HMO

SERVICE AREA:
Nationwide:
CA;

PLAN BENEFITS:
Alternative Medicine:	[ ]	Behavioral Health:	[ ]
Chiropractic:	[ ]	Dental:	[X]
Home Care:	[ ]	Inpatient SNF:	[ ]
Long-Term Care:	[ ]	Pharm. Mail Order:	[ ]
Physical Therapy:	[ ]	Podiatry:	[ ]
Psychiatric:	[ ]	Transplant:	[ ]
Vision:	[ ]	Wellness:	[ ]
Workers' Comp:	[ ]		

Other Benefits:

AIDS HEALTHCARE FOUNDATION

6255 W Sunset Blvd Ste 2100
Los Angeles, CA 90028
Phone: 323-860-5200 Fax: 323-962-8513 Toll-Free:
Web site: www.aidshealth.org

MAILING ADDRESS:
AIDS HEALTHCARE FOUNDATION
6255 W Sunset Blvd Ste 2100
Los Angeles, CA 90028

KEY EXECUTIVES:
President .... Michael Weinstein
Chief Financial Officer .... Laura Nelson
Medical Director .... Scott Howell, MD
Director of Information Technology .... Pablo Roman
Chief of Operations .... Jackie Mendelson
Chief of Marketing .... Michael O'Malley
Public Relations Director .... Ged Kenslea
Director, Human Resources .... Greg Perkins
Chief of Managed Care .... Donna Stidham
Vice President .... Peter Reis
Plan Administrator .... Scott Turner

COMPANY PROFILE:
Parent Company Name:
Doing Business As:
Year Founded: 2005 Federally Qualified: [ ]
Forprofit: [ ] Not-For-Profit: [Y]
Model Type: MIXED
Accreditation: [ ] AAPPO [ ] JACHO [X] NCQA [ ] URAC
Plan Type: Specialty HMO,
Total Enrollment:
  2001: 0 2004: 0 2007: 1,518
  2002: 0 2005:
  2003: 0 2006: 802

SERVICE AREA:
Nationwide:
CA; FL;

TYPE OF COVERAGE:
Commercial: [ ] Individual: [ ] FEHBP: [ ] Indemnity: [ ]
Medicare: [ ] Medicaid: [Y] Supplemental Medicare: [ ]
Tricare [ ]

PRODUCTS OFFERED:
Product Name:	Type:
Positive Healthcare	Medicaid
	Medicare

Managed Care Organization Profiles — CALIFORNIA

ACCESS DENTAL SERVICES

8890 Cal Center Dr
Sacramento, CA 95826
Phone: 916-563-6025 Fax: 916-646-9000 Toll-Free: 800-757-6453
Web site: www.accessdental.com

MAILING ADDRESS:
ACCESS DENTAL SERVICES
PO Box 659005
Sacramento, CA 95826

KEY EXECUTIVES:
Chief Executive Officer .... Reza Abbaszadeh, DDS
Dental Director .... Laila Baker, MD
VP & Marketing Director .... Terri Abbaszadeh
MIS Director .... Rakesh Ram

COMPANY PROFILE:
Parent Company Name:
Doing Business As:
Year Founded: 1993   Federally Qualified: [ ]
Forprofit: [Y]   Not-For-Profit: [ ]
Model Type:
Accreditation: [ ] AAPPO [ ] JACHO [ ] NCQA [ ] URAC
Plan Type: Specialty HMO, Specialty PPO,
Total Revenue: 2005: 8,819,707   2006: 34,417,458
Net Income   2005: 1,418,745   2006: 5,058,710
Total Enrollment:
   2001: 123,880   2004: 244,300   2007: 240,152
   2002: 182,918   2005: 240,070
   2003: 225,999   2006: 234,976
Medical Loss Ratio: 2005: 69.34   2006: 68.51
Administrative Expense Ratio: 2005: 16.00 2006: 18.58

SERVICE AREA:
Nationwide: N
   CA (Butte, Sacramento, Santa Cruz, Shasta, Sutter);

TYPE OF COVERAGE:
Commercial: [Y] Individual: [Y] FEHBP: [ ] Indemnity: [ ]
Medicare: [Y] Medicaid: [Y] Supplemental Medicare: [Y]
Tricare   [ ]

PRODUCTS OFFERED:
Product Name: Type:
Access Dental Plan HMO   Specialty HMO
Access Medi-Cal Risk   Medicaid

PLAN BENEFITS:
Alternative Medicine: [ ]   Behavioral Health: [ ]
Chiropractic: [ ]   Dental: [X]
Home Care: [ ]   Inpatient SNF: [ ]
Long-Term Care: [ ]   Pharm. Mail Order: [ ]
Physical Therapy: [ ]   Podiatry: [ ]
Psychiatric: [ ]   Transplant: [ ]
Vision: [ ]   Wellness: [ ]
Workers' Comp: [ ]
Other Benefits:

ACN GROUP OF CALIFORNIA - WESTERN REGION

3111 Camino Del Rio N Ste 1000
San Diego, CA 92108
Phone: 619-641-7100 Fax: 619-641-7185 Toll-Free:
Web site: www.acngroup.com

MAILING ADDRESS:
ACN GROUP OF CA - WESTERN REGN
3111 Camino Del Rio N Ste 1000
San Diego, CA 92108

KEY EXECUTIVES:
Chief Executive Officer/President .... Stephen Castro
RegionalChief Clinical Officer .... Dale Cohen

COMPANY PROFILE:
Parent Company Name: UnitedHealth Group
Doing Business As: ACN Group Inc
Year Founded: 1987   Federally Qualified: [ ]
Forprofit: [ ]   Not-For-Profit: [ ]
Model Type:
Accreditation: [ ] AAPPO [ ] JACHO [ ] NCQA [ ] URAC
Plan Type: HMO, PPO, Specialty HMO, Specialty PPO, ASO, UR,
Total Revenue: 2005: 1,666,687   2006: 3,623,943
Net Income   2005:   -342,776   2006: 1,301,629
Total Enrollment:
   2001: 0   2004: 0   2007: 848,708
   2002: 0   2005: 2,709
   2003: 0   2006: 880,730
Medical Loss Ratio: 2005: 312.25 2006: 47.27
Administrative Expense Ratio: 2005: 117.35 2006: 35.21

SERVICE AREA:
Nationwide:
   CA;

TYPE OF COVERAGE:
Commercial: [Y] Individual: [ ] FEHBP: [ ] Indemnity: [ ]
Medicare: [Y] Medicaid: [ ] Supplemental Medicare: [Y]
Tricare   [ ]

PLAN BENEFITS:
Alternative Medicine: [X]   Behavioral Health: [ ]
Chiropractic: [X]   Dental: [ ]
Home Care: [ ]   Inpatient SNF: [ ]
Long-Term Care: [ ]   Pharm. Mail Order: [ ]
Physical Therapy: [ ]   Podiatry: [ ]
Psychiatric: [ ]   Transplant: [ ]
Vision: [ ]   Wellness: [X]
Workers' Comp: [X]
Other Benefits:

AETNA HEALTH OF CALIFORNIA INC

2625 Shadelands Dr
Walnut Creek, CA 94598
Phone: 925-543-9000 Fax: Toll-Free:
Web site: www.aetna.com

MAILING ADDRESS:
AETNA HEALTH OF CALIFORNIA INC
2625 Shadelands Dr
Walnut Creek, CA 94598

KEY EXECUTIVES:
Chairman of the Board/Chief Executive Officer .... Ronald A Williams
Regional Manager-Western .... Thomas R Williams
Chief Financial Officer .... Fred Hatfield
Chief Medical Officer .... Milton Schwartz, MD
Pharmacy Director .... Yrena Friedman
Marketing Director .... John Lattig
MIS Director .... Liana Myers
Human Resources Director .... Dorian Linkogle

COMPANY PROFILE:
Parent Company Name: Aetna Inc
Doing Business As: Aetna Inc
Year Founded: 1981   Federally Qualified: [Y]
Forprofit: [Y]   Not-For-Profit: [ ]
Model Type: MIXED
Accreditation: [ ] AAPPO [X] JACHO [X] NCQA [X] URAC
Plan Type: HMO, PPO, POS, EPO, CDHP, HSA
Total Revenue: 2005: 243,728,012   2006: 1,064,583,022
Net Income   2005: 24,478,251   2006:   36,277,741
Total Enrollment:
   2001: 863,151   2004: 304,944   2007: 337,692
   2002: 523,099   2005: 294,903
   2003: 377,718   2006: 314,692
Medical Loss Ratio: 2005: 75.80   2006: 83.27
Administrative Expense Ratio: 2005: 9.86   2006: 11.91

SERVICE AREA:
Nationwide: N
   CA;

TYPE OF COVERAGE:
Commercial: [Y] Individual: [ ] FEHBP: [ ] Indemnity: [Y]
Medicare: [Y] Medicaid: [ ] Supplemental Medicare: [ ]
Tricare   [ ]

PRODUCTS OFFERED:
Product Name: Type:
US Access   HMO
QPOS   HMO
Golden Medicare   Medicare Advantage

CONSUMER-DRIVEN PRODUCTS
Aetna Life Insurance Co   HSA Company
Aetna HealthFund HSA   HSA Product
Aetna   HSA Administrator
Aetna HealthFund   Consumer-Driven Health Plan
PPO I; PPO II   High Deductible Health Plan

Managed Care Organization Profiles — ARKANSAS

KEY EXECUTIVES:

Non-Executive Chairman	Richard T Burke
Chief Executive Officer/President	Garland G Scott, III
Chief Financial Officer	Gary Charles Baker
Chief Medical Officer	Tunde Sotunde, MD
Pharmacy Director	Glenn Belemjian
Chief Information Officer	Glenn Walsh
Chief Operating Officer	Kilo Hau
Marketing Director	David T Johnson
Public Relations Director	Robert Waibel
Network/Contracts Director	Clay Bittner
Human Resources Director	James Collier
Medical Management Director	Debra Bates
Quality Assurance Director	Teresa Hill
Director of Fraud Prevention	Kristina Friberg
Director of Medicare	Lisa Lyons
Director of Operations	Kathy Jacobson

COMPANY PROFILE:
Parent Company Name: UnitedHealth Group
Doing Business As:
Year Founded: 1990　　Federally Qualified: [N]
Forprofit: [Y]　　Not-For-Profit: [ ]
Model Type: IPA
Accreditation: [ ] AAPPO [ ] JACHO [ ] NCQA [ ] URAC
Plan Type: HMO, PPO, POS, CDHP, HSA, HRA
Total Revenue　　2005: 49,153,822　　2006: 30,660,236
Net Income　　2005: 4,068,046　　2006: 3,969,188
Total Enrollment:
　　2001: 60,401　　2004: 17,859　　2007: 6,274
　　2002: 57,353　　2005:
　　2003: 37,072　　2006: 6,720
Medical Loss Ratio:　　2005:　　2006: 66.10
Administrative Expense Ratio: 2005:　　2006:

SERVICE AREA:
Nationwide: N
　　AR (Ashley, Benton, Bradley, Chicot, Cleburne, Cleveland, Columbia, Conway, Craighead, Crawford, Crittenden, Cross, Desha, Drew, Faulkner, Franklin, Garland, Grant, Hempstead, Hot Springs, Howard, Jefferson, Lincoln, Little River, Logan, Lonoke, Madison, Miller, Montgomery, Ouachita, Perry, Pike, Polk, Pope, Prairie, Pulaski; Saline, Scott, Sebastian, Sevier, Washington, White, Woodruff);

TYPE OF COVERAGE:
Commercial: [Y]　Individual: [ ]　FEHBP: [ ]　Indemnity: [ ]
Medicare: [Y]　Medicaid: [ ]　Supplemental Medicare: [ ]
Tricare [ ]

PRODUCTS OFFERED:

Product Name:	Type:
United HealthCare Select HMO	HMO
United HealthCare Select Plus	HMO + POS
United HealthCare Choice	HMO
United HealthCare Choice Plus	HMO
Preferred Provider Organizatio	PPO
Medicare Complete	Medicare

CONSUMER-DRIVEN PRODUCTS

Exante Bank/Golden Rule Ins Co	HSA Company
iPlan HSA	HSA Product
	HSA Administrator
	Consumer-Driven Health Plan
	High Deductible Health Plan

PLAN BENEFITS:

Alternative Medicine:	[ ]	Behavioral Health:	[X]
Chiropractic:	[X]	Dental:	[X]
Home Care:	[X]	Inpatient SNF:	[X]
Long-Term Care:	[ ]	Pharm. Mail Order:	[X]
Physical Therapy:	[X]	Podiatry:	[X]
Psychiatric:	[X]	Transplant:	[X]
Vision:	[X]	Wellness:	[X]
Workers' Comp:	[ ]		

Other Benefits:
Comments:
Formerly Complete Health of Arkansas.

ARKANSAS

KEY EXECUTIVES:
Chairman of the Board .... David A Jones Jr
Chief Executive Officer/President .... Michael B McCallister
Chief Financial Officer .... James H Bloem
Medical Director .... Lisa Weaver, MD
Chief Information Officer .... Bruce J Goodman
Senior VP, Human Resources .... Bonnie C Hathcock

COMPANY PROFILE:
Parent Company Name: Humana Inc
Doing Business As:
Year Founded: 1961   Federally Qualified: [Y]
Forprofit: [Y]   Not-For-Profit: [ ]
Model Type: IPA
Accreditation: [ ] AAPPO [ ] JACHO [ ] NCQA [ ] URAC
Plan Type: PPO, Specialty HMO, POS, ASO, EPO, CDHP, HDHP, HSA

SERVICE AREA:
Nationwide: N
  AR;

TYPE OF COVERAGE:
Commercial: [Y] Individual: [Y] FEHBP: [ ] Indemnity: [ ]
Medicare: [ ] Medicaid: [ ] Supplemental Medicare: [ ]
Tricare   [ ]

PRODUCTS OFFERED:
Product Name:	Type:
Humana PPO	PPO
Humana Dental	Specialty HMO

CONSUMER-DRIVEN PRODUCTS
JP Morgan Chase	HSA Company HumanaOne
HSA	HSA Product
JP Morgan Chase	HSA Administrator
Personal Care Account	Consumer-Driven Health Plan
HumanaOne	High Deductible Health Plan

PLAN BENEFITS:
Alternative Medicine:	[ ]	Behavioral Health:	[X]
Chiropractic:	[X]	Dental:	[X]
Home Care:	[ ]	Inpatient SNF:	[ ]
Long-Term Care:	[ ]	Pharm. Mail Order:	[X]
Physical Therapy:	[ ]	Podiatry:	[ ]
Psychiatric:	[X]	Transplant:	[X]
Vision:	[ ]	Wellness:	[ ]
Workers' Comp:	[X]		

Other Benefits: Long Term Disability Care

NOVASYS HEALTH NETWORK

10801 Executive Center Dr #305
Little Rock, AR 72211
Phone: 501-219-4444 Fax: 501-219-4455 Toll-Free:
Web site: www.novasyshealth.com

MAILING ADDRESS:
NOVASYS HEALTH NETWORK
PO Box 25230
Little Rock, AR 72211

KEY EXECUTIVES:
Chief Executive Officer .... John Glassford
Chief Financial Officer .... Kim Suggs
Medical Director Officer .... Roland Anderson, MD
Marketing Director .... Dwane Tankersley
VP, Information Technology .... Scott Shellabarger

COMPANY PROFILE:
Parent Company Name:
Doing Business As:
Year Founded: Federally Qualified: [ ]
Forprofit: [Y]   Not-For-Profit: [ ]
Model Type:
Accreditation: [ ] AAPPO [ ] JACHO [ ] NCQA [ ] URAC
Plan Type: PPO, CDHP, HDHP, HSA
Total Enrollment:
  2001: 36,589   2004: 56,000   2007: 0
  2002: 0   2005: 56,000
  2003: 60,000   2006:

SERVICE AREA:
Nationwide: N
  AR;

CONSUMER-DRIVEN PRODUCTS
Arkansashsa	HSA Company
NovaSys HSA PPO	HSA Product
	HSA Administrator
	Consumer-Driven Health Plan
	High Deductible Health Plan

QCA HEALTH PLAN INC

10825 Financial Centre Pky 400
Little Rock, AR 72211
Phone: 501-228-7111 Fax: 501-801-2959 Toll-Free:
Web site: www.qcark.com

MAILING ADDRESS:
QCA HEALTH PLAN INC
10825 Financial Centre Pky 400
Little Rock, AR 72211

KEY EXECUTIVES:
Chief Executive Officer/President .... Francis L Browning
Chief Financial Officer .... Michael E Stock
Medical Vice President .... Roger K Howe, MD, MMM
Chief Information Officer .... M Haley Wilson
Chief Operating Officer .... Michael E Stock
Network Development Director .... Rose Anne Catol
Vice President, Operations .... Joni S Daniels
Controller .... Randall Crow
Director of Underwriting .... Kenneth W Bowen, Jr

COMPANY PROFILE:
Parent Company Name:
Doing Business As: Qualchoice of Arkansas
Year Founded: 1996   Federally Qualified: [N]
Forprofit: [Y]   Not-For-Profit: [ ]
Model Type:
Accreditation: [ ] AAPPO [ ] JACHO [ ] NCQA [ ] URAC
Plan Type: HMO, POS, HDHP, HSA
Total Revenue: 2005: 60,478,211   2006: 60,478,211
Net Income   2005: 11,391,854   2006: 1,139,185
Total Enrollment:
  2001: 67,118   2004: 20,867   2007: 18,658
  2002: 33,686   2005: 22,201
  2003: 20,228   2006: 19,703
Medical Loss Ratio: 2005: 86.00   2006:
Administrative Expense Ratio: 2005:   2006:

SERVICE AREA:
Nationwide: N
  AR (Arkansas, Ashley, Baxter, Benton, Boone, Bradley, Calhoun, Carroll, Chicot, Clark, Clay, Cleburne, Cleveland, Columbia, Conway, Craighead, Crawford, Crittenden, Cross, Dallas, Desha, Drew, Faulkner, Franklin, Fulton, Garland, Grant, Greene, Hempstead, Hot Springs, Howard, Independence, Izard, Jackson, Jefferson, Johnson, Lafayette, Lawrence, Lee, Lincoln, Little River, Logan, Lonoke, Madison, Marion, Miller, Mississippi, Monroe, Montgomery, Nevada, Newton, Ouachita, Perry, Phillips, Pike, Poinsett, Polk, Pope, Prairie, Pulaski, Randolph, Saint Francis, Saline, Scott, Searcy, Sebastian, Sevier, Sharp, Stone, Union, Van Buren, Washington, White, Woodruff, Yell);

TYPE OF COVERAGE:
Commercial: [Y] Individual: [ ] FEHBP: [ ] Indemnity: [ ]
Medicare: [ ] Medicaid: [ ] Supplemental Medicare: [ ]
Tricare   [ ]

PRODUCTS OFFERED:
Product Name:	Type:
QCA Health Plan Inc	HMO
QCA Health Plan Inc	POS

CONSUMER-DRIVEN PRODUCTS
	HSA Company
	HSA Product
	HSA Administrator
	Consumer-Driven Health Plan
RightChoice	High Deductible Health Plan

UNITEDHEALTHCARE OF ARKANSAS

415 North McKinley Ste 300
Little Rock, AR 72205-3021
Phone: 501-664-7700 Fax: 501-664-7768 Toll-Free: 800-678-3176
Web site: www.uhc.com

MAILING ADDRESS:
UNITEDHEALTHCARE OF ARKANSAS
415 North McKinley Ste 300
Little Rock, AR 72205-3021

Managed Care Organization Profiles — ARKANSAS

COMPANY PROFILE:
Parent Company Name: Delta Dental Plan Association
Doing Business As:
Year Founded: 1982   Federally Qualified: [ ]
Forprofit: [Y]   Not-For-Profit: [ ]
Model Type:
Accreditation: [ ] AAPPO [ ] JACHO [ ] NCQA [ ] URAC
Plan Type: Specialty HMO, Specialty PPO
Total Revenue: 2005: 56,904,348   2006: 59,061,656
Net Income   2005: 4,055,117   2006: 6,692,773
Total Enrollment:
   2001: 92,759   2004: 120,280   2007: 125,524
   2002: 104,766   2005: 122,776
   2003: 114,202   2006: 122,776
Medical Loss Ratio: 2005: 78.90   2006:
Administrative Expense Ratio: 2005:   2006:

SERVICE AREA:
Nationwide: N
   AR;

TYPE OF COVERAGE:
Commercial: [Y] Individual: [ ] FEHBP: [ ] Indemnity: [ ]
Medicare: [ ] Medicaid: [ ] Supplemental Medicare: [ ]
Tricare   [ ]

PRODUCTS OFFERED:
Product Name: Type:
Delta Dental of AR   Specialty HMO

PLAN BENEFITS:
Alternative Medicine: [ ]   Behavioral Health: [ ]
Chiropractic: [ ]   Dental: [X]
Home Care: [ ]   Inpatient SNF: [ ]
Long-Term Care: [ ]   Pharm. Mail Order: [ ]
Physical Therapy: [ ]   Podiatry: [ ]
Psychiatric: [ ]   Transplant: [ ]
Vision: [ ]   Wellness: [ ]
Workers' Comp: [ ]
Other Benefits:

HEALTH ADVANTAGE

320 W Capitol Ste 900
Little Rock, AR 72201
Phone: 501-379-4600 Fax: 501-379-4659 Toll-Free: 800-843-1329
Web site: www.healthadvantage-hmo.com

MAILING ADDRESS:
   HEALTH ADVANTAGE
   320 W Capitol Ste 900
   Little Rock, AR 72201

KEY EXECUTIVES:
Chief Executive Officer/President .... David Frank Bridges
VP,Chief Financial Officer .... Steve Short
Medical Director .... Clement Fox, MD
Pharmacy Director .... Norman Canterbury
VP, Marketing .... Jim Bailey
MIS Director .... Kathy Ryan
Human Resources Director .... Richard Cooper
Regional Executive .... Jim Bailey

COMPANY PROFILE:
Parent Company Name: USABLE Corporation & Baptist Health HMO
Doing Business As: HMO Partners Inc
Year Founded: 1985   Federally Qualified: [Y]
Forprofit: [Y]   Not-For-Profit: [ ]
Model Type: IPA
Accreditation: [ ] AAPPO [ ] JACHO [ ] NCQA [X] URAC
Plan Type: HMO
Primary Physicians: 6,000   Physician Specialists:
Hospitals:
Total Revenue: 2005: 113,372,429   2006: 89,579,403
Net Income   2005: 9,128,177   2006: 9,747,146
Total Enrollment:
   2001: 0   2004: 140,000   2007: 0
   2002: 131,172 2005: 150,000
   2003: 138,463 2006: 150,000

SERVICE AREA:
Nationwide: N
   AR;

TYPE OF COVERAGE:
Commercial: [Y] Individual: [ ] FEHBP: [ ] Indemnity: [ ]
Medicare: [Y] Medicaid: [ ] Supplemental Medicare: [ ]
Tricare   [ ]

PRODUCTS OFFERED:
Product Name: Type:
Bluechoice POS   POS
HMO   Health Advantage HMO
Medipak HMO   Med Risk

PLAN BENEFITS:
Alternative Medicine: [ ]   Behavioral Health: [ ]
Chiropractic: [X]   Dental: [X]
Home Care: [X]   Inpatient SNF: [X]
Long-Term Care: [ ]   Pharm. Mail Order: [ ]
Physical Therapy: [X]   Podiatry: [X]
Psychiatric: [X]   Transplant: [X]
Vision: [X]   Wellness: [X]
Workers' Comp: [ ]
Other Benefits:

HEALTHLINK OF ARKANSAS INC

3901 McCain Park Dr Ste 201
North Little Rock, AR 72116
Phone: 501-771-2111 Fax: 501-771-1936 Toll-Free:
Web site: www.healthlink.com

MAILING ADDRESS:
   HEALTHLINK OF ARKANSAS INC
   3901 McCain Park Dr Ste 201
   North Little Rock, AR 72116

KEY EXECUTIVES:
Executive Director .... Brett Kirkman
Chief Financial Officer/VP, Marketing .... Courtney B Walter
Chief Medical Officer .... Dale Stegamen, MD
Senior VP, Network Management .... Bruce Gosser

COMPANY PROFILE:
Parent Company Name: HealthLink Inc
Doing Business As: HealthLink HMO, HealthLink PPO
Year Founded: 1985   Federally Qualified: [N]
Forprofit: [Y]   Not-For-Profit: [ ]
Model Type: MIXED
Accreditation: [ ] AAPPO [ ] JACHO [ ] NCQA [ ] URAC
Plan Type: HMO, PPO
Total Enrollment:
   2001: 0   2004: 15,076   2007: 2,751
   2002: 0   2005: 10,219
   2003: 24,525   2006: 3,020

SERVICE AREA:
Nationwide: N
   AR (Benton, Carroll, Craighead, Crawford, Garland, Independence, Jackson, Logan, Pulaski, Randolph, Saline, Sebastian, Sharp, Washington, White);

TYPE OF COVERAGE:
Commercial: [Y] Individual: [Y] FEHBP: [ ] Indemnity: [ ]
Medicare: [ ] Medicaid: [ ] Supplemental Medicare: [ ]
Tricare   [ ]

PRODUCTS OFFERED:
Product Name: Type:
HealthLink HMO   HMO
HealthLink PPO   PPO

PLAN BENEFITS:
Alternative Medicine: [ ]   Behavioral Health: [X]
Chiropractic: [ ]   Dental: [X]
Home Care: [ ]   Inpatient SNF: [X]
Long-Term Care: [ ]   Pharm. Mail Order: [X]
Physical Therapy: [X]   Podiatry: [X]
Psychiatric: [X]   Transplant: [ ]
Vision: [X]   Wellness: [X]
Workers' Comp: [ ]
Other Benefits:

HUMANA INC - ARKANSAS

500 W Main St
Louisville, KY 40201-1438
Phone: 502-580-1000 Fax: 502-580-4106 Toll-Free:
Web site: www.humana.com

MAILING ADDRESS:
   HUMANA INC - ARKANSAS
   500 W Main St
   Louisville, KY 40201-1438

ARKANSAS

CONSUMER-DRIVEN PRODUCTS

HSA Blue PPO

HSA Blue PPO Plus

HSA Company
HSA Product
HSA Administrator
Consumer-Driven Health Plan
High Deductible Health Plan

ARKANSAS COMMUNITY CARE INC

10025 W Markham St Ste 220
Little Rock, AR 72205
Phone: 201-223-9088 Fax: 510-817-1039 Toll-Free: 800-705-0766
Web site: www.arkansascommunitycare.com
MAILING ADDRESS:
ARKANSAS COMMUNITY CARE INC
10025 W Markham St Ste 220
Little Rock, AR 72205

KEY EXECUTIVES:
Chief Executive Officer/Chief Operating Officer ..... John H Austin, MD
President .... Nancy E Freeman
Chief Financial Officer .... Kenneth B Zimmerman

COMPANY PROFILE:
Parent Company Name: Arcadian Management Services Inc
Doing Business As:
Year Founded: 2005   Federally Qualified: [Y]
Forprofit: [ ]   Not-For-Profit: [ ]
Model Type:
Accreditation: [ ] AAPPO [ ] JACHO [ ] NCQA [ ] URAC
Plan Type: HMO
Total Revenue: 2005: 4,346,008   2006: 4,297,135
Net Income   2005:   -60,903   2006: -2,322,898
Total Enrollment:
  2001: 0   2004: 0   2007: 5,629
  2002: 0   2005:
  2003: 0   2006: 2,739
Medical Loss Ratio: 2005:   2006: 74.10
Administrative Expense Ratio: 2005:   2006:
SERVICE AREA:
Nationwide:
  AR (Central: Lonoke, Pulaski, Saline, White); (Northwest: Benton, Carroll, Madison, Washington);
TYPE OF COVERAGE:
Commercial: [ ] Individual: [ ]   FEHBP: [ ] Indemnity: [ ]
Medicare: [Y] Medicaid: [ ]   Supplemental Medicare: [ ]
Tricare   [ ]
PRODUCTS OFFERED:
Product Name: Type:
Arkansas Community Care   Medicare Advantage

ARKANSAS FOUNDATION FOR MEDICAL CARE

2201 Brooken Hill Dr
Ft Smith, AR 72901
Phone: 479-649-8501 Fax: 479-649-8180 Toll-Free:
Web site: www.afmc.org
MAILING ADDRESS:
ARKANSAS FNDTN FOR MED CARE
PO Box 180001
Ft Smith, AR 72901

KEY EXECUTIVES:
Chief Executive Officer/President .... Nick J Paslidis, MD, PhD, MHCM
Chief Financial Officer .... Larry Todd, CPA
Medical Director .... Michael Moody, MD
Compliance Officer .... Susie Moore

COMPANY PROFILE:
Parent Company Name:
Doing Business As:
Year Founded: 1972   Federally Qualified: [ ]
Forprofit: [ ]   Not-For-Profit: [Y]
Model Type:
Accreditation: [ ] AAPPO [ ] JACHO [ ] NCQA [ ] URAC
Plan Type: UR, PRO
Total Enrollment:
  2001: 0   2004: 0   2007: 1,200
  2002: 0   2005:
  2003: 0   2006:

SERVICE AREA:
Nationwide: N
  AR;

ARKANSAS MANAGED CARE ORGANIZATION

10 Corporate Hill Dr Ste 200
Little Rock, AR 72205
Phone: 501-225-8470 Fax: 501-225-7954 Toll-Free: 800-278-8470
Web site: www.amcppo.com
MAILING ADDRESS:
ARKANSAS MANAGED CARE ORG
10 Corporate Hill Dr Ste 200
Little Rock, AR 72205

KEY EXECUTIVES:
Chief Executive Officer/Marketing Director .... Johnna Thomas
MIS Director .... JoAnna Gist
Credentialing Manager/Provider Relations Director .... Phil Stowers
Network Development Director .... Johnna Thomas

COMPANY PROFILE:
Parent Company Name:
Doing Business As:
Year Founded: 1993   Federally Qualified: [ ]
Forprofit: [ ]   Not-For-Profit: [Y]
Model Type: NETWORK
Accreditation: [Y] AAPPO [ ] JACHO [ ] NCQA [ ] URAC
Plan Type: PPO
Primary Physicians: 5,000   Physician Specialists:
Hospitals: 100
Total Enrollment:
  2001: 175,000   2004: 200,000   2007: 200,000
  2002: 215,000   2005:
  2003: 200,000   2006: 200,000
SERVICE AREA:
Nationwide: N
  AR;
TYPE OF COVERAGE:
Commercial: [Y] Individual: [Y]   FEHBP: [ ] Indemnity: [ ]
Medicare: [ ] Medicaid: [ ]   Supplemental Medicare: [ ]
Tricare   [ ]
PRODUCTS OFFERED:
Product Name: Type:
Arkansas Managed Care Plan   PPO
PLAN BENEFITS:
Alternative Medicine: [ ]   Behavioral Health: [X]
Chiropractic: [X]   Dental: [ ]
Home Care: [X]   Inpatient SNF: [X]
Long-Term Care: [X]   Pharm. Mail Order: [ ]
Physical Therapy: [X]   Podiatry: [X]
Psychiatric: [X]   Transplant: [X]
Vision: [ ]   Wellness: [X]
Workers' Comp: [ ]
Other Benefits:
Comments:
Formerly Delta Health Alliance.

DELTA DENTAL PLAN OF ARKANSAS

1513 Country Club Rd
Sherwood, AR 72120
Phone: 501-835-3400 Fax: 501-834-6244 Toll-Free: 800-462-5410
Web site: www.deltadentalar.com
MAILING ADDRESS:
DELTA DENTAL PLAN OF AR
1513 Country Club Rd
Sherwood, AR 72120

KEY EXECUTIVES:
Chief Executive Officer/President .... Eddie A Choate
Chief Financial Officer .... Phyllis L Rogers
VP, Information Technology .... Allen Moore
Senior VP of Operations .... Lynn Harbert
VP, Sale & Marketing .... Timothy W Carney
VP, Provider Relations .... Herman E Hurd, MD
Executive Assistant .... Carla Rutherford

Managed Care Organization Profiles ARKANSAS

AETNA INC - ARKANSAS

10809 Executive Center Dr
Little Rock, AR 72211
Phone: 501-227-7776 Fax: 501-227-0581 Toll-Free: 800-821-8787
Web site: www.aetna.com
MAILING ADDRESS:
   AETNA INC - AR
   10809 Executive Center Dr
   Little Rock, AR 72211

KEY EXECUTIVES:
Chairman of the Board/Chief Executive Officer .... Ronald A Williams
Regional Manager-Southeast .... Joseph Blanford
Executive VP, Finance .... Joseph M Zubretsky
Chief Medical Officer .... Deborah Gosnell

COMPANY PROFILE:
Parent Company Name: Aetna Inc
Doing Business As:
Year Founded: 1986   Federally Qualified: [Y]
Forprofit: [Y]   Not-For-Profit: [ ]
Model Type: IPA
Accreditation: [ ] AAPPO [ ] JACHO [X] NCQA [ ] URAC
Plan Type: PPO, UR, POS, PRO, CDHP, HSA
SERVICE AREA:
Nationwide: N
   AR (Benton, Carroll, Craighead, Crawford, Crittenden, Faulkner,
   Independence, Jefferson, Logan, Lonoke, Madison, Pulaski, Saline,
   Sebastian, Washington, White);
TYPE OF COVERAGE:
Commercial: [Y] Individual: [ ] FEHBP: [ ] Indemnity: [ ]
Medicare: [ ] Medicaid: [ ] Supplemental Medicare: [ ]
Tricare   [ ]
PRODUCTS OFFERED:
Product Name: Type:
Aetna/Prudential HMO   HMO
CONSUMER-DRIVEN PRODUCTS
Aetna Life Insurance Co   HSA Company
Aetna HealthFund HSA   HSA Product
Aetna   HSA Administrator
Aetna HealthFund   Consumer-Driven Health Plan
PPO I; PPO II   High Deductible Health Plan
PLAN BENEFITS:
Alternative Medicine: [ ]   Behavioral Health: [X]
Chiropractic: [X]   Dental: [X]
Home Care: [X]   Inpatient SNF: [X]
Long-Term Care: [X]   Pharm. Mail Order: [ ]
Physical Therapy: [X]   Podiatry: [X]
Psychiatric: [X]   Transplant: [X]
Vision: [X]   Wellness: [X]
Workers' Comp: [X]
Other Benefits:
Comments:
Formerly Prudential Healthcare of Arkansas.

AETNA INC - ARKANSAS

3900 N Causeway Blvd Ste 410
Metairie, LA 70002
Phone: 504-830-5600 Fax: 504-837-6571 Toll-Free:
Web site: www.aetna.com
MAILING ADDRESS:
   AETNA INC - AR
   3900 N Causeway Blvd Ste 410
   Metairie, LA 70002

KEY EXECUTIVES:
Chairman of the Board/Chief Executive Officer .... Ronald A Williams
Regional Manager-Southeast .... Joseph Blanford
Executive VP, Finance .... Joseph M Zubretsky
Marketing Director .... David Rosenfeld
Executive Director(LA Region) .... Dean Hovencamp

COMPANY PROFILE:
Parent Company Name: Aetna Inc
Doing Business As:
Year Founded: Federally Qualified: [ ]
Forprofit: [Y]   Not-For-Profit: [ ]
Model Type:
Accreditation: [ ] AAPPO [ ] JACHO [ ] NCQA [ ] URAC
Plan Type: PPO, POS, CDHP, HSA

SERVICE AREA:
Nationwide: N
   AR (Central and Northern);
TYPE OF COVERAGE:
Commercial: [Y] Individual: [ ] FEHBP: [ ] Indemnity: [ ]
Medicare: [ ] Medicaid: [ ] Supplemental Medicare: [ ]
Tricare   [ ]
PRODUCTS OFFERED:
Product Name: Type:
Aetna US Hlthcare Golden Medic   Medicare
CONSUMER-DRIVEN PRODUCTS
Aetna Life Insurance Co   HSA Company
Aetna HealthFund HSA   HSA Product
Aetna   HSA Administrator
Aetna HealthFund   Consumer-Driven Health Plan
PPO I; PPO II   High Deductible Health Plan
PLAN BENEFITS:
Alternative Medicine: [ ]   Behavioral Health: [ ]
Chiropractic: [X]   Dental: [X]
Home Care: [X]   Inpatient SNF: [X]
Long-Term Care: [X]   Pharm. Mail Order: [X]
Physical Therapy: [X]   Podiatry: [X]
Psychiatric: [X]   Transplant: [X]
Vision: [X]   Wellness: [X]
Workers' Comp: [ ]
Other Benefits:

ARKANSAS BLUE CROSS/BLUE SHIELD A MUTUAL INSURANCE COMPANY

601 S Gaines St
Little Rock, AR 72201-2181
Phone: 501-378-2000 Fax: 501-378-3732 Toll-Free:
Web site: www.arkansasbluecross.com
MAILING ADDRESS:
   ARKANSAS BC/BS A MUTUAL INSURANCE CO
   PO Box 2181
   Little Rock, AR 72201-2181

KEY EXECUTIVES:
Chairman of the Board .... Hayes C McClerkin
Chief Executive Officer .... Robert L Shoptaw
President .... Sharon Allen
Executive VP,Chief Financial Officer .... Mark White
VP, Medical Director .... James Adamson, MD
Pharmacy Director .... Norman Canterbury
VP &Chief Information Officer .... Joseph Smith
Chief Operating Officer .... Sharon Allen
VP/Advertising & Communication .... Patrick O'Sullivan
Human Resources Director .... Richard Cooper
News Media Contact .... Max Heuer

COMPANY PROFILE:
Parent Company Name:
Doing Business As:
Year Founded: 1948   Federally Qualified: [N]
Forprofit: [ ]   Not-For-Profit: [Y]
Model Type: NETWORK
Accreditation: [ ] AAPPO [ ] JACHO [ ] NCQA [ ] URAC
Plan Type: PPO, UR, POS, CDHP, HDHP, HSA
Total Revenue: 2005: 905,658,277   2006: 951,121,311
Net Income   2005: 51,554,601   2006: 43,239,910
Total Enrollment:
   2001: 454,397   2004: 398,000   2007: 415,799
   2002: 393,923   2005: 407,061
   2003: 396,293   2006: 425,159
Medical Loss Ratio: 2005: 78.90   2006: 80.30
Administrative Expense Ratio: 2005:   2006:
SERVICE AREA:
Nationwide: N
   AR;
TYPE OF COVERAGE:
Commercial: [Y] Individual: [Y] FEHBP: [ ] Indemnity: [ ]
Medicare: [Y] Medicaid: [ ] Supplemental Medicare: [Y]
Tricare   [ ]
PRODUCTS OFFERED:
Product Name: Type:
Blue Choice POS   POS
Health Advantage HMO   HMO
Medipak HMO   Medicare

Managed Care Organization Profiles — ARIZONA

SERVICE AREA:
Nationwide: N
   AZ;

TYPE OF COVERAGE:
Commercial: [Y] Individual: [ ] FEHBP: [ ] Indemnity: [ ]
Medicare: [ ] Medicaid: [ ] Supplemental Medicare: [ ]
Tricare   [ ]

PLAN BENEFITS:
Alternative Medicine: [ ]   Behavioral Health: [ ]
Chiropractic: [ ]   Dental: [ ]
Home Care: [ ]   Inpatient SNF: [ ]
Long-Term Care: [ ]   Pharm. Mail Order: [ ]
Physical Therapy: [ ]   Podiatry: [ ]
Psychiatric: [ ]   Transplant: [ ]
Vision: [X]   Wellness: [ ]
Workers' Comp: [ ]
Other Benefits:

ARIZONA — **Managed Care Organization Profiles**

PLAN BENEFITS:
Alternative Medicine:	[ ]	Behavioral Health:	[ ]
Chiropractic:	[X]	Dental:	[X]
Home Care:	[X]	Inpatient SNF:	[X]
Long-Term Care:	[ ]	Pharm. Mail Order:	[X]
Physical Therapy:	[X]	Podiatry:	[X]
Psychiatric:	[X]	Transplant:	[X]
Vision:	[X]	Wellness:	[X]
Workers' Comp:	[ ]		
Other Benefits:			

UNIVERSITY FAMILY CARE HEALTH PLAN

2701 East Elvira Rd
Tucson, AZ 85706
Phone: 520-874-3500 Fax: 520-874-3484 Toll-Free:
Web site: www.ufcaz.com

MAILING ADDRESS:
UNIVERSITY FAMILY CARE HLTH PL
2701 East Elvira Rd
Tucson, AZ 85706

KEY EXECUTIVES:
Chief Executive Officer .... Kathy Oestriech
Chief Financial Officer .... Jody Butera
Medical Director .... William Martz, MD
Director, Planning Develop .... Mark Hillard
MIS Director .... Kathy Steiner
Credentialing Manager .... Lisa Frank
Network Development Director .... James Stover
Quality Management Manager .... Karen Geoghan
Claims Director .... Jean Wagner

COMPANY PROFILE:
Parent Company Name: University Physicians Health Plans
Doing Business As:
Year Founded: 1987   Federally Qualified: [ ]
Forprofit: [ ]   Not-For-Profit: [Y]
Model Type:
Accreditation: [ ] AAPPO [ ] JACHO [ ] NCQA [ ] URAC
Plan Type: HMO, ASO
Total Enrollment:
    2001: 15,698   2004: 15,527   2007: 7,581
    2002: 0   2005: 19,000
    2003: 0   2006: 9,800

SERVICE AREA:
Nationwide: N
AZ (Cochise, Graham, Greenlee, Pima, Pinal, Maricopa, Santa Cruz);

TYPE OF COVERAGE:
Commercial: [ ] Individual: [ ] FEHBP: [ ] Indemnity: [ ]
Medicare: [ ]   Medicaid: [Y]   Supplemental Medicare: [ ]
Tricare [ ]

PRODUCTS OFFERED:
Product Name:	Type:
University Family Care	Medicaid
University Family Care	Family Planning Ext

PLAN BENEFITS:
Alternative Medicine:	[ ]	Behavioral Health:	[X]
Chiropractic:	[X]	Dental:	[X]
Home Care:	[X]	Inpatient SNF:	[X]
Long-Term Care:	[ ]	Pharm. Mail Order:	[X]
Physical Therapy:	[X]	Podiatry:	[X]
Psychiatric:	[X]	Transplant:	[X]
Vision:	[X]	Wellness:	[X]
Workers' Comp:	[ ]		
Other Benefits:			

USA MANAGED CARE ORGANIZATION

7301 N 16th Street Ste 201
Phoenix, AZ 85020
Phone: 602-371-3880 Fax: 602-371-3889 Toll-Free: 800-872-0820
Web site: www.usamco.com

MAILING ADDRESS:
USA MANAGED CARE ORGANIZATION
7301 N 16th Street Ste 201
Phoenix, AZ 85020

KEY EXECUTIVES:
Chief Executive Officer .... George Bogle
Chief Financial Officer .... Dick Weinberger
Medical Director .... James Gerace
Chief Operating Officer .... Mike Bogle
Vice President of Sales .... Sean Dee Graff
Chief of Staff .... Donna Smith
Network Administration VP .... Tameria Scott

COMPANY PROFILE:
Parent Company Name: USA Managed Care Org Inc
Doing Business As: USA H & W Network
Year Founded: 1984   Federally Qualified: [ ]
Forprofit: [Y]   Not-For-Profit: [ ]
Model Type: MIXED
Accreditation: [ ] AAPPO [X] JACHO [ ] NCQA [ ] URAC
Plan Type: PPO, UR, EPO
Total Enrollment:
    2001: 5,200,658   2004: 0   2007: 0
    2002: 0   2005:
    2003: 0   2006:

SERVICE AREA:
Nationwide: N
AK; AL; AZ; CA; CO; CT; DC; DE; FL; GA; HI; LA; ID; IL; IN; KS; KY; LA; MA MD; MI; MN; MO; MS; NC; NE; NH; NJ; NM; NV; NY; OH; OK; OR; PA; RI; SC; TN; TX; UT; VA; WA; WI; WV;

TYPE OF COVERAGE:
Commercial: [Y] Individual: [ ] FEHBP: [ ] Indemnity: [ ]
Medicare: [ ]   Medicaid: [ ]   Supplemental Medicare: [ ]
Tricare [ ]

PRODUCTS OFFERED:
Product Name:	Type:
USA Workers Injury Network	Workers Comp PPO
USA Select Provider Accountabl	PPO
USA Genesis	Behavioral Health
USA Medicare Select	Medicare
National Utilization Managemen	UR
Footloose	Podiatric Network

PLAN BENEFITS:
Alternative Medicine:	[ ]	Behavioral Health:	[X]
Chiropractic:	[X]	Dental:	[ ]
Home Care:	[X]	Inpatient SNF:	[ ]
Long-Term Care:	[X]	Pharm. Mail Order:	[ ]
Physical Therapy:	[ ]	Podiatry:	[X]
Psychiatric:	[X]	Transplant:	[X]
Vision:	[X]	Wellness:	[X]
Workers' Comp:	[X]		
Other Benefits:			

VISION SERVICE PLAN OF ARIZONA

2111 E Highland Ave Ste B160
Phoenix, AZ 85016
Phone: 602-956-1820 Fax: 602-956-3679 Toll-Free: 800-821-8130
Web site: www.vsp.com

MAILING ADDRESS:
VISION SERVICE PLAN OF AZ
2111 E Highland Ave Ste B160
Phoenix, AZ 85016

KEY EXECUTIVES:
Chief Executive Officer .... Roger Valine
Chief Financial Director .... Patricia Cochran
Senior VP of Operations .... Gary Brooks
Senior VP of Marketing .... Don Yee
VP of Sales .... Richard W Steere
VP of Provider Relations .... Don Price
VP of Human Resources .... Walter Grubbs

COMPANY PROFILE:
Parent Company Name:
Doing Business As:
Year Founded: Federally Qualified: [ ]
Forprofit: [ ]   Not-For-Profit: [Y]
Model Type:
Accreditation: [ ] AAPPO [ ] JACHO [ ] NCQA [ ] URAC
Plan Type: Specialty HMO
Total Enrollment:
    2001: 11,872,015 2004: 7,256,286 2007: 0
    2002: 12,238,845 2005:
    2003: 11,021,559 2006:

Managed Care Organization Profiles — ARIZONA

TYPE OF COVERAGE:
Commercial: [ ] Individual: [Y] FEHBP: [ ] Indemnity: [ ]
Medicare: [ ] Medicaid: [ ] Supplemental Medicare: [Y]
Tricare [ ]
PRODUCTS OFFERED:
Product Name: Type:
Sun Health Medisun Inc   Medicare Advantage
PLAN BENEFITS:
Alternative Medicine: [ ]   Behavioral Health: [ ]
Chiropractic: [ ]   Dental: [ ]
Home Care: [X]   Inpatient SNF: [X]
Long-Term Care: [X]   Pharm. Mail Order: [ ]
Physical Therapy: [X]   Podiatry: [X]
Psychiatric: [ ]   Transplant: [ ]
Vision: [ ]   Wellness: [ ]
Workers' Comp: [ ]
Other Benefits:
Comments:
Formerly Medisun.

TOTAL DENTAL ADMINISTRATORS HEALTH PLAN

2111 E Highland Ave Ste B-425
Phoenix, AZ 85016-4735
Phone: 602-266-1995 Fax: 602-266-1948 Toll-Free: 888-422-1995
Web site: www.totaldentaladmin.com
MAILING ADDRESS:
   TOTAL DENTAL ADMN HEALTH PLAN
   2111 E Highland Ave Ste B-425
   Phoenix, AZ 85016-4735

KEY EXECUTIVES:
Chief Executive Officer/President .... Christopher A Jehle
Dental Director .... Donald J Peterson, DDS
Chief Operating Officer .... Scott E Clark
Marketing Director .... Paulette Gaffney
Director of Human Resources .... Kathy Armijo

COMPANY PROFILE:
Parent Company Name:
Doing Business As:
Year Founded: 1997   Federally Qualified: [ ]
Forprofit: [Y]   Not-For-Profit: [ ]
Model Type: IPA
Accreditation: [ ] AAPPO [ ] JACHO [ ] NCQA [ ] URAC
Plan Type: Specialty HMO, Specialty PPO, ASO, TPA
Total Enrollment:
   2001: 13,125   2004: 14,258   2007: 0
   2002: 12,299   2005: 22,309
   2003: 10,999   2006:
SERVICE AREA:
Nationwide: N
   AZ (Maricopa, Pima);
TYPE OF COVERAGE:
Commercial: [Y] Individual: [ ] FEHBP: [ ] Indemnity: [ ]
Medicare: [ ] Medicaid: [ ] Supplemental Medicare: [ ]
Tricare [ ]
PRODUCTS OFFERED:
Product Name: Type:
Total Dental Administrators   Specialty HMO
PLAN BENEFITS:
Alternative Medicine: [ ]   Behavioral Health: [ ]
Chiropractic: [ ]   Dental: [X]
Home Care: [ ]   Inpatient SNF: [ ]
Long-Term Care: [ ]   Pharm. Mail Order: [ ]
Physical Therapy: [ ]   Podiatry: [ ]
Psychiatric: [ ]   Transplant: [ ]
Vision: [ ]   Wellness: [ ]
Workers' Comp: [ ]
Other Benefits:

UNITED CONCORDIA COMPANY INC - ARIZONA

2198 Camelback Rd Ste 220
Phoenix, AZ 85016
Phone: 717-260-7500 Fax: 602-957-6686 Toll-Free: 800-998-8224
Web site: www.ucci.com
MAILING ADDRESS:
   UNITED CONCORDIA CO INC - AZ
   2198 Camelback Rd Ste 220
   Phoenix, AZ 85016

KEY EXECUTIVES:
Chief Executive Officer .... Thomas A Dzuryachko
Senior VP, Finance .... Daniel Wright
Dental Director .... Mark Schulman, DDS
Vice President, Sales & Marketing .... Nate Kleinburg
MIS Director .... Jim Robins
Director, Provider Services .... Claude Padgett, DDS
Human Resources Director .... Harlon Robinson

COMPANY PROFILE:
Parent Company Name: Highmark Inc
Doing Business As:
Year Founded: 1997   Federally Qualified: [N]
Forprofit: [Y]   Not-For-Profit: [ ]
Model Type:
Accreditation: [ ] AAPPO [ ] JACHO [ ] NCQA [ ] URAC
Plan Type: Specialty HMO, Specialty PPO, POS, TPA
Total Enrollment:
   2001: 1,175   2004: 1,096   2007: 0
   2002: 1,207   2005: 1,005
   2003: 1,048   2006:
SERVICE AREA:
Nationwide: N
   AZ; CO; HI; NV; NM; UT;
TYPE OF COVERAGE:
Commercial: [Y] Individual: [ ] FEHBP: [ ] Indemnity: [ ]
Medicare: [ ] Medicaid: [ ] Supplemental Medicare: [ ]
Tricare [ ]
PLAN BENEFITS:
Alternative Medicine: [ ]   Behavioral Health: [ ]
Chiropractic: [ ]   Dental: [X]
Home Care: [ ]   Inpatient SNF: [ ]
Long-Term Care: [ ]   Pharm. Mail Order: [ ]
Physical Therapy: [ ]   Podiatry: [ ]
Psychiatric: [ ]   Transplant: [ ]
Vision: [ ]   Wellness: [ ]
Workers' Comp: [ ]
Other Benefits:

UNITEDHEALTHCARE OF ARIZONA INC

2390 E Camelback Ste 300
Phoenix, AZ 85016
Phone: 602-244-2707 Fax: 602-651-6002 Toll-Free: 888-574-5628
Web site: www.unitedhealthcare.com
MAILING ADDRESS:
   UNITEDHEALTHCARE OF ARIZONA
   2390 E Camelback Ste 300
   Phoenix, AZ 85016

KEY EXECUTIVES:
Non-Executive Chairman .... Richard T Burke
Chief Executive Officer .... Benton Davis
Executive Director .... John Benn
Medical Director .... Robert Beauchamp, MD
Director, Provider Services .... Linda Collins

COMPANY PROFILE:
Parent Company Name: UnitedHealth Group
Doing Business As: AmeriChoice, Arizona Physicians IPA
Year Founded: 1986   Federally Qualified: [Y]
Forprofit: [Y]   Not-For-Profit: [ ]
Model Type: NETWORK
Accreditation: [ ] AAPPO [X] JACHO [ ] NCQA [ ] URAC
Plan Type: HMO, PPO, POS, TPA, CDHP, HSA, HRA
Total Enrollment:
   2001: 178,764   2004: 25,556   2007: 97,844
   2002: 138,097   2005:
   2003: 36,097   2006:
SERVICE AREA:
Nationwide: N
   AZ; NV;
TYPE OF COVERAGE:
Commercial: [Y] Individual: [Y] FEHBP: [ ] Indemnity: [ ]
Medicare: [ ] Medicaid: [ ] Supplemental Medicare: [ ]
Tricare [ ]
CONSUMER-DRIVEN PRODUCTS
Exante Bank/Golden Rule Ins Co   HSA Company
iPlan HSA   HSA Product
                                    HSA Administrator
                                    Consumer-Driven Health Plan
                                    High Deductible Health Plan

ARIZONA

MAILING ADDRESS:
PREFERRED THERAPY PROVIDERS
19820 N 7th St Ste 250
Phoenix, AZ 85024

KEY EXECUTIVES:
Chief Executive Officer/President .... Jaxene Hillebert
Director of Operations & Marketing .... Dan Sarria
Credentialing Coordinator .... Pam Carlton
Provider Relations Coordinator .... Shawna Lawrence
Credentialing Coordinator .... Pam Carlton
Vice President .... Christy Beauchamp

COMPANY PROFILE:
Parent Company Name: Preferred Therapy Providers, Inc
Doing Business As: Preferred Therapy Providers
Year Founded: 1992   Federally Qualified: [ ]
Forprofit: [Y]   Not-For-Profit: [ ]
Model Type: NETWORK
Accreditation: [X] AAPPO [ ] JACHO [ ] NCQA [ ] URAC
Plan Type: Specialty PPO
Total Enrollment:
   2001: 60,000,000   2004: 0   2007: 0
   2002: 0   2005:
   2003: 60,000,000   2006: 60,000,000

SERVICE AREA:
Nationwide: Y
  NW;

TYPE OF COVERAGE:
Commercial: [Y] Individual: [ ] FEHBP: [ ] Indemnity: [ ]
Medicare: [ ] Medicaid: [ ] Supplemental Medicare: [ ]
Tricare

PLAN BENEFITS:
Alternative Medicine: [ ]   Behavioral Health: [ ]
Chiropractic: [ ]   Dental: [ ]
Home Care: [ ]   Inpatient SNF: [ ]
Long-Term Care: [ ]   Pharm. Mail Order: [ ]
Physical Therapy: [ ]   Podiatry: [ ]
Psychiatric: [ ]   Transplant: [ ]
Vision: [ ]   Wellness: [ ]
Workers' Comp: [ ]
Other Benefits: Occupational Therapy

SECURECARE DENTAL

3625 N 16th Street Ste 206
Phoenix, AZ 85016-6447
Phone: 602-234-3266 Fax: 602-285-0121 Toll-Free: 888-256-3266
Web site: www.securecaredental.com

MAILING ADDRESS:
SECURECARE DENTAL
3625 N 16th Street Ste 206
Phoeniz, AZ 85016-6447

KEY EXECUTIVES:
Chief Executive Officer/President .... David L Popejoy
Medical Director .... Morris Bikoff, DDS
Marketing Director .... Mark D Popejoy
Director, Provider Services .... Stefanie L Triplett

COMPANY PROFILE:
Parent Company Name: SW Preferred Dental Organization
Doing Business As: SecureCare Dental
Year Founded: 1988   Federally Qualified: [ ]
Forprofit: [Y]   Not-For-Profit: [ ]
Model Type:
Accreditation: [ ] AAPPO [X] JACHO [ ] NCQA [ ] URAC
Plan Type: PPO, Specialty PPO
Total Enrollment:
   2001: 50,000   2004: 52,000   2007: 0
   2002: 1,600   2005:
   2003: 1,750   2006:

SERVICE AREA:
Nationwide: N
  AZ;

TYPE OF COVERAGE:
Commercial: [Y] Individual: [ ] FEHBP: [ ] Indemnity: [ ]
Medicare: [ ] Medicaid: [ ] Supplemental Medicare: [ ]
Tricare [ ]

PRODUCTS OFFERED:
Product Name: Type:
SW Preferred Dental Organization   Specialty PPO

PLAN BENEFITS:
Alternative Medicine: [ ]   Behavioral Health: [ ]
Chiropractic: [ ]   Dental: [X]
Home Care: [ ]   Inpatient SNF: [ ]
Long-Term Care: [ ]   Pharm. Mail Order: [ ]
Physical Therapy: [ ]   Podiatry: [ ]
Psychiatric: [ ]   Transplant: [ ]
Vision: [ ]   Wellness: [ ]
Workers' Comp: [ ]
Other Benefits:

SHPS HEALTHCARE SERVICES

9305 E Via De Ventura
Scottsdale, AZ 85258
Phone: 480-948-3105 Fax: 480-443-5302 Toll-Free: 800-333-3760
Web site: www.shps.com

MAILING ADDRESS:
SHPS HEALTHCARE SERVICES
9305 E Via De Ventura
Scottsdale, AZ 85258

KEY EXECUTIVES:
Chief Executive Officer .... Jim Beck
Medical Director .... Gerald E Osband, MD

COMPANY PROFILE:
Parent Company Name: SHPS Healthcare Services Company
Doing Business As:
Year Founded: 1991   Federally Qualified: [ ]
Forprofit: [Y]   Not-For-Profit: [ ]
Model Type:
Accreditation: [ ] AAPPO [ ] JACHO [ ] NCQA [ ] URAC
Plan Type: UR

SERVICE AREA:
Nationwide: N
  AZ;

Comments:
Formerly located in Los Angeles, CA. Formerly named Health International.

SUN HEALTH MEDISUN

13632N 99th Ave
Sun City, AZ 85351
Phone: 623-876-5432 Fax: 623-974-7439 Toll-Free: 800-446-8331
Web site: www.medisun.org

MAILING ADDRESS:
SUN HEALTH MEDISUN
13632N 99th Ave
Sun City, AZ 85351

KEY EXECUTIVES:
Chief Executive Officer .... Leland Peterson
Chief Financial Officer .... William Sellner
Medical Director .... Jack Weiss, MD
Chief Operating Officer .... Keith Dines
Marketing Director .... Kenneth Stevens
Credentialing Manager .... Mary Hickie
Public Relations Director .... Helen Bixenmann
Network Development Director .... Rick Rock
Quality Assurance Director/Credentialing Manager .... Mary Hickie
Compliance Officer .... Christine Liberato

COMPANY PROFILE:
Parent Company Name: Sun Health Corporation
Doing Business As:
Year Founded: 1985   Federally Qualified: [N]
Forprofit: [Y]   Not-For-Profit: [ ]
Model Type: IPA
Accreditation: [ ] AAPPO [ ] JACHO [ ] NCQA [ ] URAC
Plan Type: HMO
Total Enrollment:
   2001: 8,927   2004: 16,200   2007: 0
   2002: 15,000   2005:
   2003: 15,917   2006:

SERVICE AREA:
Nationwide: N
  AZ (Sun City, Northwest Valley of Phoenix);

Managed Care Organization Profiles — ARIZONA

PACIFICARE OF ARIZONA

410 N 44th St
Phoenix, AZ 85072
Phone: 602-244-8200 Fax: 602-681-7680 Toll-Free: 800-221-2462
Web site: www.pacificare.com
MAILING ADDRESS:
    PACIFICARE OF ARIZONA
    PO Box 52078
    Phoenix, AZ 85072

KEY EXECUTIVES:
Acting Chief Executive Officer .... Brendan Baker
Director of Financial Operations .... Tracy Steward
Medical Director .... Ken Davis, MD
Director of Pharmacy Services .... Cliff Hardesty
Marketing Director .... Jenny Kirges

COMPANY PROFILE:
Parent Company Name: UnitedHealth Group
Doing Business As:
Year Founded: 1985   Federally Qualified: [Y]
Forprofit: [Y]   Not-For-Profit: [ ]
Model Type: NETWORK
Accreditation: [ ] AAPPO [ ] JACHO [X] NCQA [ ] URAC
Plan Type: HMO, POS, HDHP, HSA
Total Enrollment:
    2001: 248,600   2004: 234,351   2007: 0
    2002: 229,721   2005:
    2003: 238,743   2006:
SERVICE AREA:
Nationwide: N
    AZ (Maricopa, Pima, Pinal);
TYPE OF COVERAGE:
Commercial: [Y] Individual: [ ] FEHBP: [ ] Indemnity: [ ]
Medicare: [Y] Medicaid: [ ] Supplemental Medicare: [ ]
Tricare   [ ]
PRODUCTS OFFERED:
Product Name:	Type:
Pacificare HMO	HMO
Pacificare Preferred Provider	PPO
Secure Horizons	Medicare Advantage
Pacificare POS	POS

CONSUMER-DRIVEN PRODUCTS
	HSA Company
	HSA Product
	HSA Administrator
	Consumer-Driven Health Plan
Signature Options PPO	High Deductible Health Plan

PLAN BENEFITS:
Alternative Medicine:	[ ]	Behavioral Health:	[X]
Chiropractic:	[X]	Dental:	[X]
Home Care:	[X]	Inpatient SNF:	[X]
Long-Term Care:	[X]	Pharm. Mail Order:	[X]
Physical Therapy:	[X]	Podiatry:	[X]
Psychiatric:	[X]	Transplant:	[X]
Vision:	[X]	Wellness:	[X]
Workers' Comp:	[X]		
Other Benefits:			

PHOENIX HEALTH PLAN - COMMUNITY CONNECTION

7878 N 16th St Ste 105
Phoenix, AZ 85020
Phone: 602-824-3700 Fax: Toll-Free: 800-747-7997
Web site: www.php-cc.com
MAILING ADDRESS:
    PHOENIX HEALTH PLAN/COMMUNITY CONNECTION
    7878 N 16th St Ste 105
    Phoenix, AZ 85020

KEY EXECUTIVES:
Chief Executive Officer .... Nancy Novick

COMPANY PROFILE:
Parent Company Name:
Doing Business As:
Year Founded: Federally Qualified: [ ]
Forprofit: [ ]   Not-For-Profit: [ ]
Model Type:
Accreditation: [ ] AAPPO [ ] JACHO [ ] NCQA [ ] URAC
Plan Type: HMO,
Total Enrollment:
    2001: 0   2004: 0   2007: 87.844
    2002: 0   2005:
    2003: 0   2006: 92,606
SERVICE AREA:
Nationwide:
    AZ (Gila, Maricopa, Pinal);
TYPE OF COVERAGE:
Commercial: [ ] Individual: [ ] FEHBP: [ ] Indemnity: [ ]
Medicare: [ ] Medicaid: [Y] Supplemental Medicare: [ ]
Tricare   [ ]
PRODUCTS OFFERED:
Product Name:	Type:
PHP/Community Connection	Medicaid
PHP/Community Connection	Family Planning Ext

PIMA HEALTH PLAN

3950 S Country Club #400
Tucson, AZ 85714
Phone: 520-243-8219 Fax: 520-243-8064 Toll-Free: 800-423-3801
Web site: www.pimahealthsystem.org
MAILING ADDRESS:
    PIMA HEALTH PLAN
    3950 S Country Club #400
    Tucson, AZ 85714

KEY EXECUTIVES:
Chief Executive Officer .... Mary Kaehler
Chief Financial Officer .... Donna Terry
Medical Director .... Timothy J Peterson
Pharmacy Director .... Johanna Stryker-Smit
Chief Information Officer .... Mary Kaehler

COMPANY PROFILE:
Parent Company Name: Pima Health System
Doing Business As:
Year Founded: 1983   Federally Qualified: [ ]
Forprofit: [ ]   Not-For-Profit: [Y]
Model Type:
Accreditation: [ ] AAPPO [ ] JACHO [ ] NCQA [ ] URAC
Plan Type: HMO
Total Enrollment:
    2001: 13,027   2004: 35,000   2007: 29,478
    2002: 0   2005: 31,310
    2003: 19,654   2006: 31,457
SERVICE AREA:
Nationwide: N
    AZ;
TYPE OF COVERAGE:
Commercial: [ ] Individual: [ ] FEHBP: [ ] Indemnity: [ ]
Medicare: [ ] Medicaid: [Y] Supplemental Medicare: [ ]
Tricare   [ ]
PRODUCTS OFFERED:
Product Name:	Type:
Pima Health Plan	Medicaid
Pima Health Plan	Family Planning Ext
Pima Health Plan	PC

PLAN BENEFITS:
Alternative Medicine:	[ ]	Behavioral Health:	[X]
Chiropractic:	[X]	Dental:	[X]
Home Care:	[X]	Inpatient SNF:	[X]
Long-Term Care:	[X]	Pharm. Mail Order:	[ ]
Physical Therapy:	[X]	Podiatry:	[X]
Psychiatric:	[X]	Transplant:	[X]
Vision:	[X]	Wellness:	[X]
Workers' Comp:	[ ]		
Other Benefits:			

PREFERRED THERAPY PROVIDERS OF AMERICA - CORP HEADQUARTERS

19820 N 7th St Ste 250
Phoenix, AZ 85024
Phone: 623-869-9101 Fax: 623-869-9102 Toll-Free: 800-664-5240
Web site: www.preferredtherapy.com

TYPE OF COVERAGE:
Commercial: [Y] Individual: [Y] FEHBP: [ ] Indemnity: [ ]
Medicare: [ ] Medicaid: [ ] Supplemental Medicare: [ ]
Tricare   [ ]
PRODUCTS OFFERED:
Product Name: Type:
LifeWise PPO   PPO
LifeWise Dental Standard
CONSUMER-DRIVEN PRODUCTS
HSA Bank   HSA Company
                                       HSA Product
HSA Bank   HSA Administrator
                                       Consumer-Driven Health Plan
LifeWise Fund Plans   High Deductible Health Plan
PLAN BENEFITS:
Alternative Medicine: [ ]   Behavioral Health: [ ]
Chiropractic: [X]   Dental: [X]
Home Care: [X]   Inpatient SNF: [ ]
Long-Term Care: [X]   Pharm. Mail Order: [X]
Physical Therapy: [ ]   Podiatry: [X]
Psychiatric: [X]   Transplant: [X]
Vision: [X]   Wellness: [X]
Workers' Comp: [ ]
Other Benefits:

MARICOPA HEALTH PLAN

2701 East Elvira Rd
Phoenix, AZ 85034
Phone: 602-344-8700 Fax: 520-408-4866 Toll-Free: 800-582-8686
Web site: www.mhpaz.org
MAILING ADDRESS:
   MARICOPA HEALTH PLAN
   2701 East Elvira Rd
   Phoenix, AZ 85034

KEY EXECUTIVES:
Chief Executive Officer .... Phyllis Biedes
Chief Financial Officer .... Linda Polan
Medical Director .... Mehrdad Shafa, MD
Chief Information Officer .... Rick Mitchell
Marketing Director .... Cheryl Andrews
Provider Services Director .... Gail Gibbs
Network Development Manager .... Karen Geoghan

COMPANY PROFILE:
Parent Company Name: Maricopa Health Systems (MIHS)
Doing Business As:
Year Founded: 1981   Federally Qualified: [Y]
Forprofit: [ ]   Not-For-Profit: [Y]
Model Type: NETWORK
Accreditation: [ ] AAPPO [ ] JACHO [ ] NCQA [ ] URAC
Plan Type: HMO
Total Enrollment:
   2001: 44,512   2004: 6,105   2007: 34,629
   2002: 0   2005: 240,863
   2003: 58,524   2006: 34,549
SERVICE AREA:
Nationwide: N
   AZ;
TYPE OF COVERAGE:
Commercial: [Y] Individual: [ ] FEHBP: [ ] Indemnity: [ ]
Medicare: [ ] Medicaid: [Y]   Supplemental Medicare: [ ]
Tricare   [ ]
PRODUCTS OFFERED:
Product Name: Type:
Maricopa Senior Select (MSSP)   Medicare Advantage
Maricopa Medicaid   Medicaid
Maricopa Health Plan   Family Planning Ext
Comments:
Managed by University Physicians Health Plan.

MERCY CARE PLAN

2800 N Central Ave Ste 400
Phoenix, AZ 85004
Phone: 602-263-3000 Fax: 602-263-2098 Toll-Free: 866-602-1982
Web site: www.mercycareplan.com

MAILING ADDRESS:
   MERCY CARE PLAN
   PO Box 25009
   Phoenix, AZ 85004
KEY EXECUTIVES:
Chief Executive Officer .... Stan Aronovitch
Chief Financial Officer .... Susan Karlson
Chief Medical Officer .... Martin Block, MD
Chief Operating Officer .... Mike Klimansky

COMPANY PROFILE:
Parent Company Name: Southwest Catholic Health Network Corp
Doing Business As:
Year Founded: 1985   Federally Qualified: [ ]
Forprofit: [ ]   Not-For-Profit: [Y]
Model Type: MIXED
Accreditation: [ ] AAPPO [ ] JACHO [ ] NCQA [ ] URAC
Plan Type: HMO
Total Enrollment:
   2001: 126,135   2004: 264,227   2007: 269,211
   2002: 189,000   2005:
   2003: 245,000   2006: 253,262
SERVICE AREA:
Nationwide: N
   AZ;
TYPE OF COVERAGE:
Commercial: [ ] Individual: [ ] FEHBP: [ ] Indemnity: [ ]
Medicare: [ ] Medicaid: [Y]   Supplemental Medicare: [ ]
Tricare   [ ]
PRODUCTS OFFERED:
Product Name: Type:
Mercy Care Plan   Medicaid
                                       Family Planning Ext

OUTLOOK VISION SERVICES

40 N Center St #104
Mesa, AZ 85201
Phone: 480-461-9001 Fax: 480-461-9021 Toll-Free: 800-342-7188
Web site: www.outlookvision.com
MAILING ADDRESS:
   OUTLOOK VISION SERVICES
   40 N Center St #104
   Mesa, AZ 85201

KEY EXECUTIVES:
Chief Executive Officer .... Ronald Johnson
Chief Financial Officer .... Diane Kassner
Director of Provider Services .... Sandi Coberly

COMPANY PROFILE:
Parent Company Name:
Doing Business As:
Year Founded: 1990   Federally Qualified: [ ]
Forprofit: [Y]   Not-For-Profit: [ ]
Model Type:
Accreditation: [ ] AAPPO [ ] JACHO [ ] NCQA [ ] URAC
Plan Type: Specialty PPO
Total Enrollment:
   2001: 7,000,000   2004: 0   2007: 0
   2002: 0   2005:
   2003: 0   2006:
SERVICE AREA:
Nationwide: Y
   NW;
TYPE OF COVERAGE:
Commercial: [Y] Individual: [Y] FEHBP: [ ] Indemnity: [ ]
Medicare: [ ] Medicaid: [ ]   Supplemental Medicare: [ ]
Tricare   [ ]
PLAN BENEFITS:
Alternative Medicine: [ ]   Behavioral Health: [ ]
Chiropractic: [ ]   Dental: [ ]
Home Care: [ ]   Inpatient SNF: [ ]
Long-Term Care: [ ]   Pharm. Mail Order: [ ]
Physical Therapy: [ ]   Podiatry: [ ]
Psychiatric: [ ]   Transplant: [ ]
Vision: [X]   Wellness: [ ]
Workers' Comp: [ ]
Other Benefits: Discount Vision, Pharmacy

Managed Care Organization Profiles — ARIZONA

HEALTH NET OF ARIZONA

930 N Finance Center Dr
Tucson, AZ 85710-1362
Phone: 520-751-5909 Fax: 520-733-5054 Toll-Free: 800-289-2818
Web site: www.health.net

MAILING ADDRESS:
  HEALTH NET OF ARIZONA
  930 N Finance Center Dr
  Tucson, AZ 85710-1362

KEY EXECUTIVES:
Chief Executive Officer/President .... Charles M Sowers
Chief Financial Officer .... Lorry Bottrill
VP of Medical Affairs .... Paula Mikrut, MD
Pharmacy Director .... Nick Hiner
Information Systems Director .... Stephanie Ramsey
VP Of Operations .... Robin Winskas
VP of Sales & Marketing .... Cynthia Ivan
VP of Sales & Marketing .... Matt Francis
VP of Provider Relations .... Tammy Stoltz
VP of Provider Development .... Sandra Habowski
Health Education Director .... Rose Krebs
Human Resources Director .... Lori Haygood
Medical Services Director .... Margaret Novak
Quality Management Director .... Rose Krebs
Legal & Regulatory Affairs .... Tammy Niebling

COMPANY PROFILE:
Parent Company Name: Health Net Inc
Doing Business As:
Year Founded: 1981   Federally Qualified: [Y]
Forprofit: [Y]   Not-For-Profit: [ ]
Model Type:
Accreditation: [ ] AAPPO [ ] JACHO [X] NCQA [ ] URAC
Plan Type: HMO, PPO, POS, TPA, HDHP, HSA
Total Enrollment:
  2001: 173,448   2004: 92,229   2007: 188,000
  2002: 116,859   2005: 148,242
  2003: 155,524   2006: 154,000

SERVICE AREA:
Nationwide: N
  AZ;

TYPE OF COVERAGE:
Commercial: [Y] Individual: [Y] FEHBP: [ ] Indemnity: [ ]
Medicare: [Y] Medicaid: [ ] Supplemental Medicare: [Y]
Tricare   [ ]

PRODUCTS OFFERED:
Product Name: Type:
Intergroup   Comm Group HMO
Intergroup Individual & Family   Comm Individual, Group
SeniorCare   Medicare Advantage
TRICARE HMO   HMO
TRICARE Open Network   PPO
Intercare   TPA
Interflex   POS

PLAN BENEFITS:
Alternative Medicine: [ ]   Behavioral Health: [X]
Chiropractic: [X]   Dental: [X]
Home Care: [ ]   Inpatient SNF: [X]
Long-Term Care: [ ]   Pharm. Mail Order: [X]
Physical Therapy: [X]   Podiatry: [X]
Psychiatric: [ ]   Transplant: [X]
Vision: [X]   Wellness: [ ]
Workers' Comp: [ ]
Other Benefits:

Comments:
Formerly Intergroup Healthcare Corporation.

HUMANA HEALTH CARE PLANS OF ARIZONA

20860 N Tatum Rd Ste 400
Phoenix, AZ 85050
Phone: 480-515-6400 Fax: 480-515-6681 Toll-Free: 800-288-6442
Web site: www.humana.com/arizona/home.html

MAILING ADDRESS:
  HUMANA HEALTHCARE PLANS OF AZ
  20860 N Tatum Rd Ste 400
  Phoenix, AZ 85050

KEY EXECUTIVES:
Chairman of the Board .... David A Jones, Jr
Chief Executive Officer .... Daniel Hoernke
Market President .... Jeff Montag
VP,Chief Medical Director .... Dr Mark Keffer
Chief Operating Officer .... Terry Nittle
VP of Sales .... Charles Ritz
Director of Quality Management .... Peter Metz MD
Utilization Management Associate MD .... Robert Billerbeck, MD
Quality Management Associate MD .... Thomas Davis, MD

COMPANY PROFILE:
Parent Company Name: Humana Inc
Doing Business As:
Year Founded: 1961   Federally Qualified: [Y]
Forprofit: [Y]   Not-For-Profit: [ ]
Model Type: IPA
Accreditation: [ ] AAPPO [ ] JACHO [ ] NCQA [X] URAC
Plan Type: HMO, PPO, Specialty HMO, POS, EPO, ASO, CDHP, HSA
Total Enrollment:
  2001: 21,593   2004: 303,000   2007: 303,000
  2002: 148,000   2005: 33,274
  2003: 157,400   2006:

SERVICE AREA:
Nationwide: N
  AZ;

TYPE OF COVERAGE:
Commercial: [Y] Individual: [Y] FEHBP: [ ] Indemnity: [ ]
Medicare: [Y] Medicaid: [ ] Supplemental Medicare: [Y]
Tricare   [ ]

PRODUCTS OFFERED:
Product Name: Type:
Humana Gold Plus Plan   Medicare Advantage
Humana PPO   PPO
Humana HMO   HMO
Humana Dental   Specialty HMO

CONSUMER-DRIVEN PRODUCTS
JP Morgan Chase   HSA Company
HumanaOne HSA   HSA Product
JP Morgan Chase   HSA Administrator
Personal Care Account   Consumer-Driven Health Plan
HumanaOne   High Deductible Health Plan

PLAN BENEFITS:
Alternative Medicine: [ ]   Behavioral Health: [X]
Chiropractic: [X]   Dental: [X]
Home Care: [ ]   Inpatient SNF: [ ]
Long-Term Care: [ ]   Pharm. Mail Order: [X]
Physical Therapy: [ ]   Podiatry: [ ]
Psychiatric: [X]   Transplant: [X]
Vision: [ ]   Wellness: [ ]
Workers' Comp: [X]
Other Benefits: Long Term Disability Care

LIFEWISE HEALTH PLAN OF ARIZONA

4343 N Scottsdale Rd Ste 355
Scottsdale, AZ 85251
Phone: 480-425-2300 Fax: 480-425-2400 Toll-Free:
Web site: www.lifewiseaz.com

MAILING ADDRESS:
  LIFEWISE HEALTH PLAN OF AZ
  4343 N Scottsdale Rd Ste 355
  Scottsdale, AZ 85251

KEY EXECUTIVES:
Chief Executive Officer/President .... Cliff Klima
Director of Sales .... Dan Evans, CIU
Director of Heatlhcare Delivery Systems .... Deborah Drinkwater

COMPANY PROFILE:
Parent Company Name: Premera Blue Cross
Doing Business As:
Year Founded: 1933   Federally Qualified: [ ]
Forprofit: [ ]   Not-For-Profit: [Y]
Model Type:
Accreditation: [ ] AAPPO [ ] JACHO [ ] NCQA [ ] URAC
Plan Type: PPO, CDHP, HDHP, HSA

SERVICE AREA:
Nationwide: N
  AZ;

ARIZONA — Managed Care Organization Profiles

GREAT-WEST HEALTHCARE OF ARIZONA

6909 E Greenway Pkwy Ste 180
Scottsdale, AZ 85254
Phone: 480-922-6508 Fax: 480-348-2380 Toll-Free: 800-274-4950
Web site: www.greatwesthealthcare.com

MAILING ADDRESS:
GREAT-WEST HEALTHCARE OF AZ
6909 E Greenway Pkwy Ste 180
Phoenix, AZ 85254

KEY EXECUTIVES:
Executive Director .... Roger Stinton
President .... Christopher M Knackstedt
Case Management Director .... Allan Weingarten
Network Development .... Robert Wallen
Case Management Director .... Pat Rumper

COMPANY PROFILE:
Parent Company Name: CIGNA Inc
Doing Business As: Great-West Healthcare
Year Founded: 1998   Federally Qualified: [N]
Forprofit: [Y]   Not-For-Profit: [ ]
Model Type: IPA
Accreditation: [ ] AAPPO [ ] JACHO [ ] NCQA [ ] URAC
Plan Type: HMO, PPO, POS, CDHP, HSA
Total Revenue: 2005: 1,328,804   2006: 1,328,804
Net Income   2005: 2,411,599   2006:
Total Enrollment:
  2001: 0   2004: 5,237   2007: 0
  2002: 7,119   2005: 3,582
  2003: 5,131   2006:
Medical Loss Ratio: 2005: 26.20   2006:
Administrative Expense Ratio: 2005:   2006:

SERVICE AREA:
Nationwide: N
AZ;

TYPE OF COVERAGE:
Commercial: [Y] Individual: [ ] FEHBP: [ ] Indemnity: [ ]
Medicare: [ ] Medicaid: [ ] Supplemental Medicare: [ ]
Tricare   [ ]

CONSUMER-DRIVEN PRODUCTS
Mellon HR Solutions LLC   HSA Company
                                 HSA Product
                                 HSA Administrator
                                 Consumer-Driven Health Plan
                                 High Deductible Health Plan

PLAN BENEFITS:
Alternative Medicine: [X]   Behavioral Health: [ ]
Chiropractic: [X]   Dental: [X]
Home Care: [X]   Inpatient SNF: [X]
Long-Term Care: [ ]   Pharm. Mail Order: [X]
Physical Therapy: [X]   Podiatry: [X]
Psychiatric: [X]   Transplant: [X]
Vision: [X]   Wellness: [X]
Workers' Comp: [ ]
Other Benefits:

Comments:
Acquired by CIGNA Inc April 1, 2008.

HEALTH CHOICE ARIZONA

1600 W Broadway Rd Ste 260
Tempe, AZ 85282
Phone: 480-968-6866 Fax: 480-784-2933 Toll-Free:
Web site: www.healthchoiceaz.com

MAILING ADDRESS:
HEALTH CHOICE ARIZONA
1600 W Broadway Rd Ste 260
Tempe, AZ 85282

COMPANY PROFILE:
Parent Company Name: IASIS Healthcare
Doing Business As:
Year Founded: 1998   Federally Qualified: [ ]
Forprofit: [ ]   Not-For-Profit: [Y]
Model Type:
Accreditation: [ ] AAPPO [ ] JACHO [ ] NCQA [ ] URAC
Plan Type: HMO
Primary Physicians: 500   Physician Specialists:
Hospitals:
Total Revenue: 2005: 353,200,000   2006: 353,200,000
Net Income   2005:   16,417   2006:
Total Enrollment:
  2001: 0   2004: 95,013   2007: 123,302
  2002: 0   2005: 112,259
  2003: 0   2006: 111,543

SERVICE AREA:
Nationwide:
AZ (Apache, Coconino, Gila, Maricopa, Mohave, Pima, Pinal, Navajo);

TYPE OF COVERAGE:
Commercial: [ ] Individual: [ ] FEHBP: [ ] Indemnity: [ ]
Medicare: [ ] Medicaid: [Y] Supplemental Medicare: [ ]
Tricare   [ ]

PRODUCTS OFFERED:
Product Name: Type:
Family Planning Extension   Medicaid
Health Choice Arizona   Medicaid

HEALTH MANAGEMENT NETWORK INC

1600 W Broadway Ste 300
Tempe, AZ 85282
Phone: 480-921-8944 Fax: 480-894-5230 Toll-Free: 800-448-3585
Web site: www.hma-inc.com

MAILING ADDRESS:
HEALTH MANAGEMENT NETWORK INC
1600 W Broadway Ste 300
Tempe, AZ 85282

KEY EXECUTIVES:
Chief Executive Officer .... Mark Dyer
Chief Financial Officer .... Paul Carter
Medical Director .... Wesley Romberger, MD
Pharmacy Director .... Justine Ordner
Chief Operating Officer .... Leao Light
Marketing Director .... Chris Westerman
MIS Director .... Wes Young
Credentialing Manager .... Steve DeRouin
Public Relations Director .... Curt Barker
Provider Services Supervisor .... Benjamin Newsum
Director of Network Development .... Steve DeRouin
Human Resources Director .... Curt Barker
Quality Assurance Director .... Nancy Boetcher
Credentialing Manager .... Steve DeRouin
Case Management Director .... Barbara Link
Ancillary Benefits Director .... Paul Cordes

COMPANY PROFILE:
Parent Company Name: HMA Inc
Doing Business As: Rural AZ Network, AZ Medical Network
Year Founded: 1983   Federally Qualified: [N]
Forprofit: [ ]   Not-For-Profit: [Y]
Model Type: NETWORK
Accreditation: [ ] AAPPO [ ] JACHO [ ] NCQA [ ] URAC
Plan Type: PPO, EPO
Primary Physicians: 7,000   Physician Specialists:
Hospitals:
Total Enrollment:
  2001: 0   2004: 0   2007: 0
  2002: 0   2005:
  2003: 0   2006: 1,000,000

SERVICE AREA:
Nationwide: N
NW;

TYPE OF COVERAGE:
Commercial: [Y] Individual: [ ] FEHBP: [ ] Indemnity: [ ]
Medicare: [ ] Medicaid: [ ] Supplemental Medicare: [ ]
Tricare   [ ]

PLAN BENEFITS:
Alternative Medicine: [ ]   Behavioral Health: [X]
Chiropractic: [X]   Dental: [X]
Home Care: [X]   Inpatient SNF: [X]
Long-Term Care: [ ]   Pharm. Mail Order: [ ]
Physical Therapy: [X]   Podiatry: [X]
Psychiatric: [X]   Transplant: [X]
Vision: [X]   Wellness: [X]
Workers' Comp: [X]
Other Benefits:

Managed Care Organization Profiles — ARIZONA

PRODUCTS OFFERED:
Product Name: Type:
Delta Dental Plan of AZ   Specialty PPO
PLAN BENEFITS:
Alternative Medicine: [ ]   Behavioral Health: [ ]
Chiropractic: [ ]   Dental: [X]
Home Care: [ ]   Inpatient SNF: [ ]
Long-Term Care: [ ]   Pharm. Mail Order: [ ]
Physical Therapy: [ ]   Podiatry: [ ]
Psychiatric: [ ]   Transplant: [ ]
Vision: [ ]   Wellness: [ ]
Workers' Comp: [ ]
Other Benefits:

EMPLOYERS DENTAL SERVICES INC

4720 N Oracle Rd #100
Tucson, AZ 85705
Phone: 520-696-4343 Fax: 520-696-4311 Toll-Free: 800-722-9772
Web site: www.mydentalplan.net
MAILING ADDRESS:
   EMPLOYERS DENTAL SRVS INC
   PO Box 36600
   Tucson, AZ 85705

KEY EXECUTIVES:
President .... Bruce R Hentschel
Chief Financial Officer .... Cynthia G Weeks
Dental Director .... Donald S Altman, DDS
Chief Operating Officer .... Elizabeth A Stambaugh
Director of Marketing .... Susana P Valenzuela

COMPANY PROFILE:
Parent Company Name: Principal Financial Group
Doing Business As:
Year Founded: 1976   Federally Qualified: [N]
Forprofit: [Y]   Not-For-Profit: [ ]
Model Type: IPA
Accreditation: [ ] AAPPO [ ] JACHO [ ] NCQA [ ] URAC
Plan Type: Specialty HMO
Total Revenue: 2005: 16,100,846   2006: 16,100,846
Net Income   2005:   3,876,715   2006:
Total Enrollment:
   2001: 143,370   2004: 162,942   2007: 0
   2002: 150,298   2005: 164,925
   2003: 156,028   2006:
Medical Loss Ratio: 2005: 60.70   2006:
Administrative Expense Ratio: 2005:   2006:
SERVICE AREA:
Nationwide: N
   AZ;
TYPE OF COVERAGE:
Commercial: [Y] Individual: [Y] FEHBP: [ ] Indemnity: [ ]
Medicare: [ ] Medicaid: [ ] Supplemental Medicare: [ ]
Tricare   [ ]
PLAN BENEFITS:
Alternative Medicine: [ ]   Behavioral Health: [ ]
Chiropractic: [ ]   Dental: [X]
Home Care: [ ]   Inpatient SNF: [ ]
Long-Term Care: [ ]   Pharm. Mail Order: [ ]
Physical Therapy: [ ]   Podiatry: [ ]
Psychiatric: [ ]   Transplant: [ ]
Vision: [ ]   Wellness: [ ]
Workers' Comp: [ ]
Other Benefits:

EVERCARE SELECT

3141 N Third Ave Ste 100
Phoenix, AZ 85013
Phone: 602-331-5100 Fax: 602-745-7949 Toll-Free: 800-377-2055
Web site: www.evercareonline.com
MAILING ADDRESS:
   EVERCARE SELECT
   3141 N Third Ave Ste 100
   Phoenix, AZ 85013

KEY EXECUTIVES:
Chief Executive Officer .... Marsha Smith
President .... Rhonda Brede
VP/Chief Financial Officer .... Creighton Donovan
Medical Director .... Ramona Woodriffe, MD
Operations Director .... Jenny Clark
MIS Director .... Dave Decker
Public Relations .... Michael Kennedy
Provider Relations Director .... Cathy Walbillig
Network/Contracts Officer .... Gene Dameron
Human Resources Director .... Rita Console
Medical Management/Quality Assurance Director .... Brenda Page
Fraud Prev/Invstgtn/Mem Srs D .... Dawn Barnes
Director .... John Lingenfelter MD
Director .... Henry Kaldenbaugh MD
VP/Treasurer/Secretary .... Michael Kennedy
Case Management Director .... Chris Snell

COMPANY PROFILE:
Parent Company Name: UnitedHealth Group
Doing Business As:
Year Founded: Federally Qualified: [ ]
Forprofit: [ ]   Not-For-Profit: [ ]
Model Type:
Accreditation: [ ] AAPPO [ ] JACHO [ ] NCQA [ ] URAC
Plan Type: HMO,
Total Enrollment:
   2001: 2,905   2004: 3,706   2007: 0
   2002: 2,952   2005: 4,085
   2003: 3,466   2006:
SERVICE AREA:
Nationwide: N
   AZ (La Paz, Mohave);
TYPE OF COVERAGE:
Commercial: [ ] Individual: [ ] FEHBP: [ ] Indemnity: [ ]
Medicare: [ ] Medicaid: [Y] Supplemental Medicare: [ ]
Tricare   [ ]
PRODUCTS OFFERED:
Product Name: Type:
Arizona Health Concepts   Medicaid
Comments:
Formerly known as Arizona Health Concepts.

FORTIFIED PROVIDER NETWORK INC

8096 N 85th Way Ste 103
Scottsdale, AZ 85258
Phone: 480-607-0222 Fax: 480-607-2199 Toll-Free:
Web site: www.fortifiedprovider.com
MAILING ADDRESS:
   FORTIFIED PROVIDER NETWORK INC
   8096 N 85th Way Ste 103
   Scottsdale, AZ 85258

KEY EXECUTIVES:
VP of Contracting .... Michael Olson

COMPANY PROFILE:
Parent Company Name:
Doing Business As:
Year Founded: 1997   Federally Qualified: [ ]
Forprofit: [Y]   Not-For-Profit: [ ]
Model Type: NETWORK
Accreditation: [ ] AAPPO [ ] JACHO [ ] NCQA [ ] URAC
Plan Type: PPO
Primary Physicians: Physician Specialists:
Hospitals: 400
Total Revenue: 2005:   2006:
Net Income   2005:   2006:
Total Enrollment:
   2001: 0   2004: 0   2007: 60,000
   2002: 0   2005:
   2003: 0   2006:
Nationwide:
   NW & PR;
PLAN BENEFITS:
Alternative Medicine: [X]   Behavioral Health: [X]
Chiropractic: [X]   Dental: [ ]
Home Care: [X]   Inpatient SNF: [X]
Long-Term Care: [ ]   Pharm. Mail Order: [ ]
Physical Therapy: [X]   Podiatry: [X]
Psychiatric: [X]   Transplant: [ ]
Vision: [ ]   Wellness: [ ]
Workers' Comp: [X]
Other Benefits:

CIGNA DENTAL HEALTH PLAN OF ARIZONA INC

1571 Sawgrass Corporate Pkwy
Sunrise, FL 33323
Phone: 954-514-6600 Fax: 954-514-6905 Toll-Free: 800-367-1037
Web site: www.cigna.com/dental

MAILING ADDRESS:
CIGNA DENTAL HEALTH PLAN AZ
1571 Sawgrass Corporate Pkwy
Sunrise, FL 33323

KEY EXECUTIVES:
President .... Karen S Rohan

COMPANY PROFILE:
Parent Company Name: CIGNA Corporation
Doing Business As:
Year Founded: 1995   Federally Qualified: [N]
Forprofit: [Y]   Not-For-Profit: [ ]
Model Type:
Accreditation: [ ] AAPPO [ ] JACHO [ ] NCQA [ ] URAC
Plan Type: Specialty HMO
Total Revenue: 2005: 14,730,689   2006: 14,730,689
Net Income   2005: 1,879,085   2006:
Total Enrollment:
  2001: 0   2004: 83,784   2007: 0
  2002: 108,964   2005: 77,274
  2003: 94,531   2006:
Medical Loss Ratio: 2005: 62.30   2006:
Administrative Expense Ratio: 2005:   2006:

SERVICE AREA:
Nationwide: N
AZ;

TYPE OF COVERAGE:
Commercial: [ ] Individual: [ ] FEHBP: [ ] Indemnity: [ ]
Medicare: [ ] Medicaid: [ ] Supplemental Medicare: [ ]
Tricare   [ ]

PRODUCTS OFFERED:
Product Name: Type:
CIGNA Dental Health of AZ   Specialty HMO

PLAN BENEFITS:
Alternative Medicine: [ ]   Behavioral Health: [ ]
Chiropractic: [ ]   Dental: [X]
Home Care: [ ]   Inpatient SNF: [ ]
Long-Term Care: [ ]   Pharm. Mail Order: [ ]
Physical Therapy: [ ]   Podiatry: [ ]
Psychiatric: [ ]   Transplant: [ ]
Vision: [ ]   Wellness: [ ]
Workers' Comp: [ ]
Other Benefits:

CIGNA HEALTHCARE OF ARIZONA

11001 N Black Canyon Hwy
Phoenix, AZ 85029-4754
Phone: 602-942-4462 Fax: 602-371-2998 Toll-Free:
Web site: www.cigna.com

MAILING ADDRESS:
CIGNA HEALTHCARE OF AZ
11001 N Black Canyon Hwy
Phoenix, AZ 85029-4754

KEY EXECUTIVES:
Chief Executive Officer .... H Edward Hanway
President, CHC of AZ, NV-SW Region .... Jeff Terrill
Chief Financial Officer .... Chris Gorecki
Medical Director .... Ron Ruiz, MD
Pharmacy Director .... Alicia Brockey
Chief Operating Officer .... Bob Carroll
MIS Director .... Lisa Stilwell
Public Relations Director .... Tania Graves
VP Network Operations .... Kristi Thomason
Human Resources Director .... Lane Pittman
Quality Assurance Manager .... Ann Clancy
Compliance Officer .... Diana Cerrito

COMPANY PROFILE:
Parent Company Name: CIGNA Corporation
Doing Business As:
Year Founded: 1977   Federally Qualified: [N]
Forprofit: [Y]   Not-For-Profit: [ ]
Model Type: IPA
Accreditation: [ ] AAPPO [ ] JACHO [X] NCQA [ ] URAC
Plan Type: HMO, PPO, POS, ASO, EPO, CDHP, HDHP, HSA,
Total Enrollment:
  2001: 758,381   2004: 123,342   2007: 0
  2002: 621,000   2005:
  2003: 598,000   2006:

SERVICE AREA:
Nationwide: N
AZ (Apache, Coconino, Gila, LaPaz, Maricopa, Mohave, Navajo,
Pinal, Yavapai, Yuma)

TYPE OF COVERAGE:
Commercial: [Y] Individual: [Y] FEHBP: [ ] Indemnity: [ ]
Medicare: [Y] Medicaid: [ ] Supplemental Medicare: [ ]
Tricare   [ ]

PRODUCTS OFFERED:
Product Name: Type:
CIGNA Healthcare for Seniors   Medicare Advantage
CIGNA Community Choice   Medicaid
CIGNA Healthcare of AZ   HMO
CIGNA Healthcare of AZ   POS

CONSUMER-DRIVEN PRODUCTS
JP Morgan Chase   HSA Company
CIGNA Choice Fund   HSA Product
                                 HSA Administrator
Open Access Plus   Consumer-Driven Health Plan
PPO   High Deductible Health Plan

PLAN BENEFITS:
Alternative Medicine: [ ]   Behavioral Health: [X]
Chiropractic: [X]   Dental: [ ]
Home Care: [X]   Inpatient SNF: [X]
Long-Term Care: [X]   Pharm. Mail Order: [X]
Physical Therapy: [X]   Podiatry: [X]
Psychiatric: [X]   Transplant: [X]
Vision: [X]   Wellness: [X]
Workers' Comp: [ ]
Other Benefits:

DELTA DENTAL PLAN OF ARIZONA INC

15648 N 35th Ave #111
Phoenix, AZ 85080-3000
Phone: 602-938-3131 Fax: 602-548-5099 Toll-Free: 800-352-6132
Web site: www.deltadentalaz.com

MAILING ADDRESS:
DELTA DENTAL PLAN OF AZ
PO Box 43000
Phoenix, AZ 85080-3000

KEY EXECUTIVES:
Chairman .... James P Davis
Chief Executive Officer/President .... Bernard Glossy
Chief Financial Officer .... Mark Anderson
Executive VP of Sales/Broker Relations .... Gary Feldman

COMPANY PROFILE:
Parent Company Name: Delta Dental Plan Association
Doing Business As:
Year Founded: 1972   Federally Qualified: [N]
Forprofit: [ ]   Not-For-Profit: [ ]
Model Type:
Accreditation: [ ] AAPPO [ ] JACHO [ ] NCQA [ ] URAC
Plan Type: Specialty HMO, Specialty PPO,
Total Revenue: 2005: 72,248,756   2006: 72,248,756
Net Income   2005: 22,049,541   2006:
Total Enrollment:
  2001: 0   2004: 149,159   2007: 0
  2002: 132,260   2005: 435,000
  2003: 140,139   2006:
Medical Loss Ratio: 2005: 83.40   2006:
Administrative Expense Ratio: 2005:   2006:

SERVICE AREA:
Nationwide: N
AZ;

TYPE OF COVERAGE:
Commercial: [Y] Individual: [Y] FEHBP: [ ] Indemnity: [Y]
Medicare: [ ] Medicaid: [ ] Supplemental Medicare: [ ]
Tricare   [ ]

Managed Care Organization Profiles — ARIZONA

PRODUCTS OFFERED:

Product Name:	Type:
Blue Classic	Indemnity
Blue Choice	HMO
Blue Preferred	PPO
Blue Select	HMO
Senior Security	Medicare Supplement
Senior Preferred	Medicare Supplement
Medicare Blue	Medicare

CONSUMER-DRIVEN PRODUCTS

HSA Bank	HSA Company
Blue Preferred Saver Plan	HSA Product
HSA Bank	HSA Administrator
	Consumer-Driven Health Plan
	High Deductible Health Plan

CARE 1ST HEALTH PLAN ARIZONA INC

2355 E Camelback Rd Ste 300
Phoenix, AZ 85016
Phone: 602-778-1800 Fax: 602-778-1863 Toll-Free: 866-560-4042
Web site: www.care1st.com/az

MAILING ADDRESS:
CARE 1ST HEALTH PLAN AZ INC
2355 E Camelback Rd Ste 300
Phoenix, AZ 85016

KEY EXECUTIVES:
Chief Administrative Officer .... Scott Cummings
Chief Financial Officer .... Deena Sigel
Chief Medical Officer .... David Franey, MD
Director, Pharmacy .... Jacque Griffith
Director, Sales & Marketing .... Rose Bernal
Director, Provider Network .... Sheila Jones
Director Human Resources/Facilities .... Sandra Vincent
Director, Quality Management .... Pat Seabert
Corporate Compliance Officer .... Kimulet Winzer
Director, Medicare .... Tida Garcia
Director, Utilization Mgnmnt .... Cheryl Walton, RN
Director, Claims .... Elizabeth Ohton
Director, Member Services .... Monica Husband

COMPANY PROFILE:
Parent Company Name:
Doing Business As:
Year Founded: 2003   Federally Qualified: [ ]
Forprofit: [N]   Not-For-Profit: [Y]
Model Type:
Accreditation: [ ] AAPPO [ ] JACHO [ ] NCQA [ ] URAC
Plan Type: HMO,
Total Enrollment:
    2001: 0   2004: 0   2007: 30,281
    2002: 0   2005: 30,499
    2003: 0   2006: 29,276

SERVICE AREA:
Nationwide: N
    AZ (Maricopa);

TYPE OF COVERAGE:
Commercial: [ ] Individual: [ ] FEHBP: [ ] Indemnity: [ ]
Medicare: [ ] Medicaid: [Y] Supplemental Medicare: [ ]
Tricare   [ ]

PRODUCTS OFFERED:

Product Name:	Type:
Care 1st Health Plan	Medicaid

CATALINA BEHAVIORAL HEALTH SERVICES INC

1220 Alma School Ste 109
Mesa, AZ 85210
Phone: 480-834-2700 Fax: 480-827-1551 Toll-Free: 800-977-0281
Web site: www.cbhs-az.com

MAILING ADDRESS:
CATALINA BEHAVIORAL HLTH SVCS
1220 Alma School Ste 109
Mesa, AZ 85210

KEY EXECUTIVES:
Chief Executive Officer .... Karen Smith-Hagman
Medical Director .... Robert Posner, MD
Provider Services Director .... Ray Roybal
Clinical Director-North Region .... Steve Dannenbaum
Clinical Director-South Region .... Howard Shore
Utilization Management .... Jennifer Zingsheim
Business Officer Manager .... Angie Moya

COMPANY PROFILE:
Parent Company Name: MHN
Doing Business As: Catalina Behavioral Health Services Inc
Year Founded: 1990   Federally Qualified: [N]
Forprofit: [Y]   Not-For-Profit: [ ]
Model Type: STAFF
Accreditation: [ ] AAPPO [ ] JACHO [ ] NCQA [X] URAC
Plan Type: Specialty HMO, Specialty PPO, POS
Total Enrollment:
    2001: 0   2004: 350,000   2007: 0
    2002: 0   2005:
    2003: 0   2006:

SERVICE AREA:
Nationwide: N
    Catalina Behavioral Health Services is Statewide in AZ;
    MHN is in all 50 states and Puerto Rico;.

TYPE OF COVERAGE:
Commercial: [Y] Individual: [Y] FEHBP: [Y] Indemnity: [Y]
Medicare: [Y] Medicaid: [ ] Supplemental Medicare: [Y]
Tricare   [ ]

PLAN BENEFITS:
Alternative Medicine: [ ]   Behavioral Health: [X]
Chiropractic: [ ]   Dental: [ ]
Home Care: [ ]   Inpatient SNF: [ ]
Long-Term Care: [ ]   Pharm. Mail Order: [ ]
Physical Therapy: [ ]   Podiatry: [ ]
Psychiatric: [X]   Transplant: [ ]
Vision: [ ]   Wellness: [ ]
Workers' Comp: [ ]
Other Benefits: EAP/Managed Care

CHIROPRACTIC ARIZONA NETWORK INC

3625 N 16th Street Ste 206
Phoenix, AZ 85016
Phone: 602-264-2606 Fax: 602-285-0121 Toll-Free:
Web site:

MAILING ADDRESS:
CHIROPRACTIC ARIZONA NTWK INC
3625 N 16th Street Ste 206
Phoenix, AZ 85016

KEY EXECUTIVES:
Chief Executive Officer/Chief Financial Officer .... David L Popejoy
Medical Director .... David Friedman, MD
Director, Provider Services .... Debbie Merriott

COMPANY PROFILE:
Parent Company Name: Doing Business As:
Year Founded: 1988   Federally Qualified: [ ]
Forprofit: [Y]   Not-For-Profit: [ ]
Model Type:
Accreditation: [ ] AAPPO [ ] JACHO [ ] NCQA [ ] URAC
Plan Type: Specialty PPO

SERVICE AREA:
Nationwide: N
    AZ;

TYPE OF COVERAGE:
Commercial: [Y] Individual: [ ] FEHBP: [ ] Indemnity: [ ]
Medicare: [Y] Medicaid: [ ] Supplemental Medicare: [ ]
Tricare   [ ]

PLAN BENEFITS:
Alternative Medicine: [ ]   Behavioral Health: [ ]
Chiropractic: [X]   Dental: [ ]
Home Care: [ ]   Inpatient SNF: [ ]
Long-Term Care: [ ]   Pharm. Mail Order: [ ]
Physical Therapy: [ ]   Podiatry: [ ]
Psychiatric: [ ]   Transplant: [ ]
Vision: [ ]   Wellness: [ ]
Workers' Comp: [ ]
Other Benefits:

ARIZONA — Managed Care Organization Profiles

PLAN BENEFITS:

Alternative Medicine:	[ ]	Behavioral Health:	[X]
Chiropractic:	[X]	Dental:	[ ]
Home Care:	[X]	Inpatient SNF:	[X]
Long-Term Care:	[X]	Pharm. Mail Order:	[ ]
Physical Therapy:	[X]	Podiatry:	[X]
Psychiatric:	[X]	Transplant:	[X]
Vision:	[X]	Wellness:	[ ]
Workers' Comp:	[X]		
Other Benefits:			

ASSURANT EMPLOYEE BENEFITS - ARIZONA

5353 N 16th St Ste 370
Phoenix, AZ 85016-3228
Phone: 602-308-0230 Fax: 602-263-0187 Toll-Free: 800-619-6996
Web site: www.assurantemployeebenefits.com

MAILING ADDRESS:
ASSURANT EMPLOYEE BNFTS - AZ
5353 N 16th St Ste 370
Phoenix, AZ 85016-3228

KEY EXECUTIVES:
Interim Chief Executive Officer/President ...... John S Roberts
Chief Financial Officer ...... Floyd F Chadee
VP, Medical Director ...... Polly M Galbraith, MD
Chief Information Officer ...... Karla J Schacht
Senior VP, Marketing ...... Joseph A Sevcik
Privacy Officer ...... John L Fortini
VP of Provider Services ...... James A Barrett, DMD
Senior VP, Human Resources & Dvlpmnt ...... Sylvia R Wagner
General Manager ...... Todd Boyd
National Dental Director ...... James A Barrett, DMD

COMPANY PROFILE:
Parent Company Name: Assurant Health
Doing Business As:
Year Founded: 1986   Federally Qualified: [ ]
Forprofit: [Y]   Not-For-Profit: [ ]
Model Type:
Accreditation: [ ] AAPPO [ ] JACHO [ ] NCQA [ ] URAC
Plan Type: Specialty HMO,

SERVICE AREA:
Nationwide: N
AZ;

TYPE OF COVERAGE:
Commercial: [ ] Individual: [Y] FEHBP: [ ] Indemnity: [ ]
Medicare: [ ] Medicaid: [ ] Supplemental Medicare: [ ]
Tricare [ ]

PRODUCTS OFFERED:
Product Name: Type:
                DHMO
                Vision

PLAN BENEFITS:

Alternative Medicine:	[ ]	Behavioral Health:	[ ]
Chiropractic:	[ ]	Dental:	[X]
Home Care:	[ ]	Inpatient SNF:	[ ]
Long-Term Care:	[ ]	Pharm. Mail Order:	[ ]
Physical Therapy:	[ ]	Podiatry:	[ ]
Psychiatric:	[ ]	Transplant:	[ ]
Vision:	[X]	Wellness:	[ ]
Workers' Comp:	[ ]		
Other Benefits:			

Comments:
Formerly Fortis Benefits Dental.

AVESIS INC

3724 N 3rd Street Ste 300
Phoenix, AZ 85012
Phone: 602-241-3400 Fax: 602-240-9100 Toll-Free: 800-522-0258
Web site: www.avesis.com

MAILING ADDRESS:
AVESIS INC
3724 N 3rd Street Ste 300
Phoenix, AZ 85012

KEY EXECUTIVES:
Chief Executive Officer/President ...... Alan S Cohn
Chief Financial Officer ...... Joel Alperstein
Chief Operating Officer ...... Judy Stocker
Marketing Director ...... Michael Reamer
MIS Director ...... Angela Waldron
Public Relations/Provider Relations Director ...... Anthony Girgenti
Provider Relations Director ...... Anthony Girgenti

COMPANY PROFILE:
Parent Company Name:
Doing Business As:
Year Founded: 1978   Federally Qualified: [N]
Forprofit: [Y]   Not-For-Profit: [ ]
Model Type:
Accreditation: [ ] AAPPO [ ] JACHO [ ] NCQA [ ] URAC
Plan Type: Specialty HMO, Specialty PPO, ASO, EPO, TPA
Primary Physicians: Physician Specialists: 18,000
Total Enrollment:
   2001: 0   2004: 2,000,000   2007: 0
   2002: 2,000,000 2005: 2,000,000
   2003: 0   2006: 3,000,000

SERVICE AREA:
Nationwide: Y
NW;

TYPE OF COVERAGE:
Commercial: [Y] Individual: [ ] FEHBP: [ ] Indemnity: [ ]
Medicare: [ ] Medicaid: [ ] Supplemental Medicare: [ ]
Tricare [ ]

PLAN BENEFITS:

Alternative Medicine:	[ ]	Behavioral Health:	[ ]
Chiropractic:	[X]	Dental:	[X]
Home Care:	[ ]	Inpatient SNF:	[ ]
Long-Term Care:	[ ]	Pharm. Mail Order:	[ ]
Physical Therapy:	[ ]	Podiatry:	[ ]
Psychiatric:	[ ]	Transplant:	[ ]
Vision:	[X]	Wellness:	[ ]
Workers' Comp:	[ ]		
Other Benefits: hearing			

BLUE CROSS BLUE SHIELD OF ARIZONA

2444 W Los Palmaritas Dr
Phoenix, AZ 85021
Phone: 602-864-4100 Fax: 602-864-4184 Toll-Free: 800-232-2345
Web site: www.bcbsaz.com

MAILING ADDRESS:
BC/BS OF ARIZONA
PO Box 13466
Phoenix, AZ 85021

KEY EXECUTIVES:
Executive VP, Chief Executive Officer ...... Richard Boals
Senior VP, Chief Financial Officer ...... Tony Astorga, CPA
Medical Director ...... Gary D Smethers, MD
Chief Information Officer ...... Michael J Linder
Senior VP of Marketing ...... Richard M Hannon
VP of Sales ...... Gail Damico
Senior VP Claims/Federal Programs ...... Jody Chandler

COMPANY PROFILE:
Parent Company Name: Blue Cross/Blue Shield
Doing Business As:
Year Founded: 1977   Federally Qualified: [ ]
Forprofit: [ ]   Not-For-Profit: [Y]
Model Type:
Accreditation: [ ] AAPPO [ ] JACHO [ ] NCQA [ ] URAC
Plan Type: HMO, PPO, HDHP, HSA
Total Enrollment:
   2001: 0   2004: 901,958   2007: 0
   2002: 0   2005: 1,006,509
   2003: 834,173 2006:

SERVICE AREA:
Nationwide: N
AZ;

TYPE OF COVERAGE:
Commercial: [Y] Individual: [Y] FEHBP: [ ] Indemnity: [ ]
Medicare: [Y] Medicaid: [ ] Supplemental Medicare: [Y]
Tricare [ ]

Managed Care Organization Profiles — ARIZONA

ACTION HEALTH CARE MANAGEMENT SERVICES

6245 N 24th Parkway Ste 112
Phoenix, AZ 85016
Phone: 602-265-0681 Fax: 602-265-0202 Toll-Free: 800-433-6915
Web site: www.actionhealthcare.com

MAILING ADDRESS:
    ACTION HLTH CARE MGMT SVCS
    6245 N 24th Pkwy Ste 112
    Phoenix, AZ 85016

KEY EXECUTIVES:
Chief Executive Officer .... Jean Rice
Medical Director .... Joel Brill, MD
Provider Relations .... Jeannine Boutin
Medical Management Director .... Nancy Whalley, BSN, MPA, CMAC
Case Management Director .... Cynthia Towne RN, BSN, CCM

COMPANY PROFILE:
Parent Company Name:
Doing Business As:
Year Founded: 1987   Federally Qualified: [ ]
Forprofit: [Y]   Not-For-Profit: [ ]
Model Type:
Accreditation: [ ] AAPPO [ ] JACHO [ ] NCQA [ ] URAC
Plan Type: UR
Total Enrollment:
  2001: 94,250   2004: 0   2007: 0
  2002: 105,517   2005:
  2003: 114,319   2006:

SERVICE AREA:
Nationwide: N
  NW;

TYPE OF COVERAGE:
Commercial: [Y] Individual: [Y] FEHBP: [ ] Indemnity: [ ]
Medicare: [ ] Medicaid: [ ] Supplemental Medicare: [ ]
Tricare [ ]

PRODUCTS OFFERED:
Product Name: Type:
Utilization Management
Case Management
Great Expectations
Beech St/Capp Care PPO   PPO
Hlh & Healing Trust Comp & Alt   Discount Program

PLAN BENEFITS:
Alternative Medicine: [X]   Behavioral Health: [X]
Chiropractic: [ ]   Dental: [ ]
Home Care: [X]   Inpatient SNF: [X]
Long-Term Care: [X]   Pharm. Mail Order: [ ]
Physical Therapy: [X]   Podiatry: [X]
Psychiatric: [X]   Transplant: [X]
Vision: [ ]   Wellness: [X]
Workers' Comp: [X]
Other Benefits: Pregnancy Risk/Management

AETNA INC - ARIZONA

7720 N 16th St Ste 400
Phoenix, AZ 85020
Phone: 602-427-2271 Fax: 602-427-2125 Toll-Free:
Web site: www.aetna.com

MAILING ADDRESS:
    AETNA INC - AZ
    7720 N 16th St Ste 400
    Phoenix, AZ 85020

KEY EXECUTIVES:
Chairman of the Board .... Ronald A Williams
Chief Executive Officer .... Gary M Mizell
President .... Gary M Mizell
Treasurer .... Russell P Smith
Medical Director .... Charles D Stewart
Pharmacy Director, West Regional .... Yrena Friedman
Public Relations Director .... Bobby Pena
Marketing Director .... Cindy Ryan
Head of Business Operations .... Mark T Bertolini

COMPANY PROFILE:
Parent Company Name: Aetna Inc
Doing Business As:
Year Founded: 1992   Federally Qualified: [N]
Forprofit: [Y]   Not-For-Profit: [ ]
Model Type: NETWORK
Accreditation: [ ] AAPPO [ ] JACHO [X] NCQA [ ] URAC
Plan Type: HMO, PPO, POS, CDHP, HSA
Total Enrollment:
  2001: 5,239   2004: 178,917   2007: 0
  2002: 227,079   2005: 167,952
  2003: 197,465   2006:

SERVICE AREA:
Nationwide: N
  AZ;

TYPE OF COVERAGE:
Commercial: [Y] Individual: [ ] FEHBP: [ ] Indemnity: [ ]
Medicare: [ ] Medicaid: [ ] Supplemental Medicare: [ ]
Tricare [ ]

PRODUCTS OFFERED:
Product Name: Type:
Aetna US Hlthcare Golden Medi   Medicare

CONSUMER-DRIVEN PRODUCTS
Aetna Life Insurance Co   HSA Company
Aetna HealthFund HSA   HSA Product
Aetna   HSA Administrator
Aetna HealthFund   Consumer-Driven Health Plan
PPO I; PPO II   High Deductible Health Plan

PLAN BENEFITS:
Alternative Medicine: [ ]   Behavioral Health: [ ]
Chiropractic: [X]   Dental: [X]
Home Care: [X]   Inpatient SNF: [X]
Long-Term Care: [X]   Pharm. Mail Order: [X]
Physical Therapy: [X]   Podiatry: [X]
Psychiatric: [X]   Transplant: [X]
Vision: [X]   Wellness: [X]
Workers' Comp: [ ]
Other Benefits:

ARIZONA FOUNDATION FOR MEDICAL CARE

326 E Coronado
Phoenix, AZ 85004
Phone: 602-252-4042 Fax: 602-256-7816 Toll-Free: 800-624-4277
Web site: www.azfmc.com

MAILING ADDRESS:
    AZ FOUNDATION FOR MEDICAL CARE
    326 E Coronado
    Phoenix, AZ 85004

KEY EXECUTIVES:
Chief Executive Officer .... Anthony D Mitten
President .... Maria A Verso, MD
Director/Business Relations/Communications .... Jennifer Robinson
MIS Director .... Tracy Mitchell
Credentialing Supervisor .... Barbara Keith
Director Provider Comm/Services .... Bob Smith
Director of Provider Contracting .... Bob Smith
Medical Management Director .... Kerry Kovaleski
Senior Director Administration Finance .... Sandra Flowers
Credentialing Supervisor .... Barbara Keith

COMPANY PROFILE:
Parent Company Name: Maricopa Foundation for Medical Care
Doing Business As: Arizona Foundation for Medical Care
Year Founded: 1969   Federally Qualified: [N]
Forprofit: [ ]   Not-For-Profit: [Y]
Model Type: NETWORK
Accreditation: [ ] AAPPO [ ] JACHO [ ] NCQA [X] URAC
Plan Type: PPO, UR, POS, EPO
Primary Physicians: 3,600   Physician Specialists: 5,991
Hospitals: 116
Total Enrollment:
  2001: 254,962   2004: 221,705   2007: 195,000
  2002: 207,880   2005: 221,000
  2003: 206,535   2006: 205,000

SERVICE AREA:
Nationwide: N
  AZ;

TYPE OF COVERAGE:
Commercial: [Y] Individual: [Y] FEHBP: [ ] Indemnity: [ ]
Medicare: [ ] Medicaid: [ ] Supplemental Medicare: [ ]
Tricare [ ]

PRODUCTS OFFERED:
Product Name: Type:
AZ Foundation for Medical Care PPO   PPO

Managed Care Organization Profiles

PREMERA BLUE CROSS BLUE SHIELD OF ALASKA

2550 Denali St Ste 1404
Anchorage, AK 99503
Phone: 907-258-5065 Fax: 907-258-1619 Toll-Free:
Web site: www.premera.com

MAILING ADDRESS:
    PREMERA BC BS OF AK
    2550 Denali St Ste 1404
    Anchorage, AK 99503

KEY EXECUTIVES:
Chief Executive Officer .... HR Brereton Barlow
VP, General Manager - Alaska .... Jeffrey W Davis
Executive VP, Finance/Chief Financial Officer .... Kent Marquardt
Senior VP, Chief Medical Officer .... John L Castiglia, MD
Director of Pharmacy .... Edward Wong, PharmD
Senior VP, Chief Information Officer .... Kirsten Simonitsch
Executive VP, Operations .... Karen Bartlett
Executive VP, Chief Marketing .... Heyward Donigan
Senior VP, Human Resources .... Barbara Magusin
Chief Legal/Public Policy Officer .... Yori Milo
Executive VP, Strategic Development/Health Care Sys ..... Brian Ancell
Seniorr VP, Health Care Delivery System .... Richard Maturi

COMPANY PROFILE:
Parent Company Name: Premera Blue Cross
Doing Business As:
Year Founded: 1933   Federally Qualified: [ ]
Forprofit: [ ]   Not-For-Profit: [Y]
Model Type:
Accreditation: [ ] AAPPO [ ] JACHO [ ] NCQA [ ] URAC
Plan Type: HMO, PPO, CDHP, HSA
Total Enrollment:
  2001: 0   2004: 108,000   2007: 0
  2002: 0   2005:
  2003: 108,000   2006:

SERVICE AREA:
Nationwide: N
  AK;

TYPE OF COVERAGE:
Commercial: [Y] Individual: [Y] FEHBP: [ ] Indemnity: [ ]
Medicare: [Y] Medicaid: [Y] Supplemental Medicare: [Y]
Tricare [ ]

PRODUCTS OFFERED:

Product Name:	Type:
Dimensions	PPO
Personal Dimensions	HDHP
MSC Classic Care	Medicare
Premera Blue Cross	Medicaid

CONSUMER-DRIVEN PRODUCTS

Personal Dimensions HSA	HSA Company
	HSA Product
	HSA Administrator
Dimensions	Consumer-Driven Health Plan
Personal Dimensions	High Deductible Health Plan

PLAN BENEFITS:
Alternative Medicine: [ ]   Behavioral Health: [ ]
Chiropractic: [X]   Dental: [X]
Home Care: [X]   Inpatient SNF: [ ]
Long-Term Care: [X]   Pharm. Mail Order: [X]
Physical Therapy: [ ]   Podiatry: [X]
Psychiatric: [X]   Transplant: [X]
Vision: [X]   Wellness: [X]
Workers' Comp: [ ]
Other Benefits:

Managed Care Organization Profiles **ALABAMA**

Year Founded: 1991 Federally Qualified: [ ]
Forprofit: [Y] Not-For-Profit: [ ]
Model Type:
Accreditation: [ ] AAPPO [ ] JACHO [ ] NCQA [ ] URAC
Plan Type: Specialty HMO, Specialty PPO, POS, TPA
Total Enrollment:
    2001: 0   2004: 0   2007: 0
    2002: 0   2005:
    2003: 20,000   2006:
SERVICE AREA:
Nationwide: N
    AL; AR; FL; GA; MS; NC; PR; SC; TN;
PLAN BENEFITS:
Alternative Medicine: [ ]   Behavioral Health: [ ]
Chiropractic: [ ]   Dental: [X]
Home Care: [ ]   Inpatient SNF: [ ]
Long-Term Care: [ ]   Pharm. Mail Order: [ ]
Physical Therapy: [ ]   Podiatry: [ ]
Psychiatric: [ ]   Transplant: [ ]
Vision: [ ]   Wellness: [ ]
Workers' Comp: [ ]
Other Benefits:
Comments:
For enrollment and revenue information see corporate listing, Camp Hill, Pennsylvania.

UNITEDHEALTHCARE OF ALABAMA

33 Inverness Cntr Pkwy Ste 350
Birmingham, AL 35242
Phone: 205-437-8500 Fax: 205-437-8540 Toll-Free: 800-345-1520
Web site: www.uhc.com
MAILING ADDRESS:
    UNITEDHEALTHCARE OF ALABAMA
    PO Box 830637
    Birmingham, AL 35242

KEY EXECUTIVES:
Chief Executive Officer .... Glen J Golemi
Chief Financial Officer .... Frank Ulibarri
Medical Director .... Larry B Amacker, MD
Compliance Officer .... Harry Beaudoin
Public Relations Director .... Roger Rollman
Vice President of Key Accounts .... Kim Lewis
Vice President of Small Business .... Aaron Brace
Vice President of Network Management .... Jeff Wedin

COMPANY PROFILE:
Parent Company Name: UnitedHealth Group
Doing Business As:
Year Founded: 1985   Federally Qualified: [Y]
Forprofit: [Y]   Not-For-Profit: [ ]
Model Type: IPA
Accreditation: [ ] AAPPO [X] JACHO [X] NCQA [ ] URAC
Plan Type: HMO, PPO, POS, CDHP, HSA, HRA
Total Revenue: 2005:   2006: 350,080,469
Net Income: 2005:   2006:
Total Enrollment:
    2001: 113,933   2004: 42,177   2007: 0
    2002: 87,324   2005:
    2003: 56,456   2006:
Medical Loss Ratio: 2005:   2006: 78.20
Administrative Expense Ratio: 2005:   2006:
SERVICE AREA:
Nationwide: N
    AL (Autauga, Baldwin, Barbour, Bibb, Blount, Bullock, Calhoun, Chilton, Clarke, Coffee, Colbert, Conecuh, Coosa, Crenshaw, Cullman, Dale, Dallas, Elmore, Escambia, Etowah, Franklin, Greene, Hale, Houston, Jackson, Jefferson, Lauderdale, Lawrence, Lee, Limestone, Lowndes, Macon, Madison, Marshall, Mobile, Monroe, Montgomery, Morgan, Perry, Pickens, St Clair, Shelby, Talladega, Tallapoosa, Tuscaloosa, Walker, Washington, Wilcox);
TYPE OF COVERAGE:
Commercial: [Y] Individual: [ ] FEHBP: [ ] Indemnity: [ ]
Medicare: [Y] Medicaid: [ ] Supplemental Medicare: [Y]
Tricare   [ ]
PRODUCTS OFFERED:
Product Name: Type:
Medicare Complete   Medicare Advantage
Seniors First Medicare Plan   Medicare

CONSUMER-DRIVEN PRODUCTS
Exante Bank/Golden Rule Ins Co   HSA Company
iPlan HSA   HSA Product
                                   HSA Administrator
                                   Consumer-Driven Health Plan
                                   High Deductible Health Plan
PLAN BENEFITS:
Alternative Medicine: [ ]   Behavioral Health: [ ]
Chiropractic: [X]   Dental: [X]
Home Care: [X]   Inpatient SNF: [X]
Long-Term Care: [X]   Pharm. Mail Order: [X]
Physical Therapy: [X]   Podiatry: [X]
Psychiatric: [X]   Transplant: [X]
Vision: [X]   Wellness: [X]
Workers' Comp: [ ]
Other Benefits:

VIVA HEALTH INC

1222 14th Ave S
Birmingham, AL 35205
Phone: 205-939-1718 Fax: 205-939-1748 Toll-Free: 800-294-7780
Web site: www.vivahealth.com
MAILING ADDRESS:
    VIVA HEALTH INC
    1222 14th Ave S
    Birmingham, AL 35205

KEY EXECUTIVES:
Chairman of the Board .... David Hoidal
Chief Executive Officer/President .... Arthur B Rollow
Chief Financial Officer .... Letitia E Watkins
Medical Director .... Stacy Branham, MD
Vice President, Information Systems .... Doug Cannon
Chief Operating Officer .... Letitia E Watkins
Vice President, Sales & Marketing .... Scott McDuffie
Vice President, Network Development/Provider Relations   Terry Knight
Vice President of Corp Development/Compliance .... Libba Yates

COMPANY PROFILE:
Parent Company Name: Triton Health Systems
Doing Business As:
Year Founded: 1995   Federally Qualified: [N]
Forprofit: [Y]   Not-For-Profit: [ ]
Model Type: MIXED
Accreditation: [ ] AAPPO [ ] JACHO [ ] NCQA [ ] URAC
Plan Type: HMO, ASO, EPO, TPA
Primary Physicians: 1,887   Physician Specialists: 2,771
Hospitals: 65
Total Revenue: 2005:   2006: 272,066,817
Net Income: 2005:   2006:
Total Enrollment:
    2001: 35,326   2004: 40,908   2007: 0
    2002: 39,277   2005:
    2003: 41,955   2006: 74,000
SERVICE AREA:
Nationwide: N
    AL (Autauga, Baldwin, Bibb, Calhoun, Chinton, Clarke, Conecuh, Cullman, Dale, Dallas, Elmore, Jefferson, Madison, Marion, Mobile, Monroe, Montgomery, Shelby, St Clair, Tuscaloosa, Washington Cty);
TYPE OF COVERAGE:
Commercial: [Y] Individual: [ ] FEHBP: [ ] Indemnity: [ ]
Medicare: [Y] Medicaid: [ ] Supplemental Medicare: [ ]
Tricare   [ ]
PRODUCTS OFFERED:
Product Name: Type:
Viva Medicare   Medicare
Viva HMO   HMO
PLAN BENEFITS:
Alternative Medicine: [ ]   Behavioral Health: [ ]
Chiropractic: [X]   Dental: [ ]
Home Care: [X]   Inpatient SNF: [X]
Long-Term Care: [ ]   Pharm. Mail Order: [X]
Physical Therapy: [X]   Podiatry: [X]
Psychiatric: [X]   Transplant: [X]
Vision: [X]   Wellness: [X]
Workers' Comp: [ ]
Other Benefits:

ALABAMA

Managed Care Organization Profiles

NAMCI

699 A Gallatin St
Huntsville, AL 35801
Phone: 256-532-2755 Fax: 256-532-2756 Toll-Free:
Web site: www.namci.com
MAILING ADDRESS:
  NAMCI
  PO Box 18788
  Huntsville, AL 35801

KEY EXECUTIVES:
Executive Director .... Sherree Clark
Executive Director .... David Frederick
Operations Manager .... Brenda Willoughby
Marketing & Sales Director .... Beth Couch
Credentialing/Claims Specialist .... Michelle Russell
Provider Relations Manager .... Cathy Ontiveros

COMPANY PROFILE:
Parent Company Name: Premier Health Networks of Alabama LLC
Doing Business As:
Year Founded: 1990   Federally Qualified: [N]
Forprofit: [ ]   Not-For-Profit: [Y]
Model Type: NETWORK
Accreditation: [ ] AAPPO [ ] JACHO [ ] NCQA [ ] URAC
Plan Type: PPO
Primary Physicians: 600   Physician Specialists: 985
Hospitals: 15
Total Enrollment:
  2001: 0   2004: 53,000   2007: 0
  2002: 43,617   2005: 52,000
  2003: 47,633   2006:

SERVICE AREA:
Nationwide: N
  AL; MS; TN;

TYPE OF COVERAGE:
Commercial: [Y] Individual: [ ] FEHBP: [ ] Indemnity: [ ]
Medicare: [ ] Medicaid: [ ] Supplemental Medicare: [ ]
Tricare   [ ]

PRODUCTS OFFERED:
Product Name: Type:
NAMCI PPO   PPO

PLAN BENEFITS:
Alternative Medicine: [ ]   Behavioral Health: [X]
Chiropractic: [X]   Dental: [ ]
Home Care: [X]   Inpatient SNF: [ ]
Long-Term Care: [ ]   Pharm. Mail Order: [ ]
Physical Therapy: [ ]   Podiatry: [X]
Psychiatric: [X]   Transplant: [X]
Vision: [X]   Wellness: [X]
Workers' Comp: [X]
Other Benefits: Rehab

PREFERRED HEALTH ALLIANCE

1200 Corporate Dr Ste G-50
Birmingham, AL 35242
Phone: 205-969-1155 Fax: 205-969-1199 Toll-Free:
Web site: www.whspha.com
MAILING ADDRESS:
  PREFERRED HEALTH ALLIANCE
  PO Box 382048
  Birmingham, AL 35242

KEY EXECUTIVES:
Chief Executive Officer/President .... W Hal Shepherd
Chief Financial Officer .... Ed Thomason

COMPANY PROFILE:
Parent Company Name: W H Shepherd Company
Doing Business As:
Year Founded: Federally Qualified: [ ]
Forprofit: [Y]   Not-For-Profit: [ ]
Model Type:
Accreditation: [ ] AAPPO [ ] JACHO [ ] NCQA [ ] URAC
Plan Type: TPA

SERVICE AREA:
Nationwide: N
  AL (Jefferson);

PREMIER HEALTH NETWORKS OF ALABAMA LLC

699-A Gallitin St
Huntsville, AL 35801
Phone: 256-532-2755 Fax: 256-532-2756 Toll-Free:
Web site: www.premierhealthnetwork.com
MAILING ADDRESS:
  PREMIER HEALTH NTWKS OF AL LLC
  P O Box 18788
  Huntsville, AL 35801

KEY EXECUTIVES:
Executive Director .... Sherree Clark
President/Chief Financial Officer .... David Frederick
Medical Director .... Susan Zlotnick-Hale
Operations Manager .... Brenda Willoughby
Marketing & Sales Director .... Beth Couch
Credentialing/Claims Specialst .... Nichelle Russell
Provider Relations Director .... Cathy Ontiveros

COMPANY PROFILE:
Parent Company Name:
Doing Business As: NAMCI, Comp1One,
Year Founded: 1990   Federally Qualified: [ ]
Forprofit: [Y]   Not-For-Profit: [ ]
Model Type: NETWORK
Accreditation: [ ] AAPPO [X] JACHO [ ] NCQA [ ] URAC
Plan Type: PPO
Primary Physicians: 600   Physician Specialists: 985
Hospitals:
Total Enrollment:
  2001: 0   2004: 53,000   2007: 0
  2002: 0   2005:
  2003: 42,000   2006:

SERVICE AREA:
Nationwide: N
  AL; MS; TN;

TYPE OF COVERAGE:
Commercial: [Y] Individual: [ ] FEHBP: [ ] Indemnity: [ ]
Medicare: [Y] Medicaid: [ ] Supplemental Medicare: [ ]
Tricare   [ ]

PLAN BENEFITS:
Alternative Medicine: [ ]   Behavioral Health: [X]
Chiropractic: [X]   Dental: [ ]
Home Care: [X]   Inpatient SNF: [ ]
Long-Term Care: [ ]   Pharm. Mail Order: [ ]
Physical Therapy: [ ]   Podiatry: [X]
Psychiatric: [X]   Transplant: [X]
Vision: [X]   Wellness: [X]
Workers' Comp: [X]
Other Benefits: Rehab

UNITED CONCORDIA COMPANY INC - ALABAMA

400 Vestavia Pkwy Ste 205
Birmingham, AL 35216
Phone: 205-824-1235 Fax: 205-822-1653 Toll-Free: 800-554-6155
Web site: www.ucci.com
MAILING ADDRESS:
  UNITED CONCORDIA CO INC - AL
  400 Vestavia Pkwy Ste 205
  Birmingham, AL 35216

KEY EXECUTIVES:
Chief Executive Officer/President .... Thomas A Dzuryachko
Senior Vice President, Finance .... Daniel Wright
Dental Director .... Mark Schulman, DDS
Chief Operating Officer .... Jon Seltenheim
Vice President, Sales & Marketing .... Nate Kleinberg
MIS Director .... Jim Robins
Director, Provider Services .... Ted Pesano

COMPANY PROFILE:
Parent Company Name: Highmark Inc
Doing Business As:

Managed Care Organization Profiles — ALABAMA

KEY EXECUTIVES:
Director .... Joseph Oaks
Chief Medical Officer .... Alan Goldstein, MD
Manager .... Cherie Pardi

COMPANY PROFILE:
Parent Company Name: Health Net of Alabama Inc
Doing Business As:
Year Founded: 1984   Federally Qualified: [N]
Forprofit: [ ]   Not-For-Profit: [Y]
Model Type: NETWORK
Accreditation: [ ] AAPPO [ ] JACHO [ ] NCQA [ ] URAC
Plan Type: PPO
Primary Physicians: 1,869   Physician Specialists: 2,623
Hospitals: 93
Total Enrollment:
  2001: 0   2004: 135,062   2007: 0
  2002: 169,273   2005: 165,000
  2003: 175,445   2006: 150,000

SERVICE AREA:
Nationwide: N
  Al;

TYPE OF COVERAGE:
Commercial: [Y] Individual: [ ] FEHBP: [ ] Indemnity: [ ]
Medicare: [ ] Medicaid: [ ] Supplemental Medicare: [ ]
Tricare   [ ]

PRODUCTS OFFERED:
Product Name: Type:
HealthChoice PPO   PPO

HEALTHSPRING OF ALABAMA INC

Two Perimeter Pk S Ste 300W
Birmingham, AL 35242
Phone: 205-968-1528 Fax: 205-968-2277 Toll-Free: 800-888-7647
Web site: www.myhealthspring.com/alabama

MAILING ADDRESS:
  HEALTHSPRING OF ALABAMA INC
  Two Perimeter Pk S Ste 300W
  Birmingham, AL 35242

KEY EXECUTIVES:
Chairman of the Board/Chief Executive Officer .... Herbert A Fritch
President .... Rene Moret
Chief Financial Officer .... David Beauchaine
Medical Director .... Hugh Hood, MD
Dir Medicare Compliance .... Robert Davis

COMPANY PROFILE:
Parent Company Name: New Quest LLC
Doing Business As: Healthspring of Alabama Inc
Year Founded: 1999   Federally Qualified: [ ]
Forprofit: [Y]   Not-For-Profit: [ ]
Model Type: NETWORK
Accreditation: [ ] AAPPO [ ] JACHO [ ] NCQA [ ] URAC
Plan Type: HMO,
Total Revenue: 2005:   2006: 286,085,238
Net Income   2005:   2006:
Total Enrollment:
  2001: 50,762   2004: 28,788   2007: 29,078
  2002: 26,204   2005: 36,441
  2003: 28,102   2006: 27,307
Medical Loss Ratio: 2005:   2006: 75.70
Administrative Expense Ratio: 2005:   2006:

SERVICE AREA:
Nationwide: N
  AL (Autauga, Baldwin, Bibb, Blount, Bullock, Calhoun, Cherokee, Chilton, Clarke, Coosa, Cullman, Dallas, DeKalb, Elmore, Jefferson, Lawrence, Lowndes, Macon, Marion, Mobile, Monroe, Montgomery, Russell, St Clair, Shelby, Talladega, Walker, Washington, Winston);

TYPE OF COVERAGE:
Commercial: [Y] Individual: [Y] FEHBP: [ ] Indemnity: [ ]
Medicare: [Y] Medicaid: [ ] Supplemental Medicare: [Y]
Tricare   [ ]

PRODUCTS OFFERED:
Product Name: Type:
Passport   HMO
Seniors First   Medicare
FEHBP   HMO

PLAN BENEFITS:
Alternative Medicine: [ ]   Behavioral Health: [X]
Chiropractic: [X]   Dental: [X]
Home Care: [X]   Inpatient SNF: [X]
Long-Term Care: [ ]   Pharm. Mail Order: [X]
Physical Therapy: [X]   Podiatry: [X]
Psychiatric: [X]   Transplant: [X]
Vision: [X]   Wellness: [X]
Workers' Comp: [ ]
Other Benefits:
Comments:
Formerly called "The OATH, A Health Plan of Alabama." Formerly owned by Baptist Health Systems. Purchased Merit Health Plan of Alabama.

HUMANA INSURANCE CO - ALABAMA

1100 Employers Blvd
DePere, WI 54115
Phone: 920-336-1100 Fax: 502-580-3127 Toll-Free:
Web site: www.humana.com

MAILING ADDRESS:
  HUMANA INSURANCE CO - ALABAMA
  PO Box 740036
  Louisville, KY 54115

KEY EXECUTIVES:
Chairman of the Board .... David A Jones Jr
Chief Executive Officer/President .... Michael B McCallister
Chief Financial Officer .... James H Bloem
Chief Clinical Strategy .... Jack Lord, MD
Chief Operating Officer .... Jim Murray
Chief Marketing Officer .... Steve Moya
Human Resources Director .... Bonnie C Hathcock
Senior Vice President, Strategy & Corp Develpmnt .... Tom Liston
Senior Vice President & General Counsel .... Art Hipwell
Senior Vice President, Corporate Communications .... Tom Noland
Media Relations Manager .... Mitch Lubitz

COMPANY PROFILE:
Parent Company Name: Humana Inc
Doing Business As:
Year Founded: 1961   Federally Qualified: [Y]
Forprofit: [Y]   Not-For-Profit: [ ]
Model Type:
Accreditation: [ ] AAPPO [ ] JACHO [ ] NCQA [ ] URAC
Plan Type: PPO, EPO, ASO, CDHP, HDHP, HSA,
Total Enrollment:
  2001: 0   2004: 0   2007: 0
  2002: 0   2005:
  2003: 106,000   2006:

SERVICE AREA:
Nationwide: N
  AL;

TYPE OF COVERAGE:
Commercial: [Y] Individual: [Y] FEHBP: [ ] Indemnity: [ ]
Medicare: [ ] Medicaid: [ ] Supplemental Medicare: [ ]
Tricare   [Y]

PRODUCTS OFFERED:
Product Name: Type:
Humana PPO   PPO
Humana Life   Life
Humana ASO   ASO
Humana Workers' Comp   Short Term Disabilty

CONSUMER-DRIVEN PRODUCTS
JP Morgan Chase   HSA Company
HumanaOne HSA   HSA Product
JP Morgan Chase   HSA Administrator
Personal Care Account   Consumer-Driven Health Plan
HumanaOne   High Deductible Health Plan

PLAN BENEFITS:
Alternative Medicine: [ ]   Behavioral Health: [X]
Chiropractic: [X]   Dental: [ ]
Home Care: [ ]   Inpatient SNF: [ ]
Long-Term Care: [ ]   Pharm. Mail Order: [X]
Physical Therapy: [ ]   Podiatry: [ ]
Psychiatric: [X]   Transplant: [X]
Vision: [ ]   Wellness: [ ]
Workers' Comp: [X]
Other Benefits: Long Term Disability Care

ALABAMA   **Managed Care Organization Profiles**

KEY EXECUTIVES:
Chief Executive Officer/President .... G Phillip Pope
Chief Financial Officer .... Sherrie Le Meir
Senior Vice President & Medical Director .... Patrick Ryce, MD
Vice President Operation Resources .... Terry McCartney
Senior Vice President Customer Relations .... James M Brown
Senior Vice President Health Care Networks .... Joe Bolen
Vice President Human Resources .... Richard King
Vice President Health Management .... Eddie Harris
Executive Vice President .... Terry Kellogg

COMPANY PROFILE:
Parent Company Name:
Doing Business As:
Year Founded: 1984   Federally Qualified: [ ]
Forprofit: [ ]   Not-For-Profit: [Y]
Model Type:
Accreditation: [ ] AAPPO [ ] JACHO [ ] NCQA [X] URAC
Plan Type: PPO, POS, CDHP, HDHP, HSA, UR, UMO,
Total Enrollment:
    2001: 3,108,980   2004: 3,500,000   2007: 3,600,000
    2002: 0   2005: 3,000,000
    2003: 0   2006: 2,900,000

SERVICE AREA:
Nationwide: N
    AL;

TYPE OF COVERAGE:
Commercial: [Y]   Individual: [ ]   FEHBP: [ ]   Indemnity: [ ]
Medicare: [Y]   Medicaid: [ ]   Supplemental Medicare: [Y]
Tricare [ ]

PRODUCTS OFFERED:
Product Name:	Type:
BC/BS of AL Medicare	Medicare
Health Advantage Plans	Medicare

CONSUMER-DRIVEN PRODUCTS
Mellon HR Solutions LLC	HSA Company
Preferred HSA	HSA Product
	HSA Administrator
	Consumer-Driven Health Plan
	High Deductible Health Plan

PLAN BENEFITS:
Alternative Medicine:	[X]	Behavioral Health:	[ ]
Chiropractic:	[X]	Dental:	[X]
Home Care:	[X]	Inpatient SNF:	[X]
Long-Term Care:	[X]	Pharm. Mail Order:	[ ]
Physical Therapy:	[X]	Podiatry:	[X]
Psychiatric:	[X]	Transplant:	[X]
Vision:	[X]	Wellness:	[ ]
Workers' Comp:	[X]		
Other Benefits:			

DELTA DENTAL INSURANCE COMPANY - ALABAMA

1 Perimeter Park S #420N
Birmingham, AL 35243
Phone: 205-969-5755 Fax: 205-969-5777 Toll-Free: 800-521-2651
Web site: www.deltadentalins.com
MAILING ADDRESS:
    DELTA DENTAL INSURANCE CO - AL
    1 Perimeter Park S #420N
    Birmingham, AL 35243

KEY EXECUTIVES:
President .... Tony Barth
Medical Director .... Charlotte Wiedenman, DMD
Vice President of Underwriting .... Paul Lambert
Vice President of Marketing .... Debbie Reeves
Vice President of Sales .... Dick Aracich
Provider Services Director .... Jeffrey Album
Human Resources Director .... Ruth Miller
Senior Vice President, Sales .... Belinda Martinez

COMPANY PROFILE:
Parent Company Name: Delta Dental Plan of California
Doing Business As: Delta Dental Insurance Co
Year Founded: 1970   Federally Qualified: [ ]
Forprofit: [Y]   Not-For-Profit: [ ]
Model Type:
Accreditation: [ ] AAPPO [ ] JACHO [ ] NCQA [ ] URAC
Plan Type: Specialty PPO, ASO
Total Enrollment:
    2001: 0   2004: 0   2007: 0
    2002: 0   2005:
    2003: 27,164   2006:

SERVICE AREA:
Nationwide: N
    AL;

TYPE OF COVERAGE:
Commercial: [Y]   Individual: [Y]   FEHBP: [ ]   Indemnity: [Y]
Medicare: [ ]   Medicaid: [ ]   Supplemental Medicare: [ ]
Tricare [Y]

PLAN BENEFITS:
Alternative Medicine:	[ ]	Behavioral Health:	[ ]
Chiropractic:		Dental:	[X]
Home Care:		Inpatient SNF:	[ ]
Long-Term Care:		Pharm. Mail Order:	[ ]
Physical Therapy:		Podiatry:	[ ]
Psychiatric:		Transplant:	[ ]
Vision:		Wellness:	[ ]
Workers' Comp:			
Other Benefits:			

GULF HEALTH PLANS PPO INC

2559 Emogene St
Mobile, AL 36606
Phone: 251-470-0207 Fax: 251-450-3307 Toll-Free:
Web site: www.gulfhealthplans.com
MAILING ADDRESS:
    GULF HEALTH PLANS PPO INC
    2559 Emogene St
    Mobile, AL 36606

KEY EXECUTIVES:
Chief Executive Officer/President .... Kern Wilson

COMPANY PROFILE:
Parent Company Name: Infirmary Health System
Doing Business As:
Year Founded: 1985   Federally Qualified: [N]
Forprofit: [Y]   Not-For-Profit: [ ]
Model Type: NETWORK
Accreditation: [ ] AAPPO [ ] JACHO [ ] NCQA [ ] URAC
Plan Type: PPO
Primary Physicians: 349   Physician Specialists: 836
Hospitals: 22
Total Enrollment:
    2001: 0   2004: 0   2007: 0
    2002: 97,000   2005: 90,000
    2003: 97,000   2006:

SERVICE AREA:
Nationwide: N
    AL (Baldwin, Clarke, Escambia, Mobile, Monroe, Washington); FL (Escambia, Santa Rosa); MS (George);

TYPE OF COVERAGE:
Commercial: [Y]   Individual: [ ]   FEHBP: [ ]   Indemnity: [ ]
Medicare: [ ]   Medicaid: [ ]   Supplemental Medicare: [ ]
Tricare [ ]

PRODUCTS OFFERED:
Product Name:	Type:
Gulf Health Plans PPO	PPO

PLAN BENEFITS:
Alternative Medicine:	[ ]	Behavioral Health:	[ ]
Chiropractic:	[ ]	Dental:	[ ]
Home Care:	[X]	Inpatient SNF:	[ ]
Long-Term Care:	[ ]	Pharm. Mail Order:	[ ]
Physical Therapy:	[ ]	Podiatry:	[X]
Psychiatric:	[X]	Transplant:	[X]
Vision:	[ ]	Wellness:	[ ]
Workers' Comp:	[ ]		
Other Benefits:			

HEALTHCHOICE OF ALABAMA

3201 4th Ave S
Birmingham, AL 35222
Phone: 205-715-4801 Fax: 205-715-4802 Toll-Free: 800-500-4800
Web site: www.healthchoiceofalabama.com
MAILING ADDRESS:
    HEALTHCHOICE OF ALABAMA
    PO Box 830605
    Birmingham, AL 35222

Managed Care Organization Profiles   ALABAMA

ALABAMA QUALITY ASSURANCE FOUNDATION

2 Perimeter Park S #200-W
Birmingham, AL 35243-2337
Phone: 205-970-1600 Fax: 205-970-1624 Toll-Free: 800-760-4550
Web site: www.aqaf.com
MAILING ADDRESS:
   ALABAMA QUALITY ASSURANCE FDN
   2 Perimeter Park S #200-W
   Birmingham, AL 35243-2337

KEY EXECUTIVES:
Chief Executive Officer .... Fred Ferree
President .... D Wesley Smith, MD
Chief Financial Officer .... Susan Holmes
Chief Information Officer .... Bart Prevallet
Director of Communications .... Michael Jones
Human Resources Manager .... Ruth Ann Bryant
Vice President Government Operations .... Cynthia McIntosh

COMPANY PROFILE:
Parent Company Name:
Doing Business As:
Year Founded: 1972   Federally Qualified: [ ]
Forprofit: [ ]   Not-For-Profit: [Y]
Model Type:
Accreditation: [ ] AAPPO [ ] JACHO [ ] NCQA [ ] URAC
Plan Type: UR, PRO, QIO
SERVICE AREA:
Nationwide: N
   AL;
TYPE OF COVERAGE:
Commercial: [ ]   Individual: [ ]   FEHBP: [ ]   Indemnity: [ ]
Medicare: [ ]   Medicaid: [Y]   Supplemental Medicare: [Y]
Tricare   [ ]

ASSURANT EMPLOYEE BENEFITS - ALABAMA

3595 Grandview Pkwy Ste 150
Birmingham, AL 35243
Phone: 205-909-5872 Fax: 205-909-5224 Toll-Free: 866-909-1955
Web site: www.assurantemployeebenefits.com
MAILING ADDRESS:
   ASSURANT EMPLOYEE BNFTS - AL
   3595 Grandview Pkwy Ste 150
   Birmingham, AL 35243

KEY EXECUTIVES:
Interim Chief Executive Officer/President .... John S Roberts
Chief Financial Officer .... Floyd F Chadee
Vice President, Medical Director .... Polly M Galbraith, MD
Chief Information Officer .... Karla J Schacht
Senior Vice President, Marketing .... Joseph A Sevcik
Vice President of Provider Services .... James A Barrett, DMD
SVP, Human Resources & Development .... Sylvia R Wagner
National Dental Director .... James A Barrett, DMD

COMPANY PROFILE:
Parent Company Name: Assurant Health
Doing Business As:
Year Founded: 1975   Federally Qualified: [ ]
Forprofit: [Y]   Not-For-Profit: [ ]
Model Type:
Accreditation: [ ] AAPPO [ ] JACHO [ ] NCQA [ ] URAC
Plan Type: Specialty HMO
SERVICE AREA:
Nationwide: N
   AL; LA; MS;
TYPE OF COVERAGE:
Commercial: [Y]   Individual: [Y]   FEHBP: [ ]   Indemnity: [ ]
Medicare: [ ]   Medicaid: [ ]   Supplemental Medicare: [ ]
Tricare   [ ]
PLAN BENEFITS:
Alternative Medicine: [ ]   Behavioral Health: [ ]
Chiropractic: [ ]   Dental: [X]
Home Care: [ ]   Inpatient SNF: [ ]
Long-Term Care: [ ]   Pharm. Mail Order: [ ]
Physical Therapy: [ ]   Podiatry: [ ]
Psychiatric: [ ]   Transplant: [ ]
Vision: [ ]   Wellness: [ ]
Workers' Comp: [ ]
Other Benefits:
Comments:
Formerly a Protective Life Insurance Company.

BEHAVIORAL HEALTH SYSTEMS INC

2 Metroplex Dr Ste 500
Birmingham, AL 35209-0724
Phone: 205-879-1150 Fax: 205-879-1178 Toll-Free: 800-245-1150
Web site: www.bhs-ins.com
MAILING ADDRESS:
   BEHAVIORAL HEALTH SYSTEMS INC
   PO Box 830724
   Birmingham, Al 35209-0724

KEY EXECUTIVES:
Chairman of The Board/Chief Executive Officer .. Deborah L Stephens
Chief Financial Officer .... Mark Gordon, CPA
Medical Director .... William M Patterson, MD
Chief Information Officer/MIS Director .... Paul Collins
Chief Marketing Officer .... Carol Singletary
Executive VP & Managed Care Officer .... Pat Friedley
Director, Public Relations .... Susan Levine
Director, Provider Relations .... Joyce Pullom
Director, Provider Relations .... Myles Walcott
Vice President, Clinical Services .... Beth Gregory, PhD
Director, QA Clinical Services .... Cindy Myers, MA, LPC, CHCQM
Director, Clinical Program Development .... Kyle Strange, LCSW
Executive Vice President, Managed Care Officer .... Pat Friedley
President, Safety First .... Danny Cooner
Medical Director, Safety First .... Michael Cloyd, MD

COMPANY PROFILE:
Parent Company Name:
Doing Business As:
Year Founded: 1989   Federally Qualified: [ ]
Forprofit: [Y]   Not-For-Profit: [ ]
Model Type: NETWORK
Accreditation: [ ] AAPPO [ ] JACHO [ ] NCQA [X] URAC
Plan Type: Specialty PPO, TPA, UR
Primary Physicians: 750   Physician Specialists: 6,750
Hospitals: 650
Total Revenue: 2005: 9,800,000   2006:
Net Income   2005:   2006:
Total Enrollment:
   2001: 0   2004: 225,000   2007: 0
   2002: 175,000   2005:
   2003: 200,000   2006:
SERVICE AREA:
Nationwide: N
   NW;
TYPE OF COVERAGE:
Commercial: [Y]   Individual: [ ]   FEHBP: [ ]   Indemnity: [ ]
Medicare: [ ]   Medicaid: [ ]   Supplemental Medicare: [ ]
Tricare   [ ]
PRODUCTS OFFERED:
Product Name: Type:
Behavioral Health Safety First   Drug Testing
Behavioral Health PPO   Specialty PPO
Behavioral Health Workers Comp   PPO
PLAN BENEFITS:
Alternative Medicine: [ ]   Behavioral Health: [X]
Chiropractic: [ ]   Dental: [ ]
Home Care: [ ]   Inpatient SNF: [ ]
Long-Term Care: [ ]   Pharm. Mail Order: [ ]
Physical Therapy: [ ]   Podiatry: [ ]
Psychiatric: [X]   Transplant: [ ]
Vision: [ ]   Wellness: [X]
Workers' Comp: [X]
Other Benefits:

BLUE CROSS BLUE SHIELD OF ALABAMA

450 Riverchase Pkwy E
Birmingham, AL 35244
Phone: 205-220-2100 Fax: 205-220-6477 Toll-Free:
Web site: www.bcbsal.org
MAILING ADDRESS:
   BLUE CROSS BLUE SHIELD OF AL
   PO Box 995
   Birmingham, AL 35244

Copyright MCIC -- The National Directory of Managed Care Organizations, Seventh Edition

The Solution.

When you have questions about the latest trends in managed healthcare, we have your answers!

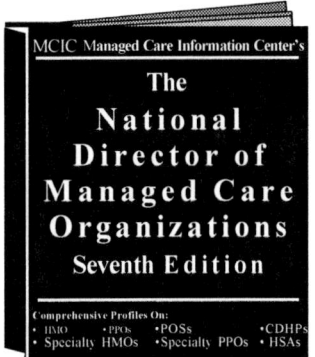
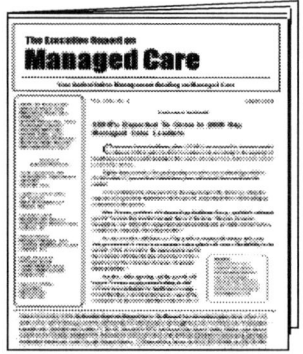
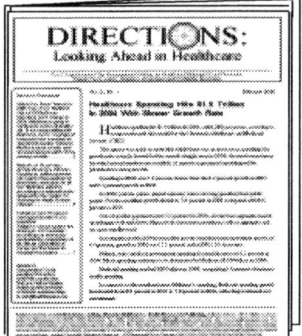
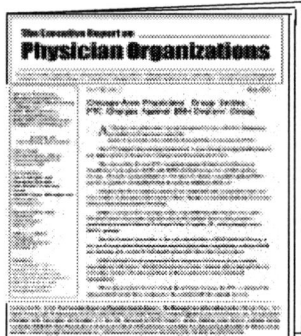
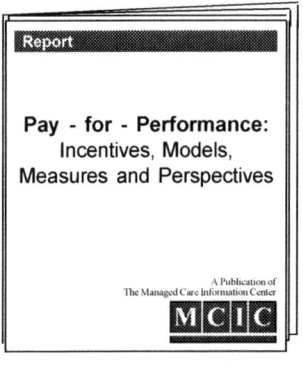
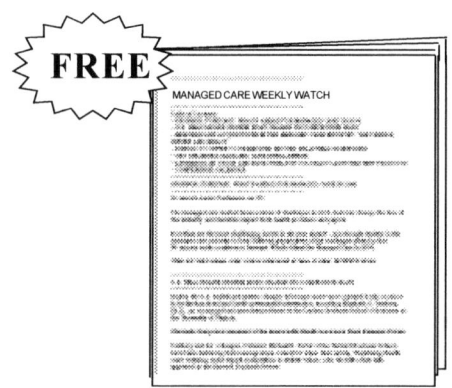

No matter what it is — managed care, integrated care, capitation, mergers & acquisitions updates, marketing strategies, management issues, monitoring of market activity — we have an advisory service or reference guide that focuses on finding solutions specifically aimed at your information needs. *The Managed Care Information Center* monitors the most critical activities affecting healthcare — Washington, D.C., on the state level, polling the experts, scouring the Internet, attending key conferences and seminars — and reports its findings to you in concise, timely executive briefings.

Whether your professional healthcare needs require you to keep pace with what is happening in your specific area of healthcare, or you need to monitor trends in various arenas of healthcare to find new areas to expand your services, you'll find your answers in one of these advisory services or reference guides. We give you the cutting-edge information on where healthcare trends are heading so you can make more informed decisions. *The Managed Care Information Center* puts the healthcare news and solutions you need at your fingertips.

Rely on the Leader . . .
Managed Care Information Center
Dept. 14D7SOLAD
PO Box 559
Allenwood, NJ 08720
Toll-Free 888-THE-MCIC
(1-888-843-6242)
Fax: 1-888-FAX-MCIC (1-888-329-6242)

Managed Care Information Center . . .
Finding the solutions you need to
plan for your organization's future.

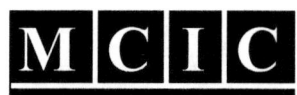

The National Directory of Managed Care Organizations • DIRECTIONS: Looking Ahead in Healthcare •
Expedite-Managed Care • ManagedCareMarketplace.com • National Directory of Medical Directors (on CD Rom) •
Pay-for-Performance: Incentives, Models, Measures and Perspectives • What's Working in Pay-for-Performance? • Managed Care Business Information Library • Managed Care Datasource • New Strategies in the Growth of Consumer Driven Healthcare

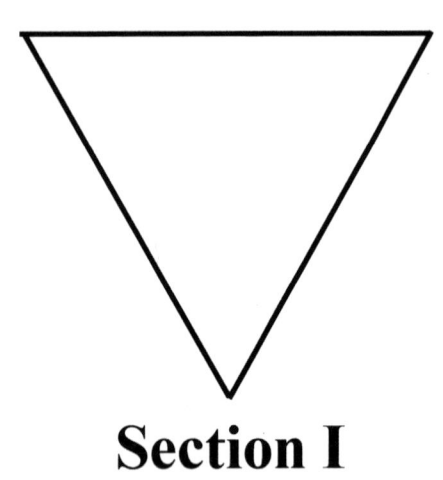

Section I

Managed Care Organization Profiles
(Alphabetically)

Section III -- Medicare Advantage Demonstration Project Participants

- The "Product Name" for the project participants operating under the Medicare Advantage Demonstration program is printed in bold type followed by a solid black line. Below the line is the organization's name that is providing services through the demonstration project followed by the company's address, the main telephone number, a toll-free number if applicable and a fax number.

- Key Organization Personnel

- Contract date, enrollment date, profit status (for-profit or non-profit), covered lives for 2000 to 2007.

Section IV -- Miscellaneous Organizations

- The "Product Name" for the participants is printed in bold type followed by a solid black line. Below the line is the organizations name followed by the company's address, the main phone number, a toll-free number if applicable and a fax number.

- Key Organization Personnel

Section V -- Directory of Healthcare Associations

Section VI -- Directory of Healthcare Resources

- Resource name, followed by a brief description of the resource along with contact information for obtaining further information or purchasing.

Indexing:

The National Directory of Managed Care Organizations incorporates 8 indexes for supplemental support of the detailed, descriptive profiles of each managed care organization. All indexes are in alphabetical order. The indexes are as follows:

        Index I   -- Managed Care Organizations

        Index II   -- Health Maintenance Organizations

        Index III -- Preferred Provider Organizations

        Index IV -- Specialty HMOs

        Index V   -- Specialty PPOs

        Index VI -- Point of Service Plans

        Index VII -- Miscellaneous Organizations

        Index VIII -- Personnel

User's Guide

The National Directory of Managed Care Organizations consists of descriptive listings grouped within separate sections by organization type. Each section is described below.

Section I -- Managed Care Organizations

- The main organization name is printed in bold type between two solid black lines at the top of each profile. Below the name is an address, the main telephone number, a toll-free number if applicable and a fax number.

- A mailing address is given which in some cases varies from that of the organization's main address.

- Key Organization Personnel includes: chief executive officer/president; chief financial officer; marketing director; MIS director; medical director; pharmacy director; contract officer; chief information officer; and director, provider services.

- Company Profile includes: parent company name; "doing business as" name -- a trade name; recognized industry name or acronym; year founded; federally qualified (Yes or No); for-profit (Yes or No); model type (applicable responses include: IPA, network, group, staff or mixed); plan type (HMO, PPO, specialty HMO, specialty PPO, CDHP, HDHP, HSA, POS, PRO, TPA, EPO, ASO, DPO or UR); integrated delivery system participation.

- Plan Statistics includes: number of primary care physicians; number of physician specialists; number of hospitals; revenues -- total revenue, net income and reporting years; type of accreditation; medical loss ratio; and administrative expense ratio.

- Enrollment demographics -- total enrollment (including dependents), enrollment by coverage, plan type and geographic breakdown.

- Type of Coverage -- an "Y" indicates affirmative and can appear in any or all of the following: commercial, individual, Medicare, Supplemental Medicare, Medicaid.

- Plan Benefits -- an "X" indicates that the benefit is offered and can appear in any or all of the following: chiropractic, dental, home care, inpatient SNF, long-term care, pharmacy mail order, podiatry, psychiatric, specialty in physical therapy, transplant, vision, wellness, worker's compensation, other (specified by survey respondent).

- Comments -- additional information pertinent to the MCO profiled.

Section II -- Benefit Management Companies contain the following data:

- Pharmacy Benefit Management (PBM)

- The main organization name is printed in bold type followed by a solid black line. Below the name organization's name is an address, the main telephone number, a toll-free number if applicable and a fax number.

- Mailing address.

services of designated physicians, hospitals or other providers of medical care. HMOs have greater control of utilization and typically use a capitation payment system that rewards providers for cost-effective management of patients.

Organizations that are designed to use the framework of a HMO, but provide the membership with healthcare benefits limited to a single area (such as dental, vision, etc.) are listed as **SPECIALTY HMOs**.

Model Types:

Group Model - An HMO model in which the physicians, employed by the HMO, are typically paid on a salary basis or fee schedule and many received in incentive payments based on their performance.

IPA Model - A type of HMO that contracts with physicians to form an independent practice association operating on behalf of the HMO. IPA physicians see members of the managed care organization through the IPA and their own patients through their medical practice.

Mixed Model - A managed care plan that mixes two or more types of delivery systems, such as an HMO and a closed and open panel system; also called a hybrid model.

Network Model - A HMO that contracts with two or more independent group practices, possibly including a staff group, to provide health services. While a network model HMO may contain a few solo practices, it is predominantly organized around group practices.

Staff Model - A HMO that delivers health services through a physician group that is controlled by the HMO entity.

Pharmacy Network

Networks of pharmacies that contract with various MCOs, such as HMOs and PBMs, to provide pharmacy services to the MCO's members.

POS: Point of Service

A type of managed care plan whereby beneficiaries have the option of choosing to obtain medical services from the provider of their choice, or through a selected primary care physician, who manages their care and refers subscribers to participating hospitals, physicians and other providers within a select network. Those who opt for care within the network receive benefits at a higher percentage of the allowable amount of covered services.

PPO: Preferred Provider Organization

A network of providers that employers contract with to provide health services to their employees. PPOs generally offer employers a reduced fee-for-service rate (or, possibly, per diem or per case payments) in return for the channeling of employees to network providers. Employees are given incentives to use network providers but may still choose to use out-of-network providers. If care is obtained outside the network, the employee pays a higher portion of the cost.

Organizations that are designed to use the framework of a PPO, but that offer benefits limited to a single are a (such as vision, pharmacy, etc.) comprise **SPECIALTY PPOs**.

PRO: Professional Review Organization

A PRO is a physician-sponsored organization charged with reviewing services provided to patients to determine if the services rendered are medically necessary; are provided in accordance with professinal criteria, norms, and standards, and are provided in the appropriate setting.

PSO: Provider Sponsored Organization

A PSO is a health plan owned and operated by providers that may be offered to Medicare beneficiaries. PSOs are authorized by the Balanced Budget Act (BBA) of 1997, which expanded the kinds of health plans available to Medicare patients as alternatives to the traditional program. PSOs are one of the health plan options available to Medicare beneficiaries under the Medicare+Choice program authorized by the BBM.

TPA: Third Party Administrator

A company designated to pay claims and to assume responsibility for managing a benefit plan for a plan owner. As a third party administrator, this service is usually performed without assuming any financial risk for the cost of claims.

UR: Utilization Review Organization

An organization that uses established benchmarks to evaluate the level, frequency, and necessity of medical care.

The National Directory of Managed Care Organizations
Introduction

The National Directory of Managed Care Organizations provides detailed profiles of health maintenance organizations (HMOs), preferred provider organizations (PPOs), specialty HMOs and PPOs, consumer-driven heatlh plans (CDHP), high deductible health plans (HDHP), health savings accounts (HSA), point of service plans (POSs), exclusive provider organizations (EPOs), peer review organizations (PROs), third party administrators (TPAs), utilization review organizations (UROs), pharmacy benefit management companies (PBMs), pharmacy networks (PNs) (See glossary included in this section for more descriptive information on these groups.)

METHODOLOGY:

The National Directory of Managed Care Organizations is drawn from a database containing more than 1,464 MCOs.

Extensive research was undertaken by the professional research staff of the Managed Care Information Center. Research efforts included verification of data through mail, fax and telephone interviews. Where possible, data was collected and verified directly by the organization's administrative office. Research included monitoring of news releases, government agency inquiries, detailed searches via the Internet, company annual reports, industry news services, attendance/monitoring of industry conferences and interviews with national trade associations.

Profiles are organized alphabetically by company name within state of origin.

ELIGIBILITY REQUIREMENTS FOR INCLUSION:

ASO: Administrative Services Only
A service under which a third party payor delivers administrative services to an employer group. The employer is at risk for the cost of healthcare services provided. This is a common arrangement when an employer sponsors a healthcare program.

CDHP: Consumer-Driven Health Plan
A healthcare model in which the consumer has more incentive to control the cost of either the health benefits or healthcare. Usually involves a a type of spending account funded partly by the employer to pay for member claims up to an annual dollar amount, combined with a health insurance policy providing coverage for services once the account is exhausted.

DPO: Dental Plan Organization
A network of dental providers that employers contract with to provide health services to their employees.

EPO: Exclusive Provider Organization
A discounted, fee-for-service physician network similar to a preferred provider organization (PPO). Whereas a PPO generally extends coverage at a lower reimbursement rate for services outside the provider network, an EPO provides coverage only for contracted providers.

HDHP: High Deductible Health Plan
A health insurance plan in which the enrollee pays a high deductible allowing them to use a health savings account. It must meet the requirements of the Medicare Prescription Drug, Improvement, and Modernization Act of 2003.

HSA: Health Savings Account
Allows individuals to pay for current health expenses through a tax-exempt savings account. You must belong to a high deductible health plan and cannot be eligible for Medicare or covered by another plan that is not a high deductible health plan or a dependent on another person's tax return. Funds carry over indefinitely during a participant's lifetime.

HMO: Health Maintenance Organization
A healthcare service plan that requires its subscribers/members, except in medical emergency, to use the

Expedite: *The Information Toolkit for Sellers of Products and Services to Managed Care...*

Target Your Managed Care Sales and Marketing efforts with "**Expedite: Managed Care**" the Information Toolkit for Sellers of Products and Services to Health and Managed Care — the most useful, comprehensive, national service that exclusively covers the rapidly changing managed care organization universe and healthcare delivery system. It includes:

- An online searchable proprietary database of more than 1,500 managed care organizations and 3,800 plan types
- Over 10,000 verified managed care key contact names
- Comprehensive profiles including enrollment figures, model types and service state
- A robust custom industry news and information not available from any other source
- Fully searchable news and company 8-year archive based on your criteria
- A special "heads up" news alert service delivered regularly to your email inbox
- Online 24x7 keyword search of information on clients, prospects, products, competitors, contracts awarded
- The most complete and current information available anywhere

The **Expedite: Managed Care** is designed to meet the needs of marketing and sales managers. Use one reliable source for your sales prospecting, marketing and market research.

Get information on significant and emerging trends in the health and managed care industry, breaking news alerts, market development information, health informatics, new software approaches, IT strategies, managed care strategic issues, technology needs and applications, mergers and acquisitions, contracts awarded, forecasts, spending, leading industry research, surveys and study results.

Business Information Tailored to Fit Your Needs

- Have access to **Expedite** from anywhere
- It's user friendly - no need for training
- The online database is continuously updated

Gather Your Team for a Real-Time Full Access Demonstration Online

The MCIC staff would be happy to walk you through **Expedite**. See for yourself how you can easily discover sales opportunities, identify market leaders, get vendor news, gather statistics and data, sales support, spot market growth, track spending forecasts, new product developments, and contracts awarded.

* *

TO SIGN UP FOR A FREE EXPEDITE DEMO

- Call The Managed Care Information Center at (888) 843-6242 today
- Download a presentation at www.managedcaremarketplace.com/paper/exped.com
- Email: expedite@themcic.com

Please reference this Code #14NRD7Expedite

Managed Care Information Center
Providing Essential Management Information to Healthcare Executives

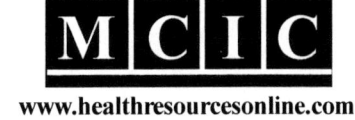

www.healthresourcesonline.com

ADVERTISERS INDEX

The Executive Report on Managed Care .... I A

Expedite: The Information Toolkit for Sellers of Products and Services to Managed Care .... I C

Managed Care Solutions 2

The National Directory of Health Systems, Hospitals and Their Affiliates 476

Pay for Performance Reporter 498

HealthResPubs Weekly E-Mail Newsletter A-141

Managed Care Weekly Watch A-142

Wellness Manager Discussion Group A-143

Managed Care Exchange Discussion Group A-144

The National Directory of Managed Care Organizations, Electronic Version .... ISFC

The National Directory of Managed Care Organizations, Online Database .... ISBC

The Managed Care Information Center .... OSBC

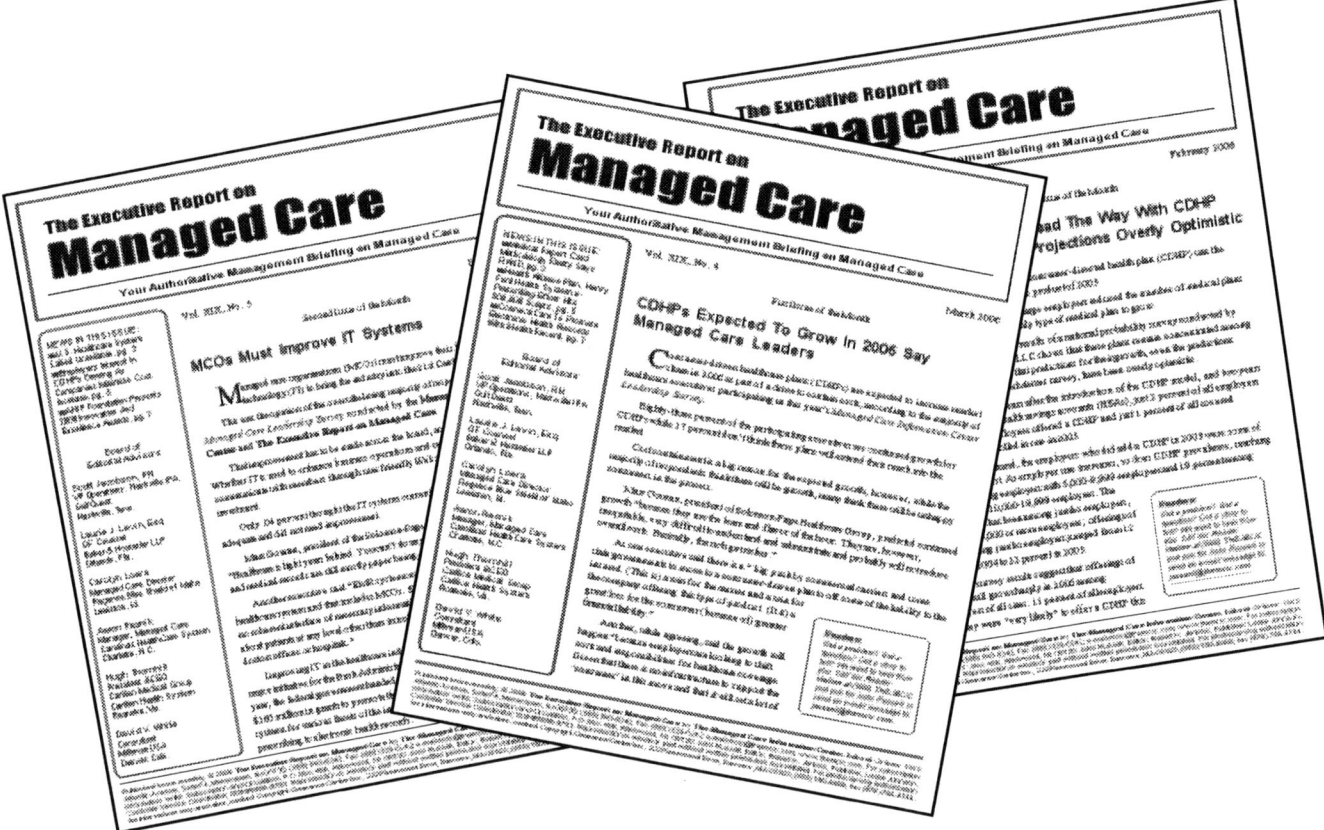

Keep on top of the latest strategic moves of managed care organizations.

The Executive Report on Managed Care is dedicated to providing up-to-date critical information for executives to evaluate and monitor managed care programs in terms of their cost-effectiveness, quality and liability. Each issue brings you the latest news on what other organizations are doing to successfully trim healthcare costs. You'll also be kept abreast of proposed and pending legislation and how these changes are expected to affect your organization.

And, right now you can take advantage of a FREE, NO-OBLIGATION, review subscription. If you find this one-of-a-kind executive advisory service doesn't meet your professional needs, you can write "cancel" on the invoice.

Call today to receive your FREE review subscription. Please be sure to reference Code: 14D7AD.

Managed Care Information Center
PO Box 456, Allenwood, NJ 08720-0456
http://www.healthresourcesonline.com

**Call TOLL-FREE
(888) THE-MCIC (888-843-6242)
Fax (888) FAX-MCIC (888-329-6242)**

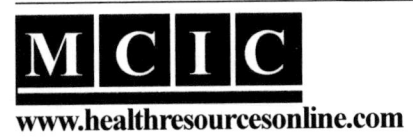
www.healthresourcesonline.com

Managed Care Information Center
Providing Essential Management Information to Healthcare Executives

> While every effort has been made to ensure the reliability of the information presented in this publication, MCIC does not guarantee accuracy of the data contained herein and will not be held liable for any misrepresentation. Errors brought to the attention of the publisher, and verified to the satisfaction of the publisher, will be corrected in future editions.

A Publication of

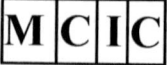

Managed Care Information Center
1913 Atlantic Ave
Suite F5
Manasquan, NJ
08736
(732) 292-1100
Fax: (732) 292-1111

Copyright 2008
Managed Care Information Center
ISBN 978-1-882364-83-1

This publication may not be reproduced, transmitted in whole or in part, or any substantial portion of it by photocopying, scanning into electronic storage, keying the contents into a storage system, or by any other means. You may key the address and telephone information in the Directory into your own company's electronic storage system for the purpose of creating mailing labels or telephone call lists for your own company's use in promoting its own products or services. However, you agree that you will not share the labels or lists you thereby create with anyone outside of your company, and that you will not use the labels for lists for the benefit of a third party. You may not include any of the contents of this Directory in any other product or material intended for resale without prior permission of **Managed Care Information Center**, 1913 Atlantic Ave., Suite F5, Manasquan, N.J. 08736

The National Directory of Managed Care Organizations Seventh Edition

---

ACKNOWLEDGMENTS

Data Compilation & Verification
Executive Editor: Phyllis J. Harris

Project Staff:
Amy Fidalgo
Donna Shadlun
Eileen Sinneck

Design & Composition:
Phyllis J. Harris

Publisher:
Robert K. Jenkins

Pharmacy Management Companies 475

Medicare Advantage Demonstration Project 497

Miscellaneous Organizations 501

Healthcare Associations 521

Directory of Healthcare Resources 525

Index I.   Managed Care Organizations A-1

      II.   Health Maintenance Organizations A-17

      III.   Preferred Provider Organizations A-27

      IV.   Specialty HMOs A-37

      V.   Specialty PPOs A-43

      VI.   Point of Service Organizations A-49

      VII.   Miscellaneous Organizations A-57

      VIII.   Personnel A-63

TABLE OF CONT

Advertisers Index I

Introduction III

User's Guide V

Plan Profiles:

Alabama 3	Puerto Rico 377
Alaska 9	Rhode Island 379
Arizona 11	South Carolina 383
Arkansas 25	South Dakota 387
California 31	Tennessee 391
Colorado 77	Texas 403
Connecticut 87	Utah 433
Delaware 95	Vermont 439
District of Columbia 97	Virginia 441
Florida 99	Washington 449
Georgia 127	West Virginia 459
Guam 135	Wisconsin 461
Hawaii 137	Wyoming 473
Idaho 141	
Illinois 143	
Indiana 157	
Iowa 169	
Kansas 177	
Kentucky 183	
Louisiana 189	
Maine 195	
Maryland 199	
Massachusetts 209	
Michigan 217	
Minnesota 233	
Mississippi 241	
Missouri 243	
Montana 253	
Nebraska 255	
Nevada 259	
New Hampshire 265	
New Jersey 267	
New Mexico 279	
New York 283	
North Carolina 309	
North Dakota 317	
Ohio 319	
Oklahoma 339	
Oregon 345	
Pennsylvania 355	